# Cancer Nursing

SEVENTH EDITION

# Cancer Nursing

## PRINCIPLES AND PRACTICE

EDITED BY

**Connie Henke Yarbro, MS, RN, FAAN**
Adjunct Clinical Associate Professor
MU Sinclair School of Nursing
University of Missouri–Columbia
Columbia, MO
Editor, *Seminars in Oncology Nursing*
Destin, FL

**Debra Wujcik, PhD, RN, AOCN®**
Director, Clinical Trials at Meharry
Vanderbilt Ingram Cancer Center
Associate Professor
Vanderbilt School of Nursing
Nashville, TN

**Barbara Holmes Gobel, MS, RN, AOCN®**
Oncology Clinical Nurse Specialist
Northwestern Memorial Hospital
Adjunct Faculty
Rush University College of Nursing
Rush University Medical Center
Chicago, IL



JONES AND BARTLETT PUBLISHERS
*Sudbury, Massachusetts*
BOSTON TORONTO LONDON SINGAPORE

*World Headquarters*
Jones and Bartlett Publishers
40 Tall Pine Drive
Sudbury, MA 01776
978-443-5000
info@jbpub.com
www.jbpub.com

Jones and Bartlett Publishers Canada
6339 Ormindale Way
Mississauga, Ontario L5V 1J2
Canada

Jones and Bartlett Publishers International
Barb House, Barb Mews
London W6 7PA
United Kingdom

Jones and Bartlett's books and products are available through most bookstores and online booksellers. To contact Jones and Bartlett Publishers directly, call 800-832-0034, fax 978-443-8000, or visit our website, www.jbpub.com.

Substantial discounts on bulk quantities of Jones and Bartlett's publications are available to corporations, professional associations, and other qualified organizations. For details and specific discount information, contact the special sales department at Jones and Bartlett via the above contact information or send an email to specialsales@jbpub.com.



The authors, editors, and publisher have made every effort to provide accurate information. However, they are not responsible for errors, omissions, or for any outcomes related to the use of the contents of this book and take no responsibility for the use of the products and procedures described. Treatments and side effects described in this book may not be applicable to all people; likewise, some people may require a dose or experience a side effect that is not described herein. Drugs and medical devices are discussed that may have limited availability controlled by the Food and Drug Administration (FDA) for use only in a research study or clinical trial. Research, clinical practice, and government regulations often change the accepted standard in this field. When consideration is being given to use of any drug in the clinical setting, the health care provider or reader is responsible for determining FDA status of the drug, reading the package insert, and reviewing prescribing information for the most up-to-date recommendations on dose, precautions, and contraindications, and determining the appropriate usage for the product. This is especially important in the case of drugs that are new or seldom used.

**Production Credits**
Chief Executive Officer: Ty Field
Chief Operating Officer: Don W. Jones, Jr.
President: James Homer
V.P., Sales: William J. Kane
V.P., Design and Production: Anne Spencer
V.P., Manufacturing and Inventory Control: Therese Connell
Publisher: Kevin Sullivan
Acquisitions Editor: Amy Sibley
Associate Editor: Patricia Donnelly
Editorial Assistant: Rachel Shuster
Senior Production Editor: Carolyn F. Rogers
Senior Marketing Manager: Rebecca Wasley
Composition: Newgen North America
Cover Design: Scott Moden
Printing and Binding: Courier Westford
Cover Printing: Courier Westford

**Library of Congress Cataloging-in-Publication Data**
Cancer nursing : principles and practice / edited by Connie Henke Yarbro, Debra Wujcik, Barbara Holmes Gobel.—7th ed.
p. ; cm.
Includes bibliographical references and index.
ISBN 978-0-7637-6357-2 (casebound)
1. Cancer—Nursing. I. Yarbro, Connie Henke. II. Wujcik, Debra. III. Gobel, Barbara Holmes.
[DNLM: 1. Neoplasms—nursing. 2. Oncologic Nursing—methods. WY 156 C2197 2010]
RC266.C356 2010
616.99'40231—dc22 2009027107

6048

Printed in the United States of America
14 13 12 11 10 10 9 8 7 6 5 4 3 2 1

# Contents

# Preface

Cancer nurses throughout the world have used *Cancer Nursing: Principles and Practice* for almost a quarter of a century. Thus, it is an honor to welcome our readers to the *Seventh Edition* of this definitive text. With this edition, we enter a new era by welcoming Debra Wujcik and Barbara Holmes Gobel as editors.

The rapid progress in the science and practice of oncology and oncology nursing has necessitated the inclusion of new topics and the extensive revision of many chapters in this edition, all of which have been updated to include the latest developments in the care of patients with cancer. Over a third of the chapters are new, with new content and new authors. The remaining chapters have had major revisions and updates.

The basic science chapters in Part I have been reorganized and updated to reflect the massive increase in scientific knowledge that has occurred in the past few years, especially as it relates to genes and cancer. The section on Prevention, Detection, and Diagnosis has had major revisions devoted to the dynamics of cancer prevention and genetic risk and hereditary syndromes. The Treatment section has a new chapter that covers the important developments of targeted therapy. The section on Cancer Symptom Management begins with a chapter on evidence-based practice. Because patients with cancer continue to encounter new problems as a result of new therapies, this edition includes two new chapters devoted to hypersensitivity reactions and mucositis. In addition, because millions of patients are cancer survivors, we felt it was important to expand the section on Dimensions of Cancer Survivorship, to not only address late effects, survivorship issues, and spiritual responses to cancer, but also to include a chapter on family and caregiver issues. The section on End-of-Life and Palliative Care, which includes chapters on the principles and issues of palliative care and the delivery of comfort care, has been continued in response to requests from our readers. The section on Professional Issues for the Cancer Nurse provides important updates on the roles of advanced practice nurses and legal issues.

Every chapter has been updated with the latest references and research studies, and many include website addresses and resources. As with previous editions, *Cancer Nursing: Principles and Practice* continues to present the most comprehensive information from leading cancer nursing experts.

We would like to extend our gratitude to the many authors whose tireless review of the literature, and whose careful writing, revising, and updating of chapters has made this book possible. The dedication of these contributors and all involved with this seventh edition will contribute to the quality of care provided to all of our patients with cancer.

The editors would like to pay a special tribute to Margaret Hansen Frogge and Michelle Goodman who have served diligently as editors of this definitive text for cancer nurses for the past 20 years. Their leadership and dedicated service have contributed to the continuing success of this book.

*Connie Henke Yarbro*
*Debra Wujcik*
*Barbara Holmes Gobel*

# The Editors

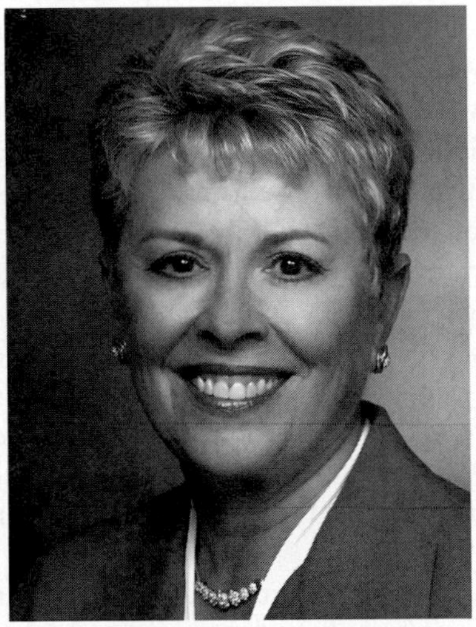

*Connie Henke Yarbro*

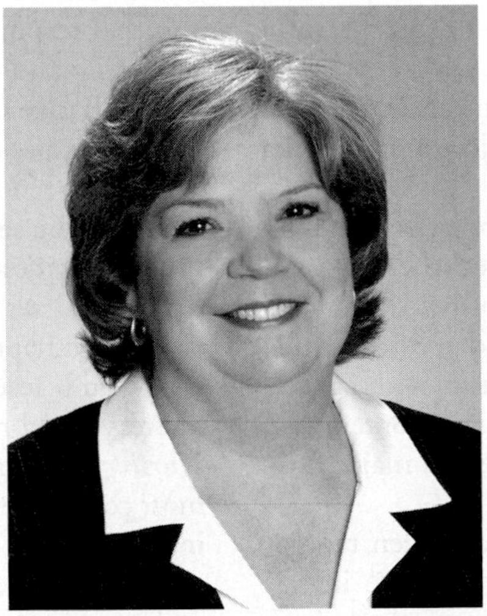

*Debra Wujcik*

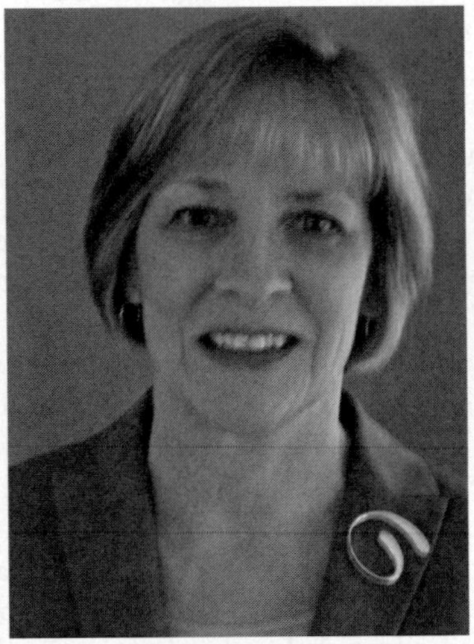

*Barbara Holmes Gobel*

# Contributors

**Lois Almadrones Cassidy, RN, MS, FNP, MPA (53)**
Retired CNS
Gynecology Oncology
Memorial Sloan-Kettering Cancer Center
New York, NY

**Lowell Anderson-Reitz, RN, MS, ANP, AOCN® (19)**
Blood and Marrow Transplant Nurse Practitioner
Baylor Blood and Marrow Transplant Program
Dallas, TX

**Terri Armstrong, PhD, ANP-BC, FAAN (49)**
Associate Professor, Dept. of Integrative Nursing Care
School of Nursing, University of Texas Health Sciences Center
Adjunct Associate Professor, Dept. of Neuro-Oncology
M.D. Anderson Cancer Center
Houston, TX

**Susan Bankston, RN, MSN, FP/MHNP-BC (26)**
Associate Professor of Nursing
Linfield-Good Samaritan School of Nursing
Portland, OR

**Susan M. Bauer-Wu, RN, PhD, FAAN (2)**
Associate Professor
Emory University
Atlanta, GA

**Susan Weiss Behrend, RN, MSN, AOCN® (13)**
Department of Radiation Oncology
Fox Chase Cancer Center
Philadelphia, PA

**Carlton G. Brown, PhD, RN, AOCN® (32)**
Assistant Professor, School of Nursing
University of Delaware
Newark, DE

**Heather L. Brumbaugh, RN, MSN, ANP, AOCN® (42)**
Nurse Practitioner
Duke University Medical Center
Durham, NC

**H. Piersol Byrnes, RN, BSN, OCN® (54)**
Nurse Clinician III
Sidney Kimmel Comprehensive Cancer Center at Johns Hopkins Hospital
Baltimore, MD

**Dawn Camp-Sorrell, MSN, FNP, AOCN® (17)**
Clinical Instructor
University of Alabama at Birmingham School of Nursing
Nurse Practitioner
St. Vincent's Hospital Adult Clinic
Birmingham, AL

**Ellen Carr, RN, MSN, AOCN® (56)**
Nurse Case Manager, Head/Neck Surgical Oncology
Moores UCSD Cancer Center
University of California–San Diego
La Jolla, CA

**Marlene Zichi Cohen, PhD, RN, FAAN (26)**
Professor and Kenneth E. Morehead Endowed Chair in Nursing
Associate Dean for Research
College of Nursing
University of Nebraska Medical Center
Omaha, NE

**Diane G. Cope, PhD, ARNP-C, AOCNP (35)**
Oncology Nurse Practitioner
Florida Cancer Specialists
Fort Myers, FL

**Regina S. Cunningham, PhD, RN, AOCN® (33)**
Senior Director, Oncology
The Tisch Cancer Institute
Mount Sinai Medical Center
New York, NY

**Georgia Decker, APRN, ANP-BC, CN®, AOCN® (24)**
Advanced Practice Nurse
Integrative Care, NP, PC
Albany, NY

**Anthony DeLaCruz, BSN, MS, RN, OCN® (10)**
Memorial Sloan-Kettering Cancer Center
New York, NY

**Barbara K. Dunn, PhD, MD (5)**
Medical Officer and Program Director
Division of Cancer Prevention
National Institutes of Health
Bethesda, MD

**Beth Eaby-Sandy, MSN, CRNP, OCN® (59)**
Nurse Practitioner
Abramson Cancer Center
University of Pennsylvania
Philadelphia, PA

**Peg Esper, MSN, MSA, RN, ANP-BC, AOCN® (74)**
Nurse Practitioner, Medical Oncology
University of Michigan Comprehensive Cancer Center
Ann Arbor, MI

**Susan A. Ezzone, MS, RN, CNP, AOCNP® (18)**
Nurse Practitioner
Blood and Marrow Transplant Program
OSUMC Arthur G. James Cancer Hospital & Solove Research Institute
Columbus, OH

**Beth Faiman, RN, MSN, APRN-BC, AOCN® (61)**
Nurse Practitioner and Predoctoral Research Fellow
Cleveland Clinic and Case Western Reserve University
Cleveland, OH

**Alecia Malin Fair, DrPH (3)**
Assistant Professor
School of Medicine, Department of Surgery
Meharry Medical College
Nashville, TN

**Barbara Felder, MSN, CRNP, AOCNP® (48)**
Nurse Practitioner
Department of Hematology/Oncology
Hospital of the University of Pennsylvania
Philadelphia, PA

**Carol Estwing Ferrans, PhD, RN, FAAN (9)**
Professor and Associate Dean for Research
Co-Director, Center for Excellence in Eliminating Health Disparities
College of Nursing
University of Illinois–Chicago
Chicago, IL

**Anne Marie Flaherty, RN, MSN, AOCNS®, APNc (41)**
Clinical Nurse Specialist
Memorial Sloan-Kettering Cancer Center
New York, NY

**Sara Bhagat Foxson, MSN, CRNP, AOCN® (48)**
Abramson Cancer Center
University of Pennsylvania Health System
Philadelphia, PA

**Janet S. Fulton, PhD, RN, ACNS-BC (76)**
Associate Professor
Indiana University School of Nursing
Indianapolis, IN

**Theresa Wicklin Gillespie, PhD, RN (11)**
Associate Professor
Department of Surgery
Emory University
Atlanta, GA

**Barbara Holmes Gobel, MS, RN, AOCN® (23, 29, 31, 38)**
Oncology Clinical Nurse Specialist
Northwestern Memorial Hospital
Adjunct Faculty
Rush University College of Nursing
Rush University Medical Center
Chicago, IL

**Tracy K. Gosselin, RN, MSN, AOCN® (12)**
Associate Chief Nursing Officer
Oncology Services
Duke University Health System
Durham, NC

**Peter Greenwald, MD, DrPH (5)**
Division Director
Division of Cancer Prevention
National Cancer Institute
National Institutes of Health
Bethesda, MD

**Nina N. Grenon, MS, ANP-BC, GNP-BC, AOCN® (58)**
Nurse Practitioner
Dana-Farber Cancer Institute
Boston, MA

**Marilyn L. Haas, PhD, CNS, ANP-BC (14)**
Nurse Practitioner
Mountain Radiation Oncology
Asheville, NC

**Eileen Danaher Hacker, PhD, APN, AOCN® (9)**
Clinical Associate Professor
Department of Biobehavioral Health Science
College of Nursing
University of Illinois–Chicago
Chicago, IL

**Ashley Somerset Harmon, MSN, APRN, ANP-BC (64)**
Adult Nurse Practitioner
Rhode Island Hospital Cancer Center
Providence, RI

**Mary B. Hodgin, MS, CMSRN (55, 63)**
Research Nurse
Department of Surgery
Surgical Nursing Administration
Johns Hopkins Hospital
Baltimore, MD

**Maureen B. Huhmann, DCN, RD, CSO (33)**
Assistant Professor
Department of Nutritional Sciences
University of Medicine and Dentistry of New Jersey
School of Health Related Professions
Clinical Dietitian
The Cancer Institute of New Jersey
New Brunswick, NJ

**Sadie P. Hutson, PhD, RN, WHNP, BC (7)**
Assistant Professor and PhD Coordinator
College of Nursing
Graduate Programs
East Tennessee State University
Johnson City, TN

**Joanne K. Itano, RN, PhD, APRN (4)**
Associate Professor and Director, Academic Affairs
University of Hawaii
Honolulu, HI

**Marcelle Kaplan, RN, MS, AOCN®, CBCN (39)**
Oncology Clinical Nurse Specialist
New York-Presbyterian Hospital
Weill Cornell Medical Center
New York, NY

**Roberta Kaplow, RN, PhD, AOCNS®, CCNS, CCRN (37)**
Clinical Nurse Specialist
Emory University Hospital
Atlanta, GA

**Meredith Wallace Kazer, PhD, APRN, A/GNP-BC (64)**
Associate Professor
School of Nursing
Fairfield University
Fairfield, CT

**AnnMarie K. McDonnell Keenan, MS, APRN-BC, AOCN® (43)**
Assistant Professor/Clinical Nurse Specialist
Adult Hematology/Oncology
Rush University Medical Center
Chicago, IL

**Linda U. Krebs, PhD, RN, AOCN®, FAAN (36)**
Associate Professor
College of Nursing
University of Colorado–Denver
Aurora, CO

**Sandra E. Kurtin, RN, MS, AOCN®, ANP-C (57)**
Hematology/Oncology Nurse Practitioner
Arizona Cancer Center
Clinical Assistant Professor of Nursing
Clinical Assistant Professor of Medicine
University of Arizona
Tucson, AZ

**Wendy Landier, RN, MSN, CPNP, CPON® (71)**
Clinical Director
Center for Cancer Survivorship
Department of Population Sciences
City of Hope Comprehensive Cancer Center
Duarte, CA

**Jennie Greco Lattimer, MSN, CRNP, AOCN® (48)**
Oncology Nurse Practitioner
University of Pennsylvania Health System
Abramson Cancer Center
Rena Rowan Breast Center
Philadelphia, PA

**Dale Halsey Lea, RN, MPH, CGC, FAAN (22)**
Health Educator
National Human Genome Research Institute
National Institutes of Health
Bethesda, MD

**Colleen O. Lee, MS, CRNP, AOCN®, CLNC (24)**
Commander, US Public Health Service
Silver Spring, MD

**Colleen Lemoine, APRN, MN, AOCN® (23)**
Clinical Nurse Specialist
Interim Louisiana State University Public Hospital
New Orleans, LA

**Victoria Wochna Loerzel, PhD, RN, OCN® (70)**
Assistant Professor
College of Nursing
University of Central Florida
Orlando, FL

**Jennifer T. Loud, RN, CRNP, DNP (7)**
Assistant Branch Chief
Clinical Genetics Branch
Division of Cancer Epidemiology and Genetics
National Cancer Institute
National Institutes of Health
Bethesda, MD

**Jean Lydon, RN, MS, AOCN® (44)**
Associate Vice President of Patient Care Services
Elmhurst Memorial Healthcare
Elmhurst, IL

**Suzanne M. Mahon, RN, DNSc, AOCN®, APNG (6, 66)**
Professor, Division of Hematology/Oncology
Department of Internal Medicine
Professor, Adult Nursing
School of Nursing
Saint Louis University
St. Louis, MO

**Sharon D. Manson, RN, MS, ACNP (60)**
Director of Nursing & Mid Level Practitioners
Acute Care Nurse Practitioner
Division of Hematology & Oncology
Rush University Medical Center
Chicago, IL

**Virginia R. Martin, MSN, RN, AOCN® (50, 62)**
Clinical Director
Ambulatory Care
Fox Chase Cancer Center
Philadelphia, PA

**Kelley D. Mayden, MSN, FNP, AOCNP® (34)**
Oncology Nurse Practitioner
Southwest Virginia Cancer Center
Norton, VA

**Mary S. McCabe, BA, RN, MA (10)**
Director, Survivorship Program
Memorial Sloan-Kettering Cancer Center
Faculty
Weill Cornell Medical College
New York, NY

**Erin McMenamin, MSN, CRNP, AOCN®, ACHPN (27)**
Oncology Nurse Practitioner
Division of Radiation Oncology
Hospital of the University of Pennsylvania
Philadelphia, PA

**Karen Meneses, PhD, RN, FAAN (70)**
Professor and Associate Dean for Research
School of Nursing
University of Alabama at Birmingham
Birmingham, AL

**Carrie J. Merkle, PhD, RN, FAAN (1)**
Associate Professor, Nursing
College of Nursing
University of Arizona
Tucson, AZ

**Marcia Mickle, RN, MSN, ACNP, AOCN® (67)**
Nurse Practitioner, GI Oncology
Northwestern Medical Faculty Foundation
Chicago, IL

**Sandra A. Mitchell, PhD, CRNP, AOCN® (30)**
Nurse Scientist
Nursing Research
NIH Clinical Center
Bethesda, MD

**Paula M. Muehlbauer, RN, MSN, AOCNS® (20)**
Clinical Nurse Specialist/Academic Educator
VA Healthcare San Diego
San Diego State University
San Diego, CA

**Laurel Northouse, PhD, RN, FAAN (72)**
Mary Lou Willard French Professor of Nursing
University of Michigan School of Nursing
Ann Arbor, MI

**Colleen O'Leary, RN, MS, AOCNS® (31, 40, 52)**
Oncology Clinical Nurse Specialist
Advocate Good Samaritan Hospital
Downers Grove, IL

**Karen Oleszewski, RN, MS, AOCN® (69)**
Senior Clinical Oncology Specialist
Genentech BioOncology
Baltimore, MD

**Judith A. Paice, PhD, RN, FAAN (75)**
Director, Cancer Pain Program
Feinberg School of Medicine
Northwestern University
Chicago, IL

**Carlene Porter, RN, MSN, ACNP (60)**
Nurse Practitioner
Elmhurst Memorial Oncology Services
Elmhurst Memorial Hospital
Elmhurst, IL

**Janice Post-White, PhD, RN, FAAN (2)**
Research Consultant in Complementary and Alternative Medicine
Adjunct Associate Professor
University of Minnesota
Minneapolis, MN

**Anna Liza Rodriguez, RN, MSN, MHA, OCN® (29)**
Director, Oncology Nursing and Service Line
Mount Sinai Hospital
Chicago, IL

**Dana N. Rutledge, RN, PhD (25)**
Professor, Nursing
California State University–Fullerton
Nursing Research Facilitator
St. Joseph Hospital
Orange, CA

**Loleta C. Samuel, RN, MSN, APRN, BC, AOCN® (46)**
Adult Nurse Practitioner
The Cancer Institute of New Jersey
Adjunct Professor, Division of Nursing
New Jersey City University
Jersey City, NJ

**Lisa C. Schulmeister, MN, APRN-BC, OCN®, FAAN (77)**
Oncology Nursing Consultant
New Orleans, LA

**Brenda K. Shelton, MS, RN, CCRN, AOCN® (28)**
Clinical Nurse Specialist
The Sidney Kimmel Comprehensive Cancer Center at Johns Hopkins
Baltimore, MD

**Gary Shelton, RN, NP, MSN, ANP-BC, AOCNP® (47)**
Oncology CNS
Adult Health NP
NYU Clinical Cancer Center
New York, NY

**Judith J. Smith, RN, MSN, AOCN® (5)**
Nurse Consultant
Lung and Upper Aerodigestive Cancer Research Group
Division of Cancer Prevention
National Cancer Institute
National Institutes of Health
Bethesda, MD

**Sonia Smith, RN, MSN, ACNP-BC (71)**
Nurse Practitioner
Prostate Cancer Survivorship Program
Center for Cancer Survivorship
Department of Population Sciences
City of Hope Comprehensive Cancer Center
Duarte, CA

**Lixin Song, PhD, RN (72)**
Postdoctoral Fellow
School of Nursing
University of North Carolina–Chapel Hill
Chapel Hill, NC

**Sharon Steingass, RN, MSN, AOCN® (45)**
Vice President
Ambulatory Care
City of Hope Comprehensive Cancer Center
Duarte, CA

**Joseph D. Tariman, APRN-BC, OCN® (61)**
Predoctoral Fellow
Biobehavioral Nursing and Health Systems Fellow, Achievement Rewards for College Scientists (ARCS) Foundation
University of Washington
Seattle, WA

**Elizabeth Johnston Taylor, PhD, RN (73)**
Associate Professor, School of Nursing
Loma Linda University
Loma Linda, CA
Research Director, Mary Potter Hospice
Wellington, Aotearoa New Zealand

**Susan Vogt Temple, RN, MSN, AOCN® (50)**
Senior Clinical Educator
GlaxoSmithKline Oncology
Seale, AL

**Peter V. Tortorice, PharmD, BCOP (15)**
Manager
Pharmaceutical Services
US Oncology
Schaumburg, IL

**Nancy D. Tsottles, RN, BSN (54)**
Senior Research Nurse/Program Coordinator
Johns Hopkins University
Baltimore, MD

**Wendy H. Vogel, MSN, FNP, AOCNP® (8)**
Oncology Nurse Practitioner
Kingsport Hematology-Oncology Associates
Kingsport, TN

**Gail M. Wilkes, MS, RN, ANP-BC, AOCN® (16, 51)**
Oncology Nurse Educator
Boston Medical Center
Boston, MA

**Laura S. Wood, RN, MSN, OCN® (65)**
Renal Cancer Research Coordinator
Cleveland Clinic Taussig Cancer Institute
Cleveland, OH

**Debra Wujcik, PhD, RN, AOCN® (21)**
Director, Clinical Trials at Meharry
Vanderbilt Ingram Cancer Center
Associate Professor
Vanderbilt School of Nursing
Nashville, TN

**Susan Germann Yackzan, RN, MSN, AOCN®, ARNP (66)**
Oncology Clinical Nurse Specialist
Central Baptist Hospital
Lexington, KY

**Connie Henke Yarbro, MS, RN, FAAN**
Adjunct Clinical Associate Professor
MU Sinclair School of Nursing
University of Missouri–Columbia
Columbia, MO
Editor, *Seminars in Oncology Nursing*

**Eric Zack, RN, MSN, ACNP-BC, AOCN® (68)**
Rush University Medical Center
Chicago, IL

# PART I

# The Cancer Problem

CHAPTER 1

Carrie J. Merkle, PhD, RN, FAAN

# Biology of Cancer

## INTRODUCTION

In his now classic writings on the origin of cancer, Sir Richard Doll[1] proposed 3 potential causative factors underlying tumor development: (1) environmental factors, particularly diet, industrial pollution, and viruses; (2) systemic factors, including breakdowns in immunosurveillance; and (3) genetic factors, such as the degree of susceptibility to cancer. Since Doll's publications in the late 1970s, the biology underlying these proposed causative factors—which were derived largely from epidemiological studies—has been carefully scrutinized to determine the causes of cancer at the biochemical, cellular, and molecular levels. Because of the intensity of biological research and the rapidity with which findings have become available, we now know that cancer is a disease resulting from the interaction of multiple factors at the cellular, genetic, immunologic, and environmental levels.

A fundamental goal of cancer research is to discern mechanisms of cancer cell development, ways that cancers grow and spread, and, finally, the means to correct abnormal mechanisms and to prevent, eradicate, and/or control cancer cell populations. This chapter reviews theories and models of tumor development, properties of cancer and transformed cells, genetic influences on cancer, the cell cycle, apoptosis, and metastasis.

## THEORIES AND RESEARCH MODELS OF TUMOR DEVELOPMENT

Several theories and hypotheses have been proposed to explain how and why cancer occurs from a continuum spanning tumorigenesis to metastasis. Many of these share similar information. Nevertheless, complete explanation of how tumors develop and how cancer progresses remain an enigma. Table 1-1 lists some of the leading theories and hypotheses of tumorigenesis and their key points.

### THEORY OF CLONAL EVOLUTION

A prevailing paradigm in tumorigenesis is that the acquisition of unlimited cellular replication, known as immortalization, is an important major step that contributes to the development of cancer.[2] Nowell's theory of clonal evolution specifies that mutant tumor cells are selected due to their growth advantages and that populations of these cells are expanded.[5] Clonal evolution theory holds that cells within a particular tumor must at some point have had the same genetic makeup and been homogeneous. Even though a carcinogen may affect a large number of cells, the resultant tumor usually represents the progeny of only a single cell or very few cells (Figure 1-1).[5,6] Initiation of this clone of cancer cells may involve a stem cell that is already dividing. During successive mitotic divisions of this cell, the lineage fails to proceed to differentiation. Uncontrolled proliferation may be accompanied by morphological and biochemical changes and/or altered gene expression in early cancer cells. Eventually, proliferation may increase and show further evidence of escape from growth-control mechanisms.

Nowell suggests that biological events in tumor progression represent effects of acquired genetic instability.[5] Each new mutation bearing a causal role would be selected for expansion if it is associated with a growth advantage.[7] Similarly, clonal expansion of partially altered cells can substantially increase the population of cells that have acquired some of the mutations critical for tumor development. This situation increases the probability that one of these cells will acquire the remaining mutations needed for neoplastic transformation.[8] Nowell's views of tumorigenesis as an evolutionary system have now been supported by over 3 decades of research,[9] though the importance of nongenetic factors such as the microenvironment and epigenetic influences are now appreciated.[3]

### RESEARCH MODELS OF TUMOR DEVELOPMENT

#### Cell culture models

Cell culture models permit investigation of cancer development at the cellular level. These models consist of cells that were obtained as primary samples of normal and cancerous tissues from humans and other animals, then serially propagated in culture. Compared with many animal models and human studies, cell culture models provide greater uniformity of the cell population, offer a higher degree of experimental control and manipulation, and are less costly.

Most normal cells proliferate for a particular number of mitotic divisions (the Hayflick limit), then attain replicative senescence.[10] Cancer cells, in contrast, typically acquire immortality and demonstrate an unlimited replicative life span. Normal cells growing in culture will sometimes spontaneously attain immortality. Furthermore, adding chemical or physical carcinogens, biological agents such as viruses, and genetic manipulation sometimes can transform normal cells into an immortal population, with or without other characteristics of tumor cells.

Transformation is the process by which a normal cell becomes a cancer cell or develops some of the properties that are typical of cancer cells. One such property is loss of contact inhibition. When normal epithelial cells grow in culture, the cells often form a continuous single layer on a plastic surface, stopping at the boundaries of the chamber; at that point the population stabilizes and cell loss approximates cell growth. In contrast, tumor cells and some transformed cells will grow in multiple layers or clusters, reaching higher densities in culture, thus losing density-dependent

**TABLE 1-1**

**Key Points of Major Theories and Hypotheses of Tumorigenesis**

| Theory or Hypothesis | Key Points |
|---|---|
| Theory of clonal expansion | See text |
| Multistep | Tumorigenesis is a multistep process that includes initiation, promotion, and progression steps. Promotion may result from factors such as inflammation. |
| Mutagenesis | Cancer is caused by changes in genetic information. Chronic insults may produce genetic mutations that cause cancer. |
| Epigenetics | Cancer can be caused by factors that do not alter the DNA nucleotide sequence. Epigenetic causes may include factors that alter the expression of genetic information at the transcriptional (eg, methylation), translational, and posttranslational (eg, micro RNA) levels. |
| Oncogene hypothesis | All cells have genes that are involved in cell proliferation and growth signaling pathways and mechanisms. Cancer may result from mutations to oncogenes and other mechanisms that lead to overactivity of these genes. |
| Tumor suppressor gene | In addition to oncogenes, there are antigrowth genes that when lost or inactivated can contribute to cancer. |
| Knudsen's two hit | Originally this held that 2 mutations (or "hits") are needed to cause the formation of a tumor, and that 1 mutation occurs on each of the 2 alleles present for a gene. It has been modified in numerous ways to include (1) allelic loss (or genetic gain) as a second hit, (2) epigenetic hypermethylation as a hit, (3) more than 2 mutations in some cancers, and in other ways. |
| Cancer stem cell hypothesis | Within tumors, there is a hierarchical organization of cells containing subpopulations of stem cell-like cancer cells with self-renewal capacity and tumor growth responsibility. Cancer stem cells are not necessarily derived from normal stem cells and are not the cell of origin of the tumor. |
| Immunosurveillance theory | Effector cells and mediators of the immune system patrol the body and function in the identification and removal of cancer cells and their precursors. |

*Source:* Data from Weinberg[2]; Visvader and Lindeman[3]; and Jaffe.[4]

contact inhibition. Another characteristic of tumor cells is anchorage independence. Normal epithelial cells will not remain viable if they become detached from the basement membrane or other substrate. Detached cancer cells, however, continue to thrive. Transformed cells may or may not be tumorigenic. The ultimate test for tumorigenicity is to inject the cells into compatible, immunosuppressed animals, to see whether tumors form.

Cancer, immortalized nontumor, and nonimmortal cell lines provide opportunities for investigation of many cellular processes and behavior. Nevertheless, extrapolation of findings from cell culture studies to cells in vivo may be inaccurate or overly simplified.

## Animal models

Animal models have made immense contributions to both the understanding of the biology of cancer and the development of cancer treatment strategies. Conventional mouse models in cancer research include inbred strains, transgenic mice, and conventional knockouts.[11] Inbred strains require multiple generations of sibling matings to develop mice that are susceptible to spontaneous or carcinogen-induced cancers. The *BALB/c* mouse, which develops plasmacytomas in response to the hydrocarbon pristane, is an example of an inbred strain. For decades, transgenic mice bearing oncogenes and "knock-out" mice missing or carrying inactive tumor suppressor genes have led to important advances in the field. These models have facilitated the development of many cancer-prone strains and provided tools for gaining insight into the roles of certain genes and the consequences of mutations in cancer development.[11]

Transgenic mice are derived from cells whose genomes have been modified by the addition of exogenous, or foreign, DNA. This DNA can comprise a manipulated sequence from the same species or from another species that has some property desirable in a particular experiment. The operational gene in the exogenous DNA is called a transgene. In studies of cancer, transgenes are typically injected into cells. The foreign DNA becomes integrated into the cells randomly, without preference for a particular chromosomal location. Three weeks after birth, the offspring are tested for the presence of transgene.

The use of transgenic adult mice in the study of cancer biology offers many benefits. Most important, this process allows the embryonic stem cells to be manipulated in

**TABLE 1-2**

**Properties of Cancer and Transformed Cells**

| Property | Characteristics of Cancer and Transformed Cells | Explanation |
|---|---|---|
| Cytological changes | Increased size and number of nucleoli | Changes reflect greater activity of tumor cells. |
| | Increased nuclear/cytoplasmic ratio | Larger nucleus reflects more activity and/or more genetic information. |
| | Altered cytoskeleton | Changes contribute to increased motility and variable sizes and shapes (pleomorphism). |
| Altered cell growth | Immortality | Normal cells senesce (remain viable but do not divide).<br>Cancer cells proliferate indefinitely, ie, become "immortal."<br>Telomeres (DNA segments at the ends of chromosomes) limit the number of cell doublings. Telomeres shorten with each chromosomal replication until reaching a threshold at which time they cause the cell to senesce.<br>Telomere stability is critical for cancer progression. Many cancers contain an enzyme, telomerase, which enables the cell to replicate indefinitely. |
| | Decreased density-dependent growth inhibition (loss of contact inhibition) | Normal cells stop growing when they contact other cells.<br>Transformed cells do not respond to physical contact with and chemical signals from neighboring cells, thereby continue to grow beyond normal limits. |
| | Decreased requirement for serum | Serum normally provides growth factors necessary for cell proliferation and survival.<br>Typically the growth factor binds to a receptor on the cell surface, which in turn activates the intracytoplasmic portion of the receptor to send a message to the nucleus (signal transduction), where an effect on gene function occurs. Sometimes, an abnormal growth factor receptor on the surface of a cancer or transformed cell can activate the signal pathway spontaneously without exposure to a growth factor.<br>Cancer and transformed cell lines may grow in media without serum, suggesting that they can synthesize and secrete their own growth factors (autocrine stimulation). |
| | Loss of anchorage-dependent growth | Cells require substrate to grow. Transformed cells do not require a solid substrate.<br>Only tumor cells grow in soft agar (no anchorage); cell growth in soft agar highly correlates with tumorigenicity. |
| | Loss of cell cycle control | Cell does not progress normally through cell cycle pathways and checkpoints. (See text.) |
| | Reduced apoptosis | Cancer cells are less susceptible to programmed death. (See text.) |
| Changes in cell membrane | New surface antigens | Cancer and transformed cells exhibit new molecules on the surface.<br>Viruses can transform and alter multiple cell surface antigens. |
| | New or altered glycoproteins (proteins complexed with polysaccharides) | Transformed cells usually have profound changes in cell-surface glycoproteins.<br>Some changes may alter cell-cell and cell-matrix adhesion.<br>Mechanism by which polysaccharides are made and attached to proteins is deranged in transformed cells. |
| | New or altered glycolipids | Content and complexity of glycolipids are reduced in transformed cell membranes.<br>Glycosphingolipid interacts with receptor proteins on the surface of normal cells to inhibit their responsiveness to growth factors.[14]<br>Transformed cells have less and/or altered glycosphingolipids on their cell surfaces, thus increasing their responsiveness to growth factors.<br>Glycosphingolipids also serve as components of surface markers involved in cell-cell recognition.[15] |

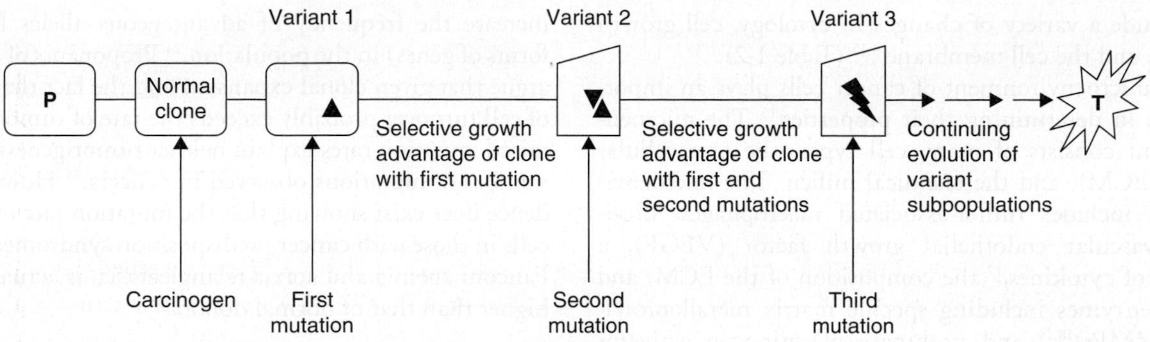


**FIGURE 1-1**

Clonal evolution in cancer. Specific generic alterations in evolving tumors may range from gene mutations to major chromosomal aberrations. This figure illustrates a carcinogen-induced genetic change in a progenitor normal cell (P), which produces a cell with selective growth advantage allowing clonal expansion to begin. In this case, gene mutations produce variant cells. Because they are at a disadvantage metabolically or immunologically, most variant cells are nonviable. If one variant has a selective advantage, its progeny become the predominant subpopulation until another variant appears. The sequential selection of variant subpopulations in each tumor (T) differs because of genetic instability, which positively or negatively affects cell proliferation. *Source*: Data from Nowell[5]; and Strachan and Read.[6]

vitro before injection into the embryo. Scientists can then produce mice with mutations in specific genes or replace a mutant gene with a wild-type (normal) gene.

Mouse models also can be problematic. Certain germline mutations can cause death during mouse embryonic stages, termed *embryonic lethality*. In addition, mutations are present in all mouse cells, not just the tissue of interest, thereby predisposing the animals to many different types of cancers that are not of interest in the particular study. These problems limit the study of sporadic cancers, which are believed to result from mutations in single cells.

Second-generation transgenic mouse models exhibit conditional gene-mutation strategies. In the commonly used *Crelloxp* recombinase system, a tumor suppressor gene may be flanked by recombinase recognition *loxP* sites (the allele is said to be "floxed"), then the *Cre* recombinase is introduced by interbreeding with transgenic mice that have tissue-specific or drug-induced *Cre*. These models avoid embryonic lethality problems and can more closely mimic the time course and tissue specificity of sporadic cancers.[11] Second-generation transgenic mice permit scientists to address higher-order questions, such as "How does angiogenesis contribute to breast cancer development and progression?"[12] Conditional mouse models, along with improved fluorescence and bioluminescence imaging mechanisms that monitor tumor development, growth, and metastasis in living mice, help address complex questions in tumor biology.

Nevertheless, differences between mice and humans exist beyond the obvious phenotypic differences. For example, mouse cells have high levels of telomerase and longer telomeres, which confer differences in the process of aging. Future models need to more closely mimic cancer development, progression, and drug actions in humans.

## PROPERTIES OF CANCER AND TRANSFORMED CELLS

Cancer cells are more autonomous than normal cells and are independent of growth-control pathways and regulatory mechanisms. Cancer cells are also less differentiated than cells of the tissue of origin and behave more like embryonic cells, which also proliferate rapidly. Despite the importance of loss of differentiation in cancer, little is known about the genetic mechanisms and biochemical pathways involved in this phenomenon. In fact, the process by which proteins that regulate gene transcription maintain the differentiation of tissues, such as the breast ductal epithelium, is just beginning to be deciphered.[13]

Some cancer cells are so poorly differentiated (or anaplastic) that the tissue of origin cannot be determined. Oncology and histology texts often present images of tumors according to degrees of abnormalities; ie, beginning with normal cells, then passing through stages of metaplasia (the presence of a cell that appears mildly less differentiated) and/or hyperplasia (more cells than normal) to dysplasia (deranged cell growth with variable shape, size, and appearance) to carcinoma in situ and finally to invasive cancer. These presentations suggest that tumors progress along a continuum from normal tissue to malignancy; however, these "distinct stopping points" in progression from normal cells to malignant have not been proven.[2] The properties of cancer and transformed cells are numerous and include a variety of changes in cytology, cell growth patterns, and the cell membrane[14,15] (Table 1-2).

The microenvironment of cancer cells plays an important role in determining their properties.[16] The microenvironment consists of many cell types, the extracellular matrix (ECM), and the chemical milieu. The microenvironment includes tumor-associated macrophages, fibroblasts, vascular endothelial growth factor (VEGF), a mixture of cytokines,[17] the composition of the ECM, and various enzymes including specific matrix metalloproteinases (MMPs)[18,19] and urokinase plasminogen activator (uPA). Differences in the microenvironment, eg, related to aging, and how these differences transform cells and promote cancer are very active areas of investigation.[20]

## GENETIC INFLUENCES ASSOCIATED WITH CANCER

### MUTATIONS

A mutation is an alteration in a DNA nucleotide sequence ie, the order of the 4 bases adenine (A), cytosine (C), thymine (T), and guanine (G). Mutations can alter both the sequence of a gene and its regulatory sites.

Germline mutations in genes that predispose the organism to cancers represent a strong risk factor for these diseases.[21] Such mutations affect genes in the ova and sperm. During meiosis, each germ cell carries 1 of the 2 copies of mutated genes present in somatic cells, resulting in a 50% chance of a child inheriting a mutated gene copy from a parent. Such mutations are transmitted from generation to generation.

#### Mutation rate and cancer

Differing schools of thought exist regarding mutation rates and cancer. The historical view is that a raised mutation rate constitutes the most important factor in tumorigenesis.[22] For example, in humans, mutations occur at a rate of 1 in 1 million genes per cell generation. Because it takes as many as 6 independent mutations in specific genes to give rise to a tumor cell, the likelihood of a tumor developing is low, though everyone has cells with mutations in at least 1 gene.[6] The perplexing question is this: How can a normal cell accumulate all of these mutations? Increased mutation rates may be more critical in the rarer cancer predisposition syndromes and in cells with reduced DNA repair capability. These cells can have a mutation rate 1000-fold higher than that in cells with intact DNA repair mechanisms.[23,24]

Another viewpoint is that a higher mutation rate may accelerate tumorigenesis, but is not necessary for it to occur.[24] The presence of cancer-causing mutations accounted for by natural selection may be more important than the mutation rate.[24] Natural selection acts directly to increase the frequency of advantageous alleles (alternate forms of genes) in the population.[24] Proponents of this view argue that given clonal expansion and the fact that the rate of cell turnover probably exceeds the rate of tumor growth, raised mutation rates explain neither tumorigenesis nor the number of mutations observed in cancers.[24] However, evidence does exist showing that the mutation rate of somatic cells in those with cancer predisposition syndromes, such as Fanconi anemia and ataxia telangiectasia, is actually much higher than that of normal donors.[25]

#### Causes of mutations

Mutations may arise spontaneously during DNA replication and recombination, or they may be caused by exogenous agents (environmental mutagens giving rise to mutations) or endogenous agents. DNA replication is a complex process resulting in the formation of identical DNA daughter strands through a process that involves complementary base pairing to the parent strand. DNA replication errors are rare due to the efficiency of the DNA polymerases and cellular strategies for identifying and removing mistakes in replication. Mutations however may arise spontaneously during DNA replication, though they are more aptly due to exogenous mutagens (environmental agents that give rise to mutations) or endogenous mutagenic agents. Frequently, DNA rearranges itself by *recombination*, a process whereby DNA is broken and rejoined to another piece of DNA. Recombination may result in loss of control of gene expression or disrupt the coding sequence of the gene.

Exogenous mutagenic agents may be environmental pollutants, pharmacological compounds, human-made chemicals (eg, pesticides, organic chemicals, alkylating agents), substances associated with unhealthy lifestyles (eg, tobacco smoke), compounds made from molds (eg, aflatoxin B1), ultraviolet (UV) radiation, and other sources. These agents may directly or indirectly damage DNA by reacting with components of the DNA or converting them to other products. Endogenous mutagenic agents include reactive oxygen species (ROS) and free radicals resulting from normal cellular metabolism. Another endogenous cause of mutation is chronic inflammation as may occur with hepatitis and human papillomavirus infections. Endogenous agents may target and damage the nitrogenous bases within the DNA structure.[2]

#### Types of mutations

Mutations commonly associated with cancer predisposition include point mutations, insertion and deletion mutations, and mutations affecting DNA repair mechanisms.

*Point mutations.* The substitution of a single base with another base is termed a point mutation. Point mutations are the most common types of mutations. Point mutations that occur in DNA sequences encoding proteins are further classified as silent, missense, or nonsense mutations.

A *silent point mutation* is a base substitution in the third position of a codon (a section of 3 DNA nucleotides that codes for an amino acid), in which the amino acid does not change. In other words, the protein product of the gene is not altered. Silent point mutations may be considered a type of "single nucleotide polymorphism (SNP)," which are described in further detail later in this chapter.

Sometimes a base substitution results in the generation of a codon that specifies a different amino acid, meaning that an amino acid is changed in the sequence of the gene product. This change is termed a *missense point mutation.* Such a mutation may or may not result in a deleterious gene product, depending on the amino acid that has been substituted. If the structure and properties of the normal and substituted amino acids are similar, no deleterious gene products will result. If the structure and properties of the 2 amino acids differ, then a deleterious gene product may result.

A *nonsense point mutation* occurs when a base substitution results in the generation of a stop codon, meaning that the gene product will be truncated and probably nonfunctional. Nonsense point mutations are deleterious mutations.

*Deletions and insertions.* Deletions or insertions occur when 1 or more base pairs are removed from or added to the DNA. This process may result in a *frameshift* mutation. If 1 or 2 bases are deleted or added, the reading frame of the sequence is altered, usually resulting in a nonfunctional gene product. Deletions of 3 nucleotides or multiples of 3 nucleotides may be less serious because they preserve the reading frame.

Combinations of insertions and deletions are possible, and sometimes an insertion mutation will restore the reading frame of a gene with a deletion mutation (and vice versa). Such a gene product would then contain a garbled amino acid sequence between the insertion and deletion, but would otherwise be correct (Figure 1-2).[26]

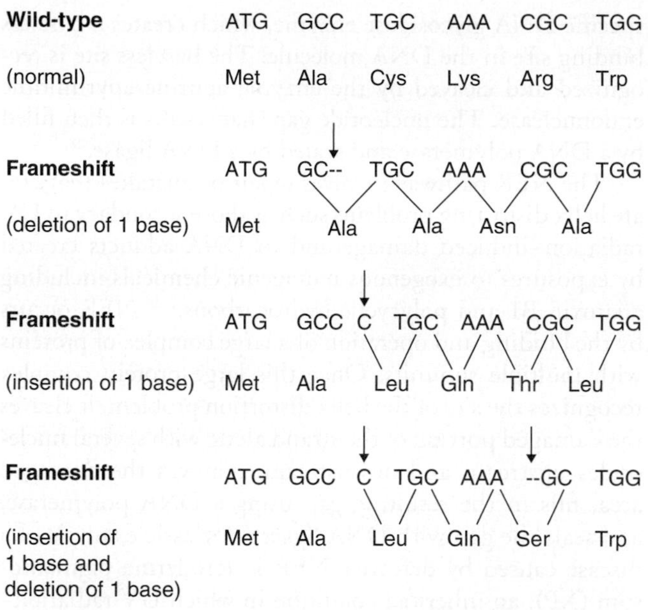


**FIGURE 1-2**

Frameshift mutations. Deletion and/or insertion of bases shifts the reading frame of the DNA sequence, thereby changing the expressed amino acids. Top rows in each set are DNA bases: A, adenine; T, thymine; C, cytosine; G, guanine. Bottom rows in each set are amino acids encoded by the bases: Ala, alanine; Arg, arginine; Asn, asparagine; Cys, cysteine; Gln, glutamine; Leu, leucine; Lys, lysine; Met, methionine; Ser, serine; Thr, threonine; Trp, tryptophan.

*Source:* Data from Loescher.[26]

## MECHANISMS TO REPAIR DNA DAMAGE

There are proofreading mechanisms that operate during DNA replication. In addition, the body contains numerous mechanisms (eg, the skin and melanin to protect from UV damage and enzymes such as superoxide dismutase that deactivate ROS to protect DNA from damage). However, DNA alterations do occur and repair is necessary. DNA repair is integral in protecting against mutations that could otherwise lead to cancer.[27] Humans have a number of mechanisms for repairing DNA damage. These include mismatch repair (MMR), base excision repair (BER), nucleotide excision repair (NER), and double-strand break repair.[2] The MMR, BER, and NER mechanisms rely on DNA being a double-stranded structure with the same information contained in both strands. When damage affects just 1 strand, it can be accurately repaired by excision and replacement, with new DNA being synthesized using the complementary strand as a template.[28]

Mismatched base pairs, as well as single-base insertions and deletions, are generally repaired by MMR. This mechanism relies on a backup signal within the DNA to distinguish between the parental strand and the daughter strand containing the replication error. In humans, a protein called MSH (MutS homolog) recognizes and binds the mismatched base pair. A protein called MLH (MutL homolog) then binds to the protein MSH. Bound to the mismatch, the MSH/MLH complex likely activates a process that unwinds DNA in the direction of the mismatch, degrades the DNA strand, and repairs the error. An example of a disease resulting from defects in MMR is hereditary nonpolyposis colorectal cancer.[2]

Base excision repair is a major repair mechanism that focuses specifically on repairing incorrect or modified bases and filling base gaps. BER removes the faulty base by a specific DNA glycosidase enzyme, which creates a baseless binding site in the DNA molecule. The baseless site is recognized and cleaved by the enzyme apurine/apyrimidine endonuclease. The nucleotide gap that results is then filled by a DNA polymerase and sealed by a DNA ligase.[28]

The NER pathway involves repair of mistakes that create helix distorting problems such as those secondary to UV radiation–induced damage and to DNA adducts created by exposures to exogenous mutagenic chemicals including aflatoxin B1 and polycyclic hydrocarbons.[2,28] NER occurs by the binding and operation of a large complex of proteins with multiple subunits. Once this large protein complex recognizes the site of the helix distortion problem, it cleaves the damaged portion of the strand along with several nucleotides upstream and downstream, removes the damaged area, fills in the resulting gap using a DNA polymerase, and seals the gap with DNA ligase.[2] A classic example of a disease caused by defective NER is xeroderma pigmentosum (XP), an inherited condition in which UV radiation–induced skin cancers result from defects in several genes in the NER pathway.[29]

The nonhomologous end-joining and homologous recombination repair pathways repair double-strand DNA breaks produced by ionizing radiation, ROS, and replication errors.[29] One of the primary activators of double-strand repair is the protein kinase ATM (for ataxia telangiectasia mutated), the deficiency of which causes the inherited disorder ataxia telangiectasia.[29]

## POLYMORPHISMS

Genetic polymorphisms, or variants, represent another influence on cancer. Polymorphisms comprise the occurrence of more than 1 allelic form or genetic variant at the same locus, with the least frequent form occurring more often (ie, > 1%) than can be accounted for by mutation alone.[30] Some polymorphisms result from the insertion or deletion of a section of DNA; these include microsatellite repeat sequences and gross genetic losses and rearrangements. The simplest types of polymorphisms, however, are SNPs. Single nucleotide polymorphism, in which a single base substitutes for another, account for 90% of all DNA polymorphisms.[31]

Although SNPs are found in regulatory regions of the gene, most occur in noncoding regions and do not alter gene expression. In some instances, SNPs may cause subtle changes in a group of genes that under normal conditions are latent, meaning that the variations are not harmful on their own (ie, they are switched "off"). With certain environmental exposures, however, they can be switched "on."[32] In other instances, the wild-type (normal) genes and the variants have dissimilar structural or functional properties. In this situation, SNPs could influence protein function, DNA repair capacity, and cancer risk.[28,33] Table 1-3 lists examples of the SNPs implicated in certain cancers. In addition to providing a source of genetic variation, a SNP when found close to a particular gene may be used as a marker for that gene. Furthermore, scientists are mapping blocks of DNA called haplotypes, which contain combinations of alleles and DNA markers that tend to be inherited together as a unit. SNPs can often be used to tag particular haplotypes and as ways to catalog unique sets of changes involved in different cancers and as potential tools to improve cancer diagnosis and treatment planning. In addition, SNPs may play a role in differing responses to treatments and individual cancer risk.[35–39] It is important however to emphasize that SNPs are only 1 type of genetic polymorphism. Others, such as restriction fragment length polymorphisms, exist and assist in describing and understanding genetic variation and cancer.

## ONCOGENES

Oncogenes are genes that encode proteins (oncoproteins) whose action may transform cells and induce cancer.[2] Oncogenes are often excessively or inappropriately active versions of normal cellular genes called *proto-oncogenes*. Oncogene activity involves "gain-of-function," such as increased cell proliferation.[29] One mechanism for overexpression of oncogenes is amplification, in which the number of copies of a gene increases, resulting in overexpression of the gene product. The gene itself may be unmodified. Oncogenes such as *MYC* and *HER2/NEU* often have amplified gene sequences that may contribute to tumorigenesis.[2,29]

Most proto-oncogenes encode for proteins in signal transduction pathways and signaling cascades that convert and amplify chemical and physical signals enabling cellular responses to be appropriate to environment changes.

**TABLE 1-3**

**Examples of Polymorphisms Implicated in Cancer**

| Gene | Polymorphism | Basic Function | Cancer Type |
|---|---|---|---|
| *OGG1* | S326C | DNA repair | Lung, prostate, esophagus |
| *XRCC1* | R14W | DNA repair | Bladder, breast, lung, etc. |
| *BRCA2* | N372H | DNA repair, etc. | Breast |
| *CYPIAI* | I462V | Detoxification | Lung (white nonsmokers) |

*Abbrevations*: *CYPIAI*, Cytochrome P450 1A1, *XRCC1*, Xray repair cross complementing protein1; *OGG1*, 8-Oxoguanine DNA glycosylase; *Source*: Data from Hussain etal[30] and Sun et al.[34]

These complex signal transduction pathways control basic cell functions such as division, motility, and survival; consequently, they need to be highly regulated. Regulation often occurs through alterations in the enzymatic activity of key proteins in the pathways and assembly of large multimolecular signaling complexes within the cell.

Signaling pathways play an important role in tumor development and cancer progression. Signaling pathways are complex and have many component signaling proteins. This may help explain the large number of identified protooncogenes. Furthermore, redundancy and interaction between the pathways and their components may explain why human cancers rarely, if ever, result from aberrant activation of a single oncogene.[29]

## Classification of oncogenes

Broad classes of oncogenes can be distinguished according to their overall function. A number of these genes encode growth factors, growth factor receptors (GFRs), signal transducing proteins (nonreceptor tyrosine kinases, serine/threonine protein kinases, and G-proteins), and transcription factors.[2,29,40]

*Growth factors.* Growth factors are proteins that influence cell growth, proliferation, and survival by binding to specific receptors in the cell membrane and, consequently, activating intracellular signal transduction pathways. Growth factor-induced signaling activity results in transmission of a signal to the cell nucleus, where genes are turned off and on. The end result is change in expression (transcription into RNA) of certain genes.

Growth factors often act by autocrine and paracrine mechanisms. In autocrine stimulation, the growth factor stimulates the cell that produced it; in paracrine stimulation, the growth factor activates adjacent cells. Oncogenic growth factors may cause tumor cell proliferation by both forms of stimulation.

Growth factor overproduction may contribute to malignant transformation,[41] though overproduction of 1 particular growth factor alone probably cannot sustain cancerous cell proliferation. For example, the oncogenes *FOS*, *JUN*, and *MYC* are early-response oncogenes that increase in activity soon after growth factor stimulation. These genes play key roles in cell proliferation. The overexpression of *MYC* coupled with the addition of fibroblast growth factor will cause DNA synthesis, whereas each alone may not. Similarly, when platelet-derived growth factor (PDGF) is combined with another growth factor such as epidermal growth factor (EGF), PDGF can stimulate cell division in cultures; it cannot accomplish this effect alone.

Overproduction of several growth factors is implicated in cancer. *Epidermal growth factor* (EGF) induces proliferation in a variety of cells such as epidermal cells, glial cells, vascular endothelial cells, and many cancer cells. It is known to protect some cancer cells from death by apoptosis. Epidermal growth factors produce a mitogenic response and other pro-oncogenic signaling pathways in cells that have the EGF receptor (EGFR). A recent report has shown that certain genetic polymorphisms in the EGF gene are associated with increased invasiveness and earlier relapse in those treated for prostate cancer.[42] *Transforming growth factor alpha* (TGF-$\alpha$) is a member of the EGF family. It can be produced by transformed cells and then cause increased cell proliferation in an autocrine manner. *Fibroblast growth factor* (FGF) stimulates the growth of fibroblasts and is released upon tissue damage, thereby stimulating tissue proliferation and healing. *Insulin-like growth factor-1* (IGF-1), which increases cell proliferation and reduces apoptosis in many cell types, has been implicated in prostate cancer development. Genetic variation in the *IGF1* gene is associated with higher levels of IGF-1.[43] Finally VEGF levels have been associated with tumor growth and in some cancers, such as breast cancer, tumor progression, and survival from the disease. Genetic variations in the VEGF have been associated with survival in those with breast cancer.[44]

*Growth factor receptors.* A second type of oncogene encodes altered growth factor receptors (GFRs), which may induce proliferative signals in the cell even in the absence of growth factors.[2] Most GFRs act through intrinsic tyrosine kinase activity, the ability to bind inorganic phosphate to the amino acid tyrosine. Increased tyrosine kinase activity leads to reactions that stimulate mitosis and can cause clonal expansion of cells. Point mutations may cause increased activity of tyrosine kinase, and deletion of the portion of the receptor that binds the growth factor may cause uncontrolled activation of the receptor. Nonmutation mechanisms for increased tyrosine kinase activity include overexpression of GFR and autocrine stimulation.

When overproduced, EGFRs are associated with poor prognosis for breast, bladder, colon, lung, and esophageal cancers.[45] *HER2/NEU* receptor (also known as *ErbB2*) overexpression is associated with poor prognosis for breast and ovarian cancers. *HER2/NEU* receptors in breast carcinoma also increase the risk of recurrence.[46]

*Signal transducers.* Many proto-oncogenes encode for proteins in cellular signal transduction pathways. These signal transducing oncoproteins can be guanine nucleotide-binding proteins (G-proteins) or nonreceptor kinase proteins. The nonreceptor kinase group can be subdivided into nonreceptor tyrosine kinases and serine-threonine kinases.

G-proteins act as signal transducers for cell-surface GFRs. An example of G-proteins is the RAS superfamily (the name RAS was derived from rat sarcoma), which includes more than 50 members. The true RAS proteins

(H RAS, K RAS, N RAS) act as signal switches at the inner leaflet cell membrane. Proteins encoded by unmutated *RAS* genes transmit stimulatory signals from GFRs to other signaling proteins. Mutated *RAS* genes cause activation of signaling pathways, even when unprompted by GFRs. Inappropriate *RAS* activation occurs in 2 ways: (1) loss of guanosine 5-triphosphate activity (through point mutations that lead to transformation) and (2) increase in G-nucleotide exchange (point mutations with a lower affinity for G-nucleotide, leading to increased turnover). Mutant *RAS* genes are found in 30% of human cancers including melanoma and pancreatic, colorectal, lung, bladder, endometrial, cervical, biliary tract, and other cancers.[47]

An example of a gene that encodes for a nonreceptor tyrosine kinase is the *SRC* proto-oncogene. This signal transducing oncogene is related to the Rous sarcoma virus in chickens, one of the first viruses implicated in cancer. *SRC* is overexpressed and has increased tyrosine kinase activity in many cancers. It has been linked to tumorigenesis, cancer progression and metastasis, and in addition to causing increased cell proliferation, *SRC* appears to promote invasion and increased cell motility, key tumor properties in metastasis.[48]

Another category of signal transducing oncogenes is one whose products are proteins with serine-threonine kinase activity. Serine-threonine kinases are centrally involved in cell cycle progression. Prototypes for the serine-threonine kinase category include the Raf-1 protein, which is activated by tyrosine kinase–associated receptors, and the mitogenic-activated protein (MAP) kinase.[29] The Raf-1 protein acts as an intermediary in the signal transduction pathway between *RAS* and the cell nucleus by activating other kinases in the MAP kinase pathway that regulates cell division. Roles for Raf-1 and the MAP kinase pathway in transformation are very important. Mutations in Raf-1 can cause most of the cell transformation characteristics seen with activation of the *RAS* oncogene. Over one-third of all cancers demonstrate deregulation of the MAP kinase pathways.[49]

*Transcription factors.* Transcription factors are proteins that activate and otherwise alter gene transcription (making of RNA from DNA). Transcription factors may bind DNA as multiprotein complexes and regulate the expression of 1 or more genes. Mutated transcription factors that regulate genes involved in cell growth and survival have been implicated in oncogenic transformation and cancer. Some oncogenic transcription factors include proteins such as Jun and Fos that are part of signal-dependent processes that control cell growth. An example of transcription factors are members of the E2F family. This is a family of proteins that activate and suppress transcription. The transcription factor E2F2 is one member that is implicated in cancer as it is overexpressed in bladder and prostate cancer.[50]

## TUMOR SUPPRESSOR GENES

Tumor suppressor genes normally suppress or negatively regulate cell growth and proliferation by encoding proteins that block the action of growth-promoting proteins. Thus, a hallmark characteristic of cancer may involve "loss-of-function" of tumor suppressor genes through inactivity due to mutation or other forms of silencing genetic information. Normally, tumor suppressor genes suppress oncogenes.[51] Tumor suppressor genes are recessive meaning that both alleles (forms of the gene) of a pair must mutate or be lost for the cancer phenotype to be expressed. In other words, loss or mutation of both copies of the gene is required for tumorigenesis. Inactivation of tumor suppressor genes is a hallmark of many cancers resulting from inherited predisposition.

Tumor suppressor genes have diverse functions. Some affect DNA transcription, such as *APC*, *MEN1*, *p53*, *RB*, and *WT1*. The tumor suppressor genes *BRCA1* and *BRCA2* have roles in DNA damage repair. The tumor suppressor genes *RB*, *p16*, and *TP53* are critical for operation of the cell cycle, suggesting that many tumor suppressor genes act as "gatekeeper" genes. Gatekeeper genes are responsible for maintaining a constant cell number by renewing cell populations or controlling proliferation in specific tissue types. A mutation in a gatekeeper gene may lead to more cell division than cell death, thereby permitting an increase in cell number and cancer cells.[52]

### Loss of heterozygosity

It is thought that the first mutation or silencing of a tumor suppressor gene affects the actual gene in 1 chromosome, and as stated above, these can be inherited (germline) and increase susceptibility to certain cancers.[2] Since tumor suppressor genes are recessive, for the cancer phenotype to be expressed, a second event, termed a loss of heterozygosity (LOH) event, occurs in the homologous chromosome. A LOH event may involve loss of a whole chromosome or loss of part of a chromosome containing the normal or wild-type gene. LOH is thought to be much more common in occurrence than mutations.[2]

### DNA methylation and epigenetic mechanisms

Another cause of tumor suppressor inactivity is a mechanism that involves a non-nucleotide alteration, hence nongenetic or "epigenetic" mechanism. One type of epigenetic mechanism that is common in cancer involves gene silencing by hypermethylation. Here methyl groups become chemically bonded to the cytosine bases in areas near the promoter region of a tumor suppressor gene and interfere with transcription of the gene. Epigenetic mechanisms are known to operate in many cancers including cancer of the colon, breast, lung, esophagus, bladder, and ovaries.[53] Epigenetic mechanisms are thought to be as important as mutations in inactivating genes and hypermethylation can serve as the second hit in Knudson's two-hit model of tumorigenesis.

## DNA REPAIR GENES

DNA repair genes are an example of "caretaker" genes, which are involved in maintaining the stability and integrity of the genome. Mutations in caretaker genes do not lead directly to cancer. Rather, mutations in these genes lead to inefficient replication or repair of DNA, which in turn allows subsequent mutations in tumor suppressor genes and proto-oncogenes to accumulate. Hence, mutations in caretaker genes increase the likelihood that additional mutations persist and facilitate tumorigenesis and cancer progression.[52]

A number of familial cancers have deficiencies in DNA repair genes, hence caretaking mechanisms, which may lead to high rates of mutations in genes that have microsatellite DNA, short stretches of DNA that include a simple repeating base sequence. The length of microsatellite DNA repeats varies in tumors and normal tissue. Microsatellite instability has been found in colorectal, gastric, breast, bladder, and nonsmall cell lung cancers and has been found to have roles in drug resistance in human tumors.[54] Though microsatellites may provide clues to gene stability, the presence of variation and mutability of microsatellite sites needs to be viewed with caution. Sites of microsatellite instability and mutability do not necessarily have roles in tumorigenesis and malignant progression.[55]

## CYTOGENETIC ABNORMALITIES

Chromosomal abnormalities are associated with cancer. The term "ploidy" refers to the number of sets of chromosomes in a cell. Normal somatic cells are diploid in that they bear 2 sets of chromosomes (1 from each parent). Normal germ cells are haploid, having only 1 chromosome. Many forms of cancer have abnormalities in ploidy as a result of the accumulation of mutations that increase chromosome missagregation. Furthermore, cancer cells typically have bizarre, unstable chromosome structure, with gains, losses, and deletions of segments, or rearrangements of chromosomes.

### Translocations and deletions

Translocations are structural abnormalities in which one part of a chromosome breaks off and fuses to another. Leukemias and lymphomas typically involve translocations. In reciprocal translocations, exchange of genetic material occurs between 2 chromosomes or within the same chromosome. For example, in chronic myelogenous leukemia, the reciprocal translocation between the q (long) arm of chromosome 9, band 34, and the q arm of chromosome 22, band 11 (9;22)(q34,q11), causes the *abl* proto-oncogene to be translocated to chromosome 22 (Philadelphia chromosome). This translocation produces a bcr-abl oncogenic protein with high tyrosine kinase activity.[56] The translocation ultimately activates numerous pathways, including Ras, and transcription factors, such as myc and nuclear factor kappa B (NF-κB).

Chromosomal deletions occur mostly in solid tumors, and commonly involve deletions of specific gene sequences (ie, loss of a chromosomal band or LOH of a specific allele). Deletions are the hallmark cancers associated with tumor suppressor gene problems; eg, retinoblastoma shows the deletion del(13)(q14q14). Deletions can inactivate tumor suppressor genes by revealing recessive mutations.

### Aneuploidy

Aneuploidy involves an abnormal chromosome number reflecting gain or loss of chromosomes. It is often seen with malignant transformation where gross changes in chromosome number occur as tumorigenesis progresses. Aneuploidy can be either random or nonrandom. In *random aneuploidy*, the change in chromosome number has no association with a tumor type; rather, it occurs late in tumorigenesis and reflects genetic instability of the tumor. *Nonrandom aneuploidy* involves a specific change in a given chromosome associated with a specific tumor. For example, trisomy 8 (3 copies of chromosome 8) is associated with acute leukemia. Nonrandom aneuploidy tends to occur earlier in tumorigenesis than the nonrandom form.

Aneuploidy as a cause or a consequence of cancer has long been debated.[57] Research suggests that the function of telomeres—chromosomal structures that determine the domain of chromosomes within a nucleus and protect chromosomes from assault from internal and external environments—may have a greater role in cancer development than aneuploidy does.[58] However, the causes, involved mechanisms, and consequences of aneuploidy are currently under intense study and this thinking may change.

## THE CELL CYCLE

Cell proliferation occurs as the result of coordinated events that include replication of DNA, mitosis, and cytokinesis. These events culminate with the division of a somatic cell into 2 daughter cells containing identical copies of the genome. The concept of a "cell cycle" to describe these events arose during the period when cell investigation relied mainly on light microscopy. Scientists could observe cycles of mitosis, a period of high activity in the cell, alternating with interphase, an inactive "resting" period.[59] After the discovery of DNA structure, further research into the biochemical events occurring in interphase elucidated several distinct phases and appreciation for the activities in interphase.

## EVENTS OF THE CELL CYCLE

The cell cycle is currently conceptualized as a 4-phase process: (1) mitosis or (M) phase; (2) gap 1 ($G_1$) phase; (3) synthesis (S) phase; and (4) gap 2 ($G_2$) phase (Figure 1-3). In the M phase, the chromatids separate to form 2 sets of chromosomes and cytokinesis occurs. Two daughter cells form, containing identical sets of chromosomes and equal amounts of cellular constituents. Following the M phase, cells either reenter $G_1$ to begin the cell cycle anew or exit the cell cycle by entering $G_0$, a state of reproductive quiescence. In the $G_1$ phase, the nucleus enlarges and transcription and translation activities occur in preparation for DNA replication. Late $G_1$ is characterized by a restriction point (R), the point at which the cell becomes committed to replicate. Normal cells will often leave $G_1$ and enter $G_0$ at the restriction point if there is a shortage of nutrients or growth factors. In the S phase, the cell replicates the DNA and forms a complementary set of chromatids. Following replication, the cell proceeds to $G_2$. Most of the cells in the adult body are in $G_0$. Cells that are highly metabolically active, such as epithelial cells in the gastrointestinal tract, stay mitotically active progressing continuously through the cell cycle.

The series of events that occur in the cell cycle is tightly controlled and regulated by proteins called *cyclins*, which combine with and activate enzymes called cyclin-dependent kinases (CDKs). Activation of cyclins and CDKs occurs at specific points in the cell cycle (see Figure 1-3).

Multiple factors in the microenvironment determine whether a particular cell will proliferate, become quiescent,

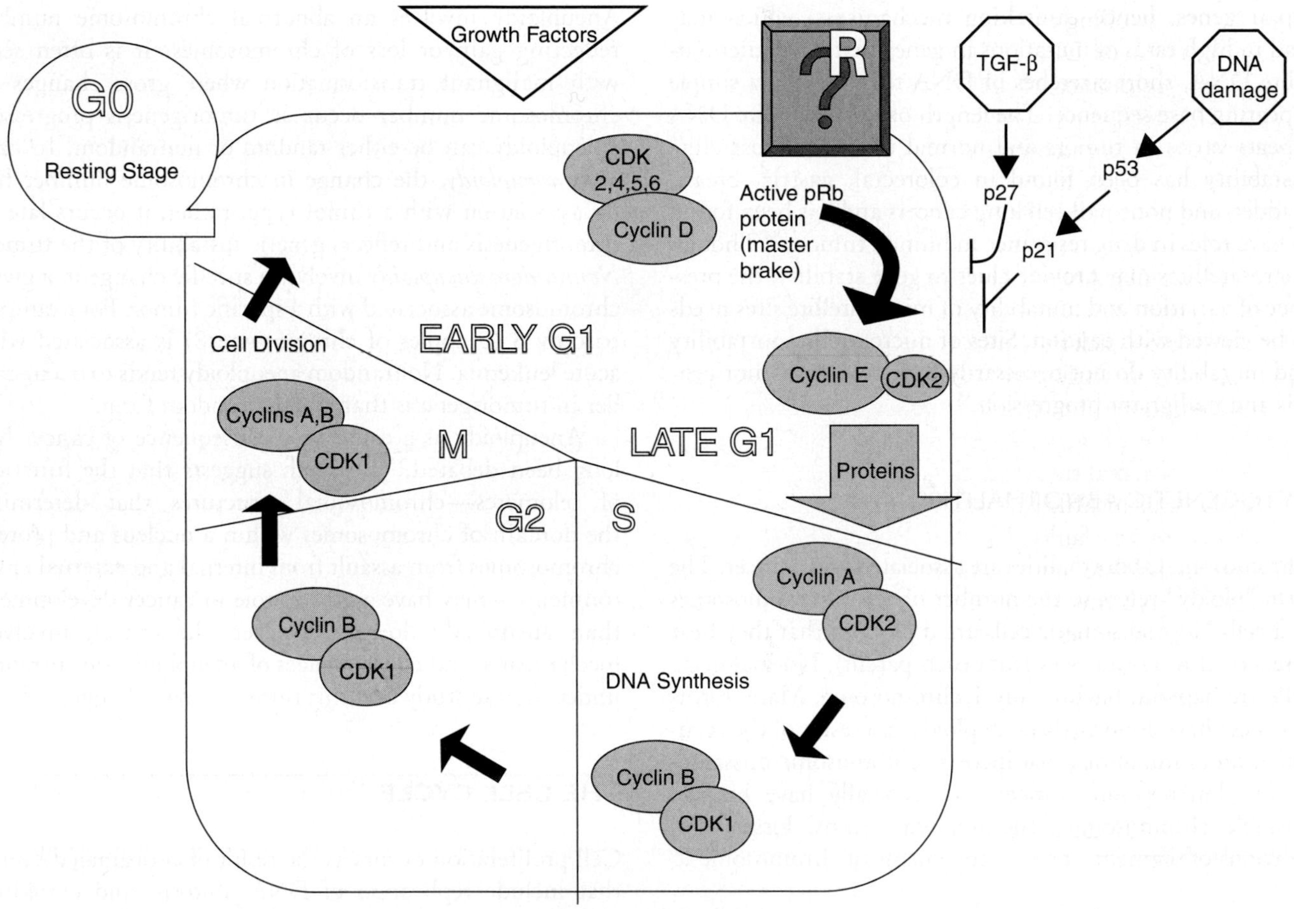


**FIGURE 1-3**

The cell cycle. The cell cycle consists of 4 phases (G1, S, G2, M) that are controlled by proteins called cyclins. The cyclins (D, E, A, B) are activated when complexed with enzymes called cyclin-dependent kinases (CDKs). Upon activation, the cyclin–CDK complex allows the cell to progress through each specific cell cycle phase. Present throughout the cell cycle, the cyclin–CDK complexes serve as checkpoints or monitors of the cell cycle. Inhibitory proteins prevent progression through the cell cycle if DNA damage is present or there is a lack of nutrients or oxygen to support cellular proliferation. Examples of inhibitory proteins include p21, p27, p53. The inhibitory proteins in turn are regulated by the presence of inhibitory growth factors and TGF-β. Once past R (the restriction point) the cell cycle is turned "on" and progression through the cell cycle is inevitable. Cyclin–CDK complexes and pRB (the "master brake") tightly regulate the R point. The stability of the inhibitory proteins and cyclin–CDK complexes are altered in cancer, thereby altering control of the cell cycle and uncontrolled cellular proliferation prevails.

or enter the postmitotic state. The retinoblastoma protein (pRb) mediates most antiproliferative signals, thereby acting as a "master brake" on the cell cycle. Hypophosphorylated pRb blocks proliferation by altering E2F transcription factors[60] that control the gene expression needed for progression from $G_1$ to the S phase. Transforming growth factor beta (TGF-β) acts to prevent phosphorylation of pRb by suppressing *c-myc* or blocking the formation of cyclin–CDK complexes. Hence, TGF-β blocks progression through $G_1$. Phosphorylation of pRb enables activation of E2F transcription factors, which in turn permit advancement through $G_1$ to S phase.

Specific biochemical checkpoints within the cell cycle ensure that the cycle proceeds in the correct sequence and that 1 event has been completed before another begins. Checkpoints exist at the decisions to enter S phase, to enter mitosis ($G_2$/M checkpoint), and to exit mitosis.[60] The checkpoint controlling entry into the S phase prevents replication of damaged DNA. The $G_2$/M checkpoint detects damaged or unduplicated DNA and unduplicated centrosomes. A checkpoint in the M phase delays chromosome segregation if all chromosomes have not become attached to the mitotic spindle fibers.[61]

## THE CELL CYCLE AND CANCER

Cancer cells often lack the ability to enter the $G_0$ (quiescent) state, a condition attributed to having a deficient amount of the pRb protein. Functional pRb may be lost through mutation of the *RB* gene. Excessive cell proliferation may involve lack of signal transduction from TGF-β because of dysfunctional or insufficient numbers of receptors.[61]

Cancer cells have faulty cell cycle checkpoints that enable them to accumulate mutations and faulty chromosome numbers.[2,62] Problems at the $G_1$/S checkpoint in human cancers currently is best understood. Loss of proper $G_1$/S checkpoint function leads to survival of genetically damaged cells and an evolutionary advantage. Research evidence indicates that dysregulation of the R point before the $G_1$/S transition accompanies the formation of most cancers.[2]

## APOPTOSIS

Apoptosis, often referred to as "programmed cell death" or "cell suicide," is a gene-directed method of cell destruction (see Figure 1-4). It can be triggered by environmental conditions, cellular receptor activation, and internal factors related to gene expression.[63,64] Apoptosis is essential for normal development, orderly cell turnover, and tissue repair and remodeling. Two principal pathways mediate apoptosis: the extrinsic and intrinsic pathways. The extrinsic pathway involves activation of cell-surface receptors; the intrinsic pathway, or "mitochondrial pathway," is responsive to internal cues such as DNA damage, which increase

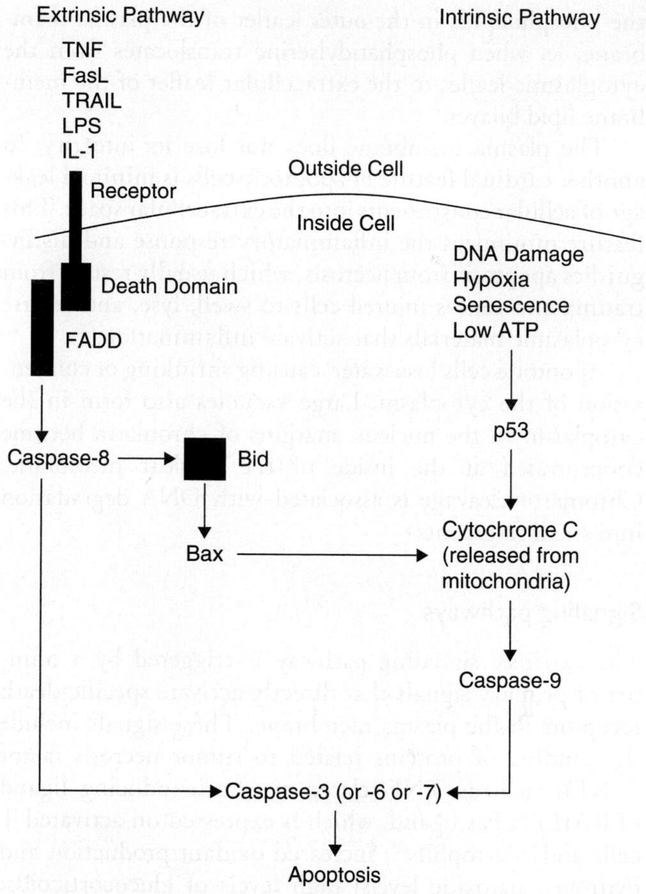


**FIGURE 1-4**

Apoptosis. The extrinsic and intrinsic pathways of apoptosis are normally activated by various cues occurring in the environment of the cell and/or within the cell. Activation of the pathways leads to activation of caspase-3 (and other executioner enzymes) which results in apoptosis. (See text for details.)

p53 protein.[63,65] Because faulty apoptotic mechanisms are important factors in tumor development and survival, many forms of anticancer therapy focus on inducing apoptosis in tumor cells.[66] Furthermore, cancer therapy-induced apoptosis of healthy cells, especially those involved in inflammation and immunity, limits the dosage of chemotherapy.

## CHARACTERISTICS OF CELLS UNDERGOING APOPTOSIS

### Structural changes

Structural changes during apoptosis include blebbing of the plasma membrane and breakage of the cell into apoptotic bodies. Apoptotic bodies help apoptotic cells to become phagocytized by cells that are not undergoing apoptosis. One way phagocytes and other healthy cells recognize apoptotic bodies is from specific changes in the composition of the phospholipids in the outer leaflet of the plasma membrane, ie, when phosphatidylserine translocates from the cytoplasmic leaflet to the extracellular leaflet of the membrane lipid bilayer.

The plasma membrane does not lose its integrity, so another cardinal feature of apoptotic cells is minimal leakage of cellular constituents into the extracellular space. This feature minimizes the inflammatory response and distinguishes apoptosis from necrosis, which usually results from trauma and causes injured cells to swell, lyse, and release cytoplasmic materials that activate inflammation.[67]

Apoptotic cells lose water, causing shrinking or condensation of the cytoplasm. Large vacuoles also form in the cytoplasm. In the nucleus, margins of chromatin become concentrated at the inside of the nuclear membrane. Chromatin cleavage is associated with DNA degradation into small fragments.

### Signaling pathways

The extrinsic signaling pathway is triggered by a number of primary signals that directly activate specific death receptors in the plasma membrane. These signals include the binding of proteins related to tumor necrosis factor (TNF), such as TNF-related apoptosis-inducing ligand (TRAIL)[68]; Fas ligand, which is expressed on activated T cells and neutrophils[63]; increased oxidant production and hydrogen peroxide levels; high levels of glucocorticoids; and presence of endotoxins, such as lipopolysaccharide.[63] Receptor activation by these primary signals triggers secondary signaling pathways that induce death. Intermediate signaling proteins activate caspase-8, which acting in concert with other caspases activates the main executioner enzyme, caspase-3.

The intrinsic (mitochondrial) pathway is activated by internal cues, such as DNA damage and hypoxia, through the p53 protein.[65] Changes in mitochondrial membrane potential release mitochondrial cytochrome *c* to the cytoplasm, which in turn leads to the activation of caspase-9. Activated caspase-9 then activates caspase-3, allowing convergence of the intrinsic pathway with the extrinsic pathway. Furthermore, the extrinsic pathway can activate the intrinsic pathway by caspase-8–induced cleavage of the protein Bid to increase the accumulation of Bax protein inside cells.[68] Bax, in turn, damages mitochondrial membrane and causes cytochrome *c* release and resultant caspase-3, -6, and -7 activation.

## GENES AND PROTEINS INVOLVED IN APOPTOSIS

Genetic alterations involving apoptosis are important factors in tumor development and biology. The *TP53* gene encodes the p53 protein, which is itself a transcription factor that helps to regulate the cell cycle, DNA repair, and apoptosis. Half of all human cancers have *TP53* mutations,[65] and more than 50 tumor types demonstrate mutated *TP53*.[69] Studies using cell lines transfected with a temperature-sensitive mutant of *TP53* have clearly shown that wild-type *TP53* function lowers the threshold for inducing apoptosis following genotoxic damage.[70]

Other genes and proteins important to apoptosis include members of the B-cell leukemia protein 2 (*Bcl-2*) gene family.[71] Certain members, including Bcl-2, $Bcl\text{-}X^L$, A1, and Mcl-1, are required for cell survival, whereas others, such as the Bax/Bak proteins, promote cell death. Overexpression of Bcl-2 on its own is weakly tumorigenic, but it is potently synergistic with other oncogenes that interfere with cell cycle control. Bax can function as a tumor suppressor and may complement the actions of *TP53*.

Members of the TNF family of ligands and receptors,[68] such as TRAIL Apo 2L/TRAIL receptors and Fas/FasL systems, also influence apoptosis.[72,73] TRAIL causes death after activation of its receptors by the extrinsic pathway, but can also trigger the intrinsic pathway by stimulating Bax-induced release of cytochrome *c* into the cytoplasm. The activation of certain TRAIL receptors recruits a Fas-associated death domain (FADD) adapter protein to form a complex containing caspase-8 and -10. This complex activates caspase-3,-6, and -7 to execute apoptosis.[68]

When FasL is present, a death-inducing signaling complex is formed, similar to that described earlier for TRAIL. Responses of this system can be controlled by the *FasL* gene, which is usually inactive but is regulated by transcription factors such as NF-κB.[74] The caspase-8 activity in the complex is regulated by a FADD-like interleukin 1B–interconverting enzyme (FLICE)-inhibitory protein (FLIP).[75] The FLIP protein can become incorporated into the death-inducing signaling complex, thereby thwarting the process.

Gene manipulation targeting apoptosis is being exploited for therapeutic purposes. For example, viral vectors are being examined to selectively destroy cells with *TP53* mutations and replace the mutated gene with nonmutated forms.[65] As a strategy to counteract drug resistance in multiple myeloma, genetic studies are focusing on perturbing NF-κB to induce apoptosis in cancer cells.[76] In studies targeting defective apoptosis signaling in cancer cells, strategies involving antisense-mediated downregulation of Bcl-2 and Bcl-XL expression and small molecules that inhibit these proteins have shown promise.[77] A problem however has been imprecise tumor cell targeting. A newer strategy under investigation employs the use of endothelial progenitor cells to specifically target the tumor and can be genetically manipulated to induce tumor apoptosis.[78]

## METASTASIS

Metastasis is the major cause of death in individuals with solid tumors. The presence of metastatic sites is an important cancer prognostic factor; unfortunately, in many cases, metastases occur before initial diagnosis of cancer. The biology of the events involved in the process of metastasis represents a fundamental area of cancer research. Strategies are being developed to disrupt the metastatic process, thereby improving outcomes of cancer care.

## FACTORS CONTRIBUTING TO METASTASIS

Metastasis is the spread of tumor cells, usually via the bloodstream or lymphatic system, from the primary tumor site to a distant site in the body. Previously the cellular and molecular steps of metastasis were thought to be similar. However, it is apparent that cancer cells use multiple strategies for invasion and colonization of distant sites.[79] Mechanisms that contribute to the process of metastasis include angiogenesis, tumor cell motility, alterations in cell adhesion, and secretion of proteolytic enzymes leading to barrier breakdown.[79] Some of these mechanisms, such as loss of cell adhesion molecules (CAMs) and increased motility, are known as the epithelial-mesenchymal transition (EMT), which is a phenotypic change in epithelial cells that facilitates invasion and metastasis by transitioning to more stem cell-like states.[79] Once in the circulation, metastatic tumor cells must escape immune surveillance, and angiogenesis must occur for the cells to establish themselves in a new tissue site. Recently, the importance of the stromal microenvironment in cancer progression and metastasis has been recognized, and its role is under investigation.[79] Recognition of the importance of the microenvironment in the ability of cancer cells to metastasize has contributed in part to revival of the so-called Soil and Seed Hypothesis originally proposed in 1889.[80] This hypothesis holds that metastasis occurs not by chance, but in organs and tissues where the environment is fertile and conducive to metastatic tumor survival and growth.

### Angiogenesis

When a tumor is only a few millimeters in diameter, its growth will remain limited unless it receives an additional blood supply. Formation of new blood vessels, a process termed *angiogenesis*, provides the nutrients and oxygen required by the growing tumor. Angiogenesis involves the migration and proliferation of endothelial cells from existing vasculature near the tumor, and possibly circulating endothelial progenitor cells.[81] Secreted MMPs promote endothelial cell proliferation by mediating degradation of the ECM and releasing specific forms of VEGF. The newly formed blood vessels provide nutrients and oxygen to the growing tumor, as well as a potential route for metastatic tumor cells to leave the primary tumor site. These blood vessels tend to be "leaky," with loose cell–cell contacts, providing an easy route by which tumor cells can enter the bloodstream for potential transport to distant sites. Tumor-associated angiogenesis also involves the lymphatics; the events of lymphangiogenesis are currently being investigated.

Both positive and negative regulators of angiogenesis exist. Tumor cells produce positive angiogenic factors such as VEGF, basic fibroblast growth factor, TNF, and angiopoietin-1, which serve as stimuli for the development of new capillaries. Angiogenic factors appear to promote locomotion and mitosis of vascular endothelium and to release endothelial growth factors, thus stimulating capillary proliferation. VEGF, which promotes growth and chemotaxis of endothelial cells in vitro, is found in high concentration in the microenvironment of many tumors. This growth factor has been proposed as the final pathway through which other angiogenic agents exert their influence.[82] Negative regulators of angiogenesis are as important as the positive stimulatory agents and include TGF-$\beta_1$, $\alpha$-interferon, angiostatin, and thrombospondin-1 and -2.[81] Transforming growth factor $\beta_1$ inhibits the proteolysis necessary for the formation of viable and effective endothelial sprouts emanating from parent vessels. Alfa-interferon, which was the first antiangiogenic substance to be used in a clinical trial, evolved following its use in the treatment of a life-threatening angioma.[82] Angiostatin, a fragment of the plasminogen molecule, generally prevents the proliferation of endothelial cells.[82] Many tumors downregulate the thrombospondins, a family of extracellular glycoproteins, during acquisition of an angiogenic phenotype.[81] Angiogenesis correlates with metastatic potential and is a prognostic factor for breast cancer.[83] Some researchers have reported that increased numbers of blood vessels associated with a tumor are the second most accurate prognostic factor, following lymph node status.[84,85]

Because many tumors remain indolent without increased vascularity, research now in progress is seeking to better understand the "angiogenic switch" that occurs in tumors. Some investigators have collected evidence for such a switch. This switch involves the production of low levels of thrombospondin-1 and -2, which interact with specific MMPs and VEGF to promote tumor-associated angiogenesis.[81] Furthermore, the use of antiangiogenic agents combined with conventional chemotherapy drugs may increase the effectiveness of the conventional agents.[86] The predicted improvement is related to a hypothesized "normalizing" process in tumor-associated vessels induced by antiangiogenic agents.[86] When the vessels become more normal, tumor pressure decreases, leading to improved uptake of chemotherapeutic agents by the tumor.

Similar to tumor development and progression, tumor angiogenesis is considered a complex process that involves contributions from other cells in the tumor microenvironment. Fibroblasts, inflammatory cells, and the ECM may all interact to control angiogenesis. Some forms of VEGF have reduced activity and are sequestered by components of the ECM. High levels of particular MMPs in the vicinity may free active forms of VEGF. Thrombospondin-1 and -2 have antiangiogenic effects when they act directly on endothelial cells, but induce angiogenic effects on these cells when they are mediated by fibroblasts and immune cells.[81]

### Motility and migration

A tumor cell must exhibit motile behavior to move from the primary tumor and enter the blood and lymph vasculature. Motogens, or motility factors, stimulate tumor cell motility. Motility factors are produced by both tumor and normal cells and include EGF and interleukins 1, 3, and 6.

Changes in the cytoskeleton that affect cell shape are associated with increased motility of tumor cells.[87] The cytoskeleton, an internal supportive structure of a cell, consists of filamentous proteins including actin, keratin, vimentin, and tubulin. The distribution of these filaments and their coexpression are associated with metastatic disease in some cancers, such as melanoma and breast and cervical cancers.[87,88]

Antimotility factors that specifically target filamentous structures of the cytoskeleton are currently in use or under investigation. Agents such as paclitaxel and colchicine work by altering microtubules. Cytochalasin D is associated with inhibition of cell motility following disruption of actin filaments. Use of many of these agents is based on the premise that tumor cells migrate as single cells that become detached from the primary tumor, enter the blood and/or lymph vasculature, exit the circulation, and seed distant organs. These individual cells have amoeboid-like and mesenchymal-type movement patterns. It is now known that cancer cells can use collective migration strategies that include movement as cellular sheets, strands, and clusters.[89] These diverse migration strategies, which entail different morphological changes and varied reliance on integrins, proteases, cadherins, and gap junctions, may explain why therapies designed to target single-cell migration have not yet demonstrated effectiveness.[89]

### Cell adhesion

Cells express surface molecules, known collectively as CAMs, that mediate both attachments to the ECM and cell–cell adhesion (Figure 1-5). Changes in the adhesive properties of cells and CAMs are thought to have an important role in the tumor development and progression. Loss of attachments to the ECM and cell–cell adhesion contributes to a more invasive phenotype, by enabling tumor cells to (1) increase their motility and leave their sites of origin, (2) degrade the ECM, and (3) invade and metastasize.[90] Families of CAMs with known roles in tumor biology and metastasis include members of the immunoglobulin (Ig) superfamily, cadherins,[91] and integrins.[90,92]

Members of the Ig superfamily are calcium-independent adhesion molecules. Cell–cell adhesion molecule 1 may be a tumor suppressor of prostate cancer, as this disease shows reduced expression of the molecule.[90] Another member of the Ig superfamily, the product of the deletion in colon cancer (*DCC*) gene, is often absent in colon cancer cells and other cancers, including prostate and bladder cancer. Loss of the *DCC* gene is associated with increased muscle invasion and recurrence.[90] The cadherins are calcium-dependent cell–cell adhesion molecules that are important in adherens junctions. Cadherin family members include epithelial- (E) and neuronal- (N) cadherins. E-cadherin-mediated cell–cell adhesion is lost in many epithelial cancers. In cancer cells that have lost E-cadherin, many times N-cadherin becomes overexpressed and the cancer cells demonstrate increased motility. This phenomenon contributes to the idea that a "cadherin switch" from E-cadherin to N-cadherin occurs during the cell's transition to EMT and an invasive phenotype.[93,94] Integrins are glycoproteins that form heterodimers of alpha ($\alpha$) and beta ($\beta$) subunits. Many combinations are possible, as 15 $\alpha$ and 9 $\beta$ forms exist. Many of the integrins function as receptors for the components of the ECM. Expression of certain integrins may be lost or gained. The integrin $\alpha_v\beta_3$, eg, is not normally expressed in epithelial cells, yet can be expressed in breast and prostate cancer cells, where it mediates invasion to bone.[95]

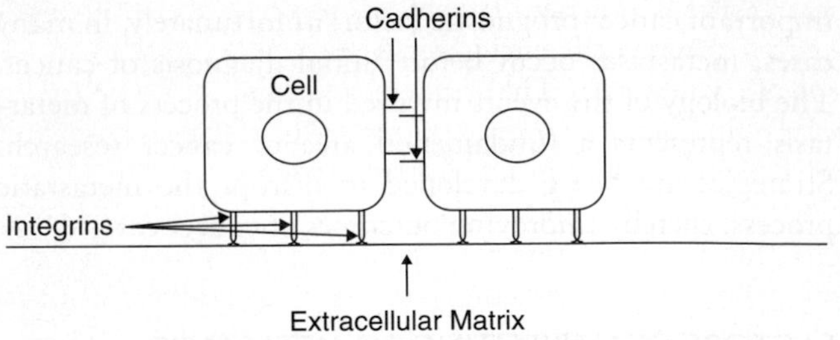


**FIGURE 1-5**

Cell adhesion. Cell adhesion molecules mediating cell–cell adhesion (cadherins) and cell–matrix adhesion (integrins) are important mediators of metastasis. Decreased cell–cell adhesion is required for the detachment of metastatic cells from the primary tumor; and decreased cell–matrix adhesion is required with decreased anchorage dependence or cell–matrix adhesion.

Many investigations of CAMs and cancer are underway. These studies concern the use of CAMs for diagnosing and staging cancers, assessing response to therapy and survival, and as potential targets for immune- and gene-based therapies.[90] Furthermore, chronic expression of CAMs, as occurs during inflammation, may facilitate metastasis.[96]

### Proteolytic enzymes

To successfully metastasize, a tumor cell must cross a number of barriers, including the ECM, connective tissue, and the endothelial barrier. The ECM serves as the first barrier that tumor cells encounter when migrating from the primary tumor site. The major components of the ECM include fibronectin, laminin, vitronectin, collagen type IV, and heparan sulfate proteoglycan. Prior to degrading the ECM, tumor cells bind components of the ECM. Integrins are a family of proteins that mediate cell–matrix interactions. Tumor cells interact with neighboring stromal cells to secrete a number of proteinases that assist with the degradation of these barriers. Once secreted, the enzymes degrade components of the ECM, permitting passage of tumor cells through the interstitium or into the circulation. Increased levels of MMPs and uPA have been associated with highly metastatic tumors.[97]

Collectively, MMPs are able to degrade every component of the ECM.[98] In healthy tissues, the expression of potentially damaging MMPs is low and remains under tight regulation of cytokines and growth factors. By comparison, the quantity of MMPs is much higher in tumors. Historically, scientists thought that the tumor cells were responsible for producing MMPs. Current data support the hypothesis that cancer cells stimulate production and release of MMPs by the neighboring stromal cells.[98] For example, certain glycoproteins in the plasma membranes of cancer cells stimulate fibroblasts in the vicinity to secrete MMPs. Furthermore, the MMPs may release growth factors sequestered by components of the ECM. Hence, the stroma and tumor microenvironment play important roles in cancer progression.

### Immunogenicity

A tumor cell's ability to elicit an immune response will determine its ability to evade the immune system. The theory of immune surveillance suggests that malignant cells develop randomly and often, but immune cells destroy cancer cells before they proliferate. Cytotoxic T lymphocytes, activated macrophages, and natural killer (NK) cells are thought to be the predominant immune cells that protect the body from cancer.[99] For cytotoxic T-cell activation, the tumor antigen must be presented by an antigen-presenting cell (APC) to the T cell. The APC cell, in turn, depends on the presentation of tumor-associated antigens on the tumor cell surface.

Natural killer cells are large, granular lymphocytes that can naturally lyse a broad range of tumor cell targets, even if they have not had prior exposure to the tumor cells. The exact mechanism of how NKs recognize tumor cells is not clear. Natural killer cells do not require APC presentation of an antigen for spontaneous cytolytic activity, but NK activation is prevented when class I MHC (major histocompatibility complex) molecules are expressed on the tumor cell surface.[99] Recent evidence in mice shows that NK cells have a lectin-like receptor NKG2D that recognizes ligands expressed by many tumor cells.[100] This mechanism is being investigated as the basis for tumor immunosurveillance.

Tumor cells evade or hide from the immune system in a multitude of ways. Many tumors downregulate MHC expression, thereby escaping detection. Other tumors secrete immunosuppressive factors such as TGF-β, which decreases T-cell proliferation. Tumor cells can release soluble antigens or intracellular adhesion molecules that block T-cell interactions with APC. Alternatively, tumor cells may develop variants with no recognizable antigenic structures. Chemotherapy and radiation treatments may depress the immune system in general.

## METASTASIS SUPPRESSOR GENES

The identification of tumor suppressor genes prompted the search for metastasis suppressor genes. A number of metastasis suppressor genes have been identified and include *NM23, MKK4, KAI1, BRMS1, KiSS1, RHOGDI2, CRSP3,* and *VDUP1.* These genes affect important signal-transduction pathways, including mitogen-activated protein kinases, RHO, RAC, and G-protein-coupled and tyrosine kinase receptors.[101]

## THE METASTATIC CASCADE

The process of metastasis is complex and involves multiple steps often referred to as the metastatic cascade. During the process, tumor cells detach from the primary tumor, become highly motile and migrate to the vasculature where they enter the blood or lymphatic circulation. If cancer cells are successful at evading the immune system, blood and lymph transport them to distant sites such as the bones, lungs, and liver. To invade normal tissues and establish metastatic colonies, the tumor cells again must attach and/or penetrate the endothelium and remain viable. Tumor cells may grow into larger colonies or remain dormant for decades before induced to proliferate.

### Steps of the metastatic cascade

*Detachment.* To invade surrounding tissues, cancer cells must detach from the primary tumor. Detachment is accomplished in part by downregulation of E-cadherin and the hypothesized "cadherin switch" to N-cadherin at the tumor cell surface.[102] This change decreases cell–cell contacts, facilitating complete detachment from neighboring tumor cells.

*Invasion.* Tumor cells can invade the surrounding tissue and enter a lymphatic vessel or a blood vessel. Invasion is facilitated by increased motility and secretion of proteolytic enzymes that are not overcome by local inhibitors. The secreted enzymes cause barrier breakdown and subsequent tumor invasion. If a tumor enters a vessel, the cells may localize at the entry site or disseminate to other destinations.

*Survival in transport.* In the bloodstream, tumor cells are at risk for destruction due to mechanical factors and attack by the immune system. It is estimated that only 1 in every 1000 tumor cells that enter the vasculature survive to give rise to a metastatic colony of cancer cells.[29] Tumor cells rely in part on survival enhancing mechanisms (see "Immunogenicity" in the previous section) to evade the immune system.

*Arrest in distant organ capillary bed.* Arrest of tumor cells in an organ capillary bed requires that they adhere to the endothelial layer or become lodged in the microcirculation as a result of the geometry of the capillary bed. To maximize their ability to adhere to a distant blood vessel, malignant cells may secrete substances that cause platelets to aggregate around them, resulting in a large, sticky mass. In turn, platelets secrete growth factors that favor continued survival of the adjoining tumor cells.

Exactly where circulating tumor cells adhere depends on certain factors that are not entirely clear at this time. Selective patterns of tumor spread are known to exist for different cancers, however. Cell-cell adhesion molecules expressed on the surface of tumor cells may influence which organs or sites certain tumors will favor, because corresponding adhesion molecules might be present within the microvasculature of distant organs. This phenomenon helps explain why prostate carcinoma cells so often go to bone and ocular melanomas arrive in the liver, while typically sparing other organs. In addition to selective target tissue adhesion, specific chemotactic factors or growth factors may attract circulating malignant cells to a particular site.

*Establishment of secondary tumor.* The formation of micrometastases and colonization of a distant site is the most complex and challenging step of the cascade.[2] The cancer cells may escape the vasculature using a diapedesis-type mechanism or begin proliferating within the microvessel. The conditions in the new microenvironment may be very different. The tumor cell may have to adapt to changes in nutrients or the presence of stimulatory growth factors. In some cancers, the metastatic cells may remain dormant for many years before proliferating into a detectable tumor. As the cells in a metastatic site are often genetically heterogeneous, evolution of metastatic ability and success may occur outside of the primary tumor site.[2]

### MODELS OF INVASION AND METASTASIS

A number of in vitro and in vivo models of metastasis have been developed and used to gain insight into the process of metastasis and to assist in the testing of agents and strategies to treat metastasis. An example of a simple test of the ability of drugs, antibodies, and genetic manipulations to perturb cancer invasiveness is the fibrin plug invasion assay, in which the endpoint is the number of cancer cells in the plug. More complex cell culture models use porous filters coated with an artificial basement membrane and suspended in a dual chamber system. The coated filter can be covered with endothelial cells, and the ability of cancer cells placed in the top chamber to cross the endothelial cells can be determined by counting the number of cancer cells that enter the bottom chamber. Newer models that employ engineered tissues are being developed.

Rodent models of metastasis also exist. Orthotopic models involve transplantation of a tumor under the skin of a rodent. Other models rely on injections of cultured cancer cells into the heart or tail vein of the animal, then monitoring metastasis. The injection of genetically engineered cells permits a high degree of experimental control and manipulation so as to gain greater insight into the mechanisms underlying the metastatic cascade. New fluorescence-labeling agents and sophisticated detection systems enable the evaluation and monitoring of metastases in living animals over time.

### TREATMENT OF METASTASIS

Tremendous progress in prolonging survival from metastatic cancer has been made in some tumor types, such as testicular cancer, whereas limited progress has been made in other tumor types, such as breast cancer. Greater emphasis is now being placed on the development of treatment strategies that abrogate various steps of the metastatic cascade and that are tailored to the gene expression profiles and targets specific to a particular tumor.

Current technology and advances in genomics now enable profiling of gene expression in tumors. In some cancers, eg, breast cancer, genetic signatures or profiles of tumors highly likely to metastasize are emerging. Such gene expression profiles will enable the development of more targeted treatments to prevent metastasis and assist in more thoroughly delineating the molecular mechanisms involved in metastasis.

## CONCLUSION

The biology of cancer is a complex, continually evolving phenomenon, and one that is difficult to keep abreast of unless immersed in cancer bioscience. Because cancer biology underlies every other aspect of cancer as a human disease, nurses need to have a basic understanding of cancer genetics, molecular and cell biology, immunology, and biochemistry. The relationships among these sciences will help us prevent and treat cancers based on knowledge of cancer development, growth, and metastasis.

## REFERENCES


1. Doll R. Introduction. In: Hiatt H, Watson JR, Winsten JA, eds. *Origins of Human Cancer.* Cold Spring Harbor, NY: Cold Spring Harbor Laboratory; 1977:1–12.
2. Weinberg RA. *The Biology of Cancer.* New York, NY: Garland Science, Taylor & Francis Group, LLC; 2007.
3. Visvader JE, Lindeman GJ. Cancer stem cells in solid tumors: accumulating evidence and unresolved questions. *Nat Rev Cancer.* 2008;8:755–768.
4. Jaffe LF. Epigenetic theories of cancer initiation. *Adv Cancer Res.* 2003;90:209–230.
5. Nowell P. The clonal evolution of tumor cell populations. *Science.* 1976;194:23–28.
6. Strachan T, Read AP. *Human Molecular Genetics.* 3rd ed. New York: Garland Science; 2004.
7. Bellacosa A. Genetic hits and mutation rate in colorectal tumorigenesis: versatility of Knudson's theory and implications for cancer prevention. *Genes Chromosomes Cancer.* 2003;38:382–388.
8. Moolgavkar SH, Luebeck EG. Multistage carcinogenesis and the incidence of human cancer. *Genes Chromosomes Cancer.* 2003;38:302–306.
9. Merlo LMF, Pepper JW, Reid BJ, Maley CC. Cancer as an evolutionary and ecological process. *Nat Rev Cancer.* 2006;6:924–935.
10. Hayflick L, Moorhead PS. The serial cultivation of human diploid cell strains. *Exp Cell Res.* 1961;25:585–621.
11. Jonkers J, Berns A. Conditional mouse models of sporadic cancer. *Nat Rev Cancer.* 2002;2:251–265.
12. Oshima RG, Lesperance J, Munoz V, et al. Angiogenic acceleration of Neu induced mammary tumor progression and metastasis. *Cancer Res.* 2004;64:169–179.
13. Kouros-Mehr H, Slorach EM, Sternlicht MD, Zerb Z. GATA-3 maintains the differentiation of the luminal cell fate in the mammary gland. *Cell.* 2006;127:1041–1055.
14. Hakomori S. Cancer-associated glycosphingolipid antigens: their structure, organization, and function. *Acta Anatomica.* 1998;161:79–90.
15. Birkle S, Zeng G, Gao L, et al. Role of tumor-associated gangliosides in cancer progression. *Biochimie.* 2003;85:455–463.
16. Bissell MJ, Radisky D. Putting tumours in context. *Nat Rev Cancer.* 2001;1:46–54.
17. Dranoff G. Cytokines in cancer pathogenesis and cancer therapy. *Nat Rev Cancer.* 2004;4:11–22.
18. Egeblad M, Werb Z. New functions for the matrix metalloproteinases in cancer progression. *Nat Rev Cancer.* 2002;2:161–174.
19. Hojilla CV, Mohammed FF, Khokha R. Matrix metalloproteinases and their tissue inhibitors direct cell fate during cancer development. *Br J Cancer.* 2003;89:1817–1821.
20. Dean JP, Nelson PS. Profiling influences of senescent and aged fibroblasts on prostate carcinogenesis. *Br J Cancer.* 2008;98:245–249.
21. Knudson AG Jr. Mutation and cancer: statistical study of retinoblastoma. *Proc Natl Acad Sci U S A.* 1971;68:820–823.
22. Jackson AL, Loeb LA. The mutation rate and cancer. *Genetics.* 1998;148:1483–1490.
23. Simpson AJ. The natural somatic mutation frequency and human carcinogenesis. *Adv Cancer Res.* 1997;71:209–240.
24. Tomlinson I, Bodmer W. Selection, the mutation rate and cancer: ensuring that the tail does not wag the dog. *Nat Med.* 1999;5:11–12.
25. Araten DJ, Golde DW, Zhang RH, et al. Quantitative measurement of the human somatic mutation rate. *Cancer Res.* 2005;65:8111–8117.
26. Loescher LJ. DNA testing for cancer predisposition. *Oncol Nurs Forum.* 1998;25:1317–1327.
27. Hoeijmakers J. Genome maintenance mechanisms for preventing cancer. *Nature.* 2001;411:366–374.
28. Hu JJ, Mohrenweiser HW, Bell DA, et al. Symposium overview: genetic polymorphisms in DNA repair and cancer risk. *Toxicol Appl Pharmacol.* 2002;185:64–73.
29. Alberts B, Johnson A, Lewis J, et al. *Molecular Biology of the Cell.* 5th ed. New York: Garland Science, Taylor & Francis Group, LLC; 2008.
30. Hussain SP, Hofseth LJ, Harris CC. Radical causes of cancer. *Nat Rev Cancer.* 2003;3:276–285.
31. Chakravarthi A. Single nucleotide polymorphisms: . . . to a future of genetic medicine. *Nature.* 2001;409:822–823.
32. Bartsch H, Rojas M, Alexandrov K, et al. Impact of adduct determination on the assessment of cancer susceptibility. *Recent Results Cancer Res.* 1998;154:86–96.
33. Miller RD, Kwok PY. The birth and death of human single-nucleotide polymorphisms: new experimental evidence and implications for human history and medicine. *Hum Mol Genet.* 2001;10:2195–2198.
34. Sun S, Schiller JH, Gadzar AF. Lung cancer in never smokers: a different disease. *Nat Rev Cancer.* 2007;7:778–790.
35. Bartsch H, Nair U, Risch A, et al. Genetic polymorphism of CYP genes, alone or in combination, as a risk modifier of tobacco-related cancers. *Cancer Epidemiol Biomarkers Prev.* 2000;9:3–28.
36. Risch A, Wikman H, Thiel S, et al. Glutathione-S-transferase M1, M3, T1 and P1 polymorphisms and susceptibility to non-small-cell lung cancer subtypes and hamartomas. *Pharmacogenetics.* 2001;11:757–764.
37. Godschalk RW, Dallinga JW, Wikman H, et al. Modulation of DNA and protein adducts in smokers by genetic polymorphisms in GSTM1, GSTT1, NAT1 and NAT2. *Pharmacogenetics.* 2001;11:389–398.
38. Vineis P, Marinelli D, Autrup H, et al. Current smoking, occupation, N-acetyltransferase-2 and bladder cancer: a pooled analysis of genotype-based studies. *Cancer Epidemiol Biomarkers Prev.* 2001;10:1249–1252.
39. Wikman H, Thiel S, Jager B, et al. Relevance of N-acetyltransferase 1 and 2 (NAT1, NAT2) genetic polymorphisms in nonsmall cell lung cancer susceptibility. *Pharmacogenetics.* 2001;11:157–168.
40. Croce CM. Oncogenes and cancer. *N Engl J Med.* 2008;358:502–511.
41. Sastry KSR, Karpova Y, Kolik J. EGF protects prostate cancer cells from apoptosis by inducing BAD phosphorylation via redundant signaling pathways. *J Biol Chem.* 2006;281:27367–27377.
42. Teixeira AL, Ribeiro R, Cardoso D. Genetic polymorphism in *EGF* is associated with prostate cancer aggressiveness and progression-free interval in androgen blockade–treated patients. *Clin Cancer Res.* 2008;14:3367–3371.
43. Johansson M, McKay JD, Wiklund F, et al. Implications for prostate cancer of *IGF1* genetic variation and circulating IGF1 levels. *J Clin Endocrinol Metab.* 2007;92:4820–4826.
44. Lu H, Shu X-O, Cui Y, et al. Association of genetic polymorphisms in the *VEGF* gene with breast cancer survival. *Cancer Res.* 2005;65:5015–5019.
45. Nicholson RI, Gee JM, Harper ME. EGFR and cancer prognosis. *Eur J Cancer.* 2001;37(Suppl 4):S9-S15.
46. Ross JS, Fletcher JA, Linette GP, et al. The Her-2/neu gene and protein in breast cancer 2003: biomarker and target of therapy. *Oncologist.* 2003;8:307–325.
47. Schubbert S, Shannon K, Bollag G. Hyperactive Ras in developmental disorders and cancer. *Nat Rev Cancer.* 2007;7:295–308.
48. Yeatman TJ. A renaissance for SRC. *Nat Rev Cancer.* 2004;4:470–480.
49. Dillon AS, Hagan S, Rath O, Kolch W. MAP kinase signalling pathways in cancer. *Oncogene.* 2007;26:3279–3290.
50. Foster CS, Falcomer A, Dodson AR, et al. Transcription factor E2F3 overexpressed in prostate cancer independently predicts clinical outcome. *Oncogene.* 2004;23:5871–5879.
51. Weinberg RA. Oncogenes and tumor suppressor genes. *CA: Cancer J Clin.* 1994;44:160–170.
52. Kinzler KW, Vogelstein B. Cancer-susceptibility genes. Gatekeepers and caretakers. *Nature.* 1997;386:761, 763.

53. Estelle M. Epigenetics and cancer. *N Engl J Med.* 2008;358: 1148–1159.
54. Picard SF, Franco N, Sergent C, et al. Analysis of microsatellite instability in acquired drug-resistance human tumor cell lines. *Oncol Rep.* 2002;9:971–976.
55. Hienonen T, Sammalkorpi H, Enholm S, et al. Mutations in two short noncoding mononucleotide repeats in most microsatellite-unstable colorectal cancers. *Cancer Res.* 2005;65:4607–4613.
56. Al-Ali H-K, Heinrich MC, Lange T, et al. High incidence of BCR-ABL kinase domain mutations and absence of mutations of the PDGFR and KIT activation loops in CML patients with secondary resistance to imatinib. *Hematol J.* 2004;5:55–60.
57. Sen S. Aneuploidy and cancer. *Curr Opin Oncol.* 2000;12:82–88.
58. Pathak S, Multani AS, Furlong CL, et al. Telomere dynamics, aneuploidy, stem cells, and cancer [review]. *Int J Oncol.* 2002;20:637–641.
59. Brown T. *Genomes.* New York, NY: Bios Scientific; 2002.
60. Hanahan D, Weinberg RA. The hallmarks of cancer. *Cell.* 2000;100:57–70.
61. Pollard T, Earnshaw W. *Cell Biology.* New York, NY: Saunders; 2002.
62. Orr-Weaver TL, Weinberg RA. A checkpoint on the road to cancer. *Nature.* 1998;392:223–224.
63. Lydon A, Martyn JA. Apoptosis in critical illness. *Int Anesthesiol Clin.* 2003;41:65–77.
64. Martin TR, Nakamura M, Matute-Bello G. The role of apoptosis in acute lung injury. *Crit Care Med.* 2003;31:S184–S188.
65. Smith ND, Rubenstein JN, Eggener SE, et al. The p53 tumor suppressor gene and nuclear protein: basic science review and relevance in the management of bladder cancer. *J Urol.* 2003;169:1219–1228.
66. Kim R, Tanabe K, Emi M, et al. Inducing cancer cell death by targeting transcription factors. *Anticancer Drugs.* 2003;14:3–11.
67. Wyllie AH. Apoptosis and carcinogenesis. *Eur J Cell Biol.* 1997;73:189–197.
68. Younes A, Kadin ME. Emerging applications of the tumor necrosis factor family of ligands and receptors in cancer therapy. *J Clin Oncol.* 2003;21:3526–3534.
69. Hollstein M, Rice K, Greenblatt MS, et al. Database of p53 gene somatic mutations in human tumors and cell lines. *Nucleic Acids Res.* 1994;22:3551–3555.
70. Lowe SW, Schmitt EM, Smith SW, et al. p53 is required for radiation-induced apoptosis in mouse thymocytes. *Nature.* 1993;362:847–849.
71. Coultas L, Strasser A. The role of the Bcl-2 protein family in cancer. *Semin Cancer Biol.* 2003;13:115–123.
72. Wajant H, Pfizenmaier K, Scheurich P. TNF-related apoptosis inducing ligand (TRAIL) and its receptors in tumor surveillance and cancer therapy. *Apoptosis.* 2002;7:449–459.
73. Nagata S. Fas-induced apoptosis. *Intern Med.* 1998;37:179–181.
74. Wajant H, Pfizenmaier K, Scheurich P. Non-apoptotic Fas signaling. *Cytokine Growth Factor Rev.* 2003;14:53–66.
75. Wajant H. Targeting the FLICE Inhibitory Protein (FLIP) in cancer therapy. *Mol Interv.* 2003;3:124–127.
76. Yang HH, Ma MH, Vescio RA, et al. Overcoming drug resistance in multiple myeloma: the emergence of therapeutic approaches to induce apoptosis. *J Clin Oncol.* 2003;21:4239–4247.
77. Shangary S, Johnson DE. Recent advances in the development of anticancer agents targeting cell death inhibitors in the Bcl-2 protein family. *Leukemia.* 2003;17:1470–1481.
78. Jarny G, Wei J, Debatin K-M, Beltinger C. Apoptosis-inducing cellular vehicles for cancer gene therapy: endothelial and neural progenitors. In: Srivastava R, ed, *Apoptosis, Cell Signaling, and Human Diseases: Molecular Mechanisms.* New York, NY: Springer-Verlag; 2007:279–302.
79. Yilmaz M, Christofori G, Lehembre F. Distinct mechanisms of tumor invasion and metastasis. *Trends Mol Med.* 2007;13:535–541.
80. Paget S. The distribution of secondary growths in cancer of the breast. *Lancet.* 1889;1:571–573.
81. Lawler J, Detmar M. Tumor progression: the effects of thrombospondin-1 and -2. *Int J Biochem Cell Biol.* 2004;36:1038–1045.
82. Folkman J, D'Amore PA. Blood vessel formation: what is its molecular basis? *Cell.* 1996;87:1153–1155.
83. Morabito A, Magnani E, Gion M, et al. Prognostic and predictive indicators in operable breast cancer. *Clin Breast Cancer.* 2003;3:381–390.
84. Sauer G, Deissler H. Angiogenesis: prognostic and therapeutic implications in gynecologic and breast malignancies. *Curr Opin Obstet Gynecol.* 2003;15:45–49.
85. Weidner N, Semple JP, Welch WR, et al. Tumor angiogenesis and metastasis—correlation in invasive breast carcinoma. *N Engl J Med.* 1991;324:1–8.
86. Jain RK. Molecular regulation of vessel maturation. *Nat Med.* 2003;9:685–693.
87. Strauli P, Haemmerli G. The role of cancer cell motility in invasion. *Cancer Metastasis Rev.* 1984;3:127–141.
88. Hendrix MJ, Seftor EA, Chu YW, et al. Role of intermediate filaments in migration, invasion and metastasis. *Cancer Metastasis Rev.* 1996;15:507–525.
89. Friedl P, Wolf K. Tumour-cell invasion and migration: diversity and escape mechanisms. *Nat Rev Cancer.* 2003;3:362–374.
90. Okegawa T, Li Y, Pong RC, et al. Cell adhesion proteins as tumor suppressors. *J Urol.* 2002;167:1836–1843.
91. Mareel M, Leroy A. Clinical, cellular, and molecular aspects of cancer invasion. *Physiol Rev.* 2003;83:337–376.
92. Mason M, Davies G, Jiang WG. Cell adhesion molecules and adhesion abnormalities in prostate cancer. *Oncol Hematol.* 2002;41:11–28.
93. Cavallaro U, Schaffhauser B, Cristofori G. Cadherins and the tumour progression: is it all in a switch? *Cancer Lett.* 2002;176:123–128.
94. Christofori G. Changing neighbours, changing behaviour: cell adhesion molecule-mediated signalling during tumour progression. *EMBO J.* 2003;22:2318–2323.
95. Cooper CR, Chay CH, Pienta KJ. The role of alpha(v)beta(3) in prostate cancer progression. *Neoplasia.* 2002;4:191–194.
96. Kobayabi H, Lin PC. Angiogenesis links chronic inflammation with cancer. *Methods Mol Biol.* 2009;511:185–191.
97. Choong PF, Nadesapillai AP. Urokinase plasminogen activator system: a multifunctional role in tumor progression and metastasis. *Clin Orthop.* 2003;415(Suppl):S46-S58.
98. Pavlaki M, Zucker S. Matrix metalloproteinase inhibitors (MMPIs): the beginning of phase I or the termination of phase III clinical trials. *Cancer Metastasis Rev.* 2003;22:177–203.
99. Diefenbach A, Jamieson AM, Lui SD, Shastrin N, Raulet DH. Ligands for the murine NKG2D receptor: expression by tumor cells and activation of NK cells and macrophages. *Nat Immunol.* 2000;1:119–126.
100. Bryceson YT, Ljunggen H-G. Tumor recognition by NK cell activating receptor NKG2D. *Eur J Immunol.* 2008;38:2927–2968.
101. Steeg PS. Metastasis suppressors alter the signal transduction of cancer cells. *Nat Rev Cancer.* 2003;3:55–63.
102. Hazen RB, Oldo R, Keren R, Badano I, Suyama K. Cadherin switch in tumor progression. *Ann N Y Acad Sci.* 2004;1014:155–163.

CHAPTER

# 2

*Janice Post-White, PhD, RN, FAAN, and Susan M. Bauer-Wu, RN, PhD, FAAN*

# Immunology

## INTRODUCTION

Through understanding the immune system and factors that affect its function, oncology nurses can play an important role in promoting optimal immunologic responses and in preventing clinical complications in patients with cancer. This chapter provides a basic review of immunology, including components of the immune system, key immunologic processes, and clinical implications. Cancer diagnosis and treatment are identified in conjunction with changes in immune function. For example, suppressed or inadequate immune processes are associated with the development of some cancers, while chemotherapeutic drugs and radiation therapy, used to treat cancer, can induce immunosuppression. Other cancer therapies, such as biotherapies, can selectively enhance the body's own immune system to fight off cancer. In addition, behavioral factors, such as nutrition, exercise, sleep, and stress, can affect immunologic functioning.

## OVERVIEW

The immune system provides the body's defense against infectious and malignant disease. It is a complex arrangement of cells, tissues, and soluble mediators. Two overall functions of the immune system are to recognize foreign substances (nonself) and to eliminate the foreign substances with restoration of homeostasis.[1] Foreign organisms that invade the body are called *antigens* and initiate immune responses.

Immune responses may be either innate or adaptive.[1] *Innate immunity*, considered the body's first line of defense, provides nonspecific responses to foreign substances. Inflammation and phagocytosis are examples of such nonspecific responses. Phagocytosis involves general recognition and engulfment of foreign organisms.

*Adaptive, or acquired, immunity* differs from innate immunity in that it is highly specific for particular antigens. This type of immunity has memory, referred to as *anamnesis*, meaning that the responses improve with each successive encounter with the same antigen.[1] Humoral and cell-mediated immune responses are interdependent functional arms that fall within the domain of adaptive immunity. The specificity and memory associated with acquired immunity form the basis of vaccination to control certain diseases.

Immune responses can be characterized as appropriate, deficient, or overreactive. An *appropriate immune response* results in the elimination of antigen and the restoration of homeostasis with memory. *Immune deficiency* is an underreactivity of the immune processes, characterized by a pattern of repeated infections with a single organism. *Overreactive or inappropriate immune responses* are classified into three categories: (1) allergy, which involves inappropriate responses to innocuous foreign substances; (2) autoimmunity, which are responses to self-tissue antigens; and (3) graft rejection, as a result of transplanted organs.[1] The quality of immune responsiveness is quite variable and depends on myriad circumstances, such as genetics, age, medications, health behaviors, and environmental factors.

## COMPONENTS OF THE IMMUNE SYSTEM

### STRUCTURES OF THE IMMUNE SYSTEM

Structures of the immune system are categorized as either primary or secondary lymphoid organs and tissues (Figure 2-1). *Primary lymphoid organs* are the anatomical locations in which lymphocytes develop immunocompetence: the bone marrow for B cells and the thymus for T cells.[1] *Secondary lymphoid organs* and tissues are where cellular and humoral responses take place. The spleen, lymph nodes, tonsils, Peyer's patches in the gastrointestinal tract, and the bone marrow are considered both primary and secondary lymphoid organs. The spleen responds to predominantly blood-borne antigens; lymph nodes mount immune responses to antigens circulating in the lymph system; and tonsils and Peyer's patches respond to antigens that have penetrated the mucosal barriers.

### CELLS OF THE IMMUNE SYSTEM

The cells of the immune system, *leukocytes*, arise from the pluripotent hematopoietic stem cells of the bone marrow, which give rise to two identified cell lines: myeloid and lymphoid (Figure 2-2). Immune cells are distinguished from one another through the expression of different surface molecules, or markers, referred to as clusters of differentiation (CD). Different markers may be characteristic of different lineages, of different stages of cell maturation, or of the presence of cell activation. An immune cell may have more than one marker, or CD number, associated with it.[1] Each immune cell has a unique function and when activated by antigen the cells release specific chemical mediators, such as inflammatory mediators and cytokines (eg, interleukins, interferons), that affect cell growth and differentiation, inflammation, and hormone production.

#### The myeloid lineage

The myeloid lineage produces monocytes, polymorphonuclear leukocytes (neutrophils, eosinophils, and basophils/mast cells), and platelets.[1] *Monocytes* in the circulation are precursors to tissue macrophages. Monocytes migrate into tissues where they develop into macrophages under the influence of macrophage colony-stimulating factor (M-CSF). Examples include Kupffer cells in the liver, intraglomerular mesangium of the kidney, alveolar macrophages

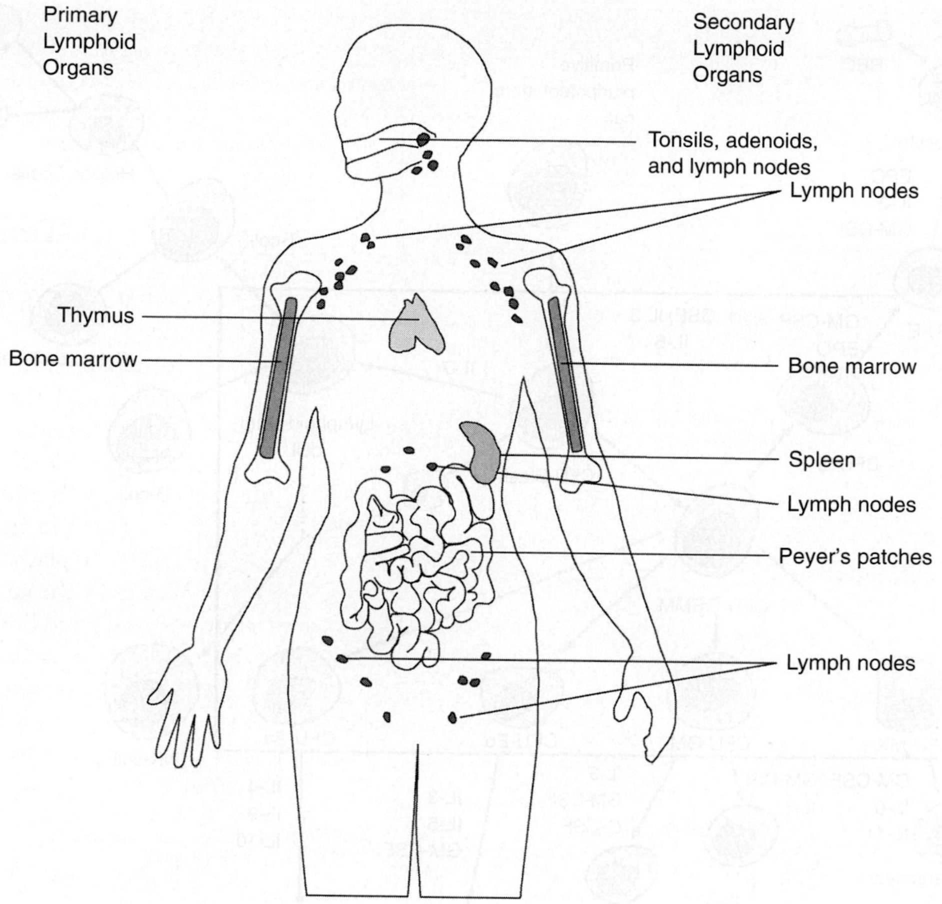


**FIGURE 2-1**

Primary and secondary lymphoid organs.

in the lung, serosal macrophages, brain microglia, spleen sinus macrophages, and lymph node sinus macrophages. Macrophages play important roles in both innate and adaptive responses and have two main functions: (1) "professional" phagocytic macrophages remove particulate antigens; and (2) antigen-presenting cells (APCs) present antigen to lymphocytes.[1] Activated macrophages kill intracellular organisms by secreting interleukin-1 (IL-1) and tumor necrosis factor-α (TNF-α), which increase the expression of adhesion molecules on endothelial cells and signal leukocytes, resulting in destruction of pathogens.

*Polymorphonuclear granulocytes* (polymorphs) make up 60% to 70% of the total normal blood leukocytes, but are also found in extravascular sites. They are rapidly produced in the bone marrow at a rate of about 80 million per minute and are relatively short-lived (two to three days) compared to monocytes/macrophages, which may live for months or years. Neutrophils constitute more than 90% of the circulating polymorphs. Their primary role is phagocytosis. *Neutrophils* are the blood cells providing the body's first line of defense. Significant loss of neutrophils, or neutropenia, can pose a serious threat to patients with cancer receiving immunosuppressive therapies.

*Eosinophils* are polymorphs that constitute 2% to 5% of blood leukocytes in healthy, nonallergic individuals. They phagocytize and kill microorganisms and are a major source of inflammatory mediators (eg, prostaglandins, leukotrienes, platelet-activating factor, cytokines). Eosinophils appear to play a specialized role in immunity to parasites and nematodes. Through a degranulating mechanism, eosinophils adhere to worm larva; granules then release a toxic protein substance.

*Basophils* constitute less than 0.2% of circulating leukocytes. *Mast cells* are indistinguishable from basophils, although mast cells are resident only in body tissues (ie, mucosal epithelia and connective tissue). Basophils and mast cells play key roles in allergic responses through a degranulation process involving the release of histamine.

Although *platelets* are not leukocytes, they are derived from the myeloid lineage (megakaryocytes) and play important roles in various aspects of the immune response, in addition to their chief role in coagulation. Following

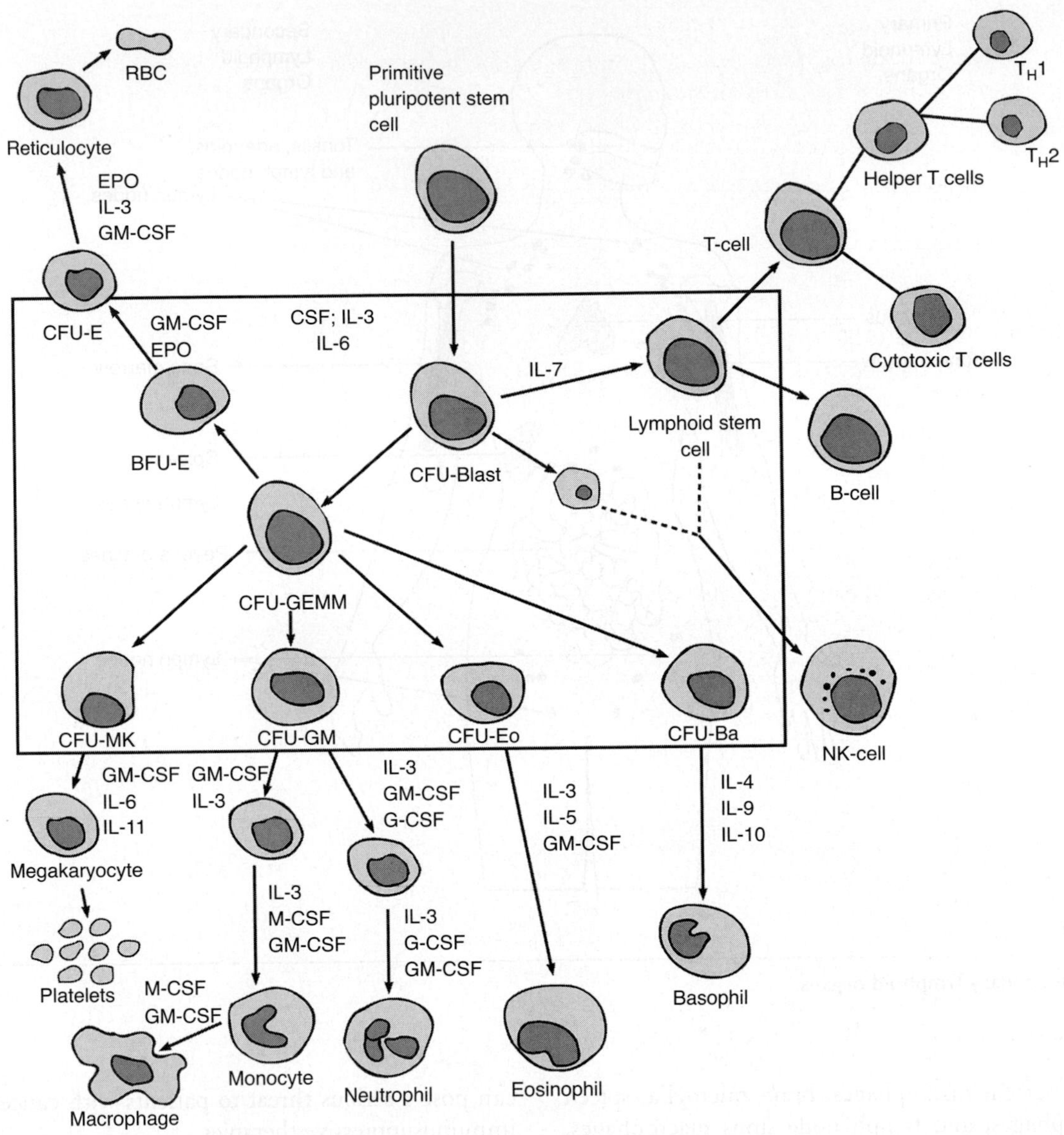


**FIGURE 2-2**

The hematologic cascade.

Abbreviations: Ba, basophil; BFU, burst-forming unit; CFU, colony-forming unit; CFU-GEMM, colony-forming unit-granulocyte/erythrocyte/monocyte/megakaryocyte; CSF, colony-stimulating factor; Eo, eosinophil; EPO, erythropoietin; G, granulocyte; GM, granulocyte/macrophage; M, macrophage; MK, megakaryocyte; NK, natural killer; RBC, red blood cells/erythrocytes; TH, helper T cells.

damage to endothelial cells, platelets adhere to and aggregate at the surface of the damaged vascular tissue. They release mediators that increase permeability and activate complement, a serum protein (described below), and therefore attract leukocytes.

## The lymphoid lineage

The lymphoid lineage produces B lymphocytes (B cells), T lymphocytes (T cells), and large granular lymphocytes (LGL) called natural killer (NK) cells. *B cells*, so named because they were originally discovered in the bursa of birds, play a major role in the humoral arm of adaptive immunity through the production of antibodies, also called *immunoglobulins*.[1] On activation, B cells become antibody-secreting plasma cells. They have a less important role in the cell-mediated arm of adaptive immunity.

*T cells*, so named because they mature in the thymus, play the major role in cell-mediated immune responses and a less important role in humoral responses. Cell-mediated immunity provides the body's defense against intracellular viruses, transplanted tissue, tumor cells, fungi, and protozoa. T cells recognize antigen not in its intact form, as it is recognized by B cells, but rather as peptide fragments that are bound to cell-surface molecules, called *major histocompatibility complex* (MHC) molecules.[1] T cells have specialized receptors that recognize the antigenic fragments bound to a MHC molecule. Two classes of the MHC molecule exist: MHC class I and MHC class II.

T cells ($CD3^+$) are divided into three general subpopulations: helper T (TH) cells, suppressor T (TS) cells, and cytotoxic T (TC) cells. Helper T cells ($CD4^+$), which are restricted to MHC class II, are differentiated into two types: TH1 cells play a role in the enhancement of cell-mediated responses, whereas TH2 cells play a role in the enhancement of antibody production in humoral responses. Suppressor T cells, in general, act to shut off TH2 when sufficient antibody has been produced. Cytotoxic T cells ($CD8^+$), which are restricted to MHC class I, are capable of recognizing and destroying specific target cells, usually virus-infected cells, through cell–cell contact. The balance of activity between the CD4 TH1 and CD4 TH2 lymphocytes is important to the overall function of the immune system. Overactive TH1 function is associated with autoimmune disease and overactive TH2 function results in allergies.

*Natural killer cells* are considered LGL because of their morphologic characteristics: distinct granules in the cytoplasm, a kidney-shaped indented nucleus, high nuclear–cytoplasmic ratio, and low density.[1] These characteristics distinguish NK cells from other lymphocytes. Natural killer cells appear to arise from stem cells other than the common lymphoid progenitors; however, this relationship is not clear. Maturation of NK cells depends on intact bone marrow but not on thymus. Although expression of a number of surface molecules has been identified on NK cells, the major marker characteristics are $CD16^+$, $CD56^+$, and $CD3^-$. Natural killer cells account for as much as 15% of peripheral blood lymphocytes. In addition to circulating in the blood, other locations of human NK cells include the spleen, tonsils, interstitial lung space, intestinal mucosa, and liver; mature NK cells are virtually absent in bone marrow. Natural killer cells, so named because of early identification of their activity of innate, non-MHC–restricted cytotoxicity of malignant and virally infected cells, play key roles in tumor surveillance and natural resistance against certain microbial infections. They secrete several cytokines (IFN-$\gamma$, IL-1, TNF-$\alpha$) that promote differentiation of cell-mediated TH1 cells and inhibition of antibody generating TH2 cells.

*Dendritic cells*, also called interdigitating reticular cells, are not lymphocytes per se, yet their activity and locations connect them to the lymphoid system. Dendritic cells are found in T-cell areas of lymphoid tissue, are potent stimulators of T-cell responses,[1] and are considered the most powerful APCs. Because dendritic cells effectively deliver tumor-specific antigens and induce tumor-specific immune responses, they are useful for cancer immunotherapy.[2] Genetically modified dendritic cell vaccination is a promising cancer treatment, with recent evidence of effectiveness for different solid tumors and hematologic malignancies.[3–6]

## SOLUBLE MEDIATORS OF IMMUNE RESPONSE

Cell-to-cell communication occurs due to the production and secretion of, and receptors for, various soluble mediators, including antibodies, cytokines, serum proteins, and prostaglandins. Cell adhesion molecules (CAMs) also play a role in cell-to-cell signaling and adhesion.

### Antibodies

Antibodies, also called immunoglobulins (Ig), are serum glycoproteins that have specificity to particular antigens. Each antibody is Y-shaped and consists of three fragments (Figure 2-3). Two identical fragments are for antigen-binding (Fab), and one crystalline fragment (Fc) is for nonspecific binding to other cells or soluble mediators of the immune system. The antibody molecule consists of four polypeptide chains: two identical light chains and two identical heavy chains. Both the light and the heavy chains are further divided into variable and constant regions. The sequencing of the amino acids, particularly with the heavy chains, determines the class of antibody, given here in decreasing order of abundance: IgG, IgA, IgM, IgE, IgD.[1] With the help of T cells, B cells rearrange their Ig genes and switch to production of IgG, IgA, or IgE.

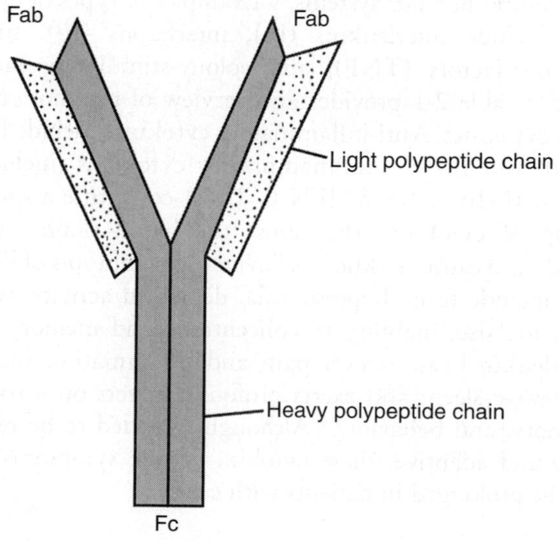


**FIGURE 2-3**

Basic antibody structure consists of a Y shape having two heavy and two light polypeptide chains, two antigen receptors (Fab), and one crystalline receptor (Fc) for binding to host cells or to soluble mediators.

IgG (γ) is the most abundant antibody, accounting for approximately 75% of serum antibodies. It is the only antibody able to cross the placenta. IgG is the major antibody produced in a secondary immune response. IgG activates complement and binds phagocytes. There are 4 subclasses of IgG: IgG1, IgG2, IgG3, and IgG4, numbered in descending order of serum concentration. IgG1 and IgG3 are most efficient at activating complement, and IgG1 and IgG3 are better mediators of antibody-dependent cellular cytotoxicity than IgG4 and IgG2.[7]

IgA (α) is present in both serum and seromucous secretions, playing a key role in secretory immunity in response to upper respiratory infections. It represents about 15% to 20% of the total serum antibody and consists of two subclasses.

IgM (μ) constitutes approximately 10% of serum antibodies. It is the major antibody expressed on B cells and the chief antibody in primary immune responses. IgM is also considered to be the most efficient activator of complement.

IgE (ε) accounts for less than 0.004% of serum antibodies. It binds to the Fc receptors on basophils and mast cells, playing the principle role in most hypersensitivity reactions.

IgD (δ) makes up less than 1% of serum antibodies. It is primarily expressed on B cells (along with IgM) and is a major B-cell activator.

## Cytokines

*Cytokines* are polypeptides produced by various immune cells. They mediate the activity of other cells, regulate immune responses, and interact with the neuroendocrine and central nervous systems.[1,8] Examples of types of cytokines include interleukins (IL), interferons (IF), tumor necrosis factors (TNF), and colony-stimulating factors (CSF). Table 2-1 provides an overview of the more common cytokines. Anti-inflammatory cytokines include IL-4, IL-10, and IL-13. Proinflammatory cytokines (including IL-1α, IL-1β, TNF-α, IFN-β, IL-6) constitute a specific group of cytokines that cross the blood–brain barrier (BBB) and cause "sickness behaviors"—symptoms of illness that include fever, hypersomnia, depressed activity, weakness, malaise, inability to concentrate, and memory loss. Interleukin-1 causes fever, pain, and inflammation; induces slow-wave sleep; and exerts profound effects on learning, memory, and behavior.[8,9] Although intended to be restorative and adaptive, these cytokines create symptoms that can be prolonged in patients with cancer.

## Serum proteins

Serum concentration levels of certain proteins increase during infection and are therefore called *acute-phase proteins.* Two key serum proteins are *C-reactive protein* (CRP) and *complement.*

C-reactive protein binds to and coats bacteria, while promoting the binding of complement and phagocytosis.[1] The complement system is a group of approximately 20 serum proteins whose overall function is to control inflammation and remove pathogens. Two mechanisms to activate the complement system exist: the alternate pathway and the classical pathway. The *alternate pathway,* which relies on CRP, is an innate, nonspecific reaction in response to antigen trigger, leading to complement coating a microorganism and subsequent uptake by phagocytes. The *classical pathway* is a specific, adaptive response activated by antibodies. The major mechanisms of the classical complement pathway include (1) opsonization (coating) of microorganisms for uptake by phagocytes; (2) chemotaxis, the attraction of phagocytes to sites of infection; (3) increased vascularity to the site of activation with increased permeability of capillaries to plasma molecules; and (4) damage to plasma membranes on cells or pathogens that have induced the activation, leading to lysis.[1]

## Prostaglandins

Prostaglandins are important mediators involved in inflammation. They are major end products of arachidonic acid metabolism produced from inflammatory immune cells, such as monocytes/macrophages and basophils/mast cells, and triggering of IL-1. Prostaglandins are thought to be the central mediators triggering central nervous system responses to inflammatory processes, as they are small and lipophilic and are able to cross the BBB. Further evidence comes from the inhibition of prostaglandins, and amelioration of the systemic sickness behaviors, produced by cyclooxygenase (COX) inhibitors.[10,11] Prostaglandins also increase platelet aggregation and inhibit the effects of heparin on smooth muscle cells and vascular endothelial cells.[7]

## Cell-adhesion molecules

Endothelial cells express immune CAMs that direct lymphocyte migration. Cell-adhesion molecules are proteins on the cell surface that act as transmembrane receptors to bind cells together or bind cells with the extracellular matrix (ECM). Most of the CAMs belong to four protein families: immunoglobulin superfamily (eg, ICAM-1, intercellular cell–adhesion molecule; VCAM-1, vascular cell–adhesion molecule), the integrins, the cadherins, and the selectins. Endothelial CAMs respond to stress and circulating IL-1 and TNF-α and play a role in signal transduction, inflammation and wound healing, and metastases of tumors.[12]

# MECHANISMS OF ADAPTIVE IMMUNITY

Humoral and cell-mediated immune responses, involving both B cells and T cells, are interdependent functional

**TABLE 2-1**

**Cytokines: Sources and Main Functions**

| Type | Source | Major Functions |
|---|---|---|
| | | **Interleukins (ILs)** |
| IL-1 (α and β) | Predominantly macrophages, TH2 | Activates T cells and B cells, inflammatory mediator (proinflammatory cytokine); crosses blood–brain barrier (BBB); ↑ glucocorticoids, ↓ dopamine, serotonin; fever and "sickness behaviors" |
| IL-2 (T-cell growth factor [TCGF]) | TH1 cells, NK cells | ↑ T-cell proliferation and differentiation; ↑ cytolytic activity of NK cells and production of LAK cells; activates B cells to ↑ Ig |
| IL-3 (multi-CSF) | Predominantly TH1 and TH2 cells | ↑ Production and differentiation of hematopoietic progenitor cells |
| IL-4 (B-cell growth factor) | TH2 cells, T cells, macrophages, mast cells, B cells, basophils | Differentiation of TH0–TH2; induces proliferation and differentiation of B cells |
| IL-6 | TH2 cells, monocytes, macrophages, fibroblasts, hepatocytes, endothelial and neuronal cells | Activates hematopoietic progenitor cells; induces maturation and ↑ platelet number; ↑ growth and/or differentiation of various cells; ↑ acute-phase protein release |
| IL-7 | Bone marrow stromal cells, fetal liver cells | ↑ Proliferation and cytotoxic activity of TC cells and LAK cells; support the growth of pre-B cells and proliferation of T cells |
| IL-8 (neutrophil chemotactic factor) | Monocytes, macrophages, endothelial cells | ↑ Chemotactic activity of neutrophils, T cells, and basophils; ↑ phagocytic activity of neutrophils |
| IL-10 (cytokine synthesis inhibitory factor [CSIF]) | TH2 cells, macrophages, B cells | ↑ Proinflammatory cytokine release of macrophages; inhibits TH1; ↑ B-cell proliferation and Ig production |
| IL-12 | Macrophages, B cells | Initiates cell-mediated immunity by inducing differentiation of TH0→TH1; ↑ growth and activity of NK and TC cells |
| | | **Interferons (IFNs)** |
| IFN-α | T cells, B cells, macrophages | Antiviral activity, modulates MHC class I and II expression on various cells; ↓ B-cell proliferation, ↓ macrophage activity and production of IL-8 |
| IFN-β | Fibroblasts, epithelial cells, macrophages | Antiviral activity; ↑ IL-6; ↓ IL-8 |
| IFN-γ | TH1 cells, T cells, NK cells | Activates NK cells antiviral activity; ↑ MHC class I and II expression on macrophages; ↑ B-cell differentiation; ↑ macrophage activity |
| | | **Tumor Necrosis Factors (TNFs)** |
| TNF-α (cachectin) | TH1 cells neutrophils, activated lymphocytes, NK cells, fibroblasts, endothelial cells, malignant cells | ↑ Macrophage activity, ↑ cytokines from NK cells, mediates expression of genes for growth factors and cytokines, inflammatory mediators, acute-phase proteins, and transcription factors |
| TNF-β (lymphotoxin) | T cells, malignant cells | Similar to TNF-α |

*(continued)*

**TABLE 2-1**

**Cytokines: Sources and Main Functions (continued)**

| Type | Source | Major Functions |
|---|---|---|
| **Colony-Stimulating Factors (CSFs)** | | |
| Granulocyte CSF (G-CSF) | T cells, macrophages, neutrophils, endothelial cells, fibroblasts | ↑ Differentiation and activation of neutrophils |
| Granulocyte-macrophage CSF (GM-CSF) | Macrophages, T cells, endothelial cells, polymorphs | ↑ Growth and differentiation of multipotential progenitor cells; stimulates all cells in myeloid lineage |
| Macrophage CSF (M-CSF) | T cells, macrophage, neutrophils, fibroblasts, endothelial cells | ↑ Growth and development of macrophage colonies; stimulates various functions of monocytes and macrophages |
| **Others** | | |
| Transforming growth factors (TGFs): α and β | Macrophages, malignant cells, other cells | Stimulates macrophages, ↑ fibroblasts, ↑ epithelial development and angiogenic activity, ↓ growth of various other cells |
| Stem cell factor (SCF) | Bone marrow stromal cells, epithelial cells, fibroblasts | Stimulates growth of myeloid, erythroid, and lymphoid progenitors; stimulates growth and proliferation of mast cells |
| Erythropoietin (EPO) | Liver, kidneys, macrophages | Stimulates growth and differentiation of erythroid progenitors; ↑ red blood cell production |

*Note:* ↑, Increased; ↓, Decreased. (See text for other abbreviations.)

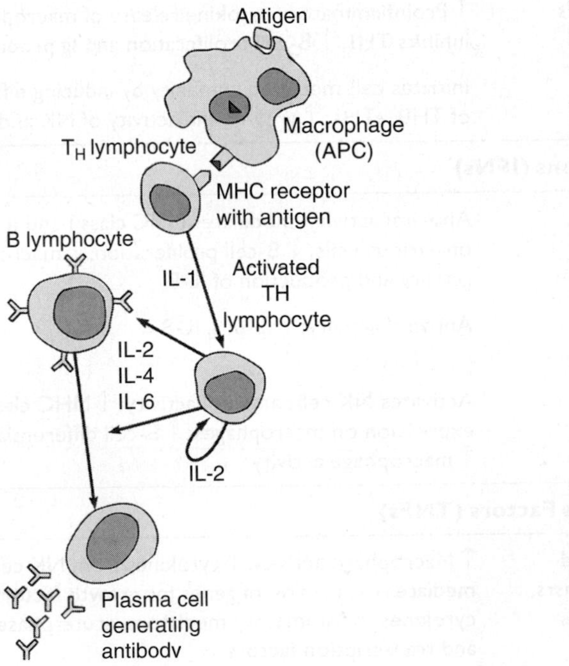


**FIGURE 2-4**

Major components of adaptive immune response.
Abbreviations: APC, antigen-presenting cell; IL, interleukin; TH, helper T lymphocyte.

arms that fall within the domain of adaptive immunity, as illustrated in Figure 2-4.

## HUMORAL IMMUNE RESPONSE

Humoral responses play important roles in the body's defense against extracellular pathogens (bacteria and some viruses) as well as in certain hypersensitivity reactions.[1] The main mechanism in humoral immune responses involves the binding of antibodies to antigens. B cells play a key role in these processes through the production of antibodies.

Two proliferative steps take place before antibody production can occur: clonal diversity and clonal selection.[1] *Clonal diversity* takes place in the bone marrow and is antigen independent and hormonally driven. It results in the generation of immature but immunocompetent B cells, with plasma-membrane receptors that can recognize any antigenic molecule. *Clonal selection*, the second step, occurs in secondary lymphoid organs such as the spleen and lymph nodes. Antigens can stimulate B cells to become antibody-producing plasma cells either with or without the help of T cells; the latter are called *T-independent antigens.*

When a B cell encounters a specific antigen, it matures and proliferates into plasma cells and a set of memory B cells. Plasma cells are active during the primary immune response; IgM is the main antibody produced during this phase. Memory B cells are active in secondary responses that occur on future exposure to the antigen and are responsible for long-term immunity. Gamma-immunoglobulin is the predominant antibody in secondary responses. Class switching of antibodies from IgG to other classes or subclasses occurs with the help of cytokines released by a type of helper T cells (TH2).[1]

### Antibody–antigen processes

An antibody circulates in the blood or in lymph fluid, or is suspended in body secretions until encountering and binding to its particular antigen. Binding of antigen (by antigenic-determinant sites) to the Fab portions of the antibody results in antigen–antibody complexes, also called *immune complexes*.[1] The class of the antibody and specific characteristics of the antigen determine subsequent processes. Most humoral immune responses are polyclonal; however, monoclonal antibodies generated in laboratories are single antibodies of known specificity that play important roles in clinical therapeutics and diagnostics of patients with cancer.

In general, antibodies function to target extracellular pathogens and their products for disposal by phagocytes, particularly macrophages and neutrophils. Antibodies play three major roles: (1) they neutralize bacterial and viral toxins; (2) they opsonize (or coat) bacteria; and (3) they activate complement.[1] In *neutralization*, antibodies bind to and neutralize toxins, thereby preventing interactions with host cells that can cause pathology. Unbound toxin can react with receptors on host cells, whereas antigen–antibody complexes cannot. These immune complexes are then typically scavenged and degraded by macrophages. In *opsonization*, an antibody literally coats an antigen, rendering it recognizable as foreign by macrophages and polymorphonuclear leukocytes. These phagocytes then destroy and ingest the antibody-coated antigen complex. Finally, bound antibodies to antigens form a receptor to activate the first protein of the complement system, C3. This activation eventually forms a protein complex on the surface of the pathogen that favors its uptake and destruction by phagocytes.[1]

## CELL-MEDIATED IMMUNE RESPONSE

T cells are responsible for cell-mediated immunity, although interaction between both T cells and B cells oftentimes occurs. Maturation and initial proliferation of T cells take place in the thymus in processes similar to clonal diversity for B cells. While journeying through the thymus, lymphocytes destined to become T cells proliferate and develop the capacity to recognize a huge spectrum of antigens that the host will encounter throughout life. Antigen cluster differentiation on the plasma membrane of the T cells takes place in the thymus. On exiting the thymus through blood and lymph vessels, T cells mature and are antigenically committed. When these immunocompetent T cells encounter a recognizable antigen in the body, they proliferate.[1]

Naïve CD8 cells leaving the thymus are predestined to become cytotoxic cells. In contrast, the differentiation of CD4 cells is much more complex. Depending on the first encounter with antigen, CD4 cells can either become type 1 helper (TH1) or type 2 helper (TH2) cells. Type 1 helper cells secrete IFN-$\gamma$, IL-2, and TNF-$\alpha$ and regulate cell-mediated immunity, whereas TH2 cell subsets regulate humoral immunity and express cytokines IL-4, IL-5, IL-6, IL-10, and IL-13.[13–15] These T-cell subsets are modulated by hypothalamus-pituitary-adrenal (HPA) axis mediators, particularly by increased circulation of the stress hormones, glucocorticoids, and catecholamines, resulting in downregulation of TH1 cell activity and enhanced TH2 humoral immune responses.[16]

### Antigen processing, recognition, and presentation

After entering the host, an antigen flows through the bloodstream, is filtered through the spleen, and enters the lymphatics. Lymph nodes and other body tissues such as the skin and mucous membranes are lined with phagocytic cells, particularly macrophages, which ingest antigen. After its ingestion by a phagocyte, the antigen is degraded. A portion of the degraded antigen is reexposed, or expressed, on the plasma membrane of the phagocyte, which "presents" it to B and T cells. This antigen–phagocyte complex, referred to as APC, is necessary to induce most immune responses.[1] Three cell types that can serve as APCs are dendritic cells, macrophages, and B cells.

The only way a T cell can recognize antigen is when it is presented in the context of "self" material, such as MHC molecules. To activate naïve T cells, APCs must be capable of processing antigen from intracellular and extracellular pathogens and presenting it on MHC class I and MHC class II molecules. The particular MHC class determines which cell will respond to the presentation of antigen. Inflammatory CD4 cells (TH1) and helper cells (TH2) both express the CD4 co-receptor and recognize antigen displayed at the cell surface by MHC class II molecules. Conversely, TC (CD8) cells kill target cells (particularly viruses) bound to MHC class I molecules at the cell surface.

T-cell receptors (TCR) are the site on T cells where APC bind. These receptors are structurally similar to the Fab portion of an antibody and are antigen specific. The two known types, TCR1 and TCR2, express different gene chains and binding patterns.[1]

Intercellular communication is dynamic during the cell-mediated immune response. Various cytokines and adhesion molecules on the surface of each cell play important roles. For example, IL-1 is produced by the APC and helps the T cell respond, while IL-2 facilitates maturation of a functional TH1 cell and binds to specific IL-2 receptors on the same cell that is producing it. This results in increased production of IL-2 and IL-2 receptor, further differentiation and proliferation of the TH1 cell, and the production of other cytokines.

## DELAYED-TYPE HYPERSENSITIVITY

Delayed-type hypersensitivity (DTH) reactions, also called type IV responses, are mediated by T cells.[1] Specifically in response to a previously responded pathogen, inflammatory (TH1) CD4 cells recognize receptors on MHC class II APCs. The TH1 cells then release inflammatory cytokines, such as macrophage chemotactic factor (MCF), TNF-α, and IFN-γ, resulting in blood-vessel permeability and fluid and protein accumulation into the tissue. This process evolves over 24 to 72 hours. Delayed-type hypersensitivity is often used as an in vivo measure of cell-mediated immunity. The prototypic DTH reaction is the tuberculin skin test.

## CELL-MEDIATED CYTOTOXICITY

Cell-mediated cytotoxicity entails the recognition and lysis of target cells (which may be tumor cells or viruses) by either TC cells or NK cells.[1] It may or may not be antibody dependent (IgG). The mechanisms of action are quite similar regardless of the type of lymphocyte or involvement of IgG. The main difference lies in the different receptors and the binding of the cytotoxic cell to the target.

Cytotoxic T cells are antigen specific and have MHC-restricted TCR. In contrast, NK cells are not antigen specific; instead, they recognize determinants expressed on neoplastic cells. Lymphokine-activated killer (LAK) cells are NK cells with enhanced cytotoxic activity due to stimulation with IL-2. These cells are used in the treatment of certain types of cancer by stimulating a patient's own NK cells with IL-2 in vitro, then returning those cells to the patient.[17]

Antibody-mediated cytotoxicity involves the binding of an effector cell, referred to as a killer (K) cell, to antigen-bound IgG. Killer cells are usually TC cells, but may also be NK cells. The K cell has Fc receptors that can bind to the Fc region of antibody that has coated a target cell. Through these receptors, the K cell can adhere indirectly to and kill an IgG-coated target.

The mechanisms involved in the killing are similar whether TC cells, NK cells, or K cells are the effectors, and no matter what kind of receptor–target interaction is responsible (Figure 2-5). First, the effector cell recognizes and makes close contact with the target cell. Upon making contact with the target cell, changes occur within the effector cell cytoplasm; specifically, the granule-containing vesicles of the Golgi apparatus fuse with the cell membrane. Through a calcium-dependent process, a protein substance called perforin is discharged from the vesicles.[18] This release of perforin causes pores to form on the target cell membrane, leading to an influx of water, electrolytes, and enzymes. Within minutes, the target cell swells and bursts. The effector cell survives this process, possibly because of a protective protein in the cell membrane called *protectin*, and continues to recognize and cause lysis of other target cells. Cytokines, particularly TNF (α and β) and IFN-γ, appear to play important roles in and are products of cell-mediated cytotoxicity.

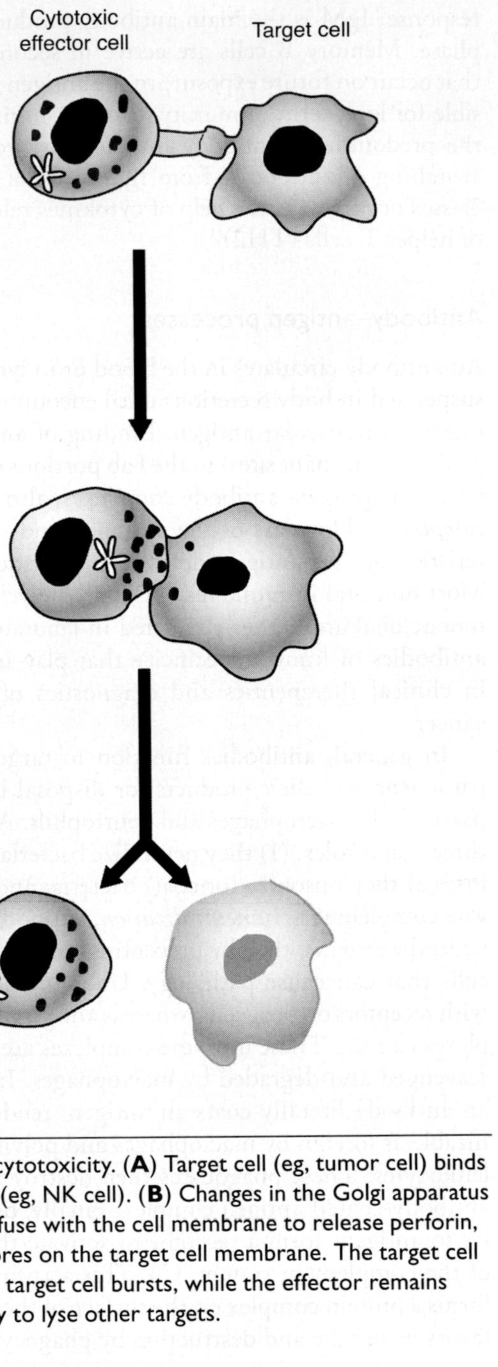


**FIGURE 2-5**

Cell-mediated cytotoxicity. (**A**) Target cell (eg, tumor cell) binds to effector cell (eg, NK cell). (**B**) Changes in the Golgi apparatus of the effector cell fuse with the cell membrane to release perforin, which forms pores on the target cell membrane. The target cell swells. (**C**) The target cell bursts, while the effector remains intact and ready to lyse other targets.

## TUMOR SURVEILLANCE

Natural killer cells lyze tumor cells without specific antigen recognition and, therefore, are important to tumor surveillance. Although it is unclear whether NK activity affects the development of cancer, some evidence supports the relationship between NK cytotoxicity and cancer recurrence and metastasis.[19–23] In addition, some studies suggest that lower NK levels at diagnosis influence prognosis and survival from cancer.[24]

In addition to NK cells, the balance between TH1 and TH2 cells and other molecular and genetic mechanisms are important for tumor surveillance. Nuclear factor-kappa B (NF-κB), a transcription factor activated by inflammatory cytokines, regulates genes involved in immune response and inflammation and contributes to tumorigenesis.[25] Growth and migration of cancer cells is dependent on a complex interplay of expression of CAMs, growth factors, hormones, neurotransmitters, cytokines, and chemokines.[15] All stress hormones influence some aspect of immunity, and immune suppression and infection often accompany increased tumor risk, indicating that tumor surveillance depends on a healthy immune system.[26,27] Stress may contribute to tumorigenesis through neuroendocrine responses that alter $T_H1$ and TH2 cells, resulting in lymphocyte apoptosis and lower NK cytotoxicity[27,28] and directly affecting genomic DNA.[29] Although not all tumors are directly responsive to immune control, innate and natural immune resistance is critical to malignant transformation of cells.[30] Some cancers may be more susceptible to stress-induced immune suppression, but all are nonspecifically responsive to NK lysis.

## TISSUE DESTRUCTION FROM IMMUNE RESPONSES

While attempting to rid the body of foreign organisms, products of certain immune processes have the potential to cause tissue damage. Specifically, neutrophils and macrophages produce toxins during inflammation and phagocytosis. For example, bacterial killing by neutrophils occurs through an oxidative process with lysosomal release of such mediators as superoxide, hydrogen peroxide, and hydroxyl radicals.[1] Fortunately, these free radicals are effective killers of pathogens. At the same time, release of these chemicals affects surrounding cells, leading to damage of healthy cells. This same mechanism supports the dietary intake of antioxidants.

## FACTORS AFFECTING IMMUNE RESPONSES

### STRESS

Stress generally refers to demands placed on the body that threaten *homeostasis* (internal stability). Stressful stimuli may be either external or internal. External stress is considered to comprise cognitive sensory stimuli because of its initial processing through the peripheral and central nervous systems; death of a loved one is an example of a cognitive stressor. Internal sensory input, or noncognitive stress, is received by the immune system, which in turn relays this information to the neuroendocrine system; viral infection is an example of noncognitive stress. Regardless of the source, stress alters the adhesive properties of leukocytes[7] and changes cytokine production, resulting in a shift away from cellular immunity (TH1) toward humoral immunity (TH2).[31] While acute or short-term stress has stimulatory effects on immune function, chronic stress consistently shows immunosuppressive effects,[31] with lower NK cell function and increased lymphocyte apoptosis, which is upregulated by endogenous opioids.[32] The hippocampus, prefrontal cortex, amygdala, and the hypothalamus respond to acute and chronic stressors and mediate these immune processes.[33]

The scientific field called psychoneuroimmunology (PNI) focuses on understanding the effects of stress on immune responses and related health outcomes through the dynamic interplay and bidirectional communication between the neuroendocrine and immune systems.[34] Substantial evidence implicates interaction of the cells of these systems in stress: (1) the immune system's interaction with the HPA axis; (2) the innervation of lymphoid organs by the autonomic nervous system; and (3) the secretion of and receptors for identical soluble mediators such as cytokines, neuropeptides, and hormones.

The field of PNI first emerged in the late 1970s and now involves interdisciplinary collaboration among professionals of various basic science, social science, and clinical disciplines. Because of the substantial body of knowledge supporting the negative effects of psychological stress on immune function,[31–34] clinical studies are attempting to evaluate and identify the benefits of stress-reducing interventions. This area holds particular interest for nurses, due to its knowledge base rooted in both basic and social sciences, and is reinforced by a holistic perspective that is at the core of the profession.[35]

#### Stress-reducing interventions

A number of stress-reducing interventions have been shown to improve neuroendocrine, immune, and overall health outcomes, including massage,[36–40] expressive or group therapies,[41,42] mindfulness meditation,[43–46] acupuncture,[47,48] music therapy,[49,50] and qi gong.[51]

### AGING

Advancing age is clearly associated with decline of immunologic functioning.[52–55] The thymus reaches its maximum size at about age 25, then begins involuting. Thymic size is only 15% of its maximum by age 50. Although numbers of T cells may not decrease with age, T-cell function does deteriorate. Older individuals (those more than 60 years of age) generally exhibit diminished responsiveness with various T-cell–mediated activities. In addition, antibody activities can decrease or become dysfunctional with increasing age, resulting in lowered resistance to infections and disease. Cytokine production also changes, with some cytokines showing no change (TNF), others increasing (IL-3, IL-4, IL-6) or decreasing (IFN-α, IL-2, TGF-β). The balance of proinflammatory and anti-inflammatory cytokines changes with age, with an anti-inflammatory phenotype (IL-4, IL-10, IL-13) correlating with longevity.[56]

## GONADAL HORMONES

Gonadal or sex hormones—specifically, estrogen, progesterone, and testosterone—are known to affect immune function. Estrogens are the most immunologically active and have mixed effects on immune function. They generally depress cellular immunity and NK cell function and increase antibody response to T-dependent antigens.[57] Testosterone is also known to be immunosuppressive, particularly for lymphocytes. While the exact mechanisms are not clear, it appears that IL-6 is central to these processes.[58,59]

## BEHAVIORAL FACTORS

Behavioral factors known to suppress immune function include alcohol, caffeine, marijuana, morphine, nutrient deficiencies, smoking, and chronic stress. Other protective factors increase immune function—some nutritional and herbal therapies, physical exercise in moderation, adequate sleep, stress-reducing interventions, mental attitude, and social support. Because changes in these behaviors are often concurrent, it is difficult to fully comprehend the individual effects of these factors. For example, individuals who are distressed may be more likely to engage in self-destructive behaviors (eg, increased smoking and alcohol/drug consumption), as well as experience changes in their appetite, energy level, and sleep pattern.

### Nutrition

Nutritional status and dietary intake can influence immunocompetence and overall health function. Protein-calorie and zinc deficiencies are associated with alterations in both innate and cell-mediated immune mechanisms, for example, while essential amino acids, the essential fatty acid linoleic acid, and certain vitamins (A, $B_6$, $B_{12}$, C, $D_3$, and E) and minerals (eg, selenium) play roles in the maintenance of healthy immune cells.[60–62] Recent studies also have demonstrated immune-related benefits of other dietary products, such as maitake[63] and *Trametes versicolor* mushrooms,[64] antioxidants (anthocyanins) in pomegranate and berries, polyphenols in resveretrol and curcumin,[65] antioxidants and catechins of green tea,[66] and select probiotic strains.[67]

### Alcohol and other CNS drugs

Consumption of alcohol (ethanol) and other CNS-acting drugs can affect immune function. Alcohol intake is associated with the suppression of NK cytotoxicity in both animal models and humans.[68,69] The deleterious effects of marijuana on NK, antibody, and cytokine production have also been documented.[70]

### Physical exercise

Although some well-designed studies show no effect,[71] changes in immune response to physical exercise have been recognized, with moderate and continued aerobic exercise having a general positive effect.[72] With vigorous aerobic exercise, changes occur in cytokines (ie, increases in CD8), hormones (ie, β-endorphin), and NK cytotoxicity. The marked increase in NK function is followed by decline, which is thought to be due to skeletal stress, inflammatory responses, or the response to catecholamines.[73–76]

### Sleep

Adequate sleep is restorative for immune function.[77,78] Growth hormone and prolactin, known to be associated with enhanced immune function, are elevated during sleep; conversely, levels of immunosuppressive corticosteroids and catecholamines are depressed. A close interaction exists between the sleep–wake cycle and melatonin. Melatonin stimulates cytokine production, enhances phagocytosis, increases NK cell activity, and increases the immune response toward a $T_H1$ profile. It also reduces NF-κB binding to DNA, which reduces the production of proinflammatory cytokines and chemokines.[79] Insomnia activates the HPA axis, thereby increasing ACTH and cortisol secretion and releasing IL-1, which induces NREM or slow-wave sleep.[80–82] In contrast, anti-inflammatory cytokines (IL-4, IL-10, and IL-13) inhibit NREM sleep.[83]

## IMPLICATIONS FOR NURSING PRACTICE

Nursing professionals strive to improve quality of life and clinical outcomes for their patients, with an emphasis toward self-care and changing behaviors. Independent nursing interventions can be educational or supportive. Educational programs and individual or group counseling sessions can be aimed at changing behaviors such as diet, exercise, sleep habits, and stress reduction. These interventions and topics are germane to nursing and ripe areas for refinement and research.

## REFERENCES


1. Murphy KM, Travers P, Walport M. *Immunobiology (Janeways Immunobiology: The Immune System)*. 7th ed. London: Garland Science/Garland; 2007.
2. Fonseca C, Dranoff G. Capitalizing on the immunogenicity of dying tumor cells. *Clin Cancer Res*. 2008;14:1603–1608.
3. Gabrilovich D. Dendritic cell vaccines for cancer treatment. *Curr Opin Mol Ther*. 2002;4:452–458.
4. Morse M, Lyerly H. DNA and RNA modified dendritic cell vaccines. *World Surg*. 2002;26:819–825.
5. Vieweg J, Dannull J. Tumor vaccines: from gene therapy to dendritic cells—the emerging frontier. *Urol Clin North Am*. 2003;30:633–643.
6. Hodi FS, Butler M, Oble DA, et al. Immunologic and clinical effects of antibody blockade of cytotoxic T lymphocyte-associated antigen 4 in previously vaccinated cancer patients. *Proc Natl Acad Sci USA*. 2008;105:3005–3010.
7. Rabin BS. *Stress, Immune Function, and Health*. New York: Wiley-Liss; 1999.
8. Besedovsky HO, Del Rey A. Cytokines as mediators of central and peripheral immune-neuroendocrine interactions. In: Ader R, Fenton DL, Cohen N, eds. *Psychoneuroimmunology*. Vol 1. San Diego, CA: Academic Press; 2001:1–20.
9. Kelley KW, Bluthe RM, Dantzer R, et al. Cytokine-induced sickness behavior. *Brain Behav Immun*. 2003;17:S112-S118.
10. Hori T, Katafuchi T, Oka T. Central cytokines: effects on peripheral immunity, inflammation and nociception. In: Ader R, Felten DL, Cohen N, eds. *Psychoneuroimmunology*. Vol 1. San Diego, CA: Academic Press; 2001:517–546.
11. Maier SF, Watkins LR, Nance DM. Multiple routes of action of interleukin-1 on the nervous system. In: Ader R, Felten DL, Cohen N, eds. *Psychoneuroimmunology*. Vol 1. San Diego, CA: Academic Press; 2001: 563–583.
12. Dittmar T, Heyder C, Gloria-Maercker E, Hatzmann W, Zänker KS. Adhesion molecules and chemokines: the navigation system for circulating tumor (stem) cells to metastasize in an organ-specific manner. *Clin Exp Metastasis*. 2008;25:11–32.
13. Curtsinger J, Schmidt C, Mondino A, et al. Inflammatory cytokines provide a third signal for activation of naïve $CD4^+$ and $CD8^+$ T cells. *J Immunol*. 1999;162:3256–3262.
14. Elenkov I, Chrousos G. Stress hormones, proinflammatory and anti-inflammatory cytokines, and autoimmunity. *Ann NY Acad Sci*. 2002;966: 290–303.
15. Murali R, Hanson MD, Chen E. Psychological stress and its relationship to cytokines and inflammatory diseases. In: Plotnikoff NP, Faith RE, Murgo AJ, Good RA, eds. *Cytokines: Stress and Immunity*. 2nd ed. Boca Raton, FL: CRC Press; 2007:29–49.
16. Eskandari F, Sternberg EM. Neural-immune interactions in health and disease. *Ann NY Acad Sci*. 2002;966:20–27.
17. Dunbar P, Chen J, Chao D, et al. Cutting edge: rapid cloning of tumor specific CTL suitable for adaptive immunotherapy of melanoma. *J Immunol*. 1999;162:6959–6962.
18. Smyth M, Thia K, Creteney E, et al. Perforin is a major contributor to NK cell control of metastasis. *J Immunol*. 1999;162:6658–6662.
19. Antoni MH. Psychoneuroendocrinology and psychoneuroimmunology of cancer: plausible mechanisms worth pursuing? *Brain Behav Immun*. 2003;17:S84-S91.
20. Menon A, Janssen-Van Rhijn C, Morreau H, et al. Immune system and prognosis in colorectal cancer: a detailed immunohistochemical analysis. *Lab Invest*. 2004;84:493–501.
21. Lotze M, Rees R. Identifying biomarkers and surrogates of tumors (cancer biometrics): correlation with immunotherapies and immune cells. *Cancer Immunol Immunother*. 2004;53:256–261.
22. Wu J, Lanier L. Natural killer cells and cancer. *Adv Cancer Res*. 2003; 90:127–156.
23. Kabingu E, Vaughan L, Owczarczak B, Ramsey KD, Gollnick SO. $CD8^+$ T cell-mediated control of distant tumours following local photodynamic therapy is independent of $CD4^+$ T cells and dependent on natural killer cells. *Br J Cancer*. 2007;96:1839–1848.
24. Fauriat C, Marcenaro E, Sivori S, et al. Natural killer cell-triggering receptors in patients with acute leukemia. *Leuk Lymphoma*. 2003;44: 1683–1689.
25. Fantini MC, Pallone F. Cytokines: from gut inflammation to colorectal cancer. *Curr Drug Targets*. 2008;9:375–380.
26. Moynihan JA. Mechanisms of stress-induced modulation of immunity. *Brain Behav Immun*. 2003;17:S11–S16.
27. Shi Y, Devadas S, Greeneltech KM, et al. Stressed to death: implication of lymphocyte apoptosis for psychoneuroimmunology. *Brain Behav Immun*. 2003;17:S18–S26.
28. Stefanek M, McDonald PG. Biological mechanism of psychosocial effects on disease: implications for cancer control. *Brain Behav Immun*. 2003;17:S2–S4.
29. Yang EV, Glaser R. Stress-induced immunomodulation: implications for tumorigenesis. *Brain Behav Immun*. 2003;17:S37–S40.
30. Sheridan J. The HPA axis, SNS, and immunity: a commentary. *Brain Behav Immun*. 2003;17:S17.
31. Segerstrom SC, Miller GE. Psychological stress and the human immune system: a meta-analytic study of 30 years of inquiry. *Psychol Bull*. 2004;130:601–630.
32. Sun E, Wei L, Roberts AI, Liu C, Shi Y. Chronic stress induces death of lymphocytes. In: Plotnikoff NP, Faith RE, Murgo AJ, Good RA, eds. *Cytokines: Stress and Immunity*. 2nd ed. Boca Raton, FL: CRC Press; 2007:157–168.
33. McEwen B. Central effects of stress hormones in health and disease: understanding the protective and damaging effects of stress and stress mediators. *Eur J Pharmacol*. 2008;583:174–185.
34. Ader R, Felten DL, Cohen N. *Psychoneuroimmunology*. San Diego, CA: Academic Press; 2001.
35. Langley P, Fonseca J, Iphofen R. Psychoneuroimmunology and health from a nursing perspective. *British J Nurs*. 2006;15:1126–1129.
36. Diego MA, Field T, Hernandez-Reif M, et al. HIV adolescents show improved immune function following massage therapy. *Int J Neurosci*. 2001;106:35–45.
37. Goodfellow LM. The effects of therapeutic back massage on psychophysiologic variables and immune function in spouses of patients with cancer. *Nurs Res*. 2003;52:318–328.
38. Ironson G, Field T, Scafidi F, et al. Massage therapy is associated with enhancement of the immune system's cytotoxic capacity. *Int J Neurosci*. 1996;84:205–217.
39. Post-White J, Kinney ME, Savik K, et al. Therapeutic massage and healing touch improve symptoms in cancer. *Integr Cancer Ther*. 2003;2:332–334.
40. Wikstrom S, Gunnarsson T, Nordin C. Tactile stimulus and neurohormonal response: a pilot study. *Int J Neurosci*. 2003;113:787–793.
41. Petrie KJ, Fontanilla I, Thomas MG, Booth RJ, Pennebaker JW. Effect of written emotional expression on immune function in patients with Human Immunodeficiency Virus infection: A randomized trial. *Psychosomatic Med*. 2004;66:272–275.
42. Bower JE, Kemeny ME, Taylor SE, Fahey JL. Finding meaning and its association with natural killer cell cytotoxicity among participants in a bereavement-related disclosure intervention. *Ann Behav Med*. 2003;25:146–155.
43. Carlson L, Speca M, Patel K, et al. Mindfulness-based stress reduction in relation to quality of life, mood, symptoms, of stress, and

immune parameters in breast and prostate outpatients. *Psychosom Med.* 2003;65:571–581.
44. Davidson RJ, Kabat-Zinn J, Schumacher J, et al. Alterations in brain and immune function produced by mindfulness meditation. *Psychosom Med.* 2003;65:564–570.
45. Witek-Janusek L, Albuquerque K, Chroniak KR, Chroniak C, Durazo-Arvizu R, Mathews HL. Effect of mindfulness based stress reduction on immune function, quality of life and coping in women newly diagnosed with early stage breast cancer. *Brain Behav Immun.* 2008;22:969–981.
46. Carlson LE, Speca M, Faris P, Patel KD. One year pre-post intervention follow-up of psychological, immune, endocrine and blood pressure outcomes of mindfulness-based stress reduction (MBSR) in breast and prostate cancer outpatients. *Brain Behav Immun.* 2007;21:1038–1049.
47. Kim CK, Choi GS, Oh SD, et al. Electroacupuncture up-regulates natural killer cell activity: Identification of genes altering their expressions in electroacupuncture induced up-regulation of natural killer cell activity. *Neuroimmunol.* 2005;168:144–153.
48. Arranz L, Guayerbas N, Siboni L, De la Fuente M. Effect of acupuncture treatment on the immune function impairment found in anxious women. *Am J Chin Med.* 2007;35:35–51.
49. Conrad C, Niess H, Jauch KW, Bruns CJ, Hartl WH, Welker L. Overture for growth hormone: Requiem for interleukin-6? *Crit Care Med.* 2007;35:2709–2713.
50. Leardi S, Pietroletti R, Angeloni G, Necozione S, Ranalletta G, Del Gusto B. Randomized clinical trial examining the effect of music therapy in stress response to day surgery. *Br J Surg.* 2007;94:943–947.
51. Lee MS, Kim MK, Ryu H. Qi-training (qigong) enhanced immune functions: What is the underlying mechanism? *Int J Neurosci.* 2005;115: 1099–1104.
52. Glaser R, MacCallum RC, Laskowski BF, et al. Evidence for a shift in the Th-1 to Th-2 cytokine response associated with chronic stress and aging. *J Gerontol Ser A: Biol Sci Med Sci.* 2001;56:477–482.
53. Kiecolt-Glaser JK, Preacher KJ, MacCallum RC, et al. Chronic stress and age-related increases in the proinflammatory cytokine IL-6. *Proc Natl Acad Sci USA.* 2003;100:9090–9095.
54. Solomon GF, Morley JE. Psychoneuroimmunology and aging. In: Ader R, Felten DL, Cohen N, eds. *Psychoneuroimmunology.* Vol 2. San Diego, CA: Academic Press; 2001:701–717.
55. Gruver A, Hudson LL, Sempowski GD. Immunosenescence of ageing. *J Pathol.* 2007;211:144–156.
56. Smith EM, Tu H, Hughes TH. Interleukin-10 and the hypothalamic-pituitary-adrenal axis. In: Plotnikoff NP, Faith RE, Murgo AJ, Good RA, eds. *Cytokines: Stress and Immunity.* 2nd ed. Boca Raton, FL: CRC Press; 2007:169–192.
57. Plotnikoff NP, Faith RE. Gender differences, stress, and immunity. In: Plotnikoff NP, Faith RE, Murgo AJ, Good RA, eds. *Cytokines: Stress and Immunity.* 2nd ed. Boca Raton, FL: CRC Press; 2007:371–385.
58. Kovacs E, Messingham K, Gregory M. Estrogen regulation of immune responses after injury. *Mol Cell Endocrinol.* 2002;193:129–135.
59. Verthelyi D. Sex hormones as immunomodulators in health and disease. *Int Immunopharmacol.* 2001;1:983–993.
60. Calder P, Kew S. The immune system: a target for functional foods? *Br J Nutr.* 2002;88:S165–S177.
61. Lopez-Varela S, Gonzalez-Gross M, Marcos A. Functional foods and the immune system: a review. *Eur J Clin Nutr.* 2002;56(suppl 3):S29–S33.
62. Mora JR, Iwata M, von Andrian UH. Vitamin effects on the immune system: vitamins A and D take centre stage. *Nat Rev Immunol.* 2008;8:685–698.
63. Kodama N, Komuta K, Nanba H. Effect of maitake (*Grifola frondosa*) D-fraction on the activation of NK cells in cancer patients. *J Med Food.* 2003;6:371–377.
64. Standish LJ, Wenner CA, Sweet ES, et al. *Trametes versicolor* mushroom immune therapy in breast cancer. *J Soc Integr Oncol.* 2008;6:122–128.
65. Clarke JO, Mullin GE. A review of complementary and alternative approaches to immunomodulation. *Nutr Clin Pract.* 2008;23:49–62.
66. Hall NS. Alternative medicine and the immune system. In: Ader R, Felten DL, Cohen N, eds. *Psychoneuroimmunology.* San Diego, CA: Academic Press; 2001:161–171.
67. Paineau D, Carcano D, Leyer G, et al. Effects of seven potential probiotic strains on specific immune responses in healthy adults: a double-blind, randomized, controlled trial. *FEDS Immunol Med Microbiol.* 2008;53:107–113.
68. Arbabi S, Garcia I, Baum G, et al. Alcohol (ethanol) inhibits IL-8 and TNF: role of the p38 pathway. *J Immunol.* 1999;162:7441–7445.
69. Ochshorn-Adelson M, Bodner G, Toraker P, et al. Effects of ethanol on human natural killer activity: in vitro and acute, low-dose in vivo studies. *Alcohol Clin Exp Res.* 1994;18:1361–1367.
70. Klein TW, Newton C, Snella E, et al. Marijuana, the cannabinoid system and immunomodulation. In: Ader R, Felten DL, Cohen N, eds. *Psychoneuroimmunology.* Vol 1. San Diego, CA: Academic Press; 2001:415–432.
71. Campbell PT, Wener MH, Sorensen B, et al. Effect of exercise on in vitro immune function: a 12-month randomized, controlled trial among postmenopausal women. *J Appl Physiol.* 2008;104:1648–1655.
72. Grant RW, Mariani RA, Vieira VJ, et al. Cardiovascular exercise intervention improves the primary antibody response to keyhole limpet hemocyanin (KLH) in previously sedentary older adults. *Brain Behav Immun.* 2008;22:923–932.
73. Nieman D, Nehlsen-Cannarella S. The immune response to exercise. *Semin Hematol.* 1994;31:166–179.
74. Shepard R, Rhind S, Shek P. Exercise and training: influence on cytotoxicity, interleukin-1, interleukin-2 and receptor structures. *Int J Sports Med.* 1994;15:154–166.
75. Shephard RJ, Shek PN. Physical activity and upper respiratory infection. In: Ader R, Felten DL, Cohen N, eds. *Psychoneuroimmunology.* Vol 2. San Diego, CA: Academic Press; 2001:511–524.
76. Hoffman-Goetz L, Pedersen BK. Immune responses to acute exercise: hemodynamic, hormonal, and cytokine influences. In: Ader R, Felten DL, Cohen N, eds. *Psychoneuroimmunology.* Vol 2. San Diego, CA: Academic Press; 2001:123–132.
77. Krueger JM, Majde JA, Obal F. Sleep in host defense. *Brain Behav Immun.* 2003;17:S41–S47.
78. Uthgenannt D, Schoolman D, Pietrowsky R, et al. Effects of sleep on the production of cytokines in humans. *Psychosom Med.* 1995;57: 97–104.
79. Szczepanik M. Melatonin and its influence on immune system. *J Physiol Pharmacol.* 2007;58(suppl 6):115–124.
80. Vgontzas AN, Chrousos GP. Sleep, the hypothalamic-pituitary-adrenal axis, and cytokines: multiple interactions and disturbances in sleep disorders. *Endocrinol Metab Clin North Am.* 2002;31:15–36.
81. Vgontzas AN, Bixler EO, Lin HM, et al. Chronic insomnia is associated with nyctohemeral activation of the hypothalamic-pituitary-adrenal axis: clinical implications. *J Clin Endocrinol Metab.* 2001;86:3787–3794.
82. Savard J, Laroche L, Simard S, Ivers H, Morin CM. Chronic insomnia and immune functioning. *Psychosom Med.* 2003;65:211–221.
83. Opp MR. Cytokines and sleep. *Sleep Med Rev.* 2005;9:355–364.

CHAPTER

3

Alecia Malin Fair, DrPH

# Epidemiology

## INTRODUCTION

Cancer epidemiology examines the frequency of cancer in populations, the role of certain risk factors that contribute to cancer rates, and the interrelationships or associations that exist between the host, the environment, and other conditions that may contribute to the development or inhibition of cancer.[1] The basic premise of epidemiology is that disease does not occur randomly, but rather in describable patterns that reflect the underlying etiology, or causes of cancer. Because disease does not occur randomly, individuals who have cancer must have been exposed to some factor, either voluntarily (through diet, medication, or smoking) or involuntarily (through factors such as cosmic radiation, air pollution, occupational hazards, or genetic constitution that contributed to the causation of disease).[2] The application of epidemiology to cancer research allows investigators to identify possible causes of disease by elucidating how those exposed and not exposed to risk factors toward cancer differ.

The first section of this chapter reviews basic epidemiological concepts. These concepts will help the reader better understand epidemiological research, identify groups at higher risk for cancer development, and learn how to conduct research in the field of cancer epidemiology. After reading this chapter, the reader should understand the major issues involved in cancer research design, assessment, and estimation of cancer risks. A brief glossary of fundamental terms used in the field of epidemiology is given in Table 3-1.[3] Table 3-2[3] includes rates and ratios frequently calculated in epidemiological research.

Subsequent sections discuss causes of cancer, risk factors that influence cancer susceptibility, and the application of epidemiological principles in nursing practice.

## BASIC CONSIDERATIONS IN EPIDEMIOLOGICAL RESEARCH

Six primary components are considered when evaluating an epidemiological research project:

- Definitions of the disease and exposures related to the research hypothesis
- Study design
- Eligibility and exclusionary criteria used to select study participants
- Definition of the source and study populations to be used in the study
- Statistical plan measuring the association between the exposures and the disease
- Identification of potential sources of bias and confounding variables.[4]

## STUDY DESIGNS

Several standard study designs are used in epidemiological research. Although this section discusses the general features of these designs, the primary emphasis is on the three designs most commonly used in epidemiological cancer research: the case-control, cohort, and clinical trial study designs. Other major study designs include experimental, ecological, and cross-sectional.[5]

In selecting the appropriate study design, several factors must be considered:

- The frequency of the disease or the exposure in the general population and the defined population to be studied
- The length of the latency period
- The anticipated size of the study sample
- The time allowed for subject recruitment
- The diagnostic characteristics of the disease and the measurability of the exposure.[4]

### Case-control studies

The case-control study design should be considered if at least one of the following criteria is met:

- The disease is rare in the general or source population (many forms of cancer meet this criterion).
- The investigation is preliminary.
- Time and funding limitations prohibit the use of larger, more expensive study designs.

The hallmark of the case-control study (as illustrated in Figure 3-1) is that it begins with people with the disease (cases) and compares them to people without the disease (controls).[6] Subjects in case-control studies are recruited on the basis of their disease status. Cases of the disease in question can be either preexisting or newly developed. Generally, a strict definition of the disease is used to identify eligible subjects. For example, pathology slides, cytology results, or medical records can be examined to identify the stage or histology of a cancer. The control subjects, or noncases,

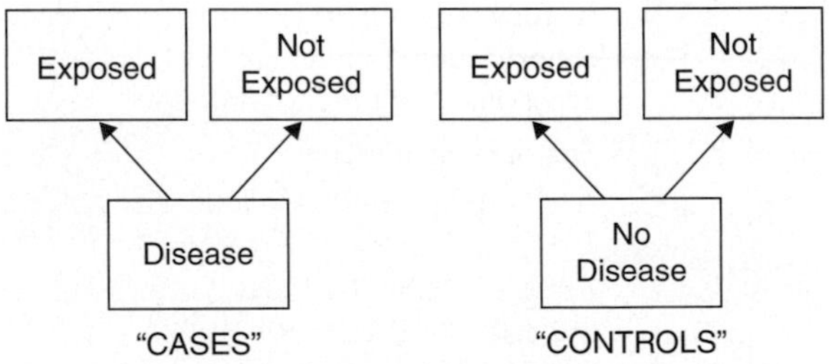


**FIGURE 3-1**

Design of a case-control study. Reprinted from Gordis,[6] Copyright 2008, with permission from Elsevier.

**TABLE 3-1**

| Glossary of Epidemiological Terms | |
|---|---|
| Association | Statistical association refers to the strength of the relationship between two variables. In epidemiological terms, association indicates the degree to which the rate of disease in persons with specific exposure is either higher or lower than the rate of disease in persons without the exposure. The strength of this dependence is greater than what would be expected by chance. |
| Bias | Selection bias results from a systematic difference in the manner in which the case and comparison groups are selected for participation in the study. This bias may produce spurious associations due to the differential inclusion or exclusion of subjects from the disease or exposure groups. |
| Case-control study | A study where individuals are selected according to the disease status of interest—those who have the disease (cases) and those individuals who do not have the disease (controls). The cases and controls are examined to ascertain which proportions were exposed to the disease risk factors and which were not. |
| Cohort study | A study where individuals are classified according to their exposure and are observed to ascertain the frequency of disease occurrence or death among those in various exposure-defined categories. |
| Confounding | The systematic overestimation or underestimation of the effect of an exposure because the influence of a disease risk factor has not been taken into account. A confounding variable is a risk factor for the disease being studied that is associated with the exposure being studied and is not an intermediate step between the exposure and the disease. |
| Epidemiological triangle | The traditional model of infectious disease causation. It consists of three components: an external agent, a susceptible host, and an environment that brings the host and the agent together. Also known as the epidemiological triad. |
| Epidemiology | Nonexperimental investigation of disease causation through observational study of human population groups. Descriptive epidemiology is the study of the frequency of occurrence of (incidence) or death from (mortality) in a disease population stratified by time, place, and/or group characteristics. Analytical epidemiology is the ascertainment of whether a particular exposure, such as a physical, chemical, or biological agent, and a specific cancer or other disease are unrelated (independent) or associated. |
| Etiology | The study of the cause of disease. |
| False negative | In analyzing the validity of a screening test for disease, those people who truly have the disease that are erroneously called "negative" by the test. |
| False positive | In analyzing the validity of screening tests for disease, those people who do not have the disease that are erroneously called "positive" by the test. |
| Historical cohort | A study using a cohort defined in the past. |
| Incidence | The number of new events or cases of disease that occur in a defined population at risk within a specified period. Incidence rates can be used to evaluate the changing patterns of disease frequency within a population and to assess the effectiveness of screening programs and treatment modalities on disease development. |
| Intervention | A study employed to test the efficacy of a preventive or therapeutic measure to knowledge about the etiology and natural history of a disease so as to formulate strategies for its prevention. Clinical trials are intervention studies that focus on the individual. They compare the outcomes in a group of patients treated with the test treatment with those observed in a comparable group of patients receiving a control or placebo treatment, where patients in both groups are enrolled, treated, and followed over the same time period. Community interventions focus on the group or community and evaluate the benefits of new policies and programs, determining which have an effect on the health of those who receive the intervention and which do not. |
| Nested case-control | A study where a series of cases are identified using a case-control approach within the confines of a well-defined cohort study. The case group consists of a representative sample of individuals, with the disease of interest occurring in the defined cohort over a specified follow-up period. |
| Population | The number of persons in a defined group who are capable of developing the disease. Can also refer to the general population; a population specifically defined by geographic boundaries, physical or social characteristics, or risk; the sampling population; and the study population. |
| Power | The probability that a study will have the statistical strength to detect relationships that exist between exposures and disease. The power of a study can be maximized by controlling for factors such as sample sizes, measurement error, and bias. |
| Prevalence | The number of new and existing cases of a given disease or condition in a defined population within a specified period of time. Point prevalence refers to prevalence at one point in time. Period prevalence refers to prevalence between two points in time. Prevalence rates can be used to compare disease frequencies across populations and to assess the magnitude of effect of certain diseases on the health status of a population. |

*(Continued)*

**TABLE 3-1**

**Glossary of Epidemiological Terms (Continued)**

| | |
|---|---|
| Rates and ratios | Calculations used to compare the frequencies of diseases in a population. Commonly used rates and ratios are given in Table 3-2, which lists the rate names. The numerator and denominator values and the population factor are used to express the rate in a standard format. |
| Risk measures | Attributable risk is the arithmetic or absolute difference between the exposed group and the nonexposed group in terms of incidence rates or death rates. It estimates the number of disease case that can be attributed to or explained by the exposure (eg, the majority of lung cancer cases can be attributed to exposure to cigarette smoking). |
| Relative risk | Relative risk (RR) is a ratio comparing the rates of a disease among the exposed group and the nonexposed group that serves as a measure of the association between the disease and the exposure. The RR is generally used in cohort studies. The formula for calculating it is $\frac{a(a+b)}{c} = (c+d)$ |
| Odds ratio | The odds ratio (OR) approximates the relative risk by comparing the rates of disease among the exposed and nonexposed groups. The OR is generally used in case-control studies with smaller sample sizes. The formula for calculating it is $\frac{ad}{cb}$<br>Both the RR and OR are expressed as ratios (eg, an OR of 1.0 means the rate of disease among the exposed group equals the rate among the nonexposed group). |
| Sensitivity | Measures the probability that a screening test will correctly classify an individual as positive for a disease when he or she actually does have the disease. |
| Specificity | Measures the probability that a screening test will correctly classify an individual as negative for a disease when he or she actually does not have the disease. |
| Spurious | As applied to associations between exposures, a false relationship produced by methodological errors or confounding variables. |
| Validity | Internal validity is the extent to which the subjects in an epidemiological study are truly comparable with respect to general characteristics (eg, if most of the cases are from an urban setting and the controls are mainly from a rural setting, the two groups are not comparable, and evaluation of the exposure–disease relationship may be affected by these differences). Internal validity is essential for the interpretability and reliability of a study.<br>External validity, or generalizability, is the extent to which the study population can be compared with a larger population (eg, the general population). External validity must be assessed before study results can be applied to a broader population (eg, a study that uses as its population a specific profession, such as nurses, may yield results that are not relevant to all woman in the general population; while the study may have strong internal validity, the participating nurses may not be representative of the women in the general population or in the nursing profession). |

*Source*: Adapted from Reid M.[4]

are defined as participants who do not have the disease at present but who, if the disease did develop, would have the same opportunity to be diagnosed as the case subjects.

The assumption that cases and controls originate from the same hypothetical source cohort is a critical issue affecting the validity of case-control data. Both cases and controls must originate from populations having similar and relevant characteristics. In this instance, the control group can be regarded as a reasonably representative sample of the case reference population. The selection of an appropriate control group represents the major challenge with case-control studies and often serves as the source of selection bias introduced into the study.[7]

The information gained from case-control studies does not establish a causal relationship between the disease and the exposure, but it does explore the concurrent association between the two. If the strength of this association is significant and supported by other studies, it can be used to justify the use of larger cohort studies or clinical trials that can investigate causative relationships.

When conducting a case-control study, be aware that cases and controls may differ in characteristics and exposures aside from the ones that have been targeted for the study. Suppose we are interested in conducting a case-control study to determine whether lung cancer was linked to cigarette smoking; with this study design, we would start with the disease outcome (eg, lung cancer) and retrospectively examine the extent of smoking among cases and controls. Age, in this instance, is related to length of smoking history

**TABLE 3-2**

**Rates and Ratios Commonly Used in Epidemiology**

| Rate Name | Rate Description | Population Factor |
|---|---|---|
| Crude birth rate | Number of live births: average or midyear population | per 1000 |
| Fertility rate | Number of live births: 15- to 41-year-old women at midyear | per 1000 |
| Crude mortality rate | Total number of deaths: total population at midyear | per 1000 |
| Age-specific mortality rate | Deaths in specific age group: midyear population in age group | per 100,000 |
| Cause-specific mortality rate | Deaths from a specific cause: total midyear population | per 100,000 |
| Infant mortality rate | Deaths of children younger than 1 year of age: number of live births | per 1000 |
| Neonatal mortality rate | Deaths of infants younger than 28 days: number of live births | per 1000 |
| Case fatality rate | Number of deaths from a disease in a given period of follow-up: number of diagnosed cases of disease at start of follow-up period | per 1000 |
| Proportional mortality rate | Number of deaths from a given cause: number of deaths from all causes | per 1000 |
| Morbidity rate | Number of cases of the disease that develop in a given period: total population at midperiod | per 100,000 |

*Source:* Adapted from Reid M.[4]

as well as to cancer of the lung. The confounding effect of age can be avoided by selecting cases and controls of the same age group or matching the two groups for age.[8]

Matching is the process of selecting controls for factors beyond the targeted factors for the study so that the controls are similar to the cases in certain characteristics, such as age, race, sex, socioeconomic status (SES), menopausal status, and occupation.[6] Two matching techniques are used in epidemiological research: frequency matching and individual matching. In frequency matching, the proportion of controls with a certain characteristic is identical to the proportion of cases with the same characteristic. In individual matching (also known as matched pairs), a control is selected for each case that is similar to the case in terms of the specific variable or variable of concern. If the first case enrolled in our study is a 50-year-old postmenopausal white woman, we would therefore seek a 50-year-old white postmenopausal control. The advantage of matching and analyzing the data for pairs of subjects is that fewer subjects are required in each group to discern a relationship between the exposure and the disease. Matching enhances the ability to substantiate a true association between exposure and disease outcome. It is useful when small numbers of case subjects with the disease are available for study and when efficiency is a major issue. Matching also provides a means for controlling potential confounding introduced by the selection of the control group.

The following example describes a case-control study that used matching to examine breast cancer and occupational exposure to electromagnetic field (EMF), an exposure for which little is known about. The cases were 6,213 patients with invasive breast cancer identified from hospitals in Massachusetts, New Hampshire, and Wisconsin that reported to their respective state cancer registry. Patients were between 20 and 69 years old. A total of 7,390 controls were identified from lists of licensed drivers and rosters of Medicare beneficiaries. The cases and controls were randomly age-matched within a five-year age strata. Data were collected through phone interviews that included questions on breast cancer risk factors such as smoking, alcohol consumption, menstrual and reproductive history, exogenous hormone use, medical history, diet, physical activity, marital status, and family history. Women were also asked to report their occupational job history beginning at age 14 for any job held for at least 1 year in which the woman worked at least 4 hours per week. Occupational categorization of EMF exposure was based on the Dictionary of Occupational Titles classification system. The results illustrated that, when compared with the referent of background exposure, the odds ratio (OR) adjusted for age and state of residence was 1.06 (95% confidence interval [CI] = 0.99–1.14) for low exposure, 1.09 (95% CI = 0.96–1.23) for medium exposure, and 1.16 (95% CI = 0.90–1.50) for high exposure. The women with high EMF exposure were 16% more likely to have breast cancer than their peers in the low and medium exposure categories, who are at 6% and 9% risk for breast cancer, respectively.[9]

Two immediate problems arise with matching. First, if an attempt is made to match too many characteristics, it may prove difficult or impossible to identify an appropriate control. Second, once cases and controls have been matched according to a given characteristic, that characteristic cannot be studied in relation to disease. Caution is advised on matching on any variable that may be of interest for exploring in a study.

## Cohort studies

A cohort study seeks to investigate whether the incidence of an event is related to a suspected exposure. That is, a cohort study is an incidence study. It starts with a group of subjects who are at risk for developing a disease, yet are free of the disease at the beginning of the study, as shown in Figure 3-2.[6] Cohort studies can be envisioned as going from cause to effect. The exposure of interest is determined for each member of the cohort, and the group is followed to document incidence of disease in the exposed and nonexposed members.

Cohort studies can be prospective, retrospective, or ambidirectional. Cohort studies are considered *prospective* or *concurrent* when the cohort is assembled at the present time and the subjects are followed concurrently through calendar time until the point at which the disease does or does not develop. The disadvantages of prospective studies relate to the amount of time needed to conduct them to determine whether the outcome of interest has developed at their usually exorbitant costs.

The Nurses' Health Study is one of the most prominent examples of a prospective cohort study.[10,11–13] Nurses between the ages of 25 and 42 years old, living in one of the 14 selected states, were enrolled in the first iteration of the study, Nurses' Health Study I, when they responded to a questionnaire about their medical histories and lifestyles in 1976. Follow-up questionnaires were sent biennially to update information on risk factors and medical events. All eligible nurses were studied for weight gain, hypertension, dietary intake, reproductive behaviors, menopausal status, family history, hormone replacement therapy (HRT), physical activity, medical history, smoking status, and alcohol consumption. Blood samples have allowed researchers to explore biomarkers and genetic factors. This study is now in its third wave of data collection, which began in 1989 with the Nurses' Health Study II (NHSII) and has addressed several hypotheses germane to women's health and female cancers, including the association of estrogens, caffeine intake, tubal ligation, folate intake, night-shift work, menopausal status, and weight gain with cancer risk.[10–13]

An alternative approach to the cohort study design is nonconcurrent cohorts, also known as *historical* or *retrospective cohort studies*. A previously defined cohort is identified and assembled in the past on the basis of existing records, and disease outcome (development or no development of disease) is ascertained at the time when the study began (Figure 3-3).[6] Nonconcurrent studies are notably less expensive and can be implemented more expeditiously than concurrent studies. Their main disadvantage is reliance on available information; consequently, the quality of exposure or outcome data is sometimes less than ideal for fulfilling the study objectives. Many occupational cohort studies are conducted retrospectively.

Case-control studies within a cohort study are known as *ambidirectional studies* or *nested case-control studies*,[11] because they combine some of the features and advantages of both cohort and case-control designs. The selection of participants is carried out using a case-control approach, as shown in Figure 3-4.[6] A nested case-control design starts with a previously established cohort and continues subject follow-up into the future. Ambidirectional designs are being used increasingly for cost-efficiency reasons when analysis of all cohort members requires substantial resources.[11]

## Clinical trials and intervention studies

A clinical trial or intervention study is a planned experiment testing medical treatments. This type of study is designed

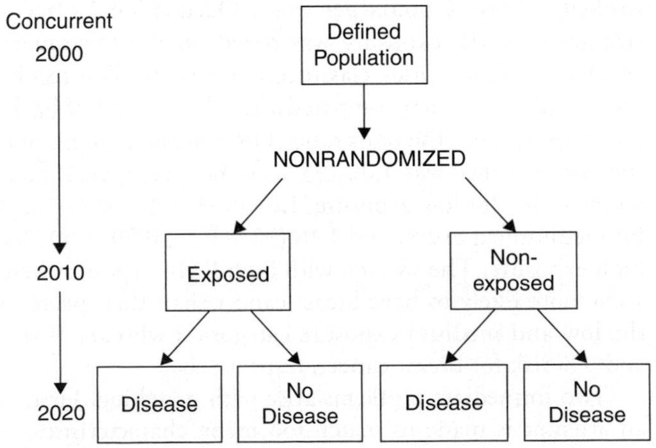


**FIGURE 3-2**

Time frame for a hypothetical concurrent cohort study begun in 2000. Reprinted from Gordis,[6] Copyright 2008, with permission from Elsevier.

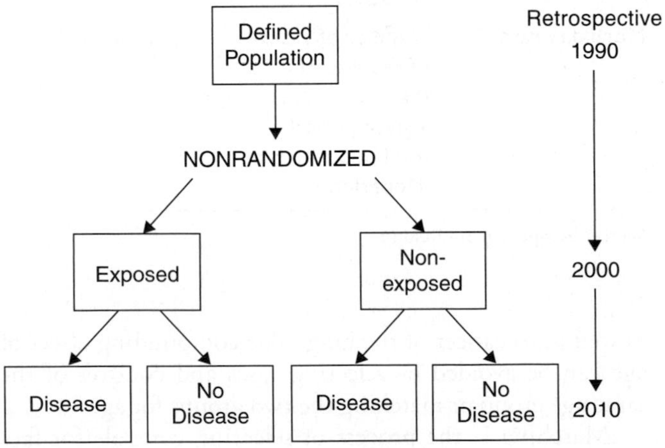


**FIGURE 3-3**

Time frame for a hypothetical retrospective cohort study begun in 2010. Reprinted from Gordis,[6] Copyright 2008, with permission from Elsevier.

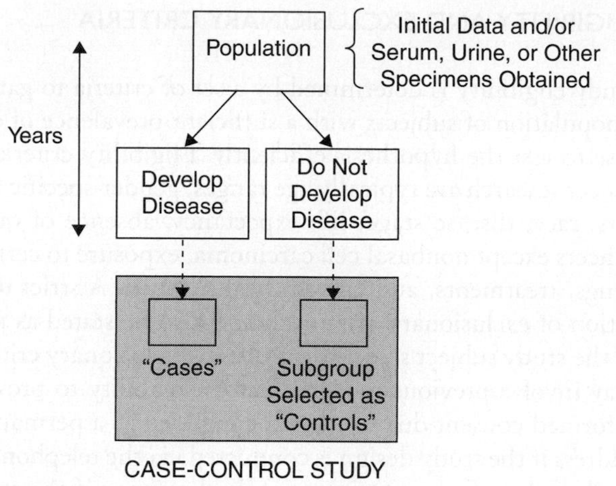


**FIGURE 3-4**

Diagram of nested case-control study. Reprinted from Gordis,[6] Copyright 2008, with permission from Elsevier.

to assess the efficacy of a treatment by comparing outcomes in a group of patients who received the test treatment with outcomes observed in a comparable group of patients who receive a control treatment. Both groups of patients are enrolled, treated, and followed over the same period.[14]

Once clinical trial patients have been screened for eligibility, they are randomly assigned to one of the study groups. There is an intervention group, which receives the test treatment, and a control group, which receives the placebo or the current therapy. A randomized clinical trial may, for example, randomly assign a group of cancer patients to a particular drug regimen and assign a similar group of cancer patients to a course of not receiving the drug. The two groups are monitored over the duration of the study, with researchers comparing the groups' survival or cure ratio of cancer.

To preserve the objectivity of the data gathered in clinical trials, the blinding approach is used. Participants are blinded as to which group assignment they will get, either the treatment or the control group. This technique prevents attrition when subjects who learn that they have been randomized to the placebo arm of the trials subsequently drop out. Additionally, the investigator can be blinded as to the subject's group assignment, creating a double-blind design. A double-blind design protects against the investigator becoming biased as to the trial's outcome, particularly if a drug manufacturer is financing the trial.[2]

A major benefit of a double-blind, placebo-controlled clinical trial is that the random assignment of treatment groups helps to distribute potential confounding variables evenly between the two groups, thereby minimizing their effects on the measurement of the association between the exposure and the disease. If this control of confounding is successful and the primary difference between the two treatment groups is the intervention, then a clinical trial can definitively evaluate the efficacy of the intervention.[15]

An example of a clinical trial is the beta-carotene and retinol efficacy trial (CARET), which used random assignment to test the efficacy of a daily combination of 30 mg of carotene and 25,000 IU of retinyl palmitate (retinol) on the incidence of lung cancers, other cancers, and death vs a placebo in 18,314 participants who were at high risk for lung cancer because of a history of smoking or asbestos exposure. Participants, who were randomly assigned to receive the active intervention, were found to have a 28% increase in incidence of lung cancer, a 17% increase in incidence of death, and a higher rate of cardiovascular disease mortality compared with participants in the placebo group. CARET was stopped ahead of schedule and participants returned the study vitamins to their study center and provided a final blood sample. CARET participants continue to be followed annually by telephone and mail self-report.[15,16]

A major limitation of the clinical trial design is that several years of subject follow-up may be required before significant changes in the rate of disease development are observed among treatment groups. The length of follow-up will depend on several factors, including the strength of the effect the treatment has on the risk of the disease. Long-term studies raise patient management issues, such as maintaining active participation of subjects, monitoring subject deaths and adverse events, and tracking subjects lost to follow-up. These factors, if unevenly distributed among the treatment groups, may confound the results of the project.

### Experimental studies

Experimental studies maintain the greatest control over the research setting. Random allocation is used to assign subjects either to receive the treatment or to not receive it or to be assigned to either the exposed or the nonexposed group. Once substantial and consistent evidence has accumulated from experimental studies, other study designs may be employed to further demonstrate the feasibility of large-scale population interventions.

The randomized control trial dominates experimental research in laboratory animals. Performing such experiments on humans does have its drawbacks; however, the most important of which are ethical. It is obviously not acceptable to expose humans intentionally to a potential carcinogenic agent in an attempt to ascertain cancer causation.[11]

### Ecological studies

Ecological studies in epidemiology occupy an intermediate position between descriptive and analytical investigations, in that they share characteristics with descriptive studies but serve etiological objectives.[11] These studies are popular because they use existing databases and can offer large exposure variation if the data arise from broad geographical areas.[17] The exposure and disease under investigation in ecological studies are not ascertained for specific individuals but rather across groups and whole populations.[18] When an exposure is fairly common, such as smoking, sunlight,[19] or fat consumption, ecological studies can elucidate the possible effects of these exposures. For example, skin melanoma is more common in geographic latitudes with more sunshine exposure, and countries with higher per capita intakes of dietary fat tend to be the same countries with high rates of breast cancer mortality.[20] The caveat of using ecological studies to prove disease causality is the phenomenon of ecological fallacy: "the bias that occurs because an association observed between variables on an aggregate level does not necessarily represent the association that exists at an individual level."[21] Specifically, there is an inability of ecological data to characterize within-area variability in exposures and confounders.

Despite their limitations, ecological studies do have merit within epidemiological research. They are quick, simple to conduct, and inexpensive. When little is known about the association between an exposure and disease, an ecological study is a reasonable place to start generating hypotheses.[2]

### Cross-sectional studies

Cross-sectional studies allow the investigator to study the relationship between an exposure (eg, EMF) and a disease outcome (eg, leukemia) by surveying a population for each participant, and determining the exposure and disease outcome simultaneously.[8] The unit of analysis in cross-sectional studies is the individual. Cross-sectional studies are referred to as "snapshot" studies because they provide a one-time view of a population's rate of existing (prevalent) cases of the disease, the degree of exposure, and other demographic characteristics of interest at a single hypothetical point in time. While cross-sectional studies cannot establish a causal relationship between the exposure and the disease, they do provide descriptive statistics for the population and are often used as the preliminary step in establishing disease or exposure status in cohort studies.

## DEFINING THE DISEASE

Defining the disease in epidemiological studies is the penultimate task in including and excluding the appropriate subjects in a study population. Disease may be defined by review of medical records, pathological results, blood test results, physical exam, histological characteristics, or results from a psychological battery of tests. To increase the rigor of this step, two different medical professionals, each unaware of the other's findings, should confirm disease status. Clearly, stating disease definition guidelines at the outset can prevent enrolling subjects who are actually ineligible for the study. Once a disease status is confirmed for each subject, he or she is eligible for study enrollment.

## ELIGIBILITY AND EXCLUSIONARY CRITERIA

Study eligibility is determined by a set of criteria to gather a population of subjects with a sufficient prevalence of disease to test the hypothesis efficiently. Eligibility criteria in cancer research are typically age ranges, gender-specific factors, race, disease stage, life expectancy, absence of other cancers except nonbasal cell carcinoma, exposure to certain drugs, treatments, and current health status. A strict definition of exclusionary criteria should also be stated as part of the study subject screening process. Exclusionary criteria may involve previous medical history, inability to provide informed consent due to mental competency, a permanent address if the study design is conducted via the telephone or mail, and proficiency in a particular language if the study materials are written and administered in one language.

Interrelated with the definition of disease is how the disease was contracted, or exposure to which factors that lead to a disease state. An exposure in epidemiology comprises the subject's contact with the variable of interest, which may influence the development or improvement in disease status. Exposures run the gamut from microenvironmental exposures on an individual level, such as nutrients, medications, physical activity, and genes, to macroenvironmental exposures, such as air pollution and environmental conditions that affect an entire community.[11] In epidemiological research, exposures are measured by their frequency and duration as well as their ability to synergistically react with one another.

Dose refers to a standardized, measured amount of exposure issued (eg, standard milligrams, as in the case of drugs; gray [Gy] for radiation; number of packs of cigarettes per year; hours of exercise; drinks of alcohol per day). It is imperative to assess whether the dose has remained constant throughout the exposure or whether certain variables or conditions have affected the dose over time. The likelihood of an association between an exposure and disease being causal is stronger if a more intense "dose" of the exposure produces higher rates of disease.

## DEFINING THE POPULATION

In addition to defining the type of study design appropriate for testing a research hypothesis and the disease/exposure, the source population for study subjects and the actual study population must be defined. This process clarifies to whom the research results can be generalized (external validity), whether the study population represents the total population and the source population, and what the overall characteristics of eligible subjects are.

The source population for the study is the larger group or population from which the study subjects are recruited. It might include, for instance, residents in a certain city or neighborhood, university students, or all patients attending a particular hospital. The source population is usually a subgroup of the total population.

The study population is the group of subjects actually recruited into the project from the source population. Recruitment into the study population, based on the defined eligibility and exclusionary criteria, is planned to access all potential subjects within the source population. It is important to review the types of subjects who were part of the source population but who were not eligible or not approached for recruitment. For example, if subjects were recruited from phone interviews, we could safely conclude that only subjects with telephones were eligible. Because the presence of a telephone in the household might be related to SES, it is possible that the study population might be biased toward subjects with a higher SES. The relationship of SES to the disease may be impossible to evaluate and may affect the results of the study.

### STATISTICAL PLAN

Epidemiological research measures disease outcomes in rates and ratios, frequencies, and distributions. Aside from these descriptive statistics, inferential statistics can be used to infer whether the exposure disease relationship that is observed in the study population is applicable to a larger population.[22,23] This premise is called *external validity* or *generalizability*. Additional factors play a role in establishing causation between exposure to risk factors and disease outcome.

### POTENTIAL SOURCES OF BIAS AND CONFOUNDING VARIABLES

To reasonably assert an uncompromised relationship between exposure and disease, we must account for any bias that exists in an epidemiological study design. The most common forms of bias in a case-control study are (1) noncases in the case series of subjects, (2) a systematic error in data collection, (3) an inordinate amount of random error in the collection of data, and (4) an inappropriate analysis of data. These types of bias result in a mistaken estimate of an exposure's effect on the risk of disease.[22]

Two primary forms of bias are encountered in epidemiological studies: selection bias and recall bias. *Selection bias* arises when the relationship between exposure and disease is different for those who participate in the study and those who would be theoretically eligible for the study but do not participate.[24] The common consequence of selection bias is that the association between exposure and outcome among those selected for analysis differs from the association among those eligible.[25] For instance, the healthy worker effect may occur in occupational cohort studies. Only employed individuals are eligible for such a study, but workers are relatively healthy people who are able to maintain employment.[2] The characteristics of these individuals are, therefore, not generalizable to the overall population. *Recall bias* results from inaccurate recall of past exposures. It is especially a concern in the context of case-control studies when cases and controls are queried for exposures in the past. Bias on the selection of subjects or the study results can lead to a spurious, or unrelated, association in contributing to the exposure–disease relationship factor.

Another concern in epidemiological studies is confounding variables. Confounding variables prevent study groups from being comparable. For instance, if a case-control study shows an association between alcohol intake and lung cancer, we must investigate whether a third factor might exist in the causal pathway of a lung cancer outcome, one that was not originally stated in the study hypothesis. Smoking is another complementary risk factor associated with drinking alcohol. Smoking in this case is a confounder. Although we were interested in the causal relationship between alcohol consumption and lung cancer, smoking is a known risk for lung cancer; it is associated with alcohol intake but is not a result of drinking alcohol.[6]

When planning an epidemiological study, consult a biostatistician or epidemiologist to help design the research protocol. Sample a large enough study group to have the ability to draw causal inferences for the general population and to perform a rigorous statistical analysis. A variety of techniques can be used to control for bias and confounding variables in epidemiological studies. Randomization, matching, and statistical analyses stratifying or controlling for confounding variables are the methods commonly used. In summary, it is advisable to retain experienced researchers to minimize potential errors at the dataset phase of the study design. Various statistical[22,23] and epidemiological texts[2,6,8,11,25] are excellent resources for fundamentals of epidemiological and statistical practice.

## CAUSES OF CANCER

### TOBACCO

The causal relationship between tobacco use and various forms of cancer has been primarily derived from epidemiological research. Epidemiological studies of tobacco have relied on mostly self-reported smoking histories. Unlike with dietary patterns, subjects participating in epidemiological research are unlikely to seriously misreport their smoking habits owing to faulty recall.[26]

Active tobacco use has been linked to many cancer types: lung; lower urinary tract, including the renal pelvis and bladder; upper aero-digestive tract, including the oral cavity, pharynx, and esophagus; and pancreas. Smoking tobacco can also cause cancer of the nasal cavity, paranasal sinuses, and nasopharynx; stomach; liver; kidney; cervix uteri; adenocarcinoma of the esophagus; and myeloid leukemia.

Cancer can be caused by smoking cigarettes, pipes, cigars, or bidis (a small amount of tobacco wrapped in the leaf of another plant, commonly used in South Asia).[2,27,28]

Given the increased bans on smoking in occupational and recreational settings, smokeless tobacco products seem like an obvious substitution for active smoking tobacco.[29] The median mortality relative risk for low-nitrosamine smokeless tobacco has been estimated to be at least 90% to 95% lower than for cigarette smoking.[30] The absence of sidestream smoke from smokeless tobacco products also reduces health risks from environmental tobacco smoke (ETS) and fire risks.[31,32]

## PASSIVE SMOKING

The carcinogenic effects of ETS or passive smoking on human lung tissues have been a hotly debated issue during the past decade. ETS can be defined as sidestream smoke and/or mainstream smoke exhaled by active smokers. Sidestream smoke consists of about 85% of total ETS, and mainstream smoke constitutes less than 15% of the overall ETS. Once released into the environment, ETS can further aggregate with existing air pollutants and change character. Therefore, the physiochemistry of ETS may be greatly different from that of mainstream smoke.[33] Both sidestream and mainstream smoke contain about 40 different chemicals that are suspected or proven carcinogens.[26,34] In 1992, the US Environmental Protection Agency (EPA) published a report that classified ETS as a group A carcinogen (known human carcinogen). Approximately 90% of the epidemiological studies on ETS focused on nonsmoking women married to smokers. The annual number of cases attributable to spousal ETS is on the order of 50 in men and more than 500 in women. The corresponding estimates for ETS exposure at the workplace are about 200 cases among men and 270 cases among women.[35] Estimates from the EPA for the U.S. population, which considered spousal and background sources of ETS, predicted in 1,930 cases among women and 1,130 cases among men. The evidence for a causal association between ETS exposure and cancer in organs other than the lung is inconclusive.[9] Being exposed to ETS in the workplace also conveys a 1.2 greater risk of developing lung cancer. Although results from studies of passive smoking and breast cancer risk have been inconclusive, new findings on active smoking status and breast cancer reveal a 1.3-fold greater risk of breast cancer in smokers compared to women who have never smoked and were not exposed to passive smoking.[36]

## DIET

More than one-half million cancer deaths occur in the United States each year, and one-third of these deaths are attributed to suboptimal diet,[37,38] which is considered a modifiable risk factor. Interest and research in the role of diet in cancer have flourished in recent years, with many micronutrients (vitamins and minerals) and some macronutrients (proteins, fats, carbohydrates) being investigated for adverse or protective effects against cancer, in both human and animal studies.[39,40] The impetus for many of these studies came from the results of ecological studies. For example, a strong positive relationship was shown between per capita fat intake and breast cancer mortality rates.[41]

### Cancer and macronutrients

*Fat intake.* Historically, results from case-control and cohort studies generally have supported high fat intake as a risk factor for colon cancer.[42–45] The role of fat in colon cancer is supported by both the rapid change in incidence with dietary change and the potential relationship of fat consumption to bile acids, which are known to be mutagenic.

Nevertheless, the relationship between fat and colon cancer has yet to be firmly established. Case-control and cohort studies on breast cancer risk and fat intake give conflicting results. A total of 14 articles have examined the relationship between breast cancer recurrence and/or survival and dietary intakes in women with diagnosed breast cancer.[46] With respect to dietary fat intake, there have been a few reports addressing this issue that describe a significant association with breast cancer outcomes. Several cohort studies found an increased risk of breast cancer death with increased fat intake.[47–49] However, the analysis of data from seven cohort studies in four countries showed no evidence of a positive association between total dietary fat and the risk of breast cancer.[50,51] Several cohort studies,[52–54] including two of the largest landmark cohort studies—the Nurses' Health Study[52] and the Iowa Women's Study[53]—showed no relationship between dietary fat intake and breast cancer risk, although some researchers suggest that this outcome may be because the range of fat intake in such studies was too small. Current dietary recommendations are for women to reduce fat intake to less than 30% of calories. The notion that fat intake may be related to breast cancer has persisted, but there has been an inability to provide individual—as opposed to national—statistics relating breast cancer to fat intake. This result has led to a wide acceptance that the relationship is not to fat but rather to total calories and especially to total calories consumed early in life.

### Cancer, micronutrients, supplements, and intake of fruits and vegetables

One of the most consistent dietary findings in analytic epidemiological studies with regard to cancer is the protective effect of fruits and vegetables.[54–56] Which particular nutrient, non-nutrient, or combination in fruits and vegetables offers protection against cancer remains under investigation. The roles of several micronutrients in cancer prevention, including the carotenoid beta-carotene, vitamin A, vitamin E, and selenium, have been extensively investigated. Relatively high levels of these four micronutrients have been found to be associated with lower cancer risk in many studies, although again not all study results are in agreement.[40,57–59]

Some have speculated that the antioxidant effect of vitamin C might play a preventive role against cancer, but this relationship has not been well established.[60–62] Various studies strongly suggest that folate has effectiveness in cancer prevention.[62] Folate is critical for both DNA synthesis and DNA methylation, and various mechanisms have been hypothesized through which folate might influence carcinogenesis. However, recent review of this association suggests that effects of folate on DNA methylation may vary by the site, dependent on cell type, stage of transformation, and the degree of duration of folate depletion.[63] Dietary and supplemental folate appear to be protective and reduce the risk of pancreatic,[64] breast,[65] colorectal,[66,67] and ovarian cancer.[68] Folate deficiency contributes to chromosomal instability and may increase susceptibility to radiation-induced DNA damage.[69] The optimal dose of folate to minimize colorectal cancer has not been established. Preliminary evidence based on pooled results from nine cohort studies suggest that intakes of approximately 400–500 μg/d may be required to minimize risk.[64]

The antioxidant effects of lycopene may explain the reduction in gastrointestinal tract, breast, and cervical cancer incidence in some populations.[70] Various observational studies have explored the role of lycopene, a carotenoid derived from tomato products like pizza, spaghetti sauce, ketchup, and salsa, in conjunction with gastrointestinal, breast, prostate, lung, and cervical cancer incidence. The mechanisms for the cancer-preventing actions of carotenoids may involve antioxidant activity, induction of detoxifying enzymes, and inhibition of cellular proliferation.[70,71]

There has been a growing interest in the preventive and therapeutic effects of phytoestrogens on various hormone-responsive cancers, such as breast, endometrial, ovarian, and prostate cancer. The phytoestrogens are compounds found in plants such as soy. The isoflavones, which show structural similarity to mammalian estrogens,[72,73] are considered to be responsible for providing the anticancer benefit. Isoflavones are present in large amounts in soybeans and soy products such as miso and tofu, kudzu root, peanuts, and lentils.[74] Their chemopreventive properties result from soy isoflavones possessing estrogenic activity, competing with estradiol for the estrogen receptor complex, and inhibiting hormone response in cancer cells and tumor growth.[75]

*Fiber intake.* A majority of studies of differing epidemiological designs support the hypothesis that high fiber intake is protective for colon cancer.[76] The well-documented relationship between meat consumption and colon cancer likely reflects the role played by animal fat consumption. The role of fiber in colon cancer has repeatedly been postulated to relate to altered transit time, altered bacterial flora in the colon, and altered exposure of the colonic mucosa to potentially carcinogenic bacterially modified bile acids. Epidemiological studies have suggested an inverse relationship between dietary fiber and colon cancer, and animal studies suggest that the type of fiber may be important,[76,77] although not all results are supportive of this position.[78,79] Vegetables as well as cereals are sources of fiber. In studies where the source of fiber has been examined, fiber from vegetables appears protective against colon cancer, whereas the data for cereal fiber are less supportive of a protective effect. According to the hypothesized mechanism, fiber affects the bile acid content of the aqueous portion of stool. These differing results may be due to the difference in composition of fiber in cereals and vegetables or to the lack of a large range in cereal fiber intake, or they may indicate that some other chemical or nutrient in vegetables is protective against colon cancer.[76–79]

*Calcium intake and vitamin D.* A protective role for high calcium intake against colon cancer has been reported in several studies[80–84] but not in all.[85] Data suggest that there is a 30% to 50% reduction in risk for developing colorectal cancer by increasing vitamin D intake to least 1000 IU/d.[86] Calcium may inhibit colorectal carcinogenesis because of its ability to bind toxic bile acids, thereby rendering them inert, or by direct effects on the cell cycle.[87] The role of calcium in colon cancer etiology is linked to vitamin D.[88] Only a few foods (oily fish and eggs) contain naturally occurring vitamin D; certain foods in the United States, including milk and orange juice, are fortified with vitamin D.[89] The major physiological function of vitamin D is to maintain blood calcium in the normal range for intestinal absorption.[90] A number of epidemiological studies have inversely linked cancer risk with dietary sources or blood levels of vitamin D with cumulative sun exposure.[91,92] In vitro animal and clinical studies strongly indicate that vitamin D may have anticancer benefits including the reduction of tumor invasion and angiogenesis[93,94] The anticancer link of vitamin D is the ability of many cells to convert 25(OH)D, the primary circulating pre-vitamin D form of vitamin D, into 1,25$(OH)_2$D, the most biologically active form of this vitamin. Vitamin D and calcium intake have been shown in negative cellular growth regulation by inhibiting cell proliferation and inducing differentiation and apoptosis in normal and malignant cells and tissues in the breast, colon, and prostate that possess the vitamin D receptor (VDR).[95] The epidemiological data for breast and prostate cancer in relation to vitamin D are promising but too sparse to draw a conclusion.[91,96] The evidence that higher 25(OH) D levels produced through sun exposure or dietary/supplement intake inhibit colorectal cancer is substantial,[97–100] although randomized intervention trials have produced mixed results.[101–104]

The available data on vitamin D, tumor biology, and cancer risk are intriguing but far from complete. At this juncture the existing evidence elicits more questions than answers, including (1) Do higher vitamin D levels alter cancer risk in humans? (2) What cancer sites are affected; if vitamin D is beneficial, what is the optimal intake and circulating concentration of 25(OH)D? and (3)What groups are at higher risk for a vitamin D deficiency?[91] Given the strong biological plausibility of the role of vitamin D and public health potential for noninvasive intervention on sun exposure and vitamin D supplementation, further research on vitamin D as a chemopreventive agent should be a priority.

Case-control and cohort studies of diet and cancer present some measurement problems:

1. The distribution of dietary components among individual foods varies greatly. The interactive roles of dietary components are not completely understood, particularly when several components are present in individual foods.[105]
2. Recall bias may be present if dietary assessment is conducted after the presentation of the disease, as in a case-control study. In essence, individuals' recall of their past diet may be affected by their knowledge that they have the disease.[106] To avoid the problems associated with self-reported dietary intake methods, direct assessment of some micronutrients has been developed, involving measuring serum micronutrient levels. Issues regarding measurement of micronutrients through biospecimens are discussed later in this chapter.

## Alcohol

Alcoholic beverages consist primarily of ethanol, water, and volatile and nonvolatile compounds. Numerous additives are also used in the production of alcoholic beverages, such as hops, synthetic flavor enhancers, preservatives, and trace elements.[107] Certain contaminants with proven mutagenic and carcinogenic properties that interfere with DNA synthesis, repair, and tumor development have been detected in alcoholic beverages, such as N-nitrosamines, asbestos, arsenic compounds, pesticides, and acetaldehyde.[108] Moderate to heavy alcohol use has been linked to cancers of the oral cavity, esophagus, larynx, bladder, rectum, distal colon,[109] and liver.[107] The association of alcohol consumption with cancers of the stomach, proximal colon, and pancreas is less well established. Rectal cancer is the exception, for it appears to be associated specifically with beer consumption.[110] Nitrosamines that are found in beer have been suggested as a possible cause for the association between rectal cancer and beer consumption.[111] Experimental evidence suggests that alcohol interferes with folate absorption, transport, and metabolism, potentially limiting tissue folate stores. Folate deficiency is implicated in carcinogenesis through interference with DNA synthesis.[112] Conflicting results have been published on the relationship of alcohol intake and breast cancer risk being reduced by adequate intake of folate,[113–116] or folate intake having no effect.[112]

Studies focusing on the relationship between alcohol and breast cancer suggest a positive but weak association. Alcohol has been well documented as a risk factor in head and neck cancer and more recently has been implicated in breast cancer,[108,117–123] although this observation remains controversial. A majority of the findings from epidemiological studies have shown a moderately increased breast cancer risk among women who consume moderate to high levels of alcohol.[108,117,118,120,122,124] Both the level of alcohol consumption required to significantly increase breast cancer risk[123] and the age at which exposure to alcohol becomes important[124] are unclear.

## Physical activity

Physical activity may protect against cancer through reduced lifetime exposure to sex steroid hormones, reduced exposure to insulin and insulin-like growth factors, and prevention of overweight and obesity, often referred to as positive energy balance.[125,126] Physical activity is[127,128] one of the few known modifiable factors, and increased exercise plays a key role in primary prevention against prostate cancer,[129,130] colon cancer,[77,131–133] precancerous colon polyps,[134] and breast cancer.[127,135–141] A emerging evidence suggests that increased physical activity is protective against ovarian[142] and kidney cancer.[143–145] There are inconsistent findings on the association between pancreatic[146] and endometrial cancer[147–150] with physical activity. Intense physical activity at the age of usual menarche may be especially important, because it can cause a delay in onset of menarche.[151] Lifetime physical activity has been proven protective against breast cancer in a large case-control study of women from Shanghai, China.[127,135,148] Graded reductions in breast cancer risk were noted in pre- and postmenopausal women who exercised in both adolescence and adulthood. These women who engaged in exercise for 16 years or longer periods reduced their risk of breast cancer by 43% and 64%, respectively.[148] The close interrelationship of physical activity with obesity and diet—two factors associated with many cancers—also makes its role in relation to cancer risk important to assess.[127]

## Occupational exposures

At least 10% of cancer deaths in the United States are attributable to workplace exposures. The reasons to study occupational causes of cancer are numerous.

1. An immense number of individuals spend large amounts of time at their jobs, and a growing repertoire

of chemicals and physical factors are found in diverse workplaces of today.

2. Workers are generally exposed to much higher levels of potentially hazardous chemical and physical factors than individuals who are exposed to similar hazards in nonoccupational settings. This phenomenon of increasing environmental cancer rates in the occupational group should be heeded by the community at large, which is itself potentially at risk.
3. Cancer stemming from occupational exposures should be considered preventable. Evidence from epidemiological research confirming causal cancer agents should prompt the removal of the agents or adequate prevention of potential exposed workers.[152]

**TABLE 3-3**

**Cancers Associated With Various Occupations and Occupational Exposures**

| Cancer Site | Carcinogenic Agent(s) |
|---|---|
| Lung | Arsenic, asbestos, bis(chloromethyl) ether, chromium compounds, coal, gasification, mustard gas, nickel refining, foundry substances, radon, soots, tars, oils, acrylonitrile, beryllium, silica, cadmium, aromatics (benzene and toluene), radon-exposed uranium, haematite and other ore miners, chloromethylmethyl ether, dioxides, creosotes, wood dust, dioxins, polycyclic aromatic hydrocarbons (PAHs), ionizing radiation |
| Bladder | Aluminum production, auramine and magenta manufacture, rubber industry, leather industry, 4-aminobiphenyl, 2-naphylamine, 4,4'-methylenebis 2-choloraniline (MOCA), chlornaphazine, benzidine, naphthylamine, arsenic, solvents, aromatic amines, petrochemicals and combustion products, mineral oils, ionizing radiation, metalworking fluids, cotton and jute spinning, coal tar creosotes |
| Nasal cavity and sinuses | Formaldehyde, isopropyl alcohol manufacture, mustard gas, nickel refining, leather dust, wood dust, chromium, metalworking fluids, mineral oils |
| Larynx | Asbestos, isopropyl alcohol, mustard gas, metalworking fluids, mineral oils, sulphuric acid exposure, rubber working, nickel refining, chemical production |
| Pharynx | Formaldehyde, mustard gas, mineral oils, wood dust, chromium, nickel |
| Mesothelioma | Asbestos, erionite |
| Lymphatic and hematopoietic system | Benzene, ethylene oxide, chlorophenols, chlorophenoxy, herbicides, x-radiation |
| Skin | Arsenic, coal tars, mineral oils, ionizing radiation, PAHs, creosotes, UV/Sun exposure |
| Soft-tissue sarcoma | Cholorophenols, cholorophenoxy, herbicide, arsenic, dioxins, ionizing radiation, vinyl chloride monomer |
| Liver | Arsenic, vinyl chloride, polychlorinated biphenyls (PCBs), ionizing radiation, trichloroethylene (TCE) |
| Brain and central nervous system | Lead, arsenic, mercury, benzene, toluene, xylene, methylene chloride, pesticides, n-nitroso compounds, ionizing radiation |
| Kidney | Arsenic, cadmium, lead, solvent exposure, petroleum products, pesticides, |
| Breast | Ionizing radiation, endocrine disrupters, solvents, polychlorinated biphenyls (PCBs), pesticides, combustion by-products, ethylene oxide |
| Bone | Ionizing radiation |
| Oesophageal | Tetrachloroethylene, metalworking fluids |
| Pancreas | Acrylamide, metalworking fluids, mineral oils |
| Prostate | Cadmium, arsenic, some pesticides, metallic dusts, metalworking fluids, PAHs, liquid fuel combustion products |
| Rectal | Metalworking fluids, mineral oils, toluene, xylene |
| Skin | UV/Sun exposure, metalworking fluids, mineral oils, arsenic, cresosote, PAHs, coal tars, ionizing radiation |
| Stomach | Metalworking fluids, mineral oils, asbestos, solvents, pesticides, gold mining industries |
| Testicle | Phtalates, PCBs, polyhalogenated hydrocarbons |
| Thyroid | Ionizing radiation |

*Source:* Data from Reid[3]; Clapp et al[153]; and International Metalworkers Federation.[154]

A summary of some occupational carcinogens that may cause cancer is found in Table 3-3.[3,153,154]

## POLLUTION

The relationship between drinking contaminated water and cancer has been established in Taiwan, where increased risk of lung cancer has been reported among people exposed to arsenic in drinking water. Trihalomethane, another more common pollutant of drinking water and in recent evidence, found in swimming pools, may be linked to rectal and bladder cancer.[155,156] These compounds are produced by the action of chlorine on organic waste.

Assessing the association of air pollution with cancer in epidemiological studies is more challenging. Specifically, it is complicated to measure past exposure to the relevant air pollution and the level of the exposure. Exposure to air pollution has been evaluated by counting the number of inhabitants in the community of residence near a major pollution source. These data mainly take into account suspended particulates, sulfur oxides, and nitrogen oxides, which are agents not responsible for the carcinogenic effect of air pollution.[11]

One type of pollution that may indirectly increase cancer risk involves chlorofluorocarbons (CFCs), which are destroying the ozone layer in the stratosphere.[157] It is predicted that this destruction will allow more ultraviolet light to reach the earth's surface, thereby increasing the risk for nonmelanoma and melanoma skin cancer. Exposure to ultraviolet-B (UV-B) radiation has been implicated by laboratory and epidemiological studies as a cause of two types of nonmelanoma skin cancers: squamous cell cancer and basal cell cancer. Studies predict that for every 1% increase in UV-B radiation, nonmelanoma skin cancer cases would increase by about 1% to 3% each year during which the condition of the deteriorating ozone exists. Recent epidemiological studies suggest that UV-B radiation plays an important role in causing malignant melanoma skin cancer; for each 1% change in UV-B intensity, the incidence of melanoma could increase from 0.5% to 1%.[158]

## VIRUSES AND OTHER BIOLOGICAL AGENTS

Viruses may contribute to approximately 15% to 20% of human cancers throughout the world.[159] Table 3-4[160] identifies viruses associated with certain cancer sites. Viruses encode proteins that reprogram host cellular signaling pathways that control proliferation, differentiation, cell death, genomic integrity, and recognition by the immune system. Both DNA and RNA viruses have been shown to be capable of causing cancer in humans. Epstein–Barr virus (EBV), human papillomavirus (HPV), hepatitis B virus (HBV), and human herpes virus-8 are the four DNA that are capable of causing the development of human cancer. Human T-lymphotrophic virus type 1 and hepatitis C virus (HCV) are the two RNA viruses that contribute to human cancers.[161] Viruses produce cancer in the host only after a substantial incubation or latency period. This latency period usually extends for years, hindering studies in linking the particular viral exposure with a particular cancer. When the initial infection with the candidate virus is subclinical, verification after clinical features emerge to establish the exact time of infection is compromised.

**TABLE 3-4**

**Cancer Types Associated With a Virus or Other Biological Agents**

| Virus or Biological Agent | Cancer |
|---|---|
| Hepatitis B virus | Hepatocellular carcinoma |
| Human papillomavirus (types 16 and 18) | Cervical cancer |
| Epstein-Barr virus | Burkitt's lymphoma |
| Human T-cell lymphotrophic virus type I | Adult T-cell leukemia/lymphoma |
| Human immunodeficiency virus | Kaposi's sarcoma: non-Hodgkin's lymphoma |
| Schistosoma | Bladder cancer |
| *Heliobacter pylori* | Gastric cancer |

*Source:* Data from the American Cancer Society.[160]

Several epidemiologists and experimental studies have established a casual role of HBV and HCV in the occurrence of hepatocellular carcinoma (HCC).[160,161] Viruses are etiologically linked to approximately 20% of all malignancies worldwide.

The EBV is a ubiquitous virus that has been linked with Burkitt's lymphoma and other B- and T-cell lymphomas, leiomyosarcomas, and nasopharyngeal carcinomas.[159] EBV has also been implicated in the development of Hodgkin's disease.[161]

The human T-cell lymphotropic virus (HTLV-1), which contributes to the development of human T-cell leukemias, is endemic to Japan, South America, Africa, and the Caribbean.[162] This virus is primarily spread from males to females, through transmission in semen, and from mother to child, with breast milk being the likely vector. After a long latent period, adult T-cell leukemia/lymphoma (ATL) occurs in 1 per 1000 carriers per year, resulting in 2500–3000 cases per year worldwide and over half of the adult lymphoid malignancies in endemic areas.[159,161]

Human immunodeficiency virus 1 (HIV-1) accounts for a significant cancer burden. Kaposi's sarcoma (KS) is a very rare tumor except after HIV-1 infection, when its incidence is greatly amplified, being magnified 70,000-fold in HIV-infected homosexual men. Human herpes virus 8 (HHV-8), which is also known as Kaposi's sarcoma-associated virus (KSHV), is an essential cofactor for the development of KS and is also believed to have a role in primary effusion lymphoma.[161] The dramatic decline of KS incidence in recent years is due to the introduction of highly active antiretroviral therapy (HAART). B-cell non-Hodgkin's lymphoma occurs as the first acquired immunodeficiency syndrome-defining diagnosis in 3% to 4% of patients infected with HIV. Hodgkin's lymphoma is also associated with HIV infection, albeit at a lower risk.

Human papillomaviruses are linked to invasive cervical cancer and anogenital cancers among patients infected with HIV. HPVs are DNA viruses that have been causally linked to cancers of the uterine cervix. Subtypes HPV-16, HPV-18, HPV-31, and HPV-45 have been linked to cervical, penile, and anal cancer. HPV DNA is found in 93% of all invasive cervical cancers, with 50% of cases being infected with subtype 16.[161]

Human endogenous retroviruses are sequences within the genome that cause malignancy via direct effects as well as through interactions with other oncogenic herpes viruses and other viruses.[159] In no case in humans, in contrast to animal and cell culture systems, has a viral infection directly produced a malignancy; in humans, cancer is a multistep process.

## RADIATION

### Ionizing radiation

The greatest source of exposure to ionizing radiation is background radiation in the environment. For U.S. residents, ionizing radiation from natural sources accounts for approximately 82% of the total exposure from all sources. Background radiation includes naturally occurring cosmic rays and radiation from ground sources, such as uranium, radon, potassium, and other substances. It is problematic to conduct epidemiological studies of potential cancer risk from naturally occurring background radiation due to the difficulty of measuring an individual's lifetime or cumulative exposure.[163]

From the standpoint of prevention, little more can be done than is already being done: minimizing exposure to man-made radiation hazards. It is notable, however, that stopping smoking has the greatest potential for preventing radiation-induced cancer of the lung, as radon exposure acts synergistically with tobacco smoke. In an Iowa-based study, multiple risk factors were examined with lung cancer risk as part of large-scale residential radon case-control study on women aged 40–84, who were residents in their homes for at least 20 years. Active cigarette smoking was the major risk factor for lung cancer in women exposed to radiation, with a 25-fold greater risk compared to never smokers (OR = 25.98; 95% CI = 17.72–38.09).[164]

In 1987, the International Agency for Research on Cancer designated radon, a radionuclide existing normally as an inert gas, as a human carcinogen. Radon exposure increases the risk of lung cancer among underground miners, and indoor radon exposure is the second leading cause of lung cancer in the United States. In 1999, the EPA released a report on the health effects of indoor radiation, integrating findings from epidemiological studies with evidence from animal experiments and other lines of laboratory investigation. This information led to investigations on the synergistic effect of smoking and radon on lung cancer risk.[165] Approximately 11,000 radon-related lung cancer deaths are estimated to have occurred in never-smokers.

Radiation exposure found in medical treatments and diagnosis largely centers on the use of x-rays or irradiation treatment for various illnesses. The therapeutic radiation dosages given to cancer patients are among the highest levels received by humans. A large body of evidence indicates that organs can develop secondary cancers caused by radiation used in the treatment of a primary cancer. Treatment with ionizing radiation for the prevention of breast cancer is a controversial issue for this reason. In a risk-vs-benefits issue, healthy women are subjected to radiation to diagnose breast cancer at an early stage through mammography, a procedure with known carcinogenic potential. Clearly, the benefits of mammography outweigh the risks, considering the reduced amount of ion radiation to which women are exposed from mammography vs the tremendous improvement in quality-control aspects of screening mammography.

Epidemiological studies of occupational exposures to radiation have been targeting radiologists since the early twentieth century. These niche groups of physicians have higher incidences of lung, pancreas, thyroid, bone, and breast cancers than practitioners in other medical specialties. Occupational exposure to ionizing radiation is highest among underground uranium miners, commercial nuclear power plant workers, fuel fabricators, physicians, flight crews and attendants, industrial radiographers, and well loggers. Other populations of interest include victims of the atomic bombings in Nagasaki and Hiroshima in World War II. The high doses of ionizing radiation contribute to cancers of the lung, breast, colon, ovary, stomach, and thyroid.

### Nonionizing radiation

Nonionizing radiation includes microwaves, radio waves, and extremely low doses of EMF. Early epidemiological studies observed that residential exposure to the weak EMF surrounding power lines was associated with a small elevated risk of childhood cancers. Among all the outcomes evaluated in epidemiological studies of EMF, childhood leukemia in relation to postnatal exposures above 0.4 μT is the one for which there is most evidence of an association. The relative risk has been estimated at 2.0 (95% confidence limit: 1.27–3.13) in a large pooled analysis. However, in this pooled analysis only 0.8% of all children were exposed above 0.4 μT. Further studies need to be designed to test specific hypotheses such as aspects of selection bias or exposure of EMF on childhood cancers.[166]

A recently updated meta-analysis of EMF, leukemia, and brain cancer revealed small increases in brain cancer and leukemia in adults with occupational EMF exposure, but noted an obvious lack in a clear pattern of exposure and risk of leukemia and brain cancer from excess occupational EMF exposure.[167]

Exposure to EMF has been hypothesized to increase the risk of breast cancer by reducing the pineal gland production of melatonin, an oncostatic hormone that may inhibit mammary carcinogenesis. Other possible mechanisms include increased proliferation of breast cancer cells, disruption of signal transduction pathways, or inhibition of cell differentiation.[168] Findings have been conflicting in this relationship with either a slight elevation in occupational exposure to EMF[168] or no association between EMF and increased breast cancer risk.[169,170]

Cell phone usage has increased to include 86.2% of all US households that have at least one cell phone up from 62% in 2002.[171] As cellular telephones are a relatively new technology, no long-term follow-up on their biological effects is possible as yet. However, the lack of ionizing radiation and the low-power frequency EMF level emitted from cell phones and absorbed by human tissues make it unlikely that these devices can cause cancer.[172] Moreover, several well-designed epidemiological studies have failed to find any consistent association between cell phone use and head and neck, brain (glioma or meningioma), or testicular cancers, from placement of the phone in the trousers pocket.[173–178] It is impossible to prove that any product or exposure is absolutely safe, especially in the absence of very long-term follow-up.

### Ultraviolet radiation

Ultraviolet-A (UV-A) radiation from sunlight can suppress cellular immunity, and the suppression of immunity has been postulated as the factor for tumor growth. UV-A is the major cause of nonmelanoma skin cancer, with cumulative exposure and number of life-time sunburns being predictive of risk. Incidence of melanoma, the most insidious form of skin cancer, is increasing worldwide more rapidly than incidence of any other cancer; mortality rates are also increasing by about 2% per year for this form of skin cancer.

Conversely, sunlight has been shown to protect against cancer development. Several lines of experimental evidence are consistent with a protective influence for vitamin D in cancer. Epidemiological studies of prostate, breast, and colon cancers suggest an inverse relationship between sunlight exposure and the incidence and mortality rates for these diseases. Sunlight activation of vitamin D has been shown to retard the growth of colon and breast cancer cells.[179]

Exposure of the skin to sunlight, especially the high-energy UVBlue (UVB) photons results in photoconversion of the cutaneous stores of a cholesterol metabolite in the skin (7-dehydrocholesterol) to provitamin D, which is then converted through a series of oxidations in the liver and kidney to its biologically active form, 1,25-dihydroxyvitamin D3 ($1,25(OH)_2D$; calcitriol) and the principal ligand of the VDR.[180,181] Vitamin D is also known to be a potent antiproliferative factor, which induces differentiation and apoptosis in cells and tissues that possess the VDR. $1,25(OH)2D_3$ may also function in apoptosis, and in the inhibition of tumor invasion and metastasis by several possible mechanisms.

Ultraviolet exposure studies showed that adults with increased melanization in the skin may be at risk for vitamin D deficiency, defined as levels ≤15 ng/mL[182] because deeply pigmented skin blocks cutaneous synthesis of vitamin D.[183] Individuals with darker skin need 10–50 times exposure to the sun vs fair skinned whites to produce the same amount of vitamin D. Individuals who do not exposure their skin to the sun and consistently wear protective clothing and sunscreen also will eliminate the cutaneous generation of vitamin D3.[183] Casual direct exposure of the skin to sunlight can generally provide sufficient vitamin D in the summer months. However, vitamin D photosynthesis is attenuated at higher latitudes, especially in winter months when little synthesis can occur through skin exposure throughout much of the United States.[181] The majority of the human requirement for vitamin D is available from adequate sun exposure. Unlike the zero tolerance given to tobacco products, it would be remiss to promulgate public health messages to completely avoid sunlight to people who have suffered little or no skin damage from UV-A/UV-B.[184]

## DRUGS

Despite the vast array of chemicals discovered to cause cancer in animals, few chemicals (other than tobacco) exist for which there is strong evidence of causation of the common cancers in humans. Medications associated with malignancies include analgesics, cyclophosphamide, and barbiturates, which have been associated with an increased risk (or, in the case of barbiturates, decreased risk) of bladder cancer. Analgesics such as phenacetin have been linked to tumors of the renal pelvis, ureter, and urinary bladder.[185] Cyclophosphamide, an immunosuppressive drug used for the treatment of non-Hodgkin's lymphoma, is prescribed to 500,000 patients annually worldwide. High relative risks have been linked to alkylating chemotherapies like cyclophosphamide specifically, which has been shown to be leukemogenic when used to treat Hodgkin's disease and other malignancies.[186] Barbiturates, such as phenobarbital, have been shown to interact negatively with smoking in bladder cancer risk.[185]

### Nonsteroidal anti-inflammatory drugs

Nonsteroidal anti-inflammatory drugs (NSAIDs) are among the most frequently used drugs in the United States. Each year, about 111 million prescriptions for NSAIDs are filled in the United States and millions of dollars are spent on over-the-counter NSAIDs.[187] NSAIDs were first introduced in 1949 for their anti-inflammatory properties in the treatment of arthritis. The term "NSAIDs" applies to all "aspirin-like" drugs that are used clinically as antipyretics, analgesics, and anti-inflammatory agents. The drugs inhibit enzymes of the cyclooxygenase (COX) family and, in doing so, prevent the production of certain eicosanoids (a large family of intracellular signaling molecules) in response to inflammatory or mitogenic stimuli.[188]

The antitumor effects of NSAIDs have been extensively studied in the past 25 years. Numerous observational and case-control studies reported since 1989 indicate that regular NSAID use is associated with a reduced risk of colorectal adenomas, cancer, and cancer mortality[189–191] Antitumor effects have been associated with NSAID-mediated inhibition of COX activity. In particular, these drugs are linked to upregulation of COX-2, an enzyme associated with tissue regulation of inflammation. COX-2 is found wherever inflammation is present; it is markedly upregulated in major epithelial cancers, including colon, esophagus, lung, breast, and prostate cancer. COX-2 may be a key component of epithelial tumorigenesis and its suppression of NSAIDs.[192,193]

Long-term use of selected NSAIDs like rofecoxib was associated with cardiovascular side effects. In 2004, Merck withdrew rofecoxib from the worldwide market because of increased cardiovascular toxicity observed in a trial designed to test the efficacy of roecoxib to prevent recurrence of colonic polyps.[194]

Observational evidence collected as part of epidemiological studies indicates that regular use of nonspecific COX-inhibiting drugs, such as celecoxib, a commonly used COX-2 inhibitor, discourages polyp and tumor growth.[195] Thought-provoking data recently emerged from a phase II study for advanced breast cancer patients on adding the COX-2 inhibitor celecoxib to a capecitabine chemotherapy regime.[196] The results revealed significantly better outcomes for those breast cancer patients whose tumors overexpressed COX-2. This data prompt the oncology community to reevaluate the prognostic and predictive potential of COX-2 expression in different cancers and the potential of COX-2 inhibition in combination with chemotherapy as a potentially effective and relatively inexpensive therapeutic strategy for appropriately selected patients.[197]

## Exogenous hormones

Combined oral contraceptives (OCs) and postmenopausal hormones are the most vital source of exogenous estrogens for women today. In the past, synthetic hormones such as diethylstilbestrol (DES) were widely prescribed for the prevention of miscarriage and to suppress lactation. Epidemiological studies of the risk of breast cancer in mothers exposed to DES during their reproductive and pregnancy years suggest a modest 20% to 50% increased risk among the exposed women, with a latency period of about 15 to 20 years.

More than 50 epidemiological studies have evaluated the relationship between OC use and breast cancer risk. Combined OCs contain ethyl estradiol and a progestin. The role of contraceptives in breast cancer risk is controversial and not clearly established, with studies showing no relationship,[198–200] a significant increase in breast cancer risk with long duration of use,[200–202] or an increased risk in breast cancer survivors.[203] The risk associated with OC use among current users was found to persist for 10 years after discontinuation, yet no risk was associated with duration of use, age at first use, or dose and formulation. The study results suggest that the pattern of risk seems incompatible with a genotoxic effect, and that OC use may act as a late-stage promoter of preexisting tumors. Case-control studies have consistently demonstrated that the use of such contraceptives reduces the risk of endometrial cancer by 50% and the risk of ovarian cancer by 40%.

The association between HRT and breast cancer is an issue of great public health importance, given the increasing size of the older female population. The composition of hormones in HRT has been classified as estrogen-only therapy, estrogen–progesterone therapy, progesterone-only therapy, estrogen–testosterone therapy, and testosterone only therapy. Data on the effect of HRT on the risk of breast cancer are inconclusive. Some risk may be associated with current or long-term HRT among women who receive it for 5 to 10 years or longer.[204,205] An elevation in risk for invasive breast cancer has been shown for women using estrogen and testosterone therapies. Estrogen and testosterone therapies could increase the risk of breast cancer indirectly through the conversion of androgens to estrogens or more directly with the effects mediated through the androgen receptor.[204] Use of estradiol administered orally (1.9 mg/d) or transdermally was associated with an appreciable risk of breast cancer after 5 years of use in a group of postmenopausal Finnish women.[206] Similar results have been found with the Million Women Study, where a 30% risk of breast cancer was found with the use of an estrogen-only regime.[207] One factor to consider in these studies is detection bias. Current users of hormones must see a physician to review prescriptions and, therefore, are more likely to be screened for breast cancer.

Tamoxifen is a nonsteroidal antiestrogen medication that has been used successfully for 15 years in the treatment of breast cancer. Because tamoxifen acts by binding to estrogen receptor sites, it has been most effective in treating postmenopausal women, who are more likely to have cancers containing estrogen receptors. In contrast to its antiestrogenic tumor-suppressor action in the case of breast cancer, this drug has been associated with the development of endometrial carcinoma.[208] The trade-off between the effective use of tamoxifen in breast cancer prevention and the higher risk of endometrial cancer leads to a recommendation for routine screening for the latter cancer in tamoxifen users.

## BIOMARKERS

As many as 80% of cancer cases are theoretically preventable because the controlling causative factors are exogenous rather than inborn or inherent. We can estimate that, in the absence of external carcinogenic exposures resulting from lifestyle, occupation, and the ambient environment, 400,000 of the annual 500,000 cancer-related deaths in the United States could be averted. More effective methods are needed to identify groups and individuals at greatest risk of cancer at a stage where intervention is possible.

The field of molecular epidemiology offers a potentially powerful tool in cancer prevention by combining biomarkers, measurement of carcinogenic dose, biological response, and susceptibility with epidemiological methods. Biomarkers offer a strategy to assess precursors of disease and identify biological markers of exposure. Traditional epidemiological tools such as questionnaires and medical records are important for measuring the external dose of a particular environmental exposure. Because these epidemiological measures rely on human recall, however, a certain amount of misclassification can be expected to occur. The magnitude and direction of the misclassification can vary from exposure to exposure. Biological measurements may be helpful in determining the accuracy of epidemiological exposure measurements and overcome the potential recall bias inherent in the use of questionnaires on diet, alcohol intake, and smoking status.[209,210]

The term *biomarker* is used to describe the application of chemical, physical, radiological, and immunobiological tests to human biological samples, such as blood, urine, and tissue. The expectation of using biomarkers in cancer epidemiology studies is that biomarkers would improve exposure assessment, document early changes preceding disease, and identify subgroups in the population with greater susceptibility to cancer, allowing investigators to identify causes and elucidate mechanisms in carcinogenesis.[211] Table 3-5 provides examples of biomarkers that measure internal dose. In biomarkers of internal dose, the investigator examines the extent to which the biomarker correlates with the epidemiological measure. The accuracy of the epidemiological exposure data can be assessed by measuring body burden levels of the actual compound or one of its stable metabolites in human tissue.[25] Examples of biomarkers include plasma or salivary cotine from cigarette smoke, urinary aflatoxin indicative of dietary exposure, and N-nitroso compounds in urine from dietary sources and cigarette smoke.[212]

**TABLE 3-5**

**Examples of Biomarkers of Internal Dose**

| Biomarker | Source of Exposure | Biological Sample |
|---|---|---|
| Aflatoxin | Contaminated food | Urine |
| Bacterial mutations | Cigarette smoke | Cervical fluids |
| Benezene, toluene | Cigarette smoke | Urine, breath concentration |
| CFA | Occupational exposure | Urine |
| Cotine | Cigarette smoke | Serum, urine, saliva |
| DNA sequences | HPV | Cervicovaginal lavage |
| Fatty acids | Diet | Subcutaneous adipose tissue, serum lipids |
| HDL, alkaline phosphatase | Alcohol | Serum |
| Mutagens | Cigarette smoke | Bone, soft tissues |
| Nitrosamino acids, NNK, NNN | N-nistroso compounds, diet, tobacco | Urine |
| Potassium | Diet | Urine |
| Selenium | Diet | Hair, toenails |
| Vitamin level | Diet | Serum |

*Abbreviations*: CFA, 3-cholro-4-fluoroaniline; HPV, human papillomavirus; HDL, high-density lipoprotein; NNK, 4-(methylnitrosamino)-1-(3-pyridyl)-1-butanone; NNN, N′-nitrosonornicotine.

*Source*: Data from Nasca[25]; Bingham[209]; and Arab and Akbar.[210]

## HOST CHARACTERISTICS INFLUENCING CANCER SUSCEPTIBILITY

### AGE

Age is a major risk factor for many health outcomes and is frequently associated with numerous exposures. Even if the effect of age is not among the primary objectives of the study, it is important to assess its relationship with exposures and outcomes, given its potentially confounding effects. As shown in Table 3-6, new cervical cancers remain high in women aged 40–59, whereas the highest distribution of new prostate cancer cases occurs in the 70 and older.[213] Because age is such an important determinant of cancer risk, it is critical in epidemiological studies to make adjustments for age in the statistical analysis, unless comparison groups have the same age distribution.

### SEX

The distributions of new cancer cases and estimated number of cancer deaths in each sex are shown in Figure 3-5. The greatest number of cancer deaths predicted for males and females in 2009 were expected from lung cancer (30% estimated deaths and 26% of estimated deaths, respectively). The leading site of new cancer cases in men is prostate cancer, followed by lung and bronchus and colorectal cancers. The leading site of new cancer cases in women is the breast, followed by lung and bronchus and colorectal cancers.[214]

**TABLE 3-5**

**Probability of Developing Invasive Cancers (%) Over Selected Age Intervals by Sex, US, 2003–2005***

| | | Birth to 39 | 40 to 59 | 60 to 69 | 70 and Older | Birth to Death |
|---|---|---|---|---|---|---|
| All sites† | Male | 1.42 (1 in 70) | 8.44(1 in 12) | 15.71 (1 in 6) | 37.74 (1 in 3) | 43.89 (1 in 2) |
| | Female | 2.07 (1 in 48) | 8.97 (1 in 11) | 10.23 (1 in 10) | 26.17 (1 in 4) | 37.35 (1 in 3) |
| Urinary bladder‡ | Male | 0.02 (1 in 4,448) | 0.41 (1 in 246) | 0.96 (1 in 104) | 3.57 (1 in 28) | 3.74 (1 in 27) |
| | Female | 0.01 (1 in 10,185) | 0.12 (1 in 810) | 0.26 (1 in 378) | 1.01 (1 in 99) | 1.18 (1 in 84) |
| Breast | Female | 0.48 (1 in 208) | 3.79 (1 in 26) | 3.41 (1 in 29) | 6.44 (1 in 16) | 12.03 (1 in 8) |
| Colon and rectum | Male | 0.08 (1 in 1,296) | 0.92 (1 in 109) | 1.55 (1 in 65) | 4.63 (1 in 22) | 5.51 (1 in 18) |
| | Female | 0.07 (1 in 1,343) | 0.72 (1 in 138) | 1.10 (1 in 91) | 4.16 (1 in 24) | 5.10 (1 in 20) |
| Leukemia | Male | 0.16 (1 in 611) | 0.22 (1 in 463) | 0.35 (1 in 289) | 1.17 (1 in 85) | 1.50 (1 in 67) |
| | Female | 0.12 (1 in 835) | 0.14 (1 in 693) | 0.20 (1 in 496) | 0.77 (1 in 130) | 1.07 (1 in 94) |
| Lung and bronchus | Male | 0.03 (1 in 3,398) | 0.99 (1 in 101) | 2.43 (1 in 41) | 6.70 (1 in 18) | 7.78 (1 in 13) |
| | Female | 0.03 (1 in 2,997) | 0.81 (1 in 124) | 1.78 (1 in 56) | 4.70 (1 in 21) | 6.22 (1 in 16) |
| Melanoma of the skin§ | Male | 0.16 (1 in 645) | 0.64 (1 in 157) | 0.70 (1 in 143) | 1.67 (1 in 60) | 2.56 (1 in 39) |
| | Female | 0.27 (1 in 370) | 0.53 (1 in 189) | 0.35 (1 in 282) | 0.76 (1 in 131) | 1.73 (1 in 58) |
| Non-Hodgkin lymphoma | Male | 0.13 (1 in 763) | 0.45 (1 in 225) | 0.58 (1 in 171) | 1.66 (1 in 60) | 2.23 (1 in 45) |
| | Female | 0.08 (1 in 1,191) | 0.32 (1 in 316) | 0.45 (1 in 223) | 1.36 (1 in 73) | 1.90 (1 in 53) |
| Prostate | Male | 0.01 (1 in 10,002) | 2.43 (1 in 41) | 6.42 (1 in 16) | 12.49 (1 in 8) | 15.78 (1 in 6) |
| Uterine cervix | Female | 0.15 (1 in 651) | 0.27 (1 in 368) | 0.13 (1 in 761) | 0.19 (1 in 530) | 0.69 (1 in 145) |
| Uterine corpus | Female | 0.07 (1 in 1,499) | 0.72 (1 in 140) | 0.81 (1 in 123) | 1.22 (1 in 82) | 2.48 (1 in 40) |

*For people free of cancer at begining of age interval.
†All sites excludes basal and squamous cell skin cancers and in situ cancers except urinary bladder.
‡Include invasive and insitu cancer cases.
§Statistic is for whites only.
American Cancer Society Surveillance and Health Policy Research, 2009
*Source*: Data from DevCan.[213]

## GENETIC PREDISPOSITION

Genetic epidemiology in cancer research is used to identify inherent susceptibility factors for primary, secondary, and tertiary prevention of cancer. The cumulative body of evidence indicates that genetic factors contribute to the development of most cancer cases, including those without a clear familial aggregation. Epidemiological studies of genetics in cancer etiology have been either family studies or genetic biomarker studies. Family studies can provide general information on the role and/or inheritance patterns of genetic factors in the etiology of cancer. Biomarker studies can target specific genetic factors suspected to be responsible for the pathology of cancer. Epidemiological investigation of genetic predisposition to cancer is increasing thanks to developments in molecular biology, which have made it possible to study genetic markers in large populations.[215] The Human Genome Project was spearheaded by the National Institutes of Health and the Department of Energy to sequence all 3 billion letters, or base pairs, in the human genome, which is the complete set of DNA in the human body. The human Genome Project's goal was to provide researchers with powerful tools to understand the genetic factors in human disease, paving the way for new strategies for their diagnosis, treatment, and prevention. The Human Genome Project was completed in 2003 and has an ambitious new initiative, the Cancer Genome Atlas, which aims to identify all the genetic abnormalities seen in 50 major types of cancer.[216]

## ETHNICITY AND RACE

The U.S. Bureau of the Census classifies race into categories such as white, African American, Asian or Pacific Islander, Mexican American, and Native American. Race is often similar to ethnicity, in that people who come from a particular racial stock may share a common ethnic identification. Caution should be used when trying to classify individuals with mixed racial parentage into a racial group

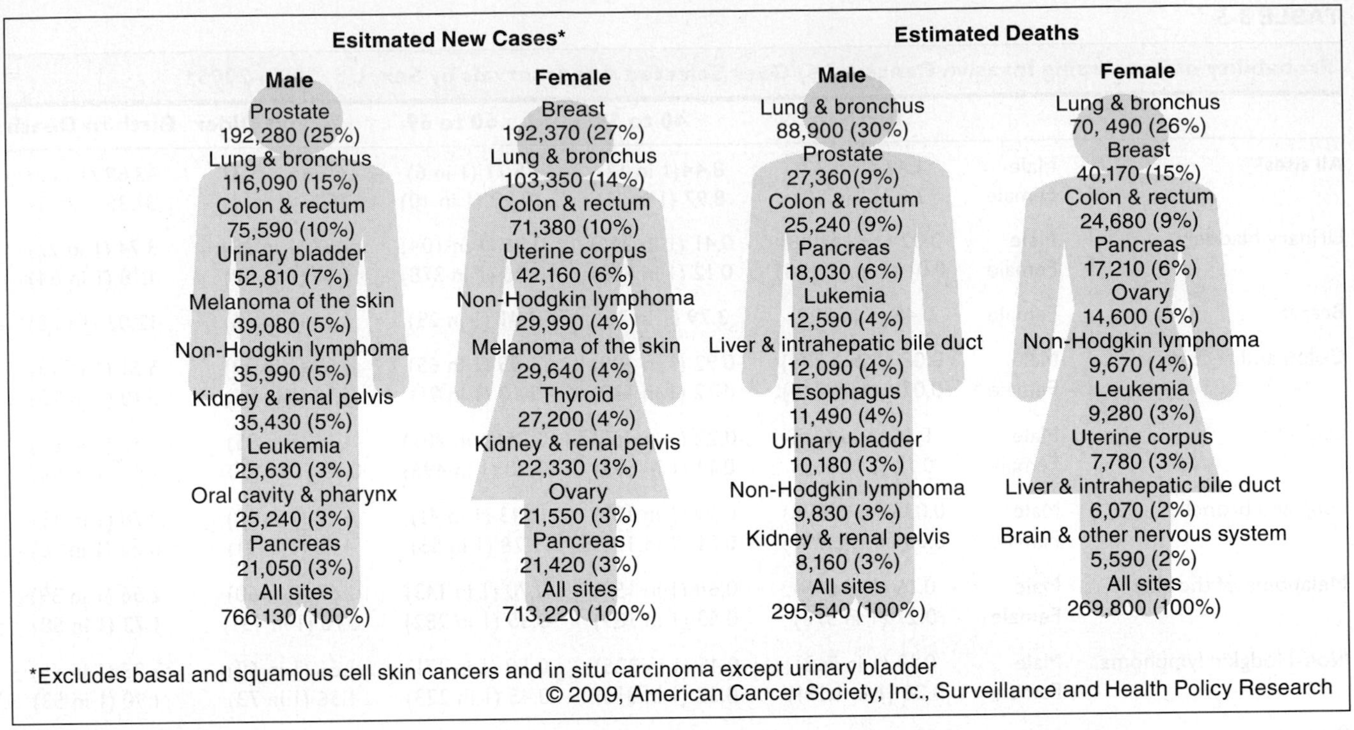

Esitmated New Cases*
Estimated Deaths
Male
Prostate
192,280 (25%)
Lung & bronchus
116,090 (15%)
Colon & rectum
75,590 (10%)
Urinary bladder
52,810 (7%)
Melanoma of the skin
39,080 (5%)
Non-Hodgkin lymphoma
35,990 (5%)
Kidney & renal pelvis
35,430 (5%)
Leukemia
25,630 (3%)
Oral cavity & pharynx
25,240 (3%)
Pancreas
21,050 (3%)
All sites
766,130 (100%)
Female
Breast
192,370 (27%)
Lung & bronchus
103,350 (14%)
Colon & rectum
71,380 (10%)
Uterine corpus
42,160 (6%)
Non-Hodgkin lymphoma
29,990 (4%)
Melanoma of the skin
29,640 (4%)
Thyroid
27,200 (4%)
Kidney & renal pelvis
22,330 (3%)
Ovary
21,550 (3%)
Pancreas
21,420 (3%)
All sites
713,220 (100%)
Male
Lung & bronchus
88,900 (30%)
Prostate
27,360(9%)
Colon & rectum
25,240 (9%)
Pancreas
18,030 (6%)
Lukemia
12,590 (4%)
Liver & intrahepatic bile duct
12,090 (4%)
Esophagus
11,490 (4%)
Urinary bladder
10,180 (3%)
Non-Hodgkin lymphoma
9,830 (3%)
Kidney & renal pelvis
8,160 (3%)
All sites
295,540 (100%)
Female
Lung & bronchus
70, 490 (26%)
Breast
40,170 (15%)
Colon & rectum
24,680 (9%)
Pancreas
17,210 (6%)
Ovary
14,600 (5%)
Non-Hodgkin lymphoma
9,670 (4%)
Leukemia
9,280 (3%)
Uterine corpus
7,780 (3%)
Liver & intrahepatic bile duct
6,070 (2%)
Brain & other nervous system
5,590 (2%)
All sites
269,800 (100%)
*Excludes basal and squamous cell skin cancers and in situ carcinoma except urinary bladder
© 2009, American Cancer Society, Inc., Surveillance and Health Policy Research


**FIGURE 3-5**

Leading sites of new cancer cases and deaths—2009 estimates.
*Source*: Data from American Cancer Society.[214]

with which they identify. Race does have implications for differences in incidence and prevalence of disease. Racial or ethnic groups may differ in their attitudes toward illness, care seeking, and prevention.

An illustration of the variation of race in cancer incidence and mortality from the Surveillance, Epidemiology, and End Results (SEER) data appears in Figure 3-7. The data on prostate cancer, which can be detected by physical exam and a prostate antigen test (PSA), reveal how cancer mortality adversely affects African Americans. Approximately 62 prostate cancer deaths per 100,000 occurred in African American males compared to approximately 25 prostate cancer deaths per 100,000 in white males.[217]

## SOCIOECONOMIC FACTORS

Socioeconomic status is determined by income, education, occupation, or percentage below the poverty level. Lower SES is related to excess mortality, morbidity, and disability rates. Higher-poverty areas are characterized by later-stage diagnosis, poorer survival, and higher mortality rates. A substantial decline in mortality over time occurs in all socioeconomic groups, but a considerable gradient is still evident where the lower-SES group has worse outcomes. Racial and ethnic disparities in cancer mortality stratified by SES has been examined by the National Cancer Institute (NCI) SEER program databases from 1990 to 2000.[218] Socioeconomic status was represented by three levels of poverty: <10% of the population in the county living below the poverty level, counties with 10% to <20% living below the poverty level, and counties with >20% living below the poverty level.[218,219] The results show that African Americans have greater disparities in cancer mortality relative to whites for each cancer site examined except for female lung cancer. The highest SES groups for both blacks and whites had declining trends in cancer mortality and the lowest SES groups had the increasing trends at each cancer site, except for female lung cancer. Other racial/ethnic groups, such as American Indian/Alaskan Natives (AI/AN) had increasing trends of cancer mortality in prostate, colorectal, lung, breast, and cervical cancer in the middle SES group (10% to <20% living below the poverty level). The dominant pattern of cancer mortality for Asians and Pacific Islanders (Asian/PIs) was the highest—SES group had the worse morality trends in all sites of male cancers, lung cancer and breast cancer. The lowest-SES groups of Asian/PIs had declining trends in prostate cancer, female colorectal cancer, and lung cancer. For Hispanics, the dominant patterns were that the middle-SES group had the best trends in all male cancers and lung cancers and female colorectal cancer and lung cancer. The patterns of cancer mortality and SES for AIs/ANs, Hispanics, and Asian/PIs indicate that mortality trends are affected by more than SES

**FIGURE 3-7**

**Cancer Incidence and Mortality Rates* by Site, Race, and Ethnicity, US, 2001–2005**

| Incidence | White | African American | Asian American and Pacific Islander | American Indian and Alaska Native† | Hispanic/Latino‡§ |
|---|---|---|---|---|---|
| All sites | | | | | |
| Male | 551.4 | 651.5 | 354.0 | 336.6 | 419.4 |
| Female | 423.6 | 398.9 | 287.8 | 296.4 | 317.8 |
| Breast (female) | 130.6 | 117.5 | 89.6 | 75.0 | 90.1 |
| Colon and rectum | | | | | |
| Male | 58.9 | 71.2 | 48.0 | 46.0 | 47.3 |
| Female | 43.2 | 54.5 | 35.4 | 41.2 | 32.8 |
| Kidney and renal pelvis | | | | | |
| Male | 18.8 | 21.3 | 9.1 | 19.5 | 17.4 |
| Female | 9.5 | 10.1 | 4.6 | 12.7 | 9.6 |
| Liver and bile duct | | | | | |
| Male | 8.2 | 13.2 | 21.7 | 14.4 | 15.0 |
| Female | 2.9 | 4.0 | 8.3 | 6.3 | 5.8 |
| Lung and bronchus | | | | | |
| Male | 79.3 | 107.6 | 53.9 | 54.3 | 44.2 |
| Female | 54.9 | 54.6 | 28.0 | 39.7 | 25.4 |
| Prostate | 156.7 | 248.5 | 93.8 | 73.3 | 138.0 |
| Stomach | | | | | |
| Male | 10.0 | 17.4 | 18.6 | 16.8 | 15.5 |
| Female | 4.7 | 8.9 | 10.5 | 7.7 | 9.5 |
| Uterine cervix | 8.2 | 10.8 | 8.0 | 6.9 | 13.2 |

| Mortality | White | African American | Asian American and Pacific Islander | American Indian and Alaska Native† | Hispanic/Latino‡§ |
|---|---|---|---|---|---|
| All sites | | | | | |
| Male | 230.7 | 313.0 | 138.8 | 190.0 | 159.0 |
| Female | 159.2 | 186.7 | 95.9 | 142.0 | 105.2 |
| Breast (female) | 24.4 | 33.5 | 12.6 | 17.1 | 15.8 |
| Colon and rectum | | | | | |
| Male | 22.1 | 31.8 | 14.4 | 20.5 | 16.5 |
| Female | 15.3 | 22.4 | 10.2 | 14.2 | 10.8 |
| Kidney and renal pelvis | | | | | |
| Male | 6.2 | 6.1 | 2.4 | 9.3 | 5.3 |
| Female | 2.8 | 2.7 | 1.2 | 4.3 | 2.4 |
| Liver and bile duct | | | | | |
| Male | 6.7 | 10.3 | 15.2 | 10.6 | 11.1 |
| Female | 2.9 | 3.9 | 6.6 | 6.6 | 5.1 |
| Lung and bronchus | | | | | |
| Male | 71.3 | 93.1 | 37.5 | 50.2 | 35.1 |
| Female | 42.0 | 39.9 | 18.5 | 33.8 | 14.6 |
| Prostate | 24.6 | 59.4 | 11.0 | 21.1 | 20.6 |
| Stomach | | | | | |
| Male | 5.0 | 11.5 | 10.1 | 9.9 | 8.7 |
| Female | 2.5 | 5.5 | 5.9 | 5.2 | 4.9 |
| Uterine cervix | 2.3 | 4.7 | 2.2 | 3.7 | 3.2 |

*Per 100,000, age adjusted to the 2000 US standard population. †Data based on Contract Health Service Delivery Areas (CHSDA), 624 counties comprising 54% of the US American Indian/Alaska Native population. ‡Persons of Hispanic/Latino origin may be of any race. §Data unavailable from the Alaska Native Registry and Kentucky. ¶Data unavailable from Minnesota, New Hampshire, and North Dakota.
American Cancer Society Surveillance and Health Policy Research, 2009

*Source*: Data from American Cancer Society,[214] and Ries LAG, Melbert D, Krapcho M, et al.[217]

factors. Culture in its many manifestations, such as access to health care on tribal reservations, acculturation to American lifestyles and diet, and cancer literacy, need to be considered in understanding the patterns seen by SES group.[218,219]

## REPRODUCTIVE HISTORY

Factors related to reproduction and sexual behaviors have been identified only for cancers in women. Earlier menarcheal age, later menopausal age, parity status, years of breast-feeding, and later age at first-live birth have been associated with breast, endometrial, and ovarian cancers.[220–225]

Cervical cancer has a very different pattern, with multiple sexual partners being identified as a major risk factor. The number of sexual partners is a measure of the likelihood that an individual has been exposed to HPV, which has been implicated as a cause of cervical dysplasia.[9,226,227]

## PSYCHONEUROIMMUNOLOGY AND CANCER RISK

### NOCTURNAL LIGHT EXPOSURE

One of the defining features of the modern work world is artificial lighting. Before industrialization and the need for electric light to push the work days longer, humans conducted their daily activities according to the sun's cycle; rising at sunrise and going to bed at sunset. These sleep rhythms were dictated by an individual's circadian rhythms following light exposure. These sleep rhythms appear more natural but essential for regulating a variety of physiological behaviors[228] in humans such as body temperature, excretion, and the production of hormones.[229] Melatonin, for example, is called the hormone of darkness, regulated via visible light exposure through the retina and secreted by the pineal gland at night when it is dark.[230] Environmental lighting powerfully alters release of melatonin, which typically peaks in the middle of the night.[231]

The benefits of electricity are obvious, although the benefit of artificial light may not be completely innocuous when exposure is inappropriately timed. Exposure to light at night in the form of occupational exposure during night shift work and as a personal choice and lifestyle is experienced by numerous night-active members of our societies.[228] Light at night, regardless of duration or intensity, inhibits melatonin secretion and phase-shifts the circadian clock, possibly altering the cell growth rate that is regulated by the circadian rhythm. Since the early 1980s evidence from experimental studies suggests a link between melatonin and tumor suppression. Reports show that melatonin is oncostatic in a variety of tumor cells. Physiological and pharmacological blood concentrations of melatonin have been shown to inhibit tumorigenesis in a variety of in vivo and in vitro experimental models of neoplasia. Several clinical studies confirm the potential of melatonin, alone or in combination with standard treatment regimes to generate more favorable response in the treatment of human cancers.[232–234]

Melatonin is a naturally produced cytotoxin, which can induce tumor cell death (apoptosis). Melatonin has been shown to inhibit the tumor's growth rate and inhibit the development of new tumor blood vessels (tumor angiogenesis), which in turn inhibits the cancer from spreading further (metastasis).[234] Melatonin is a weak preventive antioxidant which hinders tumor cells from participating in free radical damage to normal cells and consequently limits oxidative damage to DNA lipids, amino acids, and proteins. Disruption of circadian rhythm is commonly observed among cancer patients and contributes to cancer development and tumor progression. Lower levels of melatonin have been shown in advanced gastrointestinal malignancies, such as colorectal, gastric, and pancreatic cancer.[235]

The evidence from observational studies investigating the effect of occupational light exposure at night and the risk of breast cancer has been expanding in the past decade.[236] The mechanistic framework of nocturnal light exposure and breast cancer risk was refined in the classic research study by Steven and Davis[237] who purported that decreased melatonin production due to exposure to light at night led to a rise in the levels of reproductive hormones such as estrogens, thereby inducing hormone-sensitive tumors in the breast.[234,238]

Observational studies have reported on otherwise healthy women who are chronically subjected to nighttime shift work, a surrogate measure for light exposure at night and breast cancer risk. Findings have been mixed, showing meaningful increased breast cancer risk among postmenopausal women exposed to shift work.[239–242] One retrospective study of flight attendants with occupational exposure to light at night linked the employment time to an increased risk of breast cancer.[241] Nationwide record linkage studies[240,241] and one case-control study reported mixed evidence for the light-at-night hypothesis with no association between breast cancer and overall shift work (OR = 1.04; 95% CI = 0.79–1.38) or evening shift work (OR = 1.08; 95% CI = 0.81–1.44). Yet, women who had residential light-at-night exposure during sleeping hours greater than twice a week and twice/night had a 63% increased risk (OR = 1.65; 95% CI = 1.02–2.69).[242] One prospective study, The Nurses' Health Study, observed a positive association of extended periods of rotating night work and breast cancer risk for postmenopausal women with more than 30 years of rotating night work: (relative risk [RR] = 1.36; 95% CI = 1.04–1.78).[243]

There is a growing body of literature from case-control and cohort studies on subpopulations that experience increased levels of melatonin exposure on the risk of breast cancer. Higher melatonin levels have been found in blind and visually impaired people,[244–246] along with correspondingly lower incidences of cancer compared to those with normal vision, thus suggesting a role for melatonin in the reduction of cancer incidence.[246,247]

Currently, the strongest and most consistent evidence is that women with an occupational history of night shift work are at highest risk. This has resulted in a classification of shift work as a 2A probable human carcinogen by IARC.[248] There is limited but consistent evidence in support of the hypothesis that altered lighting can play a role in breast cancer causation[240,249–252] and emerging interest in light at night to other conditions such as prostate,[251] endometrial,[253] and colorectal cancer.[254]

Given the state of science, epidemiological studies are needed to determine the biological mechanisms connecting disruption of circadian rhythms, melatonin suppression, and cancer etiology. Melatonin's oncostatic properties in in vitro and in vivo models allow melatonin to be studied as a potential mediator in disease development[255,256] or through the administration of synthetic melatonin as an adjuvant therapy.[257] The long-term goal is to elicit information on melatonin mechanisms and consequences of circadian disruption from exposure to light at night for reducing health risks for night shift work which a large and increasing stratum of the population is employed.

## BIOBEHAVIORAL FACTORS AND STRESS

Epidemiological data on psychological and social characteristics may be related to cancer onset, progress, and mortality. A 2.0-fold to 9.0-fold risk of breast cancer has been found in women who experience divorce or separation from a spouse[258] to feelings of combined stress and low social support.[259] Psychoneuroimmunology evidence reconceptualizes cancer as a biological event that triggers stress responses affecting how the disease progresses. Biobehavioral factors (considered neurohormonal and neurotransmitter changes) influence multiple aspects of tumorigenesis through impact on neuroendocrine function and support a favorable physiological environment for tumor establishment and growth. Chronic perturbations such as repeated life stressors as shown in Figure 3-8 to neuroendocrine dynamics alter physiological processes in tumor pathogenesis. Response to stressors involves the central nervous system (CNS) activation of the autonomic nervous system (ANS), the hypothalamic–pituitary–adrenal (HPA) axis, and the sympathetic–adrenal–medullary (SAM) axis.[260] The production of adrenocorticotropic hormone (ACTH) by the anterior lobe of the pituitary gland results in the production of glucocorticoid hormones, such as cortisol and catecholamines (norepinephrine and epinephrine), releasing a flight or fight reaction in the ANS or defeat/withdrawal responses through activation of the HPA. These stress hormones released from the adrenal gland, brain, and sympathetic nervous system (SNS) modulate the tumor microenvironment causing promotion of tumor-cell growth, migration, angiogenesis, and invasive capacity.

Data from patients with existing tumors show cancer treatment and diagnosis cause substantial distress and has patients resorting to depressive coping methods such as hopelessness and helplessness, resulting in accelerated disease progression[261]; in contrast to cancer patient's ideation of social support-optimism as predicting longer survival.[262] Chronodisruption of circadian rhythms, such stress-related interruptions to the sleep–wake cycle, have been shown to influence the production of stress-associated hormones. Stress can disrupt circadian glucocorticoid rhythms and favor tumor initiation and progression.[260]

Animal models have provided compelling evidence regarding the effects of behavioral stress on tumorigenesis and the biological mechanisms involved. Sood et al. illustrated that when mice injected with ovarian cell lines were put under stress and exposed to catecholamines, angiogenesis was triggered, causing cellular proliferation and metastasis.[263] Further experiments were recapitulated to identify a new molecular target for halting tumor progression, which was identified as β-adrenergical receptors on the tumor cell surface.

Pharmacological interventions can potentially be used on novel targets for mitigating stress-associated influences on cancer development and progression, such agents as melatonin to reestablish circadian regulation disruption by stress-related sleeplessness. Melatonin has oncostatic properties inhibiting cellular proliferation and reducing metastatic capacity. Beta-blockers may have a role in adjuvant chemotherapy for cancer. Nonspecific beta-blockers such as propranolol may blunt the effect of the stress-generated hormones like catecholamines from promoting cellular invasion, a critical component of the metastatic cascade. Whether the agents or others can be used to reduce cancer risk through biobehavioral-related mechanisms remains to be determined.

Understanding the mechanisms responsible for ameliorating the effects of stress on human tumor biology is vital for deriving effective interventions.[260] Evidence is accumulating that a cognitive-behavioral regime integrating a cognitive technique such as cognitive-behavioral stress management (CBSM) can cause decreased expression levels of cortisol in the serum, reduced depressive mood, and increased social support. Psychosocial interventions such as meditation-based antistress procedures and guided imagery techniques can alter negative mood, modulate ANS and HPA hormonal activity, and improve sleep quality. A positive dose-response effect in stress reduction has been reported after practicing mindfulness-based stress reduction (MBSR) in breast cancer patients.[257,264,265] Psychosocial interventions with cancer as an outcome are still in the nascent stages with methodological

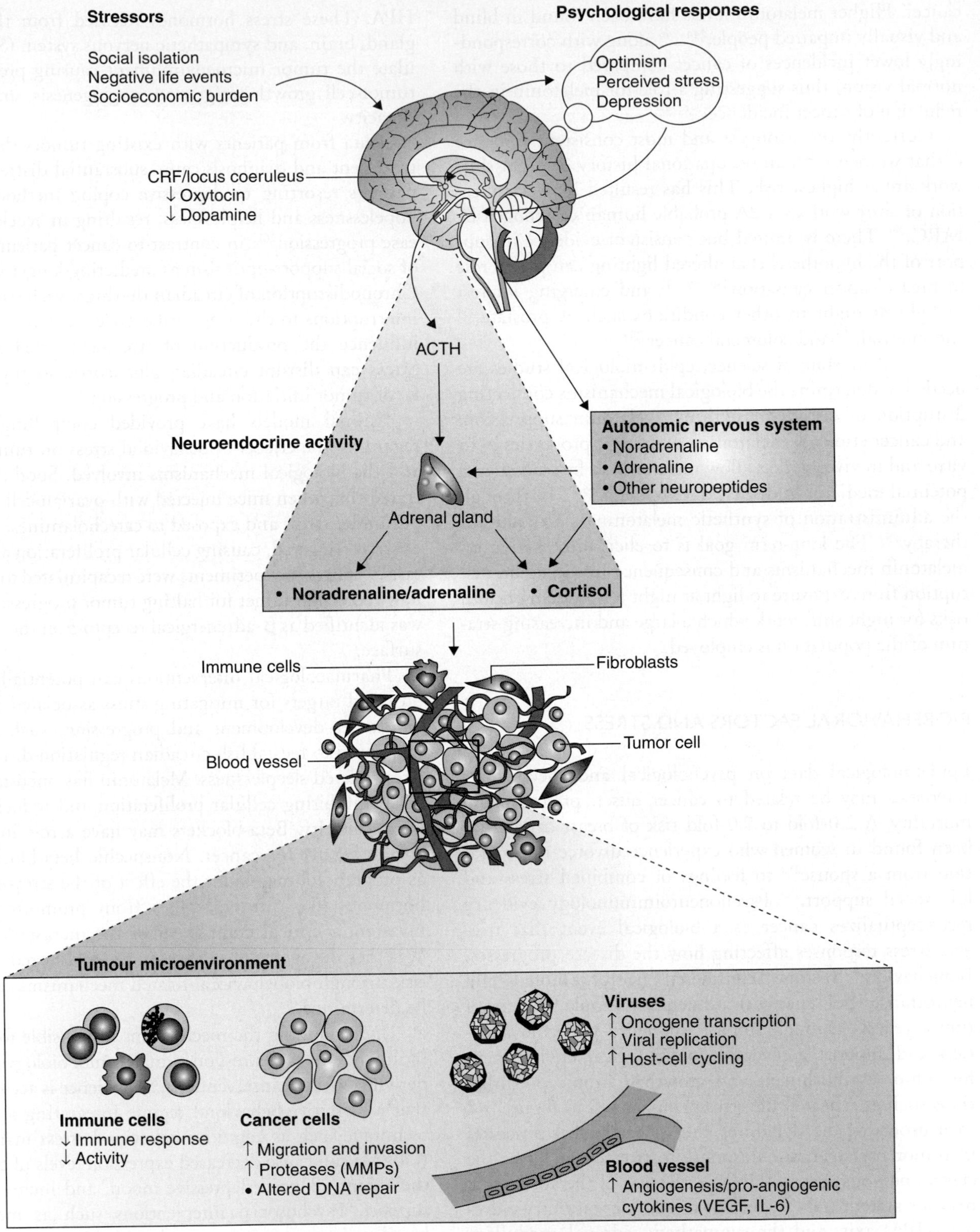


**FIGURE 3-8**

Effects of stress-associated factors on the tumor microenvironment.

*Source*: Data from Anton MH, Lutgendorf, SK, Cole SW, et al.[260]

flaws and failure to confirm a survival advantage to the treatment group.[266,267] Similar to targeted pharmacological interventions, the effectiveness of psychosocial interventions varies with the type and stage of cancer, biomedical characteristics of the patient, and social history (smoking, alcohol use, and sedentary activity). Epidemiological evidence correlating psychological and social factors (marriage/depression/social support) with cancer initiation, progression, and survival give merit to examining the biological signaling pathway and mechanisms which systematically modulate malignant potential.[268]

## APPLICATION OF EPIDEMIOLOGY TO NURSING PRACTICE

Nursing professionals play integral roles in all aspects of cancer prevention and cancer control. Nurses have played major roles in the development of effective means to educate, prevent, and detect cancers early.

Much of the progress that has been made in cancer control has stemmed from epidemiological research that aims to understand environmental, genetic, and population risks for developing specific cancer(s). Nurses are constantly challenged to construct and interpret cancer risk assessments for patients and their families. This effort demands that nurses be able to accurately interpret epidemiological studies of cancer risk.

Nurses have implemented the principles of primary, secondary, and tertiary cancer prevention through individualized cancer risk assessment and screening programs, cancer genetics counseling programs, government-sponsored programs, and programs that are offered at public events. A great need exists for nursing professionals to coordinate, implement, and help to provide cancer-control and education services.[269]

Nurses need to consider several common themes as they begin to design programs for cancer control. Some inherent cancer-control themes include consideration of the target population, resources of the institution or sponsor, opportunities for and value of collaboration, and resources for and approaches to public education, funding, marketing, and program evaluation.[270]

As cancer prevention and early detection continue to grow as a priority for oncology professionals and the institutions where they work, nurses will continue to play a critical role in the development, management, and success of cancer-control programs.

## REFERENCES


1. Trichopoulous D, Lipworth L, Petridou E. Epidemiology of cancer. In: DeVita VT, Hellman S, Rosenberg SA, eds. *Cancer Principles and Practice of Oncology.* Vol 2. 8th ed. Philadelphia, PA: Lippincott Williams and Wilkins; 2008:231–257.
2. Friis RH, Sellers TA. Overview of study designs used in epidemiology. In: Friis RH, Sellers TA, eds. *Epidemiology for Public Health Practice.* 4th ed. Gaithersburg, MD: Aspen; 2008:244–249.
3. Reid M. Cancer control and epidemiology. In: Yarbro CH, Frogge MH, Goodman M, eds. *Cancer Nursing.* 6th ed. Sudbury, MA: Jones and Bartlett; 2004:60–82.
4. Reid M. Cancer control and epidemiology. In: Yarbro CH, Frogge MH, Goodman M, Groenwald SL, eds. *Cancer Nursing Principles and Practice.* 5th ed. Sudbury, MA: Jones and Bartlett; 2000:60–82.
5. Rothman KJ, Greenland S, Lash TL. *Modern Epidemiology.* 3rd ed. Boston, MA: Little Brown; 2008.
6. Gordis L. *Epidemiology.* 8th ed. Phildelphia, PA: Elsevier; 2008.
7. Szklo M, Nieto FJ. *Epidemiology: Beyond the Basics.* 2nd ed. Gaithersburg, MD: Aspen; 2006.
8. Rothman KJ. *Epidemiology: An Introduction.* New York, NY: Oxford University Press; 2002.
9. McElroy JA, Egan KM, Titus-Ernstoff L, Anderson HA, Trentham-Dietz A, Hampton JM, Newcomb PA. Occupational exposure to electromagnetic field and breast cancer risk in a large, population-based, case-control study in the United States. *J Occup Environ Med.* 2007;49:266–74.
10. Bertone ER, Willett WC, Rosner BA, et al. Prospective study of recreational physical activity and ovarian cancer. *J Natl Cancer Inst.* 2001;93:942–948.
11. Adami H-O, Trichopoulos D. Concepts in cancer epidemiology and etiology. In: Adami H-O, Hunter D, Trichopoulos D, eds. *Textbook of Cancer Epidemiology.* 2nd ed. New York: Oxford University Press; 2008:87–109.
12. Maruti SS, Willett WC, Feskanich D, Rosner B, Colditz GA. A prospective study of age-specific physical activity and premenopausal breast cancer. *J Natl Cancer Inst.* 2008;100:728–737.
13. Tworoger SS, Gertig DM, Gates MA, Hecht JL, Hankinson SE. Caffeine, alcohol, smoking, and the risk of incident epithelial ovarian cancer. *Cancer.* 2008;112:1169–1177.
14. Piantadosi S. *Clinical Trials: A Methodologic Perspective.* 2nd ed. New York: Wiley-Interscience; 2005.
15. Goodman GE, Thornquist MD, Balmes J, et al. The Beta-Carotene and Retinol Efficacy Trial: incidence of lung cancer and cardiovascular disease mortality during 6-year follow-up after stopping beta-carotene and retinol supplements. *J Natl Cancer Inst.* 2004;96:1743–1750.
16. Bowen DJ, Thornquist M, Anderson K, et al. Stopping the active intervention: CARET. *Control Clin Trials.* 2003;24:39–50.
17. Wakefield J. Ecologic studies revisited. *Annu Rev Public Health* 2008;29:75–90.
18. Grant WB. Ecologic approach is a powerful tool for cancer research. *Eur J Cancer Prev* 2008;17:384.
19. Grant WB. Ecologic studies of solar UV-B radiation and cancer mortality rates. *Recent Results Cancer Res.* 2003;164:371–377.
20. Willett WC. Diet and breast cancer. *J Intern Med.* 2001;249:395–411.
21. Last JM: *A Dictionary of Epidemiology.* 4th ed. New York: Oxford University Press; 2000.
22. Savitz DA. *Interpreting Epidemiologic Evidence: Strategies for Study Design and Analysis.* 1st ed. New York: Oxford University Press; 2003.
23. Jewell NP. *Statistics for Epidemiology.* 1st ed. Boca Raton, FL: Chapman and Hall/CRC; 2003.
24. Hernan MA, Hernandez-Diaz S, Robins JM. A structural approach to selection bias. *Epidemiol.* 2004;15:615–625.
25. Nasca PC. Biomarkers and epidemiological studies of cancer. In: Nasca PC, Pastides H, eds. *Fundamentals of Cancer Epidemiology.* Sudbury, MA: Jones and Bartlett; 2007:109–129.
26. Nasca PC. Tobacco and cancer. In: Nasca PC, Pastides H, eds. *Fundamentals of Cancer Epidemiology.* Sudbury, MA: Jones and Bartlett; 2007:178–215.
27. Vineis P, Alavanja M, Buffler P, et al. Tobacco and cancer: recent epidemiological evidence. *J Natl Cancer Inst.* 2004;96:99–106.

28. Boffetta P, Hecht S, Gray N, Gupta P, Straif K. Smokeless tobacco and cancer. *Lancet Oncol.* 2008;9:667–675.
29. Chapman S. Should the health community promote smokeless tobacco(snus): Author's reply. *PLoS Med.* 2007;4:e299.
30. Levy DT, Mumford EA, Cummings KM, et al. The relative risks of a low-nitrosamine smokeless tobacco product compared with smoking cigarettes: estimates of a panel of experts. *Cancer Epidemiol Biomarkers Prev.* 2004;13:2035–2042.
31. Broadstock M. Systematic review of the health effects of modified smokeless tobacco products. *N Z Health Technol Assess Rep.* 2007;10(1). http://www.smokeless.com.au/media/smokeless_tobacco_2074534168.pdf. Accessed September 21, 2009.
32. Bates C, Fagerstrom K, Jarvis MJ, Kunze M, McNeill A, Ramstrom L. European Union policy on smokeless tobacco: a statement in favour of evidence based regulation for public health. *Tob Control.* 2003;12:360–367.
33. Besaratinia A, Pfeifer GP. Second-hand smoke and human lung cancer. *Lancet Oncol.* 2008;9:657–666.
34. Smith CJ, Perfetti TA, Garg R, Hansch C. IARC carcinogens reported in cigarette mainstream smoke and their calculated log P values. *Food Chem Toxicol.* 2003;41:807–817.
35. Boffetta P, Nyberg F. Contribution of environmental factors to cancer risk. *Br Med Bull.* 2003;68:71–94.
36. Khuder SA, Simon VJ. Is there an association between passive smoking and breast cancer? *Eur J Epidemiol.* 2000;16:1117–1121.
37. Mark-Wahnefried W, Rock CL, Patrick K, Byers T. Lifestyle interventions to reduce cancer risk and improve outcomes. *Am Fam Physician.* 2008;77:1573–1578.
38. Miller MF, Bellizzi KM, Sufian M, et al. Dietary supplement use in individuals living with cancer and other chronic conditions: a population-based study. *J Am Diet Assoc.* 2008;108:483–494.
39. Key TJ, Spencer EA. Carbohydrates and cancer: an overview of the epidemiological evidence. *Eur J Clin Nutr.* 2007;61(suppl 1):S112–S121.
40. Malin A, Dai Q, Shu X-O, et al. Intake of fruits, vegetables and selected micronutrients in relation to the risk of breast cancer. *Int J Cancer.* 2003;105:413–418.
41. Kesteloot HE, Zhang J. Differences in breast cancer mortality worldwide unsolved problems. *Eur J Cancer Prev.* 2006;15:416–423.
42. Sharma S, O'Keefe SJ. Environmental influences on the high mortality from colorectal cancer in African Americans. *Postgrad Med J.* 2007;83:583–589.
43. Doyle VC. Nutrition and colorectal cancer risk: a literature review. *Gastroenterol Nurs.* 2007;30:178–182.
44. Mathew A, Peters U, Chatterjee N, et al. Fat, fiber, fruits, vegetables, and risk of colorectal adenomas. *Int J Cancer.* 2004;108:287–292.
45. Robertson DJ, Sandler RS, Haile R, et al. Fat, fiber, meat and the risk of colorectal adenomas. *Am J Gastroenterol.* 2005;100:2789–2795.
46. Chlebowski R. Lifestyle change including dietary fat reduction and breast cancer outcome. *J Nutr.* 2007;137(suppl 1):233S-235S.
47. Sieri S, Krogh V, Ferrari P, et al. Dietary fat and breast cancer risk in the European Prospective Investigation into Cancer and Nutrition. *Am J Clin Nutr.* 2008;88:1304–1312.
48. Thiebaut AC, Kipnis V, Chang SC, et al. Dietary fat and postmenopausal invasive breast cancer in the National Institutes of Health-AARP Diet and Health Study cohort. *J Natl Cancer Inst.* 2007;99:451–462.
49. Boyd NF, Stone J, Vogt KN, Connelly BS, Martin LJ, Minkin S. Dietary fat and breast cancer risk revisited: a meta-analysis of the published literature. *Br J Cancer.* 2003;89:1672–1685.
50. Cho E, Spiegelman D, Hunter DJ. Premenopausal fat intake and risk of breast cancer. *J Natl Cancer Inst.* 2003;95:1079–1085.
51. Kroenke CH, Fung TT, Hu FB, Holmes MD. Dietary patterns and survival after breast cancer diagnosis. *J Clin Oncol.* 2005;23:9295–9303.
52. Willet WC, Hunter D, Stampfer MJ, et al. Dietary fat and fiber in relation to risk of breast cancer: a 8-year follow-up. *JAMA.* 1992;268:2037–2044.
53. Kushi L, Potter J, Drinkard C, et al. Dietary factors and risk of breast cancer: combined analysis of 12 case-control studies. *Cancer Epidemiol Biomarkers Prev.* 1995;4:9–11.
54. Lof M, Sandin S, Lagiou P, et al. Dietary fat and breast cancer risk in the Swedish women's lifestyle and health cohort. *Br J Cancer.* 2007;97:1570–1576.
55. Linseisen J, Rohrmann S, Miller AB, et al. Fruit and vegetable consumption and lung cancer risk: updated information from the European Prospective Investigation into Cancer and Nutrition (EPIC). *Int J Cancer.* 2007;121:1103–1114.
56. McCullough ML, Bandera EV, Patel R, et al. A prospective study of fruits, vegetables, and risk of endometrial cancer. *Am J Epidemiol.* 2007;166:902–911.
57. Kirsh VA, Hayes RB, Mayne ST, et al. Supplemental and dietary vitamin E, beta-carotene, and vitamin C intakes and prostate cancer risk. *J Natl Cancer Inst.* 2006;98:245–254.
58. Dorjgochoo T, Shrubsole MJ, Shu XO, et al. Vitamin supplement use and risk for breast cancer: the Shanghai Breast Cancer Study. *Breast Cancer Res Treat.* 2008;111:269–278.
59. Smith-Warner SA, Spiegelman D, Yaun SS, et al. Fruits, vegetables and lung cancer: a pooled analysis of cohort studies. *Int J Cancer.* 2003; 107:1001–1011.
60. Smith-Warner SA, Spiegelman D, Yaun SS, et al. Intake of fruits and vegetables and risk of breast cancer: a pooled analysis of cohort studies. *JAMA.* 2001;285:769–776.
61. Johnson LJ, Meacham SL, Kruskall LJ. The antioxidants—vitamin C, vitamin E, selenium, and carotenoids. *J Agromedicine.* 2003;9:65–82.
62. Seifried HE, McDonald SS, Anderson DE, et al. The antioxidant conundrum in cancer. *Cancer Res.* 2003;63:4295–4298.
63. Kim YI. Nutritional epigenetics: impact of folate deficiency on DNA methylation and colon cancer susceptibility. *J Nutr.* 2005;135: 2703–2709.
64. Murtaugh MA, Curtin K, Sweeney C, et al. Dietary intake of folate and co-factors in folate metabolism, MTHFR polymorphisms, and reduced rectal cancer. *Cancer Causes Control.* 2007;18:153–163.
65. Li D, Jiao L. Molecular epidemiology of pancreatic cancer. *Int J Gastrointest Cancer.* 2003;33:3–14.
66. Shrubsole MJ, Jin F, Dai Q, et al. Dietary folate intake and breast cancer risk: results from the Shanghai Breast Cancer Study. *Cancer Res.* 2001;61:7136–7141.
67. Wolpin BM, Wei EK, Ng K, et al. Prediagnostic plasma folate and the risk of death in patients with colorectal cancer. *J Clin Oncol.* 2008;26:3222–3228.
68. Tworoger SS, Hecht JL, Giovannucci E, Hankinson SE. Intake of folate and related nutrients in relation to risk of epithelial ovarian cancer. *Am J Epidemiol.* 2006;163:1101–1111.
69. Beetstra S, Thomas P, Salisbury C, Turner J, Fenech M. Folic acid deficiency increases chromosomal instability, chromosome 21 aneuploidy and sensitivity to radiation-induced micronuclei. *Mutat Res.* 2005;578: 317–326.
70. Giovannucci E. A review of epidemiologic studies of tomatoes, lycopene, and prostate cancer. *Exp Biol Med (Maywood).* 2002;227:852–859.
71. Holick CN, Michaud DS, Stolzenberg-Solomon R, et al. Dietary carotenoids, serum beta-carotene, and retinol and risk of lung cancer in the alpha-tocopherol, beta-carotene cohort study. *Am J Epidemiol.* 2002;156:536–547.
72. Fink BN, Steck SE, Wolff MS, et al. Dietary flavonoid intake and breast cancer survival among women on Long Island. *Cancer Epidemiol Biomarkers Prev.* 2007;16:2285–2292.
73. Peeters PHM, Keinan-Boker L, van der Schouw YT, Grobbee DE. Phytoestrogens and breast cancer risk. *Breast Cancer Res Treat.* 2003;77: 171–183.
74. Castle EP, Thrasher JB. The role of soy phytoestrogens in prostate cancer. *Urol Clin North Am.* 2002;29:71–81.
75. Sirtori CR, Arnoldi A, Johnson SK. Phytoestrogens: end of a tale? *Ann Med.* 2005;37:423–438.

76. Nomura AM, Hankin JH, Henderson BE, et al. Dietary fiber and colorectal cancer risk: the multiethnic cohort study. *Cancer Causes Control.* 2007;18:753–764.
77. Park Y, Hunter DJ, Spiegelman D, et al. Dietary fiber intake and risk of colorectal cancer: a pooled analysis of prospective cohort studies. *JAMA.* 2005;294:2849–2857.
78. Schatzkin A, Mouw T, Park Y, et al. Dietary fiber and whole-grain consumption in relation to colorectal cancer in the NIH-AARP Diet and Health Study. *Am J Clin Nutr.* 2007;85:1353–1360.
79. Lin J, Zhang SM, Cook NR, et al. Dietary intakes of fruit, vegetables, and fiber, and risk of colorectal cancer in a prospective cohort of women (United States). *Cancer Causes Control.* 2005;16:225–233.
80. Park SY, Murphy SP, Wilkens LR, et al. Calcium and vitamin D intake and risk of colorectal cancer: the Multiethnic Cohort Study. *Am J Epidemiol.* 2007;165:784–793.
81. McCullough ML, Robertson AS, Rodriguez C, et al. Calcium, vitamin D, dairy products, and risk of colorectal cancer in the Cancer Prevention Study II Nutrition Cohort (United States). *Cancer Causes Control.* 2003;14:1–12.
82. Cho E, Smith-Warner SA, Spiegelman D, et al. Dairy foods, calcium, and colorectal cancer: a pooled analysis of 10 cohort studies. *J Natl Cancer Inst.* 2004;96:1015–1022.
83. Terry P, Baron JA, Bergkvist L, Holmberg L, Wolk A. Dietary calcium and vitamin D intake and risk of colorectal cancer: a prospective cohort study in women. *Nutr Cancer.* 2002;43:39–46.
84. Larsson SC, Bergkvist L, Rutegard J, Giovannucci E, Wolk A. Calcium and dairy food intakes are inversely associated with colorectal cancer risk in the Cohort of Swedish Men. *Am J Clin Nutr.* 2006;83:667–673.
85. Lin J, Zhang SM, Cook NR, Manson JE, Lee I M, Buring JE. Intakes of calcium and vitamin D and risk of colorectal cancer in women. *Am J Epidemiol.* 2005;161:755–764.
86. Holick MF. Vitamin D and sunlight: strategies for cancer prevention and other health benefits. *Clin J Am Soc Nephrol.* 2008;3:1548–1554.
87. Lamprecht SA, Lipkin M. Chemoprevention of colon cancer by calcium, vitamin D and folate: molecular mechanisms. *Nat Rev Cancer.* 2003;3:601–614.
88. Boyapati SM, Bostick RM, McGlynn KA, et al: Calcium, vitamin D, and risk for colorectal adenoma: dependency on vitamin D receptor B*sm*I polymorphism and nonsteroidal anti-inflammatory drug use? *Cancer Epidemiol Biomarkers Prev.* 2003;12:631–637.
89. Holden JM, Lemar LE, Exler J. Vitamin D in foods: development of the US Department of Agriculture database. *Am J Clin Nutr.* 2008;87:1092S-1096S.
90. Welsh J, Wietzke JA, Zinser GM, et al. Impact of the Vitamin D3 receptor on growth-regulatory pathways in mammary gland and breast cancer. *J Steroid Biochem Mol Biol.* 2002;83:85–92.
91. Giovannucci E. The epidemiology of vitamin D and cancer incidence and mortality: a review (United States). *Cancer Causes Control.* 2005;16:83–95.
92. Schwartz GG. Vitamin D and the epidemiology of prostate cancer. *Semin Dial.* 2005;18:276–289.
93. Bao BY, Yao J, Lee YF. 1alpha, 25-dihydroxyvitamin D3 suppresses interleukin-8-mediated prostate cancer cell angiogenesis. *Carcinog.* 2006;27:1883–1893.
94. Nakagawa K, Kawaura A, Kato S, Takeda E, Okano T. 1 alpha,25-Dihydroxyvitamin D(3) is a preventive factor in the metastasis of lung cancer. *Carcinog.* 2005;26:429–440.
95. Uitterlinden AG, Fang Y, Van Meurs JB, Pols HA, Van Leeuwen JP. Genetics and biology of vitamin D receptor polymorphisms. *Gene.* 2004;338:143–156.
96. Lin J, Manson JE, Lee IM, Cook NR, Buring JE, Zhang SM. Intakes of calcium and vitamin D and breast cancer risk in women. *Arch Intern Med.* 2007;167:1050–1059.
97. Grant WB, Garland CF. A critical review of studies on vitamin D in relation to colorectal cancer. *Nutr Cancer.* 2004;48:115–123.
98. Giovannucci E. The epidemiology of vitamin D and colorectal cancer: recent findings. *Curr Opin Gastroenterol.* 2006;22:24–29.
99. Giovannucci E, Liu Y, Rimm EB, et al. Prospective study of predictors of vitamin D status and cancer incidence and mortality in men. *J Natl Cancer Inst.* 2006;98:451–459.
100. Wu K, Feskanich D, Fuchs CS, Willett WC, Hollis BW, Giovannucci EL. A nested case control study of plasma 25-hydroxyvitamin D concentrations and risk of colorectal cancer. *J Natl Cancer Inst.* 2007;99:1120–1129.
101. Wactawski-Wende J, Kotchen JM, Anderson GL, et al. Calcium plus vitamin D supplementation and the risk of colorectal cancer. *N Engl J Med.* 2006;354:684–696.
102. Lappe JM, Travers-Gustafson D, Davies KM, Recker RR, Heaney RP. Vitamin D and calcium supplementation reduces cancer risk: results of a randomized trial. *Am J Clin Nutr.* 2007;85:1586–1591.
103. Grau MV, Baron JA, Sandler RS, et al. Prolonged effect of calcium supplementation on risk of colorectal adenomas in a randomized trial. *J Natl Cancer Inst.* 2007;99:129–136.
104. Hartman TJ, Albert PS, Snyder K, et al. The association of calcium and vitamin D with risk of colorectal adenomas. *J Nutr.* 2005;135:252–259.
105. Nasca PC. Alcohol and cancer. In: Nasca PC, Pastides H, eds. *Fundamentals of Cancer Epidemiology.* Sudbury, MA: Jones and Bartlett; 2007:225–254.
106. Chan JM, Gann PH, Giovannucci EL. Role of diet in prostate cancer development and progression. *J Clin Oncol.* 2005;23:8152–8160.
107. Baan R, Straif K, Grosse Y, et al. Carcinogenicity of alcoholic beverages. *Lancet Oncol.* 2007;8:292–293.
108. Zhang SM, Lee IM, Manson JE, Cook NR, Willett WC, Buring JE. Alcohol consumption and breast cancer risk in the Women's Health Study. *Am J Epidemiol.* 2007;165:667–676.
109. Akhter M, Kuriyama S, Nakaya N, et al. Alcohol consumption is associated with an increased risk of distal colon and rectal cancer in Japanese men: the Miyagi Cohort Study. *Eur J Cancer.* 2007;43:383–390.
110. Simanowski UA, Homann N, Knuhl M, et al: Increased rectal cell proliferation following alcohol abuse. *Gut.* 2001;49:418–422.
111. Ferrari P, Jenab M, Norat T, et al. Lifetime and baseline alcohol intake and risk of colon and rectal cancers in the European prospective investigation into cancer and nutrition (EPIC). *Int J Cancer.* 2007;121:2065–2072.
112. Feigelson HS, Jonas CR, Robertson AS, McCullough ML, Thun MJ, Calle EE. Alcohol, folate, methionine, and risk of incident breast cancer in the American Cancer Society Cancer Prevention Study II Nutrition Cohort. *Cancer Epidemiol Biomarkers Prev.* 2003;12:161–164.
113. Baglietto L, English DR, Gertig DM, Hopper JL, Giles GG. Does dietary folate intake modify effect of alcohol consumption on breast cancer risk? Prospective cohort study. *BMJ.* 2005;331:807.
114. Jiang R, Hu FB, Giovannucci EL, et al. Joint association of alcohol and folate intake with risk of major chronic disease in women. *Am J Epidemiol.* 2003;158:760–771.
115. Sellers TA, Kushi LH, Cerhan JR, et al. Dietary folate intake, alcohol, and risk of breast cancer in a prospective study of postmenopausal women. *Epidemiology.* 2001;12:420–428.
116. Stolzenberg-Solomon RZ, Chang SC, Leitzmann MF, et al. Folate intake, alcohol use, and postmenopausal breast cancer risk in the Prostate, Lung, Colorectal, and Ovarian Cancer Screening Trial. *Am J Clin Nutr.* 2006;83:895–904.
117. Tjonneland A, Christensen J, Olsen A, et al. Alcohol intake and breast cancer risk: the European Prospective Investigation into Cancer and Nutrition (EPIC). *Cancer Causes Control.* 2007;18:361–373.
118. Li CI, Malone KE, Porter PL, Weiss NS, Tang MT, Daling JR. The relationship between alcohol use and risk of breast cancer by histology and hormone receptor status among women 65–79 years of age. *Cancer Epidemiol Biomarkers Prev.* 2003;12:1061–1066.
119. Suzuki R, Ye W, Rylander-Rudqvist T, Saji S, Colditz GA, Wolk A. Alcohol and postmenopausal breast cancer risk defined by estrogen

and progesterone receptor status: a prospective cohort study. *J Natl Cancer Inst.* 2005;97:1601–1608.
120. Deandrea S, Talamini R, Foschi R, et al. Alcohol and breast cancer risk defined by estrogen and progesterone receptor status: a case-control study. *Cancer Epidemiol Biomarkers Prev.* 2008;17:2025–2028.
121. Wayne S, Neuhouser ML, Ulrich CM, et al. Association between alcohol intake and serum sex hormones and peptides differs by tamoxifen use in breast cancer survivors. *Cancer Epidemiol Biomarkers Prev.* 2008;17:3224–3232.
122. Duffy CM, Assaf A, Cyr M, et al. Alcohol and folate intake and breast cancer risk in the WHI Observational Study. *Breast Cancer Res Treat.* 2009;116:551–562.
123. Berstad P, Ma H, Bernstein L, Ursin G. Alcohol intake and breast cancer risk among young women. *Breast Cancer Res Treat.* 2008;108: 113–120.
124. McDonald JA, Mandel MG, Marchbanks PA, et al. Alcohol exposure and breast cancer: results of the women's contraceptive and reproductive experiences study. *Cancer Epidemiol Biomarkers Prev.* 2004;13: 2106–2116.
125. Cancer prevention and management through exercise and weight control. 1st ed. Boca Raton, FL: CRC Press; 2006.
126. Fair AM, Montgomery KM. Energy balance, physical activity and cancer risk. In: Verma M, ed. *Cancer Epidemiology.* Vol 2. *Modifiable Factors.* Vol. 472. 1st ed. Totowa, NJ: Humana Press; 2009, 2008:57–88.
127. Malin A, Matthews CE, Shu XO, et al. Energy balance and breast cancer risk. *Cancer Epidemiol Biomarkers Prev.* 2005;14:1496–1501.
128. Chao A, Connell CJ, Jacobs EJ, McCullough ML, Patel AV, Calle EE. Amount, type, and timing of recreational physical activity in relation to colon and rectal cancer in older adults: the Cancer Prevention Study II Nutrition Cohort. *Cancer Epidemiol Biomarkers Prev.* 2004;13: 2187–2195.
129. Rodriguez C, Freedland SJ, Deka A, et al. Body mass index, weight change, and risk of prostate cancer in the Cancer Prevention Study II Nutrition Cohort. *Cancer Epidemiol Biomarkers Prev.* 2007;16:63–69.
130. Matthews C, Shu X-O, Jin F, et al. Lifetime physical activity and breast cancer risk in the Shanghai Breast Cancer Study. *Br J Cancer.* 2001;84: 994–1001.
131. Friedenreich C, Norat T, Steindorf K, et al. Physical activity and risk of colon and rectal cancers: the European prospective investigation into cancer and nutrition. *Cancer Epidemiol Biomarkers Prev.* 2006;15: 2398–2407.
132. Calton BA, Lacey JV, Jr., Schatzkin A, et al. Physical activity and the risk of colon cancer among women: a prospective cohort study (United States). *Int J Cancer.* 2006;119:385–391.
133. Slattery ML, Caan BJ, Benson J, Murtaugh M. Energy balance and rectal cancer: an evaluation of energy intake, energy expenditure, and body mass index. *Nutr Cancer.* 2003;46:166–171.
134. John EM, Horn-Ross PL, Koo J. Lifetime physical activity and breast cancer risk in a multiethnic population: the San Francisco Bay area breast cancer study. *Cancer Epidemiol Biomarkers Prev.* 2003;12 (Pt 1): 1143–1152.
135. Fair AM, Dai Q, Shu XO, et al. Energy balance, insulin resistance biomarkers, and breast cancer risk. *Cancer Detect Prev.* 2007;31:214–219.
136. Shin A, Matthews CE, Shu XO, et al. Joint effects of body size, energy intake, and physical activity on breast cancer risk. *Breast Cancer Res Treat.* 2009;113:153–161.
137. Kruk J. Lifetime physical activity and the risk of breast cancer: a case-control study. *Cancer Detect Prev.* 2007;31:18–28.
138. Chang SC, Ziegler RG, Dunn B, et al. Association of energy intake and energy balance with postmenopausal breast cancer in the prostate, lung, colorectal, and ovarian cancer screening trial. *Cancer Epidemiol Biomarkers Prev.* 2006;15:334–341.
139. Silvera SA, Jain M, Howe GR, Miller AB, Rohan TE. Energy balance and breast cancer risk: a prospective cohort study. *Breast Cancer Res Treat.* 2006;97:97–106.
140. Dallal CM, Sullivan-Halley J, Ross RK, et al. Long-term recreational physical activity and risk of invasive and in situ breast cancer: the California teachers study. *Arch Intern Med.* 2007;167:408–415.
141. Monninkhof EM, Elias SG, Vlems FA, et al. Physical activity and breast cancer: a systematic review. *Epidemiology.* 2007;18:137–157.
142. Olsen CM, Bain CJ, Jordan SJ, et al. Recreational physical activity and epithelial ovarian cancer: a case-control study, systematic review, and meta-analysis. *Cancer Epidemiol Biomarkers Prev.* 2007;16:2321–2330.
143. Pan SY, DesMeules M, Morrison H, Wen SW. Obesity, high energy intake, lack of physical activity, and the risk of kidney cancer. *Cancer Epidemiol Biomarkers Prev.* 2006;15:2453–2460.
144. Mahabir S, Leitzmann MF, Pietinen P, Albanes D, Virtamo J, Taylor PR. Physical activity and renal cell cancer risk in a cohort of male smokers. *Int J Cancer.* 2004;108:600–605.
145. van Dijk BA, Schouten LJ, Kiemeney LA, Goldbohm RA, van den Brandt PA. Relation of height, body mass, energy intake, and physical activity to risk of renal cell carcinoma: results from the Netherlands Cohort Study. *Am J Epidemiol.* 2004;160:1159–1167.
146. Calton BA, Stolzenberg-Solomon RZ, Moore SC, et al. A prospective study of physical activity and the risk of pancreatic cancer among women (United States). *BMC Cancer.* 2008;8:63.
147. Friedenreich C, Cust A, Lahmann PH, et al. Physical activity and risk of endometrial cancer: the European prospective investigation into cancer and nutrition. *Int J Cancer.* 2007;121:347–355.
148. Matthews CE, Shu XO, Jin F, et al. Lifetime physical activity and breast cancer risk in the Shanghai Breast Cancer Study. *Br J Cancer.* 2001;84:994–1001.
149. Colbert LH, Lacey JV Jr., Schairer C, Albert P, Schatzkin A, Albanes D. Physical activity and risk of endometrial cancer in a prospective cohort study (United States). *Cancer Causes Control.* 2003;14:559–567.
150. Friberg E, Mantzoros CS, Wolk A. Physical activity and risk of endometrial cancer: a population-based prospective cohort study. *Cancer Epidemiol Biomarkers Prev.* 2006;15:2136–2140.
151. Tehard B, Friedenreich CM, Oppert JM, Clavel-Chapelon F. Effect of physical activity on women at increased risk of breast cancer: results from the E3N cohort study. *Cancer Epidemiol Biomarkers Prev.* 2006;15:57–64.
152. Pastides H. Occupation and cancer. In: Nasca PC, Pastides H, eds. *Fundamentals of Cancer Epidemiology.* Sudbury, MA: Jones and Bartlett; 2007:158–174.
153. Clapp RW, Howe GK, Jacobs MM. Environmental and occupational causes of cancer: a call to act on what we know. *Biomed Pharmacother.* 2007;61:631–639.
154. International Metalworkers' Federation (IMF). *Occupational cancer/ Zero Cancer.* International Metalworkers' Federation (IMF); 2007.
155. Villanueva CM, Cantor KP, Grimalt JO, et al. Bladder cancer and exposure to water disinfection by-products through ingestion, bathing, showering, and swimming in pools. *Am J Epidemiol.* 2007;165: 148–156.
156. Bove GE, Jr., Rogerson PA, Vena JE. Case control study of the geographic variability of exposure to disinfectant byproducts and risk for rectal cancer. *Int J Health Geogr.* 2007;6:18.
157. Slaper H, de Gruijl F. Stratospheric ozone depletion, UV exposure and skin cancer: a scenario analysis. In: Hill DJ, Elwood JM, English DR, eds. *Prevention of Skin Cancer.* New York, NY: Springer; 2004:55–73.
158. World Health Organization. *Fluorides. Environmental Health Criteria.* Geneva, Switzerland: World Health Organization; 2002:227.
159. Laughlin-Drubin ME, Munger K. Viruses associated with human cancer. *Biochim Biophys Acta* 2008;1782:127–150.
160. American Cancer Society. *Infectious Agents and Cancer.* http://www.cancer.org/docroot/PED/content/PED_1_3X_Infectious_Agents_and_Cancer.asp. Accessed June 1 2009.
161. Liao JB. Viruses and human cancer. *Yale J Biol Med.* 2006;79:115–122.
162. Verdonck K, Gonzalez E, Van DS, Vandamme AM, Vanham G, Gotuzzo E. Human T-lymphotropic virus 1: recent knowledge about an ancient infection. *Lancet Infect Dis.* 2007;7:266–281.

163. Field RW, Krewski D, Lubin JH, et al. An overview of the North American residential radon and lung cancer case-control studies. *J Toxicol Environ Health.* 2006;69:599–631.
164. Neuberger JS, Mahnken JD, Mayo MS, Field RW. Risk factors for lung cancer in Iowa women: implications for prevention. *Cancer Detect Prev.* 2006;30:158–167.
165. Alberg AJ, Samet JM. Epidemiology of lung cancer. *Chest.* 2003;123:21S-49S.
166. Ahlbom IC, Cardis E, Green A, Linet M, Savitz D, Swerdlow A. Review of the epidemiologic literature on EMF and Health. *Environ Health Perspect.* 2001;109(suppl 6):911–933.
167. Kheifets L, Monroe J, Vergara X, Mezei G, Afifi AA. Occupational electromagnetic fields and leukemia and brain cancer: an update to two meta-analyses. *J Occup Environ Med.* 2008;50:677–688.
168. McElroy JA, Egan KM, Titus-Ernstoff L, Anderson HA, Trentham-Dietz A, Hampton JM et al. Occupational exposure to electromagnetic field and breast cancer risk in a large, population-based, case-control study in the United States. *J Occup Environ Med.* 2007;49:266–274.
169. Feychting M, Forssen U. Electromagnetic fields and female breast cancer. *Cancer Causes Control.* 2006;17:553–558.
170. Davis S, Mirick DK, Stevens RG. Residential magnetic fields and the risk of breast cancer. *Am J Epidemiol.* 2002;155:446–454.
171. Cellular-news. More Cellphone-Only Than Landline-Only Households in the USA. Cellular-News. http://www.cellular-news.com/story/26023.php. Accessed June 15, 2009
172. Frumkin H, Jacobson A, Gansler T, Thun MJ. Cellular phones and risk of brain tumors. *CA: Cancer J Clin.* 2001;51:137–141.
173. Kan P, Simonsen SE, Lyon JL, Kestle JR. Cellular phone use and brain tumor: a meta-analysis. *J Neurooncol.* 2008;86:71–78.
174. Takebayashi T, Varsier N, Kikuchi Y, Wake K, Taki M, Watanabe S. Mobile phone use, exposure to radiofrequency electromagnetic field, and brain tumour: a case-control study. *Br J Cancer.* 2008;98:652–659.
175. Hardell L, Carlberg M, Ohlson CG, Westberg H, Eriksson M, Hansson MK. Use of cellular and cordless telephones and risk of testicular cancer. *Int J Androl.* 2007;30:115–122.
176. Cook A, Woodward A, Pearce N, Marshall C. Cellular telephone use and time trends for brain, head and neck tumours. *N Z Med J.* 2003;116:U457.
177. Warren HG, Prevatt AA, Daly KA, Antonelli PJ. Cellular telephone use and risk of intratemporal facial nerve tumor. *Laryngoscope.* 2003;113:663–667.
178. Wrensch M, Minn Y, Chew T, et al. Epidemiology of primary brain tumors: current concepts and review of the literature. *Neuro-oncol.* 2002;4:278–299.
179. Robsahm TE, Tretli S, Dahlback A, Moan J. Vitamin D3 from sunlight may improve the prognosis of breast-, colon- and prostate cancer (Norway). *Cancer Causes Control.* 2004;15:149–158.
180. Abbas S, Chang-Claude J, Linseisen J. Plasma 25-hydroxyvitamin D and premenopausal breast cancer risk in a German case-control study. *Int J Cancer.* 2008;124: 250–255.
181. Egan KM, Signorello LB, Munro HM, Hargreaves MK, Hollis BW, Blot WJ. Vitamin D insufficiency among African-Americans in the southeastern United States: implications for cancer disparities (United States). *Cancer Causes Control.* 2008;19:527–535.
182. Nesby-O'Dell S, Scanlon KS, Cogswell ME, et al. Hypovitaminosis D prevalence and determinants among African American and white women of reproductive age: third National Health and Nutrition Examination Survey, 1988–1994. *Am J Clin Nutr.* 2002;76:187–192.
183. Hollis BW. Circulating 25-hydroxyvitamin D levels indicative of vitamin D sufficiency: implications for establishing a new effective dietary intake recommendation for vitamin D. *J Nutr.* 2005;135:317–322.
184. Pastides H: Ionizing, nonionizing, and solar radiation and cancer. In: Nasca PC, Pastides H, eds. *Fundamentals of Cancer Epidemiology.* Sudbury, MA: Jones and Bartlett; 2007:265–281.
185. Crallan RA, Georgopoulos NT, Southgate J. Experimental models of human bladder carcinogenesis. *Carcinogenesis.* 2006;27:374–381.
186. Mudie NY, Swerdlow AJ, Higgins CD, et al. Risk of second malignancy after non-Hodgkin's lymphoma: a British Cohort Study. *J Clin Oncol.* 2006;24:1568–1574.
187. Berardi RR. Peptic ulcer disease and NSAIDs: update on risk, risk reduction strategies, and treatment. *Rx Consultant.* 2007;18:1–8.
188. Bertagnolli MM. The potential of nonsteroidal anti-inflammatory drugs (NSAIDs) for colorectal cancer prevention. *J Surg Oncol.* 2003;84:113–119.
189. Flossmann E, Rothwell PM. Commentary: aspirin and colorectal cancer an epidemiological success story. *Int J Epidemiol.* 2007;36:962–965.
190. Routine aspirin or nonsteroidal anti-inflammatory drugs for the primary prevention of colorectal cancer: recommendation statement. *Am Fam Physician.* 2007;76:109–113.
191. Thun MJ, Henley SJ, Patrono C: Nonsteroidal anti-inflammatory drugs as anticancer agents: mechanistic, pharmacologic, and clinical issues. *J Natl Cancer Inst.* 2002;94:252–266.
192. Howe LR. Inflammation and breast cancer. Cyclooxygenase/prostaglandin signaling and breast cancer. *Breast Cancer Res.* 2007;9:210.
193. Sinicrope FA. Targeting cyclooxygenase-2 for prevention and therapy of colorectal cancer. *Mol Carcinog.* 2006;45:447–454.
194. Bresalier RS, Sandler RS, Quan H, et al. Cardiovascular events associated with rofecoxib in a colorectal adenoma chemoprevention trial. *N Engl J Med.* 2005;352:1092–1102.
195. Haller DG. COX-2 inhibitors in oncology. *Semin Oncol.* 2003;30(suppl 12):2–8.
196. Fabi A, Metro G, Papaldo P, et al. Impact of celecoxib on capecitabine tolerability and activity in pretreated metastatic breast cancer: results of a phase II study with biomarker evaluation. *Cancer Chemother Pharmacol.* 2008;62:717–725.
197. Heavey E. Start early to prevent genital HPV infection-and cervical cancer. *Nursing* 2008;38:62–63.
198. Eisen A, Lubinski J, Gronwald J, et al. Hormone therapy and the risk of breast cancer in BRCA1 mutation carriers. *J Natl Cancer Inst.* 2008;100:1361–1367.
199. Norman RJ, MacLennan AH. Current status of hormone therapy and breast cancer. *Hum Reprod Update.* 2005;11:541–543.
200. Fournier A, Berrino F, Clavel-Chapelon F. Unequal risks for breast cancer associated with different hormone replacement therapies: results from the E3N cohort study. *Breast Cancer Res Treat.* 2008;107:103–111.
201. Chen WY. Exogenous and endogenous hormones and breast cancer. *Best Pract Res Clin Endocrinol Metab.* 2008;22:573–585.
202. Collins JA, Blake JM, Crosignani PG. Breast cancer risk with postmenopausal hormonal treatment. *Hum Reprod Update.* 2005;11:545–560.
203. Anderson GL, Chlebowski RT, Rossouw JE, et al. Prior hormone therapy and breast cancer risk in the Women's Health Initiative randomized trial of estrogen plus progestin. *Maturitas.* 2006;20;55:103–115.
204. Tamimi RM, Hankinson SE, Chen WY, Rosner B, Colditz GA. Combined estrogen and testosterone use and risk of breast cancer in postmenopausal women. *Arch Intern Med.* 2006;166:1483–1489.
205. The Practice Committee of the American Society for Reproductive Medicine. Estrogen and progestogen therapy in post-menopausal women. *Fertil Steril.* 2004;81:231–241.
206. Lyytinen H, Pukkala E, Ylikorkala O. Breast cancer risk in post-menopausal women using estrogen-only therapy. *Obstet Gynecol.* 2006;108:1354–1360.
207. Beral V. Breast cancer and hormone-replacement therapy in the Million Women Study. *Lancet.* 2003;362:419–427.
208. Chasan-Taber L: Epidemiology of endogenous hormones and cancer. In: Nasca PC, Pastides H, eds. *Fundamentals of Cancer Epidemiology.* Sudbury, MA: Jones and Bartlett; 2007:389–408.
209. Bingham SA. Biomarkers in nutritional epidemiology. *Public Health Nutr.* 2002;5:821–827.
210. Arab L, Akbar J. Biomarkers and the measurement of fatty acids. *Public Health Nutr* 2002;5:865–871.

211. Vineis P, Perera F. Molecular epidemiology and biomarkers in etiologic cancer research: the new in light of the old. *Cancer Epidemiol Biomarkers Prev.* 2007;16:1954–1965.
212. Perera FP: Molecular epidemiology in cancer prevention. In: Schottenfeld D, Fraumeni JF, eds. *Cancer Epidemiology and Prevention.* 3rd ed. New York: Oxford University Press; 2006:101–115.
213. DevCan. Probability of Developing or Dying of Cancer Software, Version 6.3.0 Statistical Research and Application Branch, National Cancer Institute, 2008. srab.cancer.gov/devcan.
214. American Cancer Society: *Cancer Facts and Figures 2009.* Atlanta, GA: American Cancer Society; 2009. http://www.cancer.org/download/STT/500809web.pdf. Accessed January 1, 2010.
215. Zheng W: Epidemiological studies of genetic factors for cancer. In: Nasca PC, Pastides H, eds. *Fundamentals of Cancer Epidemiology.* Sudbury, MA: Jones and Bartlett; 2007:136–153.
216. National Human Genome Research Institute. The Cancer Genome Atlas. *J Natl Cancer Inst.* http://cancergenome.nih.gov/. Accessed January 1, 2010.
217. Ries LAG, Melbert D, Krapcho M, et al. (eds). SEER Cancer Statistics Review, 1975–2005. Bethesda, MD: National Cancer Institute; 2008. http://www.seer.cancer.gov/csr/1975_2005. Accessed January 1, 2010.
218. Chu KC, Miller BA, Springfield SA. Measures of racial/ethnic health disparities in cancer mortality rates and the influence of socioeconomic status. *J Natl Med Assoc.* 2007;99:1092–1094.
219. Singh GK, Miller BA, Hankey BF. *Area Socioeconomic Variation in US Cancer Incidence, Mortality, Stage, Treatment, and Survival, 1975–1999.* NCI cancer surveillance monograph series, NIH Publication No. 03–5417. Bethesda, MD: National Cancer Institute; 2003.
220. Baik I, Lambe M, Liu Q, et al. Birth spacing and maternal risk of invasive epithelial ovarian cancer in a Swedish nationwide cohort. *Cancer Causes Control.* 2008;*19:1131–1137.*
221. Setiawan VW, Pike MC, Kolonel LN, Nomura AM, Goodman MT, Henderson BE. Racial/ethnic differences in endometrial cancer risk: the multiethnic cohort study. *Am J Epidemiol.* 2007;165:262–270.
222. Gao YT, Shu XO, Dai Q, et al. Association of menstrual and reproductive factors with breast cancer risk: results from the Shanghai Breast Cancer Study. *Int J Cancer.* 2000;87:295–300.
223. Whiteman DC, Siskind V, Purdie DM, Green AC. Timing of pregnancy and the risk of epithelial ovarian cancer. *Cancer Epidemiol Biomarkers Prev.* 2003;12:42–46.
224. Tung KH, Goodman MT, Wu AH, et al. Reproductive factors and epithelial ovarian cancer risk by histologic type: a multiethnic case-control study. *Am J Epidemiol.* 2003;158:629–638.
225. Wise LA, Palmer JR, Harlow BL, et al. Reproductive factors, hormonal contraception, and risk of uterine leiomyomata in African-American women: a prospective study. *Am J Epidemiol.* 2004;159:113–123.
226. Castellsague X. Natural history and epidemiology of HPV infection and cervical cancer. *Gynecol Oncol.* 2008;110:S4-S7.
227. Belinson S, Smith JS, Myers E, et al. Descriptive evidence that risk profiles for cervical intraepithelial neoplasia 1, 2, and 3 are unique. *Cancer Epidemiol Biomarkers Prev.* 2008;17:2350–2355.
228. Schernhammer ES, Schulmeister K. Melatonin and cancer risk: does light at night compromise physiologic cancer protection by lowering serum melatonin levels? *Br J Cancer.* 2004;90:941–943.
229. Kuhlman SJ, Mackey SR, Duffy JF. Biological Rhythms Workshop I: introduction to chronobiology. *Cold Spring Harb Symp Quant Biol.* 2007;72:1–6.
230. Ackermann K, Stehle JH. Melatonin synthesis in the human pineal gland: advantages, implications, and difficulties. *Chronobiol Int.* 2006;23:369–379.
231. Zeitzer JM, Dijk DJ, Kronauer R, Brown E, Czeisler C. Sensitivity of the human circadian pacemaker to nocturnal light: melatonin phase resetting and suppression. *J Physiol.* 2000;526(Pt 3):695–702.
232. Vijayalaxmi, Thomas CR, Jr., Reiter RJ, Herman TS. Melatonin: from basic research to cancer treatment clinics. *J Clin Oncol.* 2002;20:2575–2601.
233. Lissoni P, Rovelli F, Brivio F, Fumagalli L, Brera G. A study of immunoendocrine strategies with pineal indoles and interleukin-2 to prevent radiotherapy-induced lymphocytopenia in cancer patients. *In Vivo.* 2008;22:397–400.
234. Blask DE, Sauer LA, Dauchy RT. Melatonin as a chronobiotic/anticancer agent: cellular, biochemical, and molecular mechanisms of action and their implications for circadian-based cancer therapy. *Curr Top Med Chem.* 2002;2:113–132.
235. Haus E, Smolensky M. Biological clocks and shift work: circadian dysregulation and potential long-term effects. *Cancer Causes Control.* 2006;17:489–500.
236. Jasser SA, Blask DE, Brainard GC. Light during darkness and cancer: relationships in circadian photoreception and tumor biology. *Cancer Causes Control.* 2006;17:515–523.
237. Stevens RG, Davis S. The melatonin hypothesis: electric power and breast cancer. *Environ Health Perspect.* 1996;104(suppl 1):135–140.
238. Cos S, Gonzalez A, Martinez-Campa C, Mediavilla MD, onso-Gonzalez C, Sanchez-Barcelo EJ. Estrogen-signaling pathway: a link between breast cancer and melatonin oncostatic actions. *Cancer Detect Prev.* 2006;30:118–128.
239. Davis S, Mirick DK, Stevens RG. Night shift work, light at night, and risk of breast cancer. *J Natl Cancer Inst.* 2001;93:1557–1562.
240. Hansen J. Increased breast cancer risk among women who work predominantly at night. *Epidemiology.* 2001;12:74–77.
241. Rafnsson V, Tulinius H, Jonasson JG, Hrafnkelsson J. Risk of breast cancer in female flight attendants: a population-based study (Iceland). *Cancer Causes Control.* 2001;12:95–101.
242. O'Leary ES, Schoenfeld ER, Stevens RG, et al. Shift work, light at night, and breast cancer on Long Island, New York. *Am J Epidemiol.* 2006;164:358–366.
243. Schernhammer ES, Laden F, Speizer FE, et al. Rotating night shifts and risk of breast cancer in women participating in the nurses' health study. *J Natl Cancer Inst.* 2001;93:1563–1568.
244. Pukkala E, Ojamo M, Rudanko SL, Stevens RG, Verkasalo PK. Does incidence of breast cancer and prostate cancer decrease with increasing degree of visual impairment. *Cancer Causes Control.* 2006;17:573–576.
245. Verkasalo PK, Lillberg K, Stevens RG, et al. Sleep duration and breast cancer: a prospective cohort study. *Cancer Res.* 2005;65:9595–9600.
246. Kliukiene J, Tynes T, Andersen A. Risk of breast cancer among Norwegian women with visual impairment. *Br J Cancer.* 2001;84:397–399.
247. Schernhammer ES, Hankinson SE. Urinary melatonin levels and breast cancer risk. *J Natl Cancer Inst.* 2005;20;97:1084–1087.
248. Straif K, Baan R, Grosse Y, et al. Carcinogenicity of shift-work, painting, and fire-fighting. *Lancet Oncol.* 2007; 8:1065–1066.
249. Blask DE, Brainard GC, Dauchy RT, et al. Melatonin-depleted blood from premenopausal women exposed to light at night stimulates growth of human breast cancer xenografts in nude rats. *Cancer Res.* 2005;65:11174–11184.
250. Stevens RG. Artificial lighting in the industrialized world: circadian disruption and breast cancer. *Cancer Causes Control.* 2006;17:501–507.
251. Kubo T, Ozasa K, Mikami K, et al. Prospective cohort study of the risk of prostate cancer among rotating-shift workers: findings from the Japan collaborative cohort study. *Am J Epidemiol.* 2006;164:549–555.
252. Caplan LS, Schoenfeld ER, O'Leary ES, Leske MC. Breast cancer and electromagnetic fields—a review. *Ann Epidemiol.* 2000;10:31–44.
253. Viswanathan AN, Hankinson SE, Schernhammer ES. Night shift work and the risk of endometrial cancer. *Cancer Res.* 2007;67:10618–10622.
254. Schernhammer ES, Laden F, Speizer FE, et al. Night-shift work and risk of colorectal cancer in the nurses' health study. *J Natl Cancer Inst.* 2003;95:825–828.
255. Travis RC, Allen DS, Fentiman IS, Key TJ. Melatonin and breast cancer: a prospective study. *J Natl Cancer Inst.* 2004;96:475–482.

256. Schernhammer ES, Berrino F, Krogh V, et al. Urinary 6-sulfatoxymelatonin levels and risk of breast cancer in postmenopausal women. *J Natl Cancer Inst.* 2008;100:898–905.
257. Srinivasan V, Spence DW, Pandi-Perumal SR, et al. Melatonin, environmental light, and breast cancer. *Breast Cancer Res Treat.* 2008;108:339–350.
258. Lillberg K, Verkasalo PK, Kaprio J, Teppo L, Helenius H, Koskenvuo M. Stressful life events and risk of breast cancer in 10,808 women: a cohort study. *Am J Epidemiol.* 2003;157:415–423.
259. Price MA, Tennant CC, Smith RC, et al. The role of psychosocial factors in the development of breast carcinoma: Part I. The cancer prone personality. *Cancer.* 2001;91:679–685.
260. Antoni MH, Lutgendorf SK, Cole SW, et al. The influence of biobehavioural factors on tumour biology: pathways and mechanisms. *Nat Rev Cancer.* 2006;6:240–248.
261. Reiche EM, Nunes SO, Morimoto HK. Stress, depression, the immune system, and cancer. *Lancet Oncol.* 2004;5:617–625.
262. Allison PJ, Guichard C, Fung K, Gilain L. Dispositional optimism predicts survival status 1 year after diagnosis in head and neck cancer patients. *J Clin Oncol.* 2003;21:543–548.
263. Sood AK, Bhatty R, Kamat AA, et al. Stress hormone-mediated invasion of ovarian cancer cells. *Clin Cancer Res.* 2006;12:369–375.
264. Smith JE, Richardson J, Hoffman C, Pilkington K. Mindfulness-Based Stress Reduction as supportive therapy in cancer care: systematic review. *J Adv Nurs.* 2005;52:315–327.
265. Shapiro SL, Bootzin RR, Figueredo AJ, Lopez AM, Schwartz GE. The efficacy of mindfulness-based stress reduction in the treatment of sleep disturbance in women with breast cancer: an exploratory study. *J Psychosom Res.* 2003;54:85–91.
266. Stefanek M, McDonald PG. *Handbook of Cancer Control and Behavioral Science: A Resource for Researchers, Practitioners, and Policy Makers.* Washington, DC: American Psychological Association; 2008.
267. Spiegel D, Giese-Davis J. Depression and cancer: mechanisms and disease progression. *Biol Psychiatry.* 2003;54:269–282.
268. Gotay CC. Behavior and cancer prevention. *J Clin Oncol.* 2005;23:301–310.
269. Mahon SM: Overview: II. Cancer prevention. In: Jennings-Dozier K, Mahon SM, eds. *Cancer Prevention, Detection and Control: A Nursing Perspective.* Pittsburgh, PA: Oncology Nursing Press; 2002.
270. Mahon SM: Overview: Section III. Cancer detection. In: Jennings-Dozier K, Mahon SM, eds. *Cancer Prevention, Detection and Control: A Nursing Perspective.* Pittsburgh, PA: Oncology Nursing Press; 2002.

# PART II

# Prevention, Detection, and Diagnosis

CHAPTER 4

*Joanne K. Itano, RN, PhD, APRN*

# Cultural Diversity Among Individuals With Cancer

## INTRODUCTION

Culture is described as the thoughts, communications, actions, customs, beliefs, values, and institutions of racial, ethnic, religious, or social groups. Culture has an impact on what is considered a health problem, how symptoms and concerns about a health problem are expressed, who should provide the treatment, what type of treatment is acceptable, and influences communication with the healthcare provider. Culture is central to the delivery of effective health care. Health care that is respectful and responsive to the health beliefs, practices, and cultural and linguistic needs of diverse patients will bring about positive health outcomes. With the growing ethnic diversity of the US population, it is essential that nurses have an understanding of cultural diversity and become culturally competent in the delivery of cancer care.[1]

### OVERVIEW

Historically, the United States has taken pride in its "melting pot," or multicultural composition of peoples from many nations. Until recently, this cultural diversity was largely limited to Caucasian immigrants from Europe, who represented the majority of the population. In the 20th century, immigration from areas such as Southeast Asia, China, Japan, Korea, the Philippines, Mexico, and the Caribbean began rapidly redefining the population composition of the United States. Projections by the US Census Bureau predict that by the year 2050, the US population will include the following distribution: Caucasian, 72.1%; Hispanic (of any race), 24.4%; African American, 14.6%; Asian, 8.0%. These projections reflect a steady decrease in the Caucasian population, from 81% of the total population in 2000 to a projected 72.1% in 2050, as compared to steady growth in the minority populations.[2] In addition, ethnic minority populations are not distributed uniformly across the United States. For example, over half (51%) of the Asians live in three states, California, New York, and Hawaii.[3]

Unfortunately, this trend of increased ethnic diversity in the US population is not matched in the composition of healthcare professionals. The percent of minority nurses reported in 2004 was 10.7%. The diversity of the RN population is far lower than that of the US population.[4] In 2004, the distribution of RNs by ethnicity (minority population is reported in the parentheses) is Hispanic or Latino with any race specified, 1.7% (13.7%); African American (non-Hispanic), 4.2% (12.2%); Asian, Native Hawaiian, or other Pacific Islander (non-Hispanic), 3.1% (4.1%), and American Indian/Alaskan Native, 0.3% (0.7%).[4]

According to an Institute of Medicine (IOM) report,[5] evidence supports the importance of increasing racial and ethnic diversity among health professionals. Greater diversity is associated with improved access to care for ethnic minority patients, including higher patient satisfaction and improved patient-provider communication. Ethnic minority healthcare providers are more likely to serve minority and medically underserved communities.

A fundamental challenge for healthcare providers is that the healthcare beliefs and practices of many ethnic groups may be incongruent with mainstream, Westernized medicine. The use of traditional healers and folk medicine, for example, often plays a major role in the provision of holistic care for African Americans, Asian and Pacific Islanders (APIs), Hispanics, and American Indians/Alaskan Natives.

This chapter provides an introduction to culture and cancer and describes the potential for oncology nurses to have a positive impact on the cancer experience of individuals and their families from different ethnic minority groups. Specific cultural information and nursing considerations for 4 ethnic minority groups (African Americans, APIs, Hispanics, and American Indians/Alaskan Natives) are addressed. The information on these 4 ethnic minority groups is limited by several factors. Foremost is the diversity within each group. African Americans, APIs, Hispanics, and American Indians/Alaskan Natives are composed of several subgroups, each with its own subculture. For example, the subgroups under the term "Hispanic" include Mexican Americans, Puerto Ricans, Cuban Americans, and Central and South Americans. Added to the existence of subgroups and their unique cultures is the inherent heterogeneity due to intragroup differences, such as socioeconomic status, education attainment level, and degree of acculturation. Most important is the individual within the group. Although profiles of ethnic minority groups are provided in this chapter, each patient must be recognized as an individual with unique needs, regardless of his or her cultural background.

### EPIDEMIOLOGY

Comparison data among the 4 major ethnic groups indicate differences in cancer incidence and morality. For example, African Americans, on the whole, have higher cancer incidence and mortality rates than do Caucasians.[6] Age-adjusted incidence and mortality rates by ethnicity are presented in Table 4-1.[7,8] There is also a difference in 5-year survival rates, in that African American men and women, American Indian/Alaskan Native men and women, and API men have lower 5-year survival rates than non-Hispanic Caucasians.[9]

#### African Americans

African Americans include immigrants from the African countries, the West Indies, the Dominican Republic, Haiti,

**TABLE 4-1**

**Cancer Incidence and Death Rates[a] by Site, Race, and Ethnicity; United States, 2001–2005**

| | Caucasian | African American | Asian American and Pacific Islander | American Indian and Alaskan Native[b] | Hispanic/ Latino[c,d,e] |
|---|---|---|---|---|---|
| **Incidence** | | | | | |
| All sites | | | | | |
| Male | 551.4 | 651.5 | 354.0 | 336.6 | 419.4 |
| Female | 423.6 | 398.9 | 287.8 | 296.4 | 317.8 |
| Breast, female | 130.6 | 117.5 | 89.6 | 75.0 | 90.1 |
| Colon and rectum | | | | | |
| Male | 58.9 | 71.2 | 48.0 | 46.0 | 47.3 |
| Female | 43.2 | 54.5 | 35.4 | 41.2 | 32.8 |
| Kidney and renal pelvis | | | | | |
| Male | 18.8 | 21.3 | 9.1 | 19.5 | 17.4 |
| Female | 9.5 | 10.1 | 4.6 | 12.7 | 9.6 |
| Liver and bile duct | | | | | |
| Male | 8.2 | 13.2 | 21.7 | 14.4 | 15.0 |
| Female | 2.9 | 4.0 | 8.3 | 6.3 | 5.8 |
| Lung and bronchus | | | | | |
| Male | 79.3 | 107.6 | 53.9 | 54.3 | 44.2 |
| Female | 54.9 | 54.6 | 28.0 | 39.7 | 25.4 |
| Prostate | 156.7 | 248.5 | 93.8 | 73.3 | 138.0 |
| Stomach | | | | | |
| Male | 10.0 | 17.4 | 18.6 | 16.8 | 15.5 |
| Female | 4.7 | 8.9 | 10.5 | 7.7 | 9.5 |
| Uterine cervix | 8.2 | 10.8 | 8.0 | 6.9 | 13.2 |
| **Mortality** | | | | | |
| All sites | | | | | |
| Male | 230.7 | 313.0 | 138.8 | 190.0 | 159.0 |
| Female | 159.2 | 186.7 | 95.9 | 142.0 | 105.2 |
| Breast, female | 24.4 | 33.5 | 12.6 | 17.1 | 15.8 |
| Colon and rectum | | | | | |
| Male | 22.1 | 31.8 | 14.4 | 20.5 | 16.5 |
| Female | 15.3 | 22.4 | 10.2 | 14.2 | 10.8 |
| Kidney and renal pelvis | | | | | |
| Male | 6.2 | 6.1 | 2.4 | 9.3 | 5.3 |
| Female | 2.8 | 2.7 | 1.2 | 4.3 | 2.4 |
| Liver and bile duct | | | | | |
| Male | 6.7 | 10.3 | 15.2 | 10.6 | 11.1 |
| Female | 2.9 | 3.9 | 6.6 | 6.6 | 5.1 |
| Lung and bronchus | | | | | |
| Male | 71.3 | 93.1 | 37.5 | 50.2 | 35.1 |
| Female | 42.0 | 39.9 | 18.5 | 33.8 | 14.6 |
| Prostate | 24.6 | 59.4 | 11.0 | 21.1 | 20.6 |
| Stomach | | | | | |
| Male | 5.0 | 11.5 | 10.1 | 9.9 | 8.7 |
| Female | 2.5 | 5.5 | 5.9 | 5.2 | 4.9 |
| Uterine cervix | 2.3 | 4.7 | 2.2 | 3.7 | 3.2 |

*Notes:*
[a]Per 100,000 population, age-adjusted to the 2000 US standard population.
[b]Data based on Contract Health Service Delivery Areas, 624 counties comprising 54% of the US American Indian/Alaskan Native population; for more information please see Espey DK et al.[7]
[c]Persons of Hispanic/Latino origin may be of any race.
[d]Data unavailable from the Alaska Native Registry and Kentucky.
[e]Data unavailable from Minnesota, New Hampshire, and North Dakota.
*Source:* Data from Ries et al[8].

and Jamaica and make up about 12% of the US population.[10] African American men have the highest overall cancer incidence rates. African Americans are more likely to die from cancer than any ethnic group. The death rate for cancer among African American men is about 37% higher than Caucasian males; for African American women, it is about 17% higher. Except for breast cancer and lung cancer incidence and death rates in women, and kidney cancer mortality rates in men, incidence and death rates for the most common cancer types are higher for African Americans than for any of the other ethnic minority groups. In addition, African Americans are less likely than Caucasians to survive 5 years after diagnosis for all sites and at all stages of diagnoses. This is likely due to diagnoses at a later stage of cancer than Caucasians, and socioeconomic factors such as access to medical care and level of education.[10,11]

### Asian and Pacific Islanders

Asian and Pacific Islanders were combined as one group until the 2000 census, which designated the Native Hawaiian and other Pacific Islanders as a separate group.[12] Asian refers to people having origins in any of the original peoples of the Far East, Southeast Asia, or the Indian subcontinent including China, Cambodia, India, Philippines, Korea, Japan, Vietnam, Laos, Thailand, Malaysia, and Pakistan. This group makes up 3.8% of the US population. More than half of all US Asians live in the western United States.[4,13]

Native Hawaiians and other Pacific Islanders refers to people having origins in any of the original peoples of Hawaii, Guam, Samoa, and other Pacific Islands (Tahitian, Northern Mariana Islander, Palauan, Fijian, or cultural groups such as Melanesian, Micronesian, or Polynesian). This group makes up 0.3% of the US population.[14]

Asian Pacific Islanders are fourth in cancer incidence, behind African Americans, Caucasians, and Hispanics, and have the lowest mortality rate compared to African Americans, Caucasians, Hispanics, and American Indians/Alaskan Natives. However, given the diversity of the group, differences in incidence and mortality rates are noted among the various subgroups of the diverse API group. For example, McCraken et al[15] reported that in California, which has the largest Asian American population of any state, Chinese Americans had the lowest incidence and death rates from all cancers combined but Chinese women had the highest lung cancer death rate. Filipinos had the highest incidence and death rate from prostate cancer and the highest death rate from female breast cancer. Vietnamese had among the highest incidence and death rates from liver, lung, and cervical cancer; and Korean men and women had the highest incidence and death rate from stomach cancer, while the Japanese had the highest incidence and death rate from colorectal cancer and among the highest death rates from breast and prostate cancer.[15]

### Hispanics

Hispanics or Latinos constitute a heterogeneous group who trace their ancestry from Mexico, Puerto Rico, Cuba, and other countries in Central and South America or other Spanish cultures. They make up about 13.7% of the US population and are the nation's fastest-growing minority group.[4] Cancer occurrence and risk factors vary among Hispanics based on their status as US or foreign born, their country of origin or heritage, their degree of acculturation, and their socioeconomic status. Hispanics have a lower incidence and mortality for all cancers combined and for the 4 most common cancers (breast, prostate, lung and bronchus, and colon and rectum) compared to non-Hispanic Caucasians. Conversely, they demonstrate higher incidence and mortality rates from cancers of the stomach, liver, cervix, gallbladder, and acute lymphocytic leukemia than non-Hispanic Caucasians.[16]

### American Indians/Alaskan Natives

The American Indian/Alaskan Native group includes people who have ancestors belonging to any of the original peoples of North, Central, and South America, and who maintain tribal affiliation or community attachment. In 2004, 0.7% of the US population was reported to be Alaskan Native or American Indian. This group generally has lower cancer rates than the non-Hispanic Caucasian population. Men and women in this group have higher incidence of liver and intrabiliary duct cancers. The men have a higher incidence and mortality of stomach cancers and women have a higher incidence of kidney cancer.[4,17]

## ETHNICITY AND CANCER

This section explores how ethnicity affects responses to the cancer experience. For each of the 4 major ethnic groups, information about health beliefs and practices, healing practices, social organization, communication, space and time, death and dying, and biologic variations is presented. Note that this information provides only a guideline for practice; each person is culturally unique. Nursing interventions that consider the patient and the family's cultural background must be based on a sound assessment and validation of the role that culture plays in the life of both patient and family.

Many subgroups exist within the 4 major ethnic groups (African American, API, Hispanic, and American Indian/Alaskan Native); however, it is beyond the scope of this chapter to provide an in-depth description of each subgroup's cultural beliefs and practices. Instead, relevant group characteristics regarding the cancer experience are presented. Various sources are available that further explore the individual subgroups.[18–23]

## AFRICAN AMERICANS

Most African Americans' ancestors were brought to the United States as slaves between 1619 and 1860 from the west coast of Africa. African Americans have also immigrated to the United States from other African countries, the West Indies, the Dominican Republic, Haiti, and Jamaica.[23] African Americans comprise about 12% of the total US population but are disproportionately represented among the poor. They account for about 24.1% of the population below the poverty level, and 19.2% are medically uninsured compared to 11.9% of Caucasians. Individuals in a lower socioeconomic group are generally at greater risk for illness, because seeking health care for early symptoms and preventive care generally are not priorities for those who struggle with day-to-day survival.[24]

### Health beliefs and practices

The health beliefs of African Americans include a tendency to categorize events as either desirable or undesirable. Illness is just another undesirable event, along with bad luck, poverty, and unemployment. Some believe illness results from their failure to live according to or to accept God's will. An individual may believe that cancer is an unnatural illness, caused by supernatural or sinful behavior, and that it cannot be treated by Western medicine.[21]

For many African Americans, a strong relationship exists between faith and healing. All blessings come from God, and only God can heal the sick. Illness may be perceived as a natural occurrence resulting from disharmony and conflict in some aspect of an individual's life, generally falling into 1 of the 3 main areas: divine punishment, impaired social relationships, and environmental hazards. Divine punishment attributes illness to sin. An example of an impaired social relationship may be a spouse leaving or parents disowning a child. Environmental hazards include being struck by lightning or bitten by a snake.[20]

Another belief among some African Americans is that everything has an opposite. For every birth, there is a death; for every marriage, there is a divorce. Some may not distinguish between physical and mental illness and spiritual problems and may, therefore, present for treatment with a combination of somatic, psychological, and spiritual complaints. The nurse must acknowledge the patient's health belief system if he or she expects the patient to participate in Western practices. Some African Americans may respond to pain stoically out of a desire to be a perfect patient; others may view pain as God's will.[20]

African Americans tend to be less knowledgeable about cancer than Caucasians. They are less likely to see a physician when experiencing warning signs or symptoms and are less aware of the benefits of specific cancer screening methods. African Americans are often more fatalistic about cancer and are less likely to believe that early detection or treatment can make a difference in the outcome of the disease. These factors lead to diagnosis at a later stage of illness, a poorer prognosis, and higher mortality rates for cancer.[25]

African Americans are more likely than Caucasians to prefer to remain ignorant of their own cancer diagnosis. They are also less likely than Caucasians to regard surgery, chemotherapy, and radiation as effective cancer treatment measures and are less optimistic about the chances of surviving cancer. In one study, 64% of African Americans believed that cancer was a death sentence, and 65% believed that cancer treatment is worse than the disease. About 80% believed that cancer was spread by surgical treatment, and 20% indicated that they would rather not know that they had cancer.[26] Thus, nurses may find African American patients unwilling, uncooperative, or apparently noncompliant partners in their treatment.

Attitudes of the African American about the US healthcare system may be explained partially by history. During slavery, African Americans received inconsistent and often barbaric healthcare treatment and developed a deep mistrust of their Caucasian masters and their harsh remedies and prescriptions. Even after slavery was abolished, African Americans often received poor health care and inferior treatment in hospitals and clinics, which merely served to reinforce their negative view of Western medicine, and led to a high level of caution and mistrust.[27] African Americans may choose not to seek care if they perceive that their values will be compromised. To work effectively with African American patients and families, the nurse will need to convey caring and understanding.

### Healing practices

Different folk healers are used by some African Americans. These healers are well-respected individuals and can be powerful resources for the healthcare team. They understand the beliefs and needs of the people they serve. Symptoms may be of minor importance. Cure may involve self-treatment or consultation with a neighbor knowledgeable in home remedies, a physician, or someone regarded to have unusual powers. Often, religion is incorporated as part of therapy. A lay-referral system typically services the health needs of the community and determines whether Western practitioners can be trusted and incorporated into the treatment. Openness, acceptance, and cooperation with this referral system by healthcare professionals may enhance acceptance and use of Western healthcare providers by African Americans.[20]

Help may be sought from an "old lady," a woman in the community who acts as a local consultant. She is knowledgeable about home remedies made from spices, herbs, and roots used to treat common illnesses. She also gives advice and makes appropriate referrals to another type of practitioner when an illness or a particular medical condition extends beyond her practice. The spiritualist is considered to have received the gift from God for healing incurable diseases or solving personal problems. This practitioner combines rituals, spiritual beliefs, and herbal medicines, and is the most prevalent and diverse type of folk practitioner. A root doctor may also meet the needs for herbs, oils, candles, and ointments. The Voodoo priest/priestess may inherit this title only by birthright and is perceived to have a special gift. Voodoo, which combines African, Christian, and magical beliefs related to religion and health care, is practiced by some African Americans. It is believed to cause, as well as prevent, the action of malevolent forces. Awareness of which home remedies have been used would help the nurse understand cultural practices and determine whether the remedies are helpful, harmful, or neutral.[20]

A treatment plan that is congruent with the patient's own beliefs has a better chance of being successful. Cultural health practices that are helpful should be encouraged. For example, use of herbal teas in place of water can serve both traditional and Western practices.

## Social organization

The history of slavery likely contributes to the large number of female-headed households among African Americans today. In 2004, 29.1% of African American women were reported as heads of households (compared to 16.4% of Hispanics, 9% of non-Hispanic Caucasians, and 7.2% of Asians).[28] The woman of the family is generally charged with the responsibility for protecting the health of family members. Family members may enter the healthcare system at the advice of the matriarch of the family. The importance of the African American woman in sharing information and helping the patient in decision making is important for the nurse to recognize.[20]

Some families have large social networks that can prove very supportive during times of illness. The added numbers may be helpful in provision of care and support but also may delay seeking help outside the network while consultation among the various members takes place. Including the members of the network in planning care may decrease the possibility of conflicting messages being given by the nurse and members of the network.[20]

The church plays an important role in the lives of many African Americans by championing their interests and providing tangible assistance during periods of economic and social instability. The church is also a source of social identity and allows escape from the harsh realities of life. It promotes self-esteem among its membership and serves as a curator for maintaining the cultures of many African Americans. Given the importance of the church in the lives of many African Americans, inclusion of the clergy in the healthcare team may be very helpful.[20]

## Communication

The dialect that is spoken by many African Americans is sufficiently different from Standard English in pronunciation, grammar, and syntax as to be classified as "African American English." The use of Standard English vs African American English varies among African Americans and is sometimes related to educational level and socioeconomic status. African American English is a unifying factor for African Americans in maintaining their cultural and ethnic identity. It is not uncommon for some African Americans to speak Standard English when in a professional capacity or when socializing with Caucasians and then revert to African American English when in African American settings. Some African Americans who have not mastered Standard English may become very quiet in settings in which they believe that Standard English is required. This may be incorrectly interpreted as hostility, submissiveness, or agreement.[20]

For more effective communication, the nurse who works with African Americans must understand as much of the context of the dialect as possible. Viewing African American English as an unacceptable form of the English language may lead to labeling and stereotyping of the patient. Chiding and correcting the speech of African Americans may result in the patient becoming quiet, passive, aggressive, or hostile. Conversely, attempting to use words common to the patient's vocabulary and mimicking the language may be interpreted as dehumanizing.

Slang also is used and may have different meanings among individuals and among cultural groups. Using words commonly understood by African Americans in place of more sophisticated medical terms might make the patient more receptive to teaching and more cooperative. Examples of such words include "miseries" for pain, "tired or low blood" for anemia, "throw up" for vomit, and "pass water," "tinkle," or "peepee" for urinate.

When working with African American patients, keep in mind that eye contact, nodding, and smiling do not necessarily mean that the African American patient is paying attention. Validation of the message is very important in improving communication. Nurses may find it difficult to communicate with African American patients who speak loudly and seem hostile and aggressive. However, it is the expressive quality of African American English that is often responsible for this behavior.[29]

## Space and time

Many African Americans have a "today" or "present" health orientation, and their approach to the prevention of cancer may be to work out problems as they occur, rather than trying to prevent them from occurring. This approach is based on the belief that planning for the future is hopeless and may reflect previous experiences with racism and discrimination. In planning nursing care for individuals with such a time orientation, explain when flexibility of time is acceptable and when a delay might result in a serious problem. Acceptance of lateness in appointments is helpful when possible.[20]

Many African Americans are highly involved people who tend to have several activities going on at the same time. This may create conflict for the nurse, who, in an effort to complete nursing care, often may be interrupted by these activities. Negotiating with the patient and family to meet the needs of both the nurse and the patient may prove helpful.

### Death and dying issues

In the African language, the primary time frames are past and present. No word exists for the distant future, as it has not yet happened. Consequently, the future and the past merge into the present. Life is viewed as cyclical in nature, and all events are given by God. Death is a natural part of the cycle of life and is unavoidable. It is familiar and near and evokes no great fear or awe.[30]

The strong family network of African Americans may be called into action when a family member is seriously ill. Care of the terminally ill is a public rather than a private undertaking, with neighbors and friends sharing resources. The family develops plans for the care of the patient, identifies tasks, and assigns family members to assume them. The home is usually viewed as the place for the ill person to spend his or her final days. Frequent visitors are common. The patient generally remains an active and vital force within the family until he or she can no longer do so. The decision as to whether to inform the patient of terminal illness is made on an individual basis.[30]

It is not uncommon for African Americans to plan their funerals and purchase grave plots long before their own deaths. Public and communal grief are openly expressed at traditional African American funerals, which are termed "home-goings." People in the congregation often respond spontaneously and out loud to the sermon. A gradual increase in emotion occurs as the funeral progresses, and many of those attending express deep emotion. Music provides a means of sending the deceased joyfully on to the next leg of his or her journey.[30]

### Biological variations

A major biological variation in African Americans relates to skin color. In other words, there is great variation in the darkness of skin color, and individuals who are fairer-skinned have a greater risk for developing skin cancers from sun exposure. A darker skin color makes the assessment of pallor, jaundice, ecchymosis, or erythema more difficult. Assessing areas of lighter melanin pigmentation such as the sclera, conjunctiva, soles of feet, and palms of the hands may be useful.

The diet of many African Americans contains little fresh produce, is highly seasoned, and includes frequent use of smoked and fatty meats as seasoning for vegetables and soups. Pork is often a staple meat. As a consequence, saturated fat intake may be high. In comparison to Caucasian women, African American women are more likely to be obese, while African American men are more likely to be underweight. The eating habits and compromised nutritional status of African Americans could be a factor in their generally higher incidence and mortality rates from cancer.[25]

Lactose intolerance affects 75% of African Americans. Affected individuals lack the enzyme to convert lactose to glucose and galactose, resulting in gastrointestinal symptoms of bloating, cramping, and diarrhea after the ingestion of milk and other products containing lactose. The intolerance tends to occur primarily in infancy shortly after weaning and in the teen years or early 20s. Treatment is to avoid milk products. As milk products are often suggested to improve nutrition for patients with cancer, awareness of possible lactose intolerance in the African American population is significant for the nurse in patient and family teaching.[20]

Alcoholism is a major health problem in the African American community and a risk factor for cancers of the mouth, larynx, tongue, esophagus, lung, and liver.[19] Factors associated with alcohol abuse include unemployment, the availability of the substance, peer pressure, a desire to escape from personal problems, and the prevalence of taverns as social centers in African American communities. Thus the causes are complex social issues and difficult to treat.[20]

## ASIAN AND PACIFIC ISLANDERS

Asian and Pacific Islanders are a heterogeneous group, composed of groups who differ in language, culture, and length of residence in the United States. This marked ethnic diversity is further compounded by inherent variations within each subgroup, such as degree of acculturation and socioeconomic status. Asian and Pacific Islanders are more likely than non-Hispanic Caucasians to have earned a college degree but are also more likely to have less than a ninth grade education. In 2001, API families were more likely than non-Hispanic Caucasians to have incomes of $75,000 and also more likely to have incomes of less than $25,000.[13,14] Because the APIs are predominately Asian, this discussion primarily addresses Asian Americans.

### Health beliefs and practices

Many Asians share traditional health beliefs and practices that are carried out in varying degrees within each group. Nevertheless, because of the common influence of Chinese culture, much similarity in beliefs and practices is noted among Asian groups. For example, one of the most common beliefs is that health is a state of harmony in body, mind, and spirit with nature and the universe.[23]

Many Asians believe that a balance between hot and cold elements is essential for good health. In the Chinese, Japanese, and Korean cultures, in particular, this balance is defined as *yin* (cold) and *yang* (hot). *Yin* and *yang* are life forces in which *yin* (cold) is characterized as female, dark, negative energy, and *yang* (hot) is male, light, positive energy. Illness is believed to result from an imbalance of these two forces. The Chinese believe that the human body, illnesses, and foods possess *yin* or *yang* characteristics, and treatment is aimed at reestablishing the balance. For example, cancer is a *yin* or cold illness and would be treated with foods, herbs, and healing ceremonies that possess "hot" properties. The Filipino, East Indian, and Southeast Asian cultures share similar beliefs about hot and cold balance and health. Other explanations for illness include an imbalance of humoral elements, an obstruction of *chi* (an essential life energy), a curse by a spirit, spiritual imbalance, punishment for immoral behavior, or an imbalance in the body caused by exposure to wind or air.[20,21]

There exists a widespread belief among some Asian groups that suffering is part of life, a philosophy that may result in postponement in seeking medical treatment, either traditional or Western. Fatalism is found in the Filipino culture where the attitude of *bahala na*—"It's in the hands of God"—exists, especially when illness and pain are seen as punishment.[22] In the Japanese culture, the term *shoganai* is used when misfortune strikes, such as an illness. Its translation, "It can't be helped," reflects an almost fatalistic view. Chinese Americans also have a fatalistic outlook on life, exemplified by their belief that they lack control over nature.[20]

Many Asians believe that blood is a life force that cannot be replaced or, if taken, will disrupt the body's balance, causing weakness and even death. Therefore, many Asians fear venipunctures. Hmong patients may be reluctant to receive blood transfusions because their perception is that the donor's spirit may enter the body via the transfusion. Chinese and Vietnamese patients may not agree to surgery when organs or body parts are to be removed because of their belief that the human body must be intact at the time of death to avoid potential adverse consequences in the afterlife. Vietnamese individuals may also avoid surgery because it is perceived as a last resort and associated with death. Hmong patients may refuse surgery because of their belief that cutting into the body releases spirits, causing an imbalance.[20,22]

### Healing practices

As part of their traditional health beliefs, Asians use herbal medications, seek out traditional healers, and perform healing ceremonies. Because Asians often employ herbal preparations concurrently with Western medicine, it is important to ascertain if, and what, herbal preparations are being used to anticipate possible drug interactions. For example, *ma huang* is a Chinese herb that contains ephedrine. Complications can arise if, in addition to the *ma huang*, the patient takes ephedrine via a Western practitioner's prescription. Ginseng, another popular herb, is considered a stimulant and has hypertensive effects. Undesirable side effects can result if the patient takes ginseng in conjunction with Western antihypertensive medication.[22]

Traditional healers among Asians include shamans (Hmong), Chinese herbalists and acupuncturists, and *faith healers (hilot) or herbalist (herbolarios)* (Filipino). These healers are often consulted before Western medical practitioners. In some cases, the perceived cause of the illness determines who is consulted first. For example, if Southeast Asians believe that an illness is organic in origin, they may seek a Western physician. Conversely, if the cause of illness is thought to be supernatural, a traditional healer would be consulted. If the illness persists after consulting with traditional healers, then Western treatment might be sought. At this point, however, the disease may be at an advanced stage and untreatable. Because Western medicine sometimes cannot cure the illness, it is therefore seen as ineffective. This pattern may reinforce the use of traditional healers. For many Asians, the Western healthcare system is foreign. Greater comfort is found in consulting a healer who understands, with whom one can communicate, and whose practice is familiar to the patient. Additionally, healers are inexpensive and have a reputation for being effective for specific conditions.[21]

Healing ceremonies or practices vary considerably across Asian groups. Examples here include coining, moxibustion, and cupping.

***Moxibustion.*** This treatment, used to restore the yin–yang balance, involves a deeply penetrating heat. Small pellets or cones made of the herb *Artemesis vulgaris* (moxa) are placed at acupuncture points on the body and are then burned. The pellets or cones are removed when the patient feels the heat. This treatment leaves small, rounded, or asymmetrical superficial burn marks. It is used in the treatment of ailments of the joints, muscles, bones, and back.[22]

***Cupping.*** Like moxibustion, cupping uses heat but in a different fashion. A material, such as alcohol-soaked cotton, is placed in a special cup and set on fire to create a vacuum in the cup. When the flame is extinguished, the cup is then placed immediately on the treatment area of the body, where it creates suction. The cup is kept there for 15 to 20 minutes or until it is easily removed. Cupping is used to treat pain, body aches, and headaches. This painful procedure sometimes leaves circular burn marks approximately 2 inches in diameter. These burn marks have been misinterpreted as child abuse in Southeast Asian children who have been treated with cupping.[18]

*Skin scraping or coining.* This treatment involves the application of a special menthol oil or ointment to the symptomatic area using a coin. With the edge of a coin, the area is then rubbed in a firm, motion away from the body. This procedure is used to treat colds, heatstroke, headache, pain, vomiting, and indigestion.[20]

### Social organization

Asians tend to have very strong, family-centered systems. The family exerts an extremely powerful force in an individual's life, and the needs of the individual are often secondary to those of the larger group. Healthcare decisions are often made by the family or social network.[20]

In many Asian groups, patrilineal authority, along with filial piety and respect for elders, often means that the eldest son or male head of the clan acts as the spokesperson for the patient. This individual is the designated family member with whom medical practitioners speak when information about the patient's condition is given or when treatment decisions need to be made.[20]

Because of the strong emphasis placed on the family, Asian family members are more likely to participate actively in the patient's daily care. Healthcare professionals need to be sensitive to these cultural needs and must support the family to prevent caregiver exhaustion, especially if one family member is the sole caregiver.[20]

### Communication

In many Asian groups, communication patterns are influenced by values that emphasize politeness, respect for authority, and avoidance of shame. These values prevent many Asians from asking health professionals questions or challenging a proposed diagnostic workup or treatment plan. Instead, an individual may nod his or her head, in what is interpreted as agreement. In reality, the patient may not necessarily agree or understand what the practitioner has said. Thus poor communication can occur between the Asian patient and the Western practitioner.[20]

In communicating with members of some Asian groups, Western practitioners may need to avoid or limit engaging in direct eye contact, as such eye contact may be perceived as being rude, challenging, or just culturally unacceptable. For example, in the Filipino culture, direct eye contact between an older man and a young woman usually implies seduction or anger. In the East Indian culture, eye contact between a woman and a man other than her husband can have sexual significance. Avoiding eye contact by the South Vietnamese is a sign of respect when talking with someone perceived to be of different rank in education, social status, age, or gender.[20]

Many Asians prefer limited or no physical contact. In some API groups, the head is sacred and touching or patting the head is perceived as a rude gesture. For some Southeast Asians, crossing the legs and pointing the foot at the individual is also considered to be insulting. Similarly, directing the sole of the shoe or foot toward Koreans is considered offensive.[20]

Many Asians do not speak English or have limited proficiency in English as their second language. Because of this language barrier, interpreters are often used. Such communication via a third party presents challenges in ensuring that the literal meaning of the conversation is translated correctly, along with the interpretation of nonverbal messages. When possible, use professional interpreters who can facilitate and ensure communication among the patient, family, and health professional.[30]

In selecting an interpreter, first ascertain the specific dialect spoken by the patient and family. For example, several dialects are spoken by Filipinos, including Visayan, Waray, Ilocano, Bicolano, Pampango, and Ibanag. Family interpreters are often used; however, the message relayed may not always be accurate. For example, if the message delivers a poor prognosis, the family member may modify it in an attempt to protect the patient. In addition, if interpreters are of the opposite sex, patients may not bring up symptoms or concerns that they perceive to be either embarrassing or culturally unacceptable to discuss in the presence of a member of the opposite sex. The traditional hierarchy in many Asian families where power and influence run from elders to youths represents another potential pitfall when using family interpreters. In some instances, especially with recent immigrants, children may be used as interpreters because they usually have a better command of English. This practice reverses the rank of the child in the family and may put undue stress on the family.[21,30]

### Space and time

Asians value privacy, and many are very modest. When physical examinations or procedures necessitate exposure of the body, it should be minimized by revealing only that part of the body that needs to be examined. Female Asian patients, such as East Indian and Chinese women, may feel more comfortable being examined by female practitioners.[21]

The concept of time varies among Asian groups. For example, Japanese patients, who are present and future oriented, are usually prompt and adhere to fixed schedules. By contrast, Chinese are more present oriented, do not necessarily adhere to fixed schedules, and may be late for appointments. Filipinos are past and present oriented and may disregard health-related matters. This time orientation is closely linked to their *bahala na* philosophy of leaving things in God's hands.[20]

### Death and dying issues

Many issues arise regarding death and dying in Asian groups. Bioethics, truth telling, the patient's right to know, and advance directive decisions are based in the tenets espoused by Western culture. It is important to be aware that patient autonomy and self-determination in Asian groups may not be culturally acceptable or valued. As discussed previously, the family or family spokesperson frequently makes decisions about the patient's care, rather than the patient.

Conflict may arise between the value in Western medicine of open disclosure of a terminal illness and the value shared by many Asian groups that "to tell someone he or she is dying is not only rude but dangerous."[31] For example, East Indians prefer not to tell patients about the seriousness of their condition or to reveal the possibility of death. They believe that "speaking of possibilities may render them too real, and a traditional Indian does not speak lightly of death;...if a patient knows the gravity of the illness, he or she will give up hope and die."[32,p.269] This concept is also seen in the Hmong culture, where the disclosure of prognosis to a terminally ill patient "is the same as wishing death upon that person and may in fact bring about that person's death."[33] Muller and Desmond further note that in many Asian groups,

> People fear that openly acknowledging an impending death is like casting a death curse upon the person; it will make the person despair and die even sooner. Thus, to engage in discussions of code status or the possibility of hospice care, interventions that can be seen as explicit preparation for death, is courting bad luck.[31,p.325]

On the other hand, although hospice care discussions may not always be encouraged, some Asians prefer to die at home rather than in the hospital. This preference is due, in large part, to the value placed on the family and

> The belief that the unfortunate who die among strangers and away from their familiar dwelling are forever condemned to wander in pain, so-called orphan souls, endlessly searching in vain for the family and home they missed when they died.[34,p.24]

Given the potential for conflict and frustration between the values of Western health care and the cultural values of various Asian groups, exploring life-support decisions with the patient and family is critical. Klessig suggests that information about the following be determined: sanctity of life, definition of death, religious background and extent of involvement, beliefs about causal agents in illness and how they relate to the dying process, social support system, and the family's decision maker.[35]

By facilitating communication about these issues between the patient, his or her family, and the healthcare team, oncology nurses can assist in narrowing the gap between these 2 value systems and support the patient and family through this phase of the cancer experience.

### Biological variations

The incidence rate for liver cancer is exceptionally high in Asian groups, particularly among the Southeast Asian groups. This increased rate is linked to the high incidence of hepatitis B infection, largely due to the fact that these groups originate from areas where hepatitis B is endemic.[36]

Lactose intolerance is also common in Asians. Milk and cheese—common foods in the mainstream American diet—may therefore be unacceptable to this group. When providing oral supplements that do not contain milk but have the appearance of a milk product, the patient and his or her family must be reassured that the supplement is not a milk product.[20]

Many Asians also have a distinguishing yellow cast to their skin that ranges in tone. This yellow cast can make the recognition of jaundice more challenging. To assess for jaundice, the sclera and excreta need to be checked.[20]

Although not a biological variation, the higher smoking rates among Southeast Asian men as compared to the general population deserve mention.[37] This is a prime area for health promotion activities. Another area of concern is that Asians had the lowest self-reported rates for Pap tests within the past 3 years. Possible reasons for this low participation rate include lack of health education programs targeted specifically at this group, fatalism belief, and decreased access to health care.[24]

## HISPANICS

Hispanics, in general, identify themselves as members of the same ethnic group—not by demographic characteristics but by their cultural values and language. *Hispanic* and Latino are used interchangeably in census 2000 and refer to people who were born in or whose ancestors came from Mexico, Puerto Rico, Cuba, Central and South America, Spain, and other Spanish-speaking communities. Whether an individual prefers to be called Hispanic or Latino is generally a matter of choice. Some have strong opinions; others do not. It may be helpful to use the name of the country of origin when referring to individuals or to a specific ethnic group.[20]

Generally, the cancer incidence and mortality rates among Hispanics rank at the median when compared to the rates among other ethnic groups.[24]

### Health beliefs and practices

For Hispanics, health often is believed to be the result of good luck or a reward from God for good behavior. The concept that a disease is God's will is widely accepted. Terminal illnesses especially are seen as the result of some indiscretion against God. Thus, health and illness in Hispanic groups have a strong religious association.

In many cases, Hispanics espouse a fatalistic belief that one is at the mercy of the environment and has little control over what happens. Personal efforts are unlikely to influence the outcome of a situation. For this reason, Hispanics often do not believe that they are personally responsible for present or future successes or failures with regard to their health and otherwise.[20]

Several categories of disease exist in the Hispanic culture. The concept of hot and cold imbalance resembles *yin* and *yang* in the Chinese culture. To ensure good health, it is believed that individuals must ingest both hot and cold foods.[23] Internal factors such as a change in body temperature and external factors such as the foods eaten can affect the hot–cold balance. Many of the disorders caused by hot and cold imbalances are digestive in nature. A stomach ulcer is a "hot illness" caused by eating too much hot food. Excesses of heat developed from within the body and extending outward are believed to be related to cancer, rheumatism, tuberculosis, and paralysis.[23]

Another group of illnesses is believed to be caused by magical interventions. *Mal ojo*, or "evil eye," occurs when someone with a powerful glance looks improperly at a child; it is believed to be a manifestation of witchcraft and, as a result, the child is said to be affected by evil spirits. Treatment entails a ceremonial ritual that includes passing an egg over the affected person's body while reciting prayers. *Susto*, or "sudden fright," occurs when an individual experiences a stressful event at some time prior to the onset of symptoms. The stressor may be the death of a significant person, a child's nightmare, or an inability to adequately fulfill social-role responsibilities. *Mal puesto* ("evil") is an illness caused by a hex bestowed by a *brujo* ("witch"), *curandero* ("folk healer"), or any other person knowledgeable about witchcraft.[23]

Hispanics commonly view cancer fatalistically as being God's will, and they believe it goes against principle to treat the disease aggressively. Family members with cancer, especially elders, often are not informed of their diagnosis, as it is believed such information will simply worsen the illness because it is considered deadly and engenders great fear. Patients often say, "I deserve to suffer." Cancer is viewed by some Hispanics as contagious and difficult to prevent because it is caused by many things. Thus going to see the doctor early serves no useful purpose. Many Hispanic patients believe that chemotherapy does not work, that radiation may cause cancer, and that cancer will remain even after surgery to remove it. Some believe that certain cancer treatments may have side effects that can be passed on to family members (eg, that family members may become radioactive if the patient receives radiation therapy).[19]

Hispanic individuals may believe that there is no need to see a physician unless a person is very ill. Hospitals are seen as places where people die. Therefore, medical attention may be sought only after symptoms develop or when the individual is too ill to be cared for by the family.[19]

Approximately 23% of Hispanics live at or below the poverty level. The cost of being sick includes not only the amount of money needed for care, but also the loss of money in time missed from work. Many Hispanics fear that because of their economic status and ethnicity, they may receive inferior care in the US medical system. Some Hispanics believe they should receive only health care that they can afford. As a consequence, if they cannot afford to pay, some Hispanic individuals may not seek care.[16,19]

In general, Hispanics are less likely than members of any other group to have medical insurance. Approximately 35% of Hispanics less than 65 years of age lack health insurance.[16] The outcome of this trend in relation to cancer is late diagnosis and higher mortality rates despite the lower overall incidence of cancer in the Hispanic population. The high percentage of Hispanics who are migrant farm workers also contributes to the overall decreased access to health care for that group.[20]

Individuals of Hispanic origin often believe that it is inappropriate to question those giving care, as they fear retaliation. Because some Hispanics believe that physical touch can promote healing, if Western providers do not touch Hispanic patients during their visit, the patients may believe that they did not derive any benefit from the visit.[19]

Martaus offers the following suggestions for assimilating Hispanic individuals to the US healthcare system:[38]

- Healthcare providers must communicate their acceptance of the person's value system to establish trust.
- Providers should incorporate a culturally relevant interview in the admission process. This practice defines the individual's perception of illness and allows the healthcare provider to establish a workable treatment plan.
- The treatment plan must include a family focus, as illness intensifies the need for family involvement.
- Many Hispanics are very religious and may view treatment without prayer as ineffective.
- Healthcare workers must take responsibility for finding common ground that incorporates traditional beliefs and modern health care.
- Many Hispanics have a great fear of authority. They may believe that disease occurs because it is God's will and may place great emphasis on treating doctors with respect.

### Healing practices

For Hispanics, home remedies represent the first line of treatment. To cure a hot or cold imbalance, the opposite quality of the causative agent is applied. For example, if the causative agent for a headache is thought to have a hot quality, cold herbs may be placed on the temples to absorb the heat. If the cause has a cold quality, hot herbs are applied. If the stool is green or yellow, the diarrhea is hot and the remedy is cold tea. If the stool is white, the diarrhea is cold and the remedy is hot tea.[20]

Usually a family folk healer, someone respected for her knowledge of folk medicine, plays a pivotal role. The healing practices are passed down in the family from mother to daughter. If home remedies do not work, Mexican Americans send for the *curandero* or *herbalista*, a traditional folk medicine healer. This person receives his or her skills through an apprenticeship or as a gift from God and is knowledgeable in the use of herbs, diet, massage, prayer, and ritual. Puerto Ricans seek out the *espiritismo*, a folk healer with the gift of contacting the spirit world and healing through the powers of spirits. Such healers analyze dreams, foretell the future, and use medals, prayers, and amulets as part of their treatment approach. The Cuban population may seek medical help from a *santero*, a medicine man who works with the spirits of good within a system to promote wellness. Animal sacrifices, rituals, chanting, and prayers are used to aid in healing. A *yerbero* is a healer who uses herbs and spices to prevent illness and enhance healing. A *brujo* uses witchcraft for healing illnesses that may be related to jealousy or envy (*envidia*). If these remedies fail, then Western physicians may be sought out for help.[20,29]

It is essential that the nurse demonstrate acceptance of the spiritual and folk basis of Hispanic people's health beliefs. Once this acceptance is conveyed, there is the potential for influencing acceptance and understanding of the rationale for modern healthcare practices, thereby gaining the community's confidence.

### Social organization

The nuclear family (parents and children) is the foundation of the Hispanic community. Men are the breadwinners, assume dominant roles in Hispanic families, and are considered to be big and strong (*macho*). The hesitancy of a woman or child to make a decision may be due to the need to inform and obtain approval of the husband and father.[29] In Hispanic culture, women have always been the primary caretakers. The extended family is valued, and the family's needs supersede those of the individual members. When a family member's illness becomes too serious for the wife and mother to handle alone, she may ask the extended family to help care for the sick individual. Family members may also speak for the patient. Because of its high value in the patient's treatment and recovery, the family should be used to help with the patient's care.

Roman Catholicism is the predominant religion among Hispanics. Because religion is such an important factor in the health beliefs of many Hispanics, the patient may turn to religious practices, such as prayer, making special devotions, visiting shrines, or lighting a candle as an act of devotion and appeal to a patron saint, to help overcome the illness. Allowing time and providing privacy for the family to practice their religion during hospitalization will be helpful to many Hispanics.[20]

### Communication

For Hispanics, Spanish is the primary language, though numerous dialectical differences exist. Many Hispanics are bilingual but have a strong preference for their native language; during times of illness, they often revert to it. There is some mistrust of Caucasians and Western medicine, especially when the healthcare provider does not speak Spanish. Language may be a barrier, and Hispanics may not let the provider know that they do not understand. Translators may be necessary.[29]

The traditional Hispanic approach to communication requires the use of much diplomacy and tactfulness. Concern and respect for another's feelings dictate that a screen always be provided to preserve the patient's dignity. The manner of expression is likely to be elaborate and indirect, so as to make a personal relationship at least appear harmonious, as respect of each person's individuality is important. Politeness and courtesy are highly regarded. Even if the Hispanic individual disagrees with another's point of view, direct argument or contradiction is considered rude and disrespectful. On the surface, he or she may seem agreeable, but only because manners dictate that his or her genuine opinions should not be expressed openly. This apparent agreement may lead to a false assumption on the part of the healthcare provider, who may believe that the patient understands and will follow through with whatever is proposed. In practice, this may not be true.[29]

Hispanics tend to view pain as a necessary part of life and enduring pain; may be viewed as a sign of strength. Pain is tolerated as long as the person can work and play. However, when pain is expressed, body language may be dramatic. Hispanics in pain may moan and groan to let those around them know they are uncomfortable and suffering.[29]

### Space and time

Adult Hispanics may be described as tactile in their relationships, yet display a high degree of modesty. This is one reason why Hispanics do not enter the US healthcare system. They generally do not like being touched by others or having to touch themselves and are not comfortable being examined by healthcare professionals of the opposite sex. Embarrassment is a common reaction to invasive procedures or body exposure during an examination.[19]

Despite the fact that Hispanics like consistent, close relationships and physical touching, female nurses should always assist a male physician when examining a female patient; likewise, a male nurse should always assist a female physician when examining a male patient. Special care should be taken to guard against exposing body parts other than those that are the focus of the examination. Male patients may refuse a complete examination because of their modesty.

Hispanics generally have a relaxed concept of time—a present orientation—and may be late for appointments. The patient may be more concerned with a current activity than with the activity of planning ahead to be on time. Such a mindset suggests a belief that future-oriented activities can be recovered and that present-oriented activities cannot. The present time orientation helps explain why Hispanics often seek out the most accessible and affordable care first (folk healing and the folk practitioner). It is therefore useful for the nurse to focus on short-term problems. For example, if a medication is not taken in a timely manner, the immediate effects should be emphasized.[20]

### Death and dying issues

The afterlife of heaven and hell exists in the Hispanic culture. As many Hispanics are Catholic, religious practices such as the sacrament of extreme unction, or anointing of the sick, are important. The family serves as a supportive network for helping the terminally ill and later their survivors. Often, the patient is not told directly by the family of his or her condition but still demonstrates some awareness of death's likelihood. Although Hispanics typically prefer to remain at home to die, dying in a hospital is an acceptable alternative. Public expression of grief is to be expected, especially among women.[21]

### Biological variations

The traditional Hispanic diet is high in fiber and carbohydrates from staples such as rice, beans, and corn. It contains few leafy, green vegetables. Beans are a source of protein and daily intake tends to be small. The use of lard and the common practice of frying foods both contribute to the high fat content of the Hispanic diet.[19]

Among the high-risk behaviors in the Hispanic population are obesity, alcohol consumption, and sexual practices. Obesity is a common problem among Hispanics in the United States due to their diet and lack of physical activity. In general, the culture accepts obesity as part of the natural aging process and does not value low body weight. To older individuals, obesity may mean health and wealth. However, obesity is a risk factor in cancers of the breast, colon/rectum, uterus, and prostate. Hispanic men tend to drink at younger ages and to consume larger amounts of alcohol and more frequently than do Caucasians. Alcohol contributes to cancers of the esophagus and pancreas. Cigarette smoking is on the rise in Hispanic adolescents, although adult Hispanics smoke less than Caucasians or African Americans. A high risk for cervical cancer is observed among Hispanic women because of sexual promiscuity and infrequent use of condoms by males, which predisposes females to sexually transmitted diseases. In addition, low socioeconomic status and low educational levels often result in infrequent Pap smears, infrequent use of barrier contraceptives, and lack of reporting of genital warts.[19]

Skin color in Hispanics can vary from a natural tan to dark brown. Those with lighter color have more Spanish ancestry, while darker-skinned individuals have more Indian ancestry.[20]

## AMERICAN INDIANS/ALASKAN NATIVES

American Indians and Alaskan Natives include natives of the continental United States, Aleuts, and Alaskan Eskimos. This very diverse group consists of many tribes and more than 560 federally recognized nations, each with its own traditions and cultural heritage. Until the 1800s, these native peoples lived in loosely formed, often nomadic bands and tribes and spoke more than 100 languages with countless dialects.[39] This section focuses on the natives of the continental United States.

The approximately 2.5 million descendants of native North American residents make up the smallest (0.9%) of the defined US minority groups. The West has the largest Indian population as a result of forced westward migration. The largest American Indian nations reported in 2000 were Cherokee, Navajo, Latin American Indian, Choctaw, Sioux, and Chippewa. The largest Alaskan Native group reported was Eskimo.[39]

American Indians who live on reservations tend to lead a more isolated, rural type of existence. Reservations have a high percentage of very young members and a growing number of members older than 55 years of age. Because reservation land cannot support a growing and increasingly concentrated population, poverty and welfare dependency are common. American Indians who relocate from reservations tend to move to urban areas away from the secure network of their family, community, and tribal lifestyle. Although lured by greater opportunities and better jobs, many experience culture shock at the significant differences in the environment. In the past 25 years, there has been an ongoing migration to urban areas. Today, nearly two-thirds of all American Indians live in nonreservation communities.[23]

Cancer is ranked as the second leading cause of death among American Indians over the age of 45 years. Because of the heterogeneity of the American Indian group, cancer rates likely vary among the tribes.[40] Native Americans with cancer have a significantly lower 5-year survival rate than other American patients with cancer; 36% as compared to 47% respectively.[41]

The Indian Health Service, through the US Public Health Service, provides inpatient facilities and outpatient clinics and serves American Indians residing on reservations in 25 states as well as the Aleut and Eskimo residents of Alaska. Although health care is available, barriers preventing American Indians from accessing it include poverty and lack of transportation. American Indians believe in living day-to-day rather than in planning for the future, so they may not have savings or insurance to pay for health care. Many live long distances from healthcare facilities and resist seeking out hospital treatment.[23]

## Health beliefs and practices

Most tribes link health beliefs and religion. To the American Indian, religion is something that surrounds an individual at all times and has a profound influence on the entire being. Wellness encompasses harmony in body, mind, and spirit as well as resilience, the ability to survive under exceedingly difficult circumstances. It is the patient's response or attitude toward circumstances that creates harmony.[20]

American Indians believe that health reflects living in harmony with nature and that humans have an intimate relationship with nature. The earth is considered a living being, the body of a higher individual with a will and desire to be well. The earth is periodically healthy or ill, just as humans are. An American Indian is expected to treat both the physical body and the earth with respect. If an individual harms the earth, he or she harms himself or herself, and vice versa. Because of this relationship between humans and nature, American Indians believe that humans should respect their bodies and nature through proper treatment.[28]

In this culture, unwellness is seen as being caused by the disharmony of mind, body, and spirit. Natural unwellness is caused by the violation of a sacred or tribal taboo. Taboos can be moral, religious, or cultural. Violations affect not only the offender but also the family.[20]

American Indians believe that illness may be caused by witchcraft as well. Evil or negative energy comes from "one who is on the bad side" or "a person who walks at night." It can be premeditated or not, so American Indians must be careful how they think or talk because bad thoughts can cause illness. Hopi Indians associate illness with evil spirits.[23] Navajos believe that witches are able to interact with evil spirits and can bring sickness and other unhappiness to those who annoy them. Traditionally, illness, disharmony, and sadness are seen by Navajos as the result of "displeasing the holy people, annoying the elements, disturbing animal and plant life, neglecting the celestial bodies, misuse of a sacred Indian ceremony, or tampering with witches and witchcraft."[42,p.21]

The cause of disease, injury, damage to property, or continued misfortune of any kind can be traced back to an action that should not have been performed, such as breaking a taboo or contacting a ghost or witch. Thus the treatment of illness must focus on external causative factors and not on the illness or injury itself.[23]

All causes of illness or disease are believed to have supernatural aspects. Treatment depends on whether the origins of bodily ailments are internal or external. External causes of illness include fractures, dislocations, wounds, and snake or insect bites. If the cause is not apparent, then it is attributed to a supernatural agency. The beliefs that illnesses are caused by germs, a malfunctioning body part, or poor nutritional intake are foreign and unacceptable to American Indians.[23]

Sickness indicates a discord with the laws of nature and, according to American Indians, is most often caused by sorcery or witchcraft, taboo violation, disease or object intrusion, spirit intrusion or being possessed by spirits, or loss of soul. Iroquois Indians also believe that unfulfilled dreams or desires can result in illness. Likewise, restriction violations are thought to cause sickness. Most tribes have prescriptions and prohibitions governing behavior and daily activities, many of which pertain to the prevention of illness. For example, a Navajo boy was diagnosed as having urinary retention caused by his urinating on an ant hill. The boy caused the ants to suffer, and the ants' revenge came in the form of an illness. The boy was out of harmony with living entities that share the universe. The cure entailed a healing ceremony involving chants, prayers, and herbs administered by a medicine man.[20]

Diseases of *object intrusion* refer to the invasion of the body by a worm, snake, insect, or small animal. This problem may be a result of witchcraft. Navajos may orally suck out the foreign object using a hollow tube or bone. *Spirit intrusion* involves being possessed by disease-causing spirits of humans and animals. The healing ceremony is an exorcism of the bad spirits. *Soul loss* usually occurs during a dream, when the soul leaves the body and travels about. Witches and evil spirits can steal a soul. It is believed that the individual is in danger of dying if the soul is not recovered.[23]

A cancer diagnosis is viewed by American Indians as a Caucasian man's disease, as punishment for their actions or a family member's actions, as a way to wear the pain to protect others in one's community, as a natural part of one's path and the lessons to learn, as the result of a curse or a personal violation of tribal mores (ie, stepping on a frog or urinating on a spider), or as the result of the contagious cancer spirit.[43]

Frequently, American Indians use traditional medicine and Western medicine, either independently of each other or simultaneously. An American Indian patient may consult both a medicine person and a Western doctor at the same time. One helps heal the individual heal by restoring harmony, while the other treats the physical disease. To treat the spirit and mind, a healer must understand why the disease occurred and begin to resolve the conflict occurring in mind, body, and spirit. In most instances, the two systems are complementary and should be encouraged.[29]

Preventive measures are generally practiced to ward off the effects of witchcraft, to reestablish harmony, or to prevent possession by an evil spirit. The medicine person may prescribe wearing a talisman, a buckskin, or cloth herbal bag that has preventive or curative powers. Removal of such items by the nurse without permission could result in serious consequences for the patient.[29]

Some tribes are not receptive to invasive bodily procedures and may agree to surgery only reluctantly. Relatives may refuse to donate blood because they fear that if the recipient dies, they may die as well. American Indians should be asked whether they wish a body part back after surgery, as some tribes believe the body must be intact for burial or that body parts can be used as a means for spirits to enter the body and cause harm.[20]

Because of their history of inconsistent care and disrespectful treatment, American Indians often are not comfortable with Western healthcare providers. Long waits in clinics, separation from their families, the unfamiliar routines of the hospital, and the often demanding and demeaning attitudes of nurses and physicians result in a variety of responses by the American Indian patient that may include silence or even leaving, never to return again.[23]

The pain threshold of American Indians is often thought to be high, as stoicism is greatly valued. This pattern stems from American Indians' tendency to look at things in totality, so that when sickness occurs it is viewed as an ailment of the whole body. Many will "grin and bear" fever and pain until the physical condition becomes disabling. Asking an American Indian, "Where does it hurt?" might commonly be responded to with "All over." It may be more useful to have the patient point to where it hurts most. When treatment is sought, medication generally is expected. If none is given, the American Indian may be disappointed, as his expectations for treatment were not met.[20]

Helpful interventions in working successfully with American Indian patients include conveying acceptance without judgment of physical appearance, beliefs, or practices; explicitly recognizing unique cultural beliefs and behaviors; and making staff and services available when the need arises rather than by scheduling appointments. An unwillingness to accept traditional healing practices may discourage many American Indians from using the Western healthcare system.[42]

## Healing practices

The traditional healer is the medicine person who is wise in the ways of the land and nature, and takes time to determine first the cause of the illness, then the proper treatment. He or she often performs special ceremonies that may take several days. These medicine men and women are "chosen"—ie, divinely inspired. They are gifted with extrasensory perception that allows them to make mythological associations, and they seek spiritual causes of illness.[23] Medicine men and women spend many years learning their skills and serving as apprentices to more experienced healers.[20]

Different types of medicine men and women play specific roles in American Indian culture. They range from those who assume a purely positive role and whose focus is to maintain cultural integration at a time of great stress, to the singer who is the medicine man and treats illnesses and disharmony.[29]

A cure often requires the involvement of several medicine men and women. Medicine people may use medicine bundles (*jish*) containing symbolic and sacred items or small jars of medicinal solutions; place red, gray, or black marks on the patient's skin; use tobacco; or burn cedar sage, grasses, or whatever is appropriate for that tribe. Bracelets of shells, seeds, beads, or arrowheads also may be used.[20]

The goal of treatment is always to enhance total healing. If an herbalist treats a patient, prayers and songs are offered in conjunction for mental and spiritual renewal. An important component of the healing is the patient's motivation for recovery. American Indians believe an individual gets back in equal proportion what he or she gives in words and actions to another.[23]

Healing ceremonies differ from tribe to tribe, and are associated with varying degrees of complexity. Most of these ceremonies take place in the home with the participation of family members and other tribal members. Supporting the use of healing ceremonies in the hospital and providing adequate space and privacy for them is helpful for the American Indian patient and family. Objects may be left in the room that were used in the ceremony. Because these objects are associated with elements identified with the cause of illness, they should not be removed without the permission of the patient and his or her family.[21]

Purification is often practiced to maintain harmony with nature and to cleanse the body and spirit. Many American Indians believe that for every natural disease, the earth provides a cure. Roots are often chewed to relieve pain, clear the mind, or treat a toothache. Herbs are viewed as being agents of nature.[23]

Traditional medicines include cedar incense (for purification) and corn pollen (for blessings). A "seat" in a sweat lodge is a type of purging that is useful for preventing and treating illness. Individuals may engage in monthly sweats because it is believed that the body periodically builds up bad or negative spirits that block energy. Note that Navajo women do not participate in sweats. Objects to guard against witchcraft may be carried by some tribes, especially at nonfamily gatherings.[20]

Western physicians are regarded by American Indians as herbalists who can cure symptoms but cannot restore the patient's harmonious relationship with nature because they lack knowledge of the important rituals. American Indians believe that a real medicine woman or man will know, without being told, what is wrong with a person. Western doctors ask many questions and often are unable to determine what is wrong. Some American Indians believe that healthcare providers from the Indian Health Service come to the reservations to "practice."[19]

### Social organization

As members of a matrilineal society, American Indian patients may not give consent for any procedure or treatment until permission is obtained from the mother, grandmother, or aunt. Sometimes consent may be obtained only after a ceremony. If it cannot be performed in the hospital, the patient may leave and return after the ceremony.[29]

The extended family is very important, especially during periods of crisis. When a family member is hospitalized, an assortment of relatives will come expecting to visit the relative. Limiting visitors to only close relatives is not relevant for American Indians, as they do not distinguish between close and distant relatives. Family members may make great sacrifices by traveling long distances to visit their family member. The hospitalized patient expects the family to visit, and the family expects to visit the patient.[21]

### Communication

Older American Indians may speak only their traditional language, and often there are no comparable medical terms in the tribal language. Although translators are needed, they must understand the nature of social, cultural, and familial lines of communication and respect. Some tribes believe that a discussion with one individual about another is a sign of disrespect and could break a cultural taboo, leaving the individual or family vulnerable to harm. For the Navajo, special emphasis is placed on individual rights. Each person speaks for himself or herself, and each individual's action should be self-initiated. In this case, trying to obtain information about another family member may be difficult. Limited ability to speak English may hamper the understanding of the patient. It is common for American Indians to be silent rather than to admit to not understanding.[20]

Making direct eye contact with an American Indian may be considered as looking into his or her soul, which could result in its loss. Consequently, American Indians who do not look directly at care providers should not be labeled as "inattentive" or "uninterested." Prolonged eye contact is considered a sign of disrespect and pointing is viewed as insulting.[29]

Interpersonal relationships are carefully spelled out among American Indian tribes. To whom one speaks, when the speaking occurs, how one speaks, and what sequence of speaking is followed are very important. For example, a mother-in-law cannot speak to her son-in-law or be in the same room with him. Awareness of these relationships is helpful to the nurse who must communicate with American Indian patients and families.[29]

The importance of observing periods of silence is a cultural trait. Silence helps formulate one's thoughts so that the spoken words will have significance. An individual who interrupts, interjects, or hurries toward abrupt conclusions is perceived to be immature. American Indians are very sensitive to body language. If a healthcare provider appears hurried, nervous, or impatient, American Indians are quick to sense these cues, and blocks to communication may occur. Because American Indians are comfortable with silence, they do not feel a need to talk constantly; as a result, continual talking by a healthcare provider trying to obtain an adequate history may not be well received.[29]

American Indians tend to be private people who do not readily volunteer information. Patients may not understand a question or may give responses they think the nurse wishes to hear, particularly if the question is regarded as inappropriate. Making a declarative statement about an obvious symptom and allowing time for the patient to respond may be a better approach.[23]

It is common for American Indians to speak in a very soft voice. The listener is expected to be attentive so as to hear what is being said. Asking for a statement to be repeated is considered rude. Thus, it is helpful to speak with an American Indian patient in a quiet setting to improve communication.[23]

Some American Indians consider a firm handshake to be a sign of aggression. Navajos extend their hand and lightly touch the hand of the person they are greeting. Knocking on the door before entering the room and introducing oneself in the native language are often appreciated.[29]

Using body language that is open, without closing or crossing the arms, is suggested. Loud speech may be viewed as rude or angry, and speaking slowly may be perceived as condescending. Note-taking is considered taboo for some American Indians, as Indian history is passed on through verbal story telling.[23]

### Space and time

Personal space is very important to some American Indians, who may have difficulty adapting to situations that place them in unfamiliar spaces such as clinics or hospitals. Hospitals may be considered a place to die, and American Indians are hesitant to be admitted or put into a room where another person has died. Some tribes would welcome having the room ritually purified before they enter it.[20]

Modesty is very significant to the American Indian; limited exposure of body parts is suggested. Permission should be asked to perform a physical examination, and American Indian women may prefer a female practitioner.[21]

American Indian time typically runs from one hour to a few days later than standard time. Homes often have no clocks. For American Indians, time is casual, present-oriented, and relative to present needs that must be accomplished within a given time frame.[20] A present time orientation may cause a Navajo patient to eat 2 meals today, 4 meals tomorrow, no meals the next day, and 3 meals the following day. This would create difficulty if the patient were instructed to take a medication 3 times a day with meals.

### Death and dying issues

Existence is circular and continuous for most traditional American Indians. They existed as spirit beings with the supreme creator before birth. At death, their spirit joins the creator and eventually returns to the physical world in another form. Death consists of joining one's ancestors, and good or bad deeds have nothing to do with this reunion.[29]

Attitudes and approaches to death and dying vary considerably among American Indian tribes. Some are very accepting of death, but others view dying people and death with fear. Some prefer that their family members die at home, while others prefer the hospital. Suffering is a major value in the American Indian culture, and dying and grief may be met with stoicism and silence. The opportunity to share feelings may be rejected by the patient or family. The family, including children, should be with the dying person, even though they often may avoid touching the dead person or articles associated with that person.[30]

### Biological variations

There is a high incidence of obesity, alcohol abuse, and domestic violence in American Indians. Some believe that the disruption and subsequent loss caused by the European settlement of North America left many American Indians feeling powerless and hopeless. These feelings may contribute to many of the social problems experienced today by American Indians.[29]

The American Indian diet has changed over time. When these peoples were nomadic, their diet was high in fiber and low in fat. Today, the diet is likely to be high in refined carbohydrates, fat, and sodium and low in fiber, meat, eggs, cheese, and milk. Obesity is a major problem in this group. Many American Indians are also lactose intolerant.[20]

## NURSING ISSUES

### CANCER, POVERTY, AND ETHNICITY

In the late 1970s, the question of poverty's role in the differences noted in cancer incidence, mortality, and survival in different ethnic groups was first raised. A landmark report by Freeman in 1989 concluded that poverty, not race, accounted for the 10% to 15% lower survival rate from cancer in many ethnic groups.[44] In particular, the disproportionate number of African Americans in the lower socioeconomic strata was found to account for the increased incidence.

The IOM released two reports, *The Unequal Burden of Cancer* (1999)[45] and *Unequal Treatment* (2003),[46] which documented the disproportionate cancer burden in African Americans. According to these reports, even at the same socioeconomic and health insurance status, African Americans are less likely to receive the most curative treatment for cancer.

According to the US Census Bureau, in the United States 35 million people (12%) are poor and 44 million (15%) are uninsured. A disproportionate number of African Americans (24%) and Hispanics/Latinos (22%) live below the poverty line compared to the Caucasians (8%).[47] Ward reports that residents who live in poorer counties have higher death rates due in part to the fact that the poor and uninsured people are more likely to be diagnosed with cancer at a later stage and are more likely to die from the disease.[24] Poverty is a significant factor in cancer disparities, being associated with a lack of resources, information, and knowledge; substandard living conditions; risk-promoting lifestyles; and diminished access to health care.[48]

The "culture of poverty" includes economic factors, such as unemployment, unskilled occupations, no savings, no health insurance, and frequent daily food purchases in small amounts; social factors, such as crowded living quarters, women as single parents, low educational attainment, and critical attitudes toward the dominant class; and psychological factors, such as feelings of helplessness, inferiority, fatalism, and dependency, and a present time orientation with an inability to defer gratification. These influences increase cancer incidence and mortality by increasing the risk factors of chronic malnutrition; occupational exposure through unskilled jobs; early initiation into sex and multiple partners; and smoking and alcoholism, contributing to cancers of the lung, oral cavity, prostate, cervix, or esophagus.[48]

Secondary prevention may be absent because of a present time orientation, where survival needs take precedence over screening and early detection. A critical attitude toward the middle class and a sense of fatalism may decrease participation in screening programs. Delayed tertiary prevention is often due to a lack of insurance, inability to pay for service, or limited care access. Emergency rooms are often used inappropriately, and referral to clinics may result in fragmented care, impersonal service, long waiting hours, and transportation and child care problems.[48]

To reduce cancer disparities based on poverty, culture, and social injustice, Freeman recommends:

- Immediate medical coverage should be provided for the uninsured and underinsured on a diagnosis of cancer to ensure that no person with cancer goes untreated.
- Geographic areas with excess cancer mortality should be delineated and targeted with an intense approach to providing culturally relevant education, appropriate access to screening, diagnosis, treatment, and an improved social support network.
- Specifically, such communities should receive funding for Patient Navigator Programs, the purpose of which is to provide personal assistance in eliminating any barriers to patients obtaining timely and adequate diagnosis and treatment.

- Systems for monitoring treatment equity according to standards of care should be established and implemented to diminish bias in the provision of health care.
- Each individual, regardless of economic status, must share in the responsibility for promoting his or her own health and well-being.
- There is a need for serious dialogue in the scientific community to elucidate how human populations really differ and how to group people for biological and clinical study. It appears that an expanded knowledge of genomics and population genetics and a more fundamental understanding of the effects of economic status and culture will be keys to this progress.
- Research studies should be supported to determine the economic cost of cancer disparities. Specifically, we must measure the cost to the nation of treating late-stage cancer to inform public policy makers about this important aspect of the economics of health care.[48]

## STRATEGIES TO ENHANCE ACCESS TO HEALTH CARE

A primary barrier to cancer care for many of the ethnic minority populations is access to health care, especially among the socioeconomically disadvantaged. Since 1989, when attention was directed to this particular need, several programs have been developed. Many of these programs focus on providing effective cancer screenings for ethnic minority populations by using culturally sensitive strategies, including (1) involvement of trusted and respected members of the community in the planning and delivery of healthcare services, (2) provision of social support by women in the social network, and (3) development of culturally sensitive patient education materials.[49]

Patient navigation is another strategy that addresses access to health care by helping patients, survivors, and their families to access and chart a course through the complex healthcare system and address obstacles to health care. Navigators are guides that understand the patients' concerns, coordinate services, and are a reliable and consistent resources for the patient.[50] Measures of success of navigation programs are increasing length of survival and improved quality of life. A study of the effect of patient navigation on women with abnormal mammograms found significant differences in diagnostic interval (fewer days for patients having a patient navigator), reduced anxiety, and increased satisfaction. The samples were mostly African American and Latino women.[51]

Mujer a Mujer: Woman to Woman is an example of a successful, culturally sensitive patient education program targeting Hispanic women. It was developed to reduce the mortality from cervical cancer in this group. Palos outlines some of the culturally appropriate strategies used in the development of this and other effective cancer-control programs:[52]

- Follow basic rules when initiating interpersonal communication, such as being courteous and respectful to establish trust or confidence.
- Use focus groups comprising grassroots (community) and professional individuals to validate promoters or barriers to attitudes, knowledge, and behavior related to cancer and its prevention.
- Use influential formal and informal leaders such as religious leaders, community gatekeepers, or opinion leaders.
- Integrate religious, cultural, and, when appropriate, traditional (folk) medicine and healing practices, beliefs, and taboos.
- Involve the family, friends, and members of other influential support systems.
- Determine a group's preferred communication process (verbal or nonverbal) as well as language preference.
- Determine an individual's degree of acculturation or assimilation, when appropriate.
- Involve paraprofessionals such as folk healers, when and if appropriate.
- Integrate cultural assessments into daily nursing practice.

## CULTURALLY APPROPRIATE PUBLIC/PATIENT EDUCATION

Ethnic minority patients with cancer are not much different from other patients with cancer in their need for basic cancer information and in their experiences of learning barriers such as anxiety and feelings of being overwhelmed about the disease and treatment. Nevertheless, ethnic minorities present certain unique challenges, such as the need to communicate in a language other than English and cultural values, beliefs, and practices that can affect the teaching/learning process.

### Strategies

Because of the challenges posed by ethnic minorities, several strategies have been identified to provide culturally sensitive patient education interventions:[52]

Keeping educational messages simple.
Determining the preferred language and learning process (eg, video vs booklets; group vs one-on-one teaching).
Identifying the preferred communication style of the individual, such as the best way to address him or her and acceptable nonverbal communication. For example, as mentioned in the description of the different ethnic groups, the appropriateness and acceptance of direct eye contact varies among cultures.

In addition, determining decision-making patterns for the particular ethnic group is important. An example of this consideration is seen in many API groups, where the family, instead of the patient, makes treatment decisions. In these situations, teaching only the patient about a proposed chemotherapy treatment may not be appropriate if the educational effort needs to be directed to the family for subsequent decision making and consent to treatment.

*Use of interpreters.* Language frequently poses a barrier to effective patient education. The use of professional interpreters, if available, is the optimal choice. Family and friends may be used, but the correct or complete message may not be relayed. This distortion or omission of parts of the message may be due to the interpreter's own skill and fluency in the language, the interpreter's subjective censoring (eg, to "protect" the patient), or the patient's comfort level in discussing personal issues in the presence of the family member or friend.[18] Recommendations for using interpreters and steps to take if no interpreter is available are listed in Table 4-2.

*Translating written materials.* Although translated cancer information materials are now available, additional resources are needed. Just as professional interpreters are desirable for clear, accurate communication, guidelines also exist for translating material. Translating material written in English into another language is not enough. To ensure that the content and tone are accurately captured and maintained throughout the translation, the newly translated material must be back-translated into English by independent translators. After making any needed text corrections, it is helpful to pilot-test the finished product with a sample of the target population for whom the translated material was created.[19]

Always assess the reading level of the original material before it is translated. Analyses of the reading levels of available cancer education materials have shown an average that is much higher than the reading level of the general population.[54] Thus the reading level of the material to be translated may need to be adjusted before it is translated. Just as literacy has been identified as a barrier to education for the general population, it also represents a challenge faced by many ethnic minority groups. The literacy level of ethnic minority groups will be influenced by whether they are literate in their native language. For example, the Hmong culture is primarily an oral culture, and many of these people who immigrated to the United States are illiterate in the Hmong language.[21]

*Preferred styles of learning.* Determining an individual's preferred style of learning is important as well. The different styles include one-to-one vs group, oral tradition, story telling, peer educators, and receiving information from "powerful others." Enlisting fellow ethnic minorities to teach their peers is the basic principle behind the peer educator's strategy. The use of "powerful others" often involves the recruitment of respected community leaders who are recognized authorities or cancer survivors from the community.[19]

Providing effective public and patient education for ethnic minority groups presents many challenges and opportunities for oncology nurses. Using the strategies presented here as well as knowledge of the individual's cultural background can help oncology nurses develop and implement successful, culturally sensitive public and patient education interventions.

## CLINICAL TRIALS AND CANCER RESEARCH

The participation of racial/ethnic minorities and other underrepresented groups in clinical trials has historically been low and this lack of diversity in randomized study populations reduces the chances for identifying effects that may be relevant to underrepresented populations. Identified barriers include lack of education about clinical trials, culturally appropriate information, ie, translated materials and knowledge about cancer.[55]

Patient-specific barriers include older age, lower socioeconomic status and ethnic/minority status, and lack/inadequate insurance. Other barriers include perceived harm from participation, loss of control over treatment choice, mistrust of research and the medical system, direct/indirect costs of participation, difficulty with transportation, time commitment, fear, and family considerations. Provider specific barriers include knowledge of and method of presenting information about the trials.[55] Blakeney suggests the following strategies to increase minority recruitment to clinical trials for cancer:

- Understand the study population
- Be sensitive to the past history of the community and the institution
- Establish trust and credibility with community
- Get study design/recruitment plan buy-in from all major stakeholders
- Identify the trusted information sources/channels in this community
- Get community-based input in the planning process
- Be clear about expectations and study limitations
- Invite past participants of clinical trials to participate in outreach activities
- Develop, pretest, and use culturally appropriate recruitment materials
- Maintain open lines of communication throughout the study and report study results.
- Maintain an "open door policy" with all stakeholders to discuss what is working and what is not during the study.[56]

In response to this under-representation of minorities and in an effort to recruit more minorities to National Cancer

**TABLE 4-2**

**Use of an Interpreter**

**Choosing an Interpreter**

- Before locating an interpreter, identify the language the person speaks at home. Be aware that it may differ from the language spoken publicly (eg, French is sometimes spoken by well-educated and upperclass members of certain Asian, African, or Middle Eastern cultures, but it is not the language spoken in the home).
- Whenever possible, use a *trained* interpreter, preferably one who knows medical terminology.
- Avoid interpreters from a rival tribe, state, region, or nation (eg, a Palestinian who knows Hebrew may not be the best interpreter for a Jewish person).
- Be aware of gender differences between interpreter and patient. In general, the same gender is preferred.
- Be aware of age differences between interpreter and patient. In general, an older, more mature interpreter is preferred to a younger, less experienced one.
- Be aware of socioeconomic differences between interpreter and patient.

**Strategies for Effective Use of an Interpreter**

- Plan what you want to say ahead of time. Meet privately with the interpreter before the interview. Avoid confusing the interpreter by backing up, hesitating, or inserting a proviso.
- Ask the interpreter to provide a line-by-line verbatim account of the conversation. Ask for a detailed interpretation when provided with brief summaries of longer exchanges between interpreter and patient.
- Be patient. When using an interpreter, interviews often take two to three times longer.
- Longer-than-expected explanatory exchanges are often required to convey the meaning of words such as *stress, depression, allergy, preventive medicine,* and *physical therapy* because there may not be comparable terms in the language the patient understands.
- When discussing diagnostic tests such as mammograms; magnetic resonance imagings (MRIs); computed tomography (CT) scans; or those involving body fluids such as blood, urine, stool, spinal fluid, or saliva, be sure to clarify the nature of the test to the interpreter. Indicate the purpose of the test, exactly what will happen to the patient, approximately how long the test will take, whether the procedure is invasive or noninvasive, and what part(s) of the body will be tested.
- Be aware that the interpreter may modify or edit some aspects of the conversation, especially if he or she thinks you might not understand the cultural context of the patient's response (eg, traditional or folk beliefs and practices related to healing).
- Avoid ambiguous statements and questions. Refrain from using conditional or indefinite phrasing such as "if," "would," and "could," especially for target languages, such as Khmer (Cambodia), that lack nuances of conditionally or distinctions of time other than simple past and present. Conditional statements may be mistaken for actual agreement or approval of a course of action.
- Avoid abstract expressions, idioms, similes, metaphors, and medical jargon.
- To ensure confidentiality and privacy, avoid using as interpreters children or strangers who may be visiting other patients.
- Be aware that an interpreter who is a nonrelative may seek compensation for services rendered. Be sure to negotiate fees ahead of time.

**Recommendations for Institutions**

- Maintain a current, computerized list of interpreters who may be contacted as needed.
- Network with area hospitals, colleges, universities, and other organizations that may serve as resources.
- Utilize over-the-telephone interpretation services provided by telephone companies. For example, since 1989. AT&T has operated the Language Line Services, which provides interpretation in more than 140 languages. Services are available around the clock every day of the year. Call (800) 628–8486 or visit http://www.languageline.com for further information on services and charges.

**Overcoming Language Barriers: What to Do When No Interpreter is Available**

- Be polite and formal.
- Pronounce name correctly. Use proper titles of respect, such as "Mr.," "Mrs.," "Ms.," "Dr." Greet the person using the last or complete name. Gesture to yourself and say your name. Offer a handshake or nod. Smile.
- Proceed in an unhurried manner. Pay attention to any effort by the patient or family to communicate.
- Speak in a low, moderate voice. Avoid talking loudly. Remember that there is a tendency to raise the volume and pitch of your voice when the listener appears not to understand. The listener may perceive that you are shouting and/or angry.
- Use any words that you might know in the person's language. This indicates that you are aware of and respect his or her culture.
- Use simple words, such as "pain" instead of "discomfort." Avoid medical jargon, idioms, and slang. Avoid using contractions (eg, don't, can't, won't). Use nouns repeatedly instead of pronouns.

Example:
Do not say: "He has been taking his medicine, hasn't he?"
Do say: "Does Juan take medicine?"

- Pantomime words and simple actions while you verbalize them.
- Give instructions in the proper sequence.

*(Continued)*

**TABLE 4-2**

| Use of an Interpreter (*Continued*) |
|---|
| Example:<br>Do not say: "Before you rinse the bottle, sterilize it."<br>Do say: "First wash the bottle. Second, rinse the bottle."<br>• Discuss one topic at a time. Avoid using conjunctions.<br>Example:<br>Do not say: "Are you cold and in pain?"<br>Do say: "Are you cold (while pantomiming)? Are you in pain?"<br>• Validate if the person understands by having him or her repeat instructions, demonstrate the procedure, or act out the meaning.<br>• Write out several short sentences in English and determine the person's ability to read them.<br>• Try a third language. Many Indochinese speak French. Europeans often know two or more languages. Try Latin words or phrases.<br>• Ask who among the person's family and friends could serve as an interpreter.<br>• Obtain phrase books from a library or bookstore, make or purchase flash cards, contact hospitals for a list of interpreters, and use both a formal and an informal network to locate a suitable interpreter. |

*Source*: Data from Jarvis.[53]

Institute (NCI)-sponsored clinical trials, NCI developed the Minority-Based (MB) Community Clinical Oncology Program (CCOP). The purpose of this program is to support research activities of physicians involved in the care of minorities who are eligible to participate in NCI clinical trials.[57]

## RESOURCES

In response to the increasing awareness of the needs of the United States' culturally diverse population and the healthcare professionals who care for them, many resources are available. Table 4-3 lists programs and organizations at the national level whose focus is to eliminate the unequal burden of cancer among ethnic minorities. Other important resources include the American Cancer Society (http://www.cancer.org) and the NCI's Cancer Information Service (http://cis.nih.gov).

Several professional organizations aim to promote cultural awareness in nurses and to provide support to ethnic minority nurses, including the Oncology Nursing Society (ONS) (http://www.ons.org) and its Transcultural Nursing Issues Special Interest Group (TNI SIG). The National Coalition of Ethnic Minority Nurse Association (NCEMNA) advocates for equity and justice in nursing and health care for ethnic minority populations. It consists of 5 national ethnic nurse associations:

- Asian American/Pacific Islander Nurses Association (AAPINA) (http://www.aapina.org)
- National Alaska Native American Indian Nurses Association (NANAINA) (http://www.nanaina.com)
- National Association of Hispanic Nurses (NAHN) (http://www.thehispanicnurses.org)
- National Black Nurses Association (NBNA) (http://www.nbna.org)
- Philippine Nurses Association of America (PNAA) (http://www.philippinenursesaa.org)

NCEMNA's goals are support for the development of ethnic nurses who reflect the nation's diversity; advocacy for culturally competent, accessible, and affordable health care; promotion of the professional and educational advancement of ethnic nurses; education of consumers, healthcare professionals, and policy makers on health issues of ethnic minority populations; development of ethnic minority nurse leaders in areas of health policy, practice, education, and research; and endorsement of best practice models of nursing practice, education, and research for minority populations.[58]

## CONCLUSION

Cultural diversity will remain a challenge in health care, as the composition of the population of the United States continues to change. The effects of cultural diversity on cancer care are multilayered. At one level, each ethnic group, with its unique values, health beliefs, and practices, responds to cancer somewhat differently. Additional factors such as degree of acculturation, socioeconomic status, and educational attainment add yet another layer to intergroup and intragroup diversity. A third level is an underlying, often negative perception among many ethnic minorities of the mainstream culture and Western medicine. This perspective primarily arises due to their history and experience with Western culture, which in turn influences their health behaviors, attitudes, and acceptance of mainstream health care.

In the midst of this diversity, one can still identify shared responses among the major cultural groups. Many of the ethnic minority groups believe in and practice folk healing, consult both traditional and Western practitioners, and use both

**TABLE 4-3**

**Selected Programs and Resources Targeting Cancer Disparities**

| Name of Program and Web Address | Sponsors/ Partners | Description |
|---|---|---|
| Intercultural Cancer Council (ICC) http://iconetwork.org | Baylor College of Medicine | The ICC established in 1995, promotes policies, programs, partnerships, and research to eliminate the unequal burden of cancer among racial and ethnic minorities and medically underserved populations in the United States and its associated territories. It prepares *Cancer Fact* Sheets that provide detailed information on cancer occurrence and risk factors among racial and ethnic minorities and the medically underserved |
| National Center on Minority Health and Health Disparities (NCMHD) http://ncmbd.nih.gov | National Institutes of Health (NIH) | The NCMHD was established in 2000. It leads and coordinates, supports, and assesses NIH efforts to reduce and ultimately eliminate health disparities |
| Center to Reduce Cancer Health Disparities (CRCHD) http//crchd.nci.nih.gov | National Cancer Institute (NCI) | The CRCHD was created in 2001 and is central to NCI's efforts to reduce the unequal burden of cancer and train the next generation of researcher funding for cancer health disparities in four years. Research will investigate social, cultural, environmental, biological, and behavioral determinants of cancer disparities across the cancer-control continuum from prevention to end-of-life care |
| Special Populations Networks for Cancer Awareness, Research and Training http//crchd.ncinih.gov/spn | National Cancer Institute (NCI) | The Special Populations Networks is a program within the CRCHD. The first projects were funded in 2001. Its purpose is to build relationships between large research institutions and community-based programs and to find ways of addressing important questions about the burden of cancer in minority communities. The major goal is to build an infrastructure to promote cancer awareness within minority and medically underserved communities, and to launch from these communities more research and cancer-control activities aimed at specific population subgroups. Currently the Special Populations Networks consists of 18 projects in 15 states. |
| Racial and Ethnic Approaches to Community Health (REACH) http://www.cdc.gov/reacch/ | Centers for Disease Control and Prevention (CDC) | The REACH program funds community coalitions to develop and implement activities to address the Healthy People 2010 goal of eliminating health disparities. The first projects were funded in 1999. The program emphasizes the importance of working more closely with communities to identify culturally sensitive implementation. |
| National Breast and Cervical Cancer Early Detection Program (NBCCEDP) http://www.cdc.gov/cancer/nbccedp | Centers for Disease Control and Prevention (CDC) | The NBCCEDP was created by Congress in 1990 to help improve access to breast and cervical cancer screening among underserved women. This program provides both screening and diagnostic services and has been implemented in all 50 states, five U.S. territories, the District of Columbia, and 12 American Indian/Alaskan Native organizations. |

*Source:* Data from Ward et al.[24]

traditional and Western medicine. Many groups also place a high value on the family. However, individual variations make it inappropriate to generalize certain group characteristics to all subgroups and to each member of each group. Regardless of ethnicity, the individual must come first.

The heterogeneity and marked cultural diversity of the US population presents many challenges for oncology nurses. Because of the inherent differences between mainstream and ethnic minority cultures and the potential for misunderstanding and conflict, continued efforts at increasing knowledge, appreciation, and understanding of each culture are needed. Our challenge is to facilitate these efforts among health professionals and in the community at large.

## ACKNOWLEDGMENT

Special thanks to Karen Taoka for her contributions to a previous edition of this chapter.

## REFERENCES


1. The Office of Minority Health. *What Is Cultural Competency?* US Department of Health and Human Services. http://www.omhrc.gov/templates/browse.aspx?lvl=2&lvlID=11. Accessed December 29, 2009.
2. US Census Bureau, 2004. US Interim Projections by Age, Sex, Race, and Hispanic Origin: 2000–2050. http://www.census.gov/population/www/projections/usinterimproj. Accessed December 29, 2009.

3. Barnes J, Bennett C. The Asian Population: 2000, US Department of Commerce, US Census 2000. 2002. http://*www.census.gov/prod/2002pubs/c2kbr01–16.pdf.* Accessed December 29, 2009.
4. US Department of Health and Human Services. *The Registered Nurse Population.* Washington, DC: US Health Resources and Services Administration; March 2004. ftp://ftp.hrsa.gov/bhpr/workforce/0306rnss.pdf. Accessed December 29, 2009.
5. Smedley BD, Butler AS, Bristol LR, eds. *In the Nation's Compelling Interest: Ensuring Diversity in the Healthcare Workforce.* Washington, DC: The National Academic Press; 2004.
6. Jemal A, Siegel R, Ward E, et al. Cancer Statistics, 2009. *CA: Cancer J Clin.* 2009;59:225–249.
7. Espey DK, Wu XC, Swan J, et al. Annual report to the nation on the status of cancer, 1975–2004. *Cancer.* 2007;110:2119–2152.
8. Ries LAG, Melbert D, Krapcho M, et al. SEER cancer statistics review, 1975–2005. Bethesda, MD: National Cancer Institute; 2008. http://seer.cancer.gov/csr/1975_2005. Accessed September 8, 2009.
9. Singh GK, Miller BA, Hankey BF, et al. *Socioeconomic Variations in US Cancer Incidence, Mortality, Stage, Treatment and Survival, 1975–1999.* NCI Cancer Surveillance Monograph Series, No. 4. NIH Publication No. 03–5417. Bethesda, MD: National Cancer Institute; 2003.
10. American Cancer Society. *Cancer Facts and Figures for African Americans, 2007–2008.* Atlanta, GA: American Cancer Society; 2007.
11. American Cancer Society. *Cancer Facts and Figures—2009.* Atlanta, GA: American Cancer Society; 2009.
12. US Department of Commerce. *Profiles of General Demographic Characteristics, 2000.* Washington, DC: US Census Bureau; 2001.
13. US Department of Commerce. *The Asian and Pacific Islanders in the US Population, 2002.* Washington, DC: US Census Bureau; 2003.
14. US Department of Commerce. *The Native Hawaiian and Other Pacific Islander Population, 2000.* Washington, DC: US Census Bureau; 2002.
15. McCraken M, Olsen M, Chen M, et al. Cancer incidence, mortality and associated risk factors among Asian Americans of Chinese, Filipino, Vietnamese, Korean and Japanese ethnicities. *CA: A Cancer J Clin.* 2007;57:190–205.
16. American Cancer Society. *Cancer Facts and Figures for Hispanics/Latinos, 2006–2008.* Atlanta, GA: American Cancer Society; 2006.
17. US Department of Commerce. *We the People: American Indians and Alaskan Natives in the US.* Census 2000. Washington, DC: US Census Bureau; 2006.
18. Andrews MM, Boyle JS, eds. *Transcultural Concepts in Nursing Care.* 5th ed. Philadelphia, PA: Wolter, Kluwer Health, Lippincott Williams and Wilkins; 2008.
19. Frank-Stromborg M, Olsen SJ, eds. *Cancer Prevention in Diverse Populations: Cultural Implications for the Multidisciplinary Team.* Pittsburgh, PA: Oncology Nursing Society; 2001.
20. Giger JN, Davidhizar RE, eds *Transcultural Nursing: Assessment and Intervention.* 5th ed. St. Louis, MO: Mosby Elsevier; 2008.
21. Lipson JG, Dibble SL, Minarik PA, eds. *Culture and Clinical Care: A Pocket Guide.* San Francisco, CA: UCSF Nursing Press; 2005.
22. Palafox N, Warren A, eds. *Cross-Cultural Caring: A Handbook for Health Care Professionals in Hawaii.* Manoa: John A. Burns School of Medicine; 1980.
23. Spector RE. *Cultural Diversity in Health and Illness.* 7th ed. Upper Saddle River, NJ: Pearson Prentice Hall; 2009.
24. Ward E, Jemal A, Cokkinides V, et al. Cancer disparities by race/ethnicity and socioeconomic status. *CA: Cancer J Clin.* 2004;54:78–93.
25. Kosary CL, Ries LAG, Miller BA, et al. *SEER Cancer Statistics Review, 1973–1992.* NIH Publication No. 95–2789. Bethesda, MD: National Cancer Institute; 1995.
26. Bloom JR, Hayes WA, Saunders F, et al. Physician induced and patient induced utilization of early cancer detection practices among black Americans. *Adv Cancer Control Innov Res.* 1989;293:279–296.
27. Winbush GB. African-American health care: beliefs, practices and service issues. In: Julia MC, ed. *Multicultural Awareness in the Health Care Professions.* Boston, MA: Allyn and Bacon; 1996:8–22.
28. US Census Bureau, Current Population Survey, Annual Social and Economic Supplement. America's Families and Living Arrangement, March 2005. http://mchb.hrsa.gov/whusa_06/popchar/graphs/0203hcV.htm. Accessed December 29, 2009.
29. Purnell LD, Paulanka BJ, eds. *Transcultural Health Care, a Culturally Competent Approach.* 3rd ed. Philadelphia, PA: FA Davis; 2008.
30. Berman B, Snyder SJ, Kozier B, Erb G, eds. *Fundamentals of Nursing.* 8th ed. Upper Saddle River, NJ: Prentice Hall Health; 2008.
31. Muller JH, Desmond B. Ethical dilemmas in a cross-cultural context—a Chinese example. *West J Med.* 1992;157:323–327.
32. Ramakrishna J, Weiss MG. Health, illness, and immigration—East Indians in the United States. *West J Med.* 1992;157:265–270.
33. Brotzman GL, Butler DJ. Cross-cultural issues in the disclosure of a terminal diagnosis: a case report. *J Fam Pract.* 1991;32:426–427.
34. Tung TM. Death, dying, and hospice: an Asian-American view. *Am J Hosp Palliat Care.* 1990;7:23–25.
35. Klessig J. The effects of values and culture on life-support decisions. *West J Med.* 1992;157:316–322.
36. Intercultural Cancer Council. *Asian Americans and Cancer.* Houston, TX. http://iccnetwork.org/cancerfacts/cfs3.htm. Accessed September 8, 2009.
37. Asian American Association for Cancer Awareness, Research and Training. *The Unequal Burden of Cancer among Asian Americans.* Sacramento, CA: UC Davis. http://www.aancart.org/unequalburden.html. Accessed September 8, 2009.
38. Martaus TM. The health seeking process of Mexican-American migrant farm workers. *Home Health Nurse.* 1986;4:32–36.
39. Ogunwole SH. *The American Indian and Alaskan Native Population: 2000.* Washington, DC: US Department of Commerce; 2000.
40. Intercultural Cancer Council. *American Indians/Alaskan Natives & Cancer.* http://iccnetwork.org/cancerfacts/ICC-CFS2.pdf. Accessed September 8, 2009.
41. American Cancer Society. *Lower Survival Rates found in Native Americans with Cancer.* 2000. Atlanta, GA: American Cancer Society. http://www.cancer.org/docroot/NWS/content/NWS_1_1x_lower_Survival_Rates_found_in_Native_Americans_with_cancer.asp. Accessed September 8, 2009.
42. Bilagody H. An American Indian looks at health care. In: Feldman R, Buch D, eds. *Ninth Annual Training Institute for Psychiatrist-Teachers of Practicing Physicians.* Boulder, CO: WICHE; 1969.
43. Burhansstipanou L, Lovato MP, Krebs LU. Native American cancer survivors. *Healthcare Women Int.* 1999;20:505–515.
44. Freeman HP. Cancer in the socioeconomically disadvantaged. *CA: Cancer J Clin.* 1989;39:266–288.
45. Institute of Medicine. *The Unequal Burden of Cancer.* Washington, DC: National Academy Press; 1999.
46. Smedley BD, Stithy AY, Nelson AR, eds. *Unequal Treatment: Confronting Racial and Ethnic Disparities in Health Care.* Washington, DC: National Academy Press; 2003.
47. Procter BD, Dalaker J. *Poverty in the US: 2002.* Washington, DC: US Government Printing Office, US Census Bureau Current Population Reports; 2003.
48. Freeman HP. Poverty, culture and social injustice, determinants of cancer disparities. *CA: Cancer J Clin.* 2004;54:72–77.
49. Burhansstipanov L, Krebs LU, Bradley A, et al. Lessons learned while developing "clinical trials education for Native Americans" curriculum. *Cancer Control.* 2003;10:29–36.
50. National Cancer Institute. NCI's *Patient navigator research program: Factsheet.* US National Institutes of Health. http://www.cancer.gov/cancer-topics/factsheet/patientnavigator. Accessed September 8, 2009.
51. Ferrante J, Chen PH, Kim S. The effect of patient navigation on time to diagnosis, anxiety and satisfaction in urban minority women with abnormal mammograms: a randomized controlled trial. *J Urban Health.* 2007;85:114–124.
52. Palos G. Cultural heritage: cancer screening and early detection. *Semin Oncol Nurs.* 1994;10:104–113.

53. Jarvis C. *Physical Examination and Health Assessment.* 5th ed. St. Louis, MO: Elsevier; 2008.
54. Chelf JH, Agre P, Axelrod A, et al. Cancer-related patient education: an overview of the last decade of evaluation and research. *Oncol Nurs Forum.* 2001;28:1139–1147.
55. Ford JG, Howerton MW, Lai GY, et al. Barriers to recruiting underrepresented populations to cancer clinical trials: a systematic review. *Cancer.* 2008;112:228–242.
56. Blakeney N. *Minority Recruitment to Cancer Clinical Trials.* University of Michigan Comprehensive Cancer Center; 2006. http://chcr.umich.edu/what_we_do/seminars/seminar.2006-02-23.6852677249. Accessed December 23, 2009.
57. Department of Health and Human Services. *Minority Based Community Oncology Program (u10).* Washington, DC. http://grants.nih.gov/grants/guide/rfa-files/RFA-CA-07-049.html. Accessed September 8, 2009.
58. National Coalition of Ethnic Minority Nurse Associations (NCEMNA). 2004. http://www.ncemna.org/ncemna/whatisncemna.asp. Accessed September 9, 2009.

CHAPTER

5

*Judith J. Smith, RN, MSN, AOCN®, Barbara K. Dunn, PhD, MD, Peter Greenwald, MD, DrPH*

# Dynamics of Cancer Prevention

## INTRODUCTION

Over the past several decades, epidemiological, basic, and clinical research have contributed to major developments in cancer prevention *science*. Although a large body of knowledge exists, we are limited in our ability to translate it into appreciable declines in nationwide cancer incidence and mortality rates for all cancers, and for all subpopulations. A coordinated effort to explore cancer risk reduction measures, through healthy lifestyle behaviors and medical interventions, is essential to establishing definitive prevention practice. This chapter presents an overview of principles, current practices, research, policy, special challenges, and responsibilities and opportunities for nurses in cancer prevention.

## CANCER PREVENTION PRINCIPLES

### CARCINOGENESIS

The transition from normal healthy tissue to invasive cancer follows a multistep process called carcinogenesis.[1–4.] The steps associated with carcinogenesis are identified as initiation, promotion, and progression, and are influenced by genetic, dietary, and environmental factors. *Initiation* occurs rapidly with exposure to a carcinogenic agent (eg, nitrosamines in tobacco smoke, ionizing radiation, oncogenic viruses), resulting in an irreversible alteration in the genotype of a cancer stem cell. During *promotion*, the cell acquires phenotypic characteristics of malignant cells, such as increased cell proliferation, disorganization, and morphological changes.[5,6] The promotion phase spans an extended period of time, up to 40 years in some cases. Reversibility is a key feature of this phase, providing an opportunity to stop, slow down, or reverse the process through an intervention such as chemoprevention.[7] Further carcinogenic exposure and multiple alterations to the cell microenvironment may lead to *progression*, the final phase of carcinogenesis. This phase occurs over a period of one or more years, is generally irreversible, and is characterized by progression of genetically altered cells to invasive malignancy.[8,9] Although the steps of the carcinogenic process provide a framework for the development of common adult epithelial cancers, a multitude of variation and overlap exists within each phase and among different cancer types. The extended period of time over which molecular alterations accumulate and the reversibility potential during the carcinogenic process have major implications for cancer prevention science.

### LEVELS OF PREVENTION

Various classification systems have been used to categorize prevention activities into different levels. To be consistent with current nursing literature, this chapter defines the levels of cancer prevention as follows: (1) *Primary* prevention refers to the decrease of cancer incidence due to behavioral or medical intervention. Such prevention strategies can be population-based or focused on specific high-risk subgroups. Adopting health-protective lifestyle behaviors that include healthy diet, physical activity, tobacco abstinence, and avoidance of excessive direct sunlight are examples of primary prevention activities that target the general population. On the other hand, chemoprevention—administration of a chemical compound or nutritional supplement, targets high-risk individuals only, and is used to prevent the development of a specific malignancy. (2) *Secondary* prevention refers to reduction in cancer mortality by means of early detection through screening. The benefits of screening include potential diagnosis of cancer at an early, preclinical stage, while an individual is still asymptomatic and treatment may be more successful. (3) *Tertiary* cancer prevention is a term that applies to prevention and reduction of morbidity and mortality of clinically evident cancer through diagnosis and treatment, and as such, is discussed elsewhere in this publication.

## CANCER PREVENTION STRATEGIES

### LIFESTYLE INTERVENTIONS

There is considerable evidence that lifestyle behaviors are responsible for approximately 70% of cancer in the United States.[10,11] Understandably, efforts by the research community to investigate the effects of nutrition, physical activity, tobacco use, and weight control on cancer incidence have flourished over the past several decades. In 2007, the World Cancer Research Fund and American Institute for Cancer Research (WCRF/AICR) published a comprehensive review of relevant evidence-based research evaluating lifestyle behaviors and cancer risk reduction.[12] The report is designed to function as a guide for future scientific research, educational programs, and most importantly, global health policy. Overall, the report advocates increased physical activity, decreased alcohol intake, limited intake of processed foods, and ingestion of a healthy well-balanced diet as the source of a combination of bioactive cancer-preventive foods (Table 5-1).[12]

#### Nutrition

Since the early 1980s, increased research efforts in biochemistry, epidemiology, molecular biology, and clinical research have explored the association between nutrition and cancer incidence. Numerous epidemiological observational studies have documented an association of diets rich in fruit and vegetable consumption with a decreased risk for a variety of cancers (pharynx, larynx, lung, esophagus, stomach, cervix, uterus, colon, and rectum).[13]

**TABLE 5-1**

| WCRF/AICR 2007 Recommendations for Decreasing Cancer Risk |
|---|
| **General Dietary Recommendations** |
| Be as lean as possible without becoming underweight |
| Be physically active for at least 30 minutes every day |
| Avoid sugary drinks |
| Limit consumption of energy-dense foods |
| Eat an increased variety of vegetables, fruits, whole grains, and legumes such as beans |
| Limit consumption of red meats (such as beef, pork, and lamb) and avoid processed meats |
| If consumed at all, limit alcoholic drinks to 2 a day for men and 1 a day for women |
| Limit consumption of salty foods and foods processed with salt |
| Do not use supplements to protect against cancer |
| **Special Population Recommendations** |
| Breastfeed exclusively up to 6 months, then add other liquids and foods |
| After treatment, cancer survivors should follow the recommendations for cancer prevention |

*Source*: Data from the World Cancer Research Fund (WCRF)/American Institute for Cancer Research (AICR).[12]

In contrast, clinical trials devoted to nutrition have focused on interventional approaches to evaluate dietary supplements and global dietary modifications for their protective effect against cancer in a controlled setting. Ideally, observational studies provide a rationale for evaluating a food component in clinical trials; however, clinical trial outcomes have not always supported results from observational studies. As an example, the Polyp Prevention Trial (PPT) and Wheat Bran Fiber Study (WBFS) were designed to validate findings from several large prospective observational studies that indicated an inverse relationship between increased fiber intake and colorectal cancer.[14,15] The PPT and WBFS evaluated the effect of diet on growth of new colorectal polyps in individuals with a prior history of polyp removal. Such clinical research investigating strategies for polyp prevention is an important avenue to pursue, as evidence shows 5% to 10% of polyps progress to malignancy if not removed. The PPT, a 4-year study, randomized over 2000 men and women to evaluate the effect of a high-fiber (18 g per 1000 calories), low-fat (20% of calories from fat), high fruit/vegetable (3.5 servings per 1000 calories) nutritional plan on polyp recurrence.[16]

Although participants in the intervention group reported a significant increased intake of fiber, fruits and vegetables, and reduced intake of fat, their risk for recurrent polyps was not significantly different from that of the control group. The PPT-Continued Follow-up Study (PPT-CFS) was initiated to provide an additional 4-year follow-up period to the original study.[17] Even with the extended follow-up period, the study failed to show any protective effect of the diet on polyp recurrence.[17] The WBFS, a 3-year study, randomized nearly 1500 men and women to evaluate the effect of increased and decreased amounts of wheat bran fiber (13.5 g per day vs 2 g per day) for protective effects against recurrent colorectal polyps.[18] Once more, results were inconsistent with observational study results, as no benefit from dietary fiber was found.

The Women's Health Initiative (WHI), a major trial sponsored by the National Institutes of Health (NIH), was designed to evaluate cardiovascular disease, cancer, and osteoporosis in postmenopausal women over a 15-year period. Initiated in 1993, the WHI accrued nearly 162,000 generally healthy postmenopausal women. Two component studies of the WHI, the dietary modification (DM) study and the calcium and vitamin D (CaD) study, are directly related to diet and nutrition.[19] The DM study randomized 48,835 females to examine strategies for preventing heart disease, as well as breast and colorectal cancers through changes in dietary patterns—low-fat intake, decreased total daily calories, increased fruit and vegetable consumption, and increased intake of grains. Results of the DM indicated that a low-fat diet did not significantly reduce the risk of breast or colorectal cancer in this cohort.[19,20] In the CaD trial, 36,282 postmenopausal women were randomized to receive 1000 mg of calcium carbonate and 400 International Units of vitamin D daily or a placebo.[21] The purpose of the study was to evaluate the effects of the supplements on risk for osteoporosis and colorectal cancer. Results indicated that supplemental intake of CaD did not decrease the incidence of colorectal cancer. Clearly, major discrepancies were found between the observational studies and the clinical trials evaluating associations between DMs and colorectal cancer risk. Instances of conflicting results between epidemiological and clinical research have been reported for other food products as well (eg, selenium, folate, and carotenoids). Reasons for discrepancies may be related to incomplete knowledge of mechanisms of the protective effects of individual nutriceuticals, aspects of trial design (eg, self-reporting vs controlled clinical trial setting) or as suggested in a recent WCRF/AICR report, a healthy well-rounded diet combining a wide array of nutrients throughout the life cycle may provide the best protective benefit, rather than inclusion or exclusion of any one individual nutrient.[12,22]

### Obesity and physical activity

Nutrition and diet are often studied in conjunction with physical activity, obesity, body mass index (BMI), and energy intake, with these factors being considered together in evaluating associations with cancer risk. A recent prospective study of 900,000 males and females evaluated BMI for association with risk of cancer-related death over a 16-year period. Findings suggested that increased body weight could account for 14% of all cancer deaths in males and 20% in females.[23] In another observational study, among men, increased BMI (greater than 5 kg/m$^2$ above average) was strongly associated with cancers of the esophagus, thyroid, colon, and kidney, with weaker associations being noted for rectal cancer and malignant melanoma.[24] The same study showed that in women similar increases in BMI were strongly associated with cancers of the endometrium, gallbladder, esophagus, and kidney. Weaker associations were observed for pancreatic, thyroid, and colon cancers, and for breast cancer in postmenopausal women only. In a recent meta-analysis by Pan and DesMeules, energy intake, physical activity, and obesity were evaluated for associations with cancer risk. Their findings support strong links between obesity and colon, rectal, kidney, postmenopausal breast, endometrial cancer, and adenocarcinoma of the esophagus.[25] Lower levels of physical activity have been shown in many studies to be a factor in weight maintenance and BMI, and to be associated with increased cancer risk. In one review for example, decreased physical activity was associated with breast cancer, especially among postmenopausal women.[26]

While the evaluation of relationships between physical activity and cancer continues in observational studies, creative interventions are being tested currently in clinical trial settings. One example is an ongoing NCI-sponsored randomized internet-based study evaluating an active lifestyle program.[27] The intervention group receives an intensive lifestyle coaching program and an individualized fitness plan, while the control group receives an educational program that describes standard health behaviors. The study stratifies participants by age ($\geq$55 vs $\leq$55 years), gender, ethnic association, and aerobic capacity. In addition to behavioral and clinical research, efforts to explore molecular pathways of carcinogenesis are underway to further the understanding of relationships among obesity, physical activity, and cancer.[28]

## Tobacco

Tobacco is the most common cause of cancer in the United States and accounts for 90% of lung cancers.[29,30] Tobacco use is responsible for approximately 160,000 cancer deaths in the United States annually.[31] Currently, an estimated 45 million American adults are habitual tobacco users, while another 45 million are former smokers. The identification of tobacco as a carcinogen reflects a major achievement in cancer prevention. Epidemiological and experimental studies in the 1950s provided strong evidence supporting tobacco exposure as an etiological factor for lung cancer.[32–34] Efforts for tobacco control began with the publication of the first Surgeon General's Report on Smoking and Health in 1964 and the National Cancer Institute's (NCI) tobacco-related research initiatives in the 1980s.[34,35] Despite a large body of behavioral and scientific evidence linking smoking and cancer, tobacco use remains the leading cause of preventable death in the United States, and it is associated with an increased risk of at least 15 cancers: cancers of the nasopharynx, nasal cavity, lips, oral cavity, pharynx, larynx, lung, esophagus, pancreas, cervix, kidney, bladder, and stomach and acute myeloid leukemia.[31,36]

Overall, cigarette consumption among American adults has been declining since the US Surgeon General's report in 1964.[11] This downward trend in cigarette consumption has led to a major reduction in lung cancer mortality rates for men. In contrast, mortality rates for women are just beginning to plateau after rising steadily for many years. This disparity between mortality trends for men and women can be explained by the fact that women started to smoke in large numbers 20 years later than men, and similarly the decrease in female smoking began to take place 20 years later. Lung cancer develops over a period of 20 years or more, explaining the differences in peak time-points for mortality rates. With this in mind, mortality rates for women are anticipated to begin decreasing over the next decade.

The harms associated with tobacco use extend beyond habitual and former tobacco users. In 2006, the US Surgeon General's Report, *The Health Consequences of Involuntary Exposure to Tobacco Smoke*, identified detrimental effects of secondhand smoke, also called side-stream smoke.[37] Secondhand smoke has been shown to increase the risk for lung cancer and coronary heart disease among nonsmoking adults. Approximately 35,000 cardiac-related deaths and 3000 lung cancer deaths occur annually among nonsmokers.[38] Secondhand smoke also has damaging effects on young children, causing a doubling of respiratory-related visits to emergency departments and a tripling of hospitalizations compared to children from nonsmoking homes.[39,40]

Teens present a unique public health problem. Approximately 3600 adolescents, younger than age 18, begin using tobacco each day; 1100 will become habitual smokers, and up to one-half ultimately will die from tobacco-related causes.[36,41,42] With such alarming statistics, national, state, local, and school initiatives are underway to educate children of all ages about the dangers associated with tobacco. The American Lung Association's Not on Tobacco (N-O-T) is a widely used national teen smoking cessation program that provides psychosocial support and guidance in a nondisciplinary manner in schools and other community settings across the country.[43] The American Lung Association's N-O-T is delivered over 10 sessions and addresses life management skills, healthy lifestyle behaviors, and decision-making strategies, in addition to teaching smoking reduction and cessation techniques. N-O-T has been implemented in 48 states and found to be cost-effective and capable of producing quit rates between 15% and 19%, the highest in the nation for teen programs.[44–48] A recent analysis of 64 controlled studies evaluating teen tobacco cessation programs showed that the most effective approaches were those presented in structured settings (eg, schools, sports clubs, community centers), consisting of up to 5 sessions, and using creative interventions (eg, games, dramatizations, Internet, and phone texting).[48] Interventions utilizing the administration of pharmacologics, specifically nicotine patches and gum, and buproprion were not found to be as effective for adolescents as other approaches. The analysis evaluated a wide variety of strategies employed to recruit adolescents to smoking cessation programs, including public announcements, incentives (money, movie tickets, gift certificates), class release time, posters, media campaigns, referrals, class credit, peer recruiters, and use of school events, and found that the most successful programs were those utilizing more than one recruitment strategy. More research is needed to evaluate efficacy of teen smoking cessation and reduction interventions in terms of successful recruitment techniques, program completion and quit rates, as well as cost-effectiveness.

Among current adult smokers, 80% report a desire to quit smoking and 70% have attempted to quit; however, the success rate remains low.[49] Although a number of smoking cessation interventions are being implemented, only a few have proved successful. Current interventions include a variety of behavioral and pharmaceutical approaches, including cessation recommendations from primary healthcare providers, group programs and classes, individual counseling sessions, pharmacological interventions, media campaigns, and worksite and statewide cessation programs.[50–52] Studies show that the most successful approaches for adult tobacco cessation result from increasing excise taxes on tobacco products, funding state and local cessation and abstinence programs adequately, implementing broad-based antismoking campaigns, and enacting comprehensive clean air and smoke-free laws.[52–55]

The Nurses' Health Study (NHS) provides interesting data regarding nurses and tobacco. The objective of the NHS was to describe smoking habits in 237,648 female registered nurses, stratified by age, between 1976 and 2003. An analysis of the NHS found that smoking trends among nurse participants mirrored smoking declines in the general population over the past several decades. In 1976, nurses participating in the study smoked at a rate of 33.2% and 13.5% by 1989. Although 79% of participants quit smoking over the duration of the study, the current smoking rate for study participants remains elevated at 8.4%.[55] By comparison, the national rate for registered nurses who are current smokers is much higher at 15%, eclipsing the smoking rate for physicians at 1%.[56] In another analysis of the NHS, nurse smokers reported lower health-related quality of life than never and former smokers.[57] Such analyses suggest critical tobacco educational deficiencies in basic nursing curricula and in continuing professional education programs. Rice and Stead conducted a comprehensive review of the literature to determine the effectiveness of nursing-delivered interventions on smoking behavior in adults. Data from 31 studies indicated that a tobacco control nursing intervention significantly increased the chance a patient would quit smoking, yet the practice of providing tobacco cessation interventions has been limited.[58,59] It is vitally important to educate nurses and nursing students about the basic mechanisms of action and physiological changes that occur in human tissue exposed to the carcinogens in cigarette smoke, as well as the availability of scientific evidence-based tobacco control interventions. Such knowledge empowers nurses with an understanding of health consequences of tobacco dependence and assists them in developing tobacco control skills for use in their personal lives and professional practice. The Tobacco Free Nurses Initiative (TFN) is a national program focused on the role of nursing in tobacco control. TFN objectives are to help nurses quit smoking and to prepare nurses to effectively promote health and wellness among their patients through strategies targeting reduction of tobacco use, increased smoking cessation, and reduced exposure to secondhand smoke.[60] The Tobacco Dependence Clinical Practice Guideline, developed by the US Public Health Service, provides a framework for TFN. The guideline is designed to present healthcare providers and administrators, insurers, and tobacco treatment specialists with evidence-based strategies and recommendations for the treatment of tobacco dependence.[61] Through a collaboration between TFN and the Public Health Service, Agency for Health-care Research and Quality (AHRQ), a new resource, "Helping Smokers Quit: A Guide for Nurses" has been developed for nurses to assist individuals with smoking cessation.[62]

The association of genetic factors with lung cancer risk is multifaceted, involving not only gene variants that modify the risk of developing lung cancer in the presence of tobacco use but also variants that influence smoking behavior.[63,64] The importance of the latter category of gene variants is evident in the positive association between lung cancer risk and number of cigarettes smoked per day. Factors that increase the amount of smoking are expected to correlate with risk. Among such factors is the rate of nicotine metabolism. The faster nicotine is metabolized, the more cigarettes must be smoked to maintain the given level in the circulation that delivers the desired psychopharmacological effect. The enzyme that metabolizes the majority of nicotine is cytochrome P450 2A6, or CYP2A6, and is coded for by the *CYP2A6* gene. In addition to the common version of this gene, in some people *CYP2A6* exists in variant, or polymorphic forms, some of which code for CYP2A6 enzymes that break down nicotine faster than normal. A high CYP2A6 activity, implying an underlying "high-activity" *CYP2A6* gene polymorphism, has been shown to correlate with increased smoking behavior. The converse is seen among Japanese who, compared to Caucasian, metabolize nicotine more slowly and, as a result, smoke fewer cigarettes per day.[63] This lower level of smoking among Japanese is believed to contribute to their lower risk of developing lung cancer. An alternate approach to exploring the relationship of nicotine to smoking behavior is seen in a study that focused on a cluster of genes (the *CHRN* genes) that encode receptors for the neuronal nicotinic acetylcholine receptor (AChR). Rather than examining the metabolic activity of a gene product, this study looked at potential associations between variants of the *CHRN* genes themselves and smoking susceptibility. Specific polymorphisms in the cluster of AChR genes that includes *CHRNA5-CHRNA3-CHRNB4* were shown to be associated with smoking quantity.[64] Overall, therefore, smoking behavior is influenced by variant forms of genes that make proteins involved in nicotine metabolism (*CYP2A6* genes) and nicotine action at its receptor (*CHRN* genes). The downstream effect of these gene polymorphisms is expected, via their impact on quantity of smoking, to influence the risk of lung cancer.

In 2009, a bill was signed into law by President Barack Obama that places the tobacco industry under the direct authority of the FDA.[65] This long-awaited and historic legislation empowers the FDA to impose potentially strict new controls on the production, sales, and marketing of tobacco products. The FDA now has the ability to reduce nicotine levels of tobacco products, administer product safety tests, and issue recalls if necessary. A new office within the FDA, the Center for Tobacco Products, will implement the statute's regulations. The main provisions of the Family Smoking Prevention and Tobacco Control Act include:

- Crack down on tobacco marketing and sales to children and adolescents
- Require more prominent, more effective health warnings on tobacco products
- Require tobacco companies to disclose the contents of tobacco products, as well as changes in products and research about their health effects
- Ban terms such as "light" and "low-tar" that mislead consumers into believing that certain cigarettes are safer
- Strictly regulate all health-related claims about tobacco products to ensure they are scientifically proven and do not discourage current tobacco users from quitting or encourage new users to start
- Empower the FDA authority to require changes in tobacco products, such as the removal or reduction of harmful ingredients.

## MEDICAL INTERVENTIONS

### Chemoprevention

The term *chemoprevention* refers to the use of natural or synthetic agents to interrupt the carcinogenic process, preventing progression to invasive cancer.[1,2,6,66] Unlike population-based lifestyle interventions (eg, diet, exercise, tobacco cessation), chemoprevention focuses more narrowly on individuals or subpopulations known to be at increased risk for developing a malignancy. Although chemopreventive agents are often nutritionally based (derived from food compounds or supplements), food components ingested as part of a regular diet are not considered chemoprevention.[2] Rather, chemoprevention refers to compounds manufactured into pill, capsule, ointment, or liquid form and administered in prescribed doses at specified frequencies. Currently, most chemopreventive agents are administered through participation in clinical trials. Table 5-2 provides a list of the current status of large chemoprevention trials in humans.[67–76]

Once identified through epidemiological, laboratory, or preclinical research, a candidate agent progresses through the well-defined clinical trials process. Although many agents enter clinical trials, few progress successfully to definitive phase III randomized controlled trials (RCTs), and fewer still find their way into standard medical practice. To date, only 3 chemopreventive agents have received approval from the Food and Drug Administration (FDA) for standard use in cancer risk management: (1) tamoxifen and (2) raloxifene—selective estrogen receptor modulators (SERMs) for use in high-risk women to lower their risk of invasive breast cancer (raloxifene is approved for postmenopausal women only), and (3) celecoxib, a selective cyclooxygenase 2 (COX-2) inhibitor indicated for the reduction of colorectal adenomas in high-risk individuals with familial adenomatous polyposis (FAP).

Chemopreventive agents are assessed for activity, safety, and efficacy in a series of phased trials, similar to chemotherapy treatment trials (Table 5-3).[77] Once the safety and efficacy of a candidate agent has been established, the agent is evaluated in long-term phase III RCTs for its ability to decrease cancer incidence. Given the rarity of cancer occurrence even among high-risk individuals, by nature these studies using cancer incidence as the primary endpoint are costly, must accrue hundreds or thousands of participants, and generally take many years to complete. In 2006, the FDA introduced the concept of *exploratory IND studies*, also called phase 0 studies or microdosing studies. The purpose of phase 0 studies is to shorten the clinical trials timeline, in part by limiting the number of subjects required for testing.[78–80] Phase 0 studies evaluate agents for pharmacokinetic (what the body does to the drug—distribution in body tissue and elimination of drug) and pharmacodynamic (what the drug does to the body—modulating biomarkers in body tissues and fluids) activity. Importantly, phase 0 studies address the ability of the agent to modulate a molecular target through administration of a one-time, subtherapeutic dose administered to a small number of subjects (10–15). If an agent exhibits the ability to modulate the target, it may be selected to advance to an accelerated phase I or IIa trial.

**TABLE 5-2**

**Selected Phase III Chemoprevention Clinical Trials**

| Clinical Trial | Target Organ | Protocol Design | N | Outcome |
|---|---|---|---|---|
| Beta-Carotene and Retinol Efficacy Trial (CARET)[67] | Lung | Four arm study: (1) beta-carotene 30 mg and retinol 25,000 IU; (2) beta-carotene 30 mg alone; (3) retinol 25,000 IU alone; (4) placebo | 18,314 | 28% increased incidence of lung cancer; 17% increased mortality in beta-carotene group |
| Alpha-Tocopherol, Beta-Carotene Prevention Trial (ATBC)[68] | Lung | Two arm study: (1) alpha-tocopherol (vitamin E) 50 mg; (2) beta-carotene 20 mg | 29,133 | No reduction in lung cancer incidence with alpha-tocopherol; 18% increased incidence of lung cancer and 8% increased lung cancer mortality rate in beta-carotene group |
| Breast Cancer Prevention Trial (BCPT)[69] | Breast | Two arm study: (1) tamoxifen 20 mg; (2) placebo | 13,388 | 49% reduction in breast cancer incidence in tamoxifen group |
| Prostate Cancer Prevention Trial (PCPT)[70] | Prostate | Two arm study: (1) finasteride 5 mg; (2) placebo | 18,822 | 25% reduction of prostate cancer in finasteride arm |
| Nutritional Prevention of Cancer (NPC)[71] | Second primary cancers in people with history of previous skin cancer | Two arm study: (1) selenium 200 μg; (2) placebo | 1312 | Increase in both basal and squamous cell skin cancer in selenium arm |
| Nutritional Intervention Studies of Esophageal Cancer (Linxian, China)[72] | Esophageal cancer | Four arm study: (1) oral vitamin C/molybdenum; (2) beta-carotene, vitamin E, selenium; (3) retinol; (4) riboflavin, niacin | 30,000 | Beta-carotene, selenium, vitamin E group experienced lower esophageal incidence and mortality |
| Adenoma Prevention with Celecoxib Trial (APC)[73] | Colorectal adenoma | Three arm study: (1) 200 mg celecoxib bid; (2) 400 mg celecoxib bid; (3) placebo twice daily (in individuals with FAP) | 2035 | 33% reduction in adenoma recurrence and advanced adenoma recurrence in participants who took celecoxib daily for 3 years compared to placebo |
| Women's Health Study[74] | All cancers by site; cancer mortality by site | Four arm study: (1) 600 IU of natural-source vitamin E on alternate days; (2) daily aspirin; (3) both; (4) placebo | 39,876 | No overall benefit for cancer or cancer mortality in healthy women; small nonsignificant reduction in lung cancer incidence in the aspirin group |
| Selenium and Vitamin E Cancer Prevention Trial (SELECT)[75] | Prostate | Four arm design: (1) vitamin E alone; (2) vitamin E and selenium; (3) selenium alone; (4) placebo | 35,000 | Selenium and vitamin E supplements, taken either alone or together, did not reduce the incidence of prostate cancer |
| Study of Tamoxifen and Raloxifene (STAR)[76] | Breast | Two arm study: (1) tamoxifen 20 mg; (2) raloxifene 60 mg | 19,747 | Raloxifene is as effective as tamoxifen in reducing the risk of invasive breast cancer |

**TABLE 5-3**

**Phases of Cancer Chemoprevention Clinical Trials**

| Trial Phase | Main Goal | Main Characteristics |
|---|---|---|
| Phase 0 (exploratory) | Assess molecularly targeted agents for proof-of-concept to determine whether further clinical development is warranted | Limited duration; agent microdose administered 1 time for pharmacokinetic and pharmacodynamic activity; performed in small number of subjects (10–15); no possibility of therapeutic benefit |
| Phase I | Assess dose-related agent safety and toxicity in preparation for more advanced clinical testing | Short duration; performed in small number of subjects |
| Phase II | Test biological activity and efficacy of agent specific to a premalignant condition | Short duration; performed in a small number of subjects; often measured against biomarkers along the carcinogenesis continuum |
| IIa | Test agent efficacy *without* placebo controls in cases where safety has been established through prior use or testing | Assess feasibility of using the agent; agents meeting criteria may bypass phase I testing and advance directly into phase IIa |
| IIb | Test agent efficacy *with* placebo controls in cases where safety of agent has been established through prior use or testing | Assess feasibility of using the agent; agents may bypass phase I testing and advance directly into phase IIb |
| Phase III | Test agents in randomized, placebo-controlled trial designed for a specific indication | Long duration; randomized clinical trials requiring large numbers of participants |

*Source*: Data from Richmond E, Viner JL.[77]

### *Agents*

As previously noted, agents used in chemoprevention may be nutritional supplements or pharmacological agents. Although no widely accepted classification system exists for chemopreventive agents, such agents fall into 2 broad categories: (1) agents that block tumor initiation and (2) agents that block tumor progression. Based on multiple mechanisms of action, a number of agents cross over into both categories and exhibit effects at different stages of carcinogenesis.[2,81]

Agents that inhibit tumor initiation are carcinogen-blocking compounds that prevent activation of carcinogens, enhance detoxification systems, or stop carcinogens before they reach their target sites. Such agents appear to react directly with initiating carcinogens. Thus, in animal models, dithiolthiones block the activation of aflatoxin; this inhibits aflatoxin-induced hepatocarcinogenesis.[82] In humans, a UV blocking agent or cream might reduce UV-induced DNA damage, and finally UV-induced skin cancer.

Agents that inhibit tumor progression are antiproliferative and act by blocking or delaying promotion and progression during the carcinogenic process.[4] Although chemopreventive agents function by various mechanisms of action, many have significant antiproliferative effects. Examples of chemoprevention agents studied in trials include (1) nonsteroidal antiinflammatory drugs (NSAIDS/COX-2 selective inhibitors) which appear to prevent the formation of colon adenomas by inhibiting the arachidonic acid pathway; (2) SERMS, including tamoxifen and raloxifene, that act as antiestrogens in the breast, thereby inhibiting ER-positive breast cancer; and (3) finasteride and flutamide that act respectively by decreasing either the production of the androgen dihydrotestosterone or by blocking the efficacy of androgens via inhibition of their action at the androgen receptor in the prostate.[83–86]

Approximately 400 compounds are currently being evaluated as potential chemopreventive agents, mainly in laboratory research. More than 60 compounds have shown early potential and are under investigation in chemoprevention clinical trials.[87] Chemopreventive agents that have shown promise and are considered priorities for investigation are listed in Table 5-4.

### *Biomarkers*

***Surrogate Endpoint Biomarkers/Intermediate Endpoint Biomarkers.*** In cancer research, biomarkers refer to substances in body tissues or fluids that are indicative of the presence of cancer. Biomarkers include genes, RNAs, proteins, and metabolites. As the molecular changes that occur during tumor development can take place over a number of years, biomarkers can be potentially used to detect cancers early, determine prognosis, and monitor disease progression and therapeutic response.

The traditional endpoint for establishing chemopreventive efficacy of an agent in large phase III RCTs is cancer incidence. Although statistics for cancer incidence and mortality in the general population might appear high, the

**TABLE 5-4**

**Chemoprevention Agents and Target Sites**

| Agent | Organ System Target |
|---|---|
| 3,3′-Diindolylmethane | Prostate |
| Acolbifene | Breast |
| Aspirin | Colon |
| Atorvastatin | Breast |
| Budesonide | Lung |
| Celecoxib | Blood, lung/bronchi |
| Celecoxib + DFMO | Colon |
| Celecoxib + Exemestane | Breast |
| Curcumin | Colon |
| DFMO | Prostate, skin |
| Erlotinib | Colon, pancreas, lung |
| Esomeprazole + Aspirin | Esophagus |
| Exemestane | Breast |
| Folic acid | Colon |
| G-2535 (Isoflavones 100) | Breast |
| Green Tea Extract | Lung |
| Lapatinib | Breast |
| Lovastatin | Skin (melanoma) |
| Lycopene | Prostate |
| Myo-inositol | Lung |
| Pioglitazone | Oral mucosa |
| Polyethylene Glycol | Colon |
| Polyphenon E | Breast, cervix, esophagus, lung, prostate |
| Resveratrol | Colon |
| S-Adenosylmethionine | Liver |
| SR13668 | Lung |
| Sulindac | Multiple sites |

risk of any one individual developing malignant disease is relatively low. Cancer incidence is therefore relatively rare, requiring large numbers of study subjects, long duration of time for follow-up, and costly investments in order to function as an endpoint in prevention studies. Consequently, cancer incidence is not an appropriate endpoint for earlier phase studies of short duration and with limited accrual. The use of biomarkers as intermediate endpoints plays an important role in such early-phase chemoprevention clinical trials; the purpose served by these biomarkers is to predict cancer occurrence.[88,89]

An intermediate endpoint biomarker, also called a surrogate endpoint biomarker, is a marker representing a biological event that takes place, ie, is "intermediate", between carcinogenic initiation and progression to invasive malignancy.[2,87,88] To be useful, a surrogate/intermediate endpoint biomarker must be reliable, highly sensitive and specific, quantitative, easily obtained from study participants, part of the causal pathway for disease, capable of being modulated by a test agent, and have high predictive value for the disease (cancer occurrence).[87] Intermediate endpoints may take the form of grossly visible lesions, some of which are premalignant lesions; examples include oral leukoplakia, colon polyps, and dysplastic nevi. Alternatively, histological markers such as hyperplasia, metaplasia, and dysplasia can also serve as intermediate endpoint biomarkers. Biochemical markers, including enzymes such as ornithine decarboxylase and prostaglandin synthetase, can also function as intermediate biomarkers. In addition, genetic abnormalities, such as DNA ploidy, oncogene activation/suppression, and micronuclei can be used for this purpose.

***Early Detection Biomarkers.*** To be useful for early detection and to serve as surrogates for preferred clinical endpoints, such as cancer incidence, biomarker tests must accurately distinguish patients with cancer from those without and be minimally invasive, cost effective, and acceptable to patients and physicians. The Early Detection Research Network (EDRN) currently has more than 120 biomarkers for most of the major adult epithelial cancers in various phases of development and validation. Biomarkers are being developed by the EDRN for prostate, colon, and breast cancer. Among biomarkers being developed for prostate cancer, for example, are assays for gene rearrangements, such as the TMPRSS2-EST gene fusions where a portion of TMPRSS is fused to a portion of an EST family gene. Other biomarkers that are being developed include RNA PCA3 (an RNA that does not code for protein), the proteins proPSA and CD90, and autoantibodies. Biomarkers for colon cancer include mutations in the oncogene *K-ras*, as well as other gene mutations and epigenetic markers in both stool and urine, and proteins CCSA-2 and CCSA-3 in blood. Biomarkers for ovarian cancer include the proteins MIF-1 and osteopontin in blood. EDRN is working toward validating a few biomarkers, such as autoantibodies against annexins and PGP9.5 for lung cancer and the proteins DCP and AFP-L3 for liver cancer.[90]

***Cancer Risk Biomarkers.*** Biomarkers that serve to establish an individual's increased risk for developing a specific cancer are called risk biomarkers. These biomarkers are, for the most part, premalignant lesions. For example, a breast biopsy that shows atypical ductal hyperplasia indicates that a female is at increased risk for developing breast cancer; just as colorectal adenomas are associated with an increased risk of colon cancer and oral leukoplakia is associated with increased risk for developing oral cancer. An important aspect of risk biomarkers is that they can be used to identify potential participants for chemoprevention clinical trials.[91] It is particularly important for cancer risk screening in normal subjects to use minimally invasive techniques that are highly specific, sensitive, and quantitative.

### Study populations

***High-Risk Individuals.*** Chemoprevention studies target only individuals at increased risk for developing a specific cancer and are not appropriate for individuals of average risk in the general population. Increased risk refers to individuals with personal or family history of the disease, known exposure to a carcinogen, or history of a prior malignancy. Studying such homogeneous increased risk cohorts allows researchers to attain statistical significance with smaller sample sizes and shorter observation periods, since an increased number of cancer events are anticipated in this group. As an example, lung cancer chemoprevention studies target smokers or former smokers, since tobacco exposure is known to increase the incidence of the disease. But again, the risk of any 1 smoker is still quite low (only 20% of smokers develop lung cancer); consequently, a thousand or more individuals may have to be screened in order to observe 100 lung cancer cases.

***Recruitment of Study Subjects.*** Recruitment of appropriate subjects to clinical trials is a major challenge for researchers. Although only 5% of adult oncology patients participate in therapeutic trials, the estimated participation of eligible individuals in prevention trials is far less.[92] Unlike treatment trials, prevention studies enroll relatively healthy individuals. Patients with cancer may be willing to tolerate moderate to high-level toxicities associated with an investigative drug if the possibility of a cure exists. In contrast, high risk but healthy individuals have a lower tolerance for even minor ongoing toxicities, for example, hot flashes, arthralgias (see Table 5-5 for key differences between chemoprevention and chemotherapy clinical trials). Recruitment of minority and underserved populations in prevention trials has posed a major challenge. Increased efforts at such recruitment in research have been an important focus of NIH since the Revitalization Act was passed by the US Congress in 1993, requiring inclusion of minorities and women in federally funded trials. The NIH established the National Center on Minority Health and Health Disparities (NCMHD) to coordinate research aimed at improving healthcare outcomes in underserved populations, "underserved" referring to specific racial and ethnic groups, and populations with lower socioeconomic status (SES).[93,94] The barriers to clinical trial participation by underserved populations reflect multilayered issues involving poor access to health care, discomfort with establishment medicine, and lack of education, as indicated in the recent literature.[95] Interestingly, low SES has been identified as a greater barrier to health care and research opportunities, than has race or ethnicity. Strategies to overcome and enhance recruitment have been developed, but few have been validated.[96]

### Chemoprevention clinical trials

***Breast Cancer Prevention Trial (BCPT).*** Results from several major clinical trials established scientific proof-of-principle for the use of chemoprevention, and demonstrated the feasibility of conducting large chemoprevention RCTs in high-risk populations. The BCPT, sponsored by the NCI and conducted by the National Surgical Adjuvant Breast and Bowel Project (NSABP), was a double-blind RCT evaluating the effectiveness of tamoxifen for breast cancer prevention in high-risk women. High-risk factors included age (women aged 60 and older or 35–59 with a risk equal to that of an average 60-year-old); personal or family history of breast cancer; history of benign breast disease;

**TABLE 5-5**

**Characteristics of Chemoprevention and Chemotherapy Clinical Trials**

| | Chemoprevention Trials | Chemotherapy Trials |
|---|---|---|
| Goals | Cancer prevention: decrease cancer incidence and mortality; prevent or reverse premalignant lesions; prevent second primaries | Cancer treatment: increase chance of cure or remission; decrease mortality and morbidity |
| Cohorts | Individuals without cancer; high-risk populations; individuals with premalignant lesions; previously treated for malignancy, but currently disease-free | Individuals with cancer |
| Biomarkers | Intermediate/surrogate endpoint biomarkers; early detection biomarkers; cancer risk biomarkers | Cancer eradication; cancer control; cancer palliation |
| Agents | Minimal toxicity profile; potentially long-term administration | Moderate to high toxicity profile is tolerated; relatively short-term administration |

hormonal functions, such as early age at menarche, late age at menopause, nulliparity, and late age at time of first birth. Tamoxifen, a SERM, was chosen to be evaluated for its antiestrogen activity in reducing the risk of breast cancer by blocking the effects of estrogen on breast tissue. The study accrued more than 13,000 participants between 1992 and 1997.[69] Subjects were randomized to receive tamoxifen 20 mg/day or placebo over a 5-year period. Women in the tamoxifen group experienced 49% fewer diagnoses of invasive and noninvasive breast cancer (eg, ductal or lobular carcinoma in situ) compared to the placebo group. Based on these findings, in October 1998 tamoxifen became the first drug ever to gain FDA approval *for* cancer risk reduction, establishing it as an effective medical intervention for breast cancer prevention in high-risk women.[97] Although the majority of adverse events associated with tamoxifen were temporary (hot flashes, vaginal dryness), several long-term and serious types of risks were identified, including increased incidence of endometrial cancer and several thromboembolic events (pulmonary embolism, deep vein thrombosis, and stroke). In 2005, after 7 additional years of follow-up, BCPT reported that women in the tamoxifen group continued to experience a decreased incidence of invasive and noninvasive breast cancer at similar rates as in the original report. This group also continued to show increased rates of endometrial cancer and thromboembolic events at a similar rate to that reported earlier. All endometrial cancers in the tamoxifen-exposed group were Stage I and therefore could be treated and "cured" with hysterectomy. Long-term follow-up continues for this important study.[98]

***Study of Tamoxifen and Raloxifene (STAR).*** Given the serious risks associated with tamoxifen, the STAR trial was designed to determine whether raloxifene, a second generation SERM, was as effective as tamoxifen in reducing breast cancer incidence, but with fewer serious adverse events. STAR enrolled 19,747 postmenopausal high-risk women from 1999 to 2004. Eligibility for STAR was restricted to postmenopausal women because raloxifene had previously been approved by the FDA for treatment of osteoporosis in this population. Nearly 50% risk reduction for invasive breast cancer was found in both groups, but women receiving raloxifene experienced 36% fewer uterine cancers and 29% fewer thromboembolic events than women receiving tamoxifen.[76] In a follow-up analysis published in 2009, results demonstrated a similar incidence of invasive breast cancer for both groups, but fewer cases of noninvasive breast cancer in the tamoxifen group, with fewer thromboembolic events in the raloxifene group.[99] The STAR trial has shown that raloxifene is as effective as tamoxifen in reducing the risk of invasive breast cancer and has a lower risk of serious adverse events, but a nonstatistically significant higher risk of noninvasive breast cancer.[99,100] This higher incidence of noninvasive cancer with raloxifene is not a major concern, as only invasive cancer metastasizes, ultimately causing death.

***Prostate Cancer Prevention Trial (PCPT).*** The PCPT was a phase III RCT evaluating the efficacy of a 5-alpha-reductase inhibitor, finasteride, for prostate cancer prevention. Finasteride inhibits the conversion of testosterone to dihydrotestosterone, which is a key promoter of prostate cancer. The study randomized 18,882 men aged 55 and older without evidence of disease, based on prostate specific antigen (PSA) ≥3.0 ng/mL, and normal digital rectal exam (DRE). Participants enrolled in the study from October 1993 to May 1997, and received finasteride 5 mg/day or placebo for 7 years.[70] The study was stopped earlier than intended when an interim analysis revealed prostate cancer incidence was lowered by 25% in the finasteride group. However, early findings also indicated those men in the finasteride group who developed prostate cancer were found to have higher-grade tumors (Gleason score 7–10) than men developing prostate cancer in the placebo group. Recent reanalysis of the original study results suggest that finasteride reduces the overall risk of prostate cancer by 30% and reduces the risk of clinically significant prostate cancer, including high-grade tumors.[101]

***Selenium and Vitamin E Cancer Prevention Trial (SELECT).*** The SELECT was designed to evaluate whether nutritional supplements, selenium and vitamin E, are effective in reducing the incidence of prostate cancer in a high-risk male population.[102] The rationale for selecting selenium and vitamin E was based on promising activity from two earlier RCTs. The selection of selenium was based on findings from the National Prevention of Cancer (NPC) trial, which found prostate cancer incidence reduced by 63% among men receiving daily selenium supplementation.[71] Vitamin E was chosen based on findings from the Alpha-Tocopherol, Beta-Carotene (ATBC) study, which indicated a 32% reduction in prostate cancer incidence and a 40% reduction in prostate cancer mortality in men taking α-tocopherol (vitamin E).[68] SELECT accrued 35,533 male subjects between 2001 and 2004 in over 400 sites across the mainland US, Canada, and Puerto Rico. Study eligibility criteria included being a male aged 55 years and older, absence of prostate cancer, serum PSA level of ≤4 ng/mL, and negative DRE. African American men, due to their increased risk of prostate cancer, were allowed to enter the trial at age 50. Participants were randomized in blinded fashion to 1 of 4 groups: (1) oral selenium (200 µg/day of L-selenomethionine) and matched vitamin E placebo; (2) vitamin E (400 IU/day of all rac-α-tocopheryl acetate) and matched selenium placebo; (3) selenium + vitamin E; or (4) 2 placebos for the 2 nutrients for a planned follow-up of at least 7 years and a maximum of 12 years. In October 2008, SELECT was stopped when results indicated that selenium and vitamin E, taken alone or together, did not reduce the incidence of prostate cancer.[75] In addition, SELECT data showed 2 trends that were concerning, though not statistically significant: (1) slight increased incidence of prostate cancer in men taking vitamin E only;

and (2) slight increased incidence of diabetes in men taking selenium only. Although SELECT was stopped early, ongoing follow-up will continue for study participants for approximately 3 years.

## Vaccines

*Infectious Agents.* Multiple epidemiological studies have reported an association between several viruses—human papillomavirus (HPV), hepatitis B virus (HBV), hepatitis C virus (HCV), and human immunodeficiency virus (HIV), and adult T-cell leukemia/lymphoma virus (HTLV-1)—and the development of various malignancies.[34,103] According to the Centers for Disease Control and Prevention, HPV is the most common sexually transmitted disease in the US, and is responsible for causing nearly all cases of cervical cancer.[104] Although only a small percentage of women with HPV develop cervical cancer, between 250,000 and 1 million American women are diagnosed with cervical dysplasia, a potential precursor to cervical cancer caused by the virus.[31] Recent evidence suggests that certain HPV types may also be associated with some head and neck cancers (eg, oropharyngeal and throat cancers).[105] Chronic HBV infection causes up to 90% of hepatocellular cancers (HCC) in adults, with HCV accounting for most of the remaining cases.[106] In 2005, HPV, HBV, and HCV were the first ever viruses identified as known human carcinogens, by the US Department of Health and Human Services National Toxicology Report.[107] These viruses and other infectious agents, such as *H. pylori*, are responsible for 10% to 20 % of cancers worldwide.

Administration of prophylactic vaccines to protect against cancer-causing viruses is a relatively new medical approach in cancer prevention, and is appropriate if (1) a microorganism is the known etiologic source of cancer; (2) vaccination can effectively prevent infection from the microorganism; and (3) prevention of infection by the microorganism can prevent cancer from developing.[108,109] Although the association between microorganisms and cancer development has been under investigation for close to half a century, only over the past several decades have vaccines slowly entered mainstream practice. Hepatitis B vaccine received FDA approval in 1982, and has proven 95% effective in preventing hepatitis B.[110] The vaccine is recommended for all infants, older children and adolescents who were not previously vaccinated, and adults employed in healthcare settings (exposure to blood). While an effective vaccine against HCV or HIV is not currently available, investigative efforts in these areas are ongoing. In 2006, the FDA approved Gardasil, the first vaccine to prevent cervical cancer caused by HPV.[111,112] Gardasil is effective against HPV types 16 and 18, which cause approximately 70% of cervical cancers, and against HPV types 6 and 11, which cause nearly 90% of genital warts. The US Centers for Disease Control and Prevention (CDC) Advisory Committee on Immunization Practices (ACIP) officially recommends that females aged 11 to 12 receive the vaccine, and further indicates that females as young as age 9 and as old as age 26 are also candidates for immunization.[113] As of late 2007, approximately 25% of US females age 13 to 17 years had received at least 1 of the 3 HPV injections. *H. pylori* is a gram negative, spiral, microaerophylic bacterium that infects more than 50% of the population worldwide, and has been associated with increased risk of gastric carcinomas and lymphomas.[114,115] Early-phase clinical trials have recently begun in small numbers of study subjects to evaluate several candidate vaccines for protective effects against *H. pylori*.

*Nicotine.* Vaccination against nicotine addiction is an innovative and appealing concept for smoking cessation, and ultimately the prevention of a variety of malignancies and chronic diseases of the heart and lung. The vaccine is thought to act by stimulating the production of antinicotine antibodies that inhibit passage of nicotine molecules across the blood/brain barrier, and consequently prevent the addiction-reinforcing characteristics of nicotine.[116] Results from early phase trials indicate smoking abstinence can occur when sufficient antibody levels in the blood are achieved and maintained. Success of an antinicotine vaccine could potentially decrease smoking and ultimately decrease lung cancer incidence and mortality worldwide.

## Screening

Screening for early detection has been an important component of cancer prevention practice since the 1940s with the development of the Papanicolaou (Pap) test for cervical cancer. The overall goal of cancer screening is to decrease cancer mortality, although not all malignancies are amenable to screening. Characteristics of malignant disease appropriate for screening are those with high rates of incidence and mortality, known natural history, high rate of prevalence in the preclinical (asymptomatic) phase, and the availability of an effective treatment should cancer be detected.[117] Ideally, an effective screening test has the following attributes: (1) the test is *sensitive*—individuals *with* cancer have a positive test; (2) *specific*—individuals *without* cancer have a negative test; and is associated with (3) high *positive predictive value*—individuals with a positive test *have cancer*; and (4) *negative-predictive value*—individuals with a negative test *do not have cancer*, for the screened malignancy.[118] Screening tests should also be safe, inexpensive, minimally invasive, and easily accessible by all populations.[119] Although the benefits of screening for early detection are well-documented, there are also associated risks that must be weighed against the benefits.[120] While the benefit of cancer screening (decreased mortality rates) is clear, the risks associated with screening are not always appreciated. Risks may include

(1) complications associated with the screening procedure itself (eg, bowel perforation associated with colonoscopy); (2) false-positive test results that lead to unnecessary anxiety and invasive diagnostic procedures, which have their own complications; (3) false-negative test results that can delay diagnosis and treatment of true disease at an early stage when cure may be more obtainable with treatment; and (4) over-diagnosis—the diagnosis and treatment of disease that otherwise may have gone undetected and remained clinically insignificant for the remainder of an individual's life. Because of these complexities which are inherent in all screening tests, individuals should discuss the benefits and risks of cancer screening with their healthcare professional prior to screening.

The most widely used screening programs have been for early detection of cancers of the cervix and breast. Since the introduction of the Pap smear in the 1940s, it has become standard screening practice. In fact, approximately 85% of women aged 18 years and older reported having had a Pap smear in the previous 3 years.[120] Prior to screening, cervical cancer was the leading cause of cancer death among women. Since that time, mortality from cervical cancer has declined sharply in the US and other developed countries, although in underdeveloped countries it remains a significant cause of cancer deaths. The identification of a causal relationship between the human papilloma virus (HPV) and cervical cancer provides one more opportunity for early detection through screening. In this case, the screen is not directly for cancer, but rather for a virus that must be present for the cancer to develop. The American College of Obstetricians and Gynecologists recommends HPV testing, in addition to Pap screening, in all women over the age of 30, although the benefits of such screening in older women have not been established.[121]

Digital mammography and magnetic resonance imaging (MRI) are examples of technological advances that enhance the ability to detect cancers at an early stage, when treatment opportunities may be more effective and allow for prolonged survival. Digital mammography is a technology that goes beyond traditional mammography in that it is capable of capturing, storing, and then manipulating electronic images for enhanced evaluation. The American College of Radiology Imaging Network (ACRIN) conducted a clinical trial, Digital Mammographic Imaging Screening Trial (DMIST), to evaluate the effectiveness of digital vs traditional film mammography. Although study results showed similar findings for both technologies in the general population, there was a suggestion that digital mammography may be beneficial in the detection and staging of breast cancers at earlier stages for women in several subgroups: (1) women under the age of 50; (2) premenopausal or perimenopausal women, and (3) women with radiographically dense breasts.[122] MRI has been tested in clinical trials, in particular for women with a familial or genetic predisposition to breast cancer.[123] Because of its high sensitivity, although accompanied by low specificity, MRI has been useful for screening in women with known genetic predisposition to cancer, such as women with *BRCA1* and *BRCA2* gene mutations.[124] The ACS recommends an annual MRI in conjunction with mammography for breast cancer screening in this high-risk population. In women at average risk, the ACS recommends clinical breast exam (CBE) at least every 3 years for women in their 20s and 30s, and annually for women over the age of 40. The ACS recommends that annual mammogram screening begin at age 40.[125] The US Preventive Services Task Force (USPSTF) recommends screening mammography, with or without CBE, every 1 to 2 years for women aged 40 and older.[126] Despite the recommendation discrepancies from these 2 groups, mammography continues to be the most widely used cancer screening test available. Biomarkers have been identified in women with a higher risk of breast cancer; molecular approaches are likely to expand in the years ahead as more is learned about the genetics of breast cancer. Molecular markers may be useful to identify women likely to benefit from specific medical interventions.

Although screening has been shown to be effective for decreasing cancer incidence and mortality rates for colorectal cancers, it has not been nearly as well accepted as screening tests for breast and cervical cancers.[127] In addition to decades of experience with Fecal Occult Blood Test (FOBT) screening for the presence of blood in the stool, several newer tests are also available. The Fecal Immunochemical Test (FIT) is similar to standard FOBT, but does not require certain food or drug restrictions that might interfere with screening results prior to testing. FIT provides superior sensitivity with similar specificity to traditional tests.[128] Stool DNA tests are also being developed to identify DNA mutations in stool samples. In addition, a recent trial comparing various colorectal screening methods reported that high-resolution computed tomography colonography (CTC) is comparable to traditional colonoscopy, with sensitivities approximately equal in identifying polyps >5 mm.[129] The NCI is conducting clinical trials to determine the most efficient and cost-effective manner to screen people for colon cancer; there are also clinical trials to determine the best population-wide strategies for improving screening participation.[130]

***Prostate, Lung, Colorectal, Ovarian (PLCO) Screening Trial.*** As with other medical prevention interventions, screening tests should be validated in phase III RCTs to determine efficacy prior to implementation in mass screening. The Prostate, Lung, Colorectal, and Ovarian (PLCO) trial is an example of a large NCI-sponsored cancer screening trial. The purpose of the PLCO is to determine whether early detection through screening effectively lowers mortality rates for cancers of the prostate, lung, colon and rectum, and ovary, which, when combined account for approximately 45% of cancer deaths in the United States annually.[31] The

PLCO screening tests include (1) chest x-ray for lung cancer and sigmoidoscopy for colon cancer for all study participants, and (2) CA125 and transvaginal ultrasound for ovarian cancer, and (3) PSA and DRE for prostate cancer. The PLCO accrued study subjects between 1993 and 2001, randomizing 155,000 males and females to 1 of 2 groups: (1) an intervention group receiving serial screening exams over 6 years, with a 7-year follow-up period; or (2) a control group receiving routine care from their healthcare providers, with follow-up for a period of 13 years. A key feature of the PLCO study design is a biorepository containing specimens obtained from study participants at baseline and throughout the study. The specimens are available to researchers throughout the country via a competitive process overseen by a PLCO review committee, to identify, develop, and validate biomarkers of risk and early detection.[131] The primary clinical endpoint of the prostate cancer screens (prostate cancer mortality) was reported; this was the first disease site to have its primary endpoint reported. Findings showed that the mortality rate from prostate cancer after 7 years of study was low overall and did not differ significantly between the intervention and control groups, despite a 22% increase in incidence in the screened group.[132] Study follow-up is ongoing to evaluate participants for quality-of-life issues surrounding diagnosis and the subsequent effects of treatment related to prostate cancer. Results from other components of this important screening study are expected to be reported over the next decade.

*National Lung Screening Trial (NLST).* Another major NCI-sponsored screening study, the NLST, is being conducted in collaboration with PLCO investigators and the American College of Radiology Imaging Network (ACRIN).[133] Although lung cancer is the leading cause of cancer mortality for men and women in the US, an effective validated screening test is not available at this time. NLST is evaluating 2 screening modalities, helical (also called spiral) CT and chest x-ray, in 53,000 smokers and former smokers over 8 years at 30 sites nationwide. Helical CT is a scanning technology in which a CT scanner rotates around a subject who is positioned on an x-ray table that passes through the center of the scanner. Helical CT allows low-resolution image of the entire thorax in a single breath-hold, reducing the chance of artifact.[134] Computer-generated images are assembled into a 3-dimensional model of the thorax using one tenth the radiation dose of a diagnostic CT scan. Earlier, results from several observational studies indicated that helical CT was able to detect tiny abnormalities in lung tissue, generally too small to be identified on chest x-ray.[135,136] However, it is unclear to the research community whether detection of such miniscule abnormalities translates into an advantage for reducing mortality. Consequently, NLST was designed as a definitive RCT to evaluate the true mortality effects of helical CT and chest x-ray. Results from NLST are expected in 2009 and could have major implications for public health policy if findings indicate a mortality benefit from lung cancer screening with helical CT.

## CANCER PREVENTION AND PUBLIC POLICY

In order to develop comprehensive and effective public health policies for cancer prevention, associations between environmental, economic, social, as well as biological factors and cancer development must be accepted by all members of society.[137] Collaborative efforts are required among policy-makers, federal agencies, industry, local governments, and communities to commit to establishing public health goals, and implementing cost-effective and safe standards for protective measures for all citizens. Ideally, a comprehensive nationwide public health prevention program encompasses tobacco control, healthy and safe food products, physical activity accommodations (eg, dedicated bike paths, publicly available swimming pools, and exercise equipment), environmental safety controls, with a special focus on a healthy lifestyle in childhood.

### TOBACCO

Tobacco use has received unprecedented attention as a result of tobacco taxes, state lawsuits against tobacco companies, and sweeping legislative proposals to reduce smoking, especially among youth. Litigation has resulted in the release of many confidential documents from tobacco companies, including unpublished research on nicotine addiction and tobacco marketing practices. It has also produced changes in the way tobacco is advertised and sold nationwide.

The state of California provides a good example of attainable progress in tobacco control strategies. California's tobacco control program was initiated in 1989, at a time when smoking prevalence in the state was approximately 11% lower than the rest of the country. By 1996, following implementation of a strict tobacco control program, the differential between California and the rest of the country had increased to 20%, and there was an overall 25% increase in smoking cessation within state.[138] California also reported an $86 billion reduction in healthcare expenditures associated with the tobacco control program over the first 5 years of program implementation.[139] The state credits dramatic declines in smoking prevalence rates primarily to strict bans on smoking in the workplace and in public areas, and increased cigarette prices.[140] Other states are resisting tobacco control interventions because of the expense involved in such projects, in part due to budget cuts, but states have also diverted tobacco settlement funds to nontobacco projects.[141] In 1998, the states received a $246 billion legal settlement from the tobacco industry for smoking cessation projects for adults and smoking prevention programs for children.[142]

A recent report indicates that over the past 10 years, the states have received $203.5 billion in tobacco-generated revenue, $79.2 billion from tobacco settlements, and $124.3 billion from tobacco taxes. Disappointingly, only 3.2% of the money has been spent on prevention and cessation programs. In addition, none of the states is funding tobacco control programs at levels recommended by the US CDC.[143] Currently, annual marketing expenditures by the tobacco industry have increased by 94% from $6.9 billion in 1998 to 13.4 billion in 2005.[142]

Recently, the US Congress considered legislation that would grant authority to the FDA to regulate tobacco products. Such regulation would restrict marketing and sales of tobacco products to adolescents, modify and enhance warning labels on cigarette packages, restrict Internet sales, and require tobacco companies to provide detailed information related to the composition of their products.

### OBESITY

In 2007, the NCI challenged researchers to explore obesity policy research, as a way to effect change in current nutritional and physical activity behaviors that contribute to the obesity epidemic. Evidence shows that obesity has the potential to profoundly affect the nation's economy, as a result of a variety of chronic conditions and illnesses, including cancer.[144] An area of growing concern is childhood obesity, with an increase of over 100% in prevalence rates since 1971.[145] Current prevalence rates for childhood overweight and obesity for children aged 2 through 5 is 12.5%, an increase from 7.2% in 1994.[145] One reason for this epidemic is related to expensive marketing campaigns for popular fast foods that target young children and adolescents, while not enough is being done by health promotion organizations (ie, CDC and NCI) to educate children about healthy food choices and other healthy lifestyle behaviors. A current study, Making Our Mealtimes Special (MOMS), is designed to evaluate 2 methods of anticipatory guidance during the first year of life to determine whether either is more effective than usual care conditions in promoting healthy eating behaviors during childhood.[145] One intervention group receives nutrition education directed toward the mother's eating behavior, while the other intervention uses an educational program that instructs mothers about healthy eating behaviors for the child. The control group receives nutritional advice that is part of a usual well-baby care visit.

### CLINICAL TRIALS

An important focus of prevention policy should be clinical trial participation in order to gain evidence-based information regarding cancer prevention and treatment. Policy to regulate payment for clinical trials would likely have a positive impact on accrual, especially for under-represented populations, which include adolescents, older adults (aged ≥65 years), individuals of low SES, individuals living in rural areas, African Americans, Latinos/Hispanics, Asian Americans and Pacific Islanders, and American Indians/Alaska Natives.[95,146] Although current regulation provides for Medicare reimbursement for routine costs associated with a study, it is not commensurate with the true cost associated with conducting a clinical trial.[141,146] Policy proposals aimed at increasing insurance reimbursement for physicians willing to participate in community clinical trials would likely improve accrual among populations covered by Medicare and Medicaid. The net result would be an acceleration of accrual, thereby decreasing the duration of what are now lengthy clinical trials. In addition, study results would be more generalizable because of the inclusion of these subpopulations.

### RECOMMENDATIONS

In a 2007 landmark report, Policy and Action for Cancer Prevention, the WCRF/AICR offered 10 comprehensive, evidence-based recommendations for global cancer prevention.[12] More recently in 2009, the WCRF/AICR went further, supplementing the recommendations with an urgent call to action at the multinational, national, state, local, and individual levels to develop, implement, and evaluate short-term and long-term health policies and prevention strategies to address the important known causes of increased cancer risk.[137] The report recommends rational policies and effective actions that could be implemented at all levels of society to achieve acceptable public health now and for future generations.

## CANCER PREVENTION CHALLENGES

As the science of prevention evolves, we are presented with a variety of challenges and opportunities. One of the primary challenges is to gain better understanding of the molecular events underlying carcinogenesis and to translate that information into clinical practice. Currently the drug development process is painstakingly slow, but the recent introduction of phase 0 trials should prove effective in shortening the time an agent spends in the clinical trials system.

Another major issue in cancer prevention is caused by misleading and confusing information. At times, conflicting accounts of the benefits and harms associated with nutritional or dietary supplements may be reported in the press simultaneously. Conflicting or partial reports contribute to confusion among information-seeking recipients and healthcare providers. Furthermore, data from observational studies have not always been consistent with findings from clinical trials. For example, numerous observational studies have reported a strong inverse association between increased intake of fruits and vegetables (rich in beta-carotene) and lung cancer incidence. Based on these data, a large RCT, the Carotene and Vitamin E Trial (CARET), was designed to evaluate and validate these supplements for lung cancer prevention. Disappointingly, increased lung cancer incidence and mortality rates were found for smokers and former smokers receiving beta-carotene.[147]

The clinical trials process presents many interesting challenges for researchers. Definitive chemoprevention trials are costly, lengthy, and require large numbers of participants, but have a great potential for public benefit. Issues related to the difficulty of conducting such large phase III trials include less than optimal numbers of individuals willing to participate in clinical trials and difficulties reaching underserved populations. Differences between chemotherapy treatment trials and chemoprevention trials underscore some of the unique challenges. Chemopreventive agents must have extremely low toxicity profiles, much lower than is acceptable in treatment trials for late stage cancers. Prevention trials utilize cancer incidence or mortality endpoints, which are more difficult to attain than the disease response endpoints that serve as a metric of success or failure in treatment trials. For this reason, surrogate endpoints, mainly biomarkers, are being developed that may serve as substitutes, but these are still in the exploratory phase. Surrogate endpoints for adverse events also would be useful. Finally, high-risk study subjects are more difficult to identify and enroll in prevention trials than are individuals with cancer.

Risks and perceptions associated with cancer screening present obstacles to successful mass screening for some diseases. For instance, despite evidence that screening reduces mortality rates for colorectal cancers, only 50% of individuals in the age group recommended for screening by the USPSTF, undergo screening.[127] Lack of insurance and access are some of the obstacles, but also the lack of educational programs and materials presented at low reading comprehension levels and in foreign languages, which often leads to a misunderstanding or lack of knowledge about available options for screening.[148] In addition, guidelines are not always consistent among organizations tasked with producing them (eg, ACS and PTSTF differ on recommended length of time between breast cancer screenings for women aged 40–50). And there are risks associated with screening tests. Because no screening test has 100% sensitivity and specificity, false-positive and false-negative readings occur. False-positive test results cause unwarranted anxiety in tested individuals while they pursue diagnostic workups. On the other hand, individuals with false-negative screening results may lose valuable diagnostic and treatment time, and therefore have lowered opportunities for survival. Finally, downstream harmful effects associated with screening tests affect not only individuals, but the healthcare community and society as well. For instance, helical CT is capable of detecting tiny lung abnormalities, an unknown number of which may never to go on to become cancers. However, once identified, the nature of a lesion must be pursued. No one can estimate the number of avoidable invasive or surgical procedures that are performed in pursuit of nonsignificant lesions identified on helical CT, associated morbidity and mortality rates, or the personal and public financial impact. For this reason, helical CT for lung cancer screening should not be implemented in the general population until results of the NLST become available. It is often difficult to convince individuals to refrain from seeking out new screening technologies until they have been validated in phase III RCTs.

## NURSING IMPLICATIONS

As the landscape of cancer prevention evolves, nurses strive to keep pace with advances in technology, medical interventions, and risk factor modifications. Nurses perform traditional cancer prevention functions such as identifying unhealthy behaviors (eg, tobacco use, obesity) and providing education and counseling related to healthier lifestyle choices and cancer screening.[149] With more than 40 million current smokers in the United States, it is vital that nurses educate themselves and other healthcare providers about tobacco dependence and evidence-based interventions to assist with smoking cessation. Nursing interventions, such as tobacco counseling, have been shown to significantly increase smoking cessation and improve outcomes. TFN and other initiatives supported by government and nongovernment organizations provide educational programs and guidelines for increasing awareness of the dangers associated with smoking and offer recommendations to lower smoking prevalence rates.

In addition to conventional responsibilities, more complex nursing roles have evolved in areas related to cancer prevention. These increased prevention-related responsibilities become more important as the demands on physician's time allows for less physician-to-patient discussions regarding healthy lifestyle modifications, screening recommendations, and chemoprevention trial options for high-risk individuals. Cancer risk assessment has become a large part of the prevention nurse's repertoire. Risk assessments include an evaluation for increased cancer risk due to behavioral, physiological, environmental, and family history and genetic factors. Nurses play an important role in identifying these high-risk individuals for inclusion in chemoprevention clinical trials. A variety of responsibilities are included in the nurse's role in clinical trials. Some nurses are involved with data collection and management and conducting data quality assurance to ensure accuracy and timeliness of the information. An important component of clinical trials nursing is identifying, reporting, and observing for trends in adverse events, especially serious adverse events. Another area of opportunity is genetics. Given the shortage of trained genetic counselors, nurses have often assumed this role in cancer settings. Nurse geneticists provide education and guidance related to the implication of genetic contributions to disease.[150] Nurses have begun to pursue graduate and doctoral degrees in greater numbers in the areas of nursing informatics, genetics, and clinical trials to support prevention science. Doctorally prepared nurses have begun teaching in subspecialty areas related to cancer prevention. In this manner nurses are gaining expertise in clinical trials, nursing informatics, genetic risk assessment, and other areas, a trend that will hopefully establish nurses as key players in the field of cancer prevention.

Organizations such the Oncology Nursing Society, International Society of Nurses in Genetics, and the National Society of Genetic Counselors provide a wealth of supportive and educational resources for nurses interested in broadening their understanding of prevention. These organizations, and others, provide professional guidelines and standards for practice, as well as online educational courses, CDs, publications, continuing education programs, and other materials related to cancer prevention and genetics-related information. The NCI Division of Cancer Prevention also provides online information regarding cancer prevention and behavioral risks, chemoprevention, screening, and descriptions of completed and ongoing clinical prevention trials.[151] In the long term, nurses can effect major changes in cancer prevention health policy by functioning as change agents and advocates for tobacco control policies, healthy school lunch programs, physical fitness curricula, diet and nutritional awareness, immunization agendas, and clean air programs in their workplaces and communities. Nurses are practicing in a new era where making appreciable changes in the lives of many individuals through cancer prevention is a reality.

## REFERENCES


1. Sporn MB. Carcinogenesis and cancer: different perspectives on the same disease. *Cancer Res.* 1991;51:6215–6218.
2. Lippman SM, Benner SE, Hong WK. Cancer chemoprevention. *J Clin Oncol.* 1994;12:851–873.
3. Greenwald P, McDonald SS, Anderson DE. An evidence-based approach to cancer prevention clinical trials. *Eur J Cancer Prev.* 2002;11(Suppl 2): S43-S47.
4. Wattenberg LW. An overview of chemoprevention: current status and future prospects. *Proc Soc Exp Biol Med.* 1997;216:133–141.
5. Lippman SM, Benner SE, Hong WK. Chemoprevention. Strategies for the control of cancer. *Cancer.* 1993;72(3 Suppl):984–990.
6. Hong WK, Sporn MB. Recent advances in chemoprevention of cancer. *Science.* 1997;278:1073–1077.
7. Kelloff GJ, Sigman CC, Greenwald P. Cancer chemoprevention: progress and promise. *Eur J Cancer.* 1999;35:2031–2038.
8. Keith L. Chemoprevention of lung cancer. *Proc Am Thorac Soc.* 2009; 6:187–193.
9. Volker DL. Carcinogenesis: application to clinical practice. *Clin J Oncol Nurs.* 2001;5:225–226, 229.
10. Peto R, Darby S, Deo H, Silcocks P, Whitley E, Doll R. Smoking, smoking cessation, and lung cancer in the UK since 1950: combination of national statistics with two case-control studies. *BMJ.* 2000;321:323–329.
11. Jemal A, Siegel R, Ward E, et al. Cancer statistics, 2008. *Cancer J Clin.* 2008;58:71–96.
12. World Cancer Research Fund/American Institute for Cancer Research. *Food, Nutrition, Physical Activity, and the Prevention of Cancer: A Global Perspective.* Washington, DC: AICR; 2007.
13. Martinez ME, Marshall JR, Giovannucci E. Diet and cancer prevention: the roles of observation and experimentation. *Nat Rev Cancer.* 2008;8:694–703.
14. Bingham SA, Day NE, Luben R, et al. Dietary fibre in food and protection against colorectal cancer in the European Prospective Investigation into Cancer and Nutrition (EPIC): an observational study. *Lancet.* 2003;361:1496–1501.
15. Peters U, Sinha R, Chatterjee N, et al. Dietary fibre and colorectal adenoma in a colorectal cancer early detection programme. *Lancet.* 2003;361:1491–1495.
16. Schatzkin A, Lanza E, Corle D, et al. Lack of effects of a low-fat, high-fiber diet on the recurrence of colorectal adenomas. Polyp Prevention Trial Study group. *N Engl J Med.* 2000;342:1149–1155.
17. Lanza E, Yu B, Murphy G, et al. The polyp prevention trial continued follow-up study: no effect of a low-fat, high-fiber, high-fruit, and -vegetable diet on adenoma recurrence eight years after randomization. *Cancer Epidemiol Biomarkers Prev.* 2007;16:1745–1752.
18. Alberts DS, Martinez ME, Roe DJ, et al. Lack of effect of a high-fiber cereal supplement on the recurrence of colorectal adenomas. Phoenix Colon Cancer Prevention Physicians' Network. *N Engl J Med.* 2000; 342:1156–1162.
19. Beresford SA, Johnson KC, Ritenbaugh C, et al. Low-fat dietary pattern and risk of colorectal cancer: the Women's Health Initiative Randomized Controlled Dietary Modification Trial. *JAMA.* 2006;295: 643–654.
20. Prentice RL, Caan B, Chlebowski RT, et al. Low-fat dietary pattern and risk of invasive breast cancer: the Women's Health Initiative Randomized Controlled Dietary Modification Trial. *JAMA.* 2006;295:629–642.
21. Jackson RD, LaCroix AZ, Gass M, et al. Calcium plus vitamin D supplementation and the risk of fractures. *N Engl J Med.* 2006;354: 669–683.
22. Temple NJ, Balay-Karperien AL. Nutrition in cancer prevention: an integrated approach. *J Am Coll Nutr.* 2002;21:79–83.
23. Calle EE, Rodriguez C, Walker-Thurmond K, Thun MJ. Overweight, obesity, and mortality from cancer in a prospectively studied cohort of US adults. *N Engl J Med.* 2003;348:1625–1638.
24. Renehan AG, Tyson M, Egger M, Heller RF, Zwahlen M. Body-mass index and incidence of cancer: a systematic review and meta-analysis of prospective observational studies. *Lancet.* 2008;371:569–578.
25. Pan SY, DesMeules M. Energy intake, physical activity, energy balance, and cancer: epidemiologic evidence. *Methods Mol Biol.* 2009;472: 191–215.
26. Monninkhof EM, Elias SG, Vlems FA, et al. Physical activity and breast cancer: a systematic review. *Epidemiology.* 2007;18:137–157.
27. National Cancer Institute PDQ. An individualized internet-based health behavior program or a standard internet-based health behavior program in preventing cancer and improving physical activity and nutrition in participants who are physically inactive with a higher body mass index. http://clinicaltrials.gov/ct2/show/NCT00128570. Accessed January 17, 2010.
28. Rogers CJ, Colbert LH, Greiner JW, Perkins SN, Hursting SD. Physical activity and cancer prevention: pathways and targets for intervention. *Sports Med.* 2008;38:271–296.
29. US Department of Health and Human Services. Tobacco information. http://www.cdc.gov/nccdphp/publications/aag/osh.htm. Accessed January 17, 2010.

30. Ezzati M, Lopez AD, Rodgers A, Vander Hoorn S, Murray CJ. Selected major risk factors and global and regional burden of disease. *Lancet.* 2002;360:1347–1360.
31. American Cancer Society. Cancer facts and figures 2009. http://www.cancer.org/downloads/STT/500809web.pdf. Accessed June 1, 2009.
32. Wynder EL, Graham EA. Tobacco smoking as a possible etiologic factor in bronchiogenic carcinoma: a study of 684 proved cases. *J Am Med Assoc.* 1950;143:329–336.
33. Doll R, Hill AB. Smoking and carcinoma of the lung: preliminary report. *Br Med J.* 1950;2:739–748.
34. Greenwald P, Dunn BK. Landmarks in the history of cancer epidemiology. *Cancer Res.* 2009;69:2151–2162.
35. US Department of Health, Education, and Welfare. Smoking and health: report of the Advisory Committee of the Surgeon General of the Public Health Service. http://profiles.nlm.nih.gov/NN/B/C/X/B/. Accessed January 17, 2010.
36. Doll R, Peto R, Wheatley K, Gray R, Sutherland I. Mortality in relation to smoking: 40 years' observations on male British doctors. *BMJ.* 1994;309:901–911.
37. US Department of Health and Human Services. *The Health Consequences of Involuntary Exposure to Tobacco Smoke: A Report of the Surgeon General.* Washington, DC: US Department of Health and Human Services; 2006.
38. Shafey O, Eriksen M, Ross H, Mackay J. *The Tobacco Atlas.* 3rd ed. Atlanta, GA: American Cancer Society; 2009.
39. Hill SC and Liang, L. Smoking in the home and children's health. Tobacco Control. 2008;17:32–37.
40. Sarna L, Bialous S. Strategic directions for nursing research in tobacco dependence. *Nurs Res.* 2006;55:S1-S9.
41. Substance Abuse and Mental Health Services Administration, Office of Applied Studies. *Results from the 2007 National Survey on Drug Use and Health: National Findings.* NSDUH Series H-34, DHHS Publication No. SMA 08–4343. Rockville, MD: Substance Abuse and Mental Health Services Administration; 2008.
42. World Health Organization. WHO report on Global Tobacco Epidemic, 2008—the MPOWER Package: tobacco facts. http://www.who.int/tobacco/mpower/en/. Accessed January 17, 2010.
43. Kohler CL, Schoenberger YM, Beasley TM, Phillips MM. Effectiveness evaluation of the N-O-T smoking cessation program for adolescents. *Am J Health Behav.* 2008;32:368–379.
44. Horn K, McGloin T, Dino G, et al. Quit and reduction rates for a pilot study of the American Indian Not On Tobacco (N-O-T) program. *Prev Chronic Dis.* 2005;2:A13.
45. Branstetter SA, Horn K, Dino G, Zhang J. Beyond quitting: predictors of teen smoking cessation, reduction and acceleration following a school-based intervention. *Drug Alcohol Depend.* 2009;99:160–168.
46. Dino G, Horn K, Abdulkadri A, Kalsekar I, Branstetter S. Cost-effectiveness analysis of the Not On Tobacco program for adolescent smoking cessation. *Prev Sci.* 2008;9:38–46.
47. Horn K, Dino G, Branstetter SA, et al. A profile of teen smokers who volunteered to participate in school-based smoking intervention. *Tob Induc Dis.* 2008;4:6.
48. Sussman S, Sun P. Youth tobacco use cessation: 2008 update. *Tob Induc Dis.* 2009;5:3.
49. Trosclair A, Caraballo R, Malarcher A, Husten C, Pechacek T. Cigarette smoking among adults—United States, 2003. *MMWR.* 2005;54:509–513.
50. Agrawal A, Sartor C, Pergadia ML, Huizink AC, Lynskey MT. Correlates of smoking cessation in a nationally representative sample of U.S. adults. *Addict Behav.* 2008;33:1223–1226.
51. Evins AE, Culhane MA, Alpert JE, et al. A controlled trial of bupropion added to nicotine patch and behavioral therapy for smoking cessation in adults with unipolar depressive disorders. *J Clin Psychopharmacol.* 2008;28:660–666.
52. Lemmens V, Oenema A, Knut IK, Brug J. Effectiveness of smoking cessation interventions among adults: a systematic review of reviews. *Eur J Cancer Prev.* 2008;17:535–544.
53. Gollust SE, Schroeder SA, Warner KE. Helping smokers quit: understanding the barriers to utilization of smoking cessation services. *Milbank Q.* 2008;86:601–627.
54. US Department of Health and Human Services. Prevention makes common "cents". Washington DC: US Department of Health and Human Services, Public Health Services. 2003. http://aspe.hhs.gov/health/prevention/index.shtml#TOBACCO. Accessed on January 17, 2010.
55. Sarna L, Bialous SA, Jun HJ, Wewers ME, Cooley ME, Feskanich D. Smoking trends in the Nurses' Health Study (1976–2003). *Nurs Res.* 2008;57:374–382.
56. Sarna L, Bialous SA, Wewers ME, Froelicher ES, Danao L. Nurses, smoking, and the workplace. *Res Nurs Health.* 2005;28:79–90.
57. Sarna L, Bialous SA, Cooley ME, Jun HJ, Feskanich D. Impact of smoking and smoking cessation on health-related quality of life in women in the Nurses' Health Study. *Qual Life Res.* 2008;17:1217–1227.
58. Rice VH, Stead LF. Nursing interventions for smoking cessation. *Cochrane Database Syst Rev.* 2008;1.
59. Sarna L, Bialous SA. Strategic directions for nursing research in tobacco dependence. *Nurs Res.* 2006;55:S1-S9.
60. Sarna L, Bialous S, Barbeau E, McLellan D. Strategies to implement tobacco control policy and advocacy initiatives. *Crit Care Nurs North Am.* 2006;18:113–122.
61. Fiore MC, Bailey WC, Cohen SJ, et al. *Treating Tobacco Use and Dependence. A Clinical Practice Guideline.* AHRQ Publication No. 00–0032. Rockville, MD: US Department of Health and Human Services; 2000.
62. US Department of Health and Human Services. US Public Health Services. Helping smokers quit: a guide for nurses. http://www.ahrq.gov/clinic/tobacco/clinhlpsmksqt.pdf. Accessed on June 22, 2009.
63. Derby KS, Cuthrell K, Caberto C, et al. Nicotine metabolism in three ethnic/racial groups with different risks of lung cancer. *Cancer Epidemiol Biomarkers Prev.* 2008;17:3526–3535.
64. Stevens VL, Bierut LJ, Talbot JT, et al. Nicotinic receptor gene variants influence susceptibility to heavy smoking. *Cancer Epidemiol Biomarkers Prev.* 2008;17:3517–3525.
65. US Department of Health and Human Services. Food and Drug Administration. FDA & tobacco regulation. 2009. http://www.fda.gov/NewsEvents/PublicHealthFocus/ucm168412.htm. Accessed on January 17, 2010.
66. Greenwald P, Kramer B, Weed D. *Cancer Prevention and Control.* New York, NY: Marcel Dekker; 1995.
67. Omenn GS, Goodman GE, Thornquist MD, et al. Risk factors for lung cancer and for intervention effects in CARET, the Beta-Carotene and Retinol Efficacy Trial. *J Natl Cancer Inst.* 1996 6;88:1550–1559.
68. The ATBC Cancer Prevention Study Group. The alpha-tocopherol, beta-carotene lung cancer prevention study: design, methods, participant characteristics, and compliance. *Ann Epidemiol.* 1994;4:1–10.
69. Fisher B, Costantino JP, Wickerham DL, et al. Tamoxifen for prevention of breast cancer: report of the National Surgical Adjuvant Breast and Bowel Project P-1 Study. *J Natl Cancer Inst.* 1998;90:1371–1388.
70. Thompson IM, Goodman PJ, Tangen CM, et al. The influence of finasteride on the development of prostate cancer. *N Engl J Med.* 2003;349:215–224.
71. Clark LC, Combs GF Jr, Turnbull BW, et al. Effects of selenium supplementation for cancer prevention in patients with carcinoma of the skin. A randomized controlled trial. Nutritional Prevention of Cancer Study Group. *JAMA.* 1996;276:1957–1963.
72. Blot WJ, Li JY, Taylor PR, et al. Nutrition intervention trials in Linxian, China: supplementation with specific vitamin/mineral combinations, cancer incidence, and disease-specific mortality in the general population. *J Natl Cancer Inst.* 1993;85:1483–1492.
73. Bertagnolli MM, Eagle CJ, Zauber AG, et al. Celecoxib for the prevention of sporadic colorectal adenomas. *N Engl J Med.* 2006;355:873–884.

74. Cook NR, Lee IM, Gaziano JM, et al. Low-dose aspirin in the primary prevention of cancer: the Women's Health Study: a randomized controlled trial. *JAMA.* 2005;294:47–55.
75. Lippman SM, Klein EA, Goodman PJ, et al. Effect of selenium and vitamin E on risk of prostate cancer and other cancers: the Selenium and Vitamin E Cancer Prevention Trial (SELECT). *JAMA.* 2009;301:39–51.
76. Vogel VG, Costantino JP, Wickerham DL, et al. Effects of tamoxifen vs raloxifene on the risk of developing invasive breast cancer and other disease outcomes: the NSABP Study of Tamoxifen and Raloxifene (STAR) P-2 trial. *JAMA.* 2006;295:2727–2741.
77. Richmond E, Viner JL. Chemoprevention of skin cancer. *Semin Oncol Nurs.* 2003;19:62–69.
78. US Department of Health and Human Services, Food and Drug Administration. Guidance for industry, investigators, and reviewers: exploratory IND studies. http://www.fda.gov/downloads/Drugs/GuidanceComplianceRegulatoryInformation/Guidances/UCM07. Accessed January 24, 2010.
79. Kummar S, Doroshow JH, Tomaszewski JE, Calvert AH, Lobbezoo M, Giaccone G. Phase 0 clinical trials: recommendations from the Task Force on Methodology for the Development of Innovative Cancer Therapies. *Eur J Cancer.* 2009;45:741–746.
80. Kummar S, Rubinstein L, Kinders R, et al. Phase 0 clinical trials: conceptions and misconceptions. *Cancer J.* 2008;14:133–137.
81. Steele VE. Current mechanistic approaches to the chemoprevention of cancer. *J Biochem Mol Biol.* 2003;36:78–81.
82. Simonich MT, McQuistan T, Jubert C, et al. Low-dose dietary chlorophyll inhibits multi-organ carcinogenesis in the rainbow trout. *Food Chem Toxicol.* 2008;46:1014–1024.
83. Bertagnolli MM, McDougall CJ, Newmark HL. Colon cancer prevention: intervening in a multistage process. *Proc Soc Exp Biol Med.* 1997;216:266–274.
84. Grubbs LM, Tabano M. Use of sunscreen in health care professionals. The health belief model. *Cancer Nurs.* 2000;23:164–167.
85. Jacoby RF, Seibert K, Cole CE, Kelloff G, Lubet RA. The cyclooxygenase-2 inhibitor celecoxib is a potent preventive and therapeutic agent in the min mouse model of adenomatous polyposis. *Cancer Res.* 2000;60:5040–5044.
86. Thompson IM, Lucia MS, Redman MW, et al. Finasteride decreases the risk of prostatic intraepithelial neoplasia. *J Urol.* 2007;178:107–109; discussion 110.
87. Greenwald P. Cancer prevention clinical trials. *J Clin Oncol.* 2002;20(18 Suppl):14S-22S.
88. Bonassi S, Neri M, Puntoni R. Validation of biomarkers as early predictors of disease. *Mutat Res.* 2001;480–481:349–358.
89. Vourlekis JS, Szabo E. Predicting success in cancer prevention trials. *J Natl Cancer Inst.* 2003;95:178–179.
90. US Department of Health and Human Services, National Institutes of Health. The Early Detection Research Network: investing in translational research on biomarkers of early cancer and cancer risk. 4th Report, January 2008. http://www.compass.fhcrc.org/edrnnci/files/pdf/edrn_4th-report_200801.pdf. Accessed October 14, 2009.
91. Kelloff GJ, Boone CW, Crowell JA, et al. Risk biomarkers and current strategies for cancer chemoprevention. *J Cell Biochem Suppl.* 1996;25:1–14.
92. Winer E, Gralow J, Diller L, et al. Clinical cancer advances 2008: major research advances in cancer treatment, prevention, and screening—a report from the American Society of Clinical Oncology. *J Clin Oncol.* 2009;27:812–826.
93. US Department of Health and Human Services, National Institutes of Health. Strategic research plan and budget to reduce and ultimately eliminate health disparities, volume I, fiscal years 2002–2006. 2002. http://ncmhd.nih.gov/our_programs/strategic/pubs/VolumeI_031003EDrev.pdf. Accessed January 22, 2010.
94. Paskett ED, Katz ML, DeGraffinreid CR, Tatum CM. Participation in cancer trials: recruitment of underserved populations. *Clin Adv Hematol Oncol.* 2003;1:607–613.
95. Ford J, Howerton M, Lai G, et al. *Barriers to Recruiting Underrepresented Populations to Cancer Clinical Trials: A Systematic Review.* Atlanta, GA: American Cancer Society; 2007:228–242.
96. Lai GY, Gary TL, Tilburt J, et al. Effectiveness of strategies to recruit underrepresented populations into cancer clinical trials. *Clin Trials.* 2006;3:133–141.
97. Lippman SM, Brown PH. Tamoxifen prevention of breast cancer: an instance of the fingerpost. *J Natl Cancer Inst.* 1999;91:1809–1819.
98. Fisher B, Costantino JP, Wickerham DL, et al. Tamoxifen for the prevention of breast cancer: current status of the National Surgical Adjuvant Breast and Bowel Project P-1 study. *J Natl Cancer Inst.* 2005; 97:1652–1662.
99. Vogel VG. The NSABP Study of Tamoxifen and Raloxifene (STAR) trial. *Expert Rev Anticancer Ther.* 2009;9:51–60.
100. Wickerham DL, Costantino JP, Vogel VG, et al. The use of tamoxifen and raloxifene for the prevention of breast cancer. *Recent Results Cancer Res.* 2009;181:113–119.
101. Lucia MS, Epstein JI, Goodman PJ, et al. Finasteride and high-grade prostate cancer in the Prostate Cancer Prevention Trial. *J Natl Cancer Inst.* 2007;99:1375–1383.
102. Dunn BK, Ryan A, Ford LG. Selenium and Vitamin E Cancer Prevention Trial: a nutrient approach to prostate cancer prevention. *Recent Results Cancer Res.* 2009;181:183–193.
103. Frazer IH, Lowy DR, Schiller JT. Prevention of cancer through immunization: prospects and challenges for the 21st century. *Eur J Immunol.* 2007;37(Suppl 1):S148-S155.
104. Dunne EF, Unger ER, Sternberg M, et al. Prevalence of HPV infection among females in the United States. *JAMA.* 2007;297:813–819.
105. zur Hausen H. Papillomaviruses in the causation of human cancers—a brief historical account. *Virology.* 2009;384:260–265.
106. Chang MH. Cancer prevention by vaccination against hepatitis B. *Recent Results Cancer Res.* 2009;181:85–94.
107. US Department of Health and Human Services, Public Health Service, National Toxicology Program. Report on carcinogens, eleventh edition. 2005. http://ntp.niehs.nih.gov/ntp/roc/toc11.html. Accessed January 17, 2010.
108. Lee WM. Hepatitis B virus infection. *N Engl J Med.* 1997;337:1733–1745.
109. US Department of Health and Human Services, Centers for Disease Control and Prevention. Viral hepatitis. http://www.cdc.gov/hepatitis/index.htm. Accessed January 17, 2010.
110. World Health Organization. Immunizations, Vaccines, and Biologics: Hepatitis B. http://www.who.int/vaccines/en/hepatitisb.shtml. Accessed January 17, 2010.
111. Hanna E, Bachmann G. HPV vaccination with Gardasil: a breakthrough in women's health. *Expert Opin Biol Ther.* 2006;6:1223–1227.
112. US Department of Health and Human Services, Food and Drug Administration. FDA licenses new vaccine for prevention of cervical cancer and other diseases in females caused by human papillomavirus: rapid approval marks major advancement in public health. http://www.fda.gov/NewsEvents/Newsroom/PressAnnouncements/2006/ucm108666.html. Accessed January 17, 2010.
113. Markowitz LE, Dunne EF, Saraiya M, Lawson HW, Chesson H, Unger ER. Quadrivalent human papillomavirus vaccine: recommendations of the Advisory Committee on Immunization Practices (ACIP). *MMWR Recomm Rep.* 2007;56(RR-2):1–24.
114. Kabir S. The current status of *Helicobacter pylori* vaccines: a review. *Helicobacter.* 2007;12:89–102.
115. Malfertheiner P, Schultze V, Rosenkranz B, et al. Safety and immunogenicity of an intramuscular *Helicobacter pylori* vaccine in noninfected volunteers: a phase I study. *Gastroenterology.* 2008;135:787–795.
116. Maurer P, Bachmann MF. Vaccination against nicotine: an emerging therapy for tobacco dependence. *Exp Opin Investig Drugs.* 2007;16:1775–1783.

117. Mandel J, Smith R. Principles of cancer screening. In: DeVita VT, Lawrence TS, Rosenberg SA, eds. *Devita, Hellman and Rosenberg's Cancer: Principles and Practice of Oncology.* Vol. 1. Philadelphia, PA: Wolters Kluwer/Lippincott Williams & Wilkins; 2008:659–670.
118. US Department of Health and Human Services, National Institutes of Health, National Cancer Institute. Cancer screening. http://www.cancer.gov/cancertopics/pdq/screening/overview. Accessed January 17, 2010.
119. Kramer BS. The science of early detection. *Urol Oncol.* 2004;22: 344–347.
120. Swan J, Breen N, Coates RJ, Rimer BK, Lee NC. Progress in cancer screening practices in the United States: results from the 2000 National Health Interview Survey. *Cancer.* 2003;97:1528–1540.
121. ACOG Committee on Practice Bulletins. AC06 Practice Bulletin: clinical management guidelines for obstetrician-gynecologists. *Obstet Gynecol.* 2003; 102:417–427.
122. Pisano ED, Gatsonis C, Hendrick E, et al. Diagnostic performance of digital versus film mammography for breast-cancer screening. *N Engl J Med.* 2005;353:1773–1783.
123. Kriege M, Brekelmans CT, Boetes C, et al. Efficacy of MRI and mammography for breast-cancer screening in women with a familial or genetic predisposition. *N Engl J Med.* 2004;351:427–437.
124. Dent R, Warner E. Screening for hereditary breast cancer. *Semin Oncol.* 2007;34:392–400.
125. Smith R, Cokkinides V, Brawley O. Cancer screening in the United States, 2009: a review of current American Cancer Society guidelines and issues in cancer screening. *CA Cancer J Clin.* 2009;59:27–41.
126. US Department of Health and Human Services, US Preventive Health Services Task Force. *Guide to Clinical Preventive Services.* Washington, DC: 1996.
127. Shapiro JA, Seeff LC, Thompson TD, Nadel MR, Klabunde CN, Vernon SW. Colorectal cancer test use from the 2005 National Health Interview Survey. *Cancer Epidemiol Biomarkers Prev.* 2008;17: 1623–1630.
128. Whitlock EP, Lin JS, Liles E, Beil TL, Fu R. Screening for colorectal cancer: a targeted, updated systematic review for the U.S. Preventive Services Task Force. *Ann Intern Med.* 2008;149:638–658.
129. Graser A, Stieber P, Nagel D, et al. Comparison of CT colonography, colonoscopy, sigmoidoscopy and faecal occult blood tests for the detection of advanced adenoma in an average risk population. *Gut.* 2009;58:241–248.
130. US Department of Health and Human Services, National Institutes of Health (NIH), National Cancer Institute (NCI). Colonoscopy or fecal occult blood test in screening healthy participants for colorectal cancer. http://www.cancer.gov/search/ResultsClinicalTrials.aspx?cdrid=644635&version=HealthProfessional&protocolsearchid=7244994. Accessed, January 20, 2010.
131. Greenwald P, Dunn BK. Do we make optimal use of the potential of cancer prevention? *Recent Results Cancer Res.* 2009;181:3–17.
132. Andriole GL, Grubb RL III, Buys SS, et al. Mortality results from a randomized prostate-cancer screening trial. *N Engl J Med.* 2009; 360:1310–1319.
133. US Department of Health and Human Services National Institutes of Health, National Cancer Institute. The National Lung Screening Trial. http://www.cancer.gov/NLST. Accessed January 17, 2010.
134. Smith JJ, Berg CD. Lung cancer screening: promise and pitfalls. *Semin Oncol Nurs.* 2008;24:9–15.
135. Henschke CI, McCauley DI, Yankelevitz DF, et al. Early Lung Cancer Action Project: overall design and findings from baseline screening. *Lancet.* 1999;354:99–105.
136. Henschke CI. Survival of patients with clinical stage I lung cancer diagnosed by computed tomography screening for lung cancer. *Clin Cancer Res.* 2007;13:4949–4950.
137. World Cancer Research Fund, Research AIfC. *Policy and Action for Cancer Prevention.* Washington, DC: American Institute for Cancer Research; 2009.
138. Bal DG, Lloyd JC, Roeseler A, Shimizu R. California as a model. *J Clin Oncol.* 2001;19(18 Suppl):69S-73S.
139. Lightwood JM, Dinno A, Glantz SA. Effect of the California tobacco control program on personal health care expenditures. *PLoS Med.* 2008;5:e178.
140. Messer K, Pierce JP, Zhu SH, et al. The California Tobacco Control Program's effect on adult smokers: (1) Smoking cessation. *Tob Control.* 2007;16:85–90.
141. Doroshow JH, Croyle RT, Niederhuber JE. Five strategies for accelerating the war on cancer in an era of budget deficits. *Oncologist.* 2009; 14:110–116.
142. Campaign for Tobacco-Free Kids. A decade of broken promises: The 1998 State Tobacco Settlement Ten Years Later. http://www.tobaccofreekids.org/reports/settlements/. Accessed October 1, 2009.
143. The Cancer Letter. Tobacco: states spent only 3.2 percent of windfall on cessation. *The Cancer Letter.* 2008;34:7–8.
144. McKinnon RA, Orleans CT, Kumanyika SK, et al. Considerations for an obesity policy research agenda. *Am J Prev Med.* 2009;36:351–357.
145. Groner JA, Skybo T, Murray-Johnson L, et al. Anticipatory guidance for prevention of childhood obesity: design of the MOMS Project. *Clin Pediatr.* 2009;48:483–492.
146. Colon-Otero G, Smallridge RC, Solberg LA Jr, et al. Disparities in participation in cancer clinical trials in the United States: a symptom of a healthcare system in crisis. *Cancer.* 2008;112:447–454.
147. Omenn GS, Goodman G, Thornquist M, et al. The beta-carotene and retinol efficacy trial (CARET) for chemoprevention of lung cancer in high risk populations: smokers and asbestos-exposed workers. *Cancer Res.* 1994;54(7 Suppl):2038s-2043s.
148. Alliance for Health Reform. Closing the gap: racial and ethnic disparities in healthcare. *J Natl Med Assoc.* 2004;96:436–440.
149. Smith JJ, Padberg RM. Dynamics of cancer prevention. In: Yarbro CH, Frogge MH, Goodman M, eds. *Cancer Nursing: Principles and Practice.* 6th ed. Sudbury, MA: Jones and Bartlett Publishers; 2005:95–107.
150. National Society of Genetic Counselors. Genetic counseling as a profession http://www.nsgc.org/about/definition.cfm. Accessed January 22, 2010.
151. US Department of Health and Human Services, National Institutes of Health, National Cancer Institute. http://prevention.cancer.gov/. Accessed January 17, 2010.

CHAPTER

6

Suzanne M. Mahon, RN, DNSc, AOCN®, APNG

# Screening and Detection for Asymptomatic Individuals

## INTRODUCTION

Improved survival from cancer has been a result of both improved treatment and the earlier detection of cancer. Oncology nurses are becoming increasingly involved in cancer prevention and detection services. This chapter provides an overview of the fundamental principles involved in the early detection of cancer, also referred to as cancer screening. Principles of cancer risk assessment will be addressed as well.

## CONCEPTUAL CONSIDERATIONS IN CANCER SCREENING

Intuitively, it makes sense to screen for and detect cancer in its earliest stages. Theoretically, treatment should be the least complicated and least toxic at this point, and there should be the greatest chance for long-term disease-free survival. Nurses are often confronted with questions about prevention, screening modalities, and the early detection of cancer. They need to be able to instruct patients and families on the principles of screening, the rationale for the different recommendations put forth by national agencies, and controversies in screening.

### DEFINITIONS

An understanding of commonly used terms for risk assessment and cancer screening is fundamental. Many of these terms are used by the public interchangeably, but there are subtle different meanings to different terms, and oncology nurses should be in a position to interpret and educate persons about cancer prevention. Oncology nurses need to be able to explain each term to patients when educating about cancer screening. Once patients understand these terms, they find it easier to make appropriate choices regarding cancer screening. Table 6-1 lists some commonly used terms and their definitions.

Cancer screening is aimed at asymptomatic persons with the goal of finding disease when it is most easily treated. It is important for patients to understand that screening is not prevention; the cancer must be measurable and present to be detected on a screening examination. True cancer prevention is aimed at keeping the cancer from ever developing. Screening tests seek to decrease both the morbidity and the mortality associated with cancer because, theoretically, at an early stage, cancer is most effectively and easily treated. This is the traditional definition of cancer

**TABLE 6-1**

**Definitions of Terms Used in Cancer Screening**

**Primary cancer prevention** includes measures to avoid carcinogen exposure, improve health practices, and, in some cases, use chemoprevention agents. Primary prevention may also include the use of prophylactic surgery to prevent or significantly reduce the development of a malignancy.

**Secondary cancer prevention** includes the identification of persons at risk for developing malignancy and the implementation of appropriate screening recommendations. Terms often used interchangeably with secondary cancer prevention are early detection and cancer screening.

**Tertiary cancer prevention** is aimed at persons with a history of malignancy and includes monitoring for and preventing recurrence and screening for second primary cancers. In many cases, those have had a diagnosis cancer and who carry a mutation in a cancer susceptibility gene are at significantly higher risk for developing a second malignancy.

**Cancer screening test** is the method to detect a specific target cancer. It may be a single modality, but often is a combination of tests. Laboratory tests of blood or body fluids, imaging tests, physical examination, and invasive procedures are all sometimes used for screening tests.

**Asymptomatic** means that the person being screened and the examiner are unaware of any signs or symptoms of cancer in the individual prior to initiating the screening test.

**Diagnostic tests** are used in those with symptoms of cancer or abnormal screening tests. The purpose of diagnostic testing is to determine the cause of symptoms or abnormal screening tests.

**Target population** is the number of persons in a defined group who are capable of developing the disease and would be appropriate candidates for screening. *Population* may refer to the general population, or a specific group of people defined by geographic, physical, or social characteristics. For example, nurses who provide cancer genetics counseling need to determine whether a person is of Ashkenazi Jewish background. This special population of Jewish people is at higher risk for three specific mutations for hereditary breast cancer.

**Mortality** is the number of persons who die of a particular cancer during a defined period of time such as one year.

**Prevalence** is the number of cancers that exist in a defined population at a given point in time.

**Outcomes** are the health and economic results that occur related to screening. Outcomes may include the benefits, harms, and costs of screening or genetic testing, and its incurred diagnostic evaluations. Outcomes may be short- or long-term in nature.

**Cost-effectiveness** is achieved if the costs of the screening program are less than the costs in the unscreened group.

screening. Some also consider screening for genetic or molecular markers, which put an individual at high risk for developing cancer, to be a form of cancer screening. This is a rapidly emerging and targeted means to better quantify risk and offer primary prevention measures (eg, prophylactic surgery).[1] Information on genetic testing is found in detail in Chapter 7. This chapter focuses on cancer screening in the more traditional sense.

## OUTCOMES

Short-term outcomes may include measures of the number of persons who are screened or who undergo genetic testing, the number of persons with abnormal screens who have further diagnostic testing, the number of cancers detected, or the cost per cancer detected and risks associated with screening. Often, healthcare providers are most focused on the short-term benefits of screening, when larger strides in decreasing the morbidity and mortality associated with cancer could ultimately be achieved with a focus on more long-term goals and an emphasis on primary prevention behaviors, especially in relation to tobacco and alcohol usage, obesity, poor dietary habits, and sedentary lifestyle.[2] Long-term outcomes may include site-specific cancers detected in the screened population, total costs, and the stage distribution of detected cancers during a specific period following an intervention.[3,4] Knowledge of outcome measures is important for nurses who provide risk assessments and cancer screening services. Goals of cancer screening are described in Table 6-2.[2,5,6] Nurses need to be able to give detailed information about the risks and benefits that can arise during the screening process and provide patients with the rationale for screening so they understand the importance of the early detection of cancer.

**TABLE 6-2**

| Goals of Cancer Risk Assessment and Screening Programs |
|---|
| • Provide accurate information on the genetic, biologic, and environmental factors related to the individual's risk for developing a cancer |
| • Formulate appropriate recommendations for primary and secondary prevention |
| • Offer emotional and psychosocial support to facilitate adjustment to the information regarding risk and promote adherence to recommendations for prevention and early detection |
| • Increase the number of individuals who are offered screening |
| • Increase the number of individuals who complete screening |
| • Assure 100% follow-up of all abnormal screens |
| • Increase the number of premalignant lesions detected |
| • Long-term goals include an earlier stage distribution of detected cancer, decreased mortality, and decreased healthcare costs |

*Source*: Data from Schottenfeld and Beebe-Dimmer[2]; Ward et al[5]; and Mahon.[6]

## CANCER RISK ASSESSMENT: THE FIRST STEP IN THE CANCER SCREENING PROCESS

A *risk factor* is a trait or characteristic that is associated with a statistically significant and increased likelihood of developing a disease.[6,7] It is important to note, however, that having a risk factor does not mean that a person will inevitably develop a disease, such as malignancy, nor does the absence of a risk factor render one immune to developing a disease or malignancy.

Basic elements of a *cancer risk assessment* may include a review of past and present medical history, a history of exposures to carcinogens in daily living, and a detailed family history. Once all information is gathered, the magnitude of the risk must be interpreted to the patient in understandable terms. Often this is accomplished by using various risk calculations such as absolute risk, relative risk, attributable risk, or specific risk models for various cancers. Lack of uniformity in how to conduct and interpret a cancer risk assessment has been a major barrier to comprehensive cancer risk assessment outside of specialized cancer risk clinics.[4] Further, it is often difficult to distinguish between hereditary risk and increased risk for the primary care provider.

Collecting enough history to construct a comprehensive cancer risk assessment is challenging. The availability of computers could potentially increase opportunities for persons to gather and store the information necessary for a cancer risk assessment. For example, "My Family Health Portrait" is available at http://www.hhs.gov/familyhistory/ and provides a tool for individuals to continually gather and update their family history in an organized fashion. The computer, however, cannot replace the judgment of a healthcare professional and interpretation of the risk assessment. The National Cancer Institute (NCI) Division of Epidemiology and Genetics also has some risk assessment tools with which patients can complete and obtain general information about their cancer risk based on a variety of risk factors. There is general risk information available as well as a tool to calculate risk of developing breast cancer and risk of developing melanoma, which is available at http://dceg.cancer.gov/tools/riskassessment. Some healthcare providers use this as a starting point to initiate a conversation about cancer risk.

### FAMILY HISTORY

A family history should focus on primary and secondary relatives. This includes an assessment of both paternal and maternal sides, as many autosomal dominant syndromes can be passed through either the father or the mother. First-degree relatives include parents, siblings, and children. Because first-degree relatives share 50% of their genes, these relatives will be the most likely to inherit similar genetic information. These families will often have multiple cases of cancer at an earlier age than expected in the general population. Information about second-degree relatives can also prove helpful. Second-degree relatives include grandparents, aunts, and uncles. Second-degree relatives have 25% of their genes in common. In particular, older second-degree relatives can provide important information about genetic risk, because they would have been expected to manifest an early-onset cancer if a hereditary trait is present in the family. The pedigree should also include nieces and nephews, because these younger family members can provide information about childhood cancers, which also has implications for the genetic risk assessment. Third-degree relatives (cousins, great-aunts and great-uncles, and great-grandparents) can be included as well, although the accuracy of reports on these relatives is not always high. These relatives share 12.5% of the same genes. Once all of this information is documented, it should be stored in a standard pedigree format. In families with multiple cases of malignancy, this pedigree can help to teach concepts of genetics, clarify relationships, and provide a quick reference. The availability of software to draw these pedigrees has greatly simplified the process of updating this information. The increased use of electronic medical records in healthcare also will potentially increase the potential for a healthcare provider to collect a family history and visually represent it in a standardized pedigree, as well as calculate risks mathematically.

Reliability of patient information should be considered both when obtaining and when communicating the risk assessment. Reports suggest that personal recall of a family history of malignancy may be inaccurate. Family reports may be inaccurate as much as 21% of the time for first-degree relatives and even more frequently for second- and third-degree relatives.[4] Further, the documentation of family history is variable in primary care settings. Although there may be a mention of family history in as many as 97% of all primary care charts, the level of detail about the family history such as specific cancer site, and age of diagnosis is insufficient and inadequate in over 65% of the cases to make an accurate risk assessment or appropriate referral for cancer genetics services.[4] With the ever increasing number of guidelines for the management of persons at increased risk for cancer because of their genetic background, it is becoming more important for providers to extract a reasonably accurate family history and refer accordingly.

Taking a family history in the primary care setting may take 15 to 30 minutes depending on the size of the family and the level of reported detail. Pursuing pathology reports to confirm diagnoses takes additional time. Interpreting that information can take even longer. Tools are being developed for providers to utilize to gather this information more efficiently. One such tool is the Genetic Risk Easy Assessment Tool (GREAT), which is an interactive computer program that collects family history and generates a pedigree.[8] Early research suggests that the tool is acceptable and, with a trend toward electronic medical records, more such tools are likely to be introduced. Such tools will only, however, be effective if the risk is interpreted to the patient and used to guide screening and prevention recommendations.

The family history provides an organized way to document the risk factors related to family history, such as whether a relative is alive or dead, age at death if applicable, significant medical diagnoses, or a diagnosis of cancer. Space can be provided to describe in detail the specific type of cancer, age at diagnosis, and other characteristics such as whether a breast cancer was premenopausal or bilateral. Specific knowledge may influence recommendations for screening. Taking a detailed family history is not only useful for cancer risk assessment, but is also the first step in identifying families with a possible hereditary predisposition to malignancy and other illnesses. Healthcare providers should ask patients about specific relatives and their health individually rather than asking a more general question such as, "Have any of your relatives been diagnosed with cancer?" After gathering the family history, it is important to recheck whether any of the patient's relatives have been diagnosed with these cancers. It is amazing how often patients forget to provide this information, and reiterating this question may unearth valuable information.

## PAST MEDICAL HISTORY/LIFESTYLE FACTORS

Assessment of past medical history and personal history factors that may increase the risk of developing cancer should be documented. Many of these risk factors are not within an individual's control and are not amenable to primary prevention efforts (eg, age at menarche). In contrast, lifestyle factors complete the risk factor assessment and are often within the control of the individual. They provide a framework for providing education about primary prevention efforts, which is discussed in more detail in Chapter 5.

Structuring the interview in more of a traditional medical history format facilitates the information gathering process. Trying to find risk factors by category or anatomical site can be confusing to the patient, resulting in a disjointed interview, and may not be as thorough as a comprehensive health history. Healthcare professionals need to realize that conducting an interview in this fashion demands that the clinician interpret the risk factors to the patient and document recommendations for cancer prevention and early detection somewhere on the chart. For that reason, specially designed forms to make documentation of risk factors comprehensive and the information easy to retrieve, update, and interpret to the patient are helpful.[6]

Past screening activities and findings from such activities contribute to the risk assessment and provide further opportunity to educate the patient about the potential strengths, benefits, and risks associated with screening. Patient's reports of these results may not be accurate. It is important to order pathology reports or actual mammograms for review before determining risk and communicating risk information to the patient. For example, there is a big difference between the risk for development of breast cancer in a woman with a biopsy-proven fibroadenoma and in a woman with biopsy-proven ductal hyperplasia with atypia. Fibrocystic disease or change is a generic term and should not be equated with an increased risk for developing breast cancer. Obtaining accurate information is necessary to develop the most accurate risk assessment possible, correct misconceptions if indicated, and make the best possible recommendations for cancer screening.

Similarly, it is often not enough to rely on an individual to provide accurate information about the last screening examinations. A large meta-analysis demonstrated that self-reported histories are often inaccurate and tend to overestimate cancer screening utilization.[9,10] Of concern regarding this overestimation is that individual patients will not be referred for cancer screening tests at an appropriate interval and nationally, such data may not provide an accurate picture of cancer screening utilization and progress toward national goals such as those set by the Healthy People 2010 program.

After all of the risk data are collected, the clinician must assimilate the risk factors mentally and provide information about them for each of the major cancers to the patient. For example, early menarche, nulliparity, and late menopause are risk factors for both breast and endometrial cancers. The communication of risk should therefore include a discussion of the risk for developing both of these cancers.

Risk can be communicated to patients in several different formats. The importance of communicating risk individually to patients should not be underestimated. A Cochrane systematic review of randomized controlled trials found that providing patients with an individualized risk estimate, as opposed to receiving general information about risk, significantly increased the probability that they will participate in a screening program.[11] Often, it is best to use several means, including absolute, relative, and attributable risk.

More recently, there has been great concern that risk assessment opportunities are often missed in primary care where practice is busy and there is limited time for health promotion activities. This may be especially true in uninsured, underinsured, and minority patients, where there are multiple barriers associated with health care.[12–14]

## ABSOLUTE RISK

*Absolute risk* is a measure of the occurrence of cancer, either incidence (new cases) or mortality (deaths), in the general population. It can be expressed either as the number of cases for a specified denominator (eg, 75 cases per 10,000 people annually) or as a cumulative risk up to a specified age (eg, 1 in 8 women will develop breast cancer if they live to age 85). Another way to express absolute risk is to discuss average risk of developing breast cancer at a certain age. For example, a woman's risk of developing breast cancer might be 2% at age 50 but 12% at age 85. Risk estimates will be much different for a 50-year-old woman than for a 85-year-old woman, as approximately 50% of the cases of breast cancer occur after the age of 65. Absolute risk factors for the major cancers are shown in Table 6-3.[15]

**TABLE 6-3**

**Lifetime Probability of Developing Invasive Cancers Over Selected Age Intervals by Sex, United States, 2002–2004**

| Site | Male | Female |
|---|---|---|
| All sites | 1 in 2 | 1 in 3 |
| Bladder | 1 in 27 | 1 in 85 |
| Breast | | 1 in 8 |
| Colon/rectum | 1 in 18 | 1 in 19 |
| Leukemia | 1 in 67 | 1 in 95 |
| Lung | 1 in 13 | 1 in 16 |
| Melanoma | 1 in 41 | 1 in 61 |
| Prostate | 1 in 6 | |
| Ovary | | 1 in 62 |
| Uterine cervix | | 1 in 142 |
| Uterine corpus (endometrium) | | 1 in 41 |

*Source*: Data from Ries et al.[15]

Patients who present for screening need to understand that certain assumptions are made to reach an absolute risk figure. For example, the "1 in 8" figure describes the "average" risk of breast cancer in Caucasian American women and takes into consideration other causes of death over the life span. By necessity, this figure will overestimate breast cancer risk for some women with no risk factors and underestimate the risk for women with several risk factors.[16] These statistics actually mean that the average woman's breast cancer risk is 0.48% to age 39; 3.86% from age 40 to 49; 3.51% from age 50 to 59; 3.21% from age 60 to 69 and 2.24% for age 70 and older.[7] The 13% or "1 in 8" risk is obtained by adding the risk in each age category (0.48 + 3.86 + 3.51 + 3.21 + 2.24 = 13.3%). When a woman who has an average risk reaches age 50 without a diagnosis of breast cancer, she has passed through 4% of her risk, so her risk to age 85 is 13% minus 4% which equals 9%. When she reaches age 70 without a diagnosis of breast cancer, her risk to age 85 is 13% – (0.48% + 3.86% + 3.51% + 3.21%) = 2.24%. Time must always be considered for the risk figure to be meaningful. For example, the average 50-year-old woman's risk is 6% to age 70 but 9% to age 80.[7] Absolute risk is helpful when a patient needs to understand the chances for all persons in a population of developing a particular disease.

Screening tests often focus on cancers with higher absolute risk because they are more common in certain populations.

## RELATIVE RISK

The term *relative risk* refers to a comparison of the incidence or deaths among those with a particular risk factor compared to those without the risk factor. By using relative risk factors, an individual can determine his or her risk factors and thus better understand personal chances of developing a specific cancer as compared to individuals without such risk factors. If the risk for a person with no known risk factors is 1.0, one can evaluate the risk of individuals with risk factors in relation to this figure. For example, for a woman whose mother had breast cancer in both breasts before age 40, the relative risk would be approximately 8.5 over her lifetime. In other words, she has eight and a half times the chance of a woman without a known family history of breast cancer.

Relative risk factors can confuse some patients. If one plans to give a patient information about his or her relative risk, it is important to specify exactly what comparison is being made. Often percentages are confusing when used with risk. If a news report states that there is a 30% to 50% increase in breast cancer risk in women who take a particular hormone therapy after menopause, it means, in absolute numerical terms, that there will be 0.6 more cases of breast cancer per 100 women from ages 50 to 70. The same concept applies if a person is informed that he or she has a 1% chance of developing cancer. This simply means that the risk has increased from 1 in 10,000 to 1.3 in 10,000.[17]

Nurses need to remember that the relative risk statistics is helpful only if it is clear what the baseline risk is. Unless the risk to the baseline group is clearly known, a comparison risk is not useful and can even prove misleading.

Relative risk can be very helpful when selecting screening recommendations. If a person's relative risk is significantly higher than most members of the general population, it will probably be necessary to modify a screening recommendation usually given in the general population.

## ATTRIBUTABLE RISK

*Attributable risk* is the amount of disease within the population that could be prevented by alteration of a risk factor. Although historically this component of risk assessment has not received much attention, assessment of attributable risk has important implications for public health policy. A risk factor could convey a very large relative risk, yet be restricted to a few individuals; as a consequence, changing it would benefit only a small group. Conversely, some risk factors that can be altered (such as cigarette smoking) could potentially decrease the morbidity and mortality associated with malignancy in a large number of people.

One clinical example involves the use of attributable risk related to smoking and lung cancers. Attributable risk could be calculated to determine how many lung cancer cases could be prevented if everyone stopped or never started smoking. Another example is the number of cases of breast cancer that might develop in women taking a particular birth control pill. A package insert might report a relative risk for developing breast cancer of 2.35 in women younger than age 35 whose first exposure to the drug was within the previous four years. Because the annual incidence rate (absolute risk) for women aged 30 to 34 is 26.7 cases per 100,000, a relative risk of 2.35 increases the possible risk from 26.7 to 62.75 cases per 100,000 women. The attributable risk of breast cancer is calculated to be 3.38 cases per 10,000 additional women per year. This slight increase in the number of cases may possibly be associated with the use of the contraceptive.

## EXPLANATION OF RISK WITH CLINICAL MODELS

More recently, models have become available with which to calculate risk for developing a specific cancer. This is a rapidly growing area especially with the increasing availability of genetic tests. Models are used not only to calculate the risk of developing a particular cancer, but also the risk of having a genetic mutation associated with hereditary risk. Most of the current models have been developed for use in women with a risk for developing breast cancer.[18–21] A list of models, the measurements they provide, and appropriate references can be found in Table 6-4.[21–38] Note that some of these models are used to calculate risk for developing a disease, whereas others are used to calculate risk of having a cancer susceptibility mutation. It is important to be careful to distinguish to patients whether the model predicts risk of developing a particular cancer or risk of having a mutation. In most cases there will be a range of risk figures. This requires the clinician to explain what the range means and that it is not an absolute figure for whether an individual has a mutation or will develop a cancer; it is an estimation of risk to guide decisions about genetic testing or screening modalities.

Each model has its own strengths and weaknesses, which must be presented to the patient. A major limitation of most of the breast models is that they do not account for mammographic density, which is a significant risk factor as well as a barrier to interpreting mammograms.[21] Some models better calculate risk at a single moment in time and others provide more cumulative risk data.[19] Many clinicians will calculate two or three models and give the individual a range of figures; this communicates that no model is perfect and may provide a better estimate of risk.[18] The purpose of calculating these models is to guide or modify screening recommendations for each individual. Other commonly cited purposes for using risk models is

**TABLE 6-4**

**Models That Predict Risk of Developing a Particular Cancer or Having a Mutation for Developing a Particular Cancer**

| Parameter | Model | References |
|---|---|---|
| Risk of developing breast cancer | Gail | 22 |
| | Claus | 23,24 |
| | Tyrer | 25 |
| Risk of a BRCA1/2 mutation | Couch | 26 |
| | Shattuck-Eidens | 27 |
| | Berry | 28 |
| | Frank | 29 |
| | Family History Assessment Tool | 30 |
| Risk of hereditary colorectal cancer mutation | Bethesda | 31 |
| | Wijnen | 32 |
| Risk of developing prostate cancer | Ohori | 33 |
| | CAPRI | 34 |
| | Eastham | 35 |
| Risk of developing melanoma | NCI Melanoma Risk Prediction Model | 36 |
| Risk of having a hereditary melanoma mutation | MELPREDICT | 37 |
| | GenoMEL | 38 |

to stratify individuals in clinical trials, estimate the cost of the disease in a population, design prevention trials, and improve decision making about genetic testing or a potential screening or prevention measure (such as prophylactic surgery) following the determination that an individual has a mutation.[20,39] For many of the major cancers, no models are available and risk assessment is less accurate.

## PRINCIPLES OF CANCER RISK COMMUNICATION

Cancer risk communication has many goals. These goals are not limited to helping people understand the risks they face.[40] Other goals include building trust, influencing public policy, fulfilling legal obligations, denying responsibility for undesirable outcomes, and justifying past actions.

Risks can be communicated to patients in numerous ways. Nurses need to be aware of the strengths and limitations of the various forms of risk communication and provide each patient with a balanced discussion of risks. Most risk discussions will include, at a minimum, a discussion of absolute risks and relative risks; in some cases, discussion of genetic risk assessment models may be warranted.

There is no perfect model that completely and accurately explains an individual's risk for developing a particular cancer.[40] Indeed, for most cancers, a portion of those cases diagnosed cannot be explained by recognized risk factors. For example, approximately 41% of breast cancer cases are attributable to later age at first birth, nulliparity, and family history of breast cancer.[7,41] Ideally, knowledge of risk factors should guide primary prevention efforts. In the case of breast cancer, however, the inability to readily alter these risk factors has limited their relevance for primary prevention. In some cancers, such as breast cancer, the central role of risk factor identification at this point is to identify women at higher risk, particularly those with a potential genetic susceptibility to breast cancer, and to screen them more aggressively. For example, women from these families may be advised to undergo mammographies at a younger age than usually recommended, or to have a clinical breast examination (CBE) twice a year instead of annually.[42]

Transmitting risk information is a central component of all screening and genetic counseling programs—a task that is much more difficult than it might appear. Risk assessment is a complex discipline that is often not fully understood by healthcare professionals and is even less clear to the lay public.[43] For professionals who practice risk assessment on a daily basis, continued debate exists over terminology and techniques.

Of course, decisions and behavior are not determined by knowledge of risk alone.[40] Being well-educated about risk and other issues offers no guarantee that good decisions will be made. Other factors may play even more powerful roles in determining how decisions about risk are made. These factors include emotions, personal values, social pressures, environmental barriers, and economic constraints.

The transmission of information about risk is also often influenced by professional judgment.[44] Many professional groups have standards of practice or position statements that influence how risks are communicated to patients. Guidelines for management of average risk and hereditary risk are provided and promoted by the American Cancer Society (ACS), National Comprehensive Cancer Network (NCCN), United States Preventive Service Task Force (USPSTF), American Society of Clinical Oncology (ASCO), Centers for Disease Control and Prevention (CDC), and a wide range of subspecialty organizations. Current guidelines can be accessed at http://www.guidelines.gov. The background for each recommendation is provided. Guidelines can also be compared at this clearinghouse.

In addition, professional opinions about emotionally charged issues such as genetic testing probably influence how risk information is communicated. These biases are probably communicated no matter how nonjudgmental a professional tries to be during a risk communication session.

Risk factor assessment is an ongoing part of oncology nursing practice. Risk factor profiles should be reviewed at least annually. Patients should be questioned about any change in their family history since the last assessment, development of any new health problems that may be associated with increased risk (eg, abnormal Pap test, a change in breast examination), and initiation of any new medications that may change the risk profile (eg, started estrogen replacement therapy or tamoxifen therapy). If significant changes have occurred, screening recommendations may need to be modified. If no significant changes have occurred, an annual review of the risk factor assessment offers an excellent opportunity to reinforce information on cancer prevention and early detection. It also communicates an ongoing concern for the patient as a dynamic individual and identifies the nurse as a resource for further information, should a problem develop.

## ORAL COMMUNICATION OF RISK

Communication of cancer risk can be challenging because it includes both qualitative and quantitative components.[44] The quantitative component is usually relatively straightforward. It typically involves sharing risk figures such as absolute or relative risk, or the probability of having a mutation in a cancer susceptibility gene. Numerical data can be presented with the understanding that some individuals have a greater capacity than others to comprehend the meaning of such data. Qualitative information should follow the presentation of quantitative data. It includes a discussion of what the quantitative data specifically mean for the individual patient. Many experts in risk communication believe that all discussions of risk should include both qualitative and quantitative components.[17]

People often hold an inaccurate assessment of their personal risk for developing cancer.[45] In other words, patients may perceive their risk to be lower or higher than it actually is. These biases may occur because persons have inaccurate information; are unable to comprehend complex, technical information; or have developed a psychologically protective coping mechanism.

An awareness of the individual's anxiety is important, because it can limit an individual's ability to actually understand his or her risk for developing cancer. The thought of cancer can be so anxiety provoking in some individuals that they fail to understand their actual risk for cancer.

Communication of risk information should reflect how much the patient or family wishes to know.[46,47] Timing may be important as well. Messages suggesting increased susceptibility to breast cancer may be less effective if delivered too soon after the breast cancer diagnosis of a close relative, but they might be appropriate several months after the diagnosis.[48]

Communication of a cancer risk assessment should be viewed as an information-sharing interview. Table 6-5 summarizes the steps involved. The manner in which the information is communicated (sometimes referred to as "framing") is also important.[49] If material is presented in a negative fashion, patients may assume that the risk is greater than it actually is. If the discussion is too positive, the magnitude of risk may be underestimated or minimized. Framing occurs with statistics, too. If an individual is told that he or she has a risk of a particular cancer of 1.4 in 10,000 compared to the general population's risk of 1 in 10,000, it will not be particularly impressive to most people. If the same risk is communicated using the format that the individual has a 40% greater risk than the general population, the situation is likely to be seen as "riskier" even though the two situations are equivalent.[47,50] Clearly, this is the most challenging aspect of cancer risk assessment communication. The goal is not to frighten a patient unnecessarily; conversely, if the risk is minimized too much, the patient may not see the value in recommended cancer prevention and screening activities.[47,51]

Achieving true informed consent may affect an individual's decision as to whether he or she truly desires to participate in cancer screening. Conveying a better understanding of one's risk for developing a particular cancer is part of this informed consent process. For example, informed consent can directly affect patient's interest and desire to undergo

**TABLE 6-5**

**Steps in Cancer Risk Communication**

1. Communication of the risk information should begin by reminding the patient of the strengths and limitations as well as the purpose of a cancer risk assessment. The patient should clearly understand that the assessment will be only as accurate as the patient provides.
2. Provide information on the risk factors for the cancer(s) for which the person desires screening.
3. Provide basic information on the cancer for which the person is at risk (eg, number of people affected annually, average age at diagnosis, clinical presentation). Information about the general population can serve as a baseline against which individuals can measure the magnitude of their increased risk.
4. A review of basic anatomy and physiology using diagrams and models may be indicated to provide necessary background information.
5. Depending on the magnitude of the risk and the ability and desire of the patient to understand the content, the discussion can be expanded to include a more detailed discussion of absolute or relative risk. Care should be given to distinguish between absolute and relative risk and reinforce the fact that risk factors do not combine in a simple mathematical fashion.
6. Information about lifestyle factors amenable to changes should be discussed.
7. Patients should receive information about the strengths and limitations of screening tools.
8. Adequate opportunity for the patient to ask questions and express concerns must be provided to make the cancer risk assessment process effective and the interview truly information-sharing.

screening. Conversely, giving more information about the benefits of a screening test when accompanied by information about personal risk may increase interest in participating in a specific screening.

Thus, the importance of communicating the risk individually should not be underestimated. A meta-analysis found that individualized risk communication generally leads to increased use of screening modalities.[52] Individualized counseling makes the risk more realistic to the individual.

## TECHNOLOGICAL COMMUNICATION OF RISK

Today, technology is affecting the means of communication of cancer risk. The use of computers in educating people about cancer risk and the management of cancer risk is relatively new. More programs are becoming available for both the public and health professionals to utilize. Little is known about the effectiveness of these programs. An advantage of using some of the newer technologies and multimedia is that by accessing the medium, patients have active—rather than passive—involvement.[53] A multimedia approach also offers the advantage of being able to deliver a consistent message to a large number of persons at a relatively low cost. Disadvantages include the difficulty of ensuring that the individual understands the meaning and implications of the risk assessment.

## VISUAL AIDS IN RISK COMMUNICATION

Graphics can be a very effective means to communicate risk. They can be especially effective in communicating numerical risk.[54] Graphics can often reveal data patterns that might otherwise go undetected. Graphs also hold people's attention for longer periods of time, which might increase the understanding of data. To be useful, they must communicate the magnitude of risk, relative risk, cumulative risk, uncertainty, and interactions among risk factors. Despite the popularity of using graphics, little research has focused on the impact of graphics in communicating risk data. In many cases, a combination of formats is used to present risk information, including numerical, visual, and explanatory formats.[50]

Several considerations do enhance the usefulness of graphs. The graph should decrease the number of mathematical computations that the user must make. In some cases, it may be best to avoid communicating small-probability events with graphs.[54] Although most persons can understand a flip of the coin (0.5 chance), it is often very difficult for persons to understand the magnitude of a small-probability event such as a 0.0003 chance. A solution to this problem is to change the probabilities to frequencies (3 out of 10,000).

The risk ladder is often used to describe environmental hazards. It displays a range of risk magnitudes by showing increasing risks as being higher on the ladder. Perceptions of risk are, therefore, influenced by the location on the ladder. The ladder helps people to anchor risk to upper and lower reference points.

Pie charts are commonly and effectively used to communicate information about proportions. Most individuals are able to understand a pie chart. These graphics can sometimes be combined to explain subcategories of data.

Histograms are also commonly used. Most individuals have some understanding of how to read a simple histogram. These illustrations will often convey the magnitude of the risk more clearly than just using numbers.[54]

## PSYCHOLOGICAL CONCERNS

Risk assessment and giving patients information about risk factors do not affect risk of developing cancer. Nevertheless, such information about risk may influence patients' choices regarding screening and may change the way in which some people think about their lives. A risk factor assessment can potentially improve patients' healthcare and ultimately their quality of life if it results in primary prevention practices and regular screenings and possibly the prevention or early detection of a malignancy. Conversely, if a person becomes distressed or upset by the information conveyed in a risk assessment, recommendations for screening may be ignored or the person may experience psychological harm and possibly increased morbidity if a malignancy is not detected early.

The psychosocial effects of risk factor communication have not received much attention.[46] Some degree of concern or anxiety about cancer might heighten an individual's vigilance and motivation to seek reassurance through repetitive screenings. Conversely, such notification may result in anxiety and cancer worries with a reduction in recommended screening. Of concern would be the potential for inappropriate decisions about the use of prophylactic surgery in persons who overestimate their risk for developing breast cancer or endometrial cancer. Clearly, the overall impact of risk assessment on quality of life is poorly understood. Similarly, it is not clear why two women with similar risk factors for developing breast cancer who receive risk factor information in a similar format can respond so differently to the information.

## DOCUMENTATION OF RISK ASSESSMENT

Documentation of a risk assessment is important and may enhance the risk communication process. The first time a patient is seen for risk assessment and screening services, information should be gathered about family history, pertinent medical background, and lifestyle factors. This information is necessary for the initial risk assessment and any subsequent reevaluation and update of the assessment. The choice of the format for documentation and risk factors to be included ultimately affect the risk assessment. For example, in a mammography center, a woman may be queried regarding risk factors for breast cancer. Some of the same risk factors may place the woman at higher risk for endometrial, ovarian, or colorectal cancer.

Few published reports describe documentation of a risk factor assessment.[6] A checklist form containing the major risk factors for the various cancers can be completed after an interview, with space being provided to encourage documentation specific to the risk factor, such as number of years of estrogen replacement therapy or number of years and packs of cigarettes a patient has smoked. Other items that should be documented are a pedigree and any numerical risk assessments that have been calculated. Components of patient education should be documented as well.

## MEASURES OF THE ACCURACY OF SCREENING TESTS

In addition to conveying information about cancer risk, nurses must communicate to patients about the accuracy of screening tests. It is not enough to simply recommend a screening test. Patients need to understand what the possibilities are regarding a truly positive or a truly negative test result.

### ACCURACY

The *accuracy* of screening tests is described using a number of terms. A *true-positive test* (TP) is a normal test for cancer in an individual who actually has cancer. In Table 6-6, the number of true-positive tests is 75. A *true-negative test* (TN) is a normal or negative screen for cancer in an individual who is subsequently found not to have cancer within a defined period after the last test. In Table 6-6, the number of true-negative tests is 775. A *false-negative test* (FN) is a normal test for cancer in an individual who actually has cancer. In Table 6-6, the number of false-negative tests is 25. A *false-positive test* (FP) is an abnormal test for cancer screening in an individual who actually does not have cancer. In Table 6-6, the number of false-positive tests is 225. An understanding of true and false test results is necessary to calculate information about sensitivity and specificity (Table 6-6). Other information about the accuracy of screening tests can be found in Table 6-7.[3]

### SENSITIVITY

The *sensitivity* of a screening test is its ability to detect those individuals with cancer. It is calculated by taking the number of TPs and dividing it by the total number of cancer cases (TP + FN). For the data in Table 6-6, sensitivity would be calculated as 75/(75 + 25) = 0.75. Most people are unwilling to accept a test with a high false-negative rate because many cancers will be missed.

**TABLE 6-6**

**Accuracy of Cancer Screening Tests**

| Results of Screening Test | Population Who Actually Have the Disease | Population Who Actually Do Not Have the Disease |
|---|---|---|
| Positive test | 75 | 225 |
| Negative test | 25 | 775 |
| Total | 100 | 1000 |

True positives = 75
True negatives = 775
False positives = 225
False negatives = 25

Sensitivity = 75/(75 + 25) = 0.75

Specificity = 775/(775 + 225) = 0.78

Positive predictive value = 75/(75 + 225) = 0.25

Negative predictive value = 775/(775 + 25) = 0.97

### SPECIFICITY

The *specificity* of a test is its ability to identify those individuals who actually do not have cancer. It is calculated by dividing the TN by the sum of the TN and FP cases. For the data in Table 6-6, specificity is calculated as 775/(775 + 225) = 0.78. A high false-positive test rate can result in unnecessary follow-up testing and anxiety in persons who have a positive screen.

### POSITIVE PREDICTIVE VALUE

The *positive predictive value* is a measure of the validity of a positive test. It is the proportion of positive tests that are TP cases. The predictive value of a test depends on the disease prevalence. As the prevalence of a cancer increases in the population, the positive predictive value of the screening tests increases, even though its sensitivity and specificity remain unchanged.[6]

### NEGATIVE PREDICTIVE VALUE

The *negative predictive value* is a measure of the validity of a negative test. It refers to the proportion of negative tests that are TNs.

**TABLE 6-7**

| Principles in Developing Cancer Screening Tests |
|---|
| • **The disease should be an important health problem.** There is little doubt that cancer is a significant health problem. Cancer is not just one disease. Some types of cancer are more significant health problems than other types. For example, the incidence of breast cancer is an estimated 194,280 new cases annually and that of lung cancer is an estimated 219,440 new cases, which make both of these cancers very significant. The mortality associated with these cancers is also high, with an estimated 40,610 deaths annually from breast cancer and an estimated 159,390 deaths annually from lung cancer. Clearly, both of these cancers are significant health problems. |
| • **The disease should have a preclinical stage before symptoms become obvious.** In breast cancer, mammography is able to detect breast cancers before the cancer is palpable. Although lung cancer has a high incidence, at present there is not an obvious preclinical stage. |
| • **The test should be treatable.** There should be a recognized treatment for lesions identified following screening. Breast cancer is a disease that responds to surgery, chemotherapy, and radiation therapy, especially when the disease is detected early. Even more important, when breast cancer is detected early, it can often be treated with less radical surgery such as lumpectomy. The same is not true of cancers such as ovarian or lung cancer. |
| • **The test must be clinically relevant.** The test must be able to detect a condition for which intervention at a preclinical stage can improve outcome. The test must be accurate. The sensitivity and specificity must be acceptable. |
| • **The test must be acceptable to individuals being screened.** Highly invasive, painful, or risky procedures are generally unacceptable. |
| • **The test must be widely available and easily accessible.** Technology has made mammography readily available. Colonoscopy is becoming increasingly available. Medicare and insurance coverage of these screening tests makes them more financially accessible to a larger group of people. |
| • **The test must be cost effective.** Measuring cost-effectiveness can be difficult. Different groups have different thresholds for what they consider to be cost-effective. |

## IMPROVING THE ACCURACY OF SCREENING

Healthcare providers can take several steps to improve the accuracy of screening tests.[55,56] Attaining certification and following federal guidelines in the area of radiology and laboratory services represent one such step. Guidelines are now in place for mammography centers and laboratories providing cancer screening services to ensure that a minimum acceptable standard is met. Certification from relevant agencies should be publicly displayed.

The person conducting the exam or interpreting the laboratory or radiological test results profoundly affects the effectiveness of a cancer screening test. For example, some healthcare professionals are clearly better at performing CBEs than others and are more likely to detect a subtle breast change. Monitoring the quality of clinical examinations is important. Monitoring and improving the quality of physical examinations in the clinical setting is far more challenging, but is nevertheless important to improve the sensitivity and specificity of the examination.[47] More recently, attention has been directed toward the quality of colorectal examinations, especially colonoscopy.[57]

Screening quality may also be improved by developing standardized instructions for patient preparation. This may not only improve patient compliance, but also help obtain the best possible screen. An example might be scheduling a breast screening a week after the menses begin, avoiding the use of deodorant prior to mammography, or instructing a patient to avoid douching for 24 hours prior to a Pap smear. The quality of the bowel preparation directly impacts the accuracy of any endoscopic evaluation of the colon.

Providers need to be continually updated on the newest guidelines and techniques for cancer screening. Such training should include a staff competency evaluation. New equipment is constantly being developed to enhance screening and diagnostic procedures. Agencies that provide screening services need to not just review such equipment, but to develop policies on how they will test and possibly eventually adapt such equipment to their specific needs. Most recently, the introduction of breast magnetic resonance imaging (MRI) for the detection of breast cancer has raised questions about the type of equipment used in breast MRI, the ability to provide biopsies, and the skill of the radiologist interpreting the examination.

## IMPLEMENTING CANCER SCREENING

A screening protocol or recommendation defines how cancer screening tests should be used. Table 6-8 illustrates the ACS recommendations for the early detection of cancer in asymptomatic individuals.[3] It is an example of a screening protocol. Such recommendations can vary among organizations and practitioners. A recommendation generally

**TABLE 6-8**

## American Cancer Society Recommendations for the Early Detection of Cancer

**Breast cancer**

- ☐ Yearly mammograms are recommended starting at age 40 and continuing for as long as a woman is in good health.
- ☐ Clinical breast exam (CBE) should be part of a periodic health exam, about every 3 years for women in their 20s and 30s and every year for women 40 and over.
- ☐ Breast self-exam (BSE) is an option for women starting in their 20s.
- ☐ Women at high risk (greater than 20% lifetime risk) should get an MRI and a mammogram every year. Women at moderately increased risk (15% to 20% lifetime risk) should talk with their doctors about the benefits and limitations of adding MRI screening to their yearly mammogram. Yearly MRI screening is not recommended for women whose lifetime risk of breast cancer is less than 15%.

**Colorectal cancer**

Beginning at age 50, both men and women at average risk for developing colorectal cancer should use one of the following screening tests. The tests that are designed to find both early cancer and polyps are preferred. Any abnormality must be further evaluated with colonoscopy. Individuals with risk factors will need more frequent screening.

*Tests that find polyps and cancer*

- ☐ Flexible sigmoidoscopy every 5 years
- ☐ Colonoscopy every 10 years
- ☐ Double contrast barium enema every 5 years
- ☐ CT colonography (virtual colonoscopy) every 5 years

*Tests that mainly find cancer*

- ☐ Fecal occult blood test (FOBT) every year
- ☐ Fecal immunochemical test (FIT) every year
- ☐ Stool DNA test (sDNA), interval uncertain

**Cervical cancer**

- ☐ All women should begin cervical cancer screening about 3 years after they begin having vaginal intercourse, but no later than when they are 21 years old.
- ☐ Screening should be done every year with the regular Pap test or every 2 years using the newer liquid-based Pap test.
- ☐ Beginning at age 30, women who have had 3 normal Pap test results in a row may get screened every 2 to 3 years.
- ☐ Another reasonable option for women over 30 is to get screened every 3 years with either the conventional or liquid-based Pap test, plus the HPV DNA test.
- ☐ Women who have certain risk factors such as diethylstilbestrol (DES) exposure before birth, HIV infection, or a weakened immune system due to organ transplant, chemotherapy, or chronic steroid use should continue to be screened annually.
- ☐ Women 70 years of age or older who have had 3 or more normal Pap tests in a row and no abnormal Pap test results in the last 10 years may choose to stop having cervical cancer screening.
- ☐ Women who have had a total hysterectomy (removal of the uterus and cervix) may also choose to stop having cervical cancer screening, unless the surgery was done as a treatment for cervical cancer or dysplasia.

**Endometrial Cancer**

- ☐ At menopause, all women should be informed about the risks and symptoms of endometrial cancer, and strongly encouraged to report any unexpected bleeding or spotting to their doctors.
- ☐ For women with or at high risk for hereditary non-polyposis colon cancer (HNPCC), annual screening should be offered for endometrial cancer with endometrial biopsy beginning at age 35.

**Prostate Cancer**

- ☐ Both the prostate-specific antigen (PSA) blood test and digital rectal examination (DRE) should be offered annually, beginning at age 50, to men who have at least a 10-year life expectancy.
- ☐ Men at high risk (African-American men and men with a strong family of one or more first-degree relatives diagnosed before age 65) should begin testing at age 45.
- ☐ Information should be provided to all men about what is known and what is uncertain about the benefits, limitations, and harms of early detection and treatment of prostate cancer so that they can make an informed decision about testing.
- ☐ Men who ask their doctor to make the decision on their behalf should be tested. Discouraging testing is not appropriate. Not offering testing is not appropriate.

**Risk Education and General Screening**

For people aged 20 or older having periodic health exams, a cancer-related checkup should include health counseling, and depending on a person's age and gender, might include exams for cancers of the thyroid, oral cavity, skin, lymph nodes, testes, and ovaries, as well as for some non-malignant (non-cancerous) diseases.

*Source*: Data based from the American Cancer Society.[3]

describes the target population to be served, the screening recommendation to be applied, and the interval at which the test should be undertaken.

## DEVELOPMENT OF SCREENING GUIDELINES

Screening guidelines change over time. The ACS, for example, has been publishing guidelines for the early detection of cancer for more than 20 years.[3] These guidelines have been revised, added, and eliminated during this time frame. This is a source of confusion for both patients and healthcare providers. In the past, the ACS has recommended screening for lung cancer using sputum cytology. Currently, the ACS does not have a recommendation for the early detection of lung cancer. All efforts are focused on prevention of and smoking cessation.[3] Although specific guidelines have changed over the years, the focus of the guidelines has changed very little. Healthcare providers are still expected to use the guidelines to select the best screening tests for an individual and to modify the guidelines in certain cases, such as if an individual has a particularly high risk for developing a specific malignancy.

Clinicians must remember that screening protocols are merely guidelines.[58] They are not practice standards to be used blindly with every individual. Many guidelines require risk assessment to apply the guidelines. This is certainly the case with colorectal cancer screening. The recommendations for screening vary depending on the risk of the individual.[57] The goal of the ACS standards is the detection of malignancy. The US Preventive Services Task Force (USPSTF) uses very strict criteria for assessing evidence of effectiveness. Cost-effectiveness of the screening recommendations is an important consideration for this group, for example. When providing information on cancer screening recommendations, nurses need to inform the individual why a certain recommendation is being made in his or her case.

Nurses will often make recommendations for various screening or detection measures, especially in persons who carry a higher risk for developing a particular cancer, based on their family history and genetic background. Nurses need to be able to accurately explain the risks and benefits of these screening tools to their patients. This requires an understanding of the measures of validity of a screening test. Specific recommendations for a screening test often vary among organizations such as the ACS, the USPSTF, or the NCI. The specific criteria that each organization uses to make recommendations may vary, which is why the recommendations are not universal and can prove very confusing to the general public. Tests are often combined to compensate for the limitations of any one test.[47] Sometimes patients must also make a choice as to what they are trying to detect. In terms of colorectal cancer screening, there are recommendations for tests that mainly detect polyps and potentially prevent cancer (such as colonoscopy) and recommendations for tests that may detect colorectal cancer (such as fecal occult blood testing).[57]

There are, however, generally agreed-upon requirements and characteristics of acceptable screening tests. When presenting screening recommendations to individuals, it is important to include the rationale and strengths and limitations of each test and to present this information in light of the individual's own risk for developing cancer. The following issues are frequently considered before recommendations for screening for the general public are made. Often those individuals with a genetic susceptibility need recommendations that are more rigorous than those for persons with an average risk.

First, nurses need to review the scientific basis for each guideline. Each agency that promulgates a guideline should make this information available. An excellent place to obtain information about the scientific basis and the review process for a guideline is from the individual agency that generates the guideline or at the National Guideline Clearinghouse (http://www.guideline.gov). It is important to note that for some guidelines, the data also only support implementation to a certain age or health parameter, such as mammography. The ACS guidelines do not give an age to stop mammography but encourage the clinician to consider the overall health of the woman when recommending the screening.[7]

Second, nurses play a key role in interpreting these data to patients. Nurses need to explain why a particular set of guidelines is being used for an individual patient. They need to remind each patient that these recommendations are guidelines and that some modifications may be made based on personal risk factor assessment and findings on a clinical examination. With some persons in failing health, it is appropriate to discuss on stopping cancer screening, although few of the guidelines provide specific direction in this area. Clearly, the benefits, risks, and potential limitations of each screening test need to be discussed individually and tailored to the risk factor assessment.

Many individuals will choose to undergo a screening examination, even if a test has a lower sensitivity and specificity, in hopes that it will prove effective for them. Screening for ovarian cancer is an excellent example. Highly specific and sensitive screening tests are currently unavailable for the early detection of ovarian cancer. Many women, however, still want an annual pelvic examination to assess for ovarian masses. This test is relatively inexpensive to perform and is usually tolerated fairly well by women. Some clinicians are better at detecting ovarian masses than others. Nevertheless, many ovarian cancers cannot be detected using this examination, even when performed by skilled clinicians. As long as a woman realizes that the test may fail to detect ovarian cancer and is willing to accept this limitation, utilizing the pelvic examination may be effective. Often women at higher risk for ovarian cancer will choose to have CA-125 antigen testing and a transvaginal ultrasound in hopes of finding early ovarian cancer. Neither of these tests has been proven to be effective in reducing the morbidity and mortality associated with ovarian cancer, yet women at higher risk continue to undergo these screening tests.

## INFORMED CONSENT

After the risk assessment is completed and its information is interpreted to the patient, a consent form should be signed for the screening procedures that the patient intends to undergo. The consent form states who will provide the screening procedure, notes that not all cancers may be detected during a screening examination, and, if the patient declines recommended screening, specifies a waiver of which recommended procedures are being declined. This consent also helps to reinforce the recommendations for screening. Table 6-9 highlights the basic elements of an individual cancer screening.

Clearly, cancer risk communication influences decisions to undergo cancer screening examinations.[52] When a healthcare provider recommends a particular screening examination, there is an increased likelihood that the individual will actually go on to have the recommended screening. Health providers can make good recommendations for screening based on the myriad of guidelines available only if they understand the biases of various guidelines and have completed an accurate assessment of risk.[55] In addition, decisions to undergo screening are influenced by how much benefit is perceived to result from undergoing the screening procedure. Such a decision must be balanced with a discussion of the risks associated with screening. Providing individuals with information about the sensitivity and specificity of a screening procedure is, indeed, challenging.

Healthcare professionals must also clarify issues when there are choices about screening. One of the most challenging screening recommendations deals with colorectal cancer screening. The ACS now distinguishes between tests that are likely to prevent cancer (through the removal of polyps) and tests likely to detect cancer. Patients must be informed of all the options. The test that prevents cancer is colonoscopy; some people are unwilling to go through the test and preparation process. As long as the patient is willing to accept the fact that a screening test to detect colorectal cancer—such as a fecal occult blood test—may not detect cancer early, they can make a decision that is congruent with their needs. Healthcare providers have a big role in providing enough information about the risks, benefits, and limitations of recommended screening tests.

## FOLLOW-UP

If the intended benefits of screening are to be realized, individuals need to have a clear understanding of the implications of tests both before they are screened and after they receive the results. The potential benefits of screening are lost if individuals are never informed of the test results or the meaning of those results. Providing patients with information about screening results generates another opportunity to reinforce the information included in the risk factor assessment. After screening tests are completed, risk may be more apparent and screening recommendations may need to be revised. For example, a 50-year-old woman may have a baseline colonosocopy examination that demonstrates a polyp that is subsequently biopsied and shows hyperplasia. Her risk for developing colon cancer is higher than initially perceived. She should be informed of this risk and be counseled about ACS's guidelines for colonoscopy following polyp removal.[3,57,59]

Nurses must also consider the various types of screening programs and identify the one which will best work in a particular environment. These options include mass screening and individual screening. To be successful, either mass screening or individual screening needs to include a strategy to follow up on both normal and abnormal test results. Procedures need to be in place to ensure that patients receive results in a timely fashion. In particular, recommendations for further follow-up or follow-up screening need to be clearly communicated to the patient.

*Mass screening* generally refers to screening programs in which large numbers of persons undergo screening, usually

**TABLE 6-9**

**Steps in a Basic Individual Cancer Screening Session**

- Complete a comprehensive health history and risk assessment.
- Communicate the risk assessment to the patient.
- Complete a physical examination of all or selected at-risk sites. This may include skin, head and neck area, breasts, abdomen, prostrate, rectum, gynecologic organs, and a survey of lymph nodes.
- Provide patient education that includes information about anatomy, physiology, risks, strengths and benefits of available screening tests, primary prevention strategies, sources for genetic counseling/testing when appropriate, early signs and symptoms of cancer, and self-examination techniques.
- Schedule and obtain appropriate laboratory and radiologic studies, including Pap test cytology and mammography. Schedule and obtain other screening tests, such as colonoscopy or endometrial biopsy.
- Ensure that the patient receives follow-up. All patients should receive the results of screening whether they are positive or negative. Patients with abnormalities should receive information about why follow-up is necessary. Those with normal screens should receive a reminder for follow-up screening in one year.

under fairly impersonal circumstances. An example would be screening 150 persons on two consecutive days for skin cancer. Workplace programs may be an effective means to increase cancer awareness and offer cancer screening to a large group of individuals.[60] This may be especially helpful in self-insured companies where there is a financial incentive to keep employees healthy. The workplace may also be an effective venue because it can provide access to large numbers of persons who are potentially a captive audience.

*Individual screening* typically includes a more traditional approach. It might include risk assessment, education about primary and secondary cancer prevention strategies, screening tests, and results-based health recommendations.

## NURSING IMPLICATIONS

### EDUCATION OF HEALTHCARE PROFESSIONALS

Risk assessment is the responsibility of many different healthcare professionals, including physicians, nurses, psychologists, and genetic counselors. Although formal and clinical education regarding risk assessment is limited in many professions,[56] historically assessment activities have received much attention in most healthcare professions. Risk factor assessment, by contrast, has received little attention in the formal educational setting. Education of healthcare professionals on techniques and tasks of risk assessment is important because healthcare professionals make initial recommendations for screening. Many oncology professionals have learned about genetics through self-study and clinical practice.[61] Although these professionals may understand oncology well, principles of risk communication may be less clear to them.

Statistics is one of the most challenging courses and a source of frustration for many nurses, both at the undergraduate level and especially at the graduate level. Many, however, do not recognize that this course has numerous ramifications for clinical practice. The challenge is for nurses to understand various statistical measures well enough to accurately critique and use existing literature and research and—more importantly—to interpret this information to patients and their families.

Educators need to consider adding information about risk factor assessment to both undergraduate and graduate curricula. In particular, these programs need to emphasize the fact that a cancer risk assessment is not merely collecting data but also communicating the meaning of those data to a patient, so that he or she can ultimately make informed decisions about cancer prevention and early detection behaviors. Specific content regarding cancer risk assessment that should be incorporated into a curriculum includes basic epidemiologic concepts, specific types of risk (absolute, relative), risk factors for specific cancers and etiologic factors (if known), basic statistics, information about cancer prevention and early detection measures, and counseling techniques.

### ADMINISTRATIVE CONSIDERATIONS

Administrators who want to introduce cancer risk assessments into a program of cancer screening or other oncology programs need to consider a number of issues. First, they must look at the rationale for implementing such a program. Often, it is just to increase awareness of cancer screening or promote a particular program. Increasing recruitment to health promotion programs is regarded as a major benefit of completing a health risk assessment. Screening programs that include risk assessments also can be incorporated into outreach programs to work site settings. Ultimately, the success of most screening programs depends on the effort taken at the beginning to completely assess the unique needs of the population or community being served.

Other important considerations include where services will be provided, marketing of services, and reimbursement issues. If the institution is unable to provide the screening that will be recommended following a risk factor assessment (eg, genetic testing), what arrangements will be made for patients who desire such services? Administrators cannot overlook the need to hire nursing or other personnel who have the expertise and skills needed to provide this essential and comprehensive service. Barriers to consider are described in Table 6-10.[6,62] Many innovative secondary cancer screening programs are described elsewhere.[62] The importance of targeting interventions that are culturally sensitive cannot be overestimated. People choose to engage

**TABLE 6-10**

| Barriers to Cancer Screening |
|---|
| **Patient factors** |
| Patient does not understand the magnitude of risk |
| Patient does not understand benefits of screening |
| Inadequate social support |
| Patient distress or misconceptions related to screening |
| Lack of financial resources to pay for screening or follow-up care |
| Lack of transportation to get to screening |
| Screening considered too uncomfortable or embarrassing |
| **Service system factors** |
| Lack of a wellness focus in healthcare system |
| Low awareness of the benefits of screening by some providers |
| Conflicting recommendations about screening |
| Lack of time to perform a comprehensive examination or risk assessment |
| Failure to recommend a screening procedure |
| Facilities may have access that is difficult or inconvenient |

*Source*: Data from Mahon[6]; Price[42]; and Stoner and Mahon.[62]

in cancer screening interventions. If an intervention is not culturally sensitive or makes an individual uncomfortable, an opportunity for screening or increasing cancer awareness may be missed.[12,63]

## ECONOMIC CONSIDERATIONS

At the clinical level, the delivery of cancer risk information takes time, and how people who provide such information should be reimbursed for their risk assessment and counseling services is unclear. Such charges may be bundled with other service charges such as mammography. Without adequate reimbursement, however, risk assessment services are unlikely to be given adequate attention or provided by people with sufficient background and expertise. When providing genetic services, many providers report that a standard protocol states that individuals or families should be seen for two visits, with each session lasting about 2 hours. In the setting of genetic risk counseling, the use of multidisciplinary teams and multiple interactions is emphasized. The underlying concern is that individuals may be "overwhelmed" by all the information provided in a single one-hour visit.[47] Such attention usually is not given to people with an average risk for developing malignancy.

Much debate focuses on how much should be spent on cancer screening. Controversy continues regarding the threshold necessary to deem a screening or treatment as cost-effective. It is difficult to find a measure that allows comparisons between healthcare interventions that save lives and those that improve quality of life.[64]

Clearly disparities exist in cancer prevention and early detection utilization. Research continues to demonstrate that a direct consequence of lack of insurance or underinsurance results in lower screening rates and limited access to primary care for prompt evaluation of symptoms. This means that this population is much more likely than those with private insurance to be diagnosed at later stages of tumor development when treatment is less likely to be effective, and is associated with increased morbidity, mortality, and economic costs. For example, 75% of women aged 40 to 64 who had private insurance had received a mammogram in the past two years, compared to 56% of women with Medicaid and 38% of women without insurance.[5] Even when programs such as the National Breast and Cervical Cancer Early Detection Program (NBCCEDP) administered by the Centers for Disease Control (CDC) are available to these groups, promoting access to these programs remains a significant challenge.

## PRACTICE CONSIDERATIONS

The cancer risk assessment begins the educational process related to cancer prevention and early detection. Without an accurate and comprehensive risk assessment, it is impossible to provide the individual with appropriate and reasonable recommendations for primary and secondary cancer prevention. The risk factor assessment provides the oncology nurse with an opportunity to teach individuals about the epidemiology, risk factors, and signs and symptoms associated with the various cancers. It transmits the framework individuals need to understand the importance and rationale for primary and secondary cancer prevention strategies as well as information about signs and symptoms that merit further evaluation.

Empowering patients with enough information in understandable terms so that they can make an informed choice about cancer screening is the ultimate goal of cancer risk counseling. When a healthcare provider simply recommends a screening test or tries to scare a patient into undergoing a screening test or genetic test by telling a poignant or compelling story, the patient may select or fail to select a screening test for the wrong reasons. Thus, it is important that providers offer balanced and accurate information. The downside of conveying a risk assessment such that the individual has enough information to make an informed decision is that it is extremely labor-intensive for the healthcare provider.[65]

Staff nurses can serve as case finders to identify individuals at increased risk (especially hereditary risk) for developing cancer who will benefit from a more detailed risk assessment, and possibly cancer genetic counseling.[66] Indeed, many staff nurses who work with patients and get to know their families are the best persons to initiate referrals and begin the cancer risk assessment process. To be an effective case finder, the nurse must understand basic cancer incidence, epidemiology, and the importance of an accurate family history.

Nurses with advance practice degrees can perform more in-depth risk assessments, recommend cancer screening procedures, explain the risks and benefits of a particular screening examination, and, in many cases, actually carry out the screening examination. They are well-suited to perform professional breast examinations, teach breast self-examination, do rectal examinations, complete a skin examination, or complete a pelvic exam, and take a Pap smear. Some advanced practice nurses with additional subspecialty training are able to perform flexible sigmoidoscopy examinations.

Oncology nurses have a major responsibility to teach the public about cancer detection and screening. Individuals need to realize that cancer screening differs from diagnostic examinations for cancer. They also need to recognize that cancer screening is not perfect and, even when conducted properly, will still fail to detect some malignancies because of the strengths and limitations associated with different screening tests.

Research continues to suggest that the single most important factor in whether an individual has ever had a screening test, or has recently had a screening test, is a recommendation from the healthcare provider.[3] When nurses recommend screening to an individual, there is a far greater chance that the individual will actually go on to have appropriate screening. This recommendation can easily come in the form of patient education about cancer prevention and early detection.

Every cancer screening program should include a significant patient education component. Increasing cancer awareness is the first step in getting individuals to engage in cancer screening. Care needs to be taken in gathering appropriate and useful materials for this purpose.[16] These materials may include brochures that may come from cancer-related organizations or that are developed specifically for an agency's population. Posters can be obtained to provide additional education and be displayed in waiting and examination areas. Bulletin boards are a relatively simple means to provide brief public education specific to a population or topic. They have the advantage of being relatively easy to produce and change to promote different cancers, risk factors, or screening events. Flip charts can be used for individual education; these can be either purchased or developed specifically for the group being served. Other educational aids might include anatomical charts and models, computer-assisted education, and professional samples (eg, sunscreen or smoking cessation kits).

When providing patients with information on cancer prevention and early detection, it is important to use educational materials that focus on wellness. More of these resources are becoming available. The NCI and the ACS have many resources for patient education that are aimed at cancer prevention and early detection. It is inappropriate to provide materials that focus on disease and treatment unless the person requests such information. In fact, some persons find them distressing. The message of education and materials should be that when detected early, cancer is associated with decreased morbidity and mortality and improved quality of life. Other examples of printed materials are readily available in the professional literature.[16]

How long a person can retain information after counseling about cancer risk factors is unclear. Information about risk and recommended screening can be reinforced by sending patients a post-visit letter that summarizes the discussion of risk and recommendations for screening or other follow-up. Consideration needs to be given to how individuals will be retained in cancer screening programs and genetic counseling programs so that risk assessments can be updated, recommendations for screening modified if needed, and regular routine screening completed. Some type of reminder is generally necessary to facilitate yearly follow-up for cancer screening in healthy individuals.

## LEGAL CONSIDERATIONS

Once cancer risks and screening recommendations are identified and communicated to the patient, the patient must make a decision as to which screening tests he or she desires. If a patient declines a recommended screening test, a waiver is signed on a consent form that acknowledges the patient was informed of the recommendation and is declining the recommended screening at that time. Information about cancer screening recommendations can be reinforced in a post-visit letter that summarizes the discussion of risk, informs the patient of the results of his or her screening tests, reiterates any recommended follow-up, and summarizes the recommendations for cancer prevention and early detection.

## INTERACTIONS WITH THE MEDIA

New risk factors seem to emerge every day. An important educational role for nurses is to help patients understand which risks they should take seriously. Most people accept a wide variety of risks (eg, driving at the posted speed limit, crossing a busy parking lot, riding a bike, flying across the country in an airplane) on a daily basis with little thought. For some reason, brief news segments about cancer risk seem to conjure up more fear. Nurses need to be aware of public news reports and go to the primary sources when new risk factors are presented so that they can interpret this information accurately to their patients. They also need to communicate concepts related to cancer risks carefully when providing information to the media. This effort may include providing the media with primary sources and reports and more integrated state-of-the-art information. Both the ACS and the other resources should be consulted prior to speaking with the media, to ensure that accurate statistics and figures are provided.

Each year the ACS publishes *Cancer Facts and Figures.*[3] Nurses can use this helpful reference to quickly gather incidence data about estimated cancer cases. The information is presented in several formats, including the estimated projected number of new cases of specific cancer (incidence) and estimated mortality rates. The incidence rates are also given by state. Oncology nurses can obtain this publication free of charge from the local unit of the ACS and may find it helpful to review so as to better understand the incidence of specific cancers in the geographical area in which they practice. The publication also offers detailed information about primary and secondary cancer prevention of the major tumors as well as projected survival data by stage. Once familiar with the format of the publication, oncology nurses will find it to be an invaluable resource. The ACS also publishes *Facts & Figures* that deal with specific cancers such as breast cancer, specific minority populations, and on cancer prevention. These are updated regularly and can be downloaded from the ACS website (http://www.cancer.org).

Another source of commonly cited data is the Surveillance, Epidemiology, and End Results Program (SEER).[15] Currently, SEER data include incidence, mortality,

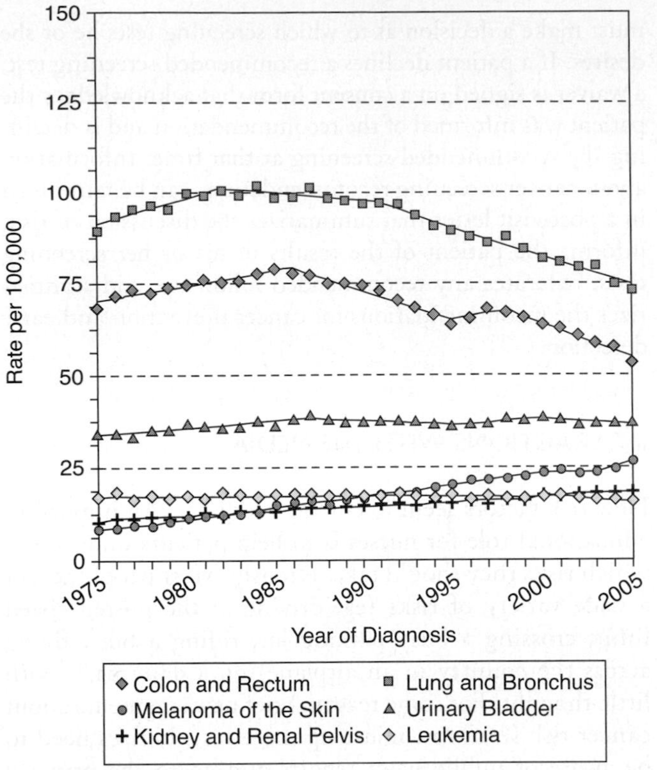


**FIGURE 6-1**

Age-adjusted SEER incidence rates by cancer site for all ages, all races, male, 1975–2005 (SEER 9).

*Incidence Source*: SEER 9 areas (San Francisco, Connecticut, Detroit, Hawaii, Iowa, New Mexico, Seattle, Utah, and Atlanta).

*Note*: Rates are per 100,000 and are age-adjusted to the 2000 US Std Population (19 age groups—Census P25-1130). Regression lines are calculated using the Joinpoint Regression Program Version 3.3, April 2008, National Cancer Institute.[15]

and survival rates from 1973 through 2004. Data from the nine SEER geographic areas are used to represent an estimated 9.5% of the US population. Currently, the database contains information on 3.1 million cases diagnosed since 1973. Approximately 125,000 new cases are added yearly. This information can be obtained easily at the NCI Web site (http://www.seer.ims.nci.nih.gov/). This database allows the user to view many different forms of data in both table and graph format and is extremely helpful when looking for trends in cancer as shown in Figure 6-1.

## FUTURE RESEARCH

Future research should evaluate the process of risk notification and its effects on knowledge, attitudes, emotions and practices, and outcomes related to health and disease status. Most of the studies of perceived risk have been cross-sectional in nature, which makes it difficult to determine whether the perceived risk is a cause or an effect in relation to cancer screening.[43] This relationship could be better understood if longitudinal studies were conducted to measure perceived risk in defined populations with different cancer screening histories that include follow-up for screening and repeated measures of risk perception. Such investigations should include controlled clinical trials to evaluate different counseling protocols. This type of research will provide information on the impact and effectiveness of cancer risk assessment and counseling.

Clearly, more information is needed on the roles played by cognition, affective state of the individual, developmental differences, and personal values and the way in which these individual qualities influence cancer risk communication.[51] More research is also needed to determine the best persons (including an interdisciplinary approach) to communicate cancer and genetic risks.[56] Likewise, information is needed on how to facilitate decision making regarding the management of cancer risks.

Prospective studies are needed to determine the psychological and behavioral implications of risk information. Little research has been done on the long-term implications of cancer screening activities.[46,67] Assessments should optimally be conducted at multiple time points and include outcome variables. More research is needed to understand why two individuals react differently to similar information regarding cancer risk. Little research has focused on how people cope with information related to their risk of disease. Models of coping with disease may not encompass the concept of coping with increased risk for developing a disease such as cancer. Coping may be influenced by the extent to which an individual believes they can control the outcome through screening.[46] People who utilized problem-focused forms of coping may be more likely to engage in screening, but this is an area of cancer screening that requires much more research. The effect of cancer risk assessment on cancer screening behaviors merits more attention.

Technical issues in cancer screening require more research. Little is known on the effectiveness of screening protocols. Clearly nurses could provide comprehensive screening services and education if there were clear guidelines or screening protocols.[68] Rising healthcare costs dictate a need for more research on the cost-effectiveness of cancer risk assessment.[69]

There is also a lack of formal education for nurses and healthcare professionals about communicating risk and genetic concepts. Future studies need to address effectiveness of this education.[42,43]

## CONCLUSION

Oncology nurses need to view risk factor assessment as a wonderful opportunity for patient education on not only cancer risk factors, but also cancer prevention and early detection activities. Cancer risk assessment can be a technical process requiring expertise. Oncology nurses have an ethical responsibility to communicate risk information in understandable terms and as accurately as possible. Indeed, risk assessment is more than collecting assessment data from the patient. A critical component of the process is communicating the information to patients in a meaningful way.

Cancer risk communication is a continuous process. The risk assessment is a large component of this process. It demands effective communication with patients so that they are informed about the best possible choices regarding cancer prevention and early detection activities. Like other components of the cancer screening process, a cancer risk assessment is most effective if it is updated and reviewed annually.

Once risk is communicated, education about cancer screening options must be provided. This effort should include accurate information about the accuracy, benefits, and risks associated with the test(s). Each individual must decide what testing her or she is willing to accept.

Once testing is completed, the results must be interpreted to the patient. Individuals with normal screening results should understand when screening is again indicated. Patients with abnormal screens need to be directed through appropriate follow-up.

Nurses need to consider epidemiological terms and calculations when conducting risk assessments. They also need to teach patients and their families about the strengths and weaknesses of various screening or surveillance strategies. This education includes a discussion of the sensitivity and specificity of various screening tests, as well as a discussion of why screening is available for some cancers and not for others. Individuals at higher risk for developing cancer because of genetic susceptibility need to understand that the screening recommendations for people of average risk, which are issued by groups such as the ACS, may be inadequate for those with higher risk.

## REFERENCES

1. Paz-Elizur T, Brenner DE, Livneh Z. Interrogating DNA repair in cancer risk assessment. *Cancer Epidemiol Biomarkers Prev.* 2005;14:1585–1587.
2. Schottenfeld D, Beebe-Dimmer J. Alleviating the burden of cancer: a perspective on advances, challenges, and future directions. *Cancer Epidemiol Biomarkers Prev.* 2006;15:2049–2055.
3. American Cancer Society. *Cancer Facts and Figures—2009.* Atlanta, GA: The author; 2009.
4. Tyler CV Jr, Snyder CW. Cancer risk assessment: examining the family physician's role. *J Am Board Fam Med.* 2006;19:468–477.
5. Ward E, Halpern M, Schrag N, et al. Association of insurance with cancer care utilization and outcomes. *CA: Cancer J Clin.* 2008;58:9–31.
6. Mahon SM. Principles of cancer prevention and early detection. *Clin J Oncol Nurs.* 2004;4:169–176.
7. American Cancer Society. *Breast Cancer Facts and Figures—2007–2008.* Atlanta, GA: The author; 2007.
8. Acheson LS, Zyzanski SJ, Stange KC, Deptowicz A, Wiesner GL. Validation of a self-administered, computerized tool for collecting and displaying the family history of cancer. *J Clin Oncol.* 2006;24: 5395–5402.
9. Rauscher GH, Johnson TP, Cho YI, Walk JA. Accuracy of self-reported cancer-screening histories: a meta-analysis. *Cancer Epidemiol Biomarkers Prev.* 2008;17:748–757.
10. Weiss NS, Bodelon C. Interview-based case-control studies of screening efficacy. *Epidemiology.* 2008;19:265–266.
11. Edwards AGK, Evans R, Dundon J, Haigh S, Hood K, Elwyn GJ. Personalised risk communication for informed decision making about taking screening tests. *Cochrane Database Sys Rev.* 2005;(4): CD001865.
12. Karliner LS, Napoles-Springer A, Kerlikowske K, Haas JS, Gregorich SE, Kaplan CP. Missed opportunities: family history and behavioral risk factors in breast cancer risk assessment among a multiethnic group of women. *J Gen Intern Med.* 2007;22:308–314.
13. Lin CJ, Block B, Nowalk MP, et al. Breast cancer risk assessment in socioeconomically disadvantaged urban communities. *J Natl Med Assoc.* 2007;99:752–756.
14. Szymczak W, Szadkowska-Stanczyk I. Cancer risk assessment: present and future. *Int J Occup Med Environ Health.* 2005;18:207–223.
15. Ries LAG, Melbert D, Krapcho M, et al. eds. *SEER Cancer Statistics Review, 1975–2005.* Bethesda, MD: National Cancer Institute; http://seer.cancer.gov/csr/1975_2005/, based on November 2007 SEER data submission, posted to the SEER Web site. Accessed June 15 2009.
16. Mahon SM. Patient education regarding cancer screening guidelines. *Clin J Oncol Nurs.* 2003;7:581–584.
17. Rothman AJ, Kiviniemi MT. Treating people with information: an analysis and review of approaches to communicating health risk information. *J Natl Cancer Inst Monogr.* 1999;25:44–51.
18. Domchek SM, Eisen A, Calzone K, Stopfer J, Blackwood A, Weber BL. Application of breast cancer risk prediction models in clinical practice. *J Clin Oncol.* 15 2003;21:593–601.
19. Fasching PA, Bani MR, Nestle-Kramling C, et al. Evaluation of mathematical models for breast cancer risk assessment in routine clinical use. *Eur J Cancer Prev.* 2007;16:216–224.
20. Freedman AN, Seminara D, Gail MH, et al. Cancer risk prediction models: a workshop on development, evaluation, and application. *J Natl Cancer Inst.* 2005;97:715–723.
21. Evans DG, Howell A. Breast cancer risk-assessment models. *Breast Cancer Res.* 2007;9:213.
22. Constantino JP, Gail MH, Pee D, et al. Validation studies for models projecting the risk of invasive and total breast cancer incidence. *J Natl Cancer Inst.* 1999;91:1541–1548.
23. Claus EB, Risch N, Thompson WD. Autosomal dominant inheritance of early-onset breast cancer: implications for risk prediction. *Cancer.* 1994;73:643–651.
24. Claus EB, Schildkraut MM, Thompson WD, et al. The genetic attributable risk of breast and ovarian cancer. *Cancer.* 1996;77:2318–2324.
25. Tyrer J, Duffy SW, Cuzick J. A breast cancer prediction model incorporating familial and personal risk factors. *Stat Med.* 2004;23:1111–1130.
26. Couch FJ, DeShano ML, Blackwood MA, et al. BRCA1 mutations in women attending clinics that evaluate the risk of breast cancer. *N Engl J Med.* 1997;336:1409–1415.
27. Shattuck-Eidens D, Oliphant A, McClure M. BRCA1 sequence analysis in women at high risk for susceptibility mutations. Risk factor analysis and implications for genetic testing. *JAMA.* 1997;278:1242–1250.
28. Berry DA, Parmigiani G, Sanchez J, et al. Probability of carrying a mutation of breast-ovarian cancer gene BRCA1 based on family history. *J Natl Cancer Inst.* 1997;89:227–238.
29. Frank TS, Deffenbaugh AM, Reid JE, Hulick M, Ward BE, Lingenfelter B, et al. Clinical characteristics of individuals with germline mutations in BRCA1 and BRCA2: analysis of 10,000 individuals. *J Clin Oncol.* 2002;20:1480–1490.
30. Gilpin CA, Carson N, Hunter AG. A preliminary validation of a family history assessment form to select women at risk for breast or ovarian cancer for referral to a genetics center. *Clin Genet.* 2000;58:299–308.

31. Lynch HT, Lynch JE. Hereditary nonpolyposis colorectal cancer. *Semin Surg Oncol.* 2003;18:305–313.
32. Wijnen JT, Vasen HF, Khan PM, et al. Clinical findings with implications for genetic testing in families with clustering of colorectal cancer. *N Engl J Med.* 1998;339:511–518.
33. Ohori M, Swindle P. Nomograms and instruments for the initial prostate evaluation: the ability to estimate the likelihood of identifying prostate cancer. *Semin Urol Oncol.* 2002;20:116–122.
34. Optenberg SA, Clark JY, Brawer MK, Thompson IM, Stein CR, Friedrichs P. Development of a decision-making tool to predict risk of prostate cancer: the Cancer of the Prostate Risk Index (CAPRI) test. *Urology.* 1997;50:665–672.
35. Eastham JA, May R, Robertson JL, Sartor O, Kattan MW. Development of a nomogram that predicts the probability of a positive prostate biopsy in men with an abnormal digital rectal examination and a prostate-specific antigen between 0 and 4 ng/mL. *Urology.* 1999;54:709–713.
36. Fears TR, Guerry IV D, Pfeiffer RM, et al. Identifying individuals at high risk of melanoma: a practical predictor of absolute risk. *J Clin Oncol.* 2006;24:3590–3596.
37. Niendorf KB, Goggins W, Yang G, et al. MELPREDICT: a logistic regression model to estimate CDKN2A carrier probability *J Med Genet.* 2006;43:501–506.
38. Goldstein AM, Chan M, Harland M, et al. Features associated with germline CDKN2A mutations: a GenoMEL study of melanoma-prone families from three continents. *J Med Genet.* 2007;44:99–106.
39. Weitzel JN, McCaffrey SM, Nedelcu R, MacDonald DJ, Blazer KR, Cullinane CA. Effect of genetic cancer risk assessment on surgical decisions at breast cancer diagnosis. *Arch Surg.* 2003;138:1323–1328, discussion 1329.
40. Weinstein ND. What does it mean to understand a risk? Evaluating risk comprehension. *J Natl Cancer Inst Monogr.* 1999;25:15–20.
41. Leventhal H, Kelly K, Leventhal EA. Population risk, actual risk, perceived risk, and cancer control: a discussion. *J Natl Cancer Inst Monogr.* 1999;25:81–85.
42. Price AS. Primary and secondary prevention of colorectal cancer. *Gastroenterol Nurs.* 2003;26:73–81.
43. Vernon SW. Risk perception and risk communication for cancer screening behaviors: a review. *J Natl Cancer Inst Monogr.* 1999;25:101–119.
44. Fischhoff B. Why (cancer) risk communication can be hard. *Natl Cancer Inst Monogr.* 1999;25:7–13.
45. Kreuter MW. Dealing with competing and conflicting risks in cancer communication. *J Natl Cancer Inst Monogr.* 1999;25:27–34.
46. Fang CY, Daly MB, Miller SM, Zerr T, Malick J, Engstrom P. Coping with ovarian cancer risk: the moderating effects of perceived control on coping and adjustment. *Br J Health Psychol.* 2006;11(Pt 4):561–580.
47. Mahon SM. Risk factors. In: Mahon SM, ed. *Breast Cancer.* Pittsburgh, PA: Oncology Nursing Society; 2007:5–25.
48. Yoder LH. Let's talk "cancer prevention." *Medsurg Nurs.* 2005;14: 195–198.
49. Salovey P, Schneider TR, Apanovitch AM. Persuasion for the purpose of cancer risk reduction: a discussion. *J Natl Cancer Inst Monogr.* 1999;25:119–122.
50. Kramer BS. Matching strength of message to strength of evidence: a discussion. *J Natl Cancer Inst Monogr.* 1999;25:85–87.
51. Maibach E. Cancer risk communication—what we need to learn. *J Natl Cancer Inst Monogr.* 1999;25:179–181.
52. McCaul KD, Tulloch HE. Cancer screening decisions. *J Natl Cancer Inst Monogr.* 1999;25:52–58.
53. Strecher VJ, Greenwood T, Wang C, et al. Interactive multimedia and risk communication. *J Natl Cancer Inst Monogr.* 1999;25:134–139.
54. Lipkus IM, Hollands JG. The visual communication of risk. *J Natl Cancer Inst Monogr.* 1999;25:149–163.
55. Foltz A. Issues in determining cancer screening recommendations: who, what and when. *Oncol Nurs Forum.* 2000;27(suppl 9):13–18.
56. Arkin EB. Cancer risk communication—what we know. *J Natl Cancer Instl Monogr.* 1999;25:182–185.
57. Levin B, Lieberman D, McFarland B, et al. Screening and surveillance for the early detection of colorectal cancer and adenomatous polyps, 2008: a joint guideline from the American Cancer Society, the US Multi-Society Task Force on Colorectal Cancer, and the American College of Radiology. *CA: Cancer J Clin.* 2008;58:130–160.
58. Beck LH. Periodic health examination and screening tests in adults. *Hosp Pract.* 1999;34:117–119, 121–122, 124–126.
59. Winawer SJ, Zauber AG, Fletcher RH, et al. Guidelines for colonoscopy surveillance after polypectomy: a consensus update by the US Multi-Society Task Force on Colorectal Cancer and the American Cancer Society. *CA Cancer J Clin.* 2006;56:143–159.
60. Bagai A, Parsons K, Malone B, Fantino J, Paszat L, Rabeneck L. Workplace colorectal cancer-screening awareness programs: an adjunct to primary care practice? *J Community Health.* Jun. 2007;32: 157–167.
61. Weitzel JN. Genetic cancer risk assessment. Putting it all together. *Cancer.* 1999;86(suppl):2483–2492.
62. Stoner C, Mahon SM. Overview section IV: cancer control—local programs. Clinical application of cancer control: case examples, In: Jennings-Dozier K, Mahon SM eds. *Cancer Prevention, Detection and Control: A Nursing Perspective.* Pittsburgh, PA, Oncology Nursing Press; 2002:769–866.
63. Albano JD, Ward E, Jemal A, et al. Cancer mortality in the United Status by education level and race. *J Natl Cancer Inst.* 2007;99:1384–1394.
64. Ubel P, Hirth RA, Chernew ME, et al. What is the price of life and why doesn't it increase at the rate of inflation? *Arch Intern Med.* 2003;163:1637–1641.
65. Edwards A, Unigwe S, Elwyn G, et al. Effect of communicating individual risks in screening programmes: Cochrane systemic review. *BMJ.* 2003;327:703–709.
66. Greco KE, Mahon S. Common hereditary cancer syndromes. *Semin Oncol Nurs.* 2004;20:164–177.
67. Gramling R, Duffy C, David S. Does providing hereditary breast cancer risk assessment support to practicing physicians decrease the likelihood of them discussing such risk with their patients? *Genet Med.* 2004;6:542.
68. Castle PE, Sideri M, Jeronnimo J, Solomon D, Schiffman M. Risk assessment to guide the prevention of cervical cancer. *Am J Obstet Gynecol.* 2007;197:356.e1–356.e6.
69. Ozanne EM, Esserman LJ. Evaluation of breast cancer risk assessment techniques: a cost-effectiveness analysis. *Cancer Epidemiol Biomarkers Prev.* 2004;13:2043–2052.

CHAPTER 7

*Jennifer T. Loud, RN, CRNP, DNP, Sadie P. Hutson, PhD, RN, WHNP, BC*

# Genetic Risk and Hereditary Cancer Syndromes

## INTRODUCTION

The clustering of cancer within families has been recognized for centuries, and over the past 30 years, scientists and geneticists actively debated whether familial cancer syndromes have an inherited genetic basis, in contrast to an environmental basis. During the past 2 decades, the elucidation of the genetic basis for many of the most prevalent and penetrant hereditary cancer syndromes seen in clinical practice has occurred. As the genetic basis of hereditary cancer syndromes is clarified, the number of hereditary cancer syndromes for which germline mutation testing for 1 or more genes is available has dramatically increased.[1] Currently, clinical genetic testing is available for more than 50 syndromes, and several online resources exist, which provide comprehensive information about the syndrome of interest (Appendix 7-1). As a result, there has been an increase in the number of genetic tests ordered for hereditary cancer risk assessment leading to an improvement in the quantification of individual hereditary cancer risk. The challenge for busy healthcare providers is to select appropriate candidates for hereditary cancer risk assessment and to provide, or identify, comprehensive cancer risk assessment and genetic counseling services for patients. As the number of candidates for genetic services increases, a diverse group of healthcare providers are called upon to integrate genetic concepts into their daily practice. Oncology nurses are at the forefront of nursing practice, integrating genetic information into patient care services.

## CANCER NURSING PRACTICE AND HEREDITARY CANCER SYNDROMES

### THE ROLE OF THE ONCOLOGY NURSE IN CANCER RISK ASSESSMENT AND COUNSELING

The need for highly educated, skilled clinicians to perform hereditary cancer risk assessment and cancer risk counseling has accelerated over the past 15 years as new cancer syndromes have been identified and clinical genetic testing becomes available. Oncology nurses with expertise in clinical cancer genetics are a key group of healthcare providers who have developed the knowledge and skills necessary to provide these services to this ever-increasing group of patients. Several nursing professional organizations have developed position statements, (Oncology Nursing Society (ONS),[2] International Society of Nurses in Genetics (ISONG),[3] American Nurses Association,[4]) and credentialing programs[3] for nurses seeking to practice in genetic health care. The ONS position statement on the role of the oncology nurse in cancer genetic counseling identifies 3 levels of oncology nursing practice in cancer genetic counseling: the general oncology nurse, the advanced practice oncology nurse, and the advance practice oncology nurse with specialty training in cancer genetics. The position statement reflects the need for oncology nurses at all levels to contribute to the following:

- Education of patients, families, and the public regarding genetic risk;
- Integration of genetic information into oncology nursing practice as new genetic information becomes available;
- Development of continuing education programs for practicing oncology nurses; and
- Collaboration with other genetic healthcare professionals and organizations to provide comprehensive care to individuals at high genetic risk of cancer.

In addition to the above, an advanced practice oncology nurse with specialty training in hereditary cancer genetics may provide comprehensive cancer genetic risk assessment services consisting of the following:

- Risk assessment;
- Pre- and post-test counseling and follow-up;
- Provision of personally tailored cancer risk management options and recommendations; and
- Psychosocial counseling and support services.

The advanced practice oncology nurse's practice must be consistent with the nurse's state nurse practice act, the nurse's educational preparation, the scope of the nurse's role, and the standards of oncology nursing practice.

International Society of Nurses in Genetics developed 2 credentialing programs for those nurses who wish to document their expertise in genetic health care:

- Nurses with a master's degree in nursing may qualify for the Advanced Practice Nurse in Genetics (APNG) credential, and
- Nurses with a baccalaureate degree in nursing may qualify for the Genetics Clinical Nurse (GCN) credential.

Both credentials document a nurse's ability to obtain a pedigree, evaluate the presence or absence of hereditary risk, assess the likelihood of the presence of a hereditary syndrome, provide genetic information and psychosocial support to individuals and families, and to provide nursing care to individuals and families affected by genetic diseases. An APNG also provides genetic counseling services including pre- and post-test counseling, facilitates genetic testing, and interprets genetic test results.[3]

## VOCABULARY OF HEREDITARY CANCER SYNDROMES FOR ONCOLOGY NURSES

The rapid increase in information about hereditary cancer syndromes has led to a challenge for oncology nurses to stay abreast of the patient care issues related to an inherited predisposition to cancer. Many complicated vocabulary terms are commonly used in the media, by researchers and healthcare professionals, and as part of daily conversations about discoveries resulting from the Human Genome Project. In order to effectively deliver care in the field of oncology, a working knowledge of the common vocabulary associated with hereditary cancer syndromes is essential. Many terms are commonly, and incorrectly, used interchangeably; it is particularly important to review and understand common terms to ensure that the appropriate information is being communicated to patients as well as other healthcare professionals. Table 7-1 includes a number of common vocabulary terms associated with hereditary cancer syndromes.

## CHARACTERISTICS OF HEREDITARY CANCER SYNDROMES

The majority of cancers are thought to be sporadic, occurring in individuals as a result of aging, and/or environmental exposures. Sporadic cancers develop because of somatic errors in DNA replication, which occur in genes (tumor suppressor genes and proto-oncogenes) that normally function to promote proper cell growth and differentiation.[5]

*Hereditary* cancers are attributable to changes (or mutations) in specific genes that are passed from either parent (mother and/or father) to their offspring. Approximately 5% to 10% of all cancers are hereditary.[1] Individuals who inherit 1 of these germline mutations will have a higher likelihood of developing cancer within their lifetime than individuals who have not inherited a germline mutation in a cancer susceptibility gene. The major individual and family features of hereditary cancer syndromes are listed in Table 7-2.[1]

A *familial* cancer pattern is characterized by an increase in the number of cancers within a family, more than what is expected by chance alone. However, the pattern of cancers observed does not fit the features of a hereditary cancer syndrome. Genetic testing for known hereditary cancer susceptibility genes is most frequently uninformative in familial cancer clusters. Cancer cases within family clusters most likely represent complex interactions of low-penetrance

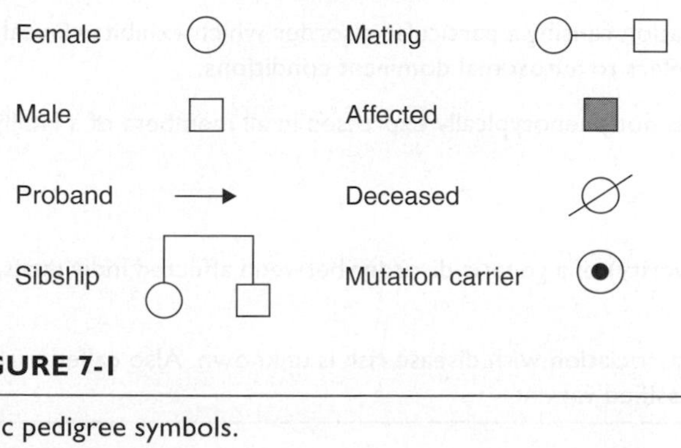


**FIGURE 7-1**

Basic pedigree symbols.

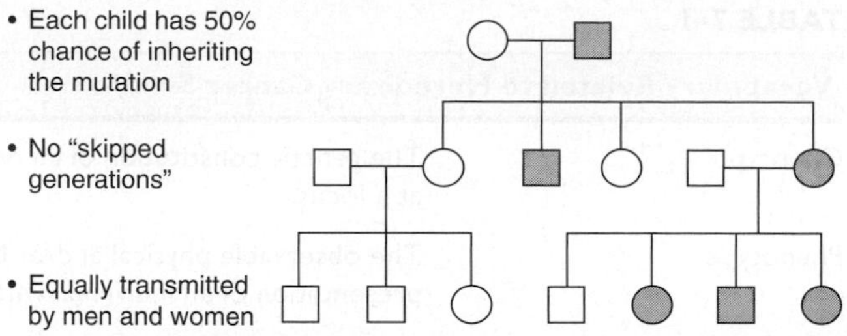

• Each child has 50% chance of inheriting the mutation
• No "skipped generations"
• Equally transmitted by men and women


**FIGURE 7-2**

Pedigree sample of autosomal-dominant inheritance (vertical pattern).

susceptibility gene(s) and/or environmental factors.[6] It is often difficult to adequately quantify the risk of developing cancer in close family members. Unaffected, close relatives are considered to be at increased risk of developing the cancers seen within the family, when compared to the general population.

## IDENTIFYING HIGH-RISK INDIVIDUALS AND FAMILIES

Identifying individuals who are at high genetic risk of cancer begins with recognizing key characteristics within an individual or family that are suggestive of a hereditary cancer syndrome. The importance of being able to construct and evaluate a 3-generation pedigree, on both the maternal and paternal lineage, cannot be overemphasized in the identification of individuals and families at risk of a hereditary cancer syndrome. Basic pedigree symbols and notations are used to construct a visual summary of the proband's and their family's health history (Figure 7-1). Dominant and recessive inheritance patterns within families can be identified during the construction of a pedigree (Figures 7-2 and 7-3). Individual and family health history information is obtained from all members

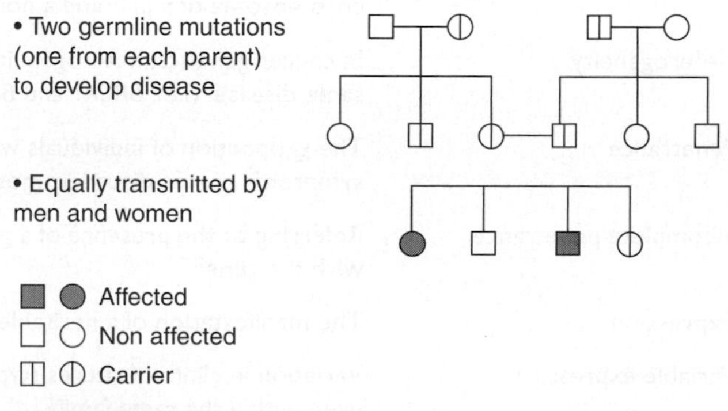


**FIGURE 7-3**

Pedigree sample of autosomal-recessive inheritance (horizontal pattern).

**TABLE 7–1**

**Vocabulary Related to Hereditary Cancer Syndromes**

| | |
|---|---|
| Genotype | The genetic constitution of an organism or cell; also refers to the specific set of alleles inherited at a locus. |
| Phenotype | The observable physical and/or biochemical characteristics of the expression of a gene; the clinical presentation of an individual with a particular genotype |
| Mutation | A mutation occurs when a DNA gene is damaged or changed in such a way that it alters the genetic code that is carried by that gene. These changes can be caused by mutagens such as chemicals, radiation, or environmental factors such as sunlight. |
| Somatic mutations | Somatic mutations can occur in any of the cells of the body except the germ cells (sperm and egg). Therefore, they cannot be passed on to children. These alterations can (but do not always) cause cancer or other diseases. |
| Germline mutations | The presence of an altered gene within the egg and sperm (germ cell) such that the altered gene can be passed to subsequent generations. |
| Sporadic mutations | An alteration in a gene that is present for the first time in 1 family member as a result of a mutation in a germ cell (egg or sperm) of one of the parents or in the fertilized egg itself. Also called de novo, or new germline mutation. An individual with a new germline mutation will lack a family history of cancer in their siblings and ancestors. However, their children will be at risk. |
| Founder mutations | A gene mutation observed in high frequency in a specific population due to the presence of that gene mutation in a single ancestor or small number of ancestors. These often arise when an ancestral population is decimated by a natural or political disaster. If a germline mutation is present among those who survive this event, it will be disproportionately more common among the descendants of the survivors. |
| Autosomal dominant inheritance | Describes a trait or disorder in which the phenotype is expressed in those who have inherited only one copy of a particular gene mutation (heterozygotes); specifically refers to a gene on 1 of the 22 pairs of autosomes (non-sex chromosomes) |
| Autosomal recessive inheritance | Describes a trait or disorder requiring the presence of 2 copies of a gene mutation at a particular locus in order to express observable phenotype; specifically refers to genes on 1 of the 22 pairs of autosomes (non-sex chromosomes) |
| X-linked inheritance | A mode of inheritance in which a mutation in a gene on the X chromosome causes the phenotype to be expressed in males who are hemizygous for the gene mutation.(i.e., they have only 1 X chromosome) and in females who are homozygous for the gene mutation (i.e., they have a copy of the gene mutation on each of their 2 X chromosomes). Carrier females who have only 1 copy of the mutation do not usually express the phenotype, although differences in X-chromosome inactivation can lead to varying degrees of clinical expression in carrier females |
| Carrier | An individual who has a recessive, disease-causing gene mutation at a particular locus on one chromosome of a pair and a normal allele at that locus on the other chromosome |
| Heterogeneity | In cancer genetics, heterogeneity refers to the presence of multiple different genes that cause the same disease, (i.e., *BRCA1* and *BRCA2* can both cause breast cancer) |
| Penetrance | The proportion of individuals with a mutation causing a particular disorder which exhibits clinical symptoms of that disorder; most often refers to autosomal dominant conditions. |
| Incomplete penetrance | Referring to the presence of a gene that is not phenotypically expressed in all members of a family with the gene |
| Expression | The manifestation of a heritable trait |
| Variable expressivity | Variation in clinical features (type and severity) of a genetic disorder between affected individuals, even within the same family |
| Variant of unknown significance | A variation in a genetic sequence whose association with disease risk is unknown. Also called variant of uncertain significance (VUS) and unclassified variant. |

**TABLE 7–2**

**Features Suggestive of a Hereditary Cancer Predisposition Syndrome**

| In the Individual Patient | In the Patient's Family |
|---|---|
| Multiple primary tumors in the same organ | One first-degree relative with the same or a related tumor and one of the individual features listed |
| Multiple primary tumors in different organs | Two or more first-degree relatives with tumors of the same site |
| Bilateral primary tumors in paired organs (e.g., bilateral breast cancer) | Two or more first-degree relatives with tumor types belonging to a known familial cancer syndrome |
| Multifocality within a single organ | Two or more first-degree relatives with rare tumors |
| Younger-than-usual age at tumor diagnosis | Two or more relatives in 2 generations with tumors of the same site or etiologically related sites |
| **Rare Histology** | |
| In the gender not usually affected (e.g., male breast cancer) | |
| Associated with other genetic traits | |
| Associated with congenital defects | |
| Associated with an inherited precursor lesion | |
| Associated with another rare disease | |
| Associated with cutaneous lesions known to have cancer susceptibility | |

*Source:* Data from Lindor et al.[1]

of the family in both the maternal and paternal lineage and includes information on race and ethnicity, current health status, current age or age at and cause of death, type of each primary cancer, age at diagnosis for each primary cancer, bilaterality for paired organs (eg, breast, eyes), and exposures (eg, tobacco exposure and asbestos) (Figure 7-4).[7,8] It is clear that family history is a powerful technique to predict disease when there are multiple family members affected, the relationship between affected relatives and unaffected relatives is close (ie, siblings or parents) and the disease occurs at an earlier age than is typically expected (Figures 7-5 and 7-6).[7] For several hereditary cancer syndromes (eg, multiple endocrine neoplasia [MEN] type 2 and familial adenomatous polyposis [FAP]), the benefits of early cancer detection and prevention have been demonstrated and it is assumed that in other syndromes significant healthcare cost-savings could be achieved by identifying high-risk individuals and intervening early.[7] Once identified, these individuals may benefit from cancer genetic risk assessment, counseling, and testing. Family members who are identified as mutation carriers can begin healthcare interventions earlier in the disease process to lower the risk of developing cancer. Family members who did *not* inherit the mutation associated with the cancers in their family will not have to undergo earlier or increased interventions to lower the risk of developing cancer.

Oncology nurses frequently identify individuals from families at high risk of a hereditary cancer syndrome. The challenge for busy clinicians is to obtain a comprehensive family history in a busy day-to-day practice. "My Family Health Portrait," a patient-oriented, family history tool was developed by the Centers for Disease Control, in conjunction with the National Institutes of Health and the US Surgeon General's office. It is available free to the public in English and Spanish at the US Surgeon General's Web site: http://www.hhs.gov/familyhistory. While it does not produce a comprehensive, 3-generation pedigree, it is simple for the lay public to complete, provides information on the individual and their close family members' health history, and alerts clinicians to possibility of the presence of a hereditary cancer syndrome. From this simple family pedigree, a more comprehensive pedigree can be developed to conduct a comprehensive cancer genetic risk evaluation.

## ETHICAL, LEGAL, AND SOCIAL IMPLICATIONS OF PREDISPOSITION GENETIC TESTING FOR HEREDITARY CANCER SYNDROMES

Genetic testing for hereditary cancer is thought to reduce cancer mortality by identifying those at high genetic risk of cancer and targeting them with increased cancer surveillance

**General medical history**
- Tobacco use, alcohol use, and exercise
- Medical conditions such as osteoporosis, thyroid disorder, hypertension, and diabetes
- Medications

**Reproductive history (female)**
- Age at menarche
- Age at menopause
- Pregnancies: including number of pregnancies, number of live births, number of therapeutic and spontaneous abortions, and age at first pregnancy
- Birth control use, in particular hormonal contraceptives (type, duration and age at time of use)
- Fertility drugs (type, duration and age at time of use)
- Menopausal hormone therapy (type and duration)

**Gynecologic history**
- Gynecologic surgeries (hysterectomy, oophorectomy, endometrial biopsies)
- History of ovarian cysts, endometriosis, and abnormal Pap smears (including colposcopy, cervical biopsy and cryosurgery, loop electrosurgical excision or cone biopsy procedures)
- Breast biopsies (including age at time of biopsy, right/left breast, results, treatment)

**Other cancer history**
- Type
- Age at diagnosis
- Treatment
  - Surgery
  - Radiation
  - Chemotherapy
  - Hormonal therapy

**Screening practices**
- Breast
  - Breast self exam (frequency)
  - Clinical breast exam (frequency)
  - Mammogram (age at baseline and frequency)
  - Ultrasound (frequency)
  - Breast MRI (frequency)
- Colon
  - Sigmoidoscopy
  - Colonoscopy (age at baseline, frequency)
- Skin
  - Biopsies
  - Frequency of exam
- Prostate
  - PSA (frequency)
  - Digital rectal exam (frequency)
- Gynecological
  - Pelvic exam (frequency)
  - Transvaginal ultrasound (frequency)
  - CA-125 (frequency)

**FIGURE 7-4**

Health information to obtain on all family members.[7,8]

*Abbreviations*: MRI, magnetic resonance imaging; PSA, prostate specific antigen.

and preventive strategies. However, genetic information has the potential to cause significant psychosocial morbidity and raise questions about the balance between the benefits of knowing one's mutation status and choosing not to know. Certainly, genetic testing for cancer susceptibility stands apart from other forms of cancer risk assessment (such as assessment of personal modifiable risk factors); there is no

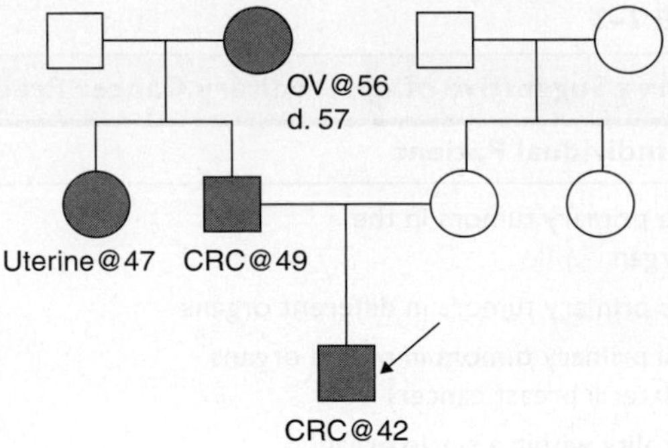


**FIGURE 7-5**

Sample Lynch syndrome pedigree.

*Abbreviations*: CRC, colorectal cancer; OV, ovarian cancer.

ability to alter one's genetic make-up. Many controversial areas exist in the ethical and social implications of testing for hereditary cancer syndromes in relation to the following:

- Who owns DNA?
- Can DNA be patented?
- Should direct-to-consumer testing be made available?
- Should children be screened for hereditary cancer syndromes that will not affect them until adulthood?

Several aspects of the ethical, legal, and social implications of genetic testing for hereditary cancer syndromes and some of the major controversies encountered in the assessment of hereditary cancer susceptibility will be considered. A list of resources on the ethical, legal, and social implications of hereditary susceptibility testing is included in Table 7-3.[8]

## ETHICAL PRINCIPLES

There are four widely accepted fundamental ethical principles to guide medical decision-making: (1) autonomy; (2) nonmaleficence; (3) beneficence; and (4) justice. These principles exist to moderate difficult decisions and to allow

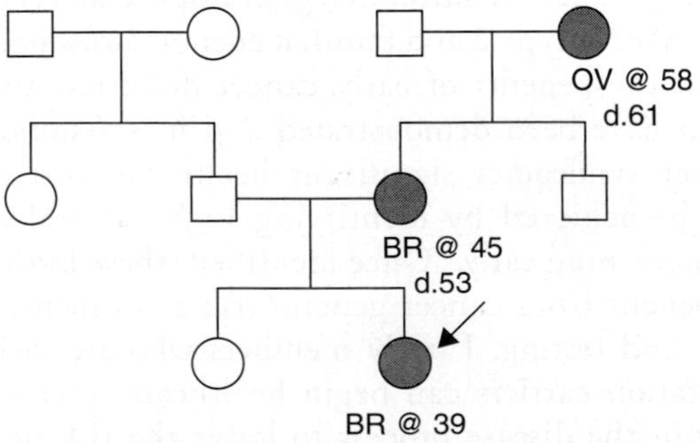


**FIGURE 7-6**

Sample hereditary breast ovarian cancer (HBOC) pedigree.

*Abbreviations*: BR, breast cancer; OV, ovarian cancer.

**TABLE 7–3**

**Resources on Ethical, Legal, and Social Implications of Cancer Genetics**

| Resource | Description |
|---|---|
| Bioethics.net<br>www.bioethics.net | Links to articles on genetics and bioethics |
| Bioethics Resources on the Web<br>http://bioethics.od.nih.gov/ | Links to bioethics resources |
| Coalition for Genetic Fairness<br>www.geneticfairness.org/ginaresource.html | Describes GINA's protections, including a history of the legislation, key examples, and definitions |
| DNA Patent Database<br>http://dnapatents.georgetown.edu/ | Searchable database of US DNA-based patents and patent applications issued by the US Patent and Patent Applications Trademark Office |
| Ethical, Legal, and Social Issues (from the Human Genome Project)<br>www.ornl.gov/sci/techresources/Human_Genome/elsi/elsi.shtml | Information, articles, and links on a wide range of issues |
| Genethics.ca<br>www.genethics.ca/ | Information on the social, ethical, and policy issues associated with genetic and genomic knowledge and technology |
| Genetics and Public Policy Center<br>www.dnapolicy.org/ | Information on public policy related to human genetic technologies for the public, media, and policy makers |
| Genome Technology and Reproduction: Values and Public Policy and Communities of Color and Genetics Policy Project<br>www.sph.umich.edu/genpolicy/ | Two subprojects combined to form a 5-year project designed to provide policy recommendations based on public perceptions and responses to the explosion of genetic information and technology |
| HumGen International<br>www.humgen.umontreal.ca/int/ | Comprehensive international database on the legal, social, and ethical aspects of human genetics |
| NCSL (National Conference of State Legislatures) Genetic Technologies Project<br>www.ncsl.org/programs/health/genetics.htm | Resources on a variety of genetics public policy and related issues for state legislators, legislative staff, and other policy makers |
| National Information Resource on Ethics and Human Genetics<br>www.genethx.georgetown.edu | Links to resources and databases on ethics and human genetics |
| National Information Resource on Ethics and Human Genetics: Annotated Bibliographies: Scope Note Series<br>www.genethx.georgetown.edu | Annotated bibliographies on various genetics and ethics issues |
| National Human Genome Research Institute (NHGRI) Policy and Legislation Database<br>www.genome.gov/PolicyEthics/LegDatabase/pubsearch.cfm | Searchable database of federal and state laws/ statutes, federal legislative materials, and federal administrative and executive materials about privacy of genetic information/confidentiality; informed consent; insurance and employment discrimination; genetic testing and counseling; and commercialization and patenting |
| National Society of Genetic Counselors (NSGC) Code of Ethics<br>www.nsgc.org/about/codeEthics.cfm | A statement to clarify and guide the ethical conduct of genetic counselors |
| The President's Council on Bioethics<br>www.bioethics.gov/ | Reports, transcripts, and background material on current bioethical issues |
| THOMAS Legislative Information (from Library of Congress)<br>http://thomas.loc.gov/ | Searchable database of US legislation (current and previous Congresses) |
| Your Genes, Your Choices<br>http://ehrweb.aaas.org/ehr/books/index.html | Description of the Human Genome Project, the science behind it, and the ethical, legal, and social issues raised by the project |

*Source:* Data from the National Cancer Institute.[8]

for a broad range in judgment. Within the realm of genetic testing and genetic information, 2 of the most important considerations are informed consent and confidentiality.[9] Many ethical dilemmas involve conflicts that arise when establishing measures of informed consent for genetic testing and in the protection of individual confidentiality. The following is a brief review of the ethical principles.

### Respect for autonomy

The principle of autonomy stands for the proposition that an adult, with the capacity to make decisions, has the right to determine what may be done to his/her body. This principle requires that even when a medical professional disagrees with a patient's informed decision, his/her opinion does not infringe upon the patient's right to choose.[9] In the field of genetics it is important to understand that we are obligated to respect the autonomy of individuals in so far as such respect is compatible with the autonomy of all. Therefore, informed consent is a central focus of autonomy when it pertains to genetic information.

### Nonmaleficence

Nonmaleficence is derived from the ancient Latin maxim *primum non nocere*, or, "first do no harm." Many medical and public health practices strive for a utilitarian approach to achieving the greatest good for the greatest number. In cancer genetics an example of a potential threat to nonmaleficence is when a clinician discloses an uninformative test result. As a consequence of an uninformative test disclosure, a patient may have a false sense of security.[10] If a patient is a member of a family with a cancer history that is suggestive of a hereditary cancer syndrome, and individual mutation testing for the appropriate syndrome(s) does not reveal a deleterious mutation, it is possible that the family's cancers are caused by a mutation that is not detectable, or is not yet discovered. Communicating the impact of an uninformative, negative genetic test result is clearly a challenge in cancer risk counseling and increases the potential for nonmaleficence on the part of healthcare providers who lack experience in interpreting genetic test results.

### Beneficence

The ethical principle of beneficence, in the context of cancer genetic susceptibility testing, can be summarized as a healthcare provider's responsibility to provide an opportunity for benefit. Given that as a society there is an underlying need for self-determination, this principle often comes into conflict with autonomy. Hence, it is not enough that nursing actions avoid harm; they must also strive to distinguish for patients the specific benefits that come from having genetic information.[11] For example, predisposition genetic testing is considered beneficent if enhanced cancer surveillance or cancer prevention strategies decrease the morbidity and mortality associated with a specific hereditary syndrome.[10] There is an ongoing need for evidence-based, safe and effective management strategies for high-risk individuals. However, the clinical validity of genetic testing and the clinical utility of many interventions for a rare hereditary cancer syndrome is based on highly selected families.[1] Until evidence of benefits in survival and decreased morbidity is established in these high-risk families, clinicians will continue to rely on cancer screening and prevention guidelines that are based on consensus expert opinion.

### Justice/equity

The principle of justice is often thought of as being synonymous with equity or fairness. Justice can be conceptualized as a balance between potential harms and benefits. Often, a decision that is equitable can still be considered unjust; it is critical to consider that what might seem just to one is contrary to that of another. A central issue of justice and equity in hereditary cancer genetics is the equitable distribution of resources to individuals. Do individuals, who might benefit from predictive genetic testing, have access to experts in cancer genetic risk assessment, counseling, and testing? Do individuals who are at high genetic risk of cancer also have the means to pay for these services? As the number of genetic tests for cancer susceptibility and other diseases increases, oncology nurses must be advocates for all patients having equal access to genetic services.

### Informed consent

Prior to obtaining informed consent for genetic testing, it is important that healthcare providers anticipate the decisions a patient may contemplate as a result of the test outcome. These include understanding the limitations of the genetic test, the accuracy and performance characteristics of the genetic test, the laboratory processing of the specimen, and implications of the results. Healthcare providers have an obligation to offer genetic testing to patients who might benefit from the results, but it is the patient who must decide what is in their own best interest. Patients have as much of a right to informed consent as they do informed refusal.[9,10,12] The requirements of informed consent include[10]:

(1) Competence to comprehend the informed consent discussion;
(2) Disclosure of known procedures, risks, and benefits;
(3) Understanding of the information presented;
(4) The voluntary nature of the decision; and
(5) Consent by the individual or appropriate surrogate.

Given the nature of genetic testing and its inherent ability to affect more than just one individual, comprehensive genetic counseling can help to ensure that patients make

**TABLE 7–4**

| Basic Elements of Informed Consent for Cancer Predisposition Testing |
|---|
| 1. Information on the specific genetic test being performed |
| 2. Implications of a positive and negative test result |
| 3. Possibility that the test will not be informative |
| 4. Options for risk estimation without genetic testing |
| 5. Risk of passing a mutation to children |
| 6. Technical accuracy of the test |
| 7. Fees involved in testing and counseling |
| 8. Psychological implications of test results (benefits and risks) |
| 9. Risks of insurance or employer discrimination |
| 10. Confidentiality issues |
| 11. Options and limitations of medical cancer risk management and strategies for prevention following testing |
| 12. Importance of sharing genetic test results with at-risk relatives so that they may benefit from this information in making their own healthcare decisions |

*Source*: Data from Knoppers et al[13]; and the American Society of Clinical Oncology.[14]

informed decisions. Table 7-4[13,14] includes a list of informed consent elements for cancer genetic testing.

## Duty to warn

In some instances, as noted above, the ethical principles of autonomy and beneficence conflict when a healthcare provider contemplates his or her duty to warn individuals of their risk of inherited cancer. Currently, the American Society of Human Genetics[13] and the American Society of Clinical Oncology[14] posit that it is the clinician's obligation to inform the proband of the risk of inherited cancer to be communicated to the biologically related family members. However, it is not a realistic expectation of the practitioner to warn all of those at risk.[15] So, what is the ethical duty to warn and the legal duty to disclose? The central difference in the case of genetics vs other instances of duty to warn is that the "victim" is not being put at risk by the proband or patient. A recent position paper by the Canadian Medical Association recommends that an intermediate position would be to respect the patient's right to confidentiality, but in exceptional circumstances a clinician may consider nonconsensual disclosure after weighing the seriousness of harm, preventability of morbidity/mortality, and the necessity of disclosure are factored into an intervention.[16] Upon deciding the best course of action, some questions for the healthcare provider to consider include the following[17]:

(1) Who is the primary client?
(2) Is there a way to satisfy all parties?
(3) What are the potential harms in disclosure/nondisclosure?
(4) What professional resources might be needed to disclose?
(5) Are there professional guidelines/position statements that may aid in the decision to disclose/not disclose?

These questions can only serve as a guide and most decisions of this nature should be reached by an interdisciplinary care team.

## The right to know or not to know

In many cases of cancer genetic testing there are individuals who want to learn their genetic status and others who do not. Again, this may bring up controversial issues in balancing the right to autonomy and privacy of individual family members. When dilemmas in balancing individual rights arise within a family, and the proband decides to undergo predictive genetic testing, a positive result will unavoidably reveal the genetic information that has profound implications for other family members. In general, when testing for hereditary cancer syndromes, an individual's right to know supersedes another individual's right not to know. It is imperative that the individual seeking predictive genetic testing be made aware of the potential for complex psychosocial consequences of testing on other family relationships.

## FAIRNESS IN USE OF GENETIC INFORMATION

One of the major controversies surrounding genetic testing for hereditary cancer involves the concept of who is entitled to access and utilize genetic information. There has been significant legislative action at the federal and state level to prohibit the use of genetic information in any aspect of employment including hiring, firing, promoting, and offering access to health insurance benefits. In 2000, President Clinton signed an executive order prohibiting federal departments and agencies from using genetic information in any hiring or promotion action.[18] Employment is only one area in which an individual's basic rights may be compromised by the use of genetic information. Other stakeholders include health and life insurance companies, judicial courts, schools, the military, and adoption agencies. So, who has the right to use a patient's genetic information? Fear of genetic discrimination is still a widespread public concern; there is potential to create a social underclass of individuals based on genetic discrimination—particularly for those who are asymptomatic. The Genetic Information Nondiscrimination Act (GINA) of 2008 was passed to protect the public against genetic discrimination.

## GENETIC INFORMATION NONDISCRIMINATION ACT OF 2008

After 13 years of congressional debate, President George W. Bush signed GINA into law on May 21, 2008. This law, which was enacted in 2009, is now the most comprehensive piece of legislation to protect individuals from genetic discrimination in employment and health insurance settings. Encompassed in this law is a definition of genetic information (including predictive genetic tests, family members' genetic tests, and family history information).[19] Essentially, GINA protects only predictive genetic information and not information from a genetic test that is directly related to an existing condition that could be reasonably detected by a healthcare provider. GINA applies to both individual and group health insurance coverage, prohibits the use of genetic information in health insurance underwriting, and bans employers and insurers from requiring genetic testing as a condition for employment or the issuance of a health insurance policy. There are some limitations to GINA; the act does not address issues pertaining to life, disability, or long-term care insurance, nor does it apply to active-duty military personnel.[19] GINA also will not mandate coverage for any particular medical tests or treatments. The most positive outcome of the GINA legislation may in fact be that patients will now partake in cutting-edge genetic technology without the fears that have discouraged predisposition genetic testing over the past decade.

## RISK ASSESSMENT OF CANCER SUSCEPTIBILITY

Families with a known hereditary cancer syndrome are human models for studying carcinogenesis and susceptibility to neoplasia including gene–gene interactions, gene–environment interactions, and environmental influences in isolation. Much of what we know about hereditary cancer syndromes today comes from the knowledge we have gained by studying highly susceptible families. Genetic risk assessment is initiated by obtaining a comprehensive individual and family history. Although it is the family history that often leads to a healthcare provider's suspicion of a hereditary cancer syndrome, there are also several important characteristics of an individual health history that can be highly suggestive of a hereditary cancer syndrome (Table 7-2). It is critical that healthcare providers ask about these characteristics, particularly if the individual is affected with cancer. The same questions can be applied to family members to obtain specific information about other individuals in the family who are affected with cancer. Pathology reports should be obtained on all reported cancer in the family to confirm the patient-reported family cancer history.

In addition to the individual and family features of the proband, the American Society of Clinical Oncology[14] recommends that the following issues be carefully considered prior to offering any genetic test:

- Evidence that a cancer susceptibility syndrome is present;
- Is the provider able to interpret the results of the genetic test being considered; and
- Certainty that the testing will yield information that will facilitate a diagnosis or be used for medical management.

## CANCER RISK ASSESSMENT MODELS

Only a small proportion of cancers can be attributed to hereditary susceptibility; cancer risk assessment models can aid healthcare providers in identifying those individuals who might be most appropriate for genetic testing or increased cancer surveillance. Current cancer risk assessment models help to (1) estimate the probability that an individual has inherited a mutation in a known hereditary susceptibility gene or (2) estimate the probability that an individual will develop cancer over a defined period of time. However, cancer risk estimate models are not substitutes for sound clinical judgment. Healthcare providers should select models that have been peer-reviewed and validated and should also consider using more than 1 risk assessment model, if available. Risk assessment models are useful tools to assist clinicians in cancer risk assessment but they are regarded as guides for, *not standards of*, cancer risk assessment, as each model comes with inherent limitations.

## GENETIC COUNSELING

The process of genetic counseling is essentially a communication process which deals with the human problems associated with the occurrence, or risk of occurrence, of a genetic disorder in a family.[13] Cancer genetic pre- and post-test counseling involves an attempt to assist the individual or family to become familiar with the following:

- Facts about the diagnosis, natural history of the disorder, and the current medical management options available, including the risk and benefits associated with genetic testing and management options.
- How heredity contributes to the disorder, and to the risk of occurrence (recurrence), in specific relatives.
- Alternatives for dealing with the risk associated with the disorder, including the risks and benefits of each alternative intervention.
- The optimal adjustment (both physiological and psychological) to the disorder in an affected family member.
- The appropriate options available (in view of their risk), their individual and family goals, and their ethical and religious beliefs, including the implications of testing and sharing of test results with other family members.

### IDENTIFYING THE OPTIMAL FAMILY MEMBER TO TEST AND INTERPRETATION OF TEST RESULTS

Genetic testing for a hereditary cancer syndrome is most informative when the test is performed in a member of the family who has had a cancer that is known to be associated with the suspected syndrome (eg, *BRCA1/2* testing in a woman with breast cancer from a family where a hereditary breast and ovarian cancer (HBOC) syndrome is suspected). If a mutation is identified in an affected family member (a "true positive" test result), genetic testing for the presence or absence of the family-specific mutation can then be offered to close, blood-line relatives. Some of the relatives may undergo testing and learn that they have not inherited the family mutation; they are said to have a "true negative" test result. In the absence of a known mutation associated with cancer in a family, a negative genetic test result (*i.e.*, no mutation detected) in a family member is considered to be "uninformative." If there are other hereditary syndromes being considered, genetic testing for the syndromes under consideration may continue in an affected family member. However, if the cancer pattern within the family is consistent with only 1 known hereditary cancer syndrome, no further testing of the unaffected family members is routinely indicated. Theoretically, it is always possible that the person selected for testing is, by chance, a sporadic occurrence of the familial cancer under evaluation. Thus, if there is a strong prior probability of a mutation being present, one may elect to test a second family member, just to be certain that a detectable syndrome has not been overlooked. Figure 7-7 represents the genetic testing algorithm for cancer susceptibility.[20]

If there is no living affected family member in a family suspected of having a hereditary cancer syndrome, consideration may be given to testing either stored tissue samples or unaffected family members. Testing stored tissue can be technically difficult and may lead to results that cannot be clearly interpreted. Testing an unaffected family member may also yield uninformative test results. Failing to detect a mutation in an unaffected individual could be because they did not inherit the mutation associated with the cancer in the family or that the mutation associated with the cancer in the family is not detectable by the technology being used. For an individual who receives an uninformative test result, the presence of a cancer susceptibility gene and an increased risk of developing cancer has not been excluded for the individual nor their family. Genetic counseling in the post-test disclosure session focuses on alternate ways to perform risk assessment, if any, and management of cancer risk based on the family's cancer history.

### GENETIC TESTING FOR CANCER SUSCEPTIBILITY IN MINORS

As noted earlier, genetic risk assessment, counseling, and testing are grounded in the ethical principles of beneficence, nonmaleficence, and respect for autonomy. A primary goal in providing genetic services to individuals and families at high genetic risk of cancer is to protect the individuals and family members from harm, including emotional harm. Family members who are minors (individuals under the age of 18) are not typically offered genetic testing for hereditary cancer syndromes until they become adults.[21,22] Many of the most common hereditary cancer syndromes are associated with cancers that do not occur until adulthood; therefore, it is appropriate to wait until an individual has reached adulthood so that they can make their own decision about genetic testing. This allows the minor to achieve majority and make an autonomous decision about whether to undergo genetic testing. However, when there is evidence of an increased risk of cancer developing in childhood (Table 7-5),[23] or there are benefits of (or consensus for) early cancer screening and prevention[23] of hereditary cancer syndromes in minors, genetic testing for the suspected cancer syndrome is appropriate in childhood.

## SELECTED HEREDITARY CANCER SYNDROMES

The following featured hereditary cancer syndromes are presented to provide information about the most commonly seen hereditary cancer syndromes for which there is clinical genetic testing available, and to provide an introduction to the management of hereditary cancer syndromes. The syndromes chosen are examples of hereditary cancer syndromes where either evidence has demonstrated that intervention improves overall survival or where there is broad consensus about the value of early cancer detection and cancer prevention interventions. A more comprehensive approach is beyond the scope of this chapter; however, several textbooks are available for those who would like to delve more deeply into hereditary cancer syndromes.[24–26]

### HEREDITARY BREAST AND OVARIAN CANCER SYNDROMES

Individuals who are at risk of carrying a mutation that predisposes them to HBOC syndrome are the most common patients referred for cancer genetic risk assessment, counseling, and testing. Approximately 7% of breast cancer cases and 10% of ovarian cancer cases are associated with a mutation in a cancer susceptibility gene.[27–29] *BRCA1* and *BRCA2* account for 84% of hereditary causes of breast and ovarian cancer.[30–34] Cowden syndrome (*PTEN*) and Li-Fraumeni syndrome (*p53*) are other hereditary cancer syndromes that are also associated with an increase in the lifetime risk of breast and/or ovarian cancer[1] and will covered later in the chapter.

*BRCA1*, located at chromosome 17q21, and *BRCA2*, located at chromosome 13q12.3, are tumor suppressor genes that are inherited in an autosomal dominant pattern.

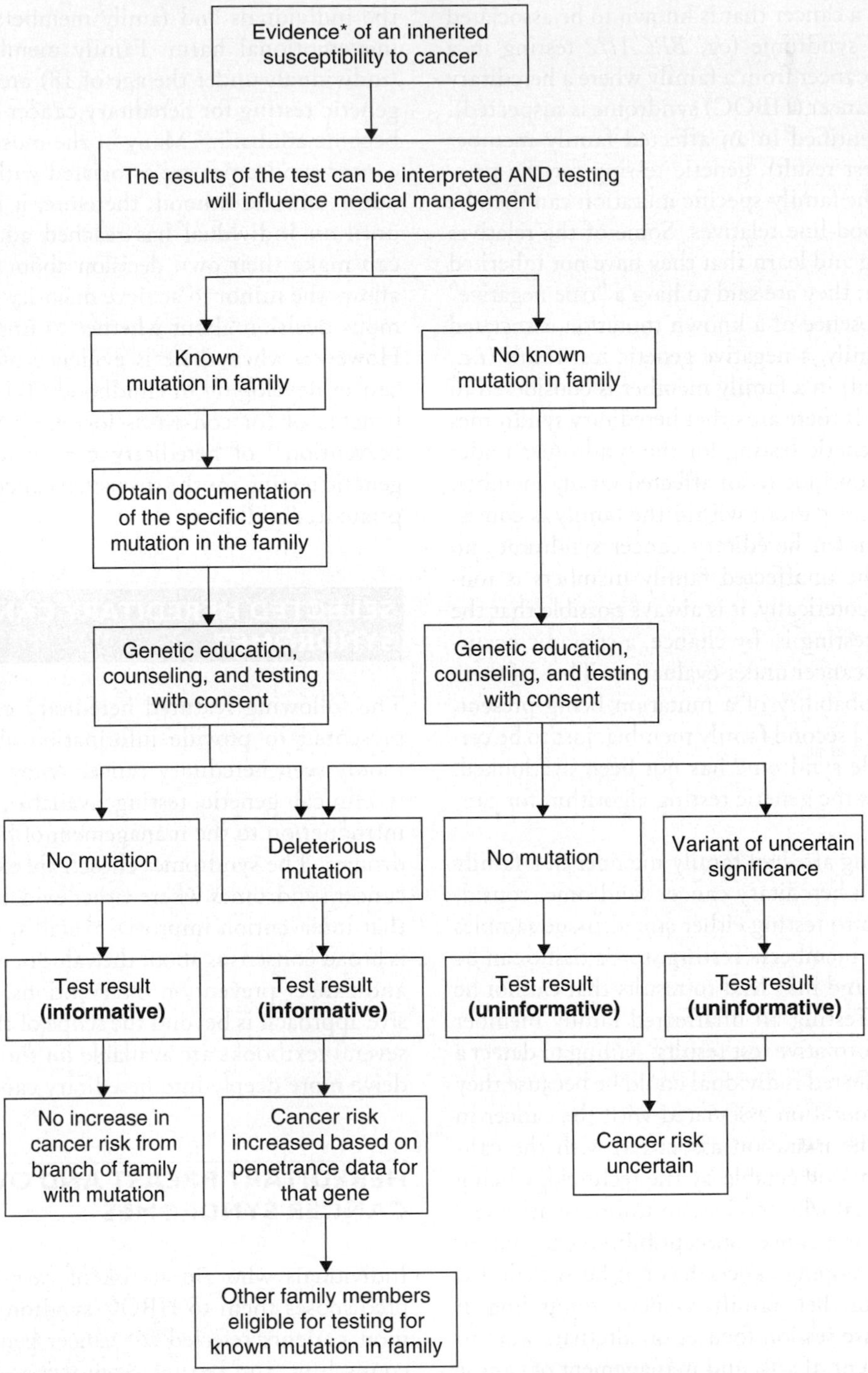


**FIGURE 7-7**

**Genetic testing algorithm for cancer susceptibility.**

*Families with evidence of an inherited susceptibility that have not had any genetic testing or in which genetic testing has not identified a mutation or families with a documented deleterious mutation.[14,20]

In normal cellular physiology, their protein products initiate response to DNA damage by slowing the cell cycle and recruiting other proteins involved in DNA damage repair.[30–34] *BRCA1* and *BRCA2* are not genetically related to one another, and each has a unique mechanism of action in repair of DNA damage. More than 1643 mutations, polymorphisms and variants have been identified.[35] There are several laboratory methods used to detect *BRCA1* and

**TABLE 7-5**

**Autosomal-Dominant Cancer Syndromes and Risk in Childhood**

| Syndrome | Probable Earliest Tumor | Risk in Childhood (%) |
|---|---|---|
| Familial adenomatous polyposis | First year | 80 |
| Neurofibromatosis | First year (meningioma) | 30 |
| von Hippel-Lindau | 1–2 yrs (retinal) | 15 |
| *MEN1* | 5 yrs | 5 |
| *MEN2A* | 3 yrs | 2.5 |
| *MEN2B* | 1 yr | <50 |
| Li-Fraumeni | First year | 30 |
| HBOC/*BRCA1* | >16 yrs | <0.1 |
| HBOC/*BRCA2* | >16 yrs | <0.1 |
| Hereditary nonpolyposis colorectal cancer | >16 yrs | <0.1 |

*Source:* Data from Eeles et al.[23]

*BRCA2* mutations and the diagnostic accuracy for each type has been reviewed.[36]

Estimates of the prevalence of the *BRCA1* mutations in the general population range from 1/312 to 1/1500.[37–40] Founder mutations in *BRCA1* and *BRCA2* have been reported in several populations.[41] In Ashkenazi Jewish (AJ) population, 3 founder mutations have been reported (*BRCA1* 185delAG, *BRCA1* 5382insC, and *BRCA2* 617delT), and together they account for 80% to 90% of all *BRCA* mutations found in AJ hereditary breast/ovarian cancer families. The mutation prevalence for 1 of the 3 AJ founder mutations is 1/40.[41]

Female carriers of a *BRCA1* mutation are at much greater risk of developing breast and ovarian cancer than individuals in the general population. They are also at higher than average risk of developing fallopian tube carcinoma and primary serous carcinoma of the peritoneum[1]. Breast cancers associated with *BRCA1* mutations tend to be estrogen-receptor negative, progesterone-receptor negative and Her2-neu negative, adenocarcinomas of the breast. Lifetime risk (to 70 years of age) of developing breast and ovarian cancer have been estimated to be 65% and 39%, respectively.[42] Other penetrance estimates have been reported and vary considerably. A large Canadian group[40] reported *BRCA1* penetrance estimates to age 80 years to be 90% for breast cancer and 24% for ovarian cancer. A meta-analysis of 10 *BRCA1* studies reported a cumulative cancer risk to age 70 years to be 57% for breast cancer and 40% for ovarian cancer.[43] In the Canadian AJ population, the penetrance of the 2 *BRCA1* mutations for breast cancer by age 70 are 64% for *BRCA1* 185delAG and 67% for *BRCA1* 5382insC. For ovarian cancer, the penetrance estimates are 14% for *BRCA1* 185delAG and 33% for *BRCA1* 5382insC by age 70. Among the US population, the penetrance estimates for breast cancer to age 70 is estimated to be 46% for breast cancer and 39% for ovarian cancer, based on 676 AJ families and 1272 families of other ethnicities.[44]

Estimates of the carrier frequency of the *BRCA2* mutation in the general population, range from 1/1453 to 1/1380.[42] Like *BRCA1* mutation carriers, *BRCA2* mutation carriers are at much greater risk of developing breast and ovarian cancer than the general population; the breast cancer risk is similar to that seen in *BRCA1* mutation carriers, but the risk of ovarian cancer is significantly lower (and the age-at-diagnosis is significantly older) than that reported for *BRCA1* carriers. Breast cancers associated with *BRCA2* mutations tend to be estrogen-receptor positive, adenocarcinomas of the breast. Lifetime estimates of developing cancer to age 70 years for *BRCA2* have been estimated to be 49% for breast cancer and 18% for ovarian cancer.[44] Penetrance estimates for the Ashkenazi *BRCA2* 6174delT mutation for breast cancer to age 70 years is 43% and 20% for ovarian cancer.[29] Male breast cancer is more common among *BRCA2* carriers; the cumulative probability to age 70 is between 6% and 6.8%.[45,46] Other cancers that have been associated with mutations in *BRCA2* include fallopian tube carcinoma, primary serous carcinoma of the peritoneum, prostate cancer, pancreatic cancer, and melanoma.[47–49]

## IDENTIFYING INDIVIDUALS AT HIGH RISK OF HBOC

Cancer genetic risk assessment and genetic counseling is indicated for individuals and families who have been identified as being at high genetic risk of HBOC. Through cancer genetic risk assessment and counseling, individuals and family members learn about hereditary cancer, the individual and family risk of cancer, and options for risk reduction, cancer screening, and cancer management. Often preliminary cancer genetic risk assessment is performed by oncology nurses, oncologists, primary care providers, and other healthcare providers, many of whom lack formal training and certification in genetic health care. In an effort to encourage busy clinicians to integrate cancer risk assessment into daily practice, guidelines to identify high-risk individuals have been developed.[50–52] These guidelines are based on the US Preventive Services Task Force clinical guidelines on genetic risk assessment and *BRCA* mutation testing for breast and ovarian cancer genetic susceptibility, include important questions to ask about the family's cancer history and suggest when to recommend genetic counseling. Once individuals from high-risk families have been identified, formal cancer genetic risk assessment and genetic counseling can be initiated. In general, breast cancer diagnosed prior to menopause (age of <50 years), ovarian cancer at any age, 2 or more primary breast cancers in the same individual, breast and ovarian cancer in the same individual, 2 or more individuals in the family with breast and/or ovarian cancer, male breast cancer, and AJ ancestry are factors that increase an individual's risk of being a *BRCA1* or *BRCA2* mutation carrier.

## *BRCA1* AND *BRCA2* CARRIER PROBABILITY

As noted earlier, mutations in *BRCA1* and *BRCA2* account for only a small proportion (approximately 5%-10%) of all breast cancers. Currently, several risk assessment tools have been published to guide healthcare providers in making decisions about when to recommend genetic testing, increased surveillance, or whether to follow consensus guidelines for syndrome-specific cancer screening for individuals who are at high genetic risk of cancer. Certainly, there are advantages to making predictions based on known hereditary patterns using family history, and pedigree construction, as a risk assessment tool. Family history can be used as a surrogate marker of shared environmental and genetic risk. Reassuringly, comprehensive cancer risk assessment was found to be a better predictor of carrier probability than computerized modeling.[53] The US Preventive Services Task Force[54] published guidelines for cancer genetic risk assessment and *BRCA* mutation testing for breast and ovarian cancer susceptibility in high-risk individuals. There are more than a dozen different models which use various statistical methods, study populations, personal and family history features, and outcomes. There are several models for estimating breast cancer risk and *BRCA1/2* carrier probability. The appropriate predictive model is chosen based on an individual's health history and the cancer pattern (and other associated features) within the family.

## MUTATION CARRIER PREDICTION MODEL: BRCAPRO

*BRCA* mutation carrier prediction models aim to identify individuals who are likely to be *carriers* of a *BRCA1* or *BRCA2* mutation. Several models are available and comparison of the different models suggested that BRCAPRO had the best performance characteristics, though all models performed adequately in clinical use.[1,55] BRCAPRO is a computerized, statistical Bayesian model that calculates *BRCA1* and *BRCA2* carrier probability based on history of breast or ovarian cancer, and age(s) at diagnosis in the proband and in the first-degree relative (FDR) and second-degree relative (SDR).[55] It also accounts for current age and age at death of unaffected relatives. The model is derived from published estimates of gene prevalence and penetrance; these are updated periodically, but estimates may be inaccurate. Other limitations include the following: (1) the model accounts only for first- and second-degree relatives of the index case; (2) it does not incorporate prostate or pancreatic cancer; and (3) it considers only the *BRCA1* and *BRCA2* genes. Therefore, some individuals with increased BRCAPRO carrier probability will have mutations in other genes but will test negative for *BRCA1* and *BRCA2*.[55,56] Healthcare providers must also take care in selecting the family member or proband who will produce the most accurate estimates based on the distribution of affected relatives. It should be noted that a recent study determined that the BRCAPRO model is highly sensitive, yet misses an estimated 15% of mutations carriers.[55] The BRCAPRO software contains the Gail and Claus models for breast cancer risk prediction embedded within its software. BRCAPRO is available at: http://astor.som.jhmi.edu/BayesMendel/brcapro.html

Recent publications have questioned the role of a number of different breast/ovarian cancer risk assessment models given that in many cases the sensitivity of the models are high while the specificity is less than 50%.[57,58] While risk assessment models can aid in determining the use of genetic testing for individuals at risk, healthcare providers must use caution when using these estimates to make clinical decisions about increased cancer surveillance and risk-reducing surgeries such as prophylactic mastectomy and bilateral salpingo-oophorectomy.[59]

## BREAST CANCER RISK: GAIL MODEL AND CLAUS MODEL

The most frequently used model for estimating breast cancer risk in clinical practice is the Gail Model.[60] The tool can be found at http://www.cancer.gov/bcrisktool and is based on a case-control analysis of the Breast Cancer Detection Demonstration Project, which was a joint American Cancer Society (ACS) and National Cancer Institute (NCI) breast cancer screening study that involved 280,000 women between the ages of 35 to 74 years. This tool takes into account variables including a woman's own personal history of prior breast biopsies and the presence of atypical hyperplasia, her reproductive history (age at menarche, and age at the first live birth of a child), and the history of breast cancer among her FDRs (mother, sisters, daughters) in order to estimate the 5-year and lifetime risk of breast cancer. Factors that correlate with an increased risk of developing breast cancer include nulliparity, early age of menarche, later age of menopause, history of previous breast biopsy, and positive family history in a FDR. The Gail Model is advantageous in that it accounts for other risk factors besides family history, and can provide comparison of risk *versus* women in the same age group from the general population. However, it does not account for paternal family history, SDRs, age-at-onset of cancer, bilateral cancers, multiple primaries, or other cancers, and does not account for the presence of inherited genetic predisposition. Thus, it is not a suitable tool for use in a family in which a *BRCA1/2* mutation is suspected. The model is most applicable to women from the general population who present for routine breast cancer screening.

In a recent study, investigators explored the impact of adding an extended family history of breast cancer to the existing Gail Model in case-control design among 1765 women recruited in Italy between 1997 and 2000.[61] The investigators modeled risk estimates based on extended family history grouped according to (1) women with no reported FDR or SDR with breast cancer; (2) women with 1 or more FDR with breast cancer; (3) women with one or more SDR with breast cancer; and (4) women with one or more FDR and/or 1 or more SDR with breast cancer. Findings demonstrated that the extended family history information could be a useful supplement to the existing standard model in predicting breast cancer risk estimates.[61]

The Claus Model is another commonly used model for estimating the cumulative probability of breast cancer.[27] The foundation for this model was a population-based case control study involving 4730 breast cancer patients. The Claus Model incorporates family history to estimate the probability that a woman will develop breast cancer. The model requires information about FDRs and SDRs who have had breast cancer, and their ages at diagnosis. It accounts for paternal contribution of breast cancer risk, which adds to the strengths of the model. Its limitations include that it does not account for bilateral cancers, multiple primaries, or other cancers, and it does not account for other breast cancer risk factors. Further, only 2 relatives can be selected to determine risk estimates, making it confusing for healthcare providers to choose the most informative case, and healthcare providers must have access to the Claus Model data tables, since this model has not been implemented as an online tool.

## *BRCA1/2* CANCER RISK MANAGEMENT

During genetic test disclosure, all *BRCA* mutation carriers are advised of the genetic risk of cancer to relatives and are strongly encouraged to alert family members to the value of genetic risk assessment. Although the major cancers associated with *BRCA* mutations are breast and ovarian, other cancers are considered to be part of the syndrome. However, for most of these cancers, no proven cancer prevention or early detection strategies are currently available. It is imperative to educate *BRCA* mutation carriers about the signs and symptoms of *BRCA*-related cancers so they do not delay seeking care for persistent symptoms which may be associated with the development of cancer.

## BREAST CANCER SURVEILLANCE IN FEMALE *BRCA1* OR *BRCA2* MUTATION CARRIERS OR IN UNTESTED FEMALES FROM FAMILIES WITH KNOWN *BRCA1* OR *BRCA2* MUTATIONS

Recommendations for breast cancer screening in women at high genetic risk include the following:[52]

- Monthly breast self-exam beginning at age 18;
- Clinical breast exam every 6 months starting at age 25;
- Screening mammogram once a year beginning at age 25; or at least 5 years before the earliest age at which breast cancer has been diagnosed in the family; and
- Breast magnetic resonance imaging (MRI) once a year starting at the same age as the mammogram.

MRI of the breast is more sensitive and highly specific as a breast cancer screening tool in young, high-risk women than mammography, breast ultrasound, or clinical breast examination.[62] MRI has also been found to detect breast cancer at an earlier stage than mammography alone.[63–65] These findings support the current recommendation to combine annual MRI with annual mammography for women who are known carriers of a *BRCA* mutation or untested women from families with a known *BRCA* mutation.[52] Data are not currently available to determine whether alternating MRI and mammography every 6 months increases or decreases the performance characteristics of these breast cancer screening modalities. In most cases, it is recommended that the imaging modalities be combined during similar time frames in order to enhance interpretation as mammography in young women can be challenging due to the density of breast tissue.

## RISK-REDUCING BILATERAL MASTECTOMY

Risk-reducing bilateral mastectomy (RRBM), the prophylactic removal of both breasts removed before a breast cancer is detected, lowers breast cancer risk by approximately 90%.[66–68] Women who are considering RRBM should discuss surgical and reconstruction options with a breast surgeon and a plastic surgeon. A small risk of breast cancer remains after this type of surgery; RRBM removes primarily visible breast tissue, leaving behind a small amount of residual breast tissue after surgery. This clinically undetectable breast tissue may give rise to a breast cancer. Although screening with mammogram and MRI are not recommended following RRBM, periodic examination of the chest can be performed.

## HORMONAL PREVENTION OF *BRCA1/2* BREAST CANCER

Bilateral oophorectomy (BO) in women who are *BRCA1* or *BRCA2* mutation carriers reduces the risk of breast cancer by approximately 50%, particularly in women who are premenopausal at the time of BO. The reduction in risk of breast cancer appears to apply to both *BRCA1* mutation carriers and *BRCA2* mutation carriers.[69,70] However, preliminary data suggest *BRCA2* mutations carriers may obtain a greater reduction in risk than *BRCA1* mutation carriers.[71]

There is limited data available to support the use of chemoprevention of breast cancer in *BRCA1* or *BRCA2* mutation carriers. A significant (approximately 50%) reduction in the risk of contralateral breast cancer was observed in *BRCA1* and *BRCA2* mutation carriers who had used tamoxifen for at least 2 years following a diagnosis of unilateral breast cancer.[72] A follow-up study to the original study confirmed a significant decrease in the risk of a contralateral breast cancer was associated with the use of tamoxifen in *BRCA1* and *BRCA2* mutation carriers.[73]

Two different medications can lower the risk of breast cancer among women at increased risk; however, they have not been adequately studied in women who have a *BRCA* mutation.[74] These medications—tamoxifen and raloxifene—belong to a class of drugs called selective estrogen receptor modulators (SERMs).

The Study of Tamoxifen and Raloxifene (STAR) compared the effectiveness of the 2 drugs among women with elevated breast cancer risk; a prior study demonstrated that tamoxifen reduced breast cancer risk by about 50%.[75] The STAR trial showed that raloxifene is as effective as tamoxifen in reducing the number of invasive breast cancer cases, and that it has fewer serious side effects. However, the benefit of these medications in unaffected women with known *BRCA* mutations is not well-established. There are no data regarding the benefits of raloxifene in *BRCA* mutation carriers, and only a limited amount of information regarding tamoxifen. The largest studies of tamoxifen as a breast cancer prevention agent in mutation carriers without a prior breast cancer diagnosis have yielded conflicting results, but there is some suggestion that there is a reduction in risk.[76,77] Therefore, tamoxifen may be a reasonable option for high-risk women to consider.

## OVARIAN CANCER SURVEILLANCE

For women with a *BRCA* mutation, who have not had their ovaries removed, the following is currently recommended:[52] transvaginal ultrasound and CA-125 blood test every 6 to 12 months, starting at age 35, or 5 to 10 years earlier than the earliest age of first ovarian cancer diagnosis in the family. However, several studies have demonstrated that screening for ovarian cancer using transvaginal ultrasound and serum CA-125 is ineffective and inefficient.[78–80] Routine use of transvaginal ultrasound and serum CA-125 does not prevent the diagnosis of late stage ovarian cancer and leads to high number of false-positive findings. For that reason, risk reducing salpingo-oophorectomy (RRSO), after childbearing is completed, is considered the most powerful intervention available to *BRCA1* or *BRCA2* mutation carriers to reduce the risk of ovarian and fallopian tube cancer.

## PROPHYLACTIC REMOVAL OF THE OVARIES AND FALLOPIAN TUBES

Risk-reducing salpingo-oophorectomy has been shown to lower the risk of developing ovarian cancer among high-risk women by 85% to 95%.[81–84] The fallopian tubes must be removed because of the increased risk of fallopian tube malignancies among *BRCA* mutation carriers.[85] It now appears that RRSO may improve both the overall and cancer-specific survival among *BRCA* mutation carriers.[84] However, the procedure does not completely protect against ovarian cancer-like malignancy. After a woman has undergone RRSO, there is still a 1% to 4% chance that she may develop a cancer in the abdomen that resembles ovarian cancer and appears to occur more frequently in *BRCA1* compared with *BRCA2* carriers.[71] Designated primary peritoneal carcinoma (PPC), this malignancy is thought to arise from other tissues in the abdomen that are related to the ovaries. There are no recommendations for routine screening following RRSO to detect PPC at this time.

Risk-reducing salpingo-oophorectomy is usually recommended starting at ages 35 to 40 years, or after finishing childbearing.[52] Before making a decision regarding RRSO, mutation carriers must engage in a thorough discussion about the age of the earliest ovarian cancer in the family, their personal reproductive plans, the degree of risk-reduction expected from RRSO, management of menopausal symptoms, and other medical conditions that may occur more frequently among women who have undergone surgical menopause. The most common symptoms associated with RRSO in premenopausal women are hot flashes and dyspareunia. Fortunately, menopausal hormone therapy (MHT), when used for short periods of time (2–3 years), has not been associated with an increased risk of breast cancer[86] and can be safely used to relieve menopausal symptoms caused by surgical menopause. Further research is needed to determine whether there are differences in the risk of developing breast cancer based on the precise hormonal preparation and duration of MHT in *BRCA1/2* mutation carriers. The Women's Health Initiative[87,88] demonstrated that women taking estrogen-only MHT did not have an increased risk of developing breast cancer. Therefore, it may be worth considering hysterectomy at the time of RRSO, in carefully-selected women, if either estrogen-only MHT is contemplated for the relief of menopausal symptoms, or if tamoxifen is being considered for breast cancer risk reduction.

## CHEMOPREVENTION OF OVARIAN CANCER

For women who are not ready to have RRSO to lower the risk of ovarian cancer, oral contraceptives pills may be considered. The use of oral contraceptive pills has been shown to decrease the risk of ovarian cancer by approximately 50% in both sporadic and hereditary ovarian cancer.[89–91] However, there appears to be an increased risk of breast cancer, in both *BRCA1* and *BRCA2* mutation carriers related to the duration of oral contraceptive use, especially if used before their first full-term pregnancy.[92] *BRCA* mutation carriers interested in using oral contraceptive pills to reduce their risk of ovarian cancer need to consider the potential increased risk in breast cancer, as well as the prevention on unintended pregnancy in weighing the relative risk and benefits associated with chemoprevention of ovarian cancer.

### CANCER RISK MANAGEMENT IN MALE *BRCA* MUTATION CARRIERS

It is recommended that male *BRCA* mutation carriers learn and perform breast self-examination monthly, undergo clinical breast examination, and consider baseline mammography. If gynecomastia or glandular breast density is seen on the baseline mammogram, annual mammography is indicated.[1,93]

Male *BRCA* mutation carriers are also at higher than average risk of prostate cancer; however, screening for prostate cancer earlier than age 50 years is of uncertain benefit. Unless there is a family history of early (age <50 years) prostate cancer, male *BRCA* mutation carriers may follow prostate cancer screening guidelines for the general population.[52,94]

## HEREDITARY COLORECTAL CANCER SYNDROMES

Colorectal cancer is the third most commonly diagnosed cancer among adults in the United States.[95] Approximately 150,000 new cases were diagnosed in 2009 and approximately 50,000 deaths occured because of the disease. The majority of colorectal cancers (75%) are the sporadic form of cancer with no evidence of an autosomal dominant inheritance pattern.[96] Among individuals diagnosed with colorectal cancer, approximately 25% have a family history of cancer that is suggestive of genetic risk or perhaps common exposures among family members associated with an increased risk of developing colorectal cancer. The hereditary colorectal cancer syndromes, Lynch Syndrome (also known as Hereditary Non-polyposis Colorectal Cancer or HNPCC) and Familial Adenomatous Polyposis (FAP) account for approximately 5%–6% of all colorectal cancers. Unique features of family history, characteristics of disease presentation and histopathological findings in tumor tissue and polyps, enhance the ability to identify family members affected by these rare syndromes. While the incidence of Lynch Syndrome (2%–3%) and FAP (1%–2%) is rare, it is important to identify mutation carriers so that early detection and cancer prevention strategies can be employed.

### LYNCH SYNDROME

Mutations associated with Lynch syndrome are inherited in an autosomal dominant pattern with incomplete penetrance. Several genes are associated with Lynch Syndrome and include: *MLH1* at 3p21.3, *MSH2* at 2p21–22, *PMS2* at 7p22, and *MSH6* at 2p16.[1] These genes function in the DNA mismatch repair complex within the cell. *MLH1* and *MSH2* are associated with over 90% of the mutations identified in Lynch syndrome families *MSH6* is associated with 7% of the mutations identified in Lynch syndrome families.[97] The syndrome is characterized by the development of colorectal cancer in the right side of the colon and several other extracolonic cancers (gastric, small intestine [ampulla of vater] biliary tract, urinary tract, ovarian, brain and endometrial) which develop at an earlier age than in the general population.[96] Turcot syndrome, consists of colorectal and brain cancer and is a variant of both Lynch syndrome and FAP. In Lynch syndrome the brain cancers tend to be glioblastomas; in FAP the brain cancers are usually medulloblastomas.[98] Another variant of Lynch syndrome, Muir-Torre syndrome, is characterized by cutaneous lesions (sebaceous adenomas, epitheliomas, carcinomas or keratoacanthomas) and other malignancies.[1] The risk of colon cancer appears to be greatest in *MLH1* mutation carriers; however, the overall risk of all cancers appears to be greatest in individuals who carry a mutation in the *MSH2* gene.[1]

Penetrance estimates for the cancers associated with Lynch syndrome by age 70 years are 24% to 75% for colorectal cancer, 27% to 71% for endometrial cancer, 3% to 13% for ovarian cancer, 2% to 13% for gastric cancer, 4% for small bowel cancer, 1% to 12% for urinary tract cancer, 4% to 7% for brain cancer and 2% for hepatobiliary cancer.[96,99] Colorectal cancer pathologic features in Lynch syndrome include a solid growth pattern, mucin production, poor differentiation and lymphoid infiltration of tumor.[98] Endometrial and ovarian cancers associated with Lynch syndrome are diagnosed an average of 10 years earlier than in the general population; however, the survival does not seem to differ significantly from the sporadic forms of cancer when matched by stage of disease at diagnosis.[99]

*Colorectal Cancer Risk Assessment: Lynch Syndrome* Identification of individuals who are likely to carry a mutation associated with Lynch Syndrome has relied on the use of family history with the Amsterdam Criteria serving as a guide. However, these criteria were initially developed for the purpose of consistent classification of research subjects.[100] The Bethesda criteria were later developed and modified to assist in identifying the risk of Lynch syndrome among patients already diagnosed with HNPCC-related tumors. Subsequently, researchers at Dana Farber Cancer Institute[31] developed a model to help healthcare professionals estimate the probability that an affected individual carries a mutation in a *MLH1* or *MSH2* gene.

### Amsterdam Criteria (revised)

The Amsterdam Criteria were originally created in 1991 and later revised after there was broad agreement that the initial criteria were too restrictive for clinical use (AC-II). The current criteria require that the following conditions be met:

- At least 3 relatives with an HNPCC-associated cancer: colorectal cancer, or cancer of the endometrium, small intestine, ureter, or renal pelvis
- One patient should be an FDR of the other two
- At least 2 successive generations should be affected
- At least 1 tumor should be diagnosed <50 years of age
- Familial adenomatous polyposis should be excluded in the colorectal cancer case (if any)
- Tumors should be verified by histopathological examination

These criteria were not intended to assist with selection of individuals for genetic testing or enhanced cancer surveillance, but instead to unify the selection of families at high-risk for research studies. It is important to note that a significant percentage of mutation positive families with Lynch syndrome do not meet the AC-II; therefore, caution must be taken when using these guidelines as there is strong suggestion that other inherited mutations may remain to be identified.

### Bethesda Criteria (modified)

The Bethesda Guidelines were developed to help identify Lynch syndrome families by categorizing colorectal cancer cases *via* molecular evaluation using microsatellite instability testing (MSI) and immunohistochemistry (IHC) analysis if criteria were met in patients already affected with HNPCC-associated malignancies.[101] The most recent guidelines posit that MSI testing of Lynch syndrome-associated tumors is indicated if any of the following criteria are met:

- The patient is younger than age 50;
- The patient has multiple HNPCC-associated tumors (metachronous or synchronous);
- The patient has at least 1 FDR who had an HNPCC-related tumor at 50 years of age or younger;
- The patient has at least 2 FDRs or SDRs with HNPCC-related tumors at any age; and
- The patient is less than 60 years and has colorectal cancer that has microscopic characteristics that are indicative of MSI.

In the clinical setting the Bethesda Guidelines constitute a useful approach to identify patients at risk of Lynch syndrome. In patients meeting the guidelines, both MSI testing and IHC staining are effective strategies (from both a clinical and economic standpoint) to further select patients who can be tested for *MSH2/MLH1* germline mutations.

### PREMM 1,2 Model

The PREMM 1,2 Model is an online risk assessment calculator designed to estimate the probability that an individual carries a mutation in *MLH1* or *MSH2*.[102] The model was derived from a logistic regression analysis of 898 patients who had submitted blood for full sequencing of the 2 genes as well as family history data. Variables included in the model were as follows:

- Diagnosis of and age at diagnosis of colorectal cancer (CRC)
- Colonic adenomas
- Endometrial cancer and other Lynch syndrome-associated cancers (ovary, stomach, kidney/urinary tract, bile ducts, small bowel, brain tumors [glioblastoma multiforme], pancreas, and sebaceous gland tumors)
- Presence of CRC or other Lynch syndrome-associated cancers in the proband's FDRs or SDRs and their ages at diagnosis

The model was later validated in a second cohort of 1016 individuals.[103] A major limitation of this model is that reported family history of cancer was not objectively verified. Further, family size and number of unaffected individuals was not taken to account for modeling; only affected individuals were known. This model does not include prediction data for mutations in *MSH6*, since routine testing for mutations in this gene was not available when the model was constructed.

### Cancer surveillance in individuals with known Lynch syndrome or in untested individuals from known Lynch syndrome families

Colorectal cancer screening guidelines for individuals who are at high genetic risk of Lynch syndrome includes colonoscopy, with removal of polyps every 1 to 2 years, beginning between ages 20 to 25 years of age, or 10 years before the earliest age of colorectal cancer in the family, whichever is younger.[99,104–106] Early and increased surveillance and removal of colon polyps has been shown to reduce the incidence of colorectal cancer in individuals with Lynch syndrome.[107]

Upper gastrointestinal and duodenal cancer screening is suggested to begin between 25 and 35 years of age and consist of an upper gastrointestinal endoscopy, to be repeated every 1 to 3 years, depending on the initial findings.[105]

### Ovarian, endometrial and urinary tract cancer risk management of Lynch syndrome

As with *BRCA1* and *BRCA2*, the efficacy of screening for ovarian cancer in Lynch syndrome has not yet been demonstrated. However, in women at high genetic risk of Lynch syndrome who are not ready for prophylactic bilateral oophorectomy, annual transvaginal ultrasound and serum CA-125 is recommended.[107,108] In the general population, oral contraceptive pills have been associated with a substantial reduction in the risk of ovarian cancer; however, this has not been demonstrated in Lynch syndrome.[1] Endometrial cancer surveillance includes: annual Pap smear, pelvic examination, annual transvaginal ultrasound, and/or endometrial biopsy and CA-125 beginning between 25 to 30 years of age. These recommendations are based on expert consensus opinion. Increased surveillance of the endometrium leads to early detection of endometrial cancer; however, whether this leads to improved survival has not yet been demonstrated.[108,109] The benefit of the prophylactic removal of the uterus and ovaries, after a woman has completed childbearing, almost completely eliminates the risk of developing ovarian and endometrial cancer[109,110] in women at high genetic risk of Lynch syndrome. Since endometrial cancer is the second most frequent malignancy occurring in Lynch syndrome, prophylactic hysterectomy after completion of childbearing warrants consideration.

The penetrance estimate for urinary tract cancers associated with Lynch syndrome is quite variable (1%–12%); however, annual urinalysis[105] is recommended in individuals who are at high genetic risk of Lynch syndrome to screen for urinary tract cancers.[110]

## FAMILIAL ADENOMATOUS POLYPOSIS

Familial adenomatous polyposis (FAP) is an autosomal dominantly inherited disorder with an incidence between 1 in 8000 to 15,000 live births.[111] Protein truncation mutations in the *APC* gene 5q21-q22 comprise 70% to 80% of reported mutations, and approximately 25% of FAP cases are due to new germline mutations (de novo mutations). Clinical diagnosis of the disease is most frequently based on the presence of large numbers (>100) of adenomatous colorectal polyps. In untreated individuals, the risk of developing colon cancer (most frequently left-sided) is nearly 100% by the fourth or fifth decade if prophylactic colectomy is not performed.[112,113] After an affected family member has tested positive for a deleterious mutation in the *APC* gene, genetic testing is offered to close family members. Colon adenomas will develop in nearly 100% of individuals who test positive for a mutation in the *APC* gene and commonly develop in the teen years. For this reason, once an informative family member has been identified, genetic testing is offered to children. When polyps are identified, risk reducing colectomy is recommended to prevent colon cancer.

Other cancers have been associated with FAP and include medulloblastoma (lifetime risk <2%), papillary carcinomas of the thyroid (lifetime risk <2%), hepatoblastoma (lifetime risk < 5%), pancreatic cancer (lifetime risk <2%) and gastric cancer (lifetime risk <1%).

Benign neoplasms have also been associated with FAP and include, congenital hypertrophy of retinal pigment epithelium (CHRPE), osteomas, supernumerary teeth, odontomas, desmoids, epidermoid cysts, duodenal and other small bowel adenomas and gastric fundic gland polyps.[1]

### Cancer risk management in FAP

For those at high genetic risk of FAP, cancer screening guidelines include early detection efforts related to cancers associated with the syndrome (see Table 7-6) and colectomy once polyps are detected. Expert guidelines for surveillance and prevention of cancers associated with FAP are updated frequently as new research about the efficacy of interventions evolves.[105] Decisions about the timing and the type of surgery are complex and require thoughtful discussions between the patient and their surgeon.

### Other colon cancer hereditary syndromes

Attenuated FAP (AFAP) is a milder form of the FAP and may be difficult to distinguish from MYH-associated polyposis and Lynch Syndrome. Carriers of a mutation in the AFAP portion of the *APC* gene (before codon 157, after 1595 and in the alternatively spliced region of exon 9),[1] develop fewer than 100 colonic adenomas and the adenomas tend to be smaller, flatter than FAP polyps and develop on the right side of the colon.[112,113] In AFAP, colorectal cancer occurs later in life, with a mean age at diagnosis of 50 to 52 years[114] If germline *APC* testing is negative in individuals who are suspected of having AFAP, genetic testing for *MYH* mutations can be contemplated.

*MYH*-associated polyposis (MAP) has an autosomal recessive inheritance pattern and homozygous mutations in the *MYH* gene have been associated with multiple colorectal adenomas with or without cancer. The *MYH* gene is located at 1p32.1-p34.3. It is a base-excision repair gene which participates in the repair of mutations caused by reactive oxygen species.[115] The incidence of the monoallelic *MYH* mutation is approximately 1% in the general population. Seven to 17% of individuals who have an FAP phenotypic expression of polyposis but without a detectable *APC* germline mutation carry biallelic mutations in the *MYH* gene.[116–119] Associated benign neoplasms include colonic and duodenal adenomas, gastric fundic gland polyps, osteomas, sebaceous gland adenomas and pilomatricomas.[120]

Cancer risk management in MAP consists of starting colonoscopy at age 25 to 30 years and repeating every 3

**TABLE 7-6**

**Summary of Cancer Risk Management**

| Hereditary Cancer Syndrome Gene (Chromosome Location) | Major Associated Malignant Neoplasms | Associated Benign Neoplasms | Primary Cancer Prevention | Cancer Syndrome Screening |
|---|---|---|---|---|
| Hereditary breast and ovarian cancer<br>AD<br>TSG<br>*BRCA1*<br>(17q21)<br>*BRCA2*<br>(13q12.3) | Breast, ovary, fallopian tube cancer, prostate<br>Basal phenotype breast cancer, pancreatic cancer<br>Estrogen receptor positive breast cancer | None known | Breast<br>– RRBM<br>– Consider chemoprevention of breast cancer<br>Ovarian<br>– Consider chemoprevention of ovarian cancer with oral contraceptives<br>Ovarian/fallopian tube<br>– RRSO (between age 35 and 40 or upon completion on childrearing) | Breast<br>– BSE training and monthly starting at age 18<br>– CBE semiannually, starting at age 25 yrs<br>– Annual mammography and breast MRI at age 25 or 5–10 yrs before the earliest breast cancer in family<br>Ovarian<br>– Twice yearly transvaginal ultrasound with CA-125 starting at age 35 yrs or 5–10 yrs prior to the earliest ovarian cancer in family<br>Male breast<br>– BSE training and monthly starting when identified as high risk<br>– Semiannual CBE<br>– Consider baseline mammogram, annual mammogram if gynecomastia or dense breasts on baseline study<br>Prostate |
| Hereditary colon cancer syndromes<br>*MLH1*, 3p21.3<br>*MSH2*, 2p21–p22<br>*PMS*, 2q31–q33<br>*PMS2*, 7p22<br>*MSH6*, 2p16<br>*MSH3*, 5q11–q12<br>AD<br>DMRG | Colorectal, endometrial, gastric, biliary tract, urinary tract, ovarian, small bowel | Sebaceous adenomas, colonic adenomas, keratoacanth-omas, Fordyce granules, epitheliomas | Endometrial/ovarian<br>– RRSO and hysterectomy after childbearing | Colon<br>– Colonoscopy and polypectomy every 1–2 yrs, starting at ages 20–25 or 10 yrs before the earliest age of CRC in family<br>Endometrial/ovarian<br>– Annual PAP smear, pelvic examination, annual transvaginal ultrasound, and/or endometrial biopsy and CA-125 |

| | | | | |
|---|---|---|---|---|
| Familial adenomatous polyposis<br>*APC*, 5q21–q22<br>AD<br>DMRG | Colon adenocarcinoma, duodenal carcinomas thyroid, brain, childhood hepatoblastoma | Adenomatous polyps of the colon, duodenal polyps, hamartomatous gastric polyps, adenomatous gastric polyps, desmoid tumors, lipomas, sebaceous or epidermoid cysts, dental abnormalities | Colorectal<br>– Colectomy after adenomas develop<br>– Consider NSAIDs on clinical trial | Colorectal<br>– Colonoscopy every 2–3 yrs beginning in late teens; annually once polyps are detected<br>Hepatoblastoma<br>– Physical examination +/or abdominal ultrasound and serum alpha-fetoprotein from birth to 6 yrs<br>Thyroid<br>– Annual palpation of the thyroid gland<br>Gastric/duodenal<br>– Esphagogastroduodenoscopy with a side-viewing endoscope by age 25 or when colonic polyps appear; repeat every 1–3 yrs; consider small bowel x-ray or CT of abdomen/pelvis every 1–3 yrs after duodenal adenomas are detected |
| Cowden syndrome<br>PTEN, 10q23.3<br>AD*<br>TSG* | Breast, thyroid, endometrial, renal | Verrucous skin lesions of the face and limbs, facial trichilemmomas, oral fibromas, hyperkeratosis, hamartomatous polyps of the stomach, small bowel and colon; lipomas, cerebellar gangliocytomtosis, hemangiomas and uterine leiomyomas; vascular abnormalities; benign breast histopathologyical findings | Breast<br>– Consider RRBM | Annual Physical Exam<br>– starting at 18 yrs or 5 yrs before the earliest cancer diagnosis in family, with attention to thyroid and breast exam<br>Breast<br>– BSE training and monthly starting at age 18<br>– CBE semiannually, starting at age 25 yrs<br>– Annual mammography and breast MRI at age 35 or 5–10 yrs before the earliest breast cancer in family<br>Endometrial<br>– Consider endometrial cancer screening starting at 35–40 yrs and participation in a clinical trial to determine the effectiveness of screening<br>Thyroid<br>– Clinical exam beginning in adolescence<br>– Baseline thyroid ultrasound at 18 yrs, consider annually<br>Renal<br>– Annual urinalysis<br>– Renal ultrasound if family history of renal cancer is present<br>Skin<br>– Consider annual dermatological exam |
| Li-Fraumeni<br>*TP53*, 17p13.1<br>AD<br>TSG | Osteogenic and chondrosarcoma, rhabdomyosarcoma, breast, brain (glioblastomas) leukemia, lymphoma, adrenocortical carcinoma | None known | Breast<br>– Consider RRBM on a case-by-case basis | Breast<br>– BSE training and monthly starting at 18 yrs<br>– CBE semi-annually starting at 20–25 yrs<br>– Mammogram and breast MRI annually starting at 20–25 yrs |

(*Continued*)

**TABLE 7-6**

**Summary of Cancer Risk Management (*Continued*)**

| Hereditary Cancer Syndrome Gene (Chromosome Location) | Major Associated Malignant Neoplasms | Associated Benign Neoplasms | Primary Cancer Prevention | Cancer Syndrome Screening |
|---|---|---|---|---|
| Multiple endocrine neoplasia type 1<br>MEN1<br>11q13<br>AD<br>TSG | Pancreatic, duodenal, gastrinomas, carcinoids of the thymus, bronchus, or stomach | Hyperparathyroidism, anterior pituitary adenomas, adrenal cortical adenomas, lipomas, collagenomas, facial angiofibromas | | Annual serum glucose, insulin, proinsulin, prolactin, IGF-1, and brain imaging every 3yrs starting at age 5<br>Age 8, start serum parathyroid hormone and ionized calcium annually; age 20 consider annual fasting serum gastrin, pancreatic polypeptide, fasting VIP and glucagons, and SRS/CT of thorax and abdomen every 2–3 yrs. |
| Multiple endocrine neoplasia type 2A/2B and familial medullary thyroid cancer (FMTC)<br>*RET*, 10q11.2<br>AD<br>OG | Medullary thyroid cancer, papillary thyroid cancer | Hyperparathyroidism (MEN2A)<br>Ganglioneuromas of the gastrointestinal tract and mucosal neuromas (MEN2B)<br>Pheochromocytomas | – Prophylactic thyroidectomy before 6 months of age for MEN2B, before 6 yrs for MEN2A and between 6 and 10 yrs for FMTC<br>– Consider the removal of 3.5 parathyroid glands at the time of thyroidectomy in MEN2A carriers | Annual screening for pheochromocytomas starting at same age as thyroidectomy; screening for hyperparathyroidism starting at 6 yrs for MEN2A carriers |
| Von Hippel-Lindau<br>*VHL*, 3p25–p26<br>AD<br>TSG | Renal carcinoma (RCC, clear cell type), pancreatic islet cell carcinomas, carcinoid (occasionally), endolymphatic sac tumors | Hemangioblastomas, retinal angiomas, pancreatic cyst, renal cyst, pheochromocytoma, adrenal adenomas, paragangliomas, epididymal cyst, hepatic cyst | | Annually:<br>Ophthalmological exam, starting by age 5 yrs<br>Physical exam, with blood pressure and neurological exam, starting at 5 yrs<br>CBC, urinalysis<br>Ultrasound of kidneys and pancreas, starting no later than 16 yrs<br>MRI imaging of CNS and spinal cord, biennially starting at 11 yrs<br>CT or MRI of kidneys and pancreas in adults, every 2–3 yrs |

[a]Or individualized based on the earliest age of onset in family.

**Abbreviations*: AD, autosomal dominant; AR, autosomal recessive; BSE, breast self-exam; CBC, complete blood count; CBE, clinical breast exam; CNS, central nervous system; CRC, colorectal cancer; CT, computed tomography; DMRG, DNA mismatch repair gene; IP, incomplete penetrance; MRI, magnetic resonance imaging; NSAID, non-steroidal anti-inflammatory drug; OG, oncogene; P, penetrance; RRBPM, risk-reducing bilateral prophylactic mastectomy; RRSO, risk-reducing bilateral salpingo-oophorectomy; SRS, somatostatin receptor scintrigraphy; TSG, tumor suppressor gene; VIP, vasoactive intestinal peptide.

*Source*: Data from Lindor, et al.[1]

to 5 years if no polyps are found. Upper gastrointestinal endoscopy with side-viewing duodenoscopy beginning at age 30 to 35 and every 3 to 5 years may also be considered. If adenomas are detected, patients should be managed according the FAP guidelines.[121] Carriers of monoallelic *MYH* mutations are recommended to begin colonoscopy at age 40 years and repeat very 5 years this suggestion is based on expert clinical judgment, ie, it is not an evidence-based recommendation.[1]

## MULTIPLE ENDOCRINE NEOPLASIA

Multiple endocrine neoplasia (MEN) syndromes are rare autosomal dominant inherited disorders that predispose individuals to benign and malignant tumors of the pituitary, thyroid, parathyroids, adrenals, endocrine pancreas, paraganglia, or nonendocrine organs. MEN type 1 (MEN1) and MEN type 2 (MEN2) are examples of classic MEN syndromes. However, von Hippel-Lindau syndrome (VHL) and Cowden syndrome may also be considered as examples of MEN.[122]

### *MEN1*

*MEN1* is caused by a mutation in the *MEN1* gene, located at chromosome 11q13. It is thought to be a regulator of gene transcription, cell proliferation, apoptosis, and genome stability.[123] The incidence of the mutation is estimated to be 1/5000 to 50,000 in Caucasian populations. Penetrance is estimated to be 80% by age 50.[122] Hyperparathyroidism is the presenting symptom or is diagnosed simultaneously as the presenting symptom in the majority of cases.[1] Cancers associated with *MEN1* mutations include parathyroid, endocrine pancreas, pituitary, adrenal, and neuroendocrine carcinoid.

Genetic testing for *MEN1* at an early age allows patients to be monitored for the development of subsequent *MEN1*-related tumors in individuals identified to be carriers of a mutation in the *MEN1* gene. Several commercial laboratories offer germline *MEN1* mutation testing for patients in whom a diagnosis of *MEN1* is suspected. Ten percent of all mutations detected are found to be de novo mutations. The efficacy, risk, and benefits of early detection in *MEN1* are unknown. Table 7-6 includes a summary of the current recommendations for early cancer detection in known carriers of a *MEN1* mutation.

### *MEN2*

MEN2 is associated with the *RET* proto-oncogene located at chromosome 10q11.2. The incidence of MEN2 is one in 30,000 births. There are 3 distinct subtypes of MEN2; MEN2A, MEN2B, and familial medullary thyroid cancer (FMTC). Each subtype has strong genotype-phenotype correlations. MEN2A is the most common subtype and is associated with medullary thyroid cancer in nearly all cases, pheochromocytoma in 50% of cases, and hyperparathyroidism in 15% to 30% of cases.[1] In MEN2B, the onset of medullary thyroid cancer is younger (<10 years), hyperparathyroidism is infrequent, and patients often have mucosal neuromas of the eyelids, lips, and tongue.[122] For individuals who are diagnosed with FMTC, medullary thyroid cancer is usually the only malignancy in the family, and the age at diagnosis is generally older than MEN2A or MEN2B.

### Cancer risk assessment and surveillance in individuals suspected of being *MEN2* mutation carriers

For affected individuals who test positive for an *MEN2* mutation, experts recommend efforts that lead to early diagnosis (Table 7-6). Genetic testing is recommended for at-risk relatives so that early cancer screening can be initiated if a mutation is detected. Most commonly, physical examination, surgery to remove at-risk organs, and biochemical screening to detect pheochromocytoma and hyperparathyroidism are included in management recommendations.

Endocrine tumors are rare in the general population, and if identified in more than 1 family member, or if more than 1 endocrine tumor is identified in an individual, formal cancer genetic risk assessment is recommended. Furthermore, certain endocrine tumors (pheochromocytoma, paraganglioma, medullary thyroid cancer, and parathyroid carcinoma) are "red flags" for a hereditary cancer syndrome. Even in the absence of a personal or family history suggestive of a hereditary cancer syndrome, individuals who are diagnosed with any one of these cancers should be referred for comprehensive cancer risk assessment.[122]

## COWDEN SYNDROME

Cowden Syndrome is a rare hereditary cancer syndrome associated with mutations in the *PTEN* gene at chromosome 10q23.3. The mode of inheritance is autosomal dominant and its incidence is estimated to be approximately 1/200,000 births.[124] Cowden disease is most commonly recognized based on clinical findings of benign skin lesions (trichilemmomas) and intestinal hamartomas.[125] Individuals who inherit a mutation in *PTEN* are at high risk of developing female breast cancer (30%-50% lifetime risk), which occurs approximately 10 years earlier than in the general population. Male breast cancer has also been reported.[1] Other cancers associated with Cowden syndrome include thyroid cancer (primarily follicular type), endometrial cancer, and renal cancer.[126] Other cancers have been reported in individuals with Cowden syndrome, but the rarity of the syndrome makes it difficult to prove the association.

### Cancer surveillance of individuals with known Cowden syndrome

Currently, the benefit of early detection and cancer prevention in Cowden syndrome is unknown.[1] However, based on expert consensus opinion, the ACS recommends annual breast MRI and annual mammography in women with Cowden syndrome. See Table 7–6 for other current recommendations for early detection and cancer prevention recommendation for individuals with Cowden syndrome.

## VON HIPPEL-LINDAU SYNDROME

Individuals who inherit a mutation in the *VHL* gene are at high genetic risk of developing renal cell carcinoma (typically, clear-cell histology) and are also at high risk of developing pancreatic islet cell carcinomas, carcinoid tumors, pheochromocytomas, endolymphatic sac tumors, and nonmalignant neoplasms including hemangioblastomas of the central nervous system and/or the retina.[1,127] The *VHL* tumor suppressor gene is located on chromosome 3p25-p26, and its incidence is approximately 1/30,000 to 40,000.[1,127] Penetrance of the diseases associated with VHL is nearly 100% by the age of 65 years. Genetic testing is available, and germline VHL mutations are detected in nearly 100% of clinically affected individuals,[1,127] which is a highly effective method to diagnose or exclude VHL in individuals who are suspected of having the disease or in individuals who have apparently sporadic VHL-related disease.[127] There are subtypes of VHL depending on the presence (VHL type 2: 7%-20% of families) or absence (VHL type 1) of pheochromocytomas within a family. VHL type 2 is further subclassified on the basis of without (2A) and with (2B) a predisposition to renal cell cancer and 2C with pheochromocytomas only within the family.[128] A series of hereditary renal cancer syndromes has been identified and their causative genes determined. Identification of these disorders has been driven by the recognition that there are numerous subtle histologic subtypes of renal cancers, each of which is associated with a different disorder.[129]

### Cancer surveillance and cancer risk assessment of individuals suspected of being VHL mutation carriers

Affected individuals suspected of being *VHL* mutation carriers are recommended to undergo comprehensive cancer risk assessment, and if a *VHL* mutation is identified, all FDRs can also be offered cancer risk assessment and genetic testing.

Cancer surveillance is initiated in childhood if an individual is identified as a *VHL* mutation carrier (see Table 7-6). The timing, duration, risks, and benefits of cancer screening for individuals at risk of VHL syndrome are not known.[128] VHL cancer screening recommendations are frequently modified and updated regularly by the VHL Family Alliance (http://www.vhl.org).

## LI-FRAUMENI SYNDROME

Li-Fraumeni syndrome is caused by a germline mutation in the tumor suppressor gene *TP53*, also known as *p53*, located at chromosome 17p13.1.[130] LFS is thought to be rare, with approximately 400 families reported in the literature. The precise incidence of the syndrome is unknown. The major cancers associated with the LFS include the following: osteosarcoma, chondrosarcoma, rhabdomyosarcoma, breast cancer, brain cancer (glioblastoma), leukemia, lymphoma, and adrenocortical carcinoma. The penetrance of the diseases associated with LFS is approximately 50% by age 30 and approach 100% by age 70.[130] The risk of developing early breast cancer among women who inherit a mutated copy of the germline *p53* gene is 100 times greater than those seen in the general population.[131] Classic LFS requires the following: one patient with sarcoma diagnosed before 45, a FDR diagnosed with cancer (any type) before age 45, and a third affected family member (FDR or SDR) with either sarcoma at any age or cancer before age 45 years.[132] Malignancies that are part of the "classic" form of LFS comprise about 80% of all cancers that occur in LFS families.[133]

### CANCER SURVEILLANCE OF INDIVIDUALS AT HIGH GENETIC RISK OF LFS

Breast cancer screening with monthly breast self-examination, every 6 month clinical breast examination, annual mammography, and breast MRI are recommended for known LFS mutation carriers and their female FDRs.[1,93] Prophylactic mastectomy can be discussed on an individual basis. The risk and benefits of screening for other malignancies associated with LFS are not known and should be tailored to the phenotype of individual families. A summary of the current cancer screening and prevention strategies for LFS are included in Table 7-6.

## FUTURE DIRECTION OF NURSING PRACTICE AND RESEARCH

Integrating rapidly emerging genetic findings into evidence-based healthcare recommendations is a challenge for all healthcare providers. Oncology nurses practice at the nexus of genetic discoveries and oncology care. They provide patient services that are driven by new discoveries leading to improvements in cancer risk prediction, prevention, and treatment. Oncology nurses work to enhance patient understanding, decision-making, and treatment outcomes in oncology by integrating genetic information into daily practice, and keeping current with evolving cancer genetic information, through ongoing continuing educational programs offered by professional groups specializing in genetics, such as the ONS, the ISONG, the American Society of Human Genetics, and the American Society of Clinical Oncology. Organizations that provide nurses the opportunity to further expand their professional practice and understanding of cancer genetics through intensive training programs include the City of Hope Cancer Center[134] and the Fox Chase Cancer Center.[135]

At the basic educational level of nursing, it is critical that registered nurses understand clinical genetics in a manner that is broader than the traditional study of Mendelian genetics. To ensure that future nurses are well educated in genetic health care, genetics, and genomics, subject-specific content has been integrated into the American Association of Colleges of Nursing document, "Essentials of Baccalaureate Education for Professional Nursing Practice" for all baccalaureate nursing programs in the United States.[136]

Changes in genetic information will continue to influence healthcare decisions and will continue to influence how nursing practice changes over time. The ONS developed position statements for oncology nurses practicing at the general oncology nurse level, the advanced practice level, and for those advanced practice nurses with specialty training in genetics to respond to this changing healthcare need. The advent of the professional credentialing process in genetics through ISONG for the generalist nurse (GN) and the APNG adds a new level of recognition to the subspecialty of genetic nursing. Again, professional nursing practice has responded to the ever-changing needs of patient care.

Oncology nurses deliver state-of-the-art oncology care by improving patient outcomes through evidence-based interventions and research to define best practices. Oncology nursing research will continue to contribute to the understanding of nursing-sensitive, patient-specific outcomes of oncology patients, and hereditary cancer genetics, including the following:

- Patient outcomes of oncology nursing interventions in providing cancer genetic services
- How healthcare systems deliver hereditary cancer genetic services
- The effects of implementing screening to identify those in need of hereditary genetic services at the population level
- How genetic information affects individuals and families
- How genetic policy affects access to health care and the use of cancer genetic services
- Whether there are barriers to, or facilitators of patient access to genetic services
- The potential risks and benefits of pharmacogenetics and pharmacogenomics in cancer care

## CONCLUSION

Oncology nurses will continue to provide state-of-the-art, cancer genetic care as new genetic information is discovered or refined. As the technologies of genomic research change, leading to new research methods that further refine our understanding of how genetic information influences health and healthcare decision-making, nurses will continue to seek and obtain education in genetics to provide excellent health care. On the near horizon, nurses must expand their understanding of genome-wide association studies and candidate gene association studies to knowledgeably participate in the broad healthcare discussion regarding:

- Whether specific genetic polymorphisms are meaningfully associated with cancer risk
- Why personal genome scans may or may not be ready for integration into healthcare decision-making[137]
- Why there may be emotional or psychological risk associated with particular findings of genetic association studies and disease prediction
- How to protect individual rights while maximizing scientific discovery
- How new genetic and genomic information affects the ethics of health care, especially related to privacy and confidentiality

Nurses will continue to advocate for high-quality patient care during the transition from pre-genomic health care to post-genomic health care. As electronic medical records improve the safety and efficiency of health care, nurses will safeguard patient privacy rights and protect against discrimination. Healthcare delivery systems will continue to change as evidence for practice is established and implemented. Nurses will continue to help patients understand and interpret complex cancer genetic information as applied to cancer diagnosis, treatment or in susceptibility testing as new genetic information emerges from research and is translated into practice. Nursing practice in genetic health care will continue to evolve in response to the needs of society and rapid changes in health care, as nursing practice has done since the beginning of the profession.

## REFERENCES

1. Lindor NM, McMaster ML, Lindor CJ, Greene MH. Concise handbook of familial cancer susceptibility syndromes. 2nd ed. *J Natl Cancer Inst Monogr.* 2008;38:1–93.

2. Oncology Nursing Society. The role of the oncology nurse in cancer genetic counseling. http://www.ons.org/publications/positions/documents/pdfs/CancerGenetic.pdf. Accessed November 23, 2009.
3. International Society of Nurses in Genetics. Provision of quality genetic services and care: building a multidisciplinary, collaborative approach among genetic nurses and genetic counselors. http://www.isong.org/about/ps_multidisciplinarygeneticcare.cfm. Accessed November 23, 2009.
4. Badzek L, Turner M, Jenkins JF. Genomics and nursing practice: advancing the nursing profession. *OJIN.* 2008;13. http://www.nursingworld.org/MainMenuCategories/ANAMarketplace/ANAPeriodicals/OJIN/TableofContents/vol132008/No1Jan08/GenomicsandAdvancingNursing. Accessed November 23, 2009.
5. Vogelstein B, Kinzler KW. The multistep nature of cancer. *Trends Genet.* 1993;9:138–141.
6. Hemminki K, Rawal R, Chen B, Bermejo JL. Genetic epidemiology of cancer: from families to heritable genes. *Int J Cancer.* 2004;111:944–950.
7. Yoon PW, Scheuner MT, Peterson-Oehlke KL, Gwinn M, Faucett A, Khoury MJ. Can family history be used as a tool for public health and preventive medicine? *Genet Med.* 2002;4:304–310.
8. National Cancer Institute. Genetics Overview (PDQ) 2008. http://www.cancer.gov/cancertopics/pdq/genetics/overview/HealthProfessional/page5 and http://www.cancer.gov/cancertopics/pdq/genetics/risk-assessment-and-counseling/HealthProfessional/page4#Section_188 Accessed November 23, 2009
9. Lowrey KM. Legal and ethical issues in cancer genetics nursing. *Semin Oncol Nurs.* 2004;20:203–208.
10. Offit K, Thom P. Ethical and legal aspects of cancer genetic testing. *Semin Oncol.* 2007;34:435–443.
11. Beauchamp TL, Childress JF. *Principles of Biomedical Ethics.* 5th ed. Boston, MA: Oxford Press; 2001.
12. Cluff CA. California Supreme Court expands the informed consent doctrine; physicians have a duty to obtain an informed refusal: Truman v. Thomas. *Brigh Young Univ Law Rev.* 1980;4:933–947.
13. Knoppers BM, Strom C, Wright Clayton E, et al. ASHG Social Issues Subcommittee on Familial Disclosure. ASHG statement: professional disclosure of familial genetic information; The American Society of Human Genetics Social Issues Subcommittee on Familial Disclosure. *Am J Hum Genet.* 1998;62:474–483.
14. American Society of Clinical Oncology. American Society of Clinical Oncology policy statement update: genetic testing for cancer susceptibility. *J Clin Oncol.* 2003;21:2397–2406.
15. Offit K, Groeger E, Turner S, Wadsworth EA, Weiser MA. The "duty to warn" a patient's family members about hereditary disease risks. *JAMA.* 2004;292:1469–1473.
16. Lacroix M, Nycum G, Godard B, Knoppers BM. Should physicians warn patients' relatives of genetic risks? *CMAJ.* 2008;178:593–595.
17. Dugan RB, Wiesner GL, Juengst ET, O'Riondan MA, Matthews AL, Robin NH. Duty to warn at-risk relatives for genetic disease: genetic counselors' clinical experience. *Am J Med Genetics* 2003; 119c: 27–34.
18. Josefson D. Clinton outlaws genetic discrimination in federal jobs. *BMJ.* 2000;320:468.
19. Leib JR, Hoodfar E, Haidle JL, Nagy R. The new genetic privacy law. *Comm Oncol.* 2008;5:351–354.
20. National Cancer Institute. Genetic testing algorithm for cancer susceptibility. http://www.cancer.gov/cancertopics/pdq/genetics/risk-assessment-and-counseling/HealthProfessional/page6. Accessed January 19, 2010.
21. Lerman C, Lustbader E, Rimer B, et al. Effects of individualized breast cancer risk counseling: a randomized trial. *J Natl Cancer Inst.* 1995;87:286–292.
22. Audrain J, Schwartz MD, Lerman C, Hughes C, Peshkin BN, Biesecker B. Psychological distress in women seeking genetic counseling for breast-ovarian cancer risk: the contributions of personality and appraisal. *Ann Behav Med.* 1997;19:370–377.
23. Eeles RA, Easton DF, Ponder BAJ, Eng C. *Genetic Predisposition to Cancer.* New York, NY: Oxford University Press; 2004.
24. Schneider K. *Counseling about Cancer: Strategies for Genetic Counseling.* 3rd ed. New York, NY: Wiley-Liss, Inc.; 2002.
25. Jenkins JF, Lea D. Nursing Care in the Genomic Eds.: A Case-based Approach. Sudbury, MA: Jones and Barlett Publishers, 2005.
26. Vogelstein B, Kinzler KW. The Genetic Basis of Human Cancer. 2nd ed. New York, NY: McGraw-Hill, Medical Pub. Division, 2002.
27. Claus EB, Risch N, Thompson WD. Autosomal dominant inheritance of early-onset breast cancer. Implications for risk prediction. *Cancer.* 1994;73:643–651.
28. King MC, Marks JH, Mandell JB. Breast and ovarian cancer risks due to inherited mutations in BRCA1 and BRCA2. *Science.* 2003;302: 643–646.
29. Antoniou AC, Pharoah PD, Narod S, et al. Breast and ovarian cancer risks to carriers of the BRCA1 5382insC and 185delAG and BRCA2 6174delT mutations: a combined analysis of 22 population based studies. *J Med Genet.* 2005;42:602–603.
30. Miki Y, Swensen J, Shattuck-Eidens D, et al. A strong candidate for the breast and ovarian cancer susceptibility gene BRCA1. *Science.* 1994;266:66–71.
31. Hall JM, Lee MK, Newman B, et al. Linkage of early-onset familial breast cancer to chromosome 17q21. *Science.* 1990;250:1684–1689.
32. Narod SA, Feunteun J, Lynch HT, et al. Familial breast-ovarian cancer locus on chromosome 17q12-q23. *Lancet.* 1991;338:82–83.
33. Wooster R, Bignell G, Lancaster J, et al. Identification of the breast cancer susceptibility gene BRCA2. *Nature.* 1995;378:789–792.
34. Wooster R, Neuhausen SL, Mangion J, et al. Localization of a breast cancer susceptibility gene, BRCA2, to chromosome 13q12–13. *Science.* 1994;265:2088–2090.
35. National Center for Biotechnology Information. Genetic database. http://www.ncbi.nlm.nih.gov/Database/. Accessed January 19, 2010.
36. Gerhardus A, Schleberger H, Schlegelberger B, Gadzicki D. Diagnostic accuracy of methods for the detection of BRCA1 and BRCA2 mutations: a systematic review. *Eur J Hum Genet.* 2007;15:619–627.
37. Whittemore AS, Gong G, John EM, et al. Prevalence of BRCA1 mutation carriers among U.S. non-Hispanic whites. *Cancer Epidemiol Biomarkers Prev.* 2004;13:2078–2083.
38. Szabo CI, King MC. Population genetics of BRCA1 and BRCA2. *Am J Hum Genet.* 1997;60:1013–1020.
39. Smith P, McGuffog L, Easton DF, et al. A genome wide linkage search for breast cancer susceptibility genes. *Genes Chromosomes Cancer.* 2006;45:646–655.
40. Risch HA, McLaughlin JR, Cole DE, et al. Population BRCA1 and BRCA2 mutation frequencies and cancer penetrances: a kin-cohort study in Ontario, Canada. *J Natl Cancer Inst.* 2006;98:1694–1706.
41. Ferla R, Calo V, Cascio S, et al. Founder mutations in BRCA1 and BRCA2 genes. *Ann Oncol.* 2007;18(Suppl 6):vi93-vi98.
42. Antoniou A, Pharoah PD, Narod S, et al. Average risks of breast and ovarian cancer associated with BRCA1 or BRCA2 mutations detected in case series unselected for family history: a combined analysis of 22 studies. *Am J Hum Genet.* 2003;72:1117–1130.
43. Chen S, Parmiginai G. Meta-analysis of BRCA1 and BRCA2 penetrance. *J Clin Oncol.* 2007;25:1329–1333.
44. Chen S, Iversen ES, Friebel T, et al. Characterization of BRCA1 and BRCA2 mutations in a large United States sample. *J Clin Oncol.* 2006;24:863–871.
45. Fentiman IS, Fourquet A, Hortobagyi GN. Male breast cancer. *Lancet.* 2006;367:595–604.
46. Tai YC, Domchek S, Parmigiani G, Chen S. Breast cancer risk among male BRCA1 and BRCA2 mutation carriers. *J Natl Cancer Inst.* 2007;99:1811–1814.
47. Cancer risks in BRCA2 mutation carriers. The Breast Cancer Linkage Consortium. *J Natl Cancer Inst.* 1999;91:1310–1316.
48. van Asperen CJ, Brohet RM, Meijers-Heijboer EJ, et al. Cancer risks in BRCA2 families: estimates for sites other than breast and ovary. *J Med Genet.* 2005;42:711–719.

49. Levy-Lahad E, Friedman E. Cancer risks among BRCA1 and BRCA2 mutation carriers. *Br J Cancer.* 2007;96:11–15.
50. Nelson HD, Huffman LH, Fu R, Harris EL. Genetic risk assessment and BRCA mutation testing for breast and ovarian cancer susceptibility: systematic evidence review for the U.S. Preventive Services Task Force. *Ann Intern Med.* 2005;143:362–379.
51. Prucka SK, McIlvried DE, Korf BR. Cancer risk assessment and the genetic counseling process: using hereditary breast and ovarian cancer as an example. *Med Princ Pract.* 2008;17:173–189.
52. National Comprehensive Cancer Network. 2008. http://www.nccn.org/professionals/physician_gls/PDF/genetics_screening.pdf. Accessed on February 2, 2009.
53. Euhus DM, Smith KC, Robinson L, et al. Pretest prediction of BRCA1 or BRCA2 mutation by risk counselors and the computer model BRCAPRO. *J Natl Cancer. Inst.* 2002;94:844–851.
54. US Preventive Services Task Force. Genetic risk assessment and BRCA mutation testing for breast and ovarian cancer susceptibility: U.S. Preventive Services Task Force recommendations. *Ann Int Med.* 2005;145:355–379.
55. Parmigiani G, Berry D, Aguilar O. Determining carrier probabilities for breast cancer-susceptibility genes BRCA1 and BRCA2. *Am J Hum Genet.* 1998;62:145–158.
56. Berry, D.A., Iversen, E.S., Gudbjartsson, D.F., Hiller, E.H., Garber, J.E., et al.. BRCAPRO validation, sensitivity of genetic testing of BRCA1/BRCA2 and prevalence of other breast cancer susceptibility genes. *J Clin Oncol.* 2002 20(1), 2701–2712.
57. Antoniou, A.C., Hardy, R., Walker, L., Evans, D.G., Shenton, A., Eeles, R. et al.. Predicting the likelihood of carrying a BRCA1 or BRCA2 mutation: validation of BOADICEA, BRCAPRO, IBIS, Myriad, and the Mancheester scoring system using data from UK genetics clinics. *JMed Genet.*2008; 45, 425–431.
58. Weitzel JN, Lagos VI, Cullinane CA, et al. Limited family structure and BRCA gene mutation status in single cases of breast cancer. *JAMA.* 2007;297:2587–2595.
59. Kauff ND, Offit K. Modeling genetic risk of breast cancer. *JAMA.* 2007;297:2637–2639.
60. Gail MH, Brinton LA, Byar DP, et al. Projecting individualized probabilities of developing breast cancer for white females who are being examined annually. *J Natl Cancer Inst.* 1989;81:1879–1886.
61. Crispo A, D'Aiuto G, De Marco M, et al. Gail model risk factors: impact of adding an extended family history for breast cancer. *Breast J.* 2008;14:221–227.
62. Lord SJ, Lei W, Craft P, et al. A systematic review of the effectiveness of magnetic resonance imaging (MRI) as an addition to mammography and ultrasound in screening young women at high risk of breast cancer. *Eur J Cancer.* 2007;43:1905–1917.
63. Kriege M, Brekelmans CT, Boetes C, et al. Efficacy of MRI and mammography for breast-cancer screening in women with a familial or genetic predisposition. *N Engl J Med.* 2004;351:427–437.
64. Warner E, Plewes DB, Hill KA, et al. Surveillance of BRCA1 and BRCA2 mutation carriers with magnetic resonance imaging, ultrasound, mammography, and clinical breast examination. *JAMA.* 2004;292:1317–1325.
65. Leach MO, Boggis CR, Dixon AK, et al. Screening with magnetic resonance imaging and mammography of a UK population at high familial risk of breast cancer: a prospective multicentre cohort study (MARIBS). *Lancet.* 2005;365:1769–1778.
66. Hartmann LC, Sellers TA, Schaid DJ, et al. Efficacy of bilateral prophylactic mastectomy in BRCA1 and BRCA2 gene mutation carriers. *J Natl Cancer Inst.* 2001;93:1633–1637.
67. Rebbeck TR, Friebel T, Lynch HT, et al. Bilateral prophylactic mastectomy reduces breast cancer risk in BRCA1 and BRCA2 mutation carriers: the PROSE Study Group. *J Clin Oncol.* 2004;22:1055–1062.
68. Hartmann LC, Schaid DJ, Woods JE, et al. Efficacy of bilateral prophylactic mastectomy in women with a family history of breast cancer. *N Engl J Med.* 1999;340:77–84.
69. Eisen A, Lubinski J, Klijn J, et al. Breast cancer risk following bilateral oophorectomy in BRCA1 and BRCA2 mutation carriers: an international case-control study. *J Clin Oncol.* 2005;23:7491–7496.
70. Kramer JL, Velazquez IA, Chen BE, Rosenberg PS, Struewing JP, Greene MH. Prophylactic oophorectomy reduces breast cancer penetrance during prospective, long-term follow-up of BRCA1 mutation carriers. *J Clin Oncol.* 2005;23:8629–8635.
71. Finch A, Beiner M, Lubinski J, et al. Salpingo-oophorectomy and the risk of ovarian, fallopian tube, and peritoneal cancers in women with a BRCA1 or BRCA2 mutation. *JAMA.* 2006;296:185–192.
72. Narod SA, Brunet JS, Ghadirian P, et al. Tamoxifen and risk of contralateral breast cancer in BRCA1 and BRCA2 mutation carriers: a case-control study. Hereditary Breast Cancer Clinical Study Group. *Lancet.* 2000;356:1876–1881.
73. Gronwald J, Tung N, Foulkes WD, et al. Tamoxifen and contralateral breast cancer in BRCA1 and BRCA2 carriers: an update. *Int J Cancer.* 2006;118:2281–2284.
74. Gulati AP, Domchek SM. The clinical management of BRCA1 and BRCA2 mutation carriers. *Curr Oncol Rep.* 2008;10:47–53.
75. Vogel VG, Costantino JP, Wickerham DL, et al. Effects of tamoxifen vs raloxifene on the risk of developing invasive breast cancer and other disease outcomes: the NSABP Study of Tamoxifen and Raloxifene (STAR) P-2 trial. *JAMA.* 2006;295:2727–2741.
76. Fisher B, Costantino JP, Wickerham DL, et al. Tamoxifen for prevention of breast cancer: report of the National Surgical Adjuvant Breast and Bowel Project P-1 Study. *J Natl Cancer Inst.* 1998;90:1371–1388.
77. King MC, Wieand S, Hale K, et al. Tamoxifen and breast cancer incidence among women with inherited mutations in BRCA1 and BRCA2: National Surgical Adjuvant Breast and Bowel Project (NSABP-P1) Breast Cancer Prevention Trial.
78. Gaarenstroom KN, van der Hiel B, Tollenaar RA, et al. Efficacy of screening women at high risk of hereditary ovarian cancer: results of an 11-year cohort study. *Int J Gynecol Cancer.* 2006;16(Suppl 1):54–59.
79. Oei AL, Massuger LF, Bulten J, Ligtenberg MJ, Hoogerbrugge N, de Hullu JA. Surveillance of women at high risk for hereditary ovarian cancer is inefficient. *Br J Cancer.* 2006;94:814–819.
80. Olivier RI, Lubsen-Brandsma MA, Verhoef S, van Beurden M. CA125 and transvaginal ultrasound monitoring in high-risk women cannot prevent the diagnosis of advanced ovarian cancer. *Gynecol Oncol.* 2006;100:20–26. *JAMA.* 2001;286:2251–2256.
81. Rebbeck TR, Lynch HT, Neuhausen SL, et al. Prophylactic oophorectomy in carriers of BRCA1 or BRCA2 mutations. *N Engl J Med.* 2002;346:1616–1622.
82. Kauff ND, Satagopan JM, Robson ME, et al. Risk-reducing salpingo-oophorectomy in women with a BRCA1 or BRCA2 mutation. *N Engl J Med.* 2002;346:1609–1615.
83. Rutter JL, Wacholder S, Chetrit A, et al. Gynecologic surgeries and risk of ovarian cancer in women with BRCA1 and BRCA2 Ashkenazi founder mutations: an Israeli population-based case-control study. *J Natl Cancer Inst.* 2003;95:1072–1078.
84. Domchek SM, Friebel TM, Neuhausen SL, et al. Mortality after bilateral salpingo-oophorectomy in BRCA1 and BRCA2 mutation carriers: a prospective cohort study. *Lancet Oncol.* 2006;7:223–229.
85. Society of Gynecologic Oncologists. Society of Gynecologic Oncologists Clinical Practice Committee: statement on prophylactic salpingo-oophorectomy. *Gynecol Oncol.* 2005;98:179–181.
86. Rebbeck TR, Friebel T, Wagner T, et al. Effect of short-term hormone replacement therapy on breast cancer risk reduction after bilateral prophylactic oophorectomy in BRCA1 and BRCA2 mutation carriers: the PROSE Study Group. *J Clin Oncol.* 2005;23:7804–7810.
87. Anderson GL, Limacher M, Assaf AR, et al. Effects of conjugated equine estrogen in postmenopausal women with hysterectomy: the Women's Health Initiative randomized controlled trial. *JAMA.* 2004;291:1701–1712.
88. Rossouw JE, Anderson GL, Prentice RL, et al. Risks and benefits of estrogen plus progestin in healthy postmenopausal women: principal

results from the Women's Health Initiative randomized controlled trial. *JAMA.* 2002;288:321–333.

89. Narod SA, Risch H, Moslehi R, et al. Oral contraceptives and the risk of hereditary ovarian cancer. Hereditary Ovarian Cancer Clinical Study Group. *N Engl J Med.* 1998;339:424–428.
90. McLaughlin JR, Risch HA, Lubinski J, et al. Reproductive risk factors for ovarian cancer in carriers of BRCA1 or BRCA2 mutations: a case-control study. *Lancet Oncol.* 2007;8:26–34.
91. Whittemore AS, Balise RR, Pharoah PD, et al. Oral contraceptive use and ovarian cancer risk among carriers of BRCA1 or BRCA2 mutations. *Br J Cancer.* 2004;91:1911–1915.
92. Brohet RM, Goldgar DE, Easton DF, et al. Oral contraceptives and breast cancer risk in the international BRCA1/2 carrier cohort study: a report from EMBRACE, GENEPSO, GEO-HEBON, and the IBCCS Collaborating Group. *J Clin Oncol.* 2007;25:3831–3836.
93. Daly MB, Axilbund JE, Bryant E, et al. Genetic/familial high-risk assessment: breast and ovarian. *J Natl Compr Canc Netw.* 2006;4: 156–176.
94. Saslow D, Boetes C, Burke W, et al. American Cancer Society guidelines for breast screening with MRI as an adjunct to mammography. *CA Cancer J Clin.* 2007;57:75–89.
95. American Cancer Society. Overview of Colon and Rectum Cancer: How many people get colon and rectum cancer? http://www.cancer.org/docroot/CRI/content/CRI_2_2_1X_How_Many_People_Get_Colorectal_Cancer.asp?sitearea=. Accessed on January 19, 2010.
96. Al-Sukhni W, Aronson M, Gallinger S. Hereditary colorectal cancer syndromes: familial adenomatous polyposis and lynch syndrome. Surg Clin North Am. 2008;88:819–844.
97. Peltomaki P, Vasen H. Mutations associated with HNPCC predisposition—update of ICG-HNPCC/INSiGHT mutation database. *Dis Markers.* 2004;20(4–5):269–276.
98. Merg A, Howe JR. Genetic conditions associated with intestinal juvenile polyps. *Am J Med Genet C Semin Med Genet.* 2004;129(1):44–55.
99. Vasen HF, Moslein G, Alonso A, et al. Guidelines for the clinical management of Lynch syndrome (HNPCC). *J Med Genet.* 2007; 44(6):353–362.
100. Vasen HF, Mecklin JP, Khan PM, Lynch HT. The International Collaborative Group on Hereditary Nonpolyposis Colorectal Cancer (ICG-HNPCC). *Dis Colon Rectum.* 1991;34:424–425.
101. Umar A, Boland CR, Terdiman JP, et al. Revised Bethesda Guidelines for hereditary nonpolyposis colorectal cancer (Lynch syndrome) and microsatellite instability. *J Natl Cancer Inst.* 2004;96:261–268.
102. PREMM 1,2 Model: Prediction Model for MLH1 and MSH2 Gene Mutations. http://www.dana-farber.org/pat/cancer/gastrointestinal/crc-calculator/. Accessed January 19, 2010.
103. Balmaña J, Stockwell DH, Steyerberg EW. Prediction of MLH1 and MSH2 mutations in Lynch Syndrome. *JAMA.* 2006;296:1469–1478.
104. Burke W, Petersen G, Lynch P, et al. Recommendations for follow-up care of individuals with an inherited predisposition to cancer. 1. Hereditary nonpolyposis colon cancer. *JAMA.* 1997;277:915–919.
105. National Comprehensive Cancer Network. Colorectal cancer screening: clinical practice guidelines in oncology. *J Natl Compr Canc Netw.* 2003;1:72–93.
106. Lindor NM, Petersen GM, Hadley DW, et al. Recommendations for the care of individuals with an inherited predisposition to Lynch syndrome: a systematic review. *JAMA.* 2006;296:1507–1517.
107. Jarvinen HJ, Aarnio M, Mustonen H, et al. Controlled 15-year trial on screening for colorectal cancer in families with hereditary nonpolyposis colorectal cancer. *Gastroenterol.* 2000;118:829–834.
108. Lecuru F, Metzger U, Scarabin C, Le Frere Belda MA, Olschwang S, Laurent Puig P. Hysteroscopic findings in women at risk of HNPCC. Results of a prospective observational study. *Fam Cancer.* 2007;6:295–299.
109. Renkonen-Sinisalo L, Kivisaari A, Kivisaari L, Sarna S, Jarvinen HJ. Utility of computed tomographic colonography in surveillance for hereditary nonpolyposis colorectal cancer syndrome. *Fam Cancer.* 2007;6:135–140.
110. Schmeler KM, Lynch HT, Chen LM, et al. Prophylactic surgery to reduce the risk of gynecologic cancers in the Lynch syndrome. *N Engl J Med.* 2006;354:261–269.
111. Gryfe R. Clinical implications of our advancing knowledge or colorectal cancer genetics: inherited syndromes, prognosis, prevention, screening and therapeutics. Surg Clin North Am 2006;86(4)787–817.
112. Merg A, Lynch HT, Lynch JF, et al. Hereditary colorectal cancer-part I. Curr Probl Surg 2005;42:195–256.
113. Merg A, Lynch HT, Lynch JF, et al. Hereditary colorectal cancer-part II. Curr Probl Surg 2005;42:267–333.
114. Bresinger JD, Laken SJ, Muce MC, et al. Variable phenotype of familial adenomatous polyposis in pedigrees with 3' mutation in the APC gene. *Gut* 1998;43:548–52.
115. Lipton L, Tomlinson I. The multiple colorectal adenoma phenotype and *MYH*, a base excision repair gene. *Clin Gastroenterol Hepatol.* 2004;2:633–638.
116. Sieber OM, Lipton L, Crabtree M, et al. Multiple colorectal adenomas, classic adenomatous polyposis, and germ-line mutations in *MYH. N Engl J Med. 2003;*348
117. Al-Tassan N, Chmiel NH, Maynard J, et al. Inherited variants of *MYH* associated with somatic G:C-T:A mutations in colorectal tumors. *Nat Genet. 2002;*30:227–232.
118. Aretz S, Uhlhaas S, Goergens H, et al. *MUTYH*-associated polyposis: 70 of 71 patients with biallelic mutations present with an attenuated or atypical phenotype. *Int J Cancer.* 2006;119:807–814.(9):791–799.
119. Sampson JR, Dolwani S, Johes S, et al. Autosomal recessive colrectal adenomatous polyposis due to inherited mutations of MYH. *Lancet* 2003;362(9377:39–41.
120. Ponti G, de Leon P, Pedroni MS, et al. Attenuated familial adenomatous polyposis and Muir-Torre syndrome linked to compound biallelic constitutional *MYH* gene mutations. *Clin Genet.* 2005:68:442–447.
121. NCCN Clinical Practice Guidelines in Oncology. Colorectal Cancer Screening, Version I.208. http://www.nccn.org/professionals/physician_gls/PDF/colorectal_screening .pdf).
122. Callender GG, Rich TA, Perrier ND. Multiple endocrine neoplasia syndromes. *Surg Clin North Am.* 2008;88:863–895.
123. Yang Y, Hua X. In search of tumor suppressing functions of menin. *Mol Cell Endocrinol.* 2007;265–266:34–41.
124. Nelen MR, Kremer H, Konings IB, et al. Novel PTEN mutations in patients with Cowden disease: absence of clear genotype-phenotype correlations. *Eur J Hum Genet.* 1999;7:267–273.
125. Schreibman IR, Baker M, Amos C, McGarrity TJ. The hamartomatous polyposis syndromes: a clinical and molecular review. *Am J Gastroenterol.* 2005;100:476–490.
126. Zbuk KM, Eng C. Cancer phenomics: RET and PTEN as illustrative models. *Nat Rev Cancer.* 2007;7:35–45.
127. Lonser RR, Glenn GM, Walther M, et al. von Hippel-Lindau disease. *Lancet.* 2003;361:2059–2067.
128. Hes FJ, van der Luijt RB, Lips CJ. Clinical management of Von Hippel- Lindau (VHL) disease. *Neth J Med.* 2001;59:225–234.
129. Rosner I, Bratslavsky G, Pinto PA, Linehan WM. The clinical implications of the genetics of renal cell carcinoma. *Uro Oncol.* 2009;27:131–136.
130. Lustbader ED, Williams WR, Bondy ML, Strom S, Strong LC. Segregation analysis of cancer in families of childhood soft-tissue-sarcoma patients. *Am J Hum Genet.* 1992;51:344–356.
131. Hwang SJ, Lozano G, Amos CI, Strong LC. Germline p53 mutations in a cohort with childhood sarcoma: sex differences in cancer risk. *Am J Hum Genet.* 2003;72:975–983.
132. Li FP, Fraumeni JF Jr. Soft-tissue sarcomas, breast cancer, and other neoplasms. A familial syndrome? *Ann Intern Med.* 1969;71:747–752.
133. Olivier M, Goldgar DE, Sodha N, et al. Li-Fraumeni and related syndromes: correlation between tumor type, family structure, and TP53 genotype. *Cancer Res.* 2003;63:6643–6650.
134. City of Hope Cancer Center. Department of Clinical Cancer Genetics. Community Cancer Genetics and Research Training. http://www.infosci.coh.org/ccgp/ Accessed on January 19, 2010.

135. Fox Chase Cancer Center. Personalized Cancer Risk Assessment: Genetics and Genomics in Nursing Practice. http://www.fccc.edu/healthProfessionals/continuingNursingEducation/index.html Accessed on January 19, 2010.
136. American Association of Colleges of Nursing. Essentials of Baccalaureate Education for Professional Nursing Practice. http://www.aacn.nche.edu/Media/NewsReleases/2008/BaccEssentials.html Accessed on January 19, 2010.
137. Khoury MJ, McBride C, Schully SD, Ioannidis JPA, Feero WG, Janssens ACJW, Gwinn M, et al. The scientific foundation for personal genomics: Recommendations from a national institutes of health-centers for disease control and prevention multidisciplinary workshop. *Gene Med* 2009;11:1–9.

Acknowledgements: Drs. Loud and Hutson wish to thank our colleague, Dr. Mark H. Greene, for his encouragement and support during the development of this manuscript. Dr. Loud's contribution to this chapter was supported by the Intramural Research Program of the National Institutes of Health and the National Cancer Institute.

**APPENDIX 7-1**

**Cancer Genetics Resources: An Organizational Guide**

| Category | Organization | Description/Materials | Contact Information |
|---|---|---|---|
| Cancer Genetics | National Cancer Institute | The official Web site of the National Cancer Institute provides a variety of resources such as the following:<br>Cancer Facts<br>Cancer Prevention, Genetics, and Causes<br>Cancer Literature<br>Clinical Trials<br>Research Programs<br>Cancer Dictionary<br>Educational Resources | www.cancer.gov |
| | Centers for Disease Control and Prevention | Office of Genomics and Disease Prevention provides information about human genomic discoveries | www.cdc.gov/genomics |
| | Gene Clinics | Genetics Web-based information resource on genetic syndromes, genetic testing, and clinical resources. | www.geneclinics.org/ |
| | OMIM™ Online Mendelian Inheritance in Man | An online catalog of information on human genes and genetic disorders | www.ncbi.nlm.nih.gov/sites/entrez?db=omim |
| | Physician's Database Query (PDQ®) | PDQ® cancer information summaries in genetics | www.cancer.gov/cancerinfo/pdq/genetics |
| | US National Library of Medicine (NLM) Genetics Home Reference | "The Genetics Home Reference: Your Guide to Understanding Genetic Conditions." Its purpose is to enhance understanding of genetic conditions and includes a glossary of genetic terms and resources and patient support | http://ghr.nlm.nih.gov/ |
| | Genetic Alliance | The nation's leading support, education, and advocacy organization for all those living with genetic conditions | www.geneticalliance.org |
| | National Society of Genetic Counselors (NSGC) | Provides information on genetic counseling, has a family tree link, lists of conferences, resources, publications, consumer information, career information, news, and a link to the *Journal of Genetic Counseling* for members. | www.nsgc.org |
| | American College of Medical Genetics (ACMG) | ACMG is the official US organization that certifies medical geneticists to practice. In addition to the usual educational content, it has sections on the Standards and Guidelines for Clinical Genetics Laboratories, the manual for reimbursement of genetic services, and a link to the journal, *Genetics in Medicine*. | http://www.acmg.net/ |
| | American Society of Human Genetics (ASHG) | This is the largest organization of human genetics researchers and clinicians. In addition to research, they are involved in applications of genetics to health care, health policy, training, and educating the public. | www.ashg.org |
| | Directory of Cancer Genetics Professionals | This directory lists professionals who provide services related to cancer genetics. These genetic counselors, nurses, and physicians have applied to and been accepted into the directory based on published eligibility criteria linked to the Web site. One may search by type of cancer, cancer syndrome, or geographic location for a provider. | http://cancer.gov/search/genetics_services/ |

(*Continued*)

**APPENDIX 7-1**

**Cancer Genetics Resources: An Organizational Guide (*Continued*)**

| Category | Organization | Description/Materials | Contact Information |
|---|---|---|---|
| | National Human Genome Research Institute (NHGRI) | This site provides information on legislation for all sites related to genetic privacy, discrimination for insurance, etc. | www.genome.gov/PolicyEthics/LegDatabase/pubMapSearch.cfm |
| | Genes and Disease | A collection of articles that discuss genes and diseases that they cause. | www.ncbi.nlm.nih.gov/disease/ |
| Resources for Genetic Nursing Practice | American Society of Clinical Oncology | The world's leading professional organization representing physicians who treat people with cancer.<br>Policy Statement Update: Genetic Testing for Cancer Susceptibility | www.asco.org |
| | International Society of Nurses in Genetics, Inc. | Statement on the scope and standards of genetics clinical nursing practice<br>Position Statements:<br>Access to genomic health care: the role of the nurse<br>Privacy and confidentiality of genetic information: the role of the nurse<br>Genetic counseling for vulnerable populations: the role of nursing | www.isong.org |
| | National Coalition of Health Care Professional Education in Genetics | Recommendations of core competencies in genetics for all health professionals. | www.nchpeg.org |
| | Oncology Nursing Society | A professional organization of nurses and other healthcare providers dedicated to excellence in patient care, education, research, and administration in oncology nursing.<br>Position Statements:<br>The role of the oncology nurse in cancer genetic counseling<br>Cancer predisposition genetic testing and risk assessment counseling | www.ons.org |

CHAPTER 8

Wendy H. Vogel, MSN, FNP, AOCNP®

# Diagnostic Evaluation, Classification, and Staging

## INTRODUCTION

The etiology of most cancers remains unknown and cancer prevention measures are complicated by multiple economic, behavioral, social, and cultural factors. The discovery of a precancerous lesion or a malignant neoplasm at its earliest stage affords the very best opportunity for cure, extended survival, less extensive treatment, and decreased cost of care. For example, the nonpalpable breast mass found on a screening mammogram or the isolated tumor found incidentally on a chest film is more likely to be diagnosed as localized disease amenable to treatment and cure.

More commonly, however, a tumor goes undetected until specific signs or symptoms become apparent, prompting the person to consult a health professional. A poor prognosis can be expected in those people who delay seeking medical evaluation at the onset of their symptoms, in those cancers for which technologic methods are unavailable to make an early diagnosis, and in people for whom the primary lesion cannot be found. For the person who presents with widespread disease, the palliative goal of treatment may direct and abbreviate an otherwise exhaustive and expensive diagnostic workup.

The workup for a suspected cancer may include tumor imaging, invasive diagnostic procedures, laboratory analysis, and genetic testing. The foundation of a cancer diagnosis remains the histopathologic identification. There are numerous diagnostic tools that augment the histopathologic workup including immunohistochemistry (IHC), flow cytometry, cytogenetic analysis, molecular diagnostics, imaging studies, and tumor biomarkers. Following diagnosis, the cancer is classified, graded, and staged, providing a comparative prognosis that will direct further management. This chapter's focus is the diagnostic approach and defining the most common tools utilized in making an oncologic diagnosis. The role of the oncology nurse throughout the diagnostic process will be discussed.

## GOALS AND FACTORS AFFECTING THE DIAGNOSTIC APPROACH

The major goals of the diagnostic evaluation for a suspected cancer are to determine the tissue type, the primary site, and the cellular characteristics of the malignancy, which help to determine the potential for tumor recurrence. The approach to the diagnostic evaluation depends on several factors:

- Presenting signs and symptoms
- Clinical status and ability to tolerate invasive procedures
- Anticipated goal of treatment once diagnosis is made
- Biologic characteristics of the suspected malignancy
- Diagnostic equipment available in the community
- Sensitivity and specificity of diagnostic tests
- Cost-effectiveness of diagnostic procedures

When cancer is not found incidentally, an individual may present with complaints of weight loss, persistent pain, unexplained fever, fatigue, or one of the seven warning signals that have brought the early detection of cancer into public awareness.[1] Table 8-1 identifies the most common warning signals of cancer, the significance of each signal or symptom, and the persons at greatest risk for developing an associated malignancy.[1–6] A patient's attitude, demographics, and behavior influence when medical attention is sought, as do geographic location, socioeconomic background, and insurance coverage. Changes in the framework of health care make it a priority to identify, address, and eliminate these potential barriers.[7]

One priority in health care is that clinicians maintain a high index of suspicion for cancer in certain high-risk groups. Those at highest risk for developing cancer at later stages when the possibility of a cure is less are the poor, the uninsured, the elderly, minorities, and those with a low-level education. Unfortunately, many of the people at greatest risk for developing later-stage cancers have an inadequate understanding of the importance of screening and early attention to symptoms, and may lack access to available resources. A study by the Center for Disease Control and Prevention[8] revealed that a significant number of older adults were unaware of colon cancer screening tests. The lack of a healthcare provider's recommendation for screening was often cited as the reason for not having testing performed, confirmed by numerous other studies.[9–12] Oncology nurses need to make a concerted effort to gather information, analyze the data, and then identify ways to increase understanding of the importance of early diagnosis, increase screening behaviors, and reduce the threat of cancer in these high-risk individuals. Nursing is well suited to provide education to laypersons about prevention measures and screening guidelines for the early detection of cancer.[13,14]

Healthcare providers can expect to see a steadily growing number of elderly patients with cancer as the US population ages and cancer incidence and mortality continue to increase.[15] Diagnosing cancer in the elderly is complicated by many issues. For example, these individuals often live alone and have limited resources. They often have a high prevalence of co-morbidities, decreasing hematopoietic reserves, cognitive impairment, functional decline, and depression. In addition, elderly patients' out-of-pocket expenses for diagnosis and treatment can be incurred at a time when their financial reserves are diminished.

## THE DIAGNOSTIC APPROACH

The "cancer-related checkup" is a periodic visit of a person who is well with a healthcare practitioner for

**TABLE 8-1**

**Seven Warning Signals of Cancer and Their Significance**

| Warning Signals | Significance of Warning Signal | Persons at Greatest Risk |
|---|---|---|
| Change in bowel and bladder habits | Changes in stool caliber and regular bowel function are frequent signs of colorectal cancer; dependent on the area of intestine involved. A change in bladder function, frequency, dysuria, retention, or hematuria may indicate prostate or bladder cancer. | *Colorectal cancer*: Over age 50, personal or family history of polyps or colorectal cancer, family history of polyposis syndromes, inflammatory bowel disease, sedentary lifestyle, obesity, high fat-low fiber diet, tobacco abuse<br>*Prostate cancer*: Over age 50, African American males, family history of prostate cancer, obesity<br>*Bladder cancer*: Tobacco abuse, males, chronic bladder inflammations, occupational exposures to benzidine, beta-naphthylamine commonly in dyes; occupations such as painters, hairdressers, machinists, printers and truck drivers; history of chemotherapy with cyclophosphamide or ifosfamide |
| Unusual bleeding or discharge | Any unusual bleeding or discharge can signify malignancy. Occult or bright red blood may be seen with colorectal cancer. Abnormal vaginal bleeding is the most frequent sign of endometrial or cervical cancer. A clear, milky, or bloody discharge from the nipple is the second-most common symptom of breast cancer. Hemoptysis is a sign of lung cancer. Hematuria is the most frequent sign of bladder cancer and is also seen in renal and prostate cancer. | *Endometrial cancer*: Postmenopausal women over age 50, family history of endometrial, ovarian or colorectal cancer; polycystic ovarian syndrome, anovulatory states, early menarche, obesity, diabetes, hypertension, unopposed estrogen exposure, nulliparity, history of tamoxifen treatment<br>*Cervical cancer*: First vaginal intercourse before age 18, more than 6 sexual partners, human papillomavirus (HPV), previous abnormal Pap smear, immunosuppressed states such as HIV, oral contraceptive use for more than 10 years, tobacco abuse |
| A sore that does not heal | Delayed healing of a sore or a change in a skin lesion's size, color, or shape, particularly on a surface exposed to ultraviolet light, can represent basal cell or squamous cell cancer. Oral lesions and leukoplakia, particularly tobacco or alcohol users, need careful follow-up. Persistent sores or itching of the vulva can indicate a preinvasive or malignant lesion. | *Skin cancer*: Excessive ultraviolet light exposure, light skin tones, blue eyes, blond or red hair, freckles or nevi, personal or family history of skin cancer, history of severe childhood sunburn(s), immunosuppression<br>*Oral cancer*: Tobacco abuse, alcohol abuse, males, excessive exposure to ultraviolet light, HPV infection, immunosuppression |
| Obvious changes in wart or mole | A change in a mole's color and pigmentation pattern, irregularities in border or surface topography, or increasing size causes suspicion of malignancy. Occurs in areas protected from or exposed to the sun. | *Melanoma and skin cancers*: Excessive ultraviolet light exposure, light skin tones, blue eyes, blond or red hair, freckles or nevi, personal or family history of skin cancer, history of severe childhood sunburn(s), immunosuppression |
| Thickening or lump in breast or elsewhere | A painless lump or mass is the most common presenting sign in cancer of the breast, testis, and soft tissue sarcoma. Persistent enlarged lymph nodes can signify lymphoma or metastatic nodal disease. | *Breast cancer*: Females, particularly over age 50, endogenous hormonal factors, personal or family history of breast or ovarian cancer, known genetic mutation (such as *BRCA 1* or *BRCA 2*), nulliparity, first full-term pregnancy after age 30, early menses, history of mantle field irradiation, atypical hyperplasia of the breast<br>*Testis*: Undescended testicle, personal or family history of testicular cancer, HIV, Caucasian race |
| Nagging cough or hoarseness | Persistent, productive cough is the most frequently reported symptom of lung cancer. Hoarseness may indicate lung, laryngeal, or thyroid cancer. | *Lung cancer*: Tobacco abuse, exposure to asbestos, radon, or secondhand smoke; radiation treatment to the lungs, personal or family history of lung cancer<br>*Head and neck cancer*: Tobacco or alcohol abuse, over age 50, males, history of Barrett's esophagus or gastroesophageal reflux disease, obesity |
| Indigestion or difficulty in swallowing | Indigestion, gastroesophageal reflux, painful "spasms" after eating or difficulty swallowing can be symptoms of cancer of the esophagus, stomach, or pharynx. | *Gastric cancer*: Helicobacter pylori infection, males, over age 50, Hispanic or African American race, diets high in nitrates, tobacco abuse, family or personal history of hereditary predisposition syndromes such as HNPCC, FAP, or HBOCS; history of Epstein-Barr virus<br>*Esophageal cancer*: Tobacco or alcohol abuse, over age 50, males, history of Barrett's esophagus or gastroesophageal reflux disease, obesity, caustic injury to esophagus |

cancer screening, risk assessment, and preventative counseling.[6] The history includes the identification of risk factors for cancer. Following a thorough history and physical exam, practitioners will offer age and gender appropriate cancer screening tests. Self-examination techniques are taught and regular performance encouraged. The cancer-related checkup is an opportunity for guidance in behavior changes as well as education regarding early signs of cancer and risk reduction strategies.

An effective clinical evaluation of the person with a suspected malignancy includes a comprehensive history with the identification of risk factors, a thorough physical examination, laboratory and imaging tests, and, perhaps most importantly, a biopsy-proven histologic verification of the malignancy. Known biologic characteristics of the suspected malignancy and the typical routes of regional and distant metastases will direct the choice of further diagnostic and staging procedures.

In the present era of cost containment in health care, the judicious selection and sequencing of diagnostic studies is stressed. The proper test is one that yields information on the suspicious site of malignancy and complements, rather than merely confirms, known information. Third-party payers, prospective payment systems, and managed care networks also play important roles as gatekeepers in the diagnostic evaluation. Due to cost-containment and insurance directives, many diagnostic evaluations are now being completed in ambulatory or outpatient facilities, unless patients are acutely ill and require hospitalization.

The selection of diagnostic tests is also based on the sensitivity and specificity of the test in question. *Sensitivity* is the percentage of people with cancer who will have positive (abnormal) test results, known as *true-positive* results. Test results of people with cancer that are negative (normal) constitute *false-negative* findings. The greater the test sensitivity, the more likely the test is to detect those with the disease. *Specificity* establishes the percentage of people without cancer who will have negative (normal) test results, known as *true-negative* results. People who are free of disease and show positive (abnormal) results are considered to have *false-positive* results. The higher the specificity of the test, the lower the likelihood of a false-positive result. A clinically useful test will detect a malignant abnormality early in its development (sensitivity) and exclude nonmalignant sources for the abnormality (specificity). In reality, many tests are highly sensitive but not very specific. The *predictive value* of a test establishes the probability that a test result correctly predicts the actual disease status.

Diagnostic testing may be performed for the purpose of screening, establishing a diagnosis, provision of prognostic information, evaluation of treatment response, or documentation of disease progression. Certain tests that are invasive or costly may be restricted to persons who have a high probability of having the disease. To achieve the expected sensitivity and specificity, the practitioner must be familiar with how the test is performed and determine whether the patient could effectively complete it. For example, a patient with claustrophobia might not tolerate conventional magnetic resonance imaging (MRI) of the head. Consideration is given to the type of abnormality suspected, the value of the information obtained, and how (or if) the results will affect decision-making.

The interpretation of diagnostic testing is examined in light of histopathologic findings, clinical presentation, patient history, and known data about the suspected tumor type. The reference ranges may vary according to patient age, gender, weight, and other factors. Even "normal" results must be interpreted collectively with other pertinent patient information. The practitioner is also cognizant of possible causes of "abnormal" test results such as medications, foods, patient's physiologic status, operator error, and instrument malfunction.

## LABORATORY ANALYSIS

Laboratory studies are performed to confirm a clinical diagnosis and to monitor the patient's response to or relapse from a specific therapy. The data provide information on the functioning of specific organs and metabolic processes that may be altered by a malignant process.

Biochemical analysis of blood, serum, urine, and other body fluids identifies chemical and hematologic values outside the normal homeostatic range. Specific malignancies characteristically alter chemical composition of the blood, but usually no single value is diagnostic for a malignancy. For example, elevated serum levels of transaminases, lactate dehydrogenase, and alkaline phosphatase are often found in individuals presenting with liver cancer and although not diagnostic, there is value in estimating prognosis.[16] Nonspecific changes such as anemia, leukocytosis or leukopenia, and thrombocytosis or thrombocytopenia also may contribute to the diagnostic evaluation.

## TUMOR MARKERS

Tumor markers (also called biomarkers or diagnostic markers) consist of proteins, antigens, ectopically produced hormones, receptors, enzymes, and genes or gene products that are *tumor derived* (expressed by the tumor) or *tumor associated* (produced by normal tissue in response to the tumor). Markers have been recognized in serum and body fluids, and in tissues at the cellular and genetic levels. Tumor markers are utilized in screening, diagnosis, staging, treatment selection, response determination, and the detection of recurrence.

Most tumor markers are not sensitive or specific enough to diagnose malignancy or to use as a screening tool. An exception is the prostate-specific antigen (PSA) used in prostate cancer screening. Tumor markers are most often used as adjuncts to diagnosis for several cancers.[17] An elevation of a tumor marker can assist in diagnosis of a tumor or to determine a recurrence. For example, an elevation of the CA (cancer antigen)-125 may increase the level of suspicion of an ovarian cancer. The carcinoembryonic antigen (CEA) is a useful tumor marker for colorectal cancer. However, like many tumor markers, the CEA lacks specificity because the antigen is expressed by benign as well as malignant cells.

The CEA may also be utilized as a prognostic indicator in colon cancer, reflecting tumor burden[17] and contributing to treatment decision making.[18] Serum $\alpha$-fetoprotein (AFP), human chorionic gonadotropin-$\beta$ ($\beta$-HCG), and lactate dehydrogenase (LDH) are tumor markers utilized in the staging of testicular cancer.[19] Evaluation of HER-2 expression (or amplification) in every breast cancer is recommended.[20] This marker predicts tumor behavior and guides treatment selection.

Most tumor markers are utilized to monitor disease progression and response to treatment. The CEA is the marker of choice in metastatic colorectal cancer to monitor treatment response.[18] A decrease in a previously elevated tumor marker may indicate a response to therapy. Serial tumor marker testing may determine disease recurrence, as with the CA 27.29 that may be elevated with recurrent breast cancer prior to any clinical indications of disease.[17,20] Early detection of recurrent cancer enables prompt treatment and perhaps improved outcomes. Table 8-2 identifies several tumor markers and indicates their clinical significance in oncologic care.[17,18,20–23]

While not yet standard of practice, there are newer biomarkers available that support treatment decision making. Pharmacogenetic testing is the identification of specific markers that enable clinicians to predict which patients will best respond to certain therapeutic regimens, allowing for individually tailored treatment selections. For example, KRAS mutation status predicts survival in patients with metastatic colorectal cancer who are treated with cetuximab.[24] The KRAS wild-type state predicts superior survival over KRAS mutants in these patients. Uridine diphosphate glucuronosyltransferase (UGT) 1A1 genetic testing can predict which patients will experience undue toxicity from irinotecan.[25] This type of testing may even have implications for preventing cancers in the future by identifying persons with certain genotypes that are more susceptible to carcinogenic influences.[26] Potential biomarkers currently under study include orotate phosphoribosyltransferase (OPRT), thymidylate synthetase (TS), thymidylate phosphorylate (TP), mismatch repair markers, and tumor suppressor p53, among many more.

Several professional organizations have developed practice guidelines for tumor marker utilization in clinical practice, including the American Society of Clinical Oncology (ASCO) and the National Comprehensive Cancer Network (NCCN).[18,19,23,27,28]

The technology involved in the recognition of tumor markers is quite complex and encompasses radioimmunoassays, monoclonal antibody production, and flow cytometry. Molecular markers are tumor markers at the molecular level and the technology includes gene studies, recombinant DNA technology, polymerase chain reaction (PCR), and automated sequencing.[17] Certain cancers have specific molecular markers that support the diagnostic process.

Techniques to produce monoclonal antibodies that detect specific tumor antigens have been important in the diagnosis, classification, localization, and treatment of several solid tumors, T- and B-cell lymphomas, and leukemia. Cell surface markers such as CD (clusters of differentiation) antigens contribute to the differentiation between hematologic malignancies.[22] For example, CD-20 is a cell surface marker of B-cell lymphoma. CD-15 is characteristic of Hodgkin's disease.

## ANALYTICAL TECHNIQUES

*Radioimmunoassay*, an important technique in the measurement of tumor markers, determines the amount of tumor antigen in a serum sample. A known amount of radiolabeled antigen, combined with antibody, is added to a serum sample. The individual's unlabeled antigen displaces the radiolabeled antigen, which permits quantification. The identification of a particular antigen will narrow the differential diagnosis.

*Immunohistochemistry* locates antigens in tissue sections by utilizing labeled antibodies and observing antigen–antibody interactions. These interactions are visualized by means of fluorescent dye, enzymes, radioactive elements, or colloidal gold. Tumor markers such as the CEA are determined by immunohistochemistry, as are estrogen and progesterone receptor and HER-2 receptor status.[29]

*Flow cytometry* rapidly measures and identifies DNA characteristics (such as ploidy) and certain cell population properties such as their distribution throughout the cell cycle.[30] Cell cycle distribution (S-phase fraction) may predict tumor behavior and correlate with patient prognosis. A *flow cytometer* measures fluorescence and light scatter as cells flow past an excitation source. In hematologic and lymphoid malignancies, fluorescent-marked antibodies directed against specific cell-surface antigens (T-cell antigens, common acute lymphocytic leukemia antigen) help to differentiate hematopoietic cell lines. Normal DNA is characterized as diploid and contrasts with abnormal, disorganized DNA, which is aneuploid. The proliferative potential of a tumor is measured by the percentage of cells in the synthesis phase of the cell cycle. Both of these factors—aneuploidy and high S-phase fraction—correlate with the biologic aggressiveness of several tumors.[30,31] DNA aneuploidy and high S-phase fraction appear to be predictors of poor prognosis in breast, bladder, and prostate

**TABLE 8-2**

**Selected Markers in the Diagnosis and Monitoring of Malignant Disease**

| Laboratory Test | Associated Malignancy | Comments |
|---|---|---|
| ***Enzymes*** | | |
| Lactic dehydrogenase (LDH) | Lymphoma, seminoma, acute leukemia, metastatic carcinoma | Elevated in 50% of patients with advanced disease, also in hepatitis and myocardial infarction |
| Prostatic acid phosphate (PAP) | Metastatic cancer of prostate, myeloma, lung cancer, osteogenic sarcoma | Elevated in 80% of patient with bone metastases from prostrate cancer, also in prostatitis, nodular prostatic hypertrophy |
| Placental alkaline phosphatase (PLAP) | Seminoma, lung, ovary, uterus | Elevated in pregnancy |
| Neuron-specific enolase (NSE) | Small cell lung cancer, neuroendocrine tumors, neuroblastoma, medullary thyroid cancer | |
| Creatine kinase-BB (CK-BB) | Breast, colon, ovary, prostate cancers, small cell lung cancer | Elevated in bowel infarction, renal failure, stroke |
| Terminal deoxynucleotidal transferase (TdT) | Lymphoblastic malignancy | Helpful in differentiating between AML and ALL |
| ***Hormones*** | | |
| Parathyroid hormone (PTH) | Ectopic hyperparathyroidism from cancer of the kidney, lung (squamous cell), pancreas, ovary, myeloma | Elevated in primary hyperparathyroidism |
| Calcitonin | Medullary thyroid, small cell lung cancer, breast cancer, and carcinoid | |
| Antidiuretic hormone (ADH) | Small cell lung cancer, adenocarcinomas | Inappropriate secretion associated with pneumonia, porphyria, CNS disease, various drugs, and endocrinopathies |
| Adrenocorticotropic hormone (ACTH) | Lung, prostate, gastrointestinal cancers, neuroendocrine tumors | Elevated in Cushing's disease |
| Human chorionic gonadotropin, beta subunit (B-HCG) | Germ cell tumors of testicle and ovary; ectopic production in cancer of stomach, pancreas, lung, colon, liver | Elevated in almost all choriocarcinoma, 60% of testicular cancer; also in pregnancy |
| ***Metabolic Products*** | | |
| 5-Hydroxindoleacetic acid (5-HIAA) | Carcinoid, lung | Drugs and diet interfere with test |
| Vanillylmandelic acid (VMA) | Neuroblastoma | Drugs and diet interfere with test; detected in ganglioneuroma |
| ***Proteins*** | | |
| Protein electrophoresis (urine—Bence Jones) (serum—immunoglobulins) | Myeloma, lymphoma | Elevated in connective tissue disease, benign monoclonal gammopathy, chronic renal failure |
| IgG | IgG myeloma | |
| IgA | IgA myeloma | |
| IgM | Waldenstrom's macroglobulinemia | |
| IgD | IgD myeloma | |
| IgE | IgE myeloma | |
| | Advanced neoplasms | |
| Beta-2 microglobulin | Myeloma, lymphoma | Invalid if patient received radioactive dyes week prior to test |
| ***Antigens*** | | |
| Alpha-fetoprotein (AFP) | Nonseminomatous germ cell testicular cancer, choriocarcinoma, gonadal teratoblastoma in children, cancer of the pancreas, colon, lung, stomach, biliary system, liver | Elevated in 80% of hepatocellular cancer, 60% of nonseminomatous germ cell cancer, also in cirrhosis, hepatitis, toxic liver injury |
| Prostate-specific antigen | Prostate cancer | Elevated in prostatitis, nodular prostatic hyperplasia |
| CA 15–3 | Breast cancer | |
| CA 27–29 | Breast cancer | |
| CA 19–9 | Pancreatic cancer | Assists in differentiating between malignant and benign pancreatobiliary disease |
| CA 126 | Ovarian cancer, pancreas, colon, lung, liver cancer | Elevated in > 80% of ovarian cancers; lesser elevations occur in endometriosis, pelvic inflammatory disease, peritonitis |

tumors, especially when correlated with other risk factors. The value of this information in solid tumors is not well established because of standardization difficulty but may be useful in the management of certain populations.[30]

Flow cytometry is largely utilized in the diagnosis and classification of acute leukemias, chronic lymphoproliferative disorders, and non-Hodgkin's lymphomas.[30] Flow cytometry enables the differentiation between myeloid and lymphoid malignancies, aids in subclassification, and identifies characteristics of malignant cells. Flow cytometry is employed in the monitoring of patients after therapy as well.

*Cytogenetics* is the analysis of cell genetic information. The entire genome with karyotype may be visualized, as well as genetic aberrations. Certain acquired genetic aberrations confirm neoplastic processes. These aberrations are found only in tumor cells (somatic mutations). The earliest example of a neoplastic genetic aberration was the notation of chromosome 22 deletion and reciprocal translocation with chromosome 9 in chronic myelocytic leukemia (the Philadelphia chromosome). Over the past 30 years, technological advances have enhanced our understanding of tumor genetics. Today cytogenetic analysis is used in diagnosis, prognostication, classification, selection of treatment, and for monitoring of disease regression or progression.[32]

The process of cytogenetic analysis may involve chromosomal banding in order to evaluate for structural and numeric chromosomal aberrations.[32] This process requires dividing cells, thus is dependent on adequate specimen processing. Fluorescence in situ hybridization (FISH) analysis (or molecular cytogenetics) uses known fluorochrome-labeled DNA sequences to hybridize to the DNA or chromosomes of the cells. Because of the tendency for a DNA strand to hybridize or bind to a matching DNA sequence, scientists may observe where a deletion, insertion, rearrangement, or translocation occurs.[32]

Polymerase chain reactions (PCR)and reverse transcription PCR (rt-PCR) are techniques that quantify relative gene expression at a particular time on a certain cell. Gene expression is the process by which genes are "turned on," thus directing some cellular activity. Older methods of visualizing this process required large amounts of RNA. PCR amplifies DNA, thus allowing visualization of gene expression from a small sample. This process allows quantification or qualification of a particular sequence in a DNA sample.

## GENETIC TESTING

Over the past decade, substantial progress has been made in the understanding of hereditary predisposition for cancer. Hereditary mutations are called germ-line mutations and are found in the DNA of the reproductive cells, and the mutation will be found in all of the offspring's cells.[33] A great deal of this progress stems from the Human Genome Project (HGP) research, which was completed in 2003.[34] As a result of rapid advances made in this area, patients and families can benefit from cancer risk assessment, undergo effective genetic testing, and consider the options for preventive therapy.

Communicating risk information to patients in a way that facilitates patient understanding and addressing the psychological issues related to the communication of cancer risk information are essential components of the cancer risk assessment. Genetic testing can assist healthcare providers in determining the probability that an individual will be diagnosed with a certain cancer in the future. Correctly estimating the risk for certain cancers is a complex endeavor, as risk estimates associated with certain mutations are changing as more information becomes available. Equally important is the nurse's sensitivity to the emotional impact of genetic information and his or her ability to support patients and families through the process.

Genetic tests for breast, ovarian, and colon cancers as well as melanoma are commercially available. Inheritance of the mutated form of the genes *BRCA1* and *BRCA2* place women up to an 87% lifetime risk for developing breast cancer and up to a 60% risk for developing ovarian cancer at a relatively young age.[33] Certain mutations in mismatch repair genes lead to a syndrome called hereditary nonpolyposis colon cancer (HNPCC). This syndrome confers up to an 80% lifetime risk of colon cancer. Women with this mutation have up to a 60% lifetime risk of endometrial cancer and 12% lifetime risk for ovarian cancer. Persons with familial adenomatous polyposis (FAP) syndromes have almost a 100% lifetime risk of having colon cancer.[33]

The American Society of Clinical Oncology recommends that clinicians offering genetic testing be able to explain the risks, benefits, and limitations of the testing procedure.[35] Once the test results become available, the clinician should discuss management options based on those results with the patient and family. Management options for persons at high risk for hereditary cancers include more aggressive screenings, prophylactic surgery, chemoprophylaxis, and risk reduction behaviors.[36]

As genetic technology evolves and knowledge of cancer genetics expands, healthcare providers must respond by informing patients, families, and the public about developments in cancer prevention, early detection, and treatment. The challenge of problem solving and knowledge application in genetic risk assessment requires that members of the health profession seek continuing education in this area. It is the position of the Oncology Nursing Society (ONS) that nurses providing comprehensive cancer genetic counseling be advanced practice oncology nurses and have specialized education in hereditary cancer genetics and oncology.[37,38]

## TUMOR IMAGING

Many diagnostic techniques and procedures are available to determine the presence of a tumor mass, localize the mass for biopsy, provide tissue characterization, and further assess or stage the anatomical extent of disease. The selection of a diagnostic test is based on the type and location of the suspected abnormality as well as the risk, discomfort, and expense to the patient. Table 8-3 identifies preferred imaging procedures for tumor definition and staging in several organ sites.[35–51] Table 8-4 elaborates on patient preparation and education for select diagnostic imaging tests.[21,47,49,52–54]

### Radiographic techniques

Radiographic studies, or x-ray films, allow for visualization of internal structures of the body. X-rays, or gamma rays, are passed through the body and are absorbed variably by tissues of differing densities; they react on specially sensitized film or fluoroscopic screens. Radiographs may be site specific, such as the standard chest film or mammogram, or they may view the dynamic function of an entire organ system. For example, in a gastrointestinal series, a continuous flow of x-rays passes through the digestive tract to assess the action of peristalsis, to detect displacement of structures, and to visualize mucosal abnormalities.

Mammographic examination is performed primarily in radiology suites dedicated solely to this procedure. These units are distinguished by the incorporation of a tissue compression device or cone that improves the quality of the image and reduces the amount of primary and scatter radiation. Mammograms detect 85% of all breast cancers, almost half of which can be visualized before they are palpable.[53] Since 1987, the American College of Radiology (ACR) has provided accreditation of mammography facilities, which has resulted in a standard of quality assurance.[52]

Diagnostic mammography is indicated when symptoms or clinical findings suggest an abnormality. The examination requires that more views be taken than those taken for the standard two-view screening mammogram. Spot compression and magnification views of suspicious areas may be indicated. Figure 8-1 is a mammogram showing a suspicious area of asymmetry with increased density. Ultrasound may also be used as an adjunct to the mammogram to determine whether a suspicious lesion is solid or cystic. Figure 8-2 is an ultrasound of the same suspicious area. Frequently, mammography is used to guide the placement of a wire, needle, dye, or catheter near a suspicious lesion in preparation for biopsy or surgery. A localizer penetrates and extends beyond the lesion for more reliable surgical excision.

Digital mammography is similar to conventional film-screen mammography, but uses a dedicated electronic detector system that captures and changes the digital image into a fixed record. The transmitted image is converted into a number of images that are transmitted as electrical signals by telephone lines, dedicated telecommunication lines, or satellite in less than 4 minutes to display the x-ray information on a computer. Digital mammography is better than conventional film mammography in pre- or perimenopausal women with dense breasts.[55]

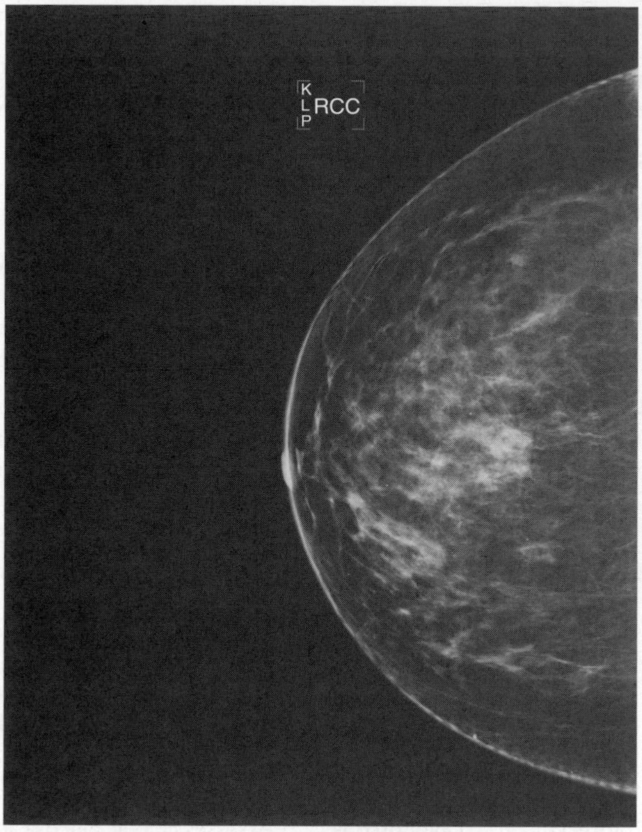


**FIGURE 8-1**

Diagnostic mammogram. Right craniocaudal view shows a 20-mm area of asymmetry with slight increased density and ill-defined margins in the upper central portion of the right breast. Ultrasound was requested to further evaluate the asymmetry.

*Source*: Courtesy of the Comprehensive Breast Center at Wellmont Holston Valley Hospital, Kingsport, TN, an American College of Radiology accredited Breast Imaging Center of Excellence.

Computerized tomography (CT) provides sectional (axial, coronal, or sagittal) views of structures in the body. After serial x-ray exposures are taken through different angles of the body, a computer analyzes the information and provides a three-dimensional, reconstructed picture of the area studied. Computerized tomography has become one of the most useful, informative, and available tests in the diagnosis and staging of malignancies.[56] Due to its profound spatial resolution, it is the diagnostic tool of choice for evaluation of the thorax, as it is capable of visualizing small lung nodules much earlier than standard imaging tests.[48] A

**TABLE 8-3**

**Imaging Procedures for Selected Sites**

| Site | Imaging Technique | Comments |
|---|---|---|
| Bladder | Cystoscopy | Test of choice for definitive diagnosis with biopsy |
| | IVP | Detects lesions >1.5–2 cm<br>Evaluates entire genitourinary system |
| | MRI | Superior to CT for soft tissue contrasting and detection of nodal metastases |
| | CT | Often used for local nodal staging and follow-up |
| | PET/CT | Excellent sensitivity for metastatic disease beyond pelvis |
| Brain | MRI | Tool of choice. Superior to CT for lesion characterization. |
| | CT | May be used to guide biopsy |
| | PET | Limited role. May be used to guide biopsy. |
| | MRA | Differentiate between tumor and aneurysm. Noninvasive. Useful in detection of vascular involvement. |
| Breast | Mammogram | Tool of choice. Digital mammography useful in pre- and perimenopausal women with dense breasts. |
| | US | Differentiates cystic from solid lesions. For mammographically negative, palpable lesions |
| | MRI | Recommended to screen high-risk women for breast cancer (such as with hereditary predisposition). Higher false-positive rate. |
| | PET | Covered for staging and restaging of distant metastases |
| | BSGI | Uses high-resolution gamma camera and Tc-Sestamibi. Equal sensitivity and greater specificity for breast tumors than MRI. Less costly than MRI. |
| Colorectal | Colonoscopy | Assesses colonic mucosa and provides a means for polyp removal and biopsy. |
| | Barium studies | Limited use, largely replaced by colonoscopy |
| | CT colonography | Noninvasive screening tool |
| | CT | Commonly used for initial staging |
| | MRI | Commonly used for initial staging. May be useful for characterization of liver lesions when CT is equivocal |
| | PET | Useful for diagnosis, staging, and restaging. Superior to CT in detecting metastases (particularly liver and nodal) in setting of rising CEA |
| Gynecologic | US | Transvaginal US useful to detect ovarian masses |
| | CT | Useful to assess extent of disease |
| | MRI | Useful to assess extent of disease |
| | PET | Provides better prognostic data, limited reimbursement coverage |
| Head and neck | CT | Superior to MRI in assessing extent of cartilage or bone involvement |
| | MRI | Used to characterize extent of primary tumor. Superior for evaluation of soft tissue lesions, tumor–tissue interface, parapharyngeal spaces |
| | PET | Increased staging accuracy. Superior to CT in determining tumor necrosis versus tumor recurrence after radiotherapy |
| | MRA | Useful in evaluating tumor involvement of vascular structures |
| Kidney | IVP | Useful in diagnosis, but largely replaced by CT |
| | CT | Test of choice for diagnosis and staging |
| | MRI | Useful when other tests are equivocal |
| Liver | CT | Test of choice for diagnosis and staging |
| | MRI | Commonly used for diagnosis |
| Lung | Chest x-ray | Useful for the detection of peripheral lesions |
| | CT | Tool of choice particularly for parenchyma and mediastinal nodes; useful solitary lung nodules |
| | MRI | Superior to CT in chest wall, hilum, and mediastinal vascular invasion; useful to evaluate for distant metastases |
| | PET | Test of choice in solitary pulmonary nodules; superior to CT for staging (non-small cell) |
| | PET/CT | Superior to PET for staging |

*(Continued)*

**TABLE 8-3**

**Imaging Procedures for Selected Sites (*Continued*)**

| Site | Imaging Technique | Comments |
|---|---|---|
| Musculoskeletal | X-ray | Malignancy must involve 30%–50% of the bone matrix to be visualized on x-ray. Skeletal survey is test of choice in detecting bone metastases from multiple myeloma |
| | Bone scan | Test of choice for detecting metastatic bone lesions (excluding purely lytic lesions) |
| | CT | Useful for detection of early metastases to bone, particularly in the spine; preferred test for intraosseous lesions |
| | MRI | Test of choice for sarcoma, evaluation of extraosseous extension of soft tissue mass into the bone, and for metastatic lytic bone lesions as in multiple myeloma |
| Pancreas | CT | Test of choice for staging and determining resectability. |
| | MRI | Alternative to CT. |
| | Abdominal US | Differentiates between cyst and solid mass. Detects presence of bile duct dilatation, masses as small as 2 cm, hepatic metastases, and extrapancreatic spread. |
| | EUS | Can enhance visualization of portal vein and regional lymph node tumor involvement |
| | ERCP | Differentiates between benign strictures and malignant strictures, and choledocholithiasis. Useful when CT is equivocal. |
| | MRA | For the evaluation of abdominal vessels |
| Prostate | TRUS | Useful to guide biopsy; contrast enhancement may be useful |
| | CT | Useful in the detection of bladder and rectal invasion, adenopathy, and distant metastases |
| | MRI | Useful in the detection of bladder and rectal invasion, adenopathy |

Abbreviations: BSGI, breast-specific gamma imaging; CT, computed tomography; ERCP, endoscopic retrograde cholangiopancreatography; EUS, endoscopic ultrasonography; IVP, intravenous pyelogram; MRA, magnetic resonance angiography; MRI, magnetic resonance imaging; PET, positron emission tomography; TRUS, transrectal ultrasound; US, ultrasound.

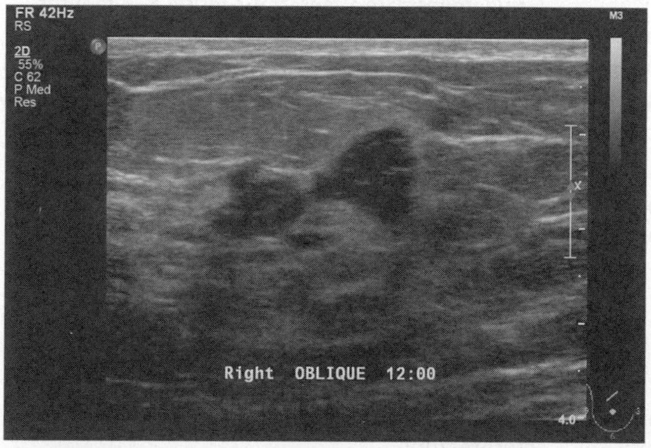


**FIGURE 8-2**

Breast ultrasound. An irregular lobular hypoechoic mass was noted correlating to the area of symmetry shown in the diagnostic mammogram, Figure 8-1. Breast-specific gamma imaging was recommended to further evaluate area of concern and to examine architecture bilaterally.

*Source*: Courtesy of the Comprehensive Breast Center at Wellmont Holston Valley Hospital, Kingsport, TN, an American College of Radiology accredited Breast Imaging Center of Excellence.

CT scan is able to detect minor differences between tissue densities in any area of the body. Computerized tomography frequently is used to direct a needle to a tumor site for percutaneous biopsy. One major disadvantage of CT is its production of artifact in areas of cortical bone content.

Computerized tomography may be completed with or without contrast agents. Imaging with contrast provides improved detection, characterization, and differentiation of various tissues and lesions.[48] Figure 8-3 demonstrates two different tumors imaged by CT with intravenous contrast. Several radiographic examinations rely on contrast materials to enhance or outline the structures to be visualized. Angiography, venography, cholangiography, and urography, in addition to CT, all rely on the intravascular administration of iodinated contrast agents for optimal visualization of body structure and function. An example is the excretory radiograph, also known as the intravenous pyelogram (IVP), which is used in the initial diagnostic evaluation of renal masses. Intrathecal contrast agents may be used in myelography and in CT. Radiographs of the subarachnoid space are taken after the injection of either an oily or a water-soluble contrast agent. The contrast agent flows only to the point of obstruction and more than one injection may be required.

**TABLE 8-4**

**Selected Diagnostic Imaging Techniques With Patient Instructions**

| Diagnostic Imaging Technique | Patient Instructions | Comments |
|---|---|---|
| Barium studies | Dietary and medication restrictions before exam<br>Laxatives/enemas to cleanse bowel prior to examination<br>Barium will taste chalky, milkshake consistency<br>Barium enema will feel cold and may cause cramping<br>Need to lie flat and secured on tilting x-ray table<br>Laxatives and fluids to clear barium after procedure<br>Time 30–60 minutes | May be exhausting for elderly patients.<br>BE must precede upper GI and small bowel series and should follow other imaging examinations.<br>Double contrast BE requires full patient cooperation due to time frame.<br>Screening recommendations for colorectal cancer include double contrast barium enema every 5 years. |
| Breast-specific gamma imaging (BSG) | Small injection of the tracing agent will be given in each arm prior to procedure.<br>Patient will sit upright and images will be taken of each breast (about 6–10 minutes each).<br>Breast will be held in place by a small panel, light pressure is applied, but breast is not compressed.<br>Time 45–60 minutes | Able to image "hard to reach" spots, such as up to the chest wall.<br>Detects early stage cancers as small as 2 mm.<br>While radiation dose to the whole body is equivalent to mammography, dose to breast is less. |
| Bone scan | No dietary restrictions, but fluids should be restricted for 4 hours prior to examination.<br>Radioactive substance will be injected into a vein before the examination and the patient must wait about 3–4 hours for the substance to accumulate in the bones. Patient will be free to move around and should void frequently.<br>Before scanning, patient should void to eliminate tracer accumulation in bladder.<br>Patient must lie still, on back during the examination.<br>Scanner may move back and forth over patient, emitting a clicking sound, usually taking about 30–60 minutes.<br>Fluid intake encouraged for 1–2 hours after examination to assist in clearance of radioisotope.<br>Patients may set off airport security systems within the first 24 hours after this procedure. If flying shortly after this procedure, adequate documentation of procedure should be brought to the airport.<br>Time 3–4 hours | Increased use of radioimmunoimaging using radiolabeled monoclonal antibodies.<br>Total amount of radiation absorbed is less than that of ordinary x-rays.<br>Results should be correlated with patient's medical history and other diagnostic studies.<br>False negatives occur in osteolytic disease, such as with multiple myeloma and renal cell carcinoma.<br>Can demonstrate a metastatic lesion 3–6 months before radiographic visualization.<br>Flare phenomenon (particularly in breast and prostate cancer) can occur during the first few months of new therapy with the appearance of increased activity or new lesions due to healing response. |
| Computed tomography (CT) | Food and fluid restriction for 4 hours prior to examination if contrast is utilized.<br>Injection of intravenous contrast may be given; a burning sensation may occur with injection, some patients may experience nausea, vomiting, flushing, itching, or bitter taste.<br>Must lie still on adjustable table while x-ray tube rotates around patient.<br>Machinery noisy | Careful history to determine whether prior adverse reaction to contrast.<br>Cost dependent on contrast use and radiologist's interpretation.<br>Careful history of kidney function and evaluation of BUN and creatinine.<br>Sedation may be needed if claustrophobic. |

*(Continued)*

**TABLE 8-4**

**Selected Diagnostic Imaging Techniques with Patient Instructions (*Continued*)**

| Diagnostic Imaging Technique | Patient Instructions | Comments |
|---|---|---|
| Computed tomography (CT) | Encourage fluids after examination to eliminate contrast<br>Time 30–60 minutes | |
| Endoscopy | Dietary restriction prior to examination<br>Conscious sedation for procedure<br>Oral:<br>• Local anesthetic sprayed in mouth<br>• Flexible tube passed through mouth to level of examination<br>• Tongue and throat may feel swollen and there may be difficulty swallowing<br>• Pressure or fullness sensations if stomach is scoped<br>Rectal:<br>• Laxative and/or enemas to cleanse bowel prior to procedure<br>• Lubricated endoscope inserted anally<br>• Feeling of coldness, urge to defecate<br>• Position change may be required during examination for scope advancement<br>Time 30–60 minutes | Endoscopic examinations provide a means for biopsies.<br>Screening recommendations for colorectal cancer include colonoscopy every 10 years or Flexible sigmoidoscopy every 5 years. |
| Magnetic resonance imaging (MRI) | Dietary restriction only if abdomen or pelvis is scanned<br>Remove anything affected by a magnet.<br>Lie still on table, secured with straps. Table will move into narrow magnet opening.<br>Contrast dye will require injection, otherwise painless.<br>Contrast may cause nausea, vomiting, or itching.<br>Time 30–90 minutes | May need sedation or alternative imaging test if patient is claustrophobic or very obese.<br>Lengthy procedure may require titration of medication for sedation or comfort.<br>Black Box Warning regarding gadolinium contrast and risk of nephrogenic system fibrosis (NSF) in patients with severe renal insufficiency. |
| Mammogram | Breast is compressed between two plates on x-ray cassette<br>Compression may feel tight and uncomfortable<br>Screening<br>• 2 views taken of each breast<br>• Time 10–15 minutes<br>Diagnostic<br>• 3 views taken of each breast<br>• Spot compression and magnification films<br>• Time 10–20 minutes | Clinical breast exam and education regarding breast self-exam should be included<br>Mammography Quality Standards Act requires that positive findings be reported to patient within days and negative findings within 30 days.<br>Accuracy may be limited by patient immobility, breast density, or venous access devices.<br>Screening recommendations include yearly mammography beginning at age 40 |
| Positron emission tomography (PET) | Patients must fast for at least 8 hours prior to the procedure and fasting blood glucose must be within a normal range.<br>Diabetic patients are not to take oral hypoglycemic agents or insulin after midnight. | May require alternative imaging test if patient is claustrophobic, unable to lie still, or very obese. |

(*Continued*)

**TABLE 8-4**

**Selected Diagnostic Imaging Techniques with Patient Instructions (*Continued*)**

| Diagnostic Imaging Technique | Patient Instructions | Comments |
|---|---|---|
| Positron emission tomography (PET) (*continued*) | Patients are to avoid vigorous exercise before examination.<br>Radiotracer will be injected, swallowed, or inhaled. It will take 30–60 minutes for absorption and patient should lie still, avoiding any activity, talking, or gum chewing.<br>All metal objects including hearing aids are removed prior to examination<br>Lie still during examination and table will move in and out of machine tunnel<br>Time 2–4 hours | Benign processes such as exercise, talking, or gum chewing cause uptake of FDG radiotracer giving a false-positive appearance.<br>Some malignant tumors (eg, well-differentiated thyroid carcinomas) have limited glucose uptake, thus giving a false-negative appearance. |
| Ultrasonogram | Dietary restrictions before exam dependent on site to be examined.<br>Full bladder for pelvic ultrasound<br>Will lie on exam table, gel applied to area to be examined, transducer will gently move over the skin, pressure may be felt, no pain.<br>Time 15–30 minutes | Transducer may be applied to body externally or internally (vaginally or rectally).<br>May be used intraoperatively or used with an endoscopic procedure.<br>Lesions or masses greater than 2 cm may be visualized. |

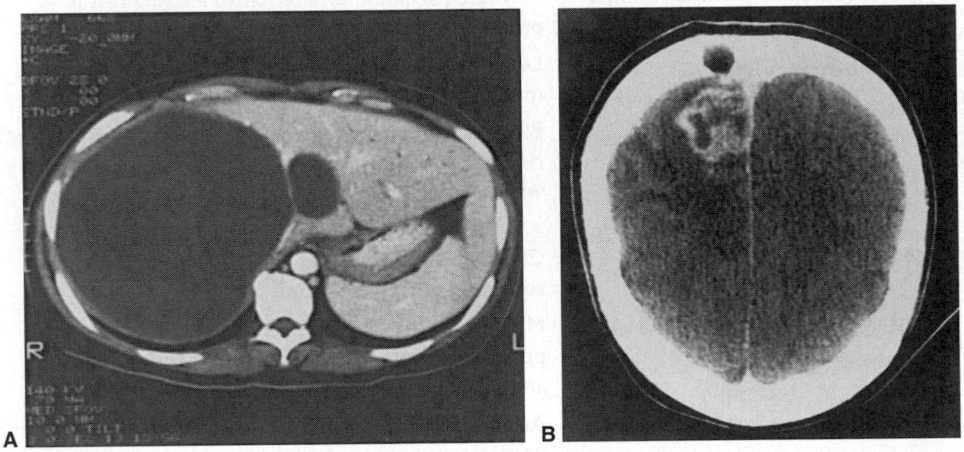

A B

**FIGURE 8-3**

Examples of contrast-enhanced CT. (**A**) CT abdominal scan revealing huge cystadenocarcinoma involving most of the liver. (**B**) CT head scan demonstrating lobular glioblastoma with peripheral rim enhancement. *Abbreviation*: CT, computed tomography.

*Source*: Courtesy of Scripps Memorial Hospital, Department of Radiology, La Jolla, CA.

Patients who undergo studies requiring iodinated contrast material can experience minor, to intermediate, to life-threatening anaphylactoid reactions.[48] When intravenous contrast is used, patients must be assessed for allergies to iodine, for venous access, and renal function. When imaging the abdomen, it is important to use oral contrast. Risks to oral contrast are the potential for aspiration and nausea. A metallic or bitter taste, becoming flushed, and a feeling of warmth all are common and transient sensations experienced during injection of contrast material. Vesicular reactions such as itching, angioedema, and mild urticaria may occur from a few minutes to several hours after contrast injection. These symptoms do not require treatment and will not progress to life-threatening reactions. There is no good predictor for severe reactions; however, patients with a history of allergic response should be considered to be at high risk, closely monitored, and premedicated. Premedication regimens using prednisone and/or diphenhydramine may be given. Occasional delayed reactions in patients have been noted from 2 to 6 hours after testing. On completion of an iodinated contrast examination, patients are instructed to drink a minimum of 8 glasses of fluid in

24 hours to prevent renal toxicity. Nonionic contrast agents are available for use with patients who have had serious reactions in the past.[21,48]

Virtual colonoscopy (VC) is a newer method for detecting colorectal polyps and cancers. Air is insufflated into a cleansed colon, and high-resolution, thinly collimated, spiral CT slices are acquired. The two-dimensional slices, as well as the post-processed "fly-through" virtual colonoscopic images, are examined for polyps and tumors. These images can be saved, manipulated to achieve better viewing angles, and reviewed after the procedure. Preparing for a VC requires administration of a laxative and insertion of a probe to push air into the colon. Moderate sedation is not required, so individuals can resume usual activities after completing a VC. The NCCN guidelines suggest that CT colonography is a reliable alternative method of colon screening,[90] particularly if colonoscopy is incomplete, unavailable, or contraindicated. In a clinical trial, 11,233 asymptomatic adults underwent both virtual and conventional colonoscopies. The sensitivity of VC for adenomatous polyps was found to be 93.8% for polyps at least 10 mm in diameter, 93.9% for polyps at least 8 mm in diameter, and 88.7% for polyps at least 6 mm in diameter. The sensitivity of optical colonoscopy for adenomatous polyps was 87.5%, 91.5%, and 92.3% for the three sizes of polyps, respectively. The specificity of VC for adenomatous polyps was 96.0% for polyps at least 10 mm in diameter, 92.2% for polyps at least 8 mm in diameter, and 79.6% for polyps at least 6 mm in diameter.[57] Indications for VC may include screening for polyps, incomplete or failed colonoscopy, and preoperative assessment of the colon proximal to an occlusive cancer.[58,59] A disadvantage of VC is that interpretation is quite time-consuming.[49]

Barium sulfate is a nonabsorbable, radiopaque agent used to enhance the contrast between the lumen of the gastrointestinal tract and adjacent soft tissues. Studies that use barium include esophagography, upper gastrointestinal (UGI) series, small bowel series, barium enema, and hypotonic duodenography. Barium is ingested or introduced into the gastrointestinal tract and allowed to coat the intraluminal surfaces. Radiographs are taken that can detect primary malignancies of the gastrointestinal organs or extrinsic compression from other tumor sites. Figure 8-4 presents a classic annular lesion of the colon imaged with radiopaque contrast. Double contrast barium enema (DCBE) uses a high-density barium suspension and air combination, whereas the single-contrast barium enema uses low-density barium suspension alone.[29] DCBE appears to be less accurate (lower sensitivity and specificity) than CT colongraphy[60,141] in the detection of colorectal polyps and adenomas less than one centimeter.[61] Complications seldom result from this examination unless there is an obstruction or a perforation of the digestive tract. Retention of the barium may cause fecal impaction and discomfort in some patients. The administration of a laxative or an enema may be necessary to assist with bowel evacuation. Today, CT, MRI, and endoscopy have now largely replaced barium studies.[56]

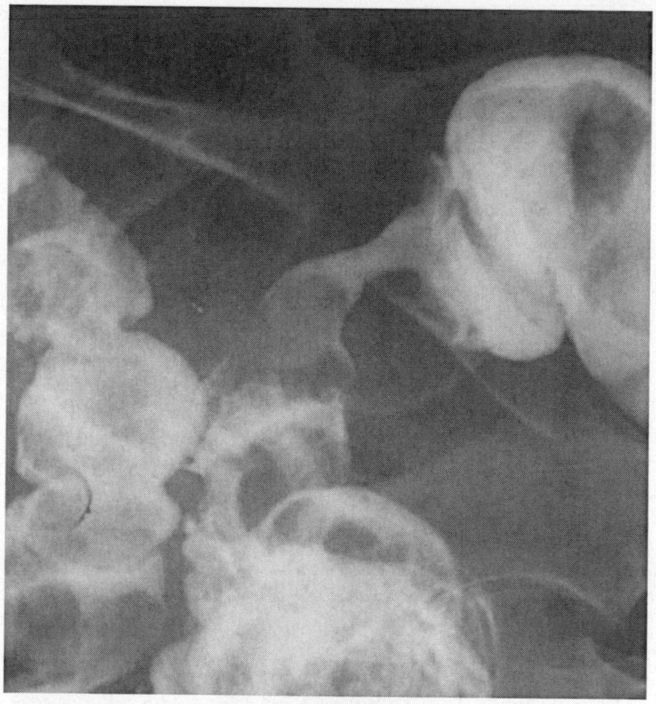

**FIGURE 8-4**

Barium enema visualizes annular, "apple core" lesion that is constricting the colon.

*Source*: Courtesy of Scripps Memorial Hospital, Department of Radiology, La Jolla, CA.

## Nuclear medicine techniques

Nuclear medicine imaging involves the intravenous injection or the ingestion of radioisotope compounds, followed by camera imaging of those organs or tissues that have concentrated the radioisotopes. Nuclear medicine studies are extremely sensitive and often will detect sites of abnormal metabolism or early malignancy several months before changes are seen on a radiograph. However, anatomic perception may be limited.[49] Because of this, almost all nuclear medicine imaging studies are interpreted in conjunction with an anatomically sensitive scan.[48] Nuclear medicine studies commonly used in oncology include bone scans, thyroid (iodine) scans, gallium scans, octreotide scans, positron emission tomography (PET) scans, and single-photon emission computed tomography (SPECT) scans.

*Bone scans* utilize the radioactive isotope Tc-diphosphonate ($^{99m}Tc$) that is given intravenously.[21] The entire body is scanned and increased uptake of the radioisotope (called a "hot spot") indicates abnormalities. Bone scans are highly sensitive for detecting malignancies and often used to evaluate patients with tumors having a propensity to metastasize

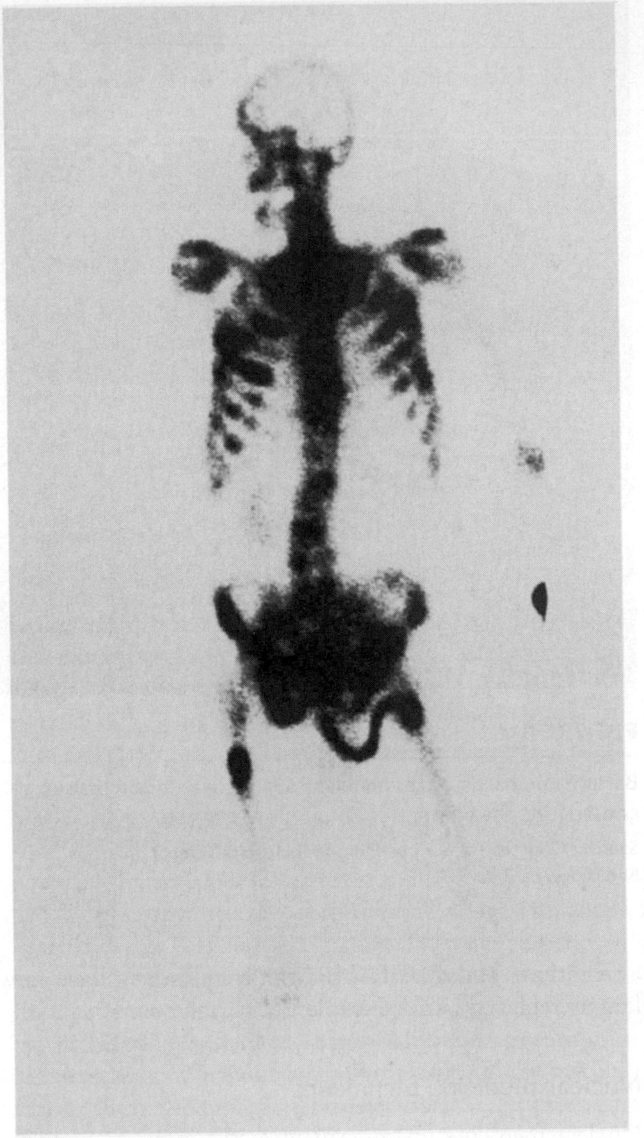

**FIGURE 8-5**

Abnormal bone scan suggesting widespread bony metastasis in central axial skeleton, pelvis, hips, and right proximal femur.

*Source*: Courtesy of Scripps Memorial Hospital, Department of Radiology, La Jolla, CA.

to the bone. Figure 8-5 shows an abnormal bone scan suggestive of widespread metastasis from prostate cancer.

*Thyroid scans* require an injection of a radioactive tracer, most commonly iodine, to evaluate the functional ability of the thyroid.[21] Increased uptake of thyroid nodules ("hot nodules") indicates thyroid hyperfunction. Decreased uptake ("cold nodules") indicates hypofunction and cold nodules are more likely to be malignant. Whole body scans utilizing $^{131}$I allow detection of metastatic thyroid cancer.

*Gallium scans* use gallium-67 citrate to visualize inflammatory lesions of the bone, bone marrow, and cartilage, breast, brain, and liver. Abnormalities of these tissues are seen as increased uptake of the radiopharmaceutical.[21] Gallium scans are particularly sensitive in detecting lymphomas, although PET scanning has largely replaced the gallium scan in these malignancies.

*Octreotide scans* are used in the diagnosis and follow-up of neuroendocrine tumors that express somatostatin receptors (such as carcinoid and islet cell tumors). The radioactive tracer utilized in octreotide scans is a somatostatin analogue. Patients currently treated with octreotide acetate (Sandostatin) will have less sensitive imaging and should discontinue therapy 24 to 48 hours prior to the scan.[21]

*Positron emission tomography* is an imaging modality that provides information based on the biochemical and metabolic activity of the tissue. Infused biochemical compounds such as glucose are tagged with radioactive particles that emit positrons detectable by gamma camera tomography. F-18 fluorodeoxyglucose (FDG) is the most widely used radiopharmaceutical. PET scanning has the ability to detect abnormal metabolic activity before morphologic changes occur.[54] Tumors have a higher rate of glycolysis, enabling FDG to trace glucose metabolism in cancerous tissues, unlike other diagnostic tests that examine only structural changes.[21,48] PET scanning is not recommended for tissue that normally takes up glucose, such as the kidney and brain. Slow-growing lesions may be difficult to detect as glucose metabolism is lower. Figure 8-6 shows a PET image demonstrating a large lung tumor. To allow maximum accumulation of FDG in cancerous tissue, patients must fast for at least 8 hours, including gum chewing, and refrain from vigorous exercise prior to the examination. Diabetic patients are asked to hold oral hypoglycemic agents or insulin after midnight.[48]

Previously used for cardiac and neurologic disorders, PET has demonstrated accuracy in a variety of cancers and is approved for reimbursement by Centers for Medicare and Medicaid Services (CMS) in breast, cervical, colorectal, esophageal, head and neck, lymphoma, melanoma, and non-small cell lung, and thyroid cancers.[62] PET is utilized in the diagnosis, prognosis, staging, and follow-up of these malignancies. It may also be used (and considered the test of choice) combined with CT in the work-up of a solitary pulmonary nodule.[63] Also, when combined with CT, PET scanning improves the accuracy of staging in many tumor types.[64,65]

The PET-CT scan is particularly useful in differentiating low-grade from high-grade tumors and in distinguishing treatment-induced tissue necrosis from recurrent tumor.[54] It has proved highly effective when evaluating patients for metastatic disease. In a study done by Zhuang et al,[66] 80 patients diagnosed with colon cancer were evaluated for recurrent disease in the liver using PET, CT scans, surgical pathology, and clinical outcome. *PET* proved more accurate than CT in diagnosing liver metastases and extrahepatic metastases. Other clinical situations where

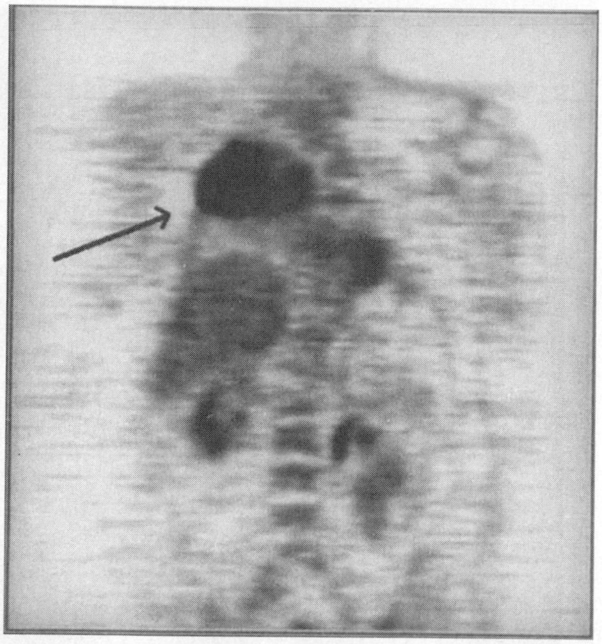

**FIGURE 8-6**

Positron emission tomography scan of lung showing large lung tumor.

*Source*: Courtesy Rush PET Center. Courtesy of Scripps Memorial Hospital, Department of Radiology, La Jolla, CA.

PET has improved diagnostic accuracy over other imaging choices include detection of head and neck cancers, staging in head and neck cancers, small cell lung cancer, and lymphomas.[67]

Limitations of the PET-CT scan include its expense, the need for a cyclotron to produce the isotopes, and the requirement that patients fast prior to the exam to allow for maximum tissue uptake of FDG. Patient movement during scanning may also create artifacts on the fused images.[54] Hip prosthesis, dental devices, and pacemakers may also interfere with imaging. There is variable physiologic FDG uptake in the digestive tract, thyroid gland, skeletal muscle, myocardium, bone marrow, and genitourinary tract. Benign pathologic FDG uptake can occur in healing bone, lymph nodes, joints, sites of infection, and sites of aseptic inflammatory response.[66,68]

Positron emission tomography and PET-CT have emerged as reliable methods for evaluating and staging recurrent disease. Additionally, it plays an important role in differentiating benign and malignant primary tumors. Although FDG has emerged as the dominant radiopharmaceutical for PET imaging in oncology, numerous other compounds are utilized in practice and in clinical trials.

Nuclear imaging with radiolabeled monoclonal antibodies visualizes microscopic sites of metastasis or suspected malignancy. This technique requires that a monoclonal antibody targeted against a specific tumor antigen be combined with trace amounts of radioactivity. After intravenous injection, the antibody binds to antigen on the tumor. Tumor sites then "light up" with imaging scanners. CYT-103 (OncoSCINT OV/ CR) is the first FDA-approved radiolabeled monoclonal antibody for diagnostic use in cancer. The indium111-labeled antibody targets the tumor-associated glycoprotein (TAG-72) found in mucin-producing adenocarcinomas. Two other FDA-approved radiolabeled antibodies include $^{90}$Y-Ibritumomab and $^{131}$I-tositumomab for the treatment of non-Hodgkin's lymphoma.[69] Although data remain limited, this type of imaging is approved for colon and ovarian cancer and plays a role in assessing occult recurrent disease.[70]

## Ultrasonography

Ultrasonography (US) is a nonradiographic and noninvasive technique for imaging deep soft-tissue structures within the body. The reflecting echoes of high-frequency sound waves directed into specific tissues are recorded on an imaging screen. The echoes are variable, depending on the tissue density, and can be used to discriminate cystic lesions from solid lesions. In oncology, ultrasonography is used most often to assess superficial structures such as the breast or thyroid to detect effusions or ascites, to evaluate organs such as the liver, ovaries, or kidneys, or to examine the vascular system.[50] It is extremely useful in the evaluation of palpable lesions, especially in the breast.[48] In interventional radiology, ultrasound often guides procedures. It is noninvasive, relatively inexpensive, and is portable. Major limitations of ultrasound are the inability to penetrate bone, fat, or air, lesser resolution when compared to CT or MRI, and lack of reproducibility.[56] Ultrasound is an important adjunct to mammography for distinguishing cysts from solid lesions with a sensitivity of about 98%.[21] It has proven useful in the evaluation of patients with dense breasts or those with breast prostheses. One of the newest applications of ultrasound, endoscopic ultrasonography (EUS), provides images during endoscopic procedures. EUS is used in screenings, improves diagnostic ability, assists in staging, and may guide biopsy procedures.[21] Contrast-enhanced ultrasound may assist in characterizing small lesions of the liver or kidney.[56]

## Magnetic resonance imaging

Magnetic resonance imaging creates sectional images of the body, similar to CT, but does not expose the patient to ionizing radiation. Images are created by placing the individual within a powerful magnetic field that aligns the body's hydrogen nuclei in one direction. Radiofrequency pulses are used to excite the magnetized nuclei and change their alignment. Between radiofrequency pulses, the nuclei return to a state of relaxation, and variable signals are transmitted on the basis of tissue characteristics. These signals are analyzed by the computer, and multiplanar (sagittal, coronal, and axial) images are produced with exquisite clarity. Magnetic resonance imaging can be enhanced with the use of a contrast agent such as gadolinium chelates.[56] Contrast agents work by reducing tissue relaxation time, thereby increasing signal intensity and image production. Adverse reactions to gadolinium, which are rare, include nausea, pain localized to the injection site, and headache occurring several hours after the examination. In 2007, the FDA required a black-box warning regarding gadolinium MRI contrast medium because of the increased risk of nephrogenic system fibrosis in patients with severe renal insufficiency.[49]

Advances in MRI technology include diffusion-weighted MRI, which compares intracellular and extracellular spaces for the degree of diffusion, enabling detection of restricted diffusion such as occurs in tumor blockages.[21] During functional MRI scanning, the patient performs certain tasks and rapid successive images are taken then compared to evaluate brain function or the auditory system. Whole-body MRI scanning has shown substantial ability to diagnose systemic primary bone malignancies, bone metastases, and other distant metastatic disease particularly from tumors that commonly spread to the liver or brain.[71,72] Perfusion MRI measures blood flow through a tumor or organ, allowing visualization of angiogenesis.[50]

Magnetic resonance imaging is the preferred imaging study when evaluating musculoskeletal tumors, the brain, and central nervous system.[49] At present, MRI enhanced with gadolinium is considered to be the best diagnostic tool for the evaluation of brain and spinal lesions[48] (Figure 8-7). MRI gives superior contrast resolution over that of CT and conventional radiography.[48] MRI is more site specific than CT because it has a smaller field of view. When examining larger areas, MRI testing time is extended.

Magnetic resonance imaging is useful in detecting cancers in women with dense breasts, whereas mammography provides less definitive results in this situation as well as in detecting residual tumor following lumpectomy.[73] Figure 8-8 demonstrates residual tumor following biopsy of suspicious mass noted in Figures 8-1 and 8-2. Findings such as this will guide the clinician in treatment decisions. MRI is appropriate for screening women at high risk for breast cancer or where a high degree of suspicion exists without evidence of disease on mammogram. In one study, the records of 367 women considered to be at high risk for breast cancer were reviewed. All had normal mammograms and underwent their first MRI of the breasts for screening due to high risk of breast cancer based on family history, previous breast cancer, or history of a precancerous lesion. (A high-risk lesion is one that can progress to cancer or is a marker for possible breast cancer in the future.) Sixty-four of the MRIs showed an abnormality that warranted a biopsy. Fifty-nine of the patients underwent the recommended

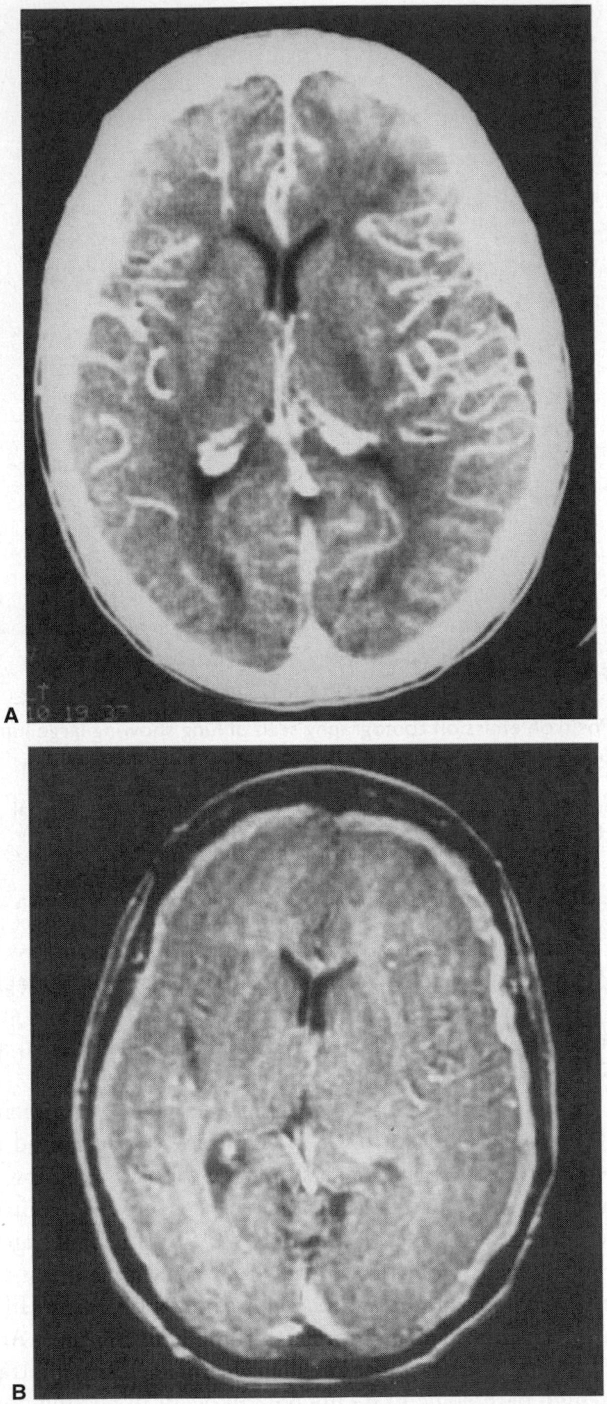

**FIGURE 8-7**

(**A**) Contrast-enhanced computed tomography (CT).
(**B**) Contrast-enhanced magnetic resonance image (MRI) of metastatic intracranial tumor. MRI shows "rind" of metastatic deposit around brain that was invisible on CT due to bone artifact.

*Abbreviations*: CT, computed tomography; MRI, magnetic resonance imaging.

*Source*: Courtesy of Scripps Memorial Hospital, Department of Radiology, La Jolla, CA.

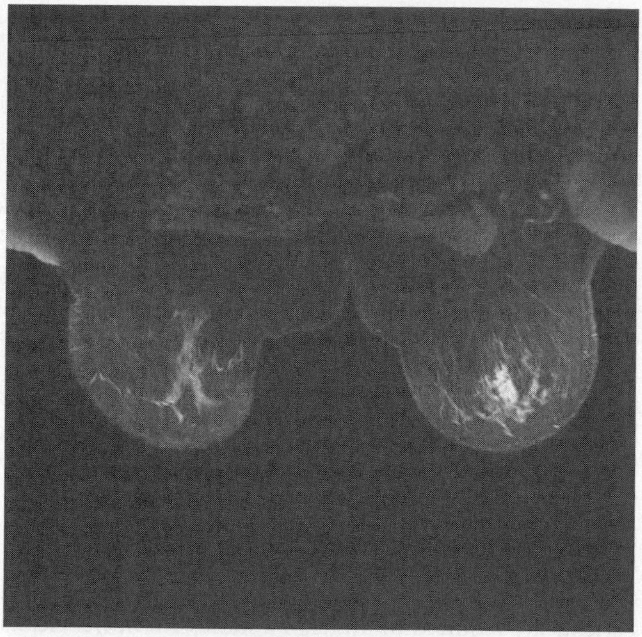

**FIGURE 8-8**

Bilateral breast MRI. After biopsy of suspicious mass noted in figures 8.1 and 8.2, bilateral breast MRI shows an irregular area of enhancement in the upper central portion of the right breast at the 12 o'clock location. These findings are consistent with residual invasive carcinoma. In the left breast, several foci of nonspecific enhancement are noted scattered in the parenchyma. These are usually benign and due to areas of adenosis.

*Source*: Courtesy of the Comprehensive Breast Center at Wellmont Holston Valley Hospital, Kingsport, TN, an American College of Radiology accredited Breast Imaging Center of Excellence.

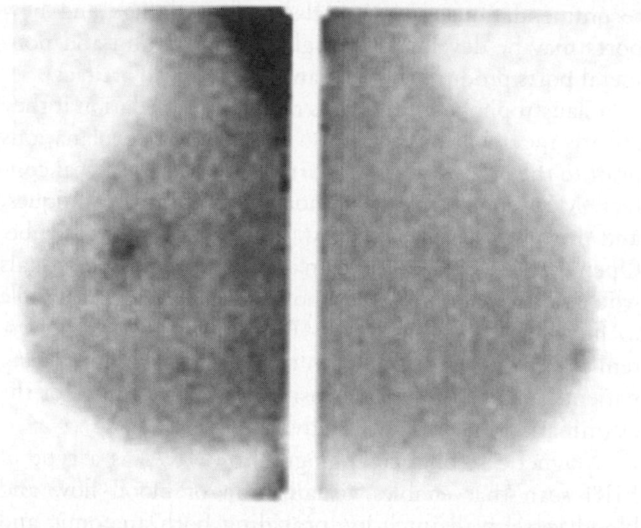

**FIGURE 8-9**

Breast-specific gamma imaging. Dense focal abnormal accumulation of radionuclide in the upper central portion of the right breast corresponds with the area of concern noted on the mammogram (Figure 8-1) and the breast ultrasound (Figure 8-2). This finding generates an extremely high degree of suspicion for infiltrating malignancy. The slight heterogeneity of the left breast is likely within normal limits. The radiologist suggested magnetic resonance imaging of the breast to determine extent of disease and possible coexisting disease prior to surgery.

*Source*: Courtesy of the Comprehensive Breast Center at Wellmont Holston Valley Hospital, Kingsport, TN, an American College of Radiology accredited Breast Imaging Center of Excellence.

biopsy; of these cases, a cancer was found in 14 patients and a high-risk lesion was seen in 13 others.[74] This study demonstrated that in these high-risk women MRI was more sensitive than mammogram in detecting early breast lesions. The NCCN recommends that high-risk women (such as those with a genetic mutation indicating hereditary predisposition for breast cancer) are screened yearly with mammography and breast MRI beginning at age 25.[75] MRI of the breast should be performed between day 6 and 16 of a woman's menstrual cycle because the luteal phase of the cycle is associated with an increase in estrogen and progesterone leading to enhancement on MRI scanning, increasing false-positive findings.[76] Hormone replacement therapy (HRT) will cause similar results and consideration should be given to scanning 2 to 3 months after discontinuation of HRT.[77]

Breast-specific gamma imaging (BSGI) may be used as an alternative to breast MRI. While breast MRI has high sensitivity in diagnosing a breast cancer, it has limited specificity. BSGI provides physiologic, nuclear medicine imaging utilizing a high-resolution, small-field of view, breast specific gamma camera.[78] It is able to diagnosis lesions as small as 2 mm. It has been shown that BSGI has equivalent sensitivity and higher specificity than breast MRI.[79] Figure 8-9 depicts abnormal activity in a breast corresponding to the suspicious mammography findings in Figure 8-1 and ultrasound findings noted in Figure 8-2.[80,81] It also has superior sensitivity for the detection of ductal carcinoma in situ when compared with breast MRI or mammography.[79]

Magnetic resonance imaging does have some limitations to its utility. A serious injury to the patient could occur from any ferrous metal in the body. This limitation could exclude use of this technology in acutely ill patients with life-support or monitoring devices. Nonferrous metallic implants may produce artifacts that distort the MRI image but are generally safe for the patient. In patients with implants that have strong ferromagnetism, MRI should be avoided.[82] The radiologist should be informed of any cardiac pacemakers, implanted cardioverter-defibrillators, implanted venous access devices, or cochlear implants, although these are rarely contraindications.[21,83] Adjustments may be made to reduce metal susceptibility artifacts by the radiologist. Patients with tattooed eyeliner may experience irritation and edema around the eye following the procedure. Camp-Sorrell identifies ports causing the least artifact but concludes that attention must be paid to the manufacturer's recommendations, as materials tend to change and new ports may be developed.[84] High-grade titanium and nonmetal ports produce the least amount of or no artifact.

Claustrophobic individuals may require sedation if they are to undergo MRI, but also benefit from explanations prior to the procedure, a support person nearby, verbal contact, MRI-compatible headphones, relaxation techniques, and prisms or mirrors to allow a view outside of the tube. Open MRI facilities offer an alternative for individuals who are claustrophobic or who are very large and unable to fit inside the cylindrical MRI tube.[85] Open MRI system places the patient between two plates, accommodating patients such as these. The cost of MRI and length of the examination may also be disadvantages.

Magnetic resonance angiography (MRA) is a type of MRI scan that enables visualization of blood flow and blood vessel wall integrity, providing both anatomic and hemodynamic information.[86] It is used to identify aneurysms, detect atherosclerosis, define injuries or disease in blood vessels, and to evaluate arteries feeding a tumor and veins draining a tumor. Contrast is often used. MRA is the preferred diagnostic test for inferior vena cava, renal, and portal vein thrombosis and has the ability to distinguish between tumor and thrombus.[87]

## INVASIVE DIAGNOSTIC TECHNIQUES

### Endoscopy

Endoscopy is a method to directly visualize the interior of a hollow viscous by the insertion of an endoscope into a body cavity or opening. The endoscope contains fiber-optic glass bundles that transmit light and then return an image to the optical head of the endoscope. The instrument may be rigid or flexible. Visual inspection, tissue biopsy, cytologic aspiration, staging the extent of disease, and excision of pathologic processes are possible through the endoscope.

By passing a flexible scope through the mouth, endoscopic examinations can visualize directly the larynx, upper airway passages and bronchial tree, esophagus, stomach, and upper duodenum. Visualization of the distal sigmoid colon, rectum, and anal canal is performed by means of a rigid scope. The entire large intestine can be viewed with a flexible colonoscope that is inserted anally. Endoscopic retrograde cholangiopancreatography (ERCP) combines the diagnostic procedures of endoscopy and contrast-enhanced radiography to evaluate biliary tract obstruction and pancreatic masses.

The endoscopic ultrasound (EUS) has proved superior to other imaging modalities for assessing direct depth of tumor invasion and local lymph node status for esophageal, gastric, and colon malignancy.[88] The EUS is capable of distinguishing benign from malignant lesions, assists in staging and in establishing operability and surgical approach, and in determining response or recurrence.[89] The best method to assess the upper GI tract for malignancy is the upper esophagogastroduodenoscopy (EGD).[88] The EGD produces excellent images and provides a means to biopsy tissues or remove polyps during this procedure. The EGD is also used for screening persons at high risk for UGI malignancy, as in Barrett's esophagus or FAP. This procedure also has therapeutic applications including dilation of strictures, stent placements, and direct tumor therapy.[88]

Colonoscopy is a fiber-optic endoscopic study that visualizes the lining of the large intestine. Evidence-based guidelines recommend colonoscopy as part of routine screening for colon cancer as noted by the American Cancer Society, the NCCN, the National Cancer Institute, as well as other professional organizations.[90–92] It also is indicated for follow-up of a positive fecal occult blood test.[21] This procedure also provides a means for biopsy or polyp removal. Patients are required to undergo a successful bowel cleansing prior to the procedure; failure to cleanse the bowel adequately makes visualization impossible.

Endoscopic retrograde cholangiopancreatography is an endoscopic procedure that uses contrast medium injected through the ampullae of Vater. This procedure examines the duodenum, and biliary and pancreatic ductal systems. More than 85% of the biliary and pancreatic ducts may be observed with this procedure.[21] In oncology, ECRP is utilized in the diagnosis as well as treatment of pancreatic and biliary cancer. ECRP can relieve biliary obstruction by providing a means of stent insertion.[88]

The cervix and vagina are directly visualized with the magnification lens of the colposcope. Peritoneoscopy or laparoscopy permits assessment of surfaces within the peritoneal cavity by the insertion of a peritoneoscope through a small incision below the umbilicus. Thoracoscopy allows visualization of the visceral and parietal pleura, mediastinum, and diaphragm by means of a thoracoscope passed through an incision in the midaxillary line of the sixth to the eighth intercostal space. The direct visualization of the tissues and organs of the mediastinum is performed by passing an endoscope into the mediastinum through a small incision above the manubrium.

### Procedures for determining extent of disease

*Laparoscopy* is a minimally invasive procedure allowing visualization inside the abdominal cavity via a laparoscope. The abdomen is insufflated with carbon dioxide and a laparoscope is inserted through an infraumbilical port. Laparoscopy has been used to diagnose, stage, and treat a wide variety of cancers, including lymphoma and gastrointestinal, urologic, and gynecologic malignancies.[93,94] The development of high resolution monitors and instrumentation as well as greater surgical experience have increased utilization of this procedure. Laparoscopy enables visualization of the abdominal cavity and lesions, and in evaluating adenopathy and liver abnormalities. It also offers the opportunity to visualize the diaphragm and peritoneal surfaces.

Patients facing a diagnosis of cancer of the pancreas, stomach, or esophagus have benefited from the use of laparoscopy rather than CT and US to determine resectability and nodal status. The surgical approach using this method decreases the need for, and may prevent an unnecessary laparotomy. Accurate diagnosis and staging of Hodgkin's lymphoma can be completed with current laparoscopic capabilities. Staging laparotomies have decreased by 70% in these patients due to the advent of laparoscopic liver and spleen biopsies.[95] Advantages of using laparoscopy include a shorter hospital stay and recovery time, which lowers costs, along with decreased pain and a quicker return to activities of daily living. The future of laparoscopy holds promise with advanced surgical training, precise instrumentation, and gathering of evidence-based data.

*Mediastinoscopy* is an invasive procedure performed under general anesthesia with a mediastinoscope inserted at the suprasternal notch along the trachea into the mediastinum. The mediastinal structure and lymph nodes are visualized and biopsies may be obtained of lymph nodes or any suspicious lesions.[21] This procedure will permit palpation of paratracheal and carinal lymph nodes as well. It is the test of choice for the evaluation of mediastinal lymph nodes for metastases in lung cancer.[96] It is often used when other diagnostic tests have failed to confirm the suspected diagnosis. It is also a means of determining stage of disease.

*Bronchoscopy* is performed by a flexible fiber-optic or a rigid metal bronchoscope.[21] Bronchoscopy will provide visualization of the larynx, trachea, and bronchi. Biopsies and bronchial washings may be obtained during this procedure. Fluoroscopy assists in the evaluation of distal lesions. Bronchoscopy is used for diagnosis, removal of tumors, and staging. It requires intravenous sedation or general anesthesia.[96]

*Video-assisted thoracoscopy* is a valuable tool for oncologic diagnosis and management.[96] This invasive procedure requires general anesthesia and single-lung ventilation, but is generally well-tolerated.[97] Video-assisted thoracoscopy provides visualization of the entire visceral and parietal pleural surfaces.[29] Video-assisted thoracoscopy is often used to diagnose malignant pleural effusions, particularly when other methods fail.

## Biopsy

A diagnosis of cancer requires histologic tissue confirmation, usually as a result of a biopsy. The importance of obtaining accurate histologic or cytologic proof of malignancy cannot be overstated. Treatment decisions for cancers arising within the same organ differ on the basis of the histopathology report. An example is the very different treatment regimens for small cell cancer of the lung and adenocarcinoma of the lung. Exactly what tissue should be biopsied depends on several factors: the clinical status of the person, his or her willingness to undergo invasive procedures, the size and location of the identified tumor, and the amount of tissue needed by the pathologist for analysis. The site selected for biopsy should be the most likely place to obtain adequate tissue and represent the least risk to the patient.[22,98] Once the pathologist has diagnosed a cancer, the practitioner examines this information in terms of the clinical presentation, known natural history of the cancer named, physical examination, patient history, adjunctive laboratory data, tumor imaging findings, and clinical judgment.

The cytologic examination of aspirated fluid, secretions, scrapings, or washings of body cavities may reveal malignant cells that have exfoliated from a primary or metastatic tumor. Tissue will not be obtained by this method, however, and the pathologist's ability to establish the primary site of the malignancy may be limited. Cancer of the cervix is one example of a malignancy that is successfully detected by the cytologic examination of cells acquired from a Papanicolaou (Pap) smear.[21]

There are several different types of biopsy procedures including fine-needle aspiration biopsy, core-needle biopsy, stereotactic biopsy, excisional and incisional biopsies, needle localization, and bone marrow biopsy.[98] The fine-needle aspiration biopsy, guided by palpation or an imaging technique, is used extensively and is available in the ambulatory setting. By removing cells from a suspicious area, this type of biopsy provides not only cytologic information but also microhistologic information if adequate tissue fragments are obtained. Accuracy rates are over 90%, but a negative biopsy does not necessarily rule out a malignancy.[98–100] Table 8-5 provides general instructions for preparing the patient for an image-guided fine-needle aspiration biopsy.[21,98]

Core-needle biopsy is retrieval of a small core of tissue, using a specialized designed spring-loaded needle.[98,100] This biopsy, like the fine-needle biopsy, may be done under local anesthesia, making it cost-effective and available in ambulatory settings. Both of these types of biopsies may still require open biopsy if pathology is inconclusive or negative.[98] At times, a vacuum-assisted core-needle biopsy is required, utilizing suction to obtain tissue samples through a probe.

Needle localization uses a small wire with a hooked end to mark a nonpalpable mass for open biopsy.[98] Stereotactic localization is another diagnostic tool that utilizes CT or MRI to establish the coordinates of a lesion and accurately position a needle for the tissue biopsy. Stereotactic breast biopsy of nonpalpable lesions is comparable to conventional needle-localization surgical biopsy, with a sensitivity of 90% to 95% for breast cancer detection.[101] Stereotactic brain biopsy of suspicious lesions is a relatively safe and

**TABLE 8-5**

| Instructions for Preparing the Patient for Image-Guided Fine-Needle Aspiration Biopsy |
|---|
| • Contrast agent may be required—intravenous or oral |
| • Intravenous line established as a precaution or for sedation |
| • Sedatives may be offered |
| • Vital signs and oximetry will be monitored if intravenous sedation is used |
| • Some pain may be experienced; local anesthetic is used |
| • Skin at biopsy site is cleansed, and the needle inserted |
| • Needle position is established by an imaging technique (eg, CT, ultrasound, or chest fluoroscopy) |
| • Syringe is attached to the needle, and the fluid and tissue are aspirated |
| • Patient is observed for infection, bleeding, or increase in pain |

quick procedure. A stereotactic head frame is fixed to the skull under local anesthesia, the lesion is scanned for localizing landmarks (including the location of arteries and vessels), a small hole is made in the skull, and the biopsy is directed by an instrument attached to the frame.

A bone marrow biopsy and aspiration is vital to the diagnostic workup of hematologic disorders and malignancies, as well as some infectious diseases. The presence, absence, and the ratio of marrow cells are examined from the specimen obtained. Diagnostic abnormal cell characteristics and patterns may identify leukemias, multiple myeloma, anemias, metastatic cancers, myeloproliferative disorders, agranulocytosis, among other disease states.

Incisional biopsy removes a part of a tumor for diagnosis. Excisional biopsy is total removal of all suspicious tissue. Incisional biopsies are generally selected for the diagnosis of large tumors that will require major surgery for complete removal. Advantages of incisional biopsy are a smaller incision site and ability to perform the procedure in an ambulatory setting with local anesthesia, although at times anesthesia may be required. Excisional biopsy may still be required following incisional biopsy if no malignancy is diagnosed but clinical suspicion of cancer remains high. Excisional biopsy is a more invasive procedure, most often requiring sedation or anesthesia and usually leaves a larger incision than with other biopsy methods.[98,100] In some cases, such as tumors of the lip, nose, ear, or breast, excisional biopsy alone will be definitive therapy. The pathologist and the surgeon will determine whether the extent of the excisional biopsy is sufficient to eliminate the possibility of residual disease or whether more extensive surgery is indicated.

Cooperation and skill are required of the nurse, surgeon, pathologist, and affiliated pathology lab to ensure that an accurate diagnosis is made. Local or topical anesthesia is commonly used. Table 8-6 describes several types of biopsies, including: (1) aspiration needles, (2) cutting or core needles, (3) large cutting needles, and (4) automated biopsy systems (biopsy guns). Some needles have carriers that shield and guide the actual biopsy needle, cup, or punch used to obtain the specimen.[98] The carrier reduces the possibility that the needle tract will become contaminated with tumor cells from the specimen as the needle is withdrawn. Fine-needle biopsy needles are usually small bore, 20 to 21 gauge. Core biopsy needles are larger, generally 14 to 16 gauge. Stereotactic biopsy usually requires 12 to 14 gauge needles.[98]

Fluoroscopy, ultrasound, or CT is often used to guide the clinician during core biopsy procedures. Local anesthesia is used. Hematoma, infection, pain, and incision site complications are post-biopsy considerations.

For a definitive diagnosis of malignancy, it is imperative that the pathologist receive an adequate, representative, and well-preserved tissue specimen. A cytologic or histologic report that is negative for malignancy may suggest a specimen inadequate for diagnostic evaluation, necessitating repeat biopsy. Only a complete excisional biopsy can exclude malignancy with certainty. When the results of a biopsy are equivocal, the specimen should be sent to an outside source for a second evaluation. The Armed Forces Institute of Pathology in Washington, D.C., is used by pathologists worldwide as a reference laboratory and for review.

Not infrequently, the biopsied tissue will confirm malignancy, but the primary site or tissue of origin cannot be established by the pathologist or the clinician. An example is the individual who undergoes biopsy of a cervical node and is diagnosed with squamous cell carcinoma but for whom a thorough examination of the chest and head and neck area fails to yield the source of the malignancy. The goals for pursuing the primary site in this situation are discussed later in this chapter in "Tumors of Unknown Origin."

### Surgical biopsy techniques

There are many different surgical biopsy techniques. Many diagnostic imaging tests may facilitate a biopsy. For example, endoscopy, as noted earlier in this chapter, may be employed to biopsy the gastrointestinal, genitourinary, or pulmonary systems. Biopsies may be guided by ultrasound, CT, or MRI.

Sentinel lymph node biopsy (SLNB) is a technique that determines metastasis to the first draining lymph node prior to surgical removal, thus avoiding the need for total regional lymph node dissection of unaffected nodes and providing staging information.[21,102] The surgeon injects a radiolabeled colloid or isosulfan blue around the tumor and then 2 to 6 hours later, lymphatic flow is followed radiographically or intraoperatively to the first draining blue or radioactive node. This lymph node is examined for the presence of metastatic disease and further lymph node dissection is based on this biopsy. The injection may be painful and patients must be prepared adequately.[103] The SLNB is used in breast, colorectal, and penile cancers and melanoma.

**TABLE 8-6**

**Approaches for Biopsy**

| Type | What Used For | Where Done | Rationale |
|---|---|---|---|
| ***Needle Biopsy*** | | | |
| *Fine-needle aspiration* (21–22 g needle 5-cc syringe): local anesthesia | Solid, palpable lesion (ie, breast mass, thyroid nodule) | Outpatient setting<br>Operating room | Involves only small amount of trauma to tissue, so if positive then surgical procedure is avoided; used when there is a high level of suspicion of malignancy |
| *Sterotaxic fine-needle aspiration* (21–22 g needle, sterotaxic equipment): local anesthesia | Solid, nonpalpable lesion (ie, mammographic abnormality) | Outpatient setting<br>Radiology center | Same as for fine-needle aspiration, but able to sample small, *nonpalpable* lesions |
| *Core-needle biopsy* (special cutting needle): local anesthesia; can use ultrasound for guidance | Solid accessible tumor | Outpatient setting | Removes larger amount of tissue than fine-needle aspiration; may allow for more information (ie, hormone receptor tests) |
| ***Surgical Biopsy*** | | | |
| *Excisional biopsy*: usually local anesthesia | Solid, palpable mass (ie, melanoma, breast mass) | Day surgery | Attempt is made to remove the whole mass only, without regard to clear margin; result should be cosmetically acceptable |
| *Incisional biopsy:* usually local anesthesia | Solid, palpable large mass (ie, large, ulcerating, or bleeding mass) | Day surgery | Biopsy is for diagnosis; mass is too large to remove without major surgery; may bleed profusely |
| *Endoscopy* (special endoscope): may use sedation | Solid mass in an accessible lumen (ie, colon, esophagus) | Outpatient setting<br>Day surgery | May be for diagnosis or treatment; avoids surgical trauma |

## SUMMARY

Rapid growth has occurred over the past few years in the technology of diagnostic imaging and biopsy procedures. This increase in healthcare technology contributes to the substantial increase in medical spending, which is largely funded by the public sector.[104] Cost constraints have required increased scrutiny and consideration of the best test or procedure for a particular clinical consideration. Clinicians must not only consider what is the most appropriate for a patient, but also which is the most cost effective.

## CLASSIFICATION AND NOMENCLATURE

### BASIC TERMINOLOGY

The terms *cancer* and *tumor* often are used interchangeably and inappropriately and can be misleading for patients, families, and professionals. A *tumor* is a swelling or mass of tissue that may be benign or malignant. *Cancer,* synonymous with *malignant neoplasm,* is an uncontrolled "new growth" capable of metastasis and invasion that threatens host survival. Cancer is caused by multiple DNA sequence changes over a period of time that result in mutations of genes that control normal cell functions.[105] These changes can occur due to hereditary predisposition, environmental disruptions, and/or carcinogens, including viruses.[106]

The term *primary tumor* is used to describe the original histologic site of tumorigenesis. A *secondary,* or metastatic, *tumor* resembles the primary tumor histologically, but sometimes may be so anaplastic as to obscure the cell of origin. A *second primary lesion* refers to an additional, histologically separate malignant neoplasm in the same patient. Although this is a relatively unusual occurrence, it must be excluded at the time of an apparent recurrence. Tables of probability for recurrence exist to guide the clinician in making these determinations. A general rule is always to biopsy the first recurrence, because it may actually represent a new, curable or treatable malignancy—for example, a patient with a history of breast cancer who presents with suspicious lymph nodes and is found on biopsy to have lymphoma. Unfortunately, some recurrences present in sites where the morbidity from biopsy is so significant that the lesion is treated without tissue confirmation—for example, a woman with breast cancer who presents with a vertebral pedicle lesion.

## BENIGN AND MALIGNANT TUMOR CHARACTERISTICS

Survival of any tissue or tumor is dependent on the balance between cell proliferation and cell death.[107] Both normal and malignant cells need oxygen and other nutrients for their survival and growth, each cell dependent for this upon nearby blood capillaries.[108] There are, however, certain biologic, histologic, and cytologic characteristics that distinguish a benign tumor from a malignant tumor. The signature property of malignant cells is the ability to metastasize and invade other cells.

In general, the following features distinguish benign tumors from those that are malignant. The *benign tumor* is relatively slow growing. Tumor stasis or regression may occur. Growth occurs as the tumor expands locally within a capsule of fibrous tissue. Benign tumors do not invade adjacent tissues, destroy normal tissue, or metastasize elsewhere in the body. Although death from a benign tumor is rare, distressing symptoms may result from a tumor's pressure on vital organs or from ectopic hormone production. Cytologic examination reveals uniform, well-differentiated cells that resemble those of the adult tissue of origin and demonstrate little or no anaplasia and rare mitoses.

In contrast, the *malignant tumor* is characterized by its generally high mitotic rate, rapid growth, and disregard for normal growth limitations. Malignant tumors are almost never encapsulated. The malignant cells invade surrounding tissue, lymphatic vessels, and blood vessels and metastasize to distant sites. The ability to metastasize to other organs causes 90% of deaths in patients with cancer.[109] Malignant cells are anaplastic, vary in morphologic characteristics within the same tumor, are more poorly differentiated, and have abnormal and inconstant numbers of chromosomes.

## TUMOR CLASSIFICATION SYSTEM

The most relevant classification systems will universally communicate clinical and prognostic information. Tumors may be classified not only by their biologic behavior (benign vs premalignant vs malignant), but also by their tissue of origin.[99]

Virtually every cell type in the body is capable of transforming into a malignant cell. It is fairly well accepted that the malignant cell derives from a postembryonic cell that is arrested in the process of differentiation.[107] Most tumors retain sufficient characteristics—such as function and structure of the normal, differentiated cell—to allow recognition of the type of tissue from which they were derived, which is the basis for the classification of human tumors by tissue type (Table 8-7).[110–112]

**TABLE 8-7**

**Selected Benign and Malignant Neoplasms Listed by Histogenic Classification**

| Tissue of Origin | Benign Neoplasm | Malignant Neoplasm |
|---|---|---|
| ***Epithelial (Endodermal)*** | | |
| Squamous | Squamous cell papilloma | Squamous cell or epidermoid carcinoma |
| Glandular | Adenoma<br>Papilloma<br>Cystadenoma | Adenocarcinoma<br>Papillary carcinoma<br>Cystadenocarcinoma |
| Respiratory tract | | Bronchogenic carcinoma |
| Renal epithelium | Renal tubular adenoma | Renal cell carcinoma (hypheremphroma) |
| Urinary tract | Transitional cell papilloma | Transitional cell carcinoma |
| Placental epithelium | Hydatidiform mole | Choriocarcinoma |
| Testicular epithelium | | Seminoma<br>Embryonal carcinoma |
| Liver | Liver cell adenoma | Hepatocellular carcinoma (hepatoma) |
| Biliary tree | Cholangioma | Cholangiocarcinoma |
| Stomach | Gastric polyp | Gastric carcinoma |
| Colon | Colonic polyp | Adenocarcinoma of the colon |
| ***Mesenchymal (Mesodermal)*** | | |
| *Connective* | | |
| Fibrous tissue | Fibroma | Fibrosarcoma |
| Adipose tissue | Lipoma | Liposarcoma |
| Cartilage | Chondroma | Chondrosarcoma |
| Bone | Osteoma | Osteosarcoma |
| *Muscle* | | |
| Smooth muscle | Leiomyoma | Leiomyosarcoma |
| Striated muscle | Rhabdomyoma | Rhabdomyosarcoma |
| *Endothelial* | | |
| Blood vessels | Hemangioma | Hemangiosarcoma |
| Lymphatic vessels | Lymphangioma | Lymphangiosarcoma |
| *Hematopoietic and lymphoreticular* | | |
| Hematopoietic cells | | Leukemias |
| Lymphoid tissue | | Lymphomas<br>Hodgkin's disease |
| Plasma cells | | Plasmacytoma (multiple myeloma) |
| ***Neural (Ectodermal)*** | | |
| Meninges | Meningioma | Meningeal sarcoma |
| Glia | Astrocytoma | Glioblastoma multiforme |
| Nerve cells | Ganglioneuroma | Neuroblastoma<br>Medulloblastoma |
| Melanocytes | Nevus | Malignant melanoma |
| ***Mixed Tissues*** | | |
| Kidney | Teratoma | Teratocarcinoma |
| Salivary gland | | Wilms' tumor |
| | Mixed tumor of salivary glands (pleomorphic adenoma) | Malignant mixed tumor at salivary gland |

### TUMORS OF UNKNOWN ORIGIN

Two to five percent of patients diagnosed with cancer each year are found to have a malignancy from an unknown primary site.[1,113] Most frequently, the histologic classification will be adenocarcinoma, but the site of origin may never be determined, even on autopsy. The prognosis in such cases is poor, primarily because predicting disease behavior and response to treatment depends on proper identification of the disease. The overall median survival of persons with an unknown primary site ranges from 9 to 12 months.[113] Investigators have found several variables that can predict prognosis in patients with tumors of unknown primary. These variables include serum albumin and lymphopenia,[114] performance status and serum LDH,[115] and presence of liver metastases.[116] Pathologic subtype is found to impact median survival time as well, with patients with adenocarcinoma having the lowest median survival time (9 months) and those with neuroendocrine carcinoma the highest median survival time (33 months).[113]

The goal of proceeding with a diagnostic investigation in this situation is to rapidly identify those malignancies, even if they are disseminated, that are potentially curable or palliated with known, effective treatment.[113] For example, lymphomas and germ-cell tumors are potentially curable with systemic chemotherapy. Lesions in the nasopharynx may be cured with radiation. Local complications such as bowel obstruction, spinal cord compression, and pathologic fractures can be palliated with surgery or radiation treatment, even when the primary site of malignancy is unknown. Hormonal therapy may be recommended if the presumptive diagnosis, based on tumor markers or hormone receptor analysis, is breast, prostate, or endometrial malignancy.

A rigorous patient history and physical examination is one of the most important tools in the workup of the patient with an unknown primary tumor. Initial laboratory evaluation includes a complete blood cell count, urinalysis, and liver function tests. Tumor markers may prove useful. Thorough pathologic evaluation, including molecular markers, is vital. Diagnostic imaging will be directed by patient history and physical examination, as well as the information gained from laboratory studies and pathologic evaluation.[113]

Patients and their families who are facing cancer from an unknown source present unique challenges for the nurse. Not only do they need information and preparation for extensive imaging and laboratory testing, but they also need support when these tests fail to yield a definitive diagnosis. It is often hoped, though does not necessarily prove true, that a known primary source of malignancy will be more treatable or curable than an unknown primary source. Coping with any cancer diagnosis is difficult. Coping with an "unknown" cancer accentuates the feelings of loss of control, anxiety, and frustration. The nurse can offer the greatest assistance by identifying psychosocial concerns and available support systems early in the diagnostic period, clarifying and reinforcing known information and the rationale for extensive testing, and providing hope and reassurance that treatment is offered for the most probable and most treatable source of malignancy.[117]

## STAGING AND GRADING CLASSIFICATIONS

### STAGING THE EXTENT OF THE DISEASE

The staging process is a method of classifying a malignancy by the extent of its spread within the body. It is a clinical and histologic determination that depends on the natural course of each particular type of cancer. Staging is based on the premise that cancers with similar histologic features and sites of origin will extend and metastasize in a predictable manner. Although most staging classifications are based on the anatomical extent of disease, other criteria are included for specific malignancies. For thyroid cancer, the age of the patient and the histologic diagnosis (papillary, follicular, medullary, or anaplastic) are included in the staging system.[19] In the staging of prostate cancer, soft-tissue sarcomas, primary malignant tumors of the bone, and brain tumors, the histopathologic grade of the tumor is significant.

There are multiple objectives of solid tumor staging, but the most important is to provide the necessary information for individual treatment planning. In addition, uniform staging procedures reveal prognosis, evaluate various treatment modalities, facilitate the exchange of information, compare mortality and morbidity statistics among various treatment centers, promote exchange of information among treatment centers, and stratify individuals who may be eligible for clinical trials.[19]

With the goal of developing an internationally consistent system of staging solid tumor malignancy, the TNM committee of the International Union Against Cancer (UICC) and the American Joint Committee on Cancer (AJCC) have agreed on the TNM staging system. This system classifies solid tumors by the anatomical extent of disease, as determined clinically and histologically. Three categories are quantified, with gradations representing progressive tumor size or involvement. First, the extent of the primary tumor (T) is evaluated on the basis of depth of invasion, surface spread, and tumor size. Second, the absence or presence and extent of regional lymph node (N) metastasis are considered, with attention to the size and location of the nodes. Third, the absence or presence of distant metastasis (M) is assessed. A three-letter abbreviation may specify the site of metastasis. For example, M1 PUL denotes pulmonary metastasis. The TNM system is further classified by whether the assessment is obtained clinically (cTNM or TNM), after pathologic review (pTNM), at the time of retreatment (rTNM), or on autopsy (aTNM). For reporting purposes, the TNM stage classification remains constant throughout the disease process. Progression of disease does not change the initial stage of disease. Table 8-8 presents the nomenclature of the TNM system for classification.[19]

It is important to distinguish the cTNM, based on a clinical exam, from the pTNM, which is determined after surgery when the true extent of the disease is known and treatment decisions can be made. This is particularly true in breast cancer, where the lymph node status (pN) is the most precise prognostic indicator and directs adjuvant therapy decisions. Oncology nurses are well aware of the support needed by the woman with breast cancer in the first 24 to 48 hours after lymphadenectomy while she is awaiting the pathologist's review of lymph nodes.[118,119] Another example occurs in the treatment of prostate cancer when the discovery of tumor in the pelvic lymph nodes (pN) at the time of surgery precludes the anticipated radical prostatectomy.

After numerical values are assigned to the T, N, and M categories, they are clustered into one of four stages (I through IV), or stage 0 for carcinoma in situ. Stage IV consistently includes distant metastases (M1) and predicts the worst prognosis. All tumor sites are grouped differently on the basis of characteristics of the disease.

Several established and accepted staging classifications other than TNM exist for particular malignancies. Melanomas have been staged not only by the level of invasion of the primary lesion but also by lesion thickness—both major determinants of prognosis. The Clark levels of invasion along with Breslow's measurement of vertical thickness are universal staging systems. The TNM system, which is now in use and highly valued in clinical practice, encompasses four stages utilizing both microstaging classifications for tumor assessment. For many years, the staging system of choice for colorectal cancer had been the Duke's system, which classifies tumors by their depth of invasion and presence of nodal metastasis. Only recently has the TNM system become widely accepted and incorporated into this medical arena. The issue of which staging system is preferred remains unresolved. The International Federation of Gynecology and Obstetrics has an accepted staging system for cervical and endometrial cancers. Hodgkin's disease and non-Hodgkin's lymphoma are routinely described by the Revised European-American Classification of Lymphoid Neoplasms (REAL) introduced by the International Lymphoma Study Group (ILSG)[19] The World Health Organization (WHO) updated its Classification of Diseases of the Hematopoietic and Lymphoid Systems and adopted the REAL classification for Lymphoid malignancies (REAL/WHO).[19] The Ann Arbor classification categorizes anatomic staging (Stages I-IV). Cancers of the brain are not entirely suited to the TNM system because there are no lymphatic structures with which to categorize nodal (N) involvement.

Nonsolid tumors do not conform to solid tumor staging principles because of their disseminated nature.

**TABLE 8-8**

**TNM Classification System for Describing the Anatomical Extent of Disease**

| | |
|---|---|
| **TNM Definitions** | |
| **T** | |
| Primary tumor | |
| TX | Primary tumor cannot be assessed |
| T0 | No evidence of primary tumor |
| Tis | Carcinoma in situ |
| T1, T2, T3, T4, | Increasing size and/or local extent of the primary tumor |
| **N** | |
| Regional lymph modes | |
| NX | Regional lymph modes cannot be assessed |
| N0 | No regional lymph node metastasis |
| N1, N2, N3 | Increasing involvement of regional lymph modes |
| **M** | |
| Distant metastasis | |
| MX | Presence of distant metastasis cannot be assessed |
| M0 | No distant metastasis |
| M1 | Distant metastasis |
| **TNM Classifications** | |
| cTNM or TNM | *Clinical classification:* Based on information obtained from the physical examination, laboratory and imaging studies, endoscopy, biopsy, and surgical exploration. Clinical staging uses all information available before the initiation of definitive treatment. |
| pTNM | *Pathologic classification:* Based on information acquired before treatment, supplemented or modified by information from surgery and the pathologic examination of a resected specimen. This includes resected tumor (pT), lymph modes (pN), and distant metastasis (pM). |
| rTNM | *Retreatment classification:* Based on all information available after a disease—free interval or at the time of a second—look surgery. The extent or absence of disease recurrence is documented before retreatment planning is begun. |
| aTNM | *Autopsy classification:* Based on all information available at the time of a postmortem examination. It is helpful in answering questions about the tumor's response to treatment, recurrence patterns, and the extent of disease at the time of death. |

Leukemias are best classified according to their predominant cell types (ie, lymphocytic or nonlymphocytic), cell maturation, and acute or chronic nature. Clinical, morphologic, histochemical, and immunologic findings help to define favorable or unfavorable prognostic categories in acute lymphoblastic leukemia. The French-American-British classification has clinical and prognostic significance in acute myeloblastic leukemia but is not a staging system. In chronic lymphocytic leukemia, two-staging systems exist: the Rai classification system and the Binet classification system. For patients with myeloma, a three-stage classification system, the Durie–Salmon staging system, correlates M proteins with myeloma cell mass to provide prognostic information.[19,120] Researchers and clinicians continue to validate current AJCC staging systems and propose modifications for the future. Changes are likely to incorporate genetic and biochemical markers as well as other prognostic indicators. Additions such as this have important implications for patients with early-stage disease (based on anatomical staging) who are actually at risk for recurrence based on other measurements of malignant potential and who will need further treatment. For example, the 30% of women with node-negative breast cancer who eventually experience a recurrence represent one subset of individuals with early-stage disease who have a less favorable prognosis. The staging system of the future will encompass an estimation of risk (of local extension and distant metastases) based on the sum of risks associated with anatomical stage, morphologic grade, biologic grade, and genetic potential.[121,122] In breast cancer, it could include the TNM stage, degree of morphologic anaplasia, estrogen and progesterone receptor status, S-phase fraction and DNA ploidy, epidermal growth factor receptors, *HER-2* or *ERB2*, and *MYC* oncogene expression.[121,122]

## PATIENT PERFORMANCE CLASSIFICATION

A multitude of factors affect treatment decisions at the time of diagnosis, with the patient's physical condition being a primary consideration. Patients who are bedridden are much less likely to respond to treatment than are those who are asymptomatic and able to maintain the activities of daily living. Performance scales that measure a person's functional status are used frequently in the eligibility criteria for cooperative group clinical trials and also periodically to evaluate the effects of treatment and disease. It is important to assess whether aggressive, toxic treatment protocols actually will permit people to feel better and to maintain their optimal functional status. The most prevalent performance scales are the Karnofsky Performance Status scale, the Eastern Cooperative Oncology Group (ECOG) scale, and the WHO scale.[123–127] The three scales are compared in Table 8-9. Nurses need to be familiar with the scoring systems, as they may be able to contribute the most accurate information to a primarily subjective rating.

## GRADING

Grading a malignant neoplasm is a method of classification based on histopathologic characteristics of the tissue. The pathologist assesses the aggressiveness or degree of malignancy of tumor cells by comparing the cellular anaplasia, differentiation, and mitotic activity with those of the cells' normal counterparts. Specific characteristics vary with each type of cancer.

The objective of grading a tumor is to quantify information so as to assist with treatment planning and prognostic determinations. For selected tumors, the grade is considered more significant than anatomical staging in terms of prognostic value and treatment. The histology of tumors that affect the brain and spinal cord is by far the most important variable with regard to prognosis, and in many cases it determines the treatment modalities that are employed. In soft tissue sarcomas, the grade is the primary determinant of stage of disease and of prognosis.

Two grading systems are commonly seen. One descriptively identifies the tumor as well-differentiated (ie, retaining most of the morphologic features and behavior of the normal cell of the tissue of origin), moderately well-differentiated, poorly differentiated, or undifferentiated. The other system numerically grades from 1 to 3 or 4, with 1 being the most differentiated and 3 and 4 being the least well-differentiated; Grade 4 applies to tumors with no specific differentiation. It is important to remember that Grade 1 well-differentiated tumor implies the best prognosis for the patient. The AJCC recommends the following grading classification:[19]

GX Grade cannot be assessed
G1 Well-differentiated
G2 Moderately well-differentiated
G3 Poorly differentiated
G4 Undifferentiated

Other grading systems under development offer more precise guidelines adding features of nuclear grade and mitotic activity to the evaluation of tissue differentiation. If there is evidence of more than one grade or of differentiation of the tumor, the least differentiated is recorded as the histopathologic grade, using only G2 through G4. For example, a colonic adenocarcinoma that is partially well-differentiated and partially moderately differentiated is coded as grade 2 (G2). The growing edge of the tumor is not generally assessed in grading because it may appear to

**TABLE 8-9**

**Comparison of Frequently Used Performance Status Scales**

| Karnofsky Scale | | ECOG Scale | | WHO Scale | |
|---|---|---|---|---|---|
| **% Score** | **Status** | **% Score** | **Status** | **% Score** | **Status** |
| 100% | Normal, no complaints; no evidence of disease | 0 | Asymptomatic | 0 | Fully active, able to carry out all predisease activities without restriction |
| 90 | Able to carry on normal activity; minor signs or symptoms of disease | 1 | Symptomatic; fully ambulatory | 1 | Restricted in strenuous activity but ambulatory and able to carry out light work or pursue sedentary occupation |
| 80 | Normal activity with effort; some signs or symptoms of disease | | | | |
| 70 | Cares for self; unable to carry on normal activity or to do active work | 2 | Symptomatic; in bed less than 50% of day | 2 | Ambulatory and capable of all self-care but unable to do any light work; up and about more than 50% of waking hours |
| 60 | Requires occasional assistance, but able to care for most needs | | | | |
| 50 | Requires considerable assistance and frequent medical care | 3 | Symptomatic; in bed more than 50% of day but not bedridden | 3 | Capable of only limited self-care; confined to bed or chair more than 50% of waking hours |
| 40 | Disabled, requires special care and assistance | | | | |
| 30 | Severely disabled; hospitalization indicated, although death not imminent | 4 | Bedridden | 4 | Completely disabled; unable to carry out any self-care and confined totally to bed or chair |
| 20 | Very sick; hospitalization necessary; active supportive treatment necessary | | | | |
| 10 | Moribund; fatal processes progressing rapidly | | | | |
| 0 | Dead | | | | |

be high grade—except in the breast, where that is the best reflection of prognosis.

For some anatomical sites, grades 3 and 4 are combined into a single grade—for example, poorly differentiated to undifferentiated (G3-G4). The combination is valid for carcinomas of the uterine corpus, ovary, prostate, urinary bladder, kidney, renal pelvis, ureter, urethra, and breast. Only three grades are used for melanoma of the conjunctiva and uvea. Grading does not apply to carcinomas of the thyroid, eyelids, and retinoblastoma or to malignant testicular tumors and melanoma of the skin.

Certain problems exist with grading classifications. Most notably, a tumor's level of differentiation may vary with time. Also, several grades of malignancy may exist within one tumor, in which case the tumor should be labeled as having the least favorable level of differentiation. It is essential that an adequate and representative biopsy specimen be obtained for a valid interpretation by the pathologist. Nurses, who are aware of the significance of a malignant tumor's grade and stage, as well as new prognostic, molecular markers, will be able to respond realistically to the patient's questions about treatment and prognosis.

## NURSING IMPLICATIONS

Many opportunities exist for nurses to promote the early detection and diagnosis of cancer. As respected members of the healthcare profession, they are consulted formally and informally about perceived signs and symptoms of cancer. Through communication, education, and intervention, nurses can increase public awareness about cancer. Nurses are well suited to provide education about prevention measures and general population screening guidelines for early detection and diagnosis of cancer. Relating principles of cancer risk assessment, discussing issues related to genetic testing, educating patients about performing self-examinations, reporting symptoms, and scheduling appropriate screening tests are some examples of their capabilities. Nurses also can facilitate entry into the healthcare system by encouraging appropriate follow-up without delay, providing accurate information on cancer detection and diagnostic procedures, clarifying misconceptions, and referring individuals to trusted healthcare providers or community programs.

Nurses are integral members of the professional team, providing information and emotional support to individuals facing the potential threat of cancer. The time elapsed between the discovery of a suspicious symptom, such as a breast lump, the seeking of medical attention, and the completion of diagnostic evaluation varies for every person and for many reasons. However, the potential for stress, disruption, anxiety, and fear always exists for individuals suspected of having cancer and for their family members.

During the prediagnostic period, a delay in seeking attention can be attributed to the perceived threat or "importance" of the symptom, the severity of the symptom, personal beliefs about cancer and treatment, and personal and financial resources. Once the individual acts on his or her concerns and seeks medical attention, the diagnostic period begins and may take several weeks before a cancer diagnosis is confirmed. Anxiety about the results of examinations and fear and curiosity regarding the technology used in procedures are common.[128] Psychological responses after receiving a diagnosis of cancer are individualized and range from suspicion, shock, denial, grief, and helplessness to loss and fear of death. Guilt feelings may be apparent if the patient did not seek attention early or if lifestyle may have contributed to the cancer.[129,130] In such situations, oncology nurses can intervene by taking time to listen to concerns, responding to questions, and providing support. Projecting optimism and hope helps to counter the worst-case scenarios often assumed by the patient and family.

Oncology nurses play a key role in providing information and support to reduce the stress of going through a diagnostic evaluation for a suspected malignancy. An accurate assessment of the individual's and family's desire to know, in addition to their ability to understand, coping abilities, and supportive resources, is the first step in providing this much-needed support. Psychological distress must be evaluated and managed before education can take place.[131] Education should be provided in a manner consistent with the cultural background and healthcare beliefs of the affected individual and his or her family. In addition, education materials provided should be language and literacy appropriate. Educational preparation for an examination should include the following elements:

1. An explanation of and necessary preparation for the procedure
2. A description of any physical sensations that might be expected, such as pain, discomfort, and facial flushing
3. The purpose of the examination, including what information can and cannot be gleaned from it
4. When and from whom the results can be expected.

Reinforcing verbal information with written materials has proved helpful.[132] Education and information sharing can also be performed via the internet or an intranet system.[133,134] Scheduling of the procedure should be done in a timely manner to decrease the patient's stress level.

Nurses also must be cognizant of any potential for complications during or after a procedure, including reactions to contrast agents, bleeding, vasovagal response, and the need for intravenous analgesia or moderate sedation. Nurses may assist with a procedure, perform the procedure, or provide postprocedure care.

Including the family members in all aspects of the diagnostic evaluation benefits the individual, the family, and the healthcare team. Families can reinforce instructions and information, assist with preparation for an examination, observe for untoward effects from procedures, and provide emotional support to the patient. An assessment of the family's ability to cope with the cancer diagnosis may prompt referrals to a variety of support services, including social services, psycho-oncology support groups, and home care agencies.

## FUTURE TRENDS

Advances in knowledge of the human genome have broadened our understanding of the variants associated with malignancy.[135,136] Future research will allow integration of genomics and proteomics into daily clinical practice, which will further our ability to accurately diagnose, prognosticate, treat, and monitor cancers in the future, allowing individualization of therapy.[137,138] Biomarker research has benefited from advances in technology such as proteomics, the study of proteins and their function. Proteomics is essential in detecting changes in protein profiles that can lead to more comprehensive understanding of the cancer process and the development and validation of new protein biomarkers.

Molecular imaging and profiling enhances the management of the patient with cancer. Combinations of various modalities of molecular imaging (such as SPECT or PET) with anatomical imaging (CT or MRI) increase the accuracy and timeliness of diagnosis and enhance staging precision. Fusion imaging combines functional radiologic imaging with metabolic studies, overcoming the drawbacks associated with these modalities. Software-based fusion of independently performed scintigraphic and radiological images has proven time-consuming and impractical for routine use. Dual-modality integrated imaging systems (SPECT/CT and PET/CT) can be particularly useful, as the anatomical images provide precise localization of the tumor and allow for the exclusion of disease in sites of physiologic tracers' accumulation for SPECT and PET findings.[139]

Results of multimodality imaging in the diagnosis of cancer have proved very encouraging, indicating that these systems are well suited for routine use in clinical practice. Fused images provide additional information that improves diagnostic accuracy and can influence patient management. The efficacy and cost-effectiveness of these multimodalities require validation and standardization for use in daily clinical practice.

## CONCLUSION

The diagnostic phase of a cancer illness is a time of adjustment, learning, anxiety, and uncertainty for both patient and family. With adequate knowledge of the symptoms of disease and of the diagnostic process required for evaluation, oncology nurses can help prepare patients, thereby easing the anxiety associated with the unknown. During this time, nurses will interact with the individual in several healthcare settings—primary clinics, inpatient and outpatient units, and extended care units—as well as in the community. Oncology nurses use their expertise to do the following:

1. Facilitate early diagnosis of cancer by promoting awareness of "warning signals" of cancer and conducting screening programs
2. Educate and prepare individuals for a diagnostic evaluation of suspicious signs or symptoms
3. Perform or assist with diagnostic procedures and interpret or clarify results
4. Counsel and support the individual and family in a therapeutic relationship
5. Prepare the individual for the possible treatment options once a definitive diagnosis is made.

Nurses have the power to promote the detection of cancer at the earliest possible stage and to assist the individual and family to regain hope, control, and quality of life once the diagnosis of cancer has been determined.

## REFERENCES


1. Jemal A, Siegel R, Ward E, et al. Cancer statistics. *CA: Cancer J Clin.* 2008;58:71–96.
2. American Cancer Society. *Cancer Facts and Figures.* Atlanta, GA: American Cancer Society; 2004.
3. Carroll-Johnson RM, ed. Cancer prevention and early detection: oncology nursing's next frontier. *Oncol Nurs Forum. 2000;*27(suppl 9):1–61.
4. Champion VL, Rawl SM, Menon U. Population-based cancer screening. *Oncol Nurs Forum.* 2002;29:853–861.
5. Newton S, Hickey M, Marrs, J. *Mosby's Oncology Nursing Advisor: A Comprehensive Guide to Clinical Practice.* St. Louis, MO: Mosby, Elsevier; 2009.
6. Smith RA, Cokkinides V, Brawley OW. Cancer screening in the United States, 2008: a review of current American cancer society guidelines and cancer screening issues. *CA Cancer J Clin.* 2008;58:161–179.
7. Eyre H, Kahn R, Robertson RM, American Cancer Society, the American Diabetes Association, and the American Heart Association Collaborative Writing Committee. Preventing cancer, cardiovascular disease, and diabetes: a common agenda for the American Cancer Society, the American Diabetes Association, and the American Heart Association. *Diabetes Care.* 2004;27:1812–1824.
8. Berkowitz Z, Hawkins NA, Peipins LA, White MC, Nadel MR. Beliefs, risk perceptions, and gaps in knowledge as barriers to colorectal cancer screening in older adults. *J Am Geriatr Soc.* 2008;56:307–314.
9. Beydoun HA, Beydoun MA. Predictors of colorectal cancer screening behaviors among average-risk older adults in the United States. *Cancer Causes Control.* 2008;19:339–359.
10. Griffith KA, McGuire DB, Rovak-Schaler R, Plowden KO, Steinberger EK. Influence of family history and preventive health behaviors on colorectal cancer screening in African Americans. *Cancer.* 2008;113:276–285.
11. Klabunde CN, Schenck AP, Davis WW. Barriers to colorectal screening among Medicare consumers. *Am J Prev Med.* 2006;30:313–319.
12. Schoenberg NE, Hopenhavn C, Christian A, Knight EA, Rubio A. An in-depth and updated perspective on determinants of cervical cancer screening among central Appalachian women. *Women Health.* 2005;42:89–105.
13. Mahon SM. Patient education regarding cancer screening guidelines. *Clin J Oncol Nurs.* 2003;7:581–584.
14. Oncology Nursing Society. Prevention and early detection of cancer in the United States. *Oncol Nurs Forum.* 2007;34:759–760.
15. Mick J. Factors affecting the evolution of oncology nursing care. *Clin J Oncol Nurs.* 2008;12:307–313.
16. Weber S, Jarnagin W, Duffy A, O'Reilly E, Abou-Alfa G, Blumgart L. Liver and bile duct cancer. In: Abeloff MD, Armitage JO, Niederhuber JE, Kastan MB, McKenna WG, eds. *Abeloff's Clinical Oncology.* 4th ed. Philadelphia, PA: Churchill Livingstone; 2008:1569–1594.
17. Sokoll LJ, Chan DW. Biomarkers for cancer diagnostics. In: Abeloff MD, Armitage JO, Niederhuber JE, Kastan MB, McKenna WG, eds. *Abeloff's Clinical Oncology.* 4th ed. Philadelphia, PA: Churchill Livingstone; 2008:277–282.
18. Locker GY, Hamilton S, Harris J, et al. ASCO 2006 update of recommendations for the use of tumor markers in gastrointestinal cancer. *J Clin Oncol.* 2006;24:5313–5327.
19. American Joint Committee on Cancer. *AJCC Cancer Staging Manual.* 6th ed. New York: Springer-Verlag; 2002.
20. Harris L, Fritsche H, Mennel R, et al. Recommendations for the use of tumor markers in breast cancer. *J Clin Oncol.* 2007;25:1–26.
21. Chernecky C, Berger B. *Laboratory Tests and Diagnostic Procedures. 5th ed.* St. Louis, MO: Saunders; 2008.

22. Lowitz BB, Casciato D. Principles of oncology. In: Casciato DA, ed. *Manual of Clinical Oncology*. 5th ed. Philadelphia, PA: Lippincott, Williams & Wilkins; 2004:3–16.
23. Ludwig JA, Weinstein JN. Biomarkers in cancer staging, prognosis, and treatment selection. *Nat Rev Cancer*. 2005;5:845–856.
24. De Roock W, Piessevaux H, De Schutter J, et al. KRAS wild-type state predicts survival and is associated to early radiological response in metastatic colorectal cancer treated with cetuximab. *Ann Oncol.* 2008;19:508–515.
25. Perera M, Innocenti F, Ratain M. Pharmacogenetic testing for uridine diphosphate glucuronosyltransferase 1A1 polymorphisms: are we there yet? *Pharmacotherapy*. 2008;28:755–768.
26. Deming S, Zheng W, Xu W, et al. UGT1A1 genetic polymorphisms, endogenous estrogen exposure, soy food intake, and endometrial cancer risk. *Cancer Epidemiol Biomarkers Prev*. 2008;17:563–570.
27. Khatcheressian JL, Wolff AC, Smith TJ, et al. American Society of Clinical Oncology 2006 update of the breast cancer follow-up and management guidelines in the adjuvant setting. *J Clin Oncol.* 2006;24:5091–5097.
28. Sturgeon C. National Academy of Clinical Biochemistry Laboratory Medicine Practice Guidelines for use of tumor markers in clinical practice: quality requirements. *Clin Chem*. 2008;54:e1–e10.
29. Viale PH. Cancer diagnosis and staging. In: Gobel BH, Triest-Robertson S, Vogel WH, eds. *Advanced Oncology Nursing Certification Review and Resource Manual*. Pittsburgh, PA: Oncology Nursing Society; 2008:77–147.
30. Borowitz MJ. Flow cytometry in oncologic diagnosis. In: Abeloff MD, Armitage JO, Niederhuber JE, Kastan MB, McKenna WG, eds. *Abeloff's Clinical Oncology*. 4th ed. Philadelphia, PA: Churchill Livingstone; 2008:241–248.
31. Mirza AN, Mirza NQ, Vlastos G, Singletary SE. Prognostic factors in node-negative breast cancer: a review of studies with sample size more than 200, follow-up more than 5 years. *Ann Surg. 2002;*235:10–26.
32. Cooley LD, Wilson KS. Conventional and molecular cytogenetics of neoplasia. In: Abeloff MD, Armitage JO, Niederhuber JE, Kastan MB, McKenna WG, eds. *Abeloff's Clinical Oncology*. 4th ed. Philadelphia, PA: Churchill Livingstone; 2008:249–263.
33. Mahon SM. Genetic risk. In: Gobel BH, Triest-Robertson S, Vogel WH, eds. *Advanced Oncology Nursing Certification Review and Resource Manual*. Pittsburgh, PA: Oncology Nursing Society; 2009:37–75.
34. Collins FS, Morgan M, Patrinos A. The Human Genome Project: lessons from large-scale biology. *Science*. 2003;300:286–290.
35. American Society of Clinical Oncology. American Society of Clinical Oncology policy statement update: genetic testing for cancer susceptibility. *J Clin Oncol*. 2003;21:2397–2406.
36. Greene H. Cancer prevention, screening, and early detection. In: Gobel BH, Triest-Robertson S, Vogel WH, eds. *Advanced Oncology Nursing Certification Review and Resource Manual*. Pittsburgh, PA: Oncology Nursing Society; 2009:1–35.
37. Oncology Nursing Society. *Cancer Predisposition Genetic Testing and Risk Assessment Counseling*. Pittsburgh, PA: Author; 2004.
38. Calzone KA, Jenkins J, Masny A. Core competencies in cancer genetics for advanced practice oncology nurses. *Oncol Nurs Forum*. 2002;29:1327–1333.
39. Dillon WP. Head and neck imaging. *Am J Neuroradiol*. 2000;21:25–28.
40. McLoud TC. Imaging techniques for diagnosis and staging of lung cancer. *Clinics Chest Med*. 2002;23:123–136.
41. Hilton S. Imaging of renal cell carcinoma. *Semin Oncol*. 2000;27: 150–159.
42. Soper JT. Radiographic imaging in gynecologic oncology. *Clin Obstet Gynecol*. 2001;44:485–494.
43. Schiepers C, Filmont JE, Czermini J. PET staging of Hodgkin's disease and non-Hodgkin's lymphoma. *Eur J Nucl Med Molec Imag.* 2003;30(suppl 1):82–83.
44. Rubin P, Bragg DG. Principles of oncologic imaging and tumor imaging strategies. In: Rubin P, ed. *Clinical Oncology: A Multidisciplinary Approach for Physicians and Students*. 8th ed. Philadelphia, PA: Saunders; 2001:241–251.
45. Brenner RJ. Interventional procedures of the breast. In: Bragg DG, Rubin P, Hricak H, eds. *Oncologic Imaging*. 2nd ed. Philadelphia, PA: WB Saunders; 2002:295–310.
46. Munden RE, Bragg DG. Primary malignancies of the thorax. In: Bragg DG, Rubin P, Hricak H, eds. *Oncologic Imaging*. 2nd ed. Philadelphia, PA: WB Saunders; 2002:313–341.
47. Skarin AT. *Atlas of Diagnostic Oncology*. 3rd ed. London: Mosby-Wolfe; 2002.
48. Bhalla S. Oncologic imaging. In: Govindan R, Arquette M, eds. *Washington Manual of Oncology*. Philadelphia, PA: Lippincott, Williams & Wilkins; 2002:533–541.
49. Wahl RL. Imaging. In: Abeloff MD, Armitage JO, Niederhuber JE, Kastan MB, McKenna WG, eds. *Abeloff's Clinical Oncology*. 4th ed. Philadelphia, PA: Churchill Livingstone; 2008:283–308.
50. Hricak H, Akin O, Bradbury M, Liberman L, Schwartz L, Larson S. Advanced imaging methods. In: DeVita VT, Hellman S, Rosenberg SA, eds. *Cancer Principles and Practice of Oncology*. 7th ed. Philadelphia, PA: Lippincott, Williams & Wilkins; 2005:589–636.
51. Newton S, Hickey M, Marrs J. *Oncology Nursing Advisor: A Comprehensive Guide to Clinical Practice*. St. Louis, MO: Mosby, Elsevier; 2009.
52. 1998 MQSA. (Mammographic Quality Standards Act) final rule released American College of Radiology. *Radiol Manage*. 1998;20:51–55.
53. Box BA, Russell CA. Breast cancer. In: Casciato DA, ed. *Manual of Clinical Oncology*. 5th ed. Philadelphia, PA: Lippincott, Williams & Wilkins; 2004:233–253.
54. Kapoor V, McCook B, Torok F. An introduction to PET-CT imaging. *Radiographics*. 2004;24:523–543.
55. Pisano ED, Hendrick RE, Yaffe MJ, et al. Diagnostic accuracy of digital versus film mammography: exploratory analysis of selected population subgroups in DMIST. *Radiology*. 2008;246:376–383.
56. Barentsz J, Takahashi S, Oyen W, et al. Commonly used imaging techniques for diagnosis and staging. *J Clin Oncol*. 2006;2:3234–3244.
57. Pickhardt PJ, Choi JR, Hwang I, et al. Computed tomographic virtual colonoscopy to screen for colorectal neoplasia in asymptomatic adults. *N Engl J Med*. 2003;349:2191–2200.
58. Ransohoff DF. Virtual colonoscopy: what it can do vs. what it will do. *JAMA*. 2004;291:1772–1774.
59. Levin B, Lieberman DA, McFarland B, et al. Screening and surveillance for the early detection of colorectal cancer and adenomatous polyps, 2008: a joint guideline from the American Cancer Society, the US Multi-Society Task Force on Colorectal Cancer, and the American College of Radiology. *CA Cancer J Clin*. 2008;58:130–160.
60. Sosna J, Sella T, Sy O, et al. Critical analysis of the performance of double-contrast barium enema for detecting colorectal polyps > or = 6 mm in the era of CT colonography. *Am J Roentgenol*. 2008;190:374–385.
61. Mahon S. Colorectal cancer screening: a review of the evidence. *Clin J Oncol Nurs*. 2004;8:536–540.
62. Centers for Medicare and Medicaid Services. Positron Emission Tomography (PET) Scans. In: *Medicare National Coverage Determinations Manual*. Baltimore, MD: Centers for Medicare and Medicaid Services; 2006:26.
63. Kim SK, Allen-Auerbach M, Goldin J, et al. Accuracy of PET/CT in characterization of solitary pulmonary lesions. *J Nucl Med*. 2007;48:214–220.
64. Antoch G, Saoudi N, Kuehl H, et al. Accuracy of whole-body dual-modality fluorine-18–2-fluoro-2-deoxy-D-glucose positron emission tomography and computed tomography (FDG-PET/CT) for tumor staging in solid tumors: comparison with CT and PET. *J Clin Oncol*. 2004;22:4357–4368.
65. Townsend D. Dual-modality imaging: combining anatomy and function. *J Nucl Med*. 2008;49:938–955.
66. Zhuang H, Purdehnad M, Duarte FS, et al. The role of positron emission tomography with fluorine-18-deoxyglucose in identifying colorectal cancer metastasis to the liver. *Nuclear Med*. 2000;219:793–798.

67. Facey K, Bradbury I, Laking G, Payne E. Overview of the clinical effectiveness of positron emission tomography imaging in selected cancer. *Health Technol Assess.* 2007;11:44.
68. Rahmim A, Zaidi H. PET versus SPECT: strengths, limitations and challenges. *Nucl Med Commun.* 2008;29:193–207.
69. Goldenberg DM, Sharkey RM, Barbet J, Chatel J. Radioactive antibodies: selective targeting and treatment of cancer and other diseases. *Appl Radiol.* 2007;36(4). http://www.appliedradiology.com/articles/Article.asp?ID=1341&IssueID=173&ThreadID=. Accessed June 18, 2009.
70. Hendee WR. New imaging techniques. In: Bragg DG, Rubin P, Hricak H, eds. *Oncologic Imaging.* Philadelphia, PA: WB Saunders; 2002:39–54.
71. Schmidt GP, Reiser MF, Baur-Melnyk A. Whole-body imaging of the musculoskeletal system: the value of MR imaging. *Skeletal Radiol.* 2007;36:1109–1119.
72. Schmidt GP, Kramer H, Reiser MF, Glaser C. Whole-body magnetic resonance imaging and positron emission tomography-computed tomography in oncology. *Top Magn Reson Imaging.* 2007;18:193–202.
73. Orell SD, Schnall MD. MR imaging of the breast for the detection, diagnosis, and staging of breast cancer. *Radiology.* 2001;220:13–30.
74. Morris EA. Screening for breast cancer with MRI. *Semin Ultrasound CT MR.* 2003;24:45–54.
75. NCCN. *NCCN Practice Guidelines in Oncology: Genetic/Familial High Risk Assessment: Breast and Ovarian*, version 1.2009. http://www.nccn.org/professionals/physician_gls/PDF/genetics_screening.pdf. Accessed June 20, 2009.
76. Rankin SC. MRI of the breast. *Br J Radiol.* 2000;73:806–818.
77. Shah SK, Shah SK, Greatrex KV. Current role of magnetic resonance imaging in breast imaging: a primer for the primary care physician. *J Am Board Fam Pract.* 2005;18:478–490.
78. Brem R, Fioerke A, Rapelyea J, Teal C, Kelly T, Mathur V. Breast-specific gamma imaging as an adjunct imaging modality for the diagnosis of breast cancer. *Radiology.* 2008;247:651–657.
79. Brem R, Fishman M, Rapelyea J. Detection of ductal carcinoma in situ with mammography, breast specific gamma imaging, and magnetic resonance imaging: a comparative study. *Acad Radiol.* 2007;14: 945–950.
80. Brem R, Petrovitch I, Rapelyea J, Young H, Teal C, Kelly T. Breast-specific gamma imaging with 99mTc-Sestamibi and magnetic resonance imaging in the diagnosis of breast cancer—a comparative study. *Breast J.* 2007;13:465–469.
81. Zhou M, Johnson N, Blanchard D, Bryn S, Nelson J. Real-world application of breast specific gamma imaging, initial experience at a community breast center and its potential impact on clinical care. *Am J Surg.* 2008;195:631–635.
82. Kumar R, Lerski RA, Gandy S, Clift BA, Abboud RJ. Safety of orthopedic implants in magnetic resonance imaging: an experimental verification. *J Orthop Res.* 2006;24:1799–1802.
83. Shinbane JS, Colletti PM, Shellock FG. MR in patients with pacemakers and ICDs: Defining the issues. *J Cardiovasc Magn Reson.* 2007;9:5–13.
84. Camp-Sorrell D. Magnetic resonance imaging and the implantable port. *Oncol Nurs Forum.* 1990;17:197–199.
85. Hailey D. Open magnetic resonance imaging (MRI) scanners. *Issues Emerg Health Technol.* 2006;92:1–4.
86. Maity A, Pruitt A, Judy K, Phillips P, Lustig R. Cancer of the central nervous system. In: Abeloff MD, Armitage JO, Niederhuber JE, Kastan MB, McKenna WG, eds. *Abeloff's Clinical Oncology.* 4th ed. Philadelphia, PA: Churchill Livingstone; 2008:1075–1136.
87. Deitcher S. Diagnosis, treatment, and prevention of cancer-related venous thrombosis. In: Abeloff MD, Armitage JO, Niederhuber JE, Kastan MB, McKenna WG, eds. *Abeloff's Clinical Oncology.* 4th ed. Philadelphia, PA: Churchill Livingstone; 2008:693–715.
88. Waxman I. Cancer diagnosis: endoscopy. In: DeVita VT, Hellman S, Rosenberg SA, eds. *Cancer Principles and Practice of Oncology.* 7th ed. Philadelphia, PA: Lippincott, Williams, & Wilkins; 2005:637–651.
89. Levy MJ, Jondal ML, Clain J, et al. Preliminary experience with an EUS-guided trucut biopsy needle compared with EUS-guided FNA. *Gastrointest Endosc.* 2003;57:101–106.
90. NCCN. *NCCN Practice Guidelines in Oncology: Colorectal Cancer Screening*, version 1.2009. http://www.nccn.org/professionals/physician_gls/PDF/colorectal_screening.pdf. Accessed June 20, 2009.
91. American Cancer Society. *American Cancer Society Guidelines for the Early Detection of Cancer.* http://www.cancer.org/docroot/PED/content/PED_2_3X_ACS_Cancer_Detection_Guidelines_36.asp. Accessed June 20, 2009.
92. National Cancer Institute. *Colorectal Cancer Screening (PDQ®).* 2008. http://www.cancer.gov/cancertopics/pdq/screening/colorectal/healthprofessional. Accessed June 18, 2009.
93. Pollock RE, Morton DL. Principles of surgical oncology. In: Kufe DW, Pollock RE, Weischelbaum R, et al, eds. *Cancer Medicine.* 6th ed. Hamilton, Ontario, Canada: BC Decker; 2003:448–458.
94. Are C, Talamini MA. Laparoscopy and malignancy. *J Laparoendosc Adv Surg Tech A.* 2005;15:38–47.
95. Lefor AT. The role of laparoscopy in the treatment of intra-abdominal malignancies. *Cancer J.* 2000;6(suppl 2):59–68.
96. Nguyen DM, Summers RM, Finkelstein SE. Respiratory tract. In: DeVita VT, Hellman S, Rosenberg SA, eds. *Cancer Principles and Practice of Oncology.* 7th ed. Philadelphia, PA: Lippincott, Williams, & Wilkins; 2005:643–651.
97. Juergens RA, Spira AI, Brahmer JR. Effusions. In: Abeloff MD, Armitage JO, Niederhuber JE, Kastan MB, McKenna WG, eds. *Abeloff's Clinical Oncology.* 4th ed. Philadelphia, PA: Churchill Livingstone; 2008:925–944.
98. Lester J. Surgery. In: Gobel BH, Triest-Robertson S, Vogel WH, eds. *Advanced Oncology Nursing Certification Review and Resource Manual.* Pittsburgh, PA: Oncology Nursing Society; 2009:187–228.
99. Illei PB, Westra W. Principles of oncology surgical pathology. In: Abeloff MD, Armitage JO, Niederhuber JE, Kastan MB, McKenna WG, eds. *Abeloff's Clinical Oncology.* 4th ed. Philadelphia, PA: Churchill Livingstone; 2008:33–239.
100. Niederhuer JE. Surgical interventions in cancer. In: Abeloff MD, Armitage JO, Niederhuber JE, Kastan MB, McKenna WG, eds. *Abeloff's Clinical Oncology.* 4th ed. Philadelphia, PA: Churchill Livingstone; 2008:407–416.
101. Liberman L. Percutaneous image-guided core breast biopsy. *Radiol Clin North Am.* 2002;40:483–500.
102. Abeloff MD, Wolff AC, Weber BL, Zaks TZ, Sacchini V, McCormick B. Cancer of the breast. In: Abeloff MD, Armitage JO, Niederhuber JE, Kastan MB, McKenna WG, eds. *Abeloff's Clinical Oncology.* 4th ed. Philadelphia, PA: Churchill Livingstone; 2008:1875–1943.
103. Fetzer S, Holmes S. Relieving the pain of sentinel lymph node biopsy tracer injection. *Clin J Oncol Nurs.* 2008;12:668–670.
104. Gazelle GS, McMahon PM, Siebert U, Beinfeld MT. Cost-effectiveness analysis in the assessment of diagnostic imaging technologies. *Radiology.* 2005;235:361–370.
105. Ford JM, Kastan MB. DNA damage response pathways and cancer. In: Abeloff MD, Armitage JO, Niederhuber JE, Kastan MB, McKenna WG, eds. *Abeloff's Clinical Oncology.* 4th ed. Philadelphia, PA: Churchill Livingstone; 2008:139–152.
106. Lambert PF, Sugden B. Viruses and human cancer. In: Abeloff MD, Armitage JO, Niederhuber JE, Kastan MB, McKenna WG, eds. *Abeloff's Clinical Oncology.* 4th ed. Philadelphia, PA: Churchill Livingstone; 2008:153–169.
107. Clarke MF, Weissman IL. Stem cells, cell differentiation, and cancer. In: Abeloff MD, Armitage JO, Niederhuber JE, Kastan MB, McKenna WG, eds. *Abeloff's Clinical Oncology.* 4th ed. Philadelphia, PA: Churchill Livingstone; 2008:95–104.
108. Jain RK, Duda DG. Vascular and interstitial biology of tumors. In: Abeloff MD, Armitage JO, Niederhuber JE, Kastan MB, McKenna WG, eds. *Abeloff's Clinical Oncology.* 4th ed. Philadelphia, PA: Churchill Livingstone; 2008:105–124.

109. Giacca AJ, Erler JT. The cellular microenvironment and metastases. In: Abeloff MD, Armitage JO, Niederhuber JE, Kastan MB, McKenna WG, eds. *Abeloff's Clinical Oncology.* 4th ed. Philadelphia, PA: Churchill Livingstone; 2008:33–47.
110. Ruddon RW. *Cancer Biology.* 3rd ed. New York: Oxford University Press; 1995:3–18.
111. Walter JB, Talbot C. *General Pathology.* 7th ed. New York: Churchill-Livingstone; 1996:471–487.
112. Chandrasoma P, Taylor CL. *Concise Pathology.* 3rd ed. Stamford, CT: Appleton and Lange; 1998.
113. Glover KY, Varadhachary GR, Lenzi R, Raber MN, Abbruzzese JL. Carcinoma of unknown primary. In: Abeloff MD, Armitage JO, Niederhuber JE, Kastan MB, McKenna WG, eds. *Abeloff's Clinical Oncology.* 4th ed. Philadelphia, PA: Churchill Livingstone; 2008:2057–2074.
114. Seve P, Ray-Coquard I, Trillet-Lenoir V, et al. Low serum albumin levels and liver metastasis are powerful prognostic markers for survival in patients with carcinomas of unknown primary site. *Cancer.* 2006;107:2698–2705.
115. Culine S, Kramar A, Saghatchian M, et al. Development and validation of a prognostic model to predict the length of survival in patients with carcinomas of an unknown primary site. *J Clin Oncol.* 2002;20:4679–4683.
116. Ponce Lorenzo J, Segura Huerta A, Díaz Beveridge R, et al. Carcinoma of unknown primary site: development in a single institution of a prognostic model based on clinical and serum variables. *Clin Transl Oncol.* 2007;9:452–458.
117. Hainsworth JD, Greco FA. Management of patients with cancer of unknown primary site. *Oncology.* 2000;12:563–567.
118. Logan J. Women undergoing breast diagnostics: the lived experience of spirituality. *Oncol Nurs Forum.* 2006;33:121–126.
119. Lacey M. The experience of using decisional support aids by patients with breast cancer. *Oncol Nurs Forum.* 2002;29:1491–1497.
120. Durie BGM, Salmon SE. A clinical staging system for multiple myeloma correlation of measured myeloma cell mass with presenting clinical features, response to treatment and survival. *Cancer.* 1975;36:842–854.
121. Kates R, Schmitt M, Harbeck N. Advanced statistical methods for the definition of new staging models. *Rec Result Cancer Res.* 2003;162:101–113.
122. Singletary SE, Connolly JL. Breast cancer staging: working with the sixth edition of the AJCC Cancer Staging Manual. *CA Cancer J Clin.* 2006;56:37–47.
123. Karnofsky DA, Abelmann WH, Craver LF, et al. The use of the nitrogen mustards in the palliative treatment of carcinoma. *Cancer.* 1948;1:634–656.
124. Oken MM, Creech RH, Tormey DC, et al. Toxicity and response criteria of the Eastern Cooperative Oncology Group. *Am J Clin Oncol.* 1982;5:649–655.
125. World Health Organization. *World Handbook for Reporting Results of Cancer Treatment.* Geneva: Author; 1979.
126. Mor V, Laliberle L, Wiemann M. The Karnofsky performance status scale: an examination of its reliability and validity in a research setting. *Cancer.* 1984;53:2002–2007.
127. Abernethy AP, Shelby-James T, Fazekas BS, Woods D, Currow DC. The Australia-modified Karnofsky performance status (AKPS) scale: a revised scale for contemporary palliative care clinical practice. *BMC Palliat Care.* 2005;4:7.
128. Boehmke M, Dickerson S. The diagnosis of breast cancer: transition from health to illness. *Oncol Nurs Forum.* 2006;33:1121–1127.
129. Vitek L, Rosenzweig MQ, Stollings S. Distress in patients with cancer: definition, assessment, and suggested interventions. *Clin J Oncol Nurs.* 2007;11:413–418.
130. Daniels J, Kissane DW. Psychosocial interventions for cancer patients. *Curr Opin Oncol.* 2008;20:367–371.
131. Stephenson P. Before the teaching begins: managing patient anxiety prior to providing education. *Clin J Oncol Nurs.* 2006;10:241–245.
132. Chelf J, Dose A, Quella S, Hillman S. Learning and support preferences of adult patients with cancer at a comprehensive cancer center. *Oncol Nurs Forum.* 2002;29:863–867.
133. Sorrentino C, Berger A, Wardian S, Pattrin L. Using the intranet to deliver patient-education materials. *Clin J Oncol Nurs.* 2002;6:354–357.
134. Clarke L. Pathways for head and neck surgery: a patient-education tool. *Clin J Oncol Nurs.* 2002;6:78–82.
135. Gomase VS, Tagore S, Kale KV, Bhiwgade DA. Oncogenomics. *Curr Drug Metab.* 2008;9:199–206.
136. Seng KC, Seng CK. The success of the genome-wide association approach: a brief story of a long struggle. *Eur J Hum Genet.* 2008;16:554–564.
137. Glinsky GV. "Stemness" genomics law governs clinical behavior of human cancer: implications for decision making in disease management. *J Clin Oncol.* 2008;26:2846–2853.
138. Lin J, Li M. Molecular profiling in the age of cancer genomics. *Expert Rev Mol Diagn.* 2008;8:263–276.
139. Rollo FD. Molecular imaging: an overview and clinical applications. *Radiol Manage.* 2003;25:28–32.
140. Ferrucci JT. Double-contrast barium enema: use in practice and implications for CT colonography. *AJR Am J Roentgenol.* 2006;187:170–173.

# PART III

# Treatment

CHAPTER 9

Carol Estwing Ferrans, PhD, RN, FAAN, Eileen Danaher Hacker, APN, RN, AOCN®

# Quality of Life as an Outcome of Cancer Care

## INTRODUCTION

Quality of life is a concept that uniquely belongs to nursing science and practice. Nurses traditionally have viewed patients from a holistic perspective, focusing not only on the length of life but also on the quality of life. Over the past 30 years, nurse scientists have been among the frontrunners in the development of quality of life as an important gauge for evaluating healthcare outcomes. Recognizing the fact that information beyond tumor response and survival time was needed, much of the ground-breaking work in the assessment of quality of life has been accomplished in oncology. In 1985, the US Food and Drug Administration identified quality of life as a key parameter for approval of new anticancer drugs for advanced metastatic disease.[1] In 1988, improvement of quality of life was identified as one of the highest priorities of the Cancer Therapy Evaluation Program of the National Cancer Institute (NCI).[2] Quality of life components now are included in many of the clinical trials conducted by the cancer cooperative groups in the United States, Canada, and Europe. In fact, the Canadian NCI requires quality of life end points to be included in all phase III clinical trials.[3] In April 2006, the importance of quality of life was further recognized by the American NCI, by instituting the Symptom Management and Health-Related Quality of Life Steering Committee, within its Coordinating Center for Clinical Trials.[4]

Quality of life issues, however, are not limited to clinical trials of therapeutic agents. Such information is critically important for the entire spectrum of cancer care, including palliative care, end-of-life care, and long-term survivorship. Oncology nurses focus on all aspects of life affected by cancer and treatment, such as physical symptoms, treatment toxicities, mental and physical functioning, body image, psychological state, work and role responsibilities, social and family life, and spiritual concerns. Because the concept of quality of life is a multidimensional construct that encompasses the whole of life, it is a useful parameter for outcomes important in oncology nursing.

## QUALITY OF LIFE AS A PROGNOSTIC INDICATOR

It has generally been presumed that the "soft," subjective measures of quality of life are inferior to "hard," clinical indicators, such as histology and weight loss. However, as the sophistication of quality of life instruments has improved over time, so has the ability to provide information of real clinical importance. In fact, patient's ratings of their quality of life before treatment have been found to be predictive of length of survival—in some cases with even more predictive power than traditional clinical indicators.

There are 22 studies in which patient's ratings of their quality of life before treatment began (at baseline) were found to be predictive of survival.[5–26] These findings also were not limited to a single type of cancer, but were found across 9 types (lung, breast, esophagus, head and neck, bladder, cervical, pancreatic, colorectal, and prostate cancer), which provides greater confidence in the findings. The quality of life scores that were predictive of survival were global quality of life, symptoms (pain, fatigue, anorexia, dyspnea), and functioning (physical, cognitive, emotional, social, and role function). Satisfaction with life was even predictive of survival in four studies. Because the studies used different instruments to measure quality of life, and patients received a wide variety of treatment regimens, they increase our confidence that a relationship between pretreatment quality of life and survival actually exists.

In some cases, the quality of life scores were even more powerful predictors than standard clinical indicators. For example, in inoperable nonsmall cell lung cancer treated by radiotherapy, Langendijk et al[9] found that global quality of life was the strongest prognostic factor of all; stronger than node classification, weight loss, or performance status. Additional clinical variables among the studies that were found to be less predictive than quality of life scores were tumor stage, disease measurability, age, gender, time since diagnosis, tumor location, number of tumor sites, tumor type, comorbidity, prior radiotherapy, hemoglobin level, bone metastasis, estrogen and progesterone receptor status, and disease-free interval.[5–26]

On the basis of the findings such as these, Ganz et al[6] recommended that patient-rated quality of life assessment should be obtained as an integral part of cancer management to serve as a guide to patient needs, as an outcome measure, and as a prognostic variable for survival time. Osoba[27] has even suggested that pretreatment quality of life ratings could be used as an eligibility criterion and stratification variable in clinical trials.

## USING QUALITY OF LIFE INFORMATION IN CANCER CARE

In large clinical trials, quality of life data have played a crucial role in the selection of therapeutic agents that have become the standard of care.[28] In addition, information about quality of life is also important for planning treatment, decision making, and providing supportive care. Table 9-1 lists examples of ways that quality of life information can be valuable in clinical practice. Such information is useful for both clinicians and patients, as well as to promote communication among them. Oncology nurses play a critical role in providing quality of life information to patients, so that they can make better-informed decisions about their treatment. Examples of quality of life studies that have contributed to cancer care are described in the following sections.

**TABLE 9-1**

| Uses of Quality of Life Information in Cancer Care |
|---|
| • Determine whether a new therapy is preferable to standard therapy |
| • Compare two standard therapies having similar survival outcomes |
| • Identify the long-term negative effects of therapy, when survival time is long |
| • Discover whether a therapeutic regimen is better than supportive care only, when survival time is short |
| • Determine the negative effects of adjuvant therapy |
| • Identify the need for supportive care |
| • Target problems and facilitate communication in clinical practice |

## NEW THERAPY vs STANDARD THERAPY

A classic use for quality of life data is to determine whether a new therapy is preferable to the standard therapy. The gold standard for these comparisons is the phase III clinical trial. An example of the importance of quality of life in a phase III study can be seen in the head-to-head comparison of a new therapy, imatinib (Gleevec), with the standard interferon-alpha plus low-dose cytarabine in patients with newly diagnosed chronic myeloid leukemia.[29] After 12 months of treatment, the imatinib group had a significantly better quality of life than the interferon/cytarabine group. In particular, the imatinib group had better daily functioning, less fatigue, fewer cognitive problems, and better social functioning. In fact, the imatinib group actually had an increase in emotional well-being as compared to base-line, as patients felt better able to cope with illness, and were less worried and sad. In addition, patients who crossed over to imatinib experienced an improvement in quality of life, as compared with patients who continued with the interferon/cytarabine regimen. As a result, these findings contributed to imatinib becoming the new standard therapy for newly diagnosed chronic myeloid leukemia.

## TWO STANDARD THERAPIES WITH SIMILAR SURVIVAL OUTCOMES

When two treatments produce similar outcomes in survival, information about differences in quality of life outcomes can help determine the best choice. An example can be found in treatment for localized prostate cancer, for which there is continuing controversy regarding whether radical prostatectomy or radiation therapy provides superior outcomes in older men.[30] In an early study comparing quality of life outcomes for men receiving radical prostatectomy or radiation therapy, Yarbro and Ferrans[31] found that those treated by surgery had significantly worse urinary and sexual functioning. Protective pads or adult diapers were worn daily by 32% of the men in the surgical group, as compared with only 6% of the radiation group. Ability to have an erection was reported to be very poor for 88% of the surgical group and for only 46% of the radiation group. In contrast, the radiation group had worse bowel functioning due to radiation damage to the rectal mucosa, although the differences between groups were smaller in this area. Diarrhea and cramping pain were problems for only a few men. Similar findings later were reported in a nationwide Prostate Cancer Outcomes Study[32,33] as well as in a prospective study.[34] These studies provide important information for older men to consider as they decide which treatment to pursue for prostate cancer.

## LONG-TERM NEGATIVE EFFECTS OF THERAPY

Quality of life information can be critically important for decision making when treatment does not clearly provide a survival advantage. For example, older men with slow-growing, early prostate cancer can choose "watchful waiting" (monitoring with no treatment), rather than prostatectomy or radiation, based on the assumption that comorbid conditions will end their lives before the cancer will. A randomized trial of watchful waiting vs radical prostatectomy found that all-case mortality was not significantly different in the two groups, even though the rate of death from prostate cancer was slightly lower in the prostatectomy group.[35] In a companion study, quality of life outcomes were assessed an average of 4 years after randomization.[36] The prostatectomy group had significantly greater urinary leakage and compromised sexual function. These results are important for older men to consider when diagnosed with prostate cancer, so that they can make informed decisions regarding treatment.

## TREATMENT vs SUPPORTIVE CARE ONLY

When survival time is expected to be short, quality of life information is critically important for clinical decision making. In these cases, quality of life data are needed to demonstrate the superiority of the treatment over supportive care alone, which would allow the last months of life to be enjoyed without the side effects of treatment. Myelodysplastic syndrome is an example of a disease that at one time had no known effective treatment and a short survival time (6–12 months median survival). Quality of life data played a significant role in establishing azacytidine as a standard therapy. In a randomized clinical trial that compared azacytidine with supportive care only, the azacytidine group had better quality of life, greater treatment response, and longer time to death or transformation to acute myeloid leukemia. This group also had less fatigue and dyspnea, better physical functioning, more positive affect, and less psychological distress, showing that azacytidine was superior to supportive care alone.[37,38]

## NEGATIVE EFFECTS OF ADJUVANT THERAPY

Quality of life concerns regarding toxicity and long-term disability have led to changes in use of adjuvant therapy. A classic example is the use of cranial radiation for central nervous system prophylaxis for acute lymphoblastic leukemia (ALL) in children, which at one time received widespread use. Hill and colleagues[39] conducted a study that demonstrated that cranial radiation contributed to deficits in attention and overall intellectual functioning in these children. Two groups of survivors of childhood ALL were compared: one group had been treated with 24 Gy of cranial radiation and intrathecal methotrexate; the other had received systemic and intrathecal methotrexate but no cranial radiation. The group who had received cranial radiation had significantly worse academic achievement and greater psychological distress. As a result, intensive efforts were made to find effective alternatives to cranial radiotherapy to prevent recurrence or relapse, such as high-dose systemic chemotherapy and intensive intrathecal therapy.[40]

## SUPPORTIVE CARE

Quality of life information can play an important role in revealing needs for supportive care, both during treatment and afterward. For example, Ganz and colleagues[41] examined the quality of life in 558 patients with breast cancer during the period of time immediately after the completion of treatment, when women need to move beyond cancer to reestablish their normal life patterns. They found that women experienced breast sensitivity, muscle stiffness, aches and pains, difficulty concentrating, and decreased energy, regardless of the type of treatment (mastectomy, lumpectomy, chemotherapy). These problems were all associated with poor physical functioning and emotional well-being. In addition, sexual functioning was worse for women who received chemotherapy, regardless of whether they underwent a lumpectomy or mastectomy. After chemotherapy, women experienced difficulties with sexual interest, lubrication, and pain with intercourse. These results are important because they target areas for intervention to help women make a smoother transition to normal life.

Quality of life issues also have been identified for long-term survivors who remain free of disease. For example, some breast cancer survivors—particularly those with mastectomies or lymphedema—continue to experience significant problems with body image, sex life, depression, and symptoms of posttraumatic stress disorder years after treatment.[42–44] In addition, long-term survivors of various cancers have been found to experience many of the same problems—namely, chronic fatigue, fear of recurrence and death, infertility, issues of control and independence, altered meaning of health, and uncertainty about the future.

Nurse-delivered interventions have been instituted to address some of these quality of life issues. For example, cancer outpatients diagnosed with major depressive disorder received a multicomponent intervention delivered by nurses.[45] The intervention was effective, in that 38.5% fewer patients in the treatment group were still depressed at the final 6-month outcome, as compared with patients who received the usual care. In another study, breast cancer patients, who were 3 to 4 months postdiagnosis, received 10 sessions of cognitive-behavioral therapy by telephone.[46] The women who received the therapy had less anxiety and confusion at the final 10-month outcome, as compared to the control group.

## USING QUALITY OF LIFE QUESTIONNAIRES IN CLINICAL PRACTICE

Originally, quality of life questionnaires were used exclusively for research. More recently, there has been growing interest in their possible contribution to routine clinical care. Studies have shown that quality of life questionnaires can be used in clinical practice to facilitate communication and identify problems that otherwise might go undetected. In a study by Detmar and colleagues,[47] chemotherapy patients completed the questionnaires in the clinic before seeing their physicians, so that the physicians had the scores in hand at the time when they met with the patients. Quality of life issues were discussed more frequently by patients who completed the questionnaires, as compared to patients who did not. In addition, the physicians identified a larger proportion of patients with moderate or severe health problems when they had the questionnaires. All physicians and 87% of the patients thought the questionnaires facilitated communication and should continue to be used. In another study, Velikova and colleagues[48] tested computerized administration of quality of life instruments in oncology clinical practice. This prospective study (28 medical oncologists and 286 patients with cancer) demonstrated that providing quality of life data to clinicians resulted in a more frequent discussion of symptoms, without prolonging the clinical encounter. Improvement of quality of life was associated with the use of quality of life data, discussion of pain, and role function. These studies demonstrate that quality of life instruments can provide useful additional information to clinicians, increase the efficiency of the clinical encounter, and result in improved outcomes for patients. Halyard and

Ferrans[49] recently published guidelines for using quality of life instruments in oncology clinical practice.

## WHAT IS QUALITY OF LIFE?

The term *health-related quality of life* commonly is used to focus on quality of life in the context of illness and treatment. Because this chapter focuses on quality of life as an outcome of cancer care, it addresses health-related quality of life. The term "health-related quality of life" is used to draw a line between the facets of life that are primarily health related and those that are not. Non-health-related quality of life typically is thought of as cultural, political, or societal types of issues that fall within the purview of fields such as economics, demography, and sociology.[50] However, because cancer has a pervasive influence on a person's life, all domains of quality of life become "health related" in this context. It is interesting to note that the World Health Organization has chosen to define *quality of life* in a comprehensive manner:

> An individual's perception of their position in life in the context of the culture and value systems in which they live and in relation to their goals, expectations, standards, and concerns. It is a broad-ranging concept affected in a complex way by the person's physical health, psychological state, level of independence, social relationships, and their relationship to salient features of their environment.[51,p.1570]

## CONCEPTUAL MODEL OF QUALITY OF LIFE

Even when we consider only health-related quality of life, we find that this term has been used to mean many different things, eg, health status, emotional adjustment, symptoms, physical functioning, well-being, life satisfaction, and happiness.[50] This ambiguity has led to a great deal of confusion, making it difficult to compare findings across studies and to apply them in clinical practice. A number of conceptual models have been developed to characterize health-related quality of life.[50] However, Wilson and Cleary[52] developed a model that is particularly helpful for clarifying the concept. Their model presents the relationships among the various types of patient outcomes that have been used to measure health-related quality of life (Figure 9-1). It focuses primarily on the 5 boxes in the center of the figure, which represent five levels of measurable patient outcomes. The first box, biological and physiological variables, focuses on the function of cells, organs, and organ systems. These are assessed through indicators such as physical assessment, laboratory tests, and histological findings. It should be noted that this first box does not actually represent a type of quality of life measure, because it is assessed using objective indicators rather than patient-reported outcomes.[53] Nevertheless, it provides an appropriate starting point for the model because it provides the basis for the following 4 boxes. Symptom status, the second box, refers to physical,

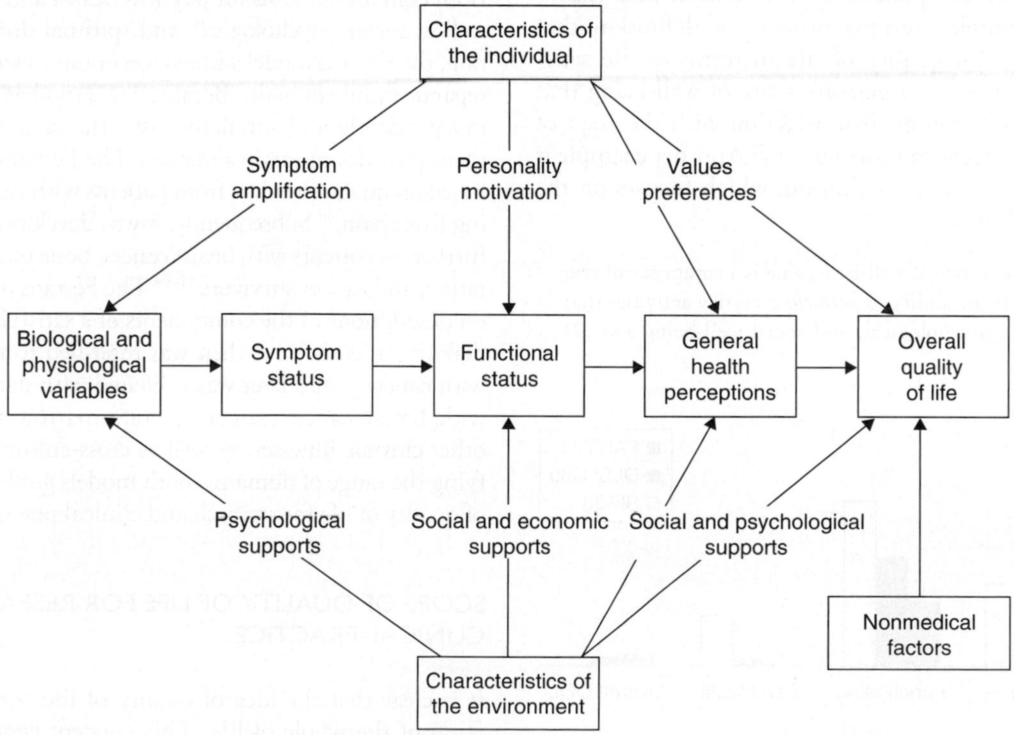


**FIGURE 9-1**

Wilson and Cleary's conceptual model for health-related quality of life.

*Source*: Reprinted with permission from Wilson and Cleary.[52] American Medical Association. 

emotional, and cognitive symptoms, which are perceived by the patient. The third box, functional status, is composed of physical, psychological, social, and role functioning. General health perceptions, the fourth box, refer to a patient's subjective rating of health. This rating provides an integration of all of the boxes that precede it in the model. The fifth box is overall quality of life—that is, how happy or satisfied someone is with life as a whole. Values and preferences of patients are characterized as contributing to general health perceptions and overall quality of life.

Wilson and Cleary's model is helpful because it clearly displays the various concepts that have been used to measure quality of life outcomes. Use of this model should help researchers and clinicians to specify what exactly is meant by the term "quality of life," which will reduce some of the current confusion. For example, Figure 9-2[28] displays the percentage of questions in the 3 most commonly used instruments in cancer clinical trials in terms of each of Wilson and Cleary's components: the FACT,[54] the EORTC QLQ-C30,[55] and the SF-36.[56] Although all 3 instruments predominantly measure symptoms and functioning, differences among the instruments are clearly apparent, with the FACT-G and EORTC QLQ-C30 primarily assessing symptoms, the SF-36 focusing mainly on functioning.[28]

Many of the definitions of quality of life that are most commonly used in health care today also can be classified in relation to the components of the Wilson and Cleary model. For example, Ferrans provides a definition that characterizes overall quality of life in terms of life satisfaction (the fifth box): "a person's sense of well-being that stems from satisfaction or dissatisfaction with the areas of life that are important to him/her."[57,p.15] Another example is provided by Gotay et al's definition, which focuses on the third and fifth boxes:

> Quality of life is a state of well-being that is a composite of two components: (1) the ability to *perform* everyday activities that reflect physical, psychological, and social well-being and (2) patient *satisfaction* with levels of functioning and the control of disease and/or treatment-related symptoms.[58,p.576]

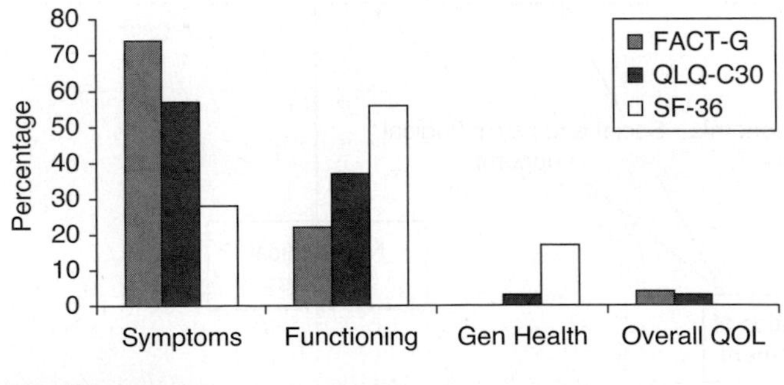


**FIGURE 9-2**

Components of health-related quality of life measured by the FACT-G, EORTC QLQ-C30, and SF-36.

*Source*: Reprinted from Ferrans,[28] with permission by Oxford Press.

Ferrans et al[53] provide further clarification of the model in terms of related theoretical frameworks that expand each of the main components of the model.

## DOMAINS OF QUALITY OF LIFE

As can be seen in the Wilson and Cleary model, quality of life is not limited to physical health status alone. There is general agreement among experts that quality of life is a multidimensional construct. As a consequence, each component of the Wilson and Cleary model should be thought of in terms of multiple domains. For example, symptom status refers to emotional and cognitive symptoms, as well as physical ones. In addition to physical functioning, functional status refers to psychological, social, and role functioning.

Leplege and Hunt[59] have criticized many of the models developed to characterize the domains of quality of life, because they were not developed based on the viewpoints of patients themselves. The 2 models of quality of life presented in this chapter were based on qualitative analysis of patients' perspectives and were validated with additional patient data. One model was developed by Ferrell and Grant (Figure 9-3) and the other by Ferrans et al (Figure 9-4 and Table 9-2). Both models are quite similar in terms of the domains identified. Both contain domains for physical health and functioning, as well as social, psychological, and spiritual domains. In addition, the Ferrans model addresses economic elements and has a separate family domain. Because the 2 models were developed independently and simultaneously, the close match between them provides mutual validation. The Ferrell et al model was based on qualitative data from patients with cancer and suffering from pain.[60] Subsequently, it was developed and validated further for patients with breast cancer, bone marrow transplantation, and cancer survivors.[61–64] The Ferrans model was based on descriptions of the components of a satisfying life given by dialysis patients.[65,66] It then was modified to include patients with cancer [57] and later was validated with data from patients with breast cancer, sarcoma, bone marrow transplant, and other chronic illnesses, as well as cross-culturally.[67] By identifying the range of domains, both models guide the assessment of quality of life for research and clinical practice.

## SCOPE OF QUALITY OF LIFE FOR RESEARCH AND CLINICAL PRACTICE

It is clear that the idea of quality of life conveys an evaluation of the whole of life. This concept generally has been addressed by including the requisite domains. However, within each domain, a question remains as to whether the scope should be limited to those things appropriately addressed by healthcare professionals. This decision depends

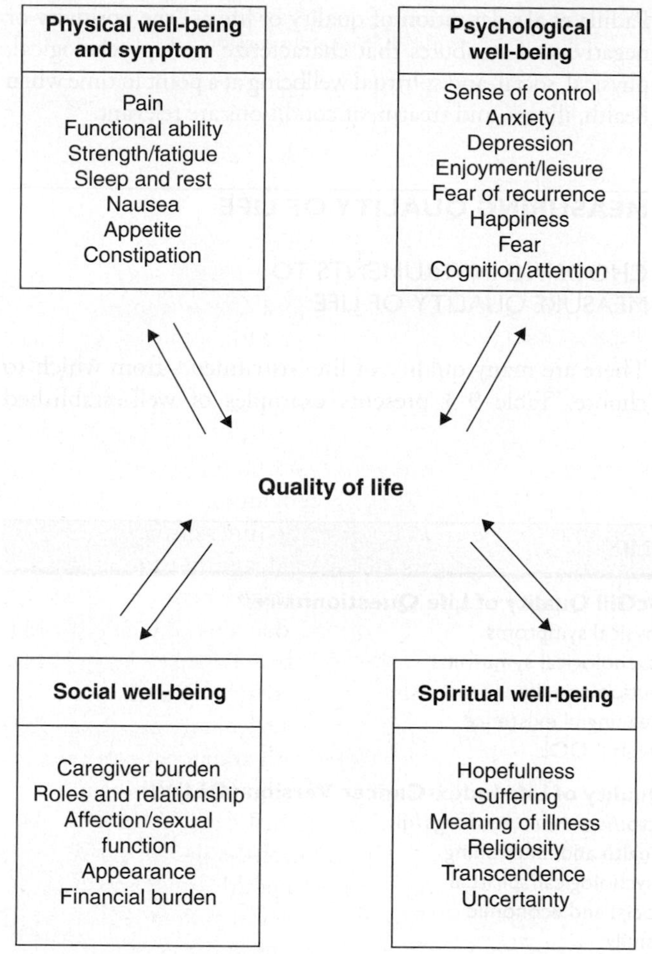


**FIGURE 9-3**

Ferrell and Grant conceptual model for quality of life.

*Source*: Reprinted with permission from Grant M and Ferrell B.[64]

on the target population and the goals to be accomplished in the particular research study or clinical practice. For example, the definition of quality of life used for a chemotherapy clinical trial might focus primarily on toxicity and interference with functioning, so it might be narrow in scope. A study in end-of-life care would require a broader definition providing a balance between physical comfort and existential concerns, such as spirituality and personal meaning.

Ferrans recently developed a taxonomy for quality of life definitions based on their scope.[50] The first level is quality of life within the commonly recognized purview of health care. This level is the most narrow, in that the healthcare system is concerned primarily with the correction of problems. These definitions highlight the negative effects of illness and treatment, such as symptoms, sexual dysfunction, or disability. An example is Schipper et al's definition: "quality of life in clinical medicine represents the functional effect of an illness and its consequent therapy upon a patient, as perceived by the patient."[68]

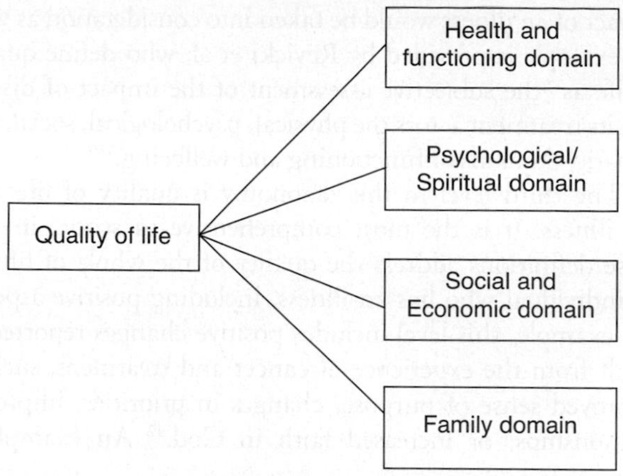


**FIGURE 9-4**

Ferrans conceptual model for quality of life.

The second level in this taxonomy is the impact of illness on quality of life. This level is broader, in that these definitions allow for consideration of the effects of illness on a wider range of aspects of life. For example, the impact of illness on a marital relationship is of interest, rather than just sexual dysfunction. Instead of focusing solely on the ability to work, the financial

**TABLE 9-2**

**Elements of the Ferrans Conceptual Model for Quality of Life**

| **Health and Functioning Domain** | **Psychological/Spiritual Domain** |
|---|---|
| Own health | Satisfaction with life |
| Pain | Happiness in general |
| Energy (fatigue) | Achievement of personal goals |
| Ability to take care of yourself without help | Peace of mind |
| Ability to take care of family responsibilities | Faith in God |
| Usefulness to others | Personal appearance |
| Worries | Satisfaction with self |
| Control over life | **Social and Economic Domain** |
| Chances of living as long as you would like | Friends |
| Chances for a happy future | Emotional support from friends |
| Sex life | Home (house, apartment) |
| Leisure time activities | Neighborhood |
| Health care | Job/unemployment |
| **Family Domain** | Ability to take care of financial needs |
| Family happiness | Education |
| Spouse, lover, or partner | |
| Children | |
| Emotional support from family | |
| Family health | |

impact of an illness would be taken into consideration as well. An example is provided by Revicki et al, who define quality of life as "the subjective assessment of the impact of disease and its treatment across the physical, psychological, social, and somatic, domains of functioning and wellbeing."[69]

The third level in this taxonomy is quality of life during illness. It is the most comprehensive in scope, in that these definitions address the quality of the whole of life for an individual who has an illness, including positive aspects. For example, this level includes positive changes reported to result from the experience of cancer and treatment, such as improved sense of purpose, changes in priorities, improved relationships, or increased faith in God.[42] An example is Padilla et al's definition of quality of life as "the positivity or negativity of attributes that characterize one's psychological, physical, social, and spiritual wellbeing at a point in time when health, illness, and treatment conditions are relevant."[70]

## MEASURING QUALITY OF LIFE

### CHOOSING INSTRUMENTS TO MEASURE QUALITY OF LIFE

There are many quality of life instruments from which to choose. Table 9-3 presents examples of well-established

**TABLE 9-3**

**Multidimensional Instruments Used to Measure Quality of Life**

**Cancer Rehabilitation Evaluation System (CARES)-Short Form**[71]
Physical
Psychosocial
Marital
Sexual
Medical interaction
Overall QOL

**EORTC Quality of Life Questionnaire (EORTC QLQ-C30)**[55,72]
http://www.eortc.be/home/qol/
Physical functioning
Pain
Fatigue
Nausea and vomiting
Overall symptoms
Role functioning
Cognitive ability
Psychological functioning
Social interaction
Finances

**Functional Assessment of Cancer Therapy (FACT/FACIT)**[54,73]
http://www.facit.org
Physical well-being
Social/family well-being
Emotional well-being
Functional well-being
Overall QOL

**Functional Living Index-Cancer (FLIC)**[74,75]
Overall QOL
Physical well-being and ability
Nausea
Hardship due to cancer
Psychological well-being
Social well-being

**McGill Quality of Life Questionnaire**[76]
Physical symptoms
Psychological symptoms
Outlook on life
Meaningful existence
Overall QOL

**Quality of Life Index-Cancer Version (QLI)**[57,65]
http://www.uic.edu/orgs/qli
Health and functioning
Psychological/spiritual
Social and economic
Family
Overall QOL

**Quality of Life Scale for Cancer (QOL-CA)**[64]
http://prc.coh.org
Physical well-being
Psychological well-being
Spiritual well-being
Social well-being
Overall QOL

**SF-36 Health Survey**[56,77]
http://www.qualitymetric.com
Physical function
Physical role function
Vitality
Bodily pain
Mental health
Emotional role function
Social function
General health perceptions

*Note*: All the instruments listed were developed for use in patients with cancer, except for the SF-36, which was designed for the general population.

instruments that were developed for use with patients with cancer (except for the SF-36, which was designed for use in the general population).[56] The domains of quality of life that each instrument measures are listed, as well as the availability of an overall quality of life score. Web sites for the instruments are identified where available; they are excellent sources for current and comprehensive information.

Many quality of life instruments were developed for specific populations and purposes, and so they may not all be equally appropriate or sensitive when used in contexts they were not originally intended for. Instruments should be selected based on the best fit with the target population and purpose for use, and a single instrument or a battery of instruments may be needed to capture the broad nature of the concept. Evidence of reliability, validity, and responsiveness/sensitivity are prerequisites for the choice of an instrument, as they provide assurance that the instrument is reasonably free of random error, measures what it was intended to measure, and is sufficiently sensitive to detect change in quality of life.

## GENERIC vs DISEASE-SPECIFIC INSTRUMENTS

A distinction made among quality of life measures is whether the instrument is generic or disease specific. Generic instruments assess all domains of quality of life, whereas disease-specific instruments target concerns that are most relevant to a specific illness and treatment. There are advantages and disadvantages for both types of instruments. Generic instruments are useful for making comparisons with the general population, which is particularly helpful for the interpretation of results. They also can be used across different treatment groups and illness populations, making it possible to compare the effectiveness of various therapies and healthcare programs. In addition, they can place symptoms within the context of life as a whole, as well as identify unanticipated adverse effects, which can help to determine the effectiveness of treatment. The major disadvantage of generic instruments is that because they are so broad, they tend to cover each area superficially, and may not address the most important symptoms. Disease-specific instruments generally tend to be more sensitive in detecting changes in symptoms and treatment effects, which gives them more statistical power. However, because of their limited scope, disease-specific instruments may miss critical aspects of quality of life. For these reasons, it is preferable to use both types of instruments whenever possible, to capitalize on the advantages of both. Many of the instruments used for cancer care are a blend of both generic and disease-specific measures. For example, the FACT/FACIT[54] and the EORTC QLQ-C30[55] are core instruments that are used for all patients with cancer. In addition, modules have been developed for use with the core instruments, which are specific for different types of cancer, such as prostate, breast, and colon cancer.

## STATUS AND EVALUATION QUESTIONS

Measures that rely on information from patients recently have become known as "patient reported outcomes" (PROs). There is general agreement that quality of life assessments, of necessity, depend on information reported by the patients themselves whenever possible. Within this subjective realm, there are actually 2 types of patient-reported information produced by quality of life questionnaires.[50] One asks for information on the state (or status) of a particular aspect of life, such as "How much pain do you have?" The other asks for an evaluation of that state, such as "How tolerable is the amount of pain that you have?" This distinction is important because the answers to these 2 types of questions (status and evaluation) provide different information. An evaluation requires additional steps in cognitive processing, because the person first must think of how much pain he or she has and then make a judgment about it—good or bad, satisfied, or dissatisfied. Some quality of life instruments are composed entirely of status questions, such as the EORTC QLQ-C30 and SF-36, whereas others are composed entirely of evaluation questions, such as the Quality of Life Index (QLI) and the Quality of Life Scale for Cancer (QOL-CA). Others contain a mixture of both status and evaluation questions, such as the Functional Assessment of Cancer Therapy (FACT/FACIT).[50]

Different information (and different scores) is produced depending on whether status or evaluation questions are asked. This consideration is important both when selecting an instrument to use and when interpreting scores from it. Evidence can be seen in studies that have used two quality of life instruments with the same sample. For example, although the FACT/FACIT scale and the QLI: Cancer Version measure many of the same domains, the correlation between the 2 instruments was only 0.41 in a sample of patients with primary brain cancer. Similarly, scores from the SF-36 and QLI were only moderately correlated, even though they measured many of the same domains, in patients with angina or HIV.[78,79]

Most definitions of quality of life used in health care today focus on the evaluative aspect of quality of life.[50] The idea of quality of life, in its essence, requires a value judgment about a person's life. It is the incorporation of a patient's values that sets it apart from measures of health status. In this way, it provides an understanding of the impact of illness from the viewpoint of the patient. However, both status and evaluation information are important for measuring outcomes in cancer care. Individuals may consider their quality of life to be good, even when faced with physical disabilities. Over time, individuals make adaptations to compensate for physical losses, in order to preserve their satisfaction with life. Covinsky et al[80] provided evidence of this adaptation in a study of 493 older patients, in which 43% of those with the worst physical functioning considered their quality of life to be good. Conversely, 15% of those with the best physical functioning considered their quality of life to be fair or poor. These findings also show that erroneous conclusions could be drawn if either the status or evaluation measures were used alone to determine the quality of life of patients in this study.

### IMPORTANCE AND PREFERENCE MEASURES

The idea of quality of life conveys a judgment about a person's life, which requires the use of values. This concept is depicted in the Wilson and Cleary model, in that values and preferences are characterized as directly influencing general health perceptions and overall quality of life (Figure 9-1).[52] This raises the question of how values are captured in quality of life instruments. As discussed previously, evaluation-type questions, by their very nature, require an additional cognitive step in that they ask for a judgment to be made, which requires the use of personal values.[50] For example, values come into play when answering questions about how distressing something is, how bothersome, or how satisfying it is. Thus, instruments that contain evaluation-type questions implicitly require the use of personal values for their questions to be answered.[50]

Some instruments incorporate values in a more structured manner. They use a variety of terms to elicit information regarding values, by asking patients to rate importance, distress, bother, or effect on quality of life. The answers are then incorporated into the quality of life scores by weighting. *Weighting* is based on the idea that highly valued areas of life have greater influence on quality of life than areas of less importance. Some instruments use ratings of importance of individual aspects of life as weights to produce scores, such as the Quality of Life Inventory (QOLI)[81] and the QLI.[58] Other instruments ask respondents to rate the importance of an entire domain, but do not use the information in a weighting scheme. Examples include the FACT (original version),[73] the WHOQOL-100 instrument,[51] and the Prostate Cancer Index (PCI).[82] All of these instruments use the values of the respondents themselves in the quality of life assessment. Other instruments use weights based on the values of the general population or values gleaned from other groups of patients, rather than the individual completing the instrument. For these instruments, a person answers status-type questions that do not ask for an evaluation, and the score is computed using values previously obtained from groups of other people. Examples of this type of instrument that have been used with patients with cancer include the EuroQol EQ-5D,[83] the Health Utilities Index,[84] and the Quality of Well-Being scale.[85] Feeny[86] provides an excellent discussion of these and other preference measures.

A different sort of preference measure that was developed specifically for cancer care is Q-TwiST (Quality-Adjusted Time without Symptoms and Toxicity).[87] With this instrument, survival time is discounted to take into consideration the effect of treatment side effects and disease symptoms, using a utility weight ranging from 0 to 1. The utility weights, which reflect preferences, were determined by the investigators themselves, rather than patients with breast cancer. Q-TwiST has been used to demonstrate the additional burden of adjuvant chemotherapy in women receiving tamoxifen.[88] However, it has been pointed out that the summary scores of instruments such as Q-TwiST do not permit identification of specific problem areas.

The question about whose values to use for quality of life measurement can be addressed by considering the purpose of the assessment. The developmental work for the WHOQOL-100[51] demonstrated that some aspects of life are of universal relevance. However, individuals and cultural groups differ from the general population in the values they attach to various aspects of life. Changes in values also occur over time, as a result of adaptation in response to significant life events. These changes, which are referred to as "response shift," can occur as a result of making accommodations to illness.[89] If the purpose is to determine the types of healthcare services that will be paid for by public resources, it has been argued that the general population's values should be used.[90] Conversely, if the purpose is to identify the needs of individual patients in clinical practice, there is no substitute for the values of the individual.

## CLINICAL SIGNIFICANCE

One important reason for assessing quality of life is to identify changes and assign meaning to these changes, whether the changes are positive or negative. In order to better understand and interpret changes in quality of life outcomes, evaluation of their significance should take place on two levels, statistical and clinical.[91] For statistical significance, researchers use inferential statistics to test hypotheses, such as comparing quality of life outcomes among patients receiving different treatments or evaluating changes in quality of life over time. Quality of life outcomes are considered statistically significant if the probability of obtaining the observed outcomes is considered unlikely by chance alone (usually less than 1 in 20 or 5%). However, a change can be statistically significant, and yet be so small that it is clinically trivial or even meaningless. For a change to be clinically significant, it must be (by definition) large or important enough to affect patient care or treatment.[91,92]

Researchers have been working to determine the clinical significance of various quality of life scores, to help users of the information interpret the clinical implications of the findings. A number of methods for determining the clinical significance of quality of life scores have been developed.[92–94] One type is an anchor-based approach, which uses other clinically relevant indicators as "anchors" for interpretation of the quality of life scores. For instance, mean score changes for the multi-item subscales of the EORTC QLQ-C30 were found to correspond with patients' ratings of change in their perceived health status.[95,96] This information led to the development of guidelines for interpreting the clinical significance of scores for the EORTC QLQ-C30. Mean score changes of 5 to 10 points are considered small clinically significant differences; mean score changes of 10 to 20 points are considered moderate differences; and changes over 20 points indicate large clinically significant differences. Thus, a 21-point difference between 2 sets of scores on the physical functioning subscale of the EORTC QLQ-C30 would be interpreted as a large, clinically significant change.

Other examples of anchor-based guidelines for interpreting scores also have been identified in the literature. For the QLI, a difference of 2 points or more in mean scores is recognized as clinically significant, based on correspondence with overall quality of life, self-image, physical symptoms, and general health.[57,97–99] For the FACT-General and Fact-Head and Neck, a change of 5% to 10% corresponds to clinically significant differences in quality of life in patients with laryngeal cancer.[100]

Distribution-based approaches for assessing clinical significance use a statistical parameter (such as variability of the quality of life scores), using group level data to determine cut points for clinical significance. Two methods have emerged as particularly useful in clinical research: the ½ standard deviation method[101] and the empirical rule effect size.[102] The ½ standard deviation method simply uses a ½ standard deviation to estimate differences in quality of life that are likely to be clinically significant. Quality of life scores that deviate from baseline scores by more than ½ standard deviation are considered to be clinically significant. The empirical rule effect size builds upon the ½ standard deviation method by incorporating effect sizes into the determination of clinical significance. Effect size is a statistical term that quantifies the strength of a relationship between two variables, and is known as the treatment effect when used with therapeutic interventions. It is important to note that all of these guidelines have been developed using group level data, and so are appropriate for interpreting quality of life outcomes from studies where the focus is on group level data. However, these guidelines may not be appropriate for interpreting clinical significance when used with individual patients, as they may not correspond to the individual patient's own threshold for clinical significance.

Multiple groups, such as patients, clinicians, and society, use information obtained from quality of life assessments to determine clinical significance.[103] The perception of the user of the information may influence whether a quality of life assessment is clinically significant. Each of these group's values and standards vary and this may result in different outcomes in relation to determination of clinical significance, so that a change that is considered clinically significant to 1 group may not be to another. For example, an individual patient may perceive a 10-point increase in fatigue as clinically significant and this may influence her decision to continue with the new treatment. The clinician, on the other hand, must weigh the benefits of treatment against the magnitude of the increase and severity of fatigue to determine whether a change in clinical practice is warranted. In the clinician's mind, a 10-point increase in fatigue may not justify changing a treatment that has a high cure rate. Society may present a third view. From a societal perspective, the productivity costs associated with a 10-point increase in fatigue due to a new treatment may be clinically significant if it causes patients to be unable to work.

A great deal of effort has been directed toward identifying the clinical significance of quality of life scores, illustrating the growing importance of the topic. An expert panel of 30 quality of life researcher published a series of 6 manuscripts detailing the state of the science of clinical significance and application of quality of life research to clinical practice, which we recommend for readers interested in learning more about the topic.[91,93,103–107]

## DATA COLLECTION IN REAL TIME

The ability to accurately assess symptoms, perceived health status, and quality of life is essential for providing quality cancer care and conducting scientifically sound research. Clinicians and researchers depend heavily on self-reported information provided by patients to guide decision-making processes. In recent years, advances have been made in methods for collecting information on patient-reported outcomes (such as quality of life). For example, several studies have demonstrated the feasibility of using computerized programs for the self-report of symptoms during scheduled clinic visits or at home, providing support for this approach.[108–110] In addition, the National Institutes of Health has sponsored a national effort to develop a computerized adaptive testing system for clinical research and practice. This will provide a common measurement system for PROs, called the Patient-Reported Outcomes Measurement Information System (PROMIS) initiative, which will be publicly available.[111]

Individuals with cancer experience a wide range of symptoms, such as fatigue, pain, nausea, vomiting and sleep disturbances, as well as changes in physical, cognitive, emotional, and social functioning. Recall bias may limit the ability to provide accurate self-report data retrieved from memory, particularly in people experiencing multiple symptoms simultaneously. Recall bias occurs when people are asked to recall events or experiences that have occurred in the past, and the memory is distorted due to cognitive restructuring of the event or experience. Cognitive restructuring can affect the patient's ability to provide accurate quality of life information, particularly health status information. Multiple factors influence the reconstruction of memories, such as length of time since the event/experience and whether the event/experience was anticipated.[112,113] Events/experiences that are fresh in the mind or novel tend to be remembered more clearly and tend to disproportionately shape the memory. For example, if a patient has been relatively pain free, but experiences 1 short-lived episode of extreme pain right before filling out a self-report questionnaire, the episode of pain is likely to play a focal role when recalling pain over the past week. Patients do not simply add up the number of painful episodes, incorporate intensity ratings, and then average them over time to produce a summary of the experiences of the past week. Other reconstruction strategies are likely to impact the patient's memory and ability to accurately recall self-report data.

Ecological momentary assessment is a methodological approach used to capture repeated real-time data in a naturalistic environment. Because patients respond in real time, it minimizes recall biases and problems with summarization processes associated with retrospective assessments.[114] The 3 components of ecological momentary assessment (real-time data collection) include (1) studying people in their natural environment, (2) collecting information regarding the person's immediate or near immediate state, and (3) sampling the phenomena under study multiple times throughout the course of the day. Thus, real-time data collection avoids problems with summarization and ensures an adequate representation of the experience over time.

Several studies have demonstrated the feasibility of using an ecological momentary approach to assess symptoms in people with cancer, including acutely ill patients.[115,116] For example, people who recently had received a hematopoietic stem cell transplant were able to provide real-time fatigue data 3 times during the course of the day, even when experiencing multiple side effects from the preparatory regimen.[116] Patients wore a device similar to a wristwatch, which signaled them when it was time to rate their fatigue. They provided the rating by pushing buttons on the device itself. Most patients reported none to mild fatigue before receiving the high-dose chemotherapy, with a shift toward moderate to severe fatigue during the immediate post-transplant period. Even though their fatigue increased substantially as they became acutely ill, the majority of patients continued to provide the fatigue ratings. Eighty-seven percent provided fatigue ratings before the stem cell transplant and 86% after transplant. This approach also has been used successfully to measure fatigue in other cancer populations, including survivors of breast cancer.[115] Real-time data collection, however, is not limited to the assessment of fatigue. Other facets of quality of life may be equally amenable to real-time data collection, such as pain and perception of health status.

## POPULATIONS PRESENTING SPECIAL CHALLENGES

### PROXY RATINGS

The term *quality of life* conveys the idea of a value judgment requiring some kind of rating, such as good/bad, high/low, or best/worst. It makes a difference who does the rating, because people use their own internal standards for what they consider a desirable or undesirable quality of life.[27] There is general agreement that quality of life is best evaluated by the patient, rather than by an outside observer. Nevertheless, in some situations the patient may not be able to provide the information needed, because of cognitive impairment, debilitating fatigue, severe nausea, pain, or other symptoms. These are often times when quality of life information is most needed, which makes the use of proxy raters appealing. A proxy rater is anyone other than the patient who evaluates the patient's quality of life.

Because patients' own perspectives differ from those of outside observers, ratings assigned by proxies may differ dramatically from the ratings patients would give themselves. These differences have been demonstrated in studies comparing patients' ratings with those of physicians, nurses, and significant others (spouse, family, friends). For example, one study reported that correlations between quality of life ratings by patients and physicians ranged only from 0.26 to 0.45, and that patient and nurse correlations were no better, ranging from 0.19 to 0.47.[117] Another review of 23 of the most methodologically sound studies found that the agreement between patients and proxies was modest to good ($r = 0.42$–$0.78$), although there were a few studies whose correlations were very low.[118] Better agreement was found for physical functioning than for other domains. This is consistent with an earlier review of 49 studies,[119] which found that proxies provided more accurate information when they assessed things that are concrete and observable, such as functional status, cigarette smoking, and consumption of food, coffee, and alcohol. Proxies provided less accurate information when they assessed things that are subjective and unobservable, such as the patient's satisfaction, pain, cognitive functioning, depression, or psychosocial adjustment to cancer.

These findings demonstrate that proxies should be used for quality of life assessment only if absolutely necessary, and with the understanding that they are an imperfect substitute for the patient. In addition, whenever possible, the level of agreement between patients and the proxies should be determined when patients are still able to answer questions. Later, when patients are no longer able to provide information, the proxy ratings can be interpreted in light of the concordance found previously between proxy and patient.

### COGNITIVE IMPAIRMENT

Cognitive impairment may make it difficult or impossible for patients to complete the response scales of many quality of life instruments. Rather than relying on proxies, there are techniques to assist patients to provide valid responses to scales with multiple categories. Patients' understanding of response choices can be improved with the use of visual aids such as histograms with bars of increasing size, which depict the response categories.[67] In addition, it can be helpful to break the cognitive task into smaller parts. For example, the QLI was administered in an interview format to patients with cognitive impairment (Mini-Mental State Examination scores ranging from 18 to 20).[120] Patients were able to provide valid responses to the 6-point response scale when it was administered in a series of dichotomous questions. They were first asked whether they were satisfied or dissatisfied with an aspect of life. Next, they were given 3 options (slightly, moderately, or very satisfied/dissatisfied) from which to choose. To facilitate the decisions, a histogram characterizing the response choices also was shown to the patients.

## CHILDREN

Work based on adults in the field of quality of life cannot be directly applied in pediatric oncology for several reasons. First, there is the complex interplay between the child's developmental stage and the experience of cancer.[121] Second, the sense of well-being in children can fluctuate in response to daily events and chronic problems, and is affected by their developing cognitive ability and personality.[122] Third, the child's quality of life has a complex interrelationship with that of the family as a unit and individual family members.[122]

For these reasons, it has been necessary to develop unique definitions, conceptual models, and instruments to address quality of life in children. Different conceptual approaches can be identified in the definitions and instruments developed. For example, the definition of quality of life of the Pediatric Oncology Group focuses primarily on functioning: "Quality of life is a multidimensional construct, incorporating both objective and subjective data, including (but not limited to) the social, physical, and emotional functioning of the child and, when indicated, his/her family. QOL measurement must be sensitive to changes that occur throughout development."[121,p.89] An alternative definition focusing on a sense of well-being is provided by Hinds et al, "an overall sense of well-being based on being able to participate in usual activities; to interact with others and feel cared about; to cope with uncomfortable physical, emotional, and cognitive reactions; and to find meaning in the illness experience."[123]

Instruments have been developed for children and adolescents with cancer that differ from each other in their conceptual approach, as shown by a qualitative analysis of their content.[124] Some measure the individual's self-assessment of functioning in physical, psychological, and social domains,[125,126] and others measure satisfaction of life in terms of the discrepancy between how life is and how one would expect it to be.[127,128] A third group of instruments measure health status.[129,130]

It is common for quality of life evaluations to be provided by parents. Unfortunately, parents are imperfect proxies for children, as shown by well-designed studies measuring quality of life. For example, using the parent and child versions of the same instrument, correlations between scores of parents and children (ages 8–11) have been found to range from 0.44 to 0.61.[131] Children reported lower quality of life in the areas of positive emotions, physical complaints, motor functioning, cognitive functioning, and autonomy.

Because children generally are recognized as the preferred source of information, a number of instruments have been developed for children to complete themselves. Touch-screen computers that speak to children can be used to administer some instruments to young children who cannot read.[125] Some instruments provide different versions for specific age groups[125] and another has been developed specifically for children with cancer, such as the Pediatric Oncology Quality of Life Scale.[132] The majority of instruments were developed for use with a wide range of pediatric and adolescent populations, although some of these have cancer-specific modules.[125,126] Additional information on defining and measuring quality of life in pediatric patients with cancer can be found in the excellent review by Hinds and colleagues.[133]

## END OF LIFE

At the end of life, cancer care focuses on promoting comfort so as to provide the best possible quality of life. Rather than tumor response and survival time, success is achieved in terms of a "good death." Recognizing this shift in emphasis, symptom management and supportive care become of paramount importance. Patients with cancer commonly experience pain, fatigue, constipation, dyspnea, and dry mouth at the end of life.[134,135] In addition to physical symptoms, Steinhauser et al[136] reported that the factors most important to patients at the end of life were mental awareness, peace with God, not being a burden to family, and feeling their life was complete. Nevertheless, the SUPPORT study, which followed approximately 4000 patients at the end of life, found that more than half had inadequate pain control, and one-fourth suffered from emotional distress, social isolation, and feelings of abandonment.[137]

What are the implications for neglecting quality of life at the end of life? For dying patients, it can lead to loss of the will to live, which can result in premature death by active suicide or passive surrender.[138] A recent report of SEER registry data found that patients with cancer have almost twice the incidence of suicide as the general population, and the highest rates are among patients with cancers of the lung and bronchus, oral cavity and pharynx, and larynx.[139] Researchers have found that the will to live is highly correlated with the sense of well-being in patients with cancer at end of life, along with depression, anxiety, and dyspnea.[140]

Measuring quality of life at the end of life presents its own set of challenges. Although physical functioning and activities of daily living are still important, these eventually become less useful to measure, because physical status deteriorates until it eventually levels off. At some point, those scores become uniformly low and so no longer provide discrimination. Instead, measures of quality of life need to capture the elements that are important to patients at the end of life, such as meaning in life, spirituality, relationship issues, and positive aspects, in addition to symptoms. Instruments have been developed expressly for the purpose of measuring these concerns, such as the Hospice Quality of Life Index,[141] McGill Quality of Life Questionnaire,[76] and Missoula-VITAS Quality of Life Index.[142] In addition, palliative care modules have been developed for general quality of life measures, such as the FACT/FACIT.[143] These instruments all elicit information directly from the patient, rather than from a proxy. Information from the patient is preferred, because proxies are less able to provide accurate information about the subjective elements that are important to patients at the end of life.[144] Because patients become unable to answer questions as death approaches, inevitably family members need to provide information about the very end of life. The Quality of Dying and Death questionnaire was developed specifically for eliciting information from family members. It was designed for use after death and asks family members to rate 31 aspects of the patient's dying experience.[145] To help clinicians and researchers find measures for use at end of life, Teno and colleagues[146] developed a Toolkit of instruments (http://www.chcr.brown.edu/pcoc/TOOLKIT.htm). The Toolkit Web site provides a review of 41 instruments they recommend to measure quality of life at the end of life, including the last month of life. It also includes reviews of numerous other instruments useful for assessing quality of life outcomes, such as pain and other symptoms, emotional and cognitive symptoms, functional status, and spirituality.

## CULTURE AND LANGUAGE DIFFERENCES

The major quality of life instruments are available in a number of languages and have been used throughout the world. When preparing the instruments for use with different cultural groups, the primary focus has been language issues. Linguistic equivalence does not necessarily ensure conceptual equivalence in terms of quality of life, an issue that often goes unaddressed.[147] Although many aspects of quality of life are universally shared, some are culturally unique.[67,148] In general, quality of life instruments have been developed based on nonminority, well-educated samples from 1 cultural group.[147] Continued work in this area is needed to provide assurance that quality of life is assessed validly for various cultural groups. Examples of instruments that have been developed expressly for cross-cultural international use include the EORTC QLQ-C30,[72] the Quality of Life Questionnaire of the EuroQol (EuroQol),[83] and the WHOQOL-100.[51]

## FAMILY CAREGIVERS

The responsibilities and experience of caring for someone with cancer can profoundly affect the quality of life of family caregivers. Quality of life is affected by 4 major characteristics of a care giving situation: (1) high care-giving demands; (2) loss of physical health for the caregiver; (3) psychological distress; (4) interference with life roles.[149] Caregivers of patients with cancer have reported that providing care introduced a "balancing act" in their lives, as they worked to provide supportive care while managing the demands of their own lives. They also reported that they felt alone in their decisions, underprepared for care giving tasks, and needed to emotionally shield the patient.[150] Because they focus on meeting the patient's needs, caregivers frequently ignore their own personal health, which can result in their own illness.[151] In a prospective, population-based study, Schultz and Beach found that the mortality rate for caregivers with mental and emotional strain was 63% higher than noncaregivers.[152] High psychological distress has been found to be 2 to 3 times higher in caregivers of patients with advanced cancer, as compared with the general population.[153] The emotional toll of care giving can result in depression, anxiety, and a feeling of burden.[151]

Researchers and healthcare providers have begun to recognize the unique needs of family caregivers and explore ways to address them. Instruments have been developed to assess various aspects of the caregiving situation, such as specific patient needs, demands on the caregiver, and the sense of burden. Two instruments for assessing the quality of life of family caregivers are the Caregiver Quality of Life Index Scale-Cancer[154,155] and the Caregiver Reaction Assessment.[156] The Caregiver Quality of Life Scale-Cancer measures burden, disruptiveness, positive adaptation, and financial concerns. The Caregiver Reaction Assessment assesses negative and positive aspects of care giving within 5 domains: caregiver esteem, lack of family support, impact on finances, impact on schedule, and impact on personal health. Other useful instruments are available to assess specific aspects of caregiving and the impact on the caregiver. They assess the amount of assistance the caregiver provides to the patient (Caregiver Assistance Scale[157]), the degree to which care giving interferes with personal aspects of life (Caregiving Impact Scale[157]), caregiver needs and activities involved in the caregiving role (Home Caregiver Need Survey[158] and the Caregiver Well-Being Scale[159]), and the intensity of the instrumental tasks of caregiving (Appraisal of Caregiving Scale[160]). Additional discussion of the quality of life issues associated with caregiving for family members with cancer, as well as instruments to assess quality of life of family caregivers, is provided by Teschendorf and Ferrans.[149]

## CONCLUSION

Over the past 30 years, quality of life has become a respected outcome for cancer care. It is recognized as a valuable supplement to standard clinical indicators, providing information about the positive and negative effects of therapy from the patient's perspective. Quality of life information provides an understanding of impact of illness from the patient's viewpoint, which is different from health status or physical functioning. Quality of life is determined by more than health problems, disabilities, or functional deficits, and people with cancer can enjoy a good quality of life even in the face of physical losses. It is the incorporation of the patient's own values that sets quality of life assessment apart from other measures of health status: it gives the patient a voice. This makes it an important tool for understanding individual differences in adapting to cancer and treatment, as well as the re-evaluation of life in the context of life-threatening disease. Quality of life assessment can provide important information for clinicians to maximize quality of life for patients, all along the cancer continuum. However, a great deal of work in this area is still needed to provide the wide range of information about quality of life outcomes required for clinical decision making, provision of supportive services, and health policy for cancer care.

## REFERENCES


1. Johnson JR, Temple R. Food and Drug Administration requirements for approval of new anticancer drugs. Cancer Treat Rep. 1985;69:1155–1157.
2. Clinical Trials Cooperative Group Program. *Cancer Therapy Evaluation Program: Guidelines.* Bethesda, MD: Division of Cancer Treatment, National Cancer Institute; 1988.
3. Osoba D. The quality of life committee of the clinical trials group of the National Cancer Institute of Canada: organization and functions. *Qual Life Res.* 1992;1:211–218.
4. National Cancer Institute. Symptom Management and Health-Related Quality of Life Steering Committee. http://restructuringtrials.cancer.gov/steering-committees/symptom-management. Accessed December 27, 2009.
5. Cella D. Changes in quality of life predict survival in NSCLC. *Oncol News Int.* 1997;6:19.
6. Ganz P, Lee J, Siau J. Quality of life assessment: an independent prognostic variable for survival in lung cancer. *Cancer.* 1991;67:3131–3135.
7. Herndon J, Fleishman S, Kornblith A, et al. Is quality of life predictive of survival among patients with advanced nonsmall cell lung cancer? *Cancer.* 1999;85:333–340.
8. Montazeri A, Milroy R, Hole D, et al. Quality of life in lung cancer patients as an important prognostic factor. *Lung Cancer.* 2001;31:233–240.
9. Langendijk H, Aaronson N, de Jong J, ten Velde G, Muller M, Wouters M. The prognostic impact of quality of life assessed with EORTC QLQ-C30 in inoperable non-small cell lung carcinoma treated with radiotherapy. *Radiat Oncol.* 2000;55:19–25.
10. Roychowdhury D, Hayden A, Liepa A. Health-related quality-of-life parameters as independent prognostic factors in advanced or metastatic bladder cancer. *J Clin Oncol.* 2003;21:673–678.
11. Monk B, Huang H, Cella D, Long H. Quality of life outcomes from a randomized phase III trial of cisplatin with or without topotecan in advanced carcinoma of the cervix: a Gynecologic Oncology Group study. *J Clin Oncol.* 2005;23:4617–4625.
12. Gupta D, Lis C, Grutsch J. The European Organization for Research and Treatment of Cancer Quality of Life Questionnaire: implications for prognosis in pancreatic cancer. *Int J Gatrointest Canc.* 2006;37:65–73.
13. Fang F, Tsai W, Chiu H, Kuo W, Hsiung C. Quality of life as a survival predictor for esophageal squamous cell carcinoma treated with radiotherapy. *Int J Radiat Oncol Biol Phys.* 2004;58:1384–1404.
14. Fang F, Liu Y, Tang Y, Want C, Ko S. Quality of life as a survival predictor for patients with advanced head and neck carcinoma treated with radiotherapy. *Cancer.* 2004;100:425–432.
15. Efface F, Biganzoli L, Piccart M, et al. Baseline health-related quality of life data as prognostic factors in a phase III multicentre study of women with metastatic breast cancer. *Eur J Cancer.* 2004;40:1021–1030.
16. Efface F, Therasse P, Piccart M, et al. Health-related quality of life parameters as prognostic factors in a nonmetastatic breast cancer population: an international multicenter study. *J Clin Oncol.* 2004;22:3381–3388.
17. Gupta D, Granick J, Grutsch J, Lis C. Prognostic association of health-related quality of life scores with survival in breast cancer. *Support Care Cancer.* 2007;15:387–393.
18. Lis C, Gupta D, Granick J, Grutsch. Can patient satisfaction with quality of life predict survival in advanced colorectal cancer. *Support Care Cancer.* 2006;14:1104–1110.
19. Lis C, Gupta D, Grutsch J. Patient satisfaction with quality of life as a predictor of survival in pancreatic cancer. *Int J Gastrointest Cancer.* 2006;37:35–43.
20. Lis C, Gupta D, Grutsch J. Patient satisfaction with health-related quality of life: implications for prognosis in prostate cancer. *Clin Genitourin Cancer.* 2008;6:91–96.
21. de Graeff A, de Leeuw JR, Ros WJ, et al. Sociodemographic factors and quality of life as prognostic indicators in head and neck cancer. *Eur J Cancer.* 2001;37:332–339.
22. Blazeby JM, Brookes ST, Alderson D. The prognostic value of quality of life scores during treatment for oesophageal cancer. *Gut.* 2001;49:227–230.
23. Maisey NR, Norman A, Watson M, et al. Baseline quality of life predicts survival in patients with advanced colorectal cancer. *Eur J Cancer.* 2002;38:1351–1357.
24. Kramer JA, Curran D, Piccart M, et al. Identification and interpretation of clinical and quality of life prognostic factors for survival and response to treatment in first-line chemotherapy in advanced breast cancer. *Eur J Cancer.* 2000;36:1498–1506.
25. Coates AS, Hurny C, Peterson HF, et al. Quality-of-life scores predict outcome in metastatic but not early breast cancer. *J Clin Oncol.* 2000;18:3768–3774.
26. Luoma ML, Hakamies-Blomqvist L, Sjöström J, et al. Prognostic value of quality of life scores for time to progression (TTP) and overall survival time (OS) in advanced breast cancer. *Eur J Cancer.* 2003;39:1370–1376.
27. Osoba D. Lessons learned from measuring health-related quality of life in oncology. *J Clin Oncol.* 1994;12:608–616.
28. Ferrans C. Differences in what quality of life instruments measure. *J Natl Cancer Inst Monogr.* 2007;37:22–26.
29. Hahn EA, Glendenning GA, Sorensen MV, et al. Quality of life in patients with newly diagnosed chronic phase chronic myeloid leukemia on imatinib versus interferon alpha plus low-dose cytarabine: results from the IRIS study. *J Clin Oncol.* 2003;21:2138–2146.
30. Moul J. Radical prostatectomy versus radiation therapy for clinically localized prostate carcinoma. *Cancer.* 2002;95:211–214.
31. Yarbro CH, Ferrans C. Quality of life of patients with prostate cancer treated with surgery or radiation therapy. *Oncol Nurs Forum.* 1998;25:685–693.
32. Potosky AL, Legler J, Albertsen PC, et al. Health outcomes after prostatectomy or radiotherapy for prostate cancer: results from the Prostate Cancer Outcomes Study. *J Natl Cancer Inst.* 2000;92:1582–1592.
33. Potosky L, Davis W, Hoffman R, et al. Five-year outcomes after prostatectomy or radiotherapy for prostate cancer: the Prostate Cancer Outcomes Study. *J Natl Cancer Inst.* 2004;96:1358–1367.

34. van Andel G, Visser AP, Zwinderman AH, et al. A prospective longitudinal study comparing the impact of external radiation therapy with radical prostatectomy on health related quality of life (HRQOL) in prostate cancer patients. *Prostate.* 2004;58:354–365.
35. Holmberg L, Bill-Axelson A, Helgesen F, et al. A randomized trial comparing radical prostatectomy with watchful waiting in early prostate cancer. *N Engl J Med.* 2002;347:781–789.
36. Steineck G, Helgesen F, Adolfsson J, et al. Quality of life after radical prostatectomy or watchful waiting. *N Engl J Med.* 2002;347:790–796.
37. Kornblith AB, Herndon JE, Silverman LR, et al. Impact of azacytidine on the quality of life of patients with myelodysplastic syndrome treated in a randomized phase III trial: a Cancer and Leukemia Group B study. *J Clin Oncol.* 2002;20:2441–2452.
38. Silverman LR, Demakos EP, Peterson BL, et al. A randomized controlled trial of azacitidine in patients with the myelodysplastic syndrome: a study of the Cancer and Leukemia Group B. *J Clin Oncol.* 2002;20:2429–2440.
39. Hill J, Kornblith A, Jones D, et al. A comparative study of the long term psychosocial functioning of childhood acute lymphoblastic leukemia survivors treated by intrathecal methotrexate with or without cranial radiation. *Cancer.* 1998;82:208–218.
40. MacLean W. Children's Cancer Group (CCG). *J Natl Cancer Inst Monogr.* 1996;20:87–88.
41. Ganz PA, Kwan L, Stanton AL, et al. Quality of life at the end of primary treatment of breast cancer: first results from the moving beyond cancer randomized trial. *J Natl Cancer Inst.* 2004;96:376–387.
42. Ferrans C. Quality of life through the eyes of survivors of breast cancer. *Oncol Nurs Forum.* 1994;21:1645–1651.
43. Kornblith AB, Herndon JE, Weiss RB, et al. Long-term adjustment of survivors of early-stage breast carcinoma, 20 years after adjuvant chemotherapy. *Cancer.* 2003;98:679–689.
44. Kornblith AB, Ligibel J. Psychosocial and sexual functioning of survivors of breast cancer. *Semin Oncol.* 2003;30:799–813.
45. Sharpe M, Strong V, Allen K, et al. Management of major depression in outpatients attending a cancer centre: a preliminary evaluation of a multicomponent cancer nurse-delivered intervention. *Br J Cancer.* 2004;90:310–313.
46. Sandgren AK, McCaul KD, King B, et al. Telephone therapy for patients with breast cancer. *Nurs Forum.* 2000;27:683–688.
47. Detmar S, Muller MJ, Schornagel JH, et al. Health-related quality of life assessments and patient-physician communication. *JAMA.* 2002; 288:3027–3034.
48. Velikova G, Booth L, Smith AB, et al. Measuring quality of life in routine oncology practice improves communication and patient well-being: a randomized controlled trial. *J Clin Oncol.* 2004;22:714–724.
49. Halyard M, Ferrans C. Quality of life assessment for routine clinical practice. *J Support Oncol.* 2008;6:221–229, 233.
50. Ferrans CE. Definitions and conceptual models of quality of life. In: Lipscomb J, Gotay CC, Snyder C, eds. *Outcomes Assessment in Cancer.* Cambridge, UK: Cambridge University Press; 2005:14–30.
51. WHOQOL Group. The World Health Organization Quality of Life Assessment (WHOQOL): development and general psychometric properties. *Soc Sci Med.* 1998;46:1569–1585.
52. Wilson IB, Cleary PD. Linking clinical variables with health-related quality of life: a conceptual model of patient outcomes. *JAMA.* 1995;273:59–65.
53. Ferrans CE, Zerwic JJ, Wilbur JE, Larson JL. Conceptual model of health-related quality of life. *J Nurs Scholarsh.* 2005;37:336–342.
54. Cella D, Bonomi A, Lloyd S, et al. Reliability and validity of the Functional Assessment of Cancer Therapy-Lung (FACT-L) quality of life instrument. *Lung Cancer.* 1995;12:199–220.
55. Aaronson NK, Cull AM, Kaasa S, et al. The European Organization for Research and Treatment of Cancer (EORTC) modular approach for quality of life assessment in oncology: an update. In: Spilker B, ed. *Quality of Life and Pharmacoeconomics in Clinical Trials.* 2nd ed. Philadelphia, PA: Lippincott-Raven; 1996:179–189.
56. Ware JE Jr, Sherbourne CD. The MOS 36-item short-form health survey (SF-36). *Med Care.* 1992;30:473–483.
57. Ferrans CE. Development of a quality of life index for patients with cancer. *Oncol Nurs Forum.* 1990;17:15–19.
58. Gotay C, Korn E, McCabe M, et al. Quality of life assessment in cancer treatment protocols: research issues in protocol development. *J Natl Cancer Inst.* 1992;84:575–579.
59. Leplege A, Hunt S. The problem of quality of life in medicine. *JAMA.* 1997;278:47–50.
60. Padilla G, Ferrell B, Grant M, et al. Defining the content domain of quality of life for cancer patients with pain. *Cancer Nurs.* 1990;13: 108–115.
61. Ferrell B, Grant M, Padilla G. Experience of pain and perceptions of quality of life: validation of a conceptual model. *Hospice J.* 1991;7: 9–24.
62. Ferrell B, Grant M, Schmidt G, et al. The meaning of quality of life for bone marrow transplant survivors. Part 1: the impact of bone marrow transplant on QOL. *Cancer Nurs.* 1992;15:153–160.
63. Ferrell B, Dow K, Leigh S, et al. Quality of life in long term cancer survivors. *Oncol Nurs Forum.* 1995;22:915–922.
64. Grant M, Ferrell B, Schmidt G, et al. Measurement of quality of life in bone marrow transplantation survivors. *Qual Life Res.* 1992; 1:375–384.
65. Ferrans CE, Powers M. Quality of Life Index: development and psychometric properties. *Adv Nurs Sci.* 1985;8:15–24.
66. Ferrans CE. Development of a conceptual model of quality of life. *Schol Inq Nurs Pract Int J.* 1996;10:293–304.
67. Warnecke R, Ferrans C, Johnson T, et al. Measuring quality of life in culturally diverse populations. *J Natl Cancer Inst Monogr.* 1996;20:29–38.
68. Schipper H, Clinch J, Olweny C. Quality of life studies: definitions and conceptual issues. In: Spilker B, ed. *Quality of Life and Pharmaeconomics in Clinical Trials.* 2nd ed. Philadelphia, PA: Lippincott-Raven; 1996:11–23.
69. Revicki D, Osoba D, Fairclough D, et al. Recommendations on health-related quality of life research to support labeling and promotional claims in the United States. *Qual Life Res.* 2000;9:887–900.
70. Padilla GV, Grant MM, Ferrell BR, et al. Quality of life—cancer. In: Spilker B, ed. *Quality of Life and Pharmaeconomics in Clinical Trials.* 2nd ed. Philadelphia, PA: Lippincott-Raven; 1996:301–308.
71. Schag C, Ganz PA, Heinrich R. Cancer Rehabilitation Evaluation System-Short Form (CARES-SF). *Cancer.* 1991;68:1406–1413.
72. Aaronson N, Ahmedzai S, Bergman B, et al. The European Organization for Research and Treatment of Cancer QLQ-C30: a quality of life instrument for use in international clinical trials in oncology. *J Natl Cancer Inst.* 1993;85:365–376.
73. Cella D, Tulsky D, Gray G, et al. The Functional Assessment of Cancer Therapy (FACT) scale: development and validation of the general version. *J Clin Oncol.* 1993;11:570–579.
74. Morrow G, Lindke J, Black P, et al. Measurement of quality of life in patients: psychometric analysis of the Functional Living Index-Cancer (FLIC). *Qual Life Res.* 1992;1:287–296.
75. Clinch J. The functional living index—cancer: ten years later. In: Spilker B, ed. *Quality of Life and Pharmacoeconomics in Clinical Trials.* 2nd ed. Philadelphia, PA: Lippincott-Raven; 1996:215–225.
76. Cohen S, Mount B, Strobel M, et al. The McGill Quality of Life Questionnaire: a measure of quality of life appropriate for people with advanced disease. *Palliat Med.* 1995;9:207–219.
77. Stewart AL, Hays RD, Ware JE. The MOS short-form general health survey. *Med Care.* 1988;26:724–735.
78. Dougherty C, Dewhurst T, Nichol P, et al. Comparison of three quality of life instruments in stable angina pectoris: Seattle Angina Questionnaire, Short Form Health Survey (SF-36), and Quality of Life Index—Cardiac Version III. *J Clin Epidemiol.* 1998;51:569–575.
79. Schlenk E, Erlen J, Dunbar-Jacob J, et al. Health-related quality of life in chronic disorders: a comparison across studies using the MOS SF-36. *Qual Life Res.* 1998;7:57–65.

80. Covinsky KE, Wu AW, Landefeld S, et al. Health status versus quality of life in older patients: does the distinction matter? *Am J Med.* 1999;106:435–440.
81. Frisch MB. The Quality of Life Inventory: a cognitive-behavioral tool for complete problem assessment, treatment planning, and outcome evaluation. *Behav Ther.* 1993;16:42–44.
82. Litwin M. Measuring health related quality of life in men with prostate cancer. *J Urol.* 1994;152:1882–1887.
83. EuroQol Group. EuroQol—a new facility for the measurement of health-related quality of life. *Health Policy.* 1990;16:199–208.
84. Feeny DH, Torrance GW, Furlong WJ. Health utilities index. In: Spilker B, ed. *Quality of Life and Pharmacoeconomics in Clinical Trials.* 2nd ed. Philadelphia: Lippincott-Raven; 1996:239–252.
85. Patrick DL, Bush JW, Chen MM. Methods for measuring levels of well-being for a health status index. *Health Serv Res.* 1973;8:228–245.
86. Feeny DH. The roles for preference-based measures in support of cancer research and policy. In: Lipscomb J, Gotay CC, Snyder C, eds. *Outcomes Assessment in Cancer.* Cambridge, UK: Cambridge University Press; 2005:69–92.
87. Gelber RP, Goldhirsch A, Cavelli F. Quality of life-adjusted evaluation of adjuvant therapies for operable breast cancer. *Ann Int Med.* 1991;114:621–628.
88. Gelber RD, Cole BF, Goldhirsh A. Adjuvant chemotherapy plus tamoxifen compared with tamoxifen alone for postmenopausal breast cancer: meta-analysis of quality-adjusted survival. *Lancet.* 1996;347:1066–1071.
89. Schwartz CE, Sprangers MAG. *Adaptation to Changing Health: Response Shift in Quality of Life Research.* Washington, DC: American Psychological Association; 2000.
90. Frost MH, Bonomi AE, Ferrans CE, et al. Patient, clinician, and population perspectives on determining the clinical significance of quality of life scores. *Mayo Clin Proc.* 2002;77:488–494.
91. Sloan JA, Cella D, Frost M, Guyatt GH, Sprangers M, Symonds T. Assessing clinical significance in measuring oncology patient quality of life: introduction to the symposium, content overview, and definition of terms. *Mayo Clin Proc.* 2002;77:367–370.
92. Wyrwich KW, Bullinger M, Aaronson N, Hays RD, Patrick DL, Symonds T. Estimating clinically significant differences in quality of life outcomes. *Qual Life Res.* 2005;14:285–295.
93. Guyatt GH, Osoba D, Wu AW, Wyrwich KW, Norman GR. Methods to explain the clinical significance of health status measures. *Mayo Clin Proc.* 2002;77:371–383.
94. Sloan JA, Frost MH, Berzon R, et al. The clinical significance of quality of life assessments in oncology: a summary for clinicians. *Support Care Cancer.* 2006;14:988–998.
95. King MT. The interpretation of scores from the EORTC quality of life questionnaire QLQ-C30. *Qual Life Res.* 1996;5:555–567.
96. Osoba D, Rodrigues G, Myles J, Zee B, Pater J. Interpreting the significance of changes in health-related quality-of-life scores. *J Clin Oncol.* 1998;16:139–144.
97. Bliley AV, Ferrans C. Quality of life after angioplasty. *Heart Lung.* 1993;22:193–199.
98. Hathaway D, Hartwig M, Milstead J, Elmer D, Evans S, Gaber A. A prospective study of changes in quality of life reported by diabetic recipients of kidney-only and pancreas-kidney allografts. *J Transpl Coord.* 1994;4:12–17.
99. Johnson C, Wicks MK, Milstead J, Hartwig M, Hathaway D. Racial and gender differences in quality of life following kidney transplantation. *Image J Nurs Sch.* 1998;30:125–130.
100. Ringash J, O'Sullivan B, Bezjak A, Redelmeier DA. Interpreting clinically significant changes in patient-reported outcomes. *Cancer.* 2007;110:196–202.
101. Norman GR, Sloan JA, Wyrwich KW. Interpretation of changes in health-related quality of life: the remarkable universality of half a standard deviation. *Med Care.* 2003;41:582–592.
102. Sloan J, Symonds T, Vargas-Chanes D, Fridley B. Practical guidelines for assessing the clinical significance of health-related quality of life changes within clinical trials. *Drug Inf J.* 2003;37:23–31.
103. Frost MH, Bonomi AE, Ferrans CE, Wong GY, Hays RD. Patient, clinician, and population perspectives on determining the clinical significance of quality-of-life scores. *Mayo Clin Proc.* 2002;77:488–494.
104. Cella D, Bullinger M, Scott C, Barofsky I. Group vs individual approaches to understanding the clinical significance of differences or changes in quality of life. *Mayo Clin Proc.* 2002;77:384–392.
105. Sloan JA, Aaronson N, Cappelleri JC, Fairclough DL, Varricchio C. Assessing the clinical significance of single items relative to summated scores. *Mayo Clin Proc.* 2002;77:479–487.
106. Sprangers MA, Moinpour CM, Moynihan TJ, Patrick DL, Revicki DA. Assessing meaningful change in quality of life over time: a users' guide for clinicians. *Mayo Clin Proc.* 2002;77:561–571.
107. Symonds T, Berzon R, Marquis P, Rummans TA. The clinical significance of quality-of-life results: practical considerations for specific audiences. *Mayo Clin Proc.* 2002;77:572–583.
108. Basch E, Artz D, Iasonos A, et al. Evaluation of an online platform for cancer patient self-reporting of chemotherapy toxicities. *J Am Med Inform Assoc.* 2007;14:264–268.
109. Karras BT, Wolpin S, Lober WB, Bush N, Fann JR, Berry DL. Electronic Self-report Assessment—Cancer (ESRA-C): working towards an integrated survey system. *Stud Health Technol Inform.* 2006;122:514–518.
110. Wilkie DJ, Judge MK, Berry DL, Dell J, Zong S, Gilespie R. Usability of a computerized PAINReportIt in the general public with pain and people with cancer pain. *J Pain Symptom Manage.* 2003;25:213–224.
111. Cella D, Yount S, Rothrock N, et al. The Patient-Reported Outcomes Measurement Information System (PROMIS): progress of an NIH Roadmap cooperative group during its first two years. *Med Care.* 2007;45(suppl 1):S3-S11.
112. Gendreau M, Hufford MR, Stone AA. Measuring clinical pain in chronic widespread pain: selected methodological issues. *Best Pract Res Clin Rheumatol.* 2003;17:575–592.
113. Stone AA, Broderick JE. Real-time data collection for pain: appraisal and current status. *Pain Med.* 2007(suppl 3):S85-S93.
114. Shiffman S, Stone AA, Hufford MR. Ecological momentary assessment. *Annu Rev Clin Psychol.* 2008;4:1–32.
115. Curran SL, Beacham AO, Andrykowski MA. Ecological momentary assessment of fatigue following breast cancer treatment. *J Behav Med.* 2004;27:425–444.
116. Hacker ED, Ferrans CE. Ecological momentary assessment of fatigue in patients receiving intensive cancer therapy. *J Pain Symptom Manage.* 2007;33:267–275.
117. Molzahn A, Northcott H, Dossetor J. Quality of life of individuals with end stage renal disease: perceptions of patients, nurses, and physicians. *ANNA J.* 1997;24:325–333.
118. Sneeuw K, Sprangers M, Aaronson NK. The role of health care providers and significant others in evaluating the quality of life of patients with chronic disease. *J Clin Epidemiol.* 2002;55:1130–1143.
119. Sprangers M, Aaronson N. The role of health care providers and significant others in evaluating the quality of life of patients with chronic disease: a review. *J Clin Epidemiol.* 1992;45:743–760.
120. Katsuno T. Dementia from the inside: how people with early-stage dementia evaluate their quality of life. *Aging & Society.* 2005;25:197–214.
121. Bradlyn AS, Pollock BH. Pediatric Oncology Group (POG). *J Natl Cancer Inst Monogr.* 1996;20:89–90.
122. Hinds PS, Hasse JE. Quality of life in children and adolescents with cancer. In: King CR, Hinds PS, eds. *Quality of Life from Nursing and Patient Perspectives, 2*nd *Ed.* Boston, MA: Jones and Bartlett; 2003:143–168.
123. Hinds P, Gattuso J, Fletcher A, et al. Quality of life as conveyed by pediatric patients with cancer. *Qual Life Res.* 2004;13:761–772.

124. Rajmil L, Herdman M, Sanmamed MJF, et al. Generic health-related quality of life instruments in children and adolescents: a qualitative analysis of content. *J Adolescent Health.* 2004;34:37–45.
125. Ravens-Sieberer U, Bullinger M. Assessing health-related quality of life in chronically ill children with the German KINDL: first psychometric and content analytical results. *Qual Life Res.* 1998;7:399–407.
126. Varni JM, Seid M, Kurtin PS. Pediatric health-related quality of life measurement technology: a guide for health care decision makers. *J Clin Outcomes Manage.* 1999;6:33–40.
127. Collier J, MacKinlay D, Phillips D. Norm values for the Generic Children's Quality of Life Measure (GCQ) from a large school-based sample. *Qual Life Res.* 2000;9:617–623.
128. Vogels T, Verrips GHW, Verloove-Vanhorick SP, et al. Measuring health-related quality of life in children: the development of the TACQOL parent form. *Qual Life Res.* 1998;7:457–465.
129. Landgraft JM, Abetz L, Ware J. *The Child Health Questionnaire User's Manual.* Boston, MA: Health Institute, New England Medical Center; 1996.
130. Starfield B, Riley A, Green B. The Child Health and Illness Profile: a population-based measure of health. *Med Care.* 1995;33:553–566.
131. Theunissen NC, Vogels TGC, Koopman HM, et al. The proxy problem: child report versus parent report in health-related quality of life research. *Qual Life Res.* 1998;7:387–397.
132. Goodwin DA, Boggs SR, Graham-Pole J. Development and validation of the pediatric oncology quality of life scale. *Psychol Assess.* 1994;6:321–328.
133. Hinds P, Burghen A, Hasse J, Phillips C. Advances in defining, conceptualizing, and measuring quality of life in pediatric patients with cancer. *Oncol Nurs Forum.* 2006;33(suppl):23–29.
134. McMillan SC, Weitzner M. How problematic are various aspects of quality of life in patients with cancer at the end of life? *Oncol Nurs Forum.* 2000;27:817–823.
135. McMillan SC, Small BJ. Symptom distress and quality of life in patients with cancer newly admitted to hospice home care. *Oncol Nurs Forum.* 2002;29:1421–1428.
136. Steinhauser KE, Christakis NA, Clipp EC, et al. Factors considered important at the end of life by patients, family, physicians, and other care providers. JAMA. 2000;284:2476–2482.
137. SUPPORT Principal Investigators. A controlled study to improve care for seriously ill hospitalized patients: the Study to Understand Prognoses and Preferences for Outcomes and Risks of Treatments (SUPPORT). *JAMA.* 1995;274:1591–1598.
138. Rummans TA, Bostwick JM, Clark MM. Maintaining quality of life at the end of life. *Mayo Clin Proc.* 2000;75:1305–1310.
139. Misono S, Weiss N, Fann J, Redman M, Yueh B. Incidence of suicide in persons with cancer. *J Clin Oncol.* 2008;26:4731–4738.
140. Chochinov HM, Tataryn D, Clinch JJ, et al. Will to live in the terminally ill. *Lancet.* 1999;354:816–819.
141. McMillan SC, Weitzner M. Quality of life in cancer patients: use of a revised hospice index. *Cancer Pract.* 1998;6:282–288.
142. Byock IR, Merriman MP. Measuring quality of life for patients with terminal illness: the Missoula-VITAS quality of life index. *Palliat Med.* 1998;12:231–244.
143. Cella D. Functional Assessment of Chronic Illness Therapy (FACIT). http://www.facit.org. Accessed November 2, 2008.
144. McPherson CJ, Addington-Hall JM. Judging the quality of care at the end of life: can proxies provide reliable information? *Soc Sci Med.* 2003;56:95–109.
145. Curtis JR, Patrick DL, Engleberg RA, et al. A measure of the quality of dying and death: initial validation using after death interviews with family members. *J Pain Symptom Manage.* 2002;24:17–31.
146. Teno JM, Byock I, Field MJ. Research agenda for developing measures to examine quality of care and quality of life of patients diagnosed with lifelimiting illness. *J Pain Symptom Manage.* 1999;17:75–82.
147. Stewart AL, Napoles-Springer A. Health-related quality of life assessments in diverse population groups in the United States. *Med Care.* 2000;38(suppl):II102-II124.
148. Meyerowitz B, Richardson J, Hudson S, et al. Ethnicity and cancer outcomes: behavioral and psychosocial considerations. *Psychol Bull.* 1998;123:47–70.
149. Teschendorf B, Ferrans C. Quality of life of family caregivers of cancer patients. In: King C, Hinds P, eds. *Quality of Life from Nursing and Patient Perspectives.* 3rd ed. Boston, MA: Jones and Bartlett. In press.
150. Teschendorf B, Schwartz C, Ferrans C, O'Mara A, Novotny P, Sloan J. Caregiver role stress: when families become providers. *Cancer Control.* 2007;14:183–189.
151. Grunfeld E, Coyle D, Whelan T, et al. Family caregiver burden: results of a longitudinal study of breast cancer patients and their principal caregivers. *CMAJ.* 2004;170:1795–1801.
152. Schultz R, Beach SR. Caregiving as a risk for mortality: the Caregiver Health Effects Study. *JAMA.* 1999;282:2215–2219.
153. Dumont S, Turgeon J, Allard P, Gagnon P, Charbonneau C, Vezina L. Caring for a loved one with advanced cancer: determinants of psychological distress in family caregivers. *J Palliat Med.* 2006;9:912–921.
154. Weitzner MA, Jacobsen PB, Wagner H, Friedland J. The Caregiver Quality of Life Index—Cancer (CQOLC) scale: development and validation of an instrument to measure quality of life of the family caregiver of patients with cancer. *Qual Life Res.* 1999;8:55–63.
155. Weitzner MA, McMillan SC. The Caregiver Quality of Life Index-Cancer (CQOLC) Scale: revalidation in a Home Hospice Setting. *J Palliat Care.* 1999;15:13–20.
156. Given CW, Given B, Stommel M, et al. The Caregiver Reaction Assessment (CRA) for caregivers to persons with chronic physical and mental impairments. *Res Nurs Health.* 1992;15:271–283.
157. Cameron JI, Franche RL, Cheung AM, Stewart DE. Lifestyle interference and emotional distress in family caregivers of advanced cancer patients. *Cancer.* 2002;94:521–527.
158. Hileman JW, Lackey NR, Hassanein RS. Identifying the needs of home caregivers of patients with cancer. *Oncol Nurs Forum.* 1992;19:771–777.
159. Berg-Weger M, Rubio DM, Tebb SS. The caregiver well-being scale revisited. *Health Soc Work.* 2000;25:255–263.
160. Oberst MT, Thomas SE, Gass KA, Ward SE. Caregiving demands and appraisal of stress among family caregivers. *Cancer Nurs.* 1989;12: 209–215.

CHAPTER 10

Anthony DeLaCruz, BSN, MS, RN, OCN®, Mary S. McCabe, BA, RN, MA

# Principles of Cancer Clinical Trials

## OVERVIEW

Scientific inquiry—and, in particular, clinical research—continues to be an incremental process, moving forward in a series of carefully planned steps. A specific type of clinical research, clinical trials, is designed to evaluate the value of new interventions in people with disease or at risk of disease. In recent years, there has been an expansion of the types of clinical trials that are conducted with greater focus on patient-centered endpoints, such as quality of life, and more evaluations of behavioral interventions, such as exercise and smoking cessation. In addition, for the treatment of many cancers, there has been a shift from non-specific cytotoxic chemotherapies to molecularly targeted therapies, used either alone or combined with traditional chemotherapies.[1] This shift presents new challenges in the design and conduct of clinical trials.

## THE CLINICAL TRIALS PROCESS AND IMPLEMENTATION

Cancer clinical trials are the prospectively designed evaluations of new interventions for the prevention, diagnosis, treatment, and/or improvement of quality of life of individuals at risk of or diagnosed with cancer. Clinical trials require careful scientific planning and rigorous review, oversight, and conduct. Such scientific evaluation includes built in safeguards for study participants who agree to participate through a process called "informed consent." The goal in conducting clinical trials is to provide answers to a well-defined question, and these studies usually proceed in a carefully planned series of steps, called phases. The process begins with small studies testing the safety of the intervention and moves to progressively larger studies testing the effectiveness of the new interventions compared to the current standard of care. In particular, treatment clinical trials are being designed with an ever increasing level of sophistication, due to the scientific community's rapidly increasing ability to apply new knowledge of cancer biology to targeted development of new agents (Table 10-1).

Specifically, recent advances in the use of biomarkers have generated new opportunities and challenges in the clinical trials process. Biomarkers are defined as characteristics used to measure and evaluate objectively normal biologic processes, pathogenic processes or pharmacological responses to a therapeutic intervention.[2] The trend is clear; biomarkers are increasingly incorporated into clinical trials each year. Biomarkers may be used for patient selection (ie, matching a patient's tumor to a specific drug), to prove that a drug engages a target and is achieving the intended pharmacologic effect, and to help avoid or attenuate toxicity by identifying patients who may be at high risk.[3]

**TABLE 10-1**

**Essential Elements in the Design of a Clinical Trial**

- Clearly stated testable hypothesis
- Well-defined primary endpoint
- Appropriate trial design
- Adequate resources to answer the study question
- Accrual of adequate number of patients to complete the study in a reasonable amount of time
- Appropriate statistical analysis of predetermined trial endpoints
- Conclusions drawn directly from the data

A critical component in the clinical trial process and design is the precise and accurate reporting of toxicities and adverse events. As clinical trials become more complex, the methods of reporting adverse events continue to evolve. The use of patient-reported outcome tools (PROs) to collect symptom measures directly from the patient is becoming more prominent. This method of reporting is intended to improve the accuracy and efficiency of subjective adverse event data reporting. PRO instruments provide a means for measuring treatment benefits by capturing concepts related to how a patient feels or functions with respect to his or her health or condition. To standardize the utilization of PRO instruments in clinical trials, the U. S. Food and Drug administration has published a guidance document for the industry to describe how the FDA evaluates PRO instruments used in studies.[4]

### TYPES OF CLINICAL TRIALS

The most common type of clinical trial is designed to evaluate new treatments. However, as cancer clinical research has evolved, studies are now being designed to develop new interventions across the entire cancer continuum, including evaluations for the prevention, detection, and improvement of quality of life of both patients and individuals at risk of developing cancer.

- *Prevention trials* are designed to evaluate interventions, such as lifestyle modifications, pharmacological agents, and dietary supplements, for the prevention of cancer in individuals at risk for cancer.
- *Screening and early detection trials* are intended to find cancer as early as possible in individuals who do not yet have a diagnosis of cancer, but who may be at risk for developing the disease.
- *Diagnostic trials* are designed to evaluate new tests, interventions, or procedures that can identify a suspected cancer earlier and more accurately. Such studies include the evaluation of tumor markers based on the molecular signature of the malignant cell.

**TABLE 10-2**

**Phases of Clinical Trials**

| | Phase 1 | Phase 2 | Phase 3 | Phase 4 |
|---|---|---|---|---|
| **Number of Participants** | 15–30 people | Less than 100 people | Generally from 100 to thousands of people | Several hundred to several thousand people |
| **Purpose** | • To find safe dosage<br>• To decide how the agent should be given<br>• To observe how the agent affects the human body | • To determine if the agent or intervention has an effect on a particular cancer<br>• To see how the agent or intervention affects the human body | • To compare the agent or intervention (or new use of a treatment) with the current standard | • To further evaluate the long-term safety and effectiveness of a new treatment |

- *Treatment trials* are designed to evaluate the safety and effectiveness of new drugs, biologics, radiation therapy techniques, surgical procedures, or new behavioural interventions in individuals who have been diagnosed with cancer.
- *Quality of life and supportive care trials* are designed to improve the comfort and domains of life that can be adversely affected by cancer and its treatment, such as physical symptoms and psychosocial functioning.

## PHASES OF CLINICAL TRIALS

Clinical trials usually proceed in four phases—1, 2, 3, and 4—and each phase is designed to answer a research question that builds on the information obtained in the previous phase of study (Table 10-2).In this section, the phases of clinical trials are explained in the context of drug treatment trials, but the same concepts generally apply to most types of clinical trials. Some basic questions are helpful in understanding the goals of the different phases of studies.

- *Phase 1 studies:* What dose is safe, how can the agent best be given, and how does the agent affect the body?
- *Phase 2 studies:* What effect does the agent have on the particular cancer, and what effect does the agent have on the body?
- *Phase 3 studies:* Is the new agent or combination better than the current standard of care?
- *Phase 4 studies:* What is the long-term safety and effectiveness of the intervention?

### Phase I trials

*Current approaches.* Frequently, phase 1 trials are designed to determine the maximum tolerated dose (MTD) and the dose limiting toxicities of a new agent. While the primary goal of a phase 1 trial is to determine toxic effects, pharmacological behavior, and recommended dosage for future studies, these studies are conducted with therapeutic intent. The dose and schedule established in these trials then determines the dose and schedule that will be used in phase 2 studies of the agent. In addition to the evaluation of previously untested, new agents ("first in human" studies), phase 1 studies are conducted to evaluate a new dose and schedule of an already approved agent in an effort to improve the efficacy and broaden the application of the agent. Later phase 1 studies may be conducted to further evaluate the agent in populations not previously studied, and some are pilot trials designed to determine the interaction of a drug with another agent.

*Patient selection.* Eligibility requirements for phase 1 studies are broad. In general, only those patients who have exhausted treatments that offer an improvement in survival can be enrolled. The consent process should clearly outline the goals of the trial and the fact that both benefit and toxicity are unknown.[5] Major organ functions must be adequate so that the drug can be metabolized and excreted normally. This helps ensure that evaluation of major organ toxicity can be determined and that patients will not be placed at even greater risk of toxicity. Study participants must have a life expectancy of at least one to two months, as this time is considered to be the minimum period required to observe toxic effects.

*Starting dose and dose escalation.* In a phase I trial of an agent that has not been administered to humans, the usual design begins with the selection of a dose presumed to be safe, based on animal studies, and gradual escalation of doses in subsequent patient cohorts.[6] The study participants are usually divided into cohorts of three to six participants. Each cohort is treated with an increased dose of the new agent, and the results obtained with early participants greatly influence the doses that subsequent participants receive. If no serious side effects are seen in the initial group after a time, usually three to four weeks, the next group of participants receives a higher dose.

Dose escalation has often followed a modified Fibonacci scheme; one in which dose levels increase by ever decreasing increments as the trial proceeds.[6] This plan sets the second dose level at double the initial dose; the third level is 67% higher than the second; the fourth is 50% higher than the third; and each subsequent level is increased by 33%. The goal is to avoid the problems of escalating the dose too rapidly (potential exposure of patients to severe toxicity) or too slowly (depriving participants of potential benefit through administration of sub therapeutic doses). The dose that is found to cause moderate, reversible toxicity in the majority of patients is recommended for further evaluation in a phase 2 trial.

*New approaches.* With the discovery of many new molecularly targeted therapies, new challenges in drug development have emerged. Unlike cytotoxic agents, most of which act on DNA or tubulin, these new therapies have a myriad of targets, including membrane receptors, components of cytoplasmic signaling pathways, cell cycle regulator proteins, and proteins or factors important in angiogenesis.[7] The antitumor behavior of these new agents will differ from traditional chemotherapeutic agents, and increasing the dose in a traditional phase 1 trial to normal tissue tolerance (MTD) may be an irrelevant end-point. Rather, the end-points of primary interest for dose determination are target or pathway inhibition.[2] This will result more and more in a shift from using the MTD as the phase 1 end-point to an approach establishing the "biologically active dose" that maximally inhibits the target or pathway.

Growing interest in the use of cancer biomarkers is emerging and possesses the potential to be useful end-points for phase 1 trials. Ideally, the use of biomarkers in early clinical trials would help predict the likelihood of success or failure of a drug in efficacy trials, guide selection of patients more likely to respond to the agent, and provide meaningful correlations with toxicity and response.[8]

## Phase 2 trials

*Current approaches.* Phase 2 trials are designed to evaluate the efficacy of the agent against specific tumors, using the dose and schedule determined to be safe in the phase 1 trials.[9] On the basis of the phase 1 study results, phase 2 studies focus on the evaluation of cancers for which no effective therapy exists and/or that are most likely to show a response to therapy.[10]

*Patient selection.* Since response rates are the primary endpoint of phase 2 trials, patients entered into these studies must all have a specific diagnosis, and, should have good performance status and minimal prior exposure to chemotherapy. Usually, one or, at most, two prior regimens are acceptable since, in patients heavily pretreated with chemotherapy, a drug may not demonstrate its true activity. The inherent problem in phase 2 trials is that individuals who have failed standard treatment may be the least likely to provide a satisfactory evaluation of the new agent. Subjects must have adequate organ function and a life expectancy of at least three months to participate. Phase 2 studies usually enroll 15 to 30 (fewer than 100) patients in a cohort group.

*Dose and schedule.* In most phase 2 studies, all participants receive the same dose of the agent (or undergo the same intervention). The new treatment is assessed for efficacy, and additional safety information is obtained. Some phase 2 studies may compare different schedules of administering the agent; at the end of the study, the most promising regimen is chosen to move into phase 3 trials. Participants in this type of phase 2 study are randomly assigned to one group or the other.

*Trial design.* Drawing conclusions regarding treatment benefit from a phase 2 single agent trial is complex. The usual measure of an agent's antitumor activity in such a trial is response rate.[11] While obtaining a response rate answers the basic question posed in the study, partial responses do not necessarily indicate patient benefit. A partial response (50% reduction in tumor mass) may be brief and complicated by toxicity. Even if the agent seems to demonstrate activity against the cancer, it usually requires further testing. Because the agent has not been compared to any other agent or intervention, its relative value is unclear, and it is impossible to rule out other factors that may have influenced its effectiveness. In addition, phase 2 studies are often too short to determine long term benefits, such as survival.

Phase 2 studies are also used to evaluate the practicality and tolerability of combination regimens. Results of this type of study are difficult to interpret, however, because often the agents under study are known to be of some benefit alone. The combination of agents must demonstrate greater activity than its most active component or greater activity than another combination. A phase 2 trial in which participants are randomized to treatment groups avoids some of these difficulties. This type of design requires simultaneously testing two or more regimens and the availability of a large number of participants. For these reasons, randomized phase 2 trials have not been common.

*New approaches.* Patient selection for study will continue to include individuals with minimal prior therapy and good performance status, but selection criteria increasingly focus on individuals with tumor types that possess the target of the new agent expressed.

There is an emerging need to change the paradigm for demonstrating anticancer agent efficacy in phase 2 trial design. End-points, such as objective response rates, that are considered standard for most phase 2 trials with traditional agents may not be adequate for targeted agents that produce growth inhibition without tumor regression.[2] Because many of these new agents may affect tumor cells by reducing proliferation, rather than by causing cell death, the impact on tumor growth may be stabilization of disease or minor tumor shrinkage. Thus, it may be argued that focusing only on establishing a response rate (based on the percent of tumor shrinkage) could result in overlooking some agents that could improve survival by causing disease stabilization.[12] A possible alternative methodological approach is the randomized discontinuation design, in which all patients initially receive the investigational agent. After a fixed period (three to four months), patients who respond to treatment continue to receive the drug; those with disease progression are taken off study, while those with stable disease are randomly assigned to continue the administration of the drug or to interrupt it (observation/placebo) for a fixed period.[13] This approach would enable the investigator to distinguish disease stabilization that may be due to the natural history of the disease from those that are a treatment effect.

Another new approach for phase 2 trials is the inclusion of patient-reported outcomes (PROs). There are at least three specific reasons one would want phase 2 PRO clinical trial data: (1) to evaluate a response to treatment in otherwise unmeasurable disease or when tumor response is not a reasonable surrogate for patient benefit; (2) to understand the impact of a toxic regimen on quality of life; and (3) to test PRO measurements for their feasibility and reliability in subsequent phase 3 trials.[14]

### Phase 3 trials

In a phase 3 trial, a new therapy is compared to a standard therapy. A new agent enters this phase of testing if it has demonstrated significant efficacy in phase 2 trials. An agent may be tested as a single agent, as part of a drug combination, or by comparing a combined modality treatment with a single modality. Phase 3 trials require hundreds to thousands of participants and are most often carried out by multiple institutions, including community settings. Because these study results guide healthcare professionals in making treatment decisions, they often include information about quality of life as well as survival.

*Patient selection.* The requirements for participation in phase 3 trials are similar to those in phase 2. Participants must have measurable disease, adequate organ function, good performance status, and little or no prior anticancer therapy. Debate has occurred regarding how narrow the eligibility criteria in phase 3 trials should be, given that narrow eligibility criteria limit the generalizability of the results.

*Trial design.* The standard design for phase 3 studies is a prospective, randomized trial. Randomization means that the participants are assigned by chance to one or the other of the agents and/or regimens being evaluated. The assignment is not biased by knowledge of specific individual characteristics. Rather, both known and unknown prognostic factors of participants are distributed randomly. This design allows results to be interpreted as being due to the therapy under evaluation, rather than due to nonrandom variations in the distribution of unknown prognostic factors.[15] Also, a randomized design is necessary to detect small, but significant differences between agents and/or regimens.

*New approaches.* As the molecular characterization of tumors continue to evolve, the design of randomized phase 3 trials evaluating the effectiveness of an agent will focus on patients expressing the molecular target. It is possible in the future, rather than studies in breast, colon, lung cancer, etc, there will be studies in patients with tumors expressing a particular target, stratifying for disease.[13]

There has been considerable progress in successfully implementing PRO end-points in phase 3 clinical trials.[16] Phase 3 studies will continue to include PRO measurements as either primary or secondary end-points and will add value by providing data from a patient's perspective.

### Phase 4 trials

Following approval by the Food and Drug Administration (FDA) of an agent or regimen, additional studies (usually considered postmarketing studies) can be and may be required to be conducted. Not all new agents will enter into phase 4 trials. The purpose of such trials is to accrue new information about any risks or side effects not previously identified. Phase 4 trials have proved extremely useful in identifying potential issues with agents that were not discovered during early-phase trials. The FDA may require such trials when approval of the new agent is based on limited data about long-term outcome, for example. For this reason, some refer to phase 4 trials as "long-term experiments."

## THE CLINICAL PROTOCOL

For each clinical trial, a formal document known as a protocol is developed to clearly describe the conduct of the research and the process of evaluation. The protocol includes a rationale for the study and provides clear, specific instructions for all individuals involved in its conduct. Each protocol includes essential elements that provide the framework for achieving the study goals (Table 10-3).[17]

## RESEARCH TEAM MEMBERS

The conduct of a clinical trial requires the collaboration of a multidisciplinary research team with each member

**TABLE 10-3**

| Elements of a Protocol |
|---|
| 1. Introduction and scientific background |
| 2. Objectives |
| 3. Selection of patients |
| 4. Design of study (including schematic diagram) |
| 5. Treatment plan |
| 6. Drug information |
| 7. Toxicities to be monitored and dosage modifications |
| 8. Required clinical and laboratory data and study calendar |
| 9. Criteria for evaluating the effect of treatment and endpoint definition |
| 10. Statistical considerations |
| 11. Informed consent and regulatory considerations |
| 12. Data forms |
| 13. References |
| 14. Study chairperson, collaborating participants, addresses, and telephone numbers |

responsible for specific functions. Typical team members include:

- Principal investigator: This individual has responsibility for overseeing all aspects of the protocol including the development of the protocol, the submission of the study to the Institutional Review Board, patient recruitment, informed consent, and data collection, analysis, interpretation and publication.
- Clinical research nurse or clinical trials nurse: This individual participates in clinical research and educates staff, participants and others involved in the clinical trial about all aspects of the study. The nurse is the communication link between the clinical setting and the principal investigator and often is responsible for the monitoring of toxicity and response, quality assurance and participates in the data collection and analysis.
- Nurse researcher: This individual is an investigator involved in conducting research directed at answering nursing related questions and mentoring other nurses in the research process. They are responsible for conducting research, analyzing data, solving clinical problems, writing grants, and publishing their findings.
- Data manager: This individual collaborates with the principal investigator and research nurse in the management of the clinical trial data. The data manager also provides data to monitoring agencies and groups and prepares data summaries for interim reports and final analyses.
- Staff physicians and nurses: members of the clinical team administer the intervention to the participants in the study as specified in the protocol; identify and record toxicities and adverse events; and provide overall clinical management.

## NONCLINICAL TRIAL ACCESS TO EXPERIMENTAL AGENTS: SPECIAL ACCESS PROGRAMS

Although only well-designed clinical trials can reliably determine whether promising agents actually help persons with cancer or at risk of developing cancer, individuals seeking access to agents being evaluated in clinical trials have specific programs available if they are not eligible for a clinical trial. These avenues include special access programs.

### GROUP C PROGRAM

In order to reduce the lag time between the date when an investigational agent was found to have anti-tumor activity and the time that the agent became available on the market, since 1976, the National Cancer Institute (NCI) has had a program (called Group C/treatment INDs) that allows early access to certain agents. These agents must be administered by properly trained physicians and cannot require specialized care facilities. Each Group C protocol specifies, eligibility, drug use and how information about the patient's use of the drug should be reported. Group C drugs are provided free of charge, and the Centers for Medicare and Medicaid Services (CMS) provides coverage for care associated with Group C therapy.

### TREATMENT REFERRAL CENTER (TRC)

TRC is another mechanism that the NCI offers to provide access to experimental agents when a patient population is identified for which an investigational agent should be available. The NCI develops and provides the TRC protocol to the requested Cancer Centers, which then may offer it to patients as a treatment option.

### SPECIAL EXCEPTION (COMPASSIONATE USE/COMPASSIONATE EXCEPTION)

People who do not meet the eligibility criteria for a clinical trial of an investigational agent may be eligible to receive the agent. The person's physician must contact the study sponsor and provides the person's medical information and treatment history. Requests are then evaluated on a case-by-case basis. To use an agent under this mechanism, there should be reasonable expectation that the agent will prolong survival or improve quality of life.

## PROTECTION OF RESEARCH PARTICIPANTS

The protection of the individuals who agree to participate in clinical research is paramount. This right has not always been respected and, in the past, there have been notorious abuses of human rights. In 1947, the post-World War II trial that led to the conviction of Nazi physicians and scientists in Nuremberg, Germany, brought international attention to the abuses of clinical research and highlighted the fact that the protection of human rights cannot be left solely to the integrity of researchers. This trial resulted in a formal statement (called the Nuremberg Code) about the ethical conduct of research in humans, which continues to form the basis for international codes of research ethics today.[18]

In the United States, a number of unfortunate, infamous clinical trials also called attention to the need for increased protection for research participants. The most notable was the Tuskegee syphilis study, in which African American men with syphilis were followed. The observational study was conducted from 1932 to 1972 without the knowledge and consent of the men who participated.[19] Even in the 1940s, after penicillin was found to be effective in the treatment of syphilis, the researchers never informed the participants or treated them with the antibiotic.

In 1974, in response to the identified need for the government to assure the protection of human subjects in research, Congress passed the National Research Act. This act required research studies involving human subjects to be reviewed by an IRB before federal grants and contracts could be funded. This requirement was then codified in the Code of Federal Regulations Title 45, Part 46 (45CFR-46), and includes the specific functions and membership of the IRB. The National Research Act also created the National Commission for the Protection of Research Subjects. This commission was extremely important in developing seminal reports on various aspects of human subject protection.[20] Most influential was the *Belmont Report,* which first identified the set of ethical principles that continue to guide the ethics of clinical research today (Table 10-4).[21] Common to these national guidelines and regulations — and others used throughout the world — are a number of agreed upon rules[22]:

- The research design must offer a high probability of generating useful knowledge.
- The probable benefits must outweigh the risks.
- The selection of subjects must be just.
- Subjects must give their informed consent.
- Subjects' rights to privacy and confidentiality must be protected.

As clinical trials methodology evolves to include more and more sophisticated therapeutic evaluations, including an understanding of molecular signatures that predispose individuals to a cancer, so does the research ethics. Greater and greater discourse is focused on how one achieves a balance between the goal of developing valuable knowledge about cancer and its treatment with the protection of those individuals who participate in these studies.[23,24]

**TABLE 10-4**

| Fundamental Principles of Biomedical Ethics |
|---|
| Respect for persons: autonomy, self-determination, the right to deliberate about personal goals and act accordingly without interference |
| Nonmaleficence: obligation to do no harm to others |
| Beneficence: obligation to do good or promote the good of others |
| Justice: fairness, equitable distribution of benefits and burdens |

## INFORMED CONSENT

The Nuremberg Code established the positive requirement that the voluntary consent of the human subject is absolutely essential. This positive rule supports the principles of respect for autonomy and respect for persons in requiring that individuals be free to choose what will happen to them.[25] This requirement has been codified in the Common Rule, which requires the informed consent of the potential research participant, or his or her legally authorized representative, along with written documentation of the consent on a form approved by an IRB. Although specific requirements govern the content of the informed consent document, it is actually the informed consent process that is of greatest importance. Legal, regulatory, medical, and ethical groups have described the process as needing to contain four essential elements: understanding, comprehension, voluntariness, and competence.[26] Table 10-5 outlines the elements required under 45CFR-46 that must be included in the informed consent document to ensure that adequate information is presented to the potential participant for consideration.

Because clinical trials are often complicated and include tests and interventions that carry risks, the manner in which the information is presented is extremely important. The information should be written and presented using clear and understandable wording, taking into consideration the educational level, language requirements, and cultural needs of the individual. Presentation of the information is necessary but not sufficient for informed consent.[27] Although it can be a challenge, it is critical that the participant comprehend the information, especially in studies where the potential

**TABLE 10-5**

**Essential Elements of Informed Consent**

- Statement that the trial involves research
- Explanation and description of the nature of the trial, purpose of the trial, duration of participation, procedures to be followed, and which procedures are experimental
- Description of foreseeable risks and discomforts
- Benefits to the participants and others
- Alternative procedures or treatments
- Description of the confidentiality of records
- Explanation of procedures if the project involves more than minimal risk (eg, compensation, availability of medical treatment)
- Contact person for questions
- Statement that participation is voluntary, that there will be no loss of benefits on withdrawal, and that the participant may withdraw at any time
- Statement that the participant's signature indicates a decision to participate, having read and discussed the information presented

for significant risk exists. Recently, attention has targeted ways to improve the informed consent process. Numerous groups, including the NCI, have developed recommendations and templates to assist investigators in developing informed consent documents.[28]

## INSTITUTIONAL REVIEW BOARD

The IRB is a uniquely important, institutionally based component of the protection system for participants in research. It is responsible for assessing the balance of risks and benefits of the clinical trials it reviews, evaluating the ethical status of the study, and, once the study is approved, monitoring the overall conduct of the clinical trial. In recent years, the deaths of clinical trials participants have spurred major changes and improvements in the institutional support for IRBs and in the degree of independent oversight that must be in place to monitor clinical trials.

Federal regulations stipulate that the composition of the IRB must include at least five people, who must come from diverse occupations and backgrounds. In addition, one member must be from outside the institution. Typically, IRBs are composed of medical specialists, nurses, other healthcare specialists, ethicists, chaplains, and lay members of the community. Since greater attention has focused on the function of IRBs, national committees and commissions have recommended that IRB membership be revised to better represent the community of potential research participants. A number of proposals and pilot studies have also evaluated the use of central—rather than institutional—IRBs as a way to improve the quality and consistency of review, given the increasing complexity of clinical trials.

## DATA MONITORING COMMITTEE

The DMC, also called the Data Safety Monitoring Board or DSMB, is an independent group (typically 3 to 7 members) of experts whose purpose is to protect the safety of trial participants, the credibility of the study and the validity of study results The NCI policy has required that Data Safety Monitoring Boards be in place for all phase 3 randomized clinical trials.

DMCs should be multidisciplinary, and should always include individuals with relevant clinical and statistical expertise. An ethicist or a representative from a patient advocacy group may also be members. The DMC will convene at predetermined intervals and review unblinded results, that is, results split by experimental and control arms. This group determines if the trial should be changed or closed. There are typically three reasons a DMC might recommend termination of the study: safety concerns, outstanding benefit, and futility.

## FEDERAL OVERSIGHT AGENCIES

Two government organizations—the Office for Human Research Protections (OHRP) in the Department of Health and Human Services and the FDA—have regulations in place to protect clinical trials participants. Some studies fall under the jurisdiction of both groups and are subject to both sets of regulations, which are basically congruent in terms of their requirements for informed consent and rules for IRBs.

### Office for Human Research Protections

Formerly known as the Office of Protection from Research Risks, the OHRP has responsibility for safe-guarding the welfare of participants in the research conducted by the 17 federal agencies and departments that come under the Common Rule. This oversight spans standards for the development of informed consent documents, the formation and function of IRBs, and rules relating to especially vulnerable populations in research, such as children and prisoners.

### Food and Drug Administration

The FDA is responsible for clinical trials of new drugs, biologics, or devices that come under its regulations, regardless of whether the studies are federally funded. The agency conducts audits of IRB operations and institutional safeguards for participants in clinical trials.

## BARRIERS TO CLINICAL TRIALS PARTICIPATION

At a time when the number of new agents to be evaluated in clinical trials is increasing, there continue to be a limited number of people who participate in these studies. No more than 5% of adults diagnosed with cancer each year will participate in a clinical trial—a figure that has not changed since the 1980s.[29,30] Several organizations have conducted surveys to understand the reason for this limited number of participants and found that the barriers to participation are multifactorial. These barriers include factors relevant to healthcare professionals, the public, and patients, especially the underserved. In surveys, physician groups state that participation is often limited by the physician's lack of awareness of appropriate trials for a particular patient population; the physician's unwillingness to "lose" control of the person's care; the common belief that standard therapy is best; the belief that participation in clinical trials adds cost and significant administrative burdens to the practice; and concerns about how the person or individual will react to the suggestion of participation in a clinical trial.

In a systematic review conducted in 2006, studies assessing barriers to participation in clinical trials were analyzed and patient identified issues were reported. The most common reasons cited included: concerns with the trial setting; a dislike of randomization; general discomfort with the research process; complexity and stringency of the protocol; presence of a placebo or no-treatment group; potential side effects; being unaware of trial opportunities; the idea that clinical trials are not appropriate for serious diseases; fear that trial involvement would have a negative effect on the relationship with their physician; and their physician's attitudes towards the trial.[31] Understanding these barriers and issues will help to develop strategies to address patients concerns and improve enrollment in clinical trials.

Unique, additional barriers exist for individuals who are members of certain ethnic groups and/or who are medically underserved. Due to past experiences, there is a long-standing fear and skepticism among some minority populations about medical research and distrust of the medical care system in general. Also, physicians may not discuss clinical trials with patients who belong to ethnic minorities out of concern of offending these individuals. The National Medical Association has created Project IMPACT (Increase Minority Participation and Awareness of Clinical Trials) to improve the use of new therapeutics in the minority community. The results of this study revealed that minority physicians are interested in participating in clinical trials, however multiple barriers exist. These include a lack of awareness and lack of access to clinical research coordinators.[32] Certainly, language and literacy barriers may make it difficult to communicate the needed information in a way that is understandable, especially the informed consent document. Costs may pose a significant barrier for the underserved, as it is most often assumed that the individual's health plan (either public or private) will cover the usual care costs. Health insurance plans vary on their coverage of clinical trials. The effort to precertify or assure this coverage can be difficult and untimely; thus it can serve as a disincentive for an individual needing immediate treatment for cancer.

Research nurses often are the first member of the research team to have comprehensive conversations with the patient about the details of a particular clinical trial. The research nurse is in an excellent position to advocate and educate their patients on available clinical trials. Strategies aimed at increasing enrollment should focus on the expertise of the research nurse.

## CANCER CLINICAL TRIALS PROGRAMS

Currently, most clinical trials are conducted by the NCI, cancer centers, and the pharmaceutical industry, often in collaboration with one another. Although in past years the NCI was the primary developer of new cancer drugs, this role has now been increasingly assumed by the pharmaceutical industry. For phase 3 randomized studies, however, the cooperative groups remain the prime entities responsible for these evaluations, and the NCI cancer centers continue to be valuable resources for the conduct of studies funded by both NCI and industry.

### NCI COOPERATIVE GROUP SYSTEM

The unique organization of the cooperative group system allows for the conduct of clinical trials in a multi-institutional setting. Established in 1955 by Congress, the cooperative groups primarily conduct large-scale studies, including combined-modality approaches and studies of cancer prevention, detection, quality of life, supportive care, and cost analysis. Currently, 10 cooperative groups are conducting studies in the United States. They include thousands of physicians and nurses in academic medical centers, hospitals, and community physician offices (Table 10-6).

### NCI CANCER CENTERS PROGRAM

The development of the NCI Cancer Centers Program began in the 1960s and was formally authorized under the National Cancer Act in 1971. This legislation, and the strong national support for it, promoted the formation of comprehensive cancer programs across the country that became national resources for research and led to the development of multidisciplinary approaches and national standards for oncology care. Cancer centers continue to be the research engines for oncology today; in

**TABLE 10-6**

**NCI-Funded Clinical Cooperative Oncology Groups**

- American College of Radiology Imaging Network
- American College of Surgeons Oncology Group
- Cancer and Acute Leukemia Group B
- Children's Oncology Group
- Eastern Cooperative Oncology Group
- Gynecologic Oncology Group
- National Surgical Adjuvant Breast and Bowel Project
- North Central Cancer Treatment Group
- Radiation Therapy Oncology Group
- Southwest Oncology Group

addition, they are developing mechanisms to better integrate their work with community programs. This integration is essential to ensure better dissemination of research results and better design of applicable research so that it will benefit the majority of patients who are not treated in cancer centers.

## CURRENT ISSUES

### ACCESS TO CLINICAL TRIALS

There has been increasing attention and interest in maximizing accrual to clinical trials and increasing access among all populations. However, disparities in access to health care among different populations ultimately lead to decreased access and participation in clinical trials. In particular, ethnic minorities are underrepresented in clinical trials, and access to expert and high-technology care is often limited.[33] Improving the communication among health care professionals and community outreach to minority populations and educating patients about clinical trials is crucial. The nurse is a key member of the research team who can assist the patient through education and structuring the questions a patient may have when considering a clinical trial. (Table 10-7)

In 2007 legislation was signed into law (Fair Access to Clinical Trials Act) to increase public access to clinical trials results reflecting increasing pressure to disclose clinical trial information to the public. The legislation is intended to standardize and centralize clinical trial disclosure and bring changes to the communication among clinical research, pharmaceutical industry, medical practitioners and the general public.

### EVALUATING A CLINICAL TRIAL

The critical evaluation of medical research and clinical trial data may appear daunting to the novice research nurse and often to a seasoned professional. Recognition of the

**TABLE 10-7**

**Questions to Ask When Considering Participation in a Clinical Trial**

**The Study**

1. What is the purpose of the study?
2. Why do researchers think the approach may be effective?
3. Who will sponsor the study?
4. Who has reviewed and approved the study?
5. How are study results and safety of participants being checked?
6. How long will the study last?
7. What will my responsibilities be if I participate?

**Possible Risks and Benefits**

1. What are my possible short-term benefits?
2. What are my possible long-term benefits?
3. What are my short-term risks, such as side effects?
4. What are my possible long-term risks?
5. What other options do people with my risk of cancer or type of cancer have?
6. How do the possible risks and benefits of these trials compare with those options?

**Participation and Care**

1. What kinds of therapies, procedures, and/or tests will I have during the trial?
2. Will they hurt, and, if so, for how long?
3. How do the tests in the study compare with those I would have outside the trial?
4. Will I be able to take my regular medications while in the clinical trial?
5. Where will I have my medical care?
6. Who will be in charge of care?

**Personal Issues**

1. How could being in this study affect my daily life?
2. Can I talk to other people in the study?

**Cost Issues**

1. Will I have to pay for any part of the trial, such as tests or the study drug?
2. If so, what will the charges likely be?
3. What is my health insurance likely to cover?
4. Who can help answer any questions from my insurance company or health plan?
5. Will there be any travel or child care costs that I need to consider while I am in the trial?

**Tips for Asking Your Doctor About Clinical Trials**

When you talk with your doctor or members of the research team:

1. Consider taking a family member or friend along, for support and for help in asking questions or recording answers.
2. Plan ahead what to ask—but don't hesitate to ask any new questions you think of while you're there.
3. Write down your questions in advance, to make sure you remember to ask them all.
4. Write down the answer, so that you can review them whenever you want.
5. Consider bringing a tape recorder to make a taped record of what is said (even if you write down answers).

limitations of the trial as well as its strengths will strengthen the credence of the data presented. To assist in the critical evaluation of research findings, the following questions have been developed. These questions will assist the nurse in determining whether the trial is valid, the strength of the results and the whether the results are applicable to an individual's practice.

1. **What is the study design?** The randomized controlled trial (RCT) is the gold standard in study design. The RCT is considered the most reliable form of scientific evidence in the medical community.
2. **What is the population being studied?** Review the inclusion and exclusion criteria of the study. Is the number of subjects adequate to answer the study question? How were participants allocated to control and experimental groups? Are all participants who entered the study accounted for in the results?
3. **Are the results statistically significant?** Are actual values presented? Are p-values reported? Are graphs and tables easy to read and understand?
4. **Were the clinical endpoints appropriate?** The choice of which endpoints to use is critical to the study design. Clinical trial endpoints are important since they are the proof that the drug does what the investigator claims. Understanding endpoints is absolutely critical to interpreting the technical medical literature. All journal articles reporting on clinical trials will report the results in terms of the endpoints which were measured.
5. **Where are the articles published?** Articles accepted in peer-reviewed journals are more credible. If the data is presented at a medical conference, the study is generally on-going and final data is unavailable.
6. **Who conducted the study?** What are the author's affiliations?
7. **Who funded the study?** Is the study sponsored by a commercial entity or from an independent grant or group of researchers?

### QUALITY OF LIFE EVALUATIONS

In recent years, more clinical trials have included quality of life endpoints in addition to the traditional end-points of response and survival as outcomes to be measured. These patient-reported evaluations of quality of life domains, which may include physical, psychosocial functioning, and symptom reduction, provide a much broader body of information about the intervention under study. The addition of such quality of life evaluations allows both clinicians and patients to weigh those items of most importance when making a decision about a particular treatment or a choice between treatments. For example, one individual may choose the therapy (based on clinical trial results) that offers the opportunity for the maximum length of survival at the price of considerable toxicity, while another individual may choose less additional survival time to forgo the toxicity of treatment with the expectation of a better quality of life during this shorter survival period.

### ECONOMIC EVALUATIONS

As a greater number of new agents and interventions undergo evaluation, there is increasing interest in including economic analyses in clinical trials. These economic evaluations form a relationship with the traditional study end points (ie, response, survival, functional status, and symptom reduction) and require new theoretical and methodologic approaches to evaluate effects such as cost-effectiveness and cost-efficiency.[34] In an economic analysis, the cost of the therapy is compared to the effect of the therapy; the overall costs are presented in financial terms, while the effects of therapy are presented in terms of a clinical measure, such as disease-free years of survival, years of life saved, or quality-adjusted years of life saved (QALY).[35] The costs to be evaluated can be medical or nonmedical, depending on the focus of the proposed evaluation. When planning for an economic evaluation, it must be first determined what type of costs will be included in the analysis. This determination will depend on whose perspective is to be considered in the study—the healthcare provider, the patient, the health plan, or society.

The integration of economics into cancer clinical trials requires close communication between economists, policymakers, and clinical researchers so that the evaluations will provide useful information that benefits patients. Including cost analyses in research studies adds a serious element to the discussion of resource allocation and must be done carefully and with objective deliberation. As we begin to utilize the knowledge of the postgenomic era, it is important to be able to explore the new targeted approaches to therapeutic development, while at the same time acknowledging the need to develop a sound financial approach to providing the most effective agents.

## FUTURE TRENDS

The completion of a clinical trial is not the end of the story in bringing new and better diagnostics, prevention strategies and therapies to the public. A critical step remains; that is, the actual introduction and use of these new interventions in the health care system. In the past, it has often taken more than a year for a scientific paper to be written and published despite the importance of the study results. But now, medical publishers have rapid alert systems for publishing immediately those studies that are of critical importance and that have potential to impact the care being given to patients. These results can be made available immediately on the internet and can then be picked up by the professional and lay press. However, the next step of incorporating the study results into the health care system can be a difficult task with multiple barriers. Although the approval process for new agents and medical devices is clearly spelled out by FDA regulations, the coverage of their costs by health plans and their use by health care providers is not assured. Better systems for the evaluation of medical evidence that lead to insurance coverage are needed as well as the broader acceptance of standards of practice which outline the most effective method of treating or preventing a particular cancer-related problem.

Many challenges lie ahead in the development of new and more effective interventions for the prevention, diagnosis, and treatment of cancer. The postgenomic era offers tremendous opportunities for applying the understanding of preclinical drug pharmacology and molecular targeting to the design and development of clinical trials.[36] There is potential for new agents entering study to have well-defined theoretical mechanisms of action, and for investigators to design studies with biochemical and molecular endpoints.[37] At the same time, as the clinical inquiry becomes more specific to the particular molecular characteristics of the individual patient's disease, it will require new trial designs focused on these characteristics rather than the more broad-based traditional approaches. Communication and education will be needed to produce effective collaboration between investigators and to ensure participant understanding about the new clinical trials designs.

Advances in monitoring therapeutic responses through enhanced imaging techniques and other biomarkers will all affect the approach investigators take in the future. For instance, the advent of new and more precise technologies has exciting implications for the use of circulating tumor cells (CTCs) as a prognostic and response to treatment indicator. Modern biological techniques now allow the isolation and characterization of CTCs with improved sensitivity and with high specificity and reproducibility, and as a result it has been possible to demonstrate that elevated CTCs are a clinically significant and statistically poor prognostic factor in women with metastatic breast cancer.[38] These new indicators will ultimately redefine how progression and treatment effects are defined.

As the use of computerized systems in clinical trials continues to evolve, the way data is stored and shared will undergo intense scrutiny. In 2007, the FDA published guidelines for industry addressing computerized systems used in clinical investigations. The document provides recommendations to investigators for maintaining and generating source data for subjects participating in a clinical trial.

Continued emphasis will be on standardizing the clinical trial process and infrastructure and enhancing the interaction between the research community and government agencies. The ever increasing knowledge of the biology of cancer will lead to an evolution of the clinical trial process to meet the demands of the future.

The trend in developing agents that have molecular targets is clear and will influence the design of randomized, controlled trials well into the future. Clinical benefits such as disease stabilization rather than reduction of disease burden will be more likely. These agents also have the potential for toxicities that are relatively less severe than traditional cytotoxic agents.

The opportunity exists to more extensively utilize patient reported outcomes, along with response and survival, in clinical trials. More patient groups and health professional organizations are working together to establish clinical outcomes of importance. The challenge of the medical, nursing, and behavioral research communities is to design trials that focus on evaluating both the effects of the intervention on the disease and its effects on the overall quality of life of the individual.

## REFERENCES


1. Le Tourneau C, Faivre S, Raymond E. New developments in multitargeted therapy for patients with solid tumors. *Cancer Treat Rev.* 2008;34:37–48.
2. Kumar S, Gutierrez M, Doroshow JH, Murgo AJ. Drug development in oncology: classical cytotoxics and molecularly targeted agents. *Brit J Clin Pharmaco.* 2006;62:15–26.
3. Chabner B. Advances and challenges in the use of biomarkers in clinical trials. *Clin Adv Hematol Oncol.* 2008;6:42–43.
4. U.S. Food and Drug Administration. Guidance for industry: Patient-reported outcome measures: Use in medical product development to support labeling claims. Dept of Health and Human Services; Washington D.C.; 2008.
5. Eisenhauer E, Bonetti M, Gelber R. Principles of clinical trials. In: Cavalli F, Hansen H, Kaye S, eds. *Textbook of Medical Oncology.* London: Martin Dunitz; 2000:99–136.
6. Dent SF, Eisenhauer EA. Phase I trial design: are new methodologies being put into practice? *Ann Oncol.* 1996;7:561–566.
7. Parulekar WR, Eisenhauer EA. Phase 1 trial design for solid tumor studies of targeted, non-cytotoxic agents: theory and practice. *J Natl Cancer Inst.* 2004;96:990–997.
8. Goulart BH, Clark JW, Pien HH, Roberts TG, Finkelstein SN, Chabner BA. Trends in the use and role of biomarkers in phase 1 oncology trials. *Clin Cancer Res.* 2007;13:6719–6726.
9. Ratain MJ, Mick R, Schilsky RL, et al. Statistical and ethical issues in the design and conduct of phase 1 and 2 clinical trials of new anticancer agents. *J Natl Cancer Inst.* 1993;85:1637–1643.
10. Simon R. Design and analysis of clinical trials. In: De Vita VT, Hellman S, Rosenberg SA, eds. *Cancer: Principles and Practice of Oncology.* 6th ed. Philadelphia: Lippincott Williams & Wilkins; 2001:521–538.
11. Thiesse P, Ollivier L, Di Stefano-Louineau D, et al. Response rate accuracy in oncology trials: reasons for interobserver variability. *J Clin Oncol.* 1997;15:3507–3514.
12. El-Maraghi RH, Eisenhauer EA. Review of phase 2 trial design used in studies of molecular targeted agents: outcomes and predictors of success in phase 3. *J Clin Oncol.* 2008;26:1346–1354.
13. Morabito A, Di Maio M, Normanno N, Perrone F. Methodology of clinical trials with new molecular-targeted agents: where do we stand? *Ann Oncol.* 2006;17(suppl 7):128–131.

14. Wagner LI, Wenzel L, Shaw E, Cella D. Patient-reported outcomes in phase 2 cancer clinical trials: lessons learned and future directions. *J Clin Oncol.* 2008;25:5058–5062.
15. Pocock SJ. Randomized clinical trials. *Br Med J.* 1977;1:1161.
16. Ganz PA, Gotay CC. Use of patient-reported outcomes in phase 3 cancer treatment trials: lessons learned and future directions. *J Clin Oncol.* 2008;25:5063–5069.
17. Spriet A, Dupen-Spriet T. *Good Practice of Clinical Drug Trials.* Farmington, CT: Karger; 1997.
18. Faden RR, Beauchamp TL. The development of consent requirements in research ethics. In: Faden RR, Beauchamp TL, eds. *A History and Theory of Informed Consent.* New York: Oxford University Press; 1986:151–199.
19. King P. The dangers of difference: the legacy of the Tuskegee Syphilis study. In: Arras JD, Steinbock B, eds. *Ethical Issues in Modern Medicine.* Mountain View, CA: Mayfield; 1995:578–584.
20. Ingelfinger FJ. Ethics of human experimentation defined by a national commission. *N Engl J Med.* 1977;296:44–45.
21. The National Commission for the Protection of Human Subjects of Biomedical and Behavioral Research. *The Belmont Report: Ethical Principles and Guidelines for the Protection of Human Subjects of Research.* Washington, DC: U.S. Government Printing Office; April 1979, 1988–201-778/80319.
22. Levine R, Lebacqz K. Ethical considerations in clinical trials. *Clin Pharmacol Ther.* 1979;25:728–749.
23. Emanuel E, Wendler D, Grady C. What Makes clinical research ethical? *JAMA* 2000;283:2701–2711.
24. Joffe S, Miller F. Bench to bedside—mapping the moral terrain of clinical research. *Hastings Center Report.* 2008;38:30–42.
25. Ramsey P. *The Patient as Person: Explorations on Medical Ethics.* New Haven, CT: Yale University Press; 1970.
26. Faden RR, Beauchamp TL. The concepts of informed consent and competence. In Faden RR, Beauchamp TL, eds. *A History and Theory of Informed Consent.* New York: Oxford University Press; 1986:274–294.
27. Daugherty CK. Impact of therapeutic research on informed consent and the ethics of clinical trials: a medical oncology perspective. *J Clin Oncol.* 1999;17:1601.
28. National Cancer Institute. Simplification of Informed Consent Documents. http://www.cancer.gov/clinicaltrials/understanding/simplification-of-informed-consent-docs. Accessed January 7, 2010.
29. Umutyan A, Chiechi C, Becket L, et al. Overcoming barriers to cancer clinical trial accrual. *Cancer* 2008;112:212–219.
30. Lippman ME, Chabner BA. *Overview of Proceedings of the NIH Consensus Development Conference on Adjuvant Chemotherpy and Endocrine Therapy for Breast Cancer NCI Monographs No. 1.* Bethesda MD: National Cancer Institute; 1986.
31. Mills E, Seely D, Rachlis B, et al. Barriers to participation in clinical trials of cancer: a meta-analysis and systemic review of patient-reported factors. *Lancet* 2008;7:141–148.
32. Powell J, Fleming Y, Walker-McGill C, Lenoir M. The project IMPACT experience to date: increasing minority participation and awareness of clinical trials. *J Natl Med Assoc.* 2008;100:178–187.
33. Petereit D, Rogers D, Govern F, et al. Increasing access to clinical cancer trials and emerging technologies for minority populations: the native American project. *JCO* 2004;22:4452–4455.
34. Integrating economic analysis into cancer clinical trials: the National Cancer Institute-American Society of Clinical Oncology economics workbook. *J Natl Cancer Inst.* 1998;24:1–3.
35. Schulman KA, Glick HA, Yabroff RK, et al. Introduction to clinical economics: assessment of cancer therapies. *J Natl Cancer Inst.* 1995;19:1–10.
36. Takimoto CH. Anticancer drug development at the US National Cancer Institute. *Cancer Chemother Pharmacol.* 2003;52(suppl 1):S29-S33.
37. Szurmomi P, Vinson V, Marshall E. Rethinking drug discovery. *Science* 2004;303:1795.
38. Smerage J, Hayes D. The prognostic implications of circulating tumor cells in patients with breast cancer. *Cancer Invest.* 2008;26:109–114.

CHAPTER

# 11

Theresa Wicklin Gillespie, PhD, RN

# Surgical Therapy

## INTRODUCTION

Surgery, whether used for diagnosis, staging, curative therapy, or palliation, remains the key component of oncology care. Surgery as the earliest form of cancer therapy dates back to the time of ancient Egypt. The first oncologic surgery of a more contemporary era occurred in 1809, when a large (22.5-lb) ovarian tumor was removed from a woman.[1] Although rudimentary, the operation was successful in that the patient survived another 30 years. Critical dates in the history of surgery as cancer therapy are listed in Table 11-1.

Currently, more than 60% of all cancers are treated with surgery, and this modality is used in diagnosis or staging of tumors in about 90% of cases.[2] The advantages of surgery include a high potential for cure when the cancer is localized and the ability to obtain tissue for initial diagnosis as well as evidence for staging of disease. The unavoidable disadvantage of cancer surgery is the need to remove normal tissue as well as malignant tissue to ensure an adequate margin of unaffected tissue when the cancer is resected. To undergo the anesthesia required for major surgery, an individual should have an acceptable performance status and organ function, especially cardiac and pulmonary.

The field of surgical oncology has progressed significantly since its inception such that surgery is now considered part of a multidisciplinary approach to cancer therapy. The thoughtful combination and careful timing of surgery along with chemotherapy, radiation therapy, immunotherapy, targeted therapies, and other novel therapeutic approaches are essential for optimal treatment planning.[3] Because the initial consultation for most patients with a possible cancer diagnosis occurs with a surgeon, surgical oncology often functions as the gatekeeper for involvement of other oncologic specialties. Therefore, to guide the treatment approach properly, surgeons must be expert not only

**TABLE 11-1**

**Critical Dates in History of Surgical Oncology**

| Date | Event | Significance in Surgical Oncology |
|---|---|---|
| 1809 | Resection of ovarian tumor | Patient survived long term postoperatively |
| 1884 | Building of first U.S. operating room in Bellevue, New York | Promoted aseptic technique and allowed more invasive surgery |
| 1889 | Introduction of x-rays in surgical practice | Allowed visualization and localization of findings prior to surgery |
| 1890 | Radical mastectomy developed by William Halstead | Demonstrated long-term control of disease through radical surgery; emphasized anatomic precision and careful handling of tissue |
| 1903 | Initiation of neurosurgery by Harvey Cushing as independent specialty | Changed approaches to endocrine tumors |
| 1975 | Initiation of first adjuvant therapy trial for early-stage breast cancer | Demonstrated survival advantage for those randomized to chemotherapy postoperatively |
| 1986 | Publication of NSABP B-06 trial | Showed equivalency of segmental mastectomy (lumpectomy) plus radiation therapy compared with mastectomy |
| 1990 | 1990 NIH Consensus Conference | Recommended 5-FU-based chemotherapy for stage III colon cancer after surgical resection |
| 1990 | Concept of sentinel lymph node introduced to Society of Surgical Oncology | Allowed resection of draining lymph node only |
| 1991 | Prospective study of resection of hepatic metastases published | Median overall survival of 3 years with resection |
| 1999 | Publication of NSABP B-24 trial | Tamoxifen after BCS and RT for DCIS reduced absolute recurrence of ipsilateral and contralateral breast cancer |
| 2007 | Emerging robotics and natural orifice transluminal endoscopic surgery in colorectal cancer | Allowed minimally invasive surgery |

*Abbreviations*: BCS, breast conserving surgery; DCIS, ductal carcinoma in-situ; 5-FU, 5-fluorouracil; NIH, National Institutes of Health; NSABP, National Surgical Adjuvant Breast and Bowel Project; RT, radiation therapy.

in the most current surgical techniques but also in the latest evidence related to other cancer therapy.[4] The initial treatment decisions by the surgical oncologist often will prove to be critical in terms of either allowing future treatment options or rendering certain therapies unfeasible.

## ROLES OF SURGERY IN ONCOLOGY CARE

### PREVENTION AND EARLY DETECTION

As knowledge of cancer genetics, genomics, and tumorigenesis has increased, understanding about interventions to prevent cancer progression and development from precancerous lesions also has advanced.[5] The roles of hereditary and susceptibility genes have been investigated to elucidate important aspects of the process of carcinogenesis, with particular emphasis on how to prevent or interrupt this process. The role of surgery as prophylaxis in asymptomatic individuals who have a genetic predisposition to certain cancers has not been evaluated through randomized clinical trials.[6] Thus careful monitoring, use of chemopreventive agents, and surgical interventions all may be options in these cases.

Evidence has demonstrated that surgical resection of premalignant lesions can effectively prevent some types of tumors from developing further into invasive cancers. The removal of precancerous lesions of the cervix, vulva, and oropharynx is a common example of the role of surgery in cancer prevention.[7] Surgery also plays a key role in the prevention of colorectal cancer. Surgical removal of noncancerous polyps detected at the time of screening or diagnostic colonoscopy effectively prevents further development of such polyps into malignancies.[8] Hereditary nonpolyposis colorectal cancer (HNPCC), familial adenomatous polyposis (FAP), and Peutz-Jeghers syndrome represent relatively rare causes of colorectal cancer. The development of colon cancer at a very early age, often before age 40, due to FAP can be prevented through a prophylactic colectomy.[9]

Barrett's esophagus is a known premalignant condition for esophageal adenocarcinoma, and its incidence has increased over the past two decades. Esophageal adenocarcinoma develops in a stepwise progression from normal tissue to dysplasia to malignancy, with the diagnosis of high-grade dysplasia (HGD) in Barrett's esophagus, and an accompanying high risk of esophageal adenocarcinoma. The management of HGD in this case is controversial, with surgical resection considered along with careful surveillance, endoscopic mucosal resection, and ablation of the mucosa.[10] Likewise, the presence of the cancer susceptibility genes *BRCA1* and *BRCA2* confers a high risk for breast and/or ovarian cancer. In such cases, prophylactic mastectomy and/or oophorectomy may be one option recommended.[11] Prophylactic surgery for individuals at high risk for developing breast and ovarian cancers may be one approach for risk reduction along with more conservative therapies.[12] The use of contralateral mastectomy in women who have had a unilateral breast cancer is also a consideration, although the impact on associated mortality is not well documented.[13]

### DIAGNOSIS

Surgery represents the primary method of obtaining tissue necessary for pathologic or cytologic diagnosis of malignancy. Common methods of biopsy for tissue diagnosis are described in Table 11-2. A tissue diagnosis is a requirement for new malignancies and generally for the first recurrence of a known primary tumor. Surgery is also used to diagnose second primary tumors and to differentiate the source of metastases if a second primary tumor is suspected. A tissue diagnosis obtained preoperatively is needed unless the surgery is planned for the purpose of diagnosis, staging, or treatment planning. A documented pathologic diagnosis is imperative in cases of extensive surgery, such as mastectomy, limb amputation, or organ removal. Pathologic diagnosis is also generally recommended for documentation of the first incidence of metastatic disease.

The location and extent of the tumor will determine which options might be pursued to obtain adequate tissue for diagnosis. Advances in interventional and guided imaging techniques have enabled clinicians to obtain necessary tissue using less invasive and often more precise procedures than open surgical approaches. CT-directed or stereotactic biopsies use computer imaging to pinpoint tumor locations and facilitate biopsy for diagnosis—for example, lung cancer and primary brain tumors. Positron emission tomography (PET) scans with [$^{18}$F]flurodeoxyglucose (FDG) imaging may detect primary, second primary, metastatic, and recurrent tumors.[14] Endoscopic evaluation provides a means to remove tissue (eg, a polyp) for diagnosis while also resecting a potentially premalignant lesion. Open biopsy may be reserved for lesions that are inaccessible by less invasive techniques, considered too risky (eg, because of the risk of pneumothorax or other complications), or best treated with debulking surgery.

Cytology, using fine-needle aspiration (FNA), may be the optimal means for diagnosis in palpable tumors. Cytologic examination often can confirm the presence of malignancy in a brief period of time. FNA may be used to obtain the initial tissue diagnosis; then additional surgical options can be explored. If complete removal of the tumor is possible, excisional biopsy with an adequate margin of tissue or more extensive surgery may be pursued following FNA diagnosis. FNA diagnosis is based on pathologic examination of cells rather than tissue, and its accuracy often depends on the sample obtained, preparation of the specimen, and the expertise of the cytopathologist interpreting the specimen. As with tissue biopsy in general, sampling error or nondiagnostic specimens may require

**TABLE 11-2**

**Surgical Techniques for Tissue Diagnosis in Cancer**

| Surgical Technique | Description | Advantages and Disadvantages |
|---|---|---|
| Fine-needle aspiration | Fine needle (21–22 gauge) inserted into palpable mass; may remove fluid and/or cells in sample | Simple procedure; results available quickly; relies on cytology review of cells obtained for diagnosis |
| Core-needle biopsy | Core/cutting needle inserted into mass and core of tissue removed | More tissue trauma than with a fine needle; obtains larger sample and tissue for histology; may be used with interventional radiology for nonpalpable mass |
| Incisional biopsy | Used for larger tumors (usually > 3 cm); piece of tumor removed from larger mass | Risk of bleeding; no information on margins of tumor; additional surgery or treatment needed for residual tumor; may be used when neoadjuvant therapy is expected |
| Excisional biopsy | Removal of entire tumor plus some additional tissue to obtain clear margins; accessible tumor usually < 3 cm | May be definitive surgery; outcome should be aesthetically acceptable; limited use if tumor is too large or defect would be too obvious |
| Needle localization biopsy | Needle or wires placed by stereotactic procedure to mark site of tumor; then tumor excised based on marker location; used for nonpalpable or hard-to-visualize tumors | Radiographic documentation that specimen was removed is necessary; possible to miss mark and remove incorrect or inadequate sample of tissue |
| Endoscopy | Tumor visualized through lighted endoscope; piece of tumor or entire tumor removed; commonly used for GI, GU, and pulmonary tumors; may be incisional or excisional | Risk of perforation and hemorrhage; increases ability to access hard-to-reach tumors; avoids surgical trauma and postoperative complications associated with open surgery |
| Laparoscopy | Tumor visualized through lighted scope; specimen can be obtained through a variety of techniques (incisional, excisional, scraping, peritoneal washing) | Useful in staging disease; risk of perforation, hemorrhage, and other postoperative complications; avoids surgical trauma and postoperative complications associated with open surgery |
| Open biopsy | Exploratory or definitive surgery to obtain primary diagnosis, perform surgical resection of disease, and note visible or palpable metastases; used to help stage disease | Allows primary access to tumor and adjacent organs affected by cancer; typical surgical risks, including trauma, postoperative complications, perforation, hemorrhage, infection, and recurrence |

*Abbreviations*: GI, gastrointestinal; GU, genitourinary.

additional interventions. Subsequent core-needle biopsy or open biopsy may be necessary to obtain adequate or precise specimens for definitive diagnosis.

Intraoperative diagnosis of tissue may be obtained using a pathologic technique termed *frozen section*. With this procedure, a sample of the mass is taken from the operating room to be interpreted immediately by a pathologist. The precise histology may not be available from this initial intraoperative interpretation, but the presence of a malignancy can be confirmed.[15] This information enables the surgeon to then pursue further surgical procedures or conclude the operation.

Although, ideally, all lesions will have either preoperative or intraoperative confirmation of malignancy, in some cases this confirmation is not possible. A classic illustration of this dilemma is the patient with jaundice and an identified mass in the head of the pancreas. Removal of the mass requires extensive surgical resection (eg, pancreatoduodenectomy, Whipple procedure), with known morbidity and mortality being associated with the intervention.[16] Unfortunately, the surgical procedure is necessary to both diagnose and treat a possible cancer in the head of the pancreas. Part of the preoperative workup for any surgery therefore must include a clear discussion of possible outcomes and complications, including the risk of more extensive surgery for what ultimately may be shown to be a benign tumor.

## STAGING OF DISEASE

Preoperative care for patients with a known or suspected diagnosis of cancer includes an adequate staging workup. The size of the tumor, as determined by clinical and radiologic evaluation, and the involvement of lymph nodes or distant sites are important factors for effective clinical decision making.[17] Preoperative staging is a critical element in deciding whether the patient would benefit from surgical approaches and what the goal of therapy might be—cure, control, or palliation. The use of CT scans, FDG-PET scans, nuclear medicine scans, mammography, and other radiologic techniques may aid in determining the extent of tumor involvement locally, regionally, and in distant organs. Although pathologic confirmation may be needed for some equivocal lesions seen on imaging exams, often these radiologic methods are sufficient to establish stage of the cancer. For example, in non-small cell lung cancer (NSCLC), involvement of the mediastinum, as seen on FDG-PET imaging to demonstrate positive lymph nodes, is a key prognostic indicator and a contraindication to surgical resection.

Pathologic examination of the tumor, lymph nodes, and any other tissue removed is crucial for effective patient management. This examination will provide pathologic staging criteria, prognostic factors, and rationale for any adjuvant therapy.[18] The stage, histologic cell type and grade of tumor, status of margins of resection (whether involved with the tumor or not), and degree of vascular invasion contribute to determination of the risk of recurrence and assessment of whether surgery is likely to represent a long-term control or cure of the malignancy. Accurate staging of disease continues to function as the principal prognostic factor for most cancers because stage of disease is often correlated directly with long-term survival. Since only a few cancers (eg, testicular) remain curable even in advanced stages, preoperative staging can assist in the decision making as to whether extensive surgical resection with the goal of cure is possible, if a neoadjuvant intervention with chemotherapy or radiation might be required to reduce the size of a larger tumor to allow resectability, or if a more palliative approach is justified.

Trends in surgical staging procedures have changed over time. Historically, the goals for staging via lymphadenectomy of regional nodes included prognosis, regional control of malignancy through removal of involved nodes, and improvement in other outcomes, including survival. However, removal of regional nodes also was associated with morbidity, reduced quality of life, loss of function, and surgical mortality.

Sentinel lymph nodes represent the initial set of nodes thought to receive drainage from a primary tumor. Thus cancer cells are theorized to metastasize first to these draining nodes, and the removal and examination of one or more identified sentinel nodes are seen as an effective approach to staging regional nodes.[19] The use of blue dye, nuclear medicine technology, and other techniques has enabled surgeons to identify one or more sentinel nodes with a high level of accuracy. If no malignant cells are found in sentinel nodes, the remaining regional nodes are usually negative as well. The traditional methods for pathologic examination of nodes also have undergone extensive revision as new laboratory methods to detect malignant involvement and micrometastases have become available. However, the prognostic significance of such newer pathologic findings as micrometastases remains to be determined. About 25% of patients with a diagnosis of breast cancer without lymph node involvement will develop metastatic spread to distant sites possibly due to micrometastatic disease. The role of micrometastases in lymph nodes and bone marrow is being investigated in multiple tumors, including breast, gynecologic, gastrointestinal, and head and neck cancers, as well as melanomas.[20]

Over the past 20 years, sentinel lymph node biopsy has replaced complete lymph node dissection as the standard of care in melanoma and breast tumors. The application of this technique remains under investigation in other solid tumors, including colorectal, gastric, gynecologic, and head and neck malignancies.[21]

## RESECTION FOR CURE

When a malignancy is diagnosed at an early or localized stage, surgical resection usually represents the best option for long-term survival and cure. The traditional surgical approach for cure has involved an open en bloc resection of the primary tumor with negative margins, along with biopsy or removal of regional or draining lymph nodes where indicated. Such techniques are being replaced by less invasive surgical approaches, including laparascopy, endoscopic microsurgery, and robotic-assisted laparascopy.[22] Early-stage solid tumors, especially in situ or encapsulated tumors where margins are clearly defined and less radical surgery is indicated, are most amenable to minimally invasive surgical resection and offer the best clinical and functional outcomes. Knowledge of the biology of the tumor and natural history of the disease is imperative when planning surgical resection. This principle is demonstrated by a comparison of two types of skin cancer: malignant melanoma, where wide resection with adequate margins is required for long-term control of disease, versus basal cell carcinoma, where less aggressive resection is often adequate for cure.[23]

Surgical resection for cure can be problematic when the tumor is large or invades vital organs or tissues with critical functions. In these cases, decision making involves both clinician and patient input regarding the risk:benefit ratio. The need for an adequate surgical margin must be weighed against potential loss of function, change in body image, and age and general health of the patient.[24] For example, surgical treatment for stage I and II NSCLC represents the standard of care.[25] With the goal of cure, the location, depth, size, and characteristics of the tumor may require different surgical approaches, including a wedge resection, a lobectomy, or pneumonectomy. In each case, the potential benefits of long-term survival resulting from removal of larger amounts of lung tissue must be judged in the context of anticipated loss of pulmonary function. Patients with head and neck cancers requiring extensive surgical resection to ensure adequate margins must be evaluated for and informed about both potential functional deficits and significant changes in self-image. In some cases, such as primary brain tumors, the location or extent of tumor involvement may be such that adequate resection is not possible without dramatic and unacceptable loss of function. In these cases, less radical surgery combined with chemotherapy or radiation delivered before or after surgery may be the optimal approach to achieve the desired treatment goals.

## RESECTION WITH MINIMAL RESIDUAL DISEASE

If the primary tumor is not amenable to complete resection with adequate margins, or if malignant cells are found in regional lymph nodes, then some form of adjuvant therapy may be considered either before (neoadjuvant) or after (adjuvant) surgery. The presence of even minimal residual disease in surgical margins or draining nodes generally indicates a high risk of recurrence. The use of adjuvant chemotherapy or radiation therapy or a combination of these modalities is often recommended pre- or postoperatively. Novel therapies such as biologic or targeted therapies also may prove to be effective in the setting of minimal residual disease. Aggressive tumor debulking may lend itself to the use of adjuvant treatment to eradicate remaining residual cancer cells. In the case of ovarian cancer, which is often diagnosed at a relatively advanced stage, cytoreduction in combination with chemotherapy can improve survival and prevent complications, such as bowel obstruction.[26] Neoadjuvant therapy may downstage the size of the tumor or even result in a pathologic complete response, with no evidence of disease, thus facilitating surgical resection and preservation of tissue or organ function.

## RESECTION IN ADVANCED DISEASE

Surgical resection of advanced disease generally is performed to achieve one of two goals: (1) resection of solitary or limited metastatic disease or (2) palliation of symptoms. Resection of a solitary metastatic lung or liver nodule is performed routinely in advanced disease to improve survival. Resectability of metastatic disease will depend on size, number, and anatomic location of the tumors; patient performance status; and the surgeon's ability to ensure negative surgical margins while leaving adequate viable tissue with reasonable organ function.[27] Preoperative use of portal vein embolization to enhance future remnant liver to the acceptable level of more than 20% of the total initial liver volume may convert unresectable disease to allow safe liver resection.[28] The most exciting advance in the surgical treatment of advanced colorectal cancer has been the ability of chemotherapy to change inoperable liver metastasis to successful resectability. Although resectability rates after neoadjuvant chemotherapy vary widely (6% to 60% based on patient selection and institution), approximately 20% of patients with colorectal cancer that has metastasized to the liver may be candidates for surgical resection. For these patients, 5-year survival rates may be greater than 50% in both single- and multicenter studies.[29] In addition, similar long-term survival is reported for surgical resection of pulmonary metastases from colorectal cancer in patients with good performance status.

Brain metastases occur in about 20% to 40% of all cancer patients.[30] For patients with a good performance status and limited or controlled systemic disease, radiosurgery alone or surgical removal of a solitary brain metastasis often in combination with whole-brain radiation can yield favorable long-term results.[30]

## RECONSTRUCTION

The goals of reconstruction in surgical oncology are fourfold: (1) restoration of function, (2) skin closure or wound covering for surgical defects, (3) restoration of cosmetic appearance (cosmesis) for improvement of body-image changes, and (4) maintenance or enhancement of quality of life. Recent advances in reconstructive surgery include the use of minimally invasive techniques to preserve function and improved ability to reconstruct surgical deficiencies. Depending on the extent of reconstruction and the specialized expertise required, reconstructive surgery may be undertaken by the primary surgeon alone or in collaboration with various other specialists, such as plastic and reconstructive surgeons, urologic surgeons, and gynecologic surgeons.[31] Consultation with other specialists in advance of the scheduled surgery promotes interdisciplinary coordination of care, facilitates the patient's comprehension of anticipated postoperative results, and enhances the patient's understanding of reconstruction options and timing.

Considerable advances in the field of reconstruction have occurred for many types of cancer. Breast cancer may have experienced the greatest changes, from the time many decades ago when wound closure following radical mastectomy was the primary goal, to current approaches including immediate reconstructive techniques, such as implants placed behind the pectoralis muscle and gradually inflated over time (expanders) and transverse rectus abdominis mocutaneous (TRAM) flap, and the more recent technique of skin-sparing mastectomy. Total skin-sparing mastectomy (TSSM) allows for immediate reconstruction, with the cosmetic appearance of the breast depending on the amount of skin that remains following mastectomy. If adequate skin is preserved, then the cosmetic appearance of the operative side is enhanced, and the need to make surgical changes on the contralateral side to achieve symmetry is reduced. Incidence rates for both local recurrence and wound complications, such as skin-flap necrosis and infections, are similar for skin-sparing mastectomy and non-skin-sparing mastectomy.[32] A nipple-sparing mastectomy (NSM) preserves the nipple-areola complex and includes intraoperative pathologic evaluation of the nipple core in combination with the surgical technique of a TSSM.[33] The type of breast reconstruction technique, timing of reconstruction (immediate or delayed), and preference for any reconstruction at all are often difficult decisions needing to be made by the woman who has experienced a recent diagnosis of cancer. Such decision making demands careful patient education, presentation of options, and provision of adequate time to consider individual preferences. Therapeutic factors, such as timing of adjuvant chemotherapy or radiation therapy, also must be discussed. Complications related to the reconstruction, such as infection or necrosis that would warrant removal of the implant or flap repair, could lead to significant delays in the delivery of adjuvant therapy.[34]

Reconstruction for head and neck cancers, depending on size, location, and extent of tumor involvement, represents a significant challenge in reconstructive surgery. Radical neck dissection, laryngectomy, and other surgeries of the oropharynx require extensive efforts to provide skin and wound closure, reasonable cosmesis, and restoration of as much function as possible. Specialists in plastic surgery, otolaryngology, medical and radiation oncology, and rehabilitation medicine all may need to be involved in treatment planning. Limited surgical defects, such as occur with a small tongue base, may undergo primary closure or be left to granulate and fill in over time. Tissue flaps have their own adequate, reliable blood supply and are composed of segments of donor tissue that match the graft site in color, texture, and often sensitivity; they are used to close larger defects. Moderate-sized surgical defects may be closed by flaps such as those from the buccal mucosa.[35] Large surgical defects require flaps, termed *pedicle flaps,* from regional muscles, including the pectoralis major or latissimus dorsi, with adequate inherent vasculature. The pectoralis major myocutaneous pedicle flap (PMMPF) has been used extensively for reconstruction after surgery for head and neck cancer. Flap procedures may be used for primary reconstruction or for second-line or "salvage" procedures to repair defects arising from surgical or flap complications. Complications of head and neck reconstruction include infection, hematoma, partial or total flap failure, dehiscence, seroma, fistula, or similar problems at the donor site.[36] Risks of complications are greater in procedures done for salvage or reconstruction of the oral cavity, and they increase with the number of comorbidities present and history of cigarette smoking. Flaps also may be used for repair of scars from previous surgery or reconstruction.[37] Examples of flaps are presented in Chapter 54. In the future, tissue engineering and cell therapy may be applied to surgical reconstructions for head and neck malignancies.

Radical surgery for gastrointestinal, urinary, and gynecologic cancers also can require attention to the needs for reconstruction and restoration of function. Tumors of the low to middle rectum may require construction of a pouch to restore function, such as reconstruction with a colonic J-pouch–anal anastomosis. Minimally invasive techniques to repair anastomotic leakage or tears without requiring creation of an ostomy include transanal endoscopic microsurgery (TEM).[38] A recent study has investigated low anterior resections for middle or distal rectal cancers performed using laparascopic techniques.[39] Where possible, bowel continuity may be restored by a colonic J-pouch–anal anastomosis or a coloplasty with coloanal anastomosis. Potential benefits of a laparascopic ultralow anterior approach include less risk of adhesions from previous abdominal surgeries.[39]

Urinary diversion and reconstruction or replacement of the bladder following cystectomy have been pursued with multiple approaches, including (1) creation of conduits to the skin using intestinal segments (conduit diversion), (2) creation of a rectal reservoir or diversion to the skin (continent diversion), (3) use of intestinal segments to replace bladder function, and (4) reconstruction of the removed bladder. In addition, laparascopic radical cystectomy is being used increasingly in many centers, with perioperative outcomes similar to those obtained with open radical cystectomy.[40] Outcomes are related to patient selection, based on assessment of comorbidities, renal status, and ability to handle the care of the diversion or reservoir postoperatively. Chronologic age or locally advanced disease is not an automatic contraindication to urinary diversion.[41]

Gynecologic malignancies often require careful reconstruction techniques because resection of these tumors may affect the function of the gastrointestinal, genitourinary, and reproductive systems. Invasive gynecologic cancer, such as cervical cancer, may call for extensive resection, including pelvic exenteration. Use of diversion techniques for urinary continence, as well as fertility-sparing surgery, require decision making relating to the patient's age, prognosis, childbearing potential, and tumor characteristics and stage.[42]

## SURGERY AS ANCILLARY INTERVENTION

Surgery plays an important role in comprehensive cancer care outside the realm of diagnosis, tumor resection, staging, and reconstruction. The surgical team, along with interventional radiology specialists in some centers, is responsible for placement of central vascular access devices (VADs). Placement of VADs may be a routine part of patient workup and staging when a diagnosis of cancer is known and the decision regarding systemic chemotherapy has been made. Placement of VADs or implantable devices for other purposes (eg, drug delivery) may occur at the time of more definitive surgery to avoid the need for additional anesthesia.[43] Other ancillary surgical procedures, including therapeutic bronchoscopy, thoracentesis for malignant pleural effusion, or repair of other complications (eg, extravasation or removal of infected catheters), may be required throughout the course of the patient's care.

## CLINICAL DECISION MAKING IN SURGICAL THERAPY

Clinical decision making in the field of surgical oncology depends on the considerable data available at the time of consultation or diagnosis. These data might encompass specific characteristics of the primary tumor or stage of disease, characteristics or desires unique to the patient, and issues pertinent to the healthcare environment. During the entire preoperative workup and treatment-planning phase, the nurse will guide and support the patient and family through an extensive and often confusing process of decisions, alternatives, and appointments. The extensive workup process can be anxiety-provoking and further complicated by overwhelming amounts of information and opinions from family and friends. The oncology nurse is in a pivotal position to help the patient and family assimilate the vast array of data and arrive at a decision of their choice.[44]

### TUMOR CHARACTERISTICS

Awareness of the differential diagnoses prior to definitive diagnosis, as well as knowledge of biologic features and natural history of specific malignancies postdiagnosis, is critical in surgery for cancer. Although general surgeons in some communities continue to perform the majority of cancer surgeries, in many settings, specialized surgeons focus only on surgical oncology. In academic centers, surgeons may specialize even further and limit their practice to certain tumor types. This specialization enables surgeons to stay current in the latest research and findings related to optimal care of specific malignancies. For example, in breast cancer, the distinctive properties of lobular carcinoma, infiltrating adenocarcinoma, and inflammatory breast cancer all require different surgical approaches to treatment. Understanding the proclivity of high-grade or aggressive cell types of tumors to proliferate more rapidly or metastasize more quickly may alter decisions regarding care. Comprehension of the concept of residual disease after primary surgical resection would lead to a referral to medical or radiation oncology for adjuvant therapy. Advances in the fields of molecular biology, genetics, and genomics have become pivotal to patient care for surgical oncologists and other providers. Knowledge of molecular prognostic indicators and predictors of disease outcomes is critical to guiding treatment decisions, including extent of surgery that might be indicated depending on biomarkers of disease and prognosis.[45]

### PATIENT CHARACTERISTICS

Although complete resection of the primary tumor for cure may be the optimal overall goal in surgical approaches, knowledge of the specific patient's medical and surgical history, prior therapies, and demographics is important in clinical decision making. Patients who have previously received radiation therapy to a tumor bed may not be candidates for surgical resection of a recurrence in the same area. Individuals with reduced pulmonary function may not be appropriate candidates for pneumonectomy but may be able to tolerate a lobectomy or wedge resection of a primary lung cancer if more conservative surgery is an alternative. Performance status and the presence of significant comorbidities, rather than chronologic age alone, are more important indicators of the ability to tolerate surgery and anesthesia. Metastatic workup and careful staging of the disease will help to determine appropriate therapeutic options.[46]

The preoperative workup should include the following elements: history and physical examination, concomitant medications, pathology of tumor (if available), staging of disease, evaluation of surgical and anesthesia tolerance, consultation by medical and/or radiation oncology as indicated, discussion of the need for preoperative or neoadjuvant therapy, documentation and communication of the goals of therapy, plans for immediate or delayed reconstruction, with consultation by plastic or reconstructive surgery, consultation with any other specialists who may need to be involved in surgery depending on the extent of resection (eg, urology in extensive colorectal or gynecologic surgeries), and plans for rehabilitation, if needed. A checklist or careful documentation in the patient's record will facilitate progression of the preoperative workup, ensure that no items are missed, and promote interdisciplinary communication and coordination of care.

### ENVIRONMENTAL FACTORS

Several environmental factors may affect the outcomes associated with the surgery: any specialized physician and nursing expertise available at the patient's selected place of care, the technology and surgical techniques to be used, the volume of cases performed by the institution and by the attending surgeon with the patient's specific tumor type/stage,[47] supportive care available (eg, hematopoietic growth factor use, antibiotics, transfusions, nutritional supplementation, and related interventions), and availability of specialized nursing care or specialty units such as critical care. Each of these environmental factors may have an effect on perioperative outcomes, from immediate postoperative morbidity and mortality to long-term rehabilitation and recovery of function.

## IMPACT OF NURSING CARE ON SURGICAL OUTCOMES

Outcomes in surgical oncology are often directly related to the quality of care provided by the entire team. Perioperative mortality may be due to wound infection, organ function (especially cardiac, pulmonary, and renal function), effects of anesthesia, anticipation and management of surgical complications, and effectiveness of patient self-care when discharged. Other outcomes may be related to postoperative changes in mobility, function, and quality of life.[48] Nursing care plays a critical role in affecting outcomes through careful assessment, intervention, and evaluation. Patient teaching, both preoperatively and postoperatively, is key to ensuring that patients and families understand anticipated procedures and effects and that desired outcomes are achieved.[49]

### SHORT-TERM OUTCOMES

*Short-term perioperative outcomes* may be defined as the events occurring preoperatively and within 30 days of surgery.[50] Serious complications that can occur during this period include life-threatening cardiac or pulmonary events, renal failure, shock, hemorrhage, infection, and the need for reoperation.[51] All patients in the postoperative setting—and cancer patients in particular—are at increased risk for thromboembolic events, including pulmonary embolism. High-risk patients, such as those with brain tumors, lung cancer, or a preexisting coagulation dysfunction, may benefit from additional interventions beyond standard antithrombolic mechanical approaches of ambulation or passive exercise. Guidelines published by the American Society for Clinical Oncology (ASCO) in 2007 recommend that patients undergoing major surgery for cancer should be considered as possible candidates for pharmacologic prophylaxis for thromboembolism, and the use of low-molecular-weight heparin (LMWH) was the preferred drug for both initial and continued treatment of patients with cancer who developed deep vein thrombosis (DVT). However, the guidelines caution that the impact of angicoagulants on long-term survival of cancer patients is not yet known.[52]

Preoperative history, staging workup, and documented comorbidities are key factors in developing a model for risk factors predicting operative mortality. Postoperative mortality for a surgical center has been associated with surgeon training, multidisciplinary care, volume of cases performed at the institution, and adherence to treatment guidelines.[53]

Surgical patients are subject to immune suppression, and cancer patients generally are already susceptible to immunosuppression as related to their disease. Nursing care in the perioperative period should be directed at assessing the causes of further depression of immune function and at facilitating approaches to boost the immune system.[54] Potential factors that may affect immune function include surgery, anesthesia, pain, opioid medications, temperature changes, blood transfusion, and physiologic and psychological stress. Although the underlying mechanism of these immune changes is not completely understood, interventions that may address immune changes include aggressive pain control, avoidance of unnecessary blood transfusions, selection of anesthetics and pain medications that may be less immunosuppressive, and conserving or limiting blood loss during extensive surgical resections.[55]

Data derived from multiple tumor types have indicated an inverse relationship between hospital volume for specific surgeries and certain outcomes and complications, including 30-day mortality.[56–59] Specialization by surgeons also has been shown to have an effect on outcomes (eg, postoperative mortality rates). Institutional volume of surgical cases and whether an institution is a teaching facility significantly affect patient survival from surgery. In a study of more than 13,000 patients with lung cancer resection, 30-day postoperative mortality rates were higher at nonteaching facilities than at teaching facilities (2.6% vs 1.1%; $P < .001$) and at low-volume centers than at high-volume centers (2.7% vs 1.6%; $P < .001$). Significant differences in mortality also were observed at 90 days postoperatively and after 5 years of follow-up.[60] Similar relationships between hospital surgical case volume and patient outcomes have been reported for head and neck cancers, breast cancer, sarcomas, and other tumors.[61] In contrast, hospital surgical volume was not shown to affect outcomes in a study of pediatric neuroblastoma and Wilms tumor. In this study, patient ethnicity, tumor stage, and use of chemotherapy were shown to be independent prognostic factors from multivariate analysis. The reasons for such differences between adult and pediatric models of cancer care are currently under investigation.[62]

### LONG-TERM OUTCOMES

Besides survival, other long-term outcomes, such as incontinence, dysphagia, or loss of mobility, as a result of surgery are important to note. Some surgically induced changes in function may recover after the immediate postoperative period, whereas other side effects may last for years or for the rest of the patient's life. Urinary incontinence and sexual impotence are two potential long-term outcomes associated with radical prostate cancer surgery, which even use of nerve-sparing surgical techniques may not prevent. Newer techniques, such as robotic-assisted laparascopic prostatectomies, have reported improved short- and long-term outcomes when compared with open radical retropubic prostatectomy, including decreased mortality, lower complications from blood loss, reduced rates of venous thrombosis, and improved patient comfort.[63] Nurses play pivotal roles in preoperative teaching and postoperative reinforcement of patient education and the need to help patients design effective strategies to address postoperative side effects.

Key long-term postoperative changes commonly occur with tumors of other sites, such as breast cancer. Lymphedema secondary to axillary lymph node dissection or more extensive surgical resection can result in loss of mobility and function in the affected arm. Although some improvement may be noted over time, often these postoperativel deficits are permanent. Other long-term outcomes associated with breast cancer and gynecologic surgery relate to reconstruction and changes in body image.[64] Even if the woman opts to undergo reconstruction immediately at the time of the surgical resection of the tumor, the reconstruction and adaptation process may take months before it is completed. Changes in body image related to surgery on the breasts or gynecologic organs can have a long-term impact on sexual functioning and self-image related to sexuality.[64]

## PREOPERATIVE TEACHING AND COUNSELING

A number of personnel may share responsibility for preoperative teaching, including surgeons, anesthesiologists, nurses, pain management teams, pharmacists, social workers, and house officers if the surgery will be performed in a teaching facility. The teaching may take place over several days or even weeks as the patient completes consultation with each specialist involved in the care. The volume of workup-related activities required to be accomplished prior to the scheduled surgery may allow only limited time for comprehensive and coordinated teaching or verification of patient understanding of the information provided. Reinforcing teaching guides and educational materials can allow patients to absorb the material at their own pace.

Preoperative teaching generally encompasses informed consent for the planned surgery, optional procedures that may be done at the time of the expected surgery, and need for blood transfusion; the type of anesthesia to be given and anticipated side effects; physical preparation for the planned surgery (eg, bowel prep); logistical information regarding the schedule of events; administration of regular medication during the perioperative period; laboratory or imaging studies required; insurance coverage; the plan for pain management; nutritional issues; and expected risks and benefits of the surgery. Patient teaching may be delivered verbally, through written pamphlets or forms, as a video, via interactive computer program, or through a combination of educational strategies. Most patients undergoing surgery for cancer want to be informed about the techniques planned and the expected short- and long-term outcomes associated with the surgery.[49] The timing of teaching may vary, although better comprehension and retention are reported when preoperative teaching takes place prior to admission for surgery.[65] Effective preoperative teaching also may serve to reduce postoperative pain and anxiety.[66]

When evaluating the effectiveness of preoperative patient teaching, the oncology nurse should be aware of the high level of anxiety commonly generated by impending hospital or day-surgery admission and surgical procedures. Individuals undergoing surgery for a known or suspected cancer diagnosis have the added burden of dealing with a potentially life-threatening disease. Consequently, comprehension and recall of teaching are often compromised.[67] Comprehension and recall may be affected by patient age, gender, educational level, stage of disease, and whether the cancer is newly diagnosed or recurrent. Patient preferences regarding the amount of information to be disclosed may vary from those desiring little or no information regarding risks, to those wanting to know of major risks, to individuals preferring to be told *all* possible risks.[68] Although individual preferences and anxiety levels should be assessed, critical and relevant information, including the potential risk of death, must be given to ensure that informed consent has been achieved.

## POSTOPERATIVE TEACHING AND COUNSELING

Knowing the purpose of the surgical intervention will help the nurse to determine the approach, content, and extent of postoperative teaching needed. It is important to know whether the surgery was performed to obtain a new diagnosis of cancer, resect with intent to cure, confirm recurrence of a previously diagnosed malignancy, or palliate the disease. The oncology nurse can tailor the information to provide education that supports the patient's and family's understanding of the goal of the surgery.

Helping patients and their families understand what to expect after an operation is critical as part of both preoperative and postoperative teaching. Often this information will need to be reinforced or modified if the extent of cancer or required surgical intervention is not known prior to surgery. Information related to pain management; wound care; restrictions on diet, exercise, or other activities; and signs and symptoms of complications in the immediate postoperative period must be explained in detail prior to discharge.

Cancer surgery, particularly for initial diagnosis, often will be performed on an outpatient basis, so limited time may be available for extensive patient teaching. In these cases, coordination between the outpatient surgery center nurses and the patient's surgeon or oncologist is imperative to ensure adequate dissemination of information. Even if the patient is admitted to the inpatient setting for more extensive surgery, the length of stay may be short and again will require careful coordination with outpatient services. A preoperative teaching checklist validating that information is given, and offering some assessment of the patient's level of understanding is helpful and may be shared among clinical sites where care is given. An example of a preoperative/postoperative patient teaching tool is provided in Figure 11-1.

Teaching patients and their families about long-term outcomes following surgery for cancer may require considerable time, repeated sessions, and the involvement of a multidisciplinary care team. For example, the relatively high incidence of urinary incontinence and sexual dysfunction following radical prostatectomy may entail postoperative teaching and intervention over an extended period of time.[69] Patients whose surgery resulted in the formation of an ostomy usually will benefit from teaching by enterostomal therapists and other specialists to help them learn to care for their ostomy, obtain and apply the needed medical devices and supplies, have nutritional counseling, and receive advice regarding potential effects of the surgery on sexuality and body image.[70]

## REHABILITATION

The need for and degree of rehabilitation following cancer surgery will depend on multiple factors: (1) the extent of surgery performed and organ preservation achieved, (2) the age and performance status of the individual, (3) comorbid conditions, (4) the patient's physical activity/mobility level prior to surgery, (5) additional treatment (eg, chemotherapy and/or radiation) given prior to or following surgery, and (6) the overall goals of therapy. Rehabilitation required for cancer surgery designed with curative intent may vary significantly from rehabilitation for surgery performed for palliation or symptom relief.

Individuals undergoing head and neck surgery may require consultation and services from specialists in fields including swallowing, audiology, speech pathology, nutrition, and plastic surgery. The amount and type of rehabilitative care required are determined by the functional abilities retained after surgery. It is important to note that more complete rehabilitation to an enhanced functional status usually translates into improved quality of life for the patient.[71] Complete discussion of tumor-specific surgeries and rehabilitation can be found in site-specific chapters throughout this book.

**Preoperative Assessment of Patient Teaching**

- □ Consultations completed
  - □ Primary surgeon
  - □ Anesthesia
  - □ Reconstruction
  - □ Other surgical subspecialty
- □ Lab work ordered and results checked
  - □ CBC
  - □ Chemistry
  - □ Anticoagulant studies
  - □ Preoperative tumor markers (CEA, CA-125, etc.)
  - □ Type and cross-match
  - □ Other
- □ Imaging studies completed
  - □ CXR, CT scan, PET
  - □ Staging studies
  - □ Tumor localization
  - □ Other ________
- □ Pathology report
  - □ Biopsy report available and reviewed
  - □ Outside consultation on slides reviewed
- □ Patient teaching
  - □ Schedule for OR, time for arrival, parking and transportation
  - □ Preoperative preparation
  - □ Medications day/night before
  - □ Medications day of surgery
  - □ Family location to wait
  - □ Contact numbers for waiting area, recovery room, ICU or patient floor
  - □ Instructions re: valuables, clothes
  - □ Review of surgery planned
  - □ Surgical consent signed and on chart
  - □ Transfusion consent signed and on chart
  - □ Other pertinent consent forms signed
  - □ Review of immediate postoperative period
  - □ Discussion of pain management
  - □ Discussion of postanesthesia management

**Postoperative Assessment of Patient Teaching**

- □ Review of findings from surgery
- □ Consultations ordered postsurgery
- □ Review of pathology
- □ Diagnosis and/or stage of disease
- □ Treatment planning
- □ Pulmonary exercises
- □ Discharge instructions:
  - □ Exercise
  - □ Nutrition
  - □ Sexual activity
  - □ Return for postoperative appointment set: ________
  - □ Signs and symptoms to watch for and report

**FIGURE 11-1**

Preoperative and postoperative patient teaching tool.

## TRENDS IN SURGICAL ONCOLOGY

Advances in oncology care and understanding of cancer biology and therapeutic implications have resulted in important developments in surgery as well as in such associated modalities as medical oncology, radiation, biotherapy, and targeted and small-molecule therapies. Recent advances in surgical oncology include a focus on organ preservation, use of neoadjuvant therapy, and expansion of the role of sentinel node mapping as a staging and prognostic tool. In addition, cancer surgery is taking on a new role of contributing to predictive markers of response to other therapies and prognostic indicators of patient outcome through accessing tissue and tumor samples used in oncogenomic analyses.

## ORGAN PRESERVATION

In the case of extensive primary disease, the use of neoadjuvant chemotherapy or radiation prior to surgery may allow for surgical resection with adequate margins along with preservation of function or improved cosmesis. Organ preservation is important in most cancers, but particularly in patients for whom retention of most of the organ tissue is critical for either function or cosmetic appearance. Such cases include cancers of the anus, rectum, or bladder; sarcomas, especially of the extremities; breast cancer; and head and neck cancers. Other types of tumors, such as lung or colon, are being investigated for their increased resectability when neoadjuvant therapy is delivered prior to surgery. Both chemotherapy and radiation, either alone or in combination, have been used in the neoadjuvant setting, reflecting their important roles in organ preservation. Hyperfractionation, or the delivery of more than one fraction of radiation per day, allows higher radiation doses to be given to tumors while sparing normal tissues. The accelerated radiation fractionation regimen also addresses the heightened malignant cell proliferation that occurs during treatment.[72] Higher doses of radiation with little increase in associated toxicity also can be achieved using three-dimensional conformal and intensity-modulated radiation therapy.[73] Novel biologic and targeted therapies, such as monoclonal antibodies, antiangiogenesis, gene therapy, vaccines, signal-transduction inhibitors, antisense technology, and small molecules, have sought to exploit advances in cancer biology. These new therapies could play a role in organ preservation because they have the potential to control or impede malignant growth.

The principles of organ preservation rely on multimodality therapy to achieve maximum shrinkage of the tumor prior to surgery (neoadjuvant) so as to render the tumor resectable while retaining organ function and possibly appearance. Response of the tumor to induction chemotherapy demonstrates its chemosensitivity and may correlate with clinical outcomes.[74] Patients may experience a complete pathologic response to neoadjuvant therapy. A less favorable response or complete lack of response indicates a poorer prognosis and the need for more radical surgery. Pathologic assessment of tumor response is also an important component in treatment planning for organ preservation. A pathologic response reflects sensitivity to the induction therapy and allows for more conservative surgery. Nevertheless, complete resection of the tumor while preserving as much organ as possible and potentially adjuvant therapy are indicated to promote long-term outcomes.

## NEOADJUVANT THERAPY

Chemotherapy for solid tumors given preoperatively (termed *neoadjuvant*) has been reported to produce significant improvements in clinical response rates as well as enhance the ability to perform organ-preserving therapy. Originally intended for large and/or locally advanced tumors, neoadjuvant therapy is increasingly being used to reduce the size of the primary tumor as part of an effort to achieve good cosmesis or improved function in organ conservation.

Adjuvant therapy in breast cancer has been used extensively for almost three decades and has demonstrated improved outcomes, including reduction in risk of recurrence and increased survival, in nearly all subsets of patients.[75] The use of neoadjuvant therapy also has shown the ability to increase clinical response rates as well as to achieve breast conservation.[76] Other advantages of neoadjuvant therapy include its use to demonstrate chemosensitivity in the presence of clinical, often measurable disease, as well as its role in allowing the analysis of biomarkers as potential predictors of response.[77] Although the prognostic significance of pathologically complete remission remains to be completely elucidated, the ability to resect tumors that otherwise would be unresectable or require much more extensive surgery generally is viewed as having a positive impact on patient outcomes and health-related quality of life.[78]

## SENTINEL NODE BIOPSY AND MAPPING

The use of sentinel lymph node (SLN) biopsy and mapping in breast cancer and many other tumors has gained considerable support. SLN biopsy is already considered the standard of care for melanoma and breast cancer in many centers with practitioners experienced in these techniques.[79] The ability to assess lymph node involvement while avoiding potential additional comorbidities associated with axillary lymph node dissection (ALND) is the major advantage of SLN mapping. The primary indication for using SLN techniques involves palpable and nonpalpable T1 and T2 tumors, with limited data supporting SLN application for other stages of disease.

SLN mapping has been associated with less morbidity compared with complete axillary node dissection in patients with primary breast cancer.[80,81] Although the specifics of procedures for lymphatic mapping, case selection, surgical techniques, pathologic analysis, definition and identification of micrometastatic disease, and related outcomes often vary by center or sometimes by practitioner, overall findings reported are similar. Experience is a prerequisite for accurate mapping, whether radioguided, blue dye, or other techniques are used. More recently, PET and FDG-PET scanning have been explored to identify SLNs and to stage cancers. In colon cancer, lymph node staging is important both for the number of lymph nodes evaluated and SLN biopsy.[82,83] Although randomized trials evaluating SLN biopsy have not yet been published in most tumor types, some groups have developed clinical practice guidelines based on currently available evidence.[84–86]

Current clinical trials, being conducted through the National Surgical Adjuvant Breast and Bowel Project (NSABP), the British Association of Surgical Oncology (BASO), the European Organization for Research and Treatment of Cancer (EORTC), and the American College of Surgeons Oncology Group (ACOSOG), are investigating associated outcomes, including survival, of both SLN-negative and SLN-positive patients who do not undergo further axillary dissection. The prognostic importance of micrometastases in lymph nodes, as well as the clinical meaningfulness of micrometastatic disease in the bone marrow at the time of diagnosis, are not known.[87,88]

## SPECIAL CONSIDERATIONS FOR NURSING CARE

### OLDER PATIENTS AND SURGICAL THERAPY

More than half of all cancers and cancer deaths occur in elderly individuals (age ≥ 65 years). The increased incidence of cancer with aging may be due to long-term accumulation of cellular and DNA mutations, heightened susceptibility of aging tissues to carcinogens, and the systemic effects of aging, including immune senescence and changes in cytokine production.[89]

An early study reporting differences in therapeutic outcomes (eg, survival) in older patients focused on age and often ignored variations in care delivery.[90] Unfortunately, clinical decision making tends to be based on chronologic age as a major criterion; however, no published data support the use of age alone as the primary means to determine contraindications to chemotherapy or optimal cancer care.[91] Lack of access to care or inadequate intensity or quality of care delivered to older patients seems to account for differences in outcomes, including survival, of older patients compared with younger cohorts.[92] Currently, no evidence exists to withhold chemotherapy or standard treatment based solely on age except in cases when the cancer is very slow growing and the individual is elderly, such as men over 75 years of age diagnosed with early-stage prostate cancer.[93] For the most part, effective therapy following standards of care can be given to elderly patients, and the outcomes and toxicities are the same as for younger patients for multiple tumor types. The use of a geriatric assessment tool can help to identify individual patients who may be too frail to tolerate standard therapy, as well as distinguish older patients with good functional status who are excellent candidates for the more intensive therapy that might be recommended for their cancer.[94]

The National Comprehensive Cancer Center Network (NCCN) formed a Breast Cancer in the Older Woman Task Force to begin to address questions about treating older women with early-stage, locally advanced, and metastatic breast cancer. This multidisciplinary group developed specific interventions and recommendations for older women with breast cancer and also identified issues requiring further investigations before recommendations could be made.[95]

More than half of all lung cancers are found in patients aged 65 years or older, yet surgical resection is performed less often in older patients than in younger individuals with NSCLC.[96] Clinical decisions to avoid surgery in such patients are often based on chronologic age rather than documented risk factors. Progress in preoperative risk assessment and surgical approaches has greatly reduced morbidity and mortality associated with lung cancer surgery in older patients.

In contrast, prostate cancer diagnosed at an early stage in elderly men, particularly those over age 75 years, who are asymptomatic with slow-growing tumors may benefit from an expectant management or medical monitoring approach rather than radical prostatectomy.[97] Treatment options, including observation, should be reviewed in the context of the biologic characteristics of the tumor and associated risk:benefit ratio, comorbidities, expected life span, and desired quality as well as quantity of life.[98]

### ONCOLOGIC EMERGENCIES

Most conditions that are classified as oncologic emergencies require immediate medical intervention. However, certain structural changes may call for emergency surgical intervention, such as spinal cord compression or increased intracranial pressure from brain tumors or brain metastases, spontaneous pneumothorax in chemosensitive tumors such as sarcoma,[99] malignant pleural effusion in lung cancer, intestinal obstruction in colon cancer, and obstructive uropathy in bladder cancer.[100] Careful assessment and rapid decision making with appropriate referral for surgical intervention or other modalities (eg, radiation therapy) are needed to relieve these life-threatening conditions and maintain optimal quality of life.[101] Nurses and other members of the healthcare team need to remember that oncologic emergencies can occur in patients who have no prior diagnosis of cancer, and the index of suspicion may be low in an individual without a known malignancy. Up to 15% of colorectal cancers may have an initial presentation as obstructive or perforated tumors, requiring emergency surgery.

Hartmann's procedure can be used to achieve a potentially curable resection even when performed as an emergency operation. A retrospective review of 50 patients who underwent emergency Hartmann's operation for obstructive or perforated left-sided colorectal cancer found an operative mortality rate of 8% and a morbidity rate of 26%.[102]

Malignant spinal cord compression is an oncologic emergency that can result in complete paralysis if not identified early with appropriate interventions performed. Similarly, superior vena cava obstruction represents a serious oncologic situation requiring rapid diagnosis and intervention. In both conditions, surgical intervention, as well as medical or radiation therapies, may be recommended. Presenting symptoms may be vague and related to numerous other conditions besides cancer. Nurses caring for patients at risk for these and other oncologic emergencies should be able to identify early signs and symptoms of these conditions and be able to conduct a thorough assessment of the patient's history and symptoms to facilitate diagnosis and prompt treatment.[103]

Patients also may be at risk for oncologic emergencies as a result of recent surgery. Such risks include life-threatening infection, hemorrhage, postoperative complications, or multiple-organ failure. Surgical nursing care in the immediate postoperative period, as well as postoperative follow-up and surveillance, should focus on assessing wound healing and function of other organ systems, management of surgical deficits or physical changes, monitoring of laboratory results, and knowledge of clinical syndromes that might be associated with the specific tumor type under treatment.[102] If an emergency event does occur in the perioperative period or the patient's condition requires unexpected surgical intervention for resolution, nurses play a pivotal role in educating patients and family members about planned procedures and in reducing anxiety associated with urgent situations.

## PERIOPERATIVE BLOOD TRANSFUSION

The need for allogeneic blood transfusion is a known risk associated with surgical procedures. The risk of requiring transfusion of red blood cells, platelets, or other blood products varies with the diagnosis, stage of disease, extent and type of surgical procedure planned, and decision to perform immediate reconstruction. Transfusion rates may be very low in some cases involving solid tumors (eg, early-stage breast cancer undergoing breast conservation) or extremely high in other procedures and tumor sites (eg, liver resection).[104] Immunosuppression associated with allogeneic transfusion, in addition to the presumed immunosuppression due to the cancer itself, is thought to be the underlying etiology for poorer outcomes reported among patients who received blood transfusion along with surgery for their cancer diagnosis. Numerous studies, including randomized trials, have reported varying results over several decades. Allogeneic blood transfusion given perioperatively for multiple tumor types has been implicated as a factor leading to important outcomes such as increased rates of postoperative infection and reduced relapse-free survival and overall survival. However, recent studies, for example, in prostate cancer, have not been associated with disease recurrence when blood transfusions were given in the perioperative period.[105] Numerous factors have been investigated to determine a possible link between perioperative blood transfusion and postoperative outcomes, including blood storage and cytokine release causing a postoperative immune or inflammatory response. Although the underlying etiology of these outcomes reported with allogeneic perioperative blood transfusion is not known, the best strategy to date seems to be blood conservation and limitation of unnecessary transfusions.[106,107]

Considerable evidence has been gathered regarding the risk of postoperative infection associated with perioperative allogeneic blood transfusion. A meta-analysis involving more than 13,000 patients who underwent surgery found that the incidence of postoperative bacterial infection associated with allogeneic blood transfusion was 3.45 (odds ratio; range 1.43–15.15).[108] Risk of infection also was increased significantly in trauma patients (odds ratio 5.263; range 5.03–5.43). Thus allogeneic blood transfusion represents a significant yet often overlooked risk factor associated with higher rates of bacterial infection postoperatively.

Nurses may play an important role in assessing risk factors prior to surgery, including anemia. Low preoperative hematocrit and low postoperative hematocrit, as well as increased blood transfusion rates, have been associated with increased mortality, increased rates of postoperative pneumonia, and increased hospital length of stay.[109,110]

## ANXIETY AND PAIN CONTROL

As with any surgical procedure, patients should be assessed carefully for pain already present prior to surgery, approaches used to control pain, effectiveness of those pain-control measures, and any adverse events associated with pain control currently in use or previously experienced. An appreciation of sources of chronic pain, in addition to the anticipated acute postoperative pain, should be part of the plan for pain control postoperatively. For major surgical procedures, a pain management team, if part of the institutional program, should be consulted preoperatively. Plans for immediate postoperative as well as postdischarge pain control should be developed and discussed with the attending physician, patient, and other members of the healthcare team.[111]

## NUTRITIONAL SUPPORT

Most types of surgery affect nutritional status to some degree, even if that impact consists of only dietary restrictions for a limited time prior to surgery. However, surgeries with known effects on patients' long-term nutrition require significant interventions before and after scheduled surgery to ensure adequate nutritional intake and to minimize any negative influence on quality of life and overall postoperative recovery. Such surgeries include radical procedures performed for pancreatic, gastric, head and neck, and colorectal cancers. In addition, surgical complications, such as infection, may increase the nutritional needs of the patient. In all these cases, consultation with appropriate nutritional support services, if available, or generation of a thoughtful plan of care prior to surgery is imperative to promote surgical healing and ensure a rapid return to preoperative quality of life.[112]

### RISK ASSESSMENT AND SURVEILLANCE AFTER SURGERY

Individuals considered at high-risk for malignancy due to a family history of the disease or other risk factors, including pathologic evidence of precancerous lesions, may be followed by surgical oncologists or other specialists for risk assessment and surveillance. Individuals in a high-risk classification may benefit from genetic counseling, participation in regular screening programs, incorporating lifestyle changes, or taking chemopreventive agents to reduce known risks of cancer. They also may need to periodically undergo biopsy or invasive tests if high-risk lesions are identified. High-risk assessment and surveillance may focus on multiple types of cancers, including breast, colorectal, pancreatic, skin, melanoma, oropharyngeal, cervical, ovarian, and lung cancer.

At completion of cancer therapy—whether surgery, chemotherapy, radiation, or combined-modality treatment—patients who are considered to be cured or in long-term remission require oversight of their subsequent care. Often, surveillance after therapy is provided by the surgeon, who may obtain periodic screening tests, biomarkers, or imaging studies, as well as perform physical examinations, to evaluate for recurrence of disease or a new primary tumor.[113] The nurse in this setting may be responsible for scheduling tests according to known patterns or recurrence or metastases, assessing patients for signs of recurrence or need for further symptom management, teaching patients and families about rehabilitative needs or adaptation after treatment, and addressing psychosocial issues related to quality of life, changes in role and functions due to the cancer or its treatment, and dealing with cancer as a chronic illness. The importance of complying with surveillance after therapy and of reporting any new physical findings to the physician or nurse should be stressed to both patients and their caregivers. A follow-up plan for patients being referred back to a primary care provider will facilitate appropriate surveillance after cancer surgery or other therapy.

## CONCLUSION

Surgery remains the cornerstone of oncology care, serving as an essential component for prevention, diagnosis, staging, therapy, and palliation of disease. Advances in surgical oncology have promoted significant improvements in organ preservation, minimally invasive approaches to surgical care, rehabilitation, and multimodality treatment planning. Nursing care affects both short- and long-term surgical outcomes in oncology by playing a critical role in perioperative assessment, teaching, symptom management, and posttreatment surveillance.

## REFERENCES


1. Scott EA (ed.). *Surgery in America: From the Colonial Era to the Twentieth Century, Selected Writings.* Philadelphia, PA: WB Saunders; 1965.
2. American Cancer Society. *Cancer Facts and Figures—2008.* Atlanta, GA: American Cancer Society; 2008.
3. Walterhouse D, Watson A. Optimal management strategies for rhabdomyosarcoma in children. *Paediatr Drugs.* 2007;9:391–400.
4. Naredi P, Leidenius M, Hocevar M, et al. Recommended core curriculum for the specialist traning in surgical oncology within Europe. *Surg Oncol.* 2008;17:277–279.
5. Ren S, Liu S, Howell P Jr, et al. The impact of genomics in understanding human melanoma progression and metastasis. *Cancer Control.* 2008;15:202–215.
6. Oseni T, Jatoi I. An overview of the role of prophylactic surgery in the management of individuals with a hereditary cancer predisposition. *Surg Clin North Am.* 2008;88:739–758.
7. Lynch HT, Silva E, Wirtzfeld D, et al. Hereditary diffuse gastric cancer: prophylactic surgical oncology implications. *Surg Clin North Am.* 2008;88:759–778.
8. Cetta F, Dhamo A. Inherited multitumoral syndromes including colorectal carcinomas. *Surg Oncol.* 2007;16:S17-S23.
9. Dionigi G, Bianchi V, Rovera F, et al. Genetic alterations in hereditary colorectal cancer. *Surg Oncol.* 2007;16:S11-S15.
10. Odze RD. Update on the diagnosis and treatment of Barrett esophagus and related neoplastic precursor lesions. *Arch Pathol Lab Med.* 2008;132:1577–1585.
11. Edlich RF, Cross CL, Wack CA, et al. Breast cancer and ovarian cancer genetics: an update. *J Environ Pathol Toxicol Oncol.* 2008;27:245–256.
12. Tutt A, Ashworth A. Can genetic testing guide treatment in breast cancer? *Eur J Cancer.* 2008;44:2774–2780.
13 Tuttle T, Habermann E, Abraham A, et al. Contralateral prophylactic mastecomy for patients with unilateral breast cancer. *Expert Rev Anticancer Ther.* 2007;7:1117–1122.
14. Wong RJ. Current status of FDG-PET for head and neck cancer. *J Surg Oncol.* 2008;97:649–652.
15. Bui MM, Smith P, Agresta SV, et al. Practical issues of intraoperative frozen section diagnosis of bone and soft tissue lesions. *Cancer Control.* 2008;15:7–12.
16. Barone JE. Pancreaticduodenectomy for presumed pancreatic cancer. *Surg Oncol.* 2008;17:139–144.
17. Patel SG, Lydiatt WM. Staging of head and neck cancers: is it time to change the balance between the ideal and the practical? *J Surg Oncol.* 2008;97:653–657.
18. Mutch MG. Molecular profiling and risk stratification of adenocarcinoma of the colon. *J Surg Oncol.* 2007;96:693–703.
19. Amersi F, Morton DL. The role of sentinel lymph node biopsy in the management of melanoma. *Adv Surg.* 2007;41:241–256.

20. Lang JE, Hall CS, Singh B, Lucci A. Significance of micrometastsis in bone marrow and blood of operable breast cancer patients: research tool or clinical application? *Exp Rev Anticancer Ther.* 2007;7:1463–1472.
21. Abu-Rustum NR, Khoury-Collado F, Gemignani ML. Techniques of sentinel lymph node identification for early-stage cervical and uterine cancer. *Gynecol Oncol.* 2008;111:S44–S50.
22. Hewett PJ, Allardyce RA, Bagshaw PF, et al. Short-term outcomes of the Australasian randomized clinical study comparing laparascopic and conventional open surgical treatments for colon cancer: the ALCCaS. *Ann Surg.* 2008;248:728–738.
23. Eggermont AM, Voit C. Management of melanoma: a European perspective. *Surg Oncol Clin North Am.* 2008;17:635–648.
24. Wasserberg N, Gutman H. Resection margins in modern rectal cancer surgery. *J Surg Oncol.* 2008;98:611–615.
25. Molina JR, Yang P, Cassivi SD, et al. Non-small cell lung cancer: epidemiology, risk factors, treatment, and survivorship. *Mayo Clin Proc.* 2008;83:584–594.
26. Bristow RE, Puri I, Chi DS. Cytoreductive surgery for recurrent ovarian cancer: a meta-analysis. *Gynecol Oncol.* 2009;112:265–274.
27. Verghese M, Pathak S, Poston GJ. Increasing long-term survival in advanced colorectal cancer. *Eur J Surg Oncol.* 2007;33:S1–S4.
28. Katz M, Vauthey JN. Potentially curable metastatic colorectal cancer. *Curr Oncol Rep.* 2008;10:225–231.
29. Gleisner AL, Choti MA, Assumpcao L, et al. Colorectal liver metastases: recurrence and survival following hepatic resection, radiofrequency ablation, and combined resection-radiofrequency ablation. *Arch Surg.* 2008;143:1204–1212.
30. Biswas G, Bhagwat R, Khurana R, et al. Brain metastasis: evidence-based management. *J Cancer Res Ther.* 2006;2:5–13.
31. Gilbert RW. Innovation in the surgical management of head and neck tumors. *Hematol Oncol Clin North Am.* 2008;22:1181–1191, viii-ix.
32. Garwood ER, Moore D, Ewing C, et al. Total skin-sparing mastectomy: complications and local recurrence rates in two cohorts of patients. *Ann Surg.* 2009;249:26–32.
33. Chung AP, Sacchini V. Nipple-sparing mastectomy: where are we now? *Surg Oncol.* 2008;17:261–266.
34. Almasad JK. Breast reconstruction in conserving breast cancer surgery. *Saudi Med J.* 2008;29:1548–1553.
35. Cordeiro PG. Frontiers in free flap reconstruction in the head and neck. *J Surg Oncol.* 2008;97:669–73.
36. Barker EV, Enepekides DJ. The utility of microvascular anastomotic devices in head and neck reconstruction. *Curr Opin Otolaryngol Head Neck Surg.* 2008;16:331–334.
37. van der Eerden PA, Lohuis PJ, Hart AA, et al. Secondary intention healing after excision of nonmelanoma skin cancer of the head and neck: statistical evaluation of prognostic values of wound characteristics and final cosmetic results. *Plast Reconstr Surg.* 2008;122:1747–1755.
38. Beunis A, Pauli S, Van Cleemput M. Anastomotic leakage of a colorectal anastomosis treated by transanal endoscopic microsurgery. *Acta Chir Belg.* 2008;108:474–476.
39. Selvindos PB, Ho YH. Multimedia article: Laparascopic ultralow anterior resectin with colonic J-pouch-anal anastomosis. *Dis Colon Rectum.* 2008;51:1710–1711.
40. Berger A, Aron M. Laparoscopic radical cystectomy: long-term outcomes. *Curr Opin Urol.* 2008;18:167–172.
41. Maffezzini M, Campodonico F, Canepa G, et al. Current perioperative management of radical cystectomy with intestinal urinary reconstruction for muscle-invasive bladder cancer and reduction of the incidence of postoperative ileus. *Surg Oncol.* 2008;17:41–48.
42. Long HJ III, Laack NN, Gostout BS. Prevention, diagnosis, and treatment of cervical cancer. *Mayo Clinic Proc.* 2007;82:1566–1574.
43. Gallieni M, Pittiruti M, Biffi R. Vascular access in oncology patients. *CA Cancer J Clin.* 2008;58:323–346.
44. Mick J. Factors affecting the evolution of oncology nursing care. *Clin J Oncol Nurs.* 2008;12:307–313.
45. Nordberg ML. Molecular pathology—translating research into clinical practice: an expanding frontier in surgical oncology. *Surg Oncol Clin North Am.* 2008;17:303–321.
46. Liombaet-Cussac A. Improving decision-making in early breast cancer: who to treat and how. *Breast Cancer Res Treat.* 2008;112:15–24.
47. du Bois A, Rochon J, Pfisterer J, Hoskins WJ. Variations in institutional infrastructure, physician specialization and experience, and outcome in ovarian cancer: a systematic review. *Gynecol Oncol.* 2009;112:422–436.
48. Michaelson MD, Cotter SE, Gargollo PC, et al. Management of complications of prostate cancer treatment. *CA Cancer J Clin.* 2008;58:196–213.
49. Barlesi F, Barrau K, Loundou A, et al. Impact of information on quality of life and satisfaction of non-small cell lung cancer patients: a randomized study of standardized versus individualized information before thoracic surgery. *J Thorac Oncol.* 2008;3:1146–1152.
50. Chiva LM, Lapuente F, Gonzalez-Cortijo L, et al. Surgical treatment of recurrent cervical cancer: state of the art and new achievements. *Gynecol Oncol.* 2008;110:S60-S66.
51. Nagai K, Yoshida J, Nishimura M. Postoperative mortality in lung cancer patients. *Am Thorac Cardiovasc Surg.* 2007;13:373–377.
52. Lyman GH, Khorana AA, Falanga A, et al. American Society of Clinical Oncology guideline: recommendations for venous thromboembolism prophylaxis and treatment in patients with cancer. *J Clin Oncol.* 2007;25:5490–5505.
53. Tekkis PP, Poloniecki JD, Thompson MR, Stamatakis JD. Operative mortality in colorectal cancer: prospective national study. *BMJ.* 2003;327:1196–1201.
54. Dionigi G, Rovera F, Boni L, et al. The impact of perioperative blood transfusion on clinical outcomes in colorectal surgery. *Surg Oncol.* 2007;16:S177-S182.
55. Szakmany T, Dodd M, Dempsey GA, et al. The influence of allogenic blood transfusion in patients having free-flap primary surgery for oral and oropharyngeal squamous cell carcinoma. *Br J Cancer.* 2006;94:647–653.
56. Zingmond D, Maggard M, O'Connell J, et al. What predicts serious complications in colorectal cancer resection? *Am Surg.* 2003;69:969–974.
57. Panageas KS, Schrag D, Riedel E, et al. The effect of clustering of outcomes on the association of procedure volume and surgical outcomes. *Ann Intern Med.* 2003;139:658–665.
58. Gutierrez JC, Perez EA, Moffat FL, et al. Should soft tissue sarcomas be treated at high volume centers? An analysis of 4205 patients. *Ann Surg.* 2007;245:952–958.
59. Cheung MD, Koniaris LG, Perez EA, et al. Impact of hospital volume on surgical outcomes for head and neck cancers. *Ann Surg Oncol.* Nov. 4, 2008 [Epub ahead of print].
60. Cheung MC, Hamilton K, Sherman R, et al. Impact of teaching facility status and high-volume centers on outcomes for lung cancer resection: an examination of 13,469 patients. *Ann Surg Oncol.* 2009;16:3–13.
61. Simunovic M, Rempel E, Theriault ME, et al. Influence of hospital characteristics on operative death and survival of patients after major cancer surgery in Ontario. *Can J Surg.* 2006;49:251–258.
62. Gutierrez JC, Koniaris LG, Cheung MC, et al. Cancer care in the pediatric surgical patient: a paradigm to abolish volume-outcome disparities in surgery. *Surgery.* 2009;145:76–85.
63. Box GN, Ahlering TE. Robotic radical prostatectomy: long-term outcomes. *Curr Opin Urol.* 2008;18:173–179.
64. Stany MP, Farley JH. Complications of gynecologic surgery. *Surg Clin North Am.* 2008;88:343–359.
65.Collins ED, Moore CP, Clay KF, et al. Can women with early-stage breast cancer make an informed decision for mastectomy? *J Clin Oncol.* 2009;27:519–525.
66. Sjoling M, Nordahl G, Olofsson N, et al. The impact of preoperative information on state anxiety, postoperative pain and satisfaction with pain management. *Patient Educ Couns.* 2003;51:169–176.
67. Spittler CA. Breast reconstruction using tissue expanders: assessing patients' needs utilizing a holistic approach. *Plast Surg Nurs.* 2008;28:27–32.

68. Dodge-Palomba S. Providing compassionate care to the pediatric patient undergoing enucleation of the eye. *Insight*. 2008;33:10–12.
69. Milne JL, Spiers JA, Moore KN. Men's experience following laparascopic radical prostatectomy: a qualitative descriptive study. *Int J Nurs Stud*. 2008;45:765–774.
70. Shaaban AA, Mosbah A, El-Bahnasawy MS, et al. The urethral Kock pouch: long-term functional and oncological results in men. *BJU Int*. 2003;92:429–435.
71. Dequanter D, Lothaire P. The role of salvage surgery in organ preservation strategies in advanced head and neck cancer. *B-ENT*. 2008;4:77–80.
72. Wickerham DL, O'Connell MJ, Costantino JP, et al. The half century of clinical trials of the National Surgical Adjuvant Breast and Bowel Project. *Semin Oncol*. 2008;35:522–529.
73. Holsinger FC. Swing of the pendulum: optimizing functional outcomes in larynx cancer. *Curr Oncol Rep*. 2008;10:170–175.
74. Scher RL, Esclamado RM. Organ and function preservation: the role of surgery as the optimal primary modality or as salvage after chemoradiation failure. *Semin Radiat Oncol*. 2009;19:17–23.
75. Herold CI, Marcom PK. Primary systemic therapy in breast cancer: past lessons and new approaches. *Cancer Invest*. 2008;26:1052–1059.
76. Garcia-Mata J, Garcia-Paloma A, Calvo L, et al. Phase II study of dose-dense doxorubicin and docetaxel as neoadjuvant chemotherapy with G-CSF support in patients with large or locally advanced breast cancer. *Clin Transl Oncol*. 2008;10:739–744.
77. Tieu BH, Sanborn RE, Thomas CR Jr. Neoadjuvant therapy for resectable non-small cell lung cancer with mediastinal lymph node. *Thorac Surg Clin*. 2008;18:403–415.
78. Wang LB, Shen JG, Xu CY, et al. Neoadjuvant chemotherapy versus surgery alone for locally advanced gastric cancer: a retrospective comparative study. *Hepatogastroenterology*. 2008;55:1895–1898.
79. Faries MB, Morton DL. Surgery and sentinel lymph node biopsy. *Semin Oncol*. 2007;34:498–508.
80. Sclafani LM, Baron RH. Sentinel lymph node biopsy and axillary dissection: added morbidity of the arm, shoulder and chest wall after mastectomy and reconstruction. *Cancer J*. 2008;14:216–222.
81. Olson JA Jr, McCall LM, Beitsch P, et al. Impact of immediate versus delayed axillary node dissection on surgical outcomes in breast cancer patients with positive sentinel nodes: results from American College of Surgeons Oncology Group Trials Z0010 and Z0011. *J Clin Oncol*. 2008;26:3530–3535.
82. Iddings D, Bilchik A. The biologic significance of micrometastatic disease and sentinel lymph node technology on colorectal cancer. *J Surg Oncol*. 2007;96:671–677.
83. Ozmen MM, Ozmen F, Zulfikaroglu B. Lymph nodes in gastric cancer. *J Surg Oncol*. 2008;98:476–481.
84. Lango MN, Myers JN, Garden AS. Controversies in surgical management of the node-positive neck after chemoradiation. *Semin Radiat Oncol*. 2009;19:24–28.
85. Scolyer RA, Murali R, Satzger I, Thompson JF. The detection and significance of melanoma micrometastases in sentinel nodes. *Surg Oncol*. 2008;17:165–174.
86. Grabau D. Breast cancer patients with micrometastases only: is a basis provided for tailored treatment? *Surg Oncol*. 2008;17:211–217.
87. Robbins KT, Shaha AR, Medina JE, et al. Consensus statement on the classification and terminology of neck dissection. *Arch Otolaryngol Head Neck Surg*. 2008;134:536–538.
88. Athanassiadou P, Grapsa D. Bone marrow micrometastases in different solid tumors: pathogenesis and importance. *Surg Oncol*. 2008;17:153–164.
89. Tew WP, Lichtman SM. Ovarian cancer in older women. *Semin Oncol*. 2008;35:582–589.
90. Carlson RW, Moench S, Hurria A, et al. NCCN Task Force report: breast cancer in the older woman. *J Natl Compre Cancer Network*. 2008;6:S1-S25.
91. Marenco D, Marinello R, Berruti A, et al. Multidimensional geriatric assessment in treatment decision in elderly cancer patients: 6-year experience in an outpatient geriatric oncology service. *Crit Rev Oncol Hematol*. 2008;68:157–164.
92. Hurria A, Wong FL, Villaluna D, et al. Role of age and health in treatment recommendations for older adults with breast cancer: the perspective of oncologists and primary care providers. *J Clin Oncol*. 2008;26:5386–5392.
93. Terret C, Zulian GB, Naiem A, Albrand G. Multidisciplinary approach to the geriatric oncology patient. *J Clin Oncol*. 2007;25:1876–1881.
94. Pasetto LM, Lise M, Monfardini S. Preoperative assessment of elderly cancer patients. *Crit Rev Oncol Hematol*. 2007;64:10–18.
95. Carlson RW, Moench S, Hurria A, et al. NCCN Task Force report: breast cancer in the older woman. *J Natl Compr Cancer Netw*. 2008;6:S1-S25.
96. Zeber JE, Copeland LA, Hosek BJ, et al. Cancer rates, medical comorbidities, and treatment modalities in the oldest patients. *Crit Rev Oncol Hematol*. 2008;67:237–242.
97. Marberger M, Carroll PR, Zelefsky MJ, et al. New treatments for localized prostate cancer. *Urology*. 2008;72:S36-S43.
98. Wedding U, Pientka L, Höffken K. Quality-of-life in elderly patients with cancer: a short review. *Eur J Cancer*. 2007;43:2203–2210.
99. Adegboye VO, Ogunseyinde AO, Obajimi MO, et al. Superior vena cava obstruction: diagnosis, management, and outcome. *East Afr Med J*. 2008;85:129–136.
100. Iversen LH, Bulow S, Christensen IJ, et al and the Danish Colorectal Cancer Group. Postoperative medical complications are the main cause of early death after emergency surgery for colonic cancer. *Br J Surg*. 2008;95:1012–1019.
101. Kawahara H, Yoshimoto K, Watanabe K, et al. Intraoperative drainage of intestinal contents in emergency surgical treatment of left-sided colonic obstruction. *Hepatogastroenterology*. 2008;55:940–942.
102. Charbonnet P, Gervaz P, Andres A, et al. Results of emergency Hartmann's operation for obstructive or perforated left-sided colorectal cancer. *World J Surg Oncol*. 2008;6:90–94.
103. Drudge-Coates L, Rajbabu K. Diagnosis and management of malignant spinal cord compression, part 2. *Int J Palliat Nurs*. 2008;14:175–180.
104. de Boer MT, Molenaar IQ, Porte RJ. Impact of blood loss on outcome after liver resection. *Dig Surg*. 2007;24:259–264.
105. Ford BS, Sharma S, Rezaishiraz H, et al. Effect of perioperative blood transfusion on prostate cancer recurrence. *Urol Oncol*. 2008;26:364–367.
106. Weber RS, Jabbour N, Martin RC II. Anemia and transfusions in patients undergoing surgery for cancer. *Ann Surg Oncol*. 2008;15:34–45.
107. Ydy LR, Slhessarenko N, de Aguilar-Nascimento JE. Effect of perioperative allogeneic red blood cell transfusion on the immune-inflammatory response after colorectal cancer resection. *World J Surg*. 2007;31:2044–2051.
108. Hill GE, Frawley WH, Griffith KE, et al. Allogeneic blood transfusion increases the risk of postoperative bacterial infection: a meta-analysis. *J Trauma*. 2003;54:908–914.
109. Sugita S, Sasaki A, Iwaki K, et al. Prognonsis and postoperative lymphocyte count in patients with hepatocellular carcinoma who received intraoperative allogeneic blood transfusion: a retrospective study. *Eur J Surg Oncol*. 2008;34:339–345.
110. Strumper-Groves D. Perioperative blood transfusion and outcome. *Curr Opin Anaesthesiol*. 2006;19:198–206.
111. Eidelman A, White T, Swarm RA. Interventional therapies for cancer pain management: important adjuvants to systemic analgesics. *J Natl Compr Cancer Netw*. 2007;5:753–760.
112. Senesse P, Assenat E, Schneider S, et al. Nutritional support during oncologic treatment of patients with gastrointestinal cancer: who could benefit? *Cancer Treat Rev*. 2008;34:568–575.
113. Klatte T, Lam JS, Shuch B, et al. Surveillance for renal cell carcinoma: why and how? When and how often? *Urol Oncol*. 2008;26:550–554.

CHAPTER 12

*Tracy K. Gosselin, RN, MSN, AOCN®*

# Principles of Radiation Therapy

- **Introduction**
- **History of Radiation Therapy**
- **Goals of Treatment Approaches**
- **Applied Radiation Physics**
- **High-Linear-Energy-Transfer and Charged-Particle Radiation Therapy**
  - *Neutron-Beam Therapy*
  - *Heavy Charged-Particle Therapy*
  - *Negative Pi-Meson Therapy*
- **Radiobiology**
  - *Cellular Response to Radiation*
    - Target theory
    - Cell cycle and radiosensitivity
    - Cell death
    - Contributing biologic factors
  - *Radiobiology of Brachytherapy*
    - Low-dose-rate brachytherapy
    - High-dose-rate brachytherapy
  - *Capitalizing on Radionuclides and Radioimmunotherapy*
- **Chemical and Thermal Modifiers of Radiation**
  - *Radiosensitizers and Radioprotectors*
  - *Combined Modality Therapy*
  - *Hyperthermia*
- **Incidental and Accidental Radiation Exposure**
  - *Chronic Low-Dose Exposure*
  - *Total-Body Radiation Syndrome*
    - Hematopoietic syndrome
    - Gastrointestinal syndrome
    - Cerebrovascular syndrome
  - *Radiation Effects on the Embryo and Fetus*
  - *Radiation-Induced Malignancies*
- **Conclusion**
- **References**

## INTRODUCTION

The role of radiation therapy in the treatment of cancer and noncancerous conditions has expanded dramatically in recent decades. Since the introduction of radiation in the early 1900s, both the field of radiation oncology and the technology used for treatment have seen many advances. Based on a greater understanding of radiobiology and physics, patients now can receive radiation as a primary treatment modality. Radiation therapy may be used alone or in combination with chemotherapy, surgery, or biotherapy. Collaboration of the multidisciplinary team is critical to ensure optimal patient outcomes.

*Radiation therapy* involves the use of ionizing radiation in the treatment of patients with benign and malignant diseases. The aim of therapy is to deliver a precisely measured dose of radiation to a defined tumor volume with as little damage as possible to surrounding healthy tissue, resulting in eradication of the tumor, high quality of life, and prolongation of survival at competitive costs.[1] Radiation therapy can be delivered to both outpatients and inpatients.

## HISTORY OF RADIATION THERAPY

Radiation occurs naturally in the environment. Although it is something we cannot see or feel, it is important to differentiate naturally occurring radiation from radiation produced by technologic means. In the course of everyday life, we are exposed to small amounts of radiation, but the amount of radiation needed to treat cancer is much larger.

The understanding and therapeutic use of radiation have evolved rapidly over the past century (Table 12-1). Wilhelm Conrad Roentgen, a German physicist, discovered the x-ray in 1895 while performing a laboratory experiment. Roentgen noticed that a cathode tube (developed by Sir William Crookes) shielded with black cardboard produced a fluorescent glow or ray after an electrical charge was passed through the tube. Roentgen eventually concluded that a new type of ray had been produced in the cathode-ray tube that could be defined based on the distance it could travel. This new ray was given the designation *X,* the scientific symbol for the unknown. In 1901, Roentgen was awarded the first Nobel Prize in Physics for this discovery.

During the same historical time frame, Antoine Henri Becquerel was in France studying the chemical properties of naturally occurring elements. He is credited with discovering radioactivity in uranium. The Curies, Pierre and Marie, further advanced Becquerel's work because Marie Curie wanted to further understand the origin of this new energy source. The Curies eventually would discover polonium and radium. For the next 35 years, Madame Curie would concentrate her efforts on the investigation of radium and radioactivity, until her death from aplastic anemia in 1934.[2]

In the early 1900s, many radiobiologic experiments were conducted in parallel with the development of radiation therapy. One of the most well-known results of the experiments was the law of Bergonié and Tribondeau,

**TABLE 12-1**

| History of Radiation | |
|---|---|
| 460 b.c. | Democritus proposes that atoms were the building blocks of all materials |
| 1600–1700s | Sir Isaac Newton and Benjamin Franklin produce developments that lead to the discovery of electricity |
| 1800s | Sir William Crookes developes the vacuum tube and cathode ray |
| 1895 | Wilhelm Conrad Roentgen discovers the x-ray |
| 1896 | Antoine Henri Becquerel discovers that uranium is naturally radioactive |
| 1897 | Professor Freund uses x-rays to make a hairy mole disappear |
| 1898 | Marie and Pierre Curie discover polonium and radium |
| Early 1900s | Law of Bergonié and Tribondeau established<br>x-rays are used therapeutically for benign and malignant diseases |
| 1920–1940s | Deep-therapy x-ray machines are developed<br>Atomic bomb developed during World War II<br>Marie Curie dies of aplastic anemia in 1934 |
| 1950s | Cobalt therapy units become available and first-generation linear accelerators are developed<br>Combined modality therapy is used |
| 1970s | The term *radiation oncology* is employed to describe the scientific as well as the therapeutic discipline |
| 1980s-early 1990s | Various treatment methods are studied in clinical trials (hyperthermia, intraoperative and radiolabeled antibodies)<br>Research is conducted with radiosensitizers and radioprotectors<br>Basic radiation metric terminology changes: gray (Gy) replaces rad |
| 1990s | Development of multileaf collimation (MLC) and intensity-modulated radiation therapy (IMRT)<br>FDA approves the first radioprotective agent—amifostine |

which states that radiosensitivity is highest in tissues with the highest mitotic index and lowest in well-differentiated tissues.[3]

Between 1920 and 1940, a series of experiments led to what we know today as *fractionation.* The development of x-ray mechanisms to treat deep tumors was under way, and brachytherapy was being performed with radium. With technological advances, the atomic bomb was developed during World War II and deployed on Hiroshima and Nagasaki, leading to radiobiologic research for decades to follow.

In the 1950s, cobalt therapy machines became a standard for treatment, and the first linear accelerators were developed. The role of combined-modality treatment was pursued in clinical trials.

In the most recent decades, both technologic and scientific advances related to radiation have occurred. The development of computers for treatment planning and dose optimization permitted the emergence of three-dimensional (3D) and 3D conformal radiation therapy (3-DCRT) treatment planning. In the 1990s, intensity-modulated radiation therapy (IMRT) and multileaf collimation (MLC) were developed to assist in minimizing treatment-related toxicity. Hyperthermia, intraoperative radiation, brachytherapy, and stereotactic radiosurgery also have undergone many refinements.

The radiation oncology team is a specialized group of healthcare providers who work collaboratively to meet patient care needs. A better understanding of radiobiology principles and the role of combined-modality treatment have provided important information about both acute and late toxicities of treatment. Ongoing research continues to assess treatment techniques, combined-modality treatment, the role of radiosensitizers and radioprotectors, and the effects of hypoxia on overall survival. The years ahead will support ongoing investigation into maximizing treatment dose without compromising quality of life and survival.

## GOALS OF TREATMENT APPROACHES

Radiation therapy plays a major role in the treatment of patients diagnosed with cancer. Approximately 60% of cancer patients will receive radiation at some point in their disease trajectory, either to cure, control, or palliate the disease.[1] If the tumor is diagnosed at an early stage, cure is possible. Patients undergoing a curative course of radiation therapy often face vigorous and lengthy treatment. In such cases, the total dose of radiation may be higher, and the toxicities of treatment may be more severe. Chemotherapy also may be used to increase the therapeutic index. Patients with early-stage Hodgkin's disease and skin cancer are often treated with radiation alone.

For certain types of cancers and those in later stages, cure or eradication is not possible. In such cases, control of the cancer with radiation therapy for periods ranging from months to years may be the goal. Recurrent breast cancer, some soft-tissue sarcomas, and lung cancer are examples of cancers controlled by radiation therapy in combination with surgery or chemotherapy.

Palliation may be another goal of radiation therapy. Relief of pain, prevention of pathologic fractures, and return of mobility can be achieved with radiation to metastatic bone lesions from primary sites such as breast, lung, and prostate. Pain relief often is dramatic, and it is not uncommon for one individual to receive multiple palliative courses to different bony structures over the course of several years. Radiation therapy contributes significantly to improved quality of life for the person with bone metastases. Palliative radiation therapy also is given for the relief of central nervous system (CNS) symptoms caused by brain metastasis or spinal cord compression. Hemorrhage, obstruction, ulceration, superior vena cava syndrome, and fungating lesions can be reduced effectively—and in some instances eliminated—by palliative radiation therapy.

*Anticipatory* palliation is an application of radiation therapy that seeks to treat potentially symptomatic lesions before they become problematic. Examples of anticipatory palliation include treatment of a mediastinal mass that threatens to produce a superior vena cava syndrome and treatment of a vertebral lesion when spinal cord compression is impending. Prophylactic treatment may be used in patients with small cell lung cancer (SCLC) who receive whole-brain irradiation to minimize their risk of developing brain metastases. In the nonmalignant setting, treatment may be given to patients who were in a accident to prevent heterotopic bone growth as well as postoperatively to patients who have undergone surgical excision for keloids to prevent recurrence.

Although treatment techniques and equipment may vary, the fundamental principles of radiobiology and radiation physics form the basis on which a course of treatment is selected and designed for each patient. Understanding these principles enables the oncology nurse to support and care for the patient receiving radiation therapy—attending to the emotional and physical needs that result from the disease and the therapy.

## APPLIED RADIATION PHYSICS

The use of ionizing radiation in the treatment of cancer is based on the ability of radiation to interact with the atoms and molecules of the tumor cells to produce specific harmful biologic effects. Ionization affects either the molecules of the cell or the cell environment.

An understanding of atomic structure is essential to understanding the ionizing effects of radiation. The atom—the basic unit of molecular structure—has two parts: (1) the nucleus, containing positively charged protons and neutrons that have mass but no charge, and (2) the shells (orbits), containing negatively charged electrons (equivalent to the number of protons). Each shell can accommodate only a certain number of electrons; if this number is exceeded, a second or third shell is established more distant from the nucleus (Figure 12-1). The negatively charged electrons orbit the nucleus and are held in place by the attractive force of the positive protons in the nucleus; thus a stable state is maintained. Certain atoms are known to be unstable, however; during the process of their decay or breakdown into a more stable state, alpha, beta, or gamma rays may be emitted. Radium, radon, and uranium are examples of unstable atoms that produce ionizing radiation.

Stable atoms also may be made to produce ionizing radiation through excitation, ionization, and nuclear disintegration. Radiation produced by these processes can be classified as electromagnetic radiation or particulate radiation. The electromagnetic spectrum can be further divided into five levels of decreasing wavelength: (1) radio waves, (2) infrared radiation, (3) visible light, (4) ultraviolet radiation, and (5) ionizing radiation.

*Ionizing radiation* has the shortest wavelength and the greatest energy of the electromagnetic spectrum and therefore is the form of energy used in radiation therapy. A classification system for ionizing radiation is shown in Figure 12-2. As seen in the figure, the terms *x-ray* and *gamma ray* both describe ionizing electromagnetic radiation. These forms differ only in their means of production. That is, x-rays are produced by specially designed equipment, and gamma rays are emitted by radioactive materials such as $^{60}Co$ undergoing nuclear transition. Both x-rays and gamma rays have no mass; rather, they are packets of available energy ready to be released on collision with a substance. Because they have no mass, x-rays and gamma rays can penetrate more deeply into tissue before releasing their energy. This process, which is commonly referred to as *photon* irradiation, is used to treat deep-seated tumors such as those located in the thoracic, abdominal, and pelvic areas. Photons are skin-sparing, so skin toxicity is minimal.

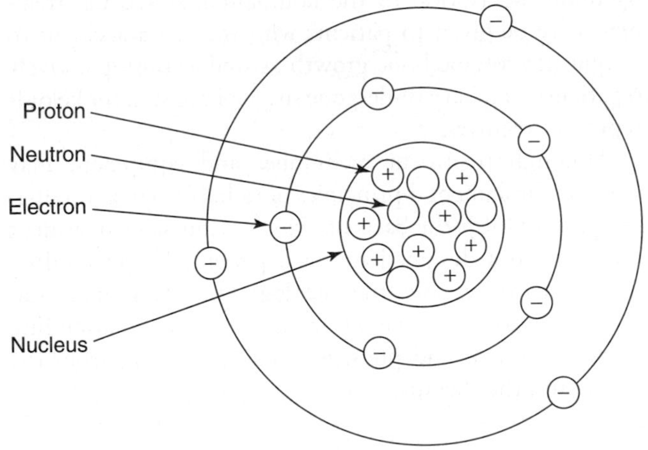


**FIGURE 12-1**

Basic structure of an atom. Protons, which are positively charged, and neutrons, which have no electrical charge, are the major components of the nucleus of an atom. The number of protons is equal to the number of negatively charged electrons orbiting the nucleus. Atoms of any given element may have different numbers of neutrons in the nucleus, thus giving atoms of the same element different atomic weights. An atom of a given element that differs only in its atomic weight is called an *isotope*.

*Particulate radiation,* by contrast, is composed of alpha and beta particles, as well as electrons and neutrons, which have mass. The relatively large size of alpha particles allows them to penetrate only a short distance into tissue before collision and energy release take place. Beta particles, which are smaller than alpha particles, penetrate more deeply but, because of their mass, do not have the ability to reach as deeply into tissues, as do x-rays and gamma rays. The significance of these variations in ability to penetrate tissue will become obvious when treatment beams and equipment are discussed in Chapter 13.

X-rays are produced when a stream of fast-moving electrons, accelerated by the application of high voltage (between the filament and the target), strikes the target, and the electrons give up their energy. This radiation loss occurs because the electron is attracted to and slowed down by the nucleus of the tungsten (target) atom. Figure 12-3 illustrates the basic structure of an x-ray tube.

In addition to x-rays, some treatment machines (eg, betatron, linear accelerator) are equipped to produce particle irradiation in the form of electrons. Electrons are small, negatively charged particles produced in an x-ray tube by bypassing one of the steps used to produce x-rays. That is, electrons from the heated tungsten filament are injected into the vacuum tube and accelerated at a high velocity; they then emerge from a window in the vacuum tube, bypassing the tungsten target and emerging as electron particles. Electrons are used to treat surface lesions and sites located a few centimeters below the skin. They also may be used at the end of treatment in what is commonly referred to as a *boost* treatment field. A boost may be administered after a course of photons has been given to treat a surgical area (usually the scar/surgical incision site) where the tumor was excised in an effort to reduce the risk of local recurrence.

Electromagnetic radiation and particulate radiation are also produced through the process of decay of radioactive elements and radioactive isotopes. This process, which produces radiation in the form of alpha, beta, or gamma rays, takes place as follows. The time required for half the radioactive atoms present at any time to decay is known as the *half-life* of that radioactive element or isotope.

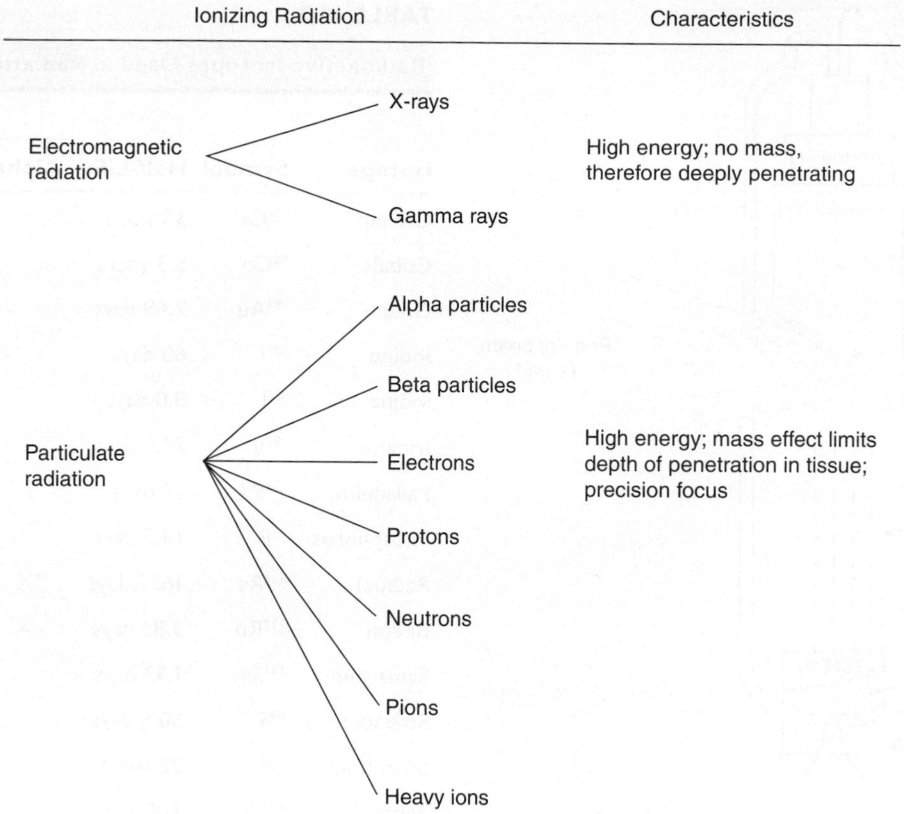


**FIGURE 12-2**

Characteristics of ionizing radiation.

Because most radioisotopes are produced by neutron bombardment of stable elements (eg, $^{60}$Co, $^{32}$P, $^{182}$Ta, and $^{198}$Au) or by nuclear fission of uranium in a nuclear reactor (eg, $^{90}$Sr and $^{137}$Cs), they are referred to as *artificial isotopes* to distinguish them from naturally occurring radioisotopes such as $^{226}$Ra and $^{222}$Rn. Radioactive isotopes are listed in Table 12-2.

## HIGH-LINEAR-ENERGY-TRANSFER AND CHARGED-PARTICLE RADIATION THERAPY

One important physical property of ionizing radiation is linear energy transfer (LET). *Linear energy transfer* describes the rate at which energy is deposited as radiation travels through matter on a given track. Electromagnetic radiation has no mass or charge and therefore is sparsely ionizing as it penetrates matter. X-rays, gamma rays, and electrons are electromagnetic and low-LET sources.

By contrast, the number of ionizing events produced by molecules of high-LET radiation is significant because of their considerable mass and charge. High-LET radiation, which includes neutron beams, heavy ions, and negative pi-mesons (pions), loses energy rapidly as it passes through matter. Multiple ionizing events occur in a relatively short distance with this type of radiation. Few high-LET radiation facilities exist, but two such centers operate at Loma Linda, California, and at the Massachusetts General Hospital, Boston. Years of research have shown that this form of therapy offers distinct advantages, yet the cost of the facilities and the technologic sophistication needed for their operation have meant that they function primarily as referral centers to treat salivary gland, prostate tumors, and certain pediatric malignancies.

High-LET radiation has several advantages over low-LET radiation:

- Greater relative biologic effectiveness (RBE)
- Reduced relative radioresistance of hypoxic cells in tumors (low oxygen enhancement ratio [OER])
- Less intertreatment recovery of tumor cells in fractionated dosage

### NEUTRON-BEAM THERAPY

Fast neutrons are produced by a *cyclotron,* equipment in which high-energy neutrons bombard targets consisting of

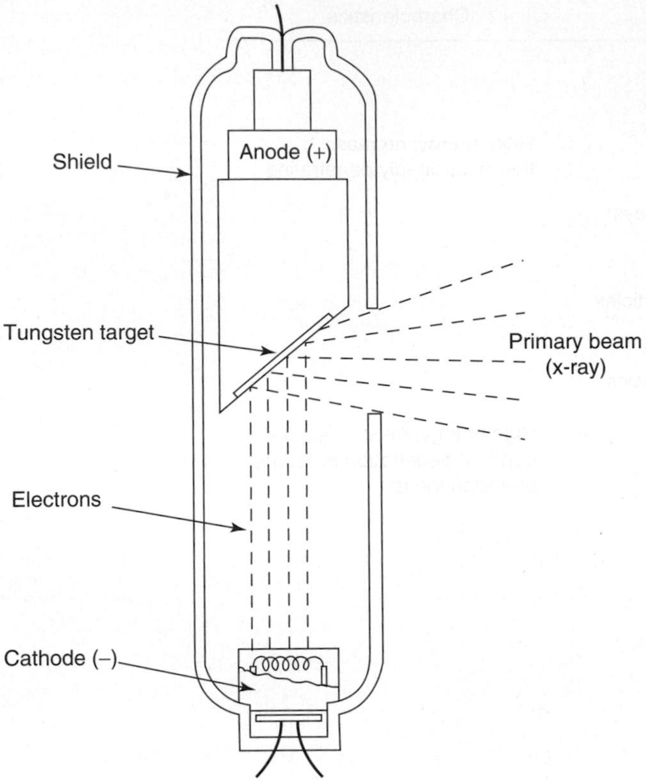


**FIGURE 12-3**

Basic structure of an x-ray tube. Electrons emitted from a heated tungsten filament are accelerated across a high-voltage source. These high-speed electrons strike a positively charged tungsten target, producing x-rays. The primary beam of radiation produced penetrates tissues. The greater the voltage, the greater is the penetrating power of the beam.

**TABLE 12-2**

**Radioactive Isotopes Used in Radiation Therapy**

| | | | Emissions | | |
|---|---|---|---|---|---|
| **Isotope** | **Symbol** | **Half-Life** | **Alpha** | **Beta** | **Gamma** |
| Cesium | $^{137}Cs$ | 30 years | | | X |
| Cobalt | $^{60}Co$ | 5.3 years | | X | X |
| Gold | $^{198}Au$ | 2.69 days | | X | X |
| Iodine | $^{125}I$ | 60 days | | X | X |
| Iodine | $^{131}I$ | 8.0 days | | X | X |
| Iridium | $^{192}Ir$ | 74.5 days | | X | X |
| Palladium | $^{103}Pd$ | 17 days | | | X |
| Phosphorus | $^{32}P$ | 14.3 days | | X | |
| Radium | $^{226}Ra$ | 1622 days | X | X | X |
| Radon | $^{222}Rn$ | 3.83 days | X | X | X |
| Samarium | $^{153}Sm$ | 1.93 days | | X | X |
| Strontium | $^{89}S$ | 50.5 days | | X | |
| Strontium | $^{90}S$ | 28 years | | X | |
| Tantalum | $^{182}Ta$ | 118 days | | X | X |
| Yttrium | $^{90}Y$ | 64 hours | | X | |

either beryllium or tritium. Neutrons have a lower OER, so the cancer cells do not need to be as well oxygenated to be damaged. Neutrons tend to be associated with less repair of both sublethal and potentially lethal damage to cells and with smaller variations in radiosensitivity according to the phase of the cell cycle.[3] Neutron therapy is less expensive than other high-LET energy producers; however, technologic problems and the low dose rate (5 to 6 cGy/minute) are among the disadvantages of this form of therapy.

## HEAVY CHARGED-PARTICLE THERAPY

Heavy ions, such as protons, helium ions, and nitrogen ions, are mainly useful for treating small tumors because the dose distribution is best for treating a small volume. As the tumor size increases, treatment volume and OER also increase. Particle beams have an inverse dose profile compared with photons: The dose increases with penetration depth, ranging from a low dose in the entrance to a sharp maximum dose at the end of the particle range.[4] This is commonly referred to as *Bragg's peak.* In the past 10 years in the United States, proton centers have started to flourish as the technology and equipment have advanced.

## NEGATIVE PI-MESON THERAPY

Negative pi-mesons (pions) are small, negatively charged particles found in the nuclei of atoms that "cement" protons and neutrons together. Pions are produced when protons are accelerated at approximately 131,000 mi/s before striking a carbon target. The pions then are collected by a system of magnets, and the beam of high-LET energy is directed at the target tissue. The first application of this form of treatment for humans took place at the Los Alamos Meson Physics Facility in Los Alamos, New Mexico, in 1974. The advantage of pion therapy, as with other forms of high-LET radiation, is that the beam can be shaped to fit the tumor precisely, thereby minimizing the amount of radiation administered to surrounding normal structures. Pions can be aimed and stopped at a specific target site by adjusting the momentum of the particles.

At Los Alamos, a number of tumor sites and histologies were treated with good local cure rates and minimal morbidity, particularly in cancers of the head and neck, lung, bladder, cervix, and prostate gland. Tumors of the large bowel, pancreas, and brain did not respond equally well. The Los Alamos program was terminated in 1981 because overall results were not impressive, and costs were prohibitive.

A second pion facility opened in 1979 in Vancouver, British Columbia, and a third opened in 1980 in Villigen, Switzerland. Approximately 500 patients were treated at Villigen, with a high incidence of long-term toxicities being noted. The severity of these late effects was attributed to the use of treatment volumes nearly three times those used by the Vancouver group. The program at Villigen was discontinued in 1993.

The Vancouver pion group completed two randomized trials in late 1995 comparing photon and pion irradiation as treatments for high-grade gliomas and advanced prostate cancers. The glioma study found no difference between the two treatment groups in terms of overall survival, time to recurrence, toxicity, and quality of life. Acute effects of pion therapy were increased over those seen with photon therapy; however, late toxicity was reduced in pion treatment.

Raju concludes that clinical results obtained with pions appear to be about equal to those achieved with photons for all sites investigated, except for the bladder.[5] Because of the cost and complexity of building and operating pion facilities, Raju also concludes that pion radiation will not likely be pursued in the future.

## RADIOBIOLOGY

The biologic effects of radiation on humans are the result of a sequence of events that follows the absorption of energy from ionizing radiation and the organism's attempts to compensate for this assault. The effects of radiation take place at the cellular level, with consequences developing in the tissues, organs, and/or the entire body depending on the treatment site. Radiation's biologic influences on these cells are mediated by a variety of biochemical, genetic, and kinetic factors. They are also affected by the dose, type, and rate at which radiation is given. The incidence and severity of these effects can be classified as acute and/or late depending on the tissue kinetics.

### CELLULAR RESPONSE TO RADIATION

#### Target theory

Radiation effects at the cellular level may be either direct or indirect, according to target theory. A direct hit occurs when any of the key molecules within the cell are damaged by energy that is directly deposited in the DNA or RNA. After high-dose radiation of DNA molecules in vitro, four types of damage are observed: (1) change or loss of a base (thymine, adenine, guanine, or cytosine), (2) breakage of the hydrogen bond between the two chains of the DNA molecule, (3) breaks in one or both chains of the DNA molecule, and (4) cross-linking of the chains after breakage. Such unrepaired breaks or alterations in a base lead to mutations that result in impaired cellular function or cell death.

An indirect hit, according to target theory, occurs when ionization takes place in the medium (mostly intracellular water) surrounding the molecular structures within the cell. Radiation absorbed by the water molecules results in the formation of a free radical when an electron is literally knocked out of orbit surrounding the ion. The free radicals produced in this way may trigger a variety of chemical reactions, producing new compounds that are toxic to the cell. Figure 12-4 illustrates the ionizing effect of radiation on the water contained within a cell.

It generally is agreed that a direct hit (ie, DNA damage and chromosomal aberrations) accounts for the most effective and lethal injury produced by ionizing radiation.[3] However, because of the relative ratio of water to DNA in a single cell, the probability of indirect damage through ionization of intracellular water is much greater than the probability of damage from a direct hit. Loss of the cell's

The final products of the ionization of water molecules (HOH) by radiation are an ion pair ($H^+$, OH-) and free radicals ($H^{\cdot}$, $OH^{\cdot}$), which are capable of damaging the cell. The ionization of water is shown in the following steps:

$$HOH \xrightarrow{radiation} HOH^+ e^-$$

The free electron ($e^-$) is captured by another available water molecule and, as shown in the next step, forms the second ion:

$$HOH + e^- \rightarrow HOH^-$$

Because the two ions ($HOH^+$, $HOH^-$) produced by these reactions are unstable, rapid breakdown occurs (in the presence of other, normal water molecules), forming yet another ion and a free radical:

$$HOH^+ \rightarrow H^{\cdot} + OH^{\cdot}$$
$$HOH^- \rightarrow OH^- + H^{\cdot}$$

Although the resulting pair of ions ($H^+$, $OH^-$) have some potential for cellular damage through chemical reactions, they are more likely to recombine and form water (HOH). The free radicals ($H^{\cdot}$, $OH^{\cdot}$) are extremely reactive, and they too may simply recombine to form water. However, free radicals appear to be more likely to undergo chemical interactions with other free radicals, forming cytotoxic agents, as shown in this reactions:

$$OH^{\cdot} + OH^{\cdot} \rightarrow H_2O_2 \text{ (hydrogen peroxide)}$$

Free radicals that result from the interaction of radiation with water are capable of triggering a variety of chemical reactions within the cell and are therefore believed to be a major factor in the production of damage in the cell.

**FIGURE 12-4**

The effect of ionizing radiation on water molecules.

reproductive capacity is considered to be the most biologically significant end point of radiation damage.[6]

In addition to the damage produced by a direct or indirect hit (Table 12-3),[7] experimental evidence shows that radiation can cause damage to proteins, carbohydrates, and enzymes within the cell. Damage to these additional molecules, as well as alterations in the permeability of the cell membrane, may contribute to the ultimate effect of radiation at the cellular level.

### Cell cycle and radiosensitivity

According to Hall and Cox, radiosensitivity appears to be maximized during the M and $G_2$ phases of the cell cycle.[3] Thus the maximum effect from radiation should occur just before and during actual cell division. In early research, Bergonié and Tribondeau suggested that the sensitivity of cells to irradiation is directly proportional to their reproductive activity and inversely proportional to their degree of differentiation.[8] A differentiated cell is one that is morphologically or functionally specialized (eg, an erythrocyte) and does not undergo mitosis. An undifferentiated cell (such as a red blood cell, stem cell, or erythroblast) has few specialized morphologic or functional characteristics, and its primary purpose is to divide and provide new cells to maintain its own population. Because the effect of radiation is known to be greatest during mitosis, undifferentiated cell populations generally are most sensitive to radiation. In contrast, well-differentiated cells are relatively radioresistant.

Changes in mitotic activity owing to radiation can be classified as either delayed onset or complete inhibition. *Delayed onset of mitosis* indicates that although damage occurred at some point during prophase, repair was accomplished, and division occurred. *Complete inhibition of mitosis,* or cell sterilization, renders the cell incapable of division, although it may continue to live in a nonreproducing state.

**TABLE 12-3**

| Biologic Effects When Cells Are Exposed to Radiation |
|---|
| Single-strand DNA damage that can be accurately repaired |
| Single-strand DNA damage that is incorrectly repaired, leading to mutations |
| Double-strand DNA damage, which usually cannot be repaired |
| Delay in mitosis to allow repair of DNA, if possible |
| Apoptosis (programmed cell death) if the DNA damage is severe and not repaired |
| Cell division and repopulation with some of the cells containing mutations |

*Source:* Reprinted with permission from Dunne-Daly C. Principles of radiotherapy and radiobiology. *Semin Oncol Nurs.* 1999;15:250–259.[7]

### Cell death

According to McBride and Withers, there are four types of cell death: (1) mitotic (or genetic), (2) interphase, (3) apoptotic, and (4) necrotic.[9] *Mitotic death* occurs after one or more cell divisions and usually with much smaller radiation doses than those required to produce interphase death. *Interphase death* occurs within 4 to 6 hours of irradiation, even with low doses of radiation. Affected cells can no longer contribute to the reproductive pool. *Apoptotic death* requires active metabolic processes and neighboring cells to phagocytose the cell remnants, with the entire process unfolding in just a few hours. *Necrotic death* involves the loss of membrane integrity, an increase in cell size, the release of lyposomal enzymes, and the generation of an inflammation response. This type of cell death also may represent a pathologic response to vascular damage as well as a default pathway for cells that lack an effective apoptotic apparatus.

### Contributing biologic factors

A number of additional factors directly affect the biologic response to radiation and, ultimately, the treatment outcome. Among these are the oxygen effect, LET, relative biologic effectiveness, dose rate, radiosensitivity, and fractionation.

*Oxygen effect.* Well-oxygenated tumors show a much greater response to radiation; that is, they are more radiosensitive than poorly oxygenated tumors. Extensive laboratory and clinical research has shown that the existence of oxygen tension from 20 to 40 mm Hg at the time of radiation greatly enhances the radiosensitivity of the cells.[3,10] One theory suggests that the mechanism of the oxygen effect is related to the ability of oxygen to combine with the free radicals formed during ionization, thereby producing new and toxic combinations. A second theory holds that the presence of oxygen at the time of irradiation prevents the reversal (and thus the repair) of some of the chemical changes that occur as the result of ionization. The clinical significance of the oxygen effect is that oxygen modifies the dose of radiation needed to produce a given degree of biologic damage. The magnitude of the oxygen effect is expressed as the oxygen enhancement ratio (OER). The OER is the ratio of radiation dose in the absence of oxygen (or hypoxia) to the radiation dose in the presence of oxygen required for the same biologic effect. Cells that are hypoxic are considered to be radioresistant and therefore limit the effectiveness of radiation therapy. Studies in head and neck and cervical cancer have demonstrated poorer survival outcomes in patients with hypoxic tumors.[11,12] It also has been noted that patients with hypoxic tumors are more likely to be anemic.[13]

*Linear energy transfer.* Linear energy transfer (LET) describes the rate at which energy is lost from different types of radiation while traveling through matter. Low-LET radiation (eg, x-rays and gamma rays) is sparsely ionizing, having a random pathway that results in few direct hits within the cell nucleus. Radiation of higher LET (eg, alpha particles, neutrons, and negative pions) has a greater probability of interacting with matter and producing more direct hits within the cell.

*Relative biologic effectiveness.* Because different types of radiation have varying rates of energy loss, the biologic responses of these treatments likewise will be different. Therefore, RBE is used to compare a dose of test radiation with a dose of standard radiation that produces the same biologic response. The following formula is used to express RBE:

$$\text{RBE} = \frac{\left(\begin{array}{c}\text{Dose of reference radiation} \\ \text{to produce a given biological effect}\end{array}\right)}{\left(\begin{array}{c}\text{Dose of test radiation} \\ \text{to produce the same biological effect}\end{array}\right)}$$

*Dose rate.* *Dose rate* refers to the rate at which a given dose is delivered by a treatment machine or equipment. Dose rate becomes particularly significant when a course of therapy is fractionated over many days and weeks, as it is in standard external-beam teletherapy. Studies have shown low dose rates to be much less effective in producing lethal cell damage than high dose rates primarily because low dose rates permit cell repair to occur before the lethal dose has been reached in fractionated teletherapy.

*Radiosensitivity.* According to Bergonié and Tribondeau, ionizing radiation is most effective on cells that are undifferentiated and undergoing active mitosis.[8] Laboratory and clinical experience has shown this relationship to hold true in most tissues.

*Fractionation.* *Fractionation* is the treatment approach that takes the total dose of radiation and divides it into equal fractions, recognizing that the dose may need to be higher owing to the plan of delivering multiple fractions. A single dose of radiation has more of a biologic effect than the same dose divided or fractionated, but that single dose will not be able to spare normal tissues and also eradicate the tumor. *Hyperfractionation* uses smaller doses per fraction, and treatment is given twice a day, separated by a minimum of 6 hours.

The four R's of radiobiology (ie, repair, redistribution, repopulation, and reoxygenation) explain the biologic and chemical effects of fractionation on tumors and normal tissues.

**Repair** of intracellular sublethal damage by normal cells between daily-dose fractions is one benefit of fractionation. The goal of fractionation is to deliver a dose sufficient to prevent tumor cells from being repaired while allowing normal cells to recover before the next dose is given. Although some tumor cells may be repaired between daily doses, they also may reoxygenate, rendering them more radiosensitive when the next dose of radiation is administered. Thus, although some degree of repair of tumor cells may occur between fractionated doses, repeated daily doses ultimately would lead to tumor control.

**Redistribution** of cell age (within the cell cycle) as a result of daily radiation is advantageous because more tumor cells are made radiosensitive. Theoretically, with succeeding daily doses of radiation, increasingly more tumor cells would be delayed in the cycle and reach the mitotic phase as the next dose is given, thereby increasing the cell kill.

**Repopulation** of normal tissues takes place through cell division at some point during the fractionated treatment. Fractionation of dose allows this repopulation to occur in normal tissues, sparing them from some of the late consequences that might arise if repopulation (new growth) was inhibited. Tumor cells that succeed in dividing while undergoing a fractionated course of radiation therapy are usually incapable of surviving because of the radiation effect. Thus fractionation favors normal tissue while eradicating tumor.

**Reoxygenation** is the fourth consideration favoring fractionation of the radiation dose. Whereas normal tissues usually are well oxygenated, tumors characteristically range from normal to hypoxic to anoxic. As discussed earlier, radiosensitivity is closely related to oxygen tension in the tumor cell; hypoxic or anoxic cells generally are radioresistant, whereas oxygenated cells are radiosensitive. Fractionating the dose allows the cells to become oxygenated as the tumor shrinks.

Tissue and organ response to radiation reflects the sensitivity of the affected cellular components. Both tissues and organs are composed of more than one cell type, with each category of cells having a different degree of radiosensitivity. Another factor that determines tissue response is related to the parenchymal versus stromal substances found in that tissue. The parenchyma is composed of cells characteristic of the tissue or organ. If those cells are radiosensitive (eg, the testis), then ionizing radiation has its greatest effect on the parenchyma. Conversely, if parenchymal tissue is relatively radioresistant (eg, the spinal cord), then radiation response in that organ is due to the indirect effects on the stromal components (especially the vasculature) that support the parenchyma. Table 12-4 lists various organs according to their degree of radiosensitivity, as measured by parenchymal hypoplasia.

**TABLE 12-4**

**Degree of Radiosensitivity of Various Organs Based on Parenchymal Hypoplasia**

| Organ | Radiosensitivity |
|---|---|
| Lymphoid organs, bone marrow, blood, testes, ovaries, intestines | High |
| Skin, cornea, oral cavity, esophagus, rectum, bladder, vagina, cervix, ureters | Fairly high |
| Optic lens, stomach, growing cartilage, fine vasculature, growing bone | Medium |
| Mature cartilage or bone, salivary glands, respiratory organs, kidneys, liver, pancreas, thyroid, adrenals, pituitary gland | Fairly low |
| Muscle, brain, spinal cord | Low |

*Apoptosis.* A major focus of research in radiobiology is currently directed toward the study of various mechanisms regulating apoptosis. *Apoptosis,* or programmed cell death, occurs in both normal and malignant cells in a process that is distinct from cellular death owing to hypoxia. Failure of the normal apoptotic process results in survival and uncontrolled proliferation of malignant cells.

As described earlier, repair of radiation injury (sublethal damage repair) takes place in healthy tissues but also may occur in the targeted malignancy, thereby reducing radioresponsiveness and diminishing the likelihood of cure. Ionization and direct damage to DNA account for the death during mitosis of most irradiated cells. It has been demonstrated that the process of apoptosis is also accelerated by radiation, particularly in lymphocytes, small-bowel crypt cells, salivary gland cells, and germ cells.[14]

The role of certain genetic, molecular, and biochemical substances (eg, *p53, pRb,* and *BCL-2*), basic fibroblast growth factors (bFGF), and protein kinase C (PKC) inhibitors, among others, at the time of irradiation is thought to be significant in radiation-induced apoptosis.[14,15] The presence or absence of these substances and many others could enhance radioresponsiveness in various cell lines. Intensive research to identify the pathways that ultimately lead to apoptosis is under way. Manipulating these pathways may hold the key to increasing the therapeutic benefit ratio in radiation oncology.[16]

## RADIOBIOLOGY OF BRACHYTHERAPY

The basic radiobiologic mechanism of cell kill in brachytherapy and teletherapy is the same because the principles described previously as the four R's of radiobiology (ie, repair, redistribution, repopulation, and reoxygenation) apply to both forms of radiation delivery. However, the temporal and spatial principles of physics are what account for the effectiveness of both brachytherapy and teletherapy.[17] Standard brachytherapy delivers continuous radiation at a low dose rate over a period of several days. Standard teletherapy delivers low-dose-rate radiation in higher doses given in daily fractions over a number of weeks.

*Brachytherapy* entails the use of implanted or injected radioactive sources, which capitalize on the effects of continuous rather than fractionated irradiation. These differences in effect occur when the dose rate is less than 5 cGy per minute.

## LOW-DOSE-RATE BRACHYTHERAPY

Low-dose-rate (LDR) brachytherapy, commonly used for gynecologic and head and neck cancers, delivers a continuous dose of radiation for as long as the source remains in place within the patient. This approach stands in contrast to the intermittent dosing that takes place when treating with fractionated external-beam teletherapy. Following doses of fractionated teletherapy, cellular sublethal damage repair (SLD-R) occurs within 1 to 4 hours following treatment, producing the initial portion of the cell-survival curve referred to as the *shoulder*. Recall that cells are most radiosensitive during the M and $G_2$ phases of the cell cycle. LDR brachytherapy increases the effectiveness of radiation by redistributing an even greater proportion of cells into the $G_2$ phase compared with fractionated treatment. Irradiated cells that manage to divide are blocked in the $G_2$ phase by continuous LDR brachytherapy.

Hypoxia in a tumor being treated with LDR brachytherapy is a less significant negative factor than it is in teletherapy. Low dose rates reduce the OER, and SLD-R is inhibited under prolonged hypoxic conditions. Thus LDR brachytherapy enhances radiation effect by taking advantage of repair, redistribution, and repopulation principles even in poorly oxygenated tissue.

## HIGH-DOSE-RATE BRACHYTHERAPY

High-dose-rate (HDR) brachytherapy is the newest delivery method for brachytherapy. HDR sources deliver more than 1200 cGy of radiation per hour, administered as single, repeated fractions rather than continuously as in LDR treatments. The equipment used for this treatment modality is highly sophisticated, with computer optimization of dose distribution and sparing of normal tissues. In addition to the advantages of outpatient treatment and reduced staff exposure to radioactivity, HDR brachytherapy has shown a lower complication rate in treatment of cervix cancer than LDR therapy, without any decrease in local control.[18]

High-dose-rate brachytherapy may be used to treat breast, gynecologic, and prostate cancers.

### CAPITALIZING ON RADIONUCLIDES AND RADIOIMMUNOTHERAPY

The development of radiopharmaceuticals dates back to the early discoveries by Becquerel and the Curies. Interest and research efforts in this area have accelerated in recent decades. Radioimmunotherapy has been studied with a variety of solid-tumor and hematologic malignancies. Among the numerous radioactive isotopes that have been administered therapeutically, $^{131}I$ and $^{90}Y$ in particular have been adopted for use in radiolabeled antibody therapy and $^{153}S$ and $^{89}S$ for bone metastases.

Radioimmunotherapy involves the fusion of a radioisotope and a monoclonal antibody through direct labeling or incorporation of an appropriate chelating agent.[19] These agents typically are administered via intravenous injection but can be given via the intrathecal, intralesional, intraarterial, or intraperitoneal route. Because radionucleotides have short half-lives, radioimmunotherapy avoids prolonged radiation exposure to healthy cells while delivering lethal or sublethal doses to the tumor. Depending on the biologic properties of the given antibody, cell kill may be based on apoptosis, antibody-dependent cellular cytotoxicity (ADCC), complement-dependent cytotoxicity (CDC), or a combination of actions.[19] Among numerous phase I, II, and III clinical trials over the past three decades, some of the more significant results have been achieved in the treatment of thyroid cancer and hematologic malignancies, particularly B-cell malignancies.[19]

A major problem in delivering the intended dose of radiation to the target site is the fact that the radiolabeled antibody is cleared rapidly from the target organ by normal blood flow, thus limiting the time of contact with the tumor target. A new delivery method has been developed and patented (U.S. Patent No. 5,424,288) that uses macroaggragated proteins injected directly into the organ site to block the rapid clearance of the radioactive substance.[20,21] This procedure, called *infusional brachytherapy,* is being employed to treat a number of advanced cancers, with the most extensive application in pancreatic adenocarcinoma.[21] Phase II multicenter trials have been initiated in the United States and Europe using macroaggragated albumin (MAA) as the blocking agent and $^{32}P$ (chromic phosphate) as the radioactive source for treatment of pancreatic cancer.[20,21]

Iodine-131 has been used historically in the treatment of neuroendocrine tumors and is referred to as *metaiodebenzylguanine* (MIBG). This isotope emits both beta and gamma rays, so patients who receive this agent are admitted to the hospital and placed on radiation precautions. Once their dose is 33 mCi or less, they may be discharged. Iodine-131 tositumomab is a conjugated monoclonal antibody attached to the radioisotope $^{131}I$. This unique compound targets a protein, the CD-20 antigen, found on the surface of malignant B cells in non-Hodgkin's lymphoma (NHL).[22] Clinical trials have demonstrated positive results in NHL patients.[23,24]

Yttrium ibritumomab tiuxetan is another radiolabeled monoclonal antibody. This beta-emitting source requires fewer precautions than $^{131}I$, which emits both beta and gamma radiation. Trials of yttrium-90 have been conducted in patients with relapsed or refractory low-grade or follicular B-cell lymphoma and have shown positive results.[25,26]

Radioimmunotherapy continues to demonstrate efficacy in cancer treatment. Radioimmunotherapy agents may be administered in nuclear medicine or radiation oncology areas depending on the practice setting. In addition to the care provided by oncologists and oncology nurses, radioimmunotherapy administration requires the services of nuclear medicine physicians and technologists or radiation oncologists, radiopharmacists, and radiation safety officers.[26]

## CHEMICAL AND THERMAL MODIFIERS OF RADIATION

### RADIOSENSITIZERS AND RADIOPROTECTORS

The goal of radiation therapy is to achieve maximum tumor cell kill while minimizing injury to normal tissues (therapeutic ratio). Local tumor failure is the cause of 40% to 60% of cancer deaths and may occur in 60% to 80% of cancer patients at the time of death.[27] Efforts to improve the therapeutic ratio have resulted in the development of certain compounds that act to increase the radiosensitivity of tumor cells or to protect normal cells from the effects of radiation. Combined-modality therapy, using both radiation and certain chemotherapeutic agents, also takes advantage of enhanced tumor cell kill. *Chemical modifiers* represent a broad class of agents that include radiosensitizers, radioprotectors, and chemotherapy agents. When used independently, radiosensitizers provide an oxygen substitute to poorly vascularized areas of the tumor that is needed at the time of radiation for the desired effect to occur.

*Radiosensitizers* are compounds that promote fixation of the free radicals produced by radiation damage at the molecular level. The mechanism of this action is similar to the oxygen effect described previously, in which biochemical reactions in the damaged molecules prevent repair of the cellular radiation damage. Free radicals (such as OH+) are captured by the electron affinity of the radiosensitizers, rendering the molecules incapable of repair.

The four most-studied sensitizers are metronidazole (Flagyl), misonidazole (RO-07–0582), etanidazole (SR-2508), and nimorazole. These agents are classified as hypoxic cell sensitizers because they replace oxygen in the chemical reaction that follows irradiation. The two most biologically active radiosensitizing compounds first tested in phase II and III studies were metronidazole and misonidazole. Major side effects of these agents were noted to relate to neurotoxicity, including peripheral neuropathies, somnolence, confusion, and transient coma. Nausea and vomiting are also frequent side effects that appear to be dose related.

Early clinical trials using misonidazole as a radiosensitizer indicated some degree of effectiveness in treatment of squamous carcinoma of the head and neck and uterine cervix. Overall results were disappointing owing to the severe toxicity and only marginal improvement in tumor control.[28] Misonidazole is the only such substance to have undergone extensive clinical trial evaluation. It has been shown to increase the cytotoxicity of alkylating agents, nitrosoureas, 5-fluorouracil (5-FU), cyclophosphamide, and melphalan. Unfortunately, the side effects commonly experienced with these agents are apparently enhanced by the addition of misonidazole. This nonselective enhancement significantly detracts from the potential benefits to be gained.

Etanidazole has been tested, with encouraging results, in early phase II and III trials. This member of the nimorazole group of compounds appears to be less toxic to the CNS tissue than misonidazole and crosses the blood–brain barrier in limited quantity. A phase III study of this agent showed an increased survival in the 2-year local control in N0 and N1 disease with 55% in the etanidazole arm and 37% in the radiation-alone arm.[29]

Nimorazole is a member of the same structural class as metronidazole but is less toxic, allowing for higher doses. A phase III study of nimorazole versus placebo in subjects with squamous cell cancer of the supraglottic larynx and pharynx demonstrated a statistically significant difference (49% versus 33%) in improvement of locoregional control at 5 years posttreatment.[30] In a phase II study of nimorazole in patients with stage III or IV squamous cell carcinoma of the head and neck who received continuous hyperfractionated accelerated radiation therapy (CHART), it was found that local control rates were higher than in other studies using CHART, suggesting a positive effect of nimorazole.[31]

Nonhypoxic cell sensitizers include the halogenated pyrimidines bromodeoxyuridine (BUdR) and iododeoxyuridine (IUdR). These agents are taken up by the DNA of rapidly dividing cells, but their mechanism of action is not completely understood. In a study by Epstein and colleagues,[32] subjects received hyperfractionated radiation with IUdR for locally advanced head and neck cancer. These researchers found a high complete response rate, but hematologic and mucosal toxicities were severe.

Hypoxic cell cytoxic agents include mitomycin-C and tirapazamine. Mitomycin-C is a bioreductive alkylating agent that has been studied in pancreatic and head and neck cancers. Tirapazamine is another bioreductive agent that is preferentially cytotoxic to hypoxic cells in vitro. It differs from oxygen-mimetic sensitizers in that it requires metabolic activation, and enhancement is seen when this agent is given prior to or after radiotherapy.[33] Studies in lung and head and neck cancers have shown positive results. Side effects include nausea, muscle cramps, and hematologic toxicities.[33,34]

Motexafin gadolinium, which is currently being studied in clinical trials, is the first in a class of pharmaceuticals known as *texaphyrins* to reach human testing. Texaphyrins accumulate inside cancer cells owing to their high rate of metabolism and induce programmed cell death. A phase I study of patients who are receiving hyperfractionated irradiation and concurrent 5-FU/cisplatin for head and neck cancer reported interim results recently. Nine of the 10 evaluable patients demonstrated a complete tumor response, and 8 of these remained in complete remission with a median follow-up of 1 year. Side effects reported include mucositis and radiation dermatitis. Motexafin gadolinium has been shown in clinical trials to have a positive impact on patients receiving whole-brain radiation therapy for brain metastasis.[35]

The utility of radiosensitizers in radiation oncology has yet to be determined definitively. Past clinical trials have demonstrated minimal to zero patient benefit and reported toxicities that adversely affected quality of life. The role of radiosensitizers in cancer care is being evaluated today both in clinical trials and in the laboratory setting. Studies are also looking at the roles of gene therapy, biologics (eg, cytokines, hormones, and growth factors), and oxygen therapy and considering how they may work in sensitizing cells.[36]

*Radioprotectors* are compounds that can protect oxygenated (nontumor) cells while having a limited effect on hypoxic (tumor) cells. This selective action serves to increase the therapeutic ratio by promoting the repair of irradiated normal tissues. Repair or return to a nondamaged state takes place through the chemical process of reduction. Free electrons are captured by the radioprotective substance, rendering them unavailable to participate in further chemical reactions that might lead to cellular damage. This process can be viewed as the opposite of what occurs when radiosensitizers are used.

The sulfhydryl groups contained in the nonprotein fraction of most cells aid in the reduction process following radiation damage. Thiophosphate compounds (eg, cysteine and cysteamine) containing sulfhydryl and aminopropyl groups were among the earliest radioprotectors synthesized.

Amifostine (WR-2721) is one of today's most widely studied radioprotectors. The US Army developed this agent initially during the cold war at Walter Reed Army Institute of Research. The project, which began in 1959, sought to identify an agent that could be used to protect military personnel in the event of nuclear warfare.[37] Amifostine selectively protects a broad range of normal tissues, including the oral mucosa, salivary glands, lungs, bone marrow, heart, intestines, and kidney. A phase III study of patients who received radiation therapy for head and neck cancer demonstrated that those who received 200 mg/m$^2$ of amifostine IVP 15 to 30 minutes prior to radiation daily had a statistically significant decrease in acute ($P \leq .001$) and late ($P \leq .0012$) grade II or higher xerostomia. Patients also experienced a statistically significant improvement ($P = .0001$) in the time to onset of grade II xerostomia (30 days versus 45 days).[38] Amifostine may be administered intravenously or subcutaneously and should be dosed daily before radiation therapy. Side effects of this agent include nausea, vomiting, and hypotension. When administered subcutaneously, the side effects may decrease, but the risk of a local injection-site reaction increases. Daily patient assessment, prompt intervention, and symptom management are essential in caring for these patients.[39] Amifostine was the first Food and Drug Administration (FDA) approved radioprotector, and use of this agent has changed over recent years in patients with head and neck cancer owing to the advent of intensity-modulated radiation therapy.

Keratinocyte growth factor (KGF) is a glycoprotein member of the fibroblast growth factor family and a potent stimulant of the proliferation of normal epithelial cells. Clinical trials have investigated its use in patients being treated for metastatic colorectal cancer and in the bone marrow transplant setting to reduce the incidence and/or severity of mucositis from chemotherapy and/or radiation therapy.[40,41] A randomized, double-blind, placebo-controlled study of 212 patients undergoing bone marrow transplant showed a significant reduction in mucositis. The study also found that patients required less use of narcotics and total parenteral nutrition. This agent is currently approved for use in patients undergoing high-dose chemotherapy and radiotherapy for hematologic malignancies.

## COMBINED MODALITY THERAPY

The role of combined modality therapy (CMT) using chemotherapy, biotherapy, surgery, and radiation in combination with one another or at alternating intervals has shown not only clinical benefit but also improvements in disease-free survival, local–regional control, and overall survival. The goal of CMT is to improve quality of life whether it is for cure, control, or palliation by maximizing tumor cell kill.

In 1999, the National Cancer Institute (NCI) announced the results of studies showing that patients who received platinum-based chemotherapy concurrently with daily radiation for cervical cancer had a 30% to 50% increase in survival. These clinical trials changed the standard of care for women receiving treatment for cervical cancer.[42–44] Other studies with chemotherapy and radiation have shown a survival advantage in patients with rectal, head and neck, and lung cancers.[45–47] Vigorous CMT also may allow for organ preservation in some cases.[48]

Chemotherapeutic agents used for their radiosensitizing effect include carboplatin, cisplatin, mitomycin C, navelbine, paclitaxel, docetaxel, and 5-FU. Other potential agents include methotrexate, doxorubicin, vinblastine, VP-16, actinomycin D, and bleomycin. Cisplatin and 5-FU are two of the most commonly used radiosensitizing agents, and temodar is used commonly in patients with brain tumors. In CMT, both radiation and certain chemotherapeutic agents are able to provide a greater cell kill than either therapy could achieve alone. However, CMT has the potential to increase both acute and late toxicities—possibilities that need to be assessed, documented, and managed promptly. It is important to know whether the chemotherapeutic agent selected has overlapping or differing toxicities than what may be expected from the radiation. Organ systems at greatest risk for acute toxicity include the gastrointestinal, integumentary, and myeloproliferative systems. Late effects typically will be experienced at the site of radiation treatment; for example, lung cancer patients may experience fibrosis and/or pneumonitis, and rectal patients may experience proctitis.

The role of targeted therapies is also starting to show promise in this field of combination regimens. Currently, cetuximab, which is a monoclonal antibody, is approved for use in patients with locally or regionally advanced squamous cell carcinoma of the head and neck in combination with radiation therapy.[49] Side effects of this agent may include acneiform rash and pruritus, as well as an infusion reaction while the agent is being administered.[50] Nurses caring for this population need to be able to distinguish between a radiation skin reaction and an acneiform rash because intervention for each of these is different. Additional studies with targeted agents are being conducted in patients with lung, colorectal, and head and neck cancers.[51] Therefore, it is important to know how these agents differ from traditional chemotherapeutic agents because their side-effect profile may not be similar.

One of the most challenging aspects of effectively combining chemotherapy and targeted agents with radiation is determining the optimal timing, sequencing, and dose of each agent/modality.[51,52] Agents may need to be given immediately before or after treatment. Many times surgery may be performed before or after chemotherapy and radiation. Induction or neoadjuvant chemotherapy is given prior to radiation and/or surgery to reduce the size of the tumor before radiation (smaller treatment field) or surgery (reduced amount of tissues removed) takes place. It may decrease the patient's risk of metastasis. Concurrent chemotherapy is given while the patient is undergoing radiation. It may include daily, weekly, or continuous infusion depending on the drug, dose, and known toxicities. Chemotherapy is used during this time to increase the cell kill and maximize the tumor response to radiation. Sequential therapy, often referred to as the *sandwich technique,* also falls under the rubric of concurrent therapy and has been used in clinical trials with lung and head and neck cancers. This approach employs a split course of radiation in which the patient is treated with chemotherapy during a planned break in the total course of radiation. Lastly, adjuvant chemotherapy can be given once a course of radiation is completed to control micrometastases and subclinical disease.

Radiation therapy also may be given preoperatively or postoperatively depending on the site of disease. Preoperative radiation assists in shrinking the tumor prior to surgery, allowing for less extensive resection and increased potential for organ preservation. The issues with this approach are that surgical staging is often affected because the tumor has shrunk, and the patient may be at risk for healing problems at the irradiated site. Postoperative radiation therapy is delivered to patients to reduce their risk of a local recurrence.

Combined modality therapy is used in the treatment of numerous cancers, including squamous cell cancer of the cervix, anus, head and neck, lung, and rectum. Cancers of the bladder, esophagus, pancreas, and stomach frequently are treated with both chemotherapy and radiation therapy in varying schedules. Vigorous CMT has enabled organ preservation for some individuals with carcinoma of the larynx, bladder, or anus.[53,54] Symptom management is critical in caring for these patients because each treatment approach has a unique side-effect profile that may prove to be synergistic or exacerbate the side effects of other treatments.

## HYPERTHERMIA

The use of hyperthermia in conjunction with other types of cancer treatment continues to be studied in clinical trials. The first references to hyperthermia occurred in an Egyptian papyrus scroll 5000 years ago.[3] Current interest focuses on the use of heat with radiation and chemotherapy and the ongoing development of treatment applicators. When hyperthermia is added to radiation, absolute complete-response rates increase 20% to 30%.[55] Hyperthermia has an additive and synergistic effect when radiation is delivered prior to treatment. Its mechanisms of action appear to be complementary to the effects of radiation with regard to inhibition of potentially lethal damage and sublethal damage repair, cell cycle sensitivity, and the effects of hypoxia and nutrient deprivation.[55] Tumor tissues appear to be preferentially sensitized compared with normal tissue. Several biologic effects support the rationale for why heat is more damaging to malignant tumors[3,56–61]:

- Heat is directly cytotoxic.
- Cells in the S phase are considered to be radioresistant and more sensitive to heat.
- The combined effects of radiation and hyperthermia produce greater cell kill than either treatment alone.
- Hypoxic cells that are typically radioresistant have been found to be thermosensitive.
- Cells that have a low pH and are metabolically deprived are more sensitive to heat. Note, however, that cells can adapt to physical changes in 80 to 100 hours and lose their thermosensitivity.
- Heat inhibits the repair of radiation damage, thereby increasing the therapeutic ratio.
- Heat preferentially damages tumor vasculature. After heating, blood flow decreases in tumors but increases in normal tissue.

Hyperthermia may be delivered locally, regionally, or systemically (whole body) depending on the malignancy. It has been used to treat cervix, head and neck, sarcoma, rectal, and breast cancers as well as melanoma. The type of treatment applicator will vary depending on the site of treatment (Figures 12-5 and 12-6). Smaller applicators are used for superficial areas, such as skin cancer, whereas regional/deep applicators are used for deep-seated tumors, such as cervix and rectal cancers.

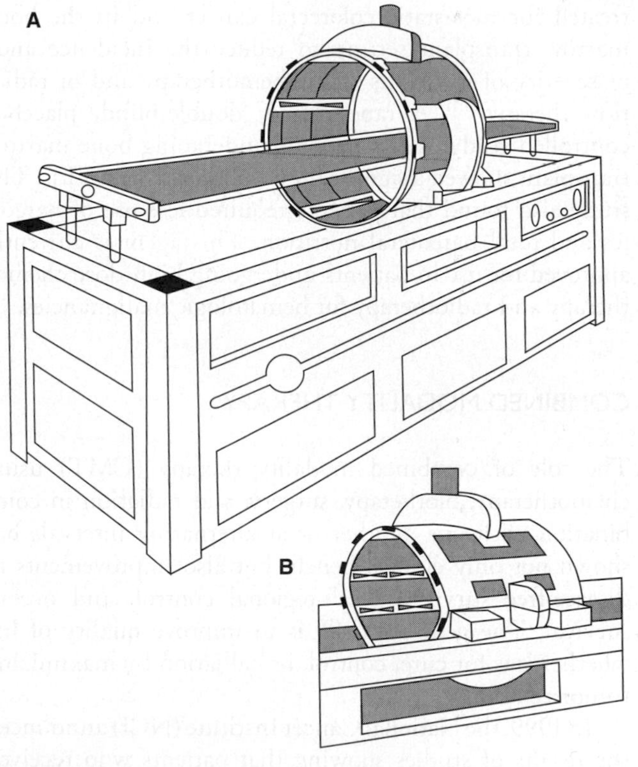


**FIGURE 12-5**

Two models of regional hyperthermia devices used for large treatment areas and tumors that are deep seated. (**A**) Using multiple antennas, widely spread applicators distribute power density and temperature. (**B**) Elliptical shape is more comfortable for the patient. Source: Reprinted with permission from Wust P, Hildebrandt G, Sreenivasa G, et al. Hyperthermia in combined treatment of cancer. Lancet Oncol. 2002;3:487–497.[61]

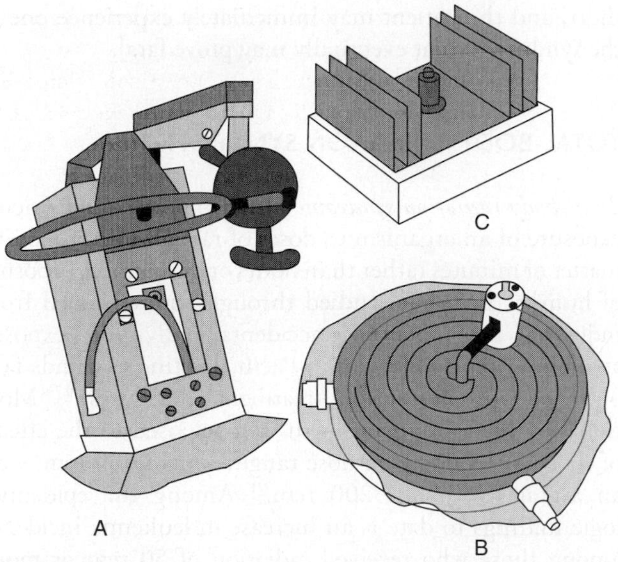


**FIGURE 12-6**

Different treatment devices are used to treat patients with small superficial lesions using local hyperthermia: (**A**) waveguide applicator; (**B**) spiral applicator; (**C**) sheet applicator. Although each device looks different, each holds a water bolus that is used to heat the respective area to be treated. Source: Reprinted with permission from Wust P, Hildebrandt G, Sreenivasa G, et al. Hyperthermia in combined treatment of cancer. *Lancet Oncol.* 2002;3:487–497.[61]

Treatment can last from 60 to 90 minutes, and the goal is to heat the tumor for 30 minutes or longer to a temperature of 40 to 43°C. Thermometry catheters are placed into the tumor itself, on the skin, and/or in a body orifice. Heating may be achieved with ultrasound, low- or high-frequency microwaves, or radiofrequencies. As temperatures increase, the first tissue reaction that occurs is increased blood flow.[55] Thermotolerance is a transient adaptation to thermal stress that renders surviving heated cells more resistant to additional heat stress; it can develop during or after heat stress and can persist for several days.[55]

Treatments may be given twice weekly, once weekly, or monthly depending on the combination with chemotherapy and radiation. Common side effects include first- or second-degree superficial or subcutaneous tissue burns. For patients receiving regional deep hyperthermia, cardiovascular stress owing to a change in pulse and blood pressure will ensue.

Hyperthermia has been shown to have additive and synergistic effects with chemotherapy and radiation therapy. A recent resurgence of interest has inspired studies that have used radiation, chemotherapy, and hyperthermia, as well as chemotherapy and hyperthermia.[58–60] Higher perfusion rates can increase drug delivery and reoxygenation, thereby increasing the efficacy of radiotherapy.[61] For most drugs (excluding 5-FU and perhaps other antimetabolites), the optimal sequence is to administer heat and the drug simultaneously or to give the drug immediately before the onset of heating.[55]

## INCIDENTAL AND ACCIDENTAL RADIATION EXPOSURE

### CHRONIC LOW-DOSE EXPOSURE

Chronic low-dose radiation exposure occurs naturally in the environment owing to background radiation from naturally occurring radioactive substances and cosmic rays. The dose of natural radiation received varies. Urban populations may receive more radiation on a yearly basis from human-made sources, including building materials.[62] It is estimated that the background dose an individual receives each year is approximately 3 mSv.[63] Table 12-5 reviews approximate societal doses of radiation. This exposure is largely unavoidable and is considered to be within safe limits as defined by federal regulations. Although radiation workers are exposed to additional ionizing radiation, the allowable limit is well below that which is known to produce ill effects. Personal dosimeters that monitor the level of exposure one may have are worn by staff working in radiation departments as well as by those who may be caring for patients receiving brachytherapy and radiopharmaceuticals.

Accidental exposure or low-dose exposure may occur in nuclear power plants or among people who handle isotopes. Accidental exposure of industrial radiation workers has been reported in the literature as case reports; in such instances, common injuries include skin changes, bone marrow changes, and chromosome translocations.[64–68]

Regulations require that institutions measure and monitor the radiation exposure to individuals and that they employ ALARA (as low as reasonably achievable) guidelines. Staff caring for patients receiving radiation therapy, as well as those working in radiology departments and on units caring for patients receiving therapy, wear film badges (personal dosimeters) that monitor exposure to radiation. Personnel handling the loading and unloading of radioactive materials may wear ring badges, and depending on the frequency of exposure, pocket ion chambers may be used.

Most of the information concerning the effects of radiation comes from reactor accidents (eg, Chernobyl) or from the atomic bombs dropped in Japan. The prodromal syndrome is immediate and follows whole-body exposure. Symptoms typically include nausea, vomiting, listlessness, headache, and hypotension. The length and severity of this syndrome depends on the amount of exposure. Treatment is primarily supportive and consists of antiemetics, intravenous fluids,

**TABLE 12-5**

**Appropriate Mean Doses Relevant to Societal Low-Dose Radiation-Risk Estimation**

| Exposure | Approximate Mean Individual Dose (mSv) |
|---|---|
| **Some Societally Relevant Exposures** | |
| Round-trip flight, New York–London | 0.1 |
| Single screening mammogram (breast dose) | 3 |
| Background dose owing to natural radiation exposure | 3/year |
| Dose (over a 70-year period) to 0.5 million individuals in rural Ukraine in the vicinity of the Chernobyl accident | 14 |
| Dose range over 20-block radius from hypothetical nuclear terrorism incident (FASEB scenario 1: medical gauge containing cesium) | 3 to 30 |
| Pediatric CT scan (stomach dose from abdominal scan) | 25 |
| Radiation worker exposure limit | 20/year |
| Exposure on international space station | 170/year |
| **Some Low-Dose Epidemiologic Studies** | |
| A-bomb survivors (mean dose in LSS cohort) | 200 |
| Medical x-rays (breast dose in scoliosis study) | 100 |
| Nuclear workers (mean dose from major studies) | 20 |
| Individuals diagnostically exposed in utero | 10 |

*Note*: Absorbed doses in milligrays are numerically the same as equivalent organ doses in millisieverts. *Absorbed dose* is the physicial quantity describing energy deposited per unit mass. For radiation-protection purposes, *equivalent dose* and *effective dose* are used, which include a radiation-dependent weighting factor. For x-rays or gamma rays, 1 mGy = 1 mSv. All doses are effective whole-body doses with the exception of the medical exposures (ie, mammography, CT scan, irradiation for scoliosis), which are to specific organs.

*Source*: Reprinted with permission from Brenner DJ, Doll R, Goodhead DT, et al. Cancer risks attributable to low doses of ionizing radiation: assessing what we really know. *PSNA*. 2003;100:13761–13766.[63]

and pain medications. The latent phase follows a variable course after the prodromal syndrome. With low-dose exposures, the latent phase may last for several weeks, whereas with higher doses, the prodromal and latent phases may be short, and the patient may immediately experience one of the syndromes that eventually may prove fatal.

## TOTAL-BODY RADIATION SYNDROME

*Total-body radiation syndrome* refers to the effects of acute exposure of an organism to doses of radiation received in a matter of minutes rather than hours or days. Acute exposure of humans has been studied through data obtained from industrial and laboratory accidents, individuals exposed at Hiroshima and Nagasaki, Pacific Testing Grounds fallout exposure, and medical treatment procedures.[69,70] More than 100,000 people in Japan were exposed to the effects of the atomic bombs in dose ranges of 0 to 600 rem, with an average of about 200 rem.[71] Among the epidemiologic findings to date is an increase in leukemia incidence among those who received radiation of 50 rem or more. This increase in incidence began 2 years following irradiation, peaked at 7 to 10 years, and returned to control levels after 20 years.[71,72] The April 1986 nuclear accident in Chernobyl, Ukraine, has yielded additional significant information about the somatic effects of exposure to high levels of radioactivity. Researchers generally agree that it takes longer for solid tumors to develop from exposure than leukemia. Total-body radiation syndrome is manifested by the critical effects seen in the hematopoietic, gastrointestinal, and cerebrovascular systems.

Doses of 15 to 200 Gy delivered to the whole body in a short time produce life-shortening or lethal damage through effects on the hematopoietic, gastrointestinal, and central nervous systems. Three types of death from total-body exposure have been delineated:

1. Doses on the order of 100 Gy or higher cause death in a matter of hours from effects on the CNS and cardiovascular collapse.
2. Intermediate doses of 10 to 20 Gy result in death within several days caused by elimination of the intestinal epithelium with intractable diarrhea.
3. Lower doses, from 1 to 5 Gy, result in depopulation of hematopoietic stem cells; death may occur several weeks after the exposure from infection or bleeding.[3]

### Hematopoietic syndrome

Total-body radiation exposure in a single dose ranging from 300 to 800 cGy leads to hematopoietic failure. Stem cells are most susceptible and are sterilized almost immediately on exposure. When the circulating cells begin to die off in a matter of a few weeks, and marrow replacement is insufficient, the crisis and symptoms appear. Generally, within 3 weeks of exposure, the patient experiences chills, fever, fatigue, petechiae, and mouth ulcerations—all symptoms of depressed blood components. Treatment typically includes transfusions, antibiotics, growth factors, and isolation. Death ensues unless marrow recovery or successful transplantation occurs. Ongoing research to treat this syndrome has focused on the use of growth factors, cytokines, and stem cell transplantation.[73]

### Gastrointestinal syndrome

Following total-body exposure to 10 Gy or more, death occurs within a few days to 2 weeks owing to the severity of gastrointestinal damage. The highly radiosensitive intestinal epithelium is essentially denuded of villi, with total loss of the normal cell-renewal mechanism. The patient suffers nausea, anorexia, vomiting, lethargy, and severe, prolonged diarrhea leading to death. Sepsis is a critical issue in this population. Treatment is primarily supportive in nature and includes antiemetics, antimotility agents, intravenous fluids, total parenteral nutrition, narcotics, and antibiotics.

### Cerebrovascular syndrome

No human has survived accidental total-body exposure to more than 10 Gy. At this dosage level, death results from the cerebrovascular consequences. Although the exact mechanism of cerebrovascular death is not clear, symptoms include disorientation, lack of coordination, seizures, visual impairment, hypotension, respiratory distress, renal failure, and coma. This syndrome has short prodromal and latent phases. At this high-dose exposure level, gastrointestinal symptoms also occur almost immediately, and death owing to neurovascular failure occurs in a matter of hours to a few days. Treatment is primarily supportive and consists of oxygen, anticonvulsants, sedatives, intravenous fluids, and narcotics. (For case descriptions of total-body radiation syndrome, see Kato and Schull[69] and Schull.[70])

## RADIATION EFFECTS ON THE EMBRYO AND FETUS

Data regarding fetal and embryonic response to radiation have been obtained primarily from laboratory animals, for the obvious reason that human experimentation is unethical. Information that has become available on human fetal exposure has been acquired from studies of the surviving children who were in utero at the time of the atomic explosions in Nagasaki and Hiroshima.[74–76] Information also has come from medical radiation exposure in the early twentieth century before the fetal dangers were recognized. Radiation is considered a teratogen, and the developing embryo/fetus is more sensitive to the damaging effects of radiation owing to its rapidly dividing cells.

Three critical periods in gestation have been identified: preimplantation, organogenesis, and the fetal period.[62] The classic triad of effects of radiation on the embryo are (1) intrauterine growth retardation (IUGR), (2) embryonic, fetal, or neonatal death, and (3) congenital malformation.[62] The frequency and severity of these effects in an irradiated population depend on a number of factors, including the stage of gestation at which irradiation occurs, the organ systems exposed, LET of the radiation, the total dose (or absorbed-dose equivalent), the dose rate, and fractionation.[62] During preimplantation or shortly afterward, radiation is almost always lethal. Surprisingly, a surviving embryo progresses to normal growth because, at this point in gestation, the only task of the cells is division, not differentiation.

During the next phase, organogenesis, the embryo is at greatest danger of developing malformations following exposure to radiation. Neonatal death is common because multiple abnormalities that result from the radiation exposure are incompatible with life. When radiation exposure occurs during the growth or fetal period (after 6 weeks in humans), the most common effects are overall growth retardation, microcephaly, and mental retardation.[77] Other reported abnormalities in humans include spina bifida, hydrocephalus, blindness, clubfoot, and scalp alopecia.[78] Radioiodine administered to the mother after the embryo/fetus's thyroid has formed may destroy thyroid function, resulting in cretinism if untreated.[79] In the postpartum period, the infant has the ability to recover partially from the growth-retarding effects of high-dose irradiation.[80]

## RADIATION-INDUCED MALIGNANCIES

The carcinogenic effects of radiation, from both chronic low-dose exposure and therapeutic radiation, are of particular interest and concern to the nurse, especially when providing support to the individual who is hesitant about accepting treatment. The key to understanding lies in the fact that acute exposure occurring in radiation accidents is rare, and chronic low-dose occupational or environmental exposure is the exception. The therapeutic doses usually prescribed (in the range of 2500 to 6500 cGy) are believed to be less carcinogenic than lower doses given over a much longer time period. Theoretically, a cell that has survived in a damaged or altered state after low-dose irradiation may undergo carcinogenic mutation in the presence of other conditional factors. At the same time, a cell that has been sterilized or destroyed by therapeutic doses of radiation should be incapable of malignant changes.

Malignancies that have been associated with radiation exposure include skin carcinoma, leukemia, sarcoma, thyroid carcinoma, and lung cancer.[3,81] Other reports have suggested the possibility of inducing breast cancer in females by frequent radiographic exposure for screening for tuberculosis, lung disease, and breast cancer itself.[3,82,83] It is also important to consider the individual factors that contribute to carcinogenesis (eg, lifestyle, geographic location, health history, and genetics). Both pediatric and adult cancer survivors are at greater risk for developing a secondary malignancy based on past treatment and genetics. Nurses caring for patients who have received radiation therapy need to encourage routine screenings and physical examinations, teach proper self-examination techniques, and assist patients in making lifestyle choices that decrease the chance of development of a secondary malignancy.

Radiation carcinogenesis depends on a number of variables but is directly related to the exposure to radiation. These factors include a latent period of 1 to 30 years, radiation dose, concomitant factors in the radiated organism's environment, and the actual fate of the cell as it responds to radiation injury.[84]

## CONCLUSION

The science of radiation oncology and medicine has achieved tremendous advances in the past century, from the early work of the Curies to the development of first-generation linear accelerators. The biologic effects of radiation therapy have long been observed, recognized, and acknowledged but not well understood. Today, researchers continue to investigate population-based exposure (Chernobyl) and the acute and late effects that patients experience while undergoing therapeutic irradiation. The recognition and pursuit of both basic and clinical radiobiologic research have led to the current emphasis on maximizing treatment outcomes while minimizing both early and late effects of treatment. This goal is being achieved with CMT, altered fractionation schedules, reduction in treatment volume and dose, and ever more sophisticated treatment planning and techniques of delivery. With the unraveling of the human genome now complete, the science behind therapy will develop at the molecular level by understanding patients' genetic makeup and tailoring treatments based on their unique profiles.

Knowledge of radiobiologic effects also has led to the expansion of radiation therapy for some nonmalignant conditions. Research in molecular and cellular biology will continue to be of primary importance in radiation oncology and improved cancer treatment.

## REFERENCES


1. Halperin EC, Schmidt-Ullrich RK, Perez CA, et al. Overview and basic science of radiation oncology. In: Perez CA, Brady LW, Halperin EC, Schmidt-Ullrich RK, eds. *Principles and Practice of Radiation Oncology.* 4th ed. Philadelphia: Lippincott Williams & Wilkins; 2004:1–95.
2. Hilderley LJ. Radiation oncology: historical background. In: Hassey-Dow K, Bucholtz J, eds. *Nursing Care in Radiation Oncology.* 2nd ed. Philadelphia: Saunders; 1997:3–5.
3. Hall EJ, Cox JD. Physical and biological basis of radiation therapy. In: Cox JD, Ang KK, eds. *Radiation Oncology.* St. Louis: Mosby; 2003:3–62.
4. Weyrather WK, Debus J. Particle beams for cancer therapy. *Clin Oncol.* 2002;15:S23-S28.
5. Raju MR. Particle radiotherapy: historical developments and current status. *Radiat Res.* 1996;145:391–407.
6. Hilderley LJ. Principles of teletherapy. In: Hassey-Dow K, Bucholtz J, eds. *Nursing Care in Radiation Oncology.* 2nd ed. Philadelphia: Saunders; 1997:6–20.
7. Dunne-Daly C. Principles of radiotherapy and radiobiology. *Semin Oncol Nurs.* 1999;15:250–259.
8. Bergonie J, Tribondeau L. Interpretation of some results of radiotherapy and an attempt at determining a logical technique of treatment. *Radiat Res.* 1959;2:587.
9. McBride WH, Withers HR. Biologic basis of radiation therapy. In: Perez CA, Brady LW, Halperin EC, Schmidt-Ullrich RK, eds. *Principles and Practice of Radiation Oncology.* 4th ed. Philadelphia: Lippincott Williams & Wilkins; 2004:96–136.
10. Gray LH. Radiobiologic basis of oxygen as a modifying factor in radiation therapy. *Am J Roentgenol Radium Nucl Ther.* 1961;85:803–815.
11. Brizel DM, Scher RI, Dewhirst MW. Oxygenation of head and neck cancer: changes during radiotherapy and impact on treatment outcome [abstract]. *Int J Radiat Oncol Biol Phys.* 1998;42:142.
12. Dunst J, Kuhnt T, Strauss HG, et al. Anemia in cervical cancer: impact on survival, patterns of replase, and association with hypoxia and angiogenesis. *Int J Radiat Oncol Biol Phys.* 2003;56:778–787.
13. Kumar P. Tumor hypoxia and anemia: impact on the efficacy of radiation therapy. *Semin Radiat Oncol.* 2000;37:4–8.
14. Dewey WC, Ling CC, Meyn RE. Radiation-induced apoptosis: relevance to radiotherapy. *Int J Radiat Oncol Biol Phys.* 1995;33:781–796.
15. Fuks Z, Haimovitz-Friedman A, Kolesnick RN. The role of the sphyngomyelin pathway and protein kinase C in radiation-induced cell kill. In: DeVita VT, Hellman S, Rosenberg SA, eds. *Important Advances in Oncology 1995.* Philadelphia: Lippincott; 1995:19–31.
16. Kim HE, Han JS, Kasza T, et al. Platelet-derived growth factor (PDGF) signaling mediates radiation-induced apoptosis in human prostate cancer cells with loss of p53 function. *Int J Radiat Oncol Biol Phys.* 1997;39:731–736.
17. Orton C. Radiobiology in brachytherapy: biologic aspects and practical applications. In: Nag S, ed. *Principles and Practice of Brachytherapy.* Armonk, NY: Futura; 1997:51–65.
18. Patel FD, Sharma SC, Negi PS, et al. Low dose rate vs high dose rate brachytherapy in treatment of carcinoma of the uterine cervix: a clinical trial. *Int J Radiat Oncol Biol Phys.* 1994;28:335–341.
19. Clapp KJ. Therapeutic aspects of radiopharmaceuticals. *Oncol Issues.* 2001;16:S9-S10.
20. Order SE, Seigel JA, Lustig RA, et al. Infusional brachytherapy in the treatment of nonresectable pancreatic cancer: a new radiation modality (preliminary report of the phase I study). *Antib Immunoconj Radiopharm.* 1994;7:11–27.
21. Westlin JE, Anderson-Forsman C, Garske U, et al. Objective responses after fractionated infusional brachytherapy of unresectable pancreatic adenocarcinomas. *Cancer.* 1997;80:S2743-S2748.
22. Benkert TA. Bexxar (tositumomab and iodine [$^{131}$I]tositumomab): an investigational drug for the treatment of low-grade and transformed low-grade non-Hodgkin's lymphoma. *Oncol Issues.* 2001;16:S18-S19.
23. Kaminski MS, Zelentz AD, Press OW, et al. Pivotal study of [$^{131}$I]tositumomab for chemotherapy-refractory low-grade or transformed low-grade B-cell non-Hodgkin's lymphoma. *J Clin Oncol.* 2001;19:3918–3928.
24. Zelentz AD, Vose JM, Knox S, et al. Iodine [$^{131}$I]tositumomab for patients with transformed low-grade non-Hodgkin's lymphoma: overall clinical trial experience [abstract]. *Blood.* 1994;94:632.
25. Witzing TE, White CA, Gordon LI. Final results of a randomized, controlled study of Zevalin radioimmunotherapy for B-cell NHL [abstract]. *Blood.* 2000;96:831.
26. Hendrick CS, de Leon C, Dillman RO. Radioimmunotherapy for non-Hodgkin's lymphoma with yttrium-90 ibritumomab tiuxetan. *Clin J Oncol Nurs.* 2002;6:144–148.

27. Wasserman TH, Chapman JD. Radiation response modulation: A. Chemical sensitizers and protectors. In: Perez CA, Brady LW, Halperin EC, Schmidt-Ullrich RK, eds. *Principles and Practice of Radiation Oncology.* 4th ed. Philadelphia: Lippincott Williams & Wilkins; 2004:663–698.
28. Brown JM. Hypoxic cell radiosensitizers: where next? *Int J Radiat Oncol Biol Phys.* 1989;16:987–993.
29. Lee DJ, Cosmatos D, Marcial VA, et al. Results of an RTOG phase III trial (RTOG 85–27) comparing radiotherapy plus etanidazole with radiotherapy alone for locally advanced head and neck carcinomas. *Int J Radiat Onco Biol Phys.* 1995;32:567–576.
30. Overgaard J, Hansen HS, Overgaard M, et al. A randomized double-blind phase III study of nimorazole as hypoxic radiosensitizer of primary radiotherapy in supraglottic larynx and pharynx carcinoma. Results of the Danish Head and Neck Cancer Study (DAHANCA) Protocol 5–85. *Radiother Oncol.* 1998;46:135–146.
31. Henk JM, Bishop K, Shepherd SF. Treatment of head and neck cancer with CHART and nimorazole: phase II study. *Radiother Oncol.* 2003;66:65–70.
32. Epstein AH, Lebovics RS, Van Waes C, et al. Intravenous delivery of 5-iododeoxyuridine during hyperfractionated radiotherapy for locally advanced head and neck cancers: results of a pilot study. *Laryngoscope.* 1998;108:1090–1094.
33. Von Pawel J, von Roemeling R, Gatzemeier U, et al. Tirapazamine plus cisplatin versus cisplatin in advanced non-small cell lung cancer: a report of the international CATAPULT I study group. Cisplatin and tirapazamine in subjects with previously untreated non-small cell lung tumors. *J Clin Oncol.* 2000;18:1351–1359.
34. Lee DJ, Trotti A, Spencer S, et al. Concurrent tirapazamine and radiotherapy for advanced head and neck carcinomas: a phase II study. *Int J Radiat Oncol Biol Phys.* 1998;42:811–815.
35. Pharmacyclics. www.pharmacyclics.com/wt/page/xcytrin. Accessed February 12, 2010.
36. Coleman CN. Chemical sensitizers and protectors. *Int J Radiat Oncol Biol Phys.* 1998;42:781–783.
37. Capizzi RL. The preclinical basis for broad-spectrum selective cytoprotection of normal tissues from cytotoxic therapies by amifostine. *Semin Oncol.* 1999;26:3–21.
38. Brizel DM, Wasserman TH, Henke M, et al. Phase III randomized trial of amifostine as a radioprotector in head and neck cancer. *J Clin Oncol.* 2000;18:3339–3345.
39. Gosselin TK, Pavilonis H. Head and neck cancer: managing xerostomia and other treatment induced side effects. *ORL Head Neck Nurs.* 2002;20:15–22.
40. Spielberger R, Emmanoulides C, Stiff P, et al. Use of recombinant keratinocyte growth factor (rHuKGF) can reduce severe oral mucositis in patients with hematologic malignancies undergoing autologous peripheral blood progenitor cell trans-plantation (auto-PBSCT) after radiation-based conditioning: results of a phase III trial [abstract]. *Proc Am Soc Clin Oncol.* 2003;22:3642.
41. Meropol NJ, Somer RA, Gutheil J, et al. Randomized phase I trial of recombinant human keratinocyte growth factor plus chemotherapy: potential role as mucosal protectant. *J Clin Oncol.* 2003;21:1452–1458.
42. Morris M, Eifel PJ, Lu J, et al. Pelvic radiation with concurrent chemotherapy compared with pelvic and para-aortic radiation for high-risk cervical cancer. *N Engl J Med.* 1999;340:1137–1143.
43. Rose PG, Bundy BN, Watkins EB, et al. Concurrent cisplatinbased radiotherapy and chemotherapy for locally advanced cervical cancer. *N Engl J Med.* 1999;340:1144–1153.
44. Keys HM, Bundy BN, Stehman FB, et al. Cisplatin, radiation, and adjuvant hysterectomy compared with radiation and adjuvant hysterectomy for bulky stage IB cervical carcinoma. *N Engl J Med.* 1999;340:1154–1161.
45. Wolmark N, Wieand HS, Hyams DM, et al. Randomized trial of postoperative adjuvant chemotherapy with or without radiotherapy for carcinoma of the rectum: National Surgical Adjuvant Breast and Bowel Project Protocol R-02. *J Natl Cancer Inst.* 2000;92:388–396.
46. Brizel DM, Albers ME, Fisher SR, et al. Hyperfractionated irradiation with or without concurrent chemotherapy for locally advanced head and neck cancer. *N Engl J Med.* 1998;338:1798–1804.
47. Lara PN, Goldberg Z, Davies A, et al. Concurrent chemoradiation strategies in the management of unresectable stage III non-small-cell lung cancer. *Clin Lung Cancer.* 2002;3:S42-S48.
48. Forastiere AA, Goepfert H, Maor M, et al. Concurrent chemotherapy and radiotherapy for organ preservation in advanced laryngeal cancer. *N Engl J Med.* 2003;349:2091–2098.
49. Bristol-Myers Squibb. http://packageinserts.bms.com/pi/pi_erbitux.pdf. Accessed February 12, 2010.
50. Bonner JA, Harari PM, Giralt J, et al. Radiotherapy plus cetuximab for squamous-cell carcinoma of the head and neck. *N Engl J Med.* 2006;354;567–578.
51. Le QT, Raben D. Integrating biologically targeted therapy in head and neck squamous cell carcinomas. *Semin Radiat Oncol.* 2009;19:53–62.
52. Coleman CN: Clinical radiosensitization: why it does and does not work. *J Clin Oncol.* 1999;17:1–3.
53. Marks L, Carroll P, Dugan T, et al. The response of the urinary bladder, urethra and ureter to radiation and chemotherapy. *Int J Radiat Oncol Biol Phys.* 1995;31:1257–1280.
54. Komaki R. Combined chemotherapy and radiation therapy in surgically unresectable regionally advanced non-small cell lung cancer. *Semin Radiat Oncol.* 1996;6:86–91.
55. Jones EL, Samulski TV, Vujaskovic Z, et al. Hyperthermia. In: Perez CA, Brady LW, Halperin EC, Schmidt-Ullrich RK, eds. *Principles and Practice of Radiation Oncology.* 4th ed. Philadelphia: Lippincott Williams & Wilkins; 2004:699–735.
56. Martin CW, Whitehead T. Radiation modifiers chemical and thermal. In: Watkins-Brumer D, Moore-Higgs G, Haas M, eds. *Outcomes in Radiation Therapy.* Sudbury, MA: Jones and Bartlett; 2001:102–120.
57. Anscher NS, Lee C, Hurwitz H, et al. A pilot study of preoperative continuous infusion 5-fluorouracil, external microwave hyperthermia, and external beam radiotherapy for treatment of locally advanced, unresectable, or recurrent rectal cancer. *Int J Radiat Oncol Biol Phys.* 2000;47:719–724.
58. Jones EL, Samulski TD, Dewhirst MW, et al. A pilot phase II trial of concurrent radiotherapy, chemotherapy, and hyperthermia for locally advanced cervical carcinoma. *Cancer.* 2003;98:277–282.
59. Blackwell K, Vujaskovic Z, Rosen E, et al. A phase I dose escalation study of liposomal doxorubicin, paclitaxel, and hyperthermia in locally advanced breast carcinoma [abstract]. *Proc Am Soc Clin Oncol.* 2002;21:200.
60. Kouloulias VE, Dardoufas CE, Kouvaris JR, et al. Liposomal doxorubicin in conjunction with reirradiation and local hyperthermia treatment in recurrent breast cancer: a phase I-II trial. *Clin Cancer Res.* 2002;8:373–382.
61. Wust P, Hildebrandt G, Sreenivasa G, et al. Hyperthermia in combined treatment of cancer. *Lancet Oncol.* 2002;3:487–497.
62. Ritenour ER. Health effects of low level radiation: carcinogenesis, teratogenesis, and mutagenesis. *Semin Nucl Med.* 1986;16:106–117.
63. Brenner DJ, Doll R, Goodhead DT, et al. Cancer risks attributable to low doses of ionizing radiation: assessing what we really know. *Proc Natl Acad Sci.* 2003;100:13761–13766.
64. Jalil A, Rab Molla MA. Accidental exposure to $^{192}$Ir source in industrial radiography: a follow-up study. *Health Phys.* 1992;62:74–76.
65. Lucas JN, Poggensee M, Straume T. The persistence of chromosome translocations in a radiation worker accidentally ex posed to tritium. *Cytogenet Cell Genet.* 1992;60:255–256.
66. Ramalho AT, Nascimento ACH, Littlefield LG, et al. Frequency of chromosomal aberrations in a subject accidentially exposed to $^{137}$Cs in the Goiania (Brazil) radiation accident: intercomparison among four laboratories. *Mutat Res.* 1991;252:157–160.

67. Raina S, Samuel AM. Isotope angiography and blood pool imaging as a procedure for assessing radiation-induced injuries to the hands. *Clin Nucl Med.* 1992;17:646–651.
68. Scott BR, Lyzlov AF, Osovets SV. Evaluating the risk of death via the hematopoietic syndrome mode for prolonged exposure of nuclear workers to radiation delivered at very low rates. *Health Phys.* 1998;74: 545–554.
69. Kato H, Schull WJ. Studies of the mortality of A-bomb survivors—Mortality, 1950–78: I. Cancer mortality. *Radiat Res.* 1982;90:395–432.
70. Schull WJ. *Effects of Atomic Radiation: A Half Century of Studies from Hiroshima and Nagasaki.* New York: Wiley-Liss; 1995.
71. Beebe GW, Kato H, Land CE. Studies of the mortality of A-bomb survivors: mortality experience of A-bomb survivors, 1950–74. Radiation Effects of Research Foundation, RERF Technical Report No. 1, 1977. http://www.rerf.org.jp/index_e.html. Accessed February 12, 2010.
72. Ishimaru T, Hoshina T, Ichimaru M, et al. Leukaemia in atomic bomb survivors—Hiroshima and Nagaski, 1 October 1950–30 September 1966. *Radiat Res.* 1971;45:216–233.
73. MacVittie TJ. Therapy of radiation injury. *Stem Cells.* 1997;15:S263-S268.
74. Wood JW, Johnson KG, Omori Y. In utero exposure to the Hiroshima atomic bomb: follow-up at 20 years. *Pediatrics.* 1967;39:385–392.
75. Otake M, Schull WJ. In utero exposure to A-bomb radiation and mental retardation: a reassessment. *Br J Radiol.* 1984;57:409–414.
76. Izumi S, Koyama K, Soda M, et al. Cancer incidence in children and young adults did not increase relative to parental exposure to atomic bombs. *Br J Cancer.* 2003;89:1709–1713.
77. Miller RW. Effects of prenatal exposure to ionizing radiation. *Health Phys.* 1990;59:57–61.
78. Dekaban AS. Abnormalities in children exposed to x-radiation during various stages of gestation: tentative timetable of radiation to the human fetus. *Int J Nucl Med.* 1968;9:471–477.
79. Glenn JE. What cancer centers should know about radioactive materials. *Oncol Issues.* 2001;16:S13-S15.
80. Arnon J, Meirow D, Lewis-Roness H, et al. Genetic and teratogenic effects of cancer treatments on gametes and embryos. *Hum Reprod Update.* 2001;7:394–403.
81. March HC. Leukemia in radiologists in a twenty-year period. *Am J Med Sci.* 1950;220:282.
82. MacKenzie I. Breast cancer following multiple fluoroscopies. *Br J Cancer.* 1965;19:1–8.
83. Myrden JA, Hiltz JE. Breast cancer following multiple fluoroscopies during artificial pneumothorax treatment of pulmonary tuberculosis. *Can Med Assoc J.* 1969;100:1032–1034.
84. Bucholtz JD. Radiation carcinogenesis. In: Hassey-Dow K, Bucholtz JD, Iwamoto R, et al., eds. *Nursing Care in Radiation Oncology.* 2nd ed. Philadelphia: Saunders; 1997:57–68.

CHAPTER 13

Susan Weiss Behrend, RN, MSN, AOCN®

# Radiation Treatment Planning

- **Introduction**
- **Overview**
- **Simulation**
  - *Treatment Simulators*
    - Fluoroscopic simulation
    - Computerized tomographic simulation
    - Magnetic resonance imaging simulation
  - *Respiratory Gating*
  - *Patient Education and Preparation*
- **Planning/Localization/Imaging**
  - *Port Films*
  - *Electronic Portal Imaging*
  - *Imaging for Target Definition*
    - Positron emission tomography
    - Multimodality fusion
    - Positron emission tomography/computed tomography fusion
    - Clinical spectroscopy in radiation oncology treatment planning
    - Prostate spectroscopy
  - *Methods of Treatment Delivery*
    - Conformal radiation therapy: 3-dimensional treatment planning
    - Intensity-modulation radiation therapy
    - Image-guided radiation therapy
    - Treatment planning computers
    - On-board imaging
    - B-mode ultrasound acquisition and targeting system
    - Cone beam imaging
    - Fiducial markers
    - Real-time tracking beacons
- **Principles of External Beam Radiation Dosing/Dosimetry**
  - *Dose Delivery of Radiation*
  - *Field-Modifying Instruments*
  - *Tissue Compensation*
- **Patient Positioning/Immobilization Techniques**
  - *Immobilization Devices*
    - Hook-and-loop tape and straps
    - Generic body supports
    - Body casts
  - *Positioning Devices*
- **Delivery of Radiation Therapy: Machines and Equipment**
  - *Linear Accelerator*
    - Collimation
  - *Orthovoltage Units*
  - *Megavoltage Units*
    - External beam units
  - *Machine Design*
  - *Proton Therapy*
- **Treatment Delivery Modalities**
  - *Stereotactic Radiosurgery*
  - *Image-Guided Cyberknife Radiosurgery*
    - Treatment procedure
    - Patient education and preparation
  - *Brachytherapy*
    - Brachytherapy equipment
  - *Unsealed Radionuclide Therapy*
  - *Radioimmunotherapy*
- **Advanced Topics: Treatment Delivery**
  - *Partial Breast Irradiation*
    - MammoSite radiation therapy system
  - *Hypofractionated Whole Breast Irradiation*
  - *High-Intensity Focused Ultrasound*
  - *Selective Internal Radiation Therapy*
- **Conclusion**
- **References**

## INTRODUCTION

Significant advances have taken place within the specialty of radiation oncology treatment planning and delivery since the previous edition of this book was published. Some of the most notable are real-time image-guided radiation therapy, computerized portal imaging systems, computerized tomographic (CT) scans, magnetic resonance imaging (MRI) scans, and positron emission tomography (PET). In addition, the fusion of PET and CT has enhanced treatment planning. Cone beam CT planning techniques are emerging that provide verification data for 3-dimensional image reconstruction. Treatment advances utilizing localization systems such as real-time tracking beacon transponders provide guidance for the identification of organ motion, thus offering enhanced treatment options.

In addition, advanced stereotactic radiosurgical techniques offer the ability to isolate and target circumscribed lesions within anatomic organs, thus providing highly targeted treatment fields. Selective internal radiation therapy (SIRT), or SIR-Spheres, is used to treat unresectable cancers such as hepatic carcinoma or liver metastasis. This treatment modality involves the injection of minute microspheres of radioactive material into arteries that surround a tumor, causing cell death. High-intensity focused ultrasound (HIFU) is another advanced modality that utilizes the technology to heat and destroy pathogenic tissue rapidly. This modality is minimally invasive and utilizes acoustic energy to ablate targeted malignant tissue.

Partial breast irradiation (PBI) and hypofractionated whole breast irradiation are treatment delivery advances with the potential to shorten overall treatment schedules for individuals with early breast cancer. At present, well-designed clinical trials are being conducted into PBI and long-term results for hypofractionation that may result in a change in the standard of care offered for this patient population. This is an exciting concept that will affect quality of life and economics and enhance utilization of radiation treatment resources.

Meticulous treatment planning in radiation oncology is paramount in the successful administration of safe and effective care for individuals receiving therapeutic radiation. It is a specialty that continues to evolve, and advances in treatment planning, delivery, equipment, and professional expertise are integral to the continuum of clinical oncology care.

Radiation oncology nurses need to understand the scientific framework of treatment as well as the equipment used to plan and deliver therapeutic radiation. Radiation therapy centers blend technological and clinical elements. Patient management issues are fundamental to the nursing process and evolve during the course of treatment. The expertise of the multidisciplinary team of radiation oncologists, nurses, medical physicists, dosimetrists, engineers, and radiation therapists is fundamental to meeting the clinical and technological challenges of radiation oncology.

## OVERVIEW

Planning for radiation therapy is a multifaceted process. Initially, a thorough consultation must occur in which the patient and family are introduced to the radiation oncologist and the radiation oncology nurse. Later, the patient meets other members of the multidisciplinary team—dosimetrists, therapists, social workers, and administrative support staff. The initial consultation includes a review of the patient's history, physical and psychosocial assessment, histological reconfirmation of the cancer diagnosis, discussion of treatment options, and educational informed consent.

Treatment recommendations are based on potential for disease response and risk of acute and long-term toxicity. A variety of radiation treatment modalities may be offered, including external beam alone or a combined regimen with internal radiation. The type and length of treatment vary according to the diagnosis, radiation sensitivity of the tumor, and patient performance status. Once these parameters have been considered, the patient is offered a therapeutic plan. Radiation oncologists, in conjunction with medical physicists, develop the radiation prescription. Treatment planning is a detailed and precise process that focuses on obtaining a series of radiographic studies to identify tumor type, size, and location. Simulation involves pretreatment filming, which, guided by a computerized planning program, circumscribes the tumor and locoregional organs and tissues. This information is used to determine the exact dose required for the target volume and surrounding normal tissues.

At the first appointment, the simulation procedure may require 1 to 2 hours. Thus, to allay anxiety, the patient should be prepared for an extended visit. At this time, the treatment field is identified and measured. Indelible small tattoos are placed on the patient's skin to mark the treatment area and enable daily replication of the target treatment field. Patients should be made aware that they will be partially disrobed during the simulation and daily treatments. The patient may be required to drink radio-opaque contrast or have intravenous contrast injected to enhance visualization of the tumor during simulation. In addition, mold-room technicians may create customized blocks and immobilization devices to shield vital organs from scattering radiation and to secure the patient's safety. At this time, the physician will obtain final informed consent. Depending on the facility's policy, the patient may be required to return for a treatment setup prior to the initial dose so that the plan can be checked methodically before actual administration. The aforementioned events can create tremendous anxiety for patients and families,[1] so it is incumbent on the professional radiation oncology nurse to provide an environment where patients feel physically comfortable and psychosocially supported.

During the initial consultation, the patient and family learn about the treatment process. The patient is required to maintain the same position throughout the treatment session. The machinery (typically a linear accelerator [LINAC]) rotates around the patient, and the average treatment time varies between 10 and 15 minutes. The radiation beam is odorless, colorless, and painless. The patient is comfortably situated alone in the treatment room and is monitored from the therapist's control station with audiovisual cameras. Some patients may require pretreatment medication with antiemetics, steroids, or analgesics. Pediatric patients may need sedation or anesthesia to diminish the risk of movement during the treatment session.[2]

The typical treatment course is daily for 5 days and varies in the total number of weeks. Frequent planning films are obtained and checked to monitor beam placement. In addition, weekly appointments are scheduled for all patients on treatment so that the radiation oncology nurse and the radiation oncologist can assess them for development of acute toxicities and overall status.

Radiation planning and simulation depend on highly accurate measurements of patient anatomy to provide for differences in dose distribution. Dosimetric planning requires expert medical physicists, dosimetrists, and equipment. The data required by the physicists to plan treatment include body contour, outline and depth of internal structures, and location and size of the target.[3] Patient contours can be determined using mechanical, optical, ultrasonic, and CT equipment. The patient's contour must be assessed in the same position as the one proposed for actual treatment. In addition, the tabletop should be included in the contour as a reference for beam angles, and bony landmarks and beam entry points should be indicated. Body contour should be continuously checked throughout the treatment in anticipation of changes due to tumor response or weight change. These quantitative data complement the qualitative diagnostic radiographic findings that are essential for the identification of realistic contours. Several radiographic techniques and devices are used for localizing internal structures to facilitate treatment planning.

Key components of the treatment planning process are as follows:

- Initial consultation—evaluating overall diagnosis and establishing goals of treatment
- Simulation—imaging and determining treatment and target volume
- Localization—identifying critical anatomic structures
- Planning/imaging/dosimetry—determining treatment volume, total dose, and fractionation schedule
- Establishing patient position and specific immobilization devices, as well as confirmation of treatment plan and delivery

Professional radiation oncology planning team members ask the following questions:

- How does radiation integrate into a multidisciplinary care plan for the patient?
- What is to be treated?
- Where is the target located?
- What critical anatomic structures surround the target?
- What is the size/volume of the target?

The team allows for planning optimal dose distribution, field delineation, and shaping.

## SIMULATION

### TREATMENT SIMULATORS

#### Fluoroscopic simulation

Traditional treatment simulators are x-ray machines that have the ability to duplicate the geometry and mechanics of radiation treatment machines. These treatment simulators display treatment fields, ensuring the location of the target volume while identifying surrounding normal tissues and thereby protecting them from excessive radiation. Conventional treatment simulators use fluoroscopy as an imaging system to visualize target and volume to enhance internal structures. Because 3-dimensional treatment planning requires a complete CT scan data set, conventional simulators have largely been replaced with CT simulators.

In the past, radiographs were taken of the treatment field, customized block templates were drawn on these films by the radiation oncologist, and mold-room technicians used these films to create customized lead blocks to protect normal tissues from the radiation beams.[4]

Simulators are critical to the delivery of radiation therapy. The use of simulators evolved for 3 reasons: the relationship between the radiation beam and external and internal anatomy cannot be assessed by diagnostic radiology; the radiographic quality of the treatment machines is not sophisticated enough to be used for precise field localization; and the use of a treatment machine for field localization is impractical and creates time constraints.

Potential problems with patient treatment setup can be identified and solved during simulation. In addition, anatomic contours and thickness relating to tissue compensators or bolus designs can be obtained during simulation. The simulator can determine the adequacy of the fabrication of shielding blocks. Laser lights, contour makers, and shadow trays are equipment accessories for simulators that facilitate these functions.[3]

#### Computerized tomographic simulation

In the past, CT and simulation were separate pretreatment planning procedures. Today, they are a combined entity for radiation treatment planning. A CT simulator is a single diagnostic treatment planning machine that combines both procedures in a single unit. In addition, CT simulation offers the advantages of increased speed, efficiency, and accuracy of treatment planning and delivery.

To accomplish this procedure, the patient is placed on the CT simulator table, and the tumor and normal structures are outlined on each CT slice. A computer performs a 3-dimensional transformation of the CT slices and creates a digitally reconstructed radiograph (DRR).[5]

The DRR resembles a normal diagnostic film, but the images are digital and can be manipulated to improve contrast and detail (Figure 13-1). Radiation oncologists draw blocks directly on the DRR to accurately differentiate the tumor from normal surrounding tissue. The mold room uses the DRR to construct blocks. The DRR and all CT slices and outlines are then digitized into the treatment planning computer. A popular mode for retrieval and monitoring of DRRs entails the use of a local area network (LAN), which enables physicians to obtain DRR and port film images on their desktop computers to ensure clinical quality assurance.[6]

Computer and other technological advances have also provided radiation oncology with the advantages of 3-dimensional conformal radiation therapy (3D-CRT).[7] The virtual simulator is used to simulate the therapy machine and operates on a digital representation of the patient. Today, virtual simulation software is widely available for clinical treatment planning.[8] The process of virtual simulation differs from that of conventional simulation, yet still accomplishes the development of a fully documented beam arrangement. Patients are immobilized in hemibody foam torso casts and custom foam head supports with thermal plastic face masks. Next, they are placed in the immobilization device and then registered electronically with the monitoring equipment on a CT scanner table. Head casts are secured to the CT table by use of a head holder. The body casts are also registered for daily alignment using lasers. A coordinate system is used to localize objects and is tailored to the individual patient (Figure 13-2).

Once the CT scans have been completed, the structures to be treated, target volumes, and surrounding anatomy to avoid are identified. Structures are outlined on a computer display of the scans. These outlines delineate the parameters for creating 3-dimensional graphical displays and for performing volume and target delineation (Figure 13-3).[9]

Virtual simulation is similar to physical simulation in that it requires a machine that can imitate the motions of the actual treatment machine. The virtual simulator display has 7 panels that provide a superset of the functions of both a conventional simulator and a treatment machine. The unit control panel provides the same functions as the traditional simulator. The table can be oriented along 3 axes, the collimator or gantry can be rotated, and the jaws of the machine can be opened or closed by operating the corresponding control with a computer mouse. Documentation of conventional simulation consists of chart notes, simulation films, and skin marks. Virtual simulation documentation is related to these parameters and includes beam parameter settings and hardcopy block templates for the

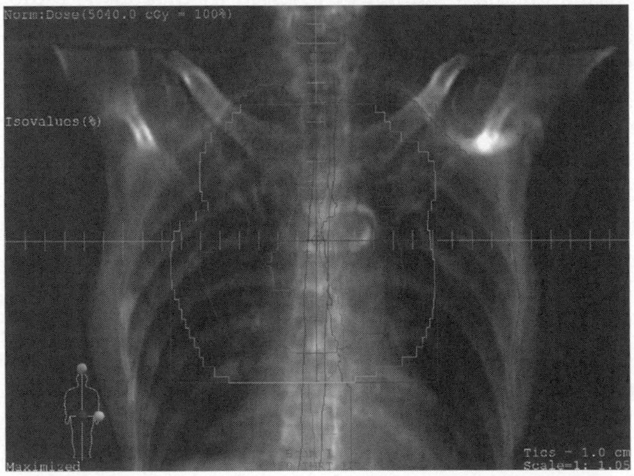


**FIGURE 13-1**

A digitally reconstructed radiograph of the chest is used for radiation therapy planning and documentation of radiation treatment fields.

*Source*: Photo courtesy of Fox Chase Cancer Center, Philadelphia, PA.

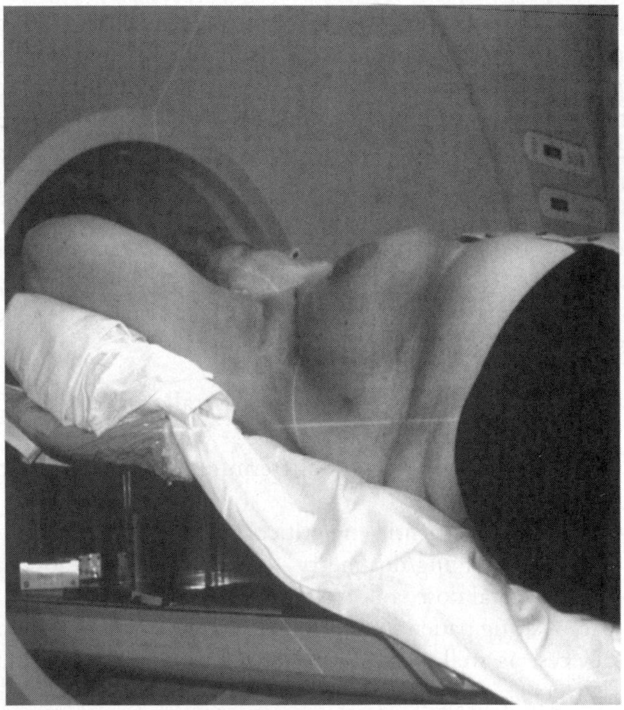

**FIGURE 13-2**

Patient in supine position for computed tomography simulation with alpha cradle immobilization and angled breast board.

*Source*: Photo courtesy of Fox Chase Cancer Center, Philadelphia, PA.

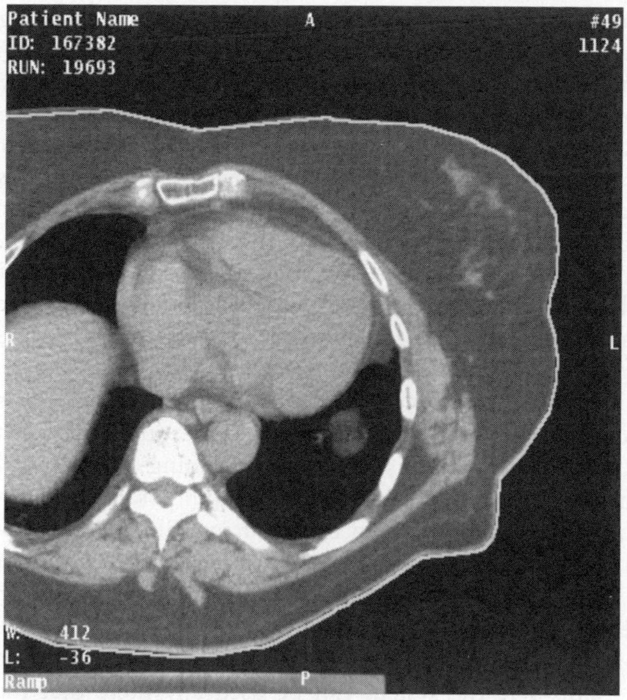


**FIGURE 13-3**

Computed tomography volume and target delineation.

*Source*: Photo courtesy of Fox Chase Cancer Center, Philadelphia, PA.

block fabrication room or multileaf collimator (MLC) parameters. These are communicated over a computerized network that controls the MLC subsystem.[10]

Virtual simulation provides for the exact identification of structures that can be visualized on CT scans as well as conformation of beam outlines to target shapes with small margins from any direction. Note that some precautions need to be considered when using this advanced practice technique. For instance, patient motion and internal organs are sometimes not visualized as clearly on virtual simulation as on fluoroscopic simulation. It is important to be aware of the potential for daily error due to the diminished visualization of structures. Virtual simulation often results in a CT study of more than 100 scans, which is a large amount of data to review to form contours of structures. In addition, virtual simulation is sometimes unable to provide a well-defined clinical target volume (CTV) for some tumor sites. In this event, it becomes necessary for radiation oncologists and dosimetrists to rely on the natural history of the patient's disease to identify the appropriate CTV. Virtual simulation is integral for conformal treatment planning and for achieving complicated configurations (Figure 13-4).

Computerized tomographic simulation is necessary for 3-dimensional treatment planning, conformal field shaping, MLC, and electronic portal imaging (EPI). CT simulators are capable of imaging patient anatomy and gross

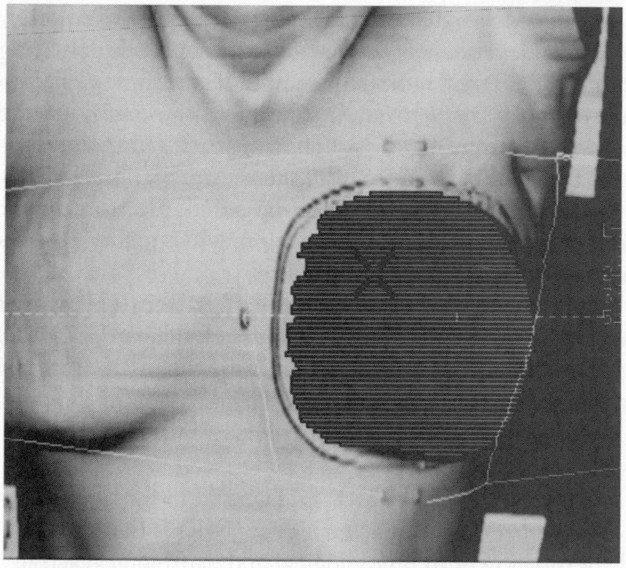

**FIGURE 13-4**

Virtual simulation used for conformal treatment planning. The target volume is the clinically defined breast tissue.

*Source*: Photo courtesy of Fox Chase Cancer Center, Philadelphia, PA.

tumor in anatomic slices. This facilitates views in multiple planes and also in 3 dimensions. CT simulators should be dedicated within radiation oncology departments because therapeutic CT simulators differ from conventional diagnostic CTs. The former use a rigid couch for reproducibility of patient position, the aperture is wider (80 cm) for flexible positioning of patients limbs if necessary, and dedicated radiation oncology therapists are trained to operate CT simulators. Proper patient alignment (using wedges or bolsters) is pivotal for exact positioning in order to determine the treatment field precisely.[11]

Computerized tomographic simulators are equipped with flat tables, laser lights for positioning, and immobilization and image registration devices. Once a CT simulation data set is generated, it provides precise localization of anatomy and tissue density. This information is key for generating treatment planning guidelines for an individual patient. The CT simulator is used to locate the target and isocenter and determine beam configurations. In addition, the CT simulator extracts the internal anatomy from 3-dimensional images, and beams are interactively visualized with a 3-dimensional display to produce a virtual simulation.

## Magnetic resonance imaging simulation

Magnetic resonance imaging simulators are now being used to enable more accurate delineation of targets and critical normal structures where clinically indicated.

Magnetic resonance imaging identifies bulk magnetization of nuclei within a given volume through the use of radiofrequency radiation and magnetic fields. A stationary magnetic field orients the spins of nuclei in the region being studied. Pulses of radiofrequency radiation are applied to perturb these magnetization states, and the nuclei acquire discrete amounts of energy. Following each pulse, the relaxation times for the spins to return to the orientation forced by the stationary magnetic field are measured. Electromagnetic radiation is emitted during relaxation. MRI quality depends on variables used during acquisition.

Magnetic resonance imaging differs from CT as it is not constrained to axial acquisition of image data. MRI has been documented as being advantageous in defining targets, with the most benefit in visualizing and targeting tumors in the central nervous system (CNS), head and neck, and prostate.[12]

Functional MRI (fMRI) is also used to facilitate radiation treatment plans. The benefit of fMRI is that it is capable of showing both physiological and neurological activity. fMRI techniques detect changes in blood flow associated with activation of specific regions of the brain. Functional imaging of the brain is capable of mapping the following important information: visual system, semantic processing areas, and sensory and motor cortex. The capability of fMRI to identify the neuropsychological activation sites prior to irradiation can significantly lower morbidity related to post-treatment function (Figure 13-5).

Magnetic resonance imaging provides better soft tissue views than CT. A CT scan is often coregistered with MRI scans in order to facilitate daily localization and position verification.[13]

## RESPIRATORY GATING

Respiratory gating is a technology that synchronizes radiation treatment regimens to the patient's respiratory cycle. It increases the accuracy of cancer radiotherapy by adjusting for tumor movements caused by respiration-induced movement. Varian Medical Systems' CT option for a real-time position management (RPM) respiratory gating system turns off the radiation beam used in therapy when a tumor moves outside the treatment area. The CT option extends gating to the CT scanner so that diagnostic imaging can be correlated with the gating system that controls the LINAC. RPM respiratory gating technology provides treatment planning information that allows for the reduction of the radiation field to avoid hitting healthy, critical tissues while delivering high doses to tumors.

High-resolution conformal radiation therapy requires accurate tumor localization for identification of distinct tumor contours. This treatment planning process will maximize the dose delivered to the tumor while minimizing the dose administered to the surrounding healthy tissue. Physiological functions such as respiration can cause a change in the tumor position during treatment, which requires the use of a larger treatment volume to compensate for tumor movement.

This versatile system can be used anywhere that the effects of respiratory motion are encountered—eg, the lung, breast, liver, pancreas, kidney, and pelvis. Respiratory gating quickly and easily monitors respiration without compromising patient comfort. A video monitoring device is used to characterize the patient's breathing pattern. The pattern is obtained by tracking the motion of a lightweight, retroreflective marker placed on the patient.[14] This respiration-related signal is derived from a transducer operated by the patient or from the CT scanner. The signal is fed into the CT system to be used as a gating mechanism for data acquisition (Figure 13-6).

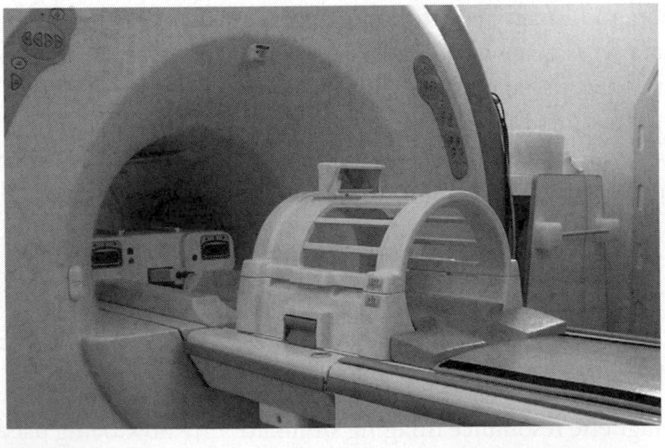

**FIGURE 13-5**

Magnetic resonance imaging simulator with head coil.

*Source:* Photo courtesy of Fox Chase Cancer Center, Philadelphia, PA.

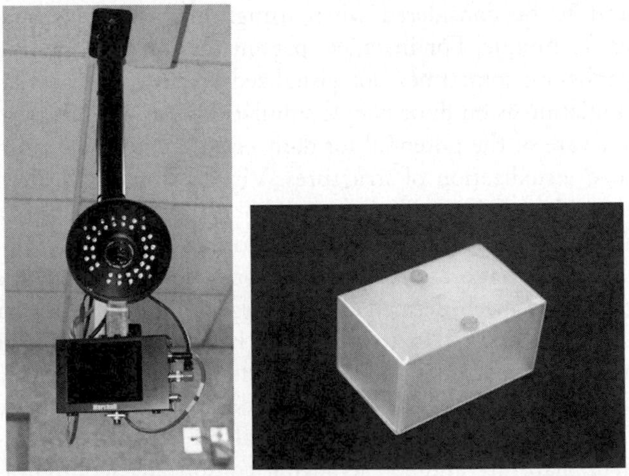

**FIGURE 13-6**

(**A**) A ceiling-mounted gating camera. (**B**) Abdominal gating sensor.

*Source:* Photos courtesy of Fox Chase Cancer Center, Philadelphia, PA.

Next, through video image analysis and signal processing, the system identifies both the full range of chest wall motion during respiration and the normal pattern of that motion. By correlating these data with the motion of the tumor in simulation, a treatment plan can be created that turns the treatment beam on only when the tumor falls within the planned beam aperture. Throughout this process, the RPM respiratory gating system allows the patient to breathe naturally and comfortably (Figure 13-7).[14]

Unanticipated patient movement during treatment such as sneezing and coughing could interfere with the normal operation of the respiratory gating system. The system, therefore, features a predictive filter that analyzes the patient's respiration, establishes a baseline respiratory pattern, and detects any deviations from the expected pattern. Deviations from this pattern result in an automatic hold of treatment delivery until the baseline respiratory pattern is reestablished.[15]

Accurate treatment gating must be supported by a LINAC with a high-speed digital control system. These features provide less than 100 millisecond beam-on times with accurate gated dose rates and uncompromised beam flatness and symmetry.[15]

The respiratory gating system should be integrated with dynamic MLC. Treatment beam gating holds the MLC motion during beam-off times, even during dynamic conformal therapy treatments and intensity-modulated radiation therapy (IMRT). Leaf motion continues during the beam-on time, with precise registration to the MLC shape defined for treatment delivery. The objective of improved patient positioning accuracy is achieved using an integrative approach to treatment planning with the RPM respiratory gating system.[14]

## PATIENT EDUCATION AND PREPARATION

Patients need to know that respiratory gating during treatment planning is available in certain centers. They should be made aware that not all individuals are candidates for this treatment planning modality. The need to comply with specific breathing instructions may preclude some individuals with compromised respiratory status from participating. No risks or side effects are inherent in this treatment planning technique, but the time required for planning using respiratory gating is longer than that for conventional treatment planning. Patients should be assessed for candidacy and should be provided with succinct, yet complete, written and verbal information regarding the details of how respiratory gating systems are used to enhance radiation treatment planning and to ultimately improve disease response.

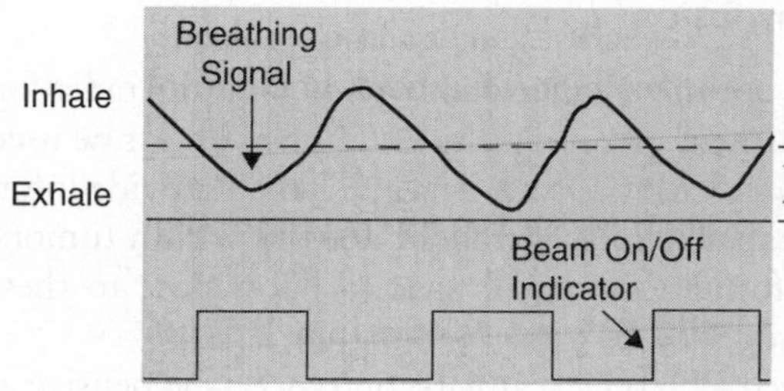


**FIGURE 13-7**

Gated treatment—synchronizing radiation beam with respiration cycles.

*Source*: Photo courtesy of Fox Chase Cancer Center, Philadelphia, PA.

# PLANNING/LOCALIZATION/IMAGING

## PORT FILMS

Port films are radiographic images taken by linear accelerators to verify treatment fields. Although these high beam energies do not produce images as detailed as standard diagnostic radiographs, they provide necessary information about treatment accuracy and quality.[4] Weekly port films should be considered mandatory for departmental quality assurance purposes. Patients frequently ask the radiation oncology nurse about the results of the "x-rays," or the port films. Nurses need to educate patients and families about the specific purpose of the port films, explaining that tumor filming for diagnostic and staging purposes occurs at the completion of treatment and beyond.

## ELECTRONIC PORTAL IMAGING

Precise imaging forms the basis for radiation oncology treatment planning. Changes and enhancements in imaging have facilitated the delivery of 3-dimensional dose distributions in radiation therapy. Imaging assesses location and extent of disease, and guides treatment planning and delivery. The most important advance in imaging is the ability to visualize patient anatomy in tomographic planes. Imaging is important to define tumor volume and shape and location of adjacent organs. CT scans provide tissue density data, and this information is used for dose calculations. Serial imaging is used to view and account for variations in tumor and normal organ position, and this facilitates complex treatment plans that spare normal tissue.[16]

Advances in radiation therapy such as IMRT and charged particle beam therapy require precise imaging of stationary and moving targets. With image-guided radiation therapy (IGRT) images are obtained daily during treatment and account for variations in organ motion and patient or plan setup.

As treatment delivery has advanced, so has the need to refine imaging techniques that account for positional and physiological variation with dynamic targets. Prescribing the appropriate dose depends directly upon sophisticated imaging capabilities to identify the target and critical surrounding tissues and structures to be spared.

Imaging is used to minimize uncertainties related to patient setup error and variations in target and organ motion. Images obtained during treatment planning are either acquired or processed. Acquired images include tomographic data such as CT scans, MRI, PET, SPECT, ultrasound (US), plane films, and electronic portal images. Processed images are derived from acquired anatomic image data. These include DRRs and volume-rendered images.[17]

## IMAGING FOR TARGET DEFINITION

### Positron emission tomography

Positron emission tomography is a nuclear medicine image that provides a 3-dimensional map of functional processes in the body. PET scanning is based on the positron-electron annihilation of photons. To obtain a PET scan, a short-lived radioactive tracer isotope is injected into the patient. This tracer is chemically incorporated into a biologically active molecule and eventually decays, emitting a positron. The molecule most commonly used is fluorodeoxyglucose (FDG) a sugar that incorporates $^{18}F$ as the positron-emitting isotope. FDG is a glucose analog that accumulates in metabolically active cells. Tumor cells are known to be active metabolically; hence, FDG uptake is positively correlated with presence of tumor cells. A waiting period of approximately 1 hour follows while the active molecule becomes concentrated in tissues before scanning occurs.[18]

As the radioisotope undergoes positron emission decay it emits a positron. Once the positron travels a few millimeters, it encounters and annihilates with an electron, producing a pair of annihilation $\gamma$-photons moving in opposite directions. These are detected when they reach a scintillator material in the scanning device, creating a burst of light. Photons that do not arrive in pairs are ignored. When the paired photons are detected, computer software reconstructs the site of the annihilation and the surrounding anatomy is imaged.[18]

Positron emission tomography scans are often read with CT or MRI scans. The fusion of either PET/CT or PET/MRI provides visualization of both anatomic and metabolic information. PET imaging has been found to be most useful together with anatomic imaging; therefore, PET scanners are now available with integrated high-end multidetector-row CT scanners. When PET and CT are done at the same time, on the same machine, the sets of images are more precisely registered, so areas of abnormality on the PET can be correlated with anatomy on the CT images.

Combining PET with CT scanning has become common practice. It is clinically advantageous to do so for the following reasons:

- It is possible to differentiate malignant tumors from normal tissue due to metabolic differences.
- PET images provide information for tumor staging.
- PET can be used to track the tumor's response to treatment.
- Simultaneous scanning does not require repositioning of the patient, which minimizes position errors.
- PET/CT fusion makes the modalities complementary.
- The resolution of the CT complements the physiological information about the tumor.

These advantages are pivotal in radiation oncology treatment planning. With fused scans the images provide high accuracy that enables the radiation oncology team to plan treatment targets in a highly efficient manner.[19]

### Multimodality fusion

The ability to correlate 3-dimensional images from various common imaging modalities (CT, MRI, and PET) has become a valuable tool in the practice of radiation oncology. Specialized computer software enables multimodality fusion and provides clinicians with the ability to identify structures in one imaging modality and then spatially register the structures in a different modality. The most frequently used 3-dimensional imaging modalities for treatment planning in radiation therapy are CT and MRI. Computerized tomography imaging is fast and cost-effective, and it provides high resolution between structures.[20]

The clinical application of multimodality image fusion will continue to be refined as imaging techniques and computer support evolve. This radiation planning technique has the potential to provide patients with the most exact treatment plan, which will enhance efficacy and minimize side effect profiles.

### Positron emission tomography/computed tomography fusion

In order to optimize the technology of PET for radiation therapy treatment planning, the PET images must be used in conjunction with CT scan data. PET data provide information on rapid cellular metabolic activity within tumors, and this information can be used to boost dose to these areas (Figure 13-8).

Combined PET/CT scanners are twice as expensive as single PET scanners. Therefore, a PET/CT scanner must be used for considerable volume to justify the cost. Scheduling of PET scans involves preapproval by insurance carriers and documentation of specific rationale for requesting a PET study. Many institutions maintain separate imaging

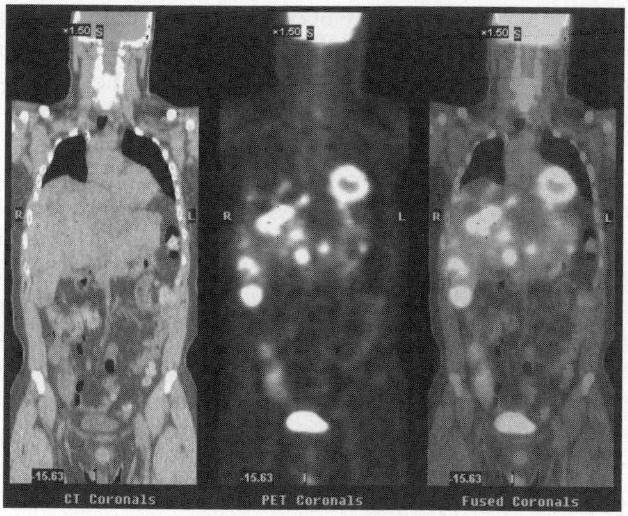


**FIGURE 13-8**

Fused positron emission tomography/computed tomography image.

*Source*: Photo courtesy of Fox Chase Cancer Center, Philadelphia, PA.

capabilities, and fusion of the images is done by specialized computer software.

Positron emission tomography/computerized tomography will continue to be used in oncology to diagnose, stage, plan, treat, and monitor response to therapy. In the future, dedicated PET cameras could be mounted in treatment rooms to record radiation dose to the tumor. Since it is known that positrons can be emitted from within irradiated tumor, detection of unstable positron nuclei may be used to monitor the location of the deposited dose of radiation to the tumor. This information may assist the radiation oncology team in the future to potentially boost the dose to the tumor site, thereby achieving higher treatment volume. This is a future application and not yet available clinically.[20]

## Clinical spectroscopy in radiation oncology treatment planning

Single photo emission computed tomography is a nuclear medicine tomographic imaging technique using xrays. SPECT provides 3-dimensional images, which distinguishes it from conventional nuclear medicine imaging. MR spectroscopy (MRS) is a relatively new imaging technique used in radiation planning. It is used to visualize brain and prostate tumors by providing clinical measurement of chemicals within these organs. Tissue sampling and the use of radioactive tracers are not required; therefore, the study is safe and can be repeated.

Spectroscopy uses gradients to produce excitement in a small volume of tissue and then records free induction decay and ultimately produces a spectrum from that voxel. A voxel is a basic unit of CT reconstruction, represented as a pixel in a CT image display. Through this mechanism certain metabolites in the brain and prostate gland can be analyzed. This produces information about tumor composition and grade and tracks changes over time.[21]

Magnetic resonance spectroscopy requires a high-strength magnet with the ability to suppress water protons, which are several thousand times higher in number than protons on other molecules. Therefore, water protons must be suppressed in order to distinguish the other metabolites in the brain. This suppression is done by the application of a very narrow bandwidth of frequency to the water proton that will suppress or spoil the signal from the water to the conducting coil. In this way, the crucial metabolites for target planning can be distinguished.[21]

There are prominent brain metabolites evaluated in proton spectroscopy are the following. *N*-acetyl-aspartate (NAA), which has a peak of 2.0 on the PPM scale, is a marker of mature neuronal density and viability. In normal tissue NAA is the highest of the peaks, and it is decreased in tumor tissue because malignant cells replace healthy neurons. Choline is a metabolite that has a peak of 3.2 on the PPM scale; it is an indicator of membrane activity and is useful for cancer detection. The third peak in the brain is that of creatinine, an energy marker, which is at 3.0 on the PPM scale. Creatinine is relatively constant throughout the brain, and it tends not to change significantly during the treatment course. Therefore, it is used as a reference marker when the levels of the metabolites are compared.[21]

Several methods exist for acquiring MRS data in radiation planning. One method is known as single voxel spectroscopy. The larger the voxel, the higher the signal. A realistic goal of patient care is to maximize the quality of the SPECT but limit the time patients are required to spend in the magnet. Spectroscopy always visualizes small areas of interest, so both diseased tissue and adjacent normal tissue are viewed together as a control.

Spectroscopy can also yield 2-dimensional and 3-dimensional views. These views allow for multiple slices in several dimensions. With multiple dimensions, more area of interest can be studied; however, because there are so many data to cover, the image takes more time to attain. Also the spectrum has a more significant signal-to-noise ratio than in single voxel or 2-dimensional spectroscopy.

In an MRS of a normal brain, a 3-dimensional scan will demonstrate peak NAA as very high, and the choline and creatinine peaks are about the same size. This is a metabolic signature spectrum of a normal brain (Figure 13-9). An MRS of a brain with metastasis will show completely different spectra, with a choline peak that has doubled and, therefore, indicates metastatic disease (Figure 13-10).

Lactate is another metabolite that is useful in evaluating intracranial malignancy. Lactate is a lipid, and the detection of it indicates that normal metabolic respiration of tissue

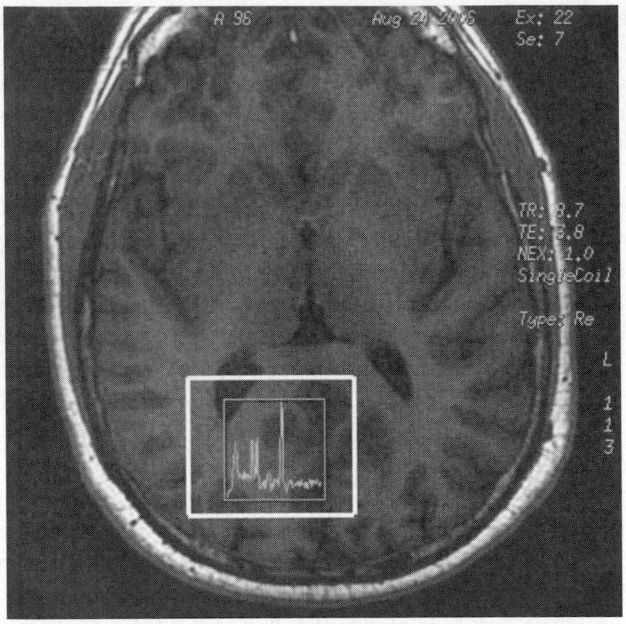


**FIGURE 13-9**

Magnetic resonance spectroscopy of a normal brain—choline and creatinine peaks are equal height, N-acetyl-aspartate (NAA) is high, this is a metabolic signature of a normal brain.
*Source*: Photo courtesy of Fox Chase Cancer Center, Philadelphia, PA.

has been altered. This may occur in highly active cellular lesions that outgrow their blood supply and enter into an anaerobic metabolic state. Necrotic tissue in tumors exhibits lipid metabolites; this can be identified with MRS.[21]

Magnetic resonance spectroscopy is a new and potentially valuable imaging technique, particularly for brain lesions. With MRS it is now possible for suspicious lesions in the brain to be closely followed before they manifest into large symptomatic tumors. Spectroscopy can map lesions that are suspicious for malignancy but may have only vascular presentations. This tracking method can be invaluable for recording potential activity of malignant lesions before symptoms are clinically established. In addition, MRS can incorporate areas of metabolic abnormality into treatment planning and provide effective target volumes with nonuniform margins that are highly targeted for treating tumor cell infiltration, rather than just providing target volumes with uniform margins. This can be very important for postoperative patients requiring treatment to a surgical bed.

## Prostate spectroscopy

In specific clinical situations prostate spectroscopy is done after MRI simulation to enhance treatment planning. First the patient has an MRI simulation using a body coil, in which a 3-mm slice thickness is obtained through the pelvic

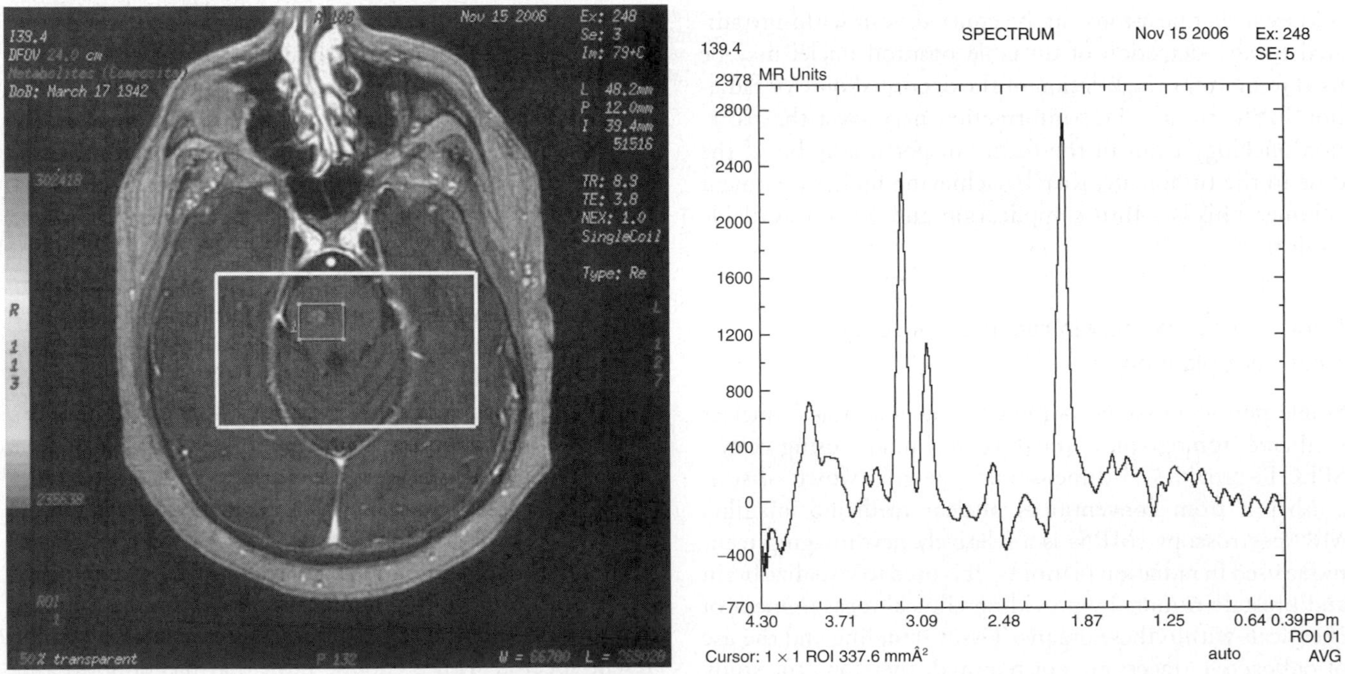


**FIGURE 13-10**

Magnetic resonance spectroscopy of brain metastasis—the choline peak doubled which is the marker for metastatic disease.
*Source*: Photo courtesy of Fox Chase Cancer Center, Philadelphia, PA.

region. This scan is then fused to a CT scan for treatment planning. Upon completion of the treatment planning the MRS occurs.

Prostate cancers usually are not distributed uniformly within the prostate gland. It is possible with IMRT and IGRT to treat irregular tumor volumes with different dose distributions within the gland. MRS has the potential to define tumor burden volume within the prostate. MRS has potential to delineate target subvolumes and predict higher risk of failure following external beam radiation therapy (EBRT). MRS has the potential to classify aggressive cancer regions within the prostate gland and to facilitate radiation therapy treatment plans and thereby function as a prognostic tool following treatment. It is not yet known whether MRI combined with magnetic resonance spectroscopic imaging (MRSI) can improve the ability to detect the extent of prostate cancer.[22]

Magnetic resonance spectroscopy of the prostate is used to image the prostate gland, the capsule, and the regional lymph nodes. MRS enables visualization of the volume of a prostate tumor and the stage, as well as a comparison of malignant to healthy tissue. Healthy prostate tissue is high in the chemical citrate and low in choline, and malignant tissue is high in choline and low in citrate (Figure 13-11). Two coils are used for prostate MRS. The patient is positioned with his pelvis on the gray coil, which is called the torso PA coil; then the physician places the endorectal coil in the patient's rectum, and the balloon surrounding the coil is inflated to secure the position.[23]

The peaks analyzed for prostate spectroscopy are citrate, choline, and creatinine. In this spectrum, the citrate is low and the choline is high, which indicates cancer. In prostate MRS, the ability to study peripheral zones surrounding the prostate can be a valuable indicator of potential surrounding target areas. With this information, radiation oncologists can adjust the treatment plans to incorporate multiple expanded target zones. On the color map, areas of high choline are visualized as red and correlate with the findings in the spectroscopy (Figure 13-11).[23]

A future implication of prostate SPECT imaging involves assessment of prostate bed fields with SPECT. This is a particular challenge for obvious reasons: The prostate has been removed, so no organ is intact to send SPECT signals, and the bladder and bone and tissue with lipids lie in the surgical bed and can compromise the line width of the SPECT peak. Future studies will focus on developing the ability to view metabolic residual diseases in the prostate bed. Another future goal of prostate SPECT is long-term follow up of patients' SPECT images to delineate trends of metabolite peaks pretreatment, post-treatment, and for long-term follow-up. In this way, SPECT imaging can be integral to providing long-term follow-up data.[23]

It is important that quality assurance studies be done on all imaging techniques in radiation oncology. This will ensure the accuracy of the equipment and technique.

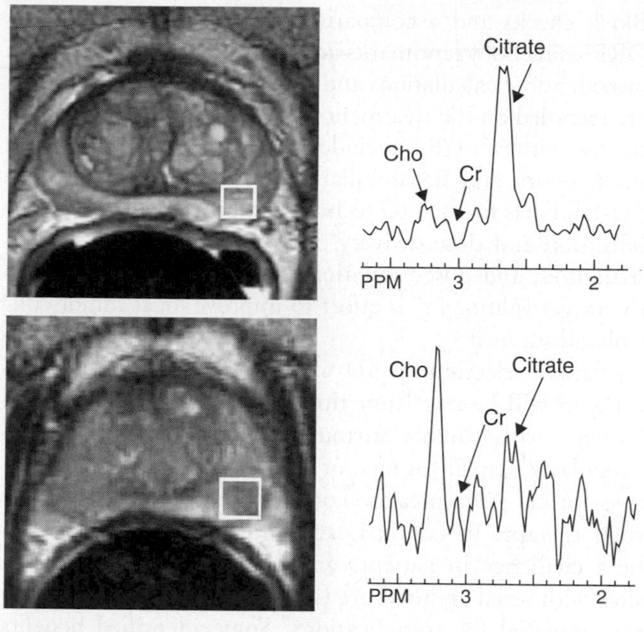


**FIGURE 13-11**

Magnetic resonance spectroscopy of prostate—top spectra is benign, bottom spectra is malignant.

*Source:* Photo courtesy of Fox Chase Cancer Center, Philadelphia, PA.

Quality assurance on SPECT is done by filling test tubes with citrate and choline, scanning them, and then measuring the peaks for exact readings.

As a relatively new imaging technique in radiation oncology, MRS has been found to be a reliable tool for investigating the metabolic state of normal and malignant tissue in vivo. MRS provides the radiation team with accurate images of tumor volume localization and therefore has the potential to improve radiation treatment planning. MRS can also function as a noninvasive technique for treatment follow-up.

## METHODS OF TREATMENT DELIVERY

### Conformal radiation therapy: 3-dimensional treatment planning

Three-dimensional treatment planning and CRT delivers a radiation dose to a target with an improved margin for sparing normal tissue compared with standard 2-dimensional treatment. The overall goal driving the research and development of this treatment advance was to create a modality that would conform the radiation prescription to the target volumes and deliver lower doses to surrounding normal structures.[10]

The process of 3D-CRT is complex and requires radiographic verification of the simulation procedure in some patients to confirm the accuracy of 3-dimensional plans.

Block checks and a comparison of portal films with the DRR using bony landmarks are performed. The dosimetrist provides dose calculations and treatment parameters, which are recorded on the treatment record. Common tumor sites treated with 3D-CRT include the prostate, lung, head and neck, brain, and hepatobiliary tract. Clinical research in 3D-CRT has focused on technical improvements in immobilization and dose delivery, reduction of dose to normal structures, and dose-escalation studies to increase dose to the target volume in an effort to improve local tumor control and survival.

Patient selection for 3D-CRT must focus on individuals who will benefit from this treatment delivery system. Patients with tumors surrounded by complex anatomy, irregularly shaped tumors, or tumors near radiation-sensitive normal structures are considered good candidates for such therapy. In contrast, achieving dose escalation can be a challenge in patients with cancers affecting certain sites with serial architecture (spinal cord and brain) due to the potential for complications. Some identified benefits of 3D-CRT include improved local tumor control due to better coverage of the target volume with a specific dose of radiation, less acute and late morbidity, the existence of dose-escalation studies, and improved survival. The efficiency of 3D-CRT is improving, and more patients are being treated using this approach.

Three-dimensional treatment planning requires precision and accuracy. It is therefore essential that a quality assurance program be designed to include the entire multidisciplinary team, be thorough, and provide for monitoring and evaluation of all parameters of these advanced treatment modalities. The testing of hardware and software and the methodical review of individual patient treatment plans must be included as part of the program. Three-dimensional physics and treatment planning includes the use of multimodality imaging to define the gross tumor volume (GTV) and CTV more precisely. MRI and PET are used to supplement CT data (Figure 13-12).

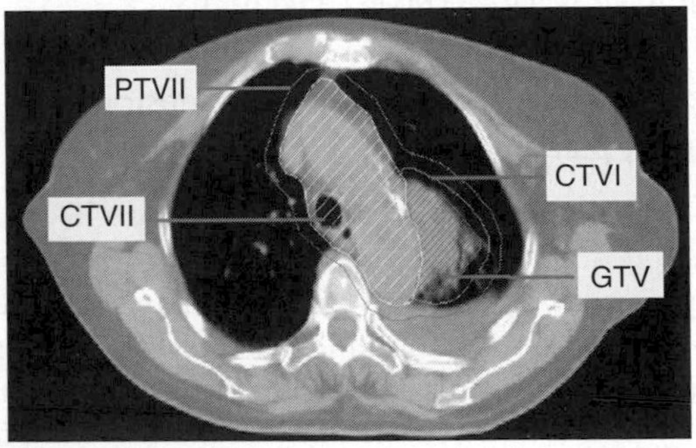


**FIGURE 13-12**

Computed tomography image: clinical target volume, gross tumor volume, and planning treatment volume.

*Source:* Photo courtesy of Fox Chase Cancer Center, Philadelphia, PA.

## Intensity-modulation radiation therapy

Intensity-modulated radiation therapy is a method of treatment delivery that utilizes varying intensities of beams, called beamlets. IMRT manipulates the intensities of radiation rays within each beam and allows increased control of radiation dose by creating custom design of optimum dose distributions. Special computer-aided optimization methods are used to set the intensities of many thousands of rays. Improvement in radiation dose conformality to treat irregularly shaped tumors and reduce toxicity has been achieved with IMRT and 3-dimensional techniques. IMRT provides precise dose conformality because the radiation field is divided into a number of beamlets with the aid of an intensity modulator and inverse treatment planning.[24] These small beamlets form a cumulative dose distribution that is contoured to the tumor. IMRT can offer differential dosing to elective nodal basins, high-risk nodal areas, and primary tumor sites.

Intensity-modulated radiation therapy can be considered a form of (3-dimensional) CRT in which a computer-aided optimization process (MLC) determines customized nonuniform dose distribution to deliver optimal dose to the target (Figure 13-13).[24]

Intensity-modulated radiation therapy is a novel technology that can deliver a precise dose of radiation to the target and spare normal surrounding tissues. The beam intensity in IMRT varies across the treatment field; IMRT irradiates the tumor using a series of small beams of different strengths. These small beams are created by the use of an MLC or a dynamic MLC.[24] The tumor receives the dose from these beams using a crossfire technique, which creates a uniform dose, sparing the surrounding tissues. The difference between IMRT and 3D-CRT is that 3D-CRT uses radiation beams of uniform strength (Figure 13-14).

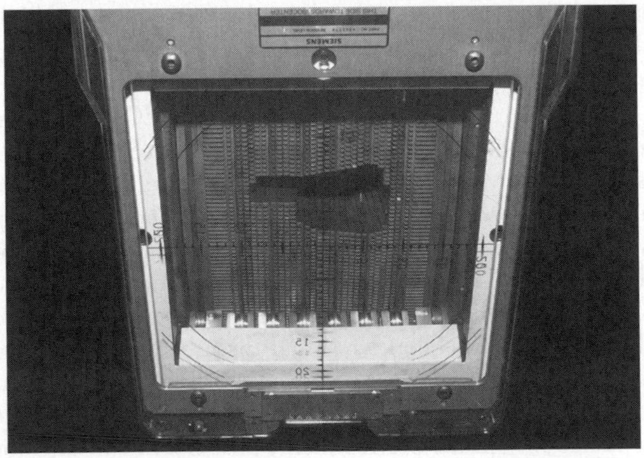

**FIGURE 13-13**

Multileaf collimator (MLC) computer-aided optimization process.

*Source:* Photo courtesy of Fox Chase Cancer Center, Philadelphia, PA.

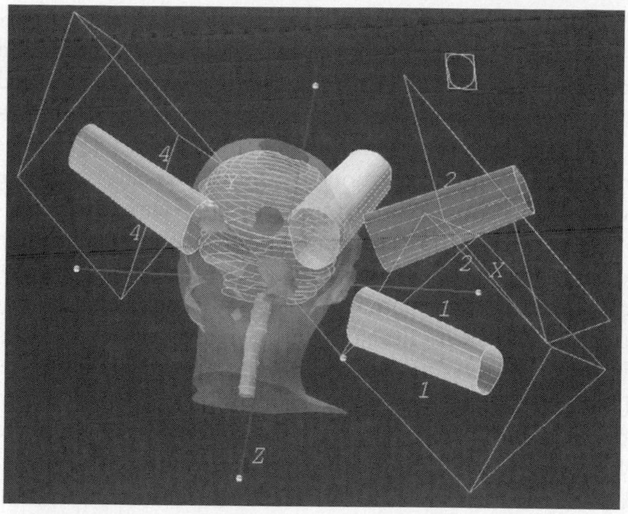

**FIGURE 13-14**

3-Dimensional conformal radiation therapy. Multiple beam arrangements.

*Source*: Reprinted with permission from Fox Chase Cancer Center, Philadelphia, PA.

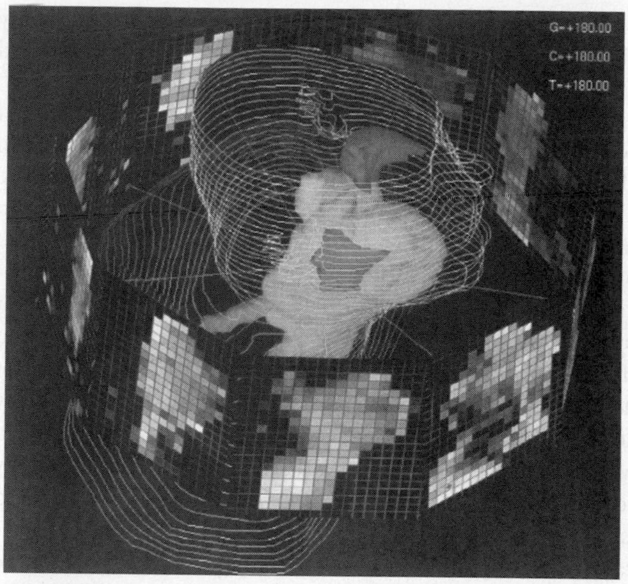


**FIGURE 13-15**

3-Dimensional view of the patient, target, volume, and parotids, and the 9 intensity-modulated radiation therapy beams used for the plan, including the intensity distributions for each beam. The parotids and PTVs are shown, as well as some of the outer contours.

*Source*: Reprinted with permission from Fox Chase Cancer Center, Philadelphia, PA.

The treatment planning software used for IMRT is based on inverse planning. The inverse planning algorithms start with the ideal distribution and then find the beam characteristics or profiles necessary to produce the intended plan. This contrasts with conventional forward planning, in which a number of beams are directed from different directions. Conventional beams cannot treat a tumor surrounding a vital organ due to their inability to avoid dosing the normal tissue. Conversely, the IMRT technology provides for separation of the tumor from adjacent structures and tissues. It is considered an advanced treatment planning system and may eventually replace 3-dimensional planning (Figure 13-15).[24]

## Image-guided radiation therapy

Image-guided radiation therapy refers to the capability of planning exquisitely complex radiation treatment with a range of imaging technologies to ensure exact treatment field targeting, reproducible patient alignment and immobilization, and responsiveness to anatomic variation. The evolution of advanced technology in radiation treatment delivery has led to the need for more precise treatment administration. The advent of IMRT provided clinicians with the skill to create conformal dosing for enhanced tumor targeting. IGRT evolved along with IMRT to provide superior imaging techniques for enhanced target localization.

Successful radiation treatment planning and delivery has always depended upon precise imaging. Imaging occurs throughout the entire course of radiation treatment. It is required during the initial diagnosis to determine location and extent of disease; during treatment planning for target volume delineation, to ensure sparing of normal tissue and organs surrounding the target; during treatment to align patients, to obtain quality assurance indicators during delivery; and at follow-up to evaluate response to treatment. So IGRT has been a long-standing premise of the practice of radiation oncology.[25] Recently, IGRT has evolved with new precision due to major innovations in 3-dimensional imaging such as CT, MRI, PET, SPECT, and US. IGRT provides innovative ways to account for challenges associated with interfractional and intrafractional anatomic variations in treatment planning and delivery.

Documentation of significant interfractional and intrafractional variations in shapes, volumes, and positions of treatment targets and the intervening and surrounding normal tissues validates the need to confirm targets through precise imaging prior to radiation delivery. The reasons for the variations are many and may include weight loss, tumor shrinkage in response to therapy, physiological functions such as respiration, and nonrigidity of soft tissue. All of these changes can affect the radiation treatment course. IGRT has the potential to target gross and microscopic disease accurately to individualize treatments, to reduce margins, to allow for the escalation of radiation dose, and to spare surrounding tissue.

Image-guided radiation therapy refers to an array of imaging technologies such as EPI, CT, MRI, and PET imaging. IGRT is divided into 2 distinct methods: 2-dimensional projection radiographs and 3-dimensional volumetric imaging. Two-dimensional imaging is used to align the patient relative to the prescribed radiation beams. This type of imaging uses megavoltage (MV) imaging and traditional x-ray films to verify setup positions. Recently, on-board imagers (OBIs) have been developed that provide diagnostic-quality x-ray images to set up the patient by alignment with the reference DRRs computed from the planning system. On-board imagers typically cannot detect soft tissue targets and are better at aligning bony landmarks or radio-opaque markers. When compared with MV images, the kV films are superior at locating bony reconstructions. Therefore, this in-room kV x-ray imaging is a major advance from traditional EPI devices. It is clinically vital to be able to visualize bony structures, and the low imaging dose is safer. For this reason, it is likely that the kV imaging system will become routine clinically for daily patient setup. This will enable the radiation delivery to localize targets with improved capabilities and to handle isocenter verification for daily setup.[25]

Three-dimensional imaging in the treatment room is the newest development of IGRT. During patient setup and immobilization on the treatment couch, true 3-dimensional imaging can be obtained with a CT scanner in the room and scanning right before the actual treatment begins. This CT capability would provide volumetric and anatomic information and be aligned with the reference CT before the start of treatment. This process provides image-guided adaptive radiotherapy by modifying plans right before and during treatment. Many forms of in-room CT scanners are available.[26]

A combination CT-LINAC system known as a "CT-on-rails" is a unique IGRT system that is a multifunctional hybrid configuration consisting of a LINAC and a diagnostic CT scanner with a sliding gantry. This configuration is a combination of a LINAC and a moveable Siemens CT scanner that slides along a pair of rails during actual treatment. The couch rotates 180° and the patient moves from the CT imaging position back to the treatment position. The first commercial CT-LINAC system in the US was installed in 2000. Recently, the system has been upgraded with a 6-degree-of-freedom couch that will permit more precise couch corrections. This system is used to treat prostate cancer, spinal metastasis, and lung cancers. Options for treatment of other disease sites is limitless, and as IGRT evolves in its complexity and differentiation clinical applications will expand greatly.[25]

The emergence of IMRT capabilities in radiation planning revolutionized conformal dose distribution techniques. This advance required more sophisticated imaging techniques in order to confirm targets as well as account for anatomic and physiological changes during actual treatment delivery. IGRT is an integral advance that dovetails perfectly with IMRT to offer highly sophisticated and precise imaging and to enhance delivery of radiation, and it has the potential to evolve as the complexities of treatment demand. This treatment planning advance brings image guidance to radiation treatment delivery, providing accurate, near-real-time target localization within the treatment room. The capability of a CT-on-rails/LINAC system provides information on the size, shape, and location of the target volume and on the location of nearby critical organs to ensure precise delivery of a prescribed course of radiation. The CT-on-rails produces accurate, virtual, real-time, diagnostic-quality images of tumors within the treatment room. This system allows patients to remain on one table while the tumor is pinpointed, and treatment is more accurately delivered.[27]

The gantry of the CT-on-rails/LINAC system moves along a series of high-precision rails that are embedded in the floor of the treatment room. The patient remains stationary on the treatment table while the CT scanner moves quickly and easily over the patient for imaging purposes. The gantry encircles the patient who is lying on the treatment table, making incremental movements during the scanning process. When image acquisition is complete, it retracts. On the basis of the updated tumor localization data, the system will then deliver the optimal radiation therapy to the tumor while providing maximal sparing of normal tissue (Figure 13-16).

Precise treatment plans and targeting abilities are the most important features associated with high doses of radiation treatment delivery. Intensity-modulated radiation therapy provides clinicians with the techniques to customize the shape of the radiation beams to the tumor, though some organs, such as the prostate, may shift positions with body movement. The CT-on-rails tracks organ movement

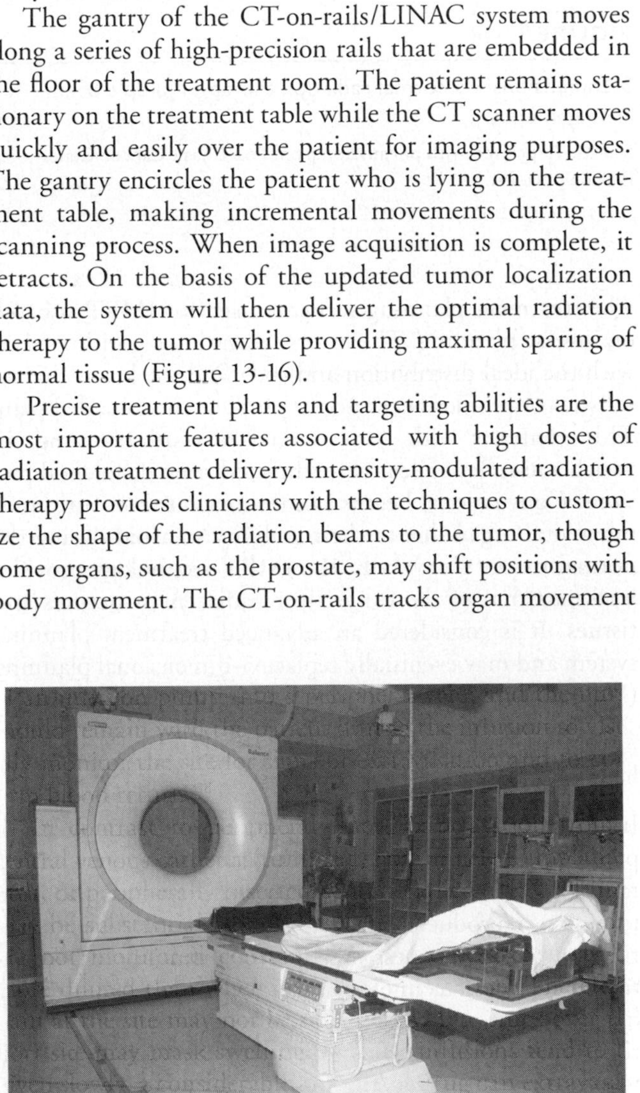

**FIGURE 13-16**

The computed tomography on rails/linear accelerator system.

*Source*: Photo courtesy of Fox Chase Cancer Center, Philadelphia, PA.

just moments before treatment and adjusts the radiation treatment plan accordingly. It allows for the precise delivery of high-dose radiation therapy. Prostate cancer illustrates the challenges facing radiation treatment planners. The gland lies between the bladder and the rectum and is subject to frequent displacement due to intermittent distention. In an attempt to target the prostate gland, urinating on command and holding back urination are difficult requests of patients who are receiving radiation treatment. Prostate gland mobility has been documented, and studies have found significant differences in marker displacements on daily images obtained by EPI during treatment sessions. This CT-on-rails permits accurate and noninvasive targeting of the prostate gland while avoiding the bladder and rectum.[28]

Computerized tomography scans are used routinely in radiation treatment planning, but the pairing of the CT scan with daily radiation treatment is unique. The CT-on-rails provides an additional technique for target localization, and in some settings is used in conjunction with US localization. The following are overall advantages offered by a CT-on-rails system:

- Fast, 3-dimensional tumor localization prior to any treatment fraction provides an opportunity to escalate dose, reduce complications, and evaluate the therapeutic effectiveness of treatment.
- Computerized tomographic functionality in the treatment room provides diagnostic-quality images with the patient in the actual treatment position, ensuring routine visualization of the tumor so as to check for anatomic movement.
- The CT scan operator in the radiation therapy department can perform the scheduling and acquisition of patients' CT image data for simulation, planning, and treatment purposes.

Image-guided radiation therapy is a new, evolving technological aspect of radiation treatment delivery. Extensive clinical trials are ongoing that will hopefully validate the clinical necessity of utilizing IGRT capabilities to treat a variety of disease sites. The attraction of IGRT is that it provides clinicians with the tools to maximize treatment planning and to achieve maximal local regional control while sparing normal tissues. Now that deformable image registration is achievable, IGRT techniques provide validation of dosing and targeting. Over the course of a patient's treatment trajectory IGRT can provide invaluable information to facilitate changes in contours, targets, and treatment beams. These are vital planning and delivery capabilities that form the basis for the future of radiation delivery.

Nurses are required to be flexible, dynamic, educated, and motivated to incorporate patient teaching materials when evolutionary equipment and treatment techniques are introduced into the radiation oncology setting. Patients must be prepared with detailed information on the rationale for the use of new equipment, the equipment itself (ie, size, sound, increased amount of time for treatment setup), the equipment's location, the personnel monitoring patient safety, and the overall role of the equipment in the treatment plan and desired therapeutic outcome.

Radiation oncology nurses must embrace the evolving science of advanced treatment planning techniques by establishing a nursing presence in the multidisciplinary planning meetings to discuss equipment purchase, rationale for incorporating the system into the treatment setting, location of equipment, and ultimate effects on the treatment plan. Invoking evidence-based practice guidelines offers a way for nurses to understand the implications of new technology and provide appropriate educational plans for patients.

## Treatment planning computers

Computerized treatment planning capabilities have revolutionized radiation treatment planning and delivery in recent years. Treatment planning computers evolved in the 1970s and replaced manual plans. These original computers provided accurate 2-dimensional plans. They accepted input from a digitizer of external patient contours, anatomic landmarks and outlines of target volumes, and of critical structures in specified planes. Today, these systems are obsolete because of the requirement to provide planning in 3 dimensions.[3]

Over the past 2 decades planning systems have become capable of 3-dimensional planning with input from patient data acquired from CT, MRI, PET, and US. Software has been revolutionized, in conjunction with hardware, to allow for complex treatments such as 3D-CRT, IMRT, IGRT, high dose rate (HDR) therapy, and brachytherapy. Inverse planning is a treatment planning algorithm that permits the planner to request a desired dose distribution and then allows the computer to generate a plan to satisfy the specifications. This capability represents the nuance of the sophistication of computerized treatment planning systems. All of these systems are commercially available and are always evolving.[3]

## On-board imaging

Accurate treatment delivery follows the scrupulous process of treatment planning. These facets of treatment are dovetailed and are subject to continuous review and analysis to ensure that the plans are exact and that the delivery is safe and effective. In the past, patient setup on the treatment couch was the one way in which reproducible plans were ensured throughout the course of treatment. Patients would be set up with the assistance of localization lasers and identification marks such as ink, tattoos, or bony landmarks drawn onto the individual patient; these markings were considered adequate as long as patients did not move and cause variations that would alter the treatment plan.

With 3D-CRT, IMRT, and IGRT, it is now necessary in contemporary practice for the patient setup and anatomy to match exactly in order to execute treatment for the entire course. Conformal plans require the most precise accuracy of patient setup. These requirements have advanced patient immobilization and dynamic targeting of planned target volume (PTV) through imaging systems mounted on the accelerators. This development is known as IGRT. Accelerator mounted imaging equipment provides online treatment plan verification and correction and dynamic targeting, synchronized with patient movement and respiratory cycles (also known as gating). These systems should consist of EPI devices (EPIDs), a peak kilovoltage ($kV_p$) source for radiographic verification of setup, an online fluoroscopic mode to permit overlaying of the treatment field aperture on to the fluoroscopy image, and cone beam CT capability for treatment plan verification.[25]

Accelerator-mounted imaging systems are required equipment in radiation oncology departments offering conformal treatment plans. Along with the sophisticated capabilities of conformal treatment comes the need to support the technology with equipment to ensure that these plans are administered. In additional, staff are required to be professionally trained to operate and monitor sophisticated machinery to deliver treatment optimally to the target volume, while sparing surrounding critical structures. Along with this training it is vital that the entire multidisciplinary team be prepared to answer patient queries about the techniques used to plan, localize, and image their treatment course.

### B-mode ultrasound acquisition and targeting system

Ultrasound is a noninvasive real-time imaging modality for targeting soft tissue structures. The primary use of US for IGRT is measurement of prostate position.[29]

The B-mode acquisition and targeting (BAT) system (NOMOS Corporation, Sewickley, Pennsylvania) is a patented US positioning system used for the delivery of radiation treatment to the prostate gland (Figure 13-17). This system provides a noninvasive way to deliver more precise radiation therapy. The BAT technology combines a US probe and a 3-dimensional positioning tool to pinpoint target organs rapidly at the time of each radiation treatment session. It dramatically reduces the need to target an extra margin of tissue around the tumor site. These extra margins have traditionally been used to compensate for errors in localization of the radiation beam. As such, BAT results in a significant reduction in the amount of healthy tissue exposed to radiation.

Preliminary feasibility trials first occurred in 1999 at the Fox Chase Cancer Center in Philadelphia and at the Cleveland Clinic. BAT is considered appropriate for any organ that can be visualized by US. Possible cancer sites for radiation treatment using this technology include the breast, liver, bladder, kidney, pancreas, and uterus. The ability of BAT to reduce treatment margins allows for more successful, higher-dose treatments while decreasing the risk of complications associated with either standard or escalated doses of radiation therapy.[29]

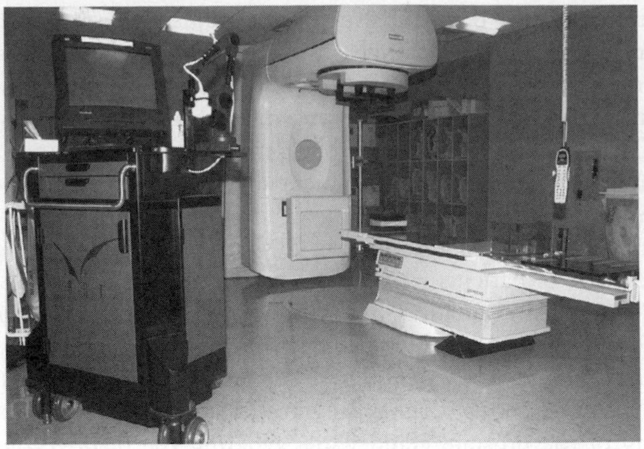

**FIGURE 13-17**

B-Mode ultrasound acquisition and targeting system.

*Source*: Photo courtesy of Fox Chase Cancer Center, Philadelphia, PA.

Ultrasound-guided imaging for radiation treatment planning has several limitations. Poor image quality and inability of radiation oncology personnel to interpret US are significant. In addition, when US is compared with CT images and implanted fiducial markers, the US localization for prostate targeting is inferior.[30] Therefore, although it is still used for prostate localization, particularly when surgical placement of fiducials is contraindicated, US is being commonly replaced by OBI with CT scan and fiducials.

### Cone beam imaging

Cone beam computed tomography (CBCT) is named for the cone-shaped beam of x-rays used to collect a complete image. Different from conventional CT, which offers a series of thin-slice x-ray images and then stacks them together to create a complete picture, CBCT produces a sophisticated image in less time with less x-ray exposure. The advantages of CBCT over standard CT are as follows: faster volume speed, efficient use of x-ray power, and sufficient data for exact 3-dimensional image reconstruction. CBCT enhances the role of treatment simulation, verification, and planning. It has the capability to reconstruct 3-dimensional volumetric data in one gantry rotation. A special computer program rapidly reconstructs the images into a 3-dimensional picture. All of this allows for more precise targeting because the image is taken with the patient in the treatment position. This allows for adjustment of the treatment plan and for the shift of internal organs.

Cone beam CT is x-ray CT scanning using a flat panel. With CBCT planar projection images are acquired from multiple directions, with the x-ray source and detector quickly rotating around the patient in approximately 1 minute.[31] CBCT systems are available as accessories to LINACs. The goal of CBCT is to acquire data for localization of soft tissues before treatment. CBCT imaging is generated using the treatment beam of the LINAC. To obtain MV CBCT imaging, a series of 2-dimensional projections around the patient are obtained. Then a 3-dimensional data set is reconstructed in a process analogous to conventional CT imaging, in which an x-ray source and a detector are mounted on a rotating gantry. Conventional CT systems use a 1-dimensional linear detector array; the CBCT system uses a 2-dimensional detector array.[32]

Cone beam CT has been used to verify patient alignment and dose. The potential benefits of MV CBCT are with imaging of head and neck, lung, and pelvic tumors. Megavoltage CBCT can identify subtle changes in target fields not seen on portal imaging.[31] Most LINACs offer gantry-mounted CBCT systems for kV systems. The images on a kV system are acquired during a 360° gantry rotation. These are then reconstructed into a 3-dimensional data set.

No clinical outcome data have been published with patients treated using kV CBCT for either setup or target localization. In a comparison of kV CBCT technologies with MV CBCT, the MV CBCT was found to offer an advantage in terms of simplicity of mechanical integration with the LINAC, and kV CBCT was found to be superior in terms of imaging of soft tissue structures and the signal-to-noise ratio per unit dose.[32]

In clinical practice, CBCT is used as an additional means of verifying the accuracy of delivery of radiation. CBCT may lead to enhanced dosing to the target with more sparing of normal structures and more precise patient positioning. CBCT is used when treating head and neck, lung, prostate, and pelvic tumors. Additional clinical applications will be forthcoming (Figure 13-18).

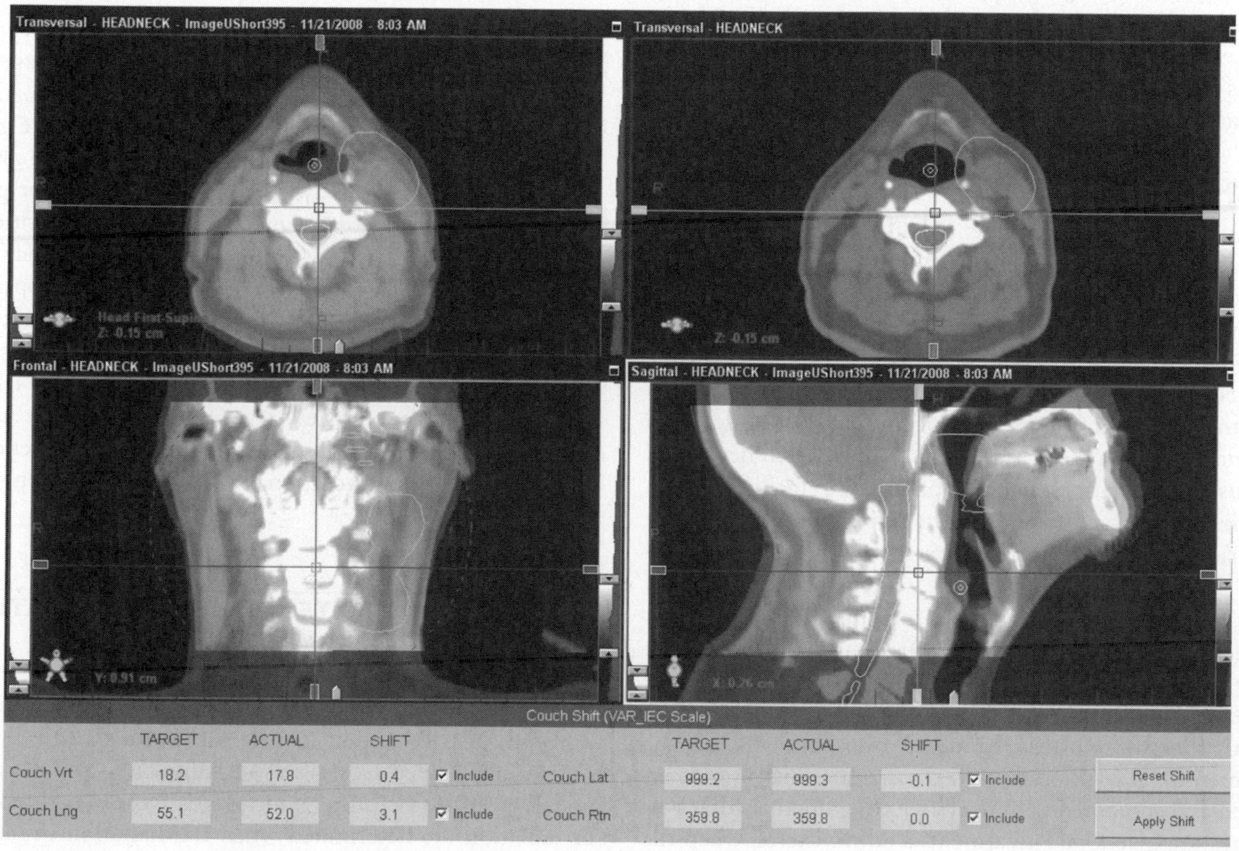


**FIGURE 13-18**

Cone beam computed tomography (CBCT). Top: axial slice superimposed on planning CT. Bottom left: coronal slice. Bottom right: saggital. Numbers are couch shifts for optimal match of CBCT and CT.

*Source*: Photo courtesy of Fox Chase Cancer Center, Philadelphia, PA.

### Fiducial markers

Prostate localization for treatment planning is a relatively new procedure that is done prior to and during external beam treatment planning for patients with localized prostate cancer and accounts for internal movement of the prostate gland during treatment. Clinical questions that have arisen regarding organ movement include the following: How much does the prostate move on a daily basis and during treatment? What is the positional relationship between the prostate and bony anatomy? Because of these queries the use of fiducial gold seed markers and daily EPI with online correction is one strategy used for treatment planning purposes to account for prostate organ movement. Many studies have documented significant prostate movement and the need to account for this during treatment planning.[33] Placement of the gold fiducial markers is done by urologists, using the same methods as a prostate biopsy. The gold fiducial markers are 2 to 3 mm in size. A transrectal US is performed to confirm and assist with placement. Prostate measurements are taken, and sometimes the prostate is anesthetized with 1.0% lidocaine. Usually 3 gold fiducial markers are inserted through a needle that is passed through the US probe. The markers are used as a fixed standard of reference during radiation.[34] The use of internal fiducial markers with EPI for patient alignment assists with precision of dose escalation in the treatment of prostate cancer.[35,36]

### Real-time tracking beacons

Organ motion is well documented during radiation therapy. A multi-institutional study demonstrated prostate organ motion during treatment fractions with variable direction. Methods used for target localization (such as fiducials), although effective, do not provide continuous real-time clinical guidance.[37] Therefore, a 4-dimensional localization system (known as Calypso 4D localization) and implanted beacon electromagnetic transponders have been developed and used in radiation oncology planning to facilitate target localization and maximize treatment planning.

Prior to patients with prostrate cancer receiving radiation, 3 tiny beacon transponders, which are made of small coils encapsulated in glass, are implanted under nuclear medicine guidance (Figure 13-19). During treatment an array placed over the patient activates the transponders through a radiofrequency signal and then listens for the signals that are returned from each transponder. Once the 3-dimensional position of each transponder has been determined and compared with the baseline geometry, shift coordinates are given, and treatment is administered when the coordinates are aligned according to exact prostate position and the target volume to their planned positions relative to the isocenter (Figure 13-20).

This localization system functions as a "global positioning system" for the body, as it displays and records prostate motion in real time using an intuitive graphical user interface. Both visual and audio cues are used to manage the motion of the gland if it moves outside of the field. Once the beacon transponders are implanted, they provide guidance to the clinician on the position of the prostate gland, and this information is used to set up and monitor prostate position during treatment delivery. This is a critically important new technology in treatment planning that provides clinicians with expanded treatment delivery options. In addition, extremely accurate localization of target volume occurs with the use of fiducials and ultimately minimizes nonionizing radiation doses to surrounding tissues and organs and maximizes target dose. Studies are under way to evaluate the use of implanted fiducials in other critical organs requiring radiation treatment, such as lung and brain.[33,38]

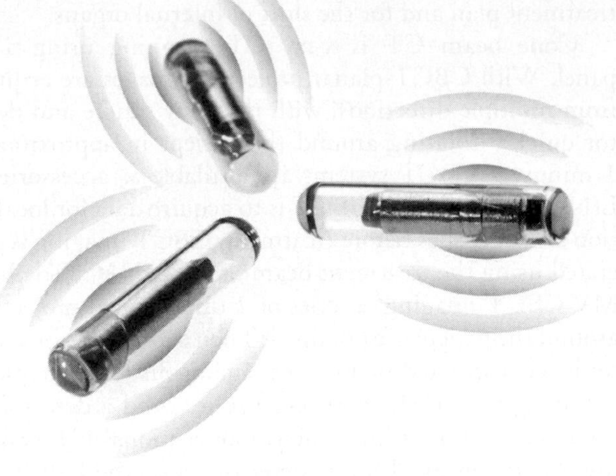

**FIGURE 13-19**

Beacon transponders for prostate localization.

*Source*: Reprinted with permission from Calypso Medical Technologies, Seattle, WA.

## PRINCIPLES OF EXTERNAL BEAM RADIATION DOSING/DOSIMETRY

Radiation dosing is a complex process based on physics. For purposes of this chapter, general definitions and key concepts are provided to serve as an adjunct to the radiation oncology nurse's clinical knowledge. Dose measurements of radiation are determined when the radiation beam hits the target (ie, the patient). These measurements depend on the depth of the calculation point below the point of entry (depth), the penetrating power of the beam (energy), the tissue type that must be penetrated (density), the distance from the radiation source to the skin surface, the size of the

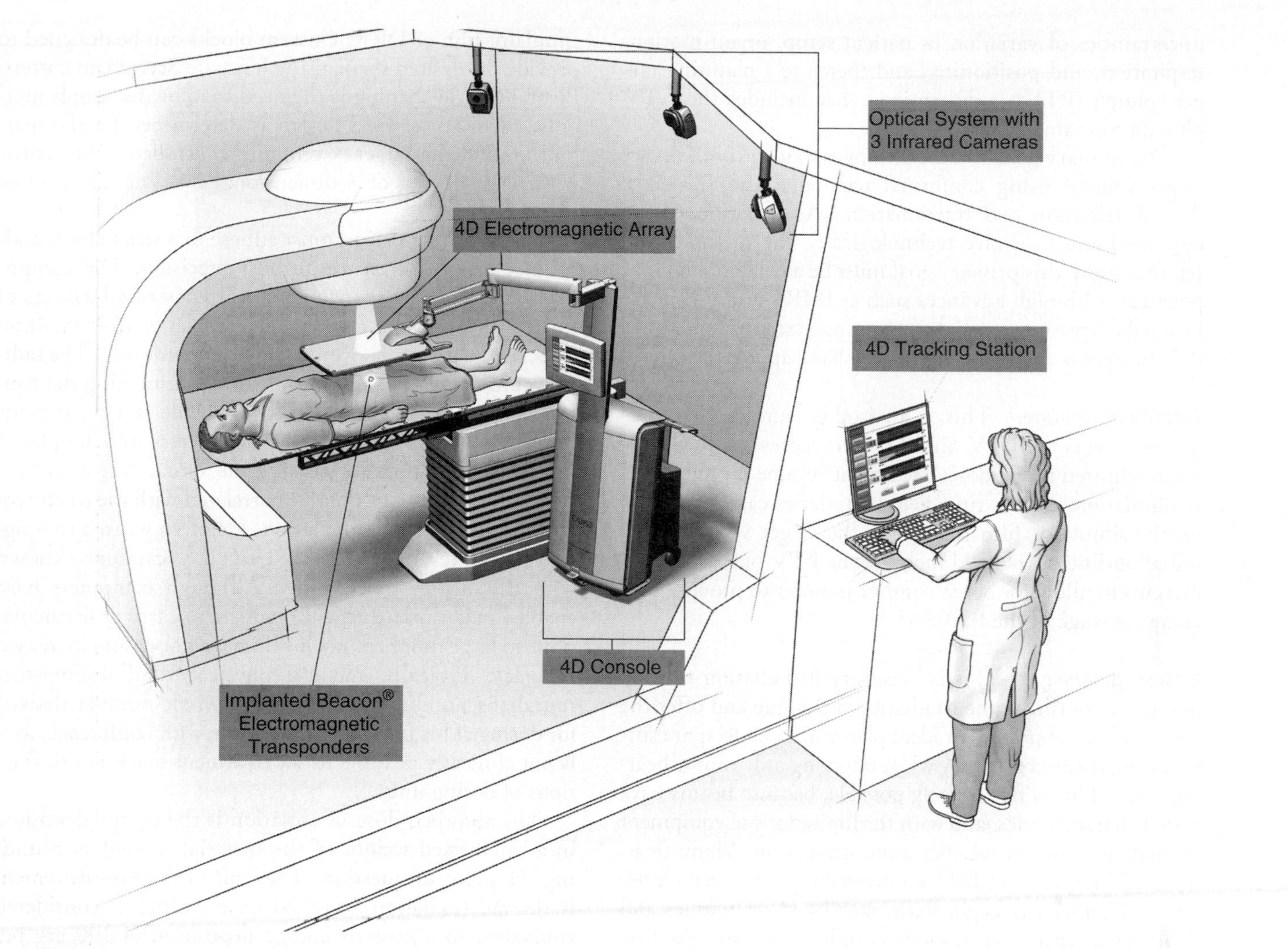


**FIGURE 13-20**

Schema of localization system for prostate cancer treatment.

*Source*: Reprinted with permission from Calypso Medical Technologies, Seattle, WA.

field on the skin surface (field size), and the type and design of the collimator.

Measured data tables are created for each treatment machine and are planned using anthropomorphic phantoms, which are commercial systems that simulate various body tissues and are used to determine dose distribution. Frequently, water is used as the phantom material because it absorbs radiation similarly to human soft tissue. Sheets of various tissue-equivalent plastics are also used for convenience. These measured data tables are referred to as dosimeters and are used by dosimetrists to quantify radiation dose distributions within phantom substances. These measurements are then used as patient controls for dose.[3]

*Target volume.* Establishing the target volume, which is the location of the tumor and the extent of it, is the first step in the treatment planning process. Target volume is the size of the tumor and approximation to surrounding critical organs. Current imaging techniques (CT, MRI, US, PET, and SPECT) are used to localize tumor target volume. These imaging systems also localize critical surrounding structures and assist in identifying sufficient margins so that the treatment field extends safely beyond the tumor volume and includes a local-regional margin. This accounts for treating microscopic spread. Target volume identification is a pivotal first step in the planning process. In order to avoid radiotherapy failures, precise tumor localization must take place.[3]

The GTV refers to the part of the tumor that is visualized with imaging. The CTV includes the entire tumor and the invisible microscopic disease that is estimated clinically. Because the CTV is a subjective clinical assessment it is necessary for the margins around the GTV to be ample in order to thoroughly treat the tumor and surrounding probable margin of disease. GTV and CTV are subject to the uncertainties of variation in patient setup, organ motion, respiration, and positioning, and therefore a planning target volume (PTV) is determined that includes the CTV plus appropriate margins.

The primary goal of radiotherapy is to identify the exact target volume using conformal technique and the right dose distribution and fractionation.[3] As radiation oncology continues to evolve technologically, the method chosen to achieve this primary goal must be available as well as practical. Although advances such as IMRT and IGRT are invaluable treatment delivery planning systems, sometimes the same goals can be achieved with basic approaches.

*Treatment volume.* This is an isodose surface that adequately covers the PTV, and the value represents the minimum required target dose. Treatment volume is established at simulation. At this time field boundaries can be marked on the simulator film to include the target volume. The initial outline of the field includes the PTV plus estimated margins to allow for beam contour in order to provide adequate coverage of the PTV.[3]

*Isodose planning.* This is necessary in radiation therapy in order to optimize the irradiation technique and offer the best dose distribution. An ideal plan would be to spare surrounding tissue completely while targeting only tumor-bearing areas. This is not entirely possible, because beams have varied characteristics, and with the limitations of equipment normal tissue often receives some irradiation. Many treatment techniques and field arrangements have been developed. Dosimetrists begin with established techniques and then adjust with modifications in order to achieve the best dose distribution for the individual patient. Sophisticated computer programs assist with isodose planning.

*Inverse planning.* This is used for isodose planning with IMRT and IGRT. With inverse planning the dosimetrist indicates the desired dose at the beginning of treatment, and then computers set the treatment machines and the dynamic (MLC) designs the optimal treatment plan.[3]

*Treatment field.* This delineation is the second most important aspect of treatment planning next to establishment of target volume. Treatment fields sometimes require shape, size, and orientation adjustment. The field has to be adequate to accommodate the isodose distribution plan. This is the time when changes to the treatment plan are often made, and sometimes, if these changes require a change in beam orientation or beam location, resimulation may need to occur. If minor treatment field adjustments are required, such as a change of margins around the target, then these can be made without resimulation.[3]

*Field shaping.* Treatment fields can be shaped in any size radiation oncologists can draw on to a beam's eye view simulator film or DRR. Custom blocks can be designed to provide the desired shape using hot-wire Styrofoam cutters. Pivotal to field shaping is the need to allow for ample margins; adequacy of field design is determined by the margins around the target. Computer-controlled MLC assists with field shaping of 3-dimensional imaging and isodose planning.[3]

The dose calculation must adhere to a strict check-and-balance system to ensure utmost precision. The components of dosing must include consistency of all aspects of the treatment machine and the data tables to avoid fatalities associated with either overdosing or underdosing. The radiation physics team is responsible for documenting the congruence of the machine settings with the treatment plans on a daily basis. Occasionally, dosimeters may be placed inside patient tissues to measure the actual dose delivered. This information can then be correlated with the treatment dose. Although dose calculations are often written to 4 significant figures, in practice the exact dose cannot be known with this degree of certainty. Although computers have enabled radiation treatment planners to carry dose calculations to large numbers, such values do not ensure increased accuracy. Typically, medical physicists and dosimetrists round the numbers to the nearest whole number derived for dosing. This practice can be done with confidence, as it is not clinically possible to set treatment machines to fractions of dosing units.[39]

The absorbed dose of radiation is the energy deposited in a small fixed weight of the material (tissue) surrounding the point in question. The unit of dose measurement is the rad (radiation absorbed dose), which is considered equivalent to a dose or energy deposition of 100 erg per gram. In clinical practice, the rad is being replaced by the gray (Gy), which is 100 times larger (1 Gy = 100 rad). One rad is, therefore, the same as one hundredth of a gray, or 1 centigray (cGy):

$$1 \text{ rad} = 1/100 \text{ Gy} = 1 \text{ cGy}$$

## DOSE DELIVERY OF RADIATION

Dose delivery of radiation involves 2 major components. The first component identifies the output of the treatment machines from a specified point in the beam, to the specific distance from the target, and through a specific medium. The second component of dosing determines the actual absorbed dose within the medium. Both of these dose delivery concepts require precise calculations and thorough knowledge of the irradiated material, the geometric relationship with the proposed beam, and the size of the irradiated field.[3]

Secondary electrons are set in motion when high-energy photon beams strike a medium. These secondary electrons have the ability to penetrate to a depth that depends on the photon energy and the composition of the medium. When the electron equilibrium is reached at this depth, the maximum dose is achieved. The maximum depth is referred to and written as *D*max; the maximum dose is also referred to and written as *D*max. These abbreviations are used interchangeably. The *D*max is the point of buildup of peak radiation dose in tissue. As the x-ray energy increases, the *D*max extends more deeply in the tissue. It is a significant measurement due to the increased skin-sparing abilities of high-energy LINAC. The buildup region comprises the difference between the surface and this depth. The dose in the buildup region increases as the electrons add to the total dose administered. This premise underlies the technology's skin-sparing capabilities. The surface layer receives a smaller dose than layers between the surface and the *D*max. If mechanical devices or the patient's clothing intercepts the beam within a few centimeters of the skin surface, the skin-sparing effect is diminished or lost. More efficient skin sparing occurs with the use of higher energies, through which the *D*max increases. The beam dose falls gradually off at higher energies due to the combination of a smaller photon supply and increased distance from the target.[40]

The percentage depth dose (%DD) is the absorbed dose at a given depth expressed as a percentage of the absorbed dose at a reference depth. This value varies according to energy, field size, skin surface distance (SSD), and change in medium. The %DD falls less rapidly with higher energy. It can be measured and plotted to form a %DD curve. As energy increases, the penetrative ability of the beam increases and the skin dose decreases.

The inverse square law of radiation states that the intensity of a radiation beam is inversely proportional to the distance from the source squared. For example, the radiation dose at 2 cm will be one fourth the dose at 1 cm. The inverse square law governs the theory of the intensity of an x-ray beam. Collimators and other scattering devices may cause deviations from the inverse square law. Consequently, the inverse square law must be checked for completeness and accuracy to avoid serious errors in dosing.

Within the body, the radiation beam must pass through tissues of different densities. The variance in lung, bone, fat, muscle, and air affects both the beam penetration and the amount of scatter. The overall effect on the dose depends on the size of the treatment volume, the tissue density, and the beam energy. This variability of irradiated media requires complex changes in dosimetry. The dose effect near the interface between layers of different densities is complex. Historically, outlining treatment borders was difficult and there were tremendous problems calculating a dose from beams that crossed inhomogeneous volumes. Now, with the use of CT to provide detailed outlines of irregularities as well as information about the density of the target, dosing capabilities have improved.[40]

Radiation doses must be measured through different media to accurately determine patient dose. Dosimetrists measure ionization of the radiation beam in air, identifying this quantity as the degree of exposure. The next steps in the process involve correcting for the presence of soft tissue and air and deriving the absorbed dose in grays.

Identification of dose variations within a field at prescribed depths is an essential component of radiation dosing techniques. The variety of clinical presentations requires that radiation treatment planning and dosing provide the capabilities to achieve a standard of safe, effective, and methodically planned treatment to targets while sparing surrounding anatomic structures. This treatment must also be reproducible daily to an exact standard, and concomitant accuracy checks and balances must be provided. Radiation oncology nurses benefit from understanding the conceptual framework that guides dosimetric treatment planning so that technical and clinical patient queries can be appropriately answered or referred.

## FIELD-MODIFYING INSTRUMENTS

Beam-modifying absorbers known as *filters* or *wedges* can be placed in the path of a beam. A typical beam-modifying filter is a wedge-shaped device made of dense material such as lead that progressively extends the beam across the field. The wedge has thick and thin sides, a shape that creates tilted isodose curves. The angle of the wedge is the angle through which an isodose curve is tilted at the central axis of the beam and at a specific depth. The degree of tilt changes with the depth; therefore, the predetermined depth is critical. Although the reference depth may vary, the wedge angle is commonly defined at the intersection of the central axis of the beam and the 50% isodose curve. The *wedge angle* refers to the tilt of the isodose curve, not the angle of the wedge filter. The wedge angle or tilt produced by a wedge has a different angle than the wedge material. Some wedge filters with standard isodose curves are prefabricated; others can be customized by technicians. In contemporary LINAC treatment units, physical wedges have largely been replaced by virtual wedges. The virtual wedge enhances efficiency and minimizes the physical workload of radiotherapists.[41]

## TISSUE COMPENSATION

When a radiation beam is projected along an irregular or sloping surface, the isodose curves bend. Such distortion may result in unacceptable nonuniformity of dose within the target and has the potential to cause excessive irradiation of sensitive structures such as the spinal cord. Several techniques are used to eliminate this problem, such as the use of wedges and the addition of bolus material or compensators. In addition, treatment fields with thinner tissue planes can be blocked for the last few treatments to reduce radiation dose.[39,42]

A bolus is a tissue-equivalent material that is put directly on the patient's skin to even the irregular contours and to create a flat surface that normalizes the radiation *z* beam. The use of a bolus differs from the application of a bolus layer, which is sufficiently thick to provide adequate dose buildup over the skin surface. A bolus layer is often referred to as a *buildup bolus.* When higher-energy beams are used, bolus application on the skin surface eliminates the skin-sparing advantage.

Compensators are designed to provide the required beam arrangement that occurs in the "missing" tissue when the body surface is irregular. The compensator is positioned at a distance from the target (15 to 20 cm away from the skin) in an effort to preserve the skin-sparing effect of the megavoltage machines. It should have adjustable dimensions and shape. The compensator must account for beam divergence, linear attenuation coefficients of the filter material and soft tissues, and the reduction in scatter at different depths. Compensators are constructed from a variety of materials to accomplish their multiple objectives. For example, compensating wedges (C-wedges) are used for oblique beam incidence or curved surfaces and are made from metals such as copper, brass, and lead. Their function is to compensate for a missing wedge of tissue in the treatment field.[39,40]

The difference between a wedge filter and a C-wedge is as follows: Wedge filters can be used as compensators, but are primarily used for tilting the standard isodose curves through a certain wedge angle in conjunction with the wedge-pair technique. In contrast, the C-wedge is used only as a compensator to facilitate the use of the standard isodose charts without modification. As such, C-wedges are more clinically practical than wedge filters as compensators because they can be used for partial-field compensation. The C-wedge is used to compensate for only a portion of the irregularly shaped contour. A wedge filter is designed to be placed in the field in a fixed position and, therefore, cannot partially compensate for the treatment field. Additional applications of compensating filters include compensators for tissue heterogeneity (for total body irradiation) and improvement of dose uniformity in fields where nonuniformity of the dose arises from sources other than contour irregularity, such as with large-mantle fields.[39,40]

## PATIENT POSITIONING AND IMMOBILIZATION TECHNIQUES

Patient positioning and immobilization are critical components of radiation treatment delivery. To achieve the goals of tumor kill and preservation of normal organs and tissues, it is mandatory that daily treatment be reproducible and accurate. If patient positioning is not exact and if immobilization devices are inadequate, lethal consequences could result. Accuracy of radiation treatment depends on both dosimetric and geometric exactness. This section focuses on the elements necessary to achieve geometric accuracy, which refers to issues of patient positioning and immobilization.

Patients must be positioned so that the target is at the isocenter.[43] The advantage of isocentric technique is that the patient is not moved between fields. If the patient lies supine on a horizontal treatment couch, a single skin mark (such as a tattoo or permanent ink) will locate the center of the target volume that imaging has shown to be at a certain depth (*d*) beneath the surface.[43]

To achieve treatment setup accuracy, continuous evaluation by the team of radiation oncology professionals is essential. Patients must also be assessed for safety and comfort. Patients will move if they are uncomfortable, and initially tense muscles may relax during the treatment process. Using wedges, pillows, and head cups can avoid this unintentional patient movement. The laser crosshair system is useful for providing additional markings for treatment setup guides that can ensure the patient is in the same position each day. Extending the skin markings as far superior and inferior to the central treatment plane as possible will improve reproducibility of beams. External anatomic landmarks should always be referred to during daily treatment setup. The distance between several visible landmarks should be calculated to determine the accuracy of the positioning. In addition, immobilization devices should be used when appropriate. These devices begin as soft, flexible materials and then become rigid sanctuaries of comfort and security for patients during daily treatment.

### IMMOBILIZATION DEVICES

Immobilization devices help keep patients in a stationary position for daily treatment. These devices also help to minimize the potential for treatment setup errors, reduce the amount of radiation to normal tissues, and ensure appropriate treatment to the target volume. Patient immobilization equipment varies in terms of construction materials and style. Some is fabricated on site; other equipment is available from commercial suppliers. Before implementing an immobilization system, it may be helpful to assess and evaluate the individual patient and treatment objectives. This inquiry can guide the radiation oncology team in creating a safe and comfortable physical environment for each patient.

The assessment begins by observing the patient's physical comfort and degree of relaxation. If the immobilization device touches the patient, it can serve as a reminder of how the position feels to the patient and, therefore, can be used to direct the therapists in replicating the setup. The patient must be secured in such a way as to preclude any movement. The immobilization equipment should be contoured to the patient's body surface. This equipment must fit the patient's anatomy properly and allow for variance in symmetry, body fat, and target location. The device should be able to position the patient in such a way as to minimize normal tissue complications. In addition, immobilization equipment should allow for unobstructed radiation beams and not interfere with the treatment plan. The material used to construct the devices should be radiotransparent, rigid, and able to be trimmed if necessary to remove sections. The devices must not cause mechanical obstruction by interfering with the LINAC gantry during beam rotation. Devices must be usable with all treatment planning systems to establish consistency for patient setup and treatment. If the radiation beam passes through the device, the effect on surface dose must be considered. Although the accumulation of surface buildup may be small, it must be documented.[43]

The immobilization device must allow sufficient space for reference marks to be seen so that patient setup can be reproduced. The immobilization device defines the patient coordinate system, which must be aligned with the room coordinate system using reference marks. This alignment is achieved through the use of treatment tables and specialized adapters.[43]

The immobilization device must be rigid and maintain its shape over time. If the device loosens over time, the patient may move within it, which could potentially flaw the setup. Radiation therapists should assess the fit of the device daily and determine normal wear and tear as well as changes in the patient's weight and environmental factors that may affect the required fit (Figure 13-21).

Every aspect of medical care has become subject to cost analysis. The costs of using complex immobilization systems must be evaluated in terms of the benefit to the

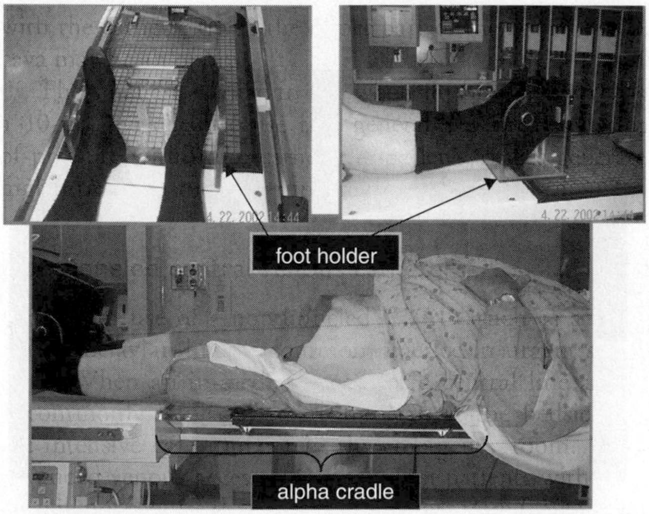


**FIGURE 13-21**

Immobilization and positioning devices.

*Source*: Photo courtesy of Fox Chase Cancer Center, Philadelphia, PA.

clinical outcome. Factors affecting the cost of an immobilization system include materials, staff time for construction and setup, supplies, potential for recycling of materials, and available storage space. Overall, immobilization devices have been identified as being beneficial and serve to enhance the administration of radiation treatments. Properly constructed immobilization devices can reduce daily setup times, increase efficiency, and reduce overall costs of treatment. Comfortable, well-fitting immobilization devices can reduce patients' fears and minimize misconceptions about treatment.[43]

Immobilization devices have been identified by category. The most common categories are discussed below.

### Hook-and-loop tape and straps

Many types of adhesive tape have been used in the past to secure patient position during treatment. Currently, straps with hook-and-loop backing are preferred to assist patient setup. Hook-and-loop tape can be affixed to the side rails of the treatment couch and then wrapped around the patient and attached to the side rail hooks. These hook-and-loop straps are padded, reusable, and much more comfortable than adhesive tape. The hook-and-loop tapes can keep both of the extremities aligned and support the chin and head and neck region.

### Generic body supports

Body supports include foam rubber wedges and supports, plastic head cups, neck rolls, knee and lumbar supports, thigh and heel stirrups, and prone face holders. This equipment provides comfort and stability during treatment. Indexed supports are a type of body support indexed by size, shape, and elevation above the treatment couch. These devices provide head and neck support as well as height and angle information for setup duplication.

### Body casts

Methods and materials used to make effective body casts have evolved over the past 2 decades due to the need to reduce patient setup errors and to allow for 3-dimensional conformal therapy treatment methods. Many of these materials originated in the specialties of orthopedics and dentistry and use modern packaging systems. For example, the Alpha Cradle (Smithers Medical Products, North Canton, Ohio) is a polyurethane foam cast that is created by placing the patient in the treatment position on a plastic bag held within a specialized form. The form is constructed of rigid polystyrene plastic blocks. When a combination of 2 chemicals known as Alpha Cradle Foaming agent is combined in the bag, the mixture reacts to form into a polyurethane foam. The foam rises and expands, supporting the patient's anatomic structures. When the foam hardens, the cast is ready to use. Alpha Cradles are effectively used for a variety of disease sites. They are rigid, are radiolucent, and fit snugly and comfortably to the patient's contours. Because they are unable to prevent patient movement and rotation, they must be used in combination with other immobilization devices. Additional methods and materials used to create body casts are vacuum bags and thermoplastics.

## POSITIONING DEVICES

Positioning devices secure patients in nontraditional positions for treatment. These devices are necessary to improve the therapeutic ratio and enhance patient comfort. Varied anatomic features coupled with nonrigid human body contours require the use of positioning devices to provide stability. Neck rolls, foam wedges, head holders, and Timo, a head and neck support (Bionix, Toledo, Ohio), are used to arrange body parts away from the path of the radiation beam and to improve positioning.

Arm boards, knee saddles, and thigh stirrups are other appliances used to position the extremities comfortably. Treating soft-tissue sarcomas of the limbs often requires careful positioning of the extremities, for example. Handgrips, overhead arm positioners, and shoulder retractors are also used to place extremities out of the path of critical treatment regions. Arms can be placed above the head or at the sides in reproducible locations with couch rail-mounted or tilt board-mounted handgrips and arm supports or with overhead arm positioners.

Patient elevation systems include tilt boards, slant boards, and breast boards. Patients who are required to maintain supine positions during treatment are often placed on tilting or slanting rigid plastic boards. These positioning devices can assist individuals who have difficulty lying supine. Tilt boards have built-in handgrips that provide comfort for arms-up treatment setups. The breast board is used most commonly for the treatment of breast cancer with parallel opposed tangential fields. It allows for arm support above the shoulders and away from the lateral field. In addition, it allows for unobstructed access to the breast by the lateral field, positions the chest wall horizontally to avoid angulation of the collimator, and by gravity pulls the large breast down for an improved treatment position. Several clinical circumstances must be considered when treating patients with breast cancer, such as stabilizing large pendulous breasts and minimizing skin reaction in the inframammary crease.[43]

Belly boards are specialized positioning devices used to support patients in prone positions that contain a window cutout for the patient's abdomen. This equipment provides comfort and stability for obese patients and minimizes the amount of intestine in the field.

The treatment chair is a positioning device that is mounted on the treatment couch. It has head and neck supports and can accommodate a variety of arm positions. The treatment chair is used for patients with respiratory compromise and for mediastinal disease, as the position minimizes the amount of normal tissue that is irradiated during treatment.

Head fixation devices are used for immobilization during stereotactic radiosurgery and for treatment of head and neck cancer. Stereotactic radiosurgery requires the use of a frame that is bolted to the patient's skull before target localization. Metal stereotactic frames are not comfortable and are used for single fraction administration only. New noninvasive, relocatable frames are now available that enhance patient comfort and facilitate precise treatment planning. Nonstereotactic head immobilization is commonly used during treatment of head and neck regions. The device is commonly made of precut thermoplastic mesh sheets that are attached to a rigid frame. Warm water softens this system and enables the thermoplastic masks to be pulled down over the patient's face, molding to the facial contours; the masks are then attached to a base plate. Bite blocks use a dental impression mouthpiece supported by a solid base plate under the patient's head, which is fastened to the treatment couch. Adjustable bite blocks are often used in conjunction with a Timo support to steady the head and neck region (Figure 13-22).[43]

Due to the enhancement of the specialty with 3-dimensional conformal therapy, dose escalation, and IMRT, it is essential that precise tumor control occur and that side effects be minimized. The ability to provide tight target margins, standardize dose, and maintain daily reproducibility is directly related to the precision of patient positioning and immobilization. Patient position has several limitations that preclude exactness: variance

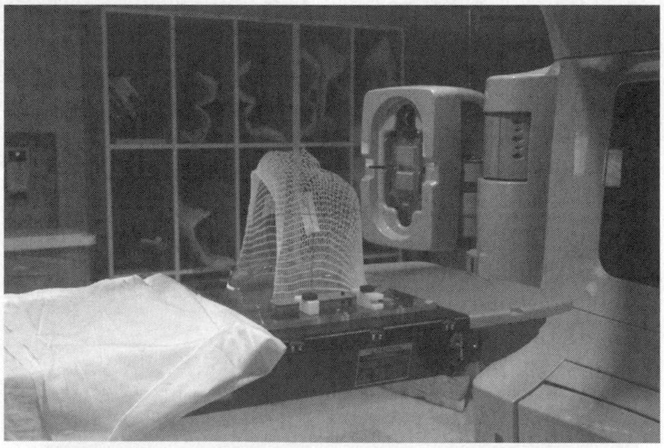

**FIGURE 13-22**

Head immobilizer attached to rigid plexiglass frame with laser coordinates for isocenter location.

*Source*: Photo courtesy of Fox Chase Cancer Center, Philadelphia, PA.

among accelerators, simulators, and treatment planning coordinate systems; daily organ movement; organ movement during the treatment processes; patient movement during treatment; rotation of the skeleton; and treatment setup errors. Appropriate patient positioning and immobilization help to diminish errors and facilitate the precise delivery of radiation. Studies have concluded that immobilization systems assist in reducing the need for large target margins.[44,45] It is pivotal that patient immobilization and positioning devices complement advanced radiation planning modalities. As treatment techniques become more precise, planning must include immobilization and positioning that can accommodate the demands of IMRT, IGRT, On-board imaging and brachytherapy protocols.

The multidisciplinary radiation oncology team must make it a priority to provide safe, secure, and comfortable surroundings for patients undergoing arduous, prolonged treatment. Nurses are in a key position to coordinate this effort by ensuring that patients are provided with comprehensive information to give informed consent about these procedures. Individuals should be encouraged to ask questions to demystify the fear of the unknown associated with radiation therapy and treatment protocols.

## DELIVERY OF RADIATION THERAPY: MACHINES AND EQUIPMENT

### LINEAR ACCELERATOR

A LINAC delivers high-energy radiation to tumors. The device uses high-frequency electromagnetic waves to accelerate charged particles, such as electrons, to high energies through a linear tube. When a beam of electrons is generated and accelerated by the LINAC, the energy increases. The electron volt (eV) is the basic unit of energy used in radiation oncology, and the escalating energy levels are kilovolts ($10^3$ eV = 1 kV) and megavolts ($10^6$ eV = 1 MeV). The electrons produced by the LINAC strike a target and produce x-rays of varying energies in the range of 10 to 30 kV; superficial units are between 30 and 125 kV. The charged electrons of the LINAC can be used to treat surface lesions as well as deep tumor targets.[4]

In lower-energy LINAC machines (6 MeV), the electrons proceed straight down a short accelerator tube to strike a target and produce x-rays. In higher-energy LINAC machines (18 MeV), the accelerator structure is longer and, therefore, must be angled to bend the electrons before striking the target.[39] An elaborate beam transport system made of specific bending magnets and focusing coils is responsible for directing the highly charged angled electrons. The LINAC treatment head consists of a thick shell of shielding material to provide protection from the danger of radiation leakage (Figure 13-23).[3]

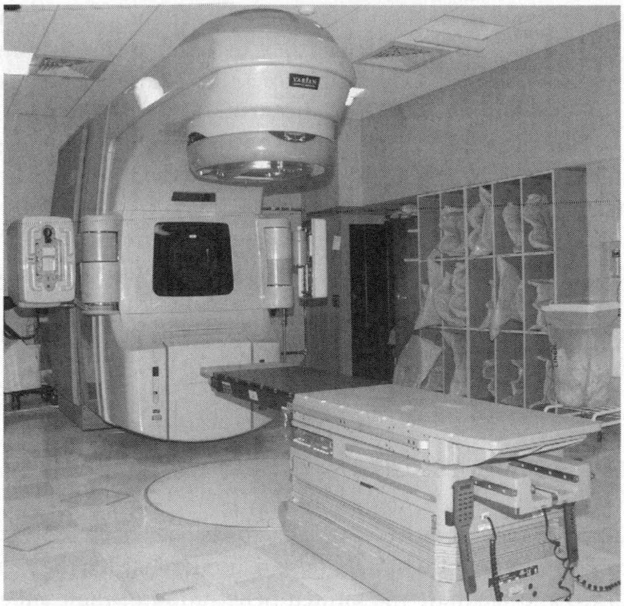

**FIGURE 13-23**

Linear accelerator uses high-frequency electromagnetic waves to accelerate charged particles.

*Source*: Photo courtesy of Fox Chase Cancer Center, Philadelphia, PA.

#### Collimation

Collimation refers to the treatment administration technique of shaping the radiation beam to the desired target. The collimator is located in the head of the LINAC. High-atomic number collimators can vary the treatment field size from 4 × 4 cm to 40 × 40 cm.[4] Electrons disperse easily in air, so the beam collimator must be approximated to the patient; 80 to 100 cm is the most common distance. The collimation system basically consists of a primary fixed collimator situated beyond the target in the direction of the beam and secondary movable collimators that shape the beam into square or rectangular fields. The 2 pairs of leaves in each secondary collimator can be moved in and out from the beam to increase or decrease the size of the treatment field. The leaves also can be closed or opened to provide the widest treatment field necessary. Various sizes of cones are attached to the collimators and extend to the skin surface of the patient. Lead cutouts at the end of the electron cone can provide additional beam shaping.[39]

The introduction of MLCs installed in the gantry of the LINAC, directly in the path of the beam, has revolutionized treatment field shaping.[39] Multileaf collimators have proved useful in providing computerized customized blocking that does not require the physical creation of a new block for each field. This advance has lessened the workload of the mold-room technicians and minimized the amount of time required for treatment planning and administration. An MLC can be programmed to change the shape of the beam to match the target shape as the beam moves around the target. This technique, called dynamic beam shaping, is considered to be clinically superior because it enhances tissue sparing.[6]

The multifaceted role of the radiation oncology nurse demands an expanded knowledge base beyond clinical management issues. It is important for the radiation oncology nurse to understand the intricacies of treatment machine options, associated costs, maintenance requirements, and pertinent information to provide patient education. This knowledge will provide a more comprehensive approach to patient care.

## ORTHOVOLTAGE UNITS

Orthovoltage units are x-ray machines that operate in the range of 150 to 500 kVp. Filters are used to harden the x-ray beam and facilitate the limited penetration of these superficial x-rays. The maximum dose from this low-energy unit is found on the surface of the patient.[39]

Although orthovoltage machines continue to be used at some radiation oncology centers to treat superficial skin lesions, the advent of electron therapy to treat superficial cancers has made this equipment obsolete. Therefore, as these units begin to require repair and maintenance, they are being replaced.

## MEGAVOLTAGE UNITS

### External beam units

***Low-energy megavoltage beams.*** Low-energy megavoltage beams (4 to 6 MV x-rays) without IMRT are used to treat shallow or moderately deep tumors such as tumors of head and neck and breast. If the low-energy machine has IMRT, the unit must have a dynamic MLC for expanded treatment plans.

***Medium- to high-energy megavoltage beams.*** These are treatment machines with energy ranges of 10 to 25 MV that are able to treat deep-seated tumors in the thorax, abdomen, and pelvis.[3] When tumors are deep seated, high-energy beams offer greater tissue sparing for all techniques, including IMRT. Electron beams in the range of 6 to 20 MeV are able to treat superficial tumors at depths of 5 cm. These are used with x-ray beams, as either a boost or mixed-beam treatment.[3] Clinical usefulness of this treatment includes: superficial cancers of the skin, lip, and chest wall, and boosts for lymph nodes and head and neck cancers. The use of electron beams to treat to this depth is extremely effective for superficial cancers and sparing of deeper normal tissues.

Equipment usage should be guided by standards in order to avoid overloaded machines and potential for compromised quality of care. The Blue Book[46] is a reference that delineates equipment usage and staffing requirements. It has been determined that megavoltage units should not exceed 20 to 30 patients treated per day. This parameter depends upon the complexity of procedures, the calibration checks, and quality assurance. Guidelines exist for calculating realistic treatment loads for megavoltage units.[3]

In recent decades, the megavoltage linear accelerator has been the machine of choice used to deliver radiation treatment. The production of x-rays with these devices is similar to that with the lower-voltage machines. The energy range of the megavoltage machines is broad: 4 to 20 MeV. The depth of the maximum dose ranges from 1.5 to 3.5 cm. The skin dose is 30% to 40% of the delivered dose. The electron beam capabilities of the megavoltage machines range from 5 to 20 MeV. An electron beam is produced by the removal of the tungsten target from the path of the beam; this beam is used for treatment purposes. The electron skin dose is high from megavoltage machines, about 80% to 95% of the delivered dose. A standard formula relating to the depth of electron penetration states that 80% of the dose is delivered at a depth (in centimeters) corresponding to one third of the electron energy in MeV. For example, a 12 MeV beam will deliver 80% of the dose at a depth of 4 cm.[4]

## MACHINE DESIGN

Radiation therapy devices are built to accommodate continual daily use for large cohorts of patients. The machines are compact and have a rotating feature that allows for 360° movement around the patient (Figure 13-24). This rotation offers a variety of options for beam

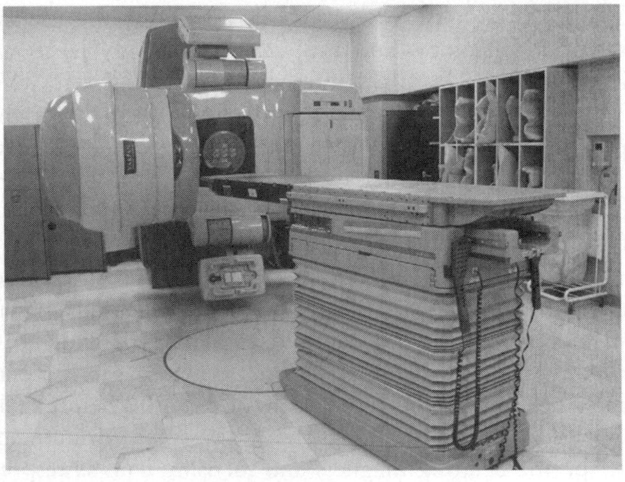

**FIGURE 13-24**

Linear accelerator in rotated position.

*Source*: Photo courtesy of Fox Chase Cancer Center, Philadelphia, PA.

angles to reach the target site. Distance must be provided between the patient and the beam-defining structures so as to allow for a safe rotation and to avoid collision with the patient and the treatment table or couch. The couch must be positioned to avoid potential interference of the beam by bars or rails. Treatment couches typically have removable sections that can be replaced either by thin polyester-film sheeting or a mesh-like insert to support the patient. The removable sections provide different options for patient treatment. First, removable side sections with a center spine for a continuous surface provide for treatment of posterior oblique fields without side rail interference. Second, a large removable center couch section allows for the treatment of a wide posterior field. Side rails are the link to support the segments of the couch, which are separated.[39]

Patient safety and comfort are priorities when treatment positioning occurs. The radiation therapists, together with the radiation nurses, must develop thorough preparatory information to ease patient fears and to ensure that a secure environment is provided throughout the treatment course. It may be appropriate to invite the patient and family to visit the treatment room to see the machines and associated equipment early in the process so that questions and concerns can be addressed prior to the actual planning and treatment sessions. Concerns about an unfamiliar environment, coupled with the multitude of anxieties associated with the entire cancer experience, can be alleviated by providing a personal introduction and tour.

## PROTON THERAPY

Proton beams consist of energized particles that are accelerated using megavoltage energy. They conform the high-dose region to the targeted volume and minimize normal tissue injury, thereby reducing treatment-related side effects. This reduction in dose to normal tissue allows for an increase of radiation dose to the target, beyond that possible with conventional radiation. Protons can be delivered to an irregular 3-dimensional volume in a variety of anatomic locations. Conforming the high-dose region of radiation beams to the tumor volume and avoiding unnecessary irradiation of normal tissue is the underlying premise of photon or electron (standard x-ray) radiation treatment. Protons have radiobiological characteristics similar to those of standard radiation.[47]

Protons were discovered in 1919 and were first accelerated to megavoltage energies in the 1930s. The clinical use of protons and the opening of treatment facilities began in the 1950s. Protons function by depositing a small portion of energy in the skin and superficial tissue, with the concentrated energy being delivered to the target volume. Protons are uniquely able to stop at the distal margin of the target, thereby sparing normal tissue.

Both conventional radiation therapy and proton beams work on the principle of selective cell destruction. A major advantage of proton treatment, however, is that the energy distribution of protons can be deposited more completely and more precisely in designated tissue than is the case with standard (photon and electron) radiation. This capability provides superior targeting and enhanced tumor control.

Protons are energized to specific velocities. These energies determine the anatomic depth of penetration of the deposited protons. As these particles travel through the body, they slow down, allowing for increased interaction with orbiting electrons. Maximum interaction with electrons occurs as the protons approach their stopping point.[47]

As noted earlier, protons release their maximum energy in the designated cancer volume. As a consequence, the surrounding healthy cells receive significantly less injury than cells in the designated target. The high-dose region of energy release occurs at a point called the Bragg peak. Protons' significant absorption characteristics result from their positive charge and heavy mass. Their energy upon entering the patient and the density of the tissue along their track determine the depth of penetration of the beam and the placement of the Bragg peak. The heavy mass results in minimal deviation and, therefore, minimal side scatter, which reduces unwanted side effects and maximizes treatment benefit.

Protons are administered through a proton accelerator. They pass through several components of the accelerator at boosted energies of 2 MeV. On their high-speed journey, they travel to and from the target about 10 million times per second. Each time they circulate, a boost of energy increases the protons' speed up to 250 MeV. These massively high energies can place the protons at any depth within the patient.[48]

A series of steering and focusing magnets guide the particles through different chambers of the accelerator. The gantries of the proton accelerator are massive and include wheels that are 35 feet in diameter and weigh approximately 90 tons. These gantries revolve around the patient and direct the beam precisely where it is needed. For their part, patients simply see a revolving cone-shaped aiming device.

The computers that control the proton facility have safety measures to ensure that patients receive their prescribed treatments. These computers verify patient identification, set operational parameters for each patient's treatment plan, and direct the host computers to deliver a specified beam.[48]

Proton particle therapy is an additional treatment modality for treating a variety of solid tumors. Currently, the clinical delivery of this therapy remains extremely limited, being restricted to only a few sites in the US and others worldwide. The installation of a proton facility poses tremendous financial and technical challenges and represents a significant limitation of this radiotherapy treatment technique.

The use of proton beam therapy remains controversial. The clinical reality of the superiority of proton therapy has not been studied in randomized clinical trials (RCTs) comparing proton beam therapy to standard x-ray therapy.

The theoretical benefits of proton therapy have been documented and are as follows: no dose to distal target volume, superior dose distribution, 2 to 3 times less energy deposited to uninvolved normal tissue, and virtually no difference in tissue response per unit dose. Clinicians aver that these aforementioned characteristics would make it unnecessary and unethical to conduct RCTs comparing standard x-ray therapy to proton therapy.[49,50]

Additional significant driving forces that limit proton use are costs, including costs of facilities, equipment, personnel, and insurance reimbursement. The costs and benefits of using proton beam therapy (PBT) to treat prostate cancer (high-volume diagnosis, focus of proton therapy centers in the US) have been assessed. PBT has been used for years to treat prostate cancer; however, although clinical efficacy has been documented, no data exist that claim PBT is superior to standard x-ray therapy.[51]

A cost analysis of intermediate-risk prostate cancer patients treated with PBT demonstrated a lack of cost effectiveness compared with standard current state-of-the-art therapy.[52] No differences in quality of life measurements were determined.[52]

Proton beam therapy is not an experimental treatment and does have advantages in treating ocular tumors, skull-based tumors, specific pediatric tumors, and prostate cancer. Of these cancers, the incidence is relatively small for all but prostate cancer. Therefore, PBT for prostate cancer will be the focus of future clinical and economic scrutiny prior to its widespread use.

## TREATMENT DELIVERY MODALITIES

### STEREOTACTIC RADIOSURGERY

Stereotactic radiosurgery is a 3-dimensional technique that delivers the entire desired dose in one fraction. Stereotactic principles guide radiosurgery and target intracranial lesions through the use of multiple beams. The concept of radiosurgery was evolved in 1951 by Lars Leksell, a Swedish neurosurgeon. His work focused on the use of a specially designed isotope unit known as the gamma knife, which was responsible for the evolution of many radiosurgical procedures. Limited availability of the gamma knife kept radiosurgery largely inaccessible until the mid-1980s,[53] when researchers began to adapt LINACs to administer radiosurgery. This made radiosurgery more widely available, as many radiation oncologists and neurosurgeons purchased hardware and software to upgrade their LINACs. Stereotactic techniques have since expanded beyond the scope of neurosurgical procedures, and are now applied to fractionated treatments, known as *stereotactic radiotherapy,* and to applications outside of the brain.[53]

Radiosurgery techniques use a stereotactic frame fixed to the patient's skull to provide accurate landmarks for localization of intracranial targets (Figure 13-25). These targets are correlated with neuroimaging studies such as MRI, CT, and angiography. The purpose of the frame is to provide a basis for target identification within an *x*, *y*, and *z*

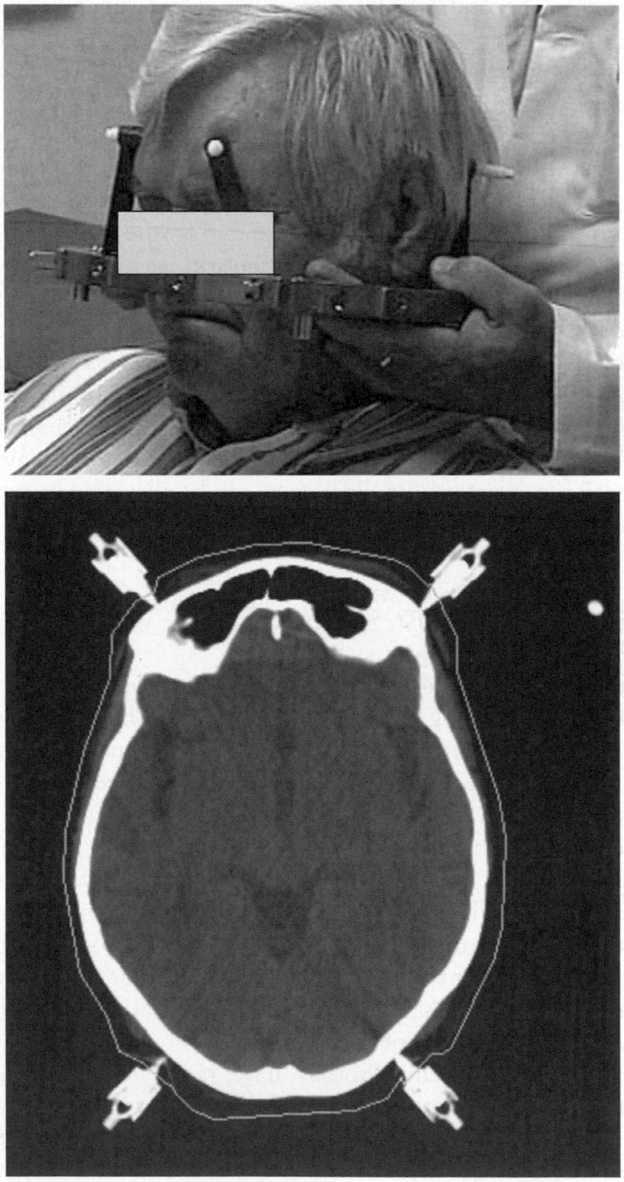

**FIGURE 13-25**

(**A**) Placement of stereotactic headframe. (**B**) Image of sterotactic headframe with bolts in place for treatment position.

*Source*: Photo courtesy of Fox Chase Cancer Center, Philadelphia, PA.

coordinate system. This system is used to define the shape and extent of the target lesion.

Radiosurgery is indicated for distinct lesions, ≤ 4 cm in size, with the potential to respond to a single fraction of radiation. Ideal targets for radiosurgery are almost entirely spherical and small (≤3 cm in maximum dimension). Irregular volumes can present the challenge of treating many isocenters to achieve conformation to the target volume. Although primary and metastatic brain tumors are most commonly treated, the greatest clinical experience has involved treatment of arteriovenous malformations (AVMs).[10]

The radiosurgery systems used are the gamma knife and the LINAC-based system. Both systems consist of a stereotactic frame, radiation delivery system, and computer hardware and treatment planning software. The radiosurgery system utilizes MRI or CT information to locate and determine target size and location, treatment planning needs, and type of radiation delivery. Although the systems vary, the clinical outcomes for treatment should be the same for similar patient groups.

The cost of the gamma knife system ranges from approximately $3.5 million to $4.2 million, including new facility construction. The cobalt sources decay after 7 years and must be replaced at a significant cost. The unit contains cobalt distributed in 201 sources over a portion of a hemisphere so that circular beams from collimators may enter the skull through a large number of evenly distributed points. The gamma knife has a permanent 18,000-kg shield surrounding a hemispheric array of cobalt sources. Four interchangeable outer collimator helmets are used to vary the target volume. Individual collimators can be plugged in to conform the dose to the target shape. The target size is about 3 to 18 mm, with a 0.1 mm degree of accuracy.[10,17]

The LINAC can be adapted to administer stereotactic radiation and is available at a much lower cost than the gamma knife. Target sizes of the LINAC range from 10 to 50 mm, with an accuracy of 0.1 to 1.0 mm. The LINAC administers radiosurgery in the following ways:

1. The gantry rotates through an arc for each of several stationary couch angles.
2. In dynamic stereotactic radiosurgery, the gantry and couch move simultaneously, and the beam of entry on the skull resembles a seam. This seam provides an advantage, in that beam entrance and exit doses do not overlap (Figure 13-26).
3. A rotating chair aligns and immobilizes the patient's head in a stationary radiation beam.

Approximately 2 to 4 months after radiosurgery, MRI is used to monitor the development of edema or potential radiation sequelae. The PET scan has emerged as a way to differentiate tumor from necrosis in previously irradiated patients.[10] Whole body stereotactic treatment is now being implemented in some centers, where appropriate.

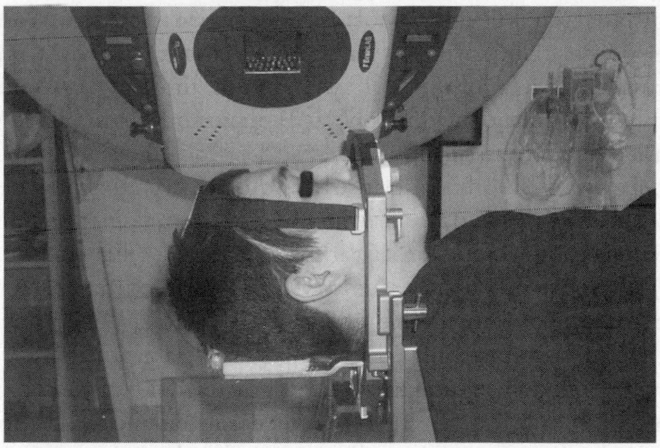

**FIGURE 13-26**

Stereotactic radiosurgery.

*Source*: Photo courtesy of Fox Chase Cancer Center, Philadelphia, PA.

## IMAGE-GUIDED CYBERKNIFE RADIOSURGERY

The cyberknife is an innovative frameless robotic radiosurgical system that is based on the original concept of frame-based radiosurgery. It includes 3 components: an advanced, light-weight LINAC, a robot, and x-ray cameras. The miniature LINAC produces high-energy (6 MeV) radiation. It is mounted on a robotic arm, which directs the LINAC to deliver radiation beams to the targeted tumor from multiple positions and angles. Image guidance cameras are used to locate the target, to take frequent pictures of the tumor during treatment, and to target the radiation beam emitted by the linear accelerator. The cyberknife uses its robotic arm to deliver highly focused beams of radiation that converge at the tumor. Thus, the tumor receives a cumulative dose of radiation to control or destroy the tumor cells, while radiation exposure to surrounding tissue is minimized. The cyberknife is able to compensate for patient movement to ensure highly accurate delivery of radiation during treatment. When patient movement occurs during treatment, the cameras detect the position change, and the robot is able to compensate for the movement by repositioning the LINAC before administering the radiation beam. This process of constantly correcting for beam placement ensures accurate tumor targeting.[54]

The first cyberknife prototype was installed for clinical use at Stanford University in 1994. Cyberknife technology was approved by the Food and Drug Administration (FDA) for general use in August 2001. Standard stereotactic techniques require that a rigid metal frame be affixed to a patient's skull for immobilization and target localization purposes. Although the frame-based systems have been effective clinically, they have many limitations, including restricting treatment fields to the brain, limiting the angles for radiation targeting, and causing patient discomfort. As an alternative to standard frame-based radiosurgical instruments, the cyberknife uses noninvasive, image-guided localization and a robotic delivery system. This technological combination enables the cyberknife to overcome the limitations of older frame-based radiosurgery equipment such as the gamma knife and LINAC.

The unique mechanism of the cyberknife provides a noninvasive, surgical-like outcome for lesions of the brain and spine. It is the first and only commercial application of robotic stereotactic radiosurgery for the spine and the spinal cord. In addition, this technology has the benefit of enabling the cyberknife system to be used for radiosurgical applications outside the brain as well as for staged radiosurgical procedures. Staged radiosurgery (ie, fractionated radiosurgery) occurs when the total dose of stereotactic radiation is divided into several smaller doses, with delivery spanning several days. The cyberknife has provided radiosurgery in utilizing 1 to 5 fractions on targets throughout the body.[54]

Cyberknife radiosurgery has also been effectively used to treat selected lung malignancies. The combination of investigational software and hardware with cyberknife technology can deliver conformal radiation to moving primary and metastatic lung tumors if surgery is not an option. The cyberknife accommodates lung and tumor motion, enabling modifications to be made so as to deliver a maximal therapeutic dose while minimizing surrounding tissue toxicity. Lung cancer patients have been treated on a dose-escalation study of 15 to 25 Gy and carefully monitored for toxicity.[55] This procedure involves a planning CT scan, foam mold construction for immobilization, and the placement of a radiographic fiducial, a gold seed that is implanted in the tumor and used for computer tracking. Once the radiation oncologist and the medical physicist design treatment plans, the patient receives the prescribed radiation treatment using the cyberknife. Its computer-controlled robotic device modifies radiation beam delivery as necessary to accommodate tumor movement. Patients are encouraged to breathe normally, as the rhythmic breathing enables the computer to track the process. The entire pretreatment evaluation and planning process spans several days. The actual treatment time is approximately 1.5 hours.[55]

### Treatment procedure

Once patients have been assessed and evaluated by the multidisciplinary team, the treatment process commences. This process involves the following 3 steps: treatment setup, treatment planning, and treatment delivery. Each of these procedures can occur either on the same day or on separate visits. Unlike with conventional stereotactic radiosurgery, the cyberknife treatment planning procedure does not require that the patient be confined in an acute care setting while the plan is formulated. Patients are ambulatory and able to return home between treatment planning appointments.

During treatment setup, the radiation oncology team plans the overall details of radiation delivery. If a cranial tumor is being treated, a custom-fit plastic mask is made for the patient. This mask serves the same purpose as the conventional metal head frame used during stereotactic radiosurgery but is noninvasive and painless. The patient has a CT scan with iodinated dye contrast (and sometimes an MRI is obtained for full visualization) with the mask in place. The CT data are then integrated into the treatment planning software, and digitally reconstructed radiographs demonstrating various patient positions are correlated with images of the target so that the computer can identify in 3-dimensional space exactly where the lesion is located.[54]

Cyberknife treatment planning utilizes the clinical experience of both the radiation oncologist and the physicist as well as the power of high-speed computers to determine the volume, dose, and pattern of radiation beam target. During this planning phase, the cyberknife performs millions of calculations to determine the most effective radiation delivery plan.

Soon after treatment planning is complete, the patient returns for treatment delivery. During treatment, the patient lies supine on the treatment table and is fitted with the appropriate immobilization device. At the beginning of the actual treatment, the imaging system acquires digital x-rays of tumor localization and patient position. This information is transmitted to the robotic arm, which is used to move the LINAC to the appropriate position. As treatment proceeds, the robot moves and retargets the LINAC at multiple positions around the patient. At each position, a small radiation beam is delivered. This process is repeated at 50 to 300 different positions around the patient to complete treatment. At various intervals, the LINAC stops and takes additional pictures, allowing the cyberknife to track and compensate for slight physical movement.

The total process takes 30 to 90 minutes to deliver radiation beams. One fraction or multiple treatments (fractionated) may be prescribed, which requires the patient to return for a repeat treatment session. The cyberknife is able to treat larger lesions than conventional radiosurgery (up to 6 cm). Typically, patients are assessed and can be discharged immediately upon completion of treatment to resume their normal activities.

### Patient education and preparation

Radiation oncology nurses assume the primary responsibility for educating patients who will undergo either standard frame-based radiosurgery or image-guided cyberknife radiosurgery. For this reason, nurses must be involved in the initial assessment of patients. Educational goals should be formulated in conjunction with the entire multidisciplinary team. Patients and families require explicit verbal informed consent accompanied by comprehensive written information and visual materials, including the option of a tour of the equipment and treatment area. Each patient must be considered individually, and an accurate assessment made about the amount of information to be provided. Nurses must ensure that educational preparation commences prior to therapy, during therapy, upon discharge, and during follow-up encounters. It is vital that patients be given adequate time for understanding advanced concepts relating to procedural details that will ensure safe and effective radiosurgical treatment outcomes.

## BRACHYTHERAPY

The goal of brachytherapy is to provide a boost dose to the tumor or tumor bed, usually postoperatively. Brachytherapy uses interstitial or intracavitary implantation of radioactive sources. Target volume localization is accomplished using clinical examination, radiographs, and CT scanning. A variety of brachytherapy planning systems are used to specify treatment dose, and computerized treatment planning systems are used to specify dosages according to isodose distribution. Computer displays during brachytherapy administration show dose distribution, which facilitates clinical evaluation.[56]

Recently, the trend in brachytherapy has been to replace low dose rate (LDR) brachytherapy, which uses manual afterloading or remote afterloading techniques, with HDR brachytherapy. HDR therapy has advantages such as outpatient treatment, flexibility of optimizing dose distribution, and personnel safety due to lower radiation exposure. Because of these advantages it is possible that HDR will replace LDR completely.[57]

Brachytherapy or implant therapy has been used clinically for more than 100 years. *Brachy* (from Greek, meaning "short distance") describes a radiation treatment in which the radiation source comes in direct contact with the tumor. With brachytherapy, dose distribution is dependent on the inverse square law, because the source is usually directly located within the tumor volume. It is, therefore, crucial that the radiation sources be placed with high precision. Brachytherapy procedures can be done with either temporary or permanent implants. Temporary implants usually have long half-lives and higher energies than permanent implants. These radiation sources can be manufactured in several forms, such as needles, seeds, and ribbons. Temporary radiation sources are inserted into catheters that are surgically placed in the tumor. A few days postoperatively, the patient is brought to the radiation department for simulation. Wires with nonradioactive metal seeds are then threaded into these catheters. Films are taken, and the image of the seed placement is digitized into a brachytherapy treatment planning computer. Once the treatment plan is complete and the optimal dose rate is selected, the radioactive sources can be inserted. The implantation occurs in the patient's room. The duration is usually 1 to 3 days. Most temporary implants are loaded interstitially.[56]

Implantation techniques may be characterized in terms of the type of surgical approach within the target volume (interstitial, intracavitary, transluminal, or mold techniques), the means of controlling the dose delivered (temporary or permanent implants), and the dose rate (low, medium, or high). Interstitial brachytherapy is the surgical implantation of small radioactive sources directly into target tissues. Permanent interstitial implants remain in place forever. The initial source strength is chosen so that the prescribed dose is fully delivered when the implanted radioactivity has decayed to a negligible level. Interstitial LDR brachytherapy is commonly used to treat cancer of the oral cavity, oropharynx, and prostate, and sarcomas. Intracavitary insertion consists of positioning applicators with radioactive sources into a body cavity close to the target tissue. The most commonly used intracavitary treatment technique entails insertion of a tandem and colpostat for cervical cancer. Intracavitary implants are temporary; they are inserted in the patient for a specified time (usually 24 to 168 hours after source insertion for LDR therapy). Transluminal brachytherapy is the insertion of a line source into a body lumen to treat its surface and adjacent tissues. Plesiocurieor mold therapy is a surface-dose application that consists of an applicator containing a variety of radioactive sources designed to deliver a uniform dose distribution to the skin or mucosal surface.[56,57]

The International Commission on Radiation Units and Measurements (ICRU) determines dose rates of implants.[58] Low dose rate implants deliver doses at a rate of 40 to 200 cGy/hour (0.4 to 2.0 Gy/hour), requiring treatment times of 24 to 144 hours. High dose rate brachytherapy delivers dose rates in excess of 0.2 Gy/minute (12 Gy/hour). Modern HDR remote afterloaders contain sources capable of delivering dose rates of 0.12 Gy/second (432 Gy/hour) at 1 cm distance, resulting in brief treatment times. A shielded vault and remote afterloading device are essential components of an HDR brachytherapy facility. LDR implant patients are confined to the hospital during treatment to manage the potential radiation safety hazard of the implant. HDR brachytherapy is performed as an outpatient procedure. Although the ultra-LDR range is not recognized by the ICRU, it is important in the implementation of treatment with permanent iodine-125 ($^{125}I$) and palladium-103 ($^{103}Pd$) seed implants. The clinical application and usefulness of radionuclides depend on physical properties such as half-life, radiation output per unit activity, specific activity, and photon energy. In the past, radium was the primary isotope used in brachytherapy. Due to its long half-life and high energy output, radium has been replaced with cesium (Cs), gold (Au), and iridium (Ir). These isotopes have shorter half-lives than radium and can be shielded more easily due to their low energies.[56,57,59]

With the use of remote afterloading devices, radiation exposure can be diminished for hospital personnel, and particularly for nursing staff, who are primarily responsible for source loading and the care of implant patients. This delivery system consists of a pneumatically or motor-driven source transport system that robotically transfers radioactive material between a shielded safe and each treatment applicator. HDR and LDR are the types of remote afterloading that can be used. The most common LDR source is $^{137}Cs$, which has a dose rate of about 1 cGy/minute. The most common HDR source is $^{192}Ir$, with a dose rate of 100 cGy/minute (Figure 13-27).[56,57]

Pretreatment brachytherapy procedures are similar to those of remote afterloading brachytherapy. The treatment plan is developed by the medical physicists and approved by the radiation oncologists, then the patient is escorted and set up in the treatment room. The source is connected to the end of a cable inside the afterloading unit. This unit has data from the planning computer. The cable is directed out of the unit into one of the patient's catheters. Several catheters can be connected to the unit. The catheters are irradiated, one at a time, until the designated dose is achieved. The motor that drives the source out of the treatment unit is connected electronically to the treatment room door. If the need arises for cessation of treatment, opening the door will cause the source to be drawn back into the unit by an interlocking system. This safety device lessens the danger of personnel exposure. This interlock is the safety advantage integral to the use of this delivery system compared with manual afterloading (Figures 13-28 and 13-29).[57]

Low dose rate remote afterloading is commonly used for intracavitary treatment of uterine cancer. All LDR procedures

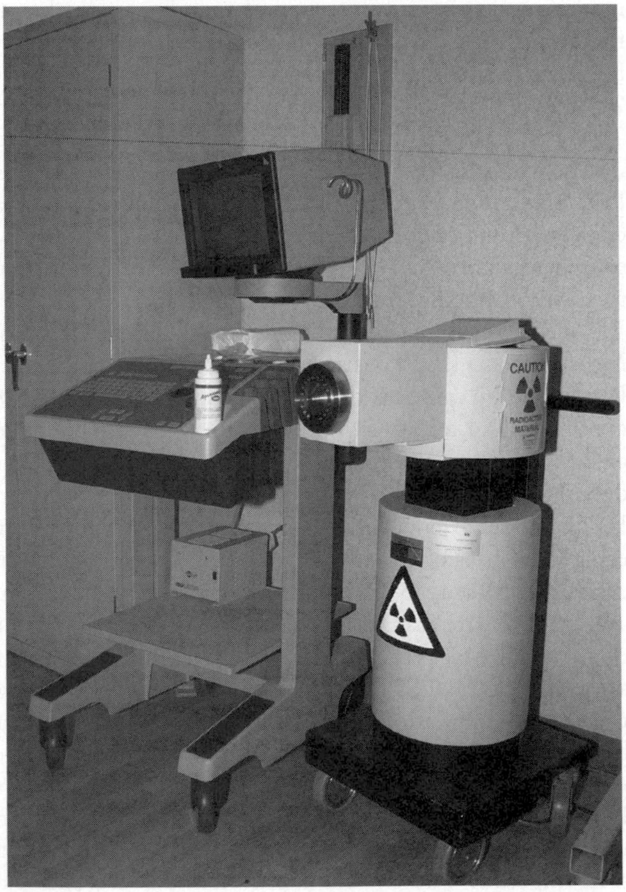

**FIGURE 13-27**

Remote afterloading equipment pneumatic source transport system.

*Source*: Photo courtesy of Fox Chase Cancer Center, Philadelphia, PA.

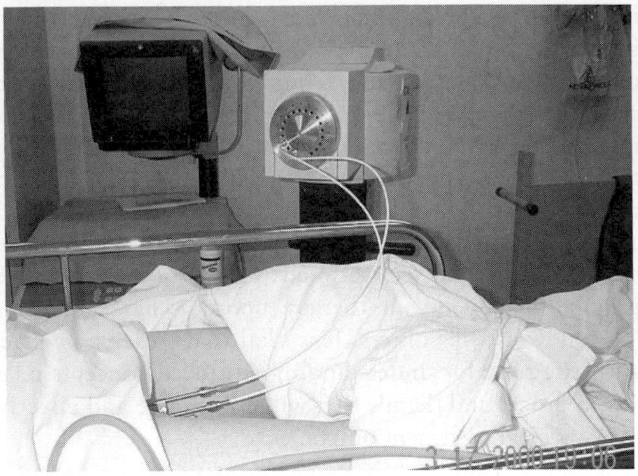

**FIGURE 13-28**

High dose rate endometrial brachytherapy.

*Source*: Photo courtesy of Fox Chase Cancer Center, Philadelphia, PA.

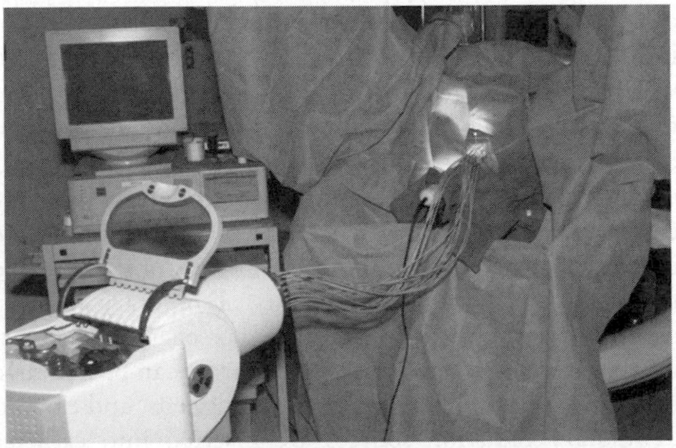

**FIGURE 13-29**

High dose rate prostate brachytherapy.

*Source*: Photo courtesy of Fox Chase Cancer Center, Philadelphia, PA.

are performed in the patient's room. The interlock is connected to the patient's door so nurses can give care and family members can visit without risk.[56] The most common applications of HDR brachytherapy include treatment of sarcomas and tumors of the vaginal apex, esophagus, lung, and floor of the mouth. Most HDR treatments are performed on an outpatient basis, which constitutes a tremendous advantage for afterloading brachytherapy.[57]

### Brachytherapy equipment

Brachytherapy is administered either alone or in conjunction with external beam treatment. Brachytherapy is indicated in the treatment of the following cancers; gynecologic, oral cavity, and prostate cancers. Most common sources are cesium-137 tubes, iridium-192 seeds contained in ribbons, iodine-125 seeds, and palladium-103 seeds. Remote afterloading units for LDR and HDR are commonly used. Departments must be equipped with computer programs to support treatment planning and administration and monitoring of Brachytherapy protocols.

## UNSEALED RADIONUCLIDE THERAPY

Unsealed radionuclide therapy is used for the treatment of benign or malignant thyroid disease, hematological disease, malignant bone disease, and benign or malignant disease within a body cavity. Strict guidelines exist for the use of these sources in women; hence, verification of a nonpregnant and nonbreastfeeding condition must be established prior to the initiation of therapy. A negative B human chorionic gonadotropin test within 48 hours before therapy, documented hysterectomy or tubal ligation, a postmenopausal state with no menstrual bleeding for 2 years, or premenarche is a sufficient clinical indicator to proceed with treatment. Breastfeeding must be stopped for 1 or 2 weeks prior to administration of an unsealed radioactive source.[10]

Specific Nuclear Regulatory Commission (NRC) guidelines must be followed for determining inpatient or outpatient dose, which is dependent on the total body burden of the radioisotope. Nurses must consistently but safely render care to patients receiving unsealed radioisotope therapy. It is essential that nurses reduce their exposure to emitted radiation by using the principles of time, distance, and shielding. Institutional policy and procedure must be in place to manage the total program and process as well as the possibility of emergency spills. Institutions administering both teletherapy and brachytherapy must have pre-established standards of nursing practice to ensure effective patient management as well as radiation safety. These nursing actions must focus on individual patient needs and provide detailed practice guidelines for both routine and emergency requirements. Table 13-1 provides an overview of nursing practice standards from a national comprehensive cancer center (Fox Chase Cancer Center, Philadelphia, Pennsylvania). These standards provide details of clinical actions for both routine and emergent situations.

Institutions administering unsealed radioactive sources must have strict quality assurance policies and procedures in place. These programs should be guided by the NRC recommendations and focus on the protection of patients, the public, and medical personnel from the potential hazards of unnecessary exposure.

## RADIOIMMUNOTHERAPY

Radioimmunotherapy (RIT) is an FDA-approved treatment modality that combines the cytotoxicity of radiation with the specificity of monoclonal antibodies for tumor cell surface antigens. RIT is a novel therapeutic modality that links radionuclides to monoclonal antibodies to form radioimmunoconjugates. Cell death occurs once the radioimmunoconjugate has become bound to the tumor cell antigen by either the antibody itself or the radiation from the radionuclide. RIT is a different approach from standard EBRT in that RIT targets radiation directly to tumor sites, potentially giving lower doses of radiation to normal tissue. Radioimmunotherapy is extremely specific and does not have the broad side effect profile associated with standard systemic or locoregional treatment modalities.

In 2002, the FDA approved ibritumomab tiuxetan (Zevalin), which is a monoclonal antibody conjugated to a molecule of yttrium-90. In 2003, tositumomab iodine-131 (Bexxar), which conjugates a molecule of iodine-131 to monoclonal antibody anti-CD20, was approved. These agents are the first to be classified as radioimmunotherapy and were approved for treatment of refractory non-Hodgkin's lymphoma.[60,61]

Oncology nurses must be knowledgeable regarding clinical trials, treatment protocols, and indications for RIT. In addition, those nurses working in radiation treatment, nuclear medicine, and medical oncology should participate in creating patient education plans for individuals receiving RIT. These educational programs should include information on background and rationale for RIT, administration information, and follow-up and safety guidelines. As RIT becomes used more frequently in the clinical setting, it is essential that nurses prioritize communication among the multidisciplinary professional team involved in RIT so that effective and safe patient administration is a reality.[62–64]

## ADVANCED TOPICS: TREATMENT DELIVERY

### PARTIAL BREAST IRRADIATION

Radiation therapy in the US has traditionally been given to patients with breast cancer daily for 5 days a week over

**TABLE 13-1**

**Standards of Nursing Practice**

Care of the patient receiving external beam radiation

1. Educate the patient with regard to the goal of therapy and treatment experiences, including simulation, setup, tattoos, blocks, and casts.
2. Be aware of the patient's treatment field and teach the patient symptom management of the associated general and site-specific reactions to the therapy. Site-specific reactions may include: diarrhea, nausea and vomiting, dysuria, dysphagia, esophagitis, mucositis, xerostomia, hair loss, and skin reactions.
3. Encourage rest periods as needed during the course of therapy to combat the anticipated side effect of fatigue.
4. Provide nutrition counseling to minimize weight loss. Encourage the patient's consumption of an appropriate diet for side effect management (eg, high protein, high calorie, low residue, or soft diet).
5. Use skin care products (ie, soaps, creams, lotions, gels) only at the recommendation of the radiation oncology staff.
6. Initiate referrals to home health services if the patient's symptoms require continued follow-up and assessment in the home.

Care of the patient receiving brachytherapy

1. Provide preimplant teaching to patients and their families to promote basic knowledge and understanding of the goals of therapy and the treatment experience.
2. Observe principles of time, distance, and shielding while caring for the implant patient. Perform patient care from behind lead shields placed at the bedside.
3. Wear a radiation film badge or direct reading dosimeter to record radiation exposure when in proximity to the implant patient.
4. Pregnant nurses are not to care for implant patients while they are loaded with radioactive sources.
5. Body fluids are not radioactive and may be disposed of according to routine institutional policy.
   *Exception*: Patients receiving systemic radioactive iodine will have contaminated body secretions. Patients' linens must remain in the room in the linen bag. Patients should be served meals with disposable utensils and paper products. The trash bin will also remain in the room until a radiation safety officer verifies it is no longer contaminated. Everything should remain in the patient's room until cleared by a radiation safety officer.
6. Check radioactive sources at the beginning and end of each shift and document the status of the implant. Applicators should have caps, and interstitial needles and catheters should be counted and observed for dislodgment.
7. If the implant becomes dislodged, the nurse will retrieve the radioactive source using the provided long forceps and place it in a source holder in the room. Notify the radiation oncologist immediately. There is a 24-hour-on-call coverage.
8. Know the correct course of action if the patient has a medical emergency.
9. Inform the patient and visitors of hospital policy regarding visitation while the patient has radioactive material in place. Children under 18 and pregnant women are prohibited from visiting. Any questions should be referred to the radiation safety officer.

*Source*: Reproduced with permission from the Department of Nursing, Fox Chase Cancer Center, Committee of Nursing Standards, Philadelphia, PA. Updated July 2008.

a 6 to 7 week course. Historically, breast cancer treatment focused on treating the entire breast to achieve local control even in patients with early stage disease. Initially the entire breast is treated for 4.5 to 5 weeks, followed by a focused boost to the area of the tumor bed for an additional 5 to 7 treatments. A total dose of 45 to 50 Gy in 25 fractions of 1.8 to 2 Gy is used. In addition, boost radiation to the site of the primary tumor is given to a dose of 10 to 16 Gy in 5 to 8 fractions.[65] Over time, local recurrences have commonly occurred in the vicinity of the surgical incision and have arisen even if the entire breast was irradiated.[66] For this reason, the focus of treatment for individuals who qualify with early stage breast cancer has changed to include the concept that PBI targeted at the lumpectomy cavity with a small surrounding margin will yield similar local control to whole breast irradiation.

Radiation treatment techniques have evolved over recent years due to 3-dimensional treatment planning, enhanced computerization, and sophisticated immobilization devices. The focus of advanced treatment delivery for qualified patients with breast cancer is to enhance quality of life by focusing on shortening the duration of treatment while retaining the same benefits of current therapy. The goal of PBI is to achieve the same success as whole breast radiation therapy. In addition, it is vital that the accelerated dosing schedules provide data that support equivalent long-term disease-free survival in appropriate patient populations, equal cosmetic result, and decreased risk of recurrence in untreated breast tissue.[67]

Breast cancer is being diagnosed earlier, and therefore women are being cured of the disease. It is important for clinicians to appreciate the changing trends with this diagnosis as it becomes a chronic process that impacts the lives of women who desire to remain both professionally and personally active during treatment and beyond. It is for these reasons that research has focused on ways to decrease treatment time for eligible individuals. Added benefits of this advanced treatment modality include economic incentives as well as increased utilization of radiation therapy resources. It is imperative that the change from conventional radiation to an accelerated schedule provide patients with the same long-term cure rates and side effect risks. Two strategies for reducing overall treatment time in early stage breast cancer are PBI and hypofractionated whole breast irradiation.

Partial breast irradiation is radiation therapy aimed directly to the area of the breast at greatest risk for local recurrence; this is the tumor bed, with a small margin, as opposed to the entire breast. is delivered twice daily with a 6-hour interval over a course of 5 days and is evolving as a potential treatment strategy for selected patients. Treatment can be administered using either invasive brachytherapy techniques such as multiple interstitial brachytherapy catheters, MammoSite balloon, or noninvasive external beam 3D-CRT. Preliminary studies have demonstrated promising results with low recurrence rates using PBI; the long-term effectiveness and side effects, as well as identification of the most eligible patients for this form of treatment, are now being studied. The most likely candidates are women with small tumors, absence of involved lymph nodes, and favorable types of breast cancer.[67]

A phase III National Surgical Adjuvant Breast Project–Radiation Therapy Oncology Group (NSABP-RTOG) intergroup trial is currently enrolling patients and is comparing conventional whole breast irradiation to partial breast irradiation.[68]

### MammoSite radiation therapy system

A targeted internal radiation therapy treatment modality referred to as MammoSite is indicated for patients with early stage breast cancer who are candidates for lumpectomy. Approved by the FDA in 2002, the MammoSite system delivers high-dose radiation directly to the site of tumor excision, targeting the area where the cancer would most likely recur and sparing approximating healthy tissue.[69]

MammoSite can be used in conjunction with conventional external beam radiation as a boost or as primary treatment for a qualified patient. The new technology reduces the length of daily radiation treatment following surgery. Patients are able to receive a higher radiation dose due to targeted concentration to one specific area. MammoSite is considered the next generation of internal radiation therapy. It is minimally invasive, has a good safety profile, and can be performed as an outpatient procedure with high patient tolerance. The overall appeal of PBI is the avoidance of interstitial brachytherapy (with its requirements of insertion of multiple needles in the breast tissue, inpatient confinement, and concomitant infection risk) as well as a reduction of required treatment time for external beam therapy and concomitant side effects.[70]

The MammoSite balloon catheter is placed at the time of lumpectomy or within 10 weeks postsurgery. Catheter placement is performed either during the surgical procedure under general anesthesia or in an ambulatory procedure room under local anesthesia. The catheter is inserted into the surgical cavity either through a separate pathway created by a trocar or through the lumpectomy scar. Its balloon end is inflated with saline and a contrast agent to allow the surrounding tissue to conform to the balloon, the exit site is dressed, and the patient is discharged.

When surgical recovery is complete (usually within 24 hours), the patient is referred to radiation oncology for treatment planning. Radiation therapy is administered on an outpatient basis. During therapy, a $^{192}$Ir seed (attached to an HDR remote afterloader) is inserted into the inflated balloon for a short duration (<10 minutes). When this is used as primary radiation therapy, 2 treatments are administered per day, for 5 days, to deliver the prescribed radiation dose (typically 34 Gy). When it is used as a boost with external beam radiation, a typical prescription requires treatment for 1 to 2 days. When the course of radiation therapy is complete, the balloon is deflated, the MammoSite catheter is removed, and no indwelling radioactive source remains (Figure 13-30).[70]

This technological advance is much more readily tolerated than conventional internal radiation therapy for breast cancer, in which radioactive seeds and multiple catheters are placed in the breast for each treatment. MammoSite is a simpler, more localized, and more effective treatment modality with a relatively low side effect profile. Brachytherapy has been used successfully to treat many solid tumors but not commonly breast cancer. Now with the development of the MammoSite radiation therapy system, which allows the use of a single, flexible catheter and outpatient treatment, brachytherapy for early stage breast cancer may eliminate the need to expose the entire breast to radiation. Currently, MammoSite is being prescribed alone and as a boost in conjunction with conventional external beam therapy. As more data are collected, the use of MammoSite without accompanying conventional EBRT may become common practice in specific clinical situations.

*Clinical data.* Data are currently available from a number of studies indicating that PBI (restricted to the tumor bed after lumpectomy) can be used safely to reduce the time and toxicity associated with traditional radiation therapy, and potentially to make the option of breast conservation more widely available. A number of institutions over the past 10 years have investigated the use of PBI as an alternative to whole breast EBRT, with favorable results. Reported local recurrence rates are low and within the recurrence rates documented for patients treated with whole breast EBRT.[71] These studies have also demonstrated good or excellent cosmetic outcomes for patients treated with PBI. Patients enrolled in these studies were carefully selected to minimize

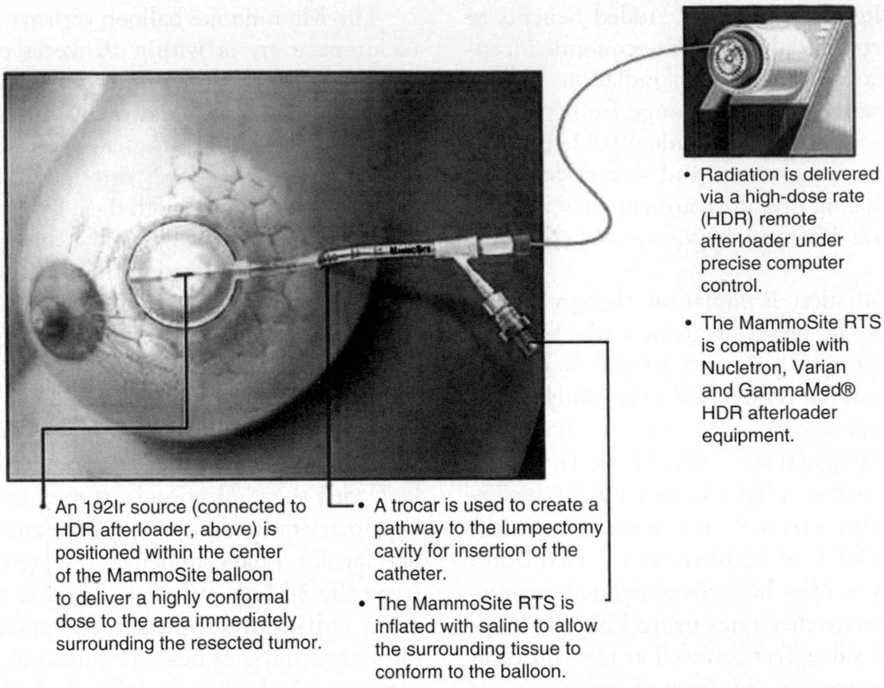

• Radiation is delivered via a high-dose rate (HDR) remote afterloader under precise computer control.
• The MammoSite RTS is compatible with Nucletron, Varian and GammaMed® HDR afterloader equipment.
• An 192Ir source (connected to HDR afterloader, above) is positioned within the center of the MammoSite balloon to deliver a highly conformal dose to the area immediately surrounding the resected tumor.
• A trocar is used to create a pathway to the lumpectomy cavity for insertion of the catheter.
• The MammoSite RTS is inflated with saline to allow the surrounding tissue to conform to the balloon.


**FIGURE 13-30**

Mammosite brachytherapy system.

*Source*: Courtesy of Hologic, Inc., Bedford, MA.

the risk of significant residual tumor surrounding the lumpectomy cavity. Appropriate patient selection is essential to successful treatment of patients with PBI as an alternative to whole breast radiation therapy. Generally, patient criteria include a diagnosis of early stage pathology of ductal carcinoma in situ (DCIS), breast cancer with tumors 3 cm or smaller in size, and age of 45 years or older.

*Patient education and practice implications.* The focus of patient care with the MammoSite system is percutaneous catheter and skin care. Nurses must assess catheters, provide routine care, and teach patients self-care. The skin at the insertion site should be assessed for erythema, edema, and exudate. Daily dressing of the entrance site includes cleansing with half-strength hydrogen peroxide and application of an antibiotic ointment and sterile dressing cover.[72] Patients are taught to keep catheters clean and dry (tub baths are permitted without submerging). Patients are taught the need for frequent temperature monitoring; an elevation of greater than 101°F, any redness or swelling of the breast, or increased tenderness or drainage from the catheter site must be reported immediately. Pain management can be assessed for and provided depending on the degree of incisional discomfort, which is usually mild.[70]

Upon completion of the final radiation therapy dose, the catheter is removed. The balloon is deflated, and then the radiation oncologist gently pulls the catheter from the breast cavity. Although it is not a painful procedure, the breast should be compressed gently over the lumpectomy site so that excess accumulated interstitial fluid is expressed. In addition, the skin should be cleansed with half-strength peroxide solution and an antibiotic ointment should be applied to the insertion site. This site should be covered with sterile gauze and redressed once daily until the skin is closed and scab formation occurs. Patients should be taught signs and symptoms of local and systemic infection and should avoid lifting the arm on the treatment side for a full 24 hours post-treatment. Side effects following MammoSite treatments have been reported as minimal and include pain, mild erythema, and dry desquamation.[73,74]

## HYPOFRACTIONATED WHOLE BREAST IRRADIATION

Hypofractionation is the delivery of more than the standard 1.8 to 2.0 Gy fraction sizes of radiation per day used to treat breast cancer. This is another method of shortening the treatment schedule. With hypofractionation, the radiation is administered in higher daily doses so that fewer days of treatment are required. Schedules of 3 to 4 weeks have been reported in Canada and the United Kingdom.[75]

Results have been superb, with the same tumor control and side effects as conventional radiation after 5 and 10 years.

The Ontario Clinical Oncology Group reported the results of a randomized trial in which 42.5 Gy in 16 fractions was given over 22 days and compared with a conventional radiation therapy course to the whole breast (50 Gy in 25 fractions over 35 days) in women with node-negative breast cancer after breast-conserving surgery. The study involved 1234 women with median follow-up of 5.8 years. The rates of local recurrence and cosmetic outcome at 5 years were equivalent. Eligibility included clear resection margins after breast-conserving surgery and large breast size (considered greater that 25 cm of tissue thickness at the midpoint of radiation fields).[76]

At the Institute of Cancer Research in the United Kingdom, 1410 women with early breast cancer were randomly assigned to 3 fractionation schedules as follows: 39 Gy in 13 fractions, 42.9 in 13 fractions, or 50 Gy in 25 fractions, all delivered over a 5-week period. At a median follow-up of 4.5 years, there was no observable difference in late radiation morbidity between 50 Gy in 25 fractions and 42.9 Gy in 13 fractions. Patients receiving 39 Gy in 13 fractions had fewer normal tissue effects that those treated with the other schedules. Local recurrence rates were not formerly reported, but local recurrence was uncommon with all 3 schedules.[77]

Concerns still exist regarding the development of long-term toxicity in patients treated with hypofractionated schedules. The concerns include potential progression of skin disease beyond 5 years and increase in local recurrence and cardiac morbidity. It is felt by many clinicians that these side effects are not likely to be more prevalent than with standard schedules of whole breast irradiation. Canada and the United Kingdom have adopted hypofractionated treatment schedules for this patient population.

At the Fox Chase Cancer Center in Philadelphia, a unique treatment schedule coupled with IMRT therapy, with a simultaneous boost to the tumor bed, offers a total treatment course in 4 weeks instead of 6 to 7 weeks. A phase II study of this treatment approach included 75 women treated with 2.25 Gy for 20 days (vs 2 Gy per day with conventional therapy) and a 2.8 Gy boost concurrently (vs sequentially delivering the boost after whole breast irradiation). The primary endpoint was acute skin toxicity. At the end of treatment, none of the women had grade 3 or 4 skin toxicity or dermatitis. Twelve percent had grade O, 65% had grade 1, and 23% had grade 2 dermatitis. All toxicity resolved within 6 weeks after treatment. In addition, no difference in cosmetic appearance was noted at 6 weeks post-treatment. Using IMRT this study examined the delivery of a higher daily dose of radiation over 4 weeks (vs a lower dose over 6 to 7 weeks). During this same time, the lumpectomy site from which the tumor was removed was treated with a high-dose radiation boost. Thus, in addition to safely increasing the dose to the entire breast over a shorter time period, this study showed the possibility of delivering the boost concurrently, eliminating an extra 2 weeks of treatment. Long-term follow-up continues in this patient population. This is a significant study because it affects patient decision making regarding commitment to treatment. This new approach of shortening a prior lengthy course of radiation will influence women's decision to choose breast-conserving treatment, which will greatly impact quality of life.[78]

Tremendous interest exists in the US currently to change the standard radiation treatment plan for eligible breast cancer patients because of the well-documented clinical studies with hypofractionation and long-term follow-up coupled with PBI protocols to study efficacy of this modality as well. Although at the present time not all centers offer IMRT and brachytherapy as treatment options, in the future this technology will become more readily available. As our society becomes increasingly cost-conscious regarding exorbitant medical costs and available treatment centers, it is probable that more practices will be offering shortened treatment courses as a viable, safe, and efficacious treatment for eligible patients with breast cancer.

## HIGH-INTENSITY FOCUSED ULTRASOUND

High-intensity focused ultrasound is a procedure that implements this technology to heat and destroy pathogenic tissue. It is a form of therapeutic US that induces hyperthermia. However, it is different from hyperthermia, as it heats more slowly and to a lower therapeutic temperature. When MRI is used with the US, the procedure is called magnetic resonance-guided focused ultrasound (MRgFUS). The MRI provides image guidance during the HIFU and is used to locate tumors prior to obliteration by US. Current clinical availability is for the treatment of uterine fibroids. FDA approval for HIFU treatment of uterine fibroids was granted in October 2004.[79] Clinical trials are ongoing to study possible efficacy of MRgFUS to treat tumors in the breast, brain, liver, and prostate as well as for palliative bone metastasis.

For purposes of treating malignant tumors, MRgFUS is being considered as an optimal noninvasive image-guided therapy for monitoring and controlling treatment. A system known as ExAblate 2000 has been developed and is the only focused US system that uses MRI guidance with HIFU beams to heat and destroy targeted tissue noninvasively. The MRI visualizes tumor targets and controls treatment by monitoring the tissue effect in real time. This is an example of an image-guided technique used to enhance visualization of a target for localization and treatment purposes.

The concept of using sound waves to ablate tumors dates back to the 1940s. However, clinical oncology implications have been limited until recently, when the addition of MRI's advanced imaging capabilities to US provided a foundation to guide and evaluate the results of this type of treatment. MRI also provides guidance of the US beam and a method to track tissue temperature and extent of tissue destruction. The uniqueness of this therapeutic approach validated the potential application in radiation oncology.[80]

Magnetic resonance-guided focused ultrasound is a diagnostic technique coupling the imaging capabilities of MRI with US, which is a form of energy that is capable of passing through skin, muscle, fat, and other soft tissue. Diagnostic US has low intensity and little or no biological effect on cells or tissues. In contrast, HIFU energy, if focused on a relatively small target, can provide a therapeutic effect by raising the tissue temperature of the target to a high enough temperature to destroy it.[81]

Ultrasound waves are emitted from a transducer (which converts electrical energy into US energy) into a small focal volume. Ultrasound beams are cone shaped and penetrate soft tissue to produce well-defined regions of protein denaturation, irreversible cell damage, and coagulative necrosis when focused at a specific target. It is important that the HIFU be tightly streamlined to limit the ablation to the intended target and spare surrounding critical and healthy tissue. The target receives multiple pulses of focused US during the treatment session; these are referred to as sonications (Figure 13-31).[81]

Magnetic resonance imaging guidance is an important element of focused US tumor ablation because MRI provides a control system for directing the energy. Essentially, MRI provides superior anatomic resolution, differentiation between treated and untreated tissue, and the ability to create real-time temperature mapping during treatment. MRI is capable of capturing 3-dimensional images displaying the tumor and surrounding organs. Patient positioning is MRI dependent, as are exact tumor targeting and beam path visualization. During MRgFUS, colored temperature maps are superimposed on the MRI, enabling a view of real-time temperature changes. This allows for adjustment of treatment parameters to ensure effective thermal ablation.[82]

The procedure involves positioning the patient on a table inside the MRI scanner. Patients are conscious but premedicated with analgesia and light sedation. Once the patient is safe and comfortable, MRI images are obtained to confirm position and optimal path for the focused US beam to be directed. The radiation oncologist uses the MRI images to identify target anatomy and to pinpoint the treatment region. Contours of the treatment area are drawn on the MRI images and verified. The MRgFUS system (ExAblate) then calculates the volume of the tissue to be treated and the number of treatment targets required. The beam path is visualized to verify that nothing interferes in any plane (Figure 13-32).[82]

Once treatment is under way, successive sonications are given to ensure tumor ablation. Phase-sensitive MRI images are acquired and real-time temperature maps are produced to confirm tissue heating. These provide feedback to the physician, who can then adjust treatment parameters to achieve optimal ablation. Between sonications, the transducer and MRI scans are automatically directed to the next area for treatment until the entire target is covered.[82]

Treatment outcome is measured by obtaining contrast MRI images to measure the degree of agent uptake. If a region does not demonstrate contrast uptake, then it has

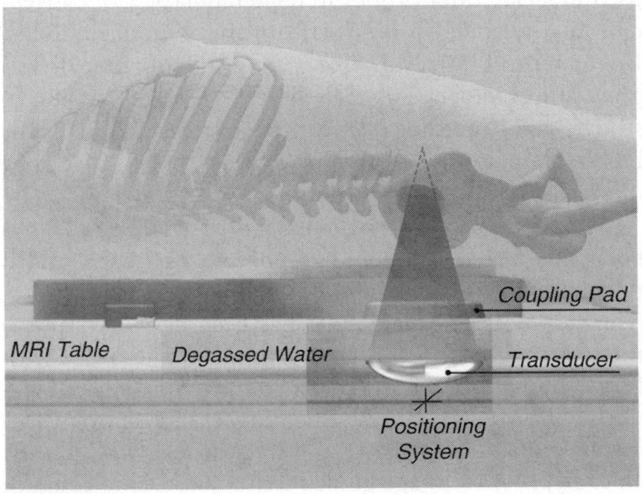


**FIGURE 13-31**

Magnetic resonance-guided ultrasound (MRgUS) for palliation of bone metastases.

*Source*: Courtesy of Insightec, Dallas, TX.

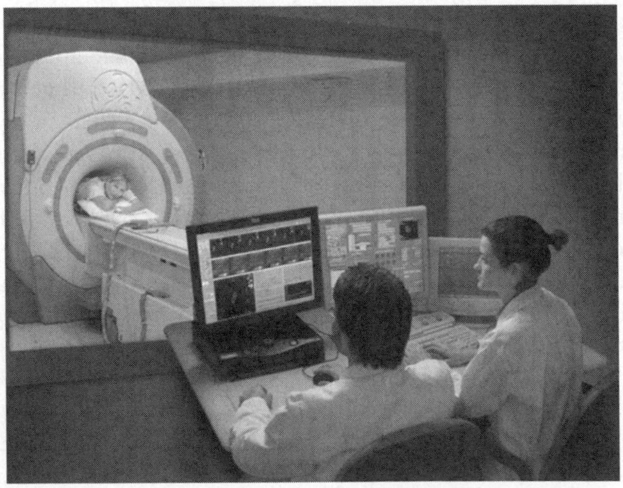

**FIGURE 13-32**

Magnetic resonance-guided focused ultrasound (MRgFUS) system combining magnetic resonance imaging with high-intensity focused ultrasound.

*Source*: Courtesy of Insightec, Dallas, TX.

been successfully ablated. If sufficient tissue needs to be treated, the radiation oncologist can repeat the procedure if deemed appropriate to do so. There is no limitation on the cumulative dose as with radiation therapy.

Clinical trials using MRgFUS in oncology are ongoing and focus on treating metastatic neoplasms of the liver and bone and primary treatment of breast cancer and prostate cancer. Focused US may be used alone or in combination with other therapies. Focused US may be feasible when conventional surgery is not an option and for salvage treatment of recurrent disease. In early trials clinical side effects included damage to tissue outside the target area.[83] Results of a European multicenter trial of focused US for prostate cancer have demonstrated that the technique is safe and may be considered in the future as primary therapy for prostate cancer.[84]

High intensity focused ultrasound has many potential future clinical applications because it may possibly be considered as both an adjunct and an alternative to conventional surgical treatment. Clinical trials using HIFU to palliate liver tumors and brain tumors and as a noninvasive alternative to surgery for small breast tumors focus on potential implications of improved local control and decreased morbidity.[85]

Palliation of pain associated with bone metastasis is unique because the acoustic absorption of bone tissue is approximately 50 times higher than that of soft tissue and the thermal conduction of bone is low. When other available treatments for bone palliation are not working, phase I/II clinical trials are being done with HIFU. Most patients studied report significant pain relief with reduced usage of analgesia following HIFU treatment.[86] Translational research will be the conduit for moving HIFU into the clinical arena.

Nursing implications of HIFU treatment involve creative clinical planning to support the experience for the patient. Prior to treatment, nurses must be prepared to answer patient questions regarding informed consent and to provide details of expectations prior to, during, and after HIFU treatment. Patients need to be informed about length of treatment, intravenous conscious sedation and recovery, foley catheter placement, and the multidisciplinary team of radiation oncology professionals who will be administering, monitoring, and documenting the treatment.

## SELECTIVE INTERNAL RADIATION THERAPY

Selective internal radiation therapy (SIRT) is a form of radiation therapy used to treat hepatic cell carcinoma or metastatic liver disease, commonly from a colorectal primary. The revolutionary aspect of SIRT is that it utilizes a new form of radiation delivery technique to treat the hepatic region, which otherwise is refractory to external beam (conventional) radiotherapy. During SIRT, millions of microscopic radioactive spheres, known as microspheres or SIR-Spheres, which are made of glass or resin, are delivered directly to liver tumors, which are selectively irradiated by the SIR-Spheres. There are 2 types of microspheres: TheraSpheres and SIR-Spheres, which differ in the radioactivity per sphere and their embolic effect. The SIR-Spheres have more embolic effect and less activity per sphere. This makes them better for certain cancers such as neuroendocrine tumors, which are highly vascular. This highly specific, locoregional, targeted form of treatment delivers a higher dose (up to 40 times greater than conventional external beam treatment) directly to the liver tumors. Side effects are specific to the liver, and treatment (both beneficial and deleterious) does not affect distant disease sites.[87]

SIR-Spheres are tiny (approximately 35 μm) polymer beads that are loaded with yttrium-90, a radioisotope that emits pure beta radiation. Yttrium-90 has a half-life of about 2.5 days, so the level of radiation falls by one half during this time frame. Radiation from yttrium-90 is confined to a tissue depth of 2 to 3 mm. The microspheres are delivered through a catheter threaded into the femoral artery and into the hepatic artery to the tumor. As liver tumors receive the majority of their blood supply from the hepatic artery, catheterization of the hepatic artery permits direct tumor targeting. The microspheres get trapped in the tumor's vascular bed, where they destroy the tumor by reducing its blood supply (embolic effect) and by causing local radiation damage to the cancer cells' DNA. The radiation is contained within the patient and continues to be delivered over 2 weeks after the procedure. After this time, the microspheres are no longer radioactive. The SIR-Spheres were granted premarket approval by the FDA in March 2002.[88]

Patients must qualify for SIRT, and prior to the procedure they are required to have a hepatic angiogram, a radiopharmacological lung scan, and a CT scan. The angiogram defines the arterial anatomy and helps the interventional radiologist embolize certain arteries that might carry the microspheres away from the target location. Lung shunting is measured with a technetium scan, and if the shunting exceeds 20% then patients are excluded from SIRT due to the risk of developing radiation pneumonitis. SIRT is commonly administered over 2 separate sessions if both lobes of the liver are to be treated.[89]

Patient outcomes, although not considered curative, have demonstrated the ability of SIRT to shrink liver tumors and therefore to increase life expectancy and improve quality of life. A landmark study published in 2006 demonstrated that the use of SIR-Spheres in patients with advanced liver disease resulted in a median survival of 10.5 months from treatment. This study followed 208 patients with unresectable liver metastases. Prior studies had shown the efficacy of SIRT, but with much smaller patient populations. Two thirds of the patients in this study were classified as responders, with a median survival rate of 10.5 months, and the remaining one third patients were nonresponders. The survival time of patients treated with SIR-Spheres was almost double that of patients treated with systemic chemotherapy. No serious side effects were reported. The researchers concluded that microspheres are a safe and effective treatment for patients with advanced unresectable liver disease.[90]

Selective internal radiation therapy administration is dependent on a multidisciplinary management team that includes specialists in medical, radiation, and surgical oncology, nuclear medicine, interventional radiology, and radiation safety. Once a patient's candidacy is established, the specific dose is determined, and it is ordered 7 to 10 days prior to the treatment date. The dose is drawn in the "hot lab" of the nuclear medicine department and is infused in the interventional radiology suite.

Criteria for patient eligibility for SIRT treatment include the following:

- Inoperable secondary liver cancer
- Liver a major disease site
- Sufficient remaining healthy liver still functioning
- Patient well enough to tolerate the implant
- Meet preselection criteria and pretreatment testing

The following are contraindications to SIRT:

- Prior EBRT to liver
- Ascites or liver failure
- Abnormal synthetic liver function tests
- Tumors surgically resectable
- More than 20% lung shunting
- Preassessment angiograms and MAA nuclear scans with reflux of hepatic arterial blood to stomach, pancreas, or bowel
- Widely disseminated or extrahepatic disease
- Treatment with capecitabine within 2 months prior to or after SIRT

Side effects following treatment may include gastritis and peptic ulceration. Therefore, preventive medications to control these symptoms are prescribed postprocedure. Lethargy, nausea, and diminished appetite may occur for a few days following the procedure. Low-grade fever may develop for up to 1 week, along with abdominal pain that subsides over time. SIRT is an outpatient procedure, and patients are discharged after a few hours of observation post-treatment, with radiation precaution teaching. Postprocedure observation may include a SPECT scan, lab tests, and PET/CT scans.

Intrahepatic carcinomas are treatable with other types of radiotherapy delivery techniques, including whole liver irradiation, partial hepatic irradiation with 3D-CRT, and stereotactic body RT. SIRT is an additional, novel approach to managing liver disease. SIRT has been administered in combination with chemotherapy to manage liver metastases from colorectal cancer. In a phase III study of 74 patients with bilobar nonresectable liver metastases from adenocarcinoma of the large bowel, a single injection of SIR-Spheres was added to a regimen of regional hepatic artery chemotherapy administered as a 12-day infusion of floxuridine and repeated at monthly intervals. When compared with chemotherapy alone, the SIR-Sphere combination was substantially more effective in increasing tumor responses and progression-free survival.[91]

Subsequent studies have demonstrated the efficacy of combining systemic treatment with SRI-Spheres for treatment of liver metastases.[92,93] IMRT is also being used to treat intrahepatic cancers. IMRT is being integrated into treatment algorithms in order to increase the dose to the tumor with less toxicity. It has been found that a significantly higher dose of radiation can be delivered safely with IMRT than with 3D-CRT. Continued research to improve radiation delivery for intrahepatic cancers involves individualizing therapy on the basis of functional imaging. The goal of this work is to determine the maximum safe dose of radiation that can be given. Veno-occlusive disease is a dose-limiting toxicity of radiation detectable about 1 month after treatment and very difficult to treat. Using dynamic contrast CT scanning, decreased blood flow in the liver can be detected during treatment, and this predicts the decrease seen 1 month after treatment. Methods to adjust the dose during treatment could individualize the course and give patients higher therapeutic doses to control disease and diminish toxicity.[94,95]

## CONCLUSION

The specialty of radiation oncology comprises a technological and clinical blend of skills and knowledge. This unique practice incorporates the talent and skills of a diverse team of professionals. Integral to the function of this complex environment is the professional oncology nurse. It is incumbent on these nurses to study, learn, and apply the scientific basis of radiation oncology practice to clinical situations. Patients treated with radiation are subject to rigorous procedures, prolonged treatment courses, and unfamiliar environments, all of which are compounded by the fear of a cancer diagnosis. Numerous questions and anxieties must be addressed. Nurses must creatively combine scientific and clinical knowledge into a pragmatic framework for patient management.

Radiation oncology continues to refine known treatment techniques and modalities and to investigate new technology. Research studies focus on the enhancement of treatment planning techniques in an effort to provide patients with the most refined modalities. Although advanced treatment planning has become popular, some institutions have not been able to implement it fully due to expense, the requirement for additional staffing, and the need for sophisticated equipment. Economic constraints continue to plague institutions and hinder the installation of state-of-the-art equipment and cutting-edge technology. By the time smaller, independent, less well-endowed radiation centers install a new technology, it may be dated. Thus, it is not the pace of discovery and application of new treatment techniques that is problematic, but rather the struggle of institutions to keep pace economically. Therefore radiation oncology professionals must advocate for the specialty so that scientific sophistication and clinical application are promoted and invoked in a timely, effective manner.

The practice of radiation oncology is constantly evolving. Hence, updating this chapter has been a process requiring much thought and reflection. This specialty is faced daily with the challenges of implementing new technology. This requires cooperation from the entire multidisciplinary team to ensure that seamless transitions and flexibility are forever in place. Fundamental principles that have been identified to assist with implementation of innovative radiation oncology delivery have been documented and are as follows: identifying a project champion; pursuing a multidisciplinary approach; showing clinical efficacy, including return on investment; and demonstrating the ability to articulate the project and celebrate success.[96]

The evolution of radiation oncology practice in the past 2 decades has included the following: IMRT; combination of RT and molecular targeted therapy; stereotactic radiosurgery; fractionated stereotactic radiotherapy; IGRT; PET/CT fusion; and virtual simulation. In order to appreciate all of the nuances of this limitless specialty, it is essential that the professional oncology nurse lead the pioneering efforts to secure a serious work ethic complemented by clinical brilliance and administrative support.

## REFERENCES


1. Ahlberg K, Ekman T, Gaston-Johansson F. Fatigue, psychological distress, coping resources and functional status during radiotherapy for uterine cancer. *Oncol Nurs Forum.* 2005;32:633–640.
2. Klosky JL, Tye VL, Tong X, et al. Predicting pediatric distress during radiation therapy procedures: the role of medical, psychosocial and demographic factors. *Pediatrics.* 2007;119:1159–1166.
3. Khan FM. Process, equipment, and personnel. In: Khan FM, ed. *Treatment Planning in Radiation Oncology.* 2nd ed. Philadelphia, PA: Lippincott, Williams & Wilkins; 2007:1–9.
4. Gazda MJ, Coia LR. Principles of radiation therapy. In: Pazdur R, Coia LR, Hosians WJ, Wagman LD, eds. *Cancer Management: A Multidisciplinary Approach.* 10th ed. New York, NY: PRR; 2007:649–660.
5. Purdy JA, Harms BS, Michalski MD, Perez MD. The CT-simulation/3-D treatment planning process. In: Purdy JA, Grant W, Palta JR, Butler EB, Perez CA, eds. *3D Conformal & Intensity Modulated Radiation Treatment; Physics and Clinical Applications.* Madison, WI: Advanced Medical Publishing; 2001:1–15.
6. Prado KL, Starkschall MR. Three-dimensional conformal radiation therapy. In: Khan FM, ed. *Treatment Planning in Radiation Oncology.* 2nd ed. Philadelphia, PA: Lippincott, Williams & Wilkins; 2007:116–141.
7. Bucci MK, Bevan A, Roach M. Advances in radiation therapy: conventional to 3D, to IMRT, to 4D, and beyond. *CA: Cancer J Clin.* 2005;55:117–134.
8. Rasch C, Steenbakkers R, Van Herk M. Target definition in prostate, head and neck. *Semin Radiat Oncol.* 2005;15:136–145.
9. Giraud P, Kanter G, Loiscan H, et al. Target definition in the thorax and central nervous system. *Semin Radiat Oncol.* 2005;15:146–156.
10. Chao KSC, Perez CA, Brady LW. *Radiation Oncology Management Decisions.* 2nd ed. Philadelphia, PA: Lippincott, Williams & Wilkins; 2001.
11. Bushberg JT, Sibert TA, Leidholt EM. *The Essential Physics of Medical Imaging.* Philadelphia, PA: Lippincott, Williams & Willkins; 2003:chap 13.
12. Chen GTY, Pelizzari CA, Rietzel ERM. Imaging in radiotherapy. In: Khan FM, ed. *Treatment Planning in Radiation Oncology.* 2nd ed. Philadelphia, PA: Lippincott, Williams & Wilkins; 2007:10–26.
13. Nelson SJ. Multivoxel magnetic resonance spectroscopy of brain tumors. *Mol Cancer Ther.* 2003;2:497–507.
14. Saw CB, Brandner E, Selvara R, Chen H, Saiful Huq M, Heron DE. A review on the clinical implementation of respiratory-gated radiation treatment. *Biomed Imaging Interv J.* 2007;3:e40.
15. Keall P, Vedam S, George R, et al. The clinical implementation of respiratory-guided IMRT. *Med Dosim.* 2006;31:152.
16. Van Elmpt W, McDermott L, Nister S, Wendling M, Philippe L, Ben M. A lit-review of electronic portal imaging for radiotherapy dosimetry. *J Eur Soc Ther Radiat Oncol.* 2008;88:289–309.
17. Herman M. Clinical use of electronic portal imaging. *Semin Radiat Oncol.* 2005;15:157–167.
18. Wahl RL. Principles of cancer imaging with fluorodeoxyglucose. In: Wahl RL, Buchanan JW, eds. *Principles and Practice of Positron Emission Tomography.* Philadelphia, PA: Lippincott, Williams & Wilkins; 2002:100–110.
19. Ciernik IF, Dizendorf E, Baument BG, et al. Radiation treatment planning with an integrated positron emission and computer tomography (PET/CT): a feasibility study. *Int J Radiat Oncol Biol Phys.* 2003;57:853–863.
20. Fox T, Elder E, Crocker I. Image registration and fusion techniques. In: Paulino A, ed. *Pet CT in Radiation Treatment Planning.* New York, NY: Saunders; 2008:38–55.
21. Maheshwari S, Mukherj S. Proton MR spectroscopy clinical applications. *Imaging Economics.* August 2002.
22. Jeffrey PI, Weinreb C. American College of Radiology Imaging Network (ACRIN) 6659 MRI and MRSI of prostate cancer prior to radical prostatectomy. A prospective multi-institutional clinico-pathological study. Paper presented at: 92nd Scientific Assembly and Annual Meeting of Radiological Society of North America (RSNA); November 28, 2006; Chicago, IL.
23. Zapotoczna A, Sasso G, Simpson J, Roach M. Current role/future perspectives of MR Spect in prostate cancer. *Neoplasia.* 2007;9:455–463.
24. Boyer AL. Intensity modulated radiation therapy. In: Khan FM, ed. *Treatment Planning in Radiation Oncology.* 2nd ed. Philadelphia, PA: Lippincott, Williams & Wilkins; 2007:142–165.
25. Dong L, Mohan R. Image-guided radiation therapy. In: Khan FM, ed. *Treatment Planning in Radiation Oncology.* 2nd ed. Philadelphia, PA: Lippincott, Williams & Wilkins; 2007:chap 12, 165–188.
26. Dawson LA, Sharpe MB. Image-guided radiotherapy, rationale, benefits and limitations. *Lancet Oncol.* 2006;7:848–858.
27. Wong JR, Cheng CW, Grim L, et al. Clinical implementation of the world's first Primatom—a combination of CT scanner and linear accelerator for precise tumor targeting and treatment. *Phys Med.* 2001;17:271–276.
28. Wong JR, Grim L, Uematsu M, et al. Image-guided radiotherapy for prostate cancer by CT-linear accelerator combination: prostate movements and dosimetric considerations. *Int J Radiat Oncol Biol Phys.* 2005;61:561–569.
29. Langen KM, Pouliot J, Anezinos C, et al. Education of ultrasound-based prostate localization for image guided radiotherapy. *Int J Radiat Oncol Biol Phys.* 2003;57:635–644.

30. Scarbrough TJ, Golden NM, Ting JY, et al. Comparison of ultrasound and implanted seed marker prostate localization methods: implications for image guided radiotherapy. *Int J Radiat Oncol Biol Phys.* 2006;65:378–387.
31. Morin O, Gillis A, Chen J, et al. Megavoltage cone-beam CT: system description and clinical applications. *Med Dosim.* 2006;31:51–61.
32. Pouliot J, Bani-Hashemi A, Chen J, et al. Low-dose megavoltage cone beam CT for radiation therapy. *Int J Radiat Oncol Biol Phys.* 2005;61:552–560.
33. Willoughby TR, Kupelian PA, Pouliot J, et al. Target localization and real-time tracking using the calypso AD localization system in patients with localized prostate cancer. *Int J Radiat Oncol Biol Phys.* 2006;65:528–534.
34. Shinohara K, Roach M. Technique for implantation of fiducial markers in the prostate. *Urology.* 2008;71:196–200.
35. Zhang M, Moiseenko V, Liu M, Craig T. Internal fiducial markers can assist dose escalation in treatment of prostate cancer result of organ motion simulations. *Phys Med Biol.* 2006;51:269–285.
36. Gladstone G, Hartford A, Marshall J, et al. Gold coils used as fiducial markers of prostate location for image-guided radiotherapy. Paper presented at: 91st Scientific Assembly and Annual Meeting of Radiological Society of North America (RSNA); 2005; Chicago, IL. [Abstract SSK 24–04].
37. Kupelian P, Willoughby T, Levine L, et al. Multi-institutional clinical experience with the Calypso System in localization and continuous real-time monitoring of the prostate gland during external radiotherapy. *Int J Radiat Oncol Biol Phys.* 2007;67:1088–1098.
38. Bauer JM, Wright JN, Newell LJ, et al. Accuracy of a wireless localization system for radiotherapy. *Int J Radiat Oncol Biol Phys.* 2005;61:933–937.
39. Bentel GC. *Radiation Therapy Planning Including Problems and Solutions.* New York, NY: McGraw-Hill; 2007:59–78.
40. Khan FM. *The Physics of Radiation Therapy.* 3rd ed. Baltimore, MD: Williams & Wilkins; 2003.
41. Mackie RT, Liu HH, McCullough EC. Treatment planning algorithms: model-based photon dose calculations. In: Khan FM, ed. *Treatment Planning in Radiation Oncology.* 2nd ed. Philadelphia, PA: Lippincott, Williams & Wilkins; 2007:63–83.
42. Ibbott G. Radiation physics. In: Haffty BG, Wilson LD, eds. *Handbook of Radiation Oncology: Basic Principles and Clinical Protocols.* Sudbury, MA: Jones and Bartlett; 2009.
43. Reinstein LE, Podgorsak MB. Patient positioning and immobilization. In: Khan FM, ed. *Treatment Planning in Radiation Oncology.* 2nd ed. Philadelphia, PA: Lippincott, Williams & Wilkins; 2007:38–62.
44. Robison B, Seibert R, Ramsey CB. Evaluation of head and neck patient set-up and immobilization errors. *Int J Radiat Oncol Biol Phys.* 2007;69:751–758.
45. Kneebone A, Gebsla V, Hogendoorn N, et al. A randomized trial evaluating rigid immobilization for pelvic irradiation. *Int J Radiat Oncol Biol Phys.* 2003;56:1105–1111.
46. Report of the Inter-Society Council for Radiation Oncology (Blue Book). Reston, VA: American College of Radiology; 1991.
47. Brada M, Pils-Johannesma M, DeRuysscher D. Proton therapy in clinical practice: current clinical evidence. *J Clin Oncol.* 2007;25:965–970.
48. Schulz-Ertner D, Tsujii H. Particle radiation therapy using proton and heavier ion beams. *J Clin Oncol.* 2007;25:953–964.
49. Gostein M, Cox JD. Should randomized clinical trials be required for proton radiotherapy? *J Clin Oncol.* 2008;26:175–176.
50. Greco C, Wolden S. Current status of radiotherapy with proton and light ion beams. *Cancer.* 2007;109:1227–1238.
51. Zietman AL. The Titanic and the iceberg: prostate proton therapy and healthcare economics. *J Clin Oncol.* 2007;25:3565–3566.
52. Knoski A, Speier W, Hanlon A, et al. Is proton beam therapy cost effective in the treatment of adenocarcinoma of the prostate? *J Clin Oncol.* 2007;25:3603–3608.
53. Bova FJ, Meeks SL, Friedman W, Wagner TH. Linac radiosurgery: system requirements, procedures and testing. In: Khan FM, ed. *Treatment Planning in Radiation Oncology.* 2nd ed. Philadelphia. PA: Lippincott, Williams & Wilkins; 2007:189–211.
54. Adler JR, Muacevic A, Romanelli P. Cyberknife radiosurgery. In: Chin L, Regine W, eds. *Principles and Practices of Stereotactic Radiosurgery.* New York, NY: Springer; 2008:171–180.
55. Rosenzweig KE. Image guided radiotherapy of lung cancer. *Int J Radiat Oncol Biol Phys.* 2008;7:957.
56. Glasgow GP. Low dose rate brachytherapy. In: Khan FM, ed. *Treatment Planning in Radiation Oncology.* 2nd ed. Philadelphia, PA: Lippincott, Williams & Wilkins; 2007:212–237.
57. Thomadsen BR. High dose rate brachytherapy. In: Khan FM, ed. *Treatment Planning in Radiation Oncology.* 2nd ed. Philadelphia, PA: Lippincott, Williams & Wilkins; 2007:240–257.
58. International Commission on Radiation Units and Measurements. *Dose and Volume Specification for Reporting Intracavitary Therapy.* Gynecology Report No. 38. Bethesda, MD: ICRU; 1985.
59. Weeks KJ. Treatment planning algorithms brachytherapy. In: Khan FM, ed. *Treatment Planning in Radiation Oncology.* 2nd ed. Philadelphia, PA: Lippincott, Williams & Wilkins; 2007:84–95.
60. Horning SJ. Future directions in radioimmunotherapy for B-cell lymphoma. *Semin Oncol.* 2003;30(6 suppl 17):29–34.
61. Vose JM. Bexxar: novel radioimmunotherapy for the treatment of low-grade and transformed low grade non-Hodgkin's lymphoma. *Oncologist.* 2004;9:160–172.
62. Hendrix C. Radiation safety guidelines for radioimmunotherapy with Yttrium 90 ibritumomab tioxetan. *Clin J Oncol Nurs.* 2004;3:31–34.
63. Riley MB, Byar K. The rationale for and background of radioimmunotherapy: an emerging therapy for B-cell non-Hodgkin's lymphoma. *Semin Oncol Nurs.* 2004;20:1–7.
64. Liebenguth P, Temple SV. Radioimmunotherapy for non-Hodgkin's lymphoma. *Semin Oncol Nurs.* 2006;22:257–266.
65. Harris JR, Hellman S. Primary radiation therapy for early breast cancer. *Cancer.* 1983;51(suppl 12):2547–2552.
66. Polgar C, Fodor J, Major T, et al. Radiotherapy confined to the tumor bed following breast conserving surgery? Current status, controversies, and future projects. *Strahlentherapie Onkologie.* 2002;178:597–606.
67. Wallner P, Arthur D, Bartelink H, et al. Workshop on partial breast irradiation: state of the art and the science. *J Natl Cancer Inst.* 2005;96:175–184.
68. Wolmark N, Curran WJ. A randomized phase III study of conventional whole breast irradiation (WBI) versus partial breast irradiation (PBI) for women with stage 0, I, or II breast cancer. NSABP B-39/RTOG Protocol 0413 Fact Sheet. April 16, 2007. Philadelphia, PA: American College of Radiology; 2007.
69. Vicini F. Limited-field radiation therapy in the management of early-stage breast cancer. *J Natl Cancer Inst.* 2003;95:1205–1211.
70. Keisch M, Vincini F, Kuske R, et al. Two year outcome with the MammoSite breast brachytherapy applicator: factors associated with optimal cosmetic results when performing partial breast irradiation. Proceedings of the 45th Annual ASTRO meeting. *Int J Radiat Oncol Biol Phys.* 2003;57:S315.
71. Calvo FA, Diaz JA, Montero A, et al. Partial breast irradiation: why and how. *Breast Cancer Res.* 2005;7(suppl):S12.
72. Hogle WP, Quinne AE, Heron DE. Advance in brachytherapy: new approaches to target breast cancer. *Clin J Oncol Nurs.* 2003;7:324–330.
73. Gordils-Perez J, Rawlins-Duell R, Kelvin JR. Advances in radiation treatment of patients with breast cancer. *Clin J Oncol Nurs.* 2003;7:629–636.
74. Moore-Higgs GJ. Radiation options for early stage breast cancer. *Semin Oncol Nurs.* 2006;22:233–241.
75. Whelan TJ. Use of conventional radiation therapy as part of breast-conserving treatment. *J Clin Oncol.* 2005;23:1718–1725.

76. Whelan TJ, Mackenzie R, Julian J, et al. Randomized trial of breast irradiation schedules after lumpectomy with lymph node-negative breast cancer. *J Natl Cancer Inst.* 2002;94:1143–1150.
77. Dewar JA, Haviland RK, Agrawal JM, et al. Hypofractionation for early breast cancer: first results of the UK standardization of breast radiotherapy (START) trials. ASCO Annual Meeting Proceedings. *J Clin Oncol.* 2007;25(suppl):18S.
78. Freedman GM, Anderson PA, Goldstein LJ, Ma CM. Four-week course of radiation for breast cancer using hypofractionated intensity modulated radiation therapy with an incorporated boost. *Int J Radiat Oncol Biol Phys.* 2007;68:347–353.
79. Leslie TA, Kennedy JE. High intensity focused ultrasound in the treatment of abdominal and gynaecological disease. *Int J Hyperthermia.* 2007;23:173–182.
80. Kopelman D, Papa M. Magnetic resonance-guided focused ultrasound surgery for the noninvasive curative ablation of tumors and palliative treatments: a review. *Ann Surg Oncol.* 2007;14:1540–1550.
81. Dubinsky TJ, Cuevas C, Dighe MK, et al. High-intensity focused ultrasound: current potential and oncologic applications. *AJR Am J Roentgenol.* 2008;190:191–199.
82. Haar GT, Coussios C. High intensity focused ultrasound: physical principles and devices. *Int J Hyperthermia.* 2007;23:89–104.
83. Halpern EJ. High-intensity focused ultrasound ablation: will image-guided therapy replace conventional surgery? *Radiology.* 2005;235:345–346.
84. Thuroff S, Chasussy C, Vallancien G, et al. High-intensity focused ultrasound and localized prostate cancer: efficacy results from the European multicentric study. *J Endourol.* 2003;226:897–905.
85. Haar GT, Coussios C. High intensity focused ultrasound: past, present, and future. *Int J Hyperthermia.* 2007;23:85–87.
86. Freedman, G. *BM-004: A Pivotal Study to Evaluate the Effectiveness and Safety of MR-Guided Focused Ultrasound treatment of Metastatic Bone Tumors for the Palliation of Pain in patients Who are not Candidates for Radiation Therapy.* Philadelphia, PA: Fox Chase Cancer Center; April 28, 2009. IRB #08–018.
87. Shepard F, Dancey J, Paul K, et al. Treatment of non respectable hepatocellular carcinoma with intrahepatic 90Y-microspheres. *J Nucl Med.* 2004;10(suppl):S107-S110.
88. Murthy R, Xiong H, Nunez R, et al. Yttrium 90 resin microspheres for the treatment of unrespectable colorectal hepatic metastases after failure of multiple chemotherapy regimens: preliminary results. *J Vasc Interv Radiol.* 2005;16:937–945; 200–205.
89. Popperl G, Helmberger T, Munzing W, et al. Selective internal radiation therapy with SIR-spheres in patients with nonresectable liver tumors. *Cancer Biother Radiopharm.* 2005;20:200–205.
90. Kennedy AS, Coldwell D, Nutting C, et al. Resin 90 Y-microspere brachytherapy for unresectable colorectal liver metastases: modern USA experience. *Int J Radiat Oncol Biol Phys.* 2006;65:412–425.
91. Gray B, Van Hazel G, Hope M, et al. Randomized trial of SIR-spheres plus chemotherapy vs chemotherapy alone for treating patients with liver metastases from primary large bowel cancer. *Ann Oncol.* 2001;12:1711–1720.
92. Van Hazel G. Selective internal radiation therapy (SIRT) plus systemic chemotherapy with FOLFOX: a phase 1 dose escalation study. Paper presented at: Gastrointestinal Cancers Symposium; January 2005; American Society of Clinical Oncology, Hollywood, FL.
93. Van Hazel G, Price D, Bower G, Blanchard KS, Steward WP, Sharma RA. Selective internal radiation therapy (SIRT) plus systemic chemotherapy with irinotecan: a phase 1 dose escalation study. Gastrointestinal Cancers Symposium; 2005; American Society of Clinical Oncology, [Abstract 265].
94. Topkan E, Onal HC, Yavuz MN. Managing liver metastases with conformal radiation therapy. *J Support Oncol.* 2008;6:9–13.
95. Lawrence TS. Radiotherapy for intrahepatic cancers: the promise of emerging sophisticated techniques. *J Support Oncol.* 2008;6:14–15.
96. The BS, Ortiz P, Paulino AC, et al. Pioneering innovative radiation oncology technology in clinics. *Biomed Imaging Interv J.* 2007;3:e57.

CHAPTER 14

Marilyn L. Haas, PhD, CNS, ANP-BC

# Radiation Therapy: Toxicities and Management

## INTRODUCTION

Approximately 60% of oncology patients will receive radiation therapy (RT) during the course of their treatment. Radiation may be administered at multiple points in the oncology continuum—as definitive, neoadjuvant, adjunctive, prophylaxis, control, or palliation.[1] Definitive therapy is prescribed as the primary radiation treatment modality which can be given with or without chemotherapy. Typically, this is prescribed for head/neck, lung, prostate, or bladder cancers. Neoadjuvant treatment is prescribed before definitive treatment. This could be a surgical procedure before radiation is administered (eg, esophageal or colon cancers). Adjunctive treatment is given after definitive therapy, either surgery or chemotherapy, to improve local control. This would include individuals who have breast, lung, or high-risk rectal cancers. Prophylactic irradiation treats asymptomatic individuals that are at high-risk for occurrence. For example, individuals who had complete response for small cell lung cancer that may receive prophylactic cranial irradiation (PCI). If the purpose is to control the cancer, radiation can limit the growth of cancer cells to extend symptom-free intervals (eg, pancreatic or even lung cancers). Palliative irradiation is given to control symptoms of bleeding, pain, airway obstruction, or neurological compromise. Examples of palliative treatments could include the following: bone metastases, blocked airways, spinal cord compression, or previously treated areas requiring retreatment. While definitive, neoadjuvant, or adjuvant is typically given over 1 treatment course, palliative treatments may occur at multiple times depending on the disease course, areas requiring additional radiation, and patient response. The purpose/goals of the therapy should be established at the onset of therapy.

Combined modality therapy with RT, chemotherapy, and/or surgery is commonly used in the treatment of cancer. The additive effect of combining these treatments with radiation generally improves outcomes, but does result in more acute and prolonged toxicities. Performance status and comorbid conditions contribute to patient tolerance of irradiation and may predispose the patient to a more difficult course of therapy. This chapter reviews the radiobiology, radiobiological rationale for radiation toxicities, site-specific acute and late toxicities, and nursing assessment and management.

## RADIOBIOLOGY

Cellular response to radiation injury is directly related to the degree of mitotic activity. Actively replicating cells have 4 stages and 1 resting phase in their life cycle:

$G_1$ The gap between the end of mitosis and the start of DNA synthesis
S DNA synthesis
$G_2$ The gap between DNA synthesis and mitosis
M Mitosis
$G_0$ Resting phase[2]

The cell is most sensitive to radiation during mitosis (M) and the $G_2$ phase, with the greatest radioresistance occurring in the DNA synthesis phase (S).[3] Today, some chemotherapy agents have their greatest direct effect on the S phase, thus arresting at different sensitive cell-cycle points as seen in Figure 14-1. This contributes to the antitumor effects of both ionizing radiation and chemotherapy.

The dose of radiation prescribed is determined by 3 main factors—radiosensitivity of the tumor, normal tissue tolerance, and the volume of tissue to be irradiated. Radiosensitivity refers to the response of tumor cells to radiation in terms of degree and speed of response. For example, poorly differentiated immature cells, rapidly proliferating cells, and cells with a high mitotic potential

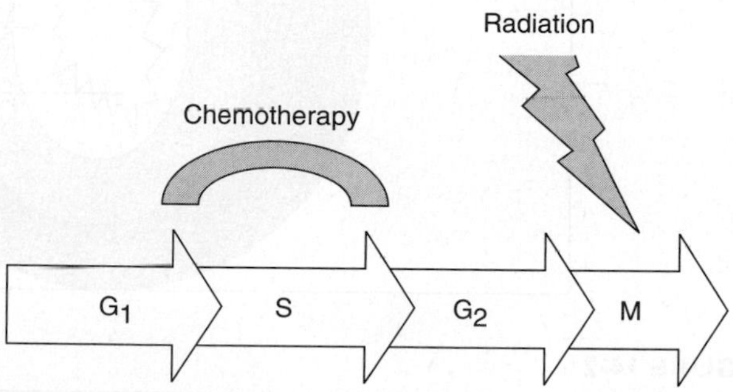


**FIGURE 14-1**

Cell life cycle sensitivity. Chemotherapy's effect on $G_1$ and S with radiation's effect on $G_2$ and M

are more radiosensitive. Tissue tolerance is the amount of radiation that adjacent structures/tissues can tolerate without being irreparably damaged. The volume of tissue, commonly referred to as target volume, includes 3 distinct volumes (boundaries)—gross tumor volume (GTV), clinical tumor volume (CTV), and planning target volume (PTV).[4] GTV is the palpable mass or extent of the growth seen on imaging studies. The CTV is the subclinical microscopic disease surrounding the GTV. The PTV is the margins surrounding the CTV to compensate the effects of tumor or organ movement. These treatment planning volumes are seen in Figure 14-2.

Radiocurability refers to local or regional eradication of tumor cells by radiation, and means that the tumor-to-normal-tissue relations are such that curative doses of radiation can be applied without excessive damage to normal tissues. Examples of radiocurable tumors include carcinomas of the cervix, larynx, breast, and prostate. The terms "radiosensitivity" and "radiocurability" are not interchangeable. For example, non-Hodgkin's lymphoma is very radiosensitive but may not be radio-curable. All tissues have a degree of radiosensitivity, but it is the effect on normal tissue surrounding the tumor that largely determines the maximum radiation dose and resulting toxicities.[5]

The goal of RT is to destroy cancer cells while maintaining the integrity of normal tissue. This range is defined as the *therapeutic ratio* (Figure 14-3).[5] Providing radiation doses within the therapeutic ratio allows for tumor eradication or reduction and minimal residual injury to surrounding normal tissues and structures. However, because ionizing radiation does not differentiate between normal cells and cancer cells, it damages both. Malignant and normal cells differ little in their overall response to ionizing radiation. Achieving the therapeutic ratio requires a delicate balance between desired treatment outcome and toxicities.

Normal cells and cancer cells undergo some degree of repair to sublethal damage between doses of radiation. A single dose of ionizing radiation will have a greater effect on cells than the same dose divided into several fractions. If the goal of radiation is maximizing tumor cell kill while sparing normal tissue, dividing the radiation into equal doses or fractions is crucial to achieving the therapeutic ratio. Radiation is most commonly administered in a daily fraction, although *hyperfractionation* (2 or more fractions per day separated by 4–6 hours) can be used in some patients. Fractionation is designed to take advantage of the "four R's" of radiobiology:

*Repair*: The ability of cells to recover from sublethal radiation injury. Repair usually occurs within 24 hours, but may occur in as little as 4 hours in some tissues. Normal cells are repeatedly repaired between daily doses. By contrast, tumor cells may be initially repaired, but as radiation continues, their repair ability decreases, increasing the radiation damage to tumor cells.

*Redistribution*: Fractionated radiation doses disrupt the cellular life cycle, causing mitotic delays in the tumor cell cycle. This disruption theoretically enhances the effects of each succeeding radiation dose because more tumor cells are likely to be in mitosis at the same time, increasing the cell kill. Tumor cells may be more subject

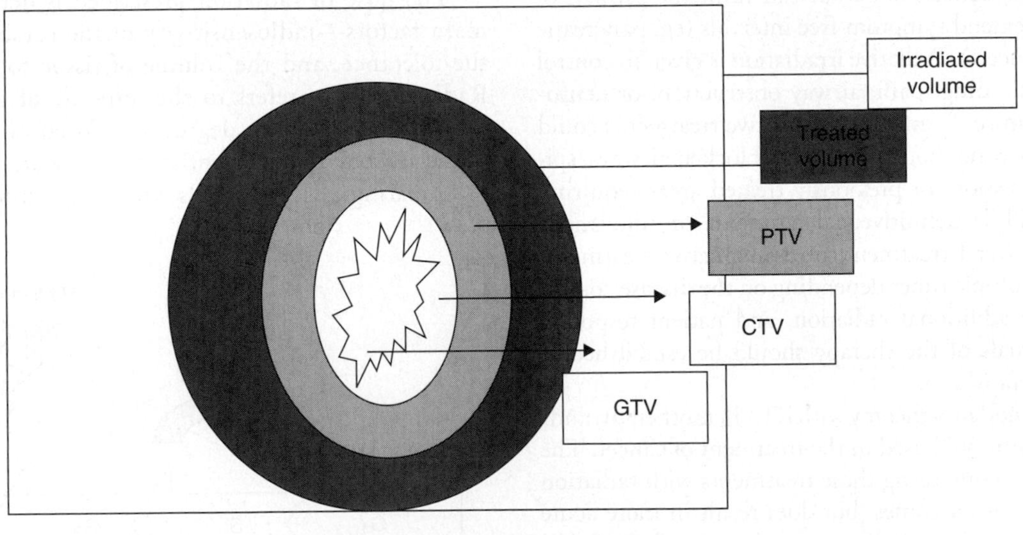


**FIGURE 14-2**

Schematic illustration of radiation treatment volumes.

*Abbreviations*: GTV, gross tumor volume; CTV, clinical tumor volume (GTV + microscopic disease); PTV, planning target volume (CTV + suspected margins).

*Source*: Data from Ibbott G (2009).[4]

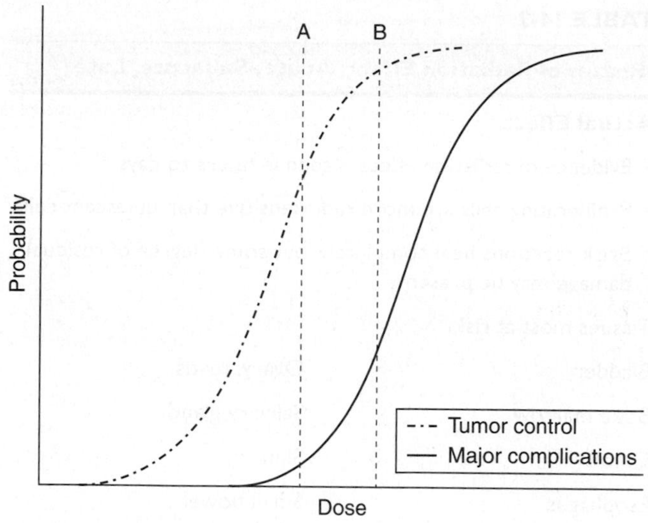


**FIGURE 14-3**

Therapeutic ratio. Sigmoid curves of tumor control and complications. (A) Dose for tumor control with minimum complications. (B) Maximum tumor dose with significant complications.

*Source*: Data from Hellman S. Principles of cancer management: radiation therapy. In: De Vita VT, Hellman S, Rosenberg SA, eds. *Cancer: Principles and Practice of Oncology*. 6th ed. Philadelphia, PA: Lippincott-Raven; 2001:265–288.

to redistribution, due in part to their erratic growth and development.

*Repopulation (regeneration)*: Irradiated normal cells are able to complete their cell cycle and undergo successful mitosis between radiation doses. Tumor cells are more likely to die after radiation injury because of the abnormal features that result from growth and mitosis. Generally, tumor cell division stays ahead of cell death or loss, which contrasts with mature normal cell growth and division that matches cell loss.

*Reoxygenation*: It is believed that well-oxygenated cells do not allow reversal and repair of the chemical changes produced by radiation. The reoxygenation process involves radioresistant hypoxic tumor cells becoming radiosensitive aerated or oxygenated cells between radiation doses. In large tumors with necrotic central components, radiation continuously destroys the outer layers (like peeling an onion), allowing the central core to be exposed to capillary oxygenation and thus becomes more radiosensitive. This theory assumes that there is adequate microcirculation of the tumor mass. Again, reoxygenation may be the most important advantage of fractionation.[5]

In summary, fractionation of the total radiation dose spares normal tissue because repair of sublethal damage allows repopulation between doses. The redistribution and reoxygenation that occur between the daily fractions increase the radiosensitivity of the tumor cells, thereby improving overall treatment outcome. The goal is to kill tumor cells and allow normal cells to regrow and repopulate surrounding tissue.[5]

## TISSUE AND ORGAN RESPONSE TO RADIATION

Normal tissue response to ionizing radiation depends on the total dose, fractionation schedule (daily dose and overall length of treatment), and volume treated (Figure 14-4).[6] This concept, which will be repeated throughout the chapter, is integral to understanding the pathophysiology and occurrence of both acute and late radiation-associated toxicities.[6] All cells and structures that lie within the path of the ionizing radiation beam are vulnerable to toxicities. Tissue and organ systems within the body are composed of multiple cellular components that have differing radiation-tolerance parameters. Normal tissue and organ tolerance determines the limit of radiation that can be safely administered to a specific target area in the body. A large body of literature has documented tolerance doses of tissues and structures within reasonably precise limits. Table 14-1 illustrates the cellular replacement times for certain body systems.[7–10]

Information on tolerance doses has been revised in recent years because of advances in combined modality therapy.

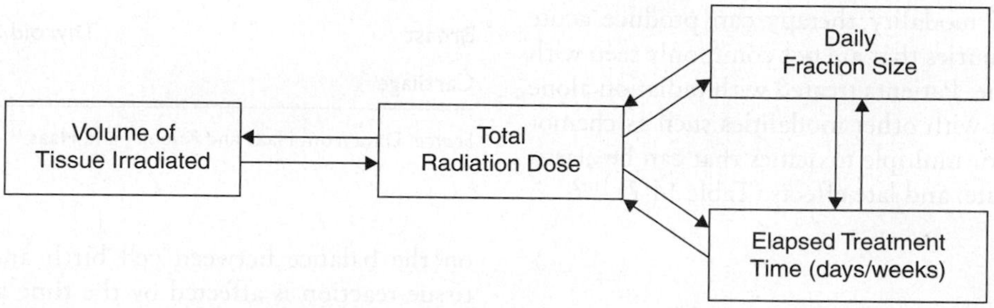


**FIGURE 14-4**

Basic factors affecting normal tissue response to radiation.

**TABLE 14-1**

**Selected Cellular Systems in Normal Tissue and Approximate Turnover/Replacement Time**

| System | Turnover/Replacement Time[a] |
|---|---|
| Integumentary | |
| Epidermis | 30 days |
| Basal cells | Nadir: 21 days<br>Re-epithelialization: 28–31 days |
| Endothelial cells | Unknown |
| Blood | |
| Red blood cells | 120 days |
| Granulocytes | 6–10 h in blood, 2–3 days in tissue |
| Lymphocytes | 100–300 + days |
| Platelets | 5–10 days |
| Respiratory tract | |
| Tracheal epithelium | 50 days |
| Lung alveolar cells | 10–30 days |
| Gastrointestinal tract | |
| Oral mucosa | 10–14 days |
| Stomach | 3–9 days |
| Small intestine | 1.5 days |
| Colon | 10 days |
| Skin | 20 days |
| Genitourinary tract | |
| Urinary bladder | 50 days |
| Testis | 20 days |
| Eye | |
| Cornea | 7 days |

[a]Turnover/replacement time is the time required for replacement of number of cells equal to that in the whole population of the system.

*Source*: Data from Coia and Myerson.[10]

**TABLE 14-2**

**Phases of Radiation Effect: Acute, Subacute, Late**

**Actual Effect**

- Evidence of radiation effect is seen in hours to days.
- Proliferating cells are more radiosensitive than quiescent cells.
- Brisk reactions heal completely, but some degree of residual damage may be present.

Tissues most at risk:

| | |
|---|---|
| Bladder | Ovary, testis |
| Bone marrow | Salivary gland |
| Colon | Skin |
| Esophagus | Small bowel |
| Lymph nodes | Stomach |
| Oral mucosa | Vagina |

**Subacute Effect**

- Evidence of damage of clinical significance is seen in weeks to a few months after completing radiation.

Tissues most at risk:

| | |
|---|---|
| Brain | Liver |
| Heart | Lung |
| Kidney | Spinal cord |

**Late Effect**

- If given sufficient doses of radiation, all tissues can manifest late effects.
- Late effects are the result of a perpetual cascade of cytokine expression causing progressive cellular and tissue destruction.
- Occurs in tissues with low cell turnover.
- Dependent on fractionation, treatment volume, and total radiation dose.

Tissue most at risk:

| | |
|---|---|
| Bile ducts | Lymph tissue |
| Bone | Pancreas (endocrine) |
| Brain | Pituitary |
| Breast | Thyroid |
| Cartilage | |

*Source*: Data from Haas and Kuehn[1]; and Haas.[12]

When chemotherapy and radiation are used concurrently, acute and late reactions in various tissues generally occur at much lower doses than when radiation is used alone. In addition, combined modality therapy can produce acute and late radiation injuries that are not commonly seen with either modality alone. Patients treated with radiation alone and in combination with other modalities such as chemotherapy are at risk for multiple toxicities that can be classified as acute, subacute, and late effects (Table 14-2).[11,12]

## ACUTE EFFECTS

Acute effects of radiation occur primarily in rapidly renewing tissues.[5] Because the response of such tissues depends on the balance between cell birth and cell death, acute tissue reaction is affected by the time allowed for repopulation and is therefore dependent on field size, daily radiation dose, and overall length of treatment (number of treatments). The concept of fractionation of RT is *crucial* to allowing normal cell repopulation (recall the four R's of radiobiology). Uninterrupted treatment would quickly overwhelm the body's ability to repair normal tissues and therefore would cause unacceptable toxicities. As a result, treatment schedules are generally 5 days per week, with 2 consecutive days of break or rest. Occasionally, treatment breaks are necessary to allow healing of normal tissue. Acute toxicities vary with each patient, are site specific and generally short term, and resolve after completion of treatment. For example, the RT nurse would expect acute oral mucositis and xerostomia when treating head/neck cancers. The time to complete resolution of acute toxicities depends on the specific tissues treated and the degree of reaction to the radiation.

### SUBACUTE EFFECTS

Subacute effects are those toxicities that are clinically evident within weeks to a few months (typically 6) after completing radiation. Examples include Lhermitte sign (tingling or shock-like sensation extending into arms or legs when the neck is flexed after receiving spinal cord radiation), pneumonitis, or rib fractures.

### LATE EFFECTS

The concern for the development of late effects is the dose-limiting factor in radiation treatment delivery.[5] The extent and degree of late effects depend on the size of the daily fraction and the total radiation dose, total treatment time, size of the treatment field, type of radiation (photons vs electrons), and concurrent chemotherapy. The mechanism of late radiation injury is not definitively known. An older paradigm described gradual ablation of the fine microvasculature leading to permanent cell/tissue death due to hypoxia. A newer model suggests that a "perpetual cascade" of cytokine (primarily the TGF family) expression causes progressive cellular and tissue death.[11] An example of an unwarranted late effect would be small or large bowel injury when treating the abdomen/pelvis.

## ROLES OF NURSING IN RADIATION ONCOLOGY

### ROLE OF THE RADIATION THERAPY NURSE

The role of the RT nurses continually evolves, in contrast to their counterpart medical oncology nurses, who have long established roles in the administration of chemotherapy and management of symptoms.[13] With increasingly aggressive cancer treatment regimens being adopted, patients are at risk for multiple toxicities, and the RT nurse must be prepared to assess and intervene as indicated. New and innovative strategies for patient teaching and managing toxicities necessitate a dialogue among all professionals involved in patient care to produce optimal outcomes. RT nurses are primarily responsible for teaching, assessing, and managing toxicities, and supporting patients through a course of irradiation.[14,15] As RT nurses longevity increased in the RT departments, other responsibilities occurred: administration, clerical, counseling, and research.[13]

Radiation therapy can engender many fears for patients, their families, and friends. Misinformation is common, and a patient's family members and friends may reinforce these concerns due to erroneous assumptions and lack of accurate information. It is essential that RT nurses are involved in education from the beginning of treatment and to include the patient, caregiver, and family members.

Having RT nurses involved in patient teaching is pivotal in patient outcomes. Hinds and colleagues[16] in earlier studies evaluated the functions and methods preferred by patients for receiving information related to RT. They concluded that RT nurses providing patient education allowed patients to be active participants in their care, reduced anxiety, and helped patients feel better prepared for the treatments. Poroch[17] demonstrated that RT patients who received structured teaching interventions, including sensory and procedural information, were significantly less anxious and more satisfied during the course of their treatment than members of a cohort control group who received standard information used in the RT department. Bennenbroek et al[18] reported on their study that evaluated the effects of 3 different audiotapes on patients' subjective understanding of RT and validation of emotions related to the cancer experience. The results indicated that the tapes had a positive effect, especially the procedural and coping tapes. These findings were similar to those in an earlier randomized study by Hagopian, who reported a benefit for patients using informational audiotapes. The conclusion was that patients who used the tapes were more knowledgeable about RT and side effects and practiced more helpful self-care measures.[19] Similar results were reported by Dunn and colleagues[20] who implemented a patient education video about RT on patients' psychological distress, knowledge about RT self-efficacy about coping with treatment and physical symptoms. While statistical significance could not be demonstrated, patients in the interventional group found the videos helpful in providing information about toxicities and would recommend others to view the video tapes. In summary, patient education should include an overview of the treatment plan, address any myths and misconceptions, information about actual treatments (including sensory information), an explanation of the simulation process, expected outcome (cure, control, or palliation), specific side effects of treatment, and symptom management. Educational resources can be located on the Internet, materials prepared and published on CDs or memory sticks that can be given to the patient for home use, or written materials still in the form of booklets and pamphlets.

The experience of cancer and its treatment generate high levels of distress and difficulty in coping. Even though cancer treatment is stressful, cessation of treatment may also be associated with emotional stress due to uncertainty about tumor recurrence.[21,22] The staff in radiation oncology departments form brief, intense relationships with patients and their families. Each individual staff member, patients, and family members deals with the ending of a course of therapy in different ways. While patients are always pleased to finish their treatment, it is important to acknowledge the ending of this portion of their cancer therapy. Often RT is the last treatment modality, after surgery and chemotherapy, and patients are indeed "finished" with treatment at the completion of the radiation course. This can be an uncertain time, with patients experiencing multiple concerns related to time to resolution of treatment-related toxicities, monitoring for cancer recurrence, and—perhaps most difficult—resuming a "normal" life. Cancer counseling or other supportive care can be extremely helpful at this point in the treatment continuum. Numerous clinical studies have followed patients after therapy and new roles may emerge for staff members in the disease trajectory of survivorship.

In general, the management of toxicities related to RT is similar to the management of chemotherapy-related side effects. It may not always be clear whether the chemotherapy or the RT is causing the specific toxicity. It is important that medical and RT nurses collaborate in planning management of side effects. While the side effects of radiation are site specific, most patients are at risk for some degree of skin reaction, fatigue, nutritional problems, and occasionally myelosuppression.

### ROLE OF THE ADVANCED PRACTICE NURSE

As the treatment complexity of RT patients has changed, the inclusion of advanced practice nurses (APNs) in the care of symptom management has evolved over recent years. More RT patients are receiving combined and strenuous chemotherapy or higher radiation doses with advanced technologies, for example, Intensity-modulated radiation therapy (IMRT), sterotactic radiation (SRS) via Cyberknife or Gamma Knife, or brachytherapy (eg, Mammosite). These procedures require more monitoring and symptom management and APNs are assisting in this managing role.[23,24] APNs are performing consultations, managing symptoms while undergoing radiation treatments, and/or following patients for recurrences and late side effects. While role responsibilities may vary between RT departments, the common denominator is patient symptom management.[25] APNs are becoming an important member of the RT team, collaborating with the radiation team and consulting services to provide evidence-based management and ensuring optimum patient care (Table 14-3).

## GENERAL SIDE EFFECTS OF RADIATION

Both the RT nurses and APNs manage patient symptoms while undergoing RT treatments. Astute skills are required to recognize early toxicities. Common general side effects that RT patients experience include the following: skin reactions (90%), fatigue (90%–100%), weight loss (prior or during), and depending on the area treated, myelosuppression.[15] If left unmanaged, quality of life for patients is diminished, possible treatment interruptions may occur, and/or the need for additional medical or surgical interventions may be required. This section will review the common side effects with a discussion of evidence-based interventions.

### SKIN REACTION (RADIODERMATITIS)

Radiodermatitis is the skin reaction that is caused by radiation to the skin tissues. Early radiation machines used much lower and less penetrating energies; therefore,

**TABLE 14-3**

**Advance Practice Nurse Reported Responsibilities From the 2006 ASTRO Workforce Survey**

| **Responsibilities** |
|---|
| New consults |
| Hospital admissions |
| Inpatient care |
| Simulations |
| Symptom management |
| Weekly treatment visits |
| Follow-up visits |
| Management involvement |
| Research |

Personal communication: Kresl and Pohar (2009)

most of the radiation dose was superficial. The degree of skin erythema was frequently used as an indication of overall radiation dose. So when the patient's skin became severely erythematous or desquamated, the radiation course ended. Modern megavoltage radiation equipment, such as the linear accelerator, is often referred to as "skin-sparing" treatment machines. Despite advanced technology in the science and delivery of radiation, the radiation beam still must first pass through the skin to reach the targeted tissue or organ. Fortunately, the dreaded and frequently severe skin reactions previously associated with RT are rarely seen with the modern treatment techniques and equipment.

Typical skin response to radiation depends on numerous radiation- and patient-related factors. Radiation factors affecting skin reaction include the following: the beam type and energy (photons or electrons), daily treatment dose (amount of gray [Gy]), tissue equivalent (bolus) material on the skin surface during treatment, accelerated dose fractionation, and location and size of the treatment fields.[15] The field location and beam arrangement (single vs opposed vs multibeam), tangential fields (higher doses received within thinner areas or parallel opposed fields [2 skin surfaces proximal to each other]) defines the skin surface(s) at risk.[15,26] Patient factors affecting skin reaction include the following: body habitus that creates significant skin folds in the treatment fields, moist areas creating friction (eg, axilla, inframammary folds, groin, or perineum), older age, nutritional status, smoking, individual radiosensitivity, and comorbid conditions and autoimmune illness (eg, lupus or scleroderma)[15,26–28] (Table 14-4). Use of concomitant chemotherapy agents can heighten the reaction (eg, doxorubicin or cetuximab). Individual skin type is not predictive of a skin reaction; therefore, it is not necessarily the case that fair-haired, light-skinned individuals are at greater risk for incurring severe skin reactions.

Skin response to radiation is dependent on dose and reflects changes in the cellular components of the epidermis, dermis, and vasculature. The epidermis and dermis are continuously renewing their cellular populations so that cell production equals cell loss. An acute skin effect is a reflection of the inability of cells in the epidermis and dermis to keep up with the accelerated loss caused by the radiation.[29,30]

## Acute skin effects

Acute skin reactions vary in intensity and duration depending on the factors mentioned earlier. The single most important factor is the location of radiation field. For example, a woman undergoing breast irradiation is at greater risk for an acute skin reaction due to the curved, tangential radiation fields that result in a higher dose to the skin surface and skin folds. In contrast, a man receiving IMRT to the pelvis (ie, advanced multi-leaf collimation and inverse treatment planning) for prostate cancer rarely experiences a skin reaction.

**TABLE 14-4**

**Overview of Factors Influencing Skin Response to Radiation**

| Radiation Related | Patient Related |
|---|---|
| • Total dose and total time | • Anatomical location of treatment field(s) |
| • Daily fraction size (Gy) | • Characteristics of skin in treatment field(s) |
| • Type of radiation beam (photon vs electrons) | • Proximity of tumor to skin surface |
| • Use of tissue-equivalent bolus material | • Concomitant conditions |
| • Size of treatment field | • Comorbid conditions |
| • Tangential/parallel opposed fields | • Nutritional status |
| • Previous irradiated fields | • Age |
| • Treatment delivery (3-D, IMRT) | |

*Source*: Data from Sparks.[29]

The degree of skin reaction can be visually assessed and may progress in a stepwise fashion from erythema to dry desquamation to moist desquamation. The stages of potential acute skin reactions are outlined in Table 14-5. It is important to understand that not all patients experience each stage of skin reaction and that some patients have several stages occurring simultaneously. Most patients demonstrate some degree of skin dryness, itching, and erythema. Erythema can progress to dermal edema and discomfort. Dry desquamation of the skin can occur as erythema resolves and the skin begins to peel. Moist desquamation of skin in the treatment field involves the epilation of the epidermis and exposure of the dermis. Patients with moist desquamation typically experience various levels of pain and may need treatment break to allow for healing.

The term *burn* is not an appropriate term to describe a skin reaction to radiation, as it implies that too much radiation was administered or that an error was made in the treatment prescription. Most RT nurses and staff avoid use of this word, although "burn" is how patients commonly describe their skin reactions. Terminology to describe radiodermatitis is depicted from National Cancer Institute (NCI) Common Terminology Criteria for Adverse Events (CTCAE) as seen in Table 14-6.[31,32] Generally, acute skin symptoms begin approximately 2 to 3 weeks into a course of treatment (20–25 Gy) and reaches maximum depletion at 50 Gy, and are confined to the treatment field.[26,33] Damage to the hair follicles and sweat glands can be permanent. Acute skin reactions usually heal completely and

**TABLE 14-5**

**Acute Effects of Radiation on Skin**

| Tissue Response | Onset/Duration | Clinical Presentation | Physiological Rationale |
|---|---|---|---|
| Early erythema | Skin reaction occurs within hours to a couple of days of starting treatments. | Faint, often unnoticed redness | Thought to be a vascular response to extracapillary cell injury |
| Prominent erythema | Skin reaction occurs 2–3 weeks into standard fractioned radiation therapy. Typically, resolves 20–30 days following last treatment | Redness that demarks treatment field and intensifies as treatment continues | Intensity greater with higher radiation doses and larger treatment fields (greater amount of vasculature). More pronounced in skin folds and moist areas. Increased blood flow through dermis from vasodilation |
| Dry desquamation | Skin reaction typically follows erythema stage, usually into 3–4 weeks of standard fractionated radiation therapy. Typically, resolves 1–2 weeks after completion of treatment | Dryness, flaking, and peeling often accompanied by itching | Each dose of radiation destroys a fixed percentage of basal cells. Surviving basal cells become conified and are shed at an increased rate. Non-cycling basal cells are stimulated and cell cycle time is shortened |
| Moist desquamation | Skin reaction occurring around 40 Gy or with trauma/excess friction/moist areas. Typically, recovery usually 2–3 weeks after completion of treatment | Brilliant erythema with sloughing of the skin where dermis is exposed and has serous exudates oozing from surface. Painful | Destruction of epithelium. All basal cells have been destroyed and no new cells are yet formed. Nerve endings in the dermis are exposed. |
| Folliculitis | Occurs most commonly when exposure exceeds 20–28 Gy | Papular erythematous rash with itching | Inflammation of hair follicules |
| Hyperpigmentation | Following 2–3 weeks of standard fractionated radiation therapy. Usually resolves 3 months to 1 year following completion of treatment but may be chronic | Tanned appearance | Comified basal cells carry more melanin into superficial layers of the epidermis and radiation stimulates tyrosinase to convert tyrosine to melanin. Increased melanocyte activity causes cells to become darker. Darker skinned people may have more hyperpigmentation because they traditionally have more melanin |

*Source*: Data from Bruner D, et al.[15]

are not always predictive of late skin manifestations. Rarely is necrosis seen as that involves damage to the deeper layers of the skin.

Concurrent chemotherapy and irradiation can result in more severe and prolonged acute skin reactions. The degree of skin effect depends on the specific chemotherapeutic agents used and the site of radiation. For example, patients receiving concurrent chemotherapy and radiation for cancers of the oropharynx, hypopharynx, or nasopharynx (skin of the neck and face), or of the anus and vulva (perianal/perineal skin) are at higher risk due to body contours that result in skin folds where the skin dose is enhanced. An erythematous skin recall reaction may occur in patients who undergo irradiation and are then given anthracyclines (eg, doxorubicin) in close proximity to completion of radiation. There are no systematic methods available to confirm skin recall, the doses of chemotherapy or radiation required, or the time interval involved. With the introduction of targeted therapies administered along with radiation, combined chemoradiation is presenting more complex dermatological side effects. Rashes that were not once present in the radiation field now occur in 45% to 100% of patients.[34] These papulopustular rashes are different from comedones or lesions associated with acne vulgaris. Evidence-based research for best management practice continues and dialogue between medical and radiation nurses is critical.

**TABLE 14-6**

| National Cancer Institute Common Terminology Criteria for Adverse Events: Dermatitis | | | | | |
|---|---|---|---|---|---|
| **Grade** | **1** | **2** | **3** | **4** | **5** |
| Rash: Dermatitis associated with radiation | Faint erythema or dry desquamation | Moderate to brisk erythema; patchy moist desquamation, mostly confined to skin folds and creases; moderate edema | Moist desquamation other than skin folds and creases; bleeding induced by minor trauma or abrasion | Skin necrosis ulceration of full thickness dermis; spontaneous bleeding from involved site | Death |

*Source*: Data from the National Cancer Institute (NCI).[32]

## Late skin effects

The late changes to skin produced by radiation can be functionally limiting if neuropathy, arthropathy, contraction, and necrosis are produced. Management of late skin effects is directed at relieving symptoms, promote healing, and surgical intervention as indicated. The late effects of radiation on the skin are dose dependent. The time interval to development of clinically evident skin changes results from the response of the cellular components in the epidermis, dermis, and microvasculature. The evolution of skin effects reflects a continuous remodeling of these cellular populations.[8]

A time period of varying length occurs in which the skin appears "normal" during radiation treatment. Then, within a period of time that may be measured in years, skin changes such as hyperpigmentation, scaling, atrophy, telangiectasias, subcutaneous fibrosis, and necrosis may develop and progress. Radiation dose schedules that produce late skin reactions are similar to those that produce acute skin reactions. Nevertheless, late effects on skin are more severe following schedules that include daily fractions of 2.5 to 3.0 Gy or higher. Most patients are treated using daily fractions of 1.8 to 2.0 Gy, thus markedly reducing the risk of late skin effects.[8] Potential late skin effects are outlined in Table 14-7.

### Skin care assessment and management

A major role performed by RT nurses is assessing skin reactions, teaching skin care, and managing skin breakdown if it occurs. Many preventive and interventional skin care regimens are currently in use, though limited scientific data support many practice interventions.[26,33] It has long been believed that skin in the treatment field should have no product (such as topical emollients) applied immediately prior to daily treatment. It is hypothesized that the product applied to the skin acts as a bolus and will enhance skin reaction. Burch et al[35] investigated what occurs on the skin surface when deodorants, powders, and creams are applied in the treatment area prior to radiation treatments. Their study was conducted using a phantom chamber to measure surface doses of radiation after various products were applied. Results showed essentially no difference in surface dose. One limitation of this study was that it was conducted using a phantom and not human subjects. Haas and Coletti[36] evaluated the affect of bolus (amount of dose the skin receives above normal dosing if dressings are kept on during RT) and compared a types of ionizing radiation beams. Eight wound dressings (soft silicone dressings, petroleum impregnated gauze, moisture vapor permeable dressing, or gel sheets) were evaluated. Two photon energy beams (6× and 15×) and 6 electron energy beams (6e-21e) were taken for each dressing. Very little bolus effect (<5%) was noted with electron therapy beams and it was more pronounced with photon beams (5%-25%). The evidence supports patients can wear dressings if receiving electron beams, but not while receiving photon beams.

At present, the optimal skin care regimen lacks evidence-based research to recommend many of the interventions or products used in the past. The goals of skin care management though remain the same—to enhance patient comfort, promote healing, and prevent infection if skin breakdown occurs.[29] Some general guidelines based on clinical experience, rather than clinical studies, are seen in Table 14-8. Major teaching points include the following: gentle skin washing with lukewarm water and mild soap in the treatment field, avoid sharp razors for shaving, wear sun-block products (SPF ≥ 30), wear loose natural fiber clothing, and implement moist wound-healing principles for the management of moist desquamation.[12,29]

Because of the lack of randomized controlled trials (RCTs) regarding the efficacy of skin care products and regimens, most skin care guidelines are institution specific and based on habit and anecdotal experience. However, there is a general agreement that hydration of the skin with an emollient, such as aloe vera, is helpful in promoting comfort and reducing pruritus. No products have been shown to definitively prevent or reliably reduce a skin reaction (refer to Table 14-9),[26,37–51] with the exception of moist

**TABLE 14-7**

**Late Effects of Radiation on Skin and Connective Tissue**

| Tissue Response | Onset/Duration | Clinical Presentation | Physiological Rationale |
|---|---|---|---|
| Photosensitivity | Begins during treatment and is lifelong | Enhanced erythema over skin exposed to UV radiation from sun and tanning beds/booths | Destruction of melanocytes in the irradiated dermis and slower melanin production following irradiation reduce the skin's ability to protect itself from UV rays. |
| Pigmentation changes: | | | |
| Hyperpigmentation | Refer to Table 14-5 | | |
| Hypopigmentation | May begin anytime following resolution of hyperpigmentation<br>Permanent | Lack of skin color | Radiation doses necessary to eradicate cancer may permanently destroy melanocytes, which results in the skin's inability to form pigment. |
| Atrophy | Following epidermal regrowth<br>Permanent | Thin and fragile epidermis | Newly formed epidermis is thinner. The epidermis thickens over time, but never attains its preirradiation thickness. |
| Fibrosis | Usually begins 4–6 months following completion of treatment<br>May worsen over time | Dense, hard, uneven skin texture<br>If extensive, may cause considerable induration and pain | Fibroblasts, responsible for producing collagen. Proliferate due to a cytokine cascade that causes increased extracellular matrix that is unchecked by normal mechanisms. Fibrotic tissue results, giving the skin an uneven texture. |
| Telangiectasia | Occurs up to 8 years following radiation therapy<br>Permanent | Purple-red spiderlike appearance of blood vessels in skin | Dose and fraction size dependent<br>Basement membrane thickening results in a decreased permeability of material through capillary walls. With capillary occlusion, there are fewer functioning small vessels and a decreased capacity for capillary regeneration. This results in increased pressure of blood flow through remaining undamaged superficial structures. |
| Ulceration and necrosis | Rare<br>May occur up to 20 years following treatment<br>Usually occurs as a result of inflammation and trauma to previously irradiated tissue. | Painful ulcers with red, raised edges and a shaggy, necrotic base.<br>Usually shows little or no tendency to epithelialize or contract.<br>Despite local treatment, ulcers tend to deepen and become more painful. | See fibrosis |

wound healing for moist desquamation. There are numerous dressings to management moist desquamation and RT nurses can consult their wound and ostomy nurses for such products.

In summary, there are no established evidence-based guidelines for skin care prevention or management. Despite various studies referenced, there is a growing body of knowledge that RT nurses are seeking to address this problem.

**TABLE 14-8**

**Suggested Skin Care Guidelines for Patients During Radiation Therapy**[a]

| What to expect when you are receiving radiation therapy? |
|---|
| • It is recommended that you pay special attention to your skin in the area being treated. Skin in the treated area will be more sensitive and can be more easily injured than usual. Skin in the treated area may become itchy, dry, red, and sore. Rarely, the skin blisters and peels. Your radiation oncology team members will be monitoring the skin. Ask questions if you have any symptoms or concerns. |
| • Most important handle skin in the treated area *gently* |
| • Do not remove temporary skin marks; tattoos are permanent and will not be affected. |
| • You will lose hair only in the immediate treated area. |
| • Wash skin in the treated area with warm—*not* hot—water. |
| • Wash—*never* scrub—the skin with care with a mild moisturizing soap (eg, Dove) and pat dry. |
| • Avoid heating pads and ice packs on the treated area. |
| • Avoid using preshave lotions and hair removal products in the treated area. |
| • If possible, do not shave the treated area. If shaving is necessary, use an electric razor. |
| • Wear loose; soft clothing over the treated area. |
| • Do not expose the treated area to the direct sun. If sun exposure is unavoidable, use sunblock having SPF. |
| • Moisturizing the skin can be helpful. Talk with your healthcare provider for a list of recommended products. |

[a]Techniques for skin care management are institution specific and not necessarily based on established data as to the optimal regimen.

*Source*: Data from Haas[12]; and Sparks.[29]

Continued research will be needed to evaluate radiation-related products to help with patient comfort, quality of life, and offering patients control over their care.

## FATIGUE

The National Comprehensive Cancer Network (NCCN) defines cancer fatigue as "a distressing, persistent, subjective sense of physical, emotional, and/or tiredness or exhaustion related to cancer or cancer treatment that is not proportional to recent activity and interferes with usual functioning".[52] Fatigue is best measured by patient self-reports of extreme tiredness, weakness, exhaustion, lack of energy, malaise, impaired ability to concentrate, and overall impaired ability to complete activities of daily living.

Fatigue during radiation is subjective reports inclusive of the above descriptors, almost universal among radiation oncology patients, and affected by multiple factors such as the extent of disease, age, concurrent chemotherapy, weight loss, pain, anemia, and length of radiation treatment. The specific etiology of radiation-related fatigue is unclear. Frequently, patients have undergone a surgical procedure(s) and received chemotherapy prior to RT. Thus, many patients come to the radiation experience familiar with fatigue and its impact on their lives.

Patients and families should be taught that fatigue is an expected effect of radiation treatments and may be further increased when receiving combined modality therapy.[53] The degree of fatigue-related symptoms increases over the course of radiation treatment.[54] During a course of fractionated RT, fatigue is often cumulative and may peak after a period of weeks. Occasionally, fatigue persists for a prolonged period after the completion of RT.

While there are numerous research studies on cancer-related fatigue, a synopsis is located on the ONS PEP-fatigue resource area and is published in ONS's publication *Putting Evidence into Practice: Improving Oncology Patient Outcomes* textbook. (http://www.ons.org/Research/PEP/Topics/media/ons/docs/research/outcomes/fatigue/samplechapter.pdf.) Radiation-induced fatigue is more site-specific which makes the management difficult. Patients can generally cope with other side effects such as nausea, vomiting, diarrhea, and skin reactions, perhaps because concrete and effective interventions are available. Fatigue, by contrast, does not lend itself to such concrete management techniques. Acknowledging fatigue as a "legitimate" toxicity of RT may be as important as making suggestions for its management. Educating patients and family members also includes helping them choose the most appropriate interventions to fight fatigue. Finding a balance of activity and energy conservation may be helpful for the chronic fatigue experienced with both chemotherapy and RT. Physical activity must be tailored to each individual, but usually includes light exercise such as walking and gardening. Mock and colleagues[55] evaluated 52 women during adjuvant chemotherapy or RT for breast cancer. They found women who exercised at least 90 minutes per week on 3 or more days significantly experienced less fatigue and emotional distress with a higher functioning ability. Yoga, a gentle form of exercise, is becoming popular and helps combat fatigue.[56,57] Whatever the form of exercise, activity has shown to increase concentration and overall ability to think clearly, which allows patients to participate more fully in their care and daily activities. Sarna and Code[58] conducted a pilot study with RT patients to describe the relationship of fatigue and physical activity. A descriptive study on 7 adult patients with various cancer sites (breast,

**TABLE 14-9**

**Description of Clinical Trials on Ointments and Creams for the Prevention and Management of Acute Radiation Skin Reactions**

| Intervention | Study (Ref.) | Study Design | No. of Patients Per Treatment Arm | Outcomes Measured | Findings |
|---|---|---|---|---|---|
| Aloe vera | Dudek et al[37] (2000) | Nonrandomized controlled | 109 (3 different commercial products of aloe vera gel)-25, 26, and 59 in each group | RTOG toxicity score, Acute Skin Reaction Index (ASRI) | No difference between groups: Aloe vera shown to be safe |
| | Heggie et al[38] (2002) | RCT | 107: aloe vera<br>101: aqueous cream | Skin toxicity, pain, itching | Higher probability of dry desquamation in aloe group; higher prevalence of dry desquamation in aloe group |
| | Olsen et al[39] (2001) | RCT | 33: mild soap + aloe<br>40: mild soap | Skin change and RTOG toxicity (erythema, skin texture, skin itch, tanning) | 69% of patients receiving aloe + soap had skin changes at <27 Gy vs 43% of soap only ($P < 0.034$) |
| | Williams et al[40] (1996) | RCT | 194: aloe vs placeho<br>108: aloe vs no treatment | Maximum dermatitis severity, time to onset of ≥ grade 2 dermatitis, duration of grade 2 dermatitis | No differences in score for all measures |
| Trolamine | Fisher et al[41] (2000) | RCT | 66: biafine<br>74: best supportive care | RN and RT grading of skin reaction | No difference in degree of skin reaction between groups |
| | Fenig et al[42] (2001) | RCT | 25: biafine<br>24: lipiderm<br>25: no treatment | Maximum skin reaction score, time to grade 2 toxicity, duration of dermatitis | No difference in degree of skin reaction between groups |
| Calendula cream | Pommier et al[43] (2004) | RCT | 126: calendula<br>128: trolamine (blafine) | Incidence, RTOG score, pain, pain and interference with ADL, treatment interruptions, product satisfaction | Reduced grade 2 or higher skin reactions ($P < 0.001$); reduced pain ($P = 0.03$) with calendula cream |
| Hyaluronic acid cream | Liguori et al[44] (1997) | RCT | 76: hyaluronic acid 0.2%<br>76: placebo | Skin reaction scale (institution based), patient tolerability, efficacy score by physician and patient | Delayed onset of skin reaction by week 3; reduced intensity and duration of skin reaction with hyaluronic acid weeks 3–7, 8, and 10 |
| Corticosteroids | Bostrom et al[45] (2001) | RCT | 25: MMF<br>25: emollient cream | Degree of erythema, pigmentation, visual skin assessment (investigator developed tool) symptom rating | 60% grade IV skin reaction in emollient group vs 35% MMF group, $P = 0.011$; no difference in pain or pruritus |
| | Schmuth et al[46] (2002) | RCT | 11: 0.5% dexpanthenol cream<br>10: 0.1% MPA<br>15: control group | Mean severity score, adverse effects (itching, burning), Skindex | No differences between groups |

(*Continued*)

**TABLE 14-9 (*Continued*)**

**Description of Clinical Trials on Ointments and Creams for the Prevention and Management of Acute Radiation Skin Reactions**

| Intervention | Study (Ref.) | Study Design | No. of Patients Per Treatment Arm | Outcomes Measured | Findings |
|---|---|---|---|---|---|
| Sulcrafate | Evensen et al[47] (2001) | RCT (patients as own control) | 60: Na SOS vs base cream | | No significant differences |
| | Maiche et al[48] (1994) | RCT (internal control method) | 44: sulcrate vs base cream | | Significant reduction in grade 2 skin reaction, more rapid healing with sulcrafate cream |
| | Wells et al[49] (2004) | RCT | 120: Aqueous cream<br>122: Sulcrate cream<br>124: No cream | | No difference in treatment arms |
| | Delaney et al[50] (1997) | RCT | 20–10% sulcrate in sorbolene cream<br>19-sorbolene cream | | No difference in pain or healing of moist desquamation |
| Barrier Films | Graham et al[51] (2004) | RCT (internal control method) | 61: No-sting vs sorbolene (30 medical application, 30 lateral) | | Reduction in frequency and duration of moist desquamation and pruritus in No-Sting group |

*Abbreviations*: ADL, activities of daily living; MMF, mometasone furoate; MPA, methylprednisolone aceponate cream; Na SOS, sodium sucrose octasulfate; RCT, randomized controlled trial; RN, registered nurse; RT, radiation therapist; RTOG, Radiation Therapy Oncology Group.

*Source*: Data from McQuestion M.[26]

lung, abdomen) were enrolled in the study and were asked to wear wrist actigraph monitors. Surprisingly, fatigue decreased with increased activity among these patients.

Other strategies to treat fatigue include modification of the patient's drug regimen, correction of metabolic abnormalities, and pharmacological treatments for anemia (eg, epoetin alfa), depression, or insomnia. Specific pharmacological approaches include psychostimulant drugs and corticosteroids. Supportive therapies may also be helpful, including the following: exercise, cognitive therapies, sleep hygiene strategies, nutritional support, and complementary approaches (eg, acupuncture, aromatherapy, and massage).[59] (See Chapter 30 for a detailed discussion of fatigue.)

## WEIGHT LOSS

A well-known important aspect of physical well-being is the ability to eat and have a good appetite.[60] This balance can be disrupted when undergoing RT. Numerous side effects from RT can place the patient at high risk for nutritional problems. Head/neck patients experience changes in their oral cavity, lung patients may experience esophagitis, or the gynecological patient experience nausea/vomiting/diarrhea.

Initiation of nutritional support begins immediately to ensure adequate oral intake as well as replacing the calories that may be lacking in their diet. Adequate hydration, maintaining or regaining previously lost weight is a primary concern during RT. Sometimes, prophylactic gastrostomy feeding tubes may be placed at the beginning of therapy to ensure adequate caloric intake. Some general nutritional hints can include the following: good oral hygiene with soft tip toothbrush; non-mint toothpaste; small, more frequent meals; and gentle exercise to stimulate hunger.[15] If the caregiver is making the meals, "gentle" encouragement is helpful and gaining weight is viewed as positive. RT nurses can direct patients to Internet nutritional resources specifically for the oncology patient (Table 14-10).

While there are several nutritional assessment tools, many are not validated in the oncology population. One valid screening nutritional tool for the oncology patient was developed by Faith Ottery, Patient-Generated Subjective Global Assessment (PG-SGA).[61] Inclusive of patient and family input, the healthcare provider can make analyses, determine the metabolic demand, and recommend

**TABLE 14-10**

**Internet Nutritional Resources for Cancer Patients and Oncology Nurses**

| Web site | URL | Contents |
|---|---|---|
| American Cancer Society | http://www.cancer.org/docroot/home/index.asp and in search box type in nutrition | On-line classes for individuals undergoing therapy, nutrition for survivors, children with cancer, with exercise and more |
| The American Dietetic Association | http://www.eatright.org/cps/rde/xchg/ada/hs.xsl/index.html and in search box type in nutrition and cancer | Journal books relating to nutrition. Also find-a-dietitian service |
| National Cancer Institute (CANCERLIT) (CancerNet) | http://www.cancer.gov/search/cancer_literature and in search box type in nutrition and cancer or CancerNet | Numerous articles with nutrition with care and prevention. Includes effects of cancer therapies and management. |
| National Coalition of Cancer Survivorship | http://www.canceradvocacy.org and in search box type in nutrition and cancer | On-line assistance for users seeking cancer resources for nutrition and other topics. |
| OncoLink (University of Pennsylvania) | http://www.oncolink.com and in search box type in nutrition and cancer | Nutritional information and supportive care strategies for cancer patients. Eating Hints for Cancer Patients booklet on-line and tips. |
| Quackwatch (Stephen Barrett, MD) | http://www.quackwatch.com | HONcode approval. Guide to health fraud, quackery, and questionable cancer therapies. |

nutritional needs.[62] Calculating ideal body weight (IBW) could be another quicker method to triage the patient[63] (refer to Figure 14-5). If further extensive medical nutritional assessment is required, a referral to the dietician can be ordered.

## MYELOSUPPRESSION

Bone marrow is an important dose-limiting cell-renewal tissue for chemotherapy, wide-field irradiation, and autologous bone marrow transplantation.[64] It is so highly radiosensitive that injury to bone marrow is produced by any dose of radiation. Following each dose of radiation, peripheral blood cells progressively decrease in number due to the destruction of both mature and precursor cells. Lymphocytes are the most sensitive cells; hence, lymphopenia develops early in the course of RT. Figure 14-6 illustrates the relative radiosensitivity of hematopoietic cell lines throughout their life cycle.[65] The radiation dose, site, and tissue volume all affect the acute response of bone marrow to therapy. When small radiation fields comprising only 10% to 15% of the bone marrow are radiated, the unexposed bone marrow responds by increasing its population of progenitor cells to meet the demands for hematopoiesis. Thus, treatment limiting myelosuppression is rarely seen unless large areas containing a substantial portion of marrow are within the radiation fields.[64] Approximately 40% of active bone marrow is in the pelvis, with the remaining 60% of active marrow distributed as illustrated in Figure 14-7.[66]

The acute effects of concurrent chemotherapy and radiation on bone marrow are complex. Any treatment regimen combining chemotherapy and RT must take into account the potential for increased dose-limiting marrow suppression.[64] Growth factors supporting the development of all hematological cell lines are seldom needed when radiation is used as a single modality. However, in combined modality therapy, growth factors are more commonly part of treatment regimens due to the increased risk of pancytopenia.

Men:
106 pounds per 5 feet in height + 6 pounds for each additional inch
Women:
106 pounds per 5 feet in height + 5 pounds for each additional inch

**FIGURE 14-5**

Calculating ideal body weight.
*Note*: For small frame: subtract 10%
For large frame: add 10%

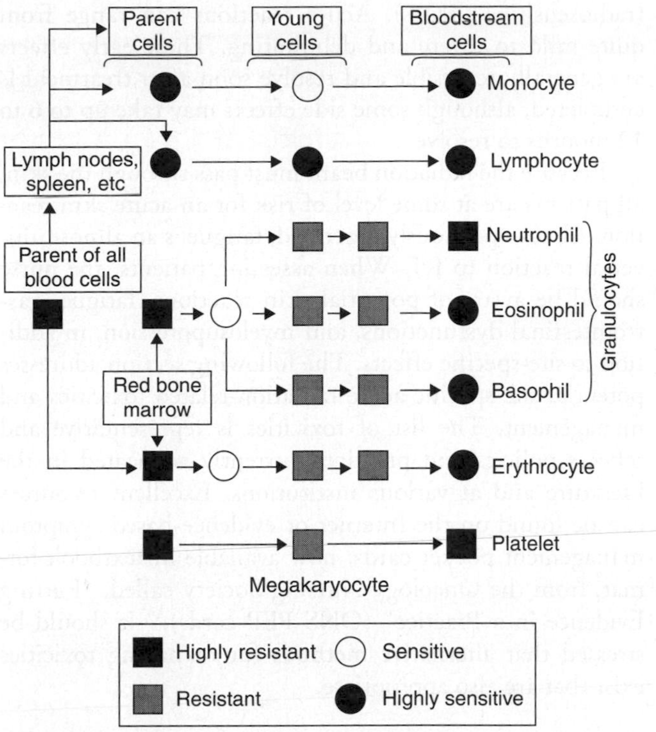


**FIGURE 14-6**

Radiosensitivity of hematopoietic blood cells. Note that lymphocytes remain highly sensitive to radiation throughout their life cycle.

Source: Adapted from Casarett.[65]

Patients at highest risk for developing cytopenias are those receiving concurrent chemoradiation, total body irradiation, extended-field (whole-abdomen) radiation, and splenic radiation. Most radiation fields are designed to limit the amount of bone marrow exposed to radiation. However, it may be necessary to irradiate marrow-producing areas in high-risk patients, such as those who have been heavily pretreated (chemotherapy and/or radiation) and those who have bony metastases that require RT for pain management. The frequency of monitoring blood counts varies by individual patient risk factors.

Chronic or late effects of radiation on bone marrow include increased hematopoietic activity in unexposed marrow segments, followed by extension of functioning marrow into previously quiescent areas such as the femora and humeri. Bone marrow regeneration is variable in each individual but generally lags behind the peripheral blood counts. Marrow recovery can occur over extended periods, with total recovery in 12 to 24 months, but this outcome depends on the volume of marrow irradiated.[64] Generally, patients are not at greater risk for infection during the chronic recovery phase.

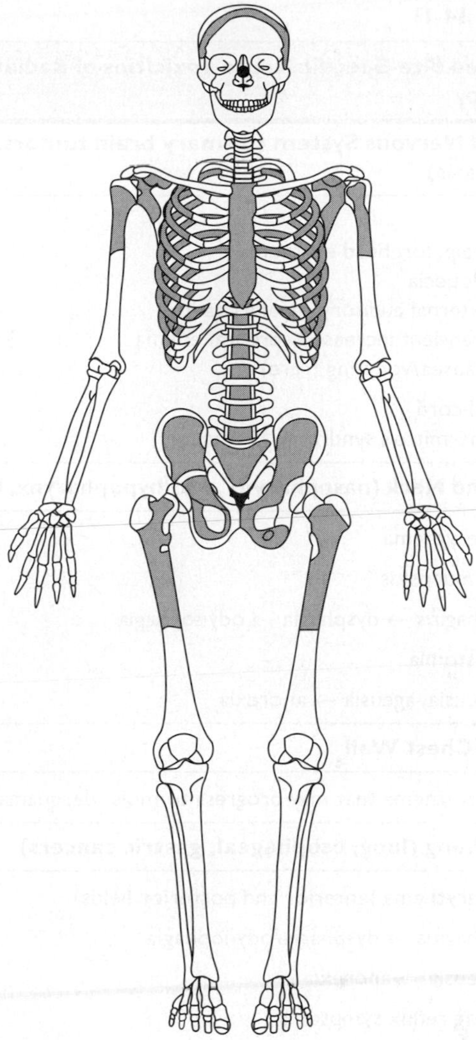

**FIGURE 14-7**

Bone marrow distribution. Bone marrow distribution in adult humans as determined by autopsy findings; active regions are shaded.

## ACUTE RADIATION TOXICITIES AND MANAGEMENT: SITE SPECIFIC

Despite the technological advances in radiation machinery and careful treatment planning to minimize radiation dose to normal tissue, patients will experience acute side effects. Radiation toxicities directly correlate with the specific normal tissues and structures within the path of the radiation beam. Table 14-11 presents a representative list of site-specific acute toxicities. The goal of radiation is to maintain the therapeutic ratio so as to achieve maximum tumor cell kill with minimal toxicity to normal tissues and structures.

Acute toxicities are dependent on the site treated, daily dose, total radiation dose, radiation energy used, and size

**TABLE 14-11**

**Selected Site-Specific Acute Toxicities of Radiation Therapy**

| |
|---|
| **Central Nervous System (primary brain tumors, brain metastasis)** |
| Brain |
| Scalp, forehead erythema |
| Alopecia |
| External auditory canal irritation |
| Transient increased cerebral edema |
| Nausea/vomiting (rare) |
| Spinal cord |
| Lhermitte's syndrome (subacute) |
| **Head and Neck (nasopharynx, oro/hypopharynx, larynx)** |
| Skin erythema |
| Oral mucositis |
| Esophagitis → dysphagia → odynophagia |
| Xerostomia |
| Dysgeusia, ageusia → anorexia |
| **Breast/Chest Wall** |
| Skin erythema that may progress to moist desquamation |
| **Chest/Lung (lung, esophageal, gastric cancers)** |
| Skin erythema (anterior and posterior fields) |
| Esophagitis → dysphagia/odynophagia |
| Dysgeusia → anorexia |
| Gastric reflux symptoms |
| Pneumonitis (subacute) |
| **Abdomen/Pelvis (gastrointestinal, genitourinary, gynecological cancers)** |
| Nausea/vomiting (radiation site dependent) |
| Diarrhea |
| Proctitis symptoms |
| Cystitis symptoms |
| Mucositis of perianal region |
| Vaginal dryness |

Acute toxicities are dependent on the site treated (the normal structures in the field), daily dose, radiation energy used, and volume treated (size of the field).

*Source*: Data from Haas.[12]

of the treatment field. Other factors would include concurrent or sequential chemotherapy, comorbid conditions, and performance status. Reactions occur as a result of 2 pathological mechanisms: inflammation of tissues and depletion of tissues with rapidly proliferating cells (radiosensitive tissues). Acute reactions can range from quite mild to severe and debilitating. These early effects are generally reversible and resolve soon after treatment is completed, although some side effects may take up to 6 to 12 months to resolve.

Because the radiation beam must pass through the skin, all patients are at some level of risk for an acute skin reaction. Also, as previously described, fatigue is an almost universal reaction to RT. When assessing patients, the nurse should be aware of potential skin reactions, fatigue, gastrointestinal dysfunctions, and myelosuppression, in addition to site-specific effects. The following section addresses potential site-specific acute radiation-related toxicities and management. The list of toxicities is representative and reflects policies and practices currently advocated in the literature and at various institutions. Excellent resources can be found on the Internet or evidence-based symptom management pocket cards, now available in textbook format, from the Oncology Nursing Society called, "Putting Evidence into Practice" (ONS PEP cards).[59] It should be stressed that alternative methods for managing toxicities exist that are also appropriate.

## BRAIN

Cranial irradiation is used to treat patients with primary or metastatic brain tumors. Primary tumors can be pilocytic or anaplastic astrocytoma, stage III/IV glioma, or central nervous system lymphoma. Metastatic tumors spread from primary sites, eg, lung, breast, renal, or colon cancers to the brain. Also, cranial irradiation can be given prophylactically for selected patients who are at high risk for developing metastatic disease, eg, patients with small cell lung cancer.

Whole or partial brain irradiation can result in the following toxicities.

### Alopecia and radiodermatitis of the scalp

Because of the high mitotic rate of hair follicles of the scalp, hair loss, referred to as alopecia, will occur when the head is irradiated. Alopecia starts approximately 2 to 3 weeks (25–30 Gy) into treatment. The extent of alopecia depends on the size of the field. If the whole brain is treated (ie, diffuse or multiple metastases), total hair loss will result. Partial brain irradiation (eg, primary brain tumor) results in alopecia that conforms to the edges of the treatment field(s). Hair almost always regrows with scalp doses of 50 to 60 Gy or less, and permanent hair loss usually occurs with doses of 60 Gy or more.[15] Regrowth of hair may take from 3 to 6 months after completion of radiation, and the new hair may be a different color and/or texture. Alopecia secondary to irradiation of the head is inevitable, and there are no proven preventive strategies. Alopecia causes a major change in self-image and is a visible reminder of the cancer experience.

When whole brain is irradiated, the skin (either the forehead or scalp) may become irritated. Excessive shedding of dead skin cells from the scalp causes pruritus. Various shades of erythema may occur and the skin can become dry, thus very itchy. This skin reaction, referred to as radiodermatitis, is managed with the same interventions discussed under acute skin effects. Patients may find anti-dandruff shampoo helpful with pruritus (eg, selsun blue family shampoo products).

*Management.* Each individual perceives hair loss differently and RT nurses should assess patient's feelings toward hair loss. Scalp irritation and erythema can be managed with gentle care to the hair and scalp. The hair should be washed beginning with a mild shampoo. Irritants such as hair dyes, hot curlers and irons, and hair dryers that can further irritate the scalp should be avoided. Patients should be encouraged to consider hair coverings (eg, wig, turban, scarf) prior to hair loss because it is much easier to match hair style and color before total alopecia occurs. The scalp tends to be sensitive after radiation-induced hair loss, especially with accompanying scalp erythema and irritation. Application of soothing moisturizing lotions or ointments may be helpful to alleviate discomfort (refer to skin care management under acute skin reactions). Some patients cannot tolerate anything on the head. Sunscreen, preferably large rimmed hats, should be worn when out in the sun.

Inform patients that significant body heat loss occurs from the head and that, without the insulation of hair, they might feel cold, especially during sleep. Tight fitting caps may help keep the exposed bald skin maintain temperature. Psychological interventions, such as support groups or patient-to-patient assistance, may help the patient cope with the effects of alopecia on self-image.

### Ear and external auditory canal irritation

If the ear is in the treatment field, the pinna and external auditory canal may become irritated, sore, and pruritic. Eustachian tubes may become swollen and interfere with hearing. Dried or dead skin within the canal may accumulate and cause pruritus.

Symptoms include feeling of ear fullness, hearing loss, itchy, and irritated inner canal. These are self-limiting and generally resolve within 1 to 2 weeks after completion of therapy.

*Management.* Instruct the patient to protect the ear from sun and cold exposure. For radiation-induced edema of the eustachian tube, over-the-counter decongestants may be prescribed. For mild discomfort in the external auditory canal, ear drops with hydrocortisone can be prescribed. Cerumen may build up and become hardened and flushing of the ear canal may be necessary. For more severe cases, steroids may be appropriate or a referral to ENT for tube placement. Most importantly, reassure the patient/family members that this is common and it should resolve after treatment.

### Cerebral edema

Increased intracranial pressure (ICP), secondary to cerebral edema, is often present at diagnosis. Radiation-induced ICP occurs, though the mechanism involved is not well understood.[67] In part, cerebral edema may be caused by the acute inflammation which causes increased permeability of the capillaries, thus causing edema and resulting in ICP. The incidence of ICP increases with the size of the initial fraction(s); for example, fractions of 2 Gy or more per day commonly result in ICP.

Symptoms include exacerbation of patients' presenting neurological symptoms, such as headache, nausea and vomiting, muscle or extremity weakness, seizures, and mental status changes. Seizures may occur, but this is rare.

*Management.* Patients with known brain tumors or metastasis are usually taking corticosteroids, and titrating the dose will often alleviate symptoms of ICP. The patient who is not taking corticosteroids and who will begin brain radiation, especially whole-brain treatment, needs to be closely monitored as cerebral edema can develop quickly. The steroid most commonly used to prevent cerebral edema is dexamethasone, which offers rapid onset of activity (peak plasma levels at 1 hour for intravenous and 1–2 hours for oral routes) and a biological half-life of 36 to 54 hours. The dose of dexamethasone varies, but a frequently used regimen is 12 to 16 mg per day (4 mg every 6–8 hours). Instruct patients not to abruptly discontinue the corticosteroid because of the risk of hypothalamic-pituitary axis (HPA) suppression, which can result in adrenal insufficiency. Symptoms of adrenal insufficiency include fatigue, nausea, vomiting, diarrhea, and weight loss.

Patients and families should be educated regarding the multiple side effects of steroids, such as gastrointestinal (GI) effects (reflux, nausea), candidiasis (especially in the oral cavity), hyperglycemia in diabetics, psychological changes such as mood swings, insomnia, and myopathy (especially proximal leg weakness). Antacid therapy (ie, $H_2$ blocker or acid-pump inhibitor) is recommended for prophylaxis of GI symptoms. Other steroid-induced toxicities are managed with medications such as lorazepam and temazepam for relaxation or sleep, systemic antifungals for candidiasis, and titration of oral antidiabetic agents or insulin for hyperglycemia.

Although steroids relieve ICP symptoms relatively quickly, most patients do not feel well while taking them and want to stop steroid therapy as soon as possible. The timing of a steroid taper varies, but generally decreasing the dose by half every 4 to 7 days will not cause exacerbation of symptoms. If symptoms recur, instruct the patient to return to the previous steroid dose. Try not to begin a steroid taper on Friday (half-life of dexamethasone is 36–54 hours) because neurological symptoms may recur on the weekend when radiation oncology staff are not as readily available.

### Nausea and vomiting

Nausea and vomiting can be caused directly from radiation, but other potential etiologies should be assessed as well. These could include chemotherapy, opioid-induced constipation, anxiety, vertigo, or delayed gastric emptying. Therefore, chronology is important. Nausea and vomiting caused by brain irradiation are short-lived effects and can be well controlled with antiemetics. Symptoms also may occur secondary to increased cranial pressure and increasing the corticosteroid dose may relieve symptoms.

*Management.* Several different antiemetics are available to control nausea/vomiting. Regimens can include the following:

Selective 5-$HT_3$ receptor antagonists
- Ondansetron 8 mg PO (tablet, oral dissolvable tablet [ODT], or oral liquid) 1 to 2 hours prior to radiation and every 8 hours prn
- Granisetron 1 mg PO (tablet) 2 tablets 1 hour prior to daily radiation or 1 tablet bid
- Dolasetron mesylate 50 to 100 mg PO (tablet) 1 hour prior to radiation

Phenothiazines
- Prochlorperazine 5 to 10 mg PO (tablet) 1 hour prior to radiation and every 6 to 8 hours prn
- Prochlorperazine 10 to 15 mg (spansules) PO approximately 1 to 2 hours prior to radiation or every 12 hours or 15 to 30 mg every am, prn
- Prochlorperazine 25 mg (suppositories per rectum) given approximately 1 to 2 hours prior to radiation or bid
- Thiethylperazine 10 mg PO (tablet) 1 hour prior to radiation and every 8 hours prn

Benzodiazepines
- Lorazepam 0.5 to 1.0 mg PO or sublingual (tablet) 3 times a day prn

Antidopaminergic (promotes gastric motility)
- Metoclopramide 10 to 20 mg PO (tablet or syrup) 4 times a day prn,

or

Corticosteroids (dosage and routes varies with individuals, refer to Physician Desk Reference)
- Dexamethosone
- Prednisone
- Prednisolone

### Somnolence syndrome (subacute)

Myelin forms a concentric sheath that surrounds the axons or nerve fibers. While totally unclear of the etiology, it is believed that RT affects myelin-producing cells, resulting in the interruption of myelin synthesis. In response, the brain produces somnolence symptoms. Somnolence syndrome is a collection of symptoms consisting of excessive sleepiness and drowsiness, lethargy and fatigue, accompanied by anorexia and occasional mild headache. This syndrome is well recognized and occurs more frequently in children than in adults. Somnolence is commonly seen in patients who receive whole brain radiation.

Symptoms occur 4 to 12 weeks after radiation is complete and can last for 2 to 8 weeks. In 1 early study, adult patients who developed somnolence syndrome after cranial irradiation for primary brain tumors identified a cyclical pattern to the symptoms.[68] Periods of drowsiness and fatigue occurred from day 11 to day 21 and from day 31 to day 35 after the completion of cranial radiation. Patients often attributed symptoms of somnolence to flu or other ailments. The unexplained and overwhelming nature of the symptoms caused anxiety.[68] Somnolence is especially distressing for children who underwent irradiation to the brain and for the caregivers.[69]

*Management.* Anticipatory guidance is a critical nursing intervention.[69] Management is directed at supportive care as the syndrome runs its course. Supportive measures include maintaining nutrition (especially in children who may sleep a greater portion of 24 hours) and prevention of problems related to prolonged immobilization, such as venous thrombosis and skin breakdown.

## HEAD AND NECK

Used in treatment for cancers of the nasopharynx, oropharynx, hypopharynx, and larynx, head and neck irradiation, especially when combined with chemotherapy, can result in multiple toxicities. Assessment and management of these toxicities present a major challenge for oncology nurses. There are numerous structures and systems in the head and neck region that result in multiple and often severe acute and late toxicities. Patients with head and neck cancer are more likely to have poor nutritional status, abuse tobacco and alcohol, and have functional deficits (ie, speech, swallowing, chewing, airway compromise). Persons with head and neck cancer need advocacy and support from all members of the cancer care team to maintain compliance with the radiation schedule, as well as to manage the toxicities and needed self-care regimens. Suspension of radiation treatment may become necessary to allow for healing of affected tissues. Irradiation to the head/neck can result in the following toxicities:

### Oral mucositis

Inflammation of the mucous membrane of the mouth is referred to as oral mucositis or stomatitis. The epithelial cells of the mucous membrane lining the oral cavity acts as a protective barrier and are highly radiosensitive.[15] The reaction of the oral mucosa from radiation can range from erythema to painful ulceration. A pseudomembrane can form and then slough off, leaving a painful, friable surface.[70] Areas of the buccal mucosa and buccal sulcus that are adjacent to metal tooth fillings are at greater risk for increased reaction due to radiation scatter from the metal filling. The onset of oral mucositis is seen approximately 2 to 3 weeks after the start of treatment. It is dose dependent and usually occurs after patients received 18 to 20 Gy.

Oral mucositis will be enhanced and prolonged in patients who have preexisting poor oral or dental hygiene, continue to smoke, use chewing tobacco, consume alcohol, and have poorly fitting dentures. Also, combined modality therapy with chemotherapeutic agents such as 5-fluorouracil, will enhance mucositis of the oropharynx. Presence of bacterial, viral, or fungal infections can compound the problem.

Symptoms generally begin as generalized oral discomfort and progress (depending on the radiation dose) to extreme pain when eating, swallowing, speaking, and sleeping. The lining of the mucosal membranes becomes raw and irritated, progressing to patchy or confluent ulcerations. Bleeding may be present and tissue necrosis can become life threatening. Any grade of oral mucositis definitely affects quality of life.[71]

Assessment for oral mucositis involves frequent inspection of the oral cavity while the patient is undergoing radiation treatments. Evaluation schedules are patient specific, though weekly inspection is adequate early in the course of treatment (first 2–3 weeks), and then as symptoms indicate. A mouth care regimen should focus on oral hygiene, dental prophylaxis, and pain control as well as nutrition.

*Management.* Management strategies are focused toward lessening the severity of oral mucositis grade (National Cancer Institute Common Toxicity Criteria clinical and functional scale—refer to Table 14-12), pain management, and ensuring nutritional needs. Prior to initiation of RT, patients should have a dental, speech, and physical therapy consults. Dental consults should include evaluation of teeth and gingival to determine if any teeth need to be extracted before beginning radiation. Fitting for fluoride trays can be molded at the same time. Swallowing problems can be identified prior to treatment by the speech therapist and physical therapists may suggest exercises to help the patient as one undergoes therapy. Recommendations should include the following: avoiding products that will further dry the mucous membranes, such as mouthwashes with alcohol and any glycerin-based product, instructing the patient to gently brush the teeth and tongue frequently with a soft toothbrush, and continue flossing the teeth as tolerated.[15] Ideally, the patient should perform oral care 4 times daily and more often once they develop thick and ropy secretions.

Mouth rinses should begin at the first day of treatment. Isotonic saline solution (swish and spit) helps loosen debris and cleanse the oral cavity. A common saline solution mixture is 1 teaspoon of salt and/or 1 teaspoon of baking soda in a quart of water. This solution is mild and rarely causes increased discomfort. Patients should be encouraged to swish and spit the solution as often as possible—ideally, every 1 to 2 waking hours. Also, a supersaturated electrolyte solution, calcium/phosphate (Caphosol) helps moisten, lubricate, cleanse the oral cavity, and decreases the severity of oral mucositis.[72–74] This solution can relieve dryness and fissuring of the oral mucosa, as well as painful tongue caused by hyposalivation.[75] Half of the combined solution should be swished for 1 minute and repeat

**TABLE 14-12**

**NCI Grading of Oral Muscositis**

| Grade | Clinical Exam | Functional or symptomatic |
|---|---|---|
| 1 | Erythema of mucosa | Minimal symptoms-normal diet |
| 2 | Patchy ulcerations or pseudomembranes | Symptomatic, but can eat and swallow modified diet |
| 3 | Confluent ulcerations or pseudomembranes; bleeding with minor trauma | Symptomatic and unable to adequately ailment and hydrate orally |
| 4 | Tissue necrosis; significant spontaneous bleeding; life threatening consequences | Symptoms associated with life threatening consequences |
| 5 | Death | Death |

Because the tolerance levels of all tissues are known, the overall risk of radiation-related late effects is very low. The percentage of risk varies by tissue site.

*Source*: National Cancer Institute (NCI).[32]

for the second minute. Patient should spit and not swallow the rinse. The patient should be instructed not to have anything to eat or drink for 15 minutes after rinsing, to be effective.

Topical anesthetics can be helpful for pain control. While there are different mixtures of what is commonly referred to as miracle mouthwash, ingredients can include a 1:1:1 mixture of liquid antacid, diphenhydramine hydrochloride, and viscous lidocaine. Patients can swish and spit/swallow 5 to 10 mL of the topical anesthetic 20 minutes prior to eating and drinking. Caution should be shared if patients are swallowing, as this could cause aspiration from the numbing effect. There are many prepared topical anesthetics available commercially (eg, OraMagic Plus, Hurricane Gel). Oral morphine sulfate rinses (2000 mg of morphine in 1000 $cm^3$ normal saline), swishing 1 tablespoon and holding for 1 to 2 minutes and spitting, 4 times a day, can decrease the pain sensation in the oral cavity.[76] Since the patient swishes and does not swallow, the typical side effects of narcotics does not occur with the morphine rinse.

Systemic analgesics are often warranted and are most convenient in liquid and transdermal patches, or forms that can be given through feeding tubes. Whenever possible, The World Health Organization ladder guidelines should be employed when managing pain.[77] Possible medications can include the following:

Morphine sulfate (MS Contin, MSIR, Avinza, Kadian)
Oxycodone (Oycontin, OxyIR, tablets with aspirin [Percodan] or acetaminophen [Roxicet, Percocet])
Hydrocodone (Hycodan, tablets with acetaminophen [Lortab, Vicodin, Vicodin ES or HP], Norco or with ibuprofen [Vicoprofen])
Oxymorphone (Opana, Opana ER)
Fentanyl (Duragesic, oral tansmucosal Actiq)

## Taste changes (dysgeusia, ageusia)

Taste buds (receptors) are primarily located on the tongue, soft palate, glossopalatine arch, and posterior wall of the pharynx. Taste sensations include sweet, sour, salty, and bitter tastes. Because the taste buds are extremely radiosensitive, symptoms are noted early in the course of treatment, often during weeks 1 and 2.[70] Patients typically describe a decrease in taste (hypogeusia) and altered taste (dysgeusia). In some patients, this effect will progress to loss of all taste (ageusia).

Taste is integrally bound to appetite. When one cannot taste food, this problem may result in progressive anorexia and weight loss. Patients may describe a sensation of the food creating a "tasteless ball of goo" in their mouth. Alteration to taste of salty or bitter foods are more pronounced and sweet taste is least affected, but each patient will report their own aversions. Add to taste changes, the symptoms of oral mucositis, acute xerostomia, or esophagitis, eating becomes an ordeal.

*Management.* Changes in taste may result in severe anorexia, therefore monitoring for weight loss is important. Encourage oral care prior to meals to help clear residual tastes and refresh the mouth for meals.[70] Rinsing with tea, ginger ale, salt/soda water before eating helps to clear the taste buds. Strategies to enhance the palatability of foods are discussed in Chapter 33 and apply to patients undergoing radiation. The loss of "salt" perception can be particularly problematic for some patients. In such a case, a dietary consult can prove very helpful. Sugarless lemon drops or mints may help get rid of unpleasant taste that lingers after eating.

## Oral candidiasis

Candidiasis is an infection of the oral mucosa with a yeast-like fungus, most commonly *Candida albicans.* In patients undergoing head and neck irradiation, candidiasis occurs frequently due to destruction of the protective oral mucosal barrier, resulting in an overgrowth of *Candida.*

The infection is characterized by white patches and clusters in the mouth. Assessment of the entire oral cavity includes the tongue, roof of mouth, and buccal sulci and membranes. Although a culture can be sent for microbiological confirmation, the diagnosis is usually made on the basis of clinical appearance.

*Management.* Antifungal medication is prescribed for oral candidiasis, commonly referred to as thrush. A variety of preparations of antifungal drugs are available, including swish-and-swallow mixtures, troches, and systemic oral agents. It is important to remember that most head and neck patients have concurrent xerostomia, so troches will be generally ineffective because they will not dissolve well, if at all. A swish-and-swallow preparation demands a compliant patient, as it must be done 4 to 5 times daily and can further irritate already painful oral mucosa. Daily oral administration of an agent such as fluconazole, which is available in liquid or tablet form, may be more appropriate for these patients. Caution is advised if patients are already on warfarin as this may increase bleeding times. Often, oral mucositis and esophagitis diminish somewhat when candidiasis is resolved. Head and neck patients endure multiple toxicities, and candidiasis is one of these many side effects if detected early, can be quickly resolved.

## Oral herpes

Distinction of the term herpes is important. There can be herpes simplex (HSV-1 transmitted orally and HSV-2 transmitted sexually) and herpes zoster shingles. Each viral infection has different presentations and interventions.

Herpes simplex virus HSV-1, is associated with oral infections. HSV-1 can affect lips, face, buccal mucosa, and throat. Oral herpetic lesions may occur with or without candidiasis. Herpes lesions appear as grouped vesicles on an erythematous base, usually the locations listed above. There may be tenderness, pain, mild paresthesia, or burning prior to the eruption of lesions. Some individuals have no prodrome. Diagnosis is made by clinical assessment, culture, and microbiological confirmation.

*Management.* Treatment of oral herpes is primarily supportive. Oral antiviral medications such as acyclovir or famciclovir are generally effective. For lesions of the lip and mouth, viscous xylocaine can be directly applied to the area or used as a rinse to facilitate eating. Application of Orabase, which is a dental protective paste, 4 times a day, can prevent irritation of lesion by the teeth. Sometimes direct ice may help with swelling and pain. Avoidance to the sun should be advised.[78]

### Acute xerostomia

Saliva plays an important role in mastication, digestion, swallowing, and speech. The mean daily salivary output ranges from 500 to 1500 mL. The average volume of saliva present in the oral cavity is approximately 1 mL.[79] More than 99% of saliva is water. Saliva also contains inorganic ions, lipids, amino acids, proteins, and traces of hormone-like substances. The proteins, including the salivary enzymes, are derived from the serum or synthesized within the parotid glands. The secretory function of the salivary glands is controlled by the autonomic nervous system and may be stimulated by the sensation of taste, smell, or chewing, and by psychological factors and stimulation, such as esophageal and gastric irritations, from other organs.[79] Saliva provides lubrication for oral tissues and protection from bacterial infections. It also inhibits enamel decalcification and provides an important excretory route for blood-borne urea, uric acid, and ammonia.

The major salivary glands (parotid, submandibular, and sublingual) are highly radiosensitive. Together, the salivary glands produce more than 1 liter of saliva per day. Typically, 60% to 65% of the total salivary volume is produced by the parotid glands, 20% to 30% by the submandibular glands, and 2% to 5% by the sublingual glands. The parotid glands are composed of serous cells and produce watery and albuminous secretions. The submaxillary and sublingual glands, composed of mixed serous cells and mucous acini, have thicker secretions.

The serous cells of the salivary glands are more radiosensitive and the mucous cells more radioresistant. A 50% or more reduction in salivary flow has been detected after the first week of fractionated RT to the head and neck area. This flow continues to decline and may become barely measurable by the end of a 6- to 8-week course of treatment. This is referred to as xerostomia, which is acute and can be chronic. Because the parotid glands (serous, watery secretions) are more affected by the radiation, the remaining saliva becomes thick and ropy.[79] Generally, patients notice the onset of dry mouth within the first 2 weeks of radiation. Xerostomia occurs at 10 Gy and is permanent at more than 40 Gy.

Clinically, xerostomia is a symptom representing subjective complaints of extremely dry mouth that is associated with mucosal inflammation, acinary atrophy, or ulceration. This condition can deteriorate to include fissures of the lips and tongue, burning sensation, and changes in the tongue surface.[80]

*Management.* Strategies for preventing oral dryness are the key. With the introduction of new technology (eg, IMRT), which is an advanced form of 3-D conformal RT, some protection of salivary function can be obtained.[81] Contouring fields to avoid the salivary glands have decreased the incidence of xerostomia. In addition, there is an FDA radioprotectant agent that has shown efficacy in preserving salivary glands, amifostine. Amifostine, first developed and referred as WR-2721 (Ethyol), contains thiol compounds and is a free-radical scavenger. Multiple studies have demonstrated its protective effects on the salivary glands during head and neck irradiation. In all studies, no tumor-protective effect by amifostine was detected.[82]

Beside technological techniques with equipment and pharmaceuticals, there are other techniques being investigated to preserve salivary function. Investigational approaches, such as transferring submandibular glands to the submental region are a surgical technique that might evidentially spare the parotid gland destruction. Also, gene therapy is being studied with this issue.

Managing oral dryness or xerostomia includes increasing oral fluids sucking on sugarless candy or gum, drinking sugarless lemon-flavored drinks, prescription medications, or over-the-counter salivary subsitutes.[15,70] Most patients find drinking water most helpful, but relief is of short duration. Sugarless products sweetened with xylitol alone or in combination with sorbital are preferred. Some data suggest that xylitol has anticariogenic properties. Xylitol is associated with a decrease in *Streptococcus mutans* levels in saliva and dental plaque.[83] Pilocarpine hydrochloride is a cholinergic stimulant that acts on postganglionic cells innervating smooth muscles and exocrine glands (ie, sweat and salivary glands).[79] Several studies have demonstrated that pilocarpine given orally can reduce the symptoms of postirradiation xerostomia in patients who have some residual salivary function.[84–87] The most common regimen consists of pilocarpine 5 mg, 4 times a day (qid), but the dose can be increased to 10 mg qid as indicated. The major side effect includes sweating, usually within 30 minutes of administration. Some data suggest that pilocarpine given concurrently and postirradiation may decrease overall postirradiation xerostomia.[87] Saliva substitutes and chemical salivary gland stimulants are available (eg, Numoisyn lozenges, either liquid 2 cm prn or 1 lozenge, prn, maximum 16 tablets a day). The so-called artificial saliva products (Oasis, Salivart,

Biotene products, Oral Balance Moisturizing Gel) are helpful for some patients, but only afford short-term relief of dryness and can be costly.

Complementary approaches can be employed.[88–90] Acupuncture has shown to increase salivary flow. The mechanism of action is unknown, but this strategy is an option for xerostomic patients. Most importantly, a dietary consult is helpful to assist patients/family members with meal planning. Changes from regular diets to soft, mechanical diets are helpful in early phases of treatments. Avoidance of caffeinated products and alcohol can lessen the severity of dry mouth.[91,92] Spicy foods, salt, and spicy herbs should be avoided.[93] Evidentially, liquid nutritional supplements (either orally or through feeding tubes) may be ordered. Supplements, such as Ensure Plus, Boost Plus, Shandi-Shake, or Juvene, are products that can provide the necessary caloric/protein intake oncology patients require to meet their nutritional needs.

### Dental caries

Dental caries technically are not an acute toxicity of head and neck irradiation, but preventive management for them during treatment is mandatory. All teeth are at risk—not just those in the path of the radiation beam. Due to xerostomia, the pH of the mouth shifts toward a highly acid oral environment, and markedly cariogenic flora develop. The teeth rapidly demineralize and enamel defects appear, especially on the cervical and incisal/occlusal surfaces. The resulting dental demineralization almost always leads to radiation-induced caries, which constitute a risk factor for osteoradionecrosis of the mandible and maxilla.[94] Osteoradionecrosis is a potentially severe chronic complication that results in bony necrosis of the jaw (primarily the mandible) and requires intensive treatment that may include surgical resection and bone grafting.

*Preventive management.* Dentulous patients must have a dental evaluation prior to starting radiation. Questionable teeth should be extracted, ideally at least 14 days prior to the initiation of irradiation. Most often, dental prophylaxis consists of daily fluoride solution or gel applied to a mold (tray) and placed on upper and lower teeth, then held in place for several minutes. Fluoride has a tendency to burn when the patient has developed oral mucositis, so the patient may hold treatments until oral mucosa heals. A home care fluoride regimen is essential, but may not be possible to maintain if severe mucositis is present. This potential complication argues for even greater compliance with the oral care regimen until fluoride prophylaxis can be resumed.

### Esophagitis and pharyngitis

The pharynx and esophagus are usually in the treatment fields for head and neck irradiation. The radiation causes inflammation and denudation of the surface epithelium of the pharynx and esophagus. The resulting mucositis leads to dysphagia (ie, difficulty swallowing) and odynophagia (ie, painful swallowing), both that can be so severe that patients may be unable to take food and fluids or swallow oral secretions.

Symptoms usually start approximately 2 weeks into a course of therapy. Often patients will complain first as "having a lump" in their throat, then as time continues swallowing becomes painful and the swallowing action more stressful. If the patient is receiving concurrent chemotherapy, symptoms may occur sooner and be more severe. As with oral mucositis, patients who continue to smoke and use alcohol are at greater risk for acute and prolonged symptoms.

*Management.* Nursing management and interventions are similar to those for oral mucositis; optimize hydration, maximize nutrition, provide comfort, and ensure safe swallowing (ie, prevention of aspiration). Esophagitis/pharyngitis is a potentially serious toxicity if patients are unable to maintain nutrition and hydration. Patients should be weighed once or twice weekly and carefully assessed as to oral intake. Enteral feeding and IV hydration are needed in many patients and should be discussed prior to initiating irradiation. When prescribing pain or other medications for the patient with odynophagia, liquids or crushable tablets should be considered. Patients quickly determine what they can swallow, and intake usually concentrates on soft to liquid foods. Soothing agents (eg, carafate slurries) or aloe-based solutions (eg, OraMagic) may be ordered. Consultation and collaboration with a dietitian may help the patient maintain the optimal protein and calorie intake.

### Laryngitis

If the larynx is in the radiation treatment field(s), patients will experience laryngitis. Radiation causes inflammation and swelling of the laryngeal cartilage, leading to decreased mobility of the vocal cords.[15] This is usually temporary and incidence varies.

The major symptom is hoarseness. Voice quality can be mild to so severe that speech sometimes becomes almost impossible.

*Management.* Interventions should be directed toward minimizing the irritation to the vocal cords. Patients should be instructed to avoid straining to speak; however, sometimes this may be difficult to accomplish. Elderly patients or those who live alone may be anxious that they will not be able to communicate their needs should they be in an emergent situation. Speech therapists can be consulted regarding assistive devices such as those that can amplify the voice during this temporary time. Warm saline gargles can be soothing. Instruct patients to avoid tobacco and alcohol. It is important to remember that compliance with abstinence from tobacco and alcohol can be difficult, if not impossible, for this group of patients, as they often have many years of dependency and use. Steroids or alpha-adrenergic agents may become necessary if edema becomes severe, but this is rare. If the airway does become compromised, a tracheostomy can be performed. Management of laryngitis is similar to management of esophagitis and focuses on nutrition, hydration, lubrication, and pain relief.

## BREAST AND CHEST WALL

Used in treatment for breast carcinoma, breast irradiation can be offered externally (teletherapy) or internally (brachytherapy). Discussion of the different modalities can be found in Chapter 13. Either modality can result in several toxicities. This discussion focuses on the effects of breast irradiation after breast-preserving surgery (ie, lumpectomy) or mastectomy. Major acute toxicities can include the following:

### Skin reactions

Skin reactions are the primary acute side effects of breast or chest wall irradiation. There was an extensive discussion presented earlier in this chapter with regard to radiodermatitis, but there are risk factors that should be considered for women undergoing breast irradiation. Women with large, pendulous breast and multiple skin folds are at higher risk for skin reactions. Combined chemotherapy and certain comorbid disease presents challenges, that is, autoimmune diseases (eg, systemic lupus erythematosis or scleroderma). Sensitive areas of breast irradiation that seem to have more skin reactions are inframammary fold, supraclavicular area, and the axillary area. When the chest wall is treated after a mastectomy, electrons beams treat more superficially, thereby causing more of a skin reaction. Changes are usually clinically evident at approximately 30 Gy with standard fractions of 1.8 to 2.0 Gy daily.[29]

All women who are receiving radiation for curative intent develop some grade of skin reaction. Appearance of skin reactions varies from light to brisk shades of erythema or hyperpigmentation. Skin reactions can progress to severe dry to moist desquamation, especially in the inframammary crease and axilla. Pruritis can occur as well.

*Management.* For management of skin reactions, refer to the acute skin effects mentioned earlier in this chapter. In addition, the patient may experience transient discomfort in the breast (ie, shooting pains, breast heaviness) and axilla during radiation. The etiology of this effect is unclear, although surgical changes and possibly radiation-related edema may be the underlying cause. Such symptoms, if long-lasting, usually respond to nonsteroidal anti-inflammatory drugs such as ibuprofen or naproxyn. Clinical studies have shown that taking glutamide, 15 mg 3 times a day, from the beginning of treatment for women with pendulous breasts may decrease overall breast swelling.[95] For severe breast edema, referral to a lymphedema specialist may be warranted.

### Esophagitis

Esophagitis may occur if the supraclavicular fossa is included in the treatment field or if the inframammary chain (IMC), which is structurally over the esophagus, is included in chest wall field. Symptoms are usually mild and limited in duration and were already described in the head/neck section.

*Management.* For the discussion and management of esophagitis and pharyngitis, please refer to the head and neck section of this chapter.

## CHEST AND LUNG

Used in treatment for lung, esophageal, gastric cancers, Hodgkin's disease, and non-Hodgkin's chest lymphoma, chest and lung irradiation results in the following toxicities:

### Esophagitis and pharyngitis

Most radiation treatment fields for treatment of lung, esophageal, and gastric cancers and some lymphomas include the mediastinum and thus affect the esophagus and hypopharynx. The resulting mucositis causes dysphagia and odynophagia that may become severe. The treatment fields are usually angled (vs initial direct anterior-posterior fields) approximately two-thirds of the way into treatment, thereby minimizing some of the dose to the pharynx and esophagus. As a consequence, symptoms lessen. Depending on the length (top to bottom) of the field and the site of esophageal or gastric cancer (eg, tumor at the gastroesophageal junction), patients may experience gastric reflux that can exacerbate esophagitis symptoms. Combined chemotherapy intensifies the reactions.

Symptoms begin usually 2 to 3 weeks after initiation of radiation, or sooner if the patient is receiving concurrent chemotherapy.[96] Patients often describe the feeling of a "lump" in the throat and a feeling of obstruction when swallowing. Patients will complain of dry or sore throat, often reporting "my throat feels like it is on fire". This can lead into a cascade of other symptoms—fatigue, depression, insomnia, or anorexia.

*Management.* Management is similar to that described under esophagitis and pharyngitis in the head and neck section of this chapter. Dietary modifications are helpful and include a soft to liquid diet and nutritional supplements. Antacid therapy or proton pump inhibitors can be started for patients who experience reflux symptoms. Pain management is essential for comfort. Close monitoring is essential, as oral intake can decrease with fluid imbalance and weight loss may occur rapidly. Patients presenting with upper gastrointestinal and lung cancers frequently already have impaired nutritional status and a history of tobacco and alcohol abuse, which can present a challenge for optimal patient management.

### Taste changes

It is unclear why patients receiving radiation to the chest experience taste changes. The cause is likely multifactorial, including prior or concurrent chemotherapy, fatigue, and medications such as opioids. Taste changes may lead to anorexia and, when combined with the previously described toxicities, can cause a cascade of effects including increased fatigue, weight loss, weakness, and delayed healing of acute side effects.

*Management.* Beside the suggestions already mentioned in the Head/Neck section, consultation with the oncology dietitian is helpful to define ways to maintain optimal nutritional status.

### Pneumonitis (subacute)

Pneumonitis is not an infectious process; indeed, *pneumonopathy* might be a more appropriate term for this toxicity. Pneumonitis is caused by a decrease in surfactant produced by the alveolar type II pneumocytes in conjunction with endothelial cell and vessel permeability that negatively affects perfusion.[15] Symptoms occur 1 to 3 months after completion of radiation (subacute toxicity) and can be seen within days after administration of certain chemotherapeutic agents, such as bleomycin, chlorambucil, the nitrosoureas, cyclophosphamide, methotrexate, and procarbazine. Symptomatic pneumonitis occurs in approximately 20% of patients, usually between 8 and 12 weeks after completing thoracic irradiation.[97]

The severity of the pneumonitis depends on the degree of pulmonary involvement, which is the amount of lung parenchyma in the treatment fields. Symptoms include low-grade fever and nonspecific respiratory symptoms such as congestion, nonproductive cough, and a feeling of fullness in the chest. If symptoms progress, the patient may experience dyspnea, pleuritic chest pain, and increasing cough that may result in small amounts of sputum with hemoptysis.

On examination, altered breath sounds are usually absent. Pleural friction rub or pleural fluid may be detected. Generally, the symptomatic phase of pneumonitis is relatively short in duration, and symptoms resolve completely.

Diagnosis of pneumonitis is made clinically with radiological studies and symptom review. A chest x-ray (CXR) may reveal a diffuse infiltrate and possibly functional lung volume loss corresponding to the radiation field. Computerized tomography (CT) scans are more sensitive in evaluating lung density. Ventilation/perfusion scans are also used for diagnosis. Pulmonary function tests (PFTs) will not demonstrate an abnormality until 4 to 8 weeks after completion of irradiation. A decrease in diffusion capacity is generally the most outstanding parameter on PFTs.[98]

*Management.* Treatment of the acute symptoms of pneumonitis includes supportive measures. This includes bed rest to conserve respiratory effort, bronchial dilators, oxygen therapy, and glucocorticoids. Treatment measures do not shorten the duration of pneumonitis; instead, they aim to palliate symptoms. In rare cases, radiation pneumonitis may be severe, with symptoms including fever and acute cor pulmonale that can lead to death. After the acute phase of pneumonitis, symptoms slowly improve, as inflammation resolves.[97]

Nursing assessment includes evaluation of symptoms and monitoring of the patient's oxygenation status and ability to complete activities of daily living. Reassurance is given to patients that this will generally resolve within 6 to 8 weeks and not to get alarmed. A physical/occupational therapy consultation can help patients adapt their daily activities to accommodate their respiratory disability.

## ABDOMEN AND PELVIS

Used in treatment for gastrointestinal, genitourinary, and gynecological cancers, the abdomen and pelvis has many radiosensitive tissues. Irradiation, either curative or palliative, can result in the following toxicities:

### Nausea and vomiting

RT is a localized treatment. As a consequence, nausea and vomiting will not occur unless radiation fields include the whole abdomen, extended pelvic fields, epigastric region, paraaortic area, or, in rare cases, the chemoreceptor trigger zone (CTZ) in the cerebral cortex.[99] Symptoms of nausea and vomiting directly related to irradiation are fairly predictable and will occur 1 to 3 hours after the daily treatment. Nausea and vomiting are influenced by multiple other factors, including medications (ie, opioids, antibiotics), chemotherapeutic agents, constipation, pain, and metabolic alterations such as hypercalcemia.[100]

*Management.* Patients who are at risk for nausea and vomiting should be premedicated with antiemetics approximately 1 hour prior to daily radiation treatment. However, timing is dependent on medication and route of administration. The goal is to prevent an initial emetic episode. Around-the-clock administration of antiemetics may be necessary if symptoms warrant. It is difficult to definitively recommend whether patients should receive daily radiation treatment with an empty or full stomach. Generally, patients feel better and have less nausea if they eat small frequent meals or snacks, including prior to daily radiation. See the discussion of nausea and vomiting in the brain section of this chapter for a brief discussion of antiemetics commonly used in RT (eg, $5HT_3$ receptor antagonists, phenothiazines, or benzodiazepines). RT nurses should review their daily intake of food and fluids when nausea/vomiting become an issue. Weight, vital signs (especially blood pressure and pulse), laboratory values all can be indicators how the patient is compensating. Sometimes distraction of music in the treatment room or patient using visual imagery can overcome the feeling of nausea. Acupressure to the wrist can help some patients decrease nausea/vomiting.[101]

### Diarrhea and proctitis

The size of the abdominal/pelvic radiation field generally determines the risk for diarrhea and proctitis. Diarrhea is a result of denuding of the intestinal mucosa, leading to decreased absorptive capacity and increased motility and peristalsis. The small bowel is much more radiosensitive than the colon or rectum, and the extent of the small bowel's involvement greatly influences the severity of the symptoms. A patient undergoing whole-abdomen radiation is at greatest risk to experience watery diarrhea and cramping, while the patient with a relatively small pelvic field (ie, radiation to the prostate cancer) will most likely have frequent soft bowel movements rather than pronounced diarrhea.

Symptoms include excessive semi-form to liquid stools. Mucous may or may not be present. Typically, blood should not be seen in the stool unless the patient has hemorrhoids. Abdominal bloating or cramping with increase flatus may occur.

Proctitis is the inflammation of the rectal mucous membranes and can be accompanied by tenesmus (spasms of the rectal area that gives a feeling of incomplete evacuation of stool). Proctitis occurs most frequently in patients receiving radiation for rectal, anal, and prostate cancers due to the location of the inferior border of the treatment fields.

Both proctitis and tenesmus are frequently painful defecation and may be accompanied by involuntary straining and other gastrointestinal symptoms. Symptoms are compounded if concurrent chemotherapy is administered.

*Management.* Assessment should start with the patient's definition of diarrhea and specific stool characteristics and frequency. Of most concern are frequent watery stools that have the potential for inducing electrolyte imbalance and dehydration. Patients most at risk for dehydration due to diarrhea or vomiting include children, the elderly, debilitated individuals, and those receiving concurrent chemotherapy (eg, 5-fluorouracil, cisplatin). It is essential to monitor weight frequently (daily if necessary), check orthostatic blood pressure, and assess skin and mucosal turgor. Some patients may require intravenous hydration and/or a break from radiation treatment.

Patients should be instructed regarding a low-residue diet and the use of antidiarrheals. A low-residue diet guideline is helpful to assist in teaching and for patient reference. Ethnic and geographic food patterns should be considered to support compliance.[100] An oncology dietitian consult can be invaluable. The patient should ideally have antidiarrheal medication (eg, loperamide or diphenoxylate/atropine) on hand in case diarrhea occurs unexpectedly. Severe or protracted diarrhea may require treatment with octreotide (Sandostatin). Octreotide, which is similar to the natural hormone sandostatin, suppresses secretions of serotonin and multiple GI peptides. It is effective in secretory-type diarrhea because it stimulates fluid and electrolyte absorption from the GI tract. This agent is administered by subcutaneous injection 1 to 3 times daily. A long-acting formulation is available as well.[102]

Proctitis symptoms can be treated with conservative management, including sitz baths and anti-inflammatory agents such as pramoxine hydrochloride 1% and/or hydrocortisone acetate 1% (cream or foam). Gastrointestinal-specific antispasmodics may decrease tenesmus symptoms. Diarrhea and frequent stools can result in painful irritation of the perianal region secondary to frequent cleansing. Helpful interventions include the following: gently cleansing the perianal region after each bowel movement with warm water using a squirt bottle, patting dry, and then applying a barrier cream and using premoistened towelettes.[15]

### Cystitis

When the bladder is totally or partially in the radiation treatment field, there is mucosal injury, initially causing inflammation to the lining. In turn, this mimics urinary tract infection symptoms. Symptoms of acute bladder irritation frequently occur 3 to 5 weeks after the initiation of RT and usually subside 2 to 8 weeks after completion of treatment. Symptoms of cystitis subside with mucosal healing, pharmacological intervention, and, if needed, a break from radiation treatment.[103]

Acute cystitis symptoms include dysuria, nocturia, hesitancy, urgency, and urinary frequency. The intensity and duration of symptoms depend on the volume of bladder in the radiation treatment field. As the radiation dose escalates, patients may experience tenesmus and bladder spasms that potentiate existing symptoms. Hematuria is uncommon.

*Management.* Pretreatment assessment of bladder function includes documentation of patterns of urinary elimination, such as symptoms of urgency, frequency, dysuria, nocturia, and past history of urinary tract infections and medications used for treatment. It is extremely important to document if the patient has urinary incontinency prior to radiation treatments.

Inflamed mucosa and ulceration of the bladder increase the potential for infection. Initial treatment consists of ruling out infection and administering antibiotic therapy if indicated. Infection often exacerbates bladder spasm and complicates delivery of radiation treatment. Antispasmodics help relieve dysuria and provide relief from bladder spasms. Optimal comfort is obtained if both infection and bladder spasm are treated simultaneously. Phenazopyridine hydrochloride is frequently used to treat dysuria symptoms. When taken orally, the majority of the drug enters the urine unchanged, where it acts as a topical analgesic within the bladder. When taking the drug, the patient's urine will be colored reddish-orange.

Symptoms such as mild urinary frequency occur due to a modest reduction in bladder capacity. To increase storage capacity, antispasmodic medications such as oxybutynin chloride and flavoxate hydrochloride may be prescribed to relax the bladder smooth muscle by inhibiting the muscarinic effects of acetylcholine. Side effects of antispasmodic therapy include hypertension, palpitation, arrhythmia, and stimulation of the central nervous system. Anticholinergic drugs should be used cautiously in patients with cardiovascular diseases and hyperthyroidism and avoided in patients with bladder outlet obstructive symptoms. Relaxation of bladder smooth muscle can also be produced by blocking the alpha-1 adenoreceptors in the bladder with medications such as terazosin and doxazocin, or alpha-IA blockers such as tamsulosin, and uroxatrol (extended release formulation) which can decrease bladder outlet obstruction without affecting contractility. Use alpha-1 blockers cautiously in patients on antihypertensive medication.[103]

Instruct patients to maintain an adequate intake of fluids to promote frequent voiding and to decrease the potential for infection by diluting the bacterial population. Recommended fluid intake is 1 to 2 L/day. If voided urine is clear to light yellow in color, hydration is probably adequate. In addition, teaching patients to avoid foods that irritate the bladder mucosa may help to delay the onset of cystitis and decrease symptoms; these foods include coffee, tea, alcohol, spices, and tobacco products.[103] Encourage patients to report any signs of bladder irritation, such as dysuria, frequency, urgency with decreased urine volume, and any signs of hematuria or excessive mucus shreds in the urine. The nurse should also be aware of the baseline hemoglobin and hematocrit values as well as any coagulation studies. Hematuria usually causes minimal blood loss and rarely anemia, but early documentation will assist in assessment of future problems. Acute cystitis symptoms cause discomfort and pain, and they may significantly disrupt the patient's life. Reassure the patient that symptoms subside gradually over 2 to 8 weeks after completion of radiation.

### Vaginal dryness/vaginitis

The most immediate response to external beam radiation and/or brachytherapy of the vagina is loss of most or all of the vaginal epithelium. This acute reaction results in vaginitis, with thinning and inflammation of the mucosa causing dryness, pruritus, and possibly a mucoid discharge.[104,105] Dyspareunia is common.

Patients report itching and discomfort, especially at the vaginal introitus, that begin at variable points in the course of treatment. Onset of symptoms is usually early and more pronounced in women who have estrogen depletion.

*Management.* Interventions are directed toward symptom relief. Women may find sitz baths cleansing and relieving of vaginal discomfort. Avoidance of irritating soaps, powders, and perfumes should be explained. Vaginal lubricants (eg, Astroglide) and vaginal moisturizers (either pectin based, such as Summer's Eve, or polycarbophil based, such as Replens) are advised to decrease discomfort and itching. Acute radiation reactions such as erythema, moist desquamation, and confluent mucositis will resolve within 2 to 3 months after completion of irradiation. Patient teaching should be offered about alternative positions for intercourse that can minimize discomfort. The American Cancer Society publishes free documents that illustrates positions and has other useful information. More detailed discussion on sexuality can be found in Chapter 36.

## EXTREMITY

Used in treatment of sarcoma and bony metastasis, radiation to the extremities, due to minimal surrounding structures, generally results in little acute toxicity. Some fields for radiation of an extremity, such as the hip or femur, include surrounding pelvic structures, so the patient will be at risk for diarrhea due to bowel sensitivity. Refer to the management of diarrhea/proctitis in the abdomen/pelvis section. Depending on the size of the field and nodal involvement, edema of extremity may occur. Dependent on the amount of bone marrow in the treatment field, patients may experience marrow suppression. Skin reactions are dependent on total dose.

*Management.* Nursing management is focused on astute nursing assessment skills. Monitoring for edema and decreased laboratory counts are important to bring to the attention of physicians or APNs. Depending on the size of the field, bone marrow suppression may occur, necessitating monitoring weekly complete blood counts. Care of the skin, when radiodermatitis develops is the same interventions listed under the section of acute skin effects.

## EYE

Used in treatment of intraocular malignancies, lymphoma and leukemia, central nervous system cancers, head and neck cancers, and thyroid eye disease (benign pathology), eye irradiation can result in conjunctival edema and tearing.

### Conjunctival edema and tearing

The eyelid, conjunctiva, cornea, sclera, and often the lacrimal gland are irradiated in treatment of ocular malignancies. Inflammatory response to radiation can occur within 24 hours following radiation, and the conjunctiva and other periocular tissues can develop edema secondary to diffuse infiltration by neutrophils. The conjunctiva will become erythematous, with periorbital edema occasionally developing within the first 24 hours after treatment.

Other acute symptoms when the eye is involved in irradiation can include transient eyelid erythema or edema, mild conjunctivitis, and loss of lashes. Patients may experience burning of the eye(s), sensation of a foreign body, diminished vision, and excessive tearing.[106] Depending on the size of the radiation field, alopecia of the eyebrow(s) may occur.

*Management.* Ocular lubrication with an artificial tears solution or ointment, patching, and antibiotic drops as indicated is helpful. Patient instructions should include toxicity time frames—symptoms peaking within 10 to 20 days, resolving within 2 to 4 weeks, and healing completely within 8 weeks.[107]

## LATE EFFECTS OF RADIATION: SITE SPECIFIC

Since the earliest application of radiation in treating cancer, providers have voiced concerns about the late effects of RT on normal tissues and organs. The inability to precisely predict manifestations of late normal-tissue injury emphasizes the importance of vigilant patient follow-up. Long-term effects occur 6 months or later after treatment is complete. Rarely do patients develop effects of doses under 2.0 Gy. Late effects are usually progressive and should be emphasized that symptom manifestations takes months to years after completion of RT. Patients are at risk for radiation-related secondary malignancies. Pediatric patient especially are at risk to develop secondary cancers after successful radiation treatments.[107]

Radiation tissue tolerance, measured in degrees ranging from minimal to maximal, can be a valuable guide for estimating long-term effects. The clinical applicability of tolerance doses has changed as a result of the introduction of agents such as biological response modifiers, chemotherapeutic drugs, new modalities (hyperthermia, high dose rate brachytherapy, and radiosurgery), and these modalities' concurrent and subsequent use with traditional irradiation, chemotherapy, and surgery.[108]

Tissue and organ tolerance is determined by the radiosensitivity of relevant stem cell subpopulations, which may not always be proliferating or dividing. Within the radiation field(s), the most radiosensitive vital cell population determines whether organ tolerance or organ failure will occur. Thus, the functional capacity of cells is often distinct from their regenerative capacity, permitting organ function to be preserved in the face of injury and allowing for recovery or repair from the radiation insult.[109] Complication probability rates have been calculated for each tissue/organ system. They define the 5% and 50% levels of a total radiation dose that are predicted to create late effects at 5 years, ie, the TD 5/5 (5% risk at 5 years) and TD 50/5 (50% risk at 5 years).[109]

All normal tissues do not follow the same behavior pattern in response to radiation. Late reactions occur in tissues that normally have low cell-cycle turnover or regeneration, (ie, endothelium and connective tissues).[108] In such tissues, the radiation produces little change in the function of mature, differentiated cells, and therefore no evidence of tissue malfunction appears until those mature cells gradually die due to normal wear and tear or additional trauma. When the tissue attempts to replace the lost cells by cellular division, the radiation damage inflicted on the tissues months or years earlier becomes manifest, as the cells are unable to produce viable new cells. In contrast, tissues in which the cells are normally replaced every few hours or days (ie, skin and mucosa) quickly recognize that cell replacement is impaired, even as treatment proceeds. These cells immediately activate compensatory mechanisms to speed up the rate of cell proliferation and thereby counteract the accelerated rate of cell loss. Molecular biology, gene expression, and cytokine cascade identification are key factors in the mechanisms responsible for late effects. Intercellular communication through autocrine, paracrine, and endocrine pathways via cytokine networks is the new pathophysiological paradigm to explain the cellular process of late radiation effects.[110]

A model to aid understanding of the clinical outcome of late effects of radiation, as described by Marks, characterizes an organ as being composed of multiple functioning subunits (FSU) that operate in 1 of 2 ways: as a parallel system or as a series system.[111] In a *parallel system*, organ function is generally maintained if damage occurs because the remaining FSUs operate independently from the damaged region, assuming there is adequate function in the remainder of the organ. Hence, part of an organ can be sacrificed or damaged beyond repair, yet the organ will continue to function adequately. The lung, liver, and kidney are highly sensitive to relatively low doses of radiation, but damage to part of these organs does not render them incapable of function. In a *series system*, damage to one portion of an organ may render the entire organ or system dysfunction because the system must work in sequence. Examples include the gastrointestinal tract and neural tissues. The series system concept can encompass organ-to-organ interactions as well. Damage produced in 1 organ can have serious consequences in another organ, such as renal failure leading to overall multisystem failure and death.[110]

Late radiation effects are now recognized as an important area of study, especially as they relate to quality of life. The dose-limiting organs in the treatment field define the amount of radiation prescribed. The risk of late effects related to radiation confirms the importance of accuracy in daily fraction dose, total radiation dose, volume treated, and patient comorbidities. Optimal dose-response curves to avoid late effects remain difficult to define, despite extensive documentation of radiation injuries in the literature. The accuracy of commonly used scales for quantification of acute and especially late reactions is important.[109] The NCI has developed a toxicity scale referred to as Common Terminology Criteria for Adverse Events (CTCAE version 4.0) http://evs.nci.nih.gov/ftp1/CTCAE/About.html. This scale provides descriptive terminology for adverse events and grading (severity) scale for each event. Grades range from 0 (no adverse event or within normal limits) to 5 (death). Most adverse events and grading criteria are applicable to any treatment modality (ie, chemotherapy, RT, or combined chemoradiation).

The morbidity and burden of specific late effects and toxicities may be perceived quite differently by patients and healthcare providers. This is especially true if the late effects and toxicities are protracted, irreversible, uncontrollable, painful, or socially disabling.[108] It is important to remember that the overall risk of late effects is very small (but never zero) and that it varies by site treated. The risk of morbidity and mortality associated with no treatment for a primary or metastatic cancer is almost always greater than the risk of late effects. Ultimately, the patient and family must decide how to weigh the risks and benefits of treatment.

In summary, late effects result from permanent damage to normal structures in the field of radiation treatments. Damage to the parenchymal cells (affects function of the organ), vasculature (affects blood supply and delivery of oxygen and nutrients to the organ), and connective tissue (affects elasticity and flexibility of underlying tissues). All of this may result in dysfunction, fibrosis, atrophy, ulceration, fistulae, and/or necrosis. Reference to the National Cancer Common Toxicities scales for grading severity for both acute and late symptoms should be used in documentation. Selected late effects on organ systems are discussed next. Table 14-13 provides a more inclusive list of site-specific late effects. The major late effects will be discussed here; onset, manifestations of symptom, and management recommendations. Most recommendations are medically related; therefore, "recognition of the late effect" is the major aspect for RT nurses.

### Radiation-induced fibrosis: subcutaneous and soft tissue

Radiation-induced fibrosis (RIF), commonly of subcutaneous and soft tissue, is defined as loss of pliability and flexibility of soft tissues down to the muscle layer. Deep tissue fibrosis involves muscle, fascia, and connective tissue down to bone. The most common regions affected are the breast, head and neck, and connective tissues. Onset is generally within 1 to 2 years after radiation. The severity of RIF can progress, and the time to onset may not plateau. Higher risk is associated with higher daily treatment doses and overall dose, combined modality therapy, and postoperative infection, seroma, wound drainage, and extensive hematoma.[112,113]

Initially there is a loss of tissue elasticity, which is followed by mild indurations. This effect can progress to rigidity of the surface skin layers and retraction of surface contours. Fibrosis can lead to disuse atrophy, ulceration/necrosis, entrapment of neurological structures (eg, brachial or lumbar plexus), and stenosis or obliteration of vital anatomy in the head and neck, chest, abdomen, or pelvis.[112,113]

*Management.* Treatment options include pharmacological agents such as pentoxifylline and vitamin E, which has shown to increase tissue pliability and arrest neurological deficits. A minimum of 3 months of treatment is needed to evaluate for response.[114] The efficacy of this regimen was examined in a RCT of women who had underwent breast irradiation and developed clinically significant RIF. A significant surface reduction of RIF was seen in the treatment group.[115] Hyperbaric oxygenation was shown to be helpful in decreasing pain and erythema. Physical therapy can be important to help preserve function, especially in those patients with restricted movement or mobility. Impedance-controlled microcurrent therapy may significantly improve range of motion in the neck and decrease pain in patients with RIF.[116]

## CENTRAL NERVOUS SYSTEM

The late effects of the central nervous system include the following:

### Brain necrosis

The onset of symptoms of brain necrosis can be as early as 6 months following radiation treatment, but the peak

**TABLE 14-13**

**Selected Site-Specific Late Effects of Radiation Therapy**

| | |
|---|---|
| **Central nervous system** | **Gastrointestinal** |
| Brain | Esophagus |
| Focal/diffuse necrosis | Dysmotility |
| Leukoencephalopathy | Dysphagia/odynophagia |
| Pituitary/hypothalamic dysfunction | Esophageal stricture/fistula |
| Cognitive dysfunction | Stomach |
| Spinal cord | Dyspepsial/gastritis |
| Myelopathy/necrosis | Contracture |
| **Head and Neck** | Small/large bowel |
| Mucosa | Mucosal injury |
| Paleness, thinning, telangiectasis | Decreased motility, malabsorption |
| Salivary gland | Obstruction |
| Chronic xerostomia | Rectum |
| Teeth/mandible | Proctitis |
| Dental caries | Fistula |
| Temporomandibular joint fibrosis | Liver |
| Osteoradionecrosis | Radiation hepatitis |
| **Thyroid** | Hepatic failure |
| Hypothyroid/hyperthyroid | **Genitourinary** |
| Thyroid cartilage necrosis | Kidney |
| Laryngeal edema | Anemia |
| **Eye** | Chronic radiation nephritis |
| Cataracts | Hypertension |
| Skin changes, loss of lashes | Bladder |
| Dry eye; corneal ulceration | Mucosal injury, hematuria |
| Visual loss/blindness | Fistula |
| **Chest** | Fibrosis |
| Lung | Prostate |
| Pneumonitis (subacute) | Impotence |
| Pulmonary fibrosis | Penis |
| Heart | Mucosal changes |
| Cardiomyopathy | Urethral stricture |
| Pericarditis | Vagina |
| Coronary artery disease | Thinning/atrophy/dry mucosa |
| Breast | Narrowing, shortening, fibrosis |
| Skin tanning, fibrosis, telangiectasias | **Reproductive** |
| Breast fibrosis, contraction, edema | Ovaries/testis |
| Increased risk of pathological rib fracture | Sterility |
| Pneumonitis (subacute) | **Hematopoietic** |
| Pulmonary fibrosis | Fibrosis |
| Pericarditis | Aplasia |
| Arm edema if axillary or supraclavicular lymph nodes treated | **Carcinogenesis** |
| **Bone** | Meningioma, nerve sheath glio |
| Necrosis of femoral head | Sarcoma bone/soft tissue |
| | Leukemias: acute myelogenous leukemia |

Because the tolerance levels of all tissues are known, the overall risk of radiation-related late effects is very low. The percentage of risk varies by tissue site.

*Source*: Reprinted with permission from Hass.[12]

time of presentation of symptoms is 1 to 2 years after completion of radiation. Brain necrosis is typically not diffuse; instead, it is focal. Symptoms of brain necrosis include manifestations of increased ICP such as headache, somnolence, intellectual and cognitive deficits, decrease in short- and long-term memory, seizures, and focal neurological deficits corresponding to the part of the brain irradiated. Magnetic resonance imaging (MRI) is the most sensitive tool available for diagnosing brain necrosis. Pathological tissue confirmation may be necessary to differentiate necrosis from recurrent tumor.[109,117] Radiation-induced brain necrosis is usually progressive and most often fatal.

*Management.* If appropriate, surgical debulking of necrosis and use of corticosteroids can offer transient symptom relief.

### Leukoencephalopathy

Leukoencephalopathy occurs almost exclusively after chemotherapy, but can occur after brain irradiation, with or without chemotherapy.[109,117] It is characterized by multiple, noninflammatory necrotic foci in the white matter of brain tissue, with demyelination and reactive astrocytosis. Symptoms of leukoencephalopathy include lethargy, seizures, spasticity, paresis, and ataxia. MRI can be helpful in the diagnosis. Leukoencephalopathy is generally irreversible.

*Management.* Treatment is limited to supportive measures, such as symptom management of seizures, and physical and occupational therapy consultations for assistance with motor dysfunction.

### Cognitive and emotional dysfunction

The incidence and extent of radiation-related cognitive and emotional dysfunction are difficult to determine due to multiple variables, including underlying disease (primary tumor, leukemia), specific brain site, increased ICP, and effects of therapies including surgery and chemotherapy. Cognitive and emotional deficits following brain radiation are well documented in children, but the contribution by radiation alone is unclear because patients often receive systemic and intrathecal chemotherapy.[109,117]

*Management.* Neuropsychiatric consultation can be valuable for behavioral and pharmacological management of specific dysfunctions. A baseline neuropsychiatric evaluation can be helpful in assessing future mental status changes.

### Pituitary and hypothalamic dysfunction

Radiation damage can affect the hypothalamic-pituitary axis and cause permanent dysfunctions. Clinical syndromes include hypothyroidism, Addison's disease, diabetes insipidus, and decreased sexual hormone levels.[117] Growth hormone is commonly affected in children and must be monitored and replaced as needed.

*Management.* Each specific syndrome is treated with replacement hormonal therapies and surveillance of hormone levels. Referrals to endocrinologists should be made once the problem is identified. Since children are particularly vulnerable, annual exams are mandatory.

### Spinal cord (myelopathies)

Myelopathies are uncommon, but not rare, complications of cancer treatment. Because the multiple signs and symptoms of radiation myelopathy can occur in variable combinations at different rates of progression, it is not possible to make the diagnosis of radiation myelopathy based on symptoms alone. The initial signs are subtle and may not be noticed by patients. Symptoms include sensory deficits (unilateral or bilateral), which are often manifested as diminished temperature sensation, leg weakness, clumsiness, and diminished proprioception. Objective signs and symptoms include changes in gait (often foot drop), spasticity, weakness, hemiparesis, Brown-Séquard syndrome (ie, a loss of motor function (paralysis and ataxia) and sensation caused by the lateral hemisection of the spinal cord), and possibly incontinence. Hyperreflexia and Babinski signs are often found on neurological examination. Pain may accompany symptoms. The patient may be asymptomatic until some trauma initiates a progressive neurological deficit. No specific combination of signs or symptoms can distinguish radiation myelopathy from myelopathies of many other etiologies.[117]

*Management.* Management of radiation-induced spinal cord myelopathy has been primarily limited to the administration of corticosteroids, with limited success. Response to corticosteroid therapy is transient with some improvement in symptoms and is likely due to a decrease in spinal cord edema. The prognosis in radiation myelopathy depends primarily on the degree to which the originally treated lesion transects the spinal cord and the anatomical level of the lesion. Complete transection of the cord is a sign of poor prognosis. Generally lesions at higher anatomical levels have a poorer prognosis than lesions at lower levels. The actuarial mortality from radiation-induced spinal cord myelopathy is 55% at 18 months for cervical lesions, and 25% at 18 months for thoracic lesions. Younger patients have a better prognosis than older patients.[116]

## HEAD AND NECK

There is the potential for multiple disabling late effects following head and neck irradiation. If the patient has also undergone surgical resection, structural dysfunction can occur in addition to the effects of irradiation. Individuals with head and neck cancer usually require extensive rehabilitation to manage alterations related to speech, eating, swallowing, and respiratory function. Late effects can include the following:

### Xerostomia and dental caries

Xerostomia persists for months to years and almost always will be present to some degree. The extent of symptoms is dependent on the volume of salivary gland tissue irradiated, the total radiation dose, and individual patient response. As a consequence, patients may experience impaired ability to swallow, chew, talk, and/or wear dentures comfortably. Most patients permanently change the nature of their diet to some degree.

Radiation-induced dental effects are indirectly produced by salivary changes that occur when the parotid glands are included in the treatment portals, and less often by direct effect of radiation on the teeth. Alteration of the normal oral microfloral balance to a more cariogenic one occurs as a result of changes in the salivary contents and a lowered oral pH. (See the discussion of xerostomia in the Head and Neck section of this chapter for a more detailed outline of salivary composition.)

Dental decay and varying degrees of dental disintegration after irradiation typically develop along the gum line.[67] Thus, patients are at high risk for dental caries, periodontal disease, stomatitis, dysphagia, and altered taste.[15] Because of changes in the oral microflora secondary to xerostomia, candidiasis and other oral infections are more common. Long-term xerostomia and dental caries can be disabling and can significantly affect quality of life.[70,79]

*Management.* Management of xerostomia is as discussed under the head/neck section of this chapter. The most important aspect of chronic xerostomia management is compliance with life-long dental surveillance and prophylaxis. Support groups may help with understanding that they are not alone and can offer suggestions of what interventions help them.

### Trismus

Tonic contractions of the jaw muscles result in fibrosis, resulting in tightness or inability to open the mouth wide. Patients often have difficulty chewing. Trismus can be painful and a long-term problem.

*Management.* At every follow-up visit, assessment includes measuring the degree of opening the patient can easily tolerate. Since changes may not be obvious immediately, measuring by millimeters is valuable in determining accuracy and changes. The key is to regularly stretch and open the mouth. Simple exercises can be taught to the patients: (1) have the person open the mouth as wide as possible for 20 times in succession, 3 times a day; (2) place heels of both hands under jaw and push up with hands while stretching the mouth open; and (3) place middle and index fingers on mandibular teeth and thumb on maxillary teeth, then use fingers in a twisting motion to pry the mouth open, holding it open as wide as possible for 2 seconds and then relax. This last exercise should be performed 10 times with each hand, and repeat 4 times a day. Supplementary devices (eg, Therabite or DynaSplit) can help patients with jaw opening exercises.

In summary, teaching patients exercises and the correct use of devices should be done at the completion of treatment. Referrals to physical or speech therapists can help manage this problem. Early interventions will avoid problems later.

### Osteoradionecrosis

Osteoradionecrosis is a serious complication secondary to the effects of xerostomia and radiation to the maxilla and mandible. Osteoradionecrosis is characterized as a hypocellular and hypovascular dissolution of bone. Osteocytes and the supporting vasculature may be irreversibly injured by radiation. Osteoradionecrosis is progressive, can lead to intolerable pain or fracture, and may necessitate surgical resection. Those patients at greatest risk are dentulous and require dental extractions after completing RT. It is neither always necessary—nor advisable—to extract all teeth before treatment as a preventive measure; however, teeth of questionable viability should be extracted prior to initiating RT.[79] Nonirritating, well-fitting dentures do not appear to increase the incidence of osteoradionecrosis. The overall risk of osteoradionecrosis is higher in patients with preexisting poor dentition, nutritional and/or immunological compromise, and smoking during radiation. Patients remain at risk for the development of osteoradionecrosis for years following RT.

Most cases of osteoradionecrosis develop in the mandible. This condition initially manifests as a nondescript erythematous change of the overlying mucosa, which then ulcerates to reveal the necrotic bone below. Necrotic bone has a dull appearance, unlike the pearly color of healthy periosteum.

*Management.* Prevention of osteoradionecrosis includes meticulous oral and periodontal hygiene, with fluoride prophylaxis and frequent dental evaluation. Oral care must be maintained indefinitely because of the impaired potential for healing in response to physical irritation, chemical agents, and microbial organisms.[79] Attempts should be made to replace or increase salivary flow. Foods and beverages containing sucrose should be avoided. If dental caries develop, removal and restoration are advised immediately. Patients are at greater risk for developing oral Candida albicans infection due to xerostomia, and prompt treatment helps maintain oral integrity. Optimal nutritional status is important for bone maintenance and healing. Head and neck cancer patients are commonly at increased risk of nutritional compromise due to poor nutritional status at diagnosis and alterations in chewing and swallowing induced by surgery and radiation.[15]

Treatment of osteoradionecrosis includes antibiotic therapy to help control acute pain, swelling, and suppuration. Surgical resection of osteoradionecrotic lesions is an option. In 1 study, 6 of 22 patients had lesions resected, with 3 patients demonstrating postsurgical recurrence. The preventive and therapeutic use of antibiotics and hyperbaric oxygenation (HBO) were effective in some cases, but clear treatment guidelines are not defined. A series of HBO treatments are recommended for post-radiation patients who must undergo dental extractions.[118]

### Hypothyroidism

Hypothyroidism is the most common clinical consequence of irradiation to the thyroid in patients who have received therapeutic doses to the neck area.[119] Patients should be monitored with periodic serum thyroid-stimulating hormone (TSH) and free thyroxin 4 (FT4) screening.

*Management.* Hypothyroidism can be effectively treated with thyroid replacement therapy. This may be managed by patient's primary care physicians or endocrinologists.

## LUNG

When treating the thoracic region, several long-term problems can arise. These include the following.

### Pulmonary fibrosis

Pulmonary fibrosis can develop insidiously in a previously irradiated lung field. Debate continues as to whether an acute phase of fibrosis, which may not be symptomatic but can be viewed radiographically, is always present. The degree of fibrosis stabilizes after 1 to 2 years. Radiation-induced lung injury is characterized by progressive fibrosis of the alveolar septa, which become thickened by bundles of elastic fibers. The alveoli subsequently collapse and are then obliterated by connective tissue. The hilum or mediastinum may become retracted with a densely contracted lung segment, resulting in compensatory hyperinflation of adjacent or contralateral lung tissue.[97] These changes can lead to the appearance (usually within 1 to 2 years after radiation) of lung scarring on CXR that corresponds to the shape of the radiation portal; CT scan may provide more definitive imaging for diagnosis.

PFTs may suggest reduced tidal volume; however, PFTs do not demonstrate significant changes when small volumes of lung are irradiated, due to functional compensation by adjacent lung regions. Thus, PFTs are not the most accurate measurement of radiation-induced lung injury. Diffusion capacity may be the best measure of total lung function, because this test is least likely to be affected by compensatory changes in unirradiated portions of the lung.[97]

Not all areas of the lung are equally functionally important. The lung bases have a greater ventilation/perfusion ratio than at the apices. Should fibrosis develop, the location of the lung treatment field serves as an important predictor of degree of respiratory symptoms. It is important to understand that all patients will develop lung fibrosis if radiation encompasses any lung tissue. Whether that fibrosis becomes clinically apparent is the issue.[120] Most patients with radiation-induced pulmonary fibrosis are asymptomatic. Symptoms are directly related to the amount of lung parenchyma involved and the patients' preexisting pulmonary reserves. Symptoms generally remain minimal if fibrosis is limited to less than 50% of 1 lung. If the volume of 1 irradiated lung exceeds 50%, the patient will likely become symptomatic to some degree. Symptoms include dyspnea on exertion, reduced exercise tolerance, orthopnea, cyanosis, and finger clubbing. In some instances, chronic respiratory failure can occur and may result in cor pulmonale and subsequent right heart failure.[97]

*Management.* Management of radiation-induced pulmonary fibrosis consists of supportive care, such as steroids, oxygen therapy, and pulmonary rehabilitation exercises to manage respiratory symptoms. Clinical trials are continuing to evaluate amifostine (Ethyol) as a pneumoprotector.[120]

## HEART

Cardiac complications are much less common in the "modern era" of radiotherapy. Most data related to heart disease after radiation has focused on childhood survivors of Hodgkin's disease. The risk of radiation-induced pericarditis, coronary artery disease, and cardiomyopathy is dramatically lower with current doses and treatment techniques. Long-term follow-up is required to confirm an actual decrease in cardiac toxicities resulting in symptomatic complications. Long-term effects include the following.

### Pericarditis

Pericarditis is a result of fibrosis in the parietal pericardium that may progress to constriction of the heart. Patients may exhibit symptoms of acute pericarditis or have a chronic pericardial effusion.[121]

*Management.* If signs of heart failure occur, treatment focuses on increasing cardiac output to maintain system perfusion. Excessive pericardial fluid may accumulate rapidly to produce cardiac tamponade, which must be relieved by pericardiocentesis or pericardiectomy. Pericardial disease may develop several months to years after RT.[121] Any signs of pericarditis should be referred to a cardiologist for further investigation and treatment.

### Cardiomyopathy

The myocardium is involved less frequently than the pericardium. The myocardium can develop patches of diffuse fibrosis affecting the anterior wall of the left ventricle and, less frequently, the anterior wall of the right ventricle.[121]

Patients present with signs and symptoms of congestive heart failure. Left ventricular ejection function (LVEF) studies can be used for monitoring during chemotherapy and radiation.[120] The combination of radiation and doxorubicin affects left ventricular systolic function and mortality more significantly than either therapy used alone.[122]

*Management.* If signs of heart failure occur, treatment focuses on increasing cardiac output to maintain system perfusion. Cardiologists should be consulted for long-term follow-up. Echocardiograms and multiple gated acquisition (MUGA) scan (noninvasive tool for assessing the function of the heart, specifically the ventricles) may be ordered to follow this condition.

### Coronary artery disease

The main types of radiation damage to arteries are intimal disruption and luminal stenosis or occlusion. Vessel changes due to atherosclerosis and with the normal aging process are produced or accelerated by radiation. Pathological changes may be difficult to distinguish from typical atherosclerotic coronary disease.[123]

*Management.* Screening and treatment are the same as they are for patients with coronary artery disease who have not had radiation. It is recommended that all cancer survivors treated with chest radiotherapy be monitored for risk factors such as obesity, hypertension, dyslipidemias, and diabetes.[122]

## BREAST/CHEST WALL

While some of the long-term effects for treating lung can apply in this section (depending on the treatment fields), more specific toxicities can include the following.

### Atrophy, fibrosis of breast tissue

The total radiation dose to the whole breast for the management of microscopic residual disease is 45 to 50 Gy. In this dose range, the incidence of late effects is very low. Higher doses to the whole breast (≥ 60–65 Gy) are associated with atrophy, fibrosis (see the earlier discussion of RIF), retraction, and telangiectasias that predispose the patient to a poor cosmetic outcome. Rarely, late effects occur that limit function, such as breast tissue contraction, necrosis, or neuropathy. Moist desquamation of the skin during radiation is not predictive of late skin effects.

*Management.* Management is directed at relieving symptoms of atrophy or fibrosis of the breast tissue. Surgical intervention may be appropriate if affecting woman's quality of life.[124,125] Surgical revision of a contracted painful breast can be difficult due to the risk of poor healing after definitive radiation doses to the breast and surrounding tissues. It must be emphasized that late effects, with a poor cosmetic outcome, are extremely rare today with the radiation doses used and modern high-energy equipment.

### Lymphedema

Lymphedema is the accumulation of fluid in the interstitial tissues that is caused by disruption of the regional lymphatic system. It may be related to radiation treatment in which scarring of the chest wall, breast, or axilla and disrupts the lymphatic circulation. Radiation-induced lymphedema is generally a late effect when majority of the lymph nodes are in the treatment field, ie, axilla. Axillary dissections can increase the risk of developing lymphedema.

*Management.* Lymphedema should be measured at the beginning of therapy and monitored appropriate throughout therapy and at follow-up visits. Early detections begin early interventions. Referrals to lymphedema specialists should be offered immediately when lympedema is suspected. Preventive measures explained by the RT nurse can include avoid wearing tight clothing, jewelry, elastic band, extreme temperatures, carrying heavy packages on affected arm, extra care while cutting nails or shaving underarms, and offering compression sleeves to anyone who plans to fly (even if patients does not demonstrate lymphedema at that time).[15]

## ABDOMEN AND PELVIS

### Small and large bowel injury

The radiation tolerance of the small and large bowel is a major dose-limiting factor in the treatment of many cancers of the abdomen and pelvis. Late radiation-related injury to the bowel is caused by intestinal wall fibrosis, vascular stenosis, and mucosal atrophy. The incidence of late effects to the bowel is 3% to 5%. Some alteration of bowel function is likely the most dominant chronic post-radiation toxicity. Interestingly, only a fraction of patients with postradiation bowel dysfunction seek medical treatment. Instead, they adjust their lifestyles to symptoms, and seem to have very little expectation for effective interventions.

Bowel late effects can be defined as symptoms altering the patient's lifestyle or hospitalization or surgical interventions.[126] Symptoms are related to malabsorption and dysmotility and include fecal frequency/urgency, tenesmus, bleeding, pain, fistula formation, and intractable diarrhea. Due to its anatomically smaller lumen size, obstruction is more common in the small bowel than in the large bowel or rectum. The most important factors contributing to the extent of bowel injury include radiation dose (the rectum is generally more tolerant than the remainder of the bowel), prior abdominal surgery, history of pelvic inflammatory disease, and concurrent chemotherapy. Some studies suggest that a history of hypertension or diabetes mellitus may be associated with a greater risk of late intestinal injury.[10,126]

*Management.* Chronic radiation injury to the small and large intestine can be managed by a low-residue diet, stool softeners, and use of loperamide or diphenoxylate with atropine. If reduced rectal sphincter compliance is a problem, fiber laxatives can be used to provide form, consistency, and softening of the stool. For diarrhea caused by small bowel injury, several studies have suggested that the use of cholestyramine might be effective. This agent presumably helps by reducing the level of intraluminal bile salts. Octreotide, now available in a long-acting formulation, offers benefits in managing secretory diarrhea. Rectal bleeding is managed with products to help improve mucosal integrity, such as sucralfate or short-chain fatty acid enemas, topical formalin, and laser cauterization.[126] Partial small bowel obstruction may be managed by bowel rest and decompression followed by dietary modification. Surgery may be necessary to relieve more extensive bowel obstruction. Nevertheless, controversy persists as to the extent of surgical resection necessary—whether all adhesions within the bowel should be lysed vs limiting the resection to the area(s) acutely involved.

Late-occurring bowel toxicities (ie, more than 10–20 years) generally have a poorer prognosis for optimal functional outcomes.[126]

## GENITOURINARY SYSTEM

Late effects regarding genitourinary system can include the following.

### Bladder injury

Most late radiation-induced complications of the bladder are related to contracture, bleeding, symptomatic cystitis, and (rarely) fistulas. Incontinence is not common, but if found is likely related to the additive effect of radiation and prior surgical manipulations of the bladder neck and urethra. The degree of late radiation-related symptoms depends on the amount of bladder included in the radiation treatment fields. Irradiation fields for prostate cancer include much less bladder volume than the treatment fields for bladder cancer.

*Management.* Treatment for late effects on the bladder is individualized, but may include drug therapy to reduce cystitis symptoms (eg, pentosan polysulfate) or surgical intervention for bleeding or to manage fistulas (eg, vesicovaginal fistula). Pelvic floor exercises, to include Kegel exercises, may be helpful.

### Vaginal changes

Chronic effects to the vagina, occurring 12 months or more after completion of radiation, include thinning and atrophy of the vaginal epithelium and development of telangiectasias. Patients may experience a decrease in size of the vaginal vault due to narrowing, shortening (made more pronounced after radical hysterectomy), paravaginal fibrosis, loss of elasticity, adhesions, and marked decrease in vaginal lubrication. All of these manifestations may result in dyspareunia. Vaginal brachytherapy can contribute to late effects.[104]

*Management.* Management begins with preradiation teaching so women know what to expect after radiation. If the female is not sexually active, vaginal dilators can be used to maintain vaginal patency. Women should begin using dilators about 2 to 4 weeks after treatment is completed. Dilators are placed in the vagina for about 20 minutes at a time, 3 times a week. If women resume regular sexual intercourse, then dilators are not necessary. Women should be instructed about the importance of keeping the vagina patent and minimizing fibrosis so as to facilitate future physical examinations essential for tumor surveillance. Problems with sexual adjustment after RT can be significant. Women may have depressive symptoms, fear of injury from intercourse, fear of recurrent cancer, poor communication with sex partner, feeling of being less feminine and desirable, and separation and loss of sex partner.[104] The RT nurse often is the most accessible and comfortable person with whom the patient can discuss this physically and emotionally complex topic.

## REPRODUCTIVE SYSTEM

Reproductive long-term effects can be very sensitive for patients to discuss openly once symptoms develop after completion of therapies. RT nurses are in excellent positions to approach these sensitive issues with the patients and not wait if the patient brings up the concern as they might be too embarrass to discuss. Long-term effects can include the following.

### Ovarian dysfunction

The probability of sterility and endocrine insufficiency is related to radiation dose, fraction size, and patient age. Definitive external pelvic irradiation of doses exceeding 24 Gy will produce permanent ovarian ablation in the adult female. If the woman is postmenopausal, few clinical consequences are likely. For the premenopausal woman, symptoms will be similar to those of menopause, including hot flashes, atrophic vulvitis, vaginitis with pruritus and dyspareunia, alterations in body fat distribution, changes in the breasts, accelerated bone demineralization, potential premature cardiovascular disease, and unpredictable effects on libido. The severity of these effects varies among individuals, based on body habitus and levels of estrogen production, both adrenal and peripheral.[104]

*Management.* Management of estrogen deficit produced by damage to the ovaries varies according to the specific cancer. Estrogen replacement in women with breast cancer is controversial and seldom advised. For women with gynecological cancers, estrogen replacement may have a role. Women are advised to discuss this issue with their oncologists. Nontraditional medicine—use of natural and herbal preparation—may be helpful in providing relief of menopausal symptoms. Women with breast cancer are generally advised to avoid all estrogens, including phytoestrogens, until more is known regarding the pathophysiology of these substances and the specific malignancy.

The premenopausal woman who requires RT that will include the ovaries may have concerns regarding conservation of potential reproductive capability. Preventing ovarian ablation is an achievable goal in patients treated with radiation. A thorough discussion of the available alternatives should occur prior to selection of a definitive plan for treatment. Strategies for conserving reproductive capability include utilization of reproductive technology such as in vitro fertilization and transplantation of one or both ovaries to sites remote from the radiation fields. If the patient is receiving high-dose chemotherapy, ovarian ablation may occur despite efforts to remove them from path of the radiation beam.[104]

### Testicular dysfunction

The testis is highly radiosensitive, and a small dose of 2 to 10 Gy or a fractionated dose of 1 to 2 Gy of radiation will cause permanent sterility. Young men who require radiation that may affect the testes should be referred for sperm analysis and sperm banking as appropriate. Although testicular shields can be used, they will not prevent internal radiation scatter; therefore, the testes will inevitably receive some radiation dose.[127]

The severity of the impairment in spermatogenesis and length of recovery depend on the radiation dose to the testis. In the typical patient receiving irradiation for a classic seminoma, the remaining testis receives a dose in the range of 0.3 to 1.8 Gy. An even greater dose is delivered to the contralateral testis if the hemiscrotum is irradiated. Radiation doses of this magnitude usually produce temporary oligospermia or azoospermia followed by recovery 18 to 24 months later.[127]

*Management.* A patient may become fertile during the recovery phase, and should be counseled regarding this possibility. Mutations induced in germinal stem cells may produce abnormal spermatozoa. Fortunately, the potentially abnormal spermatozoa arising from these mutated stem cells tend to have poor fertilization potential. The occurrence of the mutations depends on the radiation dose delivered. No genetic abnormalities from ionizing radiation have been demonstrated in humans, which perhaps reflect the body's ability to repair such damage.[127] Patients are advised to practice birth control during and after irradiation. The length of time during which birth control should be continued is not entirely clear, but generally duration of 24 months is recommended to allow for recovery of normal spermatogenesis.

### Sexual dysfunction

A comprehensive discussion of sexuality and interventions is beyond the scope of this chapter; the reader is referred to Chapter 36 for more on this topic. However, it is important to recognize that sexual dysfunction in both men and women can occur after RT for various malignancies, especially gynecological and genitourinary cancers. RT can cause significant sexual disruption. It is incumbent on RT nurses to recognize that sexual dysfunction is a problem that may be of great concern to the patient and his or her partner and therefore affect quality of life. Patients and their partners rarely verbalize issues or concerns about sexual dysfunction. Obtaining a sexual history prior to initiating treatment may allow for implementation of preventive measures that can lessen dysfunction. The direct effects of irradiation on normal tissue may progress over a number of years; thus, sexual dysfunction may be progressive and require lifelong rehabilitation and interventions.[104]

## SECONDARY MALIGNANCIES

In the retrospective evaluation of radiation-induced secondary malignancies, an important factor to remember is that many patients in the studies being reported were originally treated in the 1950s and 1960s, with some being treated as far back as 1925. Thus, patients were treated with techniques and doses different from the more refined RT currently in use.[128] Criteria for defining a second cancer include the following:

- Secondary tumors must have a different histological appearance from primary tumors.
- Both the primary and secondary tumor must be malignant.
- Both must be anatomically separate, and the second tumor cannot be a metastasis from the primary tumor.
- Secondary tumors must produce their own metastases.[128]

With increasing longevity, many patients may develop second cancers anywhere from 6 months to 20 years or longer after completion of treatment for the primary cancer. Considering the difficulty of classifying and identifying secondary cancers induced by radiation, their incidence may be higher than current studies indicate. Vigilant follow-up and surveillance are essential for recent patients to determine whether changes in therapeutic technique and radiation doses have affected the incidence of second cancers.[128]

Most solid tumors (eg, sarcoma) do not occur until 10 years or longer after radiation exposure, and for some cancer sites (eg, breast and bladder) excess risks emerge only 15 years or longer after irradiation. Radiation-induced sarcomas of bone and soft tissue are the most frequent secondary malignant neoplasms in irradiated tissues. Sarcomas have a high tendency to recur locally, metastasize, and become a fatal complication of RT.[128]

Most of the knowledge about radiation effects in humans has derived from epidemiological studies of atomic bomb survivors in Japan, occupationally irradiated workers, patients exposed to large amounts of diagnostic radiation, and patients treated with radiation for malignant and nonmalignant diseases. Studies in the atomic bomb survivors and in women treated for benign gynecological disorders have shown that the excess relative risk per gray tends to be fairly stable for at least 30 years following radiation. At present, it is not known whether the relative risk remains elevated throughout life or whether the risk for different solid tumors vs leukemia or lymphomatous cancers varies.

The risk of leukemia attributable to irradiation is observed within a few years from radiation exposure, with a peak after 5 to 9 years and a gradual decline thereafter. Continuous exposures, given at low-dose rates, are less leukomogenic than a single radiation dose. Age at exposure may be the greatest determinant of risk for radiation-induced cancer, especially in those patients who are irradiated as children or adolescents.[129]

Knowledge of the risk factors for second malignancy has made it possible to identify patient groups at high risk of developing second cancers due to treatments they received in the past. An example is the increased risk of breast cancer in women who were treated as adolescents with mantle irradiation for Hodgkin's disease. Previously irradiated patients should be closely monitored and screened as appropriate. Preventive strategies, such as smoking cessation, may substantially reduce the risk of developing a treatment-related cancer.

The issue of treatment-induced second cancers must always be viewed in relation to the dramatic improvement in survival rates for various malignancies. The carcinogenic effects of therapeutic irradiation deserve more investigation. Issues to be clarified include the shape of the radiation dose-response curve in the higher dose range, the duration of the radiation-induced cancer risk, the effects of dose fractionation, and age at radiation exposure. It is important to remember that not all second cancers are due to chemotherapy or irradiation. The occurrence of 2 primary malignancies in the same individual may reflect influences such as genetic predisposition, immunodeficiency, carcinogenic influences, clustering of risk factors, and a chance event or the interaction of multiple factors.[128] Because the mechanisms underlying the carcinogenic effects of radiation remain poorly understood, research should also focus on the identification of specific gene alterations associated with the development of radiation-induced cancer.[129]

The risk associated with cancer treatment should be weighed carefully against the consequences of not using such treatments. Changes in therapies to reduce the risk of late complications and second malignancies should be made only in the context of carefully designed clinical trials that evaluate whether the overall efficacy of treatment is maintained. In addition, for many new cancer treatments, the long-term risk of second malignancies is not known.[129]

## CONCLUSION

Cancer treatment with RT can be rigorous, with multiple acute toxicities and the risk of late effects. The global radiation oncology community is hopeful that advances in technology (eg, 3-D conformal treatment planning, IMRT, stereotactic radiosurgery, and high-dose rate brachytherapy) will result in a decreased risk of long-term morbidities, while maintaining, or improving, optimal treatment outcomes. While a toxicity-free course of radiation probably is not realistic, RT nurses are skilled at managing side effects and supporting patients through a course of therapy.

Balancing treatment outcomes with quality of life, especially when palliation is the goal, remains a priority. Radiation oncology nurses are integral in caring for cancer patients and their families at each point on the treatment continuum. Just as the RT nurses roles evolved, APN roles are developing as part of the multidisciplinary team.

APNs collaborate with the team members to assist in new consults, manage complex patients undergoing therapy or hospitalizations, and participate in follow-up visits. It is this quality of care that RT nurses/APNs make a difference in the outcomes of oncology patients.

## REFERENCES


1. Haas M, Kuehn E. Modality related outcomes: teletherapy: external radiation therapy. In: Brunner D, Moore G, Haas M, eds. *Outcomes in Radiation Therapy: Multidisciplinary Management.* Sudbury, MA: Jones and Bartlett; 2000:53–66.
2. Rosenstein B. The biologic basis of radiotherapy. In: Haffty B, Wilson L, eds. *Handbook of Radiation Oncology: Basic Principles and Clinical Protocols.* Sudbury, MA: Jones and Bartlett; 2009:41–71.
3. Hall E. *Radiobiology for the Radiologist.* New York: Lippincott-Raven; 2005.
4. Ibbott G. Radiation physics. In: Haffty B, Wilson L, eds. *Handbook to Radiation Oncology Basic Principles and Clinical Protocols.* Sudbury, MA: Jones and Bartlett; 2009:1–40.
5. Lawrence TS, Ten Haken RK, Giaccia A. . Principles of radiation oncology. In: DeVita VT, Hellman S, Rosenberg SA, eds. *Cancer: Principles and Practice of Oncology.* 8th ed. Philadelphia, PA: Lippincott-Raven; 2009: 307–336.
6. Chao KS, Perez CA, Brady LW. Fundamentals of patient management. In: Chao DS, Perez CA, Brady LW, eds. *Radiation Oncology Management Decisions.* Philadelphia, PA: Lippincott-Raven; 2001:1–13.
7. Halperin E, Perez C, Brady L, Wazer D. *Principles and Practice of Radiation Oncology.* 5th ed. Philadelphia, PA: Lippincott, Williams & Wilkins; 2007.
8. Harper J, Franklin L, Jenrette J, Aguero E. Skin toxicity during breast irradiation: pathophysiology and management. *South Med J.* 2004;97:989–993.
9. Washington D, Leaver D. *Principles and Practice of Radiation Therapy.* 3rd ed. Mosby: 2009:55–84.
10. Coia LR, Myerson RJ. Late effects of radiation therapy on the gastrointestinal tract. *Int J Radiat Oncol Biol Phys.* 1995;31:1213–1236.
11. Williams J, Chen Y, Rubin P, et al. The biological basis of a comprehensive grading system for the adverse effects of cancer treatment. *Semin Radiat Oncol.* 2003;13:182–188.
12. Haas M. Radiation therapy. In: Varrichio CG, ed. *A Cancer Source Book for Nurses.* 8th ed. Sudbury, MA: Jones and Bartlett; 2004:131–147.
13. Moore-Higgs G, Watkins-Bruner D, Balmer L, et al. The role of licensed nursing personnel in radiation oncology. Part A: results of a descriptive study. *Oncol Nurs Forum.* 2003;30:59–64.
14. Gosselin-Acomb T. Role of the radiation oncology nurse. *Semin Oncol Nurs.* 2006;22:198–202.
15. Bruner D, Haas M, Gosselin-Acomb T. *Manual for Radiation Oncology Nursing Practice and Education.* 3rd ed. Pittsburgh, PA: Oncology Nursing Society; 2005:3–10.
16. Hinds C, Streater A, Mood C. Functions and preferred methods of receiving information related to radiotherapy. *Cancer Nurs.* 1995;18:374–384.
17. Poroch D. The effect of preparatory patient education on the anxiety and satisfaction of cancer patients receiving radiation therapy. *Cancer Nurs.* 1995;18:206–214.
18. Bennenbroek FT, Buunk BP, Stiegelis HE, et al. Audiotaped social comparison information for cancer patients undergoing radiotherapy: differential effects of procedural, emotional and coping information. *Psychooncology.* 2003;12:567–579.
19. Hagopian GA. The effects of informational audiotapes on knowledge and self-care behaviors of patients undergoing radiation therapy. *Oncol Nurs Forum.* 1996;23:697–700.
20. Dunn J, Steginga S, Rose P, Scott J, Allison R. Evaluating patient education materials about radiation therapy. *Patient Educ Couns.* 2004;5:200–210.
21. Vickberg J. Fears about breast cancer recurrence. *Cancer Pract.* 2001;9:237–243.
22. Mast M. Survivors of breast cancer: illness uncertainty, positive reappraisal, and emotional distress. *Oncol Nurs Forum.* 1998;25:555–562.
23. Carper E, Haas M. Advanced practice nursing in radiation oncology. *Semin Oncol Nurs.* 2006;22:203–211.
24. Lambertz C. Advanced practice nurses in radiation oncology. In: Haas M, Hogle W, Moore-Higgs G, Gosselin-Acromb T, eds. *Radiation Therapy: A guide to Patient Care.* Philadelphia, PA: Mosby Elsevier; 2007:641–663.
25. Kelvin J, Moore-Higgs G, Maher K, et al. Non-physician practitioners in radiation oncology: advanced practice nurse and physician assistants. *Int J Radiat Oncol Biol Phys.* 1999;45:255–263.
26. McQuestion M. Evidence-based skin care management in radiation therapy. *Semin Oncol Nurs.* 2006;22:163–173.
27. Porock D. Factors influencing the severity of radiation skin and oral mucosal reactions: development of a conceptual framework. *Eur J Cancer Care.* 2002;11:33–43.
28. McQuestion M. Radiation induced skin reactions. In: Haas M, Moore-Higgs G, eds. *Principles of Skin Care and the Oncology Patients.* Pittsburgh, PA: ONS Press. In press.
29. Sparks S. Radiodermatitis. In: Haas M, Hogle W, Moore-Higgs G, Gosselin-Acomb T, eds. *Radiation Therapy: A Guide to Patient Care.* St. Louis, MO: Mosby Elsevier; 2007:511–522.
30. Hogle W. Wound issues facing oncology patients. In: Haas M, Moore-Higgs G, eds. *Principles of Skin Care and the Oncology Patients.* Pittsburgh, PA: ONS Press. In press.
31. Witt M. Radiodermatitis. In: Haas M, Hogle W, Moore-Higgs G, Gosselin-Acomb T, eds. *Radiation Therapy: A Guide to Patient Care.* St. Louis, MO: Mosby Elsevier; 2007:563–573.
32. National Cancer Institute (NCI). Common toxicity criteria for adverse events, Version 4.0. (CTAE). 2009. http://evs.nci.nih.gov/ftp1/CTCAE/About.html. Accessed 11/20/2009.
33. Main N, Hatcher A, Meeks. Dressing the discomfort: managing radiation therapy-induced dermatitis. *Ostomy Wound Manage.* 2005;51: 12–13.
34. Lacouture M. Insights into the pathophysiology and management of dermatologic toxicities to EGFR-targeted therapies in colorectal cancer. *Cancer Nurs.* 2007;30(4 Suppl 1):S17–S46.
35. Burch SE, Parker SA, Vann AM, et al. Measurement of 6-MV x-ray surface dose when topical agents are applied prior to external beam irradiation. *Int J Radiat Oncol Biol Phys.* 1997;38:447–451.
36. Haas M, Coletti J. Managing skin reaction from radiation or combined chemoradiation therapy [abstract 2642]. *Int J Radiat Oncol Biol Phys.* 2007;69:560.
37. Dudek DJ, Thompson J, Meegan MM, et al. Pilot study to investigate the toxicity of aloe Vera gel in the management of radiation induced skin reactions for post-operative primary breast cancer. *J Radiother Pract.* 2000;1:197–203.
38. Heggie S, Bryant GP, Tripcony L, et al. A phase II study on the efficacy of topical aloe vera gel on irradiated breast tissue. *Cancer Nurs.* 2002;25:442–451.
39. Olsen DL, Raub W, Bradley C, et al. The effect of aloe vera gel/mild soap versus mild soap alone in preventing skin reactions in patients undergoing radiation therapy. *Oncol Nurs Forum.* 2001;3:543–547.
40. Williams MS, Burk M, Loprinzi CL, et al. Phase III double-blind evaluation of an aloe vera gel as a prophylactic agent for radiation-induced skin toxicity. *Int J Radiat Oncol Biol Phys.* 1996;36:345–349.
41. Fisher J, Scott C, Steven R, et al. Randomized phase III study comparing best supportive care to Biafine as a prophylactic agent for radiation-induced skin toxicity for women undergoing breast irradiation: Radiation Therapy Oncology Group (RTOG) 97–13. *Int J Radiat Oncol Biol Phys.* 2000;48:1307–1310.

42. Fenig E, Brfenner B, Katz A, et al. Topical Biafine and Liperderm for the prevention of radiation dermatitis: a randomized prospective trial. *Oncol Rep.* 2001;8:305–308.
43. Pommier P, Gomez F, Sunyach MP, et al. Phase III randomized trial of Calendula Officinalis compared with Tromaline for the prevention of acute dermatitis during irradiation for breast cancer. *J Clin Oncol.* 2004;22:1447–1453.
44. Liguori V, Guillemin C, Pesce GF, et al. Double-blind randomized clinical trial comparing hyaluronic acid cream to placebo in patients treated with radiotherapy. *Radiother Oncol.* 1997;42:155–161.
45. Bostrom A, Lindman H, Swartling C, et al. Potent corticosteroid cream (mometasone furoate) significantly reduces acute radiation dermatitis: results from a double-blind randomized study. *Radiother Oncol.* 2001;59:257–265.
46. Schmuth M, Wimmer MA, Hofer S, et al. A prospective randomized, double-blind study. *Br J Dermatol.* 2002;146:983–991.
47. Eversen JF, Bjordal K, Jacobsen A, et al. Effects of Na-sucrose octasulfate on skin and mucosa reactions during radiotherapy of head and neck cancers. *Acta Oncol.* 2001;40:751–755.
48. Maiche A, Isokangas OP, Grohn, P. Skin protection by sucralfate cream during electron beam therapy. *Acta Oncol.* 1994;33:201–203.
49. Wells M, Macmillan M, Raab G, et al. Does aqueous or sucralfate cream affect the severity of erythematous radiation skin reactions? A randomized controlled trial. *Radiother Oncol.* 2004;73:153–162.
50. Delaney G, Fisher R, Hook C, et al. Sucralfate cream in the management of moist desquamation during radiotherapy. *Australas Radiol.* 1997;41:270–275.
51. Graham P, Browne L, Capp A, et al. Randomized paired comparison of No-Sting barrier film versus sorbolene cream (10% glycerine) skin care during postmastectomy irradiation. *Int J Radiat Oncol Biol Phys.* 2004;58:241–246.
52. National Comprehensive Cancer Network. Cancer-related fatigue. National Comprehensive Cancer network, Inc. 2008. http://www.nccn.org. Accessed February 20, 2010.
53. Lawrence D, Kupelnick B, Miller K, Devine D, Lau J. Evidence report on the occurrence, assessment, and treatment of fatigue in cancer patients. *J Natl Cancer Inst Monogr.* 2004;32:40–50.
54. Jereczek-Fossa B, Marsigloa H, Orecchia R. Radiotherapy-related fatigue. *Crit Rev Oncol Hematol.* 2002;41:317–325.
55. Mock V, Pickett M, Ropka M, et al. Fatigue and quality of life outcomes of exercise during cancer treatment. *Cancer Pract.* 2002;9:119–127.
56. Galantino M. Influence of yoga, walking, and mindfulness meditation on fatigue and body mass index in women living with breast cancer. *Semin Integr Med.* 2003;1:151–157.
57. Bower J, Woolery A, Sternlieb B, Garet D. Yoga for cancer patients and survivors. *Cancer Control.* 2005;12:165–171.
58 Sarna L, Code F. Physical activity and fatigue during radiation therapy: a pilot study using actigraph monitors. *Oncol Nurs Forum.* 2001;28:1043–1046.
59. Eaton L, Tipton J, eds. *Putting Evidence into Practice: Improving Oncology Patient Outcomes.* Pittsburgh, PA: ONS Press; 2009.
60. Padilla G, Preasant C, Grant M, Metter G, Lipsett J, Heide F. Quality of life index for patients with cancer. *Res Nurs Health.* 1983;6: 117–126.
61. Gupta D, Lammersfeld C, Vashi P, Dahlk S, Lis C. Can subjective global assessment of nutritional status predict survival in ovarian cancer? *J Ovarian Res.* 2008;1:5.
62. McMahon K, Decker G, Ottery F. Integrating proactive nutritional assessment in clinical practice to prevent complications and cost. *Semin Oncol.* 1998;25(2 Suppl 6):20–27.
63. Krenitsky J. Adjusted body weight, pro: evidence to support the use of adjusted body weight in calculating calorie requirements. *Nutr Clin Pract.* 2005;20:468–473.
64. Mauch P, Constine L, Greenberger J, et al. Hematopoietic stem cell compartment: acute and late effects of radiation therapy and chemotherapy. *Int J Radiat Oncol Biol Phys.* 1995;31:1319–1339.
65. Casarett GW. *Radiation Histopathology.* Vol. 1. Boca Raton, FL: CRC Press; 1980.
66. Hashimoto M. The distribution of active marrow in the bones of the normal adult. *Kyushu J Med Sci.* 1960;11:103–111.
67. Wara WM, Bauman GS, Sneed PK, et al. Brain, brain stem and cerebellum. In: Perez CA, Brady LW, eds. *Principles and Practice of Radiation Oncology.* 3rd ed. Philadelphia, PA: Lippincott; 2007.
68. Faithfull S, Brada M. Somnolence syndrome in adults following cranial irradiation for primary brain tumors. *Clin Oncol (RColl Radio).* 1998;10:250–524.
69. Ryan J. Radiation somnolence syndrome. *J Pediatr Oncol Nurs.* 2000;17:50–53.
70. Carper, E. Head and neck cancers. In: Haas M, Hogle W, Moore-Higgs G, Gosselin-Acomb T, eds. *Radiation Therapy: A Guide to Patient Care.* St. Louis, MO: Mosby Elsevier; 2007:84–117.
71. Shihn A, Miaskowski R, Dodd M, Stotts N, MacPhail C. Mechanisms for radiation-induced oral mucositis and the consequences. *Cancer Nurs.* 2003;26:222–229.
72. Haas M. Supersaturated electrolyte oral rinse aids quality of life for head/neck chemoradiation patients [abstract 2757]. *Oncol Nurs Forum.* 2008;35:505–506.
73. Haas M, Mercedes T, Manyak M. Treatment of oral mucositis by supersaturated calcium phosphate oral rinse in patients receiving chemotherapy (CT) and radiation therapy (RT). MASSC [abstract 09–090]. *Support Care Cancer.* 2008;16:673–674.
74. Haas M, Mercedes T, Manyak M. Reduction of painful oral mucositis by supersaturated calcium phosphate oral rinse in head and neck cancer patients receiving chemotherapy and radiation. [abstract 2530]. *Int J Radiat Oncol.* 2008;72(Suppl):S406.
75. Papas A, Clark B, Martuscelli G, O'Loughlin K, Johansen E, Miller K. A prospective randomized trial for the prevention of mucositis in patients undergoing hematopoietic stem cell transplant. *Bone Marrow Transplant.* 2003;31:705–712.
76. Cerchietti L, Navigante A, Bonomi M, et al. Effect of topical morphine for mucositis-associated pain following concomitant chemoradiotherapy for head and neck carcinoma. *Cancer.* 2002;95:2230–2236.
77. World Health Organization. *Cancer Pain Relief with a Guide to Opioid Availability.* 2nd ed. WHO; Geneva, Switzerland, 1996.
78. Woo S, Challacombe S. Management of recurrent oral herpes simplex infections. *Oral Surg Oral Med Oral Pathol Oral Radio Endod.* 2007;(103 Suppl):S12e.
79. Diaz-Arnold AM, Marek CA. The impact of saliva on patient care: a literature review. *J Prosthet Dentist.* 2002;88:337–343.
80. Eisbruch A, Rhodus N, Rosenthal D, et al. How should we measure and report radiotherapy-induced xerostomia? *Semin Radiat Oncol.* 2003;13:226–234.
81. Eisbruch T, Haken R, Kim H, Marsh L, Ship J. Dose, volume, and function relationships in parotid salivary glands following conformal and intensity-modulated irradiation of head and neck cancer. *Int J Radiat Oncol Biol Phys.* 1999;45:577–587.
82. Maher K. Xerostomia. In: Yarbro CH, Frogge MH, Goodman M, eds. *Cancer Symptom Management.* 3rd ed. Sudbury, MA: Jones and Bartlett; 2004:215–229.
83. Lynch H, Milgrom P. Xylitol and dental caries: an overview for clinicians. *J Calif Dent Assoc.* 2003;31:205–209.
84. Burlage F. Protection of salivary function by concomitant pilocarpine during radiotherapy: a double-blind, randomized, placebo-controlled study. *Int J Radiat Oncol Biol Phys.* 2008;70:14–22.
85. Gornitsky M, Sphenoid G, Sultanem H, et al. Double-blind randomized, placebo-controlled study of pilocarpine to salvage salivary gland function during radiotherapy of patients with head and neck cancer. *Oral Surg Oral Med Oral Pathol Oral Radiol Endod.* 2004;98: 45–52.
86. Warde P, O'Sullivan B, Aslanidis J, et al. A phase III placebo-controlled trial or oral piocarpinein patients undergoing radiotherapy for head and neck cancer. *Int J Radiat Oncol Biol Phys.* 2002;54:9–13.

87. Haddad P, Karimi P. Randomized, double-blind, placebo controlled trial concomitant pilocarpine with head and neck irradiation for prevention of radiation-induced xerostomia *Radiot Oncol.* 2002;64:29–32.
88. Johnston P, Niemtzow R, Riffenburgh R. Acupuncture for xerostomia: clinical update. *Cancer.* 2002;94:1151–1156.
89. Morganstein W. Acupuncture in the treatment of xerostomia: clinical report. *Gen Dent.* 2005;53:223–226.
90. Johnstone PA, Niemtzow RC, Riffenburgh RH. Acupuncture for xerostomia: clinical update *Cancer.* 2002;64:1151–1156.
91. Ship J, Hu K. Radiotherapy-induced salivary dysfunction. *Semin Oncol.* 2004;31:29–36.
92. Chambers M, Garden A, Kies M, Martin J. Radiation-induced xerostomia in patients with head and neck cancer: pathogenesis, impact on quality of life, and management. *Head Neck.* 2004;26:796–807.
93. Scully C, Epstein J, Sonis S. Oral mucositis: a challenging complication of radiotherapy, chemotherapy, and radiochemotherapy. Part 2: diagnosis and management of mucositis. *Head Neck.* 2004;26:77–84.
94 Murphy B, Gilbert J, Cmelak A, Ridner S. Symptom control issues and supportive care of patients with head and neck cancers. *Clin Adv Hematol Oncol.* 2007;5:807–822.
95. Rubio I, Henry-Tillman R, Klimberg V, Mancino A, Maners A, Kaufmann Y. Effects of glutamine on radiation morbidity in breast conservation therapy: P046. *Cancer J.* 2003;9:514.
96. Haas M. Lung cancer. In: Haas M, Hogle W, Moore-Higgs G, Gosselin-Acomb T, eds. *Radiation Therapy: A Guide to Patient Care.* St. Louis, MO: Mosby Elsevier; 2007:118–141.
97. Robnett T, Machtay M, Vines E, et al. Factors predicting severe radiation pneumonitis in patients receiving definitive chemoradiation for lung cancer. *Int J Radiat Oncol Biol Phys.* 2000;48:89–94.
98. Claude L, Perol D, Ginester C, et al. A prospective study on radiation pneumonitis following conformal radiation therapy in non-small-cell lung cancer: clinical and dosimetric factors analysis. *Radiat Oncol.* 2004;71:175–181.
99. Engelking C, Wickham R, Sauerland C. Radiation-induced nausea, vomiting, and diarrhea. In: Haas M, Hogle W, Moore-Higgs G, Gosselin-Acromb T, eds. *Radiation Therapy: A Guide to Patient Care.* Philadelphia, PA: Mosby Elsevier; 2007:641–663.
100. Haas M, Kuehn E. Teletherapy: external radiation therapy. In: Brunner D, Moore-Higgs G, Haas M, eds. *Outcomes in Radiation Therapy: Multidisciplinary Management.* Sudbury, MA: Jones and Bartlett; 2001:55–66.
101. Lu W. Acupuncture for side effects of chemoradiation therapy in cancer patients. *Semin Oncol Nurs.* 2005;21:190–195.
102. Benson A, Ajani J, Catalano R, et al. Recommended guidelines for the treatment of cancer treatment-induced diarrhea. *J Clin Oncol.* 2004;22:2918–2926.
103. Hogle W. Male genitourinary cancers. In: Haas M, Hogle W, Moore-Higgs G, Gosselin-Acomb T, eds. *Radiation Therapy: A Guide to Patient Care.* St. Lois, MO: Mosby Elsevier; 2007:234–266.
104. Fraunholz I, Schopohl B, Fal S, Boettcher H. Cytohormonal status and acute radiation vaginitis. In: Dorr, W. Engenhart-Cabillic, R. Zimmermann, J. eds. Normal tissue reactions in radiotherapy and oncology. *Front Radiat Ther Oncol.* 2002;37:112–120.
105. Yashar C. Basic principles in gynaecologic radiotherapy. In: DiSaia, Creasman, eds. *Clinical Gynecologic Oncology.* 7th ed. Amsterdam: Elsevier; 2007:775.
106. Kim S. Eye. In: Haffty B, Wilson L, eds. *Handbook of Radiation Oncology: Basic Principles and Clinical Protocols.* Sudbury, MA: Jones and Bartlett; 2009:343–360.
107. Chao K, Perez C, Brady, L. *Late Effects of Cancer Treatment. Radiation Oncology Management Decisions.* 2nd ed. Philadelphia, PA: Lippincott, Williams & Wilkins; 2002:103–110.
108. Moore-Higgs G. Basic principles of radiation therapy: In: Haas M, Hogle W, Moore-Higgs G, Gosselin-Acomb T, eds. *Radiation Therapy: A Guide to Patient Care.* St. Louis, MO: Mosby Elsevier; 2007:8–24.
109. Emami B, Lyman J, Brown A, Coia L, Goitein M, Munzenrider JE, Shank B, Solin LJ, Wesson M. Tolerance of normal tissue to therapeutic radiation. *Int J Radiat Oncol Biol Phys.* 1991;21:109–122.
110. Rubin P. The law and order of radiation sensitivity, absolute vs. relative. In: Vaeth JM, Meyer JL, eds. *Radiation Tolerance of Normal Tissues: Frontiers of Radiation Therapy and Oncology.* Basel, Switzerland: Karger; 1989:7–40.
111. Marks LB. The impact of organ structure on radiation response. *Int J Radiat Oncol Biol Phys.* 1996;34:1165–1171.
112. Davis AM, Dische S, Gerber L, et al. Measuring postirradiation subcutaneous soft-tissue fibrosis: state-of-the-art and future directions. *Semin Radiat Oncol.* 2003;13:203–213.
113. O'Sullivan B, Levin W. Late radiation-related fibrosis: pathogenesis, manifestations, and current management. *Semin Radiat Oncol.* 2003;13:274–289.
114. Delanian S, Balla-Mekias S, Lefaix J-L. Striking regression of chronic radiotherapy damage in a clinical trial of combined pentoxifylline and tocopherol. *J Clin Oncol.* 1999;17:3283–3290.
115. Delanian S, Porcher R, Balla-Mekias S, et al. Randomized, placebo-controlled trial of combined pentoxifylline and tocopherol for regression of superficial radiation-induced fibrosis. *J Clin Oncol.* 2003;21:2545–2555.
116. Lennox AJ, Shafer JP, Hatcher M, et al. Pilot study of impedance-controlled microcurrent therapy for managing radiation-induced fibrosis in head-and-neck cancer patients. *Int J Radiat Oncol Biol Phys.* 2002;54:23–34.
117. Knisely J, Suh J, Tsien C. Central nervous system. In: Haffty B, Wilson L, eds. *Handbook of Radiation Oncology: Basic Principles and Clinical Protocols.* Sudbury, MA: Jones and Bartlett; 2008, 221–250.
118. Andrews N. Dental implications and management of head and neck radiotherapy patients. *Ann Royal Austral Dent Surg.* 2000;15: 90–97.
119. Tell R, Lundell G, Nilsson B, Sjodin H, Lewin F, Lewensohn, R.. Long-term incidence of hypothyroidism after radiotherapy in patients with head-and-neck cancer. *Int J Radiat Oncol Biol Phys.* 2004:60:395–400.
120. Marks LB, Yu X, Vujaskovic Z, et al. Radiation-induced lung injury. *Semin Radiat Oncol.* 2003;13:333–345.
121. Adams M, Hardenbergh P, Constine L. Radiation-associated cardiovascular disease. *Crit Rev Oncol Hematol.* 2003:45:55–75.
122. Adams MJ, Lipshultz SE, Schwartz C, et al. Radiation-associated cardiovascular disease: manifestations and management. *Semin Radiat Oncol.* 2003;13:346–356.
123. Basavaraju SR, Easterly CE. Pathophysiologic effects of radiation on atherosclerosis development and progression, and the incidence of cardiovascular complications. *Med Phys.* 2002;29:2391–2403.
124. Andreassen CN, Overgaard J, Alsner J, et al. ATM sequence variants and risk of radiation-induced subcutaneous fibrosis after postmastectomy radiotherapy. *Int J Radiat Oncol Biol Phys.* 2006;64:776.
125. Anscher M. The irreversibility of radiation-induced fibrosis: fact or folklore? *J Clin Oncol.* 2005;23:8551.
126. Hauer-Jensen M, Wang J, Denham JW. Bowel injury: current and evolving management strategies. *Semin Radiat Oncol.* 2003;13:357–371.
127. King C. Testicular cancers. In: Haffty B, Wilson L, eds. *Handbook of Radiation Oncology.* Sudbury, MA: Jones and Bartlett; 2009: 557–564.
128. Haas R. Evaluating the risks of radiation-induced secondary cancers. *Radiat Ther.* 1996;4:104–112.
129. van Leeuwen FE, Travers LB. Second cancers. In DeVita VT, Hellman S, Rosenberg SA, eds. *Cancer: Principles and Practice of Oncology.* 6th ed. Philadelphia, PA: Lippincott-Raven; 2001:2939–2963.

CHAPTER 15

Peter V. Tortorice, PharmD, BCOP

# Cytotoxic Chemotherapy: Principles of Therapy

## HISTORICAL PERSPECTIVE

The term *chemotherapy* was first coined to describe the use of chemicals or drugs to treat microbial diseases and later neoplastic diseases.[1] In the 1940s, nitrogen mustard, the first cytotoxic drug, was introduced for cancer chemotherapy. Nitrogen mustard—a derivative of mustard gas, which was used as a chemical deterrent in the two world wars—was developed as an antineoplastic drug after it was learned that soldiers exposed to this drug developed reversible leukopenia. Soon after the introduction of nitrogen mustard, methotrexate, cyclophosphamide, and fluorouracil were made available for the treatment of advanced cancers. Two significant developments occurred in the 1960s and late 1970s that opened the door for modern-day cancer chemotherapy: (1) the introduction of platinum-coordinated complexes as cytotoxic therapy and (2) the practice of combining chemotherapy drugs to improve response rates and survival without significantly affecting toxicity.

The screening, synthesis, and clinical testing of new compounds or analogues of currently active agents continued through the 1970s and 1980s. Among the most useful agents discovered during this period were the semisynthetic podophyllotoxin etoposide and paclitaxel, a natural product isolated from the Western yew tree. The development of the anthracycline analogue doxorubicin also had a significant impact on the treatment of breast cancer and sarcomas. The biological response modifiers were first recognized as having antineoplastic activity in the 1980s. The search for new agents to treat cancer continues into the twenty-first century.

Current strategies being emphasized for drug development include drugs with novel mechanisms of action, monoclonal antibodies directed against specific cellular targets, drugs that modulate or reverse drug resistance, and drugs used for supportive care of the patient with cancer. Supportive therapies that have made administering and managing chemotherapy safer and easier include simple and effective antiemetic therapy and hematopoietic growth factors.

Historically, the goals of early chemotherapy were limited primarily to palliation of symptoms. An increase in available agents and more experience with cytotoxic chemotherapy produced significant tumor regression and improved control of cancer. The development and acceptance of combination chemotherapy greatly improved the outcome for otherwise incurable neoplastic diseases. This approach to cancer treatment incorporated the theoretical point that targeting multiple biochemical processes would have a greater overall effect on tumor regression and remission. Eventually, the goals of chemotherapy shifted to a curative approach for cancers in which complete responses to chemotherapy were seen. Cancers for which cures and increased survival have been accomplished using chemotherapy given alone or in combination with other modalities such as surgery and radiation therapy are listed in Table 15-1. Cytotoxic chemotherapy has produced cures in a subset of patients with cancers such as acute leukemia in children, Hodgkin's disease, and testicular tumors. Significant cure rates for the most common cancers of the breast, lung, and colon have only been achieved in the early stages of the disease with the use of adjuvant chemotherapy. Advanced stages of these diseases may be controlled with chemotherapy but are rarely cured.

The use of drugs to control or eradicate cancer has developed into the specialization of medical oncology. The treatment of individuals with cancer is one of the most rapidly expanding and dynamic fields in medicine and demands continuous reevaluation and reappraisal of both new and established therapies. To continue to develop and improve cancer treatments, more patients need to

**TABLE 15-1**

**Chemotherapy-Sensitive Tumors**

| Relative Chemosensitivity and Expected Survival Outcome | Type of Cancer |
|---|---|
| Highly sensitive: Normal survival, possible cure | Acute leukemia in children<br>Hodgkin's disease<br>Diffuse large cell lymphoma<br>Burkitt's lymphoma<br>Testicular carcinoma<br>Embryonal carcinoma<br>Ewing's sarcoma<br>Wilms' tumor<br>Skin cancer |
| Moderately sensitive: Increase in survival | Ovarian carcinoma<br>Breast carcinoma<br>Endometrial carcinoma<br>Acute leukemia in adults<br>Small cell lung cancer<br>Prostate cancer<br>Stomach cancer<br>Cervical cancer<br>Neuroblastoma |
| Minimally sensitive: Some increase in survival | Head and neck cancers<br>Gastrointestinal cancers<br>Endocrine gland tumors<br>Malignant melanoma<br>Osteogenic sarcoma<br>Soft tissue sarcoma |
| Marginally sensitive: No documented increase in survival | Bladder cancer<br>Esophageal cancer<br>Non-small cell lung cancer<br>Pancreatic carcinoma<br>Hepatocellular carcinoma |

participate in controlled clinical trials. Fewer than 10% of eligible patients actively being treated for cancer are estimated to be enrolled in clinical trials. The clinician is a key figure in encouraging cooperation not only from the patient and his or her family but also from the healthcare community, including providers and sponsors (third-party payers). Increased survival and—more important—the maintenance or improvement of quality of life for patients with cancer can be achieved with the appropriate use of cytotoxic chemotherapy.

## CANCER CHEMOTHERAPY DRUG DEVELOPMENT

Drug discovery and the eventual development of cancer treatment compounds involve numerous strategies. The most successful methods seek to combine current knowledge of the biology of cancer and the pharmacological properties of potentially therapeutic compounds. In particular, synthesis and testing of analogues of compounds with known antineoplastic activity have produced several active drugs. Synthesis of chemically or mechanistically similar compounds having different pharmacokinetic or toxic properties has yielded clinically useful new agents. Recent advances in understanding the molecular and genetic operations that neoplastic cells possess have led to the development of targeted antitumor agents—for example, angiogenesis inhibitors and oncogene suppressors. These drugs will be covered in detail in Chapter 21, Targeted Therapy, of this book.

The oncology research community is composed of national and local study groups, university-based research programs, and pharmaceutical manufacturers. The National Cancer Institute (NCI) assists in coordinating the massive efforts of researchers and clinicians in screening and developing drugs for use in cancer treatment. In addition, a significant amount of research and development, primarily by pharmaceutical manufacturers, is conducted outside the auspices of the NCI.

The drug-approval process in the US is rigorous and comprehensive. New compounds undergo extensive testing in animals (preclinical testing) and then in humans before being submitted to the US Food and Drug Administration (FDA) for approval and becoming commercially available. Because of the unique and potentially life-threatening toxicities associated with antineoplastic drugs, this approval process may become both lengthy and expensive. The average time and cost to bring a drug to market may range from 6 to 12 years and $40 million to $80 million, respectively. The FDA is committed to making changes in the drug-development process to accelerate the time necessary to make a new compound available for general use. The FDA may give a new drug orphan status if it will only benefit fewer than 200,000 Americans with a rare condition. Examples of orphan drugs are decitabine and azacitidine for myelodysplastic syndromes and pemetrexed for malignant pleural mesothelioma.

### PRECLINICAL EVALUATION

The NCI coordinates the screening of more than 10,000 compounds each year in an effort to find new and potentially useful drugs for treating cancer. Less than 1% of these screened compounds proceed to clinical trials. Compounds with known or suspected antineoplastic activity are tested in animal tumor models and human tumor cell lines. Cell lines frequently used include lung, ovarian, and renal cell cancer; malignant melanoma; brain tumors; and leukemias. Because of the interest in how drug resistance may influence chemotherapy effectiveness, multidrug-resistant (MDR) variants of human breast cancer and murine leukemia cell lines are also available for testing.

Compounds having demonstrated significant antineoplastic activity first undergo preclinical toxicology studies. The purpose of these studies is to determine a safe starting dose for use in humans. The lethal dose in 10% of animals tested ($LD_{10}$) then is used to calculate a starting dose for clinical trials. The $LD_{10}$ is usually determined in mice and dogs to avoid excessive risk to humans. Body surface area (BSA) is the preferred reference point used for making interspecies dose comparisons.

### CLINICAL TRIALS

Following the initial development and pharmaceutical preparation in the preclinical phase, new compounds must be tested in humans to evaluate their activity and toxicity in treating cancers. Table 15-2 briefly describes the phases of clinical trials conducted in the United States and lists the purpose and goals of each phase of testing. Healthy volunteers usually are recruited for phase I testing of most new drugs. However, because of the potential for significant toxicity with antineoplastic drugs, patients with advanced cancer are selected for phase I trials of these drugs. These patients also may benefit from the new therapies. The ideal patients for phase II testing are previously untreated with antineoplastic drugs, but most tend to be patients who have shown little or no response to prior chemotherapy. Usually, response rates of higher than 20% indicate that the drug may have therapeutic usefulness and warrants further clinical testing. Traditionally, response rates, duration of response, survival, and toxicity are measured, although quality of life has emerged as a focus of some clinical trials in recent years. At the conclusion of phase III testing, it should be known whether the new treatment is better than the standard therapy in terms of response, survival, and toxicity and how it affects the patient's quality of life. Phase IV studies occur after FDA approval of a drug for use in cancer and generally involve the use of drugs in combination with other therapies where cure is the goal of treatment.

## SCIENTIFIC BASIS OF CHEMOTHERAPY

Only recently have researchers begun to identify what is thought to be the primary pharmacological activity of many antineoplastic agents. The actual mechanism or combination of mechanisms responsible for killing tumor cells remains elusive. This disparity is partly a function of the lack of a clear understanding of how cancer cells originate, grow, and regress. The next section addresses tumor cell biology and examines how chemotherapeutic drugs may selectively exert their cytotoxicity.

### THE CELL CYCLE

Much of what is known regarding the effects of cytotoxic chemotherapy relies on understanding the cell cycle. The cycle consists of five phases: $G_1$, S, $G_2$, M, and $G_0$. The phases describe periods of time for different cellular processes that ultimately result in a cell's reproduction or death (Figure 15-1). In any population, only some cells are actively proliferating. The *growth fraction* is the portion of cells actively cycling compared with the entire population. Following mitosis, a cell can do any one of the following: leave the cell cycle, differentiate and eventually die, enter a resting state ($G_0$) and reenter the cycle at some later time (stem cells), or enter the $G_1$ phase and continue to cycle.

Synthesis of RNA and proteins occurs predominantly in the *$G_1$ phase.* Synthesis, or *S phase,* is when DNA is being replicated and is a relatively short period compared with the overall time a cell is cycling. The *$G_2$ phase* is also typically brief, occurring after DNA synthesis and just before cell division. Mitosis, or cell division, ensues during the *M phase,* resulting in two identical daughter cells. The time from mitosis to mitosis is described as the *cycling time.* Cells that have left the cycle to enter the *$G_0$ phase* are considered to be in a *resting* or *dormant phase.* These cells can actively synthesize RNA and proteins and differentiate. Cells in this phase are typically resistant to the cytotoxic effects of chemotherapy. *Apoptosis,* or programmed cell death, is an important cellular process that may be exploited for its antineoplastic effect by targeted chemotherapy.

**TABLE 15-2**

**Phases of Clinical Trials Conducted in the United States**

| Phase | Purpose | Goals |
|---|---|---|
| I | Determines maximum tolerated dose and describes pharmacology and pharmacokinetics in humans | Dosing starts at 10% of the $LD_{10}$ in mice<br>Determine safe dose and schedule for phase II |
| II | Determines drug activity in specific tumors | Also determines administration schedule, toxicity, supportive care |
| III | New drug or drug combinations are compared against the standard therapy | Objective criteria: Response rate, duration of response, survival, toxicity, and quality of life |
| IV | Role of drug in adjuvant/curative setting | Determines other uses, doses, schedules, and combination regimens |

*Abbreviation*: $LD_{10}$ = Lethal dose in less than 10% of animals tested.

### TUMOR CELL KINETICS

Tumor cells may be distinguished from cells of normal tissues by their loss of controlled cell division, lack of differentiation, and ability to invade surrounding tissues and establish new growth at distant sites in the body. Theoretically, most antineoplastic drugs use the rapid proliferation rate of tumor cells as a target for their cytotoxic effects. The same mechanism explains many of the toxicities seen in cells of normal tissues because these cells are also going through the cell cycle and dividing, albeit at a much slower rate. The selective effects of antineoplastic drugs on both proliferating normal and tumor cells may be explained by the following model: (1) Tumor growth is often exponential, (2) doubling times vary widely between tumors, and (3) chemotherapy-sensitive tumors tend to grow faster than slow-growing tumors that are less responsive to chemotherapy.

The doubling times of both malignant and normal tissues vary widely. Factors that affect doubling time include cell cycle time, growth fraction, and cell loss by either programmed cell death (apoptosis) or differentiation or metastasis. Cells with a rapid cycling time and a tumor with a large growth fraction should be the most responsive to cytotoxic therapy. Although tumor cells may exhibit rapid cycling, the rate is not higher than what is seen with normal renewal tissues such as bone marrow and gastrointestinal mucosa. Therefore, uncontrolled proliferation is not the sole distinguishing trait of tumor cells. Loss of homeostatic mechanisms, such as contact inhibition, cell differentiation, and maturation, leads to an increased proliferative rate, which exceeds cell death. Collectively, these processes result in the accumulation of tumor cells.

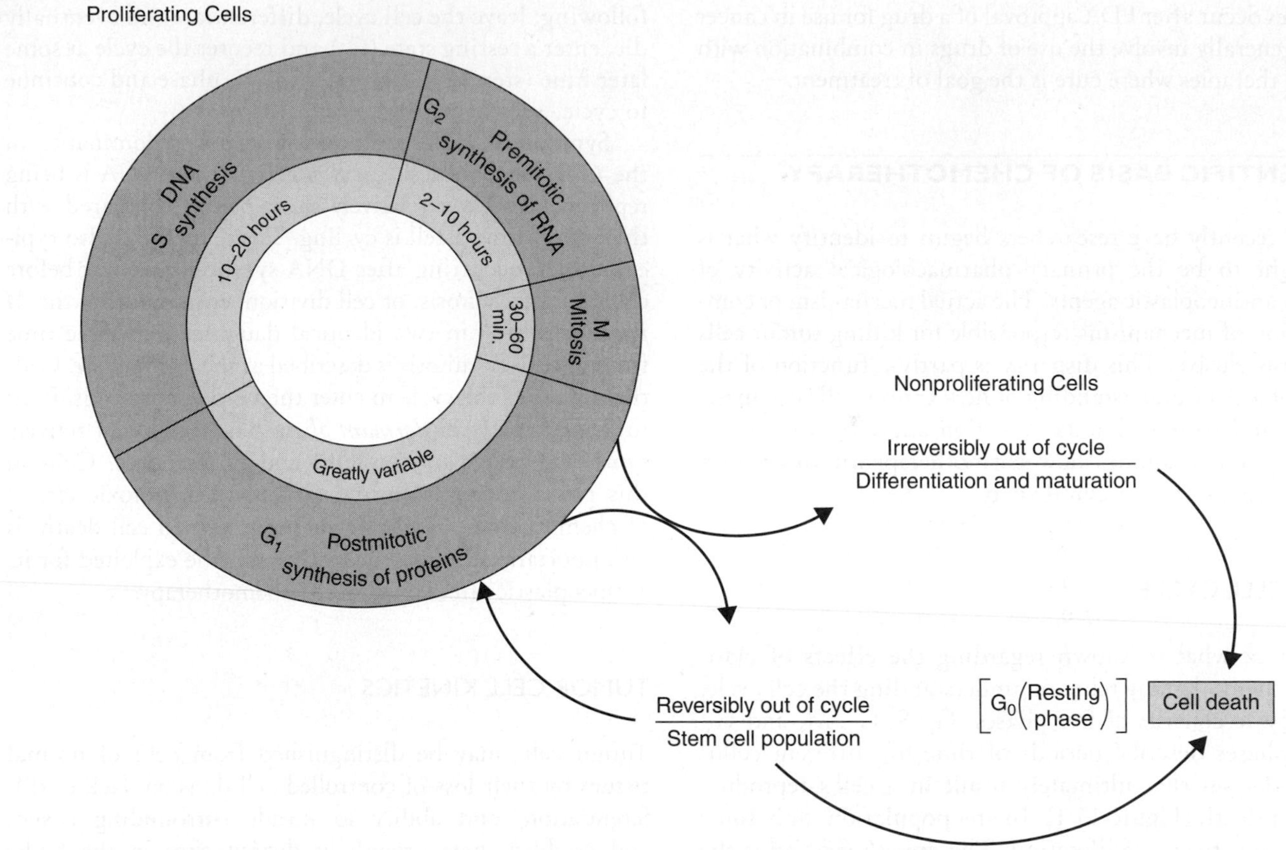


**FIGURE 15-1**

Diagrammatic representation of the life of a cell, emphasizing the relationships between the cell cycle and proliferating and nonproliferating cells.

## THE EFFECTS OF CYTOTOXIC CHEMOTHERAPY ON TUMOR CELLS

### Cell-kill hypothesis

The cell-kill hypothesis is a basic principle often used to describe the effects of cancer chemotherapy on normal and tumor cells. The hypothesis describes a first-order kinetic process that predicts the number of cells killed based on the dose of chemotherapy given. It applies only to cells that are actively proliferating and assumes that treatment sensitivity does not change and that growth rate is constant. The model is based on a log-kill relationship for dose of chemotherapy and a constant proportion of cells killed per treatment. A treatment with a 3-log kill produces a tumor reduction of 99.9%. Essentially, no treatment can bring the number of tumor cells to zero; therefore, the net effect on viable tumor cells is calculated as surviving cells plus regrowth before the next treatment. Because of these limitations, the model is not applicable to most human tumors. Malignancies that do follow this model include Burkitt's lymphoma and germ cell tumors. The cell-kill hypothesis is still used today in determining tumor cell growth inhibition of newly derived anticancer compounds.

### Gompertzian curve

The effect of antineoplastic drugs on human tumors cannot be fully explained by the cell-kill model because not all tumor cells are in a proliferative state. A Gompertzian growth curve (Figure 15-2) probably best describes the growth of human tumors and the responses observed with the administration of antineoplastic drugs.[2] Tumor growth fraction and proliferative rate are not constant but rather decrease with time as a tumor goes from a small, undetectable clump of cells to a large mass. The doubling time of a tumor increases as the mass grows in size. Eventually, the tumor reaches a growth plateau phase, where further increase in size becomes minimal because of the slower doubling time.

The Gompertzian curve also is useful in describing the observed tumor response to chemotherapy.[3] If cytotoxic chemotherapy is given in the growth phase of the tumor, the portion of cells actively proliferating, or the growth fraction, is large; therefore, a high percentage of cells will be susceptible to the effects of the drugs. In contrast, in a more advanced stage of the disease, when growth has reached a plateau, fewer cells will be dividing and therefore will be less susceptible to chemotherapy.

When surgery or radiation therapy has been used to reduce the tumor mass, chemotherapy may prove beneficial in eradicating both residual and micrometastatic disease. However, because metastatic cells often result from numerous prior divisions, the possibility that either primary or secondary drug resistance has developed is significant.

### Mechanisms and sites of action of cytotoxic chemotherapy

Chemotherapeutic drugs induce their cytotoxicity on tumor cells and normal tissue by one or more mechanisms. Figure 15-3 illustrates the potential sites and proposed mechanisms of action for many of the drugs currently available for cancer chemotherapy. Central to the diagram is the genetic machinery, considered to be the focus for most effective cytotoxic drugs.

## TARGETED THERAPIES FOR CANCER

Until recently, most cancer chemotherapy had been limited to drugs that are cytotoxic to the reproductive cycle and functions of tumor cells. A better understanding of the molecular biology of normal and tumor cells has allowed significant developments in targeting mechanisms of tumor growth, invasion, and metastasis. By targeting tumor cell growth, these types of therapies should be less toxic to normal tissues. Additionally, overall treatment of cancer may evolve from an acute tumor destruction approach to a more chronic management of malignant cells. A thorough discussion of targeted therapies for cancer can be found in Chapter 21.

## CYTOTOXIC DRUG-SELECTION CRITERIA

A wide variability in both therapeutic response and unacceptable toxicity is observed in patients receiving chemotherapy. This variability may be explained by differences in factors involving the patient with cancer, the chemotherapy being given, and the type of tumor being treated.

Patient factors include response to toxicity, organ dysfunction, previous treatment, and age. The occurrence and severity of toxicity vary widely among patients and often necessitate chemotherapy dose reductions or treatment delays. Preexisting organ dysfunction, such as renal or hepatic insufficiency, also may require dose or schedule alterations. Patients who have received chemotherapy previously may not be candidates to receive the same drug

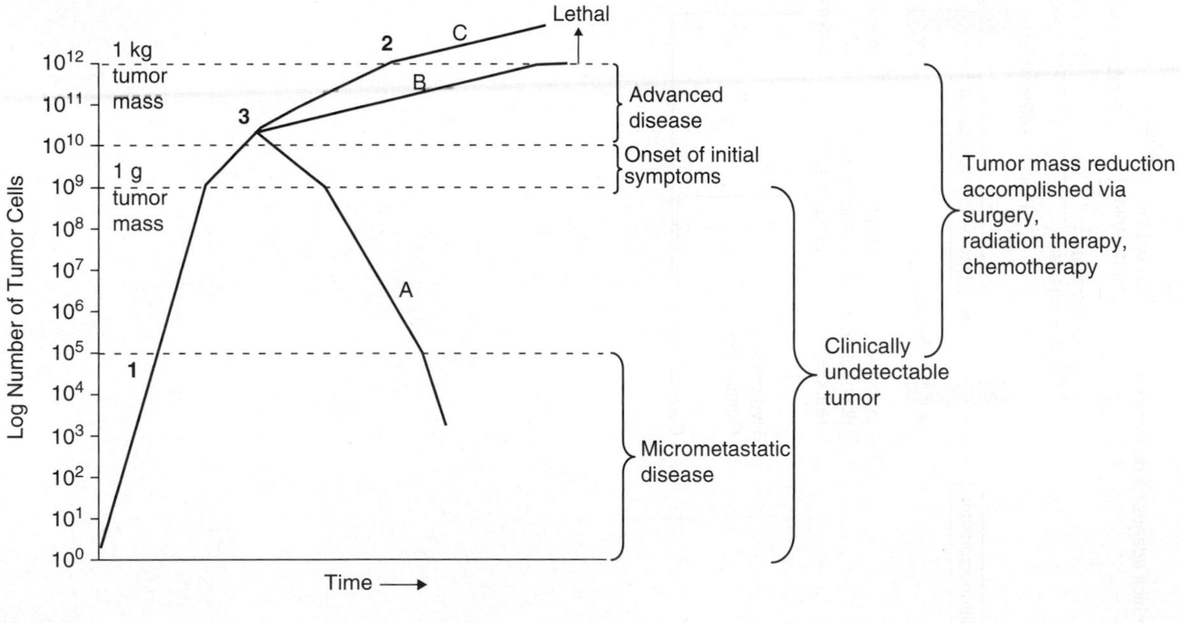


**FIGURE 15-2**

Gompertzian tumor-growth curve: Relationship of tumor mass, diagnosis, symptoms, and potential treatment regimens. Growth phases and chemotherapy response: (1) log phase (high growth fraction, short doubling time), (2) plateau phase (low growth fraction, longer doubling time), (3) initiation of chemotherapy treatments: (a) tumor cells responsive to drugs, (b) tumor exhibits initial response to treatment but develops resistance (secondary or somatic resistance), (c) tumor unresponsive to drug regimen (primary resistance).

*Source*: Data from Buick.[2]

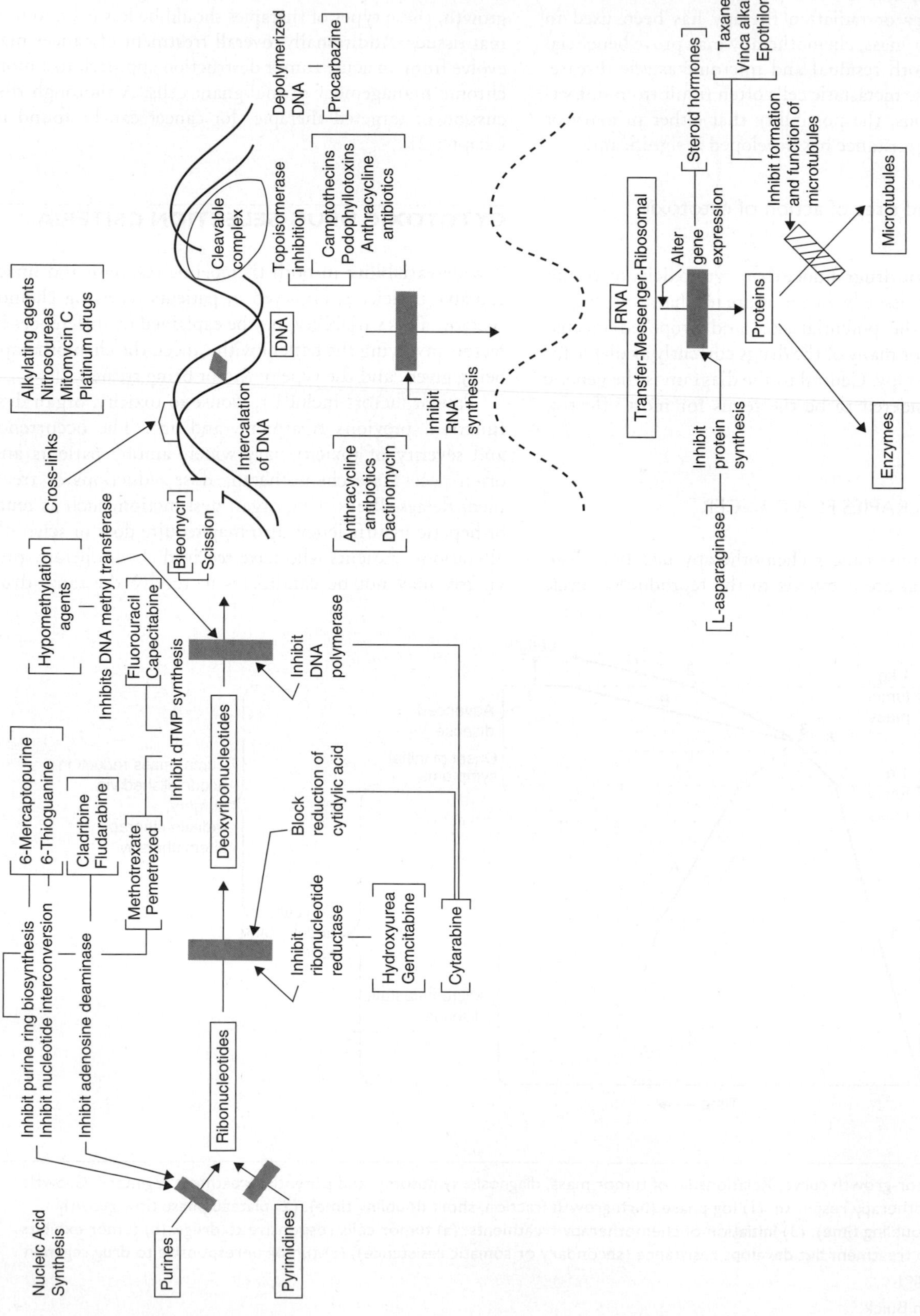


**FIGURE 15-3**
Proposed mechanisms of action of cytotoxic chemotherapeutic agents.

again or, likewise, a drug with similar toxicity. In particular, the recommended maximum lifetime dose of anthracycline drugs (eg, doxorubicin, daunorubicin, epirubicin, and idarubicin) should not be exceeded because these agents greatly increase patients' risk for developing severe cardiomyopathy. Drugs that are neurotoxic should be avoided in patients with preexisting neurological defects, such as taxane use in patients with diabetic neuropathies. Previous bone marrow transplant or the use of severely marrow-toxic drugs may preclude the future use of full doses of myelosuppressive drugs. Fludarabine is toxic to stem cells and should be avoided in patients who are candidates for autologous stem cell transplantation. All these factors may have adverse effects on a patient's response to antineoplastic drugs and the overall potential to cure or control the cancer.

Antineoplastic activity, pharmacokinetics, dose, and schedule are important drug factors that can influence chemotherapy response and toxicity. The relative cytotoxicity of any antineoplastic drug depends on the origin of the tumor and the presence of intrinsic drug resistance. Intrinsic resistance is probably a type of generic defense mechanism present in cells of certain histological types. Pharmacokinetic factors determine the ability of chemotherapeutic drugs to reach their cellular targets. Changes in these factors, such as decreased metabolic activation or increased drug clearance from the body, may decrease antitumor response. Similarly, alterations in protein binding of certain drugs, such as etoposide or teniposide, may enhance clinical toxicity. Poorly lipophilic drugs administered systemically are ineffective for tumors found in lipophilic tissues such as the central nervous system. Administration of drugs such as methotrexate or cytarabine directly into the intrathecal space will circumvent this obstacle. The ability to deliver the optimal dose of chemotherapy for a specific cancer is often limited by the patient's individualized maximum tolerated dose. The clinical use of hematopoietic growth factors, such as granulocyte colony-stimulating factor (G-CSF) and granulocyte-macrophage colony-stimulating factor (GM-CSF), has allowed the doses of myelotoxic drugs to be escalated in an attempt to improve response.

Tumor factors such as growth and size significantly influence the response to chemotherapy. Larger tumors have small growth fractions and therefore are less responsive to the cytotoxic effects of antineoplastic drugs. In addition, the ability of chemotherapy to reach large solid tumors may be hindered by inadequate blood flow. Chemotherapy response is also influenced by tumor cell histology. Table 15-1 differentiates tumor types based on their sensitivity to chemotherapy and the outcomes that may be expected in patients successfully treated with chemotherapy.

Selectivity of certain types of malignancies for specific chemotherapeutic agents is also seen. Fluorouracil is most active in cancers of endodermal tissue, such as gastrointestinal and breast neoplasms. Epithelial tumors, such as squamous cell cancers, are especially sensitive to the cytotoxic effects of bleomycin.

## MANAGING CHEMOTHERAPY RESISTANCE

In addition to the patient and drug factors that play important roles in chemotherapy response, genetic instability of the tumor cell and emergence of drug resistance are currently considered the most significant determinants of response. Although much work has focused on changing the biology or genetic composition of tumor cells, strategies for overcoming resistance need to be developed and implemented.

Cytotoxic drug resistance may be expressed as a temporary or permanent insensitivity to one or more antineoplastic drugs. Temporary or relative resistance is usually a function of the drug's inability to reach the target cells. Reasons why this could happen include poor blood supply, existence of anatomic sanctuary sites such as the testes and central nervous system, and altered pharmacokinetic parameters. Likewise, as yet undefined host defense mechanisms may have a negative effect on treatment success. In some conditions, temporary resistance may be reversed by altering drug delivery, dose, or scheduling of drug administration.

Permanent or phenotypic drug resistance is an inheritable mechanism that may result from a genetic mutation or preexisting trait.[4] This form of resistance may be present prior to treatment (*primary resistance*) or may develop after exposure to antineoplastic drugs (*secondary resistance*). *Point mutations* usually occur in a single cell and are independent of drug concentration. *Gene amplification* is influenced by drug concentration and occurs with repeated exposure over an extended period of time. For example, expression of the multidrug-resistance gene (*MDR-1*) is associated with the development of the MDR phenotype.[5]

### THEORETICAL BASIS FOR CYTOTOXIC DRUG RESISTANCE

The failure of chemotherapy to control tumor growth and induce remission from cancer is one of the most challenging problems facing the oncology clinician. Several theories and models have been developed to explain this phenomenon. The previously described cell-kill model represented an early attempt to explain neoplastic cell growth and lack of response to cytotoxic chemotherapy. According to the model, increasing the dose of a cytotoxic drug or adding other drugs results in an increase in cell kill. Therefore, the theory suggests that failure of chemotherapy to eradicate a tumor is the result of inadequate dose intensity or the presence of biochemically resistant tumor cells. Although this theory is applicable to tumor regression, clinical data do not necessarily support it.[3]

Another possible explanation for treatment failure derives from the stem cell concept. Stem cells continually produce progeny that go on to become mature cells but do not differentiate themselves. These cells constitute a small portion of the total population of cells. Therefore, eradicating the stem cell population would, in theory, eliminate the source of malignant cells and induce tumor regression. However, this must be accomplished without greatly increasing the rate of genetic mutation and producing other biochemically resistant stem cell lines.

Chemotherapy treatment failures may be explained by the development of drug resistance to specific chemotherapeutic drugs. The Goldie-Coldman theory proposes that the genetic instability of tumor cells with high mitotic rates may be responsible for the emergence of resistant clones within a population of tumor cells. Treatment failure then may be explained by the development of drug-resistant cells arising from random genetic mutations occurring prior to or during cytotoxic chemotherapy. The optimal chance for curing cancer with chemotherapy would be to apply effective drugs early in treatment so as to reduce the total number of cancer cells while preventing resistant cells from developing, thus supporting the established concepts of combination chemotherapy.[4]

Tumors that recur following effective initial treatment often present a therapeutic dilemma. Disease that recurs within 6 months usually is considered resistant to initial chemotherapy, and an alternative drug regimen is used. However, recurrence more than 6 months after treatment may be treated successfully with the same or a similar chemotherapy regimen. This phenomenon may be explained by either the reversion of resistant cells to drug-sensitive cells or the predominance of initially sensitive cells in the relapsed tumor.[3] Although the Goldie-Coldman model presents an important concept of quantitative drug resistance, the assumptions are not always applicable to human tumors. Continued diligence in exploring the mechanisms behind chemotherapy treatment failure is a goal of modern chemotherapy.

**TABLE 15-3**

**Possible Mechanisms of Cytotoxic Drug Resistance**

| Site or Type of Resistance | Mechanism of Resistance | Drugs Involved |
|---|---|---|
| Drug metabolism | Reduced drug activation | Cytarabine<br>Fluorouracil<br>6-Mercaptopurine<br>Methotrexate |
| | Increased drug deactivation | Alkylating agents<br>Cytarabine<br>Doxorubicin |
| Cytotoxic targets | Increased enzyme levels | Fluorouracil<br>Methotrexate |
| | Alteration in enzyme–substrate binding | Doxorubicin<br>Etoposide<br>Fluorouracil<br>6-Mercaptopurine<br>Methotrexate |
| Biochemical modification | Use of alternative (salvage) pathways | Cytarabine<br>Fluorouracil<br>6-Mercaptopurine<br>Methotrexate |
| | Decreased cofactor concentrations (reduced folate pool) | Fluorouracil |
| DNA repair systems | Increased DNA repair | Alkylating agents<br>Cisplatin<br>Mitomycin |
| Intracellular drug concentration | Decreased cellular uptake | Mechlorethamine<br>Methotrexate |
| | Increased efflux (P-glycoprotein-mediated) | Anthracycline antibiotics<br>Epothilones<br>Etoposide<br>Taxanes<br>Vinca alkaloids |
| Cell cycle checkpoint (failure to induce apoptosis) | *p53* mutation | Cytotoxic chemotherapy |

*Source*: Data from Buick[2]; and Goldie.[6]

## TYPES OF DRUG RESISTANCE

Table 15-3 lists possible mechanisms of resistance and the drugs most often affected.[2,6]

### Phenotypic drug resistance

Phenotypic drug resistance is believed to arise from spontaneous genetic mutations that occur regularly in a population of tumor cells.[4] The model is based on early observations of the development of acquired resistance in bacteria. A mutational origin appears to explain the development of antibiotic resistance in bacterial cells, which is analogous to the cytotoxic drug resistance observed in tumor cells. Antibiotics and cytotoxic drugs selectively kill sensitive cells and leave behind phenotypically resistant ones that reproduce and expand the volume of resistant cells.

The development of drug resistance depends on the spontaneous mutation rate of tumor cells, the timing of a significant mutation relative to the tumor's growth, and the overall tumor burden. All biological systems have an inherent probability of undergoing genetic variation from random changes. These random changes may result in minor effects, no effect, or a mutation that alters the cell's characteristics and sensitivity to cytotoxic drugs. Neoplastic cells are genetically unstable and exhibit a high rate of mutation. If mutations occur early in the growth of a population of tumor cells, a high fraction of resistant cells would result. In contrast, a mutation occurring later would produce only a small fraction of resistant clones. If no resistant cells develop prior to treatment, then a cure would be probable with the appropriate chemotherapy. Cytotoxic therapy used to treat minimal tumor burden has a much greater likelihood of proving successful.

The Goldie-Coldman model provides a strong argument for the use of adjuvant and combination chemotherapy. Adjuvant chemotherapy is used in an attempt to eradicate undetectable or micro-metastatic tumor cells. If the probability of cure decreases as the number of tumor cells or the mutation rate increases, then eliminating all possible tumor cells or clones should induce a cure or a complete response. The model also supports the use of combination chemotherapy with non-cross-resistant drugs to potentially eliminate subpopulations of resistant tumor cells. The likelihood of a cell being resistant to two or more antineoplastic drugs simultaneously is less than that of it being resistant to single agents when used alone.[4]

## Multidrug resistance

Tumor cells exposed to antineoplastic drugs sometimes develop mechanisms to protect themselves against the drug's cytotoxic effect. Resistance may result from alterations in cytotoxic drug metabolism, alterations in cytotoxic targets, biochemical cofactor presence or absence, ability of cells to repair DNA lesions, or decreased intracellular drug concentrations. Multidrug resistance (MDR) is observed in tumor cells that exhibit resistance to a group of drugs that are structurally dissimilar, have unrelated cytotoxic mechanisms, or both. Such resistance usually develops intrinsically or is acquired following exposure to a particular drug in the group.[5] It may occur as a result of overexpression of the P-glycoprotein (P-gp) membrane efflux pump, enhancements of the glutathione detoxification pathway, or alterations in topoisomerase enzyme systems. The identification and further investigation of this type of resistance and strategies to prevent MDR will have broad clinical implications for the use of chemotherapy as a form of cancer treatment.

*P-glycoprotein (P-gp)–associated MDR.* The classic form of MDR is associated with overexpression of the *MDR-1* gene, which encodes for an energy-dependent cell membrane efflux pump, P-gp. This phenomenon was first described in tumor cells selected for resistance to dactinomycin that also exhibited resistance to vinca alkaloids, daunorubicin, and mitomycin.[5] The pump naturally functions to transport toxic molecules from inside the cell to the external environment, and P-gp is found in low concentrations in normal tissues, including the renal tubules, colon, small intestine, bile canaliculi, and vascular epithelia of the brain and spinal cord.[7] Cytotoxic drugs that have entered the cell probably bind to a carrier protein before reaching their cellular targets and are transported out of the cell via the pump.[8] The actual process of drug binding and exit from the cell is unknown. The list of drugs exhibiting P-gp-associated cross-resistance includes several natural products and an antimetabolite (Table 15-4).[5]

**TABLE 15-4**

**Chemotherapeutic Drugs Exhibiting Cross-Resistance in P-Glycoprotein-Associated Multidrug Resistance**

| |
|---|
| Dactinomycin |
| Daunorubicin |
| Doxorubicin |
| Etoposide |
| Mitomycin |
| Mitoxantrone |
| Paclitaxel |
| Trimetrexate |
| Vinblastine |
| Vincristine |

*Source*: Data from Shustik et al.[5]

Detection of the *MDR-1* gene product in the cells of tumors typically resistant to chemotherapy, such as colon, kidney, liver, and pancreas, further supports the importance of P-gp in chemotherapy failure.[9] The presence of the *MDR-1* phenotype and overexpression of P-gp have been found to be predictors of poor prognosis and shortened survival in patients with acute leukemias, multiple myeloma, and malignant lymphomas.[10,11]

Several non-cytotoxic compounds are known to reverse the P-gp-mediated efflux pump *in vitro*[12] (Table 15-5).

**TABLE 15-5**

**Drugs Exhibiting Reversal of P-Glycoprotein-Mediated Drug Resistance In Vitro**

| Pharmacological Activity | Drug | Derivative |
|---|---|---|
| Cardiovascular agent | Verapamil | Dexverapamil |
| Immunosuppressant | Cyclosporine | Valspodar (PSC 833) |
| Miscellaneous | Phenothiazines | |
| | Quinidine | |
| | Reserpine | |
| | Tamoxifen | |

*Source*: Data from Thomas and Coley.[12]

However, only a few have been evaluated in clinical trials,[13–16] and none of them have been brought to the bedside successfully. Some experts believe that most trials evaluating drug-resistance-modifying agents have not been designed to evaluate all the variables of successful treatment of tumors adequately.[17,18] These variables may include: What impact does P-gp-mediated drug resistance have on treatment failure for a specific tumor? Has P-gp overexpression been demonstrated in tumor cells of study patients? Does the resistance-modifying agent affect the pharmacokinetics or pharmacodynamic of the chemotherapeutic drug?

*Other mechanisms of MDR.* Another type of MDR has been described in cells that are cross-resistant to topoisomerase drugs such as etoposide, doxorubicin, daunorubicin, and topotecan. Although most of the drugs associated with this type of MDR are also associated with P-gp-mediated MDR, the pattern of resistance is different, and cells retain sensitivity to vinca alkaloids.[19] Resistance may be conferred by the ability of tumor cells to decrease the activity of or change the binding properties of topoisomerase enzymes. Tumor cells that have developed resistance to one type of topoisomerase II drug such as intercalators like doxorubicin, may not be resistant to an alternative type, such as epipodophyllotoxins (eg, etoposide). As a consequence, resistance may be overcome by using different types of topoisomerase II drugs.

Multidrug resistance also may be demonstrated in cells with increased detoxifying systems, such as glutathione *S*-transferase (GST) enzymes, and elevated glutathione levels.[20] These enzymes catalyze conjugation of electrophilic hydrophobic compounds and their metabolites, with glutathione, which facilitates elimination from the tumor cell. Alkylating agents, their metabolites, and platinum compounds are among the most frequent substrates of these enzymes. Strategies being investigated for reversing this type of resistance include administering inhibitors of GST and glutathione synthesis such as buthionine sulfoximine (BSO).[21] Further research is needed to determine the effects of BSO on chemotherapy response rates and duration before this modulator can be used in clinical practice.

## TUMOR CELL DEATH AND CYTOTOXIC DRUG RESISTANCE

Although drugs can have numerous effects on tumor cells, the critical molecular mechanisms leading to cell death have never been clearly elucidated. For half a century, the classic belief of anticancer drug action has held that cell death is a direct consequence of a specific interaction between a cytotoxic drug and its molecular target. The last 20 years have brought a new understanding of the molecular mechanisms controlling cell cycle and programmed cell death (apoptosis). This has prompted a reexamination of the classic model of cytotoxic drug–induced cell death. Specific cytotoxic drug–target interactions are now believed to stimulate a pathway that eventually results in apoptosis. This pathway most likely involves processes or sensors that can detect an apoptotic signal, a signal-transduction network, and cell machinery that brings about cell death.[22] This pathway is complex and highly dependent on the cell type, the anticancer agent, and the drug–target interaction environment.

### *p53* and cell cycling

Cells that are undergoing replication enter the cell cycle and progress through the four phases of the cycle, resulting in the formation of two identical daughter cells. Checkpoints along the cycle ensure that DNA is undamaged before the cell is allowed to enter into DNA synthesis (S phase). The regulator protein that provides a checkpoint for cells with undamaged DNA is known as p53.[23] When cells with damaged DNA enter the cell cycle, those with nonmutated *p53* genes will be prevented from entering S phase and instead undergo apoptosis. The ability of certain tumor cells to resist or overcome the cytotoxic effects of chemotherapy is believed to result from specific mechanisms possessed by the cell and unique to a drug. Resistance is now considered more directly linked to abnormalities in the cells' genetic machinery or to alterations in critical pathways of cell-cycle control and apoptosis. In the clinical setting, support for this theory may be observed by examining the failure to overcome drug resistance when only the classic biochemical or molecular approaches to resistance are employed.

Sensitive cancer cells are killed initially in response to effective cytotoxic chemotherapy; if they survive, however, they develop resistance to further treatment. Mutations in their DNA result in dysregulation of the genetic machinery and signaling pathways that control cell cycling and apoptosis. Mutations in the *p53* gene are among the most common genetic changes observed in tumor cells and may occur in at least 50% of all human tumors.[24] p53 is a tumor-suppressor protein and critical transcriptional activator that causes both $G_1$ and $G_2$ arrest of the cell cycle and is a potent inducer of apoptosis in cells exposed to DNA-damaging drugs.[25,26] Resistance to both radiation therapy and a wide array of chemotherapy drugs has been demonstrated in *in vivo* models.[27,28] However, not all cells with *p53* mutations are resistant to various antitumor agents, thereby indicating that other factors play a role, such as the cytotoxic stimuli, differences in the overall genetic machinery, and intracellular signaling pathways.[29] An intact *p53* gene maintains the cell's genetic stability and, following exposure to DNA-damaging agents, will lead to apoptosis for the tumor cell, whereas the normal cell survives. When *p53* function is lost, the tumor cell's genomic stability decreases, the cell survives the apoptotic stimuli, and the disease progresses. The presence of a *p53* mutation usually indicates a poorer prognosis, although it does not always correlate with the ability to cure or not cure a cancer.[25]

Loss of mutation in *p53* has been found in a number of solid tumors and in chronic lymphocytic leukemia. Similarly, patients with advanced breast cancer who exhibited a poor response to doxorubicin chemotherapy and were more likely to relapse also were more likely to have *p53* gene mutations.[30] Poor responses to cisplatin chemotherapy and shorter disease-free survival were observed in 60% of patients with ovarian cancer who had inactivation of the *p53* gene. Other solid tumors with abnormal *p53* expression that show a reduced response to chemotherapy and radiation therapy include non-small cell lung cancer, gastric cancer, and colorectal cancers.[31,32] *p53* status was the strongest prognostic factor for survival in a multivariate analysis conducted in patients with B-cell chronic lymphocytic leukemia.[33]

### Other cell-cycle regulators

*p53* influences the transcriptional activation of a number of genes that are known to regulate cell-cycle checkpoint control. The cyclin-dependent kinases, when *p53* is fully active, act on other tumor suppressors to inhibit the cell from entering the S phase. The *MDR-1* gene also has been shown to be potentially influenced by *p53*. Wild-type (nonmutated) *p53* suppresses the promoter of the *MDR-1* gene, whereas the mutant protein can stimulate the promoter.[34,35]

Disregulation of the *p53* pathway leading to overproduction of gene products responsible for the cell's entry into S phase and rapid cell growth may be a significant mechanism of cytotoxic drug resistance. Resistance could be further suppressed through stimulation of the *MDR-1* gene directly by mutant *p53*.[22] Therefore, the spontaneous development of resistance and the development of MDR appear to be related more to mutations in key genes in the cell-cycle checkpoint control than to drug-specific mutations. Avoiding or reversing these genetic and molecular changes may provide an effective approach to preventing and reversing cytotoxic drug resistance.

BCL-2 and BAX are members of a large family of related proteins that control the cell's end result to enter apoptosis. The ratio of these proteins appears to be the critical determinant of whether a cell undergoes apoptosis. The BCL-2 protein blocks apoptosis, and elevated levels of it are associated with resistance to vincristine, methotrexate, fluorouracil, hydroxyurea, and cisplatin.[36] BCL-2 also can block apoptosis even in the presence of tumors with high levels of *p53* expression, which is known to promote apoptosis. Conversely, the BAX protein urges the cell to enter apoptosis and is associated with increased chemosensitivity to paclitaxel, vincristine, and doxorubicin.[37] Most of the research on ways to enhance chemosensitivity related to BCL-2 and BAX is being conducted *in vitro*. The sequencing of chemotherapy drugs to increase the phosphorylation of BCL-2 has been suggested as a way to optimize apoptosis.[38]

## CHEMOTHERAPY AS A TREATMENT FOR CANCER

### PRIMARY AND ADJUVANT CHEMOTHERAPY

Chemotherapy is considered primary treatment for cancers for which no effective alternative treatment is available or when the alternative treatment is less than optimal. *Induction* is a term used commonly to describe chemotherapy given to patients with leukemia or other advanced disease that is highly sensitive to drugs. *Neoadjuvant chemotherapy* is given prior to the standard primary therapeutic approach—usually surgery—in patients who present with locally advanced disease. Preserving organ structure and function in some tumors of the lung, colon, larynx, or breast is most appropriate for this type of cytoreductive chemotherapeutic approach. Chemotherapy given concurrently, instead of sequentially, with radiation therapy is another popular way of combining effective methods to control and potentially eradicate disease. Cancers of the head and neck are often treated in this way.

*Adjuvant* therapy is therapy following the primary treatment modality, such as surgery or radiation therapy. Adjuvant chemotherapy is a routine part of treatment for early stages of cancers of the breast, colon, and lung (non-small cell). Systemic therapy is usually given following surgical resection of the primary tumor with the intent of improving the potential for cure. Although effective chemotherapy theoretically would eradicate clinically undetected and micrometastatic disease, the overall effect on tumor recurrence has been less than dramatic for cancers of the colon and rectum. More success has been realized in patients with node-positive breast cancer.[39]

### THERAPEUTIC STRATEGIES

#### Combination chemotherapy

Administering a combination of clinically effective anticancer drugs is the standard approach for most malignancies. Although individually the drugs are biochemically and clinically active, they are rarely used alone as single agents outside metastatic disease. Combination chemotherapy was first applied with success in the treatment of leukemias and lymphomas. The objectives of combination chemotherapy are to achieve maximal tumor cell kill without excessive toxicity, to provide cytotoxic drugs that are active against

**TABLE 15-6**

**Principles for Selection of Antineoplastic Drugs for Combination Chemotherapy Regimens**

1. Choose drugs with single-agent activity. Drugs producing complete responses are preferred.
2. Avoid drugs with overlapping toxicities.
3. Administer drugs at their optimal dose and schedule as previously determined by clinical trials.
4. Give chemotherapy at regular intervals (cycles), and minimize the time between cycles.

potentially resistant heterogeneous tumor populations, and to avoid selection of resistant cell lines. Table 15-6 delineates the principles by which antineoplastic drugs are usually chosen for combination regimens.

When overlapping toxicities are unavoidable, as is often the case with marrow-suppressive drugs, administration of reduced doses or longer intervals between treatments may be necessary. Recovery time for normal tissues is typically used to determine the retreatment or cycle time. The time for the bone marrow to reach its nadir (lowest counts) and recover differs depending on which drugs are administered. Nadir and recovery periods are critical for determining the length of a treatment cycle. Therefore, chemotherapy cycles for drugs with significant myelosuppression are approximately 3 to 4 weeks. The duration or cycles administered are usually based on the response rate or a predetermined number obtained from clinical trials.

*Dose intensity.* Delivering a sufficient amount of drug over a specified period of time is of great importance in curing chemotherapy-sensitive malignancies. However, many factors may prevent the proper dose from being delivered, such as the necessity for a dose reduction or a delay in treatment because of unacceptable toxicity. Although dose reductions as small as 20% do not affect clinical response rates for most drug-sensitive tumors, curative potential may be lost. Decreasing the dose or adjusting the schedule of treatment may explain the failure of chemotherapy to cure drug-sensitive cancers.

The concept of dose intensity has been developed to assist the researcher and clinician in evaluating the effects that these changes in doses have on treatment outcomes. Dose intensity is expressed as the amount of drug delivered per unit of time (mg/m$^2$/week). The effect of a new regimen on treatment outcome can be expressed as the relative dose intensity (RDI), which is calculated by dividing the dose intensity of a test regimen by that of a standard regimen. This calculation is done for a single drug, or an average is calculated for all drugs in a regimen. The effects of dose reductions or treatment delays are best evaluated when dose intensity is based on actual or received doses instead of intended or protocol doses.

The dose intensity has been applied to a number of diseases to improve response rates. Increasing the dose has improved outcomes in lymphomas and advanced tumors of the breast, colon, and ovary.[40] Of particular interest is the demonstrated improvement in disease-free survival and overall survival with dose-dense adjuvant treatment of node-positive breast cancer.[39] Chemotherapy was given on an every-2-week schedule with hematopoietic support. High-dose chemotherapy with hematopoietic stem cell support also provides a way to administer larger doses of potentially curative therapy.

### Chemotherapy and radiotherapy protectants

Antineoplastic drugs are among the most toxic compounds administered to humans. Some toxicities, such as nausea, vomiting, mucositis, alopecia, and fatigue, affect quality of life but are rarely life-threatening. Bone marrow suppression is both common and potentially life-threatening, it is dose dependent and can be managed by reducing doses, delaying therapy, or administering hematopoietic growth factors. Prior to the introduction of drugs that increase white blood cells, including filgrastim and sargramostim, the only way to avoid life-threatening and fatal leukopenia was to reduce the chemotherapy dose or delay treatment. Filgrastim and sargramostim may be administered with the first cycle (primary prophylaxis) or subsequent cycles (secondary treatment). These drugs have been successful in reducing the time to nadir, length of nadir, and hospitalizations for febrile neutropenia.[41,42]

Several cytotoxic drugs are known to induce other life-threatening toxicities and permanent cellular injury, including kidney failure, neuropathies, and congestive heart failure. Chemoprotective and rescue agents have been developed and are under investigation for use in preventing or reversing drug-induced toxicity for selected anticancer agents, including cisplatin, cyclophosphamide, doxorubicin, ifosfamide, methotrexate, and paclitaxel. Availability of these compounds has permitted expanded clinical development and utilization of the anticancer drugs whose toxicity they ameliorate. Unfortunately, these drugs may have significant side effects of their own. Some may negatively affect the cytotoxicity of the chemotherapy, add significant cost to the treatment, or both. The American Society of Clinical Oncology (ASCO) has established guidelines for the appropriate use of chemoprotective and radioprotective drugs based on scientific evidence.[43] Table 15-7 lists currently available agents along with ASCO clinical guidelines for use, proposed mechanisms of action, and toxicities.

### High-dose chemotherapy with peripheral blood stem cell support

High-dose chemotherapy with autologous rescue (use of the patient's own peripheral blood stem cells) is considered

**TABLE 15-7**

**American Society of Clinical Oncology (ASCO) Guidelines for Use of Chemoprotective and Radioprotective Agents**

| Chemoprotective Agent | Protective Mechanism | Adverse Effects | ASCO Clinical Practice Guidelines for Use (Toxicity-, Drug-, or Disease-Based Recommendation) |
|---|---|---|---|
| Amifostine (Ethyol) | Reduces DNA damage in renal and neurological tissues | Hypotension, nausea, and vomiting | 1. Nephrotoxicity: *Consider in patients receiving cisplatin-based chemotherapy.*<br>2. Neutropenia (alkylating agents): *Alternative to dose reduction or growth factor use.*<br>3. Neurotoxicity: *Insufficient data to recommend routine use in cisplatin- or paclitaxel-induced effects.*<br>4. Thrombocytopenia: *Insufficient data to recommend use.*<br>5. Radiation-induced xerostomia: *Consider in patients undergoing fractionated radiation of the head and neck region. (Do not recommend for reduction of mucositis.)* |
| Dexrazoxane (Zinecard) | Inhibits free-radical formation in cardiac tissue | Myelosuppression, nausea and vomiting | 1. Metastatic breast cancer:<br>a. *Routine use is not recommended in patients receiving initial anthracycline chemotherapy.*<br>b. *Consider in patients who have received cumulative dose of ≥300 mg/m² of doxorubicin.*<br>2. Other tumors: *Consider in adults who have received >300 mg/m² of doxorubicin. Caution should be used if chemotherapy is known to improve survival (dexrazoxane may alter tumor-protective effects).*<br>3. Adjuvant chemotherapy: *Not recommended outside clinical trials.*<br>4. Pediatric tumors: *Insufficient evidence to recommend use with epirubicin-based regimens.* |
| Mesna (Mesnex) | Binds toxic metabolites in bladder | Nausea, vomiting, and hypersensitivity | 1. Ifosfamide chemotherapy: *Using standard doses, recommended for routine use to reduce urothelial toxicity.*<br>2. High-dose ifosfamide: *Insufficient evidence to establish guidelines for use with ifosfamide > 2.5 g/m² per day.*<br>3. High-dose cyclophosphamide: *Alternative to forced saline diuresis in stem cell transplant setting.* |

*Source:* Data from Schuchter et al.[42]

standard of care for several malignancies, including selected leukemias and lymphomas, as well as multiple myeloma.[44] This complex therapy, once available only at select treatment centers, is now available at most major medical centers and many large community hospitals. Reasons for the expansion of this form of cancer treatment include its curative potential, more experience with administering and managing this type of therapy, and advancements in supportive care for patients. The introduction of hematopoietic growth factors (HGFs), such as G-CSF (filgrastim) and GM-CSF (sargramostim), has been among the major advancements in supportive-care measures. Their availability has allowed for harvesting of hematopoietic stem cells from peripheral blood—in most situations avoiding costly and painful bone marrow harvesting. Peripheral blood stem cells (PBSCs) are committed progenitor cells existing in circulating blood that have the capacity to restore hematopoiesis.

Before receiving marrow-ablative chemotherapy, patients are given HGFs with or without chemotherapy—typically cyclophosphamide—to mobilize stem cells into the peripheral blood from the bone marrow.[45] Patients then undergo leukopheresis to remove mobilized stem cells from the peripheral blood. Leukopheresis may be performed two to six times to collect an adequate number of cells. Following high-dose chemotherapy, radiation therapy, or both—a course intended to eradicate the cancer cells and hence the bone marrow stem cells—the patient's PBSCs are reinfused. As with other forms of hematopoietic cell transplantation, infused stem cells migrate to the bone marrow and engraft. Patients who receive PBSCs typically experience fewer days of neutropenia and thrombocytopenia compared with patients who received bone marrow transplantation.

Major disadvantages of PBSC transplantation include nausea, vomiting, hypertension, hemoglobinuria, and the potential for hypersensitivity reactions associated with infusion of the large amounts of the cryopreservative dimethyl sulfoxide (DMSO) and the large volume of PBSCs.[46] Another concern is the potential to reinfuse mobilized tumor cells as well as hematopoietic stem cells. The monoclonal antibody rituximab has been used successfully to reduce the potential for recurrence following autologous PBSC transplantation. Rituximab alone or in combination with cytotoxic chemotherapy significantly depletes B cells in vivo, reducing the potential of tumor recurrence in patients treated with autologous.stem cell transplantation for follicular or mantle cell lymphoma.[44,47]

### Chemotherapy as a radiation sensitizer

The concomitant use of chemotherapy and radiation therapy has received significant attention in the literature.[48,49] The primary goal of combined-modality treatment is to increase the effectiveness of radiation and improve local–regional control of disease. A number of theoretical considerations may explain the improved results seen when chemotherapy and radiation are given concomitantly for specific tumors. The modalities affect different tumor cell subpopulations; therefore, their combined use may better eradicate otherwise resistant cells. Tumor cell regrowth following radiation therapy is slowed by the addition of chemotherapy, and cells undergoing growth are more vulnerable to the cytotoxic effects of chemotherapy. The cytoreductive effects of chemotherapy improve tumor oxygen supply, resulting in an increased susceptibility to radiation effects. In addition, direct interaction of the combined modalities, as yet undefined, may explain the improved response seen especially at a local–regional level. A *positive interaction* is defined as enhanced radiation effects in tumor cells and less observed toxicity. Significant improvement in quality of life may be achieved by using combined-modality regimens to preserve organs affected by neoplasms of the larynx, anal canal, bladder, and esophagus.[50,51]

Several large randomized trials have demonstrated that concomitant chemotherapy and radiation therapy resulted in improved survival in patients with head and neck tumors. Fluorouracil alone or in combination with cisplatin or carboplatin has been most often with added to fractionated or standard radiation therapy. Unfortunately, concomitant therapy is often accompanied by more severe treatment-related toxicity. Three cycles of fluorouracil and carboplatin along with fractionated radiation improved local–regional control, disease-free survival, and survival in patients with squamous cell carcinoma of the oropharynx.[52] A second trial also using concomitant fluorouracil and carboplatin in more advanced oropharyngeal carcinoma resulted in significantly improved 2-year disease-free survival but not overall survival for patients receiving both radiation and chemotherapy.[53] Most concomitant-therapy trials use a combination of fluorouracil and cisplatin. Patients with squamous cell carcinoma treated with a combination of fluorouracil and cisplatin along with fractionated radiation therapy had better local control and improved distant metastatic-free survival than those who were treated with radiation alone.[54] However, those receiving the chemotherapy were more likely to require feeding tubes because of the severity of mucositis. Another trial using cisplatin alone with hyperfactionated radiotherapy demonstrated improved local–regional control, relapse-free survival, and overall survival compared with radiation therapy alone.[55] Rates of leukopenia, thrombocytopenia, and hospitalization for acute toxicity also were higher in patients who received concomitant cisplatin. Patients with head and neck cancers, especially of the nasopharyngeal type, benefit from definitive radiation therapy and concomitant chemotherapy. They do so, however, not without experiencing several harsh toxicities and a decline in quality of life. The optimal combination of these two modalities remains unclear and needs to be further defined in prospective, randomized trials.

### Modulation of fluorouracil by leucovorin

Leucovorin, or folinic acid, has been developed primarily as an antidote for antifolate therapy. Another major role of leucovorin is found in its ability to modulate the cytotoxicity of fluorouracil. Although fluorouracil is the most active antineoplastic drug in cancers of the gastrointestinal tract, its ability to control progression is modest. For this reason, investigators have sought to enhance the drug's efficacy in an attempt to better control and potentially cure these cancers. In the presence of increased folate pools, the active form of fluorouracil binds more tightly to the target enzyme.[56]

The interaction of leucovorin and fluorouracil was studied in more than 650 patients, with significantly improved response rates seen with the combination compared with fluorouracil alone.[57] The optimal dose and schedule of leucovorin and fluorouracil have not been determined. However, a frequently employed schedule gives the leucovorin over 2-hours and a bolus of fluorouracil after 1 hour of the leucovorin infusion. Other drugs that have been tested but have failed as biochemical modulators of fluorouracil include methotrexate, *N*-(phosphonacetyl)-L-aspartate (PALA) and alpha interferon.

Recently, the FDA approved levoleucovorin, the pharmacologically active levo isomere of leucovorin. Levoleucovorin is dosed at one half that of racemic mixture, and is approved for reducing the systemic toxicity of antifolate therapy overdose or impaired elimination following high-dose methotrexate in osteosarcoma. Currently, levoleucovorin does not seem to offer any significant benefit over the standard racemic form of leucovorin.

## PHARMACOLOGY OF CHEMOTHERAPEUTIC DRUGS

Most drugs used to treat cancer are unique compared with drugs used to treat other illnesses such as cardiac disease, gastrointestinal disease, or neurological problems. The primary pharmacological outcome is usually cell death. Tumor cells are the intended targets; however, similarities between normal cells and tumor cells often result in destruction of healthy tissues as well as malignant cells. Understanding the pharmacology of these agents can help the researcher and clinician in optimally designing the most effective and least toxic single- and multiple-drug regimens.

The basic pharmacological principles of drugs used to treat cancer will be reviewed in this section. An explanation of the principles of pharmacokinetics and how they are applied in chemotherapy is followed by a detailed description of probable and potential drug interactions. The final parts of this section constitute an overview of the diverse pharmacological and mechanistic groups of anticancer drugs highlighting key features of individual drugs or drug classes.

## PHARMACOKINETICS OF ANTINEOPLASTIC DRUGS

*Pharmacokinetics* is the study of the movement of drugs in the body. The process may differ individually and is most closely related to the physical and chemical properties of the compound. The physical and chemical individuality of the patient and the tumor type also play an important role in determining pharmacokinetic outcomes.

### Principles of pharmacokinetics

Several parameters have been used to describe the pharmacokinetics of drugs. The serum *half-life* is the time required for the serum concentration of the drug to decrease by one-half. Knowing the half-life of a chemotherapeutic drug is of greatest interest when trying to determine the time required for elimination of an administered dose. This time period is equal to three to four half-lives of the drug.

*Clearance* is determined by blood flow to an organ, usually the kidney or liver, and the organ's efficacy in extracting the drug from the blood. If a drug is cleared from the body by more than one organ, then the total clearance is the sum of the individual clearances of the extracting organs. This pharmacokinetic parameter determines the drug's steady-state concentration and is independent of half-life. Clearance may be altered by changes in blood flow to an organ, by enzyme function, and by protein binding. For example, cyclophosphamide is highly dependent on metabolizing enzymes for activation and inactivation. Therefore, induction or inhibition of these enzymes may cause a more rapid or slower clearance of the drug.

The *volume of distribution* $V_D$ relates the amount of drug in the body to the serum concentration. This parameter differs among individuals and is a function of the drug's protein-binding capabilities and its ability to distribute to extravascular compartments (tissue binding). Changes in protein binding caused by either hypoalbuminemia or interactions with other drugs may alter the removal of highly protein-bound drugs such as etoposide or teniposide.

Variability in a drug's pharmacokinetic parameters may help to explain the differences in response and toxicity seen among patients treated with similar doses and schedules of the same chemotherapy. The basic principles of clinical pharmacokinetics may be divided into four major areas: absorption, distribution, metabolism, and elimination.

*Absorption.* Absorption from the gastrointestinal tract should be sufficient to ensure adequate bioavailability of the drug. Because the bioavailability of most anticancer drugs is poor and unpredictable, these agents are usually given parenterally to ensure accurate dosing and optimal systemic exposure. Drugs administered orally for cancer treatment include alkylating agents (eg, cyclophosphamide, chlorambucil, and melphalan), etoposide, lomustine, methotrexate, and procarbazine. Although oral absorption is less than optimal for some of these drugs, the amount that reaches systemic circulation and—more important—the tumor is sufficient to produce a response. Some drugs are available as a prodrug that is readily absorbed from the gastrointestinal tract and then converted in the body to an active cytotoxic compound. Capecitabine and temozolamide are examples of orally administered prodrugs that are transformed in vivo to biochemically equivalent forms of fluorouracil and dacarbazine, respectively.

*Distribution.* Distribution of drugs in the body is determined primarily by their ability to penetrate different tissues and their affinity for binding to plasma proteins. Drugs that are highly lipophilic tend to be more readily taken up by lipophilic tissues such as fat, bone marrow, and the central nervous system. Nitrosoureas such as carmustine and lomustine are useful for brain and hematopoietic malignancies because they readily penetrate the blood–brain barrier and bone marrow, respectively. Decreased levels of plasma proteins, especially albumin, often occur in patients with cancer. This situation may be the result of nutritional deficiencies or decreased hepatic synthesis of albumin. The cytotoxic activity of highly protein-bound chemotherapy drugs such as etoposide and teniposide may be enhanced in these patients because a greater percentage of the drug is unbound in the blood. An increase in the unbound fraction of a drug can also occur if two highly bound drugs are administered concurrently, such as etoposide with phenytoin or warfarin. Methotrexate abnormally distributes in ascites and pleural effusions, delaying clearance and enhancing hematological and mucosal toxicity.

*Metabolism.* The metabolic activation and inactivation, or catabolism, of drugs is carried out primarily by the liver. Some of these enzymatic processes are also performed in normal and tumor cells. Several chemotherapy drugs require activation systemically or intracellularly before they can

**TABLE 15-8**

**Chemotherapy Drugs That Depend on Hepatic Metabolism for Activation and Clearance From the Body**

| Chemotherapy Drug | Activation | Clearance |
|---|---|---|
| Anthracycline antibiotics | × | × |
| Capecitabine | × | × |
| Cyclophosphamide | × | × |
| Dacarbazine | × | × |
| Hexamethylmelamine | | × |
| Ifosfamide | × | |
| Ixabepilone | | × |
| Nitrosoureas | | × |
| Carmustine | | |
| Lomustine | | |
| Procarbazine | × | |
| Temozolomide | × | × |

exert their cytotoxic effects (Table 15-8). Antimetabolites such as fluorouracil and cytarabine are phosphorylated to active nucleotides in tumor cells. Cisplatin undergoes a chemical aquation or complexation with water molecules intracellularly, which generates a positively charged species that, in turn, forms adducts with DNA molecules. Cyclophosphamide and ifosfamide are transformed by hepatic microsomal enzymes into active alkylating species. Some chemotherapeutic drugs are metabolized to inactive compounds, which are then excreted by the body. The rate of metabolic conversion may be affected by a number of factors, including hepatic dysfunction (either drug-induced or tumor-induced), genetic differences in drug metabolism, or drug-induced changes in functioning of enzymes (drug interactions). Changes in liver function or metabolic enzymes may result in decreased cytotoxic activity, increased treatment-related toxicity, or both.

The cyctochrome P450 (CYP) family of microsomal enzymes is primarily responsible for the activation, degradation, or both of most therapeutic agents. The CYP subfamily, symbolized as CYP 3A4, is involved in the metabolism of several anticancer drugs, including anthracyclines, epipodophyllotoxins, ifosfamide, taxanes, and vinca alkyloids.[57] Cyclophosphamide is activated by another enzyme subfamily, CYP 2B6 and is highly inducible by antiepileptic drugs including phenobarbital and phenytoin. Genetic polymorphism exists in several CYP enzyme subfamilies, including CYP 2D6 and CYP 1A2. Three genetically distinct groups of metabolizers have been identified within the CYP 2D6 iso-enzyme group: extensive, poor, and ultrarapid metabolizers.[59] Most individuals are extensive metabolizers, but poor metabolizers make up 5% to 10% of the Caucasian population and only 1% to 2% of the Asian populations and African Americans.[59] The CYP 2D6 group metabolizes several opiate narcotics, antidepressants, and beta-blocker drugs but not any anticancer drugs known at this time; however, doxorubicin and vinblastine can competitively inhibit CYP 2D6 potentially causing a narcotic overdose.[58] Table 15-9 lists drugs known to alter microsomal enzymes and potentially affect antineoplastic drug disposition.

**TABLE 15-9**

**Drugs Known to Enhance or Inhibit CYP 3A Microsomal Enzyme Subfamily**

| Enhance | Inhibit |
|---|---|
| Cyclophosphamide[a] | Cimetidine |
| Phenobarbital | Cyclosporine |
| Phenytoin | Alfa-interferon |
| Rifampin | Ketoconazole |
| | Verapamil |
| | Aprepitant |

[a]Enhances CYP 2B6.

*Elimination.* The kidneys are primarily responsible for elimination of drugs and drug metabolites from the body. A number of anticancer drugs are highly dependent on renal function for their elimination. As a consequence, significant decreases in renal function can decrease their clearance from the body and cause excessive toxicity (Table 15-10). Cisplatin and methotrexate are both eliminated primarily by the kidneys and are nephrotoxic themselves; therefore, decreased renal function may produce enhanced toxicity and a further decline in renal function. The biliary tract is the primary route of elimination of vinca alkaloids.

## Pharmacogenomics

Some of the variability in pharmacokinetics and pharmacodynamics among patients can be explained by genetic polymorphism. Inherited differences in drug disposition and effects has been termed *pharmacogenomics* by McLeod

**TABLE 15-10**

**Chemotherapeutic Agents Requiring Dose Modification in Patients With Renal Insufficiency**

| | |
|---|---|
| Bleomycin | Cyclophosphamide |
| Carboplatin | Etoposide |
| Cisplatin | Methotrexate |
| Oxaliplatin | Streptozocin |
| | Pemetrexed |

and Evans.[60] Growing knowledge of the human genome has led the way to a better understanding and identification of nucleotide polymorphisms. Among the CYP family of microsomal enzymes, significant polymorphisms have been identified for the CYP 3A4, -2C9, and -2D6 iso-enzymes.[61]

Currently, there are only a few examples of drug-metabolizing enzyme polymorphisms with clinical applications in the area of oncology. Thiopurine-*S*-methyltransferase deficiency is inherited and confers severe intolerance to thiopurine therapy.[62] Another well-described polymorphism is a deficiency in dihydropyrimidine dehydrohenase (DPD), the rate-limiting enzyme that catabilizes fluorouracil.[63] Patients with DPD deficiency may experience severe and sometimes fatal toxicity after receiving standard doses of fluorouracil. There is now a commercially available blood test to detect DPD deficiency that can identify affected patients. These patients may be spared from receiving a pharmacologic overdose of fluorouracil. However, the broad application of this costly test would benefit only a small portion of patients.

Genetic polymorphism is not limited to describing pharmacokinetic variability but also describes pharmacodynamic differences. Tamoxifen is an antiestrogen used to reduce the risk of recurrence of breast cancer in both the adjuvant and metastatic settings. The CYP 2D6 enzyme is involved in the biotransformation of tamoxifen to its active metabolite endoxifen. There is significant genetic polymorphism of CYP 2D6, resulting in patients being poor, intermediate, or extensive metabolizers.[61] There are data now to suggest that poor metabolizers have an approximately threefold higher relative risk of breast cancer recurrence than those who are extensive metabolizers.[64] Although the data were from a retrospective analysis, they may be useful for individualization of endocrine therapy and potentially predict which patients may not benefit from tamoxifen therapy. Patients receiving concomitant drugs that are known inhibitors of CYP 2D6, such as some antidepressants (paroxetine), also may be at risk for disease recurrence because of the reduced metabolic activation of tamoxifen.

The science of pharmacogenomics will continue to expand as more studies are conducted to explain inherited differences in pharmacokinetics and pharmacodynamics among humans. These data will further contribute to our understanding of how cytotoxic drugs work and behave in patients with cancer.

## Pharmacokinetic principles applied to chemotherapeutic drugs

Chemotherapeutic drugs must reach their target site to exert their antineoplastic effects. Often targets are intracellular structures or molecules such as DNA, enzymes, and microtubules. Adequate blood supply to tumor cells is necessary for optimal delivery of chemotherapy to the drug's site of action. Then, once in the tumor microenvironment, the drug must be transported intracellularly via passive, facilitated, or active transport mechanisms. Transport mechanisms may either facilitate drug entry into the cell or hasten the drug's removal. As mentioned previously, efflux from the cell may be a major limitation of antineoplastic drug efficacy.

Systemic drug exposure is also an important parameter in ensuring the optimal cytotoxic response and minimal toxicity. The area under the serum concentration–time curve (AUC) is a measure of systemic drug exposure. Because the AUC depends on drug administration and elimination, changes in these parameters may greatly affect therapeutic outcome. Patients with a more rapid drug clearance may need larger doses than those with a slower clearance.The dose for carboplatin is usually calculated using a target AUC and the patient's individualized renal function to predict the optimal dose to be administered.

Traditionally, chemotherapy drugs are dosed based on the weight and height (body surface area [BSA]) or weight alone of the patient. Modern therapeutics emphasizes individualization of treatment regimens in an attempt to maximize therapeutic efficacy while minimizing adverse drug effects. To achieve a more individualized dosing strategy, a drug must possess specific pharmacokinetic and pharmacodynamic characteristics that can be represented by a formula that is used to calculate the optimal dose. Carboplatin is a cytotoxic drug that exhibits these principles and provides characteristics that allow the application of a nonstandard dosing approach. Carboplatin is eliminated extensively by the kidneys, and its clearance is closely correlated with the glomerular filtration rate (GFR).[64] This relatively simple kinetic model for carboplatin suggests that the therapeutic efficacy and toxicity can be explained by an area under the concentration–time curve. Therefore, dose administered and the GFR of the patient will predict the therapeutic efficacy and toxicity of carboplatin. This allows the dose of carboplatin to be adjusted based primarily on renal function and not BSA. The major hematological toxicity of carboplatin is thrombocytopenia. Unbound or free platinum AUC following a dose of carboplatin has been correlated with the thrombocytopenia nadir observed.[65] Impaired renal function is associated with more thrombocytopenia.[66] Calvert and colleagues reported on their experiences using a simple formula that is now known as the *Calvert formula* (Table 15-11) to determine carboplatin doses based on pretreatment GFR.[67] Their results suggested that a carboplatin AUC can be predicted using the Calvert formula in which the only variable is renal function. This dosing strategy avoids overdosing in patients with impaired renal function and maximizes carboplatin exposure in patients with above-average renal function who otherwise may have been underdosed.

The Calvert formula is applied widely for dosing carboplatin in adult patients with ovarian, lung, and other solid tumors. The original trial used a measured GFR that was based on $^{51}$Cr-EDTA clearance.[68] However, most

**TABLE 15-11**

**Equations Used to Calculate Creatinine Clearance and Carboplatin Dose**

| | Formula | Conditions | Equation |
|---|---|---|---|
| **Estimation of creatinine clearance, CrCl (mL/min)** | Cockcroft-Gault, modified[69] | Adult, stable renal function, "not obese"<br>For children:<br>≤1 year: (0.45 × length)/serum creatinine<br>1–20 years: (0.55 × length)/serum creatinine | Estimated CrCl = [(140—age) actual wt]/(72 × $S_{cr}$)[a]<br>Female: Multiply result by 0.85 |
| | Jelliffe[70] | Adult, stable renal function, "not obese"<br>To adjust for BSA, multiply by (BSA/1.73) | {98—[0.8 × (age—20)]}/$S_{cr}$ [a]<br>Female: Multiply result by 0.9 |
| **Dose of carboplatin based on AUC** | Calvert formula[68] | Target AUC = 5–7 for single-agent carboplatin; 4–5 for carboplatin with other myelosuppressive drugs<br>Estimated CrCl used for GFR may underestimate dose | Carboplatin dose = AUC × (GFR + 25)[b] |

[a]Age (years); wt, weight (kg); $S_{cr}$, serum creatinine (mg/dL).
[b]AUC, area under the curve (mg/mL × min); GFR, glomerular filtration rate (mL/min).

clinical applications of the Calvert formula substitute a creatinine clearance for the GFR. Creatinine clearance can be measured using a 24-hour urinary collection method, but more commonly, it is calculated using either the Cockcroft-Gault[69] or Jelliffe[70] methods (see Table 15-11). The Cockroft-Gault method is the more popular of the two methods, but all protocols for the Gynecology Oncology Group use the Jelliffe method.

Pharmacokinetic parameters should be applied routinely in clinical practice to assist in delivering the optimal dose with the least risk of serious toxicity. Interpatient variability always should be considered when evaluating therapeutic or toxic response to therapy.

## DRUG INTERACTIONS IN THE PATIENT RECEIVING CHEMOTHERAPY

A drug interaction occurs when the effects of one drug—whether therapeutic or toxic—are modified by the presence of another drug. Most of these interactions are the result of changes in the pharmacokinetics of the affected drug (object drug) induced by an interacting drug (precipitating drug). Changes in the object drug's metabolism, distribution, and elimination are most commonly the cause for the changes observed in pharmacokinetic parameters. However, a smaller number of interactions are the consequence of overlapping toxicities, such as myelosuppression or gastrointestinal intolerance. Interactions may result in a beneficial effect, such as improving therapeutic response or preventing or ameliorating toxicity. However, most of these interactions produce undesirable outcomes, such as suboptimal therapeutic response or enhanced adverse effects. Tables 15-12[58,71–80] and 15-13[71,81–84] list selected clinically significant drug interactions in patients undergoing cancer chemotherapy.

Not all drug interactions result in clinically significant or toxic outcomes. Indeed, most interactions occur only under specific pharmacologic and physiologic situations; therefore, drug interactions should be judged by their overall effect on therapeutic response and patient care. Consideration also should be given to the mechanism behind the changes in pharmacokinetics, pharmacodynamics, or both. Cyclosporine and calcium channel blockers such as verapamil are potent inhibitors of metabolic enzymes (CYP 3A4) responsible for the elimination of doxorubicin and etoposide. However, cyclosporine and verapamil are also inhibitors of the P-gp-mediated drug resistance for natural products including these same chemotherapy drugs.[58] Therefore, the overall therapeutic response or toxicity experienced is a result of both mechanisms.

The potential for serious interaction increases with the number of drugs a patient receives. The incidence of all types of drug interactions has been estimated to be between 3% and 5% in patients taking a few drugs to as high as 20% in hospitalized patients taking 10 to 20 medications.[85] Because most patients with cancer receive drugs for cancer treatment, supportive-care, and conceivably pain-management, the potential for drug interactions is relatively high. Concurrent administration of drugs with steep dose–response curves and narrow therapeutic indices further increases the chance of toxic outcomes. Up to 27%

**TABLE 15-12**

**Selected Clinically Significant Drug Interactions in Patients Receiving Cancer Chemotherapy**

| Chemotherapy Drug | Interacting Drug | Pharmacokinetic/ Pharmacodynamic Effect[a] | Management of Interaction |
|---|---|---|---|
| Arsenic trioxide | Drugs that prolong QT interval (β blockers, cisapride, dolansetron, terfenadine) | Additive toxicity | Avoid coadministration |
| Asparaginase | Methotrexate | ↓ Toxicity[b] | Give methotrexate 3–24 h prior |
| Bleomycin | Cisplatin | ↓ Renal elimination, ↑ Pulmonary toxicity | Monitor renal function in patients previously treated with cisplatin |
| | Oxygen | ↑ Risk of acute pulmonary inflammation | Avoid inspired oxygen above 25% |
| Busulfan | Phenytoin[c] | ↑ Metabolic clearance, ↓ Bone marrow cytotoxicity | Begin phenytoin therapy briefly before busulfan |
| Carmustine | Phenytoin | ↓ Phenytoin blood level, ↓ Antiseizure effect | Monitor phenytoin level and adjust dose |
| Cisplatin | Anticonvulsant drugs (carbamazepine, phenytoin, valproic acid) | ↓ Oral absorption of anticonvulsant drug, ↓ Blood levels | Monitor levels and increase dose as needed |
| | sodium thiosulfate, mesna | Chemical incompatibility, ↓ Cytotoxic and toxic effects Sodium thiosulfate may be used as an antidote for cisplatin toxicity | Do not administer in same infusion device |
| Corticosteroids (dexamethasone, hydrocortisone, methylprednisolone) | Aminoglutethimide Mitotane | ↑ Metabolic clearance, ↓ Therapeutic effect | Adjust corticosteroid dose to avoid adrenal crisis |
| | Aprepitant | ↑ Bioavailability of corticosteroids | Decrease corticosteroid dose by half |
| Cyclophosphamide | Allopurinol | ↓ Renal elimination of alkylating metabolite, ↑ toxicity | Monitor bone marrow and urological toxicity |
| CYP 3A4 metabolized drugs (docetaxel, paclitaxel, irinotecan, vinca alkaloids) | Aprepitant (Emend) | ↓ Metabolism, ↑ Cytotoxic effect | Monitor myelosuppression and other toxicities |
| Doxorubicin | Verapamil or cyclosporine | ↑ AUC, ↓ Metabolic clearance | Avoid coadministration |
| Etoposide | Highly protein-bound drugs | ↓ Protein binding, ↑ Myelotoxicity | Avoid coadministration |
| | Phenobarbital or phenytoin | ↑ Metabolic clearance | Coadminister with caution |
| Epirubicin | Paclitaxel, adminstered before epirubicin | ↑ Neutropenia, ↑ Thrombocytopenia ↑ AUC | Administer epirubicin before paclitaxel |
| Fluorouracil | Alfa-interferon | ↓ Metabolic clearance, ↑ Cytotoxicity | Monitor for severe gastrointestinal toxicity |
| | Metronidazole | ↓ Metabolic clearance, ↑ Toxicity | Coadminister with caution |

*(Continued)*

**TABLE 15-12**

**Selected Clinically Significant Drug Interactions in Patients Receiving Cancer Chemotherapy (*Continued*)**

| Chemotherapy Drug | Interacting Drug | Pharmacokinetic/ Pharmacodynamic Effect[a] | Management of Interaction |
|---|---|---|---|
| Ifosfamide | Antifungals (ketoconazole, itraconazole) | ↓ Clearance, ↑ Toxicity | Avoid coadministration |
| | Phenobarbital | ↑ Metabolic activation, ↑ Toxicity | Monitor bone marrow suppression and neurotoxicity |
| Interleukin 2 (IL-2) | Corticosteroids | Block antitumor effect, ↓ Tumor response rate | Use corticosteroids only for IL-2 toxicity management |
| Mercaptopurine | Allopurinol | ↓ Metabolic clearance, ↑ Serum levels, prolonged bone marrow suppression | Decrease dose of mercaptopurine by 75% |
| | Cotrimoxazole (trimethoprim, sulfamethoxazole) | ↑ Oral absorption, ↓ Metabolic activation | Monitor bone marrow suppression |
| Methotrexate | Cotrimoxazole | ↓ Renal clearance, additive antifolate activity, ↑ Bone marrow toxicity | Monitor methotrexate levels and toxicity |
| | Nonsteroidal anti-inflamatory drugs (NSAIDs), salicylates | ↓ Renal clearance, ↓ Protein binding, ↑ Bone marrow and gastrointestinal toxicity | Monitor methotrexate levels and toxicity (*fatal* outcomes reported in cases of oral methotrexate and NSAID use) |
| Paclitaxel | Cisplatin | ↓ Total-body clearance, ↑ Myelotoxicity | Give paclitaxel before cisplatin |
| Procarbazine | Ethanol | Blocks metabolism of alcohol, disulfiram-like reaction | Avoid coadministration |
| | Sympathomimetic drugs (ephedrine, epinephrine) Tricyclic antidepressant drugs (amitriptyline, imipramine) | MAO inhibition,[d] hypertensive crisis, tremor, excitation | Most interactions are not clinically important |
| Vinblastine | Phenytoin | ↓ Phenytoin blood level | Monitor phenytoin level and adjust dose as needed |
| Vincristine | Asparaginase | ↑ Risk of peripheral neurotoxicity | Give vincristine first |

[a]Refers to chemotherapy drug unless otherwise specified.
[b]Result of methotrexate-induced block of protein synthesis.
[c]For seizure prophylaxis for patients receiving high-dose busulfan for bone marrow transplant therapy.
[d]Monoamine oxidase inhibition decreases the metabolism of sympathomimetic drugs, neurotransmitters released by tricyclic antidepressants, and endogenous amines.

*Source*: Data from Kivisto et al[58]; Dorr and Von Hoff[71]; Hansten and Horn[72]; Balis[73]; Finley[74]; Loadman and Bibby[75]; Thyss et al[76]; Ellison and Servi[77]; Fitzsimmons et al[78]; McCrea et al[79]; and Venturini et al.[80]

of adult patients being followed in an ambulatory oncology clinic were found to have potential drug interactions.[86] Most of the interactions were of moderate severity and may have required medical treatment. Nine percent were of major severity, meaning that the outcome could lead to permanent damage or death. Chemotherapy drugs were rarely of concern; instead, drugs given for supportive care or comorbidities were more likely to be involved. Many patients with advanced disease have significant organ dysfunction, are elderly, or have concomitant illness, all of which contribute to the potential for harmful drug interactions. For patients receiving palliative care with chemotherapeutic and nonchemotherapeutic drugs, a review of clinically significant drug interactions is available.[59]

**TABLE 15-13**

**Chemotherapy Drug Interactions With Warfarin**

| Chemotherapy Drug | Possible Mechanism of Interaction | Effect on Prothrombin Time |
|---|---|---|
| Capecitabine | ↑ AUC and elimination half-life, doubling INR[a] | Prolongs |
| Folfox regimen (fluorouracil, leucovorin, oxaliplatin) | ↑ INR | Prolongs |
| Mercaptopurine | Antagonize anticoagulant effect | Shortens |
| Mitotane | ↑ Metabolic clearance | Shortens |
| Tamoxifen | Unknown; enzyme inhibition and/or protein-binding displacement | Prolongs |

[a]Observed for *S*-warfarin, not *R*-warfarin.

*Abbreviations*: AUC, area under the serum concentration–time curve; INR, international normalized ratio.

*Source*: Data from Dorr and Von Hoff[71]; Hall et al[81]; Tenni et al[82]; Camidge et al[83]; and Masci et al.[84]

## ANTINEOPLASTIC DRUGS

Cancer chemotherapeutic drugs traditionally have been classified by their mechanism of action, chemical structure, or biological source. In general, cytotoxic drugs may be grouped according to where in the cell cycle they exert their primary toxicity. Drugs that affect a specific portion of the cell cycle are often referred to as *cell-cycle-specific agents*. The larger group of drugs consists of those in which the primary toxicity cannot be attributed to effects on a specific phase of the cell cycle, and these drugs are termed *cell-cycle-nonspecific agents*.

Grouping antineoplastic drugs into categories is done primarily for convenience. Although drugs within a class share some characteristics, there are often major differences in their indications, toxicities, and pharmaceutical properties. (See Chapter 17 for detailed descriptions of chemotherapy-induced toxicities and management.) The following section will focus on cytotoxic drugs used for the medical management of cancer and associated diseases. Biological and targeted therapies are described in Chapters 20 and 21, respectively. Patients with cancer less responsive to standard treatment may receive a combination of cytotoxic, biological, and targeted therapies in an attempt to formulate highly effective and often less toxic treatments.

### Alkylating and alkylating-like agents

*Classic alkylators.* Alkylating agents were among the first drugs used to treat malignancies in humans, and they continue to play a major role in chemotherapy. This group includes a wide array of cytotoxic drugs that possess single-agent tumoricidal activity as well as play significant roles in combination chemotherapy. Alkylating agents contribute electrophilic alkyl groups ($R–CH^2–CH^2$) to attack electron-rich nucleophilic sites on biological macromolecules such as DNA. The most common site of DNA alkylation is the N-7 position of guanine. These DNA adducts may produce a variety of lesions, including strand breaks, nucleotide base deletions, and ring openings. Cytotoxicity and mutagenicity of alkylating agents usually result from these DNA adducts as well as interference with replication and transcription.[87] Many of the DNA lesions may be restored by repair enzymes; however, if the repair is only partial, additional DNA damage may result. Alkylators are non-cell-cycle-phase-specific and are most active in the resting phase ($G_0$). Most alkylating agents are considered mutagens and potentially carcinogenic; therefore, the healthcare professional should be especially careful to avoid exposure when working with these compounds.

Mechlorethamine (nitrogen mustard) was the first alkylating agent introduced for cancer therapy. The drug spontaneously undergoes molecular rearrangement in aqueous solution to form a reactive species with two chloroethyl groups available for formation of cross-links with DNA strands. Nitrogen mustard has a very short half-life and is usually undetectable in the blood within a few minutes of administration. This severe vesicant must be handled with caution to prevent exposure of the clinician and to prevent extravasation during administration. Dose-limiting toxicities are myelosuppression, which may be severe, and rapid-onset nausea and vomiting. The major therapeutic role of mechlorethamine is in the mechlorethamine, vincristine, procarbazine, and prednisone (MOPP) chemotherapy regimen for Hodgkin's disease. Other uses include topical application for mycosis fungoides or skin cancer and intracavitary instillation for malignant pleural or pericardial effusions.

Melphalan, busulfan, and chlorambucil are usually given orally. Melphalan and busulfan are currently available as injectable products for specific indications. Melphalan was developed as a targeted agent for selective uptake in tumors actively using phenylalanine and tyrosine, such as melanin-producing malignant cells. Absorption from the gastrointestinal tract is variable and is slowed when the drug is taken with food; as a consequence, this agent should be taken on an empty stomach. Melphalan may be given parenterally when the oral route is not appropriate. Parenteral melphalan is also given as a conditioning regimen in autologous stem cell transplantation when treating multiple myeloma. A 50% dose reduction should be considered in patients with significantly decreased renal function. Chlorambucil is absorbed completely from the gastrointestinal tract. It has a predictable myelotoxicity profile and is a well-established agent in the treatment of chronic lymphocytic leukemia. Busulfan is a bifunctional alkylating agent with two reactive groups on opposite ends of the molecule that form DNA adducts, resulting in cross-linked strands. In addition to its use in chronic myelogenous leukemia (CML), busulfan is part of a high-dose chemotherapy conditioning regimen for allogeneic or autologous stem cell transplantation.

Cyclophosphamide and ifosfamide undergo a multistep activation process in vivo involving both hepatic microsomal and cellular enzyme systems to generate reactive chemical species. The two active metabolites of cyclophosphamide responsible for most of the drug's cytotoxicity are phosphoramide mustard and acrolein.[88] Acrolein is also responsible primarily for inducing hemorrhagic cystitis in approximately 10% of patients. This complication may be avoided by keeping the patient adequately hydrated and encouraging frequent urination within the first 24 hours following cyclophosphamide administration. Ifosfamide administration is associated with a much higher incidence of urotoxicity than cyclophosphamide. This may be explained by an altered pharmacokinetic profile that generates more urotoxic metabolite precursors than are found with cyclophosphamide. Cystitis can be prevented by the coadministration of mesna, a compound that inactivates urotoxic metabolites in the bladder.[89] Because cyclophosphamide and ifosfamide rely on the kidneys and the liver for elimination, their toxicity may be prolonged in patients with compromised renal or hepatic failure.

Thiotepa is a polyfunctional alkylating agent that induces multiple types of DNA damage, including interstrand cross-links. It may be administered by various routes: intravenous for breast cancer, intravesical for superficial bladder cancer, intrapleural for malignant pleural effusions, and intraperitoneal for refractory ovarian cancer.

Nitrosoureas decompose in aqueous solution to form two reactive intermediates, a chloroethyldiazohydroxide and an isocyanate group. The chloroethyldiazohydroxide compound form adducts with DNA and induces interstrand cross-links. Isocyanate groups deplete glutathione and inhibit DNA repair. Nitrosoureas are distinct from other alkylators in that they are highly lipid soluble and readily cross the blood–brain barrier, so they are highly active in central nervous system (CNS) tumors. Other uses include Hodgkin's disease, non-Hodgkin's lymphoma, and malignant melanoma. Nitrosoureas may cause severe and prolonged myelosuppression because of their high lipophilicity.

Bendamustine hydrochloride (Treanda) was developed in the 1960s as an alklylating agent but was not fully evaluated as an antineoplastic drug until the 1990s. Bendamustine has a nitrogen mustard group and a unique benzimidazol ring that has a purine-analogue effect.[90] The drug exhibits partial in vitro cross-resistance with other alklylating agents.[91,92] The dose-limiting toxicity is myelosuppression, with up to 40% of patients in clinical trials experiencing grade 3 or 4 events. Hematologic nadirs are usually expected in the third week of the 28-day treatment cycle. Other adverse events include infusion reactions, anaphylaxis, severe skin reactions, and other allergic reactions. Gastrointestinal events are mild to moderate and include nausea, vomiting, and diarrhea. Patients with significant tumor burden should be monitored for the development of tumor lysis syndrome. Bendamustine is FDA approved for treatment of chronic lymphocytic leukemia and non-Hodgkin's lymphoma refractory to rituximab-based therapy.

*Platinum-containing compounds.* Cisplatin, carboplatin, and oxaliplatin make up a highly active category of antineoplastic agents used widely for cancer treatment. Platinum compounds intracellularly undergo a substitution of a water molecule ($H_2O$) for a chloride ion (aquation), thereby enabling them to react with macromolecules with strong binding sites, such as DNA. Cisplatin-induced DNA adducts and formation of intrastrand DNA cross-links correlate well with the drug's cytotoxicity and antitumor activity.[93] Although cisplatin and other platinum analogues behave similarly to alkylators, their cytotoxicity is probably the result of a combination of mechanisms of action, including inhibition of DNA and protein synthesis, alteration in cell membrane transport, and suppression of mitochondrial function.

The currently available platinum analogues are highly dependent on renal elimination as their primary route of excretion. Cisplatin is removed from the blood in both its free and protein-bound forms following a triphasic elimination model. In the first two phases, the unbound (free) form of cisplatin is eliminated. Because 90% of the drug is excreted by the kidneys, adequate renal function is important in preventing drug accumulation and excessive toxicity. Patients who previously received cisplatin may be at increased risk for toxicity with carboplatin and should be evaluated for decreased renal function. Cisplatin given intraperitoneally produces peak levels that are as much as 21 times higher than peak plasma levels using similar doses.[94] Concurrent intravenously administered sodium thiosulfate may prevent severe systemic toxicities experienced with this route of cisplatin administration. Carboplatin and oxaliplatin elimination follows a triphasic pattern similar to that of cisplatin. A formula derived by Calvert and colleagues using a patient's GFR and a desired systemic exposure (AUC) is used widely to calculate an individualized dose of carboplatin.[68] A measured or estimated creatinine clearance is commonly used for the GFR, and a target AUC is chosen based on prior and concurrent myelotoxic chemotherapy exposure. Cisplatin and carboplatin are effective in a number of similar tumors, but oxaliplatin given in combination with fluorouracil and leucovorin is the only platinum analogue with significant activity in colorectal cancer.[95]

Although the platinum analogues all possess a similar antitumor mechanism of activity, significant differences are observed in their dosing, administration, and side-effect profiles. The dose-limiting toxicity of cisplatin is nephrotoxicity. Acute renal failure may occur within 24 hours of drug administration. Patients at greatest risk for this complication are those who receive inadequate hydration. Nephrotoxicity usually may be avoided by hydrating the patient adequately and administering diuretics such as furosemide, mannitol, or both. Carboplatin and oxaliplatin, although dependent on good renal function for elimination, are not necessarily nephrotoxic and rarely require concomitant hydration and diuresis. Although nausea and vomiting are common in patients receiving any of the platinum compounds, emesis is often more severe and prolonged with cisplatin. Combination antiemetic regimens usually are necessary to prevent and treat this side effect, which is often the most feared by the patient. Dose-limiting myelosuppression is much more of an issue with carboplatin than with cisplatin. Neurotoxicity and ototoxicity are also common adverse events seen with cisplatin treatment. Oxaliplatin-induced peripheral sensory neuropathy occurred in more than 74% of patients in clinical trials. Acute neuropathies consisting primarily of peripheral sensory neuropathy and precipitated by exposure to cold temperatures were described. More persistent sensory neuropathies also were observed that lasted 2 weeks or longer and were characterized by paresthesia, dysesthesia, and numbness in the extremities and other anatomic locations.[96] The administration of magnesium and calcium immediately before and again after oxaliplatin infusion has reduced the incidence of grade 2 sensory neuropathies.[97]

*Other alkylating-like drugs.* Other drugs with alkylating-like activity include dacarbazine, temozolomide, procarbazine, and altretamine (hexamethylmelamine). These drugs, like most other alkylating agents, depend on metabolic activation for the formation of reactive species.

Dacarbazine functions primarily as an alkylating agent but also may act as an antimetabolite by inhibiting purine nucleoside incorporation into DNA. Dacarbazine does not appear to be cell cycle phase specific; it kills cells in all phases of the cycle. This drug is extremely light sensitive and will undergo spontaneous decomposition to both active and inactive compounds when exposed to light. The most significant adverse events associated with its use are nausea and vomiting, which may decrease with repeated courses. Other toxicities include a flulike syndrome, myelosuppression, and photosensitivity. Dacarbazine is also associated with hepatic venoocclusive disease characterized by fever and acute hepatic necrosis.

Temozolomide is a newer monofunctional alkylating agent that is similar to dacarbazine. It requires dealkylation to produce an unstable intermediate that decomposes rapidly to release methyldiazonium. Temozolomide is administered orally and has significant activity in patients with malignant brain tumors (eg, glioblastoma multiforme and anaplastic astrocytoma) and in advanced metastatic malignant melanoma.[98–100]

Procarbazine is administered orally in combination with other cytotoxic drugs as therapy for Hodgkin's disease and brain tumors. Two significant drug interactions are possible in patients taking procarbazine. The first relates to the drug's ability to inhibit the enzyme monoamine oxidase, which is responsible for the metabolism of amines. Inhibition of vasoactive amine metabolism may lead to hypertensive crisis, severe headache, sweating, and coma. Patients should avoid eating foods high in tyramine (eg, wine, ripe cheese, chocolate, and liver) to prevent this drug interaction. The second interaction is seen when patients on procarbazine consume alcohol. They may experience a disulfiram reaction, which is characterized by nausea, vomiting, palpitations, and sweating.

Altretamine, also known as hexamethylmelamine, is an orally administered agent FDA approved for recurrent ovarian cancer and is also used in cancer of the endometrium. The mechanism of action is unknown but is probably of an alklylating type. The most common side effects of altretamine include myelosuppression, nausea and vomiting, and peripheral neuropathy.

### Antitumor antibiotics

*Anthracycline antibiotics.* The antitumor antibiotics comprise a large and diverse group of antineoplastic drugs originally derived from natural sources. Anthracyclines are a family of highly colored compounds known as *rhodomycins,* which have both antineoplastic and antimicrobial activities. Anthracyclines (eg, daunorubicin, doxorubicin, epirubicin, and idarubicin) and the chemically related anthracenedione (mitoxantrone) have multiple mechanisms of cytotoxicity, including intercalation, covalent DNA binding, free-radical formation, and topoisomerase II enzyme inhibition. The two mechanisms now thought responsible for most of the cytotoxicity are free-radical formation and inhibition of topoisomerase II enzyme.

Anthracyclines interfere with the DNA unwinding process that is catalyzed by the nuclear enzyme topoisomerase II.[101,102] A "cleavable complex" is produced by inhibiting the enzyme's ability to reconnect DNA strands, thereby creating double-strand breaks in the DNA structure.

Anthracyclines generate oxygen radicals by donating an electron to an oxygen molecule, thereby generating a superoxide. The superoxide is converted first to hydrogen peroxide by superoxide dismutase and finally to a hydroxyl radical. Hydroxyl radicals are the most reactive compounds known and rapidly attack DNA and cell membrane lipids. An iron–anthracycline complex also may produce hydroxyl radicals from hydrogen peroxide. Most normal tissues and tumor cells possess enzymes capable of detoxifying hydrogen peroxide; heart muscle cells, however, lack these enzymes. As a result, cardiac tissue is unable to detoxify hydrogen peroxide, which then may give rise to a reactive hydroxyl radical. A substantial body of evidence suggests that the drug–iron complex plays an important role in the cytotoxicity of anthracylines.[103] Hydroxyl radical formation in cardiac tissue may be decreased significantly by the use of an edetate analogue called *dexrazoxane,* which effectively chelates iron.

Anthracyclines are metabolized to both active and inactive compounds by the liver. The major metabolites of most anthracyclines are their alcohols, such as doxorubinicinol, which have antitumor activity—albeit not as significant as that of the parent compound. The anthracycline dose should be reduced in patients with hepatic dysfunction, especially if the bilirubin level is elevated. Dose adjustment is not necessary in renal failure because renal clearance of anthracyclines is minimal.

Cardiac toxicity of anthracyclines may be manifested as acute changes in the electrocardiogram (ECG) and arrhythmias, which are more significant in patients with preexisting heart disease. However, the more common and often therapy-limiting cardiotoxicity is the development of cardiomyopathy leading to congestive heart failure. As many as 10% of patients receiving a cumulative dose of doxorubicin greater than 550 mg/m$^2$ will develop this toxicity. Cardiac function usually is monitored with serial measurements of left ventricular function and ECG. Potential strategies to prevent or lessen cardiotoxicity include prolonged infusions of doxorubicin and cardioprotective drugs such as dexrazoxane (Zinecard).[104]

Mitoxantrone may be associated with less nausea, vomiting, and alopecia. Cardiac toxicity in patients treated with this drug appears to be less than that seen with doxorubicin.[105] However, there may be no difference in the incidence of cardiomyopathy at doses equipotent to doxorubicin.

Daunorubicin, doxorubicin, epirubicin, and idarubicin are vesicants and can induce a severe extravasation injury characterized by pain, erythema, and tissue necrosis. Mitoxantrone is considered an irritant, and extravasation injury is much less common with this agent. Other toxicities of anthracyclines include mucositis, nausea and vomiting, and alopecia.

Liposomal encapsulation of doxorubicin and daunorubicin has provided two new anticancer agents with therapeutic and toxicity profiles different from those of the free forms of these drugs. The mechanism of action is believed to be unchanged; the liposomal formulation changes the pharmacokinetics, allowing for a longer half-life and increased uptake by tumor cells.[106] Liposomal daunorubicin and liposomal doxorubicin are currently established treatments for Kaposi's sarcoma in patients with acquired immunedeficiency syndrome (AIDS). Liposomal doxorubicin is also used to treat advanced breast cancer and is combined with vincristine for treating multiple myeloma. Liposomal doxorubicin is indicated for recurrent ovarian cancer. Less alopecia, nausea and vomiting, and neurotoxicity are seen with these agents than with their nonliposomal or free-drug formulations. In addition, cardiac toxicity appears to be less dose limiting with the liposomal-encapsulated drugs. Doses greater than 1000 mg/m$^2$ have been given without significant changes in left ventricular function. An infusion reaction consisting of back pain, chest tightness, and flushing has been seen in approximately 7% of patients receiving their first dose of liposomal doxorubicin.[107] This problem rarely requires discontinuing treatment and may be managed with administration of diphenhydramine and restarting the infusion at a slower rate. Palmar-plantar skin eruptions with swelling, pain, erythema, and desquamation of skin are a fairly common problem complicating therapy with liposomal doxorubicin.

*Other antitumor antibiotics.* Bleomycin is a polypeptide composed of many low-molecular-weight proteins isolated from the fungus *Streptomyces verticullus.* A drug–iron–oxygen complex binds to DNA by intercalation and generates oxygen radicals, resulting in single- and double-strand DNA breaks. Tumor cells are most sensitive to bleomycin in the premitotic, or $G_2$, phase or in the mitotic phase of the cell cycle. Bleomycin has been used to synchronize cells into the $G_2$ and S phases so that other antineoplastic agents that act in those phases may have an increased cell-kill potential. This drug also has shown efficacy in combination-chemotherapy regimens because of its lack of significant myelosuppressive effects. Bleomycin is highly dependent on renal clearance for its elimination from the body. Significant renal failure necessitates decreasing the dose by 50% to 75% of full dose. Renal function of patients previously treated with renal toxic drugs or those who are currently receiving cisplatin should be monitored closely. Pulmonary toxicity of bleomycin may present initially as cough, dyspnea, and pleuritic chest pain. Patients at higher risk for developing bleomycin-related pulmonary fibrosis include older patients (≥70 years), those with preexisting pulmonary disease, and those who have received mediastinal radiation therapy. Although a cumulative dose greater than 450 units is associated with a higher incidence of bleomycin-induced fibrosis, clinically significant pulmonary toxicity has been documented at lower doses.

Dactinomycin (actinomycin D) binds to DNA by intercalation and induces single-strand breaks similar to those seen with doxorubicin. The drug is currently limited to use in pediatric tumors and gestational trophoblastic neoplasm. Dactinomycin is not metabolized to a significant extent but instead is excreted unchanged in the urine and bile.

Mitomycin C is activated to an alkylating agent; its cytotoxicity results from formation of cross-links with DNA, leading to inhibition of DNA synthesis and cell death. The drug is preferentially activated in hypoxic tissues such as the environment common to solid tumors. Metabolism of mitomycin by the liver is poorly defined, and renal clearance plays only a minor role in total elimination. Mitomycin degrades at a pH lower than 6; therefore, when the drug is used intravesicularly for bladder cancer, a pH higher than 6 should be maintained in the bladder to ensure potency.[108] A delayed and cumulative myelosuppression is seen with mitomycin. However, the development of a hemolytic-uremic syndrome resulting in renal failure, which is rarely reversible, prompts greater concern. Mitomycin is considered a vesicant, and it is not uncommon to observe bluish streaks tracking along veins distal to the administration site.

## Antimetabolites

***Antifolates.*** Antimetabolites used in cancer chemotherapy are structural analogues of nucleotide bases, which are the building blocks of DNA and RNA. The antineoplastic effect of this group of drugs is related to their ability to inhibit nucleic acid synthesis or to falsely be incorporated into the DNA double helix. The antifolate drugs methotrexate and trimetrexate inhibit the enzyme dihydrofolate reductase (DHFR), which catalyzes the reduction of dihydrofolate (folic acid) to tetrohydrofolate (folinic acid). Reduced folates act as one-carbon donors necessary for the synthesis of purine and pyrimidine bases. Inhibition of DHFR by methotrexate depletes the intracellular reduced-folate pool, thereby blocking de novo synthesis of nucleotide bases. These compounds also inhibit other folate-dependent enzymes such as thymidylate synthase, which catalyzes uracil to thymidine. Cytotoxicity is the result of an arrest of folate-dependent enzymatic reactions, including DNA, RNA, and protein synthesis.[109]

Rapidly proliferating cells in the S phase are most susceptible to methotrexate-induced reduced folates depletion. Therefore, longer exposure of tumor cells to methotrexate will allow more cells to enter the DNA synthesis phase of the cell cycle and result in enhanced cell kill. Most cells can function with relatively small amounts of DHFR to maintain sufficient reduced-folate pools. Therefore, a high intracellular concentration of antifolate drugs should be maintained to ensure complete enzyme inhibition. This may be accomplished by administering large amounts of methotrexate, such as those seen in treatment for malignant lymphomas and sarcomas. The ability to administer such high doses is possible only with the timely administration of leucovorin (folinic acid). Leucovorin circumvents methotrexate-induced enzyme blockade and "rescues" normal cells by providing them with the reduced folates they need for nucleic acid and protein synthesis.

Methotrexate is one of the most extensively studied antineoplastic drugs for its pharmacokinetics in part because there is a simple and readily available assay to measure the blood concentration of methotrexate. This assay is frequently used to monitor for potential toxicity when administering moderate to high doses of methotrexate. The drug is well absorbed orally at moderate to low doses. Elimination occurs primarily through renal excretion via glomerular filtration and active secretion in the proximal tubule.[110] As mentioned previously, excretion is highly dependent on adequate renal function and may be inhibited by a number of compounds. Doses should be reduced in patients with decreased renal function, and blood levels should be monitored following each dose. Patients with blood levels greater than 0.5 μM at 48 hours after dosing are at increased risk for severe myelosuppression and mucositis.[111] Leucovorin therapy should be continued in these patients until methotrexate blood levels are below 0.05 μM. Patients with a creatinine clearance of 10 to 50 mL/minute should receive 30% to 50% of the original dose, and those with a creatinine clearance of less than 10 mL/minute should receive only 15% of the original dose.[110] A significant drug interaction exists between methotrexate and drugs that decrease GFR (see Table 15-12). The pharmacokinetics of methotrexate is altered by distribution into third-space fluid collections such as ascitic accumulation in the peritoneal cavity. Elimination is prolonged and toxicity is increased because of the slow redistribution of the drug from the peritoneum back into the blood.

Methotrexate-associated toxicities, besides myelosuppression and mucositis, include nephrotoxicity, hepatotoxicity, and pulmonary fibrosis. Hepatotoxicity may result from high-dose therapy and present with acute and reversible elevations in liver function enzymes. Methotrexate is useful as a treatment or prophylaxis for meningeal leukemia, but the drug is poorly distributed into the cerebrospinal fluid (CSF). For this reason, a preservative-free formulation of methotrexate must be injected directly into the CSF by lumbar puncture or intraventricular device (Ommaya reservoir). Toxicities seen with intrathecal administration include severe headache, nuchal rigidity, vomiting, and fever; in severe cases, a demyelinating encephalopathy may develop.

Pemetrexed (Alimta) is a novel antifolate that inhibits multiple enzymes involved in the synthesis of nucleotides, including thymidylate synthase, DHFR, and glycinamide ribonucleotide formyltransferase. Pemetrexed is indicated in combination with cisplatin for the treatment of unresectable malignant pleural mesothelioma and as single-agent for the treatment of recurrent non-small cell lung cancer. Severe hematologic toxicity was seen in clinical trials and correlated with poor nutritional status.[112] When patients were supplemented with folic acid and vitamin B12 during the study, significantly less toxicity was observed; therefore, all patients receiving premetrexed should receive these supplements. Other adverse events experienced include nausea, vomiting, fatigue, diarrhea, and skin rash. Dexamethasone should be given on the day before, the day of, and the day after pemetrexed administration to prevent skin rashes.[112] Pemetrexed is excreted primarily in the urine, and 70% to 90% of a dose is eliminated unchanged within the first 24 hours of administration. Patients with a creatinine clearance above 45 mL/minute do not need any dose adjustment. Coadministration of nephrotoxic drugs or renally eliminated drugs may result in a delayed clearance of pemetrexed; therefore, caution should be exercised.[113]

Raltitrexed is a quinazoline folate analogue that selectively inhibits thymidylate synthase. Raltitrexed is currently available in Canada and Europe for the treatment of colorectal cancer. The compound is under investigation in the US for mesothelioma, pancreatic cancer, head and neck cancer, and colorectal cancer.

***Pyrimidine analogues.*** The fluoropyrimidine 5-fluorouracil (fluorouracil) undergoes extensive metabolism intracellularly to evolve into an active metabolite, fluorode-oxyuridine monophosphate (FdUMP). FdUMP binds covalently with thymidylate synthase (TS) and inhibits the enzyme's ability to synthesize deoxythymidine triphosphate (dTTP), a precursor of DNA synthesis. Other metabolic pathways are conversion of fluorouracil to fluorouradine triphosphate (FUTP), which may be incorporated into RNA, and conversion of FdUMP to the triphosphate form, which may be incorporated into DNA. The cytotoxicity of fluorouracil in these metabolic pathways results in depletion of dTTP or false incorporation of other metabolites into DNA and RNA. The administration of fluorouracil and leucovorin concurrently enhances this reaction and increases the cytotoxic effect of fluorouracil (see "Modulation of fluorouracil by leucovorin" under "Therapeutic Strategies").

Rapidly cleared by the liver, fluorouracil has a plasma half-life of 6 to 20 minutes. There may be considerable variation in clearance among patients. The enzyme dihydropyrimidine dehydrogenase metabolizes fluorouracil to dihydrofluorouracil in the liver and other tissues. Patients who are deficient in this enzyme experience greatly increased fluorouracil levels and resulting toxicity.[114] When fluorouracil or floxuridine is administered directly into the hepatic artery or portal vein, hepatic metastases are exposed directly to the drug with minimal systemic exposure because of the drug's significant first-pass clearance.

The major dose-limiting toxicity of fluorouracil depends on the schedule of administration. Myelosuppression is more prominent when the drug is given by rapid bolus injection, whereas mucositis and gastrointestinal toxicity are more common with prolonged infusions over 2 to 5 days. Cholestatic jaundice and biliary sclerosis are complications of intrahepatic administration of fluoropyrimidines. Therapy with fluorouracil sometimes has caused chest pain, elevation in cardiac enzymes, and electrocardiogram (ECG) changes similar to those seen with myocardial ischemia. This syndrome may be associated with fluorouracil-induced coronary vasospasm.[115]

Orally administered fluoropyrimidines traditionally have been avoided because of the erratic bioavailability observed. Three newer approaches to orally administered fluoropyrimidines have been developed. Capecitabine is FDA approved for the treatment of patients with metastatic breast or colorectal cancer. This prodrug undergoes numerous metabolic steps in both the liver and tissues to ultimately become fluorouracil.[116] The cytotoxic metabolite is more concentrated in tumor cells than in normal cells because of the higher concentrations of thymidine phosphorylase, the enzyme responsible for the final conversion to fluorouracil. The major dose-limiting side effects include diarrhea, hand-and-foot syndrome, and stomatitis. Two other fluoropyrimidine compounds are under investigation for use in colorectal cancer. UFT is a combination of the fluorouracil prodrug ftorafur and uracil and is given orally. The pharmacokinetics of fluorouracil is significantly altered by the coadministration of 5-ethynyluracil, a potent inhibitor of dihydropyrimidine dehydrogenase that is responsible for the inactivation of fluorouracil.[117] The combination is being investigated for the oral treatment of colorectal cancer.[118]

Cytarabine was isolated originally from the sponge *Cryptothethy acrypta*. The parent drug is phosphorylated to ara-CTP, which competes with the normal substrate deoxycytidine triphosphate (dCTP) to inhibit DNA polymerase-α. DNA polymerases are critical enzymes in the synthesis and repair of DNA. The metabolite ara-CTP also may become incorporated into DNA and interfere with chain polymerization and repair of damaged DNA strands. As seen with other antimetabolites, tumor cells and normal tissues are most sensitive to cytarabine in the S phase of the cell cycle.

Cytarabine is rapidly converted to the inactive metabolite ara-U by the enzyme cytidine deaminase, which is present in many tissues, including the gastrointestinal epithelium and liver. Cytarabine is usually administered by continuous infusion. This regimen is used to maintain cytotoxic levels despite the drug's rapid inactivation and to maximally expose all cycling cells to the cytotoxic effects during the S phase of the cell cycle. Cytarabine may be used alone or in addition to methotrexate for meningeal leukemia, but direct intrathecal administration is necessary to obtain sufficient drug concentrations in the CSF. Only small amounts of cytarabine are needed intrathecally because deamination is minimal in the CSF. Toxicities of cytarabine include myelosuppression and gastrointestinal epithelial injury. When high-dose cytarabine is used for refractory acute myelogenous leukemia (AML), 20% of patients may experience a cerebral and cerebellar dysfunction. This syndrome is seen more often in individuals older than age 50 and is characterized by slurred speech, ataxia, confusion, and coma.[119] High-dose cytarabine is also associated with conjunctivitis, which usually can be prevented by giving the patient steroid ophthalmic drops.

Gemcitabine is a pyrimidine analogue of deoxycytidine that is converted intracellularly to its diphosphate and triphosphate metabolites. Gemcitabine diphosphate is an inhibitor of ribonucleotide reductase and thereby inhibits de novo nucleotide synthesis.[120] Gemcitabine triphosphate inhibits DNA synthesis by competing with the physiological substrate deoxycytidine triphosphate for DNA polymerase and incorporation into DNA. The reduction of intracellular deoxycytidine triphosphate induced by gemcitabine diphosphate enhances the incorporation of gemcitabine triphosphate into DNA, a mechanism referred to as *self-potentiation*. The half-life of gemcitabine is prolonged as a consequence of this phenomenon, so infusions should be limited to 30 minutes. Longer infusions are associated with a higher degree of myelotoxicity. Other important adverse effects include elevated liver transaminase enzymes, nausea and vomiting, and skin rash with or without pruritus.[121]

***Purine analogues.*** The thiopurines 6-mercaptopurine (6-MP) and 6-thioguanine (6-TG) are converted to their respective monophosphates, which inhibit purine synthesis and cause an accumulation of nucleic acid precursors. These precursors, in turn, facilitate the conversion of 6-MP and 6-TG to their active nucleotide forms. The triphosphate nucleotides of these drugs are incorporated into DNA and induce strand breaks, which are correlated with cytotoxicity. Methotrexate, an inhibitor of *de novo* purine biosynthesis, acts synergistically with the 6-thiopurines by blocking purine synthesis and enhancing thiopurine activation.

Fludarabine is relatively resistant to deamination (deactivation) and possesses enhanced solubility over other adenine arabinoside analogues. Following intravenous administration, the drug is rapidly dephosphorylated to F-Ara-A, which enters cells via nucleotide-specific membrane transport.[122] The primary mechanism of action is inhibition of the DNA polymerases involved in DNA synthesis and repair. Fludarabine is most active in the treatment of chronic lymphocytic leukemia and indolent non-Hodgkin's lymphoma. In the initial trials of fludarabine, doses of 75 to 150 $mg/m^2$ four times a day for 5 to 7 days produced profound neurotoxicity characterized by cortical blindness, seizures, coma, and death.[123] Subsequent trials demonstrated that fludarabine could be given safely when administered at doses between 25 and 30 $mg/m^2$ daily for 5 days.[123] At these doses, the most common toxicities are myelosuppression and immunosuppression. Patients on fludarabine also should be given prophylactic therapy for *Pneumocystis carinii*. A rare but sometimes life-threatening and potentially fatal autoimmune hemolytic anemia may occur in patients receiving fludarabine.[124] Patients rechallenged with fludarabine, whether pretreated or not with steroids, have experienced fatal outcomes.

2-Chlorodeoxyadenosine (2-CdA, Cladribine) is a deoxyadenosine purine nucleotide analogue that, like fludarabine, is resistant to deamination. Cladribine enters lymphocytes via a nucleotide transporter system and accumulates until it reaches lymphotoxic levels. Following a series of phosphorylation steps, the drug is converted to cladribine triphosphate, which is falsely incorporated into DNA, eventually interrupting DNA synthesis and repair.[125] Cladribine can produce durable complete remissions in as many as 91% of patients with hairy cell leukemia.[126,127] Responses may be seen in patients with chronic lymphocytic leukemia (CLL) and non-Hodgkin's lymphoma; however, remissions tend to be brief.[35] Myelotoxicity is dose-limiting, and recovery may take as long as 3 to 5 weeks after a single course of therapy. A severe autoimmune hemolytic anemia with fatal bone marrow aplasia has been described in CLL patients receiving repeated cycles.[128] Immunosuppression and opportunistic infections are seen less often than in patients who receive fludarabine.

Pentostatin (Nipent), or 2-deoxycoformycin, was developed as a potent inhibitor of adenosine diaminase. Blockage of this enzyme causes an accumulation of deoxyadenosine, which is mostly responsible for cladribine's cytotoxicity.[129] Pentostatin is active in a number of lymphocytic diseases, including CLL, prolymphocytic leukemia, and T-cell lymphoma. A profound immunosuppression may persist for more than a year after the drug is discontinued.[130] Other adverse events seen with pentostatin therapy include ocular complications, dermatological toxicity, and gastrointestinal toxicity.

### Hypomethylating agents

Decitabine (Dacogen) and azacitidine (Vidaza) are members of a new class of anticancer drugs known as *DNA hypomethylating agents*. They are both FDA approved for the treatment of myelodysplastic syndromes (MDSs). Hypomethylating agents exert their cytotoxic and antileukemic effects by inhibiting DNA methyltransferase.[131] In addition to these direct cytotoxic effects, phosphorylated forms of decitabine and azacitidine are incorporated into DNA, where they trap DNA methyltransferase and induce hypomethylated forms of the nucleic acid. Hypomethylation results in reexpression of tumor-suppressor genes, induction of cellular differentiation, and suppression of tumor growth.[132]

Decitabine has a dual dose-dependent mechanism of action. At higher doses, its mechanism of cytotoxicity results from covalent trapping DNA methyltransferase into DNA; at lower doses, it inhibits DNA hypermethylation and reactivates tumor-suppressor genes.[131] Decitabine is inactivated by cytidine deaminase in the liver and extrahepatically. A phase III trial in patients with MDS showed a trend toward longer median time to AML progression or death.[133] The response rate in patients who received decitabine was 17% and 0% in the supportive-care group.

Patients who experienced a response achieved a higher quality of life and became red blood cell and platelet transfusion independent. Myelosuppression was the most common adverse event; hyperbilirubinemia, pneumonia, and constipation also were seen. The optimal dosing of decitabine favors a short bolus-infusion schedule, lower doses, and a 5-day regimen to maintain dose intensity.[134]

Besides the primary antileukemic effect described earlier, azacitidine also may function as a biological response modifier by affecting cytokine cell signaling.[135] Azacitidine may be administered by subcutaneous injection or direct intravenous infusion. Azacitidine is metabolized extensively by the liver, and the intact drug and metabolites are eliminated by urinary excretion. A phase III trial comparing azacitidine with best supportive care showed a trilineage response rate (>50% normalization of all three peripheral blood cell counts and blood transfusion independence), or 23% in patients on azacitidine vs 0% in those receiving supportive care.[135] Azacitadine also was more effective in delaying AML transformation and death than supportive care. In patients who received azacitidine, myelosuppression was the most common adverse event, and treatment-related infections were seen in 20% of patients. Nausea and vomiting were reported in 4% of patients receiving azacitidine.[136]

## Natural products and analogues

Antineoplastic drugs derived from plant sources represent a large and diverse group of chemotherapeutic agents. Many of these drugs are naturally occurring compounds that were isolated from plant material (vinca alkaloids). Others are the result of synthetic and semisynthetic processes used to manufacture analogues of compounds originally extracted from plants. Examples include etoposide, docetaxel, paclitaxel, and topotecan. The discovery of new plant-derived compounds with antitumor activity is ongoing and will continue to provide important and novel agents for the treatment of cancer.

*Vinca alkaloids.* Natural alkaloids present in small quantities in the periwinkle plant play a major role in cancer chemotherapy. Although the drugs in this group are dramatically similar in chemical structure, their antitumor activity and toxicity differ greatly. Vincristine (Oncovin) has a broad spectrum of activity, leading to its use in leukemia, lymphoma, breast cancer, lung cancer, and multiple myeloma, whereas vinblastine (Velban) is used primarily in germ cell tumors and advanced Hodgkin's disease. Vinblastine is myelotoxic and neurotoxic; vincristine is also neurotoxic but has amazingly minimal myelotoxicity. Vinorelbine (Navelbine), the newest vinca alkaloid to become available in the US, is active in breast cancer and non-small cell lung cancer and is both myelotoxic and neurotoxic. Vindesine is widely available in Europe but currently not available in the US except in clinical trials.

Vinca alkaloids belong to a group of compounds known as the *tubulin-interactive agents.* They exert their cytotoxic effects primarily by interfering with normal microtubule formation and function, which is critical for the mitosis phase of the cell cycle and, ultimately, cell division. Microtubules have other important cellular functions that are affected by the vinca alkaloids, including maintenance of cell shape and intracellular transport. Vinca alkaloids bind to specific sites on tubulin, preventing formation of tubulin dimers and inhibiting the formation of microtubule structures. Although mitotic arrest is the primary mechanism of cell death, vinca alkaloids may have a cytolytic effect on resting cells in the $G_0$ phase and other cells in the $G_1$ or S phase. Cells are sensitive to low concentrations of vincristine, and duration of exposure is critical in determining the cytotoxic effect.

Despite the wide range of clinical uses of the vinca alkaloids, surprisingly little information is available on their pharmacological and pharmacokinetic profiles. This may be primarily the result of the lack of a sensitive drug assay for quantifying the low concentrations found in patients. Vincristine is highly bound to serum proteins, blood cells, and especially platelets. It is metabolized primarily by the liver and concentrates in the bile. Seventy percent of a dose is excreted in the feces, and approximately 10% is excreted in the urine.[137] Dose modification should be considered in patients with hepatic dysfunction, particularly patients with biliary obstructions. Vinblastine and vinorelbine have similar pharmacokinetic profiles, with excretion occurring primarily through the biliary tract. All the vinca alkaloids have a prolonged terminal elimination phase half-life of 1 to 4 days.

Vinca alkaloids are known for their peripheral neurotoxicity, which is frequently a cumulative dose-limiting effect. Toxicity presents initially as sensory impairment (stocking-and-glove distribution) and paresthesias. Patients later may develop neuritic pain and motor dysfunction. Loss of deep tendon reflexes, foot and wrist drop, ataxia, and paralysis may occur with continued vinca alkaloid therapy. The only effective management is discontinuation of therapy. Accidental intrathecal administration of vincristine induces an ascending paralysis resulting in death. Constipation and abdominal pain are frequent complaints of older patients on vincristine. Myelosuppression is also a dose-limiting toxicity of vinblastine and vinorelbine but not vincristine. The vinca alkaloids are vesicants, and extravasation should be avoided.

*Taxanes.* The taxanes have emerged as an extremely important group of antitumor compounds that show activity in a wide range of cancers. These complex chemical structures are difficult to synthesize in the laboratory. Extraction and isolation from the bark of the Pacific yew tree *Taxus brevifolia* was the only source for paclitaxel until the early 1990s, when a semisynthetic process using a taxane precursor was developed. Because of paclitaxel's poor water solubility, the injectable formulation must contain 50% polyoxyethylated castor oil (Cremophor EL) to maintain aqueous solubility. This vehicle creates problems with administration because Cremophor EL can leach hepatotoxic plasticizer from PVC plastic infusion devices. Cremophor EL is primarily responsible for the severe hypersensitivity reactions experienced in patients receiving paclitaxel.

Paclitaxel (Taxol) and docetaxel (Taxotere) preferentially bind to microtubules over tubulin dimers, and they inhibit microtubule disassembly, which is necessary for normal functioning of microtubule structures.[138] Cells exposed to paclitaxel display many arrays of disorganized microtubules during all phases of the cell cycle. Although taxanes have distinct antimicrotubule effects on cells, the actual mechanism of cell death remains unclear. The mechanism of action and cytotoxic effect of docetaxel are similar to those of paclitaxel.

Hepatic metabolism and biliary excretion probably constitute the major routes of elimination for paclitaxel and docetaxel.[139,140] Urinary excretion accounts for less than 5% of total-body clearance of the drugs. Paclitaxel clearance is reduced by as much as 30% when given following cisplatin.[141] This interaction results in increased peak plasma concentrations of paclitaxel and more severe myelotoxicity than is seen with the reverse administration schedule. For routine use with cisplatin or carboplatin, paclitaxel should be given first, followed by the platinum compound. Taxanes also exhibit a high degree of protein binding (90% to 95%). Among the most significant toxicities associated with taxanes are myelosuppression, neurotoxicity, hypersensitivity, total-body alopecia, and transient myalgias and arthralgias. Nail separation may occur, especially when paclitaxel is given as a weekly 1-hour infusion. Hypersensitivity reactions were seen in 10% of patients receiving paclitaxel during early clinical trials.[142] These reactions usually occur within the first 10 minutes of the initial infusion and are characterized by hypotension, bronchospasm, dyspnea, abdominal and leg pain, and severe facial flushing. Major hypersensitivity reactions may be prevented in most patients by the preinfusion administration of a corticosteroid (eg, dexamethasone), an antihistamine (eg, diphenhydramine), and an $H_2$ blocking drug. Paclitaxel may be safely given parenterally, with infusions lasting 24, 3, or 1 hour. The 3-hour infusion rate has been associated with less neutropenia than the 24-hour infusion.

The toxicity profile of docetaxel differs from that of paclitaxel.[143] The incidence of hypersensitivity reactions is lower, with severe reactions experienced in fewer than 1% of patients treated. Skin reactions, including pruritus, macular or papular lesions, erythema, and desquamation, are seen in 50% to 70% of patients treated with docetaxel. Nail changes, consisting of an orange discoloration and thickening of the nails, also were observed in many patients in clinical trials. A more significant complication is fluid retention and weight gain, which can occur in 6% of patients. A 3-day regimen of corticosteroids is useful in preventing and lessening the fluid retention, as well as for preventing hypersensitivity reactions.

A new formulation of paclitaxel is currently available in the US that is void of the solubilizer Cremophor EL base. Nanoparticle albumin–bound paclitaxel (nab-paclitaxel, Abraxane) is prepared by homogenization of paclitaxel in the presence of human serum albumin, resulting in particles of approximately 130 nm in diameter.[144] Nab-paclitaxel accumulates in tumor cells and has an AUC in tumor tissue that is 33% higher than that of Cremophor-solubilzied paclitaxel. The nanoparticles may be transported by albumin-specific gp60 receptor–mediated transcytosis, thereby increasing nab-paclitaxel uptake by tumor cells.[144] Phase I studies of nab-paclitaxel were conducted without steroid premedication and did not produce any acute hypersensitivity reactions.[145] The maximum tolerated dose in this trial was 300 mg/m$^2$, which is significantly higher than the maximum dose of conventional paclitaxel. In a phase III clinical trial in patients with metastatic breast cancer, nab-paclitaxel (ABI-007) was administered as a 30-minute infusion at a dose of 260 mg/m$^2$ vs paclitaxel in Cremophor dosed at 175 mg/m$^2$ and given over 3 hours.[146] Patients receiving nab-paclitaxel demonstrated significantly higher response rates and longer time to tumor progression than patients receiving conventional paclitaxel. Less grade 4 neutropenia and more manageable peripheral neuropathy were seen in the nab-paclitaxel-treated patients despite a 49% higher dose of paclitaxel given. No hypersensitivity reactions were seen in the nab-paclitaxel-treated subjects despite the absence of premedications and a shorter administration time. Nab-paclitaxel is FDA approved for the treatment of metastatic breast cancer following chemotherapy failure or relapse within 6 months of adjuvant therapy. Prior chemotherapy should include an anthracycline unless otherwise contraindicated.[147]

PG-paclitaxel (CT-2103, Xyotax) is a polymer–drug conjugate of polyglutamate and paclitaxel that was designed initially to overcome the poor aqueous solubility of paclitaxel and avoid the hypersensitivity reactions associated with the Cremophor solubilizer. Polymer conjugates are taken up by tumor cells and the reticuloendothelial system, and free paclitaxel is released by esterolysis intracellularly.[148] PG-paclitaxel is highly water soluble, demonstrates significantly enhanced antitumor efficacy, and is associated with improved safety compared with conventional Cremophor-based paclitaxel.[149] Tumor exposure to paclitaxel was five times greater when administered as the polyglutamate form than as the Cremophor-based form. PG-paclitaxel is being studied in large phase III trials in patients with ovarian cancer and lung cancer. The results of a trial comparing PG-paclitaxel and carboplatin with conventional paclitaxel and carboplatin in patients with NSCLC found no significant overall improvement in survival but did observe reduced incidence of side effects and a more convenient administration schedule for the polyglutamate form.[150] A subset of women in this trial faired significantly better as long as their estrogen levels were normal. Adverse effects of PG-paclitaxel were similar to those of conventional paclitaxel except for the lack of allergic reactions and only rare alopecia.

*Epothilones.* Epothilones are naturally occurring macrolides produced by the myxobacterium *Sorangium cellulosum.* They were developed initially as antifungal compounds and now have been introduced as a new class of antitumor agents. Similar to taxanes, the antineoplatic effects of epothilones probably are related to their ability to stabilize microtubules and prevent microtubule disassembly. The tubulin-binding sites of epothilones may differ from those of taxanes, and there is evidence to suggest the tubulin polymerizing activity of epothilone B is 2- to 10-fold greater than that of paclitaxel.[151] Epothilones are active in cell lines that exhibit resistance to taxanes and other chemotherapy drugs. Preclinical studies also have shown epothilones to demonstrate cytotoxic activity in chemotherapy-resistant tumor cell lines exhibiting multidrug resistance, β-tubulin mutations, and overexpression of tau protein.[152,153]

Ixabepilone (Ixempra) is the first in this family of compounds to be FDA approved for treatment of metastatic or locally advanced breast cancer. Three other epothilones are currently under clinical investigation as antineoplastic agents: patupilone (epothilone B), the first epothilone identified to posses activity in mammalian cancer cells; BMS-310705, a water-soluble epothilone; and sagopilone (ZK-Epo), an epothilone B derivative.[154] Ixabepilone is indicated for use in combination with capecitabine in tumors with inadequate response to a taxane and an anthracycline or as single agent in patients with disease that is resistant or refractory to treatment with anthracyclines, taxanes, and capecitabine. A phase III trial of ixabepilone in combination with capecitabine for metastatic or locally advanced breast cancer demonstrated a significantly longer median time to progression than in patients who received capecitabine alone (5.8 months vs 4.2 months, respectively).[155] Peripheral sensory neuropathy, fatigue, and neutropenia were the most common grade 3 and 4 adverse events in patients who received the combination. Ixabepilone is formulated in polyethoxylated castor oil (Cremophor EL), the same as paclitaxel. Therefore, the pretreatment with antihistamines (both $H_1$ and $H_2$ blockers) is recommended to prevent allergic-type reactions. Ixabepilone must be diluted in a lactated Ringer's solution before infusion.

*Epipodophyllotoxins.* Podophyllotoxin, an extract of the mandrake plant, is an antimitotic drug that binds to tubulin and inhibits microtubulin formation. This compound was not further developed as an antitumor agent because of its unacceptable toxicity in humans.

Etoposide (VP-16, VePesid, Etopophos) and teniposide (VM-26, Vumon) are glycosidic derivatives of podophyllotoxin that possess significant activity in many human tumors, such as germ cell tumors and lung cancer, but offer a more predictable and mild toxicity profile. Initially, these drugs were thought to work as antimicrotubule agents similar to podophyllotoxin and vinca alkaloids. However, they produced no effect on microtubule assembly. Cell-cycle studies demonstrated that epipodophyllotoxins induced arrest of cells in the late S or early G phase instead of the expected M-phase arrest commonly observed with antimitotic drugs. Along with the observation of drug-induced DNA strand breaks, scientists have suggested the primary cytotoxic mechanism of these compounds is inhibition of topoisomerase II.[156] Epipodophyllotoxins stabilize the enzyme–DNA complex, thereby inhibiting the reunion of the two DNA strands originally cleaved by the enzyme. Additionally, the synergy of the etoposide with antimetabolite drugs may result from inhibition of nucleoside transport into the cell.

Etoposide and teniposide are highly protein bound (94% and 99%, respectively) to the plasma protein albumin. Drugs that interfere with the protein binding of teniposide may induce greater toxicity in patients receiving both drugs (see "Drug Interactions in the Patient Receiving Chemotherapy" above). Renal clearance is the major route of elimination for etoposide, with approximately 40% to 60% of the drug being excreted unchanged in the urine. Biliary excretion and hepatic metabolism are responsible for elimination to a lesser extent. Teniposide is metabolized more extensively, with only 5% to 20% being excreted unchanged in the urine. Etoposide is available as an oral formulation, which has a bioavailability of approximately 50%.

The toxicities of both agents are similar, with myelosuppression, hypersensitivity, and infusion-related blood pressure changes being the most significant toxic effects. Both agents are also poorly water soluble, necessitating the addition of Tween 80 or Cremophor EL and other excipients to maintain the drugs in aqueous solution. The manufacturer of teniposide recommends avoiding the use of PVC plastic infusion devices to prevent exposing the patient to potentially hepatotoxic plasticizers leached from the plastic by the Cremophor vehicle.

*Camptothecin derivatives.* Camptothecin sodium was tested originally in the early 1970s as an antitumor compound. Despite the drug's significant activity in both preclinical and clinical trials, it was abandoned because of unpredictable and often severe hemorrhagic cystitis. Interest in related drugs was renewed with the introduction of two semisynthetic analogues of camptothecin, topotecan and irinotecan. Their proposed mechanism of action is inhibition of topoisomerase I, an enzyme responsible for maintaining the three-dimensional structure of DNA. Topoisomerase inhibitors bind with the DNA–enzyme complex, thereby inducing DNA strand breaks and cell death.[157]

Camptothecins appear to exist in two species in aqueous solutions: a closed lactone ring, which possesses cytotoxic activity, and an open carboxylate form, which does not. The conversion is pH dependent, with the open form predominating in an alkaline environment, and the closed, or active, form predominating in an acidic solution. Much of the unpredictable urotoxicity seen in early trials of camptothecin sodium may be explained by the lack of knowledge of the pH-dependent conversion and the shift of the equilibrium toward the active species in the acidic environment of the bladder. Irinotecan is a prodrug and must be converted to its active form via carboxylesterase in the body.[158] Myelosuppression is the major dose-limiting toxicity of topotecan, whereas diarrhea is the primary dose-limiting toxicity for irinotecan when administered on a once-weekly schedule. To manage the diarrhea associated with irinotecan effectively, patients should be instructed to start a high-dose loperamide regimen (2 mg loperamide every 2 hours) until they are diarrhea-free for 12 hours.

### Miscellaneous agents

Asparaginase (Elspar) induces a rapid and complete depletion from the blood of the amino acid L-asparagine. This biochemical process is cytotoxic to tumor cells that are highly dependent on exogenous sources of the amino acid. The major cytotoxic effect is the inhibition of protein synthesis, with a secondary effect of inhibition of nucleic acid synthesis also observed in sensitive cells. Asparaginase is considered cell-cycle-phase-nonspecific agent despite the drug's ability to block cells in the $G_1$ and S phases of the cell cycle. Its only antineoplastic use is as part of the induction and consolidation therapy for ALL in both children and adults. Asparaginase is extracted from *Escherichia coli* bacteria and is associated with a high incidence of anaphylaxis. Patients who develop severe hypersensitivity reactions to the bacterial product may receive pegaspargase, which is chemically altered to be less immunogenic. Other toxicities seen with asparaginase include hyperglycemia, hypoprothrombinemia, and neurotoxicity.

Hydroxyurea is a DNA-selective antimetabolite that inhibits ribonucleotide reductase and has minimal inhibitory effects on RNA and protein synthesis. Its major indication is in rapidly controlling blood counts in acute leukemia and other myeloproliferative diseases such as polycythemia vera and essential thrombocytosis. Allopurinol should be used in conjunction with hydroxyurea to prevent tumor lysis syndrome.

Estramustine is a unique compound made up of a molecule of estradiol phosphate combined with nitrogen mustard. Originally believed to have alkylating properties, the drug's mechanism of action is now thought to be related to antimicrotubule activity.[159] Estramustine is used in combination with docetaxel for the treatment of advanced prostate cancer.[160]

## HORMONAL THERAPY

Hormonal manipulations were among the first treatments used to control cancer. Initially, they had limited potential to induce significant response in sensitive tumors. Currently, however, they are critical components in the treatment for many different cancers. Table 15-14 lists the commonly used hormonal agents and their primary indications. Steroids, steroid analogues, and enzyme inhibitors constitute the majority of drugs used for hormonal therapy. Their mechanism of action is incompletely understood but probably involves the inhibition of stimulation of steroid-specific receptors located on the surfaces of cells. Blocking these receptors prevents the cell from receiving normal hormonal growth stimulation, thereby decreasing the growth fraction of the tumor.

### Antiestrogens

Tamoxifen is a frequently used drug in the adjuvant treatment of breast cancer and treatment of metastatic disease in estrogen-receptor-positive tumors. Its primary mechanism of action is blocking estrogen stimulation of breast cancer cells.[161] This is achieved by inhibition of both the translocation and nuclear binding of the estrogen receptor. Tamoxifen is an estrogen antagonist (blocker) in breast tissue and an estrogen agonist (stimulator) in endometrium, bone, and lipids. The most prominent toxicity is hot flashes, which affect approximately half the women who use it. Other side effects include a slightly increased incidence of thromboembolic events and endometrial cancer. In a large randomized trial comparing tamoxifen and placebo in the prevention of breast cancer in women, women at risk for developing a breast malignancy were 50% less likely to develop the disease if they took tamoxifen 20 mg daily.[162] Megestrol also has been used to treat metastatic breast cancer but now is used primarily for the treatment of anorexia-cachexia related to cancer.[163]

Fulvestrant, a monthly administered injectable antihormonal agent, is now available for patients with estrogen-receptor-positive metastatic breast cancer who have failed initial therapy with another antiestrogen (tamoxifen). Fulvestrant binds to the estrogen receptor, blocking both hormone-dependent and hormone-independent activation functions and preventing estrogen-induced cell growth.[164] Fulvestrant was found to be equivalent to anastrazole in terms of length of survival, time to progression, and tumor response in patients with locally advanced metastatic breast cancer following progression of disease while on tamoxifen or other endocrine therapies.[165] Both drugs were well

**TABLE 15-14**

**Commonly Used Hormonal Agents and Primary Indications**

| Pharmacological Class | Drug Name(s) | Primary Indication(s) |
|---|---|---|
| Corticosteroids | Dexamethasone | Leukemias |
| | Hydrocortisone | Hodgkin's disease |
| | Methylprednisolone | Malignant lymphomas |
| | Prednisone | Breast cancer |
| | | Multiple myeloma |
| Androgens | Fluoxymesterone | Breast cancer |
| | Testosterone | |
| Estrogens | Conjugated estrogens | Prostate cancer |
| | Diethylstilbesterol | Breast cancer |
| | Estradiol | |
| Antiestrogens, progestins | Medroxyprogesterone | Endometrial cancer |
| | Megesterol | Breast cancer |
| Estrogen-receptor antagonists | Tamoxifen (Nolvadex) | Breast cancer |
| | Toremifene (Fareston) | Breast cancer |
| | Fulvestrant (Faslodex) | |
| Aromatase inhibitors | Mitotane | Adrenal cancer |
| | Exemestane (Aromasin) | Breast cancer |
| | Anastrozole (Arimidex) | Breast cancer |
| | Letrozole (Femara) | Breast cancer |
| Lutenizing hormone-releasing hormone analogues | Goserelin (Zoladex) | Prostate cancer |
| | Histrelin (Vantas) | Prostate cancer |
| | Triptorelin (Trelstar) | Prostate cancer |
| | Leuprolide (Lupron) | Breast cancer |
| Gonadotropin-releasing hormone antagonist | Abarelix (Plenaxis) | Prostate cancer |
| Antiandrogens | Flutamide (Eulexin) | Prostate cancer |
| | Nilutamide (Nilandron) | |
| | Bicalutamide (Casodex) | |

tolerated, and few patients withdrew from the study due to adverse events.

## Aromatase inhibitors

Aromatase inhibitors suppress postmenopausal estrogen synthesis by inhibiting the peripheral conversion of androgens to estrogens. Aromatase is an enzyme in the CYP superfamily of enzymes and is responsible for catalyzing the final step in estrogen synthesis. Aromatase-inhibiting drugs have been developed primarily for the treatment of hormonally sensitive breast cancer. Ovarian production of estrogen is unaffected; as a consequence, these agents are useful only in postmenopausal women or oophorectomized premenopausal women. Aminoglutethamide was the first such agent available but now is used rarely because of its poor tolerance and the need to replace corticosteroids. Newer agents have been classified as steroidal inhibitors that bond irreversibly with the aromatase enzyme and nonsteroidal inhibitors that bond reversibly with the heme iron site that allows recovery of enzymatic activity when the inhibitor is removed.[166] Anastrozole and letrozole are nonsteroidal aromatase inhibitors, and exemestane is a steroidal inhibitor. All drugs are potent aromatase inhibitors and equally effective as aminoglutethamide; however, they affect the synthesis of corticosteroids, aldosterone, or thyroid hormone only minimally and therefore are associated with fewer toxicities. The nonsteroidal agents have similar toxicities that include arthralgias, loss of bone mineral density, and differential effects on lipid profile.[167] Anastozole did not show a marked effect on lipids, but letrozole increased total cholesterol and low-density lipoproteins significantly from baseline. Exemestane, a steroidal inhibitor, has a more favorable effect on bone density and may prevent bone loss. However, exemestane does posses weak androgenic properties and may cause weight gain and acne.

## Gonadotropin-releasing hormone analogues

Luteinizing hormone–releasing hormone (LH-RH) agonists are synthetic analogues of the naturally occurring hormone. Initially, these drugs induce an increase in testosterone levels secondary to their stimulation of LH release. With continued use, the pituitary gland becomes desensitized, resulting in a dramatic decrease in the production of estrogens and androgens. Leuprolide and goserelin are the most often used hormone drugs for both prostate and breast cancer. All the LH-RH agonists are available as slow-release depot injections or pellets that are administered monthly, every 3 months, every 4 months, or annually. Castration levels of testosterone are achieved within 3 to 4 weeks with leuprolide and within 1 month with goserelin.

## Antiandrogens

Antiandrogens are used in men with hormone-responsive metastatic prostate cancer either as initial therapy or in combination with a gonadotropin-releasing hormone analogue. Antiandrogens effectively prevent the flare reaction that occurs when patients with active prostate disease are initiated on LH-RH agonist drugs. Their mechanism of action is binding to the androgen receptor and blocking the effects of dihydrotestosterone on prostate cancer cells.[168] Flutamide was the first antiandrogen available; the most frequent adverse events observed with its use include diarrhea, gynecomastia, and occasionally, hepatotoxicity. Newer antiandrogens are nilutamide and bicalutamide, both of which have equivalent activity to flutamide. However, they are usually better tolerated because they produce less diarrhea and offer a simpler administration schedule.

## DIFFERENTIATION AGENTS

### Retinoids

Retinoids, a class of compounds structurally related to vitamin A (retinol), have been found to influence proliferation and differentiation of both normal and tumor cells. The two compounds most studied for their effect on controlling or preventing tumor growth are 13-*cis*-retinoic acid (isotretinoin) and all-*trans*-retinoic acid (tretinoin).[169] Isotretinoin is currently marketed as the antiacne product Accutane. Isotretinoin reverses oral leukoplakia, a premalignant state of the oral cavity in heavy tobacco smokers.[170] Other potential uses for isotretinoin include myelodysplastic syndromes and acute and chronic leukemias. Tretinoin is approved for use in induction and maintenance regimens for acute promyelocytic leukemia.

Toxicity of these compounds is similar to the pharmacological effects of hypervitaminosis A, which include dry lips and mucous membranes, skin fragility, brittle nails, photosensitivity, and conjunctivitis. Other side effects are headache, nausea and vomiting, transaminase and triglyceride elevations, arthralgia, and bone pain. Tretinoin use also has been associated with retinoic acid syndrome, characterized by severe leukocytosis, fevers, respiratory distress, pulmonary and pericardial effusions, and hypotension.[171] Retinoic acid syndrome is usually treated by withdrawing the offending agent and treating the patient with corticosteroids and supportive care. All retinoids are teratogens, so they should never be given to female patients who are pregnant or are considering becoming pregnant.

### Arsenic trioxide

Studies from China of arsenic stimulated interest in the West to further investigate this poison as a chemotherapeutic agent.[172] Arsenic trioxide induces a complete remission in a considerably higher proportion of patients with acute promyelocytic leukemia (APL) than that seen with all-*trans*-retinoic acid (tretinoin).[173] Arsenic trioxide activity in APL is associated with a partial nonterminal differentiation, degradation of the PML-RAR $\alpha$ fusion protein, and activation of capsases, leading to apoptosis.[174] The drug is generally well tolerated when administered in a low-dose daily schedule. Fatigue, light-headedness during the infusion, and characteristic maculopapular skin eruptions are common adverse events. When administered for prolonged periods, arsenic trioxide can induce a peripheral neuropathy and severe neuropathic reactions, including quadriparesis.[175] It is known to cause a prolongation of the QT interval on ECG. For this reason, patients should be monitored with weekly ECGs, and administration of other drugs known to prolong the QT interval, such as amiodarone, beta blockers, cisapride, dolaestron, quinidine, terfenadine, and tricyclic antidepressants, should be avoided. Patients on arsenic trioxide also may develop a leukocytosis and retinoic acid syndrome, as described previously for tretinoin.[176]

## CONCLUSION

Drug therapy for the control and cure of cancer has come a long way from early experimentation with mustard gas derivatives. Currently, a multitude of drugs with a variety of treatment schedules makes up the oncologist's armamentarium. Research efforts must continue to focus on improving the oncology patient's life by evaluating new drugs and therapies, as well as reevaluating old ones. Although biological agents including monoclonal antibodies and targeted therapy account for most of the new pharmaceutical agents being developed, cytotoxic therapy continues to provide the cornerstone for the medical management of patients with cancer. Further development of combining targeted therapies with biological and cytotoxic therapies may continue to change the overall treatment of cancer from a primarily acute approach to a more chronic one.

## REFERENCES


1. Kennedy BJ. Evolution of chemotherapy. *CA: Cancer J Clin.* 1991;41: 261–263.
2. Buick RN. Cellular basis of chemotherapy. In: Dorr RT, Von Hoff DD, eds. *Cancer Chemotherapy Handbook.* 2nd ed. Norwalk, CT: Appleton & Lange; 1994:3–14.
3. Gilewski TA, Norton L. The Norton-Simon hypothesis. In: Perry MC, ed. *Chemotherapy Source Book.* 4th ed. Baltimore, MD: Lippincott Williams & Wilkins; 2007:7–20.
4. Goldie JH, Coldman AJ. The genetic origin of drug resistance in neoplasms: implications for systemic therapy. *Cancer Res.* 1984;44:3643–3653.
5. Shustik C, Dalton W, Gros P. P-glycoprotein-mediated multidrug resistance in tumor cells: biochemistry, clinical relevance, and modulation. *Mol Aspects Med.* 1995;16:1–78.
6. Goldie J. Drug resistance. In: Perry MC, ed. *Chemotherapy Source Book.* 4th ed. Baltimore, MD: Lippincott Williams & Wilkins; 2007:21–29.
7. Gill DR, Hyde SC, Higgins CF, et al. Separation of drug transport and chloride channel functions of the human multidrug resistance P-glycoprotein. *Cell.* 1992;71:23–32.
8. Chu E, Devita VT. Principles of medical oncology. In: Devita VT, Hellman S, Rosenberg SA, eds. *Cancer: Principles and Practice of Oncology.* 7th ed. Philadelphia, PA: Lippincott Williams & Wilkins; 2005:295–307.
9. Goldstein LJ, Galski H, Fojo A, et al. Expression of a multidrug resistance in human cancers. *J Natl Cancer Inst.* 1989;81:116–176.
10. Dan S, Esumi M, Sawada U, et al. Expression of a multidrug-resistance gene in human malignant lymphoma and related disorders. *Leuk Res.* 1991;15:1139–1143.
11. Epstein J, Xiao HQ, Oba BK. P-glycoprotein expression in plasma-cell myeloma is associated with resistance to VAD. *Blood.* 1989;74:913–917.
12. Thomas H, Coley HM. Overcoming multidrug resistance in cancer: an update on the clinical strategy of inhibiting p-glycoprotein. *Cancer Control.* 2003;10:159–165.

13. Ozols RF, Cunnion RE, Klecker RW, et al. Verapamil and adriamycin in the treatment of drug-resistant ovarian cancer. *J Clin Oncol.* 1987;5:641–647.
14. Mross K, Bohn C, Edler L, et al. Randomized phase II study of single-agent epirubicin ± verapamil in patients with advanced metastatic breast cancer. *Ann Oncol.* 1993;4:45–50.
15. Wishart GC, Bissett D, Jodrell PD, et al. Quinidine as a resistance modulator of epirubicin in advanced breast cancer: mature results of a placebo-controlled randomized tral. *J Clin Onol.* 1994;12: 1171–1177.
16. Lhomme C, Joly F, Walker JL, et al. Phase III study of valspodar (PSC 833) combined with paclitaxel and carboplatin alone in patients with stage IV or suboptimally debulked stage III epithelial ovarian cancer or primary peritoneal cancer. *J Clin Oncol.* 2008;26:2674–2682.
17. Mross K. Multidrug-resistance modulation in metastatic breast cancer patients. *J Clin Oncol.* 1995;13:303–304.
18. Kaye SB. Reversal of drug resistance in ovarian cancer: where do we go from here? [editorial]. *J Clin Oncol.* 2008;26:2616–2618.
19. Glisson BS. Multidrug resistance mediated through alterations in topoisomerase II. *Cancer Bull.* 1989;41:37–39.
20. Mannervik B, Danielson UH. Glutathione transferases: structure and catalytic activity. *Crit Rev Biochem.* 1988;23:283–337.
21. Davies SM, Robison LL, Buckley JD, et al. Glutathione *S*-transferase polymorphisms and outcome of chemotherapy in childhood acute myeloid leukemia. *J Clin Oncol.* 2001;19:1279–1287.
22. Hickman JA. Apopotosis induced by anticancer drugs. *Cancer Metastasis Rev.* 1992;11:121.
23. Symonds H, Krall L, Remington L, et al. p53 dependent apoptosis suppresses tumor growth and progression in vivo. *Cell.* 1994;73:703–711.
24. Hollstein M, Sidransky DE, Vogelstein B, et al. *p53* mutations in human cancers. *Science.* 1991;253:49–53.
25. Reed SI. Molecular targets in oncology. Section 2: Cell cycle. In: Devita VT, Hellman S, Rosenber SA, eds. *Cancer: Principles and Practice of Oncology.* 7th ed. Philadelphia, PA: Lippincott William & Wilkins; 2005.
26. Levine AJ. p53, the cellular gatekeeper for growth and division. *Cell.* 1997;88:323–333.
27. Lowe SW, Schmitt EM, Smith SW, et al. p53 is required for radiation-induced apoptosis in mouse thymocytes. *Nature.* 1993;362:847–849.
28. Wu GS, El-Deiry WS. *p53* and chemosensitivity. *Nat Med.* 1996;2: 255–258.
29. Wahl AF, Donaldson KL, Fairchild C, et al. Loss of normal *p53* function confers sensitization to taxol by increasing $G_2$/M arrest and apoptosis. *Nat Med.* 1996;2:72–88.
30. Aas T, Borreson AL, Geisler S, et al. Specific *p53* mutations are associated with de novo resistance to doxorubicin in breast cancer. *Nat Med.* 1996;2:811–814.
31. Rusch V, Klimstra V, Venkatramen E, et al. Aberrant *p53* expression predicts clinical resistance to cisplatin based chemotherapy in locally advanced non-small cell lung cancer. *Cancer Res.* 1992;55: 5038–5042.
32. Hamada M, Fujiwara T, Hizuta A, et al. The *p53* gene is a potent determinant of chemosensitivity and radiosensitivity in gastric and colorectal cancers. *J Cancer Res Clin Oncol.* 1996;122:360–365.
33. O'Brien S, Keating MJ. Chronic lymphoid leukemias. In: Devita VT, Hellman S, Rosenber SA, eds. *Cancer: Principles and Practice of Oncology.* 7th ed. Philadelphia, PA: Lippincott William & Wilkins; 2005:2133–2143.
34. Wang Q, Beck WT. Transcriptional suppression of multidrug resistance-associated protein (*MRP*) gene expression by wildtype *p53*. *Cancer Res.* 1998;58:5768–5771.
35. Zhou G, Kuo MT. Wild-type *p53*-mediated induction of rat *mdr-1b* expression by the anticancer drug daunorubicin. *J Biol Chem.* 1998;273: 15387–15394.
36. Simonian PL, Grillot DA, Nunez G. bcl-2 and bcl-XL can differentially block chemotherapy associated cell death. *Blood.* 1997;90:1208–1216.
37. Strobel T, Swanson L, Korsmeyer S, et al. BAX enhances paclitaxel-induced apoptosis through a p53 independent pathway [abstract]. *Proc Natl Acad Sci USA.* 1996;93:14094.
38. Lictra E, Todd MB, Dipaola RS. Vinblastine or paclitaxel enhance mitoxantrone antitumor activity in a sequence dependent manner in association with BCL-2 phosphorylation [abstract]. *Proc Am Soc Clin Oncol.* 1998;17:247.
39. Citron ML, Berry DA, Cirrincione C, et al. Randomized trial of dose-dense versus conventionally scheduled and sequential versus concurrent combination chemotherapy as postoperative adjuvant treatment of node positive primary breast cancer: first report of Intergroup Trial C9741/Cancer and Leukemia Group B Trial 9741. *J Clin Oncol.* 2003;21:1431–1439.
40. Bonadonna G, Valagussa R. Dose-response effect of adjuvant chemotherapy in breast cancer. *N Engl J Med.* 1981;304:10–15.
41. Timmer-Bonte JN, deBoo TM, Smith HL, et al. Cost-effectiveness of adding granulocyte colony-stimulating factor to primary prophylaxis with antibodies in small-cell lung cancer. *J Clin Oncol.* 2006;24:2991–2997.
42. Vogel CL, Wojtukiewicz MZ, Carroll RR, et al. First and subsequent cycle use of pegfilgrastim prevents febrile neutropenia in patients with breast cancer: a multicenter, double-blind, placebo-controlled phase III study. *J Clin Oncol.* 2005;23:1178–1184.
43. Schuchter LM, Hensley ML, Meropol NJ, Winer EP. 2002 Update of recommendations for the use of chemotherapy and radiotherapy protectants: clinical practice guidelines of the American Society of Clinical Oncology. *J Clin Oncol.* 2002;20:2895–2903.
44. Schouten HC, Qian W, Kvaloy S, et al. High-dose therapy improves progression-free survival and survival in relapsed follicular non-Hodgkin's lymphoma: results form the randomized European CUP trial. *J Clin Oncol.* 2003;21:3918.
45. Cooper DL, Seropian S. Autologous stem cell transplantation. In: Devita VT, Hellman S, Rosenber SA, eds. *Cancer: Principles and Practice of Oncology.* 7th ed. Philadelphia, PA: Lippincott William & Wilkins; 2005:2414–2422.
46. Ezzone, S. Blood and marrow stem cell transplantation. In: Gobel BH, Triest-Robertson S, Vogel WH, eds. *Advanced Oncology Nursing Certification Review and Resource Manual.* Pittsburgh, PA: Oncology Nursing Society; 2009:261–303.
47. Gianni AM, Magni M, Martelli M, et al. Long-term remission in mantle cell lymphoma following high-dose sequential chemotherapy and in vivo rituximab-purged stem cell autografting (R-HDS regiman). *Blood.* 2003;102:749.
48. Salama JK, Seiwert TY, Vokes EE. Chemoradiotherapy for locally advanced head and neck cancer. *J Clin Oncol.* 2007;25:4118–4126.
49. Braendengen M, Tveit KM, Berglund A, et al. Randomized phase III study comparing preoperative radiotherapy with chemoradiotherapy in nonresectable rectal cancer. *J Clin Oncol.* 2008;26:3687–3694.
50. Rodel C, Grabenbauer GG, Kuhn R, et al. Combined-modality treatment and selective organ preservation in invasive bladder cancer: long-term results. *J Clin Oncol.* 2002;20:3061–3071.
51. Stahl M, Stuschke M, Lehmann N, et al. Chemoradiation with or without surgery in patients with locally advanced squamous cell carcinoma of the esophagus. *J Clin Oncol.* 2005;23:2310–2317.
52. Calais G, Alfonsi M, Bardet E, et al. Randomized trial of radiation therapy versus concomitant chemotherapy and radiation therapy for advanced-stage oropharynx carcinoma. *J Natl Cancer Inst.* 1999;91:2081.
53. Olmi P, Crispino S, Fallai C, et al. Locoregionally advanced carcinoma of the oropharynx: conventional radiotherapy vs accelerated hyperfractionated radiotherapy vs concomitant radiotherapy and chemotherapy—a multicenter randomized trial. *Int J Radiat Oncol Biol Phys.* 2003;55:78.
54. Adelstein DJ, Lavertu P, Saxton JP, et al. Mature results of a phase III randomized trial comparing concurrent chemoradiotherapy with radiation therapy alone in patients with stage III and IV squamous cell carcinoma of the head and neck. *Cancer.* 2000;88:876.
55. Jeremic B, Shibamoto Y, Milicic B, et al. Hyperfractionated radiation therapy with or without concurrent low-dose daily cisplatin in locally

advanced squamous cell carcinoma of the head and neck: a prospective randomized trial. *J Clin Oncol.* 2000;18:1458.
56. Bleiberg H. Role of chemotherapy for advanced colorectal cancer: new opportunities. *Semin Oncol.* 1996;23:42–48.
57. Piedbois P, Buyse M, Rustum Y, et al. Modulation of fluorouracil by leucovorin in advanced colorectal cancer: evidence in terms of response rate. *J Clin Oncol.* 1992;10:896–903.
58. Kivisto KT, Kroemer HK, Eichelbaum M. The role of human cytochrome P450 enzymes in the metabolism of anticancer agents: implications of drug interactions. *Br J Clin Pharmacol.* 1995;40:523–530.
59. Bernard SA, Bruera E. Drug interaction in palliative care. *J Clin Oncol.* 2000;18:1780–1799.
60. McLeod HL, Evans WE. Pharmacogenomics: unlocking the human genome for better drug therapy. *Annu Rev Pharmacol Toxicol.* 2001;41:101–110.
61. Flockhart DA. Clinical pharmacogenetics. In: Atkinson AJ, Daniels CE, Dedrick RL, et al, eds. *Principles of Clinical Pharmacology.* San Diego, CA: Academic Press; 2001:158.
62. Relling MV, Hancock ML, Rivera GK, et al. Mercaptopurine therapy intolerance and heterozygosity at the thiopurine S-methyltransferase gene locus. *J Natl Cancer Inst.* 1999;91:2001.
63. Diasio RB, Johnson MR. The role of pharmacogenetics and pharmacogenomics in cancer chemotherapy with 5-fluorouracil. *Pharmacology.* 2000;61:199–204.
64. Goetz M, Ames M, Filpits M, et al. Pharmacogenetic (CYP2D6) and gene expression profiles (HOXB13/IL17BR and molecular grade index) for prediction of adjuvant endocrine therapy benefit in the ABCSG 8 trial. 31st Annual San Antonio Breast Cancer Symposium; 2008; San Antonio, TX. [Abstract 57] http://www.abstracts2view.com/sabar/view.php??nu=SABC5081_1392. Accessed January 24, 2010.
65. Harland SJ, Newell DR, Tippping SJ, et al. Pharmacokinetics of cis-diammine-1,1-cyclobutane dicarboxylate phatinum(II) in patients with normal and impared renal function. *Cancer Res.* 1984;44:1693–1697.
66. Egorin MJ, VanEcho DA, Tipping SJ, et al. Pharmacokinetecs and dosage reduction of cis-diammine(1,1-cyclobutananedicarboxylato)platinum in patients with impaired renal function. *Cancer Res.* 1984;44:5432–5404.
67. Taguchi J, Saijo N, Mirua K, et al. Prediction of haematologic toxicity of carboplatin by creatinine clearance rate. *Jpn J Cancer Res.* 1987;78:977–982.
68. Calvert AH, Newell DR, Gumbrell LA, et al. Carboplatin dosage: prospective evaluation of a simple formula based on renal function. *J Clin Oncol.* 1989;7:1748–1756.
69. Cockcroft D, Gault M. Prediction of creatinine clearance from serum creatinine. *Nephron.* 1976;16:31–41.
70. Jelliffe RW. Creatinine clearance: bedside estimate. *Ann Intern Med.* 1973;79:604–605.
71. Dorr RT, Von Hoff DD, eds. *Cancer Chemotherapy Handbook.* 2nd ed. Norwalk, CT: Appleton & Lange; 1994.
72. Hansten PD, Horn JR, eds. *Drug Interactions and Updates.* Vancouver, WA: Applied Therapeutics; 1995.
73. Balis FM. Pharmacokinetic drug interactions of commonly used anticancer drugs. *Clin Pharmacokinet.* 1986;11:223–235.
74. Finley RS. Drug interactions in the oncology patient. *Semin Oncol Nurs.* 1992;8:95–101.
75. Loadman PM, Bibby MC. Pharmacokinetic drug interactions with anticancer drugs. *Clin Pharmacokinet.* 1994;26:486–500.
76. Thyss A, Milano G, Kubar J, et al. Clinical and pharmacokinetic evidence of a life-threatening interaction between methotrexate and ketoprofen. *Lancet.* 1986;1:256–258.
77. Ellison NM, Servi RJ. Acute renal failure and death following sequential intermediate-dose methotrexate and fluorouracil: a possible adverse effect due to concomitant indomethacin administration. *Cancer Treat Rep.* 1985;69:342–343.
78. Fitzsimmons WE, Ghalie R, Kaizer H. The effect of hepatic enzyme inducers on busulfan neurotoxicity and myelotoxicity. *Cancer Chemother Pharmacol.* 1990;27:27–32.
79. McCrea JB, Majumdar AK, Goldberg MR, et al. Effects of the neurokinin 1 receptor antagonist aprepitent on the pharmacokinetics of dexamethasone and methyprednisolone. *Clin Pharmacol Ther.* 2003;74:17–24.
80. Venturini M, Lunardi G, DelMastro L, et al. Sequence effect of epirubicin and paclitaxel treatment on pharmacokinetics and toxicity. *J Clin Oncol.* 2000;18:2116–2125.
81. Hall G, Lind MJ, Huang M, et al. Intravenous infusions of ifosfamide/mesna and perturbation of warfarin anticoagulant control. *Postgrad Med J.* 1990;66:860–861.
82. Tenni P, Lalich DL, Byrne MJ. Life-threatening interaction between tamoxifen and warfarin. *Br Med J.* 1989;298:93.
83. Camidge R, Reigner B, Cassidy J, et al. Significant effect of capecitabine on the pharmacokinetics and pharmacodynamics of warfarin in patients with cancer. *J Clin Oncol.* 2005;21:4719–4725.
84. Masci G, Magagnoli M, Zucali PA, et al. Minidose warfarin prophylaxis for catheter-associated thrombosis in cancer patients: can it be safely associated with fluorouracil-based chemotherapy. *J Clin Oncol.* 2003;21:736–739.
85. Nies A, Speilber SP. Principles of therapeutics. In: Brunton LL, Lazo JS, Parker KL, eds. *Goodman and Gilman's Pharmacological Basis of Therapeutics.* 11th ed. New York: McGraw-Hill; 2006:49–65.
86. Anonymous. Cancer patients at risk of drug interactions. *CA Cancer J Clin.* 2007;57:258–259.
87. Bohr VA, Phillips DH, Hanawalt PC. Heterogeneous DNA damage and repair in the mammalian genome. *Cancer Res.* 1987;47:6426–6436.
88. Hilton J. Role of aldehyde dehydrogenase in cyclophosphamide-resistant L 1210 leukemia. *Cancer Res.* 1984;44:5156–5160.
89. Schoenike SE, Dana WJ. Ifosfamide and mesna. *Clin Pharm.* 1990;9:179.
90. Barman Balfour JA, Goa KL. Bendamustine. *Drugs.* 2001;61:631–640.
91. Strumberg D, Harstrick A, Doll K, et al. Bendamustine hydrochloride activity against doxorubicin-resistant human breast carcinoma cell lines. *Anticancer Drugs.* 1996;7:415–421.
92. Friedberg JW, Cohen P, Chen L, et al. Bendamustine in patients with rituximab-refractory and alkylator-refractory, indolent, and transformed non-Hodgkin's lymphoma: results from a phase II multicenter single-agent study. *J Clin Oncol.* 2008;26:204–210.
93. Bloommaert FA, van Kijk-Knijenburg HCM, Dijt FJ, et al. Formation of DNA adducts by the anticancer drug carboplatin: different nucleotide sequence preferences in vitro and in cells. *Biochemistry.* 1995;34:8474–8480.
94. Markman M. Intraperitoneal therapy of ovarian cancer. *Semin Oncol.* 1998;25:356–360.
95. Andre T, Boni C, Mouredji-Bardint L, et al. Oxaliplatin, fluorouracil, and leucovorin as adjuvant threatment for colon cancer. *N Engl J Med.* 2004;350:2343.
96. De Gramont A, Figer A, Seymour M, et al. Leucovorin and fluorouracil with or without oxaliplatin as firstline treatment in advanced colorectal cancer. *J Clin Oncol.* 2000;18:2938–2947.
97. Nikcevich DA, Grothey A, Sloan JA, et al. Effect of intravenous calcium and magnesium (IV CaMg) on oxaliplatin-induced sensory neurotoxicity (sNT) in adjuvant colon cancer: results of the phase III placebo-controlled, double-blind NCCTG trial N04C7. [Abstract 4009]. *J Clin Oncol.* 2008;26(May 20 suppl).
98. O'Reilly SM, Newlands ES, Glaser MG, et al. Temozolomide: a new oral cytotoxic chemotherapeutic agent with promising activity against primary brain tumors. *Eur J Cancer.* 1993;29A:940–942.
99. Stupp R, Dietrich PY, Kraljevic SO, et al. Promising survival for patients with newly diagnosed glloblastoma multiforme treated with concomitant radiation plus temozolomide followed by adjuvant temozolomide. *J Clin Oncol.* 2002;20:1375–1382.
100. Middleton MR, Grob JJ, Aaronson N, et al. Randomized phase III study of temozolamide versus dacarbazine in the treatment of patients with advanced metastatic malignant melanoma. *J Clin Oncol.* 2000;18:158–166.

101. Zhang H, D'Arpe P, Liu LF. A model for tumor cell killing by topoisomerase poisons. *Cancer Cells.* 1990;2:23–27.
102. Zwelling LA. Topoisomerase II as a target of antileukemia drugs: a review of controversial areas. *Hematol Pathol.* 1989;3:101–112.
103. Takimoto CH. Topoisomerase interactive agents. In: Devita VT, Hellman S, Rosenberg SA, eds. *Cancer: Principles and Practice of Oncology.* 7th ed. Philadelphia, PA: Lippincott Williams & Wilkins; 2005:375–389.
104. Herman EH, Zhang J, Rifai N, et al. The use of serum levels of cardiac troponin T to compare the protective activity of dexrazoxane against doxorubicin- and mitoxantrone-induced cardiotoxicity. *Cancer Chemother Pharmacol.* 2001;48:297–304.
105. Fisher GR, Patterson LH. Lack of involvement of reactive oxygen in the cytotoxicity of mitoxantrone, CI941 and ametantrone in MCF-7 cells: comparison with doxorubicin. *Cancer Chemother Pharmacol.* 1992;30:451–458.
106. Forssen EA, Coulter DM, Proffitt RT. Selective in vivo localization of daunorubicin small unilamellar vesicles in solid tumors. *Cancer Res.* 1996;56:2066–2075.
107. Product information. *Doxil.* Raritan, NJ: Ortho-Biotech; 2001.
108. Issell BF, Prout GJ Jr, Soloway MS, et al. Mitomycin C intravesical therapy in non-invasive bladder cancer after failure on thiotepa. *Cancer.* 1984;53:1025–1028.
109. Kummar S, Noronha V, Chu E. Antimetabolites. In: Devita VT, Hellman S, Rosenberg SA, eds. *Cancer: Principles and Practice of Oncology.* 7th ed. Philadelphia, PA: Lippincott Williams & Wilkins; 2005:358–374.
110. Evans WE, Crom WR, Yalowich J. Methotrexate. In: Evans WE, Schentag JJ, Juskow J, eds. *Applied Pharmacokinetics: Principles of Therapeutic Drug Monitoring.* 2nd ed. Spokane, WA: Applied Therapeutics; 1986:1009–1056.
111. Stoller RG, Hande KR, Jacobs SA, et al. Use of plasma pharmacokinetics to predict and prevent methotrexate toxicity. *N Engl J Med.* 1977;297:630–634.
112. Niyikiza C. LY231514 (MTA) safety analysis, December 3, 1999. Submitted to the FDA as a Serial Number 95 to IND #40,061; on file.
113. Package insert. *Alimta (premetrexed).* Indianapolis, IN: Eli Lilly; 2005.
114. Diasio RB, Schuetz JD, Wallace HJ, et al. Dihydrofluorouracil, a fluorouracil catabolite with antitumor activity in murine and human cells. *Cancer Res.* 1985;45:4900–4903.
115. Burger AJ, Mannino S. 5-Fluorouracil-induced coronary vasospasm. *Am Heart J.* 1987;114:433–436.
116. Villalona-Calero MA, Weiss GR, Burris HA, et al. Phase I and pharmacokinetic study of the oral fluoropyrimide capecitabine in combination with paclitaxel in patient with advanced solid malignancies. *J Clin Oncol.* 1999;1915–1925.
117. Baccanari DP, Davis ST, Knick V, et al. 5-Ethynyluraci (766C85): a potent modulator of the pharmacokinetics and antitumor efficacy of 5-fluorouracil [abstract]. *Proc Natl Acad Sci USA.* 1993;90:11064.
118. Sulkes A, Benner SE, Canetta RM. Uracil-ftorafur: an oral fluoropyrimidine active in colorectal cancer. *J Clin Oncol.* 1988;16: 3461–3475.
119. Weiss RB. Adverse effects of treatment. Section 8: Miscellaneous toxicities. In: Devita VT, Hellman S, Rosenberg SA, eds. *Cancer: Principles and Practice of Oncology.* 7th ed. Philadelphia, PA: Lippincott Williams & Wilkins; 2005:2602–2614.
120. Baker CH, Banzon J, Bollinger JM, et al. 2-Deoxy-2-methylenecytidine and 2-dexoy-2, 2-difluorocytidine 5-diphosphate: potent mechansim-based inhibitors of ribonucleotide reductase. *J Med Chem.* 1991;34:1879–1884.
121. Hue YF, Reitz J. Gemcitabine: a cytidine analogue active against solid tumors. *Am J Health-Syst Pharm.* 1997;54:162–170.
122. Montgomery JA, Hewson K. Nucleosides of 2-fluoroadenine. *J Med Chem.* 1969;12:498.
123. Cheson BD, Vena D, Foss F, et al. Neurotoxicity of purine analogues: a review. *J Clin Oncol.* 1994;12:2216–2228.
124. Weiss RB, Freiman J, Kweder SL, et al. Hemolytic anemia after fludarabine therapy for chronic lymphocytic leukemia. *J Clin Oncol.* 1998;16:1885–1889.
125. Kawasaki H, Carrera CJ, Piro LD, et al. Relationship of deoxycytidine kinase and cytoplasmic 5-nucleotidase to the chemotherapeutic efficacy of 2-chlorodeoxyadenosine. *Blood.* 1994;81:597–602.
126. Estey EH, Kurzrock R, Kantarjian HM, et al. Treatment of hairy cell leukemia with 2-chlorodeoxyadenosine (2-CdA). *Blood.* 1992;79:882–895.
127. Juliusson G, Hedlal D, Hippe E, et al. Subcutaneous injections of 2-chlorodeoxyadenosine for symptomatic hairy cell leukemia. *J Clin Oncol.* 1995;13:989–999.
128. Cheson B. Immunologic and immunosuppressive complications of purine analogue therapy. *J Clin Oncol.* 1995;13:2431.
129. Plunkett W, Gandhi V. Cellular metabolism of nucleoside analogues in CLL: implications for drug development. In: Cheson BD, ed. *Chronic Lymphocytic Leukemia: Scientific Advances and Clinical Developments.* New York: Marcel Dekker; 1993:197–214.
130. Kraut EH, Neff JC, Bouroncle BA, et al. Immunosuppressive effects of pentostatin. *J Clin Oncol.* 1990;8:848–865.
131. Jabbour E, Issa JP, Garcia-Manero G, Kantarjian H. Evolution of decitabine development. *Cancer.* 2008;112:2341–2351.
132. Pinto A, Zagonel V. 5-Aza-2'-deoxycytidine (decitabine) and 5-azacytidine in the treatment of acute myeloid leukemias and myelodysplastic syndrome: past, present and future trends. *Leukemia.* 1993;7:S51-S60.
133. Kantarjian H, Issa JP, Rossenfeld CS, et al. Decitabine improves patient outcomes in myelodysplastic syndromes: results of a phase III randomized study. *Cancer.* 2006;106:1794–1803.
134. Kantarjian H, Oki Y, Garcia-Manero G, et al. Results of a randomized study of three schedules of low-dose decitabine in higher risk myelodysplastic syndrome and chronic myelogenous leukemia. *Blood.* 2007;109:52–57.
135. Silverman LR, Zinar S, Holland JF. Azacytidine acts as a biological response modifier on hematopoietic cell response to cytokines [abstract]. *Proc Am Assoc Cancer Res.* 1998;39:405.
136. Silverman LR, Demakos EP, Peterson BL, et al. Randomized, controlled trial of azacitidine in patients with the myelodysplastic syndrome: a study of the Cancer and Leukemia Group B. *J Clin Oncol.* 2002;20:2429–2440.
137. Nelson RL. The comparative clinical pharmacology and pharmacokinetics of vindisine, vincristine, and vinblastine in human patients with cancer. *Med Pediatr Oncol.* 1982;10:115–127.
138. Schiff PB, Fant J, Horowitz SB. Promotion of microtubule assembly in vitro by taxol. *Nature.* 1979;22:665–667.
139. Rowisnky EK, Burke PJ, Karp JE, et al. Phase I clinical and pharmacokinetic study of taxol. *Cancer Res.* 1989;49:4640–4647.
140. Extra JM, Rousseau F, Bruno R, et al. Phase I and pharmacokinetic study of taxotere (NSC 628503) given as a short intravenous infusion. *Cancer Res.* 1993;53:1037–1042.
141. Citardi M, Rowinsky EK, Schaefer KL, et al. Sequence-dependent cytotoxicity between cisplatin and the antimicrotubule agents taxol and vincristine [abstract]. *Proc Am Assoc Cancer Res.* 1990;31:2431.
142. Weiss RB, Donehower RC, Wiernik PH, et al. Hypersensitivity reactions from taxol. *J Clin Oncol.* 1990;8:1263–1268.
143. Chevallier B, Fumoleau P, Kerbrat P, et al. Docetaxel is a major cytotoxic drug for the treatment of advanced breast cancer. *J Clin Oncol.* 1995;13:314–322.
144. Desai N, Yao Z, Trieu V, et al. Evidence of greater tumor and red cell partitioning and superior antitumor activity of Cremophor-free nanoparticle paxlitaxel (ABI-007) compared to Taxol [abstract 348]. *Breast Cancer Res Treat.* 2003;82:S82.
145. Ibrahmin NK, Desai N, Legha S, et al. Phase I and pharmacokinetic study of ABI-007, a Cremophor-free, protein-stabilized, nanoparticle formulation of paclitaxel. *Clin Cancer Res.* 2002;8:1038–1044.
146. Gradishar WJ, Tjulandin S, Davidson N, et al. Phase III trial of nanoparticle albumin-bound paclitaxel compared with polyethylated

castor oil based paclitaxel in women with breast cancer. *J Clin Oncol.* 2005;23:7794–7803.
147. Product information. *Abraxane.* Los Angeles, CA: Abraxis Oncology; 2007.
148. Wolff AC, Donehower RC, Carducci MK, et al. Phase I study of docasahexaenoic acid–paclitaxel: a taxane fatty acid conjugate with a unique pharmacology and toxicity profile. *Clin Cancer Res.* 2003;9: 3589–3597.
149. Li C, Wallace S. Polymer-drug conjugates: recent development in clinical oncology. *Adv Drug Deliv Rev.* 2008;60:866–898.
150. Ross H, Bonomi P, Langer C, et al. Effect of gender on outcome in two randomized phase III trials of paclitaxel poliglumex (PPX) in chemo-naive patients with advanced NSCLC and poor performance status (PS2) [abstract 18S]. *J Clin Oncol, 2006 ASCO Annual Meeting Proceedings.* 2006; 24:7039.
151. Kowalski RJ, Giannakakou P, Hamel E. Activities of the microtubule-stabilizing agents epothilones A and B with purified tubulin and in cells resistant to paclitaxel. *J Biol Chem.* 1997;272:2534–2541.
152. Duran GE, Jordan MA, Sikic BI. Impaired taxane- and epothilone-driven tubulin polymerization in a non-MDR1 taxane-resistant MCF-7 breast cancer variant with reduced MAP4 and elevated MAP Tau content [abstract 3755]. *Proc Am Assoc Cancer Res.* 2006;47:47.
153. Wartmann M, Altmann KH. The biology and medicinal chemistry of epothilones. *Curr Med Chem Anticancer Agents.* 2002;2:123–148.
154. Goodin S. Novel cytotoxic agents: epothilones. *Am J Health-Syst Pharm.* 2008;65:S10-S15.
155. Thomas ES, Gomez HL, Li RK, et al. Ixabepilone plus capecitabine for metastatic breast cancer progressing after anthracycline and taxane treatment. *J Clin Oncol.* 2007;25:5210–5217.
156. Yang L, Rowe RC, Liu LF. Identification of DNA topoisomerase II as an intracellular target of antitumor epipodophyllotoxins in simian virus 40-infected monkey cells. *Cancer Res.* 1985;45:5872–5876.
157. Jones SF, Burris HA. Topoisomerase I inhibitors: topotecan and irinotecan. *Cancer Pract.* 1996;4:51–53.
158. Rothenberg ML, Kuhn JG, Burris HA, et al. Phase I and pharmacokinetic trial of weekly CPT-11. *J Clin Oncol.* 1993;11:2194–2204.
159. Stearns ME, Tew KD. Antimicrotubule effects of estramustine, an antiprostatic tumor drug. *Cancer Res.* 1985;45:3891–3897.
160. Petrylak DP, Tangen CM, Hussain MHA, et al. Docetaxel and estramustine compared with mitoxantrone and prednisone for advanced refractory prostate cancer. *N Engl J Med.* 2004;351:1513–1520.
161. Jaiyesimi IA, Buzdar AU, Decker DA, et al. Use of tamoxifen for breast cancer: twenty-eight years later. *J Clin Oncol.* 1995;13:513–529.
162. Fisher B, Costantino JP, Wickerham DL, et al. Tamoxifen for prevention of breast cancer: report of the National Surgical Adjuvant Breast and Bowel Project P-1 study. *J Natl Cancer Inst.* 1998;90:1371–1388.
163. Loprinzi CL, Ellison NM, Schaid DJ, et al. Controlled trial of megestrol acetate for treatment of cancer anorexia and cachexia. *J Natl Cancer Inst.* 1990;82:1127–1132.
164. Howell A, Osborne CK, Morris C, Wakeling AE. ICI 182,780 (Faslodex): development of a novel, "pure" antiestrogen. *Cancer.* 2000;89:817–825.
165. Robertson JFR, Osborne CK, Howell A, et al. Fulvestrant versus anastrozole for the treatment of advanced breast carcinoma in postmenopausal women. *Cancer.* 2003;98:229–238.
166. Buzdar A, Howell A. Advances in aromatase inhibition: clinical efficacy and tolerability in the treatment of breast cancer. *Clin Cancer Res.* 2001;7:2620–2627.
167. Elisaf MS, Bairaktari ET, Nicolaides C, et al. Effect of letrozole on the lipid profile in postmenopausal women with breast cancer. *Eur J Cancer.* 2001;37:1510.
168. Brogden RN, Chrisp P. Flutamide: a review of its pharmacodynamic, pharmacokinetic properties and therapeutic use in advanced prostatic cancer. *Drugs Aging.* 1991;1:104–118.
169. Lippman S, Parkinson D, Itri L, et al. 13-*cis*-Retinoic acid and interferon-α-2a: effective combination therapy for advanced squamous cell carcinoma of the skin. *J Natl Cancer Inst.* 1992;84:235–241.
170. Hong WK, Endicott J, Itri LM, et al. 13-*cis*-Retinoic acid in the treatment of oral leukoplakia. *N Engl J Med.* 1986;315:1501–1505.
171. Warrell RR. All-*trans*-retinoic acid. Paper presented at: 28th Annual Meeting of American Society of Clinical Oncology Educational Book; May 17–19, 1992; San Diego, CA.
172. Zhang P, Wang SY, Hu XH. Arsenic trioxide treated 72 cases of acute promyelocytic leukemia. *Chin J Hematol.* 1996;17:58.
173. Soignet S, Kantarjian H, Frankel S, et al. Arsenic trioxide in acute promyelocytic leukemia: results of initial U.S. pilot and multicenter trials. *Blood.* 1998;92:S483a.
174. Soignet SL, Maslak P, Wang Z-G, et al. Complete remission after induction of non-terminal differentiation and apoptosis in acute promyelocytic leukemia by arsenic trioxide. *N Engl J Med.* 1998;339: 1341–1348.
175. Westervelt P, Pollock J, Haug J, et al. Response and toxicity associated with dose escalation of arsenic trioxide in the treatment of resistant acute promyelocytic leukemia. *Blood.* 1997;90:S249b.
176. Warrel RP Jr, Chanel S, Ho R, Soignet S. Leukocytosis and retinoic syndrome in patients with acute promyelocytic leukemia treated with arsenic trioxide [abstract]. *Proc Am Soc Clin Oncol.* 1999;18:21a.

CHAPTER

16

Gail M. Wilkes, MS, RN, ANP-BC, AOCN®

# Chemotherapy: Principles of Administration

## CHEMOTHERAPY ADMINISTRATION

Chemotherapy is administered in a variety of care settings.[1] Most patients with cancer, however, receive systemic chemotherapy in a hospital-based outpatient center, physician office setting, or free-standing infusion clinic. Others may receive their chemotherapy at home. Few individuals actually require hospitalization for chemotherapy despite the fact that treatment regimens are currently more aggressive and dose intensive in nature. Hospital admission generally is reserved for patients who require intensive monitoring or who are acutely ill. However, novel areas within the hospital now serve as settings for chemotherapy administration: interventional radiology suites (eg, chemoembolization), the operating room (intraoperatively), or specialty suites such as cystoscopy.[2,3] In addition, more patients with non-cancer diagnoses, such as autoimmune diseases, are receiving treatment with chemotherapy or biotherapy.[1] Many bone marrow transplant and peripheral blood stem cell transplant programs have moved to the outpatient setting.[4] The shift to outpatient ambulatory care services has grown out of the need for more efficient and economical healthcare delivery systems as hospitals cope with a largely managed-care environment. Indeed, managed care has virtually replaced indemnity insurance reimbursement. Over the past few years, Medicare reimbursement rules and regulation changes have presented a tremendous challenge, especially in the ambulatory setting.[5] Legally responsible to follow US Food and Drug Administration (FDA)–approved labeling, Medicare and private payers use 2 compendia to evaluate whether they will reimburse for off-label uses of drugs.[5] Oncology nurses are challenged with the increased responsibility of coordinating quality patient care with limited resources and support. Through team building and collaboration with other disciplines, the nurse must effectively assess and develop a plan of care that ensures continuity regardless of the care setting. In addition, with the increased use of targeted therapies, increasingly more oral therapies are prescribed for patients, issues of nonadherence are now recognized, and standards for follow-up, monitoring, and support are just beginning to emerge.[6,7] The real challenge lies in finding ways to promote self-care in an aging population with limited personal, financial, and social resources. This chapter addresses basic and advanced principles of chemotherapy administration. It focuses on clinical practice and methods of drug delivery, including vascular access devices (VADs).

### PROFESSIONAL QUALIFICATIONS

Evidence-based guidelines for nurses administering chemotherapy are available from the Oncology Nursing Society (ONS)[1] and should be implemented in all practice settings. In 2009, the American Society of Clinical Oncology (ASCO) and the ONS developed standards for safe chemotherapy administration to adults in the outpatient setting and articulate that the practice must have processes for oversight, verification of training, and continuing education for clinical staff. These standards focus on patient safety, are applicable to diverse ambulatory and outpatient practice settings, and are measurable According to the standards, the ambulatory or outpatient practice should have a comprehensive educational program for new staff administering chemotherapy that includes a competency evaluation or an offsite program such as the ONS chemotherapy and biotherapy course that is followed by a clinical hands-on competency evaluation, and the clinical competency evaluation should be repeated annually.[7] The Infusion Nurses' Society (INS),[8] ONS,[9] and ASCO[10] all have published position statements regarding the administration of antineoplastic agents.

According to the groups just listed,[8–10] basic qualifications for nurses administering antineoplastic agents include the following:

- Current licensure as a registered nurse
- Certification in cardiopulmonary resuscitation (CPR)
- Intravenous therapy skills
- Educational preparation and demonstrated knowledge in all areas related to antineoplastic drugs (including cancer chemotherapy, targeted therapy, and biotherapy), pharmacology, drug indications, drug preparation, drug disposition, drug metabolism, elimination, drug dose calculation, symptom management, drug interactions, and side effects
- Demonstrated knowledge of prevention of medication errors, including nurse validation that the drug regimen and the doses prescribed are evidence-based and, if not, that the physician provide the evidence to support the regimen prior to mixing or administering the drug
- Demonstrated competence in the skill of chemotherapy drug administration, including patient education and assessment, monitoring, documentation, and proper use of personal protective equipment (PPE), as well as the prevention or management of hypersensitivity and extravasation during chemotherapy administration.
- Posttreatment care, management and prevention, if possible, of late and long-term side effects, and aspects of survivorship
- Demonstrated competence in patient/family education in self-care measures to minimize or prevent potential drug side effects
- Ongoing education and competency assessment
- Knowledge of policies and procedures related to chemotherapy and biotherapy administration (Table 16-1)

Formal instruction in chemotherapy administration techniques and certification programs that have both a

**TABLE 16-1**

| Institutional Policies and Procedures for Chemotherapy Administration |
|---|
| • Outcome standards |
| • Vesicant management |
| • Hypersensitivity reactions |
| • Coordination of home care |
| • Patient and family education |
| • Safe drug handling and disposal |
| • Oncology quality-improvement process |
| • Chemotherapy administration (all routes) |
| • Documentation methods (extravasation record) |
| • Management of vascular access devices (VADs) |
| • Mechanisms for prevention and reporting of drug and dosing errors |
| • Staff education for chemotherapy and other specialty procedures (ie, VADs, Ommaya reservoirs) |

didactic and clinical component are essential to ensure quality patient care as well as to achieve and maintain high safety standards.[11] Chemotherapy certification provides evidence of formalized training and skill demonstration, which is extremely important from a professional liability perspective. The ONS has established a trainer program in the administration of chemotherapy and biotherapy that prepares qualified instructors, who then can provide the program locally.[12] Nurses who successfully complete the ONS chemotherapy and biotherapy course obtain validation of their knowledge via a chemotherapy and biotherapy provider card, which is renewed every 2 years; the clinical validation of skill and ability to apply principles to practice occur most often in the clinical setting where the nurse works. Clinical competency should be validated annually.[7] Antineoplastic agents have a very narrow therapeutic window, that is, therapeutic effect without serious—even life-threatening—side effects, and it is in the best interests of the patient, nurse, and institution that educational preparation be obtained, maintained, and documented. The institution or outpatient practice setting should have established minimum qualifications for those who administer chemotherapy, as well as policies and procedures for the management of complications such as anaphylaxis and hypersensitivity. From a legal standpoint, national standards such as those developed and published by ONS and ASCO are the standards against which all nurses who administer chemotherapy are measured.[1,7] Clinically oriented policies and procedures that are part of ongoing quality improvement are necessary to provide a firm practical and legal foundation for this aspect of oncology nursing practice.

## HANDLING HAZARDOUS DRUGS

Exposure to hazardous drugs is known to be potentially dangerous to one's health.[13] Hazardous drugs may include cytotoxic, antiviral, biological, or immunosuppressive drugs. Direct exposure to cytotoxic drugs can occur during admixture, administration, or handling and involves inhalation, ingestion, or absorption. Many of the cytotoxic drugs are known to be mutagenic, teratogenic, and carcinogenic. Additionally, exposure has been reported to result in rashes, skin discolorations, scarring, blurred vision, dizziness, and possibly leukemia or other cancers in unprotected persons handling these drugs.[13] Guidelines with recommendations to prevent cytotoxic drug exposure of personnel and the environment have been established by the Occupational Safety and Health Administration (OSHA),[14] the National Institute for Occupational Safety and Health (NIOSH),[13] ONS,[15] and American Society of Health-System Pharmacists (ASHP).[16]

Each institution or practice setting should have a policy and procedure based on OSHA guidelines for use of PPE, as well as for the management of a hazardous drug spill. All drugs should be prepared under a biological safety cabinet (BSC). The nurse administering chemotherapy should wear a closed-front, fluid-impenetrable gown, 2 pairs of disposable powder-free gloves that have been tested for use with hazardous drugs, and eye goggles if an eye exposure is possible. The nurse should place an absorbent plastic-backed pad and then a gauze pad under the connection site when administering intravenous (IV)-push medications. Intermittent or bolus chemotherapy should be prepared under the BSC, and the tubing should be primed with a compatible solution not containing the chemotherapy drug. This minimizes possible exposure to the nurse when administering the drug. Alternatively, the line can be backprimed with the mainline solution. When the infusion is complete, backflush the IV tubing with the mainline solution, and administer any residual drug.[13–16]

All materials used in chemotherapy administration should be disposed of as chemotherapy waste. Gloves and gowns that are dry can be disposed of in a labeled chemotherapy waste bag, whereas needles and syringes should be discarded in a chemotherapy leakproof, puncture-proof container, as are any sharp or breakable items. The patient should be on chemotherapy precautions for 48 hours following drug administration. In the hospital, if the patient is incontinent, the caregiver should wear a chemotherapy gown and gloves in handling any excreta. The gown should be changed after use or if it becomes contaminated but should not be reused. Items such as bedpans, incontinence pads, diapers, urinals, and drainage bags used by the patient during the 48-hour period all should be disposed of as chemotherapy waste in hazardous waste containers. The waste containers should be closed and sealed when three-quarters full. Once sealed, the waste is removed by specially trained personnel who wear PPE. If the bed linens are contaminated with urine or feces, they should be prewashed by personnel wearing PPE and then rewashed with the regular wash. Thus the linens should be placed in an impervious laundry bag labeled "hazardous drug contamination" for the prewash.[14,15] In the home setting, the caregiver should be taught to wear gloves and separate the contaminated linens in a pillowcase, separate from other linen. Then the linen should be washed twice in hot water with regular detergent, separate from other household laundry.[15]

A chemotherapy spill kit is necessary in all areas where chemotherapy is administered.[15] Management of chemotherapy spills is an important area of nursing education, as well as patient education. When a hospitalized patient who is receiving chemotherapy travels to other areas of the hospitals, such as radiology, it is important that the nurse calls report to the radiology nurse; also, a spill kit may be needed. OSHA recommends the following:[14]

- *Small spills (< 5 mL or < 5 g) outside a BSC.* Wearing PPE and an N-95 respirator mask if aerosolization of drug is possible, clean the spill immediately. Use absorbent gauze pads for liquid spills and then wash the area 3 times using a detergent solution, followed by clean water. If there is broken glass, use a scoop for the broken glass, and place it in a leakproof, puncture-proof sharps container. Discard PPE, and wash hands.
- *Large spills (> 5 mL or > 5 g) outside a BSC.* Wear PPE and, if aerosolization is suspected, an N-95 respirator mask; close off the area, and then restrict the spill by placing absorbent pads on spilled liquids or damp cloths or towels over dry particles. If there is broken glass, use a scoop for the broken glass, and place it in a leakproof, puncture-proof container. Place the contaminated pads in the chemotherapy waste container, and then wash the area 3 times using a detergent solution, followed by clean water. Discard PPE, and wash hands.
- *Spills causing personnel exposure.* Immediately remove gown or gloves, and then wash the affected area with water and soap. If the eye is exposed, flood the eye at an eyewash fountain or with isotonic eyewash designated for that purpose for at least 15 minutes, and seek medical attention, such as the occupational health office or the emergency room. In addition, the spill and personnel exposure should be documented in the nurse's medical record.

Detailed drug-handling guidelines are outlined in Table 16-2.[1,13–16]

Personnel policies regarding working with chemotherapy and biotherapy during pregnancy are quite varied despite OSHA's and NIOSH's suggestion that appropriate protective practices should reduce any potential reproductive hazards.[13,14] While OSHA and NIOSH recommend that employees be informed of potential risks and, if necessary, reassigned to other duties, it is not uncommon to find institutional policies that prohibit pregnant or lactating women from working with hazardous drugs, particularly in drug preparation. These precautionary measures are undertaken to protect the mother and developing fetus from the potential effects of drug exposure and the institution from potential liability.

Another personnel issue is medical surveillance. Although the OSHA and NIOSH guidelines recommend that institutions have a medical surveillance program in place,[13,14] a survey of 263 outpatient clinic nurses revealed that only 46% of the sites reported any type of medical monitoring.[17] The most common method of surveillance identified was a pre-employment physical. See Table 16-3 for NIOSH elements of a medical surveillance program.[13]

Patient education regarding hazardous drug handling is important so that patients and family members understand why PPE is being worn and do not feel alienated by the practice. Education is a crucial element if chemotherapy is being provided in the home setting because family members need to be instructed in drug-containment practices. The patient and family should be provided with written instructions specifying vigorous handwashing before and after drug administration, wearing gloves when working with the medications, placing used materials in the provided hazardous drug containers, and avoiding direct exposure to the drugs. In addition, they should be taught safe handling of patient excreta, how to clean up spills using the provided spill kit, and to manage any direct external exposure with copious flushing and washing.[15,16] Patients receiving home chemotherapy, such as via an infusion pump, must have a chemotherapy spill kit and know how to use it.[15]

Despite proof that exposure to cytotoxic drugs can be harmful, some health professionals continue to disregard personal protective measures.[18] There appears to be a perception that low-level exposure is not harmful because no absolute scientific quantification of exposure has been defined. However, studies have consistently found evidence of work-surface contamination from chemotherapy. A study of the outer surface of an unopened package of cyclophosphamide (both blister-pack tablets and vials) as well as pharmacy work surfaces at 2 hospitals were contaminated with drug.[19] It is important to realize that the institution may incur stiff financial penalties if OSHA ascertains noncompliance with established guidelines.[14] The minimum standards to be met include (1) knowledge of the latest scientific information, (2) established policies and procedures, and (3) ongoing monitoring to ensure compliance and continuous quality improvement.[13]

**TABLE 16-2**

| Hazardous Drug Handling Guidelines |
|---|

**Preparation**

- Don a disposable gown that is lint-free, low- or nonpermeable, long-sleeved, cuffed, and solid-fronted.
- Don 2 pairs of disposable, powder-free gloves that have been tested for use with hazardous drugs, such as latex or nitrile; inner-glove cuffs should be worn under the gown cuffs, and outer-glove cuffs should extend over the gown cuffs.
- Admix all cytotoxic drugs in a class II biological safety cabinet (vertical airflow) that meets national standards and is inspected appropriately.
- Use a disposable, plastic-backed liner for the preparation area and appropriate equipment such as Luer-Loc syringes.
- Clean the cabinet daily with 70% alcohol, and decontaminate it weekly or if spills occur.
- Use aseptic technique.
- Take care to avoid drug dispersement by venting vials, handling ampules carefully, avoiding overfilling of containers, and adding diluents slowly.
- Attach and prime intravenous tubing before adding the cytotoxic drug to the intravenous (IV) solution.
- Wipe all syringes and containers, and label them appropriately, including a warning label indicating that the contents are cytotoxic.
- Do not clip or recap needles; discard all sharps in an appropriately labeled, puncture-proof container.
- Discard protective clothing and used materials in a separate trash bag labeled "Cytotoxic."
- Wash hands.
- Place prepared drug(s) in a zipper-seal plastic bag labeled as chemotherapy.

**Administration**

- Receive appropriately labeled cytotoxic drugs in clean, dry syringes or bags of IV fluids inside zipper-seal plastic bags. Inspect bags before opening to ensure no spillage in the bag.
- Wash hands. If dripping or splashing can occur, don a disposable gown that is lint-free, low- or nonpermeable, long-sleeved, cuffed, and solid-fronted.
- Don 2 pairs of disposable, powder-free gloves that have been tested for use with hazardous drugs, such as latex or nitrile; inner-glove cuffs should be worn under the gown cuffs, and outer-glove cuffs should extend over the gown cuffs.
- Place a plastic-backed absorbent pad over the work area to absorb any drips.
- Use IV administration sets and syringes with Luer-Loc fittings.
- If the administration set is not attached to the IV fluids and primed by the pharmacist, it should be attached and primed with caution to prevent exposure of the drug to the environment. It may be primed into a gauze pad inside a zipper-seal bag, or it may be piggybacked to plain fluids and primed by retrograde flow ("back primed").
- Secure all connections and Y-sites.
- Keep a gauze pad at hand to wipe droplets off Y-sites or connecting points.
- Do not expel air from syringes. If air is in a syringe, hold it in such a way that the air is up near the plunger and simply stop pushing on the plunger when all the drug is injected.
- Do not use IV bottles with venting tubes.
- Monitor administration sets and connection sites for leakage.
- Do not clip or recap needles. Discard the needle–syringe unit into a convenient and appropriately labeled, puncture-proof container.
- Discard all gauze, tubing, bags, bottles, etc. in appropriately labeled bags, and seal. Remove gown and gloves, and discard in a similar manner.
- Wash hands.

**General Handling and Disposal**

- Dispose of all sharps, containers, and cytotoxic waste according to appropriate state and federal guidelines (usually, incineration or burial in a hazardous waste landfill).

(Continued)

**TABLE 16-2**

**Hazardous Drug Handling Guidelines (*Continued*)**

**General Handling and Disposal**

- Contain all grossly contaminated linen of treated patients within 48 hours in labeled double bags, and wash twice (same procedure as for infectious wastes).
- Obtain spill kits, and place them in the admixture and administration areas.
- Clean up spills using available kits and disposable towels or sponges. For large spills, double gloving is recommended.
- If direct exposure occurs, immediately rinse the area with running water. For eye exposure, rinse with an eye wash solution or sterile saline.
- Report all episodes of exposure to employee health or the equivalent resource.

**Personnel**

- Identify all personnel who handle cytotoxic drugs.
- Educate and train personnel in proper drug handling.
- Establish a mechanism to monitor cytotoxic drug handling practices, from receipt through disposal.
- Provide ready access to information regarding hazardous drugs.
- Address pregnancy and medical surveillance issues.
- Monitor all spills and occurrences of direct exposure through a quality-improvement program.
- Develop patient education materials as needed, particularly for use in the home.
- Ensure that patients receiving chemotherapy at home have a spill kit and can verbalize its use.

*Source*: Data from the National Institute for Occupational Safety and Health[13]; Occupational Safety and Health Administration[14]; Oncology Nursing Society[15]; and American Society of Hospital Pharmacists.[16]

## PATIENT AND FAMILY EDUCATION

Educating patients and their family members about cancer is usually initiated by the physician, who explains the diagnosis of cancer, treatment options, risks and benefits of treatment, alternatives, and prognosis. Nurses are responsible for providing the patient and family with specific information about treatment side effects and self-care measures to recognize and minimize their consequences. Teaching self-care measures is critically important given the often limited resources and support services available. Patient/family teaching should be individualized and be based on principles of adult learning; in fact, when stressed by illness, a patient's reading level may fall one grade level.[20]

Principles of adult learning focus on:[20]

- Initial assessment to identify barriers to learning (such as reduced hearing or vision, ability to read, language, and ability to understand nurse's language when teaching; preferred medium to learn, such as the Internet, video, written material, spoken or face-to-face; and whether the patient has the required equipment at home, such as a DVD player if video/DVD is the preferred medium)
- Appropriate medium to teach given the patient's age, sensory perception (eg, hearing, vision, need for glasses), language, culture, and level of anxiety or depression
- Relevancy to the patient, that is, what the patient needs to know now, such as a need to know what and how to give a subcutaneous injection, and then to return the demonstration to the nurse
- Information to reinforce teaching, such as a calendar so that the patient can see the dates and timing of drug requirements

In addition, after teaching, it is important to validate the patient's recall of the teaching by asking the patient to repeat the information. Self-care guides such as those detailed by Yarbro et al. can be photocopied, individualized, and given to the patient to reinforce teaching.[21] In addition, the instruction should detail self-administration of medications that may be needed to minimize or prevent complications such as antiemetics or antidiarrheal medications and instances that require the patient to call the nurse or physician right away, such as unrelieved nausea and vomiting. It is important that the phone number for the nurse or physician be given to the patient, as well as how to contact a health professional after hours or on weekends/holidays. It is also recommended that there is follow-up of a teaching session. For example, for adult outpatients, this may mean calling the patient the next day or next week, based on when the side effects are

**TABLE 16-3**

**Elements of a Medical Surveillance Program**

- Reproductive and general health questionnaires completed at time of hire and periodically thereafter
- Laboratory evaluation (eg, complete blood count, urinalysis, possibly liver function and transaminase tests) at time of hire and periodically thereafter
- Physical examination at time of hire and as needed for workers whose health questionnaire or blood work indicates an abnormal finding
- Follow-up for workers who have health changes or have had a significant exposure (eg, substantial skin contact or cleaning a large spill)
- Review periodic health questionnaires and laboratory results for trends that may be a sign of health changes because of exposure to hazardous drugs, and if health changes are found, the employer should take the following actions:
  - Evaluate current protective measures.
    - Engineering controls (eg, biological safety cabinets, ventilation, closed-system transfer devices, closed intravenous systems)
    - Policies for the use of personal protective equipment (PPE) and employee compliance
    - Availability of appropriate PPE such as double gloves, nonpermeable gowns, respiratory protection
  - Develop an action plan to prevent further employee exposure.
  - Ensure confidential notification of any adverse health effect to an exposed worker, and offer alternative duty or temporary reassignment.
  - Provide ongoing medical surveillance of all workers at risk to determine whether the new plan is effective.

*Source*: Data from National Institute for Occupational Safety and Health.[13]

expected, and ensuring that the patient correctly recalls the instruction. For inpatients, the nurse should report on the patient's and family's response to teaching but also ask that the nurses who subsequently follow reinforce and assess the degree of learning and document this in the medical record. In the ambulatory/outpatient setting, ASCO/ONS recommend that at a minimum, the following written information be given to the patient prior to the administration of the first dose of chemotherapy[7]

- The diagnosis requiring chemotherapy, goals of therapy, planned duration of chemotherapy drugs, and schedule
- Possible short-term and long-term side effects
- Emergency contact information (eg, symptoms to report, who to call, phone number)
- Plan for monitoring and follow-up

For patients receiving oral chemotherapy, teaching should include the caregiver or family member and focus on (1) preparation and storage of drug (away from children and pets), (2) self-administration, including a calendar schedule and whether to take the drug with food and/or an antiemetic drug, and (3) disposal. Some basic steps to follow when planning and implementing patient education are listed in Table 16-4.

## SAFE PRACTICE CONSIDERATIONS

One of the primary responsibilities of the nurse in the delivery of chemotherapy is to ensure that the drug is given safely. The nurse should know the "7 rights in medication administration" and ensure that it is the *right* drug, client (2 identifiers), dose, time, route, reason, and documentation.[22] As mentioned previously, chemotherapy has a very narrow therapeutic window with potentially serious and lethal side effects. Therefore, given this high risk, nurses administering antineoplastic drugs including chemotherapy must be especially vigilant. Despite the fact that safeguards are in place, serious medication errors do occur. The oncology community has worked diligently to develop systemwide measures to reduce the chance of chemotherapy errors, which are discussed next.

As practitioners, it is important to consider the potential origins and settings in which drug errors are likely to occur. In a study of pediatric oncology patients, it was estimated that almost 6% of medication orders written for pediatric patients had errors.[23] Half the errors involved administration of the drug, such as wrong timing, omission of the drug, or improper dose. However, most often, multiple issues are involved in a drug administration error.[24] A study at the Dana Farber Cancer Institute found an overall medication error rate of 3%, with a 2% serious error rate (would have hurt the patient if carried out).[25] The most frequent medication errors were omission of dosages, incorrect dosages, and failure to discontinue orders. The authors recommended implementing standardized templates for outpatient chemotherapy to reduce the error rate.[26] Combinations of complicated regimens of drugs are currently being given in high doses in a variety of settings. Consequently, even though the healthcare professional may recognize a cumulative dose as being higher than the usual dose, he or she still may fail to question the order. In addition, institutions are being pressured to scale back costs. As resources diminish and individuals are required to do more with less, the risk of error increases. This underscores the importance of the nurse being credentialed as chemotherapy competent. Table 16-5 identifies common types of medication errors.

National standards have been advanced by ONS, ASCO, and INS, as discussed previously.[7–10] In an effort to reduce the

**TABLE 16-4**

**Chemotherapy Patient Education Guidelines**

**Preparation**

- Accompany the physician when the treatment plan is explained to the patient and family to better reinforce what they have been told.
- Identify learning needs and provide specific written instructions for the prevention and management of side effects.
- Emphasize the importance of self-care strategies, and provide the patient and family with self-care guidelines that are clearly written at a fifth-grade level of understanding.
- Determine whether audiovisuals are appropriate teaching aids. Test equipment, and establish a time for the patient and family to view the aids.
- Review policies, procedures, and documentation forms.

**Planning**

- Assess patient based on the goal of the treatment plan, and identify any barriers to learning, such as language, vision, and hearing.
- If possible, separate the teaching session from the actual drug administration procedure.
- Encourage the patient to have a family member present during instruction sessions.
- Assemble all teaching materials, including the calendar, prescriptions, drug information sheets, and other teaching materials, before you begin, to avoid interruptions.

**Presentation**

- Introduce yourself and your purpose.
- Determine if the patient has any specific questions or concerns to address before proceeding.
- Discuss the treatment process (ie, starting an intravenous infusion, administering drugs, length of time, immediate events, expected follow-up, monitoring of side effects, and home care). Describe any sensations the patient might have during the infusion/injection (eg, coolness, perirectal burning, light-headedness, nasal stuffiness).
- Describe the potential side effects and interventions to minimize their consequences. Include specific information about what to look for, what is normal, how to take a temperature, where to buy a wig, which mouth-care regimen to use, and other appropriate recommendations. Provide written information regarding when to call the physician or nurse.
- Avoid overloading the patient with information about rare or unusual risks of chemotherapy. Give written information regarding his or her treatment, and elaborate where appropriate.
- Ensure that informed consent (written or verbal) has been obtained.
- Maintain a supportive atmosphere that is open to questioning.
- Give written instructions regarding activity, diet, hygiene, medications, and other self-care behaviors for the patient to follow for the next few days or weeks.
- Recommend useful Internet sites for education reinforcement.

**Follow-Up**

- Document the encounter and the patient's response.
- Question the patient to assess his or her understanding of the information imparted.
- When possible, observe the patient to determine if his or her actions indicate an understanding of the information (eg, hydration, mouth care, medications).
- It is optimal to contact the patient within 24 hours of drug administration to determine if there are any questions or problems to be resolved, especially if the patient and nurse are no longer together in the same setting (ie, hospital or home).

risk for drug error, the following safeguards should be instituted wherever chemotherapy is admixed and administered[1,7,27–29]:

1. Chemotherapy orders for both parenteral and oral drugs must be written and signed by licensed independent practitioners whom the institution or practice site has identified as qualified. In most hospitals, physicians must apply for credentialing to prescribe chemotherapy, and this is granted only to attending-level practitioners. In academic medical centers, the institution policy may permit oncology nurse practitioners, oncology clinical nurse specialists, oncology physician

**TABLE 16-5**

**Medication Errors**

| Type of Errors | Contributing Factors | Risk Management Strategies |
|---|---|---|
| • Underdosing and overdosing<br>• Schedule and timing errors<br>• Infusion-rate errors<br>• Improper preparation<br>• Drugs given to the wrong patient | • Stress<br>• Understaffing<br>• Unclear orders<br>• Lack of experience | • Comprehensive, ongoing training<br>• Adherence to the "seven rights" of medication administration<br>• Adequate staffing<br>• At least two forms of patient identification<br>• Identify "quiet spaces" or "time out" to perform drug calculations and double checks.<br>• Develop strategies to correct prescriber poor handwriting (electronic or preprinted orders), and provide resources so that all orders can be compared with standard therapies (evidence). |

*Source*: Data from Schulmeister.[24]

assistants, and hematology/oncology fellows to write the chemotherapy orders, but the order must be signed by a credentialed attending physician. Verbal orders for chemotherapy should not be accepted.

2. The order must specify the patient's full name, unique patient identifier, full generic drug name, drug dose in milligrams per square meter ($mg/m^2$) or kilogram (kg), route of administration, total dose to be given, and date of administration. When the order specifies more than one dose, such as a daily dose for a specific number of days, the drug dose per day should be ordered. The cumulative dose for the course of treatment is not written on the order sheet to avoid the possibility of that dose being given each day by mistake. The prescriber should not use trailing zeros because 100.0 may be misread as 1000. Likewise, include a zero prior to a decimal point (0.25 mg) to avoid overdosing.
3. The generic drug name should be typed clearly and in full. Abbreviations are to be avoided, especially where drugs with similar-sounding names are concerned.
4. It is recommended that electronic order sets or preprinted order sheets be used to avoid hand-written orders that may require interpretation. The National Comprehensive Cancer Network (NCCN) has chemotherapy order templates available.[27]
5. In either the inpatient or outpatient setting, a copy of the original order or the electronic order written and signed by the credentialed physician is sent to the inpatient or outpatient pharmacy for drug verification (drug and dose are within the standard range) and preparation. In outpatient areas where nurses are preparing the drug or in the inpatient or outpatient pharmacy, the order must be double-checked against previous orders. If the drug or dose varies from the previous order, the order should be clarified with the credentialed attending physician. If the patient is on a research protocol, the nurse or pharmacy staff should have a copy of the protocol to verify the order. If the ordered regimen does not correspond to standard dosing, then the physician is contacted to provide the supporting evidence.
6. Prior to preparation, the order should be verified by 2 individuals independently as to drug name(s), drug(s) dose, volume and concentration, rate of administration, and calculation of dose. In addition, based on prior treatment history, the cumulative dose of drug should be checked, and if the individual's cumulative lifetime dose has been reached, the attending physician should be called prior to proceeding (eg, doxorubicin or bleomycin).
7. The drug must be labeled at the time of preparation by the pharmacist or nurse mixing the drug in an outpatient practice, who have demonstrated knowledge and clinical competence in mixing chemotherapy, indicating the date and time of preparation and when the drug will expire. Often computer-generated labels are used in the inpatient or outpatient pharmacy, and if so, the computer should be programmed *not* to print the label if the dose/cumulative dose are out of the ordinary and customary range. To override the computer and print the label then would require verification and authorization.
8. Prepared drugs should be dispensed in plastic zipper-lock bags identified as chemotherapy; the bags should be large enough to hold all the drugs to be given to one patient, except if a drug is intended for the intrathecal route. In that case, it should be dispensed separately. Drugs intended for one patient might be confused with another patient's order if they are not isolated in a bag. For inpatient areas, chemotherapy should not be sent by pneumatic tube to the floor. In outpatient or ambulatory areas, often the pharmacy or BSC area for preparation is right outside or in the chemotherapy treatment area. It is imperative that a system be identified so that drugs for each patient are kept separately and not mixed in with another patient's drug(s).

9. Intrathecal drug(s) should be prepared at a separate time from other chemotherapy, stored in a separate location/container, and be given to the person who will administer the drug separately from other (IV) chemotherapy.
10. The pharmacy or practice site should maintain a record including drug source and lot number, expiration date, and patient for whom the drug was prepared.
11. If the drug(s) are prepared by an outside vendor (outsourced), the ambulatory or outpatient practice must maintain a policy for quality control of chemotherapy.
12. Once the oncology nurse receives the patient's chemotherapy drug(s), the nurse and another oncology nurse or qualified clinician independently double-check the original order to ensure that the right drug and dose have been prepared. If the ordered regimen is not standard dosing, and the supporting evidence has not been obtained, the nurse contacts the physician to get the information before proceeding further. The nurse also checks the history for past cycles of chemotherapy and ensures that the appropriate time between cycles has elapsed. Prior to this, the administering nurse has verified that the patient's blood counts, liver or renal function tests, and tolerance of prior therapy are such that the patient is able to receive the prescribed chemotherapy.
13. If possible, the person preparing the drug should not be the same person double-checking the order. If a nurse is working alone in a clinic, the physician should be available to double-check the drugs prior to administration.
14. Everyone responsible for drug preparation and administration (ie, pharmacist, pharmacy technicians, and nurses) needs to be properly trained in the specialty of chemotherapy drug preparation.
15. If the patient is receiving chemotherapy at home, home-care companies that are certified to provide chemotherapy deliver the drug, manage the venous access device, and reinforce patient teaching. The nurse working in this setting should communicate patient response and any issues that arise to the prescribing physician.
16. Policies and procedures should be reviewed annually, including those for preventing and reporting drug errors, as well as those for drug preparation and administration.
17. Everyone responsible for chemotherapy drug preparation and administration should be empowered with the ability to question the order. If any question arises related to the drug, dose, route, or schedule, the individual must clarify the order and be encouraged to do so prior to the drug being administered.
18. Any protocol involving unusual dosing patterns or dose-intensive regimens should be reviewed carefully by all parties. No one should be expected to prepare or administer a drug with a dose-intensive schedule without the opportunity to review the protocol at least 24 hours in advance, especially if the protocol involves an investigational agent.
19. Establish and implement safe practice staffing guidelines.

The nurse should work with nursing management to ensure that nurses have adequate time to safely administer chemotherapy. It is not uncommon in a busy inpatient or outpatient clinic for a nurse to have no prior knowledge that a patient is beginning a new chemotherapy protocol before the patient appears in the clinic ready to be treated. This situation is not optimal because the nurse has no time to review the protocol and prepare the patient's learning packet. In addition, it is imperative that chemotherapy double-checks take place in a quiet environment with a "time out" to ensure that the double-check is carried our independently and accurately.[30] Errors can be made whenever drugs are given in a hurried and unprepared manner. Communication among the physician, pharmacist, and nurse is critical to providing a safe level of care. While chemotherapy computerized order entry has improved the prescription and delivery of chemotherapy, there continues to be need for improvement.[31] Bar coding and smart pumps into which the protocol can be loaded offer hope for improved safety.[32,33] Prospective data for these quality safety mechanisms are not yet available.

## DRUG ADMINISTRATION

### PRE-CHEMOTHERAPY PATIENT ASSESSMENT

The assessment done prior to chemotherapy administration is a critical role of the oncology nurse.[1] Chemotherapy is prescribed in cycles, and in order to derive the maximum benefit, patients should be supported with minimimal physical and psychosocial complications so that the patient can receive at least 80% relative dose intensity (receive at least 80% of the prescribed dose).[33] Prior to the patient's first cycle of chemotherapy, the patient's knowledge of the treatment goals, plan of care, and potential drug side effects is to be assessed. Many states, institutions, and outpatient physician practices require a signed consent prior to chemotherapy administration.[34] If this is the policy, then the nurse determines that a signed informed consent is in the medical record. During subsequent cycles of chemotherapy, the nurse assesses the patient's tolerance of the previous cycle of chemotherapy and discusses any needed improvements in the plan with the physician, such as an improved antiemetic plan if the patient had nausea and/or vomiting with the last treatment cycle. In addition, the nurse performs a brief focused systems assessment based on the anticipated drug's side effects.[35]

The nurse also reviews laboratory and scan data appropriate to the drugs being given, such as the multi-gated blood pool scan or echocardiogram if the first dose of doxorubicin is being given.[35] The baseline white blood cell, neutrophil, platelet, and red cell counts are assessed if bone marrow suppression is expected, as are whether growth factor support is anticipated (if the risk of febrile neutropenia is 20% or higher[36]) and liver and renal function test results if the drug is excreted via these routes. Finally, during this time, the nurse assesses the need for involvement of other members of the interdisciplinary team, such as the nutritionist or social worker.[1]

If an ideal weight table is not available,

1. Start with 100 pounds for 5 feet and add 5 pounds for each additional inch. Thus someone who is 5 feet 5 inches would ideally weigh 125 pounds.
2. Take that weight, plus their actual weight, divide by 2, which would give the weight on which to calculate the dose per square meter.
3. Example: For a patient who is 5 feet 5 inches tall and weighs 180 pounds, calculate the average, 125 lbs + 180 lbs = 305 lbs, divided by 2 = 152.5 lbs to use in the BSA calculation.

**FIGURE 16-1**

Calculation of dose adjusted for size.

*Source*: Data from Hayden and Goodman.[40]

## DOSE CALCULATION

The dose of drug to be administered generally is based on the individual's body surface area (BSA), usually expressed in milligrams per square meter or milligrams per kilogram. The patient's BSA is usually determined by a formula based on the patient's height and weight. The Mosteller equation is used most commonly:[1]

$$\text{BSA} = \frac{\sqrt{\text{height (cm)} \times \text{weight (kg)}}}{3600} \quad \text{or} \quad \frac{\sqrt{\text{height (in)} \times \text{weight (lbs)}}}{3131}$$

The question as to optimal dosing for the clinically obese patient is complex. Obesity is defined as a patient having a body mass index (BMI) of 30 or greater.[37] In a review by Hunter and colleagues, limited data were available to support empirical dose capping or reduction of the obese patient's dose, and in fact, there were negative implications for patients with treatable or curable disease who had inferior outcomes.[38] For example, Griggs and colleagues found reduced survival in obese women with breast cancer who received dose reductions.[39] This issue is of particular concern because dose reduction may compromise efficacy, which is particularly meaningful when the intent of treatment is cure. However, in situations where a dose reduction is necessary and the patient's weight is significantly greater than the ideal weight, a simple method of calculating the dose is to take the average of the ideal and actual weights (Figure 16-1).[40]

Similar issues arise in the treatment of the elderly patient, in whom chemotherapy doses may be reduced because it is assumed that the patient cannot tolerate full-dose therapy.[1] However, a number of studies are emerging showing that not only do elderly patients with a good performance status tolerate therapy similar to younger patients, but they also derive similar benefits. Folprecht and colleagues did a pooled analysis of 4 phase III trials of patients with metastatic colorectal cancer to evaluate the safety and efficacy of combination therapy (ie, irinotecan, fluorouracil, and leucovorin) with monotherapy (ie, fluourouracil or leucovorin); the authors found that patients in these studies who were aged 70 years and older had a similar benefit with similar toxicity.[41] Other studies have shown that dose reduction in older patients may in fact reduce response to therapy.[42]

In an effort to better define the individualized dose for a drug, area under the curve (AUC) dosing has emerged. This dosing method is more accurate because it takes into account the person's ability to metabolize the drug and more accurately predicts the drug serum level. Thus the dose is individualized for a particular patient's age and renal function for drugs excreted via the kidneys.[43] One example of this approach is the Calvert formula for carboplatin dosing.[44] Carboplatin is excreted by the kidneys—in particular, via glomerular filtration—with little excretion or reabsorption by the renal tubules. Therefore, pretreatment assessment of renal function or glomerular filtration rate (GFR) can be used to individualize carboplatin dose in adults. The GFR is essentially equivalent to the creatinine clearance, which can be estimated from the patient's age, serum creatinine concentration, and weight by using the Cockroft-Gault method. Another factor in the Calvert formula involves the AUC, or target drug concentration, for carboplatin. AUC is a way to estimate the amount of systemic drug exposure over time and can maximize the drug dose while minimizing toxicity. In the presence of impaired renal function, the delayed clearance of carboplatin would result in prolonged drug exposure (increased AUC); in patients with high renal clearance, decreased AUC could result in subtherapeutic dosing. Because AUC or carboplatin exposure, rather than toxicity, is the measurement, it is not influenced by concurrent myelosuppressive therapy or supportive treatment. The Calvert formula for calculating AUC is illustrated in Figure 16-2. There are two methods to determine GFR: the Cockcroft-Gault and Jeliffe methods. Whichever method is used, it should be standard in the institution because each method gives a slightly different dose.

The target AUC ranges from 1 to 8 and is selected for appropriate clinical situations. For example, if the patient

I. Calvert formula: Carboplatin dose (mg) = target AUC × (GFR + 25)

II. Calculating estimated GFR or creatinine clearance in mL/minute

A. Crockroft-Gault formula

$$\text{Males: } \frac{(140 - \text{age}) \times (\text{weight in kg})}{72 \times \text{serum creatinine (mg/dL)}}$$

$$\text{Females: } \frac{(140 - \text{age}) \times (\text{weight in kg})}{72 \times \text{serum creatinine (mg/dL)}} \times (0.85)$$

B. Jeliffe

$$\text{Males: } \frac{\{98 - [0.8 \times (\text{age}-20)]\}}{\text{Serum creatinine (mg/dL)}}$$

$$\text{Females: } \frac{\{98 - [0.8 \times (\text{age} - 20)]\}}{\text{Serum creatinine (mg/dL)}} \times 0.9$$

**FIGURE 16-2**

Calculation of the area under the curve (AUC) using the Calvert formula.

*Source*: Data from Polovich et al.[1]

has had prior treatment or is receiving carboplatin in combination with another myelosuppressive agent, an AUC of 4 to 6 might be selected. If the patient is receiving carboplatin alone and has not been treated previously with ablative chemotherapy, an AUC of 6 to 8 might be selected. If the patient is receiving the drug as a radiosensitizer, the AUC may be 2. It is important to note that doses in the Calvert method are total milligrams, not milligrams per square meter, of carboplatin.

## PRETREATMENT CONSIDERATIONS

Table 16-6 includes specific tasks involved in chemotherapy administration that are applicable in all practice settings. The treatment plan should be reviewed by the nurse in terms of drug name and dose, method of determining dose (eg, treatment protocol), route and rate of administration, frequency and/or date of administration, premedication for nausea/vomiting or hypersensitivity, and hydration if needed. Critical in error risk reduction are the 2 independent double-checks by the administering nurse together with another licensed professional who confirms dose calculation and dose appropriateness and compares the dose with the accepted standard or evidence and compares the prepared drug label with the chemotherapy order in terms of patient, dose, route, administration time, and expiration of the drug. In addition, Appendices 16A and 16B describe the dosing, efficacy, metabolism, preparation, administration precautions, and special considerations regarding the administration of the more common oral and IV chemotherapy agents. An important pretreatment consideration is the potential for infusion-related reactions, including hypersensitivity reactions and anaphylaxis. All emergency medication and equipment should be available and in good working order, and the nurse must be familiar with them. Evidence-based guidelines for emergency care should be readily available as well as appropriate personnel in the event that an emergency situation arises. In the current practice environment, it is not uncommon for one or two nurses to be the sole providers of care in an ambulatory-care setting. The physicians may see their patients and leave the clinic to do rounds in the hospital or to go to another free-standing oncology facility. The 2009 standards of practice dictate that a physician or licensed independent practitioner be immediately available when chemotherapy is administered.[7] This recommendation applies to all settings where chemotherapy drugs are administered, as well as when an experimental drug is given. The first consideration is the safety of the patient, and the policies and procedures governing the setting in which chemotherapy is given should specifically indicate that a physician or licensed independent practitioner should be physically present, not just available by phone.[7] See Chapter 31 for an in-depth discussion on hypersensitivity reactions to antineoplastic drugs.

Another pretreatment consideration involves the sequencing of various drugs to either enhance cytotoxicity or minimize toxicity to normal tissues. For example, the administration of cisplatin or carboplatin before paclitaxel induces more profound neutropenia than when the paclitaxel is given first. The incidence of neutropenia is believed to be due to the lower paclitaxel clearance rates when cisplatin or carboplatin precedes it.[45,46] Therefore, to achieve the greatest efficacy with no increase in toxicity, paclitaxel is routinely administered prior to carboplatin. According to the ONS,[1] the nurse should review the treatment plan to establish the sequence of agents. If it is not clear, then the nurse should clarify with the prescribing physician. When the patient is receiving chemotherapy on a research protocol, the protocol should be followed exactly.

Another example of the importance of sequencing in chemotherapy administration involves the administration of doxorubicin and paclitaxel. A moderate to severe mucositis can occur when paclitaxel is given prior to doxorubicin but not when it is given in the reverse sequence. The paclitaxel-related mucosal damage concomitant with neutropenia has been thought to contribute to the development of typhlitis, which can be life threatening. Pharmacokinetic data indicate that when paclitaxel is given immediately prior to doxorubicin, there is a 31.6% average decrease in the clearance of doxorubicin, which contributes greatly to profound neutropenia.[22,29] Based on this finding, the sequence of doxorubicin followed by paclitaxel is recommended.

## ROUTES OF ADMINISTRATION

Chemotherapy is a systemic treatment for cancer that has the ability to travel throughout the body via the bloodstream and damage or kill dividing cells. It is now possible

**TABLE 16-6**

**Chemotherapy Administration Guidelines**

**Professional Preparation**

- Maintain appropriate knowledge and skills regarding chemotherapy drug protocols and administration procedures.
- Review applicable policies and procedures.
- Review drug protocol and research guidelines.

**Patient Preparation**

- Verify patient identity (eg, arm band, driver's license, verbalization of name) using at least two forms of patient identification (ie, name and birth date).
- Ensure appropriate patient education.
- Confirm that appropriate laboratory tests have been completed and are within normal limits.
- Measure and record baseline vital signs, weight, and height.
- Verify patient's allergy history.
- Assess venous access device status (ie, need for VAD).
- Initiate pretreatment therapies, if ordered (eg, hydration, test dosing, antiemetics).

**Drug Preparation**

- Verify drug order (including body surface area and dosage calculations), and validate that it is standard dosing or obtain evidence to support dosing from physician.
- Obtain prepared drug, and double-check with another professional healthcare provider (eg, a nurse, physician, or pharmacist), and label for the correct drug, dose, route, and patient. If admixing, follow appropriate guidelines for cytotoxic drug admixture.
- Ensure rapid access to extravasation kit and medications necessary if hypersensitivity reaction occurs (eg, parenteral diphenhydramine hydrochloride, epinephrine, and hydrocortisone should be immediately available).
- Obtain necessary supplies and equipment for safe drug administration.
- Wash hands, and don gloves and appropriate protective clothing.

**Venipuncture Guidelines**

- Establish work area with plastic-backed pad.
- Organize materials, needle box, syringes, flush, IV start materials, and IV fluids.
- Select IV catheter size and type according to setting, patient's veins, and treatment to be administered.
- Determine appropriate site for venous access, avoiding
  - Limbs with recent venipunctures (ie, within 30 minutes)
  - Limbs with axillary node dissections, extensive radiation therapy, or obstructive process
  - Antecubital fossa (for peripheral sticks)
  - Ecchymotic or sclerosed areas
  - Bony prominences and joints
- Ensure adequate lighting and visualization of area to be accessed.
- Remove jewelry near access site.
- Select a large vein if administering drugs known to be irritating.
- Administer vesicants only at sites designated by established policies and procedures, specifically in areas with underlying subcutaneous tissue. Areas to be avoided when administering vesicants include veins over joints, bony prominences, neurovascular bundles, tendons, and areas of existing soft tissue damage.
- For peripheral sites, begin at the most distal areas, and gradually proceed proximally.
- Use an appropriate sterile technique for access.
- Achieve a "clean" venipuncture and determine patency. The IV catheter should not puncture through the back of the vein and then be resettled within the vein. There should be a brisk immediate blood return and no swelling at the IV catheter site.

(Continued)

**TABLE 16-6**

**Chemotherapy Administration Guidelines (*Continued*)**

**Venipuncture Guidelines**

- Secure IV catheter with tape, but ensure visualization of the site.
- Flush IV catheter with sterile NS or $D_5W$ to clear the line and establish patency. Observe the site at this time to ensure that swelling is not occurring at the IV catheter site.
- Use Luer-Loc fittings for IV sets and syringes; use sterile gauze or alcohol pad for priming IV sets.

**Drug Administration Guidelines**

- Check patient's condition periodically during drug administration, and explain actions being taken, when appropriate.
- Monitor the status of the venous access site periodically during the process.
- If administering a vesicant, observe the site continuously throughout the injection.
- Ensure drug containment at all times. Wipe any droplets at the connector or Y-site with a gauze pad.
- Administer IV push chemotherapy drugs as ordered, using slow, steady pressure.
- Check for a blood return every few milliliters with vesicants and before and after each drug.
- Flush between each drug with sterile NS or $D_5W$ to avoid drug admixture and potential precipitation.
- When administering short-term drips or infusions, establish the infusion, ensuring all connections securely, and set the appropriate flow rate.
- Generally, place long-term infusions on an infusion pump.
- Flush after last drug with sterile NS or $D_5W$.
- If appropriate, discontinue the IV catheter. For peripheral sites, hold pressure manually over the site for a few minutes, and then apply small, sterile dressing.
- Do not clip or recap needles.

**Post-administration Guidelines**

- Discard all materials (eg, IV cathters, syringes, bags, tubing, gown, gloves, etc.) appropriately.
- Assess patient's status and provide for follow-up:
  - *Inpatient:* Call button within reach; fluids available, etc.
  - *Outpatient:* Transportation ready; return appointment and prescriptions obtained; telephone number of physician or nurse available
  - *Home care:* Caregiver available; telephone number of nurse-on-call available
- Document all actions (flow sheets or specialized forms are recommended).

*Abbreviations:* $D_5W$, 5% dextrose in water; IV, intravenous; NS, normal saline; VAD, vascular access device.

to direct drugs systemically as well as to almost every anatomic region in the body. Intravenous chemotherapy remains the most common route of drug delivery, but other systemic routes include oral, intramuscular, and subcutaneous. Regional drug-delivery routes include topical, intraarterial, intraperitoneal, intrapleural, intravesical, intrathecal, and intraventricular. Systemic routes will be discussed first, followed by regional routes.

## Oral

A number of chemotherapy drugs are now administered orally to treat numerous types of cancer (see Appendix 16A). Weingart and colleagues studied safety practices for the use of oral chemotherapy in comprehensive cancer centers in the US and found that few of the safeguards used for IV chemotherapy administration were adopted practices for oral chemotherapy and that there was no consensus about the standards for the safe handling of oral chemotherapy.[47] The collaborative ASCO-ONS standards for safe chemotherapy administration has provided guidelines to ensure minimum standards to ensure patient safety.[7] While oral agents offer many advantages, they also present challenges, which are listed in Table 16-7. After ensuring that the patient understands the drug purpose, potential side effects, and self-care measures, nursing responsibilities for oral drug administration include safe handling and monitoring for drug adherence and side effects. When administering oral chemotherapy, the nurse should wear gloves and pour the pill into a labeled medication cup.[14] Full PPE

**TABLE 16-7**

**Pros and Cons of Oral Antineoplastic Agents**

| Advantages | Disadvantages |
|---|---|
| • Patient convenience<br>• Fewer office visits<br>• Ease of administration<br>• Eliminates the need for IV access<br>• Ability to achieve sustained blood levels | • Less professional monitoring<br>• Inconsistency of absorption<br>• Limited Medicare coverage and large co-pays<br>• Risk of overdosing or underdosing<br>• Potential for nonadherence to the treatment plan and schedule |

should be worn if a liquid is given and a splash may occur.[14] Contaminated gloves and other PPE should be disposed of in a labeled hazardous waste container or zipper-lock bag. The evidence is less clear for dry gloves and medication cups because there are no studies evaluating the true risk of inhalation or skin absorption from gloves, pill containers, or medication cups used to hold the pill prior to administration.[48] Currently, there are no standardized national guidelines for the safe handling of oral chemotherapy. If family members are administering the pill, they should wash their hands before and after, wear gloves, try not to touch the drug, and use a cup to give the pill to the patient. If the patient is self-administering the pill, he or she should try not to touch the pill or, if it is a capsule, not to open the capsule. Currently, dry gloves and medication cups are discarded in the regular trash. Oral chemotherapy should not be split or crushed because this increases the risk of drug exposure. If this must be done, it should be done by the pharmacy under a BSC.[49]

Since most patients receive oral chemotherapy as outpatients, the nurse should assess the patient's ability to adhere to the treatment regimen.[50] If the patient has difficulty remembering to take the pill, discuss strategies to remember (eg, alarm clock or alarm watch). Minimize noncompliance due to nausea by ensuring that an appropriate antiemetic is available for the patient. If the patient experiences emesis immediately after drug ingestion and the pills or capsules cannot be visualized, the drug is usually not repeated. Several oral chemotherapy drugs are also available in parenteral forms, providing an option for patients who are intolerant of or are not adherent with oral regimens. Other recommendations include the following:[1,7,31,32,51,52]

- Identify poor adherence (eg, missed appointments, lack of response to medication, and missed refills), and ask about barriers to adherence without being confrontational.
- Emphasize the importance and value of the regimen and the benefits of adherence (reinforce this at each visit).
- Ascertain the patient's feelings about his or her ability to follow the regimen, and design supports to promote adherence (enlist the patient in the decision-making process and listen to the patient so that the plan can be customized).
- Use standardized, regimen-specific preprinted forms or computer-generated forms for chemotherapy prescriptions. Each cycle of chemotherapy is to be prescribed at a time to avoid inadvertent overdosing that could be life-threatening. If the patient wishes to obtain a 90-day prescription via mail-order pharmacy because it is cheaper, discuss alternatives with the practice setting and insurance company.
- The frequency of office visits and monitoring are documented in the treatment plan, and if nonadherence or side effect management requires more frequent patient contact or monitoring, revise the plan accordingly.
- When teaching the patient the drug administration schedule, use check boxes or other strategies that the patient finds helpful; indicate whether the patient should take the drug with meals, 2 hours before or after food ingestion, or on an empty stomach based on optimal drug absorption.
- Give the patient/family education materials indicating both the generic and trade (brand) names to avoid confusion or double dosing because providers may refer to the drug as either (eg, capecitabine or Xeloda).
- Instruct the patient to maintain a record of drugs being taken, side effects that have developed, and self-care measures used to manage them.
- Simplify the regimen as much as possible.
- Encourage the use of a medication-taking system (eg, medication organizer, reminder, including blister packs, calendars, and dosage counters).
- Enlist the help of family members, friends, and community resources.
- Reinforce desirable behaviors and results when appropriate.
- Instruct the patient and family about what side effects should be reported immediately, whom to call, and the telephone number(s), and reinforce this information with written information that can be posted in the home.
- At each visit, ask the patient to bring in his or her medication bottle and drug record, and count the pills to determine adherence. If there is a discrepancy, discuss the problem(s) that have arisen and possible solutions. Review the teaching plan to see if there are ways to improve this, especially if the patient has cultural beliefs different from the nurse or speaks a different language.
- At each visit, the patient's current medications are assessed, including over-the-counter medications and complementary and alternative therapies; any changes are reviewed at the same visit to ensure compatibility. In hospital outpatient areas, compliance with medication reconciliation is an expectation of the Joint Commission.

- Provide information regarding medication assistance and medication discount programs, and refer to the social worker for assistance as needed.
- Teach the patient and family to wear nonsterile gloves when handling oral chemotherapy and to wash hands thoroughly before and after administration; the patient should not crush, chew, score, or open capsules.

It is important that the patient adhere to the treatment regimen to maximize the *goal of therapy* (ie, remission or cure). Although oral drugs give the patient control over drug administration, adherence can be a problem. Studies have reported nonadherence ranging from 26% to 59%, especially among patients older than 60 years of age.[49] Due to the side effects, a patient might decide to omit a dose to feel better temporarily. The patient needs to understand how important dosing and scheduling are and how critical it is that the prescribed regimen be followed exactly. However, if the patient is having toxicity, it is important that the patient contact the provider to discuss management because a dose modification may be indicated. With therapy such as leucovorin following methotrexate, noncompliance could be fatal. The regimen often can be modified to enhance the patient's tolerance of the side effects (eg, administering an antiemetic to minimize nausea or changing the time of dose administration).

Errors also can occur in the ambulatory and outpatient settings. In a study of outpatient medication errors in adults and children, Walsh and colleagues found the incidence of errors to be 7.1% in adult patients and 18.8% in pediatric patients. Almost half the errors had the potential to cause harm. Most of the errors involved administration (56%) or were related to confusion over two sets of orders or other communication issues.[53] In another study, the authors found that 5% of patients had chemotherapy errors in a complex regimen: incorrect administration (of oral steroids) and errors in the prescription.[54] Shulman and colleagues proposed the use of an oncology electronic health record (EHR) that controlled workflow and ensured accuracy (because no verbal or paper orders were acceptable), standardization, automation, decision support, flexibility, and reliability.[31,32] Finally, Schulmeister stated that the underlying principles for preventing chemotherapy errors include using a proactive approach, multidisciplinary participation, open communication, systems analysis, redesign of vulnerable patient systems, incorporation of safe practices, accurate and reliable information transfer, education, competency, credentialing that establishes a culture of safety, and finally, continuous quality improvement.[24]

## Intravenous

The IV route is the most common method of chemotherapy drug delivery. Detailed nursing actions concerning intravenous drug administration are included in Table 16-6 and Appendix 16B. Selection of a central venous access device (CVAD) or IV catheter will be determined by the type of therapy the patient is to receive and the condition of the patient's veins. Prior to the patient beginning chemotherapy, the nurse assesses the patient's arms for venous access, and if veins are difficult or sclerosed, then the nurse discusses with the physician or advanced practice nurse an implanted port or other CVAD for chemotherapy administration.[1,8] It is important to avoid using an existing IV catheter that is more than 24 hours old,[1] and the Infusion Nurses Society recommends a new IV line be started to administer a vesicant drug.[8] When starting a new IV line, use the smallest-gauge and shortest-length catheter that is appropriate for the patient.[8] Assess the patient's arm, starting distally and moving proximally, seeking smooth, pliable veins and avoiding injured or sclerosed veins or those that are small, fragile, or tortuous.[1,8] While metal needles (such as butterflies) were used years ago, they are now used rarely and are never used for administration of vesicant drugs.[1,8]

Choosing the appropriate device and taking the time to find the most appropriate vein are important. If a vein is not obvious, it is advisable to apply moist heat to the arms for 5 to 10 minutes and have the patient drink a warm liquid prior to attempting venipuncture.[1] If the patient is known to have small, hard-to-find veins, he or she should drink 4 to 6 glasses of fluid the morning of treatment, dress warmly, and squeeze a handball for 10 minutes prior to the nurse attempting venipuncture.[1,8] If the nurse has difficulty accessing an appropriate vein after 1 or 2 attempts, assistance should be sought. If the patient repeatedly requires more than 3 venipuncture attempts and the plan is to undergo chemotherapy for an extended period of time, a CVAD is appropriate.[1,8,55]

Another issue involves the order in which chemotherapy drugs are given. Except where sequencing is important pharmacologically, the order of drug delivery probably is not critical. When giving a vesicant chemotherapy drug, it is important for the patient to be alert and able to communicate any discomfort, stinging, or burning during the drug administration.[1,8] Many clinicians prefer to give a vesicant prior to any of the other drugs in a chemotherapy regimen because (1) venous integrity is greatest before other drugs are given, (2) the nurse's assessment skills and the patient's level of awareness and sensitivity are likely most acute at initiation of the infusion, and (3) the possibility that the vein will be irritated by other drugs or by movement is eliminated.[1] The risk of infiltration of any IV line increases over time.[8] Often, other drugs can cause venous irritation and even spasm that can result in a loss of blood return, a major assessment criterion for safe chemotherapy administration.[1,8,56]

***Vesicant extravasation issues.*** A drug is categorized according to whether it is an irritant, nonirritant, or vesicant. The most benign, local reaction to chemotherapy is a venous flare (see Color Plate 1). This reaction occurs most commonly in patients receiving doxorubicin and is characterized by localized erythema, venous streaking, and pruritus along the injected vein.[1] This localized hypersensitivity reaction is distinguishable from an extravasation by the absence of pain or swelling and the presence of ablood return. Once this important distinction is made, it is safe to continue injecting the agent. Flushing the vein with saline and slowing the injection rate appear to ease the symptoms, which dissipate without treatment within 20 to 30 minutes of the injection in most cases. However, if the flare does not resolve, administration of diphenhydramine 25 to 50 mg via IV push or hydrocortisone 25 to 50 mg via IV push is almost always effective.[1,35]

Another local tissue reaction characterized by pain, venous irritation, and chemical phlebitis can occur with certain nonvesicant chemotherapy agents.[1] These agents, which are called *irritants,* are identified in Appendix 16B. While any drug given in concentrated form in sufficient amount can cause tissue damage if infiltrated, these agents generally are not associated with ulceration unless they are very concentrated.[1] Irritants cause intravascular irritation often accompanied by pain (described as "achiness" or "tightness") only during the infusion and may, as is the case with carmustine, be a function of the diluent, which in this case is dehydrated alcohol.[57]

The most devastating skin reactions caused by chemotherapy occur when a vesicant drug is infiltrated, causing an extravasation injury. The degree of injury to local tissues is related to the vesicant properties of the drug infiltrated, the concentration of the drug, and the amount of the drug infiltrated.[56] By definition, an *extravasation* is the inadvertent infiltration of a vesicant chemotherapy drug.[1,8] A vesicant is a drug that, if infiltrated, is capable of causing pain, ulceration, necrosis, and sloughing of damaged tissue. The damage can be severe enough to result in physical deformity or a functional deficit, such as loss of joint mobility, vascularity, or tendon function (see Color Plates 2 and 3). Extravasation can occur when administering the drug peripherally or from an implanted subcutaneous port. The resulting tissue injury occurs in one of two ways, causing either direct or indirect damage. *Direct damage* occurs when the vesicant drug binds to the DNA in cells exposed to the drug, and they die, releasing substances that continue to affect neighboring cells, causing necrosis; the effect begins immediately, and examples of drugs that cause direct damage are alkylating agents such as nitrogen mustard and doxorubicin. The second type is *indirect injury*, and the drug does not bind to DNA; rather, the drug causes indirect damage to neighboring tissues, the effect may take longer to become visible, and it takes longer to heal; examples are the plant alkaloids vincristine and vinblastine.[1,56] Factors that increase the risk of extravasation are vein wall puncture, dislodgement of the catheter from the vein, administration of the drug below a recent venipuncture site, inadvertent subcutaneous or intramuscular injection, and migration or improper placement of a central line, an inadequately secured Huber needle, and the presence of a fibrin sheath or thrombus at the catheter tip.[1,8,24,56]

While a few nonantineoplastic drugs are vesicants (eg, levophed and dilantin), the number of antineoplastic vesicant drugs is significant; they are identified in Table 16-8 and Appendix 16B. In addition, there are some drugs that when diluted as in usual administration are considered to be irritants, such as paclitaxel and cisplatin, but become vesicants when they are given in concentrated doses.[1] In addition, there are some irritants that have vesicant properties, such as oxaliplatin.[1] It is critical that the nurse administering chemotherapy be aware of the drugs that are vesicants, know their antidotes, use safety measures to try to prevent extravasation, and know what to do if extravasation occurs to minimize injury. It is imperative for all institutions and ambulatory oncology practices to have policies for the preparation and competency determination of nurses who give these drugs, as well as a policy and procedure for management if extravasation of a vesicant occurs.[1,7,8,24] Although oncology nurses rarely are sued, extravasation of a vesicant is the one of the most frequent causes of litigation.[58,59] The nurse's practice is compared with the national standard, which is that described by the ONS and the INS.[1,8]

*Prevention of extravasation.* The following key points are suggested to minimize the risk of extravasation:[1,8,56]

1. Ensure that the vein or central line is patent. The peripheral IV line should be a clean stick that does not penetrate the back vein wall. The Huber needle accessing a subcutaneous implanted port should be stabilized with a securement device so that the needle cannot pull back or out. Do not start a peripheral IV line below a previous venipuncture attempt, and do not use a steel or rigid IV device.
2. Be aware of patients at increased risk for extravasation:
    a. Any patient with fragile veins or who have received sclerosing or irritating drugs previously
    b. Patients unable to communicate to the nurse about the pain of extravasation
    c. Elderly, debilitated, or confused patients with diabetes or general vascular disease.
3. Avoid infusing vesicants over joints, bony prominences, tendons, neurovascular bundles, or the antecubital fossa.
4. Never give vesicants intramuscularly or subcutaneously.
5. Avoid giving vesicant drugs in areas where venous or lymphatic circulation is poor (eg, operative side for a patient with a mastectomy or a patient with superior vena cava syndrome) or in sites that have been irradiated previously.
6. Make sure that the peripheral IV site is adequate and less than 24 hours old, or start a new IV line. A brisk

**TABLE 16-8**

**Vesicant Drugs and Management**

| Drug | Topical and Antidote Therapy | Issues/Key Points |
|---|---|---|
| Doxorubicin (Adriamycin)<br>Daurorubicin (Cerubidine)<br>Epirubicin (Ellence)<br>Idarubicin (Idamycin) | 1. Local cooling (eg, ice pack) 15 to 20 minutes at least 4 times a day for first 24 hours; remove 15 minutes prior to dexrazoxane treatment, and do not use during treatment.<br>2. Totect IV within 6 hours of extravasation daily for 3 days (at about the same time each day) in a different vein from the extravasation site.<br>• Day 1: 1,000 mg/m$^2$ IV over 1 to 2 hours<br>• Day 2: 1,000 mg/m$^2$ IV over 1 to 2 hours<br>• Day 3: 500 mg/m$^2$ IV over 1 to 2 hours<br>• 50% dose reduction if creatinine clearance < 40 mL/minute<br>3. Totect emergency treatment kit contains 10 vials of Totect 500 mg plus diluent, and if unused and expires, it will be replaced by manufacturer | Totect<br>1. Very expensive ($14,000 for regimen).<br>2. Drug is cytotoxic with additive bone marrow suppression (neutropenia, thrombocytopenia), so blood counts should be monitored posttreatment; also may cause reversible elevation of liver function tests. Drug also may cause nausea, vomiting, diarrhea, stomatitis, and burning at the IV site.<br>3. Mechanism of action of totect is unknown but may include reversal of topoisomerase II inhibition (anthracycline mechanism of action to kill cancer cells).<br>4. Drug is a hazardous drug, and safe handling PPE is required to administer the drug (mutagenic, embryotoxic, teratogenic). |
| Dactinomycin (Actinomycin D)<br>Mitomycin C (Mutamycin) | Local cooling (eg, ice pack) 15 to 20 minutes 4 times a day | 1. Potent vesicants without a known antidote<br>2. Assess area for pain, blister/ulcer formation, desquamation daily; discuss with physician or advanced practice nurse need for plastic surgery consult to excise necrotic tissue, physical therapy, or other services. |
| Vincristine (Oncovin)<br>Vinblastine (Velban),<br>Vinorelbine (Navelbine) | 1. Local warming 15 to 20 minutes 4 times a day<br>2. Teach patient to elevate extremity<br>3. Hyaluronidase (Amphadase or Hydase or Vitrase 150 units/1 mL) injected subcutaneously into subcutaneous tissue of extravasation | 1. Give 5 separate subcutaneous injections, each containing 0.2 mL of drug, changing needle with each injection.<br>2. Assess the area for pain, blister/ulcer formation, desquamation daily; ask patient to return for evaluation until stable.<br>3. Teach patient to report fever, chills, blistering, sloughing of skin over site, worsening pain, or arm or hand swelling and stiffness. |
| Mechlorethamine HCl (nitrogen mustard, Mustargen) | 1. Antidote is sodium thiosulfate that neutralizes drug<br>2. Local cooling (eg, ice pack) for 6 to 12 hours after sodium thiosulfate injection<br>3. Inject 2 mL of sodium thiosulfate for each milligram of drug thought to have extravasated | 1. Drug must be diluted to a 1/6 molar solution (mix 4 mL of 10% sodium thiosulfate with 6 mL sterile water; if 25% solution, mix 1.6 mL with 8.4 mL sterile water).<br>2. Give multiple injections into site of extravasation, changing 25-gauge needle with each injection.<br>3. Assess the area for pain, blister/ulcer formation, desquamation daily; ask patient to return for evaluation until stable.<br>4. Teach patient to report fever, chills, blistering, sloughing of skin over site, worsening pain, or arm or hand swelling and stiffness. |
| Rare vesicants:<br>Paclitaxel (Taxol)<br>Docetaxel (Taxotere) | Local cooling (eg, ice pack) 15 to 20 minutes at least 4 times a day for first 24 hours | Rare vesicants (eg, with concentrated dose), so may be given as peripheral infusion. |

*Abbreviations*: IV, intravenous; PPE, personal protective equipment.

*Source*: Data from Polovich M, et al.[1]

blood return and easy flow of fluids by gravity should be determined before administering vesicants via any IV catheter or CVAD.

7. Visualize the IV catheter or CVAD insertion site, and observe the site frequently. (Never leave the patient unattended when administering a vesicant drug peripherally.) Signs and symptoms of extravasation are any or all of the following: pain, redness, swelling, loss of blood return, and/or formation of a blister or bleb on the skin surface above the vein.
8. Give vesicants in a steady, even flow, checking frequently (every 3 to 5 mL) for a blood return. When checking for a blood return, do so gently to avoid excessive pressure on the vein. Pre-injection blood return is assessed by using a syringe at the port closest to the patient to aspirate back or by lowering the mainline IV bag below the level of the IV site and watching for a blood return. Document blood return at the beginning, during, and at the end of drug administration.
9. If in doubt whether an extravasation is occurring, treat it as an extravasation. Stop the drug immediately, aspirate any remaining drug from the tubing, and administer a local antidote or treatment. For anthracycline antibiotics (eg, daunorubicin and doxorubicin), inject dexrazoxane (Totect) if possible within 6 hours of the infiltration and apply local cooling for 20 minutes 4 times a day; for plant alkaloids (eg, vincristine, vinblastine, and vinorelbine), inject hyaluronidase and apply local heat 4 times a day; for nitrogen mustard, inject sodium thiosulfate. The antidote is injected subcutaneously into the area of infiltration using a 25-gauge needle, except for dexrazoxane, which is given daily for 3 days as an IV infusion over 2 to 3 hours.
10. If a vesicant is ordered as a continuous infusion, it is given through a central line only, and the site assessed, as well as confirmation of a blood return, per institutional policy and procedure.
11. An extravasation kit containing all the materials necessary to manage an extravasation should be available wherever vesicant drugs are administered. Include a copy of the extravasation policy and procedure in the kit.

Despite these precautions, vesicant extravasation does occur. Chemotherapy drug extravasation is a known complication of cancer treatment. The incidence of extravasation has been reported to range from 0.01% to 6% of all adverse effects associated with chemotherapy.[59]

Extravasation of a vesicant chemotherapy drug is traumatic for the patient and nurse, but it is not necessarily an act of negligence. However, to not know what to do or to ignore best practices to minimize the damage of extravasation is professional negligence or malpractice. Often the occurrence of an extravasation is more a function of venous integrity than of the administration technique. Patients should be thoroughly informed regarding the vesicant potential of the drugs they are receiving and the importance of reporting any pain, burning, or stinging during the injection. In addition, the nurse administering the drug should know the institution and national standards for managing extravasation.

*Identification of extravasation.* Detection of a vesicant extravasation in its earliest stage is most likely to result in the least possible soft tissue damage. If an extravasation is suspected but not certain, treat it as though it is an extravasation. The nurse should be aware of the following symptoms that could indicate extravasation; it is also important to note that an extravasation can occur without any immediate signs (eg, an indirect injury):[1,8,56,59]

- Swelling—bleb formation at the injection site (most common)
- Stinging, burning, or pain at the injection site (not *always* present)
- Redness (not often seen initially)
- Lack of blood return (if this is the *only* symptom, the IV line should be reevaluated; if there is still no blood return, consider other options). Lack of a blood return alone is not always indicative of an extravasation; an extravasation can occur even if a blood return is present because the IV cathter can penetrate the back wall of the vein, and the bevel can be half in and half outside the vein. Implanted ports should have a blood return, and even if the line flushes easily, further investigation should document correct catheter placement and patency via dye or flow study.[59] Whether the drug causes direct or indirect cellular injury will determine how quickly ulceration may occur (from shortly after to a month after therapy).
- Estimate the approximate volume (amount) of extravasated drug and concentration, assess the administration site (including measuring and photographing the site if possible), and assess the extremity for range of motion and discomfort with movement. Initiate treatment promprly.[1,8,59]
- The course of the progressive necrosis depends on whether the drug binds to DNA. If so, the damage is immediate, and ulceration will progress within a few days. In contrast, with the indirect damage of non-DNA-binding drugs, the damage occurs slowly, and ulceration may take weeks to months to occur after the extravasation.[1]

While generally considered a reliable and safe means of drug delivery, implanted ports and, less commonly, tunneled catheters sometimes do result in extravasation of vesicant drugs. In the case of implanted ports, the cause of drug extravasation is usually a misplaced or displaced needle.[1,56,59] In this situation, the drug extravasates into the port pocket or area surrounding the port. Another mechanism for drug extravasation from ports involves retrograde subcutaneous leakage from catheters obstructed by a fibrin sheath.[55,58] Extravasation also may occur into the subcutaneous tunnel, either from thrombosis and backtracking or from a damaged or fractured central venous catheter. Extravasation also may occur into the intrathoracic cavity as a complication of catheter placement.[55,56]

Prior to injecting or infusing a vesicant into a CVAD or a peripherally inserted central catheter (PICC), examine the exit site for leaks and the insertion site for evidence of swelling or venous thrombosis.[1,8] Catheter displacement may be evidenced by the appearance of the cuff extruding from the exit site, indicating that the catheter has been pulled or has slipped out of place.[1,8] Observe the insertion site for evidence of swelling during fluid bolus. Any evidence of swelling or subjective complaints by the patient of pain or discomfort during the fluid bolus warrants investigation.

The presence of a blood return from an implanted port or a tunneled catheter usually confirms catheter tip placement. However, it is not uncommon for a catheter to be placed properly without evidence of catheter damage and still have an absent or intermittent blood return. If the patient complains of discomfort with fluid injection or if the flow demonstrates resistance, becomes sluggish, or does not flow freely with gravity, it is possible that the catheter tip is obstructed, the catheter has drifted or migrated into a smaller ancillary vein, or it has otherwise become bent or coiled, preventing backflow of blood[1,8,56,59] (see Figure 16-3). It is important in these situations to determine catheter placement by radiological means. The injection of fluid or a chemotherapy agent should be withheld pending physician examination and patency determination by a flow or dye study. Vesicant drugs never should be given via a line or catheter without a blood return.[59]

When giving vesicant drugs through a port, whether by simple injection or by continuous infusion, it is important to use a 90-degree bent Huber-point needle that can be stabilized and secured rather than a straight needle. Straight needles can easily become dislodged because there is no way to stabilize them regardless of how brief the injection time. Patients are instructed to report any pain, burning, tightness, stinging, or discomfort over the chest area during the injection or infusion.[1] When injecting a vesicant, the blood return is assessed before, during, and at the conclusion of the injection.[1,8] During the short-term or continuous infusion of a vesicant, assessment of blood return is based on hospital policy and procedure.[1] In some situations where the patient is confused or uncooperative, it is reasonable to question whether it is safe to use a port for continuous vesicant infusions because needle dislodgment can occur even under the best conditions.

The ideal catheter for long-term cancer care and the infusion of vesicant agents in the outpatient/home environment is an implanted port, provided that the needle is stabilized adequately and the patient is capable of regularly assessing the site for proper needle placement[55,60] (see Figure 16-4). This is so because the device is totally implanted under the skin with no external parts when not being used, so the risk of infection is less (compared with other CVADs),[61] as well as the fact that patients can shower and swim and have more normal lives when the device is not accessed.[55] Alternately, the PICC line can be used, but this is intended for more short-term use (such as 4 to 6 weeks) and requires dressing changes (institution-specific but at least every 7 days).[1,8,62]

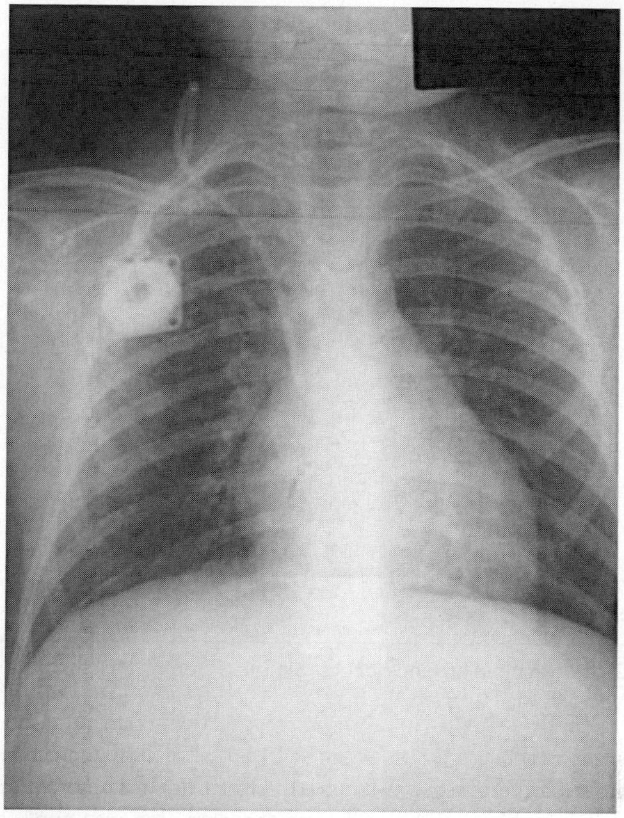

**FIGURE 16-3**

Catheter bent causing resistance during infusion and lack of blood return.

*Management of extravasation.* If a significant extravasation has occurred, it usually will be obvious to the patient and nurse at the time it occurs. In some situations, however, the actual symptoms are delayed for 24 to 48 hours.[1] The patient may report redness over the injection site that is warm to the touch. Color Plate 4 depicts a doxorubicin extravasation 12 days after drug administration. There was no pain with movement of the area, which healed spontaneously without local treatment. Color Plate 5 demonstrates erythema and edema at the injection site 1 week after doxorubicin administration. At the time of administration, blood return was lost, and the patient complained of slight pain at

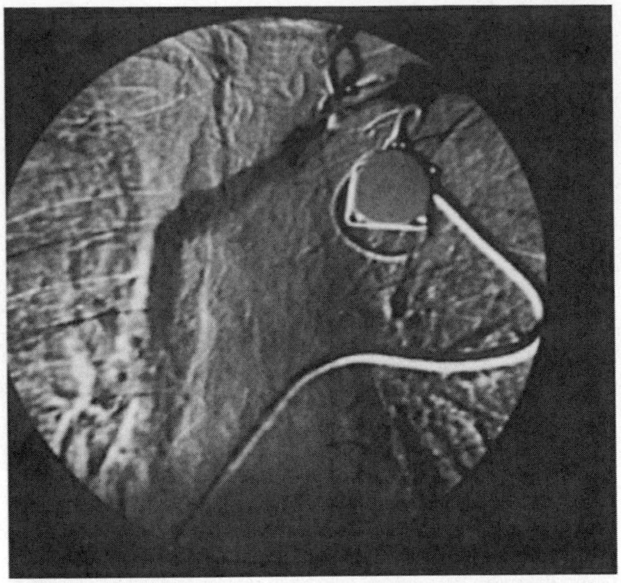

**FIGURE 16-4**

Catheter coiled around port as demonstrated by digital subtraction venogram.

the site. The drug was stopped. After flushing with saline, slight swelling was noted over the area. Ice was applied. This area progressed to blister formation in 3 weeks, with clear demarcation of the damaged area (see Color Plate 6), which was surgically excised (see Color Plate 7).

When there is cause to believe that an extravasation of a vesicant agent has occurred during drug administration, prompt nursing action, in general, will minimize tissue damage.[1,8,56,59] The nurse is responsible for ensuring that all antidotes and diluents are readily available and accessible. The management of extravasation is summarized in Table 16-8. The following steps should be taken if an extravasation is suspected:[1,8,56,59]

1. Stop the administration of the chemotherapeutic agent. If injecting through the sidearm of a free-flowing IV line, stop the fluid flow immediately; failure to do so further disperses the infiltrated drug into the tissues. Notify the physician or advanced practice nurse of the actual or potential extravasation.
2. Disconnect the IV tubing, and attach an empty small 1- to 3-mL syringe. Attempt to aspirate any residual drug from the IV device. Remove the needle.
3. If the drug has an antidote, administer it into the area of infiltration using a 25-gauge needle and syringe, changing the needle with each separate injection.
4. Dress the site with a sterile 2 × 2 gauze pad over the needle entrance site.
5. Apply local care measures, such as the application of heat or cold according to institutional policy and procedure.
6. Avoid applying direct manual pressure to the site.
7. Photograph the extravasation site prior to applying a loose sterile dressing.
8. Apply ice for 15 minutes or more every hour for 24 to 48 hours while the patient is awake, except if the extravasating drug was a vinca alkaloid (eg, vincristine, vinblastine, or vinorelbine); in this case, apply heat.
9. Instruct the patient on local care, systemic analgesics, and a plan for follow-up:
   a. Elevate the extremity for 48 hours.
   b. After the first 48 hours, the patient should be encouraged to use the extremity normally. Failure to do so may result in stiffness, neuropathy, and swelling.
   c. Arrange for a return appointment once or twice weekly depending on the amount of drug suspected to have extravasated and the patient's individual concerns.
   d. Photograph the site weekly as appropriate. Document the degree of erythema, induration, and pain and any evidence of ulceration or necrosis.
   e. If pain persists beyond 7 to 10 days, confer with the physician or advanced practice nurse regarding a plastic surgery consultation, especially if there is evidence of ulcer demarcation.
   f. Consider physical therapy consultation to encourage normal use of the extremity during healing.
   g. Promptly complete an extravasation documentation record (Figure 16-5),[62,63] paying special attention to subjective complaints and objective observations of the details immediately surrounding the extravasation event.

Paclitaxel and docetaxel are similar antineoplastic drugs that are considered to be moderate irritants with the potential to cause ulceration if concentrated amounts of the drug infiltrate. These drugs are infused routinely via peripheral veins, some with the assistance of an infusion pump. Vesicants should not administered with the force of an infusion pump into a peripheral vein, and the nurse should remain with the patient during the infusion to visually monitor the site for signs of extravasation and to confirm blood return.[1,8]

In contrast to peripheral lines, extravasation from a central venous catheter (tunneled, nontunneled, implanted port, or peripherally inserted central catheter [PICC] line) may be substantial before it is detected because infusions are not monitored constantly, and the vesicant may be more diluted than when given by IV injection. Therefore, pain at the site may not be noted early. Dressings over the port site may mask swelling. Because infusions tend to be given slowly, a considerable amount of drug can extravasate without obvious evidence of leakage. In the case of an implanted port, the cause is usually Huber needle dislodgment from the port septum.[56,59] The degree of tissue damage will depend on the concentration of the drug and the amount infiltrated. In some cases, there may be no tissue

**Documentation of Extravasation**

- Patient name, medical record number, date of drug extravasation
- Name of drug, dilution and estimated volume of extravasated drug
- Type of vascular access (eg, 22-gauge peripheral IV, PICC, implanted port and size huber needle used)
- Infusion method (eg, side-arm of freely flowing IV, direct IVP, minibag infusion, continuous infusion)
- Whether infusion pump was in use when extravasation occurred
- Pretreatment patient assessment (IV location, type and size of catheter, description and quality of blood return confirmed, and photograph if possible)
- Patient symptoms reported along with time in relation to time drug administration was initiated
- Nurse observation of extravasated area, along with photograph of area if possible. Indicate description, and dimensions of areas of edema and erythema
- Immediate nursing interventions along with time occurrence based on current standards such as hospital policy and procedure, INS and ONS standards.
- Time physician or advanced practice nurse notified, and instructions given
- Follow-up plan
  - Patient teaching, such as application of heat or cold, assessment of skin for blistering or ulceration, and temperature, and reporting any changes including onset of pain
  - Return appointment for reassessment of skin integrity, need for referral to Plastic Surgery, evaluation of limb function, and need for physical therapy referral as appropriate.

**FIGURE 16-5**

*Abbreviations:* IV, intravenous; IVP, intravenous port; INS, Intravenous Nursing Society; ONS, Oncology Nursing Society.

*Source:* Data from Polovich et al.,[1] Sauerland et al.,[55] Hayden and Goodman,[62] Schulmeister.[63]

breakdown; in others, wide excision may be required for the wound to heal.

If an extravasation is suspected from a central venous catheter, the infusion is stopped immediately, any remaining drug is aspirated, and the physician is notified. An attempt should be made to estimate the amount of drug extravasated. It may be possible to aspirate residual drug from the site. An antidote can be administered if available. Otherwise, the needle should be removed. Efforts to express fluid manually from the site should be avoided. Instead, a sterile dressing should be applied over the needle entrance site and changed frequently. Ice packs should be applied per institutional policy and procedure. Appropriate documentation (extravasation documentation record such as that depicted in Figure 16-5) should be completed, and plans for careful follow-up and additional consultation with a surgeon may be appropriate.

### Intramuscular and subcutaneous

The development of the colony-stimulating factors has increased the number of drugs given subcutaneously, whereas chemotherapy drugs such as fulvestrant (Faslodex) are given intramuscularly. Other chemotherapy drugs that may be given intramuscularly are methotrexate and asparaginase.[35] Subcutaneous injections of small volumes are given in the usual sites and should be rotated if given daily. Many drug manufacturers have distributed videos, charts, or posters that clearly outline the steps to follow for patients self-administration of subcutaneous medications. One drug that is administered subcutaneously in a rather unique way is goserelin acetate (Zoladex). This dry drug pellet is implanted in the soft tissue of the abdomen, where it is absorbed gradually over 1 to 3 months. A local anesthetic such as an anesthetic cream or ice is usually used to minimize discomfort because the needle is large (16-gauge). It is very important to remember to use safe handling precautions when administering these agents, including PPE. Syringes with needles should be dropped intact into a chemotherapy leakproof, puncture-proof bucket, and they should not be clipped because this will aerosolize the drug and increase the risk of contamination.[14]

### Intra-arterial

Intra-arterial drug administration, a drug-delivery practice that began in the early 1960s and is experiencing a resurgence in practice today, involves cannulation of the artery that provides a tumor's blood supply and subsequent administration of the drug directly through the arterial catheter to the tumor bed.[1,64] This method increases the concentration of the drug to known areas of tumor and decreases the systemic drug concentration and thus the side effects. The primary use of this route is via the hepatic artery for the management of potential or actual metastasis of colon cancer to the liver. In addition, it also has been used for hepatocellular carcinoma, as well as cancers of the brain, head and neck, and pelvis. In fact, there are exciting studies being conducted using regional chemotherapy administered in nontraditional clinical settings such as the operating room and interventional radiology suite.[2,3] Possible complications of arterial cannulation are catheter tip migration, infection, and thrombosis.[65] Antineoplastic drugs used in intra-arterial administration must show increased cell kill with increased dose and have high total-body clearance and low systemic levels, high regional extraction, and low or no regional toxicity.[65] These drugs include doxorubicin, floxuridine (FUDR), mitomycin-C, and cisplatin.[64,66] Intra-arterial chemotherapy drug delivery involves placement of a catheter into the main artery supplying the tumor for local drug therapy, long-term drug administration, or chemoembolization of the artery that then provides localized drug delivery only to the tumor and stops blood flow to the tumor.[65] Catheters can be placed by a surgeon, who uses a Silastic catheter for long-term therapy that is attached to an implanted pump; this has fewer complications, and the patient can remain an outpatient. Alternatively, catheters can be placed by interventional radiology for short-term therapy using a polyethylene catheter; this requires the patient to remain in the hospital and has more complications. For an implanted device for long-term therapy, the catheter is attached either to an implanted port or a pump. The catheter is inserted into the appropriate artery and then attached to the pump located in a surgically created subcutaneous pocket, usually in the lower abdomen or upper chest. The pump chamber is accessed via a noncoring Huber-like needle and filled with either a chemotherapeutic agent or heparinized sterile saline.[65] The flow rates depend on pump design and are either preset prior to implantation or adjustable via an external electronic wand that communicates with the internal pump. Care and maintenance of these devices by the nurse require a formalized educational program and ongoing monitoring of pump functioning.[1] The implantable pump offers patients the greatest level of freedom when receiving intraarterial chemotherapy and has lower complication rates than external methods. Nursing management includes monitoring for drug side effects and potential pump complications, such as infection, occlusion, extravasation, and malfunction.[2,3,65] Some unique nursing actions are necessary when dealing with implantable pumps, such as not aspirating the center pump septum (into which the Huber needle is placed), monitoring or establishing the pump flow rate, and detecting malfunctions. The oncology nurse is referred to the manufacturers' instructions and guidelines regarding the management of these advanced nursing responsibilities.

Nursing care of a patient receiving short-term intraarterial drug infusion via external pump is specific to the diagnosis, drug(s) being administered, and artery that is cannulated.[67] Pre-procedurally, a full chemotherapy assessment, including laboratory values, should be performed, as well as peripheral pulses using a Doppler ultrasound if necessary, teaching the patient to lie flat during the procedure, and insertion of a Foley catheter.[67] Following intraarterial line placement, the nurse must assess the patient's vital signs, level of consciousness, intraarterial line insertion site, peripheral pulses (eg, warmth and color of extremities), and signs of bleeding or hematoma at the insertion site and monitor vital signs as per institutional protocol. Potential complications include pain, bleeding, embolism, pump occlusion or malfunction, arterial injury, arterial catheter leak or break, skin reaction to the securing tape, and catheter migration or dislodgement.[1] Premedications should be administered as ordered, such as antiemetics. As discussed previously, with all chemotherapy, the drug should be double-checked independently by 2 health care professionals. Full PPE should be worn when handling the drug and caring for the patient's excreta. Duration of chemotherapy administration may be a few hours to 3 to 7 days. During drug administration, the nurse should monitor for bleeding, changes in prothrombin time/partial thromboplastin time (PT/PTT), changes in the catheter site (eg, infection or bleeding), migration/dislodgement of the catheter (eg, nausea, vomiting, diarrhea, edema, epigastric pain, diminished peripheral pulses, and inability of catheter to infuse), and catheter occlusion (eg, inability to flush or withdraw fluid from the line, abdominal pain, and change in color/pulse/temperature of involved extremity).[1,67] Following drug administration, the line is flushed with heparin solution to prevent thrombus formation, and then the line removed by the interventional radiologist.[67] Pressure is held over the site for 10 minutes, and hemostasis is obtained prior to applying a pressure dressing. Usually the patient is on bed rest for an additional 4 hours with hourly or more frequent monitoring of vital signs, peripheral pulses, and the pressure dressing. When stable and off bedrest, the Foley catheter is removed. The patient may remain in the hospital overnight to receive IV hydration and measurement of intake and output.[67]

Hepatic artery chemoembolization (HACE) is performed for patients with unresectable liver metastases, primary hepatocellular cancer, and primary carcinoid tumors. The liver receives oxygenated blood from both the left and right hepatic arteries (25% of the liver's total blood volume); in addition, the liver receives partially oxygenated blood from the portal vein that holds 75% of the liver's blood supply. While normal liver tissue receives most of its blood from the portal vein, liver tumors receive 80% of their oxygenated blood from the hepatic artery.[68] This allows effective tumor isolation and treatment (eg, embolization to stop the blood supply and local delivery of chemotherapy) without injuring normal surrounding liver tissue. The appropriate hepatic arterial branch is located and cannulated, and then the chemotherapy drug, such as doxorubicin or cisplatin, along with small particles (eg, Gelfoam [water-insoluble hemostatic device] or Ivalon [hydroxylated polyvinyl acetal sponge]) to occlude the artery and isolate the drug in the tumor are injected by IV push or short IV infusion.[65] The hepatic artery watershed area supplying the tumor is visualized radiologically during the procedure, and when the tumor blush is lost, reflecting loss of blood flow, the procedure is stopped.[65] More recently, therapeutic microspheres are used because they are more readily extracted by the tumor. The microspheres have a larger diameter than the smallest-diameter hepatic capillaries and sinusoids, so they become trapped and begin delivering drug to the targeted tumor, sparing the rest of the liver.[65] Drugs such as mitomycin-C can be incorporated into the structure of the microsphere, resulting in a high concentration of drug in the tumor bed.[63] All procedures require safe handling precautions with full PPE and management of chemotherapy waste. Finally, the microspheres also can be prepared with the radionucleotide yttrium-90, which gives off high energy up to 2 to 3 mm when the microsphere is trapped in the microcirculation. This treatment is usually given for 7 to 10 days because the nucleotide has a half-life of 64 hours.[65] This procedure requires safe handling of radioactive substances. Nursing care for patients undergoing hepatic artery chemoembolism requires (1) effective pain management during and after the treatment, (2) close monitoring of the arterial puncture site and peripheral pulses (for signs and symptoms of bleeding, nausea, vomiting, and diarrhea), vital signs, and fluid and electrolyte status, with prompt intervention if bleeding or other complications arise, and (3) laboratory monitoring (eg, hemoglobin, international normalization ratio [INR], and PT/PTT).[68]

### Intraperitoneal

Regional delivery of chemotherapy into the peritoneal space has been found to be a safe and well tolerated treatment for stage III ovarian cancer and is being studied in other solid tumors.[69] There is a resurgence of interest in the treatment of patients with surgically debulked stage III ovarian cancer using the intraperitoneal approach. Studies have shown that intraperitoneal (IP) chemotherapy extends survival (49.7 months for IV paclitaxel and cisplatin chemotherapy compared with 65.5 months with IV paclitaxel, plus IP paclitaxel and cisplatin chemotherapy; $P = 0.03$).[70] A meta-analysis of IP chemotherapy for the treatment of advanced ovarian cancer showed that both overall and disease-free survival were improved.[71] IP chemotherapy is indicated for women with stage III ovarian cancer that has less than 1 cm of residual disease after debulking surgery and is contraindicated if the peritoneal disease is adherent to the peritoneum, contains massive ascites, shows postoperative infection, or is associated gastrointestinal dysfunction or if the patient is malnourished or hypovolemic.[69,70]

The semipermeable nature of the peritoneal space allows high concentrations of the drugs to be delivered to tumor sites with lower concentrations entering the bloodstream. The procedure causes local side effects due to the large volume of fluid filling the space, such as abdominal distension, pain, and dyspnea.[69] In ovarian cancer clinical trials, women discontinued IP therapy due to issues with the IP access device, abdominal pain during the infusion, and inability to tolerate the dose of cisplatin (100 mg/m$^2$).[72] Since the tolerance of cisplatin is a rate-limiting step, Markman is investigating the use of carboplatin instead of cisplatin.[73] In addition, other toxicities were greater with the IP approach (eg, myelosuppression, emesis, and neuropathy), but although quality of life scores were lower during the first year following treatment, after 12 months, there was no difference between groups.[72]

An implanted port with a large-diameter (9.6 F) silicone catheter is the recommended peritoneal catheter, and it is subcutaneously tunneled so that the port is placed over the inferior thorax at the midclavicular line, below the bra line.[72] However, the more traditional peritoneal Tenckhoff (a type of catheter with multiple fenestrations along and at the end of the catheter) and Portacath catheters should be avoided because the fenestrations of the former may cause fibrous sheath formation and bowel adhesions and the Dacron cuff on the latter may erode into the peritoneal membrane and cause bowel obstruction.[72] The catheter can be placed at the same time as the original ovarian resection for most patients, along with a venous access device for systemic chemotherapy.[72]

Complications of the catheter include slow infusion rate of solution (related to kinks, fibrin sheath formation along the catheter, obstruction of the catheter by adhesions, or tumor), inflow failure (kinks, clot in the catheter, obstruction of catheter by adhesions, catheter migration, or tumor), outflow failure (fibrin sheath, omental adhesions, or tumor blocking catheter outflow), exit-site infection (immunosuppression or contamination of exit site), and leakage of chemotherapy (separation of the port from the catheter, dislodgement of Huber needle from the port septum, migration of the catheter out of the peritoneum, or incomplete healing of the subcutaneous tunnel).[64] In addition, peritoneal fluid can flow retrograde up the catheter into the port pocket, the catheter can kink causing fluid to flow retrograde and leak out of the port septum at the Huber-like needle, peritoneal fluid can leak from the vagina, bowel perforation may occur from the catheter, and finally, sequestering of chemotherapy may be seen in bowel adhesions.[74] Catheter troubleshooting is similar to that for subcutaneously implanted venous access ports using a dye or flow study.[72] Malfunctioning ports may need to be replaced, especially if there is fluid backflow up the catheter.

Teach patients about potential side effects and measures to reduce the risks associated with this therapy. Almadrones and colleagues have developed a patient educational tool about IP chemotherapy.[75] Potential patient side effects and nursing measures include[69,72,75,76]

- *Abdominal distension.* Instruct patients to eat a light meal prior to the treatment and to wear loose-fitting clothes. Ensure that the peritoneal cavity is completely emptied prior to infusion; use a warm intraperitoneal solution prior to treatment. Assess the abdomen and pain level before and frequently during the treatment; if pain occurs, slow the infusion until the patient is more comfortable. Administer pain medication and reassess frequently. At completion of the infusion, instruct the patient to turn side to side every 15 minutes for 1 hour. Distinguish from peritonitis (if symptoms develop immediately after drug infusion, it is likely distension), and assess for abdominal guarding on palpation, rebound tenderness, nausea, vomiting, diarrhea, fever, or leukocytosis.

- *Dyspnea.* Assess respiratory status before and regularly during the infusion. Reassure the patient that dyspnea is temporary. Increase the level of the head of the bed, and increase ambulation and sitting upright.
- *Fluid and electrolyte imbalance related to cisplatin.* Monitor electrolytes before the infusion, and replete magnesium and potassium as needed. Assess for signs and symptoms of hypomagnesemia, hypokalemia, and hypocalcemia. Instruct the patient to increase oral fluid intake to 2 L daily for 3 days (if receiving cisplatin).
- *Peripheral neuropathy (PN).* Assess risk (receiving both cisplatin and paclitaxel) and preexisting PN. Assess baseline sensory and motor function and follow serially. Instruct the patient to avoid extreme temperatures. Refer to occupational therapy for assistive devices if needed. Manage pain or discomfort in collaboration with the physician or advanced practice nurse.
- *Frequent urination.* Instruct the patient to void prior to treatment and to report difficulties resuming normal urination within 48 hours of treatment.
- *Nausea, vomiting, anorexia.* Assess baseline gastrointestinal status, nutrition, and weight. Instruct the patient to report any symptoms. Administer antiemetics prior to chemotherapy treatment, and discuss the need for adjuncts or revised regimen based on response. Instruct the patient to eat small, frequent meals, and ensure that the patient has antiemetics to take at home (delayed emesis regimen). Instruct the patient to report if the regimen is ineffective.
- *Diarrhea or constipation.* Assess baseline elimination status. Teach the patient about diet modification, and instruct the patient to increase oral fluids. If the patient has constipation, encourage a bowel regimen with increased fiber and laxatives as needed, especially if the patient is receiving opioids. If tha patient has diarrhea, teach about self-administration of antidiarrheal medicines.
- *Potential for infection, bleeding, and fatigue related to bone marrow suppression.* Monitor the complete blood count and differential, noting a shift to the left (increased number of bands) if associated with abdominal pain, and discuss the possibility of peritonitis with physician. Reinforce teaching about avoidance of infection and bleeding. Administer growth factors (eg, pegfilgrastim, darbopoetin, or erythropoietin) as ordered. Discuss dose modification with the physician if neutropenia or thrombocytopenia is present. Administer antibiotics as ordered. Assess patient's fatigue level before and during each treatment. Teach the patient strategies to minimize energy exertion and conserve energy.

Nursing care management is outlined in Table 16-9. The peritoneal catheter should be removed as soon as therapy is completed.[72]

### Intrapleural

Care of the patient with a pleural effusion traditionally involves insertion of chest tubes, drainage of the fluid, and sclerosis of the pleural space to prevent recurrence of the effusion. The pleural membranes are the visceral pleura (lines the outer surface of each lung) and the parietal pleura (lines the thoracic cavity), and pleural effusions develop between these pleural membranes. Sclerosis, or chemical pleurodesis, involves the instillation of a drug or substance that is irritating to the pleura, causing pleuritis of the pleural membranes. The inflammatory process causes the parietal and visceral pleura to stick together, thereby obliterating the pleural space and preventing any reaccumulation of pleural fluid. Over the years, many different sclerosing chemicals have been used with varying degrees of effectiveness. Bleomycin, cisplatin, tetracycline derivatives, and sterilized talc are all agents that have been used for pleural installation.[77] This insertion is accomplished by injecting the drug directly into the chest tube and clamping it for a specified time period; the evidence base for patient position change every 15 minutes for 1 to 2 hours immediately following the instillation to coat the pleural surfaces is not strong.[78] Nursing management of intrapleural chemotherapy includes patient education, safe drug handling, and side effect management. In general, nursing care focuses on emesis control, pain control, respiratory status, chest tube security, and other comfort measures, depending on the drug used[78] (see Chapter 35). For patients with recurrent pleural effusions despite pleurodesis, the use of a permanent, tunneled small-bore pleural drainage tube such as the Pleurx catheter has been successful and permits the patient to remain at home, emptying the catheter every other day or as directed. The patient is instructed not to remove more than 1 L of fluid at a time.[79]

### Intravesicular

Direct instillation of chemotherapy into the bladder has proved to be an extremely effective and simple method of controlling superficial bladder cancer and carcinoma in situ.[80] Agents such as mitomycin-C and bacillus Calmette-Guérin (BCG) have been shown to be effective, especially BCG in the adjuvant treatment of patients at significant risk of recurrence after transurethral resection of the bladder tumor (TURBT).[81] Instillation is usually weekly for 4 to 12 weeks and involves insertion of a urinary catheter, instillation of the drug (usually in 50 to 60 mL of sterile solution), and retention of the drug for 1 to 2 hours (with frequent movement to disperse the drug throughout the bladder) prior to unclamping the catheter or voiding. Some physicians prefer to have the urinary catheter remain clamped and in place for the dwell time. In this case, the fluid that drains from the catheter when it is unclamped should be contained and disposed of properly via the

**TABLE 16-9**

**Nursing Care Management of the Patient Receiving Intraperitoneal Drug Administration**

**Patient Education**

- Teach patient about the port and how to care for it prior to implantation.
- Teach patient to wear loose-fitting, comfortable clothes.
- Teach patient drug administration process, potential side effects (eg, abdominal pain, dyspnea, frequent urination), strategies to minimize side effects, chemotherapy drug side effects, and self-care measures to minimize them.
- Teach self-care measures when the patient returns home.

**Pretreatment and Site Access**

- Assess patient laboratory values (renal, electrolytes).
- Verify the drug order and drug (2 nurses independently).
- Warm IP fluid to body temperature using inline fluid warmer, or warm bags in water bath.
- Assess other treatment orders (eg, IV chemotherapy, IV hydration for IP cisplatin, IV electrolyte replacement).
- Ask patient to void, emptying bladder.
- Administer antiemetics as ordered (should be the same as if the chemotherapy was given IV).
- Gather appropriate supplies, and access port using sterile technique (19-gauge Huber needle, 1 to 1.5 inches in length), secure needle with transparent dressing. Inject 10 mL saline, attempt to aspirate ascitic return; if unable to obtain fluid, flush port again with NS; continue if able to flush without resistance and fluid flows easily with gravity flow.
- If resistance is felt or there is swelling at the port site, remove Huber needle and reprep the site. Reaccess with new sterile equipment.
- Don PPE, and attach chemotherapy infusion line(s).

**Drug Administration**

- Position patient in semi-Fowler's position.
- Open the clamp of the chemotherapy, and infuse the warmed IP fluid using gravity flow (do not use a pump); usually mixed in 2 L NS bag; allow to infuse over prescribed rate (30 minutes to several hours).
- Stop infusion immediately if severe pain is experienced, and check for catheter migration.
- Slow the rate of infusion if the patient experiences SOB or discomfort.
- Administer analgesics as needed and ordered.
- Apply blankets if the patient feels chilled.
- Close the clamp on the tubing when the infusion is completed, and encourage repositioning from side to side every 15 minutes during the dwell time (usually 2 to 4 hours).
- Monitor patient's comfort levels, SOB, abdominal discomfort, diarrhea, nausea, vomiting.
- After the prescribed dwell time, open the clamp to the drainage bag and allow the solution to drain. If flow is sluggish, check tubing for kinks, help patient roll from side to side, have patient use the Valsalva maneuver, apply manual pressure to the abdomen, or irrigate the catheter with normal saline.
- Recognize that the volume of drained fluid may be less than that infused, and reassure that the fluid will be reabsorbed and metabolized.
- Clamp tubing on drainage bag after fluid has drained (usually 30 minutes to 2 hours).
- Flush port with 10 to 20 mL saline or heparinize per hospital policy.
- Remove Huber needle and cover site with bandage or small dressing.

**Postadministration Care**

- Establish IV fluids as prescribed, or discontinue IV.
- Assess patient's status, and ensure ability to perform self-care at home as appropriate.
- Document procedure in medical record, as well as patient's response.
- Reinforce home care teaching.

*Abbreviations*: IP, intraperitoneal; NS, normal saline; IV, intravenous; PPE, personal protective equipment; SOB, shortness of breath.

toilet, with special handling by caregivers for 8 hours if the patient is incontinent. If the patient is going home with an indwelling catheter for 1 to 2 days, instruct the patient to wear gloves when handling the drainage bag and to wash his or her hands well afterward. The patient should void directly in the toilet and flush with the lid down.[82] There is no evidence that double flushing the toilet is more effective than a single flush in eliminating urine contaminated with chemotherapy, except possibly with low-volume-per-flush toilets.[1] If the physician prefers to withdraw the catheter after drug instillation and instructs the patient to void in 1 to 2 hours, instruct the patient to flush with the lid down. With BCG, a live, attenuated strain of bovine tuberculosis, patients should be taught to use bleach in toilets equal to the amount voided, letting the solution stand in the toilet for 15 minutes before flushing with the lid down.[82] Any contaminated nondisposable items are disinfected with bleach. Local side effects such as bladder irritation or, with mitomycin-C, dermatitis of the external genitalia can be experienced, and the patient is taught to wash the genital region after every urination for 6 hours to reduce skin irritation.[80] BCG causes an acute inflammatory reaction in the bladder, stimulating the immune system to attack and kill the cancer cells.[81] As a result, the side effects are painful, frequent urination and flu-like symptoms, including fever.

Nursing care management for patients receiving intravesicular chemotherapy includes patient education (stressing handwashing and personal hygiene), drug administration, side effect monitoring, and safe drug handling.[82] For most oncology nurses, it is unusual to have experience with this method of drug delivery because it is commonly performed in urologists' offices as part of a postoperative office visit.

### Intrathecal or intraventricular

Cancer cells can cross the blood brain barrier and appear in the cerebrospinal fluid (CSF), resulting in central nervous system involvement of the malignancy. This phenomenon is seen most commonly in leukemia (meningeal leukemia) and to a lesser extent in other malignancies, such as breast cancer, lymphoma, and rhabdomyosarcoma (meningeal carcinomatosis). Today, it is known that certain antineoplastic drugs cross the blood–brain barrier, such as temozolomide, irinotecan, topotecan, and at high doses, cyclophosphamide and methotrexate.[35] For tumors insensitive to these drugs, chemotherapy must be injected directly into the CSF as prophylaxis or to manage existing disease so that the drug bypasses the blood–brain barrier. The antineoplastic drugs used currently include methotrexate, and cytarabine.[83] When prepared for use by this route, the preservative-free drug is always admixed under strict sterile conditions with a preservative-free diluent such as sodium chloride USP (unpreserved) or Ringer's injection USP (unpreserved). Methotrexate is available in an unpreserved lyophilized form for intrathecal use. Cytarabine is supplied with a diluent that contains benzyl alcohol and should be replaced with an appropriate unpreserved diluent (sodium chloride or Ringer's solution).[35]

The two primary methods of instillation are intrathecal and intraventricular. The intrathecal route is achieved by performing a standard lumbar puncture using established techniques to ascertain placement and injecting 10 to 12 mL of drug, followed by withdrawal of the needle.[1] This procedure usually is performed by a physician or an advanced practice nurse on a daily to weekly basis depending on the protocol. This method is quick and easy to perform but has the disadvantage that the drug may reach only epidural or subdural spaces. Even when it reaches the subarachnoid space, therapeutic levels of the drug usually are not achieved in the ventricles. For this reason, it may be preferable to use the intraventricular route.

Central instillation of the drug into the ventricle can be achieved via an Ommaya reservoir (Figure 16-6), which is surgically implanted through the cranium. A skin flap is created, and the Ommaya reservoir is placed underneath the skin, with the catheter extending from the reservoir to the ventricle. Once the surgical site has healed, the only visible evidence of the device is a small bump on the head. Placement of this reservoir obviously involves greater risk than performance of a lumbar puncture, but it provides permanent intraventricular access for patients in whom repeated translumbar puncture is impractical. Ommaya reservoirs usually are accessed by physicians or specially trained nurses.[83]

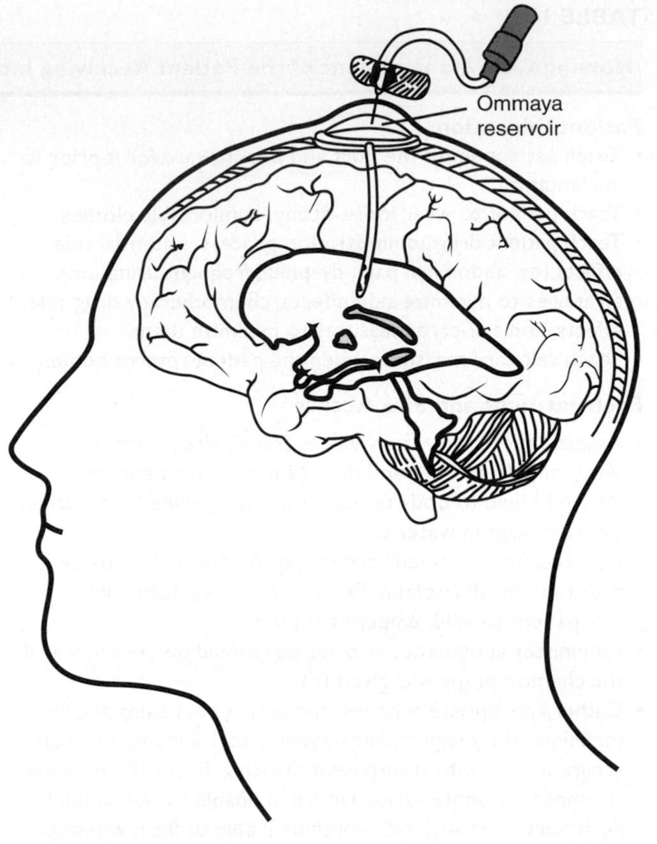


**FIGURE 16-6**

Ommaya reservoir placement.

Regardless of the specific delivery method, nursing care management includes patient education, assessment of the access site, administration (or assistance with administration) of the drug, safe drug handling, and side effect management. Even though most IV drugs do not cross the blood–brain barrier in sufficient concentration to treat meningeal disease, the intraventricular drugs are capable of entering the systemic bloodstream. Side effects of the drugs, such as nausea, stomatitis, and mild myelosuppression, are to be anticipated. Special care should be taken with methotrexate, particularly if it is given in conjunction with cranial radiation therapy, because it may result in increased central nervous system toxicity (progressive or disseminated necrotizing leukoencepthalopathy).[84] Leucovorin is no longer recommended to prevent systemic toxicity from intrathecal or intraventricular methotrexate because there is a risk at high doses of leucovorin that the efficacy of the intrathecal or intraventricular methotrexate will be significantly reduced.[85] This is because even though the leucovorin is administered systemically, a small amount crosses the blood–brain barrier into the CSF. At higher doses, the amount that crosses into the CSF may interfere with methotrexate's ability to kill tumor cells.[85] The expected side effects related to intraventricular drug administration include headache, nausea, vomiting, ataxia, and blurred vision.[83] The most serious complication is infection, which is manifested by tenderness, redness, drainage, warmth or fever, stiff neck, and headache (with or without vomiting). Acute chemical arachnoiditis characterized by headache, back pain, vomiting, fever, and nuchal rigidity has been reported.[83]

### Topical

Cutaneous malignant lesions can be treated in a variety of ways, including the topical application of antineoplastic drugs. Topical drugs are used most commonly for cutaneous T-cell lymphoma, basal cell carcinoma, Kaposi's sarcoma, and squamous cell carcinoma. The drugs used include nitrogen mustard for cutaneous T-cell lymphoma and fluorouracil for basal and squamous cell carcinomas.[86,87] The topical agent usually is applied once or twice daily until the lesions progress to the necrosis phase, which may take 1 to 3 weeks. The affected area is not washed vigorously during the treatment period. The expected result of topical antineoplastic administration is local sloughing of the affected area and eventual regranulation of normal tissue. It is normal for the treated area to become red and tender and then to form a lesion that becomes necrotic, followed by superficial sloughing of the dead tissue and regrowth of healthy skin.[87] It is unusual for the patient to experience any systemic side effects of the drugs unless most of the skin is being treated. Special nursing considerations for these patients include[86]

- Patient education, with special consideration of body-image issues
- Application of the drug using cotton swabs or nonmetal applicators
- Close attention to application only in the prescribed (affected) area
- Careful avoidance of the eyes, nose, mouth, and other areas close to mucous membranes
- Use of safe drug-handling practices (eg, gloves and strict attention to drug containment)
- When using nitrogen mustard, having sodium thiosulfate available (to neutralize the nitrogen mustard) and applying it to areas of the skin that may be exposed inadvertently (after removal of the drug)
- Application of dressings, if prescribed
- Observation for untoward sequelae (eg, severe burning or rashes, which may require discontinuation of therapy or subsequent dose reduction)

## VASCULAR ACCESS DEVICES

The development of central venous catheters (CVCs) and other types of long-term vascular access devices (VADs) has enhanced the lives of patients with cancer but added a new series of challenges for caregivers and patients. Device selection, patient selection, use, maintenance, complication management, and product development continue to be refined by practice and research. Use of VADs is not restricted to the cancer population, and the oncology nurse often serves as an expert resource for other device users. It is estimated that at least 5 million CVCs are inserted every year in the United States.[55]

Many different kinds of catheters, needles, and implantable ports are used for cancer chemotherapy delivery. Some of the major VAD types and features are outlined in Table 16-10. The nurse plays an important role in assessing the patient's vascular access needs and selecting or recommending placement of the proper device. Unfortunately, often the patient with cancer begins therapy, and then halfway through, the nurse is unable to start an IV line, and the patient requires an implanted port. The scheduling is difficult because it must be planned around the patient's nadir and risk of infection and bleeding. Long-term central lines provide a way to perform blood sampling for frequent blood tests, as well as reliable venous access for infusion of chemotherapy, fluids and electrolytes, and blood products. Thus it is important for the nurse to include vascular access in the initial patient assessment.[8] A central venous access device (CVAD) is defined as a catheter whose tip terminates in the lower third of the superior vena cava. These devices are classified as short term (1 to 3 weeks), intermediate (weeks to months), and long term (months to years).[55,60,88] The short-term CVAD is intended for hospitalized patients and is percutaneous, so the catheter is placed directly in the central vein (so it has the highest risk of infection).[55] Intermediate CVADs include the peripherally inserted central catheters or PICC lines. These catheters are inserted by specially trained IV nurses using ultrasound guidance[8] or by physicians. The FDA has approved PICC lines for placement for up to 12 months, but the life of the catheter depends on the type of catheter, the insertion technique, stabilization of the catheter, patient compliance, and nurse competence in maintaining the device.[55] PICCs are available as open-ended or valved (has a neutral displacement valve incorporated in the end of the catheter, ensuring one-way flow of blood and preventing retrograde flow of blood back into the catheter, where it can clot). In addition, PICCs are available as power injectable devices, which are able to withstand the 250 to 300 lb/in$^2$ (psi) of pressure from the radiology IV

**TABLE 16-10**

**Overview of Vascular Access Devices**

| Type | Description | Longevity | Comments |
|---|---|---|---|
| **Peripheral needle**<br>Scalp vein butterfly | Stainless steel<br>Single lumen<br>27-gauge to 19-gauge | Minutes to days | Not appropriate for vesicant injection<br>Increased risk of infiltration |
| **Peripheral catheter**<br>Intima | Catheter over needle<br>Teflon or polyurethane<br>Single and double lumen<br>26-gauge to 14-gauge | Hours to days | Excellent for multiday infusional therapy<br>Provides greater patient mobility because less likely to infiltrate |
| **Nontunneled central venous catheter** | Polyurethane or silicone<br>Single, double, and triple lumen | Hours to months | Excellent for emergency need for CVC<br>Can augment existing VAD for acute-care needs or longer-term use<br>Inserted by physician at bedside or in procedure room |
| **Peripherally inserted central catheter (PICC)** | Silicone elastomer or other polymers<br>Single and double lumen<br>24-gauge to 16-gauge<br>Available as a power injectable catheter | Weeks to months | Excellent for continuous infusion over several weeks or months<br>Can be inserted at bedside by specially trained nurse<br>Quick, easy central access without surgical procedure<br>Requires external site care and routine flushing |
| **Tunneled central venous catheter (TCVC)** | Silicone catheter with Dacron cuff<br>Single, double, and triple lumen<br>4.2 F to 19.2 F;<br>40 to 90 cm long<br>Groshong has slit valve, requiring less flushing; heparinization not required<br>Available as a power injectable catheter | Months to years | Excellent for long-term, continuous, or intermittent therapy<br>Preferred for long-term TPN administration<br>Preferred by many for vesicant infusional therapy<br>Requires external site care and routine flushing |
| **Implantable port** | Titanium, stainless steel, Silastic, or plastic portal attached to catheter<br>Single and double lumen<br>Access with noncoring needle<br>Low-profile ports available | Months to years | Excellent for long-term, intermittent infusional therapy<br>No site care required when not in use, so excellent for patients unable to perform site care<br>Surgical procedure required for removal |
| **Peripheral port** | Titanium portal attached to Silastic catheter<br>Single lumen<br>Access with noncoring 22-gauge needle | Months to years | Ideal for intermittent access, particularly for patients with active lifestyles or body image concerns<br>No external site care when not in use<br>Not ideal for blood draw due to small volume |

*Abbreviations*: CVC, central venous catheter; TPN, total parenteral nutrition; VAD, venous access device.

contrast material injector. PICCs are available as single-, double-, and triple-lumen devices. PICCs require weekly dressing changes. Clotting occurs frequently with CVADs. Long-term catheters are tunneled so that the risk of infection is reduced. Many oncology patients require complex treatment regimens and continuous infusions of vesicants or irritating drugs such as fluorouracil or have impaired venous access. As with other aspects of chemotherapy administration, education of both the nurse and the patient and family is essential when dealing with CVADs. The oncology nurse should be knowledgeable in all aspects of CVAD care. The nurse is urged to be familiar with the particular brands of devices, the manufacturers' recommendations, existing clinical practice trends, and the established policies and procedures of the employing institution.[1,8,88] Patient and family education is critical because many devices have self-care aspects that must be considered when selecting the CVAD. Many excellent booklets and videotapes have been developed by CVAD manufacturers and by hospitals and healthcare agencies, but their usefulness depends on the patient's ability to understand and comply with the actions described.[1,60]

## GENERAL MANAGEMENT

The selection, care, and maintenance of the long-term devices vary with the type of CVAD and will be addressed separately for nontunneled CVADs, tunneled CVCss, and implantable ports. Many of the major complications are handled in similar ways, so the management of complications will be addressed together for all the devices.

Most CVADs will be inserted such that the catheter tip ends in the superior vena cava, but rarely, for patients in whom this positioning is not possible, a femoral approach with the catheter tip in the upper part of the inferior vena cava may be an option.[55]

The smallest syringe to use when flushing a CVAD is a 10-mL syringe because this generates a small amount of pressure within the catheter. Smaller syringes generate higher pressure and may rupture the catheter.[8]

### Nontunneled central venous catheters

Short-term use of a nontunneled CVAD, such as a standard subclavian line, is common practice in urgent situations. When an immediate need for a central line arises, it commonly is placed by a physician at the bedside, in the intensive care unit, or in the emergency room. With advanced venous access planning, most patients with cancer will not require this type of line. Short-term CVADs are intended primarily to provide immediate access until the emergency can be resolved. The risk of infection is highest in the short-term percutaneous CVAD.[61] Dressing changes require scrupulous technique, incorporating hand hygiene, skin antisepsis with chlorhexidine gluconate, stabilization of the device to secure the line, and hub antisepsis.[89] The transparent sterile dressing over the catheter exit site is changed weekly or if nonocclusive; if the dressing is gauze, it is changed every 48 hours.[62,89] Observe the catheter insertion site for drainage, swelling, and erythema, and ask the patient if there is discomfort or pain at the site.[89]

The second type of a nontunneled CVAD is a PICC. From the patient's point of view, the PICC is the least expensive and most easily inserted intermediate- to long-term CVAD, but it requires self-care capabilities and often a caregiver because it is located at or near the antecubital fossa, and self-care has to be one-handed.[55] These small-gauge, thin-walled catheters are inserted into the basilic or cephalic vein (Figure 16-7). The procedure is performed by a physician or a specially trained nurse at the patient's bedside using ultrasound guidance.[8] PICCs are ideal for short-term access in patients with adequate antecubital veins, self-care capabilities, and the need for a wide variety of IV therapies.[8] Catheters that are 4F and larger in the internal lumen diameter are FDA approved for blood sampling and require an adequate saline flush (eg, 20 mL) following blood sampling to prevent the formation of a thrombus.[87] PICCs are now available as power-injectable PICCs, which means that the device can tolerate up to 300 psi of pressure, such as injected computerized tomography (CT) contrast dye. Thus the patient with a power PICC does not need a peripheral IV line started for the injection of IV contrast material for a radiological procedure.

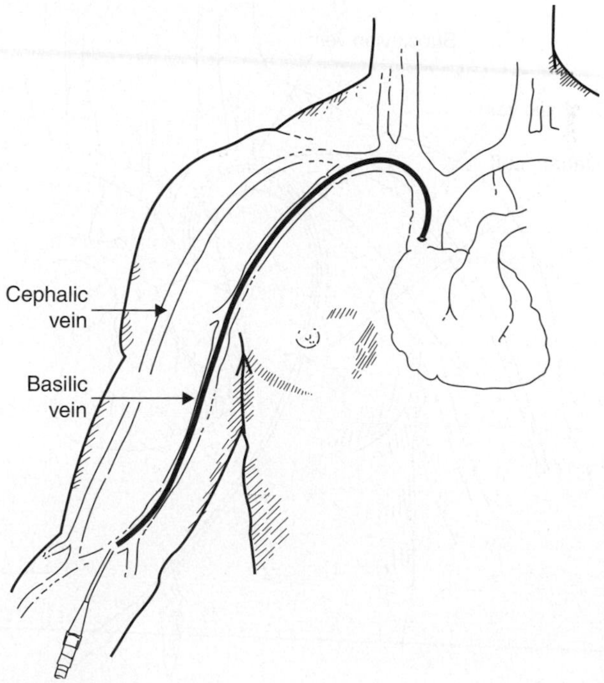


**FIGURE 16-7**

Placement of peripherally inserted central catheter (PICC).

### Tunneled central venous access devices

The tunneled CVAD (TCVADs) provides safe and reliable long-term access with a low incidence of infection, suitable for most all hematology/oncology patients.[55] The unique features of the TCVAD include a Dacron cuff around which granulation tissue forms, actually helping to hold the catheter in place, as well as reducing infection by preventing retrograde migration of bacteria.[55] The 4- to 10-inch tunnel through which the catheter is tunneled, along with the Dacron cuff that becomes overgrown with epithelial cells, serves to prevent easy passage of microorganisms from the skin along the catheter into the vein. For these reasons, tunneled catheters have been shown to have lower infection rates than the nontunneled catheters.[61] See Figure 16-8.The external portion of the TCVAD has a Luer-Loc hub (to allow direct access with an IV infusion set) or placement of an as-needed split-septum cap or valve to permit heparin locking of the device. Single-, double-, and triple-lumen TCVADs are available in various gauges and lengths.

One unique variation on the TCVAD is the Groshong catheter, which features a closed-end radiopaque tip. Flow through the catheter is achieved via a patented slit valve, which opens out into the bloodstream when fluid is infusing into the catheter, opens inward into the catheter lumen when blood is being withdrawn from the catheter, and remains closed when no pressure is being applied. Groshong catheter technology has been applied to the other VADs, and Groshong ports and PICCs are available, as well as the tunneled and nontunneled Groshong CVCs. This valved design prevents the need for regular heparinization of the catheter, which usually is flushed with sterile normal saline once a week when not in use, making it advantageous in patients for whom heparin is contraindicated.[88] Patient selection is a key issue with the TCVADs because they require regular care and maintenance. The patient or other caregiver must be willing and physically able to clean the exit site, flush the catheter, change the needleless connector (cap), and assess and report complications. The patient must have adequate insurance or be able to afford the equipment (ie, syringes, needleless connectors, heparin or saline, and dressing materials) and must have access to a clean area in the home in which to perform self-care. Body image and patient lifestyle can be issues because of the catheter exit through the chest wall, which can be distressing or embarrassing to some patients, particularly adolescents.[86] Also, whereas swimming in chlorinated pools is allowed by some practitioners, swimming in ponds, rivers, or the ocean usually is not recommended.[91]

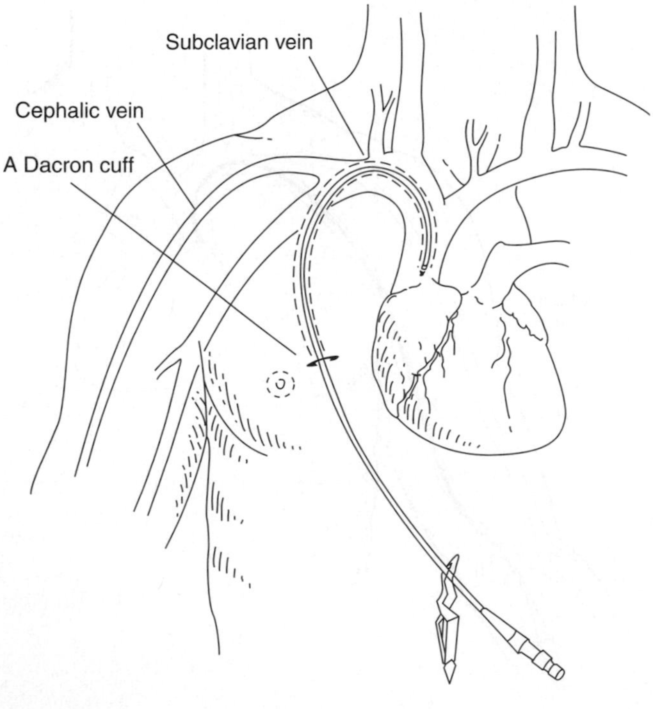


**FIGURE 16-8**

Tunneled central venous catheter placement.

The TCVAD offers several major advantages, including the elimination of needle sticks for people who have a needle phobia and the ease with which it is removed when it is no longer needed for care. It also allows for a great deal of flexibility in terms of use, being a preferred device for long-term total parenteral nutrition, vesicant infusion therapy, and continuous infusions. It also is the only long-term device that offers a triple-access option. Finally, the TCVAD is less expensive in terms of both device and insertion costs than an implantable port; however, it requires considerable more self-care activity, restrictions, and supplies. Moreover, an implanted port has a lower risk of infection with lower reported rates of catheter-related bloodstream infections[61] and allow less restricted bathing and swimming.[55]

Patients who undergo stem cell collection in preparation for high-dose chemotherapy and stem cell transplantation must have a tunneled apheresis line inserted.[92] The apheresis line has a large lumen, often 14 F, that permits pheresis of stem cells for collection in preparation for high-dose chemotherapy and stell cell rescue. The line is kept patent with heparin, although there are no clinical studies determining the correct concentration. Thus the nurse should follow the institution's policy and procedure. The heparin concentration may be as high as 1000 to 5000 units/mL times the dead space of the catheter, usually 2.3 to 2.4 mL. This heparin must be withdrawn and discarded prior to catheter use. Following use, the line is reinstilled with heparin.[8]

Insertion is not without risks, and complications include pneumothorax and arterial puncture.[93] Various techniques are used for placement, and experienced oncology nurses are beginning to work with physicians and patients prior to insertion to help select a site that is convenient when considering clothing and body contours. Adequate instruction of the patient and family both before and after placement is critical to a successful experience with a TCVAD. When developing policies and procedures governing use of TCVADs, it is recommended that the following aspects of care be included:[91,94]

- The TCVAD requires sterile site care with dressings until the formation of granulation tissue and verification of normal absolute neutrophil counts, at which time site care involves cleansing the chest wall and securing the catheter with tape to prevent dislodgment.
- When not in use, the catheter requires daily, every other day, or even weekly flushing with 3 to 5 mL of heparinized saline (10 units/mL).
- The TCVAD allows blood withdrawal for all laboratory tests that can be achieved via Vacutainer technique, if desired. The Vacutainer technique is preferred because it minimizes the risk of accidental needle sticks.
- Whenever blood has been aspirated into the catheter, it is flushed with 20 mL of saline prior to heparin locking or resuming an infusion.
- One must avoid intraluminal mixing of potentially incompatible drugs, which can be achieved by flushing with plain fluid between each drug.
- The patient must avoid scissors, sharp objects, and needles longer than 1 inch.
- Access is either direct or via an as-needed heparin-lock connector; all connections must use Luer-Locs.
- Continuous infusions should be connected directly to the catheter hub.

One unique care issue related to TCVADs is the possibility of fracture, puncture, or cutting of the external portion of the catheter. Puncture can be prevented by not using scissors or sharp objects near the catheter. It is also advisable to avoid clamping the catheter continuously or, if a clamp is used, padding and rotating the clamp site. As long as at least 2 inches of undamaged Silastic catheter exits the skin, it can be repaired using a repair kit available from the manufacturer. Most repair kits are designed only for a specific catheter, especially the double- and triple-lumen repair kits when the break occurs in the main portion of the catheter.

One major advantage of the TCVAD is the ease with which it is removed by the physician when it is no longer needed by the patient.[93] Prior to withdrawal of the catheter, some catheter manufacturers suggest a short surgical incision, under local anesthesia, to mechanically release the Dacron cuff from the subcutaneous tissue. If the cuff is not removed with the catheter, it may become infected later. Catheter removal is achieved by cleaning the exit site and manually pulling on the catheter until it loosens in the tunnel. Pressure then is applied manually over the entrance site into the vein and maintained for several minutes after catheter removal. Steady, slow pressure is applied while pulling on the catheter until the entire catheter is removed and inspected to ensure that it is intact because breakage or splintering can occur. A small dressing is applied to the exit site, if necessary.

### Implantable ports

For long-term intermittent use, implanted ports are the most widely used devices[55] and have the lowest incidence of infection.[61] The implantable port has proved to be a unique development in VADs because when it is not in use, it requires almost no care or maintenance. A *port* is a hollow housing of stainless steel, titanium, or plastic that contains a compressed latex septum over a portal chamber connected via a small catheter in the blood vessel. It is placed subcutaneously and accessed percutaneously using a special noncoring needle called a *Huber needle.* The needle has an offset bevel, which prevents coring the septum and allows 1000 to 2000 punctures per port depending on the manufacturer and needle size.[93] Ports must be implanted over a bony prominence, so they are placed most often over the bony area below the clavicle. It is imperative that the type of device and its purpose be determined prior to accessing the port. Less commonly, the port may be placed on the ribs and the catheter tunneled up to the subclavian vein. Finally, a small port can be placed on the forearm for use, with the catheter extending to the subclavian (PasPort). Most patients are given an identifying wallet card describing the date the port was implanted, the physician's name, and other information. Titanium ports are advantageous because they cause little, if any, disturbance on x-ray film during imaging procedures. Ports are available in single and double designs, with the double port having 2 distinct portal chambers to allow simultaneous administration of separate solutions.

Today, much like power-injectable PICCs, power-injectable ports are available. These allow injection of contrast material prior to CT testing because the catheter can withstand up to 300 psi of pressure; the Huber needle must be able to withstand that amount of pressure as well, so the nurse should confirm this prior to accessing the port.[95]

***Port routes.*** There are 5 major types of ports: venous, arterial, peritoneal, intrapleural, and epidural. The unique portal design allows access to more than just the vascular system. While the portal housings are all essentially the same, the catheter tip terminates in a different location. The patient should be given a card and information regarding his or her port. If that information is unavailable and the patient is unsure of the device type, then the healthcare professional must seek the operative note in the hospital chart to confirm device type and catheter route.

Nursing issues related to arterial, peritoneal, epidural, and intrapleural ports are summarized in Table 16-11 and are discussed in some detail in the earlier section of this chapter dealing with routes of drug administration.

*Port usage.* The routine care of a venous port when not being used is to flush it once every month with sterile heparinized saline (usually 5 mL of 100 units/mL solution). It is an ideal choice for patients who are receiving intermittent therapies, concerned about body image, physically active (especially if swimming in unchlorinated bodies of water), or have difficulty with self-care.[55] It also has the lowest incidence of infection of all the central lines.[60] Its major disadvantage is that it requires a needle to pass through the skin and into the port for use. The procedure of accessing the port could introduce infective organisms, cause a hematoma in a thrombocytopenic patient, cause anxiety in a patient with a needle phobia, or result in extravasation of fluid around the port if performed incorrectly, if the Huber needle is unsecured, or if the needle subsequently becomes dislodged. Nursing management of ports involves assessing the site and function of the device infusing or withdrawing fluids and flushing.

Port access usually is achieved under sterile or aseptic technique after a chlorhexidine scrub using a noncoring (Huber) needle that is bent at a 90-degree angle. The needle penetrates the septum and is advanced until it touches the bottom of the portal chamber, called the *needle stop.* The most popular access needles are actually infusion sets consisting of needle, tubing, and Luer-Loc hub and containing a Y-site and a clamp. A special power Huber needle must be used for a power port through which CT contrast material will be given.[95] These infusion sets allow great flexibility and can be left in place for as long as 7 days. For long-term access, a sterile dressing (usually transparent) is

**TABLE 16-11**

**Unique Types of Implantable Ports**

**Arterial**

- Used to administer continuous or intermittent intra-arterial chemotherapy.
- Catheter is placed into an artery, and port is usually placed on the lower rib cage.
- Accessed and managed in the usual manner, except heparinization procedure may be different, with increased frequency (ie, weekly) or higher concentrations of heparin (100 to 1000 units/mL).
- Catheter has a small lumen and seems to form clots more easily than venous catheters, hence the need for at least weekly flushing.

**Peritoneal**

- Used to administer intermittent intraperitoneal chemotherapy for ovarian or colon cancer.
- Catheter is placed in the peritoneal space, and port is usually placed on the lower rib cage but can be in the lower abdominal area.
- Accessed and managed in the usual sterile manner, except 19-gauge noncoring needles are used to facilitate large-volume infusions; the portal is flushed after use with sterile saline, and heparinization usually is not required.
- Catheter has a very large lumen with several ridges or cuffs to secure placement and multiple exit holes in the distal portion for rapid fluid infusion.

**Epidural**

- Used to administer intrathecal or epidural medications, including chemotherapy and analgesics.
- Catheter is placed into the intrathecal or epidural space and tunneled through a long subcutaneous passage from the spinal area to the side of the abdomen, where the port is placed on the lower rib cage or the abdominal area. The portal is designed with a 60 μm screen filter to remove particulate matter.
- Accessed using special 24-gauge noncoring needles, *always* with meticulous sterile technique, including sterile gloves, prep drape, and procedure tray.
- *Never to be flushed with heparin.*
- Preservative-free chemotherapy or morphine is instilled or infused into the port.
- After usage, 1 to 2 mL of sterile, preservative-free saline may be used to flush the line.
- Catheter has a small lumen (0.5-mm inner diameter), which is suitable for this type of drug delivery.

**Intrapleural**

- Used to drain pleural effusions periodically in patients who are unresponsive to sclerosing.
- Accessed with noncoring needle only.
- Patient's position is changed frequently during "tap."
- Flushed with 3 mL of saline.

placed over the site and assessed on a daily basis. Redness, rash, or blistering of the skin around the port could be indicative of an allergic reaction to the tape or dressing and is resolved by using an alternative type of tape, dressing, or skin-disinfecting agent.[8]

Several other aspects of port accessing are especially important to the patient. The area is tender and edematous for a week or so after implantation, causing manipulation of the device to be uncomfortable or even painful. When immediate use is indicated, the port should be accessed and dressed securely in the operating room. For routine use once the site is healed, the needle stick usually is not a concern to most patients and causes little discomfort. Occasionally, a patient will have a needle phobia or experience pain during insertion. An effective option is the application of an ice pack or a topical anesthetic cream (eg, ELA-Max) prior to needle access.[1,96]

*Peripheral implantable port.* A variation of the venous port is the peripherally inserted port. The PAS port (peripheral access system port) allows the peripheral insertion of a port near the antecubital fossa, along with tunneling, and the tip terminates in the lower portion of the superior vena cava.[97,98] The PAS port is about half the size of a regular port and allows patients to experience the advantages of port placement location (ie, unobtrusive long-term access and intermittent use) without having to expose the chest area to achieve access. Access is achieved through a short (½- to ¾-inch) noncoring Huber needle or infusion set. In all other aspects except placement, it is managed like other implantable venous ports.

## COMPLICATION MANAGEMENT

Occlusions, infections, and other complications can occur with all the long-term VADs. Nurses must know and assess for signs and symptoms of complications with VADs. The incidence and type of complication depend on the device, insertion technique, care regimen, and to a great extent, physiological factors inherent in the introduction of a long-term catheter into the venous system.[97,99]

### Infection

Biofilm is a bacterial film that is intended to protect the microorganisms. There are distinct stages of biofilm development: (1) initial microbial attachment to the catheter surface, (2) adhesion, growth, and grouping of cells into microcolonies, and (3) maturation and dissemination of new cells to form a new colony.[100] Microorganisms attach to the newly inserted catheter, some actually brought from the skin with the catheter as it is inserted into the vein, and they start excreting polymers that allow microbes to adhere, form a matrix, and actually change the genetic structure of the microbe.[100] This can happen within 12 minutes of catheters being introduced. Once a few microbes stick to the new catheter surface, they encourage other microbes to adhere and form a microcolony. The microbes mature and disseminate their offspring (progeny) to form new colonies.[101] The microbes are more resistant to antibiotics and host defenses because they are encased in biofilm.[100] *Staphylococcus, Candida,* and other microorganisms are well known for producing exopolysaccharide-rich slime that helps to form a microbial biofilm; other microorganisms can stick to this and survive on the surface of the catheter in the fast-moving bloodstream.[102] Circulating plasma proteins bind with biofilm, which helps to activate the coagulation cascade and complement system; this brings platelets and neutrophils, along with fibrin, to the catheter, where they also stick.[99] A fibrin sheath develops on the catheter and is made up of fibrin, neutrophils, and platelets. Clearly, biofilm is a large part of bloodstream infections related to CVADs.[99] A meta-analysis showed that CVADs impregnated with rifampicin and moncycline were effective in lowering the incidence of CVAD-associated bloodstream infections, along with cathteter microbial colonization.[103] This must be augmented by meticulous physician and nurse practice to prevent the introduction of microbes to the catheter.

The Institute for Healthcare Improvement (IHI) national campaign goal is to save 5 million lives, which includes patients who otherwise might die from a central line infection. One strategy is the "central line bundle."[102] Beginning in intensive-care units, where many short-term CVADs are used, this approach is now being applied to all CVADs and is aimed at eliminating primary catheter-related bloodstream infections. The central line bundle has 5 key components: hand hygiene, maximal barrier precautions, chlorhexidine skin antisepsis, optimal catheter-site selection (with the subclavian vein as the preferred site for nontunneled catheters), and daily review of line necessity and prompt removal of unnecessary lines.[101] In addition, as of October 2008, Medicare will no longer reimburse expenses related to central line bloodstream infections that began in the hospital.[105]

Long-term CVADs are designed to minimize the risk of infection compared with regular venous catheters, but infection still occurs in 2.7% to 60% of devices, and in the instance of long-term catheters, tunneled catheters with external hubs are more likely to develop infection (40%) than implanted subcutaneous devices, with an infection rate of 5% to 10%.[61,97] Catheter manufacturers have incorporated antibiotic formulations in their design to decrease the risk of infection, with a resulting reduction in infections and cost.[104] The widening influence of the central line bundle requiring close scrutiny and monitoring of sterility and compliance with infection control techniques during line insertion hopefully will translate into a decrease in infection rate.[101,107] Infections can occur locally (on the skin), in the catheter tunnel/port pocket, or systemically.[8] Infections are more common in patients with neutropenia (<500 granulocytes/mm$^3$), those with multilumen catheters, and those receiving total parenteral nutrition or chemotherapy. Neutropenia is an independent risk factor for catheter-related infections.[108,109] Local infections at the catheter exit site or over the skin around the port needle insertion site usually are caused by organisms on the skin, such as *Staphylococcus aureus* and *S. epidermidis.*[110] Symptoms can include redness, warmth, discomfort, and exudate.[1] Management includes culture of the area, increased frequency of dressing changes with meticulous site care, and administration of appropriate oral or IV antibiotics.[8] The needle should be removed from an implantable port if a skin infection occurs over the port, and it should not be reaccessed until the infection clears.[8]

Infections in the catheter tunnel or port pocket usually involve a variety of organisms and are manifested by redness, edema, tenderness or discomfort, exudate, skin warmth, and/or fever.[8] After cultures have been taken, including aspiration of any port-pocket exudate, appropriate IV antibiotic therapy is initiated. If the causative organism is identified and appropriate anti-infective therapy fails to resolve the infection, consideration should be given to removal of the device.[111]

Systemic infections can be thrombus related or caused by intraluminal catheter colonization with a wide variety of infective organisms.[99] Signs and symptoms include fever and chills. Blood cultures are taken through each lumen of the device as well as peripherally and can be positive either in the device only or via both routes.[112] Administration of appropriate antimicrobial therapy is initiated, and blood cultures are repeated. In addition, it may be useful to consider antibiotic lock therapy.[55] Failure to resolve the infection is cause to consider removal of the device.

Preventing infection is a primary concern when caring for all types of VADs. Attention should be focused on the techniques used in routine maintenance, and care should be taken to employ measures to minimize the risk of infection, such as decreasing catheter manipulations and ensuring aseptic handling of the hubs. In addition, use of a chlorhexidine-impregnated patch around the catheter and over the insertion site but under the transparent dressing provides continuous antisepsis to prevent the entry of microorganisms into the catheter and bloodstream and has shown a significant benefit in reducing catheter-related bloodstream infections [113]

## Occlusions

Common to all CVADs is a risk of catheter occlusions. The catheter is a foreign body, and when placed, the catheter is soon covered with plasma proteins and fibrin.[100] In addition, often the patient's malignancy is associated with hypercoaguability.[114] Within minutes, the fibrin begins to form a layer around the catheter. A fibrin tail or flap may form at the tip of the catheter, which allows outflow from the catheter, but when the nurse attempts to aspirate blood from the catheter, the fibrin tail is pulled back across the opening in the catheter tip. This is called *withdrawal occlusion.*[115] A fibrin sheath forms when the fibrin sticks to the outside of the catheter, coating it like a sock, and it may cover part or all of the catheter, including the opening of the catheter tip. A mural thrombus may form where the catheter touches and irritates the vein wall. Finally, an intraluminal thrombus forms when blood refluxes back into the catheter and attaches to the inner wall of the catheter due to improper flushing after blood sampling or after confirming a blood return or if the patient coughs.[99,116] Nurses should be vigilant and ensure that they are able to aspirate a blood return from a CVAD before administering any chemotherapy. If a blood return is not confirmed, the nurse should try repositioning the patient, and ask the patient to raise his or her arm or cough, and often this changes the intrathoracic pressure so that a blood return is achieved.[1] If not, if it is an implanted port, the Huber needle should be changed. If the nurse is still unable to aspirate a blood return, he or she should obtain an order for declotting the catheter. The line should be declotted with alteplase, a tissue plasminogen activator (tPA) (2 mg/2 mL).[95] If one attempt does not clear the line, a second instillation of alteplase can be tried. The dose of alteplase is small, and side effects are rare.[95] An occluded line can be declotted similarly.

If the line does not clear after the 2-hour dwell time of the second attempt or a blood return is not achieved, the patient should have the catheter evaluated with a flow or dye study.[59] In an attempt to prevent catheter thrombus formation, the use of low-dose warfarin has been studied. Unfortunately, a meta-analysis done by Rawson and Newburn-Cook showed that there is no apparent benefit to this practice.[114]

*Intraluminal catheter occlusion.* The complete inability to withdraw blood or infuse fluid in a VAD is most commonly the result of a blood clot within the catheter. It also can be caused by incompatible drugs or lipids that have crystallized or precipitated and have obstructed the catheter. The nurse is instrumental in assessing the catheter and its most recent usage to determine which of these causes are most likely to have occurred. Blood clots can build up over time (ie, sluggish catheter) but also can appear suddenly. Drug precipitates tend to be more directly related to a recent infusion and are seen more often with total parenteral nutrition (TPN) and lipids.[117] Measures to prevent either occurrence include the following:[1,8,89–90]

- Maintain neutral or positive pressure within the catheter, and vigorously flush the catheter, provided that no resistance is encountered. Use a push-pause motion. Intermittent resistance may mean that the catheter is

being pinched off at the level of the clavicle and first rib. Vigorously flushing in this situation can cause an aneurysm in the catheter.
- Advise the patient to avoid excessive manipulation (ie, pinching or bending) of external catheters.
- Vigorously flush with at least 20 mL of sterile normal saline after any blood is withdrawn (sampling or to check for a blood return) or infused into the catheter. This helps to prevent sludge buildup within the port.
- Document each patient's VAD experience, and discuss any changes in the care plan with the physician or advanced practice nurse. Question the patient and family regarding actual catheter maintenance activities to assess compliance with recommended care and usage.
- Flush between each drug with at least 10 mL of normal saline fluid to avoid incompatible drug admixture.
- Use correct and effective catheter flushing technique depending on the type of needleless device used. (*Negative fluid displacement devices* allow retrograde backflow of blood into the catheter, so use positive pressure to withdraw the blunt cannula while still pushing down the plunger of the flush solution or clamp the catheter at the same time. *Positive fluid displacement devices* prevent the backflow of blood into the catheter, so they do not require the positive-pressure technique. *Neutral displacement devices* can use any flush technique).

In the case of ports, the inability to infuse or aspirate typically is due to the needle being improperly placed in the septum rather than in the port. Advancing the needle into the port usually will solve the problem.[1,8] Also, if the patient has a low-profile port, the septum is not very deep, and a 1-inch Huber-point needle will result in a portion of the needle tip being occluded in the septum. When the patient has a low-profile port, a ½-inch, ¾-inch or 22-gauge Huber needle will clear the septum and function properly. Management of an occluded catheter when a blood clot is suspected involves the instillation of alteplase.[95] Certain drug precipitates can be cleared using 0.1 N hydrochloric acid for some crystals or ethanol 70% for lipid deposits.[117] Gently instill 0.2 to 1.0 mL of drug. After a dwell time of 30 to 60 minutes, an attempt is made to aspirate the catheter contents. If TPN is not involved and a specific drug is known or suspected, a pharmacist should be consulted about possible agents that might dissolve the precipitate and enable it to be aspirated from the catheter. Figure 16-9 describes a possible decision-making matrix to consider when dealing with a completely occluded catheter.

***Extraluminal catheter occlusion.*** Catheter sluggishness or partial occlusion can be due to two extraluminal phenomena: fibrin sheath formation and thrombosis. The catheter position also can affect flow, so a partial occlusion, in the absence of pain or discomfort, should be managed first by instructing the patient to change positions, raise the arms, breathe deeply, and/or cough (Figure 16-10). Each of these activities might release the open lumen of the catheter from the vein wall and allow easy flushing and blood withdrawal. If a withdrawal occlusion exists (flushes easily but backflow is sluggish or nonexistent), fibrin sheath formation or thrombosis should be considered. Fibrin sheaths can form at the catheter insertion site and float, like a sleeve, around the outside of the catheter. If the sheath extends beyond the lumen, it can cause withdrawal occlusions. Lysis of the sheath may be achieved by instilling alteplase 2 mg/2 mL into the catheter and allowing it to dwell for 2 hours or longer depending on the extent of the sheath.[93]

Venous thrombosis can be caused by a number of factors, including endothelial injury, hypercoagulability, multiple catheters, catheter stiffness (ie, polyvinyl chloride), catheter size (ie, larger bore), and catheter placement (ie, left side or in a smaller vein). The incidence of catheter thrombosis with clinical symptoms appears only to be as high as 10%.[99] Signs and symptoms are related to impaired blood flow and include edema of the neck, face, shoulder, or arm; prominent superficial veins; neck pain; tingling of the neck, shoulder, or arm; and skin color or temperature changes. A variety of radiographic studies can be used to diagnose and define the extent of the thrombosis accurately, including venogram and ultrasound.[97] Management of venous thrombosis usually involves anticoagulants or thrombolytic agents.

### Other complications

Occlusions and device malfunctions can occur for a variety of other reasons, and careful assessment of the device when occlusion occurs always should include consideration of malpositioning or breakage. Catheters can be kinked, compressed by tumor, compressed between the rib and clavicle (pinch-off sign), malpositioned due to patient manipulation (twiddler's syndrome), malpositioned for other reasons, severed, punctured, split, or separated.[55,60,118] The port access needle can be embedded in the septum, be placed inaccurately into the side of the port or catheter instead of the portal housing, or become dislodged from the port and remain under the skin.[60]

Thrombus formation can result in a retrograde flow of blood or fluid along the catheter tract with subsequent extravasation into the subcutaneous tissues.[55] Infusion of drugs into a severed, punctured, or separated catheter also can result in extravasation. Prevention of vesicant extravasation is discussed elsewhere in this chapter, but it is prudent to reiterate that all CVADs should be patent and functioning appropriately before initiating vesicant therapy.[59,119] Extravasation of vesicants into the chest wall or thorax can result in severe deformity, loss of function, or death.[119]

Manufacturers are continually developing new CVAD designs with innovative features. Oncology nurses frequently

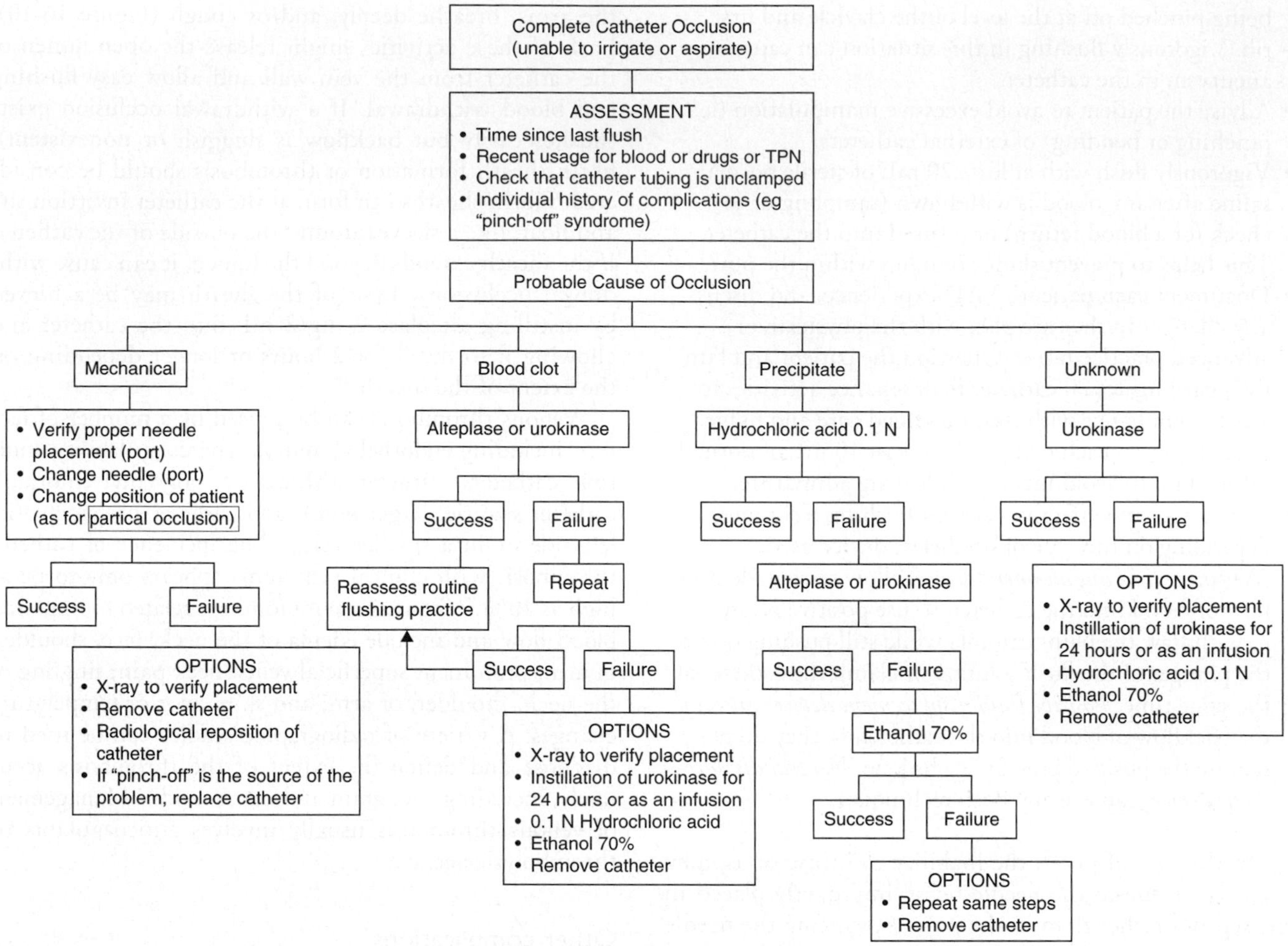


AQ: Is this partial occlusion?

**FIGURE 16-9**

Managing complete catheter occlusion.

*Abbreviation*: TPN, total parenteral nutrition.

review these new devices and are called on to evaluate their effectiveness. Cost containment is a growing concern, and the best price usually can be achieved if all the devices selected come from a limited number of vendors, thus consolidating buying power.[55] It is imperative that oncology nurses embrace the IHI's efforts to reduce bloodstream infections to zero and also act as gatekeepers and protectors of their patients' CVADs. Nurses should carefully document any issues that arise in using CVADs, whether a blood return was confirmed and if not, what was done to resolve the issue, and work to keep the device functioning effectively.

## REPORTING DEFECTS

The Safe Medical Devices Act of 1995 requires health-care facilities and manufacturers to report device-related events that did cause or could have caused serious injury or death. The MEDWatch system, enforced through the FDA, makes the reporting process simple and confidential. Forms can be obtained by calling 800-FDA-1088.[120]

## CONCLUSION

Cancer chemotherapy administration is a rapidly evolving area of oncology nursing practice that offers exciting opportunities for both beginning and seasoned oncology nurses. The level of responsibility for monitoring patients receiving chemotherapy and managing many aspects of their care continues to increase. Expanded outpatient and home-care settings, where the majority of chemotherapy is given, offer opportunities for triage assessment and nursing intervention at an increasingly autonomous level. Adherence to oral chemotherapy regimens will challenge the oncology nurse to design and individualize strategies to meet the needs of patients who have different social and economic backgrounds.[121] The technical explosions in drug-delivery systems

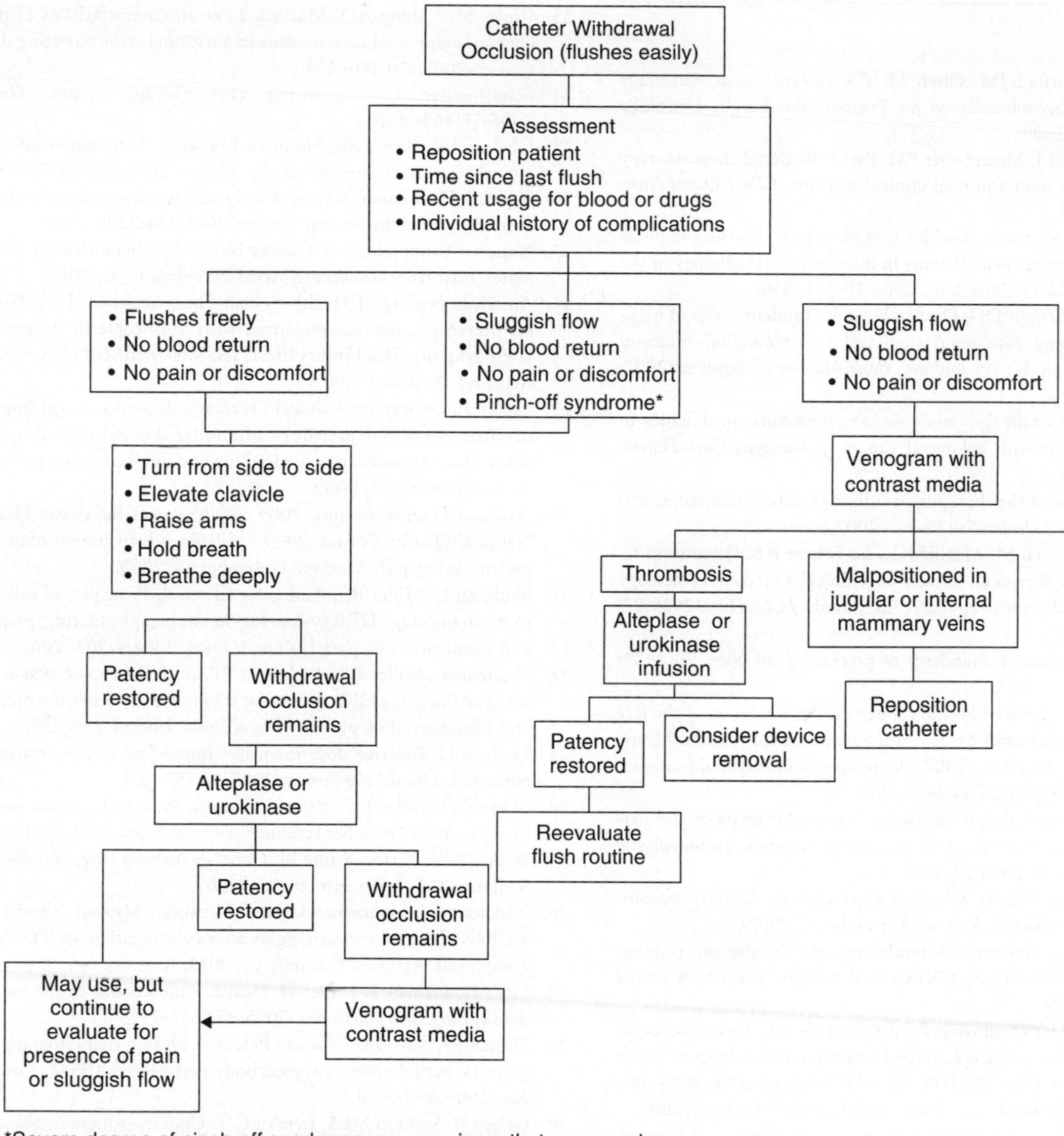


**FIGURE 16-10**

Managing catheter withdrawl occlusion.

pose a constant informational challenge, as does the process of maintaining the personal and rewarding relationships with patients for whom these advanced technologies are used.

Health care will continue to move toward more ambulatory and home care, with hospitals becoming settings where patients receiving complex regimens will receive their chemotherapy. Reimbursement, lobbying, litigation, and legislation will continue to be issues of concern in the 21st century. The oncology nurse can play a vital role in establishing effective policies and procedures by serving on institutional practice or policy committees. An oncology clinical practice committee with responsibility for reviewing and recommending procedures also can serve to evaluate new technologies. The ONS has established standards for ensuring knowledge competency and then made recommendations, as has INS, to ensure that clinical competency is determined and maintained.[1,8] While standards in ambulatory and physician office practices have been studied less intensively in the past, now standards jointly presented by the ASCO and the ONS have been advanced.[7] Patient care evaluation and quality improvement are key responsibilities recognized by The Joint Commission, which initiated clinical indicators for oncology to more closely monitor quality in the healthcare setting.

## REFERENCES


1. Polovich M, Whitford JM, Olsen M. *Chemotherapy and Biotherapy Guidelines and Recommendations for Practice.* Pittsburgh: Oncology Nursing Society; 2009.
2. Seidel GD, Locklin J, Muehlbauer PM. Part I: Regional chemotherapy clinical studies in nontraditional clinical settings. *Clin J Oncol Nurs.* 2006;10:338–344.
3. Muehlbauer PM, Klapec K, Locklin J, et al. Part II: Nursing implications of administering chemotherapy in interventional radiology or the operating room. *Clin J Oncol Nurs.* 2006;10:345–356.
4. Sanchorawala V, Wright DG, Quillen K, et al. Tandem cycles of high-dose melphalan and autologous stem cell transplantation increases the response rate in AL amyloidosis. *Bone Marrow Transplant.* 2007; 40:557–562.
5. Kaa K. Medicare challenges and solutions: reimbursement issues in treating the patient with colorectal cancer. *J Managed Care Pharm.* 2007;13:S19–S26.
6. Aisner J. Overview of the changing paradigm in cancer treatment: oral chemotherapy *Am J Health-Syst Pharm.* 2007;64:S4–S7.
7. Jacobson JO, Polovich M, McNiff KK, Le Febvre KB, Cummings C, Galioto M, et al. American Society of Clinical Oncology/Oncology Nursing Society Chemotherapy Safety Standards. *J Clin Oncol* 2009;27: 5469–5475.
8. Infusion Nurses' Society. Standards of practice. *J Inf Nurs.* 2006;29: S69–S70.
9. Oncology Nursing Society. Position statement on education of the RN who administers and cares for the individual receiving chemotherapy and biotherapy, October 2007. http://www.ons.org/Publications/Positions/RNed. Accessed October 1, 2009.
10. American Society of Clinical Oncology. Criteria for facilities and personnel for the administration of parenteral systemic antineoplastic therapy. *J Clin Oncol.* 2004;22:4613–4615.
11. Oncology Nursing Society. Chemotherapy courses. http://www.ons.org/CNECentral/Chemo, Accessed December 17, 2009.
12. Oncology Nursing Society. Chemotherapy and biotherapy training courses. http://www.ons.org/CNECentral/Chemo/Trainer, Accessed December 17, 2009.
13. National Institute for Occupational Safety and Health. Preventing occupational exposures to antineoplastic and other hazardous drugs in health care settings. NIOSH Alert, DHHS (NIOSH) Publication No. 2004–165. http://www.cdc.gov/niosh/docs/2004–165. Accessed October 1, 2009.
14. Occupational Safety and Health Administration. Technical manual, Section VI, Chapter 2. http://www.osha.gov/dts/osta/otm/otm_vi/otm_vi_2.html. Accessed October 1, 2009.
15. Polovich M, ed. *Oncology Nursing Society Safe Handling of Hazardous Drugs.* Pittsburgh: Oncology Nursing Society; 2003.
16. American Society of Health-System Pharmacists (ASHP) Guidelines on handling hazardous drugs. http://www.ashp.org/s_ashp/docs/files/BP07/Prep_Gdl_HazDrugs.pdf. Accessed October 1, 2009.
17. Martin S, Larson E. Chemotherapy handling practices of outpatient and office-based oncology nurses. *Oncol Nurs Forum.* 2003;30:575–581.
18. Gambrell J, Moore S. Assessing workplace compliance with handling of antineoplastic agents. *Clin J Oncol Nurs,* 2006;10:473–477.
19. Hedmer M, Georgiadi A, Bremberg ER, et al. Surface contamination of cyclophosphamide packaging and surface contamination with antineoplastic drugs in a hospital pharmacy in Sweden. *Ann Occup Hyg.* 2005;49:629–637.
20. Rankin SH, Stallings KD, London F. *Patient Education in Health and Illness.* 5th ed. Philadelphia, PA: Lippincott Williams & Wilkins; 2005:192–193.
21. Yarbro CH, Frogge MH, Goodman M, eds. *Cancer Symptom Management.* 3rd ed. Sudbury, MA: Jones and Bartlett; 2004.
22. Joint Commission on Hospital Accreditation. Hospitals' national patient safety goals. http://www.jointcommission.org/PatientSafety/NationalPatientSafetyGoals/06_npsg_cah.htm. Accessed October 1, 2009.
23. Rinke ML, Shore AD, Morlock L, et al. Characteristics of pediatric chemotherapy medication errors in a national error reporting database. *Cancer.* 2007;110:186–195.
24. Schulmeister L. Preventing chemotherapy errors. *Oncologist.* 2006;11:463–468.
25. Ghandi TK, Bartel SB, Shulman LN, et al. Medication safety in the ambulatory chemotherapy setting. *Cancer.* 2005;104:2477–2483.
26. Nebeker JR, Bennett CL. Reducing adverse drug events in the outpatient chemotherapy setting. *Cancer.* 2005;104:2289–2291.
27. National Comprehensive Cancer Network. Chemotherapy order templates. http://www.nccn.org. Accessed February 21, 2010.
28. American Society of Health-System Pharmacists (ASHP). Guidelines on preventing medication errors with antineoplastic agents. http://www.ashp.org/DocLibrary/BestPractices/MedMisGdlAntineo.aspx. Accessed October 1, 2009.
29. American Society for Clinical Oncology. Statement regarding the use of outside services to prepare or administer chemotherapy drugs. http://www.Asco.org/asco/downloads/OutsourcingChemotherapyDrugs.pdf. Accessed October 1, 2009.
30. National Quality Forum. 2009 Safe Practices for Better Healthcare, National Quality Forum, 2009.Available at http://www.hfap.org/pdf/patient_safety.pdf. Accessed December 16, 2009.
31. Shulman L, Miller RS, Ambinder EP, et al. Principles of safe practive using an oncology HER system for chemotherapy ordering, preparation, and administration, part 1. *J Oncol Pract.* 2008;4:203–206.
32. Shulman L, Miller RS, Ambinder EP, et al. Principles of safe practive using an oncology HER system for chemotherapy ordering, preparation, and administration, part 2. *J Oncol Pract.* 2008;4:254–257.
33. Lenhart C. Relative dose intensity: improving cancer treatment and outcomes. *Oncol Nurs Forum.* 2005;32:757–764.
34. Storm C, Casillas J, Grunwald H, et al. Informed consent for chemotherapy: ASCO member resources. *J Oncol Pract.* 2008;4:289–295.
35. Wilkes GM, Barton-Burke M. *Oncology Nursing Drug Handbook 2009.* Sudbury, MA: Jones and Bartlett; 2009.
36. National Comprehensive Cancer Network. Myeloid growth factors, V1.2009. http://www.nccn.org/professionals/physician_gls/PDF/myeloid_growth.pdf. Accessed February 21, 2010.
37. Li Z, Bowerman S, Heber D. Health ramifications of the obesity epidemic. *Surg Clin North Am.* 2005;85:1531–1543.
38. Hunter RJ, Navo MA, Thaker PH, et al. Dosing chemotherapy in obese patients: actual versus assigned body surface area (BSA). *Cancer Treat Rev.* 2009;35:69–78.
39. Griggs JJ, Sorbero MES, Lyman GH. Undertreatment of obese women receiving breast cancer chemotherapy. *Arch Intern Med.* 2005;165: 1267–1273.
40. Hayden BK, Goodman M. Chemotherapy: principles of administration. In Yarbro CH, Frogge MH, Goodman M, eds. *Cancer Nursing: Principles and Practice,* 6th ed. Sudbury, MA: Jones and Bartlett Publishers, 2005:351–411.
41. Folprecht G, Seymour MT, Saltz L, et al. Irinotecan/fluorouracil combination in first line therapy of older and younger patients with metastatic colorectal cancer: combined analysis of 2,691 patients in randomized controlled trials. *J Clin Oncol.* 2008;26:1443–1451.
42. Burdette-Radoux S, Muss HB. Adjuvant chemotherapy in the elderly: whom to treat and what regimen? *Oncologist.* 2006;11:234–242.
43. Teshima D, Maiguma T, Kaji H, et al. Estimation of the area under the curve for mycophenolic acid in adult renal transplant patients with concomitant tacrolimus using a limited sampling strategy. *J Clin Pharm Ther.* 2008;33:159–163.
44. O'Cearbhaill R, Barry A, Griffin M, et al. Evaluation of carboplatin dosage based on a body surface area adjusted four-variable modification of diet in renal disease (MDRD) equation [abstract 13524]. *J Clin Oncol.* 2008;26, Available at http://www.asco.org/ASCOv2/Meetings/Abstracts?&vmview=abst_detail_view&confID=55&abstractID=35689, Accessed December 16, 2009.
45. Jones RL, Karavasilis V, Kaye SB. Paclitaxel in the management of ovarian cancer. *Exp Rev Obstet Gynecol.* 2008;3:287–299.

46. Bristol Myers Squibb Oncology. Taxol package insert. Princeton, NJ: Bristol Myers Squibb, July 2007.
47. Weingart SN, Flug J, Brouillard D, et al. Oral chemotherapy safety practices at US cancer centers: questionnaire survey. *Br Med J.* 2007;334:407.
48. Bartel S. Safe practices and financial considerations in using oral chemotherapeutic agents. *Am J Health-Syst Pharm.* 2007;64:S8–S15.
49. Polovich M. Developing a hazardous drug safe-handling program. *Comm Oncol.* 2005;2:403–405.
50. Moore S. Facilitating oral chemotherapy treatment and compliance through patient/family-focused education. *Cancer Nurs.* 2007;30:112–122.
51. Joint Commission. National patient safety goals: Medication reconciliation in ambulatory oncology. *Joint Commission J Quality Patient Saf.* 2007;33:750–757.
52. Boyle D, Bubalo J. Enhancing patient adherence to improve outcomes with oral chemotherapy. *US Pharm.* 2007;32:1–8.
53. Walsh KE, Dodd KS, Seetharaman K, et al. Medication errors among adults and children with cancer in an outpatient setting. *J Clin Oncol.* 2009;27:891–896.
54. Hawkins DS, Taylor J, Winter L, Geyer L. Oral outpatient chemotherapy medication errors in children with acute lymphoblastic leukemia. *J Clin Oncol.* 2006;24:S9028.
55. Gallieni M, Pittiruti M, Biffi R. Vascular access in oncology patients. *Ca: Cancer J Clin.* 2008;58:323–346.
56. Sauerland C, Engelking C, Wickham R, Corbi D. Vesicant extravasation: I. Mechanisms, pathogenesis, and nursing care to reduce risk. *Oncol Nurs Forum.* 2006;33(6):1134–1141.
57. Bristol Myers Squibb Oncology. Carmustine package insert. Princeton, NJ: Bristol Myers Squibb, June 1998.
58. O'Donnell J, Carpenter LA, Gopi DA. *Drug Injury: Liability, Analysis, Prevention.* Tucson, AZ: Lawyers & Judges Publishing Co.; 2005:185.
59. Schulmeister L. Managing vesicant extravasations. *Oncologist.* 2008;13:284–288.
60. Arch P. Port navigation: let the journey begin. *Clin J Oncol Nurs.* 2007;11:485–488.
61. Maki DG, Kluger DM, Crnich CJ. The risk of bloodstream infection in adults with different intravascular devices: a systematic review of 200 published prospective studies. *Mayo Clin Proc.* 2006;81: 1159–1171.
62. Centers for Disease Control and Prevention. Guidelines for prevention of intravascular and catheter related infections. *MMWR.* 2002;51:1–29.
63. Schulmeister L. Extravasation management. *Semin Oncol Nurs.* 2007; 23(3):185.
64. Tshikawa T, Kamimura H, Tsuchiya A, et al. Clinical efficacy of intra-arterial pharmacokinetic chemotherapy with 5-fluorouracil, CDDP, gemcitabine, and angiotensin-II in patients with advanced pancreatic cancer. *Hepatogastroenterology.* 2007;54:2378–2382.
65. Ensminger W. Intra-arterial chemotherapy. In: Perry MC, ed. *Chemotherapy Source Book.* Philadelphia, PA: Lippincott Williams & Wilkins; 2007:88–89.
66. Bertino JR. Implantable pump for long-term chemotherapy administration via the hepatic artery: has it fulfilled its promise? *J Clin Oncol.* 2008;26:4528–4529.
67. Matthews E, Snell K, Coats H. Intra-arterial chemotherapy for limb preservation in patients with osteosarcoma: nursing implications. *Clin J Oncol Nurs.* 2006;10:581–589.
68. Cahill BA. Management of patients who have undergone hepatic artery chemoembolization. *Clin J Oncol Nurs.* 2005;9:69–75.
69. Marin K, Oleszewski K, Muehlbauer P. Intraperitoneal chemotherapy: implications beyond ovarian cancer. *Clin J Oncol Nurs.* 2008;11:881–889.
70. Armstrong DK, Bundy B, Wenzel L, et al. Intraperitoneal cisplatin and paclitaxel in ovarian cancer *N Engl J Med.* 2006;354:34–43.
71. Jaaback K, Johnson N. Intraperitoneal chemotherapy for the initial management of primary epithelial ovarian cancer. *Cochrane Database Syst Rev.* 2006;1:CD005340.
72. Markman M, Walker JL. Intraperitoneal chemotherapy of ovarian cancer: a review, with a focus on practical aspects of treatment. *J Clin Oncol.* 2006;24:1–6.
73. Markman M. Intraperitoneal chemotherapy in the management of ovarian cancer: focus on carboplatin. *Ther Clin Risk Manage.* 2009;5:161–168.
74. Potter KL, Held-Warmkessel J. Intraperitoneal chemotherapy for women with ovarian cancer: nursing care and considerations. *Clin J Oncol Nurs.* 2008;12:265–271.
75. Almadrones L. Evidence-based research for intraperitoneal chemotherapy in epithelial ovarian cancer. *Clin J Oncol Nurs.* 2007;11: 211–216.
76. Hydzik C. Implementation of intraperitoneal chemotherapy for the treatment of ovarian cancer. *Clin J Oncol Nurs.* 2007;11:221–225.
77. Covey AM. Management of malignant pleural effusions and ascites. *Support Oncol.* 2005;3:169–176.
78. Shuey K, Payne Y. Malignant pleural effusions. *Clin J Oncol Nurs.* 2005;9:529–532.
79. Warren W. Talc pleurodesis for malignant pleural effusions is preferred over the Pleuryx catheter (contrary). *Ann Surg Oncol.* 2007;14: 2700–2701.
80. Skinner E. Will a new intravesicular chemotherapy agent improve the treatment of non-muscle-invasive bladder cancer? *Nat Clin Pract Urol.* 2007;4:248–249.
81. McDougal WS, Shipley WU, Kaufman DS, et al. Cancer of the bladder, ureter, and renal pelvis. In: DeVita VT, Lawrence TS, Rosenberg SA, eds. *Cancer Principles and Practice.* 8th ed. Philadelphia, PA: Lippincott Williams & Wilkins; 2008:1358–1385.
82. Washburn DJ. Intravesical antineoplastic therapy following transurethral resection of bladder tumors: nursing implications from the operating room to discharge. *Clin J Oncol Nurs.* 2007;11:553–559.
83. Aiello-Laws L, Rutledge DN. Management of adult patients receiving intraventricular chemotherapy for the treatment of leptomeningeal metastasis. *Clin J Oncol Nurs.* 2008;12:429–435.
84. Pande AR, Ando K, Ishikura R, et al. Disseminated necrotizing leukoencephalopathy following chemoradiation therapy for acute lymphoblastic leukemia. *Radiat Med.* 2006;24:515–519.
85. FDA. Package insert Leucovorin calcium. Available at http://www.bedfordlabs.com/BedfordLabsWeb/products/inserts/LCV-P02.pdf , Accessed December 17, 2009.
86. Parker SRS, Bradley B. Treatment of cutaneous T-cell lymphoma, mycoses fungoides. *Dermatol Nurs.* 2006;18:566–575.
87. Snipes CJ, Sniezek PJ, Walling HW. Basal cell carcinoma responding to systemic 5-fluorouracil. *J Am Acad Dermatol.* 2006;54:1104–1106.
88. Central Venous Access Device Guideline Panel, Cancer Care Ontario. Managing central venius access devices in cancer patients: a clinical practice guideline. Evidence-based series 16–1. http://www.guidelines.gov/summary/summary.aspx?ss=15&doc_id=10160&nbr=5346. Accessed October 1, 2009.
89. Hadaway LC. Central venous access devices. *Nursing.* 2008;38: 34–40.
90. Bard Access Systems. Groshong instructions for use. Salt Lake City, UT: Bard Access Systems, 2002.
91. National Institutes of Health, Patient Information Publications. Managing your tunneled catheter. NIH Warren Grant Magnuson Clinical Center, 2003. http://www.cc.nih.gov/ccc/patient_education/pepubs/hickman.pdf. Accessed October 1, 2009.
92. Rosenthal K. Apheresis catheters: separation superstars. *Nursing Made Incredibly Easy.* 2007;5:11–14.
93. Bishop L, Dougherty L, Bodenham A, et al. Guidelines on the insertion and management of central venous access devices in adults. *Int J Lab Hematol.* 2007;29:261–278.
94. Reed WP, Newman KA, de Jongh C, et al. Prolonged venous access for chemotherapy by means of the hickman catheter. *Cancer.* 2006;52:185–192.
95. Smith LH. Implanted ports, computed tomography, power injectors and catheter rupture. *Clin J Oncol Nurs.* 2008;12:809–812.
96. Namyslowski J. Locoregional pain control: local anesthetics. In: Ray CE Jr, ed. *Pain Control and Interventional Radiology.* New York, NY: Cambridge University Press; 2008:25.

97. Pingpank JF. Vascular access and specialized techniques. In DeVita VT, Lawrence TS, Rosenberg SA, eds. *Cancer Principles and Practice.* 8th ed. Philadelphia: Lippincott Williams and Wilkins; 2008:693–701.
98. Smiths Medical. PasPort peripheral access system. http://www.smiths-medical.com/catalog/implantable-ports/p-s-port-elite.html. Accessed October 1, 2009.
99. Rosovsky RP, Kuter DJ. Catheter related thrombosis in cancer patients: pathophysiology, diagnosis, and management. *Hematol/Oncol Clin North Am.* 2005;19:183–202.
100. Ryder MA. Catheter related infections: its all about biofilm. *Topics Adv Pract Nurs eJournal.* 2005;5. http://www.medscape.com/viewarticle/508109_3. Accessed March 14, 2009.
101. Brungs SM, Render MI. Using evidence based practice to reduce central line infections. *Clin J Oncol Nurs.* 2006;10:723–725.
102. Boersma RS, Jie K-SG, Verbon A, et al. Thromotic and infectious complications of central venous catheters in patients with hematologic malignancies. *Ann Oncol.* 2008;19:433–442.
103. Falagas ME, Fragoulis K, Bliziotis IA, Chatzinikolaou I. Rifampin-impregnated central venous catheters: a meta-analysis of randomized, controlled trials. *J Antimicrob Chemother.* 2007;59:359–369.
104. Institute for Healthcare Improvement. The central line bundle. http://www.ihi.org/IHI/Topics/CriticalCare/IntensiveCare/Changes/ImplementtheCentralLineBundle.htm. Accessed October 1, 2009.
105. Department of Health and Human Services. Medicare program: changes to hospital inpatient prospective payment systems and fiscal year 2008 rates. http://www.cms.hhs.gov/AcuteInpatientPPS/downloads/CMS-1533-FC.pdf. Accessed October 1, 2009.
106. Hockenhull JC, Dwan K, Boland A, et al. The clinical effectiveness and cost-effectiveness of central venous catheters treated with anti-infective agents in preventing bloodstream infections: a systematic review and economic evaluation. *Health Technol Assess.* 2008;12:1–154.
107. Marschall J, Mermel LA, Classen D, et al. Strategies to prevent central line-associated bloodstream infections in acute care hospitals. *Infect Control Hosp Epidemiol.* 2008;29:S22–S30.
108. Howell PB, Walters PE, Donowitz GR, et al. Risk factors for infection of adult patients with cancer who have tunneled central venous catheters. *Cancer.* 2006;75:1367–1375.
109. Eagan J. Infections in the ICU. In: Kaplow R, Hardin SR, eds. *Critical Care Nursing: Synergy for Optimal Outcomes.* Sudbury, MA: Jones and Bartlett; 2007:70–71.
110. Pagani JL, Eggimann P. Management of catheter related infection. *Exp Rev Anti-infect Ther.* 2008;6:31–37.
111. Povoski SP. Long term venous access. In: Pazdur R, Coia LR, Hoskins WJ, Wagman LD, eds. *Cancer Management: A Multidisciplinary Approach.* 10th ed. Cancernetwork.com. http://www.cancernetwork.com/cancer-management/chapter43/article/10165/1243750. Accessed March 15, 2009.
112. Safdar N, Fine JP, Maki DG. Meta-analysis: methods for diagnosing intravascular device related bloodstream infection. *Ann Intern Med.* 2005;142:451–466.
113. Ho KM, Litton E. Use of chlorhexidine-impregnated dressing to prevent vascular and epidural catheter colonization and infection: a meta-analysis. *J Antimicrob Chemother.* 2006;58:281–287.
114. Rawson KM, Newburn-Cook CV. The use of low-dose warfarin as prophylaxis for central venous catheter thrombosis in patients with cancer: a meta-analysis. *Clin J Oncol Nurs.* 2007;34:1037–1043.
115. Horne MK, McCloskey DJ, Calis K, et al. Use of heparin versus lepirudin flushes to prevent withdrawal occlusion of central venous access devices. *Pharmacotherapy.* 2006;26:1262–1267.
116. Dougherty L. *Central Venous Access Devices: Care and Management.* Oxford, England: Blackwell Publishing; 2006.
117. Gupta S, Steiger E, Sands M. Vascular access for the patient receiving parenteral nutrition. In: Buchman AL, ed. *Clinical Nutrition in Gastrointestinal Disease.* Thorofare, NJ: SLACK, Inc.; 2006:414–420.
118. Forauer AR, Chen Y, Parks R. A case of posttraumatic Twidler's syndrome. *J Vasc Intervent Radiol.* 2005;16:562–563.
119. Wickham R, Engleking C, Corbi D, Sauerland C. Vesicant extravasations: II. Evidence based management and continuing controversies. *Oncol Nurs Forum.* 2006;33:1143–1150.
120. MedWatch. http://www.fda.gov/medwAtch/feedback.htm. Accessed March 15, 2009.
121. Wilson M. Readability and patient education materials used for low-income populations. *J Adv Pract Nurs.* 2009;23:33–40.

## APPENDIX 16A

**Oral Chemotherapy and Hormonal Agents**

| Drug and Disease Indications | Dose and Schedule | Side Effects: Acute or Delayed | Pharmacokinetics | Comments |
|---|---|---|---|---|
| Altretamine (Hexamethylmelamine, Hexalen)<br>Persistent or recurrent ovarian cancer | *Cap:* 50 mg and 100 mg (clear)<br>*Dose:* 260 mg/m²/day, given in 4 divided doses after meals and at bedtime, for 14–21 days in a 28-day cycle | *Nadir:* 1–28 days. Acute liver toxicity is dose limiting<br>Nausea and vomiting are dose related<br>Mild bone marrow suppression<br>Abdominal cramping, diarrhea<br>Peripheral neuropathies<br>Agitation and confusion | Variable absorption<br>Rapid metabolism<br>Urine excretion 90% in 72 hours | • Pyridoxine 50 mg/day may decrease neuropathy<br>• Take with food, prophylactic antiemetics<br>• May worsen vincristine-related peripheral neuropathy |
| Anastrozole (Arimidex)<br>Breast cancer, (adjuvant and metastatic) in hormone-positive, postmenopausal women | 1 mg PO daily (×5 years in adjuvant setting) | Hot flashes, asthenia, loss of energy<br>Vaginal dryness<br>Thrombophlebitis<br>Headache, weakness, joint disorder<br>Diarrhea, nausea | Metabolized by the liver, 70% excreted in the urine within 72 hours of taking drug | • Nonsteroidal aromatase inhibitor<br>• Well tolerated with low-toxicity profile<br>• No benefit in ER-negative women<br>• Contraindicated in pregnancy |
| Busulfan (Myleran)<br>Leukemia | *Tab:* 2 mg white<br>*Dose:* 4–12 mg/day for several weeks | *Nadir:* 10–30 days delayed marrow recovery<br>Potentially teratogenic<br>Pulmonary fibrosis with long-term use<br>Dermatologic hyperpigmentatin<br>Gynecomastia<br>Amenorrhea | Well absorbed<br>Extensive hepatic metabolism to inactive compounds<br>Renal excretion | • Bone marrow recovery may be delayed; therefore, caution is advised with long-term use. Hydration and allopurinol may be indicated to prevent hyperuricemia. Total cumulative dose: 600 mg.<br>• Long-term daily administration is not recommended due to the risk of secondary malignancies with chronic alkylating agents. |
| Capecitabine (Xeloda)<br>Metastatic breast cancer<br>Metastatic colorectal cancer | *Tab:* 150 mg light peach, 500 mg peach<br>2500 mg/m²/day ×14 days q 21 days<br>Swallow with water only; take with food | Mild BMS<br>DLT is diarrhea<br>Hand-foot syndrome, dermatitis, fatigue, anorexia, nausea, stomatitis | Metabolized to 5-FU; excreted in urine | • Administer in two oral doses, 12 hours apart, 30 minutes after a meal.<br>• Monitor coagulation profile in patients also taking Coumadin. |
| Chlorambucil (Leukeran)<br>Leukemia<br>Hodgkin's disease | *Tab:* 2 mg white<br>*Dose:* 4–8 mg/m²/day × 3–6 weeks<br>16 mg/m²/week q 4 week | *Nadir:* 7–10 days<br>Severe BMS<br>Slight nausea and vomiting<br>Occasional dermatitis<br>Abnormal liver function<br>Pulmonary fibrosis with prolonged use<br>Second malignancy<br>Sterility | Hepatic metabolism to active compound<br>Renal excretion of 50% of unchanged drug | • Good oral absorption.<br>• Concomitant barbiturate administration may enhance toxicity. Marrow suppression may be prolonged. |

(Continued)

**APPENDIX 16A**

**Oral Chemotherapy and Hormonal Agents (*Continued*)**

| Drug and Disease Indications | Dose and Schedule | Side Effects: Acute or Delayed | Pharmacokinetics | Comments |
|---|---|---|---|---|
| Cyclophosphamide (Cytoxan)<br>Breast cancer<br>Multiple myeloma<br>Small cell lung cancer<br>Malignant lymphomas<br>Leukemias | *Tab:* 25–50 mg<br>*Dose:* 1–5 mg/kg/day<br>60–120 mg/m$^2$<br>Adjust dose in the presence of renal dysfunction | *Nadir:* 7–14 days<br>Anorexia, nausea, and vomiting<br>Alopecia<br>Hemorrhagic cystitis with gross or microscopic hematuria<br>Amenorrhea<br>Sterility | Activated in the liver<br>oral absorption in 1 hour<br>30% of drug excreted unchanged in urine | • Vigorous hydration (3 L/day).<br>• Encourage frequent voiding to prevent hemorrhagic cystitis (a sterile inflammation of the urinary bladder). If patient complains of burning on urination or bladder incontinence, urinalysis may reveal occult blood. Control by withdrawal of the drug and hydration.<br>• May take pills in divided doses early in the day and with meals or all at one time. Better tolerated with cold foods.<br>• Barbiturates and other inducers of hepatic microsomal enzymes may enhance toxicity (eg, cimetidine). Allopurinol may enhance BMS. |
| Etoposide (VP-16, VePesid)<br>Lung cancer<br>Testicular cancer | *Cap:* 50 mg pink<br>*Dose:* 2 × the IV dose or 100–200 mg/m$^2$/day × 3–5 days q 3–4 weeks | *Nadir:* 7–14 days (white blood cell count)<br>Nausea and vomiting<br>9–16 days (platelets)<br>Alopecia<br>BMS is dose limiting | Renal and hepatic metabolism<br>Incomplete and variable absorption | • Nausea is mild though can be more severe with oral route than with IV route. |
| Exemestane (Aromasin)<br>Breast cancer (adjuvant and metastatic) in hormone-positive, postmenopausal women | 25 mg PO daily | Fatigue<br>Hot flashes, increased sweating<br>Pain<br>Nausea, increased appetite<br>Depression, insomnia | Rapidly absorbed from GI tract, with increased serum levels when taken with high-fat meal<br>Metabolized by CYP3A4 isoenzyme system | • Steroidal aromatase inactivator, irreversible<br>• Well tolerated with low-toxicity profile<br>• Contraindicated in pregnancy |
| Flutamide (Eulexin)<br>Prostate cancer together with an LHRH agonist | 250 mg PO every 8 hours | Decreased libido, impotence, gynecomastia<br>Hot flashes<br>Diarrhea, nausea, vomiting | Rapidly absorbed and excreted via urine | • Monitor patient closely for liver failure in first 3 months of treatment<br>• Contraindicated if severe liver dysfunction<br>• Monitor INR if on warfarin |
| Hydroxyurea (Hydrea)<br>Chronic myelocytic leukemia<br>Melanoma<br>Head and neck cancer | *Cap:* 500 mg<br>*Dose:* 80 mg/kg/day every third day<br>750–1000 mg/m$^2$/day ×5 days<br>Decrease dose in the presence of renal dysfunction<br>Store in tight container in a cool environment | *Nadir:* 13–17 days<br>Acute nausea and vomiting<br>Chronic and severe anemia<br>Neurological seizures and hallucinations<br>Dermatitis<br>Dysuria<br>Azotemia | Well absorbed<br>Hepatic metabolism<br>Renal excretion of 80% of compound in 12 hours<br>Crosses into CSF | • Concomitant radiation and/or 5-FU may enhance neurotoxicity.<br>• Dysuria and renal impairment may occur.<br>• Consider pretreatment with allopurinol. |

| | | | | |
|---|---|---|---|---|
| Letrozole (Femara)<br>Breast cancer (adjuvant and metastatic) in hormone-positive, postmenopausal women | 2.5 mg PO daily | Fatigue, hot flashes, pain<br>Nausea, vomiting, diarrhea, constipation | Rapidly absorbed; metabolized in the liver and excreted in the urine | • Nonsteroidal aromatase inhibitor<br>• Dose reduce if patient has cirrhosis and severe hepatic dysfunction |
| Lomustine (CCNU)<br>Brain cancer<br>Lymphomas | *Cap:* 100 mg/green/green, 40 mg green/white, 10 mg white<br>*Dose:* 100–130 mg/m$^2$ q 6–8 weeks | *Nadir:* 28–42 days<br>Severe cumulative BMS<br>Nausea and vomiting 4–6 hours after dosing<br>Anorexia<br>Alopecia<br>Stomatitis<br>Hepatotoxicity | Absorbed rapidly (<60 min)<br>Hepatic metabolism<br>Renal excretion of 50% in 24 hours and 75% in 96 hours<br>Crosses into CSF | • Dispense one dose at a time to prevent accidental overdose.<br>• Take on an empty stomach just before bedtime.<br>• Pretreat with aggressive antiemetics.<br>• Protect pills from heat and humidity. |
| L-phenylalanine mustard (Melphalan, Alkeran)<br>Multiple myeloma<br>Ovarian cancer | *Tab:* 2 mg white<br>*Dose:* 0.1–0.15 mg/kg/day ×2–3 week<br>Reduce dose with hepatic or renal impairment | *Nadir:* 10–18 days<br>Nausea and vomiting usually mild<br>Dermatitis<br>Pulmonary fibrosis<br>Long-term therapy can result in acute leukemia | Hepatic metabolism<br>Renal excretion 20%–35% (10% unchanged)<br>20%–50% excreted in feces within 6 days | • Protect pills from sunlight.<br>• Take on an empty stomach.<br>• BMS may be cumulative in older patients.<br>• Leukemogenic. |
| 6-Mercaptopurine (6-MP)<br>Leukemia | *Tab:* 50 mg off-white<br>*Dose:* 80–100 mg/m$^2$/day<br>Titrate dose based on blood counts<br>Reduce dose in the presence of hepatic or renal dysfunction | *Nadir:* 10–14 days<br>Nausea, vomiting<br>Mucositis<br>Diarrhea<br>Drug fever<br>Intrahepatic cholestasis<br>Pulmonary toxicity with prolonged use | Incomplete oral absorption<br>Hepatic inactivation<br>Renal excretion<br>10% unchanged in 24 hours | • Protect pills from light.<br>• Administer as single dose on an empty stomach.<br>• Increased toxicity with allopurinol (reduce dose by one-third to one-fourth of the original dose).<br>• Administer with caution to patients on sodium warfarin (Coumadin).<br>• Monitor LFTs. |
| Methotrexate<br>Squamous cell carcinoma<br>Lung cancer | *Tab:* 2.5 mg yellow<br>*Dose:* 2.5–10 mg /day PO or 15–30 mg/day PO × 5 days every 1–3 weeks | *Nadir:* 7–10 days<br>Nausea and anorexia can occur; stomatitis and ulcerations can occur, and are dose limiting. | Serum half-life is 2–4 hours<br>Excreted by the kidneys | • Dose is reduced with renal impairment; dosing on an empty stomach may enhance bioavailability. Excretion may be impaired in patients with simultaneous administration of weak acids (eg, salicylates or vitamin C); oral dosing is generally well tolerated<br>• Avoid administration with ketoprotein or probenecid as toxicity of methotrexate may be enhanced. |

(*Continued*)

**APPENDIX 16A**

**Oral Chemotherapy and Hormonal Agents (*Continued*)**

| Drug and Disease Indications | Dose and Schedule | Side Effects: Acute or Delayed | Pharmacokinetics | Comments |
|---|---|---|---|---|
| Procarbazine (Matulane)<br>Hodgkin's disease | *Cap:* 50 mg<br>*Dose:* 100 mg/m²/day ×14 days q 4 week; reduce dose in the presence of hepatic or renal dysfunction | *Nadir:* 4 weeks<br>BMS<br>Nausea, vomiting, and diarrhea gradually subside;<br>Flu-like syndrome<br>Paresthesias, neuropathies<br>Dizziness, and ataxia | Well absorbed from the GI tract<br>Metabolized in the liver with a biological half-life of about 1 hour<br>70% of the drug is eliminated by 24 hours in the urine; 5% appears as unchanged drug | • Drug and food interactions can occur.<br>• Central nervous system (CNS) depression can occur with concomitant administration of procarbazine and CNS depressants.<br>• Hypertensive crisis can occur when procarbazine is administered with certain antidepressants (tricyclics and monoamine oxidase inhibitors) and tyramine-rich foods.<br>• Severe nausea and vomiting can occur if taken with ethanol, mixed drinks, and beer. |
| Tamoxifen (Nolvadex)<br>Breast cancer (adjuvant and metastatic) in hormone-positive, postmenopausal women<br>Breast cancer prevention | 20 mg PO daily (×5 years in adjuvant setting) | Change in menses, milk production from breasts<br>Vaginal discharge<br>Hot flashes<br>Thromboembolism<br>Flare reaction | Rapidly absorbed, metabolized by CYP3A4, CYP2D6 isoenzymes in liver<br>Excreted in feces | • Nonsteroidal antiestrogen<br>• Patients should have annual gynecological exams with endometrial biopsy |
| Temozolomide (Temodar)<br>Astrocytoma | *Cap:* 5 mg green, 20 mg brown, 100 mg blue, 250 mg black<br>*Dose:* 150 mg/m²/day ×5 days q month<br>Dose escalation based on nadir counts | *Nadir:* Platelets by day 26, neutrophils by day 28<br>BMS is DLT<br>Nausea, vomiting, fatigue, and headache can be severe in 10% of cases. | Rapidly absorbed with a mean elimination half-life of 1.8 hours<br>Eliminated via the kidneys | • Take on an empty stomach at night with a glass of water.<br>• Capsules should not be opened or chewed. |
| 6-Thioguanine<br>Leukemia | *Tab:* 40 mg green/yellow<br>*Dose:* 80–100 mg/m²<br>Reduce dose if stomatitis occurs | *Nadir:* 7–28 days<br>Stomatitis<br>Diarrhea<br>Hepatotoxicity | Variable, incomplete absorption<br>Hepatic metabolism<br>Renal excretion | • Administer on an empty stomach.<br>• Does not require dose reduction when used in conjunction with allopurinol. |
| Topotecan (Hycamptin) capsules<br>Relapsed small cell lung cancer | 2.3 mg/m² PO daily ×5 consecutive days, repeated every 3 weeks | Neutropenia, anemia, thrombocytopenia<br>Nausea, vomiting, diarrhea, fatigue, alopecia | Rapidly absorbed and metabolized by hydrolysis and excreted primarily in the feces | • Crosses blood–brain barrier<br>• Neutropenia can result in neutropenic colitis<br>• Diarrhea should be aggressively managed |
| Toremifene citrate (Fareston)<br>Breast cancer, advanced | 60 mg PO daily | Menstrual irregularities<br>Hot flashes, mild fluid production in breasts<br>Vaginal discharge, bleeding<br>Flare reaction<br>Rash, alopecia | Well absorbed and highly protein bound<br>Metabolized by the liver and excreted in feces primarily | • Synthetic antiestrogen<br>• Patients should have annual gynecological exams with endometrial biopsy<br>• Monitor INR if on warfarin |

*Abbreviations*: 5-FU, 5 fluorouracil; BMS, bone marrow suppression; CSF, cerebrospinal fluid; DLT, dose limiting toxicity; ER, estrogen receptor; GI, gastrointestinal; INR, international normalization ratio; IV, intravenous; L, liter; LFTs, liver function tests; LHRH, luteinizing hormone-releasing hormone; PO, per oral.

**Intravenous Chemotherapy Agents**

| Dosage and Efficacy | Mechanism of Action and Metabolism | Administration Precautions | Side Effects |
|---|---|---|---|
| | | **ARSENIC TRIOXIDE (Trisenox)** | |
| *Dosage:*<br>• Induction: 0.15 mg/kg daily IV until bone marrow remission (not to exceed 60 doses)<br>• Consolidation: 0.15 mg/kg daily × 25 doses over 5 weeks, starting 3-6 weeks after completion of induction therapy<br>*Efficacy:*<br>• Acute promyelocytic leukemia | *Mechanism of action:*<br>• Causes morphological changes and DNA fragmentation.<br>• Damages or degrades the fusion protein PML-RAR alpha.<br>*Metabolism:*<br>• Metabolized in the liver.<br>• $t_{1/2}$ = 4–17 hours<br>• Excreted in the urine. | *Administration precautions:*<br>• Dilute in 100–250 mL of D5W or 0.9% NS and infuse over 1–2 hours. May extend infusion time up to 4 hours if acute vasomotor reactions occur.<br>• Stable at room temperature for 24 hours and 48 hours under refrigeration. | *Side effects:*<br>• Dizziness, lightheadedness, infusional hypotension, fatigue, skin reactions, musculoskeletal pain, mild hyperglycemia, nausea, vomiting, and diarrhea are the most common side effects.<br>• Peripheral neuropathy can occur.<br>• APL differentiation syndrome has been reported and can be fatal. Early signs include fever, weight gain, and dyspnea. High-dose steroids should be started immediately and continued until symptoms resolve.<br>• Can cause prolongation of the QT interval, which can lead to complete atrioventricular block. Obtain baseline EKG and monitor weekly during treatment. Potassium, magnesium, calcium, and creatinine should be monitored twice weekly during induction and weekly during consolidation. |
| | | **5-AZACYTIDINE (Vidaza)** | |
| *Dosage:*<br>• 75 mg/m² SC or IV daily × 7 days, repeated every 4 weeks × 4 or more cycles<br>*Efficacy:*<br>• Myelodysplastic syndrome | *Mechanism of action:*<br>• Hypomethylates DNA to restore function of genes responsible for cell division and differentiation<br>*Metabolism:*<br>• Rapidly absorbed; excreted in urine primarily, half-life about 4 hours | *Administration precautions:*<br>• Dose-modify based on hematological toxicity, renal function, and serum bicarbonate | *Side effects:*<br>• Neutropenia, with nadir occurring days 14–17, with recovery by day 28<br>• Nausea, vomiting, diarrhea, anorexia, stomatitis<br>• Constipation<br>• Fatigue, arthalgias, injection-site irritation |
| | | **BENDAMUSTINE (Treanda)** | |
| *Dosage:*<br>• 100 mg/m² IV infusion over 30 minutes on days 1 and 2 of a 28-day cycle × up to six cycles<br>• Dose-delay or -modify for hematological toxicity<br>*Efficacy:*<br>• Chronic lymphocytic leukemia (CLL) | *Mechanism of action:*<br>• Alkylating and purine-like (antimetabolite) action<br>• Sustainable double-strand DNA breaks and induces apoptosis, resulting in cell death<br>*Metabolism:*<br>• Highly bound to plasma proteins, hydrolyzed into low cytotoxic metabolites<br>• 90% of drug excreted via the feces | *Administration precautions:*<br>• Provide prophylaxis for tumor lysis syndrome with allopurinol first few weeks if patient at risk.<br>• Ensure WBC > 1000 cells/mm³ and platelets > 75,000 cells/mm³ for subsequent cycles.<br>• Infusion reactions common: fever, chills, pruritis, rash.<br>• Anaphylaxis may occur rarely.<br>• Use aggressive antiemetic therapy. | *Side effects:*<br>• Neutropenia<br>• Thrombocytopenia<br>• Fever, infection<br>• Discontinue for severe skin reactions<br>• Nausea<br>• Vomiting<br>• Anemia |

(Continued)

**Intravenous Chemotherapy Agents (*Continued*)**

| Dosage and Efficacy | Mechanism of Action and Metabolism | Administration Precautions | Side Effects |
|---|---|---|---|
| | | **BLEOMYCIN (Blenoxane)** | |
| *Dosage:*<br>• May be given IM, SC, IV, intratumoral, intra-arterial.<br>• 10–20 U/$m^2$ once or twice a week<br>• Intrapleural/pericardial sclerosing dose: 50-60 U/$m^2$ in 50–100 mL NS or D5W; not to exceed 40 U/$m^2$ in geriatric population<br>*Efficacy:*<br>• Cervical cancer<br>• Head and neck cancer<br>• Penis, skin, and testicular cancer<br>• Hodgkin's and non-Hodgkin's lymphoma<br>• Kaposi's sarcoma<br>• Germ cell tumors<br>Sclerosing agent for malignant pleural effusions, ascites | *Mechanism of action:*<br>• Cell-cycle phase specific for G2 and M phase. Binds to DNA.<br>• Inhibits cell progression out of G, resulting in cellular synchronization for subsequent drug therapy.<br>*Metabolism:*<br>• $t_{½}$ = 20 min<br>• Renal elimination | *Administration precautions:*<br>• Administer with caution to patients with significant pulmonary or renal disease. Prior cisplatin therapy may reduce bleomycin clearance, increasing plasma half-life and toxicity.<br>• Test dose: Bleomycin is associated with HSR and a test dose of 2 U IV in 50 mL D5W over 15 minutes followed by observation.<br>• Observe for anaphylactic reaction for 1–2 hours post-test dose.<br>• Lymphoma patients are more at risk for HSR and should be tested for the first two doses. | *Side effects:*<br>• Lifetime cumulative dose is 400 U.<br>• 25% dose reduction for creatinine clearance of 30–50 mL/minutes.<br>• 50% dose reduction for creatinine clearance of 20–30 mL/minutes.<br>• Fever occurs in approximately 50% of patients.<br>• Premedicate with acetaminophen 1g and diphenhydramine 50 mg. (Repeat 6 hours later.)<br>• Dermatological reactions such as hyperpigmentation, hyperkeratosis, and erythema on palms and fingers; urticaria, rash, mucositis, and alopecia<br>• Anorexia and mild nausea<br>• Interstitial pneumonitis and pulmonary fibrosis occur more commonly in patients who also have mediastinal radiation, are elderly, and receive higher cumulative doses. |
| | | **CARBOPLATIN (Paraplatin)** | |
| *Dosage:*<br>• IV: 360 mg/$m^2$ q 4 weeks<br>• Higher doses are given in pretransplant protocols and intraperitoneally or intra-arterially.<br>• Dose calculations are most therapeutically based on the desired serum concentration (AUC), renal status, and whether or not the patient has been previously treated with chemotherapy (Calvert method).<br>• Note that doses calculated according to the Calvert formula are total mg, not mg/$m^2$ (see text). | *Mechanism of action:*<br>• Maximal cytotoxicity occurs when cells are in the S-phase although cell kill by intrastrand DNA cross-linkage occurs throughout G1, S, and G2 phases of the cell cycle.<br>*Metabolism:*<br>• 60% eliminated unchanged in the urine.<br>• Major routes of elimination are glomerular filtration and tubular secretion.<br>• $t_{½}$ = 2.5 hours | *Administration precautions:*<br>• Available as lyophilized (powdered) form to distinguish it from cisplatin, which is available only in aqueous solution.<br>• Usually administered over 15–30 minutes in 500 mL of NS or D5W, without further hydration.<br>• May also be administered as a continuous 24 hours or longer infusion.<br>• Forms a precipitate when in contact with aluminum, causing loss of antitumor potency.<br>• Injection site irritation and erythema can occur with infiltration but no ulceration or necrosis<br>• Physically compatible with ondansetron. | *Side effects:*<br>• DLT: myelosuppression, particularly thrombocytopenia. Nadir occurs at 2–3 weeks.<br>• Nausea and vomiting are mild and rarely last beyond 24 hours.<br>• Ototoxicity and neurotoxicity (paresthesias) are uncommon.<br>• Alopecia, mucositis, and abnormal liver functions have been reported.<br>• Nephrotoxicity occurs but is less common than with cisplatin. |

*Efficacy:*
- Ovarian carcinoma
- Testicular cancer
- Head and neck cancer
- Cervical cancer
- Lung cancer

## CARMUSTINE (BiCNU)

*Dosage:*
- IV: 75–100 mg/$m^2$ IV/day × 2 days
- IV: 200–225 mg/$m^2$ q 6 weeks
- IV: 40 mg/$m^2$/day on 5 successive days, repeating cycle q 6–8 weeks
- Higher doses have been used in pretransplant protocols.

*Efficacy:*
- Brain tumors
- Multiple myeloma
- Hodgkin's disease
- Non-Hodgkin's lymphoma
- Melanoma

*Mechanism of action:*
- Inhibits enzymatic reactions involved in DNA synthesis.
- Inhibits DNA repair.
- Acts predominantly during late G and early S phase.
- Readily crosses the blood–brain barrier.

*Metabolism:*
- Metabolized by the liver.
- 80% eliminated via the kidneys.
- t½ = 15–20 minutes

*Administration precautions:*
- Soluble in water and absolute alcohol.
- Protect from light.
- Administer in 100–500 mL D5W or NS as a 1- to 2-hour infusion.
- Infusion may burn as it goes in and should be monitored closely.
- Heat provides symptomatic relief.
- Slowing the infusion rate eases vein discomfort.
- Hypotension can occur if the infusion is given rapidly.
- Facial flushing and dizziness occur infrequently.
- Compatible with ondansetron.
- Incompatible with polyvinylchloride infusion bags and with sodium bicarbonate.
- Avoid contact with skin; a brown stain may result.

*Side effects:*
- DLT: Leukopenia and thrombocytopenia occur 3–5 weeks after treatment, recovery at 8 weeks.
- Myelosuppression may be cumulative.
- Nausea and vomiting are common and require aggressive antiemetic therapy.
- Pulmonary fibrosis has been reported and generally presents as a dry cough and dyspnea.
- Alopecia is common.
- Elevation of LFTs and azotemia can occur with higher doses.
- Cimetidine has been shown to potentiate carmustine toxicity.

## CISPLATIN (Platinol) AQUEOUS SOLUTION

*Dosage:*
- IV: 50–120 mg/$m^2$ q 3–4 weeks
- IV: 15–20 mg/$m^2$ × 5 q 3–4 weeks, radio-sensitizing effect:
- IV: 15–50 mg/$m^2$ 1–3 times/week with concomitant RT

*Mechanism of action:*
- Binds to DNA affecting DNA replication.
- Forms DNA protein cross-links.
- Interacts with cellular glutathione.

*Administration precautions:*
- Dose reductions: 25% dose reduction for patients with creatinine clearance of 30–50 mL/minute and a 50% dose reduction for patients with creatinine clearance < 30 mL/minute

*Side effects:*
- Concomitant administration of probenecid enhances cisplatin renal toxicity.
- Monitor patient for HSR: tachycardia, wheezing, hypotension, and facial edema.
- Acute and delayed nausea and vomiting are preventable with aggressive antiemetics

(Continued)

Intravenous Chemotherapy Agents (*Continued*)

| Dosage and Efficacy | Mechanism of Action and Metabolism | Administration Precautions | Side Effects |
|---|---|---|---|
| **CISPLATIN (Platinol) AQUEOUS SOLUTION** (*Continued*) | | | |
| • IP: 100–270 mg/m² in 2 L of warmed NS.<br>• Infuse via gravity over 10 minutes Allow 4 hours dwell time.<br>*Efficacy:*<br>• Bladder cancer<br>• Ovarian cancer<br>• Testicular carcinoma<br>• Non-small cell lung cancer<br>• Head and neck cancer | *Metabolism:*<br>• 90% bound to plasma proteins.<br>• 20%–45% eliminated unchanged via kidney.<br>• 10% eliminated in bile.<br>• t½ = 60–90 hours | • Administer after appropriate hydration (1–2 L with mannitol).<br>• Maintain urinary output (125 mL/hour). Mixing cisplatin in 0.9% NaCl maintains drug stability.<br>• Cisplatin may react with aluminum, resulting in loss of cisplatin potency.<br>• Physically compatible with ondansetron.<br>• Sodium thiosulfate and mesna directly inactivate cisplatin.<br>• Administer with caution in patients receiving other potentially nephrotoxic drugs (aminoglycosides). | including receptor antagonists, dexamethasone, and metoclopramide.<br>• High frequency hearing loss may occur in up to 30% of patients.<br>• Tinnitis, vestibular dysfunction, and ototoxicity occur infrequently and are preventable with adequate hydration and mannitol diuresis.<br>• Peripheral neuropathy including numbness, tingling, and sensory loss occurs in arms and legs with long-term administration.<br>• Hypomagnesemia is seen with high dose (> 200 mg/m²) and is preventable with PO and IV supplements.<br>• Hemolytic anemia is seen with higher doses and responds to recombinant erythropoietin. |
| **CLADRIBINE (Leustatin)** | | | |
| *Dosage:*<br>• 0.09 mg/kg/day as a continuous infusion × 7 days (1 course only)<br>*Efficacy:*<br>• Hairy cell leukemia | *Mechanism of action:*<br>• Chlorinated purine nucleoside that accumulates in cell and interferes with DNA synthesis and repair<br>*Metabolism:*<br>• Unknown; crosses blood-brain barrier | *Administration precautions:*<br>• Unstable in 5% dextrose | *Side effects:*<br>• Neutropenia, with nadir 1–2 weeks after infusion, recovery by weeks 4–5<br>• Infection<br>• Prolonged bone marrow hypocellularity<br>• Lymphopenia<br>• Thrombocytopenia<br>• Anemia<br>• Fever, headaches, rash<br>• Diarrhea<br>• Constipation<br>• Mild nausea, vomiting |
| **CLOFARABINE (Clolar)** | | | |
| *Dosage*<br>• 52 mg/m² IV over 2 hours daily × 5, repeated after recovery of all baseline organ function, usually 2–6 weeks IV hydration during 5 days of treatment | *Mechanism of action:*<br>• Inhibits DNA synthesis and repair, causing death of actively dividing and resting cells<br>• Breaks down mitochondrial membrane releasing cytochrome C and apoptosis-inducing factor, leading to programmed cell death. | *Administration precautions:*<br>• Do not coadminister with renally toxic or hepatotoxic drugs.<br>• Provide prophylaxis for tumor lysis syndrome with allopurinol first few weeks if patient at risk.<br>• Assess for capillary leak syndrome during treatment. | *Side effects:*<br>• Severe neutropenia<br>• Infection<br>• Fever, rigors<br>• Rash<br>• Alopecia<br>• Anal mucosal irritation<br>• Fatigue<br>• Lethargy |

- Pain
- Edema
- Injection-site pain

## CYCLOPHOSPHAMIDE (Cytoxan)

*Dosage:*
- PO: 50–200 mg/m$^2$ each day × 14 days q 28 days
- IV: 400 mg/m$^2$ × 5 days
- IV: 500 mg to 1.5 g/m$^2$ q 3 week or 60 mg/kg × 2 days prior to BMT

*Efficacy:*
- Breast cancer
- Ovarian cancer
- Leukemias
- Lymphomas
- Multiple myeloma
- Lung cancer

*Mechanism of action:*
- Activated by hepatic microsomal enzymes; prevents cell division by cross-linking DNA strands.
- Non-cell cycle phase specific.

*Metabolism:*
- Metabolized in the liver.
- Excreted in the kidney (15% unchanged).
- 33% of drug is excreted unchanged in the stool.
- t½ = 3–10 hours

*Administration precautions:*
- When doses > 1000 mg are given, patients should receive hydration of 500–1000 mL NS.
- Administer IV dose slowly to prevent nasal congestion, headache, and dizziness.
- Encourage fluid intake of 3 L/day while taking cyclophosphamide.
- When taking PO doses, encourage patient to take all pills before 5 PM to minimize bladder contact with toxic metabolites.
- Phenytoin and chloral hydrate may enhance the conversion of cyclophosphamide to toxic metabolites, thereby increasing toxicity.

*Side effects:*
- Hemorrhagic cystitis occurs rarely with conventional doses.
- Hydration and mesna are indicated with high-dose and pretransplant therapy.
- SIADH can occur with high-dose cyclophosphamide.
- Nausea and vomiting are preventable with aggressive antiemetic therapy.
- Alopecia is common. Metallic taste occurs during injection and when taken orally.
- Encourage the patient to chew gum, peppermint, or lemon candy.
- Myelosuppression (leukopenia) is dose limiting.
- Amenorrhea and reversible oligospermia occur and are dose dependent.
- Cyclophosphamide 1 mg/mL is compatible with doxorubicin, cisplatin, mesna, and other drugs.
- Blurring of vision has been reported.
- Cardiac toxicity can occur with high-dose therapy, especially if given with radiation to the chest area.

## CYTARABINE (Cytosar: ARA-C Cytosine Arabinoside)

*Dosage:*
- IV: 5–10 day CI (continuous infusion) of 100-200 mg/m$^2$
- IT: 5–70 mg/m$^2$ 1–3 × /week
- SQ: 1 mg/kg 1–2 × /week or 100 mg bid × 5 days q 28 days

*Efficacy:*
- Acute leukemia
- Myeloid leukemia
- Acute nonlymphocytic leukemia
- Meningeal leukemia

*Mechanism of action:*
- Inhibits DNA polymerase causing DNA chain elongation and arrest.
- Cell cycle phase specific for the S phase.
- Antimetabolite.

*Metabolism:*
- Metabolized in the liver.
- At 24 hours, 90% of the drug is eliminated in the urine.
- t½ = 2–3 hours

*Administration precautions:*
- Given IV push or IV infusion over 30 minutes
- 5- to 10-day continuous infusions may be optimal for antitumor cytotoxicity because of the S-phase specificity.
- For IT use, mix drug with lactated Ringer's solution or NS without preservatives.
- Rotate sites for SC injections.

*Side effects:*
- Myelosuppression is the DLT. Nadir at 5-7 days, recovery in 2–3 weeks.
- Anemia is common.
- Nausea, vomiting, anorexia, stomatitis, and diarrhea are reported.
- Metallic taste
- Minimal alopecia
- Skin erythema can occur.
- Arthralgias and myalgias occur.
- After IT use, patients may experience nausea, vomiting, fever, and headache.
- Ocular toxicity: Excessive tearing, photophobia, and blurred vision
- High-dose therapy can lead to CNS toxicity: Lethargy, confusion, ataxia.
- Cytarabine may decrease the cellular uptake of methotrexate.
- Compatible with vincristine, prednisolone, sodium phosphate, and ondansetron.
- Physical changes are noted with methotrexate and 5-FU and heparin.
- Compatible with vancomycin for 4–8 hours.

(Continued)

**Intravenous Chemotherapy Agents (*Continued*)**

| Dosage and Efficacy | Mechanism of Action and Metabolism | Administration Precautions | Side Effects |
|---|---|---|---|
| **DACARBAZINE (DTIC)** | | | |
| *Dosage:*<br>• 375 mg/m$^2$ q 3–4 weeks or<br>• 150–250 mg/m$^2$/q day × 5 days q 3–4 weeks or<br>• 850 mg/m$^2$ on day 1 q 3–4 weeks<br>*Efficacy:*<br>• Malignant melanoma<br>• Soft tissue sarcomas<br>• Hodgkin's disease | *Mechanism of action:*<br>• Causes cross-linkage and breaks in DNA strands.<br>• Inhibits RNA and DNA synthesis.<br>• Cell cycle phase nonspecific, but has more activity in late G2.<br>*Metabolism:*<br>• Activated by liver microsomes.<br>• Excreted renally.<br>• t½ = 35 minutes | *Administration precautions:*<br>• Reconstitute with D5W or saline.<br>• Solution can be painful and should be administered slowly in 250–500 mL of solution over 30–60 minutes. Moist heat along the vein eases pain.<br>• Stable for 8 hours at room temperature, 72 hours if refrigerated.<br>• Drug should be protected from light.<br>• May turn a pinkish color if exposed to light.<br>• HSR can occur; hypotension occurs with high-dose therapy. | *Side effects:*<br>• DLT: moderate degree of myelosuppression.<br>• Nadir occurs at 21–25 days.<br>• Anemia can occur.<br>• Severe nausea and vomiting can occur.<br>• Aggressive pretreatment with antiemetic therapy is needed. Nausea and vomiting lessen by days 3–4 of treatment.<br>• Hepatotoxic; monitor liver functions.<br>• Flulike syndrome may occur with fever, myalgia, and malaise at about 7 days, lasting 1–3 weeks.<br>• Photosensitivity can occur; protect skin from sunlight. |
| **DACTINOMYCIN (Actinomycin D; ACT-D, Cosmegen)** | | | |
| *Dosage:*<br>• 10–15 kg/day × 5 days q 3–4 weeks or<br>• 2–4 mg/m$^2$ in divided doses over 1 week or<br>• 2 mg/m$^2$ IV q 3–4 weeks<br>*Efficacy:*<br>• Wilms' tumor<br>• Embryonal rhabdomyosarcoma<br>• Choriocarcinoma<br>• Malignant melanoma<br>• Hodgkin's and non-Hodgkin's lymphoma | *Mechanism of action:*<br>• Binds between purine-pyrimidine base pairs in DNA.<br>• Inhibits the synthesis of DNA-dependent RNA and messenger RNA.<br>• Action is cell cycle nonspecific but is more active during $G_1$ and in cells that are cycling.<br>*Metabolism:*<br>• Excreted unchanged in bile and urine. | *Administration precautions:*<br>• Reconstitute with preservative-free sterile water for injection. Preserved diluent may cause precipitation. Use drug as soon as possible.<br>• Monitor liver functions; dose reductions may be necessary.<br>• Use extreme caution during administration.<br>• Dactinomycin is a severe vesicant.<br>• Dactinomycin is compatible with ondansetron.<br>• When calculating dose, double-check the order since the drug is ordered both as μg/kg and mg/m$^2$. | *Side effects:*<br>• DLT: myelosuppression occurs within 7–10 days of dosing.<br>• Nadir may be delayed, occurring at 3 weeks.<br>• Due to its immunosuppressive effects, avoid administering dactinomycin to patients who have an active viral infection.<br>• Nausea and vomiting can be severe.<br>• Aggressive pretreatment with antiemetics is appropriate.<br>• Mucositis and diarrhea can be severe; institute preventive oral hygiene regimen.<br>• Alopecia occurs commonly.<br>• Erythema, hyperpigmentation, and an acnelike rash occur commonly.<br>• Dactinomycin can cause a radiation recall reaction.<br>• Hepatic venoocclusive toxicity manifested as elevated SGOT and bilirubin can occur. |
| **DAUNORUBICIN (Daunomycin, Cerubidine)** | | | |
| *Dosage:*<br>• 30–60 mg/m$^2$ daily × 3–5 days q 3–4 weeks<br>*Efficacy:*<br>• ALL<br>• AML<br>• Acute monocytic leukemia<br>• Acute nonlymphocytic leukemia | *Mechanism of action:*<br>• Intercalates DNA, thereby blocking DNA, RNA, and protein synthesis. It is an anthracycline antitumor antibiotic.<br>*Metabolism:*<br>• Metabolized in the liver.<br>• About 40% of the drug is eliminated via the bile. | *Administration precautions:*<br>• 20-mg vial is reconstituted with 4 mL of sterile water = 5 mg/mL.<br>• QS to 15–20 mL of NS.<br>• Stable for 24 hours at room temperature and 48 hours under refrigeration.<br>• Incompatible with heparin, 5-FU, and dexamethasone. | *Side effects:*<br>• DLT: myelosuppression.<br>• WBC nadir occurs at 7–14 days; recovery at 3 weeks.<br>• Thrombocytopenia and anemia occur.<br>• Stomatitis occurs, but is mild.<br>• Diarrhea occurs infrequently.<br>• Nausea and vomiting occur 1–5 hours after dosing but are prevented with aggressive antiemetic therapy.<br>• Alopecia is abrupt and involves all body hair. |

| | | | |
|---|---|---|---|
| | • 20%–25% is eliminated via the urine.<br>• t½ = 20–25 hours | • Compatible with ondansetron.<br>• Caution: Because the solution is red, as is doxorubicin and with a similar-sounding name, the vial should be double-checked against the order.<br>• Urine will be pink to red for 12–24 hours after administration.<br>• Daunorubicin is a severe vesicant. Extreme caution should be used in administration of this drug<br>• Administer via the side arm of a freely running IV or by the 2-syringe technique. | • Hyperpigmentation of the nails occurs.<br>• Urticaria and a generalized rash have been reported.<br>• Monitor liver functions. If elevated LFTs are noted, dose reduction is indicated.<br>• Cardiac toxicity can occur. Dose is limited to 500–600 mg/$m^2$.<br>• Manifestation of CHF is characterized by dyspnea on exertion, fatigue, and arrhythmias. |
| | | **DECITABINE (Dacogen)** | |
| *Dosage:*<br>• 15mg/$m^2$ IV continuous infusion over 3 hours, repeated every 8 hours × 3 days, repeated every 6 weeks for at least 4 cycles<br>*Efficacy:*<br>• Myelodysplastic syndrome | *Mechanism of action:*<br>• Pyrimidine analogue Prevents DNA synthesis in the S phase, leading to cell death<br>• Causes hypomethylation by trapping DNA methyltransferase, which activates genes that have been silenced.<br>• Also tumor-suppressor genes, expression of tumor antigens, and helps the cells to differentiate (mature)<br>*Metabolism*<br>• Unknown, but appears to involve deamination in the liver, other pathways | *Administration Precautions:*<br>• Dose-delay or -modify based on counts prior to the next cycle<br>• Assess CBC, differential, blood glucose, LFTs, and renal function tests prior to each cycle<br>• Assess cardiac status during treatment because MI, CHF, cardiomyopathy, and arrythmias have been reported | *Side Effects*<br>• Neutropenia,<br>• Thrombocytopenia<br>• Anemia<br>• Nausea, vomiting<br>• Stomatitis<br>• Lethargy<br>• Fever<br>• Pain<br>• Rigors<br>• Arthalgias |
| | | **DOCETAXEL (Taxotere)** | |
| *Dosage:*<br>• 60–100 mg/$m^2$ q 3 week as a 1-hour infusion<br>• 35 to 40 mg/$m^2$ IV weekly × 3 weeks, followed by 1 week rest | *Mechanism of action:*<br>• Antimicrotubule agent: a mitotic spindle poison. Enhances microtubule assembly and inhibits the depolymerization of tubulin. | *Administration precautions:*<br>• Docetaxel solution contains 2 mg (40 mg/mL) of docetaxel in polysorbate/tween 80.<br>• Refrigerated vial sits at room | *Side effects:*<br>• The DLT for docetaxel is neutropenia and thrombocytopenia.<br>• All patients receive dexamethasone 8 mg PO bid × 5 days starting 1 day prior to docetaxel |

(Continued)

**Intravenous Chemotherapy Agents (*Continued*)**

| Dosage and Efficacy | Mechanism of Action and Metabolism | Administration Precautions | Side Effects |
|---|---|---|---|
| **DOCETAXEL (Taxotere)** (*Continued*) | | | |
| *Efficacy:*<br>• Ovarian cancer<br>• Breast cancer<br>• Non-small cell lung cancer<br>• Prostate cancer<br>• Gastric cancer<br>• Head and neck cancer<br>• Small cell lung cancer<br>• Bladder cancer | This process leads to increased bundles of microtubules in the cell. The cell is then unable to divide.<br>*Metabolism:*<br>• Metabolized in the liver, excreted in the feces, and minimally excreted in the urine.<br>• t½ = 11 hours | temperature for 5 minutes. Once mixed with solvent the solution contains 10 mg/mL. The appropriate amount of docetaxel is mixed with D5W in a concentration < 1 mg/mL. Once diluted, docetaxel is stable for 8 hours at room temperature.<br>• Avoid infiltration: The drug is an irritant but can cause tissue damage depending on the concentration.<br>• Hyaluronidase SQ injections (maximum volume of 3 mL) have been recommended for treatment of infiltration. Apply cold to the site, not heat.<br>• Monitor liver functions carefully; dose adjustments are appropriate if LFTs are elevated 2.5 × normal. | to reduce the amount of fluid retention.<br>• Diphenhydramine 50 mg is also given 30 minutes prior to prevent HSRs.<br>• If mild HSR occurs with flushing, skin reactions, or pruritus, the infusion rate is slowed with observation. If the patient experiences rash, flushing, mild dyspnea, or chest discomfort, the infusion is stopped and the patient is treated with IV diphenhydramine and dexamethasone. The infusion may be resumed after symptoms abate.<br>• If severe symptoms such as generalized urticaria, angioedema, or hypotension occur, the infusion is stopped and the patient is treated with antihistamine, steroid, and if necessary epinephrine or bronchodilators. The patient may still receive the docetaxel depending on the severity of the response. If the patient reacts a second time, the patient probably should not receive the drug again.<br>• Nausea and vomiting are minimal.<br>• Alopecia occurs within 3 weeksof the first treatment.<br>• Nail separation may occur.<br>• Drug-associated fluid retention or edema including pleural effusions, ascites, and peripheral edema occur and may be managed with a diuretic, which may or may not be helpful. |
| **DOXORUBICIN (Adriamycin, Rubex)** | | | |
| *Dosage:*<br>• IV: 30–75 mg/m² q 3–4 weeks<br>• IV: 20–45 mg/m²/IV × 3 days. Higher doses are used in dose-intensive regimens. Doxorubicin may also be given intraarterially, intrapleurally, and by bladder instillation.<br>*Efficacy:*<br>• Acute nonlymphocytic leukemia<br>• ALL<br>• Wilms' tumor<br>• Neuroblastoma<br>• Soft tissue sarcoma<br>• Breast cancer<br>• Hepatocellular carcinoma | *Mechanism of action:*<br>• Binds directly to DNA base pairs and inhibits DNA, RNA, and protein synthesis. Antitumor antibiotic. Cell cycle specific for the S phase.<br>*Metabolism:*<br>• Extensively metabolized by the liver.<br>• 40%–50% of the drug is eliminated in the bile.<br>• 5% is eliminated in the urine.<br>• t½ = 18–30 hours | *Administration precautions:*<br>• Available in liquid and lyophilized forms.<br>• Reconstitute with sterile water for injection, D5W, NS to form a solution of 2 mg/mL<br>• Stable for 35 days at room temperature.<br>• Incompatible with heparin, dexamethasone, 5-FU, furosemide, and aminophylline.<br>• Compatible with cyclophosphamide, cisplatin, dacarbazine, droperidol, vinblastine, vincristine, and ondansetron.<br>• Doxorubicin turns the urine a reddish orange for 8–10 hours after administration. | *Side effects:*<br>• DLT: Myelosuppression, especially leukopenia.<br>• Nadir occurs at 10-14 days. Recovery is swift at 3 weeks.<br>• Cardiac toxicity can occur. Dose is limited to 450–550 mg/m². Doxorubicin causes damage to the myocyte of the heart, causing various degrees of damage, but manifests as CHF as the heart begins to function less efficiently as a pump.<br>• MUGA scans are done periodically to monitor left ventricular function. Early symptoms of CHF include tachycardia, dyspnea on exertion, arrhythmias, and EKG changes.<br>• Alopecia occurs predictably and is dose dependent. Doses greater than 50 mg are associated with moderate to severe loss. Doses of 90–100 mg cause hair loss in 2–5 weeks.<br>• Stomatitis is dose limiting and can be more severe with continuous infusions.<br>• Continuous infusions are only given through central lines, never through peripheral lines. |

| | | | |
|---|---|---|---|
| • Ovarian carcinoma | | • Since doxorubicin is metabolized and eliminated by the liver, LFTs are monitored frequently. Elevation in bilirubin to 1.2–3 mg/dL warrants a 50% dose reduction; bilirubin of 3 mg/dL calls for a 75% dose reduction.<br>• Administer with extreme caution. Doxorubicin is a severe vesicant. It will cause tissue damage, ulceration, and necrosis if infiltrated. Inject through the side arm of a freely running and well-established IV or by using the 2-syringe technique.<br>• Caution: It has a similar name and color to daunorubicin. Check the drug order against the vial to ensure the right dose of the right drug. | • Nail bed changes occur and include hyperpigmentation especially in blacks and in individuals of Mediterranean descent. |
| **DOXORUBICIN HYDROCHLORIDE LIPOSOME INJECTION (Doxil)** | | | |
| *Dosage:*<br>• 20 mg/$m^2$ over 30 minutes q 3 weeks<br>• 50 mg/$m^2$ q 4 weeks × 4 cycles for metastic ovarian cancer<br>*Efficacy:*<br>• AIDS<br>• Kaposi's sarcoma<br>• Ovarian cancer | *Mechanism of action:*<br>• Antitumor antibiotic binds directly to DNA.<br>• Inhibits DNA and RNA synthesis.<br>• Drug is encapsulated in stealth liposomes to prolong circulation time.<br>*Metabolism:*<br>• Slower clearance from body than doxorubicin.<br>• t½ = 55 hours | *Administration precautions:*<br>• Dilute in 250 mL 5% dextrose USP.<br>• Drug is an irritant. | *Side effects:*<br>• Acute infusion reaction may occur with flushing, shortness of breath, facial swelling, headache, chills, back pain, chest and throat tightness, and/or hypotension. Stop infusion. Restart if symptoms abate.<br>• Hand-foot syndrome may require dose reduction.<br>• Stomatitis may occur.<br>• BMS is dose limiting.<br>• Cardiac toxicity may occur.<br>• Less incidence of alopecia compared to doxorubicin. |
| **EPIRUBICIN (Ellence)** | | | |
| *Dosage:*<br>• 100–120 mg/$m^2$ IV<br>*Efficacy:*<br>• Breast cancer | *Mechanism of action:*<br>• Inhibits nucleic acid and protein synthesis.<br>• Interferes with replication and transcription of DNA. | *Administration precautions:*<br>• Administer with caution. Epirubicin is a vesicant. It can cause severe tissue damage, ulceration, and necrosis if infiltrated. | *Side effects:*<br>• Severe BMS may occur and is the dose limiting toxicity. Monitor blood counts closely.<br>• May require colony-stimulating factors to avoid dose reduction and treatment delays. |

(Continued)

**Intravenous Chemotherapy Agents (*Continued*)**

| Dosage and Efficacy | Mechanism of Action and Metabolism | Administration Precautions | Side Effects |
|---|---|---|---|
| | | **EPIRUBICIN (Ellence)** (*Continued*) | |
| | • Semisynthetic derivative of daunorubicin and a 4 -epimer of doxorubicin.<br>*Metabolism:*<br>• Rapidly and extensively metabolized by the liver.<br>• Excreted in the bile.<br>• t½ = 30–35 hours | • Refrigerate and protect from light.<br>• Inject through the side arm of a free-flowing and well-established IV line or by using the 2-syringe technique.<br>• May cause the urine to turn a pink/red color for 2 days after administration. | • Probability of developing clinically significant CHF is estimated at 3.3 % for a total cumulative dose of 900 mg/$m^2$<br>• Cardiotoxicity can occur. Do not exceed total cumulative dose of 0.9%–1 g/$m^2$.<br>• Nausea, vomiting, stomatitis, and mucositis have been reported. Premedicate with 5HT3 antagonist and dexamethasone.<br>• Amenorrhea and premature menopause may occur.<br>• Concomitant use of calcium-channel blockers requires close monitoring of cardiac function.<br>• HSRs may occur, but are rare.<br>• Discontinue cimetidine during treatment.<br>• Alopecia is common, usually after the first or second treatment, and is transient.<br>• Radiation recall may occur. |
| | | **ETOPOSIDE (VePesid, VP-16)** | |
| *Dosage:*<br>• 50–100 mg/$m^2$ IV q day × 5 (testicular cancer) q 3-4 weeks<br>• 75–200 mg/$m^2$ IV q day x 3 (small cell lung cancer) q 3–4 weeks. PO dose is twice the IV dose.<br>• 400 mg/$m^2$/day × 3 days prior to BMT<br>*Efficacy:*<br>• Small cell lung cancer<br>• Testicular cancer | *Mechanism of action:*<br>• Inhibits DNA synthesis in S and G2. Causes single-strand breaks in DNA.<br>• Cell cycle phase specific for S and G2 phases.<br>*Metabolism:*<br>• Extensively protein bound. Metabolized in the liver. Excreted in the bile and urine.<br>• t½ = 8–14 hours | *Administration precautions:*<br>• Following dilution in NS or 5% dextrose, the drug is stable for 72–96 hours at room temperature. At room temperature, stability is dependent on concentration:<br>0.6 mg/mL = 24 hours<br>1 mg/mL = 4 hours<br>2 mg/mL = 2 hours<br>• Etoposide is administered slowly over at least 30–45 minutes.<br>• Hypotension can occur if infused in less than 45 minutes. Monitor patients for drug sensitivity. | *Side effects:*<br>• DLT: Leukopenia, dose-related. Nadir occurs 7–14 days, recovery by day 21.<br>• Nausea and vomiting are uncommon.<br>• Anorexia occurs, especially with PO dosing.<br>• Alopecia occurs more commonly with IV dosing.<br>• Radiation recall and pruritus can occur.<br>• HSR is rare. |
| | | **5-FLUOROURACIL (5-FU, Adrucil)** | |
| *Dosage:*<br>• Doses vary: 300-600 mg/$m^2$ IV × 5 days q 3-4 weeks<br>• 450-600 mg/$m^2$ IV weekly<br>• 800-1200 mg/$m^2$ continuous infusion × 14-21 days to toxicity | *Mechanism of action:*<br>• Inhibits the formation of thymidine, which is necessary for DNA synthesis.<br>• Causes abnormal RNA synthesis.<br>• Acts synergistically with methotrexate.<br>• Cell cycle phase specific for the S phase. | *Administration precautions:*<br>• May be given a variety of ways: IV as a continuous infusion, IV push, arterial infusion, intracavitary, or intraperitoneally.<br>• Store at room temperature and protect from light. | *Side effects:*<br>• Myelosuppression may be dose limiting, but less common with continuous infusion.<br>• Mucositis is most common DLT with continuous infusions. Symptoms of erythema, soreness, and ulceration may begin within 5–8 days of therapy. Sucking on ice chips as tolerated may decrease PO stomatitis.<br>• Diarrhea can be severe, even life- threatening, especially when 5-FU is given in higher doses with leucovorin. |

| | | | |
|---|---|---|---|
| *Efficacy:*<br>• Breast cancer<br>• Colon cancer<br>• Rectal cancer<br>• Pancreatic cancer<br>• Stomach cancer<br>• Head and neck cancer | *Metabolism:*<br>• Poorly absorbed by mouth.<br>• After IV administration, the drug is metabolized to active metabolites.<br>• Approximately 45% of the drug is metabolized by the liver.<br>• 15% is eliminated unchanged in the urine.<br>• t½ = 10–20 minutes | • Incompatible with daunorubicin, doxorubicin, idarubicin, cisplatin, cytarabine, and diazepam.<br>• Compatible with vincristine, methotrexate, potassium chloride, and magnesium sulfate. | • Nausea, vomiting, and anorexia occur less frequently, but are more common when 5-FU is given simultaneously with radiation to the abdomen.<br>• Skin and nail bed changes occur, especially with continuous infusion. Partial nail loss can occur as well as banding. Palmar-plantar erythrodysesthesias can be severe, necessitating dose reduction and treatment delays. Hyperpigmentation and photosensitivity are common. Patients are cautioned to protect themselves from the sun.<br>• Excessive lacrimation due to tear duct stenosis and blurred vision occur in about 25% of patients.<br>• Headache, cerebellar ataxia, nystagmus, and confusion occur with higher doses.<br>• Administering 5-FU based on the patient's circadian rhythm may lessen toxicity in general.<br>• Alopecia is dose dependent.<br>• Ataxia occurs in elderly patients. Other CNS changes include headache, drowsiness, and blurred vision. |
| **FLOXURIDINE (FUDR, 5-FUDR)** | | | |
| *Dosage:*<br>• 0.1–0.6 mg/kg/day by intrahepatic infusion. Therapy is continued to toxicity, usually 7–14 days.<br>• Circadian infusion protocols have been used.<br>• IV doses range from 0.5–1.0 mg/kg/day for up to 2 weeks by continuous infusion.<br>*Efficacy:*<br>• Adenocarcinoma metastatic to the liver | *Mechanism of action:*<br>• Antimetabolite, similar to 5-FU, interrupts DNA synthesis causing cell death. Cell cycle phase specific for the S phase.<br>*Metabolism:*<br>• Metabolized to 5-FU when given IV.<br>• 70%–90% of the drug is metabolized by the liver, and metabolites are excreted by the kidneys and lungs. When given, intrahepatic FUDR has a much higher first-pass extraction rate compared to 5-FU and therefore the cytotoxic effect is more localized to the liver.<br>• t½ = 0.3–3.6 hours | *Administration precautions:*<br>• Caution should be exercised as both 5-FU and floxuridine (also called 5-FUDR) are supplied in 500-mg vials and the doses of each are dramatically different. With such similar names it is important to note that mistaking 500 mg of FUDR for 500 mg of 5-FU could be lethal.<br>• FUDR 500-mg vial of lyophilized powder is reconstituted with sterile water.<br>• Generally given via an intraarterial infusion pump.<br>• Heparin is added to the FUDR to prevent clotting of the catheter due to the slow infusion rate. | *Side effects:*<br>• When given as an intraarterial infusion an H2 antihistamine such as ranitidine may be recommended (150 mg bid) to prevent peptic ulcer disease.<br>• The intraarterial route is usually associated with less systemic toxicity.<br>• BMS is more common with IV bolus injections.<br>• Nausea, vomiting, and anorexia are common. Abdominal cramps with severe diarrhea are indications to interrupt therapy.<br>• Mucositis does not occur often. If it does occur, it is an indication to interrupt the treatment and to reduce the dose.<br>• Skin changes can occur and include edema, dermatitis, rashes, and pruritus as well as hyperpigmentation.<br>• Alopecia can occur but is usually mild. |

(*Continued*)

**Intravenous Chemotherapy Agents (*Continued*)**

| Dosage and Efficacy | Mechanism of Action and Metabolism | Administration Precautions | Side Effects |
|---|---|---|---|
| | | **GEMCITABINE (Gemzar)** | |
| *Dosage:*<br>• 800–1000 mg/m² weekly × 3 weeks q 4 weeks<br>*Efficacy:*<br>• Pancreas cancer<br>• Non-small cell lung cancer<br>• Breast cancer | *Mechanism of action:*<br>• Antimetabolite.<br>• Inhibits DNA synthesis.<br>• Cell cycle specific for the S phase.<br>*Metabolism:*<br>• Eliminated by kidneys.<br>• t½ = 20 minutes | *Administration precautions:*<br>• Reconstitute with sodium chloride to a solution containing 10 mg/mL.<br>• Dilute in 100–1000 mL of saline and infuse over 30 minutes to 3 hours.<br>• Stable at room temperature for 24 horrs. | *Side effects:*<br>• Myelosuppression, especially thrombocytopenia, can be dose limiting.<br>• Flulike syndrome with fever, mild nausea, and vomiting can occur. Fever generally occurs within 8 hours of dosing. Acetaminophen generally relieves symptoms.<br>• Rash may occur within 2–3 days of the infusion. Topical steroids may be helpful.<br>• Peripheral edema may occur. |
| | | **GEMTUZUMAB OZOGAMICIN (Mylotarg)** | |
| *Dosage:*<br>• 9 mg/m² IV of day 1and day 14<br>*Efficacy:*<br>• CD33⁺ acute myeloid leukemia | *Mechanism of action:*<br>• Causes DNA strand breakage and apoptosis.<br>• Necrotic mechanism of cytotoxicity is also suspected.<br>• Consists of an antibody and a cytotoxic antitumor antibiotic.<br>*Metabolism:*<br>• Causes hydrolytic release of a calicheamicin derivative. | *Administration precautions:*<br>• Protect from unshielded fluorescent light, direct and indirect sunlight during preparation and administration.<br>• Cover with a UV protectant bag and infuse over 2 hours.<br>• Reconstitute with 5 mL of sterile water and dilute in 100 mL of 0.9% sodium chloride solution.<br>• Must use a 1.2-micron terminal filter for administration.<br>• Can be given in an ambulatory setting. | *Side effects:*<br>• Pancytopenia is a common side effect and may be profound. Monitor blood counts very closely. Platelet and RBC transfusion are often necessary. Prophylactic antibiotics may also be helpful.<br>• Infusion reactions can be severe and usually resolve within 24 hours. Fever, chills, hypotension, and hypoxia are often seen.<br>• Premedicate with diphenhydramine 50 mg and acetaminophen 650–1000 mg PO 1 hour before, followed by two additional doses of acetaminophen at hours 4 and 8.<br>• Monitor vital signs before, during, and for the 6 hours following infusion.<br>• Observe for 4–6 hours after the completion of the infusion for side effects.<br>• Emergency equipment and medications need to be readily available.<br>• Venoocclusive disease (VOD) has been reported and can be fatal. A higher incidence has been seen with patients who have had a BMT. |
| | | **IDARUBICIN (Idamycin)** | |
| *Dosage:*<br>• 12 mg/m²/day for 3 days<br>• Doses vary<br>• Generally given in combination with other drugs<br>*Efficacy:*<br>• Acute nonlymphocytic leukemia | *Mechanism of action:*<br>• Cell cycle phase specific for the S phase.<br>• Analog of daunorubicin.<br>• Inhibits RNA synthesis.<br>*Metabolism:*<br>• Excreted primarily in the bile and urine.<br>• 25% of the drug is eliminated over approximately 5 days. | *Administration precautions:*<br>• Reconstituted with NS.<br>• Protect from light.<br>• Caution is used during administration because drug is a vesicant.<br>• Incompatible with 5-FU, etoposide, dexamethasone, heparin, hydrocortisone, methotrexate, and vincristine. | *Side effects:*<br>• DLT: Leukopenia and thrombocytopenia are expected.<br>• Urine can be pink to red for 48 hours after administration.<br>• Nausea can be mild to moderate and preventable with standard antiemetic.<br>• Diarrhea and mucositis can occur.<br>• Alopecia occurs gradually.<br>• Cumulative cardiomyopathy and CHF can occur with large cumulative doses. |

| | | | |
|---|---|---|---|
| | • Metabolized in the liver to the active form.<br>• t½ = 13–26 hours | | |
| **IFOSFAMIDE (Ifex)** | | | |
| *Dosage:*<br>• IV: 1.0–1.2 g/m²/day over a 5-day period q 3–4 weeks. Higher doses of 2.5–3.7 g/m²/day over a 2- to 3-day period.<br>• Mesna at a dose of 20% of the ifosfamide dose is given just prior to the ifosfamide and q 4 hours for 2 more doses. Mesna may be given IV or PO.<br>*Efficacy:*<br>• Testicular cancer<br>• Soft tissue sarcoma<br>• Hodgkin's and non-Hodgkin's lymphoma<br>• Acute leukemias<br>• Ewing's sarcoma<br>• Osteosarcoma | *Mechanism of action:*<br>• Ifosfamide is an alkylating agent. It is a prodrug and requires activation in the liver by microsomal enzymes.<br>*Metabolism:*<br>• Metabolized by the liver to inactive metabolites.<br>• 15%–56% of the drug is excreted unchanged in the urine.<br>• Drug elimination may be hindered by renal dysfunction.<br>• t½ = 7–15 hours | *Administration precautions:*<br>• Ifosfamide is administered over at least 30 minutes with aggressive hydration to reduce the incidence of hemorrhagic cystitis.<br>• The uroprotectant mesna is also given either as a continuous infusion or in divided doses q 4 hours × 3 doses.<br>• Ifosfamide and mesna are compatible and can be infused concurrently when high-dose ifosfamide is given. | *Side effects:*<br>• Myelosuppression is dose limiting.<br>• WBC nadir usually occurs 7–10 days posttreatment.<br>• Urinary tract toxicity is a DLT and is manifested as hemorrhagic cystitis. Patients may complain of dysuria and frequency 2–3 days after the infusion. Encourage PO intake of 2–3 L per day prior to and after dosing. Encourage patients to empty their bladders every 2–3 hours.<br>• Nausea and vomiting are common with higher doses. Symptoms are preventable with serotonin antagonist therapy.<br>• Avoid sedation with neurotoxic drugs that can exacerbate the lethargy and confusion that can occur due to the accumulation of chloracetylaldehyde, a metabolite with neurotoxic properties.<br>• Alopecia is more common with higher doses and occurs usually within 3 weeks of therapy. |
| **IRINOTECAN (Camptosar, CPT-11)** | | | |
| *Dosage:*<br>• 125–150 mg/m² IV over 90 minutes weekly × 4 weeks q 6 weeks<br>*Efficacy:*<br>• Adenocarcinoma<br>• Colon/rectal cancer | *Mechanism of action:*<br>• Topoisomerase I inhibitor.<br>• Blocks DNA and RNA synthesis in dividing cells.<br>*Metabolism:*<br>• Metabolized to its active form in liver.<br>• 20% drug excreted in the urine.<br>• 30% excreted in bile.<br>• t½ = 6–10 hours | *Administration precautions:*<br>• Dilute in 5% dextrose: stable for 24 hrs at room temperature.<br>• Drug is an irritant. | *Side effects:*<br>• Dose-limiting toxicities are diarrhea and myelosuppression.<br>• Loperamide is administered for diarrhea.<br>• Flushing and diaphoresis may occur during infusion.<br>• Moderate to severe nausea and vomiting may occur. |

(Continued)

**Intravenous Chemotherapy Agents (*Continued*)**

| Dosage and Efficacy | Mechanism of Action and Metabolism | Administration Precautions | Side Effects |
|---|---|---|---|
| | | **IXABEPILONE (Ixempra)** | |
| *Dosage:*<br>• 40 mg/m$^2$ IV over 3 hours every 3 weeks<br>• Dose-reduce if elevated ALT, AST, bilirubin<br>*Efficacy:*<br>• Breast cancer, refractory to an anthracycline and taxane | *Mechanism of action:*<br>• Microtubule inhibitor, preventing mitosis and causing cell death<br>• Semisynthetic analogue of epothilone B<br>• Activity in taxane, anthracycline, and vinca alkaloid-resistant tumors<br>*Metabolism:*<br>• Extensively metabolized in the liver via isoenzyme CYP3A4<br>• Excreted primarily in feces and to a lesser degree in the urine | *Administration precautions:*<br>• Do not administer if ANC < 1500 cells/mm$^3$ or platelet count < 100,000 cells/mm$^3$ or if bilirubin > 1 times ULN or AST or ALT > 2.5 times ULN<br>• Administered with capecitabine<br>• Assess for presence, progression of sensory peripheral neuropathy prior to each dose.<br>• Premedicate patient to prevent HSR reaction with $H_1$ (eg, diphenhydramine) and $H_2$ (eg, ranitidine) receptor antagonists. | *Side Effects*<br>• Neutropenia<br>• Thrombocytopenia<br>• Anemia<br>• Sensory peripheral neuropathy<br>• Fatigue, asthenia<br>• Myalgia, arthralgia<br>• Alopeica<br>• Nausea, vomiting<br>• Stomatitis, mucositis<br>• Diarrhea<br>• Musculoskeletal pain |
| | | **L-ASPARAGINASE (Elspar; Erwinia Asparaginase)** | |
| *Dosage:*<br>• Used in combination with other drugs in ALL 200 IU/day for 28 days, 1000 IU/kg × 10 days or<br>• 20,000 IU/m$^2$/week<br>*Efficacy:*<br>• ALL | *Mechanism of action:*<br>• Inhibits protein synthesis.<br>*Metabolism:*<br>• Biphasic elimination.<br>• Binds to vascular binding sites.<br>• May be eliminated by the liver.<br>• t½ = 4–9 hours and 1.4–1.8 days | *Administration precautions:*<br>• Dilute in NS or sterile water.<br>• Use within 8 hours.<br>• Refrigerate before and after reconstitution.<br>• Do not infuse through a filter.<br>• IV slow push over 30 minutes, or IM.<br>• Do not use if solution is cloudy.<br>• Skin test with 2 IU intradermal at least 1 hour prior to dosing.<br>• Administer subsequent doses with caution despite negative skin test. | *Side effects:*<br>• Anaphylactic reactions can occur in 20%–35% of patients.<br>• Monitor closely with appropriate support.<br>• IM use is associated with delayed allergic response.<br>• If HSR occurs, the Erwinia preparation may be used with prophylactic premedication.<br>• Urticarial eruptions are common.<br>• Incidence of reactions increases with each subsequent dosing.<br>• Slight anemia can occur; leukopenia is rare.<br>• Malaise, anorexia, nausea, and vomiting occur frequently.<br>• Hepatic toxicity is uncommon.<br>• Lethargy, somnolence, disorientation, and loss of recent memory occur with higher doses. |
| | | **MECHLORETHAMINE HYDROCHLORIDE (Nitrogen Mustard, Mustargen)** | |
| *Dosage:*<br>• IV: 6 mg/m$^2$ on days 1 and 8<br>• Topically 10 mg/60 mL ointment<br>*Efficacy:*<br>• Hodgkin's disease<br>• CML<br>• Lymphosarcoma | *Mechanism of action:*<br>• Alkylating agent results in abnormal base pairing, causing DNA miscoding, cross-linking of DNA, and strand breakage.<br>• Cell cycle nonspecific.<br>*Metabolism:*<br>• Rapidly deactivated in the blood.<br>• t½ = 15 minutes | *Administration precautions:*<br>• Once reconstituted with sterile water or NS the drug should be used within 60 minutes because of its instability.<br>• Nitrogen mustard should be administered by IV push via a freely running IV line.<br>• Administering nitrogen mustard via direct IV push technique can cause venous thrombosis and pain. | *Side effects:*<br>• Myelosuppression is the DLT.<br>• Leukopenia occurs 8–14 days following treatment. Severe thrombocytopenia may occur.<br>• Severe nausea and vomiting within 1 hour of IV administration. Patients should be premedicated with aggressive antiemetic therapy.<br>• Alopecia is common.<br>• A metallic taste is common during the injection and can be masked by encouraging the patient to chew gum or bite on a lemon rind. |

| | | | |
|---|---|---|---|
| | | • Nitrogen mustard is a severe vesicant and must be given with extreme caution.<br>• Assess for a blood return every 1 mL of injection.<br>• If extravasation occurs, inject a solution of sodium thiosulfate (1/6 molar) into the area to neutralize the drug.<br>• For 1 mg of nitrogen mustard infiltrated, inject 2 mL of the 10% thiosulfate solution.<br>• Preparation: 4 mL sodium thiosulfate injection (10%) diluted with 6 mL of sterile water for injection. | • Amenorrhea and impaired spermatogenesis occurs and is dose dependent. |
| **MELPHALAN (Alkeran, L-PAM, L-Phenylalanine Mustard)** | | | |
| *Dosage:*<br>• IV: 16 mg/m$^2$ q 3 weeks × 4 doses then q 4 weeks<br>• PO: 2 mg/kg/day × 5 days q 4–6 weeks<br>• BMT: 50–60 mg/m$^2$ IV<br>*Efficacy:*<br>• Multiple myeloma<br>• Epithelial carcinoma of the ovary<br>• BMT | *Mechanism of action:*<br>• Alkylating agent; cycle specific.<br>• Forms DNA cross-links.<br>*Metabolism:*<br>• 80%–90% of the drug is bound to plasma proteins.<br>• 10%–15% of the drug is eliminated unchanged in the urine.<br>• t½ = 1.5–4.0 hours | *Administration precautions:*<br>• Reconstitute with 10 mL of supplied diluent for a concentration = 5 mg/mL.<br>• Dilute in NS to a concentration of 0.45 mg/mL and use within 60 minutes.<br>• Do not refrigerate reconstituted product.<br>• When taken orally, peak plasma levels are reached within 2 hours. The drug is poorly absorbed when taken with food. | *Side effects:*<br>• Myelosuppression is dose limiting.<br>• GI: Mild anorexia, nausea, and vomiting when taken orally. Nausea and vomiting can be severe with higher IV doses.<br>• Mucositis, diarrhea, and oral ulceration occur infrequently.<br>• Leukopenia and thrombocytopenia peak at 2–3 weeks and may be cumulative with a prolonged recovery period of 6 or more weeks.<br>• Pruritus, dermatitis, and rash may occur.<br>• Alopecia is not common with oral dosing.<br>• Amenorrhea and oligospermia are common.<br>• Second malignancies (leukemias) have been reported. |
| **METHOTREXATE (MTX, Mexate, Amethopterin)** | | | |
| *Dosage:*<br>• IV Low: 10–50 mg/m$^2$<br>• IV Med: 100–500 mg/m$^2$<br>• IV High: 500 mg/m$^2$ and above with leucovorin rescue<br>• IT: 10–15 mg/m$^2$ in 7–15 mL of preservative-free saline<br>• IM: 25 mg/m$^2$<br>*Efficacy:*<br>• Trophoblastic neoplasms<br>• Acute leukemias | *Mechanism of action:*<br>• MTX tightly binds to dihydrofolate reductase, thereby blocking the reduction of dihydrofolate to tetrahydrofolic acid, the active form of folic acid. This process effectively arrests<br>• DNA, RNA, and protein synthesis.<br>• Antimetabolite.<br>• Cell cycle specific for the S phase. | *Administration precautions:*<br>• Lower doses (< 100 mg) are usually given IVP without leucovorin rescue<br>• When given with 5-FU for breast cancer, the MTX dose is followed in 1 hour by the 5-FU. The drugs are synergistic when given this way.<br>• Leucovorin rescue is needed because the dose of MTX is generally > 100 mg. | *Side effects:*<br>• Myelosuppression is dose limiting. Leukopenia is dose dependent and is more likely to occur with prolonged exposure.<br>• Nausea and vomiting are common with higher doses. Diarrhea can be dose limiting.<br>• Stomatitis is more common with higher doses and more lengthy infusions.<br>• Skin erythema, hyperpigmentation, photosensitivity, rash, folliculitis, and pruritus may occur. MTX can cause enhanced radiation side effects if given simultaneously. |

(Continued)

**Intravenous Chemotherapy Agents (*Continued*)**

| Dosage and Efficacy | Mechanism of Action and Metabolism | Administration Precautions | Side Effects |
|---|---|---|---|
| **METHOTREXATE (MTX, Mexate, Amethopterin)** (*Continued*) | | | |
| • Meningeal leukemias<br>• Carcinoma of the breast<br>• Osteogenic sarcoma<br>• Burkitt's lymphoma<br>• Hodgkin's disease<br>• Lung cancer<br>• CNS metastasis | *Metabolism:*<br>• MTX is distributed freely in water, which means that it will circulate in third-space fluid, increasing the toxicity of the drug since it is not being metabolized. Patients with effusions or ascites should be monitored carefully to avoid severe toxicity.<br>• MTX is highly protein bound and should not be given with acids that may compete for binding (elimination) sites, which would increase the AUC of the MTX, resulting in extreme toxicity.<br>• 90% of MTX is eliminated from the kidneys in the urine as unchanged drug.<br>• BUN and creatinine levels should be monitored regularly. If there is evidence of renal impairment, lower doses should be given with leucovorin rescue. | • Preservative-free MTX used for intrathecal injection should be prepared just prior to use.<br>• Protect infusions from light. | • Renal dysfunction is dose related and more common in patients who are dehydrated. When given in higher doses, the patient's urine pH must be > 7 to prevent precipitation of the MTX in the renal tubules, with subsequent renal damage. Administer sodium bicarbonate as directed. The BUN and creatinine are monitored prior to high-dose therapy.<br>• Neurological dysfunction can occur with IT administration, especially if cranial radiation has also been given.<br>• Photophobia, excessive lacrimation, and conjunctivitis have been noted. |
| **MITOMYCIN (Mutamycin, Mitomycin C)** | | | |
| *Dosage:*<br>• 20 mg/m$^2$ as a single dose repeated q 6–8 weeks<br>• IV: 2 mg/m$^2$ q day 5 days × or 5–20 mg/m$^2$ q 6–8 weeks<br>• Bladder instillation: 20–60 mg (1 mg/mL)<br>*Efficacy:*<br>• Adenocarcinoma of the stomach, pancreas<br>• Cancer of the bladder, breast | *Mechanism of action:*<br>• Antitumor antibiotic.<br>• Cell cycle specific.<br>• Active during the G and S phases of the cell 1 cycle.<br>• Disrupts DNA synthesis secondary to alkylation.<br>*Metabolism:*<br>• Mitomycin is inactivated by microsomal enzymes in the liver and is metabolized in the spleen and kidneys. | *Administration precautions:*<br>• Reconstitute in sterile water: 10 mL in 5 mg vial = 0.5 mg/mL. Use within 3 hours.<br>• Mitomycin is a severe vesicant. Administer with caution.<br>• Give IV push through the side arm of a freely running IV to minimize venous irritation. Assess for a blood return every 1 mL of drug. Discontinue the injection immediately if the patient complains of pain or burning. | *Side effects:*<br>• Myelosuppression is dose limiting.<br>• Leukopenia and thrombocytopenia occur late at 4–5 weeks with recovery at 7–8 weeks. Both are cumulative.<br>• Anemia and hemolytic-uremic syndrome have been reported.<br>• Nausea and vomiting are mild.<br>• Alopecia is mild; photosensitivity, skin rash, and pruritus are uncommon.<br>• VOD of the liver with abdominal pain, hepatomegaly, and liver failure occur in patients receiving mitomycin and BMT.<br>• Pulmonary fibrosis has been reported. |

| | | | |
|---|---|---|---|
| | • 10%–30% of the drug is eliminated unchanged in the urine.<br>• t½ = 0.5–1.0 hour | • Mitomycin can cause tissue damage without evidence of drug infiltration.<br>• Skin ulceration may occur at sites distant from the site of drug administration. | |
| **MITOXANTRONE (Novantrone)** | | | |
| *Dosage:*<br>• 10–12 mg/m$^2$/day × 5 days for induction of acute nonlymphocytic leukemia; 12 mg/m$^2$ q 3–4 weeks<br>*Efficacy:*<br>• Acute monocytic leukemia<br>• AML<br>• Acute promyelocytic leukemia<br>• Breast cancer<br>• Primary hepatocellular carcinoma | *Mechanism of action:*<br>• Antitumor antibiotic.<br>• Intercalates into DNA; disrupts cell division.<br>*Metabolism:*<br>• Metabolized in the liver and excreted in the bile and urine.<br>• t½ = 24–37 hours | *Administration precautions:*<br>• Dark blue solution in vials.<br>• Dilute in at least 50 mL D5W or NS.<br>• Stable for 7 days at room temperature.<br>• Administer IV over at least 5 minutes as an infusion. | *Side effects:*<br>• Leukopenia is dose limiting.<br>• Nausea and vomiting are mild and preventable.<br>• Alopecia is common.<br>• Diarrhea and stomatitis may occur.<br>• Cumulative cardiomyopathy can occur. Monitoring the left ventricular MUGA is indicated, especially in patients who are at risk for heart disease or who have received doxorubicin in the past.<br>• Blue discoloration of the sclera may occur. The urine may remain blue-green for 48 hours following treatment. |
| **OXALIPLATIN (Eloxatin)** | | | |
| *Dosage:*<br>• 85 mg/m$^2$ infusion q 2 weeks. (Given in combination with 5-FU/leucovorin)<br>*Dose Reductions:*<br>• Persistent grade 2 neuropathies: 65 mg/m$^2$<br>• Grade 3 neuropathy: Discontinue oxaliplatin<br>• Grades 3–4 GI toxicity: 65 mg/m$^2$<br>• Grades 3–4 hematological toxicity: 65 mg/m$^2$<br>*Efficacy:*<br>• Advanced colon or rectal cancer | *Mechanism of action:*<br>• Cell cycle nonspecific.<br>• Inhibits DNA replication and transcription.<br>*Metabolism:*<br>• Renal excretion is the major route of elimination.<br>• Rapid and extensive nonenzymatic biotransformation. | *Administration precautions:*<br>• Premedication with antiemetics, including 5HT, blockers with dexamethasone is recommended.<br>• Prehydration is not required.<br>• Eloxatin should not be given to patients with an allergy to platinum compounds.<br>• Never reconstitute or dilute with sodium chloride-containing solutions.<br>• Stable at room temperature for 6 hours at room temperature and 24 hours under refrigeration.<br>• Administered over 2 hours in 250-500 mL of D5W. Dilute in 500 mL if infusion pain is experienced. This drug is a severe irritant.<br>• Flush the infusion line with D5W before and after the administration of 5-FU due to incompatibility issues.<br>• Do not use aluminum needles with this drug. | *Side effects:*<br>• Neuropathy (acute and chronic persistent) are the dose-limiting toxicities. Baseline and ongoing neurological function assessment is critical.<br>• Pharyngolaryngeal dysesthesia is seen in 1%–2% of patients. This side effect is usually worse with exposure to cold.<br>• Pulmonary fibrosis has been reported and presents with unexplained respiratory symptoms.<br>• Fatigue, nausea, vomiting, diarrhea, and bone marrow suppression are commonly seen.<br>• Anaphylactic-like reactions have been reported and may occur within minutes of administration. Emergency medications including epinephrine, corticosteroids, and antihistamines should be readily available. |

(Continued)

Intravenous Chemotherapy Agents (*Continued*)

| Dosage and Efficacy | Mechanism of Action and Metabolism | Administration Precautions | Side Effects |
|---|---|---|---|
| | | **PACLITAXEL (Taxol)** | |
| *Dosage:*<br>• 200–250 mg/$m^2$ q 3 weeks or in heavily pretreated patients<br>• 135–175 mg/$m^2$ q 3 weeks or weekly in divided<br>Doses<br>*Efficacy:*<br>• Ovarian carcinoma<br>• Breast cancer<br>• Non-small cell lung cancer<br>• Head and neck cancer | *Mechanism of action:*<br>• Promotes assembly of microtubules and stabilizes them, thereby blocking mitosis.<br>• Paclitaxel also prevents transition of the cell from G0 phase to S phase by blocking cellular response to growth factors.<br>*Metabolism:*<br>• The majority of paclitaxel is protein bound.<br>• Elimination is primarily hepatic; minimal renal excretion.<br>• t½ = 1.3–8.0 hours | *Administration precautions:*<br>• Formulated in 50% polyoxyethylated castor oil (Cremophor EL) and 50% dehydrated alcohol.<br>• Administer only in glass bottles or non-PVC containers (polyolefin containers using polyethylene-lined nitroglycerin tubing sets).<br>• Cremophor-containing solutions will leach the plasticizer DEHP from PVC containers. DEHP can cause liver toxicity.<br>• Inline filtration is needed (0.02 μm) due to the natural origins of the drug.<br>• Administration rate varies from 1-3 hours to 24–96 hours. In general, the longer the infusion, the more likely the patient will experience myelosuppression that is dose limiting<br>• HSRs can occur with paclitaxel infusion and are thought to be related to the Cremophor EL. Patients are premedicated with dexamethasone 20 mg at 13 and 7 hours prior to treatment, with diphenhydramine 50 mg IV 30 minutes prior, and with an $H_2$ blocker (cimetidine 300 mg or Pepcid 20 mg) 30 minutes prior.<br>• When administering paclitaxel with doxorubicin, the doxorubicin is given first; likewise, when paclitaxel is given with cisplatin or carboplatin, the paclitaxel is given first to avoid disruption in the elimination of the platinum compound and enhanced toxicity.<br>• Synergistic with herceptin. | *Side effects:*<br>• HSRs occur infrequently with proper premedication. Most HSRs occur within the first or second dosing. Symptoms include dyspnea, urticaria, flushing, and hypotension.<br>• DLT: myelosuppression.<br>• Leukopenic nadir occurs 7–10 days after dosing, with recovery at 15 days. Anemia and thrombocytopenia occur less frequently.<br>• Peripheral neuropathy occurs more commonly in patients who are also receiving cisplatin. Hyperesthesias and burning pain in the feet may also occur.<br>• Myalgias and arthralgias occur usually 3–4 days after dosing.<br>• Alopecia is complete at 3 weeks<br>• Mucositis occurs more commonly with prolonged infusions.<br>• Nausea and vomiting are mild.<br>• Diarrhea occurs infrequently.<br>• Paclitaxel is an irritant but can cause blistering and skin breakdown if large amounts of more concentrated drug are infiltrated. |

| PACLITAXEL PROTEIN-BOUND PARTICLES FOR INJECTABLE SUSPENSION (Abraxane, nab-paclitaxel) | | | |
|---|---|---|---|
| *Dosage:*<br>• 260 $mg/m^2$ IV over 30 minutes, repeated every 3 weeks; alternative schedules are 100–125 mg IV weekly or on days 1, 8, and 15 of a 28-day cycle<br>• Dose-reduce for nadir neutopenia or severe neuropathy<br>*Efficacy:*<br>• Breast cancer refractory to combination chemotherapy | *Mechanism of action*<br>• Promotes early microtubule assembly and prevents deploymerization, so cells cannot move from G2 to M phase, and the cell dies<br>*Metabolism*<br>• Highly protein bound<br>• Metabolized by liver isoenzymes, including CYP3A4<br>• Excreted in the feces and urine<br>• More rapid and extensive distribution into tissues and longer half-life than paclitaxel | *Administration precautions:*<br>• Drug is a milky-white suspension<br>• Administer only if baseline ANC > 1500 cells/$mm^3$<br>Drug is an irritant<br>• Drug interactions include St. John's wort, drugs metabolized by the CYP2C8 and CYP3A4 isoenzymes; do not coadminister<br>• No premedication for hypersensitivity is required because drug is cremaphor-free | *Side effects:*<br>• Neutropenia<br>• Rare thrombocytopenia<br>• Sensory neuropathy, reversible<br>• Ocular and visual disturbances<br>• Rare hypotension, arrhythmia<br>• Alopecia<br>• Nausea, vomiting<br>• Diarrhea<br>• Mucositis<br>• Hepatotoxicity |
| **PEMETREXED (Alimta)** | | | |
| *Dosage:*<br>• 500 $mg/m^2$ IV (21-day cycle)<br>*Efficacy:*<br>• Malignant pleural mesothelioma | *Mechanism of action:*<br>• Disrupts the folate-dependent metabolic process essential for cell replication.<br>*Metabolism:*<br>• Eliminated by renal excretion.<br>• Elimination $t\frac{1}{2}$ = 3.5 hours | *Administration precautions:*<br>• To prevent skin rash, administer dexamethasone 4 mg po BID on the day before, day of, and day after treatment.<br>• Reconstitute in 20 mL of 0.9% NS (incompatible with diluents containing calcium). Then dilute in 100 mL of 0.9% NS and infuse over 10 minutes, then wait 30 min before infusing cisplatin at the standard rate.<br>• Administer folic acid daily of 350 ug to 1000-ug PO beginning 1 week prior to treatment, and continuing throughout and after treatment to reduce toxicity.<br>• One week prior to treatment, give 1000 ug IM injection of vitamin B12 and q 3 cycles thereafter.<br>• Stable for up to 24 hours at room temperature. | *Side effects:*<br>• Contraindicated in patients whose creatinine clearance < 45 mL/minutes.<br>• Nausea, vomiting, BMS, fatigue, stomatitis, pharyngitis, anorexia, and rash were commonly reported.<br>• Conduct periodic blood tests to evaluate renal and hepatic function.<br>• Exercise caution when administering concurrently with NSAIDs to patients with creatinine clearance < 80 mL/minutes. |

(Continued)

Intravenous Chemotherapy Agents (*Continued*)

| Dosage and Efficacy | Mechanism of Action and Metabolism | Administration Precautions | Side Effects |
|---|---|---|---|
| | | **TENIPOSIDE (Vumon, VM-26)** | |
| *Dosage:*<br>• 100 mg/m$^2$ 1–2 times weekly and 20–60 mg/m$^2$ × 5 days or 90 mg/m$^2$/day × 5 days for lung cancer<br>*Efficacy:*<br>• Relapsed or refractory acute lymphoblastic leukemia<br>• Small cell lung cancer | *Mechanism of action:*<br>• Plant alkaloid, topoisomerase II inhibitor.<br>• Phase specific, acts in late S phase and early G2 phase.<br>*Metabolism:*<br>• Bound to plasma protein; metabolized in the liver with less than 10% of the unchanged drug in feces.<br>• Eliminated in the urine.<br>• t½ = 20 hours | *Administration precautions:*<br>• Dosage is diluted in sodium chloride and is physically stable for approximately 24 hours at room temperature in glass containers. Drug may precipitate in plastic containers.<br>• Administer over at least a 45-minutes period to avoid severe hypotension.<br>• Avoid extravasation.<br>• Local phlebitis may occur.<br>• HSRs occur and include blood pressure changes, bronchospasm, tachycardia, urticaria, facial flushing, diaphoresis, periorbital edema, vomiting, and/or fever. | *Side effects:*<br>• Leukopenia is the DLT occurring at 10–14 days.<br>• Nausea and vomiting are rare.<br>• Alopecia occurs gradually.<br>• Skin rash is rare.<br>With high-dose therapy, severe skin rashes can occur.<br>• Hemolytic anemia with renal failure has occurred.<br>• HSR may be related to the Cremophor EL vehicle.<br>• Secondary malignancies occur infrequently.<br>• Hyperbilirubinemia, SGOT, and SGPT elevations can occur. |
| | | **THIOTEPA (Thioplex)** | |
| *Dosage:*<br>• 12-16 mg/m$^2$ q 1–4 weeks<br>• 900 mg/m$^2$ (transplant dose)<br>• 30–60 mg q week × 4 weeks for intravesicular use<br>• 1.0-10 mg/m$^2$ 1–2 times per week for IT use<br>*Efficacy:*<br>• Breast cancer<br>• Ovarian cancer<br>• Superficial bladder cancer<br>• Lymphoma<br>• Hodgkin's disease | *Mechanism of action:*<br>• An alkylating agent similar to nitrogen mustard<br>*Metabolism:*<br>• Variably absorbed through the bladder mucosa following intravesical injection.<br>• Metabolized in the liver.<br>• t½ = 2–3 hours | *Administration precautions:*<br>• 15-mg vial is reconstituted with 1.5 mL of sterile water and further diluted with saline for IT use (preservative free).<br>• IV and intravesical solutions may be diluted with saline, D5W, or lactated Ringer's solution and are chemically stable for at least 5 days in the refrigerator and 24 hours at room temperature.<br>• Intravesical instillation involves placement of a catheter in the bladder and instillation of the drug with retention of the liquid for up to 2 hours. The patient is repositioned q 15 minutes to maximize exposure to the tissues of the bladder.<br>• IT doses are mixed in up to 20 mL of Ringer's lactate to maximize CNS distribution.<br>• IV administration may be given IVP or as an infusion. Thiotepa is not a vesicant. | *Side effects:*<br>• Myelosuppression is the DLT and may be cumulative.<br>• Leukopenia occurs 7–10 days postinjection.<br>• Thrombocytopenia may be delayed.<br>• Nausea and vomiting are not common in nontransplant doses.<br>• Stomatitis may be severe in transplant doses.<br>• Abdominal pain, hematuria, dysuria, frequency, and urgency occur with intravesical instillation.<br>• Second malignancies have been reported. |

| | | | |
|---|---|---|---|
| **TOPOTECAN (Hycamtin)** | | | |
| *Dosage:*<br>• 1.3–1.6 $mg/m^2$ IV infusion over 30 minutes, 2 hours, or 24 hours<br>OR<br>• 1.5-2.0 $mg/m^2$/day as a 30-minutes infusion × 5 Days<br>*Efficacy:*<br>• Small cell lung cancer<br>• Ovarian cancer<br>• Esophageal cancer | *Mechanism of action:*<br>• Topoisomerase I inhibitor causes single-strand breaks in DNA, causing the cell to die during DNA replication.<br>*Metabolism:*<br>• Up to 48% of the drug is eliminated unchanged in the urine.<br>• t½ = 3 hours | *Administration precautions:*<br>• 5-mg vial is reconstituted with 2 mL of sterile water and diluted in D5W.<br>• Stable for up to 48 hours at room temperature.<br>• Given intravenously as an infusion. | *Side effects:*<br>• Leukopenia is dose limiting, and the nadir occurs at days 10-12 with recovery at 3 weeks.<br>• Thrombocytopenia and anemia occur but are not usually dose limiting.<br>• Mild to moderate nausea and vomiting may occur.<br>• Diarrhea has been reported to occur during or shortly after the infusion.<br>• Fever and mild flulike symptoms are reported.<br>• Alopecia and skin rash may occur.<br>• Elevated LFTs are common.<br>• Headache, dizziness, lightheadedness, and peripheral neuropathy have been reported. |
| **VINBLASTINE (Velban)** | | | |
| *Dosage:*<br>• 6–10 $mg/m^2$ q 2–4 weeks; 1.7-2.0 $mg/m^2$/day weekly as a continuous infusion or over a period of 96 hours<br>*Efficacy:*<br>• Hodgkin's disease<br>• Non-Hodgkin's lymphoma<br>• Testicular cancer<br>• Kaposi's sarcoma<br>• Breast cancer<br>• Melanoma<br>• Cancers of the kidney, bladder, and cervix<br>• Head and neck cancers<br>• Lung cancer<br>• Ovarian cancer | *Mechanism of action:*<br>• Cell cycle phase specific for the M phase.<br>• A plant alkaloid that binds to tubulin causing inhibition of the microtubule assembly, which inhibits mitotic spindle formation.<br>*Metabolism:*<br>• Metabolized by the liver.<br>• Less than 1% is eliminated unchanged in the urine.<br>• t½ = 20 hours | *Administration precautions:*<br>• Reconstituted with 10 mL of bacteriostatic NS to yield a concentration of 1 mg/mL.<br>• Dose may be further diluted with D5W or NS for continuous infusion.<br>• Continuous infusions may only be given through central lines because vinblastine is a severe vesicant if infiltrated.<br>• Store in the refrigerator. Stable for 14 days at room temperature and for 30 days under refrigeration. | *Side effects:*<br>• Leukopenia is dose limiting.<br>• Thrombocytopenia and anemia are less common.<br>• Nausea and vomiting, anorexia, diarrhea, and mucositis are rare.<br>• Peripheral neuropathy, constipation, paralytic ileus, and urinary retention may occur.<br>• Alopecia occurs with higher doses.<br>• Rash and photosensitivity may occur.<br>• Infiltration may cause ulceration depending on the amount of drug extravasated.<br>• Treatment with hyaluronidase and heat may minimize ulceration.<br>• Incompatible with heparin and furosemide.<br>• Compatible in solution with doxorubicin, metoclopramide, dacarbazine, and bleomycin. |

(Continued)

**Intravenous Chemotherapy Agents (*Continued*)**

| Dosage and Efficacy | Mechanism of Action and Metabolism | Administration Precautions | Side Effects |
|---|---|---|---|
| | | **VINCRISTINE (Oncovin)** | |
| *Dosage:*<br>• 0.5–1.4 mg/m$^2$ q 1–4 weeks<br>• Continuous infusion regimens of 0.5 mg/day to 0.5 mg/m$^2$/day × 4 days may be used.<br>*Efficacy:*<br>• Acute leukemia<br>• Hodgkin's disease<br>• Non-Hodgkin's lymphoma<br>• Rhabdomyosarcoma<br>• Neuroblastoma<br>• Wilms' tumor<br>• Ewing's sarcoma<br>• Melanoma<br>• Multiple myeloma<br>• Breast cancer<br>• Lung cancer | *Mechanism of action:*<br>• Plant alkaloid<br>• Binds to tubulin, causing inhibition of microtubule assembly, which inhibits mitotic spindle formation.<br>• M phase specific.<br>*Metabolism:*<br>• Metabolized by the liver.<br>• 40%–70% excreted in the bile.<br>• t½ = 70–100 hours | *Administration precautions:*<br>• Store in the refrigerator.<br>• Stable for at least 30 days at room temperature.<br>• Doses for continuous infusion are further diluted with NS or D5W.<br>• Compatible with doxorubicin, bleomycin, cytarabine, fluorouracil, methotrexate, and metoclopramide.<br>• Vincristine is a vesicant that should be given with caution and through a central line when given as a continuous infusion.<br>• Hyaluronidase plus heat to disperse the antidote are indicated if the drug should infiltrate.<br>• Greater than 2 mg total dose is usually contraindicated due to the toxicity of the drug.<br>• Vincristine is lethal if given intrathecally and should be labeled as such when dispensed by the pharmacist.<br>• Administer with caution in patients with obvious liver dysfunction. | *Side effects:*<br>• Myelosuppression is mild.<br>• Nausea, vomiting, anorexia, and diarrhea are rare.<br>• Constipation and abdominal pain may occur due to the neurological toxicity of the drug.<br>• Prophylactic stool softeners and laxatives may be indicated in patients at high risk for constipation.<br>• Alopecia is minimal.<br>• Paresthesias, ataxia, hoarseness, myalgias, headache, and seizures may occur.<br>• Severe pain in the jaw may occur. |
| | | **VINORELBINE TARTRATE (Navelbine)** | |
| *Dosage:*<br>• PO: 40-mg capsule for PO use<br>• IV: 30–40 mg/m$^2$ weekly<br>*Efficacy:*<br>• Breast cancer<br>• Ovarian cancer<br>• Head and neck cancer<br>• Esophageal cancer<br>• Non-small cell lung cancer<br>• Lung cancer<br>• Germ cell cancers | *Mechanism of action:*<br>• Cell cycle specific.<br>• Produces cell blockade in G2 and M phases.<br>• Blocks polymerization of microtubules.<br>• Impairs mitotic spindle.<br>*Metabolism:*<br>• Hepatic elimination.<br>• Binds to plasma proteins.<br>• Nonrenal elimination. | *Administration precautions:*<br>• Venous irritation occurs in about 25% of patients. Symptoms include erythema and pain at the site, vein discoloration, and tenderness along the vein.<br>• Administer drug over 6–10 minutes through the side arm of a freely running IV. Inject through the port farthest from the IV site.<br>• Follow injection with 75–125 mL of IV fluid to flush the line (peripheral IV sites only). | *Side effects:*<br>• DLT: Noncumulative neutropenia<br>• Alopecia/hair thinning after several treatments<br>• Anorexia<br>• Asthenia<br>• Peripheral neuropathy<br>• Constipation occurs in about one-third of patients and increases after several treatments<br>• Fatigue can be cumulative<br>• Arthralgias and myalgias<br>• Rash (rare)<br>• Typhlitis with abdominal pain and fever occur 3–4 days after treatment in heavily pretreated patients. |

| | | |
|---|---|---|
| | • Local tissue damage/necrosis, phlebitis may occur if the drug infiltrates.<br>• Dose reduction may be appropriate for patients with impaired liver function. If bilirubin is > 2.1, the dose of vinorelbine is reduced 50%–75% (ie, 15 to 7.5 mg/m$^2$).<br>• Pain at the tumor site can occur during administration.<br>• Vinorelbine is compatible with metoclopramide, ondansetron, chlorpromazine, promethazine, and dexamethasone.<br>• Vinorelbine is incompatible with 5-FU, thiotepa, furosemide, amphotericin, ampicillin, piperacillin, aminophylline, and sodium bicarbonate. | • Jaw pain is rare. |

*Abbreviations*: ALL, acute lymphocytic leukemia; AML, acute myelogenous leukemia; ANC, absolute neutrophil count; APL, acute promyelocytic leukemia; AUC, area under the curve; BMT, bone marrow transplant; BMS, bone marrow suppression; CHF, congestive heart failure; CI, continuous infusion; CNS, central nervous system; D5W, 5% dextrose in water; DLT, dose-limiting toxicity; EKG, electrocardiogram; 5-FU, 5-fluorouracil; 5HT3, serotonin receptor; G, gram; GI, gastrointestinal; HSR, hypersensitivity reaction; IM, intramuscular; IP, intraperitoneal; IT, intrathecal; IV, intravenous; IVP, intravenous push; IU, International unit; L, liter; LFT, liver function test; MI, myocardial infarction; MUGA, multigated acquisition scan; NS, normal saline; PML-RAR alpha, promyelocytic-retinoic acid receptor-alpha; PO, oral; PVC, polyvinyl chloride; QS, quantity sufficient; RT, radiation therapy; SC, subcutaneous; SIADH, syndrome of inappropriate antidiuretic hormone; SGOT, serum glutamic oxaloacetic transaminase; SGPT, serum glutamic pyruvic transaminase; SQ, subcutaneous; t½, half-life; U, unit; ULN, upper limit of normal; VOD, veno-occlusive disease; WBC, white blood count.

CHAPTER

17

Dawn Camp-Sorrell, RN, MSN, FNP, AOCN®

# Chemotherapy Toxicities and Management

## INTRODUCTION

Chemotherapy is administered based on a dose-response relationship (ie, the more drug administered, the more cancer cells killed). Characteristically, chemotherapeutic drugs have a narrow therapeutic index, with anticipated acute toxicities expressed in rapidly dividing normal tissues, such as bone marrow, the gastrointestinal tract, the gonads, and hair follicles. Acute and long-term toxicities from chemotherapy may also be a function of the drug's effect on specific cells of a given organ. The incidence and severity of toxicities are related to the drug's dosage, administration schedule, specific mechanism of action, as well as concomitant illness and specific measures used to prevent or minimize toxicities. Chemotherapeutic drugs cause side effects that can appear immediately or after a few days (acute), within a few weeks (intermediate), or months to years after chemotherapy administration (long-term).[1]

Because virtually every organ is affected by chemotherapy, the toxicities of the drug will commonly determine the maximum amount of drug that can be safely administered. Side effects such as stomatitis, alopecia, myelosuppression, nausea, vomiting, anorexia, and diarrhea are common, depending on the drug administered. These expected side effects can be managed effectively and generally do not warrant discontinuing the drug. *Toxic effects* refers to life-threatening, often dose-limiting effects that are characteristic of high dosages. Cumulative and irreversible damage to certain vital organs, such as the heart, limits the total dosage of chemotherapy.[2]

## PRETREATMENT EVALUATION: RISK ANALYSIS

Individuals with an overall weak physical condition and poor nutritional status are not likely to tolerate an intensive chemotherapy treatment regimen.[3] Patients previously treated with multiple chemotherapy drugs, radiation, or biotherapy may lack marrow reserve, placing them at a higher risk for infection, bleeding, or anemia. The inability or unwillingness of an individual to perform self-care may increase the severity of a side effect and delay the seeking of appropriate care from healthcare professionals.

Preexisting disorders such as hepatic or renal dysfunction can alter the absorption, distribution, metabolism, and excretion of chemotherapy, causing abnormal accumulations of the drug and its metabolites.[4] Hypovolemia due to nausea and vomiting, diarrhea, inadequate dietary intake, third spacing (a shift of fluid from the vascular space to the interstitial space), or hypoalbuminemia may increase the risk of acute renal failure. Thus, the patient could be placed at a higher risk for organ toxicities.

Because the incidence of cancer increases with age, nurses must be aware of possible additional treatment risks for the elderly. Age-related changes in physical stature, body composition, liver, kidneys, and other organs influence the pharmacokinetic and pharmacodynamic properties of chemotherapy, possibly prolonging the drug's half-life.[4] Many elderly people, especially those older than 85 years, are physically frail secondary to chronic and debilitating illness or poor nutrition or as a result of aging. Chronic illnesses such as arthritis, heart disease, diabetes, glaucoma, high blood pressure, cognitive deficits, and hearing and vision loss are common in the elderly.[4] These conditions may interfere with an individual's ability to perform basic activities of daily living. Consequently, elderly patients may be unable to perform preventive measures to minimize side effects from chemotherapy.

Gradual but substantial changes occur in body composition with age. The percentage of body fat increases with age. Decreases occur in cardiac output, kidney function, hepatic blood flow, the ability to conjugate drugs, and the effectiveness of the immune system.[4] Cardiovascular changes may include thickening of blood vessel walls, atherosclerotic plaque formation, and loss of elastin fibers. These can lead to cardiac hypertrophy, diastolic dysfunction, and myocardial ischemia.[4] With an advancing in age, the kidneys' atrophy bring subsequent decrease in renal function. Vasoconstriction of the renal vasculature decreases renal blood flow, glomerular filtration rate, and the ability to concentrate and dilute urine, resulting in a decreased creatinine clearance.[5] Bone marrow reserves decline and the ability to replicate myeloid and erythroid progenitor cells decreases. In addition, the functional ability of peripheral mononuclear cells is impaired.[4–8]

Historically, elderly patients (over 60 years) with cancer have not been treated as aggressively as their younger counterparts because it was speculated that the elderly would not be able to tolerate the side effects of chemotherapy. This trend is changing, however, and many elderly patients now receive aggressive treatment for their cancer.[6] Numerous studies have looked at the consequences of treating older patients with chemotherapy.

In general, for many solid tumors, elderly patients tolerate chemotherapy, used for either adjuvant or palliative therapy. Geriatric patients with a systemic malignancy such as lymphoma or acute leukemia usually develop more treatment-related toxicity than younger patients. Nevertheless, geriatric patients can achieve complete response from chemotherapy if they survive the intensive initial therapy.[8]

While it is critical to be knowledgeable regarding the potential problems the elderly may encounter as a consequence of physiologic aging, age alone has not been shown to be a significant factor in the incidence and severity of toxicity to chemotherapy.[4–8] Chronic illness that often accompanies longevity is a better predictor for tolerance than age alone. The one exception has been hematologic toxicity, which is probably related to decreased marrow reserve or renal function. Healthcare professionals, therefore, should monitor hematologic values closely to minimize potential ill effects. Patients older than 70 years with normal renal and hepatic function and without serious comorbid illnesses have been found to tolerate chemotherapy as well as individuals in younger populations.[4,5,7,8]

## QUALITY OF LIFE AND CHEMOTHERAPY TOXICITY

Treatment considerations include the patient's quality of life, the impact chemotherapy will have on the patient's quality of life, and the patient's physical and mental wellbeing.[9] Complications or side effects from chemotherapy are weighed against its potential antineoplastic benefits. In the past, cancer treatment was evaluated by tumor response and survival rates rather than by functional ability or quality of life.[10] Quality of life is based on the physical, psychological, social, and spiritual characteristics of what gives value in life to the individual.[10] It is recognized as an acceptable end point in clinical trials, which have been influenced by viewing cancer as a chronic condition instead of as an acute event. Cancer survivors have indicated to the healthcare community that quality of life is as important to the patient as the overall physical therapeutic effect.[11]

Physical symptoms (eg, pain, rashes, nausea, stomatitis) can result in significant distress that has a marked impact on the patient's quality of life.[12] It is important to realize that the patient's perception of cancer and chemotherapy treatment will influence how the individual reacts and ultimately adapts.[12] Side effects can impair a person's abilities to function at work or at home, maintain sexual relationships, and engage in social activities. The degree of self-reported symptoms relates to the individual's perceived quality of life, such as when an increase in symptoms correlates with a decrease in quality of life.[10–12] Feelings of helplessness are heightened because patients are dependent on healthcare professionals to deliver their treatment. Anxiety can develop at key decision points, such as diagnosis, beginning of treatment, while awaiting test results, when the treatment plan is altered, or when the chemotherapy treatment plan has been successfully completed.[9] Chemotherapy-related changes in physical appearance are often described as a distressing aspect of cancer treatment. Weight changes and alopecia commonly occur and can be especially devastating because they are physical manifestations of having cancer.[10,12]

In an effort to minimize acute and chronic toxicities, chemoprotectant agents are being developed to improve the patient's quality of life.[13,14] Agents can be given prior to the chemotherapy to decrease the incidence of the expected toxicity, such as amifostine to minimize nephrotoxicity. Other agents, such as growth factors, are given concurrently or after the chemotherapy cycle to enhance the development of normal cells, such as pegfilgrastim that stimulates neutrophil growth. Rescue agents, such as leucovorin, are given after methotrexate to help minimize acute reactions.[13]

To help the patient cope with potential side effects, it is critical to foster a trusting relationship with the patient so that communication is open and sufficient information can be provided to help the patient retain control. An important aspect of establishing a partnership with the patient and family in the pretreatment phase is knowing what concerns about the treatment need to be explored and what information needs to be provided. Such information helps patients formulate questions about available options when making difficult decisions about their care. When participating actively, the patient's feelings of control are enhanced, resulting in an improved functional status, sense of well-being, and performance of effective self-care.[15]

Patients with cancer experience a variety of distressing symptoms that usually begin prior to diagnosis and continue throughout the course of the disease and treatment. These symptoms adversely affect the patient's quality of life. Symptom clusters are defined as a group of 3 or more symptoms occurring together during cancer treatment.[12] It may be difficult to ascertain the etiology of a symptom cluster when these symptoms occur from combination treatment or from the cancer itself. For instance, a patient with esophageal cancer can experience nausea from radiation, surgical resection, or from chemotherapy. Multiple symptoms may have a more negative effect on a patent's quality of life than the experience of a single symptom.[10]

The importance of recognizing symptom clusters cannot be underestimated. Patients who experience numerous and severe symptoms experience significant decline in function compared to those with limited mild symptoms.[10] When the patient experiences multiple symptoms, each symptom will have a synergistic effect on other symptoms. Thus, by controlling one symptom, there is a potential that the other symptoms can be controlled as well.

## SELF-CARE

There is undeniable evidence that cost factors are dictating the administration of health care. Institutional, state, and federal regulatory bodies have assumed increasing jurisdiction over how and where patients will be treated. Diagnostic-related groups (DRGs) and prospective payment, cost-control measures by other insurers, and increased out-of-pocket medical expenses for consumers have all combined to create a shift from hospital-based care to outpatient and home care settings.[15] The change from inpatient to outpatient administration of chemotherapy shifts the responsibility for managing the treatment of side effects from healthcare providers to patients and their families. To facilitate self-care, nurses must understand the nature, incidence, and relative severity of each side effect, and be aware of effective self-care activities for reducing the severity of side effects.

With increasing severity of a side effect, patients may become more immobilized and may delay initiating self-care behaviors for several days. Therefore, it is critical that follow-up by the nurse be initiated within 1 to 3 days after chemotherapy to assess the patient and to determine whether side effects are being managed adequately. Patient education is essential to ensure that the patient and family understand what self-care measures need to be taken for the side effects experienced.[16] A key goal of nursing care is to minimize toxicity.

*Self-care* is any activity initiated by patient, family, or friends to alleviate or minimize a side effect.[15] Self-care activities begin before treatment and continue throughout the treatment phase to manage or minimize side effects. In situations where patients are unable or unwilling to participate, efforts must be made to include family members or visiting nurses to ensure compliance. Without compliance, the side effects can be severe and may lead to further complications, which may result in hospitalization and possibly even death. Side effects that seem to be the most distressing to patients include fatigue, nausea, vomiting, alopecia, anorexia, and mouth sores.[10] Documenting strategies that have been successful, including those suggested by the patient, can serve as a useful resource for future patient instruction.

## PATIENT EDUCATION AND FOLLOW-UP

The intent of teaching is more than simply giving information: it provides support and knowledge to empower the patient to manage self-care effectively.[16] Teaching patients about their treatment reduces fear, increases self-confidence, improves compliance, and enhances their participation in self-care.[16]

One approach to identifying the informational needs of the patient and family members is to focus on the various phases of cancer care: diagnosis, treatment, rehabilitation, survivorship, and recurrent disease. Goals of chemotherapy teaching include the following:

1. Helping the patient adjust to the treatment
2. Explaining how the treatment will affect the cancer
3. Discussing the sequence of administration
4. Recognizing and controlling side effects
5. Encouraging self-care behavior that minimize side effects
6. Listing side effects that should be reported to the health-care professional.

All information offered to the patient is documented in the patient's record (Figure 17-1) for future reference as well as to comply with professional regulations. It is important to reinforce teachings periodically, as retention without reinforcement may be short-lived.

In the outpatient setting, the nurse frequently screens phone calls and triages the patient to assist in evaluating symptoms and initiating the appropriate treatment measures. The nurse must gather sufficient data to determine whether the patient needs medical intervention and, if so, whether the patient will be cared for most appropriately in the outpatient setting or in the hospital. The nurse needs to be knowledgeable about what the patient's history is, when the last chemotherapy treatment took place, and whether this complaint is related to the treatment, is related to the disease, or is unrelated.

Objective and subjective data must be gathered methodically to formulate an opinion about the patient's experience. After consulting with the physician or advanced practice nurse, the nurse once again speaks to the patient, either to gather more information or to relay instructions to the patient or family regarding care. Examples of specific phone-triage flowcharts are included in the discussion of various chemotherapy side effects later in this chapter.

Traditionally, oncology nurses have taught patients about intravenous (IV) chemotherapy, yet this role is changing to include the administration of oral drugs. Numerous oral drugs are available, with many in clinical trials. Oral drugs provide many advantages such as patient convenience, less time away from work and family, and the elimination of the need for IV access. Yet this shift to oral drugs has created many challenges for the nurses, including patient compliance, self-assessment, management of side effects, and cost. Patient compliance is a significant concern with adherence rates to taking oral drugs for cancer being estimated at 50%, which clearly demonstrates the need for patient education. For improvement of adherence to oral drugs, patient education is imperative to reinforce follow-up visits for laboratory evaluations, reassessment, and consideration for dose adjustments.[17]

## CHEMOTHERAPY TOXICITIES

### GRADING OF TOXICITIES

Standardization of assessment and documentation of side effects are crucial in evaluating the therapeutic use of chemotherapy. Specific therapies can be assessed by comparing their benefits with toxicity occurrence. In the recognition and evaluation of toxicities, one must discriminate between an expected reaction and a toxic reaction to chemotherapy; and distinguish these from complications related to the cancer. For example, if a patient with lymphoma presents to the clinic with a complaint of paresthesias, numbness, and tingling, he or she must be evaluated for possible spinal cord compression from tumor progression and for peripheral toxicity from vincristine administration.

Using specific parameters and operational definitions to define the degree of a given toxicity ensures consistency in documenting observed reactions (Table 17-1). Toxicity grading scales have been developed by the World Health

## CHEMOTHERAPY TEACHING CHECKLIST

Patient name: ______________________

Primary nurse: ______________________

Assessment Summary:

______________________

______________________

______________________

______________________

______________________

Drugs:

______________________

______________________

| LEARNING NEED | TEACHING INITIATED (DATE & INITIALS) | KNOWLEDGE CONFIRMED (DATE & INITIALS) | COMMENTS |
|---|---|---|---|
| 1. Patient education booklets/drug cards | | | |
| 2. Viewed chemotherapy video/DVD/computer program Other: | | | |
| 3. Common side effects and treatment | | | |
| a. Nausea and vomiting — antiemetics | | | |
| b. Stomatitis — mouth care | | | |
| c. Alopecia — wigs/scarves/hats | | | |
| d. Decreased white blood cells — infection precautions | | | |
| e. Decreased red blood cells — fatigue/SOB* | | | |
| f. Decreased platelets — bleeding precautions | | | |
| g. Skin and nail bed changes | | | |
| h. Loss of appetite — nutrition | | | |
| i. Diarrhea — medication/diet | | | |
| j. Constipation — diet/medication | | | |
| k. Flu-like symptoms | | | |
| l. Urine discoloration | | | |
| m. Hemorrhagic cystitis—hydration | | | |
| n. Premedications (chemoprotectants, steroids, etc.) | | | |
| o. Cold-induced neuropathy | | | |
| p. Other | | | |
| 4. Specific teaching | | | |
| a. Subcutaneous injections | | | |
| b. Maintaining adequate nutrition | | | |

*SOB = Shortness of breath

**FIGURE 17-1**

Chemotherapy teaching checklist.

(Continued)

| LEARNING NEED | TEACHING INITIATED (DATE & INITIALS) | KNOWLEDGE CONFIRMED (DATE & INITIALS) | COMMENTS |
|---|---|---|---|
| c. Precautions to report during drug administration: | | | |
| (1) Stinging, burning pain | | | |
| (2) Flushing of face | | | |
| (3) Metallic taste | | | |
| (4) Feeling of numbness | | | |
| (5) Itching at site (or generalized itching) | | | |
| (6) Allergic reactions | | | |
| d. Reproductive changes<br>(1) Dyspareunia<br>(2) Menopausal symptoms<br>(3) Vaginal discomfort | | | |
| e. Activity | | | |
| f. Interaction with other drugs/food | | | |
| g. Vascular access device | | | |
| h. Perineal burning (Decadron) | | | |
| i. Peripheral edema | | | |
| 5. Symptoms to report to physician and/or advanced practice nurse | | | |
| a. Bleeding | | | |
| b. Prolonged nausea or vomiting | | | |
| c. Fever/chills | | | |
| d. Stomatitis | | | |
| e. Diarrhea/constipation | | | |
| f. Numbness or tingling of extremities | | | |
| g. Difficulty breathing or shortness of breath | | | |
| h. Other | | | |
| 6. Prescriptions given to patient with Instructions: ☐ Antiemetics ________________<br>☐ Wig ☐ Blood counts ☐ Other | | | |
| 7. Schedule/calendar of drug treatment | | | |
| 8. Instructions to obtain blood counts | | | |
| 9. Follow-up or referral to community resources | | | |

Comments: ____________________________________________

____________________________________________

____________________________________________

____________________________________________

Patient signature: ____________________________________________

RN signature: ____________________________________________

**FIGURE 17-1**

Chemotherapy teaching checklist.

**TABLE 17-1**

**Grading Toxicities from Chemotherapeutic Agents**

| Toxicity | Grade 0 | Grade 1 | Grade 2 | Grade 3 | Grade 4 |
|---|---|---|---|---|---|
| | | | **HEMATOLOGIC** | | |
| WBC (1000/mm³) | ≥ 4.0 | 3.0–3.9 | 2.0–2.9 | 1.0–1.9 | < 1.0 |
| Granulocytes (1000/mm³) | ≥ 2.0 | 1.5–1.9 | 1.0–1.4 | 0.5–0.9 | < 0.5 |
| Platelets (1000/mm³) | ≥ 100 | 75–99 | 50–74 | 25–49 | < 25 |
| Hemoglobin (g/100 mL) | ≥ 11 | 9.5–10.9 | 8.0–9.4 | 6.5–7.9 | <6.5 |
| Hemorrhage | None | Slight, no transfusion | Mild, 1–2 transfusions/episode | Gross, 3–4 transfusions/episode | Massive, > 4 transfusions/episode |
| Infection/fever | None | Temp: <38°C<br>No antibiotics | Temp: 38–40°C<br>Broad spectrum antibiotics | Temp: > 40°C<br>Antifungal coverage | Signs of sepsis: reevaluate medication |
| | | | **GASTROINTESTINAL** | | |
| Nausea/vomiting | None | Slight nausea, 1 episode of vomiting<br>Maintains intake | Occasional nausea, 2–5 episodes of vomiting<br>Maintains intake | Frequent nausea, 6–10 episodes of vomiting<br>Intake decreased | Constant nausea, > 10 episodes of vomiting<br>No intake |
| Diarrhea | None | 2–3 stools | 4–6 stools<br>Moderate cramps | 7–9 stools<br>Severe cramps | > 10 stools; needs rehydration |
| Constipation | None | Dry, hard passage of painful stool<br>Stool softener | No stool > 2 days laxatives | No stools > 4 days<br>Rule out obstruction or cause | — |
| Stomatitis | None | Painless ulcers, erythema, or mild soreness | Painful erythema, edema, or ulcers, but can eat | Painful erythema, edema, ulcers, cannot eat | Requires parenteral or enteral support |
| Esophagitis/Dysphagia | None | Painless ulcers, erythema, mild soreness or dysphagia | Painful erythema, edema, ulcers, or moderate dysphagia, but can eat without narcotics | Cannot eat solids, or requires narcotics to eat | As above or complete obstruction or perforation |
| Taste | Normal | Slightly altered taste, metallic taste | Markedly altered taste | — | — |
| | | | **DERMATOLOGIC** | | |
| Skin | None | Scattered macular or papular eruption or erythema; asymptomatic | Scattered macular or papular eruption, or erythema with pruritus or other associated symptoms | Generalized symptomatic macular, papular, or vesicular eruption | Exfoliative dermatitis or ulcerating dermatitis |
| Local | None | Pain | Pain and swelling with inflammation or phlebitis | Ulceration | Plastic surgery indicated |
| | | | **OTHER** | | |
| Myalgia/arthralgia | None | Mild | Decrease in ability to move | Disabled | — |

*Abbreviation*: Temp, temperature; WBC, white blood cell.

Organization, National Cancer Institute, and various cooperative study groups to provide consistency in reporting. Adequate assessment and documentation of the side effect experienced, patient's overall response to the regimen, and subsequent quality of life can be essential for evaluating the impact of treatment. Decisions regarding the need for appropriate adjustments in the treatment plan can be determined on the basis of sound, objective data documented by the nurse.[12,18]

Specific guidelines need to be taught and given in written form to the patient and caregiver to ensure that they report any type of toxicity. Misinterpretation of a patient's report can negatively affect changes made in the treatment protocol. Nurses will continue to be challenged to design effective assessment and documentation systems that ensure accurate patient observation and reporting of toxicities, especially in the home setting.

## SYSTEMIC TOXICITIES

### Bone marrow suppression

Myelosuppression is the most common dose-limiting side effect of chemotherapy and can be the most lethal.[7,8] All hematopoietic cells divide rapidly, regardless of their developmental stage, and are therefore vulnerable to the effects of chemotherapy. Proliferating progenitor cells that produce mature granulocytes, erythrocytes, and thrombocytes in the peripheral circulation are commonly destroyed by such treatment. As immature cells in the marrow and preexisting mature cells are destroyed, the nadir becomes apparent, usually 7 to 14 days after chemotherapy. At the same time, cells in the bone marrow are maturing and are ready to be released into the peripheral blood. Within a short period of time (3–4 weeks), the nadir will resolve.[19] However, when high doses of chemotherapy are administered, the stem cell population may fail to repopulate quickly enough, resulting in a prolonged nadir period.

The majority of chemotherapy drugs cause some degree of myelosuppression.[19] Agents most active against cells that are cycling or those active during a specific phase of the cell cycle can produce rapid cytopenia. Because alkylating agents and nitrosoureas affect both cycling cells and noncycling cells, these drugs are more likely to destroy the marrow stem cells. Antimetabolites, vinca alkaloids, and antitumor antibiotics are most damaging to cells that are in a specific phase of the cell cycle; thus, myelosuppression is less severe with these agents.[19] However, dose intensification and drug combinations can produce severe and prolonged neutropenia. For many drugs, myelosuppression can be the dose-limiting toxicity, especially for newer agents such as oxaliplatin, pemetrexed, decitabine, and gemcitabine.[20–22] Paclitaxel can cause neutropenia, with the severity depending on the dose, administration schedule, extent of previous treatment, and pharmacologic exposure to the drug. The neutropenic effect is not cumulative, and permanent toxicity does not occur to the bone marrow. Gemcitabine can cause myelosuppression, especially thrombocytopenia. The hematologic toxicity has been found to be cumulative with the maximum tolerated dose of 1500 mg/m$^2$/week over a 30 minute infusion. Docetaxel results in an early, short-duration type of neutropenia at a dose of 100 mg/m$^2$ or greater when infused over 1 hour every 3 weeks. The nadir usually occurs at day 8 and resolves in 1 to 2 weeks, which has not been found to be a cumulative effect. Oxaliplatin generally produces mild neutropenia and thrombocytopenia when given as a single agent. When oxaliplatin is administered in combination with 5-fluorouracil (5-FU) and leucovorin, myelosuppression can be a primary toxicity.[20]

Risk factors such as tumor cells in the bone marrow, prior treatment with chemotherapy or radiation, and a high negative nitrogen balance will compromise the marrow and increase the degree and duration of cytopenia.[19] It has been recognized that an increased risk of infection occurs among individuals suffering from protein-calorie malnutrition, which causes lymphopenia, diminished levels of the complement system, and decreased levels of certain immunoglobulins. In addition, myelotoxicity caused by chemotherapy and radiation therapy is enhanced by protein deprivation resulting from cancer cachexia. Younger patients are less likely to demonstrate severe cytopenia due to chemotherapy because their marrow is more cellular and has a decreased percentage of fat.

*Anemia.* Differences in the lengths and kinetics of the life cycles of particular blood cells account for the frequency of neutropenia, thrombocytopenia, and anemia. Maturation of cells in the bone marrow takes 8 to 10 days, with variation in the life span for each cell type. Red blood cells (RBCs) have a life span of 120 days. Chemotherapy-induced anemia occurs less frequently because the bone marrow begins to recover before the number of circulating RBCs decreases significantly. Although low hemoglobin and low hematocrit levels do not prevent administration of chemotherapy, low levels will affect how the patient feels and functions. Anemia is manifested by pallor, hypotension, headaches, irritability, and fatigue. Tachycardia and tachypnea may be present due to the hypoxic effects on the heart. Secondary problems include skin or mucous membrane breakdown arising from decreased tissue oxygenation as well as cardiopulmonary stress. The incapacitating symptoms of anemia have a profound impact on quality of life.[23,24] Anemia can usually be corrected with RBC transfusion.

Anemia of chronic disease is associated with erythroid hypoplasia of the bone marrow in underlying disease processes such as cancer, rheumatoid arthritis, and chronic infectious diseases.[23] Erythroid hypoplasia results in a slight decrease in reticulocytosis, hypoferremia, and a decrease in serum erythropoietin. Additionally, chronic inflammation and release of cytokines such as tumor necrosis factor, interferon, and interleukin 1 suppresses the production of erythropoietin, resulting in decreased RBC production. Actions of certain chemotherapeutic agents such as cisplatin may inhibit the maturation of the erythroid lineage cells in the bone marrow.[19]

Erythropoietin can be administered in an attempt to correct anemia induced by chemotherapy. This growth factor promotes erythroid progenitor cells' proliferation and maintains their survival.[24] Epoetin alfa has been available as a growth factor for RBCs for more than a decade. Initially the usual dose is 150 μ/kg subcutaneously 3 times a week until the target hematocrit is reached. Weekly epoetin alfa administration at a dose of 40,000 μ to 60,000 μ is as effective compared to 3 weekly injections.[25]

Another erythropoietin compound, darbepoietin alfa, has a prolonged half-life and increased biologic activity.[23] With the increase in serum half-life, dosing is less frequent, offering greater patient convenience, improved patient compliance, and decreased demands on healthcare professionals. The initial dose for chemotherapy-induced anemia with darbepoietin alfa is 2.25 μ/kg every week or 500 μ SQ every 3 weeks.[19] If no response appears in 4 to 6 weeks, the dose can be increased to 300 μg. The most common side effects of both erythropoietin stimulators are hypertension and pain at the injection site; for this reason, the patient's blood pressure should be monitored frequently.[19] Patients with iron deficiency require iron supplementation because adequate iron stores are necessary to support erythropoiesis. Intravenous iron has been proposed as an adjunct to erythropoietin-stimulating agents (ESAs), which has significantly improved the hemoglobin of patients with chemotherapy-induced anemia.[26] Hemoglobin and hematocrit levels should be monitored prior to ESA therapy to ensure the correct dose and the need for an injection.

Recent studies have reported decreased survival for patients with cancer receiving ESAs for correction of anemia induced by chemotherapy.[27–29] Subsequently, guidelines were developed for the use of ESAs. Erythropoietin-stimulating agents therapy is an option for patients receiving chemotherapy who have symptoms of anemia with a hemoglobin level less than 11g/dl or patients without symptoms of anemia if the hemoglobin level less than 10g/dl. The purpose of administering ESA is to avoid RBC transfusion. Continued use of ESAs for chemotherapy-induced anemia is approximately 4 weeks after treatment completion.

Emerging safety concerns such as thrombosis, cardiovascular events, tumor progression, and reduced survival prompted The Center for Medicare and Medicaid Services to make reasonable and necessary determinations on all uses of ESAs.[30] Variation in the guidelines may exist among local carriers. Several carriers have determined that ESAs are not medically necessary in chemotherapy-induced anemia if the patient's cancer is deemed curable.[30]

*Thrombocytopenia.* The life span of platelets is 7 to 10 days. Thrombocytopenia usually occurs 8 to 14 days after chemotherapy administration—in most cases, concomitantly with neutropenia. Chemotherapy may be suspended if the platelet count drops below 50,000 to 75,000 cells/mm$^3$. Thrombocytopenia is a potential or actual dose-limiting toxicity of gemcitabine, carboplatin, dacarbazine, fluorourcil, lomustine, mitomycin-C, thiotepa, and trimetrexate. A cumulative and delayed onset of thrombocytopenia has been observed with carmustine, fludarabine, lomustine, mitomycin-C, streptozocin, and thiotepa. When platelet levels are less than 50,000 cells/mm$^3$, a moderate risk of bleeding exists. As the platelet level continues to decrease below 10,000 cells/mm$^3$, a severe risk exists for fatal gastrointestinal, central nervous system, and respiratory tract hemorrhage.[19] Manifestations of thrombocytopenia are easy bruising; bleeding from gums, nose, or other orifices; and petechiae on the upper and lower extremities, pressure points, elbows, and palate (Figure 17-2). Transfusion of platelets is a common therapeutic intervention for a platelet count less than 10,000 to 20,000 cells/mm$^3$, although this step is often dependent on whether the patient is bleeding.[31]

In an attempt to minimize the occurrence of chemotherapy-induced thrombocytopenia, interleukin 11 (IL-11) has been approved as a growth factor for megakaryocytes in patients with nonmyeloid malignancies and myelosuppressive chemotherapy regimens. Interleukin 11 causes proliferation of hematopoietic stem cells and megakaryocyte progenitors and also induces megakaryocytic maturation.[32] Interestingly, IL-11 causes this effect independently of thrombopoietin. The dose of IL-11 is 50 μ/kg administered daily subcutaneously until the platelet count is greater than 50,000 cells/mm$^3$.[19] Interleukin-11 is discontinued 2 days prior to the next chemotherapy treatment. Side effects from IL-11 are thought to occur secondary to an increase in intravascular fluid from renal sodium retention and plasma volume expansion and include dyspnea, edema, and an increase in pleural effusion formation.[31,33] As a consequence, patients with a history of congestive heart failure or coronary heart disease are usually not candidates for IL-11.

Newer thrombopoietic stimulating agents have been primarily studied in the management of benign hematologic disease such as immune thrombocytopenic purpura rather than chemotherapy-induced thrombocytopenia.[32,33] Drugs currently under evaluation include eltrombopag and AKD-501 (both oral agents) and a subcutaneously administered agent, AMG-531. These drugs are thrombopoietin-receptor agonists that stimulate proliferation and differentiation of megakarocytes and progenitor cells, thus increasing platelet production. With the preliminary results in hematologic disease, hopefully the benefit will be found in chemotherapy-induced thrombocytopenia.

*Neutropenia* The life span of the granulocyte or neutrophil is 6 to 8 hours after release from the marrow. Neutropenia

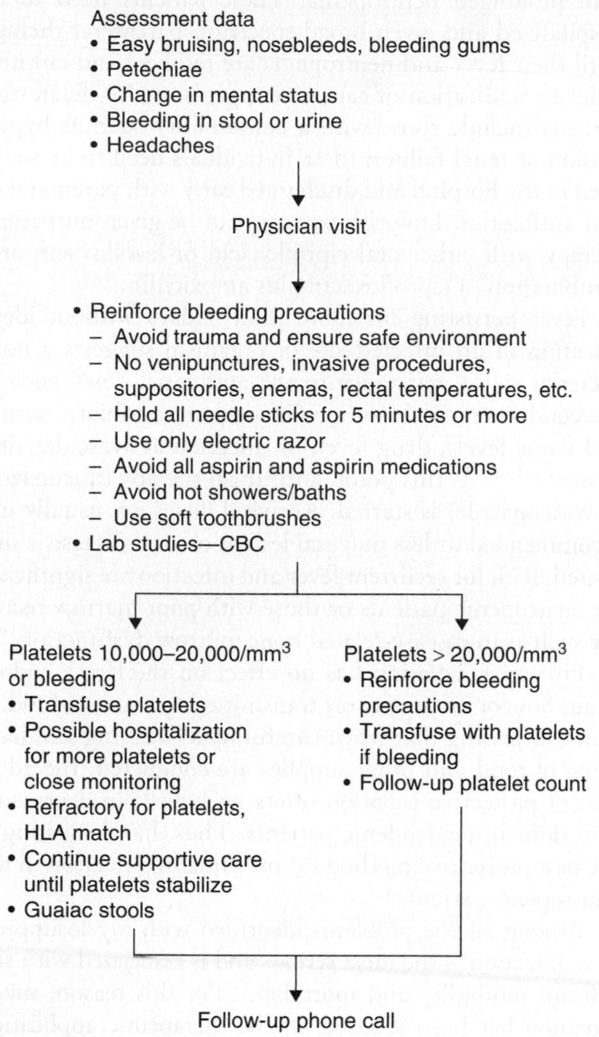
Assessment data
• Easy bruising, nosebleeds, bleeding gums
• Petechiae
• Change in mental status
• Bleeding in stool or urine
• Headaches
Physician visit
• Reinforce bleeding precautions
– Avoid trauma and ensure safe environment
– No venipunctures, invasive procedures, suppositories, enemas, rectal temperatures, etc.
– Hold all needle sticks for 5 minutes or more
– Use only electric razor
– Avoid all aspirin and aspirin medications
Avoid hot showers/baths
– Use soft toothbrushes
• Lab studies—CBC
Platelets 10,000–20,000/mm3 or bleeding
• Transfuse platelets
• Possible hospitalization for more platelets or close monitoring
• Refractory for platelets, HLA match
• Continue supportive care until platelets stabilize
• Guaiac stools
Platelets > 20,000/mm3
• Reinforce bleeding precautions
• Transfuse with platelets if bleeding
• Follow-up platelet count
Follow-up phone call

**FIGURE 17-2**

Thrombocytopenia telephone triage.

Abbreviations: CBC, complete blood count; HLA, human leukocyte antigen.

typically develops 8 to 12 days after chemotherapy, with recovery in 3 to 4 weeks. Chemotherapy is usually withheld if the patient's white blood cell (WBC) count is between 1000 and 3000 cells/mm$^3$ or if the absolute neutrophil count (ANC) is below 1500 cells/mm$^3$. Neutropenia generally is defined as an ANC less than 1500 cells/ mm$^3$. In normal individuals, neutrophils, including both the segmented and slightly less mature band forms, are found in concentrations ranging from 1830 to 7250 cells/mm$^3$. Profound neutropenia (grade 4) usually is defined as an ANC less than 500 cells/mm$^3$, and this places the patient at great risk for infection.[8,19,34,35]

It is important to note that neutropenia can occur when the total WBC count is within a normal range (4000–10,000 cells/mm$^3$). Consequently, quantifying the ANC is essential to achieve a correct assessment of neutrophil status. The ANC is calculated by multiplying the total WBC count by the differential proportion of combined band and segmented neutrophils in a blood sample:

$$\text{ANC} = \text{WBC (segmented neutrophils + band neutrophils)}$$

Thus, in a patient with a WBC count of 4000 cells/ mm$^3$, a differential of 34% segmented neutrophils plus 3% band neutrophils yields

$$\text{ANC} = 4000 \text{ cells/mm}^3 \times 0.37 = 1480 \text{ cells/mm}^3$$

The monocyte count should also be monitored because an increase in monocytes precedes and predicts resolution of neutropenia.

Because the major function of neutrophils is phagocytosis, neutropenia eliminates one of the body's prime defenses against bacterial infection. Infections, due to invasion and overgrowth of pathogenic microbes, increase in frequency and severity as the ANC decreases. In addition, risk for severe infections increases when the nadir persists for more than 7 to 10 days.[34]

Signs of an infection may not be apparent with the inhibition of phagocytic cells. The only response may be fever. It is estimated that 80% of the infections that occur arise from endogenous microbial flora of the gastrointestinal or respiratory tract.[19,36,37] When the neutrophil count is less than 500 cells/mm$^3$, approximately 20% or more of febrile episodes will have an associated bacteremia caused principally by aerobic gram-negative bacilli (eg, *Escherichia coli, Klebsiella pneumoniae, Pseudomonas aeruginosa*) and gram-positive cocci (coagulase-negative staphylococci, streptococci species, and *Staphylococcus aureus*).[38–40]

Chemotherapy-induced damage to the alimentary canal and respiratory tract mucosa facilitates the entry of infecting organisms; therefore, pneumonia and sinusitis are frequently seen. The nurse must assess for inflammation at the sites most commonly infected, including the lung, skin, anus, pharynx, perineum, periodontium, lower esophagus, and venous access exit sites. Prevention, early detection, good hand-washing technique, and prompt management of infections in patients with neutropenia are essential if sepsis and septic shock are to be avoided (Figure 17-3).[39,41]

Once appropriate cultures are obtained, broad-spectrum antibiotics are used to treat chemotherapy-induced infections (1) until cultures indicate eradication of the causative organism, (2) for a minimum of 7 days, or (3) until the neutrophil count is greater than 500/mm$^3$.[39,42] Extended-spectrum cephalosporins (ceftazidime or cefepime) and carbapenems (imipenem or meropenem) are the agents most often used for empiric monotherapy. Combination therapy with antipseudomonal third-generation cephalosporins and aminoglycosides or penicillin is generally used.[42] Other combinations include a β-lactam (ticarcillin plus clavulanate or pipercillin plus tazobactam) with an aminoglycoside (gentamycin or

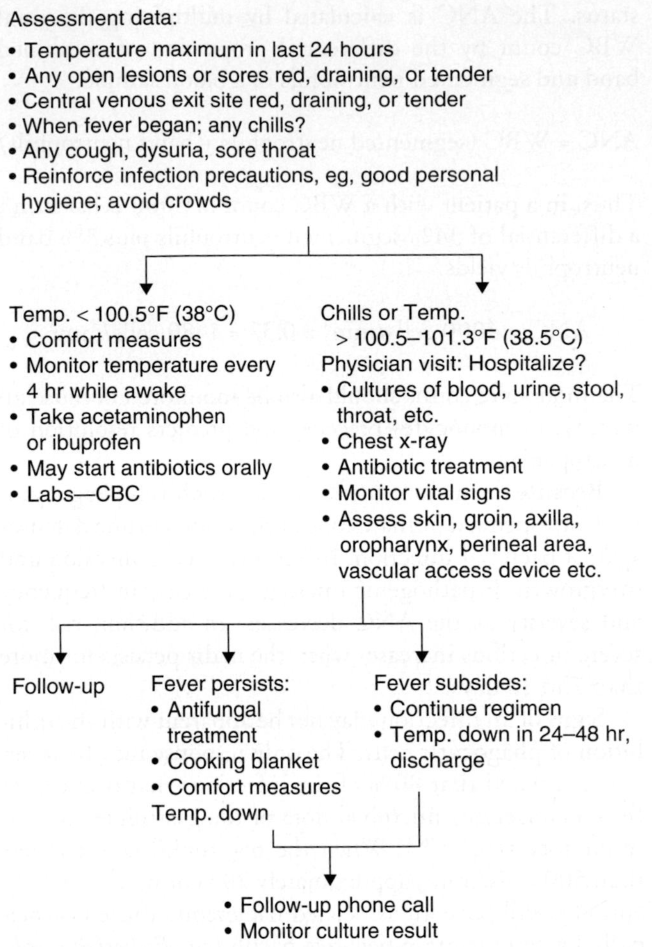
Assessment data:
• Temperature maximum in last 24 hours
• Any open lesions or sores red, draining, or tender
• Central venous exit site red, draining, or tender
• When fever began; any chills?
• Any cough, dysuria, sore throat
• Reinforce infection precautions, eg, good personal hygiene; avoid crowds
Temp. < 100.5°F (38°C)
• Comfort measures
• Monitor temperature every 4 hr while awake
• Take acetaminophen or ibuprofen
• May start antibiotics orally
• Labs—CBC
Chills or Temp. > 100.5–101.3°F (38.5°C)
Physician visit: Hospitalize?
• Cultures of blood, urine, stool, throat, etc.
• Chest x-ray
• Antibiotic treatment
• Monitor vital signs
• Assess skin, groin, axilla, oropharynx, perineal area, vascular access device etc.
Follow-up
Fever persists:
• Antifungal treatment
• Cooking blanket
• Comfort measures
Temp. down
Fever subsides:
• Continue regimen
• Temp. down in 24–48 hr, discharge
• Follow-up phone call
• Monitor culture result

**FIGURE 17-3**

Fever telephone triage flowchart.

tobramycin) or another β-lactam.[42] With the increased predominance of gram-positive organisms in febrile neutropenic patients, the use of vancomycin with an antipseudomonal β-lactam agent has been beneficial. Although effective, such combinations should not be prescribed routinely because of the potential for emergence of vancomycin-resistant organisms. Empiric use of vancomycin is recommended in patients known to be colonized with methicillin-resistant organisms, in patients with venous access devices, and in patients on quinolone prophylaxis with severe mucositis who are at risk for a streptococcal infection or positive blood cultures prior to susceptibility information.[42]

Until recently, all febrile neutropenic patients were treated with hospital-based parenteral antibiotics. Risk assessment is now used to determine the need for hospitalization and the most appropriate route of antibiotic therapy.[35,39,43] Neutropenia induced by solid tumor treatment usually lasts for less than 10 days, whereas neutropenia associated with hematologic malignancies often lasts for 15 to 20 days. High-risk patients include those with hematologic malignancies and stem cell transplant recipients with prolonged neutropenia. These patients need to be hospitalized and given broad-spectrum parenteral therapy until their fever and neutropenia are resolved and cultures indicate eradication of causative organisms. Moderate-risk patients include those with a comorbidity such as hypertension or renal failure; these individuals need to be stabilized in the hospital and discharged early with parenteral or oral antibiotics. Low-risk patients can be given outpatient therapy with either oral ciprofloxacin or levofloxacin or a combination of ciprofloxacin plus amoxicillin.[35,42,43]

Fever persisting for more than 3 days without identification of an infected site or organism suggests a nonbacterial cause, resistance to the antibiotic, emergence of a second bacterial infection, inadequate antibiotic serum and tissue levels, drug fever, or infection at avascular sites (abscess).[40,42] At this point, antifungal therapy (fluconazole or voriconazole) is started. Antiviral drugs are usually not recommended unless mucosal lesions or viral disease is suspected. Risk for recurrent fever and infection are significant for neutropenic patients or those with poor marrow recovery such as in disease-related bone marrow dysfunction.[38]

Protective isolation has no effect on the host's endogenous flora or on organisms transmitted by water or food. It is not surprising that when careful hand washing and handling of food and other supplies are conducted, the addition of protective isolation offers no benefit in decreasing infections in neutropenic patients. Thus, hand washing is the best preventive method for minimizing infection in the neutropenic patient.[41]

Among all the problems identified with myelosuppression, infection is the most serious and is associated with significant morbidity and mortality.[39] For this reason, much attention has been focused on the therapeutic application of recombinant colony-stimulating factors (CSFs) to augment neutrophil counts. Hematopoietic growth factors constitute a family of glycoprotein hormones that act as natural regulators of hematopoiesis to promote the proliferation and differentiation of hematopoietic progenitor cells along multiple pathways.[33,34,36] While hematopoietic stimulants have not changed the decline rate of granulocytes, they have shortened the duration of neutropenia, thereby dramatically reducing the morbidity and mortality from infections. Subsequently with the recovery of myelosuppression, full dosages of chemotherapy can be used in cancer therapy.

The National Comprehensive Cancer Network has developed clinical practice guidelines for appropriate use of CSFs.[3,19] After reviewing available research and literature, the following guidelines were developed to assist the practitioner in the use of CSFs. Begin by assessing for risk factors that can induce febrile neutropenia or other neutropenic events that can compromise treatment and can compromise treatment:

1. Patient risk factors comprise age greater than 65 years, female, performance status of 2 or higher, poor nutritional status, deceased immune function.

2. Comorbidities such as chronic obstructive pulmonary disease (COPD), cardiovascular disease, liver disease, or diabetes put patients at risk for neutropenic events.
3. Patients with treatment risk factors such as history of severe neutropenia with similar chemotherapy, type of chemotherapy used, planned dose of intensity, preexisting neutropenia, concurrent or prior radiation to marrow-containing bone.
4. Patients with cancer related risk such as bone marrow involvement with tumor, advanced cancer, blood-forming cancer, or lung cancer.

Inconclusive data exist on the use of CSFs with other conditions, especially febrile neutropenia. Although growth factors have made tremendous inroads on decreasing duration of neutropenia, thereby decreasing the incidence of infections, reduced efficacy occurs with multiple courses and with bone marrow depletion. Another limitation is that specific lineage growth factors may affect only a segment of one tissue compartment.[44] Three CSFs are approved to stimulate the production and activation of neutrophils.[44,45] The granulocyte colony-stimulating factor (G-CSF) recommended dose is 5 μg/kg/day for a maximum of 14 days. The granulocyte-macrophage colony-stimulating factor (GM-CSF) recommended dose is 250 $\mu g/m^2$/day for a maximum of 21 days. In general, these CSFs are initiated 24 hours after chemotherapy administration and are continued until the occurrence of an ANC greater than 10,000 cells/$mm^3$.[44] However, a shorter duration of CSF administration that is sufficient to achieve adequate neutrophil recovery is reasonable.[44,45]

Granulocyte colony-stimulating factor is available in a long-acting formulation for administration once per chemotherapy cycle.[45] Long-acting G-CSF (pegfilgrastim) is administered at a dose of 6 mg subcutaneously. This type of CSF appears to be self regulated, remaining in the blood until the postnadir ANC returns to normal. The serum concentration of the granulocyte CSF begins to decline at the onset of neutrophil recovery.[45] The most common side effects of all CSFs are mild to moderate bone pain and injection site irritation.

### Gastrointestinal tract

Chemotherapy-induced gastrointestinal toxicity can be the most devastating experience for the patient. Although numerous pharmacologic interventions have been developed to minimize these toxicities, their occurrence can lead to delay of treatment, fluid and electrolyte imbalances, weight loss, and malnutrition.

*Diarrhea.* Chemotherapy-induced diarrhea occurs due to a combination of factors, including an imbalance between absorption and secretion in the small bowel.[46–49] Diarrhea entails an increase in stool volume and liquidity, resulting in 3 or more bowel movements per day. Chemotherapy produces acute damage to the intestinal mucosa that is characterized by necrosis of the cells that line the intestinal crypt, resulting in extensive bowel wall inflammation. Without crypt cells, replacement of cells in the intestinal villi are hampered, resulting in a decreased absorptive surface. Because of the intestinal inflammation, factors such as prostaglandins and cytokines are secreted that further stimulate the secretion of intestinal fluids and electrolytes from crypt cells.[46,47,49,50]

The degree and duration of diarrhea depend on the agent, dose, nadir, and frequency of chemotherapy administration. Incidence and severity of diarrhea have increased with newer chemotherapy agents, adjunct therapies, and aggressive treatment approaches.[46] Alterations in mucosal integrity, coupled with the destruction of brush-border enzymes essential for carbohydrate and protein digestion, produce moderate to severe diarrhea immediately following chemotherapy and up to 14 days after chemotherapy. With fluorouracil and leucovorin therapy, patients may experience abdominal cramps and rectal urgency, which can evolve into nocturnal diarrhea or fecal incontinence leading to lethargy, weakness, orthostatic hypotension, and fluid and electrolyte imbalance. Without adequate management, prolonged diarrhea will cause dehydration, nutritional malabsorption, and circulatory collapse.[46,47,49,50]

Although fluorouracil is the chemotherapy drug that most commonly causes diarrhea, other agents potentially producing this effect include methotrexate, docetaxel, actinomycin D, doxorubicin, trimetrexate, irinotecan, arsenic trioxide, gefitinib, oxaliplatin, and capecitabine.[47] Combination chemotherapy and multimodal treatment can result in severe diarrhea. Antiemetics such as metoclopramide and prokinetic agents can cause diarrhea by increasing bowel transit time.[47]

Thorough evaluation to determine the cause of the diarrhea provides a firm foundation for planning interventions. Management may be limited to dietary measures, such as a low-residue, high-caloric, high-protein diet, increased fluid intake, or pharmacologic measures. Stool cultures need to be obtained initially to rule out an infectious process so that appropriate therapy can be implemented. *Clostridium difficile* has been reported in patients receiving chemotherapy who have had prior antibiotic exposure. Antidiarrheal agents should never be given to counteract diarrhea resulting from an infection, as these agents slow the passage of stool through the intestines, prolonging the mucosal exposure to the organism's toxins. When the diarrhea is a result of an infectious organism, it will typically resolve in a few days with the use of oral vancomycin or metronidazole.[51,52]

Pharmacologic interventions for diarrhea vary. Anticholinergic drugs such as atropine sulfate and scopolamine reduce gastric secretions and decrease intestinal peristalsis. Opiate therapy binds to receptors on the smooth muscle of bowel, slowing down the intestinal motility and increasing fluid absorption. Loperamide is a long-acting opioid agonist without central opioid activity. Although the recommendation is a maximum of 16 mg in 24 hours, an increase of the loperamide dose may be necessary to control irinotecan-induced diarrhea. Current recommendations for the use of loperamide for irinotecan-induced diarrhea are 4 mg initially followed by 2 mg every 4 hours until the diarrhea stops.[52] Diphenoxylate is an opiate analog that inhibits intestinal peristalsis. Because diphenoxylate has codeine-like properties, atropine has been added to decrease abuse. Atropine can be used alone in a dose of 0.25 mg to 1 mg prior to irinotecan. It is thought that irinotecan-induced diarrhea may be cholinergic mediated, thus atropine is beneficial in this setting in minimizing diarrhea.[52] Psyllium fiber supplementation has been found beneficial in treating chemotherapy-induced diarrhea. A dose of 1 to 2 teaspoons of psyllium fiber daily may help to decrease diarrhea.[52,53]

Octreotide acetate, a synthetic analog of the hormone octapeptide, inhibits the release of gut hormones, including serotonin and gastrin, from the gastrointestinal tract. It affects the gastrointestinal tract by prolonging intestinal transit time, increasing intestinal water and electrolyte transport, and decreasing mesenteric blood flow. Octreotide acetate is indicated for patients who have excessive diarrhea as a result of gastrointestinal resections or when other pharmacologic treatments have proved ineffective in managing chemotherapy-induced diarrhea.[54]

Chemotherapy usually is administered despite the occurrence of diarrhea. However, diarrhea can be severe enough to be a dose-limiting toxicity of some chemotherapeutic agents such as irinotecan, oxaliplatin, capecitabine, or combination therapy—specifically, fluorouracil and leucovorin. The nurse must carefully monitor the patient's status to provide appropriate therapy, such as antidiarrheal medications, fluid and electrolyte replacements, and perirectal care to prevent further complications (Figure 17-4).

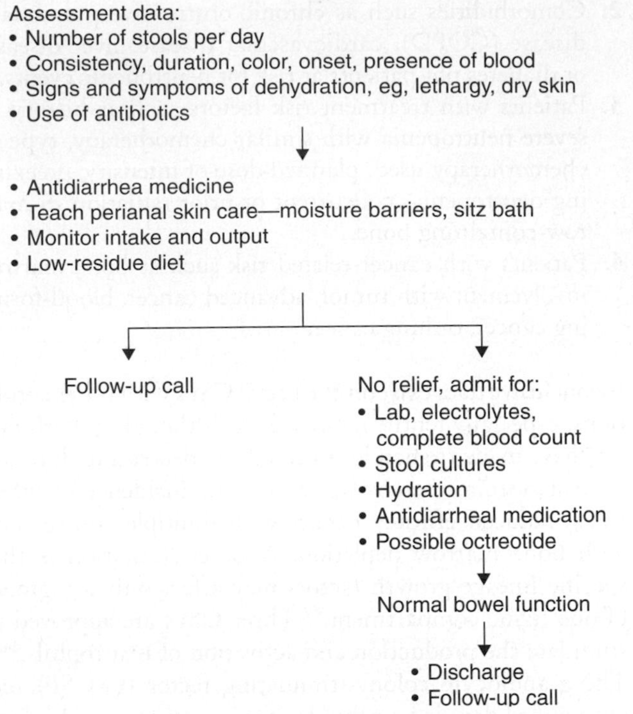
Assessment data:
• Number of stools per day
• Consistency, duration, color, onset, presence of blood
• Signs and symptoms of dehydration, eg, lethargy, dry skin
• Use of antibiotics
• Antidiarrhea medicine
• Teach perianal skin care—moisture barriers, sitz bath
• Monitor intake and output
• Low-residue diet
Follow-up call
No relief, admit for:
• Lab, electrolytes, complete blood count
• Stool cultures
• Hydration
• Antidiarrheal medication
• Possible octreotide
Normal bowel function
• Discharge
• Follow-up call

**FIGURE 17-4**

Diarrhea telephone triage flowchart.

*Constipation.* Constipation is defined as infrequent, excessively hard, and dry bowel movements resulting from a decrease in rectal filling or emptying.[49] Risk factors that contribute to constipation include narcotic analgesics, a decrease in physical activity, a low-fiber diet, a decrease in fluid intake, and bed rest. Other medications such as iron, calcium, anticholinergics, calcium-channel blockers, and anticonvulsants decrease stool frequency. Vincristine, vinblastine, and vinorelbine are the most common chemotherapy agents to cause constipation, as a result of autonomic nerve dysfunction manifested as colicky abdominal pain and ileus. Rectal emptying is specifically diminished because nonfunctional afferent and efferent pathways from the sacral cord are interrupted. Symptoms occur 3 to 7 days after drug administration and may be accompanied by evidence of peripheral nerve dysfunction.[46,55]

Even though chemotherapy is usually administered despite constipation, patients are instructed to be aware of bowel movements. If a bowel movement does not occur every other day, a laxative must be taken. If there are no results, the physician or advanced practice nurse (APN) should be consulted. Laxative therapy or prophylactic stool softener is recommended prior to the administration of drugs known to contribute to constipation, especially if the patient has a history of or is at risk for constipation. The patient should be encouraged to increase the amount of high-fiber foods in the daily diet as well as to increase fluid intake. The patient should be encouraged to increase physical activity, if that is tolerated. It should be stressed to the patient never to wait more than 3 days for a bowel movement before calling the physician or nurse, as a complication such as impaction or ileus can arise (Figure 17-5).

*Nausea and vomiting.* During the past decade, the management of chemotherapy-related nausea and vomiting has vastly improved. Understanding the pathophysiology of the symptoms, the efficacy and limitations of pharmacologic interventions, and the use of nonpharmacologictechniques is essential in minimizing nausea and vomiting. Emesis is a complicated process that requires coordination by the vomiting center (VC) in the lateral reticular formation of the medulla (Figure 17-6). The VC lies close to the respiratory center on the floor of the fourth ventricle and is directly activated by the visceral and vagal afferent pathways from the gastrointestinal tract, chemoreceptor trigger zone (CTZ), vestibular apparatus, and cerebral cortex. When the VC is

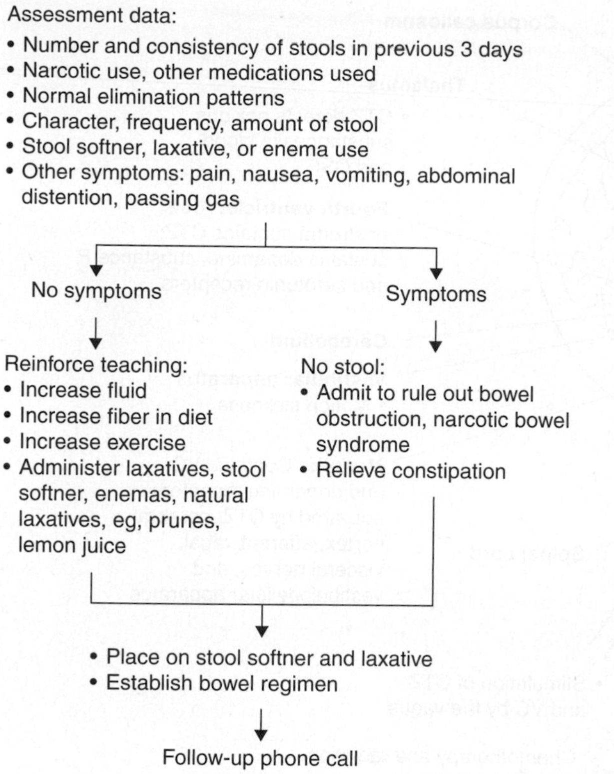
Assessment data:
• Number and consistency of stools in previous 3 days
• Narcotic use, other medications used
• Normal elimination patterns
• Character, frequency, amount of stool
• Stool softner, laxative, or enema use
• Other symptoms: pain, nausea, vomiting, abdominal distention, passing gas
No symptoms
Symptoms
Reinforce teaching:
• Increase fluid
• Increase fiber in diet
• Increase exercise
• Administer laxatives, stool softner, enemas, natural laxatives, eg, prunes, lemon juice
No stool:
• Admit to rule out bowel obstruction, narcotic bowel syndrome
• Relieve constipation
• Place on stool softner and laxative
• Establish bowel regimen
Follow-up phone call

**FIGURE 17-5**

Constipation telephone triage flowchart.

stimulated, emesis is induced via impulses to the salivation and respiratory centers and to the pharyngeal, gastrointestinal, and abdominal muscles.[56,57]

The VC is rich in neurotransmitter receptors that are sensitive to chemical toxins in the blood and cerebrospinal fluid.[56] The major receptors are dopamine, serotonin (5HT), neurokinin-1, and muscarinic cholinergic in the CTZ; muscarinic and dopamine in the VC, vestibular apparatus, and efferent vagal motor nuclei; and histamine in the VC and vestibular apparatus. Chemotherapy damages the enterochromaffin cells of the duodenal mucosa, causing serotonin release that binds to vagal afferent receptors. These afferent receptors, in turn, send impulses to the emetic center.[56]

Vestibular-cerebellar afferent pathway areas transmit impulses to the cerebellum and then to the VC, which are experienced as motion sickness. When rapid motion change occurs, the receptors of the labyrinth in the inner ear are stimulated, which is associated with nausea.[56] Obstruction, irritation, inflammation, or delayed gastric emptying may stimulate the gastrointestinal tract through vagal visceral afferent pathways.[56,57] Conditioned and anticipatory responses are controlled by the cerebral cortex and limbic system, which can be stimulated by sights, sounds, or odors that the patient associates with chemotherapy, thereby making the patient nauseated.[58]

Although nausea, retching, and vomiting commonly occur together, they are considered separate conditions.[59] *Nausea* is described as a subjective conscious recognition of the desire to vomit and is manifested by an unpleasant wavelike sensation in the epigastric area, at the back of the throat, or throughout the abdomen. It is mediated by the autonomic nervous system and accompanied by symptoms such as pallor, weakness, dizziness, tachycardia, perspiration, light-headedness, and excess salivation.

*Retching* is a rhythmic and spasmodic movement, involving the diaphragm and abdominal muscles, controlled by the respiratory center in the brain stem near the VC. Negative intrathoracic pressure and positive abdominal pressure result in unproductive retching. When the negative pressure becomes positive, vomiting occurs. *Vomiting* is a somatic process performed by the respiratory muscles causing the forceful oral expulsion of gastric, duodenal, or jejunal contents through the mouth.[58]

Nausea and vomiting can be classified as acute, delayed, and anticipatory. *Acute nausea and vomiting* occur from a few minutes to 1 to 2 hours after treatment, resolving within 24 hours. Acute onset is primarily mediated by serotonin-release.[59] The pattern is determined by the emetogenicity of the chemotherapy and pretreatment with an antiemetic agent. *Delayed nausea and vomiting* persist or develop 24 hours after chemotherapy, perhaps due to the ongoing effect that the metabolites of chemotherapy continue to exert on the central nervous system (CNS) or gastrointestinal tract. Delayed onset is mediated, in part, by substance P.[59] Although cisplatin is thought to be the main drug causing delayed nausea and vomiting, cyclophosphamide, doxorubicin, carboplatin, and ifosfamide can cause delayed nausea as well. If nausea is controlled within the first 24 hours after therapy, delayed patterns are less likely to occur. However, despite effective antiemetic regimens, patients still experience a significant amount of delayed nausea and vomiting.[59,60] *Anticipatory nausea and vomiting* occur in 25% of patients as a result of classic operant conditioning from stimuli associated with chemotherapy, usually 12 hours prior to administration of further chemotherapy. Such conditioned responses are experienced after a few sessions of chemotherapy and occur most commonly when efforts to control emesis are unsuccessful.[60] Lorazepam has been found to relieve anticipatory effects as well as delayed nausea.[61] Breakthrough nausea and vomiting can occur despite prophylactic antiemetics requiring continuous antiemetic use.[61]

It is possible to predict the degree and severity of nausea and vomiting as well as the onset and duration (Table 17-2). Mechlorethamine, for example, induces emesis within 30 minutes of IV administration, whereas other highly emetogenic drugs cause emesis at least 1 hour after infusion. With moderately to highly emetogenic drugs, emesis develops within 6 hours of administration. Drugs with low emetogenic potential usually cause emesis 12 to 48 hours after administration. The variability in their occurrence and

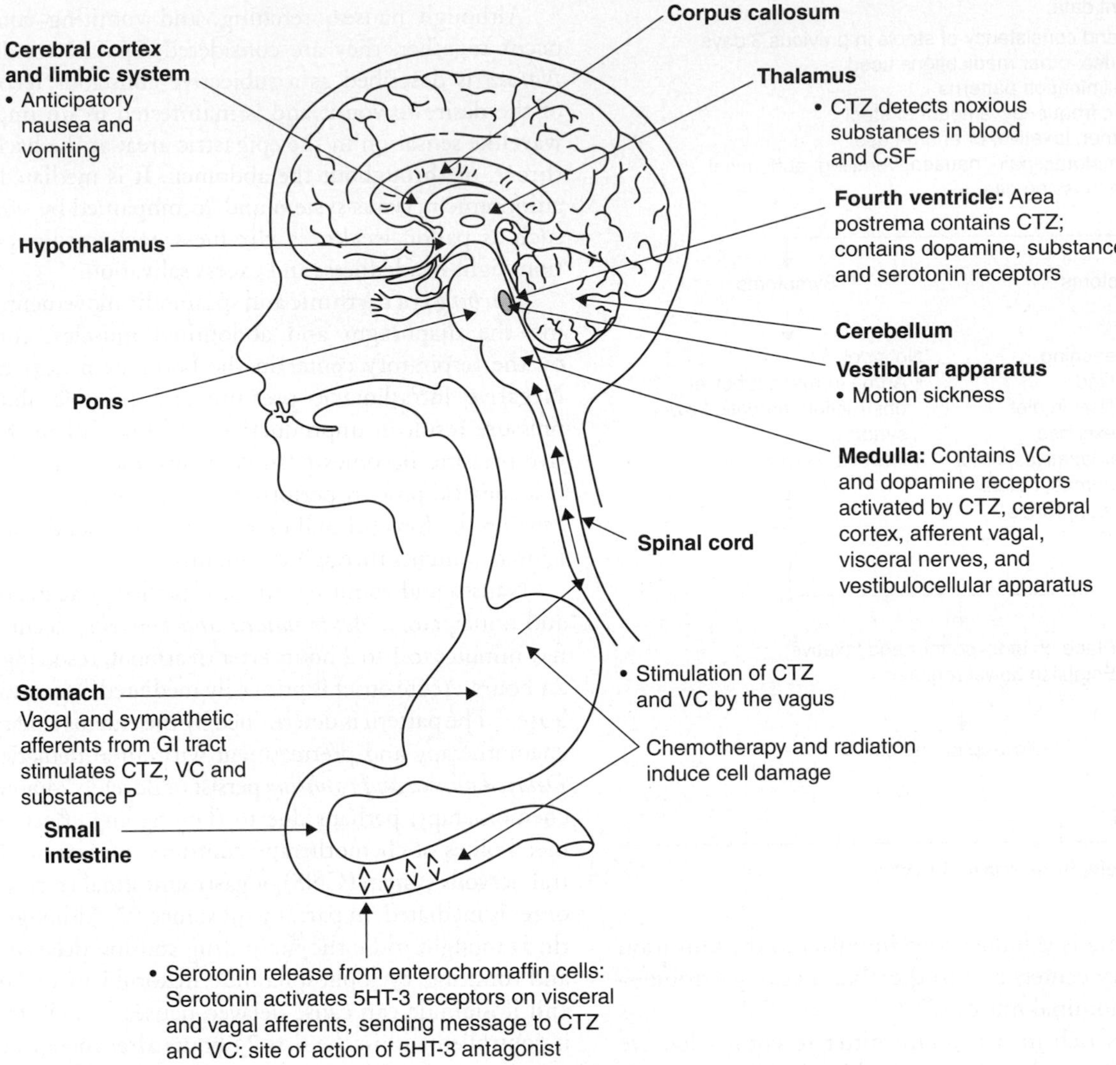


**FIGURE 17-6**

Pathways of nausea and vomiting.

*Abbreviations*: CSF, cerebrospinal fluid; CTZ, chemotherapy trigger zone; GI, gastrointestinal; VC, vomiting center.

onset suggests that each drug may cause emesis via a different mechanism or by stimulating a different pathway.[56,59,60] The rate and route of chemotherapy administration also affect emetic onset, intensity, and duration. For example, rapid infusion of cytarabine is more often associated with an earlier onset of severe emesis than is slower infusion.

Further classification has been proposed to determine the emetogenicity of combination chemotherapy (see Table 17-2). Initially, the most emetogenic drug in the combination is identified. Other drugs are then assessed for emetogenic potential with these considerations: (1) level 1 drugs do not significantly contribute to the overall emetogenicity of the combination; (2) one or more level 2 drugs increase the emetogenicity of the combination by one level greater than the most emetogenetic drugs; and (3) the emetogenicity of the combination is increased by one level per drug when a level 3 or 4 drug is added to the regimen.

Management begins with obtaining an in-depth emetic history and developing a preventive action plan with antiemetics (Table 17-3). Characteristics that affect the occurrence of nausea and vomiting include fatigue, being young, female gender, susceptibility to motion sickness, poor previous emetic control, and poor social functioning. Individuals with a heavy alcohol intake seem to have a decreased occurrence of nausea and vomiting.[56,59]

Successful antiemetic regimens interrupt the stimulation of the VC. Combination regimens must be individualized and developed according to the emetogenic

**TABLE 17-2**

**Emetogenic Potential of Chemotherapeutic Agents**

| Incidence | Level | Agent | Onset (hours) | Duration (hours) |
|---|---|---|---|---|
| Very high(> 90%) | 5 | Cisplatin (> 50 mg/m$^2$) | 1–6 | 24–48 |
| | | Dacarbazine | 1–3 | 1–12 |
| | | Mechlorethamine | 0.5–2 | 8–24 |
| | | Melphalan—high dose | 0.3–6 | 6–12 |
| | | Streptozocin | 1–6 | 12–24 |
| | | Cytarabine—high dose(> 1 g/m$^2$) | 1–4 | 12–48 |
| High (60%–90%) | 4 | Carmustine (> 600 mg/m$^2$) | 2–4 | 4–24 |
| | | Cyclophosphamide(> 600mg/m$^2$) | 4 –12 | 12–24 |
| | | Procarbazine | 24–27 | Variable |
| | | Etoposide—high dose | 4–6 | 24+ |
| | | Semustine | 1–5 | 12–24 |
| | | Lomustine | 4–6 | 12–24 |
| | | Dactinomycin | 2–5 | 24 |
| | | Plicamycin | 1–6 | 12–24 |
| | | Methotrexate—high dose | 1–12 | 12–72 |
| | | ActinomycinD | 1–12 | 24–48 |
| | | Cytarabine (500 mg/m$^2$) | 1–12 | 24–48 |
| | | Epirubicin | 6–12 | 24+ |
| | | Idarubicin | 6–12 | 24+ |
| | | Oxaliplatin | 1–6 | 24 |
| Moderate (30%–60%) | 3 | Doxorubicin (> 50–75mg/m$^2$) | 4–6 | 6+ |
| | | Mitoxantrone | 4–6 | 6+ |
| | | 5-fluorouracil | 3–6 | 24+ |
| | | Mitomycin C | 1–4 | 48–72 |
| | | Carboplatin | 4–6 | 12–24 |
| | | Daunorubicin (< 50 mg/m$^2$) | 2–6 | 24 |
| | | Asparaginase | 1–4 | 2–12 |
| | | Topotecan | 6–12 | 24–72 |
| | | Ifosfamide(1.5 g/m$^2$) | 3–6 | 24+ |
| | | Irinotecan | — | — |
| | | Epirubicin | — | — |
| | | Idarubicin | — | — |
| Low (10%–30%) | 2 | Bleomycin | 3–6 | — |
| | | Cytarabine (< 20 mg/m$^2$) | 6–12 | 3–12 |
| | | Etoposide | 3–8 | — |
| | | Melphalan | 6–12 | — |
| | | 6-Mercaptopurine | 4–8 | — |
| | | Methotrexate(< 100 mg/m$^2$) | 4–12 | 3–12 |
| | | Vinblastine | 4–8 | — |
| | | Hydroxyurea | — | — |
| | | Teniposide | — | — |
| | | Gemcitabine | — | — |
| | | Vinorelbine | — | — |
| | | Fludarabine | — | — |
| | | Hydroxyurea | — | — |
| | | Topotecan | — | — |
| | | Capecitabine | — | — |
| | | Trimetrexate | — | — |
| Very low (< 10%) | 1 | Vincristine | 4–8 | — |
| | | Chlorambucil | 48–72 | — |
| | | Busulfan | — | — |
| | | Thioguanine | — | — |
| | | Hormones | — | — |
| | | Paclitaxel | 4–8 | — |
| | | Docetaxel | — | — |
| | | Thiotepa | — | — |
| | | Temozolomide | — | — |
| | | Valrubicin | — | — |
| | | Tretinoin | — | — |

**TABLE 17-3**

**Antiemetic Therapy**

| Classification | Drugs | Availability/ Dose | Schedule | Duration | Half-Life | Comments |
|---|---|---|---|---|---|---|
| | | **Benzodiazepines** | | | | |
| *Mechanism of action* CNS depressant; interferes with afferent nerves from cerebral cortex, sedative *Common side effects* Sedation, amnesia, confusion | Lorazepam | Tablet: 1–3 mg PO or sublingual IV: 0.5–2.5 mg | q 3–4 hours | 4–8 hours | 10–15 hours | Reduces anticipatory nausea and vomiting May aggravate CNS effects of ifosfamide. Use with caution in patients with hepatic and renal dysfunction |
| | Diazepam | Tablet: 2–4 mg IV: 2–10 mg | q 4–6 hours | 4–8 hours | 30–40 hours | |
| | | **Butyrophenones** | | | | |
| *Mechanism of action* Dopamine antagonist in the CTZ, esophagus, and stomach *Common side effects* Sedation, hypotension, tachycardia, EPS | Droperidol | IM: 2.5–10 mg IV: 0.5–2.5 mg | q 3–4 hours | 2–4 hours | 10 hours | Diphenhydramine 25–50 mg PO or IV will prevent EPS. EPS more common in young patients Use caution in patients with cardiac disorders |
| | Haloperidol | Tablet: 3–5 mg IM: 1–5 mg IV: 1–3 mg | q 4 hours q 2–6 hours | 2–6 hours | 12–18 hours | |
| | | **Cannabinoids** | | | | |
| *Mechanism of action* Suppreses pathways to VC (speculated) *Common side effects* Sedation, dizziness, dysphoria, dry mouth, disorientation, impaired concentration, orthostatic hypotension, tachycardia. | Dronabinol | Tablet: 5–10 mg | q 4 hours | 4–6 hours | | May be difficult to obtain in outpatient setting Elderly patients generally do not tolerate side effects Generally used for second-line antiemetic therapy |
| | | **Phenothiazines** | | | | |
| *Mechanism of action* Blocks dopamine receptor in the CTZ; inhibits VC by blocking autonomic afferent impulses via vagus nerve | Prochlorperazine | Tablet: 5–25 mg | q4–6 hours | 3–4 hours | | Administer IV dose over 15–30 minutes EPS more common in persons < 30 years. Side effects can be cumulative in the elderly. |
| | | Sustained release: 10–30 mg PO | q10–12 hours | 10–12 hours | | |
| | | IM/IV: 20–40 mg | q3–4 hours | 3–4 hours | | |
| | | Rectal: 25 mg | q 4–6 hours | 3–4 hours | | |

*(Continued)*

**TABLE 17-3**

**Antiemetic Therapy (*Continued*)**

| Classification | Drugs | Availability/ Dose | Schedule | Duration | Half-Life | Comments |
|---|---|---|---|---|---|---|
| | | **Phenothiazines** (*Continued*) | | | | |
| *Common side effects* Sedation, orthostatic hypotension, EPS, dizziness, drowsiness | Promethazine | Tablet: 12.5–25 mg<br>IM/IV: 10–25 mg<br>Rectal: 25 mg | q4–6 hours | 3–4 hours | | Do not exceed 5 mg/minute with IV dose.<br>Dystonia can occur with chlorpromazine generally with IV dosing.<br>Chlorpromazine generally second-line antiemetic therapy.<br>Diphenhydramine can prevent EPS and dystonia.<br>Sustained-release form of prochlorperazine (currently not available) can prevent delayed nausea and vomiting. |
| | Thiethylperazine | Tablet: 10 mg<br>IM: 10 mg<br>Rectal: 10 mg | q 4–6 hours | 3–4 hours<br>6–8 hours<br>6–8 hours | | |
| | Chlorpromazine | Tablet: 25–50 mg<br>IM/IV: 25–50 mg<br>Rectal: 25–100 mg | q 4–6 hours | 3–4 hours | | |
| | Perphenazine | Tablet: 4 mg<br>IM/IV: 5 mg | q 4–6 hours | 3–4 hours | | |
| | Trimethobenzamide | Capsule: 250 mg<br>Rectal: 200 mg<br>IM: 200 mg | q 6–8 hours<br>q 6–8 hours<br>q 6–8 hours | 3–4 hours<br>3–4 hours<br>3–4 hours | | |
| | | **Substituted Benzamide** | | | | |
| *Mechanism of action* Dopamine antagonist; accelerates gastric emptying and small-bowel transit; CTZ<br>*Common side effects* Sedation, diarrhea, anxiety, EPS, fatigue, headache | Metoclopramide | Tablet: 5–10 mg<br>IV: 1–3 mg/kg | q 2–3 hours x 3–5 doses | 2–3 hours | 4–6 hours | EPS more common in young patients.<br>Administer over 15 minutes to prevent intense anxiety.<br>Use with caution in patients with renal dysfunction. |
| | | **Steroids** | | | | |
| *Mechanism of action* Antiprostaglandin synthesis activity<br>*Common side effects:* Insomnia, euphoria, anxiety, flushing | Dexamethasone | Tablet: 2–4 mg<br>IV: 10–20 mg<br>IV: 125–250 mg | q 4–6 hours<br>q 3 hours | | 2–3 hours | Rapid infusion causes perineal itching.<br>Taper dose to prevent insomnia, anxiety, and euphoria.<br>Acne may occur. |
| | | **Antihistamines** | | | | |
| *Mechanism of action* Histamine $H_1$ receptor antagonist<br>*Common side effects* Sedation, hypotension | Diphenhydramine | Tablet: 25–50 mg<br>IM/IV: 25–50 mg | q 3–4 hours | | 5–8 hours | Prevents acute dystonic reactions.<br>Use with caution in patients with hepatic dysfunction. |

(*Continued*)

**TABLE 17-3**

**Antiemetic Therapy (*Continued*)**

| Classification | Drugs | Availability/ Dose | Schedule | Duration | Half-Life | Comments |
|---|---|---|---|---|---|---|
| | | **Serotonin Inhibitors** | | | | |
| *Mechanism of action* Serotonin receptor, (5HT-3) antagonist *Common side effects* Hypotension, headache, constipation, sedation minimal | Ondansetron | IV: 16–32 mg/ 24 hours 0.15–0.18 mg/kg PO: 4 mg and 8 mg tablets. Sublingual: ODT | q 12 hours q 8 hours q 8–12 hours | 8 hours | 3–4 hours | ODT approved for days 2 and 3 after moderate chemotherapy. |
| | Granisetron | IV: 10 mcg/kg PO: 2 mg Transdermal patch 34.3 mg for 5 days | q 30 minutes prior to chemo-therapy | 12 hours | 8–10 hours | Single dose of granisetron may be sufficient for a 12 hour time period. |
| | Dolasetron | IV: 1.8 mg/kg PO: 100 mg | q 1 hour prior to chemo-therapy | 12 hours | 8–10 hours | Classification not recommended for delayed or anticipatory nausea/vomiting. |
| | Palonosetron | IV: 0.25 mg PO: 0.5 mg | 30 minutes prior to chemo-therapy | 72 hours | 40 hours | No redosing 7 days after treatment. Receptor binding affinity 30 x higher than that of other 5HT-3 antagonists. |
| | | **Anticholinergics** | | | | |
| *Common side effects* Dry mouth, sedation, blurred vision, restlessness | Scopolamine | Patch: 0.5 mg/ every 3 days | q 24 hours | 72 hours | | May irritate skin. May be difficult to obtain. |
| | | **Neurokinin 1 Receptor Antagonist** | | | | |
| *Common side effects* Constipation, diarrhea, headache, hiccups, anorexia | Aprepitant | PO: 125 mg 80 mg IV: 115 mg day 1 | q 1 hour prior to chemo-therapy Days 2 and 3 | 24 hours | 9–13 hours | Given as a part of 5HT-3 and steroid regimen. IV dose can be substituted for oral dose on day 1 |

*Abbreviations*: CNS, central nervous system; CTZ, chemoreceptor trigger zone; EPS, extrapyramidal symptoms; IM, intramuscular; IV, intravenous; LFTs, liver function tests; ODT, oral disintegrating tablet; PO, per oral; VC, vomiting center.

potential of the chemotherapy regimen, expected duration of the nausea and vomiting, and current pattern of symptoms. Numerous combinations are being investigated to eliminate the stimulation of the VC. These regimens use drugs with proven single-agent antiemetic activity, optimal doses, routes, and minimal overlapping toxicities (Figure 17-7).[56,59–62] For example, combinations of serotonin-receptor antagonists with steroids have been found to provide complete control of nausea and vomiting in as many as 100% of patients undergoing high-dose cisplatin-based regimens. Experts generally agree that nausea and vomiting occur throughout the treatment phases and no single 5HT-3 receptor antagonist is superior to another, whether given IV or orally.[56,63] A unique feature of this group of drugs is the fact that ondansetron is available as an orally disintegrating tablet (ODT). The tablet dissolves quickly when placed under the tongue, where it is directly absorbed into the bloodstream. Ondansetron ODT is approved for delayed nausea following moderately emetogenic chemotherapy. Transdermal granisetron patch is approved as a transdermal formulation offering the potential benefit of patient convenience and improved compliance.[62]

Palonosetron is a newer 5HT-3 receptor antagonist and is unique because it has a 100-fold higher receptor-binding

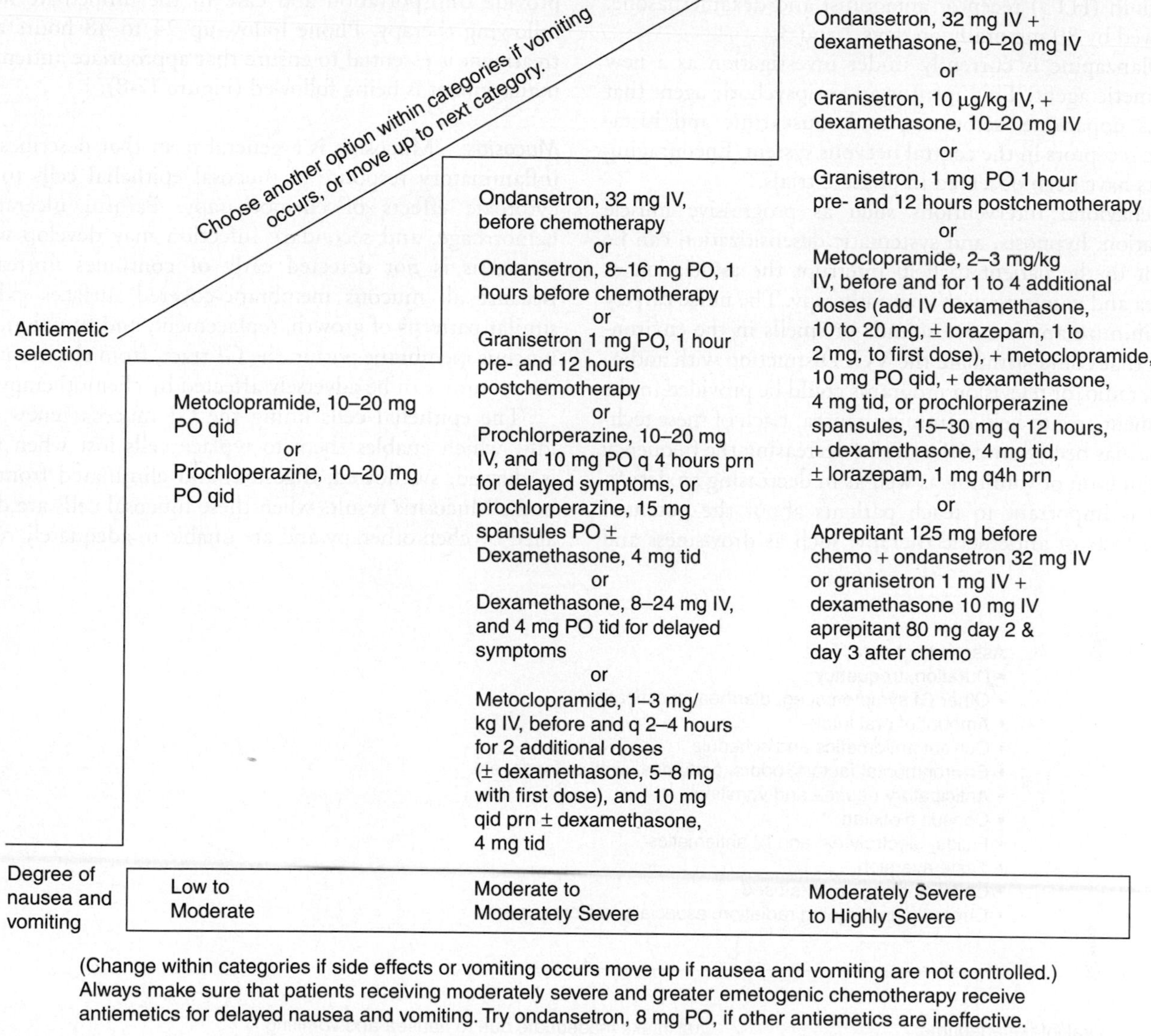
Choose another option within categories if vomiting occurs, or move up to next category.
Antiemetic selection
Metoclopramide, 10–20 mg PO qid
or
Prochloperazine, 10–20 mg PO qid
Ondansetron, 32 mg IV, before chemotherapy
or
Ondansetron, 8–16 mg PO, 1 hours before chemotherapy
or
Granisetron 1 mg PO, 1 hour pre- and 12 hours postchemotherapy
or
Prochlorperazine, 10–20 mg IV, and 10 mg PO q 4 hours prn for delayed symptoms, or prochlorperazine, 15 mg spansules PO ± Dexamethasone, 4 mg tid
or
Dexamethasone, 8–24 mg IV, and 4 mg PO tid for delayed symptoms
or
Metoclopramide, 1–3 mg/kg IV, before and q 2–4 hours for 2 additional doses (± dexamethasone, 5–8 mg with first dose), and 10 mg qid prn ± dexamethasone, 4 mg tid
Ondansetron, 32 mg IV + dexamethasone, 10–20 mg IV
or
Granisetron, 10 µg/kg IV, + dexamethasone, 10–20 mg IV
or
Granisetron, 1 mg PO 1 hour pre- and 12 hours postchemotherapy
or
Metoclopramide, 2–3 mg/kg IV, before and for 1 to 4 additional doses (add IV dexamethasone, 10 to 20 mg, ± lorazepam, 1 to 2 mg, to first dose), + metoclopramide, 10 mg PO qid, + dexamethasone, 4 mg tid, or prochlorperazine spansules, 15–30 mg q 12 hours, + dexamethasone, 4 mg tid, ± lorazepam, 1 mg q4h prn
or
Aprepitant 125 mg before chemo + ondansetron 32 mg IV or granisetron 1 mg IV + dexamethasone 10 mg IV aprepitant 80 mg day 2 & day 3 after chemo
Degree of nausea and vomiting
Low to Moderate
Moderate to Moderately Severe
Moderately Severe to Highly Severe
(Change within categories if side effects or vomiting occurs move up if nausea and vomiting are not controlled.)
Always make sure that patients receiving moderately severe and greater emetogenic chemotherapy receive antiemetics for delayed nausea and vomiting. Try ondansetron, 8 mg PO, if other antiemetics are ineffective.

**FIGURE 17-7**

Antiemetic selection for chemotherapy.

*Source*: Reprinted with permission from Wickham R. Nausea and vomiting. In Yarbro CH, Frogge MH, Goodman M, eds: *Cancer Symptom Management* (ed. 3). Sudbury, MA: Jones and Bartlett: 2004.[61]

affinity compared to earlier serotonin antagonists.[64] Also, after IV administration, this drug has a half-life of 40 hours and a duration of 7 days. Studies reveal palonosetron to be superior to similar agents in controlling delayed nausea and vomiting.[64,65] This drug is available orally in a dose of 0.5 mg administered 1 hour prior to chemotherapy.

Aprepitant is the first substance P neurokinin-1 (NK[1]) receptor antagonist. Chemotherapy-induced emesis is mediated by neurotransmitters such as serotonin, histamine, and substance P. Aprepitant prevents delayed nausea and vomiting because it effectively blocks substance P.[66] Following an oral dose, aprepitant has a half-life of 9 to 13 hours and duration of 24 hours. This drug is given in a dose of 125 mg, 1 hour prior to chemotherapy and 80 mg on days 2 and 3 after chemotherapy.[67] The drug is metabolized in the liver by CYP 3A4. Subsequently, an increase in serum concentrations of substance P may occur with drugs metabolized by this enzyme, including docetaxel, paclitaxel, etoposide, irinotecan, ifosfamide, vinorelbine, and vincristine.[67] This drug is given as 125 mg orally on day 1, together with a serotonin (HT3) receptor antagonist and dexamethasone, followed by 80 mg orally on days 2 and 3.

Olanzapine is currently under investigation as a new antiemetic agent. This agent is an antipsychotic agent that blocks dopamine, serotonin, and muscarinic and histaminic receptors in the central nervous system. Encouraging results have been observed in phase 2 trials.[68]

Behavioral interventions such as progressive muscle relaxation, hypnosis, and systematic desensitization can be taught to the patient to help interrupt the association of nausea and vomiting with chemotherapy. The nurse can try to minimize any aversive sounds or smells in the environment that could stimulate the VC. Distraction with audiotapes, radio, or television programs could be provided in the treatment area to help minimize nausea. Each of these techniques has been found effective in decreasing the frequency and duration of vomiting as well as in decreasing anxiety.[61]

It is important to teach patients about the potential side effects of antiemetic therapy, such as drowsiness and diarrhea. If the patient is returning home after an emetogenic chemotherapy treatment, ensure that someone can provide transportation and care in the immediate hours following therapy. Phone follow-up 24 to 48 hours after treatment is essential to ensure that appropriate antiemetic management is being followed (Figure 17-8).

*Mucositis.* Mucositis is a general term that describes the inflammatory response of mucosal epithelial cells to the cytotoxic effects of chemotherapy. Painful ulceration, hemorrhage, and secondary infection may develop when mucositis is not detected early or continues untreated. Because all mucous membrane-covered surfaces exhibit similar patterns of growth, replacement, and function, any mucous membrane within the GI tract, from the mouth to the rectum, can be adversely affected by chemotherapy.

The epithelial cells lining the GI mucosa renew rapidly, which enables them to replace cells lost when food is chewed, swallowed, digested, and eliminated from the body. Mucositis results when these mucosal cells are damaged by chemotherapy and are unable to adequately repair

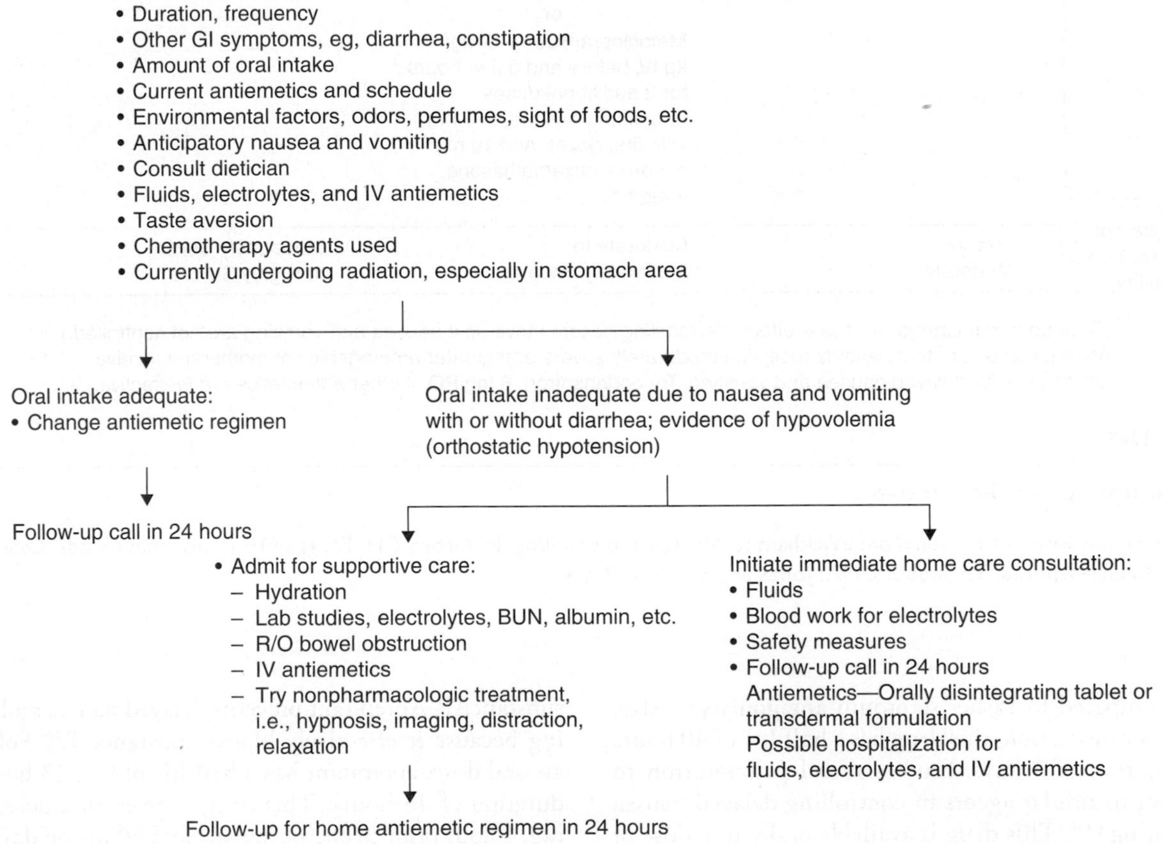
Assessment data:
• Duration, frequency
• Other GI symptoms, eg, diarrhea, constipation
• Amount of oral intake
• Current antiemetics and schedule
• Environmental factors, odors, perfumes, sight of foods, etc.
• Anticipatory nausea and vomiting
• Consult dietician
• Fluids, electrolytes, and IV antiemetics
• Taste aversion
• Chemotherapy agents used
• Currently undergoing radiation, especially in stomach area
Oral intake adequate:
• Change antiemetic regimen
Oral intake inadequate due to nausea and vomiting with or without diarrhea; evidence of hypovolemia (orthostatic hypotension)
Follow-up call in 24 hours
• Admit for supportive care:
– Hydration
– Lab studies, electrolytes, BUN, albumin, etc.
– R/O bowel obstruction
– IV antiemetics
– Try nonpharmacologic treatment, i.e., hypnosis, imaging, distraction, relaxation
Initiate immediate home care consultation:
• Fluids
• Blood work for electrolytes
• Safety measures
• Follow-up call in 24 hours
Antiemetics—Orally disintegrating tablet or transdermal formulation
Possible hospitalization for fluids, electrolytes, and IV antiemetics
Follow-up for home antiemetic regimen in 24 hours

**FIGURE 17-8**

Nausea and vomiting telephone triage flowchart.

*Abbreviations*: BUN, blood urea nitrogen; GI, gastrointestinal; IV, intravenous; R/O, rule out.

and replace normal cell loss. Manifestations of GI toxicity include mucositis in the oral cavity (stomatitis), esophagus (esophagitis), and intestines (as diarrhea; enteritis).

*Stomatitis.* Chemotherapy-induced oral complications can be acute or chronic. Acute reactions include mucosal inflammation and ulceration, infection, and mucosal bleeding. Although chronic complications can occur from chemotherapy, these changes usually result from radiation-induced changes to healthy tissue and include xerostomia, taste alterations, trismus, and soft tissue and bone necrosis.

The risk of developing stomatitis is not the same for all patients, nor is it equal for all drug regimens. Diagnosis and aggressiveness of the chemotherapy regimen are predictors of oral complications as well as prolonged or repetitive administration of lower doses of chemotherapy such as weekly fluorouracil. The frequency of oral problems is 2 to 3 times higher in patients with hematologic malignancies than with solid tumors. Stomatitis occurs more commonly in younger and elderly patients.[69]

Preexisting oral disease (dental caries, partially erupted third molars) as well as poor oral hygiene and local irritants (eg, ill-fitting dental prostheses, tobacco, alcohol) will predispose patients receiving chemotherapy to an increased risk of oral complications. Periodontitis, a common oral disease, causes a 10-fold increase in bacterial and fungal organisms in the oral cavity. Depletion of protein stores and malnutrition increases the risk of infection by altering the integrity of the epithelial barrier and depressing the immune system.[69,70]

The majority of chemotherapy drugs can cause some degree of stomatitis. Those drugs most associated with stomatitis are the antimetabolites and antitumor antibiotics—in particular, bleomycin, doxorubicin, daunorubicin, docetaxel, fluorouracil, methotrexate, and high-dose therapy with busulfan, etoposide, melphalan, and thiotepa. All-transretinoic acid and arsenic trioxide can cause cracked and inflamed lips. Mucositis is observed more often with fluorouracil when combined with other mucositis-producing drugs, such as methotrexate and doxorubicin, and when fluorouracil is given concurrently with leucovorin.

Although stomatitis is dose related and is more common with higher doses, patients who develop stomatitis with 1 cycle of therapy will almost likely develop recurrence in subsequent courses unless the drugs or doses are changed.[56,68] This is especially the case when the body is unable to adequately eliminate a stomatotoxic drug. For example, in the presence of renal dysfunction or liver dysfunction, excretion of methotrexate and doxorubicin, respectively, may be compromised.

Direct stomatotoxicity results from the cytotoxic action of drugs on the cells of the oral basal epithelium, causing a decrease in the rate of cell renewal. The sequelae include a thinned atrophic mucosa and initiation of an inflammatory response (stomatitis). Most often affected are the nonkeratinized mucosal areas, including the tongue, buccal mucosa, soft palate, and floor of the mouth. Rarely is the gingiva or hard palate involved.[50]

Histologic changes within the mouth can occur within 5 to 7 days of initial drug exposure. Dry mucosa, tongue, or lips; burning sensation in the oral cavity; and increased salivation result. Visible signs of inflammation and oral ulceration can be observed 7 to 10 days following therapy. Changes in the oral cavity correlate with the timing of myelosuppression, as leukocytes and the oral mucosal cells have similar cell renewal rates. Without complications and further insult from repeated drug administration, stomatitis is self-limiting and gradually reverses itself within 2 to 3 weeks as the granulocyte count returns to normal, often preceding bone marrow recovery by 2 to 3 days. Improvement in the status of the oral mucosa can therefore be predictive of a WBC count recovery.[68]

A baseline assessment of the oral cavity should be done prior to the initiation of treatment. Dental prophylaxis, restoration, and repair should be completed before treatment begins. Once treatment is initiated, an oral assessment should be repeated at regular intervals; outpatients should be instructed on self-assessment.[70] Nursing management of stomatitis will depend on its severity, which is often described as mild, moderate, or severe (see Table 17-1).

Oral complications can be reduced or eliminated by meticulous oral assessment with interventions before, during, and between courses of chemotherapy.[68–71] Table 17-4 describes various oral cleansing agents and devices, different means of lubricating and coating the oral cavity, and basic solutions and measures to manage oral discomfort. Developing a plan of care that the patient finds acceptable may be more beneficial than employing complicated regimens. Because reinforcement promotes compliance, nurses should continually review with the patient the individual plan for oral care and assess its continued acceptability. Generally, the recommendation is that routine oral care be performed at least after meals and at bedtime, and that the frequency increase as the severity of stomatitis increases.[71]

Mouth rinses enhance removal of loosened debris and should be nonirritating and nondehydrating. Several solutions for rinsing have been studied, including normal saline, benzydamine, sodium bicarbonate, and hydrogen peroxide, as well as several combinations of these options. Normal saline may be the least damaging. Sodium bicarbonate is effective as a cleansing agent, but some patients complain of the bad taste and a concentrated solution can change the oral cavity pH. Hydrogen peroxide breaks down new tissues and should be avoided when fresh granulation surfaces are visible in the mouth. To date, the optimal cleansing agent for stomatitis has not been determined.[69,71]

Palifermin, a recombinant keratinocyte growth factor is approved to decrease the incidence and duration of mucositis in patients undergoing hematopoietic stem cell transplantation (HSCT). This agent increases cellular proliferation of

**TABLE 17-4**

**Prevention and Management of Perioral Complications of Cancer Treatment**

| Plan/Agent | Schedule | Action | Comments |
|---|---|---|---|
| | | **Basic Oral Cleansing** | |
| **Cleansing Mouth Rinses** | | | |
| Normal saline | 4×/day | Mechanical plaque control, removes and washes away loose debris<br>Physical; moistens and soothes oral mucosa | Non-irritating and no unpleasant taste<br>Mixture preparation: 1 teaspoon salt in 1 quart warm water; use sterile saline if granulocytopenic or mouth ulcers present |
| Sodium bicarbonate solution | 4×/day | Mechanical plaque control; loosens hardened crusts and debris<br>Mucosolvent<br>Reduces acidity | Decreases odor; unpleasant taste reported<br>Mixture preparation; 1 teaspoon baking soda in 8 oz water for thick paste of sodium bicarbonate; water applied to gingival sulcus for use in mechanical plaque debridement |
| Hydrogen peroxide | 4×/day | Mechanical plaque control; loosens hardened crusts and debris | Mixture preparation; ½ water to ½ hydrogen peroxide |
| | | **Maintenance of Oral Moisture** | |
| **Oral Care** | | | |
| Orabalance | Use after rinsing mouth and after brushing | Relief of dry mouth | A non-drying moisturizing gel may be applied around the teeth and along gum line |
| Saliva substitutes | | | |
| Moi-Stir | As needed | Mouth-moistening salivary supplement | Available in oral swabsticks and spray |
| Xerolube | As needed | Mouth moisturizer; caries inhibition | Includes fluoride as an added benefit |
| Sialogogues | | | |
| Salagen | 5 mg 3×/day | Stimulates saliva production from functioning salivary glands | Contraindicated in patients with uncontrolled asthma or narrow-angle glaucoma; use caution with cardiovascular disease |
| Biotene | Use after rinsing mouth and after brushing | Relief of dry mouth | Available as mouthwash, gum, toothpaste, or oral gel |
| | | **Relief of Pain and Inflammation** | |
| **Coating Agents** | | | |
| Orabase | As needed | Topical anesthetic for localized areas of pain | Quick onset of action (30 seconds), but short duration of action (5–15 minutes)<br>Does not change consistency after application |
| Hurricane | As needed | Topical anesthetic | Available as spray, liquid, or gel<br>Onset of action, 30 seconds; Duration, 15 minutes<br>No systemic absorption |
| Oratect-gel | As needed no more than | Topical anesthetic | Gel dries in about 30–60 seconds to form a protective film<br>Maximum protection lasts about 2 hours<br>Film dissipates gradually over 6 hours<br>Do not try to mechanically remove<br>Mild, transient stinging when applied |

(Continued)

**TABLE 17-4**

**Prevention and Management of Perioral Complications of Cancer Treatment (*Continued*)**

| Plan/Agent | Schedule | Action | Comments |
|---|---|---|---|
| Zilactin | Dry lesions; apply 4×/day | Provides a protective coating and leads to pain relief | Forms protective film over oral ulcers that can last 5 hours<br>Gel forms an opaque white film inside the mouth and a transparent film extraorally when dried<br>Mild, transient burning sensation with application of gel |
| Gelclair | As needed | Moderate to severe pain | Adherent barrier forms over oral mucosa |
| **Topical Anesthetic Rinses** | | | |
| Xylocaine viscous 2% solution | 15 mL swish and swallow q3 hours, as needed | Topical anesthetic for generalized areas of pain | Onset of action is 5 minutes<br>Duration of action is approximately 20 minutes<br>Systemically absorbed<br>Watch for CNS and cardiac toxicity<br>Swish and swallow for brief pain relief (eg, before meals) |
| Dyclonine hydrochloride 0.5% or 1% solution | 15 ml swish and spit, as needed | Topical anesthetic for generalized areas of pain | Minimally absorbed<br>Decreasing potential for CNS and cardiac toxicity |
| Combination mixtures (eg, viscous xylocaine 2%, Benadryl elixir 12.5 mg/mL, Maalox) | 4×/day | Topical anesthetic for generalized areas of pain | Benadryl may exacerbate xerostomia |
| Ulcerease | 15 mL swish | Amesthetic mouth rinse | Contains no alcohol<br>Use full strength<br>May apply directly to ulcers with cotton swab after rinsing |
| Sucralfate suspension | 1 g/15 mL swish; 15 mL 4×/day | Binds to ulcerated tissue, protecting it from further insult, and may promote healing | No anesthetic action<br>Suspension may aggravate nausea |
| Vitamin E | 1 mL topically to oral lesions 2×/day | Promotes healing of mouth ulcers and controls pain | Anecdotal and research-based studies conclude vitamin E may help speed healing of chemotherapy-induced stomatitis |
| **Systemic Analgesics** | | | |
| Nonsteroidal anti-inflammatory agents (eg, Trilisate) | Depends on agent used<br>Doses vary | Mild to moderate pain | Longer duration of action than aspirin<br>No effect on platelets<br>Minimal GI side effects |
| Narcotic agents (eg, morphine) | Depends on agent used<br>Dose varies | Moderate to severe pain | |
| Capsaicin | 4×/day | Moderate to severe pain | Active ingredient in chili peppers |

epithelial cell repair. The dose is 60 μ/kg/day given IV 3 days before HSCT conditioning and continued 3 days after transplantation. Adverse events are primarily skin rash, pruritus, erythema, and taste alterations.[71–73]

Cryotherapy has been found to have a significant impact on decreasing mucositis with patients receiving 5-FU or melphalan by a rapid infusion.[69,71] Patients are to be instructed to hold ice in their mouth 5 minutes prior to infusion, during the infusion, and for 30 minutes after the infusion is completed.

The oral cavity is indirectly susceptible to infection because of chemotherapy-induced neutropenia. Chemotherapy weakens host defenses by changing the oral flora in becoming primarily gram-negative and reducing salivary and mucous gland function.[72] An overgrowth of normal oral microorganisms results in invasion of both endogenous and exogenous pathological organisms capable of producing oral infections. Mucosal disruption becomes an important portal of entry and compromises the integrity of the oral mucosa as the first line of defense. Pathogenic organisms can further contaminate the lungs and gastrointestinal tract, disseminating infection systematically.

Bacterial, fungal, and viral infections are all common in the myelosuppressed patient. Organisms such as *Streptococcus* species, *Candida* species, and herpes simplex virus (HSV) are the major oral infectious pathogens. Each infection has certain clinical features—such as the white or "cottage cheese" appearance of *Candida albicans* and the painful vesicular lesions of herpes simplex—that assist in identifying the pathogen. The proper identification of the pathogen requires a culture, and management will depend on the identified pathogen.[74–76]

The most frequent cause of oral infection is fungal. *C. albicans* is the predominate organism and pseudomembranous candidiasis (oral thrush) is the most common clinical manifestation. Oral *Candida* infections are best treated with antifungal drugs that are absorbed or partially absorbed from the GI tract. Those antifungal drugs that are absorbed from the GI tract included fluconazole, ketoconazole, and itraconazole. Those drugs that are partially absorbed from the GI tract include miconazole and clotrimazole.[77,78] A clotrimazole troche, given 5 times daily, must be sucked in the mouth until dissolved, which takes approximately 30 minutes. Long-term use of oral troches should be avoided, however, as they contain large quantities of sugar that may result in dental caries. If xerostomia is present, the troche will take longer to dissolve. Patients should be instructed to cleanse the mouth before administering the agent and not to eat or drink for at least 30 minutes after application. This regimen will permit drug contact with the mucosal surfaces to exert an antifungal effect. Denture wearers should be instructed to soak their appliance overnight with 100 mL nystatin suspension. The plastic in dentures can act as a reservoir to reinfect the treated mucosa.

Ketoconazole can be given as a 200 mg daily oral dose or fluconazole as a 100 to 200 mg oral dose daily. Absorption of ketoconazole is dependent on gastric acidity; therefore, patients are instructed to avoid the use of antacids and other medications that alter gastric pH within 2 hours of taking ketoconazole. Clotrimazole and fluconazole significantly reduce the incidence and duration of oropharyngeal candidiasis.[42,71,74] A course of low-dose IV amphotericin B is indicated for nonresponsive infection and in severe esophageal and disseminated candidal infections.[42,72,75] Antifungal drugs not absorbed from the GI tract (amphotericin B, nystatin, nystatin plus chlorhexidine, thymostimulin, amphotericin B plus nystatin, polyenes, natamycin, and norfloxacin plus amphotericin B) should not be used as studies have found that these drugs do not prevent oral candidiasis.[77,78]

Herpes simplex virus is the most common viral pathogen affecting the oral cavity. Vesicle fluid should be obtained for a culture to confirm the presence of HSV. When no vesicles are present, the base of the lesion should be swabbed using a viral culture swab. Swabs used for nasopharyngeal cultures (calcium alginate swabs) inactivate the virus and should not be used. Reactivation of latent HSV causes the majority of HSV infections.[42,75]

Immunocompromised patients who are seropositive for HSV are at risk for stomatitis. For patients with limited tissue involvement, acyclovir ointment can be applied topically every 3 to 6 hours while awake. Patients should be instructed to use gloves or cotton swabs when applying ointment, as autoinnoculation with the virus can occur. Extensive tissue involvement for disseminated herpes requires systemic acyclovir or famciclovir therapy, either orally or through IV. Antiviral prophylaxis may be used to prevent infection in selected high-risk populations, such as individuals who have undergone HSCT.[42]

Bacterial infections may affect the gingiva, mucosa, or teeth. Bacterial culture isolate and positive blood cultures confirm the diagnosis, although clinical features (pain, fever, oral lesions) may be present without positive blood cultures. Parenteral antibiotic therapy based on the causative organisms is the treatment of choice.

Oral pain is the major clinical problem associated with stomatitis. Pain results due to sloughing of the superficial epithelium, inflammation of the oral mucosa, and ulceration, making it difficult for the patient to practice adequate oral hygiene, eat properly, and communicate. Minimizing the pain can be accomplished with topical anesthetics and systemic analgesics (see Table 17-4). The latest oral pain management option is Gelclair gel. This concentrated oral base gel contains the barrier-forming ingredient polyvinylpyrrolidone and sodium hyaluronate.[56,69] An adherent barrier forms over the oral mucosa after rinsing with the gel to decrease oral pain.

Oral bleeding and hemorrhage are indirect stomatotoxic sequelae from chemotherapy-induced thrombocytopenia.

Bleeding results when the oral mucosa is traumatized or because of underlying periodontal disease; it may occur anywhere in the mouth. The lips, tongue, and gingiva are the most common sites of bleeding. For patients with a platelet count less than 20,000 cells/mm$^3$, less vigorous oral hygiene regimens should be used to clean the oral cavity. Management of bleeding with topical coagulants (thrombin-soaked gauze) and pressure is often helpful.[79]

Although the treatment of stomatitis remains palliative and symptom-oriented, ongoing studies are evaluating prophylactic measures to alleviate this side effect. Studies are underway examining the effectiveness of cytoprotective agents such as amifostine. Other agents, such as interleukin 11, keratinocyte growth factor 2, glucagonlike peptide 2, and epidermal growth factor, are also being studied. These agents stimulate growth, cellular differentiation, and cell migration of the oral epithelium.[72]

*Taste alterations.* Patients receiving chemotherapy may be susceptible to taste alterations. There can be actual or perceived changes in taste. The drugs cause direct injury to taste cells composing the taste buds, resulting in taste changes that vary widely and are highly individualized. Commonly induced changes include a lowered threshold for bitter taste, an increased threshold for sweet taste, and complaints of a metallic taste in the mouth. Chemotherapy drugs frequently associated with taste alterations include cyclophosphamide, dacarbazine, doxorubicin, fluorouracil, methotrexate, nitrogen mustard, cisplatin, and vincristine.[80]

Some agents, such as doxorubicin and methotrexate may alter taste acuity; others, such as cyclophosphamide and vincristine, can be tasted while injected. Chemotherapy-induced taste alterations can further be influenced by poor oral hygiene, infection of the oral cavity, dentures, and unpleasant odors.[80]

Unless patients are specifically questioned, taste alterations are seldom reported spontaneously. When questioned, patients may report their taste changes as reasons for their loss of appetite or decreased weight. Nursing interventions are aimed at teaching patients self-care measures to maintain optimal nutrition. Eating hints should be customized in accordance with each patient's change in taste appreciation.[81]

*Esophagitis.* Histologically, the mucosal lining of the esophagus is the same as the oral cavity. The esophagus is lined with stratified squamous epithelial cells. Destruction and inadequate replacement of these epithelial cells caused by chemotherapy agents will result in an inflammatory response called *esophagitis.* Similar to stomatitis, esophagitis can progress to ulceration, hemorrhage, and secondary infection and cause pain sufficient to make eating difficult.[50] Treatment may be discontinued temporarily to allow recovery of these cells, which parallels recovery of the WBC count.

The most common early symptoms of esophagitis include dysphagia (difficulty swallowing), odynophagia (painful swallowing), and epigastric pain. Esophageal pain that worsens and becomes continuous and substernal indicates progressive esophagitis. Any patient who develops oral mucositis following chemotherapy is at risk for spread to the esophageal mucosal tissue. Prior or concurrent radiation may exacerbate the severity and extent of mucosal injury. Some drugs, such as dactinomycin and doxorubicin, potentiate radiation injury to the esophagus; others, including fluorouracil, hydroxyurea, procarbazine, and vinblastine, produce an additive toxic effect with radiation.[56]

Although management of esophagitis varies greatly, all management is directed toward providing symptom relief and supportive care. Interventions are initiated to minimize irritation and promote comfort. This goal is best accomplished through dietary manipulation, topical anesthesia, and systemic analgesia when needed.

If nutritional status becomes compromised, patients may benefit from commercially prepared supplements. A nutritionist may be helpful in determining which products would best meet the individual needs of the patient. Some patients may require a feeding tube—usually a gastrostomy—if esophagitis is severe. Occasionally, a tube will be placed prior to initiating treatment if nutritional problems are anticipated.

Local anesthetics are often used every 3 to 4 hours as needed and prior to meals to help alleviate the pain associated with esophagitis (see Table 17-4). If topical anesthetic preparations do not relieve the discomfort, systemic narcotic analgesics may be needed. Tablets may need to be crushed and given in food. Narcotic elixirs often contain alcohol, which can further irritate the mucosa, and these may be given in foods or other nonirritating liquids.

Superimposed *Candida* infections may also present significant problems for patients with cancer.[42,72,75] Symptoms of *Candida* infection are often difficult to distinguish from treatment-induced esophagitis and may include dysphagia and pain. Prompt and appropriate medical treatment is necessary to prevent a systemic spread. Esophageal candidiasis is most commonly treated by using ketoconazole or fluconazole.[75]

### Integument

*Hyperpigmentation.* Numerous chemotherapeutic drugs are associated with hyperpigmentation (discoloration) of the skin, nails, and mucous membranes. While the etiology of hyperpigmentation is poorly understood, it is possible that the drug or a metabolic by-product of the drug stimulates melanocytes to produce increased quantities of melanin.[82] It is unclear why some drugs are associated with widespread hyperpigmentation, whereas others cause darkening confined to a specific area such as the tongue, nails, or mucous membranes. Hyperpigmentation occurs more commonly in dark-skinned individuals.

Busulfan can cause hyperpigmentation involving the neck, upper trunk, nipples, and abdomen, which is frequently associated with busulfan-induced pulmonary fibrosis. Hyperpigmentation caused by cyclophosphamide may be diffuse or confined to the palms, soles, nails, or gums. Skin contact with carmustine or nitrogen mustard can result in a contact dermatitis followed by postinflammatory hyperpigmentation.[82] After several infusions, irinotecan can cause hyperpigmentation that fades after the drug regimen is stopped. Arsenic trioxide commonly causes hyperpigmentation over the entire body surface.

Especially in those patients who receive high dose–weekly infusions with or without leucovorin, fluorouracil can cause hyperpigmentation. Hyperpigmentation occurs most readily in sun-exposed areas. Serpiginous hyperpigmented streaks overlying veins used repeatedly for fluorouracil infusions occur without any clinical evidence of cutaneous inflammation, phlebitis, or sclerosis (Figure 17-9).

Bleomycin may cause hyperpigmentation over the veins into which the drug is administered. However, bleomycin is more commonly associated with hyperpigmentation over pressure points or with linear streaks occurring in areas of intense scratching, presumably due to localized vasodilation that results in an increased bleomycin concentration in the skin (Figure 17-10).

Doxorubicin, busulfan, cyclophosphamide, fluorouracil, and etoposide have all been associated with hyperpigmentation of the oral mucosa and tongue, especially in African Americans. Doxorubicin and fluorouracil may also cause skin darkening over the interphalangeal and metacarpophalangeal joints. The mechanism of this effect is not known, but phalangeal darkening decreases once therapy is terminated.

*Miscellaneous rash.* Other drugs that can produce rash, urticaria, pruritus, or angioedema include procarbazine, cytarabine, topotecan, trimetrexate, anthracycline antibiotics, melphalan, pemetrexed, and methotrexate. All-transretinoic acid causes dry skin with mild exfoliation similar to a rash associated with pruritus.[83] Arsenic trioxide can produce urticaria, dry skin, angioedema, rash, and exfoliation of the skin.

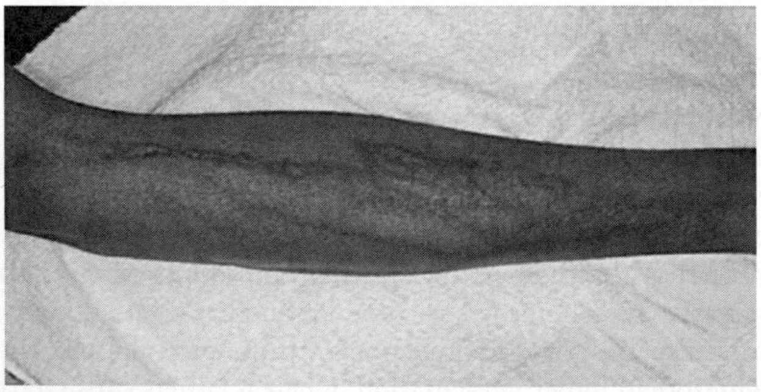

**FIGURE 17-9**

Serpiginous hyperpigmentation following 5-fluorouracil infusion.

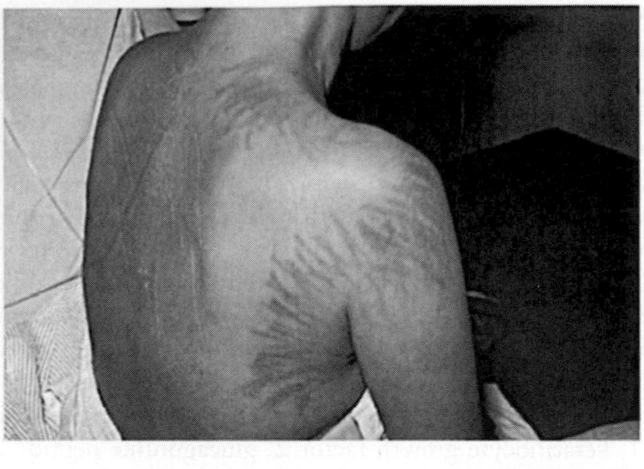

**FIGURE 17-10**

Flagellate streaks of hyperpigmentation in an Asian woman occurring in areas of intense scratching following intracavitary (intrapleural) bleomycin.

A common drug side effect is a morbilliform maculopapular rash sometimes associated with fever. The pruritic rash usually disappears and does not necessitate cessation of therapy. Rarely, it can progress and cause desquamation. Hydrocortisone may be given in higher than usual doses for the first 2 weeks of therapy in an attempt to decrease the severity of the skin rash.

Dactinomycin folliculitis presents as diffuse erythematous papules over the face and trunk, resembling acne, and appearing approximately 5 days after therapy. The rash resolves in 3 to 5 days. Folliculitis has also been reported following high-dose methotrexate.[82]

Erythema multiforme has been infrequently associated with chemotherapeutic agents. Patients receiving high-dose combination chemotherapy are at greater risk for this toxicity. The reaction is characterized by target lesions over the extremities, often involving the mucous membranes. Busulfan, etoposide, procarbazine, hydroxyurea, bleomycin, methotrexate, and cytarabine have been associated with such lesions, which occasionally develop into generalized blistering.[82,83]

Radiation recall is a type of reaction that is caused from the reactivation of inflammatory dermatitis at a site of prior radiation therapy months to years later. This reaction has been observed with the drugs gemcitabine, methotrexate, cytarabine, dactinomycin, bleomycin, lomustine, cyclophosphamide, capecitabine, doxorubicin, etoposide, fluorouracil, hydroxyurea, melphalan, and vincristine.[82] Drugs known to act as a radiosensitizer should be used with care for several weeks after radiation. Nurses must assess the radiation portal for increase skin changes.

*Acral erythema.* An intensely painful erythema, scaling, and epidermal sloughing from the palms and soles, followed by desquamation and reepithelialization of the skin, has been reported with fluorouracil, doxorubicin, paclitaxel, high-dose cytarabine, methotrexate, capecitabine, docetaxel, liposomal doxorubicin, and floxuridine. The condition, also called *palmarplantar erythrodysesthesia,* may represent a direct toxic effect on the epidermis and dermal vasculature or an accumulation of the chemotherapeutic agent in eccrine structures, causing erythema of the palms and soles where there are high concentrations of eccrine glands.[82,84,85] Initially, the patient may complain of tingling and pain of the feet and hands, which generally progress to edema, tenderness to touch, intense erythema, and desquamation. Strategies to prevent this reaction include avoiding pressure such as tight-fitting clothing over bony prominences, especially during drug infusion, and avoiding excessive heat beginning the day of infusion and for 5 days afterward. Management focuses on comfort measures.[85] Chemotherapy is usually suspended until symptoms subside and then resumes at a lower dose. However, the symptoms may recur and may necessitate cessation of therapy.

*Pruritus.* An allergic dermatitis may result from chemotherapy causing localized and generalized pruritus. Pruritus can be overwhelming and distressing to the individual, as it commonly interferes with rest and sleep and can result in skin breakdown and infection.

Assessment requires a thorough evaluation of the possible cause of the itching and any factors that might aggravate the condition. If pruritus is chemotherapy induced, the condition generally resolves when the drug is stopped or gradually dissipates following antihistamine therapy.

Nursing management focuses on skin care and comfort.[83] Medicated baths, anesthetic creams, and emollient creams may be soothing. Soaps made especially for sensitive skin should be used when skin cleansing is required. The patient is encouraged to use alternative cutaneous stimulation methods to relieve the urge to scratch, such as massage, pressure, or rubbing the area with a soft cloth. Distractions such as music, imagery, or relaxation may ease the itch sensation. Perfumes, cosmetics, starch-based powders, and deodorants should be avoided.

Environmental factors include keeping the room humidity at 30% to 40% and the room temperature cool. Cotton clothing and sheets should be washed in hypoallergenic soaps. Medications such as antihistamines or corticosteroids may be used to minimize itching.

*Photosensitivity.* Photosensitivity is an enhanced skin response to ultraviolet (UV) rays. This response may present much like a sunburn, with erythema, edema, blisters, hyperpigmentation, and desquamation or peeling. Rarely, photoallergy, similar to contact dermatitis, with immediate wheal and flare reactions or delayed reactions may occur. Photosensitivity has been reported following skin exposure to UV light after administration of fluorouracil, dacarbazine, *trans*-retinoic acid, vinblastine, and high-dose methotrexate. In general, the exposed area becomes erythematous within a few hours and gradually subsides. Dacarbazine, however, has been associated with pruritus and erythematous eruptions on the face, neck, and dorsal surfaces of both hands after sun exposure occurred within 1 to 2 hours following drug administration.[81]

Nurses must educate patients on the risk of UV light exposure. Verbal and written instructions concerning ways to reduce the risk of developing a photosensitivity reaction are given to the patient. Sun exposure, particularly between the hours of 10 AM and 3 PM, and tanning booths are to be avoided. Protective clothing and a hat should be worn even on cloudy days.

Most important, nurses should provide instructions regarding the proper use of sunscreen based on the individual's skin type. Sunscreens contain a sun protection factor (SPF) that defines the ratio of the time it takes to develop erythema with and without the sunscreen applied. For example, an individual who can be in direct sunlight for only 30 minutes without erythema may, by applying a sunscreen with an SPF of 8, remain outside for 240 minutes (30 × 8) without burning. The higher the SPF, the more complete the sun protection. Products with an SPF higher than 15 are recommended for protection following chemotherapy. Sunblocks with an SPF of 25 or higher are available and recommended for children and fair-skinned individuals. In general, the higher the SPF, the greater the chance of skin irritation. Some sunscreens are water resistant, but in general they should be applied frequently and directly to the skin. To maximize its effectiveness, the sunscreen should be applied at least 15 to 30 minutes before sun exposure and as often as indicated by activities in which the individual is engaged.

*Alopecia.* Alopecia is the most noticeable cutaneous side effect of chemotherapy and often one of the most distressing. Although certainly not a life-threatening event, loss of hair has a profound social and psychological impact on individuals and their acceptance of treatment. Some individuals may even refuse potentially curative therapy for fear of hair loss.

Chemotherapy drugs affect actively growing (anagen) hairs. Because anagen hair is the most rapidly proliferating cell population in the human body, alopecia is a common toxicity. Extent of hair loss can range from thinning of scalp hair to total body hair loss.[86] Chemotherapy causes the hair shaft to be fragile or defective and, therefore, subject to breakage with minimal trauma.

Higher doses of chemotherapy or more potent epilators cause complete mitotic arrest, resulting in atrophy of the root and loss of the hair root bulb. Hair falls out spontaneously or is lost easily when combed or washed. Drugs of less intensity temporarily inhibit or slow cellular activity, causing bulb deformity and narrowing of the hair shaft. When hair growth resumes, narrow, weakened hair shafts are prone to breakage at the point of constriction. The hair root however, remains intact and active, leaving a thinning pattern of hair loss.

With an average 85% of scalp hair follicles in the anagen phase at any given time, the most common location for hair loss is the scalp. The majority of other body hair follicles (eyebrows, axilla, pubic area) are in the less active catagen and telogen phases and, therefore, are not initially affected. However, with multiple exposures from long-term therapy, these hairs may also be lost as the hairs enter the anagen phase.[86]

Unlike natural hair loss, chemotherapy-induced alopecia occurs rapidly and usually starts 2 to 3 weeks following a dose of chemotherapy. Hair loss is usually asymptomatic; however, some patients have described intense scalp discomfort 1 to 2 days prior to and during hair shedding.

Chemotherapy-induced alopecia is temporary and reversible. After discontinuation of the drugs, regrowth is visible in 4 to 6 weeks, but complete regrowth may take 1 to 2 years. As hair grows back, alterations in hair pigmentation (lighter or darker), hair texture (finer or coarser), and hair type (straight or curly) may be evident.

The severity and duration of chemotherapy-induced alopecia are related to the type of drug, combination of drugs, dose of drug, method of administration, and pharmacokinetics. Hair loss can be described as minimal (less than 25%), moderate (25%-50%), or severe (more than 50%). Hair loss produces loss of heat or body warmth from head as well as sun exposure, which indicates the need for head covering. Chemotherapy agents most frequently associated with moderate to severe hair loss include trimetrexate, cyclophosphamide, doxorubicin, dactinomycin, daunorubicin, etoposide, idarubicin, ifosfamide, irinotecan, mechlorethamine, paclitaxel, topotecan, and vincristine. Mild hair loss is associated with bleomycin, carmustine, epirubicin, fluorouracil, methotrexate, melphalan, mitomycin, mitoxantrone, teniposide, temozolomide, and vinorelbine.

Bolus IV administration of chemotherapy results in immediate peak serum levels with subsequent exposure and damage of sensitive growing hairs, resulting in hair loss. Infusions over several hours or longer are associated with greater likelihood of alopecia. The risk of alopecia appears to be decreased with low-dose continuous infusion. This may be related to the fact that high-peak serum levels are necessary to cause hair loss.[81]

A patient-related factor that may influence the degree of scalp hair loss is the variability of scalp hair growth among individuals. Individuals who have relatively few hairs in the anagen phase will be less sensitive to the effects of chemotherapy. Another factor to consider is the condition of the patient's hair before treatment. Damaged hair (tinted, permanent use) may potentiate the risk for alopecia.

Until the early 1990s, scalp hypothermia was the technique used to prevent or minimize hair loss. However, because there was risk of scalp micrometastasis, this technique is no longer recommended.[83,84] Therefore, more emphasis needs to be placed on the psychologic support of the patient experiencing hair loss from chemotherapy and use of creative measures to preserve self-image.

It is essential that the patient and family be informed of the timing, extent, and duration of hair loss at the onset of therapy. While these factors are not always known, many times they are; for instance, when high-dose doxorubicin and cyclophosphamide are used, hair loss is nearly complete by 3 weeks. Patients should be encouraged to discuss their feelings regarding hair loss. It is often helpful for patients to prepare for alopecia by procuring a scalp prosthesis (wig or hairpiece) before it becomes necessary. This strategy often reduces the anxiety associated with the uncertain timing of hair loss and makes it easier for a stylist to match color and style. Patients should be encouraged to question their insurance carriers regarding coverage for "cranial therapeutic prosthesis" for treatment-induced alopecia. Some insurance companies will reimburse with a physician's prescription or letter.

Certain measures can be used to minimize or delay hair loss and scalp irritation. Some clinicians advise patients to cut long hair short in anticipation of hair loss. Short hair may make hair loss less noticeable, make remaining hair appear thicker, and possibly decrease the weight on the hair shaft. Once hair loss is significant, the patient may be advised to shave the remaining scalp hairs. This practice allows the hair to grow in at the same length, often permitting the patient to go without a wig sooner. In addition, shaving the head rids the patient of the problem of continuous shedding of hair. Measures to minimize hair loss include use of mild protein-based shampoos with conditioners, avoidance of daily shampooing, allowing hair to dry naturally, and grooming hair with a wide-toothed comb. Hair care practices such as blow-drying, perming, or coloring hair are controversial and areas for further nursing research. Claims have been made that these practices cause the hair to become brittle and fall out earlier during chemotherapy.

*Nails.* Changes in the fingernails and toenails are commonly seen during chemotherapy.[83] Pigmentation is seen most commonly and occurs with more regularity and intensity in blacks than in whites. The pigment generally is deposited at the base of the nail, causing transverse dark bands that correlate with the times the drug was administered. This reaction occurs most commonly with paclitaxel, docetaxel, doxorubicin, and cyclophosphamide but has been reported with melphalan, fluorouracil, daunomycin, idarubicin, and bleomycin. If continuous infusion therapy of these drugs is given, the nails darken evenly.[83]

Beau lines (transverse white lines or grooves in the nail) indicate a reduction or cessation of nail growth in response to chemotherapy. A partial separation of the nail plate (onycholysis) can be seen with fluorouracil, doxorubicin, paclitaxel, docetaxel, and bleomycin.[83]

## ORGAN TOXICITIES

Certain chemotherapy drugs may cause direct damage to specific cells of a given organ or cause indirect damage by the effects of cellular breakdown by-products. In general, organ toxicities are predictable based on the cumulative dose, the presence of concomitant organ dysfunction, the age of the patient, and the manner in which the drug is given. Of interest is the fact that the toxicity profile may be changing as a result of the more widespread use of dose-intensive regimens, multimodality treatment, chemoprotectants, and CSFs. These approaches to manage the disease are likely to result in more organ toxicities as myelosuppression becomes less prominent. Each of the major organ toxicities is discussed here. Tables 17-5 through 17-10 provide a review of major toxicities in terms of risk factors, signs of toxicity, preventive measures, grading, and management.

### Cardiotoxicity

Cardiotoxicity is described as an acute or chronic process. The acute form of cardiotoxicity consists of transient electrocardiogram (ECG) changes that occur in approximately 10% of patients receiving chemotherapy. Acute effects are immediate in onset and resolve quickly without serious complications. These effects are not dose related and are generally not an indication to stop the drug. Fewer than 5% of patients develop chronic cardiotoxicity from a cumulative drug effect that requires immediate discontinuation of the drug.[87] Chronic effects occur weeks or months after administration, involving nonreversible cardiomyopathy, presenting as a classic biventricular congestive heart failure (CHF) with a characteristic low-voltage QRS complex. Signs and symptoms are classic for CHF, including complaints of dyspnea, a nonproductive cough, and pedal edema. Generally, chronic chemotherapy-induced cardiomyopathy is poorly responsive to diuretics or digitalis and becomes progressively worse, with 60% mortality.

Anthracyclines are known to cause cardiotoxicity by directly damaging the cardiac myocyte cells. The incidence of cardiotoxicity is 10% to 26% after cumulative doses are administered.[87] However, accurately estimating the incidence of anthracycline-induced cardiotoxicity is difficult because data are primarily retrospective and long-term data is often not available. Total cumulative dosages have been established at 550 mg/m$^2$ for doxorubicin, 400 mg/m$^2$ for epirubicin, and 600 mg/m$^2$ for daunorubicin, with a decrease in dose to 450 mg/m$^2$, if mediastinal radiation has been administered.[88]

The mechanism of action related to cardiotoxicity occurs in the presence of oxygen, where the anthracyclines form a bond or union with iron or copper. These complexes inhibit lipid peroxidation, allowing free oxygen radicals to directly damage the myocyte. The results are a loss of myocardial fibrils, mitochondrial changes, and cellular destruction. As a consequence, the myocyte has limited contractility, leading to hypertrophy of the cardiac muscle, which increases the demand for oxygen.[88]

In an attempt to decrease cardiotoxicity occurrence, altering the dose and scheduling of doxorubicin to include frequent lower doses has resulted in reduction of cardiotoxicity without compromise of antitumor effects.[86] The use of liposomal doxorubicin has also demonstrated a reduction of cardiotoxicity. Chemoprotectants are being evaluated for their ability to protect the cardiac tissue by blocking damage to the myocyte. Flavonoids have been studied as possible protectants of cardiac toxicity. This class of agents has the combined ability to chelate iron and has antioxidant properties. Both in vitro and in vivo studies have shown promising results for cardio-protection.[89]

Dexrazoxane (Zinecard) is currently approved for patients with metastatic breast cancer who have received cumulative doses of 300 mg/m$^2$ of doxorubicin and are continuing treatment with doxorubicin (not for initial treatment). Patients have been able to tolerate greater cumulative doses of doxorubicin with a decreased risk of cardiac events. Dexrazoxane is administered 30 minutes prior to doxorubicin, calculated on a 10:1 ratio. Thus, with a 50 mg dose of doxorubicin, 500 mg of dexrazoxane would be administered. This compound has permitted doses of doxorubicin as high as 700 mg/m$^2$ to be administered without the occurrence of cardiotoxicity. It appears to interfere with the intracellular process responsible for anthracycline-induced cardiomyopathy.[87] Dexrazoxane has been used in other types of malignancies in adult patients who have received more than 300 mg/m$^2$ of doxorubicin.[90]

In an attempt to reduce further the cardiotoxicity from the anthracyclines, analogs that have greater antitumor activity and may have reduced cardiotoxicity have been developed. Epirubicin, idarubicin, esorubicin, and aclarubicin appear to be similar to doxorubicin, but their cardiotoxicity is significantly less. Although mitoxantrone has been associated with rare cardiac events, it is considered to be less cardiotoxic.[90] CHF has been noted to occur in patients receiving bevacizumab therapy concurrent with anthracyclines, or with a history of having receiving anthracyclines with or without left chest wall irradiation.

Acute pericarditis has been reported with high-dose cyclophosphamide therapy (90–270 mg/kg) used in the stem cell transplant (SCT) population, with subsequent pericardial effusion and cardiac tamponade.[91] Cyclophosphamide damages the myocytes in a manner similar to that seen with anthracyclines, where swelling and decreased contractility lead to less effective pumping of the heart. Hemorrhagic

**TABLE 17-5**

**Organ Toxicity of Chemotherapy Agents: Cardiotoxicity**

| Toxicity/ Symptoms | Grade | General Risk Factors | Chemotherapy Agents/Risk Factors | Mechanism of Damage | Protective/ Management Measures |
|---|---|---|---|---|---|
| • Tachycardia<br>• Dyspnea<br>• Nonproductive cough<br>• Neck vein distention<br>• Gallop rhythm<br>• Rales<br>• Pedal edema<br>• Cardiomegaly<br>• Dull or sharp precordial pain, may radiate to neck and shoulder<br>• Cardiac friction rub<br>• ST-T wave changes<br>• Supraventricular tachyarrhythmias<br>• T-wave flattening | Cardiac Dysrhythmias<br>0 = None<br>1 = Asymptomatic, transient, requires no therapy<br>2 = Recurrent or persistent, requires no therapy<br>3 = Requires treatment<br>4 = Requires monitoring hypotension ventricular tachycardia. or fibrillation<br><br>Cardiac Function<br>0 = None<br>1 = Asymptomatic decline of resting ejection by less then 20% of baseline<br>2 = Asymptomatic decline of resting ejection fraction by more than 20%of baseline<br>3 = Mild CHF, responsive to therapy<br>4 = Severe or refractory CHF | • Age, geriatric and pediatric<br>• Cumulative dose<br>• Schedule of drug administration<br>• History of cardiac disease (eg, atherosclerosis, mitral value prolapse, CHF, hypertension)<br>• Use of combination drugs<br>• Hepatic dysfunction<br>• Prior mediastinum radiation<br>• Prior anthracycline exposure | Anthracyclines<br>• Doxorubicin (> 550mg/m²)<br>• Daunorubicin (> 600 mg/m²)<br>• Dactinomycin<br>• Doxorubicin-enhanced effect with actinomycin, mitomycin, vincristine, melphalan, bleomycin, cyclophosphamide<br>• Mitoxantrone (> 160 mg/m²) | Acute Changes<br>• Hypereosinophilia of myocytes<br>Chronic Changes<br>• Loss of contractile elements<br>• Mitochondrial changes<br>• Myocyte damage | • Limit cumulative dose of doxorubicin to < 550 mg/m²<br>• Administer doxorubicin at lower doses more frequently<br>• ECG before treatment<br>• Radionuclide cardiac scan<br>• Administer dexrazoxane before anthracycline dose |
| | | | • Cyclophosphamide, high-dose (> 144 mg/kg × 4 days) | • Hemorrhagic myocardial necrosis<br>• Fibrin deposition in interstitium | • Administer calcium channel blockers before anthracycline dose |
| | | | • 5-fluorouracil | • Coronary spasm of the prinzmetal type | • Limit cumulative dose of daunorubicin to < 600 mg/m² |
| | | | • Paclitaxel | • Speculated to be related to Cremphor EL, the administration vehicle for paclitaxel that causes activation of selected cardiac histamine receptors | • Avoid alcohol, smoking, and cocaine use<br>• Moderate exercise and low-fat, low-salt diet<br>• Prevent thrombus with daily aspirin or warfarin |
| | | | • Arsenic trioxide | • Prolonged Q-T interval<br>• Premature ventricular contractions<br>• Potentially fatal<br>• Torsades-de-points<br>• Pericardial effusion | • Herceptin is not given concurrent with doxorubicin |

*Abbreviations*: CHF, congestive heart failure; ECG, electrocardiogram.

myocardial necrosis has been reported, with leakage of blood through capillaries. Transient complete heart block requiring temporary pacemaker support has been reported as well. Toxicity ranges from minor, transient ECG changes and asymptomatic elevation of cardiac enzymes to fatal myopericarditis and myocardial necrosis.[90]

Myocardial ischemia has been reported with fluorouracil infusion in patients with or without preexisting heart disease. Coronary vasospasm, with resulting angina pectoris, myocardial infarction, S-T segment elevations, and ventricular ectopy, has been described. The pathophysiology is unclear, although a direct cardiomyopathic effect from the release of vasoactive substances in the presence of fluorouracil has been suggested.[90] It has been speculated that angina is a coronary artery spasm of the Prinzmetal type that responds to nitrates. Cessation of therapy does not appear to be absolutely necessary, as patients who have such a syndrome can be pretreated with calcium channel blockers known to prevent coronary artery spasm. Case reports of patients taking capecitabine have been reported to having a myocardial infarction while on treatment.[91]

Asymptomatic bradycardia has been reported in approximately 30% of patients with ovarian cancer who have received paclitaxel. Other cardiac disturbances, which have been reported in 5% of patients, include atrioventricular conduction blocks, left bundle branch blocks, ventricular tachycardia, and symptoms of cardiac ischemia. Most paclitaxel-related cardiac disturbances were not associated with clinical symptoms and were noted incidentally during continuous cardiac monitoring. Paclitaxel infusion is not discontinued unless it is associated with progressive atrioventricular conduction disturbances. Although the mechanism is unclear, it is speculated to be the result of the administration of the drug vehicle Cremophor EL, which causes activation of selected cardiac histamine receptors. Stimulation of these receptors in the cardiac tissue increases myocardial oxygen demand and produces coronary vasoconstriction.[86] Trastuzumab has been cited as causing cardiac toxicity. The mechanism of action is not clearly understood. It appears that trastuzumab blocks the endothelial growth factor receptor pathway, which is responsible for providing regulation of cardiomyocyte growth and repair.[90,92]

Cardiac function should be evaluated throughout therapy for patients who are at high risk for cardiotoxicity or who will be receiving high dosages of paclitaxel, an anthracycline, or high-dose cyclophosphamide. Methods to evaluate cardiac function include noninvasive monitoring with ECG, echocardiography, and radionuclide cardiography. An ejection fraction less than 45% or a decrease of 5% or more from the resting value is considered abnormal. Further doses of cardiotoxic chemotherapy are not recommended.[89] Although an endomyocardial biopsy can reveal damage to the myocyte prior to clinical detection, the procedure is costly and technically difficult and requires considerable expertise.

The lifelong cardiotoxic effects of conventional anthracycline therapy highlight the need for monitoring cardiac dysfunction. Radionuclide cardiography and echocardiograms are the noninvasive methods most commonly used, despite their insensitivity for detecting early signs of cardiotoxicity.[87] Considering the occurrence of late-onset cardiac dysfunction, long-term follow-up is recommended with noninvasive testing based on the patient's risk factors and cardiac symptoms. Low-risk patients have been defined as those receiving less than 200 mg/m$^2$ of an anthracycline and no mediastinal radiation or exhibiting no cardiac abnormality. High-risk patients are considered to be those who have received more than 400 mg/m$^2$ of an anthracycline, mediastinal radiation, or have abnormal cardiac function. A follow-up evaluation 3 months after completing therapy with an echocardiogram or radionuclide angiograpy allows detection of late-developing toxicity. Long-term follow-up recommendations include a minimum of 1 echocardiogram yearly and a cardiac scan every 5 years if the patient remains asymptomatic.[88,93]

Circulating biochemical markers play a pivotal role in the diagnosis and management of cardiac toxicity. Cardiac troponin is a protein released from myocytes in response to cellular damage. The degree of troponin release has been shown to directly correlate with the degree of myocardium damage. Natriuretic peptides (BNP) are released in response to changes in circulating volume and intracardiac pressures. Their function is to reduce plasma volume through promotion of diuresis and vasodilatation. BNP levels may be useful in monitoring cardiac failure from cardiac toxicity.[2,90]

Accurate documentation and monitoring of total cumulative dosages of chemotherapy are essential. Cardiac assessment is imperative to evaluate for a third heart sound or gallop, which could indicate cardiac insufficiency. Cardiac monitoring may be necessary for administering high dosages of chemotherapy, such as cyclophosphamide. Once the patient develops chronic cardiotoxicity, nursing interventions include teaching the patient about energy conservation, managing fluid retention, and minimizing sodium in the diet. Supportive care with digitalis, angiotensin-converting enzyme (ACE) inhibitors to enhance the cardiac output, and diuretics to manage fluid should also be instituted.[88,93] Eventually, the patient may need supplemental oxygen and vasodilator medications to relieve dyspnea. Heart transplantation has become an option to treat end-stage heart disease from anthracycline cardiomyopathy.[94]

The degree of cardiac injury determines the limitations on activities of daily living that the individual will experience. Few patients are prepared for this debilitating effect, and patients and families need assistance in learning how to cope with this adverse event. Patients are also taught the importance of close cardiac follow-up, once the treatment is complete, to monitor for late cardiac effects (Table 17-5).

## Neurotoxicity

Chemotherapy-induced neurotoxicity can arise in the form of direct or indirect damage to the CNS, peripheral nervous system, cranial nerves, or any combination of the three. Although the majority of patients experience temporary neurotoxicity, some will have permanent neurological deficits. Significant neurotoxicity usually requires suspending the treatment until the symptom resolves and reinstituting therapy with a 50% dose reduction or discontinuing the drug.[95,96]

The central and peripheral nervous systems are protected against potentially neurotoxic effects by the blood-brain barrier and blood-nerve barriers. If intact, these barriers exclude most water-soluble chemotherapeutic agents and relatively large molecules. Biopsies of nerves suffering damage from chemotherapy have demonstrated a mild decrease in the number of large-diameter myelinated nerve fibers, and ultra-structural studies have shown scattered degenerating nerve fibers both in axons and in myelin sheaths. The severity of neurotoxicity is usually dose-related, with symptoms exhibited in a variable and unpredictable fashion.

The CNS consists of collections of neurons, and their connections are organized into the brain and spinal cord areas. Damage to the CNS primarily involves the cerebellum, which produces altered reflexes, unsteady gait, ataxia, and confusion. The peripheral nervous system is basically a set of communication channels located outside the CNS, consisting of the cranial and spinal nerves. Damage to the peripheral nervous system produces paralysis or loss of movement and sensation to those areas affected by the particular nerve. The autonomic nervous system (ANS) includes those peripheral nerves that regulate functions occurring automatically in the body, such as the cardiovascular, respiratory, and endocrine systems. Damage to the ANS causes ileus, impotence, or urinary retention.

Vincristine is well known for potential peripheral neuropathy characterized by myalgia and loss of the deep tendon reflex at the ankle, progressing to complete areflexia, distal symmetric sensory loss, motor weakness, foot drop, and muscle atrophy.[96] Autonomic neuropathy is characterized by ileus, constipation, impotence, urinary retention, or postural hypotension. The mechanism of damage is believed to involve disruption of the microtubule in the neural tissues, which inhibits the mitotic spindle movements necessary for the mitosis phase of cellular reproduction.[96] Vincristine doses greater than 2 mg increase the risk of neurotoxicity.

Neuropathy related to cisplatin is reversible, although cases of persistent progression after the discontinuation of the drug have been reported.[97] Cisplatin affects the large-diameter fibers of the neural tissues, resulting in sensory changes. The earliest sign of peripheral neuropathy is decreased vibratory sense, described as hand and feet paresthesias, with the classic stocking-glove distribution. Sensory loss occurs initially; without dose modification, loss of the Achilles reflex, muscle weakness, and loss of the deep tendon reflex occur. Symptoms of neuropathy are seen at cumulative doses of 300 to 500 $mg/m^2$. As the neuropathy progresses, position sense is impaired and a marked sensory ataxia develops. Peripheral neuropathy has been reported from combined therapy consisting of paclitaxel and cisplatin. Sensory-motor neuropathy occurs 1 to 21 weeks after initiation of therapy. Neuropathy appears to be progressive with additional courses, and more pronounced with higher doses of paclitaxel (cumulative dose $\geq$ 1500 $mg/m^3$).[97]

High-tone hearing loss is speculated to be related to the loss of hairs in the organ of Corti resulting from cisplatin administration. Rapid drug delivery, simultaneous administration of aminoglycosides, and dehydration seem to increase the potential for ototoxicity. Although the loss can be reversed with discontinuation of the drug, permanent damage has been reported, resulting in the need for a hearing aid.[98]

Neurotoxicity characterized by metabolic encephalopathy manifested as blurred vision, seizures, motor system dysfunction, urinary incontinence, cranial nerve dysfunction, subclinical electroencephalographic changes, or irreversible coma has been reported in 5% to 30% of patients treated with ifosfamide.[95] Signs have occurred within 2 hours of bolus administration and as long as 28 days after therapy. Within 48 to 72 hours of cessation of ifosfamide, most abnormalities spontaneously resolve. Risk factors associated with neurotoxicity include duration of administration, hepatic insufficiency, previous administration of cisplatin, presence of bulky disease, low serum albumin, and high serum creatinine.[95] Although the cause is not completely understood, the encephalopathy is thought to result from an accumulation of drug metabolites (chloracetaldehyde), which causes direct CNS damage. If the patient seems disoriented or demonstrates any neurological changes following ifosfamide infusion, subsequent doses of ifosfamide should be withheld pending further investigation. Administration of additional doses of ifosfamide to an individual already demonstrating neurotoxicity from ifosfamide can result in worsening of symptoms and seizures.

After several courses, high-dose methotrexate (>1 $g/m^2$) occasionally causes encephalopathy that usually is transient and reversible.[96] Intrathecal methotrexate may cause chemical meningitis, with fever, headache, muscle rigidity, and cerebrospinal fluid leukocytosis. This toxicity is rare, but it occurs within hours of the intrathecal injection and resolves spontaneously.

Fluorouracil may cause an acute cerebellar dysfunction, which is usually more common in the elderly. It is characterized by rapid onset of gait ataxia, dysarthria, nystagmus, diplopia, limb incoordination, and the inability to make fine, coordinated movements. Effects are reversible with drug withdrawal or dose reduction. Multifocal cerebral demyelination has been described to occur as the result of fluorouracil and leucovorin administration.[96] Symptoms that have been exhibited include acute confusion, ataxia, slurred speech, and restlessness. With steroid use and discontinuing chemotherapy, the patient's symptoms improve.

High-dose cytarabine can cause encephalopathy, leukoencephalopathy, and sometimes peripheral neuropathy with doses greater than 1.8 $g/m^2$. High doses increase the transport rate over the cell membranes, enhancing the intracellular drug concentrations and prolonging the cellular exposure to the drug's metabolites. CNS toxicity usually occurs 5 to 7 days after the start of therapy.[96] Ocular toxicity (conjunctivitis, photophobia, burning, and decreased acuity) and cerebellar and cerebral dysfunction can also occur. Once the drug is stopped, the neurological symptoms may resolve partially or completely.

Arthralgia and myalgia have been reported to occur infrequently with docetaxel administration. If symptoms occur, they are usually experienced a few days after administration and can last up to 4 days. Severity of discomfort can be reduced by the use of prophylactic analgesics such as ibuprofen. Transient arthralgia and myalgia are common after paclitaxel therapy.[95] Symptoms usually occur 2 to 3 days after treatment and resolve in approximately 6 days. The shoulder and paraspinal muscles seem to be the most common area of occurrence, but other muscle groups can be affected. All-transretinoic acid commonly causes myalgia, arthralgia, and muscle weakness.[97] Gemcitabine causes symptoms of low-grade fever, fatigue, malaise, myalgia and arthralgia with parenthesia in about 10% of patients.

One of the principal nonhematologic toxicities of paclitaxel is sensory neuropathy, which is experienced at doses of 250 mg/m$^2$ or greater. Symptoms consist of numbness, tingling, or burning pain of the lower extremities. Perioral numbness has been reported that may be asymmetrical at onset and progress in a symmetrical pattern. Neurotoxicity is typically cumulative; with large-fiber modalities (vibration, proprioception) being more frequently affected than small-fiber modalities (pain and temperature).[96] Mild symptoms improve or resolve within several months after the discontinuation of paclitaxel. Amitriptyline has been found to be show modest improvement in relieving the discomfort associated with the symptoms.[98,99] Autonomic neuropathy has been reported with high doses of paclitaxel (250 mg/m$^2$ or greater) and is manifested as paralytic ileus and orthostatic hypotension. Patients with diabetes mellitus experience this neuropathy more frequently.[100] Transient encephalopathy has been reported after paclitaxel infusion and is exhibited as confusion, word-finding difficulty, and behavioral changes. Symptoms appear 1 week after paclitaxel infusion and resolve spontaneously.[97]

Abraxene is an albumin-stabilized nanoparticle formulation of paclitaxel. Administered at a dose of 260 mg/m$^2$ as a 30-minute infusion every 3 weeks, it is associated with significantly higher incidence of peripheral neuropathy than paclitaxel.[95] Symptoms of neuropathy are sensory and similar to paclitaxel. Thalidomide is a oral immunomodulatory agent that causes peripheral neuropathy by distal axonal degeneration without demyelination. Symptoms include numbness and tingling in the hands and feet. Symptoms usually subside with discontinuation of the treatment.[97]

Docetaxel administration can produce mild sensory neuropathy. At a cumulative dose of 600 mg/m$^2$, severe and disabling neuropathy can develop. Symptoms include paresthesias, numbness, loss of sensory qualities, and a decrease in deep tendon reflexes.[97]

Oxaliplatin can induce 2 types of neurotoxicity, acute and chronic. An acute, reversible peripheral sensory neuropathy can occur within hours and as long as 2 days after infusion.[97] Symptoms may be precipitated by exposure to cold, such as cold air or cold drinks. Although discontinuation of the drug is rarely necessary, this neuropathy frequently recurs with subsequent doses. Pharyngolaryngeal dysthesia characterized by subjective sensations of dysphagia, dyspnea, or tightness in the back of throat has occurred. During this sensation, no laryngospasm or bronchospasm has been observed. Motor neuropathy can also occur, characterized by paresthesias, dysesthesia, and hypoesthesia; it may be related to a cumulative dose of 700 mg/m$^2$.[97] Patients are instructed to avoid cold drinks or exposure to cold immediately after infusion of oxaliplatin.[20]

Cognitive function can be altered with the administration of standard-dose and high-dose chemotherapy. Problems are observed in the patient's short-term memory and ability to concentrate. Cognitive deficits can continue for as long as 10 years after treatment.[101]

Chemoprotectants have been evaluated in minimizing chemotherapy-induced neurotoxicity. Amifostine has been found to decrease carboplatin and paclitaxel–based chemotherapy-induced neurotoxicity and may protect against ototoxicity.[98] Glutamine has been studied as a neuroprotective agent, and shows some benefit with use with paclitaxel-containing regimens.[102–104] Other agents have been in trials to prevent chemotherapy-induced neuropathy including acetyl-L-carnitine, alpha-lipoic acid, calcium and magnesium infusions, glutathione, recombinant human leukemia inhibitory factor and vitamin E. General use of these agents cannot be recommend because of insufficient or conflicting data.[98]

Astute neurological assessment is critical in patients receiving potentially neurotoxic agents. The baseline assessment should include gait, sensory function, motor function, range of motion, cranial nerves, and reflexes. Renal and hepatic function should be monitored closely.[100] Chemotherapy agents such as ifosfamide and cytarabine will have increased neurotoxicity with renal dysfunction. Sedatives, antiemetics, and tranquilizers, which are CNS depressants, must be used with caution because their usage may increase toxicity. In addition, other causes of these symptoms—such as electrolyte imbalances, metastasis, or other medical conditions—can cause similar effects.

Neurotoxicity will affect patients by decreasing their mobility, ability for self-care, and ability to perform fine-motor skills such as writing and buttoning a shirt. An occupational therapist may need to be consulted to help the patient adapt to loss of motor skills. Patients must be taught the importance of reporting any change in status, such as numbness and tingling of the extremities. If neurological deficits become severe, safety measures must be initiated to protect the patient from harm (Table 17-6).

### Pulmonary toxicity

Pulmonary toxicity that results from chemotherapy administration is usually irreversible and progressive. The initial site of damage seems to be the endothelial cells, with an inflammatory-type reaction resulting in drug-induced pneumonitis. Another type of damage occurs via an immunologic mechanism. Either the lung or the drug may act as

**TABLE 17-6**

**Organ Toxicity of Chemotherapy Agents: Neurotoxicity**

| Toxicity/ Symptoms | Grade | General Risk Factors | Chemotherapy Agent/ Risk Factors/ Symptoms | Mechanism of Damage | Protective/ Management Measures |
|---|---|---|---|---|---|
| Cerebellar<br>• Unsteady gait<br>• Nystagmus<br>• Ataxia<br>• Dizziness<br>• Seizures<br>• Hemiparesis<br>• Confusion<br>• Coma<br>Autonomic<br>• Ileus<br>• Constipation<br>• Impotence<br>• Urinary retention<br>• Postural hypotension<br>Peripheral/Cranial<br>• Facial palsies<br>• Diplopia<br>• Paresthesia of hands and feet<br>• Muscle atrophy<br>• Foot drop<br>• Loss of deep tendon reflexes<br>• Areflexia<br>• Sensory loss<br>• Sensory perception loss<br>• Hoarseness | Neurocerebellar<br>0 = None<br>1 = Slight incoordination dysdiadokinesis<br>2 = Intention tremor dysmetria, slurred speech<br>3 = Locomotor ataxia<br>4 = Cerebellar necrosis<br>Neurocortical<br>0 = None<br>1 = Mild somnolence or agitation<br>2 = Moderate somnolence or agitation<br>3 = Severe somnolence or agitation, confusion, disorientation, hallucination, aphasia<br>4 = Coma, seizures, psychosis<br>Neurosensory<br>0 = None<br>1 = Mild paresthesias, loss of deep tendon reflexes<br>2 = Mild or moderate objective sensory loss, moderate paresthesias<br>3 = Severe objective loss, or paresthesias that Interfere with function<br>Neuromotor<br>0 = None<br>1 = Subjective weakness<br>2 = Mild objective weakness<br>3 = Objective weakness with impairment of function<br>4 = Paralysis | • Dosage<br>• Cranial radiation<br>• Intrathecal administration<br>• Age<br>• CNS depressants (ie, antiemetics, tranquilizers,and sedatives)<br>• History of diabetes, chronic alcohol abuse | Ifosfamide<br>• High doses<br>• Cerebellar and cranial dysfunction<br>Vincristine<br>• Dose-related: > 2mg/m² of unit dose<br>• Hepatic dysfunction<br>• Autonomic, peripheral dysfunction<br>Cisplatin<br>• Dose-related<br>• Renal dysfunction<br>• Dehydration<br>• Autonomic, peripheral dysfunction<br>• Concurrent treatment with vincristine or etoposide<br>Methotrexate<br>• High dose (> 1 g/m²)<br>• Cerebellar dysfunction<br>• Concurrent cranial radiation therapy<br>• Intrathecal dose<br>• Increases effect with cytarabine, daunorubicin, salicylates, sulfonamides, vinblastine, vincristine<br>Cytarabine<br>• High doses (> 2 g/m²)<br>• Cerebellar and peripheral effects<br>5-fluorouracil<br>• Cerebellar dysfunction<br>• Dose and schedule related<br>Pemetrexed<br>• Should not be adminstered to patients with impaired creatinine clearance<br>Taxanes<br>• Peripheral neuropathies<br>• Myalgias/arthralgia<br>Oxaliplatin<br>• Peripheral neuropathy<br>• Laryngopharyngeal dysesthisia<br>Bortezomib<br>• Peripheral neuropathy | • Accumulation of drug metabolite (chloracet-aldehyde) with direct CNS effect<br>• Disrupts microtubules in the neural tissues<br>• Damages large fibers, resulting in sensory change<br>• Damage/loss of inner hair cells in the organ of Corti<br>• Demyelination of nerve fibers | • Place on bowel regimen<br>• Methylene blue infusion<br>• Oral diazepam 5 mg every 6 hours at the time of treatment, to manage muscle spasms<br>• Eliminate furosemide<br>• Avoid concurrent administration of aminoglycosides<br>• Audiometric testing for high risk<br>• Ethyol (amifostine)<br>• Withhold therapy for severe toxicity, ie, muscle weakness or pain<br>• Neurologic recovery, start drug at 50% dose reduction<br>• Monitor neurologic signs and symptoms<br>• Monitor electrolytes<br>• Institute safety measures<br>• Administer amifostine with cisplatin<br>• Glutamine and vitamin B12 with oxaliplatin may minimize symptoms<br>• Folic acid and vitamin B12 supplements reduce toxicity of pemetrexed<br>• Avoid cold drinks and cold in general with oxaliplatin |

the antigen in an allergic-type reaction.[105] Chronic exposure to chemotherapy causes an extensive alteration of the pulmonary parenchyma, with changes in the connective tissue, obliteration of alveoli, and dilatation of air spaces, known as *honeycombing.* Continuous injury and repair produce restrictive lung disease, increased work of breathing, and a functionally reduced lung volume, leading to impaired gas exchange. Hypoxemia results because oxygen does not diffuse in the damaged areas while perfusion continues.

Pulmonary toxicity usually presents clinically as mild to progressive dyspnea, unproductive cough, bilateral basilar rales, tachypnea, and low-grade fever. The chest x-ray may be within normal limits, but can show a pattern of diffuse interstitial markings. Arterial blood gases reveal hypoxia, with hypocapnea and respiratory alkalosis. The most sensitive pulmonary function test is the carbon monoxide diffusion capacity, which becomes abnormal before clinical symptoms occur.[2,106] Other pulmonary function tests can show a restrictive pattern when pulmonary fibrosis has occurred. To establish a pathological diagnosis and exclude the possibility of infection, the best method is to obtain involved tissues by an open-lung biopsy or a fiber-optic bronchoscopy. Bacterial or fungal infections and metastasis can then be ruled out.

Bleomycin is well-known to cause pulmonary toxicity. The incidence of bleomycin-induced pulmonary toxicity is 5% for a total cumulative dose of 450 units and 15% for higher dosages. Bleomycin is concentrated preferentially in the lung and is inactivated by a hydrolase enzyme. This enzyme is relatively deficient in lung tissue as compared with other tissues, such as the liver. These findings may explain the relative sensitivity of bleomycin to lung tissue, causing (1) early endothelial cell damage, (2) decrease in type I pneumocytes, with subsequent proliferation, and (3) migration of type II pneumocytes into alveolar spaces, inducing interstitial changes.[107] Following destruction of type I cells, repair is characterized by hyperplasia and dysplasia of the type II pneumocytes. Fibroblast proliferation, with subsequent pulmonary fibrosis, is probably the basis for the irreversible changes induced by bleomycin.[107]

Cytarabine exerts a direct toxic effect on the pneumocytes and capillary endothelial cells by diminishing the integrity of cell membranes and increasing capillary permeability. A capillary leak syndrome, involving primarily the lung, occurs 2 to 21 days after the first dose, resulting in pulmonary edema and respiratory failure, with features of adult respiratory disease (ARD). It appears to be related to high doses and continuous administration.[107] High-dose corticosteroids have been helpful in some cases.

Mitomycin C damage to the lung presents as diffuse alveolar damage with capillary leak and pulmonary edema. Incidence ranges from 3% to 36%, occurring 6 to 12 months after therapy. In some patients, only a brief exposure produces damage. If dyspnea occurs even with a normal chest radiograph, it may be necessary to discontinue mitomycin C from the treatment plan.[107]

Cyclophosphamide causes pulmonary fibrosis in less than 1% of patients and is associated with high doses (120 mg/kg/day for 4 days). Histological findings include endothelial swelling, pneumocyte dysplasia, edema, fibrosis, and fibroblast proliferation. The result of damage is alveolar hemorrhage and fibrin deposition.[107]

Carmustine inhibits lung glutathione disulfide reductase, which mediates the resultant cellular injury. Damage occurs after a long latency period, averaging 3 years, but may occur after only 6 weeks of therapy. High-dose carmustine has an incidence of 20% to 30% when a cumulative dose of 1500 mg/m$^2$ is given. An insidious cough with dyspnea or sudden respiratory failure occurs. It has been suggested that this reaction may be more common with co-administration of other chemotherapy, concurrent radiation and preexisting pulmonary disease.[107] Although glucocorticoid administration has improved symptoms, mortality still occurs in a small percentage of patients.

Methotrexate can also produce an acute or a chronic process related to endothelial injury.[107] Diffuse alveolar damage is characterized by the disappearance of type I pneumocytes, hyaline membrane formation, and the presence of inflammatory cells in the alveoli and interstitium. The incidence has been reported as 2% to 8% with an acute onset of pulmonary edema producing ARD or more gradual systemic toxicity (such as fever or chills), and with malaise preceding the appearance of pulmonary symptoms. Radiographic features may be unique, with pleural effusion occurring either alone or in conjunction with pulmonary infiltrates, peripheral consolidations, or chronic eosinophilic pneumonia.

An uncommon side effect of docetaxel is fluid retention. Its incidence is related to the cumulative dose. This toxicity can be disabling, worsening with higher doses. Fluid retention is exhibited peripherally, as abdominal ascites, as a pleural effusion, or as a combination of the two. The fluid retention is reversible and can be controlled with diuretics. Docetaxel has been reported to cause dyspnea and bronchospasm.[107]

All-transretinoic acid can cause a syndrome consisting of high fever, respiratory distress, pulmonary infiltrates, and pericardial or pleural effusion that occurs 2 days to 3 weeks after initiating treatment. This retinoic acid syndrome can generally be reversed with the administration of corticosteroids.[107] Irinotecan can cause dyspnea on exertion and pneumonitis with pulmonary infiltrates.[107] The pulmonary toxicity related to irinotecan is not dose-related.[107] Busulfan can cause pulmonary fibrosis when a dose exceeding 500 mg is given.[107] Lung toxicity generally occurs 3 years after initiation of busulfan but may occur after 6 weeks of therapy.

Gemcitabine can cause pulmonary symptoms ranging from mild, self-limiting dyspnea to fatal pulmonary toxicity. The signs and symptoms exhibited include tachypnea, marked hypoxemia, and interstitial infiltrates on chest x-ray consistent with pulmonary edema. Administration of corticosteroids and diuretics seems to reverse the toxicity.[107]

Because lung damage is usually irreversible and progressive, it is imperative to detect pulmonary toxicity as early as possible. The causative agent may be discontinued or the dose reduced to prevent further damage to lung tissue. High concentrations of inspired oxygen are toxic to the lungs, and the simultaneous administration of various chemotherapy drugs may induce lung damage.[107] Nurses need to be aware of this phenomenon and must monitor the patient's oxygen saturation and breath sounds closely for early signs and symptoms of pulmonary toxicity.

When oxygen saturation is compromised due to restrictive lung damage, the patient experiences dyspnea on exertion or at rest. As a result, the patient must expend increased effort to perform simple activities of daily living. Nursing care centers on teaching the patient to prioritize daily activities and to use breathing techniques such as pursed lips to lessen the effects of dyspnea. Supplemental oxygen therapy may be necessary to relieve the dyspnea. The family and patient are then taught how to administer oxygen and what safety precautions are necessary with oxygen therapy. Steroids are usually administered to lessen the pulmonary symptoms. To prevent further complications, the nurse can also teach the patient how to mobilize secretions by maintaining an adequate fluid intake and performing effective cough and deep-breathing techniques (Table 17-7).

### Hepatotoxicity

Chemotherapy agents can cause a variety of hepatotoxic reactions. The initial site of damage seems to be the parenchymal cells of the liver. Obstruction to hepatic blood flow results in fatty changes, hepatocellular necrosis, cholestasis, hepatitis, and veno-occlusive disease (VOD). Hepatotoxicity usually is diagnosed initially by transient elevations of the hepatic enzymes during treatment, which can progress to hepatomegaly, jaundice, and abdominal pain. Unless extensive fibrosis or necrosis has occurred, hepatotoxicity is reversible and nonfatal.[2,109]

Liver toxicity induced by high-dose methotrexate is transient and usually does not result in chronic liver disease. Elevation of hepatic enzyme levels is common, rising with successive courses of therapy and tending to be higher in patients treated on a daily schedule than those treated on intermittent schedules. Chronic inflammatory infiltrates in the portal tracts, focal liver cell necrosis, fibrosis, and cirrhosis may occur. However, all abnormalities usually resolve within 1 month following cessation of methotrexate therapy.[109,110]

High-dose cytarabine may induce intrahepatic cholestasis, possibly as a result of injury to the hepatocyte transport system. Changes are reversible, so they do not appear to limit cytarabine use. Fluorouracil use is also related to hepatocellular damage. These changes resolve with the discontinuation of therapy; no medical intervention is needed. Gemcitabine, irinotecan, trimetrexate, oxaliplatin, topotecan and antitumor antibiotics can cause a transient increase of hepatic enzymes that resolves after discontinuation of the drug.[2] Fluorodeoxyuridine, usually administered as a continuous arterial dose, can cause chemical hepatitis, with increases in transaminases, alkaline phosphatase, and serum bilirubin levels. In addition, stricture of intrahepatic or extrahepatic bile ducts can occur. Toxicity appears to be both time and dose dependent. Although liver function usually normalizes when the drug is discontinued, the development of biliary sclerosis is irreversible.[2]

Hepatocellular disease occurs with the administration of 6-mercaptopurine in daily doses exceeding 2 mg/kg. The histological pattern includes features of intrahepatic cholestasis and parenchymal cell necrosis. Moderate elevations occur in transaminases, alkaline phosphatase, and serum bilirubin, with episodes of jaundice occurring 30 days after initiation of therapy.[2]

Patients with underlying hepatitis B and C infections have been reported to have a reactivation of the virus during or after chemotherapy. After recovery of the immune system, viral replication can be enhanced and increases the severity of viral hepatitis. Hepatitis B has been shown to be associated with more risk of hepatotoxicity. Several chemotherapy agents have been associated with hepatitis reactivation including antitumor antibiotics, plant alkaloids, alkylating agents, antimetabolites, docetaxel, and etoposide.[111]

Although hematologic tumors, such as non-Hodgkin's lymphoma are more commonly associated with viral reactivation, patients with solid tumors have had reactivation as well. Usually the reactivation occurs after treatment; however, there are reports of reactivation during treatment and up to 1 year following treatment.[112,113]

Spontaneous resolution of the viral reactivation has been observed. Reports of lamivudine have been found to be effective in controlling viral replication during reactivation.[111] Some reports advocate giving prophylactic antiviral treatment before chemotherapy for patients who have underlying hepatitis. At this time, guidelines for patients at risk are not clearly defined.

Few guidelines exist for the use of drugs when hepatic dysfunction is present. Known hepatotoxic drugs must be avoided when liver function test results are abnormal. Impaired liver function delays excretion and results in increased accumulation of the chemotherapy in the plasma and tissues, especially with drugs such as doxorubicin, daunorubicin, paclitaxel, docetaxel, vincristine, and vinblastine, all of which are excreted primarily by the liver into the bile. It has been recommended to reduce or to not administer these agents if the serum bilirubin is between 1.5 and 3 mg/dL. If the serum glutamic pyruvic transaminase (SGOT) is between 60 and 180 international units, the dose should be reduced by 50%.[2,109]

Hepatic toxicity is uncommon, but it can be a serious consequence of chemotherapy administration, with effects

**TABLE 17-7**

**Organ Toxicity of Chemotherapy Agents: Pulmonary Toxicity**

| Toxicity/ Symptoms | Grade General | Risk Factors | Chemotherapy Agent/Risk Factors | Mechanism of Damage | Protective/ Management Measures |
|---|---|---|---|---|---|
| • Low-grade fever<br>• Nonproductive cough<br>• Dyspnea<br>• Tachycardia<br>• Diffuse basilar crackles<br>• Wheezing<br>• Pleural rub<br>• Fatigue<br>• Malaise<br>• Chest pain<br>• Night sweats<br>• Tachypnea<br>• Cyanosis<br>• Edema | Dyspnea<br>0 = None<br>1 = Asymptomatic with abnormal PFTs<br>2 = Dyspnea on exertion<br>3 = Dyspnea at normal activity<br>4 = Dyspnea at rest<br><br>Pulmonary Fibrosis<br>0 = Normal<br>1 = Radiographic changes, no symptoms<br>2 = N/A<br>3 = Changes with symptoms<br><br>Pulmonary Edema<br>0–2 = None<br>3 = Radiographic changes and diuretics required<br>4 = Requires intubation<br><br>Pneumonitis (noninfectious)<br>0 = Normal<br>1 = Radiographic change, symptoms do not require steroids<br>2 = Steroids required<br>3 = Oxygen required<br>4 = Requires assisted ventilation<br><br>Pleural Effusion<br>0 = None<br>1-4 = Present<br><br>ARDs<br>0 = None<br>1 = Mild<br>2 = Moderate<br>3 = Severe<br>4 = Life-threatening | • Age<br>• Preexisting lung disease, eg, COPD, TB<br>• History of smoking<br>• Cumulative dose<br>• Long-term therapy<br>• Mediastinal radiation<br>• High inspired concentration of oxygen<br>• Renal insufficiency | Bleomycin<br>• Synergistic with vincristine<br>• Cumulative dose > 450 mg/m²<br>• Oxygen exposure > 50% | • Initial injury to capillary endothelium cells<br>• Necrosis of type I epithelial cells<br>• Hypertrophy of type II alveolar pneumocytes<br>• Pulmonary fibrosis | • Assess for risk factors<br>• Obtain baseline pulmonary function tests<br>• Monitor cumulative dose<br>• Limit cumulative dose<br>• Limit oxygen to keep arterial $PO_2$ > 60 mm Hg<br>• Discontinue drug if dyspnea occurs<br>• Assess for pulmonary symptoms<br>• Administer steroids and oxygen<br>• Monitor activities to minimize energy<br>• Stop or reduce dose of drug<br>• Fluid restriction<br>• Administer diuretics<br>• Follow-up with PFTs |
| | | | Mitomycin C<br>• History of cyclophosphamide and/or methotrexate administration<br>• Oxygen concentrations > 50% | • Hypersensitivity reaction or immune complex related<br>• Damage similar to bleomycin<br>• Increased effect with VM-26, vincristine | |
| | | | Carmustine<br>• Dose-related (>1500 mg/m²)<br>• Concurrent administration with cyclophosphamide | • Inhibition of glutathione reductase in alveolar macrophages | |
| | | | Busulfan | • Hyperplasia and dysplasia of the type II pneumocytes | |
| | | | Cyclophosphamide<br>• High dose > 120 mg/kg/day × 4 days | • Alveolar hemorrhage and fibrin deposition<br>• Increased effect with cisplatin, VM-26, vincristine | |
| | | | Methotrexate | • Capillary leak syndrome, pulmonary edema<br>• Interstitial pneumonitis | |
| | | | Cytarabine<br>• High doses (5 g/m²) | • Capillary leak syndrome<br>• Capillary endothelial damage | |
| | | | Gemcitabine | • See cytarabine | |

*Abbreviations*: ARDS, adult respiratory distress syndrome; COPD, chronic obstructive pulmonary disorder; PFT, pulmonary function test; TB, tuberculosis.

ranging from transient enzyme elevations to permanent cirrhosis. Because many disease and treatment-related factors can be hepatotoxic, it is difficult to attribute hepatic toxicity definitively to specific agents. During chemotherapy administration, it is critical to monitor liver function tests closely, as enzymatic changes may be the first clinical evidence of hepatotoxicity.

Third spacing (the shift of fluid from the vascular space to the interstitial space) can occur as a result of hepatotoxicity. Signs of fluid shift are decreased blood pressure, increased pulse rate, low central venous pressure, decreased urine output, increased specific gravity, low levels of serum albumin, and hemoconcentration. Albumin is administered to replace the plasma protein and assist with absorption of the fluid. Fluid restriction minimizes third spacing, so this measure enhances renal blood flow, decreases systemic congestion, and improves patient comfort. Other supportive care measures include diuretics, decreased protein intake, lactulose, and emotional support (Table 17-8).

### Hemorrhagic cystitis

Hemorrhagic cystitis is a bladder toxicity resulting from cyclophosphamide and ifosfamide therapy. It ranges from microscopic hematuria to frank bleeding, necessitating invasive local intervention with instillation of sclerosing agents. Symptoms range from transient irritative urination, dysuria, and suprapubic pain to life-threatening hemorrhage. Transient cystitis has an early onset and short duration due to the direct effect of the deposition of acrolein, a by-product of metabolism, on the urothelium.[114,115] Reports of reactivation of a latent infection with a polioma or adenovirus during episodes of severe myelosuppression are thought to be involved in the pathogenesis of hemorrhagic cystitis.[114]

After oral or IV administration, cyclophosphamide is metabolized by hepatic microsomal enzymes to hydroxycyclophosphamide and later by target cells to phosphamide mustard (active) and acrolein (urinary metabolite). The binding of acrolein to the bladder mucosa results in inflammation and ulceration. Approximately 10% of people receiving cyclophosphamide experience microscopic hematuria.[115] Early diagnosis is accomplished by urine dipstick or visual observation of red-tinged urine. If necessary, a confirmed diagnosis can be accomplished by cystoscopy, which shows discrete bleeding capillaries or diffuse mucosal ulceration, hemorrhage, and necrosis.[116]

When hemorrhagic cystitis develops, drug therapy probably should be discontinued. In many patients,

**TABLE 17-8**

**Organ Toxicity of Chemotherapy Agents: Hepatotoxicity**

| Toxicity/ Symptoms | Grade | General Risk Factors | Chemotherapy Agent | Mechanism of Damage | Management Measures |
|---|---|---|---|---|---|
| • Elevated bilirubin, LDH, SGOT, alkaline phosphatase, SGPT<br>• Chemical hepatitis<br>• Jaundice<br>• Ascites<br>• Decreased albumin<br>• Cirrhosis<br>• Hepatomegaly<br>• Right upper quadrant pain<br>• Fatigue<br>• Anorexia<br>• Nausea<br>• Decreased clotting factor synthesis<br>• Hyperpigmentation of skin | Bilirubin<br>0–1 = Normal<br>2 = < 1.5<br>3 = 1.5–3.0<br>4 = > 3.0<br>SGOT/SGPT<br>0 = Normal<br>1 = < 2.5<br>2 = 2.6–5.0<br>3 = 5.1–20<br>4 = > 20<br>Alkaline Phosphatase<br>0 = Normal<br>1 = 2.5<br>2 = 2.6–5.0<br>3 = 5.1–20<br>4 = > 20<br>Liver Clinical<br>0–2 = No change<br>3 = Pre-coma<br>4 = Hepatic coma | • Prior liver damage, eg, hepatitis<br>• Dose<br>• Diabetes mellitus<br>• Tumor involvement<br>• Irradiation of liver<br>• Alcoholism<br>• Liver infections<br>• Concurrent administration or hepatotoxic drugs, eg, phenothiazines<br>• Age<br>• Hepatic dysfunction<br>• Total bilirubin > 2 mg/100 mL<br>• Obesity | • Methotrexate<br>• 6-Mercaptopurine<br>• Cytarabine<br>• Fluorodoxyuridine<br>• Nitrosoureas<br>• Etoposide, high-dose<br>• Cisplatin, high-dose<br>• Asparaginase<br>• Amsacrine<br>• Cyclophosphamide, high-dose<br>• Doxorubicin<br>• Vincristine<br>• Vinblastine<br>• Docetaxel<br>• Irinotecan<br>• Gemcitabine<br>• Trimetrexate<br>• Gefitnib<br>• Imatinib mesylate<br>• Oxaliplatin | Direct Toxic Effects<br>• Parenchymal cell damage<br>• Intrahepatic cholestasis<br>• Hepatic fibrosis<br>• Fatty changes | • Reduce dose in presence of liver dysfunction for drugs metabolized in liver, eg, vinca alkaloids or doxorubicin<br>• Avoid alcohol intake<br>• Monitor liver function tests<br>• If bilirubin > 1.5 mg, reduce dose by 50%<br>• If bilirubin > 3.0 mg, reduce dose by 75%<br>• Avoid hepatoxic drugs |

*Abbreviations*: IV, intravenous; LDH, lactic dehydrogenase; PO, per oral; SGOT, serum glutamic oxaloacetic transaminase; SGPT, serum glutamic pyruvic transaminase.

discontinuation will lead to amelioration of the symptoms without sequelae; however, microhematuria may persist long after discontinuing cyclophosphamide. When therapy is not stopped, as many as 55% of patients will have persistent symptoms. Extensive chronic bleeding and mucosal inflammation can produce long-term cystitis, irreversible bladder fibrosis, bladder contraction, and an increased risk for bladder cancer.[115] In high doses, mesna has been successful in protecting the bladder from the harmful effects of acrolein.[115]

Ifosfamide has a slower rate of metabolic activation into acrolein, allowing larger dosages to be administered as compared to cyclophosphamide. Mesna, a uroprotectant, contains a sulfhydryl group believed to bind to acrolein within the urinary collecting system and detoxifies ifosfamide. It is administered before ifosfamide and then intermittently for as long as 24 hours afterward to protect the bladder. Mesna can be administered through IV, orally, or subcutaneously.[115] Daily dose of mesna is 60% to 100% of the total daily dose of ifosfamide.

Gemcitabine can cause microscopic hematuria and proteinuria, especially with repeated cycles. In clinical trials, the occurrence was not found to be correlated with a cumulative dose or with treatment duration.[115] In a case report, temozolomide was found to cause hemorrhagic cystitis.[116] Valrubicin is a recently approved anthracycline antitumor antibiotic that is administered intravesically. The agent is excreted almost completely with voiding and can cause urinary frequency, dysuria, hematuria, and bladder pain. Hemorrhagic cystitis has been observed with dacarbazine in a patient receiving conventional doses after presenting with gross hematuria. Cytoscopy revealed inflammation and edema of the bladder mucosa.[117]

Protection of the bladder from these drugs focuses on hyperhydration, frequent voiding, and diuresis. If cystitis occurs, the treatment includes bladder irrigation through a 3-way Foley catheter to clear developing clots. The various solutions that cause a protein precipitate to form over the bleeding surfaces include saline, potassium aluminum sulfate, silver nitrate, and formalin. Vasopressins such as amino caproic acid may be administered IV or orally to decrease clotting. Cystoscopy may be necessary to cauterize bleeding vessels, if the bladder irrigations are ineffective in controlling the bleeding.[117]

Palifermin, a recombinant human keratinocyte growth factor has been used to treat hemorrhagic cystitis when supportive care alone was not effective. The growth factor was found to be beneficial in treating hemorrhagic cystitis induced from allogeneic stem cell transplant treatment.[114] Selective embolization of the internal iliac arteries with a

**TABLE 17-9**

**Organ Toxicity of Chemotherapy Agents: Hemorrhagic Cystis**

| Toxicity Symptoms | Grade | General Risk Factors | Chemotherapy Agents/Risk Factors | Mechanism of Damage | Protective/ Management Measures |
|---|---|---|---|---|---|
| • Gross hematuria<br>• Dysuria, urgency<br>• Suprapubic pain | 0 = None<br>1 = Micro only<br>2 = Gross, no clots<br>3 = Gross, with clots<br>4 = Requires transfusion | • Dose-related<br>• Pelvic radiation | Cyclophosphamide<br>• High dose (> 2.5 g) | • Drug metabolite acrolein damages bladder mucosa | • Vigorous hydration<br>• Frequent emptying of bladder, especially at night |
| | | | Ifosfamide<br>• Single high-dose versus multiple dose | Synergistic effect<br>• Cisplatin<br>• VM-26<br>• Vincristine | • Monitor urine for blood |
| | | | Gemcitabine<br>Irinotecan | | • 3-way foley irrigation with saline, alum, or formaldehyde |
| | | | Valrubucin | • Bladder wall affinity | • Administer amino caproic acid IV or PO |
| | | | | | • Mesna given in a dose of 60% total dose of ifosfamide q4h x 3 |

gelatin sponge has been found to be beneficial in controlling hemorrhagic cystitis induced after hematopoietic stem cell transplant.[119]

The nurse is in a position to monitor the urine for blood during administration of chemotherapy agents. Strict intake and output measures are imperative to ensure minimal contact of acrolein with the bladder mucosa. The patient is taught to maintain adequate hydration and to void frequently. If feasible, cyclophosphamide should be administered early in the day so that the patient can drink fluids and void frequently without interruption of sleep. Insertion of a Foley catheter may be necessary when high doses of cyclophosphamide are administered, to ensure that the agent is cleared from the bladder continuously (Table 17-9).

## Nephrotoxicity

Nephrotoxicity is a dose-limiting side effect of some chemotherapeutic drugs. Serious fluid and electrolyte imbalances that can progress to renal failure are the result of the direct and indirect effects of these drugs on the kidney. Many chemotherapy drugs are both metabolized and excreted by the kidneys; others are merely excreted as unchanged drugs including cisplatin, ifosfamide, high-dose methotrexate, mitomycin, mithramycin, and streptozocin. The manner in which chemotherapy damages the kidney varies from direct renal cell damage to an obstructive nephropathy resulting from precipitate formation. Renal failure, acid–base disorders, or electrolyte abnormalities may also occur as a result of tumor lysis syndrome or uric acid nephropathy.[2,120] When the renal clearance rate for a specific drug with linear pharmacokinetics is 35% to 40% and the patient has moderate to severe renal function, a significant increase in the drug's area under the plasma concentration curve (AUC) can occur.[2] For patients who have preexisting renal disease or who exhibit early signs of renal toxicity, the dosage may need to be reduced or the drug eliminated from the treatment plan.

Cisplatin can cause mild to severe nephrotoxicity, with specific damage occurring to the proximal and distal tubules. Platinum metal chelates in the renal tubules cause direct damage to the proximal tubular cells, injuring the tubular basement membranes, and can cause focal tubular necrosis.[116] Acute damage can occur within 3 to 21 hours after cisplatin administration, as evidenced by renal enzyme changes when precautions are not taken. Such renal dysfunction can persist for several years following cisplatin administration and may be irreversible.[121] Damage is characterized by degeneration of renal tubular epithelium, thickening of tubular basement membrane, and mild interstitial fibrosis. To avoid toxicity, patients should receive vigorous saline hydration of 1 to 2 L as well as diuresis during therapy, depending upon total cisplatin dose.

The use of mannitol in facilitating and inducing diuresis is a means of ensuring adequate urine flow. Mannitol may prevent immediate binding of cisplatin onto the renal tubules. Loop diuretics such as furosemide must be used with caution, however, as an increase in cisplatin toxicity has been reported following their administration. Frequent determinations of renal function should be obtained. If the creatinine clearance falls to less than 50 mg/mL, the drug should be withheld until renal function improves. If the serum creatinine level is elevated, cisplatin should be held. Daily magnesium supplementation may be indicated during cisplatin therapy, and electrolyte levels should be monitored frequently.[119]

Amifostine is an organic thiophosphate used to reduce the cumulative renal toxicity associated with repeated administration of cisplatin in patients with advanced ovarian or nonsmall cell lung cancer. This drug's ability to protect normal tissue without compromising tumor cell kill is attributed to its higher capillary alkaline phosphatase activity, higher pH, and better vascular bed of normal tissue as compared to cancer tissue. Other benefits seen with amifostine administration include reduced occurrence of hypomagnesemia, protection of the kidneys from nephrotoxic antibiotics, and reduced cumulative nephrotoxicity associated with cisplatin.[115]

Amifostine is dephosphorylated at the tissue site by alkaline phosphatase to form free thiol. Within the cell, thiol neutralizes the reactive components of cisplatin before damage occurs to the DNA and RNA of the normal cell. Thiol acts as a potent scavenger of free radicals and superoxide anions. This phenomenon is important because free radicals can damage cell membranes, DNA, and other vital cell components.[13,14]

Amifostine 740 mg/m$^2$ or 910 mg/m$^2$ is administered IV to the patient over 5 to 15 minutes after the patient has been given antiemetics and adequately hydrated with a minimum of 1 liter of fluid. Fifteen minutes after the amifostine is given, cisplatin is administered. The most common side effect noted has been transient systolic hypotension and nausea/vomiting, which are obstacles to convenient use. It is recommended that amifostine be administered with the patient in a supine position. Monitor blood pressure throughout the infusion and 5 minutes after the infusion. If the blood pressure drops below the threshold level from the baseline, the infusion is interrupted. The infusion can be restarted if the blood pressure returns to threshold within 5 minutes and if the patient is asymptomatic. If the blood pressure does not return to threshold, the infusion is discontinued and the next dose is reduced to 740 mg/m$^2$.[18]

Transient systolic hypotension is short term and reversible. It is treated with fluid administration and by placing the patient in the Trendelenburg position. Increased nausea and vomiting have occurred with amifostine, which may be a potentiating effect with cisplatin. Antiemetics must be given prior to amifostine administration and continued with cisplatin.[13]

Standard doses of methotrexate are not associated with renal toxicity unless the patient has preexisting renal

**TABLE 17-10**

**Organ Toxicity of Chemotherapy Agents: Nephrotoxicity**

| Toxicity/ Symptoms | Grade | General Risk Factors | Chemotherapy Agent/Risk Factors | Mechanism of Damage | Protective/ Management Measures | General Management |
|---|---|---|---|---|---|---|
| • Increased BUN, creatinine<br>• Oliguria<br>• Azotemia<br>• Proteinuria<br>• Decreased creatinine clearance<br>• Hyperuricemia<br>• Hypomagnesemia<br>• Hypocalcemia | Creatinine<br>0 = WNL<br>1 = < 1.5<br>2 = 1.5–3.0<br>3 = 3.1–6.0<br>4 = > 6.0<br><br>Proteinuria<br>0 = No change<br>1 = 1 + or < 3 g/L<br>2 = 2–3 + or 3–10 g/L<br>3 = 4 + or > 10 g/L<br>4 = Nephrotic syndrome<br><br>Hematuria<br>0 = None<br>1 = Micro<br>2 = Gross, no clots<br>3 = Gross with clots<br>4 = Requires transfusion<br><br>BUN mg%<br>0 = WNL < 20<br>1 = 21–30<br>2 = 31–50<br>3 = > 50 | • Age<br>• Dose of agent<br>• Preexisting disease of kidneys, renal insufficiency<br>• Nutritional status<br>• Duration of cancer therapy<br>• Concurrent:<br>– Aminoglycoside therapy<br>– Amphotericin-B<br>• Renal damage<br>• Dehydration<br>• Large tumor mass<br>• Ileal conduits<br>• Contrast dye<br>• History of sodium-retaining states (eg, cirrhosis, CHF, nephrosis)<br>• K+ and Mg depletion | Nitrosoureas<br>• Cumulative dose of 1200 mg/m² for carmustine and lomustine | • Direct cell damage in glomerulus<br>• Chronic interstitial nephritis<br>• Tubular atrophy | These 4 measures apply to all drugs<br>• Monitor renal function<br>• Saline diuresis<br>• Hydrate patient (3000 mL/day)<br>• Decrease uric acid production with allopurinol | • Substitute analog drug<br>• Reducedose for creatinine clearance (normal 125 mL/minute)<br><br>30–60 mL/minute:<br>Cisplatin, 50%<br>Methotrexate, 50%<br>Mitomycin, 75%<br>Nitrosoureas, hold dose<br><br>10–30 mL/minute<br>Cisplatin, hold dose<br>Mitomycin, 75%<br><br>< 10 mL/minute<br>Cyclophosphamide, 50%<br>Mitomycin, 50%<br><br>Avoid nephrotoxic drugs and contrast dye |
| | | | Mitomycin C<br>• Increased effect with vincristine and VM-26 | • Direct cell damage in glomerulus<br>• Microangiopathic hemolytic anemia | | |
| | | | Anthracyclines<br>• High dose (1.5 g/m²/week) | • Tubular atrophy | | |
| | | | Streptozocin<br>• Dose (> 1.5 g/m²/week) | • Diffuse tubulointerstitial nephritis | | |
| | | | Cisplatin<br>• Multiple doses (> 50 mg/m²)<br>• High dose<br>• Increased effect with cyclophosphamide | • Tubulointerstitial nephritis<br>• Tubular atrophy<br>• Direct cell damage in tubules<br>• Necrosis of proximal and distal renal tubules | • Stop drug if creatinine does not return to baseline<br>• Diuresis with mannitol<br>• Administer amifostine 15 minutes before administration | |
| | | | Methotrexate<br>• High dose (> 1 g/m²)<br>• Enhanced effect with cisplatin | • Precipitation of metabolites in the acid environment of the urine<br>• Obstructive nephropathy | • Maintain alkalinization of urine pH > 7<br>• Administer leucovorin<br>• Administer bicarbonate<br>• Avoid vitamin C<br>• Acids (ASA, vitamin C) compete for drug elimination sites, which increases serum concentration of methotrexate | |

*Note*: Pharmacokinetics of the following drugs suggest dose reduction when the patient has renal impairment:
Fludarabine
Carboplatin (increased thrombocytopenia with renal dysfunction)
Ifosfamide (increased CNS toxicity)
Melphalan IV
Pentostatin (increased serious toxicity)
Etoposide (increased bone marrow toxicity)
Topotecan (increased neutropenia)
Bleomycin (increased pulmonary toxicity)
Dacarbazine
Hydroxyurea (increased bone marrow toxicity)

Abbreviations: BUN, blood urea nitrogen; IV, intravenous; WNL, within normal limits.

dysfunction. High doses (> 1 g/m$^2$) can cause an obstructive nephropathy from precipitation of methotrexate or its metabolites in the renal tubules. Risk factors associated with drug-induced nephrotoxicity include low urine pH, dehydration, low methotrexate clearance, decreased urine output, and concurrent intrathecal treatment.[120] In general, urinary alkalization to maintain a urine pH greater than 7 with simultaneous administration of sodium bicarbonate or diamox prevents precipitate formation, permitting high-dose therapy to be administered. High doses of methotrexate should be accompanied by leucovorin rescue to counteract the effects of folic acid antagonists.

Streptozocin in doses exceeding 1.5 g/m$^2$ is associated with renal dysfunction in more than 65% of patients. Characteristically, streptozocin causes a tubulointerstitial nephritis and tubular atrophy due to direct damage of the tubules. This toxicity is manifested by hypokalemia, proteinuria, increased blood urea nitrogen (BUN), and increased creatinine levels.[121] Renal function tests and creatinine clearance tests should be obtained before beginning streptozocin therapy. Patients who develop an elevation of serum creatinine, even if the level subsequently returns to normal, are cautioned against receiving further streptozocin, as severe toxicity may occur.

Lomustine and carmustine can cause a delayed renal failure months or years following therapy. Azotemia and proteinuria are manifested, followed by progressive renal failure, often requiring dialysis. The incidence of renal failure appears to increase dramatically after a total dose of 1500 mg/m$^2$.[121]

Mitomycin C has been associated with a syndrome of renal failure and microangiopathic hemolytic anemia. This toxicity occurs in approximately 20% of patients who have received a cumulative dose of 100 mg or more after approximately 6 months of therapy and is characterized by an abrupt onset of microangiopathic hemolytic anemia, thrombocytopenia, azotemia, proteinuria, and hematuria.[116] Hemolytic uremic syndrome is associated with a high mortality rate of about 50%.

Nurses play a vital role in preventing nephrotoxicity. Preventive management includes aggressive hydration with hypertonic saline, diuresis, urinary alkalinization, and careful monitoring of urine output. Renal function tests, especially creatinine clearance and serum creatinine, are to be monitored before and after administering nephrotoxic drugs. Patients who must receive other nephrotoxic drugs, such as aminoglycosides or contrast dye, are monitored closely for early signs and symptoms of toxicity. Assessment of renal function should continue throughout treatment and periodically after the completion of therapy (Table 17-10).

## CONCLUSION

Advances in cancer therapy are made by continual investigations, evaluation of treatment results, and their incorporation into the practice of oncology. Successful prevention and management of toxicities of chemotherapy will occur because of research that has its origins in careful observation of patients' responses to cancer treatment. Because of the amount of time spent directly with the patient receiving chemotherapy, the nurse is often the healthcare provider best able to recognize subtle changes in the patient's status that could be indicative of pending complications from chemotherapy and therefore areas in need of research. Nursing responsibilities are expanding and multifaceted, and include patient education, ongoing physical assessments, identification of risk factors, and prompt therapeutic interventions, with continual evaluation for modification.

Occurrence of side effects does not necessarily preclude withholding of chemotherapy but instead alerts the nurse to the need for careful assessment, management, and follow-up evaluation. The nurse's assessment of a patient's response to treatment and assistance in preventing or managing side effects can make a difference in the patient's overall perceived quality of life. Once the treatment is complete, nurses can be instrumental in encouraging patients to have yearly comprehensive physical examinations to detect cancer recurrence and long-term effects of chemotherapy.

## REFERENCES


1. Gerber DE. Targeted therapies: a new generation of cancer treatment. *Am Family Physician.* 2008;77:294–296.
2. Duong CD, Loh JY. Basic review laboratory monitoring in oncology. *J Oncol Pharm Pract.* 2006;12:223–236.
3. Crawford J, Dale DC, Htoy S et al. Myeloid growth factors in cancer treatment. NCCN practice guidelines, clinical practice guidelines in oncology v. 1. 2005 http://www.nccnorg/professionals/physician
4. Balducci L. Management of cancer in the elderly. *Oncology.* 2006;20:135–143.
5. White HK, Cohen HJ. The older cancer patient. *Nurs Clin North Am.* 2008;43:307–322.
6. Ozer H. New directions in the management of chemotherapy induced neutropenia: risk models, special populations and quality of life. *Semin Oncol.* 2003;4(suppl 13):18–23.
7. Balducci L, Al-Halawani H, Charu V, et al. Elderly cancer patients receiving chemotherapy benefit from first-cycle pegfilgrastim. *Oncologist.* 2007;12:1416–1424.
8. Shayne M, Culakova E, Poniewierski MS, et al. Dose intensity and hematologic toxicity in older cancer patients receiving systemic chemotherapy. *Cancer.* 2007;110:1611–1620.
9. Iconomou G, Iconomou AV, Argyriou AA, et al. Emotional distress in cancer patients at the beginning of chemotherapy and its relation to QOL. *J. BUON.* 2008;13:217–222.
10. Given BA, Given CW, Sikosskii A. Symptom clusters and physical function for patients receiving chemotherapy. *Semin Oncol Nurs.* 2007;23: 121–126.
11. Leigh S. The changing legacy of cancer: issues of long-term survivorship. *Nurs Clin North Am.* 2008;43:243–258.
12. Honea N, Brant J, Beck SL. Treatment related symptom clusters. *Semin Oncol Nursing.* 2007;23, 142–151.
13. Schuchter LM, Hensley ML, Meropol NJ. 2002 update of recommendations for the use of chemotherapy and radiotherapy protectants: clinical

practice guidelines of the American Society of Clinical Oncology. *J Clin Oncol.* 2002;20:3895–2903.
14. Links M, Lewis C. Chemoprotectants: a review of their clinical pharmacology and therapeutic efficacy. *Drugs.* 1999;57:293–308.
15. Dodd MJ, Miaskowski C. The PRO-SELF program: a self-care intervention program for patients receiving cancer treatment. *Semin Oncol Nurs.* 2000;16:300–308.
16. Mueller PS, Glennon CA. A nurse developed prechemotherapy education checklist. *Clin J Oncol Nursing.* 2007;11:715–719.
17. Palmieri FM, Barton DL. Challenges of oral medications. *Semin Oncol Nurs.* 2007;23(suppl 2):S17-S27.
18. Joshi TG, Ehrenberger HE. Cancer clinical trials in the new millennium: novel challenges and opportunities for oncology nursing. *Clin J Oncol Nurs.* 2001;5:147–152.
19. Daniel D, Crawford J. Myelotoxicity from chemotherapy. *Semin Oncol.* 2006;33:74–85.
20. Berg D. Oxaliplatin: a novel platinum analog with activity in colorectal cancer. *Oncol Nurs Forum.* 2003;30:957–966.
21. Adams J. Proteasome inhibition in cancer: development of PS-341. *Semin Oncol.* 2001;28:613–619.
22. Deininger MW, O'Brien SG, Ford JM, et al. Practical management of patients with chronic myeloid leukemia receiving imatinib. *J Clin Oncol.* 2003;21:1637–1647.
23. Rodgers GM, Bennett CL, Chanan-Khan A, et al. Cancer and chemotherapy induced anemia. Clinical Practice Guidelines in Oncology. *J Natl Compr Canc Netw.* 2008;6:536–564.
24. Henry DH. Epoetin alfa treatment for patients with chemotherapy-induced anemia. *Support Cancer Ther.* 2007;1:78–91.
25. Spaeth D. Epoetin beta once weekly: a review of its efficacy and safety in patients with chemotherapy-induced anemia. *Expert Rev Anticancer Ther.* 2008;8:875–885.
26. Auerbach M, Ballard H. Intravenous iron in oncology. *J Natl Compr Canc Netw.* 2008;6:584–597.
27. Leyland-Jones B. Breast cancer trial with erythropoietin terminated unexpectantly. *Lancet Oncol.* 2003;4:459–560.
28. Smith R, Aapro MS, Ludwig H, et al. Darbopoetin alpha for treatment of anemia in patients with active cancer not receiving chemotherapy or radiation: results of a phase 3 multicenter randomized, double-blind, placebo controlled study. *J Clin Oncol.* 2008;26:1040–1050.
29. Thomas G, Ali S, Hoebers FJ, et al. Phase 3 trial to evaluate efficacy of maintaining haemoglobin levels above 12.0g/dl with erythropoietin vs above 10.0g/dl without erythropoietin in anemic patients receiving concurrent radiation and cisplatin for cervical cancer. *Gynaecol Oncol.* 2008;108:317–325.
30. Arbuckle RB, Griffith NL, Iacovelli LM, et al. Continued challenges with the use of erythropoiesis-stimulating agents in patients with cancer: perspectives and issues on policy guided health care. *Pharmacotherapy.* 2008;28(5 pt 2):15, 155.
31. Damron BH, Brant JM, Belansky HB, Friend PJ, Samsonow S, and Schaal A. Prevention and management of bleeding in patients with cancer. *Clin J Oncol Nurs.* 2009;13:573–583.
32. Bussell JB. Novel thrombopoietic agents: preliminary activity, potential benefit. *J Support Oncol.* 2007;5(suppl 2):63–84.
33. Smith JA. Implementation of cytokines to optimize cancer treatment outcomes. *J Support Oncol.* 2007;5(suppl 2):89–91.
34. Aapro MS, Cameron DA, Petterngell R. EORTC guidelines for the use of granulocyte colony stimulating factor. *Eur J Cancer.* 2006; 42:2433–2453.
35. Gafter-Gvili A, Fraser A, Paul M, et al. Meta-analysis: Antibiotic prophylaxis reduced mortality in neutropenic patients. *Ann Intern Med.* 2005;142:979–995.
36. Crawford J. Update on neutropenia and myeloid growth factors. *J Support Oncol.* 2007;5(suppl 2):27–29.
37. Boxer L, Dale DC. Neutropenia: causes and complications. *Semin Hematol.* 2002;39:75–81.
38. Barber FD. Management of fever in neutropenic patients with cancer. *Nurs Clin North Am.* 2001;36:631–644.
39. Rolston KV. Challenges in the treatment of infection caused by gram-positive and gram-negative bacteria in patients with cancer and neutropenia. *Clin Infect Dis.* 2005;40(suppl 4):246–252.
40. Klastersky J, Ameye L, Maertens J, et al. Bacteremia in febrile neutropenic cancer patients. *Int J Antimicrob Agents.* 2007;305:551–559.
41. Zitella LJ, Friese CR, Hauser J, Gobel BH, O'Leary C, Woolery M, et al. Putting evidence into practice: prevention of infection. *Clin J Oncol Nurs.* 2007;10:739–750.
42. Gilbert DN, Moellering RC, Ellopoulos GM, et al. *The Sanford Guide to Antimicrorbial Therapy.* 38th ed. Antimicrobial Therapy, Inc.: Hyde Park, VT; 2008.
43. Moores KG. Safe and effective outpatient treatment of adults with chemotherapy—included neutropenic fever. *Am J Health Syst Pharm.* 2007;64:717–722.
44. Dale DC. Colony-stimulating factors for the management of neutropenia in cancer patients. *Drugs.* 2002;62(suppl 1):1–15.
45. Crawford J. Safety and efficacy of pegfilgrastim in patients receiving myelosuppressive chemotherapy. *Pharmacotherapy.* 2003;23(suppl 8 pt 2):15S–19S.
46. Cope DG. Management of chemotherapy-induced diarrhea and constipation. *Nurs Clin North Am.* 2001;36:695–707.
47. Viele CS. Overview of chemotherapy-induced diarrhea. *Semin Oncol Nurs.* 2003;19(suppl 3):2–5.
48. Gwede CK. Overview of radiation and chemoradiation induced diarrhea. *Semin Oncol Nurs.* 2003;19(4)(suppl 3):6–10.
49. Gibson RJ, Keefe DMK. Cancer chemotherapy-induced diarrhoea & constipation: mechanisms of damage and prevention strategies. *Support Care Cancer.* 2006;14:890–900.
50. Stringer AM, Gibson RJ, Bowen JM, et al. Chemotherapy induced mucositis: the role of GI minoflora and mucins in the luminal environment. *Support Oncol.* 2007;5:256–267.
51. Hooker M. Clostridium difficile. *Clin J Oncol Nurs.* 2007;11: 801–804.
52. Muehlbauer PM, Thorpe D, Davis A, Drabot R, Rawlings BL, and Kiker E. Putting evidence into practice: evidence based interventions to prevent, manage, and treat chemotherapy and radiotherapy-induced diarrhea. *Clin J Oncol Nurse.* 2009;13:336–341.
53. Singh B. Psyllium as therapeutic and drug delivery agent. *Int J Pharm.* 2007;334(1–2):1–14.
54. Rosenof SH, Gabrail NY, Conklin R, et al. A multicenter, randomized trial of long-acting octreotride for the optimum prevention of chemotherapy induced diarrhea. *J Support Oncol.* 2006;4:289–294.
55. Woolery M, Bisanz A, Lyons HF, et al. Putting Evidence into Practice: evidence based interventions for the prevention and management of constipation in patients with cancer. *Clin J Oncol Nurs.* 2008;12:317–337.
56. Mitchell RP. Gastrointestinal toxicity of chemotherapy agents. *Semin Oncol.* 2006;33:106–120.
57. Herrstedt J. Antiemetics: an update and the MASCC guidelines applied in clinical practice. *Natl Clin Pract Oncol.* 2008;4:23–43.
58. Eckert RM. Understanding anticipatory nausea. *Oncol Nurs Forum.* 2001;28:1553–1558.
59. Jordan K, Sippell C, Schmoll HJ. Guidelines for antiemetic treatment of chemotherapy induced nausea vomiting: past, present and further recommendations. *Oncologist.* 2007;12:1143–1150.
60. Schwartzberg L. Chemotherapy induced nausea and vomiting: state of the art in 2006. *J Support Oncol.* 2006;4(suppl 1):3–8.
61. Wickham R. Nausea and vomiting. In Yarbro CH, Frogge MH, Goodman M, eds: *Cancer Symptom Management* (ed. 3). Sudbury, MA: Jones and Bartlett: 2004.
62. Tipton J, McDaniel R, Barbour L, et al. Putting Evidence into Practice: Evidence-based interventions for preventing and treating chemotherapy induced nausea and vomiting. *Clin J Oncol Nurs.* 2007; 11:69–78.
63. Vrabel M. Is ondansetron more effective than granisetron for chemotherapy induced nausea and vomiting? *Clin J Oncol Nurs.* 2007; 11:809–813.

64. Gralla R, Lichinitser M, Vander Vegt S, et al. Palonosetron improves prevention of chemotherapy-induced nausea and vomiting following moderately emetogenic chemotherapy: results of a double-blind randomized phase 3 trial comparing single doses of palonosetron with ondansetron. *Ann Oncol.* 2003;14:1570–1577.
65. Eisenbury P, Figueroa-Vadillo J, Zamora R, et al. Improved prevention of moderately emetogenic chemotherapy-induced nausea and vomiting with palonosetron, a pharmacologically novel 5-HT3 receptor antagonists. *Cancer.* 2003;98:2473–2482.
66. Hesketh PJ, Grunberg SM, Gralla RJ, et al. The oral neurokinin-1 antagonist aprepitant for the prevention of chemotherapy-induced nausea and vomiting: a multinational, randomized, double-blind, placebo-controlled trial in patients receiving high-dose cisplatin—the aprepitant protocol 052 study group. *J Clin Oncol.* 2003;21:4112–4119.
67. Patel L, Lindley C. Aprepitant—a novel NK1 receptor antagonist. *Expert Opin Pharmacother.* 2003;4:2279–2296.
68. Navari RM, Einhorn LH, Loehrer PJ, et al. A phase 2 trial of olanzapine, dexamethasone, and palonestron for the prevention of chemotherapy induced nausea and vomiting. *Support Care Cancer.* 2007;15: 1285–1291.
69. Bensinger W, Schubert M, Ang KK, et al. NCCN task force report: prevention and management of mucositis in cancer care. *Natl Compr Canc Netw.* 2008;6(suppl 1):S1–S30.
70. Eilers J, Million R. Prevention and management of oral mucositis in patients with cancer. *Semin Oncol Nurs.* 2007;23:201–212.
71. Harris DJ, Eilers J, Harriman A, et al. Putting evidence into practice: evidenced based interventions for the management of oral mucositis. *Clin J Oncol Nurs.* 2008;12:141–152.
72. Posner MR, Haddad RI. Novel agents for the treatment of mucositis. *J Support Oncol.* 2007;5(suppl 4):33–39.
73. Beaver AW, Shea TC. The effect of palifermin on chemotherapy and radiation induced mucositis: a review of the current literature. *Supportive Cancer Therapy.* 2007;4:188–197.
74. Hoffman HT. Oral mucositis: a challenging complication of radiotherapy, chemotherapy, and radiochemotherapy: part 1, pathogenesis and prophylaxis of mucositis. *Head Neck.* 2003;25:1057–1070.
75. Kostler WJ, Hejna M, Wenzel C, et al. Oral mucositis complicating chemotherapy and/or radiotherapy: options for prevention and treatment. *CA: Cancer J Clin.* 2001;51:290–315.
76. Lalla RV, Sonis ST, Peterson DE. Management of oral mucositis in patients who have cancer. *Dent Clin North Am.* 2008;52, 61–77.
77. Worthington HV, Eden OB, Clarkson JE. Intervention preventing oral candidiasis for patients with cancer receiving treatment [Cochrane review]. In: *The Cochrane Library*, issue 4. Oxford, UK; 2004.
78. Worthington HV, Clarkson JE. Prevention of oral mucositis and oral candidiasis for patients with cancer treated with chemotherapy. Cochrane systemic review. *J Dent Educ.* 2002;66:903–911.
79. Massler CF. Prevention and treating the oral complications of cancer therapy. *Gen Dent.* 2000;48:652–655.
80. Sherry VW. Taste alterations among patients with cancer. *Clin J Oncol Nurs.* 2001;6:73–77.
81. Ravasco P. Aspects of taste and compliance in patients with cancer. *Eur J Oncol Nurs.* 2005;9(suppl 2):S84-S91.
82. Payne AS, James WD, Weiss RB. Dermatologic toxicity of chemotherapy agents. *Semin Oncol.* 2006;33:86–97.
83. Remlinger KA. Cutaneous reactions to chemotherapy drugs. *Arch Dermatol.* 2003;139:77–81.
84. Guillot B, Bessis D, Dereurre O. Mucocutaneous side effects of antineoplastic chemotherapy. *Expert Opin Drug Saf.* 2004;3:579–587.
85. Kuruvila S, Dalal M, Sivanesan B. Bullous variant of acral erythema due to methotrexate. *Indian J Dermatol Venerol Leprol.* 2006;72: 440–442.
86. Botchkarev VA. Molecular mechanisms of chemotherapy-induced hair loss. *J Investig Dermatol Symp Pro.* 2003;8:72–75.
87. Ng R, Better N, Green N. Anticancer agents and cardiotoxicity. *Semin Oncol.* 2006;33:2–14.
88. Elliott R. Pathogenesis of cardiotoxicity induce by anthracyclines. *Semin Oncol.* 2006;33:S2-S7.
89. Bast A, Haenen GRM, Bruynzeel AME, et al. Protection by flavonoids against anthracycline cardiotoxicity: from chemistry to clinical trials. *Cardiovasc Toxiciol*, 2007;7(2)L:154–159.
90. Floyd JD, Nguyen DT, Lobins RT. Cardiotoxicity of cancer therapy. *J Clin Oncol.* 2005;23:7685–7696.
91. Manojilovic N, Babie D, Stojanovic S, et al. Capecitabine cardiotoxicity—case reports and literature review. *Hepatogastroenterology.* 2008;55:1249–1256.
92. Safra T. Chemotherapeutics and cardiac toxicity treatment considerations and management strategies. *Community Oncol.* 2007;4:540–548.
93. Viale PH,Yamamoto DS. Cardiovascular toxicity associated with cancer treatment. *Clin J Oncol Nurs.* 2008;12:627–638.
94. Grande AM, Rinaldi M, Sinelli S, et al. Heart transplantation in chemotherapeutic dilated cardiomyopathy. *Transplant Proc.* 2003;35: 1516–1518.
95. Verstappen CC, Heimans JJ, Hoekman K, et al. Neurotoxic complications of chemotherapy in patients with cancer. *Drugs.* 2003;63:1549–1563.
96. Windebauk AJ, Grisold W. Chemotherapy-induced neuropathy. *J Peripher Nerv Syst.* 2008;13:27–46.
97. Hausheer FH, Schilsky RL, Bain S, et al. Diagnosis, management and evaluation of chemotherapy induced peripheral neuropathy. *Semin Oncol.* 2006;33:15–49.
98. Visovsky C, Colins M, Abbott L, et al. Putting evidence into practice: evidence based intervention for chemotherapy induced peripheral neuropathy. *Clin J Oncol Nurs.* 2007;11:901–913.
99. Hammack J, Michalak J, Loprinzi C, et al. Phase III evaluation of nortriptyline for alleviation of symptoms of cisplatinum-induced peripheral neuropathy. *Pain.* 2002;98:195–203.
100. Wickham R. Chemotherapy-induced peripheral neuropathy: A review and implications for oncology nursing practice. *Clin J Oncol Nurs.* 2007;11:361–376.
101. Nelson CJ, Nandy N, Roth AJ. Chemotherapy and cognitive deficits: mechanisms, findings, and potential interventions. *Palliat Support Care*, 2007;5:273–280.
102. Openshaw H, Beamon K, Synold TW, et al. Neurophysiological study of peripheral neuropathy after high-dose paclitaxel: lack of neuroprotective effect of amifostine. *Clin Cancer Res.* 2004;10:461–467.
103. Stubblefield MD, Vahdat LT, Balmaceda CM, Troxel AB, Hesdorffer CS, Gooch CL. Glutamine as a neuroprotective agent in high-dose paclitaxel-induced peripheral neuropathy: a clinical and electrophysiologic study. *J Clin Oncol.* 2005;17:271–227.
104. Vahdat L, Papa Lopulous K, Lauge D, et al. Reduction of Paclitaxel-induced peripheral neuropathy with glutamine. *Clin Cancer Res.* 2001;7:1192–1197.
105. Abid SH, Malhotra V, Perry MC. Radiation-induced and chemotherapy-induced pulmonary injury. *Curr Opin Oncol.* 2001;13: 242–248.
106. Vahid B, Marik PE. Pulmonary complications of novel antineoplastic agents for solid tumours. *Chest.* 2008;133:528–538.
107. Meadors M, Floyd J, Perry MC. Pulmonary toxicity of chemotherapy. *Semin Oncol.* 2006;33:98–105.
108. Matthews, LV. Alterations in ventilation. In Itano JK, Taoka KN, eds. *Core Curriculum for Oncology Nursing.* 4th ed. St. Louis, MO: Elsevier Saunders. 2005: 347–379.
109. Rodriguez-Frias EA, Lee WM. Cancer chemotherapy: heptocellular injury. *Clin Liver Dis.* 2007;11:641–662.
110. Floyd J, Mirza I, Sachs B, et al. Hepatotoxicity of chemotherapy. *Semin Oncol.* 2006;33:50–67.
111. Yeo W, Johnson PJ. Diagnosis, prevention, and management of hepatitis B virus reactivation during anticancer therapy. *Hepatology.* 2006;43:209–220.
112. Tsutsumi Y, Kawamura R, Saitoh S, et al. Hepatitis B virus reactivation in a case of NHL treatment with chemotherapy and rituximab. *Leuk Lymphoma.* 2004;45:627–629.

113. Garcia-Rodriguez JF, Canales M, Hernandez-Maraver D, et al. Late reactivation of resolved hepatitis B virus infection. *Am J Hematology.* 2008;83:673–675.
114. Cziere A, Bruns I, Graef T, et al. Treatment of severe hemorrhagic cystitis after allogeneic stem cell transplantation with palifermin a recombinant human keratinocyte growth factor. *Biol Blood Marrow Transplant.* 2007;13:871–872.
115. Lina MV, Ferreira FV, Macedo FY, et al. Histological changes in bladders of patients submitted to ifosfamide chemotherapy even with mesna prophylaxis. *Cancer Chemother Pharmacol.* 2007;59:643–650.
116. de Jonge MGA, Verweij J. Renal toxicities of chemotherapy. *Semin Oncol.* 2006;33:68–73.
117. Islam R, Isaacson BJ, Zickerman PM, et al. Hemorrhagic cystitis as an unexpected adverse reaction to temozolomide: case report. *Am J Clin Oncol.* 2002;25:513–514.
118. Mohammadianpanah M, Shirazi M, Mosalaei A, et al. Hemorrhagic cystitis in a patient receiving conventional doses of dacarbazine for metastatic malignant melanoma. *Clin Ther.* 2007;29:1161–1165.
119. Han Y, Wu D, Sun A, et al. Selective embolization of the internal iliac arteries for the treatment of severe hemorrhagic cystitis following hematopoietic stem cell transplant. *Bone Marrow Transplant.* 2008;41:881–886.
120. Widemann BC, Adamson PC. Understanding and managing methotrexate nephrotoxicity. *Oncologist.* 2006;11:694–703.
121. Kintzel PE. Anticancer drug-induced kidney disorders. *Drug Saf.* 2001;24:19–38.

CHAPTER 18

Susan A. Ezzone, MS, RN, CNP, AOCNP®

# Principles and Techniques of Blood and Marrow Transplantation

## HISTORICAL DEVELOPMENTS

The use of human bone marrow was a treatment option for a variety of types of anemia, leukemia, and chlorosis in the late 1800s. Initially, bone marrow or spleen extract was administered by oral feedings or intramuscular injections.[1] Replacement of the bone marrow stem cells was intended to promote hematologic recovery. During the very early years, prior to the 1950s, little was understood about the advantages of this type of treatment. Later, there were several attempts to describe how shielding of the spleen from lethal irradiation in mice could allow hematologic recovery. Further attempts to describe the recovery of bone marrow function after irradiation were made using administration of syngeneic (identical twin) marrow.[2] Administration of syngeneic bone marrow was meant to promote the recovery of hematopoietic function. The first attempt to treat leukemia with high doses of chemotherapy followed by syngeneic marrow transplantation was described by Dr. E. Donnall Thomas in 1959.[3] Allogeneic transplantation using non-identical twin donors was unsuccessful due to lack of understanding of human leukocyte antigen (HLA) typing.[4] Autologous bone marrow transplantation (BMT) was first reported by Kurnick et al in 1958.[5] Infusion of autologous bone marrow allowed recovery of hematopoietic function after high-dose chemotherapy.

A successful sibling allogeneic transplant for treatment of an immune deficiency disease in an infant was performed in the late 1960s.[3] During the 1960s much emphasis was placed on improving outcomes of allogeneic transplant through gaining a better understanding of HLA typing, preparative regimens, and prophylaxis and treatment of graft-vs-host disease (GVHD).[6]

In the 1970s interest was renewed in the use of BMT for treatment of severe aplastic anemia and acute leukemia. Better overall outcomes were due to a better understanding of HLA typing, GVHD, and infection prophylaxis and treatment.[6] Improvements in use of conditioning regimens, including total body irradiation and cyclophosphamide, led to better outcomes posttransplant.[7]

In 1986, allogeneic BMT was used to treat hematologic toxicity associated with radiation exposure due to the Chernobyl nuclear reactor accident.[8] Of the 13 individuals who received a marrow transplant, only 2 were long-term survivors. Most patients developed nonhematologic toxicities due to radiation exposure. In the late 1980s interest grew in the use of autologous stem cell transplant for treatment of a variety of hematologic diseases and solid tumors. The use of autologous transplant was encouraging due to decreased posttransplant complications and earlier engraftment. Interest in use of peripheral blood stem cells (PBSCs) grew through the late 1980s for autologous and allogeneic transplantation.[9] The National Bone Marrow Transplant Donor Registry, now known as the National Marrow Donor Program (NMDP), was started in 1986 to locate unrelated donors and coordinate stem cell collection for persons who do not have an HLA-identical related donor.[10] In the mid-to late 1980s there was a growing interest in the use of stem cells collected from the umbilical cord for unrelated or related allogeneic as well as autologous stem cell transplant.

During the 1990s, interest in the use of stem cell transplant for treatment of many hematologic, nonhematologic, and autoimmune disorders continued to grow. Efforts focused on evaluating the effectiveness of a variety of preparative regimens. In addition, interest grew in methods of decreasing regimen-related toxicities. Nonmyeloablative transplant was introduced as a better-tolerated and less toxic preparative regimen. Disease was treated through the antineoplastic properties of the preparative regimen and the occurrence of GVHD, which resulted in an antitumor effect.[11]

In the 21st century, efforts to develop guidelines for evidenced-based practice were made by the American Society for Blood and Marrow Transplantation (ASBMT).[12] A consensus conference coordinated by the National Institutes of Health (NIH) published criteria for the diagnosis and management of chronic GVHD.[13]

Efforts are focused on innovative strategies to better manage acute and chronic GVHD, such as mesenchymal stem cell infusion and extracorporeal photophoresis.[14,15] Use of double umbilical cord blood (UCB) stem cell transplant continues to be evaluated.[16] Ongoing studies are using autologous, allogeneic, and nonmyeloablative transplant for treatment of a variety of hematologic and nonhematologic diseases. Efforts persist to identify the best methods of infection prophylaxis and treatment.

## HEMATOPOIESIS AND TRANSPLANT IMMUNOLOGY

The bone marrow is responsible for hematopoiesis, or production of blood cells, including the white blood cells, red blood cells (RBCs), platelets, and lymphocytes. The pluripotent or progenitor stem cell is the precursor cell for all types of blood cells and expresses CD34, a protein that is found on the surface of stem cells.[17] The CD34 protein is used to identify stem cells for collection from the autologous (self) or allogeneic (related or unrelated) donor.

The hematopoietic stem cell produces the myeloid and lymphoid stem cells, from which all white blood cells develop. The myeloid stem cells produce the granulocytes, dendritic cells, and mast cells. Granulocytes produced include neutrophils, eosinophils, basophils, and monocytes/macrophages. Although all white blood cells recognize foreign invaders, neutrophils are the most common and are the first line of defense against foreign invaders. The lymphoid stem cells produce T lymphocytes, B lymphocytes, and natural killer (NK) cells. Types of T lymphocytes include cytotoxic, helper, suppressor, and memory cells. T lymphocytes are responsible for cellular immunity. Humoral immunity, or the production of antigens, is the responsibility of B lymphocytes.

The immune system consists of a complex network of lymph nodes and organs that communicate to protect the body from foreign organisms. Immune system organs include the lymph nodes, spleen, thymus, tonsils, adenoids, abdominal Peyer's patches, bone marrow, and blood and lymphoid vessels. There are also many different lymphokines or cytokines that are secreted by many different organs or cells to initiate some type of immune response.

Immune suppression posttransplant occurs due to the immunosuppressive effects of the agents used as part of the preparative regimen. Chemotherapy agents are chosen to intentionally trigger immune suppression and eradicate disease. Immunosuppressive agents used as part of the preparative regimen are meant to suppress the recipient's immune system.

## TYPES OF TRANSPLANT

In the early years, the term bone marrow transplantation was used to describe what is now referred to as hematopoietic stem cell transplantation (HSCT). Originally, the stem cells used for autologous, allogeneic, and unrelated transplant were collected directly from the bone marrow. In the late 1980s, it was determined that stem cells could be mobilized from the bone marrow into the peripheral blood. Although the stem cells originate in the bone marrow, hematopoietic stem cells are now mobilized from the bone marrow into the peripheral blood for all types of transplant. Therefore the term HSCT is more commonly used. Although the basic types of HSCT remain the same, additional information learned has added to the complexity of each type of transplant. The three basic types of HSCT are autologous, allogeneic, and syngeneic transplantation.

### AUTOLOGOUS TRANSPLANTATION

The use of autologous HSCT for treatment of a variety of diseases (see Table 18-1) has been well described over the years. The use of bone marrow stem cells for autologous transplantation was described in 1958.[5,19] The goal of autologous stem cell transplant is to rescue the recipient's bone marrow function from the adverse effects of high-dose chemotherapy used to aggressively treat a disease.[19] Without infusion of the bone marrow stem cells, doses of chemotherapy were limited by their marrow suppressive effects. A significant challenge that has occurred as a result of high-dose chemotherapy is major organ toxicity. Over the past 20 years or more, collection, storage, and infusion of

**TABLE 18–1**

**Hematologic and Nonhematologic Conditions Treated With HSCT**

| Malignant Conditions | Nonmalignant Conditions |
|---|---|
| **Allogeneic** | **Allogeneic** |
| *Hematologic diseases* | *Hematologic disorders* |
| Acute lymphocytic leukemia | Aplastic anemia |
| Acute myelogenous leukemia | Diamond–Blackfan anemia |
| Chronic lymphocytic leukemia | Fanconi's anemia |
| Chronic myelogenous leukemia | Sickle cell anemia |
| Hodgkin's disease | Beta thalassemia major |
| Multiple myeloma | Chediak-Higashi syndrome |
| Myelodysplastic syndrome (preleukemia) | Chronic granulomatous disease |
| Non-Hodgkin's lymphoma | Congenital neutropenia |
| | Reticular dysgenesis |
| | *Congenital immunodeficiencies* |
| | SCID |
| | Wiskott-Aldrich syndrome |
| | Functional T-cell deficiency |
| | *Mucopolysaccharidoses* |
| | Hurler's disease |
| | Hunter's disease |
| | Sanfilippo's syndrome |
| | Morquio's syndrome |
| | *Lipidoses* |
| | Adrenoleukodystrophy |
| | Metachromatic leukodystrophy |
| | Caucher's disease |
| | *Miscellaneous* |
| | Osteopetrosis |
| | Langerhans cell histiocytosis |
| | Lesch-Nyhan syndrome |
| | Glycogen storage diseases |
| **Autologous** | **Autologous** |
| *Hematologic diseases* | Amyloidosis |
| Multiple myeloma | |
| Non-Hodgkin's lymphoma | |
| Hodgkin's disease | |
| Acute myeloid leukemia | |
| *Solid tumors* | |
| Neuroblastoma/glioma | |
| Ovarian cancer | |
| Germ cell tumors | |
| Sarcoma | |
| Melanoma | |
| Lung cancer | |
| Breast cancer | |

*Abbreviations*: HSCT, hematopoietic stem cell transplant; SCID, severe combined immunodeficiency.

*Source*: Data from Ezzone.[18] Used with permission from ONS Press.

PBSCs has replaced the use of stem cells collected directly from the bone marrow.

## ALLOGENEIC TRANSPLANTATION

Allogeneic stem cell transplant is described as the use of a donor for the collection and infusion of hematopoietic stem cells. As described in more detail below, stem cells may be collected from the bone marrow, peripheral blood, or umbilical cord. Identification of a suitable donor requires HLA typing of recipients and potential donors. Most commonly, donors are siblings or are identified through the volunteer unrelated donor (VUD) registry through the NMDP. In the early years of HSCT, stem cells were collected directly from the bone marrow. The bone marrow procurement was done in the operating room with the use of general anesthesia. Multiple bone marrow aspirations were done to collect sufficient stem cells for transplantation. Currently, stem cells are most often collected from the donor from the peripheral blood. Mobilization of PBSCs is accomplished through the administration of colony stimulating factor (CSF), followed by collection of PBSCs through apheresis. Stem cell collection is usually completed in 1 or 2 days.

Types of allogeneic stem cell transplant have been described as myeloablative and nonmyeloablative. Traditionally, myeloablative HSCT has been done using a conditioning regimen of chemotherapy with or without total body irradiation that has considerable treatment-related toxicities. Severe myelosuppression occurs, requiring blood and platelet transfusions. Gastrointestinal effects also occur, resulting in severe mucositis, nausea, vomiting, and diarrhea. Other potential severe organ toxicities may involve the liver, kidneys, heart, and lungs. Posttransplant immunosuppression is required to prevent GVHD. Nonmyeloablative, or reduced-intensity, HSCT uses less toxic conditioning regimens consisting of reduced doses of chemotherapy and total body irradiation. Immunosuppressive medications are used to prevent graft rejection and GVHD since both recipient and donor cells are initially present. After myeloablative and nonmyeloablative HSCT the role of GVHD in causing an antitumor effect has been described elsewhere.[20]

## SYNGENEIC TRANSPLANTATION

An identical twin sibling donor is a perfect HLA match for the other identical twin sibling recipient. Use of an identical twin donor for HSCT is called a syngeneic transplant. The conditioning regimen used for syngeneic transplant may be myeloablative or nonmyeloablative. Immunosuppressive medications are not indicated; there is no risk of GVHD with the use of syngeneic transplant, as the HLA-matched twin sibling donor is considered genotypically identical.[19]

## SOURCES OF STEM CELLS

In the early years, hematopoietic stem cells were collected directly from the bone marrow by bone marrow procurement or multiple needle aspirations. Occasionally, this process is still done for stem cell collection if other methods are not feasible. Usually, the bone marrow procurement procedure is done in the operating room while the person is under general anesthesia. Multiple needle aspirations are obtained from the bilateral posterior iliac crests. The amount of bone marrow collected is approximately 10 to 15 mL/kg and is based on the recipient's body weight.[20] Following collection, the bone marrow is filtered to remove fatty particles and bone chips. The bone marrow product is mixed with heparin to prevent clotting.

Over the years, mobilization, collection, cryopreservation, storage, and infusion of PBSCs has replaced the use of stem cells collected directly from the bone marrow. Methods to mobilize stem cells from the bone marrow into the peripheral blood have been described by many authors. The stem cell moves from the bone marrow into the peripheral blood and is collected by apheresis. Following collection, the stem cells are cryopreserved, frozen, and stored for future use. Common methods to mobilize stem cells include use of CSFs such as granulocyte CSF (G-CSF) and granulocyte-macrophage CSF (GM-CSF) or chemotherapy plus CSFs. Either method may be used for PBSC mobilization for autologous PBSC transplant, while CSFs alone are used for related or unrelated allogeneic transplantation. The most common chemotherapy agent used for autologous PBSC mobilization is cyclophosphamide, but many other regimens may be used. Apheresis usually begins on day 4 or 5 of CSF administration and approximately day 10 to 16 following chemotherapy plus CSF administration. Investigational studies continue to evaluate the most effective method of PBSC mobilization. Recently, AMD3100 or Plerixafor along with Neupogen has been used in clinical trials to successfully mobilize PBSCs.[21]

Collection of PBSCs through apheresis requires venous access either into the peripheral veins or through placement of a central venous catheter. Apheresis is done for 4 to 6 hours each day until an adequate number of stem cells have been collected. Stem cell (CD34+) targets needed for successful engraftment have been described by many authors and vary from 2 to 20 × $10^6$ CD34+ cells/kg.[20,22] Following collection by apheresis, the stem cell product is cryopreserved with dimethylsulfoxide (DMSO), frozen, and stored.

Allogeneic related or unrelated donors are given G-CSF to mobilize stem cells from the bone marrow into the peripheral blood for collection. Other bone marrow or PBSC manipulations may be done to accomplish effects such as T cell depletion to minimize GVHD or RBC depletion in ABO-mismatch transplant. Purging techniques may be used to remove tumor cells in the stem cell product prior to autologous transplant.[20]

The use of UCB stem cells for transplantation continues to evolve as an option for transplantation of autologous or allogeneic stem cell transplantation. Several UCB stem cell storage banks are available. Collection and storage of autologous UCB may be done for the purpose of saving the UCB stem cells for future use if needed. More commonly, UCB is donated to the unrelated donor registry and then used as a source of stem cells for UCB transplant. Since the dose of UCB stem cells may be low, two UCB stem cell products may be used for transplantation. Disadvantages of the use of UCB stem cells for transplantation may include delayed neutrophil or platelet recovery due to low stem cell dose infused. The use of UCB transplant may not be feasible in some adults due to the low stem cell dose obtained. Minimal acute and chronic GVHD may occur due to the immature T cells in the infused UCB.[22]

## INDICATIONS FOR TRANSPLANT AND SURVIVAL OUTCOMES (DISEASES TREATED)

The indications for use of HSCT as a treatment option continue to expand. A variety of malignant and nonmalignant conditions have been treated with HSCT (see Table 18-1).[23] The ASBMT has developed evidence-based reviews to describe when a transplant should be done for certain diseases.[12] The selected diseases described in the evidenced-based reviews are acute lymphocytic leukemia (adults and children), acute myeloid leukemia (adults and children), multiple myeloma (adults), and diffuse large B-cell non–Hodgkin's lymphoma (NHL) (adults). Although many other diseases are treated with HSCT, the evidenced-based reviews provide an important step toward consensus of an expert panel for the development of standards of practice.

## PATIENT EVALUATION

Prior to transplantation, patients must undergo thorough clinical evaluation to determine their readiness to proceed with HSCT. Most of the clinical evaluation is the same for autologous or allogeneic HSCT and includes completion of a variety of diagnostic tests for evaluation of major organ system function (see Table 18-2).[18–20] After review of the diagnostic test results, the appropriateness of proceeding with transplantation is determined. A comorbidity index (CMI) score is sometimes used in the allogeneic transplant setting to indicate risk for transplant-related complications and morbidity.[23]

Human leukocyte antigen typing must be completed to pursue allogeneic transplantation. The HLA glycoprotein is encoded by the major histocompatibility complex (MHC), which is located on chromosome 6. The HLA protein allows recognition of self and nonself. HLA typing includes identification of the class I, II, and III genes (see Table 18-3).[24,25] Serologic or molecular HLA typing is done to identify a potential donor. The NMDP has described acceptable levels of HLA matching to identify a suitable stem cell donor.[26] Although HLA matching at HLA-A, HLA-B, HLA-C, and HLA-DRB1 has shown to maximize survival, a mismatched donor may be used with acceptable outcomes.

**TABLE 18-2**

**Pretransplant Clinical Evaluation**

*Laboratory data*
Complete blood count with differential
Blood urea nitrogen, creatinine
Electrolytes, magnesium, calcium, phosphorus
Creatinine clearance
Hepatic panel
Pregnancy test
Infectious disease titers
- CMV
- EBV
- HSV
- Hepatitis B surface antigen
- Hepatitis B core antibody
- Hepatitis C antibody
- HIV
- HLLV

Prothrombin time/international normalized ratio/partial thromboplastin time
ABO/Rh typing
Tissue typing (allogeneic only)

*Diagnostic studies/consults*
Chest radiograph
Electrocardiogram
Pulmonary function test
MUGA/echocardiogram
Dental examination
Psychological evaluation
Social work evaluation

*Disease staging studies (as appropriate)*
Bone marrow biopsy and aspirate
Lumbar puncture
Myeloma survey
Myeloma blood and urine studies
24-Hour urine protein, creatinine
CT
MRI
PET or gallium scan

*Abbreviations*: CMV, cytomegalovirus; CT, computed tomography; EBV, Epstein–Barr virus; HIV, human immunodeficiency virus; HLLV, human T-cell lymphotropic virus; HSV, herpes simplex virus; MRI, magnetic resonance imaging; PET, positron emission tomography.

*Source*: Data from Ezzone[18]; Niess and Duffy[19]; and Schmit-Pokorny.[20]

**TABLE 18-3**

**HLA Typing**

| Class of HLA Antigen | Characteristics of HLA Antigen |
|---|---|
| I | Nucleated cells<br>Identified as A, B, and C loci<br>Numerous HLA alleles |
| II | B cells, macrophages, activated T cells<br>Identified as DR, DP, DQ<br>Involved in immunity and histocompatibility<br>Numerous HLA alleles |
| III | Involved in immunity<br>No role in histocompatibility |

*Abbreviation*: HLA, human leukocyte antigen.

*Source*: Data from Morishima et al[24] and Snustad and Simmons.[25]

## COMMON PREPARATIVE REGIMENS

Numerous preparative or conditioning regimens have been used over the years prior to infusion of hematopoietic stem cells. The general purposes for administration of the preparative regimens are to eradicate disease, cause myelosuppression, and cause immunosuppression. Preparatory regimens include some combination of chemotherapy and immunosuppression with or without total body irradiation (see Table 18-4).[27] Myeloablative preparative regimens aggressively treat the disease and, as an adverse effect, cause severe myelosuppression. Recovery of bone marrow function is dependent on engraftment of stem cells. Nonmyeloablative regimens treat disease less aggressively and cause myelosuppression rather than myeloablation. Hematopoietic function may be somewhat preserved, lessening the need for blood or platelet transfusion posttransplant. Immunosuppressive agents used as part of the preparative regimen are intended to prevent graft rejection. Additional immunosuppression is needed prior to and after myeloablative and nonmyeloablative transplant for prevention of GVHD. Toxicities associated with myeloablative preparative regimens may be quite severe. Symptom management of side effects such as nausea, vomiting, diarrhea, and mucositis can be quite challenging. Persistent attention to the effectiveness of strategies to manage side effects is necessary. Symptom management may include use of antiemetic agents, antidiarrheal agents, and analgesics for pain management. Mucositis may be so severe that potential airway compromise should be continuously evaluated. Hematologic effects result in the need for frequent platelet and RBC transfusion until engraftment of stem cells is achieved.

Side effects of nonmyeloablative preparative regimens are less severe and require minimal ongoing management. Although nausea, vomiting, diarrhea, and mucositis may occur, they are usually less severe, and resolution of symptoms occurs sooner. Myelosuppressive effects result in milder anemia and thrombocytopenia, reducing the need for RBC and platelet transfusions. Since engraftment occurs earlier, infectious complications may also be less common.

## TRANSPLANT COURSE

The transplant course generally contains defined time frames for administration of the preparative regimen, transplantation or infusion of stem cells, engraftment, and management of early and late side effects or complications of transplantation. The preparative regimen is administered over a specific number of days prior to transplantation. The number of days varies for each preparative regimen which is completed prior to the infusion of stem cells. Transplantation or infusion of stem cells occurs on "day zero." Methods of infusion of stem cells vary depending on the type of transplant. Autologous stem cells are collected, cryopreserved with DMSO, frozen, and stored previously. On transplant day, the cells must be thawed prior to transplantation or reinfusion. Infusion-related side effects that may occur are most often caused by the preservative DMSO but may also be related to the volume of cells infused or RBC contamination. Adverse effects may include nausea, vomiting, diarrhea, garlic-like taste, fever, chills, cough, tachypnea, facial flushing, hypertension, cardiac arrhythmias, chest tightness, and hemoglobinuria. Treatment of adverse effects with supportive care measures is usually adequate, and symptoms generally resolve within 24 to 48 hours.[27]

Allogeneic stem cells are usually infused fresh when bone marrow or PBSCs are used. Umbilical cord blood stem cells are most often cryopreserved, frozen, and stored. Infusion of fresh allogeneic stem cells is well tolerated, with few adverse effects. Blood transfusion-type side effects may occur, and symptom management successfully alleviates adverse effects. More significant adverse effects may occur in ABO mismatch transplants due to the risk of hemolysis. Premedications are given to minimize adverse effects of autologous ABO-matched and ABO-mismatched transplantation.

Hematopoietic recovery after transplant or engraftment occurs following the nadir of blood counts when the white blood cell, platelet, and RBC counts gradually increase. Engraftment is generally defined as a granulocyte count greater than $500/mm^3$ and platelet count greater than $20{,}000/mm^3$. Following autologous PBSC transplant, counts usually recover in approximately 8 to 10 days. Engraftment after myeloablative HSCT is variable but may occur at approximately day 21 for white blood cells and day 19 for platelet recovery, respectively.[28] Since blood counts do not fall as low after nonmyeloablative transplant,

**TABLE 18-4**

**Common Preparative Regimens and Indications**[a]

| Abbreviation | Regimen/Agents | Indications/Disease |
|---|---|---|
| Cy/TBI | Cyclophosphamide/total body irradiation | AML, MDS, ALL, CML, CLL, MM, HD, NHL |
| TBI/VP | Total body irradiation/etoposide | AML, ALL, NHL, HD |
| Bu/Cy | Busulfan/cyclophosphamide | AML, MDS, ALL, CML, CLL, MM, HD, NHL |
| Bu/Cy/VP | Busulfan/cyclophosphamide/etoposide | AML, MDS, ALL, CML, CLL, MM, HD, NHL |
| Cy | Cyclophosphamide | Severe aplastic anemia |
| Cy/ATG | Cyclophosphamide/antithymocyte globulin | Severe aplastic anemia |
| TBI/Mel | Total body irradiation/melphalan | MM |
| Mel | Melphalan | MM, nonmyeloablative SCT[b] |
| CTCb | Cyclophosphamide/thiotepa/carboplatin | Breast cancer |
| CT | Cyclophosphamide/thiotepa | Breast cancer |
| CEC | Cyclophosphamide/etoposide/carboplatin | Breast cancer, solid tumors |
| CBV | Cyclophosphamide/carmustine/etoposide | NHL, HD |
| BEAM | Carmustine/etoposide/cytarabine/melphalan | NHL, HD |
| MCC | Mitoxantrone/carboplatin/cyclophosphamide | Ovarian cancer |
| TBI | Total body irradiation | Nonmyeloablative SCT[b] |
| Fludara/Bu/ATG | Fludarabine/busulfan/antithymocyte globulin | Nonmyeloablative SCT[b] |
| Fludara/Cy | Fludarabine/cyclophosphamide | Nonmyeloablative SCT[b] |
| Fludara/Bu/ATG | Fludarabine/cyclophosphamide/antithymocyte globulin | Nonmyeloablative SCT[b] |
| Fludara/Mel | Fludarabine/melphalan | Nonmyeloablative SCT[b] |

[a]This list is not all-inclusive and serves only as examples of preparative regimens.

[b]These agents are currently used in clinical trials.

*Abbreviations*: ALL, acute lymphocytic leukemia; AML, acute myeloid leukemia; CLL, chronic lymphocytic leukemia; CML, chronic myeloid leukemia; HD, Hodgkin's disease; MDS, myelodisplastic syndrome; MM, multiple myeloma; NHL, non-Hodgkin's lymphoma; SCT, stem cell transplant.

*Source*: Reprinted with permission from McAdams and Burgunder.[27] Copyright © 2004 by Oncology Nursing Society.

engraftment occurs more quickly. Recovery of blood cell counts after UCB transplant occurs more slowly, at approximately day 28 for neutrophils and day 60 for platelets.[29,30] In general, engraftment after transplantation using PBSCs occurs approximately 1 week earlier than with use of stem cells collected directly from the bone marrow.

## SITE OF CARE DELIVERY

During the past several years, the site of care has gradually shifted toward an increase in outpatient care during and after transplantation. In some settings, the entire transplant experience occurs in the outpatient setting. The site of care delivery during the acute phase of the transplant experience is dependent on many factors. The outpatient care site must be capable of supporting nursing and medical care, which includes some complex aspects of care. Components of nursing care may include physical examination, intravenous (IV) fluid therapy, IV medications, central venous catheter care, medication review, and patient and family education. Medical or midlevel practitioner care may include review of chief complaint, physical examination, patient and family discussions or education, and also procedures such as bone marrow biopsy and aspirate, lumbar puncture, and skin biopsy. Outpatient lodging must be available during the weeks the patient must stay near the transplant setting. Transportation services between the hospital and outpatient lodging facility must be available. The hospital emergency room must be educated on the unique needs of the follow-up transplant patient for medical care.

## OUTPATIENT FOLLOW-UP

Posttransplant outpatient follow-up is based on institutional standards or, when applicable, research protocol requirements. In the posttransplant period, it is important to have a defined pattern of evaluation to assess disease status and for any posttransplant complications. On occasion, readmission to the inpatient transplant service is necessary to manage a posttransplant complication.

In addition, after allogeneic transplantation evaluation of conversion to donor cells is important. Chimerism is the term used to describe conversion to donor hematopoiesis posttransplant. Various types of chimerism analysis have been used over the years. Evaluation of cytogenetic or molecular tests to identify the presence of particular disease markers has been used. If a sex-mismatch transplant is done, cytogenetics for XX/CY may be done to determine presence of donor cells. Today, chimerism studies most frequently used are the CD3 (T lymphocyte) and CD33 (myeloid cell) markers. It is possible to quantify the donor vs recipient CD3 and CD33 levels. Additional donor CD3 cells may be given if conversion to donor cells does not occur. Donor CD3 cells may also be given if disease relapse occurs, with the hopes of triggering GVHD to occur along with an antitumor effect.

## FUTURE DIRECTIONS

Hematopoietic stem cell transplant continues to expand the treatment options for many malignant and nonmalignant conditions. A mix of old knowledge and new ideas shapes the role of HSCT for the treatment of many conditions. In the future, there will be continued efforts to enhance all components of the transplant experience to improve outcomes and minimize mortality.

## REFERENCES

1. Quine WE. The remedial application of bone marrow. *JAMA*. 1896;26:1012–1013.
2. Lorenz E, Uphoff D, Reid TR, Shelton E. Modification of irradiation injury in mice and guinea pigs by bone marrow injections. *J Natl Cancer Inst*. 1951;12:197–201.
3. Applebaum FR. The use of bone marrow and peripheral blood stem cell transplantation in treatment of cancer. *CA: Canc J Clin*. 1996;46:142–164.
4. Thomas E. Transplantation of hematopoietic progenitor cells with emphasis on the results in children. *Turk J Pediatr*. 1995;37:31–43.
5. Kurnick NB, Montano A, Gerdes JC, Feder BH. Preliminary observations on the treatment of postirradiation hematopoietic depression in man by the infusion of stored autologous bone marrow. *Ann Intern Med*. 1958;49:969.
6. Wingard J. Bone marrow to blood stem cells: past, present and future. In: Ezzone S, Schmit-Pokorny K, eds. *Blood and Marrow Stem Cell Transplantation: Principles, Practice and Nursing Insights*. 3rd ed. Sudbury, MA: Jones and Bartlett; 2007:1–28.
7. Thomas ED. Bone marrow transplantation. *N Engl J Med*. 1975;292:832–843, 895–902.
8. Baranov A, Gale RP, Guskova A, et al. Bone marrow transplantation after Chernobyl nuclear accident. *N Engl J Med*. 1989;321:205–212.
9. To L, Roberts M, Haylock D, et al. Comparison of haematological recovery times and supportive care requirements of autologous recovery phase peripheral blood stem cell transplant, autologous bone marrow transplants and allogeneic bone marrow transplants. *Bone Marrow Transplant*. 1992;9:277–284.
10. The National Marrow Donor Program. http://www.nmdp.org/ Accessed January 14, 2010.
11. Slavin S, Nagler A, Naparstek E, et al. Non myeloablative stem cell transplantation and cell therapy as an alternative to conventional bone marrow transplantation with lethal cytoreduction for the treatment of malignant and nonmalignant hematologic diseases. *Blood*. 1998;91:756–763.
12. American Society for Blood and Marrow Transplantation. http://www.asbmt.org/. Accessed January 14, 2010.
13. Filipovich AH, Wisdorf D, Pavletic S, et al. National Institutes of Health consensus development project on criteria for clinical trials in chronic graft-vs-host disease: I. diagnosis and staging working group report. *Biol Blood Marrow Transplant*. 2005;11:945–956.
14. Maccario R, Moretta A, Cometa A, et al. Human mesenchymal stem cells and cyclosporine A exert a synergistic suppressive effect on in vitro activation of alloantigen specific cytotoxic lymphocytes. *Biol Blood Marrow Transplant*. 2005;11:1031–1032.
15. Cristina T, Mario A, PierLuigi T, et al. Extracorporeal photochemotherapy (ECP) in patients with acute or chronic graft-vs-host disease (a/cGVHD). Clinical and immunological outcomes. *Biol Blood Marrow Transplant*. 2006;12:65.
16. Ballon KK, Spitzer TR, Yeap BY, et al. Double unrelated reduced-intension umbilical cord blood transplantation in adults. *Biol Blood Marrow Transplant*. 2007;13:82–89.
17. Williams L. Comprehensive review of hematopoiesis and immunology: Implications for hematopoietic stem cell transplant recipients. In S. Ezzone, ed. *Hematopoietic Stem Cell Transplantation: A Manual for Nursing Practice*. Pittsburgh, PA: Oncology Nursing Society; 2004:1–11.
18. Ezzone S. Blood and marrow stem cell transplantation. In: Gobel BH, Triese-Robertson S, Vogel WH, eds. *Advanced Oncology Nursing Certification: Review and Resource Manual*. ONS Press; Pittsburgh, PA, 2009:261–303.
19. Neiss D, Duffy KM. Basic concepts of transplantation. In: Ezzone S, ed. *Hematopoietic Stem Cell Transplantation: A Manual for Nursing Practice*. Pittsburgh, PA: Oncology Nursing Society; 2004:13–21.
20. Schmit-Pokorny, K. Blood and marrow transplantation: indications, procedure, process. In: Ezzone S, Schmit-Pokorny K, eds. *Blood and Marrow Stem Cell Transplantation: Principles, Practice and Nursing Insights*. 3rd ed. Sudbury, MA: Jones and Bartlett; 2007:75–107.
21. Flomenberg N, Devine SM, DiPersio JF, et al. The use of AMD3100 plus G-CSF for autologous hematopoietic progenitor cell mobilization is superior to G-CSF alone. *Blood*. 2005;106:1867–1874.
22. Chouinard M, Finn K. Understanding hematopoiesis. In: Ezzone S, Schmit-Pokorny K, eds. *Blood and Marrow Stem Cell Transplantation: Principles, Practice and Nursing Insights*. 3rd ed. Sudbury, MA: Jones and Bartlett; 2007:29–58.
23. Sorror ML, Maris MB, Storb R, et al. Hematopoietic cell transplantation (HCT)-specific comorbidity index: a new tool for risk assessment before allogeneic HCT. *Blood*. 2005;106:2912–2919.
24. Morishima Y, Sasazuke T, Inoko H, et al. The clinical significance of human leukocyte antigen (HLA) allele compatibility in patients receiving a marrow transplant from serologically HLA-A, HLA-B, HLA-DR matched unrelated donors. *Blood*. 2002;99:4200–4206.
25. Snustad DP, Simmons MJ. *Principles of Genetics*. 2nd ed. New York: John Wiley & Sons; 2000.

26. Spellman S, Setterholm M, Maiers M, et al. Advances in the selection of HLA-compatible donors: refinements in HLA typing and matching over the first 20 years of the national marrow donor program registry. *Biol Blood Marrow Transplant.* 2008;14:37–44.
27. McAdams FW, Burgunder MR. Transplant course. In: Ezzone S, ed. *Hematopoietic Stem Cell Transplantation: A Manual for Nursing Practice.* Pittsburgh, PA: ONS Publishing Division; 2004:43–49 (p. 44, Table 4–1).
28. Bensinger WJ, Martin P, Storer B, et al. Transplantation of bone marrow as compared with peripheral blood cells from HLA-identical relatives in patients with hematologic cancers. *N Engl J Med.* 2001;344:175–181.
29. Gluckman E, Roscha V, Chastang C. Allogeneic cord blood hematopoietic stem cell transplants in malignancies. In: Armitage JO, Antman KH, eds. *High Dose Cancer Therapy: Pharmacology, Hematopoietic, Stem Cells.* 3rd ed. Philadelphia: Lippincott Williams & Wilkins; 2000:211–220.
30. Rocha V, Cornish J, Sievers EL, Filipovich A, Locatelli F, Peters C. Comparison of outcomes of unrelated bone marrow and umbilical cord blood transplants in children with acute leukemia. *Blood.* 2001;97:2962.

CHAPTER 19

Lowell Anderson-Reitz, RN, MS, ANP, AOCN®

# Complications of Hematopoietic Cell Transplantation

## INTRODUCTION

Hematopoietic cell transplantation (HCT) is a widely used therapy for malignant and nonmalignant diseases. The unique and intensive nature of this treatment requires specialty care throughout the entire transplant course. Monitoring for long-term side effects can last for years after the transplant. Advances in supportive care have dramatically reduced morbidity and mortality associated with HCT. This chapter will focus on prophylactic and supportive therapies found to improve the clinical course. Evaluation and treatment of transplant related complications will also be discussed.

## PROPHYLACTIC SUPPORT

### PROPHYLAXIS OF INFECTIONS

Prevention of infections in the hematopoietic stem cell transplant patient should begin with general infection control measures. The main stay of infection control is frequent hand washing by the health care team as well as family members and caregivers. Personal hygiene by the patient is imperative for minimizing normal skin flora.[1] Meticulous oral hygiene is required, especially in those patients at risk for developing mucositis. Inpatient units should be equipped with high efficiency particulate air (HEPA) filters. Portable HEPA filters are available if patients require transfer to other units within the institution. Laminar air filtration systems are also available but effectiveness on reducing infection has not been established. Outpatient guidelines for air handling systems are ill defined and many facilities lack specific systems. Food and water guidelines are frequently set by individual institutions with little scientific evidence to support specific practices. Indwelling catheters are frequently a source of infection and meticulous care of the catheter sites dramatically decreases risks of infection.

#### Antimicrobial prophylaxis

Infections remain a significant cause of morbidity and mortality in the HCT patient despite significant strides made in terms of antimicrobial, antiviral and antifungal therapies. Infection occurrences can be stratified based on the phase of the transplant course (See Table 19-1).[2] The use of prophylactic agents remains a topic of debate due to the emergence of resistant strains of microbes. Nevertheless, the Centers for Disease Control and Prevention (CDC) recommends prophylactic antimicrobial therapy for HCT patients.

#### Bacterial prophylaxis

Bacterial infections remain the most common infections, accounting for 90% of all infections occurring during the neutropenic phase. Most gram-negative and gram-positive pathogens are endogenous and are tied to the physical barrier insults associated with the transplant process.[2] Interruptions of the skin and gut lining secondary to the conditioning regimen and indwelling catheters are the primary portals of entry.[1] Common bacterial prophylaxis includes fluoroquinolones providing both gram-positive and gram-negative coverage. Gut decontamination within the allogeneic population is frequently utilized. Trimethoprim/sulfamethoxazole is commonly used during the conditioning regimen phase for gut decontamination.[3] The fluoroquinolones continue gram-negative coverage in the subsequent neutropenic phase.

**TABLE 19-1**

**Infection Time Frame After Hematopoietic Cell Transplant**

| Days 0–30 | Days 31–100 | Day > 100 |
|---|---|---|
| Gram-positive bacteria | Gram-positive bacteria | Encapsulated organism |
| Gram-negative bacteria | Gram-negative bacteria | Pneumocystis |
| | | Varicella zoster |
| | | *Aspergillus* |
| Herpes simplex | CMV | |
| *Candida* | Varicella zoster | |
| *Aspergillus* | *Candida* | |
| | *Aspergillus* | |

*Source*: Data from Bashey[2] and Atkinson and Singhal.[3]
*Abbrevation*: CMV, cytomegalouirus.

#### Fungal prophylaxis

Fungal infections remain a major cause of morbidity and mortality in the allogeneic HCT population. *Candida* and *Aspergillus* species are the predominant cause of invasive infections.[4] Diagnosis of invasive fungal infections are difficult since they frequently do not present with specific signs or symptoms and cultures often remain negative. Owing to this fact, prevention is the focus with regard to fungal infections. Fluconazole has been the mainstay for fungal prophylaxis, reducing invasive candidal infections in the allogeneic HCT population.[5,6] Invasive candidal infections are less common in the autologous population, however fungal prophylaxis remains beneficial in reducing invasive candidal infections in the allogeneic HCT population Recent prophylactic studies evaluating broad spectrum antifungal agents such as posaconazole indicate superior results compared to fluconazole in preventing fungi not covered by fluconazole.[7] Utilization of newer azole agents with broad spectrum coverage remains debated secondary to cost of the agents and potentially significant interactions with other medications used in the allogeneic population.[4]

### Viral prophylaxis

Herpes simplex virus (HSV) infection is common in the neutropenic phase. Antiviral prophylaxis significantly reduces the reactivation rate for HSV. Acyclovir is commonly started the day following transplant and continued for at least 30 days.[1] Prophylactic use of acyclovir for Varicella-zoster virus (VZV) is commonly used for a full year following transplant. Results of studies evaluating development of resistant strains of HSV with long-term antiviral prophylaxis remain inconsistent.[8–10]

Cytomegalovirus (CMV) reactivation tends to be a late infection primarily affecting allogeneic recipients. Patients should receive irradiated/leukopoor or CMV negative blood products to help prevent CMV reactivation.[1] Although some centers have used ganciclovir or foscarnet for prophylaxis, these agents carry high risk for hematotoxicity and nephrotoxicity. These agents are, however, effective in preventing CMV reactivation. A new agent, Maribivir, has shown recent promise in preventing CMV reactivation in seropositive patients. This agent has shown significant reduction of CMV reactivation when compared to placebo and has minimal side effects.[11]

### Pneumocystis carinii prophylaxis

Allogeneic HCT recipients who require continued immunosuppression are at risk of Pneumocystis carinii pneumonia (PCP). The drug of choice for PCP is trimethoprim/sulfamethoxazole. However, due to potential marrow suppression, other agents such as dapsone or inhaled pentamidine can be utilized.[12] Prophylaxis is recommended throughout all periods of immunosuppression.[13] The safe period to discontinue prophylaxis remains under debate.

## GRAFT-vs-HOST DISEASE

Graft-vs-host disease (GVHD) remains one of the most challenging and potentially debilitating complications of allogeneic HCT. Incidence of GVHD ranges from 30% to 50% in matched sibling transplants to 50% to 80% in mismatched sibling or unrelated donor transplants.[14,15] Graft-vs-host disease is an immunological response that is mediated by the new immune system or graft, against disparate human leukocyte antigen (HLA) host cell antigens. Cells known to be involved in this process include helper T cells, cytotoxic T cells, natural killer cells, lymphokine-activated killer (LAK) cells, and antigen presenting cells.[16] Cytotoxic injury of the host tissues is the result of this activated immune response.

Discussion of prevention and prophylaxis of graft-vs-host (GVHD) disease begins with a consideration of the donor selection process. Histocompatibility with molecular matching of Classes I and II antigens is the basis for decreasing incidence of GVHD. There are numerous donor-recipient factors that affect GVHD incidence, including sex mismatch, age, and viral sero-negativity.[14,17] The intensity of the conditioning regimen is also related to GVHD. The tissue damage associated with more intense regimens causes cytokine release, which allows for alloantigen presentation for donor T cells.[18] This effect, in turn, increases the incidence of acute GVHD.

Prophylactic immunosuppression is required to prevent GVHD. Cyclosporine (CSA) and methotrexate (MTX) have been the mainstay of prophylaxis since the drug combination was shown to decrease incidence and severity of GVHD in the early 1990s.[19] Tacrolimus, also a calcineurin inhibitor like CSA, in combination with MTX has been shown to decrease grades II to IV GVHD when compared to CSA/MTX. However, tacrolimus/MTX does not show a survival benefit when compared to CSA/MTX.[20] Both regimens are used widely in clinical practice.

Multiple drug regimens for GVHD prophylaxis continue to be evaluated for effectiveness in preventing GVHD. Mycophenolate mofetil (MMF) is frequently utilized with reduced intensity regimens.[21] Regimens including antithimocyte globulin, pentostatin, sirolimus, monoclonal antibodies such as Campath (anti-CD52), intravenous immunoglobulin (IVIG), and extracorporeal photopheresis continue to be studied. No new regimens have shown enough promise in decreasing GVHD to replace CSA or tacrolimus with MTX as the primary prophylaxis regimens.

T-cell depletion (TCD) has been utilized as a means of GVHD prophylaxis for many years. GVHD can be dramatically reduced but T-cell depletion presents other limitations in terms of increased graft rejection and disease relapse.[22] Since GVHD is a result of immunocompetent donor T cells reacting to recipient alloantigens, recent work has been focused on selective donor T-cell depletion. This process aims to deplete GVHD initiating T cells while maintaining cells responsible for engraftment and graft-vs-disease effect.[22]

## VENO-OCCLUSIVE DISEASE/SINUSOIDAL OBSTRUCTION SYNDROME

Veno-occlusive disease (VOD) or sinusoidal obstruction syndrome (SOS) is a serious hepatic complication associated most commonly with high-dose chemotherapy and/or radiotherapy. Incidence is reported to range from 0% to 70% with mortality rates as high as 90%.[23] Injury of the endothelial lining of the venules and sinusoids leads to cytokine and tumor necrosis factor activation. This results in coagulation and thrombosis impairing blood flow and leads to the syndrome of VOD/SOS.[24]

Effective treatment options for VOD/SOS are absent. Due to this, much focus has been placed on prevention of VOD/SOS. Ursodeoxycholic acid (Ursadiol) has been evaluated as prophylaxis and has been shown to decrease incidence of VOD/SOS, but large randomized trials are lacking.[25] A newer agent, defibrotide, has been studied as a treatment option for VOD/SOS. More recently it has also been evaluated as a prophylactic agent and has found to be effective.[26] More study is required to better establish its usefulness as a prophylactic agent.

### MUCOSITIS

Mucositis is a general term referring to the inflammation and possible infection of mucous membranes, extending from the mouth to the anus. Chemoradiotherapy exhibits toxic effects upon rapidly proliferating cells such as the epithelial lining of the gastrointestinal tract. Oral mucositis has been reported to be one of the most distressing and toxic effects of HCT.[27] The occurrence depends on the conditioning regimen with overall incidence ranging from 75% to 99%.[27,28]

Management of mucositis in the past has primarily been supportive in nature with no preventive measures available. Cryotherapy has been attempted in the past with little positive effects. More recent studies have again evaluated this as a preventive therapy with significant improvement in oral mucositis.[29,30] Cryotherapy is now recommended for use in patients receiving high-dose melphalan.[31] Palifermin, a recombinant human keratinocyte growth factor, has also been shown to decrease incidence and duration of oral mucositis.[32] Palifermin is now recommended for use in patients receiving high-dose chemotherapy with total body irradiation (TBI) followed by autologous HCT.[31]

### NAUSEA/VOMITING

Nausea and vomiting, whether associated with chemoradiotherapy, GVHD, medications, or mucositis, remains a significant problem for HCT patients. The American Society of Clinical Oncology (ASCO) has published guidelines for prophylactic antiemetic therapy associated with high-dose chemoradiotherapy. The guidelines call for combination therapy with a first generation 5HT-3 receptor antagonist and corticosteroids during chemotherapy administration.[33] Delayed nausea and vomiting continues to be more problematic. Newer agents such as palonosetron, aprepitant, and olanzapine have been shown to be effective in controlling delayed nausea and vomiting in the general oncology population. Comparative trials evaluating these agents in the HCT population have not been conducted.

## PERITRANSPLANT SUPPORTIVE CARE

Patients undergoing HCT require intensive supportive care throughout the transplant course. Much of the supportive care required stems from side effects of the conditioning regimen administered.

### BLOOD PRODUCT SUPPORT

Pancytopenia is an expected side effect of HCT. Transfusion support with both platelets and red blood cells (RBC) is necessary. Patients undergoing fully ablative conditioning regimens have traditionally been RBC transfusion dependent requiring anywhere from 8 to 65 units of packed RBC throughout the transplant process.[34] Successful autologous transplants without blood product support for patients refusing blood for religious reasons have been reported.[35] Transfusion requirements for patients undergoing nonmyeloablative regimens are reported to be significantly less than those receiving myeloablative regimens.[36,37] Transfusion parameters vary according to the transplant center, with most maintaining hemoglobin levels above 8.0g/dL.

Platelet transfusion requirements have been reported to range from 5 to 80 units throughout the transplant course.[36] Transfusion requirements in nonmyeloablative vs myeloablative transplants are significantly reduced, with some reports indicating a near 80% decrease.[36,37] Questions regarding when platelet transfusions are required remain unanswered. Prophylactic platelet transfusions have been utilized in leukemia and HCT patients for many years. Ongoing research is required to identify safe and cost effective threshold triggers. Most centers prophylactically transfuse platelets for counts between $10 \times 10^9$/L and $20 \times 10^9$/L.[38,39] Debate also continues with regard to the type of platelet product utilized. The long standing assumption that single donor vs pooled platelet concentrates provide superior platelet increments has not been proven. Pooled platelet concentrates and single donor apheresis products have actually been shown to provide comparable increments.[40]

Blood products for all HCT patients should be irradiated and leukopoor to decrease transfusion reactions, alloimmunization, and infectious risk.[41,42] Irradiated and leukopoor blood products lessen exposure to allogeneic white blood cells, which express antigens that lead to antibody production and alloimmunization. Irradiated and leukopoor blood products also decrease possible exposure to CMV, since white blood cells harbor this virus. Patients who receive multiple transfusions throughout their treatment course can become alloimmunized despite these precautions, causing platelet refractoriness. When this situation arises patients should receive HLA matched and cross matched platelets.[42,43]

Transplant patients routinely receive hematopoietic growth factors to hasten the recovery of neutrophils and red blood cells. Both granulocyte colony-stimulating factor (G-CSF) and granulocyte-macrophage colony-stimulating factor (GM-CSF) have been shown to speed recovery of neutrophils, thereby significantly decreasing the neutropenic phase.[44,45] Specific start day for these particular growth factors remain under debate and vary from center to center.

Erythropoietin (EPO) provides stimulus for erythroid progenitors resulting in RBC production. Erythropoietin is produced by interstitial cells within the renal tubules. Since CSA and tacrolimus cause renal tubular nephrotoxicity there is decreased production of EPO. The decreased production of EPO leads to frequent longstanding anemia within the allogeneic population. Providing recombinant human erythropoietin (rHuEPO) has been shown to lower RBC transfusion requirements in the allogeneic population.[46,47] The role of rHuEPO in the autologous population has been less clear, however there are reports of its effectiveness with autologous transplant.[48,49]

### FLUID, ELECTROLYTES, AND NUTRITION

Patients undergoing HCT frequently require support with intravenous hydration. Due to complications such as nausea, vomiting, diarrhea, and mucositis, many patients are unable to adequately maintain hydration. Close monitoring of fluid balance and renal function is imperative to prevent permanent damage. Many complications along with certain medications cause electrolyte imbalances. Patients may require intravenous electrolyte supplementation with ongoing oral supplementation. Nutrition services should be consulted upon admission to establish a baseline of nutritional status. Patients have increased metabolic needs due to tissue damage, GVHD, and infection. Nutritional support such as total parenteral nutrition (TPN), enteral feedings, or simple oral dietary supplements may be required to prevent severe malnutrition.

### PAIN MANAGEMENT

Patients undergoing HCT may experience pain at various stages of the transplant process. Assessment for pain on an ongoing basis is imperative. Pain management may require both pharmacological and nonpharmacological therapies. Consultation with a dedicated pain team may be helpful for identifying alternative pain management options.

### PSYCHOSOCIAL

Much of the focus for psychosocial support has been on the post-transplant period. The peritransplant phase is intensive and stress-filled. Both patients and families need ongoing support throughout this time. Education of patients and families assists in decreasing stress and anxiety. Financial support through social services may be needed during this time. Consultation by psychiatry may be helpful in assisting with medication support.

## EVALUATION AND TREATMENT OF COMPLICATIONS

Numerous acute and chronic complications can occur with each type of transplant. The nature of some complications can be generalized to all transplant types, while others are specific to the transplant type or stem cell source. Complications are generally secondary to the conditioning regimen (chemotherapy and radiation), GVHD, the presenting disease, and the adverse effects of medications required during the transplant process. Acute complications are generally defined as those events occurring within the first 100 days after the transplant; chronic complications present after this time frame. The intricacies of both types of complications associated with stem cell transplantation present challenging management issues to the caregiver.

## ACUTE COMPLICATIONS

### ACUTE GRAFT-vs-HOST DISEASE

Acute graft-vs-host disease (AGVHD) by definition occurs within the first 100 days following allogeneic HCT. Despite advancements in prophylaxis and treatment of AGVHD, it remains one of the most challenging and debilitating complications of allogeneic HCT.

Acute graft-vs-host disease usually occurs within 2 to 5 weeks following allogeneic transplant.[50] Table 19-2 describes how these factors may affect the incidence of GVHD.[51,52]

Table 19-3 presents commonly used systems for staging and grading of AGVHD.[51,53] Grade I AGVHD has a favorable outcome and does not require treatment. Moderate disease—grade II—is associated with multi organ involvement and requires therapy to halt progression of the disease. Grade III AGVHD is severe and may lead to grade IV disease, which is life-threatening or fatal disease. Mortality rates rise significantly for patients developing moderate to severe disease due primarily to the increased risk of infection.

Acute graft-vs-host disease primarily presents in the skin, gastrointestinal tract, and liver. Skin GVHD is the most common clinical feature of AGVHD. Acute skin GVHD often presents as a pruritic or painful maculopapular erythematous rash that most commonly begins on the plantar or palmar surfaces. However, the rash can present anywhere and involve the entire body surface area. Staging of skin GVHD is based primarily on the extent of the body surface area involved (see Table 19-3).

Hepatic GVHD is the second most common manifestation of AGVHD.[54] Isolated liver AGVHD is rare, but possible. Elevated alkaline phosphatase and hyperbilirubinemia are seen first, with eventual elevation of the transaminases. Hepatomegaly and associated tenderness are late symptoms of this disease. Liver biopsy is helpful for a definitive diagnosis; however, it is not required in the face of concomitant

**TABLE 19-2**

**Influences on Incidence of Graft-vs-Host Disease (GVHD)**

| Risk Factor | Increased GVHD | Decreased GVHD |
|---|---|---|
| Donor relationship | Unrelated donor | Related donor |
| HLA match | Mismatched | Matched |
| Donor/recipient parity | Increased parity | Less parity |
| Donor/recipient age | Older | Younger |
| Donor/recipient viral seropositivity | Positive | Negative |
| Sex matched | Mismatched: female to male | Sex matched |
| TBI dose | >12 Gy | <12 Gy |
| Immunosuppressive regimen | Less intensive | More intensive |
| T-cell depletion | No T-cell depletion | T-cell depletion |

Abbreviations: HLA, human leukocyte antigen; TBI, total body irradiation.

*Source*: Data from Chao[51] and Przepiorka.[52]

skin or gastrointestinal GVHD. Staging of acute liver GVHD is based on the bilirubin level.

Gastrointestinal GVHD can present with voluminous diarrhea with bleeding and abdominal cramping. Staging for acute gastrointestinal GVHD is based on the volume of diarrhea and pain or ileus development. Upper gastrointestinal involvement is associated with nausea and vomiting, anorexia, dyspepsia, or early satiety. Endoscopy with biopsies must be completed to definitively diagnose gastrointestinal GVHD.[18] The triad of skin, hepatic, and gastrointestinal GVHD can occur independently or concomitantly.

Hyperacute GVHD also involves the previously mentioned organs, but is associated with fever, influenza-like symptoms, generalized erythroderma, and desquamation. This manifestation of AGVHD can present before signs of engraftment are clear. Biopsies of the involved organs are required for diagnosis.

The hematolymphoid system appears to be affected by AGHVD, and decreased hematopoietic precursors and low immunoglobulin production may result from this complication. Thrombocytopenia has also been reported in AGVHD.[51] These factors compound the risks associated with AGVHD and resulting infection.

### Treatment

Glucocorticoids remain the gold standard for treatment of confirmed AGVHD. Treatment is indicated for grades II to IV GVHD, consisting of the addition of glucocorticoids to

**TABLE 19-3**

**Staging and Grading of Graft-vs-Host Disease (GVHD)**

| Staging | | |
|---|---|---|
| Skin | Grade I | Maculopapular rash < 25% body surface |
| | Grade II | Maculopapular rash 25%–50% body surface |
| | Grade III | Generalized erythroderma > 50% body surface |
| | Grade IV | Generalized erythroderma with bullae formation |
| Gut | Grade I | Diarrhea < 500 mL/day or persistent nausea |
| | Grade II | Diarrhea > 1000 mL/day |
| | Grade III | Diarrhea > 1500 mL/day |
| | Grade IV | Severe abdominal cramping with or without ileus formation |
| Liver | Grade I | Bilirubin 2.0–3.0 mg/dL |
| | Grade II | Bilirubin 3.1–6.0 mg/dL |
| | Grade III | Bilirubin 6.1–15 mg/dL |
| | Grade IV | Bilirubin > 15 mg/dL |

**Overall Grade**

| Grade | Skin | Gut | | Liver |
|---|---|---|---|---|
| I | Stage I–II | None | | None |
| II | Stage I–III | Stage I | or | Stage I |
| III | Stage I–III | Stage II–III | or | Stage II–III |
| IV | Stage I–IV | Stage II–IV | or | Stage II–IV |

*Source*: Data from Chao,[51] and Przepiorka and Cleary.[53]

the ongoing prophylactic regimen. Glucocorticoids are frequently administered in doses of 1 to 2 mg/kg/day IV or by mouth with a taper schedule based on patient response.[14,52–55] Antithymocyte globulin is also commonly used as a single agent or in combination with glucocorticoids for first-line therapy.[14,50] Many of the agents used for prophylaxis are also used in the treatment of GVHD.

Steroid-refractory AGHVD carries a poor prognosis. About 60% to 75% of patients who develop grade II to IV AGVHD require additional treatment beyond corticosteroids.[56] Continuation of steroids in this population does not improve outcomes and is associated with increased infections. Recently, researchers have focused on the use of monoclonal antibodies to target specific T-cell populations (CD2, CD3, CD5, CD52) and agents that interfere or downregulate interleukin receptors.[18] Daclizumab, denileukin diftitiox, and infliximab are all monoclonal antibodies that have shown effectiveness in treating steroid refractory AGVHD.[56] Agents such as mycophenolate mofetil and pentostatin have also been evaluated in this population with positive effects.[56]

Nonpharmacological interventions such as ultraviolet A irradiation (PUVA) have been studied in steroid resistant skin AGVHD. PUVA appears to be effective in this situation, even allowing for steroids to be tapered.[57] Extracorporeal photopheresis has been studied and has shown effectiveness in both acute and chronic GVHD of the skin, liver, gastrointestinal tract, and eyes.[58] Current studies are evaluating the use of mesenchymal stem cells in the treatment of AGVHD. Mesenchymal stem cells have been shown to be effective in controlling AGVHD in the animal model and prospects appear to be favorable in humans.[59]

Patients who develop AGVHD are at high risk for infection due to the impairment of their natural barriers against infection and in association with immunosuppressive agents used to treat GVHD. Supportive care should include prophylactic antibiotic, antiviral, and antifungal therapy. Patients who develop skin GVHD should meticulously care for their external central venous catheter sites. Skin integrity and cleanliness are also critical. Lower gastrointestinal GVHD may require gut rest with hyperalimentation and pain control for abdominal cramping. Upper gastrointestinal GVHD may require a regular antiemetic regimen.

Nursing management of patients who are at risk for, or who have developed, AGVHD is complex and requires an expert knowledge base. Nursing management issues include the following concerns:

- Careful assessment and physical examination to identify early clinical signs and symptoms of GVHD
- Identification of high-risk patients
- Meticulous skin care to prevent infection
- Monitoring fluid balance—intake/output, daily weights
- Nutritional support, including monitoring of caloric intake and consulting with nutritional support team
- Monitoring serum electrolytes with appropriate supplementation
- Monitoring gastrointestinal output for signs of hemorrhage
- Pain management
- Monitoring for signs of infections, with knowledge that patients may not mount normal signs or symptoms while in an immunocompromised state
- Patient education regarding GVHD signs and symptoms and current therapies.

## INFECTION

Infections remain a significant cause of morbidity and mortality in HCT patients despite the significant strides made in terms of antimicrobial, antiviral, and antifungal therapies. Neutropenia following standard conditioning regimens lasts from 2 to 3 weeks. Data regarding neutropenia and infections following nonmyeloablative regimens are not well established. The number of patients developing neutropenia appears to range from 30% to 70%, and the duration of neutropenia ranges from 5 to 16 days.[60,61] Impairment of natural barriers—for example, mucositis development, central catheter placement, urinary catheter placement, and AGVHD—compounds the risk for infection. Likewise, humoral immunodeficiency with decreased IgG and antibody production increases the risk for infection long after transplant. Recovery of the humoral immune system occurs 3 to 6 months after autologous transplant and 6 to 12 months after allogeneic transplant. Recovery takes even longer in patients who develop GVHD and continue to require immunosuppressive agents.[1]

Patients who develop febrile neutropenia or have strong suspicion of infection after neutrophil recovery require empiric antibiotic therapy. Broad-spectrum monotherapy or multidrug treatment is required until neutrophil recovery has occurred or until signs and symptoms of infection have resolved. Antibiotics chosen for empiric therapy should be based on institutional use and identification of local resistance patterns.[62] General use of empiric vancomycin has been discouraged due to emerging resistance and its use should be based on specific clinical requirements.

Early detection of infections is important in the nursing management of HCT patients. Frequent assessment of vital signs, catheter sites, impaired skin or mucosal barriers, pulmonary status, mental status, and laboratory values should be performed.

## GASTROINTESTINAL COMPLICATIONS

The toxic effects of chemotherapy and radiation on the mucosal lining of the gastrointestinal tract lead to inflammation and ulceration of the mucosa, which is often secondarily infected. One hypothesis suggests that this chain of events is accentuated by the release of interleukin-1 and TNF-alfa.[27,63] Resulting signs and symptoms include oral tissue erythema, denudation, bleeding, pain, esophageal spasms and dysphagia, nausea and vomiting, and abdominal cramping with diarrhea. Gastrointestinal complications occurring after HCT also include AGVHD, infection, and medication side effects.

Management of oral mucositis is simply supportive, with no proven means to treat the condition. Traditionally, pain management with narcotic analgesics and routine oral care to help prevent superinfections have been the mainstays of therapy. Most centers continue to utilize bland oral rinses comprised of normal saline or sodium bicarbonate.[64]

*Candida albicans* and HSV account for most oral infections. Incidence of these infections has been significantly reduced with the adoption of prophylactic antiviral and antifungal regimens. Close observation of the oral cavity should be performed to identify possible infections without making the assumption that ulcerative changes are only secondary to chemoradiotherapy effects. Oral complications resulting from the conditioning regimen or AGVHD include altered taste and sicca syndrome. Treatment of GVHD and consultation with the nutritional support team will assist patients in combating these difficult symptoms, which can significantly affect quality of life.[65]

The etiology of abdominal cramping and diarrhea can be multifactorial. Gastrointestinal mucositis, AGVHD, infection, and medications are the most likely causative factors. Diarrhea is reported to affect 40% to 80% of HCT patients.[66,67] Management should focus on the most likely causative factor. Great care must be taken to maintain electrolyte replacements, fluid balance, and skin integrity. Antidiarrheal medications can be provided in appropriate situations.

## HEPATIC COMPLICATIONS

Numerous acute hepatic complications can arise following HCT. The most common complications include VOD/SOS, AGVHD, infection, and drug-induced injury.

The diagnosis of VOD/SOS is based on clinical findings most commonly within the first 21 days following HCT. Diagnostic criteria include two or more of the following symptoms: hyperbilirubinemia, hepatomegaly, right upper quadrant pain, and fluid retention.[23,68] Severe VOD/SOS often leads to renal insufficiency and, ultimately, multiorgan failure. Diagnostic studies to help support the presence of VOD/SOS include Doppler studies and liver biopsy. Biopsies obtained via a transjugular approach allow for measurement of hepatic venous-pressure gradients, which are increased in VOD[69]/SOS.

Most patients who develop VOD/SOS recover spontaneously. Recent studies using defibrotide have shown promise in treatment of VOD/SOS.[70] No other treatment options provide significant effects. Treatment is primarily supportive in nature, and nurses play an integral role in this care for patients. Strict fluid restriction and fluid management are essential, especially when renal function is affected. Patients may be placed on low-dose dopamine to maximize renal function. Nurses need to be cognizant of medications that are renal toxic or are cleared via the kidney so that appropriate adjustments can be made. Patients may become encephalopathic, so safety measures need to be implemented. Severe disease can lead to coagulapathies, increasing patients' bleeding risk. With severe hepatomegaly, pain management becomes imperative. The intricacies of pain management are complicated by the encephalopathy that can arise in the syndrome.

Fungal and viral infections can arise in the liver in the post-transplant period. Patients often exhibit signs of infection with fever development in the absence of another site of infection. In addition, liver function tests are often elevated. Reactivation of hepatitis B and hepatitis C can occur post-transplant. Infections are rarely severe but may cause elevation of transaminases.[71] Hepatitis C reactivation is often not seen until immune suppressants are tapered.[72] Computerized tomography, ultrasound, and liver biopsy are most commonly performed to assist with diagnosis of an infectious process.

Drug-induced hepatitis can be a common side effect with the myriad of medications that are potentially hepatotoxic. Transaminitis, mimicking viral hepatitis, is the most frequently observed sign of a hepatic inflammation. Liver biopsy is diagnostic to determine the presence of drug-induced hepatitis. The insulting drug should be identified and removed or changed if possible.

## NEUROLOGICAL COMPLICATIONS

Neurological complications in HCT patients generally arise from the underlying disease, initial treatment, conditioning regimen, immunosuppressive agents, or long-term immunosuppression.[73,74] The incidence of neurological complications ranges from 0% to 50%.[73] The most common complications are metabolic encephalopathy associated with multiorgan failure or drug toxicity and cerebrovascular events.[73,75,76] Central nervous system infections are associated with extended immunosuppression and are more common in the allogeneic transplant population.[77] Medications such as cyclosporine, tacrolimus, and corticosteroids that are required for the HCT patient can cause neurological complications including leukoencephalopathy, peripheral tremor, and steroid-induced myopathy.

Nursing management of the HCT patient should include close observation for sometimes subtle neurological changes. Rapid intervention in some situations may alleviate potentially deleterious outcomes.

## PRIMARY GRAFT FAILURE

Primary graft failure occurs if no signs of engraftment appear within the first 3 to 4 weeks following HCT. Factors that increase the risk of graft failure include T-cell depletion, reduced-intensity immunosuppressive regimen, alloimmunization by multiple blood transfusions, low donor cell count, and HLA mismatch.[78,79] Incidence of graft failure in cord blood transplants has been reported to range from 7% to 40%.[80–82] Patients experiencing primary graft failure must undergo a second transplant, which carries a high mortality rate: 70% to 80%.

## PULMONARY COMPLICATIONS

Pulmonary complications following HCT are common and are a major cause of morbidity and mortality. Such complications account for nearly 40% of all deaths following HCT.[83] Complications that occur can be classified into three primary areas: parenchymal disease, pulmonary vascular disease, and infectious complications.

Three of the more common parenchymal diseases are idiopathic pneumonia syndrome, diffuse alveolar hemorrhage, and pulmonary edema. Idiopathic pneumonia syndrome occurs in approximately 15% of patients and is characterized by fever, dyspnea, hypoxemia, and nonproductive cough.[83] Diagnosis is made in the absence of an infectious process, with radiological findings indicating diffuse alveolar infiltrates. Biopsy reveals fibrosis and inflammation most likely caused by high-dose chemotherapy and/or radiation. Although treatment has most often been corticosteroids, only anecdotal support for this therapy exists. Pulmonary edema in the post-transplant period is not well described in the literature, but has been reported in as many as 63% of patients.[83] Most patients develop pulmonary edema in the immediate post-transplant period, most likely as a result of volume overload. Patients present with classic signs of pulmonary edema, and treatment focuses on diuresis. Diffuse alveolar hemorrhage (DAH) has been reported in as many as 41% of patients.[83] This disease most often occurs within 2 weeks of HCT. Patients present with hypoxemia, dyspnea, cough, and fever, most often in the absence of hemoptysis. Radiography displays diffuse interstitial infiltrates, and histological exam identifies alveolar injury with hemorrhage.[83,84] High-dose corticosteroids are the primary treatment for DAH.[85]

Pulmonary veno-occlusive disease (PVOD) is the primary pulmonary vascular complication following HCT. This rare disease occurs 4 to 6 weeks after HCT.[83,84] Patients present with signs of pulmonary hypertension, cough, dyspnea, and possible right heart failure. Diagnosis is made by biopsy with signs of pulmonary venular thrombosis. Corticosteroids are the treatment of choice, though few hard data exist to support this choice of therapy.[86]

Infectious pulmonary complications remain the primary cause of pulmonary disease following HCT. Gram-negative bacteria are most commonly the infecting agents in the first 100 days post-HCT. Most of these infections are from endogenous sources.

Viral pneumonitis is most often caused by CMV and herpes viruses. Herpes pneumonitis usually occurs in the early post-transplant period. Cytomegalovirus infections tend to occur after engraftment and account for approximately 40% of pneumonias in this population.[83] Patients present with a nonproductive cough, fever, hypoxemia, and dyspnea. Radiographs reveal diffuse reticulonodular or "ground glass" infiltrates. Early treatment with antiviral therapies such as ganciclovir or foscarnet and corticosteroids improves survival, although mortality rates for CMV pneumonitis remain high. Viral pneumonitis can also be caused by respiratory syncytial virus, adenovirus, influenza A and B, and parainfluenza. Effective treatments and outcomes of untreated disease with these viruses remain to be identified.

Fungal pneumonia caused by the *Aspergillus* fungi remains a serious problem for HCT patients. Invasive disease is difficult to treat, although extended therapy with new antifungal agents has greatly improved outcomes.

Opportunistic infections such as *Pneumocystis carinii* pneumonia (PCP) present a risk for patients who are profoundly immunosuppressed for extended periods of time. Patients receiving immunosuppressive agents for GVHD should receive PCP prophylaxis until all immunosuppressive agents have been discontinued.

## CARDIAC COMPLICATIONS

High-dose cyclophosphamide is associated with a 5% to 10% incidence of detectable hemorrhagic cardiomyopathy in HCT patients. Clinical manifestations of this complication include congestive heart failure, pericardial effusion, loss of electrocardiogram (ECG) voltage, and cardiomegaly. Most patients experiencing cyclophosphamide-induced toxicity will experience minor ECG changes such as ST-T wave segment changes, supraventricular arrhythmias, or pericarditis without hemodynamically significant pericardial effusions. Cardiac toxicity due to cyclophosphamide is dose dependent and usually occurs acutely following administration.[87] Factors that may contribute to the development of cardiac toxicity include prior anthracycline therapy, mediastinal radiation, and total body irradiation. Anthracycline therapy prior to HCT has been shown to decrease ventricular ejection fraction prior to transplant and appears to have predictive value for those developing cardiac complications.[88]

Patients generally undergo multiple gated acquisition (MUGA) scans or echocardiograms to determine left ventricular ejection fractions prior to HCT. Most centers will exclude patients with an ejection fraction less than 50% from receiving fully ablative regimens. Patients have been found to maintain ejection fractions following HCT despite possible cardiac toxic regimens.[89]

Cardiac involvement with GVHD has been reported but is a rare but serious complication often presenting with pericardial effusion.[90]

Treatment of cardiac complications consists of symptomatic support and fluid management. Significant cardiac effusions may require surgical intervention with pericardiocentesis or pericardial window placement. Nursing management begins with identification of high-risk patients. Routine fluid management and close assessment of cardiac status during the high-risk period should be the primary focus of care.

### RENAL COMPLICATIONS

Acute renal failure (ARF) and renal insufficiency (RI) occur in 20% to 80% of HCT patients in the first 3 months following transplant.[91,92] Nephrotoxic agents and VOD/SOS are the most likely causes of ARF/RI.[91] (See Table 19-4.) Patients who experience severe VOD/SOS often develop a hepatorenal syndrome. Decreased intravascular volume and low cardiac output lead to renal hypoperfusion and RI/ARF in severe VOD/SOS.[91] Patients who are receiving nephrotoxic agents or who are developing VOD/SOS need close observation of fluid balance. Nursing management includes the administration of diuretics and evaluating responses. Patients may require hemodialysis or continuous venovenous hemodialysis for renal failure or fluid management.

## LATE COMPLICATIONS

Hematopoietic cell transplantation is becoming more common for treatment of a multitude of diseases. Advances in supportive care and development of less toxic conditioning regimens have improved the long-term survival rates

**TABLE 19-4**

| Common Nephrotoxic Agents | |
|---|---|
| Ifosfamide | Aminoglycosides |
| Foscarnet | Cyclosporine |
| Melphalan | Gancyclovir |
| Carboplatin | Acyclovir |
| Cisplatin | Amphotericin-B |
| Methotrexate | Tacrolimus |

*Source*: Data from Savdie.[91]

for patients undergoing HCT. Hematopoietic cell transplantation carries with it the possibility of many long-term complications.

### CHRONIC GRAFT-vs-HOST DISEASE

Chronic graft-vs-host disease (CGVHD) is the most common long-term complication and the major cause of mortality following allogeneic HCT.[93] Incidence of CGVHD can range from 30% to 70%, and the disease is associated with several risk factors. The degree of HLA disparity, prior AGVHD, increasing age of donor and recipient, use of an unrelated donor, donor lymphocyte infusion (DLI), shortened cyclosporine courses, and viral infections all appear to affect the incidence of CGVHD.[15,94] The effect of peripheral blood stem cells on CGVHD remains a topic of debate and is currently being studied in long-term randomized clinical trials. A recent retrospective study comparing bone marrow vs peripheral blood stem cells with regard to AGVHD and CGVHD showed a significantly higher rate of CGVHD in peripheral blood stem cell transplants.[95] Chronic GVHD can affect the skin, liver, gastrointestinal tract, oral mucosa, muscles, eyes, vagina, nerves, kidneys, lungs, and marrow function.[96,97] The grading of CGVHD is based on the extent of involvement of the affected organs and is generally of little use except to identify which patients require treatment. Patients with extensive CGVHD require treatment, whereas those with limited CGVHD may not require treatment.

Chronic GVHD occurs 100 or more days after HCT, with the highest incidence within the first 2 years posttransplant. It is important to note that symptoms of AGVHD can occur after day 100. Patients can develop CGVHD years after undergoing allogeneic HCT. Chronic GVHD that progresses directly from AGVHD is associated with the highest morbidity and mortality rates. Transplant recipients who develop CGVHD following a quiescent AGVHD period or who develop de novo CGVHD have lower morbidity and mortality rates.

Prevention of CGVHD is the same as for AGVHD. Numerous studies are investigating effective immunosuppressive regimens that could potentially lessen the incidence and severity of AGVHD and CGVHD. Currently, the treatment regimen of choice is alternating cyclosporine and prednisone every other day. Medications are then tapered based on response.[96] There are no universally accepted salvage regimens for refractory disease. Combination therapies include medications such as mycophenalate mofetil, sirolimus, thalidomide, azathioprine, pentostatin, and biological therapies such as infliximab and dacluzimab. Ultraviolet light therapy and extracorporeal photopheresis are also being studied in these patients.[98]

The most common cause of morbidity and mortality in CGVHD is infection. The combination of the immunodeficiency associated with CGVHD and the immunosuppressive agents used to treat CGVHD places these patients at high risk for incurring multiple infections. Prophylactic antibiotics, antivirals, and antifungals should be considered in profoundly immunosuppressed patients.

Nursing management of these patients is complex and requires frequent and in-depth holistic assessments. Signs and symptoms of infection may be masked by corticosteroid use and immunodeficient states. Psychosocial assessments and interventions may be required for patients who are often severely debilitated. A multidisciplinary approach to care of these patients is necessary to meet all of their complicated needs.[99]

## INFECTIOUS COMPLICATIONS

Late infectious complications following HCT are associated with several risk factors—namely, depressed T-cell and B-cell function, CGVHD, anatomical barrier impairment, and immunosuppressive agents for treatment of CGVHD. T-lymphocyte reconstitution may take months to years following HCT. There is often an inversion of the CD4/CD8 cell ratio, which may persist for a year and remain in the presence of CGVHD. B-cell/humoral immune system dysfunction usually lasts for 3 to 6 months following HCT. The recovery of immune globulin levels frequently occurs by 3 months following HCT. However, the immunosuppressive agents used to treat CGVHD disrupt T-cell development, further delaying the recovery of T cells.[2,100] Chronic graft-vs-host disease frequently damages natural anatomical barriers, leading to increased infection risk.

Bacterial infections seen in the late period are typically attributable to encapsulated organisms, due to the decreased humoral immune recovery. *Streptococcus pneumoniae* and *Haemophilus influenzae* are the most common pathogens. Although many centers have historically administered prophylaxis against these organisms, the development of resistant strains has called this practice into question.

The viral pathogen that most commonly causes infection late in the transplant course is CMV. Infections usually arise 30 to 80 days following HCT, although more CMV disease is being seen after day 100. Seropositive allogeneic HCT patients are at much higher risk for viral reactivation. Regular screening for CMV by polymerase chain reaction methods allows for early detection and therapy.[100,101] Herpes viral infections occur in 70% to 80% of seropositive patients. Active infections can be painful but, when occurring alone, pose little danger to HCT patients. In contrast, profoundly immunosuppressed patients are at risk for disseminated disease and localized infections can become superinfected, leading to higher-risk infections.[100]

*Aspergillus* infections pose the greatest risk of fungal disease late in the course of HCT. Patients who remain immunosuppressed due to CGVHD and subsequent therapy are at greatest risk for such infections. Some centers send routine fungal cultures from patients who are at high risk. Given the slow growth of fungal isolates, however, most patients will develop infection before the cultures grow.

Nonmyeloablative regimens are becoming more common for HCT. Although extensive data are not available, it appears that patients undergoing these regimens experience similar infections to those receiving myeloablative therapy, albeit with decreased incidence.[60,61]

Immunity to preventable diseases by vaccinations is lost over time following HCT, for both autologous and allogeneic transplant patients. Practices regarding vaccinations vary widely between transplant centers, and recommendations by the CDC can be followed. Vaccinations should be considered for the following diseases: diphtheria, *Haemophilus influenzae*, hepatitis B, measles, mumps, rubella, polio, tetanus, *Pneumococcus,* and seasonal influenza.[13,102] Vaccinations should be provided by one year post-transplant or when patients are no longer experiencing GVHD or receiving immunosuppression.[100,103] Nurses should maintain records detailing vaccination schedules to assure adequate immunization.

Nursing management of late infectious complications focuses on close observation of signs and symptoms of infection. Patients may not exhibit classic signs or symptoms of infection due to the use of immunosuppressive agents and their altered immune function. Patient education regarding infections is imperative, as most patients are not being observed on a daily basis.

## OPHTHALMOLOGICAL COMPLICATIONS

Cataract development and ocular GVHD are two of the most common late ophthalmological complications seen in HCT patients. Cataract development is closely associated with radiation treatments. Patients who receive a single fraction of total body irradiation (TBI) have an 80% incidence of cataracts. Onset of cataracts usually occurs within a year following HCT. Fractionated TBI carries a 50% incidence of cataracts, and fractionated TBI with doses less than 1200 cGy causes cataracts in 30% to 35% of patients.[14,104] Long-term corticosteroids and prior cranial radiation also increase the risk of cataract development. Patients receiving high-dose chemotherapy alone have a 20% incidence of cataracts. Primary treatment is standard cataract removal.

Ocular GVHD affects approximately 40% to 60% of all long-term allogeneic HCT patients. Symptoms include eye dryness with associated gritty/sandy feelings. Sicca syndrome results from the damage to the lacrimal gland.[105,106] A Schirmer's test should be performed, with at least 10 mm of wetting being found in a negative test. Isolated ocular GVHD may be treated locally with lubricating eye drops and cyclosporine eye drops. Many patients also require obstruction of the nasolacrimal duct to decrease drainage of tears. A gas-permeable sclera lens has also been recently reported to be effective in decreasing patient symptoms.[106] Patients who do not respond to local therapy or who have concomitant GVHD involvement of other organs may require systemic therapy. Patients with eye GVHD should also be treated prophylactically to prevent any bacterial ocular infections.

Nursing management of ophthalmological complications should include close observation of eye changes and patient education so that patients report any visual changes or eye symptoms.

## UROLOGICAL COMPLICATIONS

Hemorrhagic cystitis secondary to cyclophosphamide is rare late in the transplant course.[107] The cyclophosphamide metabolite acrolein can cause scarring of the bladder wall, which can, in turn, lead to protracted hematuria and urinary frequency. Bladder irrigation, cystoscopic fulguration, and—in severe cases—cystectomy are primary treatments for this diagnosis. Viral infections with CMV, BK virus, and adenovirus can also cause cystitis late in the allogeneic transplant course. No proven therapies for these infections exist, except decreasing immunosuppression. Supportive care with antispasmodics and hyperhydration help to reduce symptoms. Patients should be educated to report any urinary symptoms for prompt diagnosis and treatment.

## RENAL COMPLICATIONS

Renal insufficiency can develop late in the transplant course, due primarily to prior nephrotoxic agents and continued use of cyclosporine or tacrolimus. Renal insufficiency has been found in approximately 25% up to 10 years following HCT.[108] Identification of renal insufficiency and possible causes is important to arrest further progression. Close observation of all laboratory data is required.

## ORAL/DENTAL COMPLICATIONS

Oral GVHD is the most common cause of late oral and dental complications following HCT. Patients may experience symptoms ranging from mild tenderness and food sensitivities to severe oral pain with marked dental decay. Chronic GVHD causes decreased saliva production, leading to sicca syndrome and ensuing dental decay. Patients are often reluctant to perform good oral hygiene due to oral sensitivities, which contributes to poor dental health. Secondary fungal, bacterial, and viral infections can contribute to oral complications as well. Treatment of oral GVHD with steroid mouth washes is effective in most patients, but systemic therapy may also be required. Patients should perform meticulous oral hygiene and receive fluoride treatments to help prevent dental caries.[109,110]

## PULMONARY COMPLICATIONS

Late-onset pulmonary complications affect approximately 15% of HCT patients. Sinopulmonary infections are the most common of these complications and have been discussed previously. Interstitial pneumonitis with resulting fibrosis and bronchiolitis obliterans (BO) or bronchiolitis obliterans organizing pneumonia (BOOP) and drug-induced fibrosis are the most common pulmonary complications. High-dose carmustine (BCNU), 450 mg/$m^2$ or greater, has been associated with pulmonary fibrosis with a peak onset approximately 6 weeks following HCT. High-dose corticosteroids are effective in halting the progression and alleviating any long-term damage.

Interstitial pneumonitis, BO, and BOOP all appear to have an association with CGVHD.[111–114] Interstitial pneumonitis is also associated with prior toxicities such as radiation therapy and infectious processes, most often viral in nature. It leads to interstitial fibrosis, resulting in symptomatology of nonproductive cough with dyspnea on exertion and wheezing. High-dose corticosteroids are the treatment of choice in association with anti-infectives if secondary infections are suspected.

Bronchiolitis obliterans is a nonspecific inflammatory pulmonary injury thought to be initiated by GVHD. Histological findings are consistent with GVHD found in other organs. Patients report progressive productive cough and shortness of breath. Concurrent infections are common and may be cofactors in the development of BO. Airway obstruction is found on pulmonary function tests, with these clinical findings sufficing for diagnosis for most patients. Reported incidence is between 5% and 20%.[112] Bronchiolitis obliterans has been reported to occur from 3 months to 2 years following HCT. Mortality rates are high in severe disease, which shows little response to standard GVHD treatment. Corticosteroids with anti-infective agents are first-line therapies.

Bronchiolitis obliterans organizing pneumonia is also associated with GVHD. This condition is rarely reported, with its incidence hovering between 1% and 2%. Patients present with nonproductive cough, fever, and dyspnea. Although definitive diagnosis requires biopsies, pulmonary function tests and radiography can be suggestive of disease.[112] Prognosis is favorable, as most patients respond to corticosteroids and anti-infectives.

## ENDOCRINE COMPLICATIONS

Hypothyroidism is common following HCT. Patients receiving TBI are at highest risk of developing thyroid dysfunction, with nearly 25% of these patients requiring thyroid supplementation.[15] High-risk patients should be evaluated every 6 months, with all patients receiving routine evaluation for this potential complication every year. Thyroid supplementation should be initiated when indicated.[115]

Nursing management includes patient education regarding symptoms of hypothyroidism and close assessment to identify sometimes subtle presenting symptoms. Hypothyroidism is rarely life-threatening, but symptoms can significantly affect quality of life.

## AVASCULAR NECROSIS

Avascular necrosis (AVN) is described as nontraumatic ischemic bone necrosis. It has been reported in up to 5% of HCT patients. Patients who have required corticosteroid therapy are at highest risk for the development of AVN.[116] Although the femoral head is most commonly affected by this complication, all joints are at risk of development of AVN. Patients will report progressive joint pain, especially with activity. Primary medical treatment is joint replacement. Nurses should be aware of patient complaints of progressive joint pain with clinical courses associated with this disease, including corticosteroid use.

## SECONDARY MALIGNANCIES

The complication of secondary malignancies is increasing as patients enjoy increasingly longer lives following HCT. There appears to be a cumulative incidence effect: as survival increases, so does the risk of developing a secondary malignancy. Alkylating agents have long been associated with the development of secondary malignancies. Because most patients undergoing HCT have received alkylating agents prior to HCT, it is difficult to determine whether HCT is the greater causative effect. Secondary malignancies can be classified as one of three main types: myelodysplastic syndrome (MDS) with resulting acute myelogenous leukemia (AML), solid tumors, and post-transplant lymphoproliferative disorder (PTLD). Whereas secondary MDS and AML rarely develop following allogeneic HCT, MDS/AML occurs with some frequency following autologous HCT. The actuarial incidence of MDS has been reported to be as high as nearly 20% following autologous HCT.[117] Identification of MDS following HCT is difficult, as dysplastic changes occur following most types of chemotherapy. Treatment of secondary MDS/AML follows standard therapies, with allogeneic transplant providing the only possibility of cure.

Secondary solid malignancies more commonly develop in postallogeneic HCT patients. There appears to be a close association between these complications and radiation therapy both prior to HCT and when used as a part of the conditioning regimen. Patients who develop GVHD and require immunosuppressive therapy are also at increased risk of developing solid malignancies. Chronic GVHD is associated with increased risk of squamous cell malignancies of the buccal mucosa and skin. Age-adjusted incidence has been reported to be as high as 4.2 times higher in transplant recipients than in the general population.[14,117]

Post-transplant lymphoproliferative disorder has been well described following solid organ transplant, with incidence reaching 10% in heart/lung transplant patients. This disorder is not well described in HCT patients. Reported incidence has ranged from 0.2% to 25%; the disease has been seen in both autologous and allogeneic HCT patients, albeit with higher incidence in the allogeneic transplant population.[117] Patients who receive T cell–depleted grafts or who are treated with antithymocyte globulin or anti-CD3 monoclonal antibody are at greatest risk of developing PTLD. There is also association with Epstein–Barr viral infections. Treatment of PTLD includes combination chemotherapy and withdrawal of immunosuppression if possible.

Patients should receive ample education regarding the risk of secondary malignancies prior to undergoing HCT. Close observation for development of any secondary malignancy needs to be ongoing, as the incidence increases as survival lengthens.

## NEUROLOGICAL COMPLICATIONS

Late neurological complications are rare to nonexistent following HCT; instead, most of the neurological complications that can occur arise within the first 3 months following HCT. Magnetic resonance imaging of the brain has shown white matter lesions and brain atrophy, which were associated with CGVHD and immunosuppressive therapy. Neuropsychological testing has indicated cognitive deficits that are also associated with long-term cyclosporine use and increased age.[77] Ongoing research is being conducted to determine the effects of HCT on cognitive ability in long-term survivors.

## SECONDARY GRAFT FAILURE

Secondary graft failure (SGF) is a serious complication that occurs after initial engraftment. It has been reported in both autologous and allogeneic HCT patients. Note that improvements in HLA testing have significantly reduced SGF in the allogeneic transplant population. Historically, reported incidence has ranged from 2% to 25% depending on the donor type and HLA match.[118] Factors that affect SGF incidence include HLA disparity, T-cell depletion, related vs unrelated donor, GVHD, viral infections, inadequate donor cell counts, and stromal damage.

Treatment of SGF begins with a combination of growth factors, including G-CSF, GM-CSF, and erythropoietin. Immunosuppression should also be weaned if possible in allogeneic HCT patients. Patients who do not respond may require donor lymphocyte infusion or second transplant. Mortality rates are high if a second transplant is required.

Nursing management should focus on supportive care both physically and emotionally. Secondary graft failure is a traumatic event, and patients and families will require ample support and education to move through this time.

## GONADAL DYSFUNCTION

Gonadal dysfunction is common following HCT. Children—especially those close to puberty—experience the greatest long-term dysfunction or gonadal failure. High-dose chemotherapy can produce long-term dysfunction, and TBI has a high association with both gonadal dysfunction and failure. To date, large studies have not been completed following HCT to determine the incidence of gonadal dysfunction. Males have been reported to have fathered healthy children following HCT. Females have also been reported to have given birth to healthy children, although the number of these cases is minimal. Depending on their age, most women who undergo HCT will experience early chemical-induced menopause. Follicle-stimulating hormone and luteinizing hormone levels should be monitored to determine the need for hormone replacement therapy. Approximately 10% of males will recover spermatogenesis 2 to 5 years following HCT. Testosterone levels should be monitored in males reporting decreased libido and erectile dysfunction. Testosterone replacement therapy should be initiated in those with abnormally low levels.[115,119,120]

Nurses should have open discussions with patients and significant others regarding sexual function and fertility issues associated with HCT. Gonadal dysfunction can significantly affect quality of life, and the potential embarrassment of discussing sexual topics may keep patients from addressing these issues. Options for fertility should be discussed prior to HCT. Sperm banking may be possible if spermatogenesis remains following conventional therapies. Ovarian banking is also available, but the long-term success rate for this option is not known.

## OSTEOPOROSIS

Osteoporosis can develop late after HCT. Prolonged corticosteroid use, ovarian failure, and decreased activity increase risk for osteoporosis.[119,121] Osteopenia occurs in 50% to 60% of HCT patients, while osteoporosis occurs in 20% of HCT patients.[15,122] Bone density testing should be completed for those patients deemed at high risk for these conditions.[123] Osteoporotic patients need regular calcium supplementation, and those with severe osteoporosis should receive bisphosphonate therapy.[124] Women in chemically induced menopause should consider hormone replacement therapy. Nursing management should seek to identify patients at high risk for osteoporosis development and initiate direct testing for the disease.

## PSYCHOSOCIAL/QUALITY OF LIFE

Quality of life following HCT can be significantly affected by morbidity caused by the transplant process and subsequent long-term complications. Many studies evaluating quality of life post-transplant have already been conducted, and many more are currently enrolling patients. Quality of life has been reported to be affected for as long as 6 years following HCT.[125] Transplant centers face the challenge of developing plans of care that will improve quality of life and decrease the effects of complications on quality of life. Exercise during and following HCT has been shown to decrease the impact on quality of life and may be a simple, yet effective way to help patients recover from this life-altering therapy.[126]

Nursing management in this situation focuses on patient and family education. Providing patients with information regarding vocational counseling, financial counseling, rehabilitation programs, and support groups may help decrease the detrimental effects on quality of life.

## CONCLUSION

Hematopoietic cell transplantation is a complex process that requires the care of expert nurses. The knowledge base required to care for these patients throughout the transplant process is extensive. Patients and families rely heavily on the expert and compassionate care of nurses to help guide them through very trying times. Consequently, transplant nurses need to be equipped with adequate knowledge regarding the multitude of complications that can occur to facilitate the smooth transition from patient to successful survivor.

## REFERENCES


1. Kruger WH, Bohlius J, Cornely OA, et al. Antimicrobial prophylaxis in allogeneic bone marrow transplantation. Guidelines of the Infectious Diseases Working Party (AGIHO) of the German Society of Haematology and Oncology. *Ann Oncol.* 2005;16:1381–1390.
2. Bashey A. Infection. In: Ball ED, Lister J, Law P, eds. *Hematopoietic Stem Cell Therapy.* Philadelphia, PA: Churchill Livingstone; 2000:510–520.
3. Atkinson K, Singhal S. Bacterial infections. In: Atkinson K, ed. *Clinical Bone Marrow and Blood Stem Cell Transplantation.* New York: Cambridge University Press; 2000:716–736.
4. Robenshtok E, Gafter-Gvili A, Goldberg E, et al. Antifungal prophylaxis in cancer patients after chemotherapy or hematopoietic stem-cell transplantation: systematic review and meta-analysis. *J Clin Oncol.* 2007;25:5471–5489.

5. Goodman JL, Winston DJ, Greenfield RA, et al. A controlled trial of fluconazole to prevent fungal infections in patients undergoing bone marrow transplantation. *N Engl J Med.* 1992;326:845–851.
6. Slavin MA, Osborne B, Adams R, et al. Efficacy and safety of fluconazole for fungal infections after marrow transplantation- a prospective, randomized, double-blind study. *J Infect Dis.* 1995;171:1545–1552.
7. Ullmannn AJ, Lipton JH, Vesole DH, et al. Posaconazole or fluconazole for prophylaxis in severe graft-versus-host disease. *N Engl J Med.* 2007;356:335–347.
8. Chakrabarti S, Pillay D, Ratcliffe D, et al. Resistance to antiviral drugs in herpes simplex virus infections among allogeneic stem cell transplant recipients: risk factors and prognostic significance. *J Infect Dis.* 2000;181:2055–2058.
9. Langston AA, Redei I, Caliendo AM, et al. Development of drug resistant herpes simplex virus infection after haploidentical hematopoietic progenitor cell transplantation. *Blood.* 2002;99:1085–1088.
10. Erard V, Wald A, Corey L, et al. Use of long-term suppressive acyclovir after hematopoietic stem-cell transplantation: impact on herpes simplex virus (HSV) disease and drug-resistant HSV disease. *J Infect Dis.* 2007;196:266–270.
11. Winston DJ, Young JH, Pullarkat V, et al. Maribavir prophylaxis for prevention of cytomegalovirus infection in allogeneic stem cell transplant recipients: a multicenter, randomized, double-blind, placebo-controlled, dose-ranging study. *Blood.* 2008;111:5403–5410.
12. Wazir JF, Ansari NA. Pneumocystis carinii infection. *Archives Pathol Lab Med.* 2004;128:1023–1027.
13. Centers for Disease Control and Prevention; Infectious Disease Society of America; American Society of Blood and Marrow Transplantation. Guidelines for preventing opportunistic infections among hematopoietic stem cell transplant recipients. *MMWR.* 2000;49:1–128.
14. Tabbara I, Zimmerman K, Morgan C, et al. Allogeneic hematopoietic stem cell transplantation. *Arch Intern Med.* 2002;162:1558–1566.
15. Antin J. Long-term care after hematopoietic-cell transplantation in adults. *N Engl J Med.* 2002;347:36–42.
16. Sun Y, Tawara I, Toubai T, et al. Pathophysiology of acute graft-verus-host disease: recent advances. *Transplant Res.* 2007;150:197–214.
17. Messina C, Faraci M, de Fazio V, et al. Prevention and treatment of acute GvHD. *Bone Marrow Transplant.* 2008;41:S65-S70.
18. Davies JK, Lowdell MW. New advances in acute graft-versushost disease prophylaxis. *Transfus Med.* 2003;13:387–397.
19. Ringden O, Horowitz MM, Sondel P, et al. Methotrexate, cyclosporine, or both to prevent graft-versus-host disease after HLA-identical sibling bone marrow transplants for early leukemia? *Blood.* 1993;81:1094–1101.
20. Nash RA, Antin JH, Karanes C, et al. Phase 3 study comparing methotrexate and tacrolimus with methotrexate and cyclosporine for prophylaxis of acute graft-verus-host disease after marrow transplantation from unrelated donors. *Blood.* 2000;96:2062–2068.
21. Perez-Simon JA, Martino R, Caballero D, et al. Reduced-intensity conditioning allogeneic transplantation from unrelated donors: evaluation of mycophenalate mofetil plus cyclosporine A as graft-versus-host disease prophylaxis. *Biol Blood Marrow Transpl.* 2008;14:664–671.
22. Barrett AJ, Le Blanc K. Prophylaxis of acute GVHD: manipulate the graft or the environment? *Best Pract Res Clin Haematol.* 2008;21:165–176.
23. Senzolo M, Germani G, Cholongitas E, et al. Veno occlusive disease: update on clinical management. *World J Gastroenterol.* 2007;13: 3918–3924.
24. Kumar S, DeLeve LD, Kamath P, et al. Hepatic veno-occlusive disease (sinusoidal obstruction syndrome) after hematopoietic stem cell transplantation. *Mayo Clin Proc.* 2003;78:589–598.
25. Ohashi K, Tanabe J, Watanabe R, et al. The Japanese multicenter open randomized trial of ursodeoxycholic acid prophylaxis for hepatic veno-occlusive disease after stem cell transplantation. *Am J Hematol.* 2000;64:32–38.
26. Versluys B, Bhattacharaya R, Steward C, et al. Prophylaxis with defibrotide prevents veno-occlusive disease in stem cell transplantation after gemtuzumab ozogamicin exposure. *Blood.* 2004;103:1968.
27. Stiff P. Mucositis associated with stem cell transplantation: current status and innovative approaches to management. *Bone Marrow Transplant.* 2001;27(suppl 2):S3-S11.
28. Wardley A, Jayson G, Swindell R, et al. Prospective evaluation of oral mucositis in patients receiving myeloablative conditioning regimens and haemopoietic progenitor rescue. *Br J Haematol.* 2000;110:292–299.
29. Lilleby K, Garcia P, Gooley T, et al. A prospective, randomized study of cryotherapy during administration of high-dose melphalan to decrease the severity and duration of oral Mucositis in patients with multiple myeloma undergoing autologous peripheral blood stem cell transplantation. *Bone Marrow Transplant.* 2006;37:1031–1035.
30. Aisa Y, Mori T, Kudo M, et al. Oral cryotherapy for the prevention of high-dose melphalan-induced stomatitis in allogeneic hematopoietic stem cell transplantation. *Support Care Cancer.* 2005;13:266–269.
31. Keefe DM, Schubert MM, Elting LS, et al. Updated clinical practice guidelines for the prevention and treatment of Mucositis. *Cancer.* 2007;109:820–831.
32. Spielberger RT, Stiff P, Emmanouilides C, et al. Efficacy of recombinant human keratinocyte growth factor (rHuKGF) in reducing mucositis in patients with hematologic malignancies undergoing autologous peripheral blood progenitor cell transplantation (auto-PBPCT) after radiation-based conditioning—results of a phase 2 trial. *Proc Am Soc Clin Oncol.* 2001;20:(abstr 25).
33. Kris MG, Hesketh PJ, Somerfield MR, et al. American society of clinical oncology guidelines for antiemetics in oncology: update 2006. *J Clin Oncol.* 2006;24:2932–2947.
34. Lopez-Plaza I, Triulzi D. Transfusion support in hematopoietic stem cell transplantation. In: Ball ED, Lister J, Law P, eds. *Hematopoietic Stem Cell Transplantation.* Philadelphia, PA: Churchill Livingstone; 2000:589–597.
35. Ballen KK, Becker PS, Yeap BY, et al. Autologous stem-cell transplantation can be performed safely without the use of blood-product support. *J Clin Oncol.* 2004;22:4087–4094.
36. Weissinger F, Sandman B, Maloney D, et al. Decreased transfusion requirements for patients receiving nonmyeloablative compared with conventional peripheral blood stem cell transplants from HLA-identical siblings. *Blood.* 2001;98:3584–3588.
37. Sorror ML, Maris MB, Storer B, et al. Comparing morbidity and mortality of HLA-matched unrelated donor hematopoietic cell transplantation after nonmyeloablative and myeloablative conditioning: influence of pretransplant comorbidities. *Blood.* 2004;104:961–968.
38. Nevo S, Fuller AK, Hartley E, et al. Acute bleeding complications in patients after hematopoietic stem cell transplantation with prophylactic platelet transfusion triggers of $10x10^9$ and $20x10^9$ per L. *Transfusion.* 2007;47:801–812.
39. Lawrence JB, Yomtovian RA, Hammons T, et al. Lowering the prophylactic platelet transfusion threshold: a prospective analysis. *Leuk Lymphoma.* 2001;41:67–76.
40. Gurkan E, Patah PA, Saliba RM, et al. Efficacy of prophylactic transfusions using single donor apheresis platelets versus pooled platelet concentrates in AML/MDS patients receiving allogeneic hematopoietic stem cell transplantation. *Bone Marrow Transplant.* 2007;40:461–464.
41. Dodds A. ABO incompatibility and blood product support. In: Atkinson K, ed. *Clinical Bone Marrow and Blood Stem Cell Transplantation.* New York: Cambridge University Press; 2000:655–661.
42. Stroncek DF, Rebulla P. Platelet transfusions. *Lancet.* 2007;370: 427–438.
43. Slichter S. Platelet transfusion therapy. *Hematol Oncol Clin North Am.* 2007;21:697–729.
44. Przepiorka D, Smith T, Folloder J, et al. Controlled trial of filgrastim for acceleration of neutrophil recovery after allogeneic blood stem cell transplantation from human leukocyte antigen-matched related donors. *Blood.* 2001;97:3405–3410.
45. Wingard JR, Bartfield AA. Use of hematopoietic growth factors. In: Ball ED, Lister J, Law P, eds. *Hematopoietic Stem Cell Transplantation.* Philadelphia, PA: Churchill Livingstone; 2000:471–487.

46. Ivanov V, Faucher C, Mohty M, et al. Early administration of recombinant erythropoietin improves haemoglobin recovery after reduced intensity conditioned allogeneic stem cell transplantation. *Bone Marrow Transplant.* 2005;36:901–906.
47. Fox CP, Pacey EP, Das-Gupta NH, et al. Low dose erythropoietin is effective in reducing transfusion requirements following allogeneic HSCT. *Transfus Med.* 2005;15:475–480.
48. Marino M, Oliva E, Console G, et al. Administration of recombinant human erythropoietin alpha before autologous stem cell transplantation reduces transfusion requirement in multiple myeloma patients. *Support Care Cancer.* 2005;13:182–187.
49. Baron F, Frere P, Fillet G, Beguin Y. Recombinant human erythropoietin therapy is very effective after autologous peripheral blood stem cell transplant when started soon after engraftment. *Clin Cancer Res.* 2003;9:5566–5572.
50. Deeg HJ, Yamaguchi M. Acute graft-versus-host disease. In: Atkinson K, ed. *Clinical Bone Marrow and Blood Stem Cell Transplantation.* 2nd ed. New York: Cambridge University Press; 2000:681–699.
51. Chao NJ. *Graft-Versus-Host Disease.* 2nd ed. Austin, TX: RG Landes; 1999.
52. Przepiorka D. Prevention of acute graft-versus-host disease. In: Ball ED, Lister J, Law P, eds. *Hematopoietic Stem Cell Therapy.* Philadelphia, PA: Churchill Livingstone; 2000:452–469.
53. Przepiorka D, Cleary K. Therapy of acute graft-vs-host disease. In: Ball ED, Lister J, Law P, eds. *Hematopoietic Stem Cell Therapy.* Philadelphia, PA: Churchill Livingstone; 2000:531–540.
54. Levitsky J, Sorrell MF. Hepatic complications of hematopoietic cell transplantation. *Current Gastroenterology Report.* 2007;9:60–65.
55. Reddy P. Pathophysiology of acute graft-versus-host disease. *Hematol Oncol.* 2003;21:149–161.
56. Antin JH, Chen AR, Couriel DR, et al. Novel approaches to the therapy of steroid resistant acute graft-versus-host disease. *Biol Blood Marrow Transplant.* 2004;10:655–668.
57. Furlong T, Leisenring W, Storb R, et al. Psoralen and ultraviolet A irradiation (PUVA) as therapy for steroid-resistant cutaneous acute graft-versus-host disease. *Biol Blood Marrow Transplant.* 2002;8:206–212.
58. Couriel D, Hosting C, Saliba R, et al. Extracorporeal photopheresis for acute and chronic graft-versus-host disease: Does it work? *Biol Blood Marrow Transplant.* 2006;12:37–40.
59. Dazzi F, Marelli-Berg FM. Mesenchymal stem cells for graft-versus-host disease: close encounters with T cells. *Eur J Immunol.* 2008;38:1479–1482.
60. Mossad SB, Avery RK, Longworth DL, et al. Infectious complications within the first year after nonmyeloablative allogeneic peripheral blood stem cell transplantation. *Bone Marrow Transplant.* 2001;28:491–495.
61. Busca A, Locatelli F, Barbui A, et al. Infectious complications following nonmyeloablative allogeneic hematopoietic stem cell transplantation. *Transplant Infect Dis.* 2003;5:132–139.
62. Nichols WG. Management of infectious complications in the hematopoietic stem cell transplant recipient. *J Intensive Care Med.* 2003;18:295–312.
63. Fall-Dickson JM, Ramsay ES, Castro K, et al. Oral Mucositis-related oropharyngeal pain and correlative tumor necrosis factor-alpha expression in adult oncology patients undergoing hematopoietic stem cell transplantation. *Clinical Therapy.*2007;29 suppl:2547–2561.
64. McGuire DB, Correa MEP, Johnson J, Wienandts P. The role of basic oral care and good clinical practice principles in the management of oral mucositis. *Support Care Cancer.* 2006;14:541–547.
65. Epstein JB, Phillips N, Parry J, et al. Quality of life, taste, olfactory and oral function following high-dose chemotherapy and allogeneic hematopoietic cell transplantation. *Bone Marrow Transplant.* 2002;30: 785–792.
66. Van Kraaij M, Dekker A, Verdonck L, et al. Infectious gastroenteritis: an uncommon cause of diarrhea in adult allogeneic and autologous stem cell transplant recipients. *Bone Marrow Transplant.* 2000;26:299–303.
67. Avery R, Pohlman B, Adal K, et al. High prevalence of diarrhea but infrequency of documented *Clostridium difficile* in autologous peripheral blood progenitor cell transplant recipients. *Bone Marrow Transplant.* 1999;25:67–69.
68. Ho VT, Linden E, Revta C, et al. Hepatic veno-occlusive disease after hematopoietic stem cell transplantation: review and update on the use of defibrotide. *Semin Thromb Hemost.* 2007;33:373–388.
69. Strausser SI, McDonald GB. Gastrointestinal and hepatic complications. In: Thomas ED, Blume KG, Forman SJ, eds. *Hematopoietic Cell Transplantation.* 2nd ed. Malden, MA: Blackwell Science; 1999:627–658.
70. Richardson P, Soiffer R, Antin JH, et al. Defibrotide (DF) for the treatment of severe veno-occlusive (VOD) and multi-organ failure (MOF) post SCT: final results of a phase II, multi-center, randomized, dose-finding trial. *Blood.* 2006;108:43(abst).
71. McDonald GB. Review article: management of hepatic disease following haematopoietic cell transplant. *Aliment Pharmacol Ther.* 2006;24: 441–452.
72. Strasser SI, Myerson D, Spurgeon CL, et al. Hepatitis C virus infection after bone marrow transplantation: a cohort study with 10 year follow-up. *Hepatology.* 1999;29:1893–1899.
73. Garrick R. Neurologic complications. In: Atkinson K, ed. *Clinical Bone Marrow and Blood Stem Cell Transplantation.* 2nd ed. New York: Cambridge University Press; 2000:958–979.
74. Magalhaes-Silverman M, Hammert L. Neurologic complications. In: Ball ED, Lister J, Law P, eds. *Hematopoietic Stem Cell Transplantation.* Philadelphia, PA: Churchill Livingstone; 2000:578–588.
75. Colosimo M, McCarthy N, Jayasinghe R, et al. Diagnosis and management of subdural haematoma complicating bone marrow transplantation. *Bone Marrow Transplant.* 2000;25:549–552.
76. Denier C, Bourhis JH, Lacroix C, et al. Spectrum and prognosis of neurologic complications after hematopoietic transplantation. *Neurology.* 2006;67:1990–1997.
77. Krouwer HGJ, Wijdicks EFM. Neurologic complications of bone marrow transplantation. *Neurol Clin North Am.* 2003;21:319–352.
78. Georges G, Storb R. Failure of sustained engraftment: clinical manifestations and treatment. In: Atkinson K, ed. *Clinical Bone Marrow and Blood Stem Cell Transplantation.* New York: Cambridge University Press; 2000:662–680.
79. Chen J, Law P, Ball ED. Failure of engraftment. In: Ball ED, Lister J, Law P, eds. *Hematopoietic Stem Cell Transplantation.* Philadelphia, PA: Churchill Livingstone; 2000:521–530.
80. Schoemans H, Theunissen K, Maertens J, et al. Adult umbilical cord blood transplantation: a comprehensive review. *Bone Marrow Transplant.* 2006;38:83–93.
81. Brunstein CG, Wagner JE. Cord blood transplantation for adults. *Vox Sang.* 2006;91:195–205.
82. Narimatsu H, Kami M, Miyakoshi S, et al. Graft failure following reduced-intensity cord blood transplantation for adult patients. *Br J Haematol.* 2006;132:36–41.
83. Kreit JW. Respiratory complications. In: Ball ED, Lister J, Law P, eds. *Hematopoietic Stem Cell Transplantation.* Philadelphia, PA: Churchill Livingstone; 2000:563–577.
84. Bryant D. Pulmonary complications. In: Atkinson K, ed. *Clinical Bone Marrow and Blood Stem Cell Transplantation.* New York: Cambridge University Press; 2000:943–957.
85. Bekele A, Tefferi A, Litzow MR. Outcome of diffuse alveolar hemorrhage in hematopoietic stem cell transplant recipients. *Am J Respir Crit Care Med.* 2002;166:1364–1368.
86. Bunte MC, Patnaik MM, Pritzker MR, Burns LJ. Pulmonary veno-occlusive disease following hematopoietic stem cell transplantation: a rare model of endothelial dysfunction. *Bone Marrow Transplant.* 2008;41:677–686.
87. Kuittinen T, Husso-Saastamoinen M, Sipola P, et al. Very acute cardiac toxicity during BEAC chemotherapy in non-Hodgkin's lymphoma patients undergoing autologous stem cell transplantation. *Bone Marrow Transplant.* 2005;36:1077–1082.
88. Fujimaki K, Maruta A, Yoshida M, et al. Severe cardiac toxicity in hematological stem cell transplantation: predictive value of

reduced left ventricular ejection fraction. *Bone Marrow Transplant.* 2001;27:307–310.
89. Lehman S, Isberg B, Ljungman P, et al. Cardiac systolic function before and after hematopoietic stem cell transplantation. *Bone Marrow Transplant.* 2000;26:187–192.
90. Ueda T, Manabe A, Kikuchi A, et al. Massive pericardial and pleural effusion with anasarca following allogeneic bone marrow transplantation. *Int J Hematol.* 2000;71:394–397.
91. Savdie E. Renal complications. In: Atkinson K, ed. *Clinical Bone Marrow and Blood Stem Cell Transplantation.* New York: Cambridge University Press; 2000:930–942.
92. Chang A, Hingorani S, Kowalewska J, et al. Spectrum of renal pathology in hematopoietic cell transplantation: a series of 20 patients and review of the literature. *Clin J Am Soc Nephrol.* 2007;2:1014–1023.
93. Wingard JR. The conundrum of chronic graft-versus-host disease. *Blood Marrow Transplant.* 2002;12:3–16.
94. Bishop M. Emerging strategies in the treatment of chronic graft-versus-host disease. *Blood Marrow Transplant.* 2002;12:4–5.
95. Eapen M, Logan BR, Confer DL, et al. Peripheral blood grafts from unrelated donors are associated with increased acute and chronic graft-versus-host disease without improved survival. *Biol Blood Marrow Transplant.* 2007;13:1461–1468.
96. Volgelsang GB. How I treat chronic graft-versus-host disease. *Blood.* 2001;97:1196–1200.
97. Spiryda LB, Laufer MR, Soiffer RF, et al. Graft-versus-host disease of the vulva and/or vagina: diagnosis and treatment. *Biol Blood Marrow Transplant.* 2003;9:760–765.
98. Apisarnthanarax N, Donato M, Korbling M, et al. Extracorporeal photopheresis therapy in the management of steroid-refractory or steroid-dependent cutaneous chronic graft-versushost disease after allogeneic stem cell transplantation: feasibility and results. *Bone Marrow Transplant.* 2003;31:459–465.
99. Couriel D, Carpenter PA, Cutler C, et al. Ancillary therapy and supportive care of chronic graft-versus-host disease: National institutes of health consensus development project on criteria for clinical trials in chronic graft-versus-host disease: V. Ancillary therapy and supportive care working group report. *Biol Blood Marrow Transplant.* 2006;12:375–396.
100. Leather HL, Wingard JR. Infections following hematopoietic stem cell transplantation. *Infect Dis Clin North Am.* 2001;15:483–520.
101. Boeckh M, Leisenring W, Riddell SR, et al. Late cytomegalovirus disease and mortality in recipients of allogeneic hematopoietic stem cell transplants: importance of viral load and Tcell immunity. *Blood.* 2003;101:407–414.
102. Singhal S, Mehta J. Reimmunization after blood or marrow stem cell transplantation. *Bone Marrow Transplant.* 1999;23:637–646.
103. Ljungman P, Engelhard D, dela Camara R, et al. Vaccination of stem cell transplant recipients: recommendations of the infectious diseases working party of the EBMT. *Bone Marrow Transplant.* 2005;35:737–746.
104. Aristei C, Alessandro M, Santucci A, et al. Cataracts in patients receiving stem cell transplantation after conditioning with total body irradiation. *Bone Marrow Transplant.* 2002;29:503–507.
105. Cheok F. Eye complications. In: Atkinson K, ed. *Clinical Bone Marrow and Blood Stem Cell Transplantation.* 2nd ed. New York: Cambridge University Press; 2000:1009–1016.
106. Takahide K, Parker M, Wu M, et al. Use of fluid-ventilated, gas-permeable sclera lens for management of severe keratoconjunctivitis sicca secondary to chronic graft-verus-host disease. *Biol Blood Marrow Transplant.* 2007;13:1016–1021.
107. Bieloral B, Shulman LM, Rechavi G, et al. CMV reactivation induced BK virus-associated late onset hemorrhagic cystitis after peripheral blood stem cell transplantation. *Bone Marrow Transplant.* 2001;28:613–614.
108. Kerstino S, Hene RJ, Koomans HA, et al. Chronic kidney disease after myeloablative allogeneic hematopoietic stem cell transplantation. *Biology of Blood and Marrow Transplant.* 2007;13:1169–1175.
109. Marcellus DC, Vogelsang GB. Chronic graft-versus-host disease. In: Ball ED, Lister J, Law P, eds. *Hematopoietic Stem Cell Therapy.* Philadelphia, PA: Churchill Livingstone; 2000:614–624.
110. Carpenter PA. Late effects of chronic graft-versus-host disease. *Best Pract Res Clin Haematol.* 2008;21:309–331.
111. Wolff D, Reichenberger F, Steiner B, et al. Progressive interstitial fibrosis of the lung in sclerodermal chronic graft-versus-host disease. *Bone Marrow Transplant.* 2002;29:357–360.
112. Afessa B, Litzow MR, Tefferi A. Bronchiolitis obliterans and other late onset non-infectious pulmonary complications in hematopoietic stem cell transplantation. *Bone Marrow Transplant.* 2001;28:425–434.
113. Freudenberger TD, Madtes DK, Curtis JR, et al. Association between acute and chronic graft-versus-host disease and bronchiolitis obliterans organizing pneumonia in recipients of hematopoietic stem cell transplants. *Blood.* 2003;102:3822–3828.
114. Sakaida E, Nakaseko C, Harima A, et al. Late-onset noninfectious pulmonary complications after allogeneic stem cell transplantation are significantly associated with chronic graft-versus-host disease and with the graft-versus-leukemia effect. *Blood.* 2003;102:4236–4242.
115. Chemaitilly W, Sklar C. Endocrine complications of hematopoietic stem cell transplantation. *Endocrinol Metab Clin North Am.* 2007;36: 983–998.
116. Tauchmanova L, De Rosa G, Serio B, et al. Avascular necrosis in long-term survivors after allogeneic or autologous stem cell transplantation. *Cancer.* 2003;97:2453–2461
117. Holman PR. Myelodysplasia and second malignancies. In: Ball ED, Lister J, Law P, eds. *Hematopoietic Stem Cell Therapy.* Philadelphia, PA: Churchill Livingstone; 2000:647–657.
118. Chen J, Law P, Ball ED. Late graft failure. In: Ball ED, Lister J, Law P, eds. *Hematopoietic Stem Cell Therapy.* Philadelphia, PA: Churchill Livingstone; 2000:603–607.
119. Winters SJ, Syed M. Endocrine and metabolic complications. In: Ball ED, Lister J, Law P, eds. *Hematopoietic Stem Cell Therapy.* Philadelphia, PA: Churchill Livingstone; 2000:625–636.
120. Chatterjee R, Kottaridis PD, McGarrigle HH, et al. Management of erectile dysfunction by combination therapy with testosterone and sildenafil in recipients of high-dose therapy for haematological malignancies. *Bone Marrow Transplant.* 2002;29:607–610.
121. Cohen ML. Musculoskeletal complications. In: Atkinson K, ed. *Clinical Bone Marrow and Blood Stem Cell Transplantation.* 2nd ed. New York: Cambridge University Press; 2000:988–992.
122. Schimmer AD, Mah K, Bordeleau L, et al. Decreased bone mineral density is common after autologous blood or marrow transplantation. *Bone Marrow Transplant.* 2001;28:387–391.
123. Stern JM, Sullivan KM, Ott SM, et al. Bone density loss after allogeneic hematopoietic stem cell transplantation: a prospective study. *Biol Blood Marrow Transplant.* 2001;7:257–264.
124. Gandhi MK, Lekamwasam S, Inman I, et al. Significant and persistent loss of bone mineral density in the femoral neck after haematopoietic stem cell transplantation: long-term follow-up of a prospective study. *Br J Haematol.* 2003;121:462–468.
125. Hensel M, Erger G, Schneeweiss A, et al. Quality of life and rehabilitation in social and professional life after autologous stem cell transplantation. *Ann Oncol.* 2002;13:209–217.
126. Courneya KS, Keats MR, Turner AR, et al. Physical exercise and quality of life in cancer patients following high dose chemotherapy and autologous bone marrow transplantation. *Psychooncology.* 2000;9:127–136.
127. Bearman SI, Hinds MS, Wolford JL, et al. A pilot study of continuous infusion heparin for the prevention of hepatic venoocclusive disease after bone marrow transplantation. *Bone Marrow Transplant.* 1990;5: 407–411.
128. Attal M, Huguet F, Rubie H, et al. Prevention of hepative venoocclusive disease after bone marrow transplantation by continuous infusion of low-dose heparin: a prospective, randomized trial. *Blood.* 1992;79:2834–2840.

CHAPTER 20

Paula M. Muehlbauer, RN, MSN, AOCNS®

# Biotherapy

## INTRODUCTION

Biological therapies as cancer treatment and supportive care have evolved greatly over the past century. The development of biological agents has increased as understanding of the immune system has expanded and advances in molecular biology have allowed for the rapid production of these molecules for preclinical and clinical studies. Undeniably, biotherapy has joined the growing list of cancer therapies along with surgery, radiation therapy, chemotherapy, and targeted therapies. Biotherapy is part of the armamentarium against neoplastic diseases and as supportive care. Biological agents continue to be studied in clinical trials for a variety of cancers although limitations imposed by the use of single agent therapy mandated by the current drug development paradigm have hindered realization of the full benefit of this approach.

This chapter will provide a review of biological therapies currently approved by the US Food and Drug Administration (FDA) for cancer therapy. A separate section will address a selection of biologics currently in clinical trials.

## HISTORICAL PERSPECTIVE

Biological therapy as a potential cancer treatment dates back to the 1800s. Generally defined, biotherapy is one that uses the immune system, including the cells and molecules that act as messengers between the various immune cells, to invoke an immune response to fight cancer.[1] One of the earliest known accounts of biotherapy was reported by a New York surgeon, Dr. William Coley, who observed an association between severe infection and the regression of tumors in some of his patients. Dr. Coley developed substances called "Coley's Toxins" from attenuated or weakened forms of bacteria that he injected into solid tumors. He hypothesized that these bacterial substances would induce an immune response and produce an effect on the cancer cell similar to the natural immune response he witnessed in his infected cancer patients.[2] These toxic materials are believed to have included *Streptococcus pyogenes* with *Seratia marcesens* and *Bacillus prodigiosus*. However, in these early efforts, no standard doses, administration, or treatment duration guidelines were followed. His results were mixed and importantly, there was a lack of replication of his results. However, Dr. Coley reported long-term survival of several patients who had been inoperable.[1,3,4] The active ingredient in Coley's toxins is thought to be endotoxin from the bacterial cell wall, which induces tumor necrosis factor (TNF) and other cytokines.[5]

Despite these criticisms, his work is considered the basis of current cytokine therapy. In the early 1960s to the 1970s, clinical trials using nonspecific immune modulators such as Bacillus Calmette-Guérin (BCG), *Cornyebacterium parvum*, and levamisole were conducted in a range of tumor types. The best responses were obtained in patients with a low tumor burden and whose tumors were confined to the skin. Poor clinical outcomes were also attributed to the use of impure agents and inconsistent experimental procedures. The results were neither generalizable nor predictive of human response despite responses seen in the animal models.[1,2]

In the 1970s, a better understanding of how the human immune system works evolved leading to the discovery of certain cytokines such as the interleukins (ILs) now numbering in the range of 35 distinct molecules (Dr. John Janik, personal communication). The 1980s brought advances in biotechnology which helped advance the use of biotherapy as a viable cancer treatment. The discovery of recombinant DNA technology, the reproduction and cloning of parts of the DNA molecule, made it possible to produce large quantities of biological agents for therapeutic purposes.[1,6,7] As a result, numerous clinical trials have been initiated using various biological agents. In the past 20 years, FDA approval has been obtained for many categories of biologics. New uses for biological therapy are underway for many cancer types as well as nononcological diseases such as rheumatic disorders where inhibition of the effects of the immune system have shown great promise.[8] A timeline of the historical development of biotherapy is outlined in Table 20-1.

## IMMUNOLOGY OVERVIEW

Basic knowledge of immunology is essential when trying to understand biological therapy. Humoral (antibody-mediated or B cell) and cellular (T cell) immune system comprise the two major components of the immune system. It is believed that cell-mediated immunity provides the primary immune response in tumors responsible for tumor regression. There are two types of cellular responses: innate and adaptive immunity and both play a part in the immune response to tumors.

### INNATE IMMUNITY

Innate, or nonspecific, immunity allows the body to distinguish between normal or "self" and "nonself" such as infection, malignancies, or transplanted organs and is the first line of immunological defense. Innate immunity is not, however, antigen-specific and results in no immunological memory and no protection against a similar challenge. Innate immunity includes physical barriers (skin and mucous membranes); mechanical barriers (coughing, sneezing, and blinking); and chemical barriers (tears and sweat). Inflammatory responses are induced including production of monocytes, macrophages, large granular

**TABLE 20-1**

**Timeline of Key Events in the Development of Biotherapy**

| | |
|---|---|
| Late 1800s to mid 1900s | Impure vaccines<br>Coley's toxins<br>IFN discovered (1957) |
| 1960s to early 1970s | Clinical trials using bacterial agents to nonspecifically stimulate the immune system; examples: Bacillus Calmette-Guérin and *Cornyebacterium parvum*<br>Early immunotherapy trials<br>Limitations of studies related to:<br>Impure agents<br>Variability in experimental procedures<br>Incongruence between animal and human studies<br>Lack of generalizable results |
| Late 1970s to mid 1980s | Major technical advances<br>Increased understanding of immune system<br>Advances in genetic engineering<br>Continued advances in molecular biology<br>Ability to mass produce biological proteins and antibodies<br>Recombinant DNA technology<br>Hybridoma technology<br>Advances in laboratory methods and processes and computer systems<br>Single-agent cytokine studies initiated<br>Biological response modifier program initiated by the National Cancer Institute<br>First biological agent (IFN-α) approved by the US FDA |
| Late 1980s to present | Discovery and isolation of a variety of immune system products<br>Numerous agents recombinantly produced for clinical trials<br>Multisite clinical trials initiated; some ongoing<br>Initiation of clinical trials of combination cytokine therapy<br>Initiation of clinical trials of combination cytokine therapy and chemotherapy<br>Regulatory approval for all categories of biological agents |

*Abbreviations*: FDA, Food and Drug Administration; IFN, interferon.
*Source*: Used with permission from Rieger.[1]

lymphocytes including natural killer (NK) cells, and polymorphonuclear cells. Innate immunity also activates the complement cascade and causes production of acute-phase proteins (eg, IL-2).[9,10]

## ADAPTIVE IMMUNITY

Adaptive, or specific, immunity is the secondary line of defense. Adaptive immunity is antigen dependent and starts when the phagocytized antigen is presented to B lymphocytes or T lymphocytes. Adaptive immunity has two unique aspects: specificity and immunological memory. It requires the collaboration of B cells and T cells. The T lymphocytes recognize antigens once they are processed and presented by the antigen presenting cells (APCs). The T cells signal B cells to produce antibodies with specificity against that foreign substance. Although many cell types are involved in antitumor activity, T cells are considered to be the most important in developing antitumor activity.[1,9,11,12]

There are 3 types of adaptive immunity including humoral immunity, cell-mediated immunity, and T regulatory cells. *Humoral immunity* includes B lymphocytes, memory B cells, and plasma cells that mediate humoral immunity through the production of antibodies that recognize the antigen challenge. The result is the production of immunoglobulins. *Cell-mediated immunity* is mediated by T cells and their cytokine products. This type of immunity involves the following cell types: Cytotoxic T cells (TC) (usually CD8 positive) and Helper T cells (TH1 or TH2) (usually CD4 positive).

*T regulatory cells* (Treg) are also known as Suppressor T cells (TS). These cells display the markers CD4, CD25, and foxp3 and act to limit the activity of other immune effector cells. The primary role of Treg cells is believed to prevent the onset of immunity to normal tissues of the body and to limit the inflammatory response that can occur with infections. Animals and people without Treg cells develop a variety of inflammatory disorders primarily involving the bowel, skin, and liver.[9,10]

## CYTOKINES

Cytokines are glycoprotein products of immune cells such as lymphocytes and macrophages. Cytokines mediate effector defense functions and are usually not cytotoxic themselves. Interleukins, interferons (IFN), colony-stimulating factors, and TNF are all cytokines.

There are 2 basic principles of cytokines including the following[10,13]:

- Each cytokine may act on several different types of cells and regulate multiple immune functions. For example, IL-2 works on T cells, B cells, NK cells, and macrophages. Hence, IL-2 induces lymphocyte activation, macrophage activation, and stimulates lymphokine secretion.
- Different cytokines can have similar functions. For example, IL-1 and TNF-α are both inflammatory mediators.

## ANTIGEN PRESENTATION

Antigen presentation activates the immune pathway causing generation of a tumor specific T-cell response. Antigen is first encountered by APCs such as macrophages, dendritic cells, monocytes, Kupffer's cells, and Langerhans' cells. Of those, dendritic cells are largely responsible for initiating primary T-cell immunity. Dendritic cells capture, process, and present antigens to T lymphocytes.

This is accomplished by internalizing the antigen and splitting it into smaller fragments called peptides. These 9 to 11 amino acid peptides bind to the major histocompatibility complex (MHC) molecules in the cell and are moved to the cell surface for presentation to T cells for immune recognition. Two basic T cells, CD4+ helper T cells and CD8+ cytotoxic T cells, use a T-cell receptor (TCR) to recognize antigens on the target cell surface.[14] CD8+ cytotoxic T cells recognize antigen in conjunction with class I MHC molecules and CD4+ T helper (TH) cells in conjunction with class II MHC molecules. This activity usually occurs simultaneously. For complete T-cell activation, a co-stimulatory signal which results from the interaction of the CD28+ molecule on the T-cell surface with the ligand B7 on the APC is required. Cytokines such as IL-2 and IFN-gamma (IFN-γ) are then secreted from triggered CD4+ cells which help activated CD8+ cells to mature and differentiate into cytotoxic T cells. The cytotoxic T cells then kill target cells expressing the original antigen that elicited this response.[9,10,14]

## TUMOR ESCAPE MECHANISMS

Tumors are able to escape immune recognition for a variety of reasons. Theories describing possible mechanisms of tumor escape include variability in expression of antigen by tumors, poor antigen processing, presentation or loss of antigen expression, and induction of suppressor T cells.[15–18]

Other theories for poor immune recognition of tumors may be attributed to disease-associated alterations including apoptosis and signaling defects of T cells and immunological aging. Immunological aging involves alterations in T-cell functions causing declines in T-cell proliferation, generation of cytotoxic T cells, production of IL-2, signal transduction in lymphocytes, and an overall decline in function of other immune cells such as B cells, dendritic cells, and NK cells.

When infection is present, inflammation triggers the innate immune response activating monocytes, macrophages, and dendritic cells. Unlike an infectious process, tumors do not give off inflammatory warning signals to stimulate an immune response. Without these warning signals, termed "danger signals" the immune system may not be fully stimulated.[16,17]

Tumors have unstable genomes causing them to become heterogeneous for expressing tumor-associated antigens (TAAs) and with additional mutations escape immune recognition. This immune response to tumors is usually inadequate, known as tolerance, due to minor differences between the tumor cell and normal cell. Since the differences are slight, no immune reaction to an antigen usually occurs or the process of immune recognition may select for variants that are not as easily identified by the immune system. This is when overt tumor is recognized.[10,15,17]

Tumors produce immunosuppressive mechanisms that inhibit growth factors which would normally stimulate an immune response. One example is the production of cytokines such as IL-10 and IL-18 by tumors that limit the efficacy of immune surveillance including macrophage-mediated antigen presentation. Also, expression of Fas ligand by tumors may lead to the destruction of lymphocytes which express Fas antigen and are thereby killed when the two molecules interact allowing tumors to escape immune recognition.[15,17] A newly described molecule PD1 and its ligand PD1L also limit the effectiveness of T lymphocytes to kill tumor cells (Dr. John Janik, personal communication).

## INTERLEUKIN 2

Interleukin 2 is a cytokine produced by activated helper T cells. It was first described as a T-cell growth factor in 1976.[7] IL-2 as a cancer treatment was originally reported by Bindon and colleagues in 1983.[7,19] Natural IL-2 was used that was derived from stimulated normal lymphocytes in 2 patients with melanoma. Broad based use of IL-2 was not possible until recombinant IL-2 (rIL-2) was available. The gene for IL-2 was discovered and expressed in *Escherichia coli* producing a new molecule with properties similar to natural IL-2.[7]

Second only to the IFNs, IL-2 has been the vanguard of biological therapies.[20] IL-2 was discovered in 1976 by Drs. Gallo, Ruscetti, and Morgan.[21] A number of phase II trials demonstrated that IL-2 could induce profound, durable tumor responses in patients with metastatic melanoma and renal carcinoma resulting in the approval by the FDA for its use in the treatment of these cancers.[22–26]

## BIOLOGICAL ACTIVITY

Interleukins as a group function primarily by signaling or communicating with the various lymphocytes. Each IL is assigned a number in the order of approval by the International Congress of Immunology. The therapeutic effect of ILs is through interactions with the patient's immune system.[5,6,27]

Interleukin-2 is produced by activated T helper cells and requires 2 signals:

1. T helper cell recognition of an antigen in conjunction with the MHC antigens on an APC;
2. T helper cell interaction with co-stimulatory molecules on the APC. IL-2 is a potent immunomodulator that acts as a chemical messenger mediating the response of several other cytokines.

Interleukin 2 activates lymphocytes, macrophages, and stimulates lymphokine secretion.[10,28] Primarily, IL-2 induces proliferation of antigen-stimulated T cells, activates cytotoxic T lymphocytes (CTLs) (CD8+), NK cells and is a co-factor for the growth and differentiation of B cells. When the B lymphocytes are stimulated, immunoglobulins are produced. It also induces the release of other cytokines such as IFN-γ, granulocyte macrophage colony-stimulating factor (GM-CSF), and TNF by activated T cells.[5,21,27,29]

## INDICATIONS FOR THE USE OF IL-2

The FDA approved the use of high-dose (HD) intravenous (IV) IL-2 for the treatment of people with metastatic renal cell carcinoma (RCC) in 1992 and in 1998, for the treatment of people with metastatic melanoma.[30] Various routes and doses of IL-2 are prescribed in community settings or are under study in several clinical trials for a variety of malignancies.[20,23,31–34] Its effectiveness is based on stimulation of the host's own cytotoxic immunological response making it an ideal cytokine to test with other tumors.

Studies have indicated that IL-2 may be used to enhance the immune system as a therapeutic strategy in patients with human immunodeficiency virus (HIV).[35] People with HIV infection develop health problems when their CD4+ T cell counts decline. Interleukin 2 directly expands the CD4+ T cell pool predominantly in naive CD-4+ T cells not yet exposed to their antigen vs memory CD4+ T cells.[36–38] IL-2 can induce proinflammatory cytokine production that might enhance HIV-1 expression in latently infected cells.[38] Fauci has suggested an explanation for this paradox: latently infected cells, once stimulated, reject the virus and then undergo cell death. If IL-2 is given at the same time that highly active antiretroviral therapy (HAART) is administered, the released virus can be prevented from replicating and contaminating other cells. Therefore, over time, the reservoir of latently infected cells decreases.[38] Lu et al[37] report that the major pathogens in AIDS patients are cytomegalovirus and *Pneumocystis jiroveci,* which patients have previously been exposed to and developed memory responses. They conclude that a major benefit of IL-2 therapy may be to maintain the memory inventory as this may be sufficient for preventing opportunistic infections in most patients until the CD4+ cell count drops below 200/mm$^3$. Hence, IL-2 therapy may be beneficial if it is started in the early stages of HIV infection by maintaining and expanding the stock of CD4+ cells, thus preventing the occurrence of opportunistic infections.

Interleukin 2 is not FDA approved in the United States as treatment for HIV although it is approved for use in Europe in patients with low CD4+ cell counts. Currently, 2 ongoing phase III clinical trials are studying the clinical benefits of IL-2 in HIV. The evaluation of subcutaneous proleukin in a randomized international trial (ESPRIT) study consists of patients with initial CD4+ counts of 350/μL or higher and the subcutaneous, recombinant human interleukin 2 in HIV-infected patients with low CD4+ counts receiving active antiretroviral therapy (SILCAAT) study contains patients with initial CD4+ counts of 50 to 299/μL.[35,36,39] A meta-analysis of 3 ESPIRIT/Vanguard studies concluded that subcutaneous (SC) IL-2 at a dose of 7.5 MIU in the first 3 cycles of treatment results in greater increases in CD4 cell count after 3 cycles than occurs with doses of 4.5 MIU or 1.5 MIU.[39] These doses were administered daily for 5 days over 8 weeks for a minimum of 3 cycles. Patients randomized to each dose level of IL-2 also received HAART. Other patients were randomized to HAART alone.

Dosing of IL-2 in other clinical trials in patients infected with HIV includes SC injections of 9 to 15 MIU per day (4.5 MIU or 7.5 MIU twice daily) for 5 days every 4 to 8 weeks. If IL-2 therapy leads to prolonged increases in CD4+ cell counts, the dosing interval may be extended to 12 months or longer. Patients experience manageable toxicities that are not as severe as with higher doses. Doses less than 6 MIU/day are not as effective in raising CD4+ cell counts.[36,40] Several other studies are underway combining IL-2 with HAART.[35]

## INTERLEUKIN 2: OTHER DIRECTIONS

Many different combinations of IL-2 therapy continue to be tested. One combination that seemed promising was IL-2 plus IFN-α. Preclinical data in animals suggests that IL-2 works synergistically with IFN-α to produce greater immunological effects. French researchers Tourani and associates[41] tested the efficacy of outpatient SC IL-2 (5 days/week, 9 and 18 MIU/day) plus IFN-α (3 days/week, 6 MIU/day) over a 12-week induction period in patients with metastatic RCC in a multicenter, phase II trial ($n$ = 122). Patients with objective responses or stable disease were randomized to maintenance treatment or consolidation therapy. Forty-one patients were alive at the median 32-month follow up (range, 4 to 55+ months). The trial was closed at the 12th sequential analysis when it showed a 21% response rate which was similar to IL-2 alone. Severe toxicities resulted in treatment delay, dose reduction, or treatment termination in 27% of patients. They concluded that the combination was no better than SC IL-2 alone in patients with metastatic RCC and were consistent with other trials with similar combinations.[42–44] A review of multiple trials using similar combinations can be found in Dutcher,[45] in Noble and Goa,[28] and online at http://www.cancer.gov.

A question that has been considered for years is whether IL-2 in the adjuvant setting would be beneficial. It is generally believed that HD IL-2 would be too toxic in the adjuvant setting (Dr. Steven Rosenberg, personal communication). However, the possible synergistic combination of SC IL-2 and IFN-α may be of benefit in this setting. A study by Hauschild et al[46] investigated melanoma patients with intermediate or high-risk primary melanoma and post resection of the primary tumor. Post resection, these patients were randomized to either observation or a combination regimen of SC LD IL-2 (9 million units [MIU]/m$^2$/day) plus IFN-α (3 MIU/m$^2$/day) for 48 weeks on variable days of the week. Follow up (median 79.4) of 223 randomized patients revealed no effect on disease-free survival or overall survival (OS). At 5 years, disease-free survival in the surgery plus treatment group was 70.1% and in the surgery plus observation arm, 69.9%.

Other areas of study with IL-2 include biochemotherapy for metastatic melanoma and hematological malignancies.[47–50] Buzaid[49] reported results of 2 meta-analyses that suggest improved response rates in people with advanced melanoma using combinations involving cisplatin, IL-2, and IFN-α. The response rates in 1 analysis of 631 patients showed a 45% response rate in those treated with biochemotherapy and a 21% and 15% response rate when treated with IL-2 and IFN-α or IL-2 alone. However, there was no significant difference in survival between the groups. The other meta-analysis included 154 studies encompassing 7000 patients and reported a response rate of 47% for patients who received cisplatin, DTIC, IL-2, and IFN-α. This study did not mention OS and how it compares to IL-2 alone. Phase III studies comparing biochemotherapy to immunotherapy alone or chemotherapy alone have been conducted. Several studies have concluded these combinations do not statistically improve OS or durable responses and therefore could not be recommended as standard first-line therapy.[51–54] Toxicities are substantial and include expected side effects from IL-2 or IFN-α as well as chemotherapy-related toxicities such as peripheral neuropathy.[49]

## METHODS OF ADMINISTRATION

The only US FDA-approved regimen for IL-2 is as HD IV bolus administration, but it is also given IV in lower doses.[55] Some clinicians administer IL-2 by the SC route because of the cost and dose-limiting toxicities seen with IV infusion. Many doses in the assorted methods of administration are under investigation and the treatment of patients with regimens not approved by the FDA should be viewed as experimental. IL-2 is given alone or in combination with chemotherapy, vaccines, or other biotherapy in many clinical trials.[34]

Yang and associates[56] conducted a 3-arm randomized study comparing response rates and OS of patients with metastatic RCC receiving HD or 1 of 2 low-dose (LD) IL-2 regimens. Patients were randomized to receive 720,000 U/kg HD ($N$ = 156) IV bolus or 72,000 U/kg LD ($N$ = 150) IV bolus every 8 hours. The third arm ($N$ = 117) of LD patients consisted of SC IL-2 administration. The response rate with HD IV IL-2 was 13% and the response rate in the LD arms was similar at 10%. Patients who were complete responders in the HD IV arm had more durable responses than in the LD arms. They concluded that major tumor regression and response durability was more likely to occur in the HD IV IL-2 arm compared to either of the LD IL-2 arms. However, there was no difference in OS for patients with metastatic RCC in any arm. Yang[56] states that the LD regimens are viable options for patients with significant comorbidities and for physicians with minimal experience managing HD IV IL-2 related side effects.

Kammula et al[57] reviewed the safety trends in administering HD IV IL-2 therapy over a 12-year period. In this series, they evaluated the toxicities, the maximum number of doses of IL-2 administered, and objective response rates of 1241 patients with metastatic cancer treated with HD IV IL-2 during their first cycle of therapy. Patients were on clinical trials which may have included concurrent treatment with other cytokines, lymphokine-activated killer cells (LAK), tumor infiltrating lymphocytes (TIL), polyethylene glycol-modified IL-2 (PEG IL-2), chemotherapy, radiation, monoclonal antibodies, or cancer vaccines. Results indicated significant decreases in the number of grade 3 and 4 toxicities with the last 809 patients as compared to the initial patients. Of note, a decline in grades 3 and 4 toxicities included line sepsis (18%–4%); diarrhea (92%–12%); neuropsychiatric (Grade 4 19%–8%); pulmonary intubations (12%–3%); hypotension (81%–31%) and grade 4 cardiac ischemia (3%–0%). They surmise that these improvements are most likely reflective of better pretreatment screening strategies, improved therapeutic conditions, early recognition and treatment of toxicities, and cautious termination of dosing as toxicities warrant. This experience suggests that appropriate management of side effects and appropriate patient selection allows safe administration of HD IV IL-2.

## IL-2 SYSTEMIC SIDE EFFECTS: NURSING AND MEDICAL MANAGEMENT

The severity of side effects varies according to the route, dose, and schedule of administration.[7] Frequency of patient monitoring depends on these factors as well as how well the patient tolerates IL-2 (Table 20-2). Many side effects peak about 2 to 4 hours after dosing when IL-2 is administered as an intermittent IV bolus. Generally, the side effects diminish as time passes from the last dose. Once IL-2 therapy has been stopped, most toxicities subside and reverse within 48 to 72 hours. Although some side effects are of unknown etiology, several of the most profound toxicities are attributable to IL-2-induced capillary leak syndrome (CLS). With CLS, the production of other cytokines is stimulated including TNF-α and IL-5; generation of complement-activation; neutrophils activation; and endothelial-cell antigens stimulation. Symptoms of CLS include generalized edema, hypotension, oliguria, pleural effusions, pulmonary congestion, and ascites. These will be further explained throughout this chapter.[2,7,34,58–60] Table 20–3 provides a quick reference summary of IL-2 side effects, causes, and interventions. Clinical pathways for daily care and management of patients receiving both HD IL-2 and SC IL-2 are published elsewhere.[34]

### Constitutional symptoms

The most common side effects occurring with all methods of IL-2 administration are flulike symptoms (FLS). Within 30 minutes to 2 hours after the first dose of IL-2, patients may experience chills and rigors, which tend to abate with subsequent doses. Initially, these symptoms can be treated with warm blankets but if the chills and rigors are unrelieved, they may be treated with the administration of 25 to 50 mg of IV meperidine. Other FLS may include headaches, malaise, arthralgias, myalgias, anorexia, and abdominal discomfort. Many of these symptoms can be prophylactically treated with nonsteroidal anti-inflammatory agents (NSAIDs) such as indomethacin, acetaminophen, and ranitidine (or an equivalent) starting the night before the first dose of IL-2 and continuing until 24 hours after IL-2 therapy stops.[34,58–60] To help alleviate fatigue, patients should be encouraged to ambulate when possible and mix with periods of rest. This is especially important upon discharge. Strategies for managing cancer and treatment-related fatigue include moderate daily increases in exercise, adequate hydration and nutrition, balancing rest with activities, and possibly employing distraction techniques.[61–63] For those patients receiving SC regimens of IL-2 for longer periods of time, education and support for managing fatigue is particularly important. A comprehensive evidence-based practice guide for managing cancer-related fatigue can be found in the Oncology Nursing Society's Putting Evidence into Practice (PEP) card on fatigue (http://www.ons.org).

*Gastrointestinal.* It is not uncommon for most patients receiving IL-2 to experience some gastrointestinal (GI) distress such as nausea, vomiting, diarrhea, and anorexia. Patients experiencing these symptoms are advised not to eat or to eat small, frequent meals. Dry, cold, or salty foods tend to cause less nausea than spicy, greasy, or overly sweet foods. Nausea is treated prophylactically with antiemetics such as ondansetron or granisetron and as needed with compazine, prochlorperazine, lorazepam or phenergan for breakthrough nausea and vomiting.[2,34,58–60,64] It may take a combination of these agents to obtain relief. If initial antiemetic therapy fails, it is recommended that an agent from another class be added or that the initial agent be increased to the maximum accepted dosage range or a combination of both.[65] For example, if a patient is receiving scheduled odansetron, a 5-HT3 antagonist, and continues to experience nausea, a dopaminergic antagonist antiemetic such as prochlorperazine should be added. Another GI side effect suffered may be gastric upset, or reflux, which is managed with antacids. All patients should be placed on proton pump inhibitors or histamine blockers to prevent gastric toxicity.

Some patients experience diarrhea, which can occasionally reach grade 3 or 4 toxicity. With the first loose stool or with an increase in bowel movements, patients are given antidiarrheals such as loperamide. If the diarrhea is severe and does not abate with these medications, tincture of opium may be administered, although cautiously. A systematic review of recommendations for cancer therapy induced diarrhea can be found in Benson et al[66] and at http://www.UpToDate.com.[67] These guidelines do not specifically address IL-2-related diarrhea; however, they are still useful in this setting.

**TABLE 20-2**

**Guidelines for Monitoring Patients Receiving Interleukin 2 Therapy**

| | Frequency | | |
|---|---|---|---|
| | Inpatient | | Outpatient |
| **Parameter to Monitor** | **Not Requiring Vasopressors** | **Requiring Intensive Care Unit/Vasopressors** | |
| Vital signs | Every 4 hours | Every 1 hour | As needed |
| Intake and output | Every 8 hours | Every 1 hour | Not strictly measured |
| Weight | Daily | Daily | Daily |
| Mental status | Every 8 hours | Every 4 hours | Daily |
| IV site/injection site | Every 8 hours<br>Change peripheral IV every 3rd day | Every 8 hours<br>Change peripheral IV every 3rd day | Daily |
| Complete blood count and differential | Daily | Twice daily | Weekly |
| Electrolytes, BUN, creatinine, glucose | Daily | Twice daily | Weekly |
| AST, ALT, alkaline phosphatase, and bilirubin | Daily | Daily | Weekly |
| Albumin, $Ca^+$, $Mg^+$, and phosphorus | Daily | Daily | Each course |
| Creatinine phosphokinase | Daily | Daily | Weekly |
| Prothrombin time, partial thromboplastin time | Every 3rd day | Every 3rd day | Weekly |
| Thyroid-stimulating hormone and free T4 | Each cycle | Each cycle | Each course |
| Urinalysis | Each cycle | Each cycle | Each course |
| Electrocardiogram | Each cycle | Each cycle | Each course |
| Chest x-ray | Each cycle | Each cycle | Each course |

*Abbreviations*: ALT, alanine aminotransferase; AST, aspartate aminotransferase; BUN, blood urea nitrogen; IL-2, interluekin-2; IV, intravenous.
*Notes*: These guidelines recommend the minimum requirements. Good nursing and medical judgment will dictate more frequent monitoring as indicated.
*Source*: Used with permission from Schwartzentruber.[7]

It is essential to assess the patient's abdomen for distention, pain, and bowel sounds when using these medications since they can aggravate an intestinal ileus. Because of the psychotropic effects of tincture of opium, a neurological assessment needs to be done prior to administering and throughout treatment.[2,34,58–60] Patients are instructed to avoid caffeine, alcohol, and foods high in roughage, and to increase their intake of pectin containing foods such as peeled fruits (apples and pears) and gum fibers contained in foods such as cooked vegetables, white rice, bananas, and oatmeal.[2,34,68] Patients may rarely perforate a viscus with IL-2 therapy and patients should be closely monitored for this event.[69] A higher incidence of GI tract perforation has been noted in patients who have been treated with antibodies that bind to CTLA4, eg, ipilimumab, when they are subsequently treated with IL-2. It is recommended that patients who have received prior anti-CTLA4 antibody undergo diagnostic colonoscopy prior to the start of IL-2 therapy to rule out active chronic colitis.[70]

*Cardiopulmonary.* IL-2 administration induces a profound increase in vascular permeability known as CLS

**TABLE 20-3**

**Interleukin 2 Toxicities: Causes and Interventions**

| System | Signs/Symptoms | Pathophysiology | Interventions |
|---|---|---|---|
| Cardiovascular | Peripheral edema<br>Hypotension<br>Tachycardia<br>Weight gain<br>Ascites<br>Arrhythmias | Capillary leak syndrome (CLS): Shift of fluid from intravascular spaces to interstitial spaces induces increase in heart rate and decrease in blood pressure | Monitor blood pressure ≥ q4h<br>Fluid boluses as ordered<br>Daily weights<br>Strict intake and output (I&O)<br>Daily labs to follow electrolytes |
| Pulmonary | Crackles<br>Dyspnea/SOB<br>Increased RR<br>Hypoxia<br>Nasal/sinus congestion | CLS | Assess breath sounds q4h or more if needed<br>Assess breath sounds before and after fluid boluses<br>Baseline $O_2$ saturation and prn<br>$O_2$ therapy prn |
| GI | Anorexia<br>Nausea/vomiting<br>Mucositis<br>Diarrhea<br>Ileus | Unknown | Antiemetics: prophylactic and around the clock<br>Antidiarrheals<br>Diligent oral care<br>Perirectal care<br>H2 blocker<br>Nutrition counseling<br>Antacids |
| Renal | Oliguria<br>Increased creatinine<br>Increased BUN | 1. CLS: Decreased intravascular volume<br>2. Cumulative effect of IL-2; direct action on the kidneys | Fluid boluses<br>Dopamine at low dose (2–4 mcg/kg/min)<br>Foley catheter |
| Hematologic | Anemia<br>Thrombocytopenia<br>Lymphocytopenia | 1. Anemia partially R/T bone marrow suppression<br>2. Cumulative IL-2 doses | Daily CBC with differential<br>Assess for petechiae, bruises<br>Guiac stools, emesis as indicated<br>Monitor temperatures<br>Assess for potential sites of infection including skin, perirectal, and oral mucosa |
| Flulike symptoms | Fever<br>Chills<br>Malaise<br>Arthralgias<br>Fatigue | 1. May be R/T direct IL-2 effect on the hypothalamic regulatory centers<br>2. Fever may be caused by circulating TNF-α levels induced by IL-2 | Prophylactic anti-inflammatory agents<br>Warm blankets for chills<br>Meperidine for chills |
| Hepatic | Elevated bilirubin<br>Elevated transaminases | Manifested as reversible cholestasis | Monitor liver function tests daily |
| Integumentary | Pruritus<br>Erythematous rash<br>Skin dry, peeling and desquamation | Unknown | Nonalcohol based skin lotions<br>Oatmeal baths<br>Mild soaps<br>Anti-itching meds<br>Sunscreen when outside |
| Neurological | Confusion<br>Fatigue<br>Somnolence<br>Irritation/agitation<br>Hallucinations<br>Vivid dreams<br>Anxiety<br>Sleep disturbances | 1. IL-2 penetrates the blood–brain barrier resulting in increased brain water content<br>2. Altered sleep patterns/deprivation | Assess neuro status q8h and as needed<br>Teach relaxation techniques<br>Music therapy<br>Assess for subtle changes in personality<br>Limit antianxiety and sleep medications in later stages of treatment<br>Discontinuation of therapy<br>Airway protection if somnolent |
| Psychosocial | Fear<br>Tearfulness<br>Depression<br>Mood swings | Unknown/unclear | Emotional support<br>Teach relaxation techniques<br>Provide safe environment<br>Involve social worker and psych liaison as indicated<br>Reassure family and patient |

*Abbreviations*: CLS, capillary leak syndrome; IL-2, Interleukin-2; BUN, blood urea nitrogen; GI, gastrointestinal; SOB, shortness of breath; RR, respiratory rate; R/T, related to.

*Source*: Data from Rieger[1]; Muehlbauer[2]; Battiato[6]; Schwartzentruber[7]; and Mavroukakis, et al.[34]

which causes a shift of fluid from the intravascular space to the interstitial space.[71] As the intravascular space becomes depleted, the patient can develop oliguria, tachycardia, and hypotension. Oliguria generally precedes hypotension so accurate measurement of intake and output is essential. Because of the hypotension that occurs with IL-2, patients are encouraged to stop antihypertensive medications from the day before therapy until they have recovered from IL-2 side effects. Due to the stress placed on the cardiovascular system, patients with a history of heart disease or questionable cardiac event or those who are over the age of 50 should undergo Thallium cardiac stress testing as part of the pretreatment screening process. These precautions have all but eliminated the incidence of myocardial infarction.[57,58]

Myocarditis related to lymphocyte and eosinophil infiltration has been seen in patients receiving IL-2.[7,72] Clinically, patients may have increased creatine kinase isoenzymes with MB-band elevations. Sometimes these are not seen until 1 or 2 days post IL-2 therapy and are detected with routine daily laboratory work. Patients are usually asymptomatic but are placed on a cardiac monitor and troponin levels and electrocardiograms are done. Prior to receiving future doses of IL-2, an exercise echocardiogram (ECHO) will be performed to rule out myocardial dysfunction. If the ECHO is normal, the patient can receive future cycles of IL-2.[58,59]

Cardiac arrhythmias have been observed in 6% of patients with the majority being supraventricular (atrial fibrillation or tachycardia) in nature. These usually are short in duration and do not cause hemodynamic instability. The prime time for them to occur is at the peak of systemic toxicities when multiple fluid, electrolyte, and metabolic abnormalities occur. Treatment consists of discontinuation of therapy for that cycle, correction of electrolyte abnormalities, maintenance of good oxygenation, and diuretics for fluid overload. If indicated, interventions with agents such as digoxin, verapamil, diltiazem, or adenosine are initiated. It is safe for patients to receive subsequent cycles of IL-2 since only a minority of patients develop cardiac arrhythmias again.[7,73]

Interstitial fluid accumulates throughout the body including the skin, abdomen, and lungs leading to profound peripheral edema, ascites, and occasionally pulmonary edema. Patients require increased fluid intake to make up for losses of intravascular volume. It is not uncommon for patients' intake to exceed output by 1 to 3 L/day, causing patients to gain up to 2 kg/day.[2,7,34]

Initially, treatment of intravascular fluid loss requires replacement with IV fluids of either normal saline (NS) or lactated Ringers (LR). Colloid replacement has not been shown to provide any benefit over crystalloid.[7,74] The patient is given a fluid bolus of 250 to 500 mL until the blood pressure responds (systolic > 90) or the patient begins to experience crackles or decreased oxygen saturation. If the oxygen saturation drops below 95%, fluids should be used prudently. These respiratory symptoms indicate fluid overload and CLS-related interstitial pulmonary edema.[73] The patient may become tachypneic, dyspneic, and develop rales on auscultation. For these reasons, it is imperative to assess breath sounds both before and after administration of fluid boluses and limit fluid boluses to 1 to 2 L/day. Inability to maintain oxygen saturation above 95% on 4 L of oxygen via nasal cannula or 40% oxygen via face mask is an indication to discontinue dosing patients on HD IL-2.[7,34,59,60] As greater experience with IL-2 has been gained, the frequency for intubation for respiratory distress has decreased to about 1%. Patients with pre-existing pulmonary disease are at high risk for pulmonary complications which may require intensive care monitoring. Those patients with a history of smoking or those with large pulmonary tumor burdens should undergo pretreatment screening with pulmonary function tests.[7]

Up to 50% of patients may continue to experience hypotension and tachycardia despite fluid resuscitation, requiring vasopressor therapy.[25] The vasopressors of choice are α-adrenergic agonists such as phenylephrine, titrated to counteract the vasodilatory effects of IL-2, and beta-adrenergic agents are to be avoided due to their propensity to induce cardiac irritability and arrhythmias. The hypotensive effects of IL-2 usually peak 4 to 6 hours after dosing. If the phenylephrine can be weaned to approximately 0.5 mg/kg/min, it is generally safe to continue IL-2 dosing. Requirements of phenylephrine doses greater than 2 mg/kg/min suggest that IL-2 dosing should be discontinued.[7,34,59,60]

*Renal.* Renal dysfunction associated with IL-2 is described as prerenal azotemia. Hypotension and decreased intravascular volume result in reduced renal perfusion and oliguria.[7,59,60] Also, IL-2 appears to have a direct toxic effect on the kidneys further contributing to decreased urinary output which can result in an increase in serum creatinine and blood urea nitrogen (BUN). It has been reported that the highest mean peak creatinine value during HD IL-2 is 2.7 mg/dL.[75] Patients with RCC who have undergone a prior nephrectomy are at a greater risk for dysfunction. Other factors linked with an increased risk of nephrotoxicity include a diagnosis of RCC, older age, male gender, and pre-existing hypertension.[59] Oliguria is initially treated with fluid boluses in order to increase the circulating fluid volume. After appropriate fluid resuscitation, LD dopamine at 2 to 4 mg/kg/minute may be initiated to increase renal perfusion although the value of this intervention has never been studied. Generally, creatinine levels revert to normal within 7 to 14 days. Although patients experience these significant fluid shifts and undergo fluid replacement, electrolyte imbalances frequently occur including hypokalemia, hypomagnesemia, hypocalcemia, and hypophosphatemia. Electrolyte levels are monitored daily and replaced as needed.[58]

*Neurological.* Interleukin 2 crosses the blood–brain barrier and increases brain water content, which may cause the neurological side effects seen with IL-2.[7] These can include lethargy, anxiety, vivid dreams, confusion, sleep disturbances, decreased concentration, mood swings, combativeness, hallucinations, depression, and coma.[59,60,76,77] Contributing factors may include concomitant medications to treat other side effects such as meperidine for chills or phenothiazine or lorazepam for nausea.[59] It is important to factor these in when monitoring mental status changes. With the first sign of neuropsychiatric toxicity, IL-2 should be discontinued as these effects can worsen for several days before improving.[7] Rigorous assessment for mild mental status changes or hypodelirium is essential.

Aspiration becomes a significant threat in the presence of neurotoxicity, particularly in the obtunded or sedated patient. Occasionally, patients may require intubation to maintain a patent airway. These side effects must be closely monitored for neurological deterioration and are a prime area for nursing interventions. Reassuring patients and their families that these are normal and reversible side effects helps relieve some of the anxiety that neurotoxicities generate. Reorientation, relaxation techniques, and music therapy can help reduce patients' discomfort. Emotional support by the patient's family, healthcare providers, and social workers are imperative throughout treatment.[2,20,34,76,77] On rare occasions, more aggressive patient interventions are required to prevent self-harm, such as padding the bedrails or restraining the patient.[34] If restraints are warranted, check the institution's policy for monitoring the patient in restraints. Severe behavioral changes may require medication such as haloperidol which does not have some of the secondary side effects of other sedatives.[7]

*Integumentary.* Interleukin 2 also affects the skin and mucous membranes. Skin changes include generalized flushing or erythematous rash, pruritus, dry peeling skin, and severe itching which starts within 3 days of initiation of treatment and could continue up to 6 weeks.[59,78] Other dermatological side effects may possibly include complaints of skin burning or palmar and plantar desquamation.[7] Dermatological discomforts are managed by washing with mild soaps or cleansers and with liberal application of nonalcohol-based lotions and/or aloe vera. Topical steroids should be avoided.[2,58,59] Patients with severe, uncontrolled itching may be prescribed diphenhydramine HCL or hydroxyzine HCL. Dutcher et al[60] recommend neurontin (gabapentin) for severe pruritus since it affects peripheral nerve fibers. Patients may experience varying degrees of mucositis, glossitis, stomatitis, pharyngitis, and altered sense of taste. These symptoms are managed with frequent, meticulous mouth care including Biotene mouthwash, sodium bicarbonate mouthwash, MEDOral mouth rinse, or lidobenalox. Extremely hot, cold, or rough foods could injure oral mucosa and should be avoided. It is recommended that patients try soft or blended foods and avoid tobacco products and alcoholic beverages because these can also be irritating.[68]

*Immunological/metabolic.* Infection can be a lethal complication of IL-2 therapy as neutrophil function is impaired in patients receiving IL-2. Therefore, IV sites and all mucosal areas including the perirectal area must be assessed frequently because of the increased risk of infection during treatment. Peripheral IV sites should be routinely changed and meticulous care of central venous catheters must be maintained per the institution's policies. Prophylactic antibiotics are used for patients with central lines to prevent infection. Long-term indwelling lines are prone to infection and are not used in some institutions in patients receiving IL-2.[2,7,34]

Changes in laboratory values reflect other side effects that occur with IL-2 therapy and must be monitored regularly. Lymphocytopenia develops rapidly and persists throughout therapy, putting the patient at greater risk for developing infection. Once treatment is stopped, a rapid rebound of lymphocytes above baseline develops and persists for 3 to 7 days before returning to normal. Thrombocytopenia and anemia may occur and require assessment for petechiae, epistaxis, hematuria, guiac positive stools, and emesis for occult blood loss.[7,20,34,59,79] Elevations in the alkaline phosphatase, alanine aminotransferase (ALT), aspartate aminotransferase (AST), lactate dehydrogenase (LDH), and total bilirubin indicative of the reversible cholestasis are commonly observed in patients during IL-2 therapy.[7,20,59] Thyroid dysfunction has been reported in 13% to 41% of patients receiving monotherapy with IL-2. The majority of these irregularities have been hypothyroidism which occurs in 35% of patients and is normally subclinical. The incidence increases with the number of courses and duration of treatment. Screening of thyroid function is done routinely with each course. Moderate to severe hypothyroidism is treated with levothyroxine for up to 1 year, at which point the dysfunction typically reverses.[7]

*Hypersensitivity reactions.* Patients treated with IL-2 may develop hypersensitivity reactions to contrast dye or medications. This occurs in 10% to 28% of patients and manifests as wheezing, rash, diarrhea, chills, fever, emesis, hypotension, edema, and oliguria shortly after IV contrast.[7] Hypersensitivity reactions have also been seen with post IL-2 diuresis with drugs such as furosemide. Supportive measures and diphenhydramine are useful in alleviating symptoms. However, steroids should not be used since they block the effects of IL-2.[7]

### Subcutaneous IL-2

Overall, side effects seen in patients receiving subcutaneous IL-2 (SC IL-2) are diminished but not insubstantial. The dose-limiting toxicities observed in patients receiving SC IL-2 are similar to the profile seen in patients receiving IV IL-2 except that the overall intensity and duration of subjective side effects, such as nausea and vomiting, tends to be lower. Constitutional symptoms of fatigue, myalgias, and fever are the most common symptoms patients experience and may have more impact on their quality of life (QOL) than in patients receiving IV IL-2.[2,34,60] Yang et al[56] report that a QOL assessment obtained on patients receiving various routes of administration of IL-2 did not show a significant advantage from a QOL standpoint in patients receiving SC IL-2. The prolonged nature of the treatment (ie, 6 weeks or more) and toxicities as well as the inconvenience of SC therapy offset the more intense but shorter lived toxicities seen with IV IL-2. Fevers in the range of 38°C to 40°C (100.4°F-104°F) occur within the first 2 to 8 hours of SC administration and generally peak approximately 4 hours after each injection. Premedications commonly prescribed with IV IL-2 can be administered in the SC IL-2 population and help ameliorate these sequelae.

Mild hematological, renal, and hepatic laboratory changes are also observed. Patients' symptoms are treated with oral analgesics, antipyretics, and antiemetics and are generally not treatment limiting.[34] One recommendation is to administer the dose of IL-2 around dinnertime (6 pm) to take advantage of potential initial fever and chills prior to bedtime. The patient can then sleep throughout the night.

Other considerations for the patient receiving SC IL-2 include the patient's support systems at home; the ability to give a self-injection; the patient's overall general condition; the patient's reliability in calling the medical team when indicated, and the patient's learning abilities.[5] If the patient has been referred to a large medical center but lives in a rural area, it may limit access to immediate health care and the availability of IL-2 at the local pharmacy. All of these could factor into the ability to receive SC IL-2 as an outpatient. Several specialty home delivery pharmacies exist such as Biologics Inc. (1-800-850-4306 or http://www.biologicstoday.com) which can assist with reimbursement and getting patients prescribed medications delivered to their home.

## Eligibility for IL-2

The toxicity associated with HD IL-2 requires cautious and rigorous patient selection. Vigilant screening of IL-2 candidates must be done prior to initiating therapy. Patients with limited pulmonary function, active cardiac disease, or symptomatic brain metastases are at significant risk for serious complications and are rarely eligible for IL-2 administration. IL-2 therapy demands an intact immune system; therefore, pretreatment evaluation includes screening for HIV and other active infections, although its use in low doses is investigational in patients with HIV.[7,59,60] Since the effects of IL-2 on a fetus are unknown, women of childbearing potential undergo a pregnancy test prior to initiating therapy and are instructed in birth control measures to prevent pregnancy during therapy. Mothers are also instructed not to breastfeed during IL-2 therapy because of the unknown effects. Screening parameters are included in pretreatment evaluation in the clinical pathways. Patients are required to select a Durable Power of Attorney (DPA) since the potential neurological side effects may impair their ability to make reliable decisions during therapy.[2,34]

Acute toxicities are minimized in patients receiving LD or SC IL-2 and, therefore, more patients are eligible to receive this therapy. Patients with a poor performance status, respiratory involvement, or who for other medical reasons may be unable to tolerate HD IL-2 may be eligible to receive LD/SC IL-2. The eligibility criteria are not as clear with this regimen as they are with HD IL-2 and the decision for eligibility is primarily the responsibility of the prescribing physician.[2,34]

## Dose modification for IL-2

Patients rarely tolerate all 14 doses of HD IL-2. Therapy is routinely discontinued on the basis of dose-limiting toxicity. Doses are delayed or skipped in patients who are hemodynamically unstable or oliguric, and resumed if appropriate interventions stabilize these toxicities. The IL-2 dose should not be reduced. Toxicities which would indicate the need to stop a cycle of therapy include (1) electrocardiogram (EKG) changes indicative of ischemia, (2) ventricular arrhythmias, (3) sustained sinus tachycardia which persists after correcting hypotension, fever, and hypoxemia, (4) diarrhea greater than 1 L per 8 hours, (5) vomiting unresponsive to medication, (6) $O_2$ saturation < 94% despite oxygen therapy, (7) sustained oliguria, and (8) disorientation or hallucinations.[7,34,58–60] These side effects generally reverse within 24 hours after stopping IL-2 therapy with the exception of neurological side effects. Neurological toxicities can worsen for a few days after therapy is completed; hence, it is imperative to closely observe patients who have experienced any symptoms of neurological alterations.

Patients who receive LD IL-2 have less severe toxicities. Reasons that a patient on LD IL-2 may delay or stop therapy include a rise in creatinine to >2.5 mg/dL, shortness of breath, or constitutional symptoms that are not controlled with prophylactic medications. Major toxicities including those similar to the HD IL-2 regimen would also warrant a discontinuation of therapy.[2,34,58]

## Retreatment with IL-2

Patients may undergo a second course of IL-2 therapy if they exhibit some evidence of either stable disease or tumor regression. Retreatment cycles are administered in the same fashion as the initial cycle, although patients receiving HD IL-2 may not tolerate the same number of doses. Major responses after 2 unsuccessful courses of IL-2 are thought to be rare, although clinical trials to investigate this possibility have not been reported. Therefore, patients who have not responded after 2 courses of therapy are usually observed. Patients who respond will be offered additional courses of therapy. If a patient has a complete response, defined as a disappearance of all clinical evidence of disease, 2 additional cycles are administered in an attempt to consolidate that response. Retreatment is begun 4 to 6 weeks after the last course.[2,34,80]

### IL-2 discharge teaching

Common persistent side effects at discharge include rash, dry and peeling skin, fatigue, and anorexia. Therefore, appropriate discharge instructions are important and are delineated in Table 20-4. For patients receiving SC IL-2, self-administration of the SC IL-2 is taught with return demonstrations until the patient is comfortable. Patients are asked to keep a diary of their daily weights and temperatures, documentation that they have given themselves the IL-2 injection, and any side effects that occur during treatment.[2,34]

### Follow-up evaluation

Routine response evaluation of the patient receiving IL-2, including blood work and imaging scans outlined in the clinical pathways, should be performed 3 to 6 weeks after each course of therapy to determine retreatment options. Once treatment is concluded, regular follow-up allows assessment of OS and disease-free survival and provides the patient a significant support system. Patients with recurrent or progressive disease may benefit from other treatment interventions or may elect to pursue palliative care.[2,34]

## THE INTERFERONS

Interferons were the first identified cytokines and are a group of naturally occurring antiviral cytokines first described by Issacs and Lindenman that when induced, can inhibit the replication of other viruses.[81,82] They are named interferon because of their ability to "interfere" with viral replication.

**TABLE 20-4**

**Discharge Instructions for Patients Receiving Interleukin 2**

- Gradually increase your food intake. Continue to use high-calorie, high-protein foods until your appetite fully returns so that you get adequate nutrient intake.
- Gradually increase the variety of foods in your diet.
- Drink about 12 or more 8-ounce glasses of fluid every day. Watch the color of your urine to make sure you are getting enough fluid. Your urine should be light yellow or almost clear if you are taking enough fluids. If your urine is darker, or amber colored, increase your fluid intake.
- Nutrition tips can be found in the NCI's "Eating Hints for Cancer Patients: Before, During and After Treatment" booklet (http://www.cancer.gov/cancerinfo/eatinghints). These tips will also assist with any lingering GI side effects.
- It may take about a week before your energy is fully back. You can help regain energy by gradually increasing exercise and taking frequent rest breaks during the day. It is important that you do not sleep all day. This will make the fatigue worse. If you really cannot get your energy back, please notify your physician. Your nurse will provide a separate handout with other tips to combat fatigue.
- Sleep disturbances and unusual dreams may continue for 2 to 3 weeks after therapy.
- Use a strong sunblock with an SPF of 15 or greater even if it is cloudy or overcast.
- Wear hats with broad brims, long sleeves, and pants for extra protection against the sun.
- Skin side effects may last for 6 weeks. Continue using the creams, oils, and lotions used while in the hospital.
- Continue to use mild soaps and try to avoid swimming in chlorinated or saltwater. If you do swim, rinse off immediately and use lotions or creams on your skin.
- Do not drive for 1 week after therapy.
- Do NOT use any products containing steroids or cortisone. Many over-the-counter products including moisturizers contain these ingredients. Check with the healthcare team BEFORE using any medications, creams, or ointments.

**Symptoms to Report to the Healthcare Team**

- Nausea, vomiting, or diarrhea that lasts for more than 48 hours
- Any new onset of nausea, vomiting, or diarrhea
- Trouble with breathing
- Temperature greater than 100.8°F
- Chest pain
- Any new onset of pain including headaches

*Abbreviations*: GI, gastrointestinal; NCI, National Cancer Institute.
*Source*: Data from Muehlbauer[2]; Mavroukakis et al[34]; and Drabot.[68]

There are 3 main IFNs with clinical indications: alpha (α), beta (β), and gamma (γ). Two other IFNs, tau and omega, are not approved for therapeutic purposes in humans. In the 1970s, IFN-α was derived from donated human blood.[81–83] These early preparations were impure, but they provided a chance to test them as an anticancer therapy. As with IL-2, it was not until recombinant DNA technology was available that IFN could be produced in quantities sufficient enough to use in widespread clinical trials.[81,82] The only IFN approved for use as cancer therapy is IFN-α.

## BIOLOGICAL ACTIVITY

When a stimulus such as a virus, bacteria, parasite, or cancer activates a cell, IFN is produced. These are recognized by the body as foreign thus stimulating an immune response. Interferon binds to a cell surface receptor site and activates downstream signal transduction pathways. A signal is sent to the cell nucleus where it attaches to certain genes which then regulate cell activities including inducing apoptosis.[81,82,84] Once the signal is activated, there is significant interaction between the cytokine, hormone, and growth-factor signaling pathways which block viral and possibly cellular RNA development.[82,85]

The major actions of IFNs are antiviral, immunomodulatory, and antiproliferative. However, each IFN has similar and distinct characteristics. For example, there is evidence that IFN-α has antiangiogenic properties when given in lower doses. Endogenous IFN, a regulator of angiogenesis, inhibits endothelial cell migration as well as basic fibroblast growth factor and IL-8 both which promote tumor angiogenesis.[82,86–89] Table 20-5 summarizes the types, names, actions, and FDA-approved clinical indications of each IFN. Tayal and Kalra[13] outline a thorough overview of IFNs. Interferon-α will be the only one discussed in detail in this chapter.

## INTERFERON-α: INDICATIONS FOR USE

Studies continue to examine the effectiveness of IFN-α alone or in combination with other agents for a variety of malignancies. Clinical trials evaluating the efficacy of IFN-α alone and in combination with other drugs have been conducted for chronic myeloid leukemia (CML), follicular non-Hodgkin's lymphoma (NHL), Kaposi sarcoma, hepatocellular carcinoma, superficial bladder cancer (SBC), and RCC.[88,90–98] A selection of these trials is discussed below.

### Melanoma

Food and Drug Administration approval was obtained for high-dose IFN-α2b (HDI) as adjuvant treatment for patients with melanoma at a high risk of recurrence (American Joint Committee on Cancer [AJCC] stage IIB or IIC [thick lesions 2.01 to 4.0 mm and >4.0 mm] or stage III [lymph node positive]) in the mid 1990s. Several trials in the United States and abroad have evaluated the efficacy of IFN-α on OS and relapse-free survival (RFS).[99,100] The reason for continued studies is that the impact of HDI on long-term survival has been under scrutiny due to the cost and toxicity of the regimen as well as the absence of survival benefit in a separate trial (E1690) conducted by the Eastern Oncology Cooperative Group who did the initial trial (E1684), which was pivotal in getting HDI FDA-approved for this patient population.[99] Moschos, et al[99] report that in Europe, the Association of Dermatologic Oncologists in Germany, the Italian Melanoma Intergroup, and the Hellenic Oncology Group in Greece have only recently studied HDI. Generally, these organizations evaluated the efficacy of lower doses of IFN-α2b. Overall, study results show that lower doses of IFN-α2b show no survival benefit.[99,101–104] An overview of clinical trials can be found in Moschos et al.[99] A meta-analysis of 12 randomized clinical trials for high-risk melanoma concluded there is a significant reduction of recurrence in patients who received IFN compared with observation only.[105] Currently, there is no international consensus supporting use of HDI-α2b for high-risk melanoma.[106]

### Renal cell carcinoma

Interferon-α has a roughly 10% to 20% response rate when used alone to treat RCC. Igarahsi and colleagues[107] studied the effects of IFN-α combined with 5-Fluorouracil (5-FU). Patients received 3 MIU SC 3 times a week for 12 weeks and 600/mg/m$^2$ of 5-FU as a continuous infusion for the first 5 days followed by 600 mg/m$^2$ weekly from the third to the twelfth week. The overall response rate was 20%, which is no better than IFN alone. They concluded that this regimen has limited value for treatment of patients with advanced RCC.

Another combination studied added thalidomide, an antiangiogenic agent, to IFN-α. Investigators at Helsinki University Central Hospital hypothesized that the antiangiogenic effects of IFN-α combined with thalidomide may be enhanced. Patients were given 0.9 MU IFN-α SC 3 times a day for 1 month and then 1.2 MU IFN-α 3 times a day. The thalidomide dose was escalated from 100 mg/day for the first week to 300 mg/day thereafter. Investigators measured serum vascular endothelial growth factor (VEGF) which is a potent stimulator of tumor angiogenesis. Serum VEGF levels decreased in the patients who responded to therapy compared to those patients with stable or progressive disease. However, all responses were partial responses and the biomarkers did not correlate with significant clinical benefit.[90]

Other combinations have been tried with IFN-α in the treatment of RCC including combining IFN-α with

**TABLE 20-5**

**Interferons**

| Interferon | Actions | FDA-Approved Indications | Side Effects |
|---|---|---|---|
| IFN-α-2a and IFN-α-2b | Antiviral<br>Inhibits growth of normal and malignant cells<br>Enhances NK-cell activity<br>Enhances class I MHC expression<br>Influences differentiation of cells<br>Induces apoptosis<br>Antiangiogenic properties | IFN-α-2a<br>Chronic hepatitis C<br>Hairy cell leukemia<br>Chronic myelogenous leukemia<br>AIDS-related Kaposi sarcoma<br><br>IFN-α-2b<br>Malignant melanoma<br>Hairy cell leukemia<br>AIDS-related Kaposi sarcoma<br>Condyloma acuminata<br>Follicular lymphoma<br>Chronic hepatitis B<br>Chronic hepatitis C | Thrombocytopenia, flu-like syndrome, fatigue, neuropsychiatric symptoms (ie, depression), transaminase elevations, granulocytopenia, neutropenia, rash, alopecia, anorexia, taste changes |
| IFN-α-n3 | | Condyloma acuminate | |
| Pegylated IFN-α-2a | | Chronic hepatitis C | Fatigue, myalgias, headache, injection site reactions |
| Pegylated IFN-α-2b | | Chronic hepatitis C | |
| IFN-β-Ia and IFN-β-Ib | Antiviral<br>Enhances NK-cell activity<br>Enhances class I MHC expression<br>Induces apoptosis | Relapsing forms of multiple sclerosis | IFN-β-Ia:<br>Fever, chills, myalgia<br><br>IFN-β-Ib:<br>Injection site pain, sweating symptom, myalgia, fever, chills, asthenia |
| IFN-γ-Ib | Antiviral<br>Inhibits growth of normal and malignant cells<br>Enhances macrophage activity<br>Enhances class I and II MHC expression<br>Generates secretion of other cytokines<br>Impacts differentiation of cells<br>Enhances immunoglobulin synthesis with other cytokines<br>Induces apoptosis | Chronic granulomatous disease<br>Malignant osteoporosis | Fatigue, fever, diarrhea, headache, malaise, chills, injection site pain, rash, nausea and vomiting, arthralgia, myalgia. |

*Abbreviations*: NK, natural killer; MHC, major histocompatibility complex; IFN, interferon; AIDS, acquired immunodeficiency virus; FDA, Food and Drug Administration.
*Source*: Data from Tayal et al[13]; Cuaron et al[82]; interferon alfa (http://www.micromedex.com).[85]

retinoids. Efficacy in 2 clinical trials was minimal in terms of response rate or OS. Interferon-α has been combined separately with vinblastine, aspirin, histamine, and IFN-γ with overall mixed results. As a monotherapy, IFN-α has modest activity in metastatic RCC. Response to IFN-α correlates with characteristics such as good performance status, few metastatic sites, prior nephrectomy, and low erythrocyte sedimentation rate.[104] Patients who do achieve a durable response require ongoing therapy to maintain the remission.

## Superficial bladder cancer

Intravesical instillation of IFN-α has been studied for treatment of SBC as both a monotherapy and combined with other therapies. SBC are defined as stages Ta or Tcis (tumors confined to the mucosa) or stage T1 (tumors invading the lamina propria) which account for 80% of primary bladder tumors.[98] Clinical studies imply intravesical IFN-α has antiproliferative activity against SBC via many mechanisms including increasing production of IFN-γ, increasing the cytotoxic activity of T cells and NK cells by increasing the infiltration of these cells into the bladder wall.[97,98]

Interferon-α was not as effective as BCG in several trials as first-line therapy. However, studies indicate that IFN-α has potential as a second-line therapy for patients who did not respond to prior intravesical chemotherapy or BCG. Efficacy of intravesical IFN-α in SBC appears to be greater with higher doses such as 100 MIU.[97,98]

Ziotta and Schulman[97] report that BCG and IFN-α are biocompatible and may be used in combination intravesically as a single mixture that would produce or enhance the therapeutic response vs BCG alone. Clinical trials are underway to investigate this combination and others with chemotherapy.[97,98]

## PEG-INTERFERON-α

Pegylation of therapeutic proteins involves the addition of polyethylene glycol (PEG) to the therapeutic agent to allow for slower release of the agent. Pegylation has been done with a variety of therapeutic agents including adenosine deaminase, L-asparginase, IL-2, granulocyte colony stimulating factor, TNF-α, and human growth hormone.[108,109] Polyethylene glycol-Intron is a conjugate of recombinant IFN-α with a single straight-chain molecule of PEG and demonstrates similar biological activity compared to IFN-α2b.[108,110] The impetus in pegylating IFN-α is to provide extended half-life of IFN, thus sustaining the duration of activity of IFN-α and allowing for a once weekly injection. Other benefits of pegylation are enhanced drug solubility and lower toxicity. It is FDA approved for chronic hepatitis C infection as a monotherapy and in combination with ribavirin (Rebetol). This combination has significantly improved the elimination rate of the virus.[13,108,110] It has been investigated in patients with CML and solid tumors including melanoma and RCC. The toxicity profile has been similar for patients with CML and Hepatitis C virus (HCV) while fatigue has been reported as a dose-limiting toxicity in patients with solid tumors. Further studies are needed to determine the optimal dose and to establish if PEG Interferon-α can achieve dose intensification and improve efficacy.[108,110,111]

## INTERFERON-α: SIDE EFFECTS AND MEDICAL AND NURSING MANAGEMENT

Side effects with IFN-α are not insignificant and nursing interventions are essential in helping patients tolerate this extended therapy. Knowledge of these side effects and how to manage them will be crucial when caring for the patient receiving IFN-α. Consideration should be given to adjustment of dose or schedule of administration if the patient is experiencing unremitting toxicities.

The most common side effects reported with IFN-α include fatigue, FLS (fever, chills, myalgias, headaches, and malaise), neutropenia, anorexia, nausea/vomiting, increased liver function tests, depression, diarrhea, alopecia, and altered taste sensation.[82,112,113] Management of these symptoms necessitates a multidisciplinary approach. An overview of the more common side effects with suggested nursing management strategies is provided in Table 20-6.

### Fatigue

Fatigue, the most frequently reported symptom experienced by patients with cancer, was reported in 96% of patients receiving IFN-α2b for treatment of high-risk melanoma.[63,116,117] Fatigue is common in all treatment regimens of IFN-α but more pronounced in patients receiving doses of 10 MIU/m$^2$ or greater.[82,106] It is one of the most persistent and pervasive symptoms which can be difficult to manage and leads to dose alterations. Cancer-related fatigue is a complex, multifactorial disorder with physical, mental, and psychological dimensions and is affiliated with diminished QOL.[61–63] There is speculation that IFN-induced fatigue, appetite changes, and cognitive-emotional disorders may be the consequence of central nervous system toxicity or frontal lobe neurotoxicity.[113] Interferon potentially has a direct effect on the frontal lobe or on deeper brain structures. Central and peripheral mechanisms could be a contributory factor by releasing cytokines (ie, immunomodulators) that alter fatigue sensations.[106] Other causes of fatigue in the patient receiving IFN-α include depression, anorexia, sleep disturbances, anemia, hypovolemia, hypoglycemia, and thyroid dysfunction. Mental fatigue is affiliated with cognitive dysfunction and may persist throughout therapy. Contributing factors include the disease itself, compromised performance status, more advanced age, chronic pain, fever, and dehydration.[82,106,115,118] It is important to understand all the underlying causes of fatigue and to be able to distinguish between fatigue and depression when assisting patients in managing their fatigue.

### Flulike or constitutional symptoms

Flulike symptoms (FLS) include fevers, chills, headaches, myalgias, and malaise. These side effects develop during the first week of treatment but lessen over time because of tachyphylaxis (decreasing symptoms with increasing exposure to drug). Fevers may reach 39°C to 40°C 2 to 4 hours after IFN-α administration and last 4 to 8 hours.[2,119,120]

Body temperature is controlled by a thermoregulatory set point. The anterior hypothalamic brain centers sense deviations from a set temperature range of 36.4°C to 37.3°C and regulate thermal balance by either heat production, causing vasoconstriction and shivering or by heat loss, causing vasodilatation and sweating. Interferon fevers are a result of the release of pyrogenic factors induced by cytokine administration including the stimulation of IL-1, IL-6, and TNF. These cytokines act on thermal brain centers via prostaglandin release creating a higher body temperature setpoint, thus increasing body temperature.[7,112,119] Chills and rigors precede a rise in fever and manifest as

**TABLE 20-6**

**Interferon-α: Toxicities and Management Strategies**

| Side Effect | Nursing Interventions |
|---|---|
| Flulike symptoms | Premedicate with antipyretics and NSAIDs such as acetaminophen and indomethacin to help alleviate fever/myalgias/headaches.<br>Increase fluid intake.<br>Administer IFN before bedtime or at dinnertime (about 6 pm).<br>Layer warm blankets for chills. |
| Fatigue | Rotate periods of rest with activity.<br>Promote moderate daily exercise such as walking.<br>Use distraction techniques such as reading, watching movies, meditation, biofeedback.<br>Assist patient with time management.<br>Ensure adequate nutrition and hydration.<br>Enlist RD to assist.<br>Ask patient to keep food diary for a period of time for evaluation by RD.<br>Suggest patient drink 2 to 3 L of fluid/day.<br>Suggest patient keep a diary of activity to help identify factors contributing to fatigue.<br>Schedule activities important to patient during time of least fatigue.<br>Help patient modify activities that promote fatigue.<br>Differentiate fatigue from depression. |
| Neurological | Evaluate psychiatric history at baseline.<br>Consult with psychiatrist or psychologist if patient has a prior history of mood disorders or depression.<br>Evaluate patient on ongoing basis for symptoms of depression and other neurological changes, including mood alterations, suicidal ideations, changes in cognition.<br>Encourage support group participation.<br>Include family in education and encourage communication for signs of behavior changes.<br>Referral as indicated to psychiatrist and other support systems.<br>Patient may need medically prescribed antidepressants in some cases.<br>Use nonpharmacological interventions such as relaxation therapy and guided imagery. |
| Anorexia and weight loss | Monitor weight.<br>Promote small, frequent meals.<br>Encourage protein supplements or high-protein foods.<br>Encourage use of premade meals to conserve energy.<br>Cafeteria style restaurants allow patients to eat what they want when they want.<br>Enlist RD.<br>Medicate with antiemetics as needed.<br>Assess patient for symptoms of fluid and electrolyte imbalance. |
| Dermatological | Assess for history of dermatological problems (ie, psoriasis).<br>Assess skin at start of therapy and throughout therapy.<br>Instruct patient to use mild soaps, cleansers without a lot of fragrance.<br>Instruct patient to use fragrance-free lotions, creams, and emollients.<br>Instruct patient to use sunscreen with SPF 15 or greater every day.<br>Instruct patient to wear broad-brimmed hats and to cover exposed areas.<br>Consult with dermatologist if needed.<br>MD may prescribe histamine blockers for urticaria and rash. |

*Abbreviations*: RD, registered dietician; IFN, interferon; NSAIDs, nonsteroidal anti-inflammatory drugs.

*Source*: Data from Battiato[6]; Hauschild et al[106]; Battiato et al[112]; Dean[114]; and Kiley and Gale.[115]

muscle contractions. This increased muscle activity generates heat to change the body temperature when the thermoregulatory set point is raised. Chills, rigors, myalgias, and headaches may occur an hour before the onset of fever.[112,119] Myalgias are characterized by general muscle aches along with weakness unrelieved by rest. These can last after other FLS have abated in part because of the muscle exertion generated when a patient has chills and rigors. Rigors and chills require a large consumption of energy and oxygen. Coupled with vasoconstriction, unnecessary demands can be placed on myocardial tissue so rigors and chills need to be controlled to avoid unnecessary cardiac stress.[82,112,119]

Administration of antipyretics and NSAIDS prior to IFN-α is beneficial.[113,119] Giving IFN-α at bedtime is helpful to some patients allowing them to sleep through side effects; however, it may disrupt sleeping patterns for others.[106] A better time for these patients would be dinnertime (around 6 pm) as this allows for the worst of the initial side effects to subside prior to bedtime. If fevers persist for more than 8 hours and are unrelieved by antipyretics, the presence of infection needs to be evaluated.[2]

### Dermatological symptoms

Cutaneous reactions of varying degrees have been associated with IFN-α therapy. Alopecia, pruritus, rash, skin dryness and itching, erythema, exacerbations of herpes labialis, cutaneous vascular lesions, xerostomia, cutaneous granulomatous reactions (sarcoidosis, anular granuloma), and injection site reactions have all been reported.[106,121] Treatment varies depending on the severity but may include observation or administering topical, oral, or parenteral medication. IFN may need to be discontinued if psoriasis persists or if severe. Phototherapy or pharmacological interventions are initiated if it worsens after IFN has been discontinued.[106]

Patients should be taught to rotate injection sites to avoid injection site necrosis. Either warm or cold compresses can be applied depending on which feels better to the patient. Diphenhydramine may be helpful in reducing itching; however, its sedating effects need to be considered.[121]

Systemic steroids such as prednisone have been shown to block some antiviral activity of IFN. Therefore, systemic steroids should be avoided for the patient on IFN-α. IFN-α therapy may cause more severe cutaneous reactions in some instances necessitating holding therapy.[113,121]

Other strategies are similar to those for IL-2 including using mild soaps, using lotions, creams or ointments frequently, and encouraging adequate oral hydration. It is imperative that patients use a strong sunscreen with SPF 15 or greater, wear hats with broad brims, and cover exposed skin since photosensitivity has been reported.[2,121]

Periodic assesment of injection sites and administration techniques may be of benefit. Smaller gauge needles, room temperature solution, and slow injection of drug help alleviate injection site reactions. Other nursing considerations include ensuring that the injections are SC and not intradermal and that the correct dose and volume are being administered.[121]

### Anorexia and altered taste sensations

Weight loss from anorexia is not uncommon due to the long duration of therapy. Anorexia occurs in 43% to 69% of patients receiving higher doses of IFN-α.[82] Interferon induces secondary cytokines such as TNF-α, IL-1, IL-6, and IFN-γ that play a factor in anorexia. These cytokines alter protein, carbohydrate, and lipid metabolism by several different mechanisms. TNF-α is a cachetin that is responsible for increased muscle catabolism, lipolysis, and hyperactivation of anorexic neurons.[68,82] IL-1 breaks down adipose tissues into free fatty acids and activates anorexic neurons. IL-6 increases levels of C-reactive protein, which is associated with weight loss, anorexia, and insulin resistance. IFN-γ encourages anorexia with subsequent weight loss and breaks down protein and fat.[68]

Depression has an impact on appetite and nutritional status and is a common symptom in patients with cancer. It is estimated that 48% of patients diagnosed with cancer meet the criteria for the diagnosis of a major depressive disorder as compared to 6% of the normal population. Depression has been reported to occur in up to 40% of patients on IFN-α2b. Some symptoms of depression include decrease in appetite and weight loss.[82,106]

Taste alterations range from decreased taste to salty, bitter, or metallic taste to intolerance of sweets. Patients have reported that certain foods or beverages they enjoyed prior to IFN-α therapy are no longer appealing during therapy. A registered dietitian (RD) is helpful in assisting patients to ingest adequate calories. Interventions include small, frequent meals, high-protein supplements, premade meals, exercise prior to eating, and eating at cafeteria style restaurants where patients can choose what they are hungry for at that moment. A food diary can assist the RD in evaluation of caloric intake and breakdown of calories. Evaluation of adequate calories from protein, carbohydrates, and fat allows the RD to make suggestions to maximize calories and maintain the patient's weight.[2,121]

### Neurological symptoms

The most common neurological symptoms reported with IFN-α include mental fatigue, confusion, lack of concentration, memory problems, and depression. Patients have also complained of lack of motivation, anxiety, sleep disturbances, and decreased libido. More pronounced toxicities can occur including lethargy, somnolence, behavior changes, irritability, and confusion with higher doses of IFN-α.[106] Depression develops over a period of time while confusion manifests rapidly.[106]

There are several mechanisms that help explain the neurological toxicities. Potential contributory causes for these symptoms are a result of IFN-α, secondary cytokines, or both acting directly on the brain inducing alterations in mood and cognition. Cytokine administration alters the production of neuroendocrine hormones resulting in increased levels of cortisol, adrenocorticotrophic hormone (ACTH), and β-endorphin. IFNs are structurally similar to ACTH and β-endorphin and share a common signaling pathway. Evidence suggests that depressive symptoms are mediated by a serotonin deficiency in the brain.[122]

The single most established risk factor for neuropsychiatric effects, especially depression, is the presence of anxiety and mood symptoms prior to the start of IFN therapy. Hauschild et al[106] recommend consulting psychiatrists or psychologists prior to initiating IFN therapy in patients with a prior history of depression or mood disorders. Close observation of patients' behavior, mood, and mental status throughout therapy is imperative. IFN-α has been associated with depression, and suicidal behavior including suicidal ideation, suicide attempts, and suicide.[117] Education of the family and patient can help the healthcare provider identify mental status changes early and implement necessary interventions. Interventions may include the use of antidepressants such as selective serotonin reuptake inhibitors (SSRIs), dose delays or reduction, or referral to a psychiatrist. Other interventions include short-term administration of antianxiety agents such as lorazepam, and use of guided imagery, relaxation techniques, and participation in support groups.[82,123]

## BACILLUS CALMETTE-GUÉRIN

Bacillus Calmette-Guérin (BCG) is an attenuated strain of the mycobacterium virus which was originally developed as a vaccine against tuberculosis in the 1920s. It was noted to have antineoplastic effects under certain conditions, but the precise antitumor mechanism of action of BCG is unknown. BCG is a nonspecific immunomodulatory agent which activates various immune cells including macrophages, NK cells, T lymphocytes, and B lymphocytes.[11,123]

The FDA has approved the use of intravesical BCG (Thera Cys, Tice BCG) instillation as treatment for carcinoma in situ of the bladder. Conditions for optimal response to BCG include localized tumors, minimal tumor burden, and the direct contact of tumor cells with BCG. Bacillus Calmette-Guérin internalizes into bladder epithelial cells via a fibronectin attachment protein once it contacts the tumor cells. When BCG is instilled into the bladder, cytokines are stimulated (IL-1, IL-2, IL-6, and IL-12; IFN-γ and TNF-α) setting off a T-cell-mediated immune response that is linked to anticancer activity[123] and produces a mucosal infection that may last several months. This continued contact with the bladder and immune stimulation provides a longer duration of action than chemotherapy agents since chemotherapeutics are expelled once the patient voids. In addition, BCG penetrates into deeper layers of the bladder wall and has been detected in pelvic lymph nodes after instillation.[123]

Bacillus Calmette-Guérin should be avoided in patients who are immunocompromised, have liver disease, or have a history of tuberculosis. BCG therapy is contraindicated for the following additional reasons:[123,124]

- Urinary tract infection or hematuria
- Acute febrile illness
- For 7 to 14 days following biopsy, transurethral resection, or traumatic catheterization, since there is an increased risk for systemic BCG infection
- Active tuberculosis
- Hypersensitivity to BCG products.

### SIDE EFFECTS AND MANAGEMENT

The dosage of BCG varies but it is usually administered 2 weeks after transuretheral resection of a bladder tumor, or 7 days after a traumatic catheterization to avoid the risk of infection. Side effects are moderate and may include painful, frequent urination and flu-like symptoms including fever. Lower urinary tract symptoms appear after the third instillation of BCG in about 90% of patients and could include dysuria, hematuria, and increased frequency of urination.[123,124]

Symptoms can be managed with acetaminophen, diphenhydramine, or phenazopyridine hydrochloride. The BCG dose can be reduced in patients experiencing symptoms of increasing irritation. Fever is common in patients receiving BCG but prolonged flulike symptoms may indicate BCG infection. Urine should be treated as hazardous waste if the patient voids within 6 hours of instillation; therefore, institutional guidelines should be followed when handling body excretions or wastes.[123,124]

## IMIQUIMOD

Topical biotherapy has been used for several years to treat a variety of skin diseases. Imiquimod, an imidazoquinoline immunomodulator, is an FDA-approved topically applied agent for superficial basal cell carcinoma (BCC), external genital warts, and actinic keratosis.[125] It has also been studied for mycosis fungoides, lentigo melanoma, in combination with surgery for BCC, squamous cell carcinoma, and other disease processes. Imiquimod stimulates multiple cytokines including IFN-α, IFN-γ, TNF-α, IL-1, IL-6, IL-8, IL-10, and IL-12 and has antiviral and antitumor effects. The antiviral and antitumor effects are caused by the stimulation of immune responses in the cutaneous microenvironment and immune enhancement of viral lesions or skin tumors.[125,126] Of interest, imiquimod may reverse chronic immunosuppression caused by chronic sun exposure. This is important given the correlation between sun exposure and skin malignancies.[125]

Common dermatological side effects include application site reaction, erythema and local skin reactions. There are also reports of headache (common) and uncommonly, erythema multiforme, erythroderma, and angioedema. Imiquimod is applied in a thin layer to affected areas after cleansing and drying the area thoroughly. Contact with eyes, lips, and nostrils should be avoided and occlusive dressings should not be used. Patients need to be advised to minimize sun exposure since imiquimod may cause phototoxicity. Sexual activity should be avoided, even with condoms, when this drug is being used to treat genital warts since the cream could weaken condoms and diaphragms.[127]

## CANCER VACCINES

Vaccination is the administration of an immune stimulating agent causing an immune reaction against the foreign substances of the vaccine. These foreign substances known as antigens, will stimulate an immune response with subsequent exposures to the antigen leading the immune system to destroy the antigen. Examples of successful vaccines include polio and smallpox vaccines.[2,19,128,129]

Cancer vaccines differ from traditional or preventive vaccines in that they are considered therapeutic but not preventive. An argument can be made that preventive cancer vaccines do exist, but these are ones that are already in use to prevent a viral infection that can lead to cancer. Vaccines that can be considered prophylactic include vaccination against human papillomavirus (HPV) which has been linked to cervical cancer and vaccination against hepatitis which can lead to liver cancer.[2,15,17,114,128,130–132]

The goal of cancer vaccines is to mobilize the immune system into attacking existing cancer cells by targeting tumor-associated antigens (TAAs). TAAs are structures that are present on tumor cells but are absent or only minimally present on normal cells. These TAAs can be proteins, enzymes, or carbohydrates and they provide a target for immune system recognition and destruction.[2,11,15,18,129] TAAs are divided into different categories that are outlined in Table 20-7.

Melanoma, a highly immunogenic tumor, has been the prototype for many subsequent tumor vaccines. The most comprehensive model for TAA has been established in malignant melanoma because of its high immunogenicity.[128,131,134,135] The most common melanoma-associated antigens (MAGEs) are also expressed on normal melanocytes and include MART-1/Melan A, tyrosinase, and gp100. Other examples of TAAs that are found on normal cells include the human melanoma-associated ganglioside GD2, which is normally expressed on neural tissues, and the cancer testis antigens such as MAGE. MAGE is expressed in the testis and placenta and is not perceived as foreign by the immune system.[128,129,133]

The primary goal of cancer vaccines is to generate an immune response leading to recognition and destruction of the tumor cell. Specific antitumor T-cell immunity must occur so that the immune response can produce a clinical response. The immune system must recognize the TAA as foreign and respond with the proliferation of T cells that have the ability to recognize this specific antigen once the cancer vaccine containing the TAA is administered. These T cells circulate, find the tumor expressing the same antigen, and coordinate its destruction. Two major obstacles in developing adequate cancer vaccines include the identification of suitable antigens to target, and generating a sufficiently strong immune response against the tumor antigens that the immune system has previously been exposed to and become tolerant.[128,129,136]

### MAJOR HISTOCOMPATIBILITY COMPLEX (MHC)

T cells must be stimulated to distinguish self from nonself so that vaccines can work. T cells cannot distinguish self antigens from non-self antigens unless the antigens are presented to them in association with MHC molecules.[11,129] MHC molecules, also known as human leukocyte antigens or HLA, are unique to each person and are present on most cells in the body. The TCR on the surface of the T cell specifically interacts with a peptide/MHC complex on the tumor cell surface. If a peptide is not presented for immune recognition in the form of a peptide/MHC complex, then the desired immune response will not occur. This process is known as MHC restriction.

There are 3 classes of MHC in humans, but only classes I and II actively participate in antigen presentation. MHC class I molecules are found on nearly all nucleated cells and platelets. They restrict antigen presentation to cytotoxic T cells via interaction with the CD8+ molecule. MHC class II molecules are found on subsets of APCs such as dendritic cells, macrophages, monocytes, and B cells. MHC class II molecules restrict antigen presentation to T helper cells via interaction with the CD4+ molecule.[10]

### IMMUNOADJUVANTS

The goal of cancer vaccines is to mount an effective T-cell reaction against the tumor. Tumor cells do not produce the necessary proinflammatory cytokines and chemokines, or warning signals, necessary for the immune system to mount an adequate immune response. Cytokines are crucial in mediating T-cell activation and proliferation. Chemokines are a group of cytokines that act as chemoattractants. They are produced locally by tissues, usually when a pathogen is present, and act on leukocytes to induce immune cell activation. The necessary warning signals can be generated by adding immunoadjuvants to the vaccines. The immunoadjuvants are costimulatory molecules and may include cytokines, chemokines, or other costimulatory substances.[17,129,130]

**TABLE 20-7**

**Prospective Targets for Cancer Vaccines**

| Antigen Type | Description | Antigen (Ag) | Neoplasia |
|---|---|---|---|
| Tissue specific antigen/ differentiation antigens | Found on the tissue of origin of the tumor Examples include retina of the eye and melanocytes | Prostate-specific Ag<br>Prostate-specific membrane Ag<br>Tyrosinase<br>MART-1, gp100<br>α-fetoprotein<br>CEA | Prostate cancer<br>Prostate cancer<br>Melanoma<br>Melanoma<br>Liver cancer<br>Colon, breast, pancreas |
| Cancer testis antigen | Expressed in the testis but not in other normal tissues.<br>MAGE is expressed in placenta and is not perceived as foreign by the immune system. | MAGE-1, MAGE-3, MAGE-12, BAGE, GAGE<br>NY-ESO-1 | Melanoma, lung, gastric, head and neck, bladder<br>Melanoma, breast, lung |
| Tumor-specific antigen | These are unique antigens for individual tumors.<br>They represent normal proteins containing mutations or gene fusions that result in the generation of unique proteins. | Immunoglobin idiotype<br>TCR<br>*BCR/ABL*<br>Mutant *p53* | B-cell NHL, myeloma<br>T-cell NHL<br>CML<br>Lung, colorectal, head and neck, bladder |
| Overexpressed antigens | Antigens shared by normal tissues but overexpressed or altered on tumor cells<br>These mutations cause altered protein sequences in cancer cells making them recognizable by the immune system as foreign. | Mutated Ras<br>HER2/*neu*<br>MUC-1<br>CEA<br>Normal *p53* | Pancreas<br>Breast, ovarian, lung<br>Pancreatic, lung, breast, colorectal, other cancers |
| Viral antigens | Certain malignancies are strongly correlated with viruses.<br>Viral antigens expressed on tumor cells can serve as specific targets for immune destruction.<br>Potentially, these can be considered prophylactic cancer vaccines. | HPV<br>Hepatitis B virus<br>Epstein-Barr Virus<br>Hepatitis C Virus | Cervical<br>Hepatocellular<br>Burkitt's lymphoma<br>Hepatocellular |

*Abbreviations*: CEA, carcinoembryonic antigen; CML, chronic myeloid leukemia; NHL, non-Hodgkin's lymphoma; HPV, human papillomavirus; MAGE, RAGE, GAGE, all are melanoma-associated antigens.

*Source*: Data from Bremers et al[12]; Muehlbauer et al[129]; and Dermime et al.[133]

The role of immunoadjuvants is to promote, expedite, or lengthen the immune response to a vaccine.[137] Immunoadjuvants recruit APCs, activate nonspecific immune responses, initiate the reticuloendothelial system, and stimulate recruitment of innate immune responses. The interaction of the T cells and tumor cells in this type of environment enhances the chances of inducing cell kill by the tumor vaccine. The responses are nonspecific to cytokines and chemokines since those responses are broad. The overall immune effect is intensified by stimulating macrophages, NK cells, and T cells.[17,128,129]

Various adjuvants are used in clinical trials with vaccines. Adjuvants can be of bacterial origin (ie, BCG), cytokines such as IL-12 which activates NK cells and T cells, growth factors such as GM-CSF, or gel-type such as aluminum hydroxide which enhances the humoral response.[128,129,137]

## CANCER VACCINE STRATEGIES

A number of cancer vaccine clinical trials using various strategies exist. Multiple trials have been conducted in patients with melanoma, but several clinical trials have been conducted or are underway to test vaccination in patients with cancers of the lung, colon, stomach, prostate, and hematological malignancies.[128] This is a rapidly evolving field so no specific clinical trials will be mentioned in this chapter. An up-to-date summary can be found at http://www.cancer.gov.

The manner in which TAA is supplied or expressed by the cancer vaccine to be presented to the APC can be classified into one of several major categories. First are peptide vaccines which upon injection into the host are taken up by empty MHC molecules on the surface of the APC for presentation. The second group consists of preparations of TAA which are internalized by the APC, processed, and presented in conjunction with an MHC molecule. Vaccines in this category include tumor cells, tumor lysates, and whole tumor bodies. The third category is genetic material that is used to transduce host cells leading to endogenous expression of the TAA. Examples of these include recombinant viruses, bacteria, and naked nucleic acid molecules. A fourth category includes the administration of the APC itself expressing the appropriate TAA. Examples of this approach include dendritic cells which have been pulsed with peptides or transduced with a gene encoding the TAA.[2,11,12,15,128,129] A further overview of various cancer vaccine strategies including advantages and limitations is summarized in Table 20-8.

## HUMAN PAPILLOMAVIRUS VACCINES

The human papillomavirus (HPV) is a sexually transmitted disease that is linked to the development of genital warts, cancers of the cervix, anus, penis, vulva, and vagina. HPV goes mostly undetected and it is estimated that about 25 times more people are infected with HPV than with HIV in the United States.[155] The first FDA-approved vaccine against HPV is Gardasil which is a quadrivalent vaccine against the most common HPV types linked with cervical cancer (HPV types 6, 11, 16, 18). It is approved for the prevention of cervical cancer, genital warts, and cervical precancers in females aged 9 to 26 years old. The bivalent HPV vaccine (HPV types 16 and 18) Cervarix is under investigation in the United States but approved for use in Europe and elsewhere. Approximately 70% of cervical cancers are associated with HPV types 16 and 18. HPV types 6 and 11 are highly associated with genital warts.[156]

Both vaccines are developed from highly purified virus-like particles of the HPV types specific to each vaccine. The virus-like particles mount a humoral immune response which leads to high titers of neutralizing antibody. Gardisil clinical trial results indicated peak antibody levels at 7 months, declining levels at 24 months, and stabilization at month 36. The recommended vaccine dosing schedule is for Gardisil at months 0 (baseline), 2, and 6. It is not yet clear if additional booster vaccines will be needed. The vaccines are most effective when given prior to onset of sexual activity since they do not stimulate regression of established infection.[156–158]

Gardasil should be administered intramuscularly in the deltoid region of the upper arm or in the higher anterolateral section of the thigh. It should not be given as a SC, intradermal, or intravascular injection as it has not been studied with these methods. No dilution or reconstitution is necessary but it should be agitated well before administration.[156,158]

## NURSING MANAGEMENT

Nursing management varies depending on the route of administration. Prophylactic analgesia may be necessary for vaccines administered intradermally. Frequently, multiple injections are given over time so the sites of injections need to be monitored for redness, swelling, ulceration, tenderness, induration, and any site-specific symptoms. Some vaccines administered IV require pretreatment with antipyretics as patients can develop fever and chills; although, constitutional symptoms are generally minimal. Patients should be assessed for systemic effects regardless of the route of injection. Patients are monitored in the clinical setting for at least 15 minutes post vaccination in the event of an allergic reaction. Educating patients about side effects and what to report is necessary to monitor vaccine reactions and treat accordingly.[2,128,129]

## CURRENT STATUS/FUTURE DIRECTIONS

At this time, outcomes of clinical trials incorporating vaccines have been disappointing. Only rare and sporadic regressions of solid tumors have been reported.[159] Cancer vaccines remain under investigation but are increasingly incorporated as part of multimodality regimens including combinations with surgery, other biological agents, chemotherapy, radiation therapy, and stem cell transplantation.[129] The search for therapeutic cancer vaccines remains a major area of research. Patients who have intact immune systems and a small volume of disease may be the best candidates for cancer vaccine trials. Immunological end points may be helpful in directing efforts to optimize a vaccine strategy and its delivery. Efficacy of the vaccine will be established when clinical endpoints such as tumor shrinkage, delay in time to disease progression, or improvement in survival are measured rather than immunological endpoints.[160]

Frequently, there is no correlation with clinical regression of disease even though innate CTL can be generated against vaccines. Investigators question why the CTL activity does not overcome the targeted tumors raising the possibility that tumors resist immunotherapy because of an insufficient immune response. It is also possible that tumors adapt to the immune pressure and switch to less immunogenic phenotypes.[16]

The optimal vaccine, route, and immunization schedule remain to be determined. The most advantageous strategies for presenting antigens to the immune effecter cells continue to be explored. Progress in the ability to monitor immune response will allow greater understanding of how vaccines work and how tumors escape immune recognition.[2,16,133,147,161]

**TABLE 20-8**

**Vaccine Approaches**

| Vaccine Approach | Description | Advantages | Limitations | Diseases Targeted/Clinical Studies |
|---|---|---|---|---|
| Peptide/ Protein[129,133,138–142] | • Peptides provide the minimal target required for T-cell recognition, and vaccines using peptides can elicit T-cell-mediated immunity.<br>• Evidence shows that T-cell immunity is augmented when peptide vaccines are given with adjuvants.<br>• The immunogenicity of peptide vaccines may be improved by modifying amino acid sequences thus potentiating the interaction with HLA or with the specific TCR. | • Immune response is directed mainly against tumor cells and not normal tissues.<br>• Low toxicity profile<br>• Inexpensive to manufacture | • Peptides may not be processed naturally by APCs leading to the possibility of generating an unimportant peptide-specific response<br>• Low clinical response rates reported and possibly due to previous chemo or radiation therapy<br>• Advanced disease stage of many participants<br>• Immune escape of tumors | • The first peptide vaccines used in clinical studies were in patients with metastatic melanoma.<br>• Attempts are underway to develop peptide vaccines for common epithelial tumors such as those with mutations in the ras oncogene (pancreas, colon, and lung cancer), HER-2/*neu* oncogene (breast, ovary, and colorectal cancer), and PSA.<br>• Peptide vaccine trials directed against viruses such as HPV are also in progress. |
| Recombinant viral (poxvirus and adenovirus)/ bacterial[12,129,133,143,144] | • Recombinant techniques allow tumor antigen genes to be introduced into viruses (poxvirus or adenovirus) that attract APCs and maximize antigen presentation to the immune system.<br>• This strong immune response is generated by a viral infection which is foreign to the host and produces a significant inflammatory response.<br>• Several modalities can be utilized for generating viral cancer vaccines including:<br>  • Tumor cells may be used as the source of antigens, and adenovirus and poxvirus vectors deliver the immunomodulatory genes to the tumor cells.<br>  • One or more TAA genes can be inserted into a virus and administered as a traditional vaccine or intravenously.<br>  • Viral vaccines can be delivered by infecting dendritic cells in vitro with either recombinant poxvirus or adenoviral vectors containing tumor antigen genes or costimulatory genes. | • Recombinant gene products tend to be more immunogenic<br>• Poxviruses have a large capacity available within their genomes to insert foreign DNA and multiple genes.<br>• Poxvirus based vaccines are stable for long periods of time, safe, easy to administer, and cost-effective.<br>• Possible continuous supply of tumor antigen-derived peptides for immune presentation<br>• Accurate replication | • Require available cloned antigens<br>• Neutralizing antibodies may recognize the viral vector, especially with adenovirus | • Clinical studies with poxviruses include those directed against cancers over expressing CEA, HPV, MART, gp100, and PSA.<br>• Trials employing adenoviral vectors have been performed in patients with melanoma, breast cancer and neuroblastoma. |
| Dendritic Cell Vaccines[12,129,133,145,146] | • DCs are the most potent APCs and are found throughout the body, principally in areas that are entry sites for infectious organisms.<br>• DCs capture, process uptake antigens from tissues, and transport the antigens from peripheral to primary and secondary lymphoid sites.<br>• The DCs express high levels of MHC class I and II molecules, and high levels of costimulatory molecules necessary to signal T-cell activation. | • Hypothesized that using DCs may lead to prolonged tumor response by efficient activation of specific T cells.<br>• Generally well tolerated with few toxicities. | • Generating DCs is labor intensive, requiring large facilities to generate sufficient DCs preparation | • Several phase I and II clinical trials have been performed using DC-based vaccine therapy in an attempt to treat multiple cancers including melanoma, B-cell lymphoma, renal cell carcinoma, neuroendrocrine, brain, lung, and prostate cancer.<br>• Improving early results of DC therapy may lie in understanding the best possible routes of administration, methods to load DCs and the role of concomitant cytokine therapy. |

| | | | | |
|---|---|---|---|---|
| Dendritic Cell Vaccines (Continued) | • Primary tumors with histological evidence of infiltration with DC has been associated with prolonged patient survival and decreased metastatic disease in patients with cancers of the bladder, lung, esophagus, and nasopharynx.<br>• Conversely, a poorer prognosis has been observed in patients with tumors containing little infiltration of DC.<br>• A variety of methods have been explored to load the MHC molecules of DC with appropriate TAA including pulsing with peptides, protein, cell lysates, transfection with viral vectors and fusing with whole tumor cells.<br>• DC vaccines have been administered via a variety of routes including SC, IV, intradermal, intranodal, intralymphatic, and directly into the tumor.<br>• Optimization of DC-based therapies may be obtained by adding cytokines such as IL-2, IL-12, IL-7, IL-15, IFN-$\alpha$ or Flt-3 ligand thus increasing the immune response. | | | |
| Cellular Vaccines (Whole cell and tumor lysate) [12,15,133, 145,147–152] | • Cellular vaccines use whole tumor cells that are either irradiated or lysed by viral infection.<br>• With autologous tumor cell vaccines, tumor tissue is isolated from various sites on the patient to prepare the vaccine.<br>• Allogeneic tumor cells have been used to prepare tumor cell vaccines to overcome some of the disadvantages of autologous preparations.<br>• Allogeneic tumor cell lines need to be screened for the highest expression of TAAs to induce immune responses in the recipient.<br>• More recent clinical studies have used modified tumor cells (autologous or allogeneic or both) and genetically manipulated them to express immunostimulatory cytokines such as IL-2, granulocyte-macrophage colony-stimulating factor or IFN-$\gamma$.<br>• This diminishes the toxicities from systemic administration of these cytokines while providing the vaccine with the modulatory activity of cytokines. | • Autologous vaccines: Lack of allogeneic tissue-specific antigens that may induce unwanted immune responses in patients receiving vaccine<br>• Allogeneic tumor cell vaccines: Uses multiple established tumor cell lines with no requirement for defined tumor antigen reducing the chance of antigen selection and tumor escape. | • Autologous vaccines: During early stage of patient's disease, no tumor cells may be available. Many laborious steps necessary to prepare and standardize this type of vaccine.<br>• Allogeneic tumor cell vaccines: Moderate potency Changes of tumor cell lines in culture may result in lack of consistent antigen expression and hence stability and reproducibility of vaccine | • Clinical trials have been conducted for melanoma (ie, Melacine and CancerVax vaccines), breast, colorectal, glioblastoma, lung (ie, GVAX®), pancreas (ie, GVAX®), leukemia, sarcoma, renal, and ovarian cancers with modest results.<br>• Some clinical trials utilize cell extracts or semi-purified proteins instead of whole cells called heat shock proteins. HSP are naturally occurring intracellular substances which accompany a large variety of antigenic proteins present in the cell and channel these into MHC Class I and II pathways.<br>• HSP are also able to elicit the necessary warning signals to trigger DC mediated antigen presentation.<br>The use of DC to augment cellular vaccines is under investigation. |

(Continued)

**TABLE 20-8**

**Vaccine Approaches** *(Continued)*

| Vaccine Approach | Description | Advantages | Limitations | Diseases Targeted/Clinical Studies |
|---|---|---|---|---|
| DNA Vaccines[15,133,153–155] | • Interest in developing DNA vaccines comes from the observation that when naked DNA is injected into muscle, a powerful response is generated including cellular and humoral immunity. These vaccines may induce long lasting immune responses by the continuous expression of the tumor antigen from the DNA infected cell. | • Easy access to DNA<br>• Easy handling<br>• Low cost of production | • No good responses in humans reported.<br>• Potentially, DNA encoding self-tumor antigens could integrate into the host genome causing them to be at a high-risk for cellular transformation.<br>• Potential exists to elicit anti-DNA autoantibodies resulting in the induction or exacerbation of systemic autoimmune disease. | • Cancer clinical trials have included those directed against AIDS, hepatitis B, colon cancer, B-cell lymphoma, NHL, melanoma, and cutaneous T-cell lymphoma. |

*Abbreviations*: APC, antigen presenting cell; HSP, heat-shock protein; DC, dendritic cell; PSA, prostate-specific antigen; HPV, human papillomavirus; TCR, T-cell receptor; HLA, human leukocyte antigen; IFN, interferon; IV, intravenous; NHL, non-Hodgkin's lymphoma; MHC, major histocompatibility complex; SC, subcutaneous; TAA, tumor-associated antigen.

## ADOPTIVE CELLULAR TRANSFER THERAPY

Adoptive cell transfer (ACT) therapy is described by Rosenberg as the "transfer of immune cells with antitumor activity that can mediate, directly or indirectly, antitumor effects in the tumor-bearing host [person]."[138] The success of this treatment depends on a number of factors including lymphocyte subtype, presence of the target antigen on the tumor cell for which the lymphocytes are reactive, and the ability of the transferred lymphocytes to overcome suppressive factors that might be present in the patient's immune system or at the tumor site that would prevent the transferred cells from reacting with the tumor. Other factors include how well the lymphocytes recognize the target antigens and the ability of lymphocytes to traffic to tumor locations.[138]

Extensive work has been done in identifying and characterizing melanoma antigens because of the high immunogenicity of that tumor type. Hence, extensive studies using cell transfer therapy have been done in persons with melanoma. Various cell types have been used for this therapy including TIL, peripheral blood lymphocytes (PBL) sensitized in vitro to tumor antigens, and lymphocytes obtained from sites of tumor vaccinations. Recently, other studies have been reported using cell transfer therapy for malignancies such as nasopharyngeal carcinoma, RCC, hepatocellular cancer, pancreatic cancer, and colorectal cancer.[162–165] These studies remain experimental but many report antitumor effects in patients treated with ACT.[159,162–166]

Tumor-infiltrating lymphocytes from melanoma patients exhibit an extensive variety of MAGEs (ie, MART-1, gp100, and tyrosinase) as well as antigens that are expressed on other cancers such as the cancer testes antigen. Each of these antigens is recognized by TIL in an MHC-restricted manner.[138] Attempts at immunization against these target antigens with cancer vaccines have only rarely induced cancer regression despite the evidence that antitumor T cells which recognize tumor antigens can be generated. The generation of antitumor T cells via immunization does not appear adequate to induce regression of metastatic disease. Theoretically, the use of cell transfer therapy may overcome some of the limitations of immunization. Cell transfer therapy allows large numbers of selected cells with high affinity for recognition of tumor antigens to be administered. Reasons that make this a potentially superior therapy include the ability for the cells to be manipulated ex vivo so that they demonstrate antitumor effector function without the interference of endogenous inhibitory factors.[159,167]

The culture and growth of these TIL cells is a long, complex process taking about 5 to 8 weeks from harvest of the cells to infusion into the patient (Dudley ME, personal communication, October 10, 2008). The cells are collected either via peripheral blood or by harvesting tumor. Dudley[168] states that after immune effector cells are collected, they are then cultured ex vivo which eludes normal immune regulatory and suppressive effects. Cellular characteristics that make this therapy viable can be enhanced in cell culture. The methods applied may not be possible in vivo as the agents used to achieve the desirable cellular characteristics may be toxic or could compromise the patient's health. Once the cells have been activated and expanded, they are infused back into the patient.[168] IL-2 is generally given after infusion of adoptive TIL or PBL cells in people with melanoma. The reason is that the IL-2 causes in vivo proliferation and prolonged survival of cells. The efficacy of IL-2 has shown to be enhanced when given in conjunction with cellular therapy.[169]

The National Cancer Institute (NCI) Surgery Branch experience with ACT has been primarily in patients with metastatic melanoma and has evolved throughout the years to include other solid tumors such as breast cancer and colorectal carcinoma. Initially, nonspecific, activated lymphocytes such as lymphokine-activated killer cells (LAK) were tested. The response rates using LAK with IL-2 vs IL-2 alone in patients with metastatic melanoma or RCC were not statistically significant. These early studies indicated that tumor-antigen-specific lymphocytes were necessary for successful cell transfer cancer therapy.[159,167,170]

Currently, trials are underway that combine a lymphocyte depleting chemotherapy preparatory regimen (cyclophosphamide 60 mg/kg for 2 days then fludarabine 25 mg/m$^2$ for 5 days) followed by cell infusion and administration of HD IL-2 (720,000 IU/kg). The elimination of the patient's endogenous lymphocytes makes room for the TIL cells or genetically enhanced PBL and provides an environment for the adoptively transferred lymphocytes to survive and proliferate. Theories have been put forth that innate CD4+ T lymphocytes may suppress the antitumor effects of TIL. The elimination of CD4+CD25+ regulatory T cells with the lymphodepletive chemotherapy regimen may improve adoptive immunotherapy, although clinical trials testing this approach have not been successful to date.[170,171] The chemotherapy preparative regimen has no known effects on melanoma and its sole use is to eliminate innate T lymphocytes prior to cell transfer. These ongoing trials so far have shown ability for transferred cells to survive and grow in patients for several months after adoptive transfer. Objective response rates are reported in 21 of 43 patients (49%).[159]

Dillman and colleagues[164] report the use of autologous activated lymphocytes (AAL) for use in autolymphocyte therapy (ALT) in 47 patients with a variety of malignancies including colorectal cancer, RCC, breast, lung, pancreas, prostate, eccrine and gastric cancers, and sarcoma, melanoma. They describe autolymphocyte therapy as therapy involving helper T lymphocytes but not CTLs. Instead of using tumor as a source of lymphocytes, the lymphocytes were obtained from peripheral blood mononuclear cells (PBMC) via leukapheresis procedures. The initial leukapheresis procedure was done to obtain mononuclear cell products enriched for PBMCs enriched for lymphocytes. The cells were then washed and some were suspended in medium. These ALK cells had significant measurements of TNF-α, IL-1β, IFN-γ, and IL-6, but no IL-2. Patients then underwent up to 6 monthly leukapheresis procedures to collect PBMC for AAL. These cells were cultured in the ALK cells and resulted in increased T lymphocytes, decreased NK cells, decreased suppressor T cells, and increased helper T cells. The final product for IV infusion of AAL was placed into a 50 mL bag of 25% human albumin.

In Dillman's study,[164] patients received 600 mg of the histamine type 2 blocker, cimetidine orally every 6 hours prior to infusion of AAL and then daily until the end of treatment. Treatments were given monthly for 6 months or until disease progression in the outpatient setting. Patients did not receive IL-2 in this study. A variety of support medications were given if the patient experienced side effects such as fever or chills. They report objective tumor responses in patients with RCC and colorectal cancer.[164]

Adoptive cell transfer is evolving as more is learned about the role of the host immune environment on tumor therapy.[170,172,173] One goal is the further study of ACT in tumors other than melanoma. Researchers are looking at alternative methods for obtaining potent cells for adoptive transfer by first priming the patient with autologous tumor vaccination then expanding activated T cells in vivo that will be reinfused.[174] Concurrent vaccination after T-cell transfer has potential for improving ACT.[170] Some methods for advancing ACT include genetically modifying lymphocytes to increase antitumor effects by introducing genes encoded with cytokines, T-cell receptors, or antiapoptotic molecules; administering other cytokines to support cell growth such as IL-15; and stimulation of APCs.[159,167] A more thorough review of ACT can be found in Rosenberg et al.[159]

## CONCLUSION

Biotherapy continues to be a rapidly evolving field. As of press time, more agents and combination of agents have been studied in clinical trials than is feasible to cover in this chapter.

Nurses need to use educational strategies to stay abreast of the field. This may include online Web courses, published literature, information from conferences, and information from specialty organizations. Many, but not all, biological agents are classified as hazardous drugs. Institutional policies guide the nurse's practice in safe handling and disposal of these agents. Side effects from biological agents challenge the nurse to manage the patient for best comfort and to complete therapy.

## REFERENCES

1. Rieger P. Biotherapy: an overview. In: Rieger P, ed. *Biotherapy: A Comprehensive Overview.* 2nd ed. Sudbury, MA: Jones and Bartlett; 2001:3–37.
2. Muehlbauer PM. Biologic therapies for cancer. In: Barton-Burke M, Wilkes G, eds. *Cancer Therapy.* Sudbury, MA: Jones and Bartlett; 2006:117–180.
3. Coley WB. The treatment of inoperable sarcoma with the mixed toxins of erysipelas and *Bacillus prodigiosus. JAMA.* 1898;31:389–395.
4. Coley WB. A report of recent cases of inoperable sarcoma successfully treated with mixed toxins of erysipelas and *Bacillus prodigious. Surg Gynecol Obstet.* 1911;13:174–190.
5. Wheeler VS. Interleukins: the search for an anticancer therapy. *Semin Oncol Nurs.* 1996;12:106–114.
6. Battiato LA. Biotherapy. In: Yarbro CH, Frogge MH, Goodman, M, eds. *Cancer Nursing Principles and Practice.* 6th ed. Sudbury, MA: Jones and Bartlett; 2005:510–558.
7. Schwartzentruber DJ. Interleukin-2: clinical applications. Principles of administration and management of side effects. In: Rosenberg SA, ed. *Principles and Practice of the Biologic Therapy of Cancer.* 3rd ed. Philadelphia, PA: Lippincott Williams & Wilkins; 2000:32–50 (chap 3.1).
8. Shanahan JC, Moreland LW, Carter RH. Upcoming biologic agents for the treatment of rheumatic diseases. *Curr Opin Rheumatol.* 2003;15:226–236.
9. Janeway CA, Travers P, Walport M, Shlomchik MJ. *Immunobiology: The Immune System in Health and Disease.* 6th ed. New York and London: Garland Science; 2005.
10. Hyde RM. *The National Medical Series for Independent Study: Immunology.* 4th ed. Philadelphia, PA: Lippincott Williams & Wilkins; 2000.
11. Siemens DR, Ratliff TL. Vaccines in urologic malignancies. *Urol Res.* 2001;29:152–162.
12. Bremers AJ, Parmiani G. Immunology and immunotherapy of human cancer: present concepts and clinical developments. *Crit Rev Oncol Hematol.* 2000;34:1–25.
13. Tayal V, Kalra BS. Cytokines and anti-cytokines as therapeutics—an update. *Eur J Pharmacol.* 2008;579:1–12.
14. Darrow TL, Abdel-Wahab Z, Seigler HF. Immunotherapy of human melanoma with gene-modified tumor cell vaccines. *Cancer Control.* 1995;2:415–423.
15. Matzku S, Zoller M. Specific immunotherapy of cancer in elderly patients. *Drugs Aging.* 2001;18:639–664.
16. Marincola FM. Cancer vaccines: basic principles: mechanisms of immune escape and immune tolerance. In: Rosenberg SA, ed. *Principles and Practice of the Biologic Therapy of Cancer.* 3rd ed. Philadelphia, PA: Lippincott Williams & Wilkins; 2000:601–617.
17. Restifo NP. Cancer vaccines: basic principles: general concepts and preclinical studies. In: Rosenberg SA, ed. *Principles and Practice of the Biologic Therapy of Cancer.* 3rd ed. Philadelphia, PA: Lippincott Williams & Wilkins; 2000:571–584.
18. Schreiber H. Tumor immunology. In: Paul W, ed. *Fundamental Immunology.* 4th ed. Philadelphia, PA: Lippincott-Raven; 1999:1237–1270.
19. Bindon C, Czerniecki M, Ruell P, et al. Clearance rates and systemic effects of intravenously administered interleukin-2 (Il-2) containing preparations in human subjects. *Br J Cancer.* 1983;47:123–133.
20. Sharp E. The interleukins. In: Reiger PT, ed. *Biotherapy: A Comprehensive Overview.* Sudbury, MA: Jones and Bartlett; 1995:93–111.
21. Tushinki RJ, Mulé JJ. Biology of cytokines: the interleukins. In: DeVita VT, Hellman S, Rosenberg SA, eds. *Biologic Therapy of Cancer.* Philadelphia, PA: JB Lippincott; 1995:87–94.
22. Klapper JA, Downey SG, Smith FO, et al. High-dose interleukin-2 for the treatment of metastatic renal cell carcinoma. *Cancer.* 2008;113:293–301.
23. Rosenberg SA, Yang JC, White DE, Steinberg SM. Durability of complete responses in patients with metastatic cancer treated with high-dose interleukin-2: identification of the antigens mediating response. *Ann Surg.* 1998;228:307–319.
24. Fyfe G, Fisher RI, Rosenberg SA, Sznol M, Parkinson DR, Louie AC. Results of treatment of 255 patients with metastatic renal cell

carcinoma who received high-dose recombinant interleukin-2 therapy. *J Clin Oncol.* 1995;13:688–696.
25. Rosenberg SA, Yang JC, Topalian SL, et al. Treatment of 283 consecutive patients with metastatic melanoma or renal cell cancer using high-dose bolus interleukin 2. *JAMA.* 1994;271:907–913.
26. Atkins MB, Sparano J, Fisher RI, et al. Randomized phase II trial of high-dose interleukin-2 either alone or in combination with interferon alpha-2b in advanced renal cell carcinoma. *J Clin Oncol.* 1993;11:661–670.
27. Gale D, Sorokin P. The interleukins. In: Rieger P, ed. *Biotherapy: A Comprehensive Overview.* 2nd ed. Sudbury, MA: Jones and Bartlett; 2001:198–244.
28. Noble S, Goa KL. Aldesleukin (Recombinant Interleukin-2): a review of its pharmacological properties, clinical efficacy and tolerability in patients with metastatic melanoma. *Biodrugs.* 1997;7:394–422.
29. Durum S. Interleukins: overview. In: Rosenberg SA, ed. *Principles and Practice of the Biologic Therapy of Cancer.* Philadelphia, PA: Lippincott Williams & Wilkins; 2000:3–18.
30. Novartis Pharmaceuticals Corporation. Proleukin (aldesleukin for injection) package insert. East Hanover, NJ: Novartis Pharmaceuticals Corporation; 2007.
31. Lechleider RJ, Arlen PM, Tsang WY, et al. Safety and immunologic response of a viral vaccine to prostate-specific antigen in combination with radiation therapy when metronomic-dose Interleukin 2 is used as an adjuvant. *Clin Cancer Res.* 2008;14:5284–5291.
32. Amato RJ, Malya R, Rawat AN. Phase II study of combination thalidomide/Interleukin-2 therapy plus granulocyte macrophage-colony stimulating factor in patients with metastatic renal cell carcinoma. *Am J Clin Oncol.* 2008;31:237–243.
33. Del Monte G, Ferroni P, Mariotti S, Fossile E, Guadagni F, Roselli M. Interleukin-2 inhalation therapy in renal cell cancer: a case report and review of the literature. *In Vivo.* 2008;22:481–488.
34. Mavroukakis SA, Muehlbauer PM, White RL, Schwartzentruber DJ. Clinical pathways for managing patients receiving Interleukin-2. *Clin J Oncol Nurs.* 2001;5:207–217.
35. Temesgen Z. Interleukin-2 for the treatment of human immunodeficiency virus infection. *Drugs Today.* 2006;42:791–801.
36. Napolitano LA. Approaches to immune reconstitution in HIV infection. *Top HIV Med.* 2003;11:160–163.
37. Lu AC, Jones EC, Chow C, et al. Increases in CD4+ T lymphocytes occur without increases in thymic size in HIV-infected subjects receiving interleukin-2 therapy. *J Acquir Immune Defic Syndr.* 2003;34:299–303.
38. Morris K. HAART and host: balancing the response to HIV-1. *Lancet.* 1998;352:1686.
39. Arduino RC, Nannini EC, Rodriguez-Barradas M, et al. CD4 cell response to 3 doses of subcutaneous interleukin 2: meta-analysis of 3 Vanguard studies. *HIV/AIDS.* 2004;39:115–122.
40. Conrad A. Interleukin-2¾where are we going? *J Assoc Nurses AIDS Care.* 2003;14:83–88.
41. Tourani JM, Pfister C, Tubiana N, et al. Subcutaneous interleukin-2 and interferon-alfa administration in patients with metastatic renal cell carcinoma: final results of SCAPP III, a large, multicenter, phase II, nonrandomized study with sequential analysis design¾the subcutaneous administration Propeukin program cooperative group. *J Clin Oncol.* 2003;21:3987–3994.
42. McDermott D, Flaherty L, Clark J, et al. A randomized phase III trial of high-dose interleukin-2 versus subcutaneous IL-2 plus interferon in patients with metastatic renal cell carcinoma. *Proc Am Soc Clin Oncol.* 2001;20:172a (abstract 685).
43. Atzpodien J, Hänninen EL, Kirchner H, et al. Multi-institutional home-therapy trial of recombinant interleukin-2 and interferon-alfa in progressive metastatic renal cell carcinoma. *J Clin Oncol.* 1995;13:497–501.
44. Ravaud A, Negrier S, Cany L, et al. Subcutaneous low-dose interleukin-2 and alpha-interferon in patients with metastatic renal cell carcinoma. *Br J Cancer.* 1994;69:1111–1114.
45. Dutcher J. Current status of interleukin-2 therapy for metastatic renal cell carcinoma and metastatic melanoma. *Oncology.* 2002;16(suppl 11):4–10.
46. Hauschild A, Weichenthal M, Balda B-R, et al. Prospective randomized trial of interferon alfa-2b and interleukin-2 as adjuvant treatment for resected intermediate- and high-risk primary melanoma without clinically detectable node metastasis. *J Clin Oncol.* 2003;21:2883–2888.
47. Mitchell MS. Combinations of anticancer drugs and immunotherapy. *Cancer Immunol Immunother.* 2003;52:686–692.
48. Slavin S, Morecki S, Weiss L, Or R. Immunotherapy of hematologic malignancies and metastatic solid tumors in experimental animals and man. *Crit Rev Oncol/Hematol.* 2003;46:139–163.
49. Buzaid AC. Biochemotherapy for advanced melanoma. *Crit Rev Oncol/Hematol.* 2002;44:103–108.
50. Flaherty LE, Atkins M, Sosman J, et al. Outpatient biochemotherapy with interleukin-2 and interferon alfa-2b in patients with metastatic malignant melanoma: results of two phase II Cytokine Working Group trials. *J Clin Oncol.* 2001;19:3194–3202.
51. Atkins MB, Hsu J, Lee S, et al. Phase III trial comparing concurrent biochemotherapy with cisplatin, vinblastine, dacarbazine, interleukin-2, and interferon-alfa2b with cisplatin, vinblastine, and dacarbazine alone in patients with metastatic malignant melanoma (E3695): a trial coordinated by the Eastern Cooperative Oncology Group. *J Clin Oncol.* 2008;26:1–9.
52. Hamm C, Verma S, Petrella T, Bak K, Charette M. Biochemotherapy for the treatment of metastatic melanoma: a systematic review. *Cancer Treat Rev.* 2008;34:145–156.
53. Ives NJ, Stowe RL, Lorigan P, Wheatley K. Chemotherapy compared with biochemotherapy for the treatment of metastatic melanoma: a meta-analysis of 18 trials involving 2,621 patients. *J Clin Oncol.* 2007;25:5426–5434.
54. Bajetta E, Del Vecchio M, Nova P, et al. Multicenter phase III randomized trial of polychemotherapy (CVD regimen) versus the same chemotherapy (CT) plus subcutaneous interleukin-2 and interferon-α2b in metastatic melanoma. *Ann Oncol.* 2006;17:571–577.
55. Yang JC, Rosenberg SA. An ongoing prospective randomized comparison of Interleukin-2 regimens for the treatment of metastatic renal cell cancer. *Cancer J Sci Am.* 1997;3(suppl 1):S79-S84.
56. Yang JC, Sherry RM, Steinberg SM, et al. Randomized study of high-dose and low-dose interleukin-2 in patients with metastatic renal cancer. *J Clin Oncol.* 2003;21:3127–3132.
57. Kammula US, White DE, Rosenberg SA. Trends in the safety of high dose bolus interleukin-2 administration in patients with metastatic cancer. *Cancer.* 1998;83:797–805.
58. Schwartzentruber DJ. Guidelines for the safe administration of high-dose Interleukin-2. *J Immunother.* 2001;24:287–293.
59. Schwartz R, Stover L, Dutcher J. Managing toxicities of high-dose interleukin-2. *Oncology (Suppl).* 2002;16:11–20.
60. Dutcher J, Atkins MB, Margolin K, et al. Kidney cancer: the cytokine working group experience (1986–2001). *Med Oncol.* 2001;18:209–219.
61. Mitchell SA, Beck SL, Hood LE, Moore K, Tanner ER. Putting evidence into practice: evidence-based interventions for fatigue during and following cancer and its treatment. *Clin J Oncol Nurs.* 2007;11:99–113.
62. Curt GA. The impact of fatigue on patients with cancer: overview of FATIGUE 1 and 2. *Oncologist.* 2000;5(suppl 2):9–12.
63. Portenoy RK, Itri LM. Cancer-related fatigue: guidelines for evaluation and management. *Oncologist.* 1999;4:1–10.
64. Charland MB, Management of adverse effects associated with use of interleukin-2 in patients with HIV infection *J Assoc Nurses AIDS Care.* 2003;14:89–95.
65. ASHP therapeutic guidelines on the pharmacologic management of nausea and vomiting in adult and pediatric patients receiving chemotherapy or radiation therapy or undergoing surgery. *AM J Health Syst Pharm.* 1999;56:729–764.
66. Benson AB III, Ajani JA, Catalano RB, et al. Recommended guidelines for the treatment of cancer treatment-induced diarrhea. *J Clin Oncol.* 2004;22:2918–2926.

67. Halmos B, Krishnamurthi S. Enterotoxicity of chemotherapeutic agents. 2008. http://www.uptodate.com. Accessed January 23, 2010.
68. Drabot R. Nutrition and immunotherapy. *Oncol Nutr Connect.* 2008;16:14–19.
69. Heimann DM, Schwartzentruber DJ. Gastrointestinal perforations associated with interleukin-2 administration. *J Immunother.* 2004;27:254–258.
70. Smith FO, Goff SL, Klapper JA, et al. Risk of bowel perforation in patients receiving interleukin-2 after therapy with anti-CTLA4 monoclonal antibody. *J Immunother.* 2007;30:130.
71. Mier JW. Pathogenesis of the interleukin-2-induced vascular leak syndrome. In: Atkins MB, Mier JW, eds. *Therapeutic Applications of Interleukin-2.* New York: Marcel Dekker; 1993:363–379.
72. Kragel AH, Travis WD, Steis RG, Rosenberg SA, Roberts WC. Myocarditis or acute myocardial infarction associated with Interleukin-2 therapy for cancer. *Cancer.* 1990;66:1513–1516.
73. White RL, Schwartzentruber DJ, Guleria A, et al. Cardiopulmonary toxicity of treatment with high dose Interleukin-2 in 199 consecutive patients with metastatic melanoma or renal cell carcinoma. *Cancer.* 1994;74:3212–3222.
74. Pockaj BA, Yang JC, Lotze MT, et al. A prospective randomized trial evaluating colloid versus crystalloid resuscitation in the treatment of the vascular leak syndrome associated with interleukin-2 therapy. *J Immunother.* 1994;15:22–28.
75. Guleria AS, Yang JC, Topalian SL, et al. Renal dysfunction associated with the administration of high-dose Interleukin-2 in 199 consecutive patients with metastatic melanoma or renal carcinoma. *J Clin Oncol.* 1994;12:2714–2722.
76. Sparber AG, Biller-Sparber K. Immunotherapy and neuropsychiatric toxicity: nursing clinical management considerations. *Cancer Nurs.* 1993;16:188–192.
77. Lerner DM, Stoudemire A, Rosenstein DL. Neuropsychiatric toxicity associated with cytokine therapies. *Psychosomatics.* 1999;40:428–435.
78. Gallagher J. Management of cutaneous symptoms. *Semin Oncol Nurs.* 1995;11:239–247.
79. MacFarlane MP, Yang JC, Guleria AS, et al. The hematologic toxicity of Interleukin-2 in patients with metastatic melanoma and renal cell carcinoma. *Cancer.* 1995;75:1030–1037.
80. Proleukin (interleukin 2) [prescribing information]. East Hanover, NJ: Novartis; 2007.
81. Williams BRG. Interferon-α and -β: basic principles and preclinical studies. In: Rosenberg SA, ed. *Principles and Practice of the Biologic Therapy of Cancer.* 3rd ed. Philadelphia, PA: Lippincott Williams & Wilkins; 2000:194–208.
82. Cuaron L, Thompson J. The interferons. In: Rieger P, ed. *Biotherapy: A Comprehensive Overview.* 2nd ed. Sudbury, MA: Jones and Bartlett; 2001:125–194.
83. Cantell K, Hervonen S, Cavalletto L, et al. Human leukocyte interferon production, purification and animal experiments. In: Waymouth C, ed. *In Vitro.* Baltimore, MD: Baltimore Tissue Culture Association; 1975:35–38.
84. Clemens MJ. Interferons and apoptosis. *J Interferon Cytokine Res.* 2003;23:277–292.
85. Micromedex Health Care series online. Interferon alfa. Martindale¾the complete drug reference. 2004. http://www.micromedex.com. Accessed January 24, 2010.
86. Cáceres W, González S. Angiogenesis and cancer: recent advances. *P R Health Sci J.* 2003;22:149–151.
87. Muehlbauer PM. Antiangiogenesis in cancer therapy. *Semin Oncol Nurs.* 2003;19:180–192.
88. Krown SE, Li P, Von Roenn JH, Paredes J, Huang J, Testa MA. Efficacy of low-dose interferon with antiretroviral therapy in Kaposi's sarcoma: a randomized phase II AIDS clinical trials group study. *J Interferon Cytokine Res.* 2002;22:295–303.
89. Kerbel RS, Viloria-Petit A, Klement G, Rak J. "Accidental" anti-angiogenic drugs: anti-oncogene directed signal transduction inhibitors and conventional chemotherapeutic agents as examples. *Eur J Cancer.* 2000;26:1248–1257.
90. Hernberg M, Virkkunen P, Bono P, Maenpaa H, Joensuu H. Interferon alfa-2b three times daily and thalidomide in the treatment of metastatic renal cell carcinoma. *J Clin Oncol.* 2003;21:3770–3776.
91. Hughes TP, Kaeda J, Branford S, et al. Frequency of major molecular responses to imatinib or interferon alfa plus cytarabine in newly diagnosed chronic myeloid leukemia. *New Engl J Med.* 2003;349:1423–1432.
92. Hehlmann R, Berger U, Pfirrmann M, et al. Randomized comparison of interferon α and hydroxyurea with hydroxyurea monotherapy in chronic myeloid leukemia (CML study II): prolongation of survival by the combination of interferon α and hydroxyurea. *Leukemia.* 2003;17:1529–1537.
93. O'Brien S, Giles F, Talpaz M, et al. Results of triple therapy with interferon-alpha, cytarabine, and homoharringtonine, and the impact of adding imatinib to the treatment sequence in patients with Philadelphia chromosome-positive chronic myelogenous leukemia in early chronic phase. *Cancer.* 2003;98:888–893.
94. Allen IE, Ross SD, Borden SP, et al. Meta-analysis to assess the efficacy of interferon-α in patients with follicular Non-Hodgkins lymphoma. *J Immunother.* 2001;24:58–65.
95. Oon CJ, Chen WN. Lymphoblastoid alpha-interferon in the prevention of hepatocellular carcinoma (HCC) in high-risk HbsAg-positive resected cirrhotic HCC cases: a 14-year follow-up. *Cancer Invest.* 2003;21:394–399.
96. Yao F, Terrault N. Hepatitis C and hepatocellular carcinoma. *Curr Treat Options Oncol.* 2001;2:473–483.
97. Ziotta AR, Schulman CC. Biological response modifiers for the treatment of superficial bladder tumors. *Eur Urol.* 2000;37(suppl 3):10–15.
98. Santhanam S, Decatris M, O'Byrne K. Potential of interferon-α in solid tumors, Part 2. *Biodrugs.* 2002;16:349–372.
99. Moschos S, Kirkwood JM, Konstantinopoulos PA. Present status and future prospects of adjuvant therapy of melanoma: time to build upon the foundation of high-dose interferon alfa-2B. *J Clin Oncol.* 2004;22:11–14.
100. Masci P, Borden EC. Malignant melanoma: treatments emerging, but early detection is still key. *Cleve Clin J Med.* 2002;69:529–540.
101. Hancock BW, Wheatley K, Harris S, et al. Adjuvant interferon in high-risk melanoma: the AIM HIGH study-United Kingdom Coordinating Committee on cancer research randomized study of adjuvant low-dose extended duration interferon alfa-2a in high-risk resected malignant melanoma. *J Clin Oncol.* 2004;22:53–61.
102. Schuchter LM. Adjuvant interferon therapy for melanoma: high-dose, low-dose, no dose, which dose? *J Clin Oncol.* 2004;22:7–10.
103. Eggermont AMM, Punt CJA. Does adjuvant systemic therapy with interferon-α for stage II-III melanoma prolong survival? *Am J Clin Dermatol.* 2003;4:531–536.
104. Decatris M, Santhanam S, O'Byrne K. Potential of interferon-α in solid tumours, Part 1. *Biodrugs.* 2002;16:261–281.
105. Wheatley K, Ives N, Hancock B, Gore M, Eggermont A, Suciu S. Does adjuvant interferon-α for high-risk melanoma provide a worthwhile benefit? A meta-analysis of the randomized trials. *Cancer Treat Rev.* 2003;29:241–252.
106. Hauschild A, Gogas H, Tarhini A, et al. Practical guidelines for the management of interferon-α-2b side effects in patients receiving adjuvant treatment for melanoma. *Cancer.* 2008;112:982–994.
107. Igarashi T, Marumo K, Onishi T, et al. Interferon-alpha and 5-Flourouracil therapy in patients with metastatic renal cell cancer: an open multicenter trial. *Urology.* 1999;53:53–59.
108. Bukowski RM, Tendler C, Cutler D, Rose E, Laughlin MM, Statkevich P. Treating cancer with PEG Intron. *Cancer.* 2002;95:389–396.
109. Nuelasta (pegfilgrastim): prescribing information. Thousand Oaks, CA: Amgen; 2002.

110. Hussar DA. New drugs 2002. *Nursing.* 2002;32:56–62.
111. Michallet M, Maloisel F, Delain M, et al. Pegylated recombinant interferon alpha-2b vs. recombinant interferon alpha-2b for the initial treatment of chronic-phase chronic myelogenous leukemia: a phase III study. *Leukemia.* 2004;18:309–315.
112. Battiato LA, Wheeler VS. Biotherapy. In: Yarbro CH, Frogge MH, Goodman M, Groenwald SL, eds. *Cancer Nursing Principles and Practice.* 5th ed. Sudbury, MA: Jones and Bartlett; 2000: 543–579.
113. Tretter C, Savage PD, Muss HB, Ernstoff MD. Interferon-$\alpha$ and -$\beta$: clinical applications: renal cell cancer. In: Rosenberg SA, ed. *Principles and Practice of the Biologic Therapy of Cancer.* 3rd ed. Philadelphia, Lippincott Williams & Wilkins; 2000:252–273.
114. Dean GE. Fatigue. In: Rieger PT, ed. *Biotherapy: A Comprehensive Overview.* 2nd ed. Sudbury, MA: Jones and Bartlett; 2001:547–575.
115. Kiley KE, Gale DE. Nursing management of patients with malignant melanoma receiving adjuvant alpha interferon-2b. *Clin J Oncol Nurs.* 1998;2:11–16.
116. Hauschild A, Gogas H, Tarhini A, et al. Practical guidelines for the management of interferon-$\alpha$-2b side effects in patients receiving adjuvant treatment for melanoma. *Cancer.* 2008;112:982–994.
117. INTRON-A for Injection. Physician's Desk Reference. 2002. http://micromedex.com. Accessed October 16, 2008.
118. Cella D, Lai JS, Chang CH, Peterman A, Slavin M. Fatigue in cancer patients compared with fatigue in the general United States population. *Cancer.* 2002;94:528–538.
119. Shelton BK. Flu-like syndrome. In: Rieger PT, ed. *Biotherapy: A Comprehensive Overview.* 2nd ed. Sudbury, MA: Jones and Bartlett; 2001:519–543.
120. Kirkwood JM. Interferon-$\alpha$ and -$\beta$: clinical applications: melanoma. In: Rosenberg SA, ed. *Principles and Practice of the Biologic Therapy of Cancer.* 3rd ed. Philadelphia, PA: Lippincott Williams & Wilkins; 2000:224–251.
121. Stafford-Fox V, Guindon KM. Cutaneous reactions associated with alpha interferon therapy. *Clin J Oncol Nurs.* 2000;4:164–168.
122. Malek-Ahmadi P, Hilsabeck RC. Neuropsychiatric complications of interferons: classification, neurochemical bases and management. *Ann Clin Psychiatry.* 2007;19:113–123.
123. Kassouf W, Kamat W. Current state of immunotherapy for bladder cancer. *Expert Rev Anticancer Ther.* 2004;4:1037–1046.
124. Washburn DJ. Intravesical antineoplastic therapy following transurethral resection of bladder tumors: nursing implications from the operating room to discharge. *Clin J Oncol Nurs.* 2007;11:553–559.
125. Papadavid E, Stratigos AJ, Falagas ME. Imiquimod: an immune response modifier in the treatment of precancerous skin lesions and skin cancer. *Expert Opin Pharmacother.* 2007;8:1743–1755.
126. Martinez-Gonzalez MC, Verea-Hernando MM, Yebra-Pimentel MT, Del Pozo J, Mazaira M, Fonseca E. Imiquimod in mycosis fungoides. *Eur J Dermatol.* 2008;18:148–152.
127. Imiquimod. DrugPoint® Summary. 2008. http://micromedex.com. Accessed December 10, 2008.
128. Muehlbauer PM, Schwartzentruber DJ. Cancer vaccines. *Semin Oncol Nurs.* 2003;19:206–216.
129. Kinzler D, Brown C. Cancer vaccines. In: Rieger P, ed. *Biotherapy: A Comprehensive Overview.* 2nd ed. Sudbury, MA: Jones and Bartlett; 2001:357–382.
130. King SE. Therapeutic cancer vaccines: an emerging treatment option. *Clin J Oncol Nurs.* 2004;8:271–278.
131. Mitchell MS. Cancer vaccines, a critical review—Part I. *Curr Opin Investig Drugs.* 2002;3:140–149.
132. Lowy DR, Schiller JT. Papillomaviruses and cervical cancer: pathogenesis and vaccine development. *J Natl Cancer Inst Monogr.* 1998;23:27–30.
133. Dermime S, Armstrong A, Hawkins RE, Stern PL. Cancer vaccines and immunotherapy. *Br Med Bull.* 2002;62:149–162.
134. Boon T, Van den Eynde B. Cancer vaccines: cancer antigens: shared tumor-specific antigens. In: Rosenberg SA, ed. *Principles and Practice of the Biologic Therapy of Cancer.* 3rd ed. Philadelphia, PA: Lippincott Williams & Wilkins; 2000:493–504.
135. Nestle FO, Burg G, Dummer R. New perspectives on immunobiology and immunotherapy of melanoma. *Immunol Today.* 1999;20:5–7.
136. Borrello IM, Sotomayor EM. Cancer vaccines for hematologic malignancies. *Cancer Control.* 2002;9:138–151.
137. Salgaller ML. Cancer vaccines: basic principles: immune adjuvants. In: Rosenberg SA, ed. *Principles and Practice of the Biologic Therapy of Cancer.* 3rd ed. Philadelphia, PA: Lippincott Williams and Wilkins; 2000:584–601.
138. Rosenberg SA. Cell transfer therapy: clinical applications, melanoma. In: Rosenberg SA, ed. *Principles and Practice of the Biologic Therapy of Cancer.* 3rd ed. Philadelphia, PA: Lippincott Williams & Wilkins; 2000:322–333.
139. Disis ML. Introduction and overview. Therapeutic cancer vaccines: targeting the future of cancer treatment. *Medscape Today.* 2002. http://www.medscape.com.
140. Parmiani G, Castelli C, Dalerba P, et al. Cancer immunotherapy with peptide-based vaccines: what have we achieved? Where are we going? *J Natl Cancer Inst.* 2002;94:805–818.
141. Salit RB, Kast WM, Velders MP. Ins and outs of clinical trials with peptide-based vaccines. *Front Biosci.* 2002;7:e204–e213.
142. Rosenberg SA. Cancer vaccines: clinical applications: peptides and protein vaccines. In: Rosenberg SA, ed. *Principles and Practice of the Biologic Therapy of Cancer.* 3rd ed. Philadelphia, PA: Lippincott Williams & Wilkins; 2000:662–673.
143. Roberts B. Cancer vaccines: clinical applications: adenovirus and other viral vaccines. In: Rosenberg SA, ed. *Principles and Practice of the Biologic Therapy of Cancer.* 3rd ed. Philadelphia, PA: Lippincott Williams & Wilkins; 2000:694–705.
144. Schlom J, Panicali D. Cancer vaccines: clinical applications: recombinant poxvirus vaccines. In Rosenberg SA, ed. *Principles and Practice of the Biologic Therapy of Cancer.* 3rd ed. Philadelphia, PA: Lippincott Williams & Wilkins; 2000:686–694.
145. Kugler A, Stuhler G, Walden P, et al. Regression of human metastatic renal cell carcinoma after vaccination with tumor cell-dendritic cell hybrids. *Nat Med.* 2000;6:332–336.
146. Dallal RM, Mailliard R, Lotze MT. Cancer vaccines: clinical applications: dendritic cell vaccines. In: Rosenberg SA, ed. *Principles and Practice of the Biologic Therapy of Cancer.* 3rd ed. Philadelphia, PA: Lippincott Williams & Wilkins; 2000:705–721.
147. Mocellin S, Rossi CR, Lise M, et al. Adjuvant immunotherapy for solid tumors: from promise to clinical application. *Cancer Immunol Immunother.* 2002;51:583–595.
148. Weber J. Tumor-antigen vaccines for cancer. Therapeutics cancer vaccines: targeting the future of cancer treatment. *Medscape Today.* 2002. http://www.medscape.com.
149. Belli F, Testori A, Rivoltini L, et al. Vaccination of metastatic melanoma patients with autologous tumor-derived heat shock protein gp96-peptide complexes: clinical and immunologic findings. *J Clin Oncol.* 2002;20:4169–4180.
150. Sondak VK, Liu PY, Tuthill RJ, et al. Adjuvant immunotherapy of resected, intermediate-thickness, node-negative melanoma with an allogeneic tumor vaccine: overall results of a randomized trial of the Southwest Oncology Group. *J Clin Oncol.* 2002;20:2058–2066.
151. Sivanandham M, Stavropoulos C, Wallack M. Cancer vaccines: clinical applications: whole cell and lysate vaccines. In: Rosenberg SA, ed. *Principles and Practice of the Biologic Therapy of Cancer.* 3rd ed. Philadelphia, PA: Lippincott Williams & Wilkins; 2000:632–647.
152. Harris JE, Ryan L, Hoover HC Jr, et al. Adjuvant active specific immunotherapy for stage II and III colon cancer with an autologous tumor cell vaccine: Eastern Cooperative Oncology Group Study E5283. *J Clin Oncol.* 2000;18:148–157.
153. Morse MA. Current status of dendritic cell vaccines. Therapeutic cancer vaccines: targeting the future of cancer treatment. *Medscape Today.* 2002. http://www.medscape.com. Accessed 19 october, 2009.

154. Sundaram R, Dakappagari NK, Kaumaya PT. Synthetic peptides as cancer vaccines. *Biopolymers.* 2002;66:200–216.
155. White S, Conry R. Cancer vaccines: clinical applications: DNA vaccines. In: Rosenberg SA, ed. *Principles and Practice of the Biologic Therapy of Cancer.* 3rd ed. Philadelphia, PA: Lippincott Williams & Wilkins; 2000:674–686.
156. Tovar JM, Bazaldua OV, Vargas L, Reile E. Human papillomavirus, cervical cancer and the vaccines. *Postgrad Med.* 2008;120:79–83.
157. Schiller JT, Castellsagué X, Villa LL, Hildesheim A. An update of prophylactic human papillomavirus L1 virus-like particle vaccine clinical trial results. *Vaccine.* 2008;265:K53-K61.
158. Gardasil, Package Insert, Merck. http://www.micromedex.com. 2007. Accessed January 24, 2010.
159. Rosenberg SA, Restifo NP, Yang JC, Morgan RA, Dudley ME. Adoptive cell transfer: a clinical path to effective cancer immunotherapy. *Nat Rev Cancer.* 2008;8:299–308.
160. Simon RM, Steinberg SM, Hamilton M, et al. Clinical trial designs for the early clinical development of therapeutic cancer vaccines. *J Clin Oncol.* 2001;19:1848–1854.
161. Disis ML, Schiffman K. Issues on clinical applications of cancer vaccines. *J Immunother.* 2001;24:104–105.
162. Kondo H, Hazama S, Kawaoka T, et al. Adoptive immunotherapy for pancreatic cancer using MUC1 peptide-pulsed dendritic cells and activated T lymphocytes. *Anticancer Res.* 2008;28:379–388.
163. Weng DS, Zhou J, Zhao M, et al. Minimally invasive treatment combined with cytokine-induced killer cells therapy lower the short-term recurrence rates of hepatocellular carcinomas. *J Immunother.* 2008;31:63–71.
164. Dillman RO, Soori G, DePriest C, et al. Treatment of human solid malignancies with autologous activated lymphocytes and cimetidine: a Phase II trial of the cancer biotherapy research group. *Cancer Biother Radiopharm.* 2003;18:727–733.
165. Comoli P, De Palma R, Siena S, et al. Adoptive transfer of allogeneic Epstein-Barr virus (EBV)-specific cytotoxic T cells with *in vitro* antitumor activity boosts LMP2-specific immune response in a patient with EBV-related nasopharyngeal carcinoma. *Ann Oncol.* 2004;15:113–117.
166. Kawai K, Saijo K, Oikawa T, et al. Clinical course and immune response of a renal cell carcinoma patient to adoptive transfer of autologous cytotoxic T lymphocytes. *Clin Exp Immunol.* 2003;134:264–269.
167. Rosenberg SA, Dudley ME. Cancer regression in patients with metastatic melanoma after the transfer of autologous antitumor lymphocytes. *PNAS Early Edition.* 2004;1–7.
168. Dudley ME. Cell transfer therapy: basic principles and preclinical studies. In: Rosenberg, SA, ed. *Principles and Practice of the Biologic Therapy of Cancer.* 3rd ed. Philadelphia, PA: Lippincott Williams & Wilkins; 2000:305–321.
169. Belldegrun AS, Figlin RA, Patel B. Cell transfer therapy: clinical applications, renal cell carcinoma. In: Rosenberg SA, ed. *Principles and Practice of the Biologic Therapy of Cancer.* 3rd ed. Philadelphia, PA: Lippincott Williams & Wilkins; 2000:333–345.
170. Dudley ME, Rosenberg SA. Adoptive-cell-transfer therapy for the treatment of patients with cancer. *Nature.* 2003;3:666–675.
171. Shimizu J, Yamazaki S, Sakaguchi S. Induction of tumor immunity by removing CD25+CD4+ T cells: a common basis between tumor immunity and autoimmunity. *J Immunol.* 1999;163:5211–5218.
172. Gardini A, Ercolani G, Riccobon A, et al. Adjuvant, adoptive immunotherapy with tumor infiltrating lymphocytes plus interleukin-2 after radical hepatic resection for colorectal live metastases: 5-year analysis. *J Surg Oncol.* 2004;87:46–52.
173. Shi M, Zhang B, Tan ZR, et al. Autologous cytokine-induced killer cell therapy in clinical trial phase I is safe in patients with primary hepatocellular carcinoma. *World J Gastroenterol.* 2004;10: 1146–1151.
174. Chan B, Lee W, Hu CXL, et al. Adoptive cellular immunotherapy for non-small cell lung cancer: a pilot study. *Cytotherapy.* 2003;5:46–54.

CHAPTER

21

Debra Wujcik, PhD, RN, AOCN®

# Targeted Therapy

## INTRODUCTION

Advances in our understanding of molecular biology and carcinogenesis have changed the treatment of cancer in the last decade. Agents that interfere with specific extra and intracellular targets are now being used along with surgery, chemotherapy, and radiation therapies. Tamoxifen, heralded as the first targeted therapy, was approved in the early 1980s. Its primary mechanism of action is blocking estrogen stimulation of breast cancer cells.[1] However, trastuzumab, approved in 1997 for the treatment of metastatic breast cancer, marked the beginning of a decade of new agents approved for clinical use.[2]

The proliferation, regulation, angiogenesis, and apoptosis of both normal and cancer cells are regulated by an interconnecting network of signaling pathways. There are numerous proteins called growth factor receptors expressed or found on the cell membrane. These proteins serve as a bridge of information between the outside milieu and the intracellular environment and are essential for normal cellular growth and proliferation.[3] Alterations in genes produce variations on the cell protein population resulting in malfunction or over expressing proteins. These proteins called oncoproteins can turn healthy cells into malignant cells. Just as proteins have different functions in healthy cells, oncoproteins have similar functions in malignant cells. The DNA that regulates the oncoprotein is called an oncogene.[4]

There are 2 families of growth factor receptors of clinical significance, epidermal growth factor receptors (EGFR) and vascular endothelial growth factor (VEGF) receptors. Blocking these growth factor receptors has been the focus of drug development for cancer treatment for nearly 2 decades. More recently, other proteins found in the cytoplasm of the tumor cells have been targeted for interference such as the BCR-ABL protein, which causes chronic myeloid leukemia or the mammalian target of rapamycin (mTOR) protein, a key component in renal cell carcinoma.[5,6]

The strategies most effective for interfering with these processes are monoclonal antibodies (MoAbs) and small-molecule protein kinase inhibitors (TKIs). Monoclonal antibodies interfere with cell membrane bound targets by blocking ligand-receptor activation, antibody-dependent cellular cytotoxicity, complement-mediated cytotoxicity, and immune modulation.[7] The TKIs are effective against both membrane-bound and nonmembrane-bound targets.[8] By targeting tumor cell growth, these types of therapies should be less toxic to normal tissues than chemotherapeutic drugs. Additionally, overall treatment of cancer may evolve from an acute tumor destruction approach to a more chronic management of malignant cells.

## SIGNAL TRANSDUCTION

Signal transduction is a communication process used by regulatory molecules to mediate essential cell processes such as cell growth, differentiation, and survival. Aberrations lead to increased proliferation, sustained angiogenesis, tissue invasion, metastases, and apoptosis inhibition.[9–11]

Cell signaling begins with activation of the receptor on the cell membrane by a ligand (growth factor). The ligand binds to the receptor causing dimerization (activation). The signal crosses the cell membrane into the intracellular domain where tyrosine kinase (TK) activation occurs. This causes a downstream cascade of signaling pathways that influence cell regulation (Figure 21-1).

Cell signaling is affected by extracellular and intracellular events. The events outside the cell that turn on the signal are ligand binding and receptor over expression. Events inside the cell that turn on the signals include the binding of intracellular proteins, heterologous signals/cross talk, receptor mutation, and loss of regulatory mechanisms. Cell signaling controls proliferation, growth inhibition, and apoptosis. Genetic changes can affect the pathways in the form of oncogenes, tumor suppressor genes, and proteases (caspases).

There are a number of signaling pathways and targets that have been identified and clinical trials are underway for agents designed to exploit these pathways.[8] The focus of this chapter is on the pathways and targets that are best understood and the Food and Drug Administration (FDA) approved agents being used in clinical practice. These pathways include receptor kinases, intracellular signaling kinases, and angiogenesis (see Table 21-1). The agents include the anti-EGFR MoAbs (cetuximab, panitumumab, and trastuzumab) and small molecule inhibitors (erlotinib, gefitinib, and lapatinib), SRC-targeting small molecule inhibitor (dasatinib), mTOR inhibitors (everolimus and temsirolimus), mitogen-activated protein kinase (MAPK) pathway inhibitor (sorafenib), antiangiogenesis inhibitor MoAb (bevacizumab), and small molecule inhibitors (sorafenib and sunitimib). Agents that also target the BCR-ABL protein include dasatinib, nilotinib, and imatinib (see Table 21-2).

## RECEPTOR KINASE PATHWAYS

Receptor kinase pathways include human epidermal growth factor receptors (HERs), c-Met, and Insulin Growth Factor Pathways. Human epidermal growth factor receptors, also known as EGFRs, are a subfamily of the protein TKs. Kinases are enzymes that phosphorylate specific protein, carbohydrate, or lipid residues.[3] The super family of protein kinases is best known as regulatory signals for a variety of cellular processes such as growth and differentiation. There are 3 types of protein kinases that differ in the amino acid acting as the substrate for phosphorylation, serine, threonine, and tyrosine. There may be up to 2000 protein kinases on the human genome.[12]

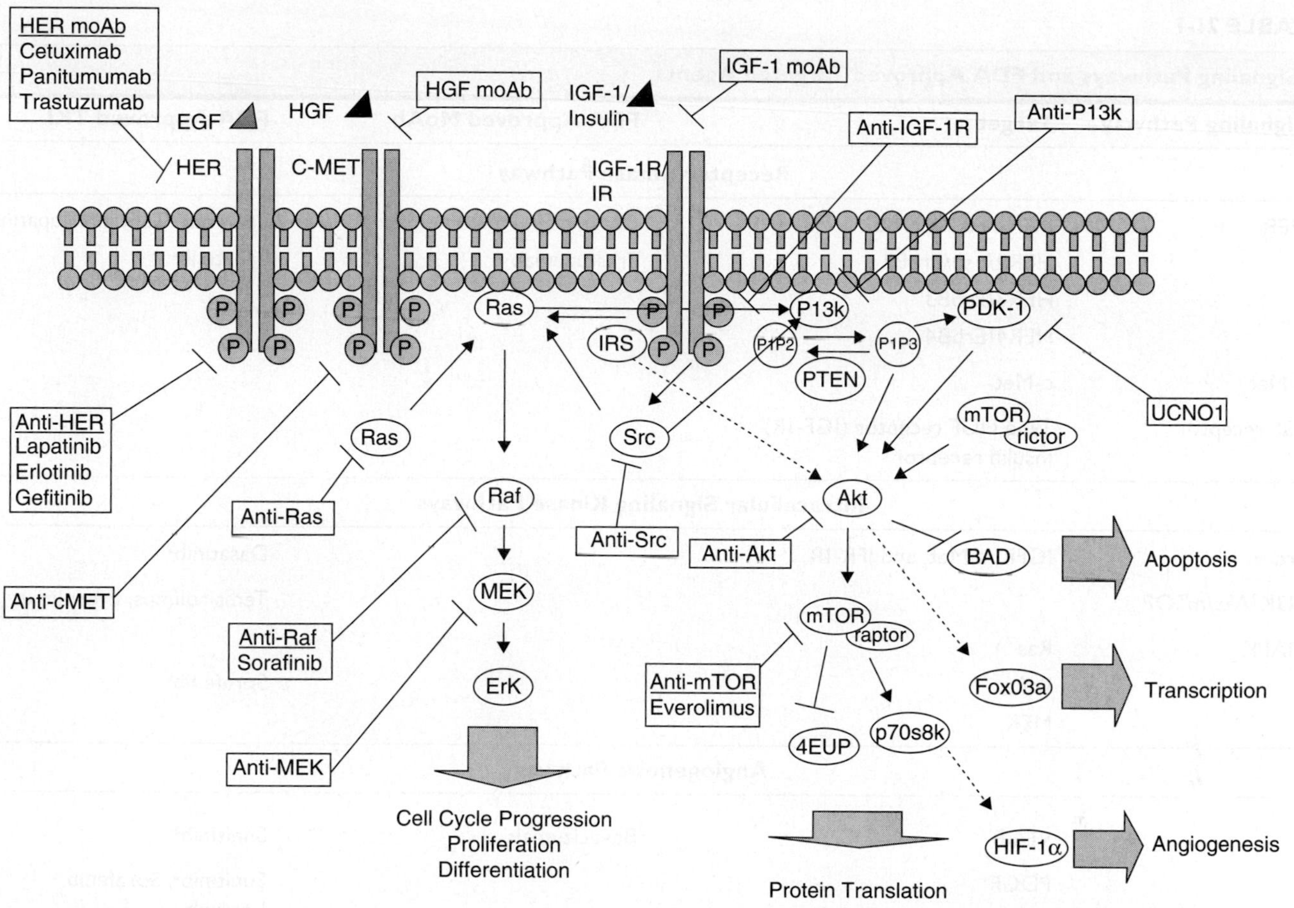


**FIGURE 21-1**

**Cellular Signaling Pathways.** Depicted are the cellular signaling pathways involved in the proliferation, angiogenesis, and differentiation in neoplasms with the targets amenable to therapeutic interventions in cancer therapy. Membrane-bound human epidermal growth factor receptors (HERs), c-MET, and insulin-like growth factor I receptor (IGF-IR) mediate mitogenic signals from extracellular ligands, such as epidermal growth factor (EGF), hepatocyte growth factor (HGF), and insulin growth factor (IGF), respectively. The Ras/Raf/MEK/Erk (mitogen-activated protein kinase, MAPK) and PI3k/Akt/mTOR pathways are major intracellular axes that regulate intracellular signaling traffic. The class and agents targeting the signaling proteins are indicated in boxes.

## HUMAN EPIDERMAL RECEPTORS

Epidermal growth factor receptors are transmembrane proteins with an extracellular ligand-binding domain joined to an intracellular tyrosine kinase domain. As a subfamily of the protein TKs, EGFRs play an important role in the regulation of cell division and growth. EGFRs are present on most cells, excluding hematopoietic cells. The HER/EGFR family members include EGFR (erbB1), HER2/*neu* (erbB2), HER3 (erbB3), and HER4 (erbB4). Note the family name (EGFR) and one of the family members are the same (EGFR).[3] All of the members are structurally related and all except HER3 contain the intracellular TK domain. All of the members, except HER2, bind to extracellular ligands. Epidermal growth factor receptors (ErbB1) is overexpressed in 25% to 77% colorectal cancer cells. HER 2 (*neu* or ErbB2) is the most well known of the HER family and it is overexpressed in 25% to 30% women with breast cancer.[10]

There are 3 areas or domains in the EGFR: 1) extracellular ligand binding domain or receptor, 2) transmembrane region, and 3) intracellular protein TK domain. Ligand binding refers to the attaching of the ligand to the receptor site. EGFR (erbB1, HER1) is the only receptor for epidermal growth factor (EGF) and transforming growth factor-alpha (TGF-α), but is not specific to these. Some other ligands are amphiregulin, heparin binding EGF, betacellulin, and epiregulin. TGF-α is the most widely expressed ligand on human tissues and is produced by both normal and malignant cells. Epidermal growth factor is found in most body

**TABLE 21-1**

**Signaling Pathways and FDA Approved Targeted Agents**

| Signaling Pathway | Target | FDA Approved MoAb | FDA Approved TKI |
|---|---|---|---|
| | | **Receptor Kinase Pathway** | |
| HER | EGFR/HER1/ErbB1 | Cetuximab, Panitumumab | Erlotinib, Gefitinib, Lapatinib[a] |
| | HER2/*neu*/ErbB2 | Trastuzumab | Lapatinib[a] |
| | HER3/ErbB3 | | |
| | HER4/ErbB4 | | |
| c-Met | c-Met | | |
| IGF receptor | Type I IGF receptor (IGF-1R)<br>Insulin receptor | | |
| | | **Intracellular Signaling Kinase Pathways** | |
| Src | IGFR, c-Met, and IFR-1R | | Dasatinib[a] |
| PI3K/Akt/mTOR | | | Temsirolimus, Everolimus |
| MAPK | Ras | | |
| | Raf | | Sorafenib[a] |
| | MEK | | |
| | | **Angiogenesis Pathway** | |
| | VEGF | Bevacizumab | Sunitinib[a] |
| | PDGF | | Sunitinib[a], Sorafenib,[a] Imatinib |
| | FLT3, cKIT | | Sunitinib,[a] Dasatinib |
| Other | BCR-ABL | | Dasatinib, Imatinib, Nilotinib |

[a]Agents with multiple targets.

*Abbreviations*: EGFR, epidermal growth factor receptor; FDA, US Food and Drug Administration; HER, human epidermal growth factor receptor; IGF, insulin-like growth factor; MAPK, mitogen-activated protein kinase; MEK, MAPK kinase; MoAb, monoclonal antibody; PDGF, platelet-derived growth factor; TKI, protein kinase inhibitor; VEGF, vascular endothelial growth factor.

fluids under normal physiological conditions and is synthesized by kidney and salivary glands.[13] ErbB2/HER2 has no natural ligand identified and therefore requires pairing with another receptor (heterodimerization) to be activated. ErbB3/HER3 receives ligand but there is no active TK domain and therefore needs another receptor partner to activate signaling.[12]

Receptor dimerization is the pairing up of 2 sides of molecules to activate the signaling pathway. Dimerization occurs across the transmembrane region, forming a signal processing layer. Homodimerization occurs when 2 identical monomers pair (eg, HER1 and HER1) and heterodimerization occurs when 2 different members of the receptor family pair (eg, HER1, HER2). A variety of ligands bind to the HER family of receptors. The most common ligands are EGF and TGF-α.[3]

The next step in the signaling pathway is the activation of the intracellular TK region. There is binding of the ATP molecule region that generates phosphorus for receptor autophosphorylation and transphosphorylation of another receptor monomer. Phosphorylation triggers intracellular paths that stimulate the cell cycle. Activation of EGFR and HER2/*neu* induces a cascade of downstream signaling though several pathways such as MAPK and PI3-kinase/Akt/mTOR, resulting in cellular proliferation, differentiation, survival, motility, adhesion, and repair.

**TABLE 21-2**

**FDA Approved Targeted Agents**

| Generic | Trade Name | Pharmaceutical Company | 1st Approval | Indication | Class | Type |
|---|---|---|---|---|---|---|
| Trastuzumab | Herceptin | Genentech | September 1997 | Breast | MoAb | Humanized |
| Imatinib mesylate | Gleevec | Novartis | April 2003 | CML, GIST | Small Molecule | TKI |
| Gefitinib | Iressa | Astra Zeneca | May 2003 | NSCLC | Small Molecule | TKI |
| Cetuximab | Erbitux | Bristol Myers Squibb | February 2004 | mCRC, SCCHN | MoAb | Chimeric |
| Erlotinib | Tarceva | Genentech | November 2004 | NSCLC, Pancreas | Small Molecule | TKI |
| Sorafenib | Nexavar | Bayer Healthcare | December 2005 | RCC, HCC | Small Molecule | Multi TKI |
| Sunitinib | Sutent | Pfizer | January 2006 | RCC, GIST | Small Molecule | Multi TKI |
| Dasatinib | Sprycel | Bristol Myers Squibb | June 2006 | CML | Small Molecule | Multi TKI |
| Bevacizumab | Avastin | Genentech | September 2006 | CRC, NSCLC, RCC | MoAb | Humanized |
| Panitumumab | Vectibix | Amgen | September 2006 | mCRC | MoAb | Fully human |
| Lapatinib | Tykerb | GlaxoSmithKline | March 2007 | Breast | Small Molecule | Multi TKI |
| Temsirolimus | Torisel | Wyeth | May 2007 | RCC | Small Molecule | mTOR |
| Nilotinib | Tasigna | Novartis | October 2007 | CML | Small Molecule | TKI |
| Everolimus | Afinitor | Novartis | Mar 2009 | RCC | Small Molecule | mTOR |

*Abbreviations*: CML, chronic myelogenous leukemia; CRC, colorectal cancer; GIST, gastrointestinal stromal tumors; HCC, hepatocellular cancer; mCRC, metastatic colorectal cancer; MoAb, monoclonal antibody; NSCLC, non-small cell lung cancer; RCC, renal cell cancer; SCCHN, squamous cell cancer head neck; TKI, tyrosine kinase inhibitor; mTOR, mammalian target of rapamycin.

Epidermal growth factor receptors are expressed in many normal epithelial tissues, including skin, hair follicles, and gastrointestinal tract and EGFR communication is essential for normal cell function. Deregulated EGFR leads to malignant cell transformation. Overexpression of normal EGFR is the result of increased transcriptional or post-transcriptional mechanisms or the consequence of gene amplification. Presence and degree of overexpression is significantly associated with increased malignancy as estimated by degree of invasiveness, frequency of relapse, and survival.

There are cellular effects of EGFR activation related to malignancy including proliferation, tumor cell motility, adhesion, and invasion. Many cancers such as colorectal and breast cancer express high levels of EGFR and EGF causing more cells to proliferate. Continuous activation of EGFR promotes tumor cell motility and lack of cell adhesion, allowing migration of tumor cells to extravascular regions. Both EGF and amphiregulin modulation are associated with invasion, especially invasion of metastatic breast cancer cells.

Signaling pathways are activated when receptors are activated by ligands. In addition, development of receptor mutants that are constitutively (continuously) active without ligands can occur. The most frequently identified mutation is EGFR VIII which has been detected in glial tumors and cancers of the breast, ovary, prostate, stomach, and non-small cell lung cancer (NSCLC).[14] Activation of normal receptors by autocrine overproduction of ligands with increased expression of EGF and TFG$\alpha$ is significant in epithelial cancers. Autocrine stimulatory loops lead to unregulated signaling, a mechanism that is useful in embryonic development but tumorogenic when no longer needed.

The level of EGFR expression may predict response to EGFR inhibitors in NSCLC and other cancer types. However, among patients with NSCLC, a greater likelihood of response to single-agent EGFR-TKIs has been found in female patients and patients with adenocarcinoma histology (especially bronchioalveolar histology), patients of Japanese origin, and patients with no previous history of smoking.[15–17]

Gene mutations are linked to a number of cancers. K-*ras* is an oncogene found on the 12p12 chromosome. Mutation of the K-*ras* oncogene results in activation of the signal transduction pathway that activates unregulated cellular proliferation and impaired differentiation. Recent evidence shows that mutations of the K-*ras* gene are good predictive markers for determining resistance to the anti-EGFR

MoAbs cetuximab and panitumumab. Mutation at key sites leads to continuous activation of K-*ras* associated signaling. Approximately 40% of patients with colorectal cancer have a K-*ras* mutation and the rest are K-*ras* wild type.[18] Due to these findings, the FDA approved changes to the product labels of cetuximab and panitumumab in July 2009. The indications for both drugs no longer include patients with K-*ras* mutations in codon 12 or 13.[19,20]

Epidermal growth factor receptors and HER2/*neu* are overexpressed or abnormally activated in a number of malignancies. The first targeted therapies approved by the FDA are anti-EGFR MoAbs such as trastuzumab for breast cancer, cetuximab and panitumumab for colorectal cancer, and small molecule inhibitors such as erlotinib, for lung and pancreatic cancers. Current research is focused on targeting more than 1 HER-family receptor simultaneously. Lapatinib is a small molecule inhibitor that targets both EGFR and HER2/*neu* receptors and is approved for the treatment of breast cancer.[21]

### C-MET PATHWAY

c-Met is another receptor kinase pathway that is involved in cellular motility, proliferation, survival, invasion, and morphogenesis.[8] The only known ligand for c-MET is hepatocyte growth factor. Oncogenic mutations of this target have been found in gastric carcinoma and hereditary papillary renal carcinoma type 1. There are currently both MoAbs and small-molecule inhibitors targeted in this pathway in clinical trials but none are FDA approved.[22–24]

### INSULIN-LIKE GROWTH FACTOR RECEPTOR PATHWAY

The insulin-like growth factor receptor pathway is similar to the EGFR pathway in that it has several circulating ligands, such as insulin-like growth factor (IGF-I), IGF-II, and insulin, and several receptors such as type I IGF receptor (IGF-1R) and insulin receptor.[25] There are several MoAbs in phase II and III trials targeting the IGF-1R receptor and small molecule inhibitors in phase I trials.[26,27]

## INTRACELLULAR SIGNALING KINASE PATHWAYS

### SRC PATHWAY

Intracellular signaling kinase pathways include Src, PI3k/Akt/mTOR, and the MAPK pathway. *c-Src* was the first proto-oncogene to be described and it is a nonreceptor TK. Src has several functional domains and mediates signals between several growth factor receptors such as IGFR, c-Met, and IGR-1R.[8] Src plays an important role in cancer cell mitosis, adhesion, invasion, motility, and progression.[28] and is important in the development and progression of breast, colorectal, lung, ovarian, and hematological malignancies. Dasatinib is the only FDA approved drug targeting this pathway and it has dual action as a Src and Abl kinase inhibitor.[29] It is approved for Philadelphia positive acute lymphoid leukemia and chronic myeloid leukemia.

### mTOR/PI3K/AKT PATHWAY

The mTOR (PI3K/AKT) pathway integrates signals from multiple receptor kinases to regulate cellular growth and metabolism.[30,31] mTOR, a serine/threonine kinase, stands for mammaliam target of rapamycin. mTOR acts at point of convergence between external growth factor signaling pathways and pathways that sense nutrient and energy (ATP) levels in the cell. The mTOR pathway has internal feedback loops and horizontal "crosstalk" pathways, including the MAPK pathway.[32] When activated by protein kinases, PI3k is a lipid kinase that generates 3-phosphoinositide (PIP3) at the cell membrane. This allows recruitment of phosphoinositide-dependent kinase 1 and AKT to the cell membrane. Phosphatase and tensin homologue (PTEN) negatively regulates PIP3.[33]

Kinases in the pathway are activated in several cancers, due to aberrant events such as loss of PTEN function, AKT amplification, or constitutive activation of kinases upstream. The downstream targets of mTOR are hypoxia inducible factor-1 (HIF-1a), which mediates cellular responses to hypoxia by increasing expression of cell survival mechanisms including angiogenic and growth factor proteins. mTOR activation increases HIF-1a gene expression through mRNA translation and protein stabilization.[34]

To date there are 2 mTOR pathway inhibitors approved for clinical use. Temsirolimus was approved in May 2007 for the treatment of advanced renal cell carcinoma.[35] Everolimus was approved in March 2009 for the treatment of patients with advanced renal cell carcinoma after failure of treatment with sunitinib or sorafenib.[36]

### MITOGEN-ACTIVATED PROTEIN KINASE

The MAPK pathway is also an intracellular signaling kinase pathway serving as a major connector between extracellular and intracellular signals. MAPK pathways connect growth factors, cytokines, and oncogenes to cellular responses such as cell adhesion, motility, proliferation and malignant transformation.[37]

Ras is a small protein that transmits signals from growth factors, cytokines, and oncogenes to Raf, and then to MAPK kinase (MEK). Ras, raf, and MEK are the main targets of the MAPK pathway.[8] Ras mutations are associated with approximately 1 in 3 human cancers: (90% pancreatic; 50% colon; 30% NSCLC). Sorafenib, a Raf inhibitor, is the only FDA approved agent targeting this pathway. It is a dual inhibitor of Raf and VEGFR.[38]

There are 2 other important TKs, c-KIT, and BCR-ABL. When the protein c-KIT develops a gene mutation, it becomes overactive, sending out a signal to keep growing. Tumors such as gastrointestinal stromal tumors (GIST) are characterized by cell surface expression of the dysregulated c-KIT TK known as CD117.[8] When c-KIT is mutated and dysregulated, it does not depend on a ligand to activate the intracellular signaling.

BCR-ABL is a protein TK formed when there is a gene translocation also known as the Philadelphia chromosome cytogenetic abnormality. This translocation is seen in 95% of patients with chronic myeloid leukemia (CML) and 15% to 30% of adult patients with acute lymphoblastic leukemia (ALL). The *BCR-ABL* oncogene is formed when the *BCR* gene on chromosome 22 is fused with the ABL gene located on the chromosome 9. The *BCR-ABL* TKs then cause dysregulation of intracellular signaling, resulting in enhanced proliferation and resistance to apoptosis of myeloid cells. There are 3 small molecule internal binding agents with targets that include the abnormal fusion protein BCR-ABL. Imatinib inhibits the TKs of *BCR-ABL*, PDGF, stem cell factor, and c-Kit in chronic myelogenous leukemia and inhibits proliferation and induces apoptosis in GIST, a disease with overexpression of the c-KIT mutation.[39] Dasatinib is a multikinase inhibitor inhibiting BCR-ABL, SRC family kinases, c-KIT, and PDGFRβ and binds to multiple conformations of the ABL kinase.[40] The third agent in this group is nilotinib, which inhibits the *BCR-ABL* kinase, binding to and stabilizing the inactive conformation of the kinase domain of the ABL protein.[41]

## ANGIOGENESIS PATHWAYS

### ANGIOGENESIS

The third pathway that has been exploited for targeted therapies is the angiogenesis pathway (Figure 21-2). Angiogenesis is the formation of new blood vessels (neovascularization) from existing vasculature. This is another normal process that becomes abnormal in malignancy. Tumors need an adequate blood supply to provide individual cells with the nutrients and oxygen required for them to grow and develop. Angiogenesis occurs as a tumor mass expands and displaces cells farther away from the primary blood source. If angiogenesis does not occur, tumor growth remains limited to a small clump of nonproliferative cells that are usually incapable of metastasizing.[42]

Several growth factors and oncogenes are known to stimulate angiogenesis. Among the most potent proteins that induce cell signaling for normal and pathological angiogenesis are VEGF and beta fibroblast growth factor (β-FGF).[43] Increased levels of VEGF are found in tumors of the lung, breast, thyroid, GI tract, kidney, bladder, ovary, cervix, and glioblastoma of the brain.[42]

Vascular endothelial growth factor promotes vascular permeability, which is important for the development of new blood vessels. Vascular endothelial growth factor binds to VEGF receptors that have an intracellular TK domain, transmitting signals from the receptor to the cell nucleus. Vascular endothelial growth factor receptors are localized primarily in endothelial cells. There are 2 main types of VEGF receptors: VEGFR-1 (Flt-1) is most important during embryonic development, but may also be involved in metastasis and other functions; VEGFR-2 (Flt-2, KDR) is the major receptor involved in pathological angiogenesis and lymphangiogenesis in tumors.[8]

Increased permeability promotes leakage of plasma proteins from small blood vessels, and that leakage provides a suitable environment for endothelial cell growth. Excessive permeability results in high interstitial pressure and uneven delivery of nutrients and oxygen to the surrounding tissue. Excessive VEGF expression in tumors promotes tumor vascular permeability, resulting in decreased efficiency in delivery of chemotherapy and other targeted therapies to tumors.

Hypoxia is known to stimulate upstream activators of angiogenesis such as HIF-1a, which induces VEGF expression. Angiogenesis activation is also caused by oncogenes, inflammatory cytokines, and growth factors such as β-FGF, and platelet derived growth factor (PDGF). TGF-α promotes expression of VEGF and increased vascular cell permeability.

Antiangiogenic agents work by blocking matrix metalloproteinases (MMPs), which degrade the vascular basement membrane and permit tumor cell invasion. Angiogenic activators such as VEGF or endothelial cells work directly or indirectly through the inhibition of endothelial cell specific integrin/survival signaling.[42,43] Antiangiogenic agents disrupt endothelial cell survival mechanisms and inhibit development of new tumor blood vessel supply. Vascular disrupting agents target abnormal epithelial cells to cause rapid and sustained inhibition of tumor blood flow. The tumor is deprived of nutrients necessary for growth and survival, causing tumor necrosis and cell death.[44] Antiangiogenic agents work in the blood by binding with VEGF.

Bevacizumab, a MoAb, targets VEGF and is approved for treatment of colorectal cancer and NSCLC.[46] Sunitinib, approved for renal cell cancer and GIST, targets VEGF, PDGF, FLT3, and cKIT.[47] Dasatinib targets FLT3 and cKIT and is approved for the treatment of CML.

## MONOCLONAL ANTIBODIES

Therapeutic use of MoAbs began in the mid 1970s after Kohler and Milstein developed hybridoma technology.

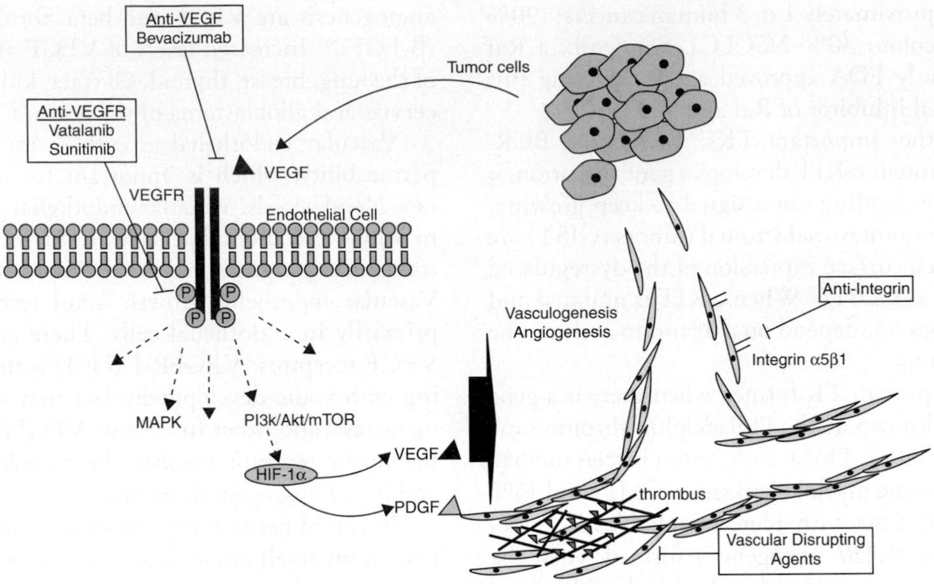


**FIGURE 21-2**

Angiogenesis pathways.

The first MoAbs used murine (mouse) antibodies that had a short antibody half life and caused reactions in humans. Further refinement of the technology has produced chimeric and humanized MoAbs that are safer and more effective in the clinical setting.[8] The mechanism of action for MoAbs includes interference with the ligand-receptor interaction, antibody-dependent cellular cytotoxicity (ADCC), complement-mediated cytotoxicity, and immune modulation.[7]

## ANTI-EGFR MONOCLONAL ANTIBODIES

Trastuzumab[2] was the first EGFR targeted drug to gain FDA approval. It is a humanized MoAb (all human) that binds to the extracellular domain of HER2/*neu*. Trastuzumab is approved for metastatic breast cancer and continues to be studied in lung, pancreas, salivary gland, colon, prostate, endometrium, and bladder cancers. In the adjuvant setting, trastuzumab is indicated for the treatment of HER2-overexpressing node positive or high-risk, node negative breast cancer. High-risk, node negative breast cancer is defined as ER/PR negative or with 1 high-risk feature. Within the adjuvant setting, 3 approved regimens are available—in combination with doxorubicin, cyclophosphamide, and either paclitaxel or docetaxel, in combination with docetaxel and carboplatin, and as a single agent treatment following multimodality anthracycline-based treatment. In the metastatic setting, trastuzumab is indicated for the treatment of HER2-overexpressing tumors in 2 regimens: in combination with paclitaxel as first line therapy, and as single agent treatment in patients who have received 1 or more chemotherapy regimens for metastatic disease. Side effects include fever and/or chills, pain, weakness, nausea/vomiting, diarrhea, headache, difficulty breathing, and rashes.

Cetuximab is a chimeric MoAb consisting of both mouse and human antibodies.[19] Cetuximab binds to EGFR and competes with ligand binding, causing decreased TK activity, decreased cell proliferation, and cell cycle arrest.[48] Cetuximab was initially approved in 2004 under accelerated approval guidelines and in 2007 received expanded labeling and regular approval for the treatment of patients with EGFR-expressing metastatic colorectal cancer after failure of both irinotecan- and oxaliplatin-based chemotherapy regimens. A loading dose of 400 $mg/m^2$ is given IV, followed by 250 $mg/m^2$ weekly. Side effects include fever, chills, asthenia, nausea, and rash.[49]

Panitumumab was approved in September 2006 for metastatic colorectal cancer following progression on prior therapy.[20] Panitumumab is a fully humanized IgG2 MoAb targeting EGFR. Due to a longer half life than other MoAbs, it can be dosed every 2 or 3 weeks. The dose is 6 mg/kg every 14 days and it is administered as an IV infusion over 60 minutes (90 minutes for doses greater than 1000 mg). A low protein binding in-filter is required. Adverse events include hypersensitivity, rash, ocular (conjunctivitis, hyperemia, increased lacrimation, and eye/eyelid irritation), mucosal, and pulmonary toxicities, and electrolyte imbalances.[50]

### ANTIANGIOGENESIS MONOCLONAL ANTIBODIES

Bevacizumab is a recombinant humanized monoclonal antibody against the VEGF molecule.[51] It is 93% human and 7% murine. Because humanized antibodies contain a much smaller percentage of mouse protein than chimerized antibodies, they are thought to be less likely to trigger an unwanted immune response. Bevacizumab recognizes all forms of VEGF and binds to the VEGF molecule with high affinity. The antibody prevents VEGF from binding to its natural receptors, thus inhibiting VEGF-induced angiogenesis. Vascular endothelial growth factor binds with bevacizumab thereby minimizing the amount of circulating VEGF available to bind to its receptors and to activate the angiogenesis process. The terminal half life of bevacizumab is 17 to 21 days.

Bevacizumab was approved in 2006 for use in first- and second-line treatment of metastatic CRC and NSCLC and in 2009 in combination with interferon alfa for patients with metastatic renal cell cancer.[46] For CRC, bevacizumab is administered as an IV infusion every 2 weeks in combination with 5-fluorouracil (5-FU) based therapy. When used in combination with bolus 5-FU, the recommended dose is 5 mg/kg; when used in combination with infusional 5-FU and oxaliplatin, the recommended dose is 10 mg/kg. For the treatment of nonsquamous, NSCLC, bevacizumab is administered on an every 3 week schedule at a dose of 15 mg/kg in combination with chemotherapy.

Because bevacizumab is a protein, it should never be mixed with a dextrose solution and should not be given IV push. The first infusion is administered over 90 minutes. If well tolerated, the second dose is administered over 60 minutes and subsequent doses over 30 minutes.[52] Bevacizumab is associated with a wide range of toxicities, some of which are disease specific. These include hemorrhage, wound healing complications, gastrointestinal perforation, hypertension, nephrotic syndrome, and proteinuria, thromboembolic events, congestive heart failure, and a rare neurological disorder called reversible posterior leukoencephalopathy syndrome (RPLS). Hemoptysis is associated with lung cancer and gastrointestinal perforation is more common in colon cancer. Hypertension and proteinuria are common in breast cancer. Patients with recent hemoptysis, brain metastases, or a history of thrombotic or hemorrhagic disorders should not receive bevacizumab because the drug may exacerbate underlying bleeding tendencies.[53]

There have been FDA black box warnings issued for bevacizumab. In August 2004 a warning was issued regarding an increase in serious arterial thromboembolic events including cerebral vascular accident, myocardial infarction, transient ischemic attacks, and angina. In September 2005, warnings were issued for increased risk of RPLS with hypertension and fluid retention. The most recent black box warning was issued in September 2007 warning of increased risk of fistula formation including tracheoesophageal, bronchopleural, biliary, vaginal, and bladder fistulas.[46]

## TYROSINE KINASE INHIBITORS

Tyrosine kinase inhibitors inhibit HER1/EGFR TK activity by preferentially occupying the ATP binding site within the intracellular TK domain. Because the TKIs bind at a higher affinity than the ATP substrate, they prevent receptor phosphorylation and signal activation. The prevention of signal transduction within the tumor cell has several potential antitumor effects; decreased activation of antiapoptotic genes with subsequent increased rate of apoptosis; decreased activation of genes promoting cell cycle progression and; reduced angiogenic signaling. The expected net effects are tumor growth inhibition and tumor shrinkage.

Although HER1 TKIs downregulate MAPK and AKT activity, they do not directly inhibit these kinases per se. They elicit their biological activity by inactivating the TK activity of HER1/EGFR, which results in the inhibition of downstream cascades such as MAPK and AKT. Tyrosine kinase inhibitors are also referred to as small molecule inhibitors because they cross the cellular membrane and act at the TK domain. TKIs are oral drugs and they all end with the suffix ib.

### ANTI-EGFR TKI

Imatinib is approved for the treatment of Philadelphia chromosome-positive CML after failure of interferon therapy.[39] In clinical trials involving interferon-refractory patients with CML treated with imatinib, 93% of patients with chronic phase CML and 68% of those with accelerated-phase CML had a complete hematologic response with a normal white blood cell and platelet count.[54,55] These patients also experienced a major cytogenetic response defined as disappearance of the Philadelphia chromosome: 61% of patients in the chronic phase and 25% of patients in the accelerated phase. This drug is also indicated in GIST that express c-KIT and are unresectable, metastatic, or both.[56] Adverse events were moderate to mild and consisted primarily of nausea, vomiting, fluid retention, and diarrhea. Fluid retention may be managed by interruption of imatinib and supportive care.

Gefitinib is a TKI approved as monotherapy for patients with locally advanced or metastatic NSCLC who have failed both platinum-based and docetaxel chemotherapy regimens.[57] Epidermal growth factor receptor is present and overexpressed in almost all NSCLC specimens. Gefitinib reversibly binds to ATP sites on TK, blocking signal transduction and resulting in decreased angiogenesis, increased apoptosis, and less tendency for invasion and metastatic potential. Two large multicenter trials of gefitinib in NSCLC demonstrated response rates of less than 20% for 2 different dose sizes.[15,16] However, those patients who did respond, experienced a rapid and marked improvement in symptoms and quality of life. The primary adverse events observed in these trials were a skin toxicity manifested as an acneiform rash and diarrhea. The addition of gefitinib to first-line chemotherapy in NSCLC showed no benefit in 2 large randomized, placebo-controlled trials.[58]

Erlotinib also targets EGFR, although the full mechanism of action is yet to be described.[59] Erlotinib is currently indicated in the treatment of both NSCLC and pancreatic cancer.[60] For NSCLC, erlotinib is used as single agent treatment of patients with locally advanced or metastatic disease who have failed at least 1 prior chemotherapy regimen. In pancreatic cancer, erlotinib is used in combination with gemcitibine for first-line treatment of patients with locally advanced, unresectable, or metastatic disease.

## MULTITARGETED TKI

Lapatinib was approved in March 2007 in combination with capecitibine for women with HER2+ advanced or metastatic breast cancers who have received prior therapy.[61,62] It is a multitargeted TKI that is an inhibitor of the ATP binding site at the TK domain of both ErbB1 and ErbB2.[63] Lapatinib is available in 250 mg tablets and the dose is 1250 mg daily on days 1 to 21 continuously in combination with capecitibine 2000 mg/m$^2$/day on days 1 to 14. Lapatinib should be taken 1 hour before or after meals while the capecitibine is taken with food or within 30 minutes of eating. Patients should have a baseline multigated acquisition scan (MUGA) and discontinue if left ventricular ejection fraction (LVEF) drops below normal. The dose must also be decreased with severe hepatic impairment so bilirubin is checked before each cycle. Because the drug is metabolized through the liver, CYP3A4 inhibitors and inducers should be avoided. Adverse events in the pivotal trial include diarrhea, palmar–plantar erythrodysesthesia (PPE), nausea and vomiting, fatigue, and cardiac changes (decreased LVEF and prolonged QT interval).[63]

Sorafinib is an oral multitargeted TKI approved in 2005 for the treatment of advanced renal cell carcinoma and in 2007 for the treatment of unresectable hepactocellular carcinoma. Sorafenib inhibits a number of TKs, including Raf kinase, VEGFR-2 and platelet derived growth factor receptor (PDGFR) beta pathways. It blocks angiogenesis and cell proliferation via the Raf pathway.[64,65]

Sorafenib is available only in 200 mg tablets and is dosed at 400 mg twice daily. It should be taken 1 hour before or 2 hours after a meal.[66] If taken with a high fat meal, bioavailability is significantly reduced. The most common side effects are diarrhea, rash, fatigue, hand–foot skin reactions, and hypertension. Sorafenib is metabolized in the liver by CYP3A4. Patients should be assessed for adverse events at 2 weeks after starting treatment. If significant adverse events are not present, patients are assessed monthly thereafter with a complete blood count and chemistry panel. Due to risk of hypophosphatemia, a phosphate level is added. Sorafenib is used cautiously in patients with QT wave prolongation, on antiarrhythmia agents, or with pre-existing cardiac disease, bradycardia, or electrolyte disturbances.

Sunitinib is indicated for treatment of patients with advanced renal cell cancer and patients with GIST after disease progression on imatinib mesylate. Sunitinib inhibits PDGFR-alpha and beta, VEGFR-1, -2, and -3, stem cell factor receptor (KIT), fms-like TK receptor-3 (FLT-3), colony stimulating factor receptor Type 1 (CSF-1R), and the glial cell-line derived neurotrophic factor receptor (RET).[67] It is available in 12.5, 25, and 50 mg tablets and is dosed for 4 weeks at 60 mg daily with or without meals, followed by a 2 week rest period.[47] Common toxicities of sunitinib include fatigue, diarrhea, nausea, mucositis, rash and skin discoloration. Sunitinib is also metabolized in the liver by CYP3A4. Patients should be monitored periodically during the first course of therapy eg, days 1, 14, and 28. The 2-week break may be extended if severe or persistent toxicities occur. A complete blood count with differential and a chemistry panel are recommended at the beginning of each cycle of sunitinib. Myelosuppression may occur but febrile neutropenia is rare. Hypothyroidism is frequently seen so regular surveillance is recommended.

Dasatinib was approved in June 2006 for adults with chronic phase, accelerated phase, or myeloid or lymphoid blast phases of CML with resistance to prior therapy including imatinib. A new dosing regimen of 100 mg orally every day was approved in November 2008; the previous dose was 70 mg twice daily.[40] Dasatinib is a multikinase inhibitor that binds to both active/open conformation and inactive/closed conformation of the ABL kinase domain BCR-ABL.[29] It is administered orally with or without a meal. Tablets should not be crushed or cut. CYP3A4 inhibitors and inducers should be avoided along with $H_2$ antagonists and antacids. If needed, antacids should not be taken within 2 hours of a dose. Myelosuppression, fluid retention, and hemorrhage may occur with dasatinib.[68]

Nilotinib was approved in October 2007 for chronic and accelerated phase Philadelphia chromosome positive CML, resistant or intolerant of prior treatment that included imatinib.[41] The target of this TKI is also the BCR-ABL protein, the most common mutation in CML. Nilotinib is not to be taken with food, so should be taken 2 hours after a meal and no food for 1 hour after the dose. The most common grades 1 and 2 toxicities includes rash, nausea, fatigue, headache, constipation, and diarrhea and grades 3 and 4 are neutropenia, thrombocytopenia, and laboratory changes (increased bilirubin, liver function tests, lipase enzymes, and blood sugar). Patients may develop QT wave elongation on electrocardiogram. Those with uncontrolled or significant cardiac disease should not receive nilotinib.[69]

### ANTI-mTOR INHIBITORS

Temsirolimus was approved in May 2007 for advanced renal cell carcinoma (RCC).[35] Temsirolimus binds to the intracellular protein FKBP12, resulting in inhibition of the mTOR pathway. This blocks downstream signaling that controls cell division. A phase III study for first-line therapy for patients with advanced RCC and 3 or more of 6 specific poor prognostic features plus metastases found improved overall median survival and median progression free survival.[70] This was the first study to show an overall advantage with single agent temsirolimus compared with interferon-$\alpha$ in patients with previously untreated RCC. The dose of 25 mg is infused over 30 to 60 minutes weekly and patients are premedicated with an antihistamine.[35] Due to hepatic metabolism of the drug, CYP3A4 inhibitors are to be avoided. The most common adverse events are asthenia, rash, nausea, anorexia, stomatitis, and peripheral edema. Laboratory abnormalities include hyperglycemia, hyperlipidemia, hypertriglyceridemia, increased alkaline phosphatase, increased serum aspartate transaminase (AST), increased creatinine, and hypophosphatemia.[71]

Everolimus, the second FDA approved mTOR inhibitor, was released in March 2009.[36] Everolimus is an oral mTOR inhibitor taken as a 10 mg daily dose. Efficacy and safety of everolimus were demonstrated in an international, double blind trial comparing everolimus to placebo in patients with advanced RCC.[72] Median progression free survival was significantly longer in the everolimus group. Common side effects (≥30%) were stomatitis, infections asthenia, fatigue, cough, and diarrhea. Common laboratory abnormalities were anemia, hyperglycemia, hypercholesterolemia, hypertriglyceridemia, lymphopenia, and increased creatinine.[64] The drug was approved for treatment of patients with advanced RCC after failure of treatment with sunitinib or sorafenib.

## NURSING MANAGEMENT

Epidermal growth factor receptor inhibitor agents have distinctly different side effects from traditional chemotherapy drugs. The most common toxicities associated with targeted therapies are dermatologic reactions and diarrhea. While rash is the most common cutaneous response, others are xerosis (dry skin), hair changes, and nail changes.[73,74] Hypersensitivity reactions are common with the monoclonal antibodies and, in rare instances, can be life threatening. Cardiac, pulmonary, metabolic, and ocular changes are less common but may be severe.[49] Oncology nurses should be aware of both the toxicities and current management standards for these adverse effects. Successful management of adverse effects benefit patients by potentially increasing quality of life and by helping patients to maintain therapy for longer periods of time, reducing dose reductions or treatment breaks.

### DERMATOLOGIC

Dermatologic toxicities are seen in more than half of patients treated with EGFR inhibitor agents and are found in 100% of patients treated for more than 6 months.[75–77] These reactions range from changes in the skin (rash, xerosis), pruritus, paronychia (fissures in the periungual regions), hair loss (alopecia) and hair growth abnormalities (trichomegaly), and telangiectasias (dilation of the capillaries).

#### Rash

*Incidence.* The skin is the largest organ in the body and it provides a number of essential functions: prevention of dehydration; protection from the environment; defense against pathogens; and thermoregulation.[78] Up to 90% of patients receiving targeted therapy experience some type of dermatologic reaction with onset in the first few weeks of treatment. Although the rash can be stressful for the patient, these reactions are not life threatening. The incidence of rash is slightly higher in patients receiving monoclonal antibodies (43%-85%)[79] than in patients receiving TK inhibitors (25%-33%).[80] Severe reactions that lead to dose modification or interruption occur in 8% to 17% of patients.[73]

*Description.* The rash caused by anti-EGFR therapy is described as acneform eruption, follicular acneform eruption, folliculitis, papulopustular rash, acneform rash, macropapular rash, or maculopustular rash. Although superficially the rash looks like acne, it is not acne and should not be described as such.[80] Acne is characterized by comedones (blackheads and whiteheads), sebaceous gland involvement, a distinct histology, and the presence of bacteria. None of these characteristics are present in anti-EGFR agent induced rash.

The anti-EGFR therapy rash contains macules that are flat, reddened lesions, papules that are solid, rounded, raised growths, and pustules that are raised and contain pus (See color plate 21-?.) The rash is often composed of more than 1 type of lesion. A macular rash has reddish, macular lesions, a mixed maculopapular rash may have some lesions flat and others raised, or present with pustular lesions.[81] Rash develops 1 to 2 weeks after treatment begins. It usually starts in the face, around the nose and cheeks, and spreads to the chest and back. In most patients the rash is confined to the face, chest and upper back and occasionally extends towards the extremities.[73] Dry skin (xerosis) occurs in 13% to 35% of patients taking gefitinib or erlotinib; rash and dry skin often develop at the same time.[80]

The rash may stabilize or periodically worsen and usually resolves completely within 2 to 3 weeks of discontinuing therapy. Although some hyperpigmentation may remain, scarring is unusual. In addition there are rare reactions such as Stevens–Johnson syndrome (hypersensitivity reaction) or a lichenoid reaction reported in patients taking imatinib.[79] The severity of the rash has not been associated with skin type or history of acne, but is associated with the agent and dose.[73]

*Grading.* Assessment and grading of the rash is essential for proper management. The National Cancer Institute Common Toxicity Grading Scale, used to assess toxicity in clinical trials is limited in ability to accurately grade/define dermatologic toxicities associated with EGFR agents. The scale has 5 levels with the difference in grades 2 and 3 being the distribution of the rash (< or > 50% of the skin surface).[82] However, clinicians found that the rash can be quite severe, yet located only on the chest or face. Through a consensus meeting, a recommendation was made for adopting a simplified and more focused scale with 3 levels to facilitate accurate grading for clinical decision making.[74] *A mild* rash is defined as a generally localized maculopapular reaction that is minimally symptomatic. A *moderate* response is a generalized papulopustular reaction accompanied by mild pruritus or tenderness. A moderate rash has minimal impact on activities of daily living and no super infection. A *severe* response is a generalized papulopustular reaction with severe pruritus or tenderness, significant impact on activities of daily living, and with potential for or existing super infection.

There is a progression of the rash. Initially patients experience sensory changes and may describe a feeling of burning on the face or upper trunk. Edema and erythema may be present. Next, a papulopustular rash erupts that contains inflammatory cells, followed by neutrophils, vasodilatation, and edema. The rash concentrates in the scalp, face, and upper body. Crusting develops as papulopustular lesions begin to dry with characteristic crusting appearance. Patients may experience dry skin with increased itching and skin changes such as telangiectasias (small blood vessels) may also appear.[78]

*Etiology.* The exact etiology by which rash develops is unknown. Epidermal growth factor receptor is a receptor involved with the normal development and function of human keratinocytes (skin) and EGFR homodimers (EGFR-EGFR) are particularly abundant in the skin.[83] The highest levels of EGFR expression are found in the basal and suprabasal layers of the epidermis and the outer root sheath of hair follicles.[84] Inhibition of EGFR at the epidermis or hair follicle can disrupt the integrity of the skin with the recruitment of inflammatory cells. Skin biopsies have been done and reveal a rash characterized by lymphocytic perifolliculitis or superficial folliculitis without an infectious process.[85] Others describe folliculits with an infectious process.[86] Vasodilatation, dermal edema, and follicular degradation are present.[78] Secondary infection is usually absent and sebaceous glands do not appear to be affected.

*Significance of rash.* Saltz et al[87] originally reported that patients with advanced colorectal cancer and EGFR+ tumors who developed rash with cetuximab and irinotecan had a higher response rate and longer survival than those who do not. Several other trials have confirmed this in other tumor types and other anti-EGFR therapies.[88–90] This may suggest that a lack of rash after a defined period of treatment can indicate failure of therapy, although data have not conclusively proved this.

*Education.* Patient education, provided at the beginning of therapy, includes written instructions and verbal discussion to ensure understanding. Helping patients to manage expectations is a key to continued compliance with therapy.[73] Patients are instructed to call the nurse as soon as symptoms appear. A prescription for clindamycin gel, a topical antibiotic with anti-inflammatory properties, to treat pustular rash and a prescription for cortisone cream to treat macular rash, are often given to the patient at the initiation of therapy to facilitate early treatment.[81]

All patients should be instructed to stay well hydrated and use water-based, nonalcohol-based skin products to minimize skin dryness. Emollient creams that contain 5% to 10% urea and water based facial cleansers are recommended.[79] Patients should avoid lotions and creams that contain irritants such as alcohol, perfume, or dyes. Patients may use camouflage makeup such as Dermablend (Dermablend Corrective Cosmetics). This product provides good results without further aggravating the rash.[79,80] Patients are also instructed to avoid sun exposure and use a broad spectrum sunscreen that contains zinc oxide or titanium dioxide.[78] Patients should bath with cool or lukewarm (instead of hot) water and use mild soaps. Sun exposure should be avoided as much as possible by wearing hats and sunscreen when outside.[91]

Patients who are still in the work force or in social settings may want to discontinue therapy due to the embarrassment of having an acne-like rash. Psychosocial support from both health-care providers and family is important. Patients may need counseling, additional support, or occasional medication breaks in order to complete therapy.[92]

*Rash management.* Currently there are no evidence-based guidelines for the management of EGFR rash. Proposed treatments are based on qualitative rather than quantitative data.[78] The rash cannot be prevented or eliminated but it can be managed successfully so that patients do not have to discontinue therapy. A severity based algorithm is recommended for management of the rash. For mild rash on the face, hydrocortisone cream (1%-2.5%) or alclometasone dipropionate cream are recommended.[78,81] Clindamycin gel (1%) can be added for pustular rash. Moderate to severe rash spreads beyond the face or begins to have drainage. Oral antibiotics are used to treat secondary infection.[80,87] The oral antibiotics minocycline or doxycycline at 100 mg orally may be added daily or twice daily for 4 to 6 weeks. These antibiotics are tetracycline based and have anti-inflammatory properties as well.[81] For patients who cannot tolerate minocycline or doxycycline, trimethoprim and sulfamethoxazole may be used.

There is a lack of data to support the use of topical and systemic steroids and a concern over potential interference with therapeutic effects of therapy. A short course of systemic steroids such as methylprednisolone are recommended for severe reactions.[78,80] No data support the use of prophylactic topical or systemic antibiotics. If there is purulent drainage or crusted scabs, infection is suspected and lesions should be cultured.

The treatment for burning and erythema is topical anesthetics such as lidocaine or pramoxine, which are both available in gel or lotion form. For a severe rash without pustules, silver sulfadiazine ointment is recommended. Grade 3 rashes using 3 levels of grading or grade 4 to 5 rashes using the NCI toxicity grading require interruption of therapy.

A mild shampoo such as baby shampoo may prevent dry skin of the scalp. Scalp lesions can be managed with clobetasol foam (Olux) or fluocinolone shampoo (Capix). Ulcers in the nares may be treated with mupirocin ointment (Bacroban).[78]

Oral antihistamines (diphenhydramine or hydroxyzine) may be needed for pruritic rash. A soothing bath in tepid water with Aveeno Colloidal Oatmeal Bath (Johnson & Johnson) may be helpful.[92]

Immunomodulatory products such as 1% pimecrolimus or 0.03% to 0.1% tacrolimus have been mentioned in the literature. Due to black box warnings in the product information regarding increased risk of skin cancer, these products should be used only in the clinical trial setting.[91,92]

Although the rash is generally managed by the oncology team, there are times when a dermatologist referral is indicated. Yellowish/brown crust overlying inflammatory lesions and significant oozing of fluid from lesions are symptoms of secondary infection. A short course of a tetracycline analogue is effective against *Staphylococcus aureus* infection. If *S. aureas* or impetigo is present, topical mupirocin is recommended. Pustule cultures are obtained if antibiotic resistance is suspected.

In addition to suspected infection, patients should be referred to the dermatologist for other indications: lesions that have uncharacteristic distribution; necrosis, blistering or petechial/purpuric lesions are present; patients with atypical dermatologic manifestations unrelated to rash.[78]

Only one study was found that addressed predictors of rash. Jatoi, et al[93] reported that men and patients <70 years were more likely to develop rash. There is emerging research testing interventions in a clinical trial setting to prevent or modify the rash. One study from the North Central Cancer Treatment Group[93] used tetracycline 500 mg orally bid for 28 days prior to the onset of rash in patients taking anti-EGFR therapy. The incidence of rash was comparable in the treatment and the placebo groups, but there was decreased severity and better scores on quality of life measures in the treatment group. Another study evaluated incidence of > grade 2 skin toxicity between patients receiving panitumumab who received prophylactic or reactive skin treatment.[94] Prophylactic therapy began 24 hours before the first dose of treatment and continued daily for 6 weeks while reactive treatment began after the first symptoms were noted. Patients receiving prophylactic treatment had > 50% reduction in the incidence of grade 2 toxicities and improved quality of life. Further studies are underway.

## Palmar–plantar erythrodysesthesia

Palmar–plantar erythrodysesthesia (PPE), also known as hand–foot syndrome, ranges from erythema, swelling, and tenderness to desquamation of skin, especially on the hands and feet. PPE occurs in 53% of patients receiving lapatinib (all grades). The pathophysiology is thought to be related to small capillaries that rupture from use, creating an inflammatory response. Early stages of PPE include numbness, dysesthesia/paresthesia, tingling, painless swelling, and discomfort of the hands and feet that does not interfere with daily activities. The PPE is grade 2 when the discomfort interferes with daily activities and grade 3 when blistering, desquamation, or severe pain is present.

There is no known prevention of PPE. A baseline skin assessment and the patient's self care ability should be documented. Patients are taught to reduce friction and heat exposure with short, tepid bathing or showers, reduce pressure on hands and feet, and apply emollients liberally. In addition, patients are reminded that changes in skin color or tenderness should be reported. The dose or frequency of lapatinib should be decreased when grades 2 or 3 develop.

Patients receiving sunitinib or sorafenib may experience acral erythema where the palms and soles of the feet become painful, edematous, and erythematous.[67] Paresthesias may occur prior to acral erythema and the condition can progress with hyperkeratosis and desquamation. This is different than the PPE associated with chemotherapy as there are more localized and hyperkeratotic lesions.[95] There are epidermal changes in the granular layer of the epidermis. Acral erythema arises 2 to 4 weeks after the start of therapy and disappears rapidly after the dose is discontinued. Tachyphylaxis can occur if the full dose is restarted after dose reduction.[79] Patients may need to use gel inserts in shoes for comfort or use loose fitting shoes or slippers. Emollient and urea based creams may soften the lesions. Analgesics may be required for moderate to severe pain. A pedicure may be recommended before starting treatment to remove any excessive calluses.[79]

### Nails

The symptoms of nail toxicity include pain, tenderness, fissuring, and paronycheal inflammation with associated swelling and friability of the lateral nail folds of toes and fingers.[96] The great toes and thumbs are most susceptible to changes. Nail toxicity occurs in 12% to 16% of patients[87] and persists throughout treatment. Symptom relief is obtained with soaks and cushioning of affected areas. Liquid cyanocrylate, Band-Aid Liquid Bandage (Johnson & Johnson), is recommended to cover fissures.[73,92]

Subungul splinter hemorrhage has also been noted in patients taking sunitinib and sorafenib.[79] This appears as black or red lines under the nail that resemble splinters and is believed to be thrombotic in origin.

### Hair

Alterations in the pigmentation of hair and skin appear at 5 to 6 weeks after treatment initiation and begin to reverse within 2 to 3 weeks after discontinuation.[96] Hair pigmentation can occur with sunitinib and imatinib possibly due to interruption of cKIT signaling involved in regulating hair pigment. Hypo and hyperpigmentation has been reported in patients taking imatinib.[79]

## INFUSION REACTIONS

Infusion reactions (IR) are much less common (3%-4%) than dermatologic toxicities (up to 90%) in patients receiving targeted therapies; however infusion reactions can be severe and cause fatal outcomes. The potential for infusion reactions with IV MoAbs decreases with immunogenicity of the compound. MoAbs are murine, chimeric, or humanized. Murine MoAbs are derived from mice and have the highest risk of causing hypersensitivity reactions. They are named with the suffix -momab. The other 3 types are engineered using lesser amounts of murine components and more human components. Chimeric MoAbs are 7% to 9% murine antibodies and named with the suffix -ximab such as cetuximab. Humanized MoAbs contain only 2% to 5% murine antibodies and are named with the suffix -zumab such as bevacizumab or trastuzumab. Fully humanized MoAbs contain only human antibodies and are named with the suffix -umab such as panitumumab. Fully humanized MoAbs have the least risk of causing hypersensitivity reactions (HSR).[97]

Infusion reactions are typically mild to moderate and develop during the infusion or several hours afterwards. They are associated with chills, fever, nausea, asthenia, headache, skin rash, and pruritus. Severe reactions may be characterized by the acute onset of bronchospasm, hypotension, urticaria, and/or cardiac arrest.[98] Drug allergy is a reaction mediated by the immune system and immunoglobulin while drug hypersensitivity is an immune mediated response to a drug in a sensitized patient.[97]

The National Cancer Institute Common Toxicity Criteria describes 2 types of reactions: HSR, a true allergic reaction, and acute infusion reaction or cytokine release syndrome (which may be reflective of MoAb reactions) (NCI/CTC). Infusion reactions are also often categorized as either anaphylactic or anaphylactoid. Although they present and are treated the same, the underlying pathology is different. Anaphylactic reactions are type I HSR that occur when antigen-specific IgE binds to mast cells and sensitizes them to the antigen.[97,98] Subsequent exposure of the sensitized mast cell to the antigen causes a series of reactions that result in the degranulation of the mast cell and release of mediators of the HSR. Symptoms include fever, nausea, vomiting, flushing, rashes, urticaria, angioedema, bronchospasm, back pain, shortness of breath, and alterations in heart rate and blood pressure. Patients express a feeling of impending doom. Since prior sensitization is required for IgE-mediated HSR, it would not be expected to occur with the first infusion.

Cytokine release syndrome is caused by elevated levels of cytokines and histamine as tumor antigen-expressing cells are destroyed. This reaction is associated with fever, chills, rigors, nausea, vomiting, dyspnea, hypotension.[97] Anaphylactoid reactions (pseudoallergic reactions) also cause symptoms similar to anaphylactic reactions, but are caused by the mediators from mast cells and basophils without specific IgE antibodies. Anaphylactoid reactions involve partial hypersensitivity, are not IgE mediated, and are generally less life threatening than anaphylactic reactions.

There is evidence that there is increased prevalence of cetuximab induced reactions in a Southern belt that includes Tennessee and North Carolina. The rate in these areas is up to 22% compared to the national average of 3%.[99] It is postulated that cetuximab IgE (C-IgE) reacts with a pre-existing IgE, present due to the high incidence of seasonal allergies in the Southern belt. Among 76 cetuximab treated patients, 25 patients had infusion reactions of any grade, 17 of the 25 had detectable C-IgE, and that group had the most severe reactions.[98]

Anaphylaxis usually describes an immediate reaction that produces symptoms such as wheezing, bronchospasm, hypotension, pruritus, urticaria, nausea, diarrhea, or sometimes cardiac effects. This reaction can be fatal for some patients if not treated appropriately. Infusion reactions are treated according to institutional protocol. For mild to moderate infusion reactions, the infusion rate is slowed and premedication with antihistamine is continued prior to future doses. Severe reactions require cessation of the agent permanently. Emergency equipment should be available and may include epinephrine, corticosteroids, IV antihistamine, bronchodilators, and oxygen.

In clinical trials, trastuzumab produced mild to moderate first infusion reactions in approx 40% of patients with infrequent reactions in subsequent infusions. Cetuximab was associated with 3% severe infusion reactions and 12% to 19% overall reactions, usually associated with the first infusion. There is a 1% incidence of infusion reaction with panitumumab which does not require premedication. Since panitumumab is a fully humanized MoAb, there is reduced potential for infusion reactions.

To prevent IR, high risk patients are identified. These are all patients during the first infusion of a MoAb. As stated previously, risk is highest with murine and chimeric MoAbs. Risk factors associated with IR in patients receiving MoAbs were history of atopy (hypersensitivity skin reactions) asthma, antihypertensive drugs (angiotensin converting enzyme inhibitors or beta-blockers), and opioid drugs.[100] In patients who developed cetuximab-induced IR, only atopic history was significantly associated with severe IR. The history included drug, food, and bee sting allergic reactions as well as comorbid conditions such as asthma, allergic rhinitis, or eczema.[99]

Since 90% of infusion reactions in the clinical trials occur with first dose of cetuximab, some clinicians have explored need for premedication. Timoney and colleagues[48] reported that 746 doses of cetuximab were given with no routine premedication of antihistamine without incident after the first and second dose was given with standard premedication. The package insert recommends the administration of an $H_1$ blocker prior to each dose. Although there are no evidence-based premedications to prevent HSR, the commonly used medications are $H_2$ antagonists (diphenhydramine) and antipyretics (acetaminophen). Corticosteroids may be added. IR are rate dependent and each MoAb has a specified starting rate based on clinical trials.

The management of infusion reactions begins with stopping the infusion at the first sign of a reaction. Once symptoms improve, the infusion may be restarted at a slower rate. Staff should be prepared in basic life support and emergency drugs and equipment should be available. Oxygen therapy is provided along with IV fluids. If an IgE mediated reaction is suspected, immediate treatment includes epinephrine, IV steroids, and antihistamine.[101] For patients having a severe reaction, the infusion is permanently discontinued. Patients with trastuzumab induced reactions have been safely rechallenged although the prescribing guidelines do not recommend it.[102] There are no data for the safe rechallenging with bevacizumab and rechallenge is not recommended after a severe reaction to cetuximab.[100]

For anaphylaxis, cease infusion immediately, maintain the IV line with normal saline solution or other appropriate solution. One nurse remains with the patient while another notifies the physician and emergency staff. The patient is placed in a supine position and the nurse continues to assess and maintain airway, breathing, and circulation. Vital signs are monitored every 2 minutes until the patient stabilizes, then every 5 minutes for 30 minutes, then every 15 minutes. Oxygen should be administered at a high flow rate and staff should be ready to perform CPR if needed.[103]

Intramuscular epinephrine (1:1000) 0.3 cc to 0.5 cc every 15 to 20 minutes as needed is given. Corticosteroids given in high IV doses early in the treatment can minimize the delayed reactions 4 to 6 hours later. $H_1$ blockers such as diphenhydramine 25 mg to 50 mg IM or slowly IV and $H_2$ blockers such as cimetidine 300 mg can be given orally, IM, or IV. Patients experiencing bronchospasm may need inhaled albuterol. The American Heart Association has noted that patients on beta blockers have a higher incidence/severity of anaphylaxis and a paradoxical response to epinephrine. Glucagon and ipratropium may be appropriate.[103,104]

## OCULAR TOXICITIES

Ocular toxicities have been studied by investigators at Northwestern University at the Skin and Eye Reactions to Inhibitors of EGFR and Kinases (SERIES) Clinic[105] where it is estimated that 1/3 of all patients receiving anti-EGFR therapy experience adverse ocular reactions. Ocular toxicities are grouped as changes in the eyelid (blepharitis, trichomegaly, meibomitis, ectropian) changes in the tear film (dysfunctional tear syndrome), and miscellaneous changes (iridocyclitis, corneal epithelial defect).

The prescribing information for gefitinib, cetuximab, and erlotinib all note some ocular toxicity. Eye pain, corneal erosions, ulcers, and some abnormal eyelash growth were reported with gefitinib.[57] Conjunctivitis and keratoconjunctivitis sicca occurred in 12% of patients with NSCLC.[66] The prescribing information for cetuximab cites grade 3 or 4 conjunctivitis in patients receiving cetuximab alone (7%) or cetuximab and irinotecan (14%) and notes the occurrence of blepharitis in some patients as well.[19] As in other targeted therapy side effects, ocular toxicity will continue to be evaluated with chronic administration of therapy.

The pathogenesis of ocular toxicities is not clearly understood. Meibomian glands are the sebaceous glands of the eye. Since these are affected in the dermis, it may be that EGFR agents target the EGFR expressing cells of meibomian glands and change the secretive function of the eye.[106]

Blepharitis is an inflammation of the eyelash follicles, along the edge of the eyelid and it is caused by an overgrowth of the bacteria that is normally found on the skin. Presentation may include itching and tearing of the eyes and lids with crusting of the lashes. Although no evidence-based management guidelines exist, general treatment includes warm compresses, eyelid scrubs, and topical antibiotic ointment. If there is no improvement, cultures may be indicated. For acute blepharitis, topical antibiotics are considered. If severe or left unchecked, blepharitis may lead to corneal infiltrates or ulcers. Although no dose reduction guidelines exist, some clinicians recommend following the package insert modification protocol for rash.[105]

Eyelid changes may be hyperemia (engorgement with blood), papulopustular rash, and crusting. For acute reactions, fluorometholone (0.1%) ophthalmic ointment may be applied to the eyelid once daily for a week, but not more than 2 weeks. An ophthalmologist should see the patient to monitor ocular pressure. For chronic reaction, apply tacrolimus (0.03%) ointment twice daily to the skin of the eyelid only. Another option is pimecrolimis twice daily to the eyelid.

Trichomegaly or elongation of the eyelashes also can occur, usually with therapy lasting longer than 2 months.[96] Some patients may experience misdirection in the growth of the eyelashes. Patients are instructed not to cut or remove eyelashes but have them evaluated by the ophthalmologist. In 1 case report of erlotinib-associated trichomegaly, successful treatment consisted of regular epilation (hair removal) and eyelash trimming. To prevent infection and protect open skin areas, follow the treatments outlined above.

Changes in the secretion of the meibomian glands also occur. Meibomian glands are located on the eyelid margin and just posterior to the base of the eyelashes; they secrete a substance that makes up part of the lipid component of tear film. This lipid component creates a barrier that helps retain the normal fluid secretions of the eye, keeping the eye moist, and helping to prevent infection. The meibomian glands may become irritated or inflamed (meibomitis or meibomian gland dysfunction) in patients receiving EGFR therapy. The irritation results in a thickened oily substance which then secondarily affects the quality of the tear film. This leads to dysfunctional tear syndrome. To treat meibomitis, patients should perform eyelid scrubs and apply warm compresses to the eyelid for at least 5 minutes daily. For severe reactions, oral doxycycline is recommended at 50 mg twice daily for 2 weeks followed by 50 mg daily for 4 weeks.[96]

Ectropion is a medical condition in which the lower eyelid turns outwards.[105] Often the condition has no symptoms, but tearing and conjunctivitis may be seen. There are no specific guidelines for management of ectropion and it may resolve with discontinuation of the drug without the need for surgical intervention.

Patient education for management of ocular toxicities includes telling patients that they may experience eye problems such as eyelid and eye irritation, oily secretions, dryness and a burning sensation in the eye, crusty skin, eyelash growth, and some vision fluctuations. Any changes should be promptly reported to the health-care team. Nurses should ask the patient if they have had any discomfort, pain, or any other problems with their eyes at each appointment.

Symptoms that require immediate referral to an ophthalmologist include sustained eye pain, vision decrease or loss, severe eye redness, photophobia (light sensitivity), and no response after a week of treatment or treatment with a topical steroid.[105]

## PULMONARY INTERSTITIAL LUNG DISEASE

Interstitial lung disease (ILD) is a rare, but potentially life-threatening complication of anti-EGFR agents. Interstitial lung disease may be related to EGFR inhibition and decreased expression of pulmonary surfactant-associated protein (SP-A). Although the pathophysiology is poorly understood, patients who experience dyspnea, cough, fever, or shortness of breath should be evaluated. Additional case reports of erlotinib-associated acute pneumonitis have been recently published. Interstitial pneumonitis has varying times of presentation (days to months) and outcomes (treatable with corticosteroids to fatal).

The incidence of ILD is 1% with gefitinib and 1/3 of the cases are fatal.[107,108] Gefitinib lung toxicity occurs within the first 90 days of treatment. Interstitial pneumonia, diffuse alveolar damage, alveolar hemorrhage and pulmonary fibrosis have been described. There is a higher incidence of ILD reported in Japanese trials (1%-2%) than US trials (.3%).[109] Risk factors include history of smoking and previous lung damage from chemotherapy, radiation, infection, or pulmonary fibrosis.[110]

Severe pneumonitis and respiratory failure resulting in death occurred in 5 patients (1%) in a phase III trial of carboplatin and paclitaxol with or without erlotinib[111] while the incidence of pneumonitis was 0.8% in another study of erlotinib in patients with previously treated locally advanced or metastatic NSCLC.[112]

Pleural effusions, pericardial effusions, and pulmonary edema develop in 2% to 6% of patients receiving imatinib.[39] The etiology of imatinib-induced pulmonary toxicity is most often related to fluid retention and pulmonary edema due to prolonged platelet-derived growth inhibition.[110] Pneumonitis develops anywhere from 10 to 282 days after treatment begins and presents with dyspnea, hypoxemia, fever, eosinophilia, and elevated KL-6 levels. Chest CT reveals diffuse or patchy ground-glass opacity.[113] Imatinib pneumonitis usually reverses with steroid treatment and often resurfaces with any attempt to rechallenge with this agent.

Trastuzumab induced pneumonitis can present with rapidly progressive pulmonary infiltrates and respiratory failure after the first dose or after 6 weeks of therapy.[110] The incidence is 0.4% to 0.6% and the mortality rate is 0.1%.[114] Approximately 15% of patients experience infusion related systems such as hypotension, angioedema, bronchospasm, dyspnea, fever, chills, and urticaria. The incidence of ILP is <0.5% with cetuximab and less than 1% with panitumumab.

Bevacizumab is associated with a 2.3% incidence of pulmonary hemorrhage and 1.6% incidence of death in patients with nonsquamous cell carcinoma.[115] The incidence is up to 31% of patients with squamous cell cancer. Hemoptysis is a common presenting symptom. There is also an increased risk of deep vein thrombosis and pulmonary embolism.[116]

Interstitial pneumonitis associated with temsirolimus has an unknown etiology and is non-dose-dependent.[117] The incidence is 1% to 36% in patients receiving 25 mg/week to 250 mg/week and the onset is within 16 weeks after treatment. Half of patients are asymptomatic with pulmonary infiltrates on chest x-ray; however symptoms include fever, cough, and hypoxemia. Risk factors may include infection, pulmonary edema, and alveolar hemorrhage.

The diagnosis of ILD is made with high resolution CT scans, which reveal the characteristic "ground glass" appearance, or surgical lung biopsy. Video assisted thorascopic procedures may also be needed. Pulmonary function tests reveal decreases in forced vital capacity (FVC), forced expiratory volume in 1 minute (FEV1), and diffusing lung capacity for carbon monoxide (DLCO). Interstitial lung disease is managed pharmacologically with high dose steroids, antibiotics, and bronchodilators and oxygen is provided. Symptoms may abate in some patients after cessation of therapy.

## CARDIAC TOXICITIES

A number of cardiac toxicities are associated with targeted therapies, including cardiac dysfunction, hypertension, congestive heart failure, arterial thromboembolic events, decreased LVEF, and prolonged QT interval.

The exact mechanism for trastuzumab cardiac dysfunction is unknown. The ErbB2 receptor is expressed on cardiomyocytes where it exerts a protective effect on cardiac function. It is postulated that cardiac toxicity is the result of trastuzumab blocking the EGFR pathway responsible for normal cardiac contractility and function.[118,119] Unlike anthracycline-induced cardiac toxicity, trastuzumab-induced cardiac dysfunction does not appear to increase with cumulative dose and is generally reversible.[120] Trastuzumab causes cardiac toxicity in 20% of patients in the metastatic setting[121] and about 5% in the adjuvant setting.[122,123]

Risk factors for trastuzumab-induced cardiac dysfunction include older age, concurrent or previous anthracycline therapy, prior chest wall irradiation, and pre-existing cardiac comorbidities. Manifestations include lowered LVEF, and symptomatic heart failure. In the adjuvant setting, 5% of patients exhibit systolic dysfunction with 1% developing symptomatic congestive heart failure (CHF).[122]

There is a black box warning for trastuzumab that calls for assessment of cardiac function before, during, and after treatment.[2] The drug is withheld for a 16% or greater absolute decrease in pretreatment LVEF. Echocardiogram or MUGA is recommended prior to treatment, every 3 months during therapy, and every 6 months for 2 years following completion of therapy.

Hypertension and heart failure are associated with angiogenesis inhibitor agents such as bevacizumab, sorafenib, and sunitinib. Hypertension occurs in 22% to 47% of patients and heart failure occurs in 3% to 8% of patients.[119] There are acute and chronic mechanisms by which VEGF-signaling pathway inhibitors cause elevations in blood pressure. Acute disruption of vasodilator production leads to vasoconstriction and chronic depletion of microvascular endothelial cells lead to an overall reduction in normal tissue microvessel density.[124]

A number of cardiovascular adverse events are associated with bevacizumab including hypertension, CHF, and arterial thromboembolic events. Congestive heart failure developed in 14% of those treated with bevacizumab and concurrent anthracyclines and 4% in those who previously received anthracyclines and then treated with bevacizumab. There is a black box warning regarding the risk of stroke, myocardial infarction, angina, reversible posterior leukoencephaly, and fatal heart disease associated with bevacizumab.[46] Risk factors for bevacizumab induced cardiac adverse events include age 65 years or older and prior arterial thromboembolic event. If uncontrolled hypertension develops, discontinuation of the drug is required.[97]

Lapatinib was associated with a decrease in LVEF in 1.3% of patients. The dysfunction was reversible and did not progress once therapy was discontinued.[89] A baseline normal LVEF is recommended before starting therapy and dose modifications for any decreased LVEF.

In phase I and II trials of patients with GIST who received sunitinib, 11% experienced cardiac events and 28% had lowering of LVEF of at least 10%.[125] Package information recommends careful monitoring of patients with prior cardiac conditions and periodic evaluation of the ejection fraction.[47] Hypertension may develop and should also be monitored aggressively.[95]

In addition, sunitinib is known to prolong the QT interval and the PR interval and to induce bradycardia and ST-T wave modifications.[126] The QT interval, which is the time between the Q and T waves on an echocardiogram, indicates the duration of ventricular depolarization and repolarization. A prolonged interval is indicative of increased risk of arrhythmia. It is recommended that patients have a baseline electrocardiogram, another 7 days after initiation of sunitinib, and at regular intervals. Patients are taught to report any new palpitations and near or full loss of consciousness (syncope).[126]

Sorafenib also causes hypertension. It is recommended that patients start therapy with BP ≤140/90 mm Hg. Blood pressure is monitored weekly for 6 weeks and the dose of sorafenib is held for increased diastolic by 20 mm Hg or reading >150/90 mm Hg.[95]

Patients receiving any of the above drugs and identified as being at risk must be monitored for signs and symptoms of early heart failure. Vital signs and weight measurement should be obtained on every visit and patients are taught to report ankle swelling, shortness of breath, and weight gain.[127]

## VASCULAR TOXICITIES

Vascular toxicities are also associated with angiogenesis inhibitors. Bleeding events include echymoses, epistaxis, hemoptysis, wound site bleeding, and menorrhagia. Although most of these events are easily treated, fatal pulmonary hemorrhage has occurred with squamous cell lung cancer patients receiving bevacizumab, sorafenib, and sunitinib.[38,128,129]

Bowel perforation has been reported in 1.5% of patients with colon cancer receiving bevacizumab.[128] Certain baseline characteristics may increase risk such as patients with the primary colon tumor intact, sigmoidoscopy/colonoscopy, or having received prior adjuvant radiotherapy. Most events occur within the first 3 months of treatment. Due to wound healing complications, bevacizumab should be discontinued prior to any planned surgery.

## ELECTROLYTE IMBALANCES

Electrolyte depletion can occur in patients receiving cetuximab alone or in combination with chemotherapy vs best standard care or chemotherapy alone.[106,130] In 244 patients, 1/2 of these patients experienced hypomagnesemia, with 10% to 15% experiencing severe hypomagnesemia. Hypomangesemia can occur days to months after initiation of therapy and electrolyte repletion is necessary in some patients. Monitoring of patients is recommended for up to 8 weeks after therapy is discontinued.

Electrolyte depletion was also seen in patients in clinical trials while receiving panitumumab. In one trial, the median magnesium levels decreased by 0.1 mmol/l with grade 3/4 patients requiring oral or IV electrolyte repletion in 4% of patients. Hypomagnesemia was seen in patients up to 6 weeks or longer after initiation of the drug. Some patients experienced hypocalcemia with hypomagnesemia. Patients should be monitored periodically during and for up to 8 weeks after completion of therapy.[130]

No guidelines exist for optimal repletion of magnesium for patients on EGFR inhibitor agents. Other drugs may cause this condition as well, including cisplatin agents and loop diuretics. Accompanying hypocalcemia may occur, but the mechanism of action is not known. Electrocardiogram changes may occur with hypomagnesemia. Adults may experience neuromuscular irritability with muscle cramps and fibrillation. Central nervous system hyperexcitability can occur. Patients may exhibit irritability, disorientation, and seizures (can occur with levels <1 mEq/L). Repletion of mild hypomagnesemia may be done orally, however severe hypomagesemia requires IV supplementation. Some patients may require both.

Tejpar and colleagues[130] recently reported on magnesium wasting with EGFR-inhibitor agents in CRC patients. Ninety-seven percent of the patients had decreasing serum magnesium concentrations. The exact mechanism is unknown, but the agents compromise the renal magnesium retention capacity. Although the study patients showed few side effects, oral repletion was usually ineffective and researchers concluded that risks and benefits of therapy should be considered for all patients receiving these agents.

Liver function abnormalities have been noted with gefitinib and erlotinib. Patients are usually asymptomatic but will present with increased liver transaminases. Laboratory values, transaminase, bilirubin, and alkaline phosphatase should be monitored regularly for changes in liver function. Medical intervention is usually not necessary; although 1 recently published case report discussed acute severe hepatitis in 1 patient receiving erlotinib monotherapy for advanced pancreatic cancer.[131]

## DIARRHEA

Diarrhea is a common side effect of the oral TKI EGFR agents as EGFR is present in the intestinal mucosa. Diarrhea is the major dose-limiting toxicity seen in the clinical trials of oral agents erlotinib and gefitinib; seen less commonly with cetuximab.[132] Patients usually present with grade 1 or 2 diarrhea and stool is often watery or loose. However, blood and mucus are usually not present. Diarrhea often occurs within 3 weeks of initiation of treatment.

The management of anti-EGFR agent induced diarrhea follows standard antidiarrhea management practice. The diarrhea often responds to loperamide treatment. Patients should be taught to take it at first sign of diarrhea and that instructions for use may vary from the package insert. Accurate grading and assessment of the diarrhea is important. The patient's baseline bowel habits should be recorded prior to start of therapy. Dietary modifications, increased fluid intake, and good perianal care are essential. Patients may need to use a diary to accurately record the diarrhea and dose reductions may be necessary.

## NAUSEA AND VOMITING

Most of the targeted therapies are fairly well tolerated with minimal nausea and vomiting. The NCCN 2007 antiemetic guidelines show imatinib in the moderate (30%-90% frequency of emesis category) and cetuximab in the low emetic risk (10%-30% frequency of emesis) category. The rest of the agents discussed in this chapter fall into the minimal emetic risk category (<10% frequency of emesis).[133] If patients require antiemetics, consider prochlorperazine or metoclopramide and lorazepam could be added as well.

## DRUG METABOLISM

Many targeted therapies are metabolized via CYP3A4 pathways. The cytochrome P450 microenzyme system accounts for 75% of total metabolism and is important for degradation of drugs. Of more than 50 human gene isoforms that exist, only a few are significant in drug metabolism. CYP1A3, CYP2C9, CYP2C19, CYP2D6, CYP3A4, and CYP3A5 metabolize 90% of drugs and CYP3A4 accounts for 60% of those metabolized in the liver.[134] Food increases the bioavailability of oral agents. Some drugs inhibit or induce CYP3A4, decreasing or increasing plasma levels of the EGFR inhibitor. This potential interaction can lead to either decreased efficacy of the agent or an increase in adverse events.[71,76] Nurses must teach patients to avoid common foods and medications such as grapefruit juice (inhibitor) and St. Johns Wort (inducer) while receiving targeted therapy. Table 21-3 provides a list of inducers and inhibitors to be considered for potential drug interactions.

## DOSE MODIFICATIONS

Dose modifications are drug specific and the prescribing information should be consulted for each. Gefitinib induced diarrhea may be successfully managed by providing a brief (up to 14 days) therapy interruption followed by reinstatement of the 250 mg dose.[57] Therapy interruption may be needed for eye symptoms so that ophthalmic intervention such as eyelash removal may occur. If pulmonary symptoms are present and worsening, therapy should be interrupted and the patient evaluated. If ILD is confirmed, therapy is permanently discontinued.

Erlotinib induced diarrhea can usually be managed with loperamide. However, if the diarrhea does not lessen/resolve with therapy or if the patient becomes dehydrated, temporary interruption of therapy may be needed. Severe skin reactions may also require dose reduction or interruption of therapy. When dose reductions are necessary, they are made in 50 mg increments. For new or progressive pulmonary symptoms, therapy is interrupted, the patient is evaluated and if ILD is confirmed, the drug is discontinued and the patient is treated as necessary.[60]

For infusion reactions due to panitumumab, the infusion rate is decreased by 50% in patients with mild/moderate reaction for duration of infusion; it is immediately discontinued permanently for patients with severe (grade 3/4) reactions. For dermatologic toxicity grade 3 or higher or intolerable, therapy is withheld. If dermatologic toxicity improves to grade 2, and the patient is symptomatically improved after withholding no more

**TABLE 21-3**

**CYP3A4 Inducers and Inhibitors**

| CYP3A4 Inducers | CYP3A4 Inhibitors |
|---|---|
| Agents that increase the enzyme action to increase the elimination of the drug, decreasing its levels and effects. | Agents that block the enzyme action to decrease the elimination of the drug, increasing its levels and effects. |
| Rifampicin | Grapefruit/grapefruit juice |
| Phenytoin | Verapamil |
| Omperazole | Erythromycin |
| Phenobarbital | Clarithromycin |
| St. John's Wort | Ketoconazole |
| | Itraconazole |
| | Voriconazole |
| | Telithromycine |
| | Troleandomycin |
| | Atanazavir Indinavir |
| | Ritonavir |
| | Saquinavir |
| | Nefazodone |
| | Ciprofloxacin |
| | Norfloxacin |
| | Fluoxetine |

than 2 doses, therapy is resumed at 50% of original dose. If toxicities recur, panitumumab is permanently discontinued. If toxicities do not recur, subsequent doses of panitumumab may be increased by increments of 25% of original dose until recommended dose of 6 mg/kg is reached.[20]

If the patient experiences a grade 1/2 infusion reaction due to cetuximab, the rate should be permanently reduced by 50%; the drug should be immediately and permanently discontinued in patients who experience severe (grade 3/4) reactions.[19] Dose modifications are recommended for severe acneform rash (grade 3/4). For the first occurrence of severe rash, the infusion is delayed for 1 to 2 weeks. If improvement is noted, the infusion is resumed at 250 mg/m$^2$. After the second occurrence, the infusion may again be delayed for 2 weeks and if improvement occurs, the infusion is restarted at 200 mg/m$^2$. After a third occurrence and delay, the infusion is restarted at 150 mg/m$^2$. If severe rash again develops after 2 dose reductions, or if there is no improvement after any dose delay, the cetuximab is discontinued. Dosage modification is not recommended for severe radiation dermatitis.

Lapatinib is discontinued for decreased LVEF that is grade 2 or higher and in patients with an LVEF that drops below the lower limit of normal. It may be restarted at a reduced dose (1000 mg/day) after a minimum of 2 weeks if the LVEF recovers to normal and the patient is asymptomatic. If there is hepatic impairment, the dose is reduced to 750 mg/day.[61]

## FUTURE IMPLICATIONS

The development of agents that exploit unique molecular targets and signaling pathways is just beginning. There are dozens of agents already in clinical trials and more anticipated in the near future.[8] Many questions remain to be answered including how to predict which patients will benefit most from EGFR therapy,[135] the significance of skin rash as a clinical surrogate marker, and the significance of high gene expression levels of EGFR ligands amphiregulin and epiregulin, and low gene expression levels of VEGF in relation to improved progression free survival in response to EGFR therapy.[136] Research is focusing on how to overcome the acquired resistance to 1 TKI can be overcome by other TKIs in the same class or other classes.[137–139] Others are redefining oncology drug development in terms of patient selection, optimal biological dose rather than maximum tolerated dose, and new definitions of response and clinical benefit.[140] Nurses must remain in the forefront of patient education and symptom management in order to keep pace with these developments; they must ensure patients are able to continue therapy with minimal delays and interruptions while maintaining their desired quality of life.

## REFERENCES


1. Fisher B, Costantino JP, Wickerham DL, et al. Tamoxifen for prevention of breast cancer: report of the National Surgical Adjuvant Breast and Bowel Project P-1 Study. *J Natl Cancer Inst.* 1998;90:1371–1388.
2. Genentech, Inc. Herceptin [Package insert]. http://www.gene.com/gene/products/information/pdf/herceptin-prescribing.pdf. Accessed February 7, 2010.
3. Wujcik D. EGFR as a target: rationale for therapy. *Semin Oncol Nurs.* 2006;22:5–9.
4. Croce CM. Oncogenes and cancer. *N Engl J Med.* 2008;358:502–511.
5. Easton JB, Houghton PJ. mTOR and cancer therapy. *Oncogene.* 2006;25:6436–6446.
6. Brugarolas J. Renal-cell carcinoma-molecular pathways and therapies. *N Engl J Med.* 2007;356:185–187.
7. Weiner GJ. Monoclonal antibody mechanisms of action in cancer. *Immunol Res.* 2007;39:271–278.
8. Ma WW, Adjei AA. Novel agents on the horizon for cancer therapy. *CA: Cancer J Clin.* 2009;59:111–137.
9. Jorissen RN, Walker F, Pouliot N, Garrett TP, Ward CW, Burgess AW. Epidermal growth factor receptor: mechanisms of activation and signaling. *Exp Cell Res.* 2003;284:31–53.
10. Barnes CJ, Kumar R. Epidermal growth factor receptor family tyrosine kinases as signal integrators and therapeutic targets. *Cancer Metastasis Rev.* 2003;22:301–307.
11. Marmor MD, Skaria KB, Yarden Y. Signal transduction and oncogenesis by ErbB/HER receptors. *Int J Radiat Oncol Biol Phys.* 2004;58:903–913.
12. Raymond E, Faivre S, Armand JP. Epidermal growth factor receptor tyrosine kinase as a target for anticancer therapy. *Drugs.* 2000;60(Suppl 1):15–23; discussion 41.
13. Pérez-Soler R, Chachoua A, Hammond LA, et al. Determinants of tumor response and survival with erlotinib in patients with non-small-cell lung cancer. *J Clin Oncol.* 2004;22:3238–3247.
14. Kuan CT, Wikstrand CJ, Bigner DD. EGF mutant receptor VIII as a molecular target in cancer therapy. *Endocr Relat Cancer.* 2001;8:83–96.
15. Fukuoka M, Yano S, Giaccone G, et al. Multi-institutional randomized phase II trial of gefitinib for previously treated patients with advanced non-small-cell lung cancer (The IDEAL 1 Trial) [corrected]. *J Clin Oncol.* 2003;21:2237–2246.
16. Kris MG, Natale RB, Herbst RS, et al. Efficacy of gefitinib, an inhibitor of the epidermal growth factor receptor tyrosine kinase, in symptomatic patients with non-small cell lung cancer: a randomized trial. *JAMA.* 2003;290:2149–2158.
17. Miller VA, Kris MG, Shah N, et al. Bronchioloalveolar pathologic subtype and smoking history predict sensitivity to gefitinib in advanced non-small-cell lung cancer. *J Clin Oncol.* 2004;22:1103–1109.
18. Jimeno A, Messersmith WA, Hirsch FR, Franklin WA, Eckhardt SG. KRAS mutations and sensitivity to epidermal growth factor receptor inhibitors in colorectal cancer: practical application of patient selection. *J Clin Oncol.* 2009;27:1130–1136.
19. Bristol-Myers Squibb Co. Erbitux [Package insert]. http://packageinserts.bms.com/pi/pi_erbitux.pdf. Accessed February 7, 2010.
20. Amgen Inc. Vectibix [Package insert]. http://www.vectibix.com/pdfs/misc/vectibix_pi.pdf. Accessed February 7, 2010.
21. Moy B, Kirkpatrick P, Kar S, Goss P. Lapatinib. *Nat Rev Drug Discov.* 2007;6:431–432.
22. Burgess T, Coxon A, Meyer S, et al. Fully human monoclonal antibodies to hepatocyte growth factor with therapeutic potential against hepatocyte growth factor/c-Met-dependent human tumors. *Cancer Res.* 2006; 66:1721–1729.
23. Gordon MS, Mendelson D, Sweeney C, et al. Interim results from a first-in-human study with AMG102, a fully human monoclonal antibody that neutralizes hepatocyte growth factor (HGF), the ligand to

c-Met receptor, in patients (pts) with advanced solid tumors [abstract]. *J Clin Oncol.* 2007;18:S3551.

24. Eder JP, Heath E, Appleman L, et al. Phase I experience with c-MET inhibitor XL880 administered orally to patients (pts) with solid tumors [abstract]. *J Clin Oncol.* 2007; 25(Suppl 18):3526.
25. Sachdev D, Yee D. Disrupting insulin-like growth factor signaling as a potential cancer therapy. *Mol Cancer Ther.* 2007;6:1–12.
26. Karp DD, Paz-Ares LG, Novello S, et al. High activity of the anti-IGF-IR antibody CP-871 in combination with paclitaxel and carboplatin in squamous NSCLC [abstract]. *J Clin Oncol.* 2008;26(Suppl):8015.
27. Tolcher A, Rothenberg M, Rodon J, et al. A phase I pharmacokinetic and pharmacodynamic study of AMG 479, a fully human monoclonal antibody against insulin-like growth factor type 1 receptor (IGF-1R), in advanced solid tumors [abstract]. *J Clin Oncol.* 2007;18:S3002.
28. Frame MC. Src in cancer: deregulation and consequences for cell behaviour. *Biochim Biophys Acta.* 2002;1602:114–130.
29. Olivieri A, Manzione L. Dasatinib: a new step in molecular target therapy. *Ann Oncol.* 2007;18 (Suppl 6):42–46.
30. Brachmann S, Fritsch C, Maira SM, García-Echeverría C. PI3K and mTOR inhibitors: a new generation of targeted anticancer agents. *Curr Opin Cell Biol.* 2009;21:194–198.
31. Wysocki PJ. mTOR in renal cell cancer: modulator of tumor biology and therapeutic target. *Expert Rev Mol Diagn.* 2009;9:231–241.
32. Meric-Bernstam F, Gonzalez-Angulo AM. Targeting the mTOR signaling network for cancer therapy. *J Clin Oncol.* 2009;27:2278–2287.
33. Granville CA, Memmott RM, Gills JJ, Dennis PA. Handicapping the race to develop inhibitors of the phosphoinositide 3-kinase/Akt/mammalian target of rapamycin pathway. *Clin Cancer Res.* 2006;12: 679–689.
34. Dutcher JP. Mammalian target of rapamycin inhibition. *Clin Cancer Res.* 2004;10:6382S-6387S.
35. Wyeth Pharmaceuticals, Inc. Torisel, Highlights of Prescribing Information. http://www.wyeth.com/content/showlabeling.asp?id=490. Accessed February 7, 2010.
36. Novartis Pharmaceuticals Corp. Afinitor [Package insert]. http://www.pharma.us.novartis.com/product/pi/pdf/afinitor.pdf. Accessed February 7, 2010.
37. Sebolt-Leopold JS, Herrera R. Targeting the mitogen-activated protein kinase cascade to treat cancer. *Nat Rev Cancer.* 2004;4:937–947.
38. Escudier B, Eisen T, Stadler WM, et al; TARGET Study Group. Sorafenib in advanced clear-cell renal-cell carcinoma. *N Engl J Med.* 2007;356:125–134.
39. Novartis Pharmaceuticals Corp. Gleevec [Package insert]. http://www.pharma.us.novartis.com/product/pi/pdf/gleevec_tabs.pdf. Accessed February 7, 2010.
40. Bristol-Myers Squibb Co. Sprycel [Package insert]. http://packageinserts.bms.com/pi/pi_sprycel.pdf. Accessed October 1, 2009.
41. Novartis Pharmaceuticals Corp. Tasigna [Package insert]. http://www.pharma.us.novartis.com/product/pi/pdf/tasigna.pdf. Accessed February 7, 2010.
42. Carmeliet P, Jain RK. Angiogenesis in cancer and other diseases. *Nature.* 2000;407:249–257.
43. Saaristo A, Partanen TA, Arola J, et al. Vascular endothelial growth factor-C and its receptor VEGFR-3 in the nasal mucosa and in nasopharyngeal tumors. *Am J Pathol.* 2000;157:7–14.
44. Cooney MM, Remick SC, Vogelzang NJ. Promising systemic therapy for renal cell carcinoma. *Curr Treat Options Oncol.* 2005;6:357–365.
45. Tozer GM, Kanthou C, Baguley BC. Disrupting tumour blood vessels. *Nat Rev Cancer.* 2005;5:423–435.
46. Genentech, Inc. Avastin [Package insert]. http://www.gene.com/gene/products/information/pdf/avastin-prescribing.pdf. Accessed February 7, 2010.
47. Pfizer Inc. Sutent. [Package insert]. http://www.pfizer.com/files/products/uspi_sutent.pdf. Accessed February 7, 2010.
48. Timoney JP, Eagan MM, Sklarin NT. Establishing clinical guidelines for the management of acute hypersensitivity reactions secondary to the administration of chemotherapy/biologic therapy. *J Nurs Care Qual.* 2003;18:80–86.
49. Kurtin SE. Targeting the epidermal growth factor receptor in colorectal carcinoma. *Cancer Nurs.* 2007;30:S1-S9.
50. Mano M, Humblet Y. Drug Insight: panitumumab, a human EGFR-targeted monoclonal antibody with promising clinical activity in colorectal cancer. *Nat Clin Pract Oncol.* 2008;5:415–425.
51. Cohen MH, Gootenberg J, Keegan P, Pazdur R. FDA drug approval summary: bevacizumab plus FOLFOX4 as second-line treatment of colorectal cancer. *Oncologist.* 2007;12:356–361.
52. Gobel BH. Nursing considerations of bevacizumab use in multiple tumor types. *Oncol Nurs Forum.* 2007;34:693–701.
53. Scappaticci FA, Fehrenbacher L, Cartwright T, et al. Surgical wound healing complications in metastatic colorectal cancer patients treated with bevacizumab. *J Surg Oncol.* 2005;91:173–180.
54. O'Brien SG, Guilhot F, Larson RA, et al. Imatinib compared with interferon and low-dose cytarabine for newly diagnosed chronic-phase chronic myeloid leukemia. *N Engl J Med.* 2003;348:994–1004.
55. Hahn EA, Glendenning GA, Sorensen MV, et al. Quality of life in patients with newly diagnosed chronic phase chronic myeloid leukemia on imatinib versus interferon alfa plus low-dose cytarabine: results from the IRIS Study. *J Clin Oncol.* 2003;21:2138–2146.
56. Demetri GD, von Mehren M, Blanke CD, et al. Efficacy and safety of imatinib mesylate in advanced gastrointestinal stromal tumors. *N Engl J Med.* 2002;347:472–480.
57. AstraZeneca. Iressa. [Package insert]. http://www1.astrazeneca-us.com/pi/iressa.pdf. Accessed February 7, 2010.
58. Cohen MH, Williams GA, Sridhara R, et al. United States Food and Drug Administration Drug Approval summary: Gefitinib (ZD1839; Iressa) tablets. *Clin Cancer Res.* 2004;10:1212–1218.
59. Perez-Solar R, HER1/EGFR targeting: refining the strategy. *Oncologist,* 2004; 9:58–67.
60. Genentech, Inc. Tarceva [Package insert]. http://www.gene.com/gene/products/information/pdf/tarceva-prescribing.pdf. Accessed February 7, 2010.
61. GlaxoSmithKline. Tykerb [Package insert]. http://us.gsk.com/products/assets/us_tykerb.pdf. Accessed February 7, 2010.
62. Crean S, Boyd DM, Sercus B, Lahn M. Safety of multi-targeted kinase inhibitors as monotherapy treatment of cancer: a systematic review of the literature. *Curr Drug Saf.* 2009;4:143–154.
63. Chowdhury S, Pickering LM, Ellis PA. Lapatinib: a novel dual tyrosine kinase inhibitor. *Target Oncol.* 2007; 2:107–112.
64. Saylor PJ, Michaelson MD. New treatments for renal cell carcinoma: targeted therapies. *J Natl Compr Canc Netw.* 2009;7:645–656.
65. Magne N, Chargara C, Castadot P. Recent advances in the treatment of renal cell carcinoma and the role of targeted therapies. *Eur J Cancer.* 2008;44:2133–2143.
66. Bayer Healthcare Pharmaceuticals, Inc. Nexavar [Package insert]. http://berlex.bayerhealthcare.com/html/products/pi/Nexavar_PI.pdf. Accessed February 7, 2010.
67. Dalgleish A, Copier J. New multitargeted treatments with antiangiogenic and antitumor activity: focus on sunitunib. *Target Oncol.* 2007;2:17–29.
68. Bryant G. A once-daily dasatinib dosing strategy for chronic myeloid leukemia. *Clin J Oncol Nurs.* 2009;13:316–323.
69. Bauer S, Romvari E. Treatment of chronic myeloid leukemia following imatinib resistance: a nursing guide to second-line treatment options. *Clin J Oncol Nurs.* 2009;13:523–534.
70. Hudes G, Carducci M, Tomczak P, et al. Temsirolimus, interferon alfa, or both for advanced renal-cell carcinoma. *N Engl J Med.* 2007;356:2271–2281.
71. Malizzia LJ, Hsu A. Temsirolimus, an mTOR inhibitor for treatment of patients with advanced renal cell carcinoma. *Clin J Oncol Nurs.* 2008;12:639–646.
72. Oudard S, Medioni J, Aylllon J, et al. Everolimus (RAD001): an mTOR inhibitor for the treatment of metastatic renal cell carcinoma. *Expert Rev Anticancer Ther.* 2009;9:705–717.

73. Sipples R. Common side effects of anti-EGFR therapy: acneform rash. *Semin Oncol Nurs.* 2006;22:28–34.
74. Eaby B, Culkin A, Lacouture ME. An interdisciplinary consensus on managing skin reactions associated with human epidermal growth factor receptor inhibitors. *Clin J Oncol Nurs.* 2008;12:283–290.
75. Lynch TJ, Kim ES, Eaby B, Garey J, West DP, Lacouture ME. Epidermal growth factor receptor inhibitor-associated cutaneous toxicities: an evolving paradigm in clinical management. *Oncologist.* 2007;12:610–621.
76. Morse L, Calarese P. EGFR-targeted therapy and related skin toxicity. *Semin Oncol Nurs.* 2006;22:152–162.
77. Osio A, Mateus C, Soria JC, et al. Cutaneous side-effects in patients on long-term treatment with epidermal growth factor receptor inhibitors. *Br J Dermatol.* 2009;161:515–521.
78. Lacouture ME. Insights into the pathophysiology and management of dermatologic toxicities to EGFR-targeted therapies in colorectal cancer. *Cancer Nurs.* 2007;30:S17-S26.
79. Robert C, Soria JC, Spatz A, et al. Cutaneous side-effects of kinase inhibitors and blocking antibodies. *Lancet Oncol.* 2005;6:491–500.
80. Pérez-Soler R, Delord JP, Halpern A, et al. HER1/EGFR inhibitor-associated rash: future directions for management and investigation outcomes from the HER1/EGFR inhibitor rash management forum. *Oncologist.* 2005;10:345–356.
81. Oishi K. Clinical approaches to minimize rash associated with EGFR inhibitors. *Oncol Nurs Forum.* 2008;35:103–111.
82. National Cancer Institute. Common Toxicity Criteria for Adverse Events v3.0. Publish date August 9, 2006. http://ctep.cancer.gov/protocolDevelopment/electronic_applications/docs/ctcaev3.pdf. Accessed October 1, 2009.
83. Laux I, Jain A, Singh S, Agus DB. Epidermal growth factor receptor dimerization status determines skin toxicity to HER-kinase targeted therapies. *Br J Cancer.* 2006;94:85–92.
84. Albanell J, Rojo F, Averbuch S, et al. Pharmacodynamic studies of the epidermal growth factor receptor inhibitor ZD1839 in skin from cancer patients: histopathologic and molecular consequences of receptor inhibition. *J Clin Oncol.* 2002;20:110–124.
85. Busam KJ, Capodieci P, Motzer R, Kiehn T, Phelan D, Halpern AC. Cutaneous side-effects in cancer patients treated with the anti-epidermal growth factor receptor antibody C225. *Br J Dermatol.* 2001;144:1169–1176.
86. Harding J, Burtness B. Cetuximab: an epidermal growth factor receptor chimeric human-murine monoclonal antibody. *Drugs Today.* 2005;41:107–127.
87. Saltz LB, Meropol NJ, Loehrer PJ, Needle MN, Kopit J, Mayer RJ. Phase II trial of cetuximab in patients with refractory colorectal cancer that expresses the epidermal growth factor receptor. *J Clin Oncol.* 2004;22:1201–1208.
88. Cunningham D, Humblet Y, Siena S, et al. Cetuximab monotherapy and cetuximab plus irinotecan in irinotecan-refractory metastatic colorectal cancer. *N Engl J Med.* 2004;351:337–345.
89. Perez-Soler R. Rash as a surrogate marker for efficacy of epidermal growth factor receptor inhibitors in lung cancer. *Clin Lung Cancer.* 2006;8(Suppl 1):S7-S14.
90. Mohamed MK, Ramalingam S, Lin Y, et al. Skin rash and good performance status (PS) predict improved survival with gefitinib for patients with advanced non-small cell lung cancer (NSCLS) [abstract 7097]. *J Clin Oncol.* 2004; 22:14S.
91. Li T, Perez-Soler R. Skin toxicities associated with epidermal growth factor receptor inhibitors. *Target Oncol.* 2009;4:107–119.
92. Esper P, Gale D, Muehlbauer P. What kind of rash is it?: deciphering the dermatologic toxicities of biologic and targeted therapies. *Clin J Oncol Nurs.* 2007;11:659–666.
93. Jatoi A, Green EM, Rowland KM, Sargent DJ, Alberts SR. Clinical predictors of severe cetuximab-induced rash: observations from 933 patients enrolled in north central cancer treatment group study N0147. *Oncology.* 2009;77:120–123.
94. Mitchell EP, Lacouture M, Shearer H, et al. Final STEPP results of prophylacatic versus reactive skin toxicity (ST) treatment (tx) for panitumumab (pmab)-related ST in patients (pts) with metastatic colorectal cancer (mCRC). *J Clin Oncol.* 2009; 27:CRA4027.
95. Wood LS, Manchen B. Sorafenib: a promising new targeted therapy for renal cell carcinoma. *Clin J Oncol Nurs.* 2007;11:649–656.
96. Lacouture ME, Boerner SA, Lorusso PM. Non-rash skin toxicities associated with novel targeted therapies. *Clin Lung Cancer.* 2006;8(Suppl 1):S36-S42.
97. Gobel BH. Hypersensitivity reactions to biological drugs. *Semin Oncol Nurs.* 2007;23:191–200.
98. Chung CH, Mirakhur B, Chan E, et al. Cetuximab-induced anaphylaxis and IgE specific for galactose-alpha-1,3-galactose. *N Engl J Med.* 2008;358:1109–1117.
99. O'Neil BH, Allen R, Spigel DR, et al. High incidence of cetuximab-related infusion reactions in Tennessee and North Carolina and the association with atopic history. *J Clin Oncol.* 2007;25:3644–3648.
100. Chung CH, O'Neil BH. Infusion reactions to monoclonal antibodies for solid tumors: immunologic mechanisms and risk factors. *Oncology.* 2009;23:14–17.
101. Khoukaz T. Administration of anti-EGFR therapy: a practical review. *Semin Oncol Nurs.* 2006;22:20–27.
102. Cook-Bruns N. Retrospective analysis of the safety of Herceptin immunotherapy in metastatic breast cancer. *Oncology.* 2001;61(Suppl 2):58–66.
103. Viale PH. Management of hypersensitivity reactions: a nursing perspective. *Oncology.* 2009;23:26–30.
104. American Heart Association: Part 10.6: anaphylaxis. *Circulation.* 2005;112:143–145.
105. Basti S. Ocular toxicities of epidermal growth factor receptor inhibitors and their management. *Cancer Nurs.* 2007;30:S10-S16.
106. Tonini G, Vincenzi B, Santini D, Olzi D, Lambiase A, Bonini S. Ocular toxicity related to cetuximab monotherapy in an advanced colorectal cancer patient. *J Natl Cancer Inst.* 2005;97:606–607.
107. Sumpter K, Harper-Wynne C, O'Brien M, Congleton J. Severe acute interstitial pnuemonia and gefitinib. *Lung Cancer.* 2004;43:367–368.
108. Nagaria NC, Cogswell J, Choe JK, Kasimis B. Side effects and good effects from new chemotherapeutic agents. Case 1. Gefitinib-induced interstitial fibrosis. *J Clin Oncol.* 2005;23:2423–2424.
109. Ohyanagi F, Ando Y, Nagashima F, Narabayashi M, Sasaki Y. Acute gefitinib-induced pneumonitis. *Int J Clin Oncol.* 2004;9:406–409.
110. Vahid B, Marik PE. Pulmonary complications of novel antineoplastic agents for solid tumors. *Chest.* 2008;133:528–538.
111. Shepherd FA, Rodrigues PJ, Ciuleanu T, et al. Erlotinib in previously treated non-small cell lung cancer. *J Clin Oncol.* 2005; 23:123–132.
112. Herbst RS, Prager D, Hermann R. TRIBUTE: a phase III trial of erlotinib hydrochloride (OSI-774) combined with carboplatin and paclitaxel chemotherapy in advanced non-small-cell lung cancer. *Clin Cancer Res.* 2005;12:679–689.
113. Lin JT, Yeh KT, Fang HY, Chang CS. Fulminant, but reversible interstitial pneumonitis associated with imatinib mesylate. *Leuk Lymphoma.* 2006;47:1693–1695.
114. Vahid B, Mehrotra A. Trastuzumab (Herceptin)-associated lung injury. *Respirology.* 2006;11:655–658.
115. Sandler AB. Nondermatologic adverse events associated with anti-EGFR therapy. *Oncology.* 2006;20:35–40.
116. Herbst RS, Sandler AB. Non-small cell lung cancer and antiangiogenic therapy: what can be expected with bevacizumab. *Oncologist.* 2004:9:S19-S26.
117. Duran I, Siu LL, Oza AM, et al. Characterisation of the lung toxicity of the cell cycle inhibitor temsirolimus. *Eur J Cancer.* 2006;42:1875–1880.
118. Safra T. 2007. Chemotherapeutics and cardiac toxicity: treatment considerations and management strategies. *Community Oncol.* 2007;4:540–548.

119. Chen MH. Cardiac dysfunction induced by novel targeted anticancer therapy: an emerging issue. *Curr Cardiol Rep.* 2009;11:167–174.
120. Perez EA. Cardiac toxicity of ErbB2-targeted therapies: what do we know? *Clin Breast Cancer.* 2008;8(Suppl 3):S114-S120.
121. Smith IE. Efficacy and safety of Herceptin in women with metastatic breast cancer: results from pivotal clinical studies. *Anticancer Drugs.* 2001;12(Suppl 4):S3-S10.
122. Hayes DF, Picard MH. Heart of darkness: the downside of trastuzumab. *J Clin Oncol.* 2006;24:4056–4058.
123. Suter TM, Procter M, van Veldhuisen DJ, et al. Trastuzumab-associated cardiac adverse effects in the herceptin adjuvant trial. *J Clin Oncol.* 2007;25:3859–3865.
124. Snider KL, Maitland ML. Cardiovascular toxicities: clues to optimal administration of vascular endothelial growth factor signaling pathway inhibitors. *Target Oncol.* 2009;4:67–76.
125. Chu TF, Rupnick MA, Kerkela R, et al. Cardiotoxicity associated with tyrosine kinase inhibitor sunitinib. *Lancet.* 2007;370:2011–2019.
126. Ederhy S, Cohen A, Dufaitre G, et al. QT interval prolongation among patients treated with angiogenesis inhibitors. *Target Oncol.* 2009;4:89–97.
127. Viale PH, Yamamoto DS. Cardiovascular toxicity associated with cancer treatment. *Clin J Oncol Nurs.* 2008;12:627–638.
128. Miller K, Wang M, Gralow J, et al. Paclitaxel plus bevacizumab versus paclitaxel alone for metastatic breast cancer. *N Engl J Med.* 2007;357:2666–2676.
129. Llovet JM, Ricci S, Mazzaferro V, et al. Sorafenib in advanced hepatocellular carcinoma. *N Engl J Med.* 2008;359:378–390.
130. Tejpar S, Piessevaux H, Claes K, et al. Magnesium wasting associated with epidermal-growth-factor receptor-targeting antibodies in colorectal cancer: a prospective study. *Lancet Oncol.* 2007;8:387–394.
131. Ramanarayanan J, Scarpace SL. Acute drug induced hepatitis due to erlotinib. *JOP.* 2007;8:39–43.
132. Sandler AB. Nondermatologic adverse events associated with anti-EGFR therapy. *Oncology.* 2006;20:S35-S40.
133. Navari RM. Overview of the updated antiemetic guidelines for chemotherapy-induced nausea and vomiting. *Community Oncol.* 2007;4:3–11.
134. Lynch T, Price A. The effect of cytochrome P450 metabolism on drug response, interactions, and adverse effects. *Am Fam Physician.* 2007;76:391–396.
135. Dei Tos AP. The biology of epidermal growth factor receptor and its value as a prognostic/predictive factor. *Int J Biol Markers.* 2007;22:S3-S9.
136. Manegold PC, Lurje G, Pohl A, et al. Can we predict the response to epidermal growth factor receptor targeted therapy? *Targ Oncol.* 2008;3:87–99.
137. Pegram M. Can we circumvent resistance to ErbB2-targeted agents by targeting novel pathways? *Clin Breast Cancer.* 2008;8(Suppl 3):S121-S130.
138. Dempke WC, Heinemann V. Resistance to EGF-R (erbB-1) and VEGF-R modulating agents. *Eur J Cancer.* 2009;45:1117–1128.
139. Bianco R, Gelardi T, Damiano V, et al. Mechanisms of resistance to EGFR inhibitors. *Targ Oncol.* 2007;2:31–37.
140. Gutierrez ME, Kummar S, Giaccone G. Next generation oncology drug development: opportunities and challenges. *Nat Rev Clin Oncol.* 2009;6:259–265.

CHAPTER 22

*Dale Halsey Lea, RN, MPH, CGC, FAAN*

# Gene Therapy

## INTRODUCTION

The diagnosis, management, and treatment of human disease are becoming individualized as a result of human genome discoveries. The new human genome era is creating increasing possibilities for genomics-based medicine called "personalized medicine."[1] Gene therapy, pharmacogenetics, and pharmacogenomics are 3 major therapeutic interventions that take into account an individual's specific genetic makeup.[2] This chapter provides an overview of current clinical applications of gene therapy and the emerging fields of pharmacogenetics and pharmacogenomics, as well as social and ethical considerations. It presents new directions for oncology nursing practice, including assessing social, cultural, and family understanding of and responses to new genetic and genomic interventions, and assuring continuity and coordination of patient and family care across the various healthcare settings.

## GENETIC DISORDERS

Genomics involves the study of genes and their surrounding DNA sequences as well as the structure and function of the human genome.[3] Genes are made up of a chemical code (DNA) particular to each gene. Human genome discoveries have revealed that approximately 25,000 genes reside in each individual's human genome.[2] The code differs in sequence from gene to gene and directs the composition and production of proteins that in turn make up living tissues and regulate all of the body's functions. Genetic disorders arise when an error in the complex, multistep process of replication and cell division occurs. The error may be slight—perhaps just one unit of the code is misspelled, repeated, or deleted—but its corresponding protein will be similarly improperly put together. When the protein is essential enough, the error may lead to a sequence of events that can cause disability or even death.[3,4]

Gene therapy interventions are being developed to treat three types of genetically caused conditions. These are single-gene, multifactorial, and acquired genetic conditions.[1] More than 10,000 genetic conditions are caused by a single altered gene. These are called *Mendelian genetic disorders* and include such conditions as cystic fibrosis, hemophilia, sickle-cell anemia, and Huntington's disease.[5] Some forms of hereditary breast and colon cancer as well as other cancers are also caused by a single-gene alteration. These and other single-gene disorders are inherited in families in either an autosomal dominant, recessive, or X-linked manner. Individually, these conditions are rare, but together they represent an important cause of disease and disability.[3] Conditions caused by a combination of genetic and environmental influences are called *multifactorial genetic disorders.* These conditions, which are more complex and less well defined than the single-gene disorders, include heart disease, high blood pressure, cancer, and mental illness. Current research efforts are providing a better understanding of the genetic susceptibility to these and other multifactorial genetic conditions. For example, a new approach to learning about the genetics of common multifactorial conditions such as cancer called Genome-Wide Association Studies (GWAS) has detected common genetic variants that contribute to small or large increases in disease risk in any one individual.[6]

*Acquired genetic conditions* are those that occur as a result of a viral infection such as hepatitis or acquired immunodeficiency syndrome. In these conditions, the disorder is caused by the new genetic information the virus carries into the host.[3]

Altogether, genetic disorders account for as much as 50% of pediatric and adult hospital admissions.[7] Gene therapy and other gene-based therapeutic interventions have the potential to offer alternative, personalized, and possibly less invasive and less expensive ways of treating genetic-related health conditions. The current concept of gene therapy is based on the premise that definitive treatment for genetic disorders should be possible by directing the treatment to the site of the defect itself—the gene mutation—rather than to the secondary effects and symptoms of the mutant gene. Newer approaches to gene therapy unite pharmacotherapeutics with genetic principles and include the use of DNA to treat disease.[8] Gene therapy represents a comprehensive range of therapeutic interventions.

## PRINCIPLES AND GOALS OF GENE THERAPY

### GENE THERAPY DEFINED

Gene therapy involves the correction of defective genes responsible for diseases such as cancer.[2] The most common gene therapy approach seeks to provide therapeutic benefit to a patient by introducing normal genes into the patient's cell nuclei to repair, enhance, replace, or compensate for an altered gene. Gene therapy strategies under investigation include inserting a new functioning gene into the cells of a patient to correct a genetic abnormality or birth defect, thereby providing a new function for the cell. Other approaches include switching the abnormal gene for a normal gene through a technique called homologous recombination; repairing the abnormal gene to return the gene to its normal function; and regulating it.[9] Gene therapy offers the potential for treating many genetic disorders as well as cancer, infectious diseases, and autoimmune disorders by genetically modifying cells in the human body.[10]

Current gene therapy initiatives are aimed at somatic cells, which are the nonreproductive cells of the body (eg, skin, muscle, bone, and liver). This type of gene therapy, called *somatic gene therapy,* can correct inherited genetic disorders and is limited to only one generation. Gene therapy aimed at altering sperm and ova (reproductive cells) is called *germ-line gene therapy.* In the United States, only somatic gene therapy has been approved for use in clinical trials. Germ-line gene therapy has been limited to animal studies and is not currently considered to be ethically acceptable in the treatment of humans. The prospect of germ-line gene therapy raises several ethical issues. The introduction of an altered gene into a fertilized egg, for example, carries the potential risk of introducing a new gene mutation that would be present in an individual at birth and could then be passed on to future generations.[11,12]

Enhancement gene therapy and eugenics are two other possible uses of gene therapy. The principle behind *enhancement gene therapy* is the placement of genes in an embryo or offspring that would improve a societally desirable trait, such as decreased weight or increased height. Gene therapy used for *eugenic purposes* involves the introduction of specific genetic traits into a population to develop "desirable" human attributes such as intelligence. These two applications of gene therapy, like germ-line gene therapy, are not considered by most to be ethically acceptable.[10,11]

## GENE IDENTIFICATION AND CHARACTERIZATION

The normal function of the gene of interest and the characterization of the protein that it makes must be completely understood before a plan for gene correction can be made. Several mechanisms can cause an altered gene to produce a defective protein or result in abnormal regulation of gene expression. For example, an alteration may occur in a gene that is critical for cell survival. Depending on where in the gene the actual defect has occurred, the resulting defective protein is either nonfunctional or poorly expressed. An example of this type of gene defect is adenosine deaminase (ADA) deficiency, in which damage to the ADA gene results in T-lymphocyte death and severe combined immunodeficiency. Individuals who have ADA deficiency have an increased risk for developing frequent and life-threatening infections.[11] An abnormality in a regulatory gene is another mechanism that can cause problems. Certain genes are responsible for controlling the production of a specific gene product. When these genes are defective, functional gene products are not produced in adequate quantities. The gene defect present in thalassemia is an example of this type of gene abnormality.[12]

## GENE TRANSFER METHODS

The most pressing technological hurdle facing gene therapy researchers is the lack of efficient methods for transferring genes into human cells.[13] Successful gene therapy requires efficient gene delivery and continuous corrective activity of the transferred gene in the patient.[13] Gene transfer methods currently under investigation include recombinant virus vectors; chemical, physical, and fusion methods; and liposomal and protein peptide transfer. Each of these techniques has demonstrated advantages and disadvantages, and each may someday find successful clinical application.[14]

Assuring that the transferred gene is integrated into the DNA of the target cell is as important as finding the proper transfer method. Stable integration of the corrected gene, for example, is critical when introducing modifications into cells that have not yet reached maturity or are rapidly dividing. These cells produce future cell populations; maintaining gene correction as the cells divide and reproduce helps to provide long-term benefit to patients. In contrast, gene insertion into nondividing and terminally differentiated tissues such as liver or skeletal muscle may not require integration as a feature of the gene transfer method.[14]

### Gene transfer in vitro and in vivo

Two general approaches—in vitro (also called ex vivo) and in vivo—have been used to transfer a corrected or altered gene to a patient.[4] The in vitro approach is used most widely in clinical trials because it has the advantage of eliminating the possibility of gene transfer into germ-line tissues. This technique is also often more efficient than in vivo transfer.

The in vitro approach requires that the defective cells or cells of interest be removed from the patient first. The corrected or marker gene is then inserted into the cells, and the altered cells are returned to the individual. The cells most commonly used for this approach include lymphocytes, skin fibroblasts, and tumor and bone marrow cells.[4] These cells are readily accessible, amenable to manipulation, and able to survive for long periods of time following reinfusion. The in vitro method has not been successful with nondividing cells such as kidney, liver, or brain cells because they cannot be grown in sufficient numbers for efficient stable gene transfer and are difficult to reimplant.

In vivo gene transfer involves the direct delivery of therapeutic genes to target body cells. This technique is more promising for its potential to directly affect disease sites with minimal risk to the individual. In vivo approaches to gene therapy have been used in clinical trials for cystic fibrosis (CF), muscular dystrophy, melanoma, and heart, lung, and metabolic conditions. With in vivo gene transfer, naked DNA can be delivered without the use of needles, using a gene gun or jet gun. Both methods use either high-pressure helium or liquid to deliver the DNA to interstitial places.[4]

Both in vitro and in vivo gene transfer methods require a carrier, or *vector*, to transfer the augmented or functional genes into the target cells. The two major vector systems currently used for gene transfer are viral and nonviral. These vectors are discussed in the next section.

## VECTORS FOR GENE TRANSFER

Effective use of gene therapy to treat inherited and acquired genetic disorders requires success in four main areas: (l) delivering the gene to the target tissue efficiently, (2) sustaining long-term gene expression, (3) ensuring that the gene transfer will not harm the patient in any way, and (4) transferring the corrected gene to nondividing cells. Another important goal is to develop a cost-effective means to manufacture the vector.[4] A variety of vector systems to deliver the genes have been developed and evaluated. These include viral vectors, such as retrovirus, adenovirus, adeno-associated virus, and herpes virus vectors. In addition, several nonviral vectors, including liposomes and protein peptides, have been created for gene transfer. Introducing a 47th chromosome into target cells is also being researched.[2] Each vector has met with some success in delivering the therapeutic gene to the target tissue, and each has distinct problems and disadvantages. The ideal vector—one that is nontoxic, nonimmunogenic, easy to produce, and efficient in delivering DNA to cells with specificity for a particular cell type—has yet to be discovered.[2]

### VIRAL VECTORS

Most current gene therapy uses viral vectors to deliver the therapeutic gene to the target tissue.[14] All viruses used have been disabled of any pathogenic effects by removing the genes required for replication of the virus and replacing them with therapeutic genes and selection markers (see Figure 22-1).[2,11] The use of viruses is a potentially powerful technique because many have evolved specific mechanisms for delivering DNA to cells. Humans, however, have an immune system designed to defend against viruses, and attempts to transfer genes by means of viral vectors have been complicated by host responses.[12]

#### Retroviral vectors

A retrovirus is composed of RNA that can insert itself readily into dividing cells. Retroviruses are considered the most promising gene transfer vehicle. These RNA viruses are able to carry out efficient gene transfer into many types of cells and can integrate into the host cell genes with stability. The therapeutic gene carried into the cell by the retrovirus will be inherited by all future generations of the cell and will provide the possibility of long-term gene expression (see Figure 22-2).[3] Retroviruses, although advantageous in many ways, pose several challenges. One major concern is that the insertion of the retrovirus will disrupt normal genes essential for proper cell function, leading to harmful physiological effects that favor cancer development. This is one of the most serious and current technical hurdles.[14]

#### Lentiviral vectors

Lentiviruses, which belong to the retrovirus family, are now being used in gene therapy because they can infect both dividing and nondividing cells and have the ability to provide long-term and stable gene expression. Human immunodeficiency virus (HIV) is the most well-known lentivirus used for gene transfer in vivo. The use of lentiviruses such as HIV as a vector for gene therapy may not cause problems, such as cancer, that have arisen with retroviral vectors.[15]

### ADENOVIRAL VECTORS

As of 2007, adenoviral gene therapy has been used in 25% of the clinical gene therapy trials worldwide.[14] Adenoviruses are a family of viruses that cause benign respiratory tract, intestinal, and eye infections in humans. They also have the capacity to infect both dividing and nondividing cells,

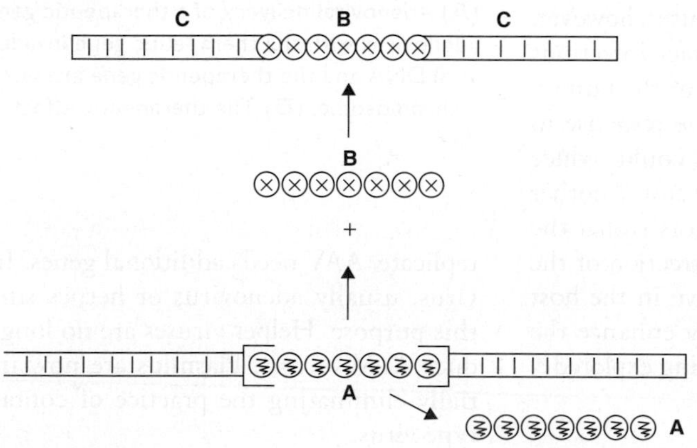


**FIGURE 22-1**

Viral vector with therapeutic gene. Viral vectors are prepared by removing the disease-producing viral-gene (**A**) and replacing it with the therapeutic gene (**B**). (**C**) Viral genes necessary for invasion of the cell are maintained.

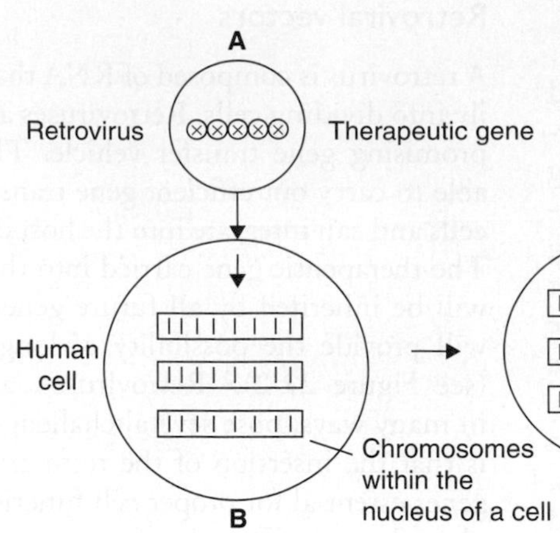


**FIGURE 22-2**

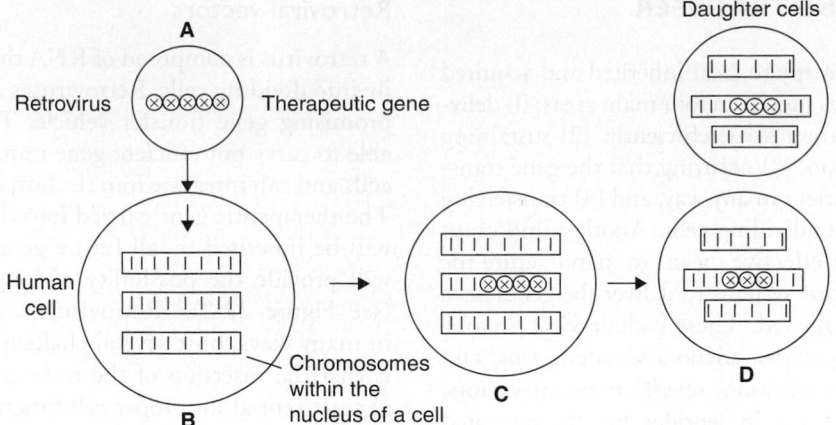

(**A**) Retroviral delivery of a therapeutic gene. (**B**) A retrovirus with the therapeutic gene invades the cell. (**C**) Reverse transcriptase makes a DNA copy of the retroviral RNA. The viral DNA and the therapeutic gene are part of the nucleus and are incorporated into one of the 46 human chromosomes. (**D**) The therapeutic effect remains if the cell replicates, providing daughter cells with a copy of the therapeutic gene.

making them useful for gene therapy. Adenoviruses are large and can hold large segments of therapeutic DNA. They can also be produced in large amounts in culture. They have been the vectors of choice for many protocols designed to treat the pulmonary complications of cystic fibrosis as well as for a variety of clinical protocols to treat cancer. In contrast to retroviruses, which contain RNA, adenoviruses contain DNA and thus do not integrate into host DNA but instead replicate themselves outside of the nucleus of the host cell. Because of this limited integration, expression of the therapeutic gene is short-lived, and regular reapplication of gene therapy using adenovirus vectors is necessary (see Figure 22-3).[2]

The potential usefulness of adenoviral vectors stems from the fact that they do not require actively dividing cells to introduce their therapeutic gene. Adenoviruses, however, are a common cause of upper respiratory tract infections in humans. As a result, unfortunately, most of the human population may experience an active immune response to antibodies from a previous infection, which could reduce the effectiveness of gene therapy using this vector. Another potential concern with using adenoviral vectors is that the integrated gene may not lead to uniform correction of the gene defect, because it may not remain active in the host cell. Other viral vectors that may potentially enhance the delivery of therapeutic genes are therefore being explored.[2]

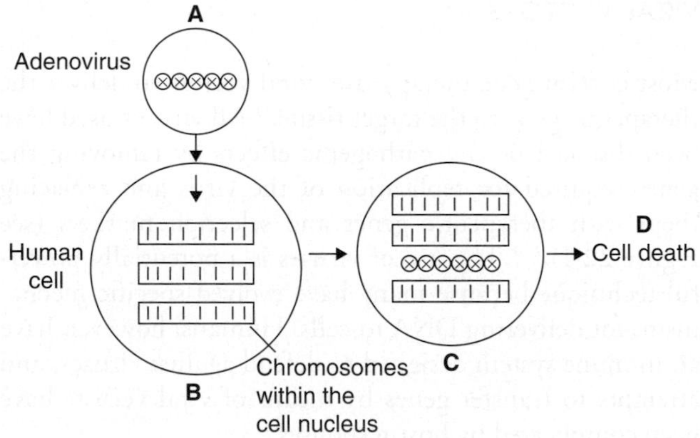


**FIGURE 22-3**

(**A**) Adenoviral delivery of a therapeutic gene. (**B**) An adenovirus with the therapeutic gene invades the cell. (**C**) The viral DNA and the therapeutic gene are not incorporated into a chromosome. (**D**) The therapeutic effect is lost when the cell dies.

## Newer adenoviral vectors

The adeno-associated virus (AAV) is one of the newer viral vectors under investigation; it is a simple, nonpathogenic virus composed of a single strand of DNA. In order to replicate, AAV needs additional genes. In the past, a helper virus, usually adenovirus or herpes simplex virus, served this purpose. Helper viruses are no longer required to produce AAV vectors. Plasmids are now used instead, essentially eliminating the practice of contaminating the wild type virus.

The AAV virus can infect a variety of types of cells, and although it appears to integrate in a nonspecific manner, it has been shown to integrate preferentially into chromosome 19. AAV gene therapy has been investigated for cystic fibrosis and for factor IX hemophilia.[16,17] Other viruses that are being considered and developed for use as vectors for gene therapy are the herpes simplex virus, which infects cells of the nervous system, and the vaccinia virus. These viral vector systems produce a transient response, and many people have an immunity to components of the virus from being infected previously.[2,14]

### NONVIRAL VECTORS

Nonviral vector delivery systems for gene transfer may provide an alternative method of efficient gene delivery. To enhance integration into the human genome, nonviral methods transfer therapeutic genes into human cells by chemical methods such as precipitation with calcium phosphate and encapsulation of therapeutic genes into liposomes or molecular conjugates (complexes of lipids and DNA). Physical methods being explored and developed include direct microinjection of DNA into cells by particle acceleration. The efficiency of this process appears to be low, but intramuscular injection of "naked" DNA has been used successfully to establish cellular and humoral responses, suggesting that simple intramuscular administration of DNA could be used to create a gene vaccine. As of 2007, the number of clinical trials using naked DNA had increased from 14% in 2004 to 18% in 2007.[14]

Nonviral gene delivery systems may provide a means for achieving short-term expression of therapeutic gene products in certain tissues with a high degree of safety. Studies to date suggest that nonviral delivery systems have toxicities and safety profiles similar to those of conventional drugs and other biological products. There have been no reports of significant toxicity involving naked DNA in animal or human studies to date. Lung, liver, and endothelial tissue appear to be particularly acceptable targets for nonviral gene therapy. Other targets include tissues that are accessible to direct interstitial injection, such as muscle, skin, and tumor masses.[14]

One of the greatest challenges for gene therapy is the development of safe and cost-effective therapeutic gene delivery systems that can be used along with conventional pharmaceutical and biological products. Current viral and nonviral vectors do not yet provide a completely satisfactory means of propagating the therapeutic genes in proliferating cells. To increase the possibilities of success, researchers are investigating the introduction of a 47th chromosome (artificial chromosome) into target cells. This method does not affect the working of the other 46 chromosomes or cause mutations. The artificial chromosome can serve as a natural human vector for therapeutic genes. Nonviral gene therapy methods offer the potential for therapeutic interventions that may be acceptable to physicians and patients and offer safety and efficiency similar to those of conventional therapeutic modalities.[2]

## FUTURE APPROACHES TO GENE THERAPY

Researchers are investigating a new approach to gene therapy called RNA interference (RNAi). RNAi is being used to block the expression of a specific gene using this mechanism as a technique for exploring gene function and for treating disease. Short interfering RNAs (siRNAs) are being used to avoid the problems with long double stranded RNA molecules that cause the interferon response in some cell types. There are currently more than 10 clinical trials using this gene therapy technique. Pharmaceutical companies are also developing RNAi-based treatments for diseases including hepatitis C, age-related macular degeneration, asthma, and Huntington Disease.[14]

Another new approach called nanotechnology is being applied in cancer diagnostics and treatments. Nanotechnology-based therapeutics approved for cancer treatment include Doxil, a liposome preparation of doxorubicin, and Abraxane, which is paclitaxel in nanoparticle formulation. Using nanoparticles, chemotherapy drugs can now be delivered directly to tumor cells and then send a signal after the cancer cells are destroyed.[18]

## CLINICAL PROTOCOLS FOR GENE THERAPY

### THE SEVERE COMBINED IMMUNODEFICIENCY DISEASE PROTOCOL

The first approved clinical protocol for gene therapy was initiated in 1990. Two girls with ADA deficiency, a rare genetic condition that produces severe immunodeficiency in children, were injected with white blood cells carrying a therapeutic gene. The clinical protocol called for inserting the ADA gene into T lymphocytes. ADA is an enzyme needed for normal immune system functioning. It prevents the buildup of deoxyadenosine, a metabolic product that becomes toxic to immune cells, especially lymphocytes, when present in high concentrations. ADA deficiency accounts for 25% of cases of severe combined immunodeficiency disease (SCID). The clinical protocol for treating ADA deficiency has served as a paradigm for both the benefits and the risks of gene therapy. It initially demonstrated the safety of retroviral gene transfer, and showed that patients could benefit from gene therapy.[19]

Treatment for ADA deficiency has also demonstrated the risks of gene therapy. In 2003, French researchers reported that two children with SCID who had been treated with retroviral gene therapy had developed a leukemia-like disorder 30 months after a single gene therapy treatment. In response to this discovery, the FDA put a hold on clinical trials that used retroviral vectors to insert the defective gene into hematopoietic cells. The American Society of Gene Therapy conducted its own investigation to determine why this occurred only in patients with SCID, and not in other

**TABLE 22-1**

**Examples of Approved Single-Gene Clinical Gene-Therapy Trials**

| Inherited Genetic Condition | Vector | Gene/Gene Product |
|---|---|---|
| Cystic fibrosis | Adenovirus, adeno-associated virus, liposomes | CFTR |
| Familial hypercholesterolemia | Retrovirus | LDL receptor |
| Severe immunodeficiency due to ADA deficiency | Retrovirus | ADA |
| Alpha-1 antitrypsin deficiency | AAV | Alpha-1 antitrypsin |
| Gaucher disease, Type 1 | Retrovirus | Glucocerebrocidase |
| Hunter syndrome | Retrovirus | Iduronate-2-sulfatase |

*Abbreviations*: ADA, adenosine deaminase; CFTR, cystic fibrosis transmembrane conductance regulator; LDL, low density lipoprotein; AAV, adeno-associated virus.

*Source*: Data from Balicki and Buetler.[23]

trials with retroviruses.[20,21] Researchers have since discovered that the retrovirus used (Moloney-murine leukemia virus, or Mo-MuLV) inserted the therapeutic genes next to a gene known to promote blood cancer. Insertional mutagenesis is a recognized complication of retroviral gene transfer attempts because gene integration occurs randomly. With Mo-MuLV, this appears to occur at the beginning of the gene, affecting how it works.[22]

Table 22-1 lists some examples of other single-gene disorders for which gene therapy is being investigated.[23]

## GENE THERAPY REGULATION

More than 700 clinical protocols have been approved throughout the world, and more than 1,300 gene therapy clinical trials have been completed, are ongoing, or have been approved worldwide.[14] Guidelines for clinical gene therapy protocols were established by the National Institutes of Health (NIH) in the document *Points to Consider in the Design and Submission of Human Somatic Cell Gene Therapy Protocols.* The guidelines require that proposals for human gene therapy go through several levels of review. Each proposed protocol must first be reviewed by local bioethics and biosafety committees and must be in accord with the standards of conventional research. The Human Gene Therapy Research Subcommittee and the Recombinant DNA Advisory Committee (RAC) then review the protocol. These two committees serve in an advisory capacity to the director of the NIH, who approves all gene transfer and gene-therapy proposals.[24] The FDA addresses the scientific methodology and preclinical safety testing and has created a set of guidelines for the initiation of gene therapy. The FDA's guidelines are separate from the Human Genome Research Subcommittee and RAC guidelines and address the characteristics, production, and certification of the biological substances being used for gene transfer. The "Points to Consider" document is updated regularly and is found as an appendix of the NIH's guidelines on recombinant DNA research.[24,25]

As of early 2008, approximately 716 clinical protocols were approved in the United States. The majority of these are for the treatment of cancer. Genetic diseases such as cystic fibrosis and other single-gene disorders make up approximately 6% of clinical gene-therapy protocols. Clinical gene-therapy trials for the treatment of infectious disease and for conditions such as peripheral artery disease, rheumatoid arthritis, and coronary artery disease also are being carried out. The majority of these approved protocols are for Phase I clinical trials.[26]

## CANCER GENE THERAPY

Treatment of cancer using gene therapy is aimed at inhibiting oncogene function and restoring tumor-suppressor function. *Proto-oncogenes* are normal cellular genes that are essential for cellular growth and development. Oncogenes stimulate neoplastic growth and are activated by proto-oncogenes that encode a growth factor or another protein and disturb normal cell development and regulation. *Antioncogenes* are those genes that block the action of growth-inducing proteins. These genes are also called tumor-suppressor genes to denote their ability to block the action of oncogenes. When functioning normally, tumor-suppressor genes and proto-oncogenes work together to enable the body to perform vital functions, such as replacing dead cells and repairing defective ones.[4]

Two types of gene transfer are used in clinical cancer–gene therapy trials: gene marking and gene therapy. *Gene marking* involves labeling cells for future identification. A gene that has been genetically marked is introduced into cells, most commonly using a retrovirus as a vector for the desired gene. This approach is being used to determine the source of relapse in individuals undergoing autologous bone marrow transplantation. Gene marking studies have been used in the treatment of melanoma, leukemia, neuroblastoma, and stem cell transplantation.[27] *Gene therapy* studies involve modification of the content or expression of altered genes in somatic cells by transferring the functional or enhanced genes.

## Cancer gene-therapy protocols

A number of protocols are investigating the transfer of genes to correct an error (gene alteration) or to add a new function (gene addition). These protocols use two general approaches. In one—a *tumor-directed* approach—the therapeutic gene is introduced into the tumor cells to destroy them. The other approach involves two forms of immunotherapy—active and adoptive. In the *active* immunotherapeutic approach, cytokines, tumor antigens, or tumor-associated antigens are introduced to stimulate the patient's immune system to mount an antitumor response. *Adoptive* immunotherapy involves the transfer of a genetically modified tumor lymphocyte to mediate tumor regression.[11,13] Such studies are founded on earlier gene-marking studies that showed that a new gene could be safely inserted into patients and followed over time.

### *Tumor-directed gene-therapy protocols*

***"Suicide gene" therapy protocols:*** These clinical trials involve the transfer of a gene that produces an enzyme whose activity converts a nontoxic prodrug to its toxic form—a "suicide gene." The gene transfer is targeted to tumor cells to make them susceptible to an agent that does not cause harm to normal cells but kills malignant cells. The suicide gene is toxic to dividing cells only, thus sparing the normal cells and nondividing tumor cells. The herpes simplex virus thymidine kinase gene (*HSV-TK*) is the one most commonly used. Any cell that incorporates the *HSV-TK* gene becomes sensitive to the antiviral drug ganciclovir and can be destroyed on exposure. Retroviral vectors transfer genes to actively dividing cells, making this type of gene therapy well suited for the treatment of brain tumors, as only the malignant cells are dividing and replicating. When a patient is treated with ganciclovir, the tumor cells are killed. Further modification of the promotor region of the vector creates tissue or organ specificity such that the suicide gene will be expressed only in cell types restricted by the specific promotor.

A new approach to suicide-gene therapy uses ultrasound and nano/microbubbles (NBs) to deliver exogenous molecules noninvasively into a specific target site. Aoi and associate researchers[28] used low-intensity pulsed ultrasound and NBs to transduce the herpes simplex thymidine kinase (*HSV-TK*) gene in vitro, leading to gene transfer. Ganciclovir (GCV) was added to the transduced cells leading to HSV-TK/GCV-dependent cell death mediated by apoptosis. This technology was assessed in mice that had subcutaneous tumors. The results were a dramatic reduction in tumor size, demonstrating the potential for using ultrasound and NBs as a new method for physical gene delivery and for cancer-gene therapy.[28]

***Tumor-suppressor gene therapy:*** The tumor-suppressor gene, *P53*, is found in approximately 50% of all cancers. In a number of clinical trials, a normal copy of the gene has been introduced to restore its function in patients with lung cancer, colorectal cancer, breast cancer, as well as many others. These treatments have met with some success. Clinical trials are now underway in which tumor suppressor–gene therapy is combined with chemotherapy to treat cancer.[29]

***Antisense oligonucleotides:*** Genetic therapies for cancer treatment are being developed that specifically target DNA and RNA. The use of specific segments of DNA—antisense oligonucleotides—is one example of this new methodology. Antisense oligonucleotides are nucleic binding agents. They are short strands of nucleotides that predictably combine with other nucleotides. This property allows for the design of a treatment drug that can recognize a unique site on a specific gene. Oligonucleotides can be inserted into cells to interfere with the translation of RNA into an oncogene protein. When transferred into patients, they prevent the oncogene's RNA message from being translated into a functional oncogene protein. This approach is being used in clinical trials of antiepidermal growth factor receptor in the treatment of head and neck squamous cell carcinoma.[30]

***Oncolytic viral gene therapy:*** Oncolytic viruses reproduce in tumor cells, causing their lyses. These viruses can be used to treat cancers with a defective *p53* pathway. In normal cells, *p53* is destroyed by adenoviruses, producing a protein called E1B 55K. This protein binds with *p53* and, in synchrony with another viral protein, directs *p53* for destruction. Researchers have been able to modify a strain of adenovirus so that it does not encode E1B 55K and lose its ability to destroy *p53*. Normally, *p53* activity causes a cascade of events that lead to the death of the affected cell, and viral replication cannot be established. In cancer cells that lack *p53*, however, the normal mechanism that leads to the death of the infected cells is abolished so that only the modified adenovirus can replicate and kill tumor cells. This approach is being used to treat head and neck cancer and, in some clinical trials, is being combined with chemotherapeutic agents.[31]

### *Active immunotherapy*

***Tumor-infiltrating lymphocytes:*** Host immunological responses can be used to alter the natural course of some cancers, especially malignant melanoma. Tumor-infiltrating lymphocytes (TILs) that are able to mediate tumor regression in patients with melanoma have been identified. Using these TILs, researchers have mapped and cloned many genes encoding shared melanoma antigens and their antigenic epitopes. Administration of an epitope in conjunction with intravenous high-dose interleukin-2 (IL-2) has been shown to mediate regression in patients with malignant melanoma. These findings have led to additional clinical trials using melanoma antigen genes to boost the immune system.[32,33]

***Cytokine genes:*** Cytokines are molecules that enhance the body's immune response to tumor antigens. Cytokine genes are being used to augment the body's ability to mount an immune response to tumor cells. Two of the most commonly used cytokine genes are IL-2 and tumor necrosis factor. These cytokine genes are modified so that they will not proliferate but can still support expression of the introduced gene products. The modified cells are then injected into the patient via subcutaneous, intradermal, or intramuscular routes.[34]

***DNA vaccines:*** Cancer vaccination is an example of an approach that is evolving into an effective and broadly applicable form of therapy. This approach circumvents the disadvantage of using common vectors such as adenovirus that cause the body to produce neutralizing antibodies or cellular immunity against the vector-derived gene products, rendering the vectors ineffective following administration. DNA vaccines that contain tumor associated–antigen genes or cytokine genes are now being used because the pure DNA encodes only the tumor associated–antigen gene. DNA vaccines are usually administered intramuscularly, alone or in combination with cytokine genes.[34]

Metastatic renal cell carcinoma is one cancer that has demonstrated responsiveness to immunotherapeutic intervention.[35,36] Therapeutic vaccine therapy is also being used in the treatment of prostate cancer. One phase 3 clinical trial used a recombinant vaccine of prostatic acid antigen. This antigen is expressed in 95% of prostate cancers. When injected with the recombinant vaccine, the circulating immune cells recognize this antigen, and the tumor response rates are boosted. Additional research is underway on tumor-specific vaccines using antigen-presenting cells such as dendritic cells to induce immune responses in T cells.[37]

*Adoptive immunotherapy.* Adoptive immunotherapy is a form of gene-transfer therapy in which the patient's own lymphocytes (peripheral blood or from TILs) are modified outside of the body with genes that enhance their antitumor activity. The modified genes are then reinfused back into the same patient. Clinical trials using anti-Epstein–Barr virus (EBV) adoptive immunotherapy have been conducted for a number of different cancers. Epstein–Barr virus is an infection associated with tumors such as lymphoproliferation, Hodgkin's disease, nasopharyngeal carcinoma, and Burkitt's lymphoma. These trials involve in vitro generation and expansion of virus specific cytotoxic lymphocytes, which can be given to patients for treatment and prophylaxis. To date, adoptive immunotherapy with EBV-specific cytotoxic T lymphocytes has been shown to be effective with immunogenic tumors such as post-transplant lymphoproliferative disease.[38,39]

***Chimeric receptors:*** Chimeric receptors are one example of adoptive immunotherapy. They consist of two different molecules brought together to form one functional molecule—an extracellular antibody molecule linked to intracellular signal domains of T-cell receptors. In this type of therapy, the patient's autologous T cells serve as the vehicle for inserted chimeric antibody molecules. The inserted antibody molecules have specificity for a tumor antigen. When transferred into patients, the modified T cells are redirected to recognize the tumor by virtue of the specific antibody on its surface. Once the tumor cells are engaged, the T cells are activated via the signaling chain and mediate antitumor activity. This approach is being used in the treatment of patients with neuroblastoma, kidney cancer, and metastatic ovarian cancer.[34,40]

***Tumor-specific T cells:*** Adoptive immunotherapy using transduction of the IL-2 gene into antitumor T lymphocytes is under investigation as a way of treating tumors and overcoming the limitation of toxicity following prolonged in vivo administration of IL-2. Transduction of an *IL-2* gene into a TIL has been used with some success in the treatment of patients with melanoma and renal cell carcinoma.[34]

## Pharmacogenetics and pharmacogenomics: Gene-based treatment of cancer

Pharmacogenetics is an emerging field of personalized treatment that deals with interindividual differences in drug response. Pharmacogenetics aims to identify the inherited basis for interindividual differences in drug response and to translate this to molecular diagnostics that can be used to individualize drug therapy. Many human genes involved in pharmacogenetic traits have now been identified, their molecular mechanisms elucidated, and their clinical use more clearly defined. Pharmacogenomics involves research to search for genetic variants that are associated with drug efficiency. The term *pharmacogenomics* comes from the terms pharmacology and genomics and is the intersection between pharmaceuticals and genomics. Pharmacogenomics leads to the development of drugs that can be adapted to each person's specific genetic make-up.[41]

One of the most well-developed examples of clinical pharmacogenetics is the genetic polymorphism of thiopurine methyltransferase (TPMT). TPMT has been associated with altered drug metabolism and increased risk for severe toxicity from the anticancer agent 6-mercaptopurine. Testing for TPMT genotypes is now used to modify doses of 6-mercaptopurine and azathioprine that are used to treat acute lymphoblastic leukemia and inflammatory bowel disease. Individuals with deficient or intermediate TPMT activity are at risk for toxicity, including fatal myelosuppression, at standard thiopurine doses. Testing for the presence of low-activity gene variants for TPMT has been done in clinical practice for more than 10 years in the United States. At present, the testing applies to Caucasian populations in which the specific variant alleles are known. Further studies are needed to identify the variants that underlie the response in different populations.[42]

A similar example of pharmacogenetics has been observed with the antineoplastic agent 5-fluorouracil. Deficiency of the enzyme dihydropyrimidine dehydrogenase leads to severe toxicity from treatment with 5-fluorouracil using the usual doses. The dose of this drug therapy is now adjusted based on the DNA sequence of drug-metabolizing enzyme genes.[43]

Treatment with trastuzumab (Herceptin) is an example of pharmacogenomics. When overexpressed, HER2, a protein located in cell surfaces, causes cancers to become more aggressive. The *HER2* oncogene is overexpressed in 20% to 30% of breast cancers, and these tumors seem to be more aggressive and somewhat more resistant to chemotherapy than those not overexpressing the oncogene. Clinical trials involving the use of gene therapy to deliver an antibody against the HER2 protein led to the creation of Herceptin, a humanized monoclonal antibody against the HER2 receptor that is linked to *HER2* overexpression. It is now standard practice to test women with breast cancer for *HER2* before initiation of treatment. Those with overexpression of *HER2* benefit from treatment with Herceptin, either alone or in combination with chemotherapy, resulting in an improved response rate and overall survival advantage. Patients with breast cancer who do not have *HER2* overexpression are prescribed alternate therapy.[44,45]

The discovery of the specific molecular defect BCR-ABL, which occurs as a result of the Philadelphia chromosome translocation, has created a new foundation for treating Philadelphia chromosome-positive leukemias. The Philadelphia chromosome translocation is present in more than 90% of patients with chronic myelogenous leukemia (CML). The translocation moves the *BCR* and *ABL* genes next to each other and causes the BCR-ABL tyrosine kinase to stay active. The activity of this kinase blocks apoptotic cell death and is the cause of chronic myeloid leukemia. The drug imatinib (Gleevec) was designed to target the molecular defect, and treatment with this specific medication has produced an 88% response in cases of Philadelphia chromosome-positive CML.[43,46]

## ETHICAL, SOCIAL, AND LEGAL ISSUES IN GENE THERAPY

As gene therapy has evolved over the last 30 years, professional and public scrutiny has focused on the ethical implications of the technology. Organized religions have taken an active part in discussions on the ethical implications of human gene therapy. The continuing dialogue among theologians, ethicists, and scientists has helped to shape and implement regulatory processes for gene therapy designed to safeguard against misuse.[47]

The NIH developed the guidelines "Points to Consider" in 1988 to solidify ethical concerns and to assist investigators and reviewers of human gene-therapy proposals in addressing difficult issues.[24,25,48] The "Points to Consider," revised in 1990, provides a foundation for current and future clinical genome research. Information from the document was condensed to form six sets of ethical guidelines:

- Concern for the clinical benefit of all persons receiving gene therapy
- Assurance of informed consent
- Fair selection of persons for gene therapy–research protocols
- Attention to the need for biosafety protocols
- Public involvement in genetic research policy
- Attention to long-term consequences of genetic research.

These considerations provide an ethical framework within which researchers and healthcare professionals can address the multitude of questions that are evolving as recombinant techniques and gene therapy become more common.[25,48]

### ASSESSING CLINICAL BENEFITS

One guideline expressed in "Points to Consider" concerns the need to assess the clinical benefits of gene therapy. This refers to the researcher's responsibility to ensure that the risk to the participant for any gene-therapy protocol is outweighed by the benefit of the treatment. To meet this responsibility, researchers must have adequate knowledge of the treatment to determine whether the participant will benefit more from the gene-therapy trial than from any alternative treatment for the condition.

In 1995, the director of the NIH convened a panel to assess the NIH's investment in gene-therapy research. The panel concluded that gene therapy had been oversold to the public and that the publicity surrounding gene therapy was already causing some patients to forgo conventional therapeutic interventions. Panel members emphasized the importance of research aimed at developing a better understanding of the underlying mechanisms that contribute to genetic disease. In October 1999, the first fatality related to gene therapy occurred and was reported. Subsequent investigations revealed the deaths of six additional gene-therapy patients that had not received the usual public disclosure. In February 2000, the United States Senate held hearings on this topic, and the heightened scrutiny and awareness has resulted in an increase in the reporting of adverse effects and renewed oversight of gene-therapy trials by both the NIH and the FDA. This kind of research and public debate conducted to support ethical and scientifically sound development and application of gene-therapy trials will better meet the needs of patients participating in the trials.[49]

## PARTICIPANT SELECTION AND INFORMED CONSENT

The "Points to Consider" document also notes that potential research subjects should choose freely to participate in gene therapy. The choice of the participants must be equitable, and candidates for gene-therapy research need to be chosen fairly from among multiple populations. Those populations considered to be vulnerable, such as prisoners, should not serve as subjects.[24,50] Participant selection also involves compassionate or "emergency" use of gene therapy. A request was made to the NIH RAC in 1993 for compassionate use of a gene-therapy protocol, for example, for a patient with limited life expectancy. The request, although finally granted, generated many questions regarding emergency access to gene therapy and fairness to other participants. If one patient is granted permission, how can a researcher turn down other applicants? How does the researcher maintain the integrity of the research data if emergency-use patients, who do not meet the clinical trial research criteria, are accepted into the protocol? These and other concerns about subject selection presented to the RAC underscore some of the inherent issues in regulating of any new and as yet unproven therapy.[51]

Clinical research always involves an informed consent process to ensure that subjects participating in the research are doing so freely and voluntarily and with full information about the risks and benefits.[52,53] This precedent does not require that protocols be completely risk free or that the benefits be unequivocally established before clinical trials are proposed. Rather, the premise of informed consent is that the risks are honestly described, and the patient considering the research ultimately decides the value of the potential benefits, weighed against the possible risks. When minors are involved as participants in clinical gene-therapy trials, the "Points to Consider" document emphasizes the need for informed consent by the minor in addition to obtaining parental permission.[24] The informed consent process for gene-therapy protocols should also include a discussion of plans for follow-up with primary-care providers, social workers, geneticists, and psychologists, in addition to the clinical investigators. Including these professionals in a follow-up plan ensures that participants will receive support in all areas of health care, including reproduction and psychological development, and normal processes that may be influenced by participation in gene therapy.

The issue of informed consent becomes more problematic when germ-line therapy is considered. Germ-line gene therapy would alter the genes of future generations and possibly create unknown long-term consequences. Germ-line gene therapy also raises the ethical concern that future unborn generations would not be able to give informed consent before gene therapy makes deliberate changes to their genetic code. For this and other ethical reasons, germ-line therapy is currently prohibited.[47]

## SAFETY ISSUES

Short- and long-term side effects and toxicities associated with new gene-therapy interventions also are of concern. Programs that implement human clinical gene-therapy trials must emphasize staff expertise, training of professional support staff, and patient and family counseling. These factors are deemed essential to ensure the safety and successful implementation of gene-therapy research.[54]

### Patient safety

To date, a number of deaths due to gene therapy have been reported, and several children undergoing gene therapy for SCID have developed a leukemia-like illness.[20–22] These toxicities have led to increased vigilance regarding patient safety. As with any research drug protocol, during administration, patients need to be observed and evaluated for an allergic reaction to the foreign protein. Common side effects reported thus far include fever, chills, headache, fatigue, myalgia, nausea, and vomiting. Less common side effects reported include anorexia, diarrhea, and central nervous system effects such as extremity weakness, anemia, and leukopenia. Table 22-2 summarizes side effects commonly reported with some of the more common vectors.[34] Researchers cannot at this time predict the long-term risks to patients undergoing gene therapy or to their children. Some adverse effects may not become apparent for years. Vigilant follow-up care is needed to identify, diagnose, and prevent side effects. Long-term follow-up care may not be built into gene-therapy protocols. Nurses caring for individuals who have undergone gene therapy must therefore be aware of this potential gap and develop a plan for following and monitoring patients.[54]

### Public safety

The safety of those working with this new method of drug delivery is a second important concern. Safety involves protecting providers, families, and the public from the possibility of infectious transmission of recombinant genes with viral vectors. To date, infectious spread of recombinant

**TABLE 22-2**

**Common Adverse Effects Reported in Worldwide Clinical Trials for Cancer Gene Therapy**

| Vector | Adverse Effect |
|---|---|
| Retrovirus | Erythema and induration, pruritus, pain, fever, elevation of liver function tests, peritumor edema, abdominal pain, diarrhea, nausea, increased local edema, seizures abducens, paresis, confusion, intratumoral hemorrhage, mild exacerbation of graft-vs-host disease |
| Adenovirus | Fever, abnormal liver function, fatigue, pulmonary infiltrate, transient lung function abnormalities |
| Liposome | Injection pain, transient pneumothorax |
| Plasmid | Fever |

*Source*: Data from Liu.[34]

viruses has not been observed, and the risk of this complication is considered to be remote. Not all gene-therapy protocols use retroviral vectors, and those that do may not all use them in the same way. Implementing universal precautions in consultation with nursing and hospital infection control officers is one safety measure that has been put in place for clinical trials using viral vectors, as these precautions are considered sufficient to prevent transmission of known pathogens such as hepatitis and HIV.[50]

## EQUAL ACCESS TO GENE THERAPY AND CONFIDENTIALITY OF GENETIC AND GENOMIC INFORMATION

As more is learned about the safety and efficacy of gene therapies to treat cancer, additional ethical issues will arise concerning the cost, availability, and allocation of these therapies.[47] It is critical to consider the ethical implications of treatments developed for individuals with end-stage disease vs research directed toward prevention and cause of disease. As with any costly treatment, access to gene therapy may be provided to only a select few. Medical centers are the only institutions that can provide gene therapies, possibly meaning additional patient expense for travel and lodging, for which insurance companies do not pay. Patients could spend large amounts of their own money just to get to and stay near their treatment location unless this cost is covered by research money. The potential for an ever-widening disparity in health and quality of life among individuals thus becomes a greater possibility than before.[47]

The potential for gene therapy as a viable intervention raises several other ethical concerns. Genetic testing and gene therapies reveal information about individuals and family members. This information has the potential to label currently healthy individuals as being "at risk." As genetic testing and therapeutics become more common, personal, and family genetic information may inadvertently become public. The Americans with Disabilities Act of 1990 offers protection against genetic discrimination in the workplace. But, until recently, many questions remained about the possibilities for genetic discrimination by insurance companies and employers.

In May 2008, a federal law called the Genetic Information Nondiscrimination Act (GINA) was signed into law. GINA prohibits group and individual health insurers and employers from discriminating against an individual based on his or her genetic information. For example, GINA prohibits health insurers from using a person's genetic information to determine eligibility or premiums and prohibits an insurer from requiring that a person undergo a genetic test. GINA also prohibits employers for using a person's genetic information in hiring, firing, job assignments, or any other terms of employment. It also prohibits employers from requesting, requiring, or purchasing genetic information about a person or his or her family members. It is important for nurses to know that GINA does not mandate coverage for any particular test or treatment, nor does it prohibit medical underwriting based on current health status. GINA, also, does not cover life, disability, or long-term care insurance.[55] Furthermore, active duty military personnel are another exception to protections against employment and insurance discrimination based on genetic information. GINA does not extend to genetic testing of active duty military personnel or genetic information obtained from active duty military personnel.[56]

Nurses must keep in mind that confidentiality, although viewed as the foundation of the patient-provider relationship, needs to be enforced in all areas of genetic testing and research. Ethical aspects of care, such as confidentiality, are core elements of professional nursing practice. The Code of Ethics for nurses created by the American Nurses Association provides an ethical foundation for nurses and a direction for practice.[57]

## EMERGING ETHICAL ISSUES IN GENE THERAPY

The RAC, which advises the NIH director on gene therapy, has engaged in discussions about fetal gene therapy. Two serious and life-threatening genetic disorders—ADA deficiency and alpha-thalassemia—are under consideration for fetal gene therapy. Current issues being debated include whether it is better to treat a disease for which backup therapies exist, as is the case for ADA deficiency, or to go forward with gene treatment for alpha-thalassemia, a blood disorder that is often fatal to fetuses. At this stage, participants in the discussions agree that more data are needed about the safety, efficacy, and cost-effectiveness of fetal gene therapy.[58] Information is available to educate the public about gene therapy and related social and

**TABLE 22-3**

**Internet Sources for Gene Therapy**

| |
|---|
| National Cancer Institute<br>http://www.nci.nih.gov |
| National Human Genome Research Institute<br>http://www.nhgri.nih.gov |
| Genetics Home Reference<br>http://ghr.nlm.nih.gov |
| U.S. Department of Energy Office of Science, Office of Biological and Environmental Research; Human Genome Project Information<br>http://www.ornl.gov/sci/techresources/Human_Genome/medicine/genetherapy.shtm |
| National Cancer Institute; Cancer Gene Therapy: Questions and Answers<br>http://www.cancer.gov/cancertopics/factsheet/Therapy/gene |
| Recombinant DNA Advisory Committee<br>http://www4.od.nih.gov/oba/rac/aboutrdagt.htm |

ethical issues. Table 22-3 lists online resources for information regarding gene therapy and the Human-Genome Project.

## PRACTICE IMPLICATIONS FOR ONCOLOGY NURSES

The evolution of genetics and genomics and their important role in health and disease is leading to continuous changes in nursing practice. To meet the changing clinical and educational needs of individuals, families, and communities, oncology nurses and the entire nursing community need to be knowledgeable and fluent in handling new genetic and genomic concepts and information.[59] Oncology nurses caring for individuals who are participating in gene-therapy trials will be involved in providing direct care, educating individuals and the public, and advocating for fair and equitable use and for the confidentiality and privacy of genetic information. Table 22-4 outlines the roles for oncology nurses providing genetic- and genomic-related health care in these areas.[60] Two emerging roles for oncology nurses are provider of genetic services and clinical investigator in nursing genetic research, as discussed in the next section.[61]

### PROVIDER OF GENETIC SERVICES

The identification of genes that predispose certain individuals to cancer and developments in gene therapy are expanding

**TABLE 22-4**

**Nursing Responsibilities in Caring for Patients and Families Undergoing Gene Therapy**

Direct Caregiver
- Provides anticipatory guidance
- Assures informed decision making/consent
- Develops treatment and management plans
- Administers gene therapy
- Observes patients for expected and unexpected side effects of treatment, including psychosocial and emotional response
- Participates in developing long-term follow-up plans
- Assures coordination and collaboration of care with all healthcare providers involved in patient/family care before, during, and after gene therapy

Educator
- Serves as an information source to patients, families, and the public
- Provides relevant, accurate, and understandable information to patients, in both written and verbal forms
- Assures that all patient/family questions are answered

Advocate
- Assures privacy and confidentiality of genetic information
- Protects against discrimination
- Advocates for fair and equitable use of gene therapies for all populations
- Promotes public understanding of somatic gene therapy

General Services Provider
- Gathers relevant family history information
- Identifies individuals and families in need of further genetic education and counseling
- Assesses psychosocial, ethnoculture, and educational background
- Provides psychosocial support in follow-up to genetic counseling

Research Investigator
- Participates in or conducts clinical-research trials in gene therapy
- Serves as a preceptor to other nurses
- Develops research protocols that will address patient/family response and adaptation to genetic information, including gene therapy

*Source*: Reprinted with permission from Lea.[60]

the role for oncology nurses as genetic service providers. Oncology nurses now have the opportunity to participate in counseling individuals and families who are at increased risk of cancer by identifying risk factors and genes associated with cancer predisposition. Although these services are not uniformly available, many centers, clinics, and community practices are increasing their activities in this area.[61]

Genetic services include identifying individuals and families in need of further genetic evaluation and testing, referring these individuals to more specialized genetics professionals, and participating in the genetic counseling process. These services are a critical component of cancer-risk assessment and treatment. Oncology nurses, by virtue of their specialized training in and knowledge of cancer and their sensitivity to the influence of family and cultural beliefs on healthcare decisions, can incorporate components of the genetic counseling process into the care of individuals receiving gene therapy and their families.[61] The Oncology Nursing Society has created a position statement titled "The Role of the Oncology Nurse in Cancer Genetic Counseling" that outlines the emerging roles for oncology nurses participating in the genetic counseling process.[62]

## NURSING RESEARCH

Gene therapy as a clinical treatment for cancer is in its early stages. Many issues regarding response to gene therapy remain for patients undergoing gene therapy. The oncology nurse needs to consider the following issues:

- The long-term physical and psychosocial ramifications of gene therapy
- How individuals and families adapt to new genetic information and therapies
- How cultural and family backgrounds may influence individuals' decision making
- What educational materials and methods are best suited for providing information about gene therapy
- How to prepare primary-care practitioners, especially nurses, to care for individuals and families throughout life following gene therapy.

Oncology nurses as direct caregivers, educators, and advocates can have an instrumental role in initiating and participating in nursing research to help address these issues.[54] They can also play a leading role in developing longitudinal research efforts focusing on the continuum of identifying individual responses and adaptation to genetic cancer risk, testing, treatment, and post-treatment. Nurses can identify fluctuations in the coping process and recognize optimal times for psychosocial interventions and support. Other areas for oncology nursing research include determining effective means of tailoring information to individuals from differing educational and cultural backgrounds, and developing nursing management approaches to address family concerns with regard to gene therapy.[54,63]

## CONCLUSION

Human-genome discoveries and the expanding roles of gene therapy, pharmacogenetics, and pharmacogenomics are leading to dramatic breakthroughs in cancer treatment. Gene therapy, pharmacogenetics, and pharmacogenomics hold the promise of increasing the ability to tailor treatments to certain populations or to individual patients, improving responsiveness to medications.[4,61] In the near future, nurses will increasingly care for patients participating in clinical trials and receiving targeted drug therapies, and will be called upon to assist families with decision making and to collaborate with other healthcare professionals to maintain continuity and coordination of care. In most acute and chronic healthcare settings, it is the nurses who have the greatest contact with patients and who will administer the gene-therapy pharmacogenetic or pharmacogenomic intervention. Nurses, as always, will have the obligation to detect changes in a patient's condition that may arise as a consequence of any of these therapies.[64]

Nurses will increasingly care for patients from diverse ethnic backgrounds and cultures. Culturally safe nursing care reflects the priorities and health needs of those receiving the care. Such care will be important with respect to gene therapy, pharmacogenetics, and pharmacogenomics. As technologies to create gene-based therapies advance, new and more individualized tools will become available that are more precise than ethnicity and will allow for culturally safe care for all populations.

Genomics research contributes to our knowledge and understanding of biology, health, and life. Although many aspects of this understanding will be of benefit to individuals, families, and communities, some applications will be controversial and will call for societal dialogues to define appropriate and inappropriate uses of genomics. Nurses need to contribute to those dialogues. As part of their responsibility to promote the health and welfare of individuals, families, and communities, oncology nurses must participate in the development of social policies regarding safety, financial, and ethical issues related to gene therapy, pharmacogenetics, and pharmacogenomics. One of the major ethical issues concerns equal access to and the affordability of health care, including reimbursement for gene-based technologies for targeted treatment. Oncology nurses are represented at the policy level on the Secretary's Advisory Committee on Genetics, Health and Society (SACGHS), which is addressing these issues. In this role, they are helping to shape new healthcare delivery options that include gene therapy, pharmacogenetics, and pharmacogenomics, to make these treatments available to all populations.[54]

Nurses are accustomed to viewing individuals in a holistic way that takes into account each person's physical, mental, spiritual, social, and cultural attributes. New genomic discoveries and technologies used to classify or categorize people by their race and ethnicity for the purpose of understanding human variation and to tailor diagnostics and therapeutics have the potential to redirect individual, family, and community identity from the social domain into the physical aspects of the body. The prominent focus on the genetic and genomic aspects may overshadow other factors, such as poverty and access to health services and the ways that each of these factors affects health and disease. Nurses and other healthcare providers will need to seek ways to utilize and interpret all aspects of health information in caring for individuals, families, and communities.

Oncology nurses practicing in all settings will be challenged as they care for individuals before, during, and after gene therapy, pharmacogenetic, and pharmacogenomic interventions. They can meet these challenges by preparing to support and facilitate patients' decision making and their adaptation to gene-based interventions, to face ethical and social issues, and to promote and advocate for the safe and fair use of this new technology. Oncology nurses can best prepare themselves for these tasks by becoming knowledgeable about all aspects of gene-therapy pharmacogenetics and pharmacogenomics and the essential nursing competencies in genetics and genomics.[65] As in any new clinical situation, a first step for oncology nurses is to examine their views and values and their role in the effective delivery of genetic health care.

## REFERENCES


1. Personalized Medicine Coalition. http://www.personalizedmedicinecoalition.org. Accessed June 15, 2009
2. U.S. Department of Energy Office of Science. Report on the Human Genome Initiative for the Office of Health and Environmental Research. http://www.ornl.gov/sci/techresources/Human_Genome/project/herac2.shtml. Accessed June 15, 2009.
3. Tefferi A. Genomics basics: DNA structure, gene expression, cloning, genetic mapping and molecular tests. *Semin Cardiothorac Vasc Anesth.* 2006;10:282–290.
4. Lashley F. *Clinical Genetics in Nursing Practice.* 3rd ed. New York, NY: Springer Publishing Company; 2005.
5. Omim. Online Mendelian Inheritance in Man. http://www.ncbi.nlm.nih.gov/omim. Accessed June 15, 2009.
6. National Human Genome Research Institute. Genome-wide association studies. http://www.genome.gov/20019523. Accessed December 23, 2009.
7. McCandless SE, Brunger JW, Cassidy SB. The burden of genetic disease on inpatient care in a children's hospital. *Am J Hum Genet.* 2003;74: 121–127.
8. Garman KS, Nevins JR, Potti, A. Genomic strategies for personalized cancer therapy. *Hum Mol Genet.* 2007;16(Review Issue 2):R226-R232.
9. Lai LW, Lein YH. Homologous recombination gene therapy. *Exp Nephrol.* 1999;7:11–14.
10. Genetics Home Reference. Gene therapy. http://ghr.nlm.nih.gov/handbook/therapy. Accessed June 15, 2009.
11. National Cancer Institute. Gene therapy for cancer: questions and answers. http://www.cancer.gov/cancertopics/factsheet/Therapy/gene. Accessed June 15, 2009.
12. Centers for Disease Control and Prevention. Blood disorders: thalassemia. http://www.cdc.gov/ncbddd/hbd/thalassemia.htm. Accessed June 15, 2009.
13. Liu K. Breakthroughs in cancer gene therapy. *Semin Oncol Nurs.* 2003; 19:217–226.
14. Edelstein MKL, Abedi MR, Wixon J. Gene therapy clinical trials worldwide to 2007—an update. *J Gene Med.* 2007;9:833–842.
15. Levine BL, Humeau LM, Boyer J, MacGregor RR, Lu X, Binder GK, et al. Gene transfer in humans using a conditionally replicating lentiviral vector. *Proc Natl Acad Sci U.S.A.* 2006;103:17372–17377.
16. Griesenbach U, Geddes DM, Alton EW. Gene therapy progress and prospects: cystic fibrosis. *Gene Ther.* 2006;13:1061–1067.
17. Chao H, Walsh CE. AAV vectors for hemophilia B gene therapy. *Mt Sinai J Med.* 2004;71:305–313.
18. Jain KK. Nonmedicine: application of nanobiotechnology in medical practice. *Med Princ Pract.* 2008;17:89–101.
19. National Human Genome Research Institute. Learning about severe combined immunodeficiency (SCID). http://www.genome.gov/13014325. Accessed June 15, 2009.
20. Noguchi P. Risks and benefits of gene therapy. *N Engl J Med.* 2003; 348:193–194.
21. Marwick C. FDA halts gene therapy trials after leukaemia case in France. *BMJ.* 2003;326:181.
22. Buckley R. Gene therapy for SCID: a complication after remarkable progress. *Lancet.* 2003;360:1185–1186.
23. Balicki D, Buetler E. Reviews in molecular medicine: gene therapy of human diseases. *Medicine.* 2002;81:69–86.
24. Jeungst E. The NIH "Points to Consider" and the limits of human gene therapy. *Hum Gene Ther.* 1990;1:425–433.
25. U.S. Department of Health and Human Services. New initiative to protect participants in gene therapy trials. March 7, 2000. http://grants.nih.gov/grants/policy/gene_therapy_20000307.htm. Accessed June 15, 2009.
26. National Institutes of Health. ClinicalTrials.gov. http://www.clinicaltrials.gov. Accessed June 15, 2009.
27. Tey SK, Brenner MK. The continuing contribution of gene marking to cell and gene therapy. *Mol Ther.* 2007;15:666–676.
28. Aoi A, Watanabe Y, Mori S, Takahashi M, Vassaux G, Kodama T. Herpes simplex virus thymidine kinase-mediated suicide gene therapy using nano/microbubbles and ultrasound. *Ultrasound Med Biol.* 2008;34:425–434.
29. Abramson Cancer Center of the University of Pennsylvania. OncoLink. http://www.oncolink.org/treatment. Accessed June 15, 2009.
30. Trojan LA, Pan Y, Szpecheinski A, Ly A, Kopinski P, Chyezewski L, et al. Antisense strategy in malignant brain tumors treatment. *Rocz Akad Med Bialymst.* 2004;49(Supplement 1, Proceedings):94–97.
31. Galanis E, Okuno SH, Nascimento AG, Lewis BD, Lee RA, Oliveira AM, et al. Phase I-II trial of ONYX-015 in combination with MAP chemotherapy in patients with advanced sarcomas. *Gene Ther.* 2005; 12:437–445.
32. National Cancer Institute. NCI Drug Dictionary. Interleukin-2 gene. http://www.cancer.gov/Templates/drugdictionary.aspx?CdrID=38045. Accessed June 15, 2009.
33. Maccalli C, Nonaka D, Piris A, Pende D, Riboltini L, Castelli C, et al. NKG2D-mediated antitumor activity by tumor-infiltrating lymphocites and antigen-specific T-cell clones isolated from melanoma patients. *Clin Cancer Res.* 2007;13:7459–7468.
34. Liu K. Breakthroughs in cancer gene therapy. *Semin Oncol Nurs.* 2003;19:217–226.
35. Vieweg J, Dunnull J. Tumor vaccines: from gene therapy to dendrite cells—the emerging frontier. *Urologic Clin North Am.* 2003;30: 633–643.
36. American Cancer Society. Cancer vaccines. http://www.cancer.org/docroot/ETO/content/ETO_1_4X_Cancer_Vaccines_Active_Specific_Immunotherapies.asp?sitearea=ETO. Accessed June 15, 2009.
37. Gemmill R, Idell CS. Biological advances for new treatment approaches. *Semin Oncol Nurs.* 2003;19:162–168.
38. Merlo A, Turrini R, Dolcetti R, Zanovello P, Amadori A, Rosato A. Adoptive cell therapy against EBV-related malignancies: a survey of clinical results. *Expert Opin Biol Ther.* 2008;8:1265–1294.
39. Dudley ME, Rosenberg SA. Adoptive cell transfer therapy. *Semin Oncol.* 2007;34:524–531.
40. Eshhar Z. The T-body approach: redirecting T cells with antibody specificity. *Handb Exp Pharmacol.* 2008;181:329–342.
41. National Human Genome Research Institute. Frequently asked questions about genetic and genomic science. http://www.genome.gov/19016904. Accessed June 15, 2009.

42. Ansari M, Krajinovic M. Pharmacogenomics in cancer treatment defining genetic bases for inter-individual differences in responses to chemotherapy. *Curr Opin Pediatr.* 2007;19:15–22.
43. Reidenberg MM. Evolving ways that drug therapy is individualized. *Clin Pharmacol Ther.* 2003;74:197–202.
44. National Cancer Institute. Trastuzumab, http://www.cancer.gov/cancertopics/druginfo/trastuzumab. Accessed June 15, 2009.
45. Piccart-Gebhart MJ, Procter M, Leyland-Jones B, Goldhirsch A, Untch M, Smith I, et al. Trastuzumab after adjuvant chemotherapy in HER2-positive breast cancer. *N Engl J Med.* 2005;353:1659–1672.
46. National Cancer Institute. Imatinib mesylate. http://www.cancer.gov/cancertopics/druginfo/imatinibmesylate. Accessed June 15, 2009.
47. Genetics Home Reference. What are the ethical issues surrounding gene therapy? http://ghr.nlm.nih.gov/handbook/therapy/ethics. Accessed June 15, 2009.
48. Points to consider in the design and submission of protocols for the transfer of recombinant DNA molecules into one or more research participants. http://oba.od.nih.gov/oba/rac/fractions/10–10-00act.pdf. Accessed on June 15, 2009.
49. Orkin SH, Motulsky AG. *Report and Recommendations of the Panel to Assess the NIH Investment in Research on Gene Therapy.* 1995. http://www.nih.gov/news/panelrep.html. Accessed June 15, 2009.
50. Subcommittee on Human Gene Therapy, Recombinant DNA Advisory Committee, National Institutes of Health. Points to consider in the design and submission of protocols for the transfer of recombinant DNA into the genome of human subjects. *Hum Gene Ther.* 1990;1:93–103.
51. Capron A, Leventhal B, Post L. Requests for compassionate use of gene therapy: Memorandum from the subcommittee to the RAC, January 13, 1993. *Hum Gene Ther.* 1993;4:199–200.
52. U.S. Surgeon General. *U.S. Public Health Service Investigation Involving Human Subjects, Including Clinical Research: Requirements for Review to Insure the Rights and Welfare of Individuals.* Public policy order no. 129, 1966.
53. Code of Federal Regulations, Title 45, Part 46. *Protection of Human Subjects* (revised March 8, 1983), 1980.
54. Reiger PT. The role of the oncology nurse in gene therapy. *Lancet Oncol.* 2001;2:233–238.
55. Hudson KL, Holohan MK, Collins FS. Keeping pace with the times—The Genetic Information Nondiscrimination Act of 2008. *N Engl J Med.* 2008;358:2661–2663.
56. Genetics and Public Policy Center. Center launches new GINA resource. http://www.dnapolicy.org/news.release.php?action=detail&pressrelease_id=101. Accessed June 15, 2009.
57. American Nurses Association. *Code of Ethics for Nurses with Interpretive Statements.* Washington, DC, American Nurses Association; 2001.
58. David AL, Peebles D. Gene therapy for the fetus: is there a future? *Best Pract Res Clin Obstet Gynaecol.* 2008;22:203–218.
59. Calzone KA, Lea DH, Masny A. Non-Hodgkin's lymphoma as an exemplar of the effects of genetics and genomics. *J Nurs Scholarsh.* 2006;38:335–342.
60. Lea DH. Gene therapy: current and future implications for oncology nursing practice. *Semin Oncol Nurs.* 1997;13:115–122.
61. Jenkins JJ, Lea DH. *Nursing Care in the Genomic Era: A Case-Based Approach.* Boston: Jones and Bartlett Publishers; 2005.
62. Oncology Nursing Society. The role of the oncology nurse in cancer genetic counseling. *Oncol Nurs Forum.* 2000;27:1348.
63. Loescher LJ, Merkle CJ. The interface of genomic technologies and nursing. *J Nur Scholarsh.* 2005;37:111–119.
64. Nicol MJ. The variation of response to pharmacotherapy: pharmacogenetics—a new perspective to "The right drug for the right person." *MEDSURG Nurs.* 2003;12:242–249.
65. Consensus Panel. Essential Nursing Competencies and Curricula Guidelines for Genetics an d Genomics. Silver Spring, MD: American Nurses Association; September 21–22, 2005.

CHAPTER

23

*Colleen Lemoine, APRN, MN, AOCN®, Barbara Holmes Gobel, MS, RN, AOCN®*

# Hematopoietic Therapy

## INTRODUCTION

Hematopoiesis is the process by which all cellular elements of the blood develop. This highly complex and tightly regulated biological function is characterized by the stimulation of the pluripotent hematopoietic stem cell by various glycoproteins known as hematopoietic growth factors (HGFs). HGFs cause stem cells to proliferate, differentiate, and ultimately, to mature into functional red blood cells, white blood cells, and platelets. Cancer and its treatments can disrupt hematopoiesis resulting in decreased numbers of circulating blood cells. In addition, increased destruction of blood cells can also contribute to clinically significant anemia, neutropenia, and thrombocytopenia. Regardless of the etiology, these side effects can affect outcomes related to therapy by interfering with dosing schedules, causing dose reductions, contributing to life-threatening complications (eg, bleeding and infection), and contributing to an impaired quality of life.

Clinical management of patients experiencing hematological complications associated with cancer and its therapy primarily involves the use of exogenous HGFs to stimulate hematopoiesis or transfusion therapy with specific blood components to replace depleted blood cell populations. Each of these therapeutic approaches involves both benefit and risk. This chapter reviews the process of hematopoiesis and discusses the indications, complications, and nursing considerations associated with both the use of recombinant HGFs and transfusion therapy in the management of cancer-associated anemia, neutropenia, and thrombocytopenia.

## HEMATOPOIETIC GROWTH FACTORS

### HEMATOPOIESIS

*Hematopoiesis* is the dynamic and delicately balanced mechanism by which the body produces the cells necessary to carry oxygen, fight infection, and promote clotting. During fetal development, the blood-forming organs include the spleen, liver, and bone marrow. The bone marrow is the primary site of hematopoiesis at the time of birth. During childhood, hematopoiesis takes place in the ribs, skull, spleen, pelvis, liver, sternum, vertebrae, and the proximal epiphyses of the long bones; all of these but the liver are involved in adult hematopoiesis. Bone marrow provides a specialized microenvironment in which hematopoietic progenitor cells proliferate and become committed to differentiation. Within the marrow, various elements—including the structural or stromal elements (fibroblasts, endothelial cells, fat cells) and the accessory cells (macrophages and lymphocytes)—interact, either to enhance or inhibit hematopoiesis.

All blood cell lines derive from a pluripotent stem cell, or common progenitor cell, which is capable of both extensive, possibly lifelong self-renewal and differentiation into all cell lineages.[1] The stem cell is not normally in an active cycle, and only a small percentage of stem cells will reproduce. When the cell must undergo division, a daughter cell leaves the stem cell pool and passes through a series of divisions and maturational changes, culminating in the formation of mature blood cells that are released into the circulating blood. The processes of proliferation, differentiation, and commitment are mediated by various humoral factors, primarily by an expanding set of HGFs. See Figure 23-1 for an outline of blood cell development and the factors that mediate this process.

Early in blood cell development, the progeny of the pluripotent stem cell form a population of multipotent progenitor cells that have not yet committed to a specific cell line and have a limited self-renewing capacity. The colony-forming unit granulocyte, erythroid, monocyte, and megakaryocyte (CFU-GEMM) is an example of the multipotent stem cell that can develop into any one of these lines. The lymphoid cell line follows a separate course of development.

As cells continue to differentiate, they become committed to specific cell lines. At this level, progenitor cells are called *unipotent* or *bipotent*, describing their ability to follow 1 or 2 cell lines, respectively. These cells include colony-forming units for granulocytes, monocytes, and macrophages (CFU-GMM); colony-forming units for eosinophils (CFU-EO); burst-forming units for erythroid (BFU-E); colony-forming units for erythroid (CFU-E); and colony-forming units for megakaryocytes (CFU-MK) and are committed stem cells.[1] Committed stem cells become increasingly differentiated and morphologically recognizable as belonging to a specific cell line. Ultimately, the cell undergoes further division and maturation and becomes a fully developed and functional component of the circulating blood.

#### Hematopoietic growth factors

Hematopoietic growth factors, known previously as colony-stimulating factors (CSFs), are a set of hormone-like glycoproteins or cytokines that mediate hematopoiesis. These endogenous glycoproteins regulate the production of blood cells at every level of development. Many unique HGFs have been identified to date. Although the complete regulatory process is not fully understood, HGFs are known to exert their effects by interacting with specific cell surface receptors found on both hematologic and nonhematologic cells.

Interleukin-3 (IL-3), also called multicolony-stimulating factor, is a growth factor for a variety of progenitor cells, as is granulocyte-macrophage colony-stimulating factor (GM-CSF). These HGFs stimulate the growth of multiple lines of the progenitor cells (*multilineage*) and cells already committed to myeloid, erythroid, or

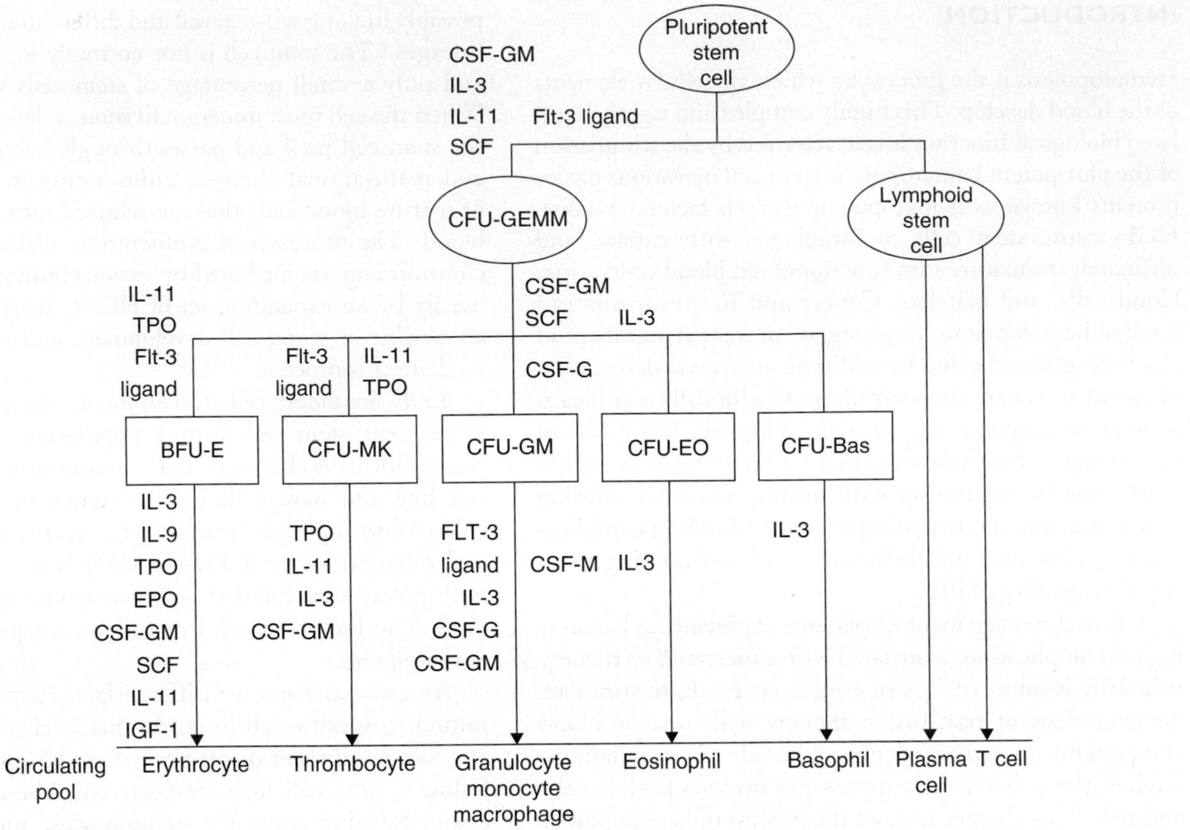


**FIGURE 23-1**

Hematopoiesis and associated growth factors.

*Abbreviations*: BFU-E, burst-forming unit for erythrocytes; CFU-EO, colony-forming unit for eosinophils; CFU-GEMM, colony-forming unit for granulocytes, erythrocytes, monocytes, and megakaryocytes; CFU-GM, colony-forming unit for granulocytes and macrophages; CFU-MK, colony-forming unit for megakaryocytes; CFU-Bas, colony-forming unit for basophils; CSF-G, colony-stimulating factor for granulocytes; CSF-GM, colony-stimulating factor for granulocytes and macrophages; CSF-M, macrophage colony stimulating factor; EPO, erythropoietin; Flt-3 ligand, FMS-like tyrosine-3 ligand; IGF-1, insulin like growth factor; IL-1, interleukin 1; IL-3, interleukin 3; IL-9, interleukin 9; IL-11, interleukin 11; SCF, stem cell factor; TPO, thrombopoietin.

megakaryocyte lines.[2] Other HGFs stimulate production of cells primarily along single blood cell lines (*lineage specific*). Granulocyte-CSF (G-CSF), macrophage-CSF, and erythropoietin (EPO) stimulate the growth predominantly of granulocytes, monocytes, and red blood cells, respectively. Although some growth factors are more lineage-specific than others, there is thought to be considerable overlap among them such that 1 growth factor can impact more than 1 cell line. In addition, there is thought to be a synergistic effect when more than 1 growth factor acts on a cell line such that the resulting cellular response is larger than the summative cellular response to each individual growth factor. Finally, many growth factors not only stimulate the production of a certain blood cell lineage but they often enhance both the function and survival of cells in that same lineage.[3]

Hematopoietic growth factors exert much of their effects by acting on various receptors that reside on the target cell membrane. The different distribution of these receptors may help to explain why certain cells are responsive to some HGFs and not others. Recent evidence suggests that HGF receptors are also present on some tumor cells. While the clinical relevance of this is yet unknown, the possibility that HGFs could potentially stimulate tumor growth must be considered and this is an active area of research.[4]

## Recombinant hematopoietic growth factors

Recombinant DNA technology has allowed for mass production of the naturally occurring HGFs for clinical use. Some of the recombinant HGFs are lineage specific, primarily stimulating only a single blood cell line. Examples of lineage-specific recombinant growth factors include EPO, which stimulates the erythroid line of blood cells, and G-CSF, which stimulates the granulocyte blood cell line. Multilineage recombinant growth factors effectively stimulate the production of more than 1 line of blood cells. An example of a multilineage growth factor is GM-CSF, which stimulates the granulocyte and the monocyte/macrophage blood cell lines.

Of the many HGFs that have been cloned over the years, only EPO, G-CSF, GM-CSF, and IL-11 (oprelvekin) have been FDA approved for clinical use. Table 23-1[5–16] lists the currently approved HGFs along with their indications. Clinical trials continue to investigate the potential for the clinical use of other HGFs such as stem cell factor (SCF) and FMS-like tyrosine-3 (FLT-3) ligand.

## Erythropoietin growth factors

Mature red blood cells develop from the common multipotential progenitor cell, the CFU-GEMM, to a committed progenitor cell known as BFU-E. Under the influence of various growth factors, including EPO, the BFU-E proliferates and differentiates into CFU-E, then into reticulocytes and ultimately into mature erythrocytes. Endogenous EPO is the only HGF that behaves as a hormone. Erythropoietin is produced primarily by the kidneys in response to hypoxia. It is secreted into the circulation and is delivered to the bone marrow via plasma. In general, plasma EPO concentration levels reflect EPO production and levels remain relatively constant until the hemoglobin level drops below 12 g/dL.[17] Erythropoietin levels can be used as a measurement to determine deficient states that may be effectively treated with recombinant EPO.[18]

*Erythropoiesis stimulating agents.* Recombinant EPO agents, now referred to as erythropoiesis stimulating agents or ESAs, were initially approved for chemotherapy-induced anemia in 1993 and are currently available in both short-acting and long-acting formulations. Short-acting formulations include epoetin alfa or EPO: Epogen and Procrit. These products are identical; however, each company retains unique marketing rights for their respective product. There are several indications for recombinant EPO that have evolved since initial approval. Currently, it is approved for the management of anemia associated with cancer chemotherapy in patients with metastatic, nonmyeloid malignancies being treated with a noncurative intent. Other indications for recombinant EPO include anemia in advanced renal disease for patients on dialysis as well as those not on dialysis, anemia related to zidovudine (AZT) therapy in HIV-infected patients, and anemia in surgical patients to reduce the need for allogeneic transfusion.

The newest ESA, FDA approved in September 2001, is the longer-acting darbepoetin alfa (Aranesp). Darbepoetin alfa is approved for the treatment of chemotherapy-induced anemia in patients with metastatic, nonmyeloid malignancies when the intent of treatment is noncurative and for the treatment of anemia associated with dialysis-dependent and dialysis-independent chronic renal failure. Darbepoetin alfa is as efficacious as epoetin alfa at decreasing the need for allogeneic transfusions but it can be administered less frequently than epoetin alfa.

The benefits of ESA therapy have been well documented and include reduced need for red blood cell transfusions and improved quality of life, most significantly, when hemoglobin levels are maintained in the 10 to 12 g/dL range.[19–24] Despite these studies, the current FDA labeling of ESAs includes verbiage that controlled trials have not demonstrated that ESA use improves symptoms of anemia, quality of life, fatigue, or patient well-being.[25]

In addition to the known benefits associated with ESAs, there are known risks that include immunogenicity (the potential to develop neutralizing antibodies to EPO resulting in a pure red cell aplasia), hypertension, and thromboembolic events. In a 2004 Cochrane review, it was concluded that although EPO and darbepoetin reduced transfusions in anemic patients with cancer, these medications increased the risk for thromboembolic complications and their effect on survival was unknown.[26] From 2003 to 2008 findings from 5 studies raised concerns about the safety of ESA use in patients with cancer, namely, the possibility of increased mortality and the potential for support of tumor growth.[27–31] As a result, in August, 2008, FDA-mandated label revisions limited the use of ESAs to patients with metastatic cancer being treated with myelosuppressive chemotherapy with a noncurative intent.[25] It is important to note that the FDA's decision was based in part on studies that had been conducted to evaluate ESA use outside of the current FDA-approved indications. In these studies, ESAs were used to treat patients with cancer and anemia who were receiving either no concurrent therapy, radiation therapy, or who were receiving chemotherapy but were being treated with ESAs to targeted hemoglobin levels above 12 g/dL, all clinical applications inconsistent with the previous FDA-approved indication of chemotherapy-induced anemia.

The present labeling for ESAs includes a blackbox warning that cautions to use the lowest dose possible to avoid transfusion due to evidence of shortened overall survival and tumor progression/recurrence associated with ESA use in some clinical trials. Further caution is given to discontinue ESA therapy following the completion of a chemotherapy course. In addition, the FDA requires that patients initiating/receiving ESA therapy be given the publication, "A Medication Guide for epoietin alfa or darbepoetin alfa" in an effort to assure that they have been made aware of the potential risks of ESA therapy.[25]

In light of the safety concerns many reviews of the evidence have been recently conducted. In 2008, an extensive review and summary of the safety of ESAs by Gascon suggested that clinical outcomes are not adversely impacted when ESAs are used within labeled indications.[32] However, the most recently published meta-analysis of randomized controlled clinical trials evaluating ESA use and mortality in patients with cancer concluded that treatment with ESAs increased mortality and worsened overall survival.[33]

**TABLE 23-1**

**FDA-Approved Hematopoietic Growth Factors for Use in the Oncology Setting**

| Agent | Generic Name | Trade Name | Indications in Cancer | Dosing | Route |
|---|---|---|---|---|---|
| G-CSF | Filgrastim | Neupogen (Amgen, Inc., Thousand Oaks, CA) | Decrease infection manifested by febrile neutropenia in patients with non-myeloid malignancies after receiving myelosuppressive chemotherapy, reduce time to neutrophil recovery in patients with AML following induction or consolidation chemotherapy, reduce duration of neutropenia and neutropenia-related sequelae after SCT for non-myeloid malignancies, mobilize hematopoietic progenitor cells in SCT PBPC[6–11] | Chemotherapy: 5 mcg/kg/day, administer 24 hours after chemotherapy, for up to 2 weeks until ANC nadir > 10,000/mm$^3$<br>Should not be administered within 24 hours of next chemotherapy dose.<br>SCT: 10 mcg/kg/day, then titrate per counts*[5]<br>SCT PBPC mobilization—10 mcg/kg/day starting 4 days before first leukopheresis and continuing through last leukopheresis | SC, IV |
| G-CSF | Pegfilgrastim | Neulasta (Amgen, Inc., Thousand Oaks, CA) | Decrease incidence of infection, as manifested by febrile neutropenia in patients with nonmyeloid malignancies receiving myelosuppressive chemotherapy[6–8] | 6 mg dose once per cycle of chemotherapy. Not in period 14 days before or 24 hours after chemotherapy | SC |
| GM-CSF | Sargramostim | Leukine (Immunex Corp., Seattle, WA) | Accelerate bone marrow recovery after SCT: in allogeneic SCT with delayed or failed engraftment; after induction therapy in AML, and in PBPC mobilization[12–14] | 250 mcg/m$^2$/day until ANC > 1500/mm$^3$ × 3 days or for a recommended maximum of 42 days | SC, IV |
| Erythropoietin alfa | Epoietin alpha | Procrit (Ortho Biotech, Inc., Raritan, NJ): Epogen (Amgen, Inc., Thousand Oaks, CA) | Treatment of anemia due to concomittantly administered chemotherapy in patients with metastatic cancer recieving myelosuppressive chemotherapy with a noncurative intent[13] | 40,000 units every week or 150 units/kg 3 times/week<br>80,000 units every 2 weeks, or 120,000 units every 3 weeks*<br>Titrate to not exceed a hemoglobin of 12 g/dL or a > 1 g/dL rise in 2 weeks<br>Titrate to the lowest dose possible to maintain RBC transfusion independence[5] | SC, IV |
| Erythropoietin alfa | Darbpoetin alfa | Aranesp (Amgen, Inc., Thousand Oaks, CA) | Treatment of anemia due to concomittantly administered chemotherapy in patients with metastatic cancer recieving myelosuppressive chemotherapy with a noncurative intent[13] | 2.25 mcg/kg every week<br>500 mcg every 3 weeks<br>100 mcg weekly*<br>200 mcg every 2 weeks*<br>300 mcg every 3 weeks*<br>Titrate to not exceed a hemoglobin of 12 g/dL or a > 1 g/dL rise in 2 weeks<br>Titrate to the lowest dose possible to maintain RBC transfusion independence[5] | SC, IV |

*(Continued)*

**TABLE 23–1**

**FDA-Approved Hematopoietic Growth Factors for Use in the Oncology Setting (*Continued*)**

| Agent | Generic Name | Trade Name | Indications in Cancer | Dosing | Route |
|---|---|---|---|---|---|
| Interleukin-11 | Oprelvekin | Neumega (Genetics Institute, Cambridge, MA) | Prevent thrombocytopenia and reduce need for platelet transfusions following myelosuppressive chemotherapy[15,16] | 50 mcg/kg/day until post-nadir platelet count is > 50,000/mm$^3$. Dose should be given 6–24 hours after chemotherapy. Should be discontinued at least 2 days before next chemotherapy treatment cycle Dosing for > 21 days is not recommended | SC |

*Abbreviations*: AML, acute myelogenous leukemia; ANC, absolute neutrophil count; G-CSF, colony stimulating factor for granulocytes; GM-CSF, colony stimulating factor for granulocytes and macrophages; IV, intravenous; PBPC, peripheral blood progenitor cell; SC, subcutaneous; SCT, stem cell transplant.

*This dose has not been FDA approved but is supported in the literature and by NCCN guidelines.

The conflicting findings and the concerns raised by these studies clearly indicate the need for further investigation and studies are currently underway to determine the safest and most appropriate strategies for ESA use.

Clinical practice guidelines for the management of anemia in patients with cancer have been published by the National Comprehensive Cancer Network (NCCN)[5] and the American Society of Clinical Oncology,[34] in conjunction with the American Society of Hematology.[35] However, only the NCCN guidelines have been formally updated since the most-recent FDA changes to the ESA labeling. The NCCN guidelines call for the evaluation of patients based on laboratory indices, as well as physical assessment findings and suggest consideration of ESAs only in patients being treated with myelosuppressive chemotherapy with noncurative intent and who are mildly symptomatic or at risk for becoming symptomatic. The guidelines recommend that other possible causes of anemia be evaluated and corrected. ESA therapy should not be initiated until the hemoglobin is ≤10 g/dL and only after critical assessment of the risks and benefits of therapy. Prior to initiating ESA therapy, laboratory evaluation of the patient's iron status, including serum ferritin and transferrin saturation, should be conducted. Oral iron supplementation is frequently necessary and parenteral iron supplementation is warranted when oral supplementation proves inadequate or in the presence of functional iron deficiencies (adequate iron stores but less than normal saturation levels). Published guidelines support the use of EPO given subcutaneously according to a number of dosing schedules for a minimum of 4 weeks.[5] ESA dosing should be adjusted to the lowest dose at which the patient can remain transfusion independent. A dose decrease is warranted once the hemoglobin concentration reaches 12 g/dL or if the hemoglobin increases by more than 1 g/dL in a 2-week period. ESA dosing should be titrated upward if an increase in hemoglobin of 1 g/dL is not realized within 4 weeks when using short-acting ESAs or within 6 weeks when using the long-acting agent. ESAs should be discontinued after 8 weeks of therapy if a hemoglobin response is not achieved or if transfusions are still required.[5]

## Myeloid growth factors

Like the erythrocyte, the monocyte/macrophage and neutrophil blood cell lineages develop from the common multipotential progenitor cell, the CFU-GEMM. Under the influence of a number of specific growth factors the CFU-GEMM further develops into the CFU-GM that ultimately differentiates into the neutrophils, monocytes, and macrophages. Granulocyte colony-stimulating factor acts on the committed granulocytes to increase their progeny. G-CSF speeds the maturation of neutrophils, promotes granulocyte survival, and decreases apoptosis of granulocytes.[1,36]

The myeloid growth factors have demonstrated enormous therapeutic value in patients with hematological diseases. The most common applications for these growth factors include myelodysplasia, stem cell transplantation, acute myeloid leukemia (AML), acute lymphoblastic leukemia (ALL), and chemotherapy-induced neutropenia.

*Granulocyte colony-stimulating factor.* The body's naturally occurring G-CSF regulates the production of neutrophils within the bone marrow, affecting proliferation, differentiation, and selected end-cell functional activation through stimulation of the neutrophil progenitor. Although G-CSF has been found to have some effect on multiple cell lines, it is generally considered to be a single-lineage growth factor.

The recombinant versions of G-CSF include filgrastim (Neupogen), FDA approved in 1991, and pegfilgrastim

(Neulasta) FDA approved in 2002. Both drugs are indicated to decrease the incidence of febrile neutropenia in patients with nonmyeloid malignancies receiving myelosuppressive cancer drug therapy. Both of these agents have demonstrated the ability to accelerate the recovery of neutrophil counts following the administration of chemotherapy for nonmyeloid malignancies and decrease the negative sequelae associated with febrile neutropenia.[6–8] Filgrastim has also been FDA approved for use in patients with AML following induction or consolidation chemotherapy to reduce the time to neutrophil recovery and the duration of fever.[9]

As with the ESAs, there is both a short-acting and a long-acting formulation of recombinant G-CSF. Although equally safe and efficacious,[6–8] the 2 agents are dosed differently due to differing pharmacokinetic properties. Filgrastim dosing is weight-based, and due to a short half-life, must be administered daily beginning 24 to 72 hours after completion of chemotherapy and continuing until postnadir neutrophil recovery. Pegfilgrastim has a longer half-life due to the addition of polyethylene glycol and dosing is fixed at 6 mg. Due to the pegylation process dosing is required only once per cycle of chemotherapy. Pegfilgrastim should not be given in the period of time from 14 days before chemotherapy until 24 hours after administration of chemotherapy. Data do not support same day dosing for either filgrastim or pegfilgrastim.[6–8,37,38]

Treatment of myeloid malignancies with G-CSF has been a concern over the years due to the thought that this agent would stimulate leukemic blast proliferation. However, the vast majority of data from controlled trials of growth factors used after induction therapy in AML have demonstrated safety of use with the treatment of AML.[6] The follow-up studies did not show any increase in the relapse rate or decreased survival among patients who went into a complete remission.

Granulocyte colony-stimulating factor use is recommended at any stage of therapy for ALL, either during induction or in subsequent intensification, as it reduces the period of neutropenia.[39] G-CSF is indicated in the stem cell transplantation setting for enhancement of neutrophil recovery and for mobilization of stem cells prior to the transplant.[10,11] The myeloid growth factors, including G-CSF, are reported to be occasionally beneficial in increasing the neutrophil count and function in patients with myelodysplasia. G-CSF is also approved for congenital, cyclic, or idiopathic neutropenia.[40]

The most frequent side effect of treatment with either version of G-CSF is bone pain that is generally responsive to nonsteroidal anti-inflammatory drugs (NSAIDs) or acetaminophen. Other side effects include lethargy, myalgia, and injection site pain. Rare but serious side effects include splenic rupture, acute respiratory distress syndrome, allergic reactions, or sickle cell crises when used in patients with sickle cell disorders.

The American Society of Clinical Oncology (ASCO) and NCCN have both published guidelines addressing the use of myeloid growth factors to reduce the incidence of febrile neutropenia associated with myelosuppressive chemotherapy regimens. ASCO recommends that primary prophylaxis with CSFs be implemented when administering chemotherapy regimens associated with a >20% incidence of febrile neutropenia.[41] In addition, ASCO guidelines recommend primary prophylaxis in patients considered to be high risk for developing febrile neutropenia based on age, comorbidities, disease characteristics, and the myelosuppressive potential of the planned chemotherapeutic regimen.

The National Comprehensive Cancer Network recommendations for CSF use vary depending on the intent of treatment—curative/adjuvant, prolong survival/quality of life, and symptom management/quality of life.[42] Risk for febrile neutropenia is determined by considering the myelosuppressive potential of the planned chemotherapy regimen and patient factors known to increase risk such as age ≥65, previous chemotherapy or radiation therapy, preexisting neutropenia, infection or open wounds, impaired hepatic or renal function, bone marrow involvement with tumor and poor functional status. NCCN guidelines strongly recommend the prophylactic use of CSFs to decrease the risk of febrile neutropenia, hospitalization and need for IV antibiotics when the risk for febrile neutropenia is >20%, and the intent of treatment is curative/adjuvant or life prolonging/quality of life. NCCN guidelines recommend considering the use of CSFs to decrease the incidence of febrile neutropenia when the risk is 10% to 20% and treatment intent is curative/adjuvant. Finally, according to the NCCN guidelines, when the intent of treatment is symptom management/quality of life, the decision to use CSFs is a difficult one and can only be made after careful discussion between physician and patient.

*Granulocyte-macrophage colony-stimulating factor.* Granulocyte-macrophage colony-stimulating factor is a multilineage growth factor that regulates proliferation and differentiation of hematopoietic progenitors of neutrophils, eosinophils, monocytes/macrophages, and myeloid dendritic cells. Megakaryocyte and erythrocyte development are also influenced by GM-CSF; however, other growth factors are necessary for final maturation of these 2 lineages. GM-CSF stimulates neutrophil production, enhances neutrophil activity, and decreases neutrophil apoptosis.[43,44] GM-CSF also stimulates the production of and enhances the activity of monocytes and macrophages, most notably, by fostering chemotaxis and phagocytosis in macrophages and the release of cytokines from monocytes that stimulates natural killer cell activity.[43] The development of dendritic cells is influenced by GM-CSF as is dendritic activity, including the movement of dendritic cells into the lymphatic system. Finally, GM-CSF influences the activity of both naïve T cells and eosinophils.[43]

The recombinant version of GM-CSF (sargramostim, Leukine) has several FDA-approved indications.

Sargramostim is approved for use in older patients with AML to enhance myeloid recovery or reconstitution following induction chemotherapy.[45,46] Sargramostim is also indicated to support patients with Hodgkin's lymphoma, non-Hodgkin's lymphoma, or acute nonmyeloid leukemia undergoing hematopoietic stem cell transplant (HSCT).[47,48] The final FDA approved indication for GM-CSF is in patients with post bone marrow transplant experiencing failure or delayed engraftment.[12–14] The incidence of graft failure is less common than in the past, due to the ability of current technologies to precisely measure the numbers of CD34-positive cells in the donor pool. The administration of GM-CSF in the HSCT setting has been shown to reduce the rate of graft failure, accelerate hematopoiesis, and help in preventing lethal complications in patients after transplantation.[13,14,47,48] GM-CSF is also used during induction or subsequent intensification therapy of ALL to help prevent life-threatening neutropenia. Like G-CSF, GM-CSF is reported to be occasionally beneficial in increasing the neutrophil count and function in patients with myelodysplasia.[49] The most prominent side effect of GM-CSF is bone pain, which is generally effectively managed with NSAIDS or acetaminophen. Other side effects include rash, fever, lethargy, myalgia, anorexia, and injection site redness.

Because of the effect that both GM-CSF and G-CSF have on immune function, there is significant research activity investigating the use of these agents within the context of vaccine development. Currently, there are phase I, II, and III vaccine trials underway across a wide variety of both solid tumor and hematological malignancies. These vaccine studies combine numerous treatment modalities including chemotherapy, biotherapy, radiation therapy, and surgery in various combinations in an attempt to identify successful prevention and treatment strategies. In the fall of 2008, the phase III VITAL-2 trial, which combined the use of the GVAX cancer vaccine with docetaxel and prednisone in patients with prostate cancer was stopped early due to the increased proportion of deaths in patients on the treatment arm.[50] Despite the numerous vaccine trials that have been undertaken, however, there have been only 2 cancer-related vaccines to receive FDA approval. These include the human papillomavirus quadrivalent (Types 6, 11, 16, and 18) vaccine, recombinant (for prevention of cervical cancer), and BCG live (for prevention of bladder cancer), neither of which incorporates the use of G-CSF or GM-CSF into the product. A vaccine that capitalizes on the immune enhancing qualities of either GM-CSF or G-CSF has yet to become commercially available.

## Multipotential growth factors

***Stem cell factor.*** Stem cell factor (SCF) is a multipotential HGF. Stem cell factor, also known as steel factor, mast cell growth factor, and kit ligand (because it binds to the c-Kit receptor that is located on many cell types including hematopoietic cells) is a normal transmembrane glycoprotein produced by the C-KIT gene.[51,52] SCF stimulates undifferentiated multipotential progenitor cells and committed cell line precursors (eg, CFU-GEMM) to further develop into mature myeloid or lymphoid blood cells.

Recombinant SCF (also known as recombinant methionyl SCF, rhSCF, r-metHuSCF, ancestim, and Stemgen) has demonstrated little colony-stimulating activity when administered alone. However, when administered along with other HGFs, particularly filgrastim, it increases the number and size of cell colonies, suggesting that it influences early progenitor activity.[53] Clinical trials involving rhSCF, most often in combination with filgrastim, have looked at its use in peripheral stem cell transplantation and have found that rhSCF may be clinically useful for the mobilization of peripheral blood progenitor cells.[54–59] Recombinant SCF is currently being studied in patients with myelodysplastic syndrome receiving lenalidomide. The main side effect of treatment with rhSCF has been mild to moderate skin rash; however, allergic reactions can occur due to the presence of c-Kit receptors on mast cells that release histamine in response to the SCF ligand.[55]

***FMS-like tyrosine-3 ligand.*** FMS-like tyrosine-3 ligand belongs to the same family of receptor tyrosine kinases as SCF.[60] It is an early-acting growth factor that stimulates proliferation of stem cells and primitive progenitor cells in combination with other growth factors. Flt-3 ligand has been shown to synergistically enhance G-CSF mobilization of hematopoietic stem cells and progenitor cells in preclinical studies.[61] Clinical trials are underway to test the effectiveness of Flt-3 ligand in mobilizing peripheral blood stem cells in humans.[62] In addition, clinical trials are ongoing looking at several tumor types (breast, colorectal, metastatic melanoma, metastatic renal cell carcinoma, acute myelogenous leukemia) in an attempt to identify the role that Flt-3 ligand may play in helping the body mount an antitumor response.

## Platelet growth factors

The mature platelet cell in the circulation derives from the megakaryocyte in the bone marrow. The megakaryocyte develops from the multipotential myeloid progenitor cell. The first committed cell is the CFU-megakaryocyte (CFU-MK). It is stimulated by various growth factors, including thrombopoietin (TPO). The CFU-MK undergoes differentiation and proliferation under the influence of GM-CSF, IL-3, IL-6, and IL-11, whereby it becomes committed to megakaryocytes that then fragment into platelets.[36]

***Interleukin-11.*** Interleukin-3, IL-6, and IL-11 are all potent stimulators of platelet precursors. However, IL-3 and IL-6 have been found to be too toxic for clinical use.

To date, only IL-11, known as oprelvekin (Neumega), has been FDA approved for the prevention of chemotherapy-induced thrombocytopenia. The use of IL-11 increases the likelihood of avoiding thrombocytopenia in patients undergoing chemotherapy and shortens the duration of the thrombocytopenia.[15,16] Two randomized controlled clinical trials of IL-11 have shown a reduction in the need for platelet transfusions in the setting of intensive chemotherapy.[63,64] However, when used in the setting of autologous transplantation, IL-11 did not reduce the need for platelet transfusion.[65]

The side effect profile of IL-11 is significant for edema and dyspnea.[1] In IL-11 trials, approximately 65% of patients experienced edema and 50% experienced dyspnea. Other adverse events included tachycardia and allergic reactions. Neither ASCO nor NCCN have published guidelines that speak to the use of IL-11 for thrombocytopenia.

*Thrombopoietin.* Two recombinant forms of TPO were studied in the 1990s and although they initially looked promising, the development of neutralizing antibodies with resulting profound thrombocytopenia caused the discontinuation of these investigations. Recently 2 new platelet production stimulating agents have been approved for the treatment of immune thrombocytopenic purpura (ITP). These agents have different mechanisms of action but are both considered to be TPO receptor agonists. They are also referred to as TPO mimetics because, although not identical to endogenous TPO, they mimic the activity of TPO. The TPO mimetics bind to and activate the TPO receptor resulting in increased platelet production. Romiplostim (Nplate) is a peptibody that shares no amino acid sequence homology with naturally occurring TPO and thus avoids the problem of developing neutralizing antibodies.[66] Eltrombopag (Promacta) is a nonpeptide, small molecule, oral agent that interacts with the transmembrane domain of the TPO receptor resulting in increased platelet production.[67] While not yet approved for any cancer-associated indications, studies are underway in solid and hematological malignancies and these agents may eventually have a role in the treatment of cancer-related thrombocytopenia.

## TRANSFUSION THERAPY

Despite the increasing use of HGFs, transfusion therapy continues to play a vital role in the care of the patient with cancer. A significant need exists for blood component therapy in the context of bleeding and/or hemorrhage, severe anemia, thrombocytopenia, and coagulation disorders caused by the disease, treatment, or both. The frequency of blood component therapy transfusions is driven by standards set in the industry regarding a safe "set point" for the need for transfusion and the individual patient's needs and tolerance of low blood counts.

Routine blood bank procedures identify most patients at risk for serious immune-mediated red-cell transfusion reactions. These procedures include major ABO typing, antibody screening, and compatibility testing. Changes in the recruiting and screening of blood donors have dramatically reduced the risk of viral transmission in blood products in the US and Europe. All units of blood in the US are tested for hepatitis B, hepatitis C, human immunodeficiency virus (HIV) 1 and 2, human T-cell lymphotrophic virus I and II (HTLV-I/II), and syphilis. In Europe and the US, nucleotide amplification testing is done for hepatitis C and HIV.

In addition to the risk for transmission of infectious diseases, transfusion therapy is also associated with acute and delayed immunological complications as well as nonimmunological complications.[68–70] Table 23-2 lists risks associated with blood component transfusion therapy. Risks associated with transfusions that can be particularly problematic for patients with cancer, especially those patients who receive large amounts of allogeneic transfusions, include the development of human leukocyte antigen (HLA) alloimmunization and graft-vs-host disease (GVHD).[71] When patients develop numerous alloantibodies, the number of units of available blood products with which they are compatible can be drastically decreased. In addition, alloimmunized patients often fail to achieve the desired therapeutic response.

In addition to concerns about the safety of transfusion therapy from the perspective of disease transmission, immunological and nonimmunological complications, new evidence suggests that transfusions may be of less therapeutic value than previously thought and could possibly cause increased risk for thromboembolic events and tumor

**TABLE 23-2**

**Risks Associated With Blood Component Transfusion Therapy**

| | Acute | Delayed |
|---|---|---|
| Immunologic | Hemolytic reactions<br>Febrile nonhemolytic reactions<br>Allergic reactions<br>Anaphylactic reactions<br>Transfusion-related acute lung injury (TRALI) | Hemolytic reactions<br>Alloimmunization<br>Post-transfusion purpura<br>Transfusion-associated graft-vs-host disease |
| Nonimmunologic | Bacterial contamination<br>Circulatory overload<br>Hypothermia<br>Metabolic complications (citrate toxicity, acidosis, alkalosis, hyperkalemia, or hypokalemia) | Disease transmission (predominantly viral and parasitic)<br>Hemosiderosis (iron overload) |

growth.[71–81] The benefits and safety profile of transfusion therapy have only been being studied in randomized controlled clinical trials since the 1980s and less than 100 have been conducted to date.[82]

In recent years, various professional societies and governmental organizations, including the American College of Physicians, the American Society of Anesthesiologists, the American Society of Clinical Oncologists, the College of American Pathologists, the NCCN, and the National Institutes of Health have developed guidelines and practice parameters as resources for the clinician to guide transfusion decision-making. These guidelines attempt to standardize the clinical criteria upon which transfusion decisions are based as well as to balance the risks and benefits of transfusions.

## RED BLOOD CELL THERAPY

Red blood cell transfusions are indicated to treat patients experiencing symptomatic anemia. Anemia is the physiological condition of too few or too small red blood cells, or a deficiency in the hemoglobin content of the blood resulting in decreased oxygen carrying capacity. Anemia is the most common hematological abnormality in patients with cancer and is frequently multifactorial, resulting from nutritional deficiencies, decreased production of red blood cells, and/or increased loss/destruction of blood cells.[83,84] Among the causes of anemia frequently seen in patients with cancer, the 2 most common are decreased red blood cell production secondary to myelosuppressive therapy and the primary disease. Common etiologies of anemia associated with cancer are listed in Table 23-3. Patients with cancer often have more slowly developing chronic anemia that is less symptomatic than rapid-onset anemia, due to the body's fluid compensatory mechanisms. Signs and symptoms of anemia, which most commonly include pallor, fatigue, tachycardia, hypotension, dyspnea, cold intolerance, and sleep disturbances, are listed in Table 23-4.

**TABLE 23-3**

**Common Etiologies of Anemia in Cancer**

| | |
|---|---|
| Decreased production | Decreased stimulatory cytokine production/activity |
| | Increased inhibitory cytokine production/activity |
| | Decreased response to stimulatory cytokines |
| | Bone marrow involvement resulting from either primary or metastatic disease |
| | Iatrogenic myelosuppression from chemotherapy known as chemotherapy-induced anemia (CIA) |
| | Iatrogenic myelosuppression from radiation therapy |
| | Iron-restricted erythropoiesis |
| | Chronic illness (anemia of chronic disease) |
| Increased destruction | Hemolysis |
| | Bleeding |
| | Erythrophagocytosis |
| | Hypersplenism |
| Nutritional deficiencies | Iron deficiency |
| | Folate deficiency |
| | Vitamin B12 deficiency |
| | General malnutrition |

**TABLE 23-4**

**Signs and Symptoms of Anemia**

| Body System | Clinical Findings |
|---|---|
| Cardiovascular | Tachycardia |
| | Palpitations |
| | Increased pulse pressure |
| | Orthostatic hypotension |
| | Cold hands and feet |
| | Cold intolerance |
| | Fainting |
| | Weakness |
| Gastrointestinal | Anorexia |
| | Nausea |
| Genitourinary | Menstrual irregularities |
| | Loss of libido |
| Immune | Impaired macrophage and T-cell functioning |
| Integumentary | Pale skin, conjunctive, and mucus membranes |
| | Skin cool to touch |
| Neurological | Fatigue |
| | Dizziness |
| | Impaired cognition |
| | Depression |
| | Headache |
| | Difficulty concentrating |
| | Sleep disturbances |
| Respiratory | Dyspnea |

The decision to transfuse with red blood cells is made within the context of the overall goals of treatment and the specific goal of the proposed transfusion. In addition, transfusion decisions are based on the clinical assessment of the patient, a review of pertinent laboratory data, and consideration of underlying disease and/or comorbidities. Rather than whole blood that contains red blood cells, white blood cells, platelets, and plasma constituents, red blood cells are usually the therapy of choice for the treatment of anemia.[85,86] The advantage of red blood cells is that depending on the preservative-anticoagulant approach used, they provide approximately 50% to 80% of the hematocrit of whole blood with only one-third of the plasma load.

Appropriate laboratory tests, including a complete blood count (CBC) and iron studies are important to the accurate diagnosis of anemia and the development of an appropriate therapeutic plan. Decreased hemoglobin and/or hematocrit levels are 2 of the most pertinent lab findings related to anemia; however, additional laboratory studies may be necessary to identify nutritional deficits or hemolytic processes that can be contributing to the anemia. Table 23-5 lists pertinent lab tests and findings associated with anemia related to cancer.[87]

Historically, the decision to transfuse with red blood cells was primarily based on hemoglobin levels varying from provider to provider. To date, controlled studies have been unable to identify the precise hemoglobin level, or "trigger" at which a transfusion is warranted.[88,89] Most practice guidelines agree that red blood cell transfusions are rarely indicated when the hemoglobin concentration is greater than 10 g/dL, but suggest that transfusions may be appropriate when the hemoglobin concentration drops to between 6 g/dL and 10 g/dL, depending on the presence of organ ischemia, actual or potential hemorrhage, intravascular volume status, and the potential complications of insufficient oxygenation.

In a retrospective study by Nordstrom and colleagues, 17.6% of patients with cancer receiving chemotherapy in 4 hospital-affiliated clinics in North Carolina received transfusions within 30 days of treatment with 78.7% being transfused at hemoglobin levels <9 g/dL and 21.3% being transfused at hemoglobin levels >9 g/dL.[90] There is movement within the medical community away from using a specific hemoglobin trigger and toward evaluating each potential transfusion using a risk-benefit analysis for the specific patient in question.

Except in life-threatening emergency situations, when transfusing red blood cells, patients must be typed and crossmatched to assure that they are ABO compatible with the donor blood and that there are no major recipient antibodies to antigens present in the donor blood. Table 23–6 highlights ABO and Rh compatibility between patient and donor blood for red blood cell transfusions. In emergency situations, O negative blood, historically known as the universal donor, can be transfused without previous typing and crossmatching, but typing and crossmatching should be done as soon as possible for future transfusion needs and to confirm the ABO and antigen–antibody compatibility of the emergently transfused unit.

The transfusion of 1 unit of red blood cells increases the hematocrit by 3% or the hemoglobin concentration by 1 g/dL in a 70 kg patient who is not bleeding. There is accumulating evidence, however, that suggests that a rise in hemoglobin and hematocrit does not directly translate into clinical benefit. It is not simply the ability of red blood cells to carry increased oxygen that confers clinical benefit, but rather, the ability of red blood cells to deliver increased oxygen to hypoxic tissue that is beneficial. A number of basic science and animal model studies have suggested various mechanisms for these findings including decreased pliability/deformability of the red blood cell related to storage conditions and duration and decreased nitric oxide content of the stored red blood cells. Current evidence suggests that the half-life of transfused red blood cells is approximately 30 days.[91]

Red blood cells can be stored for up to 5 weeks at 1°C to 6°C in solutions containing citrate, phosphate buffers, dextrose, and adenine (CPDA-1). Shelf-life is further extended if an additive solution with higher concentrations of adenine is added to the red blood cells.[71] Red blood cells with rare antigen profiles can be frozen and stored for up to 10 years. Frozen red blood cells are indicated for patients with cancer who have an alloantibody to a high-incidence antigen or have multiple alloantibodies.[71]

In order to render red blood cell products more tolerable by special populations, there are a number of postcollection/pretransfusion techniques, including leukoreduction, irradiation, and washing that can be employed. Leukocytes in red blood cell transfusions can cause reactions if the recipient has antileukocyte antibodies, which can develop following previous transfusions or pregnancies. These antigenic reactions occur much more frequently in the population of patients with cancer compared with other patient groups.[86] Transfusion of packed red blood cells in these patients can cause fever and chills, and the patient can eventually become alloimmunized or refractory to transfusions. The use of leukocyte-reduced blood component therapy is indicated for patients who have developed alloantibodies. Leukoreduction of blood products can be achieved through special processing prior to storing the blood or through the use of bedside leukocyte reduction filters at the time of administration. It is important to note, however, that when leukoreduction techniques are employed, the hematocrit of the unit is decreased by 10% to 15%.

Irradiation of red blood cells is another technique used to prevent GVHD when transfusing RBCs to an immunocompromised patient, such as a bone marrow or stem cell transplant recipient. In this population, the compromised immune system of the patient is unable to prevent the transfused lymphocytes from attacking host tissue. In an immunocompetent host, the recipient's functional immune system is able to effectively destroy transfused lymphocytes and, thus, the development of GVHD is not a concern.

Washing of red cell products with saline is a technique that can be used when the transfusion recipient has had allergic febrile reactions to previous transfusions despite prophylactic antihistamine use. The process of washing reduces plasma and plasma proteins implicated in the allergic response. Recipients who are deficient in IgA or who have antibodies to IgA can have very severe hypersensitivity reactions to red cell products containing IgA. Repeated washings can render a red cell product tolerable to these patients. The washing procedure requires the unit of red cells to be opened and thus must be used within 24 hours of the washing to minimize risk for bacterial contamination.

**TABLE 23-5**

**Laboratory Tests Pertinent to the Assessment of Anemia**

| Lab Test | Normal Value | What Is Being Measured | Variation Found in Anemia | Common Etiologies of Abnormal Findings in Cancer | What Might Affect Results |
|---|---|---|---|---|---|
| Red blood cell count (RBC) | Male: 4.2–5.4 million cells/$mm^3$<br>Female: 3.6–5.0 million cells/ $mm^3$ | The total number of red blood cells in a microliter (or cubic millimeter) of whole blood | Usually decreased, but could be normal or elevated in microcytic iron-deficiency anemia | Impaired red blood cell production, increased cell destruction, bleeding, Hodgkin's or non-Hodgkin's lymphoma, hematological malignancies, or myeloproliferative disorders | Dehydration, stress, high altitude, drugs, an insufficiently filled blood collection tube, clotting of the specimen, prolonged venous stasis, and position during venipuncture |
| Hemoglobin (Hgb) | Male: 14.0–17.4 g/dL<br>Female: 12.0–16.0 g/dL | The oxygen carrying capacity of the blood. Each gram of hemoglobin is able to carry 1.35 mL of oxygen for every 100 mL of blood. | Decreased | Impaired red blood cell production, iron deficiency, blood loss, hemolytic anemia, leukemias, Hodgkin's or non-Hodgkin's lymphoma | Very recent blood loss or transfusion, burns, high altitude, excessive fluid intake, strenuous physical exercise, and drugs. A very high white blood cell count can artificially raise the Hgb level |
| Hematocrit (Hct) | Male: 42%–48%<br>Female: 36%–48% | The mass of the red blood cells measured as a percentage of the volume of whole blood | Decreased | Impaired red blood cell production, increased cell destruction, bleeding, Hodgkin's or non-Hodgkin's lymphoma, hematological malignancies, myeloproliferative disorders, chronic disease, or hemolytic reaction | Very recent blood loss or transfusion, high altitude, dehydration |
| Mean corpuscular volume (MCV) | 82–98 fL | The average volume occupied by a single erythrocyte, measured in femtoliters (cubic micrometers) | Normocytic (normal size)<br>Microcytic (smaller than normal) <82 fL<br>Macrocytic (larger than normal) >100 fL | Acute posthemorrhagic anemia, anemia associated with bone marrow infiltration and hemolytic anemia<br>Iron deficiency anemia and anemia of chronic disease<br>Vitamin $B_{12}$ deficiency anemia, neoplastic disease | Increased reticulocytes, leukocytosis, hyperglycemia and cold agglutins can increase the MCV.<br>This value is arrived at through a calculation and it is possible to have a normocytic MCV in the presence of both microcytic and macrocytic cells |
| Mean corpuscular hemoglobin (MCH) | 26–34 pg/cell | The average weight of the hemoglobin per red blood cell measured in picograms (pg) | Increased in macrocytic anemia<br>Decreased in microcytic anemia | Vitamin $B_{12}$ deficiency anemia, neoplastic disease<br>Iron deficiency anemia and anemia of chronic disease | Hyperlipemia, cold agglutinins, and very elevated WBC (> 50,000/$mm^3$) |
| Mean corpuscular hemoglobin concentration (MCHC) | 32–36 g/dL | The average hemoglobin concentration in red blood cells measured in grams per deciliter of blood. | Decreased, indicating that a given volume of red blood cells contains less than the normal amount of hemoglobin | Iron deficiency, anemia of chronic disease, chronic blood loss | Lipemia, cold agglutinins, and rouleux (the stacking of red blood cells like coins).<br>This value is a calculated average using the weight of the Hgb in comparison to the volume of the RBC. |

(*Continued*)

**TABLE 23-5**

**Laboratory Tests Pertinent to the Assessment of Anemia (*Continued*)**

| Lab Test | Normal Value | What Is Being Measured | Variation Found in Anemia | Common Etiologies of Abnormal Findings in Cancer | What Might Affect Results |
|---|---|---|---|---|---|
| Red blood cell distribution width (RDW) | 11.5–14.5 CV of red cell size | Measures the degree of variability in the size of the RBCs (anisocytosis) and the coefficient of variation (CV) of the red blood cell size | Increased | Iron-deficiency anemia, vitamin B12 deficiency anemia, folate deficiency anemia, immune hemolytic anemia, reticulocytosis, and fragmentation of RBCs | Alcoholism and cold agglutins |
| | | | Normal | Chronic disease, acute blood loss, and aplastic anemia | |
| Reticulocyte count | 0.5%–1.5% (of RBCs) | The number of young, non-nucleated RBCs represented as a percentage of the total RBC count. | Increased (indicates the bone marrow is compensating for RBC loss) | Hemolytic anemia, post hemorrhage, following treatment of anemias | None noted |
| | | | Decreased (indicates that the bone marrow is not able to compensate for decreased RBC count) | Untreated iron-deficiency anemia, aplastic anemia, anemia of chronic disease, vitamin B12 and folate deficiency anemias, alcoholism, marrow involvement, myeloproliferative disorders, and radiation therapy | |
| | | | When < 2% reticulocyte index in the presence of anemia, it indicates the marrow is hypoproliferative<br>A reticulocyte index of > 2%–3% in the presence of anemia indicates a marrow that is increasing production. | | |
| Ferritin | Male: 20–250 mcg/L<br>Female: 10–120 mcg/L<br>Males with anemia of chronic disease: < 100 mcg/L<br>Females with anemia of chronic disease: < 20 mcg/L | The body's iron stores measured in micrograms per liter of blood. | Decreased | Iron deficiency, chronic hemorrhagic or aplastic anemia | Drugs, alcoholism (with accompanying liver disease), high red-meat consumption, hemolyzed blood specimen |
| | | | Normal | Acute hemorrhage, bone marrow aplasia or liver disease | |
| | | | Increased | Megaloblastic (pernicious), hemolytic, or sideroblastic anemias | |

| | | | | | |
|---|---|---|---|---|---|
| Serum iron | Male: 65–175 mcg/dL<br>Female: 50–170 mcg/dL | The iron bound to transferring molecules in the blood measured in micrograms per deciliter of blood. | Decreased | Iron deficiency anemia, acute and chronic blood loss, megaloblastic (pernicious) anemia and anemia of chronic illness | Drugs, hemolysis of specimen, time of day of blood draw |
| | | | Increased | Hemolytic anemia, vitamin $B_6$ deficiency, sideroblastic anemia, cancers involving the bone marrow and aplastic anemia | |
| | | | Normal | With iron deficiency anemia when the hemoglobin is > 9.0 g/dL | |
| Transferrin | Adults: 250–425 mg/dL | The amount of iron transporter molecules in the blood measured in mg per deciliter or blood. | Increased | Iron deficiency anemia | Drugs, hemolysis of specimen, time of day of blood draw |
| | | | Decreased | Microcytic anemia of chronic disease, protein deficiency, chronic infection, acute liver disease | |
| Total iron binding capacity (TIBC) | 250–450 mcg/dL | The ability of iron to bind with transferrin measured in micrograms per deciliter of blood. | Increased | Iron deficiency anemia, acute and chronic blood loss | Drugs, hemolysis of specimen, time of day of blood draw |
| | | | Decreased | Hypoproteinemia, anemia of infection and chronic disease | |
| | | | Normal | With iron deficiency anemia when the hemoglobin is > 9.0 g/dL | |
| Transferrin (or iron) saturation (TSAT) | Male: 10%–50%<br>Female: 15%–50% | The serum iron in relation to the total iron binding capacity represented as a percent. | Decreased | Iron deficiency anemia, hemorrhagic anemia, infection associated anemia and anemia of chronic disease | Drugs, hemolysis of specimen, time of day of blood draw |
| | | | Increased | Aplastic anemia and cancers involving the bone marrow | |
| Serum folate (folic acid) | 2–20 ng/mL | The unbound folate content of the blood measured in nanograms per mililiter | Decreased | Inadequate intake of folate due to poor diet, alcoholism, chronic disease, malnutrition, malabsorption or vitamin $B_{12}$ deficiency. Hemolytic anemia, vitamin $B_6$ deficiency, cancer, acute leukemias, and Crohn's disease or ulcerative colitis | Drugs, hemolyzed specimen, and iron deficiency anemia |
| RBC folate | 140–628 ng/dL | The folate associated with red blood cells measured in nanograms per milliliter of blood. | Decreased | Folate deficiency, vitamin $B_{12}$ deficiency. Tissue has been depleted of folate either due to a true folate deficiency or to a vitamin $B_{12}$ deficiency that is preventing the cells of the small intestine from being able to absorb folate. | Drugs, hemolyzed specimen, and iron deficiency anemia |
| Serum B12 (antipernicious anemia factor) | 200–835 pg/mL | The amount of vitamin $B_{12}$ measured in picograms per milliliter of blood. | Decreased | Pernicious (megaloblastic) anemia | Drugs, blood transfusion, smoking, and high intake of vitamins A and C |

*(Continued)*

**TABLE 23-5**

**Laboratory Tests Pertinent to the Assessment of Anemia (*Continued*)**

| Lab Test | Normal Value | What Is Being Measured | Variation Found in Anemia | Common Etiologies of Abnormal Findings in Cancer | What Might Affect Results |
|---|---|---|---|---|---|
| Direct Coomb's test | Negative for red blood cells | Detects the presence of antigen–antibody complexes on the surface of the red blood cell. Reported as positive if antigen–antibody complex is detected, negative if not. | Positive | Hemolytic anemia resulting from alloimmunization, transfusion reaction, and drug-related red blood cell sensitization. | Drugs |
| Indirect Coomb's test | Negative for serum | Detects the presence of serum antibodies to red blood cells but does not detect antigen–antibody complex on the red blood cell itself. Reported as positive if antibodies are detected, negative if not. | Positive | Alloimmunization, transfusion reaction, and drug-related red blood cell sensitization | None reported |
| Serum erythropoietin level | 5–36 mU/mL | The amount of circulating erythropoietin measured in milliunits per milliliter of blood. | Increased appropriately<br><br>Increased inappropriately<br>Decreased appropriately<br>Decreased inappropriately | Anemias with very low hemoglobins, iron deficiency anemia, myeloproliferative disorders, and post chemotherapy<br>Renal cell and other carcinomas<br>Cancer<br>Following bone marrow transplantation, in the presence of renal failure | Drugs, growth and thyroid stimulating hormones, transfusions |

*Source*: Data from Fischbach.[87]

**TABLE 23-6**

**ABO and Rh Compatibility for Red Blood Cell Transfusions**

| Recipient/Patient Blood Type | Compatible Donor/Unit Blood Type(s) |
|---|---|
| A+ | A+, A−, O+, O− |
| A− | A−, O− |
| B+ | B+, B−, O+, O− |
| B− | B−, O− |
| AB+ (universal RBC recipient) | AB+, AB−, A+, A−, B+, B−, O+, O− |
| AB− | AB−, A−, B−, O− |
| O+ | O+, O− |
| O− | O− |

The plus sign (+) is used to indicate the presence of the Rh antigen, referred to as Rh positive. The minus sign (−) is used to indicate the absence of the Rh antigen, referred to as Rh negative.

Washing reduces the number of red cells in the product and thus the hematocrit content will be less than in a non-washed product. In addition, although some leukocytes are removed in the washing process, the washed product is not considered to be leukoreduced; however, it may provide some protection against febrile nonhemolytic reactions.

## PLATELET THERAPY

Platelet transfusions are indicated to control bleeding in the thrombocytopenic patient or to prevent bleeding in the severely thrombocytopenic patient. The majority of platelet transfusions in the cancer population are given for treatment-induced thrombocytopenia. Thrombocytopenia is a reduction in the platelet count below the lower limit of normal, which is generally 140,000 (platelets) per cubic millimeter (/μL).

Platelet transfusions in patients with cancer are generally administered prophylactically when the platelet count falls to below 10,000/μL. Studies have found that patients receiving chemotherapy can tolerate platelet counts as low as 5000 to 10,000 μL.[92–94] The trigger at which prophylactic platelet transfusions are initiated may be higher in patients with fever, severe mucositis, or GVHD. A study by Wandt and colleagues evaluated the safety of a therapeutic transfusion strategy rather than a prophylactic approach to transfusion in patients following high-dose chemotherapy and autologous peripheral stem cell transplant. They concluded that although the number of minor bleeds was larger in the therapeutic transfusion arm, a therapeutic approach to platelet transfusion was safe and cost effective.[95] Patients with cancer undergoing invasive procedures, such as lumbar punctures, central line placement, or bone marrow aspiration, are transfused to keep the platelet count >40,000/μL.[96] In addition, when administering platelets in conjunction with invasive procedures it is important to obtain a post-transfusion platelet count to assure that an adequate increment has been achieved. When evaluating the need for platelet transfusion, it is important to consider the coagulation status of the patient as well as the platelet count because patients with plasma coagulation factor disorders are more likely to bleed at marginal platelet counts.

There are 2 ways by which platelets can be collected for transfusion. The first method involves the processing of a unit of donated whole blood into constituent parts, specifically, packed red blood cells and plasma, which is then further processed to yield a single unit of random donor platelets. One unit of platelets, collected from 1 unit of whole blood in this manner contains $\geq 5.5 \times 10^{10}$ platelets in approximately 50 mL of plasma.

The second method of platelet collection is through a process known as platelet pheresis. Using this method, an IV is established in a donor and the donor is connected to an apheresis machine, which separates the blood into its constituent parts. The platelet product yielded from this process is referred to as single donor platelets and contains $\geq 3.0 \times 10^{11}$ platelets in approximately 250 mL of plasma. A donor can be pheresed up to every other day if the donor's platelets provide the recipient/patient with good platelet count increases.

When transfusing random donor platelets, between 4 and 10 units are pooled together, which constitute an adult dose. When using single donor platelets, the product is sufficient for adult transfusion. Both random donor platelets and single donor platelets should be ABO identical when possible (particularly if patients are refractory to platelet transfusions).[85,96] When, due to a lack of Rh compatible platelets, Rh positive donor platelets are transfused to an Rh negative female of childbearing age, it is important to consider administering Rh immune globulin to prevent the development of Rh, also known as D antibodies. Table 23-7 lists the types of platelet products for transfusion along with their indications, complications, and nursing considerations. Platelets can be infused as rapidly as tolerated by the patient while being closely monitored for transfusion reactions.

Theoretically, 1 unit of platelets should increase the recipient's platelet count by 10,000 μL. However, the effectiveness of platelet transfusions is variable and depends on several factors. Failure to achieve adequate increases in the circulating platelet count may be due to fever, infection, disseminated intravascular coagulation (DIC), hypersplenism, prolonged storage of platelets, and HLA antibody grade.[85,97] Attempts should be made to lower a fever by administering acetaminophen if a patient is febrile when he or she is to receive a platelet transfusion. Fever and infection enhance the consumption of platelets and can increase the occurrence of hemorrhage. Acetaminophen, corticosteroids, and antihistamines may also be used to premedicate a patient prior to platelet therapy to minimize the chance of a febrile nonhemolytic reaction. Meperidine may be used if the patient experiences shaking chills.

Platelets are stored at room temperature (20°C–24°C), with gentle continuous agitation (to prevent the clumping of platelets in the donor product), for up to 5 days. Contaminating organisms may reach unacceptable levels beyond 5 days.

### Platelet refractory state

About 10% to 15% of patients with cancer requiring multiple platelet transfusions develop a state of platelet refractoriness, which is a failure to achieve a therapeutic increment in the platelet count following transfusion of platelets.[98] Platelet refractoriness can be due to immune or nonimmune causes such as sepsis, hypersplenism, and DIC. The most common immune cause of platelet refractoriness is the development of antibodies directed against foreign (donor) HLA types, which may result in alloimmunization. A lack of response to platelet transfusions can be associated with hemorrhagic events secondary to thrombocytopenia.

When immune-mediated platelet refractoriness is suspected, it is important to obtain a post-transfusion platelet count within 60 minutes of completion of the platelet transfusion. Post-transfusion platelet counts within this time frame most accurately reflect the impact of immune-mediated effects on platelet survival. Post-transfusion platelet counts obtained 24 hours following the completion of the platelet transfusion are more reflective of nonimmune mediated effects (such as sepsis or DIC) on platelet survival.

In order to diagnose platelet refractoriness, the patient must have failed to achieve the expected post-transfusion increment following 2 ABO-compatible transfusions of platelets that were stored for less than 72 hours. An adequate increment is generally accepted as an absolute increase in platelet count by 2000/μL per unit of platelet concentrate (random donor platelet unit) transfused.

Patients who are refractory to random-donor platelets may respond to either HLA-matched platelets or to single-donor platelet transfusions, as they significantly reduce the number of platelet and leukocyte antibodies to which the recipient is exposed. In addition, leukoreduction of platelets has been shown to decrease the incidence of HLA alloimmunization in patients who are expected to receive numerous platelet transfusions over the course of therapy. Leukocytes can be removed from platelet products by using leukoreduction techniques in the blood bank prior to storage or through the use of bedside leukocyte-reduction blood filters, or by treating the platelets with ultraviolet light (UVB).[99,100] Like red blood cell products, platelet products can also be irradiated to reduce the risk of GVHD in immunocompromised patients.

Platelet cross-matching is another method to decrease the risk of alloimmunization. Platelet cross-matching can detect antibodies in a patient's serum that will react with platelets in potential donor units, thus allowing for the selection of platelet products most likely to afford the patient a therapeutic response.[98] In patients with severe alloimmunization who fail to respond to matched platelets, prophylactic platelet transfusions have not proven to be beneficial and platelet transfusions in this population should be restricted to actively bleeding patients.

## PLASMA THERAPY

Plasma is the straw-colored, noncellular liquid component of blood that serves as the transport vehicle for the formed blood elements (red blood cells, white blood cells, and platelets). Plasma is composed predominantly of water but suspended in it are proteins (albumin and globulin antibodies such as IgA, IgG, and IgM), electrolytes (sodium, potassium, calcium, and glucose), carbohydrates, hormones, dissolved gases (oxygen, carbon dioxide, and nitrogen), clotting factors, and cellular waste.

### Thawed plasma or fresh frozen plasma

Plasma is obtained by centrifuging whole blood and it can be stored as fresh frozen plasma (FFP), FP24 (which is plasma that has been frozen within 24 hours of collection), thawed plasma, or cryoprecipitate reduced (cryo-poor) plasma. Variations in plasma products primarily involve the quantity and activity of the various clotting factors contained in the plasma. FFP is frozen to ≤–18°C within 6 to 8 hours of collection, depending on the anticoagulant used, and all clotting factors remain functional. FP24 and thawed plasma may have reduced levels of Factors V and VII. When cryoprecipitate is removed from plasma, levels of Factors VIII, XIII, von Willebrand's factor, fibrinogen, and fibronectin are decreased by 20% to 30% in the remaining plasma product.

The most common indications for plasma therapy/infusions in the cancer population include (1) the treatment of active bleeding due to multiple coagulation factor deficiencies or due to singular factor deficiencies for which no concentrated factor product is available, (2) the treatment of active bleeding associated with massive transfusion, (3) rapid reversal of warfarin therapy preprocedurally or in bleeding patients, or (4) thrombotic thrombocytopenic purpura. Fresh frozen plasma is not recommended as a volume expander, because there is a risk of transfusion-transmitted disease. Also, FFP is not recommended to treat isolated factor deficiencies because of the large volumes that would be required to attain adequate levels. A unit of FFP contains 180 to 270 mL of plasma.

Due to the presence of antibodies in plasma, FFP should be ABO compatible with the recipient.[85,96] Table 23-8 highlights ABO compatibility for plasma transfusions.

**TABLE 23-7**

**Platelet Transfusion Therapy**

| Specific Component | Concentration and Volume | General Indications | Complications | Nursing Considerations |
|---|---|---|---|---|
| **RD**<br>• Fresh—best<br>• Frozen and cryopreserved (limited application because of poor recovery) | • Multiple donors (4+) approximately 200 mL<br>• Plasma, WBCs, few RBCs | • Bleeding and bleeding prophylaxis<br>• Prophylactic for platelet count of 10,000–20,000/µL | • Exposure of patients to multiple tissue antigens, which initiates antigen–antibody formation, leading to refractoriness<br>• Hepatitis (increased risk with pooled products)<br>• Allergic reactions may be seen more often if leukocyte-reduced blood is not used | • Gently agitate bag occasionally to prevent platelet clumping<br>• Rapid infusion (per patient tolerance)<br>• Tubing should include a 170–200 µm in-line blood filter<br>• A leukocyte reduction blood filter may be required or the use of prestorage leukocyte-reduced blood<br>• Less expensive than single-donor or HLA matched platelet concentrates<br>• May require UVB irradiation if patient is severely immunosuppressed |
| **SD**<br>• Fresh (maximum effectiveness up to 6 hour) | • One donor<br>• 1 unit ∝ 300 mL<br>• Plasma, WBCs, RBCs<br>• Number of platelets in an SD unit equals approximately the number of platelets in 5 RD units | • Bleeding and bleeding prophylaxis<br>• Severe febrile reactions associated with random donor platelets<br>• Often used once a patient is refractory to random donor platelets<br>• Patients who require long-term platelet therapy<br>• Minimizes transmission of viral disease | • Refractoriness to platelets may occur over time | • Rapid infusion (generally 30 minutes +)<br>• Tubing as above<br>• Leukocyte reduction of blood as above |
| HLA matched concentrate | • 1 donor compatible at the HLA complex | • When patients become refractory to RD and SD platelets | • Minimal | • HLA-matched platelets minimize patient exposure to multiple tissue antigens (HLA complex found on all blood cells—acts as a genetic monogram)<br>• Rapid infusion (30 minutes +)<br>• Tubing as above. Generally see more effective increases in the platelet count than with RD or SD |

*Abbreviations*: HLA, human leukocyte antigen; RD, random donor; RBC, red blood cells; SD, single donor; UVB, ultraviolet light B; WBC, white blood cell.

∝ = approximately.

The amount and frequency of transfusions with plasma depend on several factors, including the severity of the deficiency, the specific factor deficiency, the size of the recipient/patient, and the severity of bleeding. Generally, diffuse bleeding due to multiple coagulation factor deficiencies should be controlled when the clotting factor levels reach 20% to 50% of normal values. Appropriate concentrations of the levels can be obtained with infusions of 2 to 6 units of plasma in a 70 kg adult.[71] Plasma and plasma factors are infused rapidly, so the maximum plasma level is reached

**TABLE 23-8**

**ABO Compatibility for Plasma Transfusions**

| Recipient/Patient Blood Type | Compatible Donor/Unit Blood Type |
|---|---|
| A | A, AB |
| B | B, AB |
| AB | AB |
| O Universal Plasma Recipient | A, B, AB, O |

before metabolic changes or degradation of the product occur (due to a short half-life).

### Cryoprecipitate

Cryoprecipitate contains fibrinogen, fibronectin, factors VIII and XIII, and some von Willebrand factor. Its use is generally limited to patients with severe hypofibrinogenemia (less than 100 mg/dL). Cryoprecipitate is obtained by thawing a unit of FFP to between 1°C and 6°C. The unthawed or cold insoluble component of the thawing FFP is the cryoprecipitate. Each unit of cryoprecipitate contains ≥150 mg fibrinogen and ≥80 IU of Factor VIII in 5 to 20 mL of plasma. The fibrinogen level should rise by approximately 8.5 mg/dL in a nonbleeding 70 kg adult per unit of cryoprecipitate. Disseminated intravascular coagulation is an oncologic emergency associated with diminished clotting factors resulting from dysregulated hemostasis. Although cryoprecipitate contains numerous clotting factors, it does not contain factor V and thus is not recommended for use alone as a treatment for DIC. Although cryoprecipitate is considered an acellular product and thus does not require compatibility testing or regard for Rh status, it is preferable to use cryoprecipitate that is ABO compatible with the patient.[85,96]

### Individual clotting factors

Purified factor preparations are usually preferred over FFP if the patient is deficient in only 1 coagulation protein, such as patients with hemophilia A (factor VIII), hemophilia B (factor IX), or acquired von Willebrand's syndrome.[85] In these cases, virally inactivated or recombinant proteins are available for use.

## TRANSFUSION REACTIONS AND COMPLICATIONS

Many risks are associated with blood component therapy, including transfusion reactions and transmission of disease.[101,102] Reactions can be acute (occurring during or within 24 hours of completion of transfusion) or delayed (occurring days to weeks later). Reactions can also be classified as immunologic or nonimmunologic in nature. Acute immunological reactions include acute hemolytic transfusion reactions (AHTRs), febrile nonhemolytic transfusion reactions, allergic and anaphylactic reactions, and transfusion-related acute lung injury (TRALI). Acute nonimmunological reactions include bacterial contamination of blood resulting in sepsis, circulatory overload, hypothermia, and metabolic complications including citrate toxicity, hypokalemia or hyperkalemia, and acidosis or alkalosis.[96,101] Delayed immunological transfusion reactions include delayed hemolytic reactions, the development of GVHD, alloimmunization, and post-transfusion purpura (PTP). Delayed nonimmunological reactions include the transmission of diseases, particularly viral diseases and iron overload. Table 23-2 lists transfusion reactions and complications, and Table 23-9 lists and explains the nursing management of transfusion reactions.

### Immediate blood transfusion reactions

*Acute hemolytic transfusion reactions.* Acute hemolytic transfusion reactions occur in 1:38,000 to 1:70,000 transfusions. These acute immunological reactions are most often the result of the transfusion of ABO-incompatible blood. Estimates for the risk of a fatal AHTR range from 1:160,000[101] to 1:1,000,000.[102] The most common cause of ABO incompatibility is a clerical error involving a misidentification of the patient. A double-check of all of the patient identifiers at every point, from collecting the specimen for type and crossmatch to dispensing the blood from the blood bank to hanging the unit of blood, is critical to avoid this type of error.

Acute hemolytic reactions commonly present with increased temperature and pulse but can also include chills, shortness of breath, flank or chest pain, hematuria, a "sense of impending doom," and shock. Changes in blood pressure are also common and vary according to the intensity of the antigen–antibody interaction as well as the body's ability to compensate. Transfusions should be started slowly and monitored closely. The transfusion should be stopped with the first signs and symptoms of an acute hemolytic transfusion reaction, minimizing the volume of incompatible blood infused.

Treatment of acute hemolytic reactions includes fluid resuscitation, cardiopulmonary support, promotion and maintenance of urine production, and transfusions with specific blood products as needed. Testing of a post-reaction blood specimen in the presence of a hemolytic transfusion reaction usually reveals hemoglobinemia, a positive direct antibody test, and increased plasma levels of lactate dehydrogenase, hemoglobin, and bilirubin.[98]

**TABLE 23-9**

**Nursing Management of Selected Transfusion Reactions**

| Type | Signs/Symptoms | Nursing Actions |
|---|---|---|
| Acute hemolytic transfusion reaction<br>• ABO incompatibility | Fever, chills, hypotension, increased pulse rate, nausea/vomiting, flushing, low back pain, decreased urine output, hematuria, dyspnea, bleeding, anaphylaxis, shock | 1. Stop transfusion<br>2. Maintain patent IV line with normal saline<br>3. Verify patient and the blood unit with another nurse (the majority of reported fatalities with an acute hemolytic transfusion reaction involve human error)<br>4. Place in supine position<br>5. Maintain open airway; provide CPR if necessary<br>6. Obtain vital signs and record<br>7. Notify physician<br>8. Monitor intake and output<br>9. Administer fluids and medications per physician order<br>10. Monitor vital signs per institutional guidelines<br>11. Obtain blood and urine specimens<br>12. Notify blood bank and return remainder of blood to blood bank<br>13. Document event<br>14. Admit patient to hospital if outpatient |
| Febrile nonhemolytic transfusion reaction (FNHTRs)<br>• Antileukocyte antibodies in the recipient directed against the donor blood | Fever (>1.8°F) ± chills, headache, hypotension, increased pulse rate, dyspnea, chest pain, nausea/vomiting | 1. Stop transfusion<br>2. Maintain patent IV line with normal saline<br>3. Obtain and monitor vital signs and record<br>4. Notify physician<br>5. Assist in ruling out infection<br>6. Administer medications and fluids per physician order; acetaminophen for fever, meperidine for chills and rigors, antihistamine for dyspnea<br>6. Obtain vital signs and record<br>7. Notify physician<br>8. Monitor intake and output<br>9. Administer fluids and medications per physician order<br>10. Notify blood bank<br>11. Document event<br>12. For patients who are known to have FNHTRs or for patients who are at high risk for FNHTRS (multiply transfused clients); acetaminophen, antihistamines and steroids may be given before the transfusion to minimize or eliminate the transfusion reaction. The use of a leukocyte-reduction filter or the use of prestorage leukocyte-reduced blood may be indicated. |
| Allergic (usually mild) reaction<br>• Recipient antibodies against immunoglobulin components or other soluble proteins in the plasma. | Hives, urticaria, cutaneous erythema; may develop severe allergic or even fatal anaphylaxis | 1. Obtain and monitor vital signs and record<br>2. Slow or stop transfusion rate, depending on symptoms<br>3. Maintain a patent IV line with normal saline<br>4. Take measures to correct shock, maintain renal circulation, and correct the bleeding, depending on symptoms<br>5. Notify physician<br>6. Administer medications per physician order. Antihistamines if reaction is mild<br>7. Treat as anaphylactic reaction if severe<br>8. Notify blood bank<br>9. Document event |
| Bacterial contamination<br>• Cold-growing organisms | Fever, chills; may result in endotoxin shock | 1. Stop transfusion<br>2. Maintain patent IV line<br>3. Take measures to correct shock and to maintain renal circulation<br>4. Obtain vital signs and record<br>5. Notify physician<br>6. Notify blood bank and return remainder of blood to blood bank<br>7. Continue transfusion if symptoms are not severe<br>8. Obtain blood and urine cultures of the patient and the unit of blood<br>9. Administer antibiotics per physician order<br>10. Document event obtain vital signs & record<br>11. Admit patient to hospital if outpatient |
| Delayed hemolytic reaction<br>• Development of alloantibodies to transfused blood | Delayed (7–10 days to weeks) decreased hemoglobin, low-grade fever, jaundice (increase in bilirubin and LDH) | Notify blood bank |

*Acute nonhemolytic febrile transfusion reactions and allergic reactions.* Febrile nonhemolytic transfusion reactions (FNHTRs) occur in about 0.5% to 6% of all RBC transfusions and 1% to 38% of platelet transfusions and are associated with a temperature increase of ≥1°C or 1.8°F either during or just after a transfusion. Shaking chills often accompany the fever. While these reactions are not dangerous, they may be a sign of a more serious reaction, such as a hemolytic transfusion reaction. Thus, any febrile reaction in a patient receiving blood products should be investigated carefully.

Febrile nonhemolytic transfusion reactions (FNHTRs) are likely caused by the presence of host antibodies to HLA-specific or leukocyte-specific antigens on white blood cells and/or platelets in the transfused product. The severity of symptoms often correlates with the number of leukocytes transfused or the rate of the transfusion. The presence of cytokines, either in the transfused product or released by the host in response to the transfused product, can also contribute to FNHTRs. These reactions are most likely to occur in patients who have become alloimmunized as a result of previous transfusions or pregnancy. Although there are no laboratory tests to predict or prevent these reactions, patients experiencing a febrile nonhemolytic reaction can generally benefit from the administration of acetaminophen for the fever, meperidine for severe rigors, and steroids for dyspnea. Patients previously experiencing febrile nonhemolytic reactions are generally premedicated with acetaminophen and steroids prior to future transfusions. In addition, reactions can generally be minimized by the use of leukocyte-reduced blood products.

Allergic reactions occur in approximately 1% to 3% of transfusions. Allergic reactions can be mild and can manifest as hives, generalized itching, or cutaneous erythema usually without accompanying fever or, in more severe cases, as wheezing, angioedema, and anaphylaxis. These reactions are immunoglobulin E (IgE) mediated and symptoms result from histamine release. Without available laboratory tests to predict or prevent allergic reactions, management consists primarily of the administration of antihistamines, corticosteroids and in severe cases, epinephrine. In cases of anaphylaxis, standard management protocols for anaphylaxis, including pulmonary and cardiovascular support, are indicated. Patients can benefit from premedication with an antihistamine and the use of saline washed products for future transfusions.

*Bacterial contamination and transfusion-related acute lung injury.* Bacterial contamination of blood, caused when bacteria enter blood bags during component preparation or from improperly cleansed skin at venipuncture sites, can result in sepsis. The incidence of bacterial contamination varies depending on the product. Red blood cells, which are stored under refrigerated conditions, have a risk for bacterial contamination of 1 in 30,000 units. Platelets, which are stored at room temperature, have a bacterial contamination rate of 1 in every 2000 to 3000 units. Bacterial contamination should be considered when patients experience a ≥2° C increase in temperature accompanied by hypotension and rigors during or shortly after a transfusion. Prompt recognition of this potential complication is critical to a successful outcome. Management strategies include the immediate discontinuation of the transfusion, prompt administration of both broad-spectrum antimicrobials and pharmacological agents that provide cardiovascular support, and an attempt to identify the causative organism (which has included both gram-positive and gram-negative microbes[103]) by culturing of patient blood, the transfused blood product, and the administration set used. Bacterial contamination, although rare, has been identified in red blood cells, platelets, and frozen products that have been thawed in a water bath.

Transfusion-related acute lung injury (TRALI) generally occurs within 6 hours of transfusion and is characterized by massive leaking of fluid and protein into the interstitial and alveolar spaces. The incidence of TRALI varies widely ranging from 1 in 500 to 1 in 190,000.[101,102] Although its etiology is not fully understood, it is thought to be the result of granulocyte activation following exposure to antigens in the donor product. The activated granulocytes migrate to the lungs where increased permeability of the microvasculature results in capillary leak and pulmonary edema.[101,102] Symptoms of TRALI include dyspnea, tachypnea, cyanosis, fever, and hypotension. Breath sounds are diminished with crackles audible throughout and fluffy diffuse infiltrates on radiographic studies reflect pulmonary edema. Management strategies for this serious, acute transfusion reaction are composed of intensive pulmonary support interventions including supplemental oxygen and mechanical ventilation. Mortality associated with TRALI is less than 10% and patients generally recover within 2 to 4 days.[102]

*Miscellaneous complications.* Other immediate complications such as circulatory overload, air embolism, hypothermia, and metabolic complications including citrate toxicity, hypokalemia or hyperkalemia, and acidosis or alkalosis may be related to the volume of blood product administered, rate of administration, administration techniques, sensitivity to additives in the blood product, or age of the blood product.[96,101,102] Management strategies are etiology-specific and can include administration of diuretics, altering the rate of infusion, prophylactic blood-warming using an FDA-approved device, use of red blood cells that are less than 10 days old, and monitoring of and when indicated, correction of electrolytes and pH.[101,102]

### Delayed blood transfusion reactions

*Graft-versus-host disease.* A serious delayed transfusion reaction in patients who are severely immunocompromised is GVHD. Patients who are at risk of developing GVHD include bone marrow transplant recipients, peripheral blood stem cell recipients, patients undergoing combination treatment for Hodgkin's and non-Hodgkin's lymphoma, and patients with leukemia who are undergoing induction therapy. This complication can occur following the transfusion of blood products containing viable T lymphocytes. The donor-competent T lymphocytes are able to mount an immune attack on immunocompromised host tissues because the recipient's weakened immune system is unable to recognize and destroy the transfused lymphocytes.[101,102] GVHD can occur in immunocompetent patients when they are transfused with blood products from a blood relative or with a blood product that is homozygous for an HLA-haplotype for which the recipient is heterozygous.[85,102] GVHD generally manifests in the skin, liver, and gastrointestinal tract and can be fatal. Post-transfusion GVHD is fatal almost 90% of the time due to the development of bone marrow hypoplasia or aplasia.[102] To prevent GVHD, it is recommended that all blood products given to severely immunocompromised patients be irradiated before transfusion with 2500 cGy to inactivate donor lymphocytes. Leukocyte reduction of blood components is not considered effective in preventing GVHD because although leukoreduction decreases the number of T lymphocytes in the donor unit, there are still sufficient numbers of viable T lymphocytes to cause GVHD.

*Transfusion-transmitted disease.* Transmission of disease, particularly viral disease, through blood products is a major concern of the public. Transmission of viral diseases has dramatically decreased over the years due to changes in the recruiting and screening of blood donors, as well as to advances in the testing of donor blood. Current estimates for the risk of transfusion-related HIV range from 1:1,450,000 to 1:660,000 units transfused.[104] With more sensitive testing capabilities currently in use, that number is likely to decrease to 1:1,900,000 units transfused.[69,105] Immunocompromised patients and splenectomized patients are most susceptible to severe infections caused by parvovirus B19, malaria, babesiosis, and cytomegalovirus (CMV).[105]

An estimated 40% to 90% of the population has been exposed to the CMV, which is a herpes virus harbored in white blood cells. Following exposure, antibodies directed against CMV develop. Estimates suggest that up to 2% of all seropositive CMV donors are actively infected, and are able to transmit a potentially serious infection to an immunocompromised person. The use of CMV-negative blood products is the standard of care for CMV-negative patients who are either severely immunocompromised or are stem cell transplant recipients.[101,104,106] The demand for CMV-seronegative blood products may exceed the supply in geographical areas where CMV-seronegative blood is limited due to high rates of CMV-seropositive individuals in the donor pool. Studies have shown that leukocyte-depleted blood products can reduce the risk of CMV transmission.[70,104,107]

*Alloimmunization.* Alloimmunization unpredictably occurs in patients who have received blood products. Through transfusions, patients are exposed to antigens on donor red blood cells, white blood cells, platelets, or plasma proteins. When alloimmunization occurs, the patient develops antibodies to these specific antigens; however, there is no clinical manifestation of this until the patient receives a subsequent transfusion with a donor product containing an antigen to which the patient has developed an antibody. Under these conditions, systemic symptoms, including fever, jaundice, and a decreasing hemoglobin level, may occur.[102]

The cellular products in the transfused unit are quickly destroyed and cleared from the circulation and the patient fails to achieve a therapeutic increment of the transfused product. Antibodies to red blood cell antigens are usually detected through the typing and crossmatching process; however, antibodies to white blood cells, platelets, or plasma-protein antigens are not detected through this routine pre-transfusion testing. Saline washing of red blood cells can decrease the risk for an allergic reaction in a patient who has developed alloimmunization. Using leukocyte reduction filters when administering platelets to patients who will likely be receiving numerous platelet transfusions over the course of therapy (ie, acute leukemia patients and patients undergoing bone marrow or stem cell transplant) can minimize the risk for the development of platelet alloimmunization or platelet-specific antibodies.

*Iron overload.* When patients with cancer receive numerous red blood cell transfusions in the absence of blood loss, iron overload can result. As the transfused red cells reach the end of their natural life span, they die and release the intracellular iron. Due to decreased red cell production, this iron is not taken up and incorporated into newly forming red blood cells but rather accumulates. Iron overload can affect cardiac, hepatic, and endocrine functioning but is not likely to be problematic until 150 to 180 mL/kg have been transfused—approximately 50 to 60 units of packed red blood cells for a 70 kg patient.[104,105,108] Treatment for iron overload involves the administration of iron chelating agents such as desferoxamine or deferasirox.[104,105]

*Post-transfusion purpura.* Post-transfusion purpura is a rare immune complication that manifests 7 to 10 days after a transfusion in patients who have an antibody to an antigen present in the transfused product. As a result of this antigen–antibody interaction, both transfused and autologous platelets are destroyed and a severe and sudden onset thrombocytopenia develops. Although the condition is self-limiting, treatment in a bleeding patient requires the administration of intravenous immune globulin (IVIG).[101,102]

## CONCLUSION

Patients with cancer, particularly patients with hematological malignancies, are often treated with therapies that cause significant alterations in their blood counts. They may face alterations in their red blood cell counts, white blood cell counts, and platelet counts. Recombinant HGFs can help prevent negative outcomes related to low blood counts and although many of these agents have been available since the early 1990s, recent safety concerns, specifically related to EPO stimulating agents, have limited their clinical application. The future of their place in the management of patients with cancer has yet to be clarified. Work continues to determine expanded roles for other HGFs, such as the role of G-CSFs in vaccine therapy.

In light of the recent developments related to ESAs, blood component therapy is experiencing resurgence as a therapeutic and supportive care intervention in the management of patients with cancer and it remains the cornerstone of treatment for the bleeding patient. The safety of blood transfusions continues to be evaluated, with regard to both the transmission of infectious diseases and the achievement of a beneficial clinical outcome. Patients with cancer frequently experience hematological abnormalities as a function of their disease, its treatment and other comorbid contributing factors and the identification of safe and effective hematopoietic therapies is essential in fostering optimal clinical outcome and maximal quality of life.

## REFERENCES


1. Kurkjian CD, Ozer H. Leukopenia anemia and thrombocytopenia. In: DeVita VT, Hellman S, Rosenberg SA, eds. *Cancer: Principles and Practice of Oncology.* 8th ed. Philadelphia, PA: Lippincott Williams & Wilkins; 2008:2617–2633.
2. Kaushansky K. Hematopoietic stem cells, progenitors, and cytokines. In: Lichtman, MA, Beutler E, Kipps TJ, Seligsohn U, Kaushansky K, Prchal JT, eds. *Williams Hematology.* 7th ed. New York: McGraw-Hill; 2006:201–220.
3. Shaheen M, Broxmeyer HE. The humoral regulation of hematopoiesis. In: Hoffman R, Benz EJ Jr, Shattil SJ, Furie B, Silberstein LE, McGlave P, Heslop HE, eds. *Hematology: Basic Principles and Practice.* 5th ed. Linn, MO: Churchill Livingstone; 2008:253–275.
4. Fandrey J. Erythropoietin receptors on tumor cells: what do they mean? *Oncologist.* 2008;13(Suppl 3):16–20.
5. Roger GM, Becker PS, Bennett CC, et al. 2009 National Comprehensive Cancer Network, Inc NCCN Clinical Practice Guidelines in Oncology: Cancer and Chemotherapy-Induced Anemia V2.2010 http://www.nccn.org/professionals/physician_gls/pdf/anemia.pdf. Accessed January 17, 2010.
6. Crawford J, Ozer H, Stoller R, et al. Reduction by granulocyte colony-stimulating factor of fever and neutropenia induced by chemotherapy in patients with small-cell lung cancer. *N Eng J Med.* 1991;325:164–170.
7. Holmes FA, O'Shaughnessy JA, Vukelja S, et al. Blinded, randomized, multicenter study to evaluate single administration pegfilgrastim once per cycle versus daily filgrastim as an adjunct to chemotherapy in patients with high-risk stage II or stage III/IV breast cancer. *J Clin Oncol.* 2002;20:727–731.
8. Green MD, Koelbl H, Baselga J, et al. A randomized double-blind multicenter phase III study of fixed-dose single-administration pegfilgrastim versus daily filgrastim in patients receiving myelosuppressive chemotherapy. *Ann Oncol.* 2003;14:29–35.
9. Heil G, Hoelzer D, Sanz MA, et al. A randomized, double-blind, placebo-controlled, phase III study of filgrastim in remission induction and consolidation therapy for adults with de novo acute myeloid leukaemia. *Blood.* 1997;90:4710–4718.
10. Linch DC, Milligan DW, Winfield DA, et al. G-CSF after peripheral blood stem cell transplantation in lymphoma patients significantly accelerated neutrophil recovery and shortened time in hospital: results of a randomized BNLI trial. *Br J Haematol.* 1998;99:933–938.
11. McQuaker IG, Hunter AE, Pacey S, et al. Low-dose filgrastim significantly enhances neutrophil recovery following autologous peripheral-blood stem cell transplantation in patients with lymphoproliferative disorders: evidence for clinical and economic benefit. *J Clin Oncol.* 1997;15:451–457.
12. Armitage JO. Emerging applications of recombinant human granulocyte-macrophage colony-stimulating factor. *Blood.* 1998;92:4491–4508.
13. Nemunaitis J, Rabinowe S, Singer J, et al. Recombinant granulocyte-macrophage colony-stimulating factor after autologous bone marrow transplantation for lymphoid cancer. *N Engl J Med.* 1991;324:1773–1778.
14. Nemunaitis J, Rosenfeld CS, Ash R, et al. Phase III randomized, double-blind placebo-controlled trial of rhGM-CSF following allogeneic bone marrow transplantation. *Bone Marrow Transplant.* 1995;15:949–954.
15. Weich NS, Neben TY, Donaldson D, et al. Effects of interleukin 11 on megakaryocytes. *Blood.* 1996;88(Suppl 1):60a.
16. Chu DT, Xu BH, Song ST, et al. Recombinant human interleukin 11 (Mega) promotes thrombopoiesis in cancer patients with chemotherapy-induced myelosuppression. *Zhongguo Shi Yan Xue Ye Xue Za Zhi.* 2001;9:314–317.
17. Finch CA. Erythropoiesis, erythropoietin and iron. *Blood.* 1982;60:1241–1246.
18. Rowe JM. Growth factors. In: Furie B, Cassileth PA, Atkins MB, Mayer RJ, eds. *Clinical Hematology and Oncology: Presentation, Diagnosis, Treatment.* Philadelphia, PA: Churchill Livingstone; 2003:419–430.
19. Henry DH, Abels RI. Recombinant human erythropoietin in the treatment of cancer and chemotherapy-induced anemia: results of a double-blind and open-label follow-up studies. *Semin Oncol.* 1994;21(Suppl 3):21–28.
20. Glaspy J, Bukowski R, Steinberg D, Taylor C, Tchekmedyian S, Vadhan-Raj S. Impact of therapy with epoetin alfa on clinical outcomes in patients with nonmyeloid malignancies during cancer chemotherapy in community oncology practice. Procrit Study Group. *J Clin Oncol.* 1997;15:1218–1234.
21. Dunphy FR, Harrison BR, Dunleavy TL, et al. Erythropoietin reduces anemia and transfusions. A randomized trial with or without erythropoietin during chemotherapy. *Cancer.* 1999;86:1362–1367.
22. Demetri G, Kris M, Wade J, Degos L, Cella D. Quality of life benefit in chemotherapy patients treated with epoetin alfa is independent of disease response or tumor type: results from a prospective community oncology study: Procrit Study Group. *J Clin Oncol.* 1998;16:3412–3425.
23. Littlewood TJ, Bajetta E, Cella D. Efficacy and quality of life outcomes of epoetin alfa in a double-blind, placebo-controlled multicenter study of cancer patients receiving non-platinum containing chemotherapy. [Abstract 2217] *Proc Am Soc Clin Oncol.* 1999.
24. Crawford J, Cella D, Cleeland CS, et al. Relationship between changes in hemoglobin level and quality of life during chemotherapy in anemic cancer patients receiving epoetin alfa therapy. *Cancer.* 2002;95:888–895.
25. US Food and Drug Administration (USFDA) Information on Erythropoiesis-Stimulating Agents (ESAs) Epoietin alfa (marketed

as Procrit, Epogen) Darbepoetin alfa (marketed as Aranesp). http://www.fda.gov/Drugs/DrugSafety/PostmarketDrugSafetyInformationforPatientsandProviders/ucm109375.htm. Accessed January 17, 2010.
26. Bohlius J, Wilson J, Seidenfeld J, et al. Erythropoietin or darbepoetin for patients with cancer. *Cochrane Database Syst Rev.* 2006;(3): CD003407.
27. Henke M, Laszig R, Rube C, et al. Erythropoietin to treat head and neck cancer patients with anemia undergoing radiotherapy: randomised, double-blind, placebo-controlled trial. *Lancet.* 2003;362:1255–1260.
28. Leyland-Jones B, Semiglazov V, Pawlicki M, et al. Maintaining normal hemoglobin levels with epoetin alfa in mainly nonanemic patients with metastatic breast cancer receiving first-line chemotherapy: a survival study. *J Clin Oncol.* 2005;23:5960–5972.
29. Wright JR, Ung YC, Julian JA, et al. Randomized, double-blind, placebo-controlled trial of erythropoietin in non-small-cell lung cancer with disease-related anemia. *J Clin Oncol.* 2007;25:1027–1032.
30. Glaspy J, Smith R, Aapro M, et al. Results from a phase III, randomized, double-blind placebo-controlled study of darbepoetin alfa (DA) for the treatment of anemia in patients not receiving chemotherapy or radiotherapy. Presented at the 98th meeting of the American Association for Cancer Research. [Abstract LB-3] Los Angeles, CA, April 14–18, 2007.
31. Overgaard JU, Hoff C, Sand Hansen H, et al. Randomized study of the importance of novel erythropoiesis stimulating protein (Aranesp®) for the effect of radiotherapy inpatients with primary squamous cell carcinoma of the head and neck (HNSCC). The Danish Head and Neck Cancer Group (DAHANCA) 10 randomized study. Presented at the 14th European Cancer Conference. Barcelona, Spain, September 23–27, 2007.
32. Gascon P. Safety update on erythropoiesis-stimulating agents: trials within and outside the accepted indications. *Oncologist.* 2008; 13(Suppl 3):4–10.
33. Bohlius J, Schmidlin K, Brillant C, et al. Recombinant human erythropoiesis-stimulating agents and mortality in patients with cancer: a meta-analysis of randomised trials. *Lancet.* 2009;373:1532–1542.
34. Rizzo JD, Somerfield MR, Hagerty KL, et al. Use of epoetin and darbepoetin in patients with cancer: 2007 American Society of Clinical Oncology/American Society of Hematology clinical practice guideline update. *J Clin Oncol.* 2008;26:132–149.
35. Rizzo JD, Somerfield MR, Hagerty KL, et al. Use of epoetin and darbepoetin in patients with cancer: 2007 American Society of Hematology/American Society of Clinical Oncology clinical practice guideline update on the use of epoetin and darbepoetin. *Blood.* 2008;111:25–41.
36. Crawford J, Blackwell S. Hematopoietic growth factors. In: Perry MC, ed. *The Chemotherapy Source Book.* 4th ed. Philadelphia, PA: Lippincott Williams & Wilkins; 2008:44–52.
37. Meropol NJ, Miller LL, Korn EL, et al. Severe myelosuppression resulting from concurrent administration of granulocyte colony-stimulating factor and cytotoxic chemotherapy. *J Natl Cancer Inst.* 1992;84:1201–1203.
38. Rowinsky EK, Grochow LB, Sartorius SE, et al. Phase I and pharmacologic study of high doses of the topoisomerase I inhibitor topotecan with granulocyte colony-stimulating factor in patients with solid tumors. *J Clin Oncol.* 1996;14:1224–1235.
39. Larson RA, Dodge RK, Linker CA, et al. A randomized controlled trial of filgrastim during remission, induction and consolidation chemotherapy for adults with acute lymphoblastic leukemia: CALGB study 9111. *Blood.* 1998;92:1556–1564.
40. Dale DC, Bonilla MA, Davis MW, et al. A randomized controlled phase III trial of recombinant human granulocyte colony-stimulating factor (filgrastim) for treatment of severe chronic neutropenia. *Blood.* 1993;81:2496–2502.
41. Smith TJ, Khatcheressian J, Lyman GH, et al. 2006 Update of recommendations for the use of white blood cell growth factors: an evidence-based clinical practice guideline. *J Clin Oncol.* 2006;24:3187–3205.
42. Roger GM, Becker PS, Bennett CC, et al. 2009 National Comprehensive Cancer Network, Inc. NCCN Clinical Practice Guidelines in Oncology: Myeloid Growth Factors V1.2009 http://www.nccn.org/professionals/physician_gls/PDF/myeloid_growth.pdf. Accessed January 17, 2010.
43. Mellstedt H, Fagerberg J, Frodin J-E, et al. Augmentation of the immune system with granulocyte-macrophage colony-stimulating factor and other hematopoietic growth factors. *Curr Opin Hematol.* 1999;6:169–175.
44. Sakamoto C, Suzuki K, Hato F, et al. Antiapoptotic effect of granulocyte colony-stimulating factor, granulocyte-macrophage colony-stimulating factor, and cyclic AMP on human neutrophils: protein synthesis-dependent and protein synthesis-independent mechanisms and the role of the Janus kinase-STAT pathway. *Int J Hematol* 2003;77:60–70.
45. Rowe JM, Rubin A, Mazza JJ, et al. Incidence of infections in adult patients (>55 years) with acute myeloid leukemia treated with yeast-derived GM-CSF (sargramostim): results of a double-blind prospective study by the Eastern Cooperative Oncology Group. In: Hiddermann W, Buchner T, Wormann B, et al., eds. *Acute Leukemias V: Experimental Approaches and Management of Refractory Diseases.* Berlin, Germany: Springer-Verlag; 1996:178–184.
46. Rowe JM, Andersen JW, Mazza JJ, et al. A randomized placebo-controlled phase III study of granulocyte-macrophage colony-stimulating factor in adult patients (>55 to 70 years of age) with acute myelogenous leukemia: a study of the Eastern Cooperative Oncology Group (E1490). *Blood.* 1995;86:457–462.
47. Greenberg P, Advani R, Keating A, et al. GM-CSF accelerates neutrophil recovery after autologous hematopoietic stem cell transplantation. *Bone Marrow Transplant.* 1996;18:1057–1064.
48. Spitzer G, Adkins D, Mathews M, et al. Randomized comparison of G-CSF + GM-CSF vs G-CSF alone for mobilization of peripheral blood stem cells: effects on hematopoietic recovery after high-dose chemotherapy. *Bone Marrow Transplant.* 1997;20:921–930.
49. Blinder VS, Roboz GJ. Hematopoietic growth factors in myelodysplastic syndromes. *Curr Hematol Rep.* 2003;2:453–458.
50. GVAX cancer vaccine fails in phase III study, RxTrials Institute Drug Pipeline Alert. *FDA News (newsletter).* 2008 Sep 2;6(3).
51. Kent D, Copley M, Benz C, Dykstra B, Bowie M, Eaves C. Regulation of hematopoietic stem cells by the steel factor/KIT signalling pathway. *Clin Cancer Res.* 2008;14:1926–1930.
52. Heinrich MC, Blanke CD, Druker BJ, et al. Inhibition of KIT tyrosine kinase activity: a novel molecular approach to the treatment of KIT-positive malignancies. *J Clin Oncol.* 2002;20:1692–1703.
53. Berstein SH, Kufe DW. Future of basic/clinical hematopoiesis research in the era of hematopoietic growth factor availability. *Semin Oncol.* 1992;19:441–448.
54. Wadhwa PD, Lazarus HM, Koc ON, et al. Hematopoietic recovery after unrelated-umbilical cord blood allogeneic transplantation in adults treated with in vivo stem cell factor (r-metHuSCF) and filgrastim administration. *Leuk Res.* 2003;27:215–220.
55. Prosper F, Sola C, Hornedo J, et al. Mobilization of peripheral blood progenitor cells with a combination of cyclophosphamide, r-metHuSCF and filgrastim in patients with breast cancer previously treated with chemotherapy. *Leukemia.* 2003;17:437–441.
56. Korper S, Hutter G, Blau O, Schrexenmeier H, Knauf W, Thiel E. Successful treatment of partial graft failure after matched unrelated donor stem cell transplantation by a combination of ancestim (stem cell factor) and granulocyte colony stimulating factor in a patient with heavily pre-treated chronic lymphocytic leukaemia. *Leuk Lymphoma.* 2008;49:2015–2017.
57. Mijovic A, Russell N, Clark RE, et al. Ancestim associated with filgrastim and/or chemotherapy can improve blood progenitor yields in patients who previously failed mobilisation. *Bone Marrow Transplant.* 2005;35:1019.
58. daSilva MG, Pimentel P, Carvalhais A, et al. Ancestim (recombinant human stem cell factor, SCF) in association with filgrastim does not enhance chemotherapy and/or growth factor-induced peripheral blood progenitor (PBPC) mobilization in patients with a prior insufficient PBPC collection. *Bone Marrow Transplant.* 2004;34:683–691.

59. To LB, Bashford J, Durrant S, et al. Successful mobilization of peripheral blood stem cells after addition of ancestim (stem cell factor) in patients who had failed a prior mobilization with filgrastim (granulocyte colony-stimulating factor) alone or with chemotherapy plus filgrastim. *Bone Marrow Transplant.* 2003;31:371–378.
60. Grundler R, Thiede C, Miething C, et al. Sensitivity towards tyrosine kinase inhibitors varies between different activating mutations of the FLT3 receptor. *Blood.* 2003;102:646–651.
61. Yoshikazu S, Shimazaki C, Ashihara E, et al. Synergistic effect of Flt-3 ligand on the granulocyte colony-stimulating factor-induced mobilization of hematopoietic stem cells and progenitor cells into blood in mice. *Blood.* 1997;89:3186–3191.
62. Lyman SD, Jacobsen SEW. C-KIT ligand and Flt-3 ligand: stem/progenitor cell factors with overlapping yet distinct activities. *Blood.* 1997;91:1101–1134.
63. Isaacs C, Robert NJ, Bailey FA, et al. Randomized placebo controlled study of recombinant human interleukin 11 to prevent chemotherapy-induced thrombocytopenia in patients with breast cancer receiving dose-intensive cyclophosphamide and doxorubicin. *J Clin Oncol.* 1997;15:3369–3375.
64. Tepler I, Elias L, Smith JW II, et al. A randomized placebo-controlled trial of recombinant interleukin 11 in cancer patients with severe thrombocytopenia due to chemotherapy. *Blood.* 1996;87:3607–3621.
65. Vredenburgh JJ, Hussein A, Fisher D, et al. A randomized trial of recombinant human interleukin 11 following autologous bone marrow transplantation with peripheral blood progenitor cell support in patients with breast cancer. *Biol Blood Marrow Transplant.* 1998;4:134–140.
66. Kuter DJ, Bussel JB, Lyons RM, et al. Efficacy of Romiplostim in patients with chronic immune thrombocytopenic purpura: a double-blind randomised controlled trial. *Lancet.* 2008;371:395–403.
67. Bussel J, Provan D, Shamsi T, et al. Effect of eltrombopag on platelet counts and bleeding during treatment of chronic idiopathic thrombocytopenic purpura: a randomised, double-blind, placebo-controlled trial. *Lancet.* 2009;373:641–648.
68. Goodnough LT. Risks of blood transfusion. *Anesthesiol Clin North America.* 2005;23:241–252.
69. Alter HJ, Klein HG. The hazards of blood transfusion in historical perspective. *Blood.* 2008;112:2617–2626.
70. Buddeberg F, Schimmer BB, Spahn DR. Transfusion-transmissible infections and transfusion-related immunomodulation. *Best Pract Res Clin Anaesthesiol.* 2008;22:503–517.
71. Madjdpour C, Spahn DR. Allogeneic red blood cell transfusion: physiology of oxygen transport. *Best Pract Res Clin Anaesthesiol.* 2007;21:163–171.
72. Almac E, Ince C. The impact of storage on red cell function in blood transfusion. *Best Pract Res Clin Anaesthesiol.* 2007;21:195–208.
73. Vincent JL, Sakr Y, De Backer D, Van der Linden P. Efficacy of allogeneic red blood cell transfusions. *Best Pract Res Clin Anaesthesiol.* 2007;21:209–219.
74. Khorana AA, Francis CW, Blumberg N, Culakova E, Refaai MA, Lyman GH. Blood transfusions, thrombosis, and mortality in hospitalized patients with cancer. *Arch Intern Med.* 2008;168:2377–2381.
75. Vamvakas EC, Blajchman MA. Transfusion-related mortality: the ongoing risks of allogeneic blood transfusion and the available strategies for their prevention. *Blood.* 2009;113:3406–3417.
76. Bennett-Guerrero E, Veldman TH, Doctor A, et al. Evolution of adverse changes in stored red blood cells. *Proc Natl Acad Sci U S A.* 2007;104:17063–17068.
77. Gonzalez AM, Yazici I, Kusza K, Siemionow M. Effects of fresh versus banked blood transfusions on microcirculatory hemodynamics and tissue oxygenation in the rat cremaster model. *Surgery.* 2007;141:630–639.
78. Atzil S, Arad M, Glasner A, et al. Blood transfusion promotes cancer progression: a critical role for aged erythrocytes. *Anesthesiology.* 2008;109:989–997.
79. Upile T, Jerjes W, Sandison A, et al. The direct effects of stored blood products may worsen prognosis of cancer patients: shall we transfuse or not? An explanation of the adverse oncological consequences of blood product transfusion with a testable hypothesis driven experimental research protocol. *Medical Hypothesis.* 2008;71:489–492.
80. Kanter J, Khan SY, Kelher M, Gore L, Silliman CC. Oncogenic and angiogenic growth factors accumulate during routine storage of apheresis platelet concentrates. *Clin Cancer Res.* 2008;14:3942–3947.
81. Dineen SP, Roland CL, Toombs JE, et al. The acellular fraction of stored platelets promotes tumor cell invasion. *J Surg Res.* 2009;153:132–137.
82. Blajchman MA. Landmark studies that have changed the practice of transfusion medicine. *Transfusion.* 2005;45:1523–1530.
83. Schwartz RN. Anemia in patients with cancer: incidence, causes, impact, management and use of treatment guidelines and protocols. *Am J Health Syst Pharm.* 2007;64(Suppl 2):s5–s13.
84. Ludwig H, Van Belle S, Barrett-Lee P, et al. The European Cancer Anaemia Survey (ECAS): a large, multinational, prospective survey defining the prevalence, incidence, and treatment of anaemia in cancer patients. *Eur J Cancer.* 2004;40:2293–2306.
85. Firestone DT, Pitocco C. Component therapy. In: Rudmann, ed. *Textbook of Bloodbanking and Transfusion Medicine.* 2nd ed. Philadelphia, PA: Elsevier Saunders; 2005:370–395.
86. King KE, Ness PM. Red cell transfusions in patients with hematologic malignancies. In: Wiernik PH, Goldman JM, Dutcher JP, Kyle RA, eds. *Neoplastic Diseases of the Blood.* 4th ed. Port Melbourne, Australia; Cambridge University Press: 2003:1017–1027.
87. Fischbach, F. Blood studies; hematology and coagulation. In *A Manual of Laboratory and Diagnostic Tests*, 7th ed. Philadelphia, PA: Lippincott Williams & Wilkins; 2004:38–162.
88. Vallet B, Adamczyk S, Barreau O, Lebuffe, G. Physiologic transfusion triggers. *Best Pract Res Clin Anaesthesiol.* 2007;21:173–181.
89. Goodnough LT. Transfusion triggers. *Surgery.* 2007;142:s67–s70.
90. Nordstrom BL, Fraeman KH, Luo W, et al. Red blood cell transfusions among cancer patients on chemotherapy: a descriptive epidemiologic study. *J Clin Oncol.* 26;(suppl):abstract 20623. 2008.
91. Klein HG, Anstee DJ, eds. *Mollison's Blood Transfusion in Clinical Medicine.* 11th ed. Malden, MA: Blackwell Publishing; 2005.
92. Rebulla P, Finazzi G, Marangoni F, et al. The threshold for prophylactic platelet transfusions in adults with acute myeloid leukemia. Gruppo Italiano Malattie Ematologiche Maligne dell'Adulto. *N Engl J Med.* 1997;337:1870–1882.
93. Navarro JT, Hernandez JA, Ribera JM, et al. Prophylactic platelet transfusion threshold during therapy for adult acute myeloid leukemia: 10,000/microL. versus 20,000/microL. *Haematologica.* 1998;83:998–1005.
94. Wandt H, Frank M, Ehninger G, et al. Safety and cost effectiveness of a $10 \times 10^9$/L trigger for prophylactic platelet transfusions compared with the traditional $20 \times 10^9$/L trigger: a prospective comparative trial in 105 patients with acute myeloid leukemia. *Blood.* 1998;91:3601.
95. Wandt H, Wendelin K, Schaefer-Eckart K, et al. A therapeutic platelet transfusion strategy without routine prophylactic transfusion is feasible and safe and reduces platelet transfusion numbers significantly: preliminary analysis of a randomized study in patients after high dose chemotherapy and autologous peripheral blood stem cell transplant. *Blood.* (ASH Annual Meeting Abstract). 2008;112:286.
96. *Practice Guidelines for Blood Transfusion: A Compilation from Recent Peer-Reviewed Literature.* 2nd ed. American Red Cross; 2007.
97. Gobel BH. Bleeding. In: Yarbro CH, Frogge MH, Goodman M, eds. *Cancer Nursing Principles and Practice.* 6th ed. Sudbury, MA: Jones and Bartlett; 2005:723–740.
98. Sloan SR, Silberstein LE. Transfusion medicine. In: Furie B, Cassileth PA, Atkins MB, Mayer RJ, eds. *Clinical Hematology and Oncology: Presentation, Diagnosis, and Treatment.* Philadelphia, PA: Churchill Livingstone; 2003:431–440.
99. The Trial to Reduce Alloimmunization to Platelets Study Group: leukocyte reduction and ultraviolet B irradiation of platelets to prevent alloimmunization and refractoriness to platelet transfusions. *N Engl J Med.* 1997;337:1861–1869.

100. Sacher RA, Kickler TS, Schiffer CA, et al. Management of patients refractory to platelet transfusion. *Arch Pathol Lab Med.* 2003;127: 409–414.
101. Firestone DT, Pitocco C. Adverse effects of blood transfusion. In: Rudmann, ed. *Textbook of Bloodbanking and Transfusion Medicine.* 2nd ed. Philadelphia, PA: Elsevier Saunders; 2005:396–418.
102. Brecher ME. Technical manual. In: *Noninfectious Complications of Blood transfusion.* 14th ed. Bethesda, MD; American Association of Blood Banks. 2002:585–612.
103. Brecher ME and , Hay SN. Bacterial contamination of blood components. *Clin Microbiol Rev.* 2005;18(1):195–204.
104. Brecher ME. Technical manual. In: *Transfusion-Transmitted Diseases.* 14th ed. Bethesda, MD: American Association of Blood Banks; 2002:613–651.
105. Dodd R. Germs, gels, and genomes: a personal recollection of 30 years in blood safety testing. In: Stramer S, ed. *Blood Safety in the New Millennium.* Bethesda, MD: American Association of Blood Banks; 2000:97–122.
106. Saavedra S, Sanz GF, Jarque I, et al. Early infections in adult patients undergoing unrelated donor cord blood transplantation. *Bone Marrow Transplant.* 2002;30:937–943.
107. Fung MK, Rao N, Rice J, et al. Leukoreduction in the setting of open heart surgery: a prospective cohort-controlled study. *Transfusion.* 2004A;44:30–35.
108. Sheth S. Transfusional iron overload. In: Simon SL, Snyder EL, Solheim BG, Stowell CP, Strauss RG, & Petrides M. eds. *Rossi's Principles of Transfusion Medicine.* 4th ed. Hoboken, NJ: Blackwell Publishing; 2009,858–869.

CHAPTER 24

Georgia Decker, APRN, ANP-BC, CN®, AOCN®, Colleen O. Lee, MS, CRNP, AOCN®, CLNC

# Complementary and Alternative Medicine (CAM) Therapies in Integrative Oncology

## INTRODUCTION

### DEFINITIONS

Professionals across multiple practice settings, including clinical practice, education, and research, contribute to the field of complementary and alternative medicine (CAM). CAM is often termed "integrative," "integrated," or "complementary" when these therapies are combined with conventional approaches and referred to as "alternative" or "unconventional" when the therapy is used instead of conventional approaches. It is the intention with which the therapy is used that often defines it. Table 24-1 provides several definitions of CAM found in the literature.[1–3] Conventional approaches, known as "standard" or "traditional" or "biomedical" approaches, are those that historically have broad application in Western medicine. To assist nurses in understanding CAM in cancer care, the Oncology Nursing Society (ONS) Position Statement entitled "The Use of Complementary and Alternative Therapies in Cancer Care" promotes standardizing terminology to enhance communication.[4] Throughout this chapter, the acronym CAM is used to refer to the broad range of complementary and alternative therapies, and the term "conventional biomedical" is used to refer to the traditional or standard approaches.

Two main approaches in categorizing CAM therapies exist. The National Center for Complementary and Alternative Medicine (NCCAM) classifies CAM therapies into five domains: (1) alternative medical systems, (2) mind–body interventions, (3) biologically based therapies, (4) manipulative and body-based methods, and (5) energy therapies.[2] The National Cancer Institute (NCI) Office of Cancer Complementary and Alternative Medicine (OCCAM)[5] expanded the NCCAM domains with 4 additional categories for clarification: nutritional therapeutics, pharmacological and biological treatments, complex natural products, and spiritual therapies.[6] *Alternative medical systems* are built upon complete systems of theory and practice. *Mind–body medicine* uses a variety of techniques designed to enhance the mind's capacity to affect bodily function and symptoms. *Biologically based therapies* in CAM use substances found in nature, such as herbs, foods, and vitamins. *Manipulative and body-based methods* in CAM are based on manipulation and/or movement of one or more parts of the body. *Energy therapies* involve the use of energy fields and are of two types: biofield therapies and bioelectromagnetic-based therapies. *Pharmacological and biological therapies* are drugs, vaccines, off-label use of prescription drugs, and other biological interventions not yet accepted in mainstream medicine. *Complex natural products* consist of crude natural substances and unfractionated extracts from marine organisms used for healing and treatment of disease. *Spiritual therapies* are interventions geared toward a connection with or source of ultimate meaning. Table 24-2 provides contemporary modalities with examples.[6]

### HISTORICAL PERSPECTIVE

Therapeutic interventions relying on natural healing (19th-century term), drugless healing (early 20th-century term), or holistic healing (1970s to present term) are not new or original in the United States as the history of complementary and/or alternative medicine dates back to the 1700s. An awareness of the historical development of CAM as a distinctive field is essential for understanding the philosophical viewpoints between and among practice disciplines.[7]

#### Ancient traditions to the 20th century

In ancient traditions, healing methods were passed on in the form of hymns, prayers, incantations, and ritual formulas containing information on how to use plants for bodily healing. The stories that formed the foundation for Ayurveda and traditional Chinese medicine remained oral for centuries before being written around 1200 BC

**TABLE 24-1**

**Definitions of Complementary and Alternative Medicine**

| Source | Definition |
|---|---|
| Ernst[1] | CAM is any approach to improve a health problem that is not used or taught routinely to conventional Western practitioners. Alternative cancer treatments are CAM therapies that reduce tumor burden or replace mainstream therapy. |
| NCCAM[2] | CAM is a group of diverse medical and healthcare systems, practices, and products that are not currently considered a part of conventional medicine. Complementary medicine is used with conventional medicine. Alternative medicine is in place of conventional medicine. Integrative medicine combines mainstream and CAM therapies for which scientific evidence of safety and efficacy exists. |
| Society for Integrative Oncology[3] | Alternative therapies are endorsed as viable options instead of conventional medicine, may be costly, not biologically active, potentially invasive, and unproven. Complementary medicine uses nonconventional therapies (that may have known efficacy) in conjunction with conventional medicine. |

**TABLE 24-2**

**Complementary and Alternative Medicine (CAM) Modalities in Clinical Trials**

| Domain | Definition | Example(s) | Modalities Studied in Clinical Trials |
|---|---|---|---|
| Alternative Medical Systems | Systems built upon well-developed systems of theory and practice | Traditional Chinese Medicine (acupuncture), Ayurveda, Homeopathy, Naturopathy, Tibetan Medicine | Traditional Chinese Medicine (acupuncture), acupressure, Homeopathy (Traumeel S®, Heel Company, Baden-Baden, Germany) |
| Energy Therapies | Therapies involving the use of energy fields | QiGong, Reiki, Therapeutic Touch, pulsed fields, magnet therapy | QiGong, Reiki, therapeutic touch |
| Exercise Therapies | Modalities used to improve patterns of bodily movement | T'ai Chi, Feldenkrais, Hatha yoga, Alexander Technique, dance therapy, Rolfing, Trager Method, applied kinesiology | T'ai Chi, Hatha yoga |
| Manipulative and Body-based Methods | Methods based on manipulation and/or movement of the one or more parts of the body | Chiropractic, therapeutic massage, osteopathy, reflexology | Therapeutic massage, reflexology |
| Mind-Body Interventions | Techniques designed to enhance the mind's capacity to affect bodily function and symptoms | Medication, hypnosis, art therapy, biofeedback, mental healing, imagery, relaxation therapy, support groups, music therapy, cognitive-behavioral therapy, psychoneuroimmunology, aromatherapy, animal-assisted therapy | Medication, art therapy, imagery, relaxation therapy, music therapy, cognitive-behavioral therapy, aromatherapy, animal-assisted therapy, narrative medicine |
| Nutritional Therapeutics | Assortment of nutrients, non-nutrients, and bioactive food components that are used as chemopreventative agents, and the use of specific foods or diets as cancer prevention or treatment strategies | Dietary regimens such as macrobiotics, vegetarian, Gerson therapy, Kelley/Gonzalez regimen, vitamins, dietary macronutrients, supplements, antioxidants, melatonin, selenium, coenzyme Q10, ephedrine, orthomolecular medicine | Selenium, curcumin, soy isoflavones, genistein, lycopene, omega-3 fatty acids, L-cartinine, alpha-lipoic acid, glutamine, coenzyme Q10, boswellia serrata, zinc, Gonzalez regimen |
| Pharmacological and Biological Treatments | Drugs, complex natural products, vaccines, and other biological interventions not yet accepted in mainstream medicine, off-label use of prescription drugs | Antineoplastons, products from honey bees, mistletoe, 714-X, low dose naltrexone, met-enkephalin, immunoaugmentative therapy, laetrile, hydrazine sulfate, New Castle Virus, melatonin, ozone therapy, thymus therapy, enzyme therapy, high dose vitamin C | Antineoplastons, ascorbic acid |
| Complex Natural Products | Subcategory of pharmacological and biological treatments consisting of an assortment of plant samples (botanicals), extracts of crude natural substances, and un-fractionate extracts from marine organisms used for healing and treatment of disease | Herbs and herbal extracts, mixtures of tea polyphenols, shark cartilage, Essiac tea, cordyceps, Sun Soup, MGN-3 | Green tea extract, Essiac tea, mistletoe, valerian, noni fruit extract, licorice root |
| Spiritual Therapies | Interventions geared toward connection with or source of ultimate meaning | Intercessory prayer, spiritual healing | Prayer |

*Source*: Adapted with permission from Lee, CO. Clinical trials in cancer Part 1: biomedical, complementary, and alternative medicine: Finding active trials and results of closed trials. *Clin J Oncol Nurs.* 2004; 531–535.[61]

into the first known texts. Important roots of what is now considered modern medicine had developed by 500–400 BC in Greece.[8] Hippocrates (460–370 BC) and later Galen of Pergamum (AD 130–200) emphasized the science of medicine and utilized animal studies to understand human disease. Improvements in medicine emerged by the Middle Ages (AD 1100–1200). Through the understanding of blood circulation, the invention of the microscope , and the humoral components of host defense, advances in medicine unfolded in the United States.[8]

Unconventional methods of disease treatment with the intent to cure prior to the 19th century were considered folk medicine or quackery. The first generation of alternative medicine in the 20th century developed from the theory and therapeutic regimens practiced in Thomsonianism, Homeopathy, Hydropathy, Mesmerism, and Eclecticism.[9] The word "allopathic," now a standard term for conventional medicine was coined by Hahnemann who founded the system of Homeopathy that became popular in the United States in the 1830s. The second generation of developing systems took place in the late 20th century, and capturing about 20% of all medical practice were the fields of Osteopathy, Chiropractic, Naturopathy, and Hydropathy. During this time, contemporary holism emerged, focusing on treating the "whole" patient and promoting the self-care philosophy, leading to the current trend of lifestyle regulation and wellness promotion. Nursing curricula designed to distinguish between analyzing patient needs and problems from a medical diagnosis began in the 1950s in the United States.[10]

## CAM UTILIZATION

Consumers continued to seek CAM despite public education, legislative action, and medical advances in the mid-1970s to 1980s. To address the mounting and significant issues, the Office of Alternative Medicine (OAM) was established in 1992, and became the NCCAM in 1998. The National Center for Complementary and Alternative Medicine(NCCAM) is one of the 27 institutes and centers that make up the National Institutes of Health (NIH), which is one of 8 agencies under the Public Health Service in the US Department of Health and Human Services. National Center for Complementary and Alternative Medicine has 4 primary focus areas: research (clinical and basic science research), training and career development (predoctoral, postdoctoral, and career researchers), outreach (conferences, educational programs and exhibits, information clearinghouse), and integration (incorporating scientifically proven CAM practices into conventional medicine).[2]

### Cancer CAM

To increase the amount of high-quality cancer research and information about CAM use, the NCI established the OCCAM in 1998. The OCCAM promotes and supports research within CAM disciplines and therapies as they relate to the prevention, diagnosis, and treatment of cancer, cancer-related symptoms, and side effects of conventional treatment. The OCCAM coordinates NCI's CAM research and informational activities and NCI's collaboration with other governmental and nongovernmental organizations on cancer CAM issues, and also provides an interface with health practitioners and researchers regarding cancer CAM issues.[5,11]

The White House Commission on Complementary and Alternative Medicine Policy (WHCCAMP) was established in March 2000 to address issues of access to and delivery of CAM, priorities for research, and the need to educate consumers and healthcare professionals (HCPs). The White House Commission on Complementary and Alternative Medicine Policy endorsed 10 principles, listed in Table 24-3.[12] A nongovernment agency established in 1970, the Institute of Medicine (IOM) of the National Academies, guarantees unbiased, evidence-based information and advice concerning health and science policy to policy-makers, HCPs, and the public. In 2003–2004, the IOM sponsored meetings to explore scientific, policy, and practice questions that arise from the increasing use of CAM by the American public. The final report of the IOM committee was released in January 2005.[13]

### Consumer issues

Issues relevant to understanding the use of CAM in the United States are as follows: the reasons for using CAM (motive), the frequency with which use occurs (prevalence), and the people who use it (patient characteristics).[14] Among the reasons for the revival of CAM in the 21st century in the United States are philosophical similarities (emphasis on holism, active patient role, natural treatments, spiritual dimension), personal control over treatment, positive relationship with therapist (time for discussion, including emotional aspects), accessibility, and increased well-being.[15] Factors that may contribute to the decreased use of conventional biomedical medicine in favor of CAM are dissatisfaction (ineffective therapies, adverse effects, poor communication with HCPs, insufficient time with HCPs, waiting lists), rejection (anti-science viewpoint), desperation, and cost of care. It is possible that the persuasive appeal of CAM is related to a perceived association of CAM with nature, a focus on energy forces promoting vitalism, intellectual traditions and sophisticated philosophies, extensive training involving complex systems and concepts, and a likely union of the physical (medical) and spiritual (truth, values, morals) realms.[14,16] Ultimately in the 21st century, patients have expressed a desire to take control of their own health, actively participate in decisions related to health and wellness, and choose treatment plans involving solely

**TABLE 24-3**

**Guiding Principles Endorsed by the White House Commisison on CAM**

- A wholeness orientation in healthcare delivery: delivery of high-quality healthcare must support care of the whole person
- Evidence of safety and efficacy: use science to generate evidence that protects and promotes public health
- Healing capacity of a person: support capacity for recovery and self-healing
- Respect for individuality: each person has the right to health care that is responsive, respects preferences, and preserves dignity
- Right to choose treatment: each person has the right to choose freely among safe and effective approaches and among qualified practitioners
- Emphasis on health promotion and self-care: good health care emphasizes self-care and early interventions for maintaining and promoting health
- Partnerships in integrated health care: good health care requires teamwork among patients, HCPs, and researchers committed to creating healing environments and respecting diversity of healthcare traditions
- Education as a fundamental healthcare service: education about prevention, healthy lifestyles, and self-healing should be part of the curriculum of all HCPs and made available to the public
- Dissemination of comprehensive, timely information: healthcare quality is enhanced by examination of the evidence on which CAM systems, practices, and products are based; this information should be widely, rapidly, and easily available
- Integral public involvement: input from informed consumers must be incorporated in proposing priorities for healthcare, research, and policy decisions

*Source*: Data from White House Commission on Complementary and Alternative Medicine Policy.[12]

conventional biomedical medicine alone, CAM alone, or a combination of both.

The first US national survey of the prevalence, cost of use, and pattern of use of CAM was published in 1993, at which time one in three respondents had used at least one "unconventional" therapy within the past year, and one-third of these respondents had sought providers for "unconventional" therapy.[17] In the early to mid-1990s, CAM surveys were not disease specific. Trends over the past decade show a gradual increase in the prevalence of CAM use among patients in the United States.[18–21] Toward the end of the 1990s, more was known about CAM use among cancer patients, rural populations, and elderly patients, and similar trends in use were seen.[22–28] Studies conducted since 2000 (sample size $N \geq 100$) show CAM use in adults with cancer as being between 25% and 80%.[29–32]

Consumers of CAM therapies are interested in choosing their providers, integrating CAM therapies into conventional care, limiting out-of-pocket expenses, and expanding insurance coverage. The amount patients are willing to pay for CAM may indicate the value they place on these therapies.[33] Given the financial investment in CAM therapies, an enduring question is whether CAM therapies can provide the beneficial health outcomes to justify the expense.[34]

## CAM REGULATION

### FDA: REGULATION OF DIETARY SUPPLEMENTS AND DEVICES

#### Dietary supplements

Confidence in the contents of a single, active molecule of a substance, such as an herb, began to emerge in the late 19th century as a result of the need to have medicines tested, standardized, and patented. Two laws, the Biologic Control Act (1902) and the Food and Drug Act (1906), formed the foundation of the present day Food and Drug Administration (FDA).[35] After multiple fatalities involving an elixir, the federal Food, Drug, and Cosmetic Act of 1938 was passed, requiring that new drugs provide evidence of safety before being placed on the market. Following another fatality in 1962, legislation was passed requiring that drug manufacturers provide evidence of efficacy before marketing a drug. The FDA governs all aspects of the development and manufacturing of drug products, product characterization, safety, efficacy, claims, and postmarket surveillance.

Prior to 1994, herbal products were not regulated; rather, they were marketed either as foods or as drugs, depending on their intended use and claims. Under the Dietary Supplement Health and Education Act (DSHEA) of 1994, a dietary supplement is now defined as a product intended to supplement the diet. A supplement may be a vitamin, mineral, herb, botanical, amino acid, or a combination of these ingredients, and may be in the form of a concentrate, metabolite, constituent, extract, a supplement to increase total daily intake, or combinations of these ingredients.[36] The product must be intended for ingestion in pill, capsule, tablet, or liquid form, must not be a conventional food or the sole item of a meal or diet, and must be labeled as a "dietary supplement." The DSHEA provides for the use of various statements on a product label that do not need preapproval, although claims must not be made about the diagnosis, prevention, treatment, or cure of a specific disease. For example, a claim for an herb cannot read, "This product will cure cancer, heart disease, and obesity." Like foods, dietary supplements must bear ingredient labeling (including the name and quantity of each ingredient) and nutrition labeling (daily consumption recommendations). Botanical and herbal products must state the part of the plant from which the ingredient originated. The DHSEA grants the FDA the authority to develop good manufacturing practices governing the preparation, packing, and holding of products. The act also created the NIH Office of Dietary Supplements to promote, collect, and compile research and maintain a database on supplements and individual nutrients. From a consumer standpoint, the DHSEA provides for over-the-counter, ready access to a wide range of products without the requirement of standardization.

### Devices

CAM providers in the United States are becoming more cognizant of the federal government's requirement for approval of any medical devices used in the treatment of patients. The FDA's legal authority to regulate both medical devices and electronic radiation-emitting products is the Federal Food, Drug, and Cosmetic Act. The FDA regulates the companies who manufacture, package, label, import, and/or sell medical devices such as lasers, x-ray systems, and ultrasound equipment. Examples of CAM devices that are currently under regulatory authority of the FDA are acupuncture needles and acupressure bands.

## PRACTICE GUIDELINES AND POSITION STATEMENTS

Presently, the WHHCAMP guiding principles and IOM model guidelines are the only widely recognized, general framework on a national level. The Society for Integrative Oncology published practice guidelines following the assembly of a panel of experts in oncology and integrative medicine.[4] The panel evaluated the current level of evidence regarding complementary therapies most commonly used by oncology patients. Although these documents provide an excellent structure for a societal, academic, and healthcare approach to CAM use, they lack detailed recommendations for nursing. The American Holistic Nurses Association and the Oncology Nursing Society (ONS) have well-developed position statements that provide guidance and competency expectations for nurses. They are: "Position on the Role of Nurses in the Practice of Complementary and Alternative Therapies" (American Holistic Nurses Association, 2007)[37] and "The Use of Complementary, Alternative, and Integrative Therapies in Cancer Care" (Oncology Nursing Society, 2009).[4] Several individual state boards of nursing have addressed the use of CAM and offered guidance to nurses such as the Maryland Board of Nursing and the California Board of Nursing (http://www.mbon.org; http://www.rn.ca.gov). CAM associations, schools, and domain-focused CAM centers have varying levels of guidelines and competency expectations.

## LICENSURE, CERTIFICATION, AND CREDENTIALING

Legal experts confirm that the doctrines that typically apply in healthcare law are applicable to the practice and integration of CAM as well as informed consent and malpractice.[39] Professional practice requirements, on the other hand, vary by the CAM modality. For example, acupuncture training that would lead to certification and licensure may take several years, while certification in therapeutic touch may only take several months. Professional licensure is governed at the state level by state law, which leaves states able to regulate the health, safety, and welfare of citizens via a medical licensing statute. This statue prohibits the unlicensed practice of medicine, which protects the public. In most states, CAM providers who lack licensure may potentially be viewed as diagnosing and perhaps treating individuals and as "practicing medicine without a license." To provide a frame of reference, osteopaths and chiropractors are licensed in all states, but naturopaths only require licensure in 15 states. Training, internship/residency, and other educational requirements also vary by state. Table 24-4 provides an overview of the licensure, certification, and training requirements for many practitioners.

## THIRD PARTY AND MEDICARE COVERAGE

Medicare and other insurers are beginning to consider CAM as a "reimbursable" expense, utilizing established billing codes for those patients who choose to use these modalities for supportive care and/or treatment. The number and scope of Current Procedural Terminology (CPT) codes for the billing of CAM services has increased in recent years. CAM services that do not have CPT codes are not considered "covered." CAM-specific codes were proposed to document services provided by CAM providers in an effort to establish a more accurate billing profile. Initially, this coding system received attention but was ultimately rejected by the Centers for Medicare and Medicaid Services.[40] The lack of reimbursement creates a challenge for conventional providers who seek to offer integrative healthcare. Current regulations require HCPs to inform patients when potential services are not "covered" and document patient awareness of these outstanding costs.[41]

# EVIDENCE-BASED PRACTICE

## THE ROLE OF EVIDENCE IN CLINICAL PRACTICE

The classification system used by the NCI Physician Data Query (PDQ) Adult Treatment Editorial Board has been adopted for use in human studies involving CAM treatments. Levels of evidence and evidence-based practice in

**TABLE 24-4**

**Licensure, Certification, and Educational Preparation for Common CAM Practitioners**

| Modality | Definition | Acronym | Licensing/Certification Body | Educational Preparation | Related Links |
|---|---|---|---|---|---|
| Acupuncture | Stimulation of anatomic points with thin metallic needles for (most commonly) the relief of pain or nausea | L.Ac. | NCCAOM | NCCAOM certification is the only nationally recognized certification available to practitioners of acupuncture and Oriental medicine; NCCAOM certification is a requirement for licensure in most states | National Certification Commission for Acupuncture and Oriental Medicine http://www.nccaom.org |
| Animal Assisted Therapy | Incorporating pets into the lives of individuals to improve health and healing | AAT | No formal credentialing or licensure process; many trained therapists (eg, physical, occupational, recreational) can incorporate AAT into their practice | The Delta Society offers a comprehensive service dog trainer curriculum according to their published "Standards of Practice in Animal-Assisted Activities and Animal-Assisted Therapy" | Delta Society http://www.deltasociety.org/index.htm |
| Aromatherapy | Use of essential oils from flowers, herbs, and trees to promote health and wellbeing | | No formal credentialing or licensure process | Many naturopaths, massage therapists, chiropractors, sports medicine therapists, and practitioners of Chinese Medicine incorporate the use of essential oils; the majority of programs are night or weekend seminars | National Association for Holistic Aromatherapy http://www.naha.org |
| Art therapy | Use of art to explore feelings, promote self-awareness, and increase self-esteem | ATR-BC | Certification is offered through the Art Therapy Credentials Board; there is no formal licensure process | Minimum educational and professional standards for the profession are established by the American Art Therapy Association, Inc., a membership and advocacy organization | Art Therapy Credentials Board, Inc. http://www.atcb.org |
| Ayurveda | Traditional Medical system that uses diet and herbal remedies that emphasize prevention and treatment of conditions of the mind, body, and spirit | BAMS, DAMS | No formal credentialing, licensure, or standard for training Ayurvedic practitioners in the US | Ayurvedic training in India is obtained with either a bachelor's degree (Bachelor of Ayurvedic Medicine and Surgery, BAMS) or doctoral degree (Doctor of Ayurvedic Medicine and Surgery, DAMS); a few states in the US have approved Ayurvedic schools as educational institutions | The Ayurvedic Institute http://www.ayurveda.com |
| Chiropratic Medicine | Whole medical system focusing on the relationship between body structure and function relying on manipulative therapy as a tool | DC | Licensure in 50 states and in the District of Columbia following a national board examination | The curriculum includes a minimum of 4,200 hours of classroom, laboratory and clinical experience | The American Chiropractic Association http://www.amerchiro.org/index.cfm |
| Healing Touch | A biofield (the magnetic field around the body) therapy that is an energy-based approach to health and healing | HT-CP | Certification may be obtained through Healing Touch International, Inc.; there is no formal licensure process | Healing Touch is a multi-level program in energy based therapy that moves from beginnig (Level 1) to advanced (Level 5) | Healing Touch Program http://www.healingtouchprogram.com |

| | | | | | |
|---|---|---|---|---|---|
| Homeopathy | Whole medical system using highly diluted quantities of medicinal substances to cure symptoms and conditions | Hom. | A diploma or certification of completion can be obtained; there is no formal licensure process | There are several homeopathic schools and programs in the US offering a range of 10-week to 3-year curriculums | Institute of Classical Homeopathy http://www.classicalhomoeopathy.org |
| Macrobiotics | Dietary and lifestyle program that includes eating more whole grains, beans, and fresh vegetables, eating regularly, and less in quantity | | No formal credentialing or licensure process | There are several macrobiotic training programs in the United States | The Kushi Institute http://www.kushiinstitute.org |
| Massage Therapy | Use of systematic manipulation of the soft tissues of the body to enhance health and healing | CMT-BC | Certification is available through the NCBTMB; massage therapists are licensed in many states | To become nationally certified: 500 hours of instruction; demonstrate mastery of core skills; pass a standardized NCBTMB exam | National Certification Board of Massage Therapy and Bodywork http://www.ncbtmb.org |
| Music Therapy | Use of music to address physical, emotional, cognitive, and social needs of individuals of all ages | MT-BC | Certification is available through the Certification Board of Music Therapy; there is no formal licensure process | Completion of an academic and clinical training program approved by the American Music Therapy Association; completion of written examination demonstrating current competency; recertification every 5 years through re-examination or 100 continuing music therapy education units | The Certification Board for Music Therapists http://www.cbmt.org |
| Naturopathy | Whole medical system that promotes the healing power of nature; treats the whole person, emphasis on prevention | ND | To date, 15 states have licensing laws for naturopaths in the US; certification can be obtained through the Naturopathic Physicians Licensing Examination Board and the North American Board of Naturopathic Examiners | Each of the six schools in North America is either accredited, or is a candidate for accreditation by an agency of the United States Department of Education | The American Association of Naturopathic Physicians http://www.naturopathic.org |

(Continued)

**TABLE 24-4**

**Licensure, Certification, and Educational Preparation for Common CAM Practitioners (Continued)**

| Modality | Definition | Acronym | Licensing/Certification Body | Educational Preparation | Related Links |
|---|---|---|---|---|---|
| Osteopathy | Whole systems approach that often uses a hands-on approach (manipulation) to assure that the body is moving freely | | Licensure occurs at the state level; Osteopaths may become certified in a specialty field | There are schools of osteopathy in the US; in addition, a 2- to 6-year residency is required within the specialty area to prepare for a board certification exam | American Academy of Osteopathy http://www.academyofosteopathy.org |
| Reflexology | Use of pressure to the feet and hand with specific thumb, finger, and hand techniques to reduce stress; based on a system of zones and reflex areas | | Certification is available through several groups such as the American Reflexology Certification Board | Educational programs vary, with introductory programs of less than 100 hours of study to advanced programs of greater than 100 hours of study | American Reflexology Certification Board http://arcb.net |
| Reiki | A Japanese technique for stress reduction and relaxation that promotes healing through "laying on hands"; based on the idea that an unseen "life force energy" flows through individuals | | Certification is available through several groups such as the American Board of Holistic Practitioners; there is no formal licensure process | Training in traditional reiki has three levels: first and second levels can be given in 8–12 hour classes over two weekends; third level training to become a certified Reiki Master may be completed in 3 days | International Association of Reiki Professionals http://www.iarp.org |
| Yoga | Yoga is the performance of poses or postures to creating balance in the body through developing both strength and flexibility | | Certification is available through Yoga Alliance; there is no formal licensure process | Yoga schools train individuals to become yoga instructors; with 200 hours instructors can become certified | Yoga Alliance http://www.yogaalliance.org |

Abbreviations: NCBTMB, National Certification Board of Massage Therapy and Bodywork; NCCAOM, National Certification Commission for Acupuncture and Oriental Medicine.

CAM are generated in the same fashion as those in conventional medicine. Angell and Kassirer assert that there cannot be two kinds of medicine, conventional and alternative.[42] They state that there is only one type of medicine: one that has been adequately tested, reasoning that once a treatment has been tested rigorously, it no longer matters whether it was considered "alternative" at the outset. If the modality is found to be reasonably safe and effective, it can be accepted into clinical practice, but assertions, speculations, and testimonials do not substitute for evidence.[42]

## INTEGRATIVE HEALTH CARE CENTERS

Integrative oncology brings together the best of complementary and conventional medicine in a multidisciplinary approach. Today, more medical centers and clinics are planning, developing, and implementing programs for cancer patients across the county. The driving forces for these programs are the development of a scientific basis for practice and promotion of open dialogue to assist patients in safe and appropriate incorporation of complementary medicine into cancer care. Five NCI Comprehensive Cancer Centers began integrative medicine clinics. These are:

- Integrative Medicine Program at the University of Texas MD Anderson Cancer Center
- The Integrative Medicine Service at the Memorial Sloan-Kettering Cancer Center
- Integrative Oncology – Leonard P. Zakim Center: The Dana-Farber Cancer Institute Experience
- The Johns Hopkins Complementary and Integrative Medicine Service
- Integrative Oncology at Mayo Clinic

Table 24-5 describes the origin, funding, and focus of each of these five NCI Designated Comprehensive Cancer Centers.[43]

## CONDUCTING AN INTEGRATED ASSESSMENT

An integrated assessment conducted by HCPs will identify relevant information regarding past and current use of CAM for cancer-related symptoms or treatment as well as comorbidities. A well-conducted integrated assessment must communicate a willingness to understand the value and significance of CAM to patients. This creates an environment that allows patients to express their willingness and desire to be a partner in decisions impacting their care. No single integrated assessment tool has been published; however, experts agree that there are core components:

- Health history basics: demographics (including insurance), chief complaint, history of present illness, past medical history, medications (including adherence), allergies, social history, immunizations and travel, family history, review of systems, labs, and diagnostics.
- Integrative assessment basics: comprehensive medication assessment,[44] previous and current CAM therapies (use, duration, reason, benefit, provider, cost, location, side effects), general well-being, nutrition, physical activity/exercise, stress management, spirituality, personal image, view toward illness state and recommended conventional therapies, and anticipated CAM use (or desire for more information).[45–47]
- Treatment plan basics: Is a safe and effective conventional therapy available? Is receiving a conventional therapy desirable to the patient? Is a safe and effective CAM therapy available? Is the population studied similar to your patient? Is there a strong belief or agreement in the rationale of the CAM therapy between the HCP and patient? Is the cost of CAM therapy low? Can the patient be monitored during the treatment period? Is there a risk of interactions between the conventional and CAM therapy? Is there a plan for consistent follow-up?[48]

A comprehensive guide to decision making in integrative oncology for nurses has not yet been developed. Nurses and other HCPs who are conducting these assessments are in a position to identify the practice issues related to care of patients with cancer who use CAM therapies. These issues include referral vs recommendation to CAM practitioners, billing issues, appropriate follow-up and communication with CAM practitioners, documentation challenges, and legal/ethical implications. A sample integrated assessment is shown in Figure 24-1.

## INTEGRATIVE ONCOLOGY: EFFICACY AND SAFETY OF COMMONLY USED MODALITIES

The Hippocratic oath "do no harm" is apropos when CAM modalities are combined with conventional biomedical interventions.[49] Concurrent use of CAM and traditional approaches requires an examination of the safety and efficacy of the CAM modality and its potential interactions with surgery, chemotherapy, radiation, and/or biologic therapies. Mandatory pathways in clinical care are (1) incorporating evidence-based practice involving the use of CAM in oncology care, (2) assessing and documenting concurrent CAM use, (3) verifying the safety and efficacy of CAM modalities under use, and (4) maintaining accountability in personal practice through proper licensure and continuing education.

Despite the fact that CAM therapies are increasingly being used in the United States and abroad, limited data are available on the safety, efficacy, and mechanism of action of many individual therapies. One must be aware of this lack of complete data when making treatment decisions. Until

TABLE 24-5

**National Cancer Institute's Comprehensive Cancer Centers with Integrative Medicine Programs**

| Program | How Program Started | Current Activities | Notes |
|---|---|---|---|
| **University of Texas, M.D. Anderson Cancer Center (MDACC)**<br>http://www.mdanderson.org/cimer | The Complementary/Integrative Medicine Education Resources (CIMER) Program started in 2002 in the Division of Cancer Medicine within the medical oncology department at MDACC<br>**Funding**: State funds, philanthropic funds, internal organization funding<br>**Education and Training** component: website, lecture series, training program<br>(1) CIMER geared toward HCP and patients<br>(2) English, Spanish, Chinese; thousands of abstracts, > 80 reviews; Web-based version for staff<br>(3) CAM elective course at University of Texas Medical School<br>(4) 3rd year medical students from Baylor rotate to *Place . . . of Wellness*<br>(5) Massage school | 100 Programs<br>Non-billable services: support groups, expressive arts, music therapy, movement, energy, relaxation/meditation, education forums, spirituality<br>Billable services: full body massage; acupuncture; physician-led comprehensive consultation service<br>**Research**: Pre-clinical and clinical in the areas of mind-body, natural products, traditional, acupuncture, traditional Chinese medicine, qualitative CAM research | **Focus:** clinical delivery, education, research<br>**Location:** Integrative Medicine Program is at the Texas Medical Center in Houston<br>http://www.mdanderson.org/departments/intmedprogram<br>Separate registration for patient with hospital and with *Place . . . of Wellness*<br>There has been development of standards of practice for common CAM modalities |
| **Memorial Sloan Kettering (MSKCC)**<br>http://www.mskcc.org/mskcc/html/1979.cfm | The Program started in 1999 as a quality of life arm of cancer care at MSKCC; program was designed to serve as a prototype<br>"Bodymindspirit" is inscribed on wall of the main MSKCC outpatient Pavilion<br>**Education and Training:**<br>(1) Integrative Oncology Fellowship Training Program to train physicians<br>(2) Medical Massage for the Cancer Patient<br>(3) Acupuncture for the Cancer Patient<br>(4) Music Therapy Program student internship programs<br>(5) About Herbs (launched 2002) with about 217 monographs | **Clinical services** for inpatients and outpatients on consult basis<br>Outpatient services are available to MSKCC patients, family members, faculty, staff, and patients from other hospitals, and the community by appointment. Fee-for-service basis: massage, music therapy, acupuncture, meditation, relaxation, fitness and nutrition, dance | **Focus:** clinical services, research, education and training, and information program<br>**Location:** Outpatient services at Bendheim Integrative Medicine Center<br>There has been development of standards of practice for common CAM modalities |
| **Dana Farber Cancer Institute DFCI**<br>http://www.dana-farber.org/pat/support/zakim/default.html | The Leonard P. Zakim Center for Integrative Therapies at Dana Farber opened in 2000<br>The Jimmy Fund Clinic clinical operations began in 2001 working closely with Center for Holistic Pediatric Education and Research at Children's Hospital, Boston<br>**Funding**: private foundations, philanthropic (70%), billable services<br>**Education and Training:**<br>(1) Arrangements with Massachusetts College of Pharmacy and Berklee College of Music<br>(2) Integrative Educational Program for patients, families, staff<br>(3) Introductory CAM lecture | **Clinical Services**: Acupuncture, massage, integrative medicine/oncology consultations, integrative nutrition counseling, TT, Reiki, and mind-body therapies for adults and patients; music therapy for pediatric patients<br>Total: 5000 encounters/year.<br>A consult service is a part of this program | **Focus:** Clinical services, education, research<br>**Location:** First located within the hospital, then re-located to a new renovated area in the hospital building complex in 2000<br>There has been development of standards of practice for common CAM modalities |

*(Continued)*

**TABLE 24-5**

**National Cancer Institute's Comprehensive Cancer Centers with Integrative Medicine Programs (Continued)**

| Program | How Program Started | Current Activities | Notes |
|---|---|---|---|
| **The Johns Hopkins Kimmel Oncology Cancer Center (JHKOCC)**<br>http://www.hopkinsintegrative.org/ | The Program began in 1999 with the hiring of an advanced practice nurse/Acupuncturist Program Manager to develop the program<br>**Funding**: billable services, philanthropic support<br>**Education and Training:**<br>(1) Mindfulness-based stress reduction<br>(2) Weekly scientific presentations<br>(3) CAM continuing medical education courses<br>(4) Lay programs | **Clinical Services:** Chinese medicine, integrative psychotherapy, acupuncture, massage<br>There is a consult service in this program | **Focus:** Research, clinical services, education, training<br>There has been development of standards of practice for common CAM modalities |
| **Mayo Clinic**<br>http://www.mayoclinic.com/health/alternative-medicine/PN00001 | In 2002, a collaborative team was created to investigate CAM modalities that oncology patients were using<br>**Education and Training:**<br>(1) Monthly seminar series<br>(2) Integrative Medicine curriculum for the Mayo Graduate School Internal Medicine Residency (2004) | **Clinical Services:** Acupuncture, massage therapy<br>There is a consult service in this program | **Focus:** Research, clinical services, and education |

Date of service: ______

Name: ______ DOB: ______

You are here today because ______

*For Office Use Only*:

**Height:** **Weight:** **Usual Weight:** **Pain (0–10):**

**T:** **P:** **B/P:** **R:** **Pulse Ox:**

**Family Medical History reviewed Y__ N __**

**Past Medical History reviewed Y__ N __**

**Current Medications/Herbs/Supplements Reviewed Y__ N__**

**Attached forms** ______

**Tobacco Use** ______

**ETOH Use** ______

**Oncology Nurse signature** ______

**Current Medical Issues** (please include symptoms)

| Medical Issue or Concern | When did it begin? | Symptom(s) |
|---|---|---|
| | | |
| | | |

**Allergies** (please include allergies to medicine, the environment, and food sensitivities)

| Medication Allergy | Environmental Allergy | Food Sensitivity |
|---|---|---|
| | | |
| | | |

**Nutrition:** What do you typically eat for breakfast, lunch, dinner, and snacks?

Breakfast ______

Lunch ______

Dinner ______

Snacks ______

What foods do you crave or dislike? ______

**Are you now receiving or have you ever received or participated in** (please circle all that apply):

Acupuncture Aromatherapy Art, Music, or Dance Therapy Reiki

Chiropractic Spinal Manipulations Counseling/Coaching Massage Yoga

Supervised Exercise Program Naturopathic/Homeopathic Medicine

Qigong or Tai Chi Therapeutic/Healing Touch Other (specify) ______

**Please list and describe the therapy, provider/geographic location, length of therapy, and experienced benefits or side effects:**

| Therapy | Provider/Location | Length of Therapy | Benefits Experienced | Side Effects Experienced |
|---|---|---|---|---|
| | | | | |
| | | | | |
| | | | | |

How may we help you **today? What information would you like to receive?** ______

What would you like us to know about you/what should we know about you that we have not asked? ______

Signature ______ Date ______

**FIGURE 24-1**

Complementary/integrative assessment. An addendum to institution/practice forms.

recently, much information available was based on theoretical or personal opinion rather than on evidence. The concept of an evidence-based approach to CAM is still in its infancy. Recommending CAM therapies remains challenging for HCPs. Eisenberg[50] offered an algorithm for advising patients regarding CAM therapies. Ernst[51] strove to establish a base of evidence for CAM and offered a direction-of-evidence model. Increasingly, HCPs encounter patients who request information regarding CAM therapies for preventing or treating medical conditions. This interest may intensify when traditional therapies are not providing the desired result.[52] This desire for CAM therapies is complicated by the amount of information, much of it inaccurate, available from a variety of sources, including the Internet and well-meaning friends and family. Opinions differ, and methods for rating therapies vary even among experts. Ernst[51] uses "direction of evidence" (clearly positive, tentatively positive, uncertain, tentatively negative, clearly negative) and "weight of evidence" (low, moderate, and high). Eisenberg[52] uses "recommend," "tolerate," and "avoid." The following discussion of therapies includes a description, evidence, contraindications, and information about practitioners.

## Acupuncture

*Description.* Acupuncture has been used by many Americans and performed by many physicians, dentists, and acupuncturists for a variety of health conditions, particularly pain. It typically involves inserting a needle into the skin in specific sites (acupoints) for therapeutic purposes. Acupoint stimulation may also be via electrical current, laser, moxibustion, pressure, ultrasound, and vibration and of Japanese, Korean, or Chinese types. The underlying principle is that *qi* (pronounced "chee" and translated as meaning "energy") is present at birth and maintained throughout life. It circulates throughout the body, and 12 meridians provide a major path for the flow of *qi*. There are approximately 350 acupoints along the 12 meridians, with additional acupoints that lie outside the meridian pathways. Health is a balance of yin and yang (opposite forces present in everyone). Disease or any medical condition is a result of imbalance, usually a result of a blockage or deficiency of energy. Acupuncture theory embraces the belief that stimulating the appropriate acupoints helps the body correct any imbalance in the flow of energy, thus restoring balance. It is also held that changes in the balance of energy and flow of *qi* may be identified before disease has developed, and therefore, acupuncture has a role in the prevention of illness and maintenance of health. It has been and is routinely used in Eastern countries. It has also been integrated with allopathic and osteopathic medicine in the United States.[53] Acupuncture has been and continues to be used for pain and other disorders of the musculoskeletal system; headaches; stress; ENT conditions, including sinusitis, tinnitus, and vertigo; allergies; dental pain; addictions; and immune system support, among others.

*Evidence.* More than 30 meta-analyses (MAs) and systematic reviews (SRs) between 1996 and 2004 examined the use of acupuncture for symptom management, mostly related to pain. The results of nearly 400 randomized controlled trials (RCTs) are reported on Medline for the same time period. There is no evidence of the physical existence of *qi* or the meridians. The effects of acupuncture are reportedly better than placebo in most trials.[51] Opioid peptides, serotonin, and other neurotransmitters are released by acupuncture.[54,55] Conclusive evidence exists that acupuncture is effective in the treatment of dental pain[56] and postoperative nausea.[57,58] The efficacy of acupuncture in relief from asthma, back pain, drug dependency, fibromyalgia, migraine and tension headaches, neck pain, osteoarthritis, and stroke is considered inconclusive by some authors.[59] Others suggest that the evidence is equivocal and/or promising for some indications, including addiction, stroke rehabilitation, postoperative and chemotherapy-related nausea and vomiting, tennis elbow, carpal tunnel syndrome, and asthma.[53]

*Contraindications.* "Needling" technique is contraindicated in those patients with severe bleeding disorders or who are at increased risk for infection, as in neutropenia, and during the first trimester of pregnancy, with the exception of treatment for nausea.[60] Patients with cardiac pacemakers should not be treated with electrical stimulation.[61] Caution is advised for the first treatment, and some authors recommend that treatment be administered with the patient in a supine position. Some patients become drowsy and should be cautioned against driving and operating machinery. Needles should not be reused, and strict asepsis is mandatory.[61] Side effects include bleeding, bruising, pain with needling, and worsening of symptoms. Reported adverse events are rare but include pneumothorax and death.[60–62]

Since the diagnostic value of acupuncture has not been established, it may constitute more risk than reward; however, it is worth consideration for a number of conditions. There is evidence that, with accurate diagnosis, it is safe and, for certain conditions, it is more effective than placebo when administered by an appropriately trained practitioner.

*Practitioners.* Nationally, acupuncturists can be certified in two ways. They can complete a formal, full-time educational program that includes both classroom and clinical hours, or they may participate in an apprenticeship program. Acupuncturists must also complete a Clean Needle Technique–approved course. Medical doctors with training in acupuncture may also obtain board certification. The National Certification Commission of Acupuncture and Oriental Medicine (NCCAOM) established standards for certification that are accepted by some states for licensure. Medical doctors must possess a valid medical license and be certified through the American Academy of Medical Acupuncture. Some states require medical referral, while others allow nonmedical practitioners to see patients without a referral. A comparison of licensed versus certified acupuncturists is available at http://www.asny.org.

### Reiki

*Description.* Reiki means "universal life energy." It is an ancient form of healing. The practitioner is the conduit for the movement of energy. It is the energy—not the healer—that influences healing. In this respect, Reiki differs from other healing systems. In other words, energy travels through the healing, not from the healer. Reiki is said to alleviate physical, emotional, and spiritual blockages.[63] The five premises of Reiki are: (1) there is an energy of unique properties applicable to physical and psychological conditions, (2) the energy has a source, (3) this source can be tapped, (4) a person can be taught to use this energy, and (5) the effects of this energy are palpable and subjective. The energy is considered pure because it is not influenced by the practitioner's faith or religion.[63] The practitioner gently places his or her hands on the client, in a particular series of positions. Typically, 5 minutes are spent on each of 12 positions, although this may vary based on the needs of the client. The client remains fully clothed at all times, and no pressure, massage, or manipulation is applied to the client. The environment is kept quiet and soothing, and the client should emerge feeling relaxed. Reiki is considered to be capable of healing anything because it works at fundamental levels of reality. The limits to Reiki seem to be in the recipient's willingness to cast off old habits and patterns, to accept change, and to accept healing.[64] Ernst considers Reiki to be a form of spiritual healing.[51]

*Evidence.* Two MAs examining Reiki (with therapeutic touch) were reported between 1999 and 2004. More than 20 RCTs are reported on Medline for the same time period. Rexilius and colleagues[65] examined the effect of massage therapy and healing touch on anxiety, depression, subjective caregiver burden, and fatigue experienced by caregivers of patients undergoing stem cell transplant. The results showed declines in anxiety scores, depression, general fatigue, motivation fatigue, and emotional fatigue for individuals in the massage therapy group only. Anxiety and depression scores decreased in the healing touch group, and fatigue and subjective burden increased but without statistical significance.[65] Reiki may be helpful in the treatment of pain,[66] mood changes,[67] and fatigue.[68] Mansour and colleagues[69] tested a standardization procedure for placebo Reiki in an effort to provide a foundation for subsequent randomized and placebo-controlled Reiki efficacy study.[69]

*Contraindications.* Reiki appears to have no adverse effects and can eventually be self-administered. Clinical trials are sponsored by the National Center for Complementary and Alternative Medicine.

*Practitioners.* Typically, Reiki is taught in three parts. Reiki Part I includes: history of Reiki, the Reiki hand positions, Reiki symbols and their names, and meditation manifestation. Part II involves intense training focusing on advanced techniques and includes a review of part I. The training for Reiki II brings knowledge of long-distance healing, scanning techniques, and the long-distance Reiki symbols and their names. Typically, there are two USUI-Reiki-Tibetan attunements at intervals throughout the course. Reiki III (Master) includes a review of previous training and practice and brings to the student knowledge for long-distance healing, scanning techniques, more meditation techniques, and an additional Reiki symbol. Typically, there is a Reiki attunement at the end of the course.

### Reflexology

*Description.* Reflexology is a therapeutic method that uses a specific type of manual pressure applied to certain areas, or zones, of the feet (and sometimes the hands or ears) that are believed to correspond to areas of the body, in order to relieve stress and prevent and/or treat physical disorders. The organs, glands, and other components of the body are represented on the foot on the same side. Examining the feet to detect imbalances or obstructions to the flow of energy, which are expressed as tenderness or feelings of crepitus or gravel at the site, assesses body health. It is believed that stimulating these areas with pressure or massage can influence bodily function. Reflexology is purported to promote homeostasis and circulation, reduce stress and eliminate toxins. Skeptics believe that reflexology has an impact because it involves caring touch.[70] From a conventional biomedical framework, there is no known neurophysiological basis for connections between organs or glands and specific areas of the feet. Three investigations into the claimed correspondences are known: reflexologists' diagnoses were no better than chance in identifying medical conditions in one blinded study whereas in another their diagnostic success was better than chance but not clinically significant.[71] Reflexology foot massage may have general health benefits independent of any correspondence of the reflex with specific organs.

*Evidence.* Nearly 20 RCTs were conducted using reflexology for the relief of cancer symptoms between 1990 and 2004. One MA reviewing the evidence on efficacy and safety of massage was completed in 2002.[72] Reflexology may involve aromatherapy massage and therapeutic touch in some trials. Key findings were (1) aromatherapy and massage may reduce anxiety for short periods of time,[73] (2) therapeutic massage and healing touch induce relaxation,[69] (3) therapeutic back massage may enhance relaxation and reduce stress in caregivers,[74] and (4) reflexology may positively influence quality of life in patients in the palliative stage of cancer.[75] In noncancer populations, several key RCTs have been reported. Reflexology may be superior to placebo reflexology for the treatment of premenstrual symptoms.[76] It may also have beneficial effects on blood glucose in diabetics.[77] An RCT in patients with multiple sclerosis showed symptomatic improvements; however, the study experienced a high dropout rate.[78] In a large observational study, 81% of patients with headaches reported themselves helped or cured at a three-month follow-up.[79]

*Contraindications.* Of concern would be conditions of the feet that might worsen or cause pain with applied pressure, such as gout and peripheral vascular disease. Some[51] suggest that reflexology may interfere with some drugs, including insulin.[80] The greatest risk would involve the use of reflexology as an alternative therapy. Reflexology should not be used alone for diagnostic purposes. When provided by an accountable practitioner, reflexology would probably do no harm and may possibly help.[51,70]

*Practitioners.* No regulatory system, licensure, or minimum training mandates exist for reflexology. Typically, healthcare professionals who may have licensure in another area, such as nursing, use it. Practitioners' backgrounds can range from self-taught to those who have attended training courses.[81]

### Aromatherapy

*Description.* Aromatherapy is the controlled use of plant essences for therapeutic purposes.[82] *Essential oil* is the aromatic essence of a plant in the form of an oil or resin derived from plant leaf, stalk, bark, root, flower, fruit, or seed. The *carrier* is the diluent used with a concentrated essential oil for application. The *neat* is the direct application of the essential oil compound (essential oil plus carrier) to the skin. The *note* is the unique aromatic variable of an essential oil used when blending combinations of essential oil compounds. The *top note* is bright, the *middle note* is lingering, and the *base note* is grounding.[83] Essential oils can be applied directly to the skin through a compress or massage, inhaled via a diffuser or steaming water, or added directly to bath water. At the present time, there are about 150 essential oils.[84] The mechanism of action in the use of essential oils begins with the olfactory sense. After sensing the smell, the limbic system is activated in retrieving learned memories. Essential oils are also absorbed via the dermal route and subcutaneous fat into the bloodstream. Entry into the body via the oral route into the digestive system is not recommended. Often, aromatherapy is practiced with massage. Aromatherapy massage is used in palliative care settings to improve quality of life for patients with cancer. Published data on dosing, comparative methods of administration, and therapeutic outcomes in the use of essential oils in aromatherapy are limited.

*Evidence.* A 2003 Cochrane Database SR was performed involving aromatherapy for dementia. Nearly 20 RCTs were reported on Medline between 1998 and 2004 for the use of aromatherapy in various clinical settings, of which four involve patients with cancer. Cooke and Ernst[85] reviewed 12 trials in an SR. Six of these trials suggested that aromatherapy massage has a relaxing effect. Louis and Kowalski[86] measured the responses of 17 patients with cancer to humidified essential lavender oil, with a positive change noted in blood pressure, pulse, pain, anxiety, depression, and sense of well-being after both the humidified water treatment and lavender treatment. Olleveant and colleagues[87] compared drop size between six different essential oils and reported that the bottles differed in their method of delivery and recommended a universal standardization of measure to ensure equity and safety in administration. Massage and aromatherapy massage offer short-term benefits for psychological well-being, with the effect on anxiety supported by limited evidence.[88] Evidence is mixed as to whether aromatherapy enhances the effects of massage. Replication, longer follow-up, and larger trials are needed to accrue the necessary evidence.[88]

*Contraindications.* Contraindications to the use of essential oils are pregnancy, contagious disease, epilepsy, venous thrombosis, varicose veins, open wounds or skin sites, and recent surgeries of any type. Essential oils should not be administered orally or applied undiluted to the skin. Possible adverse events associated with the use of essential oils are photosensitivity, allergic reactions, nausea, and headache. Many essential oils have the potential to either enhance or reduce the effects of prescribed medications, including antibiotics, tranquilizers, antihistamines, anticonvulsants, barbiturates, morphine, and quinidine.[51] Cases of potentially serious reactions involving the use of essential oils have been reported in two individuals without known allergies or sensitivities prior to exposure.[89]

*Practitioners.* Aromatherapy can be used in combination with massage therapy and holistic nursing care programs. Certification is available through the National Association for Holistic Aromatherapy (NAHA, http://www.naha.org). Schools must provide practice in the fields of aromatherapy, essential oil studies, anatomy, and physiology. Holistic nursing certification is available through the American Holistic Nurses' Certification Corporation (AHNCC, http://www.ahncc.org). Requirements include a BSN, continuing education, one year of practice, and passing a written exam. Certification in aromatherapy or holistic nursing does not qualify a nurse to work independently, nor does it necessarily meet institutional requirements for practice.[90]

Campbell and colleagues[91] and Avis[92] offer the following guidelines for integrating aromatherapy safely into clinical practice:

- Identify certified staff to serve as resources and educators.
- Conduct a patient assessment.
- Select essential oils with low known risk potential.
- Choose one supplier with stringent product testing.
- Develop a range of oils and methods of application that can be used consistently.
- When blending oils, consider symptoms, patient allergies, and preference of aroma.
- Obtain a verbal consent.
- Place the oil on a tissue for patients in semiprivate rooms.
- Document the outcome of intervention.
- Avoid vaporizers in clinical settings.

## Antioxidants

*Description.* Antioxidant vitamins—E, C, and beta-carotene—are believed to have health-promoting properties. Coenzyme Q 10 ubiquinone (CoQ10) is an antioxidant found in all living cells. It is involved in the production of energy within cells and is believed to have powerful antioxidant effects. Although the data are incomplete, up to 30% of Americans are taking some form of antioxidant supplement, and research has shown that patients with cancer take antioxidants, typically at doses higher than the recommended daily allowances (RDAs).[93] Antioxidants act by scavenging free radicals. The debate that surrounds antioxidants has focused on cancer therapies such as alkylating agents, antimetabolites, and radiation because of the purposeful creation of free radicals through cytotoxic mechanisms and, therefore, taking antioxidants could interfere in the action of these therapies. Limited research supports the belief that chemotherapy diminishes total antioxidant status,[94] but inconsistencies based on cancer site, cancer therapy, research methodologies, patient populations, variability in doses, duration of supplementation, and timing of interventions prevent the formulation of conclusions.[95]

*Evidence.* More than 45 MAs or SRs reviewing antioxidants (of which five involve patients with cancer) were reported between 1994 and 2004. More than 2000 RCTs involving antioxidants are reported on Medline during this same time period. The belief that antioxidants may interfere with the efficacy of cancer therapy is not new. The association between beta-carotene and increased risk of lung cancer in smokers is well known.[96,97] However, it has been suggested that selective inhibition of tumor cell growth is an action of antioxidants and that antioxidants may also promote cellular differentiation with enhanced cytotoxic effects.[98] Ray and colleagues[99] suggest that typically recommended doses may be insufficient to cover the higher production of reactive oxygen metabolites.[99] It has also been argued that inadequate doses may actually contribute to malignant cell proliferation.[98] Researchers have been concerned that while antioxidants may decrease some kinds of toxicity associated with cancer chemotherapy, the therapeutic benefit of the cancer therapy may be compromised. Ladas and colleagues[95] reviewed more than 100 citations on antioxidant status and cancer outcomes and antioxidant use among patients receiving chemotherapy with or without radiation therapy. Of the 52 that met their research criteria, 31 were observational studies and 21 were intervention trials. Their findings showed a decline in the total antioxidant status of patients receiving cancer therapy but conflicting and inconsistent results regarding the effect of chemotherapy on the antioxidant status of patients receiving cancer therapy. Lenzhofer and colleagues[100] found that supplementation with vitamin E altered the metabolism of doxorubicin. Landas and colleagues[95] questioned whether this means decreased treatment efficacy, arguing that adjunctive agents such as mesna and amifostine are used to reduce free radicals and do not appear to interfere with therapeutic benefit. Among patients receiving chemotherapy and total-body irradiation for bone marrow transplantation, serum vitamin E levels decreased even among those receiving total parenteral nutrition.[101] Two randomized studies treating patients with gynecologic cancers with doxorubicin; cyclophosphamide; cisplatin with melphalan; and selenium and vitamin E, or placebo demonstrated increased serum selenium levels but not increased vitamin E levels after supplementation.[102] A review of studies among patients with breast cancer revealed a possible direct effect of selenium supplementation on serum and whole blood selenium.[95] The RDAs appear to be inadequate for maintaining plasma antioxidant levels in patients receiving high-dose chemotherapy before stem cell transplant. Antioxidants may have a role in cancer prevention. Some studies suggest high vitamin C intake prior to diagnosis of breast cancer may have a positive effect on survival[103,104] and selenium and vitamin E supplementation were thought to reduce the risk of prostate cancer.[105] Variability in doses, duration of supplementation, and timing of interventions prevent the formulation of conclusions in this area of research as well. Except within the context of trials, conclusive recommendations as well as contraindications for the patient with cancer have not been established.

*Contraindications.* Contraindications exist for specific antioxidants. For example, beta-carotene increases lung cancer risk among smokers.

- *Vitamin C.* Potential interactions: aluminium antacids, cyclosporine, statins, calcium channel blockers and protease inhibitors, iron, vitamin E[106]
- *Vitamin E.* Potential interactions: cholestyramine, colestipol, mineral oil, anticonvulsants, anticoagulants, verapamil[106]

- *Beta-carotene.* Potential interactions: cholestyramine, colestipol, mineral oil, orlistat[107]

*Practitioners.* Registered dieticians have a minimum of a bachelors degree in dietetics. Certified nutritional consultants have education and training in clinical nutrition and may be nurses or other healthcare professionals. Caution should be taken when choosing a nutrition practitioner to be certain that he or she has expertise in cancer care as well as in supplements and nutrition.

## St. John's wort

*Description.* Also known as amber touch-and-heal, devil's scourge, goatweed, hypericum, Klamath weed, millepertuis, rosin rose, Tipton weed, and witch's herb, St. John's wort (SJW) is a member of the *Hypericaceae* family and contains naphthodianthrones, flavonoids, bioflavonoids, phloroglucinols, tannins, volatile oils, and xanthones. The chemical composition is dependent upon the harvesting and drying processes and storage. The biologic activity of St. John's wort is believed to be due to several of its components.[108] It has been used topically and systemically for its medicinal properties for centuries. Uses include wound healing, burns, as a diuretic, and to treat melancholia, pain, gastritis, malaria, hemorrhoids and mental illness, among others.[109] Contemporary use is almost exclusively as an antidepressant.[110] The pharmacologic actions of this herb include antiretroviral and antidepressant action. The mechanism of action is not known. Possibilities include modulation of interleukin-6 and GABA receptor binding, inhibition of serotonin reuptake, noradrenaline, and dopamine. There is some question regarding action as a MAO inhibitor. The active ingredients have not been identified, and therefore when considering safety the entire extract must be taken under consideration.[108] Some authors believe hypericin and hyperiform to be the active constituents.[110]

*Evidence.* Six MAs reviewed the efficacy of SJW in treating mild to moderate depression. More than 50 RCTs are reported on Medline between 1994 and 2004. A number of comparative RCTs have suggested this herb to be as effective as pharmaceutical antidepressants.[111–114] SJW has been shown to be as effective as light therapy in the treatment of seasonal affective disorder.[115] One study identified no antiretroviral effects in patients who were HIV positive.[116] Positive results have been reported with premenstrual syndrome,[14, 117] menopausal symptoms,[115] and depression.[117] In an open-label crossover study design, six healthy men and six healthy women ages 22 to 38 years measured plasma pharmacokinetics of alprazolam as a probe for CYP3A4 activity before and after 14 days of SJW administration. A significant decrease in CYP3A4 activity as measured by alterations in alprazolam pharmacokinetics suggests that long-term therapy with SJW may cause diminished clinical impact or increased dose requirements for all CYP3A4 substrates. This represents approximately 50% of all available medications.[118] As monotherapy, SJW has a respectable safety profile considered superior to conventional antidepressants.[110,119]

*Contraindications.* SJW is contraindicated during pregnancy and lactation. It causes photosensitivity, gastrointestinal symptoms, fatigue, and anxiety. Cases of mania, subacute toxic neuropathy, and break-through bleeding (in patients taking oral contraceptives) have been reported. Concurrent use of SJW with serotonin reuptake inhibitors can result in serotonin syndrome. An episode of transplant rejection was reported in a patient receiving cyclosporine. Additional research suggests that the use of SJW reduced plasma levels of medications metabolized by hepatic cytochrome P450, including anticoagulants, anticonvulsants, digoxin, theophylline, and protease inhibitors. A single study indicated no interaction with alcohol.[110] There is inadequate evidence for use in severe depression.

## Mindfulness meditation

*Description.* Mindfulness meditation as practiced in mindfulness-based stress reduction (MBSR) is a self-regulatory approach to stress reduction and emotion management in widespread use for the past several decades. Mindfulness is a state in which an individual is highly aware of and focused on the reality of the present moment with acceptance and acknowledgement.[120] Growing interest in the use of MBSR reflects a desire for a more holistic approach to cancer treatment and a recognition of the links between social, psychological, and physiological health determinants. MBSR programs are usually six to eight weeks in length, involving daily individual activities and group activities up to several days per week. It is anticipated that individuals will continue to practice the activities for an extended period of time following completion of the structured program for full benefit of the intervention.

*Evidence.* There are currently no published MAs involving mindfulness meditation; however, 11 RCTs were reported on Medline between 1973 and 2004. Astin and colleagues[121] tested the short- and long-term benefits of an eight-week MBSR intervention for individuals with fibromyalgia. The study results revealed no evidence that MBSR was superior to education and support as a treatment option. In a pilot study, anxiety and emotional control improved in the treatment group as compared to the control in an RCT assessing the effectiveness of an MBSR program in patients with heart disease.[122] In two RCTs involving cancer, MBSR was effective in decreasing mood disturbance and stress symptoms in both male and female patients.[123]

*Contraindications.* None have been reported.

*Practitioners.* Trained individuals may administer MBSR interventions either separately or in a group situation. It is best practiced by those licensed in counseling, psychology, or social work.

## SYMPTOM MANAGEMENT

Patients use CAM for cancer treatment and/or symptom management. Symptom management in cancer care spans the pre-diagnosis to survivorship spectrum. Tremendous advances have been made in offering relief from symptoms ranging from those that are minor inconveniences to the major debilitating aspects of symptoms associated with the disease process, its treatment, and its possible physical, emotional, spiritual, and psychological long-term consequences. Oncology nurses are experts in managing cancer symptoms by reducing the overall impact of symptoms on health outcomes.[124] Quality cancer care, as identified by the Oncology Nursing Society,[125] embraces appropriate symptom management as a supportive care component. The Priority Symptom Management "PRISM" Project developed by the ONS Foundation Center for Leadership, Information, and Research CLIR in 2000 focused on six primary symptoms: anorexia, cognitive dysfunction, depression, fatigue, neutropenia, and pain. PRISM grew to the current Putting Evidence into Practice (PEP) Project. Conventional approaches to symptom management have been enhanced in the past several years by the popularity and availability of CAM therapies although there is limited data available on safety and efficacy. Table 24-6 provides examples of CAM use for symptom management and grades the available evidence as strong, good, or unclear/conflicting.

## EDUCATION

A recent survey examining conversations between patients and their physicians regarding CAM use revealed that in spite of the acknowledged use of CAM among people age 50 or older, 69% of those individuals do not talk to their physicians about it.[126] Respondents ($N$ = 1559) to a telephone survey who were 50 years or older, most often did not discuss their CAM use with physicians because the provider never asked (42 %), the patients did not know that they should discuss it (30%), or there was not enough time during the office visit to discuss it (19%). In some settings, consumerism is encouraged with the intended outcome of a decrease in overall healthcare costs for insurers and the insured.[127] Many patients want to be involved in the processes of diagnosis, planning, and delivery of their care. To that end they are seeking information from multiple sources and willing to spend significant out-of-pocket dollars on their personal health and wellness. While in essence, self-motivated health behavior is beneficial for individuals and society, patients are sometimes seeking interventions in isolation. Open dialogue and offering to facilitate acquisition of accurate, reliable information can assist patients in making informed healthcare decisions.

## PROGRAMS FOR HEALTHCARE PROFESSIONALS

### Core competencies

A principal question that arises is to what degree is an oncology nurse responsible and accountable for baseline knowledge of CAM when patients choose to integrate conventional medicine with CAM? Compelling reasons to develop baseline knowledge include: (1) recognition and acceptance that patients use CAM and the topic must be addressed in a provider-patient partnership; (2) safe and effective CAM modalities exist for some common conditions; (3) known or suspected interactions may occur between some CAM modalities and conventional care, and these potential interactions must be addressed in a timely manner.

The development of clinical core competencies and curricula in CAM are sequential in the attainment of baseline knowledge in CAM. Knowledge could be achieved following the completion of a smaller curriculum program or a larger fellowship program that teaches the established core competencies, however, these guidelines are not yet developed and published.

CAM core competencies are fundamental skills, abilities, and/or expertise in the area of CAM and integrated medicine as applied to clinical scenarios versus the skills and abilities to deliver CAM interventions. In conceptualizing core competencies, general endpoints must be developed beginning with expanding baseline knowledge in cancer CAM, establishing standards of practice, and assisting in the design of methodologically sound, rigorous research.

### Curriculum development

Through the Consortium of Academic Health Centers for Integrative Medicine (CAHCIM), advance practice nurses can train as fellows in programs integrating biomedicine and CAM.[128] For example, a two-year distance-learning certification program at the Arizona Center for Integrative Medicine is open to nurse practitioners, physicians, and physician assistants (http://integrativemedicine.arizona.edu/education/fellowship). Nursing leaders and educators alike are seeking content and developing curriculum in CAM and integrated care.[129,130] Continuing education, not culminating in certification, is offered by several government and industry sponsors.[131–133] Self-paced learning provides a thorough review of reliable written sources of high-quality CAM information that includes conventional and alternative medicine journals, electronic media, full text databases, electronic resources and newsletters.[134]

**TABLE 24-6**

**Integrative Therapies for Cancer-Related Symptoms**

| | Strong Evidence | Good Evidence | Unclear or Conflicting Evidence |
|---|---|---|---|
| **Constipation** | *Strong:* aloe, phosphates | *Good:* flaxseed, psyllium | *Unclear or Conflicting:* barley, cascara, massage, probiotics, rhubarb |
| **Depression** | *Strong:* music therapy, St. John's wort | *Good:* art therapy, 5-hydroxytryptophan, DHEA, psychotherapy, yoga | *Unclear or Conflicting:* acupressure, acupuncture, ayurveda, folic acid, ginkgo biloba, guarana, healing touch, kundalini yoga, massage, melatonin, omega-3-fatty acids, Qi gong, reiki, relaxation therapy, vitamin $B_2$, Tai chi, vitamin $B_6$ |
| **Diarrhea** | *Strong:* There is no modality that has been tested sufficiently yet to determine if strong evidence of efficacy exists. | *Good Evidence:* saccharomyces boulardii, soy | *Unclear or conflicting evidence:* arrowroot, berberine, bilberry, goldenseal, *Lactobacillus acidophilus* |
| **Fatigue** | *Strong/Good:* There is no modality that has been tested sufficiently yet to determine if strong or good evidence of efficacy exists. | *Good:* DHEA, exercise | *Unclear or Conflicting:* shiatsu acupressure, betel nut, ginseng, glyconutrients, kiwi, physical therapy, selenium, taurine, vitamin $B_{12}$, yoga |
| **Menopausal symptoms** | *Strong:* There is no modality that has been tested sufficiently yet to determine if strong evidence of efficacy exists | *Good:* sage | *Unclear or Conflicting:* acupuncture, bilberry, black cohosh, dong quai, gamma linolenic acid, green tea, red clover, pycnogel, relaxation therapy, St. John's wort, Traditional Chinese Medicine, wild yam |
| **Mucositis** | *Strong:* There is no modality that has been tested sufficiently yet to determine if strong evidence of efficacy exists. | *Good:* acupuncture, bloodroot, borage seed oil, hypnotherapy, rhubarb, zinc | *Unclear or Conflicting:* iodine |
| **Nausea and vomiting** | *Strong:* There is no modality that has been tested sufficiently yet to determine if strong evidence of efficacy exists. | *Good Evidence:* acupuncture and acupuncture-related interventions (electroacupoint stimulation, acupressure and acustimulation wrist bands, electroacupuncture), ginger, music therapy; | *Unclear or Conflicting:* aromatherapy, (post operative nausea), ginger (post-operative nausea), TENS (post-operative nausea), hypnosis |
| **Pain** | *Strong:* There is no modality that has been tested sufficiently yet to determine if strong evidence of efficacy exists. | *Good:* comfrey, guided imagery, hypotherapy, music therapy, acupuncture | *Unclear or Conflicting:* aconite, acupressure, Transcutaneous electrical nerve stimulation (TENS) |
| **Sleep changes** | *Strong:* There is no modality that has been tested sufficiently yet to determine if strong evidence of efficacy exists. | *Good:* melatonin; music therapy, valerian | *Unclear or Conflicting:* acupuncture, guided imagery, yoga |

Adapted from *Natural Standard http://www.naturalstandard.com/*

## LOCATING RELIABLE INFORMATION

Volumes of CAM information are presented online, in the media, and in lay literature. Distinguishing high-quality from poor-quality information is critical. Web sites volunteering medical resources should openly discuss who visits the site, who pays for the site, the purpose of the site, the sources of information, how information is selected for inclusion, how recent the information is, how links to other sites are selected, what information the site collects about visitors, and how the site manages interaction with visitors.[135] Selected sponsored Web sites, peer-reviewed journals indexed in Medline, and databases are listed in Table 24-7.

**TABLE 24-7**

| Sources of Reliable Cancer CAM Information | |
|---|---|
| **Selected Sponsored Organizations** | |
| American Academy of Medical Acupuncture | http://www.medicalacupuncture.org |
| American Cancer Society | http://www.cancer.org |
| American Society for Clinical Oncology | http://www.asco.org |
| National Institutes of Health | |
| Cancer Information Service | http://cis.nci.nih.gov |
| Office of Cancer Complementary and Alternative Medicine | http://www.cancer.gov/cam |
| National Center for Complementary and Alternative Medicine | http://nccam.nih.gov |
| Office of Dietary Supplements | http://ods.od.nih.gov |
| Medline Plus | http://www.nlm.nih.gov/medlineplus/index.html |
| Cancer Patient Education Network | http://www.nci.nih.gov/cancertopics/cancer-patient-education-resource/list-serv-form |
| People Living with Cancer (ASCO) | http://www.plwc.org |
| The University of Texas MD Anderson Cancer Center (CIMER) | http://www.mdanderson.org/education-and-research/resources-for-professionals/clinical-tools-and-resources |
| The Dana-Farber Cancer Institute Zakim Center for Integrated Therapies | http://www.dana-farber.org/pat/support/zakim_about.asp |
| The Johns Hopkins Center for Complementary and Alternative Medicine | http://www.hopkinsmedicine.org/CAM |
| The Rosenthal Center for Complementary and Alternative Medicine | http://www.rosenthal.hs.columbia.edu |
| **Selected Peer-Reviewed Journals (Indexed in Medline)** | |
| Alternative & Complementary Therapies | http://www.liebertpub.com/act |
| British Medical Journal | http://www.bmj.com |
| Clinical Journal of Oncology Nursing | http://www.ons.org/publications/journals/CJON |
| Integrative Cancer Therapies | http://www.sagepub.com/journalsProdDesc.nav?prodId=Journal201510 |
| Journal of Clinical Oncology | http://jco.ascopubs.org |
| Oncology Nursing Forum | http://www.ons.org/publications/journals/ONF |
| Seminars in Oncology Nursing | http://www.elsevier.com/wps/find/journaldescription.cws_home/623110/description |
| The Journal of Alternative and Complementary Medicine | http://www.liebertpub.com/publication.aspx?pub_id=26 |
| The Journal of the American Medical Association | http://jama.ama-assn.org |
| **Selected Sponsored Databases** | |
| Clinical Trials.gov | http://clinicaltrials.gov |
| Complementary and Alternative Medicine and Pain Database (University of Maryland School of Medicine) | http://www.umm.edu/news/releases/back_pain.htm |
| Directory of Information Resources | http://dirline.nlm.nih.gov |
| Food and Drug Administration | http://www.fda.gov |
| Herbalgram.org | http://abc.herbalgram.org/site/PageServer?pagename=Homepage_2009 |
| International Bibliographic Information on Dietary Supplements | http://ods.od.nih.gov/Health_INformation/IBIDS.aspx |
| Micromedex | http://www.micromedex.com/products/hcs |
| Natural Medicine Comprehensive Database | http://www.naturaldatabase.com/(S(uk2fapn15acnul55uwmkucyh))/home.aspx?cs=CE_nodeact&s=ND |
| Natural Standard | http://www.naturalstandard.com |
| Physician's Data Query | http://1800quitnow.cancer.gov/cancertopics/pdq |
| The Cochrane Collaboration | http://www.cochrane.org |

Patients assume that healthcare decisions are firmly based on high-quality scientific research; however, in many clinical settings, treatment interventions that have not undergone clinical trial are recommended and practiced. MAs and systematic reviews (SRs) are advantageous in identifying the best available knowledge in CAM. They serve to facilitate public policy, practice decision-making, and integration into cancer and other specialty care. Bringing together research findings, appraising their quality, and synthesizing the results broadens and publicizes knowledge on which to base healthcare decisions. Since MAs and SRs are not available for all areas in cancer CAM, locating clinical trial results, unpublished data (dissertations), and case reports can be time-consuming due to various publication types and the increasing number of biomedical, social science, and nursing journals, some print based and some electronic.

EMBASE is a comprehensive biomedicine and pharmacology database that maintains a collection of more than 4,500 domestic and international journals. Searchable databases include PDQ, which offers two options: (1) PDQ under the "closed trials" option in the advanced search mechanism and (2) PDQ CAM Information Summaries. The American Society for Clinical Oncology (ASCO) sponsors the *Journal of Clinical Oncology* and the People Living with Cancer Web site, which contains abstracts and conference presentations that are viewable online. The National Library of Medicine (NLM) provides access to published results of clinical trials through (1) printed biomedical journals in the main library, (2) electronic full-text articles in publications available through Lonesome Doc, (3) PubMed or Medline searches with the "CAM" limitation for abstracts only in CAM journals (viewable under the "limits" option when searching for a topic), and (4) Medline Plus, which is a free online service of the NLM and the NIH presenting updated health information following clinical trials. Finally, a database sponsored by the University of Maryland Center for Integrated Medicine, known as the Complementary and Alternative Medicine and Pain Database (CAMPAIN), is continually expanding through a grant by the NCCAM.

## RESEARCH

### Clinical cancer CAM research

Cancer clinical trials, by definition, are research studies in humans designed to answer specific questions related to cancer. Clinical research may meet an individual's health needs in terms of quality care and treatment, although that is not the highest goal of research. Meticulously conducted cancer clinical trials are the fastest method to establishing safe and effective preventative, diagnostic, treatment, and/or supportive care interventions. Cancer CAM clinical trials are increasing in number and expanding in design. Table 24-2 provides examples of CAM clinical trials.

In tandem with increasing interest in and use of CAM in the United States, there is a growing number of research dollars dedicated to the prevention, diagnosis, and treatment of acute and chronic conditions (and their related symptoms) through the use of CAM. NIH sponsored CAM research across all institutes more than doubled ($116 million to $303 million) between 1999 and 2005.[135] In fiscal year 2005, the NCI supported approximately $121,077,000 in the form of grants, cooperative agreements, supplements or contracts representing over 400 projects related to cancer CAM.[137]

## ETHICAL CONSIDERATIONS IN RESEARCH

Ethics is a systematic method of answering questions about how and why individuals live and behave in daily life.[138] In regard to clinical research, the ethical questions include (1) *should* research be performed on human subjects? and (2) *how* should this research be performed? The primary ethical struggle in clinical research is that comparatively few individuals accept the risk of being research subjects in order to benefit others and society. Ethicists raise the point that asking subjects to bear the risk of harm for the good of others creates the potential for maltreatment or misuse. Emanuel and colleagues[139] offer a framework for ethical clinical research composed of seven requirements: social value, scientific validity, fair subject selection, favorable risk-benefit ratio, independent review, informed consent, and respect for subjects. If the research inquiry has no social value, there is no justifiable reason to subject patients to risk in a clinical trial. Further, the research must be designed and conducted with rigorous methodology to ensure the validity of its findings. Studies without scientific validity are unethical because they expose patients to risk without the possibility of generalizable knowledge. HCPs often engage in conversations with patients regarding the role of nutrition, herbal medicine, and complementary approaches in cancer care. Conversations such as these are leading HCPs to reconsider their moral, ethical, and legal obligation to remain aware of the best available evidence in CAM, to present the evidence in patient-friendly terms, and to address choices from a comprehensive perspective.[140,141] Ethical struggles in cancer CAM research surrounding informed consent, malpractice, liability, and trial design are likely to be long-term considerations.

## METHODOLOGICAL CHALLENGES

Much is lacking in the amount of available information regarding the use of some CAM modalities: the number and type of patients who use various modalities, how the practices are delivered (method, dose, etc.), how well patients respond, and side effect profiles. A common criticism of CAM by conventional biomedical practitioners is the lack of scientifically conducted research. Since the RCT is the preferred method for evaluating the efficacy of conventional biomedical interventions, many scientists, researchers, and HCPs propose that CAM modalities be evaluated in the same manner. While agreeing that the RCT is a suitable design for some CAM modalities, others suggest the use of both explanatory ("gold standard") and pragmatic RCTs.[142] Pragmatic RCTs do not require that the patient or HCP be "blind" to the modality utilized, and they consider patient preference in the delivery of the modality. Design issues related to the use of a control and methods of assessing the effects of individual differences, minimizing therapist variability, determining acceptable inclusion-exclusion criteria, and assessing treatment outcomes are ongoing considerations in pragmatic trials. The overall goal of all research in cancer CAM is to ensure methodologically rigorous trials that address the unique challenges inherent with CAM modalities without compromising the modality in a manner that is incomplete or inappropriate.[143]

An NCI-sponsored expert panel on cancer symptom research identified the following challenges in CAM research methodology:[144] (1) the development of appropriate controls, shams, and placebo interventions, (2) the development of individualized versus standardized approaches, (3) the development of new drugs within the FDA regulations, (4) the current trend toward developing phase III trials versus I/II developmental trials, (5) ethical issues, (6) the implications for statistics, and (7) tools and measurement issues. The expert panel had the following major recommendations: (1) create truly inert controls that will not cause independent beneficial or harmful effects, (2) balance the need for replication in science with the desire to study interventions in a manner that is consistent with clinical practice, and (3) obtain an investigational new drug (IND) to ensure consistency in product quality and fulfillment of pharmacology and toxicology requirements. Numerous authors[144–147] comprehensively address the methodologic issues in CAM cancer clinical research and emphasize the value in reporting all positive or negative cancer CAM trial results. Table 24-8 summarizes the pervasive methodologic challenges and offers practical solutions.

**TABLE 24-8**

**Methodologic Challenges and Proposed Solutions in Cancer CAM Research**

| Challenges | Solutions |
|---|---|
| Study accrual, adequate sample size, and randomization | Design both explanatory and pragmatic trials |
| Appropriate controls and placebo interventions | Create inert controls that do not cause independent effect |
| Individualized versus standard approaches | Combine the benefits of individualized and standardized approaches<br>Design trials considering whole alternative systems instead of a core modality<br>Design trials to study one intervention from a whole alternative system for a specific disease<br>Propose alternate study designs involving detailed case histories and case series<br>Seek a better understanding of the use of CAM by cancer patients |
| Herbs and nutritional supplements not characterized or standardized | Obtain an IND for herbs and supplements in clinical trials |
| New drug development requirements within FDA regulations | Clarify IND requirements |
| Applicability of RCTs to some CAM therapies | Use qualitative inquiry alongside quantitative measurement<br>Combine the benefits of individualized and standardized approaches<br>Seek collaboration among CAM researchers with varying approaches to design trials |
| Trial design | Conduct phase III trials vs I/II development trials |
| High-quality reporting of effectiveness | Systematically track ongoing studies<br>Report negative trial results in indexed journals |
| Generalization of results | Conduct systematic reviews and meta-analyses |
| Lack of central location in listing cancer CAM clinical trials | Conduct periodic literature reviews of locations of primary clinical trial results |
| Funding to develop and implement meticulously designed clinical trials | Obtain sustained financial support from the government, industry, advocacy groups, and the public |

*Abbreviations*: CAM, complementary and alternative medicine; FDA, Food and Drug Administration; IND, investigational new drug; RCT, randomized controlled trial.

## PATHWAYS FOR PURSUING CANCER CAM RESEARCH

Pathways toward continued research in cancer CAM are multifold. Beginning with an idea alone, the researcher may conduct a literature search to identify cancer researchers who have published on topics related to the proposed mechanism of the CAM therapy. Researchers can then initiate contact, explain the theory, and suggest collaboration. Beginning with a study population but in need of funding, researchers can submit proposals to several grant programs that offer funding, such as the NIH (NCCAM and OCCAM) and the ONS Foundation. Numerous government sources for funding are available.

Preclinical and early drug development processes assist investigators who have a product (single chemical or biological entities) for potential commercial consideration. Two such programs are the NCI's Rapid Access to Preventative Intervention Development (RAPID) and Rapid Access to Intervention Development (RAID) programs. The RAPID program provides any or all of the in vitro preclinical and phase 1 clinical developmental requirements for phase 2 clinical efficacy trials with agents that have the potential to prevent, reverse, or delay carcinogenesis. This includes preclinical pharmacology and toxicology studies, bulk supply, good manufacturing practices manufacturing and formulation, and regulatory and IND support. The RAID program assists in the translation of novel, therapeutic, and anticancer synthetic, natural product, or biologic interventions arising from the academic community to the clinic setting. This includes defining dose and schedules for in vitro and in vivo activity, assay and formulation development, IND directed in vivo toxicology, and planning of clinical trials. Single chemical or biological entities or compounds are generally always evaluated in vitro before beginning in vivo testing. Many CAM approaches are already in use with little or no preclinical or clinical research support, case reports or case series may be the only data available. The NCI Best Case Series program offers the opportunity to compile and submit case scenarios involving CAM for the treatment of cancer. A "persuasive" case is one that meets all of the following criteria: (1) a pathological diagnosis of cancer from a tissue specimen obtained prior to an alternative medicine intervention and after any conventional anticancer therapy, (2) documentation that a patient used the alternative medicine intervention under evaluation, (3) documentation of tumor regression appropriate for the disease type and location, and (4) absence of confounding and/or concurrent anticancer therapies. The medical records, radiographic imaging, and pathologic specimens are reviewed, and cases resulting in tumor regression without evidence of confounders are identified. The main goal of the review is to make an overall assessment of whether further NCI-sponsored research is warranted.[148]

## FUTURE TRENDS

### ROLE OF ONCOLOGY NURSING

Oncology nurses must become knowledgeable in understanding the role of CAM in cancer care, given the rapidly increasing use of CAM. The model for cancer CAM care begins with the nurse, the patient, and other healthcare team members and endorses three core actions: (1) distinguishing fact from fiction, (2) acknowledging misperceptions about CAM, and (3) mixing and unmixing therapies.[149] A baseline knowledge of CAM, beginning with evaluating personal

**TABLE 24-9**

| Endpoints for the Role of Nursing in Cancer CAM | |
|---|---|
| Expand individual baseline knowledge regarding cancer CAM through oral and written modes and experiential learning | Establish institution-specific standards of practice for the use of CAM therapies within specific patient populations |
| Provide high-quality patient and peer education regarding the safety and efficacy of CAM therapies | Document patient consent procedures, tolerance, and response to CAM therapy |
| Facilitate partnerships between patients, conventional HCPs, CAM providers, and colleagues to discuss knowledge and perspectives about cancer CAM | Design a new integrative care program or assist in the quality maintenance of a preestablished program |
| Seek proper training, demonstrate competency, and obtain necessary credentials if practicing a CAM therapy | Develop and update a working knowledge of cost issues and reimbursement of CAM in the community |
| Request and require informed consent (with witness) of patients receiving a CAM therapy | Collaborate in the design of methodologically rigorous cancer CAM treatment and supportive care clinical trials |
| Ensure proper credentialing of a CAM provider prior to recommending the provider to patients | Contribute to the body of nursing knowledge in cancer CAM through publications and presentations in the United States and internationally |

*Source*: Data from Lee.[149]

and professional beliefs, is mandatory. Oncology curricula in the United States guide nurses to approach cancer care using the principles and practices of conventional biomedical, "Western" medicine. Lack of content, misperceptions, and biases surrounding CAM theory and practice within nursing academic programs can leave nurses essentially unprepared to evaluate CAM clinical care options. Nursing curricula without CAM content may inadvertently communicate the notion that CAM has no valid role in health care and convey a need to minimize a patient's choice to seek CAM. Knowledgeable nurses can begin to conduct peer education and establish standards of practice in CAM therapy delivery across practice settings. Nurses must ensure that staff with proper training deliver CAM therapies and those patients sign informed consent. The medical record must contain documentation of the consent procedures, tolerance of, and response to CAM therapy. Major endpoints for the role of nursing in cancer CAM are seen in Table 24-9.

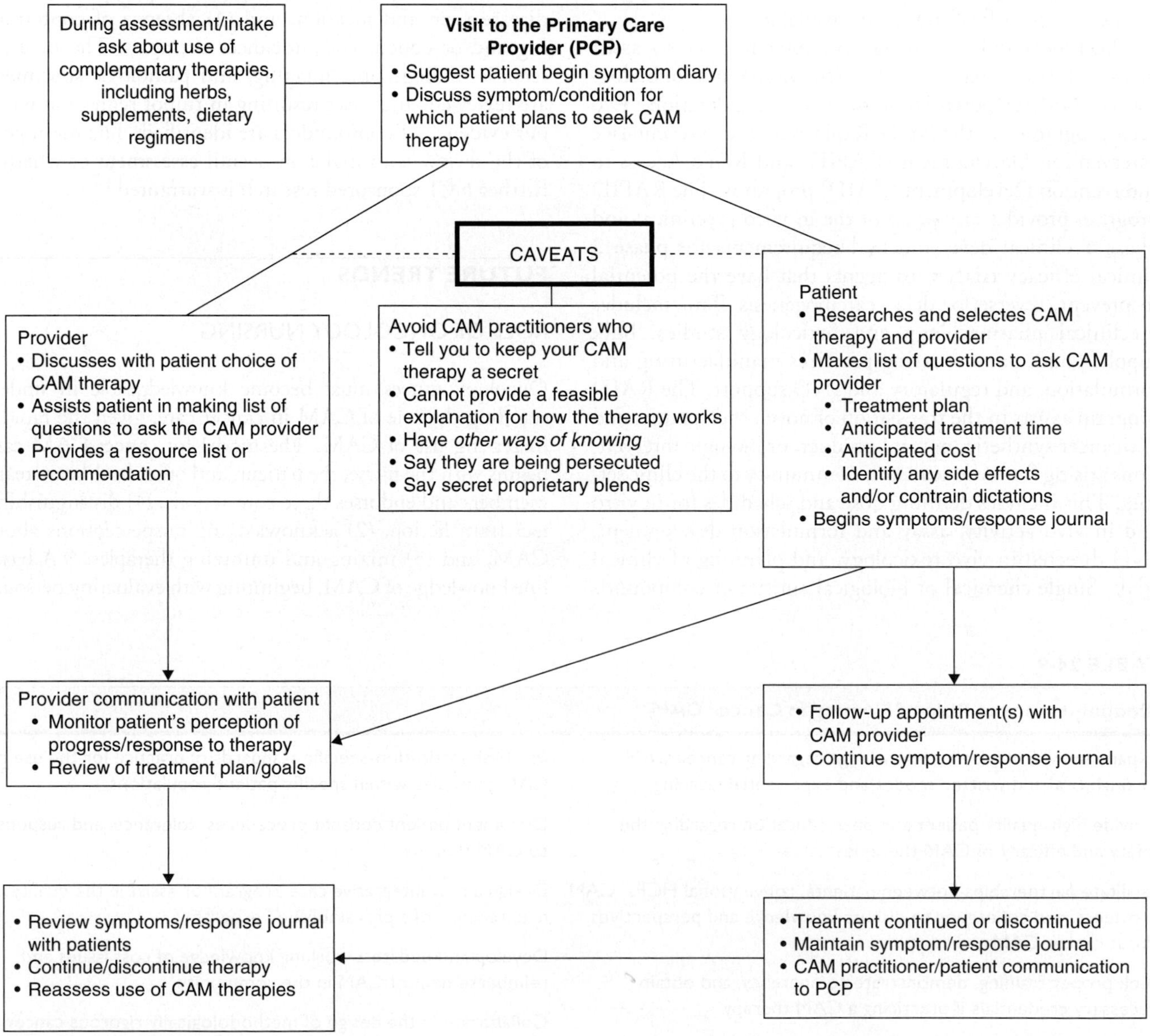


**FIGURE 24–2**

Discussing CAM therapies with patients.

*Source*: Reprinted with permission from Decker GM. Discussing CAM therapies with patients. In Buchsel PC, Yarbor CH eds. Oncology Nursing in the Ambulatory Setting; Issues and Models of Care. 2nd ed. Sadbury, MA: Jones and Bartlett; 2004:355–375.[150]

Given the widespread availability and affordability of many CAM therapies, integration of these therapies into cancer care is inevitable. To safely accomplish this integration, the clinical practice and scientific community must generate high-quality information in several ways: (1) collaborate with CAM practitioners to learn the theoretical basis for alternative systems and appropriate individualized regimens, (2) assist in the design of methodologically sound phase II and III trials, (3) perform periodic SR and MA, and (4) implement integrated curricula for students and continuing education for practitioners. Providing public education programs and forums that address the indications and contraindications creates an opportunity and arena for discussion between patients and practitioners.[150] (See Figure 24-2.)

The law does not provide a definition of complementary and alternative medicine that is inclusive and official. A number of legislative codes and judicial decisions are emerging, however. Of concern is the issue of liability when a licensed practitioner refers a patient to a CAM provider who is not licensed. To complicate matters, some practitioners may be licensed in some states and not in others (for example, massage therapists). To date, we have seen a kind of *law of the majority* influencing decisions and law making. CAM has survived and emerged from an environment of rivalry and competition. Regulatory arenas that will need to be addressed include informed consent, licensure versus certification or registration, scopes of practice, malpractice, and professional discipline. In addition, serious consideration must be given to the possible regulation of CAM as a practice discipline. Issues of reimbursement have already emerged and may be connected to informed consent as well as insurance. Some patients might prefer acupuncture to narcotic analgesia if offered the choice. If a healthcare provider fails to offer CAM therapies as a treatment option, can that be interpreted as withholding treatment? Clarification of these issues is on the immediate horizon. Many HCPs are beginning to acknowledge that health and disease are as connected to nutritional, psychological, spiritual, mind-body, and environmental factors as to physical and chemical factors. Shared perspectives will create previously unimagined possibilities for evidenced-based research and practice.

The American Holistic Nurses Association (AHNA) is the sole nursing body that offers an inclusive certification in the area of CAM. New York University School of Nursing offers an APN Practitioner program endorsed by the AHNA that provides a program of study based on the Standards of Practice for Holistic Nursing.[37] Many nurses choose to undergo training in specific areas of CAM such as bodywork or aromatherapy but these certifications focus on a specific modality versus the broad field. With increasing access to multiples sources, oncology nurses can select preferred modes of learning, and, over time, develop baseline knowledge of CAM. Nursing education and licensure provide a foundation upon which oncology nurses can pursue specialties within integrative oncology.

## REFERENCES


1. Ernst E. Alternative cancer treatments. *UpToDate Online*. 2008. http://www.utdol.com/online/content/topic.do?topicKey=genl_onc/8402&selectedTitle=7-150&source=search_result. Accessed January 2, 2010.
2. NCCAM. *National Center for Complementary and Alternative Medicine*. Bethesda, MD. 2009. http://www.nccam.nih.gov. Accessed January 2, 2010.
3. Society for Integrative Oncology. *Integrative Oncology Guidelines*. 2008. http://www.integrativeonc.org. Accessed January 2, 2010.
4. Oncology Nursing Society. *The Use of Complementary and Alternative Therapies in Cancer Care*. Pittsburgh, PA: Oncology Nursing Society; 2009.
5. OCCAM. *Office of Cancer Complementary and Alternative Medicine*. Bethesda, MD: National Cancer Institute; 2008.
6. Lee CO. Clinical Trials in Cancer Part 1: Biomedical, Complementary, and Alternative Medicine: finding active trial and results of closed trials. *Clin J Oncol Nurs*. 2004;8:531–535.
7. Whorton JC. The history of complementary and alternative medicine. In: Jonas WB, Levin JS, eds. *Essentials of Complementary and Alternative Medicine*. Philadelphia, PA: Lippincott Williams & Wilkins; 1999:16–30.
8. Swerdlow JL. *Nature's Medicine: Plants That Heal*. Washington, DC: National Geographic Society; 2000.
9. Gallin JI. A historical perspective on clinical research. In: Gallin JI, ed. *Principles and Practice of Clinical Research*. San Diego, CA: Academic Press; 2002:1–11.
10. Black JM, Matassarin-Jacobs E. Nursing process. In: Black JM, Matassarin-Jacobs E, eds. *Luckman and Sorensen's MedicalSurgical Nursing: A Psychophysiologic Approach*. Philadelphia, PA: W.B. Saunders; 1993:43–58
11. White JD. Complementary and alternative medicine research: A National Cancer Institute perspective. *Semin Oncol*. 2002;29:546–551.
12. WHCCAMP. *White House Commission on Complementary and Alternative Medicine Policy*. Washington, DC: United States Department of Health and Human Services; August 2003.
13. Institute of Medicine of the National Academies. Complementary and Alternative Medicine in the United States. 2005. http://www.iom.edu/CMS/3793/4829/24487.aspx. Accessed June 21, 2009.
14. Stevinson C. Why patients use complementary and alternative medicine. In: Ernst E, ed. *The Desktop Guide to Complementary and Alternative Medicine: An Evidence-Based Approach*. Edinburgh, Elsevier; 2001:395–403.
15. Furnham A. Why do people choose and use complementary therapies? In: Ernst E, ed. *Complementary Medicine: An Objective Appraisal*. Oxford: Butterworth Heinemann; 1996:71–88.
16. Kaptchuk TJ, Eisenberg DM. The persuasive appeal of alternative medicine. *Ann Intern Med*. 1998;129:1061–1065.
17. Eisenberg DM, Kessler RC, Foster C, et al. Unconventional medicine in the United States. Prevalence, costs, and patterns of use. *N Engl J Med*. 1993;328:246–252.
18. Eisenberg DM, Davis RB, Ettner SL, et al. Trends in alternative medicine use in the United States, 1990–1997: results of a follow-up national survey. *JAMA*. 1998;280:1569–1575.
19. Kessler RC, Davis RB, Foster DF, et al. Long-term trends in the use of complementary and alternative medical therapies in the United States. *Ann Intern Med*. 2001;135:262–268.
20. Ni H, Simile C, Hardy AM. Utilization of complementary and alternative medicine by United States adults: results from the 1999 national health interview survey. *Med Care*. 2002;40:353–358.
21. Basch E, Ulbricht C. Prevalence of CAM use among U.S. cancer patients: an update. *Cancer Integr Med*. 2004;2:13–14.
22. Ernst E, Cassileth BR. The prevalence of complementary/alternative medicine in cancer: a systematic review. *Cancer*. 1998;83:777–782.

23. Bennett M, Lengacher C. Use of complementary therapies in a rural cancer population. *Oncol Nurs Forum.* 1999;26:1287–1294.
24. Sparber A, Bauer L, Curt G, et al. Use of complementary medicine by adult patients participating in cancer clinical trials. *Oncol Nurs Forum.* 2000;27:623–630.
25. Bernstein BJ, Grasso T. Prevalence of complementary and alternative medicine use in cancer patients. *Oncology.* 2001;15:1267–1278, 1283.
26. Vallerand AH, Fouladbakhsh JM, Templin T. The use of complementary/alternative medicine therapies for the self-treatment of pain among residents of urban, suburban, and rural communities. *Am J Pub Health.* 2003;93:923–925.
27. Najm W, Reinsch S, Hoehler F, et al. Use of complementary and alternative medicine among the ethnic elderly. *Altern Ther Health Med.* 2003;9:50–57.
28. Herron M, Glasser M. Use of and attitudes toward complementary and alternative medicine among family practice patients in small rural Illinois communities. *J Rural Health.* 2003;19:279–284.
29. Ashikaga T, Bosompra K, O'Brien P, et al. Use of complementary and alternative medicine by breast cancer patients: Prevalence, patterns and communication with physicians. *Support Care Cancer.* 2002;10: 542–548.
30. Swisher EM, Cohn DE, Goff BA, et al. Use of complementary and alternative medicine among women with gynecologic cancers. *Gynecol Oncol.* 2002;84:363–367.
31. Maskarinec G, Shumay DM, Kakai H, et al. Ethnic differences in complementary and alternative medicine use among cancer patients. *J Altern Complement Med.* 2000;6:531–538.
32. Richardson MA, Sanders T, Palmer JL, et al. Complementary/alternative medicine use in a comprehensive cancer center and the implications for oncology. *J Clin Oncol.* 2000;18:2505–2514.
33. Bridevaux IP. A survey of patients' out-of-pocket payments for complementary and alternative medicine therapies. *Complement Ther Med.* 2004;12:48–50.
34. White A. Economic issues in complementary and alternative medicine. In: Ernst E, ed. *The Desktop Guide to Complementary and Alternative Medicine.* Edinburgh: Elsevier; 2001:415–422.
35. Zoon KC, Yetter RA. The regulation of drugs and biological products by the food and drug administration. In: Gallin J, ed. *Principles and Practice of Clinical Research.* San Diego, CA: Academic Press; 2002:123–132.
36. Dietary Supplement Health and Education Act of 1994, in Pub L No. 103–417 (1994).
37. American Holistic Nurses Association. *Certification in Holistic Nursing.* 2008. http://www.ahna.org/Education/Certification/tabid/1211/Default.aspx. Accessed January 2, 2010.
38. Cohen, M. Legal and ethical issues in complementary and alternative medicine. In Ernst E, ed. *The Desktop Guide to Complementary and Alternative Medicine: An Evidence-Based Approach.* Sundbury, MA: Mosby; 2003:404–411.
39. Alternative Link. *ABC Coding Solutions.* 2008. http://www.alternativelink.com/ali/abc_codes/code_mode.asp. Accessed January 2, 2010.
40. Mumber MP. Clinical decision analysis. In: Mumber MP, ed. *Integrative Oncology Principles and Practice.* New York: Taylor & Francis; 2006b:145–164.
41. White A. Economic issues in complementary and alternative medicine, in Ernst, E(ed): *The Desktop guide to Complementary and Alternative Medicine*, Edinburgh, Elsevier, 2001,pp415–422.
42. Angell M, Kassirer JP. Alternative medicine: The risks of untested and unregulated remedies. *N Engl J Med.* 1998;339:839–841.
43. Cohen L, Markman M, eds. *Integrative Oncology: Incorporating Complementary Medicine into Conventional Cancer Care.* Humana Press; 2008.
44. Lee CO. Herbs and cytotoxic drugs: recognizing and communicating potentially relevant interactions. *Clin J Oncol Nurs.* 2005;9(4): 481–487.
45. Chong OT. An integrative approach to addressing clinical issues in complementary and alternative medicine in an outpatient oncology center. *Clin J Oncol Nurs.* 2006;10(1):83–88.
46. Kenner D. Putting it all together: practicing oriental medicine. In: Cassidy CM, ed. *Contemporary Chinese Medicine and Acupuncture.* Philadelphia, PA: Churchill Livingstone; 2002:125–135.
47. Maizes V, Koffler K, Fleishman S. Revisiting the health history: an integrative medicine approach. *Adv Mind Body Med.* 2002;18(2):31–34.
48. Jonas WB, Linde K, Walach H. How to practice evidence-based complementary and alternative medicine. In: Jonas WB, Levin JS, eds. *Essentials of Complementary and Alternative Medicine.* Philadelphia, PA: Lippincott Williams & Wilkins; 1999:72–87.
49. Markel H. "I Swear by Apollo": on taking the hippocratic oath. *N Engl J Med.* 2004;350:2026–2029.
50. Eisenberg DM. Advising patients who seek alternative medical therapies. *Ann Intern Med.* 1997;127:61–69.
51. Ernst E, ed. *The Desktop Guide to Complementary and Alternative Medicine: An Evidence-Based Approach.* Edinburgh: Elsevier; 2001.
52. Eisenberg DM, Kaptchuk TJ, Laine C, et al. Complementary and alternative medicine: an Annals series. *Ann Intern Med.* 2001;135:208.
52. Mayer DJ. Acupuncture: an evidence-based review of the clinical literature. *Ann Rev Med.* 2000;51:49–63.
53. Han JS, Terenius L. Neurochemical basis of acupuncture analgesia. *Ann Rev Pharmacol Toxicol.* 1982;22:193–220.
54. Andersson S, Lundeberg T. Acupuncture—from empiricism to science: functional background to acupuncture effects in pain and disease. *Med Hypotheses.* 1995;45:271–281.
55. Ernst E, Pittler MH. The effectiveness of acupuncture in treating acute dental pain: a systematic review. *Br Dent J.* 1998;184:443–447.
56. Vickers AJ. Can acupuncture have specific effects on health? A systematic review of acupuncture antiemesis trials. *J R Soc Med.* 1976;89: 303–311.
57. Melchart D, Linde K, Fischer P, et al. Acupuncture for recurrent headaches: a systematic review of randomized controlled trials. *Cephalalgia.* 1999;19:779–786.
58. Lee A, Fan LTY. Stimulation of the wrist acupuncture point P6 for preventing postoperative nausea and vomiting. http:// www.cochrane.org/reviews/en/ab003281.html. Accessed June 16, 2009.
59. Aikins Murphy P. Alternative therapies for nausea and vomiting of pregnancy. *Obstet Gynecol.* 1998;91:149–155.
60. Ernst E, White A. Life-threatening adverse reactions after acupuncture? A systematic review. *Pain* 1997;71: 123–126
61. Kaptchuk TJ, Acupuncture: theory efficacy and practice. Ann Inter med. 2002:136:374–383.
62. Crew KD, Capodice JL, Greenlee H, et al. Pilot study of acupuncture for the treatment of joint symptoms related to adjuvant aromatase inhibitor therapy in postmenopausal breast cancer patients. *J Cancer Surviv.* 2007;1:283–291.
63. Segen JC. Dictionary of Alternative Medicine. Appleton & Lange, Stamford, 1998 Complementary, and Alternative Medicine: finding active trial and results of closed trials. *Clin J Oncol Nurs.* 2004;8: 531–535.
64. Potter P. What are the distinctions between Reiki and therapeutic touch? *Clin J Oncol Nurs.* 2003;7:89–91.
65. Rexilius SJ, Mundt C, Erickson Megel M, et al. Therapeutic effects of massage therapy and healing touch on caregivers of patients undergoing autologous hematopoietic stem cell transplant. *Oncol Nurs Forum.* 2002;29:E35-E44.
66. Olson K, Hanson J. Using Reiki to manage pain: a preliminary report. *Cancer Prev Control.* 1997;1:108–113.
67. Lafreniere KD, Mutus B, Cameron S, et al. Effects of therapeutic touch on biochemical and mood indicators in women. *J Altern Complement Med.* 1999;5:367–370.
68. Post-White J, Kinney ME, Savik K, et al. Therapeutic massage and healing touch improve symptoms in cancer. *Integr Cancer Ther.* 2003;2: 332–344.

69. Mansour AA, Beuche M, Laing G, et al. A study to test the effectiveness of placebo Reiki standardization procedures developed for a planned Reiki efficacy study. *J Altern Complement Med.* 1999;5:153–164.
70. Rosenfeld I. *Dr. Rosenfeld's Guide to Alternative Medicine.* New York: Knopf; 1996.
71. White AR, Williamson J, Hart A, et al. A blinded investigation into the accuracy of reflexology charts. *Complement Ther Med.* 2000;8: 166–172.
72. Weiger WA, Smith M, Boon H, et al. Advising patients who seek complementary and alternative medical therapies for cancer. *Ann Intern Med.* 2002;137:889–903.
73. Soden K, Vincent K, Craske S, et al. A randomized controlled trial of aromatherapy massage in a hospice setting. *Palliat Med.* 2004;18:87–92.
74. Goodfellow LM. The effects of therapeutic back massage on psychophysiologic variables and immune function in spouses of patients with cancer. *Nurs Res.* 2003;52:318–328.
75. Hodgson H. Does reflexology impact on cancer patients' quality of life? *Nurs Stand.* 2000;14:33–38.
76. Oleson T, Flocco W. Randomized controlled study of premenstrual symptoms treated with ear, hand, and foot reflexology. *Obstet Gynecol.* 1993;82:906–911.
77. Wang XM. Treating type II diabetes mellitus with foot reflexotherapy. *Zhongguo Zhong Xi Yi Jie He Za Zhi.* 1993;13:536–588.
78. Ernst E, Siev-Ner I, Gamus D. Complementary medicine — a critical review. *Isr J Med Sci.* 1997;33:808–815.
79. Launso L, Brendstrup E, Arnberg S. An exploratory study of reflexological treatment for headache. *Altern Ther Health Med.* 1999;5:57–65.
80. Jonas WB, Linde K. Conducting and evaluating clinical research on complementary and alternative medicine. In: Gallin J, ed. *Principles and Practice of Clinical Research.* San Diego, CA: Academic Press; 2002: 401–420.
81. Decker G, ed. *An Introduction to Complementary and Alternative Therapies.* Pittsburgh, PA: Oncology Nursing Press; 1999.
82. Ernst E. The current position of complementary/alternative medicine in cancer. *Eur J Cancer.* 2003;39:2273–2277.
83. Perez C. Clinical aromatherapy, Part I: an introduction into nursing practice. *Clin J Oncol Nurs.* 2003;7:595–596.
84. Thomas DV. Aromatherapy: mythical, magical, or medicinal? *Holist Nurs Pract.* 2002;16:8–16.
85. Cooke B, Ernst E. Aromatherapy: a systematic review. *Br J Gen Pract.* 2000;50:493–496.
86. Louis M, Kowalski SD. Use of aromatherapy with hospice patients to decrease pain, anxiety, and depression and to promote an increased sense of well-being. *Am J Hosp Palliat Care.* 2002;19:381–386.
87. Olleveant NA, Humphris G, Roe B. How big is a drop? A volumetric assay of essential oils. *J Clin Nurs.* 1999;8:299–304.
88. Fellowes D, Barnes K, Wilkinson S. Aromatherapy and massage for symptom relief in patients with cancer. *Cochrane Database Syst Rev.* 2004;2:CD002287.
89. Maddocks-Jennings W. Critical incident: idiosyncratic allergic reactions to essential oils. *Complement Ther Nurs Midwifery.* 2004;10:58–60.
90. Lee CO. Clinical aromatherapy, part II: safe guidelines for integration into clinical practice. *Clin J Oncol Nurs.* 2003;7:597–598.
91. Campbell L, Pollard A, Roeton C. The development of clinical practice guidelines for the use of aromatherapy in a cancer setting. *Aust J Holist Nurs.* 2001;8:14–22.
92. Avis A. Aromatherapy in practice. *Nurs Stand.* 1999;13:14–15.
93. VandeCreek L, Rogers E, Lester J. Use of alternative therapies among breast cancer outpatients compared with the general population. *Altern Ther Health Med.* 1999;5:71–76.
94. Durken M, Herrnring C, Finckh B, et al. Impaired plasma antioxidative defense and increased nontransferrin-bound iron during high-dose chemotherapy and radiochemotherapy preceding bone marrow transplantation. *Free Radic Biol Med.* 2000;28:887–894.
95. Ladas EJ, Jacobson JS, Kennedy DD, et al. Antioxidants and cancer therapy: a systematic review. *J Clin Oncol.* 2004;22:517–528.
96. Omenn GS, Goodman GE, Thornquist MD, et al. Effects of a combination of beta carotene and vitamin A on lung cancer and cardiovascular disease. *N Engl J Med.* 1996;334:1150–1155.
97. Albanes D, Heinonen OP, Huttunen JK, et al. Effects of alphatocopherol and beta-carotene supplements on cancer incidence in the Alpha-Tocopherol Beta-Carotene Cancer Prevention Study. *Am J Clin Nutr.* 1995;62(6 suppl):1427S-1430S.
98. Conklin KA. Dietary antioxidants during cancer chemotherapy: impact on chemotherapeutic effectiveness and development of side effects. *Nutr Cancer.* 2000;37:1–18.
99. Ray SD, Wong V, Bagchi D, et al. In vivo protection of DNA damage associated apoptotic and necrotic cell deaths during acetaminophen-induced nephrotoxicity, amiodarone-induced lung toxicity and doxorubicin-induced cardiotoxicity by a novel IH636 grape seed proanthocyanidin extract. *Res Commun Mol Pathol Pharmacol.* 2000;107:137–166.
100. Lenzhofer R, Ganzinger U, Rameis H, et al. Acute cardiac toxicity in patients after doxorubicin treatment and the effect of combined tocopherol and nifedipine pretreatment. *J Cancer Res Clin Oncol.* 1983;106:143–147.
101. Jonas CR, Puckett AB, Jones DP, et al. Plasma antioxidant status after high-dose chemotherapy: a randomized trial of parenteral nutrition in bone marrow transplantation patients. *Am J Clin Nutr.* 2000;72:181–189.
102. Sundstrom H, Korpela H, Sajanti E, et al. Supplementation with selenium, vitamin E and their combination in gynaecological cancer during cytotoxic chemotherapy. *Carcinogenesis.* 1989;10:273–278.
103. Holm LE, Nordevang E, Hjalmar ML, et al. Treatment failure and dietary habits in women with breast cancer. *J Natl Cancer Inst.* 1993;85:32–36.
104. Ingram D. Diet and subsequent survival in women with breast cancer. *Br J Cancer.* 1994;69:592–595.
105. Brawley OW, Parnes H. Prostate cancer prevention trials in the USA. *Eur J Cancer.* 2000;36:1312–1315.
106. Hendler SS, Rorvik D. *PDR for Nutritional Supplements.* Montvale, NJ: Thomson.
107. Skidmore-Roth,L. Mosby's Handbook Of Herbs and Natural Supplements. Mosby, 2009.
108. Fetrow C, Avila A. *A Professional's Handbook of Complementary and Alternative Medicines.* Philadephia, PA: Springhouse; 1999.
109. Ernst E. Harmless herbs? A review of the recent literature. *Am J Med.* 1998;104:170–178.
110. Ernst E. The risk-benefit profile of commonly used herbal therapies: Ginkgo, St. John's wort, ginseng, echinacea, saw palmetto, and kava. *Ann Intern Med.* 2002;136:42–53.
111. Harrer G, Schmidt U, Kuhn U, et al. Comparison of equivalence between the St. John's wort extract LoHyp-57 and fluoxetine. *Arzneimittelforschung.* 1999;49:289–296.
112. Philipp M, Kohnen R, Hiller KO. Hypericum extract versus imipramine or placebo in patients with moderate depression: randomised multicentre study of treatment for eight weeks. *Br Med J.* 1999;319:1534–1538.
113. Schrader E. Equivalence of St. John's wort extract (Ze 117) and fluoxetine: a randomized, controlled study in mild-moderate depression. *Int Clin Psychopharmacol.* 2000;15:61–68.
114. Woelk H. Comparison of St. John's wort and imipramine for treating depression: randomised controlled trial. *Br Med J.* 2000;321:536–539.
115. Wheatley D. Hypericum in seasonal affective disorder (SAD). *Curr Med Res Opin.* 1999;15:33–37.
116. Gulick RM, McAuliffe V, Holden-Wiltse J, et al. Phase I studies of hypericin, the active compound in St. John's wort, as an antiretroviral agent in HIV-infected adults. AIDS Clinical Trials Group Protocols 150 and 258. *Ann Intern Med.* 1999;130:510–514.
117. Stevinson C, Ernst E. A pilot study of Hypericum perforatum for the treatment of premenstrual syndrome. *BJOG.* 2000;107:870–876.

118. Markowitz JS, Donovan JL, DeVane CL, et al. Effect of St. John's wort on drug metabolism by induction of cytochrome P450 3A4 enzyme. *JAMA.* 2003;290:1500–1504.
119. Ernst E, Rand JI, Stevinson C. Complementary therapies for depression: an overview. *Arch Gen Psychiatry.* 1998;55:1026–1032.
120. Bishop SR. What do we really know about mindfulness-based stress reduction? *Psychosom Med.* 2002;64:71–83.
121. Astin JA, Berman BM, Bausell B et al. The efficacy of mindfulness meditation plus Qigong movement therapy in the treatment of fibromyalgia: a randomized controlled trial. *J Rheumatol.* 2003;30: 2257–2262.
122. Tacon AM, McComb J, Caldera Y et al. Mindfulness meditation, anxiety reduction, and heart disease: a pilot study. *Fam Community Health.* 2003;26:25–33.
123. Carlson LE, Ursuliak Z, Goodey E, et al. The effects of a mindfulness meditation-based stress reduction program on mood and symptoms of stress in cancer outpatients: 6-month followup. *Support Care Cancer.* 2001;9:112–123.
124. Ropka ME, Spencer-Cisek P. PRISM: Priority Symptom Management Project phase I: assessment. *Oncol Nurs Forum.* 2001;28:1585–1594.
125. Oncology Nursing Society. *Quality Cancer Care (Oncology Nursing Society Position Statement).* Pittsburgh, PA: 2009.
126. AARP: American Association for Retired Persons. *Complementary and Alternative Medicine Research Report.* 2007. http://assets.aarp.org/rgcenter/health/cam_2007.pdf. Accessed January 2, 2010.
127. Rizzo JA, Xie Y. Managed care, consumerism, preventative medicine: does a causal connection exist? *Manag Care Interface.* 2006;19(7):46–50.
128. *CAHCIM Consortium of Academic Health Centers for Integrative Medicine.* 2008. http://www.imconsortium.org/cahcim/home.html. Accessed January 2, 2010.
129. Halcón LL, Chlan LL, Kreitzer MJ, Leonard BJ. Complementary therapies and healing practices: Faculty/student beliefs and attitudes and the implications for nursing education. *J Prof Nurs.* 2003;19(6):387–397.
130. Sofhauser CD. Development of a minor in complementary health. *Nurse Educ.* 2002;27(3):118–122.
131. American Botanical Council. *The ABC Herbal Information Course.* 2008. http://abc.herbalgram.org/site/PageServer?pagename=Programs_Services#HIC. Accessed January 2, 2010.
132. CMBM Center for Mind-Body Medicine. *Science. Training. Community. Outreach.* 2008. http://www.cmbm.org/. Accessed January 2, 2010.
133. National Center for Complementary and Alternative Medicine. *Complementaryand Alternative Medicine Online Continuing Education Series.* 2008. http://nccam.nih.gov/videolectures/. Accessed January 2, 2010.
134. Lee CO. Communicating facts and knowledge in cancer complementary and alternative medicine. *Semin Oncol Nurs.* 2005;21(3):201–214.
135. National Cancer Institute: *NCI Cancer Facts Sheet: Evaluating Health Information on the Internet.* www.Cancer.gov/Cancertopics/factsheet/information/internet. Accessed January 2, 2010.
136. National Center for Complementary and Alternative Medicine. *Complementary and Alternative Medicine Funding by NIH Institute/Center.* 2008. http://nccam.nih.gov/about/budget/institute-center.htm. Accessed January 2, 2010.
137. National Cancer Institute. *NCI's Cancer CAM Research Portfolio.* 2008. http://www.cancer.gov/cam/research_portfolio.html. Accessed January 2, 2010.
138. Grady C. Ethical principles in clinical research. In: Gallin JI, ed. *Principles and Practice of Clinical Research.* San Diego, CA: Academic Press; 2002:15–25.
139. Emanuel EJ, Wendler D, Grady C. What makes clinical research ethical? *JAMA.* 2000;283:2701–2711.
140. Miller FG, Emanuel EJ, Rosenstein DL, et al. Ethical issues concerning research in complementary and alternative medicine. *JAMA.* 2004;291:599–604.
141. Cohen MH. Legal and ethical issues in complementary and alternative medicine. In: Ernst E, ed. *The Desktop Guide to Complementary and Alternative Medicine: An Evidenced-Based Approach.* Edinburgh, Elsevier; 2001:404–411.
142. Tunis SR, Stryer DB, Clancy CM. Practical clinical trials: increasing the value of clinical research for decision making in clinical and health policy. *JAMA.* 2003;290:1624–1632.
143. Smith WB. Research methodology: implications for CAM pain research. *Clin J Pain.* 2004;20:3–7.
144. Richardson MA, Straus SE. Complementary and alternative medicine: opportunities and challenges for cancer management and research. *Semin Oncol.* 2002;29:531–545.
145. Carter B. Methodological issues and complementary therapies: Researching intangibles? *Complement Ther Nurs Midwifery.* 2003;9: 133–139.
146. Hyland ME. Methodology for the scientific evaluation of complementary and alternative medicine. *Complement Ther Med.* 2003;11:146–153.
147. Ezzo J. Should journals devote space to trials with no results? *J Altern Complement Med.* 2003;9:611–612.
148. Lee CO. Translational research in cancer complementary and alternative medicine: the National Cancer Institute's Best Case Series program. *Clin J Oncol Nurs.* 2004;8:212–214.
149. Lee CO. CAM in the 21st Century in the US: role of nursing and evidence-based practice efforts. In: *4th Annual Oncology Nursing Society Institutes of Learning.* Philadelphia, PA: Oncology Nursing Society; 2003.
150. Decker GM. Discussing CAM therapies with patients. In: Buchsel PC, Yarbro CH, eds. *Oncology Nursing in the Ambulatory Setting: Issues and Models of Care.* 2nd ed. Sudbury, MA: Jones and Bartlett; 2004:355–375.

# PART IV

# Cancer Symptom Management

CHAPTER

25

Dana N. Rutledge, RN, PhD

# Evidence-Based Oncology Nursing

## INTRODUCTION

Information use in clinical decisions has to be viewed in the context of a service environment in which nurses are prevented from developing their decisions by the competing demands made on their time and skills by the sheer volume of workload. It is little wonder that nurses see clinical information use in routine decision making as a fairly low priority.[1]

On any given day, oncology nurses may face several decisions, such as:

- How to determine whether a woman with stage III breast cancer would be a candidate for exercise treatment aimed at preventing or ameliorating cancer-related fatigue.
- Whether to recommend around-the-clock dosing of a patient's pain medication.
- How best to discuss advance directives with a person newly diagnosed with metastatic lung cancer.
- A dilemma in understanding and knowing how to respond to a patient who has missed four clinic appointments.

Thus, oncology nurses, along with most nurses, need evidence to help give good patient care. A recent British study of nurses in three diverse medical surgical settings[1] found that nurses make clinical decisions in several key areas. These include decisions related to (1) type of intervention or effectiveness of an intervention; (2) choice and implementation of interventions (including their timing) to enhance benefits to patients; (3) selection of communication strategies to and from patients, families, and colleagues; (4) configuration of service organization, delivery, and management; and (5) interpretation of cues in the process of delivering patient care.

Unfortunately, oncology nurses, like the acute care nurses in the British study,[1] may not seek out the optimal evidence in making decisions regarding patient care. They may instead rely upon easily accessible evidence, which is that provided by their nursing colleagues and peers (Table 25-1). Using peers as a sole source of evidence excludes the potential effectiveness of using research-based evidence that may help nurses make decisions and use tools that optimize patient outcomes, decrease variations in care delivery, and promote patient satisfaction. In fact, evidence-based practice (EBP) has not become a reality for nurses in many areas of practice.[2–4] It is imperative that nurses go beyond easy access to find potentially important information that can enhance patient care. Practice based upon good evidence serves to improve patient care.

**TABLE 25-1**

**Advantages and Disadvantages of Information Obtained from Nursing Peers**

| |
|---|
| **Advantages** |
| Easy to access |
| Fast retrieval |
| Cheap |
| Tailored to the needs of the person asking |
| Usually easy to understand |
| Does not usually require appraisal by the person asking |
| **Disadvantages** |
| May be vague |
| May be out of date |
| May be wrong |
| May be based up on inappropriate sources |
| Nursing peers may have biases |

## EVIDENCE-BASED NURSING

What is evidence-based nursing? It is the integration of best evidence available, combined with nursing expertise and the values and preferences of the individuals, families, and communities that are served.[5] Further, evidence-based nursing is a "process of shared decision making between practitioner, patient, and others significant."[6] Evidence-based nursing requires three things: (1) that nurses have access to the evidence; (2) that a consensus of opinion exists on the implications of the evidence; and (3) that nurses in a work setting have the authority to exercise their judgment in planning and providing care. Thus, making evidence-based decisions requires access to research and other sources of evidence, the use of clinical expertise, and an understanding and acknowledgment of patient preferences.[1]

In "Nursing's Agenda for the Future,"[7] the American Nurses Association notes that decision making and positive change in nursing need to be driven by reliable data, and that selected nursing practices should lead to quality patient care. This should encourage nurses who want to deliver excellent nursing care to find out how to access all sources of evidence appropriate for their situation, and then to find out how best to implement and evaluate EBP changes or innovations.

## A FRAMEWORK: IMPLEMENTATION OF EVIDENCE-BASED PRACTICE

Out of Great Britain has come a model that seeks to explain what is necessary for EBP to occur. Basically, an EBP change is most likely to be successfully implemented when three things occur[8–10]:

- The evidence is strong and matches the professional consensus and patient need.

- The work setting or context is receptive to change, with strong leadership, decentralized decision making, and appropriate quality monitoring systems.
- The proposed change is appropriately facilitated through the system by skilled internal or external facilitators or change agents.

Evidence is defined as a combination of research, professional expertise, and patient preference.[11] Context is the environment or setting where a proposed change may be implemented. Each setting has its own organizational culture, unique leadership team and system, and degree of measurement for quality outcomes. Ideal facilitators or persons in charge of facilitating a change are clearly authorized by a system to initiate change, are credible or respected in the eyes of the users of a change, and have a flexible style of relating to others. Facilitators enable people to understand what must be changed and how to achieve the desired outcomes, to make sense of the "evidence" to be implemented[9]; to do this, they consciously use a set of interpersonal and group skills to cross professional and organizational boundaries and, eventually, to achieve the change.[8] A basic assumption of the model is that level of evidence, factors related to context, and facilitation are all important for an EBP change to occur.[10]

## BECOMING A NURSE WHO BASES CARE UPON EVIDENCE

Oncology nurses who question the way things are done, who ask themselves, "what is the best way to accomplish this goal?" and who seek to understand why patients behave the way they do are already seeking EBP. Nurses in all roles can promote and assure that EBP occurs. Roles integral to the EBP process are listed in Table 25-2.[1,12–15] Many sources of information are available to help nurses obtain the most truthful or valid information, that is, to get the evidence to answer particular questions. Several steps are involved between obtaining the evidence and implementing a practice change. Barriers to fully implementing EBP are shown in Table 25-3.[16–23] Nurses must be aware that these barriers may exist and must be addressed. Note that advanced practice nurses who are seeking evidence related to treatment decisions for individual patients may have different needs in implementing EBP. Besides those mentioned in this chapter, multiple resources related to evidence-based medicine will assist advanced practice nurses in coming up with good decisions. Some of these resources are listed in Figure 25-1.

### ASKING GOOD QUESTIONS

Oncology nurses deliver care in a multitude of environments, so their clinical questions will vary depending upon setting and other factors. Focusing an inquiry on a specific area or topic assists in finding appropriate evidence. If a search is too broad, the amount of evidence found can be overwhelming, while a too-narrow focus can lead to insufficient findings. Different types of inquiries lead to seeking different types of evidence. For example, questions such as "What works?" or "What works best?" will send nurses to sources such as experimental or clinical trial studies. On the other hand, trying to determine communication techniques to enhance adherence to oral chemotherapeutic agents may require reading findings from correlational studies (predictors of patients likely to be adherent or nonadherent) or qualitative studies (patient experiences with taking oral chemotherapy). For some clinical questions, especially those involving comparisons among strategies, oncology nurses may find it helpful to use the population, intervention, comparison intervention, outcome (PICO) method of question framing.[24] For example, if a nurse is interested in evaluating the accuracy of one tool vs another in assessing cognitive impairment in persons who have terminal cancer, PICO could be applied as follows:

- Population: terminally ill persons with cancer; the group that the question is about, the patients similar to the nurse's patients
- Intervention or tool: cognitive impairment assessment tool A, the tool the nurse is interested in or is considering
- Comparison intervention or tool: tool B, the alternate tool that can be compared with tool A
- Outcome: accuracy in measuring cognitive impairment.

The oncology nurse seeks evidence that contains all elements of PICO, when possible; for example, studies that compare the accuracy of tool A to that of tool B in terminally ill patients with cancer.

### OBTAINING EVIDENCE

Ideally, once a nurse or group of nurses determines a clinical focus, they would determine what type of evidence is necessary to help them find an answer. Besides clinical expertise and patient preferences, other types of evidence have been deemed helpful to supplement the research core of evidence.[25,26] These sources include national benchmarking data, cost-effectiveness analyses, pathophysiology texts, chart review data, quality improvement and risk management trends, standards of care, and infection control data. For a question related to central venous catheter (CVC) site care, oncology nurses would benefit by seeking out local CVC infection rates and policies or standards of care. With any search, sources of evidence must be identified and a plan for retrieval developed, including how time will be found to obtain, read, and evaluate evidence sources (see Table 25-3 for barriers related to obtaining and appraising evidence).

**TABLE 25-2**

**Potential Roles of Nurses in Evidence-Based Practice Process**

| Role | Description |
|---|---|
| Information brokers | Nurses who maintain up-to-date knowledge in a clinical area; they influence others' attitudes or behaviors in a desired manner and may be called opinion leaders.[a] Clinical nurse specialists are often information brokers. |
| Interested nurses | Nurses who want to practice from a solid evidence base will read nursing literature, particularly systematic reviews and research reports in areas of interest to them. Nurses will attend presentations where research findings are offered. Becoming a research consumer is a skill that can be taught. |
| Systems-savvy nurses | Nurses who truly understand the workings of a work setting and how changes happen there. They know who the powerful people are and the mechanisms necessary to adopt and maintain change. |
| Change agents or facilitators | Nurses who facilitate appropriate use promising new knowledge. Going beyond dissemination of new knowledge, they assist with diffusion and implementation of practices. They may serve as project leaders or may be external consultants. They flex between being nurses or patient advocates and project advocates. When successful, change agents may be considered opinion leaders. |
| Retrievers | Nurses who are experienced in using libraries and retrieving manuscripts can be vital to getting started in accessing evidence. Librarians may also be useful in this role. Manuscript retrieval can be a stumbling block early in an EBP project unless retrievers are identified. |
| Critiquers | Nurses who are excellent evaluators of nursing research have often had graduate research courses or gained much experience reading research studies. Critiquers enjoy reading and have good analytic and synthesis skills. |
| Early new practice users | Early adopters of EBP changes may tend to be leaders, although not by job description. They like learning about and trying out new ideas. Subsequently, they serve as role models for other nurses who see them using new practices. |
| Late new practice users | Nurses who follow others in using new practices may be considered early majority or late adopters. These nurses need to understand the rational behind practice changes. As early majority users adopt a practice after seeing early new practice users, diffusion of the practice amplifies, and the overall rate of adoption increases. The late majority eventually use a practice change but may need authoritative pressure to maintain it. |
| Nurse educators | EBPs can be taught by educators who emphasize the research or evidence base behind an innovation. Teaching needs to emphasize that a practice or tool has been tested and found useful, that is, its research or evidence base should include rationales for patient care practices. |

[a]Opinion leadership is the degree to which an individual is formally able to influence the attitudes and behavior of others in a specific direction and with relative frequency.[10]

*Abbreviation*: EBP, evidence-based practice.

*Source*: Data from Thompson et al[1]; Rutledge et al[12]; Rutledge[13]; Rogers[14]; and Funk et al.[15]

For any topic, finding a recent systematic review or clinical practice guideline based upon a systematic review related to the topic can help in understanding the evidence. A systematic review is an information analysis and synthesis that summarizes a body of literature, focuses on findings, and draws conclusions about the clinical implications of the findings. Systematic reviews follow particular steps, from identifying the focus area to determining what outcome data are extracted from selected studies. Using a systematic review as a starting point is efficient because reviewing primary studies takes longer and may require skills that many clinicians do not have.[27] Also, the authors of a systematic review have "already done the work of accumulating and summarizing the best of the published (and ideally unpublished) evidence," according to McKibbon and colleagues.[28] Systematic reviews may be quantitative (meta-analysis) or qualitative (narrative). In quantitative reviews, a collection of study results from individual studies is statistically analyzed in order to integrate findings. In qualitative reviews, primary study results are summarized with no statistical combination of results, but with an attempt to reduce the likelihood of bias.[29] All reviews are subject to bias and thus should be read critically. When a review is prepared carefully using specific steps, it is less likely that author bias has

**TABLE 25-3**

**Barriers to Carrying Out Research Utilization or Evidence-Based Practice**

**Seeking/Appraising Evidence Phase**
Lack of time to read research
Difficulty reading and interpreting research studies
Unclear implications for practice from research studies
Inability to find all of the relevant research studies
Lack of awareness of research findings
Staff does not see the value of research for practice
Isolation of nurses from knowledgeable colleagues with whom to discuss the research
Organizational evidence (policies, protocols, etc.) not readily available
Lack of nurse responsibility in uptake of evidence-based nursing
Heavy reliance of nurses on experiential knowledge (gained through interactions with patients/peers)

**Implementation/Evaluation Phase**
Lack of authority to change patient care
Lack of time to implement new ideas
Lack of confidence about beginning to change practice
Lack of support of administration, staff, or physicians
Research findings not generalizable to work setting
Staff unwilling to change or try new ideas
Inadequate resources for implementation of practice changes

*Source*: Data from Rutledge et al[16]; Carroll et al[17]; McCleary and Brown[18]; Nilsson et al[19]; Parahoo and McCaughan[20]; McCaughan et al[21]; and Hannes et al.[22]

Conn VS, Isaramalai SA, Rath S, et al: Beyond Medline for literature searches. *J Nurs Scholarsh* 2003; 35:177–182.

DePalma JA, McGuire DB: Research. In: Hamric AB, Spross JA, CM(eds.): *Advanced Nursing Practice: An Integrative Approach* (ed 3). Philadelphia, Saunders, 2004; 257–300.

Glanville I, Schirm V, Wineman NM. Using evidence-based practice for managing clinical outcomes in advanced practice nursing. J *Nurs Care Qual* 2000; 15:1–11.

Guyatt G, Rennie D, eds. *The Evidence-Based Medicine Working Group: Users' Guides to the Medical Literature. Essentials of Evidence-Based Clinical Practice.* Chicago, AMA Press, 2002.

Jacobs SK, Rosenfeld P, Haber J. Information literacy as the foundation for evidence-based practice in graduate nursing education: a curriculum-integrated approach. *J Prof Nurs* 2003; 19:320–328.

Jadad AR. The Cochrane Collaboration: advances and challenges in improving evidence-based decision making. *Med Dec Making* 1998; 18:2–9.

Morrisey LJ, DeBourgh GA. Finding evidence: refining literature searching skills for the advanced practice nurse. *AACN Clin Issues* 2001; 12:5760–577.

Savoie I, Helmer D, Green CJ, et al. Beyond Medline: reducing bias through extended systematic review search. *Int J Technol Assess Health Care* 2003; 19:168–178.

Soukop SM. The Center for Advanced Nursing Practice evidence-based practice model: promoting the scholarship of practice. *Nurs Clin North Am* 2000; 35:301–309.

**FIGURE 25-1**

Resources for advanced practice nurses.

occurred. When reviews are older than a couple of years, nurses should supplement their search with studies done since the oldest study cited in the review to assure the timeliness of recommendations based upon the review.

Where can systematic reviews be found? Figure 25-2 shows sources for reviews, with examples that might be of interest to oncology nurses. Reviews can also be sought by using computerized databases such as Medline and CINAHL, and limiting searches to review articles. Examples of searches using PubMed and CINAHL are given in Figure 25-3.

Some topics are of such importance to organizations that clinical practice guidelines (CPG) have been developed following a systematic review. CPGs contain recommendations based upon systematic reviews and expert consensus that aim to help healthcare providers and patients make decisions in specific clinical situations, such as when pain and other symptoms exist, when help is needed with patient-centered communication and decision making and when coordination of care may be less than optimal.[30] When done well, CPGs can be a great resource for nurses seeking answers to clinical questions. An excellent resource for those seeking CPGs is the National Guideline Clearinghouse (NGC), a public resource for evidence-based CPGs (http://www.guideline.gov). It includes guideline summaries with information about development along with available links to full-text guidelines and ordering information for print copies. The National Comprehensive Cancer Network guidelines[31] are another source of information for cancer-specific recommendations; guidelines are available for treatment of cancer by site, for detection, prevention, and risk reduction (eg, cervical cancer screening), and for supportive care (eg, adult cancer pain, venous thromboembolic disease). CPGs are developed by many different organizations and individuals, so nurses are urged to closely evaluate them for quality and appropriateness.

A new source for evidence-based recommendations is the Putting Evidence into Practice (PEP) Resources available through the Oncology Nursing Society (http://www.ons.org/research). A Nurse Sensitive Outcomes section contains information on measuring outcomes specific to oncology patients, such as pain, vomiting, peripheral neuropathies, and mucositis. Oncology Nursing Society advanced practice nurses, staff nurses, and nurse scientists developed these through the review, critique, and synthesis of appropriate literature on interventions for specific oncology patient outcomes. The resources provide recommendations for practice and include cards, definitions, evidence

**Cochrane Library Database of Systematic Reviews** (*www.thecochranelibrary.com*) This subscription-only database contains full-text reviews that are highly structured, systematically prepared, and done using meta-analyses, when possible. Done by international groups made up predominantly of physicians, the reviews may be biased toward randomized clinical trials. These reviews are also indexed in Medline and CINAHL.

*Examples*

Fellowes D, Wilkinson S, Moore P, et al. Communication skills training for health care professionals working with cancer patients, their families and/or carers. *Cochrane Database Syst Rev.* 2:CD003751, 2003.

Murray SM, Pindoria S. Nutrition support for bone marrow transplant patients. *Cochrane Database Syst Rev.* 2:CD002920, 2002.

Quigley C. Hydromorphone for acute and chronic pain. *Cochrane Database Syst Rev.* 1:CD003447, 2002.

**Database of Abstracts of Reviews of Effectiveness** (DARE) (*http://nhscrd.york.ac.uk/darehp.htm*) This is a database of quality assessed reviews, developed and updated by the National Health Service Centre for Reviews and Dissemination (CRD) at the University of York. In a search on 1/6/04 using the search terms, "sexual" and "cancer," 22 hits were obtained. The first 3 are listed as egs; structured abstracts written by CRD reviewers are linked to the titles on the DARE database.

*Examples*

Robinson JW, Dufour MS, Fung TS. Erectile functioning of men treated for prostate carcinoma. *Cancer* 1997; 79:538–544. (Record 1)

*Wessex Institute for Health Research and Development*: Psycho-social interventions in oncology: counselling services for women with breast cancer. Southampton, Wessex Institute for Health Research and Development, 1998. (Record 2)

Irwig L, Bennetts A: Quality of life after breast conservation or mastectomy: asystematic review. *Austral N Z J Surg* 67: 1997; 750–754. (Record 3)

**Online Journal of Clinical Innovations** (*www.cinahl.org*) CINAHL's online journal contains reviews of clinically relevant nursing topics that include research studies along with quality improvement and research utilization efforts. Reviews highlight analyses of innovation adoption tactics; evidence of cost, quality, or outcome improvements following implementation; and evaluation of new protocols or staff education programs. Some examples of topics are Readability of Print Materials, Fall Prevention, and Restraints in Acute Care Settings.

**FIGURE 25-2**

Sources and examples of systematic reviews.

| Database | Search Terms | Limits | Number of Hits |
|---|---|---|---|
| 1. PubMed | Gum Chewing AND Postoperative Complications | Meta-analysis | 0 |
| 2. PubMed | Gum Chewing AND Postoperative Complications | Review | 3 |
| 3. PubMed | Gum Chewing AND Postoperative Complications | Practice Guidelines | 0 |
| 4. CinahlDirect | Chewing Gum AND Postoperative Complications | Systematic Review | 0 |
| 5. CinahlDirect | Chewing Gum AND Postoperative Complications | Review | 1 |
| 6. CinahlDirect | Chewing Gum AND Postoperative Complications | Practice Guidelines | 0 |
| 7. Cochrane Library | Gum Chewing AND Postoperative Complications | | 1 protocol under development (no review completed yet) for "Chewing gum for postoperative ileus" |

**Search 2 Results**

deCastro SM, van den Esschert JW, van Heck NT, et al. A systematic review of the efficacy of gum chewing for the amelioration of postoperative ileus. *Dig Surg.* 2008;28:39–45.

Stewart D, Waxman K. Management of postoperative ileus. *Am J Ther.* 2007;14:561–566.

Gannon RH. Current strategies for preventing or ameliorating postoperative ileus: a multimodal approach. *Am J Health Syst Pharm.* 2007;64:S8–S12.

**Search 5 Results**

Leier H. Does gum chewing help prevent impaired gastric motility in the postoperative period? *J Am Acad Nurse Pract.* 2007;19:133–136.

**Search 7 Results**

Griffiths PD, Watson H. Chewing gum for postoperative ileus [Protocol]. *Cochrane Database of Systematic Reviews.* 2008;2.

**FIGURE 25-3**

Searches (6/19/08) for Effectiveness of Gum Chewing on Postoperative Complications.

tables, and references. The PEP Resource Cards can be downloaded or are available for purchase as laminated cards. Each provides the current evidence base for nursing interventions about particular topics (eg, anorexia, diarrhea, lymphedema). Recommendations for practice are categorized by color using red/yellow/green (stoplight colors). Interventions in the green have strong evidence to support consideration of using the interventions in practice. Those in the yellow indicate that there is insufficient evidence regarding the effectiveness of the interventions, yet no evidence that using them leads to harm. Interventions in the red indicate the interventions are either ineffective or may cause harm. On the Web site background information is available for each topic: definitions used in the cards, tables of evidence that show analyses of references used to support recommendations, and reference lists.

## EVALUATING THE EVIDENCE AND DETERMINING CLINICAL RECOMMENDATIONS

Evidence must be read and interpreted using some method of critical appraisal. Critical appraisal is a means of assessing the strengths and weaknesses of information in order to determine which information most reliably or "best" answers the question being posed. It is this "best" information that constitutes "evidence"; the type of information providing such evidence will depend on the question and the circumstances.[32] At this point, collaboration with others who are interested in the area can be important in assuring that the evidence is interpreted appropriately.[12] Nurses who lack expertise in evaluating research and research-based evidence can partner with others who have this knowledge or can gain expertise from courses or working with others.[27,33,34]

Desirable attributes of reviews have been determined.[32,35] These include development by a group rather than a single reviewer, indication of inclusion/exclusion criteria for the quality of the studies included, inclusion of tables with critical information for applicability, meaningful display of different aspects of the studies' findings, and communication with experts in the field by the review group.

The desirable attributes of primary studies vary with clinical questions and types of evidence. Hierarchies of quality of evidence have been developed, primarily for use in medical EBP or for questions regarding the effectiveness of treatments; these are often used to grade strength of recommendations for clinical practice guidelines (Table 25-4)[29,31,36,37]. A hierarchy developed by oncology nurses is that used in the Oncology Nursing Society Putting Evidence into Practice efforts.[29] These hierarchies typically put meta-analyses, systematic reviews, and randomized clinical trials (RCTs) as the top levels of evidence, because the degree of bias in these types of investigations is less than in other types. However, many clinical questions of interest to oncology nurses cannot be answered with clinical trials. For instance, a question related to understanding how a particular treatment (eg, cryotherapy) leads to decreased mucositis outcomes could not be addressed based upon RCT findings. The importance of context, patient characteristics, and clinical expertise are not addressed in most RCT data. Other types of studies, including qualitative ones, may be necessary to address issues of concern to nurses. For example, an ongoing problem in oncology care is providing continuity of care between hospital and non-hospital caregivers in patient transfers. Qualitative studies involving interviews with nurses involved in the discharge process[38] may give insights into expectations and satisfaction with the referral process that no clinical trial can give. In any case, nurses seeking good evidence must evaluate the quality of all studies in order to determine their usefulness in leading to practice recommendations.

A variety of tools are available to assist in appraisal. Davies and Logan[39] authored a user-friendly guide for health professionals on reading research. The guide includes helpful tips for reading both quantitative and qualitative research articles. Worksheets for critical appraisal from the guide were found useful by nurses participating in the Oncology Nursing Society Research Utilization Short Course.[27] These worksheets are also available at http://www.elseviercanada.com/ReadingResearch/stu_res6.php.

Brown's *Knowledge for Health Care Practice: A Guide to Using Research Evidence*[40] contains tools for appraising the findings of several types of studies and for summaries such as meta-analyses, integrative reviews, and clinical practice guidelines. The tools are clearly written, practical, and geared to clinicians. Brown suggests that the bottom line is whether the nurses contemplating a research-based practice change believe they should change their practice based upon the evidence reviewed and whether they can determine how patients will benefit once the practice change is made.[41]

Translating the findings from the evidence search and appraisal into practice often requires the development of written guidelines for nurses to use when learning about or implementing a new or modified procedure.[13,41] These guidelines or protocols usually give step-by-step instructions for the procedure. Brown's book *Evidence-Based Nursing: The Research-Practice Connection*[41] contains a step-by-step process for producing an evidence based–clinical practice guideline. Each work setting has norms about guideline or procedure format. As much as possible, guideline development should be driven by research findings using systems such as those in Table 25-4, with citations of key articles or sources that support the nursing practice.

## EVALUATING THE CONTEXT WHERE A CHANGE IS BEING CONTEMPLATED

Implementing and evaluating an EBP change is not a simple process. Most nurses work in organized nursing service settings, which may limit their individual adoption of many practice changes. Organizational adoption of an evidence-based change or innovation requires educating staff, disseminating policy/procedure or protocol documentation, and creating a climate that facilitates or rewards change that improves performance and outcomes.[34] The documented barriers identified in Table 25-3 were reiterated by alumni of Oncology Nursing Society-sponsored short courses aimed at assisting nurses to complete research utilization projects.[27] The alumni identified multiple barriers to project completion in nonsupportive clinical environments—specifically staffing changes, lack of administration support, high patient loads or acuity, competing time commitments, and the difficulties of staff "unlearning." Factors facilitating the successful implementation of practice changes identified by alumni were institutional and peer support, multidisciplinary support, a nursing research department in the work setting, autonomy in one's role, and access to knowledge and resources about implementing EBP change.[27] Nurses embarking upon an EBP project need to determine what barriers exist in their own work setting and to develop or gain access to resources or strategies to overcome these.

**TABLE 25-4**

**Different Systems for Establishing Evidence Decisions**

| Organization or Source | Factors Considered | Grading System | Usefulness |
|---|---|---|---|
| **Oncology Nursing Society Putting Evidence into Practice Weight of Evidence Decision Rules**[29] | Effectiveness (evidence from systematic reviews, meta-analyses, clinical trials, observational studies, consensus of experts)<br>Risk/benefit ratio | **Recommended for practice.** Interventions with demonstrated effectiveness based upon strong evidence from "rigorously designed studies, meta-analyses, or systematic reviews" (p. 2) with a good risk/benefit ratio.<br>**Likely to be effective.** Interventions with less well established evidence base than above.<br>**Benefits balanced with harms**. Interventions requiring clinician/patient determination of risk/benefit ratio in individual situations.<br>**Effectiveness not established.** Interventions without established evidence base.<br>**Effectiveness unlikely.** Interventions where evidence base less well established than for those not recommended for practice.<br>**Not recommended for practice.** Interventions with demonstrated potential for harm or to be ineffective, or with cost/burden exceeding potential benefit. | Grading nursing or medical interventions in clinical practice |
| **National Comprehensive Cancer Network Categories of Evidence and Consensus**[31] | Effectiveness (determined by strength of research evidence)<br>Consensus of clinical experts | **Category 1:** Based on high-level evidence and uniform consensus.<br>**Category 2A:** Based on lower-level evidence including clinical experience and uniform consensus.<br>**Category 2B:** Based on lower-level evidence including clinical experience and non-uniform consensus (but no major disagreement).<br>**Category 3:** Based on any level of evidence but reflects major disagreement. | Consensus-driven or collaborative reviews of evidence leading to clinical recommendations |
| **Hierarchy of Strength of Evidence for Treatment Decisions**[36] | | Systematic reviews of randomized trials<br>Single randomized trial<br>Systematic review of observational studies<br>Single observational study<br>Physiological studies<br>Unsystematic clinical observations | Grading evidence in terms of higher or lower strength |
| **Grades of Recommendation Assessment, Development, and Evaluation** (GRADE)[37] | Type of evidence<br>Limitations to study quality<br>Strength of association | **High**: Further research not likely to change confidence in estimate of effect<br>**Moderate**: Further research likely to change confidence in estimate of effect, or may change the estimate itself<br>**Low**: Further research likely to have great impact in confidence in estimate of effect; also likely to change the estimate itself<br>**Very low**: Uncertain estimate of effect | Grading nursing or medical interventions in clinical practice |

*Source*: Data from Mitchell and Friese[29]; National Comprehensive Cancer Network[31]; DiCenso et al[36]; and the GRADE Working Group.[37]

Early in the planning phase of a specific practice implementation, stakeholders for whom the practice change is important must be identified. Stakeholders are persons beyond the primary group who are in one of the following categories: (1) care whether the problem is solved; (2) may be affected by the problem or issue; (3) can help solve or address the issue; (4) bring knowledge of or skills related to the issue; (5) may benefit if the problem is solved or the issue is addressed; and (6) would bring a diverse viewpoint to the group.[42] For example, a decision to use a new dressing change procedure postcolectomy would require input from physicians, nurses, and pharmacy, with acknowledgment by the hospital supply service. A change involving the way in which the assessment of a common set of symptoms is documented in an ambulatory clinic would involve nurses, physicians, and ancillary staff, with acknowledgment from a documentation (forms) approval group. Achieving stakeholder buy-in early during implementation maximizes the chance that all aspects of the practice change will be considered.

## IMPLEMENTING AND EVALUATING AN EVIDENCE-BASED PRACTICE CHANGE

Implementation of a practice change may begin with its use on a pilot unit. Conducting a trial with a small group of patients or nurses prior to adoption by a whole system allows assessment of whether the protocol will actually work in the target setting.[13] Some types of changes lend themselves to trials better than others. For example, adopting a new skin integrity assessment tool or initiating use of hypnosis for management of anticipatory nausea can be tried on a unit or two or on a group of patients prior to general adoption.

The pilot evaluation may determine that a practice innovation is ready for implementation or that alterations are needed in the protocol, in requested resources, or in training. Once alterations occur, implementation can proceed according to the developed strategic plan. The length of time for project completion will vary with the complexity of the change involved. Implementation of strategies aimed at optimal pain management in oncology areas can take up to 2 years,[43] while changing a print pamphlet for use related to advanced directives may take little time beyond that needed for development and printing.

Evaluating evidence-based changes in work settings in which nurses are integrally involved in ongoing quality improvement processes may be easier than in settings where quality monitoring is not entrenched practice.[9] Monitoring processes of care that have been changed, along with outcomes predicted by an EBP, is necessary to determine whether a change was enacted and what its effects were. That is, if a project requires that nurses change their handwashing techniques, their compliance with the new method should be checked. Following adequate staff compliance, the potential outcomes of the change, altered nosocomial infection rates, should be monitored to make sure changes occur as predicted. Thus, it is necessary to evaluate whether the practice change has been implemented as planned as well as whether the expected outcomes have been achieved.

## CONCLUSION

Oncology nurses who seek to accomplish truly evidence-based practice must be able to identify, obtain, and evaluate information that comes in a variety of forms and formats.[44] They then must be able to inform clinical decision making and develop practical protocols following critical appraisal of the evidence gathered and read. Challenging these nurses is an educational system that may not have prepared them for seeking evidence, the pressure of time, the demands of informed patients, and the lack of role models who are "trained" in EBP.[2,45] Furthermore, these nurses must be excellent team builders who know how to rally their stakeholders in cancer care, plan strategically to implement evidence-based changes, and evaluate the processes necessary for changing practice and the desired outcomes. In order to move forward the reality of EBP, oncology nurses must demand the resources necessary to help them improve the care they deliver via incorporating evidence-based protocols into healthcare systems. Managers and administrators must ensure that giving evidence-based care is a work setting priority and they must then support nurses and others in their efforts.

## REFERENCES


1. Thompson C, McCaughan D, Cullum N, et al. *Nurses' Use of Research Information in Clinical Decision Making: A Descriptive and Analytical Study.* Centre for Evidence Based Nursing, Department of Health Studies, University of York; 2002. http://www.york.ac.uk/healthsciences/centres/evidence/decrpt.pdf. Accessed December 28, 2009.
2. Young KM. Where's the evidence? [Viewpoint]. *Am J Nurs.* 2003;103:11.
3. Leasure AR, Stirlen J, Thompson C. Barriers and facilitators to the use of evidence-based best practices. *Dimens Crit Care Nurs.* 2008;27:74–82.
4. Rolfe G, Segrott J, Jordan S. Tensions and contradictions in nurses' perspectives of evidence-based practice. *J Nurs Manag.* 2008;16:440–451.
5. Sigma Theta Tau International. STT's position statement on evidence-based nursing. http://www.nursingsociety.org/aboutus/PositionPapers/Pages/EBN_positionpaper.aspx. Accessed December 28, 2009.
6. Sigma Theta Tau International [STTI] 2005–2007 Research and Scholarship committee. STTI Position Statement on Evidence-Based Practice February 2007 summary. *Worldviews Evid Based Nurs.* 2008;5:57–59.
7. American Nurses Association. Nursing's agenda for the future. A call to the nation. http://www.nursingworld.org/MainMenuCategories/HealthcareandPolicyIssues/Reports/AgendafortheFuture.aspx. Accessed December 28, 2009.
8. Kitson A, Harvey G, McCormack B. Enabling the implementation of evidence-based practice: a conceptual framework. *Qual Health Care.* 1998;7:149–158.

9. Rycroft-Malone J, Kitson A, Harvey G, et al. Ingredients for change: revisiting a conceptual framework. *Qual Safety Health Care.* 2002;11: 174–180.
10. Kitson AL, Rycroft-Malone J, Harvey G, et al. Evaluating the successful implementation of evidence into practice using the PARiSH framework: theoretical and practical challenges. *Implement Sci.* 2008;3:1.
11. Sackett DL, Rosenberg WMC, Gray JAM, et al. Evidence based medicine: what it is and what it isn't. *BMJ.* 1996;312:71–72.
12. Rutledge DN, DePalma JA, Cunningham M. A process model for evidence-based literature syntheses. *Oncol Nurs Forum.* 2004;31: 543–550.
13. Rutledge DN. Research utilization in oncology nursing. *Oncol Nurs: Pt Treatment Support.* 1995;4:1–14.
14. Rogers EM. *Diffusion of Innovations.* New York, NY: Free Press; 1995.
15. Funk S, Tornquist EM, Champagne MT. Barriers and facilitators of research utilization: an integrative review. *Nurs Clin North Am.* 1995;30:395–407.
16. Rutledge DN, Ropka M, Greene PE, et al. Barriers to research utilization for oncology staff nurses and nurse managers/clinical nurse specialists. *Oncol Nurs Forum.* 1998;25:497–506.
17. Carroll DL, Greenwood R, Lynch KE, et al. Barriers and facilitators to the utilization of nursing research. *Clin Nurs Spec.* 1997;11:207–212.
18. McCleary L, Brown GT. Barriers to paediatric nurses' research utilization. *J Adv Nurs.* 2003;42:364–372.
19. Nilsson Kajermo K, Nordstrom G, Krusebrant A, et al. Barriers to and facilitators of research utilization, as perceived by a group of registered nurses in Sweden. *J Adv Nurs.* 1998;27:798–807.
20. Parahoo K, McCaughan EM. Research utilization among medical and surgical nurses: a comparison of their self reports and perceptions of barriers and facilitators. *J Nurs Manag.* 2001;9:21–30.
21. McCaughan D, Thompson C, Cullum N, et al. Acute care nurses' perceptions of barriers to using research information in clinical decision-making. *J Adv Nurs.* 2002;39:46–60.
22. Hannes K, Vandersmissen J, De Blaeser L, et al. Barriers to evidence-based nursing: a focus group study. *J Adv Nurs.* 2007;60:162–171.
23. Gerrish K, Clayton J. Promoting evidence-based practice: an organizational approach. *J Nurs Manag.* 2004;12:114–123.
24. Craig JV, Smyth RL, eds. *The Evidence-Based Practice Manual for Nurses.* Philadelphia, PA: Churchill Livingstone; 2002.
25. Goode CJ. What constitutes the "evidence" in evidence-based practice? *Appl Nurs Res.* 2000;13:222–225.
26. Rycroft-Malone J, Seers K, Titchen A, et al. What counts as evidence in evidence-based practice? *J Adv Nurs.* 2004;47:81–90.
27. Rutledge DN, Mooney KH, Grant M, et al. Implementation and refinement of a research utilization course for oncology nurses. *Oncol Nurs Forum.* 2004;31:121–126.
28. McKibbon A, Hunt D, Richardson S, et al. Finding the evidence. In: Guyatt GH, Rennie D, eds. *Users' Guides to the Medical Literature: Essentials of Evidence-Based Clinical Practice.* Chicago, IL: American Medical Association; 2002:21–71.
29. Mitchell SA, Friese CR. *Oncology Nursing Society Putting Evidence into Practice Weight of Evidence Decision Rules for Summative Evaluation of a Body of Evidence.* http://www.ons.org/Research/PEP/media/ons/docs/research/outcomes/weight-of-evidence-table.pdf. Accessed December, 22, 2009.
30. National Consensus Project. *Clinical Practice Guidelines for Quality Palliative Care.* Philadelphia, PA. http://www.nationalconsensusproject.org/Guideline.pdf. Accessed June 19, 2008.
31. National Comprehensive Cancer Network. NCCN categories of evidence and consensus. 2008. http://www.nccn.org/professionals/physician_gls/categories_of_consensus.asp. Accessed December 28, 2009.
32. Critical Appraisal Skills Program. Appraisal Tools. http://www.phru.nhs.uk/pages/PHD/resources.htm. Accessed December 28, 2009.
33. Barnsteiner JH. Research-based practice. *Nurs Admin Q.* 1996;20: 52–58.
34. Rutledge DN, Donaldson NE. Building organizational mechanisms for research utilization. *J Nurs Admin.* 1995;25:12–16.
35. Stetler CB, Morsi D, Rucki S, et al. Utilization-focused integrative reviews in a nursing service. *Appl Nurs Res.* 1998;11:195–206.
36. DiCenso A, Ciliska D, Guyatt G. Introduction to evidence-based nursing. In: DiCenso A, Guyatt G, Ciliska D, eds. *Evidence-Based Nursing. A Guide to Clinical Practice.* St. Louis, MO: Elsevier Mosby, 2005.
37. GRADE Working Group. Grading quality of evidence and strength of recommendations. *BMJ.* 2004;328:1490–1498.
38. Pateman B, Wilson K, McHugh G, et al. Continuing care after cancer treatment. *J Adv Nurs.* 2003;44:192–199.
39. Davies B, Logan J. *Reading research. A user-friendly guide for nurses and other health professionals.* 3rd ed. Toronto, Canada: Elsevier; 2007.
40. Brown SJ. *Knowledge for Health Care Practice: A Guide to Using Research Evidence.* Philadelphia, PA: W.B. Saunders; 1999.
41. Brown SJ. *Evidence-Based Nursing: The Research-Practice Connection.* Sudbury, MA: Jones and Bartlett; 2009.
42. Rinehart TA, Laszlo AT, Briscoe GO. *Collaboration Toolkit: How to Build, Fix, and Sustain Productive Partnerships.* Washington, DC: Department of Justice, Office of Community Oriented Policing Services; 2001.
43. Bookbinder M, Kiss M, Coyle N, et al. Improving pain management practices. In: McGuire DB, Yarbro CH, Ferrell BR, eds. *Cancer Pain Management.* Sudbury, MA: Jones and Bartlett; 1995:321–361.
44. Jacobs SK, Rosenfeld P, Haber J. Information literacy as the foundation for evidence-based practice in graduate nursing education: a curriculum-integrated approach. *J Prof Nurs.* 2003;19:320–328.
45. Rosenfeld P, Salazar-Riera N, Vieira D. Piloting an information literacy program for staff nurses: lessons learned. *Computers Inform Nurs.* 2002;20:236–241.

CHAPTER 26

*Marlene Zichi Cohen, PhD, RN, FAAN, Susan Bankston, RN, MSN, FP/MHNP-BC*

# Cancer-Related Distress

## INTRODUCTION

Cancer remains a feared diagnosis that many individuals continue to link with death despite recent and continuing advances in early detection, treatment, and survival. Although psychological distress has long been identified as a significant issue for persons with cancer, a more thorough examination reveals a continuum of vulnerable periods along the cancer trajectory, from primary prevention to tertiary prevention periods, as well as variable levels of distress in any individual at any given time. Distress related to the cancer experience is a combination of multidimensional stressors that strain individual and family coping capabilities. Coping with these stressors can range from having normal feelings of fear, sadness, and anger to meeting diagnostic criteria for adjustment or mood disorders.

The ability to successfully cope with the multitude of stressors that accompany the cancer experience often depends on intervention by the healthcare team. However, the evidence makes it clear that psychological distress is frequently undetected and, even more frequently, untreated by cancer professionals.[1,2] Recently, experts have advocated that emotional distress be considered the sixth vital sign in patients with cancer, as distress is "vital as an indicator of a patient's state of being, needs and progress through the disease."[3,4] This chapter reviews the issues involved in the detection and treatment of distress for adult individuals with cancer. While quality of life, pain, and fatigue are inextricably linked to the experience of distress, these issues receive in-depth exploration in other chapters and are only briefly reviewed here.

Psychological adaptation to the experience of cancer requires a succession of ongoing coping responses by individuals and their supportive infrastructure of family and friends. While social and cultural norms value attending to the physical symptoms of cancer to some extent, both professionals and patients continue to diminish and stigmatize the psychological symptoms of the experience.[5] Indeed, labeling symptoms "psychological" suggests that they differ from "physical" symptoms. In response to the stigmatization attached to words such as "psychiatric," "psychosocial," and "emotional," the National Comprehensive Cancer Network (NCCN) selected the word "distress" to denote the unpleasant emotional experience associated with the excessive number of stressors that people encounter along the cancer continuum.[1] These stressors include cognitive, behavioral, emotional, social, and/or spiritual issues that may interfere with the ability to successfully adjust to the demands of the disease continuum. In line with the NCCN, this chapter explores the historical perspective, language issues, current incidence, etiology of risk factors, barriers to identification and treatment, the special populations of geriatric and minority patients with cancer, clinical manifestations, assessment, and intervention strategies for distress precipitated by the numerous challenges associated with the cancer experience.

## HISTORICAL PERSPECTIVE

The notion that psychological features can cause cancer has a very long history. Hippocrates, in ancient Greece, believed that distorting the balance of humors caused disease, and that women with excess black bile in particular were melancholic and more likely to develop cancer. This connection between melancholic women and cancer was also made in 200 CE by the famous Roman doctor Galen.[6]

Early work on psychosocial factors and cancer linked anxiety and depression with cancer.[7] In addition to notions that psychological factors can cause cancer, the connection between their role and survival has also been examined. From the 1950s to 1970s, psychosocial problems were discussed in relation to cancer and survival.[8,9] However, recent findings have been mixed. A systematic review[10] found only weak evidence that psychological coping styles are associated with survival. Positive findings tended to be found in small or methodological flawed studies and those that did not adjust for potential confounding variables. Results of studies examining depression and cancer deaths are also mixed. Irwin[11] suggested that results could vary because studies include many different cancer diagnoses and types, use nonstandardized assessment of depressive symptoms, and have short follow-up time. Steel et al[12] recently examined the link between depression and survival. Among 101 patients with hepatobiliary cancer, those with depression scores of 16 or greater on the Center for Epidemiological Studies Depression Scale had a significantly shorter survival time. This study adjusted for demographic factors such as age, gender, ethnicity, and other clinical factors. They also explored potential mechanisms for the association. Depression is recognized to alter cellular immune responses with decline in natural killer (NK) cell activity, and Steel et al found declines in NK activity correlated with survival time in a small ($N = 23$) subsample of these patients.

Although evidence is accumulating that distress can alter immune function, this is not the same as, or evidence that, emotions cause the disease. One recent study found that women with depressive symptoms had a lower risk of developing breast cancer.[13] We need to be cautious that our ideas do not blame those with cancer for their disease. As Sontag[14] pointed out in her classic work, a characteristic of diseases whose causation is not understood is the idea that a disease can have a variety of causes. Indeed, cancer is actually a label for many diseases that likely have different etiologies, different courses, varied symptoms, and different effective treatments. What is important for nurses is to remember, and tend to, patients' minds, bodies, and spirits. Nightingale[15] noted, "Volumes are now written and spoken upon the effect of the mind on the body.... But I wish a little more was thought of the effect of the body on the mind." Care of the "whole" person is a central value in nursing.

## LANGUAGE

The language we use both reflects and shapes our views, and language for symptoms of distress is problematic. We chose to use the term "distress" in the title of this chapter after examining the origin of the word, which is from the Latin participial stem *distringere*, meaning "to draw asunder."[16] Distress is defined as "severe pressure of trouble, pain, sickness, or sorrow."[16] This seemed to us to reflect the experience of persons along the cancer continuum. In addition, as we discussed earlier, the NCCN panel developing standards for distress management selected the term "distress" because they viewed it as less stigmatizing and more acceptable than "psychiatric," "psychosocial," or "emotional."[1] They also noted that it sounds more "normal" and less embarrassing and can be defined and measured by self-report.

## INCIDENCE OF DISTRESS ASSOCIATED WITH CANCER

As we noted earlier, the stressors experienced along the continuum of cancer can begin even prior to diagnosis, and continue when persons have initial suspicious symptoms, await test results, have a diagnosis, are in treatment, are medically followed, have recurrences, are survivors, and have palliative care. Coping is needed from primary prevention activities through tertiary care strategies related to treatment, survivorship, and palliative care. For example, adopting or continuing unhealthy lifestyle choices (such as smoking, alcohol intake, or excessive caloric intake) can be viewed as manifestations to external and internal stressors.[17] Decisions to engage in secondary prevention activities such as early detection screening can also be significant psychological stressors for some.[18,19,20] These stressors may interfere with or impede optimal coping or adaptation.[21–23] In the past, health professionals have focused most of their attention on the active treatment period,[5,24] but susceptibility to the multiple demands of the cancer experience extends to issues of both survivorship and palliative care.[25–27]

Levels of perceived psychological distress are also significantly influenced by cancer type, stage of disease, and individual life circumstances. Although the overall rates of psychological distress were 35.1% in a large database of patients with cancer ($N = 9000$), these rates varied significantly by cancer type.[28] Patients with lung cancer reported the highest rates of psychological distress (43.4%), while those with gynecological cancers reported the lowest rates of distress (29.6%). Distress is also significantly correlated with the stage of disease in both active treatment and palliative care patients, with the prevalence of distress increasing with the stage of disease.[29–31] Finally, both the life stage of the individuals and perceptions of their support significantly influenced the level of psychological distress experienced by patients with cancer.[25,31]

## ETIOLOGY OF RISK FACTORS FOR DISTRESS

Although the incidence of psychological distress varies by type of cancer and stage of disease, individual life circumstances play a significant role in the experience of distress. These factors include the effects of prior life experiences, perceptions of social support, and the burden of physical symptoms. The next section reviews these risk factors. Specific etiologies, risk factors, and the prevalence of specific symptoms are included in the sections on these symptoms.

Current work examining whether prior experience can exacerbate symptoms in persons with cancer has had mixed results. Several studies have found that the number of lifetime stressors (such as rape and abuse) and the perceived resolution of these stressors were related to symptoms such as anger, depression, and symptom-related distress in persons with cancer and their spouses.[32,33]

Social support has been shown to mediate the effects of stress and coping on the level of distress in parents of children with cancer in Taiwan.[34] Hawkley and Cacioppo's review[35] of research linking loneliness (or social isolation, the reverse of social support) to disease suggested that loneliness can lead to altered health behaviors, excessive stress reactivity, and an inadequate or inefficient physiological repair and maintenance process. In a study of a heterogeneous sample of patients with cancer attending community cancer support groups, taking into account important demographic, medical, and group support variables, emotional suppression (inhibiting the expression of negative emotions) has been found to be significantly associated with increased mood disturbance.[36]

Evidence from autonomic, endocrine, and immune functioning suggests that these effects unfold over a long time. Therefore, providing instrumental support for the demands of coping with disease may be most clearly helpful. However, when patients and spouses were both highly distressed, they perceived little social support for either of them,[37] indicating the need to consider level of distress when providing social support. The complexity of these relationships is further indicated by the failure to find a relationship between job strain and cancer risks such as smoking, high alcohol consumption, low intake of fruits and vegetables, and lack of exercise in a study of 3309 persons in the Netherlands.[38]

## BARRIERS TO IDENTIFICATION AND TREATMENT

Studies continue to show that between 20% and 50% of patients with cancer routinely report significant levels of psychological distress, yet fewer than 10% of individuals with cancer are ever referred for psychosocial care.[23,28,31,39] Even among those identified as meeting clinical criteria for adjustment or mood disorders, few are prescribed pharmacological treatment regimens, and even fewer actually take the prescribed medication.[40] Several factors contribute to this lack of attention to psychological distress, including the reluctance of patients to report distress, clinical time constraints, and a tendency to focus on individual cancer symptoms (ie, pain or fatigue) rather than the overall impact of the combined physical and emotional stressors as individuals experience them. In this section, we review typical patient, provider, and system barriers to the recognition and treatment of psychological distress in patients with cancer.

## PATIENT BARRIERS

The reluctance of patients to report psychological distress to their healthcare providers is often influenced by an assumption that nothing can be done. Many individuals with cancer, and those in their support systems, assume that the stressors associated with the cancer experience are inevitable and are not amenable to intervention or alleviation.[5] In addition, the burden of psychological distress can impair the motivation and ability of patients to advocate for care that is not explicitly addressed by the healthcare team. Patients who are experiencing greater levels of anxiety and depression are the very individuals who are the least likely to report their psychological distress to professionals. In response, Cunningham[41] has argued that instead of waiting for patients or family to self-identify for treatment, professional advocacy is necessary for recognition and intervention.

In addition to erroneous assumptions that psychological distress is a natural by-product of the cancer experience, the inability to adapt to and cope with significant stressors continues to carry significant cultural and social stigmatization for patients with cancer. As an example of the influence of this perceived stigmatization, McLachlan and colleagues[42] analyzed the response to intervention referrals in a group of 202 patients with cancer. This intervention study assigned a triage nurse to offer appropriate referral services to meet patients' self-identified needs. The most frequently offered services were counseling (30% of referrals) and physical symptom management (20% of referrals). However, significantly more patients accepted referrals for physical symptoms than for psychological symptoms (57% vs 28%, respectively; $P = 0.0003$). Similarly, in a study of patients with cancer in palliative care, none of the patients were in favor of obtaining psychological counseling, which they regarded as an indication of their inability to cope on their own.[26] This social stigmatization is often reinforced by the supportive infrastructure of family, friends, and providers. Patients with cancer often experience considerable pressure to remain positive in the face of overwhelming physical and emotional symptoms, a perception that has been referred to by some as the "prison of positive thinking."[36,43]

Finally, many studies have reported that patients with cancer feel a need to protect their families by minimizing or masking their own negative emotions. For instance, patients in a study of relaxation therapy vs cognitive-behavioral therapy noted that either form of therapy gave them a "space" to talk about their experiences with someone outside the family.[24] This safe context applied equally to both types of therapy and was an important aspect for patients. Patients described the therapy context as a time when they could discuss negative feelings without making their family members sad. In both forms of intervention, the therapist was identified as an objective listener whose feelings were not the patient's responsibility. Similarly, palliative care patients with cancer involved in an aromatherapy massage study noted that these sessions provided an opportunity for them to talk about their concerns and fears without burdening their families.[26]

## CLINICIAN BARRIERS

Clinician barriers to the identification and treatment of psychological distress among patients with cancer are also multidimensional. A recent study found that health professionals routinely elicited only 40% of patients' key concerns.[5] Impediments to the management of psychological distress in patients with cancer include many of the same factors that impede adequate pain management.[44,45] Despite an increased recognition of distress, many healthcare professionals have inadequate knowledge concerning the manifestations of distress, conduct incomplete distress assessments, and hold misconceptions about their ability to deal with patient distress. In addition, cancer clinicians prioritize cancer cures over caring for the person with cancer. Subjective self-report of psychological distress symptoms are often minimized in comparison to objective data, such as lab values or physical findings. The clinical assessment of patient distress is often given a low priority and typically has not been a focus of ongoing assessment and monitoring efforts. In addition, clinicians are often uncertain about the clinical relevance of levels of distress and of the effectiveness of medications or psychotherapy to deal with distress, and they often have inadequate resources to address the problem.

Another common problem among professionals dealing with cancer is the use of distancing strategies designed to block patient disclosure of emotional issues. These distancing strategies typically take the form of normalization (eg, "of course you are distressed"), but these normalizing tactics typically leave patients feeling that they have no right to talk about their distress. Researchers have identified three main reasons for the use of distancing strategies by health professionals: (1) the fear of unleashing strong emotions, (2) the lack of training in communication skills, and (3) the lack of support from professional colleagues.[5]

Finally, both clinicians and researchers have focused on one symptom at a time instead of the multidimensional experience of cancer. A cluster of symptoms, including pain, fatigue, sleep disturbances, depressed mood, and cognitive dysfunction, often accompanies the experience of cancer as a normal biological response to a life-threatening illness and its treatment. Indeed, this clustering of physiological and psychological symptoms has been referred to as sickness behaviors.[46] However, while these sickness behaviors may be a normal physiological response to illness, they represent additional stressors to an individual's coping capabilities.[47] At the same time, this is a dynamic process whereby sickness behaviors increase perceived levels of distress while higher levels of distress exacerbate the physiological tolerance threshold for sickness behaviors. Only recently has there been a deliberate attempt to focus on the clustering of distressing symptoms in patients with cancer.[48]

### SYSTEM BARRIERS

A variety of system barriers noted for pain management apply equally well to distress management. These barriers include a lack of care coordination, which fragments care, and a lack of communication between specialists and primary care providers and among providers during transitions from settings, including from acute care or "cure" to hospice mode. In addition, reimbursement for symptom management is often lacking. Requiring standards for distress management may help initiate organizational changes to overcome system barriers to distress management. While pain standards, including those from The Joint Commission on Accreditation of Healthcare Organizations (JCAHO), are not sufficient to ensure adequate pain management, they have provided an important impetus for change in many organizations.[49]

## SPECIAL POPULATIONS

### GERIATRIC PATIENTS WITH CANCER

Cancer is a disease of the elderly, as 60% of all cancers and 80% of all cancer-related deaths in the US occur in those over the age of 65.[50] Considering that by 2030 nearly 1 in 5 US residents is expected to be 65 and older and that the proportion of the population aged 65 or older is expected to more than double by the year 2050,[51] and that cancer disproportionally affects older adults, lack of information concerning the impact of emotional distress in this population is surprising. This may be because the focus on the psychosocial aspects of cancer is relatively new and research is minimal.

However, preliminary information is beginning to emerge. A 2004 study by Carlson et al[52] found high levels of distress in geriatric patients with cancer including anxiety (24%), depression (30%), and symptoms of somatization (51%). Although few studies specifically focus on the epidemiology of distress in elderly patients with cancer, the fact that depression is often present in both patients with cancer and the elderly suggest that elderly patients with cancer may suffer from significant depressive disorders.[53] Using the geriatric depression scale (GDS) for screening, Repetto et al[54] found that 40% of elderly patients with cancer showed signs of depression. In breast cancer survivors age 70 or older, increasing age, fatigue, and poor physical functioning predicted high levels of depression.[55] In this population, psychosocial variables were also important, with lower levels of optimism, spirituality, and satisfaction with support associated with higher levels of depression.[55] One study found the risk of suicide was more than 4 times greater in men aged 65 and older with prostate cancer, with evidence that these men presented with more symptoms of anxiety than depression.[56]

#### Recognizing distress

Elderly patients with cancer often experience distress for the same reasons as do younger patients: confusing clinical environments, fear of treatment side effects, the recurrence of cancer, family worries, financial concerns, or termination of treatment. While the elderly may cope with chronic illness better than younger patients,[57] older patients may be less likely to report distress.

Geriatric patients who are distressed often present with somatic symptoms, which could be attributed to their cancer or side effects of treatment. However, given the high levels of untreated distress in patients with cancer,[52,58] it is recommended that somatic symptoms be considered evidence of depression despite numerous potential causes.[59] Cognitive signs of depression include increased irritability, feelings of hopelessness, worthlessness or guilt, and lack of enjoyment in previously pleasurable activities.

Elderly patients with cancer are likely to experience additional challenges common in this age group. Physiological complications of comorbidities, cognitive impairment, and functional disabilities impacting activities of daily living may all increase the difficulties of managing cancer. Older adults may have recently experienced the loss of spouse or their family support may be remote. These factors, combined with decisions regarding whether the benefits of treatment will outweigh the possible impact on quality of life, may all increase distress.[60]

The risk of distress increases with age, illnesses, and limitations in functional ability. Recently, attention has been focused on the assessment of distress in older patients with cancer with the purpose of alleviating suffering and improving outcomes. The distress of all patients with cancer should be assessed including geriatric patients. Just asking, "How is your distress on a scale of 0 to 10?"[4] can be a useful way to begin a discussion.

Recognition of emotional distress can be enhanced by the use of screening tools. The Distress Thermometer is one tool that has been recommended by the NCCN.[1] The thermometer allows patients to rate their distress on a scale from 1 to 10 and the associated problem list allows clinicians to identify sources of the distress. Considerable research has found that scores of ≥4 are associated with high levels of emotional distress.[58,61–63]

### Interventions

While studies focusing specifically on the treatment of depression in older adults with cancer are rare,[64] the overwhelming evidence suggests that patients with cancer benefit from psychosocial interventions as well as psychotropic medications. Psychotherapeutic interventions that have demonstrated effectiveness in the general cancer population include individual supportive psychotherapy, cognitive-behavioral therapies, group therapy, and psychoeducation.[65–67] Selective serotonin reuptake inhibitors (SSRIs) such as sertraline, citalopram, and paroxetine have proven helpful in the treatment of depression and anxiety.[68–70] Mirtazapine is a particularly appropriate choice to treat depressive and somatic symptoms in patients with cancer. Mirtazapine is a potent antagonist at central presynaptic $\alpha_2$-autoreceptors, postsynaptic $5HT_2$ and $5HT_3$ receptors, and $H_1$ receptor. These characteristics make it a medication that addresses many of the symptoms associated with distress in cancer treatment. It is an effective antidepressant medication, an analgesic, an antiemetic, an appetite stimulant, and a sleep aid.[71–73]

In a study of distressed elderly patients receiving palliative chemotherapy, a monthly telephone call resulted in a significant reduction in anxiety, depression, and total distress scores. When patients were asked about what was most helpful about the calls, the majority responded that a telephone call between office visits meant that somebody cared.[74] For elderly patients with cancer managing cancer treatment, evidence that the healthcare providers care about them can make an immense difference.

## MINORITIES

Health disparities exist in cancer treatment and are documented in numerous studies.[75-78] Although the overwhelming evidence suggests that interventions are effective in mitigating cancer distress, very few studies have included minorities or investigated the effect of lower socioeconomic status on psychological well-being in patients with cancer. However, some data are beginning to appear. A cross-sectional study examining coping strategies among African American, Hispanic, and non-Hispanic White women recently treated for early stage breast cancer identified differences between groups in their coping responses. Non-Hispanic White women reported more use of humor and less religious coping than did African American or Hispanic women, and venting was related to higher levels of distress in Hispanic women.[79] One randomized controlled trial investigated an uncertainty management intervention in Caucasian and African American long-term breast cancer survivors. The study evaluated a sufficient number of African American women to allow for the analysis of ethnic differences in response to the intervention. Training in uncertainty management resulted in improvements in a variety of coping skills including cognitive reframing, cancer knowledge, and patient–healthcare provider communication for the African American women. Caucasian women receiving the same intervention improved in their satisfaction with social support and use of distraction as a coping strategy.[80] The first study of a randomized support group intervention for African American women with breast cancer demonstrated that a psychoeducational support group had a positive impact on mood and noted the importance of spirituality and religion as coping strategies.[81] A later study of a small sample of African American women with breast cancer found that symptom distress and spirituality were important correlates of overall quality of life.[82]

Socioeconomic status is also associated with disparities. In Great Britain, a study of adjustment to cancer reported that initial reactions to a cancer diagnosis appeared more severe in those of a lower SES with increased depression, anxiety, and social difficulties.[83] These findings highlight the importance of culturally appropriate care to improve well-being, reduce disparities, and alleviate distress.

## CLINICAL MANIFESTATIONS OF DISTRESS

Cancer is often associated with pain, suffering, and death, and these perceptions can cause distress in patients with cancer. Distress can be manifested in a number of ways, ranging from successful coping to severe psychological distress. Our discussion of successful coping includes a continuum of distress symptoms, from mild to moderate to severe.

### SUCCESSFUL ADAPTATION

Successful coping in living with cancer is characterized by the ability to minimize disruptions to established social roles, regulate the experience of emotional distress, and maintain active engagement in meaningful life activities.[1] To successfully cope with the multiple stressors associated with the cancer experience, efforts typically focus around three categories of strategies: those that are problem-focused, those that are emotion-focused, and those that are meaning-focused. Problem-focused strategies are directed at altering problem-specific stressors. These types of stressors might include aspects of the inevitable disruptions to work or school, financial issues, transportation problems, or family care concerns. Emotion-focused strategies are directed at minimizing the degree of emotional or psychological distress related to the cancer experience—the focus of this chapter. Finally, meaning-focused strategies help individuals negotiate the spiritual or religious significance of the disease process.

## MILD DISTRESS

Mild distress is defined by the NCCN guidelines as a score of less than 4 on the distress management assessment tool (see Figure 26-1).[1] However, successful intervention to alleviate more significant levels of distress requires consideration of the many physical and psychosocial stressors associated with the cancer experience. In this section, we review the most significant physiological stressors that are typically reported by individuals with cancer. While these physiological symptoms may precipitate moderate or even severe levels of distress, we chose to address them here because they equally represent mild manifestations of distress.

### Fatigue

Fatigue is the most commonly occurring symptom among patients with cancer, significantly affecting 50% to 70% of the population.[84–86] Expert cancer professionals have

SCREENING TOOLS FOR MEASURING DISTRESS

Instructions: First please circle the number (0–10) that best describes how much distress you have been experiencing in the past week including today.

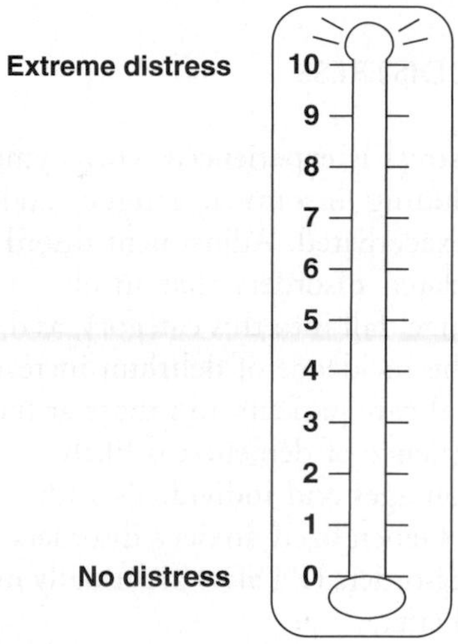


Second, please indicate if any of the following has been a problem for you in the past week including today. Be sure to check YES or NO for each.

| YES | NO | Practical Problems |
|---|---|---|
| ❑ | ❑ | Child care |
| ❑ | ❑ | Housing |
| ❑ | ❑ | Insurance |
| ❑ | ❑ | Transportation |
| ❑ | ❑ | Work/school |
| | | **Family Problems** |
| ❑ | ❑ | Dealing with children |
| ❑ | ❑ | Dealing with partner |
| | | **Emotional Problems** |
| ❑ | ❑ | Depression |
| ❑ | ❑ | Fears |
| ❑ | ❑ | Nervousness |
| ❑ | ❑ | Sadness |
| ❑ | ❑ | Worry |
| | | **Spiritual/Religious concerns** |
| ❑ | ❑ | Loss of faith |
| ❑ | ❑ | Relating to God |
| ❑ | ❑ | Loss of meaning or purpose of life |

| YES | NO | Physical Problems |
|---|---|---|
| ❑ | ❑ | Appearance |
| ❑ | ❑ | Bathing/dressing |
| ❑ | ❑ | Breathing |
| ❑ | ❑ | Changes in urination |
| ❑ | ❑ | Constipation |
| ❑ | ❑ | Diarrhea |
| ❑ | ❑ | Eating |
| ❑ | ❑ | Fatigue |
| ❑ | ❑ | Feeling Swollen |
| ❑ | ❑ | Fevers |
| ❑ | ❑ | Getting around |
| ❑ | ❑ | Indigestion |
| ❑ | ❑ | Mouth sores |
| ❑ | ❑ | Nausea |
| ❑ | ❑ | Nose dry/congested |
| ❑ | ❑ | Pain |
| ❑ | ❑ | Sexual |
| ❑ | ❑ | Skin dry/itchy |
| ❑ | ❑ | Sleep |
| ❑ | ❑ | Tingling in hands/feet |

Other problems: ______________________________

______________________________

**FIGURE 26-1**

Distress management assessment tool.

Data from National Comprehensive Cancer Network. These Guidelines are a work in progress that will be refined as often as new significant data becomes available.

The NCCN Guidelines are a statement of consensus of its authors regarding their views of currently accepted approaches to treatment. Any clinician seeking to apply or consult any NCCN guideline is expected to use independent medical judgment in the context of individual clinical circumstances to determine any patient's care or treatment. The National Comprehensive Cancer Network makes no warranties of any kind whatsoever regarding their content, use or application and disclaims any responsibility for their application or use in any way.

recently selected fatigue as one of the top symptom priorities for intervention.[87] Cross-sectional studies suggest that fatigue is a result of a combination of physical and psychological causes.[48] For example, patients with cancer who are anemic experienced statistically significant differences in fatigue compared to patients with cancer and the general US population who are nonanemic.[88] Likewise, fatigue, depression, and insomnia typically occur together in patients with cancer, suggesting a "symptom cluster" with overlapping etiologies.[89] However, preliminary data suggest that symptoms of fatigue may be ameliorated by antidepressant therapy.[90] Nevertheless, surveys consistently show that fatigue is associated with significant physical, emotional, psychological, and social consequences.

### Sleep disturbances

Individuals with cancer report significantly poorer overall sleep quality than the general population, accompanied by more daytime dysfunction.[91] An estimated 30% to 50% of patients with cancer report significant distress related to sleep disturbances, typically insomnia or disruptions in the sleep–wake cycle.[92] Inadequate sleep is strongly correlated with both fatigue and mood disorders in people with cancer.[89,92,93] Patients with cancer identified the most frequent causes of sleep disorders to be due to thoughts, concerns, and pain.[85] Left unattended, sleep disorders may progress to a chronic state, lasting several years after the initial diagnosis and treatment period ends.[94] Family caregivers have also been found to have sleep problems, which were linked with depression and fluctuated over time.[95] Benzodiazepines, hypnotics, antidepressants, antihistamines, chloral derivatives, neuroleptics, and herbal supplements are often prescribed for sleep disturbances. Likewise, sleep hygiene techniques, complementary therapies, educational interventions, and exercise have been investigated as ways to improve sleep. However, there is not sufficient evidence to definitively recommend pharmacological or nonpharmacological treatments and it is recommended that benefits vs harmful effects be considered on an individual patient basis.[96]

### Cognitive dysfunction

Cognitive dysfunction is the inability to relate current to past events or to understand experiences. Evidence from several disciplines has shown that emotions and cognitive processing are intimately linked, and recent studies have linked cognitive performance with survival.[97,98] Cognitive changes occur from both cancer and its treatment and are significantly distressing to patients, to their family members, and to nurses.[99] Subtle cognitive changes are experienced quite frequently in patients with cancer, with as many as 75% reporting mild to moderate cognitive impairment.[100] The distress that patients experience from cognitive changes occurs regardless of the degree of the impairment, which can range from subtle memory changes noticeable only to the individual to more severe memory dysfunction, including acute delirium and dementia.[101]

Many factors influence cognitive function, and it is likely that several mechanisms may be operating simultaneously. Memory and attention deficits often accompany fatigue—the most common complaint among patients with cancer.[84] Anemia, depression, and age are all associated with both cancer and the cognitive dysfunction experienced by individuals with cancer. Cognitive changes have also been linked to medication, including standard-dose chemotherapy regimens,[100] radiation therapy,[97] biological response modifiers,[102,103] and opioid use for pain management.[104] However, cognitive processing difficulties have been empirically established to occur even prior to active treatment, associated simply with the overwhelming nature of the cancer diagnosis.[21] Supporting evidence suggests that emotional distress systematically influences cognitive performance, including problem-solving abilities, working short-term memory, and the long-term consolidation of experiences.[105–107]

## MODERATE DISTRESS

Moderate distress is experienced when symptoms of mild distress, including insomnia, fatigue, and sleep disturbances, are exacerbated. Adjustment disorders, a category of anxiety-related disorders that involve difficulties coping with change, fall into this category, as do delirium and dementia. The incidence of delirium increases among the elderly, critical care patients and those at the end of life,[108] and the prevalence of dementia is likely to increase as the US population ages and individuals with chronic diseases live longer.[51] Generalized anxiety disorders and post-traumatic stress disorders (PTSDs) are usually more severe and are discussed later.

### Delirium

"Delirium," from the Latin *delirium*, meaning "deviate" or "deranged,"[16] is the diagnostic term used to describe an organic mental disorder that usually has an acute onset where both cognition and attention are disturbed. Also called acute confusional state or encephalopathy, delirium can have a short course and is reversible except when it occurs during the last 24 to 28 hours of life. Prolonged delirium may be a sign of infection or coagulopathy and is associated with increased morbidity and mortality.[109–111] Cognitive dysfunction in the form of inattention, disorientation, and impaired memory can persist for as long as one year.[112] Delirium is experienced by 15% to 40% of those with cancer and in more than 85% of those with terminal cancer.[109,113–115] Delirium causes distress in patients and caregivers, and the patient may remember some events while delirious and often want to discuss and make sense of the experience.[116]

Common causes of delirium include infection, metabolic disturbances, side effects of medications, substance withdrawal (especially alcohol and benzodiazepines), seizures, or unrelieved pain.[117,118] In advanced disease, opioid dysfunction usually is in the form of delirium.[104] Cancer therapies are also associated with delirium. Standard-dose chemotherapy has also been linked with cognitive deficits in patients with cancer.[100] Radiation therapy and combined radiation and chemotherapy are also neurotoxic.[97] Immunological therapies such as interleukin-2 and interferon-alpha are known to predispose patients to delirium.[103] A variety of risk factors for delirium have been identified in oncology patients including bone metastasis, hematological malignancies (especially lymphoma), advanced age, prior cognitive impairment, and low levels of serum albumin.[119]

### Dementia

"Dementia," from the Latin *dementare*, meaning "insane,"[16] is a chronic and irreversible cognitive disorder with more gradual onset than delirium. A simple definition of dementia is a deterioration of cognitive abilities that hinders people from performing their usual activities of daily living. Dementia is usually irreversible, may not have identified precipitating stressors, and includes impaired short- and long-term memory that causes significant social and occupational impairments. Dementia increases the risk of delirium[120] and may be the result of tumors, paraneoplastic syndromes, or cancer-related treatments on the brain.

The suspicion of dementia in a patient with cancer should prompt further evaluation as it is necessary to determine the patient's capacity to make decisions. While a diagnosis of dementia does not necessarily signify a lack of capacity, a healthcare proxy must be found if the patient cannot understand or remember information involving a particular decision or treatment.

### Adjustment disorders

Adjustment disorders are the most common mood disorders diagnosed in patients with cancer.[121] These reactions are also sometimes called "situational" or "reactive" depression. These disorders lack specific symptoms, making them difficult to diagnose and to differentiate from symptoms related to the disease process and cancer treatments. Symptoms of situational anxiety and depression may include insomnia, worry, muscle tension, restlessness, intermittent shortness of breath, palpitations, sweating, nervousness, and feeling dizzy or lightheaded. Irritability, mood swings, crying spells, poor concentration, social withdrawal, and temporary periods of hopelessness or demoralization may also be apparent.[122,123]

Screening tools often fail to differentiate distress from major depression.[124] However, adjustment disorders are usually serious enough to interfere with cancer treatments or daily functioning but not severe or pervasive enough to warrant the diagnosis of an outright anxiety or depressive disorder. Adjustment to cancer has been described as an "active psychosocial process" that may encompass both positive and negative outcomes for the individual.[125] When adjustment involves significant distress, patients with cancer may need assistance identifying coping strategies. Unstructured supportive interactions with caring providers are helpful. Providers can effectively communicate and alleviate suffering by actively listening, providing information, and exploring emotions.[126] Referral to mental health specialists is indicated if these approaches are not effective.

## SEVERE DISTRESS

### Depression

Depression is a burdensome condition that affects approximately 15% to 25% of patients with cancer.[29,127–129] As we discussed in the section on barriers, patients often mistakenly believe both that depression is normal in those with cancer and that treatment is not helpful. Litofsky and colleagues[128] found poor concordance between physician and patient ratings of depression, and few received pharmacological therapy, even when depressive symptoms were recognized by physicians. Depression affects the course of cancer by increasing morbidity and hospital stays and negatively impacting treatment compliance and possibly prognosis and mortality.[130] The symptoms of major depression are summarized in Table 26-1.[131] Depression is diagnosed in those without cancer when these symptoms last a minimum of two weeks and when the symptoms cause clinically significant distress or impairment in important areas of functioning. Of course, in those with cancer, it is important to distinguish between depression and the symptoms of cancer and cancer treatments. Many of the somatic symptoms associated with cancer and its treatment mimic the somatic symptoms of depression.[132] Consequently, the most useful symptoms to examine in making this distinction are cognitive ones, such as feelings of worthlessness, guilt, and hopelessness; thoughts of suicide; and loss of pleasure in activities.

### Anxiety

Anxiety in cancer is both common and poorly understood. This is indicated by the wide range in prevalence estimates, ranging in one literature review from 0.9% to 49%,[133] although when standardized psychiatric interviews and research diagnostic criteria are used, the range is more typically 10% to 30%.[134] Another source of variance for these estimates of prevalence is the differences in the

**TABLE 26-1**

| Diagnostic Criteria for Major Depressive Disorder |
|---|
| Five or more of the following symptoms during the same two-week depressed period represent a change from previous functioning. At least one of the symptoms represents either depressed mood or loss of interest or pleasure:<br>• Depressed mood most of the day, nearly every day<br>• Markedly decreased interest or pleasure in all or most activities most of the day<br>• Significant weight loss when not dieting, weight gain, or decrease or increase in appetite nearly every day<br>• Insomnia or hypersomnia nearly every day<br>• Psychomotor agitation or retardation (abnormal slowing) (observed by self or others)<br>• Fatigue or loss of energy nearly every day<br>• Feelings of worthlessness or excessive or inappropriate guilt nearly every day<br>• Diminished ability to think, concentrate, or indecisiveness nearly every day<br>• Recurrent thoughts of death (not just fear of dying) or suicide |

*Note*: Do not include symptoms due to general medical conditions or to substances (eg, drug abuse or medications).

*Source*: Data compiled from *DSM-IV-TR* (2000).[131]

samples studied, including differences in gender, age, type of cancer, and time since diagnosis. Patients with cancer can have one of several anxiety disorders, the most common being reactive anxiety/adjustment disorder, disease and treatment-related anxiety, substance-induced anxiety (from substances such as corticosteroids), and other anxiety disorders such as general anxiety disorders, panic, phobia, obsessive-compulsive disorder, and PTSD.

Diagnosing anxiety in patients with cancer is challenging, since the diagnosis in healthy persons is often based on somatic symptoms, including anorexia, fatigue, and weight loss, which in cancer are often symptoms of the disease itself and its treatment. The symptoms of worry, distractibility, restlessness, and fearfulness are more useful for diagnosing anxiety among patients with cancer.[135] Anxiety can be adaptive and can motivate actions to reduce the anxiety. Intervention is required when anxiety is severe or prolonged and interferes with activities of daily living and quality of life. Symptoms of anxiety result from autonomic overactivity and include intense fear out of proportion with the threat, the inability to absorb information, and the inability to cooperate with medical treatment. Somatic symptoms include shortness of breath, sweating, lightheadedness, and palpitations. Patients are generally distressed about their symptoms, and behavioral interventions and medications to treat anxiety are generally effective.

## Post-traumatic stress disorder

Post-traumatic stress disorder is a more severe anxiety-related disorder that is chronic and is the consequence of previous trauma. In 1994, the *Diagnostic and Statistical Manual*[131] added life-threatening illnesses, which had previously been explicitly excluded as stressors, to the list of factors that could precipitate PTSD. This change resulted in a great deal of attention to PTSD after a cancer diagnosis. PTSD develops in response to an unusually traumatic event that involved actual or threatened death or serious physical injury. Symptoms include feelings of intense fear combined with repeatedly reliving the event with intrusive, distressing recollections (thoughts, images); repeated, distressing dreams; and/or flashbacks, hallucinations, or illusions in which the individual acts or feels as if the event were recurring, accompanied by marked mental distress and physiological reactivity (such as rapid heartbeat and elevated blood pressure) (see Table 26-2).

Patients also repeatedly avoid stimuli related to the trauma and have a numbing of their general responsiveness, as shown by, for example, avoiding thoughts, feelings, or conversations concerning the event; avoiding activities, people, or places that recall the event; not being able to recall important features of the event; having a marked loss of interest or participation in activities important to the patient; feeling detached or isolated from other people; being restricted in the ability to love or feel other strong emotions; and having the feeling that life will be brief or unfulfilled (lack of marriage, job, children). In addition, symptoms of hyperarousal are present, as listed in Table 26-2. PTSD is diagnosed when the symptoms last longer than 1 month and cause clinically important distress or impair work, social, or personal functioning. It can occur even in very young children.[131]

Four recent reviews have examined studies of PTSD following cancer.[136–139] These studies found the incidence to range from 1.3% to 32%, with the range related to the use of more or less stringent criteria. Several studies[136–138] have also reported that between 10% and 40% of patients have intrusive and avoidance symptoms following cancer. The symptoms decline considerably for most patients within three months after diagnosis or after treatment is completed.

Several factors have been found to predict PTSD symptomatology. These include female gender, younger age at diagnosis, prior negative life stressors, history of psychological disturbance, increased distress subsequent to the diagnosis, lower education, poor social support, poor social functioning, reduced physical functioning, emotionally reactive temperament, and avoidant coping style.[140] Mixed evidence supports the role of medical variables, including type, stage, severity, and prognosis of cancer in subsequent

**TABLE 26-2**

**Diagnostic Criteria for Post-Traumatic Stress Disorder**

| The traumatic event is persistently reexperienced in one (or more) of the following ways: | Persistent avoidance of stimuli associated with the trauma and numbing of general responsiveness (not present before the trauma), as indicated by three (or more) of the following: |
|---|---|
| • Recurrent and intrusive distressing recollections of the event, including images, thoughts, or perceptions<br>• Recurrent distressing dreams of the event<br>• Acting or feeling as if the traumatic event were recurring (includes a sense of reliving the experience, illusions, hallucinations, and dissociative flashback episodes, including those that occur on awakening or when intoxicated)<br>• Intense psychological distress upon exposure to internal or external cues that symbolize or resemble an aspect of the traumatic event, and physiological reactivity upon exposure to internal or external cues that symbolize or resemble an aspect of the traumatic event | • Efforts to avoid thoughts, feelings, or conversations associated with the trauma<br>• Efforts to avoid activities, places, or people that arouse recollections of the trauma<br>• Inability to recall an important aspect of the trauma<br>• Markedly diminished interest or participation in significant activities<br>• Feelings of detachment or estrangement from others<br>• Restricted range of affect (eg, unable to have loving feelings)<br>• Sense of a foreshortened future<br>• Persistent symptoms of increased arousal<br>  • Difficulty falling or staying asleep<br>  • Irritability or outbursts of anger<br>  • Difficulty concentrating<br>  • Hypervigilance<br>  • Exaggerated startle response<br>• Duration of the disturbance (symptoms listed above) is more than one month<br>• The disturbance causes clinically significant distress or impairment in social, occupational, or other important areas of functioning |

*Source*: Data compiled from the DSM-IV-TR (2000).[131]

PTSD. Most studies have been small and cross-sectional, have relied on self-report measures, and have sampled parents of children with cancer, childhood survivors of cancer, or women with early to middle stage breast cancer, which is particularly an issue since most studies conclude that women are more likely to experience PTSD than men.

## ASSESSMENT OF DISTRESS

As is true of all symptoms, effective interventions for distress require accurate assessment, which can be accomplished only with communication among healthcare professionals, patients, and their families. While a great deal of cancer-related symptom assessment focuses on one symptom at a time, measures of multiple symptoms exist that include psychosocial symptoms.[28,141–143] However, attention to these symptoms has not always been a priority, as indicated by the fact that a stress management subscale has only recently been added to the Cancer Behavior Inventory, a measure of self-efficacy for coping with cancer.[144] The NCCN guidelines include a brief screening to assess the presence of problems and call for referral for further evaluation if the screening indicates symptoms such as delirium, dementia, mood disorders, adjustment disorders, anxiety disorder, substance abuse, and personality disorder.[1] The distress thermometer and problem list (see Figure 26-1) are brief and useful screens for distress and related problems that patients can complete in only 2 or 3 minutes.

Self-report screening instruments must be scored, evaluated, and discussed with each patient. Triage, the process of communicating screening results, discussing each patient's needs, and determining the best course of further action, is vital to successful screening. The oncology team (oncologist, nurse, palliative care specialist, social worker, and counselor) is responsible for successful triage. In fact, screening without the availability of appropriate treatment resources is considered unethical. Rapid methods of screening are needed to determine which patients need more in-depth clinical interviews for more precise diagnosis. These in-depth interviews require the skill of mental health specialists.[145] Ongoing evaluations and monitoring are also critically important.

## THERAPEUTIC APPROACHES AND NURSING CARE

The NCCN standards of care suggest that distress rated as mild might result in a referral to a local self-help group or management by the primary oncology team only. Distress rated as moderate to severe warrants referral to other appropriate professionals (psychologists, psychiatrists, social workers, palliative care specialists, or pastoral counselors), depending on the nature of the distress. In some studies, a significant percentage of patients who report moderate to high levels of distress do not get or want further assessment.[26,42] Thus, it is important to consider how the primary oncology team can introduce the need for further psychosocial assessment.

Interventions to minimize distress have focused on alleviating the physiological symptoms of cancer (ie, fatigue, pain, and insomnia), improving coping strategies with cognitive-behavioral interventions, or providing a context of supportive therapy. Recently, complementary or alternative therapies have gained attention as interventions for distress in patients with cancer. Ideally, professionals dealing with cancer should take a multifactorial approach to the alleviation of distress in cancer care. Factors associated with fatigue and pain management are found in the chapters specific to those symptoms. Here, we review some of the more recent innovative initiatives aimed at managing the cluster of distress symptoms.

## SYMPTOM MANAGEMENT STRATEGIES

Addressing the cluster of symptoms that accompany the cancer experience is an obvious focus, and an important approach, to alleviating distress. For instance, activity management—whether exercise or energy conservation—has consistently been shown to benefit the burden of fatigue.[146–148] Similarly, researchers have used cognitive-behavioral interventions to improve insomnia in women with metastatic breast cancer.[149] Both of these approaches significantly improved mood, fatigue, and quality of life.

Likewise, sensory stimulation approaches have been successful in alleviating or minimizing physiological symptoms. Cimprich and Ronis[21] have tested an environmental intervention in women newly diagnosed with breast cancer aimed at alleviating cognitive dysfunction. The intervention entailed 120 minutes of weekly exposure to an aesthetically pleasing environmental stimulus such as observing a sunset, walking through a park, or gardening. The intervention group significantly recovered their capacity to direct attention (CDA) compared to the control group, suggesting the beneficial effects of early intervention aimed at restoring cognitive functioning.

Japanese researchers have also used sensory stimulation interventions to alleviate the distress associated with chemotherapy.[150] The intervention, the Bedside Wellness System, integrates visual, auditory, and olfactory sensory stimuli and is targeted to individual preferences. Patients experienced a visual selection of a lake, a forest, or a country town. Auditory stimulation was selected and delivered by either headphones or speakers, and the system delivered a gentle, scented breeze. Each aspect (visual, auditory, and olfactory) of the sensory stimulation session was selected by the patient and lasted approximately 20 minutes. The sessions could be repeated as many times during the chemotherapy as the patient desired. The intervention had a positive effect on improving physical symptoms and decreasing negative mood states in the intervention group compared to the control group.

A recent review of massage therapy for symptom relief found some evidence that massage may be of short-term benefit in improving perceptions of well-being, including reducing pain and fatigue.[90,151] Although more rigorous studies are needed to make definitive recommendations concerning the usefulness of massage therapy to alleviate cancer symptoms, the small incidence of side effects makes it worth including in recommendations to patients.

## COGNITIVE-BEHAVIORAL STRATEGIES

Most interventions aimed at alleviating psychological distress in patients with cancer have typically focused on cognitive-behavioral interventions targeting either problem-focused or emotion-focused coping strategies. There is robust evidence that cognitive-behavioral therapy is effective for depression and anxiety.[90,152] Problem-focused coping strategies are designed to help patients manage specific problems by directly trying to alter the problem situation. Emotion-focused coping strategies are aimed at helping to regulate the experience of psychological distress.[153] The most optimal outcomes are obtained when there is a good match between the appraisal of the situation and the coping strategy selected.[154] For example, when there is a perception of high control over the situation, problem-focused coping strategies result in less psychological distress. In contrast, when the perception is that there is little control over the situation, emotion-focused coping strategies provided the best approach to alleviating distress.

As an example of a problem-focused strategy, Given and colleagues[155] randomized individuals with cancer ($N = 237$) to either a nursing intervention or the conventional care group. Individuals in the intervention group identified their unique problems with the nurse and selected specific interventions proposed by the nurse. The patient and nurse then together evaluated the outcomes of the selected interventions. Patients in the intervention group who entered the study with severe symptoms reported significantly lower severity scores at 10 and 20 weeks. Controlling for demographic and disease-specific variables did not attenuate the findings.

In contrast, emotion-focused interventions are aimed at alleviating psychological distress through stress reduction strategies. As an example, mindfulness-based stress reduction (MBSR) programs have reported significant decreases in mood disturbance and stress symptoms for up to 6 months in both male and female patients with cancer as a result of a 7-week intervention.[156] After MBSR training, oncology patients have reported a decrease in physical symptoms, improved immune function, and quality of life including more joy and less tension.[157,158] Similarly, Jacobsen and colleagues[159] compared self-administered stress management training, professionally administered stress management training, and conventional care among patients about to start chemotherapy ($N = 411$). Patients receiving professionally administered stress management training did no better than those who administered it themselves. However, both training groups did significantly better on a variety of distress measures compared to persons receiving conventional care only.

## SOMEONE WHO CARES

Several decades of research have associated levels of social support with individual coping capabilities.[154] Interventions aimed at providing a supportive environment focus on the provision of a safe, neutral context for the expression of emotions as a distress-alleviating strategy. Support groups for patients with cancer are a common intervention strategy and have shown significant results. For example, Goodwin and colleagues[27] randomized patients with metastatic breast cancer to either supportive-expressive group therapy or conventional care. The intervention consisted of weekly 90-minute sessions of 8 to 12 women and professional group leaders (psychiatrists, psychologists, social workers, or nurse clinicians). Women in the intervention arm of the study reported significantly improved mood states and decreases in perceived pain compared to the control group.

The provision of a supportive environment as a safe, neutral context takes many forms. Interestingly, MacCormack and colleagues[24] found little difference in patient perception of benefit between cognitive-emotional therapy and relaxation therapy, as long as there was nonspecific time for the patient to talk to the therapist. Likewise, relaxation and counseling were both shown to relieve psychological distress symptoms in a group of newly diagnosed patients with cancer.[160] Similarly, individuals receiving aromatherapy from a registered nurse reported significant stress-relieving benefits. Indeed, patients conveyed that the sessions provided a safe space where they could discuss their concerns and feelings without burdening their families or bothering their physicians.[26] Central to the beneficial findings in all of these studies was the opportunity to safely discuss thoughts and feelings with an attentive, empathetic, professional listener.

## COMPLEMENTARY STRATEGIES

As shown by the examples just cited, the division between professional and complementary or alternative therapies is increasingly blurred. Indeed, the importance of emotional expression has been highlighted in interventions aimed at alleviating the psychological distress of the cancer experience.[43] Supportive listening and massage therapy play a significant role in both aromatherapy[26] and reflexology.[161] Gilbar and colleagues[162] found that individuals with cancer who sought out complementary therapies in addition to conventional therapy reported significantly lower levels of distress than those individuals who did not seek outside treatment modalities, irrespective of the type of alternative treatment chosen. In contrast, Risberg and Jacobsen[163] found that, among 158 patients with cancer in Norway, those with higher levels of mental distress used more alternative medicine. Further research is needed to understand the intricacies of these approaches to alleviate distress.

## PHARMACOLOGICAL MANAGEMENT

Persons with the clinically significant distress symptoms described in this chapter may benefit from medications. The most common medications used to treat both anxiety and depression are benzodiazepines and selective serotonin reuptake inhibitors (SSRIs). In persons with physical illness, the short-acting anxiolytics (alprazolam, lorazepam, and clonazepam) are best tolerated. In addition, nonbenzodiazepines, neuroleptics, antihistamines, and SSRIs are useful in treating anxiety.[135] Medications, used to treat both anxiety and depression, include tricyclic antidepressants (TCAs), SSRIs, selective serotonin-norepinephrine reuptake inhibitors (SSNRIs), mirtazapine, beta-blockers, antihistamines, lithium, methylphenidate, monoamine oxide inhibitors (MAOIs), and central nervous system stimulants. See both Gobel[164] and Barsevick and Much[165] for a more comprehensive review of these medications, their doses, and side effects.

## CONCLUSION

The importance of alleviating physical and psychological symptoms is underscored by the finding that the burden of physical symptoms experienced by individuals with cancer is significantly correlated with the desire for a hastened death in both patients in active treatment and those receiving palliative care.[29,30] Interventions are most effective when multidisciplinary teams work together and involve patients and their families. Nurses play key roles in symptom control, education, and communication, since they have more time and develop closer relationships with patients than other professionals. The roles of psychiatrists, oncologists, clergy, and the rest of the interdisciplinary team, including social workers and psychologists, are important, as they have unique disciplinary expertise with counseling, psychotherapy, education, pastoral care, and, when indicated, medications. The need for centralized sources of information about treatment, care, and support has been recognized. An example of a program to centralize resources, described by Nemetz and Mercardante[166], was developed by a coalition of patients with cancer, volunteers, and hospital staff.

Learning from efforts to manage pain may help guide the development of effective support for symptoms of distress. The Joint Commission on Accreditation of Health Care Organizations[45] instituted pain standards in 1999, although cancer pain has long been recognized as a serious problem for persons with cancer. While relief of cancer pain remains a problem, no JCAHO standards exist for the management of distress, and many barriers exist to both effective pain and distress management. The need for systematic examination to overcome these barriers, such as staff and patient education and examination and elimination of system barriers, is important. The added burden of societal stigma of psychological problems needs to be addressed.

Recently experts have advocated that distress be considered the sixth vital sign and be assessed frequently and particularly during changes in disease status.[167] Further work is needed to establish brief but effective ways to assess distress with reliable, valid, and clinically useful measures of distress. The NCCN distress thermometer may be useful for initial screening, although research is still needed to confirm its clinical utility.[1,168] Akizuki and colleagues[169] found that one question (asking patients to rate their mood on a 0 to 100 scale) and the distress thermometer were comparable in screening for depression in individuals with cancer, but both detected less depression than the Hospital Anxiety and Depression Scale when results were compared with diagnoses made by psychiatrists using DSM IV criteria.

Interesting links between pain, disease severity, and survival are beginning to be established in both animal and clinical research. Data about these links are now conflicting, so the underlying mechanisms need to be explicated. This important beginning evidence indicates that symptom management is vital. The role of immune mediation is being explored.[170–172] Extending this research beyond pain to symptoms of distress and clarifying the "mind-body" connection will also be important in future research.

We are coming to appreciate the complexity of the experience of cancer for everyone involved. This includes those who do not have cancer but whose lifestyles make them more or less prone to the disease, patients everywhere along the trajectory of disease, their family and loved ones, and professional caregivers. Thorne and Paterson,[173] in their review of research on the elements of chronic illness experiences, noted that researchers shifted their focus in the early 1980s when the insider perspective was first obtained. Early research (1980 to 1985) focused on loss and burden (eg, suffering, sick role), and later a more optimistic perspective predominated (eg, being courageous, maintaining hope, finding meaning, and transformation). This shift was accompanied by the view of ill persons as being the experts in their own health. Thorne and Patterson appropriately caution us to remember the complexity of illness, nowhere more appropriate than with cancer, where persons experience joys and sorrows, problems, and possibilities. While patients are the experts, especially in describing their symptoms, they also need and seek the expertise of professionals. Providing a full range of resources to match needs as they change over the health and illness continuum will serve to best enable patients to live their lives as fully and productively as possible.

## REFERENCES

1. NCCN Clinical Practice Guidelines in Oncology. Distress Management (Version V.2.2009). 2009 National Comprehensive Cancer Network. http://www.nccn.org. Accessed December 28, 2009.
2. Rodin GM. Suffering and adaptation to cancer: what to measure and when to intervene. *J Psychosom Res.* 2003;55:399–401.
3. Bultz BD, Carlson LE. Emotional distress: the sixth vital sign—Future directions in cancer care. *Psychooncology.* 2006;15:93–95.
4. Holland JC, Bultz BD. The NCCN guideline for distress management: a case for making distress the sixth vital sign. *J Natl Compr Canc Netw.* 2007;5:3–7.
5. Maguire P, Pitceathly C. Improving the psychological care of cancer patients and their relatives: the role of specialist nurses. *J Psychosom Res.* 2003;55:469–474.
6. Olson J. *Bathsheba's Breast: Women, Cancer, and History.* Baltimore, MD: John Hopkins University Press; 2002.
7. Gendron D. *Enquiries into the Nature, Knowledge and Cure of Cancer.* London: J. Taylor; 1701.
8. Bard M. The sequence of emotional reactions in radical mastectomy patients. *Pub Health Rep.* 1952;76:1144–1148.
9. Renneker R, Cutler M. Psychosocial problems to adjustment to cancer of the breast. *JAMA.* 1952;148:633–638.
10. Petticrew M, Bell R, Hunter D. Influence of psychological coping on survival and recurrence in people with cancer: systematic review. *BMJ.* 2002;325:1066.
11. Irwin M. Depression and risk of cancer progression: an elusive link. *J Clin Oncol.* 2007;25:2343–2344.
12. Steel JL, Geller DA, Gamblin TC, et al. Depression, immunity, and survival in patients with hepatobiliary carcinoma. *J Clin Oncol.* 2007;25:2397–2405.
13. Nyklicek I, Louwman WJ, Van Nierop PW, et al. Depression and the lower risk for breast cancer development in middle-aged women: a prospective study. *Psychol Med.* 2003;33:1111–1117.
14. Sontag S. *Illness as Metaphor.* New York: Farrar, Straus, and Giroux; 1978.
15. Nightingale F. *Notes on Nursing: What It Is and What It Is Not.* New York: Dover; 1969.
16. Oxford University Press. *Oxford English Dictionary (Online).* http://dictionary.oed.com. Accessed December 28, 2009.
17. McEwen BS. From molecules to mind: stress, individual differences, and the social environment. *Ann NY Acad Sci.* 2001;935:42–49.
18. Klassen AC, Smith AL, Meissner HI, et al. If we gave away mammograms, who would get them? A neighborhood evaluation of a no-cost breast cancer screening program. *Prev Med.* 2002;34:13–21.
19. Smith E, Phillips JM, Price M. Screening and early detection among racial and ethnic minority women; in cultural dimensions in oncology care. *Semin Oncol Nurs.* 2001;17:190–196.
20. Phillips JM, Cohen MZ, Tarzian AJ. African American women's experiences with breast cancer screening. *J Nurs Scholarsh.* 2001;33:135–140.

21. Cimprich B, Ronis DL. An environmental intervention to restore attention in women with newly diagnosed breast cancer. *Cancer Nurs.* 2003;26:284–292.
22. Gates MF, Lackey NR, Brown G. Caring demands and delay in seeking care in African American women newly diagnosed with breast cancer: an ethnographic, photographic study. *Oncol Nurs Forum.* 2001;28:529–537.
23. Lebel S, Jakubovits G, Rosberger Z, et al. Waiting for a breast biopsy. *J Psychosom Res.* 2003;55:437–443.
24. MacCormack T, Simonian J, Lim J, et al. "Someone who cares": a qualitative investigation of cancer patients' experiences of psychotherapy. *Psychooncology.* 2001;10:52–65.
25. Cimprich B, Ronis DL, Martinex-Ramos G. Age at diagnosis and quality of life in breast cancer survivors. *Cancer Pract.* 2002;10:85–93.
26. Dunwoody L, Smyth A, Davidson R. Cancer patients' experiences and evaluations of aromatherapy massage in palliative care. *Int J Palliat Nurs.* 2002;8:497–504.
27. Goodwin P, Leszcz M, Ennis M, et al. The effect of group psychosocial support on survival in metastatic breast cancer. *N Engl J Med.* 2001;345:1719–1726.
28. Zabora J, Brintzenhofeszoc JK, Curbow B, et al. The prevalence of psychological distress by cancer site. *Psychooncology.* 2001;10:19–28.
29. Jones JM, Huggins MA, Rydall AC, et al. Symptomatic distress, hopelessness, and the desire for hastened death in hospitalized cancer patients. *J Psychosom Res.* 2003;55:411–418.
30. Kelly B, Burnett P, Pelusi D, et al. Factors associated with the wish to hasten death: a study of patients with terminal illness. *Psychol Med.* 2003;33:75–81.
31. Norton TR, Manne SL, Rubin S, et al. Prevalence and predictors of psychological distress among women with ovarian cancer. *J Clin Oncol.* 2004;22:919–926.
32. Green B, Krupnick J, Rowland J, et al. Trauma history as a predictor of psychological symptoms in women with breast cancer. *J Clin Oncol.* 2000;18:1084–1094.
33. Silver-Aylaian M, Cohen LH. Role of major lifetime stressors in patients' and spouses' reactions to cancer. *J Trauma Stress.* 2001;14:405–412.
34. Yeh CH. Psychological distress: testing hypotheses based on Roy's adaptation model. *Nurs Sci Q.* 2003;16:255–263.
35. Hawkley LC, Cacioppo JT. Loneliness and pathways to disease. *Brain Behav Immun.* 2003;17(suppl 1):S98-S105.
36. Cordova MJ, Giese-Davis J, Golant M, et al. Mood disturbance in community cancer support groups: the role of emotional suppression and fighting spirit. *J Psychosom Res.* 2003;55:461–467.
37. Baider L, Ever-Hadani P, Goldzweig G, et al. Is perceived family support a relevant variable in psychological distress? A sample of prostate and breast cancer couples. *J Psychosom Res.* 2003;55:453–460.
38. van Loon AJ, Tijhuis M, Surtees PG, et al. Lifestyle risk factors for cancer: the relationship with psychosocial work environment. *Int J Epidemiol.* 2000;29:785–792.
39. Carlson LE, Bultz BD. Cancer distress screening: needs, models, and methods. *J Psychosom Res.* 2003;55:403–409.
40. Sharpe M, Strong V, Allen K, et al. Major depression in outpatients attending a regional cancer centre: screening and unmet treatment needs. *Br J Cancer.* 2004;90:314–320.
41. Cunningham AJ. Adjuvant psychological therapy for cancer patients: putting it on the same footing as adjunctive medical therapies. *Psychooncology.* 2000;9:367–371.
42. McLachlan SA, Allenby A, Matthews J, et al. Randomized trial of coordinated psychosocial interventions based on patient self-assessments versus standard care to improve the psychosocial functioning of patients with cancer. *J Clin Oncol.* 2001;19:4117–4125.
43. Zakowski SG, Harris C, Krueger N, et al. Social barriers to emotional expression and their relations to distress in male and female cancer patients. *Br J Health Psychol.* 2003;8:271–286.
44. Jacox AK, Carr D, Payne R, et al. *Management of Cancer Pain. Clinical Practice Guideline No. 9.* AHCPR Publication No. 94–0592. Rockville, MD: Agency for Health Care Policy and Research, US Department of Health and Human Services, Public Health Service; 1994.
45. Philips DM. JCAHO pain management standards are unveiled. *JAMA.* 2000;284:428–429.
46. Kelley KW, Bluthe RM, Dantzer R, et al. Cytokine-induced sickness behavior. *Brain Behav Immun.* 2003;17:S112–S118.
47. Miller AH. Cytokines and sickness behavior: implications for cancer care and control. *Brain Behav Immun.* 2003;17:S132–S134.
48. Patrick DL, Ferketich SL, Frame PS, et al. National Institutes of Health State-of-the-Science Conference statement: symptom management in cancer: pain, depression, and fatigue, July 15–17, 2002. *J Natl Cancer Inst.* 2003;95:1110–1117.
49. Cohen MZ, Easley M, Ellis C, et al. Cancer pain management and the JCAHO's pain standards: an institutional challenge. *J Pain Symptom Manage.* 2003;25:519–527.
50. Yancik R, Ries LAG. Cancer in older persons: an international issue in an aging world. *Semin Oncol.* 2004;31:128–136.
51. U.S. Census Bureau News. An Older and More Diverse nation by Midcentury. http://www.census.gov/Press-Release/www/releases/archives/population/012496.html. Accessed December 28, 2009.
52. Carlson LE, Angen M, Cullum J, et al. High levels of untreated distress and fatigue in cancer patients. *Br J Cancer.* 2004;90:2297–2304.
53. Spoletini I, Gianni W, Repetto L, et al. Depression and cancer: an unexplored and unresolved emergent issue in elderly patients. *Crit Rev Oncol Hematol.* 2008;65:143–155.
54. Repetto L, Fratino L, Audisio RA, et al. Comprehensive geriatric assessment adds information to Eastern Cooperative Oncology Group performance status in elderly cancer patients: an Italian Group for Geriatric Oncology study. *J Clin Oncol.* 2002;20:494–502.
55. Perkins EA, Small BJ, Balducci L, Extermann M, Robb C, Haley WE. Individual differences in well-being in older breast cancer survivors. *Crit Rev Oncol Hematol.* 2007;62:74–83.
56. Llorente MD, Burke M, Gregory GR, et al. Prostate cancer: a significant risk factor for late-life suicide. *Am J Geriatr Psychiatry.* 2005;13:195–201.
57. Schnittker J. Chronic illness and depressive symptoms in late life. *Soc Sci Med.* 2005;60:13–23.
58. Graves K, Arnold S, Love C, Kirsh K, Moore P, Passik S. Distress screening in a multidisciplinary lung cancer clinic: prevalence and predictors of clinically significant distress. *Lung Cancer.* 2007;55:215–224.
59. Mulsant BH, Ganguli M. Epidemiology and diagnosis of depression in late life. *J Clin Psychiatry.* 1999;60:9–15.
60. Oncology Nursing Society. Oncology Nursing Society and Geriatric Oncology Consortium joint position on cancer care in the older adult. *Eur J Cancer Care.* 2004;13:434–435.
61. Jacobsen PB, Donovan KA, Trask PC, et al. Screening for psychologic distress in ambulatory cancer patients: a multicenter evaluation of the distress thermometer. *Cancer.* 2005;103:1494–1502.
62. Ransom S, Jacobsen PB, Booth-Jones M. Validation of the distress thermometer with bone marrow transplant patients. *Psychooncology.* 2006;15:604–612.
63. Trask PC, Paterson A, Riba M, et al. Assessment of psychological distress in prospective bone marrow transplant patients. *Bone Marrow Transplant.* 2002;29:917–925.
64. King DA, Heisel MJ, Lyness JM. Assessment and psychological treatment of depression in older adults with terminal or life-threatening illness. *Clin Psychol: Sci Pract.* 2005;12:339–353.
65. Barsevick AM, Sweeney C, Haney E, Chung E. A systematic qualitative analysis of psychoeducational interventions for depression in patients with cancer. *Oncol Nurs Forum.* 2002;29:73–86.
66. Osborn RL, Demoncada AC, Feuerstein M. Psychosocial interventions for depression, anxiety, and quality of life in cancer survivors: meta-analyses. *Int J Psychiatry Med.* 2006;36:13–34.

67. Uitterhoeve RJ, Vernooy M, Litjens M, et al. Psychosocial interventions for patients with advanced cancer: a systematic review of the literature. *Br J Cancer.* 2004;91:1050–1062.
68. Newell SA, Sanson-Fisher RW, Savolainen NJ. Systematic review of psychological therapies for cancer patients: overview and recommendations for future research. *J Natl Cancer Inst.* 2002;94:558–584.
69. Rodin G, Lloyd N, Katz M, Green E, Mackay JA, Wong RKS. The treatment of depression in cancer patients: a systematic review. *Support Care Cancer.* 2007;15:123–136.
70. Williams S, Dale J. The effectiveness of treatment for depression/depressive symptoms in adults with cancer: a systematic review. *Br J Cancer.* 2006;94:372–390.
71. Cankurtaran ES, Ozalp E, Soygur H, Akbiyik DI, Turhan L, Alkis N. Mirtazapine improves sleep and lowers anxiety and depression in cancer patients: superiority over imipramine. *Support Care Cancer.* 2008;16:1291–1298.
72. Ersoy MA, Noyan AM, Elbi H. An open-label long-term naturalistic study of mirtazapine treatment for depression in cancer patients. *Clin Drug Invest.* 2008;28:113–120.
73. Kast RE, Foley KF. Cancer chemotherapy and cachexia: mirtazapine and olanzapine are 5-HT3 antagonists with good antinausea effects: research in brief. *Eur J Cancer Care.* 2007;16:351–354.
74. Kornblith AB, Dowell JM, Herndon JE II, et al. Telephone monitoring of distress in patients aged 65 years or older with advanced stage cancer: a cancer and leukemia group B study. *Cancer.* 2006;107:2706–2714.
75. Cancer Health Disparities. *A Fact Sheet.* National Cancer Institute, 2005. http://www.cancer.gov/newscenter/benchmarks-vol5-issue6/page2. Accessed December 28, 2009.
76. Campesino M, Ruiz E, Glover JU, Koithan M. Counternarratives of Mexican-origin women with breast cancer. *ANS Adv Nurs Sci.* 2009;32:E57–E67.
77. Lisovicz N, Johnson RE, Higginbotham J, et al. The Deep South Network for cancer control; building a community infrastructure to reduce cancer health disparities. *Cancer.* 2006;107(8 Suppl):1971–1979.
78. Chu KC, Lamar CA, Freeman HP. Racial disparities in breast carcinoma survival rates: separating factors that affect diagnosis from factors that affect treatment. *Cancer.* 2003;97:2853–2860.
79. Culver JL, Arena PL, Wimberly SR, Antoni MH, Carver CS. Coping among African-American, Hispanic, and non-Hispanic White women recently treated for early stage breast cancer. *Psychol Health.* 2004;19: 157–166.
80. Mishel MH, Germino BB, Gil KM, et al. Benefits from an uncertainty management intervention for African-American and Caucasian older long-term breast cancer survivors. *Psychooncology.* 2005;14: 962–978.
81. Taylor KL, Lamdan RM, Siegel JE, Shelby R, Moran-Klimi K, Hrywna M. Psychological adjustment among African American breast cancer patients: one-year follow-up results of a randomized psychoeducational group intervention. *Health Psychol.* 2003;22:316–323.
82. Leak A, Hu J, King CR. Symptom distress, spirituality, and quality of life in African American breast cancer survivors. *Cancer Nurs.* 2008;31:E15–E21.
83. Simon AE, Wardle J. Socioeconomic disparities in psychosocial wellbeing in cancer patients. *Eur J Cancer.* 2008;44:572–578.
84. Curt GA. Impact of fatigue on quality of life in oncology patients. *Semin Hematol.* 2000;37(suppl 6):14–17.
85. Davidson JR, MacLean AW, Brundage MD, et al. Sleep disturbance in cancer patients. *Soc Sci Med.* 2002;54:1309–1321.
86. Carlson LE, Angen M, Cullum J, et al. High levels of untreated distress and fatigue in cancer patients. *Br J Cancer.* 2004;90:2297–2304.
87. Cella D, Paul D, Yount S, et al. What are the most important symptom targets when treating advanced cancer? A survey of providers in the National Comprehensive Cancer Network (NCCN). *Cancer Invest.* 2003;21:526–535.
88. Cella D, Lai J, Chang CH, et al. Fatigue in cancer patients compared with fatigue in the general United States population. *Cancer.* 2002;94:528–538.
89. Donovan KA, Jacobsen PB. Fatigue, depression, and insomnia: evidence for a symptom cluster in cancer. *Semin Oncol Nurs.* 2007;23:127–135.
90. Mitchell S, Beck S, Hood L, Moore K, Tanner E. *Putting Evidence Into Practice: What Interventions Are Effective in Preventing and Treating Fatigue During and Following Cancer and Its Treatment?* Pittsburgh, PA: Oncology Nursing Society; 2005.
91. Owen DC, Parker KP, McGuire DB. Comparison of subjective sleep quality in patients with cancer and healthy subjects. *Oncol Nurs Forum.* 1999;26:1649–1651.
92. Savard J, Morin CM, Akechi T. Insomnia in the context of cancer: a review of a neglected problem. *J Clin Oncol.* 2001;19:895–908.
93. Ancoli-Israel S, Moore PJ, Jones V. The relationship between fatigue and sleep in cancer patients: a review. *Eur J Cancer Care.* 2001;10: 245–255.
94. Morin CM, Rodrigue S, Ivers H. Role of stress, arousal, and coping skills in primary insomnia. *Psychosom Med.* 2003;65:259–267.
95. Carter P. Family caregivers' sleep loss and depression over time. *Cancer Nurs.* 2003;26:253–259.
96. Page MS, Berger AM, Johnson LB. *Putting Evidence Into Practice: What Can Nurses Do to Assist People with Cancer with Sleep-Wake Disturbances?* Pittsburgh, PA: Oncology Nursing Society; 2005.
97. Meyers C, Hess K, Yung WKA, et al. Cognitive function as a predictor of survival in patients with recurrent malignant glioma. *J Clin Oncol.* 2000;18:646–650.
98. Sherman A, Jaeckle K, Meyers C. Pretreatment cognitive performance predicts survival in patients with leptomeningeal disease. *Cancer.* 2002; 95:1311–1316.
99. Breitbart W, Gibson C, Tremblay A. The delirium experience: delirium recall and delirium-related distress in hospitalized patients with cancer, their spouses/caregivers, and their nurses. *Psychosomatics.* 2002;43:183–194.
100. Ahles TA, Saykin A. Cognitive effects of standard-dose chemotherapy in patients with cancer. *Cancer Invest.* 2001;19:812–820.
101. Cohen MZ, Armstrong T. Cognitive dysfunction. In: Yarbro CH, Frogge MH, Goodman M, eds. *Cancer Symptom Management.* 3rd ed. Sudbury, MA: Jones and Bartlett; 2004:635–650.
102. Capuron L, Ravaud A, Dantzer R. Timing and specificity of the cognitive changes induced by interleukin-2 and interferon-alpha treatments in cancer patients. *Psychosom Med.* 2001;63:376–386.
103. Lerner DM, Stoudemire A, Rosenstein DL. Neuropsychiatric toxicity associated with cytokine therapies. *Psychosomatics.* 1999;40:428–435.
104. Lawlor P. The panorama of opioid-related cognitive dysfunction in patients with cancer: a critical literature appraisal. *Cancer.* 2002;94:1836–1853.
105. Ashby FG, Isen AM, Turken AU. A neuropsychological theory of positive affect and its influence on cognition. *Psychol Rev.* 1999;106:529–550.
106. Bremner JD. *Does Stress Damage the Brain? Understanding Trauma-Related Disorders from a Neurological Perspective.* New York: Norton; 2002.
107. Storbeck J, Clore GL. On the interdependence of cognition and emotion. *Cogn Emot.* 2007;21:1212–1237.
108. Lawlor PG, Bruera ED. Delirium in patients with advanced cancer. *Hematol Oncol Clin North Am.* 2002;16:701–714.
109. Tuma R, DeAngelis LM. Altered mental status in patients with cancer. *Arch Neurol.* 2000;57:1727–1731.
110. McCusker J, Cole M, Dendukuri N, Belzile E, Primeau F. Delirium in older medical inpatients and subsequent cognitive and functional status: a prospective study. *Can Med Assoc J.* 2001;165:575–583.
111. McCusker J, Cole M, Abrahamowicz M, Primeau F, Belzile E. Delirium predicts 12-month mortality. *Arch Intern Med.* 2002;162: 457–463.
112. McCusker J, Cole M, Dendukuri N, Han L, Belzile E. The course of delirium in older medical inpatients: a prospective study. *J Gen Intern Med.* 2003;18:696–704.

113. Breitbart W, Strout D. Delirium in the terminally ill. *Clin Geriatric Med.* 2000;16:357–372.
114. Casarett DJ, Inouye SK. Diagnosis and management of delirium near the end of life. *Ann Intern Med.* 2001;135:32–40.
115. Lawlor PG, Fainsinger RL, Bruera ED. Delirium at the end of life: critical issues in clinical practice and research. *JAMA.* 2000;284: 2427–2429.
116. O'Malley G, Leonard M, Meagher D, O'Keeffe ST. The delirium experience: a review. *J Psychosom Res.* 2008;65:223–228.
117. Agar M, Lawlor P. Delirium in cancer patients: a focus on treatment-induced psychopathology. *Curr Opin Oncol.* 2008;20:360–366.
118. Han L, McCusker J, Cole M, Abrahamowicz M, Primeau F, Elie M. Use of medications with anticholinergic effect predicts clinical severity of delirium symptoms in older medical inpatients. *Arch Intern Med.* 2001;161:1099–1105.
119. Ljubisavljevic V, Kelly B. Risk factors for development of delirium among oncology patients. *Gen Hosp Psychiatry.* 2003;25:345–352.
120. Edlund A, Lundstrom M, Sandberg O, Bucht G, Brannstrom B, Gustafson Y. Symptom profile of delirium in older people with and without dementia. *J Geriatr Psychiatry Neurol.* 2007;20:166–171.
121. Miovic M, Block S. Psychiatric disorders in advanced cancer. *Cancer.* 2007;110:1665–1676.
122. Angelino AF, Treisman GJ. Major depression and demoralization in cancer patients: diagnostic and treatment considerations. *Support Care Cancer.* 2001;9:344–349.
123. Miovic M, Block S. Psychiatric disorders in advanced cancer. *Cancer.* 2007;110:1665–1676.
124. Passik S, Lundberg J, Rosenfeld B, et al. Factor analysis of the Zung self-rating depression scale in a large ambulatory oncology sample. *Psychosomatics.* 2000;41:121–127.
125. Brennan J. Adjustment to cancer—coping or personal transition? *Psychooncology.* 2001;10:1–18.
126. Angelino AF, Treisman GJ. Major depression and demoralization in cancer patients: diagnostic and treatment considerations. *Support Cancer Care.* 2001;9:344–349.
127. Bodurka-Bevers D, Basen-Engquist K, Carmack CL, et al. Depression, anxiety, and quality of life in patients with epithelial ovarian cancer. *Gynecol Oncol.* 2000;78:302–308.
128. Litofsky NS, Farace E, Anderson F, et al. Depression in patients with high-grade glioma: results of the Glioma Outcomes project. *Neurosurgery* 2004;54:358–366.
129. Lloyd-Williams M, Friedman T. Depression in palliative care patients: a prospective study. *Eur J Cancer Care.* 2001;10:270–274.
130. Pasquini M, Biondi M. Depression in cancer patients: a critical review. *Clin Pract Epidemiol Ment Health.* 2007;3:2.
131. American Psychiatric Association. *Diagnostic and Statistical Manual of Mental Disorders.* 4th ed, text revision [DSM-IV-TR]. Washington, DC: American Psychiatric Association; 2000.
132. Wedding U, Koch A, Rohrig B, et al. Requestioning depression in patients with cancer: contribution of somatic and affective symptoms to beck's depression inventory. *Ann Oncol.* 2007;18:1875–1881.
133. van't Spijker A, Trijsburg RW, Duivenvoorden HJ. Psychologic sequelae of cancer diagnosis: a meta-analytical review of 58 studies after 1980. *Psychosom Med.* 1997;59:280–293.
134. Stark D, Kiely M, Smith A, et al. Anxiety disorders in cancer patients: their nature, associations, and relation to quality of life. *J Clin Oncol.* 2002;20:3137–3148.
135. Kerrihard T, Breibart W, Dent R, et al. Anxiety in patients with cancer and human immunodeficiency virus. *Semin Clin Neuropsychiatry.* 1999;4:114–132.
136. Gurevick M, Devins GM, Rodin GM. Stress response syndromes and cancer: conceptual and assessment issues. *Psychosomatics.* 2002;43: 259–281.
137. Kangas M, Henry JL, Bryant RA. Posttraumatic stress disorder following cancer: a conceptual and empirical review. *Clin Psychol Rev.* 2002;22:499–524.
138. Neel ML. Post-traumatic stress symptomatology and cancer. *Int J Emerg Ment Health.* 2000;2:85–94.
139. Jim H, Jacobsen P. Posttraumatic stress and posttraumatic growth in cancer survivorship: a review. *Cancer J.* 2008;6:414–419.
140. Kangas M, Henry JL, Bryant RA. Predictors of posttraumatic stress disorder following cancer. *Health Psychol.* 2005;24:579–585.
141. Dugan W, McDonald MV, Passik SD, et al. Use of the Zung self-rating depression scale in cancer patients: feasibility as a screening tool. *Psychooncology.* 1998;7:483–493.
142. Kirsh KL, Passik S, Holtsclaw E, et al. I get tired for no reason: a single-item screening for cancer-related fatigue. *J Pain Symptom Manage.* 2001;22:931–937.
143. Love AW, Kissane DW, Bloch S, et al. Diagnostic efficiency of the Hospital Anxiety and Depression Scale in women with early stage breast cancer. *Austr N Zeal J Psychol.* 2002;36:246–250.
144. Merluzzi TV, Nairn RC, Hedge K, et al. Self-efficacy for coping with cancer: revision of the Cancer Behavior Inventory (version 2.0). *Psychooncology.* 2001;10:206–217.
145. Nicholas D, Veach T. The psychosocial assessment of the adult cancer patient. *Prof Psychol.* 2000;31:206–215.
146. Barsevick AM, Dudley W, Beck S, et al. A randomized clinical trial of energy conservation for patients with cancer-related fatigue. *Cancer.* 2004;100:1302–1310.
147. Nail L. Fatigue in patients with cancer. *Oncol Nurs Forum.* 2002;29:537–544.
148. Cramp F, Daniel J. Exercise for the management of cancer-related fatigue in adults. *Cochrane Database Syst Rev.* 2008;2:CD006145.
149. Quesnel C, Savard J, Simard S, et al. Efficacy of cognitive-behavioral therapy for insomnia in women treated for nonmetastatic breast cancer. *J Consult Clin Psychol.* 2003;71:189–200.
150. Oyama H, Kaneda M, Katsumata N, et al. Using the bedside wellness system during chemotherapy decreases fatigue and emesis in cancer patients. *J Med Syst.* 2000;24:173–182.
151. Wilkinson S, Barnes K, Storey L. Massage for symptom relief in patients with cancer: systematic review. *J Adv Nurs.* 2008;63:430–439.
152. Swanson S, Dolce A, Marsh K, Summers J, Sheldon LK. *Putting Evidence Into Practice: What Interventions Are Effective in Preventing Anxiety in People with Cancer?* Pittsburgh, PA: Oncology Nursing Society; 2005.
153. National Cancer Institute. Normal adjustment, and the adjustment disorders. 2008. http://www.cancer.gov/cancertopics/pdq/supportivecare/adjustment/healthprofessional. Accessed December 28, 2009.
154. Zakowski SG, Hall MH, Klein LC, et al. Appraised control, coping, and stress in a community sample: a test of the goodness-of-fit hypothesis. *Ann Behav Med.* 2001;23:158–165.
155. Given C, Given B, Rahbar M, et al. Effect of a cognitive behavioral intervention on reducing symptom severity during chemotherapy. *J Clin Oncol.* 2004;22:507–516.
156. Carlson LE, Ursuliak Z, Goodey E, et al. The effects of a mindfulness meditation-based stress reduction program on mood and symptoms of stress in cancer outpatients: 6-month follow-up. *Support Care Cancer.* 2001;9:112–123.
157. Kieviet-Stijnen A, Visser A, Garssen B, Hudig W. Mindfulness-based stress reduction training for oncology patients: patients' appraisal and changes in well-being. *Patient Educ Couns.* 2008;72:436–442.
158. Witek-Janusek L, Albuquerque K, Chroniak KR, Chroniak C, Durazo-Arvizu R, Mathews HL. Effect of mindfulness based stress reduction on immune function, quality of life and coping in women newly diagnosed with early stage breast cancer. *Brain Behav Immun.* 2008;22:969–981.
159. Jacobsen PB, Meede CD, Stein KD, et al. Efficacy and costs of two forms of stress management training for cancer patients undergoing chemotherapy. *J Clin Oncol.* 2002;20:2851–2862.
160. Petersen RW, Quinlivan JA. Preventing anxiety and depression in gynaecological cancer: a randomised controlled trial. *Br J Obstet Gynaecol.* 2002;109:386–394.

161. Milligan M, Fanning M, Hunter S, et al. Reflexology audit: patient satisfaction, impact on quality of life and availability in Scottish hospices. *Complement Ther.* 2002;8:489–496.
162. Gilbar O, Iron G, Goren A. Adjustment to illness of cancer patients treated by complementary therapy along with conventional therapy. *Patient Educ Couns.* 2001;44:243–249.
163. Risberg T, Jacobsen BK. The association between mental distress and the use of alternative medicine among cancer patients in north Norway. *Qual Life Res.* 2003;12:539–544.
164. Gobel B. Anxiety. In: Yarbro CH, Frogge MH, Goodman M, eds. *Cancer Symptom Management.* 3rd ed. Sudbury, MA: Jones and Bartlett; 2003:651–664.
165. Barsevick A, Much J. Depression. In: Yarbro CH, Frogge MH, Goodman M, eds. *Cancer Symptom Management.* 3rd ed. Sudbury, MA: Jones and Bartlett; 2003:668–684.
166. Nemetz S, Mercardante M. The evolution of a cancer support center: a work in progress. *Oncol Nurs Forum.* 2002;29:1397–1399.
167. Bultz BD, Thomas BC, Stewart DA, Carlson LE. Distress—The sixth vital sign in cancer care: implications for treating older adults undergoing chemotherapy. *Geriatrics Aging.* 2007;10:647–653.
168. Holland JC, Jacobsen P, Riba M. NCCN distress management. *Cancer Control.* 2001;8(suppl):88–93.
169. Akizuki N, Akechi T, Nakanishi T, et al. Development of a brief screening interview for adjustment disorders and major depression in patients with cancer. *Cancer.* 2003;97:2605–2613.
170. Kawashima I, Yoshida Y, Taya C, et al. Expansion of natural killer cells in mice transgenic for IgM antibody to ganglioside GD2: demonstration of prolonged survival after challenge with syngeneic tumor cells. *Int J Oncol.* 2003;21:381–388.
171. Kiecolt-Glaser J, Page G, Marucha P, et al. Psychological influences on surgical recovery. *Am Psychol.* 1998;53:1209–1218.
172. Page GG, Ben-Eliyahu S. The immune-suppressive nature of pain. *Semin Oncol Nurs.* 1997;13:10–15.
173. Thorne S, Paterson B. Shifting images of chronic illness. *Image.* 1998;30:173–178.

CHAPTER 27

Erin McMenamin, MSN, CRNP, AOCN®, ACHPN

# Cancer Pain Management

## SCOPE OF THE PROBLEM

Pain is the most feared consequence by patients with cancer. Pain has been defined as "an unpleasant sensory and emotional experience caused by actual or potential tissue damage, and defined in terms of such damage."[1] McCaffery and Pasero defined pain as "what the patient says it is, occurring when the patient says it does."[2] Many practitioners have attempted to define pain more fully, but since it is a subjective experience, the most accurate source of pain assessment is defined by those experiencing it.

Pain is multidimensional and encompasses (1) physiological (etiology of pain); (2) sensory (intensity, location, quality); (3) affective (depression, anxiety); (4) cognitive (manner in which pain influences an individual's thought processes, how the individual views self or the meaning of pain; (5) behavioral (pain-related behaviors such as medication intake and activity level); and (6) sociocultural dimensions (which includes demographic, social, and cultural characteristics that are related to the experience of pain).[3] All of these dimensions of pain are important in assessing and treating pain.

## EPIDEMIOLOGY OF CANCER PAIN

The incidence of cancer pain for all cancer diagnoses during all stages of disease is difficult to quantify because of lack of standardized definition and assessment measures. According to the International Association for the Study of Pain (IASP), pain occurs in as many as 50% of patients with cancer undergoing treatment for their disease, and more than 70% of patients experience pain towards the end of life. Cancer is a common disease and leading cause of death in the US. At least 40% of patients with cancer reported more than 1 pain site.[4] Of those cancer patients reporting pain, 42% report inadequate analgesia. In addition, as much as one-third of patients with cancer report severe pain affecting their quality of life (QOL).[5] Female gender, minority status, and advanced age are risk factors for undertreatment of pain in the adult population.[6–8] Inadequate treatment of pain may also be related to the side effects associated with the treatment of pain itself.[9] McMillan and colleagues found that unrelieved pain is also related to sleep disturbance as well as depression in patients with cancer.[10] Mao and colleagues report that as many as 34% of cancer survivors report pain.[11] In this study, pain was more frequently reported by younger survivors, those with comorbidities, and Caucasian patients.

## ETIOLOGY OF CANCER PAIN

Acute pain and chronic pain are distinctly different phenomena. Acute pain occurs when tissues are injured. Subsequent increases in blood pressure and pulse may occur, along with grimacing, pallor, diaphoresis, and dilated pupils. These are all symptoms of autonomic nervous system (ANS) stimulation. Generally, these symptoms subside over several days as the ANS accommodates to the presence of pain. Chronic pain is often not accompanied by these symptoms due to the accommodation of the ANS. Chronic pain of nonmalignant origin is often present due to changes in the brain. This pain is frequently no longer serving a purpose. Chronic pain of malignant origin is due to the disease infiltrating or compressing organs, nerves, bones, or other tissues. Additionally, the treatments for cancer may also cause pain by killing healthy cells in the mouth and gastrointestinal tract, or nerves for example. This pain, opposed to nonmalignant pain, serves a purpose, in that it is processing pain signals due to an injury to tissues that is ongoing.

There are different etiologies of pain in patients with cancer. Cancer pain can result from direct tumor involvement. For example, malignant tumors can compress or infiltrate organs, nerves, blood vessels, and connective tissue. Necrosis of tissue due to tumors can cause infection, leading to pain. Cancer pain is also associated with cancer therapy and sources of this pain can range from initial diagnostic procedures to standard therapeutic modalities (surgery, radiation therapy, chemotherapy, and targeted therapy). For example, chemotherapy can damage nerve tissue, cause painful mucositis, and other painful conditions. Radiation can cause fibrosis or strictures of the treated tissues, also resulting in pain. Pain is a significant experience for the person with cancer regardless of its cause.

## PHYSIOLOGICAL ALTERATIONS

Three specific pain syndromes occur in patients with cancer. These syndromes of somatic, visceral, and neuropathic pain are characterized by pain of different qualities, may be located in different anatomical parts of the body, and caused by different mechanisms. Distinctions between somatic and visceral pain, and neuropathic pain, reflect not only the mechanisms causing the pain but also anticipated responses to treatment. Many patients with cancer pain will have 1 or more of these 3 syndromes simultaneously and each syndrome responds differently to therapeutic modalities.

## TYPES OF PAIN

### NOCICEPTIVE PAIN

Nociceptive pain is pain that results from activation of peripheral nociceptors. There are 2 types of nociceptive pain; somatic and visceral. Somatic pain is caused by activation of the nociceptors in the periphery, such as the skin, bone, muscles, joints, or connective tissue. It is generally well localized, and often an aching, gnawing, or throbbing pain. It can be constant or intermittent. Visceral pain is caused by activation of nociceptors in the abdominal or thoracic cavities. It results from compression, infiltration, or distention of viscera.[12] It is generally a poorly localized pain, and may be described as dull, aching, or cramping.[2,13] Both types of pain respond to treatment with opioids as well as adjuvant medications.

### NEUROPATHIC PAIN

Neuropathic pain is caused by abnormal processing of input by the peripheral or central nervous system. Treede and colleagues[14] proposed redefining neuropathic pain as "pain arising as a direct consequence of a lesion or disease affecting the somatosensory system." Approximately 40% of patients with cancer report neuropathic pain.[15] It is most commonly caused by compression of a nerve by tumor or a polyneuropathy caused by chemotherapy. Neuropathic pain may be described as a shooting, burning, pins and needles, or hot or cold sensation. It is generally less responsive to opioids alone, often requiring the addition of adjuvant medications in order to obtain adequate control of pain. This is likely due to changes within the nervous system as a result of the damage. See Table 27-1 for neuropathic pain syndromes related to cancer.[16]

Many patients with cancer demonstrate mixed types of pain. For example, pain of bony origin is considered somatic pain. Bone pain may also demonstrate some characteristics associated with neuropathic pain. Neuropathic features of bone pain may result from injury and the subsequent destruction of distal sensory nerve fibers by the bone tumor cells.[9] A mixed presentation of pain may present challenges to clinicians, especially when they are not recognized and seen only as atypical for the particular pain syndrome.

## CLINICAL MANIFESTATIONS

Cancer pain generally presents in 2 patterns: persistent and intermittent or breakthrough pain (BTP). Persistent pain and BTP must be assessed and treated separately.

### PERSISTENT PAIN

Persistent pain is pain that is present most of the day (≥12 hours). Persistent pain in patients with cancer is generally managed with sustained release opioid medication administered around the clock (ATC) on a scheduled basis. This method of medication administration avoids the peaks and valleys associated with short-acting medications. In addition, ATC administration of sustained release medications allows the patient to avoid administration in the middle of the night due to the longer duration of action.

### BREAKTHROUGH PAIN

Breakthrough pain is defined as a transient exacerbation or flare of moderate to severe pain. It occurs in patients with

**TABLE 27-1**

**Neuropathic Syndromes Related to Cancer**

| Neuropathic Syndromes | Clinical Examples |
|---|---|
| Cranial nerve neuralgias<br>Postherpetic neuralgia | Base of skull or leptomeningeal metastases, head and neck cancers |
| Mononeuropathy and other neuralgias | Rib metastases with intercostal nerve injury |
| Cervical plexopathy | Head and neck cancer with local extension, cervical lymph node metastases |
| Radiculopathy | Epidural mass, leptomeningeal metastases |
| Brachial plexopathy | Lymph node metastases from breast cancer or lymphoma, direct extension of Pancoast tumor |
| Lumbosacral plexopathy | Extension of colorectal cancer, cervical cancer, sarcoma, or lymphoma; breast cancer metastases |
| Paraneoplastic peripheral neuropathy | Small cell lung cancer, antineuronal nuclear antibodies type I (ANNA-1) |
| Central pain | Spinal cord compression |
| Cachexia | Compression or entrapment neuropathies |

*Source*: Reprinted with permission from Shaiova.[16]

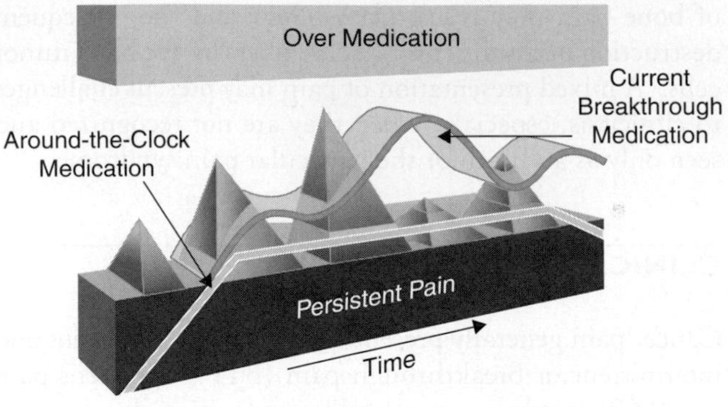


**FIGURE 27-1**

Treatment of breakthrough pain (BTP) using short-acting opioids (SAOs). The incidence of BTP is known to be very rapid at times. Typical short-acting opioids have an onset of action of approximately 20 to 30 minutes. This figure demonstrates how SAOs may have their peak effect as the BTP is decreasing.

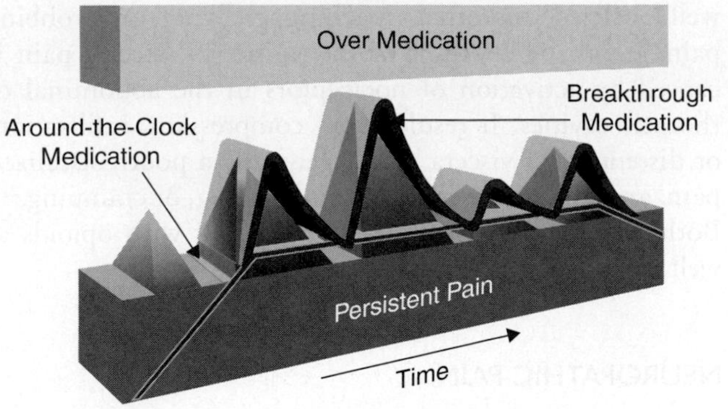


**FIGURE 27-3**

Demonstrates using opioids with a rapid onset (ROO). The ROO has an onset of action within the time frame frequently associated with BTP, resulting in adequate analgesia without sedating side effects.

otherwise stable persistent pain and is generally treated with short-acting medications.[17] Fifty-one to 89% of patients with cancer experiencing pain report BTP.[18–20] The following 3 figures show examples of persistent pain with treatment of BTP. Figure 27-1 represents treatment of BTP using short-acting opioids (SAOs). The incidence of BTP is known to be very rapid at times. Typical short-acting opioids have an onset of action of approximately 20 to 30 minutes. This figure demonstrates how SAOs may have their peak effect as the BTP is decreasing. Figure 27-2 represents BTP treated only with long-acting opioids resulting in over medication. Figure 27-3 demonstrates using opioids with a rapid onset (ROO). The ROO has an onset of action within the time frame frequently associated with BTP, resulting in adequate analgesia without sedating side effects.

Breakthrough pain has been further defined by Portenoy and colleagues[19] into 3 categories: idiopathic, incident, and end of dose failure. Idiopathic BTP is pain that has no identifiable precipitating factor and occurs spontaneously. Incident BTP is associated with specific activities and can be predictable or unpredictable. In patients experiencing predictable incident pain, specific activities that are planned such as walking are predictable in their precipitation of pain. In the case of unpredictable incident pain, events such as sneezing cannot be predicted, and are therefore, more difficult to treat in advance of the occurrence. The last type of breakthrough pain is end of dose failure. That is pain which occurs towards the end of the time interval for a sustained release medication, requiring supplementation with short-acting opioids. Common characteristics of BTP are outlined in Table 27-2.[17]

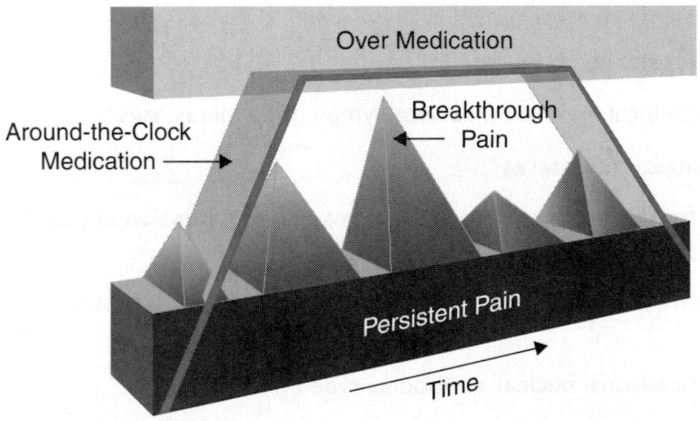


**FIGURE 27-2**

Breakthrough pain treated only with long acting opioids resulting in overmedication.

Clinicians must note the pattern of BTP medication when assessing for the need for changes in the medication regimen. In the past, clinicians were encouraged to increase the sustained release medications when the number of BTP doses exceeded 4 per day. More recent literature reveals patients experiencing incident BTP require premedication with analgesics prior to activities that exacerbate pain.[21] If patients have their sustained release medication increased in this case, they would likely become sedated, and still require BTP medications when participating in activities (Figures 27-1 to 27-3). Hagan and colleagues[22] found there was an insignificant correlation between patients' sustained release medication dose and their BTP medication dose. They found the BTP dose was higher with neuropathic pain and as much as 30% lower with increasing age.

**TABLE 27-2**

**Common Characteristics of Breakthrough Pain**

| Onset | Duration | Number of Episodes |
|---|---|---|
| As little as 3 minutes | 30 minutes | 1–5/day |

## ASSESSMENT

The most common reason for inadequate treatment of pain is lack of knowledge regarding pain. The second most common reason for inadequate treatment is lack of assessment. It is essential that nurses play a key role in assessment of pain in the patient with cancer. Nurses must present and document a concrete assessment of pain on a regular basis in order to allow clinicians making decisions regarding analgesics and other treatments to provide adequate relief for patients. Nurses must also obtain information regarding the adequacy of treatments provided to patients for the treatment of their pain and document and communicate those findings.

### PAIN HISTORY

In caring for patients, it is essential to obtain a history of the pain in order to develop a plan that meets their individual needs. The history should include when the pain first started, the pattern or time course of the pain, duration, as well as any treatments used. The effectiveness of previous treatments should be noted in order to avoid treatments the patient has attempted without success or resulted in intolerable side effects. Table 27-3 provides a list of common pain questions.

Ask the patient to describe or show you where the pain is located. If possible, have a pictorial representation of the body and have the patient color the area where they are experiencing pain. If there are multiple sites of pain, the patient can mark several areas of the body on the picture.[23]

### ASSESSMENT TOOLS

The rating of pain is very subjective. There are numerous assessment tools or pain rating scales available, however, this chapter will focus on the more commonly used scales. Scales may be unidimensional or multidimensional. Unidimensional scales have 1 measure to rate pain. These are generally pain severity scales. Multidimensional scales measure several things in addition to severity such as behavior, mood, how pain affects certain activities of daily living (ADLs), and treatments used previously. Multidimensional scales differ from each other regarding what is measured and how it is measured. There are other scales addressing special populations and/or other symptoms. Those scales are beyond the scope of this chapter.

#### Numeric scales

The most commonly used scale in adults is the numeric rating scale (NRS). Patients are instructed to rate their pain from 0 to 10, with "0" being no pain and "10" being the most severe pain they can imagine. Zero to 10 is preferable over numeric scales containing fewer or greater numbers since mild, moderate, and severe pain is well-differentiated.[24,25] In a study of patients with a wide variety of tumor types, Paice and Cohen[26] found that a verbally administered NRS was preferred over a visual analog scale (VAS) and a word descriptor scale. Farrar and colleagues[27] reported that a NRS demonstrated a clinically significant improvement in pain with a decrement of 2 or a 30% decrease in scores on a 0 to 10 scale. The decrease was consistent regardless of the severity of pain experienced by the patient.

**TABLE 27-3**

| Common Pain Assessment Questions |
|---|
| When did the pain start? |
| Where is the pain located? |
| How severe is your pain? |
| Is it constant or intermittent? |
| Does it stay constant or vary in severity? |
| How long does it last? |
| What does it feel like? |
| Does anything make it better or worse? |
| Is pain interfering with activity, mood, sleep, appetite, ability to work? |
| What treatments have you used for your pain? |
| Were they helpful? |
| Do you take the medications as prescribed? |
| Are you taking anything other than prescribed medications (eg, herbs, OTC analgesics, illicit substances)? |

*Abbreviation*: OTC, over the counter.

#### Word scales

Often referred to as the simple descriptor scale (SDS), 3 to 6 words are used to rate or describe pain in this scale. Patients are asked to rate their pain from none to severe or excruciating. The lack of consistency in the words or number of words used in this scale among practitioners has led to some difficulties in interpreting data from studies.[26] However, elderly patients with varying degrees of cognitive impairment were most often able to use the verbal scale when rating pain using a unidimensional scale.[28]

Regardless of the word scale used, it is essential that practitioners use the same words with patients using this scale in order to avoid confusion for the patient or the progress made in treating the pain. Clinicians must consider the literacy level of the patient when using word scales, as even the word moderate may be poorly understood in some patients with lower literacy levels.

## Nonverbal scales

Assessing pain in patients who have no or limited ability to communicate with practitioners regarding their pain is difficult. No scales demonstrate clinically adequate reliability and validity in patients with limited verbal abilities to communicate their pain. However, Bjoro and Herr[29] recommend the use of 5 interventions to assess this group of especially vulnerable patients. These interventions are (1) self-report, (2) the search for a cause of the pain, (3) the use of behavioral indicators of pain, (4) the use of surrogate reporters of pain, and (5) an analgesic trial to determine if behaviors that might be indicative of pain decrease after administration.

## Visual analog scale

The visual analog scale (VAS) is a scale using a 100 mm line. At each end of the line are words—no pain, and severe pain. Patients are instructed to mark an "x" on the line that corresponds with their level of pain. This scale has been validated and is used frequently in research studies.[30]

## Faces scale

The faces scale uses pictures of faces with varying levels of distress depicted from happy to crying.[31] The scale was first validated by Wong and Baker[32] for use in children with pain. Hicks et al[31] validated a revised scale for use in adults that eliminated the crying figures and adapted a more anatomically accurate picture of an adult face. It is often used as an alternative scale when patients are unable or unwilling to use the NRS or SDS. Figure 27-4 summarizes the various pain intensity scales and revised faces scale.

## Behavioral pain scale

Payen and colleagues[33] developed a pain scale for critically ill ventilated patients. The behavioral pain scale (BPS) assessed movements during procedures, facial expression, and ventilator compliance as a method to determine pain in this population of patients. The BPS reliably predicted the patient's pain when painful procedures were compared to painless procedures in a group of seriously ill patients. A higher score was predictive of more severe pain.

Holen et al[34] recommend using caution in palliative care patients when using unidimensional scales to rate pain. The authors report that multidimensional scales were preferable in this group since intensity, temporal pattern, treatment and aggravating/alleviating factors, location, and interference with health-related QOL were ranked as the most important measures in the palliative care patient by a group of surveyed experts. The authors report that most tools presently use pain intensity and interference with activity, but failed to assess temporal pattern, which was rated as the second most important item in pain assessment. Kirkova et al[35] propose that symptom rating scales should be shorter in debilitated patients. Keene and Thompson[36] found that nurses with a higher level of education were better able to assess their own ability to assess pain, but this did not result in improved treatment of patients' pain.

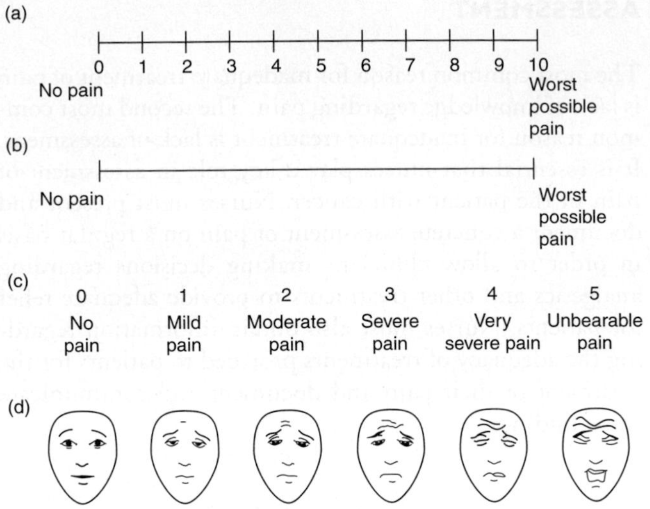


**FIGURE 27-4**

Pain intensity scales: (a) 0 to 10 numeric scale, (b) visual analog scale, (c) descriptive scale, and (d) faces pain scale—revised.
*Source:* Data from Hicks et al.[31]

## Short-form McGill Pain Questionnaire

Often, having patients describe their pain can elicit clues as to the source of the pain. For example, many neuropathic pains are described as burning or hot. Patients with incisional pain may describe their pain as sharp or stabbing. Visceral pains are often described as cramping or aching. In an attempt to provide more information regarding pain, Melzack[37] developed the Short-form McGill Pain Questionnaire (SFMPQ). The SFMPQ contains a list of 15 words that are the most commonly used words to describe pain. (See Figure 27-5). The words address the sensory as well as the affective components of pain. Using the SFMPQ, patients are asked to use the word that most accurately describes their pain. The author suggests that the SFMPQ provides more information regarding pain than a pain rating alone. In addition, the SFMPQ may be helpful in differentiating pain syndromes.

## Brief pain inventory

The brief pain inventory (BPI) assesses the effect pain has on many ADLs.[23] The patient is asked questions related

**SHORT-FORM McGILL PAIN QUESTIONNAIRE**

**PATIENT'S NAME:** ____________ **DATE:** ____________

| | **NONE** | **MILD** | **MODERATE** | **SEVERE** |
|---|---|---|---|---|
| THROBBING | 0) ___ | 1) ___ | 2) ___ | 3) ___ |
| SHOOTING | 0) ___ | 1) ___ | 2) ___ | 3) ___ |
| STABBING | 0) ___ | 1) ___ | 2) ___ | 3) ___ |
| SHARP | 0) ___ | 1) ___ | 2) ___ | 3) ___ |
| CRAMPING | 0) ___ | 1) ___ | 2) ___ | 3) ___ |
| GNAWING | 0) ___ | 1) ___ | 2) ___ | 3) ___ |
| HOT-BURNING | 0) ___ | 1) ___ | 2) ___ | 3) ___ |
| ACHING | 0) ___ | 1) ___ | 2) ___ | 3) ___ |
| HEAVY | 0) ___ | 1) ___ | 2) ___ | 3) ___ |
| TENDER | 0) ___ | 1) ___ | 2) ___ | 3) ___ |
| SPLITTING | 0) ___ | 1) ___ | 2) ___ | 3) ___ |
| TIRING-EXHAUSTING | 0) ___ | 1) ___ | 2) ___ | 3) ___ |
| SICKENING | 0) ___ | 1) ___ | 2) ___ | 3) ___ |
| FEARFUL | 0) ___ | 1) ___ | 2) ___ | 3) ___ |
| PUNISHING-CRUEL | 0) ___ | 1) ___ | 2) ___ | 3) ___ |

NO PAIN |————————————| WORST POSSIBLE PAIN

PPI

0 NO PAIN ___
1 MILD ___
2 DISCOMFORTING ___
3 DISTRESSING ___
4 HORRIBLE ___
5 EXCRUCIATING ___

**FIGURE 27-5**

Short-form McGill Pain Questionnaire (SF-MPQ). Descriptors 1–11 represent the sensory dimension of pain experience and 12–15 represent the affective dimension. Each descriptor is ranked on an intensity scale of 0 = none, 1 = mild, 2 = moderate, 3 = severe. The Present Pain Intensity (PPI) of the standard long-form McGill Pain Questionnaire (LF-MPQ) and the visual analogue (VAS) are also included to provide overall intensity scores.

*Source*: Reprinted with permission from Melzack.[37]

to activities such as interference with sleeping, eating, walking, working, etc. Many clinicians use interference with activity as a tool to measure the effectiveness of interventions for pain. The questionnaire also asks what aggravates and alleviates pain. Uncontrolled symptoms may affect survival if patients delay treatment due to unrelieved symptoms.[38] Since patients with cancer tend to experience multiple symptoms, clinicians must be cognizant of the effect the patient perceives the symptoms have on their QOL.

Practitioners should always ask patients about the psychological effects of their pain. For example, patients in whom ambulation causes severe discomfort may avoid ambulation and secondary concerns such as deconditioning will result. Additionally, these patients may become anxious about activity in general and develop a reactive depression. Caprio and colleagues reported that pain was not strongly associated with a poor QOL by family members in a group of terminal nursing home residents.[39]

## FREQUENCY OF PAIN ASSESSMENT

Insufficient assessment is a key reason for inadequate treatment of pain. Pain should be assessed on a regular basis using a standardized scale, such as a NRS or word scale.[40] The scale used to assess pain should be based on patient preference and abilities. Ongoing assessment should be performed on a regular basis to evaluate the pain intensity and the effectiveness of the interventions provided to the patient. Any change or new complaint of pain should be investigated. All assessments should be documented in an organized fashion.[41] Institutions must develop policies addressing the need for pain assessment that reflect patient needs. For example, JCAHO requires inpatient pain assessments within 24 hours of admission. However, if a patient is admitted for a pain crisis, a pain assessment must occur within a short time period after the patient arrives on the nursing unit in order to provide interventions in a timely manner. Alternatively, an outpatient who arrives for an annual physical examination requires a pain screening during the review of systems performed by the practitioner each year.

## PHYSICAL ASSESSMENT

Physical examination of the patient complaining of pain must include local examination of the painful area for discoloration, swelling, discharge, and when appropriate, function. Assessment of strength, range of motion, deep tendon reflexes, and muscle tone should be included in the initial and subsequent evaluations of patients complaining of extremity pain. Alternatively, patients complaining of abdominal pain do not require an examination of the extremities, but require thorough inspection, auscultation, palpation, and percussion of the abdomen.

## PAIN ASSESSMENT IN SPECIAL POPULATIONS

Care should be taken to provide adequate assessment of populations at risk for undertreatment of pain. These populations include those that are very young or old, women, non-English speaking, current or past substance abusers, cognitive impairment, or patients at the end of life. Each of these groups provides a separate but tangible challenge to practitioners to achieve optimal pain assessment.

### Elderly population

The elderly are at high risk for undertreatment of pain. Soscia[42] suggests that appropriate assessment is essential in treating this group effectively. Practitioners must use measures to assess pain using a scale the patient understands. Pergolizzi and colleagues[43] outline the reasons the elderly are not treated appropriately. They tend to perceive pain differently than younger patients. They may have cognitive difficulties that interfere with appropriate assessment of pain. The elderly metabolize medications differently due to changes in body composition. However, elderly patients respond to opioids and other medications for the treatment of pain. The American Geriatric Society (AGS) recommends several methods to optimize pain treatment in the elderly: use the least invasive route; use sustained release when possible; introduce 1 new agent at a time; titrate slowly with sufficient time intervals for assessment and switch opioids if necessary.[44]

### History of substance abuse

Patients with a known history of substance abuse are often undermedicated for pain. Passik and colleagues[45] studied patients with AIDS and cancer with and without a prior history of drug abuse. They found aberrant behaviors that were less likely and highly likely to be predictive of future abuse. Regardless of the severity of the behaviors, they suggest knowledge of the aberrant behavior must cue practitioners. This allows practitioners to provide the appropriate strategy to avoid the aberrant drug taking behavior and provide adequate analgesia to this challenging group of patients.

### Gender

Women are at higher risk for undertreatment of pain. Several studies have demonstrated that women with cancer are not treated with strong opioids and report lower pain relief scores compared to men with equal pain ratings.[46,47] Again, knowledge of biases is essential in preventing inadequate management of pain by practitioners.

## DOCUMENTATION OF PAIN ASSESSMENT

Pain assessment must be documented by practitioners in an organized fashion. Facilities must develop a method of documentation that meets the needs of the practitioners in the amount of information provided for future reference. In addition, care must be taken to develop a system of documentation which is not onerous to the patient or the practitioner. Simple 1 page forms are useful in clinical practice.[2] See Figure 27-6 for a sample flow sheet.

# PHARMACOLOGICAL MANAGEMENT OF PAIN

Cancer pain requires a coordinated, multimodal, and often, a multidisciplinary approach to treat pain. There are numerous interventions and techniques for managing cancer pain. Chemotherapy, radiation therapy, surgery, and hormonal therapy used to control or eradicate the tumor can also be effective in the control and palliation of cancer pain. Pharmacological management, interventional techniques to diminish or interrupt painful sensory input and nonpharmacological interventions are the focus of this chapter. It is essential that ongoing assessment for effect vs side effects of all interventions is performed when attempting to provide relief for patients in pain.

Pharmacological therapy with several classes of drugs (eg, nonopioids, opioids, and adjuvant agents) is generally considered the foundation for treating cancer pain and is employed for a wide variety of painful conditions. Nurses have a major responsibility to remain familiar with all of the pharmacological options for pain, including indications for their use, drug classifications, mechanisms and duration of action, routes of administration, usual starting doses, adverse effects and interventions to manage them, and important outcome measures for monitoring their effectiveness.

PATIENT NAME: ______

MR #: ______

WEIGHT: PRE-OP______ TODAY______ YESTERDAY______

DATE: ______

BODY SURFACE AREA: ______

**PAIN**

**Pain Characteristics**
1. Throbbing 2. Shooting 3. Stabbing 4. Sharp 5. Cramping 6. Gnawing 7. Hot-Burning 8. Aching 9. Heavy 10. Tender 11. Splitting 12. Pins & Needles 13. Numbness 14. Dull 15. Crushing

**Interventions**
1. IV Med 2. Oral Med 3. Epidural 4. PCA 5. Distraction/Relaxation 6. Warm Pack 7. Ice Pack 8. Massage 9. Position Change 10. See Notes
A. Acceptable to patient, no intervention needed
B. Patient appears to be sleeping, did not wake patient

| | | | | | | HEMODYNAMIC DATA | | | | | | | | | | PAIN | | |
|---|---|---|---|---|---|---|---|---|---|---|---|---|---|---|---|---|---|---|
| TIME | TEMP | HR / RHYTHM | RESPIRATORY RATE | BP CUFF / MEAN | BP ALINE / MEAN | RAP | PAP | PAP MEAN / WEDGE | CO / CI | SVR | $SVO_2$ | IV SITE(S) N OR Y S/S | | | LOCATION | INTENSITY | CHARAC-TERISTICS | INTER-VENTIONS |
| | | | | | | | | | | | | | | | | | | |
| | | | | | | | | | | | | | | | | | | |
| | | | | | | | | | | | | | | | | | | |
| | | | | | | | | | | | | | | | | | | |
| | | | | | | | | | | | | | | | | | | |

**FIGURE 27-6**

Sample documentation flow sheet.

Opioids are widely accepted as the primary treatment for cancer pain. However, many of the pain syndromes associated with cancer pain require a combination of medications as well as nonpharmacological therapies for effective treatment and pain relief. The explanation for this may be that cancer pain presents as a mixture of pain types in a number of cases.

## OPIOID ANALGESICS

Various patient-related factors influence the selection of a specific opioid, including pain intensity, patient age, concomitant medical illnesses, and specific drug characteristics.[48]

Additionally, there is certain critical information that nurses, physicians, and pharmacists must know before opioids are prescribed, dispensed, or administered to patients with cancer-related pain. Mechanism of action, common starting dose, equivalence to other analgesics, duration of effect, half life of the drug, available routes, and adverse effects that are common and unique to certain agents must be known. Table 27-4 contains information about the relative potencies of commonly used analgesics for severe pain.[49]

Opioids treat pain by competitively binding with opiate receptors, which block the pain impulse in the brain and spinal cord. Opioids also alter the mood, and in some cases provide patients with a sense of euphoria. The mechanism of this is not completely understood, but they alter the patient's response to the painful stimulus.[9] The following discussion reviews opioids used in the management of cancer pain.

### Morphine

Morphine is 1 of 2 opioids derived from the opium plant; codeine is the other drug obtained in this manner. Morphine is a potent analgesic with a strong affinity for the μ receptor in the brain and spinal cord. It is 3 times as potent in the intravenous (IV) vs the oral formulation. The decreased oral potency is due to the first pass effect of morphine by the liver. It is poorly absorbed from the oral mucosa. Therefore, the majority of the effect of sublingual dosing occurs from passive swallowing.

Two metabolites of morphine have been identified to have clinical activity. They are morphine 3 and 6 glucuronide. Morphine-6-glucuronide (M6G) is known to have analgesic activity that is twice as potent as morphine. Morphine-3-glucuronide (M3G) does not bind to opiate receptors, but may be responsible for some of the side effects associated with morphine. Both metabolites are excreted by the kidneys. If the metabolites are not excreted due to renal insufficiency or failure, side effects such as confusion, hallucinations and myoclonus may occur. The metabolites of morphine may not be dialyzable, leading to prolonged effect of the drug, sedation, and side effects in patients with renal insufficiency or failure.[50] Bruera and colleagues[51] report equal efficacy of morphine compared to methadone as a first-line treatment for cancer pain.

**TABLE 27-4**

**Opioid Analgesics for Severe Pain**

| Drug | Brand | Oral (mg) | Parenteral (mg) | Half life (hours) | Duration (hours) |
|---|---|---|---|---|---|
| Morphine | Generic | 30 | 10 | 2–4 | 4–5 |
| Immediate-release | MSIR, Roxanol | | | | |
| Controlled-release | MS Contin Oramorph SR. Avinza, Kadian | | | | 8–12<br>24 |
| Hydromorphone | Dilaudid | 7.5 | 1.5 | 2–3 | 3–4 |
| Levorphanol | Levo-Dromoran | 4 (acute)<br>2 (chronic) | 2 (acute)/1 (chronic) | 12–18 | 4–15 |
| Methadone | Dolophine | 10[a] | 5 | 15–100 | 6–12 |
| Oxycodone<br>Immediate-release | Roxicodone. Tylox,<br>Percocet, Percodan | 20 | – | 3–6 | 3–6 |
| Controlled-release | Oxycontin | | | | 12 |
| Oxymorphone | Numorphan | 5–10 | | 1,3–9 | 5–8 |
| Fentanyl | Duragesic patch | – | 0.1 | 30–60 | |

[a]Depends on previous dose; not recommended.

*Source*: Data from American Pain Society.[49]

Morphine is available for oral, parenteral, rectal, intraspinal, epidural, or subarachnoid administration. It is not available as a transdermal formulation. Controlled-release or long-acting morphine permits 8 to 12 hour dosing schedules as opposed to 3 to 4 hour dosing. Depending on the manufacturer, controlled- or sustained-released preparations come in multiple dosing strengths (15, 20, 30, 60, 100, and 200 mg) to allow flexibility in dosing schedules.

## Hydromorphone

Hydromorphone is a semisynthetic analog of morphine. Its relative potency is 5 to 8 times greater than morphine in the IV formulation. Hydromorphone is 5 times more potent in the IV form than the oral formulation. It is available in oral, parenteral, rectal, and spinal formulations. There is no sustained release formulation of hydromorphone available in the US at this time. As most opioids, it is metabolized by the liver. The metabolite, hydromorphone-3-glucuronide (H3G), is excreted by the kidneys. Hydromorphone-3-glucuronide has no analgesic activity and has been demonstrated to cause neuroexcitation at higher doses (>20 mg/hr IV).[52] This tends to occur more often in dialysis patients that have had infusions lasting greater than 14 days. Patients receiving dialysis have levels of H3G 4 times higher than patients with intact renal function. Patients experiencing neuroexcitation may benefit from decreasing the dose or rotating to another opioid, improving clearance of the drug, or use of adjuvant medications.[53]

## Methadone

Methadone is a μ opioid with potent analgesic properties. It is absorbed well from the gastrointestinal tract. It is metabolized by the P450 cytochrome and a large portion is excreted in the feces. Peak concentrations are reached 4 hours after ingestion. Once steady state is reached, 80% of methadone is bound to plasma proteins, which is responsible for the longer duration of action. It does not accumulate in renal failure and it is not filtered during dialysis.[54] Methadone has several unique properties including; N-methyl-D-aspartate (NMDA) receptor antagonism, serotonin and norepinephrine reuptake inhibition, and affinity for the delta receptor. These properties make it an analgesic that may be effective for patients that have not responded to other analgesics or have developed hyperalgesia in response to escalating doses of other opioids.[55] It is effectively absorbed through the oral mucosa due to its lipophilic nature.[56] The onset of action is 30 to 60 minutes after oral administration and the duration of analgesia is 6 to 12 hours. The half life of methadone may be as long as 15 to 100 hours, thus dose escalation should be implemented with caution in elderly patients.

The potency of oral methadone is approximately 50% of the parenteral dose.[57] Conversions involving methadone to or from another opioid are complex, and require experience on the part of the practitioner.[58] In addition, there are several manners in which to convert methadone,[59] none of which has proven superior over others. Methadone is metabolized by the liver, but unlike other opioids, up to 60% is excreted in the stool.[60]

Methadone may cause prolongation of the Q-T interval leading to Torsades de Pointes (TdP). While there are no clinical trials demonstrating this, it is most often reported with patients receiving greater than 200 mg, and more often with IV use.[61] A QTc (corrected) interval of 500 msec or greater has been demonstrated to be predictive of an increased risk of TdP.[62] Other risk factors for prolonged QT interval include structural heart disease, hypokalemia, other QT prolonging agents, a prolonged baseline QT (≥450 msec), family or patient history of TdP, hepatic impairment, bradycardia, and atrioventricular block.[63] Krantz and colleagues[64] found that cocaine use is also a risk factor for prolonging the QTc. They propose monitoring patients taking methadone with a baseline electrocardiogram (ECG), repeated in 1 month and annually thereafter. Patients demonstrating a QTc interval of 500 msecs or greater should discontinue methadone. Patients with a QTc of 450 but less than 500 msecs should be considered a higher risk for the development of TdP, therefore the risks and benefits of starting or continuing methadone should be considered.

Methadone is known to have potential interactions with many other medications, in part due to the cytochrome P450 activity. As a result, practitioners should exercise caution in its use. Table 27-5 describes the interaction of methadone with other drugs.[54,61]

**TABLE 27-5**

| Interactions of Methadone With Other Drugs |
|---|
| Medications whose serum levels are increased by methadone |
| Desipramine |
| Zidovudine |
| Medications associated with reduced methadone clearance |
| Acute ethanol ingestion |
| Fluconazole |
| Fluoxetine |
| Fluvoxamine |
| Ketoconazole |
| Sertraline |
| Somatostatin |
| Medications associated with increased methadone clearance |
| Carbamazepine |
| Chronic alcohol ingestion |
| Fusidic acid |
| Nevirapine |
| Olanzapine |
| Phenobarbital |
| Phenytoin |
| Resperidone |
| Rifampin |
| Ritonavir |
| Spironolactone |
| Medication associated with synergistic toxicity |
| Benzodiazepines |
| Medication associated with synergistic analgesia |
| Dronabinol |
| Ibuprofen |

*Source*: Data from Davis and Walsh[55]; and Weschules and Richeimer.[61]

## Oxycodone

Oxycodone is a semisynthetic opioid derived from morphine. It is available only as an oral analgesic in the US in a short and extended release formulation. In low doses oxycodone has frequently been used by practitioners in combination with acetaminophen. The dose of oxycodone can be escalated in a similar fashion to morphine when used without acetaminophen. It is 30% to 50% more potent than morphine.[65] The active metabolite of oxycodone is oxymorphone. Oxymorphone was found to be 8.7 times as potent as morphine for an average analgesic effect and 13 times as potent in peak effect in the intramuscular (IM) form.[65] This may explain why oxycodone is more potent than morphine. Noroxycodone is an inactive metabolite of oxycodone. The half life of immediate release oxycodone is approximately 3 hours.[65] Oxycontin, the sustained release formulation of oxycodone, has a duration of action of 12 hours.[66] The onset of oxycontin is 1 hour. Oxycontin is available in a variety of doses from 10 mg to 80 mg. It is frequently used for patients with cancer who have severe pain and require a sustained release formulation of an opioid. The side effect profile of oxycodone is similar to morphine. Hartung and colleagues[67] performed a retrospective audit of over 5000 patients receiving long-acting opioids in a state Medicaid program. The opioids included fentanyl, methadone, morphine, and oxycontin. They found that over a period of a year, patients were significantly less likely to be hospitalized or die if they received oxycontin vs morphine. Methadone and fentanyl recipients were also less likely to die than those receiving morphine, but the difference was not statistically significant. The side effect profile was less severe than morphine for all other drugs.

### Fentanyl

Fentanyl is a potent μ opioid that is highly lipophilic and a small molecule that is 75 to 100 times as potent as morphine. The side effect profile of fentanyl is similar to other opioids. The incidence of constipation is lower with fentanyl than morphine.[68] It is absorbed well through the buccal mucosa, skin, and blood–brain barrier. It is poorly absorbed through the gastrointestinal (GI) tract. When given IV, peak concentrations are reached in 3 to 5 minutes, then is rapidly redistributed into subcutaneous (SQ) tissues.

Fentanyl is well absorbed through the buccal mucosa and skin due to the high lipid solubility. Transmucosal fentanyl, a small tablet inserted in the superior portion of the buccal mucosa along the posterior of the teeth or fentanyl embedded in a sucrose base attached to a plastic handle, has been demonstrated to have an onset of effect in as little as 10 minutes.[69] Establishing an accurate equianalgesic conversion for transmucosal fentanyl has been difficult, possibly due to the rapidity of onset of action. Sixty-five percent of patients participating in titration studies of buccal fentanyl were successful in reaching a dose that effectively treated their pain with one tablet.[70]

Transdermal fentanyl, or fentanyl patch, is utilized to take advantage of the high lipid solubility of the drug. Fentanyl is absorbed through the skin and a depot is formed in the tissues. The fentanyl patch should generally be used for opioid tolerant patients with stable opioid doses. The absorption of fentanyl is variable among individuals relative to the absorption through the skin and clearance of the drug.[71] Fentanyl absorption is also dependent on complete contact with the skin, at times requiring tape around the edges of the patch. The patches are placed on the upper back, chest, or arms. Caution should be used in febrile patients as this may increase absorption of fentanyl. Patients with cachexia or anasarca may also have alterations in absorption.[72]

### Tramadol

Tramadol is a weak μ opioid receptor agonist not frequently used in cancer patients. It is a synthetic codeine analog, producing a much lower affinity for the μ receptor compared to morphine. Analgesic effect may be obtained in part from the norepinephrine and serotonin reuptake inhibition property of the medication. It is 68% bioavailable in the oral formulation, and 100% bioavailable in the IM form. Dose limitation is 400 mg per day. Duration of action is 4 hours in the short-acting formulation.[73] It is not considered a controlled substance in the US.

### Codeine

Codeine is a naturally occurring derivative of opium. Its analgesic properties are a result of binding to the μ opioid receptors, but its affinity is low, and its analgesic potency is therefore low. Codeine is metabolized by the P450 CYP2D6 cytochrome. Approximately 7% of the population lacks CYP2D6 activity, and as a result, may experience diminished efficacy when using codeine.[74] Codeine is absorbed from the gastrointestinal tract, but bioavailability may vary greatly among individuals. In most people, codeine is 60% bioavailable after taking the oral formulation of the drug. Metabolites of codeine include codeine-6-glucuronide, norcodeine, morphine, and M3G and M6G. Codeine is metabolized by the liver, 90% is excreted in the urine, and 10% is converted to morphine. Duration of action is 4 hours. Half life elimination is 2 to 4 hours.[73]

The side effect profile generated by codeine includes nausea and constipation, is dose dependent, and prohibits its use in doses sufficient to treat pain that is moderate to severe. Therefore, its use as an opioid analgesic is generally discouraged, especially in patients with cancer.

## OPIOID ANTAGONISTS

Naloxone is an opioid antagonist. Given in small doses, it reverses the effects of opioids by competitively binding with the opioid receptor. The half life of parenteral naloxone is 3.1 +/- 0.5 hours. The duration of effect is much less, commonly lasting only 30 to 60 minutes. Naloxone is often used in clinical practice inappropriately as a diagnostic tool for patients experiencing a change in mental status. It is erroneously thought to be a drug without side effects. In fact, it can have some potentially serious side effects, including pulmonary edema, seizures, ventricular tachycardia or fibrillation, and death. Practitioners must consider that change in mental status due to opioids is due to the metabolites. Naloxone does not eliminate or reverse the effects of opioid metabolites.

Appropriate use of naloxone for respiratory depression in opioid tolerant patients should include diluting 0.4 mg of naloxone in a total of 10 cc. Administer 1 cc to 2 cc every 2 minutes in divided doses until the respirations and oxygen saturation increase to an acceptable level. Cautious titration of naloxone avoids the precipitation of withdrawal in opioid tolerant patients.[75]

Methylnaltrexone has been studied in seriously ill patients with constipation. It is a μ receptor-selective antagonist. It is poorly absorbed orally, therefore it is given IV. Patients receiving SQ methylnaltrexone had a bowel movement within 4 hours more frequently than patients receiving placebo.[76] These results were repeated with repeated dosing. Methylnaltrexone is a peripheral μ receptor antagonist, therefore the analgesic effects of the opioid are not reversed by administration. Patients have not reported increased pain when receiving methylnaltrexone in the doses studied. Side effects experienced by patients receiving methylnaltrexone most commonly include abdominal cramping and flatus.[77]

Alvimopan is another peripherally acting μ receptor antagonist. It has been approved for reversal of postoperative ileus after bowel resection. It was found to decrease transit time in the bowel, but had no effect on gastric emptying. Alvimopan is administered orally. It has also demonstrated effect on laxation without effecting analgesia.[78] Both methylnaltrexone and alvimopan are being studied further to determine the effect on nausea and vomiting, cough, and urinary retention. Both showed an effect on all of the above symptoms in clinical trials.[78]

## SIDE EFFECTS OF OPIOIDS

### Respiratory depression

Respiratory depression is the most feared consequence of opioid administration. Respiratory depression occurs as a result of decreased sensitivity of the medulla to rising carbon dioxide levels, which normally prompts spontaneous respirations. This is in part because the medulla is rich in opiate receptors. Sleep can also induce a similar, but much less severe response. Respiratory depression generally does not occur in the presence of pain therefore, thoughtful, slow titration especially in opioid naïve patients is of utmost importance.[79] Patients with pre-existing pulmonary conditions, such as pneumonia and chronic obstructive pulmonary disease (COPD), are at higher risk for the development of respiratory depression. Patients receiving chronic opioid analgesics develop a tolerance to the respiratory depressant effects of opioids.

Many clinicians fear they will hasten the death of a patient at the end of life by escalating opioid doses to achieve pain control. Portenoy and colleagues[80] studied hospice patients in a variety of settings. They found that the opioid dose escalation did not correlate statistically with the timing of the death of patients. They encouraged clinicians to escalate opioid doses in order to control pain in the clinical setting. Additionally, Hall and colleagues found an inverse relationship between age and opioid dose at the end of life.[81]

### Constipation

Constipation occurs in as many as 70% of patients taking opioid analgesics.[82] Constipation is the side effect to which the body rarely accommodates in patients receiving opioid analgesics. Opioid receptors are present in the smooth muscle of the gut. In addition, opioids are involved in the neuromodulation of acetylcholine (Ach) and vasoactive intestinal peptide (VIP), both of which are involved in the regulation of peristalsis.[50] The pyloric sphincter demonstrates increased tone resulting in gastroparesis. The bowel demonstrates decreased strength of the peristaltic waves resulting in dessiccation of the stool due to the length of time the stool remains in the bowel. Anal tone is increased. In addition, the rectum demonstrates decreased sensitivity to stretching, leading to difficulty passing the stool once it reaches the rectum.

Other variables such as dehydration, advanced age, immobility, and other constipating medications may worsen the problem. Therefore, it is essential that all patients are using a scheduled bowel regimen. The bowel regimen often includes a stool softener and a laxative.[83] Table 27-6 lists laxatives that are and are not recommended for treatment of opiate-induced constipation.[56] There is a paucity of data demonstrating the efficacy of 1 laxative over another. However, Hawley and Thompson[84] reported patients receiving a senna based bowel regimen were more likely to experience laxation than those receiving a senna laxative and docusate sodium.

### Nausea

Nausea due to opioids is caused by the direct effect of the opioid on the chemoreceptor trigger zone (CTZ) in the medulla inducing vertigo, or gastroparesis. Nausea usually subsides over several days when caused by opioids. If nausea persists, dose reduction, changing route of administration, or changing opioids is recommended.[82] Antiemetics are an effective treatment for opioid-induced nausea. The additive side effects of antiemetics must be considered when choosing the appropriate nursing intervention.[85]

### Pruritus

Systemic opioids may precipitate histamine release leading to flushing and pruritus. Pruritus reportedly occurs more frequently with morphine and meperidine. Fentanyl, oxymorphone, and sufentanil do not precipitate pruritus. The effects of histamine from systemic opioids cannot be reversed with naloxone. Pruritus associated with spinal opioids can be severe and the effects can be reversed with naloxone.[86]

### Urinary retention

Urinary retention is caused by increased tone of the external sphincters and volume of the bladder. Tolerance to these effects develops over time. Urinary retention may be more severe with spinal opioids. It is also more common and more severe in men and with patients receiving morphine. Patients with spinal opioids experience urinary retention more frequently than those receiving systemic opioids.[87]

## ROUTES OF OPIOID ADMINISTRATION

A variety of routes of opioid administration are available. Individualized plans of care should be developed in

**TABLE 27-6**

**Laxatives and Opiate Use**

**A. Laxatives Used for Opiate-Induced Constipation**

| Category | Common Preparations | Mechanism of Action | Precautions |
|---|---|---|---|
| Saline | Milk of magnesia, Magnesium citrate, Sodium phosphate | Draw water into the intestinal lumen. The accumulation alters the stool consistency, distends the bowel, and induces peristaltic movements. | Repeated use can alter fluid and electrolyte balance. May cause abdominal cramping. |
| Osmotic | Lactulose, sorbitol, glycerin, polyethylene glycol | Increase volume in colon and promote water retention. | May cause flatulence. Sweet taste may cause nausea. Excessive amounts can cause diarrhea. Polyethylene glycol: better tolerated; for short-term use only; no studies performed for long-term use. |
| Stimulant | Bisacodyl, Senna, Ex Lax, Dantron | Increase motor activity of bowels by direct action on the intestines. | Bisacodyl: avoid taking within 1 hour of taking antacids, and avoid with ulcerative lesion in the colon. May cause severe cramping. Prolonged use can cause laxative dependency and loss of normal bowel function. |
| Detergent | Docusate | Reduce surface tension. | May increase the systemic absorption of mineral oil when administered together. |

**B. Laxatives Not Recommended for Opiate-Induced Constipation**

| Category | Common Preparations | Action | Reasons for Not Recommending |
|---|---|---|---|
| Bulk | Metamucil, Maltsupex Psyllium | Increase size, weight, and frequency of stool, which requires increased fluid intake. | Effectiveness and feasibility in patients is doubtful. |
| Lubricant | Mineral oil | Reduce friction and coat the stool. | Causes decreased absorption of fat vitamins. May cause incontinence. Long-term use can cause perianal irritation. |

*Source*: Data from Cahill[56]; and Thomas.[83]

collaboration with the patient and the physician. Table 27-7 briefly describes the routes of opioid administration. Continuous infusion and patient controlled analgesia (PCA) used in patients with cancer are briefly discussed.

## Continuous infusions

Continuous intravenous or subcutaneous infusions provide the patient with steady blood levels of the opioid and can avoid the potential side effects and return of pain associated with intermittent dosing. Guidelines are useful for initiating infusions and determining parameters for titrating doses. A summary of the management of continuous infusional therapy appears in Table 27-8.

Continuous subcutaneous opioid infusions provide an acceptable alternative to intravenous administration in circumstances when long-term IV access is not available or is limited. Ambulatory, computerized infusion devices have facilitated the use of subcutaneous infusions at home. Because subcutaneous infusions are relatively easy to initiate, patients can be switched over to a subcutaneous infusion in the home providing that necessary resources (drug delivery system, skilled home care professionals) are in place. The subcutaneous route avoids problems associated with IM or SQ injections.

Continuous SQ infusions of opioids are indicated for patients who (1) are unable to take oral medication due to nausea, vomiting, or a mechanical obstruction in the GI tract; (2) are unable to use alternative routes because doses may be too high; (3) have limited or no venous access; and (4) are unable to maintain control with oral administration. Care should be taken to ensure that infusions are 3 ccs/hour or less to avoid trauma to the tissues. Problems associated with SQ continuous infusions include

**TABLE 27-7**

**Routes of Opioid Administration**

| Route | Comments |
|---|---|
| Oral | Preferred in cancer pain management; effective, convenient, and safe |
| Sublingual | Used for short-term management; may yield fluctuating serum concentration with erratic pain control |
| Transmucosal | Optimal dose found via titration; available in fentanyl |
| Transdermal | Available in fentanyl; application every 3 days, 12–16 hours to achieve therapeutic effect and 18 hours to achieve a steady state |
| Rectal | Available in hydromorphone, oxymorphone, and morphine; absorption is variable |
| Topical | Lidocaine patch 12 hours on and 12 hours off; may use up to 3 patches to cover the affected area |
| Parenteral | Intramuscular administration is not recommended; clearest indication is use subsequent to an inability to tolerate oral medication |
| Intraspinal | Morphine is the gold standard; usually administrated via implantable infusion pump; may be cost-effective |

*Source*: Data from American Pain Society[49]; Cahill.[56]

local skin irritation, leakage, swelling, and discomfort at the needle site.

## Patient-controlled analgesia

The choice of opioid for patient-controlled analgesia (PCA) is guided by the same principles as the choice of any other opioid. Advances in computerized software for infusion devices have made PCA a common and acceptable method for delivering opioid analgesia through parenteral (IV and SQ) routes. Intravenous PCA for postoperative pain has become the mainstay for IV administration of opioids. Use of PCA for chronic cancer-related pain has also evolved into an effective approach for parenteral drug delivery. Patient-controlled analgesia allows patients to self-administer analgesics within a preset interval that is programmed into the infusion device. Regimens for acute pain such as postoperative pain include a self-administered or demand dose, but a continuous background infusion or basal rate of an opioid analgesic (eg, morphine, fentanyl, hydromorphone, and less often meperidine) may be added. Demand-dosing schedules usually include doses of the opioid with lock-out intervals (6–15 mins), the time allowed between doses.

**TABLE 27-8**

**Suggestions for the Management of Continuous Intravenous or Subcutaneous Infusion of Opioid Analgesics**

1. All infusions should be administered with a flow-calibrated infusion pump.
2. Convert the patient's current opioid drugs to an equal analgesic parenteral dose of the drug that will be used for the infusion.
3. If the drug to be used for the infusion is the same one the patient is currently receiving, divide the parenteral dose by 24 to determine the hourly infusion rate.
4. If the drug to be used for the infusion is a different drug, use half of the parenteral dose, and then divide by 24 to determine the hourly infusion rate.
5. Administer a loading dose at the beginning of the infusion and with each increase in the infusion rate. The amount of the loading dose depends on the patient's current opioid requirements.
6. Titrate the infusion until the patient reports pain relief or unacceptable side effects. Titration may occur the following ways:
   a. Increase the infusion rate by 10%–20% every few hours if the patient is receiving close monitoring.
   b. Administer additional doses of a short-acting opioid (preferably the same drug as the infusion) q 1–2 h parenteral (PRN) administration. Give 25%-50% of the hourly dose for PRN dosing. Increase the infusion rate q 12–24 h by the amount equal to the total number of milligrams during the preceding period divided by the number of hours in that period. Use this method if the patient is not receiving dose monitoring.
   c. If using IV/SQ for breakthrough pain, use 50%-100% of hourly rate every 6–15 min
7. Opioids with a longer half-life (methadone, levorphanol) should not be used for rapid titration.
8. Change site every 72 hours or if signs/symptoms of erythema occur at the site.
9. Limit the amount of volume to less than 5–10 mL/hr.

*Source*: Data from American Pain Society.[49]

Patients can access self-administered doses frequently to control short-term pain. This approach avoids the peaks and troughs in serum levels that are often associated with conventional as needed parenteral (PRN) administration. In contrast, PCA regimens for the management of chronic cancer pain almost always include a basal rate that is supposed to deliver the bulk of the analgesic therapy. Higher demand doses are used to supplement the basal rate. This practice is intended to prevent the patient from working too hard to maintain adequate analgesia. In general, the benefits of PCA include better overall pain control, more prompt administration of opioids to control predictable or unpredictable bouts of pain, increased onset of analgesic action, and greater patient satisfaction.

## ISSUES REGARDING OPIOID THERAPY

Despite advances in the knowledge about the use of opioids for patients with cancer pain, many healthcare professionals prescribe or administer opioids inadequately because of the needless fear that opioids will cause drug addiction. There continues to be confusion by health professionals and the public about addiction, physical dependence, and tolerance.

### Addiction

The American Pain Society (APS), the American Academy of Pain Medicine (AAPM), and the American Society for Addictive Medicine (ASAM) define addiction "as a primary, chronic, neurobiological disease, with genetic, psychosocial, and environmental factors influencing its development and manifestations. It is characterized by behaviors that include 1 or more of the following: impaired control over drug use, compulsive use, continued use despite harm, and craving."[88]

### Physical dependence

Physiological dependence to a drug results over time with continuous use of the drug. If stopped abruptly, withdrawal symptoms result. While opioid withdrawal is not life threatening, patients may experience effects such as nausea, vomiting, abdominal cramps, diarrhea, agitation, miosis, and piloerection. Patient education is important in circumventing withdrawal symptoms that may occur when patients abruptly stop medication without seeking medical advice from a practitioner.

### Tolerance

Tolerance is the diminished effect of the same amount of a drug over time. Therefore, larger doses are required for the same physiological effect of the drug and this is often necessary in patients with cancer to achieve the level of pain relief needed. The mechanism for this phenomenon is poorly understood, yet it is clinically consequential and often results in undertreatment of pain over time. Care must be taken to avoid inattention to tolerance in patients with cancer who have persistent pain.

## NONOPIOID ANALGESICS

Nonopioid analgesics are important to the successful treatment of patients with cancer pain. These drugs, acetaminophen and nonsteroidal anti-inflammatory agents, control pain independently or help reduce the dose of opioid needed for pain control.

The selection of a nonopioid drug for an individual patient is often based on the prescriber's preference and experience with particular agents. Table 27-9 lists the commonly used nonopioid agents and usual dosages.[49] The

**TABLE 27-9**

**Nonopioids Commonly Used in Analgesic Treatments of Cancer Pain**

| Name | Half-Life | Dosing Interval | Starting Dose (mg/day) | Maximum Dose (mg/day) |
|---|---|---|---|---|
| Acetaminophen | 2–3 h | q 4–6 h | 2000 | 4000 |
| Acetylsalicylic acid | 0.25 h | q 4 h | 2000 | 4000 |
| Celecoxib (Celebrex) | 11 h | q 12–24 h | 200 | 400 |
| Choline magnesium trisalicylale | 9–17 h | q 12 h | 2000 | 2000–3000 |
| Diclofenac | | q 8–12 h | 75–100 | 150 |
| Diflunisal | 8–12 h | q 8–12 h after loading dose | 500–1000 | 1500 |
| Ibuprofen | 2–2.5 h | q 4–6 h | 1600 | 2400 |
| Ketorolac (IV, PO) | 6 h | q 6 h after loading dose | 60–120 | 150 day one, 120mg thereafter |
| Naproxen | 12–15 h | q 6–8 h | 750 | 1500 |

*Source*: Data from American Pain Society[49]; Cahill.[56]

benefits of nonopioids for patients with severe pain who require higher than usual doses of opioids have not been established. Nonopioids can be considered either alone or in conjunction with an opioid when pain is mild. In summary, nonopioids are useful in the management of cancer-related pain. Optimal use of this group of drugs requires a careful medical and analgesic history.

## Acetaminophen

Acetaminophen is a nonsalicylate indicated for noninflammatory pain and for fever control. It has no anti-inflammatory action and no antiplatelet activity.[89] A proposed mechanism of action for acetaminophen is inhibition of the third isoform of cyclooxygenase (COX-3), which occurs within the CNS; it may account for the analgesic and antipyretic effects but not the anti-inflammatory action of acetaminophen.[90] Hepatic toxicity increases with dosage of greater than 4 g per day but can occur at lower doses with coexisting liver disease or regular alcohol consumption.[91] The maximum dose for long-term use is 4 to 6 g per day.[49,89] Acetaminophen is preferred to nonsteroidal anti-inflammatory drugs (NSAIDs) in the elderly because of its low GI and renal toxicity.[92] It is an under-recognized cause of excessive anticoagulation in patients taking warfarin.[93]

Acetaminophen overdose is common because this drug is found in many prescriptions and over-the-counter medications. It is important to discuss the overuse of acetaminophen with patients and their families. The opportunity for providers to educate patients about over-the-counter medications and acetaminophen is tremendous yet is often missed.[94] The maximum daily dosage of acetaminophen is 4 g for adults and 3 g for the elderly.[95] Liver damage has been reported in adults taking daily dosages as low as 6 g. Doses of 5 to 8 g every day can lead to liver failure.[95] Acetaminophen is hidden in many medications, including over-the-counter cold and cough medicines and opioid/acetaminophen combinations (Vicodin). Certain drug interactions increase the dangers of acetaminophen, such as excessive consumption of alcohol, anticonvulsants, isoniazid, and oral anticoagulants. Patients and their families should be advised that over-the-counter medications should be treated with the same care as prescribed medicines and that advice on recommended doses, contraindications, and interactions should be heeded.[96]

## Nonsteroidal anti-inflammatory drugs

Nonsteroidal anti-inflammatory drugs such as ibuprofen, naproxen, and related agents are nonselective inhibitors of both COX-1 and COX-2, which provides analgesia by inhibiting prostaglandin (PG) synthesis. Prostaglandins are present in inflammatory conditions and are therefore beneficial in several painful conditions. Nonsteroidal anti-inflammatory drugs are the most commonly used analgesic by adults and often used for mild pain. They possess analgesic, anti-inflammatory and antipyretic properties. They are an opioid sparing drug for patients with moderate to severe pain. Unlike opioids, they have a ceiling effect, but may reduce opioid requirements by as much as 30% to 50%.[97]

COX-2 selective, NSAID (celecoxib) demonstrates efficacy for persistent and background pain in the acute setting. Additionally, COX-2 NSAIDs reduce osteoclast destruction.[98] Nonsteroidal anti-inflammatory drugs are metabolized in the liver and excreted by the kidneys. One percent of patients may experience a hypersensitivity reaction to NSAIDs, which can be life threatening.

Nonsteroidal anti-inflammatory drugs do not exhibit some of the side effects common to opioids such as sedation and respiratory depression. However, there are several side effects that can be potentially life threatening. Gastric irritation can occur through 2 mechanisms. Prostaglandins inhibit the secretion of gastric acid in the stomach. In addition, direct contact with the gastric mucosa can cause irritation leading to ulceration.[99] Renal perfusion is driven by PGs. Decreased renal PGs may lead to impaired renal function. Nonselective NSAIDs inhibit platelet aggregation. COX-2 NSAID celecoxib has been found to result in an increased incidence of myocardial infarction and stroke.[100] Practitioners must determine the risk and benefit of adding a low dose aspirin to the therapy to prevent such an event in high risk patients.

## Adjuvant analgesics

Adjuvant analgesics were originally indicated primarily for uses other than pain management. "Adjuvant analgesic" can be used to describe any drug that has a primary indication other than pain but that is analgesic in some painful conditions. In patients with cancer, this type of agent is given to enhance pain relief when there is a poor response to the opioids or it becomes necessary to reduce the dose of opioids because of intolerable side effects. Antidepressants, anticonvulsants, and corticosteroids play an important role in the treatment of pain. Although several classes of adjuvant analgesics exist, only the most common agents are discussed here.

***Antidepressants.*** Tricyclic antidepressants (TCAs) have been found to be moderately effective in treating some neuropathic pains.[101,102] Several TCAs exhibit varying levels of seratonin and norepinephrine inhibition. Tricyclic antidepressants may also have some effect on sodium channels. Side effects such as confusion, dry mouth, orthostatic hypotension, constipation, and, in rare cases, cardiotoxicity have occurred with TCAs.[15] These side effects may preclude the use of TCAs in some patients. Dosages of TCAs are lower and the onset of pain relief is quicker when TCAs are used for neuropathic pain vs when they are used for depression. Newer antidepressants velafaxine and duloxetine demonstrate selective norepinephrine and serotonin reuptake inhibition. They have been found to be effective and lack the side effects associated with TCAs.[97]

*Antiepileptic drugs.* Neuropathic pain is recognized as a challenging pain to treat effectively due to neuronal hyperexcitability. The most effective drugs in treating this type of pain regulate sodium and calcium channels at the synapse. Antiepileptic drugs (AEDs) have demonstrated efficacy in the treatment of several neuropathic pain syndromes.

Gabapentin was first studied in diabetic neuropathy and postherpetic neuralgia and found to be efficacious in 60% of patients.[103] Keskinbora and colleagues demonstrated improved pain relief, less allodynia, and fewer side effects in patients with cancer with neuropathic pain receiving a combination of gabapentin and morphine vs morphine alone.[104] Caraceni and colleagues also report lower pain scores, less dysesthesia, and lower opioid doses in patients receiving gabapentin vs placebo in a group of patients with cancer.[105] Gabapentin has no known significant drug interactions. Dose limiting side effects include somnolence, dizziness, and lower extremity edema. Doses may reach 3600 mg/day in divided doses. Gabapentin may improve sleep and have a positive effect on mood. Dose reductions are required for renal impairment.

Pregabalin, a metabolite of gabapentin, was also studied in similar patient populations and found to be efficacious. It also demonstrates anxiolytic effects in generalized anxiety disorder.[106,107] The side effect profile for pregabalin is similar to gabapentin. The onset of analgesic effect is shorter since the initial dosing of pregabalin demonstrates efficacy in some patients.[108] Titration is not as lengthy a process as it may be with gabapentin. The side effects for both gabapentin and pregabalin are more tolerable than older AEDs such as phenytoin and carbemazepine.

*Steroids.* Corticosteroids may be useful in the treatment of cancer pain. Steroids provide a direct analgesic and anti-inflammatory effect leading to decreased pain.[109] In addition, steroids may improve mood, decrease nausea and vomiting, increase appetite, decrease constipation, and reverse bowel obstructions. Mercadante and colleagues[110] reported no statistical difference in pain ratings in a group of patients with cancer receiving opioids and 8 mg of dexamethasone daily compared to those receiving opioids alone. However, their effects are often demonstrated in patients experiencing a severe, intractable increase in their symptoms related to cancer and/or its treatment.

*Bisphosphonates.* Bisphosphonates clearly have palliative effects on bone pain and may improve QOL or delay its decline for patients with bone metastases. Intravenous bisphosphonates, such as pamidronate and zoledronic acid, have clinically relevant analgesic effects in patients with metastatic bone pain.[111] Baseline serum creatinine level should be measured before every dose of IV bisphosphonates, and the rate of infusion should be monitored closely.[112] Berenson reported mild to moderate elevation of serum creatinine in approximately 10% of patients receiving IV bisphosphonates.[113] Bisphosphonate administration has become the mainstay of treatment for malignancy-induced hypercalcemia because this class of drugs is well tolerated and effective.[114] Data support the usefulness of these agents for relieving bone pain and improving outcomes for patients with metastatic bone involvement.

Pamidronate has significant benefits in relieving pain from bony metastases that do not respond to NSAIDs and steroids. Small et al conducted a multicenter, randomized, placebo-controlled study of pamidronate in patients with metastatic prostate cancer.[115] Pamidronate disodium failed to demonstrate a significant benefit compared with placebo in palliation of bone pain or reduction of adverse side effects.[115] However, when Theriault et al conducted a trial on 372 females with breast cancer, they found patients who received pamidronate had less skeletal complications and longer times to the first skeletal-related events.[116] While the cost of therapy and the time necessary to administer the infusion are important to consider with pamidronate' use, economic considerations must be weighed against more costly alternatives such as surgery or radiation.[117]

Zoledronic acid, a newer-generation bisphosphonate, has been approved for patients with bone metastases secondary to prostate, lung, renal cell, and other solid tumor cancers.[112] Its indication is broader than that of pamidronate, and it is a highly potent bisphosphonate.[113] Three large, double-blind, randomized, phase III trials were conducted to investigate the efficacy of zoledronic acid.[118,119] In these trials, zoledronic acid was shown to be highly active in the treatment of bone metastasis. Saad et al conducted a study of 643 patients randomized to receive either zoledronic acid or placebo.[120] Pain scores in all patient groups increased throughout the study but were lower in the zoledronic acid group. Zoledronic acid has also been compared with pamidronate and shown to have superior efficacy.[121] The recommended dose is 4 mg IV over more than 15 minutes every 3 to 4 weeks.[122]

*Topical agents.* Capsaicin is the active ingredient in hot chili peppers. It is postulated to stimulate, then inhibit substance P in distal nerve endings, resulting in decreased pain. Substance P is essential in the transmission of pain.[123] It is applied topically, initially causing burning on application. Caution should be used to avoid open skin or the eyes when applying to the skin.[124]

Lidocaine (5%) patches are approved for the treatment of post herpetic neuralgia (PHN). Sodium builds up at the neuronal synapse in neuropathic pain states resulting in ectopic neuronal discharges. Lidoderm interferes with sodium channels at the synapse resulting in decreased pain. The side effect profile for lidocaine patches is minimal.[123] The patches are placed on the skin for 12 hours and removed for 12 hours each day. Caution should be used in overprescribing Lidoderm patches for neuropathic pain syndromes or other types of pain that have not been studied.

## DRUG THERAPY FOR THE ELDERLY

Treatment of pain in the elderly requires knowledge of their specialized needs due to the physiological and lifestyle changes that occur with aging. The application of information regarding the pharmacodynamics of analgesics is critical in selecting agents that have more benign side effect profiles. Of the aging-related pharmacokinetic changes, 2 of the most important are the decline in the glomerular filtration rates and the reduction in the activity of the cytochrome P450 system, which is responsible for the activation and metabolism of many opioids.[124] Opioids are the mainstay for treatment of cancer pain even in the elderly. Morphine was formerly the most often used opioid in the elderly. Because morphine is excreted in the kidneys and there is a decline in the glomerular filtration rate with age, neurotoxicity is likely to develop in older patients. Hydromorphone undergoes the same metabolic changes, however, toxicity due to the build up of neurotoxic metabolites occurs with high dose IV infusion in patients with renal failure. Unlike morphine and hydromorphone, fentanyl is lipophilic and suitable for transdermal administration. With chronic administration or hepatic failure, fentanyl has been reported to accumulate in the circulation due to saturation of storage sites.[125] Oxycodone is another popular opioid that is eliminated by hepatic metabolism. The fact that oxycodone's pharmacokinetics is largely independent of age, renal function, and serum albumin concentration makes this compound a favorable choice in the elderly. Meperidine is best avoided in the elderly because its metabolite normeperidine is excreted in the kidneys, accumulates in the circulation in the presence of renal insufficiency, and may cause seizures.[126] Table 27-10 outlines the important considerations for use of analgesics in the elderly.[49,92,127–131]

For the treatment of neuropathic pain, gabapentin is a valuable adjuvant agent due to its safety profile. It should be noted that this drug's pharmacokinetics is unpredictable and that gabapentin may have a prolonged half life.[49] Pregabalin, a metabolite of gabapentin, has been used in this population also. It is not FDA approved for cancer-related peripheral neuropathies, and therefore, not a first-line medication. For peripheral painful neuropathy, transdermal lidocaine may be an additional effective adjuvant treatment.

Effective treatment of pain in older patients is compelling, because pain may compromise the general health and even shorten the survival of the elderly. The assessment of pain in older patients may require a more comprehensive assessment than that in younger patients. In general, one should initiate treatment with lower doses and possibly longer dose intervals than would be used in younger patients.[125] Individual pain relief should guide dose escalation. Combination products—those that have both an opioid and a nonopioid—should be avoided because of the limited dosing available due to the ceiling dose for the nonopioid, which may lead to severe effects if excess medication is taken.[126]

## INTERVENTIONAL MANAGEMENT OF PAIN

Opioids are the foundation of pain management in patients with cancer. Unfortunately as many as 10% of patients fail to obtain adequate relief from opioid analgesics.[132] This often necessitates the implementation of alternative methods of pain control. Interventional techniques for the management of cancer pain are used for several reasons. Unwanted side effects may occur as a result of systemic opioids and/or adjuvant medications. Some patients obtain inadequate relief in spite of high dose systemic medications. Lastly, patients may obtain improved QOL when interventional techniques provide them with relief of pain not possible with systemic medications.[133,134] In a meta-analysis of the literature on intracerebroventricular (ICV), epidural (EP) and intrathecal (IT) analgesia, Ballantyne and Carwood[135] found a lack of controlled trials on the topics. Pain relief was rated highest in the ICV group, followed closely by the EP group, and then the IT group. Overall, pain relief was rated high in all 3 groups. Sedation and confusion were reported more commonly in the ICV group than the EP or IT group. Constipation was higher in the EP and IT group.

### SPINAL ANALGESIA

Spinal analgesia encompasses the administration of analgesics via both epidural and intrathecal routes and is used for patients experiencing pain below T1.[136] Opioids may be used in the spinal route more effectively with the addition of select adjuvant analgesics. Dosages vary widely among patients; therefore, careful titration and the availability of supplemental doses are essential to provide patients with adequate relief from pain.

### SPINAL OPIOIDS

Spinal opioids bind with receptors in the dorsal horn of the spinal cord. Binding with opioid receptors prevents

**TABLE 27-10**

**Special Considerations for Pain Assessment in the Elderly**

| Age-Related Changes | Specific Interventions for the Elderly |
|---|---|
| *Mental status* | |
| ↓ Mental acuity<br>Short-term memory problems<br>↓ Information processing<br>↑ Susceptibility to sedation of analgesics | • Initiate therapy with one-half of the usual starting dose for adults.<br>• Start low and go slow.<br>• Select adjuvant agents with ↓ sedating effects.<br>• Initiate safety precautions. |
| *Vision and hearing* | |
| ↓ Visual acuity and hearing | • Use pain assessment measures and teaching materials that are easy to read.<br>• Speak clearly and maintain eye contact.<br>• Avoid drugs that are contraindicated with glaucoma (agents with anticholinergic effects). |
| *Musculoskeletal* | |
| Osteoporosis<br>Joint stiffness<br>↓ Mobility | • Begin with nonopioid agents.<br>• Do not exceed the daily recommended dose of acetaminophen (>4 g/day).<br>• Use NSAIDs for inflammatory pain.<br>• Stop treatment with NSAIDs if not effective.<br>• May consider corticosteroids rather than NSAIDs for short-term use with bone pain.<br>• Encourage exercise or physical therapy. |
| *Pulmonary* | |
| COPD<br>Emphysema<br>↓ Pulmonary reserves | • Use caution with opioid and other analgesic agents that cause sedation.<br>• Initiate opioid therapy at one-half the starting dose for adults.<br>• Remember risk of respiratory depression is minimal if dosed correctly. |
| *Cardiovascular* | |
| Reduced blood volume<br>Conduction abnormalities<br>↓ Cardiac output<br>Cardiac reserve and circulation | • Drug absorption, distribution, and excretion may be altered due to aging.<br>• Administer NSAIDs cautiously to patients with congestive heart failure because a reduction in renal profusion may cause fluid retention.<br>• Avoid TCA if patients have cardiac conduction problems. |
| *Gastrointestinal* | |
| Dehydration<br>↓ Fluid intake<br>↓ Gastric emptying | • Avoid NSAIDs in patients with peptic ulcers or in patients taking anticoagulants.<br>• Use a PPI with NSAIDs.<br>• Use caution in patients who are dehydrated, as they may be more susceptible to opioid-related side effects.<br>• Use caution with TCA with ↑ anticholinergic effects (amitriptyline). |
| *Renal* | |
| ↓ Renal filtration and clearance<br>Renal insufficiency | • Obtain baseline renal function tests (BUN, creatinine, and creatinine clearance) prior to starting therapy.<br>• Consider lower doses of NSAIDs to reduce the risk of renal toxicity.<br>• Consider risk of metabolite accumulation in patients with severe renal dysfunction.<br>• Administer short-acting NSAIDs on a PRN basis rather than around the clock. |
| *Genitourinary* | |
| Urinary incontinence<br>Males: benign prostatic hypertrophy<br>Females: stress incontinence | • Patients who are opioid naïve are at greatest risk for urinary retention.<br>• Anticholinergic agents may cause urinary retention, so use caution.<br>• Instruct patients to monitor for signs of urinary tract infections. |

*Abbreviations*: ↓, decreased; ↑, increased; BUN, blood urea nitrogen; COPD, chronic obstructive pulmonary disease; NSAID, nonsteroidal anti-inflammatory drug: PPI, proton pump inhibitor; PRN, parenteral administration; TCA, tricyclic antidepressant.

*Source*: Data from American Pain Society[49]; Davis and Srivastava[92]; Gibson and Helme[127]; Fine[128]; Freedman[129]; American Geriatric Society[130]; and Levy and Cohen.[131]

transmission of painful stimuli from first to second order neurons, resulting in inhibition of nociceptive transmission. Administration of opioids via the spinal route results in opioid concentration that exceed those of plasma concentrations. An advantage of the spinal route is that other medications can be used to augment the effect of the opioids without systemic effects. For example, opioids are frequently combined with low concentrations of local anesthetics such as bupivicaine to block sensory nerve input, thereby decreasing pain more effectively without compromising motor function.[137] Epidural opioids must first pass through the dura, resulting in the availability of drug for vascular uptake. This results in a lower potency of epidural vs intrathecal opioids. This may also predispose patients to more systemic effects and side effects.

Morphine is the only opioid FDA approved for use in the intraspinal route, but several other opioids are used, including hydromorphone, fentanyl, sufentanil, meperidine, and methadone.[138] Since each of the opioids differ in the degree of lipophilicity, the spread of the drug in the intrathecal space is variable. For example, fentanyl is highly lipophilic, resulting in greater vascular uptake and resultant redistribution as well as less spread of the drug from the origin of administration in the cerebrospinal fluid (CSF).[139] Morphine is hydrophilic, poorly absorbed and spreads widely throughout the spine. This may result in better coverage of the pain regardless of the spinal level of catheter placement. Hydromorphone is also hydrophilic, spreading less than morphine but more than fentanyl.

## EPIDURAL INFUSIONS

Epidural infusions are used to infuse opioids and/or adjuvant medications into the epidural space. Epidural infusions require the insertion of a catheter into the epidural space, a space filled with fat, lymph and blood vessels, located between the dura and the connective tissues surrounding the vertebrae and ligamentum flavum. The catheter is inserted between the vertebrae at or near the level of pain experienced by the patient. Epidural catheters may be used for long-term pain management in patients with cancer, but require the insertion of a long-term silicone catheter tunneled from the insertion site to a location on the side of the body at or around the midaxillary line.[140] Tunneling of the catheter is undertaken to provide a mechanical barrier to bacteria. In addition, most catheters have a silver impregnated cuff that is bacteriocidal and promotes tissue growth to assist in anchoring the catheter. There are fewer infections with patients that had a catheter with an injection port than patients with tunneled catheters.[141]

Epidural infusions for patients with cancer may include a continuous infusion with or without a bolus. Patients experiencing incident pain with activity may require frequent BTP medication, thus the device should have the ability to deliver patient controlled boluses. To date, none of the implantable devices (intrathecal pumps) have the capability to deliver patient delivered boluses. In addition, oncology patients may require the ability to titrate frequently due to the progressive nature of the disease. Decision making

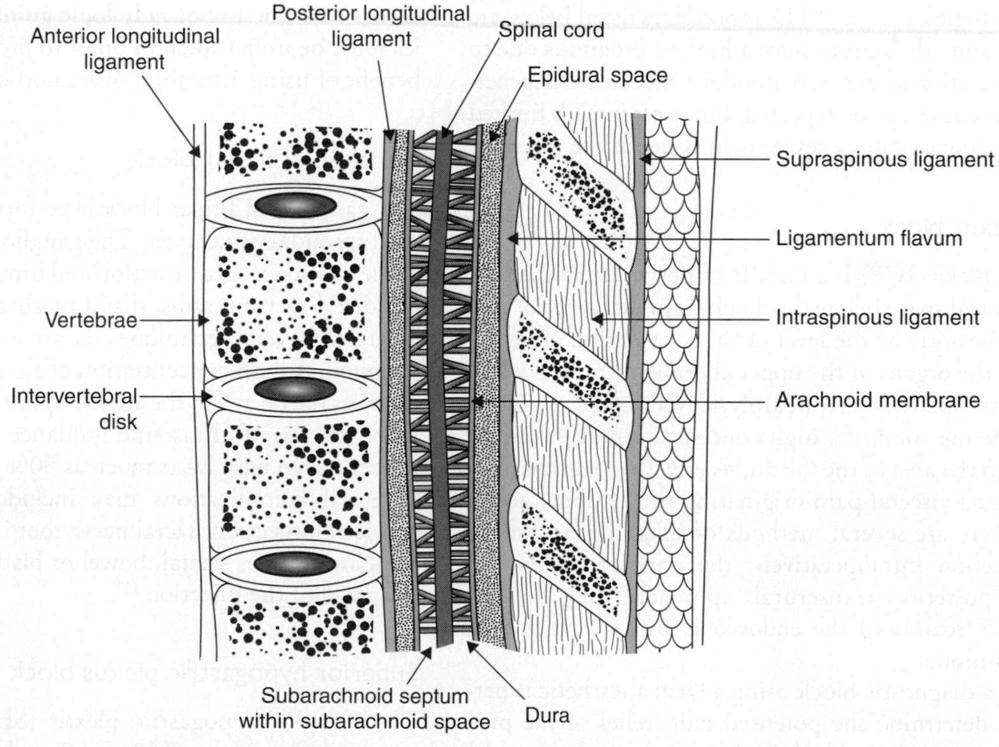


**FIGURE 27-7**

Anatomy of the spine and location of intrathecal infusions.

regarding placement of a catheter may be affected by the patient's condition. In fact, patients at the end of life may have a catheter placed in spite of potential contraindications pertinent to patients who have a longer life expectancy.[142]

## INTRATHECAL INFUSIONS

Intrathecal infusion of medications is accomplished by placing a catheter between the dura and the spinal cord (see Figure 27-7).[143] Long-term infusion of medications including opioids and adjuvant medications is accomplished by connecting the catheter to a programmable implanted pump placed in the SQ tissues in the lower abdomen.[144] These pumps hold a small volume of liquid (<20 ccs), but allow a logarithmic decrease in the amount of medication used due to the close proximity to the opioid receptors. Complications associated with intrathecal infusions include spinal headache, nerve damage, infection, pump malfunction, ineffective catheter placement, catheter kinking or breakage, injection of the medication into the SQ tissues, and granuloma formation at the tip of the catheter.[145] Pumps must be refilled every month by a skilled practitioner.

## NEUROLYTIC BLOCKS

In a small percentage of patients with cancer who have pain, the pain is optimally relieved by lysing the nerve. This is performed using high concentrations or alcohol or phenol and can provide pain relief for patients with pancreatic, colon, and gynecologic cancers.[146] The procedures listed below are used in patients thought to have a limited prognosis due to nerve regeneration after 3 to 6 months. Once nerves regenerate, the procedure can be repeated, but is often with limited success, leading to a more severe pain issue for the patient.

### Celiac plexus block

The celiac plexus (CP) is a bundle of nerves located in the retroperitoneal space below the diaphragm just anterior and lateral to the aorta at the level of the L1 vertebra. The CP innervates the organs of the upper abdomen, the left colon, rectum, and pelvis.[132] A neurolytic CP block (NCPB) involves the injection of a high concentration of phenol or alcohol into the area of the CP and is effective treatment for cancer-related visceral pain originating in the upper abdomen.[147] There are several methods of injecting, including direct injection intraoperatively, the anterior abdominal approach, posterior (transcrural) approach using fluoroscopy or CT scan, and the endoscopic ultrasound guided (EUS) technique.

Often, a diagnostic block using a local anesthetic is performed to determine the potential pain relief of the procedure. The neurolytic block is then performed using the high concentration of alcohol or phenol. Alcohol is hypobaric whereas phenol is hyperbaric. Alcohol is more likely to cause a transient neuritis when the injection is performed, but does not cause life threatening complications if injected into the vasculature. If effective, pain relief may last for several months.

Transient hypotension and diarrhea are expected side effects of the block.[148] Pneumothorax, hiccups, and hematuria are potential complications. However, there are potential serious sequelae in a small number of patients. Paraplegia may occur as a result of vasospasm or damage to the artery of Adamkiewicz.

The reported efficacy of a NCPB is variable. Many published studies are available, but there is little standardization of patient samples, limiting comparability. Patients with extensive disease or anatomic changes as a result of prior surgery may affect the outcome of the injection.[149] Yan and Myers[150] found that patients with unresectable pancreatic cancer undergoing NCPB injections had a mean improvement in pain scores of 6%. This resulted in less opioid consumption and constipation, but no significant improvement of nausea, vomiting, sedation, QOL, or survival. Zhang and colleagues[149] reported significant decrease in pain scores and opioid consumption for the patients with pancreatic cancer receiving CT guided NCPB, but no improvement in QOL in patients with early stage disease. This suggests that patients may benefit from earlier intervention. In addition, CT guidance may provide a greater benefit due to more accurate needle localization vs the method of using anatomical landmarks to guide the clinician, although there are no data to confirm better outcomes with the use of radiologic guidance.[151] Future studies must be undertaken in order to provide evidence of the benefit of using 1 method over another.

### Ganglion of Impar block

The ganglion of Impar block is performed to treat perineal pain secondary to cancer. The ganglion of Impar is located at the sacrococcygeal junction and innervates the perineum, the distal rectum, anus, distal urethra, vagina, and vulva. There are several techniques that may be used to inject the ganglion. A high concentration of alcohol or phenol is used to inject the nerves in the area. Gupta and colleagues recommend the use of ultrasound guidance for this procedure.[152] A decrease in pain by as much as 50% has been reported.[153] Potential complications may include rectal perforation, periosteal injection, sacral nerve root injury, epidural injection, and motor, sexual, bowel or bladder dysfunction due to spread of the injection.[132]

### Superior hypogastric plexus block

The superior hypogastric plexus (SHP) is a network of neuronal fibers from T10 to L2 and S2 to S4. The SHP transmits sensory input from the bladder, rectum, prostate, testes, vagina, uterus, ovaries, descending and sigmoid colon. In addition, sensory fibers are sent from the SHP to the pudendal and ilioinguinal nerves which innervate the perineum, anus, scrotum, penis, and clitoris.[134] Sympathetic input from the SHP also regulates sexual function of the pelvic organs. The primary indication for SHP is visceral pelvic pain that has been refractory to medical management.[147] An effective SHP block may provide a significant decrease in pain intensity, opioid consumption and drug related adverse events.[154]

### Stellate ganglion block

A Stellate ganglion block involves the injection of local anesthetic with or without steroid into the cervical sympathetic nerves in order to relieve neuropathic pain in the head and neck. The patient is placed supine and the needle is inserted at a ninety degree angle at the level of the sixth cervical vertebra between the cricoid cartilage and the carotid artery. Aspiration prior to injection is essential since injection of a small amount of local anesthetic into the systemic circulation can lead to immediate seizures, blindness, and loss of consciousness.[155] Generally, volumes of 5 to 10 ccs are used to obtain a sympathetic blockade while avoiding spread to unwanted structures.[156] Hardy presented 2 case studies of patients who obtained complete relief of pain due to acute herpes zoster infection in the cervical dermatomes after stellate ganglion block.[157]

### Cordotomy

A cordotomy interrupts the ascending pain pathways in the spinothalamic tract. It can be performed percutaneously or through an open surgical procedure and CT guidance is used in order to decrease the risks of adverse effects. It is generally indicated for unilateral pain below C5, inadequately treated by other methods. Cordotomy is more effective for neuropathic pain that is intermittent shooting pain and pain which can be evoked vs steady pain. Patients having a serious comorbidity are not candidates for this procedure. Complications are infrequent, but include transient bowel incontinence and worsening bladder function. Significant weakness or ataxia and respiratory failure have been reported, but are unexpected. Dysesthesias in the area of pain relief are noted in up to 10% of patients post procedure.[158]

### Spinal cord stimulation

Spinal cord stimulation uses metal contacts inserted into the dorsal column of the spinal cord. The contacts are attached to a pulse generator the size of a pacemaker to provide an electrical stimulus to the leads. The electrical pulse stimulates the larger fibers blocking the conduction of impulses along fibers in the lateral spinothalamic tract and increased stimulation of descending antinociceptive pathways. Spinal cord stimulation is useful for treatment of neuropathic pain in patients with chemotherapy-related peripheral neuropathy and those with brachial plexus lesions.[147] However, spinal cord stimulation is limited in patients with progressive disease and who require MRI for follow-up since the leads contain metal. Potential complications include infection, catheter migration or breakage.[134]

### Vertebroplasty/kyphoplasty

Vertebroplasty and kyphoplasty are performed in order to restore the height of a vertebra that is compressed due to a fracture in patients with metastatic tumors without neurological compromise. Vertebroplasty involves the injection of polymethyl methacrylate (PMMA) into the vertebra after a small hole is drilled into the vertebra. Kyphoplasty involves inflating a balloon in the compressed vertebra prior to injecting cement. Both procedures are generally performed under fluoroscopy and can be performed percutaneously or during an open procedure. Patients with neurological compromise, known infections, coagulopathies, pregnancy, a low performance status, or short life expectancy should not undergo the procedure. Potential complications of the procedure include infection, cement leakage, and neurological compromise.[159] Trout and colleagues[160] reported significant relief from pain 1 week after vertebroplasty at rest and with activity.

The nursing responsibilities for patients undergoing anesthetic and neurodestructive procedures include being knowledgeable about the (1) purpose of the procedure and how it is performed; (2) potential complications based on type of block, agent, and location; and (3) potential benefit of the procedure. An efficient way of obtaining some of this information is to participate in the explanation of the procedure to the patient and to talk with the anesthesiologist or neurosurgeon.

## NONPHARMACOLOGICAL MANAGEMENT OF PAIN

Nonpharmacological management of pain is a broad topic but an essential often overlooked component of pain. Nonpharmacological methods are most often initiated by patients. Practitioners must be cognizant of the potential benefit of nonpharmacological methods of pain management and incorporate them into their practice.

Interventions included in this approach do not generally affect the underlying pathology or alter the perception or sensation of pain, but rather help in a variety of ways to decrease patients' emotional responses to pain, enabling them to deal with it more positively and proactively. Distraction, relaxation, guided imagery, and symptom monitoring are interventions that can be taught to provide

**TABLE 27-11**

**Selected Nonpharmacological Interventions for Pain**

| Technique | Examples | Advantages | Disadvantages |
|---|---|---|---|
| Cutaneous stimulation | Superficial heating or cooling, vibration, massage | Many methods; makes pain tolerable; reduces pain, patients are receptive; can apply stimulation at site of pain or other sites; can provide distraction | Not for therapeutic or curative purposes; can damage tissue if applied incorrectly |
| Immobilization/ mobilization | Splinting, bracing, walking, exercise, rest | Decreases pain, improves range of motion, conserves energy, improves functional status, promotes relaxation | Discomfort on physical exertion; decrease in functional status |
| Distraction | *Internal:* Mental images, counting, singing silently; *external:* music, reading, television, conversation | Decreased pain intensity, increased pain tolerance; more acceptable pain sensation; greater-sense of control; improved mood | Not helpful for vigilant patients; may have no effect on pain intensity; may be hard to enact; may not "look like" they are in pain, resulting in doubt about pain and/or failure to medicate after distraction; awareness of pain and fatigue may increase irritability |
| Relaxation | Slow breathing, progressive muscle relaxation, relaxing mental imagery, repetitive activity or thought | Reduces anxiety, may reduce pain; promotes sleep; decreases fatigue and skeletal muscle tension; increases confidence in ability to handle pain | Can be time-consuming; difficult to teach, practice, and use effectively; is an adjunct method that does not directly relieve pain; often difficult to distinguish between relaxation and imagery |
| Comprehensive Models | Cognitive/behavioral interventions, psychoeducational approaches | Address multiple dimensions of pain; individualized; include patient and family; problem-focused; requires interdisciplinary team | May be difficult to assemble an appropriate interdisciplinary team depending on setting and resources can be complex and time-consuming |

*Source:* Data from McCaffery and Pasero.[2]

patients and caregivers with tools to help control the perception and experience of pain. Evidence suggests that a variety of mind–body medicine treatments can improve mood, QOL, and symptoms such as pain, nausea, and vomiting.[161] Kwekkeboom and colleagues[162] found that nurses were more likely to provide distraction and relaxation for patients than music or guided imagery techniques. However, there is a lack of data to determine the effectiveness of complementary therapies such as transcutaneous electric nerve stimulation (TENS) for cancer pain.[163] These techniques clearly serve as adjuvants to standard pharmacological therapy. Table 27-11 provides additional information about selected techniques.

## CONCLUSION

Pain assessment and management is an essential part of patient care regardless of the specialty. Oncology nurses frequently encounter the challenge of treating multiple symptoms experienced by the patients they care for on a daily basis. For that reason, it is essential that as practitioners we attempt to broaden our knowledge and skills related to pain and symptom management. By doing so, we are more able to provide the highest level of care and deliver it in the most compassionate fashion.

## REFERENCES


1. International Association for the Study of Pain Subcommittee on Taxonomy: pain terms: a list with definitions and usage. *Pain.* 1979; 6:249–252.
2. McCaffery M, Pasero C. *Pain Clinical Manual.* 2nd ed. St. Louis;MO; Mosby: 1999.
3. Coyne PJ, Watson AC, McGuire DB, Yeager KA. Assessment of cancer pain. In: Yarbro CH, Frogge MH, Goodman M, eds. *Cancer Nursing Principles and Practice.* 6th ed. Sudbury, MA: Jones and Bartlett; 2005:639–661.
4. Davis MP, Walsh D. Epidemiology of cancer pain and factors influencing poor pain control. *Am J Hosp Palliat Care.* 2004;21:137–142.

5. Ferreira KA, Kimura M, Teixeira MJ, et al. Impact of cancer-related symptom synergisms on health-related quality of life and performance status. *J Pain Symptom Manage.* 2008;35:604–616.
6. Goudas LC, Bloch R, Gialeli-Goudas M, Lau J, Carr DB. The epidemiology of cancer pain. *Cancer Invest.* 2005;23:182–190.
7. Lorenz KA, Rosenfeld K, Wenger N. Quality indicators for palliative and end-of-life care in vulnerable elders. *J Am Geriatr Soc.* 2007;55(Suppl 2):S318–S326.
8. Hanson LC, Eckert JK, Dobbs D, et al. Symptom experience of dying long-term care residents. *J Am Geriatr Soc.* 2008;56:91–98.
9. Sabino MA, Mantyh PW. Pathophysiology of bone cancer pain. *J Support Oncol.* 2005;3:15–24.
10. McMillan SC, Tofthagen C, Morgan MA. Relationships among pain, sleep disturbances, and depressive symptoms in outpatients from a comprehensive cancer center. *Oncol Nurs Forum.* 2008;35:603–611.
11. Mao JJ, Armstrong K, Bowman MA, Xie SX, Kadakia R, Farrar JT. Symptom burden among cancer survivors: impact of age and comorbidity. *J Am Board Fam Med.* 2007;20:434–443.
12. de Leon-Casasola OA. Current developments in opioid therapy for management of cancer pain. *Clin J Pain.* 2008;24(Suppl 10): S3–S7.
13. Chang VT, Janjan N, Jain S, Chau C. Update in cancer pain syndromes. *J Palliat Med.* 2006;9:1414–1434.
14. Treede RD, Jensen TS, Campbell JN, et al. Neuropathic pain: redefinition and a grading system for clinical and research purposes. *Neurology.* 2008;70:1630–1635.
15. McDonald AA, Portenoy RK. How to use antidepressants and anticonvulsants as adjuvant analgesics in the treatment of neuropathic cancer pain. *J Support Oncol.* 2006;4:43–52.
16. Shaiova L. Difficult pain syndromes: bone pain, visceral pain, and neuropathic pain. *Cancer J.* 2006;12:330–340.
17. Bennett D, Burton AW, Fishman SS, et al. Consensus panel recommendations for the assessment and management of breakthrough pain-part 1: assessment. *Pharm Ther.* 2005;30:296–301.
18. Zeppetella G, O'Doherty CA, Collins S. Prevalence and characteristics of breakthrough pain in patients with non-malignant terminal disease admitted to a hospice. *Palliat Med.* 2001;15:243–246.
19. Portenoy RK, Hagen NA. Breakthrough pain: definition, prevalence and characteristics. *Pain.* 1990;41:273–281.
20. Svendsen KB, Andersen S, Arnason S, et al. Breakthrough pain in malignant and non-malignant diseases: a review of prevalence, characteristics and mechanisms. *Eur J Pain.* 2005;9:195–206.
21. Bennett DA, Burton AW, Fishman S, et al. Consensus panel recommendations for the assessment and management of breakthrough pain-part 2: management. *Pharm Ther.* 30:354–361.
22. Hagen NA, Fisher K, Victorino C, Farrar JT. A titration strategy is needed to manage breakthrough cancer pain effectively: observations from data pooled from three clinical trials. *J Palliat Med.* 2007;10:47–55.
23. Daut RL, Cleeland CS, Flanery RC. Development of the Wisconsin Brief Pain Questionnaire to assess pain in cancer and other diseases. *Pain.* 1983;17:197–210.
24. Palos GR, Mendoza TR, Mobley GM, Cantor SB, Cleeland CS. Asking the community about cutpoints used to describe mild, moderate, and severe pain. *J Pain.* 2006;7:49–56.
25. Serlin RC, Mendoza TR, Nakamura Y, Edwards KR, Cleeland CS. When is cancer pain mild, moderate or severe? Grading pain severity by its interference with function. *Pain.* 1995;61:277–284.
26. Paice JA, Cohen FL. Validity of a verbally administered numeric rating scale to measure cancer pain intensity. *Cancer Nurs.* 1997;20:88–93.
27. Farrar JT, Young JP, LaMoreaux L, Werth JL, Poole RM. Clinical importance of changes in chronic pain intensity measured on an 11-point numerical pain rating scale. *Pain.* 2001;94:149–158.
28. Closs SJ, Barr B, Briggs M, Cash K, Seers K. A comparison of five pain assessment scales for nursing home residents with varying degrees of cognitive impairment. *J Pain Symptom Manage.* 2004;27:196–205.
29. Bjoro K, Herr K. Assessment of pain in the nonverbal or cognitively impaired older adult. *Clin Geriatr Med.* 2008;24:237–262.
30. Jensen MP. The validity and reliability of pain measures in adults with cancer. *J Pain.* 2003;4:2–21.
31. Hicks CL, von Baeyer C, Spafford PA, van Korlaar I, Goodenough B. The Faces Pain Scale—Revised: toward a common metric in pediatric pain measurement. *Pain.* 2001;93:173–183.
32. Wong DL, Baker CM. Pain in children: comparison of assessment scales. *Pediatr Nurs.* 1988;14:9–17.
33. Payen JF, Bru O, Bosson JL, et al. Assessing pain in critically ill sedated patients by using a behavioral pain scale. *Crit Care Med.* 2001;29:2258–2263.
34. Hølen JC, Hjermstad MJ, Loge JH, et al. Pain assessment tools: is the content appropriate for use in palliative care? *J Pain Symptom Manage.* 2006;32:567–580.
35. Kirkova J, Davis MP, Walsh D, et al. Cancer symptom assessment instruments: a systematic review. *J Clin Oncol.* 2006;24:1459–1473.
36. Keene PR, Thompson C. Educational implications of nurses' assessment and management of pain. *J Hosp Palliat Nurs.* 2008;10:370–375.
37. Melzack R. The short-form McGill Pain Questionnaire. *Pain.* 1987;30:191–197.
38. Cleeland CS. Symptom burden: multiple symptoms and their impact as patient-reported outcomes. *J Natl Cancer Inst Monographs.* 2007;37:16–21.
39. Caprio AJ, Hanson LC, Munn JC, et a l. Pain, dyspnea, and the quality of dying in long-term care. *J Am Geriatr Soc.* 2008;56:683–688.
40. Ferrell B, Levy MH, Paice J. Managing pain from advanced cancer in the palliative care setting. *Clin J Oncol Nurs.* 2008;12:575–581.
41. Miaskowski C, Cleary J, Burney R, et al. Guidelines for the Management of Cancer Pain. *Adults and Children.* Vol. 3. Glenview, IL; American Pain Society: 2005.
42. Soscia J. Assessing pain in cognitively impaired older adults with cancer. *Clin J Oncol Nurs.* 2003;7:174–177.
43. Pergolizzi J, Böger RH, Budd K, et al. Opioids and the management of chronic severe pain in the elderly: consensus statement of an International Expert Panel with focus on the six clinically most often used World Health Organization Step III opioids (buprenorphine, fentanyl, hydromorphone, methadone, morphine, oxycodone). *Pain Pract.* 2008;8:287–313.
44. AGS Panel on Persistent Pain in Older Persons.The management of persistent pain in older persons. *J Am Geriatr Soc.* 2002;50: S205-S224.
45. Passik SD, Kirsh KL, Donaghy KB, Portenoy RK. Pain and aberrant drug-related behaviors in medically ill patients with and without histories of substance abuse. *Clin J Pain.* 2006;22:173–181.
46. Donovan KA, Taliaferro LA, Brock CW, Bazargan S. Sex differences in the adequacy of pain management among patients referred to a multidisciplinary cancer pain clinic. *J Pain Symptom Manage.* 2008;36:167–172.
47. Cleeland CS, Gonin R, Hatfield AK, et al. Pain and its treatment in outpatients with metastatic cancer. *N Engl J Med.* 1994;330:592–596.
48. Coyle N, Cherny N, Portenoy RK. Pharmacologic management of cancer pain. In: McGuire DB, Yarbro CH, Ferrell BR, eds. *Cancer Pain Management.* 2nd ed. Sudbury, MA: Jones and Bartlett; 1993:131–158.
49. Miaskowski C, Bair M, Chou R, et al. *Principles of Analgesic Use In the Treatment of Acute Pain and Cancer Pain.* 6th ed. Glenview, IL; American Pain Society: 1–120.
50. Doyle D, Hanks G, Cherny N, Calman K. ed. *Oxford Textbook of Palliative Medicine.* 3rd ed. Oxford, UK; Oxford University Press: 2004.
51. Bruera E, Palmer JL, Bosnjak S, et al. Methadone versus morphine as a first-line strong opioid for cancer pain: a randomized, double-blind study. *J Clin Oncol.* 2004;22:185–192.
52. Wright AW, Nocente ML, Smith MT. Hydromorphone-3-glucuronide: biochemical synthesis and preliminary pharmacological evaluation. *Life Sci.* 1998;63:401–411.
53. Thwaites D, McCann S, Broderick P. Hydromorphone neuroexcitation. *J Palliat Med.* 2004;7:545–550.
54. Davis MP, Walsh D. Methadone for relief of cancer pain: a review of pharmacokinetics, pharmacodynamics, drug interactions and protocols of administration. *Support Care Cancer.* 2001;9:73–83.

55. Davis MP, Shaiova LA, Angst MS. When opioids cause pain. *J Clin Oncol.* 2007;25:4497–4498.
56. Cahill BA. Cancer pain management. In: Yarbro CH, Frogge MH, Goodman M, eds. *Cancer Nursing Principles and Practice.* 6th ed. Sudbury, MA; Jones and Bartlett: 662–697.
57. Bonica JJ. *Bonica's Management of Pain.* 3rd ed. Philadelphia, PA; Lippincott, Williams & Wilkins: 2001.
58. Guilherme L, Soares L. Methadone for cancer pain: what have we learned from clinical studies? *Am J Hosp Palliat Care.* 2005;22:223–227.
59. Weschules WJ, Bain KT. A systematic review of opioid conversion ratios used with methadone for the treatment of pain *Pain Med.* 2008:1–13.
60. Ripamonti C, Bianchi M. The use of methadone for cancer pain. *Hematol Oncol Clin North Am.* 2002;16:543–555.
61. Weschules DJ, Bain KT, Richeimer S. Actual and potential drug interactions associated with methadone. *Pain Med.* 2008;9:315–344.
62. Krantz MJ, Kutinsky IB, Robertson AD, Mehler PS. Dose-related effects of methadone on QT prolongation in a series of patients with torsade de pointes. *Pharmacotherapy.* 2003;23:802–805.
63. Gupta A, Lawrence AT, Krishnan K, Kavinsky CJ, Trohman RG. Current concepts in the mechanisms and management of drug-induced QT prolongation and torsade de pointes. *Am Heart J.* 2007;153:891–899.
64. Krantz MJ, Martin J, Stimmel B, Mehta D, Haigney MC. QTc interval screening in methadone treatment. *Ann Intern Med.* 2009;150:387–395.
65. Kalso E. Oxycodone. *J Pain Symptom Manage.* 2005;29:S47-S56.
66. Citron ML, Kaplan R, Parris WC, et al. Long-term administration of controlled-release oxycodone tablets for the treatment of cancer pain. *Cancer Invest.* 1998;16:562–571.
67. Hartung DM, Middleton L, Haxby DG, Koder M, Ketchum KL, Chou R. Rates of adverse events of long-acting opioids in a state medicaid program. *Ann Pharmacother.* 2007;41:921–928.
68. Tassinari D, Sartori S, Tamburini E, et al. Adverse effects of transdermal opiates treating moderate-severe cancer pain in comparison to long-acting morphine: a meta-analysis and systematic review of the literature. *J Palliat Med.* 2008;11:492–501.
69. Portenoy RK, Messina J, Xie F, Peppin J. Fentanyl buccal tablet (FBT) for relief of breakthrough pain in opioid-treated patients with chronic low back pain: a randomized, placebo-controlled study. *Curr Med Res Opin.* 2007;23:223–233.
70. Portenoy RK, Taylor D, Messina J, Tremmel L. A randomized, placebo-controlled study of fentanyl buccal tablet for breakthrough pain in opioid-treated patients with cancer. *Clin J Pain.* 2006;22:805–811.
71. Fitzgibbons FE. Cancer pain: management. In: Loeser JD, ed. *Bonica's Management of Pain.* 3rd ed. Philadelphia, PA; Lippincott, Williams & Wilkins: 659–703.
72. Cleary JF. The pharmacologic management of cancer pain. *J Palliat Med.* 2007;10:1369–1394.
73. Gutstein HB, Akil H. Opioid analgesics. In: Brunton LL, Lazo JS, Parker KL, eds. *The Pharmacological Basis of Therapeutics.* 11th ed. Goodman & Gilman's. New York, NY: McGraw Hill; 2006:547–590.
74. Hanks G, Cherny NI, Fallon M. *Opioid Analgesic Therapy in Oxford Textbook of Palliative Medicine.* 3rd ed. Oxford, UK; Oxford University Press; 2004:316–341.
75. Manfredi PL, Ribeiro S, Chandler SW, Payne R. Inappropriate use of naloxone in cancer patients with pain. *J Pain Symptom Manage* 1996;11:131–134.
76. Portenoy RK, Thomas J, Moehl Boatwright ML, et al. Subcutaneous methylnaltrexone for the treatment of opioid-induced constipation in patients with advanced illness: a double-blind, randomized, parallel group, dose-ranging study. *J Pain Symptom Manage.* 2008;35: 458–468.
77. Thomas J, Karver S, Cooney GA, et al. Methylnaltrexone for opioid-induced constipation in advanced illness. *N Engl J Med.* 2008;358:2332–2343.
78. Moss J, Rosow CE. Development of peripheral opioid antagonists' new insights into opioid effects. *Mayo Clin Proc.* 2008;83:1116–1130.
79. Mercadante S, Arcuri E. Pharmacological management of cancer pain in the elderly. *Drugs Aging.* 2007;24:761–776.
80. Portenoy RK, Sibirceva U, Smout R, et al. Opioid use and survival at the end of life: a survey of a hospice population. *J Pain Symptom Manage.* 2006;32:532–540.
81. Hall S, Gallagher RM, Gracely E, Knowlton C, Wescules D. The terminal cancer patient: effects of age, gender, and primary tumor site on opioid dose. *Pain Med.* 2003;4:125–134.
82. Cherny N, Ripamonti C, Pereira J, et al. Expert Working Group of the European Association of Palliative Care Network. Strategies to manage the adverse effects of oral morphine: an evidence-based report. *J Clin Oncol.* 2001;19:2542–2554.
83. Thomas J. Opioid-induced bowel dysfunction. *J Pain Symptom Manage.* 2008;35:103–113.
84. Hawley PH, Byeon JJ. A comparison of sennosides-based bowel protocols with and without docusate in hospitalized patients with cancer. *J Palliat Med.* 2008;11:575–581.
85. Ishihara M, Iihara H, Okayasu S, Matsuura K, Suzui M, Itoh Y. Pharmaceutical interventions facilitate premedication and prevent opioid-induced constipation and emesis in cancer patients. *Support Care Cancer.* 2009. Epub ahead of print.
86. Tarcatu D, Tamasdan C, Moryl N, Obbens E. Are we still scratching the surface? A case of intractable pruritus following systemic opioid analgesia. *J Opioid Manag.* 2007;3:167–170.
87. Miyoshi HR, Leekband SG. Systemic opioid analgesics. In: *Bonica's Management of Pain.* Loeser JD, Butler SH, Chapman CR, Turk DC, eds. Philadelphia, PA; Lippincott, Williams & Wilkins: 2001:1682–1709.
88. Savage S, Covington EC, Heit HA, Hunt J, Joranson D, Schnoll SH. Definitions related to the use of opioids for the treatment of pain. A consensus document from the American Academy of Pain Medicine, the American Pain Society, and the American Society of Addiction Medicine 2001. *WMJ.* 2001;100:28–29.
89. Stockler M, Vardy J, Pillai A, Warr D. Acetaminophen (paracetamol) improves pain and well-being in people with advanced cancer already receiving a strong opioid regimen: a randomized, double-blind, placebo-controlled cross-over trial. *J Clin Oncol.* 2004;22:3389–3394.
90. Chandrasekharan NV, Dai H, Roos KL, et al. COX-3, a cyclooxygenase-1 variant inhibited by acetaminophen and other analgesic/antipyretic drugs: cloning, structure, and expression. *Proc Natl Acad Sci USA.* 2002;99:13926–13931.
91. Gloth FM. Pain management in older adults: prevention and treatment. *J Am Geriatr Soc.* 2001;49:188–199.
92. Davis MP, Srivastava M: Demographics, assessment and management of pain in the elderly. *Drugs Aging.* 2003;20:23–57.
93. Hylek EM, Heiman H, Skates SJ, Sheehan MA, Singer DE. Acetaminophen and other risk factors for excessive warfarin anticoagulation. *JAMA* 1998;279:657–662.
94. Gunn VL, Taha SH, Liebelt EL, et al: Toxicity of over-the-counter cough and cold medications. *Pediatrics.* 2001;108:E52-E57.
95. Acello B. Administering acetaminophen safely. *Nursing.* 2003;33:18.
96. Bond C, Hannaford P. Issues related to monitoring the safety of over-the-counter (OTC) medicines. *Drug Saf.* 2003;26:1065–1074.
97. Guindon J, Walczak JS, Beaulieu P. Recent advances in the pharmacological management of pain. *Drugs.* 2007;67:2121–2133.
98. Colvin L, Fallon M. Challenges in cancer pain management—bone pain. *Eur J Cancer.* 2008;44:1083–1090.
99. Munir MA, Enany N, Zhang JM. Nonopioid analgesics. *Med Clin North Am.* 2007;91:97–111.
100. Silverstein FE, Faich G, Goldstein JL, et al. Gastrointestinal toxicity with celecoxib vs nonsteroidal anti-inflammatory drugs for osteoarthritis and rheumatoid arthritis: the CLASS study: A randomized controlled trial. Celecoxib Long-term Arthritis Safety Study. *JAMA.* 2000;284:1247–1255.
101. Rowbotham MC, Reisner LA, Davies PS, Fields HL. Treatment response in antidepressant-naïve postherpetic neuralgia patients: double-blind, randomized trial. *J Pain.* 2005;6:741–746.

102. McQuay HJ, Tramèr M, Nye BA, Carroll D, Wiffen PJ, Moore RA. A systematic review of antidepressants in neuropathic pain. *Pain.* 1996;68:217–227.
103. Backonja M, Beydoun A, Edwards KR, et al. Gabapentin for the symptomatic treatment of painful neuropathy in patients with diabetes mellitus: a randomized controlled trial. *JAMA.* 1998;280:1831–1836.
104. Keskinbora K, Pekel AF, Aydinli I. Gabapentin and an opioid combination versus opioid alone for the management of neuropathic cancer pain: a randomized open trial. *J Pain Symptom Manage.* 2007;34:183–189.
105. Caraceni A, Zecca E, Bonezzi C, et al. Gabapentin for neuropathic cancer pain: a randomized controlled trial from the Gabapentin Cancer Pain Study Group. *J Clin Oncol.* 2004;22:2909–2917.
106. Rickels K, Pollack MH, Feltner DE, et al. Pregabalin for treatment of generalized anxiety disorder: a 4-week, multicenter, double-blind, placebo-controlled trial of pregabalin and alprazolam. *Arch Gen Psychiatry.* 2005;62:1022–1030.
107. Montgomery SA, Tobias K, Zornberg GL, Kasper S, Pande AC. Efficacy and safety of pregabalin in the treatment of generalized anxiety disorder: a 6-week, multicenter, randomized, double-blind, placebo-controlled comparison of pregabalin and venlafaxine. *J Clin Psychiatry.* 2006;67:771–782.
108. Dworkin RH, Corbin AE, Young JP, et al. Pregabalin for the treatment of postherpetic neuralgia: a randomized, placebo-controlled trial. *Neurology.* 2003;60:1274–1283.
109. Soares LG, Chan VW. The rationale for a multimodal approach in the management of breakthrough cancer pain: a review. *Am J Hosp Palliat Care.* 2007;24:430–439.
110. Mercadante SL, Berchovich M, Casuccio A, Fulfaro F, Mangione S. A prospective randomized study of corticosteroids as adjuvant drugs to opioids in advanced cancer patients. *Am J Hosp Palliat Care.* 2007;24:13–19.
111. Van Poznak CH. The use of bisphosphonates in patients with breast cancer. *Cancer Control.* 2002;9:480–489.
112. Maxwell C, Swift R, Goode M, Doane L, Rogers M. Advances in supportive care of patients with cancer and bone metastases: nursing implications of zoledronic acid. *Clin J Oncol Nurs.* 2003;7:403–408.
113. Berenson JR: Zoledronic acid in cancer patients with bone metastases: results of phase I and II trials. *Semin Oncol.* 2001;28:(Suppl 6):25–34.
114. Viale PH, Sanchez Yamamoto D. Bisphosphonates: expanded roles in the treatment of patients with cancer. *Clin J Oncol Nurs.* 2003;7:393–401.
115. Small EJ, Smith MR, Seaman JJ, Petrone S, Kowalski MO. Combined analysis of two multicenter, randomized, placebo-controlled studies of pamidronate disodium for the palliation of bone pain in men with metastatic prostate cancer. *J Clin Oncol.* 2003;21:4277–4284.
116. Theriault RL, Lipton A, Hortobagyi GN, et al. Pamidronate reduces skeletal morbidity in women with advanced breast cancer and lytic bone lesions: a randomized, placebo-controlled trial. Protocol 18 Aredia Breast Cancer Study Group. *J Clin Oncol.* 1999;17:846–854.
117. Strong KM, McPherson ML. Pamidronate (Aredia, Ciba). *Am J Hosp Palliat Care.* 1998;15:54–55.
118. Rosen LS, Gordon D, Kaminski M, et al. Zoledronic acid versus pamidronate in the treatment of skeletal metastases in patients with breast cancer or osteolytic lesions of multiple myeloma: a phase III, double-blind, comparative trial. *Cancer J.* 2001;7:377–387.
119. Lipton A, Small E, Saad F, et al. The new bisphosphonate, Zometa (zoledronic acid), decreases skeletal complications in both osteolytic and osteoblastic lesions: a comparison to pamidronate. *Cancer Invest.* 2002;20:(Suppl 2):45–54.
120. Saad F, Gleason DM, Murray R, et al. Zoledronic Acid Prostate Cancer Study Group. A randomized, placebo-controlled trial of zoledronic acid in patients with hormone-refractory metastatic prostate carcinoma. *J Natl Cancer Inst.* 2002;94:1458–1468.
121. Major P, Lortholary A, Hon J, et al. Zoledronic acid is superior to pamidronate in the treatment of hypercalcemia of malignancy: a pooled analysis of two randomized, controlled clinical trials. *J Clin Oncol.* 2001;19:558–567.
122. Li EC, Davis LE. Zoledronic acid: a new parenteral bisphosphonate. *Clin Ther.* 2003;25:2669–2708.
123. Knotkova H, Pappagallo M. Adjuvant analgesics. *Med Clin North Am.* 2007;91:113–124.
124. Galer BS. Topical medications.In: *Bonica's Management of Pain.* 3rd ed. Loeser JD, Butler SH, Chapman CR, Turk DC, eds. Philadelphia, PA; Lippincott, Williams & Wilkins: 2001:1736–1741.
125. Balducci L. Management of cancer pain in geriatric patients. *J Support Oncol.* 2003;1:175–191.
126. Gloth FM: Pain management in older adults: prevention and treatment. *J Am Geriatr Soc.* 2001;49:188–199.
127. Gibson SJ, Helme RD. Age-related differences in pain perception and report. *Clin Geriatr Med.* 2001;17:433–56.
128. Fine PG. Opioid analgesic drugs in older people. *Clin Geriatr Med.* 2001;17:479–87.
129. Freedman GM. Chronic pain. Clinical management of common causes of geriatric pain. *Geriatrics.* 2002;57:36–41.
130. American Geriatric Society: The management of persistent pain in older persons. *J Am Geriatric Soc.* 2002;50:2–5.
131. Levy MH, Cohen SD. Sedation for the relief of refractory symptoms in the imminently dying: a fine intentional line. *Semin Oncol.* 2005;32:237–246.
132. Christo PJ, Mazloomdoost D. Interventional pain treatments for cancer pain. *Ann N Y Acad Sci.* 2008;1138:299–328.
133. Kim PS. Interventional cancer pain therapies. *Semin Oncol.* 2005;32:194–199.
134. Markman JD, Philip A. Interventional approaches to pain management. *Med Clin North Am.* 2007;91:271–286.
135. Ballantyne JC, Carwood C. Comparative efficacy of epidural, subarachnoid, and intracerebroventricular opioids in patients with pain due to cancer. *Cochrane Database Syst Rev.* 2005;1–28.
136. Ashburn MA, Lipman AG, Carr D, Rubingh C. *Principles of Analgesic Use in the Treatment of Acute Pain and Cancer Pain.* 5th ed. Glenview, IL: American Pain Society: 2003.
137. Bennett G, Serafini M, Burchiel K, et al. Evidence-based review of the literature on intrathecal delivery of pain medication. *J Pain Symptom Manage.* 2000;20:S12-S36.
138. Kedlaya D, Reynolds L, Waldman S. Epidural and intrathecal analgesia for cancer pain. *Best Pract Res Clin Anaesthesiol.* 2002;16: 651–665.
139. McQuay HJ, Sullivan AF, Smallman K, Dickenson AH. Intrathecal opioids, potency and lipophilicity. *Pain.* 1989;36:111–115.
140. Chambers WA. Nerve blocks in palliative care. *Br J Anaesth.* 2008;101:95–100.
141. de Jong PC, Kansen PJ. A comparison of epidural catheters with or without subcutaneous injection ports for treatment of cancer pain. *Anesth Analg.* 1994;78:94–100.
142. Exner HJ, Peters J, Eikermann M. Epidural analgesia at end of life: facing empirical contraindications. *Anesth Analg.* 2003;97: 1740–1742.
143. Morgan GE, Mikhail MS, Murray MJ. Clinical Anesthesiology, 4th Edition. New York, NY: McGraw Hill; 2006. http://www.accessmedicine.com. Accessed November 1, 2009.
144. Du Pen S. Complications of neuraxial infusion in cancer patients. *Oncology.* 1999;13:1–3.
145. Staats PS. Complications of intrathecal therapy. *Pain Med.* 2008;9:S102-S107.
146. Sloan PA. The evolving role of interventional pain management in oncology. *J Support Oncol.* 2004;2:491–506.
147. Fine PG, Brogan S. Interventional approaches to treating cancer pain. *ASCO Educ Book.* 2009;1:583–588.
148. Polati E, Luzzani A, Schweiger V, Finco G, Ischia S. The role of neurolytic celiac plexus block in the treatment of pancreatic cancer pain. *Transplant Proc.* 2008;40:1200–1204.

149. Zhang CL, Zhang TJ, Guo YN, et al. Effect of neurolytic celiac plexus block guided by computerized tomography on pancreatic cancer pain. *Dig Dis Sci.* 2008;53:856–860.
150. Yan BM, Myers RP. Neurolytic celiac plexus block for pain control in unresectable pancreatic cancer. *Am J Gastroenterol.* 2007;102:430–438.
151. Adolph MD, Benedetti C. Percutaneous-guided pain control: exploiting the neural basis of pain sensation. *Gastroenterol Clin North Am.* 2006;35:167–188.
152. Gupta D, Jain R, Mishra S, Kumar S, Thulkar S, Bhatnagar S. Ultrasonography reinvents the originally described technique for ganglion Impar neurolysis in perianal cancer pain. *Anesth Analg.* 2008;107:1390–1392.
153. Reig E, Abejón D, del Pozo C, Insausti J, Contreras R. Thermocoagulation of the ganglion Impar or ganglion of Walther: description of a modified approach. Preliminary results in chronic, nononcological pain. *Pain Pract.* 2005;5:103–110.
154. de Oliveira R, dos Reis MP, Prado WA. The effects of early or late neurolytic sympathetic plexus block on the management of abdominal or pelvic cancer pain pain. *Pain.* 2008;110:400–408.
155. Rosenberg M, Phero JC. Regional anesthesia and invasive techniques to manage head and neck pain. *Otolaryngol Clin North Am.* 2003;36:1201–1219.
156. Feigl GC, Rosmarin W, Stelzl A, Weninger B, Likar R. Comparison of different injectate volumes for stellate ganglion block: an anatomic and radiologic study. *Reg Anesth Pain Med.* 2007;32:203–208.
157. Hardy D. Relief of pain in acute herpes zoster by nerve blocks and possible prevention of post-herpetic neuralgia. *Can J Anaesth.* 2005;52:186–190.
158. Garber JE, Hassenbusch SJ. Neurosurgical operations on the spinal cord. In: *Bonica's Management of Pain.* 3rd ed. Loeser JD, Butler SH, Chapman CR, Turk DC, eds. Philadelphia, PA; Lippincott, Williams & Wilkins: 2001:2023–2037.
159. Bartels RH, van der Linden YM, van der Graaf WT. Spinal extradural metastasis: review of current treatment options. *CA: Cancer J Clin.* 2008;58:245–259.
160. Andrew T, Trout LAG, David F.K. Vertebroplasty in the inpatient population. *Am J Neuro Radiol.* 2005;26:1629–1633.
161. Astin JA, Shapiro SL, Eisenberg DM, Forys KL. Mind-body medicine: state of the science, implications for practice. *J Am Board Fam Pract.* 2003;16:131–147.
162. Kwekkeboom KL, Bumpus M, Wanta B, Serlin RC. Oncology nurses' use of nondrug pain interventions in practice. *J Pain Symptom Manage.* 2008;35:83–94.
163. Robb KA, Bennett MI, Johnson MI, Simpson KJ, Oxberry SG. Transcutaneous electric nerve stimulation (TENS) for cancer pain in adults. *Cochrane Database Syst Rev.* 2009;1:1–23.

CHAPTER

# 28

Brenda K. Shelton, MS, RN, CCRN, AOCN®

# Infection

## SCOPE OF THE PROBLEM

Despite tremendous progress in the management of infections in patients with cancer during recent years, infection remains one of the most significant etiologies of chemotherapy dose delays, dose reductions, morbidity, and mortality for these patients.[1–4] It is estimated that more than 25% to 44% of patients with solid tumor cancers[1–4] and nearly 70% of some with hematologic malignancies[5,6] will experience infection during the course of their treatment, and some sources suggest that the management of infectious complications accounts for 45% of inpatient care for certain patient groups.[2–7] Localized infection can result in progression to systemic dissemination of the microbes in 10% to 20% of patients and a shock response in 15% to 20% of those infected patients, which is associated with an average mortality rate of 6% to 12%.[2,4,10–15] Balducci et al suggest that older patients with cancer may have up to 30% mortality risk related to infection,[16] and studies of febrile neutropenia in children suggest a less than 10% infection-related mortality.[17,18] Although much is known about the distribution, etiology, and clinical complications associated with infection, no predictive models exist to identify which patients will develop the most life-threatening of the associated complications.[2,3,18–24] Outcomes from these infectious complications vary greatly and are dependent on individual host characteristics, type of malignancy, and organism features.

### DEFINITIONS

Infectious complications are commonly described in terms of the type of infectious microorganism, the physiological location of the infection, and the degree of tissue invasion.[8,25,26] Types of infecting microbial organisms include bacteria, fungi, viruses, and opportunistic organisms. Each of these categories includes multiple microbial species, with unique propensities to infect specific locations, and production of specific signs and symptoms. The most common microbial sources of infection and their key clinical features are described in Table 28-1.[8,27–29] In years past, the most common infections among immunocompromised patients involved gram-negative bacteria, which were thought to be primarily translocated from the gastrointestinal (GI) tract.[30–33] Today, patients at high risk for infection receive oral antimicrobial prophylaxis against gram-negative organisms, reducing the incidence of systemic gram-negative infection.[8,25,26,34–37] With the use of more invasive vascular access lines and prolonged exposure to broad-spectrum antimicrobials, gram-positive organisms are more prevalent in patients with cancer who are at risk for infection.[24,31,34,38]

Infections are also described by the specific body location that is infected. For instance, infection involving the airway is termed pneumonia, whereas the same infection affecting the meninges is termed meningitis. The specific terms and clinical manifestations of infections of different body locations are detailed in Table 28-1.[8,25–29]

The presence of microbes in and on body tissues may indicate anything from the presence of normal resident flora to the invasion of body tissues by virulent and toxic foreign microbes. Bacteria that normally reside within the body include examples such as *Escherichia coli* that are commonly found within the GI tract. These same organisms can cause infection if they are accidentally "tracked" to another part of the body. Typical normal flora and their resident human tissues are listed in Table 28-2.[39–46] It can be assumed that these normal flora are pathogenic if discovered in a different part of the body.

Infections are graded and defined according to severity based on the level of tissue penetration. When organisms are present on or in body tissues, but are not viable, multiplying, or invading the epithelial layer, the situation is termed *colonization*, a form of microbial invasion that is not usually pathogenic.[47,48] Colonization may cause infection in severely immunocompromised patients, so it is considered an aspect of the patient's clinical data that is important to follow.[44,49,50] For example, colonization of *Escherichia coli* in the GI tract of an immunosuppressed patient may result in infection. Definitions of levels of infection have been defined by the American College of Chest Physicians and Society of Critical Care Medicine,[27,47] these definitions are summarized in Table 28-3.

Infections are also defined in the context of the *chain of infection,* which relates to the spread of infection from one person to another. Not all infections are transmissible, but this theoretical model is useful for addressing all aspects of infection control for those microbial infections that can spread.[52,53] The 6-step model describes the process from microbe to clinical disease. Infectious agents (eg, bacteria, fungi, viruses, rickettsiae, parasites) are harbored in a sanctuary site called a *reservoir.* Reservoirs may comprise food, people, water, medications, equipment, or the environment. Microbes exit reservoirs by excretions, secretions, or droplets and are acquired by a host via 1 or more of the 4 modes of transmission: contact, airborne, vehicle, or vector. Microbes enter the host's body through breaks in the barrier defense or via one of the natural orifices. The susceptibility of the host is the primary variable determining whether infection will occur, and the link of transmission is the easiest to break and thereby halt the chain of infection spread.[48] Infections are described by where or how they are acquired (community acquired vs hospital acquired or nosocomial), as well as whether they are confined to the host (noncommunicable) or can spread from one person to another (communicable). Some clinical situations warrant differentiation of whether an infection is a primary (first to occur) or secondary (related to the presence or treatment of another infection). A common secondary infection in

**TABLE 28-1**

**Signs and Symptoms of Infection**

| Body System | Complication | Signs and Symptoms[a] | Infectious Organisms |
|---|---|---|---|
| Neurological | Encephalitis | Confusion, lethargy, difficulty arousing, headache, visual difficulty/photosensitivity, nausea, hypertension | *Neisseria meningitidis*, *Toxoplasma*, herpes simplex, cytomegalovirus |
| | Meningitis | Lethargy and somnolence, confusion, nuccal rigidity | *N. meningitidis*, streptococcus, *Listeria*, *Cryptococcus*, herpes simplex |
| Head/neck | Conjunctivitis | Reddened conjunctiva, excess tearing of eye, pus-like exudate from eye, blurred vision, swelling of eyelid, eye itching | Pneumococcus, streptococcus, staphylococcus, *N. meningitidis*, adenovirus, rotovirus |
| | Otitis media | Earache, difficulty hearing, itching, inner ear, ear drainage | Streptococcus, aspergillus |
| | Sinusitis | Discolored nasal mucous, nasal congestion, face pain, eye pain, blurred vision | Staphylococcus, *Haemophilus influenzae*, *Histoplasma*, aspergillus, mucor, fusarium, *Cryptococcus* |
| | Oropharyngeal infection | Oral ulcerations or plaques, halitosis, reddened gums, abnormal papillae of the tongue, sore throat, difficulty swallowing | Streptococcus, *Candida*, herpes simplex |
| | Lymphadenitis | Swollen neck lymph glands, tender lymph glands, a lump felt when swallowing | *Mycobacterium avium-intracellulare* |
| Pulmonary | Bronchitis | Persistent cough, sputum production, gurgles in upper airways, wheezes in upper airways, hypoxemia and/or hypercapnea | Streptococcus, staphylococcus |
| | Pneumonia | Chest discomfort pronounced with inspiration, persistent cough, sputum production, diminished breath sounds, crackles or gurgles, asymmetrical chest wall movement, labored breathing, nasal flaring with breathing, hypoxemia | Staphylococcus, pneumococcus, streptococcus, *N. meningitidis*, *Corynebacterium diphtheriae*, *Klebsiella*, proteus, *Pseudomonas*, actinomyces, *Nocardia*, aspergillus, *Cryptococcus*, *Blastomyces*, *Histoplasma*, cytomegalovirus, *Pneumocystis jerivichi*, legionella, mycobacterium (*Mycobacterium tuberculosis*, *M. avium-intracellulare*), *Toxoplasma*, *Haemophilus influenza*, *Candida*, herpes simplex virus, varicella simplex virus, respiratory synctival virus, adenovirus, influenza |
| | Pleurisy | Chest discomfort pronounced with inspiration, sides of chest more painful, usually unilateral discomfort, splinting with deep breaths | *Listeria, Histoplasma* |
| Cardiovascular | Myocarditis | Dysrhythmias, murmurs or gallops, elevated jugular venous pulsations, weak thready pulses, hypotension, point of maximal impulse shifted laterally | *Toxoplasma* |
| | Pericarditis | Aching constant chest discomfort unrelieved by rest or nitrates, pericardial rub, muffled heart sounds | Staphylococcus, pneumococcus, streptococcus, *N. meningitidis*, *Histoplasma* |
| | Endocarditis | Fever, tachydysrhythmias, heart murmur, hypotension, septic emboli | Streptococcus, pneumococcus, staphylococcus |
| Gastrointestinal | Gastritis | Nausea, vomiting within 30 minutes of eating, heme-positive emesis, aching stomach that initially improves by eating | Salmonella |
| | Infectious diarrhea | More than 6 loose stools per day, clay-colored stools, foul-smelling stools, abdominal cramping, abdominal distention | Staphylococcus, *Corynebacterium diphtheriae*, actinomyces, *Klebsiella*, proteus, shigella, *Pseudomonas*, legionella, cytomegalovirus, norovirus |

(*Continued*)

**TABLE 28-1**

**Signs and Symptoms of Infection** *(Continued)*

| Body System | Complication | Signs and Symptoms[a] | Infectious Organisms |
|---|---|---|---|
| | Cholelithiasis/ pancreatitis | Epigastric discomfort, intolerance to high-fat food, clay-colored stools, nausea and vomiting, hyperglycemia, hypocalcemia, hypoalbuminemia, increased lipase and amylase | *Nocardia*, *Candida*, cytomegalovirus, *Cryptosporidium* |
| | Hepatitis | Jaundice, right upper quadrant discomfort, hepatomegaly, elevated transaminases and bilirubin, fatty food intolerances, nausea and vomiting, diarrhea | Cytomegalovirus, mycobacterium (*M. tuberculosis*, *M. avium-intracellulare*), *Toxoplasma*, adenovirus, *Candida* |
| Genitourinary | Urethritis | Painful urination, difficulty urinating, itching of genitourinary orifice | *Escherichia coli*, *Candida* |
| | Cystitis | Small frequent urination (urinary urgency) feeling of fullness of the bladder | Streptococcus, *Pseudomonas*, *E. coli*, *Candida*, adenovirus |
| | Nephritis | Flank discomfort, oliguria, protein in urine | Streptococcus, *E. coli*, *Candida* |
| | Vaginitis | Itching of vaginal area, vaginal discharge | *N. meningitidis*, herpes simplex |
| Musculoskeletal | Arthritis | Joint discomfort, swollen and warm joints | Streptococcus, *Nocardia* |
| | Myositis | Aching muscles, weakness | *Candida* |
| Dermatological | Superficial skin infection | Rashes, itching, raised and/or discolored skin lesions, open draining skin lesions, patterns are unique to specific microorganism | Any organism |
| | Cellulitis | Redness, warmth, and swelling of subcutaneous tissue area, radiating pain from area toward middle of body | *Staphylococcus aureus*, streptococcus, actinomyces |
| Hematologic/ immunologic | Bacteremia | Low diastolic blood pressure, headache, confusion, oliguria, decreased bowel sounds, warmth, flushing, positive blood cultures | Any organism, although most common are those bacteria that infect the mucous membranes, lung, and GI tract, and select fungi (eg, *Candida*), viruses (eg, cytomegalovirus), and opportunistic organisms (eg, mycobacterium). |

*Note*: [a]The signs and symptoms presented in this table are unique features of each process and do not include the common constitutional signs and symptoms seen with all infections, such as fever, chills, malaise, leukocytosis, positive tissue culture for microorganisms, or increased erythrocyte sedimentation rate.

*Abbreviations*: E. coli, Escherichia coli; GI, gastrointestinal; N, Neisseria.

*Source*: Adapted with permission from Shelton BK, Friese CR. Anti-infectives. In: Gay BG, Chernecky C, eds. *Manual of Medical-Surgical Nursing*. Philadelphia, PA: WB Saunders; 2002:348–357.[28]

patients with cancer is candidal mucosal infection caused by overgrowth of normal flora when normal bacteria are suppressed by broad-spectrum antibacterial therapy.[42]

## INCIDENCE

The prevalence of specific risk factors for infection, such as neutropenia and T-cell suppression, has been a focus of research, but less information is available regarding the incidence of actual infection resulting from these risks. This may be in part due to the limitations of diagnostic procedures to validate and reveal the source of infection, or in the varied approaches to care that make data collection a difficult task.[24] In patients with fever, only 48% to 60% will have a documented infection.[14,24] Infection may be treated with intravenous antimicrobials on an inpatient basis, treated with oral antimicrobials on an outpatient basis, or not treated, allowing the body's normal immune mechanisms to overcome the microbe.

**TABLE 28-2**

**Normal Flora Within the Body**

| Body Tissue | Normal Flora at This Location |
|---|---|
| Eyes (cornea) | *Neisseria* |
| | Staphylococcus |
| | Streptococcus |
| GI tract, large intestine, rectum | *Bacteroides* |
| | *E. coli* |
| | *Enterobacter* |
| | *Klebsiella* |
| | *Proteus* |
| GI tract, small intestine | *Bacteroides* |
| | *E. coli* |
| | *Enterococcus* |
| | *Lactobacillus* |
| Oral mucosa | *Actinomyces israeli* |
| | *Candida albicans* |
| | *Entamoeba gingivalis* |
| | *Diptheroids* |
| | Streptococcus |
| | *Trichomonas tenax* |
| Reproductive system | *Candida* |
| | *E. coli* |
| | *Neisseria* |
| | Staphylococcus |
| | Streptococcus |
| Skin surface | *Candida* |
| | *Diptheroids* |
| | *Proprionibacteria* |
| | *Staphylococcus epidermis* |
| Stomach | *Candida* |
| | *Lactobacillus* |
| Upper respiratory tract | *Bronhamella* |
| | *Haemophilus* |
| | *Neisseria* |
| | Staphylococcus |
| | Streptococcus |

*Abbreviation*: *E. coli, Escherichia coli*; GI, gastrointestinal.
*Source*: Data from Fauci et al[26]; Mims et al[40]; Todar[41]; Corti et al[44]; Tuthill et al[45]; and Kontoyiannis et al.[46]

Either systemic infection (termed sepsis) or bloodstream infection (known as bacteremia) is estimated to occur in 10% to 20% of patients who have a febrile neutropenic event.[2,14,54] Bacteremia is better defined and tracked than most infections. Its incidence approaches 900,000 cases annually.[27,55] Since a specific organism may not be identified in sepsis and is not a reportable disease, it is believed to be underreported.[27] Despite this, in the United States, sepsis is still the leading cause of death in noncardiac intensive care units and the 11th leading cause of death overall in intensive care units.[55,56] Mortality associated with sepsis ranges from 28% to 55%.[27,55–57] In a study of more than 190,000 patients with severe sepsis, the additional cost of care for this complication amounted to an estimated $22,100 per case, and its annual costs exceeded $16.7 billion.[55] Although less well documented than in the critical care literature, sepsis has an estimated 25% incidence in patients with cancer, and the associated patient mortality is approximately 28%.

### ETIOLOGY AND RISK FACTORS

The causes of infection in the patient with cancer are varied, involving both host and environmental factors. To some degree, the type of invading microbe or site of infection may also be associated with specific risk factors. Examples of defective protective mechanisms and factors contributing to infection in people with cancer are listed in Table 28-4.[8,16,18,21,25,26,33–35,39,42,44,48,58–74] In some cases, specific microbial characteristics, such as extent of exposure or organism virulence, influence the incidence and severity of infection.[40–43] However, it is clear that neither the presence of a potentially pathogenic microbe nor a defined risk factor conclusively leads to infection, so other, as-yet-undefined mediating factors may exist.

## PHYSIOLOGICAL ALTERATIONS

### NORMAL ANATOMY, PHYSIOLOGY, AND SCIENTIFIC PRINCIPLES

The body's defensive systems are divided into nonspecific and specific defenses. The nonspecific defensive system of the body functions to rapidly recognize foreign antigens and mount an aggressive destruction of these proteins. It includes the skin and mucosal barriers, granulocytes, and the complement protein pathway. The specific immune system seeks to find specific antigenic material and create targeted biological agents that selectively destroy this unique substance.

The 2 systems work in an integrated fashion to produce both an immediate and a delayed response to pathogens entering the body. The specific response is a more delayed response, but is more selective in its pattern of destruction. The specific immune response is led by lymphocytes and their cytokines or immunoglobulins.

**TABLE 28-3**

**American College of Chest Physicians/Society of Critical Care Medicine Definitions of Infections and Sepsis**

*Infection*: Microbial phenomenon characterized by an inflammatory response to the presence of microorganisms or the invasion of normally sterile host tissue by those organisms.

*Bacteremia*: The presence of viable bacteria in the blood.

*Systemic inflammatory response syndrome*: The systemic inflammatory response to a variety of severe clinical insults; the response is manifested by 2 or more of the following conditions:
Temperature > 38°C or < 36°C
Heart rate > 90 beats/min
Respiratory rate > 20 breaths/min or $PaCO_2$ < 32 mm Hg (<4.3 kPa)
WBC > 12,000 cells/$mm^3$, < 4000 cells/$mm^3$, or > 10% immature (band) forms

*Sepsis*: The systemic response to infection; the response is manifested by 2 or more of the following conditions as a result of infection:
Temperature > 38°C or < 36°C
Heart rate > 90 beats/min
Respiratory rate > 20 breaths/min or $PaCO_2$ < 32 mm Hg (<4.3 kPa)
WBC > 12,000 cells/$mm^3$, < 4000 cells/$mm^3$, or > 10% immature (band) forms

*Severe sepsis*: Sepsis associated with organ dysfunction, hypoperfusion, or hypotension; hypoperfusion and perfusion abnormalities may include, but are not limited to, lactic acidosis, oliguria, or an acute alteration in mental status.

*Septic shock*: Sepsis with hypotension, despite adequate fluid resuscitation, along with the presence of perfusion abnormalities that may include, but are not limited to, lactic acidosis, oliguria or an acute alteration in mental status; patients who are on inotropic or vasopressor agents may not be hypotensive at the time that perfusion abnormalities are measured.

*Hypotension*: A systolic blood pressure < 90 mm Hg or a reduction > 40 mm Hg from baseline in the absence of other causes for hypotension.

*Multiple organ dysfunction syndrome*: Presence of altered organ function in an acutely ill patient such that homeostasis cannot be maintained without intervention.

*Source*: Reprinted with permission from Members of the American College of Chest Physicians/Society of Critical Care Medicine Consensus Conference Committee.[51]

It is divided into the primary (initial) response and the secondary response. The primary response recognizes foreign proteins and causes the release of cell killer substances termed cytokines (eg, interferon, interleukin 2), a process termed *cellular immunity.* The secondary immune response relies on the immune memory of antigens that have been previously recognized by the lymphocytes, and involves the recall of immunoglobulins that were created upon initial exposure to the antigen. This activity is also termed the *humoral immune response.*

Inadequate nonspecific immune responses (eg, breaks in the integumentary system, neutropenia, and complement deficiency) usually result in bacterial infection. In contrast, inadequate specific immune responses may result in viral or opportunistic infection. Inappropriate specific immune responses constitute a reaction that involves reaction against self or foreign substances not normally considered antigenic. This reaction may also be manifested as an allergic response or autoimmune disease.

## Integumentary, mucosal, and chemical barriers

Intact skin constitutes the most important barrier against invasion by both exogenous and endogenous organisms. The skin is made up of cornified layers of epithelial cells that cover the body and protect tissues against dehydration and invasion by harmful bacteria. When a break in the skin occurs, environmental microbes and those organisms that normally inhabit hair follicles and sebaceous glands may enter the body and cause infection.

A second major defense against infection is the mucociliary activity found in the mucous membranes. The cilia of the epithelial cells that line the respiratory tract beat rhythmically to propel mucous and entrapped foreign particles toward the nose and throat. In the GI tract, the cilia propel bacteria and waste products to be removed in the feces. Microorganisms account for as much as 60% of the weight of the stool; therefore, an intact GI mucous membrane is essential to prevent infection.

A variety of other mechanisms serve to protect the body from microbial invasion. Resident microbial flora

**TABLE 28-4**

**Characteristics and Risks for Immunocompromised Patient Populations**

| Patient Characteristics | Physiological Mechanism of Risk | Possible Consequences of Risk Factor |
|---|---|---|
| Abuse of intravenous drugs | • Chronic altered barrier defense leads to reduced WBCs and slowed phagocytic responses.<br>• Constant viral exposure may alter T-cell function. | Topical antimicrobial agents are used to prevent local infections induced by needles. Recognition of the T-cell defects and propensity for viral infections caused by IV drug abuse may allow for closer monitoring strategies and early treatment for viral infection. |
| Alcoholism | • Decreased neutrophil activity: Increased bacterial infections, more rapid dissemination of infection<br>• Hepatic/splenic congestion also slows phagocytic response. | The risk of aspiration is more common in patients who use alcohol excessively, so oral and upper GI infectious organisms are the usual suspects in patients with symptoms of pneumonia. Altered liver and spleen function may diminish immune memory and make patients prone to encapsulated organisms. |
| Antibiotics | • Destruction of normal flora, enhanced growth of resistant organism, fungal superinfection<br>• Resistant bacterial organisms emerge after normal flora are destroyed by broad-spectrum antimicrobials. | When normal bacterial flora are destroyed by the antimicrobial therapy, resistant organisms may emerge, and fungal organisms may flourish. Antifungal prophylaxis may be prescribed. More infections with resistant organisms occur. |
| Autoimmune disease | • Diseases manifested by self-rejection that implies inappropriate sensitization of foreign substances | General immunocompromised precautions are implemented in patients with poor immune recognition. These disorders are treated with immune-suppressing agents and corticosteroids, so the effects and management strategies are the same as those risk variables. |
| Blood transfusions | • Some viral illnesses are difficult to detect in blood screening, particularly in the incubation phase. Blood products infected with viruses can transmit viral disease to the recipient.<br>• Blood products that are aged, left in room air, or not handled aseptically can become contaminated with bacteria (both gram-positive and gram-negative) and be transmitted as a bacteremia. | Increased awareness of possible pathogen transmission via blood products has led more patients to donate autologous blood prior to procedures where blood transfusion is anticipated. Careful evaluation of the hematologic malignancy and transplant patient's viral status (eg, cytomegalovirus) allows for planned prophylaxis during the immunocompromised period when the patient is at greatest risk for infections. |
| Burns | • Altered barrier defenses allow pathogen entry. | Loss of integument predisposes the patient to invasion by many different microbes. The additional immunologic response of neutrophil depression adds to this risk. Specific species of microbial infection may depend on the site of injury, host colonization, or environmental factors (eg, exposure to soil). |
| Cancer | • Structural disruption may lead to bone marrow or lymphatic abnormalities.<br>• Barrier defenses are affected when tumors erode into soft tissue and mucous membranes.<br>• Certain cancers have specific immune defects (eg, diminished phagocytic activity or T-cell defects). | Cancer is a reflection of inadequate immune surveillance and abnormalities of the lymphatic system. Biological anticancer therapies are based on the premise that we can support the body's normal immune processes. Certain cancers will predispose patients to infection with normal flora from nearby tissues or organisms most likely to invade that area (eg, airborne organisms via respiratory tract). |
| | • Antineoplastic therapy can cause infection from several different mechanisms: (1) it destroys reserve of all WBCs when the bone marrow is affected; (2) it destroys the lymphatic continuum when the lymph system is affected; (3) macrophages in specific organs may be damaged by therapy; and (4) immune memory may be lost when cancer involves the B lymphocytes or when lymphocyte suppression is intended (eg, blood and marrow transplant). | Antineoplastic therapy also compromises barrier defenses and inhibits cell growth within the bone marrow, predisposing to infection. |

(*Continued*)

**TABLE 28-4**

**Characteristics and Risks for Immunocompromised Patient Populations** *(Continued)*

| Patient Characteristics | Physiological Mechanism of Risk | Possible Consequences of Risk Factor |
|---|---|---|
| Diabetes mellitus | • Decreased numbers of neutrophils and slowed phagocytic activity: More frequent infections, more disseminated infections, increased risk of infections with antimicrobial-resistant organisms<br>• Hyperglycemia causes decreased phagocytic activity and immunoglobulin defects.<br>• Neuropathy and glycosuria predispose to decreased bladder emptying and urinary tract infections.<br>• Uncontrolled hyperglycemia has been associated with poorer outcomes even independent of infection. | The extremely high risk for serious and rapidly disseminating infections prompts prophylaxis against infection for some patients, a low threshold for treatment of presumed infection, more thorough diagnostic work-ups for sources, and pathological diagnosis of infections. Patient education to help prevent infection may include foot safety, drinking plenty of fluids, and recognition of subtle symptoms. |
| Frequent hospitalizations | • Frequent exposure to environmental organisms other than one's own normal environment<br>• Exposure to other people's organisms via staff, equipment, or supplies<br>• Potential exposure to resistant organisms | Hospitalizations are avoided whenever possible to reduce the patient's exposure to foreign microbes that are more pathogenic than the ones in their normal living environment. When hospitalization cannot be avoided, careful separation of patient care items, single-patient-use items, or thorough cleaning between use reduces the transference of microbes and development of resistance microbes. |
| GI disease | • Decreased bowel motility allows normal flora to translocate across the GI wall to the bloodstream.<br>• Breaks in the mucosal integrity of the GI tract predispose patients to microbial transference into the bloodstream.<br>• Poor circulation to the GI tract causes decreased peristalsis and mucosal atrophy. Normal flora and intestinal gram-negative organisms can become pathogenic. | Maintaining minimal normal GI motility and mucosal integrity reduces the amount of infection via the GI tract. Using the gut consistently for food and fluid consumption helps maintain normal function. Enteral feeding is always attempted, if at all possible, to enhance GI integrity and function. |
| HIV disease | • Viral incorporation into the RNA, then the DNA of immune cells having the $CD8^+$ molecule disrupts normal WBC function and replication, leading to lymphopenia, lymphocyte dysfunction, and macrophage dysfunction.<br>• Disruption of these cells leads to many different infections (eg, unusual bacteria, fungi, opportunistic bacteria, viruses) and lymphoproliferative disorders/malignancies (eg, Kaposi's sarcoma, lymphoma). | HIV disease is directly treated with antiretrovirals and immune-reconstituting agents such as interleukin-2. Stabilization of lymphocyte counts reduces the risk and incidence of opportunistic infections. When the lymphocyte count drops, prophylactic antimicrobial agents specific to the organisms likely to infect these patients are prescribed in a well-defined and protocol-determined manner. Avoidance of activities likely to expose patients to infection and attempts to maintain care in the ambulatory environment may also reduce the risk of serious or resistant infections. |
| Immunosuppressive agents and corticosteroids | • Decreased phagocytic activity.<br>• Altered T-cell recognition of pathogens, especially viral.<br>• Lack of immune memory to recall antibodies to previously encountered pathogens. | Immune-suppressing agents have multiple immune-depressing functions, putting patients at risk for infection. Special precautions are implemented, and prophylactic antimicrobial agents against common opportunistic organisms may be indicated. These patients also lose immune memory and are candidates for vaccinations, provided that the vaccine does not contain live agents. Patients are taught that they will have blunted inflammatory responses and that subtle symptoms may indicate infection. Immunosuppression effects on WBC response lead to an inability to mount an inflammatory response including less ability to create a fever when infected. |

| | | |
|---|---|---|
| Indwelling intravenous catheters | • Indwelling venous or arterial access devices break the barrier defenses, with subsequent risk of microbial invasion.<br>• The presence of an intravenous device may irritate the venous wall and induce inflammatory damage, resulting in a higher risk for microbial invasion.<br>• The greater the number of providers who insert or access intravenous catheters, or the number of times the device is accessed, the higher the risk of infection. | Intravenous catheters breach the barrier defenses and increase the risk of microbial invasion into the body. Some companies have developed catheters that have been coated or treated with active antimicrobial agents such as silver ions, chlorhexidine, or heparin. Catheters have also been designed with structural variations in an attempt to reduce the irritation of veins, thereby minimizing phlebitis and infection (eg, angled catheter tips, modified catheter anchoring devices). Clinicians must choose the smallest lumen size, least number of lumens, and most appropriate permanence of a device to reduce infection rates. Heightened sterile technique when accessing these devices may also reduce the rate of associated infection.<br>Many clinical practices use dedicated venous access device teams. |
| Infants/elderly | • Immature thymus in infants: Increased viral and opportunistic infection<br>• Atrophy of thymus in the elderly: Increased viral infection<br>• Decreased antigen-specific immunoglobulins in elderly: Diminished immune memory, delayed hypersensitivity reactions<br>• Slowed macrophage activity: More fungal infection, diminished immune memory<br>• Appearance of autoimmune antibodies: Increased incidence of autoimmune disease | Immature and atrophied immune systems can lead to infection with a variety of organisms from any additional breach in the body's defenses. Frequent complex or polymicrobial infections are expected and are guarded against by careful infection prevention techniques and strategies. Recognition of the variety of infectious complications and the potential for their rapid dissemination causes increased vigilance in monitoring and early aggressive interventions for infection. Prophylactic strategies are not usually recommended in these populations, but a low threshold for treatment is implemented. |
| Invasive devices (eg, Foley catheter, nasogastric tube) | • Altered barrier defenses allow pathogen entry, especially skin organisms. | Invasive devices breach the barrier defenses and increase the risk of microbial invasion into the body. Catheters and invasive devices have been coated or treated with active antimicrobial agents such as silver ions, chlorhexidine, or heparin, in an attempt to reduce related infection. Some devices also have structural variations in an attempt to reduce the irritation or mucosal injury produced, with the hope of reducing the rate of related infection (eg, altered bluntness of the tip of a tracheal suction catheter). Infection monitoring for microbial colonization may also help detect early presence of potential pathogens in high-risk patients. |
| Malnutrition | • Inadequate WBC count<br>• Reduced neutrophil activity | Altered nutrition increases the risk of infection. Efforts to boost immune-related nutrition deficits may focus on inclusion of glutamine, arginine, and other essential amino acids in nutrient supplements as well as other measures aimed at enhancing nutrition well-being. |
| Hepatic disease | • Decreased neutrophil count<br>• Decreased phagocytic activity<br>• Lost immunoglobulin production | Hepatic disease increases the risk of bacterial infection and rapid dissemination of that infection. Loss of immunoglobulins leads to failed immune memory. Special infection precautions for immunocompromised patients are implemented. |
| Neutropenia | • Inadequate neutrophils to combat infection. | The lack of neutrophils places the patient at high risk for bacterial infections that will rapidly disseminate and potentially cause septic shock. Hematopoietic growth factors may be administered as primary or secondary prophylaxis to abrogate the severity (depth of nadir) or longevity of the period of neutropenia. |

(Continued)

**TABLE 28-4**

**Characteristics and Risks for Immunocompromised Patient Populations** (*Continued*)

| Patient Characteristics | Physiological Mechanism of Risk | Possible Consequences of Risk Factor |
|---|---|---|
| Pulmonary disease | • Inadequate oxygenation decreases neutrophil activity.<br>• Pulmonary disease may alter the person's ability to mobilize respiratory secretions.<br>• Oral secretions with non-endogenous respiratory organisms can track down the oropharynx, causing infection. | Infection risk is increased and can be decreased by implementing precautions. Excess trapped secretions can become infected, causing pneumonia. |
| Radiation therapy | • Radiation to the long bones will interfere with WBC production.<br>• Radiation in the area of certain endocrine organs can lead to endocrine failure (hypoadrenalism, hypothyroidism, pituitary dysfunction) and infection risk.<br>• Radiation damage to the barrier defenses will predispose the patient to invasion by microbes. | Destruction of stem cells and existing bone marrow reserve of hematopoietic cells is a common dose-limiting toxicity of radiation therapy involving the long bones where cells are produced. Destruction of the normal skin and soft tissue barriers is treated with specialized skin care to reduce the incidence of infection. |
| Renal disease | • Decreased neutrophil activity.<br>• Decreased immunoglobulin activity. | Patients with renal dysfunction are provided extra precautions against bacterial infection, recognizing that they may also show blunted or reduced symptoms of infection. These patients are appropriate candidates for vaccinations against many microorganisms. |
| Splenectomy | • Inability to recognize and remove encapsulated bacteria (eg, streptococci, mycobacteria). | Postsplenectomy, either functional or anatomical, the patient is at risk for specific infections. Vaccination against pneumococci is recommended for these patients. A low threshold of suspicion for streptococci with oropharyngeal or urinary tract symptoms may allow for early antimicrobial therapy. |
| Surgical procedures/ wounds | • Normal flora may be translocated by surgical procedure.<br>• Altered barrier defenses due to surgical entry.<br>• The stress of surgery or anesthetic agents may reduce neutrophil activity. | Careful surgical preparation of the planned surgical site with chlorhexidine scrubs is recommended prior to many surgical procedures. Shaving the involved area remains a debatable practice, with some believing that hair removal reduces risk, and others believing that skin nicks from the razor may increase the risk of infection. Operating room staff may also perform a surgical scrub of the site followed by placement of a clear sterile barrier film, which is subsequently cut through for the actual procedure. Conscientious postoperative care with fluids, coughing and deep breathing, and early mobility may decrease the risk of infection. Being aware of previous colonization or infection prior to surgery may assist in defining the source of fever postoperatively. |
| Traumatic injuries | • Altered barrier defenses allowing pathogen entry.<br>• Type of infection dependent on source and severity of injury (eg, soil contamination, water contamination, skin flora). | Altered barrier defenses are treated with frequent cleansing, antimicrobial cleansing, covering with sterile dressings to prevent infectious organisms from entering the bloodstream via the open wound. Antimicrobial ointments have not been proven effective. If a wound is thought to be clean and sterile, a clear protective barrier dressing may provide better occlusiveness and guard against microorganism entry. |

*Abbreviations*: GI, gastrointestinal; HIV, Human Immunodeficiency Virus; IV, intravenous; WBC, white blood cell.
*Source*: Data from Shelton,[28] Tuthill et al.[45] Allen et al,[59] Bartlett et al,[60] Crnich et al,[61] Moran et al,[66] O'Grady et al,[67] Lerman et al.[68] Shelton,[69] Yadegarynia et al,[70] and Allain et al.[73]

prevents pathogenic colonization by competing for surface-binding sites and nutrients and by producing metabolic products that are toxic to other organisms.[41] Acidic pH inhibits or prevents bacterial growth on the skin and in the stomach, bladder, and vagina. Microbicidal elements found in prostatic fluid and tears also provide a protective effect.

### Leukocytes

*Granulocytes.* Leukocytes, particularly polymorphonuclear neutrophils (PMNs), represent a significant defense against infection. Polymorphonuclear neutrophils, which are also referred to as polys or segmented neutrophils (segs), are short-lived white blood cells (WBCs) that respond quickly to bacterial invasion. They are the most numerous of the leukocytes, constituting 35% to 76% of circulating WBCs. The primary function of PMNs is the destruction and elimination of microorganisms through phagocytosis, the process of engulfing and ingesting foreign matter. In addition, PMNs secrete chemotactants, chemical substances that alert the body to the presence of an invader. Chemotactants, or monokines, stimulate increased production of PMNs, macrophages, and complement proteins and direct them to the site of invasion. Without sufficient PMNs, the body's ability to mount an inflammatory response is compromised.

*Monocytes and macrophages.* Monocytes and macrophages constitute what was previously referred to as the reticuloendothelial system. Monocytes are released from the bone marrow before they complete the maturation process; thus they are initially capable of only limited phagocytosis. After migrating into the tissues, full maturation occurs; the cells are then referred to as macrophages. Under normal conditions, more than 95% of these cells are mature tissue macrophages, while less than 2% are circulating monocytes. Monocytes represent only 1% to 10% of the circulating WBCs.

Macrophages can survive from several months to several years. They are highly phagocytic and play an important role in the inflammatory, cellular, and humoral responses. Following initial contact with a foreign protein, macrophages process and present antigens to lymphocytes, which in turn stimulate the immune response and cytokine production. Monocytes also produce specific components required for the complement cascade.[75]

*Lymphocytes.* Lymphocytes, the cells responsible for cellular and humoral immunity, provide long-term protection against a variety of microorganisms. They usually constitute 17% to 44% of the total WBC count. B lymphocytes, which are responsible for humoral immunity, produce antibodies that neutralize, destroy, or facilitate phagocytosis of foreign proteins. T lymphocytes, which provide cellular immunity, initiate a variety of activities that directly or indirectly result in elimination of microorganisms or other foreign substances. Cytokines released from T lymphocytes have direct cytotoxic activity and enhance the activity of other differentiated T lymphocytes. T-helper cells are the most numerous of the T-lymphocyte subsets, normally constituting more than 75% of total lymphocyte counts. T-helper cells serve as the principal regulators of immune function through secretion of protein mediators (cytokines) that act on other cells involved in the immune and inflammatory responses. Cytokines produced by T-helper cells include interleukin 2, 3, 4, 5, and 6; gamma interferon; and granulocyte-macrophage colony-stimulating factor (GM-CSF). See Chapter 2 for more detailed discussion of the immune response.

## PATHOPHYSIOLOGY

Once microbes invade the body's tissues, a multifaceted immune reaction occurs that involves changes in normal neurological, cardiovascular, and coagulation pathways. Even nonpathogenic endogenous microbes cause infection when translocated from one area of the body to another. A large percentage of infections in immunocompromised hosts derive from endogenous organisms.[24,31,71] Microbial tissue invasion precipitates a well-documented immunologic pathway involving cytokines and coagulation proteins. This process is a continuum that is replicated in both inflammation and infection leading to sepsis (see Chapter 40 for detailed information).

Infections occur in a defined pattern according to the immune deficit and length of immune compromise.[8,18,26,33,39,71] Bacterial infections are the usual result of granulocyte defects, although fungal infections are common after 7 to 10 days of granulocyte defects. T-cell dysfunction can result in bacterial or fungal infection, but opportunistic and viral infections are more prevalent in cellular immune defects. Infections occurring early in immune compromise are usually bacterial, with common bacteria being the infecting organisms that develop in the first 3 days, and atypical bacteria developing between days 4 and 7. The risk of fungal infection begins between day 7 and 10 after compromise occurs, and viral or opportunistic infections occur after the 10th day of immune compromise.[8]

Infection involving specific sites demonstrates characteristic pathophysiological manifestations and consequences. The most common types of infection in patients with cancer are alimentary tract (bowel, stomach, and oropharynx), blood (bacteremia), indwelling venous catheter-associated infection, pneumonia, skin, and urinary tract infections.[8,26,31,33,44,71–80]

## CLINICAL MANIFESTATIONS

The patient with cancer who is infected may not display the usual signs and symptoms of infection due to the degree of immune compromise and blunting of normal phagocytic and inflammatory responses.[74,80,81] Infection is clinically recognizable by organ-specific signs and symptoms, as well as constitutional symptoms. Multiple systemic symptoms indicate a more severe or extensive infection, with some symptoms being highly characteristic of sepsis or septic shock (Discussed in detail within Chapter 40).

The patient with localized infection will demonstrate evidence of the inflammatory response on an isolated, local level. Pain, erythema, and swelling at the site of infection are usually the first symptoms of an infection. As leukocytes respond to the infection, an exudate may form. The nature of these exudates will depend on the location of infection and on the infecting microbe. Some of these characteristics are defined in Table 28-1.[8,28,29,75–79] If the infection remains confined to the site of origin, symptoms are limited to the local level. Patients with granulocytopenia may show no localized symptoms and infection may be difficult to diagnose until it has become systemic.

When infection becomes systemic, or if a strong inflammatory response is required by the body to counteract the microbes, constitutional symptoms occur. Fever is one of the most well-recognized symptoms of infection.[8,25,81] Patients will experience rigors or shivering as the temperature begins to rise in response to a sudden presence or increase in microbes. This reaction is particularly prevalent in infections where there is periodic "showering" of microorganisms into the bloodstream, such as occurs with catheter-related infection after flushing the catheter, with administration of contaminated blood products, or with subacute bacterial endocarditis. Other systemic symptoms may include influenza-like complaints such as myalgias, arthralgias, headache, fatigue, anorexia, or nausea.[26,37,80] These symptoms are thought to be related to the cytokine response of the body to the presence of foreign microbes.

## ASSESSMENT AND GRADING

### PATIENT AND FAMILY HISTORY

Assessment for potential infection begins with evaluation of the patient's personal and family history of infections or risk factors for development of infection (see Table 28-4).[8,28,44,50,59–81] Familial risks may include inherited disorders involving any organ where immune cells are produced or stored. For example, patients with sickle cell disease experience occlusion of splenic blood-flow with sickled cells, causing auto-destruction and fibrosis of the spleen and a propensity for infection with encapsulated organisms normally detected and destroyed by the spleen.[8,26,28] Family or personal history of infections in common organs often connotes an anatomical abnormality that leads to infection of that part of the body. For example, individuals with urethral strictures or bladder abnormalities may have enhanced bladder retention of urine and will be more likely to have urinary tract infections.[26] Certain clinical diseases also place patients at risk for infection due to their interruption of various immune functions. Other variables increasing the risk of infection involve intrinsic host-related changes in health such as malnutrition or disrupted barrier defenses (eg, venous access devices). Additional factors to be considered in assessing the risk for, or type of, infection would be pets, children, recent travel, and potential airborne or ingested infectious exposures.[8,34,37,82,83] Certain characteristics of some of the risk factors defined in Table 28-4 can be further delineated to more precisely define the degree of risk for infection.[8,28,55,60,63–65,67–70] For instance, when neutropenia lasts longer than 7 days, the risk of infection increases exponentially.[2,18,25] In addition, the risk of infection due to venous access devices can be reduced by inserting cuffed permanent/semipermanent lines, using single-lumen lines, inserting catheters prior to the onset of immune suppression, or having catheters inserted and cared for by a limited number of skilled operators.[62,63,66] The evidence supporting antimicrobial or silver-coated catheters and site dressings, or antibiotic lock solutions have been inconclusive.[61–63,84,85]

Patient interview will also reveal any previous history of infections. Patients will often present repeatedly with infections in the same site or with the same microorganisms. A history of microbial colonization at a site that now presents with symptoms of infection will often be treated with the presumption that colonization has become infection.[8,28,34,37,82,86]

### PHYSICAL EXAMINATION

Physical examination for the signs and symptoms of infection requires a complete head-to-toe assessment for signs or symptoms of inflammation. Erythema, local pain, swelling, and induration may be present at the site of infection.[26,81] If the infection is systemic, the signs of compensatory hyperdynamic cardiovascular effects will be apparent, including tachycardia; warm, flushed, and dry skin; and full-bounding pulses.[28,81] The blood shunting to major organs such as the heart, lungs, and brain may result in decreased bowel sounds or oliguria.[28] Prolonged oliguria is considered a signal of infection that has progressed to sepsis.[28,82] When perfusion becomes more severely compromised, even the heart, lungs, and brain are less than optimally perfused. Altered mental status is considered an ominous sign of impending severe sepsis.[59,81,82,83,87] Breaks in the skin integrity or dark, moist, skin folds are particularly at risk for invasion by microbes. Examination of these sites for unusual skin color, texture, exudate, or lesions may yield evidence of infection. The lungs are the most common site of infection for patients with cancer; thus the nurse will perform assessment of chest excursion, breath sounds, pleural rub, and have knowledge of pulmonary diagnostic tests such as arterial blood gases.[26,44]

Vital signs, particularly the temperature, are monitored frequently. Elevated temperature may be the only sign of infection in a patient who is neutropenic, as the patient may not be able to mount an immune response. Oral temperature monitoring has been considered the most accurate for routine patient assessment.[81] Rectal probes are used infrequently due to potential injury to the rectal mucosa. Other methods of obtaining core body temperature include tympanic, temporal, and bladder thermometers.[88,89] The accuracy of tympanic thermometers is notoriously operator dependent, and bladder thermometers require insertion of a Foley catheter, although newer temporal thermometers are considered as sensitive, accurate, and easy to perform as oral and tympanic temperatures.[89,90] The temperature threshold usually defined as significant for potential infection is 38.3°C (100.9°F) orally once or 38.0°C (100.4°F) sustained for 1 hour.[39,81,83,91,92] This degree of fever is thought to demonstrate a systemic reaction to injury or microbial invasion. Not all patients will display fever, so an increase in baseline temperature of 1°C may be considered a symptom of infection in the presence of risk factors and other clinical findings.[25,81,83] Low temperatures may also occur with infections and are thought to be associated with severe lymphocyte suppression (eg, corticosteroid therapy) or the result of endotoxin release from gram-negative organisms.[8,69,87]

Fever patterns may also vary with different infecting organisms.[41,69,74] Some clinicians have suggested that bacterial infections produce high, spiking fevers with periods of return to normal. Disseminated fungal infections usually produce high, spiking fevers without any such return to a baseline. Viral infections may be characterized by low continuous fevers. Subnormal temperatures in the absence of other causes such as hypothyroidism, hypoadrenalism, anemia, or hepatic dysfunction have been linked to a greater risk for gram-negative infection.[8,41,69,74]

Most patients who have infection are tachycardic and tachypneic, except when the infection is so severe as to cause prolonged acidosis.[80] In early infection, these changes reflect compensatory increases in cardiac output and oxygen delivery. As perfusion continues to be compromised, tachypnea occurs as the body attempts to expire acid as carbon dioxide. In more severe acidosis, the heart rate decreases and heart block may occur, and respiratory efforts tire, leading eventually to a respiratory arrest.[82,87] When patients are febrile, their diastolic blood pressure also drops, causing lower mean (average) pressures. This vasodilation will first present as orthostasis, followed by systolic hypotension.[69,74]

## DIAGNOSTIC STUDIES

The gold standard for diagnosis of infection is quantitative cultures obtained from the involved body organ. These results are not usually available for 24 to 72 hours, but there are some newer rapid nucleic acid based technologies such as PCR tests for pneumocystis, leukocyte esterase for urine culture, or BAcT/ALERT for bacterial cultures that may yield more rapid results.[93–96] Performing routine surveillance cultures, including those of blood, urine, and skin surfaces is believed to potentially provide evidence of microbial infection prior to symptoms. While this practice is not routine, and there are no clear recommendations of sources or frequency, this practice remains common, particularly with patients having hematologic malignancy.[8,97] Bloodstream infections are common in patients with hematologic malignancy and the practice of paired blood cultures from venipuncture and central venous access are used without a strong evidence base to differentiate central line infection from other bacteremias.[97–99] One small study showed early detection of bacteremia in 43% of patients, showing 89% sensitivity for the central line as the source, permitting modification of clinical management prior to severe symptom onset.[97] Screening tests may be used to evaluate the probability of infection while awaiting culture results.[100] While the most common and useful test is the complete blood count, other laboratory tests that will assist in the differential diagnosis include serum chemistry (inclusive of electrolytes, creatinine, and blood urea nitrogen), bilirubin levels, hepatic transaminases, lactate (lactic acid), lactate dehydrogenase (LDH), *Legionella* antigen assay, and a galactomannin assay.[25,26,37,81,83] Some pathogens present with characteristic serum markers or antigen expression such as LDH elevations with *Pneumocystis jerivichi* or *Legionella* antigenemia *legionellosis*.[8,65,69,74] Galactomannin assays and beta-D-glucan levels are used to detect possible invasive aspergillosis.[95,100,101] Clinical markers for sepsis such as C-reactive protein and procalcitonin have been used in critically ill patients but not validated in patients with cancer.[102,103]

The complete blood count with the total WBC count and differential is the first diagnostic test used to screen for infection. White blood cells are elevated in the presence of infection. The normal WBC count is 5000 to 10,000/mm$^3$. In patients with normal immune reactions, infection causes mild to moderate elevations of 10,000 to 20,000/mm$^3$.[8,69,104,105] The extent of WBC elevation can vary depending on the specific microbe involved, severity of infection, organs involved, and the host's immune competence. Extremely high WBC counts are associated with meningitis and necrotizing organisms, or are found in children.[104,105] White blood cell counts higher than 30,000/mm$^3$ are less likely to be related to infection; and lymphoproliferative disorders are considered as part of the differential diagnosis.[69]

The WBC differential is interpreted by assessing the specific percentage of each of the major categories of WBCs: granulocytes (neutrophils, eosinophils, and basophils), monocytes, and lymphocytes. Granulocytes (inclusive of neutrophils, eosinophils, and basophils) normally account for 35% to 76% of the total WBC count, monocytes are 1% to 9%, and lymphocytes represent 17% to 44%. The only cell that will be released from the bone marrow in an immature form is the granulocyte. Granulocytes are elevated with bacterial infection or with inflammatory conditions, but immature cells are noted in the circulating serum only if infection is present. This situation is dubbed a "left shift" in the differential because there are increased numbers of immature cells.[69,104] The term "left shift" is derived from the tradition of diagramming cells on a horizontal line with immature cells on the far left and completely mature cells on the far right. Monocytes normally differentiate into tissue macrophages and are seldom present in the serum. If excessive numbers are present, then an unusual viral or opportunistic infection is most likely to blame. Lymphocytes are elevated when the body reacts to foreign antigenic agents or tissue. Elevated lymphocytes usually indicate viral infection, allergy, or rejection of transplanted tissue. Used in conjunction with risk assessment and clinical findings, the WBC count and differential can be a valuable tool in evaluating the probability of a serious infection requiring interventions such as hospitalization or intravenous antimicrobials.

Other laboratory tests that predict the risk for infection include the absolute neutrophil count (ANC), absolute lymphocyte count (ALC), and immunoglobulin levels. Recognition of low levels of these essential immune components can allow for proactive prevention of infection. An ANC of less than 2000/mm$^3$ is defined as a grade 1 neutropenia, according to the Cancer Therapy Evaluation Program. Grade 2 neutropenia is an ANC of 1000 to 1500/mm$^3$. Grade 3 neutropenia is an ANC of 500 to 1000/mm$^3$, and grade 4 toxicity is less than 500/mm$^3$.[105] The lower the neutrophil count, the greater the risk for bacterial infection. When neutrophil levels are suppressed for more than 7 days, the risk for infection increases and the scope of possible infecting organisms broadens to include atypical bacteria, fungi, viruses, and opportunistic organisms.[34,37,83] Patients are also at greater risk for infection with resistant microbes. A low ALC is common with HIV infection, although it may also occur in transplant patients or those on long-term corticosteroids. When the ALC is less than 200/mm$^3$, the patient is at risk for fungal or opportunistic organisms such as *Pneumocystis jerivichi and aspergillus*; when the ALC is less than 100/mm$^3$, infection with organisms such as *toxoplasmosis gondii* may also occur.[60,105] Immunoglobulin levels less than 300 mg/dL predispose the patient to sinus and pulmonary infections.[69] Immunoglobulin infusions are administered daily for 3 days to compensate for low immunoglobulin levels.

Radiologic tests may also be performed to screen for pockets of infection such as pneumonia or abscesses.[25] The computed tomography (CT) scan often provides useful information to aid in diagnosis of infection in most areas of the body. Some locations that are prone to motion or are dense with close organs are the abdomen and pelvis; ultrasound may be used for diagnosis of infections in these areas.[26,74] Changes in neurological tissue and joints are sensitive to magnetic resonance imaging (MRI), so MRI may be used to diagnose infections in these organs. Gallium scans have also been used for diagnosis of *Pneumocystis jerivichi*.[69]

Definitive diagnosis of infection is determined by culture for microbes. The organisms for culture will always include aerobic and anaerobic bacteria, but when infection risk has extended beyond 3 to 5 days, cultures may also include assessment for fungi, viruses, or opportunistic organisms. The technique used when obtaining culture specimens is important for attaining valid and reliable results.[26,34,37,69,83] Inadequate specimens can result in false-negative cultures. Contaminants in the culture media from lack of sterile technique can lead to false-positive cultures, although contamination is often suspected because the bacteria cultured may not be multiplying as usually seen with actual infection, and contaminants are slower to become positive.[100] Techniques for obtaining culture specimens are outlined in Table 28-5.[25,46,53,93–101,106–108] Immunocompromised patients are at high risk for polymicrobial infections and have breached mucosal barriers, necessitating a strong commitment to obtain both aerobic and anaerobic cultures.[109] Special resin-containing culture media are suggested to replace aerobic media when the patient is already receiving antimicrobial therapy.[106,110] The prevalence of infection with gram-positive organisms (approximately 75% of all infections) has led many clinicians to simultaneously obtain culture specimens for Gram stain testing.[25,26,80,111,112] Gram-positive organisms stain darkly when covered with Gram stain. After cultures are determined to be positive for the presence of a microbe, they are evaluated for sensitivity to various antimicrobial agents, a process known as "sensitivity testing." The selection of agents tested for sensitivity is based on the usual ability of those agents to destroy the microbe. Sensitivity testing reveals resistant microbial strains and permits clinicians to continually monitor the ability of common antimicrobial agents to destroy various microorganisms in their clinical region. The agent with the narrowest spectrum of activity, but with effective destruction of the infecting microbe, is chosen for treatment of the infection. This strategy limits development of antimicrobial resistance.[113]

**TABLE 28-5**

**Types of Cultures and Recommended Techniques**

| Type of Culture | Technique for Obtaining | Special Considerations/Comments |
|---|---|---|
| Blood culture, invasive line | • Assemble supplies for sterile blood drawing procedure: mask, sterile gloves, drape, hub and culture bottle disinfectant, and culture media (1 aerobic, 1 anaerobic, possibly 1 viral medium).<br>• Prepare tops of culture media bottles by thoroughly cleansing with alcohol and leaving alcohol swab on top of bottle until ready to access.<br>• Don mask, lay barrier, and don sterile gloves.<br>• Using sterile gloves, cleanse catheter connection site thoroughly with alcohol and allow to dry.<br>• Using sterile gloves, disconnect the line and cover with a sterile cap.<br>• Directly access the catheter when obtaining blood cultures.<br>• Connect blood drawing equipment (follow institutional policy for drawing a discard or not).<br>• Draw at least 5 mL for each culture bottle.<br>• Some research suggests that indwelling lines have contaminants that provide false-positive cultures. | • Some institutions recommend no blood withdrawal prior to the blood for culture; others require a waste withdrawal equivalent to at least 1.5 times the catheter volume.<br>• Some institutions suggest obtaining cultures from each line or lumen during the first fever work-up, especially if the line has been in place 7 days or longer.<br>• When using transfer devices for injecting blood into culture media, make sure the end of the syringe where air may be present is used in the aerobic bottle.<br>• If there is inadequate blood for both aerobic and anaerobic culture, blood is usually submitted for aerobic culture unless otherwise directed by the prescriber. This practice is less validated in severely immunocompromised hosts (T-cell suppression, prolonged and severe neutropenia) where gram-negative infections may have greater risk for negative outcomes.<br>• Special media may be used to enhance culture yield for mycology or viruses.<br>• Concerns about line contaminants affecting blood cultures have not been incorporated into national guidelines. |
| Blood culture, peripheral | • Assemble supplies for sterile blood drawing procedure: mask, sterile gloves, drape, skin disinfectant (chlorhexidine), culture bottle disinfectant (alcohol), and culture media (1 aerobic, 1 anaerobic, possibly 1 viral medium).<br>• Prepare tops of culture media bottles by thoroughly cleansing with alcohol and leaving alcohol swab on top of bottle until ready to access.<br>• Don mask, lay barrier, and don sterile gloves.<br>• Using sterile gloves, cleanse skin site thoroughly with chlorhexidine and allow to dry.<br>• Using sterile gloves, prepare the needle with adapter for culture bottles.<br>• Connect blood drawing equipment.<br>• Draw at least 5 mL for each culture bottle. | • Cultures should be drawn no closer than 10 minutes, and no further apart than 20 to 30 minutes.<br>• If there is inadequate blood for both aerobic and anaerobic culture, blood is usually submitted for aerobic culture unless otherwise directed by the prescriber. This practice is less validated in severely immunocompromised hosts (T-cell suppression, prolonged and severe neutropenia) where gram-negative infections may have greater risk for negative outcomes.<br>• Special media may be used to enhance culture yield for mycology or viruses. |

(Continued)

**TABLE 28-5**

**Types of Cultures and Recommended Techniques** *(Continued)*

| Type of Culture | Technique for Obtaining | Special Considerations/Comments |
|---|---|---|
| Drainage from a tube/drain (eg, biliary stent, chest tube) | • Assemble supplies for sterile blood drawing procedure: mask, sterile gloves, drape, connection hub or access port, culture bottle disinfectant, and culture media (1 aerobic, 1 anaerobic, possibly 1 viral medium).<br>• Prepare tops of culture media bottles by thoroughly cleansing with alcohol and leaving alcohol swab on top of bottle until ready to access.<br>• Don mask, lay barrier, and don sterile gloves. Using sterile gloves, cleanse connection/hub site thoroughly with alcohol and allow to dry.<br>• Using sterile gloves, disconnect the tubing and cover with a sterile cap. | • Drainage should be removed from the cleanest tubing possible. At times, it may be advisable to change to new sterile drainage tubing prior to obtaining the culture specimen. |
| Nasopharyngeal cultures | • For bacteria: Use a dry swab for each nostril and insert gently until resistance is met. Turn the swab in a complete circle and remove.<br>• For virus: With the patient leaning his or her head back slightly, instill 3 to 5 mL of preservative-free sterile water into first nostril, then have the patient lean forward and blow the nose into a sterile specimen cup without having the secretions touch the face. Repeat the procedure on the other side if the patient can tolerate it. | • Cultures for bacteria have a greater yield with simple swabbing. Upper respiratory viruses are notoriously difficult to obtain valid positive cultures. False-negative results are common. |
| Sputum culture | • Common bacterial sputum cultures require patients to attempt to cough into a sterile specimen cup, attempting not to let the sputum touch their tongue. Some institutions suggest tooth and tongue brushing prior to obtaining a specimen.<br>• Suctioned sputum culture: Using a new sterile suction catheter, the catheter is passed into the nasopharynx and can be used to obtain a specimen for culture.<br>• Induced sputum technique requires a saline neubulizer treatment followed by immediate expectoration. First morning expectoration specimens are also thought to provide best yield. | • Culture for specific organisms may require an early morning specimen to ensure a specimen from deep in the lungs and with best organism yield (eg, *Pneumocystis carinii*).<br>• Bronchodilator therapy prior to obtaining the specimen may enhance the sputum yield.<br>• A light water-soluble lubricant may be used if absolutely necessary.<br>• If there is limited sputum and it is stuck inside the suction catheter, a small amount of preservative-free sterile water can be drawn up from a sterile cup to wash the sputum from the tubing. |
| Stool culture | • Assemble sterile specimen cup, sterile gloves, and cleansing wipes.<br>• Have the patient defecate into a clean bedpan or bedside commode/toilet receptacle.<br>• Wearing clean gloves, use a wooden spatula (eg, tongue blade) to remove specimen, attempting to not touch the receptacle or to use stool that was directly touching the receptacle.<br>• Place specimen in a sterile specimen cup. | • Minimum volume is 1 ounce or approximately 1 inch. |
| Throat culture | • For bacteria: Using a dry culture swab, swipe one side across the distal pharynx on side; turn the swab over and swab the other side of the distal pharynx. | • Best yield is for bacterial infections. |

| | | |
|---|---|---|
| Urine culture | • Assemble sterile specimen cup, sterile gloves, and cleansing wipes.<br>• Cleanse the perineal area and allow to dry.<br>• Ask patient to urinate into the sterile cup (approximately 5 to 15 mL is sufficient volume).<br>• Cover quickly with the sterile cap.<br>• Obtaining a culture from a Foley catheter:<br>Don sterile gloves, and lay a sterile barrier while draining old urine down tubing.<br>Cleanse the access area with alcohol and allow to dry, with catheter access site in a level position to allow pooling of fresh urine in tubing loop.<br>Obtain needle access to the specimen port and remove 5 to 15 mL of urine.<br>Transfer urine to sterile specimen cup. | • Clean-catch midstream urine specimens for culture have not been determined to be more "sterile" than a normal urine specimen. |
| Wound culture | • If the wound is obviously dirty or contaminated, rinse it with sterile saline and pat dry prior to performing a culture.<br>• Assemble gloves, sterile drape, culture swabs, and culture media.<br>• Don sterile gloves and uncap appropriate culture swab (calcium alginate or rayon swab—*not* cotton swab).<br>• Swab with the sterile applicator in a rotary and clockwise fashion.<br>• For ulcer: Scrape into the deepest section of the wound, but do *not* culture pus, exudates, or hard eschar. | • Ensure that the wound is clean of dirt or debris that may produce false-positive culture results.<br>• Cotton swabs may leave fine fibers in the wound and worsen infection.<br>• Wide wounds may alternatively be brushed side-to-side in a Z pattern<br>• Minimum specimen is 0.25 mL. |

*Note*: Normal infection control guidelines (eg, hand washing before and after each procedure) are assumed and not defined in this table.
*Source*: Data from Schaffer et al[52]; Mayhill[53]; Bell et al[106]; Elsayed et al[107]; and Lifshitz et al.[108]

## THERAPEUTIC APPROACHES AND NURSING CARE

### PREVENTION

The most important objective in management of risk factors for infection is prevention of infection. Infection can be prevented by control of environmental exposures to microorganisms, modification of patient care routines, and primary prophylactic measures such as growth factor or antimicrobial administration.[34,113]

#### *Environmental* control

The Centers for Disease Control and Prevention (CDC) offers guidelines for construction, air handling, and water sanitation in the management of immunocompromised patients.[114–117] Construction barriers and alternative transportation routes must be provided to protect immunocompromised patients from microbes such as *Aspergillus* or *Coccidioides* that become airborne when the ground is disturbed or walls and ceilings are removed.[114] High-efficiency particulate air handling (HEPA) systems are required in the care of blood and marrow transplant patients and have proved useful in preventing fungal and opportunistic airborne infections.[34,37,83,117] All immunocompromised patients are advised to use water and ice from reliably clean sources and opt for bottled or sterile water for drinking or rinsing feeding tubes if water cleanliness cannot be verified (eg, well water).[37,117] Hospitals following the CDC guidelines for prevention of infection in immunocompromised patients have water sanitation and intermittent monitoring plans in place to assess and treat *Legionella* and *Pseudomonas* in their water systems.[117]

Although CDC guidelines do not recommend any kind of "protective" or "strict" isolation for prevention of infection, many institutions require additional protective mechanisms when caring for immunocompromised patients.[25,37,80,118,119] The CDC has carefully reviewed the scientific evidence and does not recommend barrier protection, but does emphasize that hand washing remains the single most significant measure for preventing infection.[25,34,37,83,120,121] Institutional practices vary from no special precautions, to masks only during influenza season, to full isolation barrier protection for all patient contact. At a minimum, whenever possible, immunocompromised patients should be placed in private rooms when hospitalized.[34,37,122] If this is not feasible, cohorting of immunocompromised patients is recommended.[25,34,37,80,120] Screening visitors for infection exposure or limiting children visitation may be other strategies for controlling environmental risks for infection.[25,34,37,83,117,120]

Fastidious cleaning routines for all aspects of the environment are important for prevention of infection. Regular floor cleaning, curtain cleaning, and bathroom sanitation support prevention of infection in these patients. Environmental precautions may also prohibit fresh flowers and plants.[34,37,80,83,117,121]

#### Patient care routines

Whether the granulocytes or the lymphocytes are affected, risk for infection is increased in relation to the degree of immune compromise. Patients are advised to maintain vigilant personal hygiene and to avoid exposure to people or places where communicable diseases are a prevalent issue.[34,37,83,112,121] If they have pets, patients should maintain the animals' vaccinations, cleanse them frequently, and wash after handling the animals.[34,37,83,112] When possible, patients should refrain from cleaning up their excrement.[37,83,112] If patients like to garden, they should wear good garden gloves, cover their body, and wash thoroughly after each session.[37,83,112] Patients at risk for oral mucositis should perform frequent and thorough oral care with tooth brushing and flossing to maintain optimal oral health and minimize oral microbes that can translocate through mucosal lesions or migrate into the upper respiratory tract.[34,64,121]

Particularly in the hospital, single-use and disposable items will reduce the risk of transferring infection from patient to patient.[112] Staff must be careful to follow additional precautions such as making sure their stethoscopes are cleaned between patients, and wearing cover gowns if carrying soiled linens to a hamper far away from the patient's room. Supplies should be carefully covered to prevent dust and environmental contaminants. Universal precautions are conscientiously maintained for all care delivery.

Requiring that patients eat a "low-microbial diet" has been a long-time theoretical protection to guard against infection. This diet does not permit fresh fruits, fresh vegetables, or food items such as nuts or bleu cheese. Cooked foods are permitted and assumed to protect the patient against foodborne organisms. This diet has inspired much controversy and little evidence supports its use.[37,83,112,117,121,123–127] In addition, these diets are inconsistent in their directions regarding more realistic risks such as consumption of mayonnaise that may be contaminated with *Salmonella*. General healthy eating instructions for patients should be discussed. Patients should be instructed to cook all meats thoroughly, avoid serving meat on platters where raw meat was prepared, avoid any products with eggs unless known prompt refrigeration was employed, and avoid eating any foods stored for more than 48 to 72 hours.[37,112]

#### Primary prophylaxis against infection

Primary prophylaxis involves the administration of agents in an attempt to prevent a complication of infection prior to the onset of risk. Recognition of patients at high risk for infection prior to immune suppression permits implementation of strategies to alter the course of immune suppression so as to prevent infection. Some researchers have retrospectively and prospectively studied factors that increase the risk of infection during periods of neutropenia. Three primary populations that have been studied based on the perceived high risk-benefit relationship are non-Hodgkin's lymphoma, adjuvant breast cancer, and the elderly. Risk profiles for infectious complications during neutropenia, defined by authors as models have been outlined for these populations. The presence of high-risk variables would provide data to determine best candidates for first cycle neutropenia prophylaxis with prophylactic antibiotic or growth factors. The Multinational Association for Supportive Care in Cancer (MASCC) have defined a general scoring system to identify the level of risk for serious consequences of neutropenic fever.[21] This scoring system has gained popularity due to its universality and reliability for predicting low-risk febrile patients that may have their febrile neutropenia managed as outpatients. The use of some system for assessing neutropenia risk prior to commencing chemotherapy is recommended and has been shown to reduce the incidence of hospitalization for febrile neutropenia.[128–130] The variables that increase the risk of infection during periods of neutropenia or T-cell suppressions are summarized in Table 28-6.[18,21,25,34,37,131–141]

Administration of prophylactic antimicrobial agents or growth factors prior to the onset of immune suppression are common strategies used to prevent infections in patients perceived as being at high risk for infection, particularly antineoplastic therapy-induced neutropenia.[8,12,24,54,60,142] In 3 systematic reviews of both strategies, neither intervention was deemed superior to the other.[142–145]

Antimicrobial prophylaxis is viewed as appropriate in patients with HIV infection,[142] with prolonged neutropenia, after organ or blood cell transplant,[117] with rheumatic heart disease,[8] or as a surgical adjunct in specific procedures.[25,26,34,36,37] The process of prescribing antimicrobial agents prior to chemotherapy, prior to blood cell transplant, and after severe lymphocyte depletion with HIV disease or corticosteroid administration has evolved as the natural history of infections with these disorders has become better defined. Prophylactic antimicrobial therapy is reserved for situations in which there is a high risk for infections and their associated morbidity or mortality.[8] Agents chosen as prophylactic medications should provide adequate microbial coverage with limited resistance.[25,145] Prophylaxis with antimicrobials are begun prior to the onset of immune compromise and continued until recovery. Each prophylactic strategy is targeting a specific pathogen in the susceptible population based upon their risk to develop infections with those microbes. It is common in hematologic malignancies where patients experience prolonged neutropenia to prophylaxis against gram-negative and fungal organisms.[146] Allogeneic hematopoietic stem cell transplant (HSCT) patients with lymphocyte suppression receive antibacterial, antifungal, antipneumocystis, and antiviral prophylaxis. Patients with HIV disease or receiving long-term corticosteroids will also receive antimicrobial prophylaxis based upon their ALC. In one systematic review, there was a trend toward improved outcomes in patients with hematologic malignancy or undergoing HSCT when antifungal prophylaxis is prescribed throughout the neutropenic period.[147] An overview of common antimicrobial prophylaxis regimens appears in Table 28-7.[25,29,46,49,60,117,142–145,148–153]

Hematopoietic growth factors promote the differentiation, maturation, and proliferation of hematopoietic cells within the bone marrow. These agents are used to shorten and reduce the severity of neutropenia after chemotherapy and after blood and marrow stem cell transplants.[25,31,71,112,131,142] They may also be used as priming agents prior to pheresis of hematopoietic stem cells. Specific growth factors are used to enhance growth of specific cell lines: erythropoietin for erythrocytes, and granulocyte colony-stimulating factor for granulocytes. Initially, growth factors were primarily used reactively after chemotherapy when a patient demonstrated a post-therapy febrile neutropenic event, but no clear benefit was realized in this situation. One study utilizing this strategy showed that if hematopoietic growth factors are prescribed as secondary prophylaxis (after onset of neutropenia or postchemotherapy fever), they are less cost-effective than antibiotics.[154] This practice has evolved since some of the studies used to develop risk models, and the most recent clinical guidelines suggest that it is cost-effective and clinically prudent to administer growth factors with the first cycle of therapy when the planned antineoplastic therapy is likely to produce significant neutropenia in at least 20% of patients receiving that regimen.[7,25,155,156] They may also be indicated in more moderately myelosuppressive regimens when therapy is deemed potentially curative or the dose intensity clearly influences outcomes.[8,34,37,155,156] Growth factors optimally minimize the depth and length of aplasia when administered 24 to 72 hours after the last dose of chemotherapy, although some studies of administration on the same day as chemotherapy have not shown harm and may ease patient burden.[157–161] Initial concerns and label indications prescribe that hematopoietic growth factors should not be administered to patients with myeloid malignancies due to a hypothetical risk of accelerating malignant granulocyte proliferation, but recent studies do not confirm this possibility.[162,163] Specific guidelines for administration of these agents are provided in Chapter 23.

## MANAGEMENT

The mainstay of infection management is administration of antimicrobial agents. Neutropenia or T-lymphocytic suppression increases the risk for more frequent and severe infections, so these conditions are treated aggressively. At the onset of fever in high-risk patients, aggressive treatment is implemented immediately to prevent sepsis and shock,

**TABLE 28-6**

**Models for Assessing Risk for Infection and Recommended Actions for Specific Populations**

| Patient Population | Increased Risks for Infection | Clinical Applications |
|---|---|---|
| Breast cancer, adjuvant therapy, traditional | • First-cycle ANC after treatment without prophylaxis is grade 4 toxicity level<br>• First-cycle Hgb after treatment without prophylaxis is grade 4 toxicity level<br>• Concurrent chemotherapy and radiation<br>• Previous radiation | • Growth factor prophylaxis after first-cycle assessment in patients receiving adjuvant chemotherapy |
| Elderly patients | • Age > 70 years<br>• Chemotherapy regimen with toxicity similar to CHOP chemotherapy | • Primary prophylaxis with growth factors and/or prophylactic antimicrobials in treatment regimens equivalent to CHOP chemotherapy |
| Indwelling intravenous catheters | • Large lumen<br>• Multilumen<br>• Percutaneous (not cuffed) line<br>• Line placed after the onset of immune compromise<br>• Previously infected catheter | • Choice of catheter<br>• Timing of catheter placement<br>• Catheter maintenance routine |
| Non-Hodgkin's lymphoma | • Bone marrow involvement with lymphoma<br>• Low albumin prior to chemotherapy<br>• LDH > 600 units prior to chemotherapy<br>• Poor performance status<br>• Late stage of disease | • Evaluate complete chemistry panel at the onset of chemotherapy<br>• Primary prophylaxis for selected patients |
| MASCC score index. MASCC risks for febrile neutropenia | • Severe symptoms related to infection<br>• Hypotension<br>• Presence of chronic obstructive pulmonary disease<br>• Hematologic malignancy<br>• Previous fungal infection<br>• Presenting with dehydration<br>• Inpatient at time of symptom onset<br>• Age greater than 60 years | • Using the MASCC score at the time of presentation with infectious symptoms allows for creation of a risk score. Each of the variables are phrased in a low-risk manner and have an assigned weight, although all are not equal. A maximum low-risk score is 26 points. Anyone with a score > 21 is termed low-risk for severe infectious complications. These low-risk patients are considered candidates for outpatient antimicrobial therapy or early conversion from intravenous to oral therapy with early hospital discharge. |
| Pediatric risk factors for severe sepsis | • Age ≤ 12 years<br>• Admission with infectious symptoms.<br>• C-reactive protein > 90 mg/L<br>• Admission with infectious symptoms.<br>• IL-8 ≥ 200 pg/mL<br>• 24 hour IL-8 ≥ 300 pg/mL<br>• Prolonged neutropenia (ANC < 500/mm$^3$) | • Authors suggest more routine proactive assessment of risk factors and biomarkers to detect children who are at higher risk for more severe sepsis at the onset of fever. |
| All patients with cancer to be assessed for high risk for infection prior to initiation of treatment | • Acute leukemia or allogeneic HSCT<br>• Graft vs host disease on corticosteroid receiving immunosuppressive therapy<br>• Severe neutropenia < 500/mm$^3$<br>• Prolonged neutropenia > 10 days<br>• Alemtuzumab therapy<br>• Open wounds<br>• Chronic obstructive pulmonary disease | • Risk factors are assessed prior to antineoplastic treatment and prophylactic antimicrobials or hematopoietic growth factors are initiated as indicated in those at high risk for infection. |

*Abbreviations*: ANC, absolute neutrophil count; CHOP, cyclophosphamide, doxorubicin (Adriamycin), vincristine (Oncovin), prednisone; Hgb, hemoglobin; HSCT, hematopoietic stem cell transplant; IL, interleukin; LDH, lactate dehydrogenase; MASCC, Multinational Association for Supportive Care in Cancer.

*Source*: Data from Balducci et al[131]; Balducci et al[132]; Blay et al[133]; Chang et al[134]; Garcia-Suarez et al[135]; Intraguntomchai et al[136]; Lyman[137]; Lyman et al[138]; Silber et al[139]; Silber et al[140]; and Paesmans.[142]

**TABLE 28-7**

**Antimicrobial Prophylaxis Management for Immunocompromised Patients**

| Patient Population | Specific Criteria | Organisms Likely to Lead to Infection | Suggested Antimicrobial Agents |
|---|---|---|---|
| HIV infection | All patients | Pneumococcus | Pneumovax |
| | | Influenza | Influenza vaccine—must be attenuated or dead organisms, or Amantadine |
| | | Hepatitis B | Recombivax HB or Energix B |
| | CD4 count < 200/mm$^3$ | *Pneumocystis carinii* | TMP-SMX or dapsone preferred, pyrimethamine |
| | CD4 count < 100/mm$^3$ | *Toxoplasma gondi* | TMP-SMX or dapsone, pyrimethamine |
| | | *Histoplasma*[a] | Itraconazole |
| | CD4 count < 50/mm$^3$ | *Mycobacteria avium* complex | Clarithromycin or azithromycin |
| | | *Candida*[a] | Fluconazole |
| | | *Cryptococcus*[a] | Fluconazole or itraconazole |
| | | *Coccidiomycosis*[a] | Fluconazole or itraconazole |
| | | Cytomegalovirus[a] | Ganciclovir |
| | | *Varicella*[a] | Varicella IVIG or acyclovir |
| | Positive PPD or prior positive PPD | *M. tuberculosis* | INH and pyridoxine or pyridoxine alone |
| Neutropenia | ANC < 500/mm$^3$, expected to last > 7 days | *Candida* | Fluconazole, although some alternate with itraconazole |
| | | Gram-negative bacteria | Norfloxacin or other fluoroquinolone |
| | | *C. difficile*[a] | Oral metronidazole (Flagyl) or vancomycin |
| | ANC < 500/mm$^3$ for shorter period of time but with other risk factors for infection (eg, older age, chronic lung disease) | Gram-negative and gram-positive bacteria | Norfloxacin or other fluoroquinolone |
| | Neutropenia as above and a central venous access device | Staphylococcus[b] | Broad-spectrum cephalosporin or penicillin |
| Blood and marrow transplant | All patients | Pneumococcus | Pneumovax |
| | | Influenza | Influenza vaccine—must be attenuated or dead organisms, or Amantadine |
| | | Hepatitis B | Recombivax HB or Energix B |
| | Allogeneic HSCT | *Candida*[b] | Fluconazole or itraconazole |
| | | Gram-negative organisms[b] | Norfloxacin or other fluoroquinolone |
| | Allogeneic HSCT with prior herpes simplex and (HSV+) | Herpes simplex | Acyclovir |
| | Recipients of CMV-positive graft with CMV-negative status | CMV | Acyclovir or ganciclovir with CMV immunoglobulin |

*Notes*: [a]Prophylaxis against these microbes is implemented only in the setting of significant risk and exposure; it is not implemented at all for individuals with normal immune systems.

[b]Depends on the depth and anticipated length of aplasia.

All patients with malignancy should receive influenza vaccine when possible, provided they are not neutropenic.

All patients with malignancy who are > 5 years of age, immunoglobulin deficiency, or splenic deficiency should receive pneumovax at a time when they are not neutropenic.

*Abbreviations*: ANC, absolute neutrophil count; CMV, cytomegalovirus; HIV, human immunodeficiency virus; HSCT, hematopoeitic stem cell transplant; INH, isonicotinyl hydrazine; IVIG, intravenous immune globulin; PPD, purified protein derivative; TMP-SMX, trimethoprim/sulfamethoxazole.

*Source*: Data from Shelton et al,[29] Hughes et al,[49] Bartlett et al,[60] Sullivan et al,[117]; Ellis,[149] Green et al,[150] and Furrer et al.[151]

**TABLE 28-8**

**Commonly Used Antibiotics**

| Antibiotic | Coverage | Nursing Implications |
|---|---|---|
| Aminoglycosides<br>Gentamycin<br>Amikacin<br>Tobramycin<br>Kanamycin | Most gram-negative enterobacteria (*Serratia, Proteus, Klebsiella, E. coli*), *Pseudomonas, Erwinia* | • Dose reduced in renal failure: excess serum levels are renal toxic.<br>• Long-term use causes partially reversible vestibular and auditory damage. Administering the dose more slowly may reduce incidence. Assist in hearing evaluation after course of therapy.<br>• Administered once to twice daily to decrease renal toxicity. Slower administration may reduce toxicity and does not alter antimicrobial effects, as the aminoglycoside destroys bacteria by entering the cell and killing from inside.<br>• Apply antihistamine or steroid creams if needed for rash.<br>• Alters platelet function and may enhance bleeding tendency. Avoid other anticoagulant or antiplatelet medications, such as aspirin or nonsteroidal anti-inflammatory agents.<br>• Serum blood levels are monitored for the presence of medication prior to and after a dose. These medications' toxicity is determined by persistent and high blood levels. Based on the presence of medication just before a dose is due, the dosage or frequency may be decreased. |
| Penicillins<br>Penicillin G<br>Penicillin V<br>Ampicillin<br>Amoxicillin<br>Ticarcillin<br>Pipercillin<br>Carbenicillin<br>Ticarcillin clavulanate<br>Amoxicillin clavulanate | *Actinomyces, Clostridium,* meningococcemia, *Proteus* (ampicillin), *Salmonella, Streptococcus, Staphylococcus* (second line)<br>Broader spectrum against pseudomonas | • Frequent dosing to achieve steady-state blood level.<br>• Peak-and-trough levels measured to assess whether the MIC is achieved. The MIC is the serum blood level at which specific microbes are sensitive to death for the circulating drug.<br>• Administer as rapidly as ordered to achieve a good peak blood level.<br>• Idiosyncratic glomerulonephritis may occur due to glomerular basement membrane damage.<br>• Administer antihistamine or steroid creams for itchy rash as needed (especially with ampicillin and amoxicillin).<br>• Persistent, unexplained fever may be a manifestation of hypersensitivity. Antipyretics are only partially helpful in abrogating this effect.<br>• Some hypersensitivity reactions are anaphylactoid and require emergency respiratory support, including epinephrine. The reaction does not involve the IgE antibody and, therefore, is not predictable in incidence or severity.<br>• Administer antidiarrheals as needed (especially with ampicillin).<br>• Administer with food and avoid concomitant caffeine to reduce drug-induced nausea.<br>• Alters platelet function and may enhance bleeding tendency (especially with carbenicillin and ticarcillin). Avoid other anticoagulant or antiplatelet medications such as aspirin or nonsteroidal anti-inflammatory agents.<br>• Administer potassium supplements, because most agents enhance renal excretion of potassium and cause hypokalemia.<br>• The addition of clavulanate to penicillins broadens their spectrum and provides better coverage against pseudomonas and atypical microbes. |
| **Carbapenams**<br>Imipenem cilastin<br>Meropenam | Respiratory, skin/structure, gynecological infections that are gram-positive and gram-negative | • Do not give carbenicillin or probenecid, as they interfere with absorption.<br>• May increase hepatic transaminase levels.<br>• May lower blood counts.<br>• Avoid mixing with aminoglycosides, which may be physically incompatible.<br>• The drugs are dialyzable, so administer them after dialysis treatment.<br>• The most common CNS toxicities are a lowered seizure threshold, dizziness, and confusion.<br>• Irritating to veins—give low doses over approximately 30 minutes, higher doses over 1 hour.<br>• Neuromuscular twitching may occur (especially with imipenam), and the seizure threshold may be lowered in patients with preexisting seizures. Assess for resting tremors and seizure activity. Place on seizure precautions. |

| | | |
|---|---|---|
| **Quinolones**<br>Norfloxacin<br>Ciprofloxicin<br>Ofloxacin | Resistant enterobacteria | • Administer with food and avoid concomitant caffeine to reduce drug-induced tendency to cause gastric upset.<br>• Administer acetaminophen as needed for headache.<br>• Avoid concomitant nonsteroidal anti-inflammatory agents that enhance the potential bleeding tendency.<br>• Implement safety precautions for potential dizziness or visual disturbances (blurred, diplopia).<br>• Provide an environment conducive to sleep.<br>• Perform care in increments, providing frequent rest periods due to drug-induced fatigue and malaise.<br>• Assess for depressive tendency that may be worsened by drug-related fatigue and malaise.<br>• Monitor hepatic transaminases for elevations indicating drug toxicity, or an increased risk of worsening of transaminase elevations while receiving this agent.<br>• High bioavailablity, well absorbed orally<br>• Advise patients to wear sunscreen and be aware of photosensitivity<br>• Counsel patients to contact their provider for careful monitoring if taking warfarin<br>• Monitor renal function and consider dose modification with renal impairment |
| **Other Gram-Positive Coverage**<br>Nafcillin<br>Oxacillin<br>Vancomycin | Staphylococcus, *Clostridium difficile*, *Corynebacterium diphtheriae* | • Persistent, unexplained fever may occur (especially with vancomycin). Antipyretics are only partially helpful in abrogating this effect.<br>• Administer vancomycin over at least 2 hours, as too-rapid infusion may cause warmth, flushing, tachycardia, hypertension ("red man syndrome," "Antabuse-like reaction"), or hypotension.<br>• Apply antihistamine or steroid creams if a macular, itchy rash occurs.<br>• Periodically monitor complete blood count for leukopenia (vancomycin). Drug may be discontinued if it occurs.<br>• Monitor blood levels of vancomycin for the necessary MIC of the drug against the patient's specific organism. If the organism is resistant at lower MICs, the dose may be increased as tolerated. |
| **Cephalosporins**<br>Cefamandole<br>Cefazolin<br>Cephalothin<br>Cefuroxime<br>Ceftazidime<br>Cefuraxime<br>Ceftriaxone<br>Cefepime | General enterobacter coverage (*E. coli*, *Klebsiella*, *Proteus*, *Serratia*), *Staphylococcus aureus*, *Haemophilus influenzae* | • Administer via central venous access whenever possible. Administer slowly through large peripheral vessel to reduce incidence of phlebitis.<br>• Administer antidiarrheals as needed.<br>• Hypersensitivity reactions including macular, itchy rash may occur. Apply antihistamine or steroid creams if needed.<br>• Persistent, unexplained fever may be a manifestation of hypersensitivity. Antipyretics are only partially helpful in abrogating this effect.<br>• Some hypersensitivity reactions are anaphylactoid and require emergency respiratory support, including epinephrine.<br>• Alters platelet function and may enhance bleeding tendency. Avoid other anticoagulant or antiplatelet medications such as aspirin or nonsteroidal anti-inflammatory agents (rarely occurs). |
| **Tetracyclines**<br>Tetracycline<br>Democycline<br>Monocycline | Tick fever, *Chlamydiae*, *Klebsiella* urinary tract infections, *Mycoplasma pneumoniae* (second) | • Take with food to reduce drug-related nausea.<br>• Avoid concomitant caffeine that will enhance GI upset.<br>• Implement safety precautions for potential vertigo.<br>• Administer steroid vaginal creams for itching due to vaginitis, and antifungal cream if secondary fungal vaginitis occurs.<br>• Monitor hepatic transaminases for elevations indicating contraindication for treatment or drug toxicity.<br>• Administer oral preparations with a straw to avoid teeth staining.<br>• Avoid bright lights that will hurt the eyes due to drug-related photosensitivity. |
| **Other Antibacterials** | | |
| Clindamycin | GI bacilli | • Take with food to reduce drug-related nausea.<br>• Avoid concomitant caffeine that will enhance GI upset.<br>• Administer antidiarrheals as needed.<br>• Monitor stools for quantity, fluid loss, and blood, as colitis may occur.<br>• Apply antihistamine or steroid creams if a macular, itchy rash occurs. |

(*Continued*)

**TABLE 28-8 (Continued)**

| Antibiotic | Coverage | Nursing Implications |
|---|---|---|
| **Commonly Used Antibiotics** | | |
| Erythromycin | *Campylobacter*, *Chlamydia conjunctivitis*, *Corynebacterium diphtheriae*, *Legionella*, *Mycoplasma pneumoniae* | • Administer via central venous access whenever possible. Administer slowly through a large peripheral vein to reduce incidence of phlebitis.<br>• Administer antidiarrheals as needed.<br>• Maintain good oral hygiene to reduce discomfort.<br>• If stomatitis occurs, perform oral rinsing with saline or bicarbonate rinses 4 times a day, and use oral anesthetic agents (eg, viscous xylocaine, Ulcerease) to reduce discomfort.<br>• Monitor hepatic transaminases for elevations indicating contraindication for treatment or drug toxicity.<br>• Apply antihistamine or steroid creams if a macular, itchy rash occurs.<br>• Long-term use leads to partially reversible vestibular and auditory damage. Administering the dose more slowly may reduce incidence. Assist in hearing evaluation after course of therapy. |
| Metronidazole | *Bacteroides*, various normal flora, *Clostridium difficile* | • Administer with food. Sweet hard candies may best abrogate the metallic taste.<br>• Administer acetaminophen as needed for headache.<br>• Administer via central venous access whenever possible. Administer slowly through a large peripheral vein to reduce incidence of phlebitis.<br>• Monitor peripheral sensation (soles of feet and fingertips) where peripheral neuropathies are first noted. Implement safety precautions for hands and feet, as the patient will be less aware of injury to these areas. When neuropathies occur, consider changing antimicrobial therapy.<br>• Never administer with alcohol or alcohol-based preparations (eg, many oral elixirs) due to antabuse-like reaction (warmth, flushing, tachycardia, hypertension). |
| Sulfa-trimethoprim | *E. coli* UTI, *Haemophilus influenzae*, *Shigella*, *Pneumocystis carinii*, some strains *Pseudomonas*, *Salmonella*, *Yersinia* | • Hypersensitivity reactions including macular, itchy rash may occur. Apply antihistamine or steroid creams if needed.<br>• Persistent, unexplained fever may be a manifestation of hypersensitivity. Antipyretics are only partially helpful in abrogating this effect.<br>• Some hypersensitivity reactions are anaphylactoid and require emergency respiratory support, including epinephrine.<br>• Take with food to reduce drug-related nausea.<br>• Avoid concomitant caffeine that will enhance GI upset.<br>• Periodically monitor complete blood count of leukopenia and thrombocytopenia. The drug may be discontinued if it occurs. |
| Sulfonamides (Gantricin) | Nocardia | • Hypersensitivity reactions including macular; itchy rash may occur. Apply antihistamine or steroid creams if needed.<br>• Persistent, unexplained fever may occur. Antipyretics are only partially helpful in abrogating this effect.<br>• Enhance fluid intake while on the drug to reduce the risk of crystalluria.<br>• Take with food to reduce drug-related nausea.<br>• Avoid concomitant caffeine that will enhance GI upset.<br>• Avoid bright lights that will hurt the eyes due to drug-related photosensitivity. |
| **Other Bacterials** | | |
| Azithromycin | Broad-spectrum gram-positive, gram-negative, and atypical organisms including mycobacteria that infect the oropharynx and lungs | • Administer on an empty stomach with a full glass of water<br>• Do not take within 2 hours of food<br>• Azithromycin interferes with many medications, advise patients to review medications with their provider.<br>• Counsel patients that medication may interfere with birth control pills, use alternative protection against pregnancy<br>• Patients may take acetaminophen if they experience headache<br>• Sensory changes such as taste change, tinnitus, visual blurring, or dizziness may occur and should be reported if interfere with normal activities<br>• Monitor hepatic function and presence of colestasis such as clay colored stool, dark urine |

| | | |
|---|---|---|
| **Antifungals** | | |
| Ketoconozole<br>Itraconazome<br>Voriconazole | Widely spread localized fungal infections, oral/mucotaneous *candida*; itraconazole and vorizonazole are also approved for treatment of visceral or systemic *Candida* infection | • Take with food to reduce drug-related nausea.<br>• Avoid concomitant caffeine that will enhance GI upset.<br>• Monitor hepatic transaminases for elevations indicating contraindication for treatment or drug toxicity.<br>• Prepare patient and family for altered body image (gynecomastia), secondary sex characteristics (dysmenorrhea, testes size), and decreased libido due to decreased testosterone levels.<br>• Drugs interfering with stomach acidity may alter absorption.<br>• Agents may potentiate the action of benzodiazepines.<br>• Agents may cause potassium depletion; monitor and replace potassium as needed. |
| Amphotericin-B | Topical-mucotaneous fungal infections, disseminated fungal infections (*Candida, Aspergillus, Cryptococcus*) | • Severe, high, spiking fever may occur 30 to 45 minutes into the infusion. Premedication with antipyretics is only partially helpful in abrogating this effect. Some patients require steroids to abrogate fever and chills.<br>• Rigors accompanying fever may be abrogated by covering with warm blankets or administering of intravenous morphine, demerol, or a benzodiazepine.<br>• Administer acetaminophen as needed for fever or headache.<br>• Administer potassium supplements, as renal excretion of potassium is enhanced with this agent, which causes hypokalemia.<br>• Prehydration with high-sodium fluid is thought to reduce renal toxicity.<br>• Dose should be reduced in case of renal failure.<br>• Periodically monitor complete blood count for anemia. The drug may be discontinued if it occurs.<br>• Administer via central venous access whenever possible, or give slowly through a large peripheral vein to reduce phlebitis.<br>• Tachycardia with hypertension or hypotension may occur. Monitor vital signs frequently during administration.<br>• Consider lipid formulations of the drug if renal insufficiency or severe infusional toxicity occurs. |
| Flucytosine | Disseminated or septicemic *Candida, Coccidioides, Cryptococcus* | • Administer concomitant antiemetics to abrogate nausea and vomiting.<br>• Administer with food and avoid concomitant caffeine to reduce drug-induced nausea.<br>• Apply antihistamine or steroid creams if a macular, itchy rash occurs.<br>• Monitor hepatic transminases for elevations indicating contraindication for treatment or drug toxicity.<br>• Periodically monitor complete blood count for anemia, leukopenia, and thrombocytopenia. The drug may be discontinued if they occur.<br>• Implement safety precautions and frequently check orientation, as confusion may occur with this drug. |
| Caspofungin | Disseminated *Candida* or *Aspergillus* refractory to oral therapy or amphotericin-B | • Not compatible with glucose-containing solutions; administer only with normal saline.<br>• The drug is a venous irritant, so administer cautiously through peripheral IV, slowing the hour infusion if necessary.<br>• Transient mild transaminase elevations may occur, but severe or prolonged changes warrant drug discontinuation.<br>• Hypersensitivity reactions may occur. Monitoring for itching, rash, erythema, or respiratory difficulty should be performed, being particularly vigilant during the first few doses.<br>• Assess for baseline nausea and vomiting, and manage supportively if these effects increase during therapy.<br>• Assess for baseline history of headache and advise the patient of this possible adverse effect. Discuss with the physician use of analgesic medications for management of this adverse effect. |

(*Continued*)

**TABLE 28-8 (*Continued*)**

| Commonly Used Antibiotics | | |
|---|---|---|
| **Antibiotic** | **Coverage** | **Nursing Implications** |
| **Azole antifungals** | | |
| Posaconazole | Posaconazole is indicated for prevention and treatment of invasive *Candida*, *Aspergillus*, or *Fusarium* infection | All azole antifungal agents have been associated with prolonged QT interval on ECG and increased risk of serious ventricular dysrhythmias |
| **Antivirals** | | |
| Acyclovir | Herpes simplex I and II, varicella zoster | • Administer through central venous access, if possible, to prevent irritation at the infusion site.<br>• Dose should be reduced in case of renal failure.<br>• Slower infusion rate decreases renal toxicity. Usually given intravenously over 1 hour.<br>• Monitor hepatic transaminases for elevations indicating contraindication for treatment or drug toxicity.<br>• Apply antihistamine or steroid creams if a macular, itchy rash occurs.<br>• Periodically monitor complete blood count for leukopenia and thrombocytopenia. The drug may be discontinued if either occurs.<br>• Monitor ammonia level, serum chemistry values, and glucose levels if mental status changes occur. Drug-related metabolic encephalopathy must be differentiated from clinical causes. The drug may be discontinued if it causes encephalopathy. |
| Ganciclovir | Cytomegalovirus | • Periodically monitor complete blood count for leukopenia and thrombocytopenia. The drug may be discontinued if either occurs.<br>• Apply antihistamine or steroid creams if a macular, itchy rash occurs.<br>• Monitor hepatic transaminases for elevations indicating contraindication for treatment or drug toxicity.<br>• Administer acetaminophen as needed for headache.<br>• Persistent, unexplained fevers may be partially abrogated by antipyretics.<br>• Perform frequent mental status assessment. Monitor ammonia level, serum chemistry values, and glucose levels if mental status changes occur. Drug-related metabolic encephalopathy must be differentiated from clinical causes.<br>• Assess muscle strength and motor activity. Implement physical therapy to maintain muscle tone. Myopathy occurs idiosyncratically or with long-term use. |
| Cidofovir | CMV retinitis, herpes simplex infection after failure of other agents, adenovirus | • Hazardous drug handling required<br>• Monitor for renal insufficiency<br>• Multiple drug interactions can occur.<br>• Confer with your prescriber to identify potential interactions |

| | | |
|---|---|---|
| Foscarnet | Resistant CMV or for patients who are intolerant of ganciclovir, resistant herpes simplex virus unresponsive to acyclovir | • Hazardous drug handling required.<br>• Monitor for renal insufficiency.<br>• Monitor and replace electrolytes (especially magnesium).<br>• Monitor ionized calcium that may decrease and not be evidenced by serum calcium levels.<br>• Assess for neurological changes—dizziness, tremors, and nervousness are common but not life-threatening; seizures may occur in rare circumstances.<br>• Advise patients to take acetaminophen for headache if not contraindicated.<br>• Administer antiemetics if needed. |
| Ribovirin | Respiratory synctival virus | • Hazardous drug handling required, and is challenging when giving aerosolized method of delivery—positive pressure rooms for all patients.<br>• Use scavenging system to remove aerosolize particles.<br>• PAPR protection required by caregivers.<br>• Avoid entering room within 2 hours of drug administration.<br>• Clean all room surfaces of the white powder.<br>• If given orally, administer with a high-fat food for maximal absorption.<br>• Perform pregnancy test before adminsitration.<br>• Administer antiemetics if medication causes nausea or vomiting.<br>• Monitor hepatic transaminases for toxicity.<br>• Careful monitoring for hemolysis indicative of hemolytic anemia that may occur with this agent. |

*Abbreviations*: CMV, cytomegalovirus, CNS, central nervous system; ECG, electrocardiogram; GI, gastrointestinal; IgE, immunoglobulin E; IV, intravenous; MIC, minimal inhibitory concentration; PAPR, powered air purifying respirator.

*Source*: Data from Shelton et al[29]; Allen et al[59]; and Khare et al.[166]

but lower-risk patients may be administered oral antimicrobial therapy and closely observed.[21,25,164,165] Prior to starting antimicrobial therapy, a focused physical examination for potential sites of infection is performed along with a complete culture work-up. Cultures of all excrement, wounds, lines, and drains are standard. Chest x-rays are usually ordered, but the yield is relatively low if the patient does not have accompanying respiratory symptoms; hence, this step is considered a lower priority than starting broad-spectrum antimicrobial therapy.[8] Empiric therapy is defined as initiation of antimicrobials based upon risk without clear evidence of infection and preemptive therapy is administration of antimicrobial therapy at onset of symptoms suspicious of infection. In the setting of neutropenia, the general standard of care is preemptive therapy with fever, administered within 2 hours from onset of fever.[14] This is obviously modified when patients are coming from outside the hospital. Preemptive antimicrobial agents selected for treatment may also be more broad-spectrum and comprehensive in coverage when treating immunocompromised patients.[35] Definitive, focused antimicrobial therapy may be administered if a positive culture is reported.

The National Comprehensive Cancer Network (NCCN) has defined specific thresholds and choice of agents for management of fever in neutropenic patients.[8] It recommends antimicrobial changes every 72 hours if the patient remains consistently febrile, unless there is a clear decline in the patient's stability warranting an earlier change.[25,49] This schema incorporates the conceptual belief that most initial infections are bacterial in nature, but as immune compromise and antibiotic exposure are prolonged, the spectrum of potentially infecting microbes can be broader. Common antimicrobial agents and key nursing implications are described in Table 28-8.[29,59,166]

Serious refractory infections occur in a small number of patients with cancer. Risk factors for development of refractory infection and sepsis include complex polymicrobial infections, infections lasting more than 21 days, infectious lesions larger than 5 cm, hematologic malignancy, active malignant disease, shock or respiratory distress associated with infection, and low albumin at the onset of symptoms of sepsis.[27,167]

Although many neutropenic patients who are febrile are at risk for serious infection and require hospitalization with intravenous antimicrobial therapy, approximately 2% to 15% of patients have a low risk of serious or disseminated infection, and can safely receive oral antimicrobial therapy on an outpatient basis.[164,165,168–170] Several studies have considered variables that favor successful outpatient therapy or early conversion to oral therapy with discharge from the hospital after 3 to 4 days of intravenous antibiotics. In general, although not considered mandatory or exclusive, contraindications to ambulatory oral antimicrobial therapy for treatment of fever in neutropenia include hematologic malignancy, HSCT, suspected pneumonia, history of invasive fungal infection, active malignant disease, serious comorbid health conditions, and hospital-acquired infections.[49,164,168–171]

In cases where antimicrobial therapy has failed to manage the infection, additional immune reconstitution therapies may be implemented. Studies to date have not shown proven benefit in using growth factors after the onset of infectious symptoms.[54] Immunoglobulin levels are usually normal at the beginning of the cancer illness continuum; however, in chronic disease, in children with cancer, or after hematopoietic stem cell transplant, the levels may become depleted and thus increase the risk of sinus or pulmonary infections.[171–175] Infusion of IgG may replenish immune globulins needed by the body to recognize foreign antigens.[176]

When all other supportive measures fail, infusion of granulocytes may be considered a reasonable strategy, but it is associated with significant morbidity.[8,177] A meta-analysis of articles describing the administration of granulocyte transfusions demonstrated reasonable benefit against bacterial infections in prolonged neutropenia, and refractory fungal infections.[178] Granulocytes are harvested from normal, healthy individuals and pooled in plasma for reinfusion. The patient is usually premedicated with acetaminophen, diphenhydramine, and, occasionally, corticosteroids. After baseline vital signs are taken, the infusion is started slowly, and the rate is gradually increased to a set dose per minute. The bag of granulocytes is agitated frequently to prevent rapid infusion of the cells that settle in the bottom of the bag. The patient is closely observed, as granulocytes usually go to the site of infection and can cause severe symptoms of "white-out" or diffuse infiltration of WBCs within that organ.[178]

## CONCLUSION

The clinical management of infections in the patient with cancer involves integration of a complex and dynamic body of evidence. Even as we find ourselves being able to define risk factors for severe infection and limiting exposure to antimicrobial therapy, we are challenged with new variations in microbial resistance. Currently, the most effective method of managing infection is prevention. As we look to the future, we hope to find increasing evidence-based risk models to define risk for neutropenia, risk for infection, risk for microbial resistance organisms, risk for sepsis, or risk for death. Scientists must also continue to press for more studies assessing the specific impact of infection-prevention interventions, such as low-microbial diets and specialized intravenous catheters. During the last several years the risk of death from infection has decreased approximately from 50% to less than 10%.[33] Eventually, the hope is to eradicate this complication of cancer and antineoplastic therapy.

## REFERENCES


1. Dale DC. Colony-stimulating factors for the management of neutropenia in cancer patients. *Drugs.* 2002;62(suppl 1):1–15.
2. Maxwell C, Stein A. Implementing evidence-based guidelines for preventing chemotherapy-induced neutropenia: from paper to clinical practice. *Community Oncol.* 2006;3:530–536.
3. Christaki E, Opal SM. Is the mortality rate for septic shock really decreasing? *Curr Opin Crit Care.* 2008;14:580–586.
4. Kuderer NM, Dale DC, Crawford J, Cosler LE, Lyman GH. Mortality, morbidity, and cost associated with febrile neutropenia in adult cancer patients. *Cancer.* 2006;106:2258–2266.
5. Ghalaut PS, Sen R, Dixit G. Role of granulocyte colony stimulating factor (G-CSF) in chemotherapy induced neutropenia. *J Assoc Physicians India.* 2008;56:942–944.
6. Ramzi J, Mohamed Z, Yosr B, et al. Predictive factors of septic shock and mortality in neutropenic patients. *Hematology.* 2007;12:543–548.
7. Lyman GH, Kuderer N, Greene J, et al. The economics of febrile neutropenia: implications for the use of colony-stimulating factors. *Eur J Cancer.* 1998;34:1857–1864.
8. National Comprehensive Cancer Network (NCCN). Prevention and treatment of cancer-related infections. 2008. http://www.nccn.org. Accessed November 1, 2009.
9. Pene F, Perchaeron S, Lemiale V, et al. Temporal changes in management and outcome of septic shock in patients with malignancies in the intensive care unit. *Crit Care Med.* 2008;36:690–696.
10. Da Silva ED, Koch N, Ogueira PC, Russo Zamaturo TM. Risk factors for death in children and adolescents with cancer and sepsis/septic shock. *J Pediatr Hematol Oncol.* 2008;30:513–518.
11. Schwartz JM. Toward a greater understanding: mortality of critically ill pediatric oncology patients with sepsis. *Pediatr Blood Cancers.* 2008;51:571–572.
12. Viscoli C, Castagnola E. Treatment of febrile neutropenia: what is new? *Curr Opin Infect Dis.* 2002;15:377–382.
13. Pizzo PA. Where do we go from here? *J Antimicrob Chemother.* 2009;63(suppl 1):i16-i17.
14. Courtney DM, Aldeen AZ, Gorman SM, et al. Cancer-associated neutropenic fever: clinical outcome and economic costs of emergency department care. *Oncologist.* 2007;12:1019–1026.
15. Shayne M, Curakova E, Poniewerski MS, Wolff D, Dale DC, Crawford J. Dose intensity and hematologic toxicity in older cancer patients receiving systemic chemotherapy. *Cancer.* 2007;110:1611–1620.
16. Balducci L, Al-Halawani H, Charu V, et al. Elderly cancer patients receiving chemotherapy benefit from first-cycle pegfilgrastim. *Oncologist.* 2007;12:1416–1424.
17. Basu SK, Fernandez ID, Fisher SG, Asselin BL, Lyman GH. Length of stay and mortality with febrile neutropenia among children with cancer. *J Clin Oncol.* 2004;23:7958–7966.
18. Lyman GH, Lyman CH, Agboola O; for the ANC Study Group. Risk models for predicting chemotherapy-induced neutropenia. *Oncologist.* 2005;10:427–437.
19. Blot F, Cordonnier C, Buzin A, et al. Severity of illness scores: are they useful in febrile neutropenic adult patients in hematology wards? A prospective multicenter study. *Crit Care Med.* 2001;29:2125–2131.
20. Gonzales-Barca E, Fernandez-Sevilla A, Carratala J, et al. Prognostic factors influencing mortality in cancer patients with neutropenia and bacteremia. *Eur J Clin Microbiol Infect Dis.* 1999;18:539–544.
21. Innes H, Lim SL, Hail A, Chan SY, Bhalia N, Marshall E. Management of febrile neutropenia in solid tumors and lymphoma using the Multinational Association for Supportive Care in Cancer (MASCC) risk index: feasibility and safety in routine clinical practice. *Support Care Cancer.* 2008;16:485–491.
22. Kouroukis CT, Chia S, Verma S, et al. Canadian supportive care recommendations for the mangement of neutropenia in patients with cancer. *Curr Oncol.* 2008;15(1):9–23.
23. Wilbur DW, Rentschler RE, Couperus JJ, et al. Identifying neutropenic febrile cancer patients at risk for early death. *Infect Med.* 2000;17:347–354.
24. Viscoli C; on behalf of the EORTC International Antimicrobial Therapy Group. Management of infection in cancer patients: studies of the EORTC International Antimicrobial Group (IATG). *Eur J Cancer.* 2002;38:S82-S87.
25. Kouroukis CT, Chia S, Verma S, et al. Canadian supportive care recommendations for the management of neutropenia in patients with cancer. *Curr Oncol.* 2008;15:9–23.
26. Fauci A, Braunwald E, Kasper DL, et al. Infections in patients with cancer. In: Fauci A, Braunwald E, Kasper DL, et al, eds. *Harrison's Principles of Internal Medicine.* 17th ed. New York, NY: McGraw-Hill; 2008:533–540.
27. Dellinger RP, Levy MM, Carlet JM, et al. Surviving sepsis campaign: international guidelines for management of severe sepsis and septic shock. *Crit Care Med.* 2008;36:296–327.
28. Shelton BK. Sepsis. *Semin Oncol Nurs.* 1999;15:209–221.
29. Shelton BK, Friese CR. Anti-infectives. In: Gay BG, Chernecky C, eds. *Manual of Medical-Surgical Nursing.* Philadelphia, PA: WB Saunders; 2002:348–357.
30. Openshaw PJ. Crossing barriers: infections of the lung and the gut. *Mucosal Immunol.* 2009;2:100–102.
31. Garcia-Carbonero R, Paz-Ares L. Antibiotics and growth factors in the management of fever and neutropenia in cancer patients. *Curr Opin Hematol.* 2002;9:215–221.
32. Guinan JL, McGuckin M, Nowell PC. Management of healthcare-associated infections in the oncology patient. *Oncology.* 2003;17: 415–420, discussion 423–426.
33. Morrison VA. An overview of the management of infection and febrile neutropenia in patients with cancer. *Support Cancer Ther.* 2005;2:88–94.
34. Friese C. Prevention of infection in patients with cancer. *Semin Oncol Nurs.* 2007;23:174–183.
35. Meunier F, Lukan C. The first European Conference on infections in leukemia-ECIL-1: a current perspective. *Eur J Cancer.* 2008;44: 2112–2117.
36. Moon S, Williams S, Cullen M. Role of prophylactic antibiotics in the prevention of infections after chemotherapy: a literature review. *Support Cancer Ther.* 2006;3:207–216.
37. Zitella LJ, Friese CR, Hauser J, et al. Putting evidence into practice: prevention of infection. *Clin J Oncol Nurs.* 2006;10:739–750.
38. Wisplinghoff H, Seifert H, Wenzel RP, et al. Current trends in the epidemiology of nosocomial bloodstream infections in patients with hematological malignancies and solid neoplasms in hospitals in the United States. *Clin Infect Dis.* 2003;36:1103–1110.
39. Coughlan M, Healey C. Nursing care, education and support for patients with neutropenia. *Nurs Stand.* 2008;22:35–41.
40. Mims CA, Nash A, Stephen J. *Mim's Pathogenesis of Infectious Disease.* 5th ed. San Diego, CA: Academic Press; 2001.
41. Todar K. *Todar's Online Textbook of Bacteriology, Updated 2008.* http://www.textbookofbacteriology.net/. Accessed November 1, 2009.
42. Vilanova M, Correia A. Host defense mechanisms in invasive candidiasis originating in the GI tract. *Expert Rev Anti Infect Ther.* 2008;6:441–445.
43. Brooks GF, Carroll KC, Butel JS, Morse SA. *Jawetz, Melnick, and Adelberg's Medical Microbiology.* 24th ed. New York, NY: McGraw-Hill; 2007.
44. Corti M, Palmero D, Eiguchi K. Respiratory infections in immunocompromised patients. *Curr Opin Pulm Med.* 2009;15:209–217.
45. Tuthill M, Chen F, Paston S, De La Pena H, Rusakiewicz S, Madrigal A. The prevention and treatment of cytomegalovirus infection in haematopoietic stem cell transplantation. *Cancer Immunol Immunother.* 2009:58:1481–1488.
46. Kontoyiannis DP, Lewis RE, Marr K. The burden of bacterial and viral infections in hematopoietic stem cell transplant. *Biol Blood Marrow Transplant.* 2009;15:28–133.

47. Calandra T, Cohen J. International Sepsis Forum definition of infection in the ICU Consensus Conference. The International Sepsis Forum Consensus Conference on definitions of infection in the intensive care unit. *Crit Care Med.* 2005;33:1538–1548.
48. Nirenberg A, Bush AP, Davis A, Friese CR, Gillespie TW, Rice RD. Neutropenia: state of the knowledge. part I. *Oncol Nurs Forum.* 2006;33:1193–1201.
49. Hughes WT, Armstrong D, Bodey GP, et al. 2002 guidelines for the use of antimicrobial agents in neutropenic patients with cancer. *Clin Infect Dis.* 2002;34:730–751.
50. Tsai HT, Wang JT, Chen CJ, Chang SC. Association between antibiotic usage and subsequent colonization or infection of extensive drug-resistant *Acinetobacter baumannil*: a matched case-control study in intensive care units. *Diagn Microbiol Infect Dis.* 2008;62:298–305.
51. Members of the American College of Chest Physicians/Society of Critical Care Medicine Consensus Conference Committee. Definitions for sepsis and organ failure and guidelines for the use of innovative therapies in sepsis. *Crit Care Med.* 1992;20:864–874.
52. Schaffer SD, Garzon LS, Heroux DI, et al. *Pocket Guide to Infection Prevention and Safe Practice.* St Louis, MO: CV Mosby; 1996.
53. Mayhill CG. *Hospital Epidemiology and Infection Control.* Philadelphia, PA: Lippincott, Williams & Wilkins; 2004.
54. Lyman GH, Kuderer NM. Epidemiology of febrile neutropenia. *Support Cancer Ther.* 2003;1:23–25.
55. Angus DC, Linde-Zwirble WT, Lidlicker J, et al. Epidemiology of severe sepsis in the United States: analysis of incidence, outcomes and associated costs of care. *Crit Care Med.* 2001;29:1303–1310.
56. Heron MP, Smith BL. Deaths: leading causes for 2004. *Natl Vital Stat Report.* 2007;56:1–92.
57. Girbes AR, Beishulzen A, Strack van Schijndel RJ. Pharmacological treatment of sepsis. *Fund Clin Pharmacol.* 2008;22:355–361.
58. Adib-Conquy M, Cavaillon JM. Compensatory anti-inflammatory response syndrome. *Thromb Haemost.* 2009;101:36–47.
59. Allen MA, Shelton BK. Sepsis and septic shock. In: Wright JE, Shelton BK, eds. *Desk Reference for Critical Care Nursing.* Sudbury, MA: Jones and Bartlett; 1993:1252.
60. Bartlett JG. *Johns Hopkins 2005–06 Guide to Medical Management of Patients with HIV Infection.* Philadelphia, PA: Lippincott, Williams & Wilkins; 2005.
61. Crnich CJ, Maki DG. The promise of novel technology for the prevention of intravascular device-related bloodstream infection. II. Long-term devices. *Clin Infect Dis.* 2002;34:1362–1368.
62. Eggimann P. Prevention of catheter infection. *Curr Opin Infect Dis.* 2007;20:360–369.
63. Timsit JF. Diagnosis and prevention of catheter related infections. *Curr Opin Crit Care.* 2007;13:563–571.
64. Raber-Durlacher JE, Epstein JB, Raber J, et al. Periodontal infection in cancer patients treated with high-dose chemotherapy. *Support Car Cancer.* 2002;10:466–473.
65. Bartlett JG. *Treatment of Opportunistic Infections.* Hopkins HIV Report, 2004, Vol. 16:i-iv. Atlanta, GA: Department of Health and Human Services.
66. Moran AB, Camp-Sorrell D. Maintenance of venous access devices in patients with neutropenia. *Clin J Oncol Nurs.* 2002;6:126–130.
67. O'Grady NP, Alexander M, Dellinger EP, et al. Centers for Disease Control and Prevention: guidelines for the prevention of intravascular catheter-related infections. *MMWR Recomm Rep.* 2002;51(RR-10):1–26.
68. Lerman MA, Laudenbach J, Marty FM, Baden LR, Treister NS. Management of oral infections in cancer patients. *Dent Clin North Am.* 2008;52:129–153.
69. Shelton BK. Caring for immunocompromised patients. In: Carlson K, ed. *AACN Advanced Critical Care Nursing.* Philadelphia, PA: WB Saunders; 2009:1021–1041.
70. Yadegarynia D, Tarrand J, Raad I, et al. Current spectrum of bacterial infections in patients with cancer. *Clin Infect Dis.* 2003;37:1144–1145.
71. Lyman GH, Kuderer NM. Epidemiology of febrile neutropenia. *Support Cancer Ther.* 2003;1:23–35.
72. Derr RL, Hsiao VC, Saudek CD. Antecedent hyperglycemia associated with an increased risk of neutropenic infections during bone marrow transplantation. *Diabetes Care.* 2008;31:1972–1977.
73. Allain JP, Stramer SL, Carneiro-Proietti AB, et al. Transfusion-transmitted infectious diseases. *Biologicals.* 2009;3:71–77.
74. Rolston KVI, Rubenstein EB. *Textbook of Febrile Neutropenia.* London: Martin Dunitz; 2007.
75. Shelton BK. Hematological and immune disorders. In: Sole ML, Lamborn ML, Hartshorn JC, eds. *Introduction to Critical Care Nursing.* 3rd ed. Philadelphia, PA: WB Saunders; 2001:431–432.
76. Miranda LN, van der Haijden IM, Costa SF, et al. Candida colonisation as a source for candidemia. *J Hosp Infect.* 2009;72:9–16.
77. Pedraz J, Delgado-Jimenez Y, Perez-Gala S, Nam-Cha S, Fernandez-Herrera J, Garcia-Diez A. Cutaneous expression of systemic candidiasis. *Clin Exp Dermatol.* 2009;34:106–110.
78. Choi HS, Choi JY, Yoon JS, Lee SY. Clinical characteristics and prognosis of orbital invasive aspergillosis. *Ophthal Plast Reconstr Surg.* 2008;24:454–459.
79. Maschmeyer G, Haas A, Cornely OA. Invasive aspergillosis. Epidemiology, diagnosis and management in immunocompromised patients. *Drugs.* 2007;67:1567–1601.
80. Crighton MH. Dimensions of neutropenia in adult cancer patients: expanding conceptualizations beyond the numerical value of the absolute neutrophil count. *Cancer Nurs.* 2004;27:275–284.
81. The online Merck Manual for Healthcare Professionals, 18th ed. *Manifestations of Infection.* 2008. http://www.merck.com/mmpe/sec14/ch167/ch167d.html. Accessed November 1, 2009.
82. Robson WP, Daniel R. The sepsis six: helping patients to survive sepsis. *Br J Nurs.* 2008;17:16–21.
83. Marrs JA. Care of patients with neutropenia. *Clin J Oncol Nurs.* 2006;10:164–166.
84. Ruschulte H, Franke M, Gastmeier P, et al. Prevention of central venous catheter related infections with chlorhexidine gluconate impregnanted wound dressings: a randomized controlled trial. *Ann Hematol.* 2008;88:267–272.
85. Penel N, Yazdanpanah Y. Vancomycin flush as antibiotic prophylaxis for early catheter-related infections: a cost-effectiveness analysis. *Support Care Cancer.* 2008;17:285–293.
86. Rolston KVI, Jiang Y, Matar M. VRE fecal colonization/infection in cancer patients. *Bone Marrow Transplant.* 2007;39:567–568.
87. Vincent JL, Atalan HK. Epidemiology of severe sepsis in the intensive care unit. *Br J Hosp Med.* 2008;69:442–443.
88. Hooper VD. Accuracy of noninvasive core temperature measurement in acutely ill adults: the state of the science. *Biol Res Nurs.* 2006;8:24–34.
89. Lawson L, Bridges EJ, Ballou I, et al. Accuracy and precision of noninvasive temperature measurement in adult intensive care patients. *Am J Crit Care.* 2007;16:485–496.
90. Kimberger O, Cohen D, Illievich U, Lenhardt R. Temporal artery versus bladder thermometry during perioperative and intensive care unit monitoring. *Anesth Analg.* 2007;105:1042–1047.
91. National Weather Service. Temperature conversion. 2008. http://www.wbuf.noaa.gov/tempfc.htm. Accessed November 1, 2009.
92. Marshall E, Innes H. Chemotherapy-induced febrile neutropenia: management and prevention. *Clin Med.* 2008;8:448–451.
93. Klouche M, Schroder U. Rapid methods for diagnosis of bloodstream infections. *Clin Chem Lab Med.* 2008;46:888–908.
94. Mancini N, Clerici D, Diotti R, et al. Molecular diagnosis of sepsis in neutropenic patients with haematological malignancies. *J Med Microbiol.* 2008;57:601–604.
95. Lungren B, Wakefield AE. PCR for detecting *Pneumocystis carinii* in clinical or environmental samples. *FEMS Immunol Med Microbiol.* 1998;22:97–101.
96. Kacmaz B, Cakir O, Aksoy A, Birl A. Evaluation of rapid urine screening tests to detect asymptomatic bacteriuria in pregnancy. *Jpn J Infect Dis.* 2007;59:261–263.
97. Penack O, Rempf P, Eisenblatter M, et al. Bloodstream infections in neutropenic patients: early detection of pathogens and directed

antimicrobial therapy due to surveillance blood cultures. *Ann Oncol.* 2007;18:1870–1874.
98. DesJardin JA, Falagas ME, Ruthazer R, et al. Clinical utility of blood cultures drawn from indwelling central venous catheters in hospitalized patients with cancer. *Ann Intern Med.* 1999;131:641–647.
99. Raad I, Hachem R, Hanna H, et al. Sources and outcome of bloodstream infections in cancer patients: the role of central venous catheters. *Eur J Clin Microbiol Infect Dis.* 2007;26:549–556.
100. Ben-ami R, Weinberger M, Orni-Wasserlauff R, et al. Time to blood culture positivity as a marker for catheter-related candidemia. *J Clin Microbiol.* 2008;46:2222–2226.
101. Acuna M, O'Ryan M, Cofre J, et al. Differential time to positivity and quantitative cultures for noninvasive diagnosis of catheter-related blood stream infection in children. *Pediatr Infect Dis J.* 2008;27:681–685.
102. Buyukberber N, Buyukberber S, Sevine A, Camci C. Cytokine concentrations are not predictive of bacteremia in febrile neutropenic patients. *Med Oncol.* 2009;26:55–61.
103. Sakr Y, Sponholz C, Tuche F, Brunkhorst F, Reinhart K. The role of procalcitonin in febrile neutropenic patients: review of the literature. *Infection.* 2008;36:396–407.
104. George-Gay B, Parker K. Understanding the complete blood count with differential. *J Perianesth Nurs.* 2003;18:96–117.
105. Cancer Evaluation Program. *Common Terminology Criteria for Adverse Events, v. 3.0 (CTCAE).* Bethesda, MD: DCTD, NCI, NIH, DHHS. http://ctep.cancer.gov. Accessed November 1, 2009.
106. Bell D, Leckie V, McKendrick M. The role of induced sputum in the diagnosis of pulmonary tuberculosis. *J Infect.* 2003;47:317–321.
107. Elsayed S, Gregson DB, Lloyd T, et al. Utility of Gram stain for the microbiological analysis of burn wound surfaces. *Arch Pathol Lab Med.* 2003;127:1485–1488.
108. Lifshitz E, Kramer L. Outpatient urine culture: does collection technique matter? *Arch Intern Med.* 2000;160:2537–2540.
109. Iwata K, Takahashi M. Is anaerobic blood culture necessary? If so, who needs it? *Am J Med Sci.* 2008;336:58–63.
110. Passerini R, Riggio D, Radice D, et al. Interference of antibiotic therapy on blood cultures time-to-positivity: analysis of a 5-year experience in an oncological hospital. *Eur J Clin Microbiol Infect Dis.* 2009;28:95–98.
111. Murdoch DR, Greenlees RL. Rapid identification of *Staphylococcus aureus* from BacT/ALERT blood culture bottles by direct Gram stain characteristics. *Clin Pathol.* 2004;57:199–201.
112. Shelton BK. Evidence-based care for the neutropenic patient with leukemia. *Semin Oncol Nurs.* 2003;19:133–141.
113. Mutnick AH, Kirby JT, Jones RN. Cancer Study Group. Cancer resistance surveillance program: initial results from hematology-oncology centers in North America. Chemotherapy alliance for neutropenics and the control of emerging resistance. *Ann Pharmacother.* 2003;37:47–56.
114. Kidd F, Buttner C, Kressel AB. Construction: a model program for infection control compliance. *Am J Infect Control.* 2007;35:347–350.
115. American Institute of Architects. Guidelines for design and construction of health care facilities. 2006. http://info.aia.org/nwsltr_aah.cfm?pagename=aah_gd_hospcons. Retrieved November 1, 2009.
116. Sehulster L, Chinn RY. Guidelines for environmental infection control in health-care facilities. Recommendations of CDC and the Healthcare Infection Control Practices Advisory Committee (HICPAC). *MMWR Recomm Rep.* 2003;52(RR-10):1–42.
117. Sullivan KM, Dykewicz CA, Longworth DL, et al. Preventing opportunistic infections after hematopoietic stem cell transplantation: the Centers for Disease Control and Prevention, Infectious Diseases Society of America, and American Society for Blood and Marrow Transplantation Practice guidelines and beyond. *Hematology (Am Soc Hematol Educ Program).* 2001;1:392–421.
118. Siegel JD, Rhinehart E, Jackson M, Chiarella L; for the Healthcare Infection Control Practices Advisory Committee. Guideline for isolation precautions: preventing transmission of infectious agents in healthcare settings 2007. Atlanta, GA: CDC; 2007. http://www.cdc.gov/ncidod/dhqp/gl_isolation.html. Accessed November 1, 2009.
119. Mank A, van der Lelie H. Is there still an indication for nursing patients with prolonged neutropenia in protective isolation? An evidence-based nursing and medical study of 4 years experience for nursing patients with neutropenia without isolation. *Eur J Oncol Nurs.* 2003;7:17–23.
120. Boyce JM, Didier P. Centers for Disease Control and Prevention. Guideline for hand hygiene in health-care settings: recommendations of the Healthcare Infection Control Practices Advisory Committee and the HICPAC/SHEA/APIC/IDSA Hand Hygiene Task Force. *MMWR Recomm Rep.* 2002;51(RR-16):1–44.
121. Nirenberg A, Bush AP, Davis A, Friese CR, Gillespie TW, Rice RD. Neutropenia state of the knowledge. part II. *Oncol Nurs Forum.* 2006;33:1202–1208.
122. Chaudhury H, Mahmood A, Valente M. The use of single patient rooms vs. multiple occupancy rooms in acute care environments: a review and analysis of the literature. American Institute of Architects Guidelines for design and construction of health care facilities. 2003. http://www.premierinc.com/quality-safety/tools-services/safety/topics/construction/downloads/03-review-anal-literature.pdf. Retrieved November 1, 2009.
123. Gardner A, Mattiuzzi G, Faderi S, et al. Randomized comparison of cooked and uncooked diets in patients undergoing remission induction therapy for acute myeloid leukemia. *J Clin Oncol.* 2008;26:5684–5688.
124. DeMille D, Deming P, Lupinacci P, Jacobs L. The effect of the neutropenic diet in the outpatient setting: a pilot study. *Oncol Nurs Forum.* 2006;33:337–343.
125. Mank AP, Davies M. Examining low bacterial dietary practice: a survey on low bacterial food. *Eur J Oncol Nurs.* 2008. doi:10.1016/j.ejon.2008.03.005, 1–7.
126. Moody K, Finlay J, Mancuso C, Charlson M. Feasibility and safety of a pilot randomized trial of infection rate: neutropenic diet versus standard food safety guidelines. *J Pediatr Hematol Oncol.* 2006;28:126–133.
127. Van Tiel FH, Harbers MM, Terporten PHW, et al. Normal hospital and low-bacterial diet in patients with cytopenia after intensive chemotherapy for hematologic malignancy: a study of safety. *Ann Oncol.* 2007;18:1080–1084.
128. Doyle AM. Prechemotherapy assessment of neutropenic risk. *Oncology.* 2006;20(10 Suppl Nurse Ed):32–39.
129. Te Poele EM, Tissing WJ, Kamps WA, de Bont ES. Risk assessment in fever and neutropenia in children with cancer: what did we learn? *Crit Rev Oncol Hematol.* 2009;72:45–55.
130 Mendes AV, Sapolnik R, Mendonca N. New guidelines for the clinical management of febrile neutropenia and sepsis in pediatric oncology patients. *J Pediatr.* 2007;83(2 suppl):S54-S63.
131. Balducci L, Baskin R, Cohen HJ, Engstrom PF, Ettinger DS, Kishor A; Senior Adult Oncology Guidelines Panel of National Comprehensive Cancer Networks (NCCN). Senior adult oncology, V.1. 2009. http://www.nccn.org. Accessed November 1, 2009.
132. Balducci L, Hardy CL, Lyman GH. Hematopoietic growth factors in the older cancer patient. *Curr Opin Hematol.* 2001;8:170–187.
133. Blay JY, Gomez F, Sebban C, et al. The international prognostic index correlates to survival in patients with aggressive lymphoma in relapse: analysis of the PARMA trial. *Blood.* 1998;82:3562–3568.
134. Chang J. Chemotherapy dose reduction and delay in clinical practice. Evaluating the risk to patient outcome in adjuvant chemotherapy for breast cancer. *Eur J Cancer.* 2000;36(suppl 1):S11-S14.
135. Garcia-Suarez J, Krsnik I, Reyes E, et al. Elderly haematological patients with chemotherapy-induced febrile neutropenia have similar rates of infection and outcome to younger adults: a prospective study of risk-adapted therapy. *Br J Haematol.* 2003;120:209–216.
136. Intraguntornchai T, Sutheesophon J, Sutcharitchan P, et al. A predictive model for life-threatening neutropenia after the first course of CHOP chemotherapy in patients with aggressive non-Hodgkin's lymphoma. *Leuk Lymphoma.* 2000;37:351–360.
137. Lyman GH. A predictive model for neutropenia associated with cancer chemotherapy. *Pharmacotherapy.* 2000;20(pt 2):104S-111S.

138. Lyman GH, Balducci L, Agboola Y. Use of colony-stimulating factors in the elderly cancer patient. *Oncol Spectrums.* 2001;2:414–421.
139. Silber JM, Fridman M, Shpilsky A, et al. Modeling the cost-effectiveness of granulocyte colony-stimulating factor use in early-stage breast cancer. *J Clin Oncol.* 1998;16:2435–2444.
140. Silber JH, Fridman M, DiPaolo RS, et al. First-cycle blood counts and subsequent neutropenia, dose reduction, or delay in early-stage breast cancer therapy. *J Clin Oncol.* 1998;16:2392–2400.
141. von Minckwitz G, Schwenkglenks M, Skacet T, et al. Febrile neutropenia and related complications in breast cancer patients receiving pegfilgrastim primary prophylaxis versus current practice neutropaenia management: results from an integrated analysis. *Eur J Cancer.* 2009;45:608–617.
142. Paesmans M. Risk factors assessment in febrile neutropenia. *Int J Antimicrob Agents.* 2000;16:107–111.
143. Herbst C, Naumann F, Kruse EB, et al. Prophylactic antibiotics or G-CSF for the prevention of infections and improvement of survival in cancer patients undergoing chemotherapy. *Cochrane Database Syst Rev.* 2009;21(1):CD007107.
144. Wingard JR, Elmongy M. Strategies for minimizing complications of neutropenia: prophylactic myeloid growth factors or antibiotics. *Crit Rev Oncol Hematol.* 2009;72:144–154.
145. Pascoe J, Steven N. Antibiotics for the prevention of febrile neutropenia. *Curr Opin Hematol.* 2009;16:48–52.
146. Hammond SP, Baden LR. Antibiotic prophylaxis for patients with acute leukemia. *Leuk Lymphoma.* 2008;49:183–193.
147. Falagas ME, Vardakas KZ, Samonis G. Decreasing the incidence and impact of infections in neutropenic patients: evidence from meta-analyses of randomized trials. *Curr Med Res Opin.* 2008;24:215–235.
148. Bartlett JG, ed. *Johns Hopkins POC-It Center Antibiotic Guide.* Last updated January 2, 2008. http://www.hopkins-abxguide.org. Accessed November 1, 2009.
149. Ellis M. Febrile neutropenia. *Ann NY Acad Sci.* 2008;1138:329–350.
150. Green H, Paul M, Vidal L, Leibovici L. Prophylaxis of pneumocystis pneumonia in immunocompromised non-HIV-infected patients: systematic review and meta-analysis of randomized controlled trials. *Mayo Clin Proc.* 2007;82:1052–1059.
151. Furrer H, Fux C. Opportunistic infections: an update. *J HIV Ther.* 2002;7:2–7.
152. Sepkowitz KA. Opportunistic infections in patients with and patients without acquired immunodeficiency syndrome. *Clin Infect Dis.* 2002;34:1098–1107.
153. Moore K, Crom D. Hematopoietic support with moderately myelosuppressive chemotherapy regimens: a nursing perspective. *Clin J Oncol Nurs.* 2006;10:383–388.
154. Timmer-Bonte JN, Adang EM, Termeer E, Severens JL, Tjan-Heijnen VC. Modeling the cost effectiveness of secondary febrile neutropenia prophylaxis during standard-dose chemotherapy. *J Clin Oncol.* 2008;26:290–296.
155. Smith TJ, Khatcherssian J, Lyman GH, Ozer H, Armitage JO, Balducci L. 2006 Update of recommendations for the use of white blood cell growth factors: an evidence-based clinical practice guideline. *J Clin Oncol.* 2006;24:3187–3205.
156. Eldar-Lissai A, Cosler LE, Culakova E, Lyman GH. Economic analysis of prophylactic pegfilgrastim in adult cancer patients receiving chemotherapy. *Value Health.* 2008;11:172–179.
157. Gupta NK, Thorpe S, Vanderhoff P, et al. Pegfilgrastim can be effectively administered the same day as chemotherapy to prevent neutropenia-related complications. *J Clin Oncol.* 2007;25:19571.
158. Wong MD, Hershman D, Morrison VA, Ding B, Malin JL. Use of colony stimulating factors (CSF) for primary prophylaxis of chemotherapy-induced neutropenia in community oncology practices to reduce risk of febrile neutropenia (FN). *J Clin Oncol.* 2007;25:17013.
159. National Comprehensive Cancer Network (NCCN). Myeloid Growth Factors, v. 1. 2009. http://www.nccn.org. Accessed November 1, 2009.
160. Wilson BJ, Gardner AE. Nurses' guide to understanding and implementing the National Comprehensive Cancer Network Guidelines for myeloid growth factors. *Oncol Nurs Forum.* 2007;34:347–353.
161. Lyman GH, Kuderer NM, Balducci L. Cost-benefit analysis of granulocyte colony-stimulating factor in the management of elderly cancer patients. *Curr Opin Hematol.* 2002;9:207–214.
162. Battiwalla M, McCarthy PL. Filgrastim support in allogeneic HSCT for myeloid malignancies: a review of the role of G-CSF and the implication for current practice. *Bone Marrow Transplant.* 2009;43:351–356.
163. Wadleigh M, Stone RM. The role of myeloid growth factors in acute leukemia. *J Natl Compr Cancer Netw.* 2009;7:84–91.
164. Freifeld A, Sankaranarayanan J, Ullrich F, Sun J. Clinical practice patterns of managing low-risk adult febrile neutropenia during cancer chemotherapy in the USA. *Support Care Cancer.* 2008;16:181–191.
165. Elting LS, Escalante CP, Giordano SH, et al. Outcomes and cost of outpatient or inpatient management of 712 patients with febrile neutropenia. *J Clin Oncol.* 2008;26:606–611.
166. Khare MD, Sharland M. Cytomegalovirus treatment options in immunocompromised patients. *Expert Opin Pharmacother.* 2001;2:1247–1257.
167. Baskaron ND, Adeeba K. Applying the Multinational Association for Supportive Care in Cancer risk scoring in predicting outcome of febrile neutropenia patients in a cohort of patients. *Ann Hematol.* 2008;87:563–569.
168. Nakagawa Y, Suzuki Y, Masaoka T. Evaluation of risk factors for febrile neutropenia associated with hematological malignancy. *J Infec Chemother.* 2009;15:174–179.
169. Cox H, Donowitz GR. Outpatient management of febrile neutropenia: concerns for the future. *J Support Oncol.* 2008;6:217–218.
170. Johnson TN, DeJesus Y, McMahon L, Rolston KVI, Row MB. Outpatient management of febrile neutropenia: is it safe yet? *J Support Oncol.* 2008;6:219–220.
171. Carstensen M, Sorensen JB. Outpatient management of febrile neutropenia: time to revise the present treatment strategy. *J Support Oncol.* 2008;6:199–208.
172. Cosler LE, Sivasubramaniam V, Agboola O, Crawford J, Dale D, Lyman GH. Effect of outpatients treatment of febrile neutropenia on the risk threshold for the use of CSF in patients with cancer treated with chemotherapy. *Value Health.* 2005:8:47–52.
173. Mir MA, Battiwalla M. Immune deficits in allogeneic hematopoietic stem cell transplant (HSCT) recipients. *Mycopathologia.* 2009; Jan 21 [Epub ahead of print].
174. Raanani P, Gafter-Gvili A, Paul M, Ben-Bassat I, Leibovici L, Shpilberg O. Immunoglobulin prophylaxis in haematological malignancies and hematopoietic stem cell transplantation. *Cochrane Database Syst Rev.* 2008;4.
175. Maury S, Mary JY, Rabian C, et al. Prolonged immune deficiency following allogeneic stem cell transplantation: risk factors and complications in adults patients. *Br J Haematol.* 2001;115:630–641.
176. Huang LC, Myer L, Jasper HB. The role of polyclonal intravenous immunoglobulin in treating HIV-positive children with severe bacterial infections: a retrospective cohort study. *BMG Infect Dis.* 2008;8:127.
177. Hubel K, Carter RA, Liles WC, et al. Granulocyte transfusion therapy for infections in candidates and recipients of HPC transplantation: a comparative analysis of feasibility and outcome for community donors versus related donors. *Transfusion.* 2002;42:1414–1421.
178. Massey E, Paulus U, Doree C, Stanworth S. Granulocyte transfusions for preventing infections in patients with neutropenia or neutrophil dysfunction. *Cochrane Database Syst Rev.* Jan 21(1):CD005341.

CHAPTER

# 29

*Anna Liza Rodriguez, RN, MSN, MHA, OCN®,*
*Barbara Holmes Gobel, MS, RN, AOCN®*

# Bleeding

## SCOPE OF THE PROBLEM

Hemostatic disturbances are common in patients with cancer. Bleeding in patients with cancer can result from the effects of the tumor on hemostatic mechanisms or from chemotherapy and/or radiation treatment. The resulting hemostatic disturbances significantly affect mortality and morbidity and represent one of the most complex clinical challenges in the care of the patient with cancer. The numerous and unique complications of each underlying disease, the often toxic effects of various cancer treatments, the use of drugs interfering with platelet function, complications such as fever and infection, and coagulation defects create challenges in the diagnosis and management of bleeding.[1] Multiple hemostatic abnormalities may be involved in cancer-associated bleeding. Various categories of hemostatic disturbances may be present including increased platelet aggregation, abnormal activation of the coagulation cascade, release of plasminogen activator, and decreased hepatic synthesis of anticoagulant proteins. Minor bleeding may be the initial symptom that leads to the diagnosis of cancer. More severe bleeding may indicate the onset of a progressive or terminal phase of the cancer. Because the morbidity and mortality of many bleeding problems are significant, prevention of the problem is clearly the best management plan. Rapid recognition, assessment, and knowledgeable treatment of the bleeding complications of cancer will significantly improve the patient's quality of life and potential for survival.

No specific incidence rates have been identified for this complication, as bleeding can occur with any cancer. Tumors themselves increase the risk for bleeding. Bleeding does occur more frequently in individuals with hematologic cancers compared with solid tumors. Hematologic cancers affect the bone marrow, usually resulting in thrombocytopenia or platelets with altered function. The bone marrow also becomes the target of antineoplastic therapy in these cancers, in an attempt to eradicate tumor cells. The incidence and severity of bleeding in a patient with an acute leukemia are greater than for a patient with a solid tumor. Approximately 10% of patients with acute promyelocytic leukemia (APL) suffer fatal hemorrhagic complications despite development of highly effective treatment strategies.[2] In a classic report, Dutcher et al[3] found there was a very low incidence of significant thrombocytopenia or bleeding among patients with solid tumors. However, in patients undergoing blood and marrow transplantation (BMT), hemorrhage significantly complicates survival rates as demonstrated by Bacigalupo in a study where 23% of patients receiving HLA-identical stem cells and 45% of patients receiving non-HLA identical stem cells suffered from hemorrhage.[4] Patients at risk for bleeding include those with large head and neck carcinomas, large centrally located lung cancers, refractory acute myelogenous leukemia (AML) and chronic myelogenous leukemia (CML), myelodysplasia, myeloproliferative disorder, hepatocellular carcinoma, lung cancer, metastatic tumors, BMT patients with acute graft vs host disease, and patients with disseminated intravascular coagulation (DIC).[5]

Platelets, the anucleated fragments of the megakaryocytic cytoplasm, play a critical role in hemostasis and thrombosis. The platelet count is considered to be the single most significant factor for predicting bleeding in the patient with cancer. Gaydos et al[6] first reported an association between a low platelet count and an increased risk of bleeding in 1962. It was demonstrated that for a patient with leukemia, hemorrhage rarely occurred when the platelet count remained higher than 20,000 cells/mm$^3$.

Increased bleeding may also be due to other factors, including leukostasis, leukoencephalitis, and the presence of liver metastases in patients with solid tumors.[7] Solid tumors that are more prone to having hemostatic abnormalities include the mucin-producing adenocarcinomas, including those of the lung, breast, stomach, pancreas, and prostate.[8,9] These solid tumors are more commonly associated with DIC.

This chapter reviews the processes of hemostasis and coagulation, then discusses fibrinolysis. The pathophysiology of bleeding includes platelet abnormalities and the problems associated with hypocoagulation, as well as a variety of other causes of bleeding. Care of the individual with cancer who is experiencing bleeding, including both nursing and medical support is reviewed.

## PHYSIOLOGY OF BLEEDING

### HEMOSTASIS

Hemostasis is the process by which the fluid component of blood becomes a solid clot. The hemostatic process comprises platelet aggregation, coagulation, and fibrinolysis also known as primary, secondary, and tertiary hemostasis.[10] This process is initiated by vascular or tissue injury and culminates in the formation of a firm mechanical barrier, or a clot (made up of platelets and fibrin). The sequence of events after injury includes local constriction, platelet adherence to structures in the vessel wall, aggregation of platelets to form a hemostatic plug, and coagulation or solid-clot formation.

### AGGREGATION

When blood vessel injury occurs, vasoconstriction initially provides minimal control of bleeding. Within seconds, platelets, changing from a disc shape to a compact sphere with long dendritic extensions, are attracted to and adhere to the underlying layer of collagen of the exposed subendothelial tissue (platelet adhesion). The activated platelets then release a number of granule components (platelet secretion), including calcium, serotonin, proteolytic enzymes, cationic proteins, thromboxane A, and nucleotide adenosine diphosphate (ADP).[11] ADP causes platelets to swell and become "sticky," thereby increasing their adherence to one another. Increasing levels of ADP lead to clot contraction, degranulation, and ultimately fusion of the platelets. The end result of ADP-mediated platelet accumulation is the formation of a hemostatic plug (platelet aggregation). Activated platelets also provide an anionic phospholipid surface for the clotting reactions that lead to thrombin generation, an essential precursor to fibrin. The resulting mass of platelets fills the gap in the vessel wall and arrests bleeding, usually within 5 minutes. This primary hemostatic mechanism produces only a temporary cessation of bleeding. Figure 29-1 shows the mechanism of normal blood hemostasis.

## COAGULATION

Secondary hemostasis is achieved through the sequential enzyme mediated reactions facilitating the conversion of soluble fibrinogen to the insoluble fibrin clot rapidly replacing the unstable platelet plug. When these enzymes or coagulation factors are stimulated, they become active in a sequential manner, not in numerical order (Table 29-1). This process is often referred to as the *coagulation cascade.* The coagulation cascade is initiated by 2 pathways: the *tissue factor pathway* (extrinsic pathway) triggered by release of tissue factor (TF) from the site of injury and the *contact activation pathway* (intrinsic pathway) stimulated by contact with negatively charged surfaces leading to the final common pathway.[12] These coagulation pathways were traditionally described as mutually exclusive; however, studies indicate both pathways are integrated. Multiple inhibitors and control mechanisms keep these reactions localized to the site of the injury. Figure 29-1 shows the mechanism of normal blood coagulation.

The coagulation cascade is initiated when procoagulant substances most significantly TF, are released during blood vessel injury. *Tissue factor* is a transmembrane glycoprotein present on the surface of many cell types that is not normally in contact with the circulation but is exposed to blood after vascular damage; it also plays a significant role in inflammation.[13] Upon activation, TF binds with factors VII. Factor VII is a vitamin K–dependent plasma protein

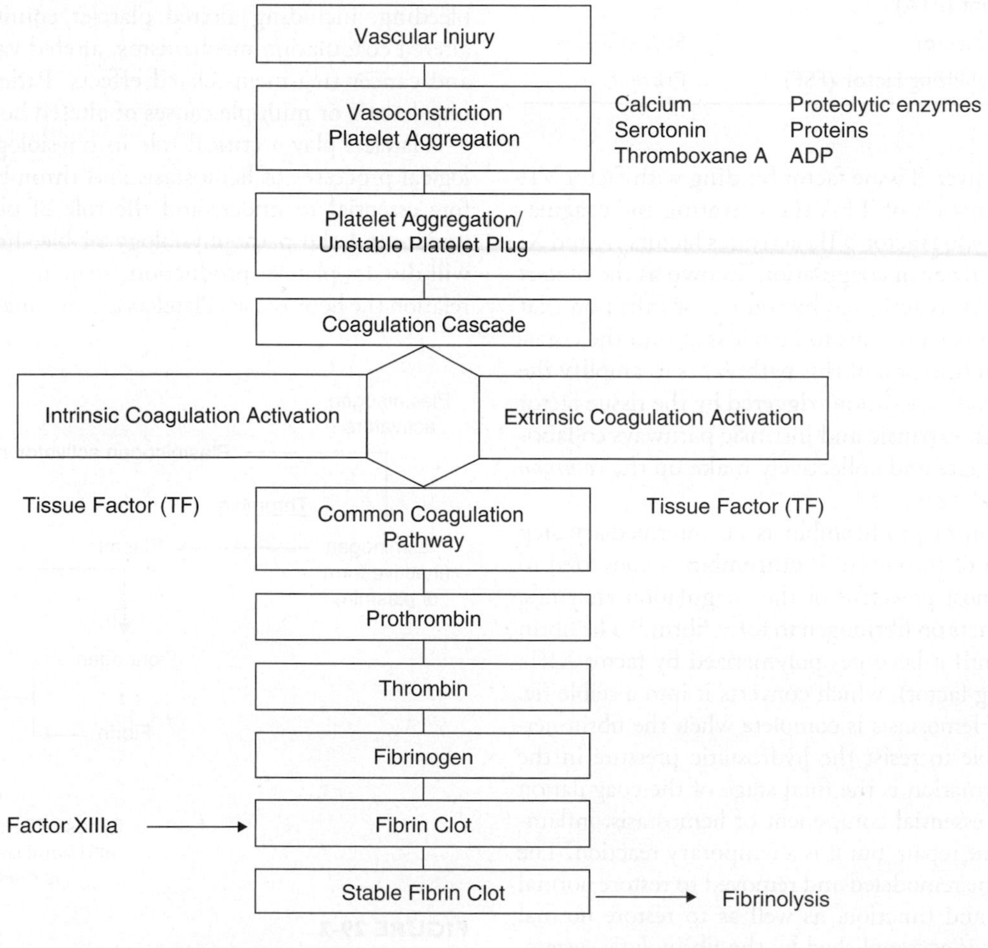


**FIGURE 29-1**

Mechanism of normal blood coagulation.

**TABLE 29-1**

**Normal Coagulation Factors**

| Factor | Factor Name | Normal Range |
|---|---|---|
| I | Fibrinogen | 142–366 mg/dL |
| II | Prothrombin | 80%–120% |
| III | Tissue factor, tissue thromboplastin (extrinsic prothrombin activator) | 80%–120% |
| IV | Calcium | 8.5–10.5 mg/dL |
| V | Proaccelerin, accelerator globulin | 50%–150% |
| VI | Not assigned | 60%–140% |
| VII | Proconvertin, serum prothrombin conversion accelerator (SPCA) | 60%–150% |
| VIII | Antihemophilic globulin (AHG), antihemophilic factor (AHF) | 60%–150% |
| IX | Plasma thromboplastin component (PTC), Christmas factor | 60%–150% |
| X | Stuart-Prower factor | 60%–150% |
| XI | Plasma thromboplastin antecedent (PTA) | 60%–135% |
| XII | Hageman factor | 50%–150% |
| XIII | Fibrin-stabilizing factor (FSF) | Present |

produced in the liver. Tissue factor binding with factor VII leads to the formation of TF-VIIa activating the coagulation cascade.[12] Tissue factor VIIa activates factors IX and X. The intrinsic pathway of coagulation, known as the *contact activation pathway*, is activated by trauma or infection that causes inflammatory proteins to be released into the circulation. The main function of this pathway is to amplify the coagulation cascade activation triggered by the tissue factor pathway.[12,14] Both extrinsic and intrinsic pathways collaborate at various stages and collectively make up the *common pathway of coagulation*.

The activation of prothrombin is an intermediary step in the activation of thrombin. Prothrombin is converted to thrombin, the most powerful of the coagulation enzymes. Thrombin then acts on fibrinogen to form fibrin.[15] The fibrin clot is soluble until it becomes polymerized by factor XIIIa (fibrin-stabilizing factor), which converts it into a stable (ie, insoluble) clot. Hemostasis is complete when the fibrin network alone is able to resist the hydrostatic pressure in the vessel. Fibrin formation is the final stage of the coagulation process. It is an essential component of hemostasis, inflammation, and tissue repair, but it is a temporary reaction. The fibrin clot must be remodeled and removed to restore normal tissue structure and function, as well as to restore normal blood flow. This is accomplished by the fibrinolytic system, which controls the enzymatic degradation of fibrin.

### FIBRINOLYSIS

*Fibrinolysis*, or clot breakdown, is initiated by enzymes known as *plasminogen activators*, which are present in most body fluids and both normal and neoplastic tissues (Figure 29-2). Plasminogen, an inactive precursor of plasmin, is activated to plasmin in the presence of thrombin. Plasmin is responsible for the lysis of fibrin clots. The breakdown of fibrinogen and fibrin results in polypeptides called *fibrin degradation products* (FDPs) or *fibrin split products* (FSPs). The FDPs are powerful anticoagulant substances that have a destructive effect on fibrin in the platelet plug. When these products are increased in the circulation, there is a predisposition to bleeding. Fibrinolysis limits clot formation and is crucial to maintaining hemostatic balance.[12]

## PATHOPHYSIOLOGY OF BLEEDING

Bleeding or hemorrhage may occur when the processes of hemostasis or coagulation are overwhelmed, such as when blood vessel injury occurs and blood escapes. Multiple mechanisms exist in a patient with cancer that may cause bleeding, including altered platelet count and function, altered coagulation mechanisms, altered vascular integrity, and cancer treatment-related effects. Patients with cancer may have 1 or multiple causes of altered hemostasis.

Platelets play a critical role in physiological and pathological processes of hemostasis and thrombosis. It is therefore essential to understand the role of platelets to better understand the pathophysiology of bleeding. This section will discuss platelet production, structure, and function in relation the hemostasis. Platelets are the smallest of the blood

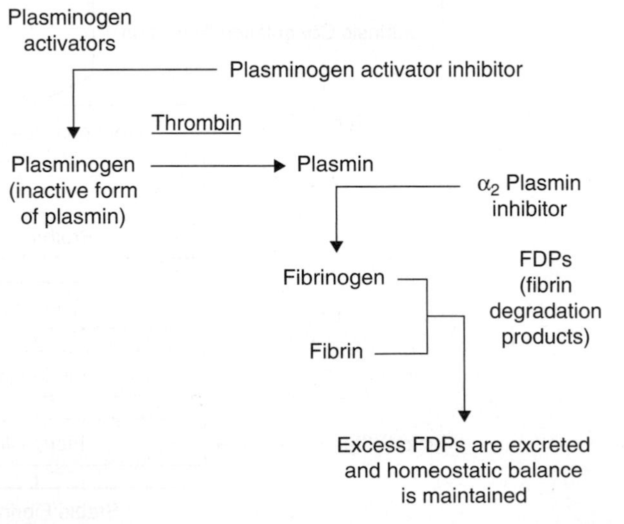


**FIGURE 29-2**

Fibrinolysis.

cells—fragments resulting from the megakaryocyte cytoplasm. Production of platelets is dependent on the proliferation and differentiation of the primitive pluripotent stem cell to the megakaryocyte lineage (thrombopoiesis). The fragmentation of the giant megakaryocyte cytoplasm into smaller platelet fragments is attributed to shear force exerted on the megakaryocyte possibly in the pulmonary circulation. Platelet production is primarily dependent on thrombopoietin; however, other cytokines such as interleukins 3, 6, and 11 and stem cell factor also play a role.[16,17] Platelets provide for the initial arrest of bleeding when a vessel wall is damaged by forming a hemostatic plug. In small wounds, the platelet plug may be sufficient in stopping bleeding; in larger wounds, fibrin stabilization of the platelet aggregate is essential for definitive hemostasis.[17] Changes in platelet production and distribution, defective platelet function, and platelet destruction can cause to thrombocytopenia potentially leading to clinically significant bleeding.

## PLATELET ABNORMALITIES

### Thrombocytopenia

*Thrombocytopenia*, a reduction in the number of circulating platelets, is the platelet abnormality most frequently associated with cancer. It may be caused by a decrease in platelet production due to myelosuppressive effects of treatment or tumor infiltration of the bone marrow, a change in platelet distribution (eg, sequestration of platelets in the spleen), platelet destruction, vascular dilution, drug therapies, or DIC (see Chapter 37).[1]

***Platelet production.*** Ineffective platelet production is attributed to failure of megakaryocytopoiesis where there is decreased available megakaryocyte cytoplasm, or failure of thrombopoiesis where the cytoplasmic development is defective.[18] This decreased production of platelets may be due to tumor invasion of the bone marrow or to acute or delayed myelosuppressive effects of chemotherapy or radiation therapy. A low platelet count is directly proportional to the degree of bone marrow infiltration by tumor cells. When tumor invasion is the cause of the decrease in platelet production, the resulting thrombocytopenia is generally a part of the total picture of pancytopenia. The degree of thrombocytopenia due to chemotherapy depends on the type of chemotherapy, dose of chemotherapy, and intervals between treatments. The extent of thrombocytopenia associated with radiation depends on the amount of bone marrow in the radiation field. In dose dense and dose intense treatments, dose limiting thrombocytopenia is encountered.[19]

***Platelet distribution.*** Thrombocytopenia due to an abnormal distribution of platelets primarily due to increased splenic platelet pooling can occur in patients with cancer, with hypersplenism. Enlargement of the spleen can be caused by infection, inflammation, autoimmune disorders, and benign or malignant neoplasms infiltrating the spleen.[20] An enlarged spleen may sequester as much as 90% of the platelet population[20] making these cells unavailable to the circulation. Tumor metastasis to the spleen, particularly due to lung, breast, colon, prostate, and stomach cancers and lymphomas, is known to cause hypersplenism and subsequent platelet sequestration. Thrombocytopenia can also be due to congestive splenomegaly related to splenic vein obstruction in pancreatic cancer.[21,22] The thrombocytopenia related to hypersplenism is generally mild to moderate (platelet count of $50 \times 10^9$/L to $150 \times 10^9$/L).[20] The absence of a palpable spleen rules out this type of thrombocytopenic disorder.

***Platelet destruction.*** Thrombocytopenia can also be due to an immune-mediated thrombocytopenia, or idiopathic thrombocytopenia purpura (ITP). The rapid destruction of platelets in ITP is caused by an autoimmune process in which antibodies are formed against the individual's own platelets. This condition results in normal or increased numbers of megakaryocytes (immature platelets) in the bone marrow and decreased numbers of circulating platelets in the general circulation. Signs and symptoms of ITP include petechiae, purpura, ecchymosis, menorrhagia, epistaxis, thrombocytopenia, and bleeding (gingival, urinary, gastrointestinal, and occasionally cerebral).[23] This autoimmune phenomenon occurs most frequently in individuals with lymphomas often preceding clinical presentation of the disease and in other lymphoproliferative disorders such as chronic lymphocytic leukemia (CLL), acute lymphocytic leukemia (ALL).[24,25] It is rarely associated with solid tumors.

***Platelet alloimmunization.*** In some patients, platelet transfusions do not always result to an increase in the post transfusion platelet count. This failure to achieve expected increments in post transfusion platelet count is referred to as platelet refractoriness. Post platelet transfusion counts are obtained 1 hour after transfusion to determine response. Patient who demonstrate platelet refractoriness achieve a post-transfusion corrected count increment of less than 5000 platelets/mm$^3$ on each of 2 sequential platelet transfusions.[26] The corrected count increment (CCI) takes into consideration the patient's body surface area (BSA in m$^2$) and platelet transfused and is calculated using the following formula:[26]

$$\text{corrected count increment} = \frac{(\text{posttransfusion} - \text{pretransfusion count}) \times (\text{BSA})}{(\text{number of platelets} \times 10^{11} \text{ transfused})}$$

Platelet refractoriness may be immune or nonimmune in nature. An example of immune platelet refractoriness is alloimmunization.

Patients who have received multiple blood transfusions may develop antibodies to human leukocyte antigens (HLAs) due to exposure to transfusion-related antigens. Platelets express HLA-A, HLA-B, and human platelet antigens (HPAs). Studies have established a strong association between the presence of HLA antibodies in the transfusion recipient and platelet refractoriness.[27] A significant percentage of chronically transfused patients develop antibodies against these foreign antigens and become alloimmunized impairing the patient's response to platelets. The use of leukoreduced platelets or HLA-matched platelets may decrease the incidence of this problem.[28]

### Thrombocythemia/thrombocytosis

Thrombocythemia and thrombocytosis are a result of overproduction of platelets. Thrombocythemia, also known as *essential* or *primary thrombocythemia*, is characterized by an abnormal expansion of the megakaryocytic progenitor cell portion of the marrow originating from a defect in a pluripotent hematopoietic stem cell.[29] It occurs in a group of related chronic myeloproliferative disorders that includes polycythemia vera, CML, agnogenic myeloid metaplasia, and idiopathic myelofibrosis.[7,29] Thrombocytosis, also known as *secondary* or *reactive thrombocytosis*, occurs in approximately 30% to 40% of patients with cancer. It is associated with hemorrhage, acute and chronic inflammatory and infectious disorders, iron deficiency, medications (vincristine, epinephrine, all-trans-retinoic acid, cytokines, and growth factors), hemolytic anemia, and splenectomized patients, and frequently occurs in individuals with widespread cancer.[29]

The major complications related to an increased platelet count are bleeding and thrombosis, albeit rarely in association with thrombocytosis. The most common sites of bleeding and potential hemorrhage associated with these conditions are the mucosa and the gastrointestinal tract. Bleeding can also occur in other sites, such as the skin and the genitourinary tract. Thrombosis may result in symptoms associated with venous thrombosis, pulmonary embolism, transient cerebral ischemia, myocardial infarction, and angina, or in portal mesenteric vein occlusion. Treatment for essential thrombocythemia includes the use of hydroxyurea or anagrelide to lower platelet levels reducing incidence of thrombosis; in contrast, patients with secondary thrombocytosis do not require platelet-lowering or antiplatelet treatment, but rather necessitates treatment of the underlying disease.[29]

### Altered platelet function

At times, patients with cancer may bleed despite normal platelet counts and coagulation factors. Alterations in platelet function may be responsible for this type of bleeding. A variety of hematologic diseases are associated with abnormal platelet function. Hemostatic abnormalities associated with abnormal platelet function include multiple myeloma, Waldenstrom's macroglobulinemia, AML, and CML.[30] Acquired platelet defects in acute leukemias and myelodysplastic syndromes are associated with reduced aggregation responses, as well as impaired procoagulant activities,[31] which is a measure of platelet factor III. Also noted in these diseases are platelets that are larger or smaller than normal, abnormally shaped platelets, and a reduced number and abnormal sizes of dense granules.[31] In addition, abnormal platelet function has been described in patients with thrombocytosis associated with the myeloproliferative disorders; this phenomenon may help to explain the increased incidence of hemorrhage in patients with an increased platelet concentration.[31,32]

## HYPOCOAGULATION

Conditions related to hypocoagulation are less common than the other types of hemostatic alterations discussed in this chapter. Although any type of coagulation abnormality can lead to bleeding, hypocoagulation disorders cause serious bleeding less frequently when they do occur. Hemorrhages tend to develop in the deeper areas of the body, such as the subcutaneous or intramuscular tissues. Bleeding into the joints, especially of the distal extremities, may occur in hypocoagulation disorders.

The most significant factor leading to a state of hypocoagulation is liver disease. Liver disease may result from infection, chemotherapy, tumor invasion, or surgical resection. Regardless of its etiology, liver disease has been reported to cause prolonged bleeding time, reduced platelet aggregation, and increased procoagulant activity.[33] Liver disease interferes with the synthesis of plasma coagulation factors I, II, V, VII, IX, and X. In addition to decreasing the production of these factors, liver disease may interfere with their functioning. Decreased liver function contributes to diminished liver clearance of FDPs and activated clotting factors, which further inhibits the coagulation mechanism.

A deficiency of vitamin K may also cause a hypocoagulation syndrome. This effect may be seen in patients with cancer who lack vitamin K in their diet, with resulting biliary obstruction, malabsorptive states, intestinal sterilization due to antibiotic administration, and impaired clotting factor synthesis due to liver disease.[34] A deficiency of vitamin K produces a greatly reduced chemical activation of vitamin K-dependent proteins, resulting in a state of decreased hemostasis.

Individuals who undergo extensive surgical procedures and receive large amounts of frozen plasma may demonstrate a prolonged prothrombin time and a prolonged partial thromboplastin time. These individuals are prone to postsurgical bleeding. Frozen plasma has deficient levels of factors V and VIII, which can also lead to a state of decreased hemostasis.

Isolated factor deficiencies are also related to cancer. Acquired von Willebrand's disease has been demonstrated to occur in solid tumors, hematologic cancers, myeloproliferative disorders, macroglobulinemia, and lymphoproliferative disorders. A small number of patients with malignant B-cell disease and Wilms' tumor have been reported to develop acquired von Willebrand's disease.[35] Patients with this syndrome demonstrate bruising, mucosal bleeding, and gastrointestinal hemorrhage. Coagulation studies show a prolonged bleeding time and diminished or absent factor VIII procoagulant activity (VIII:c), von Willebrand's factor antigen (vWF:Ag), and ristocetin cofactor activity.

## TUMOR EFFECTS

Tumor-related bleeding in cancer can occur through a variety of mechanisms. Tumor invasion in the bone marrow, due either to solid tumors or hematologic malignancies, can cause bleeding. Tumor-related bleeding may also be due to tumor extension into surrounding structures or blood vessels. Tumor-related bleeding may be manifested as DIC as well.

### Tumor invasion

Tumor invasion into the bone marrow can be caused by primary tumors in hematologic diseases that are intrinsic to the marrow or by metastatic spread of tumor to the marrow from cancers of various organs. Bone marrow failure ensues after normal hematopoietic cells are replaced usually by metastatic carcinomas.[36] This type of tumor invasion is called *myelophthisis*. Tumor invasion that causes bleeding is common in Hodgkin's and non-Hodgkin's lymphoma, leukemia, malignant melanoma, metastatic cancers, myelofibrosis, and neuroblastoma. Bleeding related to tumor invasion is also common in carcinoma of the lung, breast, prostate, thyroid, kidney, and adrenal glands.[37] Physical replacement of the marrow by the invasive tumor results in anemia, thrombocytopenia, granulocytopenia, and neutropenia. The decrease in the production of normal marrow elements is thought to comprise a response to the physiological "crowding out" of normal cells, competition for cell nutrients, and the invading cells' inhibitory factors and metabolic end products, which are toxic to normal cells.

### Tumor extension

Tumor extension may occur in surrounding structures or blood vessels. Bleeding is a common presenting symptom of cancer, generally occurring as a result of tumor and local invasion. Blood loss and the resulting iron-deficiency anemia are frequently the initial signs of lung, gynecological, genitourinary, or colorectal carcinomas. Clinically, the individual may present with symptoms ranging from minor incidents of bleeding to gross blood loss.

Frequently, the most dramatic cause of bleeding in the patient with cancer is the invasion, erosion, and sudden massive hemorrhage of the blood vessel. Any tumor involvement of vascular tissue or any tumor lying in close proximity to major vessels is seen as a risk for bleeding. Cancers of the large bronchi or lung may erode into the bronchial artery or branches of the pulmonary artery. Hemoptysis from tumor erosion into pulmonary blood vessels may appear as streaks of blood or gross blood loss. Head and neck tumors may also be associated with serious bleeding. Invasive cancers, particularly at the base of the tongue, can erode branches of the external carotid artery.

More gradual bleeding involving smaller circulatory structures is usually less obvious and therefore more difficult to diagnose. Melena due to colorectal carcinoma or the microscopic bleeding of macroglobulinemia can persist undetected until manifested by iron-deficiency anemia. A continual loss of 6 to 8 mL of blood per day will eventually precipitate classic iron deficiency, because the compensatory need for cell production exceeds the iron-producing capacity of the normal adult diet.

The homeostatic mechanisms in the body provide such remarkable compensatory adaptation that iron deficiency anemia may be quite serious before the person actually develops significant symptoms. For this reason, it is important to remember that the onset of symptoms may reflect the rate of the progression of the anemia better than the severity does. Fatigue, weakness, irritability, dyspnea, and tachycardia are typical clinical symptoms experienced by individuals with anemia.

## TREATMENT EFFECTS

Bleeding in cancer may be related to chemotherapy, biotherapy, radiation therapy, surgery, or medication effects.

### Chemotherapy/biotherapy effects

Chemotherapy is the cancer treatment most often associated with hematologic toxicity, including thrombocytopenia. The effects of chemotherapy are due in large part to the particular drugs used, dosages, schedules, routes of administration, previous cancer treatments, and any concomitant therapies. Chemotherapy-induced thrombocytopenia is usually caused by the destruction of the proliferating cells of the platelet line. As these cells are destroyed, the circulatory platelets are cleared at the end of their life span, and the nadir of a patient's blood cell count occurs. Considering that the average life span of a platelet is only 7 days, this phenomenon accounts in part for the high incidence of thrombocytopenia related to chemotherapy. Isolated thrombocytopenia with decreased megakaryocytes has been reported after chemotherapy for AML. Stem cell transplant patients particularly those receiving umbilical cord stem cells have documented delayed platelet recovery.[18]

Alkylating agents are associated with longer periods of thrombocytopenia than antimetabolites.[18,34] The chemotherapy agents mithramycin, carmustine, and daunorubicin are associated with abnormal platelet aggregation and other coagulapathies. Vincristine and vinblastine are associated with platelet dysfunction.[38]

Thrombocytopenia related to the biotherapy agents is not as common as that seen with chemotherapy. Table 29-2 lists chemotherapy, biotherapy, and radiotherapy agents associated with moderate to severe thrombocytopenia. Reducing the intensity of the chemotherapy or biotherapy for patients suffering from severe or prolonged thrombocytopenia is appropriate. Altering doses of these agents has important implications for treatment outcomes.

## Radiation therapy effects

Radiation therapy can cause hematologic toxicity, particularly when large areas of bone marrow are treated. The most significant factor that determines the risk of bone marrow suppression related to radiation therapy is the volume of productive bone marrow in the radiation field. Megakaryocytes are affected 1 to 2 weeks after exposure to the radiation, and they take about 2 to 6 weeks to recover from such damage. Radiation therapy is local treatment, except for total nodal or total body irradiation, and rarely causes the nadirs in

**TABLE 29-2**

**Chemotherapeutic, Biotherapy and Radiotherapy Agents Associated With Significant Thrombocytopenia**

| Chemotherapeutic Agent | Degree of Suppression | Nadir (days) | Recovery (days) |
|---|---|---|---|
| Busulfan | Moderate | 21–28 | 42–56 |
| Carmustine | Severe | 28–42 | 35–42 |
| Chlorambucil | Moderate | 21–28 | 42–56 |
| Cladribine | Moderate | 14 | 60 |
| Cyclophosphamide | Moderate (dose-related—100 mg/m$^2$) | 7–14 | 21 |
| Cytarabine | Severe | 10 | 21 |
| Dacarbazine | Marked (dose-related—200 mg/m$^2$ IV daily × 5 days) | 10–14 | 21–28 |
| Dactinomycin | Severe | 14 | 21–28 |
| Daunorubicin hydrochloride | Severe | 10 | 21–28 |
| Docetaxel | Moderate to severe | 8 | 14 |
| Doxorubicin | Moderate to severe (dose-related) | 10–14 | 21 |
| Epirubicin hydrochloride | Moderate | 10–14 | 21 |
| 5-Flurouracil | Moderate (dose-related—12–15 mg/kg) | 9–21 | 21 |
| Gemcitabine | Moderate | | |
| Gemtuzumab ozogamicin | Moderate to severe | | Prolonged |
| Hycamptin | Moderate | 10–12 | 15–21 |
| Hydroxyurea | Moderate | 7 | 14 |
| Ibritumomab tiuxetan | Moderate to severe | 7–14 | 14–21 |
| Idarubicin | Moderate | 10–15 | 25 |
| Irinotecan | Severe (rare) | | |
| Lomustine | Severe | 21–28 | 42 |
| Mechlorethamine | Moderate | 10–14 | 21–28 |
| Methotrexate | Moderate (dose-related—100 mg/m$^2$) | 10 | 14 |
| Mitomycin C | Severe | 21–28 | 42–56 |
| Oxaliplatin | Moderate | | |
| Paclitaxel | Severe | 8–15 | 21 |
| l-Phenylalanine | Moderate | 14–21 | 21–28 |
| Plicamycin | Moderate | 14 | 21 |
| Procarbazine | Moderate | 14 | 21–28 |
| Rituximab | Moderate to severe (rare) | | |
| Streptozocin | Moderate | | |
| 6-Thioguanine | Moderate to severe | 14–28 | 28–35 |
| Tositumomab | Moderate to severe | 7–14 | 14–42 |
| Triethylenephosphoramide | Moderate | 14–21 | 40–50 |
| Vinblastine | Moderate to severe | 10 | 21 |
| Vinorelbine | Mild to moderate | 14 | 21 |

blood counts seen with chemotherapy. The localized nature of this treatment generally allows the untreated marrow to compensate for the damage to the treated marrow.

Radiolabeled monoclonal antibodies have a therapeutic radioisotope that is chemically bound to the antibody. The advantage of using radiolabeled monoclonal antibodies is that the antibodies deliver the radiation primarily to the tumor cells with less radiation to the normal cells.[39] Side effects associated with radiolabeled monoclonal antibodies include reversible decreases in blood counts, including anemia, leukopenia, and thrombocytopenia.[40] Table 29-2 lists the radiolabeled monoclonal antibodies associated with moderate to severe thrombocytopenia.

### Surgical effects

Bleeding may result from surgery performed in an attempt to manage the cancer itself. For example, carotid artery rupture could potentially occur after a radical neck dissection for the treatment of head and neck cancer. Carotid artery rupture occurs more frequently when the patient has received prior radiation therapy. Prophylactic arterial ligation may be performed to minimize the risk of a carotid hemorrhage. The patient who undergoes a ligation of the external carotid arteries runs the risk of a stroke. Small transient bleeding usually occurs before any vessel rupture. Careful observation can assist in predicting and controlling such a complication.

### Medication effects

Numerous drugs are known to affect platelet number and function. Thrombocytopenia is the most common of the drug-induced blood dyscrasias, as any drug can cause unexpected thrombocytopenia.[41] Drug-induced thrombocytopenia may be caused by immune-mediated suppression or destruction of platelets, decreased production of platelets, or a nonimmune direct effect on circulating platelets (such as occurs with the use of heparin). Quinine and quinidine are drugs known to produce drug-induced immune thrombocytopenia.[42] When patients have been sensitized to the use of these drugs, their platelet count may drop rapidly, with bleeding occurring within hours or days of ingestion. Many drugs can cause a decreased production of platelets, including thiazide diuretics as well as furosemide, phenothiazines, antimetabolites, antimitotic agents, antitumor antibiotics, benzene and benzene derivatives, ionizing radiation, nitrogen mustard, estrogens, tricyclic antidepressants, and alcohol. If bleeding or prolonged thrombocytopenia becomes a problem, these medications should be stopped or altered. Drug-induced thrombocytopenia is confirmed when platelet counts recover within 5 to 6 days after a suspected drug is withdrawn.[17]

Heparin is the most common cause of drug-induced thrombocytopenia; this problem may arise either due to a direct aggregating effect of heparin, leading to reversible platelet clumping in which complications are unlikely, or due to heparin-induced thrombocytopenia (HIT). The latter condition is more serious and can lead to bleeding. Heparin-induced thrombocytopenia can be immune or nonimmune mediated. In nonimmune-mediated HIT, there is a slight decrease in platelet count usually occurring within less than 5 days after initiation of heparin therapy. In immune mediated HIT, the decrease in platelet count is usually moderate to severe with 30% to 50% reduction from baseline platelet count and occurs within 5 to 14 days of heparin therapy.[43] In HIT, heparin binds to platelet factor 4 forming a highly immunogenic membrane surface which triggers antibody development. The heparin–platelet factor 4–antibody complex activates platelets later destroyed by the reticuloendothelial system resulting to lower peripheral platelet count.[43] In addition, the platelet activation results in platelet clumping contributing to a thrombotic state. Low-molecular-weight heparins are associated less often with HIT.[44]

Many drugs are known to affect platelet aggregation, as demonstrated by a prolonged bleeding time. Nevertheless, only aspirin has been shown to cause a significant increased risk of bleeding. Aspirin works primarily by inactivating platelet cyclooxygenase. Inactivation of cyclooxygenase decreases platelet aggregation, prevents release of vasoactive substances, and prolongs the bleeding time.[31,45] This platelet aggregation abnormality is so characteristic that abnormal platelet aggregation patterns of any etiology are often termed *aspirin-like*. The bleeding time can be prolonged for as long as 4 days after a single dose of aspirin, until normal platelet turnover results in a significant number of new platelets with normal function. The mechanism of action of several other nonsteroidal antiinflammatory drugs (NSAIDs), including indomethacin, ibuprofen, sulfinpyrazole, meclofenamic acid, phenulbutazone, and sulindac, appears to be similar to that of aspirin inhibition of platelet cyclooxygenase.[31] However, these drugs have only a short-lived and reversible effect, causing inhibition only as long as the active drug remains in the circulation. The newer class of NSAIDs (COX-2 inhibitors) have minimal platelet effects and are an important option for patients with cancer.[46]

Antibiotics are frequently associated with causing bleeding. High-dose β-lactam antibiotics (eg, carbenicillin, ticarcillin, penicillin, ampicillin, nafcillin, cloxacillin, mezlocillin, oxacillin, and piperacillin) inhibit platelet aggregation and secretion responses and platelet adherence to the exposed subendothelial structure resulting to dose- and time-dependent prolonged bleeding time.[31] Maximal platelet dysfunction occurs 3 to 5 days after initiation of therapy and resolves within 3 to 4 days after therapy is stopped.[47] The cephalosporins and maxalactam may cause a similar pattern of platelet dysfunction. Vitamin K may be given parenterally to counter this effect.

Herbal supplements are also known to possess antiplatelet activity, and when used concomitantly with NSAIDs increase the risk of bleeding. Herbal supplements possessing antiplatelet activity include ginkgo, garlic, ginger, bilberry, dong quai, feverfew, turmeric, meadowsweet, and willow.[48] Chamomile, motherworth, horse chestnut, fenugreek, red clover, and tamarind also increase the risk of bleeding.

### INFECTION-RELATED EFFECTS

Infections caused by viruses, mycoplasmas, bacteria, mycobacteria, rickettsiae, or protozoal parasites can result to thrombocytopenia due to platelet phagocytosis[20] or decreased platelet production.[18] Localized infections, including viral and bacterial infections that occur at sites of blood vessels, may cause cavitational or local ulcerations that lead to bleeding. Systemic infections—particularly gram-negative bacteremias—can stimulate DIC, which can result in life-threatening bleeding and thrombosis.

### MISCELLANEOUS EFFECTS

The production of high-viscosity proteins in multiple myeloma and Waldenstrom's macroglobulinemia can cause bleeding. Although rare, this overproduction of abnormal proteins has been identified in 2% to 6% of patients with multiple myeloma with a reported incidence of 4.2% particularly in patients with immunoglobulin G (IgG) myeloma.[49] In multiple myeloma and other conditions such as amyloidosis, plasma cell leukemia, lymphoma, or Waldenstrom macroglobulinemia, the platelet dysfunctions manifested as prolonged bleeding time, abnormal platelet retention and aggregation, and reduced platelet procoagulant activity are attributed to binding of monoclonal immunoglobulins produced by abnormal plasma cells and lymphoid neoplasm (paraproteins) to the platelet membrane.[31,32] A clinical triad of symptoms is associated with this hyperviscosity syndrome—namely, bleeding, visual changes, and neurological deficits. Bleeding usually occurs in the nose, gastrointestinal tract, gingivae, vagina, and uterus.[50] Thrombocytopenia associated with multiple myeloma usually occurs following chemotherapy or radiation therapy. Thrombocytopenia may also be seen when the myeloma expands within the marrow, further contributing to the risk of bleeding. Moreover, a qualitative defect in platelet function can occur, as the M protein (myeloma protein or malignant protein of myeloma) coating the platelet interferes with its function.[30]

## ASSESSMENT FOR BLEEDING

Assessment for bleeding in the patient with cancer begins with a thorough history and physical examination. The assessment may be comprehensive, as when interviewing a person suspected of having cancer, or cursory, as when caring for an individual with acute blood loss due to cancer. A number of laboratory screening tests provide information about the risk of bleeding, measure actual blood loss, and help to determine the pathophysiology of the bleeding. Diagnostic tests may also be ordered to evaluate internal hemorrhage, including magnetic resonance imaging and angiography (MRI/MRA) scans, computerized tomography (CT) scans, plain film radiographs, and ultrasound. The information gathered in the assessment of bleeding is critical in preparing an appropriate plan of care.

### PATIENT/FAMILY HISTORY

The patient/family history is a vital component of a complete assessment. Because bleeding is a common problem in many malignancies, it is important to remain alert to findings that suggest bleeding disorders. Key aspects of a comprehensive history for the individual at risk for bleeding include the following:

- Bleeding history. Bleeding tendencies, including easy bruising, excessive nosebleeds, gingival bleeding, presence of petechiae, change in color of stools or urine, stomach discomfort, vision problems, and painful joints. Describe pattern and extent of bleeding. Understanding the pattern of bleeding is essential in differential diagnoses of various bleeding disorders such as hemophilias, leukemias, and von Willebrand disease. Obtain history of previous hospital or physician visit for bleeding, laboratory tests and results, and treatments received (blood product administration).
- History of and current signs or symptoms of anemia, which may signify undetected long-term bleeding.
- Medications, including antibiotics, chemotherapy or any over-the-counter medications (including herbal medications) that might interfere with the coagulation mechanism or that might uncover an important symptom for which the person is taking medication.
- Acute bacterial or viral infections that may affect platelet production or increase the risk of DIC.
- General performance status that helps to identify the effects of the disease or the presence of complications.
- Transfusion history, including blood components required and the response to therapy (may provide information regarding potential risk of alloimmunization to prior blood products).
- Nutritional status, to identify vitamin K or vitamin C deficiency or generalized malnutrition or malabsorption that will affect the person's hematologic system.
- Immunological disorders, such as ITP, that increase the risk of bleeding.
- Family history of any bleeding abnormalities.

## PHYSICAL EXAMINATION

Physical examination of the patient with actual or potential bleeding requires a thorough head-to-toe approach. Diagnostic signs can be subtle, including skin petechiae or superficial ecchymoses noticed while bathing the patient, gingival bleeding as the patient brushes his or her teeth, and oozing from venipuncture sites or sites of injections. Other manifestations include mucosal or cutaneous bleeding, bullous buccal hematomas, or petechiae. Such observations can lead to early diagnosis of bleeding problems and might prevent an incident of spontaneous hemorrhage.

The major problem associated with active bleeding is hemorrhage. Although bleeding can occur from any part of the body, common sites of hemorrhage include the gums, nose, brain, bladder, and the gastrointestinal tract. An examination of all body systems is done on a routine basis for any patient known to have a bleeding disorder (Table 29-3).[51,52] Table 29-4[53,54] describes grading of the severity of hemorrhage or bleeding.

## SCREENING TESTS

Several screening tests provide information about hemostatic function, more specifically about the phases of hemostasis and fibrinolysis. The hematologic alterations leading to bleeding are complex, and test results vary depending on the degree of the original coagulation dysfunction and the cascading effect of related hemostatic mechanisms. Some of the most common screening tests of hemostatic functions are discussed next. A listing of tests of hemostasis is found in Table 29-5. Table 29-6[55-57] provides possible differential diagnoses based on results of initial hemostatic tests.

## COMPLETE BLOOD COUNT AND PERIPHERAL BLOOD SMEAR

Complete blood counts can establish isolated thrombocytopenia or general myelosuppression. The peripheral blood smear findings can detect abnormal size and defective platelet morphology. The presence of schistocytes (RBC fragmentation) in the peripheral blood smear is often associated with thrombotic thrombocytopenic purpura, hemolytic uremic syndrome, or DIC.

### Platelet count

The platelet count is the best indicator of potential risk of bleeding in a patient with cancer. Normal platelet counts are considered to be 150,000 to 400,000 cells/mm$^3$; platelet counts below 100,000 cells/mm$^3$ are considered indicative of thrombocytopenia. Spontaneous hemorrhage generally is not a concern until the platelet count drops below 15,000 cells/mm$^3$. Thrombocytosis occurs when the count rises above 400,000 cells/mm$^3$. Table 29-7[53,54] lists platelet count grading scales.

### Bleeding time

This test measures the time it takes for a small skin incision to stop bleeding. Small incisions on the forearm are created after which a sphygmomanometer is placed around the arm and inflated to 40 mm Hg. The time until bleeding ceases is measured. The results depend on the platelet number and function and the ability of the capillary wall to vasoconstrict. A normal bleeding time varies from 1 to 9 minutes. The bleeding time is prolonged when platelets are lacking or with a severe factor deficiency. Examples of disease states in which a prolonged bleeding time may be found include thrombocytopenia, von Willebrand's disease, infiltration of the marrow by tumor, and consumption of platelets in DIC. A prolonged bleeding time is also found with drugs that affect platelet function, such as aspirin.

### Bone marrow aspirate

In most cases, the definitive test to determine the etiology of thrombocytopenia is the bone marrow aspirate. If the platelet count is low, the bone marrow aspirate will demonstrate few megakaryocytes because of underproduction of cells. This may occur when there is crowding of the marrow by disease. The bone marrow aspirate will demonstrate adequate to increased levels of megakaryocytes if the platelets are being destroyed in the peripheral blood by the immune system. This may occur with diseases such as ITP or as a result of marrow toxic therapy.

### Partial thromboplastin time (activated)

A normal activated partial thromboplastin time (aPTT) is approximately 30 to 40 seconds. The aPTT screens for coagulation deficiencies in the intrinsic and common pathways of coagulation. A prolonged aPTT is evidenced when any clotting factor, except for factors VII or XIII, exists in inadequate quantities. A prolonged aPTT may be seen with DIC, liver disease, biliary obstruction, and with circulating anticoagulants such as heparin. There is a risk of spontaneous hemorrhage if the aPTT is greater than 100.

### Prothrombin time

The prothrombin time (PT) screens for coagulation deficiencies along the extrinsic or common pathways of coagulation. The PT is prolonged when clotting factors I, II, V, VII, or X are deficient due to decreased synthesis of 1 or more coagulation proteins, proteolytic consumption, or presence of antibodies against coagulation factors.[58] Prolonged PT values are seen in liver disease (hepatitis

**TABLE 29-3**

**Physical Examination and Care of the Patient With Actual or Potential Bleeding**

| System | Physical Examination | Management |
|---|---|---|
| Central nervous system | Mental status changes including confusion<br>Lethargy<br>Restlessness<br>Changes in cognition<br>Alteration in level of consciousness<br>Obtundation<br>Seizures or coma<br>Changes in neurological signs including widening pulse pressure, pupil size, and reactivity, motor strength and coordination, speech and paralysis<br>Complaints of headache | Head CT scan for accurate diagnosis of intracranial bleeding<br>Monitor vital signs<br>Blood product transfusion maintaining platelet level above 20,000 $mm^3$<br>Administer corticosteroids or mannitol to decrease intracranial pressure<br>Instruct patient to avoid Valsalva maneuver<br>Administer pain medication for severe headache<br>Administer cough medicine as needed to patients to prevent further spontaneous bleeding due to forceful coughing |
| Eyes and ears | Visual disturbances including diplopia, blurred vision, and partial field loss<br>Increased injection on the sclera<br>Periorbital edema<br>Subconjunctival hemorrhage (homogenous red color that is sharply outlined on the sclera)<br>Eye or ear pain | Blood product transfusion<br>Artificial tears to provide lubrication and relieve burning and itching from the eye irritation |
| Nose, mouth, and throat | Petechia on nasal/oral mucosa<br>Ulcerations<br>Gingivitis or mucous membrane bleeding<br>Epistaxis | Maintain good oral hygiene.<br>Instruct patient to:<br>• use soft bristled toothbrush<br>• use alcohol-free mouthwash<br>• avoid using ill-fitting dentures<br>Apply topical thrombin/hemostatic agents on bleeding oral lesions<br>Avoid forceful blowing of nose<br>Manage epistaxis:<br>• position patient high Fowler's<br>• apply direct pressure on nares<br>• apply cold compress for vasoconstriction<br>• topical epinephrine or silver nitrate<br>• nasal packing with amicar saturated dressing<br>• apply direct pressure with balloon catheters (balloon Foley) |
| Cardiovascular system | Changes in vital signs, color, and temperature of all extremities<br>Changes in peripheral pulses<br>Tachycardia<br>Hypotension | Observe for angina<br>Monitor vital signs<br>Blood product transfusion<br>Hemodynamic support with fluids or vasopressors |
| Pulmonary system | Respiratory rate and depth: dyspnea, tachypnea, shortness of breath<br>Crackles, wheezing, stridor<br>Orthopnea<br>Hemoptysis (usually bright red in color and frothier than hematemesis)<br>Cyanosis | Thoracentesis for pleural effusions<br>Sclerosis of bleeding site<br>Suctioning as needed<br>Administer:<br>• codeine or hydrocodone to control coughing<br>• glucocorticoids to control bleeding<br>• oxygen therapy for shortness of breath<br>• antianxiety medication<br>Position the patient high Fowler's to relieve dyspnea<br>Intubation for severe bleeding |

*(Continued)*

**TABLE 29-3**

**Physical Examination and Care of the Patient With Actual or Potential Bleeding (*Continued*)**

| System | Physical Examination | Management |
|---|---|---|
| Abdominal system | Pain (location, occurrence, duration, quality)<br>• Right upper quadrant pain and abdominal distention may be indicative of hepatomegaly<br>• Left flank or shoulder pain may be indicative of splenomegaly<br>• Vague abdominal pain may be indicative of retroperitoneal bleeding<br>Palpable spleen<br>Blood around rectum<br>Tarry stools<br>Frank or occult blood in stool<br>Hematemesis | Administer<br>• antiemetics<br>• antacids<br>• $H_2$ blockers<br>• intravenous DDAVP for massive esophageal varices bleeding<br>• antibiotics<br>• sulcrafate to coat mucosal lining<br>• stool softeners<br>Gastric decompression to prevent nausea and vomiting from accumulated blood in the stomach<br>Avoid rectal manipulation (rectal thermometer, suppositories, and rectal tubes)<br>Blood product support<br>Possible surgery for ruptured spleen |
| Genitourinary system | Blood in urine (measure for frequency and size of clots)<br>Dysuria, burning, frequency, and pain on urination<br>Decreased urine output<br>Character and amount of menses | Administer cytoprotectants such as mesna prior to high dose chemotherapy<br>Continuous bladder irrigation<br>Instruct patient to void frequently if without indwelling foley catheter<br>Administer:<br>• phenazopyridine hydrochloride for pain and burning<br>• oxybutynine chloride to relieve spasms<br>Bladder sclerosis with formalin, silver nitrate or prostaglandin for uncontrolled bladder hemorrhage<br>Monitor menstrual bleeding (number of saturated sanitary pads used)<br>Administer hormone therapy for uncontrolled heavy menses<br>Blood product transfusion |
| Musculoskeletal system | Warm, tender, swollen joints with diminished mobility for active and passive range of motion indicating bleeding into the joints | Correct coagulation deficits by vitamin K administration, plasma product transfusion<br>Pain medication as needed for joint pain |
| Integumentary system | Bruising, petechia, purpura, ecchymoses, hematomas<br>Acrocyanosis (irregularly shaped cyanotic patches on the periphery of the arms and legs associated with bleeding due to DIC)<br>Pallor and jaundice<br>Oozing from venipuncture or injection sites, biopsy sites, central lines, catheters, or nasogastric tubes | Direct pressure on site of bleeding<br>Apply cold compress to promote vasoconstriction<br>Apply topical absorbable hemostats: collagen, fibrins |

*Abbreviation*: DIC, disseminated intravascular clotting; DDVAP, desmopressin acetate.

*Source*: Data from Gobel[51]; and Friend and Pruett.[52]

and tumor involvement), in obstructive biliary disease (eg, bile duct obstruction secondary to tumor), and with coumarin, heparin, streptokinase, and urokinase ingestion.[59]

Taken together, the aPTT and the PT can give a fair indication of the nature of the clotting defect. If both the aPTT and the PT are normal and the patient is bleeding, the vessels or platelets are probably defective. Likewise, if either the aPTT or the PT is prolonged and the patient is bleeding, the defect is likely in the clotting mechanism.

## International normalized ratio

The effects of anticoagulation therapy are often measured by the international normalized ratio (INR). The INR is

**TABLE 29-4**

**Hemorrhage/Bleeding Toxicity Criteria**

**Hemorrhage Toxicity Criteria**

| Organization | Grade 1 | Grade 2 | Grade 3 | Grade 4 |
|---|---|---|---|---|
| WHO, ECOG, SWOG | Mild, no transfusion | Gross, 1–2 units transfusion per episode | Gross, 3–4 units transfusion per episode | Massive, >4 units transfusion per episode |
| NCI CTCAE v3 | Mild, minimal/microscopic bleeding, intervention not indicated | Symptomatic and medical intervention or minor cauterization indicated | Transfusion, interventional radiology, endoscopic, or operative intervention indicated, radiation therapy (ie, hemostasis of bleeding time) | Life-threatening consequences; major urgent intervention indicated |

*Abbreviations*: ECOG, Eastern Cooperative Oncology Group; SWOG, Southwestern Oncology Group; WHO, World Health Organization.

*Source*: Data from National Institutes of Health[53]; and Comis.[54]

the desired patient/mean normal PT ratio.[58] The normal INR is less than 2.0. An INR greater than 2.0 is considered anticoagulated (eg, for the treatment of deep-vein thrombosis or pulmonary embolus).

## Factor assays

Measurement of specific factors identifies specific factor deficiencies, which may help in the diagnosis of bleeding.

## Fibrin degradation products test and the D-dimer assay

The measurement of fibrinogen degradation products (FDPs) provides an indication of the activity of the fibrinolytic system. Agglutination is demonstrated if the patient's blood contains degradation fragments or products. Levels of FDP greater than 10 g/mL indicate increased fibrinolysis, as seen in DIC and primary fibrinolytic disorders. The D-dimer is a neoantigen formed as a result of plasmin digestion of fibrin. This test also measures the amount of FDPs in the blood.[60]

**TABLE 29-5**

**Tests of Hemostasis**

| Test | Measures | Normal Value |
|---|---|---|
| | **Platelet Function** | |
| Platelet count | Number of circulating platelets | 150,000–400,000 cells/mm$^3$ |
| Bleeding time | Platelet plug formation; response of small vessels | 1–9 min |
| Bone marrow biopsy | Etiology of thrombocytopenia | Megakaryocytes present |
| | **Coagulation** | |
| Activated partial thromboplastin time (aPTT) | Intrinsic and common pathways of coagulation cascade | Varies, compare with normal control (usually 30–40 sec) |
| Prothrombin time (PT) | Diminished or absent coagulation factors | Varies, compare with normal control (approximately 70%–130%) |
| International normalized ratio (INR) | Coagulation state | < 2; > 2 show anticoagulation |
| Thrombin time | Fibrinogen concentration; structure of fibrinogen; presence of inhibitors | Varies: compare with normal value (approximately 200–400 mg/dL) |
| Specific factor assays | Concentration of functional factors in plasma | 50%–150% activity in pooled normal plasma |

**TABLE 29-6**

**Differential Diagnosis Using Initial Hemostasis Test Results**

| PT | APTT | Bleeding | Related Disorder |
|---|---|---|---|
| Normal | ↑ | Yes | Deficiencies of factors VIII, IX, XI<br>Inhibitors of factors VIII, IX, XI<br>Hemophilia A or B<br>von Willebrand disease<br>Heparin therapy |
| Normal | ↑ | No | Isolated factor deficiency (VIII, IX, XI, XII, contact pathway protein)<br>Lupus inhibitor<br>Heparin |
| ↑ | Normal | Yes | Severe factor VII deficiency<br>Dyfibrinogenemia due to liver disease<br>Warfarin therapy<br>Factor deficiencies due to liver disease<br>Factor deficiencies due to vitamin K deficiency<br>DIC<br>Paraproteinemia |
| ↑ | Normal | No | Mild factor VII deficiency<br>Vitamin K deficiency<br>Use of oral anticoagulants<br>Sepsis |
| ↑ | ↑ | Yes | Dysfibrinogenemia<br>Severe deficiencies of factors II, V, VIII, X<br>Factor deficiencies due to liver disease<br>Deficiency of vitamin K–dependent factors<br>DIC<br>Paraproteinemia<br>Amyloidosis,<br>Heparin therapy |
| ↑ | ↑ | No | Hypofibrinogenemia<br>Mild deficiencies of Factors II, V, X<br>Lupus anticoagulants<br>Heparin therapy<br>Warfarin therapy<br>Vitamin K deficiency<br>Liver disease |
| Normal | Normal | Yes | Thrombocytopenia<br>Von Willebrand disease<br>Factor XIII deficiency<br>Platelet inhibitory drugs<br>Thrombolytic drugs |

*Abbreviations*: APTT, activated partial prothrombin time; PT, prothrombin time.
*Source*: Data from Data Konkle[55]; Deloughery[56]; and Seligsohn and Kaushansky.[57]

## THERAPEUTIC APPROACHES AND NURSING CARE

### PREVENTION OF BLEEDING

#### General measures

Bleeding precautions are instituted for any patients at risk for bleeding to maintain their physical safety. These measures are taught to both the patient and the family so that they are aware of the potential risks of bleeding. Table 29-8 presents a care plan for a patient experiencing thrombocytopenia or bleeding. Environmental safety is critical in patients at risk for bleeding; bumps or falls can be dangerous and even fatal.

Diligent measures to maintain skin integrity are instituted. Personal hygiene is essential for maintaining skin integrity. The use of a good emollient lotion helps

**TABLE 29-7**

**Toxicity Criteria**

**Platelets/Thrombocytopenia Toxicity Criteria**

| Organization | Grade 1 | Grade 2 | Grade 3 | Grade 4 |
|---|---|---|---|---|
| World Health Organization (WHO), Eastern Cooperative Oncology Group (ECOG) | 75.0–normal | 50–74.9 | 25–49.9 | < 25 |
| National Cancer Institute (NCI) Common Terminology Criteria for Adverse Events (CTCAE) version 3 | < LLN-75,000/mm$^3$ | < 75,000–50,000/mm$^3$ | < 50,000–25,000/mm$^3$ | < 25,000/mm$^3$ |

*Abbreviation*: LLN, lower limit of normal.

*Source*: Data from National Institutes of Health[53]; and Comis.[54]

to minimize dryness and potential breaks of the skin. In addition, paper tape or similar tapes should be used rather than adhesive tape to avoid trauma to the skin. Patients are advised to wear slippers or shoes at all times to minimize risk for injury.

All unnecessary procedures are avoided in the patient at risk for bleeding, including intramuscular or subcutaneous injections, rectal temperatures or suppositories, and indwelling catheters. If the patient requires parenteral administration of medications, the intravenous route is used whenever possible. Intramuscular and subcutaneous injections place the patient at risk for the development of hematomas, which can become sites of infection when granulocytopenia is present. If injections are unavoidable, the smallest-gauge needle possible is used. Pressure to the injection site is applied for several minutes, followed by the application of a pressure bandage to avoid a hematoma. Cold compresses may be used to assist in vasoconstriction. Similar care is taken at venipuncture sites.

The mouth and gums are easily damaged when the platelet count is low, and they become an excellent potential source of bleeding and infection. A systematic mouth care regimen should be instituted to minimize this problem. A lubricant to the lips, gums, and tongue will help avoid dryness and cracking. Soft-bristled toothbrushes help avoid trauma to sensitive gums. If the platelet count drops below 20,000 to 30,000 cells/mm$^3$ or if the gums and mouth are bleeding, bristled toothbrushes should be avoided and mouth swabs or Toothettes used. Most commercial mouthwashes should be avoided, as they contain a high alcohol content that is irritating and drying to the gums and mouth. When the gums and mouth are irritated, dentures should not be replaced, particularly if they fit poorly. Patients requiring oxygen via nasal cannula or endotracheal tube are assessed for irritation to the mucosa. A lubricant may need to be applied to the nares to minimize drying and cracking.

Prevention of forceful coughing, sneezing, nose blowing, or vomiting can be critical in a patient at risk for bleeding. Reducing the risk of bleeding helps to avoid increased intracranial pressure, which is critical in preventing intracranial hemorrhage in patients with low platelet counts.[52,61] Cough medications, especially those containing codeine or hydrocodone, may help to minimize bleeding related to coughing. For significant hemoptysis, in addition to cough suppressants the patient may need anxiolytics to promote decreased anxiety during this frightening event. Teaching the patient to gently clean the nares with tissue or a cotton swab dipped in saline may minimize bleeding related to nose blowing. Antiemetics minimize the potential of nausea and vomiting as well as keeping gastric juices from irritating the esophagus. The risk of upper gastrointestinal bleeding is minimized by treating patients who are on corticosteroids with $H_2$ blockers or proton pump inhibitors.

Persistent and severe headaches need to be assessed further. Referral for further diagnostic testing is essential to rule out any neurological conditions predisposing the patient for an intracranial hemorrhage. Patients with severe headaches experiencing coughing episodes should be managed as described above.

Bowel strain caused by constipation can initiate rectal bleeding. Laxatives and stool softeners may be necessary to avoid constipation. Instruction regarding proper diet and exercise to avoid constipation is also appropriate. The Valsalva movement that may be used by patients with hard stool may increase intracranial pressure, which may in turn lead to intracranial hemorrhage.

### Prophylactic blood component therapy transfusions

Transfusions of red blood cells (RBCs), platelets, and plasma may be administered to prevent bleeding in the thrombocytopenic patient. Red blood cell transfusions are generally given prophylactically when the hemoglobin level drops below 8 g/dL. To date, no controlled studies have been done to determine the hemoglobin concentration at which RBC transfusions improve clinical outcomes.

Prophylactic platelet transfusions are important in managing patients at risk for bleeding considering the critical role

**TABLE 29-8**

**Care Plan for the Patient at Risk for Bleeding Related to Thrombocytopenia**

| Patient Problem | Expected Outcomes | Nursing Interventions |
|---|---|---|
| Potential for bleeding related to thrombocytopenia | The patient will have minimal or no bleeding.<br>The patient/significant other will be able to state signs/symptoms indicative of bleeding.<br>The patient/significant other will be able to demonstrate knowledge of their understanding of bleeding precautions. | 1. Monitor platelet count and other coagulation tests and report abnormal values.<br>2. Assets vital signs q4h or as indicated.<br>3. Hold myelosuppressive agents as indicated<br>4. Test all excreta for occult blood and report positive results.<br>5. Assess patient for any signs/symptoms of bleeding (see Table 29-3).<br>6. Teach patient/significant other about the signs/symptoms of bleeding.<br>7. Maintain and reinforce bleeding precautions when the patient's platelet count is ≤ 20,000 cells/mm³ or the patient is bleeding.<br>a. Use an emollient lotion on patient's skin.<br>b. Use only electric razor.<br>c. Use soft bristled toothbrush or moistened cloth to clean teeth.<br>d. Use only alcohol-free mouthwash.<br>e. Avoid use of dental floss and toothpicks.<br>f. Avoid venipuncture, invasive procedures, rectal thermometers or suppositories, and indwelling catheters.<br>g. Apply pressure to puncture sites for at least 5 min<br>h. Avoid forceful coughing, sneezing, nose blowing, or nausea/vomiting.<br>i. Avoid constipation; may require laxatives and/or stool softeners.<br>j. Avoid cutting toenails and fingernails.<br>k. During menses, monitor pad count.<br>l. Avoid aspirin or any medications that may cause/aggravate thrombocytopenia.<br>m. Avoid tight-fitting or constrictive clothing.<br>n. Use only humidified oxygen.<br>8. Administer recombinant thrombopoietin (rhIL-II) as indicated.<br>9. Administer platelet transfusion if ordered.<br>a. Premedicate patient as indicated.<br>b. Use leukocyte reduction filter on platelet transfusion as indicated.<br>c. Use HLA-matched platelets, if refractory to platelets.<br>d. Monitor, document, and notify physician if any allergic reaction (fever, chills, rash, hives, skin flushing) occurs.<br>e. Obtain post-transfusion platelet count. |

platelets play in primary hemostasis.[62–64] A recent American Society of Clinical Oncology (ASCO) Platelet Transfusion Expert Panel recommendation regarding prophylactic platelet transfusions identified a platelet threshold of 10,000 cells/mm³ in adult patients receiving therapy for acute leukemia.[28] Prophylactic platelet transfusions at higher threshold levels of 15,000 to 20,000 cells/mm³ may be needed in patients with signs of hemorrhage, high fever, hyperleukocytosis, or rapid fall of the platelet count in cases of coagulation abnormalities, and in patients undergoing invasive procedures or in circumstances in which platelet transfusions may not be readily available.[28] A threshold platelet count of 50,000 cells/mm³ is indicated for patients undergoing invasive procedures while a threshold of 100,000/mm³ is recommended for patients undergoing neurosurgical procedures.[65] Plasma transfusions are generally given in patients with coagulation abnormalities who require surgical procedures.

## Colony-stimulating factors

The use of recombinant colony-stimulating growth factors to accelerate hematologic recovery following intensive chemotherapy or radiation therapy continues to be an area of intensive investigation. Studies in both animals and humans have clearly shown that the administration of growth factors can reduce the hematopoietic toxicities that follow exposure to chemotherapy and radiation therapy. For a more thorough discussion of these factors, see Chapter 23.

*Recombinant human interleukin 11 (rhIL-11).* Several different cytokines or growth factors have been evaluated for their ability to stimulate megakaryocyte proliferation and maturation in patients undergoing chemotherapy.[66–68] The dose-dependent effect of using rhIL-11 increases the likelihood of avoiding thrombocytopenia in patients undergoing chemotherapy and shortens the duration of the thrombocytopenia.[69] Phase I/II clinical trials in the 1990s demonstrated rhIL-11 efficacy in the prevention of severe thrombocytopenia following myelosupressive chemotherapy in adults with solid tumors and lymphoma at high risk for this toxicity.[65,70–72] A recent study of rhIL-11 use in patients with AML demonstrated a shortened the duration of severe thrombocytopenia and the number of platelet transfusions although there was no significant effect on overall survival.[73] A phase II study using low-dose rhIL-11 in patients with MDS demonstrated clinical evidence of increased platelet counts and reduced platelet transfusion requirements.[74] Another recent study also demonstrated a reduced platelet recovery time and reduced number of platelet transfusions following chemotherapy in children with recurrent/refractory solid tumors or lymphoma.[75] The reduction of treatment-associated thrombocytopenia and need for platelet transfusions in patients who receive dose-intensive chemotherapy may allow for chemotherapy to be administered at the intended doses as planned preventing dose delays. To achieve maximum benefit, rHIL-11 must be started within 24 hours of chemotherapy completion and continued for at least 10 days postchemotherapy for a maximum of 21 days to increase platelet levels within 5 to 9 days of administration to coincide with the expected chemotherapy induced platelet nadir.[76]

*Erythropoietin.* The hematopoietic growth factor that regulates the proliferation, differentiation, and viability of erythrocyte progenitor cells and mature erythrocytes is erythropoietin (EPO). Erythropoietin (also known as epoietin alpha) has been shown to be an effective treatment for anemia associated with cancer and chemotherapy-associated anemia in some patients. A 10% to 20% increase in circulating platelets is documented in patients with long-term use of EPO.[77] Cloning of the *EPO* gene was accomplished in 1985,[78,79] which allowed for large-scale production of this growth factor using recombinant DNA technology. Darbepoietin alfa is a novel erythropoiesis-stimulating protein developed for the treatment of anemia. Because of its longer half-life, compared to EPO, it is given less frequently than EPO (once weekly vs 3 times weekly).[80]

Erythropoietin administration is well tolerated and effective in the management of anemia associated with cancer and cancer chemotherapy. The administration of EPO increases the hemoglobin concentration and reduces red cell transfusion requirements (thereby decreasing exposure to donor blood products) in patients with cancer who receive chemotherapy and are anemic. There are limited studies demonstrating the role of EPO in platelet activity. Studies however present favorable findings demonstrating the need in further investigating EPO's use in thrombocytopenia. A study by Tang et al[81] showed recombinant human EPO (rHuEpo) at the 400 U/kg dose attenuated the effects of aspirin on bleeding time and increased the platelet count. Homoncik et al[82] demonstrated increased platelet counts and platelet reactivity in patients with alcoholic liver cirrhosis treated with EPO.

*Recombinant thrombopoietin.* First generation thrombopoietic agents, recombinant (rHuTPO) and pegylated human megakaryocyte growth factor (PEG-rHUMGDF), initially introduced in the late 1990s were successful in increasing platelet counts within days after administration in patients after nonmyeloablative therapy.[83] The platelet response however was not as favorable in patients after myeloablative treatment. In addition, side effects of these first generation thrombopoietic agents included development of antibodies to endogenous thrombopoietin causing refractory thrombocytopenia in healthy volunteers.[83–85] Second generation thrombopoietic agents romiplostim (AMG531) and eltrombopag are expected to receive Food and Drug Administration (FDA) approval for use in ITP and clinical trials are currently underway investigating use in chemotherapy-induced thrombocytopenia.[86] Preliminary studies suggest these new thrombopoietic agents appear to be safe, tolerable, and very effective in regulating megakaryopoiesis.

### Chemotherapy protectors

Another approach to preferentially protecting normal tissues from the toxicities of chemotherapy entails the administration of cytoprotectant agents before the cancer treatment. Some of these agents have been used for many years, including leucovorin (prevents myelosuppression and mucositis associated with high-dose methotrexate) and mesna (prevents hemorrhagic cystitis associated with cyclophosphamide and ifosfamide). Saline diuresis or forced saline diuresis is also recommended to decrease the incidence of hemorrhagic cystitis associated with high-dose cyclophosphamide in the setting of stem cell transplantation.[87] Amifostine administered in combination with pentoxifilline, ciprofloxacin, and dexamethasone reverses cytopenias, including thrombocytopenia, in patients with MDS and AML.[88] Amifostine stimulates proliferation of normal hematopoiesis.

## MANAGEMENT OF BLEEDING

Various measures are available to maintain hemostasis including mechanical, thermal, or chemical techniques. Mechanical techniques include applying direct pressure, fabric pads, gauze, sponges, or blood component transfusion.[89] Thermal techniques such as electrocautery are available but infrequently used for patients with cancer. Chemical techniques used include pharmacological agents such as epinephrine, Vitamin K, protamine, desmopressin, aminocaproic acid, and topical hemostats.

## General measures

If acute bleeding occurs, direct measures to stop the bleeding are instituted immediately. Application of direct, steady pressure at the site of bleeding is the first step in controlling bleeding. Mechanical pressure, such as is produced by the insertion of an occlusion balloon catheter into the bronchus or the use of nasal packing during epistaxis, can be applied if the site of bleeding is not directly exposed. Care should be exercised when removing or replacing the nasal packing to avoid dislodging the clot. For epistaxis, the patient is placed in high Fowler's position. Gentle, steady pressure on the nares and a cold compress to constrict the bleeding vessels generally helps to stop the bleeding. Other measures implemented to stop the bleeding may include topical thrombin, topical epinephrine, and silver nitrate to the affected nares.[90]

Hemostatic bioabsorbable dressings may be applied to stop bleeding on peripheral and central venous catheter sites, and phlebotomy sites in addition to direct mechanical pressure. Topical hemostatic agents include absorbable gelatin, collagen, cellulose, fibrin sealants, and alginates.[89]

Iced saline gastric lavages or enemas may help to control gastrointestinal bleeding. Hypovolemic shock is to be avoided in situations of acute hemorrhage. Control of life-threatening hemorrhage is generally achieved with a combination of packed red cells with crystalloids or albumin as opposed to whole blood.

Intracranial bleeding in the thrombocytopenic patient may occur due to increased intracranial pressure from coughing, sneezing, or vomiting, or related to a valsalva maneuver. The immediate action with an intracranial bleed is to transfuse platelets. Corticosteroids are also given to decrease the concomitant intracranial edema and resultant increase in intracranial pressure.[52,61] Close monitoring of the patient with increased intracranial pressure is imperative, along with frequent vital sign and neurological monitoring and serial head CT scans to monitor resolution or progression of bleeding.

Minor vascular bleeding due to capillary destruction is best controlled by treating the underlying malignancy. If iron-deficiency anemia arises, oral or parenteral iron supplements are indicated. Oral iron supplements are often recommended because they are safe and usually correct the anemia within 6 weeks, but therapy generally continues for 4 to 6 months to adequately replace the iron stores.[91] Parenteral iron supplements may be given if the patient cannot tolerate oral therapy or has a malabsorption problem. Iron dextran, generally given intravenously, requires a test dose because it is associated with a small risk of anaphylaxis.[91]

Physical and emotional rest are essential when the patient is bleeding. Rest helps to decrease pulse rate and blood pressure, allowing for clot formation. A state of active bleeding is frightening and anxiety-producing for the patient and family. A calm approach and reassurance are essential when managing an individual who is actively bleeding. Sedation can also be used to decrease anxiety and the metabolic rate.

## Thrombocytopenia

Although thrombocytopenia may be the immediate cause of bleeding in individuals with platelet disorders, therapy must address the underlying cause of the decreased platelet level. When decreased platelet production results from tumor infiltration of marrow, the best therapy is treatment of the tumor itself. The hematologic complications will remain or worsen as long as marrow involvement persists. Platelet transfusions are often given to maintain a safe level of circulating thrombocytes until tumor regression occurs and marrow function returns. If platelet production has been depressed by chemotherapy or radiation therapy, in addition to platelet support the dosage or administration schedule of the treatment can be altered to maintain safe levels of platelet production.[92]

*Platelet distribution.* Thrombocytopenia related to platelet sequestration due to an enlarged spleen is treated most effectively by aggressive tumor therapy. Chemotherapy and radiation therapy are usually most effective for this condition. Sequestration of platelets is sometimes reversible with epinephrine, which causes a release of trapped platelets from an enlarged spleen. Transient control of platelet sequestration has also been achieved with corticosteroid therapy. Steroids have a capillary-stabilizing effect that is important in minimizing the bleeding potential of thrombocytopenia. Splenectomy may be considered if other methods fail to control the sequestration of platelets. Kauffman et al[93] investigated the use of partial splenic embolization (PSE) to reduce splenic parenchymal volume. The researchers demonstrated that PSE significantly reduced splenic platelet sequestration evidenced by increase platelet counts post embolization.

*Platelet destruction.* Individuals with asymptomatic ITP may be followed closely with no treatment. Oral corticosteroids are the standard initial treatment for ITP. Platelet transfusions are seldom indicated for patients with ITP because the survival time of transfused platelets is shortened. Intravenous immunoglobulin therapy plays an important role in managing acute bleeding by stimulating rapid platelet increases. The efficacy of platelets has been found to be improved immediately after an infusion of intravenous immunoglobulin. Patients who are refractory to steroids and high-dose intravenous immunoglobulins may also benefit from anti-D immunoglobulin.[94] In patients refractory to steroids and IVIG, treatments to prevent or delay splenectomy include high-dose dexamethasone, intermittent anti-D immunoglobulin infusions, and rituximab.[95,96] Other ongoing clinical trials for the treatment of ITP include the use of thrombopoietin receptor agonists.[95]

Splenectomy was used for the management of ITP for many years before the advent of glucocorticoids. The decision to perform splenectomy for the treatment of ITP is determined by the course and severity of the disease. Splenectomy may be done early on in the course of severe thrombocytopenia that is unresponsive to prednisone, or it may be undertaken after several months if disease remission cannot be attained.[97] If patients fail prednisone therapy or show no response to splenectomy, other treatments include splenic radiation or partial splenic embolization, vincristine, vinblastine, bleomycin, danazol, colchicine, anti-D antibody, and alfa-interferon.[98,99]

*Altered platelet function.* Drug-induced platelet abnormalities must be assessed carefully in the context of the patient's total clinical profile. Aspirin has been demonstrated to increase the risk of bleeding. For this reason, the patient with cancer should avoid taking aspirin or any compounds containing aspirin. The clinical risk for bleeding associated with NSAIDs is much less than the risk associated with aspirin ingestion. However, the former drugs should be used cautiously in patients with preexisting thrombocytopenia. The potential for β-lactam-induced bleeding generally does not prohibit patients from being treated with appropriate antibiotic coverage; these patients need to be monitored closely for any signs or symptoms of bleeding. Platelet transfusions may be used during periods of thrombocytopenia to avoid hemorrhage as well as during periods of acute bleeding.

### Hypocoagulation

Effective tumor therapy is the best means to control abnormalities related to hypocoagulation. Plasma and plasma derivative therapy may be used discriminately in specific clinical situations. Replacement of specific diminished factors is difficult because of the complex nature of these abnormalities. Generally, the treatment of specific inhibitors of coagulation factors depends on the severity of the abnormality.

Liver disease associated with bleeding and clotting can be treated with infusion of fresh-frozen plasma or prothrombin complex concentrate (which contains prothrombin and factors VII, IX, and X) when rapid correction of abnormalities is required. Prothrombin complex may also be given when attempting to shorten a prolonged prothrombin time, such as before a needle biopsy of the liver. Albumin can be used as a volume expander in cases of active bleeding. Albumin is safer than plasma because it carries no risk of hepatitis transmission. It may, however, precipitate congestive heart failure in patients with compromised cardiovascular function. When albumin is used as a volume expander, the patient's cardiac and renal status must be monitored closely. Desmopressin acetate (DDAVP) may be infused when the patient with liver disease has a prolonged bleeding time, with mild to moderate amounts of bleeding.[100,101] DDAVP increases von Willebrand factor (vWF) and factor VIII.[102] DDAVP is administered intravenously (0.3 μg/kg body weight) or by concentrated nasal spray (1.5 mg/mL)

Vitamin K is essential in maintaining normal biological activities of clotting factors II, VII, IX, and X.[102] Generally, subcutaneous vitamin K (menaphthone, AquaMEPHYTON) is administered to correct the protein defects when this vitamin is deficient, as demonstrated by prolonged prothrombin and bleeding times. Vitamin K is also administered orally (2.5 mg) or intravenously (5–10 mg).[103] The patient is also instructed about consuming dietary sources of vitamin K if absorption of the vitamin is not a problem. The major sources of dietary vitamin K are liver, broccoli, and spinach.[104] Prothrombin complex concentrates or fresh-frozen plasma can be used in situations of vitamin K deficiency with concomitant severe bleeding.

Isolated factor deficiencies are best treated with specific plasma components if they can be identified. Patients with acquired von Willebrand's disease are generally treated when they experience bleeding or when they require an invasive procedure. The severity of the bleeding dictates the type and amount of therapy used. Treatment for bleeding due to this syndrome includes fresh-frozen plasma, cryoprecipitate, packed RBCs and platelet concentrates, along with high-dose corticosteroids, factor VIII concentrates, desmopressin infusions, epsilon-aminocaproic acid (amicar), intravenous gammaglobulin, and extracorporeal immunoabsorption.

## BLOOD COMPONENT THERAPY

In recent years, several professional societies and governmental organizations, including the American Society of Anesthesiologists, ASCO, and the College of American Pathologists, have developed "guidelines" and "practice parameters" for the use of blood component therapy. These guidelines have been prompted by the recognition that even though blood component administration has clearly accepted benefits, it still has significant complications, including transfusion reactions, transmittal of bacterial or parasitic diseases, immunosuppression, and high cost. Table 29-9[28] summarizes the ASCO clinical practice guidelines.

### Platelet therapy

Platelet transfusions have proved to provide tremendous therapeutic value in controlling and preventing hemorrhage

**TABLE 29-9**

**Summary of the ASCO Platelet Transfusion Clinical Practice Guidelines**

| Guideline for Platelet Transfusion | Recommendation | Level of Evidence* |
|---|---|---|
| Platelet product | Single donor platelet concentrates or random donor pooled platelets can be used interchangeably | I |
| Prophylactic vs therapeutic platelet transfusion | Administer prophylactic platelet transfusion for thrombocytopenic patients with impaired bone marrow function when platelet count is below predetermined threshold level | IV and expert consensus |
| Acute leukemia | Platelet level of 10,000/mm$^3$ | I |
| Hematopoietic stem cell transplantation | Follow guidelines for acute leukemia | III |
| Patients with chronic severe thrombocytopenia | No prophylactic transfusion recommended. Observe patient. Administer platelets for episodes of hemorrhage or when receiving active treatment | IV |
| Patients with solid tumors | Platelet level of 20,000/mm$^3$ | IV |
| Prevention of alloimmunization to RhD antigens | Exclusive use of platelets from RhD negative donors or anti-D immunoprophylaxis should be considered for RhD-negative children and women of child-bearing age | IV |
| Prevention of alloimmunization using leukoreduced blood products | Administer leukoreduced blood products to patients with AML and for patients expected to receive multiple platelet transfusions during their treatment course | I |
| Diagnosis of refractoriness to platelets | Post-transfusion platelet count should be obtained after all transfusions whenever possible. Additional transfusions should be administered if post-transfusion count is less than the platelet trigger. Diagnosis of refractoriness made if platelet increment remains poor after transfusion of 2 ABO-compatible platelets stored less than 72 hours | V |
| Management of refractoriness to platelet transfusion | Administer HLA-compatible platelets if available, or administer crossmatched platelets | III |

*Level I, evidence from meta-analysis; Level II, evidence from one well designed experimental study; Level III, evidence from well designed quasi-experimental studies; Level IV, evidence from well designed non-experimental studies; Level V, evidence from case reports and clinical examples.

*Source*: Data from Schiffer et al.[28]

in patients undergoing chemotherapy for leukemia and other cancers.[28] Platelets transfused are either single donor platelets (obtained via apheresis from single donors) or pooled platelet concentrates (pooled from 6 random donor whole blood units). Comparative studies established similar results with either platelet concentrate product in terms of post transfusion increments, hemostatic benefits, and side effects.[28] Numerous studies established platelet transfusion threshold levels dependent on patient's diagnosis, clinical condition, and treatment modality. American Society of Clinical Oncology recommends a threshold of 10,000/mm$^3$ for prophylactic transfusion in adults receiving therapy for acute leukemia and hematopoietic stem cell transplantation, and solid tumors with suggested increased threshold of 20,000/mm$^3$ for patients receiving aggressive bladder cancer treatment.[28] Theoretically, 1 unit of platelets should increase the recipient's platelet count by 6,000 to 10,000 cells/mm$^3$.[90] In reality, the effectiveness of platelet transfusions is variable and depends on several factors. Platelet refractoriness or failure to achieve adequate increases in the circulating platelet count after transfusion may be due to fever; infection; hypersplenism; DIC; previous administration of drugs including amphotericin B, vancomycin, ciprofloxacin, and heparin; prolonged storage, and HLA antibody grade.[48,105]

Fever and infection enhance the consumption of platelets and can increase the occurrence of hemorrhage. Patients with fever or sepsis may require more frequent platelet transfusions to maintain adequate platelet counts. Patients with fever can be premedicated with antipyretics prior to platelet

**TABLE 29-10**

**Practical Considerations in Platelet Transfusions**

**Types of Platelet Concentrate (PC)**

| PC Type | Method of collection | Benefit/Indication |
|---|---|---|
| Platelet concentrates from whole blood | Pooled from 4 to 6 random donor whole blood units | |
| Apheresis platelet concentrates | Apheresis collected from a single donor | Reduces risk for transfusion related infections and platelet alloimmunization |
| Crossmatched platelets | Testing recipient plasma from alloimmunized patient against previously collected platelets | Alloimmunized patients with rare HLA type |
| HLA-typed platelets | Identifying the HLA-type of the recipient and transfusing platelets with matched antigens | Alloimmunized patients |

**Special Handling**

| Special Handling | Rationale | Indication |
|---|---|---|
| Leukoreduction | Reduces alloimmunization<br>Prevents cytomegalovirus (CMV) transmission<br>Reduction in febrile transfusion reactions | Indicated for AML patients, HSCT patients, and patients expecting multiple platelet transfusions [14] |
| Gamma irradiation | Prevents transfusion related graft-vs-host-disease (GVHD) | Allogeneic stem cell transplant patients<br>Severely immunocompromised patients |
| CMV-negative | Prevents CMV infections | Severely immunocompromised patients |
| Volume reduced | Concentrated platelets with reduced volume via centrifugation | Severely fluid overloaded patients |

**Complications of Platelet Transfusion**

| Complication | Cause/Description | Prevention |
|---|---|---|
| Infection | Transmission of blood borne pathogens from Infected/contaminated donor | Screening and testing of donors, administration of CMV-negative platelet concentrates |
| Febrile transfusion reactions | Transfusion of leukocyte rich platelets. Patients present with fever, chills, rigors, and nausea[65] | Leukoreduction, premedication with acetaminophen and diphenhydramine |
| Anaphylactic reactions | Antibodies in patients reacting with IgA | Premedication with acetaminophen, diphenhydramine, and hydrocortisone. For documented anaphylactic transfusion reactions, platelets may need to be washed |
| Alloimmunization | Chronically transfused patients develop antibodies to HLA class I antigens expressed by platelets resulting to refractoriness or decreased post transfusion platelet increments.[107] | Leukoreduction via filtration and UVB irradiation of platelet concentrate; transfusion of HLA-compatible and crossmatched platelets to alloimmunized patients[14]<br>For severely alloimmunized patients with rare HLA types, the following are administered to increase platelet response: IVIG, vinblastine, staphylococcal protein A, cyclosporin A[107] |
| Graft-vs-host disease | Engraftment of donor leukocytes in severely immunocompromised patients | Irradiation of platelets |

*Source:* Data from Mackman et al[14]; Schiffer et al[28]; Slichter[65]; Slichter et al[106]; and Stroneck and Rebulla.[107]

transfusion in an attempt to minimize platelet destruction; premedication may also consist of corticosteroids and antihistamines. Demerol may be given if the patient is having shaking chills.

Patients with hypersplenism who are receiving platelet transfusions will have a reduced recovery of circulating platelets that is generally proportionate to the size of the spleen. If platelets are transfused while the patient is actively bleeding, increased increments will not be detectable in blood counts. Instead, the effectiveness of platelet transfusions is determined by clinical improvement and control of the bleeding.

The preparation and storage of platelets are also important factors in determining the quality of the platelet transfusion. To be most effective, platelets must be fresh and metabolically active. Maximum effectiveness remains for as long as 6 hours after platelets are obtained. When platelets are properly collected and preserved, however, they can be stored for as long as 5 days.[28]

The responses to platelet transfusion measured are platelet increments, intervals during platelet transfusion, and platelet refractoriness.[106] Platelet increments are usually measured at 60 minutes after the transfusion.[27] Table 29-10[17,28,65,106,107] details the practical aspects of platelet transfusion. Table 29-11[67,108] describes management of platelet transfusion reactions. For patients with active bleeding persistently with poor platelet increments despite strategies such as transfusion of HLA-compatible or cross matched patients, the following

**TABLE 29-11**

**Management of Platelet Transfusion Reaction**

| Reaction Type | Onset | Pathophysiology | Symptoms | Management |
|---|---|---|---|---|
| Acute intravascular hemolytic reaction | Within 15 minutes | Immune-mediated lysis of transfused red cells due to major blood incompatibility | Fever<br>Chills/rigors<br>Dyspnea<br>Hypotension<br>Tachycardia<br>Flushing<br>Vomiting<br>Lower back pain<br>Oliguria<br>Hemoglobinuria<br>Shock | 1. Stop transfusion immediately.<br>2. Notify physician.<br>3. Obtain vital sign and pulse oximetry.<br>4. Maintain airway<br>5. Administer epinephrine, corticosteroids, or antihistamines for allergic reactions<br>6. Administer 0.9 NaCl fluid diuresis to prevent acute oliguric renal failure<br>7. Administer vasopressors for blood pressure support.<br>8. Administer bronchodilators and oxygen therapy for respiratory support.<br>9. Follow institution protocols for transfusion reaction work-up |
| Febrile nonhemolytic transfusion reaction | Immediate to 6 hours post transfusion | Reaction to leukocytes contaminating platelet product | Fevers<br>Rigors/chills<br>Pallor<br>Flushing | • Perform clerical check comparing patient name, medical record number, to platelet unit<br>• Return remaining platelet product to blood bank for further testing<br>• Draw blood for repeat compatibility testing<br>• Send urine for hemoglobinuria<br>10. Monitor renal status, BUN, creatinine |
| Anaphylactic reaction | Immediate to 1 hour post transfusion | Plasma components sensitization such as immunoglobulin A, cytokines | Hives<br>Pruritus<br>Dyspnea<br>Wheezing<br>Bronchospasm<br>Hypotension<br>Tachycardia<br>Shock | 11. Monitor coagulation status<br>12. Monitor for signs of hemolysis<br>For future platelet transfusions, the following may be considered:<br>1. Premedication with acetaminophen 650 mg, diphenhydramine 25–50 mg 30 minutes prior to platelet transfusion<br>2. Premedicate with hydrocortisone 100 mg 30 minutes for patients with anaphylactic reaction to platelets<br>3. Administer washed platelets (anaphylactic reaction, severe NHTR) |

*Source*: Data from Konkle[55]; and Stroneck and Rebulla.[107]

strategies are useful: frequent platelet transfusions every 4 to 6 hours, administration of IgG, fibrinolytic inhibitors, and recombinant factor VIIa.[106]

### Red blood cell therapy

In any patient, the clinical concern for the adverse physiological effects of anemia is usually the basis for considering RBC replacement. Generally, the decision to transfuse is based on the overall clinical picture, including any underlying cardiac or pulmonary conditions or any concurrent conditions that might impair the patient's tolerance of anemia. The usual transfusion threshold for RBC replacement in the bleeding patient is a hematocrit below 30%. Among the causes of anemia frequently seen in patients with cancer, the 2 most common are decreased RBC production secondary to myelosuppressive therapy and the primary disease process.

The transfusion of 1 unit of red blood cells increases the hematocrit by 3% or the hemoglobin concentration by 1 g/dL in a 70 kg nonbleeding patient. Packed erythrocytes are typically the therapy of choice. The advantage of packed red blood cells is that they provide more than 70% of the hematocrit of whole blood with only one-third of the plasma. Their use prevents unnecessary volume, electrolyte load, and anticoagulants that might otherwise be transfused.

### Plasma therapy

Human plasma, derived from whole blood products or plasmaphereis, is used to correct coagulopathy. Plasma proteins such as albumin and cryoprecipitate can be isolated and removed from plasma. Plasma derived and stored within 6 to 8 hours are referred to as fresh frozen plasma (FFP).[109] FFP, the most frequently used of the plasma products, contains all of the labile clotting factors and the plasma proteins.[43] FFP is generally administered for patient INR levels >2.0 with abnormal aPTT level. Cryoprecipitate is derived from thawed FFP where the white precipitate that adhered to the walls of the bag is resuspended and refrozen.[103] Cryoprecipitate contains vWF, factors VIII and XIII, and fibrinogen, and is administered for fibrinogen level less than 125 mg/dL. A pool of 8 bags of cryoprecipitate increase fibrinogen levels by 50 mg/dL.[103] Plasma component therapy is also administered for shock, severe bleeding, bleeding associated with infections, and management of acute DIC. Fresh frozen plasma is generally not the treatment of choice for replacing most individual clotting factors, because large volumes would be required to obtain adequate factor levels. The patient's cardiovascular and pulmonary status may preclude the use of large amounts of plasma.[105]

The amount and frequency of transfusions depend on several factors, including the severity of the deficiency, the specific factor deficiency, and the severity of bleeding. Another important dosing consideration in plasma therapy is the metabolic half-life of the plasma and plasma derivatives. Replacement therapy is given in doses high enough to compensate for the decrease in plasma level as it is metabolized. The metabolic half-life varies for each of the factors. Typically, plasma and plasma factors are infused rapidly so that the maximum plasma level is reached before metabolic changes or degradation occurs.

## CONCLUSION

Bleeding associated with cancer presents a complex clinical challenge to the nurse. It can occur as a result of the cancer itself or as a complication of the treatment of the cancer. Bleeding can be occult and chronic, or acute and life-threatening. Nurses who work with patients with cancer must be prepared to meet the complex needs of these patients. Early detection of the signs and symptoms of bleeding allows for prompt diagnosis and treatment of the bleeding, thereby preventing further complications. Management of bleeding is often as complex as the bleeding process itself. A variety of medications may be used to prevent and treat bleeding disorders. The cornerstone therapy in the prevention and management of bleeding is blood product transfusion therapy. An important adjunct to blood transfusion therapy in preventing and treating a bleeding problem is recombinant colony-stimulating factors. Exciting research continues in this area to identify as yet unknown CSFs that may benefit the patient with bleeding.

## REFERENCES


1. Avvisati G, Tirindelli MC, Annibali O. Thrombocytopenia and hemorrhagic risk in cancer patients. *Crit Rev Oncol Hematol.* 2003; 48(Suppl):S13–S16.
2. Arbuthnot C, Wilde J. Haemostatic problems in acute promyelocytic leukaemia. *Blood Rev.* 2006;20:289–297.
3. Dutcher JP, Schiffer CA, Aisner J, et al. Incidence of thrombocytopenia and serious hemorrhage among patients with solid tumors. *Cancer.* 1984;53:557–562.
4. Bacigalupo A. Haemopoietic stem cell transplants: the impact of haemorrhagic complications. *Blood Rev.* 2003;17:S6–S10.
5. Prommer E. Management of bleeding in the terminally ill patient. *Hematology.* 2005;10:167–175.
6. Gaydos LA, Frierich EJ, Mantel N. The quantitative relation between platelet count and hemorrhage in patients with acute leukemia. *N Engl J Med.* 1962;266:905–909.
7. Arnold SM, Patchell R, Lowry AM, et al. Paraneoplastic syndromes. In: DeVita VT, Hellman S, Rosenberg SA, eds. *Cancer Principles and Practice of Oncology.* 6th ed. Philadelphia, PA: Lippincott Williams & Wilkins; 2001:2511–2536.
8. Avances C, Oumaya C, Granger V, et al. Prostate cancer and acute disseminated intravascular coagulation. Therapeutic management based on three cases. *Prog Urol.* 2003;2:303–312.
9. Gobel BH. Disseminated intravascular coagulation. In: Yarbro CH, Frogge MH, Goodman M, eds. *Cancer Nursing Principles and Practice.* 5th ed. Sudbury, MA: Jones and Bartlett; 2000:869–875.

10. Stassen JM, Arnout J, Deckmyn H. The hemostatic system. *Curr Med Chem.* 2004;11:2245–2260.
11. Jurk K, Kekrel BE. Platelets: physiology and biochemistry. *Semin Thromb Hemost.* 2005:31:381–392.
12. Norris LA. Blood coagulation. *Best Pract Res Clin Obstet Gynecol.* 2003; 17:369–383.
13. Versteeg HH, Peppelenbosch MP, Spek CA. The pleiotropic effects of tissue factor: a possible role for factor VIIa-intracellular signaling? *Thromb Haemost.* 2001;89:592–593.
14. Mackman N, Tilley RE, Key NS. Role of extrinsic pathway of blood coagulation in hemostasis and thrombosis. *Arterioscler Thromb Vasc Biol.* 2007;27:1687–1693.
15. Howell DC, Laurent GJ, Chambers RC. Role of thrombin and its major cellular receptor, protease-activated receptor-1, in pulmonary fibrosis. *Biochem Soc.* 2002;30(part 2):211–216.
16. George JN, Colman RW. Overview of platelet structure and function. In: Colman RW, Clowes AW, Goldhaber SZ, et al, eds. *Hemostasis and Thrombosis: Basic Principles and Clinical Practice.* 5th ed. Philadelphia, PA: Lippincott Williams & Wilkins; 2006:437–442.
17. George JN. Platelets. *Lancet.* 2000;355:1531–1539.
18. Opalinska JB, Gewirtz AM. Thrombocytopenia due to decreased platelet production. In: Hoffman R, Benz EJ, Shattil SJ, Furie B, Cohen JH, Silberstein LE, McGlave P, eds. *Hematology: Basic Principles and Practice.* 4th ed. New York: Churchill Livingstone; 2005:321–327.
19. Blayney DW, McGuire BW, Cruickshank SE, et al. Increasing chemotherapy dose density and intensity: Phase I trials in non-small cell lung cancer and non-Hodgkin's lymphoma. *Oncologist.* 2005;10:138–149.
20. Warkentin TE, Kelton JG. Thrombocytopenia due to platelet destruction and hypersplenism. In: Hoffman R, Benz EJ, Shattil SJ, Furie B, Cohen JH, Silberstein LE, McGlave P, eds. *Hematology: Basic Principles and Practice.* 4th ed. New York: Churchill Livingstone; 2005:2305–2440.
21. Yamakado K, Nakatsuka A, Tanaka N, et al. Malignant portal venous obstructions treated by stent placement: significant factors affecting patency. *J Vasc Intern Radiol.* 2001;12:1407–1415.
22. Yamakado K, Nakatsuka A, Tanaka N, et al. Portal venous stent placement in patients with pancreatic and biliary neoplasms invading portal veins and causing portal hypertension: initial experience. *Radiology.* 2001;220:150–156.
23. Lynch MP. Idiopathic thrombocytopenic purpura. In: Lynch MP, ed. *Clinical Manual for the Oncology Advanced Practice Nurse.* Pittsburgh, PA: Oncology Nursing Press; 2001:689–691.
24. Hauswirth AW, Skrabs C, Schutzinger C, et al. Autoimmune thrombocytopenia in non-Hodgkin's lymphomas. *Haematologica.* 2008; 93:447–450.
25. Saitoh T, Matsushima T, Saito Y, et al. Hodgkin's lymphoma presenting with various immunologic abnormalities including autoimmune hepatitis, Hashimoto's thyroiditis, autoimmune haemolytic anemia, and immune thrombocytopenia. *Clin Lymphoma Myeloma.* 2008;8:62–64.
26. Kickler TS. Principles of platelet transfusion therapy. In: Hoffman R, Benz EJ, Shattil SJ, Furie B, Cohen JH, Silberstein LE, McGlave P, eds. *Hematology: Basic Principles and Practice.* 4th ed. New York: Churchill Livingstone; 2005:2433–2440.
27. Stroncek DF, Rebulla P. Platelet transfusions. *Lancet.* 2007;370: 427–438.
28. Schiffer CA, Anderson KC, Bennett CL, et al. Platelet transfusion for patients with cancer: clinical practice guidelines of the American Society of Clinical Oncology. *J Clin Oncol.* 2001;19:1519–1538.
29. Schafer AI. Thrombocytosis. *N Engl J Med.* 2004;350:1211–1219.
30. Munshi NC, Tricot G, Barlogie B. Plasma cell neoplasms. In: DeVita VT, Hellman S, Rosenberg SA, eds. *Cancer Principles and Practice of Oncology.* 6th ed. Philadelphia, PA: Lippincott Williams & Wilkins; 2001:2465–2499.
31. Rao KA. Acquired qualitative platelet defects. In: Colman RW, Clowes AW, Goldhaber SZ, et al, eds. *Hemostasis and Thrombosis: Basic Principles and Clinical Practice.* 5th ed. Philadelphia, PA: Lippincott, Williams, & Wilkins; 2006:1045–1060.
32. Liebman HA. Hemostatic defects associated with dysproteinemias. In: Hoffman R, Benz EJ, Shattil SJ, Furie B, Cohen JH, Silberstein LE, McGlave P, eds. *Hematology: Basic Principles and Practice.* 4th ed. Churchill Livingstone; 2005:2183–2188.
33. Gralnick A, Ginsberg D. Von Willebrand's disease. In: Beutler E, Lichtman MA, Coller BS, Kipps TJ, eds. *Williams Hematology.* 5th ed. New York: McGraw-Hill; 1995:1458–1480.
34. Patel P. Vitamin K deficiency. Updated June 20, 2006. http://www.emedicine.com/MED/topic2385.htm. Accessed February 2, 2010.
35. Kumar S, Pruthi RK, Nichols WL. Acquired von Willebrand disease. *Mayo Clin Proc.* 2002;77:181–187.
36. Makoni SN, Laber DA. Clinical spectrum of myelophthisis in cancer patients. *Am J Hematol.* 2004;76:92–93.
37. Elting LS, Rubenstein EB, Martin CG, et al. Incidence, cost, and outcomes of bleeding and chemotherapy dose modification among solid tumor patients with chemotherapy-induced thrombocytopenia. *J Clin Oncol.* 2001;19:1137–1146.
38. Smith MR, Khan N. Transfusion therapy, bleeding, and clotting. In: Skeel RT, ed. *Handbook of Cancer Chemotherapy.* 5th ed. Philadelphia, PA: Lippincott Williams & Wilkins; 1999:63–143.
39. Idec Pharmaceuticals Corporation. *A Practical Guide for the Healthcare Professional.* San Diego, CA: Author; 2002.
40. Tuinstra N. Outpatient administration of radiolabeled monoclonal antibodies. *Clin J Oncol Nurs.* 2003;7:106–108.
41. Drews RE. Critical issues in hematology: anemia, thrombocytopenia, coagulation, and blood product transfusion in critically ill patients. *Clin Chest Med.* 2003;24:607–622.
42. Reddy JC, Shuman MA, Aster RH. Quinine and quinidine-induced thrombocytopenia: a great imitator. *Arch Intern Med.* 2004;164:218–220.
43. Cooney MF. Heparin-induced thrombocytopenia: advances in diagnosis and treatment. *Crit Care Nurse.* 2006;26:30–36.
44. Hirsh J, Heddle N, Kelton JG. Treatment of heparin-induced thrombocytopenia: a critical review. *Arch Intern Med.* 2004;164:361–369.
45. PDR Nurses Drug Handbook. Clifton Park, NY: Delmar Learning, a division of Thomson Learning; 2003.
46. Verburg KM, Maziasz TJ, Weiner E, et al. COX-2-specific inhibitors: definition of a new therapeutic concept. *Am J Ther.* 2001;8:49–64.
47. Cotran RS, Kumar V, Collins T. Red cells and bleeding disorders. In: Cotran RS, Kumar V, Collins T, eds. *Pathological Basis of Disease.* 6th ed. Philadelphia, PA: WB Saunders; 1999:601–643.
48. Abebe W. Herbal medications: potential for adverse reactions with analgesic drugs. *J Clin Pharm Ther.* 2002;27:391–401.
49. Park MS, Kim BC, Kim IK, et al. Cerebral infarction in IgG multiple myeloma with hyperviscosity. *J Korean Med Sci.* 2005;20:699–701.
50. Mullen E, Mendez N. Hyperviscosity syndrome in patients with multiple myeloma. *Oncol Nurs Forum.* 2008;35:350–352.
51. Gobel BH. Bleeding. In: Yarbro CH, Frogge MH, Goodman M, eds. *Cancer Nursing: Principles and Practice.* 6th ed. Sudbury, MA: Jones and Bartlett; 2005:723–740.
52. Friend PH, Pruett J. Bleeding and thrombotic complications. In: Yarbro CH, Frogge MH, Goodman M. *Cancer Symptom Management.* 3rd ed. Sudbury, MA: Jones and Bartlett; 2004:233, 251.
53. National Institutes of Health. Common terminology criteria for adverse events (CTCAE) version 3.0. http://ctep.cancer.gov/protocol Development/electronic_applications/docs/ctcaev3.pdf. Accessed February 12, 2010.
54. Comis R. ECOG Common toxicity criteria. Updated June 15, 2007 http://ecog.dfci.harvard.edu/general/ctc.pdf. Accessed February 13, 2010.
55. Konkle BA. Clinical approaches to the bleeding patient. In: Colman RW, Clowes AW, Goldhaber SZ, et al, eds. *Hemostasis and Thrombosis: Basic Principles and Clinical Practice.* 5th ed. Philadelphia, PA: Lippincott Williams & Wilkins; 2006:1147–1158.
56. Deloughery TC. Management of acute hemorrhage. In: Colman RW, Clowes AW, Goldhaber SZ, et al, eds. *Hemostasis and Thrombosis: Basic Principles and Clinical Practice.* 5th ed. Philadelphia, PA: Lippincott Williams & Wilkins; 2006:1159–1172.

57. Seligsohn U, Kaushansky K. Classification, clinical manifestations, and evaluations of disorders of hemostasis: overview. In: Lichtman MA, Beutler E, Kipps TJ, et al, eds. *Williams Hematology.* 7th ed. McGraw Hill Companies; 2006:1741–1748.
58. Rand JH, Senzel L. Laboratory evaluation of hemostatic disorders. In: Hoffman R, Benz EJ, Shattil SJ, Furie B, Cohen JH, Silberstein LE, McGlave P, eds. *Hematology: Basic Principles and Practice.* 4th ed. New York: Churchill Livingstone; 2005:2001–2010.
59. Furie B. Presentation of bleeding disorders. In: Furie B, Cassileth PA, Atkins MB, Mayer RJ, eds. *Clinical Hematology and Oncology.* Philadelphia, PA: Churchill Livingstone; 2003:265–271.
60. Bick RL. Disseminated intravascular coagulation: pathophysiological mechanisms and manifestations. *Semin Thromb Haemost.* 1998;24:3–18.
61. Damron BH, Brant JM, Belansky HB, Friend PJ, Samsanow S, Schaal A. Putting evidence into practice: prevention and management of bleeding in patients with cancer. *Clin J Oncol Nurs.* 2009;13:573–583.
62. Reed E. Critical issues in hematology: anemia, thrombocytopenia, coagulopathy, and blood product transfusions in critically ill patients. *Clin Chest Med.* 2003;24:607–622.
63. Pisciotto PT, Benson K, Hume H, et al. Prophylactic versus therapeutic platelet transfusion practices in hematology and/or oncology patients. *Transfusion.* 1995;35:498–502.
64. Norfolk DR, Ancliff PJ, Contreras M, et al. Consensus conference on platelet transfusion. Royal College of Physicians of Edinburgh, 27–28 November, 1997. *Br J Haematol.* 1998;101:609–617.
65. Slichter SJ. Evidence-based platelet transfusion guidelines. *Hematology.* 2007; 2007:172–178.
66. Demetri GD. Pharmacologic treatment options in patients with thrombocytopenia. *Semin Hematol.* 2000;37(Suppl 4):11–18.
67. Reid TJ, Rentas FJ, Ketchum LH. Platelet substitutes in the management of thrombocytopenia. *Curr Hematol Rep.* 2003;2:165–170.
68. Vadhan-Raj S. Clinical experience with recombinant human thrombopoietin in chemotherapy-induced thrombocytopenia. *Semin Hematol.* 2000;37(Suppl 4):28–34.
69. Chu DT, Xu BH, Song ST, et al. Recombinant human interleukin 11 (Mega) promotes thrombopoiesis in cancer patients with chemotherapy-induced myelosuppression. *Zhongguo Shi Yan Xue Ye Xue Za Zhi.* 2001;9:314–317.
70. Gordon MS, McCaskill-Stevens WJ, Battiato LA, et al. A phase I trial of recombinant human interleukin-11 (Neumega rhIL-11 growth factor) in women with breast cancer receiving chemotherapy. *Blood.* 1996;87:3615–3624.
71. Orazi A, Copper RJ, Tong J, et al. Effects of recombinant human interleukin-11 (neumega rhIL-11 growth factor) on megakaryocytopoiesis in human bone marrow. *Exp Hematol.* 1996;24:1289–1297.
72. Isaacs C, Robert NJ, Bailey FA, et al. Randomized placebo-controlled study of recombinant human interleukin-11 to prevent chemotherapy-induced thrombocytopenia in patients with breast cancer receiving dose-intensive cyclophosphamide and doxorubicin. *J Clin Oncol.* 1997;15:3368–3377.
73. Cripe LD, Rader K, Tallman MS, et al. Phase II trial of subcutaneous recombinant human interleukin-11 with subcutaneous recombinant granulocyte-macrophage colony stimulating factor in patients with acute myeloid leukemia (AML) receiving high-dose cytarabine during induction: ECOG 3997. *Leuk Res.* 2006;30:823–827.
74. Montero AJ, Estrov Z, Freireich EJ, et al. Phase II study of low dose interleukin-11 in patients with myelodysplastic syndrome. *Leuk Lymphoma.* 2006;47:2049–2054.
75. Cairo MS, Davenport V, Bessmertny O, et al. Phase I/II dose escalation of recombinant human interleukin-11 following ifosfamide, carboplatin and etoposide in children, adolescent, and young adults with solid tumors or lymphoma: a clinical, haematological and biological study. *Br J Haematol.* 2004;128:49–58.
76. Bhatia M, Davenport V, Cairo MS. The role of interleukin-11 to prevent chemotherapy-induced thrombocytopenia in patients with solid tumors, lymphoma, acute myeloid leukemia and bone marrow failure syndromes. *Leuk Lymphoma.* 2007;48:9–15.
77. Jelkman W. Erythropoietin: structure, control of production, and function. *Physiol Rev.* 1992;72:449–489.
78. Erslev AJ. Erythropoietin. *N Engl J Med.* 1991;324:1339–1344.
79. Erickson N, Quesenberry PJ. Regulation of erythropoiesis. *Med Clin North Am.* 1992;76:745–755.
80. Cases A. Darbepoietin alfa: a novel erythropoiesis-stimulating protein. *Drugs Today.* 2003;39:477–496.
81. Tang YD, Rinderm HM, Katz SD. Effects of recombinant human erythropoietin on antiplatelet action of aspirin and clopidogrel in healthy subjects: results of a double-blind, placebo-controlled randomized trial. *Am Heart J.* 2007;154:494.e1–494.e7.
82. Homoncik M, Jilma-Stohlawetz P, Schmid M, et al. Erythropoietin increases platelet reactivity and platelet counts in patients with alcoholic liver cirrhosis: a randomized, double-blind, placebo-controlled study. *Aliment Pharmacol Ther.* 2004;20:437–443.
83. Levy B, Arnason JE, Bussel JB. The use of second-generation thrombopoietic agents for chemotherapy-induced thrombocytopenia. *Curr Opin Oncol.* 2008;20:690–696.
84. Andemariam B, Psaila B, Bussel JB. Novel thrombopoietic agents. *Hematology.* 2007;2007:106–113.
85. Peeters K, Stassen J-M, Collen D, et al. Emerging treatments for thrombocytopenia: increasing platelet production. *Drug Discov Today.* 2008;13:798–806.
86. George JN, Terrel DR. Novel thrombopoietic agents: a new era for management of patients with thrombocytopenia. *Haematologica.* 2008;93:1445–1449.
87. Schuchter LM, Hensley ML, Meropol NJ, et al. 2002 Update of recommendations for the use of chemotherapy and radiotherapy protectants: clinical practice guidelines of the American Society of Clinical Oncology. *J Clin Oncol.* 2002;20:2895–2903.
88. Erikci AA, Ozturk A, Karagoz B, et al. Results of combination therapy with amifostine, pentoxifylline, ciprofloxacin and dexamethasone in patients with myelodysplastic syndrome and acute myeloid leukemia (Abstract). *Hematology.* 2008;13:289–292.
89. Samudrala S. Topical hemostatic agents in surgery: a surgeon's perspective. *AORN J.* 2008;88:S2–S11.
90. Pereira J, Phan T. Management of bleeding in patients with advanced cancer. *Oncologist.* 2004;9:561–570.
91. Jayakumar S, Jayakumar S. Iron-dextran anaphylactic-like reaction with a negative test dose and subsequent successful administration of 3 doses. *Dialysis Transpl.* 2000;29:198, 200.
92. Camp-Sorrell D. Chemotherapy: toxicity management. In: Yarbro CH, Frogge MH, Goodman M, eds. *Cancer Nursing Principles and Practice.* 5th ed. Sudbury, MA: Jones and Bartlett; 2000:444–486.
93. Kauffman CR, Mahvash A, Kopetz S, et al. Partial splenic embolization for cancer patients with thrombocytopenia requiring systemic chemotherapy. *Cancer.* 2008;112:2283–2288.
94. Longhurst HJ, O'Grady C, Evans G, et al. Anti-D immunoglobulin treatment for thrombocytopenia associated with primary antibody deficiency. *J Clin Pathol.* 2002;55:64–66.
95. Rodeghiero F. First line therapies for immune thrombocytopenic purpura: re-evaluating the need to treat. *Eur J Hematol. Suppl.* 2008;69:19–26.
96. Arnold DM, Kelton JG. Current options for the treatment of idiopathic thrombocytopenic purpura. *Semin Hematol.* 2007;44: S12–S23.
97. Zimmer J, Andres E, Noel E, et al. Current management of adult idiopathic thrombocytopenia purpura in practice: a cohort study of 201 patients from a single center. *Clin Lab Haematol.* 2004;26:137–142.
98. Maloisel F, Andres E, Zimmer J, et al. Danazol therapy in patients with idiopathic thrombocytopenia purpura: long-term results. *Am J Med.* 2004;116:590–594.
99. Stasi R, Provan D. Management of idiopathic thrombocytopenia purpura in adults. *Mayo Clin Proc.* 2004;79:504–522.
100. Carpenter CL. Platelet disorders: acquired and congenital. In: Furie B, Cassileth PA, Atkins MB, Mayer RJ, eds. *Clinical Hematology and Oncology Presentation, Diagnosis, and Treatment.* Philadelphia, PA: Churchill Livingstone; 2003:485–497.

101. Kessler CM, Tfayli A. Coagulation disorders: acquired and congenital. In: Furie B, Cassileth PA, Atkins MB, Mayer RJ, eds. *Clinical Hematology and Oncology Presentation, Diagnosis, and Treatment.* Philadelphia, PA: Churchill Livingstone; 2003:498–510.
102. Chiu J, Ketchum LH, Reid TJ. Transfusion-sparing hemostatic agents. *Curr Opin Hematol.* 2002;9:544–550.
103. Green D. Management of bleeding complications of hematologic malignancies. *Semin Thromb Hemost.* 2007;33:427–434.
104. Johnson SR, Ernst ME, Graber MA. Commonly overlooked sources of Vitamin K. *Ann Pharmacother.* 2003;37:302.
105. Perrotta PL, Synder EL. Transfusion therapy. In: DeVita VT, Hellman S, Rosenberg SA, eds. *Cancer Principles and Practice of Oncology.* 6th ed. Philadelphia, PA: Lippincott Williams & Wilkins; 2001:2753–2766.
106. Slichter SJ, Davis K, Enright H, et al. Factors affecting posttransfusion platelet increments, platelet refractoriness, and platelet transfusion intervals in thrombocytopenic patients. *Blood.* 2005;105:4106–4114.
107. Stroncek DF, Rebulla P. Platelet transfusions. *Lancet.* 2007;370:427–438.
108. Wu Y, Snyder EL. Transfusion reactions. In: Hoffman R, Benz EJ, Shattil SJ, Furie B, Cohen JH, Silberstein LE, McGlave P, eds. *Hematology: Basic Principles and Practice.* 4th ed. New York: Churchill Livingstone; 2005:2515–2526.
109. Stanworth SJ. The evidence-based use of FFP and cryoprecipitate for abnormalities of coagulation tests and clinical coagulopathy. *Hematology.* 2007;2007:179–176.

CHAPTER 30

*Sandra A. Mitchell, PhD, CRNP, AOCN®*

# Cancer-Related Fatigue

## SCOPE OF THE PROBLEM

Cancer-related fatigue (CRF) is a prevalent and disabling symptom experienced by both patients with cancer and cancer survivors. Studies suggest that CRF is a multifaceted condition characterized by diminished energy and an increased need to rest, disproportionate to any recent change in activity level, and accompanied by a range of other characteristics, including generalized weakness, diminished mental concentration, insomnia or hypersomnia, and emotional reactivity.[1] Decrements in physical, social, cognitive, and vocational functioning,[2–5] adverse mood changes,[6] sleep disturbances,[7–9] treatment noncompliance,[10] and emotional and spiritual distress for both the patients and their family members[9,11–13] are among the consequences of CRF.

However, studies suggest that the identification, and evaluation of fatigue in patients with cancer is suboptimal; that fatigue is undertreated; and that healthcare professionals may not fully appreciate the degree of distress and functional loss that fatigue produces.[14–16] Identified barriers to communication between patients and their clinicians about fatigue include the clinician's failure to offer interventions (47%), patients' lack of awareness of effective treatments for fatigue (43%), a desire on the patient's part to treat fatigue without medications (40%), and a tendency to be stoic about fatigue to avoid labeling as a "complainer" (28%).[2,17] Other barriers to the recognition and management of fatigue may include the fact that fatigue is largely invisible and not life-threatening, and a tendency for clinicians and patients to view CRF as an inevitable consequence of illness.

This chapter reviews the state of the science concerning CRF, and offers guidance for practice, education, and research. Four major content areas relative to CRF are addressed: (1) definition, incidence, etiology; (2) pathophysiological aspects; (3) screening and evaluation of the patient with CRF; and (4) evidence-based pharmacological and nonpharmacological interventions to prevent and manage fatigue during and following cancer and its treatment.

## DEFINITION

Though many different definitions of CRF have been proposed, the National Comprehensive Cancer Network (NCCN) defines CRF as a distressing, persistent, and subjective sense of tiredness or exhaustion related to cancer or cancer treatment that is not proportional to recent activity and interferes with usual functioning.[18] Based on the 10th International Classification of Disease (ICD-10) criteria for the diagnosis of CRF (see Table 30-1), CRF is of a markedly different quality and severity from ordinary fatigue, adversely impacts function, and is unrelieved by rest or sleep.[19] To make the diagnosis of CRF, fatigue must be persistent, and be accompanied by associated symptoms such as increasing need for rest, limb heaviness, diminished concentration, inertia, emotional lability, and postexertional malaise. One must also be fairly certain that the underlying cause is cancer or its treatment.

**TABLE 30-1**

**International Classification of Diseases (10th Edition) ICD-10 Criteria for Cancer-Related Fatigue**

Six (or more) of the following symptoms have been present every day or nearly every day during the same 2-week period in the past month, and at least one of the symptoms is (A1) significant fatigue.

A1. Significant fatigue, diminished energy, or increased need to rest, disproportionate to any recent change in activity level
A2. Complaints of generalized weakness or limb heaviness
A3. Diminished concentration or attention
A4. Decreased motivation or interest to engage in usual activities
A5. Insomnia or hypersomnia
A6. Experience of sleep as unrefreshing or nonrestorative
A7. Perceived need to struggle to overcome inactivity
A8. Marked emotional reactivity (eg, sadness, frustration, irritability) to feeling fatigued
A9. Difficulty completing daily tasks attributed to feeling fatigued
A10. Perceived problems with short-term memory
A11. Postexertional malaise lasting several hours
B. The symptoms cause clinically significant distress or impairment in social, occupational, or other important areas of functioning.
C. There is evidence from the history, physical examination, or laboratory findings that the symptoms are a consequence of cancer or cancer therapy.
D. The symptoms are not primarily a consequence of comorbid psychiatric disorders such as major depression, somatization disorder, somatoform disorder, or delirium

*Source*: Cella et al.[1] Used with permission.

The clinical expression of CRF is multidimensional, making evaluation of a patient experiencing fatigue challenging. An inherently subjective condition, fatigue may be experienced and reported differently by each individual. Qualitative studies of fatigue underscore the fact that the cancer fatigue experience is unlike any other fatigue they have previously experienced, and suggest that its unpredictability and refractoriness to self-management strategies contribute to the distress associated with CRF.[20,21] Personality and coping style may also influence the experience of CRF.[22] Some patients identify the main features of their fatigue as a loss of efficiency, mental fogginess, inertia, and that sleep is not restorative, while others describe an excessive need to rest, the inability to recover promptly from exertion, or muscle heaviness and weakness. Further research is needed to determine whether these represent variable features of fatigue, suggest the presence of fatigue subtypes, or are the cause or sequelae of fatigue.[23,24] Efforts continue to be directed toward clarifying what are the defining features of fatigue[25] and determining how CRF may be distinguished from syndromes such as depression, cognitive dysfunction, or asthenia that have overlapping symptoms[26–31] or may share neurophysiological mechanisms.[32,33]

## INCIDENCE

Fatigue is one of the most commonly reported symptoms experienced by patients receiving treatment for cancer, and it often persists beyond the conclusion of active treatment and at the end of life.[10,16,19,34,35] Depending upon how CRF is defined and measured, prevalence estimates across the disease trajectory range from 25% to 99%.[36] A recent survey of more than 500 patients and nearly 100 clinicians found that across all cancer types, fatigue is ranked as the most important symptom or concern.[37] Longitudinal and comparative studies indicate that fatigue may also be a significant problem for cancer survivors, with many survivors reporting fatigue scores higher than that of an age matched general population.[7,35,38–41] In the setting of advanced cancer, almost 60% of patients experience fatigue, with one quarter reporting severe fatigue.[42] Fatigue may occur as an isolated symptom or as one component within a cluster of other symptoms, including depression, pain, sleep disturbance, and menopausal symptoms.[43–48]

## ETIOLOGY AND RISK FACTORS

The etiology and risk factors for CRF are multifactorial. Though the relationships between fatigue and treatment with radiation, chemotherapy, hematopoietic stem cell transplantation, hormonal, and biological agents have been explored, few consistent relationships between fatigue and treatment-related variables such as dose-intensity, radiation fractionation schedule, and time since treatment completion have been observed.[35] Associations between the occurrence and severity of CRF and demographic variables such as gender, age, marital status, employment status have also not been identified consistently. Studies suggest that fatigue may be related to anemia, myeloid suppression, mood disorder, concurrent symptoms such as pain, sleep disturbances, electrolyte disturbances, cardiopulmonary, hepatic or renal dysfunction, hypothyroidism, hypogonadism, adrenal insufficiency, infection, malnutrition, deconditioning, and the side effects of drugs that act on the central nervous system.[36,49–57] Accumulating evidence also suggests that gene polymorphisms, altered circadian rhythmicity, immune dysregulation, and proinflammatory cytokine activity[58-65] may directly or indirectly contribute to CRF.

## PSYCHOPHYSIOLOGICAL MODELS OF CRF

Several different explanatory models of the psychophysiology of CRF have been proposed. Many of these models utilize similar constructs. These conceptual models can be organized into 4 thematic groups: (1) energy balance/energy analysis models, (2) fatigue as a stress response models, (3) neuroendocrine-based regulatory fatigue models, and (4) hybrid models.

*Energy balance/energy analysis models* depict energy as the major variable in fatigue and alterations in the balance among intake, metabolism, and expenditure of energy as factors in producing fatigue. Examples of this thematic group of models include Piper's integrated fatigue model,[66] Irvine's energy analysis model,[67] and Winningham's psychobiological entropy model.[68] *Fatigue as a stress response models* posit that tiredness, fatigue, and exhaustion form an adaptational continuum of response to stress. Each state along this continuum from tiredness to exhaustion may be distinguished by different behavioral and symptom characteristics. Examples of models included in this thematic class include fatigue models proposed by Aistairs,[69] Rhoten,[70] Glaus,[71] and Olson.[72,73] *Neuroendocrine-based regulatory fatigue* models hypothesize that the multiple dimensions of fatigue are explained by dysregulation in the function of neuroendocrine-based regulatory systems including the hypothalamic-pituitary axis (HPA), circadian rhythms, and neuroimmune system transmitter secretion and function. Examples of models based on neuroendocrine dysregulation include those that have been proposed by Lee,[33] Payne,[74] and Schubert.[62] More recently, 2 models that represent *hybrid* approaches have been proposed. Based on their earlier work, Olson et al[73] have recently proposed a model of CRF proposing that stressors associated with cancer and its treatment trigger declines in 4 systems—cognitive function, sleep quality, nutrition, and muscle endurance—and that these declines impair adaptation. Their model suggests that an understanding of the characteristics and etiologic mechanisms of CRF will emerge through study of the interactions among these 4 systems. Al-Majid and Gray[75] have also recently developed a model incorporating the biological, psychobehavioral, and functional variables implicated in the induction of CRF, and suggest the application of this model to elucidate the mechanisms by which exercise may ameliorate CRF. Models in all 4 thematic classes may be helpful in guiding the development and evaluation of interventions to limit and manage fatigue and to reduce its deleterious impact on health-related quality of life. These models may also contribute to defining a minimum data set for studies of CRF and to generating testable hypotheses for continued research into the problem of CRF.

## EVALUATION OF THE PATIENT WITH CANCER-RELATED FATIGUE

Evaluation of the patient at risk for or experiencing CRF can be separated into 2 aspects: (1) routine, periodic screening of all patients to identify the presence of CRF and gauge its severity; and (2) in patients with moderate or severe CRF, a detailed evaluation of the characteristics, consequences, and potential contributing factors. A wide range of approaches to the assessment of CRF are available, including single items that gauge fatigue severity; instruments that were designed specifically to evaluate CRF from a multidimensional perspective; and single items or subscales that measure relevant aspects of the fatigue experience that have been drawn from measures of quality of life, psychosocial adjustment, mood or self-reported health status.

Screening patients with CRF is fundamental to improving fatigue management and is a key component of care quality. Although there is currently no consensus concerning the optimal method or frequency to screen for CRF in the clinical setting, the high prevalence of CRF supports a conclusion that routine screening for CRF should occur at regular intervals throughout treatment, initial post-treatment follow-up, long-term follow-up during survivorship, and at the end-of-life. There is accumulating evidence to suggest that single-item measures to screen for fatigue are rapid and sensitive, and can be applied efficiently in the clinic to identify individuals who would benefit from more systematic evaluation.[76–79] In selecting a measure for screening, consideration must be given to what response frame (ie, past 24 hour, past 7 days, past month) has the most clinical relevance for a specific patient population and will be least affected by biases of recall or by transient changes in CRF severity. Technological advances in item-banks, computerized-adapted testing, and other digital formats[80–83] may contribute in improving the efficiency, precision, and ease of interpretation of screening measures for CRF.

Although a single-item measure may provide rapid assessment of general fatigue or serve as a screening tool, evidence suggests that single-item measures do not fully capture all the dimensions of fatigue.[84] There is good consensus in the literature that the experience of fatigue can be separated into a sensory dimension (eg, fatigue severity, persistence), a physiological dimension (eg, leg weakness, diminished mental concentration), an affective dimension (eg, sadness, depression, fear), and a behavioral dimension (eg, reduction in the performance of needed or valued activities). More than 20 self-report measures (including single item measures, multi-item unidimensional scales, and multidimensional inventories) have been developed to measure fatigue in patients with cancer.[85–87] Unidimensional fatigue measures typically focus on the severity of fatigue, although multi-item unidimensional scales may also ask about the severity of other symptoms such as exhaustion, tiredness, or weakness. Examples of unidimensional measures of fatigue include quality-of-life measures such as the Functional Assessment of Cancer Therapy Fatigue (FACT-F) and the fatigue subscale of the European Organization for Research and Treatment of Cancer Quality-of-Life Questionnaire (EORTC-QLQ-C-30). Measures of symptoms, health, mood state, or psychosocial adjustment such as the Medical Outcomes Study Short Form-36 (SF-36), Profile of Mood States, Rotterdam Symptom Checklist, Brief Symptom Inventory, and Symptom Distress Scale also include single items that address fatigue or have subscales that reflect fatigue, vigor, or vitality. When selecting a measure of fatigue, it is important to keep in mind that other descriptions of fatigue such as weakness, tiredness, or the absence of vigor may not necessarily be equated with fatigue. Multidimensional fatigue measures provide information about this full range of characteristics beyond fatigue presence and intensity. Table 30-2 summarizes the included dimensions, number of items, scaling, and other features for several of the most commonly used unidimensional and multidimensional measures of cancer-related fatigue.

Consideration of the measurement properties and strengths and limitations of these instruments including reliability, validity, specificity, sensitivity to change, recall period, respondent burden, translation in multiple languages, and the availability of normative values to aid interpretation should be used to guide decisions about the utility of a measure for specific clinical or research purposes.[28,51,103–106] Ecological momentary assessment (a technique that elicits a repeated, real-time measurement of behaviors or experiences as they occur in the naturalistic setting of an individual's day-to-day life) may overcome methodological limitations including recall bias and the influence of current context on self-report of fatigue. This technique has been recently applied to assess fatigue outcomes in a research context.[107,108]

The NCCN guidelines recommend that CRF be assessed using a 2-tiered approach.[109] Every patient should be screened for the presence of fatigue, and if present, fatigue should be assessed quantitatively on a 0 to 10 scale (0 = no fatigue and 10 = worst fatigue imaginable). Those patients with a severity of more than 4 should be further evaluated by history and physical examination.

As outlined in Table 30-3, a detailed history includes the presence, intensity, and pervasiveness of fatigue, its course over time, the factors that exacerbate or relieve fatigue, and the impact of fatigue on functioning and level of distress. Clinicians can obtain valuable information about the consequences of CRF by exploring the effects of CRF on self-esteem, mood, and the ability to perform activities of daily living, fulfill important roles as parent, spouse, and worker, and relate to family and friends. Inquiring about the self-management interventions the patient has tried for fatigue, and their effectiveness can be helpful in tailoring recommendations for fatigue management.

In evaluating the patient with CRF, it is also important to screen for etiological or potentiating factors that may contribute to CRF. These are summarized in Table 30-4 and include hypothyroidism, hypogonadism, adrenal insufficiency, cardiomyopathy, pulmonary dysfunction, anemia, neutropenia, sleep disturbance, fluid and electrolyte imbalances, emotional distress, and uncontrolled concurrent

**TABLE 30-2**

**Instruments to Measure Cancer-Related Fatigue**

| Measure | Dimensions of Fatigue Evaluated | Number of Items | Scaling | Features | Source for More Information |
|---|---|---|---|---|---|
| Brief fatigue inventory | Severity and impact of fatigue | 9 | 11 point Likert scale | Available in multiple languages | Mendoza et al 1999[88] |
| Fatigue numerical scale | Severity of fatigue | 2 | 100 mm linear analogue scale | | Okuyama et al[89] |
| Cancer-related fatigue distress scale | Consequences of fatigue relative to physical, social, psychospiritual distress | 20 | 11 point Likert scale | | Holley[90] |
| Chalder fatigue scale | Fatigue severity, associated distress, self-efficacy for coping, and the extent to which fatigue was overwhelming, uncontrollable, unpredictable, and abnormal. | 7 | 100 mm linear analogue scale | | Armes et al[91] |
| Functional assessment of cancer therapy fatigue | Physical, affective and cognitive dimensions of fatigue and consequences for daily functioning | 13 | 5 point Likert scale | Available in multiple languages; Norms for comparison with health and cancer samples available | Yellen et al[92] |
| Cancer fatigue scale | Physical, affective, and cognitive dimensions of fatigue | 15 | 5 point Likert scale | Available in multiple languages | Okuyama et al[89] |
| Fatigue symptom inventory | Severity, frequency, daily pattern of fatigue and its interference with quality of life | 13 | 11 point Likert scale | | Hann et al[93] |
| Fatigue severity scale | Single item fatigue severity score and impact of fatigue on daily functioning | 10 | 7 point Likert scale for impact items; single item 100 mm linear analogue scale for severity | | Krupp et al[94] |
| Fatigue scale adolescent | Multiple dimensions of fatigue including affective, behavioral, somatic, and cognitive aspects of fatigue and consequences for daily functioning | 14 | 5 point Likert scale | | Hinds et al[95] |
| Multidimensional fatigue symptom inventory | Multiple dimensions of fatigue: global experience, somatic symptoms, cognitive symptoms, affective symptoms, and behavioral symptoms | | | | Stein et al[96] |
| Multidimensional fatigue inventory | Multiple dimensions of fatigue: global experience, somatic symptoms, cognitive symptoms, affective symptoms and behavioral symptoms | 20 | 5 point Likert scale | Available in multiple languages | Smets et al[97] |
| Multidimensional assessment of fatigue | Fatigue severity, timing, distress and interference | 16 | 100 mm linear analogue scale; 2 additional items are multiple choice | | Belza[98] |

*(Continued)*

**TABLE 30-2**

**Instruments to Measure Cancer-Related Fatigue (*Continued*)**

| Measure | Dimensions of Fatigue Evaluated | Number of Items | Scaling | Features | Source for More Information |
|---|---|---|---|---|---|
| Piper fatigue scale—revised | Multiple dimensions of fatigue including severity/behavioral, sensory, affective/meaning, cognitive/mood | 22 | 11 point Likert scale | | Piper et al[99] |
| Rhoten fatigue scale | Fatigue severity | 1 | 11 point linear analogue scale | | Schneider[100] |
| Schwartz cancer fatigue scale | Physical and perceptual fatigue | 6 | 5 point Likert scale | | Schwartz[101] |
| Lee fatigue scale | Fatigue, energy | 18 | Linear analogue scale scaled from 0–10 | | Lee et al[102] |

symptoms. Evaluation should also include whether disease progression or recurrence could be among the causes of fatigue. The medication profile should also be reviewed to identify specific classes of medications (including over-the-counter medications) with a sedative side-effect profile. Medications with a sedative side effect profile may include opioid analgesics, sedative–hypnotic agents such secobarbital, benzodiazepines such as lorazepam, and anxiolytics such as buspirone. A number of antidepressant agents, antiemetics, antihistamines, and anticonvulsant agents such as gabapentin, phenobarbital, or tegretol also have the potential to produce sedation and daytime sleepiness and fatigue. Certain cardiac medications such as beta-blockers may contribute to fatigue by causing bradycardia, while corticosteroids may cause fatigue by disrupting sleep or by creating proximal muscle weakness. Coadministration of multiple agents with sedative, cardiac, or sleep disrupting side effects may significantly compound fatigue symptoms.

## INTERVENTIONS FOR FATIGUE

Because fatigue typically has several different causes in any one patient, the treatment plan must be multidimensional and individually tailored. It is helpful to work with the patient and their family members to improve the assessment of fatigue and identify management strategies. Open communication between the patient, family, and caregiving team will facilitate discussion about the experience of fatigue and its effects on daily life. General supportive care recommendations for patients with fatigue include encouraging a balanced diet with adequate intake of fluid, calories, protein, carbohydrates, fat, vitamins and minerals, and balancing rest with physical activity and attention restoring activities such as exposure to natural environments, and pleasant distractions such as music.[18] There have been more than 150 empiric studies of pharmacological and nonpharmacological interventions to reduce or manage CRF, and several recent meta-analyses or systematic reviews have recently been published.[111–115] For some interventions, there is strong and consistent evidence to support effectiveness, while for other interventions, only preliminary data are available. The results of studies examining the impact of pharmacological and nonpharmacological interventions on fatigue outcomes during and following cancer and its treatment are summarized in Tables 30-5 and 30-6, and selected findings are discussed below.

### SCREEN FOR, AND MANAGE AS INDICATED, MECHANISMS OR COMORBIDITIES CONTRIBUTING TO FATIGUE

There is expert consensus that patients with fatigue should be evaluated for potentially treatable etiologic factors contributing to fatigue,[18,206] and managed as indicated. Examples include endocrinopathies (hypothyroidism, hypogonadism, adrenal insufficiency), cardiopulmonary dysfunction, impaired sleep quality, medications with fatigue or sedation as side effects (eg, opiates, antidepressants, antiemetics, antihistamines), deconditioning, asthenia, and sarcopenia, and concurrent symptoms such as pain, nausea, or depression.

### EXERCISE

Deconditioning related to decreased activity is common among patients with cancer and can cause or intensify fatigue from other causes. Meta-analyses of randomized

**TABLE 30-3**

**Assessment of Characteristics and Consequences of Cancer-Related Fafigue**

**Severity**
- On a scale of 0–10 where zero is no fatigue and 10 is the worst fatigue imaginable, how severe has your fatigue been in the past 7 days:
- Would you say that your fatigue is mild, moderate or severe?

**Persistence/Frequency/Temporal Features**
- When did the fatigue start? ____________________
- Frequency of fatigue: ____ days during past week or hours per day _________

**Factors Associated with Fatigue**
- What makes your fatigue better?
- What makes your fatigue worse?
- Does rest relieve your fatigue?
- Do you feel weak?
- Do you have any trouble sleeping?
- Do you have daytime sleepiness (likely to doze off during quiet activities such as reading, watching TV, sitting quietly after lunch)?
- Do you have other symptoms such as pain, difficulty breathing, nausea, and vomiting?
- Do you experience anxiety? If yes, how often?
- Do you feel discouraged, blue, or sad? If yes, how often?
- Do you feel bored? If yes, how often?

**Interference/Distress**
- As a result of fatigue, to what extent have you:
  - limited your social activity,
  - had difficulty getting things done,
  - felt like fatigue was making it difficult to maintain a positive outlook?
- To what extent does fatigue interfere with relationships or fulfilling responsibilities at work or in the home?

**Self-Management**
- What do you do to help with fatigue or manage fatigue?
- Have you discussed your fatigue with anyone on your healthcare team?
- Have you ever been given any recommendations for managing your fatigue?

trials support the benefits of exercise in the management of fatigue during and following cancer treatment for patients with breast cancer, solid tumors, or undergoing hematopoietic stem cell transplantation, although effect sizes are generally small and positive results for the outcome of fatigue have not been observed consistently across studies. The exercise modalities that have been tested differ in content (walking, cycling, swimming, resistive exercise, or combined exercise), frequency (ranging from 2 times per week to 2 times daily), intensity (with most programs at 50% to 90% of the estimated $VO_2$ maximum heart rate), degree of supervision (fully supervised group vs self-directed exercise), and duration (from 2 weeks up to 1 year). Additional empiric knowledge about the type, intensity, and duration of physical exercise most beneficial in reducing fatigue at different stages of disease and treatment is not known,[207] and more research is needed to systematically assess the safety of exercise (both aerobic exercise and strength training) in cancer subpopulations. Patients require formal practical guidance about how to begin, maintain, and advance an exercise program. Referral to a rehabilitation professional such as physical therapy can be helpful in providing specific and detailed recommendations about the type, intensity, and frequency of exercise in which the patient should engage, and ongoing follow-up by rehabilitation professionals can be helpful in strengthening motivation and adherence and in advancing the exercise program as functional capacity improves.

## PSYCHOEDUCATIONAL AND SELF-MANAGEMENT INTERVENTIONS

A growing body of evidence that includes several adequately powered randomized controlled trials suggest that educational interventions and psychological support play an important role in supporting positive coping in patients with fatigue. Psychoeducational interventions that have been shown to be effective include anticipatory guidance about patterns of fatigue and recommendations for self-management, counseling and supportive psychotherapy, and coordination of care. Across studies, a number of common elements were incorporated into the psychoeducational

**TABLE 30-4**

**Etiological Factors for CRF**

- Advanced/metastatic disease or cancer recurrence
- Cancer treatment (chemotherapy, radiation, surgery, biological agents, hormonal agents, molecularly targeted agents)
- Anemia
- Neutropenia
- Hypothyroidism
- Adrenal Insufficiency
- Hypogonadism
- Infection
- Malnutrition
- Depletion of vitamins $B_1$, $B_6$, and $B_{12}$
- Electrolyte disturbances (calcium, magnesium, phosphorus)
- Cardiopulmonary, hepatic, or renal dysfunction
- Sarcopenia, asthenia, deconditioning
- Proinflammatory cytokine expression associated with generalized inflammation
- Medications with sedating side effects (eg, narcotics, anxiolytics, antiemetics, antidepressants), or medications with fatigue as part of the side effects profile (eg, beta-blockers) of medications
- Concurrent symptoms (eg, pain, dyspnea, nausea, diarrhea)
- Impaired sleep quality
- Psychological distress (depression, anxiety)

*Source*: Based on information from Radbruch et al.[110]

interventions. These included anticipatory guidance about patterns of fatigue, tailored recommendations for self-management of fatigue, including increased activity/exercise and measures to address sleep dysregulation, coaching to enhance motivation and empower self-care and active coping, and praise and encouragement to promote self-efficacy and augment feelings of control. Other elements of effective psychoeducational interventions for fatigue included supportive counseling (to support in coping with fear of disease recurrence and to augment social support in patients with low social support), the use of a fatigue diary to record the affective consequences of fatigue, and cognitive restructuring to help normalize CRF and restructure catastrophizing thought patterns (eg, this fatigue is so terrible, I can't cope, I am helpless, there is nothing I can do) that diminish mood and interfere with goal setting, self-efficacy, and incremental goal attainment. Principles of patient and family education concerning CRF are outlined in Table 30-7.

Energy conservation and activity management (ECAM) is a self-management intervention that teaches patients to apply the principles of energy conservation and activity management and provides coaching to integrate these activities into their daily lifestyle. ECAM has been found to have a modest but significant effect in a large, multisite RCT in patients (predominantly with breast cancer) initiating chemotherapy or radiation and in a small pilot study using historical controls. The principles of delivering an ECAM intervention are summarized in Table 30-8.

Studies also indicate that cognitive-behavioral interventions designed to improve sleep quality also have a beneficial effect on fatigue. These interventions to improve sleep quality can be delivered individually or in a group setting, and include relaxation training, along with sleep consolidation strategies (avoiding long or late afternoon naps, limiting time in bed to actual sleep time), stimulus control therapy (go to bed only when sleepy, use bed/bedroom for sleep and sexual activities only, consistent time to lie down and get up, avoid caffeine and stimulating activity in the evening) and strategies to reduce cognitive-emotional arousal (keep at least an hour to relax before going to bed and establish a presleep routine to be used every night). Cognitive-behavioral self-management strategies to improve sleep quality are summarized in Table 30-9.

Cognitive-behavioral therapy (CBT) for treating concurrent symptoms such as pain or depression may also produce beneficial effects on CRF. Although outcomes of a randomized controlled trial of CBT for cancer pain in 131 patients demonstrated improvement in the outcomes of pain, the differences in fatigue were not statistically significant.[136] However, 2 RCTs ($n$ = 200 patients with cancer with major depressive disorder[208] and $n$ = 45 women with metastatic breast cancer[138]) and a small case series ($n$ = 6 women with metastatic breast cancer[137]) demonstrated that a CBT intervention for depression also resulted in statistically significant improvements in fatigue.

## STRUCTURED REHABILITATION

Several trials[153,173,209,210] and a systematic review[211] suggest that structured rehabilitation programs result in statistically significant and sustained improvements in fatigue, particularly in patients who have completed treatment and are in the survivorship phase. The rehabilitation interventions studied were multicomponent interventions comprised of a structured combination of intensive exercise, physical training, sports, psychoeducation, and physical modalities such as massage, mud packs, and manual lymph drainage. In some studies these therapies were delivered over the course of a several week inpatient rehabilitation hospital stay.

Though a fairly consistent pattern of improved fatigue outcomes has been demonstrated across this broad array of rehabilitative, psychoeducational, and supportive care interventions, many rehabilitation, psychoeducational, and supportive care programs that have been research-tested are not routinely available in general oncology programs. Moreover, a deliberative selection of management strategies and tailoring of the program based on the patient's current level of energy, attention, motivation, and stage on the treatment trajectory appear to be essential since at least

**TABLE 30-5**

**Pharmacological Interventions for Fatigue During and Following Cancer and Its Treatment**

| Intervention(s) | Design and Sample | Effect on Fatigue | Source |
|---|---|---|---|
| ATP (adenosine 5′-triphosphate) infusion | RCT, *N* = 58 patients with lung cancer | Improvement | Agteresch et al[116] |
| Bupropion sustained release | 2 single-arm pilot studies, *N* = 36 patients with mixed tumors | Improvement | Moss et al[117]; Cullum et al[118] |
| Donepezil | 2 single-arm open label pilot studies, *N* = 62 patients with mixed tumors | Improvement | Shaw et al[119]; Bruera et al[120] |
| Methylphenidate (patient-controlled administration) | RCT, double-blind, placebo-controlled, *N* = 112 patients with advanced cancer and moderate to severe fatigue | No improvement | Bruera et al[121] |
| Methylphenidate | 5 single-arm, open label studies, *N* = 102 patients with mixed solid tumors, some at the end of life and some receiving active treatment | Improvement | Hanna et al[122]; Bruera et al[120]; Schwartz et al[123]; Sugawara et al[124]; Sarhill et al[125] |
| Modafinil | 2 single-arm pilot studies (*N* = 20 and *N* = 19) in patients with lung cancer or mixed tumor types and a systematic review | Improvement | Blackhall et al[126]; Cooper et al[127]; Spathis et al[128] |
| Paroxetine | 3 RCTs, *N* = 624 patients, most with breast cancer | No improvement | Roscoe et al[129]; Morrow et al[130]; Capuron et al[26] |
| Paroxetine | Single-arm pilot study, *N* = 13 patients with localized breast cancer who were post-treated and experiencing hot flashes | Improvement | Weitzner et al[131] |
| Essiac supplementation | Retrospective cohort study, *N* = 510 randomly selected women from a primary breast cancer registry with primary breast cancer | No improvement | Zick et al[143] |
| Ginseng | Dose-finding, double-blinded RCT (*N* = 290) in adults with mixed tumors | Trend toward improvement at higher dose levels | Barton et al[144] |
| Lectin-standardized mistletoe extract | Observational cohort analysis with parallel groups, *N* = 689 women with breast cancer in 27 centers, who had been treated with surgery and were receiving chemotherapy, radiation therapy or hormone therapy | Improvement | Schumacher et al[145] |
| L-carnitine supplementation | Four open label phase I-II trials, (*N* = 172) in patients with mixed advanced solid tumors | Improvement | Gramignano et al[146]; Cruciani et al[147]; Cruciani et al[148]; Graziano et al[149] |
| High-dose vitamin C supplementation | Single-arm, open label trial, *N* = 39 terminally patients with advanced malignancies | Improvement | Yeom et al[150] |
| Omega-3 fatty acid supplementation | RCT (*N* = 91) in patients with advanced mixed tumors; open-label phase II trial (*N* = 23) in patients initiating chemotherapy for advanced colorectal cancer | No improvement | Bruera et al[120]; Read et al[151] |
| **Combination:** diet with high polyphenols content (400 mg), antioxidant supplementation, supplementation with EPA, DHA, medroxyprogesterone and celecoxib | Open label, early-phase II study, Simon 2-stage design, in *N* = 39 patients with advanced malignancy of mixed solid tumor types | Improvement | Mantovani et al[152] |

*Notes*: Effect on fatigue: Improvement = statistically significant improvement in fatigue; no improvement = no statistically significant improvement in fatigue.

*Abbreviations*: DHA, docosahexaenoic acid; EPA, eicosapentaenoic acid; RCT, randomized controlled trial.

**TABLE 30-6**

**Nonpharmacological Interventions for Fatigue During and Following Cancer and Its Treatment**

| Intervention(s) | Design and Sample | Effect on Fatigue | Source |
|---|---|---|---|
| Acupuncture (traditional chinese) | Single-arm pilot study, *N* = 37 patients with unspecified tumor types | Improvement | Vickers et al[132] |
| Acupuncture-like transelectrical nerve stimulation | Double-blinded RCT, *N* = 15 patients with mixed tumors at the end of life | Improvement | Gadsby et al[133] |
| Cognitive-behavioral treatment for insomnia, depression or other distressing symptoms | 4 RCTs (*N* = 345) and 5 uncontrolled trials (*N* = 76) in patients with mixed tumor types undergoing active treatment, follow-up or at the end of life | 3 RCTs demonstrated improvement; three uncontrolled trials demonstrated improvement | Gielissen et al[134]; Savard et al[135]; Dalton[136]; Levesque et al[137]; Savard et al[138]; Quesnel et al[139]; Berger et al[140]; Berger et al[141]; Davidson et al[142] |
| Energy conservation and activity management (ECAM) | Single-arm study (*N* = 38) and RCT (*N* = 396) in patients undergoing active treatment for mixed tumor types | Improvement | Barsevick et al[157]; Barsevick et al[158] |
| Exercise | 11 meta-analyses or systematic reviews, *N* = 257 studies in patients with breast cancer and other solid tumors, some with advanced disease, and others who were undergoing active treatment, long-term follow-up or were at the end of life | 10 meta-analyses or systematic reviews demonstrated improvement; one showed no improvement | Markes et al[159]; Kirschbaum[160]; McNeely et al[161]; Conn et al[162]; Knols et al[163]; Schmitz et al[164]; Galvao et al[165]; Oldervoll et al[166]; Stevinson et al[167]; Stricker et al[168]; Courneya et al[169] |
| Expressive writing | Pilot study RCT, *N* = 42 patients with newly diagnosed metastatic renal cell carcinoma undergoing active treatment | Improvement in vigor | de Moor et al[170] |
| Group psychotherapy ± exercise | 2 RCTs (*N* = 341) in patients with solid tumors undergoing active treatment, long term follow-up and at the end of life | No improvement with psychotherapy alone; addition of exercise to psychotherapy produced improvement | Courneya et al[171]; Goodwin et al[172] |
| Intensive rehabilitation | Single-arm trial, *N* = 72 patients with mixed solid tumors, primarily breast cancer who are post-treatment | Improvement | van Weert et al[173] |
| Massage therapy | 2 RCTs (*N* = 264) and 1 retrospective review (*N* = 1290) in patients with mixed tumor types and undergoing active treatment | Improvement | Cassileth et al[174]; Post-White et al[175]; Ahles et al[176] |
| Mindfulness-based stress reduction intervention | Single-arm trial, *N* = 63 patients with mixed tumors | Improvement | Carlson et al[177] |
| Music therapy | RCT, *N* = 63 patients undergoing radiation therapy with curative intent | No improvement | Clark et al[178] |
| Polarity therapy | RCT, *N* = 15 patients with breast cancer undergoing active treatment | Improvement | Roscoe et al[179] |
| Progressive muscle relaxation | Two RCTs (*N* = 142) and a meta-analysis (*N* = 2 studies where fatigue outcomes were measured) in patients with mixed tumor types undergoing active treatment | One RCT demonstrated improvement, 1 RCT and meta-analysis demonstrated no improvement | Haase et al[180]; Decker et al[181]; Luebbert et al[182] |

*(Continued)*

**TABLE 30-6**

**Nonpharmacological Interventions for Fatigue During and Following Cancer and Its Treatment (*Continued*)**

| Intervention(s) | Design and Sample | Effect on Fatigue | Source |
|---|---|---|---|
| Psychoeducational | 10 RCTs (*N* = 1076), 2 single-arm studies (*N* = 118) and a matched pairs design (*N* = 101) in patients with mixed tumor types at all phases across the disease trajectory | Seven RCTs, the matched pairs design, and both single-arm studies demonstrated improvement; 3 RCTs demonstrated no improvement | Brown et al[183]; Godino et al[184]; Ream et al[185]; Vilela et al[186]; Boesen et al[187]; Lindemalm et al[188]; Williams et al[189]; Yates et al[190]; Allison et al[191]; Given et al[192]; Kim et al[193]; Fawzy[194]; Fawzy et al[195] |
| Reiki | Counterbalanced crossover trial, *n* = 16 patients with colorectal, breast, lung, or gastric cancer who had recently completed treatment | Improvement | Tsang et al[196] |
| Relaxation breathing and yoga-like positioning | RCT, *n* = 35 patients with hematologic malignancies and undergoing stem cell transplantation | Improvement | Kim et al[197] |
| Virtual reality distraction | 4 RCTs (*N* = 189) and 1 single-arm pilot study (*N* = 22) in patients with solid tumors undergoing chemotherapy | Three RCTs demonstrated no improvement; 1 RCT and single-arm pilot study demonstrated improvement | Schneider et al[198]; Schneider et al[199]; Schneider et al[200]; Oyama et al[201]; Oyama et al[202] |
| Yoga | 2 RCTs (*N* = 77) in patients with breast cancer or lymphoma and a single-arm pilot study (*N* = 18) | Two RCTs demonstrated no improvement; single-arm pilot study demonstrated improvement | Carson et al[203]; Culos-Reed et al[204]; Cohen et al[205] |
| **Combination:** Individualized inpatient rehabilitation incorporating manual lymph drainage, exercise, massage, counseling, relaxation, carbon dioxide baths and mud packs | Single-arm trial, *n* = 149 women with breast cancer who had undergone either mastectomy or breast conserving surgery in combination with chemotherapy, radiation therapy, and hormonal therapy | Improvement | Strauss-Blasche et al[153] |
| **Combination:** Aromatherapy, footsoak, and reflexology | Single-arm open label, *n* = 20 patients with advanced cancer at the end of life | Improvement | Kohara et al[154] |

*Note*: Effect on fatigue: improvement = statistically significant improvement in fatigue; no improvement = no statistically significant improvement in fatigue.

*Abbreviation*: RCT, randomized controlled trial.

one study suggests that programs that are too intensive or demanding programs may actually worsen CRF.[183]

## CORRECTION OF ANEMIA LESS THAN 10 G/DL

Data from 7 systematic reviews[212–218] suggest that patients receiving recombinant human erythropoietin to correct anemia less than 10 g/dL may experience increased vigor and diminished fatigue. However, there is only limited evidence that erythropoietin improves fatigue when anemia is less severe. Data suggest that a target hemoglobin level of 11 to 12 g/dL will produce the greatest gains in fatigue and other quality-of-life outcomes.[219] Although both epoietin and darbepoietin are generally well-tolerated, the use of these agents specifically for the management of fatigue must be considered in light of safety issues, including a small increased risk of thrombotic events, hypertension,

**TABLE 30-7**

**Components of Patient and Family Education About Fatigue**

- Encourage patient to differentiate facets of the fatigue experience (fatigue, tiredness, weakness, cognitive slowing)
- Explain the multifactorial causes of fatigue, including:
  - Side effects of treatment
  - Psychosocial stressors
  - Concurrent symptoms
  - Imbalance of rest and activity
  - Insufficient sleep
  - Inadequate nutrition
  - Muscle weakness/deconditioning
  - Sedating/fatiguing side effects of medications
  - Proinflammatory cytokine release
  - Anemia/neutropenia
- Offer anticipatory guidance about possible patterns of fatigue onset occurrence (eg, at nadir, with conclusion of radiotherapy, and in association with boredom, excess activity, impaired sleep quality or stress)
- Explain that fatigue can develop or worsen as a direct result of treatment, and that this does not necessarily indicate that a treatment is ineffective or that the disease is progressing.
- Suggest a journal, log or diary of activities, fatigue severity, associated feelings/symptoms, and an evaluation of self-care actions
- Develop and tailor an individualized plan for fatigue management
- Inform patient and family that interventions such as energy conservation, exercise, relaxation and stress management, psychosocial support, and measures to optimize sleep quality and reduce concurrent symptoms have been shown to be effective in limiting the severity of fatigue during treatment
- Teach energy conservation strategies and principles of cognitive-behavioral self-management to improve sleep quality, and provide coaching to integrate these into daily patterns
- Affirm the benefits of open communication between patient, family, and caregiving team to facilitate discussions about the experience of fatigue and its effects on daily life
- Encourage attention restoring activities such as exposure to natural environments and pleasant distractions such as music
- Provide information concerning the importance of a balanced diet with adequate intake of fluid, calories, protein, carbohydrates, fat, vitamins and minerals
- Teach diversional techniques, relaxation procedures, and distraction/diversion
- Encourage patient to implement a gentle exercise program (walking, stretching)
- Offer information and referrals to counseling or support groups

pure red cell aplasia, and theoretical concerns that epoietin may support or extend tumor growth in certain disease tumor types.[219–222] Overall, better quality evidence is needed to unequivocally support the use of recombinant human erythropoietin solely as an intervention to improve patient reported outcomes such as fatigue.[212,223] National clinical practice guidelines[224–225] and the guidance of the US Food and Drug Administration should be used to inform the management of patients receiving ESAs, including decisions about patient monitoring, treatment thresholds, dose reductions, treatment discontinuation, and the use of supplemental iron for patients receiving ESAs.

## PHARMACOLOGICAL MEASURES

Several pharmacological agents (paroxetine, methylphenidate, donepezil, bupropion, and modafinil) have been evaluated for their effectiveness in reducing fatigue during and following cancer treatment.[114] Although 4 trials have examined the effectiveness of paroxetine in treating fatigue during and following cancer treatment, the results have been mixed. In 2 large multicenter, randomized, double blinded placebo controlled trials, paroxetine 20 mg po daily did not have an effect on fatigue, although improvements in depression and overall mood were noted in the paroxetine treatment group. However, 2 small trials have shown a trend towards a possible benefit for paroxetine in treating fatigue in 2 distinct subpopulations: women experiencing hot flashes and patients receiving interferon alpha. One randomized controlled trial, and 5 open label, single-arm trials with small samples have examined the use of methylphenidate in reducing fatigue. Although the 5 open label single-arm trials reported improvements in fatigue in most of their participants as a result of the methylphenidate intervention, a randomized controlled trial of a patient-controlled dosing schedule for methylphenidate did not demonstrate

**TABLE 30-8**

**Principles of Energy Conservation and Activity Management for CRF**

Energy conservation is recommended to help patients examine their daily routines and find ways to: (a) reduce the amount of effort needed to perform certain tasks, (b) eliminate tasks, and (c) alternate periods of rest and activity throughout the day to limit bursts of activity and discourage physical inactivity.

The following are suggestions to recommend to plan, prioritize, pace, and modify activities:

**Arrange the Environment**

- Keep frequently used items in easily accessible places
- Adjust work spaces, such as raising a tabletop, to eliminate awkward positions and improve mechanics
- Sit rather than stand whenever possible: while preparing meals, washing dishes, ironing, etc
- Use adaptive equipment (such as a jar opener, a reacher, a shower chair)
- Use prepared foods when possible
- Get a rolling cart to transport things around the house, rather than carry them
- See if your grocery store will deliver your groceries
- Use store-provided wheelchairs or scooters when you shop

**Plan Ahead**

- Gather all the supplies you need for a task or project before starting, so everything is in one place.
- Call ahead to stores to make sure the items you need are available.
- Cook in larger quantities and refrigerate or freeze extra portions for later.
- Work rest breaks into activities as often as possible. Take a break before you get tired.
- Schedule enough time for activities—rushing takes more energy.
- Try keeping a daily activity journal for a few weeks to identify times of day or certain tasks that result in more fatigue.

**Prioritize**

- Eliminate or reduce tasks that aren't that important to you.
- Delegate tasks to friends or family members who offer help.
- Consider hiring professionals, such as a cleaning or lawn care service, to cut down your workload
- Invite family members' energy-saving ideas

**Alternate Activity with Rest**

- Rest before becoming too tired, and avoid bursts of activity or prolonged activity that induces severe fatigue
- With permission your healthcare team, begin a program of physical activity such as walking or cycling. Begin with 5 or 10 minutes twice daily, and increase the time by 1 minute a day
- Do not be tempted to perform excessive exercise, but rather strive for consistency in implementing a daily exercise program

improvement in the outcome of fatigue. Moreover, in one study,[125] more than half of the patients experienced side effects such as insomnia, agitation, anorexia, nausea, and vomiting or dry mouth.

Small open label trials also suggest that donepezil at a dose of 5 to 10 mg/day or bupropion sustained release at a dose of 100 to 150 mg/day may be effective in limiting fatigue. However, controlled studies are necessary to establish the efficacy of these pharmacological agents in larger and more homogeneous samples of patients with cancer, and to determine whether the effects of bupropion are separate from its action as an antidepressant. Several trials also suggest that modafinil at a dose of 100 mg BID may be effective in treating fatigue and improving daytime wakefulness and cognitive function in patients during and following cancer treatment.[209–211,226]

Several trials suggest that levocarnitine supplementation in patients who have low serum carnitine levels[146–149] and treatment with ginseng[144] are safe and potentially efficacious in treating CRF. Although interpretation of the results of these studies is limited by the small sample size, and in the case of levocarnitine supplementation by the absence of a double-blinded randomized control design, results are encouraging and suggest that levocarnitine supplementation and ginseng should receive further study.

## COMPLEMENTARY THERAPIES

There is preliminary evidence to support the efficacy of yoga, relaxation, healing touch, massage, a mindfulness-based stress reduction intervention, acupuncture, and several combined modality interventions that include aromatherapy, lavender footsoak, and reflexology in the management of CRF. The design of these studies was open labeled and/or uncontrolled, with no random assignment,

**TABLE 30-9**

**Elements of Cognitive Behavioral Therapy to Improve Sleep Quality**

- **Cognitive behavioral therapy** (CBT) helps to change the thoughts and actions that interfere with the ability to get restful sleep. The approach is based on the idea that how one thinks (cognition) and acts (behavior) affects the way one feels.
- The **cognitive** portion of CBT teaches the patient to recognize and change false beliefs that affect their ability to sleep. Cognitive therapy also deals with misperceptions about the amount of time actually spent sleeping.
  - For example, a person may believe that they must get 8 h of sleep every night to function, when in fact, 7 h of sleep may be adequate for them.
  - People with insomnia often sleep more than they realize.
- The **behavioral** portion of CBT helps reprogram the part of the brain that governs the sleep-wake cycle. It targets specific behaviors —what sleep experts call "sleep hygiene"—that negatively affect sleep.
  - Such behaviors include failing to exercise or drinking beverages that contain caffeine just before bedtime.
- CBT works on multiple levels and contains 1 or more of the following elements:

| | |
|---|---|
| 1. Cognitive control and psychotherapy | This type of therapy helps control or eliminate negative thoughts and worries that keep the patient awake. It may also involve eliminating false or worrisome beliefs about sleep, such as the idea that a single restless night will make them sick or unable to function |
| 2. Sleep restriction | This approach tries to match the time spent in bed with the patient's actual sleep requirement. Reducing the amount of time spent in bed without sleeping will actually increase the desire to sleep. |
| 3. Remain passively awake | Called paradoxical intention, this involves avoiding any effort to fall asleep, with the goal of eliminating any anxiety the patient may feel about falling asleep easily. |
| 4. Stimulus control | This method helps disassociate any negative cues attached to the bedroom environment and condition a positive response with getting into bed. For example, the patient might be coached to use the bed only for sleep and sex. |
| 5. Sleep hygiene | This method of therapy involves correcting basic lifestyle habits that influence sleep, such as smoking or drinking too much coffee or alcohol late in the day and failing to exercise regularly. It also includes tips that help the patient prepare to sleep better, such as winding down an hour or 2 before bedtime with a warm bath. |
| 6. Relaxation training | This method helps induce relaxation to reduce or eliminate the arousal that disturbs sleep. Approaches include meditation, hypnosis, and muscle relaxation. |

- When used as an insomnia treatment, CBT may take several weeks of steady practice to become fully effective, and usually requires four to eight 30-minute sessions with a behavioral sleep therapist, such as a nurse, psychologist, or other professional.

and with sample sizes that were extremely small, making it difficult to draw firm conclusions about efficacy. Of note, the studies evaluating acupuncture and the combined aromatherapy, footsoak, and reflexology intervention included patients with advanced cancer and at the end of life. If found to be effective in larger randomized controlled trials, these approaches may offer treatment options for patients with advanced cancer and those at the end of life for whom other fatigue interventions such as exercise may not be feasible.

## CONCLUSION AND FUTURE DIRECTIONS

Fatigue continues to be the most common symptom experienced by patients with cancer on therapy and in cancer survivors. With continued progress in delineating the pathophysiology and etiology of CRF, we have also made gains in identifying interventions that are effective for this distressing symptom. However, the challenge in improving CRF outcomes remains that the causative factors are distinct and evolving and treatment approaches are largely empiric. Thus, the intervention approach for each patient is symptom-oriented, and must be individualized and regularly revised. A multimodal approach that includes exercise, psychoeducational interventions, efforts to manage concurrent symptoms, and interventions to improve sleep quality, together with judicious use of medications such as modafinil, methylphenidate, and complementary therapies such as relaxation, massage, healing touch, or acupuncture offers the greatest likelihood of success, and is consistent with evidence-based guidelines from the National Comprehensive Cancer Network[206] and the Oncology Nursing Society.[115]

In summary, a wide range of pharmacological and non-pharmacological interventions have been studied, though several recent systematic reviews[112–115] concluded that many have only been tested in uncontrolled or pilot studies. Interventions for fatigue that are supported by one or more well-designed randomized trials include exercise, psychoeducational interventions, measures to optimize sleep quality, as well as relaxation, massage, and healing touch. A consensus of expert opinion strongly supports the importance of screening for and correcting reversible causes of fatigue. There is preliminary evidence to suggest that pharmacological agents including paroxetine, methylphenidate, donepezil, buproprion sustained release, modafinil, ginseng, and levocarnitine have a role in the management of fatigue, though systematic drug development studies are needed to define the optimal dosing, gauge the toxicity profile, and determine the effectiveness of these agents in specific populations. Interventions for which there is also preliminary evidence of effectiveness include individual and group psychotherapy and complementary therapies such as yoga and acupuncture. Rigorously designed and adequately powered randomized controlled trials of therapies for fatigue that have shown initial promise are urgently needed. Research focused on developing and testing interventions specifically for patients with fatigue in the setting of advanced cancer and at the end of life is an imperative. The role of strategies such as motivational interviewing and nurse coaching in helping patients to make behavior and lifestyle changes also deserve exploration. With a substantial body of evidence now available in support of rehabilitative, supportive care, and psychoeducational interventions that are effective for CRF, questions remain concerning about how to best disseminate these research-tested interventions, how to educate and support providers for widespread delivery of these interventions in the community, and how to target the patient population and phase in the illness trajectory at which they will be most effective.

## REFERENCES


1. Cella D, Peterman A, Passik S, Jacobsen P, Breitbart W. Progress toward guidelines for the management of fatigue. *Oncology (Williston Park).* 1998;12:369–377.
2. Curt G. Impact of fatigue on quality of life in oncology patients. *Semin Hematol.* 2000;37(4 suppl 6):14–17.
3. Curt G, Johnston PG. Cancer fatigue: the way forward. *Oncologist.* 2003;8(suppl 1):27–30.
4. de Jong N, Candel MJ, Schouten HC, Abu-Saad HH, Courtens AM. Course of the fatigue dimension "activity level" and the interference of fatigue with daily living activities for patients with breast cancer receiving adjuvant chemotherapy. *Cancer Nurs.* 2006;29:E1–E13.
5. Mallinson T, Cella D, Cashy J, Holzner B. Giving meaning to measure: linking self-reported fatigue and function to performance of everyday activities. *J Pain Symptom Manage.* 2006;31:229–241.
6. Dimeo F, Schmittel A, Fietz T, et al. Physical performance, depression, immune status and fatigue in patients with hematological malignancies after treatment. *Ann Oncol.* 2004;15:1237–1242.
7. Andrykowski MA, Curran SL, Lightner R. Off-treatment fatigue in breast cancer survivors: a controlled comparison. *J Behav Med.* 1998;21:1–18.
8. Lindqvist O, Widmark A, Rasmussen BH. Meanings of the phenomenon of fatigue as narrated by 4 patients with cancer in palliative care. *Cancer Nurs.* 2004;27:237–243.
9. Magnusson K, Moller A, Ekman T, Wallgren A. A qualitative study to explore the experience of fatigue in cancer patients. *Eur J Cancer Care (Engl).* 1999;8:224–232.
10. Rao AV, Cohen HJ. Fatigue in older cancer patients: etiology, assessment, and treatment. *Semin Oncol.* 2008;35:633–642.
11. Mystakidou K, Parpa E, Katsouda E, Galanos A, Vlahos L. The role of physical and psychological symptoms in desire for death: a study of terminally ill cancer patients. *Psychooncology.* 2006;15:355–360.
12. Servaes P, Verhagen S, Bleijenberg G. Determinants of chronic fatigue in disease-free breast cancer patients: a cross-sectional study. *Ann Oncol.* 2002;13:589–598.
13. Wang XS, Giralt SA, Mendoza TR, et al. Clinical factors associated with cancer-related fatigue in patients being treated for leukemia and non-Hodgkin's lymphoma. *J Clin Oncol.* 2002;20:1319–1328.
14. Hockenberry-Eaton M, Hinds PS. Fatigue in children and adolescents with cancer: evolution of a program of study. *Semin Oncol Nurs.* 2000;16:261–272; discussion 272–268.
15. Knowles G, Borthwick D, McNamara S, Miller M, Leggot L. Survey of nurses' assessment of cancer-related fatigue. *Eur J Cancer Care (Engl).* 2000;9:105–113.
16. Vogelzang NJ, Breitbart W, Cella D, et al. Patient, caregiver, and oncologist perceptions of cancer-related fatigue: results of a tripart assessment survey. The fatigue coalition. *Semin Hematol.* 1997;34(3 suppl 2): 4–12.
17. Passik SD, Kirsh KL, Donaghy K, et al. Patient-related barriers to fatigue communication: initial validation of the fatigue management barriers questionnaire. *J Pain Symptom Manage.* 2002;24:481–493.
18. NCCN. Cancer-related fatigue (version 1.2009), 2009 publication. http://www.nccn.org/professionals/physician_gls/PDF/fatigue.pdf. Accessed November 13, 2009. .
19. Cella D, Lai JS, Chang CH, Peterman A, Slavin M. Fatigue in cancer patients compared with fatigue in the general United States population. *Cancer.* 2002;94:528–538.
20. Glaus A, Crow R, Hammond S. A qualitative study to explore the concept of fatigue/tiredness in cancer patients and in healthy individuals. *Eur J Cancer Care (Engl).* 1996;5(2 suppl):8–23.
21. Wu HS, McSweeney M. Cancer-related fatigue: "It's so much more than just being tired". *Eur J Oncol Nurs.* 2007;11:117–125.
22. Andrykowski MA, Schmidt JE, Salsman JM, Beacham AO, Jacobsen PB. Use of a case definition approach to identify cancer-related fatigue in women undergoing adjuvant therapy for breast cancer. *J Clin Oncol.* 2005;23:6613–6622.
23. Sadler IJ, Jacobsen PB, Booth-Jones M, Belanger H, Weitzner MA, Fields KK. Preliminary evaluation of a clinical syndrome approach to assessing cancer-related fatigue. *J Pain Symptom Manage.* 2002;23:406–416.
24. Tchekmedyian NS, Kallich J, McDermott A, Fayers P, Erder MH. The relationship between psychologic distress and cancer-related fatigue. *Cancer.* 2003;98:198–203.
25. Jacobsen PB, Donovan KA, Weitzner MA. Distinguishing fatigue and depression in patients with cancer. *Semin Clin Neuropsychiatry.* 2003;8:229–240.
26. Capuron L, Gumnick JF, Musselman DL, et al. Neurobehavioral effects of interferon-alpha in cancer patients: phenomenology and paroxetine responsiveness of symptom dimensions. *Neuropsychopharmacology.* 2002;26:643–652.
27. Hinshaw DB, Carnahan JM, Johnson DL. Depression, anxiety, and asthenia in advanced illness. *J Am Coll Surg.* 2002;195:271–277.
28. Lai J-S, Cella D, Dineen K, et al. An item bank was created to improve the measurement of cancer-related fatigue. *J Clin Epidemiol.* 2005;58: 190-197.

29. Reuter K, Harter M. The concepts of fatigue and depression in cancer. *Eur J Cancer Care (Engl).* 2004;13:127–134.
30. Valentine AD, Meyers CA. Cognitive and mood disturbance as causes and symptoms of fatigue in cancer patients. *Cancer.* 2001;92(6 suppl):1694–1698.
31. Van Belle S, Paridaens R, Evers G, et al. Comparison of proposed diagnostic criteria with FACT-F and VAS for cancer-related fatigue: proposal for use as a screening tool. *Support Care Cancer.* 2005;13:246–254.
32. Bower JE, Ganz PA, Aziz N. Altered cortisol response to psychologic stress in breast cancer survivors with persistent fatigue. *Psychosom Med.* 2005;67:277–280.
33. Lee BN, Dantzer R, Langley KE, et al. A cytokine-based neuroimmunologic mechanism of cancer-related symptoms. *Neuroimmunomodulation.* 2004;11:279–292.
34. Ahlberg K, Ekman T, Gaston-Johansson F, Mock V. Assessment and management of cancer-related fatigue in adults. *Lancet.* 2003;362:640–650.
35. Prue G, Rankin J, Allen J, Gracey J, Cramp F. Cancer-related fatigue: a critical appraisal. *Eur J Cancer.* 2006;42:846–863.
36. Servaes P, Verhagen C, Bleijenberg G. Fatigue in cancer patients during and after treatment: prevalence, correlates and interventions. *Eur J Cancer.* 2002;38:27–43.
37. Butt Z, Rosenbloom SK, Abernethy AP, et al. Fatigue is the most important symptom for advanced cancer patients who have had chemotherapy. *J Natl Compr Canc Netw.* 2008;6:448–455.
38. Andrykowski MA, Carpenter JS, Greiner CB, et al. Energy level and sleep quality following bone marrow transplantation. *Bone Marrow Transplant.* 1997;20:669–679.
39. Bower JE, Ganz PA, Desmond KA, et al. Fatigue in long-term breast carcinoma survivors: a longitudinal investigation. *Cancer.* 2006;106:751–758.
40. Hjermstad MJ, Oldervoll L, Fossa SD, Holte H, Jacobsen AB, Loge JH. Quality of life in long-term Hodgkin's disease survivors with chronic fatigue. *Eur J Cancer.* 2006;42:327–333.
41. Young KE, White CA. The prevalence and moderators of fatigue in people who have been successfully treated for cancer. *J Psychosom Res.* 2006;60:29–38.
42. Johnsen A, Petersen M, Pedersen L, Groenvold M. Symptoms and problems in a nationally representative sample of advanced cancer patients. *Palliat Med.* 2009;23:491–501.
43. Beck SL, Dudley WN, Barsevick A. Pain, sleep disturbance, and fatigue in patients with cancer: using a mediation model to test a symptom cluster. *Oncol Nurs Forum.* 2005;32:542.
44. Bender CM, Ergyn FS, Rosenzweig MQ, Cohen SM, Sereika SM. Symptom clusters in breast cancer across 3 phases of the disease. *Cancer Nurs.* 2005;28:219–225.
45. Chow E, Fan G, Hadi S, Filipczak L. Symptom clusters in cancer patients with bone metastases. *Support Care Cancer.* 2007;15:1035–1043.
46. Francoeur RB. The relationship of cancer symptom clusters to depressive affect in the initial phase of palliative radiation. *J Pain Symptom Manage.* 2005;29:130–155.
47. Glaus A, Boehme C, Thurlimann B, et al. Fatigue and menopausal symptoms in women with breast cancer undergoing hormonal cancer treatment. *Ann Oncol.* 2006;17:801–806.
48. Walsh D, Rybicki L. Symptom clustering in advanced cancer. *Support Care Cancer.* 2006;14:831–836.
49. Iop A, Manfredi AM, Bonura S. Fatigue in cancer patients receiving chemotherapy: an analysis of published studies. *Ann Oncol.* 2004;15:712–720.
50. Morrow GR, Shelke AR, Roscoe JA, Hickok JT, Mustian K. Management of cancer-related fatigue. *Cancer Invest.* 2005;23:229–239.
51. Nail LM. Fatigue in patients with cancer. *Oncol Nurs Forum.* 2002;29:537.
52. Nail LM. My get up and go got up and went: fatigue in people with cancer. *J Natl Cancer Inst Monogr* 2004;32:72–75.
53. Paddison JS, Temel JS, Fricchione GL, Pirl WF. Using the differential from complete blood counts as a biomarker of fatigue in advanced non-small-cell lung cancer: an exploratory analysis. *Palliat Support Care.* 2009;7:213–217.
54. Stasi R, Abriani L, Beccaglia P, Terzoli E, Amadori S. Cancer-related fatigue: evolving concepts in evaluation and treatment. *Cancer.* 2003; 98:1786–1801.
55. Strasser F, Palmer JL, Schover LR, et al. The impact of hypogonadism and autonomic dysfunction on fatigue, emotional function, and sexual desire in male patients with advanced cancer: a pilot study. *Cancer.* 2006;107:2949–2957.
56. Tavio M, Milan I, Tirelli U. Cancer-related fatigue (review). *Int J Oncol.* 2002;21:1093–1099.
57. Wagner LI, Cella D. Fatigue and cancer: causes, prevalence and treatment approaches. *Br J Cancer.* 2004;91:822–828.
58. Ancoli-Israel S, Liu L, Marler MR, et al. Fatigue, sleep, and circadian rhythms prior to chemotherapy for breast cancer. *Support Care Cancer.* 2006;14:201–209.
59. Bower JE, Ganz PA, Dickerson SS, Petersen L, Aziz N, Fahey JL. Diurnal cortisol rhythm and fatigue in breast cancer survivors. *Psychoneuroendocrinology.* 2005;30:92–100.
60. Collado-Hidalgo A, Bower JE, Ganz PA, Cole SW, Irwin MR. Inflammatory biomarkers for persistent fatigue in breast cancer survivors. *Clin Cancer Res.* 2006;12:2759–2766.
61. Massacesi C, Terrazzino S, Marcucci F, et al. Uridine diphosphate glucuronosyl transferase 1A1 promoter polymorphism predicts the risk of gastrointestinal toxicity and fatigue induced by irinotecan-based chemotherapy. *Cancer.* 2006;106:1007–1016.
62. Schubert C, Hong S, Natarajan L, Mills PJ, Dimsdale JE. The association between fatigue and inflammatory marker levels in cancer patients: a quantitative review. *Brain Behav Immun.* 2007;21:413–427.
63. Wood LJ, Nail LM, Gilster A, Winters KA, Elsea CR. Cancer chemotherapy-related symptoms: evidence to suggest a role for proinflammatory cytokines. *Oncol Nurs Forum.* 2006;33:535–542.
64. Berger AM, Farr LA, Kuhn BR, Fischer P, Agrawal S. Values of sleep/wake, activity/rest, circadian rhythms, and fatigue prior to adjuvant breast cancer chemotherapy. *J Pain Symptom Manage.* 2007;33:398–409.
65. Fernandes R, Stone P, Andrews P, Morgan R, Sharma S. Comparison between fatigue, sleep disturbance, and circadian rhythm in cancer inpatients and healthy volunteers: evaluation of diagnostic criteria for cancer-related fatigue. *J Pain Symptom Manage.* 2006;32:245–254.
66. Piper B, Lindsey A, Dodd M. Fatigue mechanisms in cancer patients: developing nursing theory. *Oncol Nurs Forum.* 1987;14:17–23.
67. Irvine D, Vincent L, Graydon JE, Bubela N, Thompson L. The prevalence and correlates of fatigue in patients receiving treatment with chemotherapy and radiotherapy. A comparison with the fatigue experienced by healthy individuals. *Cancer Nurs.* 1994;17:367–378.
68. Winningham ML. Strategies for managing cancer-related fatigue syndrome: a rehabilitation approach. *Cancer.* 2001;92(suppl 4): 988–997.
69. Aistars J. Fatigue in the cancer patient: a conceptual approach to a clinical problem. *Oncol Nurs Forum.* 1987;14:25–30.
70. Rhoten D. Fatigue and the postsurgical patient. In: Norris C, ed. *Conceptual Clarification in Nursing.* Rockville, MD: Aspen; 1982:277–300.
71. Glaus A. Fatigue in patients with cancer: analysis and assessment. *Recent Results Cancer Res.* 1998;145:1–172.
72. Olson K. A new way of thinking about fatigue: a reconceptualization. *Oncol Nurs Forum.* 2007;34:93–99.
73. Olson K, Turner AR, Courneya KS, et al. Possible links between behavioral and physiological indices of tiredness, fatigue, and exhaustion in advanced cancer. *Support Care Cancer.* 2008;16:241–249.
74. Payne JK. A neuroendocrine-based regulatory fatigue model. *Biol Res Nurs.* 2004;6:141–150.
75. Al-Majid S, Gray DP. A biobehavioral model for the study of exercise interventions in cancer-related fatigue. *Biol Res Nurs.* 2009;10:381–391.
76. Danjoux C, Gardner S, Fitch M. Prospective evaluation of fatigue during a course of curative radiotherapy for localised prostate cancer. *Support Care Cancer.* 2007;15:1169–1176.

77. Hwang SS, Chang VT, Kasimis BS. A comparison of three fatigue measures in veterans with cancer. *Cancer Invest.* 2003;21:363–373.
78. Kirsh KL, Passik S, Holtsclaw E, Donaghy K, Theobald D. I get tired for no reason: a single item screening for cancer-related fatigue. *J Pain Symptom Manage.* 2001;22:931–937.
79. Temel JS, Pirl WF, Recklitis CJ, Cashavelly B, Lynch TJ. Feasibility and validity of a one-item fatigue screen in a thoracic oncology clinic. *J Thorac Oncol.* 2006;1:454–459.
80. Carpenter JS, Rawl S, Porter J, et al. Oncology outpatient and provider responses to a computerized symptom assessment system. *Oncol Nurs Forum.* 2008;35:661–669.
81. Cella D, Gershon R, Lai JS, Choi S. The future of outcomes measurement: item banking, tailored short-forms, and computerized adaptive assessment. *Qual Life Res.* 2007;16(suppl 1):133–141.
82. Jones JB, Snyder CF, Wu AW. Issues in the design of Internet-based systems for collecting patient-reported outcomes. *Qual Life Res.* 2007; 16:1407–1417.
83. Lind L, Karlsson D. A system for symptom assessment in advanced palliative home healthcare using digital pens. *Med Inform Internet Med.* 2004;29:199–210.
84. Banthia R, Malcarne VL, Roesch SC, et al. Correspondence between daily and weekly fatigue reports in breast cancer survivors. *J Behav Med.* 2006;29:269–279.
85. Minton O, Stone P. A systematic review of the scales used for the measurement of cancer-related fatigue (CRF). *Ann Oncol.* 2009;20: 17–25.
86. Mota DD, Pimenta CA. Self-report instruments for fatigue assessment: a systematic review. *Res Theory Nurs Pract.* 2006;20:49–78.
87. Wagner L, Cella D. Cancer related fatigue: clinical screening, assessment and management. In: Marty M, Pecorelli S, eds. *ESO Scientific Updates: Fatigue, Asthenia, Exhuastion and Cancer.* 5th ed. Oxford, England: Elsevier Science; 2001:201–214.
88. Mendoza TR, Wang XS, Cleeland CS, et al. The rapid assessment of fatigue severity in cancer patients: use of the Brief Fatigue Inventory. *Cancer.* 1999;85:1186–1196.
89. Okuyama T, Akechi T, Kugaya A, et al. Factors correlated with fatigue in disease-free breast cancer patients: application of the Cancer Fatigue Scale. *Support Care Cancer.* 2000;8:215–222.
90. Holley SK. Evaluating patient distress from cancer-related fatigue: an instrument development study. *Oncol Nurs Forum.* 2000;27: 1425–1431.
91. Armes J, Chalder T, Addington-Hall J, Richardson A, Hotopf M. A randomized controlled trial to evaluate the effectiveness of a brief, behaviorally oriented intervention for cancer-related fatigue. *Cancer.* 2007;110:1385–1395.
92. Yellen SB, Cella DF, Webster K, Blendowski C, Kaplan E. Measuring fatigue and other anemia-related symptoms with the Functional Assessment of Cancer Therapy (FACT) measurement system. *J Pain Symptom Manage.* 1997;13:63–74.
93. Hann DM, Jacobsen PB, Azzarello LM, et al. Measurement of fatigue in cancer patients: development and validation of the Fatigue Symptom Inventory. *Qual Life Res.* 1998;7:301–310.
94. Krupp LB, LaRocca NG, Muir-Nash J, Steinberg AD. The fatigue severity scale. Application to patients with multiple sclerosis and systemic lupus erythematosus. *Arch Neurol.* 1989;46:1121–1123.
95. Hinds PS, Hockenberry M, Tong X, et al. Validity and reliability of a new instrument to measure cancer-related fatigue in adolescents. *J Pain Symptom Manage.* 2007;34:607–618.
96. Stein KD, Martin SC, Hann DM, Jacobsen PB. A multidimensional measure of fatigue for use with cancer patients. *Cancer Pract.* 1998;6:143–152.
97. Smets EM, Garssen B, Bonke B, De Haes JC. The Multidimensional Fatigue Inventory (MFI) psychometric qualities of an instrument to assess fatigue. *J Psychosom Res.* 1995;39:315–325.
98. Belza BL. Comparison of self-reported fatigue in rheumatoid arthritis and controls. *J Rheumatol.* 1995;22:639–643.
99. Piper BF, Dibble SL, Dodd MJ, Weiss MC, Slaughter RE, Paul SM. The revised Piper Fatigue Scale: psychometric evaluation in women with breast cancer. *Oncol Nurs Forum.* 1998;25:677–684.
100. Schneider RA. Reliability and validity of the multidimensional fatigue inventory (MFI-20) and the Rhoten Fatigue Scale among rural cancer outpatients. *Cancer Nurs.* 1998;21:370–373.
101. Schwartz AL. The Schwartz cancer fatigue scale: testing reliability and validity. *Oncol Nurs Forum.* 1998;25:711–717.
102. Lee KA, Hicks G, Nino-Murcia G. Validity and reliability of a scale to assess fatigue. *Psychiatry Res.* 1991;36:291–298.
103. Meek PM, Nail LM, Barsevick A, et al. Psychometric testing of fatigue instruments for use with cancer patients. *Nurs Res.* 2000;49: 181–190.
104. Schwartz AH. Validity of cancer-related fatigue instruments. *Pharmacotherapy.* 2002;22:1433–1441.
105. Varricchio CG, ed. *Measurement and assessment: What are the issues?* Sudbury, MA: Jones and Bartlett; 2000.
106. Wu HS, McSweeney M. Measurement of fatigue in people with cancer. *Oncol Nurs Forum.* 2001;28:1371–1384; quiz 1385–1376.
107. Curran SL, Beacham AO, Andrykowski MA. Ecological momentary assessment of fatigue following breast cancer treatment. *J Behav Med.* 2004;27:425–444.
108. Hacker ED, Ferrans CE. Ecological momentary assessment of fatigue in patients receiving intensive cancer therapy. *J Pain Symptom Manage.* 2007;33:267–275.
109. Mock V, Atkinson A, Barsevick AM, et al. Cancer-related fatigue. Clinical practice guidelines in oncology. *J Natl Compr Canc Netw.* 2007;5:1054–1078.
110. Radbruch L, Strasser F, Elsner F, et al. Fatigue in palliative care patients—an EAPC approach. *Palliat Med.* 2008;22:13–32.
111. Cramp F, Daniel J. Exercise for the management of cancer-related fatigue in adults. *Cochrane Database Syst Rev.* 2008;(2):CD006145;
112. Jacobsen PB, Donovan KA, Vadaparampil ST, Small BJ. Systematic review and meta-analysis of psychological and activity-based interventions for cancer-related fatigue. *Health Psychol.* 2007;26:660–667.
113. Kangas M, Bovbjerg DH, Montgomery GH. Cancer-related fatigue: A systematic and meta-analytic review of non-pharmacological therapies for cancer patients. *Psychol Bull.* 2008;134:700–741.
114. Minton O, Richardson A, Sharpe M, Hotopf M, Stone P. A systematic review and meta-analysis of the pharmacological treatment of cancer-related fatigue. *J Natl Cancer Inst.* 2008;100:1155–1166.
115. Mitchell S, Beck S, Hood L, Moore K, Tanner E. Putting evidence into practice (PEP): evidence-based interventions for fatigue during and following cancer and its treatment. *Clin J Oncol Nurs.* 2007;11: 99–113.
116. Agteresch HJ, Dagnelie PC, van der Gaast A, Stijnen T, Wilson JH. Randomized clinical trial of adenosine 5'-triphosphate in patients with advanced non-small-cell lung cancer. *J Natl Cancer Inst.* 2000;92:321–328.
117. Moss EL, Simpson JS, Pelletier G, Forsyth P. An open-label study of the effects of bupropion SR on fatigue, depression and quality of life of mixed-site cancer patients and their partners. *Psychooncology.* 2006;15: 259–267.
118. Cullum JL, Wojciechowski AE, Pelletier G, Simpson JS. Bupropion sustained release treatment reduces fatigue in cancer patients. *Can J Psychiatry.* 2004;49:139–144.
119. Shaw EG, Rosdhal R, D'Agostino RB, Jr., Lovato J, Naughton MJ, Robbins ME, et al. Phase II study of donepezil in irradiated brain tumor patients: effect on cognitive function, mood, and quality of life. *J Clin Oncol.* 2006;24:1415–1420.
120. Bruera E, Strasser F, Shen L, Palmer JL, Willey J, Driver LC, et al. The effect of donepezil on sedation and other symptoms in patients receiving opioids for cancer pain: a pilot study. *J Pain Symptom Manage.* 2003;26:1049–1054.
121. Bruera E, Valero V, Driver L, Shen L, Willey J, Zhang T, et al. Patient-controlled methylphenidate for cancer fatigue: A double-blind, randomized, placebo-controlled trial. *J Clin Oncol.* 2006;24:2073–2078.

122. Hanna A, Sledge G, Mayer ML, Hanna N, Einhorn L, Monahan P, et al. A phase II study of methylphenidate for the treatment of fatigue. *Support Care Cancer.* 2006;14:210–215.
123. Schwartz A, Thompson J, Masood N. Interferon-induced fatigue in patients with melanoma: a pilot study of exercise and methylphenidate. *Oncol Nurs Forum.* 2002;29:E85–90.
124. Sugawara Y, Akechi T, Shima Y, Okuyama T, Akizuki N, Nakano T, et al. Efficacy of methylphenidate for fatigue in advanced cancer patients: a preliminary study. *Palliat Med.* 2002;16:261–263.
125. Sarhill N, Walsh D, Nelson KA, Homsi J, LeGrand S, Davis MP. Methylphenidate for fatigue in advanced cancer: a prospective open-label pilot study. *Am J Hosp Palliat Care.* 2001;18:187–192.
126. Blackhall L, Petroni G, Shu J, Baum L, Farace E. A pilot study evaluating the safety and efficacy of modafinal for cancer-related fatigue. *J Palliat Med.* 2009;12:433–439.
127. Cooper MR, Bird HM, Steinberg M. Efficacy and safety of modafinil in the treatment of cancer-related fatigue. *Ann Pharmacother.* 2009;43:721–725.
128. Spathis A, Dhillan R, Booden D, Forbes K, Vrotsou K, Fife K. Modafinil for the treatment of fatigue in lung cancer: a pilot study. *Palliat Med.* 2009;23:325–331.
129. Roscoe JA, Morrow GR, Hickok JT, Mustian KM, Griggs JJ, Matteson SE, et al. Effect of paroxetine hydrochloride (Paxil) on fatigue and depression in breast cancer patients receiving chemotherapy. *Breast Cancer Res Treat.* 2005;89:243–249.
130. Morrow GR, Hickok JT, Roscoe JA, Raubertas RF, Andrews PL, Flynn PJ, et al. Differential effects of paroxetine on fatigue and depression: a randomized, double-blind trial from the University of Rochester Cancer Center Community Clinical Oncology Program. *J Clin Oncol.* 2003;21:4635–4641.
131. Weitzner MA, Moncello J, Jacobsen PB, Minton S. A pilot trial of paroxetine for the treatment of hot flashes and associated symptoms in women with breast cancer. *J Pain Symptom Manage.* 2002;23: 337–345.
132. Vickers AJ, Straus DJ, Fearon B, Cassileth BR. Acupuncture for postchemotherapy fatigue: a phase II study. *J Clin Oncol.* 2004;22: 1731–1735.
133. Gadsby JG, Franks A, Jarvis P, Dewhurst F. Acupuncture-like transcutaneous electrical nerve stimulation within palliative care: A pilot study. *Complement Ther Med.* 1997;5:13–18.
134. Gielissen MF, Verhagen S, Witjes F, Bleijenberg G. Effects of cognitive behavior therapy in severely fatigued disease-free cancer patients compared with patients waiting for cognitive behavior therapy: a randomized controlled trial. *J Clin Oncol.* 2006;24:4882–4887.
135. Savard J, Simard S, Ivers H, Morin CM. Randomized study on the efficacy of cognitive-behavioral therapy for insomnia secondary to breast cancer, part I: Sleep and psychological effects. *J Clin Oncol.* 2005;23:6083–6096.
136. Dalton JA, Keefe FJ, Carlson J, Youngblood R. Tailoring cognitive-behavioral treatment for cancer pain. *Pain Manag Nurs.* 2004;5: 3–18.
137. Levesque M, Savard J, Simard S, Gauthier JG, Ivers H. Efficacy of cognitive therapy for depression among women with metastatic cancer: a single-case experimental study. *J Behav Ther Exp Psychiatry.* 2004;35: 287–305.
138. Savard J, Simard S, Giguere I, et al. Randomized clinical trial on cognitive therapy for depression in women with metastatic breast cancer: psychological and immunological effects. *Palliat Support Care.* 2006;4:219–237.
139. Quesnel C, Savard J, Simard S, Ivers H, Morin CM. Efficacy of cognitive-behavioral therapy for insomnia in women treated for nonmetastatic breast cancer. *J Consult Clin Psychol.* 2003;71:189–200.
140. Berger AM, VonEssen S, Kuhn BR, Piper BF, Agrawal S, Lynch JC, et al. Adherence, sleep, and fatigue outcomes after adjuvant breast cancer chemotherapy: results of a feasibility intervention study. *Oncol Nurs Forum.* 2003;30:513–522.
141. Berger AM, VonEssen S, Khun BR, Piper BF, Farr L, Agrawal S, et al. Feasibility of a sleep intervention during adjuvant breast cancer chemotherapy. *Oncol Nurs Forum.* 2002;29:1431–1441.
142. Davidson JR, Waisberg JL, Brundage MD, Maclean AW. Nonpharmacologic group treatment of insomnia: A preliminary study with cancer survivors. *Psychooncology.* 2001;10:389–397
143. Zick SM, Sen A, Feng Y, Green J, Olatunde S, Boon H. Trial of essiac to ascertain its effect in women with breast cancer (TEA-BC). *J Altern Complement Med.* 2006;12:971–980.
144. Barton DL, Soori GS, Bauer BA, et al. Pilot study of Panax quinquefolius (American ginseng) to improve cancer-related fatigue: a randomized, double-blind, dose-finding evaluation: NCCTG trial N03CA. *Support Care Cancer.* 2009, May 06, 2009 E. Pub Ahead of Print.
145. Schumacher K, Schneider B, Reich G, Stiefel T, Stoll G, Bock PR, et al. Influence of postoperative complementary treatment with lectin-standardized mistletoe extract on breast cancer patients. A controlled epidemiological multicentric retrolective cohort study. *Anticancer Res.* 2003;23:5081–5087.
146. Gramignano G, Lusso MR, Madeddu C, et al. Efficacy of L-carnitine administration on fatigue, nutritional status, oxidative stress, and related quality of life in 12 advanced cancer patients undergoing anticancer therapy. *Nutrition.* 2006;22:136–145.
147. Cruciani RA, Dvorkin E, Homel P, et al. Safety, tolerability and symptom outcomes associated with L-carnitine supplementation in patients with cancer, fatigue, and carnitine deficiency: a phase I/II study. *J Pain Symptom Manage.* 2006;32:551–559.
148. Cruciani RA, Dvorkin E, Homel P, et al. L-carnitine supplementation for the treatment of fatigue and depressed mood in cancer patients with carnitine deficiency: a preliminary analysis. *Ann N Y Acad Sci.* 2004;1033:168–176.
149. Graziano F, Bisonni R, Catalano V, et al. Potential role of levocarnitine supplementation for the treatment of chemotherapy-induced fatigue in non-anaemic cancer patients. *Br J Cancer.* 2002;86:1854–1857.
150. Yeom CH, Jung GC, Song KJ. Changes of terminal cancer patients' health-related quality of life after high dose vitamin C administration. *J Korean Med Sci.* 2007;22:7–11.
151. Read JA, Beale PJ, Volker DH, Smith N, Childs A, Clarke SJ. Nutrition intervention using an eicosapentaenoic acid (EPA)-containing supplement in patients with advanced colorectal cancer. Effects on nutritional and inflammatory status: a phase II trial. *Support Care Cancer.* 2007;15:301–307.
152. Mantovani G, Maccio A, Madeddu C, Gramignano G, Lusso MR, Serpe R, et al. A phase II study with antioxidants, both in the diet and supplemented, pharmaconutritional support, progestagen, and anti-cyclooxygenase-2 showing efficacy and safety in patients with cancer-related anorexia/cachexia and oxidative stress. *Cancer Epidemiol Biomarkers Prev.* 2006;15:1030–1034.
153. Strauss-Blasche G, Gnad E, Ekmekcioglu C, Hladschik B, Marktl W. Combined inpatient rehabilitation and spa therapy for breast cancer patients: effects on quality of life and CA 15–3. *Cancer Nursing.* 2005;28:390–398.
154. Kohara H, Miyauchi T, Suehiro Y, Ueoka H, Takeyama H, Morita T. Combined modality treatment of aromatherapy, footsoak, and reflexology relieves fatigue in patients with cancer. *J Palliat Med.* 2004;7:791–796.
155. Cerchietti LC, Navigante AH, Peluffo GD, Diament MJ, Stillitani I, Klein SA, et al. Effects of celecoxib, medroxyprogesterone, and dietary intervention on systemic syndromes in patients with advanced lung adenocarcinoma: a pilot study. *J Pain Symptom Manage.* 2004;27:85–95.
156. Jensen MB, Hessov I. Randomization to nutritional intervention at home did not improve postoperative function, fatigue or well-being. *Br J Surg.* 1997;84:113–118.
157. Barsevick AM, Dudley W, Beck S, Sweeney C, Whitmer K, Nail L. A randomized clinical trial of energy conservation for patients with cancer-related fatigue. *Cancer.* 2004;100:1302–1310.

158. Barsevick AM, Whitmer K, Sweeney C, Nail LM. A pilot study examining energy conservation for cancer treatment-related fatigue. *Cancer Nurs.* 2002;25:333–341.
159. Markes M, Brockow T, Resch KL. Exercise for women receiving adjuvant therapy for breast cancer. *Cochrane Database Syst Rev.* 2006:CD005001.
160. Kirshbaum MN. A review of the benefits of whole body exercise during and after treatment for breast cancer. *J Clin Nurs.* 2007;16(1): 104–21
161. McNeely ML, Campbell KL, Rowe BH, Klassen TP, Mackey JR, Courneya KS. Effects of exercise on breast cancer patients and survivors: a systematic review and meta-analysis. *CMAJ.* 2006;175:34–41.
162. Conn VS, Hafdahl AR, Porock DC, McDaniel R, Nielsen PJ. A meta-analysis of exercise interventions among people treated for cancer. *Support Care Cancer.* 2006;14:699–712.
163. Knols R, Aaronson NK, Uebelhart D, Fransen J, Aufdemkampe G. Physical exercise in cancer patients during and after medical treatment: a systematic review of randomized and controlled clinical trials. *J Clin Oncol.* 2005;23:3830–3842..
164. Schmitz KH, Holtzman J, Courneya KS, Masse LC, Duval S, Kane R. Controlled physical activity trials in cancer survivors: a systematic review and meta-analysis. *Cancer Epidemiol Biomarkers Prev.* 2005;14:1588–1595.
165. Galvao DA, Newton RU. Review of exercise intervention studies in cancer patients. *J Clin Oncol.* 2005;23:899–909.
166. Oldervoll LM, Kaasa S, Hjermstad MJ, Lund JA, Loge JH. Physical exercise results in the improved subjective well-being of a few or is effective rehabilitation for all cancer patients? *Eur J Cancer.* 2004;40:951–962.
167. Stevinson C, Lawlor DA, Fox KR. Exercise interventions for cancer patients: systematic review of controlled trials. *Cancer Causes Control.* 2004;15:1035–1056.
168. Stricker CT, Drake D, Hoyer KA, Mock V. Evidence-based practice for fatigue management in adults with cancer: exercise as an intervention. *Oncol Nurs Forum.* 2004;31:963–976.
169. Courneya KS, Friedenreich CM. Physical exercise and quality of life following cancer diagnosis: a literature review. *Ann Behav Med.* 1999;21:171–179.
170. de Moor C, Sterner J, Hall M, Warneke C, Gilani Z, Amato R, et al. A pilot study of the effects of expressive writing on psychological and behavioral adjustment in patients enrolled in a Phase II trial of vaccine therapy for metastatic renal cell carcinoma. *Health Psychol.* 2002;21: 615–619.
171. Courneya KS, Friedenreich CM. Physical exercise and quality of life following cancer diagnosis: a literature review. *Ann Behav Med.* 1999;21:171–179.
172. Goodwin PJ, Leszcz M, Ennis M, Koopmans J, Vincent L, Guther H, et al. The effect of group psychosocial support on survival in metastatic breast cancer. *N Engl J Med.* 2001;345:1719–1726.
173. van Weert E, Hoekstra-Weebers J, Otter R, Postema K, Sanderman R, van der Schans C. Cancer-related fatigue: predictors and effects of rehabilitation. *Oncologist.* 2006;11:184–196.
174. Cassileth BR, Vickers AJ. Massage therapy for symptom control: outcome study at a major cancer center. *J Pain Symptom Manage.* 2004;28:244–249.
175. Post-White J, Kinney ME, Savik K, Gau JB, Wilcox C, Lerner I. Therapeutic massage and healing touch improve symptoms in cancer. *Integr Cancer Ther.* 2003;2:332–344.
176. Ahles TA, Tope DM, Pinkson B, Walch S, Hann D, Whedon M, et al. Massage therapy for patients undergoing autologous bone marrow transplantation. *J Pain Symptom Manage.* 1999;18:157–163.
177. Carlson LE, Garland SN. Impact of Mindfulness-Based Stress Reduction (MBSR) on sleep, mood, stress and fatigue symptoms in cancer outpatients. *Int J Behav Med.* 2005;12:278–285.
178. Clark M, Isaacks-Downton G, Wells N, Redlin-Frazier S, Eck C, Hepworth JT, et al. Use of preferred music to reduce emotional distress and symptom activity during radiation therapy. *J Music Ther.* 2006;43:247–265.
179. Roscoe JA, Matteson SE, Mustian KM, Padmanaban D, Morrow GR. Treatment of radiotherapy-induced fatigue through a nonpharmacological approach. *Integr Cancer Ther.* 2005;4:8–13.
180. Haase O, Schwenk W, Hermann C, Muller JM. Guided imagery and relaxation in conventional colorectal resections: a randomized, controlled, partially blinded trial. *Dis Colon Rectum.* 2005;48:1955–1963.
181. Decker TW, Cline-Elsen J, Gallagher M. Relaxation therapy as an adjunct in radiation oncology. *J Clin Psychol.* 1992;48:388–393.
182. Luebbert K, Dahme B, Hasenbring M. The effectiveness of relaxation training in reducing treatment-related symptoms and improving emotional adjustment in acute non-surgical cancer treatment: a meta-analytical review. *Psychooncology.* 2001;10:490–502.
183. Brown P, Clark MM, Atherton P, et al. Will improvement in quality of life (QOL) impact fatigue in patients receiving radiation therapy for advanced cancer? *Am J Clin Oncol.* 2006;29:52–58.
184. Godino C, Jodar L, Duran A, Martinez I, Schiaffino A. Nursing education as an intervention to decrease fatigue perception in oncology patients. *Eur J Oncol Nurs.* 2006;10:150–155.
185. Ream E, Richardson A, Alexander-Dann C. Supportive intervention for fatigue in patients undergoing chemotherapy: a randomized controlled trial. *J Pain Symptom Manage.* 2006;31:148–161.
186. Vilela LD, Nicolau B, Mahmud S, Edgar L, Hier M, Black M, et al. Comparison of psychosocial outcomes in head and neck cancer patients receiving a coping strategies intervention and control subjects receiving no intervention. *J Otolaryngol.* 2006;35:88–96.
187. Boesen EH, Ross L, Frederiksen K, Thomsen BL, Dahlstrom K, Schmidt G, et al. Psychoeducational intervention for patients with cutaneous malignant melanoma: a replication study. *J Clin Oncol.* 2005;23:1270–1277.
188. Lindemalm C, Strang P, Lekander M. Support group for cancer patients. Does it improve their physical and psychological wellbeing? A pilot study. *Support Care Cancer.* 2005;13:652–657.
189. Williams SA, Schreier AM. The role of education in managing fatigue, anxiety, and sleep disorders in women undergoing chemotherapy for breast cancer. *Appl Nurs Res.* 2005;18:138–147.
190. Yates P, Aranda S, Hargraves M, Mirolo B, Clavarino A, McLachlan S, et al. Randomized controlled trial of an educational intervention for managing fatigue in women receiving adjuvant chemotherapy for early-stage breast cancer. *J Clin Oncol.* 2005;23:6027–6036.
191. Allison PJ, Edgar L, Nicolau B, Archer J, Black M, Hier M. Results of a feasibility study for a psycho-educational intervention in head and neck cancer. *Psychooncology.* 2004;13:482–485.
192. Given B, Given CW, McCorkle R, Kozachik S, Cimprich B, Rahbar MH, et al. Pain and fatigue management: results of a nursing randomized clinical trial. *Oncol Nurs Forum.* 2002;29:949–956.
193. Kim Y, Roscoe JA, Morrow GR. The effects of information and negative affect on severity of side effects from radiation therapy for prostate cancer. *Support Care Cancer.* 2002;10:416–421.
194. Fawzy FI. A short-term psychoeducational intervention for patients newly diagnosed with cancer. *Support Care Cancer.* 1995;3: 235–238.
195. Fawzy FI, Cousins N, Fawzy NW, Kemeny ME, Elashoff R, Morton D. A structured psychiatric intervention for cancer patients. I. Changes over time in methods of coping and affective disturbance. *Arch Gen Psychiatry.* 1990;47:720–725.
196. Tsang KL, Carlson LE, Olson K. Pilot crossover trial of Reiki versus rest for treating cancer-related fatigue. *Integr Cancer Ther.* 2007;6:25–35.
197. Kim SD, Kim HS. Effects of a relaxation breathing exercise on anxiety, depression, and leukocyte in hemopoietic stem cell transplantation patients. *Cancer Nurs.* 2005;28:79–83.
198. Schneider SM, Prince-Paul M, Allen MJ, Silverman P, Talaba D. Virtual reality as a distraction intervention for women receiving chemotherapy. *Oncol Nurs Forum.* 2004;31:81–88.

199. Schneider SM, Ellis M, Coombs WT, Shonkwiler EL, Folsom LC. Virtual reality intervention for older women with breast cancer. *Cyberpsychol Behav.* 2003;6:301–307.
200. Schneider, S.M. and L.E. Hood, Virtual reality: a distraction intervention for chemotherapy. *Oncol Nurs Forum*, 2007: 34(1): 39–46.
201. Oyama H, Kaneda M, Katsumata N, Akechi T, Ohsuga M. Using the bedside wellness system during chemotherapy decreases fatigue and emesis in cancer patients. *J Med Syst.* 2000;24:173–182.
202. Oyama H, Ohsuga M, Tatsuno Y, Katsumata H. Evaluation of the psycho-oncological effectiveness of the bedside wellness system. *Cyberpsychol Behav.* 1999;2:81–84.
203. Carson JW, Carson KM, Porter LS, Keefe FJ, Shaw H, Miller JM. Yoga for women with metastatic breast cancer: results from a pilot study. *J Pain Symptom Manage.* 2007;33:331–341.
204. Culos-Reed SN, Carlson LE, Daroux LM, Hately-Aldous S. A pilot study of yoga for breast cancer survivors: physical and psychological benefits. *Psychooncology.* 2006;15:891–897.
205. Cohen L, Warneke C, Fouladi RT, Rodriguez MA, Chaoul-Reich A. Psychological adjustment and sleep quality in a randomized trial of the effects of a Tibetan yoga intervention in patients with lymphoma. *Cancer.* 2004;100:2253–2260.
206. Cheville, A. (2009). Cancer-related fatigue. Physical Medicine and Rehabilitation Clinics of North American, 2009; 20: 405–416.
207. Humpel N, Iverson DC. Review and critique of the quality of exercise recommendations for cancer patients and survivors. *Support Care Cancer.* 2005;13:493–502.
208. Strong V, Waters R, Hibberd C, et al. Management of depression for people with cancer (SMaRT oncology 1): a randomised trial. *Lancet.* 2008;372:40–48.
209. Heim ME, v d Malsburg ML, Niklas A. Randomized controlled trial of a structured training program in breast cancer patients with tumor-related chronic fatigue. *Onkologie.* 2007;30:429–434.
210. Korstjens I, Mesters I, van der Peet E, Gijsen B, van den Borne B. Quality of life of cancer survivors after physical and psychosocial rehabilitation. *Eur J Cancer Prev.* 2006;15:541–547.
211. van Weert E, Hoekstra-Weebers JE, May AM, Korstjens I, Ros WJ, van der Schans CP. The development of an evidence-based physical self-management rehabilitation programme for cancer survivors. *Patient Educ Couns.* 2008;4:4.
212. Bohlius J, Wilson J, Seidenfeld J, et al. Recombinant human erythropoietins and cancer patients: updated meta-analysis of 57 studies including 9353 patients. *J Natl Cancer Inst.* 2006;98:708–714.
213. Bottomley A, Thomas R, van Steen K, Flechtner H, Djulbegovic B. Human recombinant erythropoietin and quality of life: a wonder drug or something to wonder about? *Lancet Oncol.* 2002;3:145–153.
214. Cella D, Dobrez D, Glaspy J. Control of cancer-related anemia with erythropoietic agents: a review of evidence for improved quality of life and clinical outcomes. *Ann Oncol.* 2003;14:511–519.
215. Djulbegovic B. Erythropoietin use in oncology: a summary of the evidence and practice guidelines comparing efforts of the Cochrane Review group and Blue Cross/Blue Shield to set up the ASCO/ASH guidelines. *Best Pract Res Clin Haematol.* 2005;18:455–466.
216. Jones M, Schenkel B, Just J, Fallowfield L. Epoetin alfa improves quality of life in patients with cancer: results of metaanalysis. *Cancer.* 2004;101:1720–1732.
217. Littlewood TJ, Cella D, Nortier JW. Erythropoietin improves quality of life. *Lancet Oncol.* 2002;3:459–460.
218. Wilson J, Yao GL, Raftery J, et al. A systematic review and economic evaluation of epoetin alfa, epoetin beta and darbepoetin alfa in anaemia associated with cancer, especially that attributable to cancer treatment. *Health Technol Assess.* 2007;11:1–220.
219. Stasi R, Amadori S, Littlewood TJ, Terzoli E, Newland AC, Provan D. Management of cancer-related anemia with erythropoietic agents: doubts, certainties, and concerns. *Oncologist.* 2005;10:539–554.
220. Glaspy JA. The development of erythropoietic agents in oncology. *Expert Opin Emerg Drugs.* 2005;10:553–567.
221. Littlewood T, Collins G. Epoetin alfa: basic biology and clinical utility in cancer patients. *Expert Rev Anticancer Ther.* 2005;5:947–956.
222. Steensma DP, Loprinzi CL. Erythropoietin use in cancer patients: a matter of life and death? *J Clin Oncol.* 2005;23:5865–5868.
223. Bottomley A, Thomas R, Van Steen K, Flechtner H, Djulbegovic B. Erythropoietin improves quality of life—a response. *Lancet Oncol.* 2002;3:527.
224. NCCN. Cancer- and chemotherapy-induced anemia (version 2.2010) publication. http://www.nccn.org/professionals/physician_gls/PDF/anemia.pdf. Accessed November 13, 2009.
225. Rizzo JD, Somerfield MR, Hagerty KL, et al. Use of epoetin and darbepoetin in patients with cancer: 2007 American Society of Hematology/American Society of Clinical Oncology clinical practice guideline update. *Blood.* 2008;111:25–41.
226. Kohli S, Fisher SG, Tra Y, et al. The effect of modafinil on cognitive function in breast cancer survivors. *Cancer.* 2009;115:2605–2616.

CHAPTER

31

Barbara Holmes Gobel MS, RN, AOCN®, Colleen O'Leary RN, MS, AOCNS®

# Hypersensitivity Reactions to Antineoplastic Drugs

## SCOPE OF THE PROBLEM

Hypersensitivity reactions related to antineoplastic drugs can be potentially life-threatening. Nearly all of the chemotherapy and biotherapy drugs used today in cancer treatment have the potential to cause hypersensitivity reactions. These reactions can range from a single wheal at an injection site to anaphylaxis and death. Certain groups of antineoplastic drugs are frequently associated with hypersensitivity reactions, which include the taxanes, asparaginases, platinum compounds, epipodophyllotoxins, procarbazine, and murine and chimeric monoclonal antibodies.

Most hypersensitivity reactions are immune (immunoglobulin) mediated reactions that are the result of the release of histamines and cytokines. Some reactions are nonimmune mediated as many patients can tolerate re-exposure to a drug if it is readministered slowly after pretreatment with steroids and antihistamines.[1] Almost all hypersensitivity reactions related to antineoplastic drugs are associated with the parenteral administration of the drug. Most hypersensitivity reactions related to chemotherapy and biotherapy occur within minutes to hours after the administration of the drug, but some reactions can be delayed by 1 or 2 days.[1]

It is critical to be able to recognize and manage hypersensitivity reactions to chemotherapy and biotherapy, particularly as these reactions can be life-threatening in nature. Knowledge of the drugs that have a high risk of causing a hypersensitivity reaction is required to assist the nurse in the prevention, early recognition, and appropriate management of hypersensitivity reactions.

## DEFINITIONS

The terms "drug reaction," "drug allergy," and "drug hypersensitivity" are often used synonymously in the literature and in clinical practice. *Drug reaction* includes all adverse drug events related to that drug's administration, regardless of etiology.[2] Most drug reactions are caused by predictable nonimmunological effects, such as the development of a dry mouth from the administration of antihistamines. Immune-mediated drug reactions account for about 5% to 10% of all drug reactions and include drug allergy and drug hypersensitivity reactions.[3] A *drug allergy* is a reaction specifically mediated by the immune system and immunoglobulin E (IgE). *Drug hypersensitivity* is an immune-mediated response to a drug in a sensitized patient. The reaction may be localized or systemic, and results in local tissue injury or changes throughout the body in response to an antigen or foreign substance.[1,3,4]

Many biological agents cause an acute infusion reaction described as a *cytokine release syndrome*.[5] This syndrome is a drug reaction that is more specific to drugs directed against immune system targets, such as anti-CD20 antibodies. As a result of this drug reaction, there is a release of cytokines, including tumor necrosis factor-alpha (TNF-$\alpha$), interleukin-6 (IL-6), and interferons.

*Anaphylactic reactions* are allergic reactions that are mediated by IgE, which can result in a life-threatening response. Anaphylactic reactions usually develop rapidly and can have cutaneous, respiratory, cardiopulmonary, and gastrointestinal manifestations. *Anaphylactoid reactions* are hypersensitivity reactions that are not IgE mediated.[6] Both types of reactions are generally referred to as anaphylaxis as they have similar pathophysiological processes and clinical manifestations.[7]

## INCIDENCE

Severe hypersensitivity reactions to chemotherapy and biotherapy are rare, with an overall incidence rate of about 5%.[8] The incidence rate of mild-to-moderate hypersensitivity reactions is cited to be between 5% and 15%; however, the exact incidence rates to individual drugs vary and may be higher.[8] It is thought that the incidence of these reactions is underestimated in the oncology community.[9] See Tables 31-1 and 31-2[10,11] for a list of chemotherapy and biotherapy drugs with a high risk of hypersensitivity reactions.

Of the 3 formulations of asparaginase (the original *Escherichia coli* derivative, L-asparaginase, and the *Erwinia chrysanthemi* derivative), the incidence of hypersensitivity reactions is similar with the asparaginase and *Erwinia*-derived products. The risk of hypersensitivity reactions to these formulations is 5% to 8% and increases with cumulative dosing. Up to 33% of patients experience a hypersensitivity reaction by the fourth dose.[12] Another approach to decrease the risk of a hypersensitivity reaction is to switch to a polyethylene glycol-modified *E. coli* asparaginase (ie, PEG-asparaginase), but reactions can still occur with this formulation.

Procarbazine has long been known to cause hypersensitivity reactions. Reactions have been reported in 30% to 50% of patients treated for brain tumors and in 5% to 10% of patients treated for Hodgkin's lymphoma.[13,14]

Both of the epipodophyllotoxins, teniposide and etoposide, are associated with a high risk of hypersensitivity reactions. Teniposide causes hypersensitivity reactions in approximately 6% of patients, although the incidence of reactions varies depending on the tumor being treated. For example in patients with neuroblastoma, the incidence of hypersensitivity reactions can increase to 13%.[15] The incidence rate of etoposide is reported to be between 1% and 3%.[16] One study reported an incidence rate of 51% when etoposide was used in a chemotherapy regimen for the treatment of Hodgkin's lymphoma.[17] Most reported hypersensitivity reactions to epipodophyllotoxins have

**TABLE 31-1**

**Immediate Hypersensitivity Reactions: Predicted Risk of Chemotherapy Data from Gobel[4]**

**High Potential**
- Asparaginase
- Taxanes

Paclitaxel
  - Docetaxel
- Platinum compounds
  - Cisplatin
  - Carboplatin
  - Oxaliplatin
- Epipodophyllotoxins
  - Etoposide
  - Teniposide
- Procarbazine

**Occasional Potential**
- Anthracyclines
  - Doxorubicin
  - Daunorubicin
  - Idarubicin
  - Epirubicin
- Mercaptopurine
- Azathioprine

**Rare Potential**
- Bleomycin
- Chlorambucil and melphalan
- Cyclophosphamide and ifosfamide
- Cytarabine and fludarabine
- Dacarbazine
- Dactinomycin
- 5-fluorouracil
- Hydroxyurea
- Methotrexate
- Polyethylene glycol-modified *E. coli asparaginase*
- Vincristine and vinblastine

*Source*: Data from Gobel.[11]

**TABLE 31-2**

**Biotherapy Drugs Associated with Hypersensitivity Reactions and Cytokine-Release Syndromes**

**Interferon**
- Interferon alfa
- Interferon beta (1A and 1B)
- Interferon gamma

**Interleukin**
- Aldesleukin
- Denileukin diftitox

**Monoclonal antibodies (murine)**
- Ibritumomab tiuxetan
- Tositumomab

**Monoclonal antibodies (chimeric)**
- Cetuximab
- Rituximab

**Monoclonal antibodies (humanized)**
- Alemtuzumab
- Bevacizumab
- Gemtuzumab ozogamicin
- Trastuzumab

**Monoclonal antibodies (fully human)**
- Panitumumab

*Source*: Data from Lentz[8]: Gobel.[11]

been mild and are associated with the intravenous (IV) formulations of these drugs.[18] No hypersensitivity reactions to oral etoposide have been reported.

The incidence of severe hypersensitivity reactions to the platinum compounds, taxanes, and monoclonal antibodies are similar and are reported to be between 2% and < 10%.[18–23] The reported incidence of any grade hypersensitivity reaction to carboplatin or oxaliplatin is approximately 12% to 19%.[9,20,24,25] The reported incidence rate for paclitaxel and docetaxel are between 8% and 45% and 5% and 20%, respectively.[26,27] Mild-to-moderate hypersensitivity reactions occur frequently in monoclonal antibodies, particularly during the first infusion. Hypersensitivity reactions occur in up to 26% of patients receiving tositumomab and in about 10% of patients receiving the first dose of ibritumomab tiuxetan.[11,28] The incidence rate of hypersensitivity reactions to rituximab is 77%, 16% to 19% with cetuximab, and up to 40% with trastuzumab.[29–31] Hypersensitivity rates of 5% are even seen with the newest fully human monoclonal antibody, panitumumab.[32,33]

## RISK FACTORS

Nearly all chemotherapy and biotherapy drugs have the potential to cause hypersensitivity reactions. Although the risk of hypersensitivity reactions increases with certain groups of drugs (eg, asparaginases, taxanes, platinum compounds, epipodophyllotoxins, and murine and chimeric monoclonal antibodies), there are other factors that will increase the risk of a patient developing a hypersensitivity reaction. The risk of hypersensitivity reactions and anaphylaxis increases when drugs are given at high doses (eg, high dose etoposide), drugs given via the IV route, drugs derived from bacteria (eg, asparaginase), rapid administration of the drug (eg, IV push vs slow infusion), drugs given as crude preparations (eg, those drugs used in phase I studies), and when there is a failure to administer known effective prophylactic medications for high-risk drugs.[4,34]

Other risk factors that increase the risk of development of hypersensitivity reactions include female gender and history of prior allergic reactions to food, insulin, opiates, penicillins, bee stings, blood products, and radiologic contrast media.[35]

Patients may react to the first exposure to a chemotherapy drug, such as with paclitaxel, but previous exposure to certain chemotherapy drugs increases the risk for hypersensitivity reactions. The likelihood of hypersensitivity reactions increases with repeated exposure to the asparaginases, the platinum compounds (including oxaliplatin), and with the epipodophyllotoxins.[36–38] The nitrosoureas (eg, carmustine and lomustine) are the only class of chemotherapy drugs that have never been documented to cause a hypersensitivity reaction.[34]

All types of biotherapies have been implicated in the development of hypersensitivity reactions, yet there is an increased risk particularly with some of the monoclonal antibodies. There are 4 types of monoclonal antibodies and their structure is a factor in their influence on the development of hypersensitivity reactions. (Figure 31-1 depicts the 4 types of monoclonal antibodies.) Murine monoclonal antibodies are derived completely from mice antibodies and have the highest risk of developing hypersensitivity reactions. The names of murine monoclonal antibodies end in the suffix "-momab" and include drugs such as tositumomab and ibritumomab tiuxetan. Chimeric monoclonal antibodies are made up of a combination of human antibody and about 7% to 10% of mouse antibody. The names of chimeric monoclonal antibodies end in the suffix "-ximab" and include drugs such as rituximab and cetuximab. Because these drugs also have high mouse antibody content they place the patient at risk for hypersensitivity reactions. Humanized monoclonal antibodies have only about 2% to 5% of mouse antibody, thus decreasing their potential for causing hypersensitivity reactions. The names of humanized monoclonal antibodies end in the suffix "-zumab" and include drugs such as trastuzumab, bevacizumab, gemtuzumab, and alemtuzumab. The first fully human monoclonal antibody, panitumumab, has no murine component and ends with the suffix "-umab." As it is fully human it has the decreased potential to cause immunogenicity and infusion reactions, although the risk of hypersensitivity reactions with this drug is still about 5%.[32,33,39]

Other factors that increase the risk of hypersensitivity reactions or cytokine release syndrome in patients receiving monoclonal antibodies include first infusion of a monoclonal antibody and patients with high circulating lymphocyte counts (25,000/mm$^3$).[40]

In recent years, specific populations of patients have been found to have a higher average incidence of reactions to certain monoclonal antibodies. Three different studies demonstrated a higher incidence of reactions to cetuximab in the southeastern portion of the United States.[41,42,43] O'Neill and colleagues reported on 88 patients in clinical trials in North Carolina and Tennessee, who were treated with cetuximab for a variety of tumor types, who experienced a hypersensitivity reaction (grade 3 or grade 4) rate of 22%. All patients who experienced a reaction did so with their first dose of the drug. The researchers found a strong relationship between prior allergy history and a high risk of hypersensitivity reactions. They suggest that there may be a preexisting IgE antibody that is directed against cetuximab and that this response could be caused by regional plants or tree pollens.[41] Owera and colleagues also found a high incidence of hypersensitivity reactions (24.6%) to cetuximab infusions in Missouri. They also identified a strong association between prior allergy history and a high risk of hypersensitivity reactions.[42] In a retrospective database review of 54 patients in Arkansas who received cetuximab for the first time, Makhou et al found a 19% hypersensitivity reaction rate that was classified as severe or life-threatening. This group also found that race may be associated with a higher risk of hypersensitivity reactions: 24% of Caucasians in the group

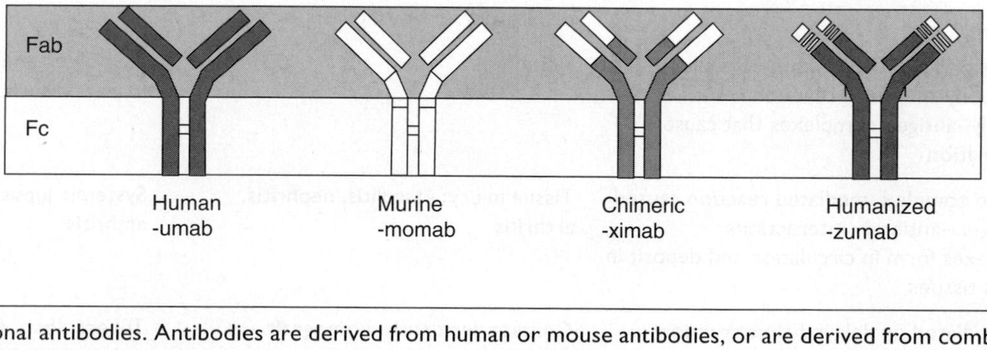


**FIGURE 31-1**

Types of monoclonal antibodies. Antibodies are derived from human or mouse antibodies, or are derived from combinations of both. The Fab portion of the antibody is the variable portion of the antibody that recognizes and binds to a specific antigen. The Fc portion of the antibody is the stem of the antibody that signals the immune system to destroy the cell to which it becomes bound.

had a first infusion reaction vs 0% of African Americans, although this finding was not statistically significant.[43]

## PHYSIOLOGICAL ALTERATIONS

### PATHOPHYSIOLOGY

#### Hypersensitivity reactions related to chemotherapy

There are 4 categories of hypersensitivity reactions: type I is an immediate IgE-mediated immune reaction that can result in anaphylaxis; type II is an immunoglobulin G (IgG) or immunoglobulin M (IgM)-mediated reaction that results in antibody–antigen complexes; type III is an immune complex–mediated reaction that is caused by antigen–antibody interactions, in which the complexes form in the circulation and deposit in various tissues; and type IV is a cell-mediated or delayed-type reaction that involve sensitized T lymphocytes. (See Table 31-3 for a classification of hypersensitivity reactions.[34,44–46]) Most reactions to chemotherapy drugs are consistent with type I reactions, although there are case reports of types II, III, and IV to chemotherapy.[18]

Type I reactions occur following exposure to a foreign substance or antigen (eg, the chemotherapy drug or chemotherapy drug metabolite). The antigen exposure results in the formation of IgE antibodies, which bind to receptors on the mast cells in tissues or basophils in the peripheral blood. Upon subsequent exposure to the antigen, the antigen then attaches to the IgE antibody, which induces mast cells to degranulate, releasing the chemical mediators of these reactions into the surrounding tissue and blood. These chemical mediators include histamines, leukotrienes, prostaglandins, and chemotactins.[6] The signs and symptoms of type I hypersensitivity reactions are the result of the effects of the mediators on the target organs including the skin, lungs, heart, bladder, ureters, and gastrointestinal tract. These effects result in the local or systemic reactions that characterize type I reactions. Type I reactions are characterized by rapid smooth muscle contraction and dilation of capillaries that result in rash, urticaria, angioedema, bronchospasm, and hypotension. See Table 31-4 for a list of the clinical features of hypersensitivity reactions.[4,8,34,47,48] There are a number of factors that impact the development and degree of a type I reaction including the antigen's route of entry (anaphylaxis is more common with the IV route of administration), the amount of antigen introduced (risk of reaction increases as the amount of antigen that is introduced increases), and the rate of the antigen absorption (faster infusion times increase the risk of a reaction).[44] In addition to chemotherapy, other causes of type I hypersensitivity reactions include pollens, food allergies, and allergies to IV dye.

Some type I hypersensitivity reactions to chemotherapy are considered to be anaphylactoid instead of anaphylactic. Anaphylactoid reactions occur when the patient has not been previously exposed to the chemotherapy. The chemotherapy, their metabolites, or drug vehicles interact directly with mast cells and basophils inducing the chemical mediators of type I hypersensitivity reactions.[18] An anaphylactoid response is indistinguishable from an IgE-mediated response.

**TABLE 31-3**

**Types of Hypersensitivity Reactions**

| Type | Mechanism of Action | Signs and Symptoms | Examples |
|---|---|---|---|
| I | Immediate immunoglobulin E-mediated reaction. Mediator release from basophils and mast cells | Fever, rash, nausea, vomiting, flushing, urticaria, bronchospasm, hypotension, angioedema, feeling of impending doom, respiratory and cardiovascular collapse | Anaphylaxis to chemotherapy, biotherapy, food, and bee stings |
| II | Immunoglobulin G or immunoglobulin M antibody-mediated reaction results in antibody–antigen complexes that cause inflammation | Hemolysis | Hemolytic anemia, hemolysis from transfusion |
| III | Immune complex–mediated reaction caused by antigen–antibody interactions<br>Complexes form in circulation and deposit in various tissues | Tissue injury; vasculitis, nephritis, arthritis | Systemic lupus, rheumatoid arthritis |
| IV | Cell-mediated or delayed-type reaction due to sensitized T lymphocytes that interact with antigen | Contact dermatitis, homograft rejection, granuloma formation | Tuberculosis, granulomas, poison ivy |

*Source*: Data from Gobel[4]; Myers[34]; Labovich[44]; Ream[45]; and Thomas.[46]

**TABLE 31-4**

**Clinical Signs and Symptoms of Hypersensitivity Reactions**

| System | Signs or Symptoms |
|---|---|
| General | Fever, chills, flushing, rigors, sweating, fatigue, agitation, metallic taste |
| Cutaneous | Rash, urticaria (hives, welts, wheals), pruritis, angioedema (including face, lips, or eyelids) |
| Respiratory | Dyspnea, wheezing, stridor, rhinitis, repetitive cough, chest tightness, throat tightness, change in voice quality (from laryngeal edema) |
| Cardiovascular | Tachycardia, hypotension/hypertension |
| Gastrointestinal | Nausea, vomiting, diarrhea, abdominal cramping |
| Renal | Flank pain, back pain, hematuria |
| Neurological | Headache, dizziness, tunnel vision, "feeling of impending doom" |

*Source*: Data from Gobel[4]; Lenz[8]; Myers[34]; National Cancer Institute[47]; and Van Gerpen.[48]

### Hypersensitivity reactions related to biotherapy

Treatment with biotherapy, particularly the monoclonal antibodies, has been associated with infusion reactions. The National Cancer Institute Common Toxicity Criteria (NCI-CTC) distinguish between hypersensitivity reactions and acute infusion reactions induced by cytokine release[47] (Table 31-5). Although cytokine release syndrome can present almost identical to type I hypersensitivity reactions (and can progress to anaphylaxis-like symptoms), it is felt that these reactions are not induced by IgE antibodies.[49] Although the exact mechanism for infusion reactions is not well understood, cytokine release syndrome is related to elevated levels of cytokines and histamines that are released as tumor antigen–expressing cells are destroyed. These effects can be demonstrated after the administration of monoclonal antibodies, interferon, and immune-response modifiers. Elevated cytokine levels induce a variety of symptoms that are similar to hypersensitivity reactions and include fever, chills, rigors, nausea, vomiting, dyspnea, and hypotension.[50] A cytokine release syndrome does not depend on prior sensitization, thus this syndrome most commonly occurs with the first infusion of monoclonal antibodies and decreases with subsequent infusions.[49,51]

## CLINICAL MANIFESTATIONS

The clinical signs and symptoms related to hypersensitivity reactions and cytokine release syndrome to chemotherapy and biotherapy can range from localized symptoms such as itching or a wheal at an injection site to overwhelming anaphylaxis that may result in cardiovascular collapse and death. Type I reactions may present as a local reaction and then progress to systemic anaphylaxis, or the initial presentation may be anaphylaxis. The most common signs and symptoms of hypersensitivity reactions include dyspnea, agitation, and hypotension. Other symptoms include fever, nausea, vomiting, flushing, back pain, angioedema, dyspnea, stridor, bronchospasm, "feeling of impending doom," and alterations in heart rate and blood pressure.[52] Table 31-5 lists the grading of hypersensitivity reactions based on the NCI-CTC. Mild-to-moderate reactions (grades 1 and 2) are characterized by fever, rash, chills, rigors, flushing, dyspnea, and mild hypotension. Severe reactions (grades 3 and 4) associated with bronchospasm, hypotension, cardiac dysfunction, and anaphylaxis require emergent treatment.[8]

## CHEMOTHERAPY DRUGS FREQUENTLY ASSOCIATED WITH HYPERSENSITIVITY REACTIONS

### Asparaginase

Asparaginase has long been associated with a high risk of hypersensitivity reactions. Asparaginase is a bacterial polypeptide protease derived from *E. coli*. The risk of hypersensitivity reactions increases significantly with cumulative dosing of the drug: the risk for the initial doses is 5% to 8% per administered dose with the risk increasing to 33% by the fourth dose.[12] The clinical manifestations of reactions to asparaginase are demonstrated as type I reactions, which can progress from localized symptoms to full blown anaphylaxis. Reactions are more common with IV injections vs intramuscular or subcutaneous injections, as well as with intermittent (eg, weekly or monthly) vs continuous (eg, daily) schedules.[1] Reactions to asparaginase may occur several hours after administration of the drug.[53] Retreatment with asparaginase is frequently associated with an increased risk of reaction.[54] Potential substitutes for asparaginase to decrease the

**TABLE 31-5**

**Grading of Hypersensitivity Reactions According to the NCI Common Terminology Criteria for Adverse Events v 3.0**

| HSRs | Grade 1 | Grade 2 | Grade 3 | Grade 4 | Grade 5 |
|---|---|---|---|---|---|
| Hypersensitivity (allergic reaction) | Transient flushing or rash; drug fever 38°C (<100.4°F) | Rash; flushing; urticaria; dyspnea; drug fever ≥38°C (≥100.4°F) | Symptomatic bronchospasm, with or without urticaria; parenteral medication(s) indicated; allergy-related edema/angioedema; hypotension | Anaphylaxis | Death |
| Acute infusion reaction (cytokine release syndrome) | Mild reaction; infusion interruption; intervention not indicated | Requires therapy or infusion interruption but responds promptly to symptomatic treatment (eg, antihistamines, NSAIDS, narcotics, IV fluids); prophylactic medication indicated for ≥24 hours | Prolonged (ie, not rapidly responsive to symptomatic medication and/or brief interruption of infusion); recurrence of symptoms following initial improvement; hospitalization indicated for other clinical sequelae (eg, renal impairment, pulmonary infiltrates) | Life-threatening; pressor or ventilator support indicated | Death |

*Abbreviations*: HSRs, hypersensitivity reactions; NCI, National Cancer Institute; NSAIDs, nonsteroidal anti-inflammatory drugs.
*Source*: Data from the National Cancer Institute.[47]

risk of hypersensitivity reactions include *E. chrysanthemi* (derived from a plant pathogen) and PEG-modified asparaginase or pegaspargase. The antileukemia effect of the *E. chrysanthemi* may be inferior to asparaginase. Although any of the 3 formulations of asparaginases can potentially cause a hypersensitivity reaction, the pegaspargase is the least immunogenic.[3]

## Taxanes

Paclitaxel and docetaxel are commonly used drugs to treat breast cancer, non-small cell lung cancer, and gynecological cancers. Severe hypersensitivity reactions occur in about 2% to 4% of patients treated with paclitaxel and in about 1% to 3% of patients treated with docetaxel.[8] Up to 41% of patients experienced any grade of hypersensitivity reactions to paclitaxel in clinical trials. Clinical manifestations of reactions to these drugs are demonstrated as type I reactions and can include rash, erythema, dyspnea, flushing, chest pain, angioedema, and/or bronchospasm. Severe reactions can cause cardiopulmonary collapse and death. Most reactions occur within the first hour of infusion. Because most reactions occur with the first or second dose of the drug, it is thought that these reactions are anaphylactoid in nature and are not caused by an IgE-mediated response.[55,56] Instead, these reactions may be caused by direct effects on immune cells or other mechanisms.

The antigen that is most likely responsible for hypersensitivity reactions to paclitaxel is not the drug itself, but the excipient found in paclitaxel. This excipient, Cremophor EL (polyoxyethylated castor oil), has been shown to induce histamine release and hypotension.[16,57] This same excipient is found in teniposide, vitamin K, and cyclosporine. An albumin-bound form of paclitaxel that does not contain Cremophor EL has been found to cause little to no incidence of severe hypersensitivity reactions.[58] The excipient in docetaxel is polysorbate 80 (Tween 80), and this drug too is associated with severe hypersensitivity reactions.[59]

## Platinum compounds

Hypersensitivity reactions to platinum compounds, including cisplatin, carboplatin, and oxaliplatin, are generally consistent with type I IgE-mediated reactions, as they generally occur after prolonged use.[24,25] These drugs are used frequently to treat a variety of cancers including bladder cancer, gynecological tumors, adenocarcinoma of the lung, and metastatic colon cancer. Combined, these drugs are associated with a high risk of hypersensitivity reactions (10% to 27%) and have been documented to occur with all routes of administration including IV, intraperitoneal, and intravesicular.[60–62] More than 50% of patients who develop reactions to the platinum compounds develop at least moderately severe hypersensitivity reactions.[20] Delayed reactions may also be seen with this group of drugs.

The incidence of hypersensitivity reactions to cisplatin has decreased over time, possibly due to the routine use of premedications (eg, corticosteroids and antihistamines) before administration of the drug. In early clinical trials, the incidence of hypersensitivity reactions to cisplatin was reported to be between 5% and 20%.[63–65] The highest rate of reactions related to cisplatin administration is with multiple-dose intravesicular administration for bladder cancer (10% to 25%).[34]

The incidence of severe hypersensitivity reactions to carboplatin is about 2%. The reactions can demonstrate as a rash, urticaria, erythema, pruritis, and even bronchospasm and hypotension. These reactions have been documented to occur most often after 6 to 8 cycles of the drug.[20,66]

Oxaliplatin is also associated with hypersensitivity reactions after repeated dosing of the drug. The incidence of hypersensitivity reactions is about 10% to 12% with a median administration of 10 doses.[55,59] No reactions with the first infusion of oxaliplatin have been documented.[16] Delayed reactions to oxaliplatin have been documented, but the symptoms of hypersensitivity reactions are similar whether they are immediate or delayed and may include erythema of the hands and face accompanied by pruritis of the hands.[67] The incidence of severe hypersensitivity reactions is 2% to 3%.[68] The clinical manifestations related to these reactions are similar to cisplatin and carboplatin.

### Epipodophyllotoxins

The epipodophyllotoxins are used to treat a variety of cancers. Etoposide is used to treat small cell lung cancer, refractory testicular cancer, neurological cancers, and occasionally hematologic cancers. Teniposide is used primarily to treat hematologic cancers in children. Combined, these drugs have a hypersensitivity reaction incidence of 6% to 41% and an anaphylaxis incidence of 0.7% to 14%.[69] Reactions are consistent with type I IgE-mediated reactions, as reactions can occur with any dose of the drug, and may occur after only a few milligrams of the drug have been administered. Most reported hypersensitivity reactions to these drugs have been mild.[18] Clinical manifestations may include fever, chills, urticaria, dyspnea, and possibly bronchospasm.

The incidence of hypersensitivity reactions related to etoposide is estimated to be 1% to 3%.[16] Most reactions occur with the first or second dose of the drug. No hypersensitivity reactions have been reported related to the oral administration of etoposide.

Teniposide causes hypersensitivity reactions in about 6% of patients. The rate of reactions is reported as higher in patients with neuroblastoma.[15] Reactions may occur with any dose of the drug, including the initial dose. Teniposide is solubilized in the excipient Cremophor EL, but there is no available data that identify this excipient as the causative agent in hypersensitivity reactions to teniposide.[1]

### Procarbazine

Hypersensitivity reactions to procarbazine have been reported in 5% to 10% of patients with Hodgkin's lymphoma and in 30% to 50% of patients with brain tumors.[13,14] One of the reasons for the variation may be that patients with brain tumors are most often taking anticonvulsants, which may enhance the cytochrome P450 enzyme pathway thereby increasing the risk for hypersensitivity reactions.[70] The clinical manifestations most commonly related to reactions to procarbazine include diffuse, pruritic, erythematous, and maculopapular rash. Also reported are high fever, urticaria, and angioedema.[71]

## BIOTHERAPY DRUGS FREQUENTLY ASSOCIATED WITH HYPERSENSITIVITY REACTIONS AND CYTOKINE RELEASE SYNDROMES

### Interferons

A variety of interferons (alfa, beta, and gamma interferons) are available to treat a variety of cancers as well as other diseases. Common infusion-related side effects of the interferons include fever, chills, rigors, and diaphoresis.[72] These symptoms are often described as "flulike" symptoms that generally occur 1 to 2 hours after a dose and may persist for up to 18 hours. These symptoms occur regardless of dose, route, or schedule of the drugs given.[73]

### Interleukins

The flulike symptoms of chills, fever, and rigors are common with the administration of aldesleukin and denileukin diftitox.[74,75] These symptoms can be experienced as both an immediate and a delayed reaction to denileukin diftitox. Acute hypersensitivity reactions have been reported in 69% of patients treated with denileukin diftitox in clinical trials.[73] Reported symptoms included rash, back pain, chest pain, chest tightness, shortness of breath, dysphagia, tachycardia, syncope, and anaphylaxis. Anaphylaxis was reported in 1% of patients receiving this drug in clinical trials.[74,75]

### Monoclonal antibodies

The murine monoclonal antibodies, *ibritumomab tiuxetan* and *tositumomab*, are well known to cause both hypersensitivity reactions and infusion-related reactions. The most common symptoms related to the use of both of these drugs include fever, chills, and rigors. The reactions generally occur with the first infusion of the drugs and the incidence decreases with subsequent infusions. Infusion-related symptoms generally resolve with slowing of the infusion. Other reported reactions that are similar to hypersensitivity reactions include nausea, vomiting, hypotension, hypertension, wheezing, rhinitis, dyspnea, dizziness, bronchospasm, and angioedema.[76,77] Anaphylaxis has been reported in less than 1% of patients treated with ibritumomab tiuxetan.[78]

Of the 2 chimeric monoclonal antibodies, *rituximab* and *cetuximab*, rituximab is known to cause infusion-related reactions more frequently. Infusion-related reactions occur in 80% of patients during the first infusion of rituximab, and this decreases to 30% during the fourth infusion and 14% with the eighth infusion.[16] The most common symptoms related to both these drugs are fever, chills, and rigors. These symptoms generally occur in the first 30 minutes to 2 hours of the drug infusion. Infusion-related reactions generally resolve with slowing or stopping of the infusion and symptomatic treatment of the patient. These flulike symptoms occur in about 15% of patients treated with cetuximab.[11]

Severe infusion-related reactions occur in about 10% of patients receiving rituximab.[72] Symptoms that are significant for severe reactions include nausea, vomiting, flushing, pruritis, urticaria, dyspnea, rhinitis, hypotension, stridor, bronchospasm, angioedema, and cardiac arrest.[21,29] Severe infusion-related reactions occur in about 2% of patients treated with cetuximab, and 90% of these severe reactions occur during the first infusion of the drug.[30]

The humanized monoclonal antibodies are made up of about 2% to 5% murine antibody, thus have the potential to cause hypersensitivity reactions. These monoclonal antibodies cause hypersensitivity reactions less often than do the murine or chimeric monoclonal antibodies. *Alemtuzumab* is a humanized monoclonal antibody that targets the Cluster of Differentiation (CD) 52 antigen present on the surface of most B and T lymphocytes, as well as malignant B and T lymphocytes. Infusion-related reactions are common as cytokines are on the surface of T lymphocytes. The most frequent infusion-related symptoms include rigors, fever, nausea, vomiting, rash, urticaria, dyspnea, pruritis, and hypotension.[79]

*Bevacizumab* is a humanized monoclonal antibody that targets vascular endothelial growth factor. Infusion reactions (of any grade) occur in about 3% of patients and are severe in about 1% of patients. Infusion-related reactions to bevacizumab tend to be mild and self-limiting and include fever, chills, rigors, and myalgias.[80] These reactions are more common with the first infusion of the drug and can generally be managed by slowing the infusion of the drug.[30] Clinical manifestations evident of a more severe reaction include hypertension, hypertensive crises, wheezing, oxygen desaturation, hypotension, bronchospasm, chest pain, and angioedema.[81]

*Gemtuzumab ozogamicin* is a humanized monoclonal antibody that targets the CD33 antigen expressed on the myeloblast cell in patients with acute myeloid leukemia. It is a drug that is combined with the cytotoxic antibiotic calicheamicin. Infusion-related reactions occur in about 30% of patients during the first infusion, which decreases to about 10% with subsequent infusions.[82] The most common infusion-related reactions include fever, chills, nausea, vomiting, headache, and hypotension. The symptoms generally occur within the first 2 hours after the administration of the drug, but they can occur within 24 hours after completion of the drug. Severe hypersensitivity reactions and anaphylaxis have been reported associated with gemtuzumab ozogamicin.[82,83]

*Trastuzumab* is a humanized monoclonal antibody that targets the human epidermal growth factor receptor (EGFR) 2 protein (*HER-2*). The incidence of infusion-related reactions to trastuzumab is reported to be between 20% and 40%, occurring during the initial infusion of the drug.[84] The incidence of infusion-related reactions decreases with subsequent infusions of the drug. Most reactions are mild and symptoms include fever and chills. Other reported symptoms include rash, rigors, nausea, headache, abdominal pain, dyspnea, dizziness, and hypotension. Severe or anaphylactic reactions occur in less than 1% of patients treated with trastuzumab.[22,31]

Fully human monoclonal antibodies target EGFR on cells. *Panitumumab* is the first fully human monoclonal antibody available to treat cancer. During clinical trials, 3% of patients experienced an infusion-related reaction and 1% of patients experienced severe or anaphylactic reactions.[85]

## THERAPEUTIC APPROACHES AND NURSING CARE

### PREVENTION

Because there is a potential for hypersensitivity reactions with almost any chemotherapy or biotherapy drug, it is imperative for the nurse to be prepared to identify and manage these reactions. The nurse must have knowledge of the drug being administered and the risk of hypersensitivity reaction associated with the particular drug. An initial step before beginning any antineoplastic regimen is to complete a detailed history of allergies including any reactions to previous drugs. A previous history of hypersensitivity reactions, even to structurally unrelated drugs, is important since it increases the patient's risk of subsequent reactions.[42] A complete baseline assessment should be performed on each patient before initiation of an infusion to include vital signs, lung sounds, cardiovascular status, and any skin rashes or breakdown. When educating the patient about the potential side effects of the drug that they will be receiving, it is important to include the potential for hypersensitivity reactions. The education should include the symptoms associated with hypersensitivity reactions and the importance of reporting any unusual symptoms promptly.

Pharmacological prophylaxis before the administration of drugs with a high risk of reaction or for patients with a history of hypersensitivity is recommended.[4,18] Premedication can help to prevent or reduce the severity of hypersensitivity reactions. Medications commonly used to prevent reactions include corticosteroids such as dexamethasone; histamine receptor 1 ($H_1$) antagonists such as diphenhydramine; histamine receptor 2 ($H_2$) antagonists such as cimetidine, famotidine, and ranitidine; and antipyretics such as acetaminophen.[8]

Despite the use of preventative measures, hypersensitivity reactions can occur at any time. Therefore, the nurse needs to be prepared for a potential hypersensitivity reaction during each administration of chemotherapy or biotherapy, particularly drugs with a high risk of reactions. Patients' vital signs should be monitored before, during, and after the infusion.[47] In addition, patients should be observed for signs or restlessness, fidgeting, scratching, changes in mood, and frequent position changes. Patients may not interpret these signs as abnormal or associated with a potential hypersensitivity reaction.[86]

It is widely recommended in the literature that standing orders be in place to allow immediate intervention if a reaction occurs. Emergency medications and equipment needed for resuscitation should be readily available. This includes pharmacological agents such as epinephrine and aerosolized bronchodilators, as well as oxygen tanks, oxygen masks and nasal cannula, Ambu bag, oral airways, tracheostomy equipment, and a defibrillator.[8]

### Asparaginase

Intradermal skin testing is recommended before the first dose of asparaginase to identify those patients who are likely to experience a hypersensitivity reaction to the drug. Additional skin testing should be performed whenever an interval of 1 week or more has elapsed between doses.[87,88] A positive test is defined as a wheal or erythema appearing at the site of injection within 1 hour after administration of the test dose. It is important to note that there is no standardization to this testing and reactions can occur in patients who have had a negative skin test. Therefore, clinicians should be prepared for the development of hypersensitivity reactions including anaphylaxis throughout all administrations of asparaginase.[87] If the test is positive, there are 3 options for patients to continue treatment. One option is for the patient to undergo desensitization to the drug. A desensitization protocol can either be based on escalating doses of the drug or switching from a bolus IV dose or intramuscular dose to a slow, continuous infusion.[89]

Another option for the patient who is sensitive to asparaginase is to use the polyethylene glycolated (PEG) form of the drug, pegaspargase, which provides for extended uptake of the drug. If given intramuscularly, approximately 70% of patients who previously had a reaction to asparaginase tolerate the PEG form vs 90% of patients with no history of sensitivity to the unpegylated form. When given intravenously, however, the tolerance decreases to 40% for sensitive patients vs 90% for those with no known sensitivity to L-asparaginase.[87]

Finally, asparaginase is derived from *E. coli*. Another formulation is made from *E. chrysanthemi*, a parasitic bacterium. The 2 formulations have been shown to be immunologically distinct.[90] In a study of 21 patients who had severe reactions to asparaginase, 20 were switched to the *Erwinia* asparaginase and 18 of the 20 were able to complete treatment.[87]

### Taxanes

Both paclitaxel and docetaxel require interventions to reduce the incidence and severity of hypersensitivity reactions. Common preventive measures in the past included an administration time over 24 hours. Premedication with corticosteroids and antihistamines have allowed for faster infusion times (between 1 and 3 hours) and has reduced the rate of severe reaction to 2% to 4%.[49,91] Most patients who experience mild-to-moderate reactions during the first exposure will tolerate readministration of the drug using a slower infusion rate and further premedication after all symptoms have resolved.[8] Premedication typically includes corticosteroids, an $H_1$ antagonist, and a $H_2$ antagonist administered intravenously 30 minutes before the administration of the taxanes.[92]

Patients who have experienced sensitivity to paclitaxel generally tolerate docetaxel. However, reactions have also been noted with docetaxel, so premedication with steroids and antihistamines is still recommended.[93] There is no clear understanding of why patients may be able to tolerate docetaxel over paclitaxel. One explanation may be that docetaxel is a semisynthetic taxane while another explanation may be the lack of cross-sensitivity between the 2 drugs.[4] Desensitization protocols modifying infusion times have been used with success to reduce the risk of second reaction to paclitaxel.[8] Protocols are based on reinstating treatment at low concentrations and progressively increasing the concentration of the drug over extended infusion times, while continuing to premedicate patients with corticosteroids and antihistamines.

### Platinum compounds

There are no standard prophylaxis protocols for use with the platinum compounds. Most antiemetic regimens for the platinum compounds include corticosteroids, therefore adding some potential prophylaxis for hypersensitivity reactions as well. It is recommended to add some prophylaxis against hypersensitivity reaction in patients who will receive more than 4 to 5 courses of the platinum compounds. However, in a series of patients who received high-dose steroids and antihistamines before re-exposure to oxaliplatin, the majority of the patients (5 of 6) experienced a hypersensitivity reaction of the same severity as with a previous exposure to the drug.[9] There is some data that suggests that increasing the length of the infusion time with oxaliplatin will decrease the incidence of hypersensitivity reactions.[9,94,95]

No common strategy for resuming treatment after discontinuation after an episode of hypersensitivity is agreed upon. Premedication, desensitization, and replacement with a different platinum compound have all been used with some degree of success.[96] However, cross-reactivity to other platinum compounds must be considered with any subsequent treatment. Skin testing has been used to determine sensitivity and cross-sensitivity in patients receiving platinum compounds. Skin testing has shown a positive predictive value in several studies not only in identifying those at risk for hypersensitivity reaction, but also in cross-sensitivity following a hypersensitivity reaction to 1 platinum compound.[18,20,96] No standard strategy currently exists for skin testing patients for the potential for a hypersensitivity reaction.

### Epipodophyllotoxins

There is no standard prophylaxis protocol for preventing hypersensitivity reactions related to the administration of etoposide or teniposide.[4] One study has shown that rechallenge following a hypersensitivity reaction to either etoposide or teniposide preceded by premedication including steroids and antihistamines, as well as using a slowly titrated infusion could be successful.[69]

### Procarbazine

There are no standard prophylaxis protocols for preventing hypersensitivity reactions related to procarbazine. Many patients who receive procarbazine as part of the mechlorethamine, vincristine, procarbazine, and prednisone (MOPP) regimen for Hodgkin's lymphoma also receive a corticosteroid as part of their treatment regimen. In addition, the patients with brain tumors being treated with procarbazine are commonly also receiving steroid treatment. These regimens may preclude the need for additional prophylaxis.

### Biotherapy drugs

There is currently no premedication prophylaxis protocol based on research that is considered standard in preventing hypersensitivity reactions to biotherapy drugs. Histamine-2 receptor antagonists, such as diphenhydramine, and antipyretics, such as acetaminophen, are routinely ordered to decrease the potential of reaction with those drugs that carry a high risk of reaction. These drugs include the monoclonal antibodies with a high murine component, the interferons or the interleukins. Regularly scheduled antipyretics are often prescribed to minimize the side effects of fever and chills when using interferons and interleukins.

Each monoclonal antibody also has a specified infusion rate determined through clinical trials. Studies have shown that when these drugs are given at a slower rate there is generally a lower incidence of hypersensitivity reactions. An example of this is the standard infusion protocol for rituximab. The initial infusion is started at 50 mg/hour; the rate is then increased by 50 mg/hour every 30 minutes to a final rate of 400 mg/hour as long as the patient tolerates it. If the patient tolerates the first infusion, then subsequent infusions are started at 100 mg/hour and increased every 30 minutes by 100 mg/hour to a final rate of 400 mg/hour. Often, if patients do experience a hypersensitivity reaction, they can continue the infusion at the last tolerated rate once all symptoms have subsided. Published recommendations are to restart the infusion at half the rate before the reaction occurred.[29]

## NURSING CARE AND MANAGEMENT

Prompt recognition and immediate medical attention are crucial to reducing the risk of negative outcomes related to hypersensitivity reactions. Initial interventions should focus on preventing hypersensitivity reactions including anaphylaxis, which is manifested by increased capillary permeability, vasodilatation, and smooth muscle contraction. Oncology nurses administering medications with a risk of hypersensitivity reaction should have knowledge of and access to protocols that outline the management of hypersensitivity reactions. These protocols allow for immediate intervention by the nursing staff if a reaction occurs.

The first intervention in managing a suspected hypersensitivity reaction is to stop the drug infusion. The IV line should be maintained with normal saline or another appropriate solution. The nurse should stay with the patient while the physician is being notified. The patient should be placed in supine position to promote organ perfusion. Vital signs are monitored every 2 minutes until stable, then every 5 minutes for 30 minutes, and then every 15 minutes. It is essential to maintain the airway, providing oxygen if the patient experiences respiratory difficulty.

Emergency medications are necessary when hypersensitivity reactions continue to progress despite stopping the infusion. (See Table 31-6 for an outline of drugs used in the treatment of a hypersensitivity reaction of anaphylaxis.[49]) The first-line medication, used to manage a severe hypersensitivity reaction is epinephrine. Epinephrine can be given via the following routes: subcutaneous, intravenous, sublingual, intramuscular, and via the endotracheal tube. The route of administration generally depends on what form of the drug is immediately available; however, the subcutaneous route is preferred. There is no standard dose of epinephrine that is accepted, but a suggested protocol is 0.3 mg to 0.5 mg subcutaneously of a 1:1000 aqueous epinephrine solution diluted in 10 mL of normal saline. The dose may be repeated depending on the patient's condition.[52] Epinephrine is used to slow the absorption of the antineoplastic drug that caused the reaction, thus

**TABLE 31-6**

**Drugs Used in the Treatment of a Hypersensitivity Reaction of Anaphylaxis**

| Drug | Dose/Route | Action |
|---|---|---|
| Epinephrine | 0.1–0.5 mg (1:10,000) IV<br>0.2–0.5 mg (1:1000) subcutaneous (preferred) | Slow absorption of drug; counteracts effects of HSR: bronchodilation, peripheral vasoconstriction; increases cardiac contractility and heart rate |
| | | **Antihistamines** |
| H-1 antagonists | | Reduces multiple histamine effects: inhibits respiratory, vascular, and GI smooth muscle constriction; decreases capillary permeability; manages urticaria |
| Diphenhydramine | 25–50 mg IV | |
| H-2 antagonists | | |
| Cimetidine | 300 mg IV | |
| Famotidine | 20 mg IV | |
| Ranitidine | 50 mg IV | |
| Aminophylline | 5 mg/kg IV over 30 minutes | Bronchodilation |
| Dopamine | 2–20 mcg/kg/min IV | Increases cardiac output, blood pressure, and organ perfusion |
| Corticosteroids | | |
| Dexamethasone | 10–20 mg IV | Slows or halts the inflammatory process, decreases vascular permeability, blocks production of prostaglandins and leukotrienes, and enhances therapeutic effect of epinephrine |
| Hydrocortisone | 30–60 mg IV | |
| Methylprednisolone | 100–500 mg IV | |

*Abbreviations*: GI, gastrointestinal; HSR, hypersensitivity reaction; IV, intravenous.
*Source*: Reprinted with permission from Van Gerpen.[48]

counteracting the effects of hypersensitivity reactions. This occurs through bronchodilation, peripheral vasoconstriction, and increasing cardiac contractility and heart rate.[34,44,86]

Antihistamines are used to counteract the dyspnea and wheezing associated with hypersensitivity reactions. This is accomplished by reducing multiple histamine effects, thus inhibiting respiratory, vascular, and gastrointestinal smooth muscle contraction. Antihistamines also decrease capillary permeability and manage urticaria associated with hypersensitivity reactions.[44,86] The first-line antihistamine used is the $H_1$ antagonist diphenhydramine given intravenously 25 to 50 mg. $H_2$ antagonists, including cimetidine, famotidine, or ranitidine intravenously, can also be used in combination with diphenhydramine as second-line therapy. If diphenhydramine is ineffective, then aminophylline can be given intravenously over 30 minutes for bronchodilation.[34,97]

Large volumes of crystalloid fluids, either normal saline or Lactated Ringer's, are required to restore intravascular volume loss. During hypersensitivity reactions, especially during severe reactions, intravascular fluid shifts from the intravascular space to the extravascular space. Fluids are infused rapidly to help restore and maintain blood pressure.[52]

If hypotension persists despite fluid resuscitation, vasopressors such as dopamine are used to increase cardiac output, blood pressure, and organ perfusion.[44,52,10] Dopamine is generally the vasopressor of choice and is given at a rate of 2 to 20 mcg/kg/minute and is adjusted to the patient's response to the drug.[52] Corticosteroids such as dexamethasone, hydrocortisone, and methylprednisolone are used to slow or halt the inflammatory process, decrease vascular permeability, and block the production of prostaglandins and leukotrienes. Corticosteroids also enhance the therapeutic effect of epinephrine.[34,44] Corticosteroids may also prevent delayed or recurrent symptoms of hypersensitivity reactions. Beta-adrenergic blockers, angiotensin-converting enzyme inhibitors, monoamine oxidase inhibitors, or tricyclic antidepressants may interfere with the effectiveness of epinephrine and the body's compensatory mechanisms.[44] Intravenous glucagon, 1 to 2 mg over 5 minutes or 1 mg in 1000 mL of dextrose 5% in water at 5 mL to 15 mL/min, has been proven effective in some patients on beta-blockers who have experienced a hypersensitivity reaction.

In most cases of mild-to-moderate hypersensitivity reactions, the symptoms will resolve after a brief interruption of the infusion and administration of supportive medications. Patients who experience mild-to-moderate reactions to taxanes and monoclonal antibodies with the first exposure can often tolerate readministration of the drug at a slower rate once supportive medications are administered and symptoms have resolved.[8,49] However, rechallenge after a severe initial hypersensitivity reaction is discouraged. Thus, it is critical for accurate grading of infusion reactions.

Desensitization protocols have been used effectively to allow patients who have experienced a hypersensitivity reaction to continue treatment with drugs vital to their regimen. Desensitization protocols have been used for asparaginase, taxanes, platinum compounds, and monoclonal antibodies. Rapid desensitization protocols involve reintroduction of the drug beginning at low doses and increasing to their full therapeutic dose over a much shorter period of time; typically 4 to 14 hours.[86] Rapid desensitization protocols have been used successfully with carboplatin and oxaliplatin.[49] Any desensitization should only be performed in settings that can provide continuous observation and in which emergency resources are readily available.

## CONCLUSION

Hypersensitivity reactions to chemotherapy and biotherapy drugs are potentially life-threatening. Although any chemotherapy or biotherapy drug has the potential to cause hypersensitivity reactions, there are certain classes of drugs that put the patient at higher risk of developing a hypersensitivity reaction. These classes of drugs include the asparaginases, taxanes, platinum compounds, epipodophyllotoxins, procarbazine, and monoclonal antibodies with a high murine content. It is critical for nurses to be aware of these drugs and other risk factors to be able to effectively prevent hypersensitivity reactions, and to act promptly if these reactions do occur. Medical management with pharmacological intervention providing the ABCs of resuscitation can help to prevent the negative outcomes related to a hypersensitivity reaction. The development of a hypersensitivity reaction is often an anxiety provoking situation, thus it is critical for the nurse to provide emotional support to the patient and his/her family. Finally, all signs and symptoms of the hypersensitivity reactions and interventions should be thoroughly documented in the patient's record.

## REFERENCES


1. Shepherd GM. Hypersensitivity reactions to drugs: evaluation and management. *Mount Sinai J Med.* 2003;70;113–125.
2. Riedl MA, Casillas AM. Adverse drug reactions: types and treatment options. *Am Fam Physician.* 2003;68:1781–1790.
3. Weiss RB. Adverse effects of treatment: miscellaneous toxicities. In: DeVita VT, Hellman S, Rosenberg SA, eds. *Cancer: Principles and Practice of Oncology.* 7th ed. Philadelphia, PA: Lippincott Williams & Wilkins; 2005:2964–2976.
4. Gobel BH. Chemotherapy-induced hypersensitivity reactions. *Oncol Nurs Forum.* 2005;32:1027–1035.
5. Winkler U, Jensen M, Manzke O, et al. Cytokine-release syndrome in patients with B-cell lymphocytic leukemia and high lymphocyte counts after treatment with an anti-CD20 monoclonal antibody (rituximab, IDEC-C2B8). *Blood.* 1999;94:2217–2224.
6. Joint Task Force on Practice Parameters. The diagnosis and management of anaphylaxis: an updated practice parameter. *J Allergy Clin Immunol.* 2005;3(Suppl. 2):S438–S524.
7. Tang AW. A practical guide to anaphylaxis. *Am Fam Physician.* 2003;68:1325–1332, 1339–1340.
8. Lenz HJ. Management and preparedness for infusion and hypersensitivity reactions. *Oncologist.* 2007;12:601–609.
9. Brandi G, Pantaleo MA, Galli C, et al. Hypersensitivity reactions related to oxaliplatin (OHP). *Br J Cancer.* 2003;89:477–481.
10. Polovich M, Whitford JM, Olsen M, eds. *Chemotherapy and Biotherapy Guidelines and Recommendations for Practice* (3rd ed.) Pittsburgh, PA; Oncology Nursing Society: 2009.
11. Gobel BH. Hypersensitivity reactions to biological drugs. *Semin Oncol Nurs.* 2007;23:191–200.
12. Dellinger CT, Miale TD. Comparison of anaphylactic reactions to asparaginase derived from *Escherichia coli* and from *Erwinia* cultures. *Cancer.* 1976;38:1843–1846.
13. Sandberg-Wollheim M, Malmstrom P, Stromblad LG, et al. A randomized study of chemotherapy with procarbazine, vincristine, and lomustine with and without radiation therapy for astrocytoma grades 3 and/or 4. *Cancer.* 1991;68:22–29.
14. Coyle T, Bushunow P, Winfield J, Wright J, Graziano S. Hypersensitivity reactions to procarbazine with mechlorethamine, vincristine, and procarbazine chemotherapy in the treatment of glioma. *Cancer.* 1992;69:2532–2540.
15. O'Dwyer PJ, King SA, Fortner CL, Leyland-Jones B. Hypersensitivity reactions to teniposide (VM-26): an analysis. *J Clin Oncol.* 1986;4:1262–1269.
16. Kingsley CD. Hypersensitivity reactions. In: Perry MC, ed. *The Chemotherapy Source Book.* 4th ed. Philadelphia, PA: Lippincott Williams & Wilkins; 2008:152–173.
17. Hudson MM, Weinstein HJ, Donaldson SS, et al. Acute hypersensitivity reactions to etoposide in a VEPA regimen for Hodgkin's disease. *J Clin Oncol.* 1993;11:1080–1084.
18. Zanotti, KM, Markman M. Prevention and management of antineoplastic-induced hypersensitivity reactions. *Drug Saf.* 2001;24:767–779.
19. Thomas RR, Quinn MG, Schuler B, et al. Hypersensitivity reactions to chemotherapy drugs. *Alergol Immunol Clin .* 2000;15:161–181.
20. Markman M, Kennedy A, Webster K, et al. Clinical features of hypersensitivity reactions to carboplatin. *J Clin Oncol.* 1999;17:1141–1145.
21. Coiffier B, Lepage E, Briere J, et al. CHOP chemotherapy plus rituximab compared with CHOP alone in elderly patients with diffuse large-B-cell lymphoma. *N Engl J Med.* 2002;346:235–242.
22. Cook-Bruns N. Retrospective analysis of the safety of Herceptin® immunotherapy in metastatic breast cancer. *Oncology.* 2001;61 (Suppl 2):58–66.
23. Gomes ER, Demoly P. Epidemiology of hypersensitivity drug reactions. *Curr Opin Allergy Clin Immunol.* 2005;5:309–316.
24. Polyzos A, Tsavaris N, Kosmas C, et al. Hypersensitivity reactions to carboplatin administration are common but not always severe: a 10-year experience. *Oncology.* 2001;61:129–133.
25. Gowda A, Goel R, Berdzik J, et al. Hypersensitivity reactions to oxaliplatin: incidence and management. *Oncology (Williston Park).* 2004;18:1671–1675; discussion 1676, 1680, 1683, 1684.
26. Taxol® (paclitaxel) Injection [package insert]. Princeton, NJ: Bristol-Myers Squibb Company; March 2003.
27. Taxotere® (docetaxel) Injection Concentrate [package insert]. Bridgewater, NJ: Sanofi-Aventis; 2006.
28. Kaminski MS, Zelenetz AD, Press OW, et al. Pivotal study of iodine I-131 tositumomab for chemotherapy-refractory low grade or transformed low-grade B-cell non-Hodgkin's lymphoma. *J Clin Oncol.* 2001;19:3918–3928.
29. Rituxan® (rituximab) [package insert]. South San Francisco, CA: Genentech, Inc and Cambridge, MA: Biogen Idec Inc; February 2006.
30. Erbitux® (cetuximab) [package insert]. New York: ImClone Systems Inc and Princeton, NJ: Bristol-Myers Squibb Company; March 2006.

31. Herceptin® (trastuzumab) [package insert]. South San Francisco, CA: Genentech, Inc; February 2005.
32. Peeters M, Van Cutsem E, Siena S, et al. A phase III, multicenter, randomized controlled trial (RCT) of pantitumumab plus best supportive care (BSC) vs BSC alone in patients (pts) with metastatic colorectal cancer (mCRC). *Proc Am Assoc Cancer Res.* 2006;47:Abstract CP-1.
33. Vectibix™ (pantitumumab) [package insert]. Thousand Oaks, CA: Amgen Inc; September 2006.
34. Myers JS. Complications of cancer and cancer treatment. In: Langhorne ME, Fulton JS, Otto SE, eds. *Oncology Nursing.* 5th ed. St. Louis, MO: Mosby; 2007:402–453.
35. Grosen E, Siitari E, Larrison E, Tiggelaar C, Roecker E. Paclitaxel hypersensitivity reactions related to bee-sting allergy [research letters]. *Lancet.* 2000;355:288–289.
36. Stahl M, Koster W, Wilke H. Reaction after oxaliplatin—prevention with corticosteroids? *Ann Oncol.* 2001;12:874.
37. Brandi G, Pantaleo MA, Galli C, et al. Hypersensitivity reactions related to oxaliplatin (OHP). *Br J Cancer.*2003;89:477–481.
38. Lee C, Gianos M, Klaustermeyer WB. Diagnosis and management of hypersensitivity reactions related to common cancer chemotherapy agents. *Ann Allergy Asthma Immunol.* 2009;102:179–187; quiz 187–189, 222.
39. Wilkes GM. Chemotherapy and biotherapy. In: Gobel BH, Triest-Robertson S, Vogel WH, eds. *Advanced Oncology Nursing Certification Review and Resource Manual.* Pittsburgh, PA: Oncology Nursing Society; 2009:149–185.
40. Breslin S. Cytokine-release syndrome: overview and nursing implications. *Clin J Oncol Nurs.* 2007;11(Suppl 1):37–42.
41. O'Neil BH, Allen R, Spigel DR, Stinchcombe TE, Moore DT, Berlin JD, et al. High incidence of cetuximab-related infusion reactions in Tennessee and North Carolina and the association with atopic history. *J Clin Oncol*, 2007; 25:3644–3648.
42. Owera R, Gill A, Haddadin. High incidence of hypersensitivity reactions to cetuximab infusions in mid-Missouri: association with prior history of atopy. [abstract 20747], *J Clin Oncol*, 2008; 26; (May 20 Suppl.).
43. Makhoul I, Siegel E., Hutchins L. Cetuximab-related first infusion reaction (FIR) in colorectal cancer (CRC) and other cancer (CA) in patients (Pts). [abstract 381], presented at ASCO 2008 Gastrointestinal Cancers Symposium.
44. Labovich TM. Acute hypersensitivity reactions to chemotherapy. *Semin Oncol Nurs.* 1999;15:222–231.
45. Ream M, Tunison D. Hypersensitivity reactions. In: Yasko JM, ed. *Nursing Management of Symptoms Associated with Chemotherapy.* 5th ed. Bala Cynwyd, PA: Meniscus Limited; 2001:271–282.
46. Thomas M. *Treatment-Related Hypersensitivity Reactions to Antineoplastic Agents: Recognition, Prevention, and Management* [Continuing education monograph and self-test]. Skillman, NJ: American Academy of Continuing Medical Education; 2004.
47. National Cancer Institute. Common Terminology Criteria for Adverse Events v3.0 (CTCAE). Published date August 9, 2006. http://ctep.cancer.gov/protocolDevelopment/electronic_applications/docs/ctcaev3.pdf. Accessed January 18, 2010.
48. Van Gerpen R. Chemotherapy and biotherapy-induced hypersensitivity reactions. *J Infus Nurs.* 2009;32:157–165.
49. Cheifetz A, Smedley M, Martin S, et al. The incidence and management of infusion reactions to infliximab: a large center experience. *Am J Gastroenterol.* 2003;98:1315–1324.
50. Yeung S, Escalante CP. Oncologic emergencies. In: Kufe DW, Pollock RE, Weichselbaum RR, et al, eds: *Holland-Frei Cancer Medicine.* 5th ed. Hamilton, Ontario: BC Decker Inc; 2000:2659–2670.
51. Chung CH. Managing premedications and the risk for reactions to infusional monoclonal antibody therapy. *Oncologist.* 2008;13:725–732.
52. Drain KL, Volcheck GW. Preventing and managing drug-induced anaphylaxis. *Drug Saf.* 2001;24:843–853.
53. Truini Pittman L, Rosseto C. Pediatric considerations in tumor lysis syndrome. *Semin Oncol Nurs.* 2002;18(Suppl 3):17–22.
54. Muller HJ, Beier R, Loning L, et al. Pharmacokinetics of native *Escherichia coli* asparaginases (Asparaginase medac) and hypersensitivity reactions in ALL-BFM 95 reinduction treatment. *Br J Haematol.* 2001;114:794–799.
55. Feldweg AM, Lee C-W, Matulonis UA, et al. Rapid desensitization for hypersensitivity reactions to paclitaxel and docetaxel: a new standard protocol used in 77 successful treatments. *Gynecol Oncol* 2005;96:824–829.
56. Ardavanis A, Tryfonopoulos D, Yiotis I, et al. Non-allergic nature of docetaxel-induced acute hypersensitivity reactions. *Anticancer Drugs.* 2004;15:581–585.
57. Reimann HJ, Schmal A, Dormann P, et al. Histamine release in dogs by Cremophor EL and its derivatives: oxethylated oleic acid is the most effective constituent. *Agents Actions* 1977;7:63–67.
58. Gradishar WJ. Albumin-bound paclitaxel: a next-generation taxanes. *Expert Opin Pharmacother.* 2006;7:1041–1053.
59. Markman M. Managing taxanes toxicities. *Support Care Cancer.* 2003;11:144–147.
60. Blumenreich MS, Needle B, Yagoda A, Sogani P, Grabstald H, Whitmore WF Jr. Intravesical cisplatin for superficial bladder tumors. *Cancer.* 1982;50:863–865.
61. Denis L. Anaphylactic reactions to repeated intravesical instillation with cisplatin [letter]. *Lancet.* 1983;1:1378–1379.
62. Shukunami K, Kurokawa T, Kawakami Y, Kubo M, Kotsuji F. Hypersensitivity reactions to intraperitoneal administration of carboplatin in ovarian cancer: the first report of a case. *Gynecol Oncol.* 1999;72:431–432.
63. Cheng E, Cvitkovic E, Wittes RE, Golbey RB. Germ cell tumors (II): VAB II in metastatic testicular cancer. *Cancer.* 1978;42:2162–2168.
64. Anderson T, Javadpour N, Schilsky R, Barlock A, Young RC. Chemotherapy for testicular cancer: current status of the National Cancer Institute combined modality trial. *Cancer Treat Rep.* 1979;63:1687–1692.
65. Gralla RJ, Casper ES, Kelsen DP, et al. Cisplatin and vindesine combination chemotherapy for advanced carcinoma of the lung: a randomized trial investigating two dosage schedules. *Ann Intern Med.* 1981;95:414–420.
66. Paraplatin (carboplatin aqueous solution) Injection [package insert]. Princeton, NJ: Bristol-Myers Squibb Company; 2004.
67. Sorich J, Taubes B, Wagner A, Hochster H. Oxaliplatin: practical guidelines for administration. *Clin J Oncol Nurs.* 2004;8:251–256.
68. Thomas RR, Quinn MG, Schuler B, et al. Hypersensitivity and idiosyncratic reactions to oxaliplatin. *Cancer.* 2003;97:2301–2307.
69. Kellie SJ, Crist WM, Pui CH, et al. Hypersensitivity reactions to epipodophyllotoxins in children with acute lymphoblastic leukemia. *Cancer.* 1991;67:1070–1075.
70. Lehmann DF, Hurteau TE, Newman N, Coyle TE. Anticonvulsant usage is associated with an increased risk of procarbazine hypersensitivity reactions in patients with brain tumors. *Clin Pharmacol Ther.* 1997;62:225–229.
71. Glovsky MM, Braunwald J, Opelz G, Alenty A. Hypersensitivity to procarbazine associated with angioedema, urticaria, and low serum complement activity. *J Allergy Clin Immunol.* 1976;57:134–140.
72. Wilkes GM, Barton-Burke M, eds. *Oncology Nursing Drug Handbook.* Sudbury, MA: Jones and Bartlett; 2009.
73. Fischer DS, Knobf MT, Durivage HJ, et al, eds. *The Cancer Chemotherapy Handbook.* 6th ed. Philadelphia, PA: Mosby; 2003.
74. Foss FM, Bacha P, Osann KE, et al. Biological correlates of acute hypersensitivity events with DAB (389) IL-2 (denileukin diftitox, ONTAK) in cutaneous T-cell lymphoma: decreased frequency and severity with steroid premedication. *Clin Lymphoma.* 2001;1:298–302.
75. Olsen ED, Duvic M, Frankel A, et al. Pivotal phase III trial of two dose levels of denileukin diftitox for the treatment of cutaneous T-cell lymphoma. *J Clin Oncol.* 2001;19:376–388.

76. Wiseman GA, White CA, Witzig TE, et al. Radioimmunotherapy of relapsed non-Hodgkin's lymphoma with zevalin, a 90Y-labeled anti-CD20 monoclonal antibody. *Clin Cancer Res.* 1999;5:3281s–3286s.
77. Kaminski MS, Tuck M, Estes J, et al. Pivotal study of iodine I131 tositumomab for chemotherapy-refractory lowgrade or transformed low-grade B-cell non-Hodgkin's lymphomas. *J Clin Oncol.* 2001;19:3918–3928.
78. DeNardo G. Treatment of non-Hodgkin's lymphoma (NHL) with radiolabeled antibodies (mAbs). *Semin Nucl Med.* 2002;35:202–211.
79. LaCasce AS, Castells MC, Burstein H, Meyerhardt JA. Infusion reactions to therapeutic monoclonal antibodies used for cancer therapy. http://www.uptodate.com. Accessed January 18, 2010.
80. Hurwitz H, Fehrenbacher L, Novotny W, et al. Bevacizumab plus irinotecan, fluorouracil, and leucovorin for metastatic colorectal cancer. *N Engl J Med.* 2004;350:2334–2342.
81. Avastin® (bevacizumab) [package insert]. South San Francisco, CA: Genentech, Inc; June 2006.
82. Larson RA, Boogaerts M, Estey E, et al. Antibody-targeted chemotherapy of older adults with acute myeloid leukemia in first relapse after Mylotarg (gemtuzumab ozogamicin). *Leukemia.* 2002;16:1627–1636.
83. Sievers EL, Larson RA, Stadtmauer EA, et al. Efficacy and safety of gemtuzumab ozogamicin in patients with CD33-positive acute myeloid leukemia in first relapse. *J Clin Oncol.* 2001;19:3244–3254.
84. Cobleigh M, Vogel CL, Tripathy D, et al. Multinational study of the efficacy and safety of humanized anti-HER2 monoclonal antibody in women who have HER2-overexpressing metastatic breast cancer that has progressed after chemotherapy for metastatic disease. *J Clin Oncol.* 1999;17:2639–2648.
85. Hecht JR, Patnaik A, Berlin J, et al. Panitumumab monotherapy in patients with previously treated metastatic colorectal cancer. *Cancer.* 2007;110:980–988.
86. Carr BW, Burke C. Outpatient chemotherapy: hypersensitivity and anaphylaxis. *Am J Nurs.* 2001;101(Suppl):27–30.
87. Shepherd GM. Hypersensitivity reactions to chemotherapeutic drugs. *Clin Rev Allergy Immunol.* 2003;24:253–262.
88. Elspar® (Asparaginase) product information. http://www.merck.com/product/usa/pi_curculars/e/elspar_pi.pdf. Published 2005. Accessed January 18, 2010.
89. Rodriguez T, Baumgarten E, Fengler R, et al. Long-term infusion of L-asparaginase—an alternative to intramuscular injection? *Klin Padiatr.* 1995;207:207–210.
90. Stone HD Jr, DiPiro C, Davis PC, et al. Hypersensitivity reactions to *Escherichia coli*-derived polyethylene glycolate-asparaginase associated with subsequent immediate skin test reactivity to *E. coli*-derived granulocyte-colony stimulating factor. *J Allergy Clin Immunol.* 1998;101:429–431.
91. Seidman AD, Hudis CA, Albanel J, et al. Dose-dense therapy with weekly 1-hour paclitaxel infusion in the treatment of metastatic breast cancer. *J Clin Oncol.* 1998;16:3353–3361.
92. Myers JS. Hypersensitivity reaction to paclitaxel after acute hypersensitivity reactions. *J Clin Oncol Nurs.* 2000;4:161–163.
93. Berstein BJ. Docetaxel as an alternative to paclitaxel after acute hypersensitivity reactions. *Ann Pharmacother.* 2000;34:1332–1335.
94. Dold F, Hoey D, Carberry M, et al. Hypersensitivity in patients with metastatic colorectal carcinoma undergoing chemotherapy with oxaliplatin [abstract 1478]. *Proc Am Soc Clin Oncol.* 2002;21:370a.
95. Giachetti S, Perpoint B, Zidani R, et al. Phase III multicenter randomized trial of oxaliplatin added to chronomodulated fluorouracil-leucovorin as first-line treatment of metastatic colorectal cancer. *J Clin Oncol.* 2000;18:136–147.
96. Leguy-Sequin V, Jolimy G, Coudert B, et al. Diagnostic and predictive value of skin testing in platinum salt hypersensitivity. *J Allergy Clin Immunol.* 2007;119:726–730.
97. Lieberman P, Kemmp SF, Oppenheimer J, et al. The diagnosis and management of anaphylaxis: an updated practice parameter. *J Allergy Clin Immunol.* 2005;115(3 Pt 2):S483–S523.

CHAPTER

32

Carlton G. Brown, PhD, RN, AOCN®

# Oral Mucositis

## SCOPE OF THE PROBLEM

Mucositis is a common symptom reported by patients undergoing chemotherapy or radiation treatment for cancer.[1–5] Sometimes referred to as *stomatitis,* mucositis is one of the most painful, incapacitating, and menacing side effects associated with the treatment of cancer. In a study by Borbasi and colleagues, one participant stated that "mucositis is the worst thing that happened" to the patient during treatment.[6,p.1054]

Because mucositis is considered to be an inflammatory and ulcerative response to some forms of cancer treatment, virtually all tissue of the gastrointestinal (GI) tract is potentially damaged in the form of open sores. Historically, mucositis was divided into two major categories: oral and GI.[7] While this chapter will recognize both forms of mucositis, the primary focus will be on oral mucositis.

Patients with oral mucositis (OM) sometimes have mouth sores, oral pain, difficulty eating and swallowing, dry mouth, and difficulty talking. In fact, approximately 80% of patients with OM have oral pain.[2] Sometimes the oral pain is so significant that patients must take some form of pain medication, often an opioid analgesic, for pain relief. Further, some patients find OM so painful that they prematurely withdraw from their cancer therapy.[8] Sonis and colleagues estimated that approximately 30% of patients with OM discontinued treatment completely; 60% of patients with OM had subsequent treatment delays.[8] Elting and colleagues noted that the risk of dose reduction of chemotherapy doubled when OM was present.[9]

Infection is another major problem for patients with OM. Because of ulcerative damage to the mucosal tissue, an "open window" for microorganisms (bacteria and fungi) is sometimes created, placing patients at risk for numerous opportunistic and systemic infections. The impact of OM should not be underestimated and, if untreated, affects treatment schedules, quality of life, and aspects of daily living. Unfortunately, to date, despite a recent increase in research and attention to this troublesome side effect, there are very few clinical outcomes based in research that are successful in preventing or lessening OM.

Oral mucositis is multifactorial in nature. This chapter will review the pathophysiology of oral mucositis, along with the risk factors, clinical manifestations, and assessment. Care of the patient with OM will be reviewed with a specific focus on interventions to alleviate or lessen this debilitating problem for patients treated for cancer.

## DEFINITIONS

*Mucositis* refers to an inflammatory process involving the mucous membranes of the oral cavity and GI tract.[10] As discussed previously, the terms *mucositis* and *stomatitis* historically have been used to signify tissue damage specific to the oral cavity. However, damage to the GI tract actually begins at the lips of the oral cavity and ends at the rectum. Therefore, new terminology has been suggested that terms all mucositis as *alimentary mucositis* while using the more specific terms *oral mucositis* to refer to the oral cavity and *gastrointestinal mucositis* to refer to the rest of the GI tract. It is suggested that the continued use of these newer terms by healthcare providers will improve overall communication of the type of mucositis being discussed and assist in clear verbalization of interventions for both prevention and treatment.[10]

## INCIDENCE

It is estimated that 400,000 people each year develop OM due to cancer treatments.[11] There is significant variability in the incidence of OM depending on several factors, including age, diagnosis, level of oral health prior to and during treatment, and dose and frequency of the respective cancer therapy.[12] Specific ranges of OM incidence will be discussed in more detail later in this chapter, but in general, the incidence of OM in patients treated for cancer ranges from 30% to 100%. Virtually every patient with head and neck cancer treated with radiation will endure some degree of OM.[13] Patients who receive radiotherapy and chemotherapy concurrently for head and neck cancer also have marked OM.[14]

There is quite a bit of variability in OM in relation to the administration of chemotherapy. Approximately 75% of patients undergoing high-dose chemotherapy during stem cell transplantion experience OM. Further, allogeneic transplants are associated with higher levels of OM than autologous transplants.[15] In a more recent study, Brown and colleagues found that 50% of patients receiving outpatient chemotherapy complained of some level of sore mouth, an indicator of OM.[16]

## ETIOLOGY AND RISK FACTORS

Are there factors that place a patient at heightened risk for OM? Why do some patients experience more severe OM than others? Interestingly, the incidence and severity of OM vary depending on numerous patient-related (Table 32-1) and treatment-related risk factors (Table 32-2).[17,18]

### Patient-related factors

Both age and gender appear to play a potential role in the development of OM, yet according to Barasch and Peterson, it is uncertain how these variables influence OM.[18] When compared with adults, children and the elderly seem to be at a higher risk for OM. Cheng and Chang noted that OM was one of the most distressing side effects for pediatric patients treated with chemotherapy.[19]

**TABLE 32-1**

**Patient-Related Risk Factors for the Development of Oral Mucositis**

| | |
|---|---|
| Age | Children/elderly are at greater risk. |
| Oral health/hygiene | Poor oral health/hygiene increases risk of OM. |
| Salivary secretion function | Reduced salivary flow increases susceptibility to OM. |
| Genetic factors | Patients who express high levels of cytokines may be at higher risk for OM. |
| BMI | Low BMI (<20 for males and <19 for females) increases the risk of OM. |
| Renal function | Decreased renal function increases the risk of OM. |
| Smoking | Patients who smoke may be at higher risk of OM. |
| Previous cancer treatment | Patients treated previously for cancer may be at higher risk for OM. |
| Oral microflora | Higher incidence of OM in patients with higher levels of microflora. |
| Inflammation | Role of inflammation in development of OM unclear but suspect. |
| Gender | Women greater than men. |

*Abbreviations*: BMI, body mass index; OM, oral mucositis.

*Source*: Based on data from Avritscher et al[17] and Barasch and Peterson.[18]

**TABLE 32-2**

**Treatment-Related Risk Factors for the Development of Oral Mucositis**

| | |
|---|---|
| Chemotherapy agent | 5-FU, methotrexate, and etoposide produce high rate of OM. |
| Chemotherapy dosage | High-dose chemotherapy regimens are associated with higher incidence and severity of OM. |
| Type of SCT | Allogeneic SCT recipients experience higher rates of mucositis than autologous SCT recipients. |
| Radiation site | Radiation administered directly to the head and neck, thorax, and abdomen produce higher rates of OM. |
| Combined modality | The use of chemotherapy in conjunction with RT is associated with increased risk and severity of OM. |

*Abbreviations*: OM, oral mucositis; RT, radiation therapy; SCT, stem cell transplant; 5-FU, 5-fluorouracil.

*Source*: Based on data from Avritscher et al[17] and Barasch and Peterson.[18]

Zalcberg and colleagues compared levels of OM in three patient groups, those 60 years old and younger, those 61 to 69 years old, and those 70 years old or older, and found that older age was significantly correlated with OM, especially in the group over 70 years of age.[20] In another study, patients with GI cancer over 50 years of age developed more severe and longer-lasting OM, and the researchers from this study suggested that a decrease in renal function might be the etiology for increased OM.[21] When renal function is decreased, it takes longer for chemotherapy to be eliminated from the body. Higher levels of circulating chemotherapy might be a potential cause of more significant OM in the elderly population.

Gender also seems to be a potential risk factor for a higher incidence and severity of OM. In a study of adult patients receiving 5-fluorouracil, women in the study reported OM more frequently (women 63%, men 52%; $P = 0.002$) and with a greater severity.[22] In another two studies, women were reported to have a higher incidence of OM when compared with men.[20,23] In contrast, Chiara and colleagues reported a significantly higher incidence of OM in males.[24] Future research could clarify if gender is a specific risk factor for OM.

Salivary function, condition of the oral cavity prior to treatment, and level of oral hygiene are also patient-related factors that appear to play some role in OM. In a study of 63 adult patients receiving 5-fluorouracil, xerostomia (dry mouth) was a significant predictor of OM both prior to and during treatment.[25] It is hypothesized that saliva in the mouth helps to protect and wash the oral cavity; thus, when there is an absence of saliva, levels of OM appear to worsen.

Perhaps one of the most significant risk factors associated with the potential development of OM is preexisting oral or dental illness.[26,27] Given that approximately 80% of Americans have some level of periodontal disease,[21] many patients are already at risk for OM before cancer treatment even begins. While not completely supported with evidence, there is a belief among OM researchers that intensive oral hygiene during treatment helps to lessen the problem of OM.

Patients with poor nutritional status and lower body mass may be at higher risk for OM. Raber-Durlacher and colleagues concluded that a body mass index less than 20 for males and less than 19 for females is a significant predictor of OM.[21] Since appropriate nutritional status leads to proper healing, poor nutritional status prior to and during treatment could be related to more difficulty with OM. Poor nutritional status during treatment may be exacerbated because many patients find OM so painful that they often have difficulty eating or swallowing. Another patient-related factor that puts patients at higher risk for OM is genetics. Sonis and Fey hypothesize that proinflammatory cytokines play an important role in the pathogenesis of mucositis.[28] Some patients are genetically predisposed to produce higher levels of cytokines, which increases their risk of OM.

Patients who smoke or have smoked tobacco products in the past are at higher risk for developing OM.[29,30] It is hypothesized that smoking affects tissue healing, creating an environment where healing is less than optimal. Finally, patients who have had previous treatment for cancer, especially when the treatment consisted of several modalities, such as radiation and chemotherapy together, have a higher risk of developing OM.[30]

### Treatment-related factors

*Radiation.* Radiation-induced OM is the hallmark acute symptom in patients treated for head and neck cancer.[26] Gastrointestinal mucositis is also a problem, but to a lesser extent, when radiation is administered to the head and neck. When patients receive radiation therapy (RT) for the treatment of cancer, the overall goal is to cause permanent cell damage to the DNA, thus resulting in death of the cancer cells.[31] Unfortunately, other healthy cells that fall within the beam of RT are also damaged, which causes significant amounts of mucositis, especially in patients treated for head and neck cancer. Researchers estimate that almost all recipients of RT for head and neck cancer will experience OM to some degree.[32]

In a retrospective study investigating OM in patients receiving RT for head and neck cancer, Elting and colleagues reported that 91% of all patients in the study experienced some degree of OM.[32] Of that group, 66% had OM that was considered severe (rated grade 3 to 4). Of interest, participants in this study who experienced OM were significantly more likely to experience OM-related pain and weight loss.

According to Dodd, degree and duration of OM depend on four important factors that include radiation source, cumulative dose, dose intensity, and volume of radiated tissue.[33] Many patients who undergo RT treatment receive their therapy 5 days per week for numerous weeks (4 to 6 weeks), and their OM is almost always correlated with the number of treatments and the amount of radiation they have received. The more doses of RT a patient receives, the higher the incidence and severity of OM. Thus, by the final weeks of a patient's treatment, he or she is likely to experience the worst levels of OM severity over the entire treatment. Shih and colleagues note that damaging changes in the epithelium of the oral membrane often occur at a total dose level of 1600 to 2200 cGy when radiation is administered at a rate of 200 cGy per day.[31] These same researchers note that the worst total mucosal damage occurs at 5,000 to 6,000 cGy. Radiation therapy–induced OM is usually dose limiting; thus, when the RT is completed, partial healing begins almost immediately. Unfortunately, there are long-term sequelae associated with RT treatment, which may include permanent tissue damage and xerostomia, or absence of saliva.[33]

*Chemotherapy.* Numerous chemotherapeutic agents cause OM.[34] Table 32-3 presents those chemotherapy drugs with a higher affinity for the development of OM. A group of researchers conducted a review of 338 research studies that reported results of recent chemotherapy and radiation regimens with associated grade 3 and 4 OM.[8]

In a study of patients receiving standard-dose chemotherapy over a 2-week interval, 32% of participants reported experiencing OM, and 69% of those same participants considered OM to be an important toxicity associated with chemotherapy administration.[35] Raber-Durlacher and colleagues determined in a retrospective study of patients receiving chemotherapy for a variety of solid tumors that

**TABLE 32-3**

**Chemotherapeutic Agents With a Tendency to Cause Oral Mucositis**

| | |
|---|---|
| 5-Fluorouracil[a] | Etoposide |
| 6-Mercaptopurine | Floxuridine |
| 6-Thioguanine | High-dose methotrexate |
| Actinomycin D | Hydroxurea |
| Bleomycin | Mechlorethamine[a] |
| Busulfan[a] | Melphalan |
| Capecitabine[a] | Mitomycin |
| Cyclophosphamide[a] | Mitoxantrone |
| Cytosine arabinoside | Paclitaxel |
| Daunomycin | Procarbazine |
| Daunorubicin | Thiotepa |
| Docetaxel | Vinblastine |
| Doxil[a] | Vinorelbine |
| Doxorubicin | |

[a]Most commonly implicated in the development of oral mucositis.

*Source*: Based on data from Wilkes.[34]

approximately 31% of the patients developed mucositis.[21] Of that 31%, 11% had slight OM, 17% had mild to moderate OM, and only 4% had moderate to severe OM. Of interest, none of the patients in this study reported severe OM. Zalcberg and colleagues conducted a study of 444 patients who either received raltitrexed or 5-fluorouracil/leucovorin for colorectal cancer.[20] There was a statistically significant higher incidence of mucositis ($P < 0.001$) in the group receiving 5-fluorouracil (22%) vs those who received raltitrexed (2%). This study supports the idea that 5-fluorouracil, especially given continuously for several days, is a risk factor for the development of OM.

In general, the incidence and severity of OM often are related to the dose and frequency of administration of chemotherapy agents to patients with cancer.[33] For example, patients receiving high-dose chemotherapy for stem cell transplantation and certain leukemia regimens are at higher risk for OM. As with RT treatment, chemotherapy-induced OM is dose related; when the chemotherapy treatment is terminated, the oral mucosa begins to heal. While the long-term effects of chemotherapy on mucosal tissue are unknown in relationship to permanent damage, it appears that chemotherapy does not cause as much long-term permanent damage as RT.

It is also suggested that patients who receive chemotherapy continuously, as is the case for some patients with colon cancer who receive 5-fluorouracil, have a higher severity of OM. Finally, in many instances, for patients who receive several cycles of chemotherapy consecutively, OM severity tends to worsen with each cycle, suggesting a cumulative effect of these agents on OM.

*Combination therapy.* When certain chemotherapy agents and RT treatments are combined or used sequentially, OM is an even more serious problem. Perhaps the issue is that in some instances mucosal tissue exposed to the effects of one treatment never completely heals before the next therapy is initiated. Mucosal tissue that has been irradiated almost never recovers completely and thus is more susceptible to damage by future treatments of chemotherapy.[31]

Shih and colleagues estimate that when RT and chemotherapy are used concurrently, OM increases from 60% to 100%.[31] In a previously mentioned study, Elting and colleagues found that patients with oral cavity or oropharynx cancer who received both chemotherapy and RT together had significantly higher levels of OM than those who had RT alone (98% vs 85%; $P = 0.002$).[9]

*Stem cell transplantion.* Oral mucositis is a frequent symptom of patients undergoing stem cell transplantation (SCT). McGuire and colleagues found that 86% of patients undergoing allogeneic and autologous SCT experienced OM.[2] In a pilot study of SCT patients, 70% reported mild to moderate oral pain described as "tender," "irritating," and "sore." Patients who received high-dose chemotherapy followed by SCT reported OM as the most debilitating side effect associated with that treatment.[1] The conditioning regimen for patients undergoing SCT includes chemotherapy in high doses, often several times greater than the standard dose of chemotherapy for solid-tumor malignancies.[17] Some SCT patients receive treatments that consist of high-dose chemotherapy and total-body irradiation (TBI), which places them at even higher risk for mucositis. There seems to be some variability in OM depending on the type of transplant a patient receives. Sonis and colleagues found that more patients (35%) receiving allograft transplants had grade 3 OM than patients receiving autograft transplants (21%).[15]

Oral mucositis in the transplant population is a particular concern. The oral mucosa serves as a barrier for many bacterial, viral, and fungal microorganisms. During periods of OM, it is common to have sores or breaks in the oral mucosa that provide an entry way for microorganisms. Many patients undergoing SCT have a reduced infection-fighting capacity. Thus patients with OM undergoing transplant are at a very high risk for systemic infections, which could lead to eventual sepsis.

## PHYSIOLOGICAL ALTERATIONS

### PATHOGENESIS OF ORAL MUCOSITIS

Historically, it was hypothesized that OM was the result of nonspecific damage to the epithelium caused solely by radiation and chemotherapy injury.[36] While damage to the epithelium is still believed to be part of the problem, Sonis and colleagues[36] have proposed a theoretical model for the development and resolution of OM that is a complex process and includes 5 phases: (1) initiation, (2) primary damage response, (3) signaling and amplification, (4) ulceration, and (5) healing. Figure 32-1 presents an abbreviated path of the phases of OM.

#### Phase I: Initiation

Almost immediately following exposure to chemotherapy or ionizing radiation, the initiation phase begins. DNA and non-DNA are damaged, resulting in a distinct injury to the cells of the submucosa and basal epithelium. While the mucosa appears completely normal, it is the damage to the cells of the underlying submucosa that begins a downward spiral of overall tissue injury.

#### Phase II: Primary damage response

After initiation, numerous individual biological actions happen that create further damage. Apoptosis (programmed cell death) happens to the cells of the epithelium. The transcription factor nuclear factor kB (NF-kB) is activated, thus controlling some 200 genes closely associated with toxicity of the

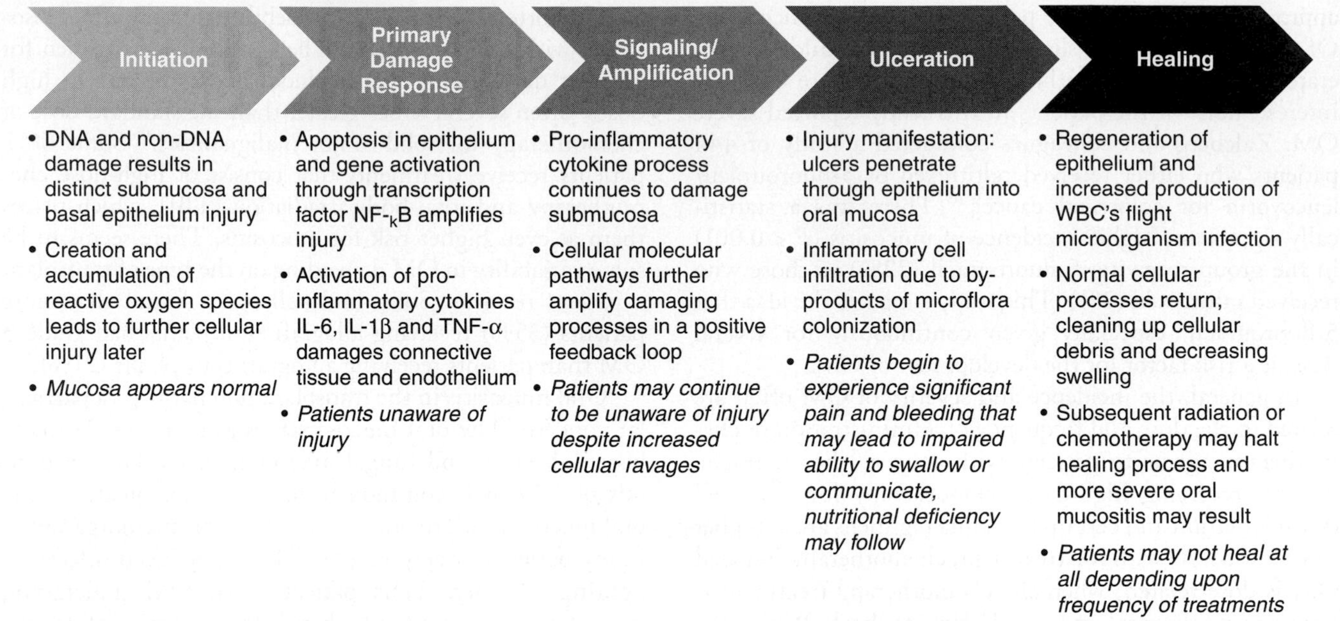


**FIGURE 32-1**

The five biological phases of mucositis.

*Abbreviations*: IL, interleukin; NF, nuclear factor; TNF, tumor necrosis factor; WBC, white blood cell.

*Source*: Based on data from Sonis.[36]

mucosa.[36] As these genes, which are present in the endothelium, fibroblasts, macrophages, and epithelium, become activated, they cause an amplification of injury. Sonis hypothesizes that at this point proinflammatory cytokines including interleukin 6 (IL-6), IL-1β, and tumor necrosis factor-α (TNF-α) become activated, causing early damage to connective tissue and endothelium.[36] Further, the proinflammatory cytokines are believed to initiate mesenchymal-epithelial signaling, reduce epithelial oxygenation, and ultimately result in injury and subsequent death of epithelial basal cells. Of interest, patients are not likely to be aware of the damage that is occurring during this phase of mucositis.

### Phase III: Signaling and amplification

In this phase, proinflammatory cytokines and other proteins continue to barrage tissue of the submucosa, thereby causing further damage. In addition, molecular pathways are activated that amplify mucosal injury through a positive-feedback loop. Amazingly, even in the first few phases of OM, patients still may not feel the effects of the ongoing mucosal damage.[36]

### Phase IV: Ulceration

The ulceration phase may be the most complex and symptomatic for the patient.[36] As the biological cascade begins to take its toll on the oral mucosa, injury is manifested in the form of ulceration, which penetrates through the epithelium into the submucosa. In addition, significant inflammatory cells infiltrate, in part, as a result of the metabolic by-products of colonizing microflora.[37] It is during this phase that OM greatly affects the patient's well-being by causing painful lesions.[38] Patients may begin to feel significant pain and have loss of full swallowing effect that may lead to nutritional deficiencies. Also during this phase, patients may experience decreased ability to communicate and increased amounts of bleeding.

### Phase V: Healing

This phase of the development of OM is characterized by direct healing of the epithelium through regeneration. As the epithelium heals, there is also an increased production of white blood cells, which help to fight infection from bacteria and other harmful microorganisms. It is important to remember that if a patient is receiving subsequent cycles of chemotherapy or radiation, the underlying cells and tissues of the mucosa may not return immediately to their original healed state. If subsequent treatments of radiation or chemotherapy are indicated, the stage may be set for more severe OM in future cycles related to incomplete healing.

## CLINICAL MANIFESTATIONS

In patients receiving chemotherapy, inflammation may occur between 2 and 14 days following drug administration.[39]

In chemotherapy-related OM, lesions usually are located on the nonkeratinized surfaces of the soft palate, buccal mucosa (inside of cheek), and lateral and ventral sides of the tongue.[40] Oral mucositis in patients receiving chemotherapy can last up to 28 days. If numerous cycles of chemotherapy are being administered, OM associated with subsequent cycles of chemotherapy may have a longer duration related to the lack of time for cellular recovery and adequate healing.[39]

In patients receiving RT, OM usually begins the second week following treatment or after a dose of 2000 cGy and continues for up to a few weeks after RT is completed. Patients with head and neck cancer are usually treated for 5 to 7 weeks and receive approximately 200 cGy/day with a treatment regimen of 5 days per week. Oral mucositis in patients receiving RT usually worsens as treatment continues and is specifically related to the beam of the radiation. Healthy tissue that falls within the beam of radiation will be affected, whereas tissue outside the beam generally is spared damage. Patients will develop severe OM after receiving more than 5000 cGy of RT.[40] Patients suffering from radiation-induced OM also experience pain and varied levels of xerostomia.

Each patient experiences OM differently depending on numerous risk factors previously discussed that include type of treatment (RT/chemotherapy) and dosage administered. Oral mucositis usually starts with asymptomatic erythema and redness of the oral cavity.[26] Eventually, erythema is replaced by erosion and eventual ulceration, which is often covered with a white fibrinous pseudomembrane.[37] It is not usually until the ulceration phase that patients begin to feel pain associated with OM.[36] The eventual ulcerations can become significantly painful, and patients sometimes describe OM as the worst symptom associated with their respective treatment. In general, OM begins to heal once chemotherapy and RT are terminated, yet long-term effects, such as xerostomia, will plague some patients for the rest of their lives.

## ASSESSMENT AND GRADING

Numerous scales are available to assess the severity and other aspects associated with OM. Unfortunately, a big impediment to OM research has been the absence of a validated scoring assessment tool. Perhaps the simplest and easiest-to-use tool is the World Health Organization (WHO) scale that grades OM on a scale of 0 to 4. A WHO score of 0 equals no OM, whereas a score of 4 equals the presence of ulcers and alimentation that is not possible due to mucositis.[41]

The Oral Assessment Guide (OAG), designed by Eilers and associates,[42] has been used in several research studies.[3,27,43,44] The OAG is fairly simple to use, has a limited number of items on the tool, and takes approximately 3 to 4 minutes to complete.[43] The OAG, shown in Table 32-4, explores changes in the oral cavity using 8 parameters—voice, swallow, lips, tongue, saliva, mucous membranes,

**TABLE 32-4**

**Oral Assessment Guide (OAG)**

| | Score | | |
|---|---|---|---|
| **Item** | **1** | **2** | **3** |
| Voice | Normal | Deeper or raspy | Difficulty talking or painful |
| Swallow | Normal swallow | Some pain on swallowing | Unable to swallow |
| Lips | Smooth and pink and moist | Dry or cracked | Ulcerated bleeding |
| Tongue | Pink and moist and papillae present | Coated or loss of papillae with a shiny appearance with or without redness | Blistered or cracked |
| Saliva | Watery | Thick or ropy | Absent |
| Mucous membrane (buccal mucosa, palate) | Pink and moist | Reddened or coated (increased whiteness) without ulceration | Ulceration with or without bleeding |
| Gingiva | Pink and stippled and firm | Oedematous with or without redness | Spontaneous bleeding or bleeding with pressure |
| Teeth or dentures | Clean with no debris | Plaque or debris in localized area (between teeth if present) | Plaque or debris generalized along gum line or denture bearing area |

*Source*: Used with permission from Eilers, Berger, and Peterson.[42]

gingiva, and teeth or dentures—and has an adequate validity (content, construct) and reliability (interrater).[42,43]

The Oral Mucositis Assessment Scale (OMAS) focuses on erythema and ulceration throughout the oral cavity.[45] The Eastern Cooperative Oncology Group (ECOG) scale is another toxicity criteria-rating scale that can be used to assess the severity of OM.[46] Other assessment tools include the Oral Mucosa Rating Scale (OMRS),[47] the Oral Mucositis Index (OMI),[48] and the OM rating tool created by the Western Consortium for Cancer Nursing Research.[49] Regardless of the assessment tool that is used, it is imperative that caregivers use a tool that is reliable, valid, and *clinically* useful. According to McGuire, "Without consistent oral assessment, caregivers cannot know the characteristics or extent of oral complications, nor can they monitor progress and outcomes following treatment."[50 p.437]

Usually, patients are acutely aware of any changes in their own oral cavity. The oral cavity in a healthy individual is moist, clean, pink, and intact. Abnormal assessment findings include changes in moisture (dryness and decreased amounts of saliva), color (pallor, erythema, white patches), cleanliness (odor and accumulation of debris), integrity (ulcers, cracks, lesions), and perception (pain, hoarseness, difficulty swallowing).[39] It is recommended that all patients with cancer receive a systematic assessment of their oral cavity. The patient should be asked about ill-fitting dentures or other appliances, current oral pain, changes in saliva and swallowing, obvious lesions, and any other changes to the oral mucosa. It is also helpful to understand the patient's current oral care practices.

It is critical for nurses or other health care professionals to conduct an oral assessment prior to treatment and, depending on the risks for OM, more frequently (daily) during treatment.[51] According to Beck,[39] the assessment should be conducted in an area with natural light to allow for better observation, and the assessment generally takes only a minute or two to conduct. Prior to assessment, equipment that will be used during the oral assessment should be gathered, including nonsterile gloves, tongue blade, dental mirror, and gauze. Before beginning the assessment, the patient removes any partial plates or full dentures. During inspection, the nurse should observe the outer lips, teeth, gums, tongue, inside the cheek area, and hard and soft palate. Particular attention should be focused on inspection of the floor of the oral cavity under the tongue and to the upper and lower cheeks and tissue close to the gums. Sometime during the oral assessment, the nurse should ask the patient to rate his or her oral pain using a 0 to 10 scale. The nurse then uses both patient report and physical findings from the oral examination to guide interventions for the patient experiencing OM. Following the oral assessment, the nurse should document findings in the patient record. The patient should be referred to a dentist if a more thorough examination is warranted. It may be helpful for patients to have a full dental examination by a dentist prior to starting any type of cancer therapy if time allows.[51]

## THERAPEUTIC APPROACHES AND NURSING CARE

Over the last decade, numerous interventions in the form of rinses, mouthwashes, and other pharmacological medications have been used to prevent or treat OM. Unfortunately, to date, very few interventions have been tested adequately to show evidence to support future use. Researchers and health care providers from the Mucositis Study Group of the Multinational Association of Supportive Care in Cancer (MASCC) and the International Society of Oral Oncology (ISOO) published an evidence-based clinical practice guideline for the prevention and management of OM.[52,53] Additionally, two recent Cochrane Reviews focused on interventions for the treatment and prevention of OM.[54,55] Harris and colleagues published "Putting Evidence into Practice (PEP): Evidence-Based Interventions for the Management of Oral Mucositis" that was a review of empirical evidence related to OM interventions.[51,56,57] Each of these guidelines and reviews identified interventions that were either recommended for practice or not recommended for practice. *Recommended for practice* is described as "effectiveness demonstrated by strong evidence from rigorously designed studies, meta-analyses, or systematic review. Expected benefit exceeds expected harm."[51,p.142] *Not recommended for practice* is defined as "ineffectiveness or harm clearly is demonstrated, or cost or burden exceeds potential benefit."[51,p.142] Those interventions will now be discussed, followed by a short section that identifies other interventions where evidence of "effectiveness is not established," usually as a result of research with inadequate sample sizes or other methodological problems.

### RECOMMENDED FOR PRACTICE

#### Oral care

While not specifically supported by randomized clinical trials, it is generally hypothesized that basic oral care is an important element in preventing and managing OM.[51,53,58] Dodd and colleagues[27] noted that there was a reduction in the incidence of OM from an a priori estimate of 44% to less than 26% in patients treated for cancer who received a standard oral care protocol consisting of tooth brushing, flossing, vigorous mouth washing several times per day, and using a mouth moisturizing product. The weakness of the Dodd study was that the standard oral care protocol was only one of the variables studied because they also investigated two different mouthwashes to see if either affected OM. Unfortunately, to date, the study by Dodd and colleagues was the only research that investigated the role of oral care in decreasing OM. McGuire and colleagues commented, "despite lack of evidence, the value of basic oral care in maintaining mucosal health, integrity, and function and in reducing risk of dental complications . . . is commonly accepted by clinicians."[59,p.542] Oral care is thought to prevent infection and decrease the hazard of future dental complications, plus decrease pain, bleeding, and elevated levels of microbial flora.[51,53,60]

According to Harris and colleagues, basic components of an oral care protocol include an assessment, patient education, tooth brushing, flossing, and use of an oral rinse.[51] The OM PEP resource also presented recommendations, based on "expert opinion," specifically for patients presented in Table 32-5.[51] Harris and colleagues also make the following recommendations, also based on "expert opinion" for clinicians[51]: (1) work with a multidisciplinary team throughout treatment, (2) assess the oral cavity using an appropriate tool daily or at each visit, (3) teach patients when to report self-assessment findings to the health care provider, and (4) provide patients with written instructions and education and verify their understanding.

### Palifermin

Recombinant human keratinocyte growth factor (KGF1, fibroblast growth factor 7), or palifermin, is recommended for use in patients with hematological malignancies who are receiving high-dose chemotherapy and TBI with autologous stem cell transplantation.[52] The recommended dose is 60 μg/kg per day for 3 days prior to conditioning treatment and for 3 days after transplantation for the prevention of OM. In 2 randomized controlled studies, palifermin was well tolerated and decreased the severity and duration of OM.[61,62]

**TABLE 32-5**

**Core Elements of an Oral Care Protocol for Patients**

1. Brush all tooth surfaces for at least 90 seconds using a soft toothbrush twice daily.
2. Allow the toothbrush to air dry before storing, and replace it on a regular basis.
3. Floss at least once daily or as advised by a clinician.
4. Rinse the mouth four times daily (with a bland mouthwash such as normal saline) or as advised by a clinician.
5. Avoid tobacco, alcohol, and irritating foods.
6. Use water-based moisturizers to protect lips.
7. Maintain adequate hydration.

*Source*: Used with permission from Harris et al.[51]

### Cryotherapy

Cryotherapy involves using ice chips or cold water to help with the prevention of OM during chemotherapy administration. Patients are to hold ice chips or cold water in their mouth, which causes vasoconstriction of the oral cavity, thus resulting in less exposure from chemotherapy to the tissue of the mouth.[63] Cryotherapy is supported for use when patients are receiving high-dose melphalan,[64] bolus doses of edatrexate, and bolus administration of 5-fluorouracil.[51,52] The MASCC guidelines recommend that the patient suck on ice chips for 30 minutes during administration of the chemotherapy agents just discussed. The ONS PEP resource recommendations are similar, but they are more specific in recommending cryotherapy 5 minutes prior to infusion, during, and 30 minutes following the infusion. Cryotherapy is not recommended for continuous infusion of 5-fluorouracil.[57]

## NOT RECOMMENDED FOR PRACTICE

### Growth factor mouthwash

Granulocyte-macrophage colony-stimulating factor (GM-CSF) is a hematopoietic growth factor that has been added to a mouthwash. It is hypothesized that GM-CSF promotes neutrophil development while regulating leukocytes and macrophages in the submucosa.[65] Two studies showed no benefit in the use of GM-CSF mouthwash in treating OM.[66,67] Therefore, GM-CSF is not recommended for practice for OM prevention.[51,52]

### Sucralfate

Sucralfate is a mucosal coating agent that was hypothesized to protect oral mucosa. Dodd and colleagues conducted research using sucralfate in patients receiving radiation and found no benefit in the treatment of OM.[68] The MASCC guidelines[52] recommend that sucralfate not be used due to a lack of evidence of effectiveness.

### Chlorhexidine

Chlorhexidine is an oral rinse initially thought to benefit patients who were experiencing chemotherapy-induced OM by decreasing oral flora buildup. However, chlorhexidine's benefit was not established in research.[69] There are reports that chlorhexidine causes discomfort, teeth staining, and alterations in taste.[43,44,70] Given these potentially negative outcomes of chlorhexidine, it is not recommended for use.[51,52]

## EFFECTIVENESS NOT ESTABLISHED

Numerous other interventions may be helpful in the prevention and treatment of OM; however, effectiveness has not yet been established. According to Harris and colleagues, effectiveness not established is defined as "data currently insufficient or are of inadequate quality."[51,p.142] These interventions include allopurinol, amifostine, anti-inflammatory rinses, antimicrobial agents, benzydamine, flurbiprofen tooth patch, granulocyte colony-stimulating factor (G-CSF) (subcutaneous), GM-CSF (subcutaneous), immunoglobulins, glutamine, low-level laser therapy, multiagent rinses ("magic/miracle" mouthwash), oral aloe vera, pilocarpine, povidine-iodine (oral), tetracaine, and zinc supplementation.[51] It is imperative to point out that some of these interventions may be useful in preventing or lessening OM, but more reliable controlled, randomized clinical trials are needed to describe the potential benefit of each respective intervention.[51]

## CONCLUSION

Patients describe OM as one of the most painful and debilitating symptoms associated with cancer treatment. Unfortunately, there are very few interventions that can help to alleviate or lessen OM in patients receiving chemotherapy and RT for the treatment of cancer. By alleviating or lessening OM, patients may be able to receive the needed dosage of radiation or chemotherapy to cure or control their respective cancer.

Oncology nurses stand in the forefront of care for patients suffering with OM. It is the nurse who spends the most time with patients and hears from patients about their painful symptoms of OM. Nurses can make a difference by following the clinical guidelines and teaching patients to use a basic oral care plan of proper brushing, flossing, and rinsing of the oral cavity. Nurses also can lead the way toward future randomized clinical trials that test both the effectiveness of basic oral care and other interventions to prevent or manage OM. Finally, nurses can assist patients to manage oral pain and other side effects that will lead to better nutritional intake, potential elimination of infection, and improved quality of life both during treatment and long after their respective cancer therapy has ended.

## REFERENCES


1. Bellm LA, Epstein JB, Rose-Ped A, et al. Patient reports of complications of bone marrow transplantation. *Support Care Cancer.* 2000;8:33–39.
2. McGuire DB, Altomonte V, Peterson DE, et al. Patterns of mucositis and pain in patients receiving preparative chemotherapy and bone marrow transplantation. *Oncol Nurs Forum.* 1993;20:1493–1502.
3. McGuire DB, Yeager KA, Dudley WN, et al. Acute oral pain and mucositis in bone marrow transplant and leukemia patients: data from a pilot study. *Cancer Nurs.* 1998;21:385–393.
4. Papas AS, Clark RE, Martuscelli G, et al. A prospective, randomized trial for the prevention of mucositis in patients undergoing hematopoietic stem cell transplantation. *Bone Marrow Transplant.* 2003;31:705–712.
5. Rose-Ped AM, Bellm LA, Epstein JB, et al. Complications of radiation therapy for head and neck cancers. *Cancer Nurs.* 2002;25:461–469.
6. Borbasi S, Cameron K, Quested B, et al. More than a sore mouth: patients' experience of oral mucositis. *Oncol Nurs Forum.* 2002;29:1051–1057.
7. Keefe DM. Intestinal mucositis: mechanisms and management. *Curr Opin Oncol.* 2007;19:323–327.
8. Sonis ST, Elting LS, Keefe D, et al. Perspectives on cancer therapy-induced mucosal injury: pathogenesis, measurement, epidemiology, and consequences for patients. *Cancer.* 2004;100:1995–2025.
9. Elting LS, Cooksley C, Chambers M, et al. The burdens of cancer therapy: clinical and economic outcomes of chemotherapy-induced mucositis. *Cancer.* 2003;98:1531–1539.
10. Eilers J, Million R. Prevention and management of oral mucositis in patients with cancer. *Semin Oncol Nurs.* 2007;23:201–212.
11. American Cancer Society. Mouth sores painful for patients: new scoring system to aid in treating mouth sores. http://www.cancer.org/docroot/NWS/content/NWS_1_1x_Mouth_Sores_Painful_for_Patients.asp. Accessed December 26, 2009.
12. Miaskowski C, Dodd M, Lee K. Symptom clusters: the new frontier in symptom management research. *J Natl Cancer Inst Monogr.* 2004;32:17–21.
13. National Cancer Institute. Oral complications of chemotherapy and head and neck radiation. http://www.cancer.gov/cancertopics/pdq/supportivecare/oralcomplications/healthprofessional. Accessed December 26, 2009.
14. Peterson DE, Cariello A. Mucosal damage: a major risk factor for severe complications after cytotoxic therapy. *Semin Oncol.* 2004;31:35–44.
15. Sonis ST, Oster G, Fuchs H, et al. Oral mucositis and the clinical and economic outcomes of hematopoietic stem-cell transplantation. *J Clin Oncol.* 2001;19:2201–2205.
16. Brown CG, McGuire DB, Peterson DE, et al. The experience of a sore mouth and associated symptoms in patients with cancer. *Cancer Nurs.* 2009;32:259–270.
17. Avritscher EB, Cooksley CD, Elting LS. Scope and epidemiology of cancer therapy-induced oral and gastrointestinal mucositis. *Semin Oncol Nurs.* 2004;20:3–10.
18. Barasch A, Peterson DE. Risk factors for ulcerative oral mucositis in cancer patients: unanswered questions. *Oral Oncol.* 2003;39:91–100.
19. Cheng KKF, Chang AM. Palliation of oral mucositis symptoms in pediatric patients treated with cancer chemotherapy. *Cancer Nurs.* 2003;26:476–484.
20. Zalcberg J, Kerr D, Seymour L, et al. Haematological and non-haematological toxicity after 5-fluorouracil and leucovorin in patients with advanced colorectal cancer is significantly associated with gender, increasing age and cycle number. *Eur J Cancer.* 1998;34:1871–1875.
21. Raber-Durlacher JE, Weijl NI, Abu Saris M, et al. Oral mucositis in patients treated with chemotherapy for solid tumors: a retrospective analysis of 150 cases. *Support Care Cancer.* 2000;8:366–371.
22. Sloan JA, Loprinzi CL, Novotny PJ, et al. Sex differences in fluorouracil-induced stomatitis. *J Clin Oncol.* 2000;18:412.
23. Vokurka S, Bystrická E, Koza V, et al. Higher incidence of chemotherapy induced oral mucositis in females: a supplement of multivariate analysis to a randomized multicentre study. *Support Care Cancer.* 2006;14:974–976.
24. Chiara S, Nobile NT, Sanguineti O, et al. Oral mucositis in advanced colorectal cancer patients receiving continuous 5-fluorouracil (5-FU) infusions (c.i.) + oral leukovorin (L-LV). *Support Care Cancer.* 1996;4:238.
25. McCarthy GM, Awde JD, Ghandi H, et al. Risk factors associated with mucositis in cancer patients receiving 5-fluorouracil. *Oral Oncol.* 1998;34:484–490.
26. Brown CG, Wingard J. Clinical consequences of oral mucositis. *Semin Oncol Nurs.* 2004;20:16–21.
27. Dodd MJ, Larson PJ, Dibble SL, et al. Randomized clinical trial of chlorhexidine versus placebo for prevention of oral mucositis in patients receiving chemotherapy. *Oncol Nurs Forum.* 1996;23:921–927.
28. Sonis ST, Fey EG. Oral complications of cancer therapy. *Oncology (Williston Park, NY)* 2002;16:680–686.

29. Dodd MJ, Miaskowski C, Shiba GH, et al. Risk factors for chemotherapy-induced oral mucositis: dental appliances, oral hygiene, previous oral lesions, and history of smoking. *Cancer Invest.* 1999;17:278–284.
30. McGuire DB. Mucosal tissue injury in cancer therapy more than mucositis and mouthwash. *Cancer Pract.* 2002;10:179–191.
31. Shih A, Miaskowski C, Dodd MJ, et al. Mechanisms for radiation-induced oral mucositis and the consequences. *Cancer Nurs.* 2003;26: 222–229.
32. Elting LS, Cooksley CD, Chambers MS, et al. Risk, outcomes, and costs of radiation-induced oral mucositis among patients with head-and-neck malignancies. *Int J Radiat Oncol Biol Phys.* 2007;68:1110–1120.
33. Dodd MJ. The pathogenesis and characterization of oral mucositis associated with cancer therapy. *Oncol Nurs Forum.* 2004;31:5.
34. Wilkes JD. Prevention and treatment of oral mucositis following cancer chemotherapy. *Semin Oncol.* 1998;25:538–551.
35. Goldberg SL, Chiang L, Selina N, et al. Patient perceptions about chemotherapy-induced oral mucositis: implications for primary/secondary prophylaxis strategies. *Support Care Cancer.* 2004;12:526–530.
36. Sonis ST. The pathobiology of mucositis. *Natl Rev Cancer.* 2004;4: 277–284.
37. Lalla RV, Sonis ST, Peterson DE. Management of oral mucositis in patients who have cancer. *Dent Clin North Am.* 2008;52:61–77.
38. Sonis ST. Mucositis as a biological process: a new hypothesis for the development of chemotherapy-induced stomatotoxicity. *Oral Oncol.* 1998;34:39–43.
39. Beck SL. Mucositis. In: Yarbro CH, Frogge MH, Goodman M, eds. *Cancer Symptom Management.* 3rd ed. Sudbury, MA: Jones and Bartlett; 2004:276–287.
40. Lalla RV, Peterson DE. Oral mucositis. *Dent Clin North Am.* 2005;49:167–184.
41. World Health Organization. *Handbook for Reporting Results of Cancer Treatment.* Geneva, Switzerland: WHO; 1979.
42. Eilers J, Berger AM, Peterson MC. Development, testing, and applications of the oral assessment guide. *Oncol Nurs Forum.* 1988;15:325.
43. Cheng KKF, Chang AM, Yuen MP. Prevention of oral mucositis in paediatric patients treated with chemotherapy: a randomised crossover trial comparing two protocols of oral care. *Eur J Cancer.* 2004;40:1208–1216.
44. Dodd MJ, Dibble SL, Miaskowski C, et al. Randomized clinical trial of the effectiveness of 3 commonly used mouthwashes to treat chemotherapy-induced mucositis. *Oral Surg Oral Med Oral Pathol Oral Radiol Endod.* 2000;90:39–47.
45. Sonis ST, Eilers JP, Epstein JB, et al. Validation of a new scoring system for the assessment of clinical trial research of oral mucositis induced by radiation or chemotherapy. Mucositis Study Group. *Cancer.* 1999;85:2103–2113.
46. Eastern Cooperative Oncology Group. ECOG: Common toxicity criteria. http://www.ecog.org/general/ctc.pdf. Accessed December 26, 2009.
47. Kolbinson DA, Schubert MM, Flournoy N, et al. Early oral changes following bone marrow transplantation. *Oral Surg Oral Med Oral Pathol.* 1988;66:130–138.
48. Schubert MM, Williams BE, Lloid ME, et al. Clinical assessment scale for the rating of oral mucosal changes associated with bone marrow transplantation. *Cancer.* 1992;69:2469–2477.
49. Western Consortium for Nursing Research. Priorities for cancer nursing research: a canadian replication. *Cancer Nurs.* 1987;10:319–326.
50. McGuire D. Barriers and strategies in implementation of oral care standards for cancer patients. *Support Care Cancer.* 2003;11:435–441.
51. Harris DJ, Eilers J, Harriman A, et al. Putting evidence into practice: evidence-based interventions for the management of oral mucositis. *Clin J Oncol Nurs.* 2008;12:141–152.
52. Keefe DM, Schubert MM, Elting LS, et al. Updated clinical practice guidelines for the prevention and treatment of mucositis. *Cancer.* 2007;109:820–831.
53. Rubenstein EB, Peterson DE, Schubert M, et al. Clinical practice guidelines for the prevention and treatment of cancer therapy-induced oral and gastrointestinal mucositis. *Cancer.* 2004;100:2026–2046.
54. Clarkson JE, Worthington HV, Eden OB. Interventions for treating oral mucositis for patients with cancer receiving treatment. *Cochrane Database Syst Rev.* 2007;2:CD001973.
55. Worthington HV, Clarkson JE, Eden OB. Interventions for preventing oral mucositis for patients with cancer receiving treatment. *Cochrane Database Syst Rev.* 2007;4:CD000978.
56. Harris DJ, Eilers J, Harriman A, et al. *Putting Evidence into Practice: Mucositis.* Pittsburgh: Oncology Nursing Society; 2007.
57. Harris DJ, Eilers J. Mucositis. In: Eaton LH, Tipton JM, eds. Putting evidence into practice improving oncology patient outcomes, Pittsburgh, PA: *Oncology Nursing Society.* 2009:201–209.
58. Karagözoğlu S, Filiz Ulusoy M. Chemotherapy: the effect of oral cryotherapy on the development of mucositis. *J Clin Nurs.* 2005;14:754–765.
59. McGuire D, Correa M, Wienandts P. The role of basic oral care and good clinical practice principles in the management of oral mucositis. *Support Care Cancer.* 2006;14:541–547.
60. Cawley MM, Benson LM. Current trends in managing oral mucositis. *Clin J Oncol Nurs.* 2005;9:584–595.
61. Meropol NJ, Somer RA, Gutheil J, et al. Randomized phase I trial of recombinant human keratinocyte growth factor plus chemotherapy: potential role as mucosal protectant. *J Clin Oncol.* 2003;21:1452–1458.
62. Spielberger R, Stiff P, Bensinger W, et al. Palifermin for oral mucositis after intensive therapy for hematologic cancers. *N Engl J Med.* 2004; 351:2590–2598.
63. Lilleby K, Garcia P, Gooley T, et al. A prospective, randomized study of cryotherapy during administration of high-dose melphalan to decrease the severity and duration of oral mucositis in patients with multiple myeloma undergoing autologous peripheral blood stem cell transplantation. *Bone Marrow Transplant.* 2006;37:1031–1035.
64. Aisa Y, Mori T, Kudo M, et al. Oral cryotherapy for the prevention of high-dose melphalan-induced stomatitis in allogeneic hematopoietic stem cell transplant recipients. *Support Care Cancer.* 2005;13: 266–269.
65. Shih A, Miaskowski C, Dodd MJ, et al. A research review of the current treatments for radiation-induced oral mucositis in patients with head and neck cancer. *Oncol Nurs Forum.* 2002;29:1063–1080.
66. Dazzi C, Cariello A, Giovanis P, et al. Prophylaxis with GM-CSF mouthwashes does not reduce frequency and duration of severe oral mucositis in patients with solid tumors undergoing high-dose chemotherapy with autologous peripheral blood stem cell transplantation rescue: a double blind, randomized, placebo-controlled study. *Ann Oncol.* 2003;14:559–563.
67. Valcárcel D, Sanz MA, Sureda A, et al. Mouth-washings with recombinant human granulocyte-macrophage colony stimulating factor (rhGM-CSF) do not improve grade III-IV oropharyngeal mucositis (OM) in patients with hematological malignancies undergoing stem cell transplantation: results of a randomized double-blind placebo-controlled study. *Bone Marrow Transplant.* 2002;29:783–787.
68. Dodd MJ, Miaskowski C, Greenspan D, et al. Radiation-induced mucositis: a randomized clinical trial of micronized sucralfate versus salt and soda mouthwashes. *Cancer Invest.* 2003;21:21–33.
69. Scully C, Sonis S, Diz PD. Oral mucositis. *Oral Dis.* 2006;12: 229–241.
70. Eilers J. Nursing interventions and supportive care for the prevention and treatment of oral mucositis associated with cancer treatment. *Oncol Nurs Forum.* 2004;31:13.

CHAPTER 33

Regina S. Cunningham, PhD, RN, AOCN,® Maureen B. Huhmann, DCN, RD, CSO

# Nutritional Disturbances

## SCOPE OF THE PROBLEM

In the United States, recognition of the relationship between cancer and nutrition began in the 1930s[1] and became the subject of systematic research in the 1970s.[2] Two major areas of investigation have emerged; these include the following: (1) the relationship of nutrient intake to the development of cancer, and (2) cancer-induced nutritional disturbances and their management, which is the primary focus of this chapter.

Undernutrition is the most common nutritional alteration associated with both pediatric and adult malignancies.[3,4] However, the evidence that both undernutrition and overnutrition negatively affect morbidity, survival, and quality of life[4–6] emphasizes the need for oncology nurses to evaluate the nutritional status of all individuals to whom they provide care.

## DEFINITIONS

The 2 opposite endpoints of the malnutrition continuum in individuals with cancer are obesity and cancer cachexia. *Obesity* is frequently defined as a body mass index (BMI) of greater than 30 kg/m$^2$, but this definition can be misleading. While obesity is associated with surplus fat, weight above the normal range can occur secondary to increased muscle mass or fluid retention. As such, evaluation of body composition should be made when weight tables are used to diagnose obesity.

Terms used to describe nonmalignant nutritional deficiencies, and occasionally malignant starvation, are *kwashiorkor* (protein malnutrition with an adequate caloric intake), *marasmus* (simple starvation with protein-calorie malnutrition), and *inanition* (progressive deterioration with muscle wasting and energy loss). *Cachexia,* a general term meaning ill health, can occur in non-neoplastic diseases, such as sepsis, cardiac failure, and starvation. The term *cancer anorexia-cachexia syndrome* (CACS) is often used to refer to cachexia in individuals with cancer. Cancer cachexia is characterized by anorexia, weight loss, skeletal muscle atrophy, and asthenia (loss of strength). Other symptoms of cancer cachexia include early satiety, edema, anemia, reduced attention span, organ dysfunction, metabolic abnormalities, and susceptibility to other diseases.

## INCIDENCE

Neither the incidence nor the prevalence of malnutrition is accurately documented in patients with cancer. Most individuals with cancer develop some degree of malnutrition during their illness. The exact incidence of malnutrition in specific cancer types is difficult to quantify for several reasons. First, nutritional status is rarely assessed when cancer is diagnosed, especially in the obese. Because assessment of nutritional status frequently is delayed, the opportunity to find more easily treated, minimal nutrient deficiencies in early stages is often lost. Second, no consensus exists regarding which indicators of nutritional status should be routinely assessed in patients with cancer. Although weight is universally accepted as an essential component of nutritional assessment, there is little agreement on which other parameters must be included. Recommendations vary from nutritionally focused clinical examinations to the use of an array of laboratory tests.[7] There is also no agreement on how the severity of malnutrition should be graded. In clinical trials, study groups have developed toxicity scales for weight change and anorexia; however, these scales are better suited to determining side effect profiles rather than malnutrition levels. The American Dietetic Association is in the process of developing nutrition diagnosis categories and labels to be used in classifying alterations in nutrition status.[8]

Overnutrition is most commonly documented in breast cancer. The incidence of obesity among women recently diagnosed with breast cancer ranges from 24% to 36%.[9,10] In addition, 40% to 100% of women with breast cancer receiving adjuvant chemotherapy gain weight, and some become obese.[11,12] Concern about weight change arises not only because of cardiac or quality of life issues, but also because studies suggest that women with breast cancer who are obese have poorer survival rates than women who are not obese.[13] However, specific characteristics that predispose patients with cancer to weight gain are still being sorted out. Borugian et al[13] found that obesity, as evidenced by an elevated waist-to-hip ratio, was linked to increased mortality in postmenopausal patients with estrogen receptor–positive breast cancer, but there was no such effect in premenopausal women. Overnutrition can exist in other cancers as well. Whether increased weight has negative consequences in types of cancer other than breast cancer is not clear.

## RISK FACTORS

Individuals who are nourished adequately at the time of the cancer diagnosis have fewer problems with both the cancer and its treatment. The body's response to the tumor and the tumor-initiated metabolic changes are significant sources of malnutrition in patients with cancer.[14] In addition, treatment imposes a burden by requiring repair of treatment-induced damage and by reducing the ability of the body to absorb nutrients.

### External and internal factors

External factors include the environmental and social contexts within which an individual exists. These contexts encompass the overall health of the country's economy, which has an impact on transportation, access to food shopping, availability of different nutrients, adequacy of housing and food preparation facilities, and availability of programs that offer food assistance. Environmental factors influence the individual, who possesses cultural beliefs and attitudes about nutrition and eating behaviors. Internal factors that influence a person's tendency to develop nutritional deficiencies include age, body image, past history of food fads or eating disorders, social support, educational level, alcohol or tobacco intake, and presence of comorbid diseases. Much more research in this area is needed before individuals at risk can be reliably identified.

### Cancer-related factors

The type of cancer affects the probability of malnutrition. Individuals with breast cancer or leukemia are at low risk, whereas 31% to 48% of patients with non-Hodgkin's lymphoma have significant weight loss. Moreover, unfavorable histologies are correlated with higher weight loss.[3] Individuals with cancers of the aerodigestive (upper respiratory and digestive) and gastrointestinal (GI) tracts are at special risk for undernutrition from mechanical obstruction and physiological dysfunction due to local tumor compression.[15] Host responses to the cancer and the cancer itself cause changes in metabolism and energy needs and may explain why those individuals with advanced disease are more likely to have nutritional problems.[6]

### Treatment-related factors

All cancer therapies have the potential to cause nutritional deficiency. The magnitude of the treatment-related risk depends on the area of treatment, type of treatment, number of therapeutic modalities used, dosages of therapy used, and length of treatment.

*Surgery.* The effects of surgery on an individual's nutritional status depend on the extent of the procedure as well as the anatomical site of the operation. Complications associated with surgery also are related to the nutritional status of the individual prior to the operation. Malnourished individuals have a higher incidence of morbidity and mortality than do those patients who are adequately nourished.[16] This fact has particular relevance for individuals with cancers of the aerodigestive or GI tract. These patients may come to surgery with nutritional deficits because of cancer-related disruption of intake or absorption. In addition, they often have undergone multiple tests requiring restricted diets.

Surgery itself alters function. Major aerodigestive resections may produce taste alterations, dysgeusia, or impaired swallowing, resulting in reduced intake. Rearranged anatomy, which is common with esophageal, gastric, pancreatic, and intestinal resections, can create multiple lesions affecting nutrition. Patients with abdominal and pelvic incisions may experience an ileus after surgery, complicating the ability to consume adequate nutrition postoperatively.[17] Resections of large segments of the bowel can lead to malabsorption of fat, inadequate caloric intake, vitamin $B_{12}$ deficiency, anemia, and fluid-electrolyte imbalance.[15] These problems can become chronic, resulting in reliance on enteral or parenteral feedings to provide adequate caloric support.

For individuals with cancers affecting other sites, nutritional problems resulting from surgery are often limited to the immediate perioperative period. Interruption of oral intake is usually minimal. Use of antibiotics in the perioperative period, although disruptive to digestive processes that utilize intestinal bacteria, can be offset by intake of acidophilus-containing products such as yogurt. Surgical procedures create the same response to injury as does surgery for nonmalignant diseases. This stress is added to the psychological stress of dealing with a cancer diagnosis. Catecholamine, glucocorticoid, and glucagon outputs increase, resulting in increased energy needs, loss of nitrogen, and water and sodium retention. Surgery can increase energy requirements. For this reason, surgical candidates must be assessed carefully prior to treatment so that any nutritional deficiencies can be addressed proactively.[18]

*Radiation.* Radiation therapy can alter nutritional status by exerting both systemic and local effects. The extent of the alteration varies with the area of the body being treated, the size of the area being treated, and the duration of treatment.[19] Radiation alters function in the treatment area and poses particular problems for patients with aerodigestive or GI cancers. Acute effects are transient and include anorexia, diarrhea, bleeding, nausea, vomiting, weight loss, mucositis, esophagitis, gastritis, xerostomia, and changes in taste. Local desquamation reactions can temporarily increase energy needs. Some of these changes—especially xerostomia, taste changes, and diarrhea—can become chronic.[19]

Indirect effects of radiation can also influence nutritional status. Fatigue and appetite changes commonly occur among individuals receiving radiation therapy. These symptoms can alter the person's desire and ability to procure, prepare, and ingest food. Delayed effects of radiation, such as intestinal strictures, fibrosis or obstruction, fistulas, and hepatic or pulmonary fibrosis, may cause mechanical problems in gut function and oxygenation. These, in turn, interrupt the person's ability to absorb, process, and ingest food and may necessitate long-term management.

*Chemotherapy.* Chemotherapy has a number of direct and indirect effects on nutrition. Direct effects include alteration of the absorptive surface of the GI tract, excitation of the chemoreceptor trigger zone and true vomiting center, and interference with specific metabolic and enzymatic reactions. The majority of chemotherapeutic agents, because of the damage they cause to frequently reproducing cells, alter the length and surface area of intestinal villi. The reduced ability of the gut to absorb nutrients and water production that results can induce diarrhea and malabsorption.

Direct excitation of the centers for nausea and vomiting occurs to varying degrees with the majority of chemotherapy drugs.[20] This variability is dependent upon both patient- and regimen-related risk factors. The most salient risk factor for the development of chemotherapy-induced nausea and vomiting is the emetogenic potential of the particular agent or combination of agents being administered. Patient-related risk factors include age, gender, prior experience with chemotherapy, a history of nausea and vomiting during pregnancy, and stress.[21] In addition to these nonspecific changes in nutritional intake, some drugs cause specific nutritional problems. For example, cisplatin can cause magnesium wasting, which may require replacement therapy.

Indirect effects of chemotherapy on nutrition status may occur as a result of symptoms that interfere with intake. Common symptoms in patients receiving chemotherapy include anorexia, nausea, vomiting, fatigue, constipation, taste changes, food aversions, anxiety, and depression. The number and magnitude of these effects depend on the specific antineoplastic agent; and the dose, frequency, and duration of drug administration. Although these side effects clearly alter nutrient intake during treatment, their significance to overall nutritional status has not been adequately studied.

*Biotherapy/immunotherapy.* The effects of biotherapy on nutritional status are both direct and indirect. Agents such as the interferons and interleukins cause anorexia, malaise, mucositis, nausea, and vomiting. Biotherapy-induced fevers directly increase energy and fluid requirements. Indirect influences, such as fatigue and flu-like symptoms, can make food procurement and preparation difficult. The magnitude and duration of these side effects are variable and may decrease over time. Their clinical effect on nutritional status is not well documented.

*Targeted therapies.* Targeted therapies now represent a major line of defense in the therapeutic armamentarium of cancer treatments. These therapies have evolved as a result of advances in the field of molecular biology. Signal transduction is the biological process of cellular communication. Cells receive both internal and external messages that control specific biological functions such as growth, differentiation, and apoptosis. Targeted therapies aim to interfere with cell signaling patterns that support cancer growth and development. Several therapies that target key molecular pathways have been developed. Growth factors and their receptors have been extensively investigated, including epidermal growth factor receptor (EGFR), vascular endothelial growth factor (VEGF), vascular endothelial growth factor receptor (VEGFR), and human epidermal receptor 2 (HER2). Drugs that inhibit EGFR cause mechanism-based side effects, which include GI alterations such as diarrhea and, to a lesser extent, nausea and vomiting. Some targeted therapies (eg, cetuximab) can also cause magnesium wasting.[22–24]

Many targeted therapies have demonstrated improved outcomes either alone or in combination with chemotherapy in selected patients.[25,26] Additional research is clearly needed to understand the full effects of these agents on nutritional status. As research in this area evolves, it will be essential to consider how targeted therapies influence patient's ability to consume adequate nutrition.

*Multimodality therapy.* Patients with cancer often receive therapeutic modalities in combination. Patients with early-stage breast cancer, eg, typically require care that includes surgical intervention followed by chemotherapy and radiation. Patients with lung cancer or GI malignancies are often treated with multimodality therapy. When such combinations are part of the therapeutic regimen, the patient's risk for nutritional disturbance is increased.

## NORMAL NUTRITIONAL PHYSIOLOGY

Several models depict the complex relationships influencing nutrition; those used in much of the cancer literature are specific to the disease state.[27] Simply stated, weight gain and loss are directly related to the ratio of the amount of energy, quantified as calories, consumed and expended. The amount of calories consumed can be calculated from oral, enteral, and parenteral intake. The quantity of energy expended is more difficult to quantify.

Energy is obtained through the ingestion, digestion, and metabolism of macronutrients (carbohydrates, protein, lipids, and water) and micronutrients (minerals and vitamins). Optimal energy retention and absorption requires an intact GI tract, including proper secretory and motility function. Multiple factors can affect a patient's ability to meet energy needs orally. Physiological (eg, growth factors, insulin, glucose, thyroxine, smell/taste transmitters), psychological (eg, body image, self-esteem, meaning/sight/smell of food), and cultural (eg, acceptable foods, eating patterns, social importance of food) factors can have beneficial or detrimental effects on intake.

Energy expenditure refers to both the minimum amount of energy required for basic body functioning, known as the basal metabolic rate, as well as energy expended for activity and digestion. Energy expenditure is affected by certain medications, stress, and injury. Basal metabolic rate can be measured through indirect calorimetry, which will be described later in this chapter.

Body composition is affected by a surplus or deficit of energy intake. Body composition is often described in terms of body compartments. Body compartments include fat, protein (skeletal muscle, viscera, plasma, bone, cartilage, collagen), glycogen, minerals, and water (intracellular and extracellular). The percentage of each of these components varies with genetics, gender, and age. Methods for measuring these compartments are described in the Anthropometrics section of this chapter. The interplay among the compartments, in the setting of an adequate nutrient intake, results in sufficient body storage for energy needs and protection from illness.

## PATHOPHYSIOLOGY

Cancer, host response, and cancer treatment all alter normal physiology. Alterations in energy intake and expenditure affect nutritional status. These alterations result in modified body storage, with the potential for development of obesity, weight loss, or cachexia.

### CANCER-INDUCED ALTERATIONS IN NUTRIENT INTAKE

#### Changes in appetite

*Anorexia.* Anorexia is defined as a loss of desire to eat that is accompanied by diminished intake.[28] Anorexia often occurs in concert with a number of other symptoms that can exacerbate diminished food intake and are associated with central nervous system regulation of energy intake, such as smell and taste alterations, early satiety, and nausea and vomiting. In cancer, anorexia is most frequently associated with cachexia (often referred to as the anorexia-cachexia syndrome), but it is important that anorexia be recognized and addressed as an independent symptom. Anorexia is present in close to half of patients with cancer at the time of diagnosis and in later stage disease, the prevalence of this symptom approaches 80%. Anorexia can lead to malnutrition, decreased ability to tolerate treatment, increased toxicity, debilitation, and decreased quality of life.[28]

Anorexia is regulated by numerous physiologic, GI, metabolic, and endocrine mechanisms. Evidence suggests that loss of appetite is likely the result of the effects of hormones (eg, leptin, ghrelin), neuropeptides, and cytokines produced by the cancer and the host in response to the disease.[28,29] Cytokines, including tumor necrosis factor-$\alpha$ (TNF-$\alpha$), interferon-$\gamma$, leukemia inhibitory factor (LIF), interleukin 1 and 6, and ciliary neurotrophic factor (CNTF), are thought to play a pivotal role in the stimulation of anorexigenic and orexigenic circuits that regulate intake and body weight.[28] TNF-$\alpha$ produces anorectic effects by acting directly on the central nervous system. The hypothesized mechanism appears to be modulated through effects on neural activity of glucose sensitive neurons within the lateral hypothalamic area. Mechanisms underlying the anorectic effects of interleukin-1 have not been clearly elucidated, but are thought to be related to the early development of satiety.[30] Elevated levels of interleukin-6 have been associated with weight loss in patients with lymphoma, lung, and colorectal cancers.[31] Cytokines can also induce tumor products such as lipid-mobilizing factor and proteolysis-inducing factor (PIF), which can directly affect tissue metabolism.[32] Some evidence also supports an effect of neurotransmitters such as serotonin and dopamine on appetite suppression, although this effect is believed to be interrelated with the effects of hormones and cytokines.[14] Animal studies support the importance of serotonin and ammonia as anorectics in cancer; to date, studies in humans have been limited.[28]

Loss of appetite may be precipitated by cancer-induced psychological distress as well. Depression, anxiety, pain or pain medications, or situational factors (isolation, dislike of hospital food) may negatively influence food intake. Cancer-related fatigue, the most commonly reported symptom in patients with cancer, has also been associated with diminished intake. Fatigue often interferes with activities of daily living and may limit the patient's ability to procure and prepare food. This problem may linger long after cancer treatment has been completed.

*Increased appetite.* Increased appetite has been reported among women with breast cancer. Investigators suggest that increased as well as decreased appetite may occur as a function of psychological distress.[11,12] Many healthy women regularly limit their food intake. Following a breast cancer diagnosis, these women may lose their restraint, eat more, and gain weight. It has been suggested that extremes in diet, sometimes seen in the breast cancer population, may be associated with poor survival.[33] Additional studies in this area are needed.

#### Changes in taste and smell

Altered taste and smell sensors, with loss of taste and olfactory cues, change the normal references that are part of appetite and intake. Physiological increases in the recognition thresholds for sweet, sour, and salty and decreases in the recognition levels for bitter are common in cancer. These threshold changes can lead to meat and other food aversions, which in turn can diminish food intake and lead to malnutrition among patients with cancer. Psychological factors may also contribute to food aversions. The hedonistic component of eating can be negatively influenced by alterations in taste or smell, leading to a reduced interest in eating and loss of appetite.

Taste alterations are defined as changes in the usual patterns of taste perception that are unique to the person experiencing the changes.[34] These alterations are common in patients with cancer, but may be overlooked because of more pressing consequences of disease and treatment. As a result, data on incidence and prevalence, as well as the effects of these symptoms on the etiology of nutritional alterations, are limited. One recent study in subjects with advanced cancer reported that 86% of patients reported some type of chemosensory alteration.[35]

Taste is a chemical sense that is detected through taste buds. Taste buds are located in the tongue, between the hard and soft palate, and in the throat. Taste buds contain receptor sites for sweet, sour, salty, and bitter sensations. Cranial nerves innervate these areas and route taste information to the medulla and, ultimately, the cortex. Somatosensory sensations such as touch, temperature, irritation, and pain also contribute to taste perception. Taste and smell are tightly integrated. Unlike taste buds, the receptors for olfaction are not located on discrete anatomical structures; they are found on the ciliated dendrites of olfactory neurons. Air entering the nostrils ascends to the top of the nasal cavity and enters the olfactory cleft where it comes in contact with the olfactory receptors. During eating, the pressure gradient created by chewing and swallowing pushes air from the mouth into the nose. Once the olfactory receptors are stimulated, the signal is carried through cranial nerve I to the cortex and subcortex. Changes in taste and smell may be caused by direct tumor invasion; cancer-induced deficiencies of zinc, copper, nickel, vitamin A, and niacin; specific anticancer medications; or cytokine activity. Distorted taste perceptions (dysgeusia) are often described by patients as rancid, bitter, salty, or metallic. Other taste alterations experienced include enhanced taste sensitivity (hypergeusia), diminished taste sensitivity (hypogeusia), or complete absence of taste (aguesia). Distorted perception of smell (dysosmia) is categorized according to whether it is preceded by something in the environment (parosmia) or happens spontaneously (phantosmia). Dysosmia is often unpleasant and is frequently described by patients as rancid.[35]

## Early satiety

Early satiety has been correlated with other nutrition-impact symptoms including anorexia.[36] Early satiety is defined as the desire to eat without the ability to consume foods because of a sense of fullness.[37] Sometimes considered a silent or orphan symptom, early satiety is under-recognized and under-reported. Patients often do not spontaneously offer information about this experience and many assessment tools used in clinical practice settings do not specifically ascertain information on this symptom. When specifically asked about the symptom however, patients do report that it is common. In a recent prospective evaluation of symptoms in more than 1000 patients with advanced cancer, early satiety ranked among the 10 most common symptoms experienced. Further analysis of this dataset demonstrated that early satiety clustered with anorexia, weight loss, and taste changes.[36] Early satiety occurs in patients with all types of malignancies and is more frequently associated with advanced disease; it is also more common in women and does not appear to be related to radiation or chemotherapy administration. Walsh et al[38] reported that early satiety contributes to decreased intake and has been identified as an independent prognostic variable.

Both central and peripheral pathophysiologic mechanisms contribute to the development of early satiety. Central influences include alterations in smell and taste, food aversions, and diurnal variations in food intake. Satiety is less pronounced during the early hours of the day. Peripheral mechanisms underlying early satiety include gastric dysmotility and accommodation as well as the influence of specific gastric and small bowel hormones. Ghrelin is a growth hormone that stimulates gastric motility. Ghrelin levels correlate with both anorexia and cachexia in advanced cancer. Cholecystokinin, which is released from the small bowel in response to protein and fat intake, produces satiety and diminishes food intake. Bombesin, a gastrin inhibitory peptide, both releases cholecystokinin and inhibits gastric emptying.[36]

## Cancer cachexia

Cachexia represents one of the most profound nutritional alterations seen in patients with cancer. This syndrome is characterized by marked weight loss, anorexia, asthenia, and muscle wasting. Complications associated with the development of the cachectic state affect physiological and biochemical outcomes, influence the efficacy of cancer treatment, and result in substantially decreased survival.[39] At a metabolic level, this condition causes myriad derangements in lipid, protein, and carbohydrate synthesis, storage, and degredation.

Glucose is the most important energy substrate of the human body; it is required to support all essential organ functions. In patients with cancer, the intake of glucose as a source of energy can be severely reduced by anorexia, nausea, early satiety, or other symptoms. An inadequate supply of glucose to support cellular function initiates gluconeogenesis, or the production of glucose from lactate, muscle amino acids, and free fatty acids. The cycle that converts lactate to pyruvate and then to glucose is called the Cori cycle. In cachectic patients, Cori cycle activity is increased from 20% (the amount typically seen in healthy subjects) to 50%. Moreover, this increased production of glucose is associated with diminished production of insulin and the development of insulin resistance.[40]

Cachexia is also associated with dramatic decreases in white adipose tissue, which results primarily from diminution of lipoprotein lipase (LPL) activity and an increase in the activity of hormone-sensitive lipase. LPL is responsible for the cleavage of triacylglycerols into glycerol and fatty acids. When its activity is decreased, fat is not developed or stored properly and patients lose substantial amounts of body fat. This is exacerbated by profound changes in lipid metabolism that subsequently interfere with almost all metabolic pathways associated with fat accretion and mobilization. Historically, adipose tissue was considered a dormant reservoir of fat. More recent studies, however, have indicated that fat cells, or adipocytes, are involved in key aspects of body weight regulation. Adipocytes are capable of manufacturing, storing, and secreting biologically active substances, including cytokines, that have important effects on specific target tissues. This understanding has led to the hypothesis that the fat loss experienced by cachectic patients may be accountable for other metabolic changes that lead to muscle wasting and ultimately death.[39]

Steadily progressive depletion of muscle mass is a characteristic feature of cancer cachexia. The preferential depletion of skeletal muscle is the result of an imbalance between the rate of protein synthesis and degradation. Proteolysis-inducing factor (PIF) is a biologically active glycoprotein secreted by cachexia-inducing tumors that can induce breakdown of lean muscle mass. PIF increases protein degradation and decreases protein synthesis. Moreover, PIF is involved in hepatic gene expression, which in turn influences the production of specific cytokines that are hypothesized to play a pivotal role in the development of cachexia. Intracellular protein degradation is dependent on several proteolytic systems; these include the acidic lysosomal, the calcium-dependent, and the ubiquitin-dependent pathways.[14,41]

The precise mechanisms underlying the development of cancer cachexia are far from being clearly understood. The syndrome is believed to occur as a result of circulating factors produced by the tumor or by the host in response to the tumor. The hypothesized pathophysiology is fairly complex. Cytokines are thought to play a key role in influencing many of the metabolic changes seen in patients with cachexia; however, no single cytokine is believed to be primarily responsible. Instead, there are a number of different cytokines that work in concert to induce cachexia-related inflammation and the acute-phase response. There are a number of proinflammatory cytokines that can modulate gastric motility and emptying either directly through the GI tract, or by altering efferent signals that regulate satiety. Tumor necrosis factor-α, or cachectin, produces reduction in food intake and wasting. Interferon-γ is produced by activated NK cells and has biological functions that overlap with those of TNF. Ciliary neurotrophic factor (CNTF) is produced by the glial cells of the peripheral nervous system and is expressed in skeletal muscle. CNTF has been shown to induce cachectic effects and produce acute-phase proteins. Leukemia inhibitory factor (LIF) and transforming growth factor-β are also thought to be mediators of cachexia.[42–44]

Although highly complex, it is essential to understand the molecular mechanism of cachexia. This knowledge will drive the design of rational therapeutic strategies for the future. Currently, woefully few of the interventions available to treat this condition are effective.

### Changes in electrolyte balance

Alterations in micronutrient availability occur in paraneoplastic syndromes. Cancer can cause hypercalcemia and hypocalcemia, hyponatremia, or hyperphosphatemia and hypophosphatemia. Some of these abnormalities are caused by tumor-produced hormones and can be life-threatening. For example, anticancer therapies such as cisplatin and procarbazine can cause wasting of magnesium and potassium leading to abnormal serum levels. They also cause altered mental status as well as taste changes, with associated problems in intake and adherence to treatment regimens.

## CANCER-INDUCED CHANGES IN ENERGY BALANCE

### Changes in energy expenditure

Patients with cancer frequently experience alterations in basal energy expenditure. These alterations are often hard to predict. Patients may have reduced, normal, or increased energy expenditure.[1–4] The variability is partly caused by the heterogeneity of "cancer," as well as the impact of the patient's physiological responses to tumor such as infection, elaboration of an acute-phase reaction, and organ-specific reactions.[1,14]

Proposed mechanisms for those patients who do have increased energy expenditure include heightened cytokine activity, especially TNF and interleukin-6, increased use of futile metabolic cycles, and inappropriate energy production in response to decreased intake.[14] Patients with cancer can also have increased energy needs initiated by cancer-induced sepsis, fistulas, or lesions. These energy demands can produce malnutrition in some patients, but they are not responsible for cachexia. Although early research suggested that cachexia results from tumor-driven increases in energy expenditure, data in this area are inconsistent and a definitive etiology for cancer cachexia has not been explicated.

Decreases in energy expenditure can lead to weight gain in patients with cancer. This may be due to a decrease in basal metabolic rate resulting from a loss of muscle mass secondary to deconditioning during hospitalizations. It can also occur from a decrease in physical activity secondary to treatment induced fatigue.

## Changes in nutrient metabolism

Cancer, even in its early stages, and prior to the development of cachexia, can be associated with abnormalities in carbohydrate, protein, and lipid metabolism. Changes in carbohydrate metabolism include increased Cori cycle activity, altered peripheral utilization of glucose, increased glucose turnover, and glucose intolerance.[45,46] Glucose intolerance has been linked to insulin resistance, delayed glucose clearance, reduced glucose uptake in skeletal muscles, and an inability to produce glycogen in muscle. Unlike diabetics, individuals with cancer have normal plasma insulin levels. It is not known whether patients with cancer also have normal insulin secretion. Although the origin of the glucose intolerance remains unknown, researchers have suggested that some cases may result from the cytokines produced by the host in response to the tumor.[45] Indirect effects of cancer that alter glucose metabolism include reduced activity and infection.

Increased hepatic glucose production has been reported in both undernourished and normal-weight patients with cancer.[45,46] The elevated glucose level is one of the features that differentiates cancer starvation/cachexia from normal starvation responses. In normal starvation, hepatic glucose production falls; this effect does not occur in cancer cachexia. The lack of a normal response to decreased intake may be related to the reliance of cancer on glucose or it may be the product of a cancer-associated abnormal growth hormone.

Individuals with cancer may develop altered protein metabolism. Some studies indicate that tumors preferentially take up nitrogen-containing materials.[45,46] The shunting of needed proteins to the cancer, increased muscle breakdown and hepatic protein activity may occur.[15] Despite the increased hepatic activity, protein synthesis does not match protein catabolism. The net result is increased whole-body protein turnover. However, not all researchers have observed increased protein turnover, especially among patients with cancer who are maintaining their weight.[39]

Abnormal lipid metabolism noted in cancer includes increased lipid mobilization and turnover, elevated triglyceride levels, decreased lipogenesis, altered glycerol transport, and decreased LPL activity.[14,46] To some degree, the alteration in fat metabolism may be related to insulin resistance, with preferential oxidation of fat rather than carbohydrates.

## Changes in the gastrointestinal tract

The balance of energy intake and expenditure is heavily dependent on an intact GI system. Cancer can produce direct negative effects on the digestive system. Cancers of the aerodigestive structures can cause primary reduction in food and nutrient intake associated with the following problems:

- Difficulty chewing or swallowing
- Partial or complete obstruction
- Dysmotility
- Inactivation of bile salts or pancreatic enzymes
- Blind loop syndrome
- Fistulas
- Interference associated with pain (eg, ulceration, nerve compression)
- Bowel wall and mesenteric infiltration
- Protein-losing enteropathy

The type and magnitude of the nutritional deficit depend on the tumor site and size. Nongastrointestinal cancers can cause alterations in nutritional status by physically interfering with food intake or increasing energy demand. Examples of these types of direct and indirect interference with intake include pain, dyspnea, blockages of mesenteric or peritoneal lymphatics, paraneoplastic syndromes that alter fluid or mineral balance, and altered cognitive function. Ulcerated lesions, both external and internal, increase nutrient need.

## Changes in body storage

The degree of body storage alteration varies along the continuum of malnutrition. With small changes in nutrient intake or absorption, there may be no obvious change in body composition. In patients with weight gain, the compartment in which the change occurred should be determined. The most commonly affected compartments are the extracellular fluid and adipose tissue compartments.

The most striking change in body composition is seen in cachexia. The total body fat and skeletal muscle components can decrease by as much as 85% and 75%, respectively.[14] Reduction in intracellular water and mineral supplies also occurs, albeit not to the same degree. Feedback signals from the body storage compartment are deranged, reflecting the effect of cytokine activity and metabolic dysfunction. The altered feedback perpetuates the nutritional deficiencies, making this condition extremely difficult to treat.

Individuals who gain weight during treatment experience changes in body storage. The observation in hormone-sensitive tumors, such as breast and prostate, is gain[9,10] or redistribution of body fat to a sarcopenic distribution.[9] Sarcopenic obesity refers to the presence of weight gain in addition to loss or maintenance of lean body mass.[8] It has been postulated that this may be due to a combination of a decrease in physical activity level and the failure to reduce energy intake to compensate for this.[12,13] Studies indicate that the decrease in resting energy expenditure is not a direct result of the chemotherapy, as similar changes are seen in placebo groups.[9]

## TREATMENT-INDUCED ALTERATIONS TO NUTRIENT INTAKE

### Changes in appetite

Just as cancer causes changes in appetite, so can therapy. Depressed appetite can be caused by biotherapeutic agents—notably, TNF, interferon, and the interleukins.[22–24] Psychological responses to having and being treated for cancer with any modality may alter mood and change appetite. Medications prescribed for treatment may also affect mood and appetite. Some drugs produce increased—rather than decreased—appetite or nutrient intake. For example, corticosteroids, which are prescribed in both pediatric and adult populations, can increase appetite.

Surgical anesthesia and radiation produce indirect effects on appetite through the induction of treatment-related side effects such as nausea, vomiting, and food aversions. Anticipatory nausea and vomiting may develop if emetic control is poor during early cycles of chemotherapy. This conditioned response may have a substantial effect on appetite. The clinical significance of these changes is unclear, because some patients alter their choice of foods and eating patterns but not their total intake when faced with these symptoms.[47]

A number of chemotherapeutic agents are associated with the development of taste and smell alterations in patients with cancer; these include the following: cisplatin, doxorubicin, carboplatin, methotrexate, 5-fluorouracil, levamisole, and cyclophosphamide.[48] In addition, antineoplastic drugs target rapidly dividing cells such as mucosal cells and taste and olfactory receptors (which regenerate every 10 and 30 days, respectively). Cellular damage to these areas can contribute to or exacerbate changes in taste or smell and decreased intake. The effects of chemotherapy on taste may be immediate (during the administration of the drug) and short-lived, or they may last for several weeks. Some chemotherapeutic agents can be tasted or smelled because they pass into the saliva. Radiation therapy can also damage taste and olfactory receptors, as well as decrease salivary function. This may diminish the flow of saliva to the extent that tastants do not reach the olfactory receptors, rendering food tasteless. Xerostomia may also occur in these patients, further exacerbating alterations in taste and smell, and subsequently diminishing food intake.

Taste changes are associated with head and neck surgery as well as radiation. In addition, such changes may result from oral infections, use of antibiotics, or administration of other medications. These changes may be temporary and are sometimes related to zinc deficiency. In contrast, radiation and surgical alterations in gustatory and olfactory structures can be permanent. This change may result in an alteration of the normal references for food acceptability or in a general reduction in intake over time.

## TREATMENT-INDUCED CHANGES IN ENERGY BALANCE

### Changes in energy expenditure

Treatment can affect energy needs both directly and indirectly. Some biotherapeutic agents elicit shaking chills and fever, which increase energy demands. Increased energy needs from fever and infection can also accompany bone marrow suppression. Moreover, antifungal agents administered to immunocompromised patients may produce fever and chill responses. Nutritional needs increase as the body responds to repair damage induced by surgery, radiation, or chemotherapy. Energy requirements are related to the type and magnitude of the treatment.

### Changes in the gastrointestinal tract

Surgical resection removes or bypasses areas of the aerodigestive or GI tract, causing a number of nutritional lesions. Chemotherapy and radiation cause direct injury to the intestinal villi, reducing the absorptive surface. Secondary candidiasis throughout the GI tract can occur following antibiotic therapy associated with any treatment. These problems represent major threats to the proper absorption of both macronutrients and micronutrients. Side effects of treatment include anorexia, nausea, vomiting, lactose intolerance, diarrhea, and constipation, all of which can create obstacles to normal gut function and intake. In addition, chronic changes can occur. Total bowel resection, bone marrow transplant-induced graft-vs-host disease, and radiation enteritis can lead to long-term patient dependence on parenteral nutritional support.

## CLINICAL MANIFESTATIONS

The most common clinical manifestation identified with cancer is cancer cachexia, which is characterized by skeletal muscle wasting, weight loss, and reduced function. The patient may complain of loss of appetite, inability to eat, or early satiety. Because the nutrient deficiencies occur along a continuum, however, nutritional deficits can exist without these cardinal or extreme signs and symptoms. This is especially true of obese individuals, in whom weight loss can be overlooked. Fluid changes, such as edema or effusions, can mask protein and fat loss. The fact that nutritional disturbances can be subtle and are frequently nonspecific renders the need for assessment that much more important.

It is clear that patients with cancer experience changes in body weight. Patients with lung, GI, and head and neck tumors experience not only weight loss exceeding 10% of total body weight, but also loss of both muscle and fat. Individuals with GI malignancies experience the largest decreases (>50%) in muscle mass and protein content, as well as 30% to 40% loss of body fat. However, even patients who experience severe wasting retain some body fat. Visceral muscle is also preserved to some extent, whereas skeletal muscle loss is the primary form of lean body mass loss. A recent study revealed that patients with solid tumors could lose as much as 1.34 kg of fat-free mass (FFM) in as little as 4 weeks.[49]

## SCREENING, ASSESSMENT, AND GRADING

The goal of screening in nutrition is to identify those persons who are at risk of developing nutritional problems associated with their cancer. Nutrition assessment is an in-depth evaluation that incorporates medical history, a detailed dietary history, physical examination, anthropometric measurements, and laboratory data.[10] The purpose of nutrition assessment is to plan nutrition interventions. Although nurses play an integral part in accurate nutritional assessment, registered dietitians and nutritionists are more frequently responsible for the nutritional assessment. Nurses should enlist the aid of trained dietary specialists to assist with this aspect of nutritional care. Nurses often conduct screening for, and early detection tests of, nutritional deficits or excesses. For this reason, the discussion here concentrates on screening and anthropometrics. For more detailed information on assessment, the reader is referred to other sources.[50–52]

### NUTRITIONAL SCREENING

The Joint Commission on Accreditation of Healthcare Organizations' (JCAHO) standards require the identification of clients who are nutritionally at risk by means of an initial screening mechanism. This screening must be completed within 24 hours of admission to a hospital, within 14 days of admission to a long-term care facility, or within a facility-defined period of time in ambulatory care and home care settings.[53] The American Society for Parenteral and Enteral Nutrition (ASPEN) published guidelines for nutritional screening in 2002. These guidelines state that a nutritional screen should include the following items: height, weight, weight change, primary diagnosis, and presence of comorbid conditions.[54] In 2003, the American Dietetic Association implemented its Nutrition Care Process model, which is intended to direct the nutritional care of individuals with and without complex disease states. Nutritional screening is an essential preliminary step on which the success of an effective nutritional care plan depends.[8]

The need to assess nutritional status quickly and efficiently has inspired the development of a number of screening instruments. The Patient-Generated Subjective Global Assessment (PG-SGA) is currently endorsed by the American Dietetic Association for oncology patients and has been used by oncology nurses in a variety of settings. The PG-SGA was modified by Ottery from the Subjective Global Assessment of Nutritional Status (SGA), an instrument with proven sensitivity and specificity.[55,56] Both the SGA and PG-SGA evaluate weight change, dietary intake changes, GI symptoms lasting more than 2 weeks, and activity levels. The PG-SGA includes cancer-specific symptoms and a refinement of the activity-level estimation. The patient is able to complete a portion of the assessment, thereby decreasing the amount of clinician time required for data collection. The clinician, taking into consideration the diagnosis, stage of cancer, estimated treatment- and tumor-associated metabolic demand, and findings from a focused physical examination, determines a rating of well-nourished, moderately (or suspected) malnourished, or severely malnourished. The PG-SGA takes only a few minutes to complete, making it a practical screening tool in a busy clinical setting. PG-SGA forms and additional information about scoring can be found on the Society for Nutritional Oncology and Adjuvant Therapy's (NOAT) Web site (http://www.ctrf.org/history.cfm).

A number of formulas integrate several objective measures into assessment of prognosis (Table 33-1), including the Nutritional Index (NI), the Prognostic Nutritional Index (PNI), the Hospital Prognostic Index (HPI), and the Nutrition Risk Index (NRI). These indices are especially helpful in identifying which individuals undergoing head and neck or GI surgery might benefit from nutritional intervention before and after surgery.[17] The HPI and NRI utilize measures that are commonly used and readily available.

### NUTRITIONAL ASSESSMENT

Nutritional assessment has historically been performed by a registered dietitian (RD). The nutritional care provided by an RD is often termed medical nutrition therapy (MNT). MNT is defined by the 2001 Medicare MNT benefit legislation as "nutritional diagnostic, therapy, and counseling services for the purpose of disease management which are furnished by a registered dietitian or nutrition professional."[8]

In 2003, the American Dietetic Association published the Nutrition Care Process (NCP) model. The NCP provides a structure for the provision of nutrition care to all

**TABLE 33-1**

**Prognostic Nutrition Assessment Formulas**

| Nutritional Formula | Formula | Key to Formula |
|---|---|---|
| Nutritional index (NI) | 1.9579 − 0.0017 × (IgM × prealbumin) − (0.0075 × complement factor C3) − (0.0066 × fibrinogen) + (0.033 × cholesterol) − (0.1858 × vitamin A–binding protein) + (0.6636 × thyroxine-binding globulin) | IgM, complement, fibrinogen, cholesterol, vitamin A–binding protein, and thyroxine are measured in mg/dL |
| Prognostic nutritional index (PNI) | 158 − (16.6 × albumin) − (0.78 × triceps skin-fold) − (0.2 × transferrin) − (5.8 × delayed hypersensitivity reaction) | Albumin is measured in g; triceps skin-fold in mL; transferrin in mg/dL; delayed hypersensitivity as 0 (nonreactive), 1 (< 5 mm reactivity), or 2 (≥ 5 mm reactivity) |
| Hospital prognostic index (HPI) | (0.91 × albumin) − (1.00 × delayed hypersensitivity) − (1.44 × sepsis rating) + (0.98 × diagnosis rating) − 1.09 | Albumin is measured in g; delayed hypersensitivity as 1 (positive to 1 or more antigen) or 2 (nonreactive); sepsis as 1 (present) or 2 (absent); diagnosis as 1 (cancer present) or 2 (cancer not present) |
| Nutrition risk index (NRI) | (15.19 × albumin) + (0.417 × % usual body weight) | Albumin is measured in g; % usual body weight is actual weight/usual weight × 100 |

patients and provides a framework by which the RD can think critically and make decisions regarding medical nutrition therapy. There are 4 steps to the process: nutritional assessment, nutritional diagnosis, nutritional intervention, and nutritional monitoring and evaluation.[8] The *nutritional assessment* is a comprehensive evaluation of a client's nutrition status, performed by an RD. Components of the assessment include medical, social, nutritional, and medication history; physical examination; anthropometric measurements; and laboratory data. The nutritional assessment builds on the information collected as part of the nutritional screening.[57] Its goal is to develop an effective nutrition plan of care that can address issues identified as part of the assessment and screening.[7] On the basis of the assessment, a decision about the individual's nutritional diagnosis is made. A *nutritional diagnosis* describes "an actual occurrence, risk of, or potential for developing a nutritional problem that dietetics professionals are responsible for treating independently."[8] *Nutritional intervention* is the activity intended to address that problem. The effects of this intervention are then monitored and evaluated, with changes being made as necessary.

## Anthropometrics

*Anthropometrics*, the measurement of the weight, size, and proportions of the body, commonly includes height, weight, and skin-fold thickness. Serial weight measurement is perhaps the single most important indicator of nutritional status for the clinician, although its importance is often underemphasized. Weights need to be measured from a reliable baseline using instruments that are periodically calibrated to maintain their accuracy and precision. Serial weight measurement is also the anthropometric measure most often performed in the clinical oncology settings. Standard weight measurement is inexpensive, quick, and practical.

Weight should not be considered the sole determinant of nutritional status, however, as weight alone does not reveal body composition. Weight among individuals with cancer may reflect tumor mass or fluid retention while masking loss of lean body mass. For example, children with abdominal masses are at risk for being considered at normal weight for height, despite loss of lean body mass. Adults with ascites are at similar risk. Attempts have been made to improve body composition determination through a variety of measures: ultrasound, computerized tomography, magnetic resonance imaging, dual-photon and dual-energy radiographic absorptiometry, neutron activation, total body potassium, total body water, and bioelectrical impedance. These techniques vary in their invasiveness, availability, and expense. Currently, the primary use of these measures is in research, not routine clinical practice. For the most part, clinical body composition estimates utilized in daily patient care rely on weight measures coupled with additional anthropometrics, such as height or skin folds.

Bioelectrical impedance analysis (BIA) provides an estimate of total body water (TBW) via a measure of electrical impedance within the body. Using values of TBW derived from BIA, one can estimate FFM and body fat. BIA is based on the principle that the body is a biological circuit, such that a fixed, low-voltage, high-frequency current introduced into the human body is conducted almost completely through the greater electrolyte content of the fluid compartment of FFM. It is assumed that the total conductive volume of the body is equivalent to TBW. The opposition to the flow of this current, called resistance (R), is measured.[58,59] The measured resistance is approximately equivalent to that of muscle tissue. Impedance measures vary with the frequency of current used. The current typically used with single-frequency BIA (SFBIA) is 50 kHz, the characteristic frequency for skeletal muscle tissue.[59] BIA has the potential to provide valuable information about changes in oncology patients' body composition. This technology is inexpensive, does not require specific operator skills, and provides no burden to the subject.[60] Studies of ambulatory normal-weight and underweight patients with cancer have concluded that the SFBIA parameter ht$^2$ R is highly correlated with TBW in this population. Note that BIA systematically overestimates TBW in underweight patients (BMI < 19.6) by 5.0% when a prediction model that was developed for normal-weight healthy subjects is used.

Weight combined with height measurement, or ideal body weight (IBW), is an indirect indicator of body composition. It can be used to screen for both undernutrition and overnutrition. The Metropolitan Life Insurance Company Height-Weight Table was used at one time as such a screening device.[61] Because of its possible inaccuracy, stemming from (1) its use of clinician estimation rather than calculation of frame size and (2) its reliance on data from white, insured persons aged 25 to 59 as the basis of the table, concerns have arisen about using the Metropolitan table. Although Metropolitan standards have been shown to be applicable to non-Caucasian US populations, few comparisons have been made with African American women and the majority of Asian Pacific populations. Moreover, considerable controversy continues over what should be considered the normal range of age-related weight increases. Thus, the Metropolitan tables should be used in conjunction with other measures to determine nutritional status and with an understanding of their limitations.

Another method of calculation of ideal body weight more commonly utilized is the Hamwi method. This method estimates weight for height based on frame size.[62] It provides only a rough estimate of ideal body weight, however, and it does not take into account age, race, and the differences in body composition that occur in athletes.[48]

- **Males**
  - Medium frame: 106 pounds for the 1st five feet, plus 6 pounds for every inch over.
  - Small frame: Subtract 10% from the medium-frame number.
  - Large frame: Add 10% to the medium-frame number.
- **Females**
  - Medium frame: 100 pounds for the first 5 feet, plus 5 pounds for every inch over.
  - Small frame: Subtract 10% from the medium-frame number.
  - Large frame: Add 10% to the medium-frame number.

Weight and height can also be used to calculate the BMI. The BMI (Table 33-2) is considered a more accurate estimation of total body fat than the Metropolitan weight tables. The BMI has limited utility in individuals with increased lean muscle mass or with large frames, as well as individuals with ascites or fluid overload. It is also more relevant for determining obesity than for assessing undernutrition. The formula for BMI calculation is

$$\frac{\text{Weight in kilograms}}{\text{height in meters squared}}$$

OR

$$\frac{\text{Weight in pounds}}{\text{height in inches squared}} \times 704.5$$

In an oncology population a weight measure that is more important than ideal body weight is the percent of usual body weight (UBW). This calculation determines the change in an individual's weight over time, using that individual as a standard to which measurements are compared. The degree of change in body weight is used to assess the degree of malnutrition. Table 33-3 provides a description of how change in usual body weight is classified.

Despite the overall importance, practicality, and clinical relevance of weight and height measurements in nutritional assessment, the reliability of both measures is questionable when calibration checks of scales and uniform measuring methods are not practiced. Clearly articulated policies and procedures outlining the process for obtaining heights and weights should be available. Scales should be calibrated regularly. Self-calibrating scales also should be tested periodically. The use of patient-reported weight and height should be discouraged. Training in accurate measurement and monitoring for quality assurance could improve the assessment process.

Additional anthropometrics used in nutritional assessment include skin-fold thickness and body-part circumferences to assess fat and muscle compartments. The assumptions underlying the use of skin-fold measures in

**TABLE 33-2**

**Classification of Body Mass Index in Adults**

| | Degree of Adiposity (kg/m$^2$) |
|---|---|
| Underweight | < 18.5 |
| Normal weight | 18.5–24.9 |
| Overweight | 25–29.9 |
| Obesity (class 1) | 30–34.9 |
| Obesity (class 2) | 35–39.9 |
| Extreme obesity (class 3) | ≥ 40 |

*Source:* Data from National Institutes of Health.[63]

**TABLE 33-3**

**Categories of Weight Loss and Malnutrition**

| | |
|---|---|
| *Degree of Malnutrition* | |
| Mild | 85%–90% UBW |
| Moderate | 75%–84% UBW |
| Severe | < 74% UBW |
| *Significant Weight Loss* | |
| 5% loss in 1–3 months | |
| 7.5% loss in 3–6 months | |
| 10% loss in 6 or more months | |
| *Severe Weight Loss* | |
| > 5% loss in 1 month | |
| > 7.5% loss in 3 months | |
| > 10% loss in 6 months | |

*Abbreviation*: UBW, usual body weight.
*Source*: Data from Blackburn and Bistrian.[64]

this way remain the subject of debate, as do the number and specific skin-fold measures that should be included in assessment. In addition, reliability of measurement is dependent on training and quality control. For these reasons, skin-fold measures are rarely used in clinical practice; when cause for their use presents itself, the procedure is best performed by a registered dietitian or nutritionist.

## CALCULATING ENERGY NEEDS

Another important function of the anthropometric measures of height and weight relates to their use in calculating an individual's energy needs. Currently, a very accurate assessment of energy needs can be obtained via indirect measurement of energy expenditure. Indirect calorimetry is one example of such an assessment. Indirect calorimetry requires the measurement of an individual's oxygen and carbon dioxide content of expired and inspired breath. It can be expensive and is not always practical in ambulatory settings. Much research has been devoted to creating equations that generate estimates of energy needs similar to those obtained through indirect calorimetry. To date, more than 200 equations have been designed for estimating the nutritional needs of various patient groups. A small representation of these equations is presented in Table 33-4. Caloric prescriptions for individuals with cancer are frequently based on the Harris-Benedict (HB) equation. Another equation used in critically ill oncology patients is the Ireton-Jones equation. The American Dietetic Association recently undertook an evaluation of multiple studies which sought to identify energy needs for patients with cancer in order to develop evidence-based guidelines. The conclusion of the evaluation was that there was no method, at this time, that consistently predicted the energy needs of patients with various types of cancer.[11]

These equations indicate the number of calories expended while the individual is at rest, or the *resting energy expenditure* (REE). This number is corrected for the level of required energy and varies according to activity, treatment, and comorbid condition (Table 33-5). Activity levels and stress need to be considered as well.[20] However, few estimates have focused on the energy required by individuals with cancer; those that are available suggest that determining the appropriate caloric need is difficult. Luthringer[19] found that although 66% of patients with colon cancer expended less than their estimated basal energy postoperatively, they also lost weight, indicating that providing adequate nutrition based on HB estimates did not translate into weight maintenance.

## LABORATORY TESTS

Laboratory tests are commonly used to evaluate nutritional status.[47,51] It is important to remember that most laboratory tests are nonspecific for malnutrition. Example test results include low blood count, decreased lymphocyte count, and delayed hypersensitivity testing, all of which can be affected by both cancer and cancer treatment. In addition, the tests are often not sensitive to nutritional deficiencies. For example, severe nutritional deficiencies may exist before albumin levels fall. Serum albumin is a poor marker for screening or early detection purposes but an excellent indicator of prognosis. Because laboratory parameters can be influenced by a number of other factors, it is essential that all values be considered within the patient's specific clinical context.[68]

## PHYSICAL EXAMINATION

Physical examination is limited in its ability to distinguish between the effects of cancer and the effects of nutritional deficiency. The fact that physical changes such as glossitis, muscle wasting, or diarrhea exist in many patients with cancer secondary to their disease or treatment does not minimize these changes' usefulness as indicators of problems in energy intake, absorption, or need. The patient's general appearance is important. The level of mobility may provide information about functional status; fat and muscle status can be assessed by visualizing the posterior ribs, scapula, or spine. Skin tone and turgor should be noted. Scaling skin may indicate vitamin (niacin) or trace element (zinc) deficiencies. An assessment of fluid status should also be conducted.[68] In addition, physical examination may identify other cancer-related changes, such as fevers, fistulas, or external lesions, that influence the intake or expenditure of energy.

**TABLE 33-4**

**Selected Adult Nutritional Assessment Equations**

| Nutritional Assessment Method | Formula | History |
|---|---|---|
| Calorie per kilogram | 25–35 Calories/kg | Extrapolated from the WHO calculations. Estimate based on nonobese population. ASPEN recommends that predictive energy requirements should fall within the range of 20–35 Calories/kg. |
| World Health Organization (WHO) | Women:<br>18–30 years = 15.3 (weight in kg) + 679<br>30–60 years = 11.6 (weight in kg) + 879<br>> 60 years = 8.8 (weight in kg) + 1128 (height in m)−1071<br>Men:<br>18–30 years = 14.7 (weight in kg) + 496<br>30–60 years = 8.7 (weight in kg) + 829<br>> 60 years = 9.2 (weight in kg) + 637 (height in m)−302 | Developed by FAO/WHO in 1974 for a healthy population.[65] |
| Harris-Benedict | Women:<br>REE = [655 + 9.6 (weight in kg) + 1.7 (height in cm)] + 4.7 (age in years)<br>Men:<br>REE = [66 + 1.37 (weight in kg) + 5 (height in cm)] + 6.8 (age in years) | Developed in 1919 from studies of indirect calorimetry of 239 men and women. Random error calculations female equation ($r^2 = 0.53$), male calculation ($r^2 = 0.75$).[57,61] |
| Ireton-Jones | Ventilator dependent:<br>EEE = 1784−11(a) + 5(w) + 244(s) + 239(t) + 804(b)<br>Spontaneous breathing:<br>EEE = 629−11(a) + 25(w)−609(o)<br>a = age (years)<br>w = body weight (kg)<br>s = sex (male = 1, female = 0)<br>t = trauma (present = 1, absent = 0)<br>b = burn (present = 1. absent = 0)<br>o = obesity [BMI > 27] (present = 1, absent = 0) | Developed for critically ill and hospitalized patients using indirect calorimetry.[61] |
| Mifflin–St. Jeor | Women:<br>REE = −161 + 10 (weight in kg) + 6.25 (height in cm)−5 (age)<br>Men:<br>REE = 5 + 10 (weight in kg) + 6.25 (height in cm)−5 (age) | Developed in 1990 from studies of 247 women and 251 men ($r^2 = 0.71$). |
| Dietary reference intake for energy | Women:<br>EEE = 354−6.91 (age) + PA [9.36 (weight in kg) + 726 (height in m)]<br>Men:<br>EEE = 662−9.53 (age) + PA [9.36 (weight in kg) + 539.6 (height in m)]<br>PA (physical activity coefficient):<br>Sedentary = 1.00<br>Low active =1.11<br>Active = 1.25<br>Very active = 1.48 | Developed in 2002 by the Institute of Medicine from studies of doubly labeled water for use in a healthy population.[66] |

*Abbreviations*: ASPEN, American Society for Parentral and Enteral Nutrition; EEE, estimated energy expenditure; FAO, Food and Agricultural Organization; REE, resting energy expenditure.

**TABLE 33-5**

**Correction Factors for Use with Measures of Resting Energy Expenditure**

| | Energy Correction Factor |
|---|---|
| *Activity Factors* | |
| Confined to bed | 1.2 × REE |
| Sedentary | 1.4–1.9 × REE |
| Active | 2.0–2.4 × REE |
| *Stress Factors* | |
| Fever | 1.0 + 0.13 per 1°C > 37°C × REE |
| Elective surgery | 1.0–1.1 × REE |
| Sepsis | 1.2–1.4 × REE |
| Multiple trauma | 1.4 × REE |
| Cancer | 1.1–1.45 × REE |
| Burns | 1.5–2.1 × REE |
| Infection with trauma | 1.3–1.55 × REE |
| Severe infection | 1.2–1.6 × REE |

*Abbreviations*: REE, resting energy expenditure.
*Source*: Data from Edel J, Murray M, Schurer W, et al.[67]

## DIETARY INFORMATION

Dietary intake information is used to identify existing and potential nutritional excesses and deficits. In a full diet history, information that reflects both diet and general health is included. General questions alert the nurse to the need for more in-depth study of dietary intakes. Dietary information is obtained by using a number of approaches: 24-hour recall surveys, food frequency measures, diet diaries, calorie counts, or monthly purchase records. The last method is rarely used in clinical practice. Any of the types of food intake recordings provide information about energy, nutrient, vitamin, and mineral intakes. Obtaining this information requires variable amounts of time to input the data into nutrient analysis programs. The need for this depth of assessment will depend on the setting. Full dietary assessments are usually conducted by registered dietitians or nutritionists. However, the nurse should be alert to nursing assessment items of weight change, recent changes in intake, symptoms that influence eating or food preparation, and indications that alternative or complementary nutritional products are being used.

## FUNCTIONAL ASSESSMENT

Assessment of the ability to perform the activities of daily living, especially in the areas of food procurement and preparation, are part of a thorough nutritional assessment. For the past 2 decades, performance level assessments have also been used to determine the relationship of nutrition to function.[69,70] The use of more specific measures, such as muscle strength, have likewise been suggested as sensitive indicators of both positive and negative changes in food intake.[71,72] However, the use of such measures remains uncommon except in research situations.

## NUTRITION-RELATED SYMPTOM ASSESSMENT

Assessment of symptoms that interfere with intake is part of an oncological nutritional assessment. Many symptoms have the potential to influence nutritional intake. These may include, but are not limited to, anorexia, nausea, vomiting, diarrhea, constipation, mouth sores, dry mouth, pain when eating or swallowing, other pain, taste change, fatigue, difficulty in swallowing, indigestion, early satiety, cramping, or bloating. Effective management of nutrition-impact symptoms relies on a proactive approach that includes anticipating those symptoms that are associated with the patient's particular disease and treatment. Assessment of the nutritional impact of symptoms should be systematic and include the use of tools that have been designed for this purpose. Linear analog self-assessment, Likert-type, or narrative grading scales may be useful in identifying the severity of the problem and the effectiveness of intervention[73] (Figure 33-1). The National Cancer Institute's Common Terminology Criteria for Adverse Events (CTC-AE) version 3.0 is a descriptive terminology tool that may also be useful.[74] Many nutrition-impact symptoms are included in this tool. In addition, both weight gain and weight loss are listed under constitutional symptoms within this reference. One caveat when using this tool is that the severity scores assigned

**Linear Analog Self-Assessment**
During the last week, I was nauseated
not at all ———————————— all the time

**Likert Scale**

| | | | | | |
|---|---|---|---|---|---|
| Nausea | 1 | 2 | 3 | 4 | 5 |
| | No problem | | | | As sick as I could be |

**Objective Scale**

| | | | | |
|---|---|---|---|---|
| Nausea | 0 | 1 | 2 | 3 |
| | None | Able to eat reasonable intake | Intake significantly decreased, but able to eat | No significant intake |

**FIGURE 33-1**

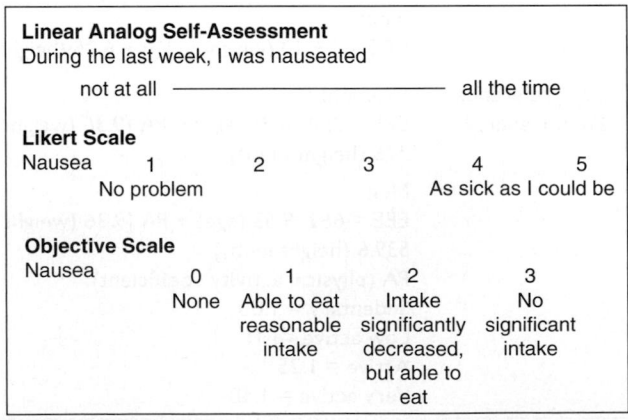

Examples of nutritionally linked symptom measurement.

to weight gain and weight loss outcomes are quite lenient. Weight loss, for example, is not considered severe (grade 3) until patients have lost ≥ 20% of their baseline weight. Systematic interventions to prevent or minimize weight loss associated with nutrition-impact symptoms need to start well in advance of this point. Proactive monitoring and early intervention is the most effective means of minimizing the negative effects of symptoms on nutritional status.[68]

## THERAPEUTIC APPROACHES AND NURSING CARE

Because malnutrition is associated with poor outcomes, including increased morbidity and mortality and decreased quality of life,[3,24,43] interventions that might prevent or minimize nutritional problems represent a worthy goal. Ongoing research in this area is exploring nutritional manipulation in cancer prevention, as an adjunct to standard cancer treatment and as a mode of therapy. In addition, continuing studies are examining interventions that could minimize the threats of treatment to the host's nutritional status.[75] Optimal nutrition planning utilizes a nutritional team with expertise in cancer-associated malnutrition. When such a program is not available, a general nutritional support team may be of assistance. Development of a nutritional care plan may require the collaboration of nurses, physicians, dietitians, pharmacists, speech therapists, and social workers. The patient and family or significant others are an integral part of this effort. Without their participation in goal setting and method choice, it is unlikely that any intervention will succeed.

Interventions must also be based on realistic goals and ethical considerations. Goals may target specific or general dietary components to influence morbidity, mortality, appetite, function, or well-being. For patients in whom response to treatment is expected or for whom morbidity will be reduced, intervention is a sound practice. Goal setting within an ethical context can be more difficult for individuals with progressing disease, anorexia, and weight loss. Often, family members concentrate on reversing the patient's lack of appetite and weight loss, which can put undue stress on the patient and the family relationship. Since eating is often a major source of comfort and enhances quality of life, the use of interventions that improve appetite and alter the metabolic abnormalities should be considered where appropriate. In situations where the patient is in the terminal stages of illness and unable to eat or drink fluids, then allowing dehydration to proceed is ethically and legally acceptable.[75]

Oncology nurses play a key role in assessing nutritional issues across the continuum of cancer care. Nurses should be knowledgeable about nutritional issues commonly encountered in the cancer population and anticipate those issues in patients for whom they provide care.

## NUTRITIONAL INTERVENTIONS

The nutritional assessment, described previously and performed by members of the nutritional team, provides the basis for the nutritional prescription and development of intervention strategies. Possible prescriptions range from oral supplementation or deletion of specific nutrients to institution of total parenteral nutrition. Strategies include verbal counseling to alter intake or manage symptoms, prescription of medications to minimize side effects, and identification of resources to facilitate treatment with oral supplements, tube-administered enteral nutrition, or total parenteral nutrition. The level of intervention and accompanying strategy are dictated by the patient's baseline nutritional state, disease status, risks for malnutrition from treatment, anticipated response to therapy, and resources. Algorithms for individuals at normal weight and those who are undernourished are provided in Figures 33-2 and 33-3.

### NUTRITIONAL PRESCRIPTION

#### Alteration in specific dietary components

The development of some nutrient deficiencies is common across diseases. For example, low serum iron and potassium are not unusual in a number of chronic diseases. In patients with cancer, these deficits arise from a combination of chemotherapy-related effects on bone marrow, anemia of chronic disease, medications for comorbid conditions, and antibiotic use. Other deficiencies that are more specific to cancer include hypomagnesemia related to platinum chemotherapy; hyponatremia and hypercalcemia, resulting from paraneoplastic syndromes; and zinc deficiency accompanying head and neck cancers. Intervention with parenteral fluids or supplements may be required for some patients; in others, oral mineral supplementation is used to control these problems. Educating the patient about foods that are good sources of the deficient mineral may also be helpful.

In addition to reversing known deficiencies, supplemental nutrients are given to minimize the side effects and maximize the therapeutic effect of standard treatment. The role of immunonutrition, or specific nutrients, such as arginine, omega-3 fatty acids, and glutamine, in the diet remains controversial. Consensus recommendations, published in 2001, concluded that immune-enhancing diets containing arginine, glutamine, omega-3 fatty acids, and RNA nucleotides are beneficial to severely malnourished patients undergoing major surgery. Subsequent analysis indicated a possible benefit in critically ill patients and no

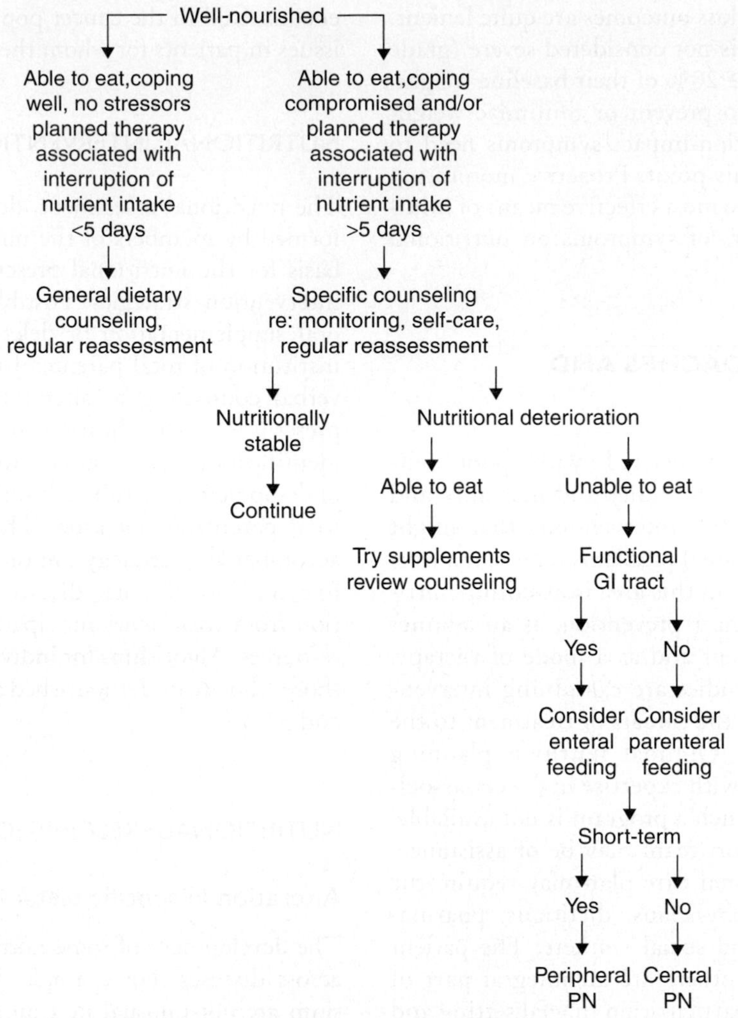


**FIGURE 33-2**

Nutritional support algorithm for individuals well-nourished at baseline. *Abbreviations*: GI, gastrointestinal tract; PN, parenteral nutrition.

benefit in the postoperative period.[76,77] Glutamine supplementation may provide the benefits of protection from chemotherapy-induced mucositis, diarrhea, neuropathy, hepatic venoocclusive disease, and cardiotoxicity. Oral glutamine supplementation may also protect normal tissues from, and sensitize tumor cells to, radiation therapy.[78] The increased use of these approaches depends on additional study to verify their effectiveness, target population, dosages, and scheduling.

Similarly, reduction of specific macronutrients has been the target of nutritional intervention. Dietary fat intake has become a target for specific treatment, especially among patients with breast cancer.[13] Clinical trials indicate that verbal counseling results in significantly decreased fat intake within 3 months among patients with breast cancer.[79] The altered intake pattern is sustained past the period of counseling. Several of the trials have found documented increased survival among participants.[80] Reduction of fat in combination with other diet manipulations are also being tested.

## Alteration in general intake

A more traditional nutritional goal has been the improvement of the patient's overall intake to aid general nutritional status, minimize treatment side effects, and maximize treatment delivery. Increases in nutrient intake can significantly reduce the morbidity and mortality among severely malnourished patients in certain settings. However, the complex interaction of nutrition, cancer, and host can alter the usual response to increased intake. Investigators report that increased caloric intake may neither reverse weight loss nor

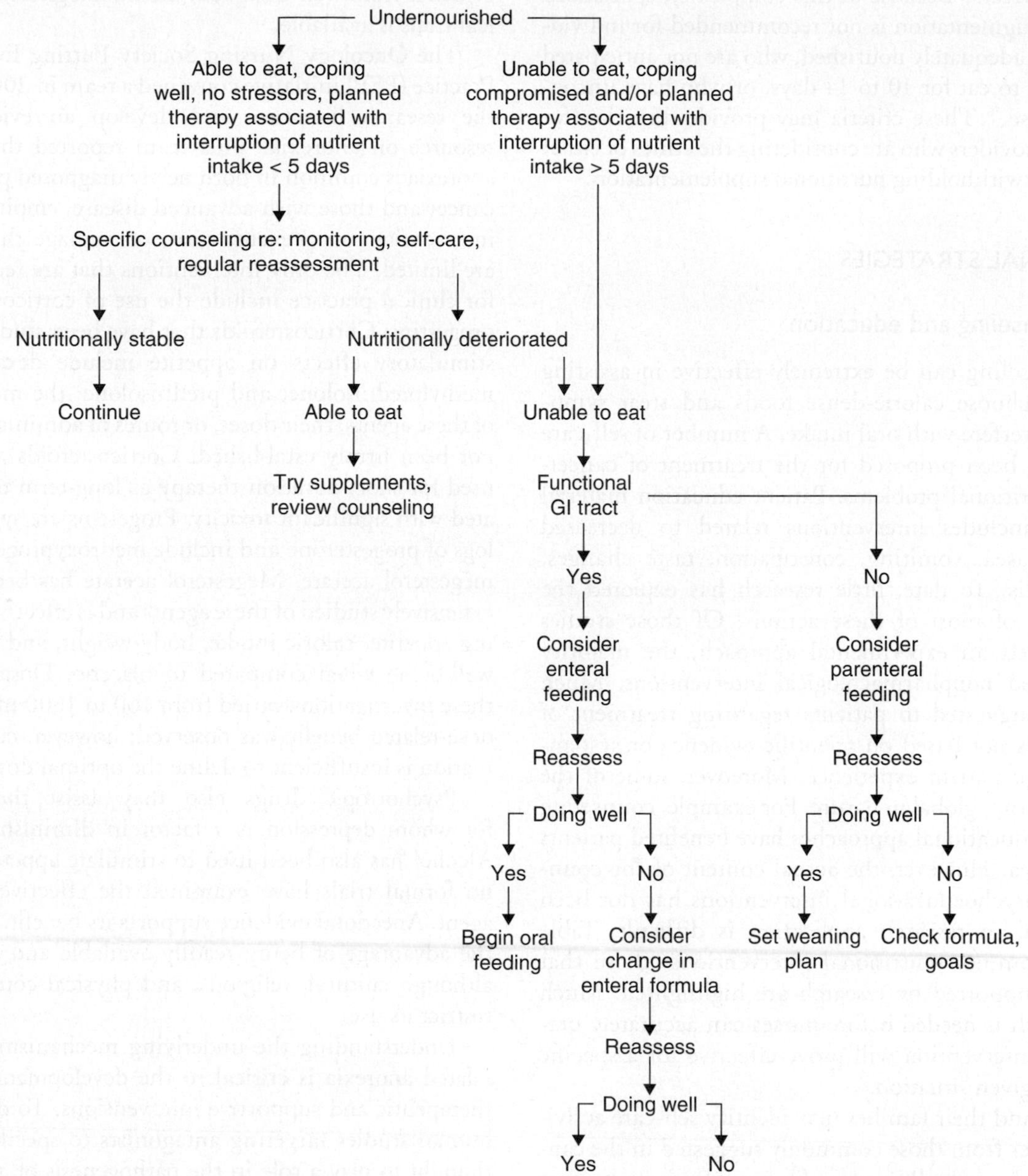


**FIGURE 33-3**

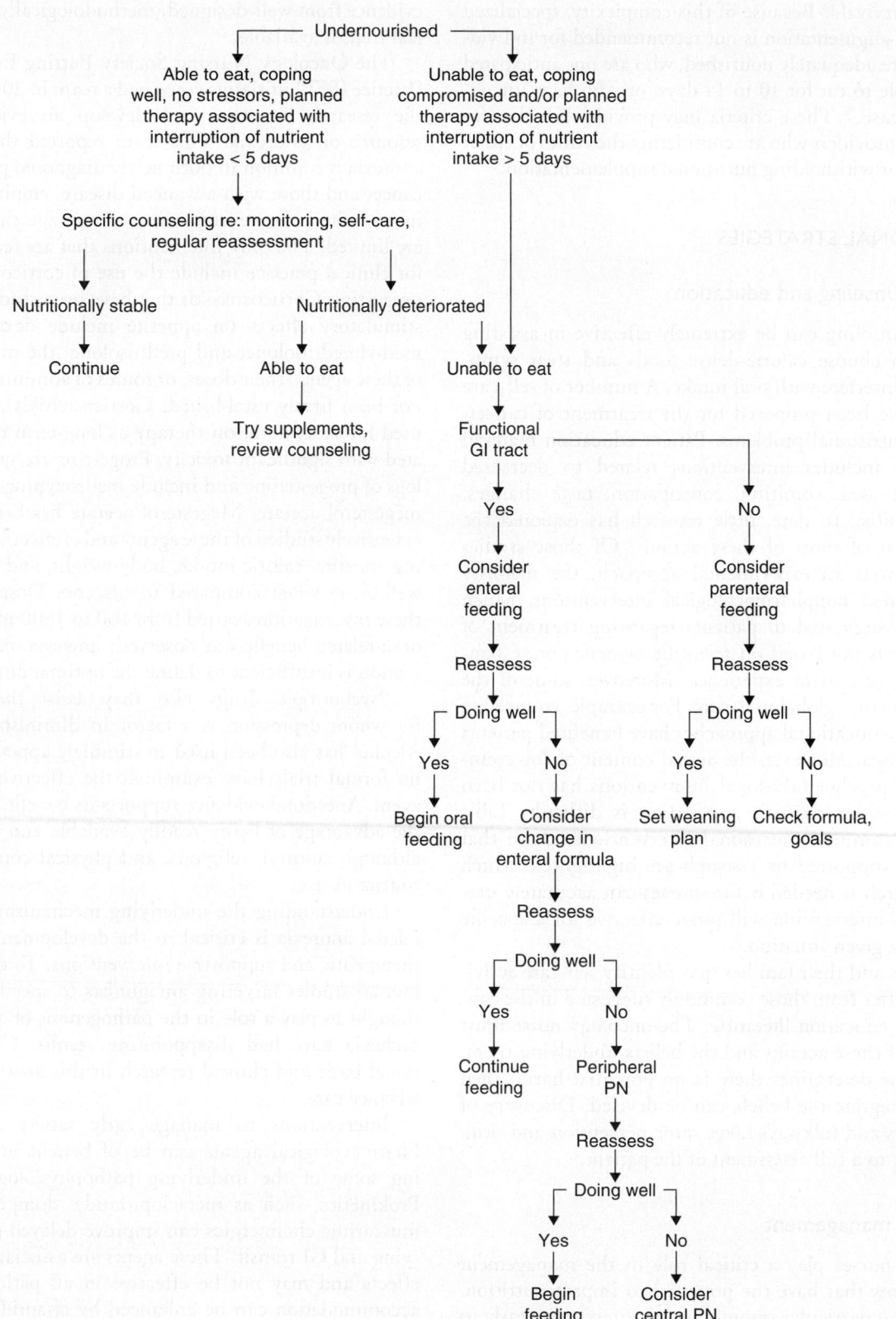

Nutritional support algorithm for individuals undernourished at baseline. *Abbreviations*: GI, gastrointestinal tract; PN, parenteral nutrition.

improve survival.[14] Because of this complexity, specialized nutritional augmentation is not recommended for individuals who are adequately nourished, who are not anticipated to be unable to eat for 10 to 14 days, or who have uncontrolled disease.[76] These criteria may provide direction for healthcare providers who are considering the ethics of either supplying or withholding nutritional supplementation.

## NUTRITIONAL STRATEGIES

### Verbal counseling and education

Verbal counseling can be extremely effective in assisting patients to choose calorie-dense foods and treat symptoms that interfere with oral intake. A number of self-care actions have been proposed for the treatment of cancer-induced nutritional problems. Patient education material commonly includes interventions related to decreased appetite, nausea, vomiting, constipation, taste changes, and mucositis. To date, little research has explored the effectiveness of most of these actions. Of those studies that employed an experimental approach, the majority have included nonpharmacological interventions. Much of what is suggested to patients regarding treatment of side effects is not based on scientific evidence or systematic review of patient experience. Moreover, some of the interventions are global in nature. For example, counseling and psychoeducational approaches have benefited patients having nausea. However, the actual content of the counseling and psychoeducational interventions has not been standardized, so research application is difficult. Table 33-6 lists common nutritional interventions; those that have been supported by research are highlighted. Much more research is needed before nurses can accurately predict which intervention will prove effective for a specific patient in a given situation.

Patients and their families may identify self-care activities that differ from those commonly suggested in the cancer patient education literature. The oncology nurse must be aware of these actions and the beliefs underlying them. If the nurse determines there is no potential harm, then ways to integrate the beliefs can be devised. Discovery of such beliefs and folkways takes some perception and skill, but is basic to a full assessment of the patient.

### Symptom management

Oncology nurses play a critical role in the management of symptoms that have the potential to impact nutrition. Anticipating particular symptoms and intervening early to prevent or minimize these issues is a key strategy to optimize nutritional intake. Symptom management is typically a large part of the nutrition care plan, as many symptoms can greatly impact ability to eat. Symptom management interventions should be evidence based to the extent that evidence from well-designed, methodologically sound clinical trials is available.

The Oncology Nursing Society Putting Evidence into Practice (PEP) initiative convened a team in 2008 to review the research literature and develop an evidence-based resource on anorexia. This team reported that although anorexia is common in both newly diagnosed patients with cancer and those with advanced disease, empirically based interventions to prevent, treat, or manage this symptom are limited. The only interventions that are recommended for clinical practice include the use of corticosteroids and progestins. Corticosteroids that have been studied for their stimulatory effects on appetite include dexamethasone, methylprednisolone, and prednisolone; the most effective of these agents, their doses, or routes of administration have not been firmly established. Corticosteroids are typically used for short-duration therapy as long-term use is associated with significant toxicity. Progestins are synthetic analogs of progesterone and include medroxyprogesterone and megesterol acetate. Megesterol acetate has been the most extensively studied of these agents and is effective in increasing appetite, caloric intake, body weight, and sensation of well-being when compared to placebo. Dosages used in these investigations varied from 160 to 1600 milligrams. A dose-related benefit was observed; however, current information is insufficient to define the optimal dose.[81]

Psychotropic drugs also may assist those patients for whom depression is a factor in diminished appetite. Alcohol has also been used to stimulate appetite although no formal trials have examined the effectiveness of this agent. Anecdotal evidence supports its benefit. Alcohol has the advantage of being readily available and inexpensive, although cultural, religious, and physical conditions may restrict its use.

Understanding the underlying mechanisms of cancer-related anorexia is critical to the development of rational therapeutic and supportive interventions. To date, the few human studies targeting antagonists to specific cytokines thought to play a role in the pathogenesis of anorexia and cachexia have had disappointing results. Clearly, additional basic and clinical research in this area is needed to advance care.

Interventions to manage early satiety are limited. Pharmacological agents can be of benefit in counteracting some of the underlying pathophysiological effects. Prokinetics, such as metaclopromide, domperidone, and muscarinic cholinergics can improve delayed gastric emptying and GI transit. These agents are associated with side effects and may not be effective in all patients. Gastric accommodation can be enhanced by cisapride, sumatriptan, clonidine, and sildenafil. Smaller, more frequent meals and cooler food temperatures (to minimize food aversions) may also be of benefit. Dietary fat can reduce satiety, so increasing the fat content of foods consumed may be helpful. Appetite stimulants are not recommended; increasing

**TABLE 33-6**

**Suggested Interventions for Nutrition-Related Side Effects**

| Side Effects | Suggested Interventions |
|---|---|
| Appetite change | After food choice, increase oral hygiene; avoid sight, smell of food; eat sour foods; eat cold foods; use straw; increase seasoning; use plastic utensils; small amount of alcohol. |
| Constipation | Increase liquid intake; eat more fiber; eat more fruit; exercise; take laxative; drink hot beverages; add bran to foods. |
| Diarrhea | Take medicine; increase fluids; drink rehydration fluids; low-residue diet; avoid spices and caffeine, avoid milk products; take soluble-fiber supplement; eat low-fat diet. |
| Dry mouth | Take medicine (pilocarpine, saliva substitutes in xerostomia); increase fluids; chew gum; suck on sugarless candy; blend foods; avoid acid, salty, or spicy foods; moisten food, humidify air; apply oil to oral cavity. |
| Early satiety | Eat frequently, eat small meals; drink between meals; limit liquids at meals. |
| Mucositis | Take medicine (sucralfate, capsaicin, GSF, antibiotic pastilles, interleukin 1); apply cold (ice) to oral cavity during chemotherapy administration; increase oral hygiene; drink liquids; use soft toothbrush; avoid spicy food; humidify air, avoid use of gravy; use baking soda mouthwash; apply mucosa-adhesive film, avoid alcohol and tobacco; use straws; use supplements; use glutamine. |
| Nausea | Take medicine; alter diet, practice relaxation; listen to music; rest after meals; avoid sight, smell of food; eat cold foods; increase oral hygiene; eat small frequent meals; eat slowly; get fresh air; drink clear liquids; keep busy/distracted; chew food well; drink between meals; eat crackers; breathe through the mouth: eat sour foods; eat low-fat foods; avoid spicy foods; eat sweet foods. |
| Conditioned nausea | Practice relaxation or deconditioning imagery, self-hypnosis; take medication. |
| Taste change | Alter food choice; increase oral hygiene; avoid sight, smell of food; eat sour foods; eat cold foods; increase seasoning; use straw, avoid tart foods; chew sugarless gum; eat less fat; use plastic utensils. |
| Vomiting | Take medicine; practice relaxation; rest after meals; drink clear liquids; avoid sight, smell of food; eat slowly; eat crackers; eat cold foods; get fresh air; chew mint candy; eat room-temperature foods; alter diet; increase oral hygiene; eat small frequent meals; eat low-fat diet; avoid spicy foods. |

*Note*: Boldface type indicates that research support exists for the intervention.
*Abbreviation*: GSF, granulocyte-stimulating factor.

appetite in the context of decreased ability to consume may actually worsen early satiety.[36,82] Additional research is needed in the area in order to more precisely define the underlying pathophysiologic mechanisms and to identify optimal supportive interventions.

Empirical evidence on effective strategies to manage taste and smell alterations experienced by patients with cancer is severely lacking. In a review of the literature, no investigations testing specific interventions for either taste or small alterations were identified. Several descriptive studies suggested interventions that may be of benefit; these included providing relevant anticipatory information to patients,[83,84] avoiding foods with strong tastes or odors, marinating foods, using smaller portions, brushing teeth before eating, consuming more water with foods, and using spices and condiments.[84]

## Pharmacological interventions

Medications are used by patients to prevent or treat a number of nutrition-related problems. Taking medicine is the most effective self-care technique reported in controlling constipation, diarrhea, nausea, vomiting, and mucosal irritation.[85] In addition to improving appetite and early satiety, medications may be prescribed to increase nutrient intake, offset cancer-induced metabolic disturbances, and limit or reverse losses of lean body mass.

Metoclopramide has been used to improve oral intake based on its effect on nausea, gastric motility, early satiety, and reflux. The usual dose is 10 mg taken orally before meals and at bedtime. Very few trials have been performed to study the drug's effect on intake and weight, and more studies are needed.

Dronabinol, like metoclopramide, has been explored largely in terms of its effect on chemotherapy-induced nausea and vomiting. Few randomized trials have investigated the effect of the drug on intake. Increases in weight have been reported at doses ranging from 2.5 mg twice per day to 15 mg per day. Changes in weight may be related to fluid retention or fat rather than increased lean body mass. Dronabinol's effectiveness may be greater in individuals who have used the drug before. Side effects are more common in older persons, especially at higher doses, but may be reduced with timing administration of the drug after a meal. Cost and concerns about the abuse of cannabinoids may limit its acceptance, even though abuse of dronabinol is not common.[86]

Eicosapentaenoic acid (EPA) is an essential fatty acid, most abundantly found in fish oils and plant sources such as algae, flaxseed, and walnuts. EPA has been substantially researched as a potential weapon in the fight against cancer-induced weight loss. Multiple studies have utilized liquid nutritional supplements as a vehicle for administration of 1 to 2 g of EPA to patients with weight loss or cachexia. The majority of the research with EPA has involved patients with pancreatic cancer. Results indicate slowing or reversing of weight loss in most studies; however, there is no impact on lean body mass. In addition, the cost of the supplements is often prohibitive. Noncompliance with the regimen is a commonly cited problem.[81]

Several drugs have been tested for their normalizing effect on metabolism, including insulin, hydrazine sulfate, and pentoxifylline. Unfortunately, clinical trials suggest that these drugs are not useful. Insulin use is complicated by the difficulties of side effect management. Hydrazine sulfate and pentoxifylline showed promise in early trials, but placebo-controlled studies have indicated that neither offers a significant benefit. Additional drugs being tested in the cachectic AIDS population include thalidomide and melatonin, both of which have been associated with weight stabilization or reduced weight loss. Preliminary studies in patients with cancer indicate reduced weight loss and some gain in lean body mass.[87]

Drugs that have been investigated for their ability to maintain lean body mass include the anabolic steroids fluoxymesterone, nandrolone, and oxandrolone and the growth hormone rhGH. Available research indicates that nandrolone is associated with significant improvements in weight, lean body mass, and quality of life in patients with AIDS but not in patients with lung cancer. Oxandrolone induces weight gain or maintenance in 81% of patients with cancer cachexia.[88] Growth hormone use results in short-term conservation of protein in patients with AIDS.[89] Studies in more diverse cancer populations and with rigorous designs are needed before the use of these drugs can be supported as routine care.

## ENTERAL AND PARENTERAL NUTRITION

When severe malnutrition exists or oral intake is threatened for longer than a week, alternative methods of intake should be explored. Table 33-7 provides guidelines for the use of nutritional support in patients with cancer.

If the GI tract is functioning, enteral feeding is the intervention of choice. It is crucial for individuals with aerodigestive or upper GI surgery. Enteral feeding assists in the

**TABLE 33-7**

**Guidelines for the Use of Nutrition Support in Patients With Cancer**

*ADA Goals of Medical Nutrition Therapy*[90]

- Maintain adequate intake of calories and protein.
- Select foods to limit the side effects of treatments.
- Maintain stable weight.
- After treatments, adopt healthy eating plans.

*2002 ASPEN Guidelines*[54]

- Specialized nutrition support is appropriate in patients receiving active anticancer treatment who are malnourished and are anticipated to be unable to ingest and/or absorb adequate nutrients for a prolonged period of time.
- Preoperative specialized nutrition support may be beneficial in moderately or severely malnourished patients if administered for 7–14 days preoperatively, but the potential benefits of nutrition support must be weighed against the potential risks of the nutrition support itself.
- Specialized nutrition support should not be used routinely in patients undergoing major cancer operations. Use of nutrition support in patients undergoing major cancer operations does not improve surgical outcome.
- Specialized nutrition support should not be used routinely as an adjunct to chemotherapy.
- Specialized nutrition support should not be used routinely in patients undergoing head and neck, abdominal, or pelvic irradiation.
- The palliative use of specialized nutrition support in terminally ill patients with cancer is rarely indicated.

*NCI Contraindications to Enteral Nutrition Support*[91]

- Malfunctioning gastrointestinal tract.
- Malabsorptive conditions.
- Mechanical obstructions.
- Severe bleeding.
- Severe diarrhea.
- Intractable vomiting.
- Gastrointestinal fistulas in locations difficult to bypass with an enteral tube.
- Inflammatory bowel processes:
  - Prolonged ileus.
  - Severe enterocolitis.
- Overall health prognosis not consistent with aggressive nutrition therapy.

*NCI Contraindications to Parenteral Nutrition Support*[91]

- Functional gut.
- Limited life expectancy (<40 days)
- Lack of adequate vascular access.
- Lack of severe nutritional deficit such as temporary inability to eat (eg, postsurgery).

*Abbreviations*: ADA, American Dietetic Association; ASPEN, American Society for Parenteral and Enteral Nutrition; NCI, National Cancer Institute.

maintenance of GI digestive and absorptive function and is very effective for individuals with GI obstructions that can be bypassed by tube placement. This feeding option, especially in the upper GI tract, maintains the normal stimulation of enzymatic and mucosal activity in the gut, an important attribute when oral feeding is to be resumed.[45,92]

For individuals without a functioning GI tract, total parenteral nutrition (TPN) may be the nutritional treatment of choice. A number of studies have reported the effect of TPN on the morbidity and mortality in malnourished patients undergoing surgery and have been critically reviewed.[92] Total parenteral nutrition has been associated with reduced morbidity in bone marrow transplant treatment when administered either before cytoreduction or when GI reaction denudes the gut mucosa.[92] Patients with significant GI malfunction, but otherwise with cured, controlled, or indolent disease, may also benefit from parenteral feeding. The largest group of patients with cancer receiving home parenteral nutrition are those with chronic small or large bowel obstruction.[78]

Other uses of aggressive nutritional support remain controversial, in part because of problems of design or methodology in the extant research. Many of the relevant studies have small sample sizes. Studies also frequently have different nutritional outcomes, differing patient populations, and different feeding formulas. They reveal that although subsets of patients benefit from nutritional repletion, aggressive nutritional intervention does not alter morbidity or mortality for the majority of individuals with cancer. In addition, the risks associated with the various treatments must be considered. The problems and common solutions associated with enteral and parenteral nutritional interventions are listed in Tables 33-8 and 33-9. The role of aggressive nutritional intervention in cancer treatment clearly requires more study. As the nutritional abnormalities created by cancer are better understood, more appropriate interventions will be developed.

## PHYSICAL ACTIVITY

Physical inactivity can lead to muscle atrophy, contributing to loss of cardiorespiratory fitness and fatigue. Weight loss that occurs secondary to catabolic activity or cytokine-mediated changes in metabolism or corticosteroid use can also contribute significantly to decreased muscle mass. The structure and function of muscle and bone depend on physical activity combined with appropriate nutritional intake and a hormonal milieu that supports anabolism.[93] An evolving body of knowledge supports the role of physical activity in enhancing a number of clinical outcomes. Improvements have been documented in functional capacity, fatigue, medication requirements, self-esteem, mood, sense of control and well-being, and immunological

**TABLE 33-8**

**Common Enteral Feeding Problems and Solutions**

| Problem | Solution |
|---|---|
| Diarrhea | Give formula at room temperature; use lactose-free formula; add fiber, add antidiarrheal medicine; reduce rate of feeding; reduce volume or use continuous feeding schedule; reduce strength of formula; review other potential sources (medications, treatment) |
| Regurgitation | Check tube placement; check residuals and withhold feedings if more than 100–200 mL; keep in Fowler's position; use small bore tube; place tube distally (jejunum, duodenum); consider drugs to increase motility |
| Nausea | Check tube placement; reduce rate; reduce anxiety; change formula; review other potential sources (infection, medications, treatment) |
| Distention | Use low-fat or hydrolyzed formula; encourage activity; review other potential sources (obstruction, constipation, organomegaly) |
| Dehydration | Increase water intake to ensure adequate amounts (usually 1 mL/kcal); control (diarrhea, nausea); watch for glucosuria |
| Fluid overload | Reduce water intake; use concentrated formula |
| Constipation | Increase water; increase fiber; increase activity |
| Local irritation | Clean area around tube; apply skin-protecting agents; monitor for otitis media if using nasal tubes |
| Mouth dryness | Frequent mouth rinsing; use xerostomia products; sugarless gum or mints if medically allowed |
| Tube obstruction | Use room-temperature feedings; irrigate with water; use pump with high-density formulas (>1.5 kcal/mL) or small-bore tubes; use liquid medicines rather than crushing pills whenever possible |
| Metabolic imbalance | Monitor carbon dioxide levels; reduce carbohydrate in formula; monitor glucose; monitor potassium and supplement if needed |

**TABLE 33-9**

**Parenteral Feeding Considerations**

*General Indications*: Nonfunctioning gastrointestinal tract; unable to begin enteral feedings for 7 or more days; high-output fistulas; in combination with enteral feedings for some bowel resections; severe radiation enteritis with or without malignant disease: temporary malabsorption secondary to aggressive therapy (eg, bone marrow transplant); obstructed bowel but otherwise acceptable quality of life; pancreatitis.

**Common Parenteral Feeding Problems and Solutions**

| Problem | Solutions |
|---|---|
| Pneumo-hemothorax | Put patient in Trendelenburg position for line placement; check x-ray postprocedure |
| Embolism | Follow flushing regimen; avoid use of small-diameter syringes when flushing; avoid exposure to free air |
| Obstruction | Flush per protocol; check for flow per protocol; treat with antiembolics per institutional protocol |
| Dislodgment | Assess for patency; be alert to patient complaints of pain or swelling in area of catheter insertion |
| Metabolic abnormalities | Monitor levels of glucose, ammonia, phosphate, liver enzymes, magnesium, potassium, hemoglobin/hematocrit |
| Infection | Perform careful site care and evaluation; monitor temperature, glucose levels, glucosuria |
| Trace element deficiency | Monitor vitamin and trace element |
| Bleeding | Monitor vitamin K administration |

parameters.[94] Physical activities might include walking programs, stretching, use of resistance bands, swimming, cycling, or dancing, as tolerated.

## COMPLEMENTARY AND ALTERNATIVE NUTRITIONAL INTERVENTIONS

Selected traditional cancer centers are engaging in rigorous study of complementary and alternative medicine (CAM). This interest arises from at least 2 factors. First, research has shown that 20% to 66% of individuals with cancer combine conventional and alternative or complementary therapies.[95,96] Nutritional approaches are the most commonly used complementary treatments. Second, a growing body of evidence has demonstrated the effectiveness of some of the products used in CAM. These elements make it essential for nurses to understand both the benefits and the disadvantages of CAM. CAM is reviewed in depth in Chapter 24.

## CONCLUSION

Nutrition influences carcinogenesis itself, as well as the quantity and quality of life, once the disease exists. The nurse's ability to take full advantage of nutritional interventions is hampered by insufficient understanding of the pathophysiology of the tumor–host relationship. Without this knowledge, it is difficult to match a specific intervention with a specific nutritional problem.

This lack of knowledge emphasizes the importance of nursing care. Nurses are in the best position to detect undernutrition and overnutrition among individuals with cancer across the cancer care trajectory. The nurse attends to basic nutritional information during the diagnostic process: height, weight, recent weight change, eating problems, unhealthy and healthful food choices, social situations that interfere with food procurement, and psychological responses that may alter intake. Given this base, the nurse can work with other care providers to prioritize and define nutritional care. The nurse continues the assessment function throughout the patient's treatment and follow-up. Nutritional intervention can be devised in the overall context of the clinical situation and in accordance with the patient's beliefs, cultural context, and desires.

Although the scientific information is still far from complete, early nutritional intervention—when the tumor burden is relatively small—has the best chance to alter patient outcomes. This is particularly true for those undergoing surgery. Appropriate nutritional intervention reduces morbidity, length of hospital stay, and possibly mortality in these patients. For some patients, the need for nutritional support will continue for a period following hospitalization. Understanding the limitations of nutritional interventions is important for both nurses and patients. Assisting patients to make the best decisions for themselves may reduce frustration and minimize use of questionable methods (See Table 33-10).[97,98,99,100,101]

Nurses also should be attuned to newer approaches in the use of nutrition as therapy. Determining what role nutritional interventions will play in the cancer armamentarium needs additional study. Further, nurses have an obligation to continue research into the self-care actions routinely prescribed in dealing with nutritional disturbances. Many of the actions commonly suggested are based solely on

**TABLE 33-10**

**Questionable Dietary Treatments for Cancer**

| Diet/Additive | Proposed Activity | Comments/Side Effects |
|---|---|---|
| Antineoplastin/ Burzynski therapy[97,98] | Antineoplastons are described as amino acid derivatives, peptides, and essential amino acids present in the diet of all biological organisms. Antineoplastons are theorized to interrupt the activity of the *ras* oncogene, which causes cells to divide endlessly. At the same time, antineoplastons stimulate *p53* tumor suppressor genes, which induce apoptosis. Healthy cells remain unaffected under these processes. It is usually given by injection. The length of treatment is usually between 4 months to a year, depending on how the person responds. | Side effects include nausea, vomiting, stomach gas, chills, rashes, fever, joint pain, changes in blood pressure, and body odor during treatment. |
| Cancell/Cantron/ Protocel[99] | According to manufacturers, this product causes cancer cells to become completely primitive (residual aerobic metabolism is inhibited and they produce energy solely by glycolysis). The resulting primitive cells are then seen by the body as foreign and destroyed. The exact composition of Cancell/Cantron/Protocel is unknown. The FDA lists the ingredients as inositol, nitric acid, sodium sulfite, potassium hydroxide, sulfuric acid, and catechol. It has been administered orally, rectally, and topically. | Side effects include temporary, moderate fatigue during the first few weeks of treatment and nausea. There are no human studies published at this time. |
| Gerson Diet[100] | Originally developed to treat migraines, the Gerson diet consists of a strict raw vegetarian diet, 13 glasses of raw fruit and vegetable juices (prepared from fresh, organic produce), dietary supplements (pepsin, potassium, niacin, an iodine solution called Lugol, Vitamin B12, potassium, thyroid hormone, an injectable crude liver extract, and pancreatic enzymes), and 3–4 coffee enemas daily. Salt, spices, and aluminum cookware or utensils are not allowed in food preparation. | A component of the diet that included the consumption of raw calf's liver has been eliminated secondary to illness. |
| Macrobiotic Diet[101] | Macrobiotic diets are based on whole grains and cereals, vegetables, seaweed, beans, fermented soy products, fruits, nuts, seeds, soup made from these ingredients and teas. Diets are individualized and based on the tumor types category of "yin" or "yang." The diet is a nutritional attempt to balance "yin" and "yang"—forces that the Chinese believed must be kept in harmony to achieve good health | Diet can be very labor intensive and low in protein if not planned properly |
| Gonzalez Diet[98] | Also called the Kelley-Gonzalez diet, patients with cancer are assigned to a metabolic type and a diet is designed for that type. Gonzalez felt that pancreatic enzymes could act like chemotherapy and kill cancer cells. The regimen includes pancreatic enzymes orally every 4 hours and at mealtime. Includes dietary supplements such as magnesium citrate, papaya plus, vitamins, minerals, trace elements, and animal glandular products. Coffee enemas are included daily. | Individuals are required to take 130–160 supplements daily. Risk of perforation and infection associated with coffee enemas.<br>A 5-year phase III clinical trial at Columbia University comparing gemcitabine and the Gonzalez therapy in patients with pancreatic cancer was closed early for poor accrual. |

anecdotal evidence. Much more study is needed before a nurse can accurately predict which self-care actions will be effective for a given patient. With the base of nursing research added to that of other disciplines, oncology nurses can positively influence the incidence and prevalence of nutritional deficiencies in cancer.

## REFERENCES

1. Warren S. The immediate causes of death in cancer. *Am J Med Sci.* 1932;184:610–615.
2. Schattner, M. & Shike, M. In Shils ME, Shike, M. Rose, RC, Caballero, B, Cousins RJ, Eds. *Modern Nutrition in Health and Disease* 10th Ed. Philadelphia, PA: Lippincott Williams&Williams; 2006, 1290–1313.

3. Bozzetti F. Screening the nutritional status in oncology: a preliminary report on 1,000 outpatients. *Support Care Cancer.* 2009;17:279–284.
4. Mosby T, Day S, Challinor J, Hernández A, García J, Velásquez S. Nutritional issues in pediatric oncology: an international collaboration between the Central American nurses cooperative group and U.S.-based dietary and nursing experts. *Pediatr Blood Cancer.* 2008;50: 1298–1300.
5. Caro MM, Laviano A, Pichard C. Nutritional interventions and quality of life in adult oncology patients. *Clin Nutr.* 2007;26:289–301.
6. Herman DR, Ganz PA, Petersen L, Greendale GA. Obesity and cardiovascular risk in younger breast cancer survivors: the Cancer and Menopause Study (CAMS). *Breast Cancer Res Treat.* 2005;93:13–23.
7. Anthony PS. Nutrition screening tools for hospitalized patients. *Nutr Clin Pract.* 2008;23:373–382.
8. Lacey K, Pritchett E. Nutrition care process and model: ADA adopts road map to quality care and outcomes management. *J Am Diet Assoc.* 2003;103:1061–1072.
9. McTiernan A, Rajan KB, Tworoger SS, et al. Adiposity and sex hormones in postmenopausal breast cancer survivors. *J Clin Oncol.* 2003; 21:1961–1966.
10. Harvie M, Hooper L, Howell AH. Central obesity and breast cancer risk: a systematic review. *Obes Rev.* 2003;4:157–173.
11. Harvie MN, Campbell IT, Baildam A, Howell A. Energy balance in early breast cancer patients receiving adjuvant chemotherapy. *Breast Cancer Res Treat.* 2004;83:201–210.
12. Campbell KL, Lane K, Martin AD, Gelmon KA, McKenzie DC. Resting energy expenditure and body mass changes in women during adjuvant chemotherapy for breast cancer. *Cancer Nurs.* 2007;30:95–100.
13. Borugian M, Sheps S, Kim-Sing C, et al. Waist to hip ratio and breast cancer mortality. *Am J Epidemiol.* 2003;158:963–968.
14. Tisdale MJ. Protein metabolism in cachexia. In: Mantovani G, Anker SD, Inui A, et al, eds. *Cachexia and Wasting: A Modern Approach.* Milan, Italy: Springer-Verlag Italia; 2006:185–190.
15. Sungurtekin H, Sungurtekin U, Balci C, Zencir M, Erdem E. The influence of nutritional status ion complications after major abdominal surgery. *J Am Coll Nutr.* 2004;23:227–232.
16. dos Santos Junqueira JC, Soares EC, Correa Filho HR, et al. Nutritional risk factors for postoperative complications in Brazilian elderly patients undergoing major elective surgery. *Nutrition.* 2003;19:321–326.
17. Feo CV, Romanini B, Sortini D, et al. Early oral feeding after colorectal resection: a randomized controlled study. *ANZ J Surg.* 2004;74:298–301.
18. Hurst JD, Gallagher AL. Energy, macronutrient, micronutrient and fluid requirements. In: Elliott L, Molseed LL, McCallum PD, eds. *The Clinical Guide to Oncology Nutrition.* Chicago, IL: American Dietetic Association; 2006:54–71.
19. Luthringer S. Nutritional implications of radiation therapy. In: Elliott L, Molseed LL, McCallum P, eds. *The Clinical Guide to Oncology Nutrition.* Chicago, IL: American Dietetic Association; 2006:88–93.
20. Wickham R. Nausea and vomiting. In: Yarbro CH, Frogge MH, Goodman M, eds. *Cancer Symptom Management.* 3rd ed. Sudbury, MA: Jones and Bartlett; 2004:187–214.
21. Cunningham RS, Rittenberg C. Chemotherapy-induced nausea & vomiting. *Clin J Oncol Nurs.* 2005;9:257–260.
22. Kurtin SE. Targeting the epidermal growth factor receptor in colorectal carcinoma. *Cancer Nurs.* 2007;30(suppl. 4S):1–9.
23. Khoukaz T. Administration of anti-EGFR therapy: a practical review. *Cancer Nurs.* 2006;22:20–27.
24. Thomas M. Cetuximab: adverse event profile and recommendations for toxicity management. *Clin J Oncol Nurs.* 2005;9:332–338.
25. Herbst RS, Arquette M, Shin DM, et al. Epidermal growth factor receptor antibody cetuximab and cisplatin for recurrent and refractory squamous cell carcinoma of the head and neck: a phase II, multicenter study. *J Clin Oncol.* 2005;23:1–10.
26. Veronese ML, O'Dwyer PJ. Monoclonal antibodies in the treatment of colorectal cancer. *Eur J Cancer.* 2004;10:1292–1301.
27. Bossola M, Pacelli F, Tortorelli A, Doglietto GB. Cancer cachexia: it's time for more clinical trials. *Ann Surg Oncol.* 2006;14:276–285.
28. Laviano A, Meguid MM, Fanelli FR. Anorexia. In: Montovani G, Anker SD, Inui A, et al, eds. *Cachexia and Wasting: A Modern Approach.* Milan, Italy: Springer-Verlag Italia; 2006:139–148.
29. Dahele M, Fearon KC. Research methodology: cancer cachexia syndrome. *Palliat Med.* 2004;18:409–417.
30. Ramos EJ, Suzuki S, Marks D, Inui A, Asakawa A, Meguid MM. Cancer anorexia-cachexia syndrome: cytokines and neuropeptides. *Curr Opin Clin Nutr Metab Care.* 2004;7:427–434.
31. Rubin H. Cancer cachexia: its correlations and causes. *Proc Natl Acad Sci USA.* 2003;100:661–671.
32. Laviano A, Rossi-Fanelli F. Pathogenesis of cancer anorexia: still doubts after all these years? *Nutrition.* 2003;19:67–68.
33. Goodwin PJ, Ennis M, Pritchard KI, et al. Diet and breast cancer: evidence that extremes in diet are associated with poor survival. *J Clin Oncol.* 2003;21:2500–2507.
34. Sherry VW. Taste alterations among patients with cancer. *Clin J Oncol Nurs.* 2002;6:73–77.
35. Hutton V, Baracos W, Wismer WV. Chemosensory dysfunction is a primary factor in the evolution of declining nutritional status and quality of life in patients with advanced cancer. *J Pain Symptom Manage.* 2007;33:156–165.
36. Davis MP, Walsh D, Lagman R, Yavuzsen T. Early satiety in cancer patients: a common and important but underrecognized symptom. *Support Care Cancer.* 2006;14:693–698.
37. Sarhill N, Christie R. Early satiety in advanced cancer: a common unrecognized symptom (letter)? *Am J Hosp Palliat Care.* 2002; 19:305.
38. Walsh D, Donnelly S, Rybicki L. The symptoms of advanced cancer: relationship to age, gender, and performance status in 1000 patients. *Support Care Cancer.* 2000;8:175–179.
39. Argiles JM, Lopez-Soriano FJ, Busquets S. Novel approaches to the treatment of cachexia. *Drug Discov Today.* 2008;13:73–78.
40. Maccio A, Madeddu C, Mantovanni G. Glucose metabolism. In: Mantovani G, Anker SD, Inui A, et al, eds. *Cachexia and Wasting: A Modern Approach.* Milan, Italy: Springer-Verlag Italia; 2006:477–482.
41. Muscaritoli M, Bossola M, Doglietto GB, Fanelli FR. The ubiquitin/proteasome system in cancer cachexia. In: Mantovani G, Anker SD, Inui A, et al, eds. *Cachexia and Wasting: A Modern Approach.* Milan, Italy: Springer-Verlag Italia; 2006:503–508.
42. Mantovani G, Madeddu C. Proinflammatory cytokines: their role in multifactorial cancer cachexia. In: Mantovani G, Anker SD, Inui A, et al, eds. *Cachexia and Wasting: A Modern Approach.* Milan, Italy: Springer-Verlag Italia; 2006:477–482.
43. Tan BH, Fearon KC. Cachexia: prevalence and impact in medicine. *Curr Opin Clin Nutr Metab Care.* 2008;11:400–407.
44. Tan BH, Deans DA, Skipworth RJ, Ross JA, Fearon KC. Biomarkers for cancer cachexia: is there also a genetic component to cachexia? *Support Care Cancer.* 2007;16:229–234.
45. Bosaeus I. Nutritional support in multimodal therapy for cancer cachexia. *Support Care Cancer.* 2008;16:447–451.
46. Morley JE, Thomas DR, Wilson MM. Cachexia: pathophysiology and clinical relevance. *Am J Clin Nutr.* 2006;83:735–743.
47. Cooley ME, Short TH, Moriarty HJ. Symptom prevalence, distress, and change over time in adults receiving treatment for lung cancer. *Psychooncology.* 2003;12:694–708.
48. Bernhardson BM, Tishelman C, Rutqvist LE. Olfactory changes among patients receiving chemotherapy. *Eur J Oncol Nurs.* 2009;13:9–15.
49. Pia de la Maza M, Agudelo GM, Yudin T, et al. Long-term nutritional and digestive consequences of pelvic radiation. *J Am Coll Nutr.* 2004;23:102–107.
50. Duguet A, Bachmann P, Lallemand Y, Blanc-Vincent MP. Summary report of the standards, options, and recommendations for malnutrition

and nutritional assessment in patients with cancer (1999). *Br J Cancer.* 2003;89(suppl 1):592–597.
51. Unsal D, Mentes B, Akmansu M, Uner A, Oguz M, Pak Y. Evaluation of nutritional status in cancer patients receiving chemotherapy. *Am J Clin Oncol.* 2006;29:183–188.
52. van Bokhorst-de van der Schueren MA. Nutritional support strategies for malnourished cancer patients. *Eur J Oncol Nurs.* 2005;9:S74-S83.
53. Joint Commission on Accreditation of Healthcare Organizations (JCAHO). *Accreditation Program: Ambulatory Health Care: Provision of Care, Treatment, and Services.* Oakbrook Terrace, IL: JCAHO. http://www.jointcommission.org/AccreditationPrograms/Hospitals/Standards/09_FAQs/PC/Nutritional_+Functional_Pain_+Assessments.htm. Accessed February 12, 2010.
54. Huhman M, August DA. American Society for Parenteral Enteral Nutrition (ASPEN): guidelines for the use of parenteral and enteral nutrition in adult and pediatric patients. *J Parenteral Enteral Nutr.* (in press).
55. Isenring E, Bauer J, Capra S. The scored patient-generated subjective global assessment (PG-SGA) and its association with quality of life in ambulatory patients receiving radiotherapy. *Eur J Clin Nutr.* 2003;57:305–309.
56. McCallum PD. Nutrition screening and assessment in oncology. In: Elliott L, Molseed LL, McCallum P, eds. *The Clinical Guide to Oncology Nutrition.* Chicago, IL: American Dietetic Association; 2006:44–53.
57. Hammond K. Dietary and clinical assessment. In: Mahan L, Escott-Stump S, eds. *Krause's Food Nutrition and Diet Therapy.* 11th ed. Philadelphia, PA: W.B. Saunders; 2003:407–435.
58. Bauer J, Capra S, Davies PS. Estimation of total body water from foot-to-foot bioelectrical impedance analysis in patients with cancer-related cachexia-agreement between three prediction methods and deuterium oxide dilution. *J Hum Nutr.* 2005;19:433–446.
59. Buchholz AC, Bartok C, Schoeller DA. The validity of bioelectrical impedance models in clinical populations. *Nutr Clin Pract.* 2004;19: 433–446.
60. Toso S, Piccoli A, Gusella M, et al. Bioimpedance vector pattern in cancer patients without disease versus locally advanced or disseminated disease. *Nutr Cancer.* 2003;19:510–514.
61. Robinett-Weiss N, Hixson ML, Keir B, Sieberg J. The metropolitan height-weight tables: perspectives for use. *J Am Diet Assoc.* 1984;84:1480–1481.
62. Hamwi G. Changing dietary concepts. In: Danowski T, ed. *Diabetes Mellitus: Diagnosis and Treatment.* vol 1. New York: American Diabetes Association; 1964:73–78.
63. National Institutes of Health. *Clinical Guidelines on the Identification, Evaluation, and Treatment of Overweight and Obesity in Adults: The Evidence Report.* Bethesda, MD: National Institutes of Health. http://www.nhlbi.nih.gov/guidelines/obesity/ob_gdlns.htm. Accessed November 1, 2009.
64. Blackburn G, Bistrian B. Nutritional and metabolic assessment of the hospitalized patient. *J Parenteral Enteral Nutr.* 1977;1:11–22.
65. World Health Organization. *Energy and Protein Requirements. Report of a Joint FAO/WHO/UN Expert Consultation.* Geneva, Switzerland: Author; 1985.
66. Food and Nutrition Board Institute of Medicine. Energy. In: Institute of Medicine, ed. *Dietary Reference Intakes for Energy, Carbohydrates, Fiber, Fat, Protein, and Amino Acids.* Washington, DC: National Academy Press; 2002:1–79.
67. Edel J, Murrey M, Schurer W, et al. Nutrition assessment of adults. In: Rychlec 6th ed. *Manual of clinical Dietetics,* Chicago, IL. American Dietetic Association, 2000:3–38
68. Cunningham RS. The anorexia-cachexia syndrome. In: Yarbro CH, Frogge MH, Goodman M, eds. *Cancer Symptom Management.* 3rd ed. Sudbury, MA: Jones and Bartlett; 2003:137–167.
69. Davies M. Nutritional screening and assessment in cancer-associated malnutrition. *Eur J Oncol Nurs.* 2005;9:564–573.
70. Toliusiene J, Lesauskaite V. The nutritional status of older men with advanced prostate cancer and factor affecting it. *Support Care Cancer.* 2004;12:716–719.
71. Robinson SM, Jameson KA, Batelaan SF, et al. Diet and its relationship with grip strength in community-dwelling older men and women: the Hertfordshire Cohort Study. *J Am Geriatr Soc.* 2008;56:84–90.
72. Norman K, Kirchner H, Freudenreich M, Ockenga J, Lochs H, Pirlich M. Three month intervention with protein and energy rich supplements improve muscle function and quality of life in malnourished patients with non-neoplastic gastrointestinal disease—a randomised controlled trial. *Clin Nutr.* 2007;27:48–56.
73. Naliboff BD. Choosing outcome variables: global assessment and diaries. *Gastroenterology.* 2004;126(suppl 1):S129-S134.
74. Common Terminology Criteria for Adverse Events (CTCAE) version 3.0. http://ctep.cancer.gov/protocolDevelopment/electronic_applications/docs/ctcaev3.pdf. Accessed December 23, 2009.
75. Mirhosseini N, Fainsinger RL, Baracos V. Parenteral nutrition in advance cancer: indications and clinical practice guidelines. *J Palliat Care Med.* 2005;10:914–918.
76. Macfie J. European round table: the use of immunonutrients in the critically ill. *Clin Nutr.* 2004;23:1426–1429.
77. Sax HC. Immunonutrition and uppergastrointestinal surgery: what really matters. *Nutr Clin Pract.* 2005;20:540–543.
78. Savarese DM, Savy G, Vahdat L, et al. Prevention of chemotherapy and radiation toxicity with glutamine. *Cancer Treat Rev.* 2003;29: 501–513.
79. Rock CL, Flatt SW, Thomson CA, et al. Effects of high-fiber, low-fat diet intervention on serum concentrations of reproductive steroid hormones in women with a history of breast cancer. *J Clin Oncol.* 2004;22: 2379–2387.
80. Rock CL. Diet and breast cancer: can dietary factors influence survival? *J Mammary Gland Biol Neoplasia.* 2003;8:119–132.
81. Adams LA, Caruso RA, Shepard NE, Norling MJ, Blair H, Cunningham RS. Putting evidence into practice: evidence-based interventions to prevent and manage anorexia. *Clin J Oncol Nurs.* 2009;13:95–102.
82. Strasser F. The silent symptom early satiety: a forerunner of distinct phenotypes of anorexia/cachexia syndromes. *Support Care Cancer.* 2006;14:689–692.
83. Bertereteche MV, Dalix AM, Cesar d'Ornono AM, Bellisle F, Khayat D, Faurion A. Decreased taste sensitivity in cancer patients under chemotherapy. *Support Care Cancer.* 2004;12:571–576.
84. Rehwaldt, M. Wickham, R. Purl, S. et al. Self-care strategies to cope with taste changes after chemotherapy. *Oncol Nurs Forum.* 2009; 36(2): E47-E56.
85. Epstein JB, Schubert MM. Managing pain in mucositis. *Semin Oncol Nurs.* 2004;20:30–37.
86. Wilson MM, Philpot C, Morley JE. Anorexia and aging in long term care: is dronabinol an effective appetite stimulant? *J Nutr Health Aging.* 2007;11:195–198.
87. Khan ZH, Simpson EJ, Cole AT, et al. Oesophageal cancer and cachexia: the effect of short-term treatment with thalidomide on weight loss and lean body mass. *Aliment Pharmacol Ther.* 2003;17:677–682.
88. Von Roenn J, Tchekmedyian S, Hoffman R, et al. Safety of oxandrolone in cancer-related weight loss [abstract]. *Proc Am Soc Clin Oncol.* 2003;22:749.
89. Mulligan K, Schambelan M. Anabolic treatment with GH, IGF-1, or anabolic steroids in patients with HIV-associated wasting. *Int J Cardiol.* 2002;85:151–159.
90. Luthringer S. Cancer (medical) medical nutrition therapy protocol. In: Gilbreath J, Inman-Felton AE, Johnson EQ, Robinson G, Smith KG, eds. *Medical Nutrition Therapy Across the Continuum of Care.* 2nd ed. Chicago, IL: American Dietetic Association; 1998:1–15.
91. National Cancer Institute. Nutrition in cancer care. http://www.cancer.gov/cancertopics/pdq/supportivecare/nutrition/healthprofessional/allpages Accessed February 12, 2010.

92. Wolfe RR. The underappreciated role of muscle in health and disease. *Am J Clin Nutr.* 2006;84:475–482.
93. Ottery F, Kasenic SR, Cunningham RS. Multimodality approaches to optimize survivorship outcomes: body composition, exercise, and nutrition. *Issues in Nutrition and Cancer: Update 2004.* 2004;19:11–14.
94. Fairey AS, Courneya KS, Field CJ, et al. Effects of exercise training on fasting insulin, insulin resistance, insulin-like growth factors, and insulin-like growth factor binding proteins in postmenopausal breast cancer survivors: a randomized controlled trial. *Cancer Epidemiol Biomarkers Prev.* 2003;12:721–727.
95. Navo MA, Phan J, Vaughan C, et al. An assessment of the utilization of complementary and alternative medication in women with gynecologic or breast malignancies. *J Clin Oncol.* 2004;22:671–677.
96. Henderson JW, Donatelle RJ. Complementary and alternative medicine use by women after completion of allopathic treatment for breast cancer. *Altern Ther Health Med.* 2004;10:52–57.
97. NCI. Cancer Facts: Antineoplastons. http://www.cancer.gov/cancertopics/pdf/cam/antineoplastons/Healthprofessional. Accessed February 12, 2010.
98. Vickers A. Alternative cancer cures: "unproven" or "disproven"? *CA: Cancer J Clin.* 2004;54:110–118.
99. NCI. Cancell/Cantron/Protocel (PDQ®) http://www.cancer.gov/cancertopics/pdq/cam/cancell/HealthProfessional/page2. Accessed February 12, 2010.
100. NCI. Gerson Therapy. http://www.cancer.gov/cancertopics/pdf/cam/gerson/Healthprofessional. Accessed February 12, 2010.
101. Agency BC. Macrobiotic Diets/ Zen Macrobiotics. http://www.bccancer.bc.ca/PPI/UnconventionalTherapies/MacrobioticDietsZenMacrobiotics.htm. Accessed February 12, 2010.

CHAPTER 34

Kelley D. Mayden, MSN, FNP, AOCNP®

# Paraneoplastic Syndromes

## INTRODUCTION

Paraneoplastic syndromes (PNSs) have been reported as far back as the 18th century.[1] They are a rare, heterogeneous group of disorders that are a result of cancer or its metastases. Although a direct result of malignancy, signs and symptoms related to PNSs occur at sites distant from the primary tumor or its metastases.[2] Virtually any body system may be affected and the manifestations of this syndrome may be seen in the endocrine, neuromuscular, renal, hematologic, cardiovascular, cutaneous, musculoskeletal, gastrointestinal, or rheumatologic systems. Early recognition of PNS is of paramount importance, as they often present well in advance of a primary malignancy and may allow for earlier cancer detection.

The true etiology of PNS is yet to be fully understood. One or more of the following mechanisms are thought to be involved with PNS development: (1) tumor production of bioactive substances such as growth hormones, cytokines, and/or growth factors, (2) total body depletion of normal substances resulting in disturbance of metabolic or steroid metabolism, or (3) host autoimmune response triggered by tumor-produced antibodies.[2,3] The exact incidence of PNS is unknown but is estimated to occur in 10% to 20% of all patients with cancer. Many consider tumor fever, anemia of malignancy (AOM), and cancer-related anorexia-cachexia as PNS. Inclusion of these events would mean that, at some point, almost every patient with cancer experiences at least one of the PNSs.

Although observed with all types of histological lung cancer, small cell lung cancer (SCLC) is most often associated with PNSs, particularly neurological syndromes with a 3% to 5% observance rate.[4] There is no documented predilection to age, race, or sex. Children may also experience PNS prior to malignancy. The most common childhood malignancies associated with any syndrome are neuroblastoma and Wilms' tumor. Several case reports suggest paraneoplastic pemphigus as a precursor to the diagnosis of Castleman's disease in children.[5,6]

Despite their infrequent occurrences, an awareness of the presentation and manifestation of PNSs is essential as it may lead to earlier cancer detection. Over the past 20 years, research has led to the discovery of an association between many PNSs and antineuronal antibodies (ANAs) resulting in earlier recognition and more informed treatment.[7] Some PNSs produce proteins that can be used as tumor markers that help monitor patients prior to and after therapy. The effects of PNSs can be devastating and debilitating. In general, treatment is aimed at the underlying malignancy, but many PNSs will not respond to treatment.[2]

## NEUROLOGICAL PARANEOPLASTIC SYNDROMES

### SCOPE OF THE PROBLEM

Paraneoplastic neurological disorders (PNDs) consist of a group of neurological syndromes associated with malignancy but are unrelated to direct tumor invasion, metastases, side effects of therapy, coagulopathy, infection, or metabolic disruptions.[8] PNDs are rare and occur in less than 1% of patients with cancer.[9] Lambert-Eaton myasthenic syndrome (LEMS) affects approximately 3% of patients with SCLC. Myasthenia gravis (MG) is seen in 15% of patients with thymoma and demyelinating peripheral neuropathy and is present in 3% to 10% of B-cell or plasma-cell neoplasms. In other cancers, such as breast and ovarian, the incidence of PNDs is below 1%.[10,11]

These disorders can be subacute or acute in nature, tend to have a debilitating course, and are usually triggered in the early stages of cancer when tumors are undetectable.[11] PNDs can attack any part of the central or peripheral nervous system from the cerebral cortex to the retina.[12] Some PNDs affect only a single cell type or area whereas others involve multiple levels of the nervous system. The true pathogenesis of PNDs remains unknown. It is generally believed that PNDs are immune-mediated and are the end result of an antigen–antibody interaction. In other words, tumors, or their metastases, ectopically express proteins normally found in the nervous system. The immune system then mounts an attack response to the tumor-generated antigens, thus forming an antigen–antibody complex. Unfortunately, cross-reactivity occurs within the nervous system leading to discrete or multifocal areas of degeneration resulting in diverse symptoms and deficits. It is important to note that not all PNDs are a result of this type of humoral immune response. Some PNDs are mediated by a T-cell immune response to target antigens of accompanying antibodies.[12,13] At autopsy, brain tissue of patients with PNDs revealed large amounts of T lymphocytes.[14]

The recognition of the immune system's role in the development of PNDs has become important diagnostically. Many syndromes are associated with unique ANAs found in the serum and cerebrospinal fluid (CSF) of patients and are used as markers in identifying specific syndromes or cancers (see Table 34-1). In as many as 60% of patients with PNDs, highly specific ANAs are isolated and two-thirds of patients may experience symptoms up to 4 years before tumor diagnosis.[15] Antibodies may not be pathonomic or always correlate with a particular syndrome.[16] Some PNDs show CSF evidence of inflammation, suggesting an immune response, but have no known specific ANAs.[12] Diagnosis of PNDs can occur independently of ANAs and their presence does not always signal the presence of a disorder.[14]

Traditionally, PNDs have been categorized according to anatomic location, either central nervous system or peripheral nervous system. However, more recently, with the association between antibodies and PNDs, many neurologists and oncologists advocate a new classification system using the categories of definite and possible.[8] Paraneoplastic cerebellar degeneration (PCD), paraneoplastic limbic encephalitis (PLE), paraneoplastic opsoclonus-myoclonus (POM), paraneoplastic sensory neuronopathy (PSN), LEMS, and

**TABLE 34-1**

**Well-Characterized Antibodies and Paraneoplastic Syndromes**

| Antibodies | Syndrome |
|---|---|
| Anti-Hu | PLE, POM, PSN |
| Anti-MA2 | PLE, POM |
| Anti-CRMP5/CV2 | PLE, POM, PSN |
| VGPC | PLE |
| VGCC | LEMS, PCD |
| Anti-Zic | POM, PCD |
| Anti-Yo | POM, PCD |
| Anti-Ri | POM, PCD |
| Anti-Tr | PCD |
| Anti-AchR | MG |

*Abbreviations*: LEMS, Lambert-Eaton myasthenic syndrome; MG, myasthenia gravis; PCD, paraneoplastic cerebellar degeneration; PLE, paraneoplastic limbic encephalitis; POM, paraneoplastic opsoclonus-myoclonus; PSN, paraneoplastic sensory neuronopathy; VGCC, voltage-gated calcium channel; VGPC, voltage-gated potassium channel.
*Source*: Data from Bataller and Dalmau.[12]

MG are the most recognized PNDs and are discussed in greater detail in the following sections.

## Definitions

*Paraneoplastic cerebellar degeneration* (PCD) is characterized by subacute pancerebellar dysfunction manifested as ataxia, dysarthria, and/or nystagmus.[17] Other symptoms may include nausea, diplopia, or lightheadedness. PCD is generally symmetric and can evolve rapidly or over a period several days to weeks. The hallmark of PCD is irreversible loss of Purkinje cells and cerebellar atrophy. It often precedes the diagnosis of cancer and is associated with SCLC, ovarian cancer, breast cancer, and Hodgkin's lymphoma.[18]

*Paraneoplastic limbic encephalitis* (PLE) is defined by mental status changes such as confusion, delirium, dementia, hallucinations, or short-term memory loss. Patients may be very anxious or depressed. In its most severe form, seizures can occur. The onset may be insidious or acute and can easily be mistaken for viral syndromes such as herpes simplex encephalitis.[12]

*Paraneoplastic opsoclonus-myoclonus* (POM) is characterized by abnormal ocular motility and typically demonstrates a severe clinical course. Chaotic, arrhythmic, multidirectional eye movements occur in all fields of gaze without a movement interval.[19] These symptoms are often accompanied by myoclonus and truncal ataxia.[12]

*Paraneoplastic sensory neuronopathy* (PSN) involves the dorsal root ganglia. Sensory deficits can be asymmetric and nonlength dependent and usually evolve over weeks to months.[17] Patients with PSN experience pain, numbness, sensory ataxia, and decreased or absent reflexes. Other sensory deficits can affect limbs, trunk, and cranial nerves with resultant hearing loss. Although PSN can occur in isolation, it often accompanies paraneoplastic encephalomyelitis, a PNS involving the central nervous system, including the brain stem, cerebellum, spinal cord, and limbic system.[12]

*Lambert-Eaton myasthenic syndrome* (LEMS) is a disorder of the neuromuscular junction, is autoimmune in nature, and is a peripheral antibody-mediated defect in neuromuscular transmission.[20] Consequently, there is impaired acetylcholine release from the presynaptic motor terminal.[11] Antibodies against voltage-gated calcium channels (VGCCs) are usually present.[17] Symptoms include fatigue, myalgias, muscle stiffness, lower extremity weakness, gradual onset of hip girdle weakness, and upper extremity weakness. The weakness tends to follow a caudocranial pattern with decreased reflexes. Sweating, dry mouth, and constipation are frequently seen, as is erectile dysfunction in male patients.[21]

*Myasthenia gravis* (MG) results from the development of autoimmune antibodies to the acetylcholine receptor on postsynaptic neuromuscular junctions, resulting in abnormal neuronal transmission. Blurred vision, diplopia, fatigue, dysphagia, dysarthria, muscular weakness, and respiratory failure are the clinical features of the disease.[11] This paraneoplastic disorder is most often associated with thymoma, a rare, indolent tumor with malignant potential.[22]

## Incidence

Paraneoplastic cerebellar degeneration (PCD) is rare and occurs in approximately 2 out of every 1000 patients with cancer. There are roughly 300 cases reported in the literature.[17] PCD has been associated with most tumor types but is more commonly found in lung, breast, and gynecological cancers as well as lymphoma.[19] It is present more frequently in women.[23]

Paraneoplastic limbic encephalitis (PLE) is rare and the exact incidence is unknown. It occurs alone but more often in association with cerebellar symptoms or brain dysfunction. Fifty percent of patients with PLE have SCLC and 20% have testicular cancer.[8] Typically, PLE precedes a cancer diagnosis.

Paraneoplastic opsoclonus-myoclonus (POM) has been described in adult patients and is most commonly found in SCLC. Case reports also exist for breast, bladder, thymus, thyroid, and gynecological cancers.[24] In children, most cases of POM accompany the diagnosis of neuroblastoma.[12] Paraneoplastic sensory neuronopathy (PSN) can be one of the earliest clues to an underlying lung malignancy. It presents in over 80% of patients diagnosed with SCLC. PSN may develop 42 months prior to diagnosis.[11]

Lambert-Eaton myasthenic syndrome (LEMS) is the most common of the PNDs. It is most frequent in SCLC with an incidence of 3%. It may be discernible 2 years before diagnosis.[23] In a few cases, it has been seen in patients with carcinoid or large-cell neuroendrocrine carcinoma.[11]

Myasthenia gravis (MG) is present in approximately 50% of cases of thymoma and the majority of patients with MG have some thymic abnormality. At least 15% of patients with MG have a thymoma that is unrecognized when MG is diagnosed.[17] It was once thought that MG associated with thymoma was of negative prognostic significance, but recent reports contradict this association.[11]

### Etiology and risk factors

The etiology of PNDs is not fully understood. Purported causes have included toxic substances, bacteria, viruses, and metabolic changes. It is thought that the majority of PNDs are immune-mediated. With documented evidence of ANAs in the serum of patients with PNDs, an autoimmune pathogenesis is plausible.[17] Both humoral and cell-mediated immunity play a role in the development of PNDs and cellular autoimmunity serves as a primary mediator of neuronal damage in PNDs.[16,25] Clearly, lung cancers, especially SCLC, carry the greatest risk of PND development, either prior to or in conjunction with the diagnosis of cancer.

## PATHOPHYSIOLOGY

As tumors mature, they ectopically express neuronal proteins referred to as onconeural antigens, or ANA. Similar antigens are normally expressed in the brain and testes making the tumor antigens appear similar to neural antigens. Once the immune system recognizes the tumor antigens as foreign, it mounts an aggressive assault as a means of tumor control. Consequently, this aids in the control of cancer growth and it is believed, in some cases, to obliterate the disease. Symptoms of PNDs develop once cytotoxic T cells and antibodies cross the blood–brain barrier and react with onconeural antigens.[25] In many cases, this immune response produces specific ANAs that are used to help diagnose some PNDs ( see Table 34-1).[12]

Paraneoplastic cerebellar degeneration (PCD) is related to a near complete or complete loss of Purkinje cells and is immune-mediated. With PCD, thinning of the molecular layer within the cerebral cortex is observed.[26] Inflammatory changes occur in the surrounding white matter but are less pronounced in the Purkinje layer.[2] Like PCD, PLE is immune in nature. Pathology results from alterations in limbic and basal ganglia structures including neuronal cell loss, perivascular lymphocytic infiltration, and reactive microglial proliferation.[26]

The pathophysiology of POM is poorly understood. Disinhibition of the fastigial nucleus of the cerebellum has been suggested. Antibodies against postsynaptic antigens are the most compelling finding associated with POM.[27] A hallmark of PSN is infiltration by lymphocytes and macrophages in the dorsal root ganglia. In some instances, no sensory neurons remain. Axonal degeneration can be seen in the dorsal root ganglia and posterior spinal cord. Motor neurons and nerve roots are often unaffected with PSN.[17]

Classic findings in LEMS support a cause of presynaptic neuromuscular dysfunction in which a decrease in small compound muscle action potentials are noted with low frequency stimulation, but increase with high frequency stimulation. Antibodies against VGCCs are usually present.[17,26] MG is an immune process with symptoms resulting when antibodies are formed against nicotinic acetylcholine receptors.

## CLINICAL MANIFESTATIONS

Early on, PCD may be heralded by nausea, vomiting, or dizziness. An unsteady gait usually follows and may be accompanied by diplopia, dysphagia, vertigo, or nystagmus. Patients can become disabled, immobile, and severely dysarthric within a few weeks of diagnosis. Although asymmetry has been observed, PCD is usually symmetrical.[26] Other neurological symptoms such as sensorineural hearing loss or peripheral neuropathy may occur. Once symptoms peak in severity, they tend to stabilize. Despite treatment, the neurological symptoms are often permanent.

Paraneoplastic limbic encephalitis presents with anxiety, depression, irritability, amnesia, and possibly seizures. Recent memory is impaired and progression to dementia can be observed. With treatment of the underlying tumor, improvement can occur.[28] Patients who have antibodies against voltage-gated potassium channel (VGPC) antibodies respond better to immunotherapy.[12]

In POM, eye movements are involuntary, irregular, chaotic, and alternating horizontally, vertically, and around the line of sight. This is often accompanied by involuntary limb jerking, cerebellar ataxia, tremor, or encephalopathy.[29]

Patients with PSN experience a pure sensory loss involving all sensory modalities, usually in the upper and lower extremities, but rarely in the face.[17] Initial complaints usually involve paresthesia followed by pain, extremity ataxia, and slow, involuntary, wormlike movements.[8]

Fatigue, muscle pain, lower extremity weakness, and indistinct paresthesias are early findings in LEMS. Subjective reports of dry eyes and mouth, impotence, dizziness, or sweating may be elicited. MG features extremity weakness and fatigue and is also characterized by ptosis, diplopia, dysarthria, and respiratory compromise.[11]

## ASSESSMENT

### Diagnostic studies

The appearance of neurological symptoms in patients with and without cancer warrants an immediate and thorough investigation. PNDs should always be part of the differential diagnosis until proven otherwise. It is not uncommon to see a diagnostic delay due to the rarity of PNDs. A missed diagnosis is common because many disorders share common features.[12] Two presenting features shared by most PNDs are rapid onset and inflammation in the CSF, including lymphocytosis, pleocytosis, elevated protein, increased IgG index, and oligoclonal bands.[30] Therefore, CSF studies are needed not only to diagnosis PNDs, but also to rule out other causes such as infection or meningitis.

Although the results of neuroimaging studies are usually normal in early PNDs, brain computed tomography (CT) scans and magnetic resonance imaging (MRIs) are useful to show that there is no evidence of stroke, hemorrhage, or metastatic cancer. In later stages, hypothalamic or basal ganglia changes are seen and inflammatory infiltrates can be demonstrated as gadolinium-enhancing abnormalities. A very late finding related to PND is cerebellar atrophy. CT of the chest can be useful if a primary lung cancer is suspected and, in women with PNDs, mammogram and pelvic ultrasound may be needed as breast and gynecological cancers are associated with PNDs. Because of its high negative predictive value and sensitivity, positron emission tomography (PET) is becoming the test of choice for detection of occult malignancy.[31]

If a PND is suspected, the CSF and serum of patients should be examined for the presence of ANAs. (See Table 34-1) These can be present in the serum of patients with cancer that do not have PNDs, but the titers are usually lower than those with PNDs. It is important to note that the discovery of any ANA in a patient with neurological symptoms is highly predictive of underlying malignancy.[12]

Antibodies commonly found in PCD include anti-Yo, anti-Ri, anti-Tr, anti-Zic, and most notably VGCC antibodies. Up to 40% of patients with PCD do not harbor antibodies. Since approximately 40% of patients with PLE are seronegative, the remaining 60% are positive for anti-Hu, anti-MA2, anti-CRMP5/CV2, and less often VGPC antibodies. With POM, the majority of patients do not harbor ANAs. A minority will have anti-Hu, anti-Ri, anti-CRMP5/CV2, anti-Zic, anti-Yo, and anti-MA2. The presence of anti-Ri antibodies should prompt investigation for breast, lung, or gynecological cancer. No serum antibodies are detectable in 18% of patients with PSN. However, when present, they include anti-Hu and anti-CRMP5/CV2 antibodies.[12] LEMS is confirmed by the presence of P/Q type VGCC antibodies. Anti-AChR is a paraneoplastic marker for MG.[17]

Electrophysiological testing of the peripheral nervous system can be helpful in PNDs such as LEMS and MG. Repeated nerve stimulation will cause an increase in muscle action potential, resulting in a temporary increase in muscle strength in LEMS. On the contrary, patients with MG will experience a progressive decrease in muscle response. In some cases, muscle biopsy can help establish nonneoplastic syndromes.

## THERAPEUTIC APPROACHES AND NURSING CARE

The primary nursing intervention for patients with PNDs includes maintaining and supporting maximal neurological function. Frequent assessment of vital signs and neurological status is imperative and prompt reporting of new signs and symptoms, as well as minute changes, can prove to be life-saving actions. Patients and families often require significant support, and a multidisciplinary approach is best, including psychiatric and rehabilitative services.

Treatment of the underlying malignancy is the mainstay of therapy for PNDs. Patients treated early in their disease state tend to stabilize and respond most positively. Overall, despite an immune etiology, PNDs are resistant to immunomodulatory treatment.[26] However, there is evidence to suggest that, in certain cases, immune therapy is appropriate. It was once theorized that immunosuppression would hasten tumor growth, but there continues to be a lack of evidence to support such a theory.[12]

In the early stages, PLE and POM do respond to corticosteroids. LEMS has also demonstrated a response to steroids, plasma exchange, and immune globulin.[26] Drugs that promote acetylcholine release from the nerve terminal, such as 3,4-diaminopyridine and guanidine, often are used in LEMS and may result in alleviated symptoms with minimal side effects.[2] In those patients that present with MG and thymoma, surgical resection of tumor often results in a significant improvement or resolution of symptoms.[22]

# ENDOCRINE PARANEOPLASTIC SYNDROMES

## SCOPE OF THE PROBLEM

Endocrine paraneoplastic syndromes (EPSs) are a direct result of ectopic hormone release (see Table 34-2). These hormones are the end products of various cytokines, proteins, hormone precursors, and growth factors inappropriately produced by tumors; lung cancers are a frequent culprit. Many of these hormones have autocrine stimulatory effects. While the molecular mechanisms of EPSs are not clear, they present a wide array of signs and symptoms. Treatment of the underlying malignancy usually results in

**TABLE 34-2**

**Endocrine Paraneoplastic Syndromes**

| Syndrome | Hormone | Associated Malignancy | Clinical Presentation | Comments |
|---|---|---|---|---|
| HHM | PTHrP | Lung<br>Renal<br>Breast<br>Ovarian<br>Lymph system<br>Multiple myeloma<br>Head and neck | Confusion<br>Weakness<br>Lethargy<br>Apathy<br>Nausea<br>Vomiting<br>Constipation<br>Anorexia<br>Polyuria<br>Polydyspia | Symptom severity correlates with degree and rate of onset |
| EAS | ACTH | SCLC (6%)<br>Carcinoid<br>Pancreas<br>Thymus<br>Pheochromocytoma | Hypokalemia<br>Muscle weakness/ atrophy<br>Weight loss<br>Hyponatremia<br>Edema<br>Fatigue<br>Glucose disturbance<br>Buffalo hump<br>Purple striae | |
| SIADH secretion | Nonpituitary arginine vasopressin (AVP) | SCLC (80%)<br>Head and neck<br>Brain<br>Pancreas<br>Prostate<br>Lymph system<br>Duodenum | Water intoxication<br>Excess water retention<br>Dilutional hyponatremia | |

*Abbreviations*: ACTH, adrenocorticotropic hormone; EAS, ectopic adrenocorticotrophic syndrome; HHM, humoral hypercalcemia of malignancy; PTHrP, parathyroid hormone–related protein; SCLC, small cell lung cancer; SIADH, syndrome of inappropriate antidiuretic hormone.

resolution of the symptoms and syndromes.[2] EPSs are well defined, with descriptions dating back to the early 1900s. The most common and best understood EPSs are paraneoplastic ectopic adrenocorticotrophic syndrome (EAS), syndrome of inappropriate antidiuretic hormone (SIADH), and humoral hypercalcemia of malignancy (HHM).

## Definitions

*Ectopic adrenocorticotrophic syndrome* (EAS) causes an increased production of ectopic adrenocorticotrophic hormone (ACTH) that produces signs and symptoms typically associated with Cushing's syndrome (CS), which occurs in the presence of excess ACTH production. EAS occurs in the absence of pituitary neoplasm or hyperplasia.[23] *Syndrome of inappropriate antidiuretic hormone* (SIADH) is a form of hyponatremia characterized by an excess of water in relation to sodium in the extracellular fluid.[32] With SIADH, there is a resultant increase in urine osmolality.[33] *Humoral hypercalcemia of malignancy* (HHM) results from ectopic secretion of parathyroid hormone–related protein (PTHrP) by malignant cells. Normally, it is produced in cells such as the skin, brain, kidney, and parathyroid. In HHM, calcium levels exceed the upper level of normal, a value of around 11 mg/dL by most standard laboratory analyses.

## Incidence

Ectopic adrenocorticotrophic syndrome (EAS) accounts for 10% to 20% of all cases of CS. The presence of EAS predicts a poorer prognosis. The majority of cases are associated with neuroendrocrine tumors such as SCLC, carcinoid tumors, thymic tumors, islet cell tumors, and pheochromocytoma.[34] Fifty percent of cases occur in patients diagnosed with SCLC but only about 2% to 10% of these patients are clinically diagnosed with a significant form of the disease.[23]

Syndrome of inappropriate antidiuretic hormone is seen with many types of malignancy such as head and neck cancer but is most commonly associated with lung cancer, and most notably SCLC. Circulating levels of ADH are measured in up to 75% of patients with SCLC but only 7% to 11% of these patients develop clinically significant SIADH.[23] In the hospital setting, the incidence of SIADH may be as high as 35%.[33]

Hypercalcemia is reported to be present in up to 30% of patients with cancer at some time during the course of their illness.[35] In those with solid tumors and hypercalcemia, 80% have an increase in serum concentrations of PTHrP.[36] The incidence of HHM is much less. For example, at the time of diagnosis, less than 1% of patients with lung cancer have incidences of HHM.[23] Common tumor types associated with hypercalcemia and malignancy include lung, renal, breast, ovarian, lymphoma, multiple myeloma, and squamous cell cancer of the head and neck.[19]

### Etiology and risk factors

Cancer is the most common etiology of all EPSs. Abnormal hormone secretions and metabolic disturbances are common to all. EAS results from the abnormal production of ACTH or ACTH-like substances that lead to adrenal hyperplasia and hypercortisolism.[2] The prognosis for patients with this condition is poor due to the fact that ACTH may function as a growth factor for neoplastic cells and excessive cortisol levels suppress immune function, thus leading to an increased risk of infection, especially infections of a fungal nature.[37] The median survival time for SCLC patients with EAS is 3 to 7 months.[38] Patients with SCLC, islet cell tumors, and carcinoid tumors have the greatest risk of developing EAS.[39]

Ectopic ADH has no regard for normal endocrine feedback mechanisms. In SIADH, abnormal production of ADH, also known as arginine vasopressin, results in dilutional hyponatremia and water excess. Cancers of the brain, pancreas, prostate, duodenum, and lymph system have been associated with SIADH but the majority of cases occur in SCLC with an average incidence of clinical SIADH in 4% of newly diagnosed SCLC patients.[40] Older patients, and those being treated with drugs, such as carboplatin, cisplatin, vinca alkaloids, and ifosfamide, are at greater risk of developing SIADH.

Hypercalcemia in malignancy can be a direct result of focal bone destruction. Focal bone destruction is mediated by tumor cells, cytokines, and growth factors that act on osteoclasts directly or interact with osteoblasts to up-regulate osteoclast activity. Regardless, the end result is bone invasion, bone destruction, and hypercalcemia.[2] Although hypercalcemia, as a result of bone metastases, is well defined clinically, the predominant cause of HHM is the ectopic secretion of PTHrP. At least 80% of patients with hypercalcemia have increased serum levels of the ectopic hormone. It produces not only humoral effects, but also plays a role in osteolysis and bone metastases.[36] Patients at greatest risk are those with cancers of the lung, breast, kidney, multiple myeloma, and head and neck. Severe hypercalcemia is a poor prognostic sign.[2]

## PATHOPHYSIOLOGY

In cancer, ectopic hormone production results in abnormal physiological responses in metabolic function. Normal metabolic pathways disregard regulating endocrine feedback loops. Ectopic hormone production not only alters physiological pathways but can also directly stimulate the release of other hormones, cytokines, and growth factors that, in turn, enhance their activity. Rarely, cancer will metabolize steroids to an active form leading to the development of EPSs.[2]

In patients with EAS, there is an increased production by tumors of ACTH, ACTH precursor propiomelanocortin (POMC), and increased conversion of POMC to ACTH.[24] Genetic cloning of POMC has revealed that it contains not only ACTH but melanocyte-stimulating hormone, β-lipotropin, endorphins, and enkephalins.[2] These exert ectopic action on the adrenal glands leading to hyperadrenalism and hyercortisolism.

Syndrome of inappropriate antidiuretic hormone is the result of abnormal (nonpituitary) production of ADH. The unregulated ADH binds to receptors in the renal collecting system and ascending loop of Henle with a consequential reabsorption of water and increased delivery of sodium to the distal tubule. As intravascular volume increases, so does renal perfusion while proximal tubular resorption of sodium decreases.[2] Pathological expression of excess water retention and dilutional hyponatremia are the main clinical features of SIADH.

Under normal circumstances, PTHrP is produced in the body and is responsible for signaling at local tissue sites with little systemic effects.[23] In HHM, PTHrP can activate parathyroid hormone receptors and cause hypercalcemia. But HHM can occur independent of parathyroid hormone secretion.[41] PTHrP can stimulate interleukin 1 (IL-1), interleukin 6 (IL-6), prostaglandin E, and tumor necrosis factor-alpha (TNF-α), all of which contribute to hypercalcemia. PTHrP is believed to promote tumor progression and bone metastases by offsetting the normal osteoclastic and osteoblastic bone modeling pathway.[2] PTHrP also has a phosphaturic action and increases renal tubular resorption of calcium, thereby aggravating hypercalcemia.[36] The true prognostic significance of the presence of PTHrP in primary tumor cell is not known but is currently under investigation.[42]

## CLINICAL MANIFESTATIONS

The clinical presentation of EAS is often influenced by an underlying tumor. Patients with SCLC develop symptoms of mineralocorticoid excess, such as edema and hypokalemia, early in their course of illness. Long-term effects of EAS consist of fatigue, hypertension, refractory hypokalemia, hirsutism, glucose disturbance, metabolic alkalosis, moon facies, muscle weakness or wasting, truncal obesity, weight loss, peripheral edema, hyperpigmentation, and late in the course, purple striae and buffalo hump.[23]

In SIADH, many patients are asymptomatic and the severity of symptoms correlates with the level of sodium decline.[32] When sodium levels are maintained at approximately 125 mmol/L, milder symptoms such as headache, weakness, fatigue, dysgeusia, impaired concentration, poor memory, and muscle cramps have been reported. As the serum sodium falls below 125 mmol/L, life-threatening conditions tend to develop within 48 hours. These include confusion, hallucinations, respiratory compromise, decerebrate posture, seizures, coma, and death. It is unclear why, but the threshold for serum sodium levels at which neurological complications occur is higher among females than males.[32]

Signs and symptoms in HHM are related to the magnitude of hypercalcemia and the rate of rise from the serum calcium [43] In mild to moderate HHM, when calcium levels fall between 10.5 and 14.0 mg/dL, symptoms include polyuria, polydipsia, fatigue, apathy, and mild confusion.[23] Anorexia, constipation, nausea, and vomiting are also common and result from depression of neuromuscular transmission to the gastrointestinal tract. Severe hypercalcemia, when serum calcium is >14.0 mg/dL, presents with extreme confusion, lethargy, or coma. Bradycardia and dysrhythmias occur due to depressed cardiac contractility. In the setting of volume depletion, renal failure is likely.[43]

## ASSESSMENT

### Diagnostic studies

When a paraneoplastic condition is suspected, it is important to distinguish EAS from the clinically classic and more common CS.[44] Initially, screening for cortisol excess may include a 24-hour urine sample for urinary-free cortisol or more commonly an ACTH plasma level (ACTHpl). In adrenal-driven diseases, the ACTHpl is low. In contrast, with EAS, which is not adrenal driven, the ACTHpl is elevated. If elevated levels are present, then a high-dose dexamethasone suppression (HDDS) test should follow.[2] Because cortisol production is pituitary-independent, suppression by high-dose dexamethasone will not be seen and the test will be negative.[45] False positives can occur and some in the medical profession have questioned the accuracy of the HDDS test. The metyrapone and corticotrophin-releasing hormone stimulation tests can be used. In these tests, patients with CS show increased ACTH production, whereas patients with EAS do not.[2] In the clinical trial setting, newer diagnostic modalities like plasma calcitonin, plasma gastrin, urinary 5-hydroxyindoleacetic acid, and inferior petrosal sinus sampling are being investigated.[46,47] If EAS is diagnosed, further tests to isolate a tumor are needed. Newer imaging studies such as PET and improved MRI and CT scanning have increased the accuracy with which occult tumors are discovered.[44]

Prior to establishing a diagnosis of SIADH, other causes of hyponatremia such as hyperglycemia, excessive water intake, heart failure, cirrhosis, and medications should be considered.[48] With SIADH, the classic finding of inappropriate water reabsorption leads to a decrease in serum sodium and serum osmolality. Potassium, calcium, and magnesium are decreased while blood urea nitrogen (BUN) and creatinine remain normal. Despite a low serum sodium, renal perfusion and excretion of sodium continue and an increase in urine sodium results. Urine osmolality is also increased due to reabsorption at the tubules. In selected cases, supplemental diagnostic testing, such as a water-loading test, may prove helpful.[49] As well, serum ADH is elevated and uric acid levels are low. Imaging is not usually required to make the diagnosis of SIADH but may be helpful in isolating the primary cancer.[33]

The presence of an elevated calcium level is one element of HHM. However, calcium levels must always be evaluated with respect to a patient's albumin level because calcium is bound to albumin; thus, if the albumin is low the calcium level may appear to be falsely high. A formula for corrected serum calcium exists, but is not always precise. A measurement of serum ionized calcium is accurate and reliable and should be ordered whenever there is doubt concerning the true total calcium level.[35] Other tests helpful in HHM include the serum phosphorus (decreased), BUN and creatinine (increased), and urinary calcium (increased) due to renal excretion of an increased calcium load. A baseline electrocardiogram may show QT abnormalities, increased PR intervals, or dysrhythmias.[50]

## THERAPEUTIC APPROACHES AND NURSING CARE

Most patients with EPSs are anxious and demonstrate altered levels of functioning. Therefore, nursing care is focused on psychological support of the patient and family. Ensuring patient safety and educating patients about their disease process and treatment options are of chief importance. Frequent monitoring of vital signs, mental status, intake and output, and cardiac function cannot be understated. A multidisciplinary approach is needed.

Surgery is the optimal treatment for EAS, but many patients presenting with this do so after tumor metastases is already established, thereby rendering surgery ineffective. However, in patients with metastases limited to the liver, resection of the cancer may produce cure. In all other patients, systemic treatment must be initiated as severe hypercortisolism leads to infection, hypokalemia, cognitive impairment, thromboembolism, and excessive mortality.[51,52] Treatment of the underlying cancer is important and should be augmented by drug therapy; an adrenal enzyme inhibitor is the drug of choice. Ketoconazole (400–1200 mg/day) works by effectively blocking corticosteroid production thereby inhibiting 17-hydroxylase and 11-hydroxylase.[23] Treatment with ketoconazole results in biochemical improvement for most patients but places the patient at risk for adrenal insufficiency. In this population, replacement corticosteroids should be considered and moderate- to high-dose steroids can be administered if patients experience increasing stressors such as surgery, trauma, or additional metabolic disturbances. Aminoglutethimide and metyrapone are other agents that may be used to treat EAS.[53] Even though expensive, octreotide, a long-acting somatostatin, quickly reduces ectopic ACTH. Typically, octreotide is given twice daily or as a monthly injection. It has activity alone or in combination with ketoconazole. At least one case report exists of a patient successfully treated off-label for 9 weeks with mifepristone.[54] In refractory cases, bilateral adrenalectomy is used, but is rare in application.[23]

In 80% of patients with SCLC, treatment of the underlying malignancy with chemotherapy is associated with dramatic improvement of SIADH and symptoms within 6 weeks of treatment. During this time, additional measures such as free water fluid restriction (500–1000 mL/day) and pharmacological support can impart stability.[23] Demeclocycline (600–1200 mg/day) interferes with ADH's action on the renal tubules, lithium (600–900 mg/day) decreases renal sensitivity to ADH, and urea (30–60 g/day) promotes osmotic diuresis, all of which result in decreased water resorption and work toward restoration of a normal sodium level (135–145 mmol/L). In severe SIADH, where altered mental status is observed, urgent treatment with 3% saline and furosemide may be warranted. The administration rate should not exceed 1 mEq/L/hour and should take place in the ICU setting.[23] Vasopressin receptor antagonist, a new class of drugs, also known as Vaptans, have been developed and continue to be studied in clinical trials for the treatment of SIADH.[55]

Treatment of HHM alone fails to increase overall survival of those who suffer from it. As with other EPSs, therapy of the underlying malignancy is imperative. At times, when death is eminent, withholding antihypercalcemic therapy that leads to coma and death may be appropriate. Hypercalcemia leads to dehydration and patients require fluid replacement with normal saline. Once adequately hydrated, loop diuretics such as furosemide may be given to increase renal excretion of calcium. Thiazide diuretics are contraindicated as they stimulate, rather than inhibit, renal calcium reabsorption.[35] Perhaps the backbone of current management of HHM is the use of bisphosphonate therapy. Bisphosphonates interfere with osteoclast function and block calcium release from the bone; examples include pamidronate, etidronate, and zoledronate. The newer agent, zoledronate, appears to have increased activity and ease of administration compared to older agents. In refractory cases of HHM, calcitonin (6–8 IU/kg) given SQ or IM every 6–12 hours can be administered. A nasal form of calcitonin is also available. In the most intractable cases, plicamycin (1.5–2.0 mg IV) or gallium nitrate (250 mg/m$^2$/day over 24 hours) may be needed.[23]

## HEMATOLOGIC PARANEOPLASTIC SYNDROMES

### SCOPE OF THE PROBLEM

Clinically significant hematologic and thrombotic disorders are common among patients with cancer. They can be mild or life-threatening and impact length and quality of life. They are often a complication of cancer therapy or the result of invasive disease to the bone or bone marrow. Although still poorly understood, it is thought that hematologic disorders do occur as PNSs driven by cytokines, growth factors, impaired hematopoiesis, hormones, free radicals, or as an autoimmune response to cancer. Common hematologic PNSs include anemia, granulocytopenia, erythrocytosis, granulocytosis, eosinophilia, or thrombocytopenia. Thrombotic syndromes such as Trousseau's syndrome (TS), marantic endocarditis, disseminated intravascular coagulation, arterial thrombosis, or thrombotic microangiopathy may precede the diagnosis of cancer by months or years.[56,57] Anemia, eosinophilia, and TS will be discussed in more detail in the following sections.

#### Definitions

In the purest sense, anemia is defined as a decrease in hemoglobin (Hgb) or hematocrit (Hct).[58] Among patients with cancer, anemia is common and often expected as a side effect of chemotherapy, iron or B12 deficiency due to poor nutrition, or marrow replacement by metastases. Pure red cell aplasia, autoimmune hemolytic anemia, and microangiopathic hemolytic anemia are more rare forms of anemia. *Paraneoplastic anemia of malignancy* (AOM) is the most common anemia in patients with cancer. It is normochromic and normocytic in nature, characterized by low erythropoietin, a low serum iron level, normal iron stores, low reticulocyte count, normal to increased ferritin, and normal soluble transferring receptor.[59] *Eosinophilia* is a marked and persistent increase in the number of blood eosinophils ( $>1.5 \times 10^9$/L) for more than 6 months.[60]

Clinical databases clearly document an increased risk of cancer diagnosis after an episode of venous thromboembolism. The correlation between malignancy and venous thrombosis was first recognized by Trousseau more than 100 years ago.[61] *Trousseau's syndrome* (TS) is a rare, migratory thrombophlebitis that is recurrent and usually involves superficial veins. Veins in the arms and of the chest are most often affected. A tumor may not be detected at presentation, but a visceral cancer may be observed months to years later.[62]

### Incidence

Anemia is underreported and is more common than previously realized. Data from the National Center for Health Statistics reveals that approximately 3.4 million Americans suffer from anemia. Women, African Americans, low income groups, and the elderly are disproportionately affected.[63] Anemia of chronic disease, of which AOM is a part, is prevalent, second only to iron deficiency.[59] Anemia due to cancer or cancer treatment varies according to tumor type and stage of disease. For example, in SCLC, anemia is present in 30% to 60% of patients.[63] The true incidence of AOM is underreported and unknown and this is also true of eosinophilia.

Thromboembolism is present in up to 11% of patients with cancer and is the second leading cause of death among patients with cancer. The percentage of individuals hospitalized with an initial thrombotic event is higher in those with malignant disease vs nonmalignant disease: 0.60% vs 0.57%, respectively. Up to 10% of patients with pancreatic carcinoma develop TS. Pancreatic tumors are most commonly associated with TS followed respectively by lung, prostate, stomach, acute leukemia, and colon cancer. Data support an increased incidence of clotting in those individuals with cancer and factor V Leiden or prothrombin 20210A mutation.[64]

### Etiology and risk factors

The etiology of AOM is multifactorial. Altered function of the reticuloendothelial system, response to tumor cytokines, damage from free radicals, premature apoptosis of red blood cells, and a blunted response to erythropoietin all contribute to the pathology of AOM. Bone marrow invasion by tumor or bone marrow damage from cytotoxic treatment and comorbidities such as infection, human immunodeficiency virus (HIV), hepatitis C, and malaria (very rarely) can complicate AOM.[59] Poor nutrition, advanced age, advanced disease, and renal insufficiency increase the risk for AOM.

Eosinophilia is commonly linked to allergic disease, immune dysfunction, parasitic infections, or medications. Eosinophilia can be paraneoplastic and is most frequently a precursor to leukemia or lymphoma. It is also documented in solid tumors such as breast, lung, liver, thyroid, genitourinary, and gastrointestinal. An exact mapping of its pathogenesis has yet to be discovered, but evidence suggests that it is cytokine and immune-driven.[65]

Thromboembolism and TS result from tumor-induced alterations in the coagulation cascade that lead to hypercoagulability, vessel wall damage, and vessel stasis.[66]

Patients with tumors of the lung, pancreas, ovary, and prostate are at greatest risk for thrombotic events. Carriers of the prothrombin 20210A and factor V Leiden mutation have up to an 18-fold increased risk of clotting.[67] Other factors that increase the risk of thrombosis include the use of growth factors, chemotherapy (platinum, tamoxifen, fluorouracil, mitomycin), and central venous catheters.[68]

## PATHOPHYSIOLOGY

In AOM, ectopic secretion of proinflammatory cytokines, such as IL-1 and TNF-α, lead to a disturbance in iron homeostasis. The reticuloendothelial system increases uptake and storage of iron. This results in a decreased availability of circulating iron that is necessary for complete erythropoiesis; in addition, excess stored iron limits erythropoiesis. IL-1 and TNF-α also inhibit erythropoietin expression and through erythrophagocytosis decrease erythrocyte half-life.[59] To complicate matters, hepcidin, an acute phase protein produced in the liver, elevates in response to IL-6 and results in decreased iron release from enterocytes, hepatocytes, and macrophages. The resultant initial decrease in available iron for bacteria and tumor cells may be protective, but in the long run induces hypoferremia and worsens AOM.[69]

Normally, eosinophil development requires 3 cytokines: granulocyte-macrophage colony stimulating factor, interleukin 3, and interleukin 5 (IL-5). Lymphoma and leukemic cells can overproduce IL-5, thereby producing hypereosinophilia. Monocolonal T-cell populations can overproduce IL-5 with the same result. T-cell lines with abnormal chromosomes have an increased affinity for neoplastic transformation.[70] Myeloproliferative clones that result from defects in normal suppressive regulation of eosinophilopoiesis and defects in signal transduction from the receptors that regulate eosinophilopoiesis, result in an overproduction of eosinophils.[71]

With TS and thromboembolism, cancer itself is often the underlying mechanism. As malignant cells collide with immune surveying monocytes and macrophages, cytokines such as IL-6 and IL-1, along with TNF-α, induce endothelial damage and cause shedding of endothelial cells. This results in a resurfacing of the vascular lining into a thrombotic plane. Accordingly, platelets, factor X, and factor XII become activated and this leads to formation of thrombin and ultimately thrombosis. Procoagulant substances from tumor cells have thromboplastin-like activity. They can directly stimulate the activation of factor X to factor Xa or cause direct activation of factor VII to factor VIIa. Mucins from adenocarcinomas can activate factor X.[68]

## CLINICAL MANIFESTATIONS

Clinical signs and symptoms of the normochromic, normocytic AOM can be mild or severe. Common symptoms include weakness, fatigue, headache, muscle cramps, mood disturbance, and cognitive dysfunction. More severe symptoms include dyspnea on exertion, orthostatic lightheadedness, tachycardia, tachypnea, cardiac disturbance, and syncope. Patients often report decreased activity tolerance, decreased performance status, and decreased quality of life.[72] Objective measurements include, but are not limited to, pallor, tachycardia, cyanosis, clubbing, hypoxia, splenomegaly, decreased red cell indices, and orthostatic hypotension.

Clinical features of eosinophilia may precede its discovery. These features include rash, cough, fever, fatigue, angioedema, retinal lesions, muscle pains, and breathlessness. Prolonged eosinophilia can lead to target organ damage and coagulation disorders. Hepatomegaly, splenomegaly, and gastroenteritis are common complications related to eosinophilia. Neurological manifestations involving both the central and peripheral nervous systems can result in encephalopathy or polyneuropathy. As a cardiac complication, endomyocardial fibrosis is a serious, generally irreversible complication of eosinophilia.[60]

Superficial thrombophlebitis is the hallmark of TS. Erythema and swelling may be noted in the upper and lower extremities. Clinical characteristics of TS can include thrombocytopenia, disseminated intravascular coagulation (DIC), arterial emboli, and warfarin resistance.[66] Anxiety, dyspnea, chest pain, or hypotension is indicative of pulmonary thrombosis. It is important to note that some patients will have no presenting symptoms.

## ASSESSMENT

### Diagnostic studies

Anemia of malignancy is normochromic and normocytic. Laboratory profiling usually reveals a Hgb level around 10 mg/dL and a normal mean corpuscular volume. Classically, patients have a low reticulocyte count (indicates underproduction of red blood cells), reduced transferring saturation, reduced serum iron, normal to elevated serum ferritin, normal soluble transferring receptor, and low erythropoietin levels.[59] Bone marrow aspiration and biopsy may be needed to rule out marrow infiltration as a source of anemia. Abdominal ultrasound or CT scan may identify liver or spleen enlargement that can contribute to red blood cell sequestration and destruction.

Identification of eosinophilia is fairly straightforward. Increased numbers appear in the differential of the complete blood count and peripheral smear. Bone marrow biopsy, with chromosomal analysis and staining for reticulin fibrosis, reveals increased eosinophils, and in some cases, atypical mast cells. Chromosome studies are normal in the majority of cases. CT scans can identify organ damage, lymphadenopathy, or splenomegaly.[60]

Duplex venous ultrasonography is the initial and recommended imaging modality for diagnosis of deep venous thrombosis. It is cost-effective and noninvasive. If a clinical suspicion of pulmonary embolism (PE) exists, CT angiography is needed for evaluation. Chest x-rays and EKGs lack the sensitivity or specificity to diagnose PE. D-dimer testing is not recommended in the diagnosis of PE.[66]

## THERAPEUTIC APPROACHES AND NURSING CARE

There is an association between uncorrected anemia and worsened clinical outcomes. Treatment of AOM can result in decreased morbidity and mortality and result in an increase in quality of life. Nurses provide supportive care, education, and delivery of transfusions, iron, erythropoietin, oxygen, and chemotherapy to treat an underlying cancer. Transfusion with one unit of packed red blood cells can increase Hgb by 1 g/dL and result in a rapid increase in Hgb and Hct that alleviates symptoms such as dyspnea and fatigue.[72] The risks associated with red cell transfusions include congestive heart failure, infection, transfusion-related reactions, and iron overload. It may be comforting to patients to know that, since 1984, heightened screening of blood products has greatly reduced the incidence of transfusion-related infections.[73]

Administration of erythropoietin has been widely recommended to increase the hemoglobin level and results in a decrease in transfusion requirements in patients undergoing chemotherapy, while increasing quality of life. It is important to note that in March 2007, the Food and Drug Administration (FDA) mandated a black box warning advising that erythropoietin replacement should be given to maintain the lowest Hgb level necessary to avoid transfusions. In March 2008, that warning was strengthened when data review indicated an increased risk of tumor progression and shortened survival in patients with advanced breast, head and neck, lymphoid, and non-SCLCs when Hgb levels exceeded 12 g/dL. This, along with other data, guided a revision in the National Comprehensive Cancer Network (NCCN) guidelines for anemia that state, "An FDA cancer advisory committee has recommended that erythropoietin should not be used in cancer patients receiving potentially curative treatments or among patients with breast, head and neck, and non-small cell lung cancers."[72]

Treatment of eosinophilia is aimed at the underlying malignancy. Supportive measures such as oxygen and emotional support may be required for respiratory compromise. Patient education will help decrease anxiety, especially if the cause is not yet known.

Warfarin is an option for patients with cancer and thrombosis. However, in the case of TS, many patients will not respond to warfarin and heparin may be needed. Unfractionated heparin rapidly interrupts thrombosis by inactivating factor Xa and platelet activation. It has long been the preferred treatment in TS due to its multiple actions. Recently, low–molecular weight heparins (LMWH) have become popular due to decreased incidence of heparin-induced thrombocytopenia and a daily dosing schedule.[62] These are safe and effective, but care should be taken when giving LMWH to patients with renal insufficiency as they have an increased risk of bleeding with standard dosing.[66] Teaching patients to avoid sharp objects, report bleeding, self-injection, and environmental safety should be nursing priorities. Nursing assessment and reporting of patients' prothrombin time (PT) or partial thromboplastin time (PTT) is central to successful management of patients with TS on anticoagulants. Patient self-monitoring is being increasingly observed and nurses have the prime responsibility of educating patients on the correct procedure for home management.[74]

## RENAL PARANEOPLASTIC SYNDROMES

### SCOPE OF THE PROBLEM

Renal complications are common in patients with cancer and include tumor infiltration of the kidney, urethral obstruction, renal vein thrombosis, fluid and electrolyte imbalances, and glomerular abnormalities. Radiation, chemotherapy, and support medications all impact renal function. Renal complications also occur due to paraneoplastic presentations. Hemolytic uremic syndrome, membranoproliferative glomerulonephritis, amyloidosis, and nephrotic syndrome are rare PNSs. Nephrotic syndrome will be discussed in greater detail below.

#### Definition

*Nephrotic paraneoplastic syndrome* (NPS) results from damage to the renal glomerulus. This may be from renal lesions, obstruction by tumor products, or may be caused by idiopathic tumor factors. Edema, proteinuria, hypoalbuminemia, hypertension, and dyslipidemia are typically the end result of NPS. Like other PNSs, NPS often occurs prior to the cancer being diagnosed and may herald tumor recurrence.

#### Incidence

The true incidence of NPS is uncertain, but it is considered rare and has a poor prognosis. It is more likely to occur in patients with lung cancer, leukemia, melanoma, Hodgkin's disease, and non-Hodgkin's lymphoma. Cases have been reported in thyroid, colon, breast, pancreatic, and ovarian cancer.[1] The incidence of NPS is unusual in patients with skin cancer, but it will rarely coincide with pheochromocytoma.[75] Although NPS can occur at any point in the course of disease, the majority of cases are diagnosed concurrently with the disease or within a year's time.

#### Etiology and risk factors

In most cases of NPS and malignancy, the lesion most often isolated in patients is membranous glomerulonephropathy (81%). This has supported the hypothesis that NPS is immune-mediated.[76] Secondary amyloidosis, immunoglobulin, complement, and sedimentation of immunocomplexes in the nephron result in filtration unit damage. Tumor-specific antigens and associated tumor antigens play an ill-defined role. Malignant hypoalbuminemia further reduces albumin synthesis thereby complicating the clinical picture.[1] Occult malignancy is the largest risk factor for NPS, but it is thought to be limited largely by host immune responses.

### PATHOPHYSIOLOGY

Undetected tumors produce antigens (fetal, viral, and autologous nontumor) that incite an immune response. The resultant immune-mediated immunoglobulin and complement complexes deposit in the glomerulus. Once this occurs, subepithelial deposits can be detected by electron microscopy. This is the pathological hallmark of NPS.[2] Damage to the endothelial surface and glomerular basement membrane leads to increased glomerular permeability followed by hyperalbuminuria, hypoalbuminemia, decreased plasma colloid osmotic pressure, and edema.[77] Urinary loss of antithrombin III and plasminogen stimulate an increased production of clotting factors resulting in an increased predisposition to thrombosis in patients with NPS. Fibrin formation within the glomeruli also increases this risk of thrombosis.[78]

### CLINICAL MANIFESTATIONS

Clinical symptoms are a direct result of the altered physiological processes that characterize NPS. Frothy urine, weakness, fatigue, and abdominal pain may be early symptoms. Advanced findings are severe proteinuria, hypoalbuminemia, and hypertension. A compensatory increase in liver protein synthesis, including lipoproteins, occurs due to hypoproteinemia. This, along with decreased lipid catabolism due to low plasma levels of lipoprotein lipase, results in elevated serum lipids. Late effects of NPS are malignant ascites and pleural effusions.[77] Arterial or venous thromboembolism can precede or accompany NPS.

### ASSESSMENT

#### Diagnostic studies

Initially, a 24-hour urine sample is needed and classic finding include proteinuria, hematuria, and elevated urinary albumin. A high ratio of urinary albumin to globulin is common and the amount of protein excreted can range from 1 to 20 g, with the majority ranging from 4 to 7 g. In preliminary stages, blood chemistries may show normal renal function but as the disease progresses, a rise in serum creatinine is expected. A complete blood count may reveal elevated Hgb and Hct values secondary to contracted plasma volume that accompanies hypoalbuminemia. The serum albumin level correlates with the severity of proteinuria and is generally less than 2.5 g/dL, but can be as low as 0.5 g/dL. The lipid profile is in opposition to serum albumin concentrations. Low-density lipoproteins and very low-density lipoproteins are elevated, whereas high-density lipoproteins are low. Secondary expressions of the hyperlipidemia include hyponatremia and low serum osmolality. Hypocalcemia is common but ionized calcium levels, which correct for low albumin, are normal to low normal.[79]

Imaging studies are not routinely recommended as diagnosis is largely based on clinical findings. Nevertheless, renal ultrasound may be used to confirm the presence of two kidneys while testing for renal enlargement, cysts, lesions, or hydronephrosis. Chest x-ray and abdominal ultrasound can reveal effusions and ascites. In rare cases, a renal biopsy may be needed to determine the cause.[79]

### THERAPEUTIC APPROACHES AND NURSING CARE

NPS has been known to resolve with treatment of the underlying malignancy.[2] Resolution can occur rapidly provided the tumor responds to therapy. Management of NPS centers on symptomatic treatment with appropriate diuretic therapy (furosemide or spironolactone), treatment of electrolyte disturbances, control of hypertension, and avoidance of nephrotoxic agents. Intravenous albumin may be needed but should be given cautiously to avoid pulmonary edema. Salt poor albumin accompanied by furosemide usually proves to be the most effective treatment. Albumin may also delay response to treatment and worsen glomerular damage. Another mainstay of therapy is glucocorticoids in high doses followed by a taper regimen. If infection occurs due to lowered immunity, oral penicillin is an excellent choice unless the patient is allergic to this drug.[78] Fluid restrictions are not usually necessary. A high protein diet, with salt reduction, may help reduce symptoms of edema. Thoracentesis and paracentesis can improve symptoms of respiratory distress and abdominal discomfort, but can further cheat the body of albumin. Hospitalization is not usually required but may be necessary in the presence of rapid deterioration.

## MISCELLANEOUS PARANEOPLASTIC SYNDROMES

### CUTANEOUS PARANEOPLASTIC SYNDROMES (CPSs)

Although rare, CPSs can develop as a result of cancer and present before it is diagnosed. Common examples of CPS include acanthosis nigricans, acquired ichthyosis, acrokeratosis paraneoplastica, phemphigus, extramammary Paget's disease, Sweet's syndrome, and others (See Table 34-3). Some CPSs can occur together as in Sign of Leser-Trelat, which is a rapid increase in the number and size of seborrheic keratoses. It is often associated with thickened, velvety palms or florid cutaneous papillomatosis. Common clinical entities such as itching and herpes zoster can mimic symptoms of an underlying cancer. CPSs have been reported across the cancer continuum and case reports exist for not only solid tumors, such as adenocarcinomas, but for other illnesses such as AIDS, systemic lupus erythematosus, sarcoidosis, endocrine abnormalities, and massive infections.[80]

The pathophysiological mechanisms by which CPSs arise remain undiscovered. These phenomena are thought to result from an interaction among the tumor, some mediating factors, and the target tissue involved.[81] Mediators may include polypeptide hormones, cytokines, enzymes, prostaglandins, antibodies, and growth factors, which act by disrupting communication between cells, thereby producing either abnormal or increased cellular activity.[82]

Because CPSs can manifest ahead of, concurrent with or after cancer, once identified, complete systemic investigation is needed to isolate the cause. History, physical exam, laboratory studies, and radiological testing are part of the initial work-up. In cases where the CPS is not known to be directly associated with certain types of tumors, a PET scan may prove useful.

Treatment of CPSs is directed at the underlying malignancy. In the majority of cases, this results in improvement of skin lesions. Supportive measures include analgesics for pain relief, antihistamines to treat pruritus, and both systemic and topical steroids to reduce inflammation and block tumor production of prostaglandins thought to sensitize peripheral nerve endings to substances that cause itching.[83] Topical or systemic antibiotics may be used to treat cutaneous superficial infections. Nursing care is supportive and includes education, dressing changes, medication management, maintaining skin integrity, and emotional support.

### CANCER ANOREXIA-CACHEXIA SYNDROME

Anorexia is defined as a decreased desire for food. Its prevalence varies with different cancers and stage of disease but can be as high as 74% in patients with cancer.[84] It is

**TABLE 34-3**

**Paraneoplastic Cutaneous Syndromes**

| Disorder | Clinical Presentation | Associated Malignancy | Comments |
|---|---|---|---|
| *Pigmented Legions* | | | |
| Acanthosis nigricans | Velvety brown, symmetrical legions with hyperkeratosis that occur primarily in flexural areas—axilla, posterior neck, perineum, umbilicus | 90% of cases associated with malignancy<br>60% gastric carcinoma<br>5% lung carcinoma | Usually associated with advanced disease |
| Sign of Leser-Trelat | Multiple seborrheic (wartlike) lesions | Adenocarcinomas<br>Non-Hodgkin's lymphoma<br>GI malignancies—43% | Rapid development signals malignancy<br>Pruritic |
| Sweet's Syndrome (acute febrile neutrophilic dermatosis) | Painful erythematous plaques covering arms, head and neck | 10%–15% of cases associated with malignancy, usually hematologic, leukemias (AML) myeloma | |
| Bazex's Syndrome | Scaly, pruritic psoriasiform rash affecting nails, nose, ears, elbows, knees, fingers, and toes | GU, GI, breast—less common<br>Squamous cell carcinomas of head and neck, esophagus, lung<br>Vulvar, esophageal, and uterine carcinomas | Males ordinarily affected<br>Females less common<br>100% associated with malignancy |
| *Erythemas* | | | |
| Erythema gyratum repens (*repens* is Latin for "to crawl or creep") | Expanding, scaly, concentric bands (tyri) with a "wood grain" pattern | 32% lung carcinoma<br>Breast<br>Esophagus<br>Uterine | Pruritic<br>Moves rapidly across skin surface—about 1 cm/day<br>2:1 male to female ratio<br>100% association with malignancy<br>Tumor resection results in complete resolution within 6 weeks |
| Glucagonoma syndrome (necrolytic migratory erythema) | Erythematous patches<br>Stomatitis | Islet cell tumors of pancreas | Tumor resection results in clearance of the eruption within 48 hours |
| *Endocrine/Metabolic Lesions* | | | |
| Porphyria cutanea tarda | Early photosensitive subepidermal vesicles, fragile skin hyperpigmentation<br>Late alopecia, scarring, sclerodermoid changes | Liver carcinoma | Often painful, pruritic |
| Systemic nodular panniculitis | Fever, erythematous SQ nodules, fat necrosis of bone marrow, lungs, and other organs; abdominal pain | Pancreatic adenocarcinoma | Occurs rarely, also associated with benign pancreatic disease |
| *Miscellaneous* | | | |
| Pruritus | Generalized itching with areas of excoriation from scratching<br>Chronic, intensive itching of nostrils associated with advanced brain tumors | Hodgkin's and T-cell lymphomas<br>Polycythemia vera<br>CNS malignancies | 25% of Hodgkin's lymphoma patients experience generalized itching<br>May be presenting system of malignancies |

(*Continued*)

**TABLE 34-3**

**Paraneoplastic Cutaneous Syndromes (*Continued*)**

| Disorder | Clinical Presentation | Associated Malignancy | Comments |
|---|---|---|---|
| Hypertrichosis lanuginosa (malignant down) | Fine, silky hair occurring primarily on forehead and ears | Lung, colon carcinomas, also bladder, uterine | Rapid onset<br>90% association with malignancy |
| HPO | Painful, symmetric arthropathy involving fingers, wrists, elbows, and knees caused by periostitis | Intrathoracic malignancies, primarily lung carcinomas (88%)<br>Most common histologies are large cell and adenocarcinoma of the lung | Associated with clubbing of fingers and toes<br>May resemble rheumatoid arthritis<br>Usually precedes diagnosis of malignancy |

*Abbreviations*: AML, acute myeloid leukemia; CNS, central nervous system; GI, gastrointestinal; GU, genitourinary; HPO, hypertrophic pulmonary osteoarthropathy; SQ, subcutaneous.

most common in cases of gastrointestinal malignancies and advanced disease.[84] Cachexia is a debilitating state of involuntary weight loss involving both adipose tissue and skeletal muscle.[85,86] Patients with cancer are affected by both and together they are known as the cancer anorexia-cachexia syndrome (CACS). CACS is the most common paraneoplastic phenomenon among all tumors.[23] Wasting is not attributed to malnutrition that results in lipid depletion from fat stores, but results from the interaction of several factors whose end is anemia, insulin resistance, immunosuppression, increased basal energy expenditure, and inflammation.[86]

Multiple cytokines are thought to induce anorexia and increase resting energy expenditure. They include TNF-α, IL-1-β, IL-6, serotonin, and interferon. Evidence supports the belief that proteolysis-inducing factor, lipid-mobilizing factor, and the ATP-ubiquitin-proteasome pathway also play a role in the disturbed metabolism of proteins, lipids, and carbohydrates. As caloric supply decreases, the demand for gluconeogenesis increases leading to protein catabolism, muscle and weight loss, and a negative nitrogen balance. This is followed by tissue wasting and compromised immunity.[23]

Weight loss is the most common clinical finding in CACS. More than 15% of patients with cancer will experience a 10% or greater weight loss.[23] Associated symptoms include nausea, vomiting, constipation, mouth pain, dysphagia, depression, fatigue, weakness, and changes in performance status.[84] It is not surprising that CACS is associated with a poorer prognosis, lower response rates to treatment, disease progression, and death.[87]

Nursing management begins with a thorough review of diet history and documentation of height, weight, and body mass index. In certain cancers such as head and neck, where oral intake is compromised, and in those with good life expectancy, feeding via the gastrointestinal tract may be started. This is the preferred route since it is both physiologically beneficial and cost-effective. Total parenteral nutrition may be an option in persons who are potentially curable but has no role in patients with CACS and advanced disease.[23]

Clinical trials have examined several pharmacological agents for use in CACS. The most widely studied and most commonly used agents are corticosteroids, such as dexamethasone, and progestational agents, such as megestrol acetate. Other agents such as cannabinoids and serotonin antagonists are also used. To date, none of these agents have demonstrated benefits in terms of prolonged survival or improvement in global quality of life. They do temporarily improve appetite and this is often important for the patient and family. Current clinical trials are investigating many new agents like thalidomide, growth hormone, and melatonin that may prove useful in the future treatment of CACS.[88,89]

## MUSCULOSKELETAL/RHEUMATIC PARANEOPLASTIC SYNDROMES

Paraneoplastic musculoskeletal disorders (PMDs) and paraneoplastic rheumatic disorders (PRDs) can precede cancer and some have the potential for malignant transformation. PMDs may involve muscles, joints, or bones. The best described of the PMDs are dermatomyositis and polymyositis. Both are inflammatory, systemic myopathies that result in proximal muscle weakness and can involve the heart, joints, lungs, and gastrointestinal tract. A heliotrope rash over the face, knees, elbows, or knuckles is a classic cutaneous finding related to PMDs. Lung and breast tumors are most commonly associated with PMDs.[2]

Like PMDs, the pathogenesis of PRDs is poorly understood. It is postulated that malignant transformation occurs as a result of immune dysregulation. Strong evidence exists to support the theory that rheumatoid arthritis, systemic lupus erythematosus, systemic sclerosis, Sjögren's syndrome, sarcoidosis, and ankylosing spondylitis can be premalignant conditions. Most all patients with these conditions have an increased risk of lymphoma and those with lupus have an increased risk of lung and hepatobiliary cancers.[90]

Immunosuppressants and immune modulators are the mainstay of treatment for musculoskeletal and rheumatic disorders. The course of disease for these PNSs is unpredictable. Cases exist from 2 to 20 years before malignancy is confirmed.[90] Although extensive testing of tumor markers and total body scanning at initial presentation of a rheumatic or musculoskeletal disorder is cost prohibitive, when symptoms arouse suspicion, an extensive search for cancer should be conducted. Nurses play a key role in assessment and support of these at-risk patients.

### TUMOR FEVER

Fever is common in the cancer population and may be due to infection, neutropenia, drug use, or administration of blood products. Fever can also present as a PNS. Paraneoplastic tumor fever (PTF) is the second most common cause of fever in the patient with cancer.[91] PTF is commonly seen in leukemia, lymphoma, renal cell carcinoma, and gastrointestinal malignancy, including hepatoma. It occurs more often in the evening and follows a continual-remittent pattern. It results from the release of endogenous pyrogens (cytokines) and may be associated with disorders of steroidogenesis.[1]

Paraneoplastic tumor fever signals a poor prognosis.[91] The primary therapy for PTF involves treatment of the underlying cancer. Supportive measures include maintaining adequate hydration, assessing for underlying infection, and minimizing the discomfort of the fever and associated fatigue and chills. Commonly used antipyretics such as acetaminophen or salicylates can be used, but may cause nausea. Nonsteroidal anti-inflammatory drugs, such as ibuprofen, are most often used to treat fever resulting from cancer. They too can cause nausea or renal insufficiency. For unresponsive fevers, a short course of corticosteroids may be useful.

## CONCLUSION

Paraneoplastic syndromes are a heterogeneous group of disorders and often result from the presence of malignancy at sites distant to the source. They can affect any body system, are rare, differ from person to person, and have variable outcomes. Nursing management of these syndromes is complex and dependent on the systems affected by the cancer itself. Regarding treatment, a multidisciplinary approach is best. Nurses should operate from an in-depth knowledge base and employ evidence-based guidelines in caring for patients with PNSs. As the genetic and molecular revolution continues to expand, more information about cytokines, tumor biology, and immune response will hopefully lead to a better understanding of the intricate pathophysiology of PNSs and culminate in better methods for early detection and curative treatments.

## REFERENCES


1. Santacroce L. Paraneoplastic syndromes. *EMedicine*. http://emedicine.medscape.com/article/280744-overview. Accessed November 1, 2009.
2. Arnold SM, Lieberman FS, Foon KA. Paraneoplastic syndromes. In: DeVita VT, Hellman S, Rosenberg SA, eds. *Cancer Principles and Practice of Oncology*. Philadelphia, PA: Lippincott Williams & Wilkins; 2005:2189–2211.
3. Collins LG, Haines C, Perkel R, Enck RE. Lung cancer: diagnosis and management. *Am Fam Physician*. 2007;75:56–63.
4. Dalmau J, Rosenfeld MR. Paraneoplastic syndromes of the CNS. *Lancet Neurol*. 2008;7:327–340.
5. Hung J, Lin JJ, Yang CP, Hsuen C. Paraneoplastic syndrome and intrathoracic Castleman disease. *Pediatr Blood Cancer*. 2006;47:616–620.
6. Lane JE, Woody C, Davis LS, Guill MF, Jerath RS. Paraneoplastic autoimmune multiorgan syndrome (paraneoplastic pemphigus) in a child: case report and review of literature. *Peds*. 2004;114:513–516.
7. Karim A. An introduction to paraneoplastic neurological antibodies. *BMS*. 2006;966–969.
8. Honnorat J, Antoine JC. Paraneoplastic neurological syndromes. *Orphanet J Rare Dis*. (2007, February). http://www.ojrd.com/content/2/1/22. Accessed November 1, 2009.
9. Antoine JC, Camdessanche JP. Peripheral nervous system involvement in patients with cancer. *Lancet Neurol*. 2007;6:75–86.
10. Latov N. Pathogenesis and therapy of neuropathies associated with monoclonal gammopathies. *Ann Neurol*. 1995;378(supp 1):32–42.
11. Rudnicki SA, Dalmau MD. Paraneoplastic syndromes of the spinal cord, nerve, and muscle. *Muscle Nerve*. 2000;23:1800–1818.
12. Bataller L, Dalmau JO. Paraneoplastic disorders of the central nervous system: update on diagnostic criteria and treatment. *Semin Neurol*. 2004;24:461–471.
13. Zasshi N. Pathophysiology of paraneoplastic neurological syndromes: role of cellular immunity. *Intern Med*. 2008;97:1816–1822.
14. Albert ML, Austin LM, Darnell RB. Detection and treatment of activated T cells in the cerebrospinal fluid of patients with paraneoplastic cerebellar degeneration. *Ann Neurol*. 2000;47:9–17.
15. Linke R, Schroeder M, Helmberger T, Voltz R. Antibody-positive paraneoplastic neurological syndromes: value of CT and PET for tumor diagnosis. *Neurology*. 2004;63:282–286.
16. Vernino S, O'Neill BP, Marks RS, O'Fallon JR, Kimmel DW. Immunomodulatory treatment trial for paraneoplastic neurological disorders. *Neuro-Oncol*. 2004;6:55–62.
17. Fong CS. Recent advances in immunological tests in paraneoplastic neurological syndromes. *Acta Neurol Taiwan*. 2005;14:29–35.
18. Hagler KT, Lynch JW. Paraneoplastic manifestations of lymphoma. *Clin Lymphoma*. 2004;5:29–36.
19. Dalmau J, Rosenfeld MR. Paraneoplastic neurological syndromes. In: Abeloff MD, Armitage JO, Niederhuber JE, Kastan MB, McKenna WG, eds. *Clinical Oncology*. Philadelphia, PA: Elsevier; 2004:993–1006.
20. Monstad SE, Drivsholm L, Storstein A, et al. Hu and voltage-gated calcium channel (VGCC) antibodies related to the prognosis of small-cell lung cancer. *J Clin Oncol*. 2004;22:795–800.
21. Weimer MB, Wong J. Lambert-Eaton myasthenic syndrome. *Curr Treat Options Neurol*. 2009;11:77–84.
22. Riedel RF, Burfeind WR. Thymoma: benign appearance, malignant potential. *Oncologist*. 2006;11:887–894.

23. Thomas L, Kwok Y, Edelman MJ. Management of paraneoplastic syndromes in lung cancer. *Curr Treat Options Oncol.* 2004;5:51–62.
24. Graus F, Keine-Guibert F, Rene R, et al. Anti-Hu associated paraneoplastic encephalomyelitis: analysis of 200 patients. *Brain.* 2001;124:1138–1148.
25. Darnell RB, Posner JB. Paraneoplastic syndromes involving the nervous system. *N Engl J Med.* 2003;349:1543–1554.
26. Ress JH. Paraneoplastic syndromes: when to suspect, how to confirm, and how to manage. *J Neurol Neurosurg Psychiatry.* 2004;75(supp 2):43–50.
27. Bataller L, Rosenfeld MR, Graus F, et al. Autoantigen diversity in the opsoclonus myoclonus syndrome. *Ann Neurol.* 2003;53:347–353.
28. Dalmau J. Clinical and immunological diversity of limbic encephalitis: a model for paraneoplastic neurological disorders. *Hematol Oncol Clin North Am.* 2006;20:1319–1335.
29. Baets J, Pals P, Bergman B, et al. Opsoclonus-myoclonus syndrome: clinicopathological confrontation. *Acta Neurol Belg.* 2006;106:142–146.
30. DeGraaf MT, Smitt PA, Sillevi PA. Paraneoplastic syndromes associated with MCUOS. In: Wick MR, ed. *Metastatic Carcinomas of Unknown Origin.* New York: Demos Medical; 2008:27–72.
31. Patel RR, Subramaniam RM, Mandrekar JN, Hammack JE, Lowe VJ, Jett JR. Occult malignancy in patients with suspected paraneoplastic neurological syndromes: value of positron emission tomography in diagnosis. *Mayo Clin Proc.* 2008;83:917–922.
32. Ellison D. Berl T. The syndrome of inappropriate antidiuresis. *N Engl J Med.* 2007;356:2064–2072.
33. Dambro M. *Griffith's 5 Minute Clinical Consult.* Philadelphia, PA: Lippincott Williams & Wilkins; 2006:586–587.
34. Strewler GJ. Hormonal manifestations of malignancy. In: Kronenberg HM, Melmed S, Polonsky KS, Larsen PC, eds. *Kronenberg: Williams Textbook of Endocrinology.* Philadelphia, PA: Elsevier Health Sciences; 2007:1812–1815.
35. Stewart AF. Hypercalcemia associated with cancer. *N Engl J Med.* 2005;352:373–379.
36. Strewler GJ. The physiology of parathyroid hormone-related protein. *N Engl J Med.* 2000;342:177–185.
37. Beuschlein F, Hammer GD. Ectopic pro-opiomelanocortin syndrome. *Endocrinol Metab Clin North Am.* 2002;31:191–234.
38. Marchioli CC, Graziano SL. Paraneoplastic syndromes associated with small-cell lung cancer. *Chest Surg Clin North Am.* 1997;7:65–80.
39. Aniszewski JP, Young WF, Thompson GB, et al. Cushing syndrome due to ectopic adrenocorticotropic hormone secretion. *World J Surg.* 2001;25:934–940.
40. Langfeldt LA, Cooley ME. Syndrome of inappropriate antidiuretic hormone secretion in malignancy. *Clin J Oncol Nurs.* 2003;7:425–430.
41. Nussbaum SR, Gaz RD, Arnold A. Hypercalcemia and ectopic secretion of parathyroid hormone by an ovarian carcinoma with rearrangement of the gene for parathyroid hormone. *N Engl J Med.* 1990;323:1324–1328.
42. Nishihara M, Kamematsu T, Taquchi T, Razzaque MS. PTHrP and tumor genesis: is there a role in prognosis. *Ann N Y Acad Sci.* 2007; 1117:385–392.
43. Moe S. Disorders involving calcium, phosphorus, and magnesium. *Prim Care.* 2008;35:215–237.
44. Isidori AM, Kaltasa GA, Pozza C, et al. The ectopic adrenocorticotropin syndrome: clinical features, diagnosis, management, and long-term follow-up. *J Clin Endocr Metab.* 2006;91:371–377.
45. Pivonello R, DeMantino MC, Deleo M, Lombardi G, Colao A. Cushing's syndrome. *Endocrinol Metab Clin North Am.* 2008;37:135–146.
46. Nieman LK, Ilias I. Evaluation and treatment of Cushing's syndrome. *Am J Med.* 2005;118:1340–1346.
47. Salgado LR, Fragoso MC, Knoepfelmacher M, et al. Ectopic ACTH syndrome: our experience with 25 cases. *Eur J Endocrinol.* 2006; 155:725–733.
48. Adrogue HJ, Madias NE. Hyponatremia. *N Engl J Med.* 2000;342: 1581–1589.
49. Williams H, Elisaf M. Hyponatremia and SIADH. *CMAJ.* 2002; 167:450.
50. Wald DA. ECG manifestations of selected metabolic and endocrine disorders. *Emerg Med Clin North Am.* 2006;24:145–157.
51. Fareau GG, Vassilopoulou-Sellin R. Hypercortisolemia and infection. *Infect Dis Clin North Am.* 2007;21:639–657.
52. Lindholm J, Jorgensen JO, Astrup J, et al. Incidence and late progression of Cushing's syndrome: population based study. *J Clin Endocrinol Metab.* 2001;86:117–123.
53. Vaughan ED, Blumenfield JD. Pathophysiology, evaluation, and medical management of adrenal disorders. In: Wein AJ, Karoussi LR, Novick AC, Partin A, Peters CA, eds. *Campbell-Walsh Urology.* Philadelphia, PA: Saunders; 2007:1836–1837.
54. Johanssen S, Allolio B. Mifepristone (ru 486) in Cushing's syndrome. *Eur J Endocrinol.* 2007;157:561–569.
55. Ali F, Guglin M, Vaitkevicius P, Ghali JK. Therapeutic potential of vasopressin receptor antagonist. *Drugs.* 2007;67:847–858.
56. Bolt E, Decandin D, Veyradier A, Bardier A, Zagame OL, Pouillart P. Cancer related microangiopathy secondary to von Willebrand factor-cleaving protease deficiency. *Thromb Res.* 2002;106:127–130.
57. Rak J, Klement P, Yu J. Genetic determinants of cancer coagulopathy, angiogenesis and disease progression. *Vnitr Lek.* 2006;52(supp 1): 135–138.
58. Munker R. Anemias. In: Munker R, Hiller E, Glass J, Paquette R, eds. *Modern Hematology.* Totowa, NJ: Humana Press; 2007:83–99.
59. Weiss G, Goodnough LT. Anemia of chronic disease. *N Engl J Med.* 2005;353:1011–1023.
60. Roufosse FE, Goldman M, Cogan E. Hypereosinophilic syndromes. *Orphanet J Rare Dis.* 2007;2:37.
61. Sorensen HT, Mellemkjoer L, Olsen JH, Baron JA. Prognosis of cancers associated with venous thromboembolism. *N Engl J Med.* 2000;343: 1846–1850.
62. Varki A. Trousseau's syndrome: multiple definitions and multiple mechanisms. *Blood.* 2007;110:1723–1729.
63. Nissenson AR. Anemia: not just an innocent bystander. *Arch Intern Med.* 2003;163:1400–1404.
64. Phom C, Shen Y. Antiphospholipid antibodies and malignancy. *Hematol Oncol Clin North Am.* 2008;22:121–130.
65. Samyn I, Fontaine C, Tussenbroek FV, Pipeleers-Marichal M, Greve JD. Paraneoplastic syndromes in cancer. *J Clin Oncol.* 2004;22: 2240–2242.
66. Wagman LD, Baird MF, Bennett CL, et al. Venous thromboembolic disease. NCCN clinical practice guidelines in oncology. *J Natl Compr Canc Netw.* 2008;6:716–753.
67. Blom JW, Dogger CJ, Osanto S, Rosendaal FR. Malignancies, prothrombotic mutations, and the risk of venous thrombosis. *JAMA.* 2005;293:715–722.
68. Bick RL. Cancer-associated thrombosis. *N Engl J Med.* 2003;349:109–111.
69. Malyszko J, Mysliwiec M. Hepcidin in anemia and inflammation in chronic kidney disease. *Kidney Blood Press Res.* 2007;30:15–30.
70. Schwartz RS. The hypereosinophilic syndrome and the biology of cancer. *N Engl J Med.* 2003;348:1199–1200.
71. Ackerman SJ, Bachner BS. Mechanisms of eosinophilia in the pathogenesis of hypereosinophilic disorders. *Immunol Allergy Clin North Am.* 2007;27:357–375.
72. Rodgers GM, Becker PS, Bennett CL, et al. NCCN clinical practice guidelines in oncology: cancer and chemotherapy induced anemia. http://www.nccn.org. Accessed August 10, 2009.
73. Dodd RY. Current risk for transfusion transmitted infections. *Curr Opin Hematol.* 2007;14:671–676.
74. Gardiner C, Longair I, Prescott MA, et al. Self monitoring of oral anticoagulation: does it work outside clinical trial conditions? *J Clin Pathol.* 2009;62:168–171.
75. Tirri R, Casiere D, Mattera E, Guarino G, Iacono G, Federick P. The nephritic syndrome and pheochromocytoma. A report of a rare clinical case. *Clin Ter.* 1994;145:199–203.

76. Russo, GE, Morgia, A, Cavallini, M. Glomerulonephritis. *Clin Ter.* 2007;158:495–496.
77. Agraharkar M. (2007, February). Nephrotic syndrome. *EMedicine.* http://emedicine.medscape.com/article/244631-overview. Accessed November 1, 2009.
78. Lizakowski S, Zdrojewski Z, Jagodzinski P, Rutkowski B. Plasma tissue factor and tissue factor pathway inhibitor in patients with primary glomerulonephritis. *Scand J Urol Nephrol.* 2007;41:237–242.
79. Travis L. Nephrotic syndrome. *EMedicine.* http://www.emedicine.com/med/topic1564.htm. Accessed August 25, 2008.
80. Levin WJ, Raugi GJ. Paraneoplastic diseases. *EMedicine.* http://www.emedicine.com/DisplayTopic.asp?bookid=2&topic=552. Accessed September 11, 2008.
81. Weiss P, O'Rourke MF. Cutaneous paraneoplastic syndromes. *Clin J Oncol Nurs.* 2000;4:257–262.
82. Zumsteg MM, Casperson DS. Paraneoplastic syndromes in metastatic disease. *Semin Oncol Nurs.* 1998;14:220–229.
83. Wilcock A, Twycross RG. Symptom management in palliative care: optimizing drug treatment. *Br J Hosp Med.* 2006;67:400–403.
84. Dy SM, Lorenz KA, Naeim A, Sanati H, Walling A, Asch SM. Evidence-based recommendations for cancer fatigue, anorexia, depression, and dyspnea. *J Clin Oncol.* 2008;26:3886–3895.
85. Davis MP, Dreicer R, Walsh D, Lagman R, LeGrand SB. Appetite and cancer-associated anorexia: a review. *J Clin Oncol.* 2004;22:1510–1517.
86. Chamberlain JS. Cachexia in cancer—zeroing in on myosin. *N Engl J Med.* 2004;351:2124–2125.
87. Jatoi A. Pharmacologic therapy for the cancer anorexia/weight loss syndrome: data-driven practical approach. *J Support Oncol.* 2006;4:499–502.
88. Gordon JN, Trebble TM, Ellis RD, Duncan HD, Johns T, Goggin PM. Thalidomide in the treatment of cancer cachexia: randomized placebo controlled trial. *GUT.* 2005;54:540–545.
89. Perboni S, Bowers C, Koijima S. Growth hormone releasing peptide 2 reverses anorexia associated with chemotherapy with 5-fluoruracil in colon cancer cell-bearing mice. *World J Gastroenterol.* 2000;14:6303–6305.
90. Naschitz JE, Rosner I. Musculoskeletal syndromes associated with malignancy (excluding hypertrophic osteoarthropathy). *EMedicine.* http://www.medscape.com/viewprogram/8735_pnt. Accessed February 24, 2010
91. Penel N, Fournier C, Clisant S, et al. Fever and solid tumor: diagnostic value of procalcitonin and c-reactive protein. *Rev Med Interne.* 2001;22:706–714.

CHAPTER 35

Diane G. Cope, PhD, ARNP-C, AOCNP®

# Malignant Effusions

## INTRODUCTION

An effusion is an accumulation of fluid in body tissue or cavities. Malignant effusions are the accumulation of fluid caused by a neoplastic process and are associated with morbidity and mortality in the patient with cancer. Malignant effusions can be a presenting sign and symptom at the time of diagnosis but are more often seen in patients with advanced metastatic disease.[1,2] Overall, the prognosis of patients with malignant effusions is poor. The types of malignant effusions most frequently encountered are pleural, pericardial, and peritoneal.

## PLEURAL EFFUSIONS

### SCOPE OF THE PROBLEM

Malignant pleural effusions are the accumulation of excess fluid in the pleural space. They can occur as the result of a neoplastic process due to direct pleural invasion or secondary to impaired pleural lymphatic drainage from a mediastinal tumor.

Approximately 40% to 50% of pleural effusions are due to malignancy and, in patients older than 50 years of age, cancer is the second leading cause of pleural effusion.[3,4] As a result of the increasing incidence of breast and lung cancer, an estimated 200,000 to 250,000 new cases of malignant pleural effusions are identified annually,[5] affecting approximately 1.3 million individuals.[6] The most common cancers associated with malignant pleural effusion are lung cancer, breast cancer, and lymphoma, accounting for approximately two-thirds of all malignant pleural effusions.[2] In male patients, approximately 50% of malignant effusions are caused by lung cancer, 20% by lymphoma or leukemia, 7% by gastrointestinal primaries, 6% by genitourinary primaries, and 11% by tumors of unknown primary sites. In female patients, about 40% of malignant effusions are caused by breast cancer, 20% by gynecological tumors, 15% by lung primaries, 8% by lymphoma or leukemia, 4% by gastrointestinal primaries, and 9% by tumors of unknown primary sites.[7]

### PHYSIOLOGIC ALTERATIONS

The pleurae are composed of mesothelial cells that envelop the lungs. They encompass the visceral pleura, the outer lining of the lung, and the parietal pleura, the inner lining of the thoracic cavity (Figure 35-1).[8] The pleural space is between the visceral and parietal pleura and normally contains 5 to 15 mL hypoproteinemic plasma at one time, although 100 to 200 mL of fluid moves through the pleural space in a 24-hour period.[9]

Normally, a dynamic balance between the osmotic and hydrostatic pressures controls the secretion and reabsorption of pleural fluid. Alterations in fluid movement and changes in capillary permeability, hydrostatic and colloidal osmotic pressures, and lymphatic drainage can be caused by several neoplastic processes—for example, pleural implantation of cancer cells, lymphatic obstruction, venous obstruction, and tumor cell shedding.[1,2] Pleural implantation occurs when cancer cells seed or become implanted on the pleural surface, causing increased capillary permeability and inflammation of the pleural surface with leakage of fluid into the pleural space. This phenomenon is most commonly seen in patients with lung cancer. Lymphatic obstruction occurs when pulmonary lymphatic drainage becomes obstructed, causing alterations in fluid and protein reabsorption. This problem may occur with bulky tumor obstruction or lymph node involvement and is most commonly seen with lymphomas and metastatic breast and lung cancer. Pulmonary venous obstruction causes alterations in hydrostatic pressure, resulting in decreased fluid reabsorption. It may be seen with lung cancer. Tumor cell shedding into the pleural space decreases osmotic pressure, resulting in decreased

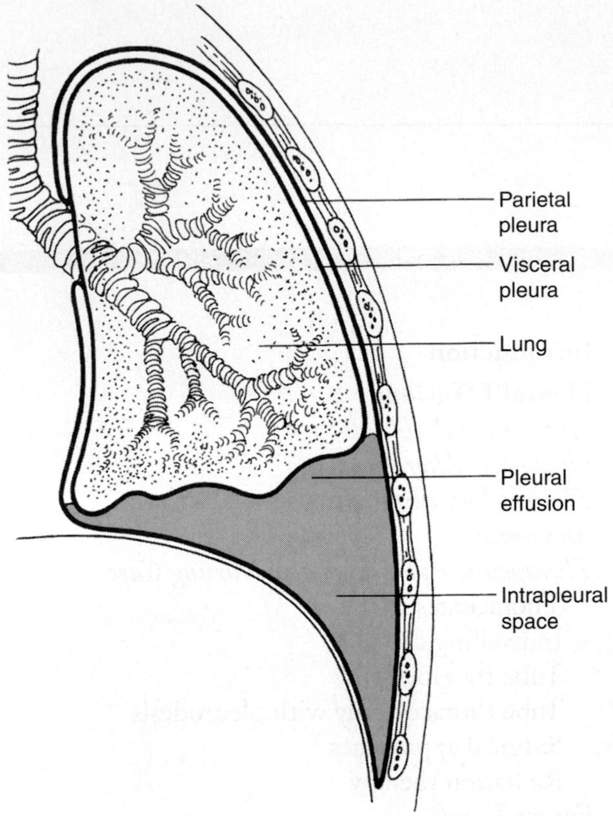


**FIGURE 35-1**

In the lung, fluid is constantly being filtered across the intrapleural space from the parietal pleural surface and reabsorbed through the visceral pleura. When obstruction by malignant processes prevents reabsorption, fluid accumulates in the intrapleural space and a pleural effusion results.

fluid reabsorption; it may be seen with lung and breast cancers.[1,7]

## CLINICAL MANIFESTATIONS

Decreased respiratory function depends on the amount and rate of pleural fluid accumulation and the patient's baseline pulmonary status. Fluid accumulation restricts lung expansion, reduces lung volume, alters the ventilation and perfusion capacity, and results in abnormal gas exchange and hypoxia. Malignant pleural effusions usually develop slowly, in contrast to other etiologies that cause rapid onset with sudden dyspnea. Patients may be asymptomatic with malignant pleural effusions and become apparent as an incidental finding on imaging studies although presenting symptoms typically include cough, severe dyspnea, especially with exertion, and chest discomfort that can range from dull ache to sharp pleuritic pain.[2,10] The dyspnea progresses to orthopnea as the effusion increases.

## ASSESSMENT

A thorough history and physical examination with diagnostic studies are critical in guiding the evaluation and diagnosis of a malignant pleural effusion, because several other conditions can produce pleural effusion and must be included in a differential diagnosis list. These alternative etiologies may include trauma, tuberculosis, renal failure, benign pleural effusion, congestive heart failure, coronary artery bypass graft surgery, acute bacterial pneumonia, pulmonary embolism, cirrhosis with ascites, pancreatitis, superior vena cava syndrome, collagen vascular disease, and chemotherapy-induced effusions.[6] Definitive diagnosis of malignant pleural effusion is based on a positive cytological analysis of pleural fluid, although fluid analysis is diagnostic in only 50% of individuals with malignant pleural effusion.[2]

A patient's history should focus on pulmonary complaints (Table 35-1). Cough associated with pleural effusion is described as a dry, nonproductive cough that increases with activity, conversation, or deep inspiration. Chest discomfort is usually present near the involved lung. The patient may also report decreased appetite and oral intake as well as excessive fatigue.

A patient's physical examination should include baseline vital signs, patient appearance, mental status, and lung assessment (Table 35-2). Alterations suggestive of pleural effusion may include hypertension, tachycardia, tachypnea, cyanosis, weight gain, low-grade fever, shortness of breath with conversation or exertion, decreased level of consciousness, intercostal prominence, dullness on percussion, decreased tactile fremitus, and decreased breath sounds.[4,5]

Diagnostic studies for pleural effusions include a posterior–anterior chest film, a lateral decubitus film, a contrast-enhanced chest computed tomography (CT), a positron emission tomography (PET) with fluorine-18-deoxyglucose (FDG), and arterial blood gases or oxygen saturation evaluation. Posterior–anterior chest x-rays with effusion will reveal costophrenic angle blunting and an opaque shadow in the involved lung (Figure 35-2). A lateral decubitus will identify small effusions less than 200 mL.

A chest CT may reveal possible primary tumors such as a breast or lung mass. Furthermore, chest CT includes images of the upper abdomen that may identify adrenal or hepatic metastases.[10] Chest CT findings that are suggestive of malignant pleural effusion include circumferential pleural thickening, nodular pleural thickening, parietal pleural thickening >1 cm, and mediastinal pleural involvement.[10,11]

A PET-FDG scan has a reported sensitivity that approaches 100% for malignant pleural disease. Fused images of PET-FDG and CT scans facilitate the identification of PET abnormalities for needle guided biopsies.[10] Oxygen saturation may be compromised with pleural effusions. However, oxygen saturation provides limited diagnostic data and should be used as a supplement to other more definitive assessment data for malignant pleural effusion.

Further diagnostic testing includes a thoracentesis with pleural fluid analysis. Pleural fluid analysis requires a sample of at least 25 to 50 mL for adequate analysis and evaluates for transudate vs exudate, color (bloody, turbid, milky, or straw-colored), glucose, protein, lactate dehydrogenase (LDH), and

**TABLE 35-1**

| Patient History and Assessment: Pleural Effusion |
|---|
| 1. When did the shortness of breath begin? |
| 2. Are you able to carry on your normal activities? |
| 3. Are you able to lay flat or supine to sleep? |
| 4. Do you need several pillows to sleep? |
| 5. Is your cough dry or productive? |
| 6. Have you seen any blood in your sputum? |
| 7. Do you have any chest discomfort or pain and, if so, where is it located? |

**TABLE 35-2**

| Physical Examination for Pleural Effusion |
|---|
| Weight: increased |
| Baseline vital signs: blood pressure, pulse, respiratory rate, temperature |
| Patient appearance: color, respiratory patterns, pain |
| Mental status: level of consciousness, orientation |
| Lung assessment: diaphragmatic alterations, percussion, auscultation |

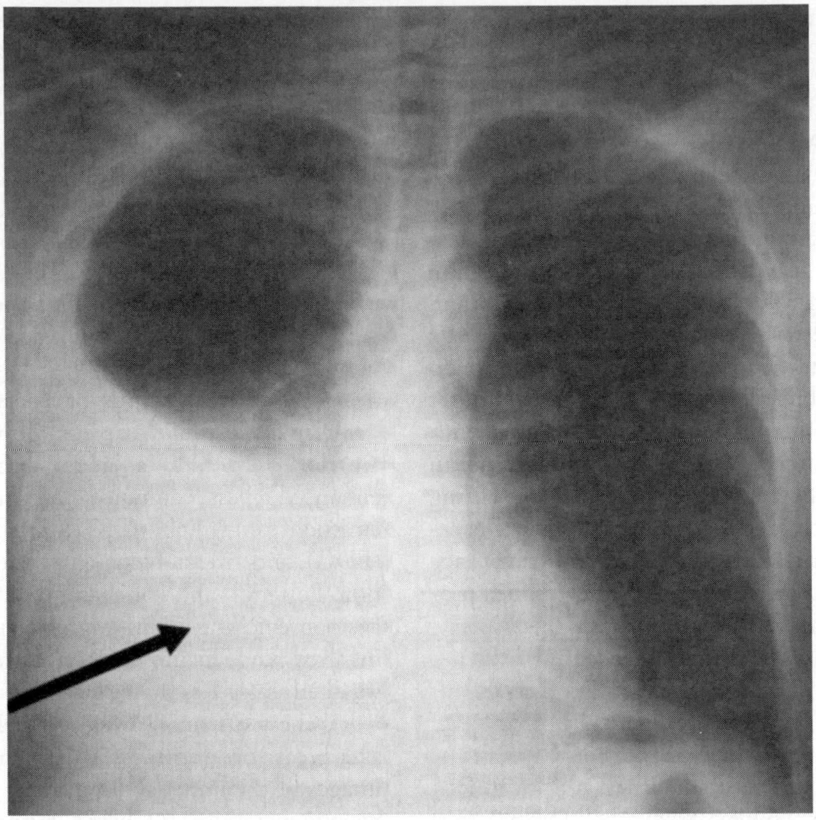

**FIGURE 35-2**

Chest x-ray film showing right pleural effusion.

*Source*: Courtesy of Rush University Medical Center, Chicago, IL.

lymphocyte content and cytology.[1] Fluids termed *transudate* are low in protein and are clear, watery, or lightly straw colored. By contrast, fluids termed *exudates* are high in protein and are dark yellowish, cloudy, or bloody in appearance. Positive pleural fluid cytologic analysis is found in approximately 50% of patients with pleural effusions, with an additional 20% being diagnosed as positive with repeat thoracentesis.[2] A therapeutic thoracentesis is usually performed at the same time as the diagnostic thoracentesis to provide immediate relief of symptoms.

The majority of malignant pleural effusions are classified as exudates. Pleural fluid consistent with malignancy characteristically is blood-tinged or grossly bloody, secondary to the disruption of capillaries or venules by direct tumor invasion, is hypercellular with leukocytes (predominantly lymphocytes and monocytes), and possesses an elevated LDH level, low pH, and a low glucose level (Table 35-3). Tumor marker concentrations in pleural fluid have been evaluated for their significance in determining benign vs malignant pleural effusion. Tumor markers such as carcinoembryonic antigen (CEA), carbohydrate antigen 15-3, cytokeratin 19 fragments, and cancer antigen 125 (CA 125) may be detected by electrochemiluminescence and microparticle enzyme immunoassays of pleural fluid. At present, no tumor markers have been proven useful as a diagnostic study.[10]

**TABLE 35-3**

| Characteristics of Malignant Pleural Fluid | |
|---|---|
| Color | Cloudy, straw-colored, bloody, or purulent |
| pH level | < 7.3 |
| LDH level | > 1000 IU/L |
| Glucose level | < 60 mg/dL |

*Source*: Data from Heffner and Klein.[10]

## THERAPEUTIC APPROACHES AND NURSING CARE

The approach to the treatment of a malignant pleural effusion depends on the type of tumor and previous therapy that the patient has had (Figure 35-3). Patients with chemosensitive tumors, such as small cell lung cancer and high-grade non-Hodgkin's lymphomas, and small, asymptomatic

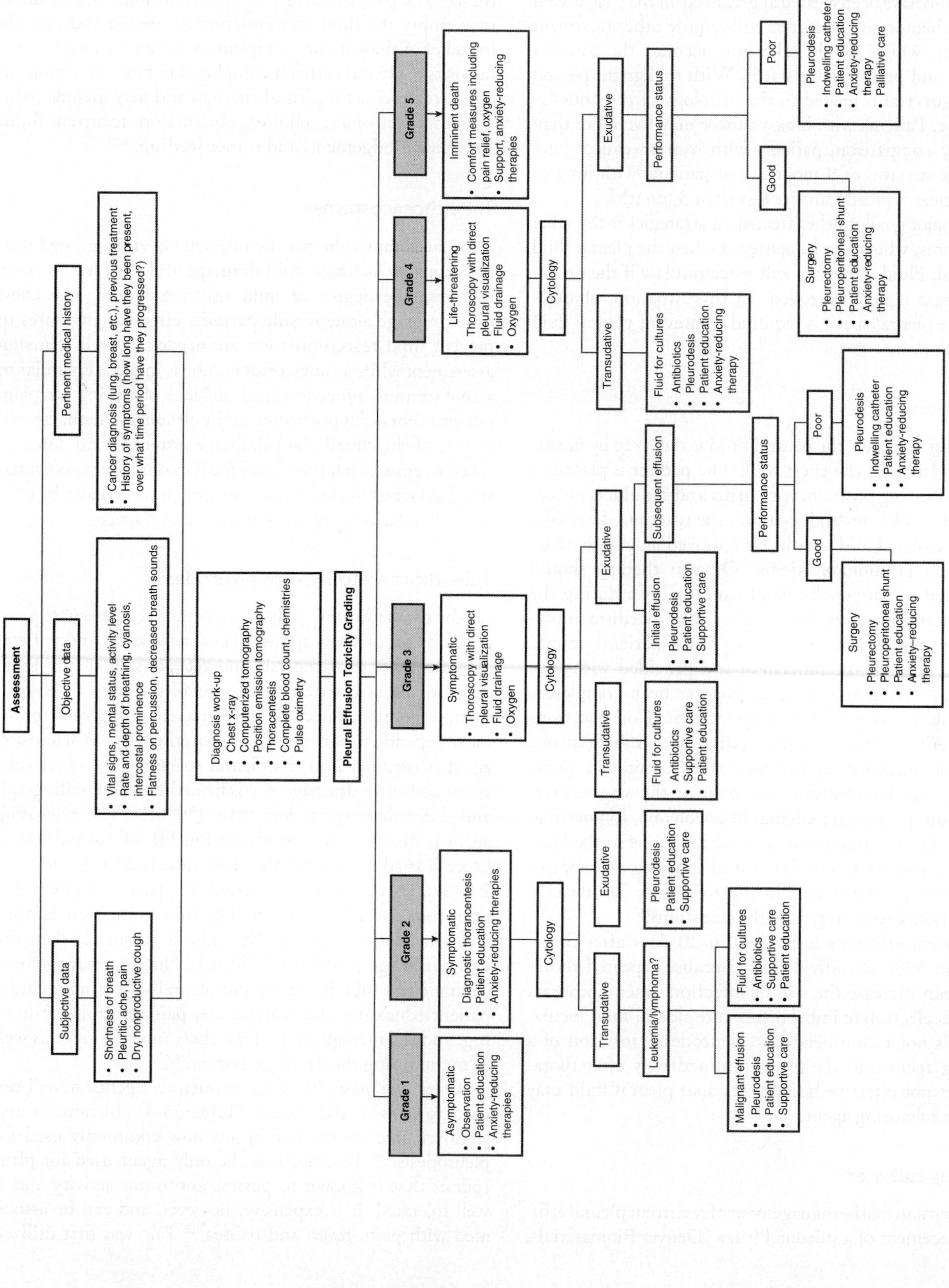


**FIGURE 35-3** Algorithm for the management of pleural effusion.

effusions will usually respond to systemic chemotherapy or hormonal therapy. If a patient possesses a chemosensitive tumor and is asymptomatic, proceeding with chemotherapy or hormonal therapy may be an initial treatment option. Patients who have been treated aggressively in the past or who possess a chemoresistant tumor will require other treatment approaches, which should take into account the patient's prognosis and performance status. With malignant pleural effusion, survival is related to the histology of the underlying disease. Patients with breast cancer may live more than 1 year; by comparison, patients with ovarian cancer have an average survival of 9 months and patients with lung or gastric cancer typically survive less than 3 months.[12]

The major goal of other treatment strategies is the relief of symptoms, which can be achieved when the pleural fluid is removed. Fluid, however, will reaccumulate if the underlying disease is not controlled. In this situation, obliteration of the pleural space is required to prevent pleural fluid reaccumulation.

### Thoracentesis

With a thoracentesis, the pleural fluid is removed by needle aspiration through the chest wall. The patient is placed in an upright sitting position, with arms and shoulders raised. This position elevates and separates the ribs to make needle insertion easier. Fluid should be removed slowly to avoid reexpansion pulmonary edema. Oxygen therapy should be provided to patients by nasal cannula both during the procedure and for several hours after the procedure to prevent hypoxemia.[6] Prior to thoracentesis, patients should be educated about the procedure and provided with supportive care. After the thoracentesis has been completed, they should be assessed for complications. Complications of thoracentesis may include bleeding with subcutaneous hematoma, infection of the pleural space or soft tissue overlying the thoracentesis site, pain at the site, vasovagal reaction, pulmonary edema, hypovolemia, hypoxemia, splenic or hepatic laceration, adverse reactions to the local anesthetic, pain from reexpansion of the lung and apposition of pleural surfaces, and, in approximately 5% of cases, pneumothorax requiring tube thoracostomy.[6]

Recurrent effusions occur within 30 days after thoracentesis in 97% of individuals.[10] Because repeated thoracentesis can increase the risk of infection, pneumothorax, empyema, electrolyte imbalances, and pleural fluid loculations, it is not recommended.[10] Pleurodesis, infusion of a sclerosing agent into the pleura, immediately after thoracentesis is not effective because residual pleural fluid may dilute the sclerosing agent.[2]

### Indwelling catheter

Another option for the management of recurrent pleural effusion is placement of a silicone Pleurx (Denver Biomaterials, Golden, CO) catheter. This catheter is ideal for patients with recurrent effusions unresponsive to therapy and is intended for long-term use. An externally draining catheter is surgically placed in the pleural space under local anesthesia. The patient, family caregiver, or home health nurse may empty the fluid accumulation as needed and provide for relief of the patient's symptoms without repeated hospital visits.[13] Pleural catheter complication rates are similar to other treatments for pleural effusion and may include pain, bleeding, empyema, cellulitis, obstruction, recurrent fluid, catheter dislodgement, and tumor seeding.[10,14]

### Tube thoracostomy

A thoracostomy tube may be inserted via video-guided thoracoscopy to facilitate fluid drainage and then left in place to assess the degree of fluid reaccumulation. The chest tube drainage alone is only partially effective: measures to prevent fluid reaccumulation are needed as well. Nursing assessment while a thoracostomy tube is in place is similar to a thoracentesis procedure and includes observing for pain, pneumothorax, hypotension, and pulmonary edema as well as care of the closed-chest drainage system.[15] Care must be taken to ensure that the chest tube remains patent, as exudative fluid tends to clot. Thoracostomy tubes can also be used to instill sclerosing agents into the pleural space.

### Tube thoracostomy with pleurodesis

A tube thoracostomy is placed to completely evacuate pleural fluid and to allow apposition of the visceral and parietal pleura after a thoracentesis and reexpansion of the lung. A chest tube is inserted at the level of the sixth or seventh intercostal space laterally and directed posteriorly to the most dependent portion of the pleural cavity.[2] A sclerosing agent is instilled into the pleural space via the chest tube when complete drainage is confirmed by chest radiograph and daily drainage is less than 150 mL. The sclerosing agent is dissolved in 100 mL to 150 mL of normal saline. Once it is administered, the chest tube is clamped for 1 to 2 hours. During this time period, the patient rotates positions to distribute the agent. The tube is then unclamped and attached to suction. The tube is removed when the daily drainage is less than 150 mL. Nursing management during chest tube insertion and pleural sclerosing includes patient education and reassurance, pain control, positioning, and the management of the chest tube drainage as well as maintaining the drainage system.[16,17]

Over the past 50 years, numerous agents have been used to achieve pleurodesis (Table 35-4). Bleomycin and sterilized talc are the two agents now commonly used for pleurodesis.[2,18] Bleomycin is the only agent used for pleurodesis that is known to possess antitumor activity and is well tolerated. It is expensive, however, and can be associated with pain, fever, and nausea.[1,2] Talc was first utilized

**TABLE 35-4**

| Sclerosing Agents Commonly Used to Treat Pleural Effusion |
|---|
| Talc |
| Bleomycin |
| Tetracycline |
| Doxycycline |
| Quianacrine |
| Nitrogen mustard |
| Minocycline |
| Mitomycin |

in 1950 and has been shown to be superior to other sclerosing agents, including tetracycline, doxycycline, and bleomycin.[2,18,19] Talc possesses a 71% to 96% success rate and is cost-effective, with minimal side effects that include fever, dyspnea, chest pain, atelectasis, pneumonia, arrhythmias, empyema, and acute respiratory failure.[10]

Biologic response modifiers have been used as a sclerosing agent to treat malignant pleural effusions because of their antitumor activity. Biological response modifiers—interferons and interleukin-2—must be given in high systemic doses and are associated with severe side effects, such as fever, pruritus, skin rashes, flulike syndromes, and transient increase in pleural effusion.[3,18] These agents have not been compared with talc in large randomized trials and are not routinely administered for malignant pleural effusions.[10]

### Surgical approaches

If a pleural effusion persists after other treatment methods have been performed, surgery is another option for patients with good performance status and longer life expectancy. Pleurectomy—stripping of the parietal pleura and obliterating the pleural space—is 100% effective in controlling malignant pleural effusion[2] and is used as the primary therapeutic modality for patients with some types of mesothelioma that are frequently associated with the development of pleural effusions.[19] More recently, pleurectomy via video-assisted thoracoscopic surgery rather than thoracotomy has been performed.[19] Despite recent surgical advances, pleurectomy possesses significant morbidity and mortality rates.[2]

Another surgical option for therapeutic management of malignant pleural effusion is the pleuroperitoneal shunt. The shunt is used for patients with recurrent effusions that are refractory to tube thoracostomy and pleurodesis or for patients with malignant pleural effusions associated with trapped lung.[2] (A trapped lung is a fibroelastic peel that covers the visceral pleura on part or all of a lung lobe. The lobe cannot expand, which causes negative pressure between the chest wall and the nonexpanding lung. Fluid can enter into the pleural space, causing a pleural effusion. Trapped lung can be caused by empyema, malignancy, postcardiac and pericardial surgery, hemothorax, and tuberculosis.) The shunt is composed of a silicone rubber conduit with a unidirectional valved pump chamber that connects to pleural and peritoneal catheters. The pumping chamber, implanted into a subcutaneous pocket or placed as an external pumping chamber, requires active pumping at least 400 times a day. Patients who are unable to compress the pumping chamber, have pleural infection, multiple loculations, short-life expectancy, or an obliterated peritoneal space are not candidates for this procedure.[2] Shunt complications that require shunt revision or replacement occur in approximately 15% of patients and involve infection, skin erosion, and clotting of the catheter and shunt obstruction.[20]

### Radiation therapy

Radiation therapy is indicated for treatment of the underlying disease, although it is not recommended for first-line management of malignant pleural effusions. Radiation used to treat the mediastinal tumors seen with lymphoma and lung cancer has been effective in decreasing obstruction due to bulky tumor, thereby improving pleural fluid reabsorption. Side effects of radiation therapy to the lung field include cough, radiation pneumonitis, and increased sputum production.

## FUTURE TRENDS

Overall, the prognosis for patients with malignant pleural effusion is poor, with 65% dying within 3 months and 80% dying within 6 months.[2] Treatment for malignant pleural effusion at present focuses on the treatment of underlying malignant disease and palliation of symptoms. Recently gained knowledge into the molecular mechanisms involved in pleural inflammation has focused attention on new substances, such as transforming growth factor beta and vascular endothelial growth factor, as possible sclerosing agents for the future. More studies are needed to elucidate the potential use of these substances. Further research is also needed to investigate procedures that are cost-effective and produce minimal side effects with consideration of patients' quality of life, performance status, and activity levels.

# PERICARDIAL EFFUSIONS

## SCOPE OF THE PROBLEM

Pericardial effusion is an accumulation of excess fluid in the pericardial sac that can result from infection, inflammation, or metastatic or primary disease. Pericardial effusion is the most common cardiac complication associated with cancer

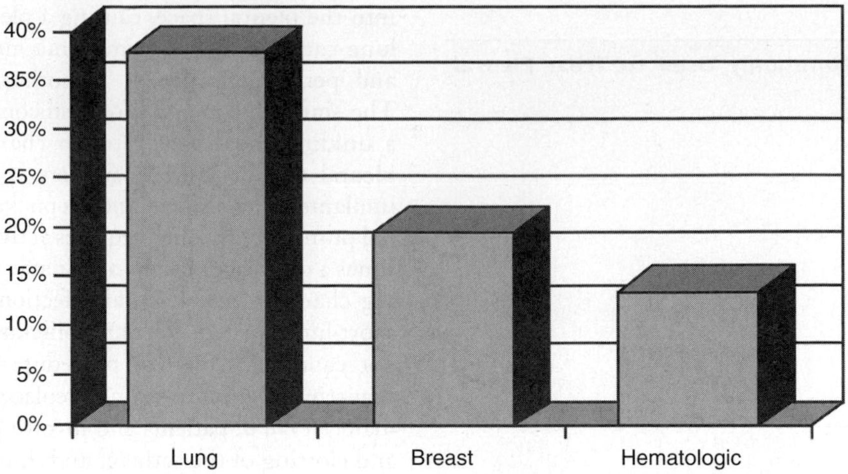


**FIGURE 35-4**

Tumor types associated with pericardial effusions. Incidence is illustrated as a percent of all pericardial effusions.
*Source*: Data from Taubert.[22]

and indicates a poor prognosis, with patients generally surviving less than 6 months after its occurrence regardless of treatment.[2]

Pericardial effusions are present in approximately 5% to 15% of patients with cancer at the time of autopsy.[21] Approximately 50% of pericardial effusions in patients with cancer are malignant.

Malignant pericardial effusion is most often associated with lung (36.5%) and breast (22.3%) cancers. However, other malignancies are also associated with increased risk of pericardial effusion, such as leukemia and lymphoma (17.2%), sarcoma (3.5%), and melanoma (2.7%) (Figure 35-4).[22] Patients with cancer may develop pericardial effusion as a result of direct tumor extension with lung or esophageal cancers or as a result of chemotherapy-induced pericarditis or anthracycline therapy. Radiation therapy greater than 4000 cGy to the mediastinal area involving at least 33% of the heart can lead to radiation-induced pericarditis.[23] In addition, pericardial effusions can be related to hypothyroidism, hypoalbuminemia, renal failure, collagen vascular disease, chest trauma, aneurysm, uremia, autoimmune disorders, improper insertion or placement of central venous catheters, or viral, fungal, or bacterial infection-related pericarditis.[1,24]

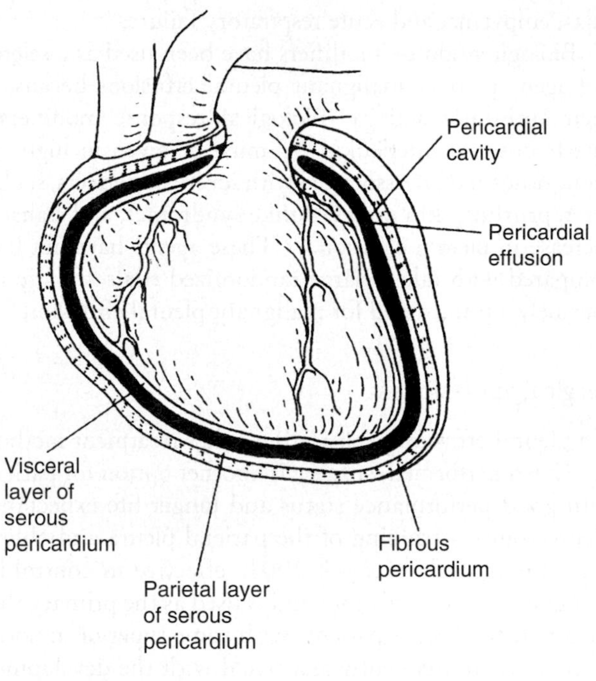


**FIGURE 35-5**

Structure of the pericardium with effusion present.

## PHYSIOLOGIC ALTERATIONS

The heart is surrounded by the pericardium, a thin, fibrous sac composed of two membranous layers, the visceral pericardium and the parietal pericardium (Figure 35-5). The visceral pericardium is the inner membrane that is connected to the surface of the heart. The parietal pericardium is the outer fibrous membrane that is in direct contact with the chest wall and provides structure and protection for the heart. The pericardial sac between the two membranes normally contains 15 to 50 mL of clear, serous, lubricating fluid that decreases friction during cardiac contraction. This pericardial fluid is produced by the lymphatic channels surrounding the heart and is reabsorbed by the lymphatic system into the mediastinum and right heart cavities.

Malignant pericardial effusions occur as a result of excess fluid accumulation from obstruction of the venous and lymphatic drainage by direct tumor invasion or from lymphatic or hematogenous spread. The majority of malignant pericardial effusions result from blockage of the lymphatic drainage of the heart. The effects of pericardial effusion accumulation depend on the rate of fluid accumulation, the physical compliance capacity of the pericardial cavity, ventricular function, myocardial size, and blood volume. If the fluid accumulation is gradual, the pericardium is able to stretch and accommodate as much as 2 liters of fluid without symptoms.[14] However, normal compensatory mechanisms are unable to adapt, with rapid fluid development of only 150 to 200 mL resulting in severe cardiac compromise and symptoms.[25]

## CLINICAL MANIFESTATIONS

Symptoms associated with pericardial effusion are related to the rate of effusion accumulation. The most common symptoms include cough, fever, dyspnea, orthopnea, chest pain, and edema, although patients may also report weakness, dysphagia, syncope, and palpitations.[2,21] The most common signs of pericardial effusion are rales, tachypnea, tachycardia, hypotension, peripheral edema, paradoxical pulse, distant heart sounds, and pericardial rub.[21]

## ASSESSMENT

In most patients with cancer, malignant pericardial effusions may be asymptomatic and go undiagnosed until the late stages of the disease.[1,2] Although the symptoms of pericardial effusion—dyspnea, cough, orthopnea, and chest pain—can be related to numerous other etiologies, the clinician should have a high index of suspicion for pericardial involvement whenever patients with cancer present with cardiovascular symptoms.

The physical assessment should include a thorough examination focusing on the cardiac system. This examination should include blood pressure, pulse, respiratory rate, color, breath sounds, jugular venous distention, peripheral pulses, heart sounds, and abdominal girth. Physical exam findings consistent with pericardial effusion include cyanosis, narrowing pulse pressure, pulsus paradoxus in which the pulse becomes weaker with inhalation and stronger with exhalation, jugular venous distention, weak distant heart sounds with arrythmias and possible friction rub, weak peripheral pulses, and increased abdominal distention.

Initial diagnostic studies should include an echocardiogram, an electrocardiogram(ECG), and an anterior–posterior chest film. The echocardiogram is the most commonly used diagnostic tool because it is a reliable, noninvasive test that can evaluate the effect of a pericardial effusion on ventricular function.[2] The gold standard for the diagnosis of pericardial effusion is the two-dimensional echocardiography that can identify the location and amount of effusion and the presence of pericardial or intracardiac masses.[2,26] Changes on the electrocardiogram associated with pericardial effusion include tachycardia, atrial and ventricular arrhythmia, low QRS voltage, ST elevations, and T-wave inversion.[21] Chest radiographic changes associated with pericardial effusion include cardiomegaly, bilateral pleural effusions, mediastinal widening, and hilar lymphadenopathy. The heart may have a "water-bottle" appearance that is indicative of a large pericardial effusion.[21] Computed tomography scan of the chest can identify pericardial fluid, as minimal as 50 mL, as well as pericardial thickening and masses.[2,27] CT scans may be more time consuming and provide similar information as the echocardiography and therefore is not the preferred study for diagnosing pericardial effusion.

Pericardiocentesis is another diagnostic tool; albeit one that requires an invasive procedure. For this reason, its use is reserved for individuals who are symptomatic from a large effusion. While the patient is sitting at a 30° to 45° angle to allow for pericardial fluid to pool inferiorly, a local anesthetic is administered. The pericardial sac is entered by passing an 18- or 19-gauge needle attached to a large syringe cephalad at an angle of approximately 45° and directed at the patient's scapula. The fluid is analyzed to determine whether it is a transudate or an exudate, and is sent for bacterial, fungal, and mycobacterial cultures and cytology. Malignant pericardial fluid is exudative or bloody in appearance. Positive cytologic examination is confirmed in only 50% to 60% of pericardial effusions in patients with cancer.[2] Complications associated with pericardiocentesis are myocardial puncture, coronary artery or vein laceration, hemopericardium, laceration of the internal mammary artery, pneumothorax, and liver and aortic injury.[21]

## THERAPEUTIC APPROACHES AND NURSING CARE

The goals of treatment for pericardial effusion are relief of symptoms, identification of positive cytology and prevention of fluid reaccumulation. The patient's diagnosis, stage of disease, and performance status should be considered in determining treatment approaches (Figure 35-6).

Pericardiocentesis can be used as a diagnostic tool but is most frequently performed in symptomatic patients as a therapeutic procedure. Although it has a high success rate, fluid reaccumulation occurs in approximately 50% of patients; therefore, other definitive medical or surgical treatment is necessary to prevent recurrence.[28]

Nursing care during the pericardiocentesis includes explanation of the procedure to the patient; positioning the patient in a semi-Fowler's position; maintaining asepsis; and having available a defibrillator, oxygen, and emergency

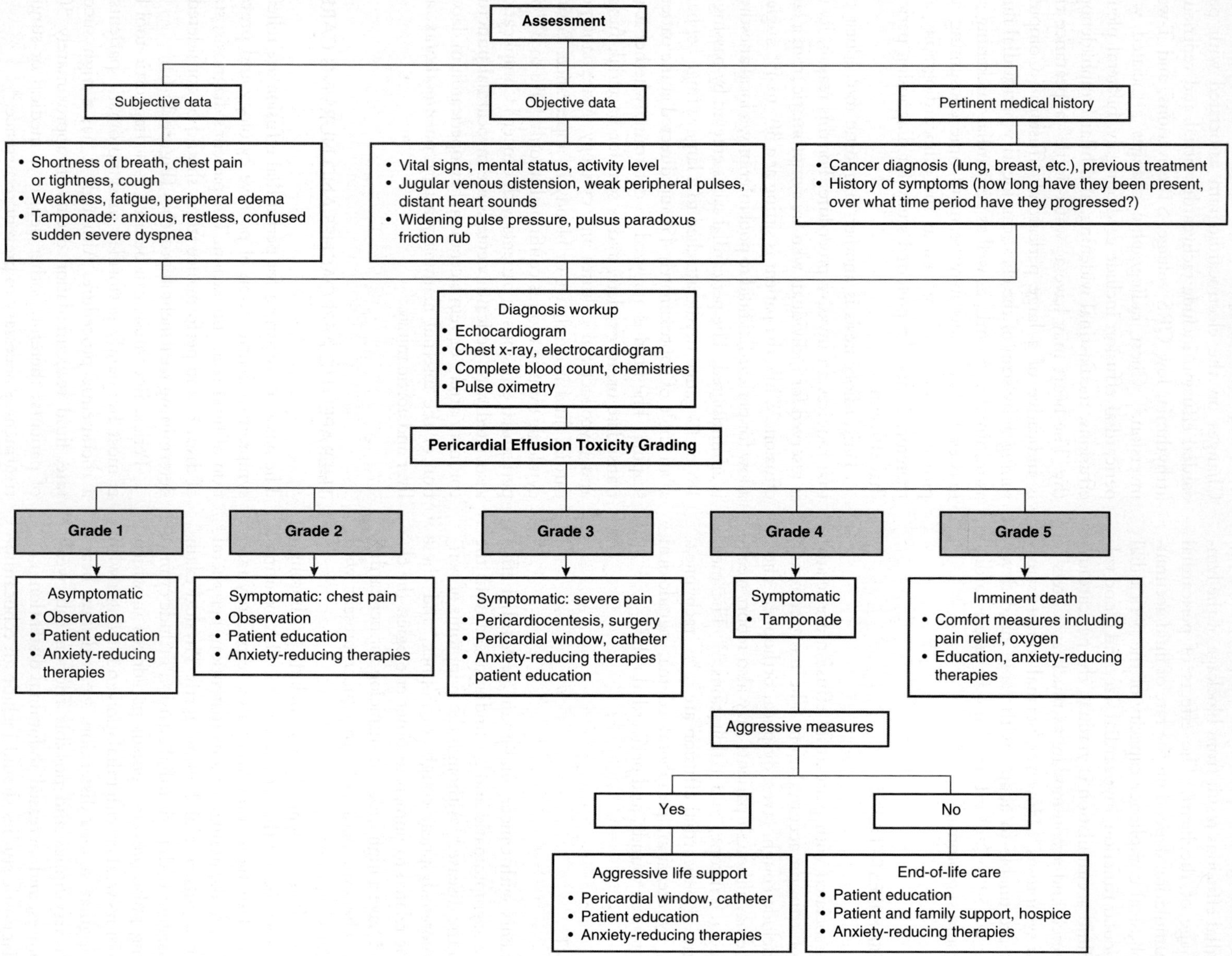
Assessment
Subjective data
Objective data
Pertinent medical history
• Shortness of breath, chest pain or tightness, cough
• Weakness, fatigue, peripheral edema
• Tamponade: anxious, restless, confused sudden severe dyspnea
• Vital signs, mental status, activity level
• Jugular venous distension, weak peripheral pulses, distant heart sounds
• Widening pulse pressure, pulsus paradoxus friction rub
• Cancer diagnosis (lung, breast, etc.), previous treatment
• History of symptoms (how long have they been present, over what time period have they progressed?)
Diagnosis workup
• Echocardiogram
• Chest x-ray, electrocardiogram
• Complete blood count, chemistries
• Pulse oximetry
Pericardial Effusion Toxicity Grading
Grade 1
Grade 2
Grade 3
Grade 4
Grade 5
Asymptomatic
• Observation
• Patient education
• Anxiety-reducing therapies
Symptomatic: chest pain
• Observation
• Patient education
• Anxiety-reducing therapies
Symptomatic: severe pain
• Pericardiocentesis, surgery
• Pericardial window, catheter
• Anxiety-reducing therapies patient education
Symptomatic
• Tamponade
Imminent death
• Comfort measures including pain relief, oxygen
• Education, anxiety-reducing therapies
Aggressive measures
Yes
No
Aggressive life support
• Pericardial window, catheter
• Patient education
• Anxiety-reducing therapies
End-of-life care
• Patient education
• Patient and family support, hospice
• Anxiety-reducing therapies

**FIGURE 35-6**

Algorithm for management of pericardial effusion.

medications. The nurse must continuously monitor the patient and the ECG during the pericardiocentesis and after the procedure to detect any cardiac or pulmonary abnormalities.

### Subxiphoid pericardiostomy

Subxiphoid pericardiostomy (pericardial window) is the most commonly performed procedure for pericardial effusions and can be performed under local anesthesia. A small, vertical skin incision is made in the subxiphoid region. The anterior pericardium is incised, and fluid is drained. Next, the pericardium is explored and a sample is obtained for pathologic studies. A pericardial tube is then placed in the upper abdominal wall into the pericardial space to allow for drainage. For subxiphoid pericardiostomy, the overall mortality rate is approximately 46%, the overall morbidity rate is approximately 1.53%, and the recurrence rate for effusion is approximately 3.5%.[2] Nursing care is the same as for the pericardiocentesis.

### Balloon pericardiotomy

Balloon pericardiotomy is a nonsurgical procedure that is performed to create a pericardial window. After percutaneously accessing the pericardial space, a guide wire is threaded into the pericardium. A balloon-dilating catheter is then inserted and inflated to create a pericardial window for fluid drainage. This procedure has been found to be helpful in the management of massive pericardial effusions in patients with poor performance status.[29]

### Pericardiocentesis with sclerosing agent instillation

Pericardiocentesis with the instillation of sclerosing agents has been used to obliterate the pericardial space by inducing an inflammatory response with resultant fibrosis and sclerosis in the pericardium. Sclerosing agents used in the management of pericardial effusions have included tetracycline, doxycycline, thiotepa, bleomycin, minocycline, 5-fluorouracil, cisplatin, and nitrogen mustard; of these options, tetracycline and doxycycline have been the most extensively evaluated sclerosing agents.[2] This treatment approach controls the pericardial effusion for longer than 30 days in more than 90% of patients. Other sclerosing agents found to be associated with minimal side effects while controlling malignant pericardial effusions include carboplatin[30] and cisplatin.[31,32]

### Surgery

Surgical intervention, including transthoracic pericardial window via thoracotomy and pericardiectomy, is generally reserved for individuals who require repeated pericardiocentesis and are medically appropriate patients because general anesthesia and thoracotomy are required. Patients undergoing transthoracic drainage are at increased risk for complications including pneumonia, pleural effusion, respiratory failure, cardiac arrhythmia, deep-vein thrombosis, and pulmonary embolism. In comparison to thoracotomy, a preferred option is video-assisted thoracoscopy, which is less invasive.[2,33]

### Radiation therapy

Radiation therapy is generally indicated for patients with leukemia/lymphoma or breast carcinoma.[2] Radiation therapy is associated with several weeks of daily treatments or prolonged hospitalization, and can potentially cause acute pericarditis or myocarditis. The usual dose for palliative radiotherapy is 100 to 200 cGy daily for approximately 3 to 4 weeks.[24]

### FUTURE TRENDS

At the present time, subxiphoid pericardial window is the preferred surgical treatment for pericardial effusion. Further research is needed to investigate sclerosing agents, patient characteristics, and less-invasive, cost-effective procedures that may enhance patients' quality of life.

## MALIGNANT PERITONEAL EFFUSIONS

### SCOPE OF THE PROBLEM

Malignant peritoneal effusion, commonly termed ascites, is fluid accumulation in the peritoneal cavity, a sac located between the parietal and visceral peritoneum. The most likely cause of ascites in a patient with known intra-abdominal cancer is spread of disease. This condition is associated with a poor prognosis. Treatment is usually aimed at palliative care, with survival typically lasting only a few months.

Although ascites may occur with many types of carcinomas, its exact incidence is not well documented. Ascites is most often associated with ovarian cancer, with approximately 33% of patients having ascites at presentation and more than 60% having ascites at the time of death.[34] Malignant ascites can also occur commonly in patients with lymphoma, mesothelioma, ovarian, breast, gastric, hepatic, pancreatic, and colon carcinomas.[34,35]

### PHYSIOLOGIC ALTERATIONS

The peritoneal cavity is covered by a serous lining composed of the visceral peritoneum, which lines and supports the abdominal organs, and the parietal peritoneum. The parietal peritoneum covers the abdominal and pelvic walls

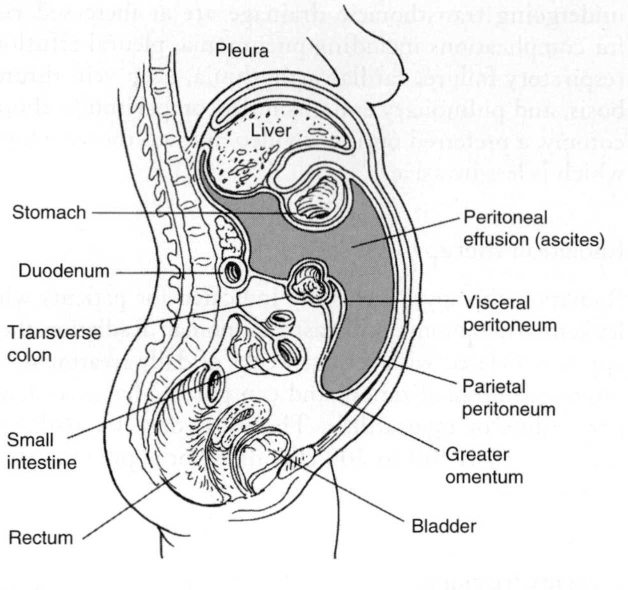


**FIGURE 35-7**

The peritoneal cavity is covered by the visceral peritoneum that lines and supports the abdominal organs, and the parietal peritoneum that covers the abdominal and pelvic walls and the undersurface of the diaphragm. If, due to malignant processes, the volume of fluid accumulating in the peritoneal space exceeds the capacity of lymphatic channels to drain the cavity, ascites develops.

and the undersurface of the diaphragm (Figure 35-7). Normally, a small amount of fluid is present to lubricate the cavity. Malignant ascites occurs when the fluid production exceeds the ability of the lymphatic channels to drain the cavity, because of increased peritoneal fluid production or lymphatic obstruction with decreased fluid reabsorption.

Enck has defined four types of malignant ascites.[36] The first and most common type is peripheral ascites. With peripheral ascites there is mechanical interference with venous and lymphatic drainage, which produces ascites and accounts for approximately 50% of all cases.

The second type is central ascites and occurs in approximately 20% of all cases. Portal and lymphatic flow is compromised as a result of hepatic metastases, and hypoalbuminemia—frequently seen in the patient with cancer—produces decreased oncotic pressure. Both of these pathophysiologic mechanisms increase ascites.

The third type is mixed ascites and occurs in approximately 20% of all cases. Malignant ascites is the result of both peripheral and central ascites with tumor involving the liver and peritoneal surface. The fourth type is chylous ascites and occurs with retroperitoneal metastasis that obstructs lymphatic drainage. This type is less common than the first three types of ascites.

Peripheral ascites can be caused by tumor seeding of the peritoneum, resulting in obstruction of the diaphragmatic and abdominal lymphatics. This phenomenon occurs primarily with gynecological cancers.[8] Widespread peritoneal carcinomatosis or tumor seeding results in damaged capillary endothelium and increased capillary permeability with increased peritoneal fluid formation. Tumors may also produce humoral factors that cause increased capillary leakage of proteins and fluids into the peritoneum. Tumor obstruction of the main thoracic duct or of the hepatic venous system will result in blockage of the lymphatic channels and impair normal lymphatic drainage. Patients with diffuse hepatic metastases and venous obstruction may develop a transudative ascites, as this condition is caused by hypoalbuminemia and increased portal vein pressure.

Additional factors that may facilitate the development of malignant ascites are now being explored. Vascular permeability factor (VPF) and vascular endothelial growth factor (VEGF) have been shown to increase microvascular endothelial cell permeability to plasma proteins, contributing to the development of malignant ascites.[37–40]

## CLINICAL MANIFESTATIONS

Symptoms of ascites vary depending on the amount of peritoneal fluid present. As the amount of ascitic fluid increases, its pressure on abdominal organs and visceral structures becomes restrictive. The abdomen is distensible and able to accommodate large volumes of ascitic fluid. Patients may become symptomatic when the fluid amount present is ≥500 mL.[8]

## ASSESSMENT

A detailed history should include the patient's recent dietary intake, urinary and bowel patterns, and abdominal complaints. Symptoms associated with ascites include abdominal distention, weight gain, indigestion, dyspnea, orthopnea, early satiety, anorexia, fatigue, abdominal or back pain, constipation, and urinary urgency, urinary frequency, and decreased output. In severe cases, massive ascites can cause intestinal obstruction, resulting in nausea and vomiting, and lower extremity lymphatic obstruction with the development of peripheral edema.

The physical examination should focus on a detailed abdominal and respiratory assessment. With malignant peritoneal effusion, the abdomen is usually distended with tightly stretched, shiny skin, and bulging flanks. The abdominal girth should be obtained as a baseline. Abdominal percussion reveals tympany in the upper and mid-abdominal regions and dullness over the flanks.[8] A Sister Mary Joseph nodule, a firm nodule located in the umbilicus, may be present and is suggestive of peritoneal carcinomatosis associated with gastric, pancreatic, or primary hepatic malignancy.[41] A fluid wave may also be present and may be elicited by placing the ulnar surface of the hand on the midline of the patient's abdomen and applying pressure, producing movement or a wave of the fluid. Bowel sounds may be high-pitched, diminished, or absent, depending on the amount of ascitic fluid. Ascites may also involve the respiratory system, with physical findings revealing diaphragm elevation and pleural effusions. The presence of pleural effusions will produce dullness upon percussion over the involved lung fields, with diminished breath sounds upon auscultation.

The presence of malignant ascites is assessed by several diagnostic studies, including abdominal x-ray, ultrasound, and CT scan, and paracentesis with fluid evaluation. An abdominal x-ray may reveal a generalized ground-glass appearance, with central positioning of the small bowel loops and separation of the bowel loops by ascitic fluid. Abdominal ultrasound and CT scan are very sensitive examinations to detect amounts of fluid as small as 5 to 10 mL.[41] A thickened caking of tumor noted on the omentum and peritoneal surfaces may be seen in patients with malignant ascites.[35] A paracentesis should be performed to confirm the diagnosis and provide relief of symptoms.

The fluid appearance can provide important information regarding the etiology of the fluid accumulation. Normal ascitic fluid is translucent yellow in appearance.[35] Bloody ascites, likely characterized as exudate, is often seen in ovarian or hepatocellular carcinoma but may also be associated with peritoneal carcinomatosis. Chylous ascites or a milky appearance may result from obstruction of the thoracic duct by lymphoma. Serous fluid may be suggestive of congestive heart failure or nephrotic syndrome. A cloudy appearance may be due to an infectious process. The fluid should be cultured for bacterial, fungal, and mycobacterial organisms and analyzed for protein, glucose, LDH, and amylase levels. Malignant ascites usually reveals elevated total protein and LDH levels.[35]

Baseline serum laboratories should be obtained to assess the metabolic and organ function of the patient. Laboratory studies include complete blood count, complete metabolic panel, prothrombin and partial thromboplastin times, urinalysis and tumor markers such as CA-125, CEA, CA 19–9, and CA 27–29.[42]

## THERAPEUTIC APPROACHES AND NURSING CARE

Malignant ascites is usually difficult to control in those individuals who develop fluid accumulation rapidly and are refractory to treatment. The majority of therapeutic approaches for malignant ascites focus on palliative care and symptom management (Figure 35-8).[43] Goals of nursing care are the maintenance of fluid and electrolyte balance, comfort measures, and early recognition of complications.

### Diuretics and albumin administration

The role of loop and aldosterone-inhibiting diuretics is unclear because of the limited number of randomized trials comparing diuretics with other treatment modalities and the limited data supporting the effectiveness of diuretics in controlling malignant ascites.[35] In addition, the administration of albumin has not been shown to delay fluid reaccumulation.

### Fluid removal—paracentesis

Removal of peritoneal fluid by paracentesis is useful as a diagnostic tool but has little therapeutic benefit because the fluid reaccumulates rapidly without other interventions. Removal of 2 to 3 liters of fluid and repeated paracentesis procedures can lead to infection, severe protein depletion, postural hypotension, intraperitoneal visceral injury, and electrolyte abnormalities.[35] Unlike ascites secondary to other etiologies, malignant ascites may be removed in large volumes, approximately 5 liters, without altering hemodynamic equilibrium.

### Obliteration of the intraperitoneal space

Intracavity therapy has included the instillation of a radioactive colloid suspension (no longer in favor) or a chemotherapeutic agent. The chemotherapy instillation is designed to provoke an inflammatory response, leading to sclerosis of the peritoneal space membranes. Modest responses to bleomycin instillation for palliation have been reported with no significant side effects.[44] Doxorubicin, cisplatin, carboplatin, etoposide, nitrogen mustard, and tetracycline have also been used as intraperitoneal sclerosing agents. Biologic response modifiers have been used as an alternative to chemotherapeutic agents, although further research is needed to elucidate their effectiveness.[32,44,45]

Obtaining access to the peritoneal cavity for drug administration is an important technical problem. The peritoneum can be entered on a temporary basis with various catheters, but repeated puncture of the abdominal wall and peritoneum can lead to increased risk of adhesions, bowel perforation, and peritonitis. Placement of a long-term catheter, such as a Tenckhoff, Pleurx, or Groshong catheter is often used to provide access for repeated paracentesis. The catheter can remain in place indefinitely and allows for peritoneal fluid sampling, fluid removal, and drug instillation. The catheter needs to be monitored for patency and signs of infection. In general, however, indwelling catheters enhance patient comfort by alleviating symptoms and reducing the need for repeated percutaneous paracentesis.[34,46,47]

## FUTURE TRENDS

At present, no definitive management guidelines for malignant ascites exist, although the mainstays of treatment include

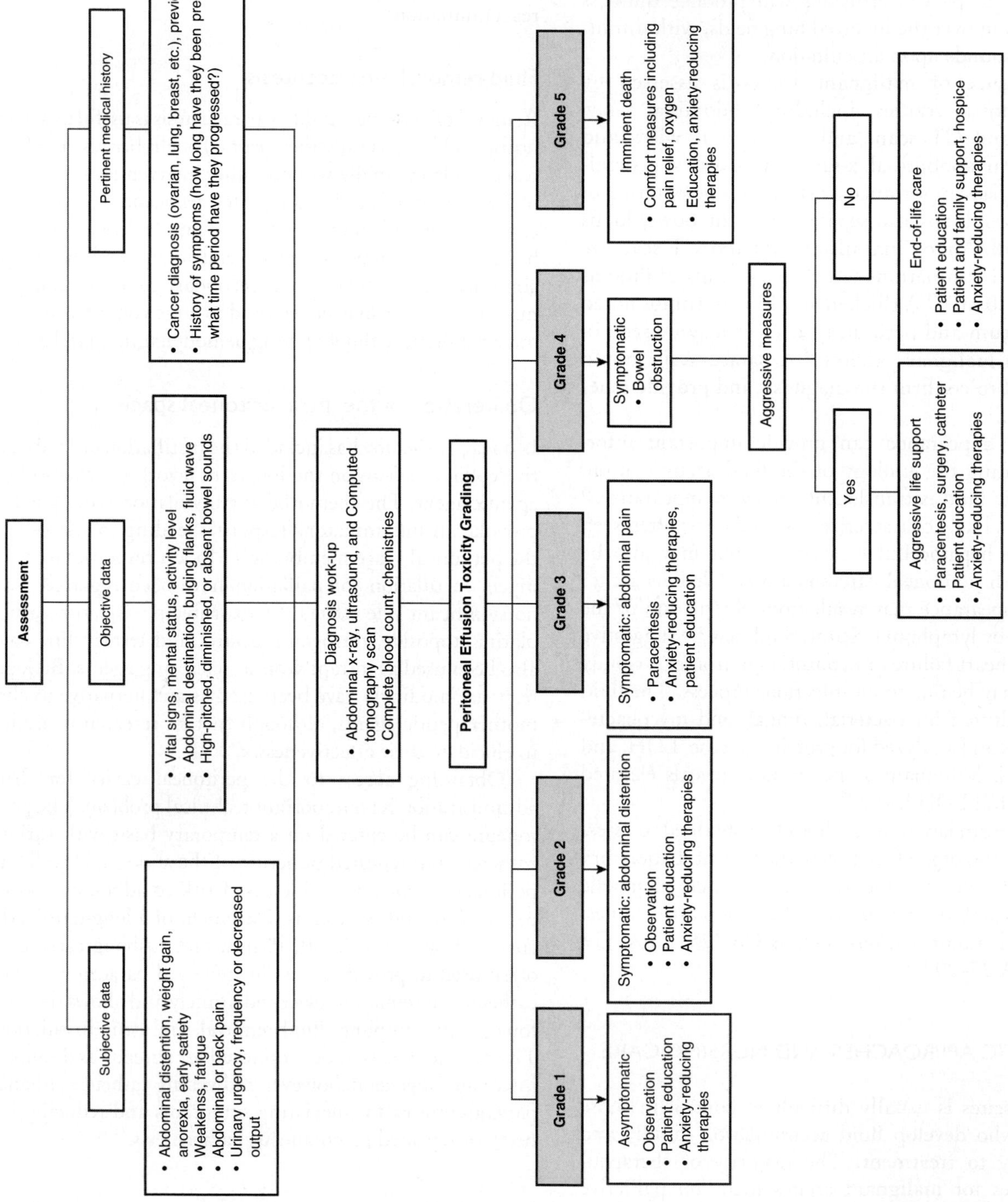

Assessment
Subjective data
• Abdominal distention, weight gain, anorexia, early satiety
• Weakenss, fatigue
• Abdominal or back pain
• Urinary urgency, frequency or decreased output
Objective data
• Vital signs, mental status, activity level
• Abdominal destination, bulging flanks, fluid wave
• High-pitched, diminished, or absent bowel sounds
Pertinent medical history
• Cancer diagnosis (ovarian, lung, breast, etc.), previous treatment
• History of symptoms (how long have they been present, over what time period have they progressed?)
Diagnosis work-up
• Abdominal x-ray, ultrasound, and Computed tomography scan
• Complete blood count, chemistries
Peritoneal Effusion Toxicity Grading
Grade 1
Asymptomatic
• Observation
• Patient education
• Anxiety-reducing therapies
Grade 2
Symptomatic: abdominal distention
• Observation
• Patient education
• Anxiety-reducing therapies
Grade 3
Symptomatic: abdominal pain
• Paracentesis
• Anxiety-reducing therapies, patient education
Grade 4
Symptomatic
• Bowel obstruction
Aggressive measures
Yes
Aggressive life support
• Paracentesis, surgery, catheter
• Patient education
• Anxiety-reducing therapies
No
End-of-life care
• Patient education
• Patient and family support, hospice
• Anxiety-reducing therapies
Grade 5
Imminent death
• Comfort measures including pain relief, oxygen
• Education, anxiety-reducing therapies

**FIGURE 35-8** Algorithm for the management of malignant peritoneal effusion.

*Source:* Data from US Department of Health and Human Services.[43]

diuretics and recurrent large-volume paracentesis. Recent evidence suggests that immune modulators, vascular permeability factors, and metalloproteinases may be significant contributing factors in the pathophysiologic process of malignant ascites.[37–40,47,48,49] Based on this rationale, new, more targeted therapies, such as matrix metalloproteinase inhibitors and VEGF antagonists, may offer better management of malignant ascites. Further research is needed to investigate these novel therapies.

## CONCLUSION

Malignant effusion, as a presenting sign or symptom or with advanced metastatic disease, is associated with a poor prognosis for patients with cancer. The goal of treatment is symptom relief and treatment of the underlying malignant disease; however, fluid often reaccumulates, producing significant morbidity. New therapies, such as vascular endothelial growth factor, matrix metalloproteinase inhibitors, and vascular endothelial growth factor antagonists, have been suggested but further research is needed to validate these therapies as future sclerosing agents to improve patients' quality of life.

## REFERENCES


1. Goldman D. Effusions. In: Yarbro CH, Frogge MH, Goodman M, eds. *Cancer Symptom Management.* 3rd ed. Sudbury, MA: Jones and Bartlett; 2004:420–439.
2. Nguyen DM. Malignant effusions of the pleura and the pericardium. In: DeVita VT, Lawrence TS, Rosenberg SA, eds. *DeVita, Hellman and Rosenberg's Cancer: Principles and Practice of Oncology.* 8th ed. Philadelphia, PA: Lippincott, Williams & Wilkins; 2008:2523–2532.
3. Schrump DS, Nguyen DM. Malignant pleural and pericardial effusions. In: DeVita VT, Hellman S, Rosenberg SA, eds. *Cancer: Principles and Practice of Oncology.* 6th ed. Philadelphia, PA: Lippincott, Williams & Wilkins; 2001:2729–2744.
4. Walker DL, Casciato DA. Malignant effusions. In: Haskell CM, ed. *Cancer Treatment.* 5th ed. Philadelphia, PA: W.B. Saunders; 2001:1578–1590.
5. Light RW. Pleural effusion. *N Engl J Med.* 2002;346:1971–1977.
6. Abrahamian FM. Pleural effusion. *eMedicine.* http://www.emedicine.com/emerg/topic462.htm. Accessed January 10, 2010.
7. Pass HI. Malignant pleural and pericardial effusions. In: DeVita VT, Hellman S, Rosenberg SA, eds. *Cancer: Principles and Practice of Oncology.* 5th ed. Philadelphia, PA: Lippincott-Raven; 1997:2586–2598.
8. Works C, Maxwell MB. Malignant effusions and edema. In: Yarbro CH, Frogge MH, Goodman M, Groenwald SL, eds. *Cancer Nursing: Principles and Practice.* 4th ed. Sudbury, MA: Jones and Bartlett; 2000:813–830.
9. Cope DG. Pleural effusions: Malignant. In: Chernecky CC, Murphy-Ende K, eds. *Acute Care Oncology Nursing.* 2nd ed. St. Louis, MO: Elsevier/Saunders; 2008:435–441.
10. Heffner JE, Klein JS. Recent advances in the diagnosis and management of malignant pleural effusions. *Mayo Clin Proc.* 2008;83:235–250.
11. Yilmaz U, Polat G, Sahin N, Soy O, Gulay U. CT in differential diagnosis of benign and malignant pleural disease. *Monaldi Arch Chest Dis.* 2005;63:17–22.
12. Fenton KN, Richardson JD. Diagnosis and management of malignant pleural effusion. *Am J Surg.* 1995;170:69–74.
13. Brubacher S, Gobel BH. Use of the Pleurx pleural catheter for the management of malignant pleural effusions. *Clin J Oncol Nurs.* 2003;7:35–38.
14. Stather DR, Tremblay A. Use of tunnelled pleural catheters for outpatient treatment of malignant pleural effusions. *Curr Opin Pulm Med.* 2007;13:328–333.
15. Shuey K, Payne Y. Malignant pleural effusion. *Clin J Oncol Nurs.* 2005;9:529–532.
16. Spiea AI, Brahmer JR. Effusions. In: Abeloff MD, Armitage JO, Niederhuber JE, et al, eds. *Clinical Oncology.* New York: Churchill Livingstone; 2004:1179–1212.
17. Marchi E, Teoxeora R, Vargas FS. Management of malignancy associated pleural effusion: current and future treatment strategies. *Am J Respir Med.* 2003;3:261–273.
18. Shaw P, Agarwal R. Pleurodesis for malignant pleural effusions. *Cochrane Database System Rev.* 2004;1:CD002916.
19. Nakas A, Martin Ucar AE, Edwards JG, Waller DA. The role of video-assisted thoracoscopic pleurectomy/decortication in the therapeutic management of malignant pleural mesothelioma. *Eur J Cardiothorac Surg.* 2008;33:83–87.
20. Genc O, Petrou M, Ladas G, Goldstraw P. The long-term morbidity of pleuroperitoneal shunts in the management of recurrent malignant effusions. *Eur J Cardiothorac Surg.* 2000;18:143–146.
21. Venugopalan P. Pericardial effusion, malignant. *eMedicine.* http://www.emedicine.com/ped/topic1764.htm. Accessed January 10, 2010.
22. Taubert J. Management of malignant pleural effusion. *Nurs Clin North Am.* 2001;36:665–683.
23. Shelton BK. Pericarditis/pericardial effusion/pericardial tamponade. In: Camp-Sorrell D, Hawkins RA, eds. *Clinical Manual for the Advanced Oncology Nurse.* 2nd ed. Pittsburgh, PA: Oncology Nursing Press; 2006:369–383.
24. Bullock B. Altered cardiac function. In: Bullock B, Henze R, eds. *Focus on Pathophysiology.* Philadelphia, PA: Lippincott; 2000:455–502.
25. DeMichele A, Glick J. Cancer-related emergencies. In: Lenhard R, Osteen R, Gansler T, eds. *Clinical Oncology.* Atlanta, GA: American Cancer Society; 2001:733–764.
26. Palacios IF. Pericardial effusion and tamponade. *Curr Treat Options Cardiovasc Med.* 1999;1:79–89.
27. Retter A. Pericardial disease in the oncology patient. *Heart Dis.* 2002;4:387–391.
28. Spodick DH. Acute cardiac tamponade. *N Engl J Med.* 2003;329: 684–690.
29. Wang HJ, Hsu KL, Chiang FT, et al. Technical and prognostic outcomes of double-balloon pericardiotomy for large malignancy-related pericardial effusions. *Chest.* 2002;122:893–899.
30. Moriya T, Takiguchi Y, Tabeta H, et al. Controlling malignant pericardial effusion by intrapericardial carboplatin administration in patients with primary non-small cell lung cancer. *Br J Cancer.* 2000;83:858–862.
31. Maisch B, Ristic AD, Pankuweit S, et al. Neoplastic pericardial effusion. Efficacy and safety of intrapericardial treatment with cisplatin. *Eur Heart J.* 2002;20:1625–1631.
32. Tomkowski WZ, Wisniewska J, Szturmowicz M, et al. Evaluation of intrapericardial cisplatin administration in cases with recurrent malignant pericardial effusion and cardiac tamponade. *Support Care Cancer.* 2004;1:53–57.
33. Lin JC, Hazelrigg SR, Landreneau RJ. Video-assisted thoracic surgery for diseases within the mediastinum. *Surg Clin North Am.* 2000;80:1511–1533.
34. Iyengar TD, Herzog TJ. Management of symptomatic ascites in recurrent ovarian cancer patients using an intra-abdominal semi-permanent catheter. *Am J Hosp Palliat Care.* 2002;1:35–38.
35. Kammula US. Malignant ascites. In: DeVita VT, Lawrence TS, Rosenberg SA, eds. *DeVita, Hellman and Rosenberg's Cancer: Principles and Practice of Oncology.* 8th ed. Philadelphia, PA: Lippincott, Williams & Wilkins; 2008:2533–2544.
36. Enck RE. Malignant ascites. *Am J Hosp Palliat Care.* 2002;19:7–8.

37. Zebrowski BK, Liu W, Ramirez K, et al. Markedly elevated levels of vascular endothelial growth factor in malignant ascites. *Ann Surg Oncol.* 1999;6:673.
38. Hicklin DJ, Ellis LE. Role of the vascular endothelial growth factor pathway in tumor growth and angiogenesis. *J Clin Oncol.* 2005;5:1011–1027.
39. Mesiano S, Ferrara N, Jaffe RB. Role of vascular endothelial growth factor in ovarian cancer: inhibition of ascites formation by immunoneutralization. *Am J Pathol.* 1998;153:1249.
40. Tamsma JT, Deizer HJ, Meinders AE. Pathogenesis of malignant ascites: starling's law of capillary hemodynamics revisited. *Ann Oncol.* 2001;12:1353.
41. Shah R. Ascites. *eMedicine.* http://www.emedicine.com/med/topic173.htm. Accessed January 10, 2010.
42. Murphy D. Malignant ascites. In: Chernecky CC, Murphy-Ende K, eds. *Acute Care Oncology Nursing.* 2nd ed. St. Louis, MO: Elsevier/Saunders; 2008:26–34.
43. US Department of Health and Human Services. *Common Terminology Criteria for Adverse Events (CTCAE)* v3.0. Bethesda, MD: National Institutes of Health/National Cancer Institute; 2003. http://ctep.cancer.gov/protocolDevelopment/electronic_applications/docs/ctcaev3.pdf. Accessed January 10, 2010.
44. Parsons SL, Watson SA, Steele JC. Malignant ascites. *Br J Surg.* 2005;1:6–14.
45. Lissoni P, Mandala M, Curigliano G, et al. Progress report on the palliative therapy of 100 patients with neoplastic effusions by intracavitary low-dose interleukin-2. *Oncology.* 2001;60:308–312.
46. Lee A, Lau TN, Yeong KY. Indwelling catheters for the management of malignant ascites. *Support Care Cancer.* 2000;6:493–499.
47. Richard HM, Coldwell DM, Boyd-Kranis RL, et al. Pleurx tunneled catheter in the management of malignant ascites. *J Vasc Intervent Radiol.* 2001;3:373–375.
48. Smith EM, Jayson GC. The current and future management of malignant ascites. *Clin Oncol.* 2003;15:59–72.
49. Aslam N, Marino CR. Malignant ascites: new concepts in pathophysiology, diagnosis, and management. *Arch Intern Med.* 2001;22:2733–2737.

CHAPTER 36

Linda U. Krebs, PhD, RN, AOCN®, FAAN

# Sexual and Reproductive Dysfunction

## SCOPE OF THE PROBLEM

Although increasingly recognized as consequences of cancer or cancer therapy, sexual and reproductive dysfunctions often have been dismissed as normal side effects about which the caregiver can do little or nothing. Indeed, these dysfunctions frequently have gone underdiagnosed, underrated, or both, because of lack of concern, information, or knowledge on the part of the caregiver, or because of fear, lack of knowledge, or embarrassment on the part of the patient or family. Often, problems related to sexuality and reproduction are not addressed unless the patient is extremely assertive or presents to the healthcare provider in a crisis situation. However, linking sexuality with health, initiating discussion of potential sexuality-related issues and concerns, and conducting a brief sexual assessment may prevent or minimize future complications.[1] Of all the complications associated with cancer, difficulties in the ability to feel comfortable with one's own sexuality and body image, to be sexually intimate, and to bear children have remained major concerns that affect all aspects of the patient's and his or her family's lives. For some patients, sexual or reproductive dysfunctions may be temporary, with full recovery expected when therapy is completed. For many others, alterations in sexual or reproductive function are permanent, requiring adaptations in management of intimate relationships and lifelong plans to bear and raise children. Even short-term, temporary alterations can have long-term effects on the patient and family, influencing lifestyles and life choices.

Sexuality and reproductive ability are intrinsic components of every individual, involving every facet of who we are as an individual.[2] The sexuality and reproductive capacity of the individual with cancer may be affected by a variety of factors, including the biological process of cancer, the effects of treatment, additional health problems and medications, and the psychological and social issues, such as religious and cultural norms, surrounding the patient and family.[3] Physiological problems of infertility and sterility, changes in body appearance, and the inability to have intercourse are exacerbated by the psychological and psychosexual issues of alteration in body image, fear of abandonment, loss of self-esteem, alteration in sexual identity, and concerns about self. Without appropriate education, counseling, and support, it may be difficult for the patient and family to adapt to the alterations that cancer can produce.

## PHYSIOLOGICAL ALTERATIONS

The pituitary and the hypothalamus regulate gonadal function. The pituitary is divided into two distinct parts—the anterior and posterior portions—and is attached to the hypothalamus by the pituitary or hypophysial stalk, through which runs a minute blood vessel system, the hypothalamic-hypophysial portal vessels.[4,5]

Hypothalamic-releasing or hypothalamic-inhibiting hormones are secreted within the hypothalamus and then spread via the portal vessel system to the anterior pituitary, where they act to influence glandular secretion. When produced in appropriate amounts, these hormones institute a feedback mechanism that shuts off hormonal secretion at the hypothalamus and pituitary level.[4,5]

In gonadal function, luteinizing hormone-releasing hormone (LHRH) or gonadotropin-releasing hormone (GnRH) is secreted by the hypothalamus and stimulates the anterior pituitary to produce luteinizing hormone (LH) and follicle-stimulating hormone (FSH). Luteinizing hormone and FSH stimulate the testis and ovary to produce the appropriate hormones. When blood levels of these hormones are adequate, the hormones exert a negative feedback on the pituitary, thereby decreasing glandular secretion.[4,5]

Follicle-stimulating hormone and LH play major roles in the control of male sexual function. Luteinizing hormone acts on the interstitial Leydig cells to produce testosterone; FSH, in conjunction with testosterone, is responsible for the conversion of spermatogonia into spermatocytes. A reciprocal inhibition of hypothalamic/anterior pituitary secretion of gonadotropic hormones by testicular hormones keeps the level of hormones stable. In this system, the hypothalamus secretes GnRH, which causes the anterior pituitary to secrete LH. In turn, LH stimulates the Leydig cells to produce testosterone. The testosterone then negatively feeds back to the hypothalamus, inhibiting production of GnRH. Spermatogenesis is controlled in much the same manner, with FSH stimulating the Sertoli cells to convert spermatids into sperm. The Sertoli cells then secrete a hormone called *inhibin* that, through negative feedback, causes a decrease in FSH production, thus keeping spermatogenesis at a constant rate.[4,5]

The female hormonal system, like its male counterpart, consists of 3 levels of hormones: GnRH from the hypothalamus, LH and FSH from the anterior pituitary, and estrogen and progesterone from the ovary. In the nonpregnant female, monthly rhythmic changes in the rates of secretion of female hormones and responding changes in the sexual organs result in the female sexual (menstrual) cycle. As a result, a single mature ovum is released from an ovary, and the endometrium of the uterus is prepared for implantation. Follicle-stimulating hormone is responsible for growth of the ovarian follicle, which eventually will become the mature ovum. At the beginning of menstruation, FSH and LH increase, causing rapid cellular growth in about 20 follicles. Eventually, one follicle begins to outgrow the others, causing atresia of the remaining follicles. During follicle growth, estrogen is secreted, probably causing a positive feedback mechanism that results in a surge of LH. This surge of LH, which occurs 2 days before ovulation, is necessary for follicular growth and ovulation.

Around the time of ovulation, the ruptured follicle, under the stimulation of LH, becomes the corpus luteum, which secretes both estrogen and progesterone. After several days, the estrogen and progesterone create negative feedback, decreasing secretion of FSH and LH. The corpus luteum, which also secretes inhibin, slowly degenerates, leading to a loss of the feedback mechanism and an associated rise in secretion of FSH and LH, beginning a new ovarian cycle, and leading to menstruation.[4,5]

Ovarian failure and germinal aplasia can occur as a result of disease, therapy, nutritional status, psychological factors, or any combination of these. Ovarian failure also is related to age; as women near menopause, ovarian failure is more likely. In ovarian failure, damage to ovarian follicles causes decreased levels of estrogens and progesterones, which results in increased levels of LH and FSH with no compensating feedback mechanism. In addition, inhibin may be produced and may react further to alter FSH production. Ovulation ceases, menstruation becomes erratic or ceases, and early menopause often results.[4,5] In the male, damage to the Leydig cells results in decreased testosterone production; LH and FSH levels will be elevated. Initially, Leydig cell activity may be sufficiently compensated to produce adequate amounts of testosterone, but continued damage results in temporary, but more often permanent, sterility.[4,5]

## CLINICAL MANIFESTATIONS: EFFECT OF CANCER THERAPY ON GONADAL FUNCTION

### SURGERY

Some surgical procedures for cancer of the gastrointestinal and genitourinary tracts cause sexual dysfunction through the removal of sexual organs, damage to nerves that enervate sexual organs, or alteration of normal function. In addition, surgery for cancers of the head and neck and the breast, and amputation alter body image and may affect sexual identity. Organ dysfunction, either through loss of or alteration in normal function, is most common in cancers of the colon, rectum, bladder and associated urinary structures, and male and female genital tracts. Even when organs are not removed, normal function may be disrupted through removal of tumor tissue surrounding an organ, lymph node dissection, or associated physiological and psychological abnormalities related to the type of surgery required.

#### Cancer of the colon and rectum

Surgery for cancer of the colon and rectum may cause sexual dysfunction in both men and women. In general, sexual dysfunctions in women are more commonly related to psychosocial issues, whereas dysfunctions in men may be both physical and psychosocial. The most common surgery for colon cancer is some degree of colectomy, with or without a colostomy. Previously cancer of the rectum and anus often required an anterior or an abdominoperineal resection (APR), sphincter-preserving surgery without need for an ostomy is now the most common surgical procedure for rectal cancer.[6,7] The use of the laparoscopically assisted rectal resection offers some hope for a decrease in sexual morbidity and may be particularly useful in those who are obese or who have had previous abdominal surgery with adhesions. Schmidt and colleagues[8] noted an increased dysfunction in men receiving this procedure as compared to the more standard anterior resection or APR. However, Selvindos and Ho[9] noted that sexual dysfunction appeared to be more related to adjuvant chemotherapy than to the surgery. Techniques that save the sphincter may cause less sexual dysfunction due to improved body image and a sense of control; however, the surgery is associated with increased bowel frequency, a sense of urgency, fecal leakage, rectovaginal fistula and bladder, and erectile dysfunction in many patients.[10,11]

For those patients in whom an APR is necessary, sexual dysfunction may be related to the placement of the colostomy, removal of or interference with sexual organ function, or some combination of the two. A colostomy can be associated with sexual dysfunction because of negative changes in the patient's body image and self-esteem as well as the responses of family and friends. In an extensive review of quality of life literature focusing on patients with and without a stoma, the majority of patients with a stoma had some type of sexual dysfunction. The most common complaints were erectile dysfunction and ejaculatory dysfunction in men and dyspareunia and orgasmic dysfunction in women. As a group, individuals with a stoma were less sexually active and experienced more generalized distress than those without a stoma. Of additional importance was the finding that all patients with colorectal cancer experienced some degree of sexual dysfunction and decreased quality of life, regardless of the type of therapy.[12–14]

For the woman with an APR, the ovaries or uterus may be removed at the time of surgery in addition to the colostomy being performed, causing dysfunction from primary inability to bear children or alterations in normal hormonal patterns. In addition, women may have part of the vagina removed, or healing of the perineal wound may result in vaginal scarring that causes painful or incomplete vaginal intercourse. A decreased incidence of orgasm and vaginal lubrication, reduced libido, decreased sexual satisfaction, and dyspareunia has also been noted, but these outcomes are much less common, occurring alone or in combination in 5% to 10% of women undergoing an APR.[7,13–15]

For the man who has an APR, sexual dysfunction is more severe, with 11% to 73% having erectile dysfunction, and 21% to 90% experiencing ejaculatory dysfunction.[16] Age appears to be a factor, with the older patient being more likely to suffer complete or incomplete erectile dysfunction.[16,17] This effect is most likely due to damage to the parasympathetic and sympathetic nerves that control both erection and ejaculation. In addition to erectile dysfunction, decreased amount and force of ejaculation, or retrograde ejaculation may occur. This result, which may be temporary or permanent, adds to the trauma of surgery for the patient because the outcome is unpredictable. For all patients, damage to nerves enervating the pelvic plexus appears to be the most common denominator in organic sexual dysfunction. If a complete nerve-sparing procedure is undertaken successfully, erectile and ejaculatory functions are maintained and the majority of men are able to have sexual intercourse and achieve orgasm. Indeed, sexual dysfunction was significantly decreased in those with sigmoid colon cancer receiving a laparoscopic nerve-sparing procedure during the anterior resection with less than 10% experiencing problems with either erections or ejaculation.[15,18] The use of sildenafil (Viagra) has been shown to be effective in reversing or improving erectile dysfunction in 79% of patients who underwent rectal excision for either cancer or inflammatory bowel disease.[19] In addition, intracavernosal injection of prostaglandin $E_1$ has also been proven beneficial, with 70% of users having an erection sufficient for vaginal penetration.[14]

## Cancers of the genitourinary tract

***Bladder cancer.*** The treatment of bladder cancer may alter sexual function in both men and women. Repeated cystoscopy for local treatment of transitional cell cancer has been noted to cause pain with coitus for women, transient pain during erection and ejaculation in men, and temporary decrease in desire for both. Transurethral resection or partial cystectomy may result in mild pain or dyspareunia; however, normal sexual function should not be altered. For some patients, urinary incontinence may cause cessation of normal activities for fear of having an accident. In addition, body image and self-esteem may be altered due to the need to use incontinence pads or other protective materials.

Radical cystectomy results in sexual dysfunction for both men and women because of organ removal and damage to nerves.[20–24] Erectile dysfunction occurs in approximately 86% of men undergoing radical cystectomy.[20] Orgasm may be experienced but is usually less intense and without ejaculate.[21] Sexual interest and penile sensation are not altered.[21] For the woman who undergoes a radical cystectomy, the surgery usually includes removal of the bladder and urethra, uterus, ovaries, fallopian tubes, and anterior portion of the vagina. Although vaginal reconstruction typically is performed, the resulting vagina may be more narrow and shallow and provide less lubrication than before surgery, leading to difficulty with penetration. In addition, the removal of the ovaries, with associated estrogen loss, leads to dryness, inelasticity of the vagina, dyspareunia, and menopausal symptoms. Vaginal dilation and the liberal use of lubrication may provide relief.[13,21]

For both sexes, urinary diversion is a necessity with radical cystectomy; this may result in alterations in self-esteem and body image and lead to a decrease or cessation of all sexual activities[21,22], with women reporting decreased desire and feelings of decreased attractiveness.[21,] In the past, the ileal conduit, which necessitated the continuous use of an ostomy appliance, was the most common method for urinary diversion. Today, the surgical development of a Koch or Indiana pouch, or continent reservoir, has become more widely employed, resulting in overall improved sexual adjustment due to decreased odor and leakage.[25] Most recently, the construction of a neobladder, made from the ileum and the large intestine, has allowed patients to maintain bladder function and normal voiding patterns.[24,25] While most commonly used in men, women also may benefit from this technique; however, many may experience voiding problems and maintaining continence.[25] In studies comparing the neobladder to the ileal conduit, improved quality of life and decreased alterations in sexual functioning were noted in both men and women who had bladder substitution.[24,25] Those who are older are more likely to experience incontinence, primarily due to muscular weakness. In potency-sparing or sexuality preserving cystectomy where the prostate is spared and a neobladder is created, potency is maintained in 75% to 100% and daytime continence is 95% to 100%. Nighttime continence may be decreased for some (0%–69%).[26] An additional concern noted when the ileum is used as a conduit or to form a neobladder is the potential for metabolic abnormalities including hyperchloremic acidosis and vitamin B12 malabsorption. The former can be managed with sodium bicarbonate and the latter with vitamin B12 injections.[26]

***Penile cancer/cancer of the male urethra.*** Cancer of the penis and male urethra are rare. Primary treatment is total or partial penectomy although a number of methods for conservative surgery, from circumcision to wide local excision and skin grafting have been identified.[27] The degree of limitation primarily relates to the amount of tissue removed and psychosocial issues related shame and stigma from having penile cancer.[13,28] Partial penectomy does not result in loss of erectile, ejaculative, or orgasmic abilities, whereas erectile ability obviously is absent with total penectomy.[13,29] Desire remains, and stimulation of the remaining genital tissue can produce orgasm.[19,29,30] Ejaculation, through the perineal urethrostomy, should continue. Techniques to create a penis have been identified. Phalloplasty, which is used in female-to-male transsexual surgery, has been used for penile insufficiency and may be of benefit in this population.[31] Insertion of a semirigid or inflatable prosthesis restores the ability to have intercourse and has been reported to increase erectile ability, libido, and frequency of intercourse.[32] Those patients treated with radiation therapy had significantly fewer concerns related to sexual dysfunction than those undergoing partial or total penectomy, although erectile dysfunction is seen in 20% to 30%.[33] More recently, laser surgery has been employed with the result that sexual satisfaction and sexual dysfunction are only minimally affected. Painful intercourse, which frequently occurs in those with partial penectomy, was reduced to 10%.[30]

*Testicular cancer.* The treatment of testicular cancer includes an orchiectomy and typically retroperitoneal lymph node dissection (RPLND) and removal of a pelvic mass, usually followed by chemotherapy or radiation therapy. Unilateral orchiectomy will not result in infertility or sexual dysfunction, providing that the contralateral testis is normal and the individual is fertile at diagnosis. Infertility before any definitive therapy begins is well documented and may be related to hormonal imbalance or result from subacute chronic illness.[34] If bilateral orchiectomy is performed, sterility and decreased libido, related to loss of testosterone, will result. Retroperitoneal lymph node dissection done for staging or as treatment may result in temporary or permanent loss of ejaculation, whereas potency and the ability to have an orgasm remain.[13,35] Whenever possible, nerve-sparing RPLND should be done, as this procedure is associated with preservation of ejaculatory function and fertility.[13] In some individuals, retrograde ejaculation has been noted. In addition, decreased libido and arousal, decreased pleasure and intensity of orgasm, and erectile dysfunction have been described.[13,21] Between 10% and 25% of those patients undergoing retroperitoneal surgery experience complete absence of ejaculation, while erectile dysfunction is rare in those treated solely with unilateral orchiectomy.[36] For most patients, discussions about sexuality before, during, and following treatment are crucial. Prior to therapy, an important aspect of discussion should involve providing information about sperm banking, including issues of feasibility due to prior pre-existing fertility problems, cost, timing and possible treatment delay.[21]

*Prostate cancer.* Therapy for prostate cancer consists of various combinations of surgery, chemotherapy, radiation therapy, and hormonal manipulation, all of which have a potential to alter sexual function. Surgical treatment of prostate cancer includes prostatectomy or bilateral orchiectomy, although locally advanced prostate cancer may be treated with cryosurgery. Transurethral resection of the prostate generally does not cause erectile dysfunction; however, retrograde ejaculation occurs in approximately 90% of all patients. Transabdominal resection of the prostate results in retrograde ejaculation in 75% to 80% of patients and may cause erectile dysfunction.[37] However, with newer techniques, including the ability to separate sperm from urine, sterility in individuals with retrograde ejaculation is not as frequent.

The perineal approach, or radical prostatectomy, may result in permanent damage to erectile function with concomitant loss of emission and ejaculation.[19,37] While alterations in desire, penile sensation, and the ability to reach orgasm should not occur, many men have reported feeling less masculine, more uncomfortable with sexual intimacy, and experiencing less sexual enjoyment following prostatectomy.[38]

Preserving the cavernous nerves is most important for postprostatectomy erectile function recovery.[39] Nerve-sparing or potency-sparing surgery was developed by Walsh in the 1980s and, according to Church,[40] probably has been the most significant surgical development in the treatment of prostate cancer. Prior to the development of this procedure, 2% to 15% of patients experienced urinary incontinence, and 80% to 90% experienced erectile dysfunction. Current techniques, including the use of laparoscopic and robot-assisted approaches, have decreased the incidence of erectile dysfunction; however, the exact percentage of those experiencing erectile dysfunction varies among individual reports and by whether the patient had a non-nerve-sparing, unilateral nerve-sparing, or bilateral nerve-sparing procedure.[21,23,36,41]

Because radical prostatectomy still results in a significant level of erectile dysfunction, a number of new procedures are being tested to maintain potency. Among them are intraoperative cavernous nerve stimulation and nerve grafting. The CaverMap surgical probe allows identification of the cavernous nerves, whose preservation relates to maintenance of potency. Results of studies to date have been conflicting, but some evidence indicates that potency can be maintained in as many as 70% of patients for at least 1 year following radical prostatectomy.[37] In addition, cavernous nerve reconstruction has been undertaken to preserve spontaneous erectile function, with potency and the ability to have intercourse being maintained in 33% to 43% of patients.[39,41,42]

Bilateral orchiectomy causes sexual dysfunction through gradual diminution of libido, erectile dysfunction, gynecomastia, penile atrophy, and body image changes.[36,37] Testicular implants filled with saline may be of benefit in managing body image changes. Various methods, including the use of penile prostheses, suction or vacuum devices, intracorporeal injections of papaverine hydrochloride or prostaglandin $E_1$, insertion of transurethral alprostadil (MUSE) and medications such as yohimbine hydrochloride, have been used to restore erectile potential.[21,23,36,43,44] Sildenafil citrate (Viagra), vardenafil (Levitra), and tadalafil (Cialis), all PDE5 (phosphodiesterase type 5) inhibitors have been tried to manage erectile dysfunction in men who have had radical prostatectomy.[21,36,43] Sildenafil and vardenafil each have a half-life of 4.5 to 6 hours, while tadalafil has a half-life of 16 to 18 hours, allowing for longer potential for erection and intercourse.[45] Kendirci and colleagues[43] noted that nightly use of 50 mg to 100 mg of sildenafil was of significant use in reducing the incidence of erectile dysfunction by promoting surgical site healing and reducing scar tissue formation. Vardenafil at doses of 10 mg to 20 mg per night improved erections on 60% to 70% of those who took the drug for 12 or more weeks following radical retropubic prostatectomy.[36] Multiple studies have shown the benefit of including the PDE5 inhibitors in postoperative prostatectomy care. Each drug has its own particular risks and benefits which should be discussed with the patient prior to prescribing. In addition, education about the use of these drugs should include the need for sexual stimulation to attain erection and information that generally multiple sexual attempts are needed to be successful.[21,36,43]

Psychological issues also play a role in erectile dysfunction with fear of failure being very common. A variety of approaches to decreasing the emphasis on intercourse and increasing the focus on sexual intimacy have been used with success.[21,36,37] The recognition that return of full erection potential may take as long as 2 years is important in counseling the patient. The use of postoperative PDE5 inhibitors appears to shorten this timeframe and may decrease some psychological manifestations.[43]

## Gynecologic malignancies

Surgical management of gynecologic malignancies includes surgery of the vulva, vagina, uterus and uterine cervix, ovary, and fallopian tube, and pelvic exenteration. Although the majority of gynecologic surgeries are invisible assaults to femininity, sexual identity and sexual functioning are often permanently affected. It is imperative that sexual and reproductive counseling be provided to the patient and family before surgical intervention, because most surgeries permanently alter fertility and may alter sexuality. Studies have shown that women treated for gynecologic malignancy are likely to experience alterations in sexuality and sexual functioning, including decreased desire, dyspareunia, recurrent vaginal infections, vaginal atrophy and dryness, decreased sense of feeling feminine, cessation of all sexual activities, and difficulties related to menopausal symptoms and infertility.[13,46–49]

***Vulvar cancer.*** Vulvar cancer was commonly believed to be a disease of those over the age of 60.[13] More recently, vulvar intraepithelial neoplasia (VIN) has been diagnosed in much younger women, with a tripling of disease in women younger than 50, over the past 2 decades.[50] Of these women, 8% to 19% will be diagnosed with concomitant invasive disease, most commonly in those who are older or have a larger lesion. Treatment of VIN may include laser removal, simple excision of the lesion or more complex surgery including vulvectomy and clitoris removal.[50,51] Treatment for VIN and invasive vulvar cancer will not alter fertility but may affect sexuality. In general, good cosmetic results occur with treatment of early disease except for the simple vulvectomy, which removes the labia and subcutaneous tissue, but generally retains the clitoris. Introital stenosis may result but may be easily managed through the use of lubrication and vaginal dilators. Whenever possible, conservative therapy should be employed to minimize cosmetic alterations, maintain body image, and minimize sexual dysfunction. However, scarring may occur that may affect both body image and sensation.[50,51]

Radical vulvectomy frequently results in delayed wound healing, altered body image, abnormalities in sensory perception of the genital area, leg edema, decreased range of motion in lower extremities, altered orgasmic potential, and introital stenosis.[46,52] Evaluation of lymph nodes prior to radical surgery may allow for more limited surgeries with less compromise to sexuality[13] Newer use of sentinel lymph node biopsy to assess spread of disease has resulted in decreased use of lymphadenectomy and minimized associated side effects.[13] In those women who undergo radical pelvic surgery, generalized sexual dysfunction, including pain, anxiety, and decreased desire, is common, occurs earlier, and persists unless appropriately treated. In general, if cure is a possibility, women have been willing to live with sexual dysfunction and body image changes, provided adequate information and discussion about causes of dysfunction and alternative methods of sexual satisfaction are given.[13,50,51] All women need education on the effects of removal of tissue and on body image prior to surgery to promote self-esteem, function, and compliance with care.

***Vaginal cancer.*** Vaginal cancer is rare. Surgery for the majority of gynecological cancers results in some abnormality and need for reconstruction of the vagina. Potential sexual side effects include alterations in body image and loss of femininity and body image.[46] A shortened vagina can cause considerable sexual dysfunction because of decreased vaginal length and width, lack of lubrication, and pain on intercourse. Total vaginectomy without reconstruction precludes vaginal intercourse; however, multiple techniques for vaginal reconstruction exist. Reconstruction can be accomplished using the large or small bowel, the umbilicus, gracilis or rectus musculocutaneous flaps, or a pedicle graft from the greater omentum.[53–55] In 30% to 70% of patients who do have reconstruction, there is a return of orgasmic sensations if they existed before surgery. Despite this finding, reconstruction should not be considered a panacea for sexual dysfunction, as some women complain that the new vagina is too large, is too small, or has a persistent, annoying discharge.[53,54,56]

***Cervical cancer and endometrial cancer.*** Surgical treatment for cervical intraepithelial neoplasia and carcinoma in situ includes conization, laser therapy, cryosurgery, loop electrosurgical excision (LEEP), or simple hysterectomy.[57] All but the last usually have no effect on fertility (conization may result in cervical stenosis or incompetence), nor should they cause any physiological sexual dysfunction.

Simple hysterectomy precludes further childbearing but should not affect sexual functioning. Early-stage disease may be treated with radical trachelectomy and pelvic lymphadenectomy to preserve fertility.[57] Sides effects of trachelectomy include neocervical stenosis, menstruation difficulties, dyspareunia, vaginal scarring and possibly subfertility. Cervical dilation in the clinic or office may reduce the incidence of these difficulties.[58]

Treatment for invasive disease is usually radical hysterectomy, with or without bilateral salpingo-oophorectomy. If oophorectomy is included, menopausal symptoms, with hot flashes and decreases in vaginal lubrication and elasticity, may severely alter sexual functioning.[56] Approximately 50% of patients treated for early-stage cervical cancer have a marked decrease in their sexual relationships and experience extreme fatigue, lack of energy, depressed mood, weight gain, and anxiety,[59,60] with additional complaints of dyspareunia and decreased frequency of intercourse seen in 10% to 20% of women.[61]

In women with endometrial cancer, effects of treatment and uncertainty about the future increase sexual difficulties.[49,62] However, in a review of studies, consensus has shown that the majority of women experience no lasting sexual side effects, although grieving for lost fertility and inability to bear children is of concern.[63] Of those satisfied with their current sexual functioning, the majority noted that return to normalcy occurred gradually over a prolonged period.

Although sexual feelings should not be altered after a radical hysterectomy, delayed bowel and bladder function may occur and necessitate discharge from the hospital with a urinary catheter. Long-term catheter placement may alter body image and affect sexuality. Intercourse can be accomplished by securing the catheter to the abdomen and making changes in coital position.[62,64] It also should be remembered that many women measure femininity by the ability to bear children. If this ability is removed, sexual dysfunctions may occur even in the absence of organic cause.

*Ovarian cancer.* Initial treatment for ovarian cancer is surgery, usually consisting of a radical hysterectomy with bilateral salpingo-oophorectomy and omentectomy. Fertility is lost and the associated menopausal symptoms occur. In addition, alterations in body image, decreased sense of desirability, and vaginal dryness may occur, resulting in decreased sexual interest.[65,66] In the young woman with ovarian teratoma or borderline malignant epithelial neoplasia, it is possible to maintain fertility if disease is confined to one ovary and is of low grade. Adequate staging is essential, and the patient must be willing to comply with all follow-up recommendations.[65,67] Treatment usually continues with combination chemotherapy, further compounding sexual and reproductive dysfunctions, including alterations in libido, frequency of intercourse, and desire for close physical contact.[65,67,68]

### Pelvic exenteration

Although pelvic exenteration may be performed in the man or woman with advanced colorectal or bladder cancer, the most common indication for this procedure is a locally advanced gynecologic malignancy. Surgery is undertaken with curative intent, with more than 95% surviving the surgery and 40% to 50% alive at 5 years post surgery.[69] Current use of laparoscopic procedures has reduced both mortality and morbidity.[69] An anterior pelvic exenteration preserves the rectum, whereas a posterior exenteration preserves the bladder. A total pelvic exenteration involves removing the vagina, uterus, ovaries, fallopian tubes, bladder, and rectum; in the man, the prostate, seminal vesicles, and vas deferens are removed.[57,70] In patients with total pelvic exenteration, a urinary conduit and colostomy are created and a neovagina may be constructed.[69,70] In the woman, reproductive and sexual dysfunctions are profound. Dysfunction related to removal of all pelvic organs with resulting ostomies is obvious. An Indiana pouch, a continent urinary pouch made from a piece of bowel and placed behind the umbilicus, requires catheterization, but may decrease some body image alterations.[71] In addition, body image, sexual identity, and self-esteem are disturbed, and appropriate interventions and education need to be provided. In the woman with vaginal reconstruction, intercourse may be possible; however, the physiological and psychological ramifications of this surgery may result in inability and lack of desire to participate in sexual activities.[56,67]

### Breast cancer

Although some surgeries may not be strictly related to sexual functioning, they may cause dysfunction as a result of the psychological issues related to the particular body part. The most likely assault to body image and sexual identity with resultant sexual dysfunction is surgical removal of all or part of the breast. Although fertility is not altered by mastectomy or lumpectomy, the inability or difficulty in breast-feeding should pregnancy be accomplished may be a major assault to the woman's femininity. Removal or partial removal of a breast may result in sexual dysfunction because of fear of rejection, physical discomfort, anxiety about initiating sexual activities, feelings of being defective or different, or any combination of these factors.[72] In addition, if lymphedema occurs, body image alterations as well as difficulty with clothing, and the potential for infection are enhanced.[73]

Having the ability to choose the type of therapy does not appear to play a role in overall sexual adjustment; however, Pelusi noted that while women generally have fewer body image concerns following breast conservation surgery, they are more likely to be fearful of recurrence which eventually may result in increased body image issues.[74]

In general, breast reconstruction does not appear to influence overall sexual adjustment following mastectomy although it does appear to positively affect overall psychosocial and body image adjustment. Atisha and colleagues noted that these benefits continue and actually increase with time,[75] while Warren et al[76] note that breast reconstruction is occurring during a paradigm shift in breast cancer treatment. This includes the increased use of breast conservation surgery, the common inclusion of sentinel lymph node biopsy, and oncoplastic surgery that includes breast reduction and breast remodeling techniques to improve cosmetic results without compromising treatment outcomes.[76] Whenever possible, surgical options, including breast reconstruction, should be made available to the woman with breast cancer, since being able to make decisions about the type of surgery does appear to impact overall satisfaction with surgical outcomes regardless of which procedure is chosen.[77]

An additional, but rarely discussed, issue is that of the man diagnosed with breast cancer. Male breast cancer is rare, but appears to be increasing. Treatment is similar to that in women, with surgery as the initial form of treatment. Little research has been conducted with this population, particularly in the area of psychosexual concerns. Breast cancer is generally considered to be a woman's disease; men often feel less masculine and resultant scarring from surgical removal can affect both body image and sexual intimacy. Men frequently do not discuss their breast cancer, further compromising psychosexual adjustment. Sexual dysfunction associated with male breast cancer would benefit from further research to minimize potential sexual side effects.[78]

### Head and neck cancer

Although not generally considered an area responsible for sexual dysfunction, surgical treatment for cancers of the head and neck region is responsible for varying degrees of alteration in body image, leading to changes in sexuality and intimacy. Results of disease and treatment are readily apparent. Even with reconstructive surgery or the use of prostheses to ameliorate deformities, sexuality may be affected by the alterations in sensation, breathing, and voice; by the ability to use the mouth and tongue for activities such as chewing, swallowing or kissing; or because of dental problems or similar abnormalities. Difficulty with arousal and orgasm and cessation of sexual activities have been reported.[13,62,79] In addition, in those with radical neck dissection, nerve damage and cosmetic defects result in further assaults to body image and may affect sexual function.[73] Presurgical counseling and long-term follow-up may be necessary for sexual rehabilitation.

## RADIATION THERAPY

Radiation therapy can cause sexual and reproductive dysfunction through primary organ failure (eg, ovarian failure and testicular aplasia), alterations in organ function (eg, decreased lubrication and erectile dysfunction), and the temporary or permanent effects of therapy not associated with reproduction (eg, diarrhea and fatigue). Permanent effects most commonly are related to total dose, location, length of treatment, age, and prior fertility status.[36,49,80] In women, fertility depends on follicular maturation and ovum release. Radiation therapy to the ovaries has its most direct effect on the intermediate follicles. If these follicles are damaged by radiation and insufficient small follicles remain, permanent sterility results. In men, although the Leydig cell and mature sperm are relatively radioresistant, immature sperm and spermatogonia are extremely radiosensitive. Small doses of radiation will begin the process of infertility, which, depending on total dose, may be permanent.[81]

In women, temporary or permanent sterility is related to the dose of radiation, the volume of tissues radiated, the time period during which the ovaries are exposed to radiation, and age.[80,81] Because a woman has fewer oocytes as she nears menopause, radiation injury at that point in the life span is more likely to be permanent. A radiation dose of 600 to 1200 cGy is capable of inducing menopause. Younger women appear to be more resistant to this effect and may not experience permanent sterility until a dose of greater than 2000 cGy. In women older than 40, a dose of 600 cGy often is associated with subsequent menopause and the associated menopausal symptoms of hot flashes, amenorrhea, dyspareunia, loss of libido, and vaginal atrophy.[82] For some women, the use of exogenous estrogens may alleviate these side effects.

Movement of the ovaries out of the radiation field (oophoropexy), with appropriate shielding, has helped maintain fertility even when relatively high doses of radiation have been given. Ovaries can be moved to the midline of the uterus or to the iliac crests. In young women or those desiring to maintain both reproductive capacity and hormonal function, ovarian transposition, with the ovaries moved to the upper abdomen, can be undertaken. Menstrual function is preserved in approximately 50%[80] Successful pregnancies, without evidence of fetal congenital anomalies, have been reported following oophoropexy.[82]

In addition to sterility or transient infertility, radiation therapy can produce other sexual dysfunctions, which may be temporary or permanent. Decreases in sexual enjoyment, ability to attain orgasm, libido, and frequency of intercourse and sexual dreams, as well as vaginal stenosis or shortening, vaginal irritation, increased risk of infection, and decreased lubrication and sensation have been reported in women treated with radiation therapy. Painful intercourse and menstrual changes have also been reported.[3,83–86] Vistad and colleagues[87] reported increased incidence of dyspareunia, vaginal dryness, and discomfort with sexual activity leading to altered sexual activity in survivors of cervical cancer treated with radiation therapy. Chronic fatigue played an important role in altered sexual activity, but lack of a partner was noted as the primary cause.[87] A small, handheld device called Eros Therapy has been used with some benefit in women experiencing severe sexual dysfunction following radiotherapy for stage I and II cervical cancer. The Eros Therapy device increases blood flow to the clitoris and surrounding tissues. After 3 months of use, all participants noted a significant improvement in sexual desire, arousal, lubrication, and satisfaction as well as a decrease in dyspareunia.[88]

In men, temporary or permanent azoospermia is a function of age, dose, tissue volume, and exposure time. When the testis is exposed to radiation, a reduction in sperm count begins within 6 to 8 weeks and continues for up to 1 year after completion of therapy. Doses less than 500 cGy usually are associated with temporary sterility, whereas doses greater than 500 cGy typically result in permanent sterility.[81,82] The return of normal spermatogenesis is related to total testicular dose, with a dose of less than 100 cGy taking 9 to 12 months for recovery, whereas recovery from 200 to 300 cGy may take 2 to 3 years and 400 to 600 cGy takes 5 years or more.[89–91]

Below-diaphragm irradiation for Hodgkin's disease (HD) and testicular cancer has been associated with long-term azoospermia. Sperm counts generally reach their lowest level by 6 months and for some patients will return to baseline levels over a 2-year period.[91] Generally, shielding the testicle results in a mean dose of less than 44 cGy to the testicle. Thus, for those patients not requiring primary testicular irradiation, adequate testicular shielding may alleviate the sequelae of infertility. In addition, repositioning the unaffected testicle to the groin to allow for shielding may preserve testosterone production, thus preserving fertility.[92]

The majority of men treated by external beam for prostate cancer experience temporary or permanent erectile dysfunction. Erectile dysfunction is believed to be caused by fibrosis of pelvic vasculature or radiation damage of pelvic nerves. In addition to erectile dysfunction, patients experience decreased frequency of ejaculation and libido. Those who receive irradiation to the whole pelvis are likely to experience more severe side effects.[93] Interstitial therapy appears to decrease the incidence of erectile dysfunction, although bowel, bladder and some level of erectile dysfunction, ranging from 6% to 90%, still occur.[94–96] Morillo and colleagues reported that 71% of their patients maintained potency at 4 years following $^{125}$I seed implantation.[97] Increased doses to the proximal penis appear to be associated with a higher incidence of erectile dysfunction.[98] Newer radiation delivery methods, such as three-dimensional conformal radiation therapy (3D-CRT), and use of smaller radiation therapy ports have decreased the incidence of erectile dysfunction in patients with prostate cancer, although the addition of hormone therapy may negate this decrease. Erectile dysfunction appears to stabilize by 18 to 24 months following 3D-CRT.[99,100] In addition to difficulty in gaining or maintaining an erection, a decreased libido, inability to ejaculate, inability to lubricate, inability to achieve orgasm or reduced intensity of orgasm, and decreased sexual pleasure are common findings in men who receive radiation to the pelvis. The addition of phosphodiesterase 5 inhibitors, such as sildenafil, may help to preserve potency.[101–105]

Along with direct assaults to sexual and reproductive function, the general side effects and accompanying psychological effects of radiation therapy frequently can alter sexual function. Mild to severe fatigue is reported to occur in as many as 80% of those patients receiving radiation therapy.[106] Severe fatigue can limit all activity. Nausea, vomiting, and diarrhea can decrease energy, sexual desire, and feelings of desirability and can interfere with a sense of general well-being. Inflammation, pain, and limited range of motion may make sexual activities difficult or impossible. In addition to physical limitations, fear, depression, anxiety, stress, body image alterations, and lowered self-esteem may be burdens. The appropriate use of energy-conserving strategies, medications, lubricants, dilators, prostheses, time, and counseling may alleviate side effects, promote a sense of well-being, and improve sexual function.[81,101]

## CHEMOTHERAPY

Chemotherapy-induced reproductive and sexual dysfunction is related to the type of drug, dose, length of treatment, age and sex of the individual receiving treatment, and length of time after therapy. In addition, the use of combination therapy, with multiple agents and drugs given to combat side effects of chemotherapy, plays a role in infertility or sexual dysfunction.

Infertility and sterility after chemotherapy have been noted since the early 1970s, with reports of amenorrhea and azoospermia after single-agent or combination therapy. Adult men are more likely to experience long-term side effects regardless of age, whereas women are more apt to have permanent cessation of menses as they near age 40. Newer targeted treatments or those of shorter duration appear to have fewer long-term side effects.[80,90,107–119] The principal drugs that induce infertility are the alkylating agents, but others have been implicated—in particular, cytosine arabinoside, 5-fluorouracil, vinblastine, vincristine, cisplatin, and procarbazine. Combinations of these drugs appear to prolong infertility[110–119] (Table 36-1).

### Men

Infertility occurs in men primarily through depletion of the germinal epithelium that lines the seminiferous tubules. On testicular biopsy, the interstitial Leydig cells appear normal, whereas the tubules are abnormal, contain Sertoli cells, and have depleted or absent germinal epithelium. Clinically, testicular volume decreases, oligospermia or azoospermia

**TABLE 36-1**

**Chemotherapeutic Agents Affecting Sexual or Reproductive Function**

| Agent | Complication |
|---|---|
| **Alkylating Agents** | |
| Altretamine<br>Busulfan<br>Carboplatin<br>Chlorambucil<br>Cisplatin<br>Cyclophosphamide<br>Estramustane<br>Ifosfamide<br>Melphalan<br>Nitrogen mustard<br>Oxaliplatin | Azoospermia, decreased libido, ovarian dysfunction, erectile dysfunction, testicular atrophy, gynecomastia |
| **Antimetabolites** | |
| Capecitabine<br>Cytosine arabinoside<br>5-fluorouracil<br>Fludarabine phosphate<br>Gemcitabine<br>Methotrexate<br>Trimetrexate | Same as for alkylating agents |
| **Antitumor Antibiotics** | |
| Daunorubicin<br>Doxorubicin<br>Dactinomycin<br>Epirubicin<br>Idarubicin<br>Plicamycin | Same as for alkylating agents |
| **Plant Products** | |
| Vincristine<br>Vinblastine | Retrograde ejaculation, erectile dysfunction |
| Vinorelbine | Decreased libido, ovarian dysfunction, erectile dysfunction |
| **Miscellaneous Agents** | |
| Abarelix | Gynecomastia, erectile dysfunction, hot flashes |
| Aminoglutethimide | Masculinization (women) |
| Androgens | Masculinization (women) |
| Antiandrogens | Decreased libido, erectile dysfunction, gynecomastia, breast tenderness, hot flashes |
| Antiestrogens | Gynecomastia, erectile dysfunction, menstrual irregularities, hot flashes |
| Corticosteroids | Irregular menses, acne |
| Estrogens | Decreased libido, erectile dysfunction |
| Interferon | Transient erectile dysfunction, amenorrhea, pelvic pain |
| Leuprolide | Decreased libido, amenorrhea, gynecomastia, erectile dysfunction |
| Nonsteroidal aromatase inhibitors | Hot flashes, vaginal dryness, decreased libido |
| Procarbazine | As for alkylating agents |
| Progestins | Menstrual abnormalities, change in libido |

*Source*: Data from Wilkes and Barton-Burke[110]; Otto[111]; Cleri and Haywood[112]; Gullatte[113]; Chu and DeVita[114]; Braun-Inglis[115]; Blecher[116]; Gobel[117]; Krebs[118]; and Orbaugh.[119]

occurs, and infertility results.[120–122] Leydig cell dysfunction, manifested by a raised LH level and low or normal testosterone level, is usually seen.[80,121–123] Following drug-induced azoospermia, the process of spermatogenesis must start all over, as if the patient were going through puberty. Initially, the germ stem cell must repopulate the testicle, then spermatogenesis should occur. This process may take several years.[121,124,125]

Both single-agent and combination chemotherapy have been reported to cause germinal aplasia, with alkylating agents being the most extensively studied in terms of this effect. Cumulative doses of greater than 400 mg/m$^2$ of cisplatin have been associated with irreversible damage to gonadal function, while cyclophosphamide in doses >300 mg/kg caused gonadal dysfunction in more than 80% of patients.[121] Huddart and colleagues[109] reported on sexual dysfunction and fertility alterations in 680 men treated for testicular cancer at the Royal Marsden Hospital. All patients were more than 5 years from initial diagnosis and treatment. Of these patients, 351 had received either chemotherapy alone or a combination of chemotherapy and radiation therapy. While satisfaction with sexual relationships was reported in 83%, many experienced decreased interest in sex and decreased sexual activity. All experienced some level of gonadal dysfunction with decreased testosterone and increased FSH levels. Approximately 30% attempted to conceive post treatment, with an approximately 70% success rate.[109] Bohlen and colleagues reported on 59 patients treated with 2 cycles of platinum, vinblastine and bleomycin and did not see an adverse effect in either future fertility or in sexual activity.[126] Fertility appears to improve over time in patients who had initially been rendered azoospermic or oligospermic following combination chemotherapy for testicular cancer, with reports describing slow recovery of spermatogenesis, culminating with the ability to father children.[80,90,109,121,122]

Hormonal manipulation and treatment with estrogens are well known as a cause of sexual dysfunction. The majority of patients who receive androgen-ablative therapy experience a major reduction in interest in sexual intercourse and are unable to attain or maintain an erection.[125,127] The incidence of hot flashes in men with prostate cancer treated with GnRH analogs, antiandrogens, or estrogens ranges from 10% to 45%. Hot flashes may be managed with drugs such as transdermal estradiol, diethylstilbesterol, oral progesterones, or venlafaxine.[128] In some instances, the addition of finasteride has been shown to maintain potency while maintaining the androgen-ablative effect.[114] Gynecomastia and decreases in libido, sexual excitement, and the ability to achieve sexual fulfillment are significant problems.[110,112,114]

Other potential side effects of chemotherapy include partial or total erectile dysfunction, ejaculatory difficulties, and decreased desire, arousal, and orgasmic ability. Semen cryopreservation prior to initial therapy should be considered for all men interested in fathering a child.[21,23,36,129]

### Women

Women experience sexual and reproductive dysfunction from chemotherapy as a result of hormonal alterations or direct effects that cause ovarian fibrosis and follicle destruction. Previous sexual health may also play a role. Follicle-stimulating hormone and LH levels are elevated and the estradiol level is decreased, leading to amenorrhea, menopausal symptoms, dyspareunia, and vaginal atrophy and dryness.[80,90,110,120]

Like men, women experience reproductive dysfunction from both single-agent and combination chemotherapy. However, age appears to play a more significant role in infertility in women than in men, with women younger than 30 years able to tolerate much higher doses of chemotherapy without resultant permanent amenorrhea and premature menopause.[80,90,130] However, a more recent study suggests that in women with HD, premature ovarian failure although it is delayed in younger women. Amenorrhea has been noted in women treated with combination chemotherapy for a variety of malignancies including breast cancer, HD, melanoma and leukemia, particularly when the regimen contained an alkylating agent.[108,110,131,132] Women with ovarian germ cell tumors treated with fertility-sparing surgery followed by platinum-based chemotherapy also reported amenorrhea, although less frequently than those receiving true alkylating agents.[133] In those patients experiencing temporary amenorrhea, menstruation returns in approximately 50% of those younger than 40 years of age within 15 months.[131] Permanent amenorrhea may be evident by cessation of therapy but often occurs gradually over time.[80,90] In younger women, permanent amenorrhea may appear in 6 to 16 months, in women closer to normal menopause, amenorrhea may occur in only 2 to 4 months. Schover noted that amenorrhea occurred more commonly in women older than 35 to 40 and that the ovarian failure rate was correlated with receiving alkylating agents or taxanes, particularly at higher cumulative doses.[132] Ovarian dysfunction occurs at all ages but is more frequently reported and diagnosed in women closer to menopause. Indeed, it has been suggested that for each month a woman receives chemotherapy, 1.5 years of reproductive life are lost.[132] However, it should be noted that even with decreased numbers of ovarian follicles, pregnancy can occur.[108]

It appears that any combination of drugs containing an alkylating agent is apt to cause infertility, and as women near menopause, permanent cessation of menses becomes more likely. When hormonal manipulation includes androgens, not only sexual and reproductive function but also body image and feelings of sexual identity are affected. Chemotherapy contributes significantly to sexual dysfunction through menopausal symptoms as well as through increased risk of urinary tract infections and candida infections, vaginal irritation, exacerbations of genital herpes and human papillomavirus, and alterations in desire and arousal due to decreases in circulating androgens. In addition, the use of hormonal therapies, such as tamoxifen, aminoglutethimide, and letrazole, has been associated with menopausal symptoms and decreased sexual desire.[110,132] Appropriate support and counseling should be provided to affected individuals. More research into the best methods to decrease menopausal side effects in patients with cancer needs to be undertaken. In addition, long-term survivors have noted lack of sexual interest, difficulty reaching orgasm, and inability to relax and enjoy a sexual encounter.[134]

### Children/adolescents

The effect of chemotherapy on gonadal function in children and adolescents has been extensively studied.[108,122] Primary effects include delayed sexual maturation and alterations in reproductive potential. While chemotherapy affects girls and boys differently, the primary effects appear to be age-related. Prepubescent boys seem to be minimally affected by chemotherapy and progress into and through puberty without major difficulty.[122] Young men treated during puberty appear to be more likely to have gonadal dysfunction, with profound effects on both germ cell production and Leydig cell function, resulting in increases in FSH and LH and a decrease in testosterone levels.[122,135] In a study of 77 men who had been treated for childhood cancer more than 13 years previously, 63% were found to be normozoospermic, while 20% had oligospermia and 17% had azoospermia.[136] The reserve supply of spermatogonia in young men is much smaller than in adults; however, chemotherapy has the potential to significantly alter spermatogenesis. This effect cannot be easily assessed until puberty.[122] The majority of girls treated with combination therapy appear to have normal ovarian function, although long-term follow-up is needed to assess whether these individuals will experience premature menopause.[108,132]

In reviews of female and male participants of the Childhood Cancer Survivor Study, no adverse pregnancy outcomes were found for either the women or the partners of men who had received chemotherapy when children.[137,138] Of importance, many children who receive therapy for childhood cancer experience decreased quality of life, including lower rates of marriage and parenthood, and fears about their reproductive capacity.[139–141]

### Other issues

Drugs used to manage chemotherapy side effects can alter sexual function. Erectile dysfunction, decreased sexual desire, decreased sense of sexual fulfillment, and decreased ability to achieve orgasm all have been associated with these agents (Table 36-2).[110–114]

## BIOLOGICAL RESPONSE MODIFIERS

Although frequently used in the adjuvant setting and for treatment of early-stage disease, biological response modifiers (BRMs) have not yet been studied sufficiently with regard to their sexual side effects. Most changes in sexuality are related to known BRM side effects, including fatigue, mucous membrane dryness, flulike symptoms, and body image changes.[142] Some information is available on the use of the interferons—in particular, alfa-interferon—alone or in combination with other agents. Decreased libido, amenorrhea, pelvic pain, uterine bleeding, and erectile dysfunction have been reported with alfa-interferon, and animals exposed to all interferons have demonstrated an increased rate of spontaneous abortion.[110–113,142] Likewise, the retinoids have been associated with spontaneous abortion and fetal malformation.[142] In addition to drug-induced dysfunction, the usual side effects of fatigue and flulike symptoms affect interest in and comfort with sexual activities.[143] No studies have examined the effects of BRMs on human pregnancy and lactation; information often is extrapolated from animal data. The use of these agents during pregnancy and while lactating is contraindicated. Future research on the subject of gonadal dysfunction related to BRMs is extremely important.

## TARGETED THERAPIES

Use of the novel anticancer therapies that inhibit cancer cell growth is increasing. These agents affect specific molecular targets that are responsible for the growth of tumors. Among

**TABLE 36-2**

**Cancer-Associated Drugs That Affect Sexual and Reproductive Function**

| Agent | Complication |
|---|---|
| **Antidepressants** | |
| Amitriptyline<br>Bupropian hydrochloride<br>Clonazepam<br>Duloxetin hydrochloride<br>Imipramine<br>Selective serotonin reuptake inhibitors (SSRIs)<br>Venlafaxine hydrochloride | Erectile dysfunction, altered libido, irregular menses, anorgasmia |
| **Antiemetics/Sedatives/Tranquilizers** | |
| Chlorpromazine<br>Diazepam<br>Lorazepam<br>Metochlopramide<br>Prochlorperazine<br>Scopolamine | Sedation, orgasm without ejaculation, erectile dysfunction, decreased sexual interest, decreased intensity of orgasm, gynecomastia |
| **Antihistamines** | |
| Diphenhydramine | Sedation, decreased sexual interest |
| **Steroids** | |
| (See Table 36-1) | |
| **Narcotics** | |
| Codeine<br>Fentanyl<br>Hydromorphone<br>Methadone<br>Morphine | Decreased libido, sedation, impaired potency |
| **Miscellaneous** | |
| Celexa | Decreased libido, anorgasmia, erectile dysfunction |
| Cimetadine | Erectile dysfunction |
| Dronabinol | Altered libido, sedation |
| Gabapentin | Amenorrhea, erectile dysfunction, vaginal hemorrhage |
| Ketoconazole | Decreased libido, gynecomastia, oligospermia, erectile dysfunction |

*Source*: Data from Wilkes and Barton-Burke[110]; Otto[111]; Cleri and Haywood[112]; Gullatte[113]; and Chu and DeVita.[114]

these are epidermal growth factor tyrosine kinase inhibitors (ie, gefitinib, imatinib), fusion proteins (eg, denileukin diftitox), and antiangiogenic agents (ie, bevacizumab, thalidomide). The sexual side effects related to these agents are unclear; however, rash, fatigue, diarrhea, and the potential for severe birth defects are well documented with many of these agents.[144] The use of thalidomide requires 2 types of contraception and pregnancy tests prior to each cycle due to the potential for fetal malformations. Currently, all of these agents are contraindicated during pregnancy and breastfeeding.[110,144–148]

### STEM CELL AND MARROW TRANSPLANTATION

As long-term survival from transplantation increases, issues related to sexuality and sexual dysfunction have become more evident. The late effects of bone marrow transplantation (BMT) include chronic fatigue, body image alterations, gonadal dysfunction, and infertility. Women experience decreased sexual desire and satisfaction, vaginal atrophy and decreased vaginal lubrication, premature menopause, failure to achieve orgasm, and painful intercourse, as well as feelings of loss of femininity.[149–151] Partnered women were generally more satisfied with their sex lives and sexual partners than single women; however, in a study by Tierney et al, a depressed libido was seen in 73% of women and 54% reported avoiding intimacy.[151] Men frequently experience ejaculatory difficulties, while long-term consequences may include decreased desire, body image alterations, and erectile dysfunction most often related to arteriogenic insufficiency.[150,152,153] Other side effects may include gynecomastia, Leydig cell insufficiency, and decreased libido.[154] The hospitalization often required in conjunction with transplantation can affect sexuality and intimacy due to lack of privacy and limited physical contact. The combination of high-dose chemotherapy and total body irradiation (TBI) exacerbates sexually related side effects, with women having more long-term sequelae than men.[149,150,152,155]

Primary gonadal dysfunction has been described in all transplant patients, whether or not the patients received TBI. Recovery of gonadal function is rare in both men and women (<10%) and is related to age as well as the use of TBI and combination vs single agent chemotherapy.[149,150,156,157] Nevertheless, successful pregnancy has been reported following transplantation. Increasing age and the use of TBI seemed most integral to the inability to conceive or father a child.[157] Assisted reproduction techniques have been shown to benefit those individuals desiring a child following transplant.[158] The use of testosterone and/or sildenafil has been shown to be of benefit in decreasing or preventing erectile dysfunction,[153] while the use of leuprolide acetate has been tested to protect ovarian function in young women undergoing SCT with mixed results. The addition of hormone replacement therapy post transplant has led to resumption of menses and to successful pregnancies in some patients.[158]

Numerous authors have investigated quality of life in survivors of BMT.[151,155,156,158] Major concerns included decreased energy, moderate to severe fatigue, infertility, inability to perform sexually, and alterations in sexual intimacy, pleasure, and ability to achieve orgasm and an erection.[149–151,155,156,158] Other potential side effects include anxiety, depression, and current life stressors.[149] Sexual and reproductive implications of treatment should be discussed and counseling provided prior to, throughout, and following treatment.

## ASSESSMENT

Although not always accurately portrayed, sexuality is more than the act of intercourse. It includes intimacy, touching, a multitude of activities to show affection, and a variety of methods to communicate with others. Cancer and treatment may disrupt or permanently alter one's ability to maintain previous sexual patterns or may cause infertility; at the same time, cancer cannot alter the fact that one is a sexual being. This information, along with treatment and side effect information, needs to be reiterated and reinforced to the patient and family.[3,159–162]

Although not every nurse can be a sexual counselor, listening to the concerns of the patient and family, presenting factual information in a nonthreatening manner, managing noncomplex disease- and treatment-related symptoms, and providing appropriate referrals can be easily incorporated into routine care. Many healthcare providers rarely discuss issues related to sexual and reproductive concerns for a variety of personal and professional reasons. Primary reasons cited include personal discomfort, lack of training or knowledge, and fears of embarrassing themselves or their patients. Additional reasons include lack of time, concerns about the appropriateness of such discussions when dealing with a life-threatening illness, and the belief that these subjects are not part of the nurse's job description.[3,48,159–161,163,164] A common concern is that of "opening a can of worms" in which the nurse does not feel adequately prepared to discuss the issues of sexuality or reproductive dysfunction and thus fears that by broaching the topic she/he may create more problems for the patient, including increasing the patient's anxiety and treatment decision making.[165]

### ASSESSMENT STRATEGIES

To effectively assess a patient for alterations in sexuality, the nurse must understand the patient's medical, psychiatric, and psychosexual status; evaluate present relationships; and provide recommendations and encouragement.[56,159–161] Nurses should include sexuality in their assessment of all patients and should provide hope, reassurance, and basic information.[159–161,166] While all patients should be assessed, it is important to recognize those who may be at high risk for sexual dysfunction. Characteristics include advancing age; surgery or radiation therapy to the pelvis; higher doses of chemotherapy; the use of medications for pain, hypertension, and nausea; and alterations in body image and self-esteem (see Table 36-3).[160,161,167]

To conduct an effective assessment, the nurse should use an array of models, discussion questions and/or evaluation tools to assess the patient's potential and current sexual dysfunction. Depending on the type of patient interaction, the relationship the nurse has with the patient and family, and the patient's medical condition and needs, the assessment can be brief or intensive. Topics discussed may include current level of sexuality and intimacy, present relationships, current and future childbearing desires, methods of communication, and coping skills. Additional topics could include contraceptive techniques, social support, cognitive function, and any history of rape, domestic violence, or abuse.[160,161]

## Assessment models

Multiple models have been developed to assess sexuality and intervene in sexual and reproductive concerns. While not necessarily developed for patients with cancer, all can be used effectively by the nurse or sexual counselor to evaluate sexuality issues. The models can generally be divided into 3 categories: pure assessment models (ALARM,[56] Auchincloss,[166] and Schover[168]); pure intervention models (PLISSIT[169] and Ex-PLISSIT[170,171]); and models that allow for both assessment and intervention (BETTER[172] and PLEASURE[173]).

The assessment models were developed in the 1990s for use with patients with cancer. Each assessment model allows for a discussion of current sexual activities and concerns coupled with an understanding of the patient's current medical treatments and status. In addition to medical issues, Schover's model does include identifying the patient's sexual desires, goals and knowledge as a major component.[168] The assessment models tend to be more medically focused, with questions about the sexual response cycle and medical comorbidities, and may seem too limited for the practicing nurse who wants to provide support and relief of concerns within the frequently limited nursing encounter.[160,161]

The intervention models focus on methods to alter current or potential sexual dysfunction. These models assume the nurse has already completed a sexual assessment prior to model use and that the interventions will be individualized for each patient. The PLISSIT model was developed by Annon in the 1970s and has been used with patients with all types of illnesses since that time. The primary components include Permission (to be sexually active), Limited Information (about disease and treatment effects on sexuality and reproduction), Specific Suggestions (strategies to overcome or manage any dysfunction) and Intensive Therapy (psycho- or sex therapy). It is generally suggested that most nurses can effectively manage the first 3 steps of these models while the final step will require a trained, licensed sexual therapist; however, referral at any time point is appropriate.[169] Davis and Taylor[170,171] expanded the PLISSIT model by adding permission-giving to each step and also incorporating both a personal reflection by the nurse on the interaction with the patient and a review of the interaction and any specific interventions with the patient at the end of each interaction. Expansion of PLISSIT should

**TABLE 36-3**

**Sexual and Reproductive Dysfunction: High-Risk Characteristics**

| Characteristic | Women | Men |
|---|---|---|
| Age | Over age 30 | Post-puberty |
| Surgery | Gynecologic surgeries<br>Abdominal-perineal resection<br>Pelvic exenteration | Prostate, orchiectomy<br>Abdominal-perineal resection<br>Pelvic exenteration |
| Radiation therapy | Pelvic | Pelvic |
| Medications | Antidepressants, antihistamines, antihypertensives, antiemetics, antiestrogens, narcotics, sedatives, tranquilizers, alcohol | Antidepressants, antihistamines, antihypertensives, antiemetics, estrogens, narcotics, sedatives, tranquilizers, alcohol |
| Psychosocial issues | Alterations in body image and self-esteem, decreased sense of femininity | Alterations in body image and self-esteem, decreased sense of masculinity |
| Comorbidities | Arthritis, COPD, dementia, depression, diabetes, myocardial infarction, spinal cord injury | Arthritis, COPD, dementia, depression, diabetes, myocardial infarction, spinal cord injury |

*Source*: Data from Krebs.[160,161,167]

allow for introduction of assessment throughout the levels of the original model, making it more useful for nursing practice.

The combination models allow for both assessment and intervention, incorporating an evaluation of sexual concerns with individualized methods to manage each issue. These may be more comfortable for the novice nurse to use on a daily basis. These models assume that the patient is a sexual being and will have sexual concerns that may or may not be openly addressed. By combining assessment and intervention, these models allow the nurse to more effectively intervene in a shorter time, if needed. However, the PLEASURE model, developed by Schain in the 1980s and focusing primarily on psychosexual issues (Partner, Lovemaking, Emotions, Attitudes, Understanding, Reproduction, and Energy), has been infrequently cited in the literature and does not appear to have been updated or evaluated in the past decade.[173] More recently, the PLISSIT model has been expanded by some healthcare professionals for both assessment and intervention through incorporating permission to discuss sexual issues into the initial permission component (permission to be sexually active) first described by Annon.[159,160]

In a review of the intimacy and sexuality literature, Hordern[174] provides a critical analysis of 3 of the models noted previously, ALARM, PLISSIT and BETTER. She notes that the ALARM model focuses on a penetrative, orgasmic perspective rather than looking at the entire continuum of sexuality for the patient. She believes that this model (and most likely any of this specific type), supports the often unspoken idea that healthcare providers do not have a role, or have only a limited role, in discussing sexuality outside of sexual intercourse and reproduction. In terms of the PLISSIT model, Hordern notes that most current discussions of the model do not incorporate the potential for referral throughout each level as was inherent in Annon's original intent. In addition, the model is neither cancer-site-specific nor does it rely on patient–provider reflection on the interaction for evaluation.[174] She does not discuss the Ex-PLISSIT model, which was intended to alter this particularly glaring lack of patient-provider interaction and reflection. Finally, Hordern discusses the BETTER model, which she feels promotes improved interaction between the nurse and patient and promotes discussion of the entire continuum of sexuality and insists upon accurate recording of the interaction in the patient's medical record. Her primary criticism is that the model does not acknowledge the need for nurses to be educated to discuss sexuality issues particularly as they relate to the nurse's own personal beliefs and suppositions. She states it is imperative to discuss any assumptions with each patient to assure their validity before interventions are undertaken.[174] The models most commonly identified in the literature (ALARM, PLISSIT, and BETTER) as well as the expanded PLISSIT model (Ex-PLISSIT) are described in Table 36-4.

## Assessment methods

To maintain integrity and to improve quality of life, it is essential that all patients receive counseling about sexual dysfunction, that open communication be encouraged, and that interventions be individualized and valued by the participants. Assisting patients and families with sexual alterations is congruent with and integral to the nurse's role in providing holistic care. Many simple, easy-to-follow methods exist, but for nurses to provide assistance, they must first understand their own sexual identity, what constitutes acceptable sexual patterns and practices, as well as the sociocultural, environmental, and other beliefs that may influence how the nurse interacts with others as sexual beings. Being comfortable with one's own sexuality as well as having basic knowledge about sexual issues and concerns facilitates providing assistance.[3,159–161,175] In discussing how to include sexual assessment in nursing practice, Shell[176] focuses on the importance of ensuring privacy during discussions and maintaining confidentiality about issues discussed, the need to begin discussions as early as possible, and to continue the discussions throughout treatment and into follow-up, the importance of identifying the patient's goals and focusing any intervention on meeting them, prevention of any overreaction to issues discussed, and the importance of timely and appropriate referrals.

**TABLE 36-4**

**Models for Sexual Assessment and/or Intervention**

| ALARM Model | PLISSIT | Extended PLISSIT (Ex-PLISSIT) | BETTER |
|---|---|---|---|
| **A**—Activity (Sexual) | **P**—Permission | PLISSIT model plus | **B**ring up sexuality |
| **L**—Libido/desire | **LI**—Limited Information | Permission giving throughout | **E**xplain role of sexuality in QOL |
| **A**—Arousal/orgasm | **SS**—Specific Suggestions | Interactions reviewed with patient at each assessment point | **T**ell about/facilitate resources |
| **R**—Resolution/release | **IT**—Intensive Therapy | Nurse reflection throughout | **T**iming critical |
| **M**—Medical data | | | **E**ducate patient/partner |
| | | | **R**ecord in health record |

*Source*: Data from Andersen and Lamb[56]; Annon[169]; Davis and Taylor[170]; and Mick et al.[172]

Asking about the patient's sexual practices early in the clinical assessment legitimizes and normalizes the subject and gives patients permission to discuss sexual issues. Current practices, cultural and religious beliefs, and general intimacy issues should be incorporated in the discussion. Questions such as frequency of sexual activity, satisfaction with sexual response or asking how the patient and partner are communicating and responding to sexual concerns are all appropriate during the assessment. In addition, males should be asked whether they are experiencing any erectile dysfunction and females should be asked about menopause/ menopausal symptoms. As trust is gained, and when deemed appropriate, more sensitive questions, such as "Do you use sexual aids or participate in oral or anal sex?" can be included in the discussion.[21,36,160,161] Whenever possible and appropriate, the patient's partner should be included.[3,160,161,175]

When conducting an assessment, it is important for the nurse to act in a professional manner, speaking in a straightforward and matter of fact manner. When culturally appropriate, eye contact should be maintained and whenever possible, the nurse should sit rather than stand. Medical jargon and value-oriented terminology should be avoided, and questions and responses should acknowledge the subject and related concerns as being normal and important. It is important to keep all questions neutral to gender and sexual orientation, and to avoid cultural stereotyping or assumptions about sexual orientation. Topics should move from areas of less sensitivity to more sensitive areas and patients should be given permission to discuss or not discuss each area. Questions should move normally from one topic to another rather than being a "laundry list" of issues. Verbal and nonverbal communication should be assessed, with clarifying questions and reflection on information shared provided throughout. When the assessment is complete, a plan of care should be developed with the patient that will both address the patient's sexual concerns and provide continual follow-up for evaluation and addressing any new issues.[160,161]

## THERAPEUTIC APPROACHES AND NURSING CARE

### INTERVENTION STRATEGIES

Providing an individualized patient intervention requires not only that the nurse be comfortable in discussing sexuality issues and reproductive concerns, but also that the nurse has the factual information and skills to do so. The nurse must be knowledgeable about the patient's type of cancer and potential treatment and the possible alterations to sexual and reproductive function that may occur. The nurse also needs to know how to access resources and support to effectively intervene.[160,161]

Katz[13] and Krebs[159–161] note that it is essential to understand your own beliefs about sexual issues as these beliefs may hamper your ability to discuss sexuality or intervene appropriately. Wilmoth identified 4 processes that she believes are key to discussing sexual issues with patients: 1) attaining an appropriate level of comfort to discuss sexuality with patients, 2) learning how to communicate effectively, 3) enhancing one's personal knowledge about potential sexual dysfunction in those with cancer, and 4) being able to identify and facilitate the patients use of appropriate resources.[177] Finally, Mick, developer of the BETTER model suggests 10 strategies for the nurse to improve sexuality assessment. In addition to those already identified above, Mick adds encouraging the patient to ask questions about sexuality, using current practice standards, listening objectively, and the need to conduct an independent sexual assessment that goes beyond the questions asked on a standard intake assessment form and incorporates the nurse's individual skills and knowledge.[178]

Components of the intervention should include factual information about disease, treatment, and potential side effects. Discussing potential alterations in sexual functioning, including fertility issues, prior to or early in treatment and continuing these discussions well into the follow-up phase, is essential. Information is needed to dispel myths, decrease anxiety, minimize embarrassment, provide a basis for alternative strategies, and open lines of communication between the patient and others.[3,160,161]

Managing the side effects of cancer and treatment is also integral to the nurse's role. Offering simple suggestions and appropriately managing side effects may be sufficient for most patients to continue or reinstitute sexual activities and enhance intimacy. In addition to management of such traditional symptoms as pain, nausea, vomiting, and bone marrow depression, nurses should provide information and strategies about less commonly recognized symptoms that affect sexual function, such as peripheral neuropathies, malnutrition, stomatitis, fatigue, hand-foot syndrome, and incontinence.[110,160,161] They also should stress the importance of communication and openness; potential alterations in body image and self-esteem; the need for exercise, rest, and adequate nutrition; the use of contraception; setting the stage for sexual activities (candles, music, sexy clothing); experimentation with alternative methods of intimacy; and the liberal and adequate use of lubricants, foreplay, and more comfortable positions. Energy conservation techniques and information on the timing of medications and methods to maintain cleanliness and personal hygiene are important as well.[3,160–162,169]

Knowing when to make referrals and recognizing appropriate community resources are essential. Areas of referral include hormonal therapies, vacuum devices, or medications to manage erectile dysfunction, sperm banking and other fertility-preserving options, and reconstructive surgery and prostheses. Some patients will require psychosexual counseling; others will not. Individualization of education and counseling is important for each patient. It is crucial that the nurse (or others) not invent sexual concerns for those who do not have them; rather, the nurse anticipates, recognizes, advocates, and assists those who do.[21,36,160,161]

Of particular importance is being able to integrate the topic of alterations in sexual and reproductive function into one's practice. Doing so requires many skills that most nurses do not obtain in basic nursing education, although this does appear to be changing. Participating in continuing education programs and in journal clubs focused on sexually related issues and the use of role models can provide the novice nurse with initial skills for sexual assessment. Continuing education programs should focus on skills acquisition and values clarification through the use of both didactic and interactive components such as small group discussions and role playing. Additional skills can be gained through continual incorporation of sexuality assessment and counseling into daily nursing practice, attending advanced seminars, taking part in values clarification exercises, and participating in interdisciplinary rounds and educational offerings. In addition, work sites can amend or add standards of care that include provision for sexual assessment and intervention.[160,175,176]

## FERTILITY CONSIDERATIONS AND PROCREATIVE ALTERNATIVES

Fertility and pregnancy following cancer diagnosis are fraught with a multitude of concerns, particularly the ability to conceive, carry to term, and deliver a healthy newborn with no congenital abnormalities and no increased risk for future malignancies because of either parent's previous diagnosis and treatment for cancer. Radiation therapy and chemotherapy, alone or in combination, have the potential to induce infertility. Proved fertility is measured by pregnancy rates. Even when fertility is preserved, conception may be delayed. Information about procreative alternatives, the potential for infertility, and issues related to genetic inheritance, mutagenicity, and timing of pregnancy must be thoroughly discussed with potential parents prior to their attempting conception.[179,180]

Individuals are considered to be clinically infertile if they are unable to conceive after a minimum of 1 year of unprotected intercourse occurring during the fertile phase of a woman's menstrual cycle. Approximately 1% of the general population is believed to be infertile, with fertility declining with age after the late thirties for men and late twenties for women. Compromises to fertility in cancer survivors are related to type and dose of treatment, age and pretreatment fertility.[180,181]

Multiple authors have reviewed fertility concerns related to cancer and cancer therapy.[135,181–188] Problems with fertility in women are related to premature menopause, a compromised ability to carry a pregnancy to term, or total loss of fertility related to organ removal, while men experience compromised sperm production; DNA damage to sperm; a decrease in sperm's quality, quantity, or motility; organ removal; or nerve damage to reproductive organs. In addition to surgical consequences, chemotherapy and radiotherapy can affect fertility. With chemotherapy, the type of drug, dose and treatment schedule, and/or drug combinations can affect fertility; the overall dose, fractionation, and treatment site can affect fertility in those treated with radiotherapy. It is well recognized that the alkylating agents, particularly at high doses, can affect fertility.[135,180,181,183–185] Total body irradiation, field size and higher doses of radiation therapy, particularly to the pelvis, can cause infertility, with doses as low as 2.5 Gy to the testicles or doses to the whole abdomen in women of ≥6 Gy causing the highest risk. Younger men and women can tolerate higher doses than adults, with prepubertal children at the lowest risk. In addition, whole brain radiation in doses ≥40 Gy can affect fertility, most likely by damaging the hypothalamic-pituitary axis.[135,180–185] Fertility effects of the BRMs and targeted therapies remain unclear and will need further evaluation as these drugs are more heavily utilized.

It is suggested that many men and women are infertile or subfertile at the time of cancer diagnosis, although until recently, few patients, and in particular women, had actually had their fertility assessed prior to initiation of cancer therapy. Methods to evaluate fertility include semen, sperm, and hormonal analyses in men and hormonal analyses and ultrasound of the ovaries in women.[135,180,181,184,187]

As the field of infertility medicine has improved its methods of enhancing fertility, these successes have been more commonly employed in patients with cancer hoping to preserve their fertility while undergoing cancer treatment. Multiple methods have been identified to attempt to preserve fertility, although not all have been entirely successful. Movement of the ovaries out of the radiation field (oophoropexy or ovarian transposition) for those women receiving pelvic or whole abdomen radiation has met with some success, while fertility sparing surgery (trachelectomy for cervical cancer or removal of only one ovary and maintaining the uterus for those with early stage ovarian cancer), has been beneficial in young woman wishing to maintain fertility. Embryo, egg, and ovarian tissue cryopreservation are also being used with varying levels of success. For men, sperm banking and testicular shielding have been the primary methods, while testicular transposition to protect from radiation therapy damage has recently been used with some success. Testicular tissue freezing remains experimental, but has been successful in animal models. Most recently, studies using GnRH analogs such as leuprolide to preserve ovarian function in young women have been given concomitantly with chemotherapy. Results have been mixed and the treatment remains controversial.[178,180,184,188,189]

### Mutagenicity

*Mutagenicity* is the ability to cause an abnormality in the genetic content of cells, resulting in cell death, alteration(s) in growth and replication, or no noticeable alteration in cell function. Although chromosomal alterations have been noted in patients who have recently completed cancer therapy, possible germ cell mutations may not be evident for generations of offspring.[135,190]

Numerous researchers have investigated the offspring of individuals exposed to chemotherapy or radiation therapy as children, adolescents, or young adults as a method to adequately assess mutagenicity following therapy.[182,186,187,191–193] While several specific instances of fetal wasting or congenital malformations, such as an increase in first pregnancy miscarriages[191,193] and congenital cardiac abnormalities,[192] were identified, no statistical difference in congenital malformations, stillbirths, or low birth weights was seen.[186,191,192] Edgar and colleagues[187] identified several large international studies providing a pool of more than 25,000 childhood survivors for evaluation of mutagenicity. They noted that no increased risk of genetic abnormality was identified in the offspring of survivors. Indeed, in a study by Fossa and Dahl,[135] there were no increased incidences of birth defects in the offspring of cancer survivors when compared to their nontreated siblings; while Hansen, et al[194] reported no congenital malformations in the 22 children conceived after their fathers received treatment for testicular cancer In addition, no increased risk of genetic disease was identified in more than 4500 children of adult survivors of childhood cancer.[195] Meistrich and Byrne[196] evaluated the 2 most comprehensive studies of genetic abnormalities in the offspring of cancer survivors. Findings showed no statistically significant difference in the percentage of offspring with a genetic abnormality in those treated with potentially mutagenic therapy, less or no mutagenic therapy or nontreated sibling controls, although there was a marginally significant difference in the percentage of children with genetic abnormalities born to those given low/no-mutagenic treatments. They postulate this may be due to chance or to therapies that are not yet known to be mutagenic, may be mutagenic in combination or may somehow damage the uterine lining resulting in abnormalities. They reported no difference in the types of genetic abnormalities between the groups; however, they did note an alteration in male to female gender ratio in the offspring of women treated with highly mutagenic therapies with a significant decrease in the number of male offspring. In all studies, it has been difficult to specifically implicate germ cell mutations as the cause of adverse outcomes of pregnancy. Follow-up over several generations of patients and their offspring will be needed before definitive answers are obtained.

### Teratogenicity

*Teratogenicity* is the ability of a toxic compound to produce alterations in an exposed fetus. Both chemotherapy and radiation therapy are known to have teratogenic effects on the fetus, causing spontaneous abortion, fetal malformation, or fetal death, especially during the first trimester. Low-dose radiation has also been implicated in fetal malignancy.[197–199]

Radiation exposure during the first trimester represents the greatest risk to the fetus, with an exposure of 100 cGy or more resulting in fetal death, microcephaly, eye anomalies, and intrauterine growth retardation. In the second or third trimester, fetal death is unlikely, but growth retardation, sterility, and cataracts are common findings. As one progresses into the third trimester, the potential deleterious effects are less apparent; however, the potential for development of cancer during the first decade of life is elevated with a 40% increase when the fetus is exposed to a total dose of 0.01 Gy.[186,200]

Chemotherapy, particularly when received during the first trimester, has been related to congenital abnormalities, with approximately 10% of fetuses experiencing some type of anomaly. In general, the alkylating agents and antimetabolites have been most often associated with fetal malformations. Chemotherapy during the second or third trimester may cause premature birth, intrauterine growth retardation, or low birth weight, but congenital abnormalities are not increased over the incidence with normal pregnancy.[160,197,200–202] The timing of chemotherapy is critical. Therapy given prior to the fifth week of gestation is most likely to result in spontaneous abortion if severe damage to the blastocyst occurs. Between the fifth and twelfth weeks, structural damage is most common and congenital malformations tend to occur. After the twelfth week, fetal growth restriction is most common. Effects may be related to drug dose, length of exposure, frequency of administration, and type and number of drugs administered as well[186,200] (Table 36-5).

### Reproductive counseling

While it is recognized that reproductive counseling about fertility preservation should occur for all patients with cancer desiring future childbearing, many healthcare providers state they do not have accurate, up to-date knowledge about potential alterations to fertility and/or knowledge about where to refer patients for preservation procedures and thus are less likely to discuss the topic or provide a referral to an appropriate facility.[203,204] These findings were supported by a study by King and colleagues,[205] in which nurses were asked to identify barriers to discussing fertility preservation with their patients. While it was believed that nurses had a responsibility to discuss such measures with their patients and, in fact, were in an ideal position to do so, the participants cited a lack of knowledge about procedures and facilities, ethical concerns such as religion or what to do with unused embryos or sperm, lack of time and the belief that these discussions should be initiated by

**TABLE 36-5**

**Teratogenetic Effects of Chemotherapy**

| Agent | Complication |
|---|---|
| | **Alkylating** |
| Altretamine<br>Busulfan<br>Chlorambucil<br>Cyclophosphamide<br>Dacarbazine<br>Ifosfamide<br>Nitrogen mustard<br>Nitrosoureas<br>Temozolomide | Spontaneous abortions, skeletal malformations |
| | **Antimetabolites** |
| Capecitabine<br>Cytosine arabinoside<br>6-mercaptopurine<br>5-fluorouracil<br>Gemcitabine<br>Methotrexate<br>Pemetrexed<br>Raltitrexed<br>Trimetrexate | Spontaneous abortions, skeletal malformations |
| | **Miscellaneous Agents** |
| Angiogenesis inhibitors | Skeletal malformations |
| Antitumor antibiotics | Spontaneous abortions |
| Arsenic trioxide | Skeletal malformations |
| Asparaginase | Skeletal malformations |
| EGRF inhibitors | Malformations, spontaneous abortions |
| Glucocorticoids | Spontaneous abortions |
| Hydroxyurea | Spontaneous abortions |
| Imatinib mesylate | Malformations |
| Irinotecan | Spontaneous abortions |
| Procarbazine | Atrial/septal defects |
| Retinoids | Spontaneous abortions, malformations |
| Revlimid | Skeletal malformations |
| Thalidomide | skeletal malformations |
| Vinblastine | Spontaneous abortions, malformations |
| Vinorelbine tartrate | Malformations |

*Source*: Data from Wilkes and Barton-Burke[110]; Otto[111]; Cleri and Haywood[112]; Chu and DeVita[114]; Blecher[116]; Krebs[118]; Rieger[142]; Remer[144]; Green et al[192]; Robinson and Krebs.[197]

physicians were all cited as barriers to fertility preservation discussions.[205]

Discussions concerning fertility and reproduction issues need to be held prior to the onset of therapy and should continue well into post treatment and follow-up. Current fertility status, desire for future childbearing, and contraception practices should be investigated during the initial assessment. Potential alterations should be openly discussed and referrals made as appropriate. Counseling for possible risks of mutagenicity, increased cancer risk, and unknown sequelae of treatment for progeny should be included.[125,132,203,204,206–208] Birth control methods need to be implemented to minimize the possibility of an unplanned pregnancy during therapy. In addition, methods to maintain fertility during therapy should be investigated.

Patients should be encouraged to ask questions about their sexuality and fertility prior to and throughout the treatment continuum. Questions should include the potential of a particular treatment to alter sexual or reproductive function, how fertility might be protected, potential risks to future children, and resources for fertility preservation and counseling/support services.

Methods have been identified that may preserve fertility during cancer treatment. For those patients receiving radiation therapy, appropriate shielding of the testes or ovaries or oophoropexy to position the ovaries outside the radiation field may be of benefit.[180,207,208] Birth control pills in women and GnRH analogs in men and women have been postulated to protect the germ cells from damage by chemotherapeutic agents. However, studies evaluating treatment of men with GnRH analogs have been disappointing despite initial optimism from animal studies[208]; while in women, results have been inconsistent.[207]

Because it is often difficult to predict when an individual receiving chemotherapy is infertile, it is extremely important that methods to prevent pregnancy be discussed and appropriate contraceptive drugs or devices be provided. It has been suggested that following cancer therapy an individual should wait a minimum of 2 years before attempting conception. This suggestion is made both to prevent pregnancy during the time when recurrence is most likely and to allow for the recovery of spermatogenesis or ovarian function if it has been temporarily altered by therapy.[13,197,206,209] It should be noted, however, that this time frame may be too long for some women at risk for early menopause and that no benefit is known to be derived from a prolonged waiting time.[179] In these individuals, it is suggested that a minimum wait of at least 6 months is needed to decrease the potential for birth defects and miscarriage.[3,209]

Many methods to preserve fertility remain under investigation.[180,183,210–213] These measures include ovarian tissue transplantation,[180,183,210,211,214] oocyte harvesting and cryopreservation[162,180,183,210–212]; the use of progestins in young women with endometrial cancer[215]; the use of GNRH analogues as an ovarian protectant for women receiving adjuvant chemotherapy for breast cancer[180,183,207,209,213]; and ovarian and testicular tissue cryopreservation.[162,180,183,210–212] In addition, harvesting of spermatogonial stem cells from the immature testicle of prepubertal boys has been suggested; these studies are still in preclinical study.[216,217] All of these procedures are still being evaluated.

In 2006, the American Society of Clinical Oncology developed recommendations for fertility preservation for individuals with cancer. A panel identified the scientific literature on current fertility options. Options considered as standard of care for men include semen cryopreservation, gonadal shielding, testicular cryopreservation and testicular xenografting, while standard procedures for women include embryo cryopreservation, gonadal shielding, oophoropexy and conservative gynecologic surgery, such as trachelectomy. Oocyte and ovarian tissue cryopreservation, spermatogonial isolation and GNRH analogue suppression of ovaries or testes remain investigational.[181]

Of note, any discussion of fertility preservation using cryopreserved tissue (embryos, oocytes, sperm and ovarian or testicular tissue) should include a discussion of disposition of these tissues should the patient not survive or otherwise be unable to use them. This discussion would optimally take place at the preservation procurement facility and should be outlined and legally agreed upon by all parties. For procedures involving children, parents should evaluate the nature of the potential procedure and assure the child's assent prior to proceeding.[180]

Although some successes have been seen with most methods, no individual method appears to be successful for each person, treatment regimen, or tumor type. Discussions of alternative methods of parenting such as surrogacy, adoption or step-parenting should be discussed as appropriate.

## Semen cryopreservation and sperm recovery

Semen storage for use in artificial insemination has been available for many years, with the first pregnancy from frozen sperm reported in 1953.[218] Although initially used to establish pregnancy in infertile couples, sperm banking has more recently been used to preserve procreation abilities in men undergoing cancer therapy. Unfortunately, the option to bank sperm will not be available to every man undergoing cancer therapy. Many men will be subfertile or infertile at the time of diagnosis, particularly those with testis cancer or HD.[184,212] Although techniques such as mapping and fine-needle aspiration of the testis to recover sperm after treatment can be used, sperm banking is most effective when completed prior to initiation of therapy. Thus, anyone with rapidly progressing disease cannot delay the start of therapy to complete the cryopreservation process. Even so, cryopreservation of sperm has provided a viable option for improving fertility prospects in men with various forms of cancer,[121,122,184,212,218] and any semen sample that contains even 1 motile or viable sperm can be preserved.[184,212,218]

Cryopreserved samples can be used in a variety of ways. The initial technique is usually intrauterine insemination (IUI), in which the thawed and washed semen samples are introduced into the partner's uterus around the time of ovulation. More technical procedures, such as in vitro fertilization (IVF) or intracytoplasmic sperm injection (ICSI), in which a single sperm is injected into a single egg, will be tried if this procedure is unsuccessful, or if the number of cryopreserved semen samples is inadequate, or the samples do not contain sufficient numbers of viable sperm.[184,219] In a study of 28 young men who had cryopreserved semen prior to chemotherapy, Agarwal and colleagues noted that a total of 87 assisted reproduction technique cycles (using IUI, IVF, or ICSI) were performed. In 18% of the cycles, pregnancy resulted, with 75% of the pregnancies resulting in a live birth.[220] In addition, sperm may be obtained through testicular sperm extraction (TESE) and testicular sperm aspiration (TESA).[216,221] However, Agarwal et al suggest that these latter methods could potentially result in genetic risk to future children.[212]

Even if artificial insemination is never completed, the knowledge that semen has been banked and is available when needed can provide a significant psychological boost for the man undergoing cancer therapy.[122,221] All aspects of the sperm-banking process, from the initial visit through the completion of insemination, should be fully discussed with the patient so that informed decisions can be made.

For those men who have maintained some degree of fertility but experience retrograde ejaculation, a trial of a sympathomimetic agent may prove beneficial. If this procedure is not helpful, sperm can be harvested from urine, washed, and used for insemination. For true ejaculation, a rectal probe that electrically stimulates the vas deferens, seminal vesicle, and prostate to initiate the ejaculatory reflex may be of benefit. In addition, some men will benefit from sperm aspiration from the vas deferens or epididymis, followed by ICSI.[121,212,218] Finally, scientists are investigating the potential for restoration of spermatogenesis through transplantation of the male germ cell.[212,216,218]

## In vitro fertilization/embryo transfer

In vitro fertilization, used for male infertility due to low sperm counts or for female infertility due to severe endometriosis, immunological infertility, or absent or damaged fallopian tubes, has experienced remarkable technological advances. In the past 12 years, there has been a doubling of the number of procedures, with more than 122,000 IVF cycles performed every year in the US.[222,223] This technique requires ovarian stimulation followed by ova retrieval via ultrasound-guided needle aspiration of the preovulatory follicles. Laparoscopy also may be used. The retrieved oocytes are then incubated with sperm for 5 to 26 hours. Following incubation, the embryos are transferred to the uterus and released. The rate of successful pregnancy with IVF is approximately 43%.[222] The process for ICSI is the same except that a single sperm is injected directly into the oocytes.[219,223] The use of ICSI has increased the rate of successful fertilization, thereby increasing the potential for a successful pregnancy[218,223]; however, there is concern that while safe, both IVF and ICSI are complicated by multiple gestations and a higher risk of congenital abnormalities.[223]

### Embryo, oocyte, and ovarian tissue cryopreservation

Human embryo cryopreservation has been used for more than 25 years and is considered a routine procedure. The process of retrieval is the same as with IVF and ICSI. For women about to undergo gonadotoxic cancer therapy, ovarian stimulation to retrieve oocytes which are then fertilized using a partner's or donor's sperm has been most successful in preserving fertility in young women. However, for those without a partner or donor or for prepubertal girls, this method may not be satisfactory. In addition, concerns have been raised about the use of stimulation agents in those with estrogen-sensitive tumors. Alternative stimulation agents, such as the aromatase inhibitors or tamoxifen have been successfully used without adding undue risk.[180,183,209,211,212]

Researchers are investigating new techniques to cryopreserve oocytes that can later be autotransplanted into the infertile woman or isolated and allowed to mature in vitro. Concerns about the best methods for cryopreservation, implantation and the potential for reintroduction of malignant cells have affected the use of these approaches although the thawed oocytes appear to be viable and the procedure promising. The use of the process of vitrification, or ice-free cryopreservation done by ultra rapid cooling, has resulted in oocytes survival rates of almost 100% with fertilization rates of approximately 90% and successful pregnancy rates of 33% to 57%. Previous rates for the standard slow cooling method that results in ice crystal formation in the oocytes has significantly lower survival and fertilization and pregnancy rates.[210,212,224] Porcu and colleagues describe the birth of healthy twins following oocytes cryopreservation in a young woman treated for ovarian cancer. She underwent 2 separate ovariectomy procedures, but was able to undergo oocyte procurement prior to removal of the second ovary. The oocyte were frozen for 4 years, then 3 were thawed, fertilized, and implanted. A twin pregnancy occurred resulting in the birth of 2 apparently healthy females delivered by cesarean section at 38 weeks.[225]

Investigation continues with cryopreservation of ovarian tissue. This procedure may be the most appropriate for prepubertal girls. There is, however, concern that cancer cells could be implanted with transplantation of the ovarian tissue. Thorough assessment of the tissue prior to implantation is essential.[180,183,210–212] Demeestere et al[226] reported the successful transplantation of cryopreserved ovarian tissue in a young woman who underwent a bone marrow transplant for HD. After the first cycle of her conditioning regimen, she underwent unilateral ovariectomy. Following removal, the ovarian cortex was divided into 40 pieces which were cryopreserved. After successful recovery from her HD, the patient underwent transplantation of her 3 pieces of ovarian tissue. Ovarian function was restored and a pregnancy ensued, but resulted in a miscarriage at 7 weeks. One year later, 4 pieces of ovarian cortex were thawed and implanted. Approximately 4 months later pregnancy was confirmed, resulting in delivery of a healthy female at 41 weeks gestation.[226]

## SEXUAL DYSFUNCTION IN SPECIAL POPULATIONS

### Adolescents/young adults

Adolescents and young adults (AYAs) with cancer remain a unique challenge when addressing the sexual and reproductive needs of patients with cancer. As noted by Bolte and Zebrack,[227] adolescence and young adulthood is a time of developing one's own self and personal identity and laying the groundwork for intimate relationships in the future. A diagnosis of cancer can affect these critical developmental activities by creating isolation and alienation from the AYA's peer group through absences from school or work, missing out on normal life experiences such as dating, the need to be protective of one's health, being seen or seeing the self as different, and/or through dealing with issues of grief, loss and death if cancer becomes untreatable.

While dealing with cancer and cancer treatment, the AYA may find it difficult to access appropriate sexual health knowledge, manage a changing body image, and effectively deal with interpersonal relationships. Because of illness, the AYA may obtain sexual information differently from peers or at a time when cognitively the patient is less able to understand the short- and long-term ramifications of sexual dysfunction and potential infertility.[13,227,228] Discussions with providers and parents may be couched so that potential problems are minimized and cultural, environmental and other biases may prevent full discussion of potential sexual or reproductive alterations, or possible solutions such as sexual education or counseling, or fertility preserving activities such as sperm banking and egg harvesting.

Katz[13] and Evan and colleagues[228] suggest that AYAs particularly need to be supported through the cancer experience so that sexual identity, self-esteem, and the ability to process and manage future sexuality and fertility issues can be appropriately and adequately addressed. Providing support includes such activities as establishing trust, allowing choice, addressing myths and providing sexual resources. It is important not to assume sexual identity or presence or lack of previous sexual activity. Based on the age of the patient as well as patient preference, discussions can be held with family or independently. For all procedures, patient assent as well as appropriate parental consent should be obtained.

Based on the identified need to provide education and counseling about sexuality to AYAs in order to decrease the possibility of long-term sexual impairment, Canada and colleagues[229] evaluated a program to enhance psychosexual development of AYAs. The program consisted of 2 individual counseling sessions during which the impact of cancer on sexual development, sexual functioning, fertility, and relationships were discussed. Interactive exercises were included as part of each session. Patients were randomized to either take part in the intervention immediately or to take part at a later date. Following the intervention participants had increased knowledge and body image and decreased concerns about romantic and sexual relationships. These gains were maintained at 3 months following the intervention. Programs such as this need further evaluation, but appear to be a good beginning at managing the unique issues of sexuality in AYAs with cancer.

### Older adults/elderly

Managing sexuality issues in the older adult with cancer is fraught with the complexities of integrating a cancer diagnosis, comorbidities, aging, partner availability, social isolation, and alterations in housing and lifestyle. While sexual activities generally decrease with advancing age, changes in physical (cancer treatment side effects) and mental ("chemo brain") conditions related to cancer or cancer treatment coupled with comorbidities such as arthritis or dementia particularly can impact both an interest in and the ability to take part in previous sexual activities.[230]

Factors most commonly associated with changes in sexuality in older adults are ill health or lack of a partner. Many continue to have active and satisfying sex lives late in life, although they may substitute intimacy, touching, kissing, and cuddling for previous penetrative activities. Alterations in lifestyle such as moving to assisted living or living with family members can affect function due to lack of privacy or permission to be sexually active, while changes in a partner's desire or ability to be sexually active will affect overall function.[13,49,230,231]

For healthcare providers, it is essential to remember that advancing age does not equate with a lack of interest in sexual expression. It is important to ask about sexuality, albeit gently, and be prepared with answers. Ensuring privacy and confidentiality and recognizing that many have nontraditional relationships are crucial for any comprehensive discussion. As with any sexual assessment, the provider should move from less to more sensitive areas, focus on goals important to the patient, include the partner when possible and permissible, and avoid any overreaction or appearance of being bored. Providing appropriate education based on the patient's desire and level of need and offering resources for information and counseling are critical.[13,49,230,231] In addition, it is becoming more common for older adults to enter into new relationships following the death or separation from a previous partner. Education about sexually transmitted disease as well as methods to share a cancer diagnosis and associated treatment with a new partner should be included in sexuality discussions.[230]

### Gay, lesbian, bisexual, and transgender individuals

As Dibble and colleagues[232] have noted, nurses are caring for gay, lesbian, bisexual and transgender (GLBT) individuals in all practice settings. Unfortunately, many of these patients remain somewhat to totally invisible as most nurses and others assume or at least function as though there are only 2 genders (male and female) and that patients generally are heterosexual. Because sexual orientation or gender identity is not always easily identifiable, providers need to ask; indeed, most GLBT patients prefer that they do.

In order to provide culturally appropriate care, use of the ASK (Awareness, Sensitivity, and Knowledge) framework is suggested. In this framework, providers should be aware of their own actual or potential biases towards GLBTs, should be sensitive in their approach to these individuals, and should use current and appropriate knowledge to inform their practice. This is especially true when assessing for sexual and reproductive dysfunction associated with cancer and cancer treatment as one of the barriers to discussing sexuality is discordance between the provider's and the patients gender or sexual identity.[232–234]

Few studies have specifically evaluated the impact of cancer on the sexuality of GLBTs. Blank[235] described the impact of prostate cancer on gay men, noting that erectile dysfunction can have very different implications for gay men. He also commented that most discussions of erectile dysfunction are focused on vaginal intercourse for those in long standing, opposite-sex, partnered relationships. Blank also suggests that gay men may need different support services and evaluation of psychosexual needs; 2 services not always provided. Arena and colleagues[236] evaluated lesbian and heterosexual women with breast cancer, identifying that lesbians had less disruption in sexual activity, fewer sexual concerns, and were more likely to use their current support systems to effectively manage the cancer experience. They note that further research is needed to understand differences and similarities in order to provide comprehensive care.

As previously noted, essential to any sexual discussion is providing confidentiality and privacy, but establishing trust so that sexual orientation and gender identity can be disclosed is paramount. Questions should be asked from a neutral or inclusive stance including asking about relationship rather than marital status and identifying sexual partners by asking who the patient has sex with (exclusively women, mostly women, both, mostly men, or exclusively men) rather than assuming a particular orientation. Whether the patient wants this information in the medical record or not also should be assessed and the request honored. In addition, a positive environment that is free from overt or covert bias or comments and that includes supplying appropriate resources should be provided in order to promote discussion and assure quality care.[13,232,234]

### Terminally ill/palliative care

Unfortunately, many providers do not think of discussing sexuality or supporting sexual issues as patients near the end of life. However, the need to be sexually intimate, to feel close, to touch and be touched and to feel cared for, not only do not lessen as life nears its end, but even may become more important.[237] Indeed, as noted by Shell,[237] sexual expression at the end of life (or at any time) is the patient's right and should be encouraged; however, providers, facilities, employees, family members, and others may make it difficult if not impossible to fulfill the patient's desire for sexual expression.

The factors that affect sexuality for the terminally ill are essentially the same as for those going through cancer treatment, although the focus may be different and the potential for returning to normalcy no longer exists. Issues of privacy and the ability to lie with one another may be impacted by moving to a healthcare facility or having family, friends, and providers coming in and out. Permission may need to be given to sexually active and other methods of sexual expression may need to be explored. Comprehensive symptom management (for pain, nausea, difficulty breathing, vaginal dryness, etc.) and strategies to conserve energy are essential, while appropriate education, including contraceptive use, should be provided as appropriate. When death is imminent, the patient and partner should be encouraged to express intimacy in whatever way is possible and comfortable, including touching, kissing, and verbalization of endearments.[13,237,238]

## PREGNANCY AND CANCER

Although pregnancy complicated by a diagnosis of cancer is a rare event, it creates multiple problems for all concerned. Uncertainty about the prognosis of mother and fetus, the rigors of treatment, and the long-term sequelae of cancer for patient, infant, and family compound events that normally are surrounded by a myriad of conflicting emotions. Only with comprehensive care by many healthcare and ancillary individuals can a positive outcome for mother, fetus, and family be anticipated.

Cancer is the second leading cause of death during the reproductive years. It is estimated that cancer complicates about 1 in 1000 pregnancies and that approximately 1 in 118 women with cancer has a concomitant pregnancy. The most commonly associated cancers are lymphoma, leukemia, malignant melanoma, and cancers of the breast, cervix, ovary, and colorectum—the cancers with the highest incidence during the reproductive years.[239–242]

In general, most cancers do not adversely affect a pregnancy, nor does pregnancy adversely affect the cancer outcome, although the treatment necessary to manage the cancer may potentially have an adverse effect on the pregnancy. Therapeutic abortion has not been shown to be of benefit in altering disease progression and should not be considered unless continued pregnancy will compromise treatment and thus prognosis. The wishes of the patient and family must be considered, with therapeutic options, including prognosis for mother and fetus, being fully explained.

In the past, it was believed that cancer associated with pregnancy was more aggressive and that the outcome for all patients was dismal. Today, it is recognized that delay in diagnosis may be a more likely cause of advanced disease at the time of diagnosis. Diagnosing cancer during a pregnancy is difficult, and signs and symptoms of the disease may be misconstrued or underestimated. Treatment options should be evaluated as though the patient were not pregnant and therapy instituted when appropriate.[197,239,242–245]

## MEDICAL MANAGEMENT OF COMMONLY ASSOCIATED CANCERS

### Breast cancer

Breast cancer is the cancer most commonly associated with pregnancy, occurring in 1 of every 1500 to 1 in every 4000 pregnancies, or in approximately 10% to 20% of women of childbearing age.[197,222,243–246] Among all women with breast cancer who are still in their childbearing years, 1 in 3 will be pregnant at the time of diagnosis[197,239]; of those younger than age 40, about 1 in 200 is at risk of developing breast cancer.[131]

Breast examination should be part of the initial prenatal visit, and any woman 40 or older who is planning a pregnancy should consider having a screening mammography prior to attempting conception.[247] Although breast enlargement during pregnancy makes examination difficult, it is essential that all women have a thorough examination. If a mass is felt, prompt evaluation is necessary. Although a mammogram is difficult to interpret because of the density of the breast, it may be safely undertaken if appropriate fetal shielding is used.[243–245] Even if a mammogram shows negative results, a breast mass must be investigated until a definitive diagnosis is made.[243–245]

Treatment of breast cancer in the pregnant woman should be the same as in the nonpregnant woman. Initial diagnosis should be attempted by fine-needle aspiration, followed by open biopsy if a definitive diagnosis cannot be made.[243–245] Biopsy with the patient under local anesthesia has not been shown to cause fetal harm and should be performed without delay.[243–245] Once a definitive diagnosis is made, further therapy can be tailored to time of gestation, physician recommendations, and patient wishes. In general, modified mastectomy with lymph node sampling is the standard treatment for early disease. The use of sentinel lymph node biopsy is controversial, with particular concern about the risk of fetal radiation exposure related to the use of 99mTc-sulfur colloid and the use of ososulfan blue dye that is classified as a category C drug, and thus should not be used in pregnant patients.[243] Depending on gestational age, adjuvant chemotherapy can often be delayed until after delivery. For the woman desiring breast-conserving surgery, lumpectomy with lymph node sampling may be done if she is close to term, with radiation therapy and chemotherapy being delayed until after delivery. For advanced disease, surgery and chemotherapy should be undertaken without delay. Therapeutic abortion may be suggested during the first trimester to prevent chemotherapy exposure to the fetus; however, as noted, therapeutic abortion does not alter disease outcome and should not be recommended to increase chances of survival.[243–245,248] Chances for survival have been considered poor; however, when patients are matched stage for stage with nonpregnant control subjects, there appear to be no differences in survival rates.[243–245,248] It should be noted, however, that Rodriguez and colleagues noted a 14% increased risk of death when pregnant patients were compared to nonpregnant patients after controlling for race, hormone receptor status, and stage of disease.[249] Delay in diagnosis, often for more than 3 months, may be the most important factor leading to decreased survival.

Pregnancy safety following cancer treatment has been extensively evaluated, particularly for women treated for breast cancer.[250] There appears to be no decrease in survival for women who become pregnant following breast cancer treatment.[245,248,251] It is even possible that a further pregnancy may actually protect against recurrence. In reality, there may be inherent differences between those able to conceive and those unable to conceive, which may alter the survival statistics for this population.[245,248,251] While increasing, the number of reported pregnancies remains small and thus most likely represents a select and nongeneralizable subset of women with breast cancer. For those desiring future pregnancies, a wait of 1 to 5 years following cessation of all treatment, including adjuvant tamoxifen or similar drugs, is recommended.[245,248,251] Women who are known to be *BRCA1* positive should consider seeking genetic counseling prior to attempting conception.

Breastfeeding after a breast cancer diagnosis has been the subject of much debate. For the woman who has received primary breast radiation, it has been suggested that breast-feeding occur only on the nonirradiated side, primarily because of the possible increase in mastitis associated with breast-feeding in the irradiated breast but also because of diminished or absent lactation.[206,248] Pregnancy subsequent to breast irradiation often results in breast asymmetry, with little enlargement of the irradiated breast and minimal to no lactation from the radiated side.

## Cancer of the cervix

The second most common cancer during pregnancy is cancer of the cervix, which occurs in 1 in 400 pregnancies. Approximately 1 in every 100 women diagnosed with cervical cancer will be pregnant at the time of diagnosis. Carcinoma in situ is most commonly found, with invasive disease seen in only 2% to 5% of all patients. Signs and symptoms of cervical cancer are similar to those found in the nonpregnant patient, with the majority of pregnant patients experiencing vaginal bleeding or discharge.[252–254] Diagnosis is most commonly made by Papanicolaou smear. If the smear is abnormal, colposcopy with appropriate biopsies should be undertaken. Cone biopsy is rarely indicated but may be used to confirm a diagnosis of microinvasion. However, it is not without risks and is associated with a 30% complication rate, including hemorrhage, premature delivery, and infection.[137,196,206,253,254] More recently, loop electrode excision has been proposed to minimize the potential complications of conization; this type of excision does not appear to improve disease-free surgical margins; it is associated with an increased incidence of cervical hemorrhage[137,206,253,254]; and women who have a loop excision are more likely to have preterm births and low-birth-weight infants.[255] Laser vaporization may be of benefit but has not been tested in pregnancy. Importantly, it does not affect subsequent pregnancies, as is common with conization.[137,206,253,254]

In patients with cervical intraepithelial neoplasia (CIN 2–3), the pregnancy may be allowed to continue. Cytology and colposcopy should be repeated every 6 to 10 weeks and, unless progression occurs, definitive therapy should be delayed until after delivery.[256] If frank invasion is found, treatment consistent with standard practice for nonpregnant women should not be delayed. During the first 2 trimesters, surgery or radiation therapy without therapeutic abortion is usually undertaken. Early-stage disease (IA and IB) may be treated with radical hysterectomy and pelvic lymph node dissection; in advanced disease, radiation therapy is the most common treatment. During the third trimester, fetal viability usually can be awaited and the baby can be delivered by cesarean section, after which the appropriate cancer therapy is given.[206,252–254,257] For some patients with invasive disease, treatment with radical trachelectomy, rather than radical hysterectomy, has resulted in the ability to conceive and carry the pregnancy to a viable birth, with 1 study reporting 22 pregnancies in 18 patients, 12 full-term births, and 6 preterm births, most commonly due to premature rupture of membranes.[258] However, while this procedure has been used during pregnancy, it is noted to be complicated by a high likelihood of extreme blood loss and the significant potential for fetal loss and is not suggested at this time.[252,259]

Controversy exists over the safety of vaginal delivery. Some believe vaginal delivery would disseminate the cancer or cause hemorrhage or infection; as a result, cesarean section was recommended. Others have suggested that vaginal delivery may be associated with an improved overall survival and should be allowed if possible.[252,253] Recurrence in the episiotomy has been reported following vaginal delivery.[260] Careful follow-up for recurrence is essential. The definitive approach remains unclear.

### Ovarian cancer

Ovarian masses are common during pregnancy, occurring once in every 81 pregnancies. In general, only 2% to 6% of these masses are malignant, for an estimated 1:9000 to 1:32,000 case ratio. Most patients are asymptomatic, with an adnexal mass being noted at the first prenatal visit.[197,252,253,261,262] There are a variety of ways to approach a pelvic mass during pregnancy, including the use of ultrasonography and magnetic resonance imaging.[252,253,262,263] In general, any mass that is unilateral, greater than 6 cm, and solid, and that lasts into the second trimester must be evaluated.[252,253,262] Surgical delay until the second trimester is recommended since the spontaneous abortion rate is approximately 10% when abdominal surgery is performed in the first trimester.[261]

If malignancy is diagnosed, treatment should proceed as in the nonpregnant woman. Early-stage disease (IA) with low-grade histological findings can be managed by unilateral oophorectomy and biopsy of the other ovary. The pregnancy may be allowed to continue.[264] For all other stages, standard therapy of radical hysterectomy, omentectomy, node biopsy, and peritoneal washings are generally carried out, although Behtash and colleagues suggest that a hysterectomy is primarily indicated if it is required for adequate tumor debulking.[261] If the woman is near term, a cesarean section, followed by the appropriate therapy, may be performed. Unfortunately, 30% to 50% of all women will be diagnosed with stage III or IV disease. Although recent management approaches for stage III disease have resulted in improved survival, in general the prognosis for long-term survival is poor.[252,253,262] As in the treatment of all cancers, the wishes of the patient must be considered. It is not uncommon for a pregnant woman with advanced disease to delay treatment until the fetus is viable. Palliative treatment should be instituted at the earliest possible time.

### Malignant melanoma

Malignant melanoma is one of the most rapidly increasing cancers. It occurs most often in a preexisting mole in fair-haired individuals with blue or green eyes and an inability to tan when exposed to the sun; the peak incidence is during the third and fourth decades. Melanoma is expected to increase during pregnancy as women delay childbearing until late in life, when melanoma is more common.[242,265]

Melanoma arising during pregnancy has been postulated to be associated with poor prognosis because it is hormonally influenced and thus exacerbated by pregnancy. At present, this hypothesis does not appear to be true.[266] What is known is that melanoma that occurs during pregnancy more often is found on the trunk, a site associated with a poor prognosis. Also, these melanomas tend to be thicker, which is also synonymous with a poor prognosis.[242] In addition, all pigmented areas darken during pregnancy, making diagnosis of early changes more difficult. Biopsy and removal of questionable lesions are indicated. There appears to be no difference in survival between the pregnant and nonpregnant woman with melanoma.[242,265–267]

Treatment consists of wide excision with skin graft if necessary. While lymph node dissection remains controversial, sentinel node biopsy is recommended.[266] It should be noted, however, that some authors suggest that sentinel lymph node biopsy is permissible during pregnancy, many consider it to be controversial.[199,242,243] Adjuvant therapy, including the use of melanoma vaccines, remains under investigation, but no definitive answers are available for the pregnant patient. The benefits of chemotherapy and BRMs remain unclear.[198,266,268] While chemotherapy regimens can be safely administered during the second and third trimesters,[198,268] it has been standard to delay the adjuvant use of alfa-interferon until postpartum due to the increased rates of fetal and maternal complications associated with high-dose regimens. However, Egberts and colleagues[267] presented a case report in which a pregnant woman received 3 MIU of alfa-interferon 3 times weekly from weeks 8 to 36 of her pregnancy. Although the authors note that the product information states that pregnant women should not receive interferon, the patient continued to receive interferon and delivered healthy twins at 36 weeks gestation.[267] For individuals with advanced disease, therapeutic abortion followed by palliative chemotherapy is advised; however, the wishes of the patient should be weighed against potential outcomes if the pregnancy is allowed to progress. For the individual with brain metastasis, surgery or radiation therapy with appropriate fetal shielding may be undertaken. The use of MRI and CT for metastatic work-up is known to be safe, while the use of the PET scan during pregnancy is not indicated.[269–271]

Malignant melanoma is known to metastasize to the placenta and fetus. The placenta should be carefully evaluated at delivery and the infant monitored for development of melanoma.[242,265,267] Further pregnancies should not be undertaken until at least 2 years after diagnosis and treatment, due to the increased risk of recurrence during this time for all patients with malignant melanoma.[242,265]

### Lymphomas

Both non-Hodgkin's lymphoma (NHL) and HD may occur during pregnancy, although the incidence is rare, with HD occurring in 1 in 6000 pregnancies and NHL rarely associated.[201,272,273] Hodgkin's disease usually occurs as asymptomatic lymphadenopathy of the cervical, supraclavicular, or mediastinal regions. Disease confined to the neck or axilla usually can be treated with radiation therapy combined with fetal shielding. Because more extensive disease requires combination chemotherapy, a therapeutic abortion is suggested if treatment is needed during the first trimester. During the second and third trimesters, therapy will be defined by the stage of the pregnancy. If fetal viability is imminent, therapy may be delayed or single-drug treatment instituted and delivery awaited. For rapidly progressing disease, combination chemotherapy should be instituted immediately. Pregnancy does not appear to negatively affect the clinical course of HD.[202,272,273]

Fewer than 100 cases of NHL and pregnancy have been reported in the literature. In general, pregnant patients tend to be diagnosed later and have a poor prognosis with increased risk of relapse after remission.[202,272] For those with indolent lymphomas, treatment may be delayed until after the first trimester; while those with more aggressive disease should be treated promptly with combination therapy. Rituximab has been given during pregnancy without adverse fetal outcome; however no recommendation can be made assuring safety. Although NHL is known to metastasize to the placenta and fetus, only 8 cases of placental and/or fetal spread have been documented in the past 15 years. Of these cases, 25% of the infants and two-thirds of the mothers have died of lymphoma or its complications. The placenta requires careful observation at delivery.[198,272]

### Leukemia

Leukemia occurs in 1 in 75,000 pregnancies. Diagnosis is often made on routine complete blood count. Treatment should be instituted immediately unless the fetus is viable or near viability. If the fetus is viable, delivery should not be delayed. If the fetus is near viability, leukapheresis may be utilized until delivery is possible. Combination chemotherapy has been administered safely in the second and third trimesters, with no increased incidence of neonatal birth defects.[202,274] Improved treatment and supportive care regimens have decreased the incidence of life-threatening complications and increased remission induction rates; as a consequence, initial survival of the pregnant woman and her fetus is common.[202,274] Therapeutic abortion is suggested in the first trimester to avoid fetal exposure to chemotherapy.[202,274]

## EFFECTS OF TREATMENT AND MALIGNANCY ON THE FETUS

### Surgery

Maternal surgery can be safely accomplished with minimal risk to the fetus.[186,200,206,268,270] Pelvic surgery is more easily accomplished during the second trimester and is associated with a lower rate of preterm birth, as first trimester rates of fetal death have been estimated to range between 8% and 11%.[200,275] There is little risk to the fetus from short exposure to anesthetic agents after the first trimester; however, longer exposure may lead to decreased birth weight.[275] Adequate ventilation and prevention of hypotension are of prime importance. As long as competent surgeons and anesthesiologists with appropriate fetal monitoring equipment are available, no harm to the fetus should occur.[186,200,248,252,268] MRI and ultrasound can safely be used to evaluate presurgical conditions.[263,270,271,276]

### Radiation

Radiation doses of greater than 250 cGy during pregnancy have been associated with fetal damage—for example, mental retardation, skin changes, and spontaneous abortions (depending on stage of gestation). Low doses of radiation associated with diagnostic x-ray studies (<0.5 cGy) are probably not harmful if adequate fetal shielding is provided.[199,277] Radioisotope scans and radiation to the pelvis should be avoided.[199,200,270,271] Endoscopy can be undertaken, but with minimal or no sedation; radiation exposure should not cause teratogenicity. Little is known about potential adverse effects of bowel cleansing regimens.[278] Lethal effects are greatest during preimplantation (conception to day 9 or 10), while during organogenesis (weeks 3 to 12) retarded growth, microcephaly, and ocular problems can occur. Weeks 20 to 25, the fetal period, are associated with functional abnormalities of the liver, kidney, and bone marrow, and sterility.[186,199,245,271,279] Because fetal death, malformation, and mental retardation are associated with doses of 100 to 200 cGy and higher, as long as fetal doses remain less than 100 cGy, therapeutic abortion need not be considered.[280] Long-term effects of low dose radiation remain unknown, but the concerns about chromosomal aberrations and increased rates of childhood cancer in children exposed in utero remain. Follow-up over many generations may be necessary to determine the exact effects.[186,199]

### Chemotherapy

Chemotherapy has been administered prior to and concurrent with pregnancy. As previously noted, chemotherapy during the first trimester has been associated with fetal wastage, malformations, and low birth weights. Many studies indicate that the incidence of fetal malformation is low (<10%) and may be minimized or avoided with careful selection of agents and delay of treatment until the second trimester. Latent effects are still unknown, and offspring need continuous evaluation.[167,198,206,248,281,282]

The majority of information is for single-agent chemotherapy with less information available for combination therapy and the biologics. Mir and colleagues[283,284] described the use of taxanes, vinorelbine and epirubicin during breast cancer. They noted that when given during the second and third trimester, toxicities were minimal. However, they noted that trastuzumab when given during any trimester was associated with anhydraminos in the mother and altered kidney development in the fetus.[283,284] Others[198,268,285] have noted that the biologics have the potential to cause fetal abnormalities similar to chemotherapy, and thus should be avoided during pregnancy if at all possible. However, treatment as close to that used in the nonpregnant patient should be administered whenever possible to increase the potential for long-term remission/cure.[248]

Pereg and colleagues note that the pharmacokinetics of chemotherapeutic agents may be altered by the normal physiological changes of pregnancy. These may include increased hepatic oxidation and renal clearance, problems related to amniotic fluid third spacing, and increased plasma volume.[186] As a result, monitoring for unexpected toxicities or altered response patterns is of extreme importance. Delivery should be delayed for 2 to 3 weeks post-treatment to allow for bone marrow recovery and fetal excretion of drugs through the placenta. Regardless of when the chemotherapy has been given prior to delivery, evaluation of the newborn for toxicities is paramount. Both neonatal metabolism and drug excretion may be suboptimal, and the placenta, which is the normal mechanism for excretion, has been eliminated, increasing the risk of neutropenia and other treatment related toxicities.[167,186,198,206,248,268,281,282]

### Maternal-fetal spread

Only a few cancers spread from the mother to the fetus, with melanoma, NHL, and leukemia being the most common.[242,265,267,272,286] Because few studies have been compiled, the exact incidence is unknown. Dildy and colleagues reviewed literature related to maternal malignancy metastatic to the fetus and reported on 53 cases.[287] The most common cancer was malignant melanoma; metastasis to the placenta occurred in 12 patients and spread to the fetus in 7 cases. The second most common cancers were hematological malignancies (leukemia and lymphoma), involving 8 instances of placental spread and 4 cases of fetal spread. Breast and lung cancers were the next most common, although no cases of spread to the fetus have been reported. In most instances, the cancer spreads to the placenta but no fetal involvement ensues, although reports have noted the infrequent development of cancers in infants of mothers with aggressive metastatic disease.[242,272] There is no evidence that fetal malignancy spreads to the mother.[281]

Because of the rare incidence of metastatic involvement affecting the infant, evaluation of the placenta and fetus is essential in women with disseminated cancers, in additional to a full physical exam of the newborn.[198,242,265,267,272,281] If there is no incidence of spread to the newborn, prophylactic treatment should not be undertaken, but close follow-up is needed.[281]

## NURSING MANAGEMENT OF THE PREGNANT PATIENT

Nursing management of the pregnant patient with a concomitant diagnosis of cancer can be extremely complicated. Interventions including psychosocial, educational, and ethical considerations must be developed and implemented. It has been suggested that pregnancy and cancer be treated as a high-risk event with all the associated needs.[206,239,266] Careful explanations of all aspects of care, with special emphasis on support of the patient and her family, need to be provided. Normal activities of pregnancy may be delayed or prevented by disease or treatment, and fears of fetal demise, cancer therapy, and death may prevent resolution of ambivalence toward pregnancy and establishment of emotional affiliation to the growing child. Ethical considerations become apparent as plans for pregnancy are contrasted with needs for therapy. In some instances, therapeutic abortion may be necessary for optimal treatment; in other instances, therapy delays may be requested to provide for the safety of the fetus. Nonjudgmental care by healthcare personnel is essential during these difficult times.

Nursing care of the woman with cancer and her baby is extremely complex and of utmost importance. With a focus on educational interventions, psychological support, and coordination of care, the nurse has an important role in the final outcome. Treatment plans; coordination of follow-up; education about cancer, pregnancy, and treatment; and emotional support of the patient and significant others are integral components of the comprehensive care needed by the pregnant woman with cancer. Without these essential elements, it may not be possible to provide the necessary care that will ensure a positive or improved maternal and fetal outcome.

## CONCLUSION

Sexual and reproductive dysfunction in patients with cancer occurs much more frequently than previously recognized. Almost every patient exposed to cancer or cancer treatment may experience some form of sexual dysfunction at some point during his or her illness. With cancer survival rates improving, and with the understanding that sexual and reproductive function are important to all individuals, it is essential that sexuality and sexual function be assessed and evaluated prior to therapy and that appropriate interventions be implemented throughout treatment and the follow-up period.

## REFERENCES


1. McKee AL Jr, Schover LR. Sexuality rehabilitation. *Cancer.* 2001;92:1008S-1212S.
2. Tierney DK. Sexuality: a quality-of-life issue for cancer survivors. *Semin Oncol Nurs.* 2008;24:71–79.
3. Nishimoto PW. Sexuality. In: Gates RA, Fink RM, eds. *Oncology Nursing Secrets.* 3rd ed. St. Louis, MO: Mosby; 2008:488–501.
4. Deneris A, Huether SE. Structure and function of the reproductive systems. In: Huether SE, McCance KL, eds. *Understanding Pathophysiology.* 4th ed. St. Louis, MO: Mosby; 2008:821–847.
5. Marieb EN. *Human Anatomy and Physiology.* 6th ed. Menlo Park, CA: Benjamin/Cummings; 2004:1030–1077.
6. Schmidt CE, Bestmann B, Kuchler T, Longo WE, Rohde V, Kremer B. Prospective evaluation of quality of life of patients receiving either abdominoperineal resection or sphincter-preserving procedure for rectal cancer. *Ann Surg Oncol.* 2005;12:117–123.
7. Berg DT. *Pocket Guide to Colorectal Cancer.* Sudbury, MA: Jones and Bartlett; 2003.
8. Schmidt CE, Bestmann B, Kuchler T, Kremer B. Factors influencing sexual function in patients with rectal cancer. *Int J Impotence Res.* 2005;17:231–238.
9. Selvindos PB, Ho YH. Laparoscopic ultralow anterior resection with colonic j-pouch-anal anastomosis. *Dis Colon Rectum.* 2008;51:1710–1711.
10. Chatwin NA, Ribordy M, Givel JC. Clinical outcomes and quality of life after low anterior resection for rectal cancer. *Eur J Surg.* 2002;168:297–301.
11. Nicoletti S, Young J, Levitt M, King M, Chidlow C, Hollingsworth S. Bowel problems, self-care practices, and information needs of colorectal cancer survivors at 6 to 14 months after sphincter-saving surgery. *Cancer Nurs.* 2008;31:389–398.
12. Cotrim H, Pereira G. Impact of colorectal cancer on patient and family: implications for care. *Eur J Oncol Nurs.* 2008;12:217–226.
13. Katz A. *Breaking the Silence on Cancer and Sexuality.* Pittsburgh, PA: Oncology Nursing Society; 2007.
14. da Silva GM, Hull T, Roberts PL, et al. The effect of colorectal surgery in female sexual function, body image, self-esteem and general health: a prospective study. *Ann Surg.* 2008;248:266–272.
15. Chorost MI, Weber TK, Lee RJ, et al. Sexual dysfunction, informed consent and multimodality therapy for rectal cancer. *Am J Surg.* 2000;179: 271–274.
16. Schmidt CE, Bestmann B, Kuchler T, Longo WE, Rohde V, Kremer B. Gender differences in quality of life of patients with rectal cancer. A five-year prospective study. *World J Surg.* 2005;29:1630–1641.
17. Kim NK, Aahn TW, Park JK, et al. Assessment of sexual and voiding function after total mesorectal excision with pelvic autonomic nerve preservation in males with rectal cancer. *Dis Colon Rectum.* 2002;45: 1178–1185.
18. Liang JT, Lai HS, Lee PH, Chang KJ. Laparoscopic pelvic autonomic nerve-preserving surgery for sigmoid colon cancer. *Ann Surg Oncol.* 2008;15:1609–1616.
19. Lindsey I, George B, Kettlewell M, et al. Randomized, double-blind, placebo-controlled trial of sildenafil (Viagra) for erectile dysfunction after rectal surgery for cancer and inflammatory bowel disease. *Dis Colon Rectum.* 2002;45:727–732.
20. Davila HH, Weber T, Burday D, et al. Total or partial prostate sparing cystectomy for invasive bladder cancer: long-term implications on erectile function. *BJU Int.* 2007;100:1026–1029.
21. Albaugh A, Kellogg-Spadt S, Krebs LU, Lewis JH, Kramer-Levien D. Sexual function and sexual rehabilitation with GU cancer: what patients want to know. In: Held-Warmkessel J, ed. *Site-Specific Cancer Series: Urologic Cancers.* Pittsburgh, PA: Oncology Nursing Society; 2009;121–148.
22. Martis G, D'Elia G, Diana M, Ombres M, Mastrangeli B. Prostatic capsule-and nerve-sparing cystectomy in organ-confined bladder cancer: preliminary results. *World J Surg.* 2005;29:1277–1281.
23. Galbraith ME, Crighton F. Alterations of sexual function in men with cancer. *Semin Oncol Nurs.* 2008;24:102–114.
24. Horenblas S, Meinhardt W, Ijzerman W, et al. Sexuality-preserving cystectomy and neobladder: initial results. *J Urol.* 2001;166:837–840.
25. Nieuwenhuijzen JA, de Vries RR, Bex A, et al. Urinary diversions after cystectomy: the association of clinical factors, complications and functional results of four different diversions. *Eur Urol.* 2008;53: 834–844.
26. Puppo P, Introni C, Bertolotto F, Naselli A. Potency-preserving cystectomy with intrafascial prostatectomy for high-risk superficial bladder cancer. *J Urol.* 2008;179:1727–1732.
27. Antunes AA, Dall'Oglio MF, Srougi M. Organ-sparing treatment for penile cancer. *Urology.* 2007;4:596–604.
28. Korets R, Koppie TM, Snyder ME, Russo P. Partial penectomy for patients with squamous cell carcinoma of the penis: The Memorial Sloan-Kettering experience. *Ann Surg Oncol.* 2007;14:3614–3619.
29. Romero FR, Romero KR, Mattos MA, Garcia CR, Fernandes Rde C, Perez MD. Sexual function after partial penectomy for penile cancer. *Urology.* 2005;66:1292–1295.
30. Windahl T, Skeppner E, Andersson S-O, Fugl-Meyer KS. Sexual function and satisfaction in men after laser treatment for penile carcinoma. *J Urol.* 2004;172:648–651.
31. Lumen N, Monstrey S, Selvaggi G, et al. Phalloplasty: a valuable treatment for males with penile insufficiency. *Urology.* 2008;71:272–277.
32. Moncada I, Martinez-Salamanca JI, Allona A, Hernandez C. Current role of penile implants for erectile dysfunction. *Curr Opin Urol.* 2004;14:375–380.
33. Mosconia AM, Roilaa F, Gattab G, Theodorec C. Cancer of the penis. *Crit Rev Oncol/Hematol.* 2005;53:165–177.
34. Nonomura N, Nishimura K, Takaha N, et al. Nerve-sparing retroperitoneal lymph node dissection for advanced testicular cancer after chemotherapy. *Int J Urol.* 2002;9:539–544.
35. Joly F, Heron JF, Kalusinski L, et al. Quality of life in long-term survivors of testicular cancer: a population-based case-control study. *J Clin Oncol.* 2002;20:73–80.
36. Bruner GW, Calvano T. The sexual impact of cancer and cancer treatments in men. *Nurs Clin North Am.* 2007;42:555–580.
37. Montorsi F, Salonia A, Zanoni M, et al. Counselling the patient with prostate cancer about treatment-related erectile dysfunction. *Curr Opin Urol.* 2001;11:611–617.
38. Davison BJ, So AI, Goldenberg SL. Quality of life, sexual function and decisional regret at 1 year after surgical treatment for localized prostate cancer. *BJU Int.* 2007;100:780–785.
39. Darst EH. Sexuality and prostatectomy: nursing assessment and intervention. *Urol Nurs.* 2007;27:534–541.
40. Church PA. Prostate cancer. In: Steele G, Cady B, eds. *General Surgical Oncology.* Philadelphia, PA: Saunders; 1992:275–285.
41. Kim RD, Nath R, Kadmon D, et al. Bilateral nerve graft during radical retropubic prostatectomy: 1-year followup. *J Urol.* 2001;165:1950–1956.
42. Chang DW, Wood CG, Kroll SS, et al. Cavernous nerve reconstruction to preserve erectile function following non-nerve-sparing radical retropubic prostatectomy: a prospective study. *Plast Reconstr Surg.* 2003;111:1174–1181.
43. Kendirci M, Bejma J, Hellstom WJ. Update on erectile dysfunction in prostate cancer patients. *Curr Opin Urol.* 2006;16:186–195.
44. Miranda-Sousa AJ, Davila HH, Lockhart JL, Ordorica RC, Carrion RE. Sexual function after surgery for prostate or bladder cancer. *Cancer Control.* 2006;13:179–187.
45. Kunthe A. Phosphodiesterase 5 inhibitors in male sexual dysfunction. *Curr Opin Urol.* 2003;13:405–410.
46. Gossfield LM, Cullen ML. Sexuality and fertility. In: Moore-Higgs GJ, ed. *Women and Cancer: A Gynecologic Oncology Nursing Perspective.* 2nd ed. Sudbury, MA: Jones and Bartlett; 2000:466–500.
47. Stilos K, Doyle C, Daines P. Addressing the sexual health needs of patients with gynecologic cancers. *Clin J Oncol Nurs.* 2008;12:457–463.

48. Krychman ML, Pereira L, Carter J, Amsterdam A. Sexual oncology: sexual health issues in women with cancer. *Oncology.* 2006;71:18–25.
49. Barton-Burke M, Gustason CJ. Sexuality in women with cancer. *Nurs Clin North Am.* 2007;42:531–554.
50. Likes W, Stegbauer C, Tillmanns T, Pruett J. Pilot study of sexual function and quality of life after excision for vulvar intraepithelial neoplasia. *J Reprod Med.* 2007;52:23–27.
51. Likes W, Stegbauer C, Tillmanns T, Pruett J. Correlates of sexual function following vulvar excision. *Gynecol Oncol.* 2007;105:600–603.
52. Door A. Less common gynecologic malignancies. *Semin Oncol Nurs.* 2002;18:207–222.
53. Abd El-Aziz S. Vaginal reconstruction using the ileocecal segment after resection of pelvic malignancy. *J Egypt Natl Cancer Inst.* 2006;18:1–7.
54. Imparato E, Alfei A, Aspesi G, Meus AL, Spinillo A. Long-term results of sigmoid vaginoplasty in a consecutive series of 62 patients. *Int Urogynecol J.* 2007;18:1465–1469.
55. Soper JT, Secord AA, Havrilesky LJ, Berchuck A, Clarke-Pearson DL. Comparison of gracilis and rectus abdominis myocutaneous flap neovaginal reconstruction performed during radical pelvic surgery: flap-specific morbidity. *Int J Gynecol Cancer.* 2007;17:298–303.
56. Andersen BL, Lamb M. Sexuality and cancer. In: Murphy GP, Lawrence W, Lenhard RE, eds. *American Cancer Society Textbook of Clinical Oncology.* 2nd ed. Atlanta, GA: American Cancer Society; 1995:699–713.
57. Schlaerth JB, Spirtos NM, Schlaerth AC. Radical trachelectomy and pelvic lymphadenectomy with uterine preservation in the treatment of cervical cancer. *Am J Obstet Gynecol.* 2003;188:29–34.
58. Carter J, Sonoda Y, Chi DS, Raviv L, Abu-Rustum NR. Radical trachelectomy for cervical cancer: postoperative physical and emotional adjustment concerns. *Gynecol Oncol.* 2008;111:151–157.
59. Wilmoth MC, Spinelli A. Sexual implications of gynecologic treatments. *J Obst Gynecol Neonatal Nurs.* 2000;29:413–421.
60. Bergmark K, Avall-Lundqvist E, Dickman PW, et al. Patient rating of distressful symptoms after treatment for early cervical cancer. *Acta Obstet Gynecol Oncol.* 2002;81:443–450.
61. Jongpipan J, Charoenkwan K. Sexual function after radical hysterectomy for early-stage cervical cancer. *J Sex Med.* 2007;4:1659–1665.
62. Shell JA. Sexuality. In: Langhorne ME, Fulton JS, Otto SE, eds. *Oncology Nursing.* 5th ed. St. Louis, MO: Mosby; 2007:546–564.
63. Porter S. Endometrial cancer. *Semin Oncol Nurs.* 2002;18:200–206.
64. Shell JA. Body image and sexual functioning. In: Dow KH, ed. *Nursing Care of Women with Cancer.* St. Louis, MO: Mosby; 2006:264–281.
65. DeGaetano C. Ovarian cancer—it whispers…so listen. *Nurs Spectr.* 2001 Jan; 28–32.
66. Stead ML, Fallowfield L, Selby P, Brown JM. Psychosexual function and impact of gynaecological cancer. *Psychol Issues Obstet Gynaecol.* 2007;21309–320.
67. Fitch MI. Psychosocial management of patients with recurrent ovarian cancer: treating the whole patient to improve quality of life. *Semin Oncol Nurs.* 2003;19(suppl 1):40–53.
68. Sun CC, Ramirez PT, Bodurka DC. Quality of life for patients with epithelial ovarian cancer. *Nat Clin Pract Oncol.* 2007;4:18–29.
69. Ferron G, Querleu D, Martel P, Letourneur B, Soulie M. Laparoscopy-assisted vaginal pelvic exenteration. *Gynecol Oncol.* 2006;100:551–555.
70. Goldberg GL, Sukumvanich P, Einstein MH, Smith HO, Anderson PS, Fields AL. Total pelvic exenteration: The Albert Einstein College of Medicine/Montefiore Medical Center experience (1987 to 2003). *Gynecol Oncol.* 2006;101:261–268.
71. Fischer M. Cancer of the cervix. *Semin Oncol Nurs.* 2002;18:193–199.
72. Amichetti M, Caffo O. Quality of life in patients with early-stage carcinoma treated with conservation surgery and radiotherapy: an Italian monoinstitutional study. *Tumori.* 2001;2:78–84.
73. Fialka-Moser V, Crevenna R, Korpan M, Quittan M. Cancer rehabilitation, particularly with aspects on physical impairments. *J Rehabil Med.* 2003;35:153–162.
74. Pelusi J. Sexuality and body image. *AJN.* 2006;106(3 suppl):32–38.
75. Atisha D, Alderman AK, Lowery JC, Kuhn LE, Davis J, Wilkins EG. Prospective analysis of long-term psychosocial outcomes in breast reconstruction. *Ann Surg.* 2008;247:1019–1028.
76. Warren AG, Morris DJ, Houlihan MJ, Slavin SA. Breast reconstruction in a changing breast cancer treatment paradigm. *Plast Reconstr Surg.* 2008;121:1116–1126.
77. Temple WJ, Russell ML, Parsons LL, et al. Conservation surgery for breast cancer as the preferred choice: a prospective analysis. *J Clin Oncol.* 2006;24:3367–3373.
78. Donovan T, Flynn M. What makes a man a man? *Cancer Nurs.* 2007;30:464–470.
79. Bjordal K, Ahlner-Elmqvist M, Hammerlid E, et al. A prospective study of quality of life in head and neck cancer patients. *Laryngoscope.* 2001;111:1440–1452.
80. Brydoy M, Fossa SD, Dahl O, Bjoro T. Gonadal dysfunction and fertility problems in cancer survivors. *Acta Oncologica.* 2007;46:480–489.
81. Iwamoto RR, Maher KE. Radiation therapy for prostate cancer. *Semin Oncol Nurs.* 2001;17:90–100.
82. Rubin A, Williams JP. Principles of radiation oncology and cancer radiotherapy. In: Rubin A, ed. *Clinical Oncology: A Multidisciplinary Approach for Physicians and Students.* 8th ed. Philadelphia, PA: Saunders; 2001:99–125.
83. Jensen T, Groenvald M, Klee MC, et al. Longitudinal study of sexual function and vaginal changes after radiotherapy for cervical cancer. *Int J Radiat Oncol Biol Phys.* 2003;56:937–949.
84. Bakewell RT, Volker DL. Sexual dysfunction related to the treatment of young women with breast cancer. *Clin J Oncol Nurs.* 2005;9:697–702.
85. Maher EJ, Denton A. Survivorship, late effects and cancer of the cervix. *Clin Oncol.* 2008;20:479–487.
86. White ID. The assessment and management of sexual difficulties after treatment for cervical and endometrial malignancies. *Clin Oncol.* 2008;20:488–496.
87. Vistad I, Fossa SD, Kristensen GB, Dahl AA. Chronic fatigue and its correlates in long-term survivors of cervical cancer treated with radiotherapy. *BJOG.* 2007;114:1150–1158.
88. Goodman A. In small study, hand-held device offers hope for women alleviating radiation-induced sexual dysfunction in women. *Oncol Times.* 2002 Dec:44–46.
89. Rowly MJ, Leach DR, Warner GA, et al. Effects of graded doses of ionizing radiation on human testes. *Radiat Res.* 1974;59:665–678.
90. Tomao F, Miele E, Spinelli GP, Tomao S. Anticancer treatment and fertility effects. Literature review [Review]. *J Exp Clin Cancer Res.* 2006;25:475–481.
91. Revel A, Revel-Vilk S. Pediatric fertility preservation: is it time to offer testicular tissue cryopreservation? *Mol Cell Endocrinol.* 2008;282:143–149.
92. Gruschow K, Kyank U, Stuhldreier G, Fietkau R. Surgical repositioning of the contralateral testicle before irradiation of a paratesticular rhabdomyosarcoma for preservation of hormone production. *Pediatr Hematol Oncol.* 2007;24:371–377.
93. Akbal C, Tinay I, Simsek F, Turkeri LN. Erectile dysfunction following radiotherapy and brachytherapy for prostate cancer: pathophysiology, prevention and treatment. *Int Urol Nephrol.* 2008;40:355–363.
94. Merrick GS, Wallner KE, Butler WM. Permanent interstitial brachytherapy for the management of carcinoma of the prostate gland. *J Urol.* 2003;169:1643–1652.
95. Beard CJ. The risk of bladder, bowel, and sexual dysfunction after radiation therapy: what data tell us and how we can use it to counsel our patients. *Cancer J.* 2005;11:106–109.
96. Katz A. Quality of life for men with prostate cancer. *Cancer Nurs.* 2007;30:302–308.
97. Morillo V, Guinot JL, Tortajada I, et al. Secondary effects and biochemical control in patients with early prostate cancer treated with $^{125}I$ seeds. *Clin Transl Oncol.* 2008;10:359–366.
98. Merrick GS, Butler WM, Wallner KE, et al. The importance of radiation dose to the penile bulb vs crura in the development of postbrachytherapy erectile dysfunction. *Int J Radiat Oncol Biol Phys.* 2002;54:1055–1062.

99. Valicenti RK, Bissonette EA, Chen C, et al. Longitudinal comparison of sexual function after 3-dimensional conformal radiation therapy or post brachytherapy. *J Urol.* 2002;168:2499–2504.
100. Van der Wielen GJ, van Putten WLJ, Incrocci L. Sexual function after three-dimensional conformal radiotherapy for prostate cancer: results from a dose-escalation trial. *Int J Radiat Oncol Biol Phys.* 2007;68:479–484.
101. Stipetich RL, Abel LJ, Blatt HJ, et al. Nursing assessment of sexual function following permanent prostate brachytherapy for patient with early-stage prostate cancer. *Clin J Oncol Nurs.* 2002;6:271–274.
102. Valicenti RK, Choi E, Chen CT, et al. Sildenafil citrate effectively reverses sexual dysfunction induced by 3-dimensional conformal radiation therapy. *Urology.* 2001;57:769–773.
103. Stipetich R, Abel L, Anderson RL, Butler WM, Wallner KE, Merrick GS. Nursing considerations in brachytherapy-related erectile dysfunction. *Urol Nurs.* 2005;25:249–254.
104. Teloken PE, Ohebshalom M, Mohideen N, Munhall JP. Analysis of the impact of androgen deprivation therapy on sildenafil citrate response following radiation therapy for prostate cancer. *J Urol.* 2007;178:2521–2525.
105. Incrocci L, Slob AK, Hop WC. Tadalafil (Cialis) and erectile dysfunction after radiotherapy for prostate cancer: an open-label extension of a blinded trial. *Urology.* 2007;70:1190–1193.
106. Jereczek-Fossa BA, Marsiglia HR, Orecchia R. Radiotherapy-related fatigue. *Crit Rev Oncol Hematol.* 2002;41:317–325.
107. Chapman RM. Effect of cytotoxic therapy on sexuality and gonadal function. *Semin Oncol.* 1982;9:84–94.
108. Davis M. Fertility considerations for female adolescent and young adult patients following cancer therapy: a guide for counselling patients and their families. *Clin J Oncol Nurs.* 2006;10:213–219.
109. Huddart RA, Norman A, Moynihan C, et al. Fertility, gonadal and sexual function in survivors of testicular cancer. *Br J Cancer.* 2005;93:200–207.
110. Wilkes GM, Barton-Burke M. *2008 Oncology Nursing Drug Handbook.* Sudbury, MA: Jones and Bartlett; 2008.
111. Otto S. Chemotherapy. In: Langhorne ME, Fulton JS, Otto SE, eds. *Oncology Nursing.* 5th ed. St. Louis, MO: Mosby; 2007:262–276.
112. Cleri LB, Haywood R. *Oncology Pocket Guide to Chemotherapy.* 5th ed. Philadelphia, PA: Mosby; 2002.
113. Gullatte MM, ed. *Clinical Guide to Antineoplastic Therapy: A Chemotherapy Handbook.* Pittsburgh, PA: Oncology Nursing Society; 2001.
114. Chu E, DeVita VT. *Physicians' Cancer Chemotherapy Drug Manual 2001.* Sudbury, MA: Jones and Bartlett; 2001.
115. Braun-Inglis C. Chemotherapeutic agents. In: Newton S, Hickey M, Marrs J, eds. *Mosby's Oncology Nursing Advisor: A Comprehensive Guide to Clinical Practice.* St. Louis, MO: Mosby; 2009:197–198, 223–238.
116. Blecher CS. Chemotherapeutic agents. In: Newton S, Hickey M, Marrs J, eds. *Mosby's Oncology Nursing Advisor: A Comprehensive Guide to Clinical Practice.* St. Louis, MO: Mosby; 2009:198–223.
117. Gobel BH, Mast D. Chemotherapeutic agents. In: Newton S, Hickey M, Marrs J, eds. *Mosby's Oncology Nursing Advisor: A Comprehensive Guide to Clinical Practice.* St. Louis, MO: Mosby; 2009:238–263.
118. Krebs LU. Chemotherapeutic agents. In: Newton S, Hickey M, Marrs J, eds. *Mosby's Oncology Nursing Advisor: A Comprehensive Guide to Clinical Practice.* St. Louis, MO: Mosby; 2009:263–286.
119. Orbaugh K. Hormonal therapy agents. In: Newton S, Hickey M, Marrs J, eds. *Mosby's Oncology Nursing Advisor: A Comprehensive Guide to Clinical Practice.* St. Louis, MO: Mosby; 2009:317–325.
120. Schilsky RL, Lewis BJ, Sherins RJ, et al. Gonadal dysfunction in patients receiving chemotherapy for cancer. *Ann Intern Med.* 1980;93:109–114.
121. Schmidt KL, Carlsen E, Andersen AN. Fertility treatment in male cancer survivors. *Int J Androl.* 2007;39:413–419.
122. Bashore L. Semen preservation in male adolescents and young adults with cancer: one institution's experience. *Clin J Oncol Nurs.* 2007;11:381–386.
123. Howell SJ, Radford JA, Smets EM, et al. Fatigue, sexual function and mood following treatment for haematological malignancy: the impact of mild Leydig cell dysfunction. *Br J Cancer.* 2000;82:789–793.
124. Gospodarowicz M. Testicular cancer patients: considerations in long-term follow-up. *Hematol/Oncol Clin North Am.* 2008;22:245–255.
125. Thaler-deMers D. Endocrine and fertility effects in male cancer survivors. *AJN.* 2006;106:66–71.
126. Bohlen D, Burkhard FC, Mills R, et al. Fertility and sexual function following orchiectomy and 2 cycles of chemotherapy for stage 1 high-risk nonseminomatous germ cell cancer. *J Urol.* 2001;165:441–444.
127. DiBlasio CJ, Malcolm JB, Derweesh IT, et al. Patterns of sexual and erectile dysfunction and response to treatment in patients receiving androgen deprivation therapy for prostate cancer. *BJU Int.* 2008;102:39–43.
128. Spetz A-C, Zetterlund E-L, Varenhorst E, et al. Incidence and management of hot flashes in prostate cancer. *J Supportive Oncol.* 2003;1:263–273.
129. Vogel WH. Alterations in sexuality. In: Newton S, Hickey M, Marrs J, eds. *Mosby's Oncology Nursing Advisor: A Comprehensive Guide to Clinical Practice.* St. Louis, MO: Mosby; 2009:340–343.
130. Kurebayashi J. Adjuvant therapy for premenopausal patients with early breast cancer. *Curr Opin Obstetr Gynecol.* 2008;20:51–54.
131. Minton SE, Munster PN. Chemotherapy-induced amenorrhea and fertility in women undergoing adjuvant treatment for breast cancer. *Cancer Control.* 2002;9:466–472.
132. Schover LR. Premature ovarian failure and its consequences: vasomotor symptoms, sexuality and fertility. *J Clin Oncol.* 2008;26:753–758.
133. Gershenson DM, Miller AM, Champion VL, et al. Reproductive and sexual function after platinum-based chemotherapy in long-term ovarian germ cell tumor survivors: a Gynecologic Oncology Group study. *J Clin Oncol.* 2007;25:2792–2797.
134. Broeckel JA, Thors CL, Jacobsen PB, et al. Sexual functioning in long-term breast cancer survivors treated with adjuvant chemotherapy. *Breast Cancer Res Control.* 2002;75:241–248.
135. Fossa SD, Dahl AA. Fertility and sexuality in young cancer survivors who have adult-onset malignancies. *Hematol/Oncol Clin North Am.* 2008;22:291–303.
136. Relander T, Cavallin-Stahl E, Garwicz S, et al. Gonadal and sexual function in men treated for childhood cancer. *Med Ped Oncol.* 2000;35:52–63.
137. Green DM, Whitton JA, Stovall M, et al. Pregnancy outcome of female survivors of childhood cancer: a report from the childhood cancer survivor study. *Am J Obstet Gynecol.* 2002;187:1070–1080.
138. Green DM, Whitton JA, Stovall M, et al. Pregnancy outcome of partners of male survivors of childhood cancer: a report from the childhood cancer survivor study. *J Clin Oncol.* 2003;21:716–721.
139. Langeveld NE, Stam H, Grootenhuis MA, et al. Quality of life in young adult survivors of childhood cancer. *Support Care Cancer.* 2002;10:579–600.
140. van Dijk EM, van Dulmen Broeder E, Kaspers GJL, van Dam EWCM, Braam KI, Huisman J. Psychosexual functioning of childhood cancer survivors. *Psycho-Oncology.* 2008;17:506–511.
141. Mattsson E, Lindgren B, Von Essen L. Are there any positive consequences of childhood cancer? A review of the literature. *Acta Oncologica.* 2008;47:199–206.
142. Rieger PT. Patient management. In: Rieger PT, ed. *Biotherapy: A Comprehensive Overview.* 2nd ed. Sudbury, MA: Jones and Bartlett; 2001:461–503.
143. Rothaermel JM, Baum B. Biological response modifiers/biological response modifier agents. In: Newton S, Hickey M, Marrs J, eds. *Mosby's Oncology Nursing Advisor: A Comprehensive Guide to Clinical Practice.* St. Louis, MO: Mosby; 2009:161–182.
144. Remer SE. Targeted therapy/targeted therapy agents. In: Newton S, Hickey M, Marrs J, eds. *Mosby's Oncology Nursing Advisor: A Comprehensive Guide to Clinical Practice.* St. Louis, MO: Mosby; 2009:287–313.

145. Krozely P. Epidermal growth factor receptor tyrosine kinase inhibitors: evolving role in the treatment of solid tumors. *Clin J Oncol Nurs.* 2004;8:163–168.
146. Walker PL, Dang NH. Denileukine diftitox as novel targeted therapy in non-Hodgkin's lymphoma. *Clin J Oncol Nurs.* 2004;8:169–174.
147. Schmidt KV, ed. Emerging therapies. *Semin Oncol Nurs.* 2003;1:153–229.
148. Birner A. Pharmacology of oral chemotherapy agents. *Clin J Oncol Nurs.* 2003;7:11–19.
149. Tierney DK. Sexuality following hematopoietic cell transplantation. *Clin J Oncol Nurs.* 2004;8:43–47.
150. Lee HG, Park EY, Kim HM, et al. Sexuality and quality of life after hematopoietic stem cell transplantation. *Korean J Int Med.* 2002;17:19–23.
151. Tierney KD, Facione N, Padilla G, Blume K, Dodd M. Altered sexual health and quality of life in women prior to hematopoietic cell transplantation. *Eur J Oncol Nurs.* 2007;11:298–308.
152. Chatterjee R, Andrews HO, McGarrigle HH, et al. Cavernosal arterial insufficiency is a major component of erectile dysfunction in some recipients of high-dose chemotherapy/chemo-radiotherapy for haematological malignancies. *Bone Marrow Transplant.* 2000;25: 1185–1189.
153. Chatterjee R, Kottaridis PD, McGarrigle HH, et al. Management of erectile dysfunction by combination therapy with testosterone and sildenafil in recipients of high-dose therapy for haematological malignancies. *Bone Marrow Transplant.* 2002;29:607–610.
154. Harris E, Mahendra P, McGarrigle HH, et al. Gynaecomastia with hypergonadotrophic hypogonadism of high dose chemotherapy or chemo-radiotherapy. *Bone Marrow Transplant.* 2001;28:1141–1144.
155. Syrjala KL, Kurland BF, Abrams JR, Sanders JE, Heiman JR. Sexual function changes during the 5 years after high-dose treatment and hematopoietic cell transplantation for malignancy, with case-matched controls at 5 years. *Blood.* 2008;111:989–996.
156. Hammond C, Abrams JR, Syrjala KL. Fertility and risk factors for elevated infertility concern in 10-year hematopoietic cell transplant survivors and case-matched controls. *J Clin Oncol.* 2007;25:3511–3517.
157. Tauchmanova L, Alviggi C, Foresta C, et al. Cryptozoospermia with normal testicular function after allogeneic stem cell transplantation: a case report. *Hum Reprod.* 2007;22:495–499.
158. Liu J, Malhotra R, Voltarelli J, et al. Ovarian recovery after stem cell transplantation. *Bone Marrow Transplant.* 2008;41:275–278.
159. Krebs L. What should I say? Talking with patients about sexuality issues. *Clin J Oncol Nurs.* 2006;10:313–315.
160. Krebs LU. Sexual assessment: research and clinical. *Nurs Clin North Am.* 2007;42:515–529.
161. Krebs LU. Sexual assessment in cancer care: concepts, methods and strategies for success. *Semin Oncol Nurs.* 2008;24:80–90.
162. Thaler-DeMers D. Intimacy issues: sexuality, fertility and relationships. *Semin Oncol Nurs.* 2001;17:255–262.
163. Hautamaki K, Miettinen M, Kellakumpu-Lehtinen P-K, Aalto P, Lehto J. Opening communication with cancer patients about sexuality-related issues. *Cancer Nurs.* 2007;30:399–404.
164. Katz A. The sounds of silence: sexuality information for cancer patients. *J Clin Oncol.* 2008;23:238–241.
165. Gott M, Galena E, Hinchcliff S, Elford H. "Opening a can of worms": GP and practice nurse barriers to talking about sexual health in primary care. *Fam Pract.* 2004;21:528–536.
166. Auchincloss S. Sexual dysfunction after cancer treatment. *J Psychosoc Oncol.* 1991;9:23–42.
167. Krebs LU. Sexual and reproductive issues. In: Yasko JM, ed. *Nursing Management of Symptoms Associated with Chemotherapy.* 5th ed. West Conshohocken, PA: Meniscus; 2001:205–214.
168. Schover LR. Sexual dysfunction. In: Holland JC, ed. *Psycho-oncology.* New York: Oxford University Press; 1998:494–499.
169. Annon JS. *The Behavioral Treatment of Sexual Problems.* Honolulu, HI: Mercantile Printing; 1974:43–47.
170. Davis S, Taylor B. From PLISSIT to Ex-PLISSIT. In: Davis S, ed. *Rehabilitation: The Use of Theories and Models in Practice.* Edinburgh: Elsevier; 2006:101–129.
171. Taylor B, Davis S. Using the extended PLISSIT model to address sexual healthcare needs. *Nurs Stand.* 2006;21:35–40.
172. Mick J, Hughes M, Cohen MZ. Using the BETTER model to assess sexuality. *Clin J Oncol Nurs.* 2004;8:84–86.
173. Schain W. A sexual interview is a sexual intervention. *Innov Oncol Nurs.* 1988;4:2, 3, 15.
174. Hordern A. Intimacy and sexuality after cancer: a critical review of the literature. *Cancer Nurs.* 2008;31:E9–E17.
175. Wilmoth M, Bruner DW. Integrating sexuality into cancer nursing practice. *Oncol Nurs Patient Treatment Support.* 2002;8:1–14.
176. Shell JA. Including sexuality in your nursing practice. *Nurs Clin North Am.* 2007;42:685–696.
177. Wilmoth MC. Life after cancer: What *does* sexuality have to do with it? *Oncol Nurs Forum.* 2006;33:905–910.
178. Mick JM. Sexuality assessment: 10 strategies for improvement. *Clin J Oncol Nurs.* 2007;11:671–675.
179. Nicholson HS, Byrne J. Fertility and pregnancy after treatment for cancer during childhood or adolescence. *Cancer.* 1993;71(suppl): 3392–3399.
180. Fallat ME, Huttner J. Preservation of fertility in pediatric and adolescent patients with cancer. *Pediatrics.* 2008;121:1461–1469.
181. Lee SJ, Schover LR, Partridge AH, et al. American Society of Clinical Oncology recommendations on fertility preservation in cancer patients. *J Clin Oncol.* 2006;24:2917–2931.
182. Kalapurakal JA, Peterson S, Peabody EM, et al. Pregnancy outcomes after abdominal irradiation that included or excluded the pelvis in childhood Wilms tumor survivors: a report from the National Wilms Tumor Study. *Int J Radiat Oncol Biol Phys.* 2004;58: 1364–1368.
183. Maltaris T, Seufert R, Schaffrath M, Pollow K, Koelbi H, Dittrich R. The effects of cancer treatment on female fertility and strategies for preserving fertility. *Eur J Obstet Gynecol Reproduct Biol.* 2007;130:148–155.
184. Leonard M, Hammelef K, Smith GD. Fertility considerations, counselling and semen cryopreservation for males prior to initiation of cancer therapy. *Clin J Oncol Nurs.* 2004;8:127–147.
185. Yap JKW, Davies M. Fertility preservation in female cancer survivors. *J Obstet Gynaecol.* 2007;27:390–400.
186. Pereg D, Koren G, Lishner M. Cancer in pregnancy: gaps, challenges and solutions. *Cancer Treatt Rev.* 2008;34:302–312.
187. Edgar AB, Wallace HB. Pregnancy in women who had cancer in childhood. *Eur J Cancer.* 2007;43:1890–1894.
188. Hart R. Preservation of fertility in adults and children diagnosed with cancer. *BMJ.* 2008;337:a2045–a2051.
189. Kim SS. Fertility preservation in female cancer patients: current developments and future directions. *Fertil Steril.* 2006;85:1–11.
190. Byrne J. Fertility and pregnancy after malignancy. *Semin Perinatol.* 1990;14:423–429.
191. Hawkins MM. Is there evidence of therapy-related increases in germ cell mutation among childhood cancer survivors? *J Natl Cancer Inst.* 1991;83:1643–1650.
192. Green DM, Zevon MA, Lowrie G, et al. Congenital anomalies in children of patients who received chemotherapy for cancer in childhood and adolescence. *N Engl J Med.* 1991;325:141–146.
193. Robinson LL, Green DM, Hudson M, et al. Long-term outcomes of adult survivors of childhood cancer: results from the Childhood Cancer Survivor Study. *Cancer.* 2005;104(11 suppl):2557–2564.
194. Hansen PV, Glavind K, Panduro J, et al. Paternity in patients with testicular germ cell cancer: pretreatment and posttreatment findings. *Eur J Cancer.* 1991;27:1385–1389.
195. Byrne J, Rasmussen SA, Steinhorn SC, et al. Genetic disease in offspring of long-term survivors of childhood and adolescent cancer. *Am J Hum Genet.* 1998;62:45–52.

196. Meistrich ML, Byrne J. Genetic disease in offspring of long-term survivors of childhood and adolescent cancer treated with potentially mutagenic therapies. *Am J Hum Genet.* 2002;70:1069–1071.
197. Robinson WA, Krebs LU. Oncologic disease. In: Abrams R, Wexler P, eds. *Medical Care of the Pregnant Patient: Concepts and Management.* Boston, MA: Little, Brown; 1983:307–319.
198. Leslie KK, Koil C, Rayburn WF. Chemotherapeutic drugs in pregnancy. *Obstet Gynecol Clin North Am.* 2005;32:627–640.
199. Kal HB, Struikmans H. Radiotherapy during pregnancy: fact and fiction. *Lancet Oncol.* 2005;6:328–333.
200. Moran BJ, Yano H, Al Zahir N, Farquharson M. Conflicting priorities in surgical intervention for cancer in pregnancy. *Lancet Oncol.* 2007;8:536–544.
201. Zemlickis D, Lishner M, Degendorfer P, et al. Fetal outcome after in utero exposure to cancer chemotherapy. *Arch Intern Med.* 1992;152:573–576.
202. Hurley TJ, McKinnell JV, Irani MS. Hematologic malignancies in pregnancy. *Obstet Gynecol Clin North Am.* 2005;32:595–614.
203. Vadaparampil ST, Clayton H, Quinn GP, King LM, Nieder M, Wilson C. Pediatric nurses' attitudes related to discussing fertility preservation with pediatric cancer patients and their families. *J Pediatric Oncol Nurs.* 2007;24:255–263.
204. Quinn GP, Vadaparampil ST, Bell-Ellison BA, Gwede CK, Albrecht TL. Patient-physician communication barriers regarding fertility preservation among newly diagnosed cancer patients. *Soc Sci Med.* 2008;66:784–789.
205. King L, Quinn GP, Vadaparampil ST, et al. Oncology nurses' perceptions of barriers to discussion of fertility preservation with patients with cancer. *Clin J Oncol Nurs.* 2008;12:467–476.
206. Krebs LU. Cancer and pregnancy. In: Gates RA, Fink RM, eds. *Oncology Nursing Secrets.* 3rd ed. St. Louis, MO: Mosby; 2008:563–569.
207. Leonard M. Fertility preservation options for women with cancer. *Curr Topics Cancer Fertil Oncol Nurs.* 2006;1:1–2, 6.
208. Schover LR. The impact of cancer on men's fertility. *Curr Topics Cancer Fertil Oncol Nurs.* 2006;1:3, 6.
209. Lostritto K. Fertility considerations for women with breast cancer. *Curr Topics Cancer Fertil Oncol Nurs.* 2006;1:4–6.
210. Tao T, Valle AD. Human oocytes and ovarian tissue cryopreservation. *J Assist Reprod Genet.* 2008;25:287–296.
211. Stern CJ, Toledo MG, Gook DA, Seymour JF. Fertility preservation in female oncology patients. *Aust N Z J Obstet Gynecol.* 2006;46:15–23.
212. Agarwal A. Technical and ethical challenges of fertility preservation in young cancer patients. *Reprod Biomed Online.* 2008;16:784–791.
213. Recchia F, Saggio G, Amiconi G, et al. Gonodotropin-releasing hormone analogues added to adjuvant chemotherapy protect ovarian function and improve clinical outcomes in young women with early breast carcinoma. *Cancer.* 2006;106:514–523.
214. Lee DM, Yeomann RR, Battaglia DE, et al. Live birth after ovarian tissue transplant. *Nature.* 2004;428:137–138.
215. Gotlieb WH, Beiner ME, Shalmon B, et al. Outcome of fertility-sparing treatment with progestins in young patients with endometrial cancer. *Obstet Gynecol.* 2003;102:718–725.
216. Revel A, Revel-Vilk S. Pediatric fertility preservation: is it time to offer testicular tissue cryopreservation? *Mol Cell Endocrinol.* 2008;282:143–149.
217. Orwig KE, Schlatt S. Cryopreservation and transplantation of spermatogonia and testicular tissue for preservation of male fertility. *J Natl Cancer Inst Monogr.* 2005;34:51–56.
218. Anger JT, Gilbert BR, Goldstein M. Cryopreservation of sperm: indications, methods and results. *J Urol.* 2003;170:1079–1084.
219. Leonard M, Hammelef K, Smith GD. Fertility considerations, counseling, and semen cryopreservation for males prior to the initiation of cancer therapy. *Clin J Oncol Nurs.* 2004;8:127–131.
220. Agarwal A, Ranganathan P, Kattal N, et al. Fertility after cancer: a prospective review of assisted reproductive outcome with banked semen specimens. *Fertil Steril.* 2004;81:342–348.
221. Salihu HM, Aliyu MH. Sperm retrieval in infertile males: comparison between testicular sperm extraction and testicular sperm aspiration techniques. *Wiener Klinisch Wochenschrift.* 2003;115:370–379.
222. Robins JC, Carson SA. Female fertility: what every urologist must understand. *Urol Clin North Am.* 2008;35:173–181.
223. Alukal JP, Lamb DJ. Intracytoplasmic Sperm Injection (ICSI)—what are the risks? *Urol Clin North Am.* 2008;35:277–288.
224. Cobo A, Domingo J, Perez S, Crespo J, Remohi J, Pellicer A. Vitrification: an effective new approach to oocyte banking and preserving fertility in cancer patients. *Clin Transl Oncol.* 2008;10:268–273.
225. Porcu E. Healthy twins delivered after oocyte cryopreservation and bilateral ovariectomy for ovarian cancer. *Reprod Biomed Online.* 2008;17:265–267.
226. Demeestere I, Simon P, Emiliani S, Delbaere A, Englert Y. Fertility preservation: successful transplantation of cryopreserved ovarian tissue in a young patient previously treated for Hodgkin's disease. *Oncologist.* 2007;12:1437–1442.
227. Bolte S, Zebrack B. Sexual issues in special populations: adolescents and young adults. *Semin Oncol Nurs.* 2008;24:115–119.
228. Evan EE, Kaufman M, Cook AB, Zeltzer LK. Sexual health and self-esteem in adolescents and young adults with cancer. *Cancer.* 2006;107(7 suppl):1672–1679.
229. Canada AL, Schover LR, Li Y. A pilot intervention to enhance psychosexual development in adolescents and young adults with cancer. *Pediatr Blood Cancer.* 2007;49:824–828.
230. Kagan SH, Holland H, Chalian AA. Sexual issues in special populations: geriatric oncology-sexuality and older adults. *Semin Oncol Nurs.* 2008;24:120–126.
231. Shell JA. Sexuality care of the older adult with cancer. In: Cope DG, Reb AM, eds. *An Evidence-Based Approach to the Treatment and Care of the Older Adult with Cancer.* Pittsburgh, PA: Oncology Nursing Society; 2006:439–464.
232. Dibble SL, Eliason MJ, Christiansen MAD. Chronic illness care for lesbian, gay & bisexual individuals. *Nurs Clin North Am.* 2007;42:655–674.
233. Lipson JG, Dibble SL. Providing culturally appropriate health care. In: Lipson JG, Dibble SL, eds. *Culture and Clinical Care.* San Francisco, CA: UCSF Nursing Press; 2005:xi–xviii.
234. Dibble S, Eliason MJ, DeJoseph JF, Chinn P. Sexual issues in special populations: Lesbian and gay individuals. *Semin Oncol Nurs.* 2008;24:127–130.
235. Blank TO. Gay men and prostate cancer: invisible diversity. *J Clin Oncol.* 2005;23:2593–2596.
236. Arena PL, Carver CS, Antoni MH, Weiss S, Ironson G, Duran RE. Psychosocial responses to treatment for breast cancer among lesbian and heterosexual women. *Women Health.* 2007;44:81–102.
237. Shell JA. Sexual issues in the palliative care population. *Semin Oncol Nurs.* 2008;24:131–134.
238. Morriss BB, Pace JC. Sexuality. In: Esper P, Kuebler KK, eds. *Palliative Practices from A-Z for the Bedside Clinician.* 2nd ed. Pittsburgh, PA: Oncology Nursing Society; 2008:235–240.
239. Krebs LU. Pregnancy and cancer. *Semin Oncol Nurs.* 1985;1:35–41.
240. Waalen J. Pregnancy poses tough questions for cancer treatment. *J Natl Cancer Inst.* 1991;83:900.
241. Ward RM, Bristow RE. Cancer and pregnancy: recent developments. *Curr Opin Obstet Gynecol.* 2002;14:613–617.
242. Leachman SA, Jackson R, Eliason MJ, Larson AA, Bolognia JL. Management of melanoma during pregnancy. *Dermatol Nurs.* 2007;19:145–161.
243. Barnes DM, Newman LA. Pregnancy-associated breast cancer: a literature review. *Surg Clin North Am.* 2007;87:417–430.
244. Ring A. Breast cancer and pregnancy. *Breast.* 2007;16:S155-S158.
245. Molckovsky A, Madarnas Y. Breast cancer in pregnancy: a literature review. *Breast Cancer Res Treat.* 2008;108:333–338.
246. Petrek J, Seltzer V. Breast cancer in pregnant and postpartum women. *J Obstet Gynaecol Canada.* 2003;25:944–950.

247. Hindle WH, Gonzalez S. Diagnosis and treatment of invasive breast cancer during pregnancy and lactation. *Clin Obstet Gynecol.* 2002;45:770–773.
248. Rimes S, Gano J, Hahn K, Ramirez M, Milbourne A. Caring for pregnant patients with breast cancer. *Oncol Nurs Forum.* 2006;33:1065–1069.
249. Rodriguez AO, Chew H, Cress R, et al. Evidence of poorer survival in pregnancy-associated breast cancer. *Obstet Gynecol.* 2008;112:71–78.
250. Dow KH, ed. *Pocket Guide to Breast Cancer.* 2nd ed. Sudbury, MA: Jones and Bartlett; 2002:231–255.
251. Maltaris T, Weigel M, Mueller A, et al. Cancer and fertility preservation: fertility preservation in breast cancer patients. *Breast Cancer Res.* 2008;10:206–216.
252. Amant F, Van Calsteren K, Vergote I, Ottevanger N. Gynecologic oncology in pregnancy. *Crit Rev Oncol/Hematol.* 2008;67:187–195.
253. Latimer J. Gynaecological malignancies in pregnancy. *Cur Opin Obstet Gynecol.* 2007;19:140–144.
254. Kyrgiou M, Koliopoulos G, Martin-Hirsch P, Prendiville W, Paraskevaidis E. Obstetric outcomes after conservative treatment for intraepithelial or early invasive cervical lesions: systematic review and meta-analysis. *Lancet.* 2006;367:489–498.
255. Crane JM. Pregnancy outcome after loop electrosurgical excision: a systematic review. *Obstet Gynecol.* 2003;103:1058–1062.
256. Vlahos G, Rodolakis A, Diakomanolis E, et al. Conservative management of cervical intraepithelial neoplasia (CIN (2–3)) in pregnant women. *Gynecol Obstet Invest.* 2002;54:78–81.
257. Charkviani L, Charkviani T, Natenadze N, et al. Cervical carcinoma and pregnancy. *Clin Exper Obstet Gynecol.* 2003;30:19–22.
258. Bernardini M, Barrett J, Seaward G, et al. Pregnancy outcomes in patients after trachelectomy. *Am J Obstet Gynecol.* 2003;189:1378–1382.
259. Plante M, Renaud M-C, Hoskins IA, Roy M. Vaginal radical trachelectomy: a valuable fertility-preserving option in the management of early-stage cervical cancer. A series of 50 pregnancies and review of the literature. *Gynecol Oncol.* 2005;98:3–10.
260. Goldman NA, Goldberg GL. Late recurrence of squamous cell cervical cancer in an episiotomy site after vaginal delivery. *Obstet Gynecol.* 2003;101:1127–1129.
261. Behtash N, Zarchi MK, Gilani MM, Ghaemmaghami F, Mousavi A, Ghotbizadeh F. Ovarian carcinoma associated with pregnancy: a clinicopathologic analysis of 23 cases and review of the literature. *BMC Pregnancy Childbirth.* 2008;8:3–9.
262. Leiserowitz GS. Managing ovarian masses during pregnancy. *Obstet Gynecol Surv.* 2006;61:463–470.
263. Kilpatrick CC, Monga M. Approach to the acute abdomen in pregnancy. *Obstet Gynecol Clin North Am.* 2007;34:389–402.
264. Schilder JM, Thompson AM, DePriest PD, et al. Outcome of reproductive age women with stage IA or IC invasive epithelial ovarian cancer treated with fertility-sparing therapy. *Gynecol Oncol.* 2002;87:1–7.
265. Wiggins CL, Berwick M, Newton Bishop JA. Malignant melanoma in pregnancy. *Obstet Gynecol Clin North Am.* 2005;32:559–568.
266. Katz VL, Farmer RM, Dotters D. Focus on primary care: from Nevus to neoplasm: myths of melanoma in pregnancy. *Obstet Gynecol Surv.* 2002;57:112–119.
267. Egberts F, Lischner S, Russo P, Kampen WU, Hauschild A. Diagnostic and therapeutic procedures for management of melanoma during pregnancy: risks for fetus? Case report and review of the literature. *J Dtsch Dermatol Ges.* 2006;4:717–720.
268. Lenhard MS, Bauerfeind I, Untch M. Breast cancer and pregnancy: challenges of chemotherapy. *Clin Rev Oncol/Hematol.* 2008;67:196–203.
269. Nicklas AH, Baker ME. Imaging strategies in the pregnant cancer patient. *Semin Oncol.* 2000;27:623–632.
270. Chen MM, Coakley FV, Kaimal A, Laros RK. Guidelines for computed tomography and magnetic resonance imaging use during pregnancy and lactation. *Obstet Gynecol.* 2008;112(2, pt 1):333–340.
271. Patel SJ, Reede DL, Katz DS, Subramaniam R, Amorosa JK. Imaging the pregnant patient for nonobstetric conditions: algorithms and radiation dose considerations. *RadioGraphics.* 2007;27:1705–1722.
272. Pereg D, Koren G, Lishner M. The treatment of Hodgkin's and non-Hodgkin's lymphoma in pregnancy. *Hemotologica.* 2007;92:1230–1237.
273. Patel A, Camacho J, Stevenson J. Hodgkin's lymphoma during pregnancy. *Comm Oncol.* 2008;5:389–391.
274. Chelghoum Y, Vey N, Raffoux E, et al. Acute leukemia during pregnancy: a report on 37 patients and a review of the literature. *Cancer.* 2005;104:110–117.
275. Jenkins TM, Mackey SF, Benzoni EM, et al. Non-obstetric surgery during gestation: risk factors for lower birthweight. *Aust N Z J Obstet Gynaecol.* 2003;43:27–31.
276. Kawabata I, Takahashi Y, Iwagaki S, et al. MRI during pregnancy. *J Perinatal Med.* 2003;31:449–458.
277. Damilakis J, Perisinakis K, Prassopoulos P, et al. Conceptus radiation dose and risk from chest screen-film radiography. *Eur Rad.* 2003;13:406–412.
278. O'Mahony S. Endoscopy in pregnancy. *Best Pract Res Clin Gastroenterol.* 2007;21:893–899.
279. Dow KH. Pregnancy and breast cancer. *J Obstet Gynecol Neonatal Nurs.* 2000;29:634–640.
280. Kusama TOK. Radiological protection for diagnostic examination of pregnant women. *Congen Anomalies.* 2002;42:10–14.
281. Leslie KK. Chemotherapy and pregnancy. *Clin Obstet Gynecol.* 2002;45:153–164.
282. Hahn KME, Johnson PH, Gordon N, et al. Treatment of pregnant breast cancer patients and outcomes of children exposed to chemotherapy in utero. *Cancer.* 2006;107:1219–1226.
283. Mir O, Berveiller P, Ropert S, et al. Emerging therapeutic options for breast cancer chemotherapy during pregnancy. *Ann Oncol.* 2008;19:607–613.
284. Mir O, Berveiller P, Rouzier R, Goffinet F, Goldwasser F, Treluyer JN. Chemotherapy for breast cancer during pregnancy: is epirubicin safe? *Ann Oncol.* 2008;19:1814–1815.
285. Robinson AA, Watson WJ, Leslie KK. Targeted treatment using monoclonal antibodies and tyrosine-kinase inhibitors in pregnancy. *Lancet Oncol.* 2007;8:738–743.
286. Tolar J, Neglia JP. Transplacental and other routes of cancer transmission between individuals. *J Pedtr Hematol Oncol.* 2003;25:430–434.
287. Dildy GA, Moise KJ, Carpenter RJ, et al. Maternal malignancy metastatic to the products of conception: a review. *Obstet Gynecol Surv.* 1989;44:535–540.

# PART V

# Oncologic Emergencies

CHAPTER 37

Roberta Kaplow, RN, PhD, AOCNS®, CCNS, CCRN

# Cardiac Tamponade

## SCOPE OF THE PROBLEM

Cardiac tamponade is one of several life-threatening complications that patients with cancer may develop. It results as a side effect of antineoplastic therapy or from the cancer itself. It is essential that the oncology nurse promptly identify the signs and symptoms of cardiac tamponade and intervene so as to mitigate morbidity and mortality.

### DEFINITIONS

Cardiac tamponade results from an excess accumulation of fluid in the pericardial sac, which presents as a pericardial effusion. This fluid collection increases the hemodynamic pressure around the heart, gradually causing compression of the heart and a diminished flow of blood to the ventricles.[1–5] The net effect is a decrease in cardiac output (the amount of blood ejected by the heart each minute) and impaired cardiac function. The body tries to compensate for the heart's inability to pump by stimulating the sympathetic nervous system, resulting in an increase in myocardial workload. Eventually, compensatory mechanisms fail, which leads to cardiovascular collapse, shock, cardiac arrest, and death.[6] Cardiac tamponade is a life-threatening complication of cancer and is present when the pericardial effusion evolves into the aforementioned hemodynamic instability and compensatory mechanisms are no longer effective.[5,7]

### INCIDENCE

The diagnosis of cardiac tamponade is often missed because many patients with pericardial effusions are asymptomatic.[1,8] Patients with pericardial effusions are at risk for developing cardiac tamponade if those complications are left untreated, due to the increase in pressure in the pericardial space. Malignancies are the most common cause of cardiac tamponade,[2] occurring in as many as 13% to 23% of individuals with cancer.[8] Pericardial effusions have occasionally been reported as the initial manifestation of cancer.[9,10]

### ETIOLOGY AND RISK FACTORS

Patients with cancer may develop a pericardial effusion due to a variety of reasons. They may arise secondary to metastatic disease of the pericardium, metastatic disease to the heart, or primary heart malignancies. Metastatic disease of the pericardium has been reported as a sequela to mesotheliomas, sarcomas, and teratomas. Metastatic disease to the heart occurs most often with breast and lung cancers, leukemia, and lymphoma. It is seen less often in melanoma, liver, gastric, esophageal, and pancreatic cancers.[4–6,7,11,12] Pericardial effusions have also been reported in a patient with advanced thymic carcinoma as well as a rare manifestation of metastatic adenocarcinoma of the vagina.[13,14]

When tumors metastasize to the pericardium or myocardium, obstruction of venous and lymphatic drainage occurs and an excess amount of pericardial fluid accumulates, resulting in a pericardial effusion. Cardiac tamponade (hemodynamically significant compression of the heart by pericardial fluid)[15] can also result from constriction of the pericardium by tumor or postradiation pericarditis. Individuals who have received more than 4000 cGy of radiation therapy to areas surrounding the heart (eg, those with breast cancer) may develop a pericardial effusion.[16] The incidence of this complication is reported as rare.[17] Radiation to the mediastinal areas or thyroid can also lead to the development of cardiac tamponade as a result of radiation pericarditis. In these instances, the pericardial effusion and cardiac tamponade are felt to be due to substitution of the normal adipose tissue of the outer layer of the heart with thick collagen and fibrin.[18] Certain antineoplastic agents, such as anthracyclines, cytarabine, cyclophosphamide, and all-trans retinoic acid, may also cause pericardial effusions due to their effects on cardiac tissues.[19]

Small effusions usually do not cause signs and symptoms, so patients with cardiac tamponade may be challenging to identify in the early stages of this condition.[20] Clinical manifestations are often vague or attributed to other causes. In particular, many of the symptoms associated with the presence of cardiac tamponade are not specific to that disorder and may be related to other unrelated conditions. This uncertainty poses a challenge for the nurse and other members of the healthcare team. Knowing that cardiac tamponade is a potential complication of both the cancer and cancer treatment enables the nurse to identify the early and subtle changes in a patient's vital signs and clinical status, signaling the need for prompt and aggressive treatment so that the life-threatening complications of cardiac tamponade may be averted.

## PHYSIOLOGICAL ALTERATIONS

### NORMAL ANATOMY AND PHYSIOLOGY

The pericardium is a thin, double-layered sac surrounding the heart. The outer layer is the parietal pericardium and the inner layer is the visceral pericardium or epicardium,[5] see Figure 37-1. The pericardium lubricates and protects the heart from infection, secures the heart in the mediastinum, and prevents the heart from significant dilation in response to acute changes in volume.[5,21,22] Approximately 50 mL of low-protein fluid in the pericardium helps attain these functions.[5,20,23]

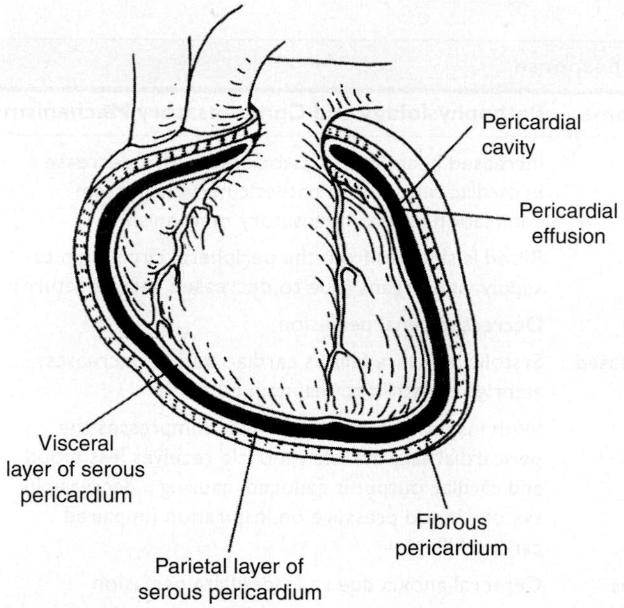


**FIGURE 37-1**

The pericardial sac.

Normally, intrapericardial pressure is lower than ventricular diastolic pressure and is equal to pleural pressure. This normal pressure gradient between the heart chambers and the pericardium allows the heart chambers to fill.

## PATHOPHYSIOLOGY

The amount of fluid surrounding the heart in an individual with pericardial effusion can range from 50 mL to greater than 1 L.[2,22,24] As the fluid accumulates, the ventricle's ability to fill during diastole becomes impaired. The degree of pathophysiological changes that occur depends on how quickly the excess fluid builds up.[2–4] When fluid accumulates gradually, the pericardium has time to compensate for the increased volume by expanding before a tamponade (decreased cardiac output) occurs. When fluid accumulates rapidly, intrapericardial pressure rises. This increase in pressure accounts for the hemodynamic instability and impaired cardiac function associated with cardiac tamponade.[20,21]

When an excess amount of fluid fills the pericardial sac, the heart is unable to fill during diastole and pump adequately.[26] Right ventricular filling is contingent upon the existence of a gradient between central venous pressure and right ventricular diastolic pressure. The increase in intrapericardial pressure that results from the excess fluid accumulation affects this gradient, such that right ventricular filling cannot be adequately sustained. Decreased right ventricular filling and compression of the right ventricle result in a decrease in blood leaving that chamber. Thus, a smaller amount of blood enters and leaves the left side of the heart.[2,3,11] The compression also causes an increase in intracardiac diastolic pressures on the right and left sides of the heart as well as equalization of filling pressures in each of the heart chambers.[5] Hence, the development of cardiac tamponade from a pericardial effusion is based on the compliance of the pericardium, the rate of accumulation of fluid, and the amount of fluid that accumulates.[4]

Compensatory mechanisms include an increased production of endogenous catecholamines from the sympathetic nervous system.[25] Catecholamine production results in tachycardia, increased contractility, and increased peripheral vasoconstriction of the arterial and venous beds. If the tamponade is severe, compensatory mechanisms include an increase in systemic vascular resistance (SVR)—the amount of work the heart has to do to eject blood. It is essential that the oncology nurse be aware that the presence of tachycardia is indicative of depletion of compensatory mechanisms. The patient has an altered hemodynamic status secondary to the effusion, and hemodynamic collapse may be forthcoming.[25] If rapid fluid accumulation occurs, the pericardium will not stretch, compensatory mechanisms cannot be activated, and hemodynamic instability ensues.[5]

## CLINICAL MANIFESTATIONS

The signs and symptoms of cardiac tamponade are variable and depend on the rate and amount of pericardial fluid accumulation, etiology of the tamponade, and the patient's age.[1,2,11,23,26] A summary of the signs and symptoms appears in Table 37-1. Patients with mild cardiac tamponade are usually asymptomatic. However, patients with moderate or severe cardiac tamponade will usually manifest a variety of symptoms.[20] The most frequently reported signs and symptoms are tachycardia, dyspnea, elevated jugular venous pressure, and pulsus paradoxus.[5,11] If fluid accumulation occurs slowly, signs and symptoms may include fatigue, shortness of breath, nausea, vomiting, diarrhea, hepatomegaly, and abdominal distention. As the amount of fluid increases, cardiovascular signs and symptoms become more prominent. One of the earliest noted signs of cardiac tamponade is an elevation in central venous pressure, which results from the increase in intrapericardial pressure caused by the fluid accumulation.[11] Elevation in central venous pressure may be indicated by neck vein distention. Ordinarily, when a person inspires, there is a decrease in intrathoracic pressure with a resultant increase in blood return to the heart and collapse of neck veins. When an individual has cardiac tamponade, blood cannot return to the heart and neck vein distention occurs.[11]

Other signs and symptoms of increased fluid accumulation in the pericardial space include the presence of distant

**TABLE 37-1**

**Cardiac Tamponade: Clinical Presentation and Pathological Response**

| Pathology | Clinical Presentation: Signs and Symptoms | Pathophysiology and Compensatory Mechanisms |
|---|---|---|
| Decrease in cardiac output | Tachycardia | Increased heart rate is associated with a decrease in cardiac output (sympathetic nervous system stimulation as a compensatory mechanisms) |
| | Peripheral vasoconstriction causing cyanosis | Blood is shunted from the peripheral circulation to supply vital organs (due to decreased venous return) |
| | Decreased urinary output (oliguria or anuria) | Decreased renal perfusion |
| | Narrowing pulse pressure, hypotension, increased systemic vascular resistance | Systolic pressure falls as cardiac output decreases; arteries constrict to maintain perfusion |
| | Pulsus paradoxus | With inspiration, the diaphragm compresses the pericardial sac; the left ventricle receives less blood and cardiac output is reduced, causing a decrease in systolic blood pressure on inspiration (impaired cardiac filling) |
| | Anxiety, restlessness, confusion, mental status changes, dizziness, lightheadedness, agitation, fatigue | Cerebral anoxia due to inadequate perfusion |
| | Symptoms of shock | Cardiac decompensation; compensatory mechanisms have been exhausted/failed |
| | Dyspnea, tachypnea, orthopnea, shortness of breath, air hunger | Hemodynamic changes/instability and decreased cardiac output result in hypoxia |
| | Weakness, fatigue, cool extremities | Decreased cardiac output causes decreased peripheral perfusion, visceral congestion, venous stasis, and hepatic and visceral congestion |
| | Kussmaul's sign | A rise in venous pressure with spontaneous inspiration; present only in patients with constrictive pericarditis |
| Compression of heart and structures in chest | Dysphagia, cough, retrostemal chest pain and heaviness, hoarseness, hiccups | Fluid collection around heart compresses the trachea, esophagus, and adjacent nerves and bronchi |
| Venous congestion | Peripheral edema, jugular venous distention | With decrease in ventricular filling, venous return is reduced, causing vascular congestion |
| Distention and filling of pericardial sac | Dullness to percussion, weak heart sounds, chest fullness/discomfort | With decrease in ventricular filling, venous return is reduced, causing vascular congestion |
| Increase in central venous pressure | Nausea, vomiting, diarrhea, hepatojugular reflux, hepatomegaly, abdominal distention | Increase in pericardial pressure causes increase in central venous pressure |

or muffled heart sounds, decreased or absent apical pulse, and decreased cardiac output. Distant or muffled heart sounds are the result of fluid surrounding and compressing the heart and are not an essential component of a cardiac tamponade diagnosis. The patient may or may not have a pericardial friction rub due to the effusion separating the pericardial surfaces.[11]

If fluid accumulation is rapid, the body does not have time to develop compensatory mechanisms.[5] The resultant clinical signs include an increase in ventricular diastolic and pulmonary venous pressures, and a decrease in stroke volume (the amount of blood ejected by the heart with each beat), cardiac output, and arterial blood pressure. These signs of hemodynamic compromise are accompanied by tachypnea, dyspnea, and orthopnea. Other signs related to rapid fluid accumulation include hypotension and tachycardia.[27] Individuals may also develop chest pain or heaviness if fluid accumulation is large or rapid. Chest pain is enhanced when the patient is supine but decreases when the patient leans forward because of compression of the heart.[11] (See Table 37.2 for a discussion about the symptoms of cardiac tamponade based on the rate of fluid accumulation.)

**TABLE 37-2**

**Cardiac Tamponade: Symptoms Based on Rate of Fluid Accumulation**

| Gradual Accumulation of Fluid | Acute Accumulation of Fluid |
|---|---|
| Tachycardia | Hemodynamic instability |
| Increased cardiac contractility | Impaired cardiac function |
| Increased peripheral vasoconstriction of arterial and venous beds | Chest pain or heaviness |
| Fatigue | Increased ventricular diastolic and pulmonary venous pressures |
| Shortness of breath | Decreased stroke volume |
| Nausea | Decreased cardiac output |
| Vomiting | Hypotension |
| Diarrhea | Tachypnea |
| Hepatomegaly | Dyspnea |
| Abdominal distention | Orthopnea |
| **As Fluid Increases** | Tachycardia |
| Increased central venous pressure | Cyanosis |
| Neck vein distention | **As Fluid Increases** |
| Distant, muffled heart sounds | Increased systemic vascular resistance |
| Diminished or absent apical pulse | Narrowing pulse pressure |
| Decreased cardiac output | **If Hypotension Is Prolonged** |
| | Oliguria and anuria |
| | Weakness |
| | Fatigue |
| | Increased dyspnea |
| | Cool and clammy extremities |
| | Hepatojugular reflux |
| | Mental status changes |
| | Apprehension |
| | Cough |
| | Hiccups |
| | Hoarseness |
| | Dysphagia |

Most patients with cardiac tamponade report dyspnea. Dyspnea is indicative of hemodynamic compromise from the effusion.[5,25] Tachypnea and dyspnea on exertion can progress to air hunger at rest. Rapid, progressive dyspnea is usually due to cardiac compression.[11,20] Tachypnea may also be a result of a decrease in cardiac output and resultant hypoxia. Cyanosis results from the decrease in venous return and venous hypertension. No adventitious sounds are audible with the disorder, as no pulmonary congestion is present.[25]

Individuals with cardiac tamponade often have a pulsus paradoxus: a decrease in systolic arterial blood pressure of greater than 10 mm Hg during inspiration.[3,4,11,25] Individuals with cardiac tamponade may also have Kussmaul's sign, which is a rise in venous pressure with spontaneous inspiration.[4] Kussmaul's sign may only present in patients with constrictive pericarditis.[5] The etiology of pulsus paradoxus is believed to be due to impaired cardiac filling, and this condition should be suspected when a palpated pulse decreases in intensity or disappears upon inspiration.[5,25] It is important to remember that pulsus paradoxus, like other signs and symptoms of cardiac tamponade, is not specific to tamponade. Pulses paradoxus can also be found in patients with obesity, chronic obstructive pulmonary disease, massive pulmonary embolism, right ventricular infarction, constrictive pericarditis, heart failure, mitral stenosis, severe hypovolemic shock, tense ascites, and restrictive cardiomyopathy.[5,20] Similarly, some conditions may mask the presence of pulsus paradoxus. These conditions include hypotension, aortic regurgitation, atrial septal defects, pericardial adhesions, and right ventricular hypertrophy.[20]

To measure the extent of a pulsus paradoxus, the blood pressure cuff should be inflated above the level of the individual's systolic pressure and deflated at a rate of 3 mm Hg/second. The first systolic pressure reading heard only during exhalation should be noted. This sound disappears upon inspiration. The systolic pressure reading that is audible during both inspiration and exhalation is then noted. If the difference between the two systolic pressure sounds is greater than 10 mm Hg, the individual has a pulsus paradoxus. Presence of a pulsus paradoxus may provide the clinician with an idea of the degree of hemodynamic compromise associated with cardiac tamponade.[5] There is a normal decrease in blood pressure and stroke volume associated with inspiration due to negative intrapleural pressure. In cardiac tamponade, high pericardial pressure compresses the heart. As a result, during inspiration left heart filling is more dramatically restricted by right heart filling.[27]

As the cardiac tamponade increases, stroke volume continues to decrease, SVR increases, systolic blood pressure falls, diastolic blood pressure increases, and pulse pressure (the difference between the systolic and diastolic blood pressures) narrows. The "classic" signs of cardiac tamponade—distant heart sounds, hypotension, and increased jugular venous distention—constitute "Beck's triad."[3,5] It has been reported, however, that most patients with cardiac tamponade do not manifest this combination of symptoms.[4]

Individuals with cardiac tamponade may also present with mental status changes, anxiety, dizziness, lightheadedness, and agitation. These signs and symptoms result from the hemodynamic instability, decreased cardiac output, and hypoxia.[12] Individuals may also exhibit hepatojugular reflux, an increase in jugular venous pressure of 1 cm Hg or more.[28] To determine whether hepatojugular reflux is present, the individual is placed in a supine position with the head of the bed elevated so that jugular venous palpations are discernible. Pressure is exerted for 30 to 60 seconds over the right upper quadrant of the abdomen. The test is positive if an elevation in the jugular venous pressure occurs when pressure is exerted on the abdomen. Such a result is due to the elevation of central venous pressure. Gastrointestinal side effects may include nausea and vomiting due to visceral congestion and venous stasis.[29]

Prolonged periods of hypotension cause hypoperfusion to the kidneys, which can result in oliguria or anuria.[30] Prolonged hypotension and decreased cardiac output may also result in decreased peripheral perfusion, which may be manifested as weakness, fatigue, dyspnea, and cool, clammy extremities.[11] Other findings may include apprehension, cough, hiccups, hoarseness, and dysphagia.[2,11] The latter symptoms are thought to be related to compression of the esophagus.[5] Less common signs and symptoms of cardiac tamponade include peripheral edema, low-grade fever, abdominal pain, and nausea.[1,5,11,25,26] The latter two symptoms are believed to be due to hepatic and intestinal congestion. Presence of a fever usually indicates the presence of an infectious process.[5]

## ASSESSMENT

### PHYSICAL EXAM

Any of the aforementioned clinical manifestations may be noted on physical exam, depending on the rate of accumulation of the fluid, the amount of fluid accumulated, and the baseline cardiac function of the individual (see Figure 37-2). Conversely, assessment for physical findings alone is not adequate, as patients may be asymptomatic.[20,25]

### DIAGNOSTIC TESTS

Several tests and procedures aid in the diagnosis of cardiac tamponade. These include 2-dimensional echocardiography, chest radiograph, computerized tomography (CT) scan, magnetic resonance imaging (MRI), pulmonary artery catheterization, electrocardiogram (ECG), and pericardiocentesis with pericardial fluid evaluation.

*Echocardiography.* Two-dimensional echocardiography is the most sensitive and precise method for the diagnosis of cardiac tamponade. It is considered the "gold standard" for diagnosis.[1,2,7,11,26] During an echocardiogram, ultrasonic waves are produced via a probe placed on the chest wall.[23] These waves create a picture of the heart and can depict heart functioning. An echocardiogram will reveal fluid in the pericardial sac, compression of the right ventricular free wall during early diastole, inspiratory changes in ventricular size, mitral valve motion abnormalities, dilated inferior vena cava, swinging heart, and collapse of the right atrial and ventricular free walls during diastole in individuals with cardiac tamponade.[11,26] Because the right side of the heart contains less myocardium than the left side, the pressure being exerted by the pericardial fluid can cause the right side to collapse. Echocardiographic findings indicating the presence of a pericardial effusion coupled with hemodynamic compromise will help lead the clinician to a diagnosis of cardiac tamponade.[5]

In addition to pericardial fluid, an echocardiogram can reveal a low ejection fraction and, possibly, a pericardial mass. Quantification of the pericardial fluid is also possible.[20,22] Similarly, echocardiography may prove helpful in the assessment of hemodynamic effects of the tamponade.[22] A 2-dimensional echocardiography is useful for the detection of fluid as well as for selecting the appropriate site to perform a pericardiocentesis. Use of 3-dimensional echocardiography is reported to have more appreciable images of the changes in heart chamber size and shape in comparison to 2-dimensional echocardiogram.[31]

*Radiograph.* Chest radiograph is not a definitive diagnostic method for cardiac tamponade because fluid may not appear radiographically if the effusion is small. Nevertheless, cardiac tamponade may be suspected if the chest radiograph reveals cardiomegaly, increased mediastinal width, normal lung patterns, prominence of the superior vena cava (due to elevated central venous pressure), and dilated cardiac silhouette.[3,5,11,25] The cardiac silhouette will appear enlarged only after at least 200 mL to 250 mL of pericardial fluid has accumulated.[23] In affected patients, a pleural effusion may have the appearance of a "water bottle-shaped heart." Lung fields are usually clear in individuals with cardiac tamponade unless pulmonary disease is present. A confirmation of the diagnosis must be made with echocardiography, ultrasound, MRI, or CT scan. Each of these imaging techniques can show fluid in the pericardium better than an ordinary radiographic study.

*Computerized tomography.* A CT scan may indicate the presence of a cardiac tamponade, and it is useful for determining the pericardial thickness and presence of a pleural effusion or masses.[1,23] Cardiac tamponade will appear on CT scan with the presence of a large pericardial effusion with distension of the superior and inferior vena cavae, deformity and compression of heart chambers, and other intrapericardial structures.[15] As a diagnostic test, however, a CT scan has limited usefulness. The continuous heart motion produces a blurring of pericardial contents, making the images of a CT scan less useful for screening.[32] CT scan will not provide data on how well the heart is functioning.[17]

*Magnetic resonance imaging.* Magnetic resonance imaging also has limited usefulness in the diagnosis of cardiac tamponade. While MRI does afford the clinician a more defined view of the myocardium compared to CT, it offers no benefit over echocardiography.[1] It will detect effusions, masses, and pericardial thickening. Like a CT scan, an MRI will not provide data on how well the heart is functioning.[16]

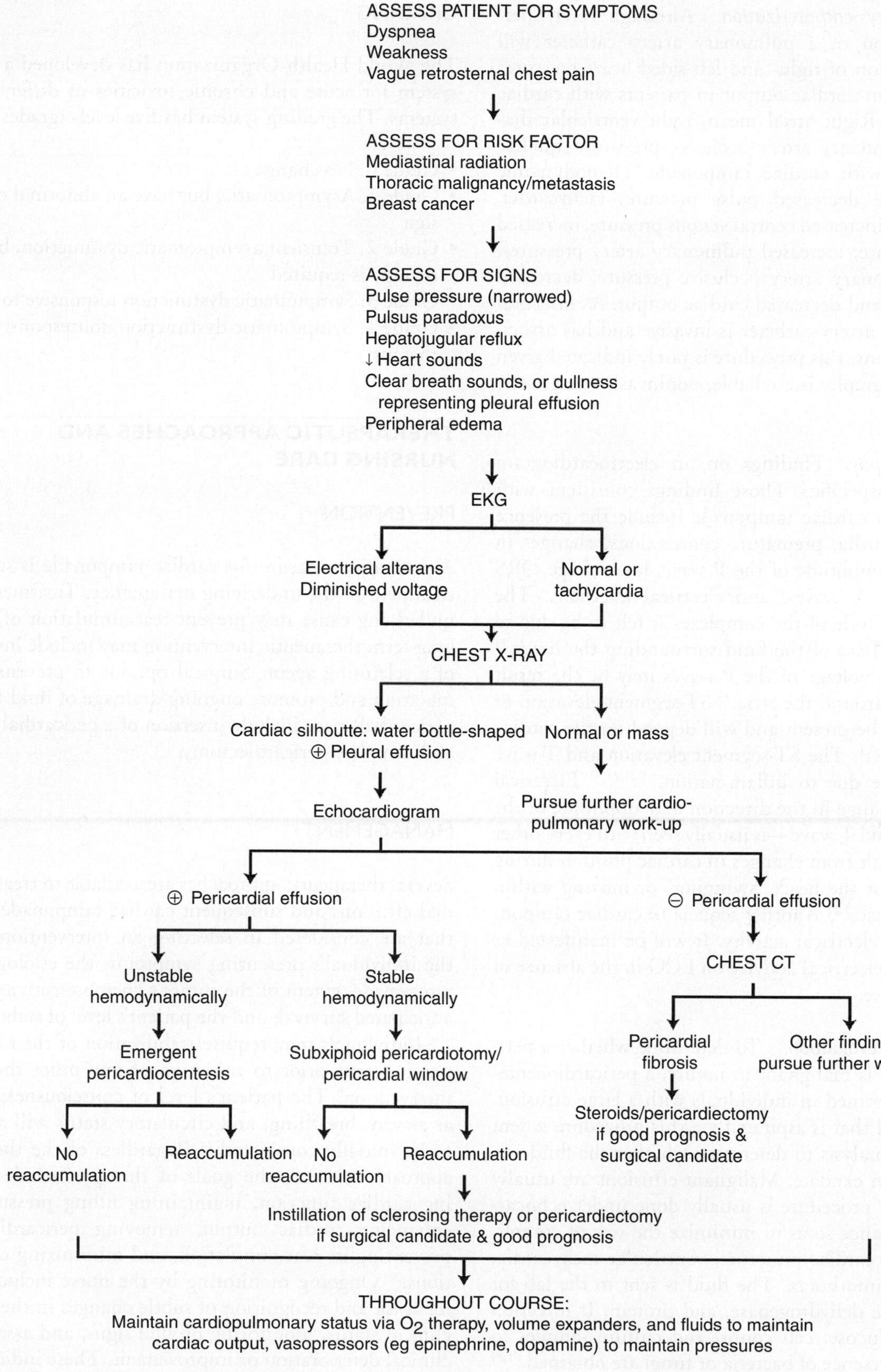


**FIGURE 37-2**

Clinical pathway for cardiac tamponade.

*Abbrevations*: CT, chest tomogram; ECG, electrocardiogram; $O_2$,oxygen.

*Pulmonary artery catheterization.* Although rarely performed, insertion of a pulmonary artery catheter will reveal equalization of right- and left-sided heart pressures and a decrease in cardiac output in patients with cardiac tamponade.[1,5,32] Right atrial mean, right ventricular diastolic, and pulmonary artery occlusive pressures equalize in individuals with cardiac tamponade. Hemodynamic changes include decreased pulse pressure, tachycardia, increased SVR, increased central venous pressure, increased left atrial pressure, increased pulmonary artery pressures, increased pulmonary artery occlusive pressure, decreased blood pressure, and decreased cardiac output. As insertion of a pulmonary artery catheter is invasive and has associated complications, this procedure is rarely indicated given that echocardiography is a reliable, noninvasive diagnostic method.[32]

*Electrocardiography.* Findings on an electrocardiogram (ECG) are nonspecific.[5] Those findings consistent with the diagnosis of cardiac tamponade include the presence of sinus tachycardia, premature contractions, changes in the shape and amplitude of the P wave, low-voltage QRS complexes, and T waves, and electrical alternans. The change in amplitude of the complexes is felt to be due to the insulation effect of the fluid surrounding the heart.[24] The decrease in voltage of the P waves may be the result of lack of fluid around the atria.[33] ST-segment elevation or depression may be present and will depend on the cardiac lead being viewed. The ST-segment elevation and T-wave changes may be due to inflammation.[3,5,21,22,33] Electrical alternans—a change in the direction and amplitude of the QRS complex and T wave—is usually seen with every other beat. It may result from changes in cardiac position during depolarization or the heart "swinging" or moving within the pericardial sac.[3,22] Another sequela to cardiac tamponade is pulseless electrical activity. It will be manifested as the presence of electrical activity on ECG in the absence of a detectable pulse.

*Pericardial fluid evaluation.* To determine whether a pericardial effusion is malignant in nature, a pericardiocentesis may be performed in individuals with a large effusion. Pericardial fluid that is aspirated via this procedure is sent to the lab for analysis to determine whether the fluid is a transudate or an exudate. Malignant effusions are usually exudates.[34] The procedure is usually done under echocardiography guidance so as to minimize the risk of complications such as cardiac puncture, ventricular tachycardia, or tension pneumothorax. The fluid is sent to the lab for cytology, lactate dehydrogenase, and protein. If infection is suspected, glucose, cell count, and culture samples to assess for the presence of bacteria or fungi are obtained.[31,34] Malignant effusions appear bloody or serosanguinous in 76% of cases, or serous in 24% of cases as opposed to straw-colored, normal pericardial fluid.[31]

### GRADING

The World Health Organization has developed a grading system for acute and chronic toxicities of different body systems. The grading system has five levels (grades 0–4):

- Grade 0: No change
- Grade 1: Asymptomatic, but have an abnormal cardiac sign
- Grade 2: Transient asymptomatic dysfunction, but no therapy is required
- Grade 3: Symptomatic dysfunction responsive to therapy
- Grade 4: Symptomatic dysfunction nonresponsive to therapy

## THERAPEUTIC APPROACHES AND NURSING CARE

### PREVENTION

A preventive measure for cardiac tamponade is successful treatment of the underlying malignancy. Treatment of the underlying cause may prevent reaccumulation of fluid. A long-term therapeutic intervention may include instillation of a sclerosing agent. Surgical options to prevent reaccumulation and promote ongoing drainage of fluid from the pericardial space include insertion of a pericardial window and complete pericardiectomy.

### MANAGEMENT

Several therapeutic approaches are available to treat pericardial effusions and subsequent cardiac tamponade. Factors that are considered in selecting an intervention include the individual's presenting symptoms, the etiology of the tamponade, extent of the tumor's chemosensitivity, overall anticipated survival, and the patient's level of stability.[1,17,35]

Individuals may require stabilization of their hemodynamic status prior to initiation of any other therapeutic intervention. The patient's level of consciousness, as well as airway, breathing, and circulatory status will also need to be initially considered.[24] Regardless of the therapeutic approach selected, the goals of therapy include enhancing cardiac function, maintaining filling pressures, and enhancing cardiac output, removing pericardial fluid, preventing its reaccumulation, and minimizing complications.[26] Ongoing monitoring by the nurse include assessment for and recognition of subtle changes in the patient's clinical status, monitoring of vital signs, and assessing for clinical deterioration or improvement. These indicators are essential, as a patient's level of stability is a primary factor in determining what and when treatment procedures are performed.

## Supportive care

Prior to treatment for cardiac tamponade, individuals can be stabilized with oxygen to reduce cardiac workload, anxiety, and respiratory distress; with aggressive fluid volume resuscitation; and with administration of inotropic agents to enhance cardiac output and prevent cardiovascular collapse.[3,26] Patients with cardiac tamponade with no or mild hemodynamic compromise can be managed with the administration of isotonic intravenous fluids (eg, normal saline), blood, plasma, or dextran to avoid volume depletion while treating the underlying cause of the tamponade.[36] Volume repletion is considered a temporizing measure and may only be effective in patients who are hypovolemic. Attainment of a systolic blood pressure of 90 mm Hg or higher will improve ventricular filling pressure. Titration of inotropic agents such as dopamine, norepinephrine, or dobutamine, all of which stimulate $beta_1$ receptors, may be employed to enhance contractility and cardiac output. The latter agent, dobutamine, is suggested as the preferred inotrope for hypotension associated with cardiac tamponade. The use of inotropes is reported as controversial but should be considered in patients who do not respond to fluid resuscitation alone.[7,36] Inotropes are administered to improve contractility and cardiac output. When the heart is compressed, as with cardiac tamponade, stimuli to increase the force of contractions will not be effective as the external force will impede the desired effects. In addition, some inotropes (eg, norepinephrine, high dose dopamine) cause an increase in SVR (the amount of work the heart must do to eject blood). Administration of agents that increase SVR will decrease cardiac output further. Lastly, inotropes typically cause tachycardia, which can aggravate symptoms of cardiac tamponade. If inotropes are to be used to help treat hypotension, selection of an agent that does not increase SVR (eg, dobutamine) is suggested. The nurse will then monitor for tachycardia and note any hemodynamic effects related to the increase in heart rate.[37]

Agents that stimulate alpha-receptors, thereby causing vasoconstriction, will increase the amount of work the heart must do to eject blood and decrease cardiac output. Conversely, use of arterial vasodilators such as nitroprusside will decrease the amount of work the heart must do to eject blood and may help increase blood pressure.[26] Abrupt changes in filling pressures with vasodilators and vasoconstrictors should be avoided in patients with cardiac tamponade. Patients with cardiac tamponade are very sensitive to changes in filling pressures and can sustain a rapid clinical decline.[26] Administration of diuretics will decrease circulating volume, thereby decreasing ventricular filling; for this reason, these agents should not be given. Use of positive-pressure ventilation should, ideally, be avoided, as it is associated with an increase in intrathoracic pressure and subsequent decrease in cardiac output.[26] Maintaining the individual on bed rest in semi-Fowler's position may be helpful, as it further decreases cardiac workload.

## Pericardiocentesis

Echocardiogram-guided pericardiocentesis is considered the best initial treatment for cardiac tamponade when patients have hemodynamic compromise.[1,7,38] Pericardiocentesis entails an aspiration needle being inserted into the pericardial sac for the removal of fluid.[1,3,21] It relieves the increased end diastolic pressure and decreased ventricular filling. Improvement in clinical status (eg, decreased central venous pressure and pulsus paradoxus; increased cardiac output and blood pressure; and pressures of the right and left ventricles no longer being equalized) is usually seen after as little as 25 mL to 50 mL of fluid is removed.[20]

Pericardiocentesis can be performed at the bedside with cardiac monitoring available. If not clinically contraindicated, assessment and any correction of the individual's coagulation status should be attempted prior to performing a pericardiocentesis. The individual is placed in a semi-Fowler's position with the head of bed elevated 30° to 45°, the site is cleansed with an antibacterial solution, and local anesthesia is injected into the site. The semi-Fowler's position is assumed so that most of the fluid will be in the most dependent position. Using sterile technique, a 16- to 18-gauge intracardiac needle attached to a 30 to 50 mL syringe is inserted into the pericardial sac using a subxiphoid approach under ultrasound guidance of 2-dimensional echocardiography or with ECG monitoring.[31–36] When using ECG monitoring, alligator clamps are attached to the hub of the needle and to a V-lead on the ECG machine.[31] When the needle comes in contact with the pericardium, the QRS voltage will increase. If it comes in contact with the epicardium, the individual may develop ectopic beats (premature atrial or ventricular contractions) or ST-segment elevation.[36] The needle should be withdrawn if ectopy or ST-segment elevation is observed. When the needle reaches the pericardial sac, the patient may experience a vasovagal response necessitating administration of intravenous atropine.[36] Once the needle is inside the pericardial sac, fluid is gradually aspirated with the syringe.

As most effusions recur, when the pericardiocentesis is completed, a catheter may be inserted into the site. This catheter may be left in place and the effusion allowed to drain until the output is less than 25 mL to 30 mL in 24 hours.[31,39]

Nursing care during the pericardiocentesis procedure is reviewed in Table 37-3. Several complications may occur during the procedure, including dysrhythmias, pneumothorax, laceration of the coronary arteries, myocardial puncture, trauma to abdominal organs (especially the liver), and hypotension.[31] A rare complication reported is acute left ventricular failure with pulmonary edema.[39] Nursing monitoring for signs and symptoms of any of these complications is important. The incidence of these complications is decreased when the procedure is conducted under direct visualization or electrocardiographic guidance. Given the decreased morbidity associated with direct visualization and guidance, unguided pericardiocentesis procedures are recommended in emergent situations only.[31]

Frequent monitoring of vital signs, hemodynamic status (ie, central venous pressure), and assessment for the presence of dysrhythmias, and complications during and following the procedure are essential. Hemodynamic status should improve following adequate fluid removal. As fluid reaccumulation is likely to occur,[31] monitoring for signs of symptoms of buildup is vital.[16,40] Administration of analgesics will likely be required postprocedure. The sterility of any remaining catheters or drains is essential.

## Pericardiocentesis with sclerosing

Patients may experience reaccumulation of pericardial fluid after pericardiocentesis.[31] Up to a 50% recurrence rate has been reported in patients who have not been treated for the underlying malignancy.[16] In an attempt to prevent reaccumulation of fluid, management of cardiac tamponade includes instillation of a sclerosing agent into the pericardial sac every 1 to 2 days via the pericardiocentesis catheter. This procedure is done once pericardial fluid output is reduced to 50 mL to 100 mL in 24 hours.[41] The sclerosing agent selected is based on antitumor activity. Nitrogen mustard and thiotepa were used as sclerosing agents in the 1970s. Instillation resulted in significant pain and bone marrow suppression, which led to the discontinuation of these agents. Doxycycline, which replaced tetracycline, bleomycin, and cisplatin are used as sclerosing agents. Data suggest lower complication rates and decreased hospital stay in patients who have received bleomycin vs doxycycline.[35] Immunotherapy with agents such as interleukin 2 (IL-2) and OK-432 have been used as sclerosing agents.[42] Preliminary data of pericardial instillation of $^{125}I$ being tagged to a monoclonal antibody (HMF-G2) suggest positive results. This technique is still under investigation.[31] Instillation of a sclerosing agent into the pericardial sac creates an irritation to the pericardium. This response bonds the two layers of the pericardium, thereby obliterating the pericardial space.[31] Reports have cited a success rate greater than 70% with sclerosing therapy as measured in terms of morbidity, mortality, and fluid reaccumulation.[31,43] Side effects of administration of sclerosing agents include pain, fever, nausea, and arrhythmias.[16] A rare report of constrictive pericarditis appears in the literature.[31] Nursing care of individuals undergoing pericardiocentesis with sclerosing is similar to that described for individuals undergoing pericardiocentesis. A proactive approach to pain management following instillation of a sclerosing agent is vital.[16]

**TABLE 37-3**

**Pericardiocentesis: Nursing Care**

**Preprocedure**
- Describe possible sensations that may be experienced by the patient during the procedure (initial stick of the small needle for administration of the local anesthetic, burning during administration of the local anesthetic, pressure sensation during insertion of the pericardiocentesis needle, and some pain if the needle touches the pericardium during the procedure [the pericardium, which has nerve endings, is not anesthetized by the local anesthesia])
- Procure all needed equipment
- Supportive therapy with oxygen, aggressive fluid resuscitation, and administration of vasoactive agents, as clinically indicated and prescribed
- Assess for signs and symptoms of cardiac tamponade and obtain baseline hemodynamic parameters
- Ensure that signed consent has been obtained
- Explain procedure to individual
- Ensure IV access
- Position supine with HOB elevated 30° to 45°, as tolerated and suggested by physician performing procedure.
- Connect to cardiac monitor, ECG machine, noninvasive blood pressure monitoring device, and pulse oximeter
- Administer sedation/anxiolytics, as prescribed
- Connect alligator clamp to hub of intracardiac needle and to V-lead on ECG machine or cardiac monitor

**During Procedure**
- Monitor cardiac rhythm, vital signs, and hemodynamic status
- Observe for complications related to procedure
- Monitor amount and characteristics of drainage being aspirated
- Administer sedation or anxiolytics as needed

**Postprocedure**
- Assess for complications
- Assess for improvement in hemodynamic status and resolution of other signs and symptoms of cardiac tamponade
- Assess amount and characteristics of drainage if catheter left in place
- Ascertain that pericardial fluid specimens are sent to the lab for analysis
- Document vital signs, medications administered, and response to the procedure according to institutional policy and procedure

*Abbreviations*: HOB, head of bed; EKG, electrocardiogram.

## Percutaneous balloon pericardiotomy

Pericardiocentesis usually provides only temporary relief from signs and symptoms of cardiac tamponade until the underlying malignancy is treated. A percutaneous balloon pericardiotomy is an alternative method undertaken to prevent the reaccumulation of fluid[9] and is considered less invasive and more effective than other procedures for refractory pericardial effusion management.[12,44] It involves incision of the pericardium and insertion of a balloon catheter into the pericardial sac. By decreasing the potential space, it minimizes the risk of fluid accumulation. The balloon creates an opening in the pericardium, allowing for internal drainage and reabsorption of any fluid that may accumulate. Once in place, the balloon is dilated to form a pericardial window, enabling pericardial fluid to drain.[43]

Nursing care of the individual undergoing pericardiotomy includes aggressive pain management as postprocedure pain is common, drainage measurement, and monitoring for complications.[17] Success rates of percutaneous balloon pericardiotomy is reported at 96%.[43]

### Pericardial window

A pericardial window (partial pericardiectomy) is usually performed on individuals for whom other interventions have not been effective and have a good long-term survival expectation.[31] It is most often performed in the operating room under general anesthesia. A pericardial window can also be performed using local anesthesia in approximately 30 to 45 minutes.[31]

This procedure involves removal of a piece of the pericardium.[16,21] The purpose of a pericardial window is to drain the fluid from the pericardial sac if the effusion and tamponade are recurrent.[1,3,7] A small opening is made in the pericardium and is sutured to the lung. Pericardial fluid can then drain into the lung. A pericardial window should be considered when other procedures have not been successful in managing pericardial effusions, and long-term survival is anticipated.[16] As this procedure is not well tolerated in a critically ill person, stabilization should be accomplished before it is undertaken.

A pericardial window can also be performed using a video-assisted thoracoscopic surgery (VATS) to manage chronic pericardial effusions. Using a VATS procedure, a thorascope is inserted and a pericardial window is performed under thoracoscopic vision. Long-term success rates with no significant morbidity or mortality are reported related to this procedure.[16]

Postprocedure prevention of complications is essential. Patency of the drainage catheter must be maintained. The pericardial space must remain decompressed with suction until there is less than 50 mL of drainage in 24 hours.[31]

Data suggest that the performance of a laparoscopic pericardio-peritoneal window may have some advantages over a thoracoscopy pericardial window. By creating a "window," pericardial fluid is drained and absorbed by the peritoneal cavity. Advantages reported include no need for postprocedure pleural drainage or intubation and the use of reverse Trendelenburg (vs lateral decubitus) position for the laparoscopic procedure. (The latter position is associated with prolonged anesthesia time). Symptomatic relief with no effusion recurrence in patients with malignant effusions have been reported related to this procedure.[45]

### Pericardiectomy

Pericardiectomy is the excision of part or all of the pericardium.[1] It involves a thoracotomy or median sternotomy. The pericardium is resected to facilitate drainage of fluid into the pleural space. This procedure is performed in the operating room under local or general anesthesia; general anesthesia is used for individuals with hemodynamic stability. As with a pericardial window, pericardiectomy can be considered when other management strategies for pericardial effusion have not been effective and long-term survival is expected.[16] Reported advantages of a pericardiectomy include low morbidity and mortality rates and instant relief of a cardiac tamponade. The reported success rate is 83%.[31] Reported complications include wound infection and pulmonary complications.[46]

### Chemotherapy, radiotherapy, and immunotherapy

Treatment of the underlying malignant process may help to prevent recurrence of cardiac tamponade. Administration of systemic chemotherapy and radiotherapy for disease in the pericardium has been effectively used to control pericardial effusions.[1,7,11]

Use of external beam radiotherapy to the heart, pericardial structures, and lower mediastinum has also been reported in the management of pericardial effusions. Radiotherapy is indicated for the individual with radiosensitive malignancies such as lymphoma or leukemia who has not received radiotherapy in the past.[16,31] Another treatment reported in the literature includes immunotherapy, including administration of autologous tumor-infiltrating lymphocytes (TILs) into the pericardial cavity.[38]

Tumor-infiltrating lymphocytes are a type of adoptive immunotherapy. They are isolated from tumor tissue, cultured with lymphokines (eg, IL-2), and then reinfused into the patient. It is felt that infusion of TILs may induce tumor regression and possibly decrease cardiac tamponade if caused by malignant pericarditis.[47,48]

Nursing care of individuals receiving systemic chemotherapy, radiotherapy, or immunotherapy for cardiac tamponade includes providing patient education materials to facilitate the decision-making process regarding treatment options and specific information related to antineoplastic toxicities. Fluid reaccumulation rates are reported at 31%[43] for these antineoplastic therapies.

Cardiac tamponade is a life-threatening oncologic emergency that can cause anxiety for the patient and family. This may be related to the significance of the presence of the tamponade with respect to disease progression or complications of treatment. Emotional support is pivotal. Once fluid has accumulated and interventions are required, emotional support must be provided to combat the fear and anxiety associated with experiencing a life-threatening emergency.[49] The acute onset of the signs and symptoms as well as the need for possible admission to a critical care unit are additional sources of anxiety.

Providing an explanation of anticipated interventions and allowing the individual to verbalize concerns are essential. In addition to the reduction in psychosocial distress, support may result in a concomitant decrease in cardiac workload. As part of their patient care management, nurses should assess signs of ineffective coping and depression.[50]

Patients should be prepared for the procedures that they will undergo as treatment for the cardiac tamponade. An explanation of the sensations that they will feel during and after the procedure may help allay some of the anxiety associated with this complication. Individuals and families must be educated about signs and symptoms of recurrence and actions to take in the event of recurrence.[49] Early intervention is pivotal in trying to decrease complications and improving individual outcomes. Educational endeavors should also include information about the diagnostic and therapeutic interventions the individual will be experiencing. Other education should focus on signs and symptoms and complications to observe for and report once the patient has been discharged from the hospital.[50]

## CONCLUSION

Cardiac tamponade is a life-threatening oncologic emergency that requires immediate management. Signs and symptoms may occur slowly, over time, or acutely. Patients require ongoing monitoring of their hemodynamic status to ensure that the appropriate therapies are implemented. No one therapeutic intervention is preferred in the management of cardiac tamponade. The decision for treatment is based on numerous factors, including the individual's disease type and clinical status. Despite the high level of acuity that the patient may present, prompt and accurate nursing recognition and intervention based on knowledge of the etiology, signs and symptoms, pathophysiology, and management of the problem are essential to decrease the morbidity and mortality associated with this oncologic emergency.[16]

## REFERENCES


1. Halfdanarson TR, Hogan WJ, Moynihan TJ. Oncologic emergencies: diagnosis and treatment. *Mayo Clin Proc.* 2006;81:835–848.
2. Grannis FW, Cullinane CA, Lai L. Fluid complications. In: Pazdur R, Coia LR, Hoskins WJ, et al, eds. *Cancer Management: A Multidisciplinary Approach.* 9th ed. Lawrence, KS: CMP Healthcare Media; 2007:1035–1049.
3. Brown H. Cardiac tamponade. *Nursing.* 2005;35:88.
4. El Fortia M, El Gatit A, Bendaoud M. Metastatic pericardial effusion and cardiac tamponade. *Internet J Cardiol* [serial online]. 2006;3:9. http://www.ispub.com. Accessed March 2, 2010.
5. Roy CL, Minor MA, Brookhart MA, Choudhry NK. Does this patient with pericardial effusion have cardiac tamponade? *JAMA.* 2007; 297:1810–1818.
6. Forauer AR. Pericardial tamponade in patients with central venous catheters. *J Infusion Nurs.* 2007;30:161–167.
7. Higdon ML, Higdon JA. Treatment of oncologic emergencies. *Am Fam Phys.* 2006;74:1873–1880.
8. Levy PY, Corey R, Berger P, et al. Etiologic diagnosis of 204 pericardial effusions. *Medicine (Baltimore).* 2003;82:385–391.
9. Vega E, Rondon FP, Lopez F, et al. Tumor-associated significant pericardial effusions: analysis of 18 cases. *Revista Clinica Espanola.* 2004;204:260–263.
10. Imazio M, Demichelis B, Parrini I, et al. Relation of acute pericardial disease to malignancy. *Am J Cardiol.* 2005;95:1393–1394.
11. Morris JC, Holland JF. Oncologic emergencies. In: Kufe DW, Pollack RE, Weichselbaum RR, et al, eds. *Cancer Medicine.* 6th ed. Ontario, Canada: BC Decker; 2003:2433–2453.
12. Furnkawa A, Itoh A, Nakamura T, et al. Efficacy of percutaneous balloon pericardiotomy and intrapericardial instillation for the management of refractory pericardial effusion: a case report. *J Cardiol.* 2007;50:389–395.
13. Cheng M, Tsai C, Chiang P, Lee H. Cardiac tamponade as a manifestation of advanced thymic carcinoma. *Heart Lung.* 2005;34:136–141.
14. Nagarsheth NP, Harrison M, Kalir T, Rahaman J. Malignant pericardial effusion with cardiac tamponade in a patient with metastatic vaginal adenocarcinoma. *Int J Gynecol Cancer.* 2006;16:1451–1456.
15. Restrepo CS, Lemos DF, Lemos JA, et al. Imaging findings in cardiac tamponade with emphasis on CT. *Radiographics.* 2007;27:1595–1610.
16. Hillis LD, Lange RA, Winniford MD, Page RL. Radiation-induced pericardial and myocardial diseases. In: Hillis LD, Lange RA, Winniford MD, Page RL, eds. *Manual of Clinical Problems in Cardiology.* Philadelphia, PA: Lippincott Williams & Wilkins; 2002:281–283.
17. Watson AC. Urgent syndromes at end of life. In: Ferrell B, Coyle N, eds. *Textbook of Palliative Nursing.* New York: Oxford University Press; 2005:443–466.
18. Corey GR. *Etiology of Pericardial Disease.* http://www.utdol.com. Accessed March 2, 2010.
19. Chan K-S, Sham MM, Tse DM, et al. Palliative medicine in malignant respiratory diseases. In: Doyle D, Hanks G, Cherny N, Calman K, eds. *Oxford Textbook of Palliative Medicine.* 3rd ed. New York: Oxford University Press; 2005:587–597.
20. Hoit BD. Pericardial disease and pericardial tamponade. *Crit Care Med.* 2007;35:S355–S364.
21. Zeller JL, Lynm C, Glass RM. Pericardial effusion. *JAMA.* 2007;297: 1844.
22. Humphreys M. Pericardial conditions: signs, symptoms and electrocardiogram changes. *Emerg Nurse.* 2006;14:30–37.
23. Beste Jones L, Lome B. Delayed cardiac tamponade following blunt chest trauma. *Adv Emerg Nurs J.* 2006;28:275–283.
24. Morgan E. Pericardial tamponade. *Nursing.* 2006;36:88.
25. Goldstein JA. Cardiac tamponade, constrictive pericarditis, and restrictive cardiomyopathy. *Curr Probl Cardiol.* 2004;29:503–567.
26. Cousineau A, Cavitsky E. Cardiac tamponade presenting as an apparent life-threatening event. *Pediatr Emerg Care.* 2005;21:104–108.
27. Fowler NO. Physiology of cardiac tamponade and pulsus paradoxus. I: Mechanisms of pulsus paradoxus in cardiac tamponade. *Mod Concepts Cardiovasc Dis.* 1978;47:109–113.
28. Starley BQ, Rohrer MS, Harrison EA. Cardiac tamponade: a rare complication of interferon-induced hypothyroidism. *Resid Staff Phys.* 2007;53:18–23.
29. DeGowin RL, LeBlond RF, Brown OD. Chest signs. In: DeGowin RL, LeBlond RF, Brond OD, eds. *DeGowins's Diagnostic Examination: The Complete Guide to Assessment, Examination, Differential Diagnosis.* New York: McGraw-Hill; 2004:440.
30. Plurad D, Brown C, Chan L, Demetriades D, Rhee D. Emergency department hypotension is not an independent risk factor for post-traumatic acute renal dysfunction. *J Trauma.* 2006;61:1120–1128.

31. D'Cruz IA, Khouzam RN, Minderman D. Three-dimensional echocardiographic appearances of pericardial effusion with tamponade. *Echocardiography.* 2007;24:162–165.
32. Ruckdeschel JC, Moores DW. Management of advanced lung disease including pleural and pericardial effusions. In: Berger AM, Shuster JL, Von Roenn JH, eds. *Principles and Practice of Palliative Care and Supportive Oncology.* Chicago, IL: Lippincott Williams & Wilkins Wolters Kluwer; 2006:309–326.
33. Medias JE. The importance of the P waves in the differentiation of attenuation of the QRS voltage due to pericardial effusion versus due to peripheral edema. *J Card Fail.* 2008;14:55–60.
34. Corey GR. *Diagnosis and Treatment of Pericardial Effusion.* http://www.utdol.com. Accessed March 2, 2010.
35. Thai V, Oneschuk D. Malignant pericardial effusion treated with intraperitoneal bleomycin. *J Palliat Med.* 2007;10:281–282.
36. Becker RC. Pericardiocentesis. In: Irwin RS, Rippe JM, Lisbon A, Heard SO, eds. *Procedures, Techniques, and Minimally Invasive Monitoring in Intensive Care Medicine.* Chicago, IL: Lippincott Williams & Wilkins Wolters Kluwer Health; 2007:80–86.
37. Sahjian M. Post-cardiac surgery tamponade. *Air Med J.* 2007; 26:188–190.
38. Toh U, Fujii T, Seki N, Nilya F, Shirouzu K, Yamana H. Characterization of IL-2-activated TILs and their use in intrapericardial immunotherapy in malignant pericardial effusion. *Cancer Immunol Immunother.* 2006;55:1219–1227.
39. Shabatai R. *Technique of Pericardiocentesis.* http://www.utdol.com. Accessed March 2, 2010.
40. Aghassi P, Markowitz DH. Pericardiocentesis. In: Irwin RS, Rippe JM, eds. *Manual of Intensive Care Medicine.* 4th ed. Philadelphia, PA: Lippincott Williams & Wilkins; 2005:32–35.
41. Martinoni A, Cipolla CM, Cardinale D, et al. Long-term results of intrapericardial chemotherapeutic treatment of malignant pericardial effusions with thiotepa. *Chest.* 2004;126:1412–1416.
42. Mentzer SJ. Surgical palliative care in thoracic diseases. *Surg Clin North Am.* 2005;8:315–328.
43. Shabestari M, Dadgar AA, Danesh SH, Alizadeh I, Tayeo M, Dehestani GH. Percutaneous balloon pericardiotomy in a patient with recurrent pericardial tamponade. *Med J Mashhad Univ Med Sci.* 2004;47:210–216.
44. Swanson N, Mirza I, Wijesinghe N, Derlin G. Primary percutaneous balloon pericardiotomy for malignant pericardial effusion. *Catheter Cardiovasc Interv.* 2008;71:508–509.
45. Staltari D, Diaz A, Capellino P, et al. Laparoscopic pericardio-peritoneal window: an alternative approach in the treatment of recurrent pericardial effusion, in-hospital evolution and survival. *Surg Laparosc Endosc Percutan Tech.* 2007;17:116–119.
46. Tiruvoipati R, Naiki RD, Loubani M, et al. Surgical approach for pericardiectomy: a comparative study between medial sternotomy and left anterolateral thoracotomy. *Interact Cardiovasc Thorac Surg.* 2003;2:322–326.
47. National Cancer Institute. *NCI Dictionary.* http://www.cancer.gov/Templates/drugdictionary.aspx?cdrID=41004. Accessed January 13, 2010.
48. Tuh U, Fujii T, Seki N, et al. Characterization of IL-2-activated TILs and their use in intrapericardial immunotherapy in malignant pericardial effusion. *Cancer Immunol Immunother.* 2005;55:1219–1227.
49. Kaplow R, Reid MM. Oncologic emergencies. In: Schell HM, Puntillo KA, eds. *Critical Care Nursing Secrets.* 2nd ed. St. Louis, MO: Elsevier; 2006:398–414.
50. Flounders JA. Cardiovascular emergencies: pericardial effusion and cardiac tamponade. *Oncol Nurs Forum.* 2003;30:E48–E55.

CHAPTER 38

*Barbara Holmes Gobel, MS, RN, AOCN®*

# Disseminated Intravascular Coagulation

## SCOPE OF THE PROBLEM

### DEFINITIONS

Disseminated intravascular coagulation (DIC) is an oncologic emergency that is characterized by inappropriate and exaggerated overstimulation of normal coagulation, in which thrombosis and then bleeding occurs. This seemingly paradoxical situation results in hypercoagulation, in which multiple small clots are formed in the microvasculature, and fibrinolysis, in which there is consumption of clots and clotting factors. Ultimately, the body becomes unable to respond to vascular or tissue injury through stable clot formation and hemorrhage occurs. The hemorrhage associated with DIC may be profound, but it is the intravascular coagulation that leads to irreversible morbidity and mortality in this population of patients.[1] The resulting thrombosis of DIC leads to ischemia, impairment of blood flow, and end-organ damage. DIC is the most common serious thrombotic state that occurs in individuals with cancer.

Disseminated intravascular coagulation can be chronic or acute in nature. If only a minor imbalance is present related to the intravascular coagulation, the syndrome may be chronic. Chronic DIC generally presents as localized thrombotic events, eg, deep vein thrombosis. Acute DIC, which can be life-threatening, occurs when the intravascular coagulation becomes overwhelming to the body.[2] Acute DIC is seen in certain defined clinical situations such as sepsis, acute leukemia, and tumor lysis. This chapter will deal with the acute form of DIC.

### INCIDENCE

Although DIC is considered to be a problem commonly associated with cancer, its incidence is difficult to estimate as it varies depending on the type of associated neoplasm and concomitant disorders (eg, sepsis). Abnormal blood coagulation studies that demonstrate laboratory evidence of DIC are frequently reported in patients with disseminated solid malignancies (particularly the mucin-secreting adenocarcinomas) and leukemia (particularly acute promyelocytic leukemia [APL]).[3–5] DIC is estimated to occur in 10% of all patients with solid tumor malignancies,[5] and in as many as 85% of patients with APL.[3] Although significant bleeding is the predominant clinical finding in APL, severe thrombotic events can be observed at diagnosis and throughout treatment.[6,7]

### ETIOLOGY AND RISK FACTORS

Disseminated intravascular coagulation in the cancer population is always secondary to either the malignancy itself or to an underlying condition. Activation of the coagulation system in cancer can result from specific cancers themselves, infection, liver abnormalities, intravascular hemolysis, metabolic acidosis, and the use of certain prosthetic devices. Table 38-1 lists common causes of DIC in cancer. The most common cancers associated with acute DIC include acute leukemia and the mucin-producing adenocarcinomas.

Acute promyelocytic leukemia is the cancer most commonly associated with DIC. DIC associated with APL can occur before and in conjunction with chemotherapy administration. APL cells express procoagulant substances including tissue factor (TF) and cancer procoagulant (CP).[8,9] TF is the physiologic activator of coagulation in normal tissues and is an important activator of coagulation in cancer. The procoagulant activity of TF is largely dormant and generally occurs when there is cell death or apoptosis, such as during chemotherapy or radiation therapy. APL cells also contain an abnormally high level of annexin II. This phospholipid-binding protein is found on the surface of endothelial cells (including cerebral microvascular endothelial cells) and serves to bind plasminogen

**TABLE 38-1**

**Common Causes of Disseminated Intravascular Coagulation in Cancer**

**Neoplasms**
- Leukemia—acute myelomonocytic, acute promyelocytic, acute myelogenous, chronic myelogenous, acute lymphoblastic
- Solid tumors—lung, breast, ovary, renal, stomach, pancreas, prostate, melanoma, gallbladder

**Infections**
- Gram-negative bacteria—meningococcus, pseudomonas, salmonella, haemophilus, enterobacteriaceae
- Gram-positive bacteria—pneumococcus, staphylococcus, hemolytic streptococci
- Viremias—hepatitis, varicella, cytomegalovirus, human immunodeficiency virus
- Septic shock

**Liver Disease**
- Obstructive jaundice
- Fulminant hepatic failure

**Intravascular Hemolysis**
- Acute hemolytic transfusion reaction
- Multiple transfusions of whole blood
- Minor hemolysis

**Prosthetic Devices**
- Peritoneovenous shunts
- Aortic balloon-assist devices

**Metabolic Acidosis**

and its activator, tissue-type plasminogen activator (tPA).[10] Increased levels of annexin II lead to increased production of plasmin, with resultant bleeding from unopposed fibrinolysis.[11] With the introduction of all-transretinoic acid in the late 1980s and its routine use in the management of all newly diagnosed patients with APL, the disease-free survival related to this disease has decreased dramatically.[12,13] Unfortunately, the early death rate in patients with APL has not changed significantly, with hemorrhage being a significant cause of early death.[14,15]

The solid tumors that are most commonly associated with DIC are the mucin-producing adenocarcinomas, including those of the lung, breast, stomach, pancreas, and prostate. Of these solid tumors, breast and prostate cancers are probably the most common cancers related to DIC.[16] (The incidence of these cancers is significantly higher than the incidence of APL.) In addition to an unidentified procoagulant substance thought to be released from these cancers directly stimulating the coagulation system, tumors may release necrotic tissue or tissue enzymes into the circulation, thereby activating the coagulation mechanism.[17]

Infection and sepsis associated with cancer are the most common causes of acute DIC, and can be associated with a variety of bacterial, fungal, and viral infections. Sepsis, especially from meningococcemia and other gram-negative bacteria, is the most frequent cause of DIC. In fact, DIC may occur in 30% to 50% of patients with sepsis.[18,19] It is believed that bacterial endotoxins released from gram-negative bacteremia activate one of the clotting factors (factor XII) of the clotting cascade. Endotoxin also induces release of tumor necrosis factor-alpha (TNF-α), interleukin 1 (IL-1), and complement activation, all leading to endothelial damage and endothelial permeability leading to multi-end-organ damage.[1] Activation of factor XII can initiate coagulation as well as stimulate fibrinolysis (the breakdown of clots), thus setting up DIC.

Gram-positive organisms are thought to initiate coagulation by a similar mechanism as gram-negative bacteremia.[1] The triggering mechanism associated with viruses, including varicella, hepatitis, cytomegalovirus (CMV), or human immunodeficiency virus (HIV) is unclear. Antibiotic therapy can also initiate DIC. Antibiotic therapy may alter intestinal flora, which is a source of vitamin K, thereby altering the coagulation process.[20]

Primary liver disease, liver metastasis, or liver damage due to chemotherapy or radiation therapy can increase the risk of DIC. The liver replaces clotting factors and inhibitors as they are consumed. The liver also clears activated coagulation factors and fibrinolytic degradation products from the systemic circulation. Hepatic failure then disrupts the normal balance of coagulation, which can lead to DIC.[1]

Hemolytic transfusion reactions may be complicated by shock, renal failure, and DIC with severe bleeding. These reactions are probably due to generalized endothelial injury caused by activated complement, cytokines, and neutrophil products occurring during acute hemolytic transfusion reactions.[1] Also during hemolysis, there is a release of adenosine diphosphate (ADP) or red cell membrane phospholipoprotein that activates the procoagulant system, which may account for the DIC.[21] DIC may also occur after massive transfusions, but its etiology is unknown.

Prosthetic devices, such as aortic-balloon assist devices and peritoneovenous shunts may activate the coagulation system. Peritoneovenous shunts are used to shunt ascitic fluid into the systemic circulation. Ascitic fluid contains collagen and other procoagulant substances. When these substances are shunted into the general circulation, DIC can be triggered.[22]

Activation of the procoagulant system related to metabolic acidosis can occur as a result of endothelial sloughing with activation of factor XII to XIIa, activation of XI to XIa and platelet release reaction. In addition, cytokine release during metabolic acidosis can activate the coagulation system with resultant fibrin deposition.[1] Acidosis along with cytokine release can inhibit thrombin-mediated activities, some of which are antithrombotic in nature, thus resulting in increased thrombus formation.[23]

## PHYSIOLOGICAL ALTERATIONS

### PATHOPHYSIOLOGY

Although DIC is triggered by a number of defined clinical events such as infection or the cancer itself, once initiated the pathophysiology is similar in all disorders. When one of these events occurs, the coagulation system is activated, thus activating thrombin and eventually activating the fibrinolytic system with the production of plasmin.[2] As discussed in Chapter 29 on Bleeding Disorders, in which there is a thorough discussion of the physiology of coagulation, thrombin is the central proteolytic enzyme of blood coagulation. The presence of thrombin is also necessary for the breakdown of clots, or fibrinolysis.

In DIC there is an excess of thrombin formation that results from an overstimulation of the coagulation system, in which there is a disruption in the balance of coagulation and fibrinolysis. The excess formation of thrombin in DIC is driven by a transmembrane glycoprotein, called tissue factor (TF), and activated factor VIIa of the extrinsic coagulation pathway.[24] Tissue factor is present on the surface of many cell types (including endothelial cells, macrophages, and monocytes) and is exposed to the general circulation after vascular damage. It is released in response to exposure to cytokines, endotoxin, and TNF, which plays a major role in the development of DIC in septic conditions.

The excess formation of fibrin (the end result of coagulation is a stable fibrin clot) that occurs in patients with DIC results from excess circulating thrombin, suppression of the anticoagulation mechanisms, and impaired removal of fibrin.[25] The alterations in these processes are mediated by several proinflammatory cytokines, including interleukin 6 (IL-6) and TNF-α. There are several mechanisms that normally inhibit the coagulation cascade that are largely defective in DIC including the tissue factor pathway inhibitor (TFPI), activated protein C, and antithrombin III (AT III).[25] Protein C deficiency occurs with sepsis, promotes thrombin formation in the microvasculature, and may increase inflammation and endothelial cell dysfunction.[19]

Excess circulating thrombin yields fibrinogen, which leaves behind fibrin monomers that polymerize into fibrin clots in the circulation.[1] These excess clots trap platelets that lead primarily to microvascular thrombosis, but can also lead to macrovascular thrombosis with subsequent ischemic impaired organ perfusion and end-organ damage.[1,2] This entrapment of platelets also leads to a worsening of the thrombocytopenia, which is generally seen with acute DIC. As this process continues, clotting factors are consumed, overwhelming their potential for production. At the time of maximal coagulation during DIC, the fibrinolytic system is largely suppressed.[26] This inhibition is caused by high levels of plasminogen activator inhibitor type 1, which is the main inhibitor of fibrinolysis. This impairment of fibrin removal creates increased fibrin levels in the microvasculature and macrovasculature leading to further damage.[25]

Eventually, the excess circulating thrombin also assists in the conversion of plasminogen to plasmin, causing fibrinolysis, which in turn results in increased amounts of fibrin degradation products (FDPs) that have strong anticoagulant properties, leading to hemorrhage. Excess plasmin can inactivate clotting factors, but it can also activate the complement and kinin systems. Activation of these systems can lead to increased vascular permeability, hypotension, and shock. The clinical picture of acute DIC is a hemodynamically unstable patient who is experiencing a combination of extreme thrombosis and bleeding. Figure 38-1 depicts the process of DIC.

## CLINICAL MANIFESTATIONS

Signs and symptoms of acute DIC are variable and complex. Recognizing this syndrome in its early phase and treating it promptly are crucial to the prognosis of the affected patient. Unfortunately, DIC is often a fatal process as it frequently goes unrecognized until severe hemorrhage occurs.

Thrombus formation often occurs early, and can occur simultaneously with bleeding in DIC. Thrombi generally form in the superficial and smaller veins, and may be clinically undetectable. Subtle signs and symptoms of thrombi

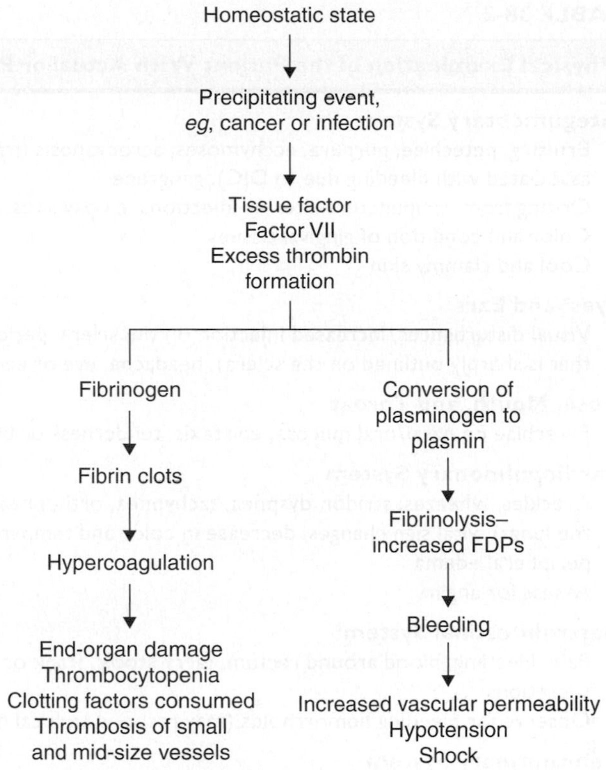


**FIGURE 38-1**

The process of disseminated intravascular coagulation.

*Abbreviation*: FOPs, fibrinogen degradation products.

include red indurated tender areas indicating ischemia, found over organ sites. When more significant thrombosis occurs, the clots may obstruct the microvascular system and large vessels, thereby decreasing organ function.[27] The signs and symptoms of widespread thrombosis may include focal ischemia, acrocyanosis, superficial gangrene, frank gangrene, altered sensorium, ulceration of the gastrointestinal tract (including stress ulcers with frank gastrointestinal bleeding), jaundice due to the release of excess bilirubin during hemorrhage, decreased urinary output if the renal system is affected,[1] and dyspnea (that can lead to acute respiratory distress syndrome). Widespread thrombosis (purpura fulminans—irregular hemorrhagic skin lesions) and significant bleeding can occur simultaneously.

Bleeding is the most obvious sign of a hemorrhagic disorder and can occur from any orifice or opening on the surface of the skin. Patients may ooze blood from surgical, venipuncture, or wound sites. Symptoms of bleeding may include purpura, petechiae, ecchymoses, hematomas, and acrocyanosis can be readily apparent.[20] Overt hemorrhage involving multiple unrelated sites is not uncommon in the patient with acute DIC. See Table 38-2 for the physical examination of the patient with actual or potential bleeding. Hemoptysis, intraperitoneal hemorrhage, and intracranial bleeding all pose life-threatening events for the patient with DIC.

**TABLE 38-2**

**Physical Examination of the Patient With Actual or Potential Bleeding**

**Integumentary System**
- Bruising, petechiae, purpura, ecchymoses, acrocyanosis (irregularly shaped cyanotic patches on the periphery of arms and legs associated with bleeding due to DIC), gangrene
- Oozing from venipuncture sites or injections, biopsy sites, central lines, catheters, or nasogastric tubes
- Color and condition of gingival tissues
- Cool and clammy skin

**Eyes[a] and Ears**
- Visual disturbances, increased injection on the sclera, periorbital edema, subconjunctival hemorrhage (homogeneous red color that is sharply outlined on the sclera), headache, eye or ear pain

**Nose, Mouth, and Throat**
- Petechiae on nasal/oral mucosa, epistaxis, tenderness or bleeding from gums or oral mucosa

**Cardiopulmonary System**
- Crackles, wheezes, stridor, dyspnea, tachypnea, orthopnea, hypoxia, cyanosis, and hemoptysis (all possible signs of bleeding in the lungs), vital sign changes, decrease in color and temperature of all extremities, decreased peripheral pulses, tachycardia, peripheral edema
- Assess for angina

**Gastrointestinal System[b]**
- Pain, bleeding, blood around rectum, tarry stools, frank or occult blood in stools, dysphagia, hematemesis, blood-tinged secretions
- Observe for bleeding hemorrhoids (may respond to local measures)

**Genitourinary System**
- Bleeding, character, and amount of menses
- Monitor intake and output (if urine drops below 30 mL/hour it may be due to acute tubular necrosis secondary to thrombi, bleeding, or hypovolemia

**Musculoskeletal System**
- Check for complaint of painful joints while performing active or passive range of motion, which may indicate bleeding into the joint

**Central Nervous System**
- Mental status changes, including restlessness, confusion, lethargy, dizziness, obtundation, seizures, or coma (may indicate intracranial hemorrhage or impaired tissue perfusion)
- Headache, nausea/vomiting, retching

[a]Bleeding in the optic fundus could lead to permanent visual impairment.
[b]Guaiac all excreta for blood.

Systemic signs and symptoms of DIC are based on the underlying pathophysiology of this process. The signs and symptoms can include fever, hypoxia, acidosis, hypotension, and proteinuria. If severe, the patient may demonstrate a clinical picture of shock.[28]

## ASSESSMENT

### HISTORY

A thorough history should include a review of any risk factors associated with an increased risk of DIC as outlined in Table 38–1. The history should also include information about medications that the patient is taking (including any over-the-counter medications), nutritional status (indicating a potential vitamin K deficiency), any prior bleeding tendencies, bleeding episodes, or history of blood clots.[29]

### PHYSICAL EXAMINATION

The physical examination of a patient suspected for DIC should include evaluation of any signs and symptoms related to bleeding and thrombosis. See Table 38-2 for the physical examination of the patient with actual or potential bleeding. Each organ system is evaluated for the presence of bleeding or thrombosis—eg, signs of bleeding and/or clotting in the CNS may include headache, nausea, vomiting, retching, and mental status changes. Gastrointestinal bleeding and/or clotting may be manifested by gastrointestinal pain, hematemesis, and frank or occult blood in the stool.

## DIAGNOSTIC TESTS

There is no specific laboratory finding that is absolutely diagnostic of DIC. A battery of lab tests in conjunction with the patient's history and clinical evidence must be used to confirm the diagnosis, as well as to monitor response to treatment. A number of clinical conditions will affect these tests, which makes their interpretation difficult—eg, multiple blood product transfusions will dilute clotting factors or platelets, and liver disease with portal hypertension can lead to thrombocytopenia and the activation of the fibrinolytic system.

The platelet count and the plasma fibrinogen level (long used to help determine the diagnosis of DIC) are almost always decreased in the presence of DIC. Neither of these tests is sensitive nor specific for DIC, but normal levels exclude the possibility of DIC.[30] The presence of schistocytes, or red cell fragments, in the blood smear is a frequent but nonspecific finding for acute DIC. The presence of schistocytes supports the diagnosis of chronic DIC more significantly, as they are found in almost all such cases. Other coagulation studies often done to support the diagnosis of DIC are the prothrombin time (PT), activated partial thromboplastin time (aPTT), and the international normalization ratio (INR).[3,31] All of these global clotting times are expected to be prolonged in DIC; they are nonspecific as they can be shortened or normal in the presence of DIC. Table 38-3 describes laboratory studies for DIC.

Two of the newer and more sophisticated tests that are done to help determine a diagnosis of DIC include the D-dimer assay and the Fibrin Degradation Product titer or the FDP titer. These tests can be performed alone or in combination. The D-dimer is a neoantigen formed as a result of plasmin digestion of fibrin. This test is specific for FDPs, which are found in increased levels in acute DIC.[1] Likewise, the FDP assay tests for increased levels of FDPs; FDP assays are also elevated in acute DIC. These tests reflect the microangiopathy of DIC and have been

**TABLE 38-3**

**Laboratory Studies for Disseminated Intravascular Coagulation**

| Test | Result | Comments |
|---|---|---|
| D-dimer assay | Elevated | Neoantigen formed when plasmin digests fibrin<br>Specific for increased fibrin degradation products |
| Fibrin Degradation Product (FDP) titer | Elevated | Increased consumption of clots<br>Specific for increased fibrin degradation products |
| Platelet count | Decreased | Frequent, but nonspecific finding in DIC |
| Fibrinogen | Decreased | Nonspecific in DIC |
| Prothrombin time | Prolonged | Nonspecific in DIC; can be prolonged, shortened, or normal |
| Activated partial thromboplastin time | Prolonged | Nonspecific in DIC; can be prolonged, shortened, or normal |
| International normalization ratio | Prolonged | Nonspecific in DIC; can be prolonged, shortened, or normal |
| Peripheral smear | Schistocytes | Frequent, but nonspecific finding in DIC |
| Antithrombin III level | Decreased | Demonstrates accelerated coagulation |
| Protein C | Decreased | Demonstrates accelerated coagulation |
| Protein S | Decreased | Demonstrates accelerated coagulation |
| Fibrinopeptide A level | Elevated | Reflects the rate of fibrin formation, demonstrates accelerated coagulation |
| Prothrombin fragments (F1 and F2) | Elevated | Reflects the rate of thrombin formation, demonstrates accelerated coagulation |
| Thrombin–antithrombin (TAT) complexes | Elevated | Reflects the rate of thrombin formation, demonstrates accelerated coagulation |
| Plasminogen levels | Decreased | Suggests hyperfibrinolysis |
| α2-antiplasmin levels | Decreased | Suggests hyperfibrinolysis |

found to be sensitive, specific, and efficient in the diagnosis of DIC.[31]

Other tests may be done to document accelerated coagulation and accelerated fibrinolysis, which may also help to support a diagnosis of DIC. A decreased level of antithrombin III (AT III) demonstrates accelerated coagulation, which is suggestive for DIC. Decreased levels of Protein C and Protein S also demonstrate accelerated coagulation that can occur with DIC.[32] Measuring the products of coagulation factor activation provide more information about the dynamics of DIC. Other tests that may be done to determine accelerated coagulation include the plasma level of fibrinopeptide A, levels of prothrombin activation peptide (F1 and F2), and thrombin-antithrombin complexes (TAT).[33]

In addition to FDP titers and the D-dimer assay tests to detect accelerated fibrinolysis in DIC, plasminogen and α2-antiplasmin levels may be drawn. The presence of lower or falling levels of plasminogen and α2-antiplasmin levels suggests hyperfibrinolysis.[14] These tests also help to support the diagnosis of DIC.

The Scientific Subcommittee on DIC of the International Society on Thrombosis and Haemostasis has published a diagnostic set of criteria for DIC. This diagnostic algorithm designates a score based risk assessment for DIC and on the severity of the platelet count, fibrin-related monomers, PT, and fibrinogen level. A score of 5 or greater on this algorithm is compatible with overt or acute DIC.[34] The use of this algorithm has been found to be sensitive and specific for the diagnosis of DIC, and has been found to be useful in clinical practice.[35,36] Figure 38-2 provides a review of this algorithm.[37]

## THERAPEUTIC APPROACHES AND NURSING CARE

### PREVENTION OF COMPLICATIONS

Disseminated intravascular coagulation related to cancer cannot necessarily be prevented, as it often occurs as a result of the cancer itself or treatment of the cancer (eg, administration of chemotherapy or blood products). The potential for preventing DIC related to infection may result from aggressive management of the neutropenic patient. Early detection of the signs and symptoms of DIC allows for the best chance for prompt diagnosis and treatment, resulting in a better prognosis for the patient with DIC.

Prevention of complications of DIC includes a focus on any activities or interventions that may prevent further bleeding or thrombosis. It is important to remove any tight or restrictive clothing. If edema is present, it should be measured daily. Elastic support stockings may help to minimize stasis and promote venous return. Other measures to decrease stasis and promote venous return include assisting the patient with leg lifts or elevating the legs to 15 to 20 degrees at intervals, and teaching the patient to wiggle his or her toes and perform ankle circles frequently while in bed. Compression to the knee vessels is minimized by avoiding placing anything under the knees while in bed (pillows, knee gatches), by avoiding crossing of the knees or legs, and by avoiding dangling the legs over the side of the bed.[20]

### MANAGEMENT

Treatment of the underlying etiology is critical in the management of DIC. Until the underlying stimulus of DIC is managed successfully, all other therapies will merely provide an interval of symptomatic relief. The patient with DIC can become unstable very quickly because of the complications of bleeding and thrombus formation, and must be supported hemodynamically to alleviate shock. The patient with DIC must be monitored closely for signs and symptoms of bleeding. A thorough review of organ systems must be done to minimize blood loss.

When DIC is suspected oxygen therapy is initiated immediately for the hypoxia and associated acidosis. Fluid replacement therapy must also be initiated promptly, as the patient can quickly become hypovolemic with significant bleeding. Fluid replacement therapy will help manage the associated proteinuria (from thrombosis occuring in the kidneys) and hypotension. Fluid replacement may include simple crystalloids such as Ringer's lactate, artificial colloids such as dextran and hydroxyethyl starch, or human albumin.[38] The administration of plasma substitutes (dextran, hydroxyethyl starch, or plasma proteins) may result in adverse reactions ranging from allergic urticarial reactions to life-threatening anaphylaxis.[38] The administration of blood components such as red blood cells, platelets, and fresh-frozen plasma (FFP) may also double for use as replacement fluids. Caution must be used in treating the bleeding patient to avoid fluid overload and complications such as congestive heart failure.

Education is a necessary component of care when a patient is at risk for or is experiencing DIC. Patients and families are taught to report any bleeding or unusual symptoms. They are taught to save all excreta for the nurse to examine for blood. The patient and family will also need excellent psychosocial support should the patient develop this paradoxical situation of hemorrhage and thrombus formation.

#### Managing intravascular clotting

Although the bleeding associated with DIC is obvious and may be dramatic, it is the thrombotic process that has the greatest impact on morbidity and mortality in patients with DIC. Thus, an anticoagulant such as heparin may be initiated to stop the intravascular clotting process. Heparin acts to inhibit further thrombogenesis, prevent reaccumulation of

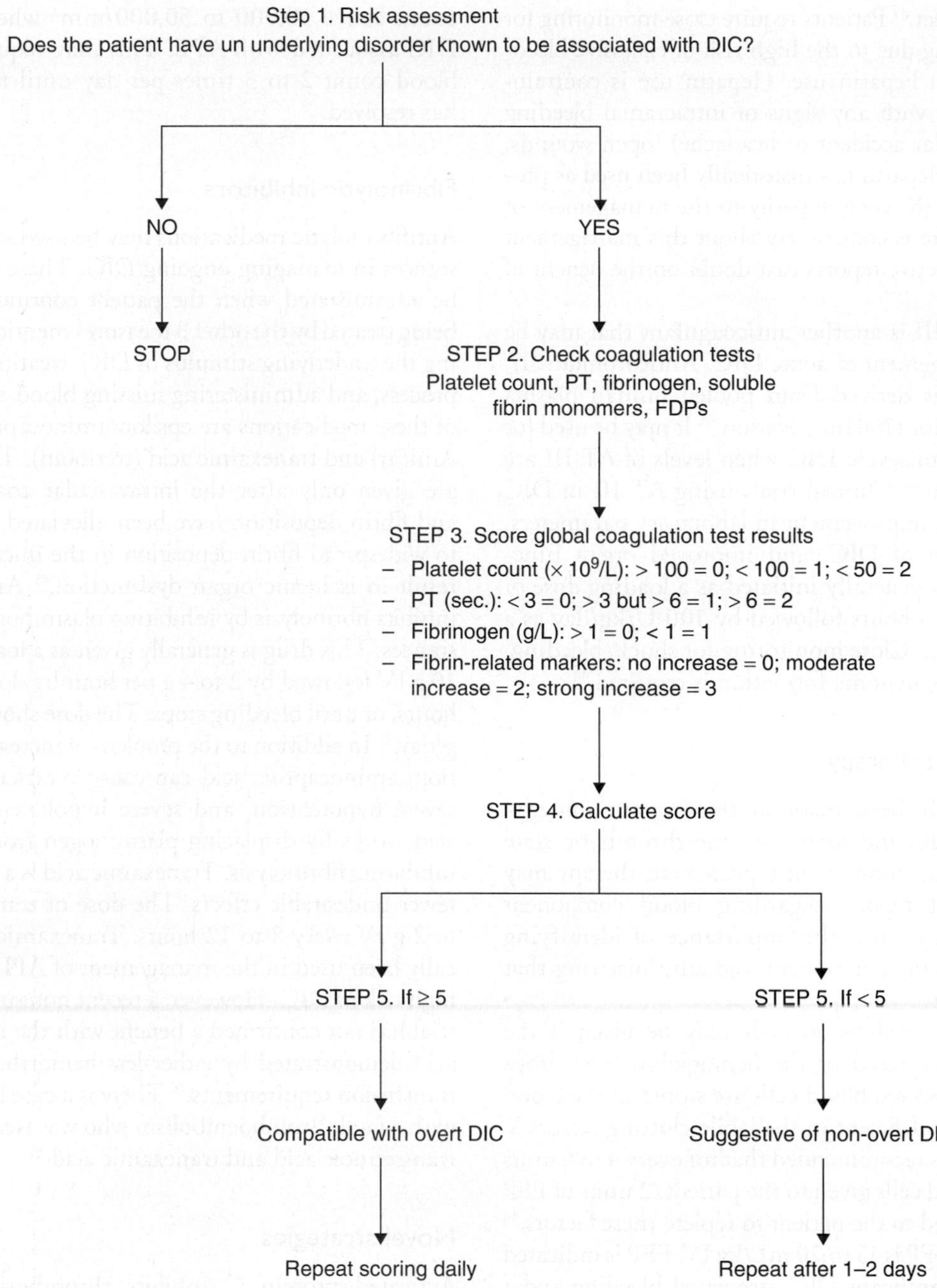

Step 1. Risk assessment
Does the patient have un underlying disorder known to be associated with DIC?
NO
YES
STOP
STEP 2. Check coagulation tests
Platelet count, PT, fibrinogen, soluble fibrin monomers, FDPs
STEP 3. Score global coagulation test results
– Platelet count (× 10⁹/L): > 100 = 0; < 100 = 1; < 50 = 2
– PT (sec.): < 3 = 0; > 3 but > 6 = 1; > 6 = 2
– Fibrinogen (g/L): > 1 = 0; < 1 = 1
– Fibrin-related markers: no increase = 0; moderate increase = 2; strong increase = 3
STEP 4. Calculate score
STEP 5. If ≥ 5
STEP 5. If < 5
Compatible with overt DIC
Suggestive of non-overt DIC
Repeat scoring daily
Repeat after 1–2 days

**FIGURE 38-2**

Diagnostic algorithm and scoring system for disseminated intravascular coagulation.

*Abbreviations*: FDPs, fibrin degradation products; PT, prothrombin time.

Reprinted from open access article that permits unrestricted use, distribution, and reproduction from Franchini M, Lippi G, Manzato F. Recent acquisitions in the pathophysiology, diagnosis, and treatment of disseminated intravascular coagulation. *Thromb J*. 2006;4:4.[37]

a clot, and reduce the consumption of platelets and clotting factors. Adequate prophylaxis is also needed to eliminate the risk of venous thromboembolism. Patients with DIC are usually given relatively low doses of heparin, such as 80 to 100 U/kg subcutaneously every 4 to 6 hours or 20,000 to 30,000 U/day as a continuous infusion.[27] Effectiveness of low-dose heparin is generally seen within about 3 to 4 hours after initiation of therapy, first by correction of lab values and then by a cessation of clinically significant bleeding and thrombosis. Low-molecular-weight heparin (LMWH) may be an alternative to unfractionated heparin. LMWH has higher bioavailability, a longer half-life, and a more predictable antithrombotic effect.[39] Patients require close monitoring for evidence of bleeding due to the high risk of excessive bleeding associated with heparin use. Heparin use is contraindicated in patients with any signs of intracranial bleeding (eg, cerebral vascular accident or headache), open wounds, or recent surgery. Heparin has historically been used as prophylaxis to control the coagulopathy in the management of APL; however, there is controversy about this management strategy as retrospective reports cast doubt on the benefit of this practice.[40,41]

Antithrombin III is another anticoagulant that may be used for the management of acute DIC. Antithrombin III, alpha-2-globulin, is derived from pooled human plasma and is heat treated for viral inactivation.[42] It may be used for moderately severe to severe DIC when levels of AT III are markedly depressed.[43] Clinical trials using AT III in DIC have demonstrated improvement in laboratory parameters, shortened duration of DIC, and improved organ function.[43] This drug is generally initiated as a loading dose of 100 U/kg IV over 3 hours followed by 100 U/kg/day as a continuous infusion. Close monitoring for shock, bleeding, hypotension, and hematoma formation is required.[44]

### Blood component therapy

After attempts have been made at treating the underlying stimulus of DIC and managing the thrombotic state of the patient, blood component replacement therapy may be initiated. Most reports regarding blood component replacement therapy stress the importance of identifying the missing or lacking component and administering that specific component.

Washed, packed red blood cells may be given if the patient continues to bleed or the hemoglobin level drops below 8 g/dL. When red blood cells are stored in the blood bank, they become deficient in the labile clotting factors V and VIII. Thus, it is recommended that for every 4 to 6 units of banked red blood cells given to the patient, 2 units of FFP also be administered to the patient to replete these factors.[38] The usual dose of FFP is 15 to 20 mL/kg IV. FFP is indicated in patients with significant DIC-associated bleeding and a fibrinogen level below 100 mg/dL.[37] The use of FFP in the management of DIC is somewhat controversial because FFP contains fibrinogen, which can potentially create higher levels of FDPs that will further impair hemostasis.[1]

Cryoprecipitate (a concentrated source of fibrin and factor VIII) may be used to treat the severely bleeding patient who is hypofibrinogenemic, yet it too may create increased levels of FDPs. Transfusions of cryoprecipitate are generally given at 1 U/10 kg to maintain a fibrinogen level above 100 to 150 mg/dL until the coagulopathy resolves.[37] Platelets may be given if the platelet count drops below 20,000 cells/mm$^3$ or if the patient is actively bleeding. Stein et al[4] stress the importance of aggressive blood product support including platelet transfusions to maintain the platelet count above 30,000 to 50,000/mm$^3$ when managing the DIC associated with APL. This may require checking the blood count 2 to 3 times per day until the coagulopathy has resolved.

### Fibrinolytic inhibitors

Antifibrinolytic medications may be used in specific circumstances in managing ongoing DIC. These medications may be administered when the patient continues to bleed after being treated by the other 3 measures mentioned earlier: treating the underlying stimulus of DIC, treating the thrombotic process, and administering missing blood components. Two of these medications are epsilon-aminocaproic acid (EACA, Amicar) and tranexamic acid (tretinoin). These medications are given only after the intravascular coagulation process and fibrin deposition have been alleviated, as they can lead to widespread fibrin deposition in the microcirculation and result in ischemic organ dysfunction.[45] Aminocaproic acid inhibits fibrinolysis by inhibiting plasminogen activator substances. This drug is generally given as a loading dose of 5 to 10 g IV followed by 2 to 4 g per hour by slow IV push for 24 hours, or until bleeding stops. The dose should not exceed 30 g/day.[27] In addition to the problem of increased fibrin deposition, aminocaproic acid can cause ventricular arrhythmias, severe hypotension, and severe hypokalemia.[1] Tranexamic acid works by displacing plasminogen from fibrin, thereby inhibiting fibrinolysis. Tranexamic acid is a newer agent with fewer undesirable effects. The dose of tranexamic acid is 1 to 2 g IV every 8 to 12 hours. Tranexamic acid has historically been used in the management of APL, where there is a high risk of DIC. However, a recent nonrandomized clinical trial has not confirmed a benefit with the use of tranexamic acid demonstrated by either less hemorrhage or decreasing transfusion requirements.[46] There is a case report of a patient with a fatal thromboembolism who was treated with both all transretinoic acid and tranexamic acid.[47]

### Novel strategies

Activated protein C inhibits thrombosis and promotes fibrinolysis. Recombinant human activated protein C (drotrecogin alpha) has been reported to reduce mortality in patients with severe sepsis.[48] Drotrecogin alpha also has been found to inhibit thrombosis, promote fibrinolysis, and exert antiinflammatory effects.[44] The dose of drotrecogin alpha is 24 mcg/kg/hour continuous IV infusion over 96 hours.[27] Bleeding may be significant with this drug and should be discontinued with clinically significant bleeding.

## CONCLUSION

Acute DIC related to cancer can be due to a number of causative factors, including the cancer itself or a process such as infection. The primary management of patients with acute DIC is to treat the underlying pathology creating the DIC condition. Patients may also be treated aggressively to maintain their hemodynamic status, as well as with a variety of medications and blood components.

Because DIC contributes greatly to morbidity and mortality in patients with cancer, nurses play a valuable role in the prompt recognition of its signs and symptoms. Early recognition of the signs and symptoms of bleeding or clotting can lead to prompt treatment of this challenging problem. It is hoped that future research will identify more clearly the most appropriate treatment for acute DIC.

## REFERENCES


1. Bick RL. Disseminated intravascular coagulation: current concepts of aetiology, pathophysiology, diagnosis, and treatment. *Hematol Oncol Clin North Am.* 2003;17:149–176.
2. Furlong MA, Furlong BR. *Disseminated Intravascular Coagulation.* http://www.emedicine.com/emerg/topic150.htm. Accessed December 31, 2009.
3. Ezzone SA. Disseminated intravascular coagulation. In: Camp-Sorrell D, Hawkins RA, eds. *Clinical Manual for the Oncology Advanced Practice Nurse.* 2nd ed. Pittsburgh, Oncology Nursing Society; 2006:823–829.
4. Stein E, McMahon B, Kwaan H, Altman JK, Frankfurt O, Tallman MS. The coagulopathy of acute promyelocytic leukaemia revisited. *Best Pract Res Clin Haematol.* 2009;22:153–163.
5. Gouin-Thibault I, Achkar A, Samama MM. The thrombophilic state in cancer patients. *Acta Haematol.* 2001;106:33–42.
6. Dally N, Hoffman R, Haddad N, et al. Predictive factors of bleeding and thrombosis during induction therapy in acute promyelocytic leukemia—a single center experience in 34 patients. *Thromb Res.* 2005;116:109–114.
7. Goldschmidt N, Gural A, Ben Yehuda D. Extensive splenic infarction, deep vein thrombosis and pulmonary emboli complicating induction therapy with all-trans-retinoic acid (ATRA) for acute promyelocytic leukemia. *Leuk Lymphoma.* 2003;44:1433–1437.
8. Falanga A, Consonni R, Marchetti M, et al. Cancer procoagulant and tissue factor are differently modulated by all-transretinoic acid in acute promyelocytic leukemia cells. *Blood.* 1998;92:143–151.
9. Falanga A, Alessio MG, Donati MB, et al. A new procoagulant in acute leukemia. *Blood.* 1988;71:870–875.
10. Hajjar KA, Menell JS. Annexin II: a novel mediator of cell surface plasmin generation. *Ann NY Acad Sci.* 1997;811:337–349.
11. Menell JS, Cesarman GM, Jacovina AT, et al. Annexin II and bleeding in acute promyelocytic leukemia [see comments]. *N Engl J Med.* 1999;340:994.
12. Fenaux P, Castaigne S, Dombret H, et al. All-transretinoic acid followed by intensive chemotherapy gives a high complete remission rate and may prolong remissions in newly diagnosed acute promyelocytic leukemia: a pilot study on 26 cases. *Blood.* 1992;80:2176–2181.
13. Tallman MS, Andersen JW, Schiffer CA, et al. All-trans-retinoic acid in acute promyelocytic leukemia. *N Engl J Med.* 1997;337:1021–1028.
14. Tallman MS, Andersen JW, Schiffer CA, et al. All-trans retinoic acid in acute promyelocytic leukemia: long-term outcome and prognostic factor analysis from the North American Intergroup protocol. *Blood.* 2002;100:4298–4302.
15. Sanz MA, Martin G, Gonzalez M, et al. Risk-adapted treatment of acute promyelocytic leukemia with all-trans-retinoic acid and anthracycline monochemotherapy: a multicenter study by the PETHEMA group. *Blood.* 2004;103:1237–1243.
16. Avances C, Oumaya C, Granger V, et al. Prostate cancer and acute disseminated intravascular coagulation. Therapeutic management based on three cases. *Prog Urol.* 2003;13:308–312.
17. Gobel BH. Disseminated intravascular coagulation. In: Yarbro CH, Frogge MH, Goodman M, eds. *Cancer Nursing Principles and Practice.* 6th ed. Sudbury, MA: Jones and Bartlett; 2005:869–875.
18. Levi M, de Jonge E, van der Poll R, Ten Cate H. Advances in the understanding of the pathogenic pathways of disseminated intravascular coagulation result in more insight in the clinical picture and better management strategies. *Semin Thromb Hemost.* 2001;27:569–575.
19. Ezzone SA. Disseminated intravascular coagulation. In: Kaplan M; ed. *Understanding and Managing Oncologic Emergencies: A Resource for Nurses.* Pittsburgh, PA: Oncology Nursing Society; 2006:31–49.
20. Gobel BH. Disseminated intravascular coagulation in cancer: providing quality care. *Top Adv Pract Nurse J.* 2002;2. http://www.medscape.com/viewarticle/442737. Accessed December 31, 2009.
21. Bick RL. Disseminated intravascular coagulation: objective clinical and laboratory diagnosis, treatment and assessment of therapeutic response. *Semin Thromb Hemost.* 1996;22:69–88.
22. Staudinger T, Locker GJ, Frass M. Management of acquired coagulation disorders in emergency and intensive-care medicine. *Semin Thromb Hemost.* 1996;22:93–104.
23. Bouchama A, Hammami M, Haq A, Jackson J, al-Sedairy S. Evidence for endothelial cell activation/injury in heatstroke. *Crit Care Med.* 1996;24:1173–1178.
24. Carey MH, Rogers GM. Disseminated intravascular coagulation: clinical and laboratory aspects. *Am J Hematol.* 1998;59:65–73.
25. Levi M. Current understanding of disseminated intravascular coagulation. *Br J Haematol.* 2004;124:567–576.
26. Levi M, Ten Cate H. Disseminated intravascular coagulation. *New Engl J Med.* 1999;341:586–592.
27. Cope DG. Metabolic emergencies. In: Gobel BH, Triest-Robertson S, Vogel W, eds. *Advanced Oncology Nursing Certification Review and Resource Manual.* Pittsburgh, PA: Oncology Nursing Society; 2009:547–598.
28. Lin EM. Oncologic emergency: case 3. In: Lin EM, ed. *Advanced Practice in Oncology Nursing Case Studies and Review.* Philadelphia, PA: W.B. Saunders; 2001:312–319.
29. Friend PH, Pruett J. Bleeding and thrombotic complications. In: Yarbro CH, Frogge MH, Goodman M, eds. *Cancer Symptom Management.* 3rd ed. Sudbury, MA: Jones and Bartlett; 2004:233–251.
30. Mammen EF. Disseminated intravascular coagulation (DIC). *Clin Lab Sci.* 2000;13:239–245.
31. Yu M, Nardella BS, Pechet L. Screening tests of disseminated intravascular coagulation: guidelines for rapid and specific laboratory diagnosis. *Crit Care Med.* 2000;28:1777–1780.
32. Fourriei F, Chopin C, Goudemand J, et al. Septic shock, multiple organ failure, and disseminated intravascular coagulation. Compared patterns of antithrombin III, protein C, and protein S deficiencies. *Chest.* 1992;101:816–823.
33. Wada H, Sakuragawa N, Nori Y, et al. Hemostatic molecular markers before the onset of disseminated intravascular coagulation. *Am J Hematol.* 1999;60:273–278.
34. Taylor FB, Toh CH, Hoots WK, Wada H, Levi M. Towards definition, clinical and laboratory criteria, and a scoring system for disseminated intravascular coagulation. *Thromb Haemost.* 2001;86:1327–1330.
35. Bakhtiari K, Miejers JCM, de Jonge E, Levi M. Prospective validation of the International Society of Thrombosis and Haemostasis scoring system for disseminated intravascular coagulation. *Crit Care Med.* 2004;32:2416–2421.
36. Sivulla M, Tallgren M, Pettila V. Impact of scoring system for DIC in the critically ill [Abstract]. *Criti Care Med.* 2004;32(Suppl. 12):A78.
37. Franchini M, Lippi G, Manzato F. Recent acquisitions in the pathophysiology, diagnosis, and treatment of disseminated intravascular coagulation. *Thromb J.* 2006;4:4.
38. Letsky EA. Disseminated intravascular coagulation. *Best Pract Res Clin Obstet Gynaecol.* 2001;4:623–644.

39. Dolovich LR, Ginsberg JS, Douketis JD, et al. A meta-analysis comparing low-molecular-weight heparins with unfractionated heparin in the treatment of venous thromboembolism. *Arch Intern Med.* 2000;1603:181–188.
40. Rodeghiero F, Avvisati G, Castaman G, et al. Early deaths and antihemorrhagic treatments in acute promyelocytic leukemia. A GIMEMA retrospective study in 268 consecutive patients. *Blood.* 1990;75:2112–2117.
41. Goldberg MA, Ginsburg D, Mayer RJ, et al. Is heparin administration necessary during induction chemotherapy for patients with acute promyelocytic leukemia? *Blood.* 1987;69:187–191.
42. Harper JL. *Antithrombin III deficiency.* http://www.emedicine.com/ped/topic119.htm. Accessed December 31, 2009.
43. Levi M. Current understanding of disseminated intravascular coagulation. *Br J Haematol.* 2004;124:567–576.
44. Becker JU, Wira CR. *Disseminated intravascular coagulation.* (2008, March). http://www.emedicine.com/emerg/topic150.htm. Accessed October 1, 2009.
45. Wilkes GM, Ingwersen K, Barton-Burke M, eds. Molecularly targeted therapies. In: *Oncology Nursing Drug Handbook.* Sudbury, MA: Jones and Bartlett; 2003:394–483.
46. Sanz MA, Montesinos P, Vellenga E, et al. Risk-adapted treatment of acute promyelocytic leukemia with all-trans retinoic acid and anthracycline monochemotherapy: long-term outcome of the LPA 99 multicenter study by the PETHEMA Group. *Blood.* 2008;112:3130–3134.
47. Hashimoto S, Koike T, Tatewaki W, et al. Fatal thromboembolism in acute promyelocytic leukemia during all-trans retinoic acid therapy combined with antifibrinolytic therapy for prophylaxis of hemorrhage. *Leukemia.* 1994;8:1113–1115.
48. Bernard GR, Vincent JL, Laterre PF, et al. Efficacy and safety of recombinant human activated protein C for severe sepsis. *N Engl J Med.* 2001;344:699–709.

CHAPTER 39

Marcelle Kaplan, RN, MS, AOCN®, CBCN

# Hypercalcemia of Malignancy

- **Scope of the Problem**
  - *Definition*
  - *Incidence*
  - *Etiology and Risk Factors*
- **Physiological Alterations**
  - *Normal Bone Homeostasis and Bone Remodeling*
  - *Normal Calcium Homeostasis*
    - Determining plasma calcium levels
  - *Regulation of Normal Calcium Homeostasis*
    - Role of parathyroid hormone
    - Role of the calcium-sensing receptor
    - Role of calcitonin
    - Role of vitamin D
    - Role of the kidneys in calcium homeostasis
    - Renal contributions in hypercalcemia
  - *Etiology of Hypercalcemia of Malignancy*
    - Humoral hypercalcemia of malignancy
  - *Nonmalignant Causes of Hypercalcemia*
- **Clinical Manifestations of Hypercalcemia**
  - *Gastrointestinal Effects*
  - *Renal Effects*
  - *Neurological Effects*
  - *Cardiac Effects*
  - *Musculoskeletal Effects*
- **Assessment**
  - *Blood Chemistry Measurements*
    - Serum calcium
    - Serum electrolytes
    - iPTH, PTHrP, and calcitriol levels
  - *Other Studies*
- **Grading Hypercalcemia in Malignant Disease**
  - *Mild Hypercalcemia*
  - *Moderate Hypercalcemia*
  - *Severe Hypercalcemia*
- **Therapeutic Approaches**
  - *Principles of Antihypercalcemic Treatment*
    - General measures
    - Antineoplastic therapy
    - Extracellular fluid volume expansion and calciuresis
    - Loop diuretics
    - Calcitonin
  - *Antiresorptive Therapy: Bisphosphonates*
    - Overview
    - Osteonecrosis of the jaw
    - Pamidronate
    - Zoledronic acid
    - Ibandronate
    - Clodronate
  - *Other Antihypercalcemic Therapies*
    - Plicamycin
    - Gallium nitrate
    - Corticosteroids
    - Phosphate replacement
    - Dialysis
    - Mobilization and dietary restriction
  - *Future Directions in the Management of Hypercalcemia of Malignancy*
- **Nursing Management**
  - *Overview*
  - *Patient and Caregiver Education*
  - *End-of-Life Considerations*
- **Conclusion**
- **References**

## SCOPE OF THE PROBLEM

### DEFINITION

Hypercalcemia is the most common life-threatening metabolic complication of malignancy, occurring in 10% to 20% of all patients with cancer. In spite of its frequency, diagnosis of hypercalcemia of malignancy (HCM) is often delayed or unrecognized, due to the nonspecificity of symptoms that are often attributed to the underlying disease process or treatment effects.[1–3] Most patients are diagnosed with HCM at an advanced stage of disease, and the diagnosis portends a poor prognosis and a limited life expectancy, often only a matter of weeks.[2,4] Several pathological mechanisms contribute to the development of HCM; however, the final common mechanism is tumor-induced destruction of bone. Clinical manifestations of HCM are reflected in the renal, skeletal, neuromuscular, gastrointestinal (GI), and cardiovascular systems, but correlations between presenting symptoms and serum calcium concentrations are weak.[4,5] Knowledge of the types of malignancies commonly associated with the development of HCM, an understanding of the pathophysiological mechanisms generating the hypercalcemia, and alertness to the early manifestations of hypercalcemia will guide the oncology nurse in preventing, recognizing, and implementing care of patients at risk for and experiencing HCM. Early initiation of appropriate treatment strategies and active palliation measures may increase patient survival and improve end-of-life quality.

### INCIDENCE

The frequency with which HCM occurs varies considerably among tumor types. HCM most often develops in solid tumors, especially breast cancer of all types and squamous cell carcinoma of the lung. It occurs in approximately 30% of patients with advanced breast cancer and up to 20% of patients with lung cancer.[6] Less common squamous cell carcinomas that are frequently associated with HCM include head, neck, renal, esophageal, cervix, and vulvar carcinomas, as well as such uncommon tumors as small-cell carcinoma of the ovary and cholangiocarcinoma.[2,7] Among hematological malignancies, HCM occurs in 20% to 40% of patients with multiple myeloma and in patients with a variety of lymphomas, especially adult T-cell lymphoma.[6,8] Surprisingly, no direct relationship exists between the presence of bone metastases and the development of hypercalcemia. HCM is rare in certain cancers that frequently metastasize to bone, such as small-cell lung cancer, prostate cancer, and adenocarcinomas of the lung, colon, and stomach. It is also rare in primary bone cancers, such as osteogenic sarcoma.[5,9] Table 39-1 lists the incidence of HCM and bone metastases for malignancies frequently associated with hypercalcemia.[8–15]

### ETIOLOGY AND RISK FACTORS

Hypercalcemia associated with malignant disease results from a combination of complex pathophysiological events

**TABLE 39-1**

**Incidence of Hypercalcemia of Malignancy and Bone Metastases**

| Malignancy | Incidence of Hypercalcemia of Malignancy | Incidence of Bone Metastases |
|---|---|---|
| Breast cancer (with bone metastases) | 30%–40% | 65%–75% |
| Multiple myeloma | 20%–40% | 70%–90% |
| Squamous cell carcinoma of lung | 12.5%–35% | 30%–40% |
| Squamous cell carcinoma of head and neck | 2.9%–25% | Uncommon |
| Renal cell carcinoma | 3%–17% | 20%–25% |
| Lymphomas: | | |
| Hodgkin's disease | 0.6%–5.4% | Rare |
| Non-Hodgkin's, high-grade | 14%–33 % | |
| T-cell lymphoma (human T-cell lymphotrophic virus type 1) | 50% | |
| Other malignancies: Ovary, liver, pancreas, esophagus, cervix | 7% | |
| Unknown primary | 7% | |

*Source*: Data from Heys et al[8]; Grill and Martin[9]; Coleman and Rubens[10]; Kaplan[11]; Kvols[12]; Mundy[13]; Munshi and Anderson[14]; and Yeung and Gagel.[15]

that affect the movement of calcium in the body, primarily from bone, but also across the kidney and GI tract.[11] The skeletal complications of malignancy primarily result from the interaction between systemic and/or local biochemical agents and bone that result in destruction of bone.[16] In patients with solid tumors, HCM is most commonly mediated by systemic humoral factors secreted by tumor cells, and thus is called humoral hypercalcemia of malignancy (HHM). Metastatic disease to bone contributes to the development of hypercalcemia through the release of local tumor-induced inflammatory cytokines that stimulate bone breakdown (osteolysis). This type of local osteolytic hypercalcemia (LOH) is often associated with carcinoma of the breast and multiple myeloma,[17] and with lymphoma and leukemia.[5] The factor common to both mechanisms is inhibition of bone formation and increased bone breakdown (resorption) that releases large quantities of calcium into the circulation, which overwhelms the renal capacity to excrete calcium. The kidneys have the capacity to reabsorb about 600 mg of calcium a day, equivalent to a 150% increase in bone breakdown over bone formation, before renal clearance mechanisms are overwhelmed.[5] Increased synthesis of vitamin D (calcitriol) is another mechanism associated with the risk for hypercalcemia, notably in patients with Hodgkin's lymphoma. Calcitriol acts to increase calcium absorption from the GI tract and to increase calcium reabsorption in the kidneys.[17] The status of renal function plays an important role in the etiology of HCM. Conditions that compromise adequate renal function, such as dehydration or fluid volume depletion that occur due to disease or treatment effects (eg, fever, nausea, vomiting, anorexia, mucositis, or dysphagia), can potentiate or exacerbate the development of HCM in at-risk patients.[11] A brief review of normal bone remodeling and calcium homeostasis follows to enhance understanding of the underlying pathologies associated with the development of HCM.

## PHYSIOLOGICAL ALTERATIONS

### NORMAL BONE HOMEOSTASIS AND BONE REMODELING

The skeleton is both a structural support and a metabolic organ. It is the main storage organ for calcium and phosphorus, and regulates these ions in the serum in response to a finely balanced interaction between the gut, kidneys, parathyroid glands, and the skeleton itself. Disturbances in this complex interactive system that cause changes in serum calcium levels lead to alterations in bone structure to assist in maintaining calcium equilibrium.[18]

Skeletal bone in the adult consists of two types: dense, compact cortical bone that comprises 85% of total bone; and spongy, cancellous (trabecular) bone that comprises the remaining 15% of the skeleton. The proportions of the two types of bone differ at various sites in the skeleton; cancellous bone is located predominately in the epiphyses of the long bones, and cortical bone in the shafts of long bones.[17] Cancellous bone is most prominent in the vertebral column and is the type of bone most often involved in malignancy-induced bone destruction.[13] The marrow within the bone is the site of hematopoietic stem cells, stromal cells, and immune cells. Circulating hematopoietic stem cells give rise to osteoclasts, which are giant, multinucleated bone cells that mediate bone breakdown (resorption). Osteoblasts are bone forming cells derived from stromal cells in the marrow. Normal bone is a dynamic tissue, continuously being remodeled or "turned over" in response to a large number of regulatory mechanisms, including hormones, cytokines, and changes in mechanical forces, so that over a span of 40 to 50 years the normal skeleton is completely renewed.[18] In young adults, the processes of bone breakdown and bone formation are balanced under the control of a highly complex process called coupling. With age, and with certain disease states, an imbalance develops favoring bone destruction over formation. Bone mass is lost, as occurs with osteoporosis. Cancer alters the normal actions of cells involved in bone remodeling and uncouples the balance between bone resorption and formation.[10,13,18]

### NORMAL CALCIUM HOMEOSTASIS

Calcium is an inorganic element essential to many fundamental metabolic processes in the body. The adult human body contains approximately 1 kg of calcium, of which 99% is stored in bone. The 1% of body calcium outside of bone is predominantly found in the plasma. Minute concentrations of calcium are present in cells and are vital to maintaining normal cellular function and control of essential physiological functions including formation and maintenance of bones and teeth, contractility of muscle (cardiac, smooth, and skeletal), transmission of nerve impulses, normal blood clotting, hormone secretion, and cellular permeability.

Normal calcium homeostasis is maintained by a dynamic equilibrium between intestinal absorption of calcium, bone resorption and formation, and renal excretion of calcium. Distribution of calcium within the body is dependent on the balance between calcium intake and calcium loss. Although bone is a massive storage site for calcium, normally there is very little transfer of calcium between bone and the plasma. Calcium that is absorbed from food within the intestine enters the circulation and is filtered by the kidney. Around 98% of the filtered calcium is reabsorbed in the proximal renal tubules and the rest is excreted in the urine.[5,6]

Outside of bone, the extracellular calcium circulating in the plasma is divided into two major fractions. One fraction, which equals approximately 50% of total plasma

**Formula:**
Corrected serum calcium (mg/dL) = measured total serum calcium (mg/dL) + [4.0 (low normal value for albumin) – patient's serum albumin level (g/dL)] × 0.8

**Example:** Laboratory values: albumin = 2.3 g/dL
calcium = 10.5 mg/dL

1. Determine decrease in albumin from normal level:
   4.0 g/dL (low normal)
   – 2.3 g/dL (measured level)
   1.7 g/dL
2. Estimate and correct underreported serum calcium:
   a. 0.8 mg/dL : 1 g/dL = *X* mg/dL : 1.7 g/dL
   *X* = 0.8 x 1.7 = 1.36 mg/dL calcium
   b. 10.5 mg/dL + 1.36 mg/dL = 11.86 mg/dL calcium
3. 11.86 mg/dL = Hypercalcemia
   (corrected serum calcium is > 10.5 mg/dL)

**FIGURE 39-1**

Formula for "corrected" ionized serum calcium (adjusted for decreases in serum albumin).

calcium, circulates as free (ionized) calcium and is the only form of calcium that has physiological effects. The other fraction, about 40% of total plasma calcium, is nonionized and is mainly bound to albumin, but occasionally is bound to other proteins such as globulin and paraproteins. The remaining 10% of plasma calcium is bound with anions such as citrate, bicarbonate, and phosphorus. Ionized calcium represents the biologically active fraction of total calcium; the nonionized, protein-bound fraction is not biologically active and has no clinical significance.[5,11,17]

## Determining plasma calcium levels

Serum calcium levels are tightly controlled within a narrow range, usually 8.5 to 10.5 mg/dL, depending on laboratory reference values.[7,17] Most often the level of total calcium is measured and used to infer the level of ionized calcium. This method is usually fairly accurate except when hypoalbuminemia is present, which may occur in a patient with cancer as a result of cachexia or anorexia.[3,11] Thus, it is important to accurately determine the ionized serum calcium concentration based on the correlation between serum albumin and serum calcium. Any decrease in serum albumin results in an increase in the percentage of active, freely circulating ionized calcium, in contrast to the fraction of protein-bound (inactive) calcium, which declines. The increase in the serum ionized calcium can be "corrected" for the albumin level by using a simple formula that adds 0.8 mg/dL of ionized calcium for every 1 mg decrease in serum albumin below 4 mg/dL (see Figure 39-1). This estimation may not be accurate in certain conditions such as with the presence of elevated serum paraproteins, as occurs in multiple myeloma, with hyperphosphatemia, and with acid–base disorders. These conditions may warrant a direct measurement of serum ionized calcium. Metabolic acidosis causes less calcium to become bound to albumin, increasing the fraction

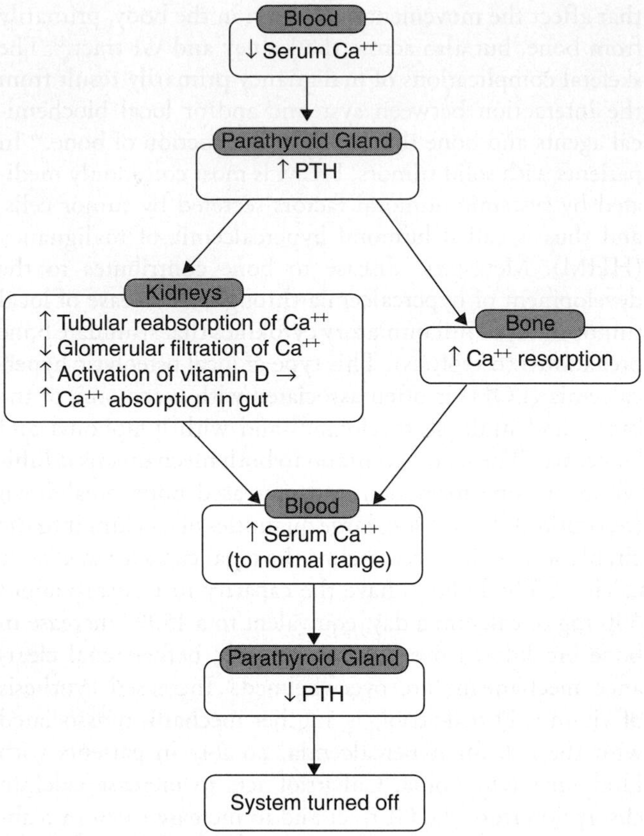


**FIGURE 39-2**

Negative feedback mechanisms for calcium regulation.
*Abbreviations*: PTH, parathyroid hormone; $Ca^{++}$, calcium.

of active ionized serum calcium; metabolic alkalosis is associated with more calcium being bound to protein, decreasing the ionized fraction of serum calcium.[3,12,17]

# REGULATION OF NORMAL CALCIUM HOMEOSTASIS

Calcium homeostasis is tightly controlled. Alterations in these homeostatic mechanisms lead to disorders of calcium metabolism that are reflected in the effects on multiple processes in the body, including muscle contractility, nerve conduction, blood clotting, cell permeability, and bone formation. Essential cellular functions are dependent on maintaining the serum calcium concentration within a narrow physiologic range that is maintained by moving calcium between the plasma, bone, kidney, and GI tract. A sensitive negative feedback loop that is controlled by the concentration of serum ionized calcium and the actions of three major hormones, parathyroid hormone (PTH), calcitonin, and calcitriol (the active form of vitamin D), regulates the movements of calcium ions. Figure 39-2 depicts the negative feedback process involved in calcium homeostasis.

### Role of parathyroid hormone

Parathyroid hormone (PTH) is the major hormone regulating the extracellular concentration of ionized calcium. PTH is released in response to a decrease in ionized calcium and acts to achieve calcium homeostasis through direct and indirect effects on three organ systems: bone, kidney, and gut. Direct actions of PTH include increased bone resorption leading to the release of both calcium and phosphorus into the circulation and increased renal reabsorption of calcium and urinary excretion of phosphorus. Indirectly, PTH acts to increase absorption of ingested calcium from the gut and stimulate the kidneys to convert vitamin D to calcitriol, the biologically active form of vitamin D. Parathyroid hormone regulates calcium and phosphorus in inverse proportion to one another; mechanisms that decrease one ion (eg, excretion) will increase the other ion (eg, reabsorption). For this reason, serum phosphate and calcium levels should always be evaluated together.[11] Restoration of serum calcium to normal levels signals the parathyroid glands to suppress PTH secretion, completing the typical endocrine negative feedback loop.

### Role of the calcium-sensing receptor

Minute-to-minute secretion of PTH is under the control of the extracellular calcium-sensing receptor (*CaSR*).[5,17] The *CaSR* is a G protein-coupled receptor that is expressed in many normal tissues, including the parathyroid gland, thyroid gland, and kidneys, and has an essential role in calcium homeostasis. The *CaSR* senses the serum calcium concentration and acts to restore ionized calcium to normal levels by regulating the secretion of PTH from the parathyroid glands, reabsorption of calcium from the renal tubules, and secretion of calcitonin. High levels of ionized serum calcium activate the *CaSR* and leads to suppression of PTH secretion.[19,20] Inherited defects in the *CaSR* gene can result in three uncommon disorders: familial benign hypocalciuric hypercalcemia, in which high serum calcium is unable to activate the *CaSR* in the renal tubules and the *CaSRs* function as if blood calcium levels were low; neonatal severe hyperparathyroidism; and autosomal dominant hypocalcemia with hypercalciuria.[21,22]

### Role of calcitonin

Calcitonin is a hormone produced by the thyroid gland that participates in calcium and phosphorus metabolism. It is released from parafollicular C cells of the thyroid gland in response to elevated serum calcium levels and has effects antagonistic to those of PTH.[4] Calcitonin decreases blood calcium levels primarily through its effects on bone, where it inhibits bone resorption by osteoclasts, and promotes bone formation by osteoblasts.[18] In the kidneys, calcitonin increases the excretion of calcium and phosphorus by inhibiting their tubular reabsorption. Calcitonin secretion also increases briefly after meals.[19] Although calcitonin has an important role in calcium homeostasis in some animal species and in fish, its role in humans is uncertain. Alterations in calcium balance are rarely seen in conditions where calcitonin is absent (following total thyroidectomy) and where calcitonin might be elevated, as seen in pregnancy and in patients with medullary carcinoma of the thyroid. The effects on plasma calcium levels in humans are mainly seen in response to pharmacological doses of calcitonin.

### Role of vitamin D

Vitamin D is not actually a vitamin, but is a fat-soluble steroid hormone. Several steps of activation are required before vitamin D is converted to the biologically active metabolite, 1,25-dihydroxyvitamin $D_3$ (calcitriol), which can act on target tissues. The vitamin D precursor is synthesized in the skin through exposure to sunlight or ingested in fortified foods, particularly dairy products and some cereals. Activation begins in the liver with conversion to 25-hydroxyvitamin $D_2$, called calcidiol.[17] Further conversion to the active form 1,25-dihydroxyvitamin $D_3$ (calcitriol) takes place in the kidney, mediated by an enzyme in the proximal nephron, 1α-hydroxylase (CYP27B1).[19] Parathyroid hormone, which is in the circulation in response to low levels of calcium and phosphorus, stimulates CYP27B1 to convert vitamin $D_2$ to calcitriol in the kidneys. Calcitriol acts to increase plasma concentrations of calcium and phosphorus in several ways: it increases absorption of calcium and phosphorus from the GI tract, stimulates maturation of osteoclast precursor cells to bone destroying osteoclasts, and enhances the effects of PTH on calcium reabsorption in the renal tubules. The presence of calcitriol inhibits the activity of CYP27B1 in the nephrons, thus providing the negative feedback loop that regulates calcitriol synthesis.[17,19] In the setting of tumor-induced hypercalcemia, vitamin D metabolism and intestinal absorption of calcium are typically suppressed due to negative feedback mechanisms stimulated by increased serum calcium levels; exceptions are certain lymphomas, in which increased activation of calcitriol causes hypercalcemia. Dietary intake of calcium should be avoided in this situation.[11,17] In addition to its humoral effects on calcium homeostasis, there is recent evidence that receptors for vitamin D are found in multiple genes and organ systems and are responsible for several nonendocrine effects of vitamin D, including cell differentiation and proliferation, immune functions, and resisting infections.[17]

### Role of the kidneys in calcium homeostasis

The kidneys play a major role in maintaining levels of ionized serum calcium within physiological range. The kidney normally filters about 10 g of calcium from the serum daily. Most of the filtered calcium (60%-70%) is reabsorbed from the proximal convoluted tubule, independent of hormonal control but driven by the gradient generated by reabsorption of sodium and water.[17] Another 25% of calcium is reabsorbed in the Loop of Henle. Regulation of calcium excretion occurs in the distal tubules and collecting ducts of the kidney, fine-tuned by negative feedback mechanisms involving PTH. Low levels of ionized serum calcium stimulate increased tubular reabsorption of calcium so that minimal calcium is lost in the urine. In contrast, even a tiny elevation in serum calcium causes greatly increased urinary calcium excretion and reduced intestinal absorption of calcium.[17] The normally functioning kidney has great adaptive capacity and can increase daily calcium excretion up to 5 times normal, up to approximately 600 mg of calcium per day, before an increased calcium load overwhelms renal compensatory mechanisms and hypercalcemia develops.[5]

## Renal contributions in hypercalcemia

Impaired renal function is rarely the initiating factor in HCM, but the kidneys can contribute to and exacerbate hypercalcemia. The presence of excessive serum calcium interferes with the ability of the renal system to concentrate urine, which is regulated by antidiuretic hormone (ADH). The distal tubules and collecting ducts become resistant to the actions of ADH and impermeable to water. Instead of being reabsorbed, water remains in the tubular lumen and is excreted as large volumes of dilute urine (polyuria), which in turn stimulates excessive thirst (polydipsia). Both polyuria and polydipsia are hallmark signs of hypercalcemia.[23] Even with the powerful stimulus of thirst, the hypercalcemic patient may be unable to replace the lost fluid, due to symptoms that result from hypercalcemia, including nausea, vomiting, confusion, and stupor. In addition, common side effects of the disease process or of cytotoxic therapy, such as anorexia, nausea, vomiting, mucositis, dysphagia, and fever, can contribute to fluid and sodium loss. The ensuing dehydration triggers the kidneys to increase the reabsorption of sodium and water in the proximal tubules; calcium follows closely. Another consequence of fluid volume depletion is reduced blood flow through the kidneys and reduced glomerular filtration that results in less calcium filtration from the plasma for excretion in the urine. The effects of increased tubular reabsorption of calcium and decreased calcium filtration in the kidneys contribute to developing hypercalcemia that in turn exacerbates hypovolemia and can lead to progressive renal failure. In summary, any condition that contributes to, or exacerbates dehydration and fluid volume depletion, triggers a response by the kidneys that potentiate existing hypercalcemia. Figure 39-3 illustrates the reciprocal effects between hypercalcemia and the kidneys.

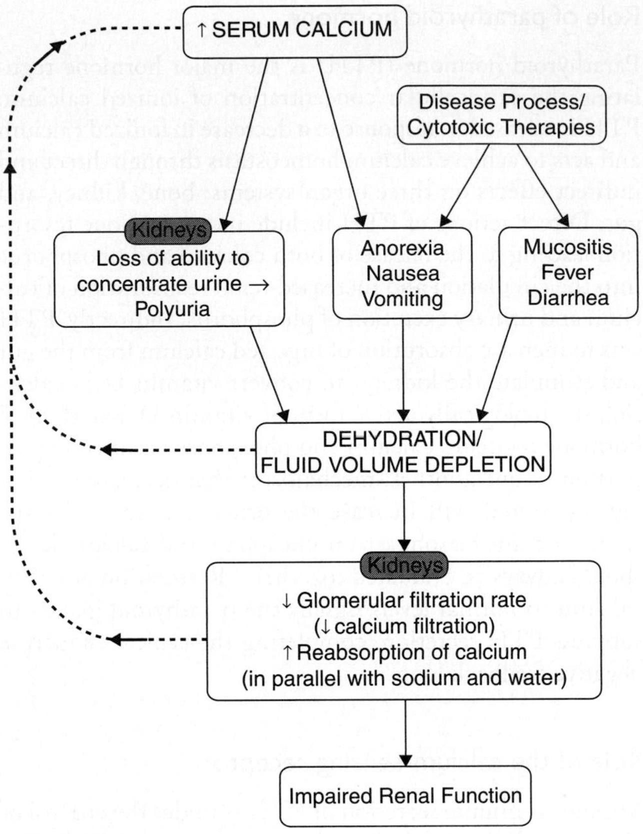


**FIGURE 39-3**

Role of kidneys in hypercalcemia.

## ETIOLOGY OF HYPERCALCEMIA OF MALIGNANCY

An understanding of normal calcium homeostasis illustrates that there are three mechanisms that can contribute to the development of HCM: (1) calcium in bone can be released in quantities sufficient to overwhelm the renal excretory mechanism, (2) calcium reabsorption in the kidneys can be inappropriately increased or excretion can be decreased, and (3) calcium absorption in the gut can be inappropriately enhanced.

Advances in molecular biology have led to increased understanding of the etiology of HCM. Initially, HCM was thought to be a direct consequence of bone destruction caused by local extension of tumor into bone or through distant metastasis to bone, but this has not been found to be consistent with the true clinical picture of HCM. The presence of hypercalcemia does not correlate with the amount of bone destroyed in all circumstances; about 15% of patients with malignancy-associated hypercalcemia have little or no evidence of bone destruction. It is recognized that HCM can result from different mechanisms depending on the type of malignancy. The mechanism in common is excessive increase in osteoclastic activity that causes bone destruction. A humoral component is instrumental in the etiology of each type of HCM: (1) circulating factors secreted by tumor cells stimulate osteoclastic resorption of bone and lead to HHM, (2) metastatic invasion to bone releases and activates local humoral substances that stimulate increased osteoclastic activity and cause local osteolytic hypercalcemia, and (3) increased production of 1,25-dihydroxyvitamin $D_3$ (calcitriol) that stimulates GI absorption of calcium, and enhances PTH and osteoclastic activity.[4,9,17]

## Humoral hypercalcemia of malignancy

*Parathyroid hormone–related protein.* In 1987, a polypeptide hormone similar to PTH was isolated from tumors in patients with HCM. Because of its similarity to PTH in both structure and actions, the substance was called parathyroid hormone–related protein (PTHrP). Since then, PTHrP has been identified as the major humoral factor responsible for HCM.[5,9,20] Parathyroid hormone–related protein is secreted by malignant tumor cells and mimics the physiological activity of PTH by binding to the same receptors on skeletal and renal target tissues, but is not affected by normal PTH negative feedback mechanisms that regulate calcium and phosphorus homeostasis. The unregulated hormonal actions of PTHrP stimulate increased bone resorption and increased calcium reabsorption accompanied by decreased phosphate reabsorption in the renal tubules. The result is hypercalcemia and hypophosphatemia.[17,24]

Humoral hypercalcemia of malignancy occurs most frequently in solid tumors, including cancers of the breast, lung, kidney, and head and neck, which together account for approximately 80% of the total incidence of hypercalcemia.[23] Immunoassays used to distinguish PTHrP from PTH have also detected PTHrP expression in melanoma, skin tumors, neuroendocrine tumors, and medullary thyroid cancer. Circulating levels of PTHrP have been detected in 100% of patients who have solid tumors complicated by HCM in the absence of bone metastases, and in up to two-thirds of hypercalcemic patients who have bone metastases.[9,20,24] High circulating PTHrP levels have been revealed in most of the patients with adult T-cell leukemia/lymphoma who have developed hypercalcemia. Parathyroid hormone–related protein has been detected to a lesser extent in hypercalcemic patients with non-Hodgkin's lymphoma (NHL), especially the B-cell type, and in patients with multiple myeloma.[25]

*Calcium-sensing receptor.* Over the past 10 years, research into the actions of the extracellular CaSR has demonstrated that the CaSR has an essential role in the etiology of HHM. The CaSR directly regulates the secretion of PTHrP in both normal and malignant cells and has been shown to be overexpressed in several types of cancer, including breast and prostate cancer. The CaSR contributes to HHM by inappropriately stimulating secretion of PTHrP in response to increased calcium levels. In addition, the CaSR regulates cellular processes that are important to survival of both normal and malignant cells, such as the processes of proliferation, chemotaxis, apoptosis, and differentiation. Animal models have shown that the CaSR promotes growth and survival of cancer cells by activating multiple signaling pathways to stimulate cellular proliferation and reduce apoptosis.[20]

*Local osteolytic hypercalcemia.* Bone is unique among target tissues affected by cancer because it is a dynamic tissue, constantly being remodeled in a cycle of bone disposal and renewal. Metastasis to the skeleton unbalances the normal bone remodeling process and stimulates the creation of two types of lesions, osteolytic or osteoblastic. Osteolytic lesions are the most common form of bone metastasis and are characterized by bone loss that is not balanced by bone formation. Local osteolytic hypercalcemia is typically associated with cancers that have significant osteolytic bone involvement, particularly breast cancer and multiple myeloma, but also leukemia and lymphoma, particularly Hodgkin's disease. In breast cancer, osteolytic lesions are found in 80% of patients with metastatic disease, but up to 15% of patients have osteoblastic lesions or a mix of the two types. Osteolytic bone destruction is also common in patients with advanced lung cancer and multiple myeloma, both of which are associated with increased incidence of hypercalcemia. Metastatic osteoblastic bone disease, in which formation of abnormal bone predominates over bone resorption, is much less common, and occurs most frequently in advanced prostate cancer that is rarely complicated by HCM.[5,20,23,26]

The bone microenvironment, which is rich in growth factors and cytokines, provides a fertile soil for tumor invasion and growth. As demonstrated in metastatic breast cancer, tumor cells that are deposited in bone secrete PTHrP that acts to increase osteoclastic bone resorption and to mediate the release and activation of multiple growth factors and cytokines that are stored within the matrix of normal bone. This group of humoral agents includes transforming growth factor (TGF)-β, insulin-like growth factor (IGF)-I and -II, fibroblast growth factor (FGF)-1 and -2, and platelet-derived growth factors (PDGFs), and bone morphogenetic proteins. Release and activation of these factors enhance survival and growth of metastatic cancer cells and contribute to cancer spread and bone destruction, creating a vicious cycle of metastasis and bone pathology.[10,26–29]

*RANK, RANKL, and OPG.* Identification of a cytokine system that plays a key role in the interactions between osteoblasts and osteoclasts has increased understanding about local control of normal bone remodeling. The osteoblasts have been revealed as the key to normal bone remodeling because their actions control the maturation and activity of the osteoclasts.[18,30,31] The presence of tumor cells in bone subverts this normal process. Metastatic cells release PTHrP that binds with and activates normal PTH receptors on osteoblasts and bone marrow stromal cells. Activation of the

PTH receptor stimulates the expression of a cell surface protein on the osteoblast, called the receptor activator of nuclear factor-kB (RANK) ligand, or RANK-ligand (RANKL). RANKL is a member of the tumor necrosis factor superfamily and is a powerful mediator of osteoclast differentiation and function.[5,27,30–32] RANKL stimulates osteoclast activity by binding to its related receptor, RANK, located on undifferentiated, precursor osteoclastic cells. When RANKL activates the RANK receptors the preosteoclasts fuse and differentiate into mature multinucleated osteoclasts that resorb bone.[15,31] In the normal regulation of bone remodeling, the process of osteoclast activation and ensuing bone resorption is inhibited by another cytokine, called osteoprotegerin (OPG). OPG is a soluble, free-floating "decoy" receptor produced and secreted by the osteoblast that counteracts the effects of RANKL by binding with it, thus blocking further osteoclastic maturation and halting excessive bone resorption. The balance that is maintained between RANKL and OPG, regulated by systemic hormones and local bone cytokines, determines osteoclastic functions. Figure 39-4 depicts the

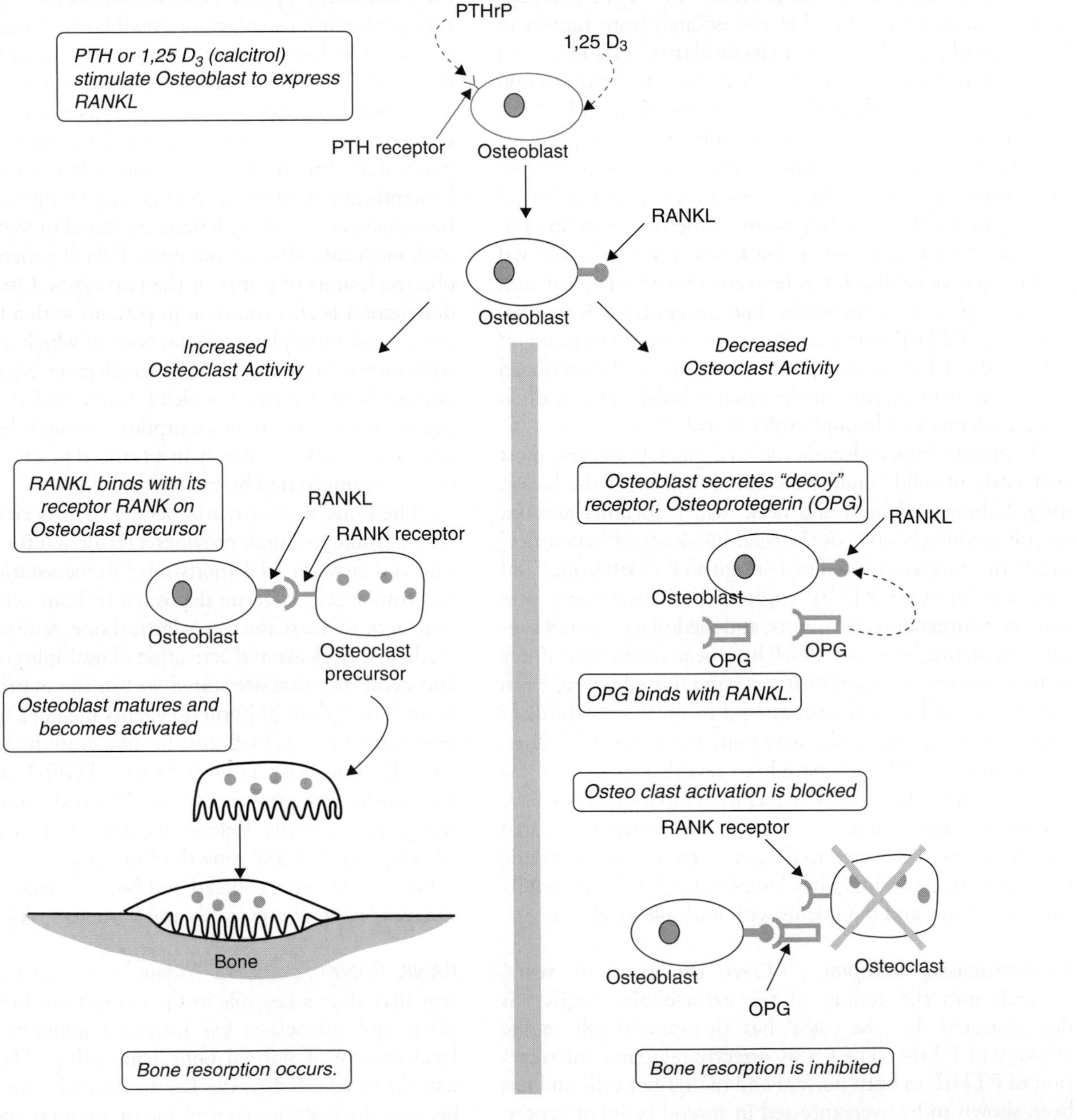


**FIGURE 39-4**

Normal bone remodeling: a balanced process.

*Abbreviations*: OPG, osteoprotegerin; PTH, parathyroid hormone; RANK, receptor activator of nuclear factor κB; RANKL, receptor activator of nuclear factor κB ligand.

interactions underlying normal bone remodeling.[10,15,27,29,31,32] When invaded by cancer cells, the normal bone microenvironment becomes deregulated and an imbalance develops in the RANKL/OPG ratio which favors RANKL expression and leads to increased bone destruction.[27,32] Overexpression of RANKL contributes to the hypercalcemia that occurs in more than 50% of patients with adult T-cell lymphoma, a disease strongly associated with human T-cell lymphotropic virus type 1 (HTLV-1). In this disease, studies show that RANKL is expressed in response to macrophage inflammatory protein-1α that also stimulates maturation of osteoclasts and bone resorption.[5]

*RANKL and multiple myeloma.* Multiple myeloma, a cancer of plasma cells, is the most common primary cancer of the skeleton. Hallmark features of myeloma are widespread tumor-induced osteolytic bone destruction and renal failure. Hypercalcemia occurs in at least one-third of patients with multiple myeloma most often in those with the greatest volume of tumor, and it can be life-threatening. Renal dysfunction is common in patients with multiple myeloma, and it contributes to hypercalcemia by decreasing renal calcium excretion secondary to reduced glomerular filtration.[5,14,33] PTHrP overexpression is not typically associated with hypercalcemia in multiple myeloma. Instead, extensive osteolysis is induced by potent osteoclast-activating cytokines that are expressed or locally secreted by the myeloma cells. RANKL is known to be the final common mediator of osteoclastic bone resorption in myeloma, but macrophage inflammatory protein-1α, tumor necrosis factors, and the interleukins also contribute.[34] Myeloma cells in the bone marrow are able to secrete RANKL, or interact with bone marrow stromal cells to markedly stimulate RANKL expression, while downregulating OPG expression. The resulting imbalance between RANKL and OPG counteracts normal inhibition of osteoclastic overactivity; formation and activation of osteoclasts is promoted and osteolytic bone destruction occurs.[33–36] Targeting RANKL and other molecular and signaling pathways involved in osteolysis may lead to the development of novel therapeutic strategies in myeloma bone disease and myeloma-associated hypercalcemia.

*Calcitriol (1,25-dihydroxyvitamin D3).* Levels of 1,25-dihydroxyvitamin $D_3$ (ie, calcitriol), the active metabolite of vitamin D, are low in most cases of tumor-induced hypercalcemia, but in the setting of Hodgkin's disease and NHL, calcitriol acts as a humoral mediator of hypercalcemia.[9,15] Hypercalcemia occurs in the absence of osteolytic bone lesions because macrophages that are in close proximity to the lymphoma cells stimulate the metabolism of 25-hydroxyvitamin $D_2$ to its active form 1,25-dihydroxyvitamin $D_3$. Calcitriol acts directly on the intestines to increase calcium absorption from the diet, on the kidneys to increase filtered calcium reabsorption, and on the bones to enhance osteoclastic bone resorption resulting in hypercalcemia. Elevated serum calcitriol levels are seen in approximately 50% of patients with lymphoma complicated by hypercalcemia. The rest have elevated concentrations of PTHrP.[5] The incidence of hypercalcemia associated with Hodgkin's disease is low, ranging from 1.6% to 5.4%, mostly in older patients with stage III/IV bulky disease below the diaphragm. In patients with NHL, HCM occurs most often in those with aggressive histologies. The characteristic clinical features of calcitriol-mediated hypercalcemia include an absence of bone metastases, suppressed serum PTH, undetectable PTHrP, normal or slightly increased serum phosphate levels, elevated calcitriol level, and hypercalciuria.[15]

## NONMALIGNANT CAUSES OF HYPERCALCEMIA

Aside from malignancy, hypercalcemia can be caused by a variety of conditions affecting bone metabolism, especially primary hyperparathyroidism. Malignancy and hyperparathyroidism together account for 90% of the diagnosed cases of hypercalcemia.[4,7] In recent years malignancy has exceeded primary hyperparathyroidism as the most frequent cause of hypercalcemia.[17] The incidence rate of primary hyperparathyroidism is 25 cases per 100,000 among the general population of the US, but is much higher for older women and hospitalized patients.[36] Hypercalcemia associated with primary hyperparathyroidism tends to be mild and prolonged, and is often asymptomatic and undiagnosed until routine blood tests are performed. The abnormal parathyroid tissue causes increased secretion of PTH and increased renal production of calcitriol, which lead to increased serum calcium concentration. However, despite over secretion of PTH, bone formation and bone breakdown are balanced in primary hyperparathyroidism so that bone mass may remain normal for decades. In general, serum calcium levels that are mildly elevated over a long period of time are due to nonmalignant conditions; rapidly rising calcium levels are more likely to indicate malignancy.[21] It is not unusual for primary hyperparathyroidism or other benign causes of hypercalcemia, such as vitamin D excess, granulomatous, genetic, endocrine, or drug-induced etiologies, to coexist with malignancy.[11] The challenge for healthcare providers is to differentiate the etiology of the hypercalcemia so that prognosis and optimal treatment can be determined and initiated early. Table 39-2[3,4,6,11,17] lists nonmalignant conditions associated with hypercalcemia.

## CLINICAL MANIFESTATIONS OF HYPERCALCEMIA

Hypercalcemia of malignancy frequently presents insidiously and is often unrecognized because many symptoms are vague or nonspecific and are attributed to the underlying disease process or to the effects of therapy. Symptom

**TABLE 39-2**

**Nonmalignant Causes of Hypercalcemia**

**Altered Parathyroid Gland Function**
Primary hyperparathyroidism associated with:
- Hyperplasia, adenoma, or carcinoma of the parathyroid glands
- Multiple endocrine neoplasia (*MEN TypeI* and *MEN Type II*) (*MEN* syndromes represent hyperfunction of two or more endocrine glands)

**Granulomatous Disorders**
Sarcoidosis, tuberculosis, leprosy, histoplasmosis, coccidiomycosis

**Renal Failure**
- Acute renal failure: recovery phase
- Chronic renal failure

**Drug-Induced**
- Thiazide diuretics
- Lithium
- Vitamin D intoxication (usually from excessive over-the-counter supplementation)
- Vitamin A (retinol) intoxication (due to excessive dietary supplementation or analogs used to treat acne)
- Aluminum toxicity (from aluminum-containing antacids)
- Tamoxifen
- Hormonal therapy: estrogens, antiestrogens, androgens, and progestins
- Total parenteral nutrition
- Theophylline toxicity
- Milk-alkali syndrome

**Endocrine disorders**
- Hyperthyroidism (thyrotoxicosis)
- Adrenal insufficiency (Addison's disease)
- Acromegaly
- Pheochromocytoma

**Genetic disorders**
- Familial hypocalciuric hypercalcemia (dominantly inherited defect in calcium-sensing receptor)

**Immobilization**
- Prolonged immobilization (especially in the young and those with underlying Paget's disease of bone)

*Source*: Data from National Cancer Institute[3]; Carroll and Schade[4]; Morton and Lipton[5]; Kaplan[11]; and the Moe.[17]

severity depends on the magnitude of hypercalcemia and the rate of rise in serum calcium although there is much individual variation regardless of serum calcium levels. Multisystem clinical manifestations become apparent as serum calcium concentration increases and reflect the depressant effects of elevated serum calcium on nerve tissue excitation and on the contractility of cardiac, skeletal, and smooth muscle.[11] Although HCM affects the renal, GI, neurological, cardiovascular, and musculoskeletal systems, the effects are especially profound in the renal and

**TABLE 39-3**

**Clinical Manifestations of Hypercalcemia of Malignancy**

**Gastrointestinal**
Early: Anorexia, nausea, vomiting, constipation, vague abdominal pain, weight loss, peptic ulcers, acute pancreatitis

Late: Atonic ileus, obstipation

**Renal**
Early: Polyuria, polydipsia, nocturia, dehydration, decreased glomerular filtration, hypercalciuria, kidney stones, renal insufficiency

Late: Renal failure

**Neurological**
Early: Drowsiness, lethargy, weakness, decreased deep tendon reflexes, apathy, restlessness, irritability, depression, confusion, personality changes, cognitive dysfunction, disorientation, delirium, psychotic behavior, visual disturbances

Late: Seizures, stupor, coma

**Cardiovascular**
Early: Electrocardiographic changes indicating slowed conduction, prolonged P-R interval, widened QRS complex, shortened Q-T interval, shortened or absent S-T segments; digitalis sensitivity, broadened T wave, sinus bradycardia, arrhythmias

Late: Heart block, cardiac arrest

**Musculoskeletal**
Early: Muscle weakness, fatigue, hypotonia, bone pain

Late: Ataxia, pathological fractures

**Other**
Pruritis

Calcium precipitates in cornea (band keratopathy)

Soft tissue calcifications (calciphylaxis)

*Note*: There is significant individual variation regardless of serum calcium levels.

*Source*: Data from the National Cancer Institute[3]; Kaplan[11]; Pearson[37]; and Richerson.[38]

neurological systems.[21] See Table 39-3[3,11,37,38] for a list of clinical manifestations of increased serum calcium.

## GASTROINTESTINAL EFFECTS

Gastrointestinal symptoms are present in most patients with HCM, and are related to the depressive effects of elevated serum calcium on the autonomic nervous system, and the resulting hypotonicity of smooth muscle in the GI tract. The most common GI manifestations are nausea, vomiting, anorexia, and constipation caused by delayed gastric emptying and slowed GI motility.[5,17] Cramping abdominal pain may occasionally be present and complete ileus can occur with very high calcium levels. Rarely, peptic ulcer disease may develop in response to increased gastrin release stimulated by prolonged hypercalcemia, and acute pancreatitis may develop secondary to phospholipase activation by calcium.[3,11]

### RENAL EFFECTS

Hypercalcemia is toxic to the renal tubules. The urine-concentrating ability of the kidneys becomes impaired, causing some of the hallmark clinical manifestations of HCM: polydipsia, polyuria, and nocturia.[11] Calcium deposition within the renal tubules inhibits the action of ADH in concentrating urine and nephrogenic diabetes insipidus develops with diuresis of large volumes of dilute urine.[23] Anorexia and vomiting, early GI manifestations of hypercalcemia, overcome the stimulus of thirst and severe dehydration ensues. Volume depletion causes the glomerular filtration rate to fall, decreasing calcium excretion, worsening the hypercalcemia, and leading to acute renal failure. Prolonged hypercalcemia may be associated with kidney stones that develop secondary to hypercalciuria, and with calcium deposition in soft tissues in the body, especially when hyperphosphatemia related to renal failure is present.[21] The degree of renal impairment frequently determines the course of hypercalcemia; increasingly severe renal dysfunction often portends a fatal outcome.

### NEUROLOGICAL EFFECTS

Central nervous system changes reflect the direct depressant effect of hypercalcemia on the transmission of nerve impulses. Neurological symptoms include fatigue, apathy, lethargy, depression, difficulty concentrating, hyporeflexia, and muscle weakness. Extreme muscle weakness can confine the patient to bed, further enhancing hypercalcemia.[5] As calcium levels increase, alterations in mental status progress to confusion, psychotic behavior, seizures, coma, and ultimately death.[3,11]

### CARDIAC EFFECTS

High serum calcium levels depress the electrical conduction system of the heart, and increase cardiac muscle contractility and irritability. Electrocardiographic changes, such as shortened QT interval and prolonged PR and QRS intervals, reflect slowed conduction through the heart. Cardiac arrhythmias are rare and may result from decreases in serum potassium and magnesium or from digitalis toxicity as increasing serum calcium concentration potentiate the effects of digitalis.[4,17] Clinical effects related to arrhythmias range from feeling lightheaded, to fainting, to sudden death if serum calcium rises acutely.[3] Hypertension may be present, caused by the vasoconstricting effect of calcium on arterial smooth muscle, but is more often associated with hypercalcemia from nonmalignant causes.[11]

### MUSCULOSKELETAL EFFECTS

Elevation of serum calcium levels decreases neuromuscular excitability causing hypotonicity of smooth and striated muscle. Proximal muscle weakness, easy fatigability, and atrophy of muscles may be striking.[22] Neuromuscular manifestations are usually more marked in older patients. Bone pain may be present regardless of the extent or absence of metastatic bone involvement because calcium has neurosensitizing actions that diminish the pain threshold. Pathological fractures and skeletal deformities may develop with progressive disease.[3]

## ASSESSMENT

Evaluation of a patient presenting with hypercalcemia begins with a careful history and physical examination focusing on clinical manifestations of hypercalcemia, risk factors for malignancy, and potentially causative dietary supplements or medications, such as vitamins D or A, calcium-containing antacids, or thiazide diuretics. For patients with a known history of malignancy, an understanding of which tumor types are associated with increased risk of hypercalcemia will help raise awareness to the nonspecific, early symptoms of HCM that typically include fatigue, anorexia, nausea, vomiting, thirst, muscle weakness, polyuria, and constipation.

### BLOOD CHEMISTRY MEASUREMENTS

#### Serum calcium

In a patient with known malignant disease, the first step in the diagnostic evaluation is to determine the serum calcium level. Total calcium and albumin are generally measured in tandem and a correction formula is used to arrive at the estimated corrected value for ionized serum calcium, as discussed earlier (see Figure 39-1). However, in asymptomatic patients with multiple myeloma and hypercalcemia, measures of ionized calcium are more appropriate to obtain.[6] Urinary calcium measurements may also be useful because increases in calcium excretion may be detected before serum calcium rises.[5]

#### Serum electrolytes

Appropriate laboratory measurements include blood urea nitrogen and creatinine concentrations to provide information about renal function, as well as phosphorus, magnesium, and potassium.[3,5,39] Phosphorus and calcium have an inverse relationship regulated by PTH, and should be evaluated together. Serum phosphorus levels may be low or normal, or elevated in the presence of widespread bone metastasis.[40] Low magnesium levels may aggravate the neuromuscular effects of hypercalcemia.[12] Serum alkaline phosphatase may also be elevated in patients with breast cancer metastatic to bone reflecting increased osteoblast activity.[13] Hypokalemia may be revealed, and may relate to inadequate dietary intake of potassium.[39] Serum chloride levels usually are elevated in primary hyperparathyroidism and decreased in other forms of hypercalcemia.[4,17]

### iPTH, PTHrP, and calcitriol levels

Determination of plasma immunoreactive parathyroid hormone (iPTH) levels may be useful to rule out nonmalignant causes of hypercalcemia. In the setting of HCM, the plasma iPTH is typically decreased or undetectable; in hyperparathyroid disease iPTH is often increased. Assays for PTHrP are available and may be needed when the cause of hypercalcemia is obscure. Circulating PTHrP levels are undetectable or low in normal individuals and elevated in most patients with HHM. Plasma calcitriol levels should be measured when a granulomatous disorder, such as sarcoidosis, or a lymphoma, especially Hodgkin disease, is considered.[3,7,22,40] See Table 39-4[7,11,19,22,36] for the differential diagnosis of hypercalcemia.

**TABLE 39-4**

**Differential Diagnosis of Hypercalcemia**

| | Primary Hyperparathyroidism | Humoral Hypercalcemia of Malignancy |
|---|---|---|
| **Plasma** | | |
| Calcium | High | High |
| Phosphate | Low | Low |
| Chloride | High | Low |
| Bicarbonate | Low | High |
| Calcitriol 1,25-dihydroxyvitamin $D_3$ | High | Low or undetectable (except in calcitriol-mediated HCM) |
| iPTH | High | Low or undetectable |
| PTHrP | Undetectable | High |
| pH | Metabolic acidosis | Metabolic alkalosis |
| **Renal** | | |
| Nephrogenous cAMP | High | High |
| Phosphate | High | High |
| Calcium | High | Higher than with PHP |
| **Bone** | | |
| Resorption | Increased | Increased |
| Formation | Increased | Decreased |

*Abbreviations*: cAMP, cyclic adenosine monophosphate; HCM, hypercalcemia of malignancy; iPTH, immunoreactive parathyroid hormone; iPTHrP, immunoreactive parathyroid hormone-related protein; PHP, primary hyperparathyroidism.

*Source*: Data from Stewart[7]; Kaplan[11]; Mundy and Guise[19]; Potts[22]; and Hemphill.[36]

### OTHER STUDIES

Hypercalcemia may produce electrocardiogram abnormalities that affect conduction time through the heart. A shortened QT interval is common and the PR interval may be prolonged. When serum calcium levels are very high, the QRS interval may lengthen, T waves may flatten or invert, and a variable degree of heart block may develop.[22,36] Orthostatic hypotension and signs of dehydration may indicate compromised renal function. A mild metabolic alkalosis may accompany HHM.[5] No imaging studies can definitively diagnose hypercalcemia but radiographic imaging, isotope bone scans, and skeletal surveys (in the case of myeloma) may demonstrate the presence of malignancy such as lung cancer, breast cancer, myeloma, or bone metastases.[3,7,36]

## GRADING HYPERCALCEMIA IN MALIGNANT DISEASE

Hypercalcemia may be graded into categories of mild, moderate, and severe based on corrected serum calcium levels; however, there is often a lack of correlation between symptom severity and serum calcium levels. In general, the severity of symptoms is most closely associated with the rapidity of onset of hypercalcemia, the degree of serum calcium elevation, and the age and performance status of the patient.[11] Patient prognosis depends on how quickly the hypercalcemia can be recognized and treated. Early intervention can help prevent secondary organ damage. Older adults or debilitated patients, such as patients with late stage disease, may become symptomatic with only a slight rise in ionized calcium, especially if it is rapid. Patients with HCM often have greater symptomatology for any given rise in calcium level in contrast to patients with primary hyperparathyroidism who are able to tolerate quite high serum calcium levels with few symptoms.[3] There are no formal guidelines for classifying the levels of severity of hypercalcemia; however, the grading categories discussed in this section are used frequently in the clinical setting.[2,7]

### MILD HYPERCALCEMIA

Asymptomatic patients with a corrected serum calcium concentration of 10.5 mg/dL to 11.9 mg/dL are considered to have mild hypercalcemia. Hypercalcemia of malignancy is frequently detected as part of routine laboratory testing during an outpatient visit. Although patients may not require intervention beyond close monitoring, oral hydration, and ambulation, the occurrence of HCM may indicate a diminishing response to antineoplastic therapy or recurrence of disease.[11,38,41] Over time, the HCM can be expected to increase in severity, especially if renal function becomes compromised by continuing fluid losses and/or the introduction of nephrotoxic agents.[5]

### MODERATE HYPERCALCEMIA

A corrected calcium concentration of 12 mg/dL to 13.9 mg/dL indicates moderate hypercalcemia. These patients may still be asymptomatic but the HCM can readily progress to a more serious problem.

### SEVERE HYPERCALCEMIA

Hypercalcemia of malignancy is considered severe at levels ≥14.0 mg/dL. However, regardless of the measured increase in serum calcium, any patient who has symptoms clearly related to HCM is considered to have severe HCM and should be treated as an acute medical emergency.[5,40] Patients with corrected serum calcium concentrations >14 mg/dL are invariably symptomatic and the situation can be life-threatening; without proper intervention, almost 50% of hypercalcemic patients will die as a consequence of either renal failure, coma, or cardiac arrest.[11,39]

## THERAPEUTIC APPROACHES

### PRINCIPLES OF ANTIHYPERCALCEMIC TREATMENT

#### General measures

The goals of antihypercalcemic therapy include improving renal function, and mental status, and prolonging life, while waiting for antitumor therapy to become effective at controlling the underlying malignancy. The therapeutic approach varies for each patient and is based on multiple factors: elevation of serum calcium, severity of symptoms, individual tumor type, status of disease, and prognosis for survival. The initial therapy selected depends on the severity of the HCM. Patients with mild hypercalcemia (<12 mg/dL corrected serum calcium), who are asymptomatic and receiving antineoplastic therapy, may only require careful observation and oral hydration plus a variety of preventive measures. Preventive measures include increasing oral fluid intake to 3 L per day to expand the intravascular fluid volume, controlling nausea and vomiting to prevent dehydration, and promoting ambulation and weight-bearing activities to decrease bone resorption. Medications that might potentiate hypercalcemia, such as thiazide diuretics that decrease renal excretion of calcium, and nonsteroidal anti-inflammatory drugs that inhibit renal blood flow should be avoided, as well as oral supplementation of vitamins A and D, and calcium-containing supplements and antacids. Calcium should be removed from parenteral and enteral feeding solutions. Dietary calcium restriction is generally unnecessary because GI absorption of calcium is very low, except in the case of some lymphomas in which HCM is mediated by calcitriol. Use of sedating medications should be minimized to enhance the patient's mental clarity and to be able to promote weight-bearing ambulation. Adequate salt intake is encouraged to help expand fluid volume.[3,7,11,39]

In cases of more severe hypercalcemia, when serum calcium concentration exceeds 12 mg/dL, or the patient manifests symptoms, hospitalization is required and aggressive therapies instituted to relieve acute symptoms and prevent progression to a life-threatening emergency.[2,22] The more severe the hypercalcemia, the greater the number of treatment approaches that need to be implemented to provide both rapid correction and long-lasting results. See Table 39-5[3,5,22–24,41–48] for an overview of antihypercalcemic therapy.

#### Antineoplastic therapy

Cancer-induced hypercalcemia is a reflection of tumor activity. The most effective long-term treatment of HCM is directed at decreasing the tumor burden and abolishing the mechanisms initiating the hypercalcemia. Antineoplastic therapy, whether surgical, radiotherapeutic, chemotherapeutic, or biological, designed to ablate tumor growth is an essential addition to initial antihypercalcemic measures. Treatment of HCM should be vigorous for patients with severe hypercalcemia who are likely to respond to antitumor therapy while waiting for antineoplastic therapy to become effective. However, the benefits of antineoplastic therapy need to be weighed against the patient's clinical condition. Many patients who develop HCM have advanced disease and a life expectancy of only a few weeks. In some cases, allowing the patient to return home with therapies aimed at ameliorating the distressing symptoms of hypercalcemia may be preferable to initiating aggressive antihypercalcemic treatment.

#### Extracellular fluid volume expansion and calciuresis

Hypercalcemia invariably leads to dehydration due to the combined effects of polyuria, vomiting, anorexia, and defects in urinary concentrating ability.[11,23] Thus, the

**TABLE 39-5**

**Overview of Therapeutic Interventions for Hypercalcemia of Malignancy**

| Treatment Modality | Mechanism of Action | Dosage | Management/Side Effects |
|---|---|---|---|
| | **Tumor-Specific Therapy** | | |
| **Treat underlying malignancy:** Surgery, chemotherapy, radiation therapy, hormonal therapy, immunotherapy, biotherapy | Goal of antineoplastic therapy is to ablate disease and abolish precipitating factors | | Chemotherapy and hormonal therapies may be effective in producing normocalcemia in patients with multiple myeloma or breast cancer<br>Tamoxifen for breast cancer bone metastases may cause transient increased serum calcium ("flare" reaction) |
| | **General Measures** | | |
| **Identify patients at risk** | Certain cancers are associated with increased risk for hypercalcemia of malignancy (see Table 39-1) | | Emphasize need for adequate oral hydration<br>Perform serial checks of serum calcium, phosphorus, and albumin levels |
| **Water and electrolyte repletion:**<br>Oral fluids<br>Saline hydration and sodium diuresis | Expands fluid volume; reverses dehydration; improves renal function<br>Calcium is excreted in the urine alongside sodium | Oral hydration: 3–4 L/day<br>Initial IV: 0.9% NaCl 100–300mL/hour<br>Maintenance IV: 2.5–4 L/day | Encourage oral fluids<br>Monitor renal and cardiac function and intake and output for fluid overload<br>Monitor electrolytes<br>Patients may need replacement of potassium and magnesium to prevent cardiac arrhythmias, especially with digitalis |
| **Forced diuresis:**<br>Saline plus loop diuretic (furosemide) | Blocks calcium and sodium reabsorption in Loop of Henle | Given after rehydration IV: 20–40 mg q 12 hours<br>Aggressive therapy, IV: 80–100 mg q 2–4 hours | Administer diuretics after rehydration is achieved<br>Monitor intake and output and electrolytes<br>Requires intensive care setting to monitor central venous pressure and electrolytes<br>Therapy can cause hypovolemia and life-threatening decreases in potassium, phosphorus, magnesium |
| **Mobilization** | Weight-bearing activities decrease bone resorption | | Ambulate TID if possible<br>Initiate active resistive exercises with pain management for patients on bed rest<br>Evaluate for pathological fracture if bone pain is present |
| **Drugs to avoid:**<br>Thiazide diuretics<br>NSAIDS, $H_2$-receptor agonists<br>Vitamins A and D | Increase renal calcium absorption<br>Inhibit renal blood flow<br>Increase bone resorption | | Withhold drugs that may potentiate hypercalcemia |
| **Dietary recommendations:**<br>Maintain salt intake<br>Dietary calcium restriction usually not necessary | Sodium promotes fluid volume expansion<br>Calcium is poorly absorbed from the gut | | Encourage adequate salt intake<br>Exception is hematological malignancies that increase vitamin D synthesis |
| | **Agents to Inhibit Bone Resorption** | | |
| **Bisphosphonates** | All drugs in this class inhibit osteoclastic activity and bone resorption | | All bisphosphonates are potentially nephrotoxic<br>Administer saline hydration to maintain urine output at 2 L/day throughout treatment for all bisphosphonates |

*(Continued)*

**TABLE 39-5**

**Overview of Therapeutic Interventions for Hypercalcemia of Malignancy (Continued)**

| Treatment Modality | Mechanism of Action | Dosage | Management/Side Effects |
|---|---|---|---|
| Pamidronate (Aredia) | Second generation<br>Approved for HCM<br>Also indicated for osteolytic bone lesions in multiple myeloma and breast cancer in conjunction with standard antineoplastic therapy | HCM:<br>IV: Single dose of 60–90 mg over 2–24 hours; dose may be repeated after a minimum of 7 days<br>Osteolytic lesions:<br>IV: 90 mg over 2 hours every 3–4 wks:<br>IV: 90 mg over 4 hours monthly | Monitor serum creatinine prior to each dose to assess renal status and need for dose adjustment<br>Fever, infusion site reaction, nausea<br>Mild decrease in phosphorus, potassium, magnesium<br>Osteonecrosis of the jaw<br>Ocular inflammation (eg, uveitis and scleritis) is an infrequent finding |
| Zoledronate (zoledronic acid, Zometa) | Third generation<br>High potency<br>Approved for HCM; also indicated for multiple myeloma and bone metastases from solid tumors in conjunction with standard antineoplastic therapy | HCM:<br>IV: Single dose of 4 mg over no less than 15 minutes<br>Dose may be repeated after a minimum of 7 days<br>Multiple myeloma and bone metastases:<br>IV: Single dose of 4 mg over no less than 15 minutes every 3–4 weeks | Monitor serum creatinine prior to each dose to assess renal status and need for dose adjustment<br>Fever, flu-like syndrome nausea, vomiting, infusion site reaction, mild decreased potassium, phosphorus, magnesium<br>Osteonecrosis of the jaw<br>Ocular inflammation (eg, uveitis or scleritis) is an infrequent finding |
| Ibandronate (Bondronat) | Third generation<br>Licensed in Europe for HCM<br>Also indicated for bone metastases and prevention of skeletal events with breast cancer | HCM:<br>IV: Single dose of 2–4 mg over 1 hour | Favorable renal safety profile; mandatory monitoring of renal function not required<br>Dose adjustments only required with severe renal impairment<br>Drug-induced fever |
| Clodronate (Bonefos)<br>Available worldwide; not commercially available in the US | Second generation<br>Non-nitrogen containing | IV: 300–500 mg/day over 4 h for 3–7 days; or 1500 mg dose over 4 h<br>PO: 1600–2400 mg/day<br>In palliative setting can be given as SQ infusion | Mild local reaction<br>Increased creatinine<br>Decreased phosphorus |
| Calcitonin (Calcimar or Miacalcin) | Thyroid hormone<br>Rapid action; direct inhibition of osteoclast receptors; increased renal calcium excretion<br>Small analgesic effect | SQ or IM:<br>4–8 IU/kg q 6–12 hours for 2 days | Safe in dehydrated patients and with preexisting renal failure<br>Brief effect; resistance develops<br>Useful as rapid-acting adjunct in severe HCM, nausea, hypersensitivity |
| Plicamycin (Mithramycin) | Direct toxic effect on osteoclasts; blocks RNA synthesis | IV: 25 mcg/kg/day over 4–6 hours for 3–8 doses (ideally through central line) | Irritant drug<br>Nausea, vomiting; bone marrow, renal, hepatic, and neurological toxicities<br>Used when HCM is resistant to safer drugs |

(Continued)

**TABLE 39-5**

**Overview of Therapeutic Interventions for Hypercalcemia of Malignancy (Continued)**

| Treatment Modality | Mechanism of Action | Dosage | Management/Side Effects |
|---|---|---|---|
| Gallium nitrate (Ganite) | Inhibits osteoclastic activity | Given after adequate rehydration<br>IV: 200 mg/m$^2$/day continuous for 5 days | Renal toxicity<br>Saline hydration to maintain urine ouput at 2 L/day throughout treatment |
| | | **Other Hypercalcemic Therapies** | |
| **Dialysis** | Rapidly lowers serum calcium concentration but is short-acting | | Used for select patients with preexisting renal failure who can't tolerate saline diuresis |
| **Corticosteroids** | Therapy of choice for steroid-sensitive, calcitriol-mediated cancers: multiple myeloma, lymphomas<br>Inhibits vitamin D conversion to calcitriol | PO Prednisone: 40–100 mg/day<br>IV Hydrocortisone: 100–300 mg/day for 3–7 days | Long-term use of steroids can cause hyperglycemia, hypokalemia, immunosuppression,Cushingoid symptoms, gastritis, osteoporosis, muscle wasting<br>Has no role in solid tumors |
| **Phosphates**<br>Neutra-Phos | Used to correct hypophosphatemia, which stimulates increased calcium resorption from bone | PO: 250–375 mg 4 times a day | Oral use: diarrhea<br>IV phosphates are toxic; reserved for life-threatening HCM when oral or nasogastric administration is not possible<br>Severe hypocalcemia, acute renal failure, soft tissue calcifications |

*Note*: ; Based on information from Carroll and Schade[4]; Morton and Lipton[5]; Potts[22]; Fojo.[23]

*Abbrevations*: HCM, hypercalcemic of malignancy; $H_2$, histamine 2 receptors; IM, intramuscular; IU, international unit; L, liter; NSAIDs, nonsteroidal anti-inflammatory drugs; SQ, subcutaneous.

*Source*: Adapted with permission from Kaplan.[11] Copyright © 2006 by the Oncology Nursing Society.

cornerstone of antihypercalcemic treatment is extracellular fluid volume (ECF) expansion in amounts sufficient to reverse the typical effects of hypercalcemia: (1) dehydration, (2) depletion of intravascular volume, and (3) decrease in glomerular filtration.

Rehydration helps decrease the calcium level through dilution and through expansion of extracellular volume that restores the glomerular filtration rate and increases renal calcium excretion.[36] Oral hydration with 3 to 4 L of fluid per day may be sufficient to restore normal fluid volume in the patient who is asymptomatic or has mild hypercalcemia. However, the symptomatic patient requires aggressive rehydration with intravenous normal saline to stimulate urinary calcium loss because the renal tubules excrete sodium and calcium in parallel. Normal saline is administered at a rate between 200 and 500 mL per hour based on the severity of hypercalcemia, the level of dehydration and renal function, cardiovascular status, and degree of mental impairment.[7,17,22] Care must be taken to prevent volume overload in elderly patients and in patients with poor cardiac reserve as severe congestive heart failure may develop.[5,36]

During rehydration, the patient is assessed for fluid overload and renal function by monitoring fluid intake and output and laboratory values for blood urea nitrogen, creatinine, sodium, potassium, calcium, and magnesium.[11,38] Sodium diuresis can increase renal excretion of potassium and magnesium and patients may require supplementation of these electrolytes to prevent cardiac arrhythmias, especially if they are taking digitalis.[3,17] During volume expansion, dependent edema may occur in patients who have hypoalbuminemia due to advanced malignant disease.[5] Calcium-containing renal calculi are also a potential complication of saline diuresis.[22]

After restoration of normal ECF volume, a daily maintenance infusion of 2.5 to 4 L of normal saline will induce continued mild diuresis of sodium and calcium. Fluid and electrolyte status are closely monitored and the patient is encouraged to drink freely and increase oral fluid intake.[5,22,38] Although rehydration is effective at increasing urinary output and renal calcium excretion, achieving normocalcemia through saline diuresis alone is unlikely.

### Loop diuretics

Once the hypercalcemic patient has been rehydrated sufficiently to maintain a urine output between 3 and 4 L per day, a loop diuretic, such as furosemide, may be added to force additional renal excretion of calcium. Loop diuretics block calcium and sodium reabsorption in the Loop of Henle and can increase calcium excretion by as much as 30%.[5] Loop diuretics should not be administered until the patient has been fully hydrated as they can create more dehydration by decreasing glomerular filtration and calcium excretion, thus worsening hypercalcemia.[5,7] Moderate doses of furosemide (20–40 mg intravenously every 12 hours) are used to prevent or to manage fluid overload in adequately hydrated patients. The urinary output in response to a given dose of furosemide is difficult to predict and careful assessment of intake and output is necessary to determine the optimal dose.[17] Thiazide diuretics are contraindicated because they stimulate renal calcium reabsorption and may exacerbate hypercalcemia.[7,11,38] In life-threatening HCM, aggressive therapy using high doses of furosemide or other powerful loop diuretics may be necessary. Intravenous furosemide administered in large doses of 80 to 100 mg every 2 hours can lead to significant reductions in serum calcium levels but requires the facilities of an intensive care unit.[5,22] Accurate measurements of central venous pressures, urine volumes (bladder catheterization may be necessary), and plasma and/or urine electrolytes are mandatory with this aggressive therapy to identify developing hypovolemia, which can exacerbate hypercalcemia, and electrolyte losses that can lead to hypokalemia, hypophosphatemia, and hypomagnesemia, which can become life-threatening.[3,22] The use of loop diuretics is limited to acute situations; forced diuresis is difficult to sustain even in patients with good cardiopulmonary and renal function, and diuretics have no effect on bone resorption, the primary cause of HCM.[22]

### Calcitonin

Calcitonin, a peptide hormone secreted by the thyroid gland, is especially safe in the acute management of hypercalcemia in patients with renal or cardiac failure who cannot tolerate large sodium loads.[9,42] It can induce renal calcium excretion within a few hours of administration by inhibiting calcium reabsorption in the distal tubules. Osteoclastic bone resorption is also blocked.[22] Calcitonin has a rapid onset of action with maximum response occurring within 12 to 24 hours, but its use is limited by short duration of action and the development of drug resistance.[7,17] It is administered either by a subcutaneous or intramuscular route in doses of 4 to 8 U/kg body weight every 6 to 12 hours for 2 to 3 days.[36,41] Although its effects are transitory, calcitonin can be useful for severe life-threatening hypercalcemia as a rapid-acting bridge therapy in association with intravenous bisphosphonates, which produce delayed but prolonged effects.[5,23,49] Common side effects of calcitonin include rash, nausea, flushing, and malaise.[39] Randomized controlled trials have shown that calcitonin provides an analgesic effect in reducing the pain associated with acute vertebral fractures, phantom limb pain, and possibly metastatic bone pain.[50]

## ANTIRESORPTIVE THERAPY: BISPHOSPHONATES

### Overview

Rehydration and forced diuresis are important initial approaches to treating hypercalcemia but administration of bisphosphonates provides the most effective and sustained therapeutic effects in managing HCM. Intravenous bisphosphonate therapy, in conjunction with volume repletion, has supplanted all other drug therapies in the treatment and prevention of malignancy-associated hypercalcemia; the exception being steroid-sensitive malignancies, such as myeloma and lymphoma.[23,24] Bisphosphonates are low-molecular-weight molecules that have a composition similar to pyrophosphate in bone. They are potent inhibitors of osteoclast activity and work by blocking osteoclast-mediated bone resorption, which is the final common mechanism in both humoral and local osteolytic hypercalcemia.[5,7,17] Serum calcium levels can be normalized within 4 to 7 days of initiation of bisphosphonate therapy in 60% to 90% of patients with responses lasting 1 to 3 weeks.[7,40] Bisphosphonates are delivered solely through the intravenous route in treating HCM. Oral doses are poorly absorbed from the GI tract; if taken with food the bioavailability of bisphosphonates is reduced to nearly zero.[5,7]

Nephrotoxicity is the most significant side effect of bisphosphonate therapy. Bisphosphonates are cleared from the body via renal excretion and patients require close monitoring of renal function during treatment. Serum creatinine levels prior to initiation of bisphosphonate therapy and prior to each dose are mandatory. Specified infusion times for each agent cannot safely be shortened.[43] All patients receiving bisphosphonates should be vigorously hydrated to maintain a daily urine output of 2 L throughout treatment.[44,45,51] In general, bisphosphonate infusions are well tolerated. Transient low-grade fevers, myalgias, arthralgias, malaise, and local infusion reactions may occur with the first dose but diminish with subsequent treatments and are not an indication to discontinue drug treatment. In most cases, the symptoms are self-limiting and subside after 24 to 48 hours.[44,45] Hypocalcemia occurs in up to 50% of patients treated with bisphosphonates for HCM, although symptomatic hypocalcemia is rare.[49] Hypophosphatemia requiring supplementation may develop with bisphosphonate use. The mechanisms of phosphate imbalance are unclear but may include preexisting nutritional deficiency aggravated by volume expansion, renal phosphate wasting in association with PTHrP activity, and increased normal PTH activity as normocalcemia or mild hypocalcemia follows therapy.[5] Ocular adverse effects, such as scleritis, have been reported with intravenous bisphosphonate exposure.[43]

In the US, 2 bisphosphonates, pamidronate and zoledronate, are approved by the Food and Drug Administration (FDA) for the acute management of mild-to-severe HCM, and are currently the agents of choice for this complication. Both these bisphosphonates begin to reduce the serum calcium concentration within 12 hours of initiation. Serum calcium levels decrease to normal or near-normal range within approximately 4 to 7 days and remain there for 1 to 3 weeks, allowing time for antineoplastic treatments to be instituted against the precipitating malignancy.[7] Ibandronate and clodronate are two other bisphosphonates that are widely used outside the US to treat HCM. Etidronate was the first bisphosphonate approved by the FDA for HCM therapy but has been replaced by these newer, more potent bisphosphonates.

### Osteonecrosis of the jaw

Osteonecrosis of the jaw (ONJ) is an uncommon but potentially serious risk of intravenous bisphosphonate therapy in patients being treated for cancer. ONJ is associated with exposed necrotic bone in the jaw, occurring in the mandible more frequently than the maxilla. Symptoms may include local pain, numbness, soft tissue swelling, drainage, tooth mobility, suprainfection and poor healing.[52] Reports of this complication first appeared in the literature in 2003. Since then the incidence of bisphosphonate-related ONJ in patients with malignancy has been reported to range between 1% and 10%, but the true incidence is unknown.[52,53] Patients with breast cancer and multiple myeloma seem to be affected predominantly.[52,54] The manner in which bisphosphonate therapy contributes to ONJ is unclear because other therapies are commonly used concurrent with or prior to the development of ONJ, including chemotherapy, radiotherapy, and corticosteroids. Precipitating factors have been associated with the state of oral and dental health, including invasive dental procedures that require bone healing (eg, tooth extractions and implants), periodontal disease, and poor oral hygiene.[43–45,55] However, a recent retrospective study of patients treated with intravenous bisphosphonates for metastatic bone disease did not find that corticosteroid use or dental and oral health status were predictors of risk for ONJ. Instead, factors such as cancer type (breast and multiple myeloma especially, followed by prostate cancer), duration of exposure to bisphosphonate therapy, and comorbid osteoarthritis or rheumatoid arthritis were significantly associated with increased risk for ONJ.[52] Several observational studies have reported that exposure to zoledronic acid has been associated with a higher risk of ONJ than therapy using sequential pamidronate followed by zoledronic acid, or pamidronate alone, in descending order of risk.[49,52] Animal models have shown that bisphosphonates may exert antitumor effects on multiple myeloma and cancers of the breast and prostate by inhibiting angiogenesis, which also has an essential role in wound healing and bone remodeling.[52] It may be that the antiangiogenic effects of the bisphosphonates contribute to ONJ risk in certain situations. In recent years, several medical, dental, and bone organizations have studied the etiology of ONJ to develop guidelines for prevention and clinical management of this problem. Effective management strategies remain to be determined and all professional groups recommend prevention of bisphosphonate-associated ONJ as the best approach. Prevention strategies include recommending that patients have a comprehensive dental examination and necessary dental work completed prior to initiating bisphosphonate therapy. Active oral infections should be treated, and sites at high risk for infection should be eliminated. There is no evidence that interrupting bisphosphonate therapy to perform invasive dental procedures will lower the risk of ONJ.[43–45,53,55]

### Pamidronate

Pamidronate (Aredia), the first of the more potent group of nitrogen-containing bisphosphonates (aminobisphosphonates), received FDA approval for treatment of HCM in 1991. In comparison studies pamidronate was proven more effective than clodronate or etidronate, restoring normocalcemia in 90% patients for a significantly longer period.[5] A 60 mg dose of pamidronate administered as a single-dose IV infusion over 2 to 24 hours is effective for patients with moderate hypercalcemia. For more severe cases, and those with a humoral component, a single dose of 90 mg is infused over 2 to 24 hours.[23] Serum creatinine is monitored before each dose to assess renal function and urine output is maintained at 2 L per day throughout treatment. Pamidronate decreases serum calcium levels by more than 1 mg/dL per dose. A minimum of 7 days should elapse to allow for full response to the initial dose of pamidronate before retreatment at the same dosing schedule is considered.[44] Fever is a frequent side effect, and induration and pain at the injection site are common with the 90 mg dose. Transient decreases in serum levels of potassium, phosphate, and magnesium may occur, but are rarely of clinical significance.[38,41,51] Osteonecrosis of the jaw may develop, as described above. Ocular adverse effects from pamidronate, such as uveitis and conjunctivitis, are infrequent but well-recognized complications.[49]

### Zoledronic acid

Zoledronic acid (Zometa) is a third-generation aminobisphosphonate that currently is the most potent bisphosphonate in use in the US. Zoledronic acid received FDA approval for treatment of HCM in 2001. It is indicated for use in patients with multiple myeloma and in patients with documented bone metastases from solid tumors in conjunction with standard antineoplastic therapy. Patients with prostate cancer should have demonstrated disease progression after treatment with at least one hormonal agent before beginning zoledronic acid.[45] In comparison with pamidronate, zoledronic acid has the advantage of rapid and simpler administration (15 minutes vs 2 hours for infusions), and studies have shown that zoledronic acid is significantly more effective than pamidronate in achieving normocalcemia, providing a higher response rate and faster onset and longer duration of action.[5,7]

Zoledronic acid is excreted intact primarily via the kidney and is associated with renal toxicity that may be greater in patients with impaired renal function. Treatment in patients with severe renal impairment is not recommended; careful consideration of the risks and benefits of instituting bisphosphonate therapy is required for patients with HCM complicated by severe renal impairment. Renal function is carefully monitored in all patients by obtaining serum creatinine levels before each dose of zoledronic acid and urine output is maintained at 2 L per day throughout treatment. Dose adjustments are not necessary prior to treatment initiation in patients with mild-to-moderate renal impairment (serum creatinine < 4.5 mg/dL).[45] The maximum recommended dose of zoledronic acid for HCM therapy is 4 mg delivered as a single-dose IV infusion over no less than 15 minutes. Retreatment with the 4 mg dose may be considered after a minimum period of 7 days to allow for full response to the initial dose. Dose reduction or withholding of zoledronic acid is based on the extent of renal dysfunction as indicated by increases in serum creatinine; special attention should be paid to geriatric patients because renal dysfunction occurs more commonly in the elderly.[45] Standard hypercalcemia-related metabolic parameters, such as serum levels of calcium, phosphate, and magnesium, should be monitored regularly following initiation of therapy with zoledronic acid. Hypocalcemia, hypophosphatemia, or hypomagnesemia may occur and may require short-term supplemental therapy. Side effects associated with zoledronate infusion include flu-like syndrome consisting of fever, chills, flushing, bone pain and/or arthralgias, and myalgias, and occasionally infusion site reaction. Ocular inflammation such as uveitis and scleritis has been reported.[45,49]

Osteonecrosis of the jaw has increasingly been reported in association with intravenous bisphosphonates, most commonly with zoledronic acid. Prevention measures are recommended. See above discussion of ONJ. Severe and occasionally incapacitating bone, joint, and/or muscle pain have also been reported. The time to onset of pain symptoms varied from 1 day to several months after starting bisphosphonate infusions; severe symptoms required discontinuation of therapy.[45]

## Ibandronate

Ibandronate (Bondronat) is a third-generation aminobisphosphonate and is a derivative of pamidronate that was licensed in the European Union in 1997 for treatment of HCM.[48,56] A comparative study demonstrated that ibandronate was at least equal to pamidronate in terms of efficacy in decreasing serum calcium and was associated with a longer duration of response than pamidronate. The doses recommended depend on the baseline serum calcium level: 2 mg for patients with moderate hypercalcemia and 4 mg for those with severe hypercalcemia in a single 1-hour IV infusion. A phase II study comparing the renal safety profiles of ibandronate 6 mg infused over either 15 minutes or 60 minutes found that a single infusion of 6 mg over 15 minutes every 3 to 4 weeks is effective and well tolerated (indicated by serum creatinine and creatinine clearance levels) as a treatment for hypercalcemia and other complications of malignant bone disease, such as fractures and bone pain.[48] The time to normalization of the serum calcium concentration varies between 2 and 7 days, with 4 days being usual in most patients. The median time to relapse, indicated by increasing serum calcium concentration, is 26 days and is similar for all doses. Patients with local osteolytic tumors, such as breast cancer and multiple myeloma, had a better hypocalcemic response to ibandronate than patients with predominantly humorally induced hypercalcemia.[24] Tolerability to ibandronate is excellent. The renal safety profile is similar to that of placebo so that mandatory monitoring of renal function prior to each ibandronate infusion is not required. Only patients with severe renal impairment require dose reductions.[43,48,56] Adverse reactions are minor and rarely require treatment. Reported side effects include fever, hypocalcemia, and hypophosphatemia, and less commonly, flu-like symptoms and GI disturbance.[42]

## Clodronate

Clodronate (Bonefos) is a first generation nonnitrogenous bisphosphonate (in the same family as etidronate) and possesses intermediate potency. Except in the US, clodronate is approved worldwide for oral or IV administration to treat tumor-induced osteolysis and hypercalcemia and to decrease bone pain.[43,46] Compared with the nitrogenous amino-bisphosphonates (pamidronate and zoledronic acid), clodronate appears to suppress bone remodeling by a different mechanism and is not usually associated with ONJ. Clodronate has a very high affinity for bone tissue, and is rapidly absorbed onto the bone surface. About 50% of the drug is excreted unchanged by the kidney and therapy should be discontinued if renal function deteriorates during treatment.[57] Clodronate is administered as an intravenous infusion of 300 mg over no less than 2 hours once a day; rapid infusions may compromise renal function in patients with diminished renal reserves.[5] The drug may be given daily for up to 7 days, but normal calcium levels are generally achieved with 2 to 5 days of treatment. A single dose of 1500 mg infused over 4 hours has been found to be as effective as daily 300 mg infusions repeated for 5 days.[5,24,46] Treatment with oral clodronate following intravenous infusion has been found to prolong the duration of action. Oral clodronate is taken at least 2 hours before or after meals in doses of 1600 mg to 2400 mg in 1 or 2 divided doses per day, not to exceed a daily dose of 3200 mg.[46] An advantage of clodronate is that it can be given as a subcutaneous infusion for bone pain in the palliative care setting.[58] The principal side effect of clodronate is mild local reaction; hypophosphatemia has also been reported.[23]

Failure to respond to bisphosphonate therapy is a poor prognostic feature in the treatment of HCM, but older antihypercalcemic agents that were commonly used before the advent of bisphosphonates may be attempted.

## OTHER ANTIHYPERCALCEMIC THERAPIES

### Plicamycin

Plicamycin (Mithramycin), a cytotoxic antibiotic, was the mainstay of therapy for tumor-induced hypercalcemia before the bisphosphonates became available. Now its toxicity profile and low efficacy restrict its use to patients with HCM who have failed to respond to IV bisphosphonates or their use was contraindicated.[5,17,49] Plicamycin is more potent than calcitonin, producing a direct toxic effect on osteoclasts by blocking RNA synthesis. The usual dose is 25 mcg/kg/day infused slowly over 4 to 6 hours for 3 to 8 doses.[4] Plicamycin is an irritant drug, and is ideally administered through a central IV line.[41] It reduces serum calcium levels within 12 hours of treatment, producing a peak effect at 48 hours.[23] It is used with caution because it has significant cumulative side effects, including thrombocytopenia, nausea and vomiting, hypotension, and renal, hepatic, and neurotoxicities.[9]

### Gallium nitrate

Gallium nitrate was originally developed as a chemotherapy agent and was found to produce hypocalcemic effects in people being treated for lymphoma. Researchers do not fully understand its mechanism of action, but it appears to have multiple effects on the skeleton without being cytotoxic to bone.[47] Randomized studies have shown that gallium nitrate has high efficacy in the treatment of HCM and is significantly superior to calcitonin, etidronate, and pamidronate, restoring normocalcemia in 75% to 85% of patients.[42,47,49] The drug is initiated only after the patient has been rehydrated to maintain urinary output at 2 L per day throughout treatment. Gallium nitrate is administered by continuous IV infusion over 5 days in a daily dose of 200 mg/m$^2$.[5,59] Renal toxicity, which occurs in 10% of patients, is the major side effect; concurrent use of nephrotoxic drugs should be avoided. The usefulness of gallium nitrate is limited by the need for continuous intravenous administration over a period of 5 days and the potential for nephrotoxicity. It can be used effectively in patients who are refractory to the bisphosphonates, particularly those with recurrent HCM.[23,49] It may be a more effective antihypercalcemic agent for cancers associated with higher levels of PTHrP[5] and may be used in treating hypercalcemia associated with tamoxifen flare.[59]

### Corticosteroids

Glucocorticoids are effective as first-line agents in calcitriol-mediated hypercalcemia associated with steroid-sensitive hematological malignancies, such as lymphoma, leukemia, and multiple myeloma.[41] They act to decrease 1,25-dihydroxyvitamin $D_3$ production, negating calcitriol-induced calcium absorption from the gut and increasing urinary calcium excretion. The glucocorticoids are also incorporated into antineoplastic regimens for lymphoid malignancies and multiple myeloma, blocking production of those factors responsible for the hypercalcemia. They have no role in treating HCM in patients with solid tumors.[5] The minimum effective dose is uncertain, but generally between 40 and 100 mg oral prednisone per day is used.[5,17] Intravenous hydrocortisone (100–300 mg daily) for 3 to 7 days may also be an option.[40] Long-term use of steroids can produce undesirable side effects, including immunosuppression, hyperglycemia, hypokalemia, GI hemorrhage, bone destruction, and muscle wasting.[41]

### Phosphate replacement

Most patients with HCM will develop hypophosphatemia at some point during the course of the hypercalcemia due to several factors, including decreased food intake, saline diuresis, use of loop diuretics, PTHrP-stimulated renal phosphate excretion, and the hypercalcemia itself. Hypophosphatemia contributes to hypercalcemia by stimulating increased osteoclastic activity and release of calcium from bone. Elevating serum phosphorus levels helps to lower the serum calcium concentration because calcium and phosphorus are regulated in inverse proportion to one another.[22]

Phosphorus is replaced orally or administered through a nasogastric tube as neutral phosphate with the goal of maintaining the serum phosphorus concentration in the range of 2.5 to 3.0 mg/dL.[7] Oral phosphate is usually taken in doses of 250 to 375 mg 4 times a day to minimize the potential for hyperphosphatemia and is contraindicated with renal failure. Diarrhea is a dose-limiting side effect of oral phosphate administration but initially may counteract the constipation that patients experience secondary to hypercalcemia.[42] Patients should avoid magnesium- and aluminum-containing antacids during phosphate replacement because they bind to phosphate.[21] Intravenous phosphorus replacement is very effective at rapidly decreasing serum calcium levels, but the treatment is toxic and very dangerous. Its use should be reserved for severe life-threatening HCM when oral or nasogastric administration is not possible. Phosphorus infusion can cause severe hypocalcemia, acute renal failure, hypotension, seizures, and precipitation of calcium-phosphate complexes in tissues throughout the body.[7,22]

### Dialysis

Patients with HCM, renal failure, and/or severe congestive heart failure who cannot handle aggressive saline hydration may be appropriate candidates for treatment with either hemodialysis or peritoneal dialysis to correct the hypercalcemia.[7,22,36] In general, dialysis is considered as an initial hypocalcemic therapy only for those patients whose malignancies are expected to respond favorably to antineoplastic treatments. Peritoneal dialysis with calcium-free dialysis fluid can remove 200 to 500 mg of calcium in 24 to 48 hours, which lowers serum calcium concentration by 3 to 12 mg/dL. Along with calcium, large quantities of phosphate are lost during dialysis, so serum phosphate levels should be measured after each dialysis session and supplemented in the dialysate fluid or diet as needed.[22,42] Occasionally, patients with severe acute HCM may require emergency dialysis to quickly lower serum calcium levels and prevent cardiac arrhythmias or severe neurological complications.

### Mobilization and dietary restriction

Whenever possible, weight-bearing ambulation is encouraged to counteract the effects of immobility on bone that include increased bone resorption and release of calcium into the circulation. For patients who must remain in bed, active resistive exercises coupled with a pain management program may be helpful in controlling loss of calcium from bone. Dietary restriction of calcium is usually not necessary in treating HCM because negative feedback mechanisms reduce calcium absorption from the gut in most hypercalcemic patients. The exception is patients experiencing calcitriol-mediated hypercalcemia, in which case, patients should avoid dietary calcium.

## FUTURE DIRECTIONS IN THE MANAGEMENT OF HYPERCALCEMIA OF MALIGNANCY

Although bisphosphonates have supplanted all other therapeutic agents and can normalize calcium in more than 90% of patients with HCM, their efficacy is reduced when hypercalcemia recurs. Therapies that focus on inhibiting tumor-induced bone resorption by interrupting the RANKL/RANK signaling pathway and neutralizing the effects of PTHrP are being studied in mouse models or early clinical trials.[5,15,32] One approach under investigation is the use of soluble recombinant OPG. OPG is the natural decoy receptor for RANK and a powerful inhibitor of bone resorption. It prevents RANKL from binding with its receptor (RANK) to signal increased osteoclastic activity. OPG has been shown to reverse HHM in a mouse model. No human clinical trials of OPG in treating HCM have been reported. However, a phase I study in patients with bone metastases from myeloma or breast cancer demonstrated potent antiresorptive effects of OPG on bone and decreased serum calcium concentration.[5] Targeting RANKL or PTHrP with monoclonal antibodies may be promising approaches to counteracting mechanisms responsible for HCM. Denosumab, a new fully human monoclonal antibody that specifically targets RANKL, is being studied in patients with normal serum calcium levels who have breast cancer, prostate cancer, other solid tumors, or multiple myeloma as a therapy to prevent skeletal-related events and in patients with breast and prostate cancers as a treatment for existing bone metastases.[5] Denosumab is in early trials in patient with them that has not responded to intravenous bisphosphonates.[60] In mouse studies, antibodies directed against PTHrP were effective in reversing HHM and improving nutritional status.[5,15] Monoclonal antibodies have the advantage of being administered subcutaneously and do not produce renal side effects, but antibodies against them may develop with prolonged use. Currently, antibodies are being studied in humans in relation to limiting bone destruction by metastatic tumors.

Another approach that holds potential for treating HHM is to target the CaSR. The CaSR contributes to HHM by mediating growth signals between tumor and bone that leads to osteolysis.[21] Two classes of agents that antagonize or neutralize the CaSR have been developed. The first class of drugs is the calcimimetics, including cinacalcet, which binds to the receptor and increases the sensitivity of the CaSR to extracellular calcium. PTH secretion diminishes and serum calcium levels are lowered.[20,36] Calcimimetics have been approved for the treatment of hyperparathyroidism in end-stage renal disease and for parathyroid cancer. A second class of drugs that targets the CaSR is the calcilytics. Calcilytic agents have been proposed as an anabolic therapy for osteoporosis and act similarly to injectable PTH, though these drugs have not yet been approved for clinical use. By preventing calcium-stimulated activation of the CaSR and subsequent release of PTHrP by tumor cells, calcimimetics and calcilytics may interrupt the cycle of bone destruction and are potentially useful for the prevention and treatment of bone metastases.[26]

## NURSING MANAGEMENT

### OVERVIEW

Nursing management in the care of patients with HCM is multifaceted and is directed at prevention, early detection, treatment and side effect management, safety measures, quality of life issues, and support of patients and family. Table 39-6[3,5,37,38] presents an overview of nursing management. It is essential that nurses know what types of cancers

**TABLE 39-6**

**Nursing Management of Hypercalemia of Malignancy**

| Issue | Nursing Measures |
|---|---|
| **Early detection of HCM** | Identify patients at risk: Obtain history related to type of cancer, presence of bone metastases, and treatment regimens |
| | Check vital signs, serum electrolytes and blood chemistries (with particular attention to calcium, phosphorus; albumin, BUN, creatinine levels); urinary calcium, and electrocardiogram, if done |
| | Review medications and supplements to identify drugs and vitamins that may contribute to hypercalcemia and should be discontinued (eg, thiazide diuretics, vitamins A and D) |
| | Evaluate for early signs of hypercalcemia (see Table 39-3) |
| | Conduct physical assessment, looking for signs of dehydration: poor skin turgor, dry mucous membranes, rapid, weak pulse, weight loss, orthostatic hypotension |
| | Assess muscle strength, neurological, and mental status; record baseline |
| | **Prevention measures for high-risk patients** |
| **Hydration** | Explain need for maintaining oral fluid intake of 3 L per day |
| **Mobilization** | Emphasize importance of weight-bearing activity |
| | Coordinate an activity and exercise regimen based on the patient's physical ability and the physician's orders; patients unable to ambulate can be helped to stand at the bedside 4–6 times a day |
| | Encourage patients who are at home to ambulate as much as possible |
| | Provide assistive devices as necessary: eg, cane, walker, handrails |
| | Patients on bedrest: Provide active resistive exercises every hour while awake; couple with a pain management program if necessary |
| | Pain management: Achieve a narcotic-sedation level that promotes increased physical activity, rather than oversedation |
| **Supportive nursing care** | Supportive care for patients with HCM focuses on:<br>Evaluating treatment effectiveness and side effects |
| | Managing fluid and electrolyte imbalances |
| | Assessing mental status changes, gastrointestinal disturbances, alterations in renal and cardiac function |
| | Instituting safety measures, pain management, comfort measures |
| | Providing emotional support to the patient and caregivers |
| **Antihypercalcemic therapy** | Administer fluids and hypocalcemic agents as ordered and observe for side effects (see Table 39-5) |
| | Monitor daily serum calcium levels to evaluate treatment response |
| | Observe for clinical manifestations related to HCM (see Table 39-3) |
| | Assess for bone pain and pathological fractures; administer analgesics as ordered |
| **Fluid and electrolyte balance** | Mild HCM:<br>Encourage oral fluid intake of 2–4 L/day if possible |
| | Correction of fluid volume depletion: administer saline infusion as ordered; monitor blood pressure, pulse, breathe sounds throughout infusion period; measure intake and output q 2 hours for first 24 hours, then every 4–8 hours; check for signs of fluid overload (rales, shortness of breath, weight gain, peripheral edema, distended neck veins) every 4 hours and as necessary |
| | Record daily weights |
| | Administer loop diuretics after rehydration, as ordered; thiazide diuretics are contraindicated, as they impair renal excretion of calcium |
| | Monitor electrolytes daily for decreases in serum calcium, sodium, potassium, phosphorus, and magnesium |
| | Report and correct hypokalemia, hypophosphatemia, and hypomagnesemia, as ordered |
| **Renal function** | Assess for declining renal function: increases in BUN and creatinine; oliguria, and anuria |

*(Continued)*

**TABLE 39-6**

**Nursing Management of Hypercalemia of Malignancy (Continued)**

| Issue | Nursing Measures |
|---|---|
| **Cardiac changes** | Monitor heart rate and rhythm for bradycardia and arrythmias; observe electrocardiogram for delayed cardiac conduction<br>Reduce digoxin doses as ordered |
| **Mental status alterations** | Monitor for lethargy, restlessness, disorientation, personality changes, progressive changes in level of consciousness<br>Institute falls, safety, and seizure precautions as per protocols |
| **Gastrointestinal disturbances** | Administer antiemetics for nausea and vomiting and stool softeners and laxatives for constipation, as ordered |
| **Patient and family teaching and advocacy** | Teaching focuses on several areas of self-care, including: understanding preventive measures (ie, ensuring adequate fluid and salt intake, maintaining weight-bearing activities), and the importance of early therapeutic interventions; recognizing and reporting conditions that prevent oral intake or increase fluid loss (eg, vomiting, diarrhea, fever); recognizing and reporting manifestations of HCM (eg, anorexia, lethargy, nausea, vomiting, constipation, excessive thirst); understanding the importance of following prescribed medical regimens; avoiding drugs and supplements that potentiate HCM and nephrotoxicity; and adhering to follow-up schedules; managing pain and coping with changes in mental status<br>Nurses provide emotional support, help to identify and support coping strategies, communicate acceptance of patients' beliefs, and act as patient advocates in discussions related to discontinuing antihypercalcemic therapies, and instituting palliative and comfort care, as appropriate |

*Note*: Based on information from National Cancer Institute[3]; Morton and Lipton[5]; Kaplan.[11]
Abbreviations: BUN, blood urea nitrogen; HCM, hypercalemia of malignancy; L, liter.
*Source*: Adapted with permission from Kaplan.[11] Copyright © 2006 by the Oncology Nursing Society.

are associated with elevated risks for HCM so they have a raised awareness when a patient with a cancer history demonstrates nonspecific signs and symptoms that may indicate early HCM. Those patients require continual assessment of their physical, mental, and renal status, and frequent monitoring of their serum calcium and albumin levels in order to distinguish between disease and treatment effects and the manifestations of developing hypercalcemia. Although cancer-induced hypercalcemia may not be preventable, early recognition and prompt treatment may prevent it from becoming a life-threatening oncologic emergency.

Patients with mild or asymptomatic HCM and those who have achieved normocalcemia may be followed on an outpatient basis. Renal function and serum calcium levels of patients receiving antihypercalcemic therapy are monitored daily until the calcium concentration normalizes, and then weekly (or more frequently, as needed) to assess the need for further treatment. Serum concentrations of potassium, magnesium, and phosphate may decline steeply as calcium levels are corrected and are monitored to determine the need for supplementation.[5,11,39] The need for other laboratory tests depends on the individual's clinical condition and response to therapy.

Supportive nursing care of the patient with hypercalcemia is multifocal. Nurses are responsible for managing fluid and electrolyte imbalances, evaluating treatment effectiveness and side effects, and monitoring and managing changes in mental status, GI disturbances, and alterations in renal and cardiac function. They also coordinate appropriate weight-bearing or exercise regimens for patients, institute safety measures and falls prevention strategies, manage pain, and provide comfort and emotional support to patients and caregivers.[11,37]

## PATIENT AND CAREGIVER EDUCATION

Education of patients and caregivers is directed toward providing them with information needed to prevent, recognize, and manage the manifestations of HCM in their loved one. Nurses teach them to (a) practice preventive measures, such as maintaining adequate hydration and safe weight-bearing activities; (b) recognize and report any condition, such as diarrhea or vomiting, which can contribute to fluid loss and exacerbate dehydration; and (c) recognize and report the nonspecific manifestations of hypercalcemia, such as anorexia, nausea, constipation, and lethargy. Essential information is provided about safety precautions, including falls prevention strategies, the need for close observation of confused or restless patients, and the need for careful movement and transfers of bed-bound patients to decrease the risk of pathological fractures. Patients and caregivers receive instructions about the importance of taking medications as prescribed, avoiding drugs and vitamin supplements that can potentiate hypercalcemia, and methods for managing pain, ideally without oversedating hypercalcemic patients, who may already be lethargic or confused.

## END-OF-LIFE CONSIDERATIONS

Patients and caregivers may have to face profound decisions regarding initiating or continuing antihypercalcemic treatment. Treatment may not be indicated for all patients with tumor-induced hypercalcemia as some may be close to the end of life. Patients and their caregivers may have to cope with difficult decisions between beginning antihypercalcemic treatment, or allowing the patient to return home at the end of life with palliative measures to manage the side effects of hypercalcemia.

In the situations where hypercalcemia develops after antineoplastic therapies have been completed, or where antineoplastic therapies were not effective in controlling the precipitating malignancy, hypercalcemia is likely to recur as the disease progresses. The patient usually dies from renal failure or cardiac arrhthymias secondary to hypercalcemia or from progressive disease.[15] Severe hypercalcemia depresses cerebral function and leads to coma. The decision not to begin treatment or to discontinue treatment may be appropriate in order to spare the patient from further suffering and futile treatments, especially if the patient is expected to soon become comatose and die.

Palliative bisphosphonate therapy can be instituted at the end of life to ameliorate or reverse the many unpleasant and distressing side effects that accompany the hypercalcemic state, such as anorexia, nausea, vomiting, constipation, and confusion. The bisphosphonates and calcitonin also provide an analgesic effect that reduces bone pain.[58] If the patient's response to bisphosphonate therapy is inadequate, alternative antiresorptive therapy can be attempted using gallium nitrate or plicamycin.[5] Second-line, noninvasive therapies, such as subcutaneous calcitonin and oral bisphosphonates, are also an option in the palliative care setting and their use can improve end-of-life quality.[58] Nurses can provide patients with comfort measures to alleviate distressing symptoms while offering their caregivers continuing support, reassurance, and solace as they cope with decisions about continuing treatment and face the progressive deterioration and the end of their loved one's life.

## CONCLUSION

Tumor-induced hypercalcemia results from disruption of normal calcium homeostasis and impaired renal excretion of calcium. Early signs and symptoms of HCM are general and nonspecific and can be difficult to distinguish from disease- or treatment-related side effects. It is essential that nurses recognize which malignancies are associated with increased risk and understand the pathological mechanisms that can precipitate and/or contribute to HCM. Successful clinical management depends on correcting the abnormalities of bone, kidney, and intestinal calcium absorption associated with HCM while waiting for antineoplastic therapies to take effect. Essential components of antihypercalcemic treatment include instituting preventive measures, controlling the precipitating malignancy, reversing dehydration, and inhibiting bone resorption. Knowledge of the rationales for the various treatment modalities will assist nurses in implementing antihypercalcemic treatments, evaluating treatment effectiveness and side effects, and instituting pain management and safety and comfort measures. Although tumor-induced hypercalcemia may not be preventable, early recognition and appropriate treatment may deter it from becoming a life-threatening oncologic complication.

## REFERENCES


1. Lamy O, Jenzer-Closut A, Burckhardt P. Hypercalcemia of malignancy: an undiagnosed and undertreated disease. *J Intern Med.* 2001; 250:73–79.
2. Jibrin IM, Lawrence GD, Miller CB. Hypercalcemia of malignancy in hospitalized patients. *Hosp Phys.* 2006;42:29–35.
3. National Cancer Institute. Hypercalcemia (PDQ): 2008. http://www.cancer.gov/cancerinfo/pdq/supportivecare/hypercalcemia/HealthProfessional. Accessed January 15, 2010.
4. Carroll MF, Schade DS. A practical approach to hypercalcemia. *Am Fam Phys.* 2003;67:1959–1966.
5. Morton AR, Lipton A. Hypercalcemia. In: Abeloff MD, Armitage JO, Niederhuber JE, Kastan MB, McKenna WG, eds. *Abeloff: Abeloff's Clinical Oncology.* 4th ed. Philadelphia, PA: Churchill Livingstone/Elsevier. 2008:739–748.
6. Mundy G. Hypercalcemia. In: Mundy G, ed. *Bone Remodeling and Its Disorders.* 2nd ed. London: Martin Dunitz; 1999:107–122.
7. Stewart AF. Hypercalcemia associated with cancer. *N Eng J Med.* 2005;352:373–379.
8. Heys SD, Smith IA, Eremin O. Hypercalcemia in patients with cancer: aetiology and treatment. *Eur J Surg Oncol.* 1998;24:139–142.
9. Grill V, Martin TJ. Hypercalcemia of malignancy. *Rev Endocr Metabolic Disord.* 2000;1:253–263.
10. Coleman RE, Rubens RD. Bone metastases. In: Abeloff MD, Armitage JO, Niederhuber JE, Kastan MB, McKenna WG, eds. *Clinical Oncology.* 3rd ed. Philadelphia, PA: Elsevier Churchill Livingstone; 2004:1091–1128.
11. Kaplan M. Hypercalcemia of malignancy. In: Kaplan M, ed. *Understanding and Managing Oncologic Emergencies: A Resource for Nurses.* Pittsburgh, PA: Oncology Nursing Society; 2006:51–97.
12. Kvols LK. Neoplasms of the diffuse endocrine system. In: Kufe DW, Pollock RE, Weichselbaum RR, et al, eds. *Holland-Frei Cancer Medicine.* 6th ed. Hamilton, ON: BC Decker; 2003:1275–1323.
13. Mundy GR. Metastasis to bone: causes, consequences and therapeutic options. *Nat Rev Cancer.* 2002;2:584–593.
14. Munshi NC, Anderson KC. Plasma cell neoplasms. In: DeVita VT, Hellman S, Rosenberg SA, eds. *Cancer: Principles and Practice of*

*Oncology*. 7th ed. Philadelphia, PA: Lippincott Williams & Wilkins; 2005:2160–2164.
15. Yeung S-C J, Gagel RF. Endocrine complications and paraneoplastic syndromes. In: Kufe DW, Pollock RE, Weichselbaum RR, et al, eds. *Holland-Frei Cancer Medicine*. 6th ed. Hamilton, ON: BC Decker; 2003:2609–2622.
16. Bone H. Bone disease and malignancy. In: Hosking D, Ringe J, eds. *Treatment of Metabolic Bone Disease: Management Strategy and Drug Therapy*. London: Martin Dunitz; 2000:57–74.
17. Moe SM. Disorders involving calcium, phosphorus, and magnesium. *Prim Care Clin Office Pract*. 2008;35:215–237.
18. Adler C-P. Bones and bone tissue. In: Adler C-P, ed. *Bone Diseases: Macroscopic, Histological, and Radiological Diagnosis of Structural Changes in the Skeleton*. Berlin and New York: Springer; 2000:1–11.
19. Mundy GR, Guise TA. Hormonal control of calcium homeostasis. *Clin Chem*. 1999;45:1347–1352.
20. Chattapadhyay N. Effects of calcium-sensing receptor on the secretion of parathyroid hormone-related peptide and its impact on humoral hypercalcemia of malignancy. *Am J Physiol Endocrinol Metab*. 2006;290:E761–E770.
21. Agraharkar M, Dellinger DO. Hypercalcemia. 2006. http://www.emedicine.com/med/topic1068.htm. Accessed January 15, 2010.
22. Potts JT Jr. Diseases of the parathyroid gland and other hyper- and hypocalcemic disorders. In: Fauci AS, Braunwald E, Kasper DL, et al, eds. *Harrison's Principles of Internal Medicine*. 17th ed. New York, NY: McGraw-Hill Medical; 2008:2377–2396.
23. Fojo AT. Metabolic emergencies. In: DeVita VT, Hellman S, Rosenberg SA, eds. *Cancer: Principles and Practice of Oncology*. 7th ed. Philadelphia, PA: Lippincott Williams & Wilkins; 2005:2292–2300.
24. Body JJ. Hypercalcemia of malignancy. *Semin Nephrol*. 2004; 24:48–54.
25. Ikeda K, Ohno H, Hane M, et al. Development of a sensitive two-site immunoradiometric assay for parathyroid hormone-related peptide: evidence for elevated levels in plasma from patients with adult-T-cell leukemia/lymphoma and B-cell lymphoma. *J Clin Endocrinol Metab*. 1994;79:1322–1327.
26. Kingsley LA, Fournier PGJ, Chirgwin JM, Guise TA. Molecular biology of bone metastases. *Mol Cancer Ther*. 2007;6:2609–2617.
27. Lerner UH. New molecules in the tumor necrosis factor ligand and receptor superfamilies with importance for physiological and pathological bone resorption. *Crit Rev Oral Biol Med*. 2004;15:64–81.
28. Phadke PA, Mercer RR, Harms JF, et al. Kinetics of metastatic breast cancer cell trafficking in bone. *Clin Cancer Res*. 2006;12:1431–1440.
29. Roodman GD. Mechanisms for bone metastases. *N Eng J Med*. 2004;350: 1655–1664.
30. Davis EO. Stuck on the TRAIL of osteoclast differentiation. *Blood*. 2004;104:1914–1915.
31. Teitelbaum SL. Bone resorption by osteoclasts. *Science*. 2000;289: 1504–1508.
32. Hofbauer LZ, Schoppet M. Clinical implications of the osteoprotegerin/RANKL/ RANK system for bone and vascular diseases. *JAMA*. 2004;292:490–495.
33. Oyajobi BO. Multiple myeloma/hypercalcemia. *Arthritis Res Ther*. 2007;9(suppl 1):S4. http://arthritis-research.com/content/9/S1/S4. Accessed January 15, 2010.
34. Sezer O, Heider U, Zavrski I, Kuhne CA, Hofbauer LC. RANK ligand and osteoprotegerin in myeloma bone disease. *Blood*. 2003;101: 2094–2098.
35. Kyle RA, Rajkumar SV. Drug therapy: multiple myeloma. *N Eng J Med*. 2004;351:1860–1873.
36. Hemphill RH. Hypercalcemia. 2007. http://www.emedicine.com/emerg/topic260.htm. Accessed January 15, 2010.
37. Pearson KE. Tumor-induced hypercalcemia. In: Chernecky CC, Murphy-Ende K, eds. *Acute Care Oncology Nursing*. 2nd ed. St. Louis, MO: Saunders/Elsevier; 2009:284–297.
38. Richerson MT. Electrolyte imbalances: hypercalcemia. In: Yarbro CH, Frogge MH, Goodman M, eds. *Cancer Symptom Management*. 3rd ed. Sudbury, MA: Jones and Bartlett; 2004:440–453.
39. Morton AR, Ritch PS. Hypercalcemia. In: Berger AM, Portenoy RK, Weissman DE, eds. *Principles and Practice of Palliative Care and Supportive Oncology*. 2nd ed. Philadelphia, PA: Lippincott Williams & Wilkins; 2002:493–507.
40. Khosla S. Hypercalcemia and hypocalcemia. In: Fauci AS, Braunwald E, Kasper DL, et al, eds. *Harrison's Principles of Internal Medicine*. 17th ed. New York, NY: McGraw-Hill Medical; 2008:285–287.
41. Davidson TG. Conventional treatment of hypercalcemia of malignancy. *Am J Health Syst Pharm*. 2001;58(suppl 3):S8-S15.
42. Hussein M, Cullen K. Metabolic emergencies. In: Johnston PG, Spence RAJ, eds. *Oncologic Emergencies*. Oxford: Oxford University Press; 2002:51–73.
43. Kyle RA, Yee GC, Somerfield MR, et al. American Society of Clinical Oncology 2007 Clinical Practice Guideline update on the role of bisphosphonates in multiple myeloma. *J Clin Oncol*. 2007;25:2464–2472.
44. Aredia (pamidronate). [package insert]. East Hanover, NJ: Novartis Pharmaceuticals; 2008.
45. Zometa (zoledronic acid). [package insert]. East Hanover, NJ: Novartis Pharmaceuticals; 2008.
46. Cancer Care Ontario, Canada. http://www.cancercare.on.ca/pdfdrugs/clodronate.pdf. Revised 2006/2007. Accessed January 15, 2010.
47. Leyland-Jones B. Treating cancer-related hypercalcemia with gallium nitrate. *J Support Oncol*. 2004;2:509–516.
48. Von Moos R, Caspar CB, Thürlimann B, et al. Renal safety profiles of ibandronate 6 mg infused over 15 and 60 min: a randomized, open-label study. *Ann Oncol*. 2008;19:1266–1270.
49. Pecherstorfer M, Brenner K, Zojer N. Current management strategies for hypercalcemia. *Treat Endocrinol*. 2003;2:273–292.
50. Visser EJ. A review of calcitonin and its use in the treatment of acute pain. *Acute Pain*. 2005;7:185–189.
51. Spratto GR, Woods AL. *PDR: Nurses Drug Handbook*. 2008 ed. Montvale, NJ: Thomson Healthcare; 2007.
52. Estilo CL, Van Poznak CH, Williams T, et al. Osteonecrosis of the maxilla and mandible in patients with advanced cancer treated with bisphosphonate therapy. *Oncologist*. 2008;13:911–920.
53. Khosla S, Burr D, Cauley J, et al. Bisphosphonate-associated osteonecrosis of the jaw: report of a task force of the American Society for Bone and Mineral Research. *J Bone Min Res*. 2007;22:1479–1489.
54. Hoff AO, Toth BB, Altundag, K, et al. Frequency and risk factors associated with osteoporosis of the jaw in cancer patients treated with intravenous bisphosphonates. *J Bone Min Res*. 2008;23:826–836.
55. Ruggiero S, Gralow J, Marx RE, et al. Practical guidelines for the prevention, diagnosis, and treatment of osteonecrosis of the jaw in patients with cancer. *J Oncol Pract*. 2006;2:7–14.
56. Henrich D, Hoffmann M, Uppenkamp M, Bergner R. Ibandronate for the treatment of hypercalcemia or nephrocalcinosis in patients with multiple myeloma and acute renal failure: case reports. *Acta Haematol*. 2006;116:165–172.
57. Diel IJ, Fogelman I, Al-Nawas B, et al. Pathophysiology, risk factors and management of bisphosphonate-associated osteonecrosis of the jaw: is there a diverse relationship of amino- and non-aminobisphosphonates? *Crit Reviews Hematol Oncol*. 2007;64:198–207.
58. Kovacs CS, MacDonald SM, Chik CL, Bruera E. Hypercalcemia of malignancy in the palliative care patient: a treatment strategy. *J Symptom Manage*. 1995;10:224–232.
59. Arumugam GP, Sundravel S, Shanthi P, Sachdanandam P. Tamoxifen flare hypercalcemia: an additional support for gallium nitrate usage. *J Bone Miner Metab*. 2006;24:243–247.
60. Study of Denosumab in the treatment of hypercalcemia of malignancy in sublects with elevated serum calcium. http://clinicaltrials.gov/ct2/show/NCT00896454. Updated December 10, 2009. Accessed January 15, 2010.

CHAPTER 40

Colleen O'Leary, RN, MSN, AOCNS®

# Septic Shock

## SCOPE OF THE PROBLEM

There are 5 types of shock: hypovolemic, cardiogenic, anaphylactic, neurogenic, and septic shock. Hypovolemic shock is a result of decreased intravascular volume. Cardiogenic shock results from the heart's impaired ability to pump blood adequately. Anaphylactic, neurogenic, and septic shock are all considered distributive or vasogenic in that they are the result of an abnormality in the vascular system. Septic shock is a complex condition occurring when overwhelming infection leads to low blood pressure, low blood flow, altered coagulation, and impaired clot breakdown. With the highest mortality rate of any type of shock, septic shock is a potentially life-threatening oncologic emergency that leads to inadequate tissue perfusion, cellular ischemia, cellular hypoxia, and organ or system failure.

### DEFINITIONS

The classic definitions of the spectrum of sepsis were developed by Roger C. Bone and associates of the American College of Chest Physicians (ACCP) and the Society of Critical Care Medicine (SCCM) in 1992.[1] Although still widely held, an attempt to update these definitions was completed in 2001 by the SCCM, ACCP, European Society of Intensive Care Medicine (ESICM), American Thoracic Society (ATS), and the Surgical Infection Society (SIS) to reflect a better understanding of the pathophysiology of this syndrome.[2] This spectrum of sepsis includes the continuum of infection/bacteremia, systemic inflammatory response syndrome (SIRS), sepsis, severe sepsis, septic shock, and multiple organ dysfunction syndrome (MODS) (see Table 40-1). The first stage, *infection*, is defined as a microbial phenomenon caused by the invasion of normally sterile tissue, fluid, or body cavities by pathogenic or potentially pathogenic microorganisms.[2] *Bacteremia* is the presence of one of these viable bacteria in the blood. The next stage, SIRS, is a continuum of escalating stages in response to a variety of severe clinical insults. This response is manifested by 2 or more specific physical and laboratory findings. These findings include temperature greater than 100.4°F or less than 96.8°F, heart rate greater than 90 beats per minute, respiratory rate greater than 20 breaths per minute or $PaCO_2$ less than 32 mm Hg, and white blood cell count greater than 12,000 cells/mm$^3$ or less than 4000 cells/mm$^3$ or greater than 10% immature cells (bands).[2] Investigators have also detected elevated circulating levels of interleukin (IL)-6, adrenomedullin, extracellular phospholipase A2, and C-reactive protein in patients meeting the SIRS criteria.[2] With additional epidemiological studies using these criteria, it may be possible in the future to use more strict biochemical and/or immunological, rather than clinical, criteria to identify the inflammatory response.

**TABLE 40-1**

**Spectrum of Sepsis**

**Infection:** Inflammatory response by host to invading microorganism.

**Bacteremia:** The presence of viable bacteria in the blood.

**Systemic Inflammatory Response Syndrome (SIRS):** The systemic inflammatory response to severe clinical insults, manifested by 2 or more of the following:

- Temperature > 100.4°F or < 96.8°F
- Heart rate > 90 beats/min
- Respiratory rate > 20 breaths per min
- White blood count > 12,000/mm$^3$, < 4000/mm$^3$ or > 10% bands

**Sepsis:** A systemic response to infection. It is identical to SIRS except that there is a known documented infection.

**Severe Sepsis:** Sepsis complicated by organ dysfunction, hypoperfusion, or hypotension. Hypoperfusion and perfusion abnormalities may include lactic acidosis, oliguria, or acute alterations in mental status.

**Septic Shock:** Sepsis with persistent hemodynamic instability despite aggressive fluid challenge unexplained by other causes.

**Multiple Organ Dysfunction Syndrome (MODS):** A continuation of the sepsis syndrome characterized by the presence of altered organ function of more than 1 organ such that homeostasis cannot be maintained without immediate intervention.

*Source*: Data from Bone[1]; and Levy et al.[2]

However, no large prospective studies currently support this conclusion. SIRS can and does occur in the absence of infection as in the case of patients with burns, pancreatitis, and other disease states. *Sepsis*, then, is the systemic response to infection. It is identical to SIRS, except that it must result from infection. Severe sepsis is defined as sepsis complicated by organ dysfunction, hypoperfusion, or hypotension. Hypoperfusion and perfusion abnormalities may include lactic acidosis, oliguria, or acute alterations in mental status. Septic shock is sepsis with persistent hemodynamic instability despite aggressive fluid challenge unexplained by other causes.[2] Multiple organ dysfunction system is a continuation of the sepsis syndrome characterized by the presence of altered organ function of more than 1 organ such that homeostasis cannot be maintained without immediate intervention.

### INCIDENCE

Septic shock is the most common cause of noncoronary intensive care deaths in the US with the incidence increasing over the past 20 years.[3] Between 1979 and 2000 there was an increase in the incidence of sepsis of 8.7%, from about 164,000 cases to nearly 700,000 cases.[3,4] Sepsis occurred in nearly 2% of all acute-care hospitalizations in the US and resulted in close to 350,000 deaths annually.[3–6] Patients with cancer are 5 times more likely to develop sepsis and 3 times more likely to be hospitalized for severe sepsis than the overall population with 4.9% of all patients with cancer experiencing sepsis.[2] Incidence rates for patients without cancer consistently increase with age. Mortality rates for hospitalized patients with sepsis fell from 27.8% during the period from 1979 through 1984 to 17.9% during the period from 1995 through 2000, yet the total number of deaths continues to rise.[4] Mortality related to sepsis was highest among African American men. Organ failure contributed cumulatively to mortality with improvements in survival among patients with fewer than 3 failing organs.[4] The rate of sepsis due to fungal organisms has increased by 20% and is associated with significant mortality. Gram-negative bacteria were responsible for 50% to 60% of all cases of septic shock from 1979 through 1987 but that has decreased to 40% in recent years.[4] Since 1987, gram-positive bacteria have become the more predominant pathogens.[4] This is most likely due to the extensive use of central venous access devices as well as mucosal toxicities of cytotoxic regimens placing patients at a greater risk.[4] In an estimated 20% of cases of septic shock an initiating organism is never identified.[4]

## ETIOLOGY AND RISK FACTORS

The patient populations most susceptible to sepsis include those with the following characteristics: age younger than 1 year old or older than 65 years, chronic illness, immunosuppression, broad-spectrum antibiotic use, and exposure to infection associated with surgical and invasive procedures, indwelling devices, organ related disease, long intensive care stays, and loss of skin or mucosal injury (see Figure 40-1).[8–11] Advanced age is related to a decline in immune function.[9] Studies have shown that age-related changes in the immune system leads to T-cell and B-cell impairment. Physical deficits that contribute to the high risk of sepsis in the elderly include dementia, decreased gag and cough reflex, immobility, skin breakdown, poor urinary bladder emptying, and obstruction leading to infection.[10]

Patients with cancer have been shown to have the highest rate of sepsis and are among those with the worst outcomes. They are 5 times more likely to develop sepsis compared with patients who do not have cancer and their mortality rate is 55% higher compared with patients without cancer.[11] Cancer being a strong independent predictor of mortality from sepsis may be due to one of several reasons. Patients may be immunocompromised due to the use of chemotherapy, radiation, or other immune modulating therapy or they may have impaired leukocyte function secondary to the malignancy itself. Patients with cancer are also more prone to having additional chronic comorbid medical conditions further compromising their ability to combat sepsis. Granulocytopenia related to disease such as leukemia or lymphoma, treatments such as chemotherapy, biotherapy, and radiation therapy, and bone marrow infiltration by solid tumor; is the single most important risk factor in the development of sepsis in the patient with cancer.[11] Patients with cancer may also experience malignancy-related immunosuppression. This can be in the form of modified humoral immunity or modified cellular immunity. Humoral immunity is seen when the B lymphocytes produce antibodies to foreign antigens. In patients with multiple myeloma, chronic lymphocytic leukemia, Waldenström's macroglobulinemia and those who are asplenic and receiving cytotoxic regimens, humoral immunity can be modified or compromised. Patients with humoral immune deficiencies are susceptible to fulminant infections caused by *Streptococcus pneumoniae* and other encapsulating organisms that require

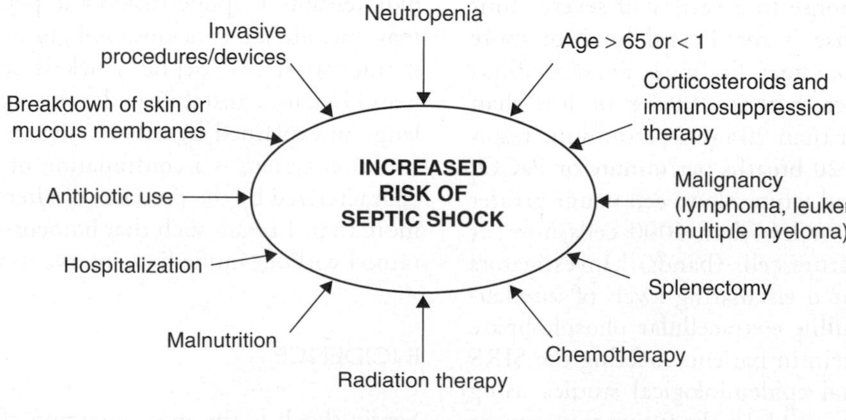


**FIGURE 40-1**

Risk factors for septic shock.

complement for elimination placing them at greater risk for sepsis.[12] Cellular immunity serves to eliminate pathogens, malignant cells, and viruses via monocytes and T lymphocytes. In patients with Hodgkin's disease, acute leukemia, advanced lung cancer as well as those patients undergoing stem cell transplant, cellular immunity may be modified or compromised placing them at a greater risk for sepsis.[12]

## PHYSIOLOGICAL ALTERATIONS

### NORMAL PHYSIOLOGY

In an intact immune system, when a foreign intruder such as bacteria, fungus, or virus invades the body, white blood cells recognize it as foreign and an immune response follows. Neutrophils, macrophages, lymphocytes, and antibodies are released to phagocytize the intruder and prevent colonization. However, if the virulence of the invading microbe exceeds the capabilities of the host immune system, sepsis may follow. Because patients with cancer have a compromised immune system, they are at greater risk for this to occur.

### PATHOPHYSIOLOGY

The current prevailing theory is that septic shock is actually a demonstration of an uncontrolled inflammatory response.[11] Initially, sepsis may be characterized by increases in inflammatory mediators; but as sepsis persists, there is a shift toward an anti-inflammatory immunosuppressive state.[13] If the pro-inflammatory and anti-inflammatory responses are imbalanced, widespread system infection and septic shock can occur. An anti-inflammatory state may increase the immunocompromised state of many patients with cancer. This can lead to delayed hypersensitivity, inability to clear infection, and a predisposition to nosocomial infections.[13]

Endotoxins from gram-negative bacteria and exotoxins from gram-positive bacteria are released into the blood stream as bacterial pathogens are phagocytized. The macrophages respond by releasing vasoactive mediators in the form of cytokines. These cytokines can be either inflammatory or anti-inflammatory. The inflammatory cytokines include tumor necrosis factor alpha (TNF-$\alpha$), histamine, kinins, interferon-gamma (IFN-$\gamma$), and both IL-1 and IL-2. Anti-inflammatory cytokines include IL-4, IL-10, and transforming growth factor-beta (TGF-$\beta$). The factors that determine which type of cytokine is released are unknown but may be influenced by the type of pathogen, the size of the bacterial inoculum, and the site of infection.[13] Inflammatory cytokines, especially IL-1 and TNF-$\alpha$, are potent mediators of inflammation. Their release stimulates the release of additional inflammatory mediators such as IL-6, IL-8, thromboxanes, leukotrienes, platelet-activating factor, prostaglandins, and complement.[14] This inflammatory cascade leads to fever, chills, vasodilatation, and hypotension.

The anti-inflammatory cytokines suppress gene expression and synthesis of IL-1 and TNF. When working synergistically, these anti-inflammatory cytokines can help to reduce the vasodilatory and pyrogenic characteristics of IL-1 and TNF. However, in the patient with sepsis, these functions are often overwhelmed by the inflammatory responses.

Septic shock is the most common cause of circulatory collapse in patients with cancer. The principle feature of sepsis, hemodynamically, is arterial vasodilatation. The release of inflammatory cytokines such as bradykinin, histamine, and serotonin cause increased capillary permeability. This increased permeability and subsequent decreased peripheral vascular tone forces the body to be dependent on cardiac output to maintain an efficient blood pressure. In an attempt to increase cardiac output, vasodilatation occurs. If a sufficient rise in cardiac output is not achieved to compensate for the vasodilatation, hypotension and shock may occur.

When endotoxins and exotoxins are initially released the endothelium itself is altered. These endothelial changes cause microthrombi to form that activates the complement, coagulation, and fibrinolytic systems. Simultaneously, the endothelium responds to endotoxins with the release of endothelium-derived relaxing factor, or nitric oxide, which causes further vasodilatation and decreased arterial and venous tone. Increased capillary permeability also renders vessels porous to fluids and solutes resulting in hypovolemia via capillary leak and third spacing. This combination of increased capillary permeability with subsequent cytokine release is exhibited as hypovolemia, hypotension, hypoxia, tissue ischemia, disseminated intravascular coagulation (DIC), ileus, oliguria, and liver failure that accompany septic shock.

## CLINICAL MANIFESTATIONS

Sepsis, in general, initially appears as fever, shaking chills, hypotension, tachycardia, tachypnea, and mental status changes. However, symptoms are often subtle and due to the immunocompromised state of patients with cancer, and fever may be the only recognizable symptom. Fever is defined as a single oral temperature of 100.9°F (38.3°C) or higher or a temperature of 100.4°F (38.0°C) sustained for 1 hour or longer.[15] Fever may be absent, especially in elderly patients.[15] Therefore, close attention must be paid to all clinical changes in order to recognize and treat the syndrome of sepsis. Throughout the spectrum of sepsis, the clinical presentation represents the results of each stage of the syndrome (see Table 40-2). Sepsis/SIRS are manifested by such things as fever, tachycardia, tachypnea, and increased white blood

**TABLE 40-2**

**Clinical Manifestations of Organ Dysfunction in Septic Shock**

| Organ System | Severe Sepsis | Septic Shock |
|---|---|---|
| Central nervous system | Apprehension<br>Confusion<br>Disorientation<br>Agitation | Obtundation<br>Coma |
| Cardiovascular | Sinus tachycardia<br>Cardiac output normal to increased<br>BP < 90 mm Hg or 40 mm Hg baseline<br>Systemic vascular resistance | Acrocyanosis<br>Tachycardia<br>Dysrrhythmias<br>Hypotension<br>Cardiac output normal or high<br>Systemic vascular resistance or shortness of breath |
| Pulmonary | Tachypnea<br>Shallow breaths<br>Hypoxic on room air<br>Respiratory and metabolic acidosis<br>Breath sounds and crackles | Refractory hypoxemia<br>Respiratory and metabolic acidosis<br>Breath sounds, crackles, and wheezes<br>Pulmonary edema<br>Acute respiratory distress syndrome |
| Renal | Urine output<br>Increased osmolality | Oliguria<br>Anuria<br>BUN<br>Creatinine<br>Acute renal failure |
| Hematology | Leukopenia or leukocytosis<br>Thrombocytopenia<br>PT/PTT prolonged<br>Fibrinogen<br>Fibrin degradation products | Leukopenia or leukocytosis<br>Thrombocytopenia<br>Anemia<br>PT/PTT prolonged<br>Fibrinogen<br>Fibrin degradation products |
| Metabolic and electrolyte | Temperature > 100.4°F or < 96.8°F<br>Lactic acidosis<br>Hyperglycemia | Temperature > 100.4°F or < 96.8°F<br>Lactic acidosis<br>Hyperglycemia<br>Albumin<br>Potassium<br>Sodium<br>Calcium<br>Magnesium<br>Phosphate |
| Integument | Dry, warm, and flushed skin | Cold, pale, and clammy skin |
| Gastrointestinal | Nausea and vomiting<br>GI motility | GI motility<br>GI bleeding<br>Liver function tests<br>Jaundice |

*Abbreviations*: BUN, blood urea nitrogen; GI, gastrointestinal; PT, prothrombin time; PTT, partial thromboplastin time.

cells. In severe sepsis, the patient may display symptoms of organ dysfunction, hypoperfusion, and hypotension associated with lactic acidosis, oliguria, and mental status changes. Mental status changes can range from simple apprehension to agitation, withdrawal, confusion, and obtundation. These changes may result from hypoperfusion, cerebral edema, or metabolic abnormalities. Mental status changes often precede fever or hypotension. Therefore close attention and regular assessment of mental status changes is crucial in the early identification of sepsis in high-risk patients.

Septic shock is seen as severe sepsis along with the presence of perfusion abnormalities. Shock is caused by hypoperfusion with lactic acidosis and tissue damage. Organ dysfunction associated with septic shock is manifested throughout the body systems (see Table 40-2). In the cardiovascular system, hypoperfusion is associated with tachycardia and increased cardiac output, decreased systemic vascular resistance, hypovolemia, hypotension, widened pulse pressure, arrhythmias, and decreased ejection fraction.[16] Typically shock is defined as a systolic blood pressure of less than 90 mm Hg that is unresponsive to fluids or requires vasoactive drugs.[1] The use of fluids and vasoactive drugs often restores the blood pressure to normal even though the underlying defect remains unchanged. Therefore, it is critical to use measures other than blood pressure alone to identify septic shock.

Pulmonary symptoms may be the first alert to the onset of septic shock. Almost all patients exhibit dyspnea and tachypnea resulting in respiratory alkalosis from the hyperventilation. Hypoxemia, pulmonary edema, acute respiratory distress syndrome (ARDS), respiratory acidosis, and ultimately respiratory failure will follow if the escalation of septic shock is not prevented.[16] Acute respiratory distress syndrome occurs most frequently in patients with gram-negative infections. The development of ARDS increases mortality in sepsis up to 80% to 90%. Concomitant thrombocytopenia raises the morbidity even higher.[14] In the renal system transient oliguria related to hypotension is often seen. This is generally resolved with fluid resuscitation. Anuria is rare in septic shock.

Hematologic changes are seen throughout the spectrum of sepsis. Elevation of white blood cells, leukocytosis, results from increased neutrophil production, and movement into the circulating blood in response to invading organisms. In contrast, leukopenia may be seen due to consumption, sequestration, or decrease in the number of white blood cells resulting from the underlying malignancy. Thrombocytopenia may be seen as a result of decreased production, increased destruction, pooling, and sludging of platelets in the microvasculature. Granulocytopenia in septic shock generally correlates with a poor prognosis.[16] Slight increases in prothrombin time (PT) and partial thromboplastin time (PTT) is a common subclinical sign. Disseminated intravascular coagulation (DIC) can be seen septic shock and the presence of DIC doubles the risk of death in patients with septic shock.[16] Clinical indications of DIC include thrombosis, ischemia, and bleeding (see Chapter 38). Anemia is commonly seen in septic shock as a result of hemodilation, hemorrhage, and shortened red blood cell survival.[16]

Hyperglycemia is present in both sepsis and severe sepsis. The sympathetic nervous system releases endogenous catecholamines, epinephrine, norepinephrine, glucocorticosteroids, and simultaneous gluconeogenesis all cause a sharp rise in blood glucose levels. In prolonged septic shock hypoglycemia may be seen that indicates hepatic failure and loss of compensatory mechanisms.[16] Other metabolic changes include elevated serum lactate levels that reflects anaerobic metabolism in response to tissue hypoxia which occurs early in the spectrum of sepsis. In addition lowered levels of albumin, sodium, potassium, calcium, and magnesium are often seen.[16] The skin and extremities are initially warm, dry, and flushed due to massive vasodilatation. As septic shock progresses, the skin becomes cold, pale, and clammy as a result of altered blood flow.[16]

Because the gastrointestinal (GI) tract is so highly vascularized, it is sensitive to ischemic conditions that are present in the sepsis. Ileus is typically seen for 1 to 2 days with septic shock.[16] Later in septic shock, stress ulcers and GI bleeding can occur as a result of coagulopathies and tissue injury. Hyperbilirubinemia and transaminase elevations are commonly seen in septic shock; however, frank liver failure is rare.[16]

## ASSESSMENT AND GRADING

### PATIENT HISTORY AND PHYSICAL EXAM

A thorough patient history is essential in attempting to identify a patient at risk for potentially manifesting signs of the spectrum of sepsis. The initial evaluation focuses on determining the potential sites and causative organisms of infections and assessing the patient's risk of developing infection. Knowledge of a past treatment including chemotherapy, radiation therapy, steroid use, or other immunosuppressive drugs can be critical information when attempting to diagnose and treat sepsis. The use of any indwelling devices, prior infections, and antibiotic use may provide clues to the development of secondary infections or resistant organisms. Individuals with age younger than 1 year old or older than 65 years, chronic illness, immunosuppression, broad-spectrum antibiotic use, and exposure to infection associated with surgical and invasive procedures, indwelling devices, organ related disease, long intensive care stays, and loss of skin or mucosal injury are at a significant risk for sepsis and septic shock.[9–11]

A physical exam with focus on high-risk sites of infection is critical. Common sites of infection include the respiratory tract, GI tract, genitourinary tract, skin including the perianal region, and mucous membranes.[17] Since almost every organ system is affected during sepsis and septic shock, an assessment of all areas with knowledge of potential manifestations of sepsis and septic shock is important (see Table 40-2).

### DIAGNOSTIC STUDIES

Diagnostic studies are used to determine the severity of septic shock and identify the source of infection. Initial laboratory/radiology evaluation should include a complete blood count with differential analysis, platelets, blood urea nitrogen, creatinine, electrolytes, total serum bilirubin, liver associated enzymes, and renal function tests.[18] Chest radiographs should be done for all patients with respiratory symptoms. Blood cultures should be drawn promptly. Two blood samples should be cultured. There are 3 options for obtaining blood cultures: (1) one set can be drawn peripherally and one set from a central venous catheter (CVC) if present, (2) both sets can be drawn peripherally, or (3) both sets can be drawn from the CVC.[19] The positive predictive value of a culture retrieved from a catheter is less than a culture retrieved from a peripheral site. Obtaining cultures from both a peripheral and central site may help to determine whether the CVC is the site of infection based on the differential time to positivity.[19] The National Comprehensive Cancer Network (NCCN) advisory panel on infection states that the volume of blood obtained is the most important aspect of blood culturing and agrees that the use of sites remains unclear.[19]The only way to establish a definitive diagnosis of central line infection is removal of the catheter for culture. Thus, if the CVC is suspected for infection it should be removed and sent for culture.[18]

Cultures of body fluids such as urine, stool, sputum, or other exudate should be collected as clinically significant. Cultures should be repeated at least every 24 hours if sepsis continues. Echocardiogram, computerized tomography (CT), ventilation/perfusion scans, and angiography may be performed to further evaluate organ function.

Acquired protein C deficiency is prevalent in > 85% of patients with sepsis and is predictive of increased morbidity and mortality.[8] The protein C pathway regulates one of the major regulatory systems of hemostasis. Protein C has been shown to be higher in patients with sepsis than in patients with shock resulting from other causes. Serial protein C measurements may be helpful in determining sepsis from other causes of shock.

## THERAPEUTIC APPROACHES AND NURSING CARE

### PREVENTION AND DETECTION

The key to preventing progression of infection to sepsis and septic shock is early identification and intervention. Patients should be educated on the signs and symptoms of infection and the importance of reporting these promptly. The progression of infection to sepsis and septic shock is often preceded by hours or even days by abnormalities in routine observations. Although the measurement of vital signs has been standard practice for over a century, few attempts have been made to quantify what vital signs truly mean in terms of clinical performance related to sepsis. In 1999, the Audit Commission in London reported that the effectiveness of critical care services varied between hospitals and recommended the development of early warning systems (EWSs) to help staff identify when to call for specialist advice related to changes in vital signs and declining physical status.[20]

#### Acute physiology and chronic health evaluation system

The Acute Physiology and Chronic Health Evaluation (APACHE) system was introduced in the early 1980s, and although minor modifications have been made over the years, only 3 major revisions have occurred since that time. The most recent tool, the APACHE IV, was published in May 2006. Although not the most current version, the APACHE II tool is the most widely used prognostic scoring tool used in intensive care units (ICU) in the United States.[21] The APACHE II tool is widely available, easily accessible to clinicians, and is free of charge online. One simply has to input the vital signs and other parameters measured and the tool automatically calculates a score. On the other hand, the APACHE III and APACHE IV tools are proprietary commercial products that must be purchased for use and are generally hand calculated.

The APACHE II ICU prognostic scoring system was based on data from 42 ICUs in the United States and has been in use since 1991. The APACHE II is first calculated based on 12 physiological variables, whereas the APACHE III and IV have 17 variables. The additional variables in the more current versions include albumin, bilirubin, glucose, BUN, and urine output. Points are added for age and the presence or absence of comorbid conditions. Subsequently, consideration of the diagnosis that led to the ICU admission and the source of admission enable a prediction of mortality to be calculated based on the APACHE II score.[21–23] (see Table 40-3). The APACHE II is used during the first 24 hours of an ICU admission. In general, the higher the APACHE score, the greater the chance of mortality. Since this instrument was designed to only deal with ICU patients, it lacks sensitivity and cannot be used to rule out severe illness. Thus, the APACHE II score is used to help determine the aggressiveness of therapy.

#### Modified early warning score

In 1999, a modification of Morgan's Early Warning Score called the Modified Early Warning Score (MEWS) was proposed.[24] The MEWS has been used to assess acutely ill general medical patients. The MEWS was evaluated on 206 surgical patients over 9 months.[20] The purpose of the MEWS is to facilitate prompt communication between nursing and medical staff when deterioration in a patient's condition first becomes apparent. The authors intended this system to result in earlier intervention in the general medical setting so that transfer to a critical care facility is either prevented or occurs without unnecessary delay. A MEWS

**TABLE 40-3**

**Acute Physiology and Chronic Health Evaluation (APACHE) System**

| APACHE II | APACHE III |
|---|---|
| Temperature | Temperature |
| Heart rate | Heart rate |
| Respiratory rate | Respiratory rate |
| Blood pressure | Blood pressure |
| Hematocrit | Hematocrit |
| White blood count | White blood count |
| Serum sodium | Serum sodium |
| Serum potassium | Serum potassium |
| Serum sodium bicarbonate | Serum sodium bicarbonate |
| Creatinine | Creatinine |
| $PaO_2$ or $FIO_2$ | $PaO_2$ or $FIO_2$ |
| pH and $pCO_2$ | pH and $pCO_2$ |
| | Albumin |
| | Bilirubin |
| | Glucose |
| | BUN |
| | Urine output |

**Additional Variables Measured Include**

Age
Glascow coma score
Admission diagnosis (50 types: APACHE II; 78 types: APACHE III)
Type of admission
Prior treatment location (APACHE III only)

| APACHE Score | Approximate Death Rate (%) |
|---|---|
| 0–4 | 4 |
| 5–9 | 8 |
| 10–14 | 15 |
| 15–19 | 25 |
| 20–24 | 40 |
| 25–29 | 55 |
| 30–34 | 75 |

**Comorbid Conditions Considered in Scoring**

| APACHE II | APACHE III |
|---|---|
| AIDS | AIDS |
| Immunosuppression | Immunosuppression |
| Lymphoma | Lymphoma |
| Leukemia/multiple myeloma | Leukemia/multiple myeloma |
| Hepatic failure | Hepatic failure |
| Cirrhosis | Cirrhosis |
| Chronic renal insufficiency | Chronic renal insufficiency |
| Chronic cardiac insufficiency | Chronic cardiac insufficiency |
| Chronic respiratory insufficiency | Chronic respiratory insufficiency |
| | Metastatic cancer |

*Abbreviations*: AIDS, acquired immunodeficiency syndrome; APACHE, acute physiology and chronic health evaluation; BUN, blood urea nitrogen; $FIO_2$, fraction of inspired oxygen; $PaO_2$, partial pressure of oxygen, arterial; $pCO_2$, partial pressure of carbon dioxide.

*Source*: Data from Holmes et al[22]; and Knaus et al.[23]

score of > 4 is associated with an increased risk of death and indicates an urgent need for intensive care (see Table 40-4).[20,24,25] Use of the MEWS on surgical wards has been shown to decrease APACHE II scores on admission to the intensive care.[25]

## MANAGEMENT

Management of patients with sepsis and septic shock includes treatment of infection, treatment of inflammation, hemodynamic support, fluid resuscitation, vasopressor and inotropic support, and oxygenation support. The Surviving Sepsis Campaign (SSC), along with the Institute for Healthcare Improvement (IHI) developed a "bundle" of management strategies for severe sepsis with the aim being to decrease the relative mortality from sepsis by 25% by 2009.[26,27] A bundle is a group of interventions related to a disease process that, when executed together, result in better outcomes than when implemented individually. The individual bundle elements are built upon evidence-based practices. Generally, the science behind the elements of a bundle is so well-established that their implementation should be considered a generally accepted practice.

The SSC and IHI developed 2 distinct bundles in relation to sepsis. The 2 bundles are the severe sepsis resuscitation bundle (SSRB) and the sepsis management bundle[28] (see Table 40-5). The SSRB describes 7 tasks that should begin immediately, and must be accomplished within the first 6 hours of presentation for patients with severe sepsis or septic shock. Some items may not be completed if the clinical conditions described in the bundle do not prevail in a particular case, but clinicians must assess for them. The goal is to perform all indicated tasks 100% of the time within the first 6 hours of identification of sepsis.[28]

Measuring serum lactate is the first task in the SSRB. Lactate is elevated (>4 mmol/L) in patients with severe sepsis who demonstrate poor tissue perfusion. Even with a normal blood pressure, severe sepsis causes problems with oxygen delivery to the tissues and vital organs. Obtaining serum lactate is essential to identifying tissue hypoperfusion in patients who are not yet hypotensive but who are at risk for septic shock.[28] Collecting blood cultures is the second task in the SSRB. Positive blood cultures are seen in 30% to 50% of patients presenting with a clinical syndrome of severe sepsis or shock. Therefore, blood should be obtained for culture in any critically ill septic patient.[28] Collecting blood cultures prior to antibiotic administration provides the best chance of identifying the organism that caused severe sepsis in an individual patient. Failure to check blood cultures prior to antibiotic infusion may affect the growth of any blood borne bacteria and prevent a culture from becoming positive later. The third

**TABLE 40-4**

**Modified Early Warning Scoring System (MEWS)**

| | 3 | 2 | 1 | 0 | 1 | 2 | 3 |
|---|---|---|---|---|---|---|---|
| Temperature (°F) | | < 96.8 | | 96.8–100.4 | | > 100.4 | |
| Heart rate (per minute) | | < 40 | 41–50 | 51–100 | 101–110 | 111–129 | > 129 |
| Respiratory rate (per minute) | < 10 | | | 10–20 | 21–24 | 25–28 | > 28 |
| $SpO_2$ in % | < 91 | | 91–94 | 95–100 | | | |
| Systolic blood pressure (mm Hg) | < 81 | 81–90 | 91–100 | 101–160 | 161–170 | 171–180 | > 180 |
| Dyspnea | Observed SOB | Verbal C/O | | | | | |
| Urine output (ml/kg/hour) | Nil | < 0.5 | | | | | |
| Mental status | New MS changes | | | Alert | Reacting to voice | Reacting to pain | Unresponsive |
| Total = | | | | | | | |

*Notes*: The scores for each parameter are recorded at the time that observations are taken. If total is 4 or more, further action is required.
*Abbreviations*: C/O, complaints of; MEWS, modified early warning scoring system; MS, mental status; SOB, shortness of breath; $SpO_2$, saturation of peripheral oxygen.
*Source*: Data from Audit Commission[20]; Stenhouse et al[24]; and Kellett et al.[25]

task is early administration of broad-spectrum antibiotics to treat the underlying infection. Early administration of appropriate antibiotics reduces mortality in patients with gram-positive and gram-negative bacteremias thus improving survival benefits for patients with sepsis and septic shock.[28] If the patient is hypotensive or the serum lactate level is >4 mmol/L, the next task is to deliver an initial fluid bolus followed by administration of vasopressors for hypotension not alleviated by fluid resuscitation. Fluid resuscitation should be started as soon as possible in patients with septic shock, even before ICU admission. Fluid resuscitation should be clearly defined and understood as not equivalent to increasing maintenance fluids. A typical fluid resuscitation is given over a short period of time, 10 to 15 minutes, with the purpose of expanding the patient's intravascular volume. Fluid resuscitation quickly restores the patient's intravascular volume, whereas increasing maintenance fluids would take hours to achieve the same result.[28] When an appropriate fluid challenge fails to restore an adequate arterial pressure and organ perfusion, therapy with vasopressor agents should be started.[28] The final task in the SSRB is to achieve central venous pressure (CVP) of >8 mm Hg and a central venous oxygen saturation ($ScVO_2$) of >70%. To maintain an appropriate CVP, a central venous catheter is placed and fluid resuscitation is repeated until the target value is achieved.[28] Two techniques are used to maintain $ScVO_2$. Once the patient has achieved a CVP of >8, if they remain hypovolemic and the hematocrit is <30%, it is appropriate to transfuse packed red blood cells. This may help to increase the $ScVO_2$ due to increased oxygen delivery to ischemic tissue beds and to keep the CVP >8 for a longer period of time than using fluids alone.[28] When the patient's cardiac output remains insufficient to meet metabolic needs of certain tissue beds despite increasing the circulating fluid volume, administration of inotropic medications beginning with dobutamine is used to maintain $ScVO_2$.[28]

The sepsis management bundle lists 4 management goals. Efforts to accomplish these tasks should also begin immediately, but these interventions must be completed within 24 hours of presentation for patients with severe sepsis or septic shock.[28] The first goal is the administration of low-dose corticosteroids. Intravenous corticosteroids are recommended in patients with septic shock who despite adequate fluid replacement require vasopressor therapy to maintain adequate blood pressure.[28] The use of corticosteroids is based on the role that they play in the stress response to infection and the anti-inflammatory effects that they exert. However, the use of corticosteroids in the treatment of infection is not without controversy. This aspect is discussed further in a subsequent section. The second goal in the sepsis management bundle is the administration of drotrecogin alfa also known as recombinant human activated protein C (rhAPC). Drotrecogin alfa is recommended in patients at high risk of death as determined by

**TABLE 40-5**

**Sepsis Bundles**

**Sepsis Resuscitation Bundle (6-Hour Bundle)**

1. Serum lactate measured
2. Blood cultures obtained before antibiotic administration
3. From the time of presentation, broad-spectrum antibiotics administered within 3 hours for ED admissions and 1 hour for non-ED admissions
4. In the event of hypotension and/or lactate > 4 mmol/L (36 mg/dL)
   - Deliver an initial minimum of 20 mL/kg of crystalloid or colloid fluid equivalent
   - Apply vasopressors for hypotension not responding to initial fluid resuscitation to maintain mean arterial pressure of > 65 mm Hg
5. In the event of persistent hypotension despite fluid resuscitation (septic shock) and/or lactate > 4 mmol/L (36 mg/dL)
   - Achieve central venous pressure of > 8 mm Hg
   - Achieve $ScVO_2$ of > 70%

**Sepsis Management Bundle (24-Hour Bundle)**

1. Low-dose steroids administered for septic shock in accordance with a standardized ICU policy
2. Drotrecogin alfa (activated) administered in accordance with a standardized ICU policy
3. Glucose control maintained greater than lower limit of normal but < 150 mg/dL (8.3 mmol/L)
4. Inspiratory plateau pressures maintained < 30 cm $H_2O$ for mechanically ventilated patients

*Abbreviation*: ED, emergency department; ICU, intensive care unit; $ScVO_2$, central venous oxygen saturation.

*Source*: Data from Institute for Healthcare Improvement.[28]

an APACHE II score of >25, sepsis-induced multiple organ failure, septic shock or sepsis-induced ARDS. In addition, because of the high risk of bleeding associated with rhAPC, the patient must have no absolute contraindication related to bleeding or a relative contraindication that outweighs the potential benefit of rhAPC.[28] The third goal of the sepsis management bundle is to maintain glucose greater than the lower limit of normal but <150 mg/dL. Insulin treatment has reduced the number of deaths from multiple organ failure with sepsis, regardless of whether there was a history of diabetes or hyperglycemia.[28] The final goal is to maintain an inspiratory plateau pressure <30 cm $H_2O$ for mechanically ventilated patients. Most mechanically ventilated patients with severe sepsis and/or septic shock will meet criteria for lung injury or ARDS and could benefit from inspiratory plateau pressures <30 cm $H_2O$.[28]

Studies have shown that compliance with the 6 hour sepsis bundle was associated with a more than 2-fold decrease in hospital mortality (23% vs 49%), and compliance with the 24 hour bundle showed a trend to reduced mortality.[28] Although the trend is showing reduced mortality using sepsis bundles, the original goal of the SSC and IHI to decrease the relative mortality from sepsis by 25% by 2009 has not been fully realized.[3–6]

## Treatment of infection

The most important intervention in the management of septic shock is immediate treatment with intravenous antibiotic therapy.[29] According to the sepsis resuscitation bundle, antibiotics should be administered within 3 hours from the time of presentation for emergency department admissions and within 1 hour from the time of presentation for non-emergency department admissions.[28] Making a microbiological diagnosis in sepsis is important to ensure that effective antimicrobial therapy is given. However, blood cultures are positive in only one-third of sepsis cases.[30] Gram-positive bacteria now account for 60% to 70% of microbiologically documented infections.[30] Both the NCCN and the Surviving Sepsis Campaign Guidelines (SSCG) recommend that 1 or more antimicrobial drugs are started empirically that would be effective against both fungal and bacterial microbes and would most likely be able to target the source of infection.[19,26] The choice of empiric antimicrobials should depend on the patient's history, including drug intolerances, underlying disease, and the clinical syndrome.[19,26] In general, any antibiotic that was recently administered to the patient should be avoided. The susceptibility patterns and prevalence of pathogens in a particular setting should be taken into consideration. For instance, the recent prevalence of oxacillin (methacillin)-resistant *Staphylococcus aureus* (ORSA or MRSA) as well as the increased virulence of these pathogens should be considered before starting a patient on an antimicrobial that may add to this phenomena. The NCCN recommends initial antimicrobial therapy with single-agent cefepime, imipenem, meropenem, piperacillin/tazobactam or combination therapy with an aminoglycoside + cefepime, or ciprofloxacin + antipseudomonal penicillin for patients at high risk with neutropenia.[18] The antimicrobial regimen should be assessed daily to optimize activity, prevent the development of resistance, reduce toxicity, and reduce costs.[19,26]

The use of vancomycin, linezolid, or daptomycin is not routinely recommended.[19,26] Vancomycin should be used initially if (1) line sepsis is strongly suspected; (2) there is a high rate of nosocomial infection in the hospital with MRSA, or the patient has a known MRSA colonization; (3) the patient is in shock with respiratory distress and there are strong reasons to suspect hemolytic viridans streptococcal bacteremia; or (4) the patient is at high risk for endocarditis.[8] In patients with sepsis or septic shock the addition of fluconozole should be considered, especially in patients not receiving antifungal prophylaxis.[19,26]

## Treatment of inflammation

The rationale for using corticosteroids in the management of septic shock stems from the understanding of septic shock as a profound inflammatory reaction to infection. Chronic inflammation is characterized by the overexpression of many inflammatory genes. The main effect of corticosteroids is to turn off these inflammatory genes that include cytokines, chemokines, adhesion molecules, inflammatory enzymes, receptors, and proteins. The use of corticosteroids in the treatment of many chronic inflammatory conditions has become the mainstay of therapy. However, no studies exist that target severe sepsis in the absence of shock and offer support for use of stress doses of steroids in this patient population.[26] Several meta-analyses have consistently shown that treatment with high doses of glucocorticoids (up to 42,000 mg of hydrocortisone) have been ineffective or harmful in the treatment of sepsis and septic shock, including an increase in the number of secondary infections with slower resolution and an increased mortality from these infections.[31–33] The general consensus from these meta-analyses was that the high doses of corticosteroids actually failed to decrease the inflammatory response sufficiently and, in fact, induced immunosuppression. Therefore, the use of corticosteroids for the treatment of sepsis in the absence of shock is not recommended.[26] Steroids may be indicated in the presence of a history of steroid therapy or adrenal dysfunction.

## Activated protein C

Recombinant human activated protein C, an anticoagulant, is the first anti-inflammatory agent that has proved effective in the treatment of sepsis.[13,26] In patients with sepsis, administration of rhAPC resulted in a 19.4% reduction in the relative risk of death and an absolute risk reduction of 6.1%.[13,26,34] Recombinant human activated protein C inactivates factors Va and VIIIa, thereby preventing the generation of thrombin. Inhibition of thrombin generation by rhAPC decreases inflammation by inhibiting platelet activation, neutrophil recruitment, and mast-cell degranulation. A major risk with the use of rhAPC is hemorrhage. In a study of rhAPC, 720 patients were initially enrolled to evaluate the effectiveness of rhAPC in the treatment of severe sepsis and septic shock. The study was subsequently revised to exclude patients who received bone marrow or solid organ transplants or had metastatic cancer or pancreatitis. Because of these changes, which were made in a blinded manner, the study population changed to include patients with less severe underlying disease and more acute infectious illnesses.[35] Study results showed that 3.5% of patients treated with rhAPC had serious bleeding described as intracranial hemorrhage, a life-threatening bleeding episode, or a requirement for 3 or more units of blood, as compared with 2% of patients who received placebo.[35] Caution is advised in the use of rhAPC in patients with a platelet count of <30,000/mm$^3$. Currently, rhAPC is approved only for use in patients with sepsis who have the most severe organ compromise and the highest likelihood of death. The use of rhAPC is suggested only for patients with an APACHE II score of > 25, multiple organ failure, or high risk of death.[13,19,26,35]

## Hemodynamic support

Septic shock alters tissue perfusion, causing a reduction in the delivery of oxygen and other nutrients to the tissues, resulting in cellular and then organ dysfunction. The goals of hemodynamic therapy are to restore effective tissue perfusion and therefore normalize cellular and organ function. Early goal-directed therapy is now routinely used in ICUs for the management of severe sepsis and septic shock. This involves adjustments of cardiac preload, afterload, and contractility to balance oxygen delivery with oxygen demand. Endpoints include normalization of mixed venous oxygen saturation, arterial lactate concentration, base deficit, and pH.

## Fluid resuscitation

The goal of fluid resuscitation is restoration of tissue perfusion. Volume replacement results in increased cardiac output and oxygen delivery. Fluid resuscitation can be achieved with either colloids (eg, albumin) or crystalloids (eg, normal saline, lactated ringers). There is no evidence for the use of one type of fluid over another.[26] It is recommended that fluid resuscitation initially target a CVP of ≥ 8 mm Hg (12 mm Hg in mechanically ventilated patients) and continue as long as the hemodynamic improvement continues.[26] Fluid challenge in patients with suspected hypovolemia should be started with ≥ 1000 mL of crystalloids or 300 to 500 mL of colloids over 30 minutes. More rapid administration and greater amounts of fluid may be needed in patients with sepsis-induced tissue hypoperfusion.[26] A patient's response to a fluid challenge must be closely monitored in order to avoid the development of pulmonary edema. This can be done by using a fluid challenge in which a large amount of fluid is administered over a limited period of time.[26] The degree of intravascular fluid deficit in patients with severe sepsis varies. Most patients in septic shock experience varying degrees of venous dilation and ongoing capillary leak, thus most patients will require continuing aggressive fluid resuscitation during the first 24 hours of management.

## Blood product administration

Blood product administration is generally not considered during initial fluid resuscitation, but does have therapeutic value under certain conditions. It is generally agreed upon in the critical care literature that a hemoglobin of between

7 and 9 g/dL does not increase mortality when compared to higher hemoglobin levels between 10 and 12 g/dL. In patients with sepsis, red blood cell transfusions increases oxygen delivery but does not usually increase oxygen consumption.[26] Therefore, it is recommended that a target hemoglobin in patients with sepsis be 7 to 9 g/dL and that red blood cell transfusions should occur when the hemoglobin decreases to <7.0 g/dL.[26]

### Vasopressors and inotropic support

If fluid resuscitation fails to restore organ perfusion the use of vasopressors is required. Even if hypovolemia has not been restored, vasopressors may be needed when the patient is experiencing life-threatening hypotension in order to maintain perfusion. Perfusion becomes more dependent on pressure once the mean arterial pressure (MAP) falls to critical low levels, as the body can no longer autoregulate its vascular beds. Therefore, patients may require vasopressor therapy to achieve the minimal perfusion pressure and to maintain adequate blood flow. A MAP of ≥65 mm Hg should be maintained.[26,36] A MAP of <60 mm Hg is associated with compromised autoregulation in coronary, renal, and cerebral vascular beds with elderly patients requiring higher pressures to maintain adequate perfusion.[29]

There is no high-quality evidence to recommend one catecholamine over another.[26] Human and animal studies suggest some advantages of norepinephrine and dopamine over epinephrine and phenylephrine.[26] Both dopamine and norepinephrine increase the MAP. Dopamine works by increasing stroke volume and heart rate thus increasing MAP and cardiac output. However, it also causes more tachycardia and arrhythmias. Because of its effect on the stroke volume and cardiac output, dopamine may be particularly effective in patients with altered systolic function. Alternately, norepinephrine has vasoconstrictive properties that raises the MAP but exerts little effect on stroke volume or heart rate. Although either drug may be used to correct hypotension in sepsis, norepinephrine is much more potent than dopamine, thus may be more effective in correcting hypotension in patients with septic shock. Epinephrine has a potential for tachycardia, as well as negative effects on splenic circulation and may produce hyperlactemia. However, there is no clinical evidence that epinephrine results in worse clinical outcomes. Therefore, it should be the first alternative agent when blood pressure is poorly responsive to norepinephrine or dopamine.[26] Phenylephrine works by decreasing stroke volume and is the adrenergic agent least likely to produce tachycardia.

Dopamine increases MAP and cardiac output, primarily due to an increase in stroke volume and heart rate. If a patient is experiencing low cardiac output despite adequate left ventricular filling pressure, dobutamine would be the first choice of an inotropic agent.[26] Even after fluid resuscitation patients who are septic may remain hypotensive with varying degrees of cardiac output. Therefore, treatment with a combined inotrope/vasopressor, such as norepinephrine or dopamine, is recommended especially when initiating therapy prior to admission to the ICU when cardiac output may not be measured.[26] It is recommended that an arterial catheter is placed as soon as practical if resources are available.[26]

### Oxygen therapy

As interstitial and alveolar edema worsens in sepsis and septic shock, ventilation/perfusion mismatch occurs taxing the respiratory effort and increasing oxygen demand. Oxygen therapy should be initiated with a nasal cannula at the first indication of dyspnea or increased respiratory effort. Increased use of oxygen therapy should be based on oxygen saturation, arterial blood gas levels, and lactate levels as well as patient complaints of dyspnea. Respiratory complications of sepsis include ARDS, which is a severe form of acute lung injury (ALI) in the cascade of respiratory dysfunction.[8] The mortality associated with ALI and ARDS is about 40%.[37] Early endotracheal intubation and mechanical ventilation are encouraged to increase oxygen delivery and decrease oxygen demand until the results of septic shock can be reversed.[37] The use of mechanical ventilatory support with ARDS reduces the work of breathing for the patient and allows for increased blood flow to other essential organs.

### Supportive therapy

The nursing management of a patient within the spectrum of sepsis is extremely complex and challenging. Fundamental supportive care is important to the care of the patient throughout the spectrum of sepsis. Nutritional support, prevention of nosocomial infections, pressure ulcers, skin breakdown, and deep vein thrombosis (DVT) may play an important role in the outcome of sepsis and septic shock. Protein and calorie requirements are much higher in patients with sepsis. Enteral nutrition is the preferred method of nutrition in critically ill patients when possible. Parenteral nutrition should be reserved for those patients who cannot tolerate enteral nutrition or in the presence of other comorbidities such as bowel ischemia or obstruction.[29] Patients with sepsis who are immunocompromised have a predisposition to nosocomial infections. Maintaining an aseptic environment including hand washing and universal precautions for all patients can be a key in caring for the patient with sepsis. Awareness of the necessity for thorough skin assessment is imperative to managing the patient with sepsis. Frequent turning, specialty beds, and skin care products can assist in preventing pressure ulcers that could easily lead to worsening infection. Unless otherwise contraindicated, the use of low molecular weight heparin or low-dose unfractionated heparin should be used to prevent DVT.[26] In patients for whom anticoagulation is contraindicated, mechanical methods such as intermittent compression devices or graduated compression stocking are recommended.[26,38,39]

### Glucose control

Patients with sepsis may develop hyperglycemia due to a combination of factors. Stress induces an elevation in plasma levels of hormones such as catecholamines, glucagon, cortisol, and growth hormones that usually help to regulate blood glucose levels. Insulin resistance, which is proportional to the severity of the stress response, also comes into play with changes in glucose levels in patients with sepsis. In addition, treatments such as the use of glucocorticosteroids may contribute to the development of hyperglycemia in the patient being treated for septic shock. Several studies have shown that reducing blood glucose levels in patients with sepsis has proven to reduce organ dysfunction, decrease overall length of stay, and decrease mortality rates.[40,41] However, more recent randomized controlled studies (RCT) of intensive insulin therapy, failed to demonstrate improvement in mortality.[42,43] It is therefore recommended that patients with severe sepsis and hyperglycemia who are admitted to the ICU receive insulin therapy to reduce blood glucose levels to < 150 mg/dL.[26]

### Renal replacement

Renal replacement therapy is often necessary in the patient with severe sepsis when acute renal failure occurs. Research has been conducted to determine whether the use of continuous or intermittent methods of replacement is superior in improving outcomes. Numerous studies including nonrandomized controlled studies, randomized controlled studies and 2 meta-analyses have failed to show any significant difference in outcomes or tolerance of therapy related to the use of either continuous or intermittent renal replacement.[44,45] In addition, the Veterans Administration/National Institutes of Health Renal Failure Trial Network supported these results. The findings of this study, which included 1124 patients, concluded that continuous renal support in critically ill patients with acute kidney injury did not decrease mortality, improve recovery of kidney function, or reduce the rate of nonrenal organ failure as compared to less-intensive therapy involving intermittent hemodialysis.[46] Therefore, the SSC guidelines suggest that continuous renal replacement therapies and intermittent hemodialysis are equivalent in patients with severe sepsis and acute renal failure.[26]

### Control of stress ulcers

Conditions such as coagulopathy, hypotension, and mechanical ventilation have been shown to benefit from stress ulcer prophylaxis. Since many patients with severe sepsis and septic shock exhibit these same conditions, it is recommended that stress ulcer prophylaxis also be used in patients with severe sepsis or septic shock.[26] Recommendations include the use of histamine 2 blockers or proton pump inhibitors for the stress ulcer prophylaxis in reducing GI bleeding.

## CONCLUSION

Understanding of sepsis has improved dramatically since the development of an expert consensus definition more than 15 years ago. We now have a better understanding of the factors that influence the risk of sepsis and subsequent, relevant clinical outcomes. Advances have been made in understanding the pathophysiology of sepsis, which has translated into more effective therapies.

It is recognized that not all patients with infection will develop the sequelae of sepsis. Studies aimed at identifying genetic factors that may predispose patients to increased mortality from sepsis are ongoing. The allele, tumor necrosis factor 2 (TNF2), is responsible for the generation of TNF-$\alpha$ that plays a central role in the development of septic shock. Mutations of TNF2 have been identified as potentially affecting the risk and progress of infection.[8]

Diverse new agents have shown efficacy in clinically relevant animal models and offer hope as well as new insight into sepsis. IL-12 has been shown to reduce mortality from subsequent sepsis when administered after burn injury.[13] Excessive production of the complement-activation product C5a causes neutrophil dysfunction with loss of bacterial killing, platelet activation, and direct or indirect microvascular damage. Therefore, administration of antibodies directed against complement-activation product C5a decreased the frequency of bacteremia, prevented apoptosis, and improved survival.[13,47] Studies have shown that high concentrations of macrophage inhibitory factor were present in patients with sepsis and that the administration of antibodies against macrophage migration inhibitory factor protected mice from peritonitis.[13,47] Strategies that block apoptosis of lymphocytes or GI epithelial cells have improved survival in experimental models of sepsis.[13] Thus, a variety of agents hold promise as effective new therapies for sepsis.

Although the incidence of sepsis approaches 800,000 cases per year, the overall fatality rate has been decreasing on an annual basis to less than 20% for patients with sepsis, 30% for patients with severe sepsis, and 50% for patients with septic shock.[3] However, despite the decline in fatality rates, sepsis continues to be the tenth leading cause of death overall in the United States and the most common cause of noncoronary ICU deaths.[3] Given these facts, septic shock remains a significant oncologic emergency. Early recognition and treatment of sepsis have shown improved outcomes. These interventions along with education about the risk factors, manifestations of illness, and pathophysiology may promote better patient care. The oncology nurse plays a leading role in the early detection, monitoring, and treatment of patients throughout the spectrum of sepsis. Education, use of protocols for early detection, and improved management and monitoring allow healthcare professionals to work together to positively impact critically ill patients with sepsis and septic shock.

## REFERENCES


1. Bone RC. The sepsis syndrome: definition and general approach to management. *Clin Chest Med.* 1996;17:175–182.
2. Levy M, Fink M, Marshall JC, et al. *Crit Care Med.* 2003;31:1250–1256.
3. Danai P, Martin GS. Epidemiology of sepsis: recent advances. *Curr Infect Dis Rep.* 2005;7:329–334.
4. Martin GS, Mannino DM, Eaton S, et al. The epidemiology of sepsis in the United States from 1979 through 2000. *N Engl J Med.* 2003;348:1546–1554.
5. Angus DC, Linde-Zwirble WT, Lidicker J, et al. Epidemiology of severe sepsis in the United States: analysis of incidence, outcomes, and associated cost of care. *Crit Care Med.* 2001;29:1303–1310.
6. Centers for Disease Control and Prevention. National center for health statistics: faststats death and mortality. http://www.cdc.gov/nchs/fastats/deaths.htm. Accessed September 25, 2009.
7. Williams MD, Braun LA, Cooper LM, et al. Hospitalized cancer patients with severe sepsis: analysis of incidence, mortality and associated costs of care. *Crit Care.* 2004;8:R91–R98.
8. Moore S. Septic shock. In: Yarbro CH, Frogge MH, Goodman M, eds. *Cancer Nursing: Principles and Practice.* 6th ed. Sudbury, MA: Jones and Bartlett; 2005:895–908.
9. Hachem R, Raad I. Prevention and management of long term catheter related infections in cancer patients. *Cancer Invest.* 2002;20:1105–1113.
10. Girard T, Wesley E. Insights into severe sepsis in older patients: from epidemiology to evidence-based management. *Clin Infect Dis.* 2005;40:719–727.
11. Martin GS, Mannino DM, Moss M. The effect of cancer on risks and outcomes in sepsis [Abstract]. *Am J Respir Crit Care Med.* 2003;167:A549.
12. Shelton BK. Infection. In: Yarbro CH, Frogge MH, Goodman M, eds. *Cancer Nursing: Principles and Practice.* 6th ed. Sudbury, MA: Jones and Bartlett; 2005:698–722.
13. Hotchkiss RS, Karl IE. The pathophysiology and treatment of sepsis. *N Engl J Med.* 2003;348:138–150.
14. Myers JS. Septic shock. In: Langhorne ME, Fulton JS, Otto SE, eds. *Oncology Nursing.* 5th ed. St. Louis, MO: Mosby; 2007:436–453.
15. National Comprehensive Cancer Network Panel Members. Myeloid growth factors: NCCN practice guidelines in oncology. v.1.2009. Jenkintown, PA: National Comprehensive Cancer Network. http://www.nccn.org/professionals/physician_gls/PDF/myeloid_growth.pdf. Accessed January 13, 2010.
16. Dellinger R. Cardivascular management of septic shock. *Crit Care Med.* 2003;31:946–955.
17. Gobel B, O'Leary C. Bone marrow suppression. In: Langhorne ME, Fulton JS, Otto SE, eds. *Oncology Nursing.* 5th ed. St. Louis, MO: Mosby; 2007:488–504.
18. Raad I, Hanna HA, Alakech B, et al. Differential time to positivity: a useful method for diagnosing catheter-related bloodstream infections. *Ann Intern Med.* 2004;40:18–25.
19. National Comprehensive Cancer Network Panel Members. Prevention and treatment of cancer related infections. NCCN practice guidelines in oncology. v.1.2008. Jenkintown, PA: National Comprehensive Cancer Network. http://nccn.org/professionals/physician_gls/PDF/infections.pdf. Accessed January 13, 2010.
20. Audit Commission. *Critical to Success: The Place of Efficient and Effective Critical Care Services within the Acute Hospital.* London: Audit Commission; 1999.
21. Keegan MT, Harrison BA, Brown DR, et al. The acute physiology and chronic health evaluation III outcome prediction in patients admitted to the intensive care unit after pneumonectomy. *J Cardiothorac Vasc Anesth.* 2007;21:832–837.
22. Holmes CL, Gregore G, Russell JA. Assessment of severity of illness. In: Hall JB, Schmidt GA, Wood LDH, eds. *Principles of Critical Care.* 3rd ed. Columbus, OH: McGraw Hill; 2005:63–78.
23. Knaus WA, Draper EA, Wagner DP, et al. APACHE II: a severity of disease classification system. *Crit Care Med.* 1985;13:818–829.
24. Stenhouse C, Coated S, Tivey M, et al. Prospective evaluation of a modified early warning score to aid earlier detection of patients developing critical illness on a general surgical ward [Abstract]. *Br J Anaesth.* 1999;84:663.
25. Kellett J, Deane. The simple clinical score predicts mortality for 30 days after admission to an acute medical unit. *QJM.* 2006;99:771–781.
26. Dellinger RP, Mitchell M, Cartlet JM, et al. Surviving sepsis campaign: international guidelines for management of severe sepsis and septic shock: 2008. *Crit Care Med.* 2008;36:296–327.
27. Zambon M, Ceola M, Almeida-de-Castro R, et al. Implementation of the surviving sepsis campaign guidelines for severe sepsis and septic shock: we could go faster. *J Crit Care.* 2008;23:455–460.
28. Institute for Healthcare Improvement. Sepsis. http://www.ihi.org/IHI/topics/CriticalCare/sepsis. Accessed January 13, 2010.
29. Zimber N, Campbell A. Sepsis, SIRS, and MODS. *Surgery.* 2004;22:73–76.
30. Hughes WT, Armstron D, Bodey GP, et al. 2002 Guidelines for the use of antimicrobial agents in neutropenic patients with cancer. *Clin Infect Dis.* 2002;34:730–751.
31. Keh D. Corticosteroid therapy in sepsis: where are we? *Adv Sepsis.* 2006;5:138s–140s.
32. Annane D, Bellissant E, Bollaert PE, et al. Corticosteroids for treating severe sepsis and septic shock. *Cochrane Database Syst Rev.* 2004;(1):CD002243.
33. Minneci PC, Deans KJ, Banks SM, et al. Meta-analysis: the effect of steroids on survival and shock during sepsis depend on the dose. *Ann Intern Med.* 2004;141:47–56.
34. Bernard GR, Vincent JL, Laterre PF, et al. Efficacy and safety of recombinant human activated protein C for severe sepsis. *N Engl J Med.* 2001;344:699–709.
35. Warren HS, Suffredini AF, Eichacker PQ, et al. Risks and benefits of activated protein C treatment for severe sepsis. *N Engl J Med.* 2002;347:1027–1030.
36. Hollenberg SM, Ahrens TS, Annane D, et al. Practice parameters for hemodynamic support of sepsis in adult patients: 2004 update. *Crit Care Med.* 2004;32:1928–1948.
37. Zambon M, Vincent JL. Mortality rates for patients with acute lung injury/ARDS have decreased over time. *Chest.* 2008;133:1120–1127.
38. Geerts W, Cook D, Shelby R, et al. Venous thromboembolism and its prevention in critical care. *J Crit Care.* 2002;17:95–104.
39. Attia J, Ray JG, Cook DJ, et al. Deep vein thrombosis and its prevention in critically ill adults. *Arch Intern Med.* 2001;161:1268–1279.
40. Van den Berghe G, Wouters P, Weekers F, et al. Intensive insulin therapy in critically ill patients. *N Engl J Med.* 2001;345:1359–1367.
41. Van den Berghe G, Wilmer A, Hermans G, et al. Intensive insulin therapy in the medical ICU. *N Engl J Med.* 2006;354:449–461.
42. Brunkhorst FM, Kuhnt E, Engel C, et al. Intensive insulin therapy in patients with severe sepsis and septic shock is associated with an increased rate of hypoglycemia—results from a randomized multicenter study (VISEP). *Infection.* 2005;33:19–20.

43. Preiser JC. Intensive glycemic control in med-surg patients (European Glucontrol trial). Program and abstracts of the society of critical care medicine 36th critical care congress. Orlando, FL; 2007 February 17–21.
44. Kellum JA, Angus DC, Johnson JP, et al. Continuous versus intermittent renal replacement therapy: a meta-analysis. *Intensive Care Med.* 2002;28:29–37.
45. Tonelli M, Manns B, Feller-Kopman D. Acute renal failure in the intensive care unit: a systematic review of the impact of dialytic modality on mortality and renal recovery. *Am J Kidney Dis.* 2002;40:875–885.
46. Palevsky PM, Hongyuan Z, O'Connor TZ, et al. Intensity of renal support in critically ill patients with acute kidney injury. *N Engl J Med.* 2008;359:7–20.
47. Huber-Land MS, Sarma JV, McGuire SR, et al. Protective effects of anti-C5a peptide antibodies in experimental sepsis. *FASEB J.* 2001;15:568–570.

CHAPTER

41

Anne Marie Flaherty, RN, MSN, AOCNS®, APNc

# Spinal Cord Compression

- **Scope of the Problem**
  - *Definition*
  - *Incidence*
- **Pathophysiology**
  - *Anatomy of the Spinal Cord*
  - *Etiology*
  - *Pathogenesis*
  - *Site of Compression*
- **Clinical Manifestations and Physical Assessment**
  - *Back Pain*
  - *Motor Weakness and Motor Loss*
  - *Sensory Disturbances and Sensory Loss*
  - *Autonomic Dysfunction*
- **Diagnostic Evaluation**
  - *Plain Films and Bone Scans*
  - *Magnetic Resonance Imaging*
  - *Myelogram with Computerized Tomography*
- **Therapeutic Approaches and Nursing Care**
  - *Medical Management*
    - Steroids
    - Radiation
    - Surgical interventions
    - Chemotherapy
  - *Symptom Management*
    - Pain
    - Mobility
    - Bowel and bladder dysfunction
    - Skin care
- **Conclusion**
- **References**

## SCOPE OF THE PROBLEM

### DEFINITION

Although rare, malignant spinal cord compression (MSCC) is a devastating complication of cancer. It is a malignant process that causes disruption in neurological function when a tumor and its destructive effects on the spinal cord compress neural tissue or interfere with its blood supply.[1] MSCC can be defined clinically as well as radiographically and includes involvement of both the spinal cord and the cauda equina. The clinical definition includes both compression of the thecal sac and the cord or equina to result in symptoms, whereas the radiographic definition can be only indentation of the dural lining of the thecal sac at the level of disease.[2]

### INCIDENCE

Spinal cord compression occurs in approximately 5% of patients with cancer and is the second most common neurological complication of cancer.[3] These data are based on autopsy results, inpatient studies and few studies on defined populations.[2,4,5] More than 12,700 cases of spinal cord compression are diagnosed annually, about twice the number of traumatic spinal cord injuries.[6] The incidence of spinal cord compression may actually be increasing due to improved treatments and prolonged survival currently seen in various cancers such as breast and prostate cancers, improved quality and availability of diagnostic tests, and earlier screening.[1,7] Spinal cord compression is now referred to as a skeletal-related event or a consequence of bone metastases, reflecting the fact that almost 90% of cases are due to involvement of the vertebral column with metastatic disease. The majority of spinal cord compressions in these cases are due to cancers of the lung, breast, and prostate. Approximately 20% of patients present with spinal cord compression as their initial symptom of cancer, and half of those patients will ultimately be diagnosed with lung cancer.[8]

In this chapter, the discussion is primarily related to metastatic epidural spinal cord compression and not primary spinal cord tumors, as less than 5% of cases are related to primary spinal cord tumors. Oncology nurses are in the best position to identify those individuals at risk to develop spinal cord compression and those with early-stage spinal cord compression so that treatment is instituted prior to neurological deterioration. The primary goal is to preserve and maintain the neurological status of the individual, thereby maintaining the patient's quality of life. The most important prognostic factor in MSCC is the neurological function prior to the initiation of treatment. In the classic study by Gilbert and colleagues, the majority of those patients who were ambulatory prior to treatment remained so after its completion.[9]

## PATHOPHYSIOLOGY

### ANATOMY OF THE SPINAL CORD

The spinal cord consists of ascending and descending nerve tracts that carry impulses to and from the brain and peripheral nerves. These impulses result in sensory information and motor ability.[10] The spinal cord is protected and cushioned by 3 connective tissue membranes known as the leptomeninges: (1) pia mater, the innermost layer; (2) arachnoid, the middle layer; and (3) dura mater, the outermost layer. See Figure 41-1(A).These layers comprise a compartment that surrounds the cord known as the thecal sac and the area outside the outer most layer of the sac is the epidural space.[11] Between the arachnoid and pia mater layers circulates the cerebrospinal fluid.

The spinal cord is surrounded by the vertebral column—a bony structure that consists of stacked vertebrae and provides flexibility and support.[11] Each vertebra consists of a vertebral body, two laminae, two pedicles, and a spinous process. See Figure 41–1(B). The spinal cord starts at the

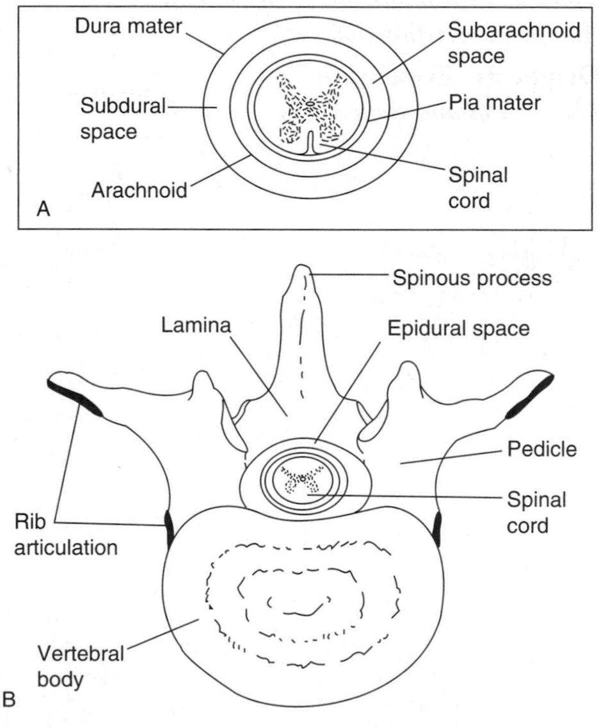


**FIGURE 41-1**

(**A**) This cross section illustrates the leptomeninges or membranes surrounding the spinal cord and spaces between the membranes. (**B**) Cross section of vertebra and spinal cord. The vertebra consists of the vertebral body, pedicles, laminae, and spinous process. The spinal cord spans the length of the vertebral column in the canal formed by the vertebrae.

base of the brain and ends in the space between the first two lumbar vertebrae. The cauda equina refers to a group of lumbar and sacral nerve roots emerging from the end of the spinal cord. The spinal cord is larger in the cervical and lumbar regions and consequently these vertebrae are also larger to accommodate the cord. At each vertebral body level, dorsal and anterior nerve roots exit from the spinal cord via the intervertebral foramina and continue on to form spinal nerves. The spinal cord is arranged into several distinct regions. The butterfly-shaped gray matter has anterior horns controlling motor function, lateral horns controlling autonomic functions, and posterior horns related to sensation. The lateral and anterior spinal cord white matter includes corticospinal tracts and additional nerve tracts that control fine motor control and tone. The spinocerebellar tracts are associated with muscle stretch and tone sensation. The lateral spinothalamic tract carries pain fibers, and the dorsal columns transmit fine touch and positional sense (Figure 41-2).[12]

## ETIOLOGY

Spinal cord compression can arise from either a primary tumor within the spinal cord and its protective layers or as a result of metastatic disease. Primary tumors of the spine that arise within the cord itself are called *intramedullary;* those that develop within the leptomeningeal layers are called *extramedullary intradural.* These tumors include malignancies such as ependymoma, astrocytoma, oligodendroglioma, and meningioma.[10]

Metastasis to the spine can be classified as intramedullary (within the spine itself), leptomeningeal (within the lining of the spinal cord), and epidural (outside the lining of the spinal cord). Intramedullary and leptomeningeal metastases are rare and arise from hematogenous spread via paravertebral and extradural vessels as well as growth along nerve roots from paravertebral tumors. Intramedullary metastases are most often associated with breast and lung cancer, whereas leukemia and lymphoma are more likely to result in leptomeningeal carcinomatosis.[13,14] Epidural metastasis—the most common type of metastasis to the spine—occurs because of the extension of a tumor or bone from the vertebral column, extension of a tumor through the intervertebral foramina, or direct tumor deposits in the epidural space (Figure 41-3). Eighty-five percent of cases of epidural metastasis involve the vertebral column, whereas 10%-15% of cases develop compression from paravertebral tumors that extend through the foramina. Direct epidural metastasis is rather uncommon and accounts for less than 5% of cases.[15]

The skeleton is the third most frequent site of metastasis after the lung and liver, and the vertebral column is the most common site for skeletal metastasis.[16] The vertebral body—rather than the pedicles or laminae—is most often involved. The vertebral column is rich with growth factors,

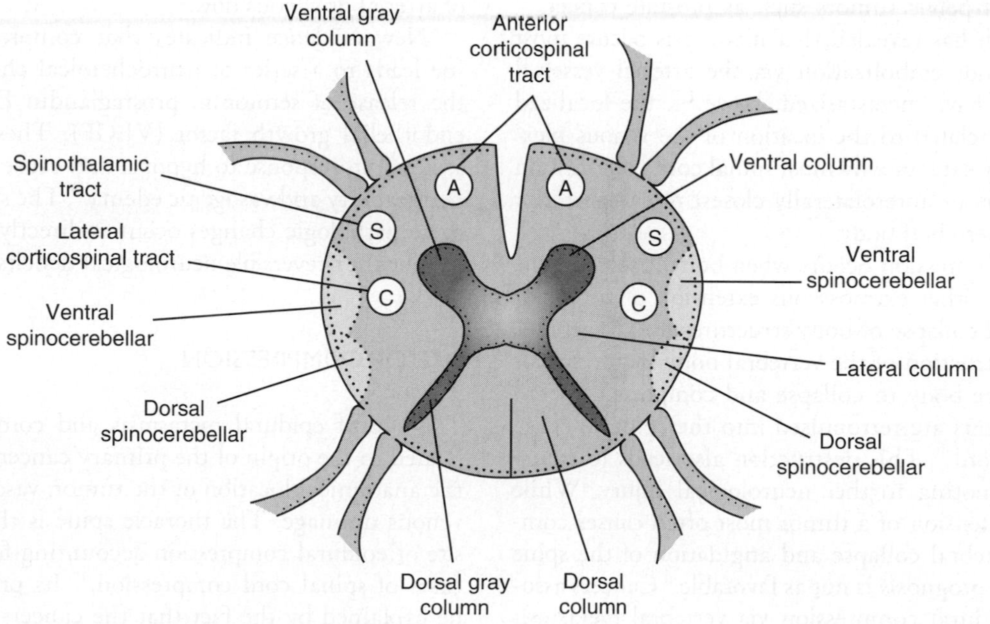


**FIGURE 41-2**

Cross section of spinal cord and spinal tracts.

*Abbreviations*: A, anterior; C, corticospinal; S, spinothalamic.

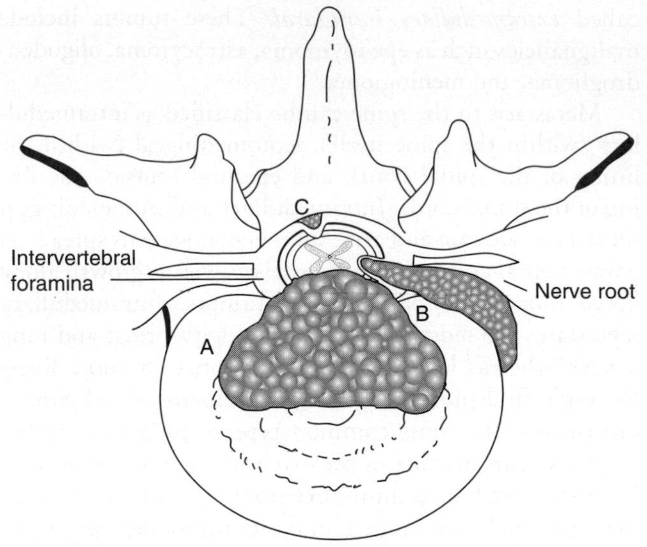


**FIGURE 41-3**

Primary types of epidural metastases: (**A**) tumor extension from vertebral body; (**B**) tumor traveling along nerve root into intervertebral foramina; (**C**) direct epidural metastasis.

which are present in the bone marrow and help to support malignant growth. Another factor encouraging metastatic growth in the vertebral column is its blood supply. The vertebrae also have a large bed of capillaries with vessel walls that are irregularly shaped allowing for stasis of blood and harboring of tumor cells.[16]

The venous plexus is the primary mechanism involved in metastasis of pelvic tumors such as prostate cancer. [15] Animal research has revealed that metastasis occurs most often from tumor embolization via the arterial vessels.[17] Once the cells have metastasized, however, the localized spread may be related to the location of the venous plexuses, which may explain why most spinal cord compression occurs anteriorly or anterolaterally closest to the posterior portion of the vertebral body.

Epidural compression occurs when bony disease in the vertebra causes either extraosseous extension of tumor or destruction and collapse of bony structures into the epidural space.[18] Destruction of the vertebral body by the tumor causes either the body to collapse and compress the cord or bony fragments are retropulsed into the epidural space and onto the cord.[19] This destruction also leads to spinal instability promoting further neurological injury. While extraosseous extension of a tumor most often causes compression, if vertebral collapse and angulation of the spine are present, the prognosis is not as favorable.[6] Cancers associated with epidural compression via vertebral metastasis include cancers of the breast, lung, prostate, kidney, and multiple myeloma and melanoma.[20]

While vertebral metastasis is the most common mechanism for spinal cord compression, tumors can compress the cord by direct extension through the intervertebral foramina.[18] Lymphomas and neuroblastoma travel through this space and may compress the spine without invasion of the bony structures. Some tumors (eg, colon, kidney, prostate, and head and neck) can extend directly into the vertebral structures or epidural space without metastases.[21]

Although this chapter reviews metastatic spinal cord compression, epidural catheters and medications administered epidurally can result in a nonmalignant cord compression. The epidural route of analgesic administration is often used in the oncologic population postoperatively as well as a method of controlling chronic pain. Cases have been reported where hematoma or infection as a result of immunocompromise, coagulopathy or an epidural catheter has caused cord compression.[22,23] Precipitate from medication administered epidurally has also resulted in spinal cord compression.

## PATHOGENESIS

Early in spinal cord compression, compression of the epidural venous plexus or direct mechanical injury causes venous congestion, vasogenic edema, white matter edema, and axonal swelling.[18] Further compression leads to ischemia, conduction block, and demyelination of mostly white matter.[16] This loss of myelin sheath insulating the nerves affects conduction of signals, resulting in neurological deficits. Demyelination is regulated by lipid peroxidation and lipid hydrolysis. As the compression progresses, additional white matter is injured and the cord may infarct due to lack of arterial or venous flow.[19]

New evidence indicates that compressed neural tissue leads to a series of neurochemical changes caused by the release of serotonin, prostaglandin E2, and vascular endothelial growth factor (VEGF). These mediators are secreted in response to hypoxia and cause further vascular permeability and vasogenic edema.[18] The speed with which these pathologic changes occur is directly related to more significant irreversible neurological deficits. [22,24]

## SITE OF COMPRESSION

The site of epidural metastasis and cord compression is related to the origin of the primary cancer and depends on the anatomical location of the tumor, vascular supply, and venous drainage. The thoracic spine is the most frequent site of epidural compression accounting for about 70% of cases of spinal cord compression.[25] Its predominance can be explained by the fact that the cancers most frequently associated with bone metastases—breast, lung, and prostate—most often cause thoracic compression. In addition, there are more thoracic vertebrae than lumbosacral or cervical vertebrae. Although lumbosacral metastases are more commonly seen on autopsy, they are asymptomatic and often go undetected.[4] About one-third of all patients with spinal cord compression will have multiple noncontiguous sites of metastases.[26]

## CLINICAL MANIFESTATIONS AND PHYSICAL ASSESSMENT

It is not clear which specific pathophysiologic changes cause each of the clinical manifestations associated with spinal cord compression. These manifestations of cord compression depend on the level of the lesion and compression but not necessarily on which part of the cord—anterior, posterior, or lateral—is actually compressed.[25]

The symptoms of cord compression usually start as mild and noncontributory, but eventually become more pronounced. These symptoms most often follow a progressive pattern that the clinician must recognize to diagnose cord compression early and preserve neurological function. The initial symptom is back pain that is accompanied or followed by motor weakness and decreased sensation. This weakness then progresses to motor and sensory loss, and loss of proprioception, vibratory sense, and bowel and bladder function.[27]

### BACK PAIN

Back pain is the presenting symptom in more than 95% of individuals with spinal cord compression. Approximately one-third of individuals who present with back pain have significant spinal cord compression despite a normal neurological exam.[28] Central back pain is caused by mechanical distortion via vertebral collapse or bone marrow disease that causes stretching of the periosteum of the involved bony structure or invasion of soft tissue.[18] The pain is localized within 1 or 2 vertebrae of the compression in about half of the cases of epidural compression that involve one vertebra.[12] The pain, however, can occur in multiple areas in cases that involve multiple noncontiguous areas of vertebral metastases.

Back pain can also be radicular in nature, meaning that the pain moves or radiates from one location to another. Such a pattern is caused by the tumor irritating the nerve roots such that the pain follows the distribution of the nerve. Radicular pain with cervical and lumbosacral compression is usually unilateral, whereas thoracic compression is usually associated with bilateral pain.[27] Radicular pain with thoracic compression is described as a constrictive-band-like pain; in contrast, cervical and lumbosacral compression may cause pain that radiates to a limb. Radicular pain is more common in lumbar and cervical spinal cord compression.[25]

Back pain often heralds an impending cord compression and can be present a few days to months before diagnosis of this oncologic emergency. The pain is similar to that associated with degenerative disease or herniated disc in that it can be elicited with cough, movement, Valsalva maneuver, and straight leg raising or neck flexion. Back pain from cord compression differs from degenerative disease in that lying supine does not alleviate the pain. Lying down can increase venous congestion and edema, both of which exacerbate pain. Individuals complain of being unable to sleep at night and feel more comfortable in a recliner or chair. Epidural compression can occur at any level in the spine, whereas degenerative changes are most often seen in the cervical and lumbar spine.[16] Sometimes it may be difficult to distinguish pain related to spinal cord compression, but suspicion should be raised when the nature, intensity, or location of back pain changes in a patient with cancer. Pain with any movement can represent an unstable spine with pathologic vertebral collapse and should evoke even more a sense of urgency for diagnosis and intervention before severe spinal injury results.[18]

The clinician tries to elicit the back pain by percussing the vertebrae and having the patient perform leg raising or neck flexion. This motion will cause further stretching of the periosteum and induce pain. Where the patient experiences pain can help identify the level of the spinal cord compression because the abnormality will cause discomfort at that location. The assessment also includes a description of the nature and character of the pain, its intensity, and alleviating as well as aggravating factors.

### MOTOR WEAKNESS AND MOTOR LOSS

In general, muscle weakness follows pain as cord compression progresses. Rarely is weakness, which is a prelude to loss of motor function, the only presenting symptom of cord compression. Approximately three-fourths of affected individuals are obviously paraparetic at the time of diagnosis, and even more cases are identified during a neurological exam. The weakness is usually described as a heaviness or stiffness and involves proximal muscles that are used to climb stairs or get out of a chair.[29]

Roughly 95% of patients who have weakness have a significant compression of the spinal cord.[9] On physical exam, the strength of the extremities and gait are assessed to determine motor loss. This step is important in identifying early neurological deficits that represent a more urgent clinical condition. Ambulation at the time of diagnosis is critical because less than 25% of paralyzed patients will regain their ability to ambulate after treatment of spinal cord compression.[30] See Table 41-1 for a discussion about the relationship of pretreatment neurological status to ambulation after treatment.[31]

Motor weakness is evaluated by having the patient get out of a chair, walk, and push an extremity against a resisting force. The clinician carefully observes for any gait disturbances. Sometimes back pain will be accompanied by

**TABLE 41-1**

**Relationship of Pretreatment Neurological Status to Ambulation After Treatment**

| Pretreatment Neurological Status | Treatment | Posttreatment Neurological Status |
|---|---|---|
| 52% of patients ambulatory with minimal impairment | Dexamethasone 10 mg IV followed by 4 mg q 6 hours | 94% of patients ambulatory |
| 39% of patients paraparetic and nonambulatory | Radiation 200–300 cGy every day for a total of 2000–3000 cGy | 60% of patients ambulatory |
| 9% of patients paraplegic | | 1% of patients ambulatory |

*Source:* Data from Maranzano and Latini.[31]

ataxia, which is caused by compression of the spinocerebellar tracts.[30] This ataxia is unrelated to other neurological findings and may be confused with central nervous system pathology. In addition to muscle strength and gait, muscle tone is assessed for spasticity and flaccidity, which reflects further progression of the cord compression.

Reflexes are also evaluated: tendon reflexes in elbow, knee, and ankle; Babinski sign; and abdominal reflexes. Early in spinal cord compression, reflexes are decreased or absent but as the compression progresses, they may become hyperactive.[16]

### SENSORY DISTURBANCES AND SENSORY LOSS

Sensory changes are less common than motor weakness, but early complaints include numbness or paresthesia. The sensory loss ascends from the toes to the level of the compression as it progresses and can correspond to within 2 vertebral bodies of the site of the lesion. Clinicians should be aware that this finding is not always reliable because multiple lesions may be present and multiple dermatomes may be affected. In addition, many sensory and motor pathways cross and overlap, making identification of the level of the lesion extremely difficult. In cauda equine compression, sensory loss involves the perianal region, or lateral or posterior thighs, and is dermatome specific and usually bilateral.[15]

As the compression progresses, sensory loss is accompanied by loss of proprioception, position sense, vibration, temperature sense, and deep pressure.[32] Loss of pain and temperature sensation below a specific dermatome indicates disruption of the spinal thalamic pathway in the lateral column of the spinal cord's white matter. Loss of vibration accompanies sensory loss and is associated with disruption in the posterior spinocerebellar pathways or posterior columns.[32] Deep-tendon reflexes may be decreased at the level of the lesion and hyperactive below that level.[33]

On physical exam, the clinician assesses for any numbness or paresthesia by testing for light touch with a cotton-tipped applicator, pain with a pin-prick technique, and proprioception by moving the big toe and fingers in various positions. For an accurate assessment of spinal cord disease, the clinician begins at the feet and works upward to determine the highest level of intact sensory function.[32]

### AUTONOMIC DYSFUNCTION

Autonomic dysfunction includes an array of bowel and bladder disturbances that are due to disruption in lower motor neuron function.[27] This late sign of spinal cord compression includes sphincter problems that result in bowel and bladder incontinence or retention. The individual may experience difficulty initiating urinary flow, sometimes in conjunction with retention, frequency, or incontinence. Urinary retention is defined as a post-void residual of greater than 150 mL when one is catheterized after micturition.

Early bowel problems may be present when the individual complains of difficulty expelling stool and experiences loss of feeling. This problem may eventually lead to constipation or incontinence. Poor sphincter tone is a late sign of autonomic dysfunction and is a poor prognostic sign.[30] Those individuals who have autonomic dysfunction are usually nonambulatory and rarely regain the ability to ambulate.

## DIAGNOSTIC EVALUATION

### PLAIN FILMS AND BONE SCANS

The type of evaluation for spinal cord compression is dictated by the clinical condition of the patient. If the patient presents with vague complaints that do not help direct the evaluation, a bone scan and plain films will assist the practitioner in ordering further appropriate diagnostic studies. Plain radiological films of the painful area of the vertebral column will demonstrate vertebral body collapse, pedicle erosion, and osteolytic or osteoblastic lesions in more than 80% of cases of epidural metastasis.[33] The degree of vertebral destruction caused by metastatic disease as seen on plain films may be directly related to the incidence of spinal cord compression. For plain films to demonstrate osteolytic osseous destruction, more than 50% of bone must be affected.[34] While a bone scan is more sensitive than x-rays, it is often not as helpful as plain films in diagnosing areas of potential cord compression. Bone scans pinpoint the area of disease but do not identify the degree of bone destruction or epidural cord compression. Also, if widespread disease is present, many vertebral bodies may be positive and the level or degree of actual compression not identified.

## MAGNETIC RESONANCE IMAGING

Magnetic resonance imaging (MRI) has emerged as the safest and preferred tool for the diagnosis of spinal cord compression.[15] This noninvasive technique provides a variety of images to help visualize different abnormalities in the spinal cord and surrounding structures. While it is equivalent to a myelogram with computerized tomography (CT) scan in diagnosing cord compression due to extradural masses, MRI is far superior in diagnosing paravertebral masses, intramedullary disease, and bone metastases.[15] The cost of diagnosing MSCC without the use of MRI has been found to be significantly more expensive than if MRI is used.[35] An MRI is performed with and without gadolinium, as paravertebral masses, leptomeningeal disease, and intramedullary tumors are better visualized with gadolinium. Based on the bone scan, spine films, and clinical presentation, the site of compression can be generally identified. If only a specific area of the spine is examined by MRI, additional sites of compression may not be identified and go untreated. Given that 10%-30% of patients with clinical symptoms of spinal cord compression have multiple lesions, the entire spine should be imaged to identify additional areas that are not near the symptomatic lesion. A sagittal MRI survey of the entire spine can be obtained to identify sites of compression, and then more detailed images at that level can aid in further visualizing the type and degree of compression.[6]

Individuals who suffer from claustrophobia may not be able to tolerate the MRI exam. In such a case, patients may be referred to an "open" MRI facility or a sedative such as lorazepam may be given prior to the exam. Persons who have a pacemaker or metal implantation near the area to be imaged cannot undergo an MRI, nor can patients with a very large body habitus.

## MYELOGRAM WITH COMPUTERIZED TOMOGRAPHY

If an MRI cannot be performed, myelography with CT scan is comparable in adequately diagnosing spinal cord compression. With CT guidance, contrast is injected via a lumbar puncture into the subarachnoid space, and flow is observed to identify any defects. If a complete block is found, a cervical or cisternal puncture is required to determine the upper level of the block. If multiple complete blocks are suspected, then additional punctures are required. Cerebrospinal fluid (CSF) withdrawn prior to the instillation of contrast is analyzed for malignant cells, cell count, glucose, and protein. Presence of malignant cells in the CSF confirms leptomeningeal carcinomatosis or tumor in the lining or meninges.

Myelography is not without risks. An invasive procedure, it requires proper coagulation as well as adequate renal function for the use of contrast. The MRI technique is preferred if available to the patient because of its lower cost, greater convenience, and better anatomical detail. The positron emission tomography (PET) scan has emerged as a useful tool in staging and evaluation of malignant diseases and often provides early identification of vertebral or spinal disease. The combination of $^{18}$F or positron-emitting radioactive isotope fluorine-18, with FDG or 2-fluoro-2-deoxy-D-glucose is the radionucleotide used in PET. PET/CT superimposes the PET scan over the CT and adds another dimension in that it has better specificity for detection of spinal involvement and allows for precise localization of disease and soft tissue involvement of the spine, nerve roots and cauda equina(n). One small study of 51 patients concluded that PET/CT had better specificity than PET alone and was very helpful in optimal treatment planning and the differentiation between pathological and osteoporotic compression fractures.[36] Several algorithms have been developed to aid clinicians in promptly diagnosing spinal cord compression (Figure 41-4).[16] It is critical to identify all areas of disease, distinguish which areas may cause neurological sequelae, and identify adequate treatment ports for radiation. The goal is to accomplish this in the most efficient and cost effective manner. If the clinical condition demonstrates obvious signs of epidural compression, however, then MRI with gadolinium is warranted. In addition, if other areas of early cord compression are not identified, they may go untreated and become symptomatic with neurological deterioration.[16]

Talcot and colleagues developed a predictive model for spinal cord compression based on a regression analysis of various patient and clinical factors.[37] Table 41-2 outlines these 6 factors that can be used to predict which patients are at highest risk to develop metastatic spinal cord compression. They found that the presence of all factors predicted an 87% risk versus 1 factor, which was associated with a 4% risk. Interestingly, back pain alone failed to predict MSCC and is not one of the factors.

# THERAPEUTIC APPROACHES AND NURSING CARE

## MEDICAL MANAGEMENT

Epidural spinal cord compression is a life-threatening condition requiring immediate intervention so that the patient's neurological condition is at least preserved; ideally it is improved. Disease progression can cause rapid deterioration and paraplegia, quadriplegia, and even respiratory arrest if the cervical spine is involved. The major therapeutic approaches include steroids, radiation

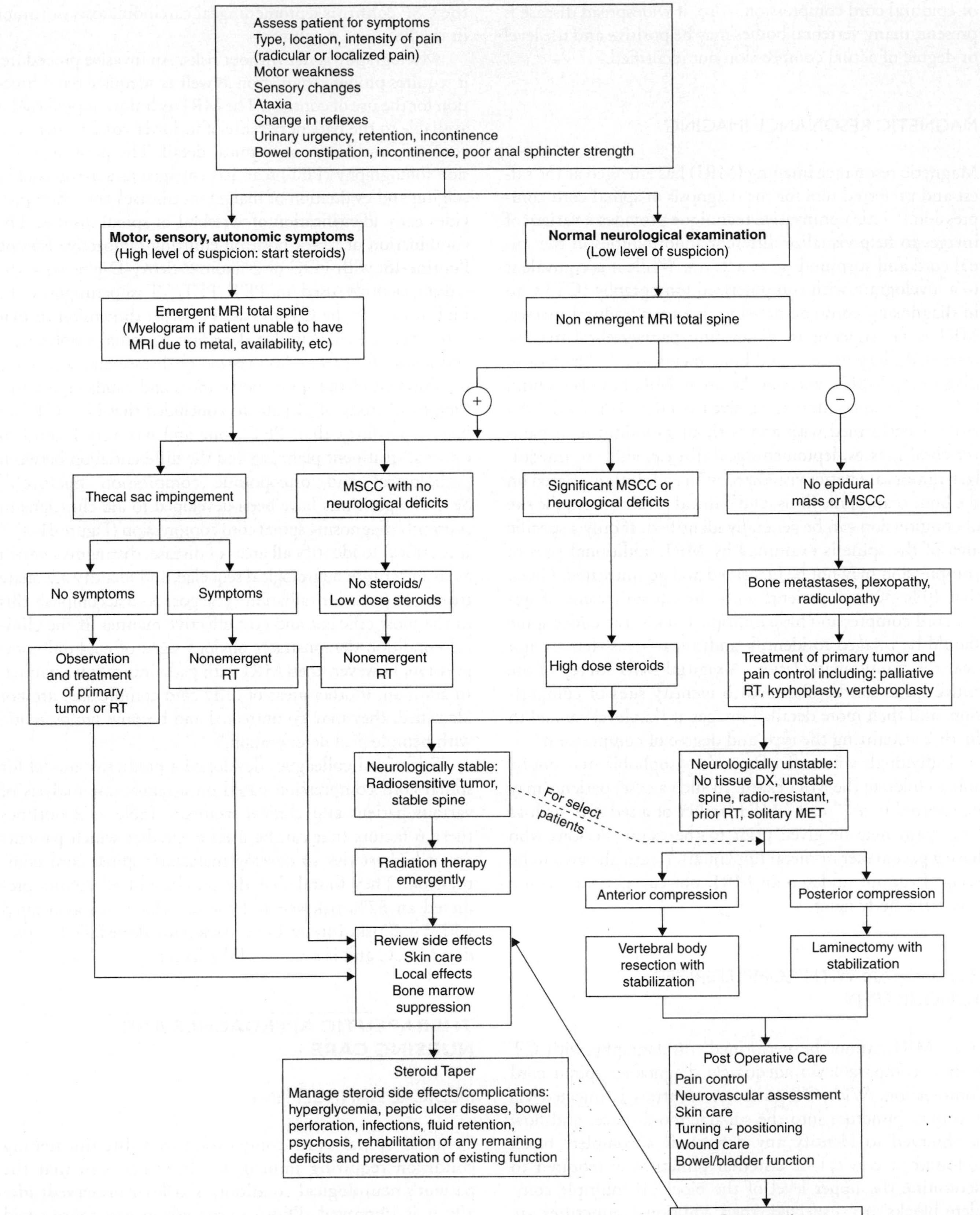


**FIGURE 41-4**

Clinical pathway for spinal cord compression.

*Abbreviations*: DX, diagnosis; MET, metastasis; MSCC, malignant spinal cord compression; RT, radiation therapy.

**TABLE 41-2**

**Predictive Risk Factors for Malignant Spinal Cord Compression**

- Inability to walk
- Increased deep tendon reflexes
- Compression fractures on spine films
- Presence of bone metastatsis
- Bone metastasis diagnoses of more than 1 year
- Patient age less than 60 years

*Source*: Data from Talcott et al.[37]

therapy, and surgery, including either laminectomy or vertebral body resection with spine stabilization and chemotherapy. While controversy exists over which treatment or combination of treatments is the best approach, post-treatment neurological status is most directly related to pretreatment neurological status.[28,38] The goals of treatment include decompression of neural tissue, eradication of tumor, relief of pain, preservation of neurological function and stability of spine, and prevention of recurrence and progression.[25]

## Steroids

The usual treatment for spinal cord compression, regardless of the type of cancer, comprises steroids combined with radiotherapy. Steroids are instituted when there is a high level of suspicion of spinal cord compression and prior to definitive treatment because they relieve pain and improve neurological function by reducing spinal cord edema. The one exception occurs when spinal cord compression is the presenting symptom of cancer and lymphoma is suspected. Due to the oncolytic effect of steroids, tissue diagnosis may be difficult with concomitant use of steroids.[16,39] Steroids reduce the release of total free fatty acids that prevents lipid hydrolysis and peroxidation, thus reducing injury to the spinal cord. They also inhibit Prostaglandin E2 (PGE2) that is related to prostaglandin synthesis and down regulate VEGF, thereby preventing certain effects on vascular permeability and reducing edema.[40,41]

The dosing of steroids is not standardized, and experts differ on the proper starting dose. The traditional dosing for steroids is either moderate dose, consisting of a bolus of dexamethasone 10 mg intravenously (IV) followed by 4 mg every 6 hours, or high dose, consisting of a bolus of 100 mg followed by 24 mg every 6 hours. One non-randomized study compared high-dose dexamethasone to a lower dose and found no difference in overall neurological recovery.[42] Higher doses of steroids should be reserved for those patients with significant neurological symptoms or rapidly progressing symptoms, as higher doses are associated with more significant side effects.[14]

Steroid therapy continues during the early phase of definitive treatment and may begin to be tapered if the individual's neurological status improves or is stabilized. The taper continues unless symptoms worsen, in which case doses should be increased until improvement and tapered again after restabilization.[14] Tapering is a priority to avoid the long-term side effects of steroid therapy, such as hyperglycemia, psychosis, gastric ulceration, immunosuppression and opportunistic infections, and proximal muscle weakness, in an already compromised individual. One steroid complication that is unique to patients with spinal cord compression is gastrointestinal perforation from straining with constipation.[21] Complications associated with steroid use are more common when serum albumin is low, length of administration is longer than 3 weeks, and the cumulative dose is high.[16] One study looked at eliminating the use of steroids completely in patients who had normal neurological function and minor compression of the cord at the time of diagnosis. In this group of patients, steroids were not required during the course of treatment with radiation.[43]

## Radiation

Radiation therapy is the standard treatment for spinal cord compression due to epidural metastasis. The radiation port is identified by MRI and extends 2 vertebrae above and below the level of the compression. This field ensures that the metastatic disease is fully treated and prevents nearby recurrences. The usual dosage range is 20–40 Gy given in 5–20 fractions over 2–4 weeks.[25] The dose of radiation and length of treatment are determined partly by histology, as most solid tumors respond at 30 Gy delivered in 10 fractions. Neuroblastoma and lymphoma have favorable histologies and respond to 20–30 Gy, whereas more radiation-resistant tumors such as melanoma require more than 30 Gy. Overall, breast and prostate cancer, myeloma, and lymphoma respond to radiation better than melanoma, sarcoma, lung, colon and renal cell cancer.[43]

As demonstrated in Table 41-1, the degree of neurological impairment prior to initiating treatment is predictive of recovery of ambulation post-treatment. In a classic study, Maranzano and Latini evaluated the effect of radiation and steroids on neurological status in cord compression.[44] The majority of individuals were ambulatory (52%), and 94% of these patients remained so post treatment. Patients who were paraparetic or paralyzed did not respond as well, with only 60% and 11%, respectively, being ambulatory after treatment. Median survival time was longer for females, those patients who remained ambulatory, and for those individuals with favorable histologies such as myeloma and breast and prostate cancers. Again, the major conclusion drawn from this study is the importance of early diagnosis.

In a study at a cancer center, the outcome status of 166 patients with spinal cord compression was evaluated by looking at performance and neurological status.[45] More than 90% of the patients received radiation therapy; neurological status improved in 20% of patients, while performance status improved in only 16%. The majority of patients stayed the same, but 25% were worse after treatment. Radiation therapy, however, is quite effective in relieving pain. The Maranzano and Latini study found that pain was relieved in 85% of patients who received such treatment.[44]

Newer approaches to radiation therapy in the treatment of spinal cord compression include intensity-modulated radiotherapy, short-course radiotherapy, and stereotactic radiosurgery. Intensity-modulated radiotherapy and stereotactic radiosurgery are techniques that are geared toward treating the tumor while sparing surrounding healthy tissue.[46] High-dose, single-fraction image-guided intensity-modulated radiotherapy for metastatic spinal lesions was evaluated for toxicity and efficacy in 103 patients at a major cancer center.[47] This noninvasive intervention used an average dose of 24 Gy and was found to be safe while providing effective palliation with an overall control rate of 90% at a median follow-up of 15 months. Short-course radiotherapy includes 1 or 2 fractions of 8 Gy and has been found to be an effective treatment with tolerable side effects.[48] It is indicated for palliation and pain relief in those patients who have been paralyzed more than 24 hours and who have a very short life expectancy. Stereotactic surgery, widely used for intracranial lesions has recently been investigated for its usefulness with metastatic spinal lesions.[49] Spinal radiosurgery can achieve rapid and durable pain relief and presents a viable treatment option for single spinal metastasis.[50] Additional research is needed to fully evaluate these newer approaches and define their roles in the treatment of spinal cord compression.

Approximately 10% of individuals with spinal cord compression will experience a local recurrence, the majority within a couple of vertebrae of the initial site of cord compression.[33] Additional radiation may or may not be an option given the maximum amount the spinal cord can tolerate without injuring the healthy neural tissue. If excessive radiation is given, the cord may become damaged and result in further weakness, sensory changes, or autonomic dysfunction. The likelihood of radiation-induced myelopathy depends on the dose of radiation per fraction, total dose, size or volume of the field, and amount of time between courses of radiation.[43] If near maximum doses of radiation have been reached, then stereotactic radiosurgery or intensity-modulated single-fraction radiotherapy may be indicated.

The side effects of radiation are minimal and relate to where on the spinal column the radiation is directed. Radiation is generally well tolerated, but patients with preexisting bone metastasis and less than optimal bone marrow function may incur pronounced myelosuppression due to radiation effects. Skin reactions are usually mild, and doses are delivered in such a fashion that surrounding tissue is minimally affected.

### Surgical interventions

In the past, surgery was indicated only for those patients with neurological deficits that progressed during radiation or that presented acutely with rapid deterioration, with spinal instability, or with local recurrence after completion of radiation. The development of MRI, which provides detailed imaging of the tumor and neural structures, and new spine stabilization techniques have made surgery a more effective and earlier option. Historically, surgery involved a laminectomy with a posterior approach because surgeons were unable to adequately stabilize the vertebral body, which would be required with an anterior approach. The laminectomy procedure partially resects the tumor and decompresses the cord or nerve roots, but the outcome has proved to be no more effective than radiation alone.[51] Most spinal cord metastases are located anteriorly, anterolaterally, or posterolaterally, and this surgical approach precludes complete resection.

A newer surgical approach, called circumferential decompression, completely resects the tumor, frees the thecal sac and nerve roots of malignant compression, and reconstructs the spine so that stability is achieved.[46] To accomplish this, surgery may include multiple approaches. Because the majority of tumors are anterior, an anterior approach is most often required. The diseased vertebral body is resected (corpectomy) and reconstructed with methylmethacrylate or other material, then the spine is further stabilized with either anterior or posterior devices that attach to healthy adjoining vertebral bodies. The spine can also be stabilized with bone grafting or fusion posteriorly. The anterior approach requires a thoracotomy for thoracic and some cervical vertebrae. For lumbar resection, a retroperitoneal approach is often used, whereas an anterolateral approach is required for most cervical lesions.[46]

The first study comparing circumferential surgery followed by radiation versus radiation alone was stopped prematurely because the results were so positive in the surgery arm.[52] Patients in the surgery arm were able to walk for a median of 126 days versus 35 days in the radiation therapy arm. In addition, more than 50% of the nonambulatory patients in the surgical arm regained the ability to walk compared to 19% in the radiation therapy arm. The surgical patients maintained continence and performance status significantly longer than the patients who received radiation therapy. Pain was also significantly less in the surgery arm. While length of survival was not significantly longer, quality of life was maximized. Surgery is usually followed by radiation therapy to achieve maximal results. Because radiation will interfere with bone grafting and wound healing, it must be timed appropriately and radiation should not be given before surgery if possible.[53]

Surgery, while it has many advantages, is not without risk. Surgical morbidity with resection and stabilization has been estimated to be as high as 48% and mortality to be about 6%.[52] Complications encountered postoperatively include wound dehiscence, infection, CSF leakage, progression of neurological deficits, instrumentation or stabilization failure, and hemorrhage.[53,54] Some tumors, such as sarcomas and renal and thyroid cancers, are particularly vascular and require preoperative embolization prior to surgery to reduce the risk of bleeding.[7]

Surgery must be carefully considered on a case-by-case basis, and the indications for this treatment approach are outlined in Table 41-3. Two important factors are the performance status of the individual prior to surgery and whether the benefit outweighs the risk. Surgery is indicated when tissue is needed for histologic diagnosis, especially if this is the only accessible area of disease. Extensive bone destruction, vertebral collapse, and spine instability (particularly when accompanied by intractable pain) may be best treated with a surgical approach but requires healthy adjoining vertebrae to attach stabilization rods or cages.[52,55] Paravertebral tumors, which are most common in lung cancer, are also best treated with a surgical approach. In addition, if the patient is currently receiving steroid and radiation therapy and experiences rapid neurological deterioration, surgery may be warranted but must be performed within 24 hours.[53] Paralysis beyond 24 hours eliminates surgery as an option. Surgery should also be considered in those cases of solitary recurrence in the spinal cord, given that intact surrounding vertebrae are required for the attachment of stabilization instruments. New techniques related to the attachment of these instruments, known as cages, are being investigated as part of surgery for patients with multilevel spinal metastases.[29] The desire to maintain and improve the quality of life for those patients with metastatic cancer initially motivated the use of this aggressive approach, which is now considered both effective and safe.

**TABLE 41-3**

| Indications for Surgical Management of Spinal Cord Compression |
|---|
| • Intractable pain |
| • Solitary metastasis |
| • Radioresistant tumor |
| • Prior radiation to the site |
| • Histological diagnosis required |
| • Compression of the spinal cord by bone |
| • Neurological deterioration despite radiation |
| • Spinal instability caused by pathological fracture |

*Source*: Data from Gerstzen and Welch[7]; and Meyers.[10]

## Chemotherapy

Chemotherapy may be a treatment option in chemosensitive tumors such as Hodgkin's and non-Hodgkin's lymphoma, small cell lung cancer, neuroblastoma, and germ cell tumors.[6,21,56] It may also be used as an adjuvant therapy to surgery and radiation, but it has a limited role and usually is not the primary treatment in an acute situation. Hormone therapy is another option for those patients with prostate and breast cancer. These patients may have had the disease a long time, have been treated with hormone manipulation, and may be resistant. The hormone-sensitive cases may benefit from a trial in addition to standard therapy for spinal cord compression.[20]

A new therapy that has emerged as a preventive measure for spinal cord compression is the administration of bisphosphonates. Bisphosphonates are bone resorption inhibitors that have been traditionally used to treat osteoporosis. They work by inhibiting osteoclast-mediated bone resorption, which slows bone remodeling and increases bone mineral density.[57]

Recent research has shown that bisphosphonates delay the onset and reduce the frequency of skeletal-related episodes (SREs) such as pathologic fractures, bone pain, hypercalcemia, and spinal cord compression.[58,59] They also reduce the need for palliative radiotherapy and orthopedic surgery. When they were first introduced, these agents were used primarily with bone metastases from breast cancer and multiple myeloma. Bisphosphonate administration has since expanded to other cancers that have metastasized to bone, such as renal cell, prostate, and lung cancers. While bisphosphonates have improved quality of life, prolonged survival has not been associated with their addition to supportive care.[60] Both pamidronate and zoledronic acid are FDA approved to treat bone metastases in the United States. They are associated with renal toxicity, which can be minimized by adhering to recommended dosing and infusion times.[61] If renal dysfunction does develop, bisphosphonates should be held until renal function is restored. Hypocalcemia may develop as a result of the administration of bisphosphonates, so calcium supplements with Vitamin D may be required. Mild side effects of bisphosphonates include arthralgias, myalgias and fever lasting about 48 hours.[62]

Zoledronic acid has emerged as the bisphosphonate of choice overall because its administration time is significantly shorter than that of pamidronate, 15–30 minutes versus 2 hours, and this nitrogen containing bisphosphonate is more potent and durable than pamidronate.[57] Few long-term effects have emerged with pamidronate — specifically, ocular effects, mild anemia and thrombocytopenia.[60]

Since zoledronic acid has been used as a standard of care in patients with bone metastasis, some new toxicities have emerged with its widespread use. Osteonecrosis of the jaw (ONJ) leading to oral infections as well as tooth and bone loss have been observed primarily in patients on long-term therapy with zoledronic acid although it can occur with any bisphosphonate. The incidence of ONJ is 1%-10% in the oncology population and is seen more often in patients with breast cancer who received pamidronate followed by zoledronic acid. It is also more common in patients with nonmalignant hematologic diseases and those with rheumatoid or osteoarthritis.[63]

Overall, bisphosphonates have had a profound impact on bone metastases and their effects on patients with cancer, but currently no evidence indicates that they reduce the incidence of spinal cord compression.[64]

## SYMPTOM MANAGEMENT

The nursing care of the individual experiencing spinal cord compression is primarily focused on early detection and symptom management. Clinical problems evolve from the rapidity of onset, level and degree of compression, presenting symptoms, as well as type and response to treatment. Assessment is crucial throughout this emergency for evaluation of neurological status and preservation of maximal function. Assessment includes monitoring of sensory and motor function as well as of bowel and bladder function. Table 41-4 lists the problems most frequently associated with epidural spinal cord compression and management goals with interventions to help direct care.

### Pain

Because more than 95% of patients with spinal cord compression have pain, knowledge of pain management is essential in caring for these individuals. Pain assessment is crucial to help identify intensity, location, factors that help or exacerbate pain, and other symptoms that accompany pain. Oncology nurses need extensive knowledge of the principles of analgesia, opioids, equianalgesia, cost analyses of various regimens, and nonpharmacological approaches. In addition, adjunct agents such as nonsteroidal anti-inflammatory drugs (NSAIDs), anticonvulsants, and antidepressants may be helpful in pain management.

An "analgesic ladder" approach has been developed by the Cancer Pain Relief and Palliative Care Program of the World Health Organization.[65] This approach helps clinicians select agents based on the patient's severity of pain and provides a standard for pain management. Many large institutions have "pain teams" that act as consultants for individuals with unusual or refractory pain and for whom standardized approaches, as outlined in the analgesic ladder, are ineffective.

NSAIDs are very useful in managing bone pain, but bleeding and renal problems may occur and individuals require close monitoring when these agents are used on a regular basis. Recently, anticonvulsants and antidepressants have emerged as useful agents to treat neuropathic pain that occurs when peripheral nerves or their roots are compressed or infiltrated.[66] This type of pain typically does not readily respond to opioids and requires adjunct agents for management. Epidural cord compression may also cause spastic reactions below the level of the compression and require the use of benzodiazepines. With affected patients, effective analgesia is established early and adjusted as steroids and radiation relieve pain. A variety of agents and types of administration are available to provide comfort.

Two new approaches to establish spine stabilization and pain relief in metastatic spinal disease are vertebroplasty and kyphoplasty. Both of these procedures have specific indications and contraindications, but offer an approach that may be adjunct to the traditional treatment for spinal cord compression. These procedures are indicated for patients with chronic pain and vertebral instability who are not neurologically compromised or have epidural compression. Further research is needed to define their particular roles in conjunction with other modalities..

Vertebroplasty is a minimally invasive procedure performed under CT guidance or fluoroscopy in which a needle is inserted into the vertebral body and polymethylmethacrylate (PMMA) is injected. Once the vertebral body is strengthened and fortified, the patient experiences relief of pain and greater mobility. Theories as to how this procedure relieves pain include immobilization of microfractures, reduction of mechanical forces, destruction of nerve endings by PMMA, and a possible antitumor effect of PMMA. The complication rate for vertebroplasty is about 10%, and the major complications are related to trauma to surrounding vessels or organs and cement leakage.[67]

Kyphoplasty evolved from vertebroplasty and also uses PMMA to strengthen the vertebral body. This procedure, however, uses a balloon that is inserted into the vertebral body and slowly inflated to restore the height of that vertebral body. Once this is accomplished, PMMA is injected into the space created by the balloon using cement filler. The advantage of this procedure is that it restores vertebral body height in addition to providing pain relief and stabilization.[68]

Vertebroplasty is used primarily for vertebral stabilization and pain relief while kyphoplasty restores height in the vertebral body as well as allow some tumor to be removed.. It is preferred over vertebroplasty when there is more that a 20 degree deformity in the spine and the posterior cortex of the vertebra is involved.[69] The interventions are used primarily for stabilization and pain relief in those patients who are poor surgical candidates.

### Mobility

Quality of life is deeply affected by changes in one's ability to ambulate and function independently. It is crucial; therefore, that the oncology nurse identifies any motor or sensory changes early, before more profound loss is encountered. Preserving and maximizing function are a priority

**TABLE 41-4**

**Symptom Management**

| Problem | Patient Goals | Intervention |
|---|---|---|
| Pain due to irritation and compression of nerve roots and neural tissue and/or stretching of the periosteum, as evidenced by localized or radicular pain | Maximum comfort as reported on a pain scale during rest and activity by appropriately using various types of analgesics and nonpharmacological interventions | • Opioids—time release, immediate, transdermal release<br>• Dexamethasone<br>• NSAIDs<br>• Anticonvulsants/antidepressants<br>• Complementary medicine: capsicum cream, hydrotherapy<br>• Vertebroplasty, kyphoplasty |
| Immobility due to edema and ischemia of neural tissue, motor neurons, as evidenced by proximal muscle weakness that progresses to motor loss | Maintain optimal level of mobility, range of motion, and strength through an activity and exercise program | • Referral to physical therapy<br>• Obtain equipment and devices to preserve alignment, enhance mobility, and stabilize spine<br>• Assist home-care agency in organizing environment to be conducive to mobility |
| Risk of injury due to sensory loss, which includes paresthesia and loss of temperature, position and vibratory senses, and light touch | Safety will be preserved at all times | • Assess degree of sensory changes: touch, temperature, paresthesia<br>• Assess environment for physical, thermal, and chemical hazards and organize environment to minimize hazards<br>• Assist patient with ADLs as indicated |
| Bladder dysfunction due to disruption of lower motor neurons (autonomic function), as evidenced by incontinence, frequency, and/or retention | Maintain adequate urinary elimination with early identification and treatment of urinary tract infections | • Fluid intake greater than 2 quarts/day<br>• Adequate intake of juices to maintain acidity (eg, cranberry)<br>• Straight catheterization/indwelling catheter to maintain continence and empty bladder<br>• Change indwelling catheter each week<br>• Urinalysis/urine culture for pain, burning, foul-smelling/cloudy urine, fever, increased WBC count<br>• Prompt treatment of UTI with antibiotic sensitive to the organism identified<br>• Daily perineal hygiene |
| Bowel disturbances due to opioid use and disruption of lower motor neurons (autonomic function), as evidenced by constipation, incontinence, and/or difficulty expelling stool | Maintain adequate bowel elimination and prevent impaction from constipation | • Establish bowel regimen including stool softener (ie, docusate sodium), intestinal lubricants, mineral oil, laxatives, senna products, magnesium-based products (eg, milk of magnesia, magnesium citrate), miralax, or polyethylene glycol 3350<br>• Dietary recommendations include fresh fruits, vegetables, and high-fiber cereals<br>• Adequate fluid intake greater than 2 quarts/day<br>• Provide periodic perineal hygiene |

*Abbreviations*: ADL, activities of daily living; NSAID, non-steroidal anti-inflammatory drug; UTI, urinary tract infection; WBC, white blood cell.
*Source*: Data from Wilkes.[27]

because many patients have rehabilitative potential after treatment is initiated.

If spine and vertebral instability is present at diagnosis, the patient should be fitted for a stabilization brace to provide support until surgery can be performed. This brace is worn whenever the patient is moved or gets out of bed and postoperatively until the stabilization materials or bone grafts heal and strengthen the structures surrounding the spine. If the patient undergoes a thoracotomy for anterior resection or a 2-step procedure of anterior and posterior resection, postoperative care includes turning and positioning with special attention to preserving alignment and spine stabilization during recovery. Neurological assessment is critical in the postoperative phase as well as pain control, wound care, and preliminary rehabilitation.[70]

Physical therapy is essential for patients who experience any motor weakness and can be beneficial to all with regard to strength and conditioning. If recovery is realistic, therapy is directed toward regaining full mobility and strength. If there is permanent weakness or motor loss, the goals of therapy include maintaining existing function, strength, and range of motion. Assistive devices such as walkers, commodes, wheelchairs, and transfer boards may be required to maximize the patient's mobility. This equipment can be individualized to the patient's needs and physical environment.

### Bowel and bladder dysfunction

Autonomic disturbances include bowel and bladder incontinence and retention. Weakness of sphincters can lead to incontinence, whereas paralysis of muscles associated with emptying the bladder and rectum can lead to retention and constipation. Establishment of daily elimination regimens will help manage any bowel and bladder dysfunction.

If a patient is dexterous with a good prognosis, intermittent self-catheterization is the most effective method for urinary continence. It provides control and continence, offers ease of mobility without external devices, and reduces the incidence of urinary tract infections (UTI's). A recent review by the Cochrane group concluded that there is not enough reliable evidence to recommend sterile vs. nonsterile technique, type of catheter or strategies to prevent infection.[71] However, Medicare recently approved reimbursement for individual sterile disposable catheters for patients who require self catheterizations in an effort to prevent chronic UTI's in this population.[72] Conversely, patients with advanced cancer would benefit from an indwelling urinary catheter. Appropriate maintenance of an indwelling catheter is now a priority since Medicare will no longer reimburse for UTI's that develop while a patient is hospitalized with an indwelling urinary catheter.

Fluid intake, daily perineal hygiene, and catheter care with scheduled changes will reduce the incidence of urinary tract infections associated with indwelling catheters.[73] Fluid intake should exceed 2 liters per day and contain liquids that maintain acidity (eg, cranberry juice). Nurses must be vigilant about early diagnosis of urinary tract infections by watching for such symptoms as foul-smelling or cloudy urine, elevated white count on complete blood count (CBC), and fever. Treatment with a fluoroquinolone or sulfa-based antibiotic will usually cover most common organisms associated with urinary infections.[74]

Bowel control can be established with the appropriate use of diet, stool softeners, lubricants, and laxatives. In addition to maintaining fluid intake, dietary adjustments to help reduce constipation and establish a regular pattern include increasing fiber consumption. For patients with cancer, however, these goals may be difficult to accomplish due to anorexia and fatigue. A bowel regimen will reduce the incidence of constipation as well as establish continence. Stool seepage is less likely if the rectum is evacuated on a regular basis. If muscle tone and sphincter control are disrupted, medication can assist in developing regular bowel habits.[75]

Many lubricants and laxatives are available. Compliance, ease of use, and individual preference are factors to consider when selecting laxatives and lubricants for each individual. The regimen usually consists of a stool softener and laxative. Lubricants (eg, mineral oil) are essential if the patient has refractory constipation or impaction.

Laxatives are classified as saline, osmotic, or stimulant. Saline-type laxatives include magnesium citrate and magnesium hydroxide. The most common osmotic laxatives are polyethylene glycol 3350 (miralax), lactulose and sorbitol. Senna products, bisacodyl (dulcolax), and cascara are stimulant laxatives that are frequently prescribed.[76] A combination of these types of laxatives may be required to adequately establish regularity. Usually rectal suppositories and enemas are reserved for impaction and severe cases of constipation. In spinal cord compression, however, rectal suppositories may be needed to stimulate the intestinal nerve plexus so as to evacuate the rectum.[76]

### Skin care

Skin care is essential during radiation therapy, particularly if the patient is receiving higher doses or treatment to a large port. The radiation oncology nurse performs routine assessment so that skin problems are identified promptly. During radiation therapy, skin should be washed with a mild soap, the use of a plain, nonscented, lanolin-free hydrophilic cream may be useful in preventing radiation skin reaction. Usual skin reactions are redness and mild discomfort similar to sunburn. While skin reactions from spine irradiation are rare, biofine cream or calendula can be applied if an open area develops, although validated recommendations are lacking today.[77]

## CONCLUSION

Spinal cord compression is one of the most common neurological emergencies facing the individual with cancer. Prompt recognition and treatment may preserve neurological function and prevent permanent deficits, such as paraplegia and bowel and bladder incontinence. MRI has emerged as the safest and most clinically useful diagnostic tool in spinal cord compression. Although radiation therapy has been the primary treatment, new surgical techniques are emerging as feasible options to restore ambulation and relieve pain.

Nurses play a pivotal role in identifying those patients at risk and early cases of spinal cord compression. Early identification is facilitated by nurses educating patients about the early signs and symptoms of MSCC, particularly in those patients with malignancies that have a tendency to metastasize to the bone.[19] One study that followed patients who were diagnosed with spinal cord compression until 1 month after treatment reinforced prior findings that those patients who are ambulatory before treatment, 65% remain so after treatment, whereas 69% of patient who were walking with assistance or unable to walk required long term facility care. Interestingly, despite the physical disabilities associated with MSCC, the majority of patient rated their quality of life positively and few rated high for anxiety or depression. This tells us that physical distress does not preclude emotional well being and patients require highly effective interventions to prevent and treat MSCC.[78]

## REFERENCES


1. Quinn JA, DeAngelis LM. Neurologic emergencies in the cancer patient. *Semin Oncol.* 2000;27:311–321.
2. Loblaw DA, Laperriere NJ, Mackillop WJ. A population-based study of malignant spinal cord compression in Ontario. *Clin Oncol (R Coll Radiol).* 2003;15:211–217.
3. Byrne TN. Metastatic epidural cord compression. *Curr Neurol Neurosci Rep.* 2004;4:191–195.
4. Barron KD, Hirano A, Araki S, Terry RD. Experiences with metastatic neoplasms involving the spinal cord. *Neurology.* 1959;9:91–106.
5. Back F, Larsen BH, Rohde K, et al. Metastatic spinal cord compression, occurrence,symptoms, clinical presentations and prognosis in 398 patients with spinal cord compression. Acta Neurochir. 1990;107:37–432.
6. Abrahm JL. Assessment and treatment of patients with malignant spinal cord compression. *J Support Oncol.* 2004;2:377–388, 391; discussion 377–388.
7. Gerszten PC, Welch WC. Current surgical management of metastatic spinal disease. *Oncology.* 2000;14:1013–1024.
8. Levack P, Graham J, Collie D. et al. Scottish Cord Compression Study Group. Don't wait for a sensory level—listen to the symptoms: a prospective audit of the delays in diagnosis of malignant cord compression. Clin Oncol (R Coll Radiol). 2002;14:472–480..
9. Gilbert RW, Kim JH, Posner JB. Epidural spinal cord compression from metastatic tumor: diagnosis and treatment. *Ann Neurol.* 1978;3:40–51.
10. Meyers JS: Complications of cancer and cancer treatment. In Langhorn ME, Fulton JS, Otto SE, eds *Oncology Nursing,* ed 5. St. Louis, Mosby; 2007:402–453.
11. Moore KL, Dalley AF. *Clinically Oriented Anatomy,* ed 4. Philadelphia, Lippincott, Williams and Wilkins;1999:1093–1096.
12. Henze R. Traumatic and vascular injuries of the central nervous system. In Bullock B, Henze R, eds. *Focus on Pathophysiology.* Philadelphia, Lippincott; 2000:938–978.
13. Byrne TN, Waxman SG. Spinal cord compression: diagnosis and principles of treatment. In *Contemporary Neurology Series,* vol. 33. Philadelphia, FA Davis; 1990:66.
14. Byrne TN. Spinal cord compression from epidural metastases. *N Engl J Med.* 1992;327:614–619.
15. Schiff D. Clinical features and diagnosis of neoplastic epidural spinal cord compression, including cauda equina syndrome. http://www.utdol.com/online/content/topic.do?topicKey=genl_onc/5033&selectedTitle=1-96&source=search_result. Accessed November 8, 2009.
16. Weinstein SN. Management of spinal cord and cauda equina compression. In Berger A, Shuster JL, Von Roenn JH. *Principles And Practice Of Palliative Care and Supportive Oncology.* Philiadelphia: Lippincott, Williams and Wilkins; 2007:415–424.
17. Arguello F, Baggs RB, Duerst RE, Johnstone L, McQueen K, Frantz CN. Pathogenesis of vertebral metastasis and epidural spinal cord compression. *Cancer.* 1990;65:98–106.
18. Cole JS, Patchell RA. Metastatic Epidural Spinal Cord Compression. http://neurology.thelancet.com Vol 7 May 2008. Accessed October 8, 2009.
19. Drudge-Coates L, Rajbabu K. Diagnosis and management of malignant spinal cord compression: part 1. *Int J Palliat Nurs.* 2008;14:110–116.
20. Osowski M. Spinal cord compression: An obstructive oncologic emergency. http://www.medscape.com/viewarticle/442735 Accessed August 10, 2009.
21. Deangelis LM, Posner JB: Neurologic complications. In Holland JF, Frei E, Bast RC, et al, eds. *Cancer Medicine* ed 5. Baltimore, Williams and Wilkins; 2001:2451–2467.
22. Smitt PS, Tsafka A, Teng-van de Zande F, et al. Outcome and complications of epidural analgesia in patients with chronic cancer pain. *Cancer.* 1998;83:2015–2022.
23. Coffey RJ, Burchiel K. Inflammatory mass lesions associated with intrathecal drug infusion catheters: report and observations on 41 patients. *Neurosurgery.* 2002;50:78–86; discussion 86.
24. Gledhill RF, Harrison BM, McDonald WI. Demyelination and remyelination after acute spinal cord compression. *Exp Neurol.* 1973;38: 472–487.
25. Spinazzé S, Caraceni A, Schrijvers D. Epidural spinal cord compression. *Crit Rev Oncol Hematol.* 2005;56:397–406.
26. Helweg-Larsen S, Hansen SW, Sørensen PS. Second occurrence of symptomatic metastatic spinal cord compression and findings of multiple spinal epidural metastases. *Int J Radiat Oncol Biol Phys.* 1995;33: 595–598.
27. Wilkes GM: Spinal cord compression. In: Yarbro CH, Frogge MH, Goodman M, eds. *Cancer Symptom Management.* ed 3. Sudbury, MA, Jones and Bartlett; 2004:359–373.
28. Helweg-Larsen S, Sørensen PS, Kreiner S. Prognostic factors in metastatic spinal cord compression: a prospective study using multivariate analysis of variables influencing survival and gait function in 153 patients. *Int J Radiat Oncol Biol Phys.* 2000;46:1163–1169.
29. Sun H, Nemecek AN. Optimal management of malignant epidural spinal cord compression. *Emerg Med Clin North Am.* 2009;27:195–208.
30. Posner JB: *Neurologic Complications of Cancer.* Philadelphia, FA Davis; 1995:135–145.
31. Maranzano E, Latini P, Beneventi S, et al. Radiotherapy without steroids in selected metastatic spinal cord compression patients. A phase II trial. *Am J Clin Oncol.* 1996;19:179–183.
32. Hickey JV: *The Clinical Practice of Neurological and Neurosurgical Nursing,* ed 6. Philadelphia, Lippincott, Williams and Wilkins; 2003:427–435.
33. Huff SJ: Neoplasms, spinal cord. *eMedicine Journal* 2, 2001. *www.emedicine.com/emerg/topic337.htm.* Accessed February 20, 2009.
34. Schiff D. Spinal cord compression. *Neurol Clin.* 2003;21:67–86.
35. Jordan JE, Donaldson SS, Enzmann DR. Cost effectiveness and outcome assessment of magnetic resonance imaging in diagnosing cord compression. *Cancer.* 1995;75:2579–2586.
36. Metser U, Lerman H, Blank A, Lievshitz G, Bokstein F, Even-Sapir E. Malignant involvement of the spine: assessment by 18F-FDG PET/CT. *J Nucl Med.* 2004;45:279–284.
37. Talcott JA, Stomper PC, Drislane FW, et al. Assessing suspected spinal cord compression: a multidisciplinary outcomes analysis of 342 episodes. *Support Care Cancer.* 1999;7:31–38.
38. Byrne TN: Metastatic epidural spinal cord compression. In Black PH, Loeffler JS, eds. *Cancer of the Nervous System.* London, Blackwell Scientific;1997:664–673.
39. Bilsky MH, Lis E, Raizer J, Lee H, Boland P. The diagnosis and treatment of metastatic spinal tumor. *Oncologist.* 1999;4:459–469.
40. Amar AP, Levy ML. Pathogenesis and pharmacological strategies for mitigating secondary damage in acute spinal cord injury. *Neurosurgery.* 1999;44:1027–39; discussion 1039.
41. Hayashi T, Sakurai M, Abe K, Sadahiro M, Tabayashi K, Itoyama Y. Expression of angiogenic factors in rabbit spinal cord after transient ischaemia. *Neuropathol Appl Neurobiol.* 1999;25:63–71.
42. Vecht CJ, Haaxma-Reiche H, van Putten WL, de Visser M, Vries EP, Twijnstra A. Initial bolus of conventional versus high-dose dexamethasone in metastatic spinal cord compression. *Neurology.* 1989;39:1255–1257.
43. Janjan NA, Delclos ME, Ballo MT, et al. Palliative care. In Cox JD, Ang KK, eds, *Radiation Oncology,* ed 8. St. Louis, Mosby; 2003:954–986.

44. Maranzano E, Latini P. Effectiveness of radiation therapy without surgery in metastatic spinal cord compression: final results from a prospective trial. *Int J Radiat Oncol Biol Phys.* 1995;32:959–967.
45. Cowap J, Hardy JR, A'Hern R. Outcome of malignant spinal cord compression at a cancer center: implications for palliative care services. *J Pain Symptom Manage.* 2000;19:257–264.
46. Klimo P, Kestle JR, Schmidt MH. Treatment of metastatic spinal epidural disease: a review of the literature. *Neurosurg Focus* 15, 2003. www.medscape.com/viewarticle/465359. Accessed November 8, 2009.
47. Yamada Y, Bilsky MH, Lovelock DM, et al. High-dose, single-fraction image-guided intensity-modulated radiotherapy for metastatic spinal lesions. *Int J Radiat Oncol Biol Phys.* 2008;71:484–490.
48. Maranzano E, Latini P, Perrucci E, Beneventi S, Lupattelli M, Corgna E. Short-course radiotherapy (8 Gy x 2) in metastatic spinal cord compression: an effective and feasible treatment. *Int J Radiat Oncol Biol Phys.* 1997;38:1037–1044.
49. Finn MA, Vrionis FD, Schmidt MH. Spinal radiosurgery for metastatic disease of the spine. *Cancer Control.* 2007;14:405–411.
50. Ryu S, Jin R, Jin JY, et al. Pain control by image-guided radiosurgery for solitary spinal metastasis. *J Pain Symptom Manage.* 2008;35:292–298.
51. Young RF, Post EM, King GA. Treatment of spinal epidural metastases. Randomized prospective comparison of laminectomy and radiotherapy. *J Neurosurg.* 1980;53:741–748.
52. Patchell R, Tibbs P, Regine WF, et al. Randomized trial of direct decompressive surgical resection in the treatment of spinal cord compression caused by metastatic cancer. *The Lancet.* 2005;366:643–648.
53. Ghogawala Z, Mansfield FL, Borges LF. Spinal radiation before surgical decompression adversely affects outcomes of surgery for symptomatic metastatic spinal cord compression. *Spine.* 2001;26:818–824.
54. Villavicencio AT, Oskouian RJ, Roberson C, et al. Thoracolumbar vertebral reconstruction after surgery for metastatic spinal tumors: long-term outcomes. *Neurosurg Focus.* 2005;19:E8.
55. Witham TF, Khavkin YA, Gallia GL, Wolinsky JP, Gokaslan ZL. Surgery insight: current management of epidural spinal cord compression from metastatic spine disease. *Nat Clin Pract Neurol.* 2006;2:87–94; quiz 116.
56. Daw HA, Markman M. Epidural spinal cord compression in cancer patients: diagnosis and management. *Cleve Clin J Med.* 2000;67: 497–504.
57. Viale PH, Yamamoto D. Bisphosphonates: expanded roles in the treatment of patients with cancer. *Clin J Oncol Nurs.* 2003;7:393–401.
58. Ali SM, Esteva FJ, Hortobagyi G, et al. Safety and efficacy of bisphosphonates beyond 24 months in cancer patients. *J Clin Oncol.* 2001;19:3434–3437.
59. Van Poznak CH. The use of bisphosphonates in patients with breast cancer. *Cancer Control.* 2002;9:480–489.
60. Pavlakis N, Schmidt RL, Stockler M. Bisphosphonates for breast cancer. *Cochrane Database Syst Rev.* 2005:CD003474.
61. Major P. The use of zoledronic acid, a novel, highly potent bisphosphonate, for the treatment of hypercalcemia of malignancy. *Oncologist.* 2002;7:481–491.
62. Zolidronic Acid Lexi-Drugs online http://online.lexi.com/crlsql/servlet/crlonline. Accessed November 8, 2009.
63. Estilo CL, Van Poznak CH, Wiliams T, et al. Osteonecrosis of the maxilla and mandible in patients with advanced cancer treated with bisphosphonate therapy. *Oncologist.* 2008;13:911–920.
64. Penas-Prado M, Loghin ME. Spinal cord compression in cancer patients: review of diagnosis and treatment. *Curr Oncol Rep.* 2008;10:78–85.
65. Ashby M, Jackson K. When the WHO ladder appears to be failing: approaches to refractory or unstable cancer pain. In Sykes N, Fallon MT, Patt RB, eds. *Clinical Pain Management: Cancer Pain.* New York, Oxford University Press; 2003:143–156.
66. National Pain Foundation: Neuropathic Pain. http://www.nationalpainfoundation.org/articles/357/medications?PHPSESSID=b317b1269b597e016649cbbba20b847e. Accessed November 8, 2009.
67. Pilitsis JG, Rengachary SS. The role of vertebroplasty in metastatic spinal disease. *Neurosurg Focus.* 2001;11:e9.
68. Linville DA. Vertebroplasty and kyphoplasty. *South Med J.* 2002;95: 583–587.
69. Victor T. Spinal metastasis and metastatic disease to the spine and related structures: treatment & medication. http://emedicine.medscape.com/article/1157987-treatment. Accessed November 8, 2009.
70. Wiggins GC, Mirza S, Bellabarba C, West GA, Chapman JR, Shaffrey CI. Perioperative complications with costotransversectomy and anterior approaches to thoracic and thoracolumbar tumors. *Neurosurg Focus.* 2001;11:e4. www.medscape.com/veiw article/421505. Accessed November 8, 2009.
71. Moore KN, Fader M, Getliffe K. Long-term bladder management by intermittent catheterisation in adults and children. *Cochrane Database Syst Rev.* 2007:CD006008.
72. Coloplast: Continence Care: Fact Sheet for Intermittent Catheter Medicare Policy Change. http://www.coloplastmediakit.com/pdf/Colplast_ContinenceCare_MedicareFactSheet.pdf. Accessed March 10, 2010.
73. Cochran S. Care of the indwelling urinary catheter: is it evidence based? *J Wound Ostomy Continence Nurs.* 2007;34:282–288.
74. Lajiness MJ. Medication minute. Common antibiotics for the treatment of urinary tract infections.*Urol Nurs.* 2008;28:387–389.
75. Preziosi G, Emmanuel A. Neurogenic bowel dysfunction: pathophysiology, clinical manifestations and treatment. *Expert Rev Gastroenterol Hepatol* 2009;3:417–423.
76. Gardner NM, Cope DG. Symptom management of diarrhea and constipation. In Cope DG, Reb AM. eds. *An Evidence Based Approach to Treatment and Care in the Older Adult with Cancer.* ONS, Pittsburgh; 2006:67–389.
77. Bolderston A, Lloyd NS, Wong KS, Holden L, Robb-Blenderman L. The prevention and management of acute skin reactions related to radiation therapy: a systematic review and practice guideline. *Support Care Cancer.* 2006;14:802–817.
78. Conway R, Graham J, Kidd J, Levack P. Scottish Cord Compression Group. What happens to people after malignant cord compression? Survival, function, quality of life, emotional well-being and place of care 1 month after diagnosis. *Clin Oncol (R Coll Radiol).* 2007;19:56–62.

CHAPTER

42

*Heather L. Brumbaugh, RN, MSN, ANP, AOCN®*

# Superior Vena Cava Syndrome

## SCOPE OF THE PROBLEM

### DEFINITIONS

Superior vena cava syndrome (SVCS) develops as a result of obstruction or compression of the superior vena cava (SVC). SVCS is an obstruction of blood flow through the SVC, the major vein that carries blood to the heart from the arms, upper chest, head, and neck. The obstruction can be caused by intrinsic or extrinsic factors to the SVC. Intrinsic factors include intraluminal tumor or thrombosis in the SVC. Tumor and enlarged lymph nodes are the most common cause of extrinsic compression of the SVC. Whether the cause is intrinsic, extrinsic, or a combination, it causes impairment of the venous return to the heart, resulting in increased venous pressure and decreased cardiac output. The onset of signs and symptoms varies from gradual to rapid depending on the cause. SVCS becomes an oncologic emergency when respiratory distress and cerebral edema occur.[1]

### INCIDENCE AND ETIOLOGY

Approximately 15,000 people in the United States develop SVCS each year.[2] SVCS was first described by William Hunter in 1757 in a patient who had a syphilitic aneurysm involving the ascending aorta.[3] In 1954, over 40% of SVCS cases were a result of syphilitic aneurysms and tuberculous mediastinitis.[4] Presently, the most common cause of SVCS is malignant disease, accounting for 70% to 80% of cases.[5]

In the adult population, a malignancy in the mediastinal area causing obstruction of upper venous blood return to the heart is the most common cause of SVCS[5,6] (Table 42-1). The most frequent occurrence of SVCS is in men ages 50 to 70 years with primary or metastatic tumors of the mediastinum.[6,7] Lung cancer is the most common malignancy that causes SVCS, accounting for over 75% of cases.[5–7] Small cell lung cancer (SCLC) is the most common histology, causing up to 65% of all cases of SVCS, even though it comprises only 15% to 20% of all newly diagnosed lung cancers. This is likely due to the tendency of SCLC to occur in the central part of the lung and involve the mediastinal lymph nodes. Squamous cell carcinoma is the second most common lung histology. Right-sided lung cancers are more likely to cause SVCS. Despite lung cancer being the leading malignant cause of SVCS, only 3% to 10% of patients with lung cancer will develop SVCS.[1,6,7]

The next most common malignant cause of SVCS is non-Hodgkin's lymphoma. The subtypes of non-Hodgkin's lymphoma associated with SVCS are diffuse large cell and lymphoblastic lymphomas, both of which often have mediastinal involvement.[5] Although Hodgkin's lymphoma commonly involves the mediastinum, it rarely results in SVCS.[1,5] Metastatic cancers cause SVCS in approximately 5% to 10% of cases. Breast cancer is the most common metastatic etiology of SVCS. Any cancer that metastasizes to the mediastinum can cause SVCS, with other reported types including sarcomas, thymoma, Kaposi's sarcoma, germ cell tumors, and gastrointestinal cancers.[1,5,6]

**TABLE 42-1**

**Cancer Etiology of Superior Vena Cava Syndrome**

| Type of Cancer | Percentage |
|---|---|
| Lung cancer | 52–81 |
| Lymphoma | 2–21 |
| Metastatic breast cancer | 3–11 |

From 22% to 40% of cases of SVCS are due to nonmalignant causes. Intravascular devices such as pacemakers and central venous catheters are the most common nonmalignant causes of SVCS (70%) as a result of thrombus formation, and they account for 3% to 5% of all cases of SVCS.[6,8,9] The second most common nonmalignant cause of SVCS is mediastinal fibrosis. Mediastinal fibrosis can be from previous radiation to the mediastinum or as a result of infection from histoplasmosis or tuberculosis.[7,10] Other rare benign causes of SVCS include retrosternal goiters, *Norcardia* infection, thoracic aortic aneurysms, and congestive heart failure.[1,9,10]

SVCS is rare in the pediatric population and most frequently a result of iatrogenic causes secondary to cardiovascular surgery for congenital heart disease or ventriculoatrial shunts for hydrocephalus.[10] Thrombosis from venous access catheters is the most common cause of nonmalignant SVCS in children.[11] The most common malignant cause of SVCS in pediatric patients is non-Hodgkin's lymphoma. Other malignant causes are acute lymphoblastic leukemia, Hodgkin's lymphoma, neuroblastoma, and yolk sac tumors.[10,12]

### RISK FACTORS

Based on the etiology of SVCS, the most significant risk factor for the development of SVCS is having a malignancy. The most common malignancy that results in increased risk for SVCS is lung cancer that commonly occurs in older patients with a history of smoking. Breast cancer is the most common metastatic cause of SVCS; thus patients with a history of breast cancer are at increased risk as well. Other tumor types that commonly involve the mediastinum are also risk factors, including non-Hodgkin's lymphoma, thymoma, and germ cell tumors. Patients with cancer often have vascular access devices for treatment purposes, and this also increases their risk for developing SVCS. Despite this, only 3% to 4% of people with cancer develop SVCS.[5,8]

## PHYSIOLOGICAL ALTERATIONS

### NORMAL ANATOMY AND PHYSIOLOGY

The SVC is the major vessel located in the middle mediastinum. It is a formed by the junction of the right and left brachiocephalic (or innominate) veins at the level of the sternal angle. The brachiocephalic veins are formed by the joining of the internal jugular and subclavian veins (Figure 42-1). As a result, the SVC carries venous drainage from the head, neck, upper extremities, and upper thorax to the right atrium of the heart, which is approximately one-third of the venous return. The SVC descends 6 to 8 cm on the right side of the ascending aorta into the pericardial sac, where it is in a fixed position and empties into the right atrium. Other rigid structures in this area of the mediastinum include the sternum, trachea, pulmonary artery, right main stem bronchus, vertebrae, and perihilar and paratracheal lymph nodes. Although the SVC is a relatively large vessel (1.5 to 2 cm in diameter), unlike other structures in the mediastinum, it has thin walls and a low intravascular pressure, allowing it to be compressed easily. The SVC is completely surrounded by chains of lymph nodes that drain the structures of the right thoracic cavity and lower left thorax (Figure 42-2). The azygous vein carries blood from the posterior torso and empties into the SVC at the level of the right main stem bronchus (Figure 42-3). The azygous vein is an important collateral pathway if a blockage to the SVC occurs above its entrance.[5]

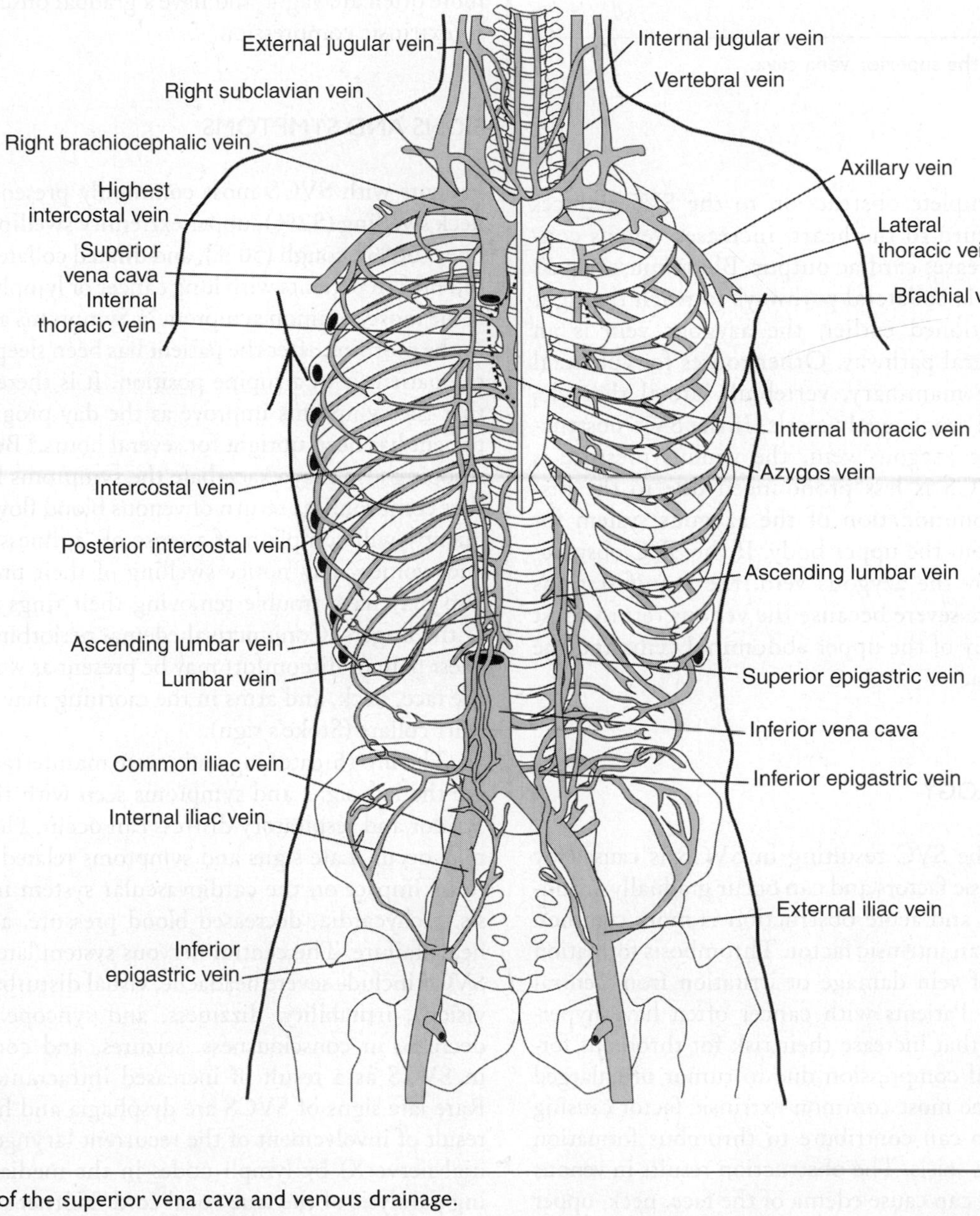


**FIGURE 42-1**

Anterior view of the superior vena cava and venous drainage.

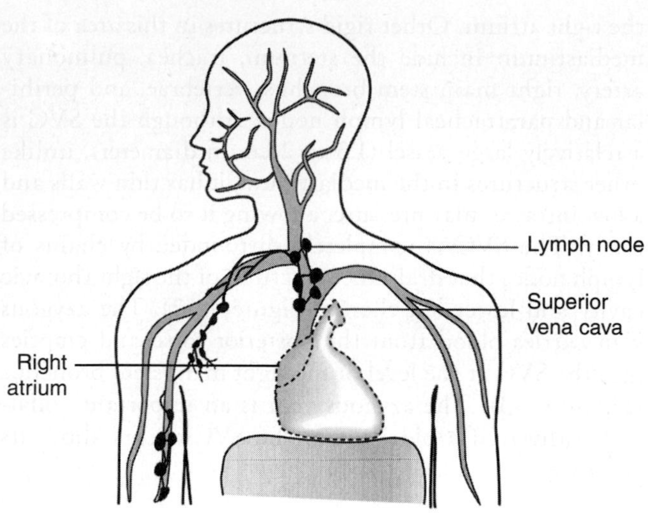


**FIGURE 42-2**

Lymph nodes near the superior vena cava.

Partial or complete obstruction to the SVC reduces venous blood return to the heart, increases venous congestion, and decreases cardiac output. Blood must bypass the obstruction via collateral pathways to reach the right atrium. As mentioned earlier, the azygous vein is an important collateral pathway. Other routes for collateral flow include the mammary, vertebral, lateral thoracic, paraspinous, and esophageal vessels. If the SVC obstruction is above the azygous vein, the venous pressure is less, and the SVCS is less pronounced due to the distension and accommodation of the azygous system for venous return from the upper body. If the SVC obstruction occurs below the azygous vein, the manifestations of SVCS are more severe because the venous return must be shunted by way of the upper abdominal veins and the inferior vena cava.[5]

### PATHOPHYSIOLOGY

Obstruction of the SVC resulting in SVCS is caused by extrinsic or intrinsic factors and can occur gradually or suddenly.[7] Complete and acute obstruction is more common with thrombosis, an intrinsic factor. Thrombosis formation can be a result of vein damage or irritation from central venous catheters. Patients with cancer often have hypercoagulable states that increase their risk for thrombus formation.[10] External compression due to tumor or enlarged lymph nodes is the most common extrinsic factor causing SVCS, but it also can contribute to thrombus formation by causing venous stasis. The obstruction results in venous hypertension that can cause edema of the face, neck, upper thorax, and upper extremities. Pleural and pericardial effusions also can develop as a result of decreased venous blood return.

## CLINICAL MANIFESTATIONS

The clinical manifestations of SVCS are affected by the obstruction of the venous drainage in the upper body, the underlying disease process, and the rapidity of onset. Often, collateral circulation develops, and symptoms actually may improve. The urgency of intervention is determined by the severity of symptoms, with sudden onset requiring more rapid intervention. As mentioned previously, a thrombus is more likely to result in complete obstruction, causing sudden onset of symptoms. The initial signs and symptoms more often are vague and have a gradual onset when caused by extrinsic compression.[7]

### SIGNS AND SYMPTOMS

Patients with SVCS most commonly present with face or neck swelling (82%), upper extremity swelling (68%), dyspnea (66%), cough (50%), and dilated collateral chest veins (38%).[6] In patients with lung cancer or lymphoma, dyspnea is the most common symptom.[5,6] Symptoms are often worse in the morning after the patient has been sleeping and when the patient is in a supine position. It is therefore common that the symptoms improve as the day progresses and the patient has been upright for several hours.[8] Bending over or stooping also may exacerbate the symptoms because it further compromises return of venous blood flow. Patients frequently will complain of a sense of "fullness" in the head, and women may notice swelling of their breasts. Patients also may have trouble removing their rings due to edema of the fingers. Conjunctival edema, periorbital edema, and chest pain or discomfort may be present as well. Swelling of the face, neck, and arms in the morning may result in tight shirt collars (Stoke's sign).

The life-threatening and severe manifestations of SVCS are the late signs and symptoms seen with this syndrome. Stridor and respiratory distress can occur. Hemoptysis also may occur. Late signs and symptoms related to SVCS due to its impact on the cardiovascular system include cyanosis, tachycardia, decreased blood pressure, and congestive heart failure. The central nervous system late symptoms of SVCS include severe headache, visual disturbances (blurred vision), irritability, dizziness, and syncope.[13] Confusion, decrease in consciousness, seizures, and coma can occur in SVCS as a result of increased intracranial pressure.[2,10] Rare late signs of SVCS are dysphagia and hoarseness as a result of involvement of the recurrent laryngeal nerve (cranial nerve X) by lymph nodes in the mediastinum, causing paralysis of the true vocal cord. Horner's syndrome (ie,

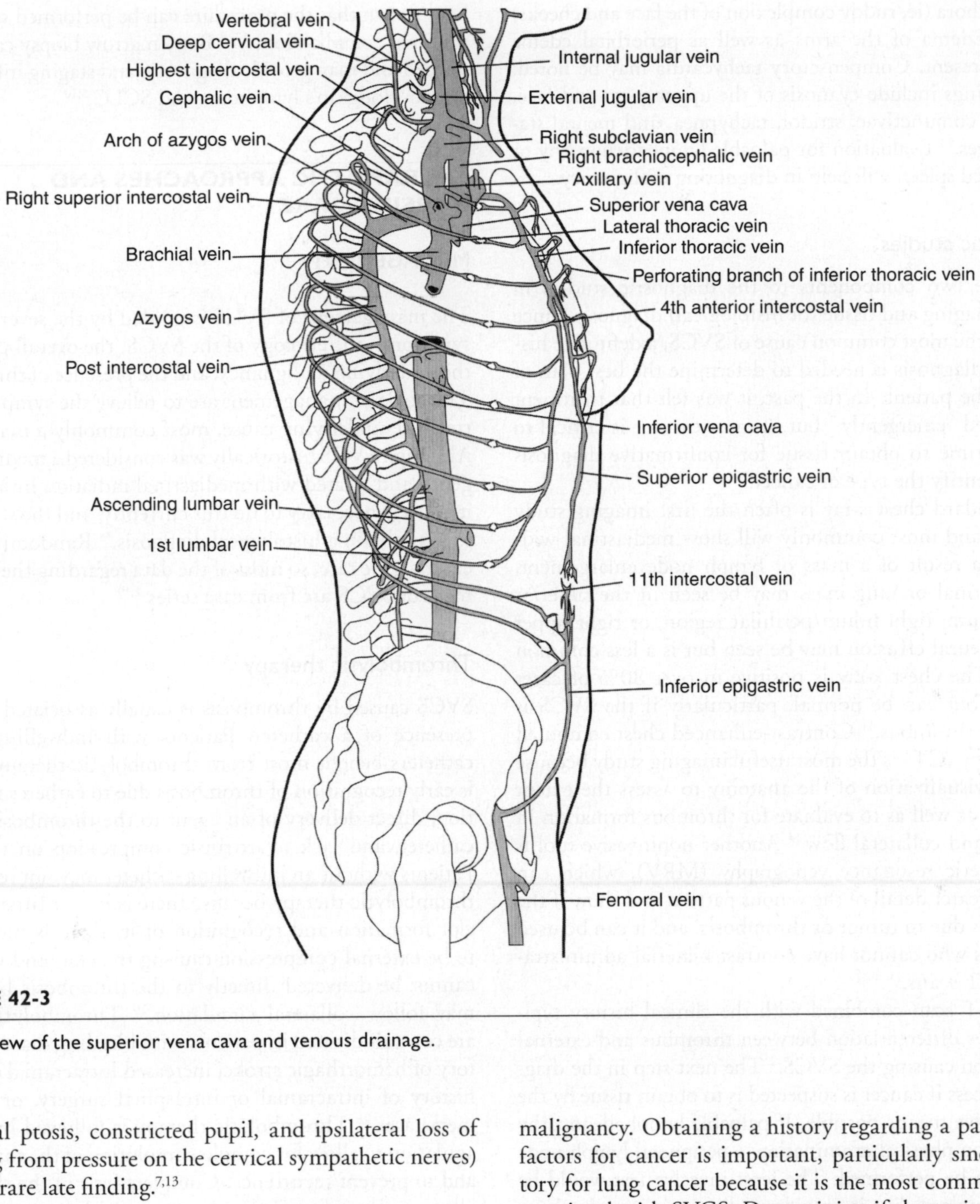


**FIGURE 42-3**

Lateral view of the superior vena cava and venous drainage.

unilateral ptosis, constricted pupil, and ipsilateral loss of sweating from pressure on the cervical sympathetic nerves) is also a rare late finding.[7,13]

## ASSESSMENT

### Patient history

History-taking is an important aspect of evaluating the patient suspected of having SVCS. Evaluating the duration of symptoms is important to determine the urgency for intervention. Since SVCS is most commonly caused by malignancy, a thorough history regarding any cancer diagnosis is critical.[5–7] SVCS can be the initial presentation of a malignancy. Obtaining a history regarding a patient's risk factors for cancer is important, particularly smoking history for lung cancer because it is the most common cancer associated with SVCS. Determining if the patient has any intravascular devices such as central venous catheters or pacemakers is necessary because thrombus is the most common benign cause of SVCS.[6] Another risk factor is a previous history of mediastinal radiation, so the patient should be asked about any treatment with radiation in the past.[2]

### Physical examination

The physical examination findings of SVCS are specific to the syndrome. Most patients with SVCS will have dilated neck and/or chest wall veins and facial edema.[2,8] Often facial plethora (ie, ruddy complexion of the face and cheeks) is seen. Edema of the arms as well as periorbital edema may be present. Compensatory tachycardia may be noted. Late findings include cyanosis of the upper torso and face, engorged conjunctivae, stridor, tachypnea, and mental status changes.[13] Evaluation for palpable lymphadenopathy or an enlarged spleen will help in diagnosing malignancy.

### Diagnostic studies

There are two components to the diagnostic studies in SVCS, imaging and tissue (or histological) diagnosis. Since cancer is the most common cause of SVCS, a definitive histological diagnosis is needed to determine the best plan of care for the patient. In the past, it was felt that treatment was needed "emergently," but in most cases it is critical to take the time to obtain tissue for confirmative diagnosis and to identify the type of cancer.[1,10]

A standard chest x-ray is often the first imaging study obtained and most commonly will show mediastinal widening as a result of a mass or lymph node enlargement. A mediastinal or lung mass may be seen in the superior mediastinum, right hilum/perihilar region, or right upper lobe. A pleural effusion may be seen but is a less common finding. The chest x-ray is positive in over 80% of cases of SVCS but can be normal, particularly if the SVCS is caused by thrombus.[11] Contrast-enhanced chest computed tomography (CT) is the most useful imaging study because it allows visualization of the anatomy to assess the extent of disease as well as to evaluate for thrombus formation in the SVC and collateral flow.[14] Another noninvasive tool is the magnetic resonance venography (MRV), which can provide greater detail of the venous pattern and show if the blockage is due to tumor or thrombosis, and it can be used in patients who cannot have contrast material administration for CT scans.[15]

The CT scan combined with the clinical history typically allows differentiation between thrombus and external compression causing the SVCS.[2] The next step in the diagnostic process if cancer is suspected is to obtain tissue by the least invasive means possible. If palpable lymphadenopathy is present on physical examination, a peripheral lymph node biopsy can be performed. The least invasive test would be sputum cytology, but it provides a diagnosis in only about 50% of patients with lung cancer.[5] If a pleural effusion is present, thoracentesis can be considered, although the diagnostic yield related to the cancer diagnosis is also only 50%.[16] Bronchoscopy, particularly in SCLC, will lead to a diagnosis in up to 70% of patients. Mediastinoscopy, while more invasive, has a diagnostic yield of over 90% and may be needed to obtain adequate tissue specifically in lymphoma, where a lymph node is needed to determine the subtype.[17] In the past, there was concern that mediastinoscopy would have a higher rate of complications (such as bleeding due to increased venous pressures) in patients with SVCS, but recent studies have shown that the procedure can be performed safely with minimal complications.[17,18] Bone marrow biopsy can be performed and may provide diagnostic and staging information in non-Hodgkin's lymphoma and SCLC.[5,10]

## THERAPEUTIC APPROACHES AND NURSING CARE

### MANAGEMENT

The management of SVCS is guided by the severity of the symptoms, the etiology of the SVCS, the overall prognosis, the underlying malignancy, and the presence of thrombosis. The goals of management are to relieve the symptoms and treat the underlying cause, most commonly a malignancy. Although SVCS historically was considered a medical emergency and treated with mediastinal radiation immediately, it is rarely necessary to do this currently, and the standard is to first obtain a histological diagnosis.[18] Randomized clinical trials are rare, so most of the data regarding the management of SVCS are from case series.[2,19]

### Thrombolytic therapy

SVCS caused by thrombosis is usually associated with the presence of a catheter. Patients with indwelling venous catheters benefit most from thrombolytic therapy if there is early recognition of thrombosis due to catheter malfunction, direct delivery of an agent to the thrombosis via the catheter, and lack of extrinsic compression on the SVC. Patients without an indwelling catheter may not respond to thrombolytic therapy because there is longer time between clot formation and recognition of it, there is more likely to be external compression causing the clot, and the agent cannot be delivered directly to the thrombosis because it may follow collateral circulation.[20] Thrombolytic agents are contraindicated in patients with bleeding disorders, history of hemorrhagic stroke, increased intracranial pressure, history of intracranial or intraspinal surgery, or cerebral metastases.[21] Thrombolytic therapy is followed by anticoagulation to allow for complete resolution of the thrombosis and to prevent recurrence. Complete lysis of the thrombus allows catheter function to be preserved.[20]

Thrombolytic therapy is used to dissolve the thrombus by activating plasminogen to plasmin. Plasmin in the proximity of a thrombus degrades fibrin to soluble peptides.[21] Agents that have been used for thrombolysis are streptokinase, urokinase, and tissue plasminogen activator (alteplase [tPA]).[21,22] Thrombolytic agents are given intravenously through the catheter if possible, or a peripheral venipuncture site can be just as effective. Intravenous infusion of thrombolytic agents causes activation of fibrinolysis in more than 90% of patients, resulting in thrombolysis throughout the vasculature. For a thrombus in the SVC, an initial bolus is given, followed by an infusion over 8 to 48 hours.[8,20,22] Tissue plasminogen activator appears to be more fibrin specific than streptokinase or urokinase, so it requires a shorter infusion time.[21] All the agents, though, can cause lysis of fresh platelet–fibrin plugs and result in bleeding anywhere in the vasculature. Extravasation of the agent can cause inflammation and/or ecchymosis. If this occurs, the infusion should be stopped and restarted at another site. Ice or cold packs can be applied to the extravasation site.[21] Studies have shown that therapy should be initiated within 5 days of the onset of symptoms to be effective, and urokinase was more efficacious than streptokinase.[21,22]

Tissue plasminogen activator has been associated with febrile reactions, but these can be managed with acetaminophen. Anaphylaxis and angioedema also have been seen in patients receiving tPA for the management of acute thrombotic (ischemic) stroke and myocardial infarction.[23] These severe reactions are uncommon and likely a result of activation of the complement and kinin cascades during the infusion. Concurrent use of angiotensin-converting enzyme (ACE) inhibitors may increase the risk of this complication based on case reports.[24] Patients receiving tPA should be monitored for signs of angioedema or anaphylaxis during and immediately after the infusion.[23,24] If anaphylaxis occurs, standard emergency care should be given. Angioedema should be treated with ranitidine, diphenhydramine, and epinephrine at the first signs of throat or tongue swelling. Assessment of the tongue and oropharynx should be done every 30 to 45 minutes at the start of the infusion. In the case reports of angioedema associated with tPA, the tongue swelling initially was unilateral and then progressed to involve the entire tongue and oropharynx.[24]

Following lysis of the thrombus by a thrombolytic therapy, anticoagulation should be given to prevent recurrence. Unfractionated heparin or low-molecular-weight heparin (LMWH) should be continued for at least 5 days after thrombolytic therapy. Oral anticoagulation (warfarin) should overlap the heparin or LMWH for at least 4 to 5 days. Once the international normalized ratio (INR) is therapeutic (between 2 and 3) for 2 consecutive days, the heparin or LMWH can be stopped. Continued LMWH is the treatment of choice for patients with warfarin hypersensitivity or pregnancy or patients who cannot be monitored adequately on warfarin.[21]

Bleeding precautions are an important nursing function during thrombolytic and anticoagulation therapies. Assessment for bleeding and vital sign monitoring are needed. Venous hypertension due to SVCS can cause increased intracranial pressure and increase the risk of intracranial hemorrhage. Laboratory monitoring for patients receiving thrombolytics includes a baseline complete blood count (CBC) and activated partial thromboplastin time (aPTT) prior to initiation of therapy and every 6 hours during the infusion. Once the patient is on anticoagulation, unfractionated heparin is monitored with an aPTT, LMWH is monitored by LMWH or enoxaparin level, and warfarin is monitored by the INR.[21] If the patient is continued on warfarin, he or she will need education that any change in medications requires monitoring of the INR.

### Chemotherapy

Since cancer is the most common cause of SVCS, treatment of the cancer also can treat SVCS. For cancers that are highly chemosensitive, chemotherapy is an appropriate treatment measure. Complete relief of symptoms can be obtained in 80% of patient with non-Hodgkin's lymphoma and SCLC.[8,25] Germ cell tumors also respond well, and even up to 40% of non-small cell lung cancer patients will respond to chemotherapy.[8,10,25] Multiagent or combination chemotherapy is the standard.

In SCLC, chemotherapy is the preferred treatment, even in the presence of SVCS.[10,25] The prognosis of patients with SCLC is not adversely affected by the presence of SVCS. Treatment is usually cisplatin or carboplatin based and combined with other agents such as etoposide, ifosfamide, cyclophosphamide, doxorubicin, vincristine, taxanes, or gemcitabine.[26] Most patients will have improvement in their symptoms in 7 days and complete resolution within 2 weeks.[8,10] In contrast to SCLC, patients with non-small cell lung cancer who have SVCS tend to have a poorer prognosis but still may respond to chemotherapy for palliative intent.[10,27]

Patients with non-Hodgkin's lymphoma typically are treated with chemotherapy because it is a chemosensitive disease. As in SCLC, presenting with SVCS in non-Hodgkin's lymphoma does not indicate a poorer prognosis, and patients can be cured. The presence of hoarseness, stridor, or dysphagia and short symptom duration do indicate poorer prognosis in this population.[5] Histological diagnosis is important in non-Hodgkin's lymphoma to select the appropriate chemotherapy regimen. Lymphoma regimens commonly include cyclophosphamide, doxorubicin, vincristine, prednisone, rituximab, or fludarabine.[7]

Chemotherapy also may be used in combination with radiation therapy to provide quicker relief of symptoms in some patients. Patients with SVCS may require a central line through the femoral vein for safe drug delivery. Venous stasis in the upper thorax from the SVCS could result in concentration of the chemotherapy if the agents are delivered via the upper extremities.[7] Other nursing care depends on the chemotherapeutic agents given. If chemotherapy is combined with radiation therapy, there will be increased risk for neutropenia and esophagitis. Other considerations are nausea and vomiting, stomatitis, myelosuppression, and alopecia. It is also important to remember that SVCS can be the initial presentation of malignancy, so patient education and emotional support regarding the disease process also may be needed.

### Radiation therapy

Radiation therapy is used to treat symptomatic patients with SVCS and is effective in most tumor types if the clinical status deteriorates requiring emergent intervention.[2,28] Radiation therapy is the treatment of choice in patients with non-small cell lung cancer.[25] Recent studies indicate that endovascular stenting should be considered as a sequential or simultaneous treatment to provide rapid relief and allow for histological diagnosis.[28,29] Case series of patients receiving radiation therapy for SVCS show a 31% resolution of obstruction and 23% partial improvement on serial venograms. Autopsy studies showed 14% complete patency and 10% partial patency of the SVC. Although significant blockage remained, 85% of these patients reported symptom relief.[30] The findings suggest that the development of collateral circulation contributes to improvement in symptoms and confirms that emergent therapy is not a necessity, emphasizing the importance of histological diagnosis and use of chemotherapy in chemosensitive tumors.[2]

Determination of the dose of radiation is based on tumor histology, history of previous mediastinal radiation, extent of tumor, and the patient's performance status. The initial 2 to 3 days are usually higher-dose fractions around 4 Gy to obtain a more rapid response. The subsequent fractions are at 1.8 to 2 Gy daily over 2 to 5 weeks until completion of the prescribed dose.[2,31] Standard doses generally total 30 to 50 Gy but can be as high as 60 to 70 Gy depending on tumor type. Lymphoma is more radiosensitive and requires lower doses. The radiation field for mediastinal involvement typically includes mediastinal, hilar, and supraclavicular nodes. Improvement in symptoms from venous congestion can be seen in 3 to 4 days, with maximum symptom relief in 3 weeks. Results are better in patients with lymphoma than in those with lung cancer.[2,8,28]

Nursing care of patients receiving radiation therapy is related to the side effects. Side effects vary based on the total dose, the fraction (daily) dose, the amount of normal tissue in the radiation field, and whether concomitant chemotherapy is given. Short-term or early side effects occur in the first month and include fatigue, nausea, cough, dysphagia, heartburn, esophagitis, and skin irritation. Long-term side effects of radiation are pneumonitis/interstitial lung changes, esophageal stenosis, pulmonary fibrosis, cardiac changes, and spinal cord myelopathy.[31]

### Stent placement

Another possible intervention for SVCS is percutaneous placement of an endovascular stent to bypass the obstruction. This approach provides rapid relief of symptoms, usually within 48 hours, and can be done prior to tissue diagnosis. It is therefore recommended as a first choice for palliation in cancer while the etiology is being determined and appropriate staging and treatment plans are made.[6,30,32,33] Stent placement should be considered for tumors that do not respond well to chemotherapy or radiation therapy, such as mesothelioma or lung cancer.[2] Stent placement is still possible with total occlusion of the SVC, and repeat stenting may be feasible if needed.[34,35] Resolution of headache and edema is seen within days, and 68% to 100% of patients report resolution of symptoms.[25] Complication rates are 3% to 7% for stent placement in patients with SVCS and include infection, bleeding, stent migration, stent occlusion, hematoma at the insertion site, pulmonary embolus, and very rarely, perforation.[30,35–38] Stent placement is contraindicated when tumor invasion of the vessel is present.[36]

The self-expanding wire stent is placed under local anesthesia by interventional radiology. Venous access to the obstruction for stent placement is through the basilic, subclavian, jugular, or femoral vein. The obstruction is transversed by a guidewire, and the stent is placed. Angioplasty may be needed to allow complete expansion of the vessel.[36] There is no consensus on anticoagulation therapy after stent placement. Some studies recommend full anticoagulation for patients with an underlying malignancy, others use antiplatelet agents alone, and still others suggest low-dose warfarin (1 mg/day) to maintain an INR of less than 1.6.[32,34,36,38]

Nursing care after stent placement involves assessing for complications such as hematoma, infection, deep venous thrombosis, or pulmonary embolism. Pleuritic chest pain or shoulder pain may require analgesics. Deep venous thrombosis presents with unilateral swelling of the extremity and can lead to pulmonary embolism. Pulmonary embolism can present with dyspnea, decrease in oxygen saturation, and chest pain. Localized hematoma, hypotension, and tachycardia can indicate bleeding.

### Surgical bypass

Surgical bypass has a limited role in the management of SVCS, particularly when it is from a malignant cause. It can be considered for symptomatic patients refractory to chemotherapy and radiation therapy with a life expectancy of greater than 6 months.[39] For SVCS of benign etiology, surgical bypass may be used to relieve obstruction resulting from an anterosternal goiter, aortic aneurysm, or fibrosing mediastinitis.[40] Surgical bypass can be accomplished with synthetic grafts, autologous pericardium, or saphenous vein graft.[40,41] The saphenous vein graft is preferred because of its better potential for long-term patency. The saphenous vein is slit longitudinally and wrapped around a stent (usually a chest tube) of the desired diameter; then the edges are joined by continuous suture to form a large-bore conduit. The bypass then is formed between the brachiocephalic or left internal jugular vein and the right atrium using an end-to-end anastomosis.[39,41] Surgical bypass is used only when other management techniques have failed to relieve the symptoms of SVCS.[5,8,39]

### Nursing care

Nursing management of the patient with SVCS involves assessment of cardiac, pulmonary, and neurological status to detect worsening of symptoms that would warrant intervention. Promoting oxygenation and perfusion is important through the use of oxygen therapy, elevation of the head of the bed, and anxiety management.[1] Comfort measures to relieve dyspnea will decrease anxiety of both the patient and family members. Activity may need to be limited to decrease exertion. Ongoing assessment of vital signs, oxygen saturation, activity, and mental status is needed. Signs of bronchial compression, laryngeal edema, or alterations in neurological status require emergent intervention.

Fluid balance is important in this patient population. Loop diuretics and low-sodium diets often are prescribed to reduce edema, even though efficacy is not confirmed in studies.[2,6] Careful monitoring of intake and output is needed to avoid dehydration, which can increase the risk of thrombus formation. Overhydration will exacerbate the symptoms of SVCS.[5] Avoidance of the Valsalva maneuver is essential in patients with SVCS. The Valsalva maneuver increases venous pressure, and the use of stool softeners for bowel management, as well as cough suppressants for cough, is useful.

Steroids are used commonly in patients with SVCS despite no evidence to support their use. It is thought that they may improve symptoms by decreasing the inflammatory reaction to the tumor or radiation therapy, but no controlled studies have been done to evaluate this.[5,6] Steroids may have some benefit in SVCS patients with non-Hodgkin's lymphoma because the disease is steroid responsive, but there is limited to no value in other etiologies.[2,8,25]

Oncology nurses can be of great help to patients with SVCS by helping to manage anxiety and providing education. In many patients, the initial presentation of cancer may be SVCS, and in others, it can indicate recurrence of the disease process. Emotional support for the patient and family members is an essential role for the oncology nurse. Changes in physical appearance may be present due to facial and periorbital edema. Providing reassurance that this will improve with treatment will help to decrease anxiety and fear. Head congestion and breathlessness also will increase the patient's anxiety, and a calm, restful setting can help to ease some of the anxiety. Anxiolytics may be needed and prescribed in patients with SVCS symptoms.

## CONCLUSION

Superior vena cava syndrome results from obstruction of blood flow to the SVC. The presentation can be dramatic, with facial, periorbital, and upper extremity edema, but it is rarely a true emergency. Most cases are caused by cancer, specifically lung cancer and non-Hodgkin's lymphoma. Establishment of a histological diagnosis is critical for treatment planning and prognosis. If life-threatening symptoms are present, endovascular stent placement can provide rapid relief and allow time for obtaining a tissue diagnosis. Early recognition of signs and symptoms is important to allow for evaluation, initiation of therapy, and prevention of the need for emergent intervention. Therapy is directed at the underlying condition, typically cancer, and includes chemotherapy, radiation, thrombolytic therapy, stenting, and rarely, bypass surgery. Patients presenting with SVCS still can be cured, depending on the underlying cause, and relief of symptoms is possible for most patients.

## REFERENCES


1. National Cancer Institute. Cardiopulmonary syndromes, 2005. http://www.cancer.gov/cancertopics/pdq/supportivecare/cardiopulmonary/HealthProfessionals/page5. Accessed January 16, 2010.
2. Wilson LD, Detterbeck FC, Yahalom J. Superior vena cava syndrome with malignant causes. *N Engl J Med.* 2007;356:1862–1869.
3. Hunter W. History of an aneurysm of the aorta, with some remarks on aneurysms in general. *Med Observ Inquir.* 1757;1:323–357.
4. Schechter MM. The superior vena cava syndrome. *Am J Med Sci.* 1954;227:46.
5. Yahalom J. Oncologic emergencies: superior vena cava syndrome. In: DeVita VT, Hellman S, Rosenberg SA, eds. *Cancer: Principles and Practice of Oncology.* 7th ed. Philadelphia, PA: Lippincott, Williams, & Wilkins; 2005:2273–2280.
6. Rice TW, Rodriguez RM, Light RW. The superior vena cava syndrome: clinical characteristics and evolving etiology. *Medicine.* 2006;85: 37–42.
7. Flounders JA. Oncology emergency modules: superior vena cava syndrome. *Oncol Nurs Forum Online.* 2003;30:E84–E88. Available at http://onlinelexi.com. Accessed March 3, 2010.
8. Cheng S. Superior vena cava syndrome: a contemporary review of a historic disease. *Cardiol Rev.* 2009;17:16–22.
9. Schifferdecker B, Shaw JA, Piemonte TC, et al. Nonmalignant superior vena cava syndrome: pathophysiology and management. *Cathet Cardiovasc Intervent.* 2005;65:416–423.
10. Johnson DH, Laskin J, Cmelak A, et al. Superior vena cava syndrome. In: Abeloff MD, Armitage JO, Niederhuber JE, et al, eds. *Abeloff's Clinical Oncology.* 4th ed. New York, NY: Churchill-Livingstone; 2008:803–812.
11. Journeycake J, Buchanan GR. Thrombotic complications of central venous catheters in children. *Curr Opin Hematol.* 2004;10:369–374.
12. Piastra M, Caresta E, Ruggiero A, et al. Management of critically ill children with mediastinal neoplasms: a 6-year survey from a single institution. *Med Pediatr Oncol.* 2003;40:329–331.
13. Hunter JC. Structural emergencies. In: Itano JK, Taoka KN, eds. *Core Curriculum for Oncology Nursing.* 4th ed. Philadelphia, PA: Elsevier/Saunders; 2005:422–439.
14. Eren S, Karaman A, Okur A, The superior vena cava syndrome caused by malignant disease: imaging with multi-detector row CT. *Eur J Radiol.* 2006;59:93–103.
15. Lin J, Zhou KR, Chen ZW, et al. Vena cava 3D contrast-enhanced MR venography: a pictorial review. *Cardiovasc Intervent Radiol.* 2005;28:795–805.
16. Rice TW, Rodriguez RM, Barnette R, et al. Prevalence and characteristics of pleural effusions in superior vena cava syndrome. *Respirology.* 2006;11:299–305.
17. Dosios T, Theakos N, Chatziantoniou C. Cervical mediastinoscopy and anterior mediastinoscopy in superior vena cava obstruction. *Chest.* 2005;128:1551–1556.

18. Porte H, Metois D, Finzi L, et al. Superior vena cava syndrome of malignant origin: which surgical procedure for which diagnosis? *Eur J Cardiothorac Surg.* 2000;17:384–388.
19. Wilson P, Bezjak A, Asch M, et al. The difficulties of a randomized study in superior vena caval obstruction. *J Thorac Oncol.* 2007;2:514–519.
20. Escribano JF, Anton RF, Rubio AC, et al. Superior vena cava syndrome with central venous catheter for chemotherapy treated successfully with fibrinolysis. *Clin Transl Oncol.* 2007;9:198–200.
21. Hyers TM, Agnelli G, Hull RD, et al. Antithrombotic therapy for venous thromboembolic disease. *Chest.* 2001;119:176S–193S.
22. Morales M, Comas V, Trujillo M, et al. Treatment of catheter-induced thrombotic superior vena cava syndrome: a single institution's experience. *Support Care Cancer.* 2000;8:334–338.
23. Chodirker WB. Reactions to alteplase in patients with acute thrombotic stroke [comment]. *CMAJ.* 2000;163:387–389.
24. Hill MD, Barbar PA, Takahashi J, et al. Anaphylactoid reactions and angioedema during alteplase treatment of acute ischemic stroke [comment]. *CMAJ.* 2000;162:1281–1284.
25. Rowell NP, Gleeson FV. Steroids, radiotherapy, chemotherapy and stents for superior vena caval obstruction in carcinoma of the bronchus: a systematic review. *J Clin Oncol.* 2002;14:338–351.
26. Spira A, Ettinger DS. Multidisciplinary management of lung cancer. *N Engl J Med.* 2004;350:379–392.
27. Kvale PA, Selecky PA, Prakash UB. Palliative care in lung cancer: AACP evidence-based clinical practice guidelines (2nd ed.). *Chest.* 2007;132:368S–403S.
28. Mose S, Stabik C, Eberlein K, et al. Retrospective analysis for the superior vena cava syndrome in irradiated cancer patients. *Anticancer Res.* 2006;26:4933–4936.
29. Bierdrager E, Lampmann LE, Lohle, PN, et al. Endovascular stenting in neoplastic superior vena cava syndrome prior to chemotherapy or radiotherapy. *Neth J Med.* 2005;63:20–23.
30. Ahmann FR. A reassessment of the clinical implications of the superior vena caval syndrome. *J Clin Oncol.* 1984;2:961–969.
31. Anderson PR, Coia LR. Fractionation and outcomes with palliative radiation therapy. *Semin Radiat Oncol.* 2000;10:191–199.
32. Lanciego C, Chacon JL, Julian A, et al. Stenting as first option for endovascular treatment of malignant superior vena cava syndrome. *AJR.* 2001;177:583–593.
33. Schainfeld RM. Turning the old school on its head: Stenting as the therapy of choice for SVC syndrome. *Cathet Cardiovasc Intervent.* 2005; 65:424–426.
34. Lee-Elliott CE, Abubacker MZ, Lopez AJ. Fast-track management of malignant superior vena cava syndrome. *Cardiovasc Intervent Radiol.* 2004;27:470–473.
35. Tzifa A, Marshall AC, McElhinney DB, et al. Endovascular treatment for superior vena cava occlusion or obstruction in a pediatric and young adult population. *J Am Coll Cardiol.* 2007;49:1003–1009.
36. Uberoi R. Quality assurance guidelines for superior vena cava stenting in malignant disease. *Cardiovasc Intervent Radiol.* 2006;29:319–322.
37. Smayra T, Otal P, Chabbert V, et al. Long-term results of endovascular stent placement in the superior vena caval venous system. *Cardiovasc Intervent Radiol.* 2001;24:388–394.
38. Nagata T, Makutani S, Uchida H, et al. Follow-up of 71 patients undergoing metallic stent placement for the treatment of a malignant obstruction of the superior vena cava. *Cardiovasc Intervent Radiol.* 2007;30: 959–967.
39. Panneton JM, Andrews JC, Hofer JM. Superior vena cava syndrome: relief with a modified saphenojugular bypass graft. *J Vasc Surg.* 2001;34:360–363.
40. Kalra M, Gloviczki P, Andrews JC, et al. Open surgical and endovascular treatment of superior vena cava syndrome caused by nonmalignant disease. *J Vasc Surg.* 2003;38:215–223.
41. Doty JR, Flores JH, Doty DB. Superior vena cava obstruction: bypass using spiral vein graft. *Ann Thorac Surg.* 1999;67:1111–1116.

CHAPTER 43

AnnMarie K. McDonnell Keenan, MS, APRN-BC, AOCN®

# Syndrome of Inappropriate Antidiuretic Hormone

## SCOPE OF THE PROBLEM

Syndrome of inappropriate antidiuretic hormone (SIADH) is a paraneoplastic endocrine disorder associated with several malignancies, particularly lung carcinomas. Typically, the disorder results from tumor secretion of an endocrine peptide (vasopressin) unrelated to tissue invasion or metastases. Besides ectopic vasopressin secretion by tumors, inappropriate eutopic secretion of vasopressin from the posterior pituitary gland may result from intrathoracic infection, positive-pressure ventilation, central nervous system disorders, acquired immune-deficiency syndrome (AIDS), and a variety of drugs. Although SIADH is frequently classified as an oncologic emergency, most patients present with asymptomatic hyponatremia that is discovered on routine chemistry evaluation before or at the time of a cancer diagnosis or during the course of treatment. Alternatively, some patients may develop chronic SIADH with exacerbations relating to progression of the malignancy.

### DEFINITIONS

Schwartz and colleagues originally described 2 patients with bronchogenic carcinoma who developed hyponatremia with elevated urine sodium levels hypothesized to be due to inappropriate secretion of antidiuretic hormone (ADH).[1] Subsequently, researchers suggested that tumor-derived ADH may cause SIADH.[2] *Syndrome of inappropriate antidiuretic hormone* is currently defined as the inappropriate production and secretion of ADH, also known as its biologically active form *arginine vasopressin* (AVP), causing a syndrome of hyponatremia, urine osmolality disproportionately higher than plasma osmolality, and elevated urinary sodium concentrations. The term *inappropriate* refers to ADH release causing increased water reabsorption in the patient categorized as euvolemic. In other words, the nonosmotic release of ADH is not stimulated by physiological mechanisms required for homeostasis, for example, hemodynamic changes.

Although ADH is the primary endocrine peptide involved in SIADH, the ectopic production of atrial natriuretic peptide (ANP) by cardiac atrial cells or tumor cell lines may cause SIADH independently.[3–5] In some patients, both ectopic ADH and ANP secretion may contribute to the etiology of SIADH. The relative contribution of ANP in producing hyponatremia in lung cancer has not been clearly defined.[4]

### INCIDENCE

Syndrome of inappropriate antidiuretic hormone is primarily associated with bronchogenic carcinoma, particularly small cell lung cancer (SCLC), which accounts for approximately 15% of new lung cancer cases annually in the US.[3] Reports indicate that 15% to 50% of patients with SCLC will develop SIADH.[3,6] Patients may exhibit no symptoms or, alternatively, present with signs and symptoms that range from anorexia, nausea, and weakness to life-threatening seizures and coma. The presence of SIADH is unrelated to the stage and prognosis of disease.[3]

## ETIOLOGY AND RISK FACTORS

Syndrome of inappropriate antidiuretic hormone is caused by the ectopic production of vasopressin by malignant cells. While structurally identical to normal ADH, the synthesis and release of ectopic ADH is unregulated. In an earlier study involving 263 patients with lung cancer, 21 of the 133 patients with SCLC were hyponatremic. Eleven of these patients had tumor cell lines assayed for the presence of ADH and ANP. Nine patients' tumors produced ANP, seven produced ADH, and five produced both ANP and ADH.[7] The more severe cases of hyponatremia are associated with ectopic ADH rather than ANP production.[8]

Apart from a paraneoplastic origin, SIADH is associated with pain, stress, nausea, surgery, pulmonary disease (eg, pneumonia, tuberculosis, and aspergillosis), central nervous system disorders (eg, head trauma, acute psychosis, and peripheral neuropathy), physical and emotional stress, and pharmacological agents (particularly narcotics), including many chemotherapy drugs. The list of drugs associated with SIADH continues to expand. Commonly prescribed antidepressants, selective serotonin reuptake inhibitors (SSRIs) and serotonin and norepinephrine reuptake inhibitors (SNRIs), are increasingly reported to cause SIADH, especially in the elderly. Collectively, these nonparaneoplastic causes of SIADH may either increase eutopic ADH secretion or potentiate its effect.[5,9–14] The data indicate that patients with AIDS frequently exhibit hyponatremia, with SIADH as the underlying cause in up to 66% of these patients.[15] Table 43-1 identifies nonparaneoplastic causes of SIADH..

Patients with cancer who are at risk for developing SIADH are primarily those with lung carcinomas, especially SCLC. Other patients at risk include those with head and neck carcinomas, particularly following neck dissection.[3,10] Melanoma and gastrointestinal, gynecological, prostatic, hematological, and neurological malignancies are also associated with SIADH; however, case reports include very few patients.[5,16–19] The patients at highest risk are those with tumors of squamous cell or neuroendocrine histology. Malignancies associated with SIADH are listed in Table 43-2.

## PHYSIOLOGICAL ALTERATIONS

### NORMAL PHYSIOLOGY AND SCIENTIFIC PRINCIPLES

Important aspects relevant to the maintenance of body fluid balance include distribution of total-body water

**TABLE 43-1**

**Nonparaneoplastic Causes of Syndrome of Inappropriate Antidiuretic Hormone**

**Pulmonary**
- Infection (tuberculosis, lung abscess, pneumonia, empyema)
- Chronic obstructive pulmonary disease
- Positive pressure ventilation

**Central Nervous System**
- Trauma (subdural hematoma, skull fracture, concussion, stroke, subarachnoid hemorrhage, cerebral vascular thrombosis)
- Intracranial space-occupying lesions (primary or metastatic tumors)
- Infection (encephalitis, meningitis)
- Guillain-Barré syndrome
- Vasculitis (lupus)
- Acute intermittent porphyria
- Pain and emotional stress
- Nausea

**Drugs**
- Chemotherapeutic agents (vincristine, vinblastine, vinorelbine, cyclophosphamide, ifosfamide, cisplatin, docetaxel)
- Narcotics (morphine, barbiturates)
- General anesthesia
- Nicotine
- Chlorpropamide (Diabinese)
- Carbamazepine (Tegretol)
- Tricyclic antidepressants
- Selective serotonin reuptake inhibitors (floxenine, sertraline, paroxetine, fluvoxamine, citalopram, escitalopram)
- Serotonin and nonadrenaline reuptake inhibitor (venlafaxine)
- Immunoglobulin therapy

**Surgery**
- Neck dissection
- Mitral stenosis correction

**Other**
- AIDS

*Source*: Data from Heideman et al[5]; Turchin et al[9]; Zacay et al[10]; Langer-Nitsche et al[11]; Kao et al[12]; Kuroda et al[13]; Romero et al[14]; Berl et al.[15]

(TBW), mechanisms of sodium and water regulation, and the effect of ADH on the kidney. Total-body water is distributed between intracellular (IC) and extracellular (EC) spaces in a 2:1 ratio. Extracellular fluid is further divided between intravascular (approximately 35% of the EC fluid) and interstitial (approximately 65% of the EC fluid) spaces. Small amounts of water are also present in bone, digestive secretions, and cerebrospinal fluid.[20] In adults, water accounts for 45% to 65% of body weight; variations are due to age, gender, muscle mass, and fat content. Women and obese individuals have less body water because they have a higher fat content than men and lean individuals, who have a lower fat content.

**TABLE 43-2**

**Malignancies Associated With Syndrome of Inappropriate Antidiuretic Hormone**

- Lung cancer
  - Small cell
  - Non-small cell
- Head and neck carcinoma
- Duodenal and pancreatic carcinoma
- Melanoma
- Prostate carcinoma
- Lymphomas (Hodgkin's and non-Hodgkin's)
- Leukemias
- Gynecologic
  - Ovarian carcinoma
  - Cervical (small cell)
  - Ovarian teratoma (germ cell)
  - Papillary serous carcinoma peritoneum
- Neuroblastoma
- Thymoma

*Source*: Data from Johnson et al[13]; Heideman et al[6]; Galesic et al[16]; Thompson and Adlam[17]; Bogdanos et al[18]; and Robertson.[19]

Constant regulation of body water between IC and EC fluid compartments is achieved because of solute-impermeable but water-permeable membranes.[21] Water readily diffuses across membranes to maintain an equal concentration of solutes (dissolved substances contained in water) inside and outside cells. Sodium, an important solute, is referred to as a physiologically "effective" osmole because it does not freely cross the membrane. In contrast, physiologically "ineffective" osmoles freely cross cell membranes and do not contribute to osmolality.[5] Sodium is restricted predominantly to the EC space and thus is the dominant EC cation, closely reflecting plasma osmolality, the ratio of solute to free water. In SIADH, a quick estimate of osmolality may be made by doubling the serum sodium level. A more reliable formula commonly used is:[5]

$$\text{Osmolality} = 2(\text{Na}) + \frac{\text{Glucose}}{18} + \frac{\text{BUN}}{2.8}$$

Normally, renal reabsorption or excretion of solute-free water maintains a plasma osmolality of 275 to 290 mOsm/kg. Constant regulation of osmolality within this narrow range occurs primarily because sensitive hypothalamic osmoreceptors sense volume changes. Secondarily, stimulation of cardiovascular and pulmonary baroreceptors is involved in the control of plasma osmolality. Osmoreceptor and baroreceptor stimulation ultimately leads to the release or inhibition of the critical hormone arginine vasopressin in response to clinical changes in plasma osmolality. Arginine vasopressin, synthesized in large neuronal cells of the hypothalamus, is stored in the posterior pituitary gland (neurohypophysis).[20,22] In the presence of ADH, water is reabsorbed, resulting in concentrated urine. In the absence of ADH, water is excreted, and thus urine is dilute.[23] Arginine vasopressin acts specifically on the principal cells of the renal collecting duct, a location within the renal tubular system where the final steps in urine concentration occur. The classic G-protein-regulated signal casade involving cyclic adenosine monophosphate (cAMP) as the second messenger and protein kinase A (PKA) triggers the phosphorylation of a water channel know as *aquaporin-2* (AQP2). Aquaporin-2 is expressed exclusively in the collecting duct. The facilitation of water reabsorption ultimately occurs due to insertion of AQP2 water channels on the principal cells of the luminal (apical) membrane, along with AQP3 and AQP4 at the basolateral membrane (bloodstream)[24–26] (Figure 43–1). Conditions that increase plasma osmolality, stimulating ADH release, include dehydration, positive-pressure breathing, and vasodilation. Plasma osmolality below 280 mOsm/kg inhibits ADH release, resulting in reabsorption of less free water and therefore a dilute urine. Cold temperatures, recumbancy, and negative-pressure breathing inhibit ADH release. The release of ADH is also regulated by neurotransmitters and neuropeptides such as angiotensin II, histamine, and bradykinin. On the other hand, dopamine, norepinephrine, and serotonin inhibit AVP release.[15] Although ADH plays a crucial role in regulating osmolality, the thirst stimulus provides another less sensitive means for the body to maintain water balance by facilitating oral intake of free water.[21]

## PATHOPHYSIOLOGY

The ability of neoplastic cells to autonomously synthesize, store, and release ADH results in excessive amounts of this circulating hormone. The presence of unregulated ADH causes water to be conserved at the kidney, with production of a concentrated urine (urine osmolality > 100 mOsm/kg in adults).[27] The increase in free water in the extracellular fluid (ECF) leads to plasma hypoosmolality and dilutional serum hyponatremia. It is interesting to note that in most cases of hyponatremia, the underlying problem is due to water excess, not sodium loss. Renal sodium loss in SIADH is due to activation of secondary natriuretic mechanisms in response to the minimal increase in extracellular volume; regulatory mechanisms handling sodium are therefore intact.[28] Sodium continues to be excreted from the kidney in parallel to the sodium intake. Intracellular edema occurs as the plasma water follows an osmotic gradient, moving from EC to IC.[21] Cerebral edema occurs because of cell

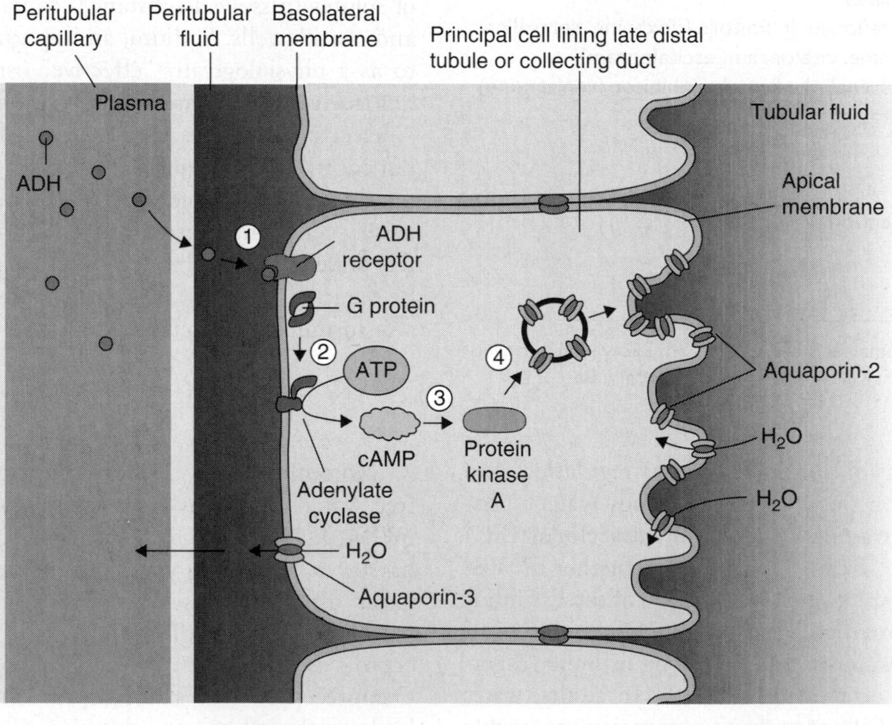


**FIGURE 43-1**

Effects of ADH on principal cells of the renal collecting duct. (1) ADH binds to receptors on basolateral membrane. (2) Via activation of G protein, adenylate cyclase is activated, catalyzing the formation of cAMP and leading to (3) activation of protein kinase A that (4) stimulates insertion of aquaporin-2 water channels into the apical membrane.

swelling that leads to varying levels of disruption in neural function and in severe cases may cause death.

## CLINICAL MANIFESTATIONS

Water excess accounts for the symptomatology of SIADH. Since the excess water is distributed primarily to the IC fluid compartment with only a minimal expansion of the intravascular volume, patients are categorized as euvolemic with no evidence of clinical edema. Clinical manifestations vary greatly among patients, and levels of serum sodium do not consistently correlate with signs and symptoms of hyponatremia. Hyponatremia with a serum sodium level of 121 to 134 mEq/L may cause headache, nausea, weakness, anorexia, fatigue, and muscle cramps. These vague, nonspecific complaints can be attributed easily to the primary malignancy or treatment regimens and often are not identified as early signs of hyponatremia. Since the signs and symptoms that a patient exhibits may not reflect the level of hyponatremia, clinicians must evaluate other factors. Perhaps the most important variable that determines symptom severity is related to whether the patient experienced an acute or chronic onset of hyponatremia. Rapid-onset hyponatremia, defined as occurring in less than 48 hours, typically is associated with the most severe symptomatology. Elderly patients have been reported to tolerate acute hyponatremia better than younger individuals because brain atrophy associated with aging allows more room for swollen brain cells.[20]

As hyponatremia worsens, especially with an acute onset, symptoms may progress to include changes in mental status, such as confusion, lethargy, combativeness, or psychotic behavior. Severe neurological symptoms typically do not appear unless the serum sodium level is less than 120 mEq/L.[20] Signs and symptoms result from brain cell edema. Severe hyponatremia (reported levels vary from less than 110 mEq/L to less than 125 mEq/L) may be associated with generalized seizures and coma, although patients with a sodium value of 124 mEq/L may be asymptomatic or, alternatively, exhibit moderate symptoms.[29]

## ASSESSMENT AND GRADING

Assessment of the patient with SIADH focuses on a skillful neurological examination. *Mild to moderate hyponatremia* is defined as a serum sodium of 121 to 134 mEq/L and *severe hyponatremia* is defined as a serum sodium of less than 120 mEq/L. Due to the nonspecificity and vagueness of the symptoms related to hyponatremia, SIADH may go undiagnosed until the hyponatremia becomes severe, and cerebral edema produces neurological changes. With regard to patients with SCLC, the presence of SIADH does not appear to negatively correlate with the stage of disease, response to chemotherapy, or survival.[3]

The diagnosis of SIADH is often made concurrently with discovery of the malignancy. SIADH is a diagnosis of exclusion. Other nonmalignant etiologies must be ruled out, such as infection, central nervous system disorders, and drug-related SIADH. The diagnosis of SIADH requires the presence of hyponatremia in addition to decreased plasma osmolality and inappropriately concentrated urine (Table 43–3). Plasma osmolality must be less than 275 mOsm/kg with a concurrent spot urine indicating a sodium level greater than 30 mEq/L.[27,30] If the patient is sodium depleted, urine sodium values may be slightly lower, that is, 20 to 30 mEq/L. Supportive laboratory results include a decreased uric acid level and a normal or decreased blood urea nitrogen (BUN).[27] The uric acid level is a more reliable indicator because BUN levels are affected by dietary protein intake. Both uric acid and BUN levels reflect a dilutional effect as a result of a modest increase in intravascular volume. Measurement of serum and urine AVP levels is possible by radioimmunoassay but is rarely performed because these levels are an unreliable indicator of changes in secretion or plasma concentration of the hormone.[6] Clinicians currently use a comparison between serum and urine osmolality as a replacement to the measurement of AVP levels.[26]

## THERAPEUTIC APPROACHES AND NURSING CARE

The only potential cure for SIADH is successful treatment of the underlying malignancy. In the meantime, stabilization of the patient and correction of the hyponatremia are essential. The degree and rate of development of the hyponatremia, along with the presence or absence of symptoms, determine the specific treatment of SIADH (Figure 43-2). Free-water restriction, however, is the initial treatment of choice for most patients with SIADH.[20] In many cases, reducing oral fluid intake to 500 to 1000 mL/

**TABLE 43-3**

| Criteria for the Diagnosis of Syndrome of Inappropriate Antidiuretic Hormone |
|---|
| Serum osmolality (< 275 mOsm/kg) |
| Serum sodium (< 135 mEq/L) |
| Urine osmolality (urine osmolality > serum osmolality) |
| Urinary sodium (> 30 mEq/L) |
| Euvolemia |
| Decreased levels of uric acid, blood urea nitrogen |
| Absence of edema |
| Normal renal, adrenal, and thyroid function |

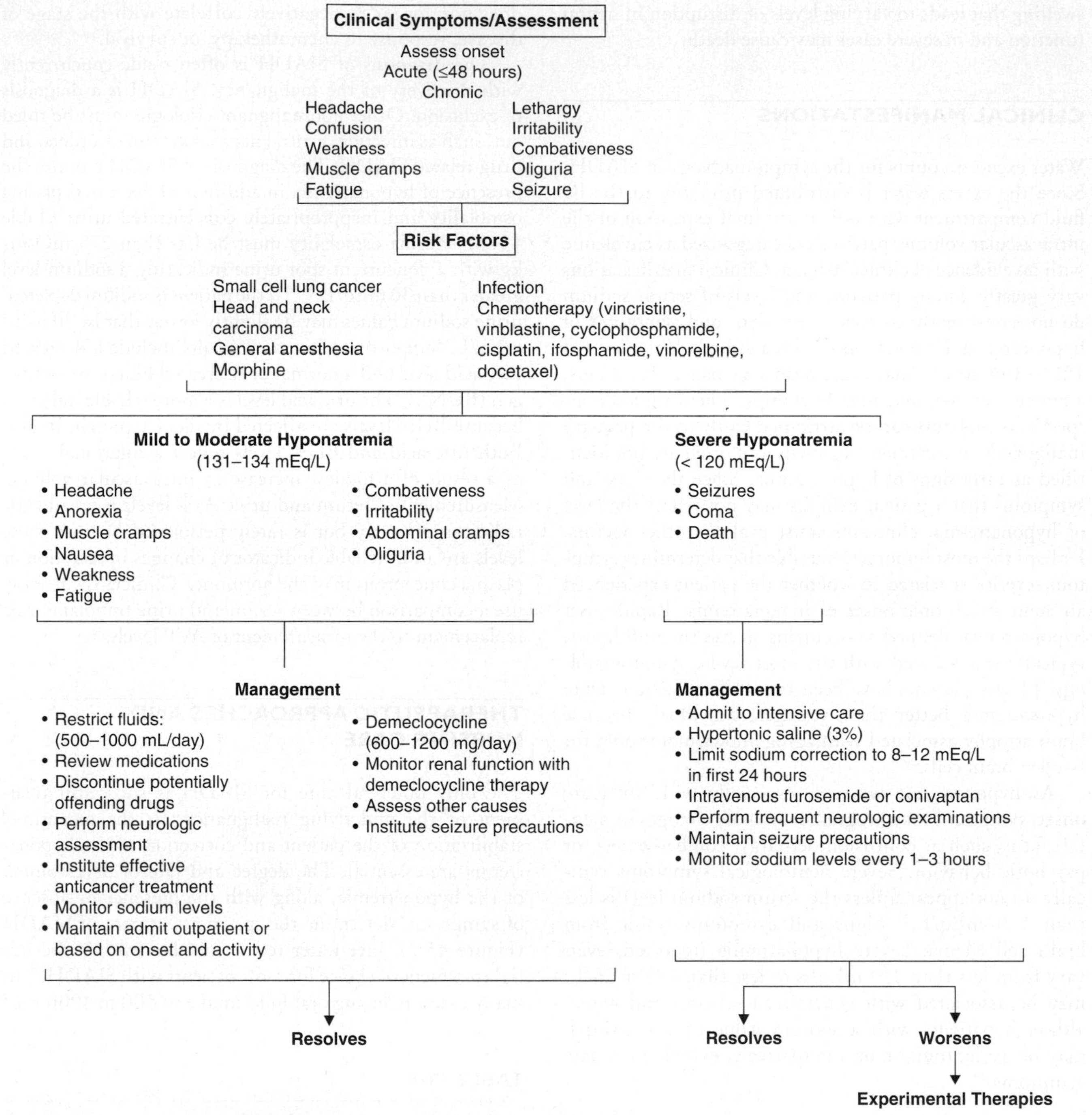


**FIGURE 43-2**

Management of syndrome of inapproprate antidiuretic hormone.

day may be the only required therapy. Fluid restriction allows the plasma osmolality and sodium level to increase gradually through eventual loss of free water, generally over a period of 3 to 5 days.

Severe, symptomatic acute hyponatremia (serum sodium concentration <110 to 115 mEq/L) resulting from SIADH is an oncologic emergency requiring immediate attention. Seizure precautions should be instituted for sodium levels less than 120 mEq/L. During the first few hours of correction, hypertonic (3%) saline is given intravenously,[19] along with intravenous furosemide (1 mg/kg), to expedite water loss.[20] Such therapeutic endeavors are instituted only in carefully controlled settings. The patient must be monitored carefully, and the serum sodium level and electrolytes must be checked frequently, at least every 1 to 3 hours. Frequent neurological assessments of the severely hyponatremic patient are essential. These assessments should include an evaluation of mental status and level of consciousness. Restriction of oral fluids also should be instituted. The patient's fluid balance is monitored, including daily weights. The rate of total serum sodium correction should not exceed more than 8 mEq/L per day.[20] Initial therapy is discontinued once the patient becomes mildly hyponatremic (serum sodium level = 125 to 130 mEq/L) in an effort to avoid iatrogenic neurological complications. Rapid correction of the serum sodium level may cause neurological damage from brain cell dehydration, potentially leading to an irreversible neurodegenerative disorder called *osmotic demyelination syndrome* (ODS), previously known as *central pontine myelinolysis*.[21] Originally this complication of rapid correction was thought to involve the pons, but more recently, lesions characterized by disruption of myelin also have been identified in extrapontine areas.[20] Symptoms of osmotic demyelination typically appear 1 to 6 days following seemingly effective treatment. Patients may exhibit delayed progressive neurological dysfunction, including palsies and spastic quadriparesis that do not respond to treatment.[21] Patients with chronic hyponatremia are at significant risk of developing ODS after rapid correction of the serum sodium level because once brain adaptation to a hypoosmolar state has occurred, rapid increases in serum sodium are not well tolerated.[21]

If chemotherapeutic treatment aimed at tumor control can be instituted immediately, pharmacological interventions may be unnecessary. In most cases, however, pharmacological therapy is employed, particularly in chronic hyponatremia. Oral medications traditionally used to treat SIADH include demeclocycline, lithium, and urea. The preferred drug, demeclocycline (600 to 1200 mg/day administered in divided doses), is a tetracycline derivative that stimulates diuresis by inhibiting the effect of AVP on the renal tubule, causing a nephrogenic form of diabetes insipidus.[27] Treatment continues for several days, allowing for maximal diuresis. Demeclocycline often allows a normal daily intake of water and other fluids. Reversible azotemia, the most common side effect of demeclocycline therapy, necessitates frequent evaluation of renal function. The expense, delayed onset, and long duration of action of demeclocycline are reported to limit its effectiveness.[20] Lithium is an alternative oral agent that also antagonizes the effects of ADH, although the effects are inconsistent. Since lithium has a low therapeutic index, toxicity can occur at blood levels that are only slightly beyond therapeutic levels. Even at therapeutic levels, significant side effects occur, limiting the usefulness of this drug.[27] Urea, available both orally and intravenously, has been used extensively in Europe. The drug acts to increase solute-free water excretion and decrease urinary sodium excretion. Poor palatability, gastrointestinal side effects, and azotemia are disadvantages to using urea.[20,27]

Novel targeted approaches to treat SIADH involve the use of AVP-receptor (AVPR) antagonists, collectively known as *vaptans*. Conivaptan, the only Food and Drug Administration (FDA) approved agent in this class, is currently indicated for the short-term treatment of both euvolemic and hypervolemic hyponatremia.[31] In the treatment of SIADH, this drug likely will be used more often in the setting of acute hyponatremia. Conivaptan is a nonselective nonpeptide AVPR antagonist that binds to $V_{1a}$ and $V_2$ receptors.[23] Both receptor subtypes cause physiological effects at various target tissues where these receptors are located. For example, $V_2$ receptors, primarily expressed on the principal cell of the renal collecting duct, when activated by ADH, stimulate the insertion of AQP2 channels, allowing reabsorption of solute-free water. Conivaptan, a $V_2$ antagonist, inhibits the action of ADH by preventing the formation of AQP2 channels, thus allowing for the excretion of solute-free water. No loss of sodium accompanies this effect. Other target tissues and functions of vasopressin subtypes are listed in Table 43-4.[27,32] Although no significant effects have been reported related to $V_2$ antagonism,

**TABLE 43-4**

**Description of AVP Receptor Subtypes and Conivaptan Effect**

| Subtype | Location | Function | Antagonistic Effect |
|---|---|---|---|
| $V_{1a}$ | Vascular smooth muscle | Vasoconstriction | Vasodilatation |
| | Platelets | Platelet aggregation | Inhibits platelet aggregation |
| $V_2$ | Renal collecting duct | Insertion of AQP2 channels | Inhibits formation of AQP2 channels |
| | Vascular endothelium | Releases von Willebrand factor and Factor 8 | Inhibits release of von Willebrand Factor and Factor 8 |
| | Vascular smooth muscle | Vasodilatation | Vasodilatation |

*Abbreviations*: AVP, arginine vasopressin; AQP2, aquaporin-2.
*Source*: Modified from Chen et al.[32]

it is important to monitor adverse effects such as bleeding complications that potentially may occur because vascular endothelium contains $V_2$ receptors. Inhibition of $V_2$ receptors in vascular endothelium is known to prevent the release of both von Willebrand's factor and Factor 8.[32] Conivaptan is available only for intravenous (IV) administration. The oral formulation has been withdrawn from clinical use because of potential drug interactions that may occur with extended use. Conivaptan is a potent inhibitor of the cytochrome p450 isoenzyme 3A4 that is responsible for the metabolism of multiple drugs. The drug therefore will be metabolized slowly and potentially interact with many drugs also metabolized by 3A4, including statins, ketoconazole, itraconazole, clarithromycin, ritronavir, and indinivir.[32,33] Dosing recommendations begin with a loading dose of 20 mg IV over 30 minutes. The loading dose is followed by 20 mg/day in 250 mL of 5% dextrose as a continuous infusion for up to 4 days. If the serum sodium level rises in a shorter period of time, the drug is discontinued. If adequate correction is not achieved in the first day, the dose may be increased to 40 mg/day. It is recommended to limit the correction of serum sodium to no more than 12 mEq/L in the first 24 hours. The half-life of conivaptan is 5 to 9 hours.[27,34] The most common adverse effects that have been reported include mild infusion-site phlebitis and pain. Less common adverse effects associated with conivaptan are headache, hypokalemia, thirst, and othostatic hypotension.[32]

A number of clinical trials testing oral vaptans have been preformed recently. Tolvaptan, lixivaptan, and satavaptan are selective $V_2$-receptor antagonists that are anticipated to have an important role in the management of chronic SIADH. These agents, like conivaptan, will decrease the need for fluid restriction in many cases, hopefully resulting in a simpler and more effective therapy.[27]

Obtaining a comprehensive patient history, conducting a careful nursing assessment, and reviewing serum chemistries may facilitate early diagnosis. Patients and their family members are instructed regarding the symptoms of hyponatremia (ie, nausea, weakness, muscle cramps, confusion, and lethargy) and are encouraged to report these symptoms promptly. Communication between nurses in the inpatient and ambulatory settings regarding the hospitalization course, current medications, and status at discharge is essential to optimize therapeutic outcomes.

## CONCLUSION

Syndrome of inappropriate antidiuretic hormone is a paraneoplastic endocrine syndrome primarily associated with SCLC that most frequently follows a chronic course but can present as an oncologic emergency. Nurses caring for patients with cancer, especially those with SCLC, must have a high index of suspicion for the presence of SIADH. Early intervention can prevent serious complications resulting from hyponatremia.

## REFERENCES


1. Schwartz WB, Bennett W, Curelop S, et al. A syndrome of renal sodium loss and hyponatremia probably resulting from inappropriate secretion of antidiuretic hormone. *Am J Med.* 1957;23:529–542.
2. Amatruda TT, Mulrow PJ, Gallagher JC, et al. Carcinoma of the lung with inappropriate antidiuresis: demonstration of an antidiuretic-hormone-like activity in tumor extract. *N Engl J Med.* 1963;269: 544–550.
3. Johnson DH, Blot WJ, Carbone DP, et al. Cancer of the lung: non-small cell lung cancer and small cell lung cancer. In: Abeloff MD, Armitage JO, Niederhuber JE, et al, eds. *Abeloff's Clinical Oncology.* 4th ed. Philadelphia: Churchill-Livingstone/Elsevier; 2008:1307–1366.
4. Radulescu D, Bunea D, Pripon S, et al. Severe paraneoplastic hyponatremia in a patient with small-cell lung carcinoma: syndrome of inappropriate antidiuretic hormone secretion versus atrial natriuretic peptide or both? *Clin Lung Cancer.* 2007;8:392–395.
5. Heideman, RL, Heideman NH. Hyponatremia. In: Abeloff MD, Armitage JO, Niederhuber JE, et al, eds. *Abeloff's Clinical Oncology.* 4th ed. Phildelphia: Churchill-Livingstone/Elsevier; 2008:749–758.
6. Jameson JL, Johnson BE. Paraneoplastic syndromes: endocrine/hematologic. In: Fauci AS, Braunwald E, Kasper DL, et al, eds. *Harrison's Principles of Internal Medicine.* 17th ed. New York, NY: McGraw Hill; 2008:617–623.
7. Gross AJ, Steinberg SM, Reilly JG, et al. Atrial natriuretic factor and arginine vasopressin production in tumor cell lines from patients with lung cancer and their relationship to serum sodium. *Cancer Res.* 1993;53:67–74.
8. Marchioli CC, Graziano SL. Paraneoplastic syndromes associated with small cell lung cancer. *Chest Surg Clin North Am.* 1997;7:65–80.
9. Turchin A, Seifter JL, Seely EW. Clinical problem solving: mind the gap. *N Engl J Med.* 2003;349:1465–1469.
10. Zacay G, Bedrin L, Horowitz Z, et al. Syndrome of inappropriate antidiuretic hormone or arginine vasopressin secretion in patients following neck dissection. *Laryngoscope.* 2002;112:2020–2024.
11. Langer-Nitsche C, Luck HJ, Heilmann M. Severe syndrome of inappropriate antidiuretic hormone secretion with docetaxel treatment in metastatic breast cancer [letter]. *Acta Oncol.* 2000;39:1001.
12. Kao CD, Chen JT, Wu ZA, et al. SIADH and seizures associated with immunoglobulin therapy [letter]. *Eur J Neurol.* 2003;10:748–749.
13. Kuroda H, Kawamura M, Hato T, et al. Syndrome of inappropriate secretion of antidiuretic hormone after chemotherapy with vinorelbine. *Cancer Chemother Pharmacol.* 2008;62:331–333.
14. Romero S, Pintor L, Serra M, et al. Syndrome of inappropriate secretion of antidiuretic hormone due to citalopram and venlafaxine. *Gen Hosp Psychiatry.* 2007;29:81–84.
15. Berl T, Verbalis J. Pathophysiology of water metabolism. In: Brenner BM, ed. *The Kidney.* 7th ed. Philadelphia: Saunders; 2004:865–919.
16. Galesic K, Krizanac S, Vrkljan M, et al. Syndrome of inappropriate secretion of antidiuretic hormone due to malignant thymoma. *Nephron.* 2002;91:752–754.
17. Thompson M, Adlam DM. Syndrome of inappropriate antidiuretic hormone secretion associated with oral squamous carcinoma. *Br J Oral Maxillofac Surg.* 2002;40:216–219.
18. Bogdanos J, Karamanolakis D, Milathianakis C, et al. Syndrome of inappropriate antidiuretic hormone secretion in a patient with hormone refractory prostate cancer. *Anticancer Res.* 2003;23:1775–1756.
19. Robertson GL. Neuroendocrinology: antidiuretic hormone, normal and disordered function. *Endocrinol Metab Clin North Am.* 2001;30:671–694.

20. Sterns RH. Renal function and disorders of water and sodium balance. In: Dale DC, Federman DD, eds. *ACP Medicine.* 3rd ed. New York, NY: WebMD, Inc.; 2007:1975–1993.
21. Lin M, Liu SJ, Lim IT. Disorders of water imbalance. *Emerg Med Clin North Am.* 2005;23:749–770.
22. Lingappa VR. Disorders of the hypothalamus and pituitary gland. In: McPhee SJ, Lingappa VR, Ganong WF, eds. *Pathophysiology of Disease: An Introduction to Clinical Medicine.* 4th ed. New York, NY: Lange Medical Books/McGraw-Hill; 2003:531–555.
23. Schrier RW, Berl T. The patient with hyponatremia or hypernatremia. In: Schrier RW, ed. *Manual of Nephrology.* 7th ed. Philadelphia, PA: Wolters Kluwer/Lippincott Williams & Wilkins; 2009:22–37.
24. Molina PE. The hypothalamus and posterior pituitary gland. In: Molina PE, ed. *Endocrine Physiology.* New York, NY: Lange Medical Books/McGraw-Hill; 2004:27–47.
25. Lien YHH, Shapiro JI. Hyponatremia: clinical diagnosis and management. *Am J Med.* 2007;120:653–658.
26. Hoorn EJ, Zietse R. Hyponatremia revisted: translating physiology to practice. *Nephron Physiol.* 2008;108:46–59.
27. Verbalis JG, Goldsmith SR, Greenberg A, et al. Hyponatremia treatment guidelines 2007: expert panel recommendations. *Am J Med.* 2007;120:S1-S21.
28. Boyiadzis M, Lieberman FS, Geskin LJ, Foon KA. Paraneoplastic syndromes. In: DeVita VT, Lawrence TS, Rosenberg SA, eds. *Cancer: Principles and Practice of Oncology.* 8th ed. Philadelphia, PA: Wolters Kluwer/Lippincott Williams & Wilkins; 2008:2446–2455.
29. Ellison DH, Berl MD. The syndrome of inappropriate antidiuresis. *N Engl J Med.* 2007;356:2064–2072.
30. Decaux G, Musch W. Clinical laboratory evaluation of the syndrome of inappropriate secretion of antidiuretic hormone. *Clin J Am Soc Nephrol.* 2008;3:1175–1184.
31. Metzger BL, DeVita MV, Michelis MF. Observations regarding the use of the aquaretic agent conivaptan for treatment of hyponatremia. *Int Urol Nephrol.* 2008;40:725–730.
32. Chen S, Jalandhara N, Battle D. Evaluation and management of hyponatremia: an emerging role for vasopressin receptor antagonists. *Nat Clin Pract Nephrol.* 2007;3:82–95.
33. Yeates KE, Morton AR. Vasopressin antagonists: role in the management of hyponatremia. *Am J Nephrol.* 2006;26:348–355.
34. U.S. Food and Drug Administration. Vaprisol, 2007. http://www.fda.gov/medwatch/safety/2007/Feb_PI/Vaprisol_PI.pdf. Accessed January 16, 2010.

CHAPTER 44

Jean Lydon, RN, MS, AOCN®

# Tumor Lysis Syndrome

## SCOPE OF THE PROBLEM

### DEFINITION

Tumor lysis syndrome (TLS) is a metabolic complication of cancer therapy that occurs when large numbers of tumor cells are destroyed rapidly. Tumor-cell destruction causes high levels of intracellular components—primarily potassium, phosphorus, and nucleic acids—to be released into the bloodstream. Metabolic abnormalities associated with TLS include hyperuricemia, hyperkalemia, hyperphosphatemia, and hypocalcemia. This syndrome can lead to life-threatening complications, including cardiac arrhythmias, renal failure, and acute respiratory distress syndrome. Although the most frequent cause of TLS is the administration of systemic chemotherapy, any form of cancer therapy that causes rapid cell lysis and necrosis of a tumor mass can induce this syndrome.

### INCIDENCE

The true incidence of TLS is not known. Since its first description in 1980 as a potential oncologic emergency,[1] several case reports and studies have been carried out to determine its incidence in children and adults. In a study of 1791 pediatric patients with non-Hodgkin's lymphoma (NHL), 78 children (4.4%) developed TLS. In a specific subgroup of patients with either Burkitt's ALL (B-ALL) or Burkitt's lymphoma, the rate of TLS was 8.4%. When reviewing patients in the B-ALL subgroup only, the rate of TLS was 26.4%, suggesting that these patients are at the highest risk of developing TLS.[2] In a retrospective review of 766 adult and pediatric patients with acute lymphoid leukemia (ALL), acute myeloid leukemia (AML), and NHL, the incidence of TLS was 5.3% despite preventative measures in many patients.[3] In a study of 194 patients, aged 18 to 86 years with AML or advanced MDS undergoing induction chemotherapy, 19 patients or 9.8% of patients developed TLS.[4]

Tumor lysis syndrome occurs more frequently in patients with aggressive hematological malignancies, particularly acute leukemias and high-grade lymphomas, than in those patients with solid tumors. It is, therefore, not surprising that this syndrome occurs more frequently in the pediatric population. Hematological malignancies commonly associated with TLS include high-grade lymphomas, particularly Burkitt's lymphoma and diffuse large B-cell lymphoma, ALL, and AML. This syndrome is observed less frequently in other hematological malignancies including chronic lymphocytic leukemia (CLL), chronic myelogenous leukemia (CML), and NHL.[5–9] TLS has also been observed in patients with advanced myeloma, myelodysplastic syndrome (MDS), and refractory anemia.[10] Although rare in patients with solid tumors, TLS has been reported in a variety of solid tumors, including breast cancer, testicular cancer, medulloblastoma, small cell and non-small cell lung cancer, Merkel cell carcinoma, hepatocellular carcinoma, sarcoma, melanoma, colorectal cancer, gastric cancer, prostate cancer, vulvar carcinoma, ovarian cancer, neuroblastoma, thymoma, and germ cell tumors.[11,12] In a review of the literature between the first reported case in 1977 and 2002, a total of 45 cases of TLS were reported in solid tumors. When these cases are reviewed with respect to growth kinetics and sensitivity to antineoplastic therapy, only small cell lung cancer and germ cell tumors share similar characteristics with hematological malignancies—yet the data does not reveal an increased incidence in these types of tumors when compared to other solid tumors.[12] In fact among these cases, 37 occurred in tumors sensitive to chemotherapy, whereas 8 occurred in tumor types relatively insensitive to chemotherapy.[11] Although it is thought that early recognition and prophylactic treatment have decreased the incidence and severity of TLS, particularly in high-risk patients, the incidence of TLS may increase as more sophisticated and targeted therapies are developed to manage previously untreatable diseases.[5]

### ETIOLOGY AND RISK FACTORS

The risk of developing TLS is influenced by several tumor-related and host-related factors. Tumor-related factors include a large tumor burden, a high tumor cell proliferation rate, tumor chemosensitivity, elevated levels of lactate dehydrogenase (LDH), and elevated white blood cell (WBC) count (>50,000/mm$^3$). TLS occurs most frequently in Burkitt's lymphoma, ALL, and diffuse large B-cell lymphoma. These malignancies are characterized by high nucleic acid and phosphorus content, very active purine metabolism, and tumor chemosensitivity.[5–9] In a study of 772 adult patients with AML receiving induction chemotherapy, an analysis of risk factors for clinical tumor lysis syndrome (CTLS) and laboratory tumor lysis syndrome (LTLS) revealed that impaired renal function, high WBC count, and high serum levels of uric acid and LDH at presentation were the main risk factors for both forms of TLS. In addition, the study showed that high pretreatment LDH and creatinine were associated with the development of LTLS and CTLS.[13] In solid tumors, the presence of liver metastasis seems to predispose patients to TLS either due to high purine pools, increased tumor burden, or impaired uric acid metabolism.[12]

Host-related factors include preexisting uremia or hyperuricemia, decreased urinary flow, acidic urine, dehydration, oliguria, anuria, and renal insufficiency or renal failure.[5–10,14] Patients with pretreatment renal impairment as a result of dehydration, metabolic disturbances, or obstruction are at greater risk for TLS because they are less able to clear the products of cellular breakdown. Patients with preexisting metabolic disturbances are at increased risk for TLS. Significant hyperphosphatemia, hyperuricemia, and/or hyperkalemia may exist prior to initiating cytotoxic therapy.[10,14–17] For example, the lymphoblasts of leukemia patients contain four times more phosphate than do normal mature lymphoblasts. Thus, the phosphate metabolism is increased in patients with high levels of lymphoblasts, causing significant hyperphosphatemia before initiating treatment.[15] Serum uric acid and uric acid excretion can be affected by the degree of elevation in the WBC count; the degree of enlargement of the lymph nodes, spleen, and liver; dehydration; baseline renal insufficiency; acidic urine; and decreased urinary flow rate 24 hours prior to treatment.[15–17] In the patient with cancer, hyperkalemia may be present before initiating cytotoxic therapy, due to renal insufficiency, dehydration, adrenal insufficiency, acidosis, and/or medications.[10]

The increase in knowledge of both tumor- and host-related risk factors has led to the development of scoring systems that can be used as a predictive model in estimating the risk of TLS in certain populations, as well as an individual's risk for the development of TLS.[4,13] In a multivariate analysis of 194 patients with AML or advanced MDS undergoing induction chemotherapy, 6 significant predictors of TLS were found: elevated prechemotherapy values for uric acid, creatinine, LDH, and white blood cell count; male sex; and history of chronic myelomonocytic leukemia (CMML) (with preinduction uric acid and LDH levels and gender being independent predictors for TLS). The authors designed a scoring system based on these factors that then serve as a predictive model for identifying patients at risk for TLS. The authors report that their analysis could be used to develop guidelines for TLS management for AML or advanced MDS patients.[4] In another multivariate analysis of 772 adult patients receiving induction chemotherapy for AML, the following risk factors for TLS were identified: pretreatment LDH above normal, creatinine > 1.4 mg/dL, uric acid > 7.5 mg/dL, and WBC counts > 25 × $10^3$/L. A scoring system based on pretreatment WBC counts, LDH, and uric acid levels was used and found to be accurate in predicting TLS.[13] Further studies are needed to develop predictive scoring systems for CTLS in other patient populations, which may then serve as a useful tool in selecting high-risk patients that should receive a risk-adjusted prophylaxis regimen.[13]

A panel of experts in pediatric and adult hematological malignancies and TLS utilized risk factors for TLS to stratify patients into high-, intermediate-, and low-risk groups. Stratification was based on type of malignancy, WBC counts, and type of therapy. High-risk patients are defined as those having Burkitt's lymphoma, lymphoblastic lymphoma, and B-cell ALL. Patients with intermediate risk are those having diffuse large-cell lymphoma or other rapidly proliferating malignancies. Low-risk patients are those with indolent NHL or other slowly proliferating malignancies. Patients with ALL, CML, and AML are stratified by WBC counts (Table 44-1).[5] The primary treatment-related cause of TLS is chemotherapy. Specific chemotherapeutic agents more commonly associated with TLS include cisplatin, etoposide, cytosine arabinoside, paclitaxel, fludarabine, intrathecal methotrexate, and hydroxyurea. Immunotherapy such as interferons, interleukins, and tumor necrosis factor, as well as monoclonal antibodies including rituximab, gemtuzumab, alemtuzumab, and imatinib mesylate have been associated with this syndrome. Additionally, radiation therapy, chemoembolization, surgery, hormone therapy, particularly tamoxifen, and corticosteroids, either alone or in combination, have been shown to induce TLS.[8,10,15,16]

**TABLE 44-1**

**Patient Stratification by Risk**

| | Risk | | |
|---|---|---|---|
| **Type of Cancer** | **High** | **Intermediate** | **Low** |
| NHL | Burkitt's, lymphoblastic, B-ALL | DLBCL | Indolent NHL |
| ALL | WBC ≥ 100,000/mm$^3$ | WBC 50,000–100,00/mm$^3$ | WBC ≤ 50,000/mm$^3$ |
| AML | WBC ≥ 50,000/mm$^3$, monoblastic | WBC 10,00–50,000/mm$^3$ | WBC ≤ 10,000/mm$^3$ |
| CLL | | WBC 10,000/mm$^3$–100,000/mm$^3$ Tx w/fludarabine | WBC ≤ 10,000/mm$^3$ |
| Other hematological malignancies (including CML and multiple myeloma and solid tumors) | | Rapid proliferation with expected rapid response to therapy | Remainder of patients |

*Abbreviations*: ALL, acute lymphoblastic leukemia; AML, acute myeloid leukemia; B-ALL, Burkitt's acute lymphoblastic leukemia; CLL, chronic lymphocytic leukemia; CML, chronic myeloid leukemia; DLBCL, diffuse large B-cell lymphoma; NHL, non-Hodgkin's lymphoma; Tx, treatment.

*Source*: Data from Coiffier et al.[5]

Spontaneous tumor lysis syndrome (STLS) has been described as electrolyte abnormalities and renal dysfunction that occurs in the presence of rapid cell turnover or cellular death before the administration of cytotoxic therapy. Spontaneous tumor lysis syndrome is thought to be due to the spontaneous necrosis of malignant cells. The actual incidence of acute STLS is difficult to ascertain, but is considered to be a rare clinical syndrome that is most often seen in patients with Burkitt's lymphoma, leukemias, and in patients with AML.[17–19] In a retrospective chart review of all patients with acute renal failure who developed acute TLS, 10 out of 926 patients or 1.08% developed STLS-induced acute uric acid nephropathy.[19] In a study of 772 adult patients with AML receiving induction chemotherapy, 25% of the cases of TLS (8 cases with CTLS and 24 cases of LTLS) occurred before the induction of chemotherapy.[13] Only 7 cases of STLS have been reported in solid tumors.[20] The important distinction between STLS and acute TLS is the lack of hyperphosphatemia in STLS. It is postulated that in STLS the tumor is able to reutilize phosphate released by the lysed cells, whereas in post-treatment ATLS there is not enough viable cells to reutilize the large amounts of phosphates released.[19,21] In summary, cytotoxic therapy in the patient with pretreatment hyperphosphatemia, hyperuricemia, and/or hyperkalemia increases the risk of TLS.[5,8,10]

## CLASSIFICATION AND GRADING

Tumor lysis syndrome has been broadly defined as the metabolic abnormalities caused by the rapid release of cellular components into the blood after lysis of tumor cells. Although there is a general agreement on the definition of TLS, there is currently no universally accepted classification and grading system.[9]

Cairo and Bishop developed a classification system that aids in the rapid assessment of TLS. According to the Cairo and Bishop risk-classification grading system, LTLS is defined as 2 or more serum values of uric acid, potassium, phosphate, or calcium that are more than or less than normal at presentation or if they change by 25% within 3 days before or 7 days after initiation of treatment (Table 44-2).[7,9] CTLS requires the presence of LTLS plus one or more of the following clinical complications: renal insufficiency, cardiac arrhythmias/sudden death, and seizures (Table 44-3).[9] This system defines three groups of patients: no TLS, LTLS, and CTLS. In addition, Cairo and Bishop developed a grading system for TLS based on the presence and severity of renal, cardiac, and neurological clinical manifestations (Table 44-4).[9] The Cairo and Bishop classification and grading system is currently being used in the Children's Oncology Group study ANHL01P1 of patients with advanced B-cell lymphoma.[9] Development of a standardized classification and grading system for TLS would increase our knowledge of the incidence, tumor types, risk factors, and morbidity and mortality rates associated with this syndrome. Furthermore, specific prevention and treatment programs based on classification and grade of TLS could be developed and evaluated.

**TABLE 44-2**

**Cairo–Bishop Definition of Laboratory Tumor Lysis Syndrome (LTLS)**

| | |
|---|---|
| Uric Acid | $x \geq 476$ μmol/L or 25% increase from baseline |
| Potassium | $x \geq 6.0$ mmol/L or 25% increase from baseline |
| Phosphorous | $x \geq 2.1$ mmol/L (children), $x \geq 1.45$ mmol/L (adults) or 25% increase from baseline |
| Calcium | $x \geq 1.75$ mmol/L or 25% increase from baseline |

Modified from Hande and Garrow.[7]

*Note*: Laboratory tumor lysis syndrome is defined as either a 25% change or level above or below normal, as defined above, for any two or more serum values of uric acid, potassium, phosphate, and calcium within 3 days before or 7 days after the initiation of chemotherapy. This assessment assumes that a patient has or will receive adequate hydration (± alkalinization) and a hypouricaemic agent(s).

*Source*: Reprinted with permission from Cairo and Bishop.[8]

## PHYSIOLOGICAL ALTERATIONS

The kidneys regulate fluid and electrolyte balance by filtering essential substances from the blood—selectively

**TABLE 44-3**

**Cairo–Bishop Definition of Clinical Tumor Lysis Syndrome (CTLS)**

1. Creatinine[a]: $x \geq 1.5$ ULN[b] (age > 12 years or age adjusted)
2. Cardiac arrhythmia/sudden death[a]
3. Seizure[a]

Modified from Hande and Garrow[7].

*Notes*: Clinical tumor lysis syndrome (CTLS) assumes the laboratory evidence of metabolic changes and significant clinical toxicity that requires clinical intervention. CTLS is defined as the presence of LTLS and any one or more of the above-mentioned criteria.

[a]Not directly or probably attributable to a therapeutic agent (eg, rise in creatinine after amphotericin administration).

[b]Creatinine levels: patients will be considered to have elevated creatinine if their serum creatinine is 1.5 times greater than the institutional upper limit of normal (ULN) below age/gender defined in ULN. If not specified by an institution, age/sex ULN creatinine may be defined as: > 1< 12 years, both male and female, 61.6 μmol/L; ≥ 12 < 16 years, both male and female, 88 μmol/L; ≥ 16 years, female, 105.6 μmol/L; ≥ 16 years, male, 114.4 μmol/L.

*Source*: Reprinted with permission from Cairo and Bishop.[8]

**TABLE 44-4**

**Cairo–Bishop Grading Classification of Tumor Lysis Syndrome**

| | Grade 0[a] | Grade I | Grade II | Grade III | Grade IV | Grade V |
|---|---|---|---|---|---|---|
| LTLS | — | + | + | + | + | + |
| Creatinine[b,c] | < 1.5 × ULN | 1.5 × ULN | > 1.5–3·0 × ULN | > 3.0–6.0 × ULN | > 6.0 ULN | Death[d] |
| Cardiac arrhythmia[c] | None | Intervention not indicated | Non-urgent medical intervention indicated | Symptomatic and incompletely controlled medically or controlled with device (eg, defibrillator) | Life-threatening (eg, arrhythmia associated with CHF, hypotension, syncope, shock) | Death[d] |
| Seizure[c] | None | — | One brief generalized seizure; seizure(s) well controlled by anticonvulsants or infrequent focal motor seizures not interfering with ADL | Seizure in which consciousness is altered; poorly controlled seizure disorder; with breakthrough generalized seizures despite medical interventions | Seizures of any kind which are prolonged, repetitive or difficult to control (eg, status epilepticus, intractable epilepsy) | Death[d] |

*Note*: Clinical tumor lysis syndrome (CTLS) requires one or more clinical manifestations along with criteria for laboratory tumor lysis syndrome (LTLS). Maximal CTLS manifestation (renal, cardiac, neuro) defines the grade.

[a]No laboratory tumor lysis syndrome (LTLS).

[b]Creatinine levels: patients will be considered to have elevated creatinine if their serum creatinine is 1.5 times greater than the institutional upper limit of normal (ULN) below age/gender defined ULN. If not specified by an institution, age/sex ULN creatinine may be defined as: > 1 < 12 years, both male and female, 61.6 umol/L; ≥ 12 < 16 years, both male and female, 88 umol/L; ≥ 16 years, female, 105.6 umol/L; ≥ 16 years, male, 114.4 umol/L.

[c]Not directly or probably attributable to a therapeutic agent (eg, rise in creatinine after amphotericin administration).

[d]Attributive probably or definitely to CTLS.

*Source*: Reprinted with permission from Cairo and Bishop.[8]

reabsorbing needed fluid and electrolytes and excreting those not needed into the urine. Normally, small and controlled amounts of potassium, phosphorus, and uric acid are present in the blood. In the intracellular fluid, potassium is the major cation and phosphorus is the major anion. When cells are destroyed or lysed, the DNA in the nucleus of the cell is released into the blood, and the purines (nucleic acid) are converted in the liver to uric acid. Uric acid production requires cell catabolism but relies on the kidney for excretion. At normal rates of production and excretion, excesses of potassium, phosphorus, and uric acid do not occur.[22] When massive amounts of cells are destroyed, however, these substances are released into the blood, causing abnormally high levels of these minerals. An inverse relationship exists between phosphorus and calcium whereby if one mineral increases the other decreases in the same proportion. Thus, when tumor cells lyse, which results in the release of large amounts of phosphorus into the blood, there is a proportional decrease in serum calcium, resulting in hypocalcemia.[9,16,23]

Although TLS can occur spontaneously prior to treatment, it is more commonly seen after the initiation of cytoxic chemotherapy. Patients with tumors that have a high proliferative rate, a large tumor burden, and a high sensitivity to cytotoxic therapy are at greater risk for the development of this syndrome. Effective cancer therapy—usually chemotherapy—can initiate TLS by causing the cell membrane to rupture, releasing the intracellular contents into the extracellular fluids and subsequently into the bloodstream. TLS usually occurs 6 to 72 hours following chemotherapy and lasts for 5 to 7 days. It is during this post-therapy time that increased tumor lysis occurs. Pathophysiologically, these events can lead to acute renal failure and cardiac conduction abnormalities.[9,24,25]

Acute renal failure secondary to TLS is primarily due to hyperuricemia and hyperphosphatemia. Uric acid nephropathy is a complication that can occur secondary to hyperuricemia whereby uric acid crystals form in the collective ducts of the kidneys and ureters. These crystallizations lead to obstructive uropathy, resulting in decreased glomerular filtration, increased hydrostatic pressure, obstructed urine flow, and eventually acute renal failure. Similarly, calcium phosphate salts secondary to hyperphosphatemia may precipitate in the renal tubules and cause renal failure. Although the kidneys normally can accommodate moderate elevations in uric acid and phosphorus by increasing excretion, continued tumor lysis overwhelms the body's homeostatic mechanisms, ultimately resulting in acute renal failure. Renal insufficiency in turn exacerbates the existing hyperkalemia and hypocalcemia.[9,16,23,24]

The cardiac conduction abnormalities related to TLS are due primarily to hyperkalemia. Around 98% of the body's potassium is in the intracellular compartment. When cell lysis occurs, potassium is released from the intracellular compartment to the extracellular compartment and serum potassium levels increase. Hyperkalemia has a major depressant effect on cardiac function, resulting in bradycardia, heart block, and asystole. Electrocardiogram changes reveal widening of the QRS complex, elevated T waves, and flat or absent P waves. At serum potassium concentrations of >9 mEq/L, conduction is so delayed that the heart becomes flaccid and, if not recognized and treated immediately, cardiac arrest will result.[9,165,24,25]

## CLINICAL MANIFESTATIONS

The four major metabolic abnormalities responsible for the clinical manifestations of TLS are hyperuricemia, hyperkalemia, hyperphosphatemia, and hypocalcemia. These manifestations may occur individually or in combination. The severity of these metabolic alterations is related to tumor burden and renal dysfunction, which determine the signs and symptoms observed in TLS.

The early manifestations of TLS include fatigue/lethargy, nausea, vomiting, anorexia, diarrhea, cloudiness of urine, flank pain, muscle weakness, and cramps. These initial symptoms can be vague, mild complaints easily attributed to a side effect of treatment. As the potassium level increases, elevations in blood pressure and heart rate may occur. A patient in the early phase of TLS may exhibit minimal renal symptoms. As the metabolic abnormalities increase, however, the patient will become more symptomatic and exhibit further TLS-related symptoms. Gastrointestinal symptoms will increase in severity, and the patient may experience severe abdominal cramping and pain. Neuromuscular symptoms will also increase from mild paresthesias and muscle irritability to tetany and convulsions. Specific electrocardiogram (ECG) changes are evident in the early and late phases of TLS. Prolongation of the QT interval and ST segment, as well as lowering and inversion of the T wave are early ECG changes associated with TLS. Late TLS-associated ECG changes include elevated T waves, shortened QT interval, widened QRS, loss of P wave, and sine wave. Initially, the patient may exhibit an increase in blood pressure and heart rate, but as these metabolic disturbances continue, a decrease in blood pressure and heart rate occurs. Persistent hypocalcemia and hyperkalemia result in neurological changes, including memory loss, delirium, and hallucinations. Severe azotemia, which generally presents as increased serum urea and creatinine levels, and anuria due to progressive renal impairment are seen in the later phases of TLS. If TLS is unrecognized, untreated, or continues despite treatment, anuria, cardiac arrest, and death may occur. In summary, the physical consequences of TLS affect all body organs and frequently result in severe systemic effects. Figure 44-1 provides an overview of early and late signs and symptoms of TLS by body systems.[9,16,24–26]

## ASSESSMENT

The diagnosis of TLS is based primarily on laboratory and clinical findings of four metabolic abnormalities: hyperuricemia, hyperkalemia, hyperphosphatemia, and hypocalcemia. An accurate assessment of the patient prior to initiating cytotoxic therapy is necessary to rule out pretreatment TLS and to establish baseline laboratory and clinical data. Initially, a complete history and physical is performed and risk factors for TLS are identified. In taking the patient's history, the healthcare provider will obtain information regarding weight, nutritional and hydration status, past and current medications, and history of chronic health problems, allergies, or organ dysfunction. Assessment of risk factors is necessary for the prevention and management of TLS but can also determine the best setting for initiating cytotoxic therapy. Patients at high risk of developing TLS (eg, those with high-grade lymphoma, acute leukemia, preexisting renal impairment, or elevated LDH pretreatment) may require hospitalization for their treatment, whereas those patients at low risk (eg, those with a solid tumor, low-grade lymphoma, adequate renal function, or normal pretreatment LDH) can be treated on an outpatient basis. Specific laboratory parameters evaluated prior to, during, and after treatment include serum potassium, phosphorus, calcium, uric acid, blood urea nitrogen (BUN), creatinine, LDH, complete blood count (CBC), platelet count, and urinary pH and specific gravity. Assessment of the physical signs and symptoms of TLS related to gastrointestinal, neuromuscular, neurological, cardiovascular, and renal function is critical to TLS management (see Figure 44-1).[9,16,24–26] Renal function is closely monitored by analyzing serum electrolytes, BUN, creatinine, urinary pH and osmolality, urine specific gravity, and intake and output.[8,24] Occasionally, a renal ultrasound or other radiologic procedures are ordered to rule out other renal dysfunctions not caused by hyperuricemia such as a lymphoma pressing on the kidneys or the renal tubules.[8,27] Cardiac function is evaluated by frequent vital signs, ECG,

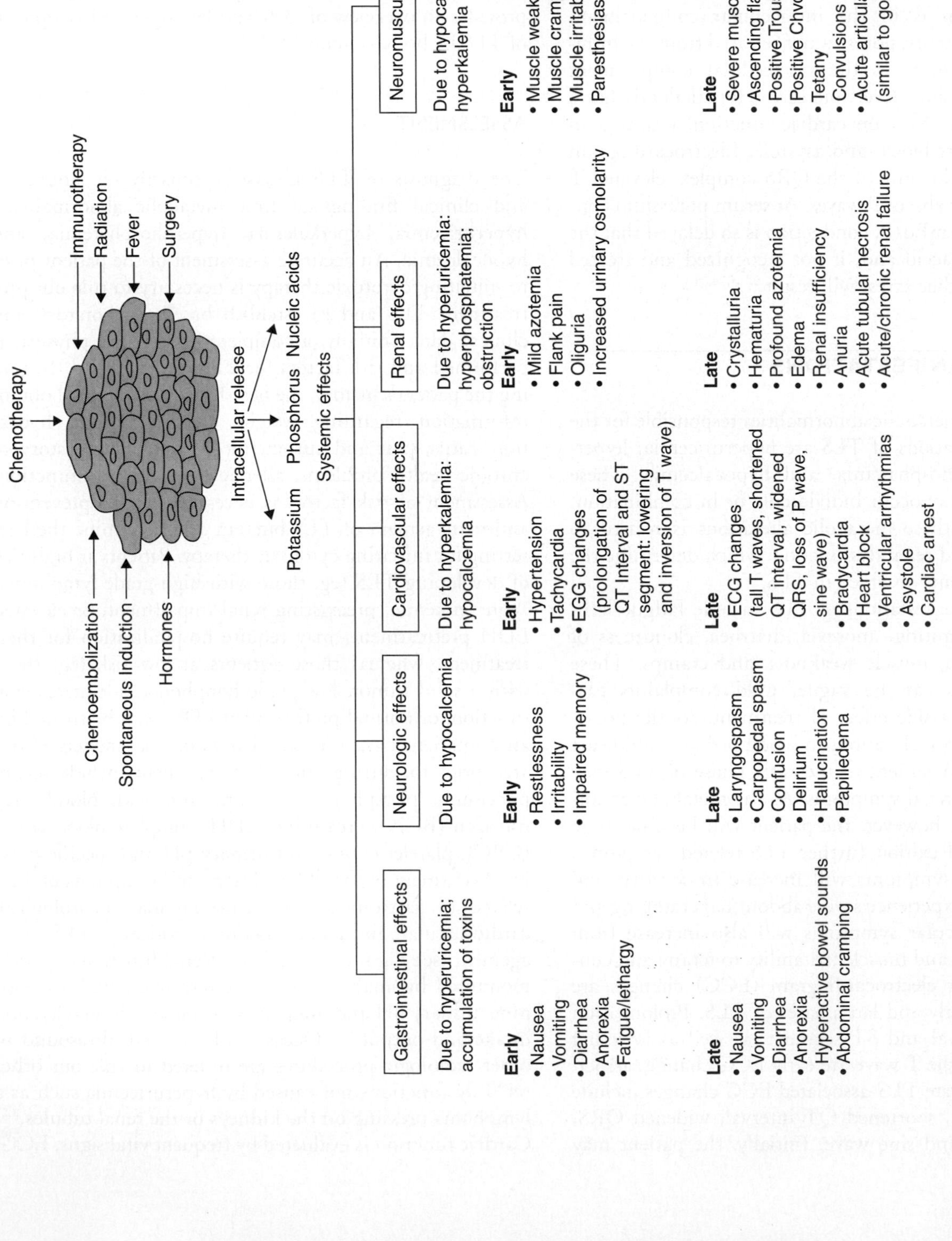


**FIGURE 44-1**
Systemic effects of tumor lysis sydrome occurring early and late in the disease.

and, if necessary, a chest x-ray and multigated acquisition heart scan (MUGA) to assess for fluid overload and the heart's left ventricular ejection fraction (LVEF).[9,16,26]

## THERAPEUTIC APPROACHES AND NURSING CARE

The primary goal of TLS management is prevention. Recognition of patients at risk for this syndrome allows preventive measures to be instituted 24 to 48 hours prior to treatment, thereby decreasing the risk of severe electrolyte imbalances. Early identification of TLS requires frequent laboratory assessment of electrolytes and renal function, as well as careful assessment of the signs and symptoms associated with each metabolic abnormality. Laboratory evaluation of patients with TLS or at high risk of developing TLS requires monitoring of LDH, potassium, sodium, uric acid, BUN, creatinine, phosphorus, and calcium prior to therapy and every 4 to 6 hours for the first 48 to 72 hours after the initiation of treatment.[6] Therapies and/or medications that could contribute to the electrolyte abnormalities associated with TLS should be minimized or eliminated. For example, ACE inhibitors, angiotensin II receptor blockers, heparin, and exogenous potassium sources such as oral supplements and dietary intake can contribute to hyperkalemia and therefore should be avoided where appropriate. While it is important to minimize or eliminate medications or conditions that could contribute to TLS, the implementation of prophylactic treatment regimens is crucial to preventing this syndrome.[24,25,28]

The established key elements of TLS prevention and intervention are aggressive hydration and diuresis, administration of prophylactic allopurinol, and for certain high-risk patients, the administration of rasburicase for the prevention and treatment of hyperuricemia. Alkalinization of the urine although widely used in the past is now controversial.[5–9,29] The rationale, use, and considerations for each of these elements will be discussed.

### HYDRATION

One of the most important mechanisms for preventing uric acid nephropathy and acute renal failure is by aggressively hydrating a patient with at least 2 to 3 liters/m$^2$/day with either normal saline or 5% dextrose solution.[5,6,9,16,19] Potassium, calcium, and phosphate should be withheld initially from hydration fluids due to the concurrent risk of hyperkalemia, hyperphosphatemia, and/or calcium phosphate precipitation. Expansion of plasma volume through aggressive hydration is an important intervention to induce diuresis, thereby decreasing renal insufficiency. Urine output needs to be maintained within a range of 150 to 200 mL/hour and must be closely monitored.[25] Urine specific gravity should be maintained at <1.010 and closely monitored.[5] If there is no evidence of acute obstructive uropathy and/or hypovolemia, diuretics may be used to maintain this urinary flow rate and prevent renal tubular damage.[5,9] Diuretics (loop or osmotic) are often used to maintain this urinary flow rate and to prevent renal tubular damage. The use of diuretics is particularly important for elderly patients and those at risk for fluid overload, such as patients with a large abdominal tumor or large mediastinal mass, or those with superior vena cava syndrome.[29,30] These measures improve glomerular filtration; enhance excretion of potassium, phosphate, and uric acid; and inhibit calcium reabsorption. If necessary, dopamine at low doses (5 µg/kg/min) can be given to further improve renal perfusion. It is important that aggressive hydration, with or without diuretics, begin 24 to 48 hours prior to treatment and continue for several days post treatment.[5–10]

### MEDICATIONS

Allopurinol administration is another key element of TLS prevention and intervention. Allopurinol blocks the conversion of the enzymes xanthine and hypoxanthine to uric acid. Since its introduction in 1965, allopurinol has been shown to decrease the formation of uric acid and reduce the incidence of obstructive uropathy caused by uric acid precipitation in patients at risk of developing TLS.[5] Allopurinol can be given orally (PO) or intravenously (IV). In a retrospective review of 1172 patients treated with IV allopurinol, the efficacy, administration schedule, and adverse effects were similar to the oral formulation.[31] The guidelines for allopurinol dosages and administration for pediatric and adult patients are the same. Allopurinol is administered at a dose of 50 to 100 mg/m$^2$ every 8 hours orally with a maximum dose of 300 mg/m$^2$/day. Intravenous administration of allopurinol is given at a dose of 200 to 400 mg/m$^2$/day in 1 to 3 divided doses with a maximum dose of 600 mg/day.[31] Treatment with allopurinol should be started 1 to 2 days before the start of induction chemotherapy and continued for up to 3 to 7 days after the therapy, depending on the uric acid levels, tumor burden, WBC and other laboratory values, and ongoing risk of developing TLS.[5]

Because allopurinol acts by decreasing the formation of uric acid, it is ineffective in reducing preexisting uric acid. The reduction in urate levels occurs slowly, beginning 1 to 3 days after initiation of the drug and reaches maximum efficacy after 7 to 10 days. Because it may take several days for uric acid levels to be reduced, delays in cytotoxic therapy may be necessary. Allopurinol can increase the serum levels of the purine precursors xanthine and hypoxanthine. Because xanthine is less soluble in urine, xanthine crystal deposition in the renal tubules can occur, resulting in acute obstructive uropathy.[5,6,9,10] Another limitation of allopurinol is that it reduces the clearance of other purine-based chemotherapeutic agents such as 6-mercaptopurine (6-MP) and azathioprine that are frequently used in the treatment of leukemia. A dose reduction of 65% to 75% of these agents is recommended when used concomitantly with allopurinol.[5,9] In addition, allopurinol can interfere with the metabolism of several drugs, including cyclophosphamide, 6-mercaptopurine, azathioprine, cyclosporin, chlorpropamide, dicumarol, and thiazide diuretics.[10] Allopurinol is contraindicated in patients receiving capecitabine.[29] Allopurinol is generally well tolerated, but hypersensitivity reactions have been reported in a minority of patients, with skin rash and fever being the most frequent side effect.[29] If allergic side effects occur, it is recommended that allopurinol be discontinued immediately. Because allopurinol is excreted in the kidney, the dose of allopurinol should be adjusted in patients with renal impairment.[9] A 50% dose reduction is recommended in patients with renal insufficiency.[5]

Rasburicase (elitek) a recombinant urate oxidase, converts uric acid into allantoin, which is a by-product of uric acid. Allantoin is 5 to 10 times more soluble than uric acid and is therefore rapidly excreted by the kidneys.[5,9] The results of early studies of this drug using a nonrecombinant urate oxidase demonstrated the effectiveness of urate oxidase in rapidly reducing urate levels and decreasing the need for dialysis during the early management of TLS. However, this form of urate oxidase was associated with a 5% rate of acute hypersensitivity reactions, including life-threatening anaphylaxis.[32–34] Thus, a recombinant form of urate oxidase was developed. It is produced from a modified strain of *Saccharomyces cerevisiae* cloned with a DNA from a strain of *Aspergillus flavus*. Several studies have demonstrated that rasburicase can significantly decrease uric acid levels more rapidly and to a greater degree than allopurinol in both children and adults.[3,35–38]

The GRAAL (Groupe d'etude des lymphomes de l'adulte trial on rasburicase activity in adult lymphoma) study provided evidence of the efficacy and safety of the prophylactic use of rasburicase in 100 adults with aggressive NHL during the first course of chemotherapy. All patients had a decrease in uric acid levels within 4 hours after the first dose of rasburicase and normalization of phosphorus, potassium, and calcium levels.[37] A compassionate use trial conducted in the United States and Canada included 682 children and 387 adults with hematological malignancies associated with a high tumor burden and/or high leukocyte counts. The data revealed a significant reduction in uric acid levels from a median of 10.9 to 0.7 mg in patients with elevated uric acid levels.[38]

Rasburicase is approved for the initial management of hyperuricemia in pediatric patients receiving treatment for hematological malignancies or solid tumors who are at risk for hyperuricemia and/or TLS. Rasburicase was recently approved for the initial management of plasma uric acid levels in adults with leukemia, lymphoma, and solid tumors receiving anticancer therapy expected to result in tumor lysis.[39] The approved dose of rasburicase is 0.15 to 0.2 mg/kg dose IV over 30 minutes once a day for 5 days, with the first dose administered 4 to 24 hours before starting chemotherapy.[40] Tumor Lysis Guidelines by a panel of experts recommend a rasburicase dose of 0.10 to 0.2 mg/kg daily depending on whether it is being given for prevention or treatment of TLS. Duration of treatment can range from 1 to 7 days with the average of 3 days. However, specific recommendations of rasburicase administration is related to the control of plasma uric acid levels and therefore clinical judgement should be utilized to determine dose, length of treatment, or need to increase the administration schedule to twice daily.[5] Rasburicase is recommended for the initial management of patients considered to be at high risk for TLS. There was no consensus in the treatment approach for intermediate risk patients but a single dose of rasburicase might be considered in the initial management. It is noted by the panel that rasburicase has been used in the initial management of both high-risk and intermediate risk patients in Europe. For low-risk patients, rasburicase is not recommended and a watch-and-wait approach with close observation and monitoring is suggested.[5]

Due to the high cost of rasburicase, alternative dosing schedules have been used and there is now evidence from several trials for use of shorter length of treatment and at lower doses than the approved dose and treatment schedule. Studies using single dose rasburicase, lower doses, and shorter course of treatment (2–3 days vs 5 days) have all demonstrated efficacy in both the prophylaxis and treatment of TLS.[41–46] The correct dosing of rasburicase in obese patients is not known, as there have been no clinical trials to evaluate rasburicase dosing in the obese. A case report in the literature revealed that a single dose of rasburicase based on ideal body weight (IBW) was effective in preventing TLS and normalizing the uric acid level within 4 hours. The pharmacokinetic profile and mechanism of action of rasburicase suggest that dosing obese patients based on IBW appears reasonable but further studies are needed.[47]

In general, rasburicase is well tolerated, with the most frequently reported side effects including headache, nausea, vomiting, fever, and diarrhea.[46] The most serious adverse reactions are rare (<1% of patients) and include rash, anaphylaxis, hemolysis, and methemoglobinemia.[39,46,48] Other serious adverse reactions include neutropenia (with or without fever), respiratory distress, mucositis, and sepsis. In approximately 5% to 15% of patients, anti-rasburicase antibodies develop.[10] Time to detection of antibodies can range from 1 to 6 weeks after administration. However, it is not known if the antibodies are neutralizing antibodies, and the clinical significance and relationship to adverse events has not been established.[8]

Rasburicase is contraindicated in patients with known glucose-6-phosphate dehydrogenase (G6PD) deficiency that is seen in some patients of African, Mediterranean, or Southeast Asian descent. Patients with G6PD deficiency cannot break down hydrogen peroxide, a by-product of rasburicase, which can cause severe hemolysis. It is not known if a history of asthma or allergy should be a contraindication for the administration of rasburicase.[15,46,48] Anecdotal evidence suggests that rasburicase can be used in patients with a history of allergy but further research is needed.[5]

In summary, rasburicase provides an effective but costly alternative for the prevention and treatment of hyperuricemia and TLS.[5,9,10,49] Rasburicase differs from allopurinol as it can affect existing plasma uric acid and quickly decrease uric acid levels prior to or during cytotoxic therapy. In addition, because clearance of rasburicase is independent of renal and hepatic function, it can be used safely in elderly patients and patients with impaired renal or liver function.[40] The cost-effectiveness between allopurinol and rasburicase whereby the cost of the drug is compared with the costs associated with hospital days, treatment in an intensive care unit, and dialysis must be considered. Significant costs are associated with the complications of hyperuricemia and TLS such as acute renal failure, dialysis, and death. A study by Candrilli et al[50] evaluated the medical resources and costs associated with renal complications in patients with hematological malignancies. Patients who developed acute renal failure requiring dialysis had an average length of stay of 21 days with an average total cost per discharge of $51,990. Patients who developed acute renal failure but did not require dialysis had an average length of stay of 13 days and an average cost of $25,575. In comparison, patients who did not have any renal complications had an average length of stay of 7 days and an average cost of $9,978 (all costs in 2002 US dollars).

## URINARY ALKALINIZATION

Alkalinization of the urine (urine pH >7.0) has historically been recommended for the prevention and/or treatment of TLS.[5,9] Urinary alkalinization increases the solubility of uric acid, thereby promoting the excretion of uric acid in the urine.[5,9,24] The practice of urinary alkalinization is controversial because complications of urinary alkalinization include an increased precipitation of calcium phosphate in the renal microvasculature and tubules that can lead to obstructive nephropathy and increased risk of renal failure. Furthermore, urinary alkalinization can cause hypocalcaemia and increase the risk for xanthine nephropathy.[5,9] Recently, a consensus panel of experts recommended that alkalinization only be used for patients with metabolic acidosis. However, the panel did not reach consensus regarding urinary alkalinization for patients who will receive allopurinol. In making their recommendations, the panel cited that there was lack of evidence of benefit, and that there are potential complications associated with alkalinization of the urine in the prevention of TLS. Urinary alkalinization is not required in patients receiving rasburicase.[5] Therefore, urinary alkalinization measures to prevent renal complications secondary to TLS must be individualized and used cautiously. Alkalinization of the urine can be achieved by adding 50 to 100 mEq of sodium bicarbonate to each liter of IV hydration and/or administering acetazolamide, 250 to 500 mg IV daily.[5,10,24,29] Early identification and correction of electrolyte imbalances is the key component of TLS prevention and management. Accurate phone triage is critical to the management of TLS on an outpatient basis (see Figure 44-2).[6,9,28,29] Prompt recognition and treatment of these metabolic abnormalities often reduces the need for hospitalization by preventing the development of TLS. However, if metabolic abnormalities related to TLS and/or clinical symptoms persist for 48 to 72 hours despite aggressive preventive and treatment measures, hospitalization is necessary. Hospitalization is recommended for adult and pediatric patients at high risk of developing TLS with induction chemotherapy.[5]

## DIALYSIS

Laboratory values and the patient's clinical condition can change quickly over a few hours, necessitating more intensive monitoring and treatment. The patient will be admitted to the intensive care unit if the laboratory and/or clinical signs and symptoms of TLS continue to worsen despite preventive and treatment measures, or if the patient develops renal, respiratory, or cardiac failure. These patients often require aggressive hemodynamic monitoring and mechanical ventilation. If the electrolyte abnormalities of TLS cannot be corrected or if renal failure worsens despite aggressive management, dialysis should be promptly instituted. Dialysis has been particularly successful in treating obstructive nephropathy, acute renal failure, and accompanying metabolic abnormalities associated with TLS. Dialysis is also recommended for patients with fluid volume overload, renal insufficiency, or symptomatic hypocalcemia, and for those patients who do not respond to other corrective treatment measures.[5,8,9,24] Hemodialysis, peritoneal dialysis (PD), continuous renal replacement therapies (CRRT), and new hybrid therapies, such as sustained low efficiency dialysis and extended daily dialysis, have been used in the treatment for both children and adults with TLS. Unfortunately, data comparing the various modalities are sparse. In general, hemodialysis is preferred because it can rapidly correct life-threatening electrolyte disturbances. Compared to hemodialysis, peritoneal dialysis is much less efficient in correcting metabolic abnormalities and can be technically difficult when hepatosplenomegaly or a large abdominal tumor is present.[8,9,16] The duration of dialysis should be every 12 hours until renal function, metabolic abnormalities, and urinary volume are corrected. Repeated dialysis procedure at 12- to 24-hour intervals may be necessary in patients with a large phosphate burden.[24] TLS resulting in renal failure and the requirement of dialysis has been reported to occur in 15% to 30% of cases when standard therapy was utilized in the prevention or treatment of TLS.[48]

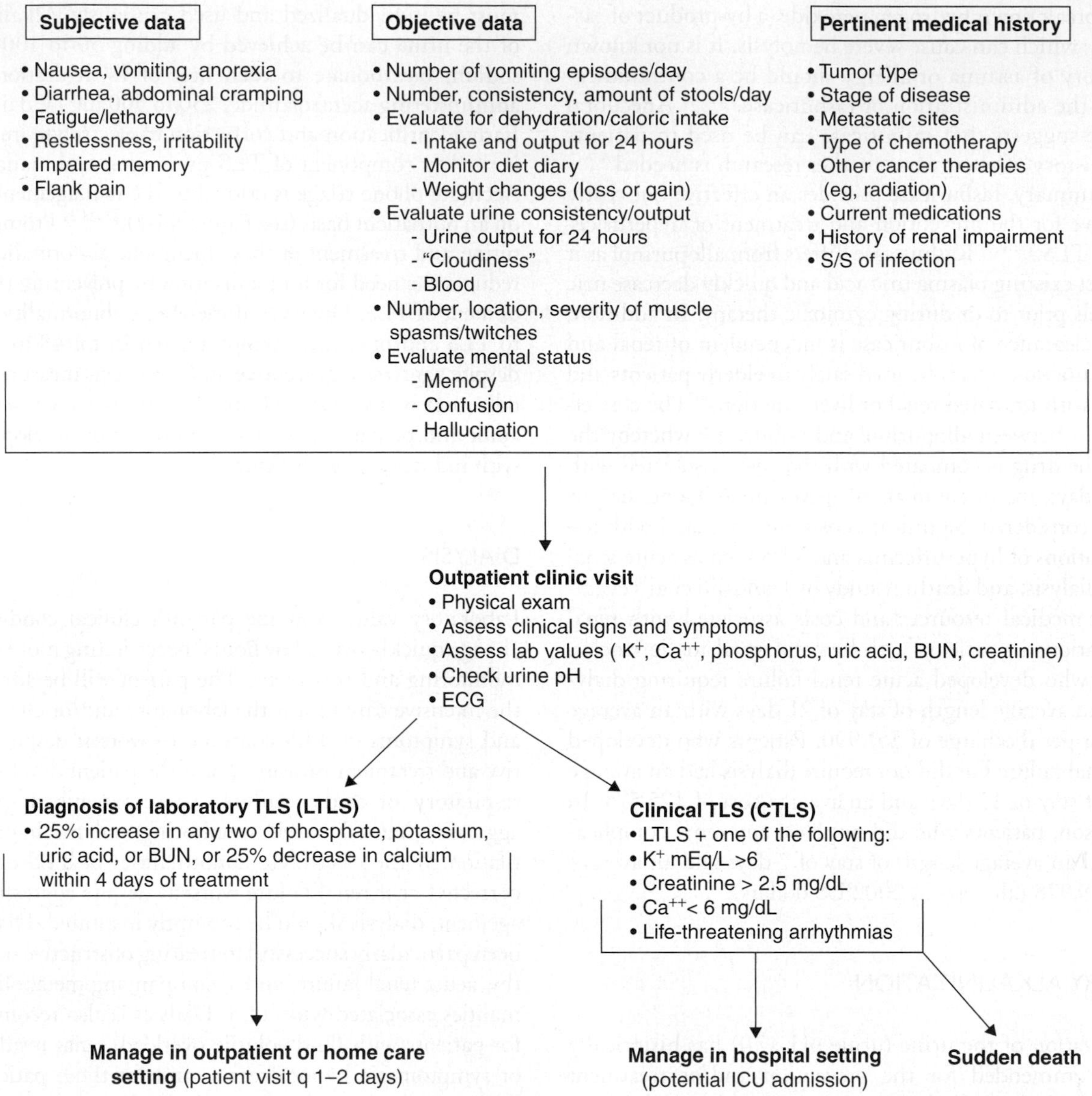
Subjective data
• Nausea, vomiting, anorexia
• Diarrhea, abdominal cramping
• Fatigue/lethargy
• Restlessness, irritability
• Impaired memory
• Flank pain
Objective data
• Number of vomiting episodes/day
• Number, consistency, amount of stools/day
• Evaluate for dehydration/caloric intake
- Intake and output for 24 hours
- Monitor diet diary
- Weight changes (loss or gain)
• Evaluate urine consistency/output
- Urine output for 24 hours
- "Cloudiness"
- Blood
• Number, location, severity of muscle spasms/twitches
• Evaluate mental status
- Memory
- Confusion
- Hallucination
Pertinent medical history
• Tumor type
• Stage of disease
• Metastatic sites
• Type of chemotherapy
• Other cancer therapies (eg, radiation)
• Current medications
• History of renal impairment
• S/S of infection
Outpatient clinic visit
• Physical exam
• Assess clinical signs and symptoms
• Assess lab values ( K+, Ca++, phosphorus, uric acid, BUN, creatinine)
• Check urine pH
• ECG
Diagnosis of laboratory TLS (LTLS)
• 25% increase in any two of phosphate, potassium, uric acid, or BUN, or 25% decrease in calcium within 4 days of treatment
Clinical TLS (CTLS)
• LTLS + one of the following:
• K+ mEq/L >6
• Creatinine > 2.5 mg/dL
• Ca++< 6 mg/dL
• Life-threatening arrhythmias
Manage in outpatient or home care setting (patient visit q 1–2 days)
Manage in hospital setting (potential ICU admission)
Sudden death

**FIGURE 44-2**

Phone triage assessment of tumor lysis syndrome and patient disposition.

*Abbreviations*: BUN, blood urea nitrogen; CTLS, clinical tumor lysis syndrome; ECG, electrocardiogram; ICU, intensive care unit; LTLS, laboratory tumor lysis syndrome; S/S, signs and symptoms; TLS, tumor lysis syndrome.

However, the rate of need for dialysis in studies with the use of rasburicase ranged from 0% to 4%.[14]

## SPECIFIC ELECTROLYTE MANAGEMENT

Successful treatment of TLS is also dependent on the prompt identification and treatment of hyperkalemia, hyperphosphatemia, and hypocalcemia. Hyperkalemia, defined as a potassium level greater than 6.0 mEq/L is one of the earliest life-threatening complications of TLS.[12] Hyperkalemia can be managed with the use of sodium polystyrene sulfonate, IV calcium gluconate, IV calcium chloride, IV glucose and insulin infusion, loop diuretics, or dialysis. The specific intervention is dependent on the potassium level, clinical findings, and/or the patient's symptoms. For a serum potassium level greater than 7.0 to 7.5 mEq/L and/or significant EKG changes, immediate intervention is indicated with rapid acting insulin and glucose infusion. For the treatment of life-threatening arrhythmias such as bradycardia, IV calcium gluconate can be given slowly with EKG monitoring. For asymptomatic patients (and a potassium of <6.5 mEq/L), sodium polystyrene sulfonate should be administered orally or by retention enema.[28] Loop diuretics can be given to decrease potassium by increasing urinary potassium excretion.[5,12] Electrolytes, ECG, and cardiac rhythm should be closely monitored. Supplemental oral and IV potassium should be avoided.[5,51] If these therapeutic measures fail to correct the hyperkalemia, dialysis would be required.[5,12]

Hyperphosphatemia, defined as a phosphorus level of 6.5 mg/dL in children and 4.5 mg/dL in adults should be treated as this should also correct hypocalcaemia due to the inverse relationship between phosphorus and calcium. Hyperphosphatemia can be managed with eliminating other sources of phosphorus (diet, IV solutions, and medications), oral phosphate binders (eg, aluminum hydroxide), or hypertonic dextrose and insulin.[5] Patients with hyperphosphatemia should not receive calcium infusions.[8] Phosphorus and calcium levels should be closely monitored. If hyperphosphatemia persists despite these measures, hemodialysis should be considered. Phosphate clearance is significantly better with hemodialysis as compared with peritoneal dialysis or continuous venous hemofiltration.[5,9]

Hypocalcemia, defined as $\leq$ 7.0 mg/dL, may or may not be treated. In general, treatment of asymptomatic hypocalcemia is not recommended.[5,9,12] In patients with symptomatic hypocalcaemia, intravenous calcium gluconate, administered slowly with ECG monitoring, may be necessary to correct the clinical symptoms. However, since this may increase the risk of calcium phosphorus deposition and obstructive uropathy, close monitoring of calcium and phosphorus levels, clinical symptoms, and EKG must be done.[6,8] Management and potential outcomes of TLS are presented in Figure 44-3.[5–10,12,16,29]

## NURSING CARE

When caring for a patient at risk for TLS, a nurse's goal is prevention and minimizing the consequences of TLS. Prevention, early identification, and intervention for the metabolic abnormalities of TLS require knowledge of risk factors, laboratory and clinical signs and symptoms of each metabolic abnormality, and treatment measures. Identification of patients who are at risk based on the type of malignancy, extent of disease, preexisting clinical condition, and baseline laboratory values can lead to a proactive management approach and implementation of preventive measures. Whether TLS is a potential problem for an individual or has already occurred, two major nursing responsibilities are education and assessment. Education of the patient and family regarding the risk factors, clinical manifestations, possible treatment measures, and when to seek medical help is the key in preventing TLS.[51] All patients at risk for TLS should receive both verbal and written information regarding the syndrome. Educating and encouraging patients and families to be involved in the prevention and treatment of TLS can increase the patient's sense of control, as well as highlight the importance of family involvement in caring for their loved one. The importance of educating patients and family members regarding the complications of cancer therapy has become increasingly clear, as the majority of cancer therapies are given on an outpatient basis and the complexity of cancer therapies has increased.

Another major responsibility of the nurse is the accurate and continual assessment of the patient before, during, and after cancer therapy. Baseline and ongoing assessment of laboratory parameters and clinical manifestations will help to detect subtle clinical changes, thereby preventing serious and life-threatening complications of TLS. A thorough physical assessment is conducted prior to, during, and after cancer therapy to determine the effect of the metabolic abnormalities on many organ systems. Certain diagnostic tests such as Chvostek's sign (elicited by tapping the cheek below the temple near the facial nerve; positive sign if lip or nose twitches on the side of the tap), Trousseau's sign (elicited by using a blood pressure cuff to occlude arterial flow in the arm for 1 to 3 minutes; positive sign if the thumb adducts and the fingers extend or the muscles of the hand or forearm spasm), deep tendon reflexes (elicited by mildly stretching a muscle and tapping a tendon; provides data about the integrity of sensory and motor pathways of the reflex arc and specific spinal cord segments), and ECG are useful in monitoring the clinical status of a patient with potential or actual TLS.[52,53]

The medical management of TLS requires active participation of nurses in various healthcare settings. Nurses are primarily responsible for the day-to-day management of the patient. The development of new cancer therapies, prophylactic/therapeutic regimens for TLS, and alternative routes of administration for medications will significantly affect patient outcomes associated with TLS. Participation in research studies may lead to a better understanding of the incidence, prevention strategies, and management of this syndrome. Since patients with potential or actual TLS often traverse different healthcare settings in the treatment of their disease, the nurse serves as the liaison or coordinator to ensure continuity of care. Communication of all patient-related findings to physicians and other healthcare providers is necessary for prompt recognition and treatment of TLS. The importance of providing emotional support to the patient and family cannot be understated. It is often difficult for patients and families to understand how such a severe and life-threatening complication can occur when the treatment is working well against the disease.

## SPECIAL CONSIDERATIONS IN THE ELDERLY

Since the majority of cancers occur in adults over the age of 65 and with approximately 70% of all cancer deaths in this population, the prevention and management of TLS in the elderly requires special consideration. Although the identification of patients at risk and the initiation of prophylactic

**Management of Hyperuricemia**

- Administer allopurinol
  - 50–100 mg/m² q 8 hours PO (maximum dose 800 mg/day)
  - 200–400 mg/m²/day in 3 divided doses IV (maximum dose 600 mg/day)
  - Reduce dose by 50% or more in renal failure
  - Reduce 6-mercaptopurine and/or azathioprine by 65%–75% with concomitant allopurinol
- Increase or continue allopurinol until uric acid is normal
- Administer elitek (rasburicase)
  - 0.15–0.2 mg/kg IV over 30 minutes daily for 5–7 days (FDA recommendation); alternative doses and schedules have been utilized
- IV hydration 2–3 L/m²/day of normal saline or 15% dextrose solution
- Urinary alkalinization is controversial: 50–100 mEq/L of sodium bicarbonate to maintain pH > 7.
- Administer acetazolamide 250–500 mg/IV/day if volume load a problem or hyperuricemia refractory to above measures
- Initiate low-dose dopamine (0.5–3 mcg/kg/minute) for oliguria or preexisting fluid retention

**Management of Hypocalcemia**

- Monitor ECG
- Institute seizure precautions
- If symptomatic, administer 10% IV calcium gluconate in D5W solution slowly, 1–3mL/ minute with ECG monitoring for severe changes
- Administration of $CA^{++}$ supplements is controversial
- No treatment if asymptomatic

**General Principles—Management**

- Identify high risk patients for TLS and implement prophylactic treatment regimen
- Withhold further antitumor therapy until TLS resolves
- Review medications/conditions that could contribute to TLS
- Assess clinical signs and symptoms
- Monitor electrolytes and renal function q 6–12 hours for LTLS and q 2–4 hours for CTLS
- Ensure hydration of 2–3 L/m²/day
- Administer appropriate dose of allopurinol
- Administer appropriate dose of rasburicase
- Alkalinization of urine is controversial and not recommended in management guidelines; however, individualized approach should be used
  - Administer sodium bicarbonate (50–100 mEq/L) IV to maintain pH > 7
  - Monitor urine pH 3–4 times/day for LTLS and q 4 hours for CLTS
- Force diuresis by administering non-thiazide diuretic if urinary output < 100cc/hour
- Monitor I & O
- Weigh daily
- Monitor ECG—reporting changes immediately
- Monitor arterial blood gas
- Follow specific dietary restrictions where appropriate
- Document all assessments, interventions and evaluations in medical record

**Management of Hyperkalemia**

- Review medications contributing to ↑ $K^+$, provide alternatives when possible
- Restrict dietary $K^+$
- Assess clinical signs and symptoms
- Monitor ECG
- Administer sodium polystyrene resin 15–30 g orally or rectally for $K^+ < 7$ and no ECG change
- Administer sodium polystyrene sulfonate 10–30 g over 1–5 minutes orally or retention enema for mild $K^+$ (< 6.5mEq/L)
- Administer 10% IV calcium gluconate (10 mL) in D5W solution slowly, 1–3 mL/minute with ECG monitoring for $K^+ > 7$ and ECG changes
- Administer sodium bicarbonate 50–100 mEq/L IV
- Administer furosemide (0.5–1.0 mg/kg) or mannitol (0.5 mg/kg) IV. For severe oliguria or anuria, administer a single dose of furosemide (2–4 mg/kg)
- Administer 10–20 units of regular insulin in D10W IV over 1 hour in patient who is oliguric

**Management of Hyperphosphatemia**

- Administer phosphate binding antacids (aluminum hydroxide 30 cc PO TID or potassium and sodium phosphate 2 tabs PO TID)
- Eliminate other sources of phosphorous (diet, medications)
- Administer hypertonic glucose and insulin infusion
- Monitor calcium

**FIGURE 44-3**

Principles of management of TLS.

*Abbreviations*: CTLS, clinical tumor lysis syndrome; ECG, electrocardiogram; FDA, Food and Drug Administration; g, grams; I&O, intake and output; LTLS, laboratory tumor lysis syndrome; TLS, tumor lysis syndrome.

measures are the same for the elderly, the management of TLS in the elderly may be complicated by the following: renal and heart senescence, presence of multiple comorbid conditions, polypharmacy, and difficulties with adherence to complex medication and dietary regimens.[30]

Chronic renal failure is frequently seen in the elderly and often is associated with malignancy.[30] Renal failure results in abnormalities in extracellular fluid balance, electrolyte levels, and acid–base balance. The reduced functioning of the kidney as evidenced by decreased glomerular filtration rate, renal blood flow, renal clearance, and renin and aldosterone can contribute to increased risk of hyperkalemia, hyperphosphatemia, hyperuricemia and therefore TLS. Aging is also associated with extensive changes throughout the cardiovascular system that can substantially decrease cardiovascular reserve and predispose patients to develop heart failure. Additionally, hypertension and coronary artery disease are increased in the elderly.

In addition to changes in the renal and cardiovascular systems, there are several other conditions commonly seen in the elderly that could affect the management of TLS. Comorbidities in the elderly may include altered hepatic metabolism, diabetes, obesity, insulin resistance, benign prostatic hypertrophy, high serum triglycerides, cholesterol, and/or low-HDL cholesterol. These factors place patients at risk for impaired renal function, electrolyte disturbances, hypotension, and orthostatic intolerance.

The elderly patient is often on several medications to prevent or treat multiple health conditions. The polypharmacy and the increased complexity of medications and dietary regimens can result in lack of compliance, limited success of controlling the condition, and increased susceptibility to side effects of medications. In addition, many drugs commonly taken by the elderly including digitalis, beta blockers, ace-inhibitors, antipsychotics, and diuretics can increase serum uric acid, leading to an increased risk of TLS.

The management of TLS, particularly in the areas of hydration, metabolic abnormalities, and supportive treatment of renal failure need special consideration. Due to age-associated changes in the renal and cardiovascular systems, the elderly patient is at greater risk of volume overload when aggressive fluid administration is utilized. Blood pressure, urinary output, renal function, and serum electolytes, particularly potassium must be closely monitored during treatment. Hyperkalemia must be corrected quickly before potential fatal ventricular arrhythmias occur. Administration of 10% calcium gluconate is recommended for treatment of severe hyperkalemia. Sodium bicarbonate should be administered judiciously in elderly patients or in patients with renal failure, since it can lead to inappropriate volume expansion. Hyperphosphatemia in the elderly must be treated quickly to avoid hypocalcemia, nephrocalcinosis, nephrolithasis, and acute obstructive uropathy.[30] If severe hyperphosphatemia continues despite oral aluminum hydroxide therapy, then hemodialysis is required.[5,9,30]

In summary, the elderly patient is at greater risk for the development of metabolic abnormalities and the severity of complications associated with TLS. The oncology nurse needs to understand how age-related changes in the renal and cardiovascular systems, the presence of multiple comorbidities, medications, and diet of the elderly patient could impact the development and management of TLS. With this knowledge, the oncology nurse will be better able to identify subtle changes in laboratory values and/or clinical conditions that require immediate attention by the healthcare team.

## MORBIDITY AND MORTALITY

Precise morbidity and mortality rates for patients who develop TLS are not known. Some authors report resolution of TLS with treatment, while others report death despite appropriate treatment. In a report of adverse consequences of TLS in patients with CLL treated with Fludarabine, the authors state that although the overall incidence of TLS was low (0.4%), the outcome was extremely poor with 30% of patients requiring dialysis and 40% of patients who died.[11] In a multicenter retrospective chart review of 766 patients with ALL, AML, or NHL, 7 patients died from a TLS-related cause accounting for 0.9% of the total sample studied and 17.5% of patients were affected by TLS.[3] In a single center retrospective chart review of 614 consecutive patients undergoing induction chemotherapy for AML, the TLS-related morbidity and mortality was 5% and 2%, respectively. Although there was no correlation between LTLS and death rate, CTLS was associated with a higher death rate, mostly due to hemorrhage.[13] The mortality rate among patients with TLS in solid tumors is higher than among those with hematological malignancies, presumably due to the heightened awareness of this syndrome, the institution of prophylactic measures, and the close monitoring of patients with hematological malignancies. In addition, the mortality rate is higher in patients with solid tumors even after correction and resolution of metabolic and renal problems.[11,12] A review of the literature of 45 patients with solid tumors who developed TLS found that 16 out of the 45 patients, or one-third of the patients, died as a result of TLS due to either cardiac arrythmias or acute uremia.[11] Further studies are needed to define the morbidity and mortality associated with TLS. It seems likely, however, that the occurrence and resolution of TLS depend not only on specific risk factors but also on the early identification and initiation of preventive measures.

## CONCLUSION

Although our knowledge of TLS risk factors, prevention measures, and management strategies has increased, the results of current studies indicate that despite available preventive measures, TLS and its associated complications still occur. With advances in cancer therapy, particularly newer and more targeted therapies, the incidence of TLS may increase. The major clinical consequences, significant costs, and morbidity and mortality associated with TLS warrant the need for more effective preventive measures and treatment. Further study will be required to establish the role and cost effectiveness of rasburicase in the prevention and treatment of hyperuricemia, whereby the costs associated with hospital days, treatment in an intensive care unit, and dialysis are evaluated. The Cairo–Bishop classification and grading system and the current guidelines for the management of pediatric and adult patients with TLS will assist in the future use of prophylactic measures and the appropriate treatment necessary to manage TLS in specific subpopulations at risk for the development of this syndrome. The oncology nurse plays a critical role in the prevention and management of TLS through assessment, careful monitoring, implementation of prophylactic treatment regimens, and collaboration with other members of the healthcare team. Oncology nurses' early recognition of TLS and prompt intervention may prevent this serious complication.

## REFERENCES


1. Cohen LF, Balow JE, Magrath IT, et al. Acute tumor lysis syndrome: a review of 37 patients with Burkitt's lymphoma. *Am J Med.* 1980;68:486–491.
2. Wossmann W, Schrappe M, Meyer U, Zimmerman M, Reiter A. Incidence of tumor lysis syndrome in children with advanced stage Burkitt's lymphoma/leukemia before and after introduction of prophylactic use of urate oxidase. *Ann Hematol.* 2003;82:160–165.
3. Annemans L, Moeremans K, Lamotte M, et al. Pan-European multicentre economic evaluation of recombinant urate oxidase in prevention and treatment of hyperuricaemia and tumour lysis syndrome in haematological cancer patients. *Support Care Cancer.* 2003;11:249–257.
4. Mato AR, Riccio BE, Qin L, et al. A predictive model for the detection of tumor lysis syndrome during AML induction therapy. *Leuk Lymphoma.* 2006;47:877–883.
5. Coiffier B, Altman A, Pui CH, et al. Guidelines for the management of pediatric and adult tumor lysis syndrome: an evidence based review. *J Clin Oncol.* 2008;26:2767–2778.
6. Hochberg J, Cairo MS. Tumor lysis syndrome: current perspective. *Hematologica.* 2008;93:9–13.
7. Hande RR, Garrow GC. Acute tumor lysis syndrome in patients with high-grade non-Hodgkin's lymphoma. *Am J Med.* 1993;94:133–139.
8. Tosi P, Barosi G, Lazzaro C, et al. Consensus conference on the management of tumor lysis syndrome. *Haematologica.* 2008;93:1877–1885.
9. Cairo MS, Bishop M. Tumour lysis syndrome: new therapeutic strategies and classification. *Br J Haematol.* 2004;127:3–11.
10. Navolanic PM, Pui C-H, Larson RA, et al. Elitek rasburicase: an effective means to prevent and treat hyperuricemia associated with tumor lysis syndrome, a meeting report, Dallas, Texas, January, 2002. *Leukemia.* 2003;17:499–514.
11. Baeksgaard L, Sorensen JB. Acute tumor lysis syndrome in solid tumors—a case report and review of the literature. *Cancer Chemother Pharmacol.* 2003;51:187–192.
12. Gemici C. Tumour lysis syndrome in solid tumours. *Clin Oncol.* 2006;18:773–780.
13. Montesinos P, Lorenzo I, Martin G, et al. Tumor lysis syndrome in patients with acute myeloid leukemia: identification of risk factors and development of a predictive model. *Haemotologica.* 2008;93:67–74.
14. Sood AR, Burry LD, Cheng DK. Clarifying the role of Rasburicase in tumor lysis syndrome. *Pharmacotherapy.* 2007;27:111–121.
15. Bessmertny O, Robitaille LM, Cairo MS. Rasburicase: a new approach for preventing and/or treating tumor lysis syndrome. *Curr Pharm Des.* 2005;11:4177–4185.
16. Davidson MB, Thakkar S, Hix JK, et al. Pathophysiology, clinical outcomes and treatment of tumor lysis syndrome. *Am J Med.* 2004;116: 546–554.
17. Riccio B, Mato A, Olson EM, et al. Spontaneous tumor lysis syndrome in acute myeloid leukemia. *Cancer Biol Ther.* 2006;5:1614–1617.
18. Ahamed SM, Varma RS, Hamide TM, et al. Spontaneous tumor lysis syndrome associated with non-Hodgkin's lymphoma—a case report. *Indian J Pathol Microbiol.* 2006;49:26–28.
19. Hsu HH, Chan YL, Huang CC. Acute spontaneous tumor lysis presenting with hyperuricemic acute renal failure: clinical features and therapeutic approach. *J Nephrol.* 2004;17:50–56.
20. Agnani S, Gupta R, Atray NK, et al. Marked hyperuricemia with aute renal failure: need to consider occult maligning and spontaneous tumor lysis syndrome. *Int J Clin Pract.* 2006;60:364–366.
21. Vaisban E, Braester A, Mosenzon O, et al. Spontaneous tumor lysis syndrome in solid tumors: really a rare condition? Am J Med *Sci.* 2003; 325:38–40.
22. Reilly RF, Bulger RE, Kriz W. Structural-functional relationships in the kidney. In: Schrier RW, ed. *Diseases of the Kidney and Urinary Tract.* Philadelphia, PA: Lippincott, Williams & Wilkins; 2007:2–53.
23. Bellinghieri G, Santoro D, Savica V. Pharmacological treatment of acute and chronic hyperuricemia in kidney diseased patients. In: Ronco C, Rodeghiero F, eds. *Hyperuricemic Syndromes: Pathophysiology and Therapy.* Basel, Switzerland: Karger; 2005:149–160. *Contributions to Nephrology*; vol. 147.
24. Rampello E, Fricia T, Malaguarnera M. The management of tumor lysis syndrome. *Nat Clin Pract Oncol.* 2006;3:438–447.
25. Hagmeister F, Huen A. The status of allopurinol in the management of tumor lysis syndrome: a clinical review. *Cancer J.* 2005;11:S1-S10.
26. Tiu R, Mountantonakis SE, Dunbar AJ. Tumor lysis syndrome. *Semin Thromb Hemost.* 2007;33:397–407.
27. Yarpuzlu AA. A review of clinical and laboratory findings and treatment of tumor lysis syndrome. *Clin Chim Acta.* 2003;333:13–18.
28. Gobel BH. Tumor lysis syndrome. In: Kaplan M, ed. *Understanding and Managing Oncologic Emergencies: A Resource for Nurses.* Pittsburgh, PA: Oncology Nursing Society; 2006:285–306.
29. Coffier B, Riouffol C. Management of tumor lysis syndrome in adults. *Expert Rev Anticancer Ther.* 2007;7:233–239.
30. Pumo V, Sciacca D, Malaguarnera M. Tumor lysis syndrome in elderly. *Crit Rev Oncol Hematol.* 2007;64:31–42.
31. Smalley RV, Guaspari A, Hasse-Statz S, et al. Allopurinol: intravenous use for prevention and treatment of hyperuricemia. *J Clin Oncol.* 2000;18:1758–1763.
32. Pui CH. Urate oxidase in the prophylaxis or treatment of hyperuricemia: the United States experience. *Semin Hematol.* 2001;38: 13–21.
33. Pui CH, Relling MV, Lascombes F, et al. Urate oxidase in prevention and treatment of hyperuricemia associated with lymphoid malignancies. *Leukemia.* 1997;11:1813–1816.
34. Patte C, Sakiroglu C, Ansorborlo S, et al. Urate oxidase in the prevention and treatment of metabolic complications in patients with B-cell lymphoma and leukemia, treated in the So′ Francaise d′ Oncologie Pediatrique LMB89 protocol. *Ann Oncol.* 2002;13:789–795.
35. Trifilio S, Gordon L, Singhal S, et al. Reduced dose rasburicase in adult cancer patients with hyperuricemia. *Bone Marrow Transplant.* 2006;37:997–1001.

36. Goldman SC, Holcenberg JS, Finklestein JZ, et al. A randomized comparison between rasburicase and allopurinol in children with lymphoma or leukemia at high risk for tumor lysis. *Blood.* 2001;97:2998–3003.
37. Coiffier B, Mounier N, Bologna S, et al. Efficacy and safety of rasburicase for the prevention and treatment of hyperuricemia during induction chemotherapy of aggressive non-Hodgkin's lymphoma: results of the GRAAL1 (Groupe d'Etude des Lymphomes de l'Adulte Trial on Rasburicase Activity in Adult Lymphoma) study. *J Clin Oncol.* 2003;21:4402–4406.
38. Jeha S, Pui CH. Recombinant urate oxidase (Rasburicase) in the prophylaxis and treatment of tumor lysis syndrome. *Contrib Nephrol.* 2005:147:69–79.
39. FDA approval for rasburicase www.cancer.gov/cancertopics/druginfo/fda-rasburicase. Accessed January 15, 2010.
40. Elitek (prescribing information). Bridgewater, NJ: Sanofi-Aventis US; 2007.
41. Lee ACW, Li CH, So KT, et al. Treatment of impending tumor lysis with single-dose rasburicase. *Ann Pharmacother.* 2003;37:1614–1617.
42. McDonnell AM. Single-dose rasburicase 6 mg in the management of tumor lysis syndrome in adults. *Pharmacotherapy.* 2006;26:806–812.
43. Hummel M, Buchheidt D, Reiter S, et al. Successful treatment of hyperuricemia with low doses of recombinant urate oxidase in four patients with hematologic malignancy and tumor lysis syndrome. *Leukemia.* 2003;17:2542–2444.
44. Hummel M, Buchheidt D, Reiter S, et al. Recurrent chemotherapy-induced tumor lysis syndrome with renal failure in a patient with chronic lymphocytic leukemia: successful treatment and prevention of TLS with low-dose rasburicase. *Eur J Hematol.* 2005;75:518–521.
45. Jeha S, Kantarjian H, Irwin D, et al. Efficacy and safety of rasburicase, a recombinant urate oxidase (Elitek), in the management of malignancy-associated hyperuricemia in pediatric and adult patients: final results of a multicenter compassionate use trial. *Leukemia.* 2005;19:34–38.
46. Ueng S. Rasburicase (Elitek): a novel agent for tumor lysis syndrome. *Proc (Bayl Univ Med Cent).* 2005;18:275–279.
47. Arnold TM, Reuter JP, Delman BS, et al. Use of single-dose rasburicase in an obese female. *Ann Pharmacol.* 2004;38:1428–1431.
48. Pui CH, Jeha S, Irwin D, et al. Recombinant urate oxidase (rasburicase) in the prevention and treatment of malignancy-associated hyperuricemia in pediatric and adult patients: results of a compassionate use trial. *Leukemia.* 2001;15:1505–1509.
49. Annemans L, Moeremans K, Lamotte M, et al. Incidence, medical resource utilization and costs of hyperuricemia and tumour lysis syndrome in patients with acute leukaemia and non-Hodgkins lymphoma in four European countries. *Leuk Lymphoma.* 2003;44:77–83.
50. Candrilli S, Bell T, Irish W, et al. A comparison of inpatient length of stay and costs among patients with hematological malignancies (excluding Hodgkins disease) associated with and without acute renal failure. *Clin Lymphoma Myeloma.* 2008;8:44–51.
51. McGraw B. At an increased risk: tumor lysis syndrome. *Clin J Oncol Nurs.* 2008;12:563–565.
52. Myers JS. Complications of cancer and cancer treatment. In: Langhorne ME, ed. *Oncology Nursing.* 5th ed. St. Loius, MO: Mosby Elsevier; 2007:402–453.
53. Neel E. Health assessment and physical examination. In: Potter PA, Perry AG, eds. *Fundamentals of Nursing.* 7th ed. St. Louis, MO: Mosby Elsevier; 2009:552–640.

# PART VI

# The Care of Individuals with Specific Cancers

CHAPTER 45

*Sharon Steingass, RN, MSN, AOCN®*

# AIDS-Related Malignancies

## INTRODUCTION

Human immunodeficiency virus (HIV) is a lentivirus that can lead to acquired immune-deficiency syndrome (AIDS). HIV and AIDS are not synonymous terms. The term *AIDS* was first used in 1981 when a group of young men in Los Angeles were reported to have a rare type of pneumococcal pneumonia associated with profound immunosuppression. This same picture then was observed across the United States and Europe over the next 5 years. AIDS is used to describe the severe clinical conditions that may occur along the continuum of HIV infection. The continuum of HIV infection spans from a symptom-free period, which may range for 10 or more years, where CD4+ T-cell counts are greater than 500/mm$^3$ to clinically apparent disease states that may include candidiasis (oral or genital), cervical dysplasia, herpes zoster, pelvic inflammatory disease, cancer, and CD4+ T-cell counts that are less than 200/mm$^3$.[1]

HIV infection in humans is now pandemic. As of January 2007, the Joint United Nations Programme on HIV/AIDS (UNAIDS) and the World Health Organization (WHO) estimated that worldwide there were 33.2 million persons living with HIV infection.[2] HIV primarily infects cells in the immune system: helper T cells (specifically CD4+ T cells), macrophages, and dendritic cells. The HIV lentivirus, on entry into the target cell, converts the RNA genome to a double-stranded DNA by a virally encoded reverse transcriptase that is present on the virus particle. The viral DNA then is integrated into the cellular DNA by a virally encoded integrase along with host cellular cofactors.[3] The viral infection can become latent, which allows the infected cells to function normally, or it can become active and replicate, and then a large number of virus particles is liberated and can infect other cells. When the virus is highly active, the viral infection leads to low CD4+ cells through three main mechanisms: by killing infected CD4+ cells, by CD8+ cells that recognize and kill infected cells, and by increasing apoptosis in infected cells.[4] The decrease in CD4+ cells to a critical level results in a loss of cell-mediated immunity, which puts the body at higher risk for opportunistic infections. Without treatment, about 9 of every 10 persons with HIV infection will progress to AIDS after 10 to 15 years.[5] Although much has been learned about the treatment and prevention of HIV, developing countries in Africa and Asia continue to struggle to educate their populations about prevention and control strategies.

The introduction of highly active antiretroviral therapy (HAART) in 1995 began to change the course and prognosis of HIV infection. Antiretroviral medications are classified by the phase of the retrovirus life cycle that the drug inhibits. A summary of these classifications can be found in Table 45-1. Treatment guidelines for HAART set by the

**TABLE 45-1**

**Antiretroviral Medication Classification and Mechanism of Action**

| Classification | Example Medications | Mechanism of Action |
|---|---|---|
| Nucleoside and nucleotide reverse-transcriptase inhibitors (NRTIs) | Abacavir<br>Didanosine<br>Emtricitabine<br>Entecavir<br>Lamivudine<br>Zidovudine | Inhibit reverse transcription by being incorporated into the newly synthesized viral DNA and preventing further elongation |
| Non-NRTIs | Delavirdine<br>Efavirenz<br>Emtricitabin<br>Nevirapine<br>Tenofovir | Inhibit reverse transcriptase directly by binding to the enzyme and interfering with enzyme function |
| Protease inhibitors | Amprenavir<br>Fosamprenavir<br>Indinavir<br>Ritonavir | Target viral assembly by inhibiting the activity of protease, an enzyme used by HIV to cleave proteins for final assembly |
| Integrase inhibitors | Raltegravir | Inhibit integrase enzyme, which is responsible for the integration of viral DNA into the DNA of an infected cell |
| Entry inhibitors or fusion inhibitors | Maraviroc | Interfere with finding, fusion, and entry of HIV-1 into the host cell by blocking one or more targets |
| Maturation inhibitors | | Inhibit last step in viral processing; This classification of medications is currently under investigation. |

**TABLE 45-2**

**Guidelines for use of HAART**

- History of AIDS-defining illness or severe symptoms of HIV infection regardless of CD4+ T-cell counts
- Asymptomatic patients with CD4+ T-cell counts of less than 200/μL
- Asymptomatic patients with CD4+ T-cell counts of between 201 and 350/μL should be offered therapy.
- Asymptomatic patients with CD4+ T-cell counts of greater than 350/μL and plasma HIV RNA viral load of greater than 100,000/mL may be considered.
- Defer therapy for patients with CD4+ T-cell counts of greater than 350/μL and HIV RNA viral load of less than 100,000/mL

*Abbreviation*: HAART, highly active antiretroviral therapy.
*Source*: Data from US Department of Health and Human Services.[6]

US Department of Health and Human Services are listed in Table 45-2. Preferred initial treatment regimens are efavirenz + zidovfudine + lamivudine, efavirenz + tenofovir + emtricitabine, or lopinavir boosted with ritonavir + zidovudine + lamivudine.[6] Certain antiretroviral medications are not recommended for use during pregnancy. Because of the side effects of HAART, adherence can be a challenge. Patients need to be actively involved in the selection of the agents and instructed on the common side effects. In addition to the adverse effects of the medications, other reasons for nonadherence may include complexity of the regimen (pill burden, food drug interactions, and dosing), difficulty in swallowing large pills, and pill fatigue. Common side effects of antiretroviral medications include but are not limited to hepatotoxity, hyperglycemia, hyperlipidemia, lactic acidosis, osteonecrosis, osteopenia, osteoporosis, pancreatitis, peripheral neuropathy, and skin rashes.

## HIV DISEASE AND CANCER

Case reports of Kaposi sarcoma (KS) among men who had sex with men in San Francisco and New York in 1981, followed by the sudden increase in the incidence of KS in the United States during the 1980s, as well as the increased severity of KS in Africa, began to demonstrate the link between HIV-infected individuals and cancer. The widespread use of HAART in developing countries has prolonged the lifespan of HIV-infected patients, resulting in a large number of older individuals living with HIV/AIDS.[7] The prolonged lifespan may not be true in other countries, where access to modern health care is not prevalent. Thus cancer is a growing concern for HIV-infected patients, and close to 30% of all contemporary deaths in HIV-infected patients are cancer-related.[8] AIDS-related malignancies are a group of cancers that are diagnosed in people with HIV/AIDS.[9] Kaposi sarcoma, non-Hodgkin's lymphoma, and cervical cancer are AIDS-defining malignancies (ADMs). HIV-infected individuals are also known to have a higher incidence of other types of non-AIDS-defining malignancies (NADMs), including anal cancer, Hodgkin's disease, and lung, liver, and head and neck cancers. Table 45-3 provides a summary of ADM and NADM. The increased incidence of cancer in HIV-infected individuals also may be a result of a higher number of cancer risk factors, including cigarette use, alcohol use, and virus coinfections such as human papilliomavirus, herpes simplex, hepatitis B and C, and Epstein–Barr virus.[10–15]

Patel and colleagues from the Centers for Disease Control and Prevention (CDC) studied cancer rates in two large U.S. cohorts of people with HIV/AIDS.[16] This prospective observational analysis included HIV-positive patients in the Adult and Adolescent Spectrum of Disease (AASD) Project and the HIV Outpatient Study (HOPS) between 1992 and 2003. Standard rate ratios (SSR) were calculated to compare cancer incidence in the HIV population and the general population. The results of this study demonstrated that 80% of the HIV population had ADMs and 20% had NADMs.[16] The study also demonstrated that the overall incidence of ADMs has decreased since the advent of HAART, as well as the specific incidence rates of certain types of ADMs such as KS, non-Hodgkin's lymphoma, and primary central nervous system lymphoma, whereas the incidence rates

**TABLE 45-3**

**AIDS-Defining and Non-AIDS-Defining Malignancies**

| AIDS-Defining Malignancies | Non-AIDS-Defining Malignancies |
|---|---|
| • Non-Hodgkin's lymphoma<br>• Kaposi sarcoma<br>• Cervical cancer | • Anal cancer<br>• Hodgkin's lymphoma<br>• Head and neck cancers<br>• Liver cancer and other gastrointestinal cancers<br>• Lung cancer<br>• Melanoma<br>• Renal<br>• Urogenital cancers<br>• Multiple myeloma |

of several NADMs have increased because HIV-positive individuals are living longer and therefore have more time to develop cancer.[17–19] The NADMs that have increased include anal cancer (59 times more common), vaginal cancer (20 times more common), Hodgkin's lymphoma (18 times more common), and liver cancer (7 times more common).[16]

## NON-HODGKIN'S LYMPHOMA

Lymphomas are a group of cancers of the immune system that manifest as involvement in lymph nodes and tissues with spread to other organs. Several types of lymphoma are present in the HIV-infected population, including systemic non-Hodgkin's lymphoma (NHL), primary central nervous system NHL (also referred to as *primary brain lymphoma* or *cerebral lymphoma*), and primary effusion lymphoma (PEL). The diagnosis of AIDS precedes the onset of NHL in approximately 57% of the patients, but in 30% of the patients the diagnosis of AIDS is made at the time of the diagnosis of NHL and HIV positivity.[20] Most AIDS-related lymphomas are of B-cell origin and can range from being indolent to aggressive.[21] The roles of Epstein-Barr virus (EBV) and two types of herpes simplex virus have been studied, and they may play a role in the development of HIV-related lymphoma.[22]

### EPIDEMIOLOGY

Approximately one year (1982) after the first descriptions of *Pneumocystis carinii* pneumonia (PCP) and KS, the CDC reported on a small group of homosexual men with Burkitt's-like lymphoma.[23] AIDS-related lymphoma was first incorporated into the CDC case definition of AIDS in 1985.[24] NHL is the second most common tumor in people with AIDS.[25] Surveillance, Epidemiology, and End Results (SEER) study data indicate that NHL incidence (per 100,000) in white men rose gradually from 10.4 in 1973 to 14.5 in 1983 before the onset of the AIDS epidemic and then increased more rapidly to a peak of 2.1 in 1995.[26] The incidence of NHL in the HIV-infected population, however, has decreased with the introduction of HAART regimens for both systemic and central nervous system lymphomas. Tumors of high clinical grade (with the exception of lymphoblastic lymphoma) are designated as *AIDS defining* and include small noncleaved lymphoma (Burkitt's or non-Burkitt's), large cell lymphoma, immunoblastic lymphoma, and primary central nervous system (PCNS) lymphoma.[27,28] The risk factors for AIDS-associated lymphoma are poorly understood, but the absolute risk increases with age and is higher in men and in whites.[29] The introduction of HAART regimens in 1996 changed the spectrum of the HIV disease, but the distribution of lymphomas remains the same in the post-HAART era.[30]

### ETIOLOGY AND PATHOPHYSIOLOGY

AIDS-related NHL is more likely to occur when there is significant immune suppression,[31] with CD4+ cell counts below 200/mm$^3$, and a history of prior AIDS-defining illness. Grulich and colleagues[31] indicated that B-cell stimulation and prolonged immunodeficiency are risk factors for lymphoma development in the HIV-1 infected individuals because the HIV infection induces chronic B-cell stimulation, proliferation, and activation. Patients with AIDS have an increased risk of an immunoblastic lymphoma and a higher incidence of diffuse large B-cell lymphoma (DLBCL) than the general population.[32,33] Analysis of Ig variable (V) gene use from circulating B cells of HIV-1 infected individuals demonstrated aberrant and unstable expression of Ig genes, providing strong evidence for a dysregulated humoral immune system in HIV-1 infection.[34] AIDS-related lymphoma is an aggressive widespread disease that involves extranodal sites, including bone marrow, liver, and the gastrointestinal (GI) tract.[35–37]

### PREVENTION AND EARLY DETECTION

Screening programs for HIV-associated lymphoma do not exist. Early detection is important and should be an element of patient education. Patients who are HIV-positive should be taught to report any rapidly enlarging peripheral lymph nodes so that a biopsy can be performed and diagnosis obtained.

### CLINICAL MANIFESTATIONS

Patients commonly present with systemic B symptoms, including unexplained fever, malaise, weight loss (10% loss of weight within the last 6 months), and drenching night sweats. Enlarged lymph glands may be present in the axilla, groin, or cervical area, but the absence of enlarged lymph nodes does not mean that lymphoma is not present. Bone marrow involvement is diagnosed in approximately 20% of patients at the initial presentation, and greater than 50% marrow involvement is associated with a decreased survival.[31] Extranodal GI presentation is most common, occurring in up to 27% of patients, with stomach involvement being the most predominant, followed by oral cavity, esophagus, small and large bowel, and anal presentations.[32]

### ASSESSMENT AND DIAGNOSIS

Lymphadenopathy, which is commonly present, must be assessed carefully regarding the time of presentation, the number of enlarged nodes, and changes in the nodes over time because lymphadenopathy already may be present as a result of HIV infection. Physical examination should include determination of performance status and assessment of the liver and spleen because the patient may present with jaundice, abdominal pain, and/or anorexia.

CT scanning is helpful in determining areas of generalized or local lymphadenopathy, and gallium scans assist in identifying lesions that have not yet caused specific organ or nodal involvement.[38] A fine-needle aspiration (FNA) alone of a lymph node may not provide enough information to make a definitive diagnosis of lymphoma; thus an excisional biopsy is preferred. Immunohistochemical studies will help to determine the lymphoma subtype, and molecular genetic analysis will assist in detecting antigen–receptor gene rearrangement. Routine complete blood count (CBC) commonly demonstrates anemia, thrombocytopenia, and leukopenia. Other blood work commonly done at the point of diagnosis includes lactate dehydrogenase (LDH) level and uric acid level, both of which may be elevated. Assessment of the viral load and presence or absence of other viral pathogens will assist with treatment planning and patient management because certain viruses such as hepatitis B virus (HBV) and EBV may become reactivated during treatment. Bone marrow aspiration and biopsy also should be included in the initial staging workup to determine the presence or absence of marrow involvement. Although not routine in patients with *de novo* lymphoma, patients with systemic AIDS-related lymphoma should undergo diagnostic lumbar puncture at the time of the initial staging evaluation.[38] Approximately 20% of patients demonstrate lymphoma in the cerebrospinal fluid (CSF) and do not demonstrate any clinical sign of CNS involvement.[39]

The overall prognosis of AIDS-related NHL has improved in the era of HAART in part due to the higher mean CD4+ counts at the time of diagnosis.[40,41] Higher CD4+ counts allow the patient to better tolerate chemotherapy. Overall prognosis of the patient with AIDS-related lymphoma is associated with the stage of the disease, for example, extent of extranodal involvement, LDH level and bone marrow involvement, age, severity of the underlying immunodeficiency, history of or current opportunistic infection, and performance score.[35] The Ann Arbor staging system is used to stage AIDS-related lymphoma.[42]

## THERAPEUTIC APPROACHES

Chemotherapy is the mainstay of treatment for the patient with AIDS-related lymphoma and may be given either in standard dose or low-dose combination regimens. Prior to the availability of HAART, the use of standard-dose multiagent chemotherapy was associated with increased toxicity without an increase in response rates or survival when compared with low-dose regimens.[43] Thus low-dose regimens of cyclophosphamide, doxorubicin, vincristine, and prednisone (CHOP) or methotrexate, bleomycin, doxorubicin, cyclophosphamide, vincristine, and dexamethosone (m-BACOD) were recommended. The combinations of chemotherapy were changed once HAART was introduced and demonstrated prolonged survival in patients with AIDS-related lymphoma. The National Comprehensive Cancer Network (NCCN)-recommended treatment regimens for AIDS-related lymphoma are listed in Table 45-4.[44] Patients should receive granulocyte colony-stimulating factors during chemotherapy to decrease prolonged periods of neutropenia and prevent opportunistic infections.[44] The NCCN guidelines also recommend the use or continuation of antiviral therapy during chemotherapy.[44] However, the relationship between the use of HAART and multiagent chemotherapy and the outcomes of treatment have not been well studied.

The addition of rituximab to the CHOP regimen in elderly patients with *de novo* diffuse large B-cell lymphoma (DLBCL) has been associated with improved response and overall survival.[45] Based on these data, the use of rituximab also was studied in patients with AIDS-related DLBCL. A phase III randomized study conducted by the AIDS Malignancy Consortium (AMC) that compared CHOP with or without rituximab demonstrated improved tumor responses (57.6% versus 47%; $P = .147$), but infectious deaths offset any gain (14% versus 2%).[46] Patients with CD4+ counts of less than 50 cells/mm$^3$ are at higher risk of dying; thus clinicians should implement infection prophylaxis for the management of febrile neutropenia and *Pneumocystis* pneumonia. Patients also must be assessed carefully for bacterial, parasitic, fungal, and viral infections.

### Relapsed or refractory disease

Relapsed and refractory AIDS-related lymphoma has been treated with high-dose therapy and autologous peripheral blood stem cell transplantation with successful outcomes.[47,48] Patients with active opportunistic infections are excluded as transplant candidates. Patients are required to have an undetectable or at least stable viral load at the time of transplantation. HAART commonly is held during the neutropenic period until engraftment of the stem cells is documented. Infectious complications encountered prior to count recovery are fairly similar to those seen in HIV-negative patients and consist of gram-positive and -negative bacterimia and, less frequently, fungal pneumonia.[49] Determination of viral load and close observation for infection are essential in this patient population during the transplant phase and after discharge.

## NURSING CARE

Patients with AIDS-related lymphoma need to be assessed routinely for signs and symptoms of infection, symptoms of tumor lysis syndrome in patients with bulky disease,

**TABLE 45-4**

**Chemotherapy Treatment Guidelines for AIDS-related B-Cell Lymphoma**

| Diagnosis | Regimen | Treatment Regimen and Schedule |
|---|---|---|
| Burkitt's lymphoma CD4+ > 100/mm$^3$ | CODOX-M/IVAC | Cyclophosphamide 800 mg/m$^2$ on day 1 and 200 mg/m$^2$ on days 2 to 5<br>Vincristine 1.5 mg/m$^2$ on days 1, 8, and 15 during cycle 2<br>Doxorubicin 40 mg/m$^2$ on day 1<br>High-dose methotrexate 1200 mg/m$^2$ over 1 hr followed by 240 mg/m$^2$ over 23 hr; alternate with ifosfamide 1500 mg/m$^2$ on days 1 to 5<br>Etoposide 60 mg/m$^2$ on days 1 to 5<br>High-dose cytarabine 2000 mg/m$^2$ every 12 hr on days 1 and 2 (total 4 doses) |
| | CDE | Cyclophosphamide 200 mg/m$^2$/day × 4 days<br>Doxorubicin 12.5 mg/m$^2$/day × 4 days<br>Etoposide 60 mg/m$^2$/day × 4 days (continuous IV infusion over 96 hr) |
| | EPOCH | Etoposide 50 mg/m$^2$ on days 1 to 4 (continuous IV infusion over 96 hr)<br>Vincristine 1.4 mg/m$^2$ on days 1 to 4 (continuous IV infusion over 96 hr)<br>Doxorubicin 10 mg/m$^2$ on day 1 to 4 (continuous IV infusion over 96 hr)<br>Cyclophosphamide 375 mg/m$^2$ on day 5<br>Prednisone 60 mg PO on days 1 to 5 |
| Burkitt's lymphoma CD4+ <100/mm$^3$ | EPOCH | Same as above except dose adjustment of cyclophosphamide to 186 mg/m$^2$ on day 5 |
| | CHOP | Cyclophosphamide 375 mg/m$^2$<br>Doxorubicin 25 mg/m$^2$<br>Vincristine 1.4 mg/m$^2$ (maximum 2 mg)<br>Prednisone 100 mg PO on days 1 to 5 |
| Diffuse large B-cell lymphoma | EPOCH | Same as above except dose adjustment to cyclophosphamide<br>See Burkitt's lymphoma with CD4+ < 100/mm$^3$. |
| | CDE | Cyclophosphamide 200 mg/m$^2$/day × 4 days<br>Doxorubicin 12.5 mg/m$^2$/day × 4 days<br>Etoposide 60 mg/m$^2$/day × 4 days (continuous IV infusion over 96 hr) |
| | CHOP | Cyclophosphamide 375 mg/m$^2$<br>Doxorubicin 25 mg/m$^2$<br>Vincristine 1.4 mg/m$^2$ (maximum 2 mg)<br>Prednisone 100 mg PO on days 1 to 5 |
| Primary central nervous system lymphoma | | High-dose methotrexate 3 g/m$^2$ every 14 days<br>Radiotherapy alone—resistant disease |

*Source:* Data from *NCCN Practice Guidelines.*[44]

and assessment of psychosocial and functional status. A detailed assessment of current medications, including dose and schedule, is required because antiviral medications may be reduced or held during neutropenic periods, and prophylactic anti-infective agents may be initiated.

Education is essential, and areas for nurses to cover in their discussions with patients include the nature of the disease and treatment, management of side effects, how to prevent infections, and the signs and symptoms of infection and when to report those symptoms. The nurse, along with the physician and pharmacist, must ensure that the home medication instructions are clear and comprehensive and reviewed at each patient encounter. The number and types of oral medications required to prevent infection and manage postchemotherapy side effects, as well as the HIV-related antiretrovirals, may make medication compliance difficult. The nurse can assist by helping the patient to establish a medication record that defines medication dosages and schedules. During treatment, the nurse also may be involved in the coordination of ancillary care in the home if the patient requires additional assistance with self-care and the activities of daily living. Once treatment is completed, nurses play an active role in ensuring that the patient continues to be followed by either the oncologist or the primary care physician.

## PRIMARY CENTRAL NERVOUS SYSTEM LYMPHOMA

Primary central nervous system lymphoma (PCNSL) is an extranodal non-Hodgkin's lymphoma that arises from the brain parenchyma, eyes, mengies, or spinal cord in the absence of systemic lymphoma. PCNSL is rare, accounting for fewer than 5% of primary brain tumors, but the risk is heightened in patients who are infected with HIV.[50]

## EPIDEMIOLOGY

PCNSL is diagnosed in at least 2% of HIV-infected individuals and is an AIDS-defining illness.[50] SEER data demonstrated a threefold increase of PCNSL in HIV-infected patients.[26] The incidence is higher in patients older than 60 years of age. In the period before HAART, the relative risk of PCNSL was estimated to be over 1000 to 3600 times greater in HIV-infected individuals.[51] The use of HAART has decreased the overall incidence of PCNSL but has not had a dramatic impact on overall survival.[52,53]

## PATHOPHYSIOLOGY

PSNCL in immunosuppressed patients is commonly associated with a latent infection of neoplastic B cells by EBV. Infected B cells are able to replicate spontaneously, and proliferation is not controlled by normal immune system regulation. The pathogenesis of this disease is not well understood. Several possible pathogenic mechanisms may include (1) systemic B-cell lymphoma seeds multiple organs, but the tumors develop only in the central nervous system (CNS), (2) a benign inflammatory process of the CNS attracts the polyclonal B cells, from which a monoclonal B-cell lymphoma arises, and (3) B-cell molecules adhere to the CNS environment, where proliferation results and a lymphoma arises.[54]

## CLINICAL PRESENTATION

The clinical presentation depends on the site of CNS involvement, and the location of the mass determines the presenting signs and symptoms. Altered mental status, including confusion, lethargy, memory loss, coordination deficiencies, aphasia, headache, visual disturbances, and/or seizures, may be the presenting sign. The clinical course is rapid and the median survival in untreated patients is measured in days to weeks.

## STAGING

Neurologic staging is important in patients with PCNSL and should include the following: cranial magnetic resonance imaging (MRI) with contrast enhancement, spine MRI with contrast enhancement (if spinal symptoms present), lumbar puncture for CSF cytology, and slit-lamp examination. CSF should be evaluated for cytology and total protein concentration. In addition to these neurologic examinations, a computed tomography (CT) scan of chest, abdomen, and pelvis and a bone marrow biopsy should be included to determine the presence or absence of systemic lymphoma. Testicular ultrasound may be considered in older men to exclude an occult testicular lymphoma with brain metastasis.[54]

## THERAPEUTIC APPROACHES AND NURSING CARE

Historically, PCNSL was treated with radiotherapy alone, which produces an initial response but a high rate of recurrence. Standard therapy for NHL such as the use of CHOP was associated with only a transient response and added no benefit over radiotherapy alone.[55] High-dose methotrexate (3 $mg/m^2$ every 14 days) should be used at the time of initial diagnosis, and radiotherapy should be reserved for relapsed or chemoresistant disease.[38,39,54] Both radiotherapy and high-dose methotrexate can cause progressive dementia, psychomotor slowing, memory dysfunction, behavioral changes, ataxia, and incontinence. Patients with PCNSL need to be assessed for issues related to safety.

# KAPOSI SARCOMA

Kaposi sarcoma (KS) was first described in 1872 by the Hungarian dermatologist Moritz Kaposi. Until the AIDS/HIV disease became endemic, KS was a rare tumor. There are four separate classifications of KS, which include (1) classic, (2) African, (3) transplant-related or iatrogenic, and (4) disseminated or HIV-associated KS. Classic forms of KS were seen in Europe and North America in elderly men of Italian or eastern European Jewish ancestry. Classic KS is more common in men than in women and is a relatively benign disease with an indolent course of 10 to 15 years. Lesions usually appear on the lower extremities, and the disease lacks visceral involvement. African KS was recognized as endemic in native Ugandan males in 1950.[56] Transplant-related KS was recognized in 1969 when renal transplant patients developed KS. The medial time to develop KS following a renal transplant was 16 months, and the disease usually remains localized, involving only the skin.[57] In 1981, a fulminate and disseminated form of KS in young homosexual or bisexual men was identified as a part of an epidemic now known as AIDS.[28,58] Of all four classifications of KS, the endemic or AIDS-related form is the most aggressive. In all four clinical categories, the tumor represents aberrant angiogenesis or lymph-angiogenesis through proliferation of spindle-shaped endothelial cells that line vascular structures.[59]

## EPIDEMIOLOGY

Young homosexual or bisexual men were first reported as a part of the epidemic now known as AIDS when they presented with the disseminated form of KS.[58] Approximately 95% of all cases of epidemic KS in the United States have been diagnosed in homosexual or bisexual men.[16] Other risk groups include HIV-positive drug abusers and hemophiliacs. The proportion of HIV-infected patients with KS has decreased steadily since the epidemic was first identified in 1981 and fell dramatically during 1993–2003.[16] The use of HAART has been associated with a sustained and substantial decline in the incidence of KS.[41,60–62] Even with the declining incidence, KS still remains a common HIV-associated malignancy and may present as either a primary or secondary diagnosis after another AIDS-defining condition.[25,26,28] Presently, most patients who develop KS while taking HAART show evidence of virologic treatment failure.[60]

## ETIOLOGY

Risk factors for the development of KS include sex, age, drug use, geographic location, ethnicity, and HLA type. The incidence of KS in men is higher than in women due to the risk factor of men who have sex with men. Recreational use of amyl nitrate may alter T-cell function, thus increasing the vulnerability to infectious agents and perhaps the expression of angiogenic vascular endothelial growth factor (VEGF).[63,64] African and Mediterranean countries demonstrate an increased incidence of African and classic KS that may be linked to environmental exposure and genetic predisposition.

## PREVENTION, SCREENING, AND EARLY DETECTION

Prevention of KS is achieved by preventing the exposure to HIV through sexual abstinence, monogamy, condom use, and avoidance of intravenous drug abuse. For patients who are HIV positive, the decreased risk of KS may be achieved by the use of HAART. Presentation of KS by age varies based on the type of KS as follows: AIDS-related KS commonly occurs in middle-aged adults age 20 to 54 years, classic KS in patients aged 50 to 70 years, and African KS in patients aged 35 to 40 years.[28] In HIV-infected individuals, a full-body assessment including oral assessment is essential to screen for any KS lesions. This screening becomes more important during times of profound immunosuppression. Compliance with and the maintenance of HAART are essential to lower the risk of occurrence of KS in HIV-infected individuals.

## PATHOPHYSIOLOGY

The histopathology of the different types of Kaposi tumors is essentially identical in all forms of KS. A key element present in the pathogenesis was the discovery of a gamma herpesvirus, human herpesvirus type 8 (HHV-8).[65] Overwhelming molecular and serologic evidence now has accrued to qualify KS-associated herpesvirus (KSHV), also called *human herpesvirus* (HHV-8), as the causal agent of the clinical forms of KS.[65] Histologically, KS presents as an antiproliferative disease characterized by neoangiogensis and infiltrates of plasma cells, lymphocytes, and other inflammatory cells, as well as the hallmark spindle cells.[66] The pathogenesis of KS represents a complex chain of events that involves the interaction of immunosuppression, dysregulated cytokine production, the action of HIV proteins, and infection by a sexually transmitted virus like the HHV-8 virus.[66]

## CLINICAL MANIFESTATIONS

KS usually presents with the appearance of a single or multiple pink, red, or violet macular papules or nodules that are nonblanching, painless, nonpruritic, and palpable.[66,67] The lesions may be difficult to distinguish from other skin abnormalities, especially in dark-skinned individuals, because the lesions may appear as faint light-brown or pink macules.[67] These lesions are most commonly present on the upper body and face (particularly the nose and retroauricular area), the trunk, and the lower extremities.[67] Early lesions may be palpable before they are visible. Cutaneous lesions, particularly those associated with rapidly progressive KS, may be surrounded by a halo or yellowish discoloration.[67] Cutaneous KS may cause edema of the extremities due to tumor impingement on lymph nodes. Edema is a hallmark symptom of advanced KS and the edema most commonly involves the lower extremities. In rare occurrences, the skin over the KS lesions may break down resulting in bleeding and open wounds. Extracutaneous sites for AIDS-related KS involve the mucous membranes, GI tract, lung, liver, spleen, adrenal gland, pancreas and testis.[67] Oral cavity involvement is common and the lesions may occur on the palate, tongue, lips and tonsils.[67] Advanced GI mucosal involvement may result in pain, bleeding or obstipation.

## ASSESSMENT AND DIAGNOSIS

A complete history should include a review of past drug use, sexual practices, past illnesses, and ethnic ancestry. Physical examination should include a comprehensive skin assessment, including observation of the oral cavity and sclera, and total-body assessment. Diagnosis is confirmed by a punch biopsy of an accessible lesion, which is the gold standard. In developing countries, where punch biopsy is not available, FNA can be used for diagnosis. The FNA specimen is submitted for cytology to confirm the presence or absence of HHV-8.[67] Patients also may present with other symptoms, such as cough or chest pain (occurs in pulmonary KS), stomach or intestinal pain, and/or unexplained rectal bleeding (associated with GI KS). Patients whose presentation suggests involvement of other organs will need additional diagnostic testing that may include chest radiographs, thallium or gallium scans, and/or endoscopic procedures with biopsy to determine the cause of the presenting symptoms. Laboratory work will include viral load and assessment. Staging will depend on CD4+ lymphocyte count.

## PROGNOSTIC INDICATORS

Patients are placed in a good- or poor-risk category based on the extent of the disease, immune status, and presence of HIV-associated systemic illness. In a cohort group of epidemic KS patients, prognostic factors were identified as prior or coexisting opportunistic infection (OI), presence of B symptoms (ie, weight loss, fever, and night sweats), and an absolute CD4+ cell count of less than 300 cells/µL.[68] Of these three factors, the most important is OI, which was associated with a median survival of only 7 months versus 20 months for patients without prior OI.[68] Patients with visceral disease, tumor-associated edema, and CD4+ cell counts of less than 200 cells/µL are classified as poor risk.

## CLASSIFICATION AND STAGING

There is no official accepted staging system for HIV/AIDS-related KS. In 1989, the AIDS Clinical Trial Group (ACTG) developed a staging system called the *TIS system* to describe the tumor extent (T), immune system status (I) as measured by CD4+ T-lymphocyte count, and presence of HIV-associated systemic illness (S).[69] Within each of these three components of the system, there are two subgroups: good risk or poor risk. Table 45-5 is a summary of the TIS system.[69] The usefulness of this TIS system has been questioned with the addition of HAART. Known and colleagues[70] validated the ACTG staging classification as a predictor of survival in pre-HAART patients, with CD4+ T-lymphocyte count and tumor stage being the most predictive elements. Guglielmo and colleagues[71] evaluated the usefulness of the staging classification in the post-HAART era and found that tumor extension (T) and HIV-related systemic illness (S) were still important predictive factors, but the CD4+ cell count (I) did not correlate with survival predictions. Thus it has been eliminated as a prognostic determinant.

**TABLE 45-5**

**TIS System for AIDS-Related Kaposi Sarcoma Staging**

| | Good Risk (0) | Poor Risk (1) |
|---|---|---|
| Tumor (T) | • Confined to the skin and/or lymph nodes and/or minimal oral disease | • Tumor-associated edema or ulceration; extensive oral or GI KS |
| Immune (I) system | • CD4+ cell count ≤ 200/mm³ | • CD4+ cell count < 200/mm³ |
| Systemic (S) illness | • No systemic illness present<br>• No presence of B symptoms<br>• Karnofsky performance status (KPS) 70 or higher | • History of systemic illness and/or thrush<br>• One or more B symptoms present (eg, fever, weight loss, night sweats)<br>• KPS < 70<br>• Other HIV-related illness present |

Good risk = 0 subscript: T0, I0, S0; poor risk = 1 subscript: T1, I1, S1.
*Abbreviations*: GI, gastrointestinal; KPS, Karnofsky performance status; KS, Kaposi sarcoma.

*Source*: Data from Aversa et al.[69]

## THERAPEUTIC APPROACHES

Treatment for HIV-related KS commonly includes antiretroviral treatment to control the viral disease as well as local or systemic treatments to address the KS. The major goals of treatment for patients with KS are the palliation of symptoms and shrinkage of the lesions to prevent organ compromise, edema, and disease progression. The principal factors implicated in the selection of therapy are based on the extent and rate of tumor growth, the presence or absence of visceral involvement, tumor-associated symptoms, immune status, and history of OIs.[66] Table 45-6 includes a summary of treatment options for patients with KS.[67]

## HAART

Durable suppression of HIV replication by HAART has been important in the recovery of CD4+ cells and decreased morbidity and mortality due to OIs and HIV-related cancers.[71] HAART is important in the management of KS in that it decreases inflammatory cytokines and indirectly improves immune function. Protease inhibitors have been reported to have a direct antiangiogenetic activity, which is important in the pathogenesis of KS.[72]

### Localized treatment

Local therapy is best suited for patients who require palliation of locally advanced symptomatic disease, for patients

**TABLE 45-6**

**Treatment Considerations for Kaposi Sarcoma**

| Tumor | Viral Load | Treatment Recommendations |
|---|---|---|
| Minimal, nonprogressive | Undetectable | • Radiation therapy<br>• Interferon |
| Extensive mucocutaneous, no edema | Undetectable | • Interferon<br>• Chemotherapy<br>• Consider clinical trial |
| Extensive mucocutaneous | Detectable | • Antiretroviral therapy<br>• Chemotherapy<br>• Thalidomide |
| Symptomatic mucocutaneous disease with or without visceral or pulmonary disease | Detectable | • Liposomal anthracyclines<br>• Paclitaxel for resistant disease<br>• Antiretroviral therapy<br>• Thalidomide<br>• Clinical trial |

*Source*: Data from Von Roenn.[67]

who have cosmetically unacceptable lesions, for patients who have significant comorbid illness, or for patients who have systemic disease that is refractory to systemic treatment. Localized therapy also can be used to achieve better cosmesis and control bulky lesions that may cause bleeding, edema, or pain. Localized therapies for KS include radiation therapy, intralesional or topical therapy, cryosurgery, laser surgery, excisional surgery, and electrocauterization.

Radiation therapy is the most common form of local treatment, resulting in response rates of 90% in lesions that are cosmetically disturbing, bulky, painful, or obstructive.[73] Electron-beam therapy is used for lesions with limited dermal penetration, and conventional radiation therapy is used for bulky or deep lesions. Electron-beam therapy is usually given once weekly in 4 Gy fractions. Recurrence may occur in adjacent, untreated areas. Patients with widespread skin involvement will be treated with extended-field electron-beam therapy. Treatment is given in weekly fractions of 4 Gy for a total of 6 to 8 weeks.

Intralesional injections may be used in a limited fashion for patients with classic KS. Agents that have been used to treat oral and cutaneous KS include vinblastine, 3% sodium tetradecyl sulfate, and/or interferon-alpha.[67] Concentrations of intralesional vinblastine vary from 0.1 to 0.6 mg/mL, with higher doses recommended for oral lesions or larger papulonodular lesions.[74] Treatment is done every 3 to 4 weeks. Pain and ulcer formation occur after the treatment but usually resolve within 1 week.

Topical therapy was approved in 1999 with the introduction of Alitretionin gel 0.1% (9-*cis*-retinoic acid).[75] Alitretionin is a naturally occurring retinoid that both binds to retinoic acid receptors and regulates cell proliferation and differentiation. A phase III study demonstrated that most patients require a 4- to 8-week treatment before responses have been seen.[75] The initial dose of the gel is 0.1% applied twice daily for 2 weeks and then increased to four times daily. Common side effects include local inflammation and depigmentation of the skin.

Cryosurgery or cyoablation involves the application of liquid nitrogen to freeze and kill the cancerous cells and is used for small facial lesions that are less than 1 cm in diameter. Following application, a blister of the affected area forms, followed by sloughing or shedding of the dead tissue, and a scar may remain. Hypopigmentation of the skin may occur following the use of cryotherapy. The advantages of cryotherapy include minimal discomfort, short duration of treatment, and treatment in the outpatient setting in combination with other types of therapy. Surgical excision of the lesion and surrounding tissue is commonly done for a single or localized lesion. Surgical excision also can be used for patients with visceral crises such as obstruction or bleeding due to KS lesions.

## Systemic treatment

Chemotherapy is commonly reserved for use in patients with extensive disease because it will further compromise immune function. Candidates for systemic chemotherapy include patients with rapidly progressing KS, patients with visceral or pulmonary KS, and patients with significant lymphedema. Even though chemotherapy is not considered curative, remission can be achieved with the combination of chemotherapy and HAART. Three single agents have been approved by the Food and Drug Administration (FDA) for the management of AIDS-related KS: liposomal doxorubicin, liposomal daunorubicin, and paclitaxel.[67] Clinical trials of the liposomal anthracyclines of doxorubicin and daunorubicin in patients with disseminated disease demonstrated superiority over conventional chemotherapy regimens of bleomycin and vincristine and/or doxorubicin, bleomycin, and vincristine.[76,77] Liposomal compounds can reliably shrink the tumor, lessen edema, and cause the color of lesions to fade. Paclitaxel is used in patients with anthracycline-resistant disease.[78] The dose of paclitaxel is 100 mg/m$^2$ over 3 hours every 2 weeks, and this treatment regimen has demonstrated a partial response in 56% of patients with a median duration of 8.9 months[78] Although well tolerated in most patients, the resulting high prevalence of alopecia with these agents may be added stress for an already altered body image. Paclitaxel is also associated with myalgia/arthralgia and bone marrow suppression. Docetaxel also has been studied in patients with recurrent or refractory KS. Docetaxel administered at 25 mg/m$^2$ intravenously every 8 weeks demonstrated a 42% partial response in 10 patients with a median time to disease progression of 26 months.[79]

### Interferon

Interferon-alpha was the first agent approved for AIDS-related KS. Mechanisms of action for both type 1α and 1β include antiviral, antiproliferative, antiangiogenesis, and immune modulation, all which are important in the control of KS. Interferons have been known to inhibit HIV replication *in vitro*.[80] The combination of interferon with antiviral agents was tested in the 1980s. Dosages of 1 million units subcutaneously daily demonstrated response rates in an average of 6 to 12 months with minimal toxicity.[67] As a result of the long time to response (8 to 12 weeks), interferon is not a treatment choice for patients with rapidly progressive KS or KS with debilitating symptoms or visceral disease.[67]

### Thalidomide

Thalidomide-induced regression of KS has been documented by several studies.[81–83] Thalidomide has been shown to clear the HHV-8 DNA from the blood and reduce the viral load in tumors.[82] Doses begin at 200 mg orally given once daily and are escalated to 1,000 mg nightly based on patient tolerance. Depression, fever, rash, and neurologic toxicity are common side effects of this medication.

## NURSING CARE

Patient education is a primary element of the plan of care for patients with KS. The education should include teaching about skin assessment and management, treatment schedules, related toxicities, and management of functional or daily activities. Patients must be taught to report new lesions as they develop, as well as any potential skin breakdown. As KS progresses, lymphedema may develop, resulting in skin breakdown as well as decreased mobility. Measures to prevent skin breakdown are important and the involvement of wound care experts may be needed. Decreased functional ability may require physical therapy to ensure safety and preserve mobility. Because of the compromised immune function and the use of HAART, patients may be at higher risk for infection. Thus, patients must understand preventive measures, the signs and symptoms of infection, and when to report symptoms.

Depending on the location of the KS lesions, body image may be a major concern of the patient and an important element of the plan of care. Lesions that occur on the face or upper extremities may be of great concern, and patients may need to understand how to camouflage these lesions. The appearance of lesions may cause family and/or friends to withdraw from the patient, resulting in isolation and depression of the patient. Involvement of interdisciplinary care members such as social work, psychology, and/or clergy may assist in the management of these feelings.

Nurses should perform a visual skin assessment on a routine basis to assess for new lesions and/or skin breakdown. Open skin lesions put the patient at higher risk for systemic infections and must be kept clean and dry. Areas in the perineal area may be difficult to manage, and involvement of the wound, ostomy, and continence nurse (WOCN) may be essential in the management of skin lesions.

Pulmonary KS can lead to severe respiratory compromise and place the patient at higher risk for pulmonary infiltrates and infection. Assessment should include auscultation of the lung fields as well as assessment of oxygenation status. Patients who are at home should be taught to report any signs of respiratory distress and symptoms of cough, fever, shortness of breath, and/or dyspnea on exertion.

Patients who are receiving systemic chemotherapy will need ongoing education and support to manage both the side effects of the treatment and the disease. Additional medications to manage nausea may add to the complexity of an already complicated pill regimen, so reeducation and assistance in putting together a medication calendar may be important to ensure that the patient is talking all the required medications at the prescribed intervals. The nurse also should assess for any drug–drug interactions and complete medication reconciliation at each outpatient visit. Patients may be at increased risk for systemic infection during periods of neutropenia and must be educated about the signs and symptoms to report.

## CERVICAL CANCER

Invasive cervical cancer was included as an AIDS-defining diagnosis in 1993, and there is good epidemiologic evidence that the precursor lesions, cervical intraepithelial neoplasia (CIN) and squamous intraepithelial lesions (SILs), also occur more frequently in women with HIV infection.[84] CIN is the growth of precancerous cells on the cervix, which can progress to invasive cervical cancer as they grow deeper into the layers of the cervix. CIN is classified histologically as mild dysplasia (CIN 1), moderate dysplasia (CIN 2), and severe dysplasia or carcinoma *in situ* (CIN 3). CIN is common in HIV-infected women because both HIV and human papilliomavirus (HPV) are sexually transmitted. HIV-infected women are more likely to have persistent HPV infections, and persistent infection with one or more oncogenic HPV subtypes is a major factor in the pathogenesis of premalignant and malignant cervical disease.[85,86]

## EPIDEMIOLOGY

In the United States, 81% of HIV-infected women have annual Pap smear tests and 94% of the tests detected early precancerous changes.[87] Most women with AIDS have been infected through contaminated needles during intravenous drug use or though heterosexual contact with multiple partners (more than six).[88] Several studies have been conducted to determine the risk factors among HIV-infected women to determine if HIV has an independent risk for developing cervical cancer. One of these studies, the Women's Interagency HIV Study (WHIS), evaluated cytology and cervicovaginal HPV in both HIV-infected and noninfected women. At baseline, there was a significantly higher rate of cervicovaginal HPV in the HIV-infected women (63% versus 30%).[89] In the HIV-infected population, those who were at greatest risk for HPV coinfection were women with CD4+ cell levels less than 200/μL and an RNA viral load greater than 20,000 copies per milliliter.[89] Other identified independent risk factors for HPV coinfection included being of African-American descent and being a current smoker.[89]

## ETIOLOGY

The progression from CIN to invasive cancer in HIV-positive women is slow, often taking several years, but the progression is more rapid in HIV-infected women than in noninfected women. The CDC reports multiple risk factors for the development of CIN and cervical cancer in the HIV-infected woman, including early age of first intercourse, multiple sex partners, sex with men who have had sex with multiple partners, cigarette smoking, use of oral contraceptives, immunosuppression, lack of access to health care, and history of sexually transmitted diseases, especially HPV.[90]

## PREVENTION, SCREENING, AND EARLY DETECTION

Prevention strategies for cervical cancer include limiting the number of sexual partners, use of a condom during sexual intercourse, and vaccination with the HPV vaccine. In 2006, a vaccine (Gardasil) was approved by the FDA for the prevention of four strains of HPV. Most HPV infections are asymptomatic and transient, but four HPV strains (6, 11, 16, and 18) are responsible for 70% of all cervical cancers and 90% of genital warts.[90] Gardasil is administered in three intramuscular injections over a 6-month period. The second and third doses should be given 2 and 6 months after the initial dose. The vaccine is indicated for female patients between the ages of 9 and 26 years and is not recommended to be given during pregnancy. If the vaccine is given prior to the individual engaging in sexual activity, it helps in the prevention of HPV and cervical cancer. The American College of Obstetrics and Gynecology recommends use of the vaccine to decrease the incidence of cervical cancer.[91]

Screening and early treatment are important in the prevention of cervical cancer in both HIV-positive and noninfected women. Many women with early-stage cervical cancer are asymptomatic; thus screening examinations are extremely important. The transformation zone is an area of changing cells, and it is the most common place on the cervix for abnormal cells to develop. The location of the transformation zone varies among women. In teenage girls, the transformation zone is on the immature cervix's outer surface and is more susceptible to infection than in adult women. In older women, the transformation zone may be higher in the cervical canal. The performance of cervical cytology assessment is a relatively reliable primary screening tool for cervical neoplasia in HIV-infected women.[92] Cost, lack of trained personnel, inadequate laboratory facilities, and lack of follow-up by women have an impact on the effectiveness of cervical screening. It is recommended that HIV-infected women should receive a Pap smear every 6 months, and in women with high CD4+ cell counts who have had at least two normal tests, the interval can be lengthened to once per year.[93] In patients with abnormal Pap smear results, a colposcopy (examination of the cervix under magnification following the application of acetic acid or Lugol's iodine solution) and/or biopsy of the affected area may assist with definitive diagnosis. HPV DNA testing is recommended for high-risk types of HPV when Pap smears reveal abnormal squamous cells.[94] Blood tests for high-risk HPV strains (HPV-16 and HPV-18) are highly sensitive and less dependent on the skill of healthcare or laboratory staff.

## CLINICAL MANIFESTATIONS

CIN has no presenting signs and symptoms and thus may go undetected in women who do not have routine physical examinations and Pap smears. Presenting signs and symptoms for cervical cancer may include bloody spotting between menstrual periods; menstrual bleeding that is longer and heavier than usual; bleeding after sexual intercourse, douching, or pelvic examination; pain during or following sexual intercourse; and increased vaginal discharge. HIV-infected women also may demonstrate other inflammatory changes, including hyperkeratosis, parakeratosis, trichomoniasis, herpetic changes, and HPV-related changes.[74]

## ASSESSMENT

A complete history of patients with risk factors for cervical cancer should include the following: date of last physical examination and Pap smear, date of last menses, changes in menses since last physical examination, incidence of vaginal discharge or bleeding between normal cycles, incidences of sexually transmitted diseases, use of birth control measures, number of sexual partners, frequency of unprotected intercourse, and in young women, history of receiving HPV vaccination. Higher rates of concomitant vaginal infections in seropositive women may obscure smears and lead to incomplete or inaccurate readings. Physical examination should include both a pelvic examination and a Pap smear. The ThinPrep method of preparing cervical cytology smears appears to have increased sensitivity and specificity over conventional smears.[95] Patients with an abnormal or suspicious Pap smear should be followed with repeat Pap smear and colposcopy. Colposcopy has a higher sensitivity for detecting cervical abnormalities than conventional Pap smear (94%) but has a much less lower specificity (48%).[94] Colposcopic evaluation should view the entire lower genital tract, including the cervix, vagina and vulva, because dysplasia in the entire lower genital tract is increased in HIV-infected women.[96] Colposcopy is more expensive and time-consuming and, if accompanied with a biopsy, is more uncomfortable for the women. The cost and fear of discomfort may lead to lack of compliance with regular screening examinations.

### PROGNOSIS

Surveillance after treatment is recommended for all patients who have cervical cancer because 35% of all cervical cancer patients will have persistent or recurrent disease.[95] Management of HIV-positive patients with invasive cervical cancer is complicated by the fact that patients are younger and may present with more advanced disease.[74] Women who are HIV positive with cervical cancer have a significantly higher mortality rate than HIV-negative patients. Patients with advanced cervical cancer commonly die of their cervical carcinoma rather than from the HIV infection. Data show that the mortality rate for cervical cancer in HIV-infected women was 14.6 per 100,000 with a relative risk of 5.5 compared with uninfected individuals with an age range of 25 to 44 years.[97]

### STAGING

Cervical cancer is staged according to the standards of the International Federation of Gynecology and Obstetrics (FIGO), which also applies to patients with AIDS. The staging sequence ranges from stage 0 to stage IV depending on the extent of tissue or organ involvement[98] (see Chapter 50).

### THERAPEUTIC APPROACHES AND NURSING CARE

The goal for women with histologically confirmed CIN 3 or preinvasive disease is to prevent the development of cervical cancer. Most CIN lesions are found in the transformation zone. Thus the treatment approach includes either removal or destruction of the abnormal epithelium in the transformation zone. Treatment modalities include cryocoagulation, laser evaporation or excision, and cone biopsy or large loop excision of the transformation zone (LEEP). Following localized treatment, women should be followed closely with surveillance and repeat cytology at 4- to 6-month intervals for up to 2 years and then yearly.[99,100] Surveillance should include cytology as well as colposcopy to detect recurrent or persistent disease. Women who are negative at 24 months may return to a routine screening program.

The same treatment principles used for patients with cervical carcinoma apply to patients with AIDS. Treatment may include surgery, radiation therapy, and chemotherapy. Ablative therapies including cryotherapy and laser therapy are acceptable for patients with clearly defined lesions on the endocervix. Patients with microinvasive disease can be treated surgically with a hysterectomy. Patients who have extracervical disease (eg, pelvic lymph node involvement or parametrial involvement) are treated with radiation therapy and/or cisplatin-based chemotherapy. Patients with HIV-related recurrent disease are treated in the same manner as patients without HIV infection (see Chapter 50).

Education about HPV as a sexually transmitted disease and the risk of cervical cancer is an important element of nursing care. Table 45–7 includes educational pointers for the prevention of HPV and cervical cancer. Education about prevention and vaccine administration also should include the parents of children under 18 years of age. Parental consent will be needed for administration of the vaccine as well as preventive education. In addition to educating patients about HPV and prevention strategies, nurses can assist in ensuring that women are scheduled for and follow through with routine screening examinations. Education also should include teaching women how to perform self-examination for vulvar irritation or genital warts. Women with HIV-related cervical cancer have a high likelihood of recurrence. Once a patient has an abnormal Pap smear, the nurse is responsible to ensure that the patient understands the implications for routine and regular follow-up. Emotional support and counseling should be a component of the nursing care plan because some women may experience anger and/or shame from the diagnosis of a sexually transmitted disease. Fulcher and colleagues[101] followed a cohort of 127 HIV-infected women with cervical dysplasia as well as 193 matched women who were HIV negative. All patients received either ablative or excisional treatment. Within 3 years of treatment, 62% of the HIV-infected population demonstrated recurrence, and of the patients who required additional treatment, 50% went on to develop additional recurrences.[101]

## NON-AIDS-DEFINING MALIGNANCIES

Other malignancies not included in the CDC case definition of *AIDS-defining* include anal cancer, Hodgkin's

**TABLE 45-7**

**Education Pointers for Prevention of Human Papilliomavirus (HPV) Infection and Cervical Cancer**

- Genital HPV is transmitted through direct skin-to-skin contact most common in penetrative genital contact (vaginal or anal).
- Protective measures such as abstinence and monogamy have been demonstrated to lower incidence of sexually transmitted disease.
- Use of latex condoms demonstrates lower incidence of cervical cancer, but condoms may not eliminate the risk of HPV transmission.
- Vaccine administration does not prevent all types of HPV infections.
- Vaccine administration is not intended to treat cervical cancer; its goal is to prevent the development of cervical cancer.
- Vaccine is not a live vaccine; thus no one can get infected with HPV from the vaccine.

disease, head and neck cancer, testicular cancer, basal cell and squamous cell cancer of the skin, and melanoma.[102] An analysis of cancer death rates among people infected with HIV disease from 1990 to 1995 showed a significant increase in the relative risk of dying from a non-AIDS-defining cancer.[97] Several of the more common non-AIDS-defining cancers will be discussed briefly.

## ANAL CANCER

The incidence of anal cancer has increased in the past decade in certain population subgroups of HIV-positive men and in men who have sex with men. Although not an AIDS-defining malignancy, the incidence of anal cancer has increased in the post-HAART era. The incidence of anal intraepithelial neoplasia (AIN) was found to be higher in HIV-positive individuals than in seronegative individuals before the advent of combination antiretroviral therapy.[103] Anogenital human papillomavirus infection and HPV-related AIN are the precursors of anal cancer. Recent evidence suggests that anal infection with HPV is strongly associated with subsequent development of anal cancer.[104–106]

### Epidemiology

The incidence of anal cancer seems to be increasing, and it may be due to the extended life of HIV-positive individuals. The incidence of anal cancer is reported to be two-fold higher in HIV-infected men who have sex with men (MSM) than in HIV-seronegative MSM.[107–112] The relative risk of anal cancer in HIV-positive men and HIV-positive MSM was 37- to 59-fold higher than in the general population.[96] Anal cancer is 14 to 175 times more frequent in HIV-infected patients than in the general population, and the prevalence of HPV infection is also higher in this population.[111,112] In the post-HAART era, HIV-positive men had a fourfold higher incidence of anal cancer than in the pre-HAART era.[109,113] Anal cancer is diagnosed at a younger age in HIV-infected patients, particularly in men, whereas in the general population, anal cancer is more frequent in women and usually occurs in the sixth decade of life.[114]

### Etiology

The increased incidence of anogenital cancer in the HIV-positive population is common given what is known about the causal role of HPV in the immune-suppressed population. Receptive anal intercourse (RAI) may increase the likelihood of anal cancer, but it is not a prerequisite for anal HPV infection or dysplasia. Risk factors include unprotected RAI, multiple partners, and RAI with individuals who have had multiple partners. HIV-positive persons are two to six times more likely than HIV-negative persons to have detectable anal HPV infection regardless of sexual practices.[110,115] HIV-infected patients demonstrate a higher incidence of precancerous lesions, a higher incidence of high-grade lesions, lower CD4+ cell counts, and a higher overall incidence of HPV infection.[74]

### Prevention, screening, and early detection

Prevention of HPV infection as a result of anal sex is difficult because latex barriers may be only partially effective and do not protect contact outside the area that is covered by the barrier. Understanding this history and potential exposure to HPV infections is important in the screening and early detection of HIV-related anal cancer. Cytologic screening programs and guidelines for people at risk for AIN and HPV infection need to be developed.[109,110,116] Recommendations have been made to develop guidelines that vary between homosexual and heterosexual men. Abramowitz and colleagues[110] recommended the following guidelines: regular screening exams for all HIV-positive men regardless of CD4+ cell count or antiretroviral therapy with an emphasis on men who have frequent sexual activity or a history of anal HPV lesions. Screening examinations should include cytology examination using Pap smears and colposcopy for magnification or anoscopy. Examination should include assessment for lesions, masses, and condylomata. Individuals with abnormal cytology should be referred for high-resolution anoscopy and biopsy to grade the lesion.

### Clinical manifestations

Patients with early anal dysplasia are usually asymptomatic. Patients with invasive anal cancers may present with bleeding from the anus or rectum, pain or pressure in the area around the anus, itching or discharge from the anus, a lump near the anus, or a change in bowel habits.

### Assessment and staging

A complete history should include screening for perianal warts (known risk factors for anal HPV infection in both male and female adolescents), number of sexual partners, and previous history of HPV anal infection. Patients with the symptoms discussed previously may require a variety of diagnostic procedures, which may include digital rectal examination, anoscopy, proctoscopy, endoanal or endorectal ultrasound, and/or biopsy. Most anal carcinomas are of the squamous cell type. Results from the physical assessment and screening are categorized as normal, atypical, low-grade squamous intraepithelial lesions (LSIL), or high-grade squamous intraepithelial lesions (HSIL). Terminology for anal cancer staging is AIN I (equivalent to LSIL) and AIN II or carcinoma *in situ* (equivalent of HSIL).

### Therapeutic approaches and nursing care

The goal of treatment is to prevent progression to invasive anal cancer. Although not currently available, vaccine treatments for the prevention of anal cancers associated with HPV are being evaluated. Optimal treatment for high-grade dysplasia is not known, and specific treatment may depend on the size, location, and extent of the lesion. Topical therapy using 80% trichloracetic acid or liquid nitrogen has been demonstrated to be successful in small intraanal lesions.[117] Infrared coagulation also has been shown to have promising results and can be done easily as an outpatient procedure. Large or extensive lesions may require surgical resection, local radiation therapy, and/or chemotherapy, and treatment is similar to that of patients who are HIV-negative. Combined modality treatment has replaced abdominal pelvic resection and includes radiation therapy in combination with 5-fluorouracil and cisplatin.

Prevention strategies for anal cancer should be emphasized in high-risk patients, and these include minimizing the risk of exposure by limiting the number of sexual partners, use of condoms during sexual activity, avoiding anal intercourse with HIV-positive partners, and routine examinations for the early detection of precancerous lesions. High-risk patients also should be taught the signs and symptoms of anal cancer and the importance of reporting these symptoms in a timely manner.

## HODGKIN'S LYMPHOMA

Although the incidence of Hodgkin's lymphoma in HIV-infected persons has increased in the era of HAART,[118] when compared with population-based expectations, the disease is classified as a non-AIDS-defining illness. Hodgkin's disease is the most common type of non-AIDS-defining tumor that occurs in the HIV-infected population.[119] Decreasing CD4+ T-lymphocyte counts are associated with an increased incidence of NHL, whereas the opposite is true in Hodgkin's lymphoma, where an increased risk is associated with increased CD4+ cells.[118] Patients with HIV-related Hodgkin's lymphoma tend to have symptomatic stage IV disease at the time of diagnosis, with bone marrow involvement in approximately 40% to 60% of patients.[120–122] In HIV-infected patients, noncontiguous spread of tumor may be observed (eg, liver involvement without spleen involvement or lung involvement without mediastinal node involvement).[123] Because of the systemic nature of the disease at the time of presentation, most patients are not candidates for radiation therapy alone and require systemic chemotherapy. Treatment options include doxorubicin, bleomycin, vincristine, and dacarbazine[122] and the Stanford V[123] regimen of nitrogen mustard, doxorubicin, vinblastine, vincristine, bleomycin, and prednisone. The main problem associated with systemic chemotherapy is immunosuppression, which puts the patient at further risk for OIs. Myelosuppression thus leads to dose reduction and places the patient at risk for decreased response. The role of HAART during chemotherapy treatment is still unknown. The AIDS Clinical Study[122] did not include the use of antiretroviral therapy, but it was used in the trial of the Stanford V regimen.[123] Patients who received HAART during the Stanford V regimen did not have increased toxicity and demonstrated an overall reduction in OIs.[123]

## LUNG CANCER

Lung cancer is one of the most frequent non-AIDS-defining malignancies in the post-HAART era.[124] The incidence is two to four times higher in the HIV-infected population than in the general population.[125] The relationship of tobacco use, which is traditionally high in the HIV-infected population, is difficult to disentangle for lung cancer and HIV infection. In the HIV-infected population, lung cancer is commonly diagnosed late, and the prognosis is poorer than in other patients.[126] Once diagnosed, there is no evidence-based argument to treat HIV-infected patients differently than noninfected patients.[124]

## CLINICAL TRIALS AND HIV

The National Institutes of Health (NIH) and the FDA historically have excluded vulnerable study participants in clinical research unless there were compelling scientific and ethical grounds for inclusion.[126] Individuals who are HIV positive commonly have been excluded from cancer clinical trials due to their vulnerability and the potential risk of the trial. Understanding the spectrum of HIV disease helps to understand why these individuals may be suitable participants in clinical trials. Improvements in HIV treatment have lead to a reevaluation of this issue. The Cancer Therapy Evaluation Program (CTEP) and the NCI now state that HIV-positive individuals should not be excluded arbitrarily from participation in clinical trials. The rationale for inclusion of these individuals includes an improved understanding of how to treat cancer in HIV-infected persons, assurance that research findings from cancer treatment are generalizable to representative populations, and enabling novel treatments to be available clinically and effective for all individuals.[127] Since chemotherapy has a similar effect on lymphocyte counts regardless of HIV status, the risk for inclusion in antineoplastic clinical trials is not valid. Infectious complications can be avoided with rigorous monitoring and the appropriate use of anti-infective therapy.

**TABLE 45-8**

**Current Knowledge of AIDS-Related Malignancies**

- HAART should aim at reaching and maintaining a CD4+ > 500 cells/mm$^3$ to prevent the occurrence of all cancers.
- Most neoplasms in patients with HIV infection are linked to other viral diseases (EBV linked with lymphoma, HHV-8 linked with KS, HPV linked with cervical and anal cancer, HCV and HBV linked with liver cancer).
- Prophylaxis of OIs has to be done while patients are receiving chemotherapy, even with CD4+ cells > 200 cells/mm$^3$.
- Factors related to neoplasms rather than HIV variables are the main predictors of treatment response and outcome.
- All HIV patients with lymphoma (Hodgkin's and non-Hodgkin's) should be treated with chemotherapy and HAART simultaneously.
- Rituximab significantly improves survival of patients with HIV-related non-Hodgkin's lymphoma without increasing mortality from infections.
- CNS prophylaxis should be only done in patients with the greatest risk for developing neurologic disease, such as patients with Burkitt's lymphoma, those with stage IV disease, or those with ORL lymphoma
- In HIV-infected patients with refractory or relapsed lymphoma, if the clinical situation is good enough and salvage therapy is to be used, consideration should be made for autologous hematopoietic stem cell transplantation.
- In HIV-infected individuals, there is an increased risk of several other cancer types, mainly lung cancer and Hodgkin's lymphoma.

*Abbreviations*: CNS, central nervous system; EBV, Epstein-Barr virus; HAART, highly active antiretroviral therapy; HCV, hepatitis C virus; HHV, human herpesvirus; HPV, human papilliomavirus; KS, Kaposi sarcoma; OI, opportunistic infection; ORL, oral, rhino, loryngeal.
*Source*: Data from Persad et al.[128]

Inclusion of patients with HIV infection in clinical trials requires planning[127] because certain HIV-specific vulnerabilities such as erratic antiretroviral therapy require additional safeguards. Appropriate criteria for the assessment of HIV-positive patients should be carefully developed and described in the clinical trial.

## CONCLUSION

The introduction of HAART has greatly increased survival of HIV-infected individuals, making HIV a chronic illness. The current knowledge of AIDS-related malignancies is summarized in Table 45-8.[128] Patients are living longer with HIV, and the incidence and patterns of AIDS-related malignances, as well as potential comorbid conditions, require a comprehensive patient-centered approach to care. Health care today is in the hands of subspecialists, which has the potential to result in fragmented care. Nurses often help to ensure continuity of care and access to physiologic and psychosocial resources are a part of the plan of care. Nurses also play an important role in the education of patients and their caregivers to adequately provide care for patients between clinical assessments and/or treatments. In addition to providing care to patients with AIDS- related malignancies, nurses may assist in providing education to the HIV-positive population regarding the risk factors and important prevention strategies relating to AIDS-related malignancies.

## REFERENCES

1. Borchardt KA, Noble MA. *Sexually Transmitted Diseases: Epidemiology, Pathology, Diagnosis and Treatment.* Boca Raton, Fla.: CRC Press; 1997.
2. Joint United Nations Programme on HIV/AIDS (UNAIDS) and World Health Organization (WHO). *AIDS Epidemic Update.* Geneva, Switzerland: UNAIDS; 2007.
3. Smith J, Rene D. Following the path of the virus: the exploitation of host DNA repair mechanisms by retrovirus. *ACS Chem Biol.* 2006;1:217–226.
4. Ameisen JC. Programmed cell death (apoptosis) and cell survival regulation: relevance to AIDS and cancer. *AIDS.* 1994;8:1197–1213.
5. Buckbinder SP, Katz MH, Hessol NA, O'Malley PM, Holmberg SD. Long-term HIV-1 infection without immunologic progression. *AIDS* 1994;8:1123–1128.
6. Guidelines for the Use of Antiretroviral Agents in HIV-1 Infected Adults and Adolescents, US Department of Health and Human Services. http://www.cdc.gov/mmwr/preview/mmwrhtml/rr5107a1.htm. Accessed January 19, 2010.
7. Silverberg MJ, Abrams D. AIDS-defining and non-AIDS-defining malignancies: cancer occurrence in the antiretroviral therapy era. *Curr Opin Oncol.* 2007; 9:446–451.
8. Bonnet F, Lewden C, May T, et al. Malignancy-related causes of death in human immunodeficiency virus-infected patients in the era of high active antiretroviral therapy. *Cancer.* 2004;101:317–324.
9. AIDS-related cancers. Detailed Guide: HIV Infection and AIDS. American Cancer Society. http://www.cancer.org/docroot/CRI/content/CRI_2_4_4x_AIDS-Related_Cancers_78.asp?sitearea=. Accessed September 19, 2009.

10. Clifford GM, Polesel J, Rickenbach M, et al. Cancer risk in the Swiss HIV Cohort Study: associations with immunodeficiency, smoking and highly active antiretroviral therapy. *J Natl Cancer Inst* 2005;97:425–432.
11. Murillas J, Del Rio M, Riera M, et al. Increased incidence of hepatocellular carcinoma (HCC) in HIV-1 infected patients. *Eur J Intern Med.* 2005;16:114–115.
12. Hessol NA, Seabery EC, Preston-Martin S, et al. Cancer risk among participants in the Women's Interagency HIV Study. *J Acquir Immun Defic Syndr.* 2004;36:987–985.
13. Martin JN, Ganem DE, Osmond DH, et al. Sexual transmission and the natural history of human herpes virus B infection. *N Engl J Med.* 1998;338:948–954.
14. Phelps RM, Smith DK, Heilig CM, et al. Cancer incidence in women with or at risk for HIV. *Int J Cancer.* 2001;94:753–757.
15. Evans AS, Kaslow RA. *Viral Infections of Humans.* New York: Plenum Medical Book Co.; 2006.
16. Patel P, Hanson, DL, Sullivan PS, et al. Incidence of types of cancer among HIV-infected persons compared with the general population in the United States, 1992–2003. *Ann Intern Med.* 2008;148:728–736.
17. Bower M, Palmieri C, Dhillon T. AIDS-related malignancies: changing epidemiology and the impact of highly active retroviral therapy. *Curr Opin Oncol.* 2008;19:14–19.
18. Ledergerber B, Telenti A, Effer M. Risks of HIV-related Kaposi's sarcoma and non-Hodgkin's lymphoma with potent antiretroviral therapy: prospective cohort study. *BMJ.* 1999;319:23–24.
19. Mocroft A, Katama C, Johnson AM, et al. AIDS across Europe, 1994–1998: the Euro SIDA study. *Lancet.* 2000;356:291–296.
20. Stebbing J, Gizzard B, Mandilia S, et al. Antiretroviral treatment regimens and immune parameters in the prevention of systemic AIDS-related non-Hodgkin's lymphoma. *J Clin Oncol.* 2004;22:2177–2183.
21. AIDS-related lymphoma treatment (PDQ): health professionals' version, National Institutes of Health. http://www.cancer.gov/cancertopics/pdq/treatment/AIDS-related-lymphoma/healthprofessional Accessed September 19, 2009.
22. Simonelli C, Spina M, Cinelli R, et al. Clinical features and outcome of primary effusion lymphoma in HIV-infected patients: a single-institution study. *J Clin Oncol.* 2003;21:3948–3954.
23. Centers for Disease Control and Prevention. Diffuse undifferentiated non-Hodgkin's lymphoma among homosexual males—United States. *MMWR Morb Mortal Wkly Rep.* 1982;31:277–279.
24. Kristal AR, Nasca PC, Burnett WS, Miki J. Changes in the epidemiology of non-Hodgkin's lymphoma associated with epidemic human immunodeficiency virus (HIV) infection. *Am J Epidemiol.* 1988;128:711–718.
25. Mbulaiteye SM, Parkin DM, Rabkin CS. Epidemiology of AIDS-related malignancies: an international perspective. *Hematol Oncol Clin North Am.* 2003;17:673–696.
26. Eltom MA, Jemal A, Mbulaiteye SM, Devesa SS, Bigger RJ. Trends in Kaposi's sarcoma and non-Hodgkin's lymphoma incidence in the United States from 1973 through 1998. *J Natl Cancer Inst.* 2002;94:1204–1210.
27. Centers for Disease Control and Prevention. 1993 Revised classification system for HIV-infection and expanded surveillance case definition for AIDS among adolescents and adults. *JAMA.* 1993;269: 729–730.
28. Centers for Disease Control and Prevention. 1993 Revised classification system for HIV infection and expanded surveillance case definition for AIDS among adolescents and adults. *MMWR Recomm Rep.* 1992;41:1–19.
29. Biggar RJ, Rabkin CS. The epidemiologic of acquired immunodeficiency syndrome-related lymphomas. *Curr Opin Oncol.* 1992;4:883–893.
30. Sparano JA. Clinical aspects and management of AIDS-related lymphoma. *Eur J Cancer.* 2001;37:1296–1305.
31. Grulich AE, Wan X, Las MD, et al. B-cell simulation and prolonged immune deficiency are risk factors for non-Hodgkin's lymphoma in people with AIDS. *AIDS.* 2000;14:133–140.
32. Cote TR, Biggar RF, Rosenberg PS, et al. Non-Hodgkin's lymphoma among people with AIDS: incidence presentation and public health burden. *Int J Cancer.* 1997;73:645–650.
33. Biggar RJ, Rosenberg PS, Cote T. Kaposi's sarcoma and non-Hodgkin's lymphoma following the diagnosis of AIDS. *Int J Cancer.* 1996;68:754–755.
34. Bessudo A, Cherepakhin V. Johnson TA, Rassenti LA, Kipps, JG. Favored use of immunoglobulin V(H)4 genes in AIDS-associated B-cell lymphoma. *Blood.* 1996;88:525–560.
35. Bower M. Gazzard G, Mandalia S, et al. A prognostic index for systemic AIDS-related non-Hodgkin lymphoma treated in the era of highly active antiretroviral therapy. *Ann Intern Med.* 2005;143;265–273.
36. Senevirarne L, Tulpule A, Espina BM, et al. Clinical, immunologic and pathologic correlates of bone marrow involvement in 291 patients with AIDS-related lymphoma. *Blood.* 2001; 98:2358–2363.
37. Friedman SL. Gastrointestinal hepatobiliary neoplasms in AIDS. *Gastroenterol Clin North Am.* 1998;17:465–486.
38. Levine AM. AIDS-related lymphoma. *Semin Oncol Nurs.* 2006;22:80–89.
39. Levine AM. Acquired immunodeficiency syndrome-related lymphoma [Review]. *Blood.* 1992;80:8–20.
40. Besson C, Goubar A, Gabarre J, et al. Changes in AIDS-related lymphoma since the era of highly active antiretroviral therapy. *Blood.* 2001;98:2339–2344.
41. Tam HK, Zhan ZF, Jacobson LP, et al. Effect of highly active antiretroviral therapy on survival among HIV-infected men with Kaposi's sarcoma and non-Hodgkin's lymphoma. *Int J Cancer.* 2002;98:916–922.
42. Lymphoid neoplasms. In: *American Joint Committee on Cancer: AJCC Cancer Staging Manual.* 6th ed. New York: Springer; 2002:393–406.
43. Kaplan LD, Straus DJ, Testa MA, et al. Low dose compared with standard dose mBACOD chemotherapy for non-Hodgkin's lymphoma associated with human immunodeficiency virus infection. National Institute of Allergy and Infections Diseases AIDS Clinical Trials Group. *N Engl. J Med.* 1997;336:1641–1648.
44. AIDS-Related B-cell lymphoma. In: *NCCN Practice Guidelines.* Version 3, April 2008. http://www.nccn.org/index.asp. Accessed September 19, 2009.
45. Coiffier B, Lepage E, Brfiere J, et al. CHOP chemotherapy plus rituximab compared with CHOP alone in elderly patients with diffuse large B-cell lymphoma. *N Engl J Med.* 2002;346:235–242.
46. Kaplan LD, Lee JY, Ambinder RF, et al. Rituximab does not improve clinical outcome in a randomized phase 3 trial of CHOP with or without rituximab in patients with HIV-associated non-Hodgkin's lymphoma: AIDS-Malignancies Consortium Trial 010. *Blood.* 2005;106:1538–1543.
47. Serrano D, Carrioin R, Balsalobre P, et al. HIV-associated lymphoma successfully treated with peripheral blood stem cell transplantation. *Exp Hematol.* 2005;33:284–494.
48. Benicchi T, Ghidini C, Allessandro RE, et al. T-cell immune reconstitution after hematopoietic stem cell transplantation for HIV associated lymphoma. *Transplantation.* 2005;80:673–682.
49. Wagner-Johnston ND, Ambinder R. Blood and marrow transplant for lymphoma patients with HIV/AIDS. *Curr Opin Oncol.* 2008;10:201–205.
50. Kasamon Y, Ambinder RF. AIDS-related primary central nervous system lymphoma. *Hematol Oncol Clin North Am.* 2005;19:665–687.
51. Cole, TR, Manns A, Hardy CR, et al. Epidemiology of brain lymphoma among people with or without acquired immunodeficiency syndrome. AIDS/Cancer Study Group. *J Natl Cancer Inst.* 1996;88:675–679.
52. Conte S, Masocco M, Pezzotti P, et al. Differential impact of combined antiretroviral therapy on the survival of Italian patients with AIDS-defining illnesses *J Acquir Immun Defic Syndr.* 2000;25:451–458.
53. Sacktar N, Lynes, RH, Skolasky R, et al. HIV-associated neurologic diseases incidence and changes: Multicenter AIDS Cohort Study, 1990–1998. *Neurology.* 2001;56:257–260.

54. Iwamoto F, DeAngelis L. An update on primary central nervous system lymphoma. *Hematol Oncol Clin North Am.* 2006;20:1267–1285.
55. Mead GM, Gleehen NM, Gregor A, et al. A medical research council randomized trial in patients with primary cerebral non-Hodgkin's lymphoma: cerebral radiotherapy with and without cyclophosphamide, doxorubicin, vincristine, and prednisone chemotherapy. *Cancer.* 2000;89:556–564.
56. Taylor JF, Templeton AC, Vogel CL, et al. Kaposi's sarcoma in Uganda: a clinicopathologic study. *Int J Cancer.* 1971;8:122–135.
57. Penn I. Kaposi's sarcoma in organ transplant recipients: report of 20 cases. *Transplantation.* 1979;27:1:8–11
58. Kaposi's sarcoma and *Pneumocystis* pneumonia among homosexual men—New York and California. *MMWR.Morb Mortal Wkly Rep* 1981;30:305–308.
59. Coleman R, Blackbourn D. Risk factors in the development of Kaposi's sarcoma. *AIDS.* 2008;22:1629–1632.
60. Portsmouth S, Stebbing J, Gill J, et al. A comparison of regimens based on nonnucleoside reverse transcriptase inhibitors or protease inhibitors in preventing Kaposi's sarcoma. *AIDS.* 1993;17:17–22.
61. Dupont D, Vasseur E, Beauchet A, et al. Long-term efficacy on Kaposi's sarcoma of highly active antiretroviral therapy in a cohort of HIV-positive patients. *AIDS.* 2000;17:987–993.
62. Carrieri MG, Pradler C, Piselli P, et al. Reduced incidence of Kaposi's sarcoma and of systemic non-Hodgkin's lymphoma in HIV-infected individuals treated with highly active antiretroviral therapy. *Int J Cancer.* 2003;103:142–144.
63. Goedhert JJ, Neuland CY, Wllen WE, et al. Amyl nitrite may alter T-lymphocytes in homosexual men. *Lancet* 1982;1:412–416.
64. Fung HL, Tran DC. Effects of inhalant nitrites on VEGF expression: a feasible link to Kaposi' sarcoma. *J Neuroimmune Pharmacol.* 2006;1:317–322.
65. Schulz TF. The pleiotropic effects of Kaposi's sarcoma herpesvirus. *J Pathol.* 2006;208:187–198.
66. Aversa SML, Cattelan AM, Salvagno L, et al. Treatments of AIDS-related Kaposi's sarcoma. *Crit Rev Oncol Hematol.* 2005;53:253–265.
67. Von Roenn J. Clinical presentations and standard therapy for AIDS-associated Kaposi's sarcoma. *Hematol Oncol Clin North Am.* 2003;17:747–762.
68. Cachoua A, Kreigel R, Lafleur F, et al. Prognostic factors and staging classification of patients with epidemic Kaposi's sarcoma. *J Clin Oncol.* 1989;7:774–780.
69. Known SE, Metroka C, Wenz JC. Kaposi's sarcoma in the acquired immune deficiency syndrome: a proposal for uniform evaluation, response and staging criteria. *J Clin Oncol.* 1989;7:1201–1207.
70. Known SE, Testa MA, Huang J. AIDS-related Kaposi's sarcoma: prospective validation of the AIDS Clinical Trials Group staging classification. *J Clin Oncol.* 1997;15:3085–3092.
71. Guiglielmo N, Renato T, Antinori A, et al. AIDS-related Kaposi's sarcoma: evaluation of potential new prognostic factors and assessment of the AIDS Clinical Trial Group staging system in the HAART era. The Italian Cooperative Group on AIDS and tumors and the Italian Cohort of patients naive from antiretrovirals. *J Clin Oncol.* 2003;21:2876–2882.
72. Ensoli B, Stirzl M. Kaposi's sarcoma: a result of the interplay among inflammatory cytokines, antigenic factors and viral agents. *Cytokine Growth Factor.* 1998;9:63–83.
73. Swift PS. Radiation therapy in the management of HIV-related KS. *Hematol Oncol Clin North Am.* 1996;10:1069–1080.
74. Escalon MP, Hagmeister FB. AIDS-related malignancies. In: Kantarjian HM, Wolff RA, Koller CA, eds. *MD Anderson Manual of Medical Oncology.* New York: McGraw-Hill; 2006:903–910.
75. Walmaley S, Northlel DW, Melosky B, et al. Treatment of AIDS-related cutaneous Kaposi's sarcoma with topical Alitretionin gel. *J Acquir Immun Defic Syndr Hum Retrovirol.* 1999;22:235–246.
76. Gill PS, Wentz J, Scaddem DT, et al. Randomized phase III trial of liposomal daunorubicin versus doxorubicin, bleomycin and vincristine in AIDS-related Kaposi's sarcoma. *J Clin Oncol.* 1996;14:2353–2364.
77. Northfelt DT, Dezube BJ, Thommes JA, et al. Pegylated-liposomal doxorubicin versus doxorubicin, bleomycin and vincristine in the treatment of AIDS related Kaposi's sarcoma. *J Clin Oncol.* 1998;18:2445–2451.
78. Gill PS, Tulpule A, Espina GM, et al. Paclitaxel is safe and effective in the treatment of advance AIDS-related Kaposi's sarcoma. *J Clin Oncol.* 1997;17:1876–1883.
79. Lim ST, Tupule A, Espina BM, Levine AM. Weekly docetaxel is safe and effective in the treatment of advanced-stage acquired immunodeficiency syndrome-related Kaposi sarcoma. *Cancer.* 2005;103:417–421.
80. Ho DD, Harshon KL, Rota TR, et al. Recombinant human interferon alpha-A suppresses HIV-III replication *in vitro. Lancet.* 1985;1(8429): 602–604.
81. Soler RA, Howard M, Brink NS, et al. Regression of AIDS-related Kaposi's sarcoma during therapy with thalidomide. *Clin Infect Dis.* 1996;23:501–503.
82. Fife K, Howard MR, Gracia F, et al. Activity of thalidomide in AIDS-related Kaposi's sarcoma and correction with HHV-8 titter. *J STD AIDS.* 1998;9:751–755.
83. Little RF, Wyvill KM, Pluda J, et al. Activity of thalidomide in AIDS related Kaposi's sarcoma. *J Clin Oncol.* 2000;18:2593–2602.
84. Ellebrock TV, Chiasson MB, Gush TJ, et al. Incidence of cervical squamous intraepithelial lesions in HIV infected women. *JAMA.* 2000;283:1031–1037.
85. Strickler, HD, Burk RD, Fazzari M, et al. Natural history and possible reactivation of human papilliomavirus in human immunodeficiency virus-positive women. *J Natl Cancer Inst.* 2005;97:577.
86. Clifford GM, Goncalves MA, Franceschi S. Human papilliomavirus types among women infected with HIV: a meta-analysis. *AIDS.* 2006;20:2337.
87. Franceschi S, Jaffe H. Cervical cancer screening of women living with HIV infection: a must in the era of antiretroviral therapy. *Clin Infect Dis.* 2007;45:510–517.
88. Gallagher B, Want Z, Schymura MJ, Kahn A, Fordyce EJ. Cancer incidence in New York State acquired immunodeficiency syndrome patients. *Am J Epidemiol.* 2001;154:544–556.
89. Palefsky JM, Minkoff H, Kalish LA, Levine A, Sacks HS, Garcia P, et al. Cervicovaginal human papilliomavirus infection in human immunodeficiency virus-1 HIV positive and high risk HIV-negative women. *J Natl Cancer Inst.* 1999;91:226–236.
90. Centers for Disease Control and Prevention. HPV vaccine information for clinicians. http://www.cdc.gov/std/HPV/STDfact-HPV-vaccine-hcp.htm. Accessed September 19, 2009.
91. American College of Obstetrics and Gynecology. HPV vaccine—ACOG recommendations. http://www.acog.org/acog_districts/dist9/quadrivalentHPV.pdf. Accessed September 19, 2009.
92. Robinson WR, Luck MB, Kendall MA, Darragh TM. The predictive value of cytologic testing in women with the human immunodeficiency virus who have low-grade squamous cervical lesions: a substudy of a randomized phase III chemoprevention trial. *Am J Obstet Gynecol.* 2003;188:896.
93. Highleyan L. Human papilliomavirus. In: *Beta Bulletin of Experimental Treatments for AIDS: A Publication of the San Francisco AIDS Foundation.* Summer 2007:35–39.
94. Wright JR, Cox TC, Massad L, et al. 2001 consensus guidelines for the management of women with cervical cytological abnormalities. *JAMA.* 2002;287:2120–2129.
95. Steir E. Cervical neoplasia and the HIV-infected patient. *Hematol Oncol Clin North Am.* 2003;17:873–887.
96. Frish M, Bigar JR, Goedert JJ. Human papilliomavirus associated cancers in patients with human immunodeficiency virus infection and acquired immunodeficiency syndrome. *J Natl Cancer Inst.* 2000;92:1500–1510.
97. Selik RM, Rabkin CS. Cancer death rates associated with human immunodeficiency virus in the United States. *J Natl Cancer Inst.* 1998:90:1300–1302.
98. Pecorelli S, Zigliani L, Odicino F. Revised FIGO staging for carcinoma of the cervix. *Int J Gynecol Obstet.* 2009;105:107–108.

99. Zielinski GD, Bais AG, Helmerhorst TJ, et al. HPV testing and monitoring of women after treatment with CIN3: review of the Literature and meta-analysis. *Obstet Gynecol Surv.* 2004;59:543–553.
100. O'Meara A. Present standards for cervical screening. *Curr Opin Oncol.* 2002;14:505–511.
101. Fruchter RG, Maiman M, Sedlis A, Bartley L, et al. Multiple recurrences of cervical intraepithelial neoplasia in women with the human immunodeficiency virus. *Obstet Gynecol.* 1996; 87:338–344.
102. Cooley T. Non-AIDS-defining cancer in HIV-infected people. *Hematol Oncol Clin North Am.* 2003;17:889–899.
103. Palefsky JM, Holly EA, Hogeboon CJ, Ralston ML, DaCosta MM, Botts R, et al. Virologic, immunologic and clinical parameters in the incidence and progression of anal squamous intraepithelial lesions in HIV-positive and HIV-negative homosexual men. *J Acquir Immun Defic Syndr Hum Retroviral.* 1998;17:314–319.
104. Fox PA. Human papilliomavirus and anal intraepithelial neoplasia. *Curr Opin Infect Dis.* 2006;19:62–66.
105. Frisch M, Glimelius B, van de Brule AJ, et al. Sexually transmitted infection as a cause of anal cancer. *N Engl J Med.* 1997;337:1350–1358.
106. Bjorge T, Engeland A, Luostarinen T, et al. Human papilliomavirus infection as a risk factor for anal and perianal skin cancer in a prospective study. *Br J Cancer.* 2002;87:61–64.
107. Goedert JJ. The epidemiology of acquired immunodeficiency syndrome malignancies. *Semin Oncol.* 2000;27:390–401.
108. Klencke B, Palefsky J. Anal cancer: an HIV-associated cancer. *Hematol Oncol Clin North Am.* 2003;17:859–872.
109. D'Souza G, Wiley D, Xiuhong K, et al. Incidence and epidemiology of anal cancer in the multicenter AIDS cohort study. *J Acquir Immun Defic Syndr.* 2008;48:491–499.
110. Abramowitz L, Benadberrahumane D, Ravud P, et al. Anal squamous intraepithelias lesions and condyloma in HIV-infected heterosexual men, homosexual men and women; prevalence and associated factors. *AIDS* 2007;21:1457–1465.
111. Bower M, Powles T, Newsm-Davis T, Thirlwell C, Stebbing J, Mandalia S, et al. HIV-associated anal cancer: has highly active antiretroviral therapy reduced the incidence or improved the outcome? *J Acquir Immun Defic Syndr.* 2004;37:1563–1565.
112. Frish M, Biggar RF, Engles EA, Goedert JJ. Association of cancer with AIDS-related immunosuppression in adults. *JAMA.* 2001;285:1736–1745.
113. Horster S. Is anal carcinoma a HAART-related problem? *Eur J Med Res.* 2003;8:142–146.
114. Chiao EY, Giordano TP, Richardson P, El-Serag HB. Human immunodeficiency virus-associated squamous cell cancer of the anus: epidemiology and outcomes in the highly active antiretroviral therapy era. *J Clin Oncol.* 2008;26:464–479.
115. Palesky JM, Holly EA, Ralston ML Jay N, Berry JM, Darragh TM. High incidence of anal high-grade squamous intra-epithelial lesions among HIV-positive and HIV-negative homosexual and bisexual men. *AIDS* 1998;12:495–503.
116. Goldie SJ, Kunz KM, Weinstein MC, Freedberg KA, Palefsky JM. Cost-effectiveness of screening for anal squamous intraepithelial lesions and anal cancer in human immunodeficiency virus negative homosexual and bisexual men. *JAMA* 1999;281:1822–1829.
117. Chin-Hong PV, Palerfisky JM. Natural history and clinical management of anal human papilliomavirus disease in men and women infected with human immunodeficiency virus. *Clin Infec Dis.* 2002;35:1127–1134.
118. Biggar RG, Feffe ES, Goedert J, et al. Hodgkin lymphoma and immunodeficiency in persons with HIV/AIDS. *Blood.* 2006;108:3786–3791.
119. Spina M, Massimiliano B, Tirelli U. Hodgkin's disease in HIV. *Hematol Oncol Clin North Am.* 2003;17:843–858.
120. Vaccher E, Spina M, Tirelli U. Clinical aspects and management of Hodgkin's disease and other tumors in HIV-infected individuals. *Eur J Cancer.* 2001;37:1306–1315.
121. Pelstring RJ, Zellmer RB, Sulak LE, et al. Hodgkin's disease in association with human immunodeficiency virus infection: pathologic and immunologic features. *Cancer.* 1991;67:1865–1873.
122. Levine AM, Li P, Cheung T, et al. Chemotherapy consisting of doxorubicin, bleomycin, vinblastine, and dacarbazine with granulocyte colony-stimulating factor in HIV-infected patients with newly diagnosed Hodgkin's disease: a prospective, multi-institutional AIDS Clinical Trials Group study (ACTG 149). *J Acquir Immun Defic Syndr.* 2000;15:444–450.
123. Spina M, Gabarre J, Rossi G, Fasan M, Schiantarelli C, Nigra E, et al. Stanford V regimen and concomitant HAART in 59 patients with Hodgkin disease and HIV infection. *Blood.* 2002;100:1984–1988.
124. Bonnet F, Chene G. Evolving epidemiology of malignancies in HIV. *Curr Opin Oncol.* 2008;20:534–540.
125. Herida M, Mary-Krause M, Kaplan R, et al. Incidence of non-AIDS defining cancers before and during the high active antiretroviral therapy in a cohort of human immunodeficiency virus-infected patients. *J Clin Oncol.* 2003;21:3447–3453.
126. Tireli U, Spina M, Dandri S, et al. Lung carcinoma in 36 patients with human immunodeficiency virus infection: the Italian Cooperative Group on AIDS and Tumors. *Cancer.* 2000;88:563–569.
127. Emanuel EJ, Wendier D, Grady C. What makes clinical research ethical? *JAMA.* 2000;283:2701–2711.
128. Persad G, Little RF, Grady C. Including persons with HIV infection in cancer clinical trials. *J Clin Oncol.* 2008;26:1027–1032.
129. Ortega ME. AIDS-related malignancies—a new approach. *AIDS Rev.* 2008;10:125–126.

CHAPTER 46

Loleta C. Samuel, RN, MSN, APRN-BC, AOCN®

# Bone and Soft Tissue Sarcomas

## INTRODUCTION

Sarcomas are a heterogeneous family of rare solid tumor cancers primarily of mesenchymal origin, which have distinct clinical and pathological features in more than 50 histological subtypes.[1,2] There are 2 main categories of sarcomas. These include bone sarcomas, and soft tissue sarcomas. Bone sarcomas arise from bone tissues. Soft tissue sarcomas arise in tissues, which support, connect, or surround body organs and structures. These include soft tissues of fat, nerves, muscle, blood vessels, fibrous tissue, synovial tissues, nerve sheath, and other connective tissues.[2] Soft tissue sarcomas are usually named by the type of tissue in which they arise (see Table 46-1).

Soft tissue and bone sarcomas affect both genders, and all age groups. A multidisciplinary team approach to care is essential to guide the patient and family through diagnosis and treatment. Team members should include surgical subspecialties such as orthopedics, vascular, thoracic, and plastics/reconstructive as well as medical oncologist, pathologist, physical therapist, nurse, social worker, occupational therapist, rehabilitation physician, and prosthetist. Advances in the understanding of the biology of sarcomas, new surgical techniques, improvements in radiological imaging and an interdisciplinary approach to treatment have improved outcomes for the sarcoma patient. A systematic biological understanding of the interaction between the tumor, host, and environment is essential not only to help identify populations at risk, but for better prevention and treatment strategies.[1]

## EPIDEMIOLOGY

Primary sarcomas account for approximately 1% of all adult malignancies and 15% of pediatric malignancies.[1] Malignant bone and soft tissue tumors that present as primary tumors are exceptionally small in number. The American Cancer Society, which keeps track of newly diagnosed cases and deaths by cancer type, estimated 2570 new cases of bone and joint cancer in 2009, with a slightly higher proportion of males than females. The estimate for soft tissue (including heart) cancer was approximately 10660, again with a slightly higher proportion of males. The number of deaths was estimated to be 1470 from bone and joints and 3820 from soft tissues.[3]

## ETIOLOGY

Although most sarcomas are etiologically indeterminate, some genetic alterations, environmental, and host-related factors have been identified as potential etiologies. Risk factors have been isolated in some instances, and can be delineated as host vs environmental. (Table 46-2).

**TABLE 46-1**

**Classification of Sarcoma Tissue Subtypes**

| Tissue Origin | Sarcoma Subtype Examples |
|---|---|
| Blood and lymph vessels | Angiosarcoma (malignant hemangioendothelioma)<br>Kaposi sarcoma<br>Lymphangiosarcoma<br>Hemangioendothelioma |
| Bone and cartilage | Chondrosarcoma<br>Ewing's sarcoma<br>Osteosarcoma |
| Fat (adipose tissue) | Liposarcoma<br>Atypical lipoma |
| Fibrous<br>(Hold muscles, bones, and organs in place) | Fibrosarcoma<br>Dermatofibrosarcoma protuberans (DFSP)<br>Malignant fibrous histiocytoma (MFH)<br>Myxofibrosarcoma |
| Mesencyhmal cells<br>(develops into blood vessels, connective tissue, lymphatic tissue) | Gastrointestinal stromal tumor (GIST)<br>Malignant mesenchymoma |
| Neural/peripheral nerves | Malignant granular cell tumor<br>Malignant peripheral nerve sheath tumor (MPNST)—also called malignant schwannoma or neurofibrosarcoma |
| Perivascular<br>(near or around blood vessels) | Glomangiosarcoma<br>Malignant hemangiopericytoma |
| Skeletal muscle | Rhabdomyosarcoma |
| Smooth muscle<br>ie: uterus | Leiomyosarcoma |
| Synovial tissue<br>(lines joints, tendon sheaths, and fluid sacs between tendons and bones) | Synovial sarcomas |
| Other<br>(specific tissue origin unknown) | Alveolar soft part sarcoma<br>Clear cell sarcoma<br>Desmoplastic small cell tumor<br>Epithelioid sarcoma<br>Malignant extrarenal rhabdoid tumor<br>Malignant fibrous mesothelioma |

Some identified host risk factors include a diagnosis of Ollier's disease, which involves multiple enchondromas, may deteriorate to a low-grade chondrosarcoma. Neurofibromatosis carries a low but very real risk of neurofibrosarcoma. Paget's disease has been linked to osteosarcoma. Environmental

**TABLE 46-2**

**Some Risk Factors for Sarcomas**

| | |
|---|---|
| Environmental exposure | |
| radiation | Radiotherapy used to treat malignancies |
| chemicals | Polyvinyl chloride (PVC)<br>Arsenic<br>Thorotrast<br>Androgenic-anabolic steroids<br>Hemochromatosis<br>Copper exposure<br>Dioxins<br>Chlorophenoles<br>Benzophenone<br>O-Nitrotoluene |
| Host-related | Immune suppression: EBV, HHV8<br>Acquired immune deficiency syndrome (AIDS)<br>Solid organ transplantation<br>Chronic tissue irritation from inflammation or foreign body: lymphedema after radiation |
| Genetic: Hereditary genes<br>*p-53*<br>*NFI*<br>*RbI* | Genetic alterations-fusion genes<br>Familial gastrointestinal stromal tumors (GIST) syndrome<br>Hereditary leiomyomatosis and renal cell syndrome<br>Li-Fraumeni syndrome<br>Neurofibromatosis type I (Von Recklinghausen disease)<br>Hereditary reinoblastoma (Rb)<br>Mutations in RBI tumor suppressor gene<br>Werner syndrome (WS)<br>Rothmund–Thompson syndrome (RTS)<br>Bloom syndrome (BS) |

*Abbreviations*: EBV, Epstein Barr virus; HHV8, human herpesvirus 8.

*Source*: Data from Lahat, et al.[1]

risk factors related to sarcomas include pollutants, smoking, chemicals, infectious disease, and radiation. Factors such as tobacco use, physical inactivity, and a diet high in saturated fat and low in fiber have a greater influence on an individual's risk of cancer than low concentrations of pollutants in the air, food, or drinking water.[4] Smoking, diet, and inactivity are controllable variables. Exposure in the workplace to higher concentrations of certain chemicals, metals, and ionizing radiation provides a greater risk, which increases substantially with prolonged exposure, more intense exposure, and higher concentrations of pollutants. Examples of workplace carcinogens include radon and asbestos. Tobacco use greatly increases these risks.

Chemical risk factors include Agent Orange (a defoliant used in the Vietnam War), vinyl chloride gas, dioxin, and arsenic. Also, prior cancer treatment with high-dose radiation has been associated with the development of both bone and soft tissue sarcomas. Alkylating agents used in chemotherapy have also been associated with the development of sarcomas.

Molecular genetics may provide clues to the underlying cause of sarcomas. Some neoplasms are thought to originate from genetic alterations. In general, cancer as a whole is viewed as a sequence of genetic alterations that influence the loss of tumor-suppressor genes (TSG) function, and result in damage to cell growth regulation.[1] TSGs often serve as cell-cycle regulators.[5] The TSG *p53* and the retinoblastoma (Rb) gene are often mutated in osteosarcoma. The cell-cycle regulator Rb has the capability to induce programmed cell death or apoptosis. It can trigger the repair of genetic damage or cause apoptosis in the cell if restoration is not feasible. A flaw in this gene or its protein could possibly lead to an explosion of DNA-damaged progeny.[5,6] The *p53* gene is thought to be the predominant gene that is altered in human cancers.[1] These genetic alterations are thought to be the origin of neoplasms.

## SCREENING AND EARLY DETECTION

Due to their rarity, there is no routine health maintenance screening tool to detect these conditions, as is done for prostate cancer or breast cancer. Patients with a family history of sarcomas should be aware of presenting symptoms for sarcomas and should be certain that their routine physicals are comprehensive.

Li-Fraumeni syndrome is a primarily inherited familial cancer syndrome that is identified by the early development of tumors. Routine radiographs are generally not recommended as a screening tool. The only exception to this principle would be a chest x-ray at the discretion of the physician during a comprehensive physical examination. Symptoms such as unexplained bone pain, especially at night, or a palpable mass should be investigated, even if there is no family history of cancer.

## PATHOPHYSIOLOGY

Primary bone and soft tissue tumors originate from the mesoderm germ layer of the cell. These tumors are characterized by their ability to form certain types of cells. Collagen-producing tumor cells structure the osteogénic, chondrogenic, and fibrogenic tumors. Osteosarcoma is characterized by the formation of bone or osteoid. Primary chondrosarcoma is characterized by the formation of cartilage by tumor cells. Marrow tumors or round-cell tumors are composed of densely packed small cells with rounded nuclei. Ewing's sarcoma falls into this category. Vascular tumors, such as angiosarcomas, are characterized by asymmetric vascular channel formations. These channels are lined with atypical epithelial cells and solid accumulations of poorly differentiated cells. The vascular formations can occur in any of the blood vessels of the bone.

Bone and soft tissue tumors can affect almost the entire skeleton and adjacent soft tissues. The knowledge that certain tumors have a predilection for certain bones and locations can serve as a diagnostic aid for the healthcare provider. Soft tissue tumors occur most often in the extremities. They are also found in the head, neck, and abdominal and retroperitoneal areas. Bone and soft tissue sarcomas most commonly metastasize to the lungs. This is theorized to be a phenomenon in which there is microinvasion of cancer cells into the venous system, and subsequent circulation to other lungs. The lymphatic system, bone, soft tissues, and liver are other sites of metastatic disease. The detection of pulmonary metastases is mainly related to the sensitivity of the imaging method used, but in general, a nodule cannot be detected until it reaches 3 mm.[5] Chest computed tomography (CT) is used to diagnose the presence of distant disease.

## CLINICAL MANIFESTATIONS

Bone and soft tissue tumors can present as one or more of the following:

- A palpable mass, with or without associated pain
- Pain that wakes the patient at night
- Alterations in function or mobility of the affected area.

## ASSESSMENT

A comprehensive assessment is essential to ensure a timely work up and treatment. The assessment should include a history of present illness, past medical history, past surgical history, family history, social history, risk factors for cancer, physical examination, and diagnostic and pathologic study results.

### PATIENT AND FAMILY HISTORY

Family history or worsening physical symptoms are often the defining motivation for a patient and may include pain, a palpable mass, or alteration in function. Pain evaluation is important in ruling out the suspected differential diagnoses. Pain that alters in intensity, worsening at night or at rest, is often a signal of a malignant process. Pain is usually the initial symptom of Ewing's sarcoma. The presenting pain symptom is often associated with minor trauma, and has not improved over time.[7] A change in function is often another symptom that motivates a patient to consult a physician. In the case of bone tumors, microfractures through the involved portion of the bone or the compression of juxtaposed neurovascular structures may be the cause of pain.[5] The clinical picture may also involve a palpable mass, which may be masked in an area such as the pelvis or groin area.

The patient's age and diagnostic imaging findings are helpful components in narrowing down the differential diagnoses. In the evaluation of a bone lesion in a patient, male or female, over the age of 40, metastatic disease is the likely diagnosis. Bone tumors tend to develop in a span of approximately 2 decades. Osteosarcoma usually develops between the ages of 10 and 30, while Ewing's sarcoma generally occurs between the ages of 5 and 15.

Some sarcomas tumors affect one sex more commonly than the other. Osteosarcomas occur more frequently in males, with a ratio varying from 1.3 to 1.7 to 1. The exception is pariosteal osteosarcoma, which has a female-to-male ratio of 2 to 1.[8]

Soft tissue sarcomas often present as a painless mass that increases in size. As the mass increases in size, pain may be experienced as the tumor impinges on surrounding neurovascular structures. It is important to evaluate the patient's account of when the mass was initially found, and how rapidly it enlarged. A family history of cancer, its treatment; and outcome is of importance to the emerging clinical picture. Additional signs such as café-au-lait spots, hemangiomas, or asymmetrical edema can be beneficial in the diagnostic process. Prior illnesses conditions (ie, Paget's disease, neurofibromatosis, or Ollier's disease) fever, other areas of pain, and exposure to known carcinogens; and other systemic symptoms must be noted.

During the diagnostic phase, it is critical at this time to evaluate for immediate or potential concerns regarding the patient's social and financial support systems. The inability to pursue one's livelihood as well as leisure activities can be of great importance to a patient facing a life-threatening diagnosis. If a patient is the carrier of the primary medical insurance, the inability to work can be very stressful. The continued dignity of a patient and family is an important facet in the patient's treatment and overall wellbeing. Educating the patient concerning the diagnosis is important; this education will need to be reinforced and expanded as the treatment evolves. It is crucial for a patient to receive accurate explanations from all involved healthcare professionals.

### PHYSICAL EXAMINATION

Although a comprehensive review of systems, past medical history, past surgical history, social history, and history of present illness are necessary, a detailed physical exam may provide important clinical clues to diagnosis. The physical examination of the patient with an alleged bone or soft tissue sarcoma entails detailed inspection, and palpation of the affected region and comparison with the contra lateral region for symmetry. Findings may be nonspecific, but, when combined with radiographic findings, could lead to a more complete diagnostic picture.

An evident mass may be fixed or mobile, firm, and/ or associated with a locally elevated temperature and possibly a network of dilated superficial veins. (See Figure 46-1). Physical inspection may also reveal café-au-lait spots or hemangiomas. The patient may report some form of neurological deficit, which is likely the result of the tumor exerting pressure on surrounding nerves and vessels. Unilateral edema may result from a bone tumor's expansive spread to soft tissue.

Joint involvement may result in limited range of motion, and subsequent muscle atrophy. If one of the lower extremities is involved, the patient may favor the affected limb, which would result in an antalgic gait or limp. The physician should also assess for adenopathy or hepatomegaly. A soft tissue mass would also be assessed for any appreciable bruit or thrill, which would indicate vascular involvement.

## DIAGNOSTIC STUDIES

Although laboratory tests are routinely ordered to assist in a diagnostic work up; they have been found to have limited value in the diagnosis and staging of both bone and soft tissue sarcomas. A differential diagnosis must be formed using every feasible diagnostic tool. Some useful laboratory tools include erythrocyte sedimentation rate (ESR), alkaline phosphatase. Complete blood count (CBC), comprehensive metabolic panel (CMP), and prothrombin time (PT) to evaluate hemodynamic stability if a biopsy is planned.

Erythrocyte sedimentation rate is a somewhat vague value that is usually found to be elevated in the presence of infection, pregnancy, or recent surgery.[8] Tumors that affect the bone marrow cells such as Ewing's sarcoma, multiple myeloma, lymphoma of the bone, leukemia, and histiocytosis often show a marked increase in the ESR value. Patients who are diagnosed with Ewing's sarcoma or lymphoma and are found to have an elevated ESR generally have a poor prognosis.[8]

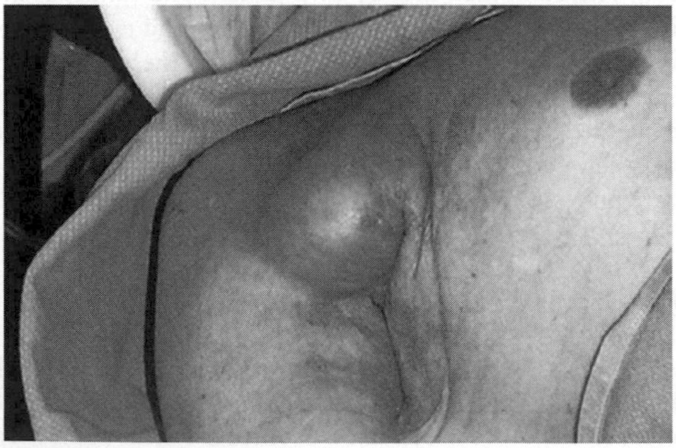

**FIGURE 46-1**

Leiomyosarcoma soft tissue mass with superficial veins.

An elevated alkaline phosphatase level is often evident in approximately one half of osteosarcoma patients. In other primary malignant bone tumors, this level is smaller. The prognostic value of this test has been widely debated due to natural variations related to adolescent growth surges, and the peak age for developing osteosarcoma. The possibility of Paget's disease and metastatic osteosarcoma must also be examined when this test is used to aid diagnosis.

Radiographic correlation is a very important aspect of the diagnostic process. The multidisciplinary collaboration among the surgical oncologist, medical oncologist, radiologist, and pathologist provides the primary expertise needed for the proper diagnosis and treatment of both bone and soft tissue sarcomas. The patient's history and physical exam findings are used in conjunction with a diversity of imaging modalities such as CT, magnetic resonance imaging (MRI), plain x-ray radiographs, bone scans, positron-emission tomography (PET) in the diagnostic work up, treatment follow up and surveillance for bone and soft tissue sarcomas. Each of these imaging modalities have their own dedicated diagnostic value for sarcomas.

Plain x-rays or conventional radiographs are first line imaging modality.[9,10] A vast majority of bone sarcoma diagnoses are made with plain radiographs alone. They are cost-conscious, have superior spatial resolution imaging for trabecular bone detail, and thus can provide a valuable characterization of the intraosseous extent of a bone tumor, except when there is a rather vague zone of transition that makes the medullary extent of the tumor difficult to determine. If the zone of transition is narrow or well demarcated, the host bone responds by forming new bone in reaction to the lesion. In this instance, the lesion is most likely benign.[8,9]

Plain radiographs also produce evidence as to the distinction between ossification and calcification. The mineralization of matrix is ossification, which has a semblance of order. Calcification is viewed as chaotic mineralization with a compressed and random appearance. Lesions with calcified areas usually indicate a cartilaginous process. Ossification in the substance of the lesion indicates bone formation by a tumor.[8] Cortical destruction or periosteal formation of new bone is considered a red flag for an aggressive tumor. (See Figure 46-2 and Figure 46-3.)

CT scans are noninvasive rapid acquisition cross sectional images. Recent advances in CT imaging with the introduction of thin-section multi-detector scanners, have improved image resolution and quality.[9] They are less expensive than MRI and can provide valuable characterization of

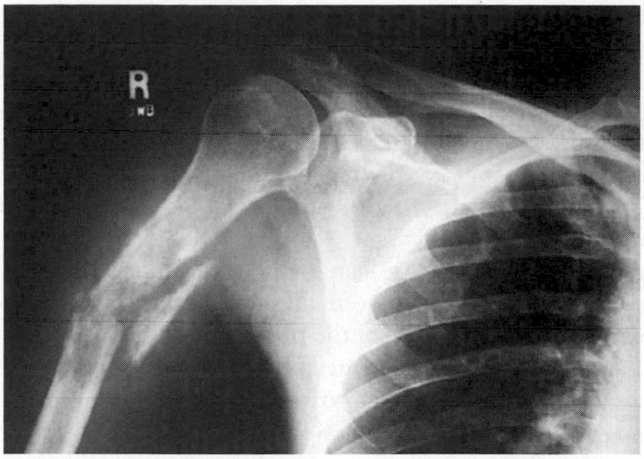

**FIGURE 46-2**

A destructive lesion is producing bone in the metaphysis of the humerus. There is a pathologic fracture at the tumor site.

the primary tumor mass such as its intraosseous extent—in the case of primary bone sarcoma; and the destruction of bone cortex in the case of a soft tissue sarcomas. CT scans show mineralization fractures, and calcification or ossification of bone better than MRI scans do.[9] They also show heterogeneous fat density, which is invaluable in the diagnosis of soft tissue tumors (ie, liposarcoma). CT angiography is an evolving imaging modality for sarcomas. It allows enhanced visualization of the degree of vascularity, as well as delineation of the tumor size, extent and source.[9] CT scans are useful to diagnose metastatic disease to the lungs, pelvis, and abdomen, as well as potential tumor recurrence when MRI is contraindicated by the presence of hardware. The disadvantages of CT imaging include radiation exposure; risk of allergic reaction, or contrast nephropathy.[9]

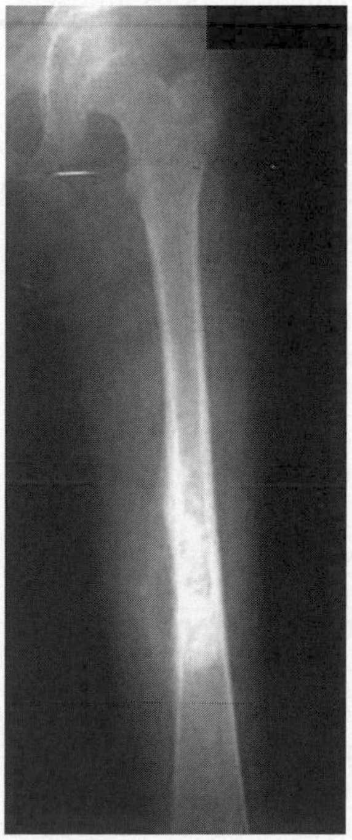

**FIGURE 46-3**

Midshaft femur osteosarcoma with cortical destruction.

MRI offers high-resolution cross-sectional imaging superior to CT scans in the diagnosis of soft tissue sarcomas, in that it is the best modality for observing the relationship among the tumor anatomy, intramedullary extent and neurovascular structures that aids in delineating tumor characteristics and locally affected tissue such as compartmental involvement of the tumor in the muscles, fascia, bones and joint.[9] This information provides a blueprint of information about the extent of the disease by which, the surgical oncologist can then plan for surgical options such as biopsy, limb salvage, and amputation.[9] MRI is excellent for demonstrating the relationship between a soft tissue mass and the cortex of a bone in that, it offers a concise picture of cortical and medullary bone, corruption of an immediate joint, visualization of soft tissue involvement, tumor necrosis, and its relationship to local neurovascular structures. Postoperatively, MRI is the modality of choice for delineating residual or recurrent tumor and postoperative fibrosis or inflammation. It is thought to be the optimal choice for staging pelvic tumors. The axial views provide the optimal perspective.[5,10] MRI can also be used to monitor locoregional tumor response to neoadjuvant chemotherapy, because it can help to estimate the percentage of tumor necrosis, which can then predict treatment outcome.[9] The disadvantages of MRI include lengthy procedural time, and concerns for claustrophobia, which sometimes creates an indication for sedation. Due to the strong magnetic field, MRI is absolutely contraindicated in the presence of cardiac pacemaker, defibrillator, aneurysm clips, carotid artery vascular clamp, neurostimulator, implanted drug infusion device, cochlear or otologic or ear implant, bone growth or fusion stimulator.[9]

Bone scintigraphy or bone scan does not provide any conclusive diagnostic information with regard to soft tissue sarcomas. It allows for whole body imaging, and can detect functional changes before structural alterations occur with metastatic bone lesions. (See Figure 46-4.) It is useful in accentuating abnormal bone, although it does not differentiate between a benign and malignant process; nor will it provide the specifics of the dimension or extent of tumors; but can provide an indication of bone metastasis, which is prevalent with bone sarcomas.[11] It also competes with MRI for cost, imaging time and patient comfort during exam.[11]

Positron-emission tomography is a noninvasive, whole-body imaging modality. It enables the evaluation of the metabolism and physiology of both normal and diseased tissues. A radio labeled tracer is injected into the patient.

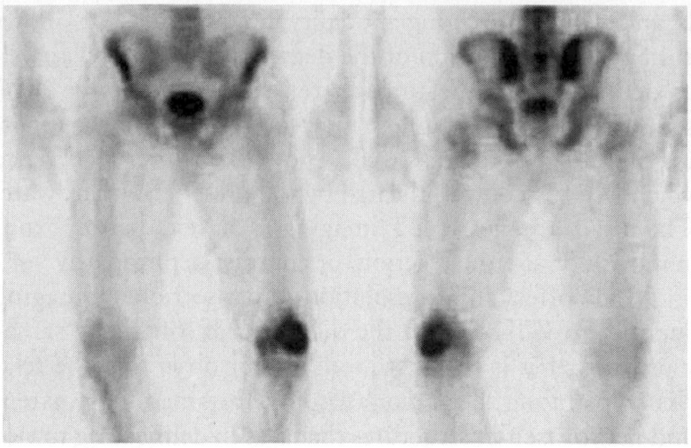

**FIGURE 46-4**

Bone scan of a distal femur osteosarcoma.

The most commonly used radiotracer in PET imaging is F-18 fluorodeoxyglucose (FDG), which is a glucose analog that accumulates in cells in proportion to the rate of glucose metabolism by the cells.[9,12] The degree of metabolic activity in a region of interest is quantified by a measure of the FDG in standard uptake value (SUV).[9] Malignant cells often feature increased metabolism, and the FDG tracer has been shown to accumulate in certain cancer tissues. Although PET imaging is reliable for targeting high yield sections of a tumor mass for biopsy, as well as predicting drug-induced tumor necrosis after neoadjuvant chemotherapy, and staging for distant metastases,[9,12] it does not allow for the histological prediction of a mass and it has poor spatial resolution compared to MRI and CT. Thus PET imaging should be interpreted in conjunction with a cross-sectional study such as CT.[9,12] Studies have suggested that chest CT is more sensitive than PET in detecting pulmonary metastases from bone and soft tissue sarcomas.[13] This is thought to be related to the physical limitations of the PET technology, that relate to the concept that lung metastases do not appear to have as good vascular supply as their original tumors until they reach a certain size, therefore tumor blood flow and possible altered glucose metabolism or reduced number of glucose transporter proteins to the metastases affect PET imaging. Further, today's thin slice CT scans can detect sub centimeter lesions that may be under the spatial resolution of the PET imaging.[13] Fluoroscopy is another tool used to pinpoint bony lesions during a biopsy. This ensures a more accurate biopsy.

Utilization of all of the appropriate modalities available to the oncology team is essential for accurate staging of the bone or soft tissue tumor. These tools are all employed to differentiate among potential diagnoses before a biopsy is performed. Tumors that are large and deep are more likely to have a malignant diagnosis. It is critical that a surgical oncologist perform the biopsy. In the best scenario, the biopsy and definitive surgery would be performed by the same surgeon.

Biopsies can be performed in a variety of ways, but are generally classified as open vs closed. The importance of performing a biopsy correctly cannot be stressed enough. An open biopsy is performed open, with an incision; whereas a closed biopsy uses needles or a special biopsy instrument used for bone or soft tissue. A properly placed incision may prevent a postoperative hematoma or infection. This may mean the difference between salvaging the limb and amputation or the recurrence of the tumor.[14–16]

Biopsies can be performed in a variety of ways. Closed needle biopsies have approximately an 84% accuracy rate.[17] It is crucial to obtain diagnostic tissue—viable tumor cells, not necrotic tissue. A fine needle aspiration (FNA) is one type of closed biopsy. Its major limitation is that it provides only cells, not tissue samples. A nondiagnostic or inconclusive specimen may warrant a repeat procedure. Another mode of closed biopsy is the image-guided core needle biopsy as may be done with CT, MRI, or ultrasound. This technique provides an excellent avenue for the diagnosis of bone and soft tissue tumors in that it allows for accurate penetration into the desired tissue and the ability to avoid critical structures.[18] Further, the core needle biopsy provides actual tissue samples vs only cells as with the FNA. If closed biopsies are nondiagnostic or inconclusive, an open biopsy, considered the gold standard, is then scheduled.

Open biopsies can be incisional or excisional. The surgeon may take two types of sections during an open biopsy: frozen and permanent sections and send for pathological evaluation. Frozen sections are usually done while the patient is still on the procedure table, and offer an immediate opinion as to possible tissue pathology. This is deemed preliminary as snap-freezing may alter the look of the cells under scrutiny. The frozen section offers the surgeon aid to the final plan for surgery with regards to how much margin is to be obtained when the tumor is removed based on the malignancy and grading if possible. The final diagnosis is not rendered until the permanent section, which has been embedded in paraffin, has been evaluated. It should be noted that bone specimens take more time to diagnose, due to the need to decalcify the specimen and evaluate the tumor cells.

## PROGNOSTIC INDICATORS

The prognosis for patients with a bone or soft tissue sarcoma is determined by the tumor characteristics such as size, location, histological grade, and presence or absence of distant metastasis. Large tumors that are deep, with distant metastasis, have a much poorer prognosis. Metastasis often occurs in the lungs, in the lymph nodes, and in other bones.

## CLASSIFICATION AND STAGING

Classification of sarcoma tissue subtype is usually based on tissue origin (See Table 46-1).[19] The staging process begins at the time that a tumor is diagnosed as malignant. Staging for sarcomas is important for treatment decisions and prognosis. Currently, staging is accomplished by diagnostic evaluation of variables such as tumor size (T), tumor grade (G), lymph node involvement (N) and the presence or absence of metastasis (M). Ultimately, the goal of staging for sarcomas is to present a portrait of the anatomic location and extent of disease upon initial diagnosis; and therefore, identify patients who may benefit from single modality therapy such as surgery, or multimodality therapy such as surgery with radiation and/or systemic therapy.[19,20]

The first important component in the staging of a sarcoma is the size of the mass (T).[19–21] Larger tumors have a greater risk for local recurrence and for distant metastasis.[20] Considerations for treatment are also influenced by these variables (see Tables 46-3 and 46-4). A soft tissue sarcoma tumor that is larger than 5 cm or bone sarcoma tumor that is larger than 8 cm is thought to have a poorer prognosis than one that is smaller.[20, 22] Masses that grow quickly are more likely to be malignant and possibly higher grades than slower growing tumors. The anatomical location of the tumor, in conjunction with the size, influences treatment and outcome.[2,20] Soft tissue sarcomas of the proximal extremities and retroperitoneum are often large, whereas the distal extremity tumors are often small.[2]

Tumor grade (G) is a histological calculation of a tumor and the tendency of the tumor to metastasize.[15,20] This information is the foundation of clinical decision-making about treatment options and help ascertain prognosis.[19] Some sarcomas can be assigned a definitional grade by subtype, but due to the rarity of soft tissue tumors, there is no allowance for separate grading criteria for each subtype.[19] Historically, grading schemes for sarcomas have attempted to correlate with prognosis, recurrence, progression free survival, and overall survival.[19] Enneking and colleagues provided a classic staging system for sarcomas that designate 2 histological grades: G1, which is low grade, and G2 which is high grade.[23] In this system, the higher the grade, the greater potential for metastasis. A second staging system, developed by the American Joint Committee on Cancer, designates a 4-tiered grading system for sarcomas.[20] If the grading cannot be assessed, the tumor is labeled GX. Well-differentiated sarcomas are graded as G1. Moderately well-differentiated sarcomas are designated as G2. Poorly differentiated sarcomas are designated as G3, and undifferentiated sarcomas as G4 (see Tables 46-3 and 46-4). In the AJCC staging system, Ewing's sarcoma is classified as G4.[20] The final and most significant component in the staging process is the presence or absence of metastases (M). A patient who presents with metastatic disease at the initial diagnosis has a poorer prognosis.[20] Restaging may

**TABLE 46-3**

**AJCC Staging for Soft Tissue Sarcoma**

| | |
|---|---|
| **Primary Tumor (T)** | |
| TX | Primary tumor cannot be assessed |
| T0 | No evidence of primary tumor |
| T1 | Tumor 5 cm or less in greatest dimension |
| T1a | Superficial tumor* |
| T1b | Deep tumor* |
| T2 | Tumor more than 5 cm in greatest dimension |
| T2a | Superficial tumor* |
| T2b | Deep tumor* |

*Superficial tumor is located exclusively above the superficial fascia without invasion of the fascia; deep tumor is located either exclusively beneath the superficial fascia, superficial to the fascia with invasion of or through the fascia, or both superficial, yet beneath the fascia. Retroperitoneal, mediastinal, and pelvis sarcomas are classified as deep tumors.

| | |
|---|---|
| **Regional Lymph Nodes (N)** | |
| NX | Regional lymph nodes cannot be assessed |
| N0 | No regional lymph node metastasis |
| N1+ | Regional lymph node metastasis |

Presence of positive nodes (N1) is considered stage IV.

| | |
|---|---|
| **Distant Metastases (M)** | |
| MX | Distant metastasis cannot be assessed |
| M0 | No distant metastasis |
| M1 | Distant metastases |
| **Histological Grade** | |
| GX | Grade cannot be assessed |
| G1 | Well differentiated |
| G2 | Moderately differentiated |
| G3 | Poorly differentiated |
| G4 | Poorly differentiated or undifferentiated (4 tiered systems only) |

**Stage Grouping**

| | | | | | | |
|---|---|---|---|---|---|---|
| Stage I | T1a, 1b, 2a, 2b | N0 | M0 | G1—2 | G1 | Low |
| Stage II | T1a, 1b, 2a | N0 | M0 | G3—4 | G2—3 | High |
| Stage III | T2b | N0 | M0 | G3—4 | G2—3 | High |
| Stage IV | Any T | N1 | M0 | Any G | Any G | High or Low |

*Source*: Data from Green FL, Page DL, Fleming JD, et al.[20]

take place if the sarcoma recurs or metastasis is discovered. The purpose of this restaging is to change the treatment if needed or to direct the patient to clinical trials.

## THERAPEUTIC APPROACHES AND NURSING CARE

Treatment strategies for patients with bone or soft tissue sarcomas may include a variety of supportive therapies in combination with complete surgical excision with adequate margins if possible, along with selective radiotherapy and chemotherapy based on the tumor size, grade and margins of resection. The medical regimen for sarcoma is a specialized program: each bone and soft tissue sarcoma has an individualized protocol for treatment. The ultimate treatment goal for any patient with a primary bone or soft tissue sarcoma is long-term survival. This would be accomplished by the complete eradication of the tumor to maintain optimal function and the best quality of life. This goal may or may not include amputation. Amputation may provide a more desirable level of function than a resection would. It should not be viewed as a failure in treatment, but as the best-informed choice for the patient's particular circumstance.

## SURGERY

### BONE

The decision as to the type of surgery to perform is based on the tumor histopathology, dimensions, anatomical site, and on the specific neurovascular structures involved. The anatomical site is divided between intracompartmental and extracompartmental; these data are obtained from radiographic studies. The histopathological characteristics of the primary bone or soft tissue sarcoma and its dimensions are also a primary concern. Critical data obtained from radiographic studies, lab studies, the history, and the physical examination of the patient are all incorporated into the decision making process to provide the best strategy for surgery.

Prior to the 1970s, amputation or disarticulation was the accepted treatment for primary bone tumors. These surgeries provided a very poor survival rate of 10% to 20%.[5,24] The treatment was aimed at completely eliminating the tumor, hence the acceptance of amputation or disarticulation. Anatomically nonresectable tumors in locations such as the pelvis, spine, and skull were treated in a palliative manner. These locations included the pelvis, spine, and skull. Because such tumors were difficult to eradicate completely, they could recur or metastasize.

The 1970s and 1980s brought chemotherapy, which provided an improved efficacy in the treatment of primary bone sarcomas. A combination of improved protocols and

**TABLE 46-4**

**AJCC Staging for Bone Cancer**

| | |
|---|---|
| **Primary Tumor (T)** | |
| TX | Primary tumor cannot be assessed |
| T0 | No evidence of primary tumor |
| T1 | Tumor 8 cm or less in greatest dimension |
| T2 | Tumor more than 8 cm in greatest dimension |
| T3 | Discontinuous tumors in the primary bone site |
| **Regional Lymph Nodes (N)** | |
| NX | Regional lymph nodes cannot be assessed |
| N0 | No regional lymph node metastasis |
| N1 | Regional lymph node metastasis |

*Note*: Because of the rarity of lymph node involvement in sarcomas, the designation **NX** may not be appropriate and could be considered **N0** if no clinical involvement is evident.

| | |
|---|---|
| **Distant Metastases (M)** | |
| MX | Distant metastasis cannot be assessed |
| M0 | No distant metastasis |
| M1 | Distant metastases |
| M1a | Lung |
| M1b | Other distant sites |
| **Histological Grade** | |
| GX | Grade cannot be assessed |
| G1 | Well differentiated—low grade |
| G2 | Moderately differentiated—low grade |
| G3 | Poorly differentiated—high grade |
| G4 | Undifferentiated—high grade |

**Stage Grouping**

| | | | | | |
|---|---|---|---|---|---|
| Stage IA | T1 | N0 | M0 | G1, 2 | Low grade |
| Stage IB | T2 | N0 | M0 | G1, 2 | Low grade |
| Stage IIA | T1 | N0 | M0 | G3, 4 | High grade |
| Stage IIB | T2 | N0 | M0 | G3, 4 | High grade |
| Stage III | T3 | N0 | M0 | Any G | |
| Stage IVA | Any T | | N0 | M1a | Any G |
| Stage IVB | Any T | | N1 | Any M | Any G |
| Any T | Any N | | M1b | Any G | |

*Source*: Data from Green FL, Page DL, Fleming JD, et al.[20]

chemotherapeutic agents provided the patient and surgeon with the option of limb preservation.[25]

When deciding whether to perform limb-sparing surgery, the surgical team must take certain considerations into account. The incidence of recurrence of the tumor should be no greater than it would be with amputation. Patient survival should be equal between both types of surgeries, and the initial surgery and any treatment of complications should in no way hinder the resumption of adjuvant chemotherapy. Additionally the function of the limb should be comparable to the function of the limb with an amputation. A patient may choose amputation over sparing the limb or vice versa depending on occupation, lifestyle, or self image.[21,26] It is important to maintain both a sensate and functional limb.[14] Contraindications exist that may preclude a limb salvage surgery, such as (1) a tumor that involves a neurovascular bundle that cannot be reconstructed; (2) surgical margins that do not include a cuff of normal tissue; (3) pathological fractures with a hematoma; (4) limb length discrepancy of more than 8 cm, usually in children under the age of 10 years; (5) severe infection within the area of surgery; (6) expansive implication of soft tissue or muscle; (7) a biopsy that was performed in an inferior fashion, or one with complications; and (8) a meager response to neoadjuvant chemotherapy.[24,27]

### Radical resection with reconstruction: limb salvage

A radical resection with a reconstruction is a long surgical process that will be unfamiliar to the patient and family. Therefore they must be provided a clear and concise picture of the surgery, postoperative management, and rehabilitation. Patients must be aware of the possibility of needing further surgeries for complications, such as implant failure, infection, and the possible need for amputation. The postoperative course is directly related to the severity of the resection in terms of the amount of soft tissue and bone involved. The management of physical therapy, mobility, the necessity for bracing equipment, and the progression of recovery depends on the individual surgery. Radical resections may involve the complete resection of major muscle groups, as well as reconstruction of a joint and soft tissue. Any limitation of motion, whether related to the surgery or to lack of resected tissue, must be dictated by the surgeon. Figure 46-5 illustrates intraoperative placement of a megaprosthesis following resection of an osteosarcoma of the distal femur.

Radical reconstructive surgeries are lengthy procedures due to the extensive reconstruction of bone, connective tissue, and vascular structures. These complex procedures require an extensive perioperative period, which requires the patient to be under anesthesia for an extended period. Complications of these lengthy surgeries include pulmonary problems as well as possible venous stasis.

Venous stasis may lead to deep vein thrombosis and pulmonary embolism. The physician may require the patient to wear sequential stockings and elastic antiembolic hose postoperatively. A low-molecular-weight heparin may also be initiated to prevent blood clots while the patient is hospitalized and warfarin for another 6 weeks after discharge.

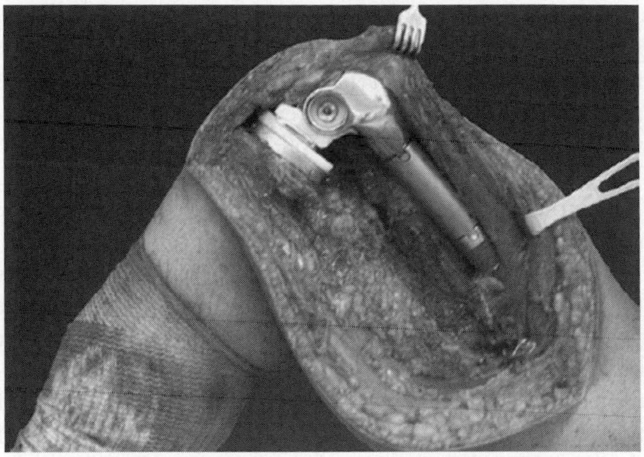

**FIGURE 46-5**

Megaprosthesis placement intraoperatively following the resection of osteosarcoma of the distal femur.

Pulmonary complications may involve atelectasis, and related fevers, as well as pneumonia. These complications are often preventable if the healthcare team is vigilant in its preoperative baseline assessment and follow-up care. Pulmonary toileting must be stressed to the patient to facilitate the healing process.

An ongoing assessment by the physician as well as the nurse and physical therapist is critical to evaluate the progress of motor function and any changes in sensation of the operative limb. The nature of the reconstruction may alter or damage the neurovascular structures, and it is imperative to observe the patient for any changes, positive or negative.

Lengthy surgeries may also result in extensive blood loss that may lead to anemia. Ferrous sulfate may be requested to help increase red blood cells. These patients may also have had neoadjuvant chemotherapy, which affects their healing and laboratory values. It is very important to observe for low hematocrit and infection, both of which are complications that may be evident after chemotherapy and extensive surgery. Patients with anemia may require blood transfusions postoperatively to normalize their hematocrit. This helps patients have the stamina to participate in physical therapy and rehabilitation in a productive manner. Oncology patients, by nature of their illness, are unable to donate autologous blood. Patients may choose to have their family and friends donate blood or to utilize the hospital's blood bank program. Orthopedic oncology surgeries may require 2 to 6 units of blood, as well as fresh frozen plasma in some cases.

Radical reconstructive surgeries may involve the resection of extensive amounts of bone and soft tissue, which may leave large deficits in the operative field. Drainage tubes are placed during surgery to prevent seromas and hematomas, which may lead to complications such as infection. These tubes are left in place until the drainage is minimal. While these drainage tubes are intact, an antibiotic may be administered to prevent infection complications.

Radical reconstructive surgeries may involve restrictions regarding mobility of the affected limb; these may include position, flexion, elevation of the limb, and precautions for limb extension, and weight bearing. These are all determined by the surgeon, with the goal of optimal function of the surgical limb. These restrictions vary with the nature of the surgery and the extent of the resection. Pain management for the patient is handled by the pain service team, if available, and the surgical team. Surgical pain may be initially managed by an epidural, patient-controlled analgesic pump (PCA), peripheral nerve sheath catheter, or a combination of these. As the pain decreases, the intravenous/epidural narcotic analgesic is discontinued and oral narcotic analgesics are initiated. Patients are discharged to rehabilitation or to their homes with oral medications prescribed. Patients may also experience nerve pain, which is managed in a different manner than surgical pain. Gabapentin and amitriptyline are medications used to control nerve pain, which includes phantom pain in amputees.

An essential member of the multidisciplinary team is the plastic/reconstructive surgeon. The treatment of the patient may include chemotherapy and/or radiation therapy. These modalities may lead to the complication of insufficient soft tissue coverage due to wound necrosis or the resection of radiated tissue. Plastic surgeons utilize local or free muscle flaps and split-thickness skin grafts to provide adequate soft tissue coverage.(See Figures 46–6A-C.) The tibia is a common location for lower extremity sarcomas. This location has been particularly problematic due to poor soft tissue coverage. Wound necrosis and infection can occur in the flaps used to close the surgical wound. This problem is exacerbated by irradiated skin, which is more fragile than healthy tissue.

Surgical procedures are sometimes performed in stages, with the soft tissue coverage occasionally occurring 2 to 3 days after the initial surgery. A wound vacuum may be used to granulate the tissue before the grafts are secured. Wound care is managed by the plastic surgeon. Complications may include wound necrosis, infection, seromas, and hematomas. Preoperative radiation therapy and neoadjuvant chemotherapy used in the treatment of sarcomas, compromises the patient's immunity, and predisposes the patient to infection. Wound infection is a prime concern of the surgeon. Metallic implants and allografts are used to replace the bone and joint that has been resected to remove the tumor. Deep infections following these surgeries may require the removal of the metallic hardware and possibly an amputation if the infection cannot be treated. If the infection can be identified and treated, antibiotic treatment is initiated. Intravenous antibiotic therapy usually is conducted for at least 6 weeks and as long as a year or more. Additional surgeries may include irrigation and debridement of the affected limb and may be performed in stages. It is critical that the patient be educated to watch for the signs and symptoms of infection and to report these immediately to the physician.

The primary goal of the surgical oncologist is to preserve life, followed by preservation of the affected limb. Preoperative education about the postoperative functional independence of the patient is critical. A patient's needs after surgery vary greatly with the type and extent of the surgical procedure. The patient may need braces and assistive walking devices, which may be permanent or temporary, and shoe lifts to compensate for discrepancies in limb length. Physical and occupational therapists, as well as prosthetists and orthotists, are instrumental in the rehabilitation of the surgical oncology patient. Social workers, psychologists, and support groups can contribute to the patient's emotional growth and well-being.

The reconstruction of a limb may involve an arthroplasty, which utilizes allografts and metal implants that replace the bone and the involved joint.[27] The allograft, which is procured from deceased donors, is selected by the surgeon according to the dimensions of the resected bone that it is to replace. The prosthesis is cemented, which permits a speedier rehabilitation and recovery. Complications include implant fracture and loosening, infection, and nonunion. This option does not permit the patient to engage in repetitive activities such as jogging due to the artificial joint. Intercalary allograft reconstruction is another method that surgeons utilize. These allografts are secured with plates and screws that ensure the stability of the reconstruction.

The third most utilized method of reconstruction is the arthrodesis or fusion. It provides a stable and durable joint, but one that is stiff. This surgical option is achieved with the use of an intercalary allograft, metallic implants, and possibly hardware to stabilize the joint. It is an excellent option for geriatric patients due to a lower expenditure of energy necessary for gait. Complications include nonunion and infection.

One newer limb salvage technique is hyperthermic isolated limb perfusion with tumor necrosis factor alpha and melphalan with or without radiotherapy.[28]

There are nursing standards of care for these varied surgeries. The assessment of neurovascular function in a reconstructed limb is of the utmost importance. Nerves may be sacrificed during the tumor resection. Patients must be aware of the possibility of insensate areas that may or may not be permanent. The patient may also experience referred pain or sensation related to transposed muscle in flaps. The viability of resected tissues must be constantly monitored to assess for wound necrosis and infection. Radical resections

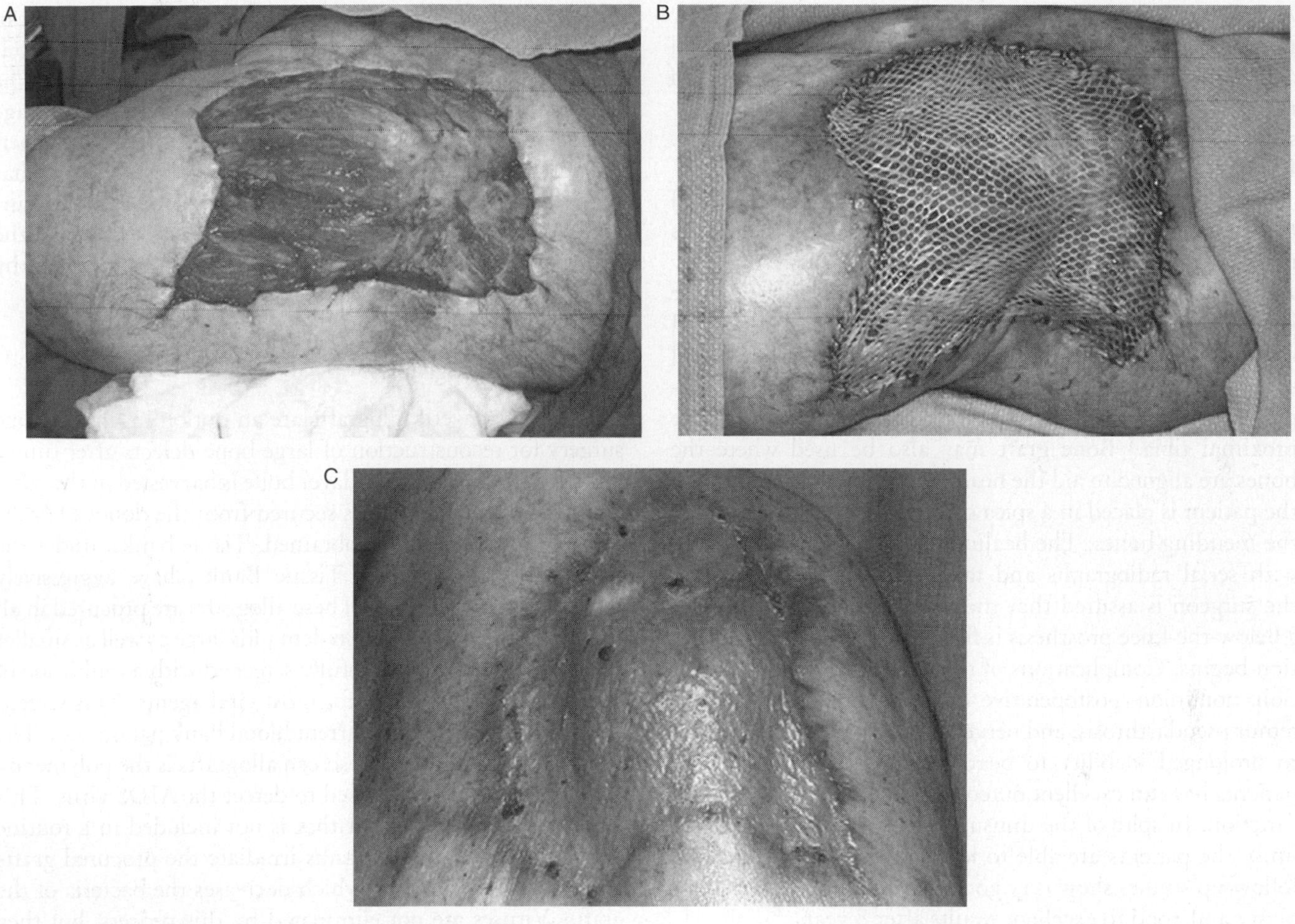

FIGURE 46-6

**(A)** Shoulder with soft tissue mass excision. **(B)** Skin graft covering the surgical defect after the excision. **(C)** Skin graft healing.

may make patients prone to hematomas and seromas, which could lead to infection. This infection could lead to further surgeries, including amputation. Another consideration with respect to surgical wound healing is the resumption of chemotherapy and radiation therapy. The surgeon has the final say as to when a wound is ready for radiation and chemotherapy. Follow-up appointments with the orthopedic oncology surgeon include possible serial plain x-rays to evaluate bone healing, wound evaluation and staple removal, and the progression of physical or occupational therapies.

## Rotationplasty

Children present a challenging dilemma to the surgeon. Due to the fact that children are skeletally immature, surgery options for them are unique. One option is the Van Nes rotationplasty.[29] Rotationplasties in the lower extremities were first utilized in the treatment of infections and then with congenital deformities. The rotationplasty demands special planning and preparation by the entire surgical team. The first step is to fully educate the patient and family about all the options available to the patient; these include amputation or the use of an expandable prosthesis. One valuable mode of education is the use of videos to show other patients who have had the surgery and how they have adapted to everyday life. This is especially critical to young patients who still have the desire to have a more active lifestyle. The optimal educational tool is to have the patient personally meet other rotationplasty patients. This meeting allows a question and answer exchange that may help to put many concerns to rest. The patient is able to view firsthand how a prosthesis will fit and how well he or she will ambulate.

When the patient and family have made a firm decision to have the rotationplasty, the intensive planning begins. The surgical team must calculate the length of both lower limbs; this measurement is essential to ensure minimal length discrepancy. The child's age is added to the equation since this varies with the amount of growth remaining.

Another consideration by the surgeon is that the sciatic nerve must be salvageable. Vascular structures are preserved and coiled, but can be reconstructed if necessary. After a transtibial and transfemoral incision is made, the soft tissues are resected, maintaining the neurovascular bundle. Figure 46-7 shows the incision sites for a rotationplasty.

The malignant tumor in the distal femur and proximal tibia is removed by means of an osteotomy and the tibia is rotated 180 degrees. The calculations previously made by the surgeons become critical to ensure that the rotated ankle is at a similar level as the contralateral knee.[27] The rotated ankle now becomes the new knee joint, which in time will support a prosthesis. The osteotomy is secured with a compression plate and screws, aligning the distal femur to the proximal tibia.[8] Bone graft may also be used where the bones are aligned to aid the healing process. Postoperatively, the patient is placed in a spica cast to ensure stabilization of the mending bones. The healing of the bones is monitored with serial radiographs and takes about 12 weeks. After the surgeon is assured that the bone is sufficiently healed, a below-the-knee prosthesis is fitted and the long rehabilitation begins. Complications of this procedure include infection, nonunion, postoperative vascular occlusions, tibial to femur pseudarthrosis, and nerve palsies or osteopenia related to prolonged inability to bear weight on the leg.[30] Most patients have an excellent outcome with a very good level of function. In spite of the unusual appearance of the rotated limb, the patients are able to lead an active life. Extended follow-up studies show very good durability of the rotationplasty and good to excellent results after 8 years.[29]

## Prosthetics

One challenge that the pediatric patient presents is that growth is still an ongoing process. To compensate for the length discrepancy between the operative and nonoperative limb, the expandable prosthesis was developed. One type of expandable prosthesis developed more than 20 years ago is the Lewis Expandable Adjustable Prosthesis (LEAP).[31] The lengthening process is accomplished in steps; the average lengthening is 1.5 to 2 cm. The technology needed to perfect this type of prosthesis is still evolving. This surgery has many disadvantages, including the need for multiple surgeries, loosening or failure of the prosthesis, collapse of the prosthesis, nerve palsy, flexion contractures, and a lengthy rehabilitation.[8,24]

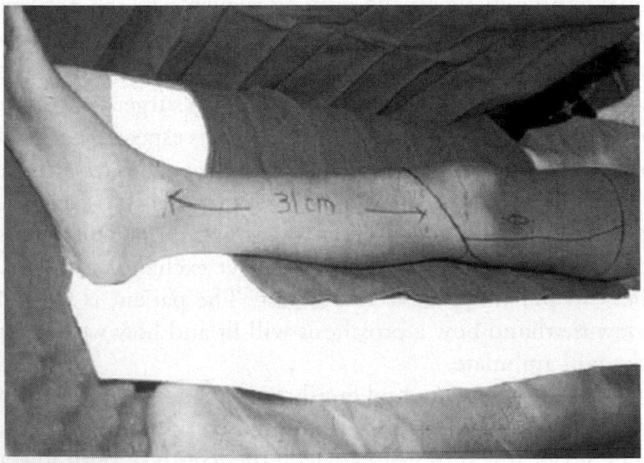


**FIGURE 46-7**

Incision planning for a rotationplasty.

## Allografts/autographs

Structural cadaveric allografts are an option in limb salvage surgery for reconstruction of large bone defects after tumor resection.[32] Allograft or cadaver bone is harvested in the operating room after consent is secured from the donor's family, just as organ donation is obtained. Tissue banks, under the American Association of Tissue Banks, have aggressively pursued bone donations.[8] These allografts are procured in all sizes; skeletal reconstruction demands large as well as smaller allografts. Donors are carefully screened with a multitude of serologic tests that screen for most viral agents. This screening is done according to current blood bank parameters. The one additional test used to screen allografts is the polymerase chain reaction, which is used to detect the AIDS virus. This test is an added safety test that is not included in a routine antibody screen. Tissue banks irradiate the procured grafts with low-dose radiation, which decreases the bacteria of the grafts. Viruses are not eliminated by this process, but they are significantly reduced. HIV transmission is approximately the same in allografts as in blood: about 1 in every 500,000 units of blood.[8,33] Allografts are not tissue typed and have a very low rejection rate.

Allografts, by nature of the availability of various sizes, are very adaptable to the needs of the tumor surgeon. The surgeon must determine the strength and size needed for the bone replacement. Freeze drying of the bone, as well as irradiation, affects the overall strength and torsion strength to some degree. The function of allografts is to heal the bone graft by the host bone to incorporate both bone elements into 1 union. The surgeon may use the allograft as an intercalary graft, which is secured between 2 sections of host bone by metallic screws and plates. These sections eventually heal to the allograft to form 1 contiguous bone. Studies involving the allograft replacement of long bones have met with encouraging results.[33–35] Alloprosthetic composite reconstruction is usually done after resection of the proximal portions of the femur, tibia, and humerus. This provides the advantage of a biological anchor for attachment of the host tendons, and ultimately improved functional outcomes for mobility.[32]

When cadarevic allografts are not readily available, autografts of tumor bearing bone can be done as a cost-effective alternative, after careful selection of patients.[32]

This procedure involves the reimplantation of structurally sound bone after it has been resected and autoclaved for 10 minutes at 120 degrees.[32] Infection was the most common complication.[32]

Patients who have had a metallic implant as well as allograft surgery have similar restrictions. Weight-bearing restrictions are surgery specific, but the ability to bear weight is limited, and the surgery eliminates the possibility of high-impact exercise. During the healing period, the patient's mobility may be limited by a specialty brace or a cast. This healing process may take as long as a year. The complications of both procedures include infection, nonunion, and fracture at the site of the allograft. The reported incidence of infection is approximately 1 in 20 cases.[36] Oncology patients who must undergo chemotherapy may take longer to heal and have an increased risk of complications. Chemotherapy may lead to increases in infection and wound healing problems, but the use of allografts is a promising alternative in tumor surgery.

### Radical resection without reconstruction

Sarcomas in bones that are not essential for structure or stability are resected without the necessity of reconstruction. These bones include the clavicle, areas of the pelvis, and the fibula. The difference between this type of resection surgery and surgery with reconstruction is that nonreconstructive surgery lacks implants. The concern for infection is therefore less, as are other considerations related to implant surgery.

One difference between amputation and limb salvage is the difference in gait. Gait analysis is measured by the level of oxygen consumption during ambulation and the amount of muscle strength. Studies have shown that patients who have had limb salvage surgery involving the knee have a lower expenditure of energy than do patients with amputations.[37] Another consideration is the rate of complications in limb-sparing surgeries as opposed to amputation. One study found that complications occur in limb-sparing surgeries 3 to 4 times more often than in amputations.[38] Limb-sparing surgeries may eventually lead to amputation, if the complications are significant.

### Amputation

Once a patient has been diagnosed and staged, the decision is made with the patient as to which type of surgical intervention should be performed. The decision to undergo an amputation is an extremely difficult one. The patient is faced with the prospect of possible death, disability, and body image disturbance. The decision is irreversible and may affect the patient's ability to earn a living, interact socially, or engage in recreational activities. Many patients may have problems with depression, anxiety, and low self-esteem. It is important to address these prospective problems before the day of surgery. Amputation must be viewed as an option and not as a failure; it is often the best choice when the involved limb would be flaccid or nonfunctioning if it was salvaged.[27]

When amputation is the surgical choice, the goal is to achieve wide margins in the surgical resection and to reconstruct the residual limb to provide optimal function. Amputation in a lower extremity is performed in 1 of 5 ways; transtibial amputation (below the knee amputation, or BKA), knee disarticulation, transfemoral amputation (above the knee amputation, or AKA), hemipelvectomy, and hip disarticulation. The bulk of amputations are of the AKA variety, due to the predilection of bone sarcomas for the distal femur.[27] Function is a prime concern in surgery, and the lower the amputation, the better the limb function; therefore, transtibial amputations have a better functional outcome than transfemoral amputations.[39–43]

Patients who must undergo a hemipelvectomy for tumors of the pelvis have special concerns regarding basic function, ambulation, and physical and emotional issues. Surgery varies from an internal hemipelvectomy, or partially resected pelvis, to a radical hemipelvectomy. These surgeries can produce a significant disability to the patient with regard to joint stability and compromised hip function. They present a special challenge to the prosthetist with regard to creating a prosthesis or a customized hip brace. Prosthetic devices have improved dramatically in both appearance and function. It is important that the patient meet with his or her prospective prosthetist before surgery. It is also beneficial for the patient to meet other patients with a similar amputation who have learned to cope with the challenges involved. Personal concerns regarding sexual adequacy and function must also be addressed. The age of the patient and the type of surgery will affect sexual function, as will nerve damage or resection. The alteration of the blood supply during surgery may also affect function, if only temporarily. Pregnancy and a vaginal delivery are possible after a hemipelvectomy, but the patient will not be able to use her prosthesis during pregnancy due to increased edema. Her gait and balance will also be altered due to her increasing girth. It is important that the patient discuss any concerns with regard to prospective pregnancies with her obstetrician.

Obtaining a prosthesis can be a costly undertaking. Children constantly need their prostheses revamped due to growth. Many patients wish to return to the very active lifestyle that they enjoyed prior to their surgery. Patients must understand their limitations and use any adaptive devices that may make their lives as active as possible. Many amputees enjoy downhill skiing, cycling, basketball, soccer, and even karate with their prosthesis or a specialized recreational prosthesis. The range of recreational sporting activities enjoyed by amputees is growing. Many amputees participate in sporting activities, including organized competition. An amputation provides a special challenge to the elderly because of decreased strength and possible associated medical conditions. These patients may need to use adaptive devices, such as canes or walkers and even wheelchairs on a regular basis.

The social worker who is involved with the oncology group can provide the patient with answers regarding financial resources, rehabilitation programs, and support groups. Examples of these support groups include associations such as the American Cancer Society and the American Handicapped Association.

Rehabilitation is a crucial piece in the patient's recovery and return to a fulfilling and productive life. Physical and occupational therapy is a long process, requiring extensive physical energy, dedication, and a positive attitude. The patient must be certain to keep the avenues of communication open with all of the professionals involved in his/her care. Progress in rehabilitation depends on a prosthesis that is comfortable and on having enough physical reserves to participate in a demanding physical therapy program. A patient who has undergone chemotherapy or is still receiving therapy must relay any physical problems to his/her medical oncologist so that they can be addressed.

*Phantom limb phenomenon.* Patients who are scheduled for an amputation must be educated about phantom limb sensation and pain. This phenomenon is caused by the nerve pathway that has been transected during surgery. This transection results in the transmission of abnormal impulses. Patients may feel pain, burning, itching, cramping, and throbbing sensations in the limb that has been amputated. This is a strange and somewhat disconcerting experience that may occur approximately 1 to 4 weeks postoperatively. Phantom pain usually decreases substantially during the first year; however, some patients are troubled with it for years.[27] Any pain must be evaluated to differentiate between phantom pain and a possible neuroma, which is a possible complication of surgery. Phantom sensation can be exacerbated by stress, fatigue, and emotional stressors. It is managed in a variety of ways, including with a variety of medications. Gabapentin, which is an antiseizure medication, is prescribed postoperatively. Muscle relaxants and tranquilizers have also been used. Chronic pain specialists may be consulted to manage any ongoing problems. At times, simple measures such as the use of a stump shrinker which exerts pressure, heat packs, or distraction measures may reduce or eliminate the problem. If the problem cannot be resolved, additional surgery may be warranted. The stump may need revision or possibly a higher-level amputation.

*Amputation of the lower extremity.* During the preoperative visit, the patient is told what to expect after surgery. Patients who are having a hemipelvectomy must have a bowel preparation to thoroughly clean the bowel to prevent contamination during surgery. Patients will have a urethral catheter placed to measure urine output. Pain will be managed with an epidural, patient-controlled analgesic pump, peripheral nerve sheath catheter, or a combination of these methods. Compressive embolic devices, antiembolic stockings, and prophylactic anticoagulants are utilized postoperatively. Hospital beds should be equipped with a trapeze to aid the patient with mobility and strengthening in preparation for the use of crutches or a walker.

Prosthetic fitting may take place immediately postoperatively or may be delayed. The immediate postoperative fitting uses a fixed dressing and a cast. This type of prosthesis is utilized with younger, healthier patients, not the elderly or vascularly impaired patient. A pylon prosthesis is attached to the molded cast to provide stump shaping with appropriate compression.

If a delayed prosthesis is chosen as the better option, the patient will emerge from surgery with a compressive dressing and an Ace elastic wrap. The residual limb is kept wrapped and the patient is taught how to care for the limb until the postoperative edema has decreased. An early postsurgical fitting takes place 3 to 6 weeks after surgery and the patient works with a physical therapist who will help with gait training. A permanent prosthesis is fitted approximately 3 months after surgery if there are no postoperative complications. A prosthesis may need adjustment related to ongoing chemotherapy, which may affect the residual stump size, to weight gain or loss, or to other health-related problems.

Each type of prosthesis, immediate and delayed, has advantages and disadvantages. Postoperatively, the stump needs careful assessment related to neurovascular function and possible infection. It needs to be elevated to curtail edema and to encourage venous return. Care must be taken to prevent contractures of the hip. This is done by encouraging the patient to lie prone every 6to 8 hours and to sleep in this position. Physical therapy can encourage muscle tone, reduce edema, and strengthen the affected limb as well as the upper extremities for ambulation and can encourage range of motion of the hip and knee, if applicable.

Care of the amputated limb involves wrapping the stump with an Ace wrap or using an elastic stump shrinker to mold the stump and control edema. Physical therapists will work on the first day postoperatively to help the patient sit on the side of the bed and possibly stand with the aid of a walker or crutches and transfer to a chair. Patients who have had the more radical hemipelvectomy usually work with physical therapists on the third day after surgery, or earlier if the patient is progressing well. Hospital stays vary depending on the nature of the surgery, generally 2 days for BKA surgery, 3 days for AKA surgery, and 5 days for hip disarticulations and hemipelvectomy. These are estimates and are based on there being no postoperative complications.

Pelvic resections are divided into 4 different types. Type I includes the ilium, type II the acetabulum, type III the ischium, and type IV the sacrum. These types may be combined and in such cases are identified by both numbers. The resection of the pelvis is a challenge to the prosthetist due to the removal of the ischium, which is necessary for sitting balance. A patient who has undergone a hemipelvectomy must have a bucket prosthesis fashioned. This allows the patient to sit more comfortably without exerting undue pressure on the surgical region. Until the prosthesis is made, the surgical region is elevated with pillows or other nonirritating padding. Adults often do not use a prosthesis for ambulating but will wear one for cosmetic reasons. Children and more active younger adults are more likely to use a prosthesis. Care should be taken to encourage patients to take advantage of a prosthesis, if they are able to use one.[8]

The optimal progression of care after an amputation and hospital stay is for the patient to go to a rehabilitation hospital. The main focus of the rehabilitation stay is on mobility, to prevent complications that may develop with prolonged bed rest, such as deep vein thrombosis and muscle atrophy. Intensive education and training regarding gait, transfers, maneuvering stairs, muscle strengthening, and range of motion are all included in the postoperative period. Depending on the type of surgery, a patient may have special restrictions or a brace that requires special training for the activities of daily life. This training helps ensure that the patient adheres to all prescribed restrictions while taking care of daily activities. It also provides the opportunity to procure equipment that may be needed at home or at the patient's place of work. The return to work and to a more stable financial future provides a great incentive for the patient. This equipment may include environmental adaptive devices such as ramps, grab bars, elevated commode seats, and bathtub seats to ensure patient safety.[14]

Patients must also be taught to care for the stump. They must be taught to wash the stump with mild soap and water and to inspect the area for problems. Skin irritations, blisters, or abrasions could delay the wearing of the prosthesis. Patients need to avoid alcohol, which is drying, and skin creams or oil. Elastic wraps or stump socks should be fitted to ensure proper compression and should be changed daily. Patients need to be instructed in the importance of keeping edema at a minimum by wearing their prosthesis as soon as they rise in the morning. They will gradually increase their wearing time, which will also help keep edema at a minimum. During their hospital stay, patients should also be instructed in how to care for a prosthesis if it is an immediate rather than delayed one. Any malfunctions or discomfort in the prosthesis should be reported to the prosthetist, who should make any necessary adjustments. A patient's prosthesis is ordered via a prescription from the physician to the prosthetist. The prosthetist evaluates the patient physically and determines the patient's expectations regarding lifestyle needs. It is important to have a prosthetist who is certified by the American Board for Certification of Prosthetists to ensure optimal treatment. Prosthesis fitting is a dynamic endeavor that may need periodic adjustments. A lower extremity prosthesis has components that usually consist of a socket, knee joint, ankle joint, and various suspension systems. These suspension systems may involve a waistband and latex or suction sleeves that cover the stump sock. A wide variety of components provide the patient with many options. Gait is a very important element in the construction of the prosthesis. Mechanical or hydraulic knee joints control the elements of walking and ensure standing stability. A variety of prosthetic feet are available that aid in a smoother gait. The prosthesis is assembled and adjusted to fit the patient and to ensure as smooth a gait as possible. These various components may add additional weight, be costly, and increase maintenance problems. Careful thought must be given to the design and construction of the prosthesis. Variables include the patient's age, physical health, occupation, financial considerations, comfort, fit, alignment, appearance, and the user-friendliness of the prosthesis. This information is gathered by the healthcare professional, patient, and prosthetist.

Patients should be made aware of other outpatient programs that may prevent or improve some chronic problems, such as lymphedema and soft tissue and joint contractures. Patients who are troubled with chronic pain should be evaluated and treated by pain management specialists. Other issues that may be addressed include scar massage, special exercises focusing on flexibility and endurance, and the protection and assessment of insensate skin. The final intervention may include counseling to cope with the patient's new lifestyle and necessary adaptations.

Rehabilitation is a long process, and it may take many months for the patient to complete physical therapy, prosthesis adjustment, and other medical treatments so that he or she can declare independence and satisfaction with his or her new body.

***Amputation of the upper extremity.*** The patient who is about to undergo an upper extremity amputation faces many of the same concerns as a lower extremity amputee; however, the psychological impact of losing an arm is greater than that of losing part of a lower extremity. Preoperative and postoperative guidelines are similar, but the rehabilitation process presents some additional considerations. Lower limb prostheses are far superior to those available for the upper extremity amputee. Positive outcomes are directly influenced by the level of amputation necessary to resect the tumor with adequate margins. It is critical to retain adequate soft tissue coverage and stump length. The primary concern is to eradicate the tumor and then to provide a stump that is sufficient in length to accommodate a prosthesis. A prosthesis with a longer stump has better function than one with a shorter stump.

Body-powered components use the mechanical transmission of muscular exertion (myoelectric transmission) that originates from another area of the body, not the amputation site. An active muscle provides a small amount of electrical potential, which acts as the source of control. This potential is electronically processed and is used to start the controller that sends power to the electric motor. This motor drives the prosthetic device. Electrodes on the surface of the body are used to pick up the electrical signal. These electrodes must be worn daily and for extended periods of time, meaning that the patient must be able to tolerate these electrodes without irritation. Testing is performed on the patient to evaluate the ability to produce and control myoelectric signals. Externally powered components use battery-powered electronic devices when the use of body power is not feasible or the power is insufficient. These units provide the best cosmetic appearance with less energy depletion, but they tend to be costly. Other problems pertain to electrical interference and involuntary muscle contractions (coughing, sneezing, or stretching) that interfere with function.

Although upper extremity prostheses are improving with regard to function and appearance, lower extremity prostheses are still superior. Function is often sacrificed for cosmetics, and vice versa. It is crucial that patients have all their questions answered and have the opportunity to see what options are available to them. Prosthetic rehabilitation is a long process, and it is important for the patient to understand what is involved. Questions are best addressed by a certified prosthetist, who can show the patient different options and explain their advantages and disadvantages.

Upper extremity amputations are very similar to lower extremity amputations with regard to postoperative care. The prosthesis can be applied directly after the amputation (immediate) or as a delayed procedure. Stump care is the same as in a lower extremity amputation, including compression and a soft dressing with an elastic bandage. The postoperative hospital stay depends on any complications and the age and medical condition of the patient, but is usually 1 to 2 days. Home nursing may be needed for stump care, assessment, and occupational therapy for activities of daily living. The patient will also need vocational rehabilitation, which is usually a community resource, for possible employment changes or adjustments.

## SOFT TISSUE SURGERY

Dramatic strides have been made in the treatment of soft tissue sarcomas. Advances in imaging and meticulous biopsy techniques have improved the diagnostic process. MRIs are the preferred modality for imaging soft tissue sarcomas.[9] The treatments for soft tissue sarcomas include adjuvant radiation therapy, surgery, brachytherapy, postoperative radiation, neoadjuvant chemotherapy, and adjuvant chemotherapy. These techniques are used in combination; not all treatments are necessarily effective with all soft tissue sarcomas. In general, large (>5cm), deep (down to superficial fascia), high grade, high risk histological subtype sarcomas have a poorer prognosis.[21,22] This is thought to be due in part to the compromise of neurovascular structures and the ability of the tumor to cause more harm with its increasing size.

The goal of the oncologic surgeon is to resect the soft tissue tumor with a clear margin of tissue and to save and protect the surrounding tissue from contamination. Function of the limb is protected, but not at the expense of the patient's survival. The resection of a large portion of a major muscle group is not uncommon to achieve tumor-free margins. Large tumors demand a sizable resection, which leaves a huge defect. The defect may need coverage by a plastic surgeon after the resection of the tumor. If the margins of the resection are suspect, brachytherapy may be used to eradicate the remaining tumor.[21]

The biopsy is a crucial element in the diagnosis of a soft tissue mass. A poorly placed biopsy, with inadequate hemostasis, will cause a larger excision and a more extensive defect. The diagnostic process is also crucial and, together with the biopsy, may mean the difference between a functioning limb and one that is suboptimal.[21]

## METASTATIC SARCOMA

Metastatic disease is the spread or dissemination of cells from a primary tumor to local tissues through the vascular and lymphatic systems. The cells then lodge in distant organs and bones, where they establish a blood supply, and undergo numerous mutations to survive and thrive. Metastatic disease from bone and soft tissue sarcomas is a major clinical problem. Local treatment failure rates have decreased due to advances in local therapeutics, however, distant metastatic lesions are seldom amenable to curative treatment as well as there are low efficacy rates—30%—with conventional chemotherapy, and no improvement in overall survival.[28]

Bone and soft tissue sarcomas often metastasize hematogeneously through systemic venous circulation of the tumor cells. They have a predilection for the pulmonary system as the most common site of metastasis, and less frequently, the liver and bone. Lymphangitic spread is uncommon.[8,21,28] In general, the incidence of pulmonary metastases within each histological subgroup of sarcomas is related to the incidence of high grade tumors within that group, with undifferentiated tumors having the highest percentage of pulmonary metastases.[28]

Surgical resection is the treatment of choice for pulmonary metastasis,[28] however multiagent chemotherapy is also employed. Approximately 20% of patients who initially present with a high-grade bone or soft tissue sarcoma have metastatic pulmonary disease. The prognosis for these patients is very poor if not treated. Untreated patients usually die within 18 months.[28] Surgical management consists of a wedge resection or video-assisted thoracic surgery (VATS). The cardiothoracic surgeon reviews the CT scan of the chest to determine whether surgery is a viable alternative and to decide which procedure is indicated. Another very critical factor is the control of the primary tumor. If the pulmonary surgery is to be effective, the primary tumor must be under control before the pulmonary nodules are resected. During surgery, the lungs are salvaged and the nodules resected. Patients who have pulmonary metastatic disease that has been successfully resected have a more promising survival rate at 5 years. Favorable survival variables after resection of pulmonary metastases for sarcoma patients are the following: possibility of complete resection of the metastases; presence of unilateral vs bilateral metastases; 3 or fewer metastatic lesions to be resected; longer disease free interval between primary therapy and appearance of metastases.[28] Conversely, negative prognostic variables with pulmonary metastases from sarcomas include the following: the presence of greater than 3 metastatic nodules; largest metastasis greater than 2 cm; high-grade primary tumor histology.[28]

Chemotherapeutic management of recurrent or metastatic sarcoma is done to palliate symptoms and prolong survival. Studies of single agent drugs such as doxorubicin and ifosfamide have demonstrated encouraging results.[28] However, the standard of therapy is a combination regimen with mesna, (a uroprotectant against hemorrhagic cystitis from ifosfamide) doxorubicin, ifosfamide, and dacarbazine (DTIC) (MAID), which showed higher response rates and longer time to disease progression, but requires colony stimulating factor support due to increased myelotoxicity.[28,44] Beyond MAID, phase II trials have reported encouraging response rates for comparison combinations of mesna, doxorubicin, ifosfamide (MAI), vs mitomycin, doxorubicin and cisplatin (MAP), with response rates of 34% and 32% respectively.[28] Further, gemcitabine, and docetaxel combination have also showed increased progression free survival rates in metastatic disease.[28,44] Pegylated liposomal doxorubicin is also considered as a reasonable second or third line agent. Temozolomide has been evaluated in phase II trial of metastatic soft tissue sarcoma, and is thought a good consideration for second or third line therapy, especially for leiomyosarcoma patients who never received DTIC as part of initial chemotherapy. Temozolomide works to kill the tumors through breaking down to 5–3-methyl-1-trizenolimidazole-4-carboxamide, which is an active metabolite of DTIC.[28]

Patients with bone and soft tissue sarcomas have a CT scan of the chest at the initial staging and then every 3 months for the first 2 years. Musculoskeletal radiologists compare the scans to evaluate for metastatic disease and to follow the lesions that are less than 5 mm. These lesions are considered nonspecific until they are larger than 5 mm and deemed unresectable. Biopsies are performed only if these small lesions increase in size or multiply. Sarcomas that have a low potential for pulmonary metastasis are followed with plain chest x-rays instead of the more costly CT scan.

## RADIOTHERAPY

Radiation therapy for sarcomas has its limits. Malignant bone sarcomas are less radiosensitive than are soft tissue sarcomas. Ewing's sarcoma is the exception as it is susceptible to radiation. Radiation therapy is used in the palliative treatment of metastatic bone tumors and is also used adjuvantly for high-grade sarcomas. It is also used in conjunction with both surgery and chemotherapy.[45] Radiation therapy uses high energy x-rays to kill local malignant cells or cause tumor growth cessation, For sarcomas, it can be used in the neoadjuvant, adjuvant and metastatic settings sometimes in combination with surgery and/or chemotherapy to maximize local disease control and functional outcomes, but provides no benefit for distant metastases or overall survival.[45] It is based on the premise that radiation will cause enough of a mutagenic effect on the malignant tumor cells to prevent repair and regrowth. The dosage of radiation must be sufficient to kill a significant number of the cells. High doses can cause severe injury to normal healthy tissue, and are unlikely to produce tumor control. A balance must be sought to maintain healthy tissue and at the same time destroy malignant tissue. High-dose radiotherapy treatment has proved less effective than fractionated small dose treatment. Treatment consists of an initial consultation, simulation, and the actual treatment. While the main modes for delivery of radiation therapy are internal or external, there are multiple delivery methods within these modes.

External beam radiation therapy (EBRT), also called teletherapy, delivers the radiation to the tumor from outside of the body. EBRT is the most commonly used type of radiation therapy. It is used for curative as well as palliative treatment of sarcomas. Positioning of the patient is crucial for effective treatment. The patient feels no heat, pain, tingling, or burning during treatment. Any discomfort felt by the patient is due mostly to the positioning. The radiation oncologist checks the periodic beam radiographs against the original simulation radiographs to ensure accuracy. Studies have shown that adjuvant brachytherapy gives acceptable morbidity as well as local control similar to that of external beam radiation.[45,46] Linac-based intensity modulated radiation therapy (IMRT), and 3-D conformal are types of EBRT that are also used in sarcomas.[45] Intensity modulated radiation therapy enables a precise conformal (approximating the shape of the tumor) dose of radiation to be distributed to a targeted area, so a higher dose of radiation can be given to the tumor after immobilization of the affected area, without delivery to normal tissue. This delivery method can allow fractionated dosing given multiple times per day or once daily to reach the tumor cells in different stages of growth and therefore cause more tumor kill. IMRT can be used to treat recurrent tumors in patients who have previously received maximum dosage by conventional radiotherapy. 3-D conformal therapy is CT-guided IMRT, also called TomoTherapy in which a CT scan of the treatment area is taken daily before the dose of radiation is delivered. This allows comparison to baseline for the size, shape and location of tumors, to ensure accurate delivery of the radiation, or to modify the treatment.

With internal radiation therapy, the radiation is delivered to the tumor directly using needles, seeds, wires, or catheters that are placed directly into the tumor cavity (intracavitary) or tissues (interstitial). Brachytherapy can be interstitial, or intracavitary in high dose rate or low dose rate). Brachytherapy is a type of internal radiation therapy. It permits the delivery of localized high-dose radiation directly to the tumor bed and ensures radiation of the margins while protecting adjacent structures. This method is often used in previously radiated sites, with positive results.[45] The advantages of brachytherapy are that the overall treatment time is short, the radiation is restricted to the smallest and most efficacious area, and the treatment is made to the affected area when it remains well-oxygenated.[45,47]

In addition to the above techniques, radiotherapy has been delivered concurrently with chemotherapy, in efforts to improve resectability in sarcomas deemed unresectable at presentation, however, there is no evidence to show efficacy with tumor downsizing enough to allow resection, or prolonged local control.[45]

Preoperative radiation for sarcomas is done to reduce the tumor bulk, thus improving tumor respectability while preserving neurovascular structures, and provide adequate surgical margins. This may determine whether the mass is resectable. Preoperative radiation has the highest post-operative wound healing complication rate, approximately 30%, secondary to the tissue damage, such as fibrosis, burns or infection, induced by the radiation therapy.[45,47] Further, the postradiation effect on the tissues can also complicate pathological evaluation of the surgical specimen.[45] Complications are site dependent, and may postpone the planned surgical procedure. Surgery should be scheduled 3 to 4 weeks after radiation treatment is completed, to allow for soft tissue healing and before fibrosis sets in. Tissue fibrosis would make resecting the vessels and nerves adjacent to the tumor more difficult, due to loss of pliability.[45]

Soft tissue tumors are far more radiosensitive than bone tumors. Radiation is often utilized in pelvic tumors that are not resectable. Due to necrosis, these tumors form a covering or rind that aids the surgeon in the resection. Radiation of tumors is diagnosis specific, and the efficacy of treatment depends on this diagnosis.[45]

Nursing care of the patient who is undergoing radiation therapy is dependent on the type of therapy. A patient who is receiving brachytherapy must be isolated in a specially constructed room, and both staff and visitors must observe radiation precautions. Education of the patient and family is an important aspect of treatment. It is important to maintain these precautions without making the patient feel isolated and alone. The side effects of radiation should be discussed with the patient before the start of therapy. Patients have varying degrees of side effects, especially skin reactions. These include itching, erythema, dryness, wet desquamation (similar to a second-degree burn), rash, loss of hair, radiation-induced necrosis, and general discomfort.[46,47] Posttherapy skin care must also be reviewed with the patient. The patient must protect his or her skin from sunlight; wear loose fitting clothing; avoid alcohol, which is drying to the skin; use mild soap and water and a water-soluble moisturizer; and avoid cornstarch powder, which provides an excellent medium for fungus. The skin condition must be evaluated by the surgeon before the tumor can be resected. There is usually a 3- to 4-week hiatus between radiation therapy and surgery, which allows the skin to heal.

## CHEMOTHERAPY

More than one-half of sarcoma patients die of disease within 5 years of diagnosis.[44] Traditional treatment for sarcomas has been surgery with or without radiotherapy. Chemotherapy has proven effective in the treatment of some types of soft tissue sarcomas, osteosarcoma and Ewing's sarcoma, but not chondrosarcoma. The use of adjuvant chemotherapy in soft tissue sarcomas remains controversial due to the rarity of sarcomas, and the heterogeneity of histological subtypes, that has left gaps in accrual of patients to large randomized clinical trials, Further, adjuvant chemotherapy has not been shown to increase overall survival in soft tissue sarcoma patients.[28,44,48]

Responses rates in bone and soft tissue sarcomas have shown marked improvement with the introduction of multiagent therapy instead of the use of a single agent. A careful balance between efficacy in long term or progression free survival and minimizing toxicity is the goal during treatment. Chemotherapy is administered intravenously; intra-arterial dosing remains controversial. The duration of therapy ranges from 6 to 12 months, depending on the diagnosis and treatment plan. Protocols have been developed through careful monitoring of patients and their response to prescribed agents. The Children's Oncology Group uses multiagent chemotherapy, with cisplatin, doxorubicin, high-dose methotrexate, and ifosfamide.[28,44,49]

Neoadjuvant chemotherapy is given before surgery to shrink the primary tumor and sterilize the microscopic tumor foci in the reactive zone around it with the desired effect of reducing tumor load and eliminating micrometastasis. If this goal is realized, limb salvage is more likely. Neoadjuvant chemotherapy also allows adequate time for surgical planning, allograft procurement and fabrication of prosthesis if indicated.[50] After the prescribed cycles of neoadjuvant chemotherapy, new radiological scans are taken to evaluate the effectiveness of the therapy. The definitive result of the chemotherapy cannot be evaluated until the tumor has been resected and the pathologist determines the extent of tumor kill/tumor necrosis. The amount of tumor necrosis after chemotherapy is an important long-term prognostic indicator.[50] Tumor necrosis of 90% carries a better prognosis.[44,48]

The side effects of chemotherapy are far-reaching. Cells with a rapid turnover (skin, hair, mucous membranes, and hematopoietic stem cells) are affected. Skin reactions are usually temporary; erythema, pruritus, hyperpigmentation, photosensitivity, and dry desquamation are known side effects. Major side effects include mucositis, myelosuppression (neutropenia, thrombocytopenia, anemia), infection, and renal and neurological toxicity with the alkylating agent, ifosfamide, and cardiac toxicity with the anthracycline doxorubicin at cumulative doses over 450mg/mm$^2$. These conditions are all closely monitored and doses may need to be adjusted. General physical well-being is also affected, with fatigue, constipation, and loss of appetite being reported.

## TARGETED THERAPY

The rarity, heterogeneity, wide range of tumor types with different therapeutic approaches for bone and soft tissue sarcomas have presented challenges in developing systemic therapy options for patients. Recent advances have been made in the identification of pathological molecular alterations in sarcomas. These alterations have been shown to be responsible for how sarcomas phenotypically develop, proliferate, survive, invade tissues, spread, and create blood supply for tumors. Molecular targeted therapy is a current therapeutic approach concept that aims to inhibit molecular alterations and reverse the biology of tumor formation by specifically targeting key molecules of cancer cells or neovascular cells with little or no effect on normal cells/tissues. Ultimately, this approach could offer another modality of systemic treatment, based on the biological characteristics of sarcoma tumors, and thus will allow more specific interventions for the subtypes. Currently there are a number of targeted drug therapies in clinical trials for sarcomas. See Table 46-5.

Some current examples of molecular targets identified in sarcomas include epidermal growth factor receptor/human epidermal growth factor receptor 2 (EGFR/EGFR2), insulin-like growth factor receptor (IGF-1R), fibroblast growth factor receptor 1 (FGF1), and vascular endothelium growth factor (VEGF), *Ras/Raf* kinase gene mutations, among others. (See Table 46-5.)

## DESCRIPTION OF SELECTED SARCOMAS

### OSTEOSARCOMA

Osteosarcoma is the most common primary malignant bone tumor. It originates from mesenchymal tissue that produces bone, is usually high grade, highly aggressive, and rapidly metastasizes to distant sites. The lungs are the most common sites of metastases and lymphatic spread is rare.[50] It has a peak prevalence in the second decade of life, with a second peak in the seventh decade.[50] An increased prevalence has been noted in patients with Paget's disease of the bone; history of retinoblastoma, and previous radiation therapy, as well as family history of Li-Fraumeni syndrome.[50] Osteosarcomas can occur in any bone, but 80% to 90% occur in areas of rapid skeletal growth such as the metaphyses of long bones and extend into the epiphyses, The most frequent locations include the distal femur, proximal tibia, and proximal humerus.[50]

Pain is the most prevalent presenting symptom of osteosarcoma.[50] The pain is often exacerbated by activity, and sometimes occurs at night. Patients may also associate noticing the onset of pain after an episode of minor trauma. The pain is thought to be related to possible microfractures in the affected bone as well as compression or stretching of adjacent anatomic structures.[50] Other symptoms may include a palpable mass, limping gait, weakness, decreased range of motion of the affected joints, edema, venous engorgement, and elevated serum LDH.[50]

After the history and physical, the diagnostic workup for osteosarcoma is followed with laboratory assessment, and radiological imaging followed by biopsy if indicated. Laboratory values have a very limited value in the diagnosis of osteosarcoma, but can serve as prognostic indicators of response to treatment.[32,50] Serum LDH and alkaline phosphatase should be drawn at baseline for comparison once intervention with chemotherapy and surgery has begun. Serum alkaline phosphatase, which measures osteoblastic activity, is elevated in some individuals with osteosarcoma. This level decreases postoperatively after the sarcoma resection. As a child matures and grows, these levels are normally elevated, so this laboratory value can be somewhat ambiguous. There does seem to be a correlation between patients who present with elevated serum alkaline phosphatase levels to more than twice the normal and a higher recurrence rate.[32,50]

Radiological imaging during the workup should begin with plain film x-rays of the affected part. These may show lytic and/or blastic areas of bone destruction in both the cortex and cancellous bone, and usually a soft tissue mass with fluffy irregular densities. Further, the cortical margins

**TABLE 46-5**

**Targeted Therapy for Sarcoma**

| Molecular Target | Category | Function of the Target | Current Drug Available for Target | Sarcoma Activity Evidence |
|---|---|---|---|---|
| c-kit | Signal transducer | Activates KIT protein transmembrane receptor tyrosine kinase to signal cell proliferation and enhanced survival | Imatinib (Gleevec)<br>• Inhibits certain tyrosine kinases, including KIT | Metastatic gastrointestinal stromal tumor (GIST)<br>• 65%–70% partial response.<br>• 15%–20% stable disease. |
| VEGF (Vascular endothelium growth factor) | Growth factor receptors/antagonists | Angiogenesis: stimulates new blood vessel formation for tumor | Bevacizumab (Avastin)<br>• Inhibits VEGF | Metastatic soft tissue sarcomas (STS) in combination with doxorubicin<br>• 12% response rate<br>• 65% stable disease |
| Raf-1<br>VEGFR-2<br>VEGFR-3<br>PDGR<br>FLt-3<br>c-kit | | Angiogenesis | Sorafenib (Nexavar)<br>• Inhibits receptor tyrosine kinases involved in tumor angiogenesis.<br>Sunitinib (Sutent)<br>• Antiangiogenesis | Ongoing phase II studies for locally advanced and metastatic soft tissue sarcomas.<br>• Approved for second-line therapy in GIST.<br>• Ongoing phase II trials for soft tissue sarcomas |
| VEGF | Growth factor receptors/antagonists | Angiogenesis | Thalidomide (Thalomid)<br>• Antiangiogenesis | Non-AIDS related Kaposi's sarcoma |
| Her2/EGFR | Growth factor receptors/antagonists | | Lapatinib<br>• Active against EGFR and HER2 | Some efficacy in metastatic carcinoma but needs further study since HER2 expression in sarcomas. |
| IGF-1R | Growth factor receptors/antagonists | Tyrosine kinase surface cell receptor | AEW541<br>• Inhibits receptor, induces apoptosis | Studies suggest efficacy in Ewing's sarcoma |

of the tumor may show Codman triangles—triangular shaped areas of reactive periosteal new bone formation that happens with an aggressive bone process.[50] Patients with osteosarcoma who have a pathological fracture at initial diagnosis have a decreased survival rate compared to patients without such a fracture.[51] Figure 46-8 depicts the destructive nature of osteosarcoma of the humerus. If osteosarcoma is suspected, further imaging should include an MRI of the entire affected bone to determine the local extent of the disease including the condition of the bone marrow, presence of skip metastases (foci of the tumor outside the reactive area in the same bone), associated soft tissue mass, and status of nearby neurovascular structures and adjacent joint. CT scans of the chest are required to assess for pulmonary metastases. Bone scintigraphy or PET scan can also be done as indicated for staging of primary involvement, and distant osseous metastases.[9,11,12,50] Gross pathological evaluation of osteosarcoma shows soft tissue mass that originated in the medullary canal of the bone and extends beyond the cortex, with its innermost portions heavily mineralized.[50] Histological examination reveals pleomorphic, mitotic, malignant cells producing osteoid in a predominantly fibrous or chondroid background stroma.[50] Some areas may exhibit tumor necrosis. Periosteal and parosteal osteosarcomas occur on the surface or juxtacortical surface of the bone. Parosteal lesions occur in the distal femoral metaphysis and appear on x-rays as radiodense lesions. These lesions have a predilection for females between 20 and 40 years of age.[5] These tumors are usually low grade and can be treated with surgery only and no chemotherapy. The long-term prognosis is very favorable, at 93%.[52] Periosteal osteosarcoma is diagnosed as an intermediate-grade tumor with a preponderance for the diaphyseal portion of the tibia. The histological composition of the tumor is osteoid with a chondroid background.[5] Treatment usually consists of wide excision.[5]

Osteosarcoma metastasizes to the lungs more often than to any other site. Chest CT scans are therefore performed

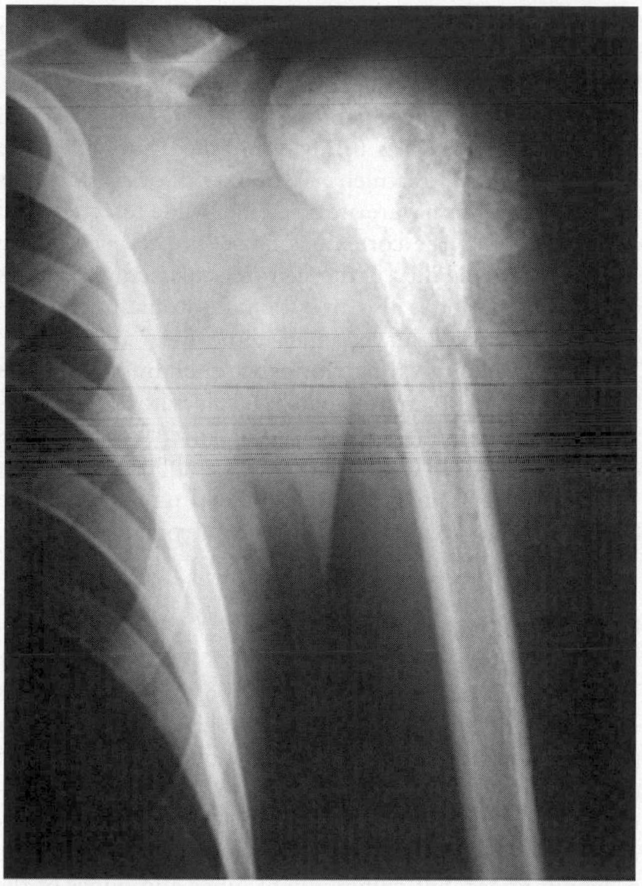

**FIGURE 46-8**

The destructive nature of osteosarcoma of the humerus is depicted on plain x-ray.

on a routine basis, usually every 3 months until 5 years after the initial diagnosis. The first 2 years are the critical period when lung metastatic disease usually occurs. Patients with osteosarcoma who have a pathological fracture with their initial presentation or during chemotherapy have a decreased survival rate and an increased rate of local recurrence.[51] This factor must be evaluated with regard to limb salvage. Such factors as the patient's response to chemotherapy and whether the fracture has attained union are important in the patient's treatment plan.

The optimal treatment regimen for osteosarcoma is neoadjuvant chemotherapy, followed by surgery for wide resection limb-sparing or amputation, and then adjuvant chemotherapy.[50] Additional surgeries and alternative chemotherapy treatments are possible in the event of a recurrence. Radiation therapy is not a recognized treatment for osteosarcoma. It is only used in cases that present as inoperable. After a preoperative chemotherapy regimen, surgery is performed and the tumor is evaluated for tumor kill, or tumor necrosis, which indicates the effectiveness of the chemotherapy. Tumor necrosis of 90% carries a better prognosis. The effectiveness of chemotherapy, the lack or presence of pulmonary metastasis, and the possibility of a pathological fracture are considerations for the surgeon when considering limb salvage vs amputation. Chemotherapy, if effective, can reduce the soft tissue involvement of the tumor. It is also effective in destroying microscopic disease after the spread of tumor cells to the lungs. Chemotherapy may be important in treatment after lung resections for metastatic nodules. Current chemotherapeutic regimens for osteosarcoma are multiagents that include doxorubicin, high dose methotrexate, cisplatin, and ifosfamide.[50]

The main goal of surgery for osteosarcoma is to obtain wide surgical margins with removal of the tumor. Either limb sparing or amputation accomplishes this. Limb sparing is indicated if wide margins and sparing of major nerves are attainable with residual soft tissue coverage for flaps and without rendering the limb nonfunctional. Further, major vessels would need to be preserved or reconstructed, and the end result of the overall reconstruction should be equal or better than prosthesis after amputation.[50] Important poor clinical prognostic indicators for long-term survival in osteosarcoma include the following: the presence of detectable metastases, especially skip metastases, at presentation; poor tumor necrosis after neoadjuvant chemotherapy (<90%); elevated alkaline phosphatase levels more than twice the normal before chemotherapy with continued elevation post-chemotherapy before surgery. Further, elevated LDH and tumor locations in the pelvis, proximal femur and proximal humerus also indicate poor prognosis.[32,50]

NCCN guidelines 2008, for osteosarcoma surveillance after initial treatment, recommend physical exam with functional assessment, chest imaging (CT if indicated), plain film of the extremity (bone scan if indicated), every 3 months for 2 years, then every 4 months for next year, then every 6 months for 2 years, then annually 5 years.[2]

## CHONDROSARCOMA

Chondrosarcoma is a malignant lesion composed of cartilage cells with a mesenchymal origin. This diagnosis is more prevalent in the middle decades of life. Histologically, the tumor appears very mitotic with plump nuclei and sheets of spindle cells that encompass lobules of chondroid.[53] It may arise from benign lesions that exist in the bones, from exostosis, and occasionally from an enchondroma. Tumors cells form cartilage cells that are of a higher cellularity and a greater pleomorphism than a benign chondroma. Nearly 75% of chondrosarcomas are primary lesions not associated with preexisting lesions, and 25% are secondary tumors, originating from benign preexisting cartilage lesions. Secondary tumors are related to diagnoses of Ollier's disease and Maffucci's syndrome, which are multiple enchondromatosis. An association exists between secondary tumors and multiple hereditary exostoses, Paget's disease, and fibrous dysplasia. Radiographically, the lesion is seen as a thick, irregular cartilage cap with an irregular pattern of mineralization. A cartilage cap thickness of more than 2 cm is considered a sign of malignancy in those patients with secondary exostoses.

Chondrosarcomas are also designated as central or peripheral. A central chondrosarcoma has its origin within the medullary cavity of the bone. A peripheral chondrosarcoma originates on the outer surface of the bone cortex. The majority of primary chondrosarcomas, approximately 75%, are of the central variety. Secondary chondrosarcomas are classified mostly as peripheral tumors. Patients who present with a secondary chondrosarcoma have a significantly better survival rate than patients with a primary diagnosis.[53]

Chondrosarcoma occurs, in most cases, in the shoulder girdle, hip girdle, and trunk. The pelvis accounts for approximately 30% of the reported cases, the femur about 20%, the shoulder girdle about 15%, and the ribs and sternum about 10%. The remaining cases are distributed among various bones.[8] The size of the tumor depends on the location; the pelvis has the largest tumors, which may grow for years before they are diagnosed. The grade is higher among the myxoid chondrosarcomas, dedifferentiated chondrosarcomas, and mesenchymal chondrosarcomas. There is a higher correlation between tumors with a higher grade and distant metastasis. In turn, distant metastasis increases the risk of death.

The treatment for chondrosarcoma is surgical resection, with the goal of adequate resection in conjunction with wide margins of normal tissue. Chemotherapy and radiation therapy used in the neoadjuvant or adjuvant mode have been shown to be ineffective.[54] These treatment modes are used only for patients with dedifferentiated chondrosarcoma or mesenchymal chondrosarcoma, or in patients with a poor surgical outcome.

When a patient presents to the physician, it is usually with the complaint of pain, which may be intermittent and aching. Laboratory findings are usually normal, although occasionally the ESR may be elevated. All other lab values of serum and urine should present as normal. The physical examination may show subtle abnormalities, such as a mild antalgic gait and a possible decrease in the range of motion of adjacent joints. The affected extremity may also demonstrate mild atrophy.[55]

Primary central chondrosarcoma usually arises in the metaphysis, but it can also arise in the long bone diaphysis. Plain x-rays show bone destruction, with periosteal reaction and intralesional calcifications. Periosteal reaction is circumferential, and the cortex is thinned in an unequal fashion. CT scans are utilized to evaluate the intralesional calcifications. In a patient with a diagnosis of dedifferentiated chondrosarcoma, the aggressive nature of the disease is evident in the rapid rate of its growth and its destructive nature. An extraosseous portion of the tumor is often evident and can be detected by an MRI. MRIs are best for visualizing the intramedullary portion of the tumor, which is evident on the T2-weighted image. It presents as a bright signal, which is the norm for cartilage.

Diagnosis can be established with a biopsy. When a definitive diagnosis is firmly established, surgery is the accepted form of treatment. Extremity chondrosarcomas that are central in nature are treated by wide resection and reconstruction if the cortex has not been breached. Limb salvage is a possibility if the neurovascular component is intact. Amputation is also an option if it would not be possible to reconstruct the extremity to provide a useful limb.

The 5-year survival rate for pelvic chondrosarcoma has been shown to be approximately 65%, with a 54% survival at 10 years. Chondrosarcoma of the entire skeleton is approximately 67% to 79% at 5 years and 50% to 66% at 10 years. Patients diagnosed with chondrosarcoma have a better prognosis than those with osteosarcoma.

## FIBROSARCOMA

Fibrosarcomas occur in deep fibrous soft tissue that holds muscles, bones and organs in place. They show no gender predilection, but commonly occur in middle-aged and older adults. They account for 1% to 5% of adult sarcomas; usually involve the deep soft tissues of the extremities, trunk, head, and neck. Further, they rarely metastasize to lymph nodes, but commonly to lungs and bones of the axial skeleton. The only presenting symptom may be a nonpainful mass. Five-year survival rates approximate 50%.[19] Historically, this type has been one of the most common of the adult soft tissue sarcomas; however, in recent decades, diagnostic criteria have become more standardized, and it has been replaced by malignant fibrous histiocytoma (MFH). Histopathologically, the diagnosis of fibrosarcoma is now reserved for those tumors displaying the herringbone pattern of interlacing fascicles of spindle cells that have tapered, darkly staining nuclei, scant cytoplasm, and variable, but almost always present mitotic activity. Higher grade tumors stain more densely and can display multinucleated cells.[19] The more common MFH cells demonstrate significant pleomorphism in whorled pattern.[19]

## EWING'S SARCOMA

Ewing's sarcoma is a family of primarily bone tumors, with a relatively small percent occurring in the soft tissues. They include the subtypes of Ewing's sarcoma, primitive neuroectodermal tumor (PNET), Askin's tumor, PNET of bone, and extraosseous Ewing's sarcoma.[19,26] They are the second most common primary malignant bone tumor in children and young adults.[19] Males under the age of 20 years account for a significant number of Ewing's sarcoma patients. This malignancy can occur in any bone, but the majorities are in the long bones of the lower extremities (femur), and the pelvic girdle and bones of the chest wall.[19,26] They commonly metastasize to the lungs and bone marrow.[19,26] Evidence of metastasis at presentation indicates a poor prognosis.[19] A fast growing palpable mass, localized pain and swelling are often the initial presenting signs. They may be accompanied by systemic symptoms such as edema, fever, fatigue weight loss, anemia, as well as laboratory values demonstrating leukocytosis, an elevated ESR, and elevated LDH.[19,26]

Diagnostic workup for Ewing's sarcoma should include plain film x-rays and MRI of the primary site as well as CT, bone scan or PET to evaluate the local and distant extent of the disease; possible bone marrow biopsy. Laboratory tests include CBC, differential, LDH, ESR, and cytogenetic studies for t(11;22) (q24;q12) translocation.

The radiographic appearance of Ewing's sarcoma demonstrates an extensive destructive bone lesion that includes the diaphyseal or metadiaphyseal section of the long tubular bone. An "onion skin" mottled appearance on the periosteum is a common characteristic.[26] There is often a soft tissue component of varying size and extent. This component is best visualized with an MRI. Bone scans to evaluate the possibility of multiple sites; CT scans of the chest to evaluate for metastatic disease, and a bone marrow aspiration are all performed as part of the diagnostic process. Ewing's sarcoma is often mistaken for an infection; needle biopsy specimens will even have the appearance of pus. It is crucial to have a frozen section evaluated, as well as to test cultures for infection.

Histopathologically, Ewing's sarcoma tumors microscopically demonstrate highly compressed cellular masses in diffuse sheets, of uniform small round blue cells with sparse intercellular stroma; clear or bubbly cytoplasm in alternating patterns of dark and light; and low mitotic activity.[5,8,19] Further, tumorigenesis in this family of tumors is genetically noted to be from a fusion of 2 translated protein molecules that lead to abnormal DNA regulation. Specifically, when DNA transcription factor *EWS* gene on chromosome 22 joins to RNA binding factor *FLII* gene on chromosome 11. This is called a t(11; 22)(q24;q12) translocation, which can be identified in molecular cytogenetic studies.[5,8,19]

In general, primary treatment for Ewing's sarcoma is a 4-agent combination chemotherapeutic regimen with myeloid growth factor support for a period of 12 to 24 weeks. Chemotherapeutic agents used include ifosfamide and/or cyclophosphamide, doxorubicin, etoposide, and vincristine.

The treatment for Ewing's sarcoma includes local and systemic control with chemotherapy, radiation, and surgical resection, depending on the tumor location. The outcome of the operative treatment of Ewing's sarcoma that has not metastasized depends on the histological response to preoperative chemotherapy and the size of the primary tumor. These outcomes should be used to identify patients who are at higher risk, so that they can look to a more aggressive approach or even clinical trials.[54–57] Neoadjuvant chemotherapy is used to address micrometastases in the lungs and bone and to shrink the tumor prior to surgery. Current studies in the administration of chemotherapeutic agents have focused on a more intensive therapy over a shorter period and on intensifying the alkylating agents (cyclophosphamide). The chemotherapeutic regimen includes vincristine, actinomycin D, cyclophosphamide, and doxorubicin. Ifosfamide and etoposide may also be added to increase the response rate. The treatment course is usually from 6 months to a year. Surgery and/or radiation are performed depending on the location of the tumor. Pelvic tumors are often treated with chemotherapy and radiation only.

The 5% to 10% of patients who present with a pathological fracture pose a unique dilemma: fracture hematoma. Fracture displacement may influence the possibility of limb-sparing surgery. Preoperative chemotherapy and the response of the tumor will be the determining factors in limb-sparing surgery for patients with pathological fractures.

Ewing's sarcoma is extremely radiosensitive. Radiation therapy may be used in conjunction with chemotherapy as the only treatment. Doses of 45 to 60 Gy are used to shrink tumors. The higher doses may cause fibrosis of the soft tissues and of the joints and may compromise pediatric growth plates. The combination of chemotherapy, radiation, and surgery with negative margins is the treatment used for cure. The patient who relapses is treated with an alkylating agent, ifosfamide, as a single-agent therapy.

The treatment needed to provide a cure for Ewing's sarcoma involves a multidisciplinary approach; the orthopedic oncology surgeon, medical oncologist, and radiation oncologist are critical to the care of the patient. NCCN guidelines recommend follow-up surveillance with a physical exam, local imaging, chest imaging every 2 to 3 months, with increased time intervals after 2 years, and annually after 5 years.

## SOFT TISSUE SARCOMAS

Soft tissue sarcomas have their origin in the mesenchymal tissue of connective tissue, blood vessels, muscles, joints and fat. Classifications of soft tissue sarcomas have been dramatically transformed in the last 30 years. These changes are due mainly to the use of the electron microscope, histological analysis, and immunohistochemistry by the experienced pathologist.[37] The new classification system is based on the cell origin. The goal is to identify the patient population that may need more intensive therapy or less aggressive treatment. These finite classifications help to differentiate soft tissue sarcomas with a low metastatic potential from those with a higher potential for metastasis.

One study looked at cases diagnosed between 1972 and 1994 and reviewed the pathology in accordance with the modern sarcoma classification system. The original recurrent diagnoses were MFH at 26%, liposarcoma at 21%, fibrosarcoma at 11%, and leiomyosarcoma at 10%. The diagnoses using the new classification showed a dramatic swing in the proportions. Leiomyosarcomas increased to 20%, liposarcomas decreased to 17%, synovial sarcomas totaled 14%, and finally the sarcomas "not otherwise specified" (NOS) were at 11%. Of the original cases, 57% had a change in diagnosis. The diagnosis of fibrosarcoma decreased from 32 cases to 6, and the diagnosis of MFH was dramatically reduced from 72 cases to 2. The remaining cases included 22 that were renamed as myxofibrosarcomas, and another 20 (7%) were determined not to be sarcomas.[58] These changes were made due to advances in immunohistochemistry (IHC) in addition to the alterations in nomenclature. The World Health Organization (WHO) published a classification of soft tissue sarcomas in the fall of 2002.[59] This classification recognizes the inclusion of IHC in the diagnosis; in addition, molecular genetic results are often included.[58]

Patients with a soft tissue mass present with a palpable mass but with little or no pain. Function of the affected area is usually not altered significantly. Benign soft tissue masses out number sarcomas at a ratio of 100 to 1. One half of sarcomas are found in the extremities, with those in the lower extremities outnumbering those in the upper extremities. Soft tissue sarcomas are also found in the retroperitoneum, head, and neck. Plain x-rays have little value in the diagnosis of soft tissue sarcomas. Masses should be evaluated with a physical examination using percussion, which evaluates for a Tinel's sign (a lesion that involves a nerve will cause a tingling sensation distally). Auscultation can assess for a bruit, which would indicate an aneurysm.[9] Ultrasound may be utilized to evaluate the depth and dimensions of the tumor and whether it is a solid mass or cystic. Bone scans are used to reveal bone metastasis. CT scans are used to provide the physician with information regarding the local extent of the tumor. They provide critical data with regard to adjacent anatomy, showing fat densities and cortical integrity of bone. MRIs are an excellent mode of imaging to demonstrate neurovascular involvement and the relationship to the tumor. They are capable of providing axial, sagittal, and coronal images, which produce different views of the tumor. The signals are weighted as T1 or T2, which also provide different data, aiding the physician in the diagnostic process.[9] MRI is the best imaging modality for the evaluation of soft tissue masses.[9]

The most critical portion of the diagnosis is the biopsy, which is performed after the scans are completed. A biopsy that is performed properly is paramount in the treatment of the patient. An improperly placed biopsy that is not a longitudinal incision will most certainly have an adverse affect on the patient. A biopsy that does not include meticulous hemostasis may contaminate the area and necessitate more extensive surgery. An inferior biopsy may also make determining of the margins of the original mass very difficult. When the pathology is finalized, the treatment plan is implemented. It should be noted that in some cases a biopsy may need to be repeated if the specimen is insufficient or nondiagnostic.

Soft tissue tumors are divided into groups according to their histogenetic origins.[8] The most common types include leiomyosarcoma, liposarcoma, synovial sarcoma, rhabdomyosarcoma, and malignant fibrous histiocytoma. Fibrosarcoma was closed among the soft tissue sarcomas until the reclassification changed many of the former diagnoses. (See Table 46-1 and Table 46-2)

Leiomyosarcoma is a sarcoma that arises from smooth muscle fibers. It is usually seen in the viscera, but it is also seen in the extremities that arise from the walls of the major vessels. Liposarcoma arises from adipose tissue. The thigh is a common site; less common are the omentum, breast, and chest wall. Synovial sarcomas are histologically similar to normal or reactive synovium, but they do not arise from synovial tissue. Approximately 70% of synovial sarcomas occur in the lower extremities, 25% of patients present with upper extremity masses, and the remaining 5% are located in the trunk.[8] Rhabdomyosarcoma, the most common childhood soft tissue sarcoma, is often located in the head and neck (40%) and in the trunk and extremities (25%). The remaining tumors are found in the retroperitoneum and genitourinary tract. These tumors arise from striated muscle. Malignant fibrous histiocytoma arises from fibrous tissue. It is usually found in the lower extremities, often the thigh. These tumors are often large at diagnosis, from 5 cm to 30 cm.[2]

Treatment for soft tissue sarcomas may include chemotherapy, radiation therapy, and surgical excision. The chemotherapy agents doxorubicin, cyclophosphamide, etoposide, and high-dose methotrexate are utilized in the treatment of soft tissue sarcomas. Ifosfamide has also been used. Surgical resection includes the resection of the tumor, including any contaminated tissue and an uncontaminated margin. If the margins are smaller than 3 cm or are questionable, radiation is used to control the disease. The timetable for treatment depends on whether radiation is necessary. Radiation is given prior to surgery and the skin must then heal for 3 to 4 weeks before surgery can be performed. Wound complications are a significant concern when radiation is performed preoperatively. The rationale for preoperative radiation is to shrink the tumor and ensure a more definitive resection. If the surgical margins are not optimal, postoperative radiation may be ordered. Intraoperative radiation or brachytherapy may be ordered to ensure that the tumor bed and nearby neurovascular structures are disease free. This is especially effective for large, deep tumors. Metastasis in soft tissue sarcomas has a hematogenous behavior. The primary site of metastasis is the lungs, with the liver and bone being only occasional sites. Lymph nodes are not common metastatic sites; the exception is in certain subtypes of synovial sarcomas, rhabdomyosarcomas, and epithelioid sarcoma. Lymph node involvement, larger masses, and deep or high-grade tumors have a poorer prognosis.

## METASTATIC BONE TUMORS

Malignant tumors have the capability of spreading to distant sites and growing at those sites. It is difficult to determine the volume of cells that escape from the primary tumor in relation to the number that are able to thrive and form a clinical metastatic focus. The process of metastasis is accomplished in a progressive effect. First, the cells leave the primary tumor and invade adjacent normal tissue. The tumor cells then must invade a blood or lymphatic vessel and travel to a distant part of the vascular system. Therefore, the tumor cell must be capable of finding its way through the vessel wall and invading the nearby tissue. When the tumor cell reaches this tissue, it must establish its own blood supply and begin to divide. Metastases typically disseminate via a hematogenous route.

Patients with a history of cancer of the lung, breast, kidney, thyroid, or prostate commonly present with skeletal pain. The metastatic sites are the proximal long bones (femur and humerus), spine, pelvis, ribs, and skull. A patient who is over 40 years of age and who presents with skeletal pain and a prior history of cancer will have a bone scan to establish any other sites of disease. Pathological fractures are a serious risk at any site of metastasis. Diagnosis is established with a biopsy and radiographic imaging. CT scans are valuable for evaluating cortical destruction. MRI scans are useful for evaluating compression fractures of the spine.

When the sites of metastasis are identified, the surgeon evaluates the risk of fracture. One treatment option includes the use of bisphosphonates, compounds that inhibit osteoclast-mediated bone reabsorption.[60] Preventing this mechanism decreases the likelihood of pain and pathological fractures.[61] Pamidronate is usually prescribed for breast cancer patients with bone metastasis. The bisphosphonate, zoledronic acid or Zometa, has provided encouraging results for certain types of metastatic lesions.[61]

External beam radiation therapy is a palliative treatment for pain in metastatic disease. It has been found to be more effective for patients with lung or breast cancer than those with renal cell carcinoma. Newer technology in radiation oncology has provided the possibility of more-focused and directed doses, which allows a varying dose of fractionated treatments. This may allow the protection of the soft tissues that surround the targeted lesion. The question then arises as to which lesions should be radiated and which need surgical intervention. CT scans are a useful tool for evaluating bone destruction.

Surgical intervention for bone metastasis is palliative. One advancement is in the use of radiofrequency ablation (RFA), which is especially effective in spine metastasis. Radiofrequency ablation is an outpatient, minimally invasive, developing approach, currently being used to treat osteoid osteomas, but may also be able to treat metastatic sarcoma to the lungs and spine.[28,61] This approach uses thermal electrical energy in a heated probe or needle guided by CT scan, to destroy metastatic lesions in a defined area.[28] This therapy seems to have few adverse neurological effects at present.[61] Surgery would include curettage of the lesion, possible cementation (polymethylmethacrylate or PMMA), and fixation of the lesion with nails, screws, and plates. Joint replacements are also performed for pain relief and to reestablish mobility. One concern of the surgical team is whether enough healthy bone exists to anchor the hardware. Intramedullary nails and rods are used in upper extremity procedures. Proximal femurs and hip surgeries make use of long-stemmed prostheses.

The optimal outcome for the patient with metastatic disease is the reduction of pain and the stabilization of the affected areas. This may be accomplished with medications, radiation, surgery, or a combination of these modalities. Pain management may be an ongoing and evolving process for the patient and his/her healthcare team.

## SYMPTOM MANAGEMENT AND SUPPORTIVE CARE

### PAIN

Bone sarcomas often cause pain, which often interferes with a patient's daily activities. Soft tissue sarcomas may present with pain when the mass exerts pressure on surrounding tissue. Patients will start their pain management with over-the-counter medications such as ibuprofen, aspirin, or acetaminophen. The newer nonsteroidal antiinflammatory medications may provide some pain relief for a period of time. Patients may later be obliged to seek stronger medications to control their pain. Physicians may prescribe mild opiates, such as codeine, for this purpose. As the patient's treatment progresses, stronger medications, including opiates, would be utilized. Multidisciplinary treatment may reduce pain; eg, radiation treatments may shrink tumors and, as a result, decrease pain. This also presents the challenge of which physician will handle the patient's pain management needs. As the patient pursues treatment, it is important to provide him/her with as much independence as possible. This may be accomplished with the use of mobility aids, such as a cane, walker, wheelchair, or motorized scooter, if applicable. The patient may need to see a social worker to assist with everyday responsibilities such as transportation or child care.

### LIMITATIONS OF MOBILITY

The physician may instruct the patient not to place any weight on the affected limb to prevent further injury or pain. The patient may find it necessary to use crutches, a walker, or even a wheelchair for lower extremity protection. An upper extremity tumor may limit mobility and necessitate a sling or splint. Day-to-day activities may present a challenge for the patient during treatment. Impaired mobility, fatigue, and pain may also impede the patient's ability to continue a normal life. The patient may find it necessary to call upon friends and family to provide both emotional and physical support. Patients may benefit from assistive measures such as obtaining handicap parking permits, reducing work hours, and collecting disability insurance benefits.

## CONTINUITY OF CARE: NURSING CHALLENGES

One of the greatest challenges facing both the patient and the orthopedic oncology team is the complex system of healthcare insurance. Health care is becoming more specialized, and patients with special needs will seek out those specialists. Many insurance companies penalize customers for seeking care that is out of their network. Oncology treatments are extremely costly and many are experimental, causing insurance companies to deny payment. Other logistical problems, such as allowing surgery at a tertiary facility but denying laboratory or radiographic studies at the same institution, cause needless delays in treatment. Problems may extend to rehabilitation care and home care after surgery, which may be denied by insurance companies. It is important to be certain that patients fully understand what benefits their insurance provides.

Hospital stays for complicated surgeries are becoming briefer. Insurance companies are encouraging shorter hospital stays, with possible skilled nursing or rehab stays afterward. Treatments such as radiation and some chemotherapy infusions are now performed on an outpatient basis. This provides the patient with the comfort of staying at home but presents the logistical problem of how to get to treatments once and sometimes twice a day. Continuity of care is crucial and must be stressed to the patient and family members; appointments must be kept to advance the progression of care in a positive direction.

Many insurance companies will provide home care for dressing changes, medication infusion, central venous line care, wound assessment, and physical and occupational therapy for a limited time. The ideal plan, according to the insurance companies, is to teach family members to assume these tasks after a short period of time. As was stated earlier, some insurance plans do not provide home care or any outpatient services. It is important that the healthcare team maintain an open line of communication with the patient to answer questions regarding pain, wound care, and any follow-up care that may be necessary.

## FUTURE TRENDS

Advances in the diagnosis and treatment of a very complex and often enigmatic disease have made great strides in the past few decades. The improvements in surgical techniques, neoadjuvant and adjuvant chemotherapy, and radiation therapy have contributed to a better prognosis for cancer patients. Impressive surgical advances such as limb salvage and the use of prosthetic implants have given patients the possibility of a fuller and longer life. Research in chemotherapy, advances in radiation therapy and new modalities from clinical trials provide additional hope in the treatment of sarcoma patients and in their long-term survival. Further research into cytogenetic abnormalities may help to define similarities relevant for tumor diagnostics, prognosis, and may provide insight to develop novel therapeutic strategies.[62]

## REFERENCES


1. Lahat G, Lazar A, Lev D. Sarcoma epidemiology and etiology: potential environmental and genetic factors. *Surg Clin North Am.* 2008;88:451–481.
2. Soft Tissue Sarcoma Clinical Practice Guidelines in Oncology (Version 2.2008). 2006 National Comprehensive Cancer Network, Inc. http://www.nccn.org. Accessed January 6, 2010.
3. American Cancer Society. *Cancer Facts and Figures 2009.* Atlanta, GA: Author; 2009.
4. Jemal A, Siegel R, Ward E, et al. Cancer statistics, 2009. *CA: Cancer J Clin.* 2009;58:225–249.
5. Gibbs CP, Weber K, Scarborough MT. Malignant bone tumors. *Instr Course Lect.* 2002;51:413–428.
6. Wang LL. Biology of osteogenic sarcoma. *Cancer J.* 2005;11: 294–305.
7. Widhe B, Widhe T. Initial symptoms and clinical features in osteosarcoma and Ewing's sarcoma. *J Bone Joint Surg Am.* 2002;82:667–674.
8. Simon MA, Springfield DS, eds. *Surgery for Bone and Soft Tissue Tumors.* Philadelphia, PA: Lippincott-Raven; 1998.
9. Fadul D, Fayad LM. Advanced modalities for the imaging of sarcoma. *Surg Clin North Am.* 2008;88:521–537.
10. Anderson SE, Steinbach LS, Schlicht S, Powell G, Davies M, Choong P. Magnetic resonance imaging of bone tumors and joints. *Top Magn Reson Imaging.* 2007;18:457–465.
11. Wang K, Allen L, Fung E, Chan CC, Griffith JF. Bone scintigraphy in common tumors with osteolytic components. *Clin Nucl Med.* 2005;30:655–671.
12. Hawkins DS. Positron emission tomography in musculoskeletal sarcomas. *Curr Opin Orthop.* 2006;17:573–577.
13. Iagaru A, Chawla S, Menendez L, Conti PS. 18F-FDG PET and PET/CT for detection of pulmonary metastases from musculoskeletal sarcomas. *Nucl Med Commun.* 2006;27:795–802.
14. Yasko AW, Reece GP, Gillis TA, et al. Limb-salvage strategies to optimize quality of life: the M.D. Anderson Cancer Center experience. *CA: Cancer J Clin.* 1997;47:226–238.
15. Peabody TD, Gibbs CP, Simon MA. Current concepts review: evaluation and staging of musculoskeletal neoplasms. *J Bone Joint Surg Am.* 1998;80:1204–1218.
16. Mankin HJ, Mankin CJ, Simon MA. The hazards of the biopsy, revisited. Members of the Musculoskeletal Tumor Society. *J Bone Joint Surg Am.* 1996;78:656–663.

17. Springfield DS, Rosenberg A. Biopsy: complicated and risky. *J Bone Joint Surg Am.* 1996;78:639–643.
18. Issakov J, Flusser G, Kollender Y, et al. Computed tomography guided core needle biopsy for bone and soft-tissue tumors. *Isr Med Assoc J.* 2003;5:28–30.
19. Wu JM, Montgomery E. Classification and pathology. *Surg Clin North Am.* 2008;88:483–520.
20. Greene FL, Page DL, Fleming ID, et al, eds. *AJCC Cancer Staging Manual.* 6th ed. New York: Springer-Verlag; 2002:187–200.
21. Hueman MT, Thornton K, Herman JM, Ahuja N. Management of soft tissue sarcomas. *Surg Clin North Am.* 2008;88:539–557.
22. Rydholm A, Gutafson P. Should tumor depth be included in the prognostication of soft tissue sarcoma? *BMC Cancer.* 2003;3:17.
23. Enneking WF, Spanier SS, Goodman MA. A system for surgical staging of musculoskeletal sarcoma. *Clin Orthop.* 1980;153:106–120.
24. DiCaprio MR, Friedlander GE. Malignant bone tumors: limb sparing versus amputation. *J Am Acad Orthop Surg.* 2003;11:25–37.
25. Eilber FR, Eckhardt J, Morton DL. Advances in the treatment of sarcomas of the extremity: current status of limb salvage. *Cancer.* 1984;54(Suppl 11):2695–2701.
26. Bone Cancer Clinical Practice Guidelines in Oncology (Version 1.2008). 2006 National Comprehensive Cancer Network, Inc. http://www.nccn.org. Accessed January 6, 2010.
27. Nagarajan R, Neglia J, Clohisy DR, et al. Limb salvage and amputation in survivors of pediatric lower-extremity bone tumors: what are the long-term implications? *J Clin Oncol.* 2002;20:4493–4501.
28. Thornton K, Pesce CE, Choti MA. Multidisciplinary management of metastatic sarcoma. *Surg Clin North Am.* 2008;88:661–672.
29. Hanlon M, Krajbich JI. Rotationplasty in skeletally immature patients: long term follow-up results. *Clin Orthop.* 1999;358:75–82.
30. Ozaki T, Nakatsuka Y, Kunisada T, et al. High complication rate of reconstruction using Ilizarov bone transport method in patients with bone sarcomas. *Arch Orthop Trauma Surg.* 1998;118:136–139.
31. Kenan S, Bloom N, Lewis MM. Limb-sparing surgery in skeletally immature patients with osteosarcoma: the use of an expandable prosthesis. *Clin Orthop.* 1991;270:223–230.
32. Lewis VO. What's new in musculoskeletal oncology. *J Bone Joint Surg Am.* 2007;89:1399–1407.
33. Greenwald AS, Boden SD, Goldberg VM, et al. Bone-graft substitutes: facts, fictions, and applications. *J Bone Joint Surg.* 2001;83A(Suppl 2, part 2):98–103.
34. Wallace RD, Davoudi MM, Neel MD, et al. The role of a pediatric plastic surgeon in limb salvage surgery for osteosarcoma of the lower extremity. *J Craniofac Surg.* 2003;14:680–686.
35. Deijkers RLM, Bloem RM, Kroon HM, et al. Epidiaphyseal versus other intercalary allografts for tumors of the lower limb. *Clin Orthop.* 2005;439:151–160.
36. Dion N, Sim FH. The use of allografts in orthopedic surgery, part I: the use of allografts in musculoskeletal oncology. *J Bone Joint Surg.* 2002;84:644–654.
37. Gebhardt MC. What's new in musculoskeletal oncology. *J Bone Joint Surg Am.* 2002;84:694–701.
38. Renard AJ, Veth RP, Schreuder HW, et al. Function and complications after ablative and limb-salvage therapy in lower extremity sarcoma of bone. *J Surg Oncol.* 2000;73:198–205.
39. Thomas MD, Epps CH. Complications of amputation surgery. In: Epps CH, Bowen JR, eds. *Complications in Pediatric Orthopedic Surgery.* Philadelphia, PA: Lippincott; 1995:817–830.
40. Perrson B. Lower limb amputation, part 1: amputation methods—a 10-year literature review. *Prosthet Orthot Int.* 2001;25:7–13.
41. Geertzen J, Martina J, Rietman H. Lower limb amputation. Part 2: rehabilitation—a 10-year literature review. *Prosthet Orthot Int.* 2001;25:14–20.
42. Leung E, Rush P, Devlin M. Predicting prosthetic rehabilitation outcome in lower limb amputee patients with the Functional Independence Measure. *Arch Phys Med Rehabil.* 1996;77:605–608.
43. Treweek S, Condie M. Three measures of functional outcome for lower limb amputees: a retrospective review. *Prosthet Orthot Int.* 1998;22:178–185.
44. Thornton K. Chemotherapeutic management of soft tissue sarcoma. *Surg Clin North Am.* 2008;88:647–660.
45. Kaushal A, Citrin D. The role of radiation therapy in the management of sarcomas. *Surg Clin North Am.* 2008;88:629–646.
46. Alektiar KM, Leung D, Zelefsky MJ, et al. Adjuvant brachytherapy for primary high-grade soft-tissue sarcoma of the extremity. *Ann Surg Oncol.* 2002;9:48–56.
47. Crownover RL, Marks KE. Adjuvant brachytherapy in the treatment of soft-tissue sarcomas. *Hematol Oncol Clin North Am.* 1999;13:595–607.
48. Halpern JL, Gilbert J, Holt GE, Schwartz HS. Chemotherapy for soft tissue sarcoma. *Curr Opin Orthop.* 2007;18:604–610.
49. Hawkins DS, Arndt CAS. Pattern of disease recurrence and prognostic factors with osteosarcoma treated with contemporary chemotherapy. *Cancer.* 2003;98:2447–2456.
50. Gibbs CP Jr, Weber K, Scarborough MT. Malignant bone tumors. *J Bone Joint Surg.* 2001;83-A:1728–1745.
51. Scully SP, Ghert MA, Zurakowski D, et al. Pathological fracture in osteosarcomas: prognostic importance and treatment implications. *J Bone Joint Surg Am.* 2002;84:49–57.
52. Sheth DS, Yasko AW, Raymond AK, et al. Conventional and dedifferentiated parosteal osteosarcoma: diagnosis, treatment, and outcome. *Cancer.* 1996;78:2136–2145.
53. Pring ME, Weber KL, Unni KK, et al. Chondrosarcoma of the pelvis. *J Bone Joint Surg Am.* 2001;83:1630–1642.
54. Bacci G, Forni C, Longhi A, et al. Long-term outcome for patients with non-metastatic Ewing's sarcoma treated with adjuvant and neoadjuvant chemotherapies. 402 patients treated at Rizzoli between 1972 and 1992. *Eur J Cancer.* 2004;40:73–83.
55. Grier HE, KrailoMD, Tarbell NJ, et al. Addition of ifosfamide and etoposide to standard chemotherapy for Ewing's sarcoma and primitive neuroectodermal tumor of bone. *N Engl J Med.* 2003;348:694–701.
56. Kolb EA, Kushner BH, Gorlick R, et al. Long-term event free survival after intensive chemotherapy for Ewing's family of tumors in children and young adults. *J Clin Oncol.* 2003;21:3423–3430.
57. Miser JS, Krailo MD, Tarbell NJ, et al. Treatment of metastatic Ewing's sarcoma or primitive neuroectodermal tumor of bone: evaluation of combination ifosfamide and etoposide— a childrens's cancer group and pediatric oncology group study. *J Clin Oncol.* 2004;22:2873–2876.
58. Daugaard S. Current soft-tissue sarcoma classifications. *Eur J Cancer.* 2004;40:543–548.
59. Fletcher CDM, Unni KK, Mertens F, eds. *Pathology and Genetics of Tumours of Soft Tissue and Bone (World Health Organization Classification of Tumours).* Lyon, France: IARC Press; 2002.
60. Green J. Bisphosphonates in cancer therapy. *Curr Opin Oncol.* 2002;14:609–615.
61. Weber KL, Gebhardt MC. What's new in musculoskeletal oncology. *J Bone Joint Surg Am.* 2003;85:761–767.
62. Eisenberg BL. Soft tissue sarcomas:opportunities for defining the molecular phenotype of a solid tumor malignancy. *Curr Opin Oncol* 2005;17:355–356.

CHAPTER 47

*Gary Shelton, RN, NP, MSN, ANP-BC, AOCNP®*

# Bladder Cancer

## INTRODUCTION

Bladder cancer incidence rates have leveled off in recent years, which may be a result of the decrease in smoking, the most significant risk factor.[1] Almost one-quarter of those diagnosed with bladder cancer will succumb to their disease. Without effective screening, the diagnosis of bladder cancer generally awaits the onset of symptoms.

## EPIDEMIOLOGY

Approximately 70,980 Americans were diagnosed with bladder cancer in 2009.[1] It is the fourth most common cancer and the eighth leading cause of cancer deaths in men. Approximately 14,330 men and 10,180 women will die of bladder cancer in 2009.[2] Men have nearly 3 times the incidence of bladder cancer as compared to women (52,810–18,170). It occurs over twice as often in white men, than in African American men.[1] It was previously thought that women had a protective effect from hormones, but more recent data demonstrate that women are as susceptible as men when known to have similar environmental and work-related risk factors.[3] Bladder cancer is generally considered a disease of the older population (median age 65) and rarely diagnosed in men and woman in young adulthood.

## ETIOLOGY

Smoking is the most important exogenous risk factor for bladder cancer. It is estimated that a smoking history is present in up to 50% of those diagnosed with this disease.[4] The exact mechanism of carcinogenesis is unknown. Smoking cessation decreases the risk of bladder cancer up to 40% in 1 year; however, former smokers continue to have a higher incidence of bladder cancer than nonsmokers up to 35 years after cessation.[5] Approximately 48% of bladder cancer death rates in men and 28% in women are due to smoking.[1]

Occupational exposures to aniline dyes and aromatic amines, most commonly beta-naphthylamine and benzidine, have also been identified as risk factors for bladder cancer. A recent prospective study, looking at lifetime exposure of a heterocyclic aromatic amine pesticide (eg, Imazethapyr, used in the US since 1989), a widely used crop herbicide, found an excess risk for both bladder cancer and colon cancer compared to those not exposed.[6] Exposure to chemicals used in the manufacturing of aluminum, petroleum, dyes, paint, rubber, leather, and textiles, as well as long-term exposure to diesel fumes (truck drivers) and older hair dyes (barbers and hair dressers) increase the risk of bladder cancer.[4,5] The latency period between exposure and tumor development is often prolonged. Ingestion of other physical agents, such as coffee, alcohol, saccharin, and phenacetin, has also been proposed as risk factors. Studies have shown inconclusive results related to increased risk of bladder cancer from consumption of coffee and artificial sweeteners. A recent European review reports no strong association between coffee consumption and the risk of bladder cancer. This group also reports no association between alcohol consumption and the risk of bladder cancer.[7] Data questioning the risk of bladder cancer from the consumption of dairy foods has been inconsistent. A recent study from Sweden found an inverse protective effect from consuming 2 or more servings of cultured milk (yogurt or sour milk), daily.[8]

Several compounds found in nature and as a result of industrial waste have been reported to increase the risk of bladder cancer. Arsenic is found in abundance in nature, generally carried in water. Nitrates, often resulting from nitrogen-based pesticides, are often present in ground water. Epidemiological studies report an increased risk of bladder cancer secondary to consumption of arsenic and nitrates.[9,10] A recent study reported that the consumption of well water was linked to a higher incidence of bladder cancer in women but mortality was alike in both sexes.[9] However, studies have not always included data on age, sex, and cigarette smoking among the populations investigated.[5,9,10]

Additional risk factors include repeated chronic irritation of the urothelial lining due to infections, infusions of cyclophosphamide or ifosphamide especially with a history of hemorrhagic cystitis, and long-term indwelling catheters.[4,5] A high incidence of squamous cell carcinoma of the bladder in many African countries, most notably Egypt, is linked to exposure to the parasite *Schistosoma haematobium*, which can be found in the water of these countries.

The familial risk of bladder cancer is not well understood. Lin et al[11] noted that smoking may increase the risk of bladder cancer in individuals with a family history of bladder cancer. Siblings of hereditary colorectal cancer who have an MSH2 mutation, a repair protein, seem to be at risk for both colon and transitional cell carcinomas (TCCs).[12] Knowledge of the risks factors associated with prior cancer treatments and the awareness of the hypothesis of prolonged contact with carcinogens to the urothelial mucosa alerts oncology nurses to identify populations and follow them more closely.

## PREVENTION, SCREENING, AND EARLY DETECTION

The best preventive strategy to reduce the risk of bladder cancer is to never start smoking. Efforts to assist current smokers to stop smoking may rely solely on healthcare professionals. Identification of past smokers at risk for bladder cancer can facilitate preventive screening and early detection strategies. Nurses who are uncomfortable or less knowledgeable about smoking cessation programs (both behavioral and chemical) should refer smokers to reliable sources for assistance or to a smoking cessation program.

It has been hypothesized that the risk of bladder cancer may be related to the concentration of carcinogens in urine and the amount of time urothelial tissue is exposed to these carcinogens. A prospective study of 47,000 healthy men supports the exposure hypothesis. Health professionals consuming > 1440 mL of water daily had a significantly decreased risk of bladder cancer as compared to those consuming < 240 mL of water daily.[13] Thus, increased fluid intake causing increased urination may be a preventive measure for bladder cancer. A recent study found a protective effect from nocturia, dilution of urine from increased fluids, and diminished exposure by more frequent urination.[14]

Dietary intake continues to be explored with conflicting data supporting the preventive effects of cruciferous vegetables consumed as a form of bladder cancer prevention. A recent report suggests prevention benefit from the consumption of raw cruciferous vegetables, even with populations of smokers.[15] Increasing consumption of cultured dairy products to 2 or more servings of sour milk or yogurt daily does appear to reduce the risk of bladder cancer.[8]

Bladder cancer allows for relatively easy and noninvasive screening strategies, such as microscopic urinalysis, dipstick evaluation, urine cytology, bladder tumor antigen (BTA), nuclear matrix protein (NMP22) immunoassay testing, and serum genetics. Cystoscopy can be done in the outpatient clinic to allow inspection and sampling of urothelial tissue. Studies are being conducted to find more sensitive and specific, and therefore more predictive evaluations to screen for bladder cancer. However, there are no current screening guidelines for use in the asymptomatic population.[16,17]

Current early detection methods include the microscopic examination of cells in urine and the examination of bladder wall epithelium via cystoscopy. These tests are not recommended for screening and early detection of individuals with average risk factors, but for those with increased risk factors secondary to exposures. Individuals with known diagnoses of bladder cancer are offered early detection methods for surveillance of their disease and for the evaluation of recurrence.[17]

## PATHOPHYSIOLOGY

The most common type of bladder cancer is TCC of the urothelium. More than 90% of bladder cancers diagnosed in the US originate in the urinary bladder, 8% in the renal pelvis, and 2% in the urethra or ureter.[18] The urinary bladder is composed of 3 distinct layers: epithelium, muscularis, and perivesical fat.[19] TCC can originate anywhere transitional epithelium exists; from the renal pelvis, ureter, bladder, and upper portion of the urethra. Urothelial tumors presenting with mixed histology, but predominantly TCC, are generally treated as urothelial carcinomas.[18] Only 5% of bladder cancers are either squamous cell or adenocarcinomas.[18] Adenocarcinomas may develop in the dome of the bladder but are rare cancers that may respond to treatments typically prescribed for gastrointestinal cancers. An even more rare subtype of bladder cancer is small cell, which can present with or without a paraneoplastic syndrome.

Bladder cancers are generally considered to belong to 1 of 3 categories: (1) superficial noninvasive tumors, (2) invasive lesions into the muscle, and (3) metastatic with spread beyond the bladder urothelium. These categories differ in prognosis and therapeutic goal, dependent on growth rate, grading, and staging. TCC spreads by local extension through the basement membrane into the muscularis and into the perivesicular fat. Migration into the muscle allows for vascular and lymphatic invasion and distant spread. Superficial lesions in the epithelial layer can remain indolent for many years. The most common sites of hematogenous spread are lung, bone, liver, and brain.

## CLINICAL MANIFESTATIONS

Diagnosing bladder cancer early can be problematic as presenting symptoms can be considered as benign conditions. Urinary tract infections, interstitial cystitis, prostatitis, and the passing of kidney stones can imitate manifestations of bladder cancer. Signs of cancer may also be intermittent and otherwise overlooked.[20]

Hematuria is the most common presenting symptom. The amount of blood noted in the urine may not be predictive or prognostic. Microscopic hematuria may be detected from routine urinalysis and should be considered significant. Gross hematuria, although potentially painless and intermittent, occurs in 80% to 90% of patients who are ultimately diagnosed with bladder cancer.[21] The presence of unexplained gross hematuria in all patients denotes a urothelial cancer until proven otherwise.[21]

Other presenting symptoms may include dysuria, urinary frequency, urgency, and urinary tract infections. Painful urination is often secondary to locally advanced disease. Flank, pelvic, rectal or bone pain, anorexia, fatigue, weight loss, and lower extremity edema may indicate metastatic cancer. More ominous presentations signaling probable advanced disease and a poor prognosis include fatigue, weight loss, anorexia, and failure to thrive.

## ASSESSMENT

### DIAGNOSTIC STUDIES

Bladder cancer is rarely found during a physical examination. A full urological evaluation is indicated for those at risk or suspected of bladder cancer, which includes cystoscopy, urinary cytology, and an evaluation of the upper tracts since urothelial cancers can occur anywhere between the renal pelvis and proximal urethra. Imaging studies that may be ordered include excretory urogram, intravenous pyelogram (IVP), retrograde pyelogram, renal ultrasound, computed tomography (CT) scan, and magnetic resonance imaging (MRI).

Urine cytology may diagnose noninvasive bladder cancers, for example, carcinoma in situ, but overall sensitivity is low. Thus, urine cytology is not used as a routine screening method. Several noninvasive urinary antigen tests have been evaluated but their sensitivity is low and may result in false-positive and false-negative results.[22] These include bladder tumor antigen (BTA, TRAK, BTA stat) and nuclear matrix protein (NMP22) assays. Fluorescence in situ hybridization (FISH) has been reported to have greater sensitivity than urine cytology in the detection of TCC of the bladder; however, a prospective study by May et al[23] reported that urine cytology was superior to FISH.

Flow cytometry can assist in the diagnosis of bladder cancer by evaluating urine cells stained with DNA-specific fluorescein dye, allowing for the determination of cell ploidy and DNA clustering. Detecting DNA aneuploid cells by flow cytometry may be more accurate than urine cytology in diagnosing bladder cancer. However, urine for flow cytometry must be obtained via catheter rather than a voided specimen.

Cystoscopy is the standard method for the diagnosis of bladder cancer. This procedure can be done in the office, where available and appropriate, and is useful for observation as well as biopsy of urothelial tissue. If a lesion is seen, the patient should be scheduled for a transurethral resection of the bladder tumor (TURBT) to confirm the diagnosis of cancer and help determine the extent of disease within the bladder. If the tumor appears to be solid (sessile), high-grade, or invading the muscle, a CT scan of the abdomen and pelvis is recommended prior to the TURBT. For those patients whose disease appears purely papillary or in cases where only mucosa appears abnormal, CT scans are not indicated.[18]

If the patient has an elevated alkaline phosphatase or bone pain, a bone scan should also be a part of the diagnostic workup. Treatment and management decisions are made after considering the extent of disease within the 3 general categories noted previously: noninvasive, invasive, and metastatic.

### PROGNOSTIC INDICATORS

The probability of recurrence or disease progression is related to (1) depth of invasion, (2) size of tumor, and (3) histological grade. Carcinoma in situ (CIS or Tis) commonly progresses to muscle invasion and there is a 50% to 90% chance of recurrence in 5 years.[18] A number of laboratory tests have been used to prognosticate progression of bladder tumors: Thompson-Friedenreich (T) antigen expression, lectin-binding carbohydrate structures, ABH blood antigen groups, and epidermal growth factor receptors; however, these tests have not been used to direct treatment decision-making.[24] The clinical benefit of ploidy, vascularity, p53 status, chromosomal alterations by FISH is uncertain, and should not be used to guide decision-making outside research settings.[18]

## CLASSIFICATION AND STAGING

The classification and staging of bladder tumors provide information to estimate prognosis and to help in treatment decision-making. Cancers of the bladder are classified as being either low grade or high grade, replacing a former system categorizing tumors as being low, intermediate, or high grades.[25] The histological grade examines the degree to which tumor cells resemble normal tissue architecture and is most important to characterize or prognosticate noninvasive tumors because almost all muscle-invasive tumors are high-grade. Low-grade tumors are less likely to invade muscle and stay superficial. Carcinoma in situ, which is seen as flat, nonpapillary, inflammatory and may be of low-grade, has a high potential to invade muscle and recur.[26] The stage of disease is the most important independent prognostic factor and most important in establishing a diagnosis and plan of care. The most commonly used staging system for bladder cancer is the tumor, node, metastases (TNM) staging system developed by the American Joint Committee on Cancer (AJCC) (Table 47-1).[19]

Treatment decisions are made after determining the stage and histological grade of bladder cancer. These decisions are based on the depth of invasion and the extent of known or predicted disease. Tis, Ta, and T1 stages indicate superficial cancer; T2 represents muscle-invasive disease; T3 is categorized as extravesical cancer; and T4 is metastatic disease. The 5-year survival for patients with superficial or localized cancers is $> 90\%$; for those with muscle-invasive disease it is 44%, and 6% for those with distant metastasis.[27] Figure 47-1 identifies the extent of primary bladder cancer.

## THERAPEUTIC APPROACHES AND NURSING CARE

Current approaches for the therapeutic management of bladder cancer depend on the stage of disease. Treatment options include cystoscopic excision for localized noninvasive cancers, intravesical therapy, segmental bladder resection with pelvic lymphadenectomy, irradiation, neoadjuvant and/or adjuvant chemotherapy, radical surgery,

**TABLE 47-1**

**AJCC TMN Staging Classification**

| | |
|---|---|
| **T: Primary tumor** | |
| TX: | Primary tumor cannot be assessed |
| T0: | No evidence of primary tumor |
| Ta: | Noninvasive papillary carcinoma |
| Tis: | CIS |
| T1: | Tumor invades subepithelial connective tissue |
| T2: | Tumor invades muscle |
| T2a: | Tumor invades superficial muscle (inner half) |
| T2b: | Tumor invades deep muscle (outer half) |
| T3: | Tumor invades perivesical tissue |
| T3a: | Microscopically |
| T3b: | Macroscopically |
| T4: | Tumor invades any of the following—prostate, uterus, vagina, pelvic, or abdominal wall |
| T4b: | Tumor invades prostate, uterus, or vagina |
| T4b: | Tumor invades pelvic or abdominal wall |
| **N: Regional lymph nodes** | |
| NX: | Regional lymph nodes cannot be assessed |
| N0: | No regional lymph node metastasis |
| N1: | Metastasis in a single lymph node 2 cm or smaller (largest dimension) |
| N2: | Metastasis in a single lymph node 2–5 cm or multiple lymph nodes less than 5 cm in greatest dimension |
| **M: Distant metastasis** | |
| M0: | No distant metastasis |
| M1: | Distant metastasis |

*Abbreviations*: AJCC, American Joint Committee on Cancer; CIS, carcinoma in situ.

and palliation. Radical cystectomy with pelvic lymphadenectomy remains the standard treatment for muscle-invasive urothelial tumors. Metastatic disease is treated for control and palliation with various clinical trial options. See Table 47–2 for an overview of bladder cancer treatment.[18,28]

Nursing management of the patient with bladder cancer encompasses all aspects of care. An assessment of the patient throughout the continuum of care is of utmost importance. As noted, the expectations of therapeutic management are dependent on the stage of disease. Patient education and preparation are dictated by the patient's assessed needs.

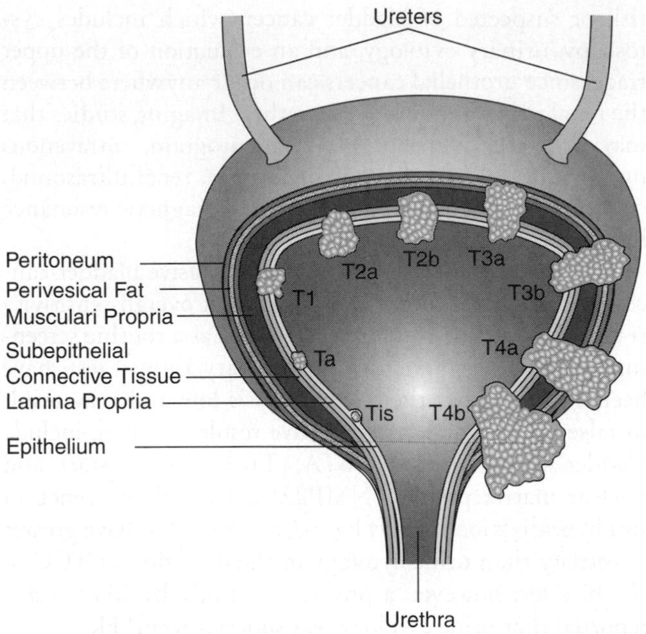


**FIGURE 47-1**

Bladder cancer staging diagram.

## NON–MUSCLE-INVASIVE CANCER/SUPERFICIAL

Non–muscle-invasive neoplasms of the bladder are divided into noninvasive papillomas or carcinomas (Ta), CIS or Tis, and those invading the lamina propria (T1). Overall, these tumors have been called superficial but this is no longer descriptive or prognostic. CIS tumors have a high potential to both recur and to become high grade.[18] Carcinoma in situ appears as a flat nonpapillary lesion that can also be associated with noninvasive papillary tumors. Standard treatment for noninvasive disease is transurethral resection (TUR) and intravesical bladder instillations, with aggressive and frequent follow-up.[29]

### Transurethral resection of bladder tumor

Surgical procedures continue to be integral in the management of bladder cancer despite advances in medicine, radiation, molecular, and biological investigation. Transurethral resection is most effective in diagnosing and evaluating recurrence of noninvasive bladder cancer.[29] Low-grade Ta tumors are generally treated with TUR, alone. Depth of invasion, determined by TUR specimens, may dictate additional therapy including intravesical instillations. Those with higher risk tumors, T1 and Tis, should expect TUR with intravesical administration within 24 hours of surgery.[29,30]

**TABLE 47-2**

**Overview of Bladder Cancer Management**

| Cancer Stage and Grade | Probable Therapy |
|---|---|
| Noninvasive/superficial (Tis, Ta, T1; N0, M0) | TURBT, instillation of intravesical BCG, radical cystectomy for recurrent superficial cancers |
| Muscle-invasive (T2a, T2b; N0, M0) (T3a, T3b, T4a; N0, M0) | Radical cystectomy; potential for neoadjuvant chemotherapy |
| Metastatic (T4b; N0, M0) (Any T, N1,2,3, M0) (Any T, any N, M1) | Systemic chemotherapy with M-VAC; or CG; or Clinical trial |

*Abbreviations*: BCG, Bacillus Calmette-Guérin; CG, cisplatin plus gemcitabine; M-VAC, methotrexate, vinblastine, doxorubicin, and cisplatin; TURBT, transurethral resection of the bladder tumor.
*Source*: Data from National Comprehensive Cancer Network[18]; and the National Cancer Institute.[28]

## Partial cystectomy

In a very select number of patients, a partial cystectomy may be appropriate; tumors that are solitary and invading the posterior lateral wall of the bladder or dome, those with a diverticular lesion, those with unresectable tumors away from the base or bladder neck, and those who have not responded to intravesical instillations. Such patients may be free of disease after a partial cystectomy. Within this select group of patients, recurrence is not uncommon. Close follow-up, at least every 3 months, is recommended.

## Intravesical therapy

Intravesical therapy with immunotherapeutic and chemotherapeutic agents has been shown to be effective in the treatment of superficial bladder cancer. Bacillus Calmette-Guérin (BCG), a live attenuated strain of *Mycobacterium bovis* is the standard treatment for superficial bladder cancer.[18] Treatment with BCG has delayed progression of disease, reduced recurrence, and prolonged survival. BCG is instilled into the bladder cavity via catheter, once weekly for 6 consecutive weeks followed by a 6-week rest and repeated. Urine cytology and cystoscopy are carried out every 3 months to evaluate therapy and to both remove disease and diagnose recurrence.

BCG can cause local inflammation, frequent and painful urination, and flu-like symptoms within 24 to 48 hours of dosing. BCG should not be used in patients with gross hematuria or active cystitis and especially not in the immune compromised population. BCG instillations may cause TB-like infections that should be treated as such. Patients are told to immediately report high fevers, shaking chills, hypotension, and cough, as these may be signs of systemic illness and sepsis. Interferon may also be used in combination with BCG.

Most patients tolerate BCG therapy fairly well. Table 47–3 provides information for patients undergoing BCG therapy.[31] Because of the side effect profile of most chemotherapy medications, their use is not as common as with the immunotherapeutic agents. Valrubicin has been approved for patients with CIS disease when there has been documented failure to BCG.[32] Mitomycin C and thiotepa as well as doxorubicin or epirubicin are used in patients with less risk of recurrence. Mitomycin C has few systemic side effects; however, thiotepa, doxorubicin, and epirubicin can cause myelosuppression.[33] Recent evidence suggests that a single instillation of mitomycin C within 24 hours of surgery and repeated once every 3 months is equivalent to weekly intravesical instillations.[34] Oncology nurses must assure that patients are taught the side effects of these medications, as well as to provide a framework for assessment and management of possible side effects. Safe handling of these agents, administration, and disposal must be directed by policy and procedure.[35] See Table 47–4 for a list of agents for intravesical therapy.[33]

**TABLE 47-3**

**Intravesical BCG: What You Need to Know**

- Do not drink liquids for 4 hours prior to your appointment.
- Empty your bladder prior to the treatment.
- The medication must stay in your bladder for 2 hours.
- Speak to your doctor if you cannot hold the medication for 2 hours.
- You should turn from side to side during the time the medication is in your bladder so that all the surfaces have contact with the medication.
- You should sit to urinate to get the medication out of your body (avoid splashing).
- Put 2 cups of chlorine bleach in the toilet following urination. Close the lid and wait 15 minutes before flushing.
- Clean your genital area and hands carefully with soap and water each time you urinate.
- Unless medically contraindicated, drink plenty of fluids to flush your system for at least 6 hours following your treatment.
- Talk to your doctor or the nurse about any concerns that you have during your treatment.

*Abbreviation*: BCG, Bacillus Calmette-Guérin.
*Source*: Adapted from Wood and Calabrese.[31]

**TABLE 47-4**

| Agents for Intravesical Therapy |
|---|
| BCG |
| BCG + interferon |
| Doxorubicin |
| Epodyl |
| Gemcitabine |
| Interferon |
| Mitomycin C |
| Thiotepa |
| Valrubicin |

*Abbreviation*: BCG, Bacillus Calmette-Guérin.
*Source*: Data from Grossman et al.[32]

Patients who recur after 2 cycles of intravesical immunotherapy or chemotherapy should be considered for cystectomy or a clinical trial. Studies are underway to evaluate the role of chemoradiation therapy in patients who have failed repeated BCG therapy, in an attempt to either stave off further disease progression or to spare patients from cystectomy.[36] For patients on follow-up, it is recommended that repeat cystoscopies with cytology be performed every 3 months for the first 2 years, every 6 months for the next 2 years, and then annually. Supporting patients through the anxieties of repeat exams and fear of potential recurrence is of utmost importance.

## MUSCLE-INVASIVE CANCER

The muscularis is invaded in patients with T2a and T2b disease. These lesions are considered invasive but without "proven" spread to lymph nodes or distant metastasis. For this population of patients, a decision must be made to either totally remove the bladder surgically, or partially remove it if overall survival is not compromised. The standard surgical approach for T2 lesions remains a radical cystectomy with pelvic lymph node dissection. T2 tumors have a better prognosis than those that have invaded the perivesical fat (T3).[18] A recent analysis of data linking the Surveillance, Epidemiology, and End Results (SEER) database to the Medicare database reveals increased mortality in patients in whom a delay of more than 12 weeks occurred from diagnosis of muscle-invasive bladder cancer and timing of their cystectomy.[37]

In a small percentage of the bladder cancer population, with a suspected single nodule, a partial or segmental cystectomy may be performed.[18] For these patients, adjuvant radiotherapy or chemotherapy will be considered. For all surgical candidates, surgical pathology will dictate whether adjuvant treatment is warranted.[18]

### Radical cystectomy

Radical cystectomy with bilateral lymphadenectomy is the standard treatment for muscle-invasive bladder cancer. It is considered the most effective treatment for the local control of tumor recurrence, precise pathological staging, and optimal survival. In men, the removal of the bladder may also include a prostatectomy and removal of the prostatic urethra and seminal vesicles. Often, loss of sexual function is a consequence. In women, a radical cystectomy includes removal of the bladder with perivesical fat, peritoneal attachments, proximal urethra, ovaries, fallopian tubes, uterus, cervix, anterior vaginal vault, and lymph nodes. As with any form of surgery, there are risks associated with the procedure, healing, and other potential complications. Such major surgeries, though potentially curative, remove organs that imply changes that should be addressed before and certainly after therapy.

### Cystectomy with urinary diversion

Following the removal of the patient's bladder, a urinary diversion needs to be created to manage the flow of urine. These diversions can either be incontinent (ileal conduit) or continent (orthoptic).[31]

*Ileal conduit.* The ileal conduit has been the mainstay for bladder cancer surgeries since the 1950s. In this procedure, a section of ileum is removed to make a pathway from the ureters to the outside of the abdomen, via a stoma. Urine flows into the ileal conduit with peristalsis moving urine out through the stoma into an external appliance that continually collects urine.

*Nursing care.* The stoma needs to be assessed frequently for viability during the immediate postoperative period. Normal stoma color is a beefy, dark red. A stoma with a dusky appearance, ranging from purple to black, indicates circulatory impairment and should be reported immediately to the surgeon as reoperation to restore circulation may be indicated.

Stoma edema is normal in the immediate postoperative period due to surgical manipulation, but the edema should not interfere with the stoma function. The size of the stoma will decrease as the edema subsides. The pouch size will need to be adjusted as this occurs, so as to prevent urinary leakage and/or peristomal skin irritation.

An enterostomal therapist (ET) is a valuable resource to assist the patient and family in learning to manage the care of the ileal conduit. Some patients may become upset when they first view the stoma because of the change in body image. As the patient is physically and psychologically able, he or she should be encouraged to first observe the stoma care, and then begin to assist with the care. Ultimately, the goal is to have the patient assume care under supervision and then independently. Instructions should be given to the patient on management of the peristomal skin, equipment to use, how and where to get supplies, and how to reach the resource person if questions or problems arise. The United Ostomy Association and the American Cancer Society are additional resources for the patient.

Complications that may occur following the creation of an ileal conduit include ureteral stenosis, ureteral obstruction, and lithiasis. Regular evaluation and assessment can identify emerging problems, allowing for ready intervention to preserve kidney function.

There also needs to be a periodic evaluation of the stoma, the peristomal skin, and the stoma functioning. Potential problems may include a stoma that recedes (difficulty keeping an appliance intact without leakage), irritated or macerated peristomal skin (caused by an improperly fitting appliance), or encrustations around the stoma (due to alkaline urine). Stomal stenosis or narrowing interferes with urinary drainage and can lead to urinary stasis and/or infection. Education regarding potential problems is necessary so that appropriate interventions can be instituted to avoid long-term sequelae.

*Continent/orthoptic urinary diversions.* In recent years, continent urinary diversions have become the procedure of choice for total cystectomy in order to have a diversion that functions more like the original bladder. Creating reservoirs to collect urine inside the body allows for less change in body image. As with the conduit, a section of bowel is used to create the pouch or reservoir to hold up to 400 mL of urine. Depending on the surgical procedure and surgical candidate, the new bladder can be connected to the urethra or to include a continent stoma, for exiting through the abdomen.

Following surgery for a continent urinary diversion (catherizable stoma or orthoptic neobladder), the patient remains hospitalized for 7 to 10 days. In addition to routine postoperative care, the patient needs to learn to irrigate the tubes placed in the continent reservoir so as to facilitate drainage of urine and keep the reservoir empty. Irrigation is important because the bladder should not be overly distended until healing has occurred. The tubes that the patient has will vary according to physician preference, but may include stents, a suprapubic tube, as well as a catheter through the stoma (Indiana pouch) or a Foley catheter (orthoptic neobladder). See Table 47-5 for care of the abdominal tube and foley catheter.

Approximately 3 weeks after surgery, the patient should have an x-ray of the bladder to assess healing. If no extravasation of contrast occurs, the patient will proceed to learn how the new bladder will function.

The patient with a catherizable stoma will be taught to intubate the reservoir with a 14 or 16 Fr. catheter. Once the

**TABLE 47-5**

**Abdominal Tube and Foley Catheter Care**

The purpose of the abdominal tube and Foley catheter (if present) is to keep the neobladder empty until it has healed following surgery. Inspect the skin and sutures around the abdominal tube daily.

- Wash the surrounding skin with mild soap and water, and dress with a gauze pad daily.
- Irrigate this tube with 30–60 mL normal saline every 3–4 hours. Irrigation may need to be repeated if the solution is not returning freely.
- It may be necessary to use gentle suction to remove the fluid, mucus plug, or blood clots.
- The tubes need to be irrigated at least once during the night.
- It is important to drink at least 6 8-ounce glasses of fluids each day. Your tubes may have better drainage if at least half of your liquid intake is water.
- If you are unable to irrigate either of the tubes or if the fluid does not drain out, call your doctor's office.

*Source:* Data from Woods and Calabrese.[31]

patient is comfortable with this procedure, the tubes will be removed, and the patient will intubate the pouch according to a set schedule, increasing the time between intubations by an hour each week. The patient should not go longer than 5 to 6 hours between intubation procedures.

With an orthoptic neobladder, the patient is instructed on voiding technique. He or she is instructed to void by sitting on the commode, bearing down, and applying gentle pressure on the lower abdomen (Credé maneuver). The patient should begin a toileting regimen of voiding every 2 hours and increasing the time interval by 30 to 60 minutes per week (Table 47-6).

Following the removal of the tubes, patients with an orthoptic neobladder can expect to be incontinent for a period of time. Many products are available to help the patient manage the leakage until urinary control returns, including guards, undergarments, and briefs (diapers). Each person regains urinary control at a different rate. Control during the daytime usually returns first, and approximately 90% of patients eventually obtain complete urine control during the day. Complete nighttime control returns in approximately 80% of patients, while the other 20% experience some amount of incontinence during the night.[38] Emptying the bladder at bedtime (either by voiding or by doing self-catheterization) or setting the alarm to awaken once during the night may help to alleviate the incontinence.

The next follow-up appointment for the patient usually is in 4 to 5 weeks. At that time, the patient will have blood work to evaluate kidney function and an imaging study of the upper urinary tract to evaluate for hydronephrosis.

**TABLE 47-6**

**Orthoptic Neobladder: Instructions After the Tubes Are Removed**

- Urination is done slightly differently now. You should sit on the toilet, relax your pelvic muscles, and bear down using your abdominal muscles to empty your bladder. You may also use gentle pressure on your bladder with your hands to help empty the bladder. In time, this will become "second nature" to you.
- Follow this schedule for voiding:
  - First week: Void every 2 hours during the day and every 3 hours at night
  - Second week: Void every 3 hours during the day and every 4 hours at night
  - Third week: Void every 4 hours during the day and every 4–5 hours at night.
  - Fourth week and thereafter: Void every 4–5 hours during the day and every 4–6 hours at night.
- It is important to drink 6 to 8 8-ounce glasses of fluids each day. Make it a habit to drink a glass of fluids with each meal and 1 glass of fluids between each meal every day for the rest of your life.
- You will leak urine when your Foley catheter is removed. Be patient with yourself. As your body heals, you will begin to regain urine control.
- You will always have mucus in your urine because your bladder is made from intestine. You will learn what is a normal amount of mucus for you.
- If something does not seem right to you, call your doctor's office.

Cancer follow-up evaluations with CT scans are per the physician's usual protocol.

Complications of continent urinary diversions can include metabolic and nutritional disorders (related to the part of the bowel that is used), pyelonephritis and renal deterioration (manifested by hydronephrosis or an increasing serum creatinine), and formation of renal or bladder calculi. The latter complication is related to persistent infection. Some patients may need suppressive antibiotics for the remainder of their lifetime.

Oncology nurses work collaboratively with social workers, home-health nurses, sex therapists, physician assistants, and physicians, to best provide overall care for patients. Postoperative care must be explained to minimize complications, promote healing, and acceptance of body changes.

### Radiation therapy

In select patients, radiation therapy may be a treatment option allowing for preservation of bladder function. Radiation therapy may be offered for patients with muscle invading disease without lymph node involvement, or for those with poor performance status or comorbid conditions.[18,31] Ongoing studies by the Radiation Therapy Oncology Group (RTOG) are investigating bladder preservation approaches with radiation therapy alone or with sensitizing chemotherapy.[39]

### Chemotherapy

The presence of unknown or occult micrometastases at the time of radical cystectomy will devalue the surgery and allow for local and distant failures in patients otherwise candidates for curative surgery.[40–43] Less than 50% of patients with advanced node positive bladder cancer will survive if treated by surgery alone.[4] Thus, neoadjuvant chemotherapy is the standard of care for patients with muscle-invasive disease.[40] For patients who are not surgical candidates or have refused radical cystectomy, neoadjuvant chemotherapy with or without radiation therapy may lead to favorable outcomes.[40,42,43] There is less definitive evidence to support waiting until after cystectomy for adjuvant chemotherapy.[18,41–43]

Neoadjuvant chemotherapy may shrink the tumor and enhance resectability. Recent studies using neoadjuvant therapy with a cisplatin-based chemotherapy regimen suggests significant benefits in overall survival and 5-year disease-free survival.[28,29,44,45]

Whether chemotherapy is initiated prior to surgery or postoperatively, the regimens used are the same. Methotrexate, vinblastine, doxorubicin, and cisplatin (M-VAC) was the standard chemotherapy regimen for bladder cancer; however, it has been largely replaced with the use of cisplatin plus gemcitabine (CG), which is equivalent in effectiveness and less toxic.[44,46–48] Either chemotherapy regimen alerts nurses to prepare patients for potential toxicities.

## METASTATIC DISEASE

### Surgery

A recent study conducted by the European Association of Urology (EAU) suggests a benefit in cancer control and potential cure in a subset of patients with limited disease when surgical resection of minimal metastatic sites was combined with systemic chemotherapy.[49] Surgical interventions, therefore, have only been done for debulking of disease and for palliation.[18]

### Chemotherapy

Bladder cancer that has metastasized or is diagnosed as T4 disease with lymph node involvement is not curable with current treatment options. Treatment considerations include systemic chemotherapy and entry on a clinical trial. Chemotherapy discussions must include strategies for safety and risk reduction as well as provisions for managing side effects.

Cisplatin-based chemotherapy, as noted for locally advanced bladder cancer, is the standard of care for this population of patients.[21,48] Both M-VAC and CG have similar response rates, with 5-year overall survival at 11% to 15%.[50] Because CG has similar survival outcomes and is less toxic it has become the standard of care for patients with metastatic disease.[21]

Alternatives to platinum-based therapies are necessary for patients who are unable to tolerate platinum as well as for those patients who have failed prior platinum-based regimens. Emerging evidence holds promise for improved treatment of patients with metastatic disease who have already received platinum agents.[51] Several agents are being investigated as single agents or in combination with other agents and include paclitaxel, docetaxel, gemcitabine, ifosfamide, and carboplatin.[52,53] Novel agents in clinical trials with promising results include halichondron, bevacizumab, vinflunine, sunitinib, and sorafinib.[54] As these and other agents become approved for use, oncology nurses will be instrumental in transporting the state of the science and evidence to the bedside, thus allowing for safe and improved patient outcomes for this potentially deadly disease.

## SYMPTOM MANAGEMENT AND SUPPORTIVE CARE

Sexual functioning can be affected following removal of the bladder. Men may be impotent even if the procedure is a nerve-sparing one. Treatment options for these patients are the same as for men undergoing a radical prostatectomy. For women, the removal of the tubes and ovaries can lead to vaginal dryness, decreased libido, and discomfort with intercourse (because part of the vagina is removed). There can also be a psychological component to the changes in sexual functioning. A change in body image can affect the person's relationship with others.

Patients may not be open or comfortable discussing urinary issues. Sensitivity by the nurse of a patient's culture, body image, self-awareness, and esteem may facilitate a more relaxing and beneficial discussion of urinary tract issues and sexual function.

## CONCLUSION

Bladder cancer is a disease that affects individuals in the prime of their lives. Nurses working with these patients are in a unique position to help the patient, significant other, and family through major surgery and the changes that come along with the cystectomy and urinary diversion. By being open to the issues and concerns that patients voice, nurses can provide suggestions on how to deal with these issues and improve their quality of life. Oncology nurses are integral in transporting evidenced-based care to the bedside.

## REFERENCES


1. American Cancer Society. *Cancer Facts and Figures 2009.* Atlanta, GA: American Cancer Society; 2009.
2. Jemal A, Siegel R, Ward E, Hao Y, Xu J, Thun MJ. Cancer statistics, 2009. *CA: Cancer J Clin.* 2009;59:225–249.
3. Castelao JE, Yuan JM, Skipper PL, et al. Gender and smoking-related bladder cancer risk. *J Natl Cancer Inst.* 2001;93:538–545.
4. Creel P. Bladder cancer: epidemiology, diagnosis, and treatment. *Semin Oncol Nurs.* 2007;23:4(suppl 3):S3-S10.
5. Leppert JT, Shuarts O, Kawaoka K, et al. Prevention of bladder cancer: a review. *Eur Urol.* 2006;49:226–234.
6. Koutros S, Lynch CF, Ma X, et al. Heterocyclic aromatic amine pesticide use and human cancer risk: results from the U.S. agricultural health study. *Int J Cancer.* 2009;124:1206–1212.
7. Pelucchi C, LaVecchia C. Alcohol, coffee, and bladder cancer risk: a review of epidemiological studies. *Eur J Cancer Prev.* 2009;18:62–68.
8. Larsson SC, Andersson SO, Johansson JE, Wolk A. Cultured milk, yogurt, and diary intake in relation to bladder cancer risk in a prospective study of Swedish women and men. *Am J Clin Nutr.* 2008;88:1083–1087.
9. Colli JL, Knox M, Clayton D, Martin B, Waits J, Amling CL. Bladder cancer incidence and mortality rates compared to ecological factors in the United States. *J Urol* [Abstract 460]. 2009;181(Suppl):65.
10. Steinmaus C, Yuan Y, Bates MN, Smith AH. Case-control study of bladder cancer and drinking water arsenic in the western United States. *Am J Epidemiol.* 2003;158:1193–1201.
11. Lin J, Spitz MR, Dinney CP, Etzel CJ, Grossman HB, Wu X. Bladder cancer risk as modified by family history and smoking. *Cancer.* 2006;107:705–711.
12. Skeldon S, Semotiuk K, Gallinger S, Cotterchio M, Jewett M, Zlotta A. MSH2 mutations and bladder cancer risk: family members of hereditary nonpolyposis colorectal cancer (HNPCC) patients with MSH2 mutations are at increased risk not only for upper urinary tract transitional cell carcinoma (TCC) but also bladder cancer. *Eur Urol* [Abstract 876]. 2008;7(Suppl.):290.
13. Geoffroy-Perez B, Cordier S. Fluid consumption and the risk of bladder cancer: results of a multicenter case-controlled study. *Int J Cancer.* 2001;93:880–887.
14. Silverman DT, Alguacil J, Rothman N, et al. Does increased urination frequency protect against bladder cancer. *Int J Cancer.* 2008;123:1644–1648.
15. Tang L, Zirpoli GR, Guru K, et al. Consumption of raw cruciferous vegetables is inversely associated with bladder cancer risk. *Cancer Epidemiol Biomarkers Prev.* 2008;17:938–944.

16. Leppert JT, Shuvarts O, Kawaoka K, et al. Prevention of bladder cancer: a review. *Eur Urol.* 2006;49:226–234.
17. U.S. Preventive Services Task Force (USPSTF). *Screening for Bladder Cancer in Adults: Recommendation Statement.* Rockville, MD: Agency for Healthcare Research and Quality (AHRQ); June 2004. http://www.ahrq.gov/clinic/3rduspstf/bladder/blacanrs.htm. Accessed July 9, 2009.
18. National Comprehensive Cancer Network. NCCN practice guidelines in oncology. Vol. 1, 2009. http://www.nccn.org/professional/physician_gls/f_guidelines.asp. Accessed October 23,2009.
19. Urinary bladder. In: Greene FL, Page DL, Fleming ID, et al, eds. *AJCC Cancer Staging Manual.* 6th ed. New York: Springer; 2002:335–340.
20. Khadra MH, Pickard RS, Charlton M, et al. A prospective analysis of 1,930 patients with hematuria to evaluate current diagnostic practice. *J Urol.* 2000;163:524–527.
21. Steinberg GD, Kim HL, Sachdeva K, et al. Bladder cancer. eMedicine Web site. http://www.emedicine.com/MED/topic2344.htm. Accessed July 9, 2009.
22. Black PC, Brown GA, Dinney CP. Molecular markers of urothelial cancer and their use in the monitoring of superficial urothelial cancer. *J Clin Oncol.* 2006;24:5528–5535.
23. May M, Hakenberg OW, Gunia S, et al. Comparative diagnostic value of urine cytology, UBC-ELISA, and fluorescence in situ hybridization for detection of transitional cell carcinoma of urinary bladder in routine clinical practice. *Urology.* 2007;70:449–453.
24. Jafri SZ, Dinan D, Francis IR, et al. Follow up imaging of bladder carcinoma. National Guideline Clearinghouse. http://www.guideline.gov. Accessed September 23, 2009.
25. Epstein JI, Amin MB, Reuter VR, Mostofi FK. The World Health Organization/International Society of Urological Pathology consensus classification of urothelial (transitional cell) neoplasms of the urinary bladder. Bladder Consensus Conference Committee. *Am J Surg Pathol.* 1998;22:1435–1448.
26. Smith D, Montie J, Sandler H. Carcinoma of the bladder. In: Abeloff M, Armitage J, Niederhuber J, Kastan M, McKenna W, eds. *Abeloff's Clinical Oncology.* 4th ed. Philadelphia: Elsevier; 2008:1635–1649.
27. Ries LAG, Melbert D, Krapcho M, et al, eds. *SEER Cancer Statistics Review, 1975–2004.* Bethesda, MD: National Cancer Institute. http://seer.cancer.gov/csr/1975_2004/. Accessed July 9, 2009.
28. National Cancer Institute, U.S. National Institutes of Health. Bladder cancer PDQ®. http://www.cancer.gov/cancertopics/pdq/treatment/bladder/healthprofessional/allpages. Accessed January 17, 2009.
29. Parekh DJ, Bochner BH, Dalbagni G. Superficial and muscle-invasive bladder cancer: principles of management for outcomes assessments. *J Clin Oncol.* 2006;24:5519–5527.
30. Gudjonsson S, Adell L, Merdasa F, Olsson R, Larsson B, Davidsson T. Should all patients with non-muscle-invasive bladder cancer receive early intravesical chemotherapy after transurethral resection? The results of a prospective randomised multicentre study. *Eur Urol.* 2009;55(4)773–780.
31. Wood LS, Calabrese D. Bladder cancer and kidney cancer. In: Yarbro CH, Frogge MH, Goodman M, eds. *Cancer Nursing, Principles and Practice.* 6th ed. Sudbury, MA: Jones and Bartlett; 2005:1005–1021.
32. Grossman HB, O'Donnell MA, Cookson MS, Greenberg RE, Keane TE. Bacillus Calmette-Guerin failures and beyond: contemporary management of non-muscle-invasive bladder cancer. *Rev Urol.* 2008;10:281–289.
33. Lamm DL, McGee WR, Hale K. Bladder cancer: current optimal intravesical treatment. *Urol Nurs.* 2005;25:323–326, 331–332.
34. Herr H, Konety B, Stein J, Sternberg CN, Wood DP. Optimizing outcomes at every stage of bladder cancer: do we practice it? *Urol Oncol.* 2009:27:72–74.
35. Washburn DJ. Intravesical antineoplastic therapy following transurethral resection of bladder tumors: nursing implications from the operating room to discharge. *Clin J Oncol Nurs.* 2007;11:553–559.
36. Wo JY, Shipley WU, Dahl DM, et al. The results of concurrent chemoradiotherapy for recurrence after treatment with bacillus calmette-guerin for non-muscle-invasive bladder cancer: is immediate cystectomy always necessary? *BJU Int.* 2009;104(2):179–183.
37. Gore JL, Lai J, Setodji CM, Litwin MS, Saigal CS. Mortality increases when radical cystectomy is delayed more than 12 weeks: results from a Surveillance, Epidemiology and End Results-Medicare analysis. *Cancer.* 2009;115:988–996.
38. Montie JE, Marcovich R. Selecting and counseling patients for cystectomy or cystoprostatectomy. In: Kursh ED, Ulchaker JC, eds. *Office Urology: The Clinician's Guide.* Totowa, NJ: Humana Press; 2001:203–212.
39. Kaufman DS, Winter KA, Shipley WU, et al. Phase I-II RTOG study (99–06) of patients with muscle-invasive bladder cancer undergoing transurethral surgery, paclitaxel, cisplatin, and twice-daily radiotherapy followed by selective bladder preservation or radical cystectomy and adjuvant chemotherapy. *Urology.* 2009;73:833–837.
40. Calabro F, Sternberg CN. Neoadjuvant and adjuvant chemotherapy in muscle-invasive bladder cancer. *Eur Urol.* 2009;55:348–358.
41. Sonpavde G, Amiel GE, Mims MP, Hayes TG, Lerner SP. Neoadjuvant chemotherapy preceding cystectomy for bladder cancer. *Expert Opin Pharmacother.* 2008;9:1885–1893.
42. Yafi FA, Steinberg JR, Kassouf W. Contemporary management of muscle-invasive bladder cancer. *Int J Clin Oncol.* 2008;13:504–509.
43. Stenzl A, Cowan NC, DeSantis M, et al. The updated EAU guidelines on muscle-invasive and metastatic bladder cancer. *Eur Urol.* 2009;55(4)815–825..
44. Grossman HB, Natale RB, Tangen CM, et al. Neoadjuvant chemotherapy plus cystectomy compared with cystectomy alone for locally advanced bladder cancer. *N Engl J Med.* 2003;349:859–866.
45. Cohen SM, Goel A, Phillips J, Ennis DE, Grossbard ML. The role of perioperative chemotherapy in the treatment of urothelial cancer. *Oncologist.* 2006;11:630–640.
46. Sherif A, Holmberg L, Rintala E, et al. Neoadjuvant cisplatinum based combination chemotherapy in patients with invasive bladder cancer: a combined analysis of two Nordic studies. *Eur Urol.* 2004;45:297–303.
47. Winquist E, Kirchner TS, Segal R, et al. Neoadjuvant chemotherapy for transitional cell carcinoma of the bladder: a systematic review and meta-analysis. *J Urol.* 2004;171:561–569.
48. von der Maase H, Sengelov L, Roberts JT, et al. Long-term survival results of a randomized trial comparing gemcitabine plus cisplatinum with methotrexate, vinblastine, doxorubicin, plus cisplatinum in patients with bladder cancer. *J Clin Oncol.* 2005;23:4602–4608.
49. Lehmann J, Suttmann H, Albers P, et al. Surgery for metastatic urothelial carcinoma with curative intent: the German experience (AUO AB 30/05). *Eur Urol.* 2008;55:1293–1299.
50. Garcia JA, Dreicer R. Systemic chemotherapy for advanced bladder cancer: update and controversies. *J Clin Oncol.* 2006;24:5545–5551.
51. Shelton G. Introduction. *Semin Oncol Nurs.* 2007;23:4(suppl 3):S1-S2.
52. Kaufman DS. Challenges in the treatment of bladder cancer. *Ann Oncol.* 2006;17(suppl 5):v106-v112.
53. Bamias A, Tiliakos I, Karali MD, et al. Systemic chemotherapy in inoperable or metastatic bladder cancer. *Ann Oncol.* 2006;17:553–561.
54. Manchen E. Emerging agents for the treatment of advanced bladder cancer. *Semin Oncol Nurs.* 2007;23:4(suppl 3):S11-S14.

CHAPTER 48

Sara Bhagat Foxson, MSN, CRNP, AOCN®
Jennie Greco Lattimer, MSN, CRNP, AOCN®
Barbara Felder, MSN, CRNP, AOCNP®

# Breast Cancer

## INTRODUCTION

Breast cancer is the most frequently diagnosed cancer in women, accounting for 27% of all new cases of cancer among females in 2009. It is the leading cause of death due to cancer for women aged 20 to 59 and is second to lung cancer as the leading cause of cancer deaths in women of all ages. Also, it is estimated that in 2009, 1,910 males will be diagnosed with breast cancer, and 440 will die from the disease.[1] The incidence of breast cancer has risen steadily for decades, but 2008 marked the first decrease in breast cancer incidence since 1980, particularly for small (<2 cm), estrogen receptor (ER) positive tumors.[2] Research indicates that these trends correlate with increasing rates of mammography screening and decreasing use of postmenopausal hormone replacement therapy (HRT). Mammography screening increased from 1980 to 1993 but has leveled off since then; HRT increased from 1988 to 2002 and then dropped by 75%. The incidence of large tumors or advanced-stage disease did not decline during this same time period.[3]

## EPIDEMIOLOGY

Currently, in the US, a woman's lifetime risk for developing breast cancer is 12.8%, or 1 out of every 8 women will be diagnosed with the disease in her lifetime. The incidence of breast cancer increases with age, increases more slowly between the ages of 45 and 50, and then rises steadily with each year to the age of 85. More than 50% of all breast cancers occur in women over the age of 61.[4]

Caucasian women over the age of 40 have a higher incidence of breast cancer than African American women. African American women under the age of 40 have a higher incidence of breast cancer than Caucasian women and are more likely to die from breast cancer at any age. Caucasian women tend to be diagnosed with small (<2 cm), local tumors. Women from racial and ethnic groups other than Caucasian or African American have a lower incidence of breast cancer, but women from all minority groups tend to be diagnosed with advanced or metastatic disease and have a higher mortality rate.[2]

The death rate from breast cancer in women has declined steadily since 1990.[5] The number of breast cancer deaths among women in 2009 is estimated to be 40,170.[1] Currently, the 5-year survival rate of women with breast cancer is 89%, an increase of 12% since 1975. The survival rate at 10 years after diagnosis is 81% and at 15 years is 73%.[2] The decrease in both incidence and mortality of female breast cancer can be attributed to a better understanding of risk factors and prevention, improved screening methods, and the development of new treatments. However, the mortality rate for breast cancer in African American women of all ages is higher than that of Caucasian women, and the 5-year survival rate for African American women with all stages of breast cancer is lower than Caucasian women.[5] These factors and the recent drop in the rate of mammography screening provide opportunities and direction for oncology nurses to educate and care for their patients.[6]

The interdisciplinary team utilizes a variety of clinical, histological, and pathological findings to define, as precisely as possible, the particular characteristics of a breast cancer that will determine the most appropriate treatment plan for a given patient. This approach integrates the physical examination with the histopathological characteristics of the tumor, and it incorporates the patient's personal bias based on her emotional needs and physical preferences. As a member of this team, the nurse must be aware of the factors affecting the selection of the treatment plan and appropriately educate the patient regarding the various treatment strategies in an effort to prevent and manage complications of the disease and its treatment.

## ETIOLOGY

The etiology of breast cancer is thought to be multifactorial, with genetic and nongenetic, and modifiable and nonmodifiable components. As populations with a higher incidence of breast cancer are studied, potentially causative genetic, hormonal, or biochemical factors may emerge. Such epidemiological features, when statistically correlated with incidence of disease, identify risk factors for the disease. Hormone exposure (endogenous and exogenous), family or personal history of breast cancer, lifestyle factors, and exposure to radiation are broad categories that are associated with an increased risk for breast cancer.[7] These include modifiable and nonmodifiable factors. See Table 48-1[8] for established breast cancer risk factors.

### HORMONAL FACTORS

Exposure to ovarian hormones has long been recognized as a major factor in the development of breast cancer. This relationship is well demonstrated in that gender is the most significant risk factor for the development of the disease. Women are 100 times more likely to develop breast cancer than men.[9]

Age is the second most significant risk factor for the development of breast cancer.[4] This correlates with length of exposure to ovarian hormones. Breast cancer rarely occurs in women younger than 20 and then steadily advances with age. The current lifetime risk for a woman living in the US to be diagnosed with breast cancer is 12.3% (1 in 8). The lifetime risk for the disease in the 1970s was 1 in 11. This increase is thought to be due to a longer life expectancy, increased use of hormone replacement therapy (HRT) during most of this period, and the increasing prevalence of obesity.[4]

**TABLE 48-1**

**Established Breast Cancer Risk Factors**

| Risk Factor | Magnitude of Risk | Notes |
|---|---|---|
| Age ≥ 50 vs < 50 | 6.5 | The strongest risk factor |
| Number of first-degree relatives with breast cancer | 1.4–13.6 | Family history is the second strongest risk factor after age |
| Age at menarche < 12 vs ≥ 14 | 1.2–1.5 | Menarche at ages 12–13 has a smaller effect and is not listed |
| Age at menopause (≥ 55 vs < 55) | 1.5–2.0 | Years from menarche measures long-term estrogen exposure |
| Age at first live birth > 30 vs < 20 | 1.3–2.2 | First live birth at ages 20–30 has a smaller effect and is not listed |
| Previous breast biopsy (whether positive or negative) | 1.5–1.8 | |
| Lobular carcinoma in situ | 5.4–11 × general population; 18% after 20 years | A risk factor and nonobligate precursor for invasive or intraductal carcinoma |
| At least 1 biopsy with atypical hyperplasia | 4.0–4.4 | |
| Hormone replacement therapy | 1.5 | |
| Radiation to chest area | Up to 20-fold increase at age 32 | Data from A-bomb survivors<br>Radiation for Hodgkin's disease also increases risk |
| High mammographic breast density | 1.8- to 6-fold | May be hereditary, a Claus risk assessment may be worthwhile |
| Alcohol use > 15 g/day | 2.5-fold | |
| Alcohol 1.5 drinks per day | 1.3 | |
| Postmenopausal BMI | 1.19 for each 5 kg/m rise in BMI | Perhaps attributed to associated increase in estrogen, especially bioavailable estradiol |

*Abbreviation*: BMI, body mass index.

*Source*: Reprinted with permission from Hulka and Moorman.[8]

The total duration of exposure to endogenous estrogen and its metabolites seems to significantly increase the risk for breast cancer.[10] Consequently, early menarche (<12 years), late menopause (>55 years), nulliparity or older age at first full-term pregnancy (>30 years), and fewer full-term pregnancies increase a woman's exposure to reproductive hormones and her risk of breast cancer.[7] Breast feeding, particularly of longer duration, has been shown to decrease breast cancer risk. There is no evidence to indicate that induced abortion increases risk of breast cancer.[8,11]

Exogenous hormones present in HRT have been implicated in increasing the risk of breast cancer. The combination of estrogen and progesterone was frequently used through the late 1990s to treat the symptoms of menopause and is likely associated with the increased incidence of breast cancer during that period.[10] The Women's Health Initiative (WHI) is a large, ongoing, randomized study to investigate strategies to reduce heart disease, breast cancer, colorectal cancer, and fractures in postmenopausal women (161,809 women aged 50 to 79). The study is divided into several trials focusing on low-fat dietary patterns, calcium and vitamin D intake, and hormone use—2 trials involving (1) either 0.625 mg estrogen plus 2.5 mg progestin or placebo (for women with a uterus) and (2) either estrogen alone or placebo (for women with a hysterectomy). The estrogen and progestin arm (16,608 women) was stopped after 5.2 years due to a small but statistical increased risk of breast cancer, coronary heart disease (CHD) events (fatal and nonfatal), stroke, and pulmonary embolism. Although there was a reduction in fractures and colorectal cancer and a smaller reduction in endometrial cancer, the results indicated that combined HRT is not a recommended intervention for primary prevention. Note that the increased risk in breast cancer applies only to current HRT users and those who stopped taking HRT less than 5 years earlier. The risk of breast cancer for women who stopped HRT use more than 5 years earlier is no different than that for women who never used HRT.[12,13] The estrogen-only trial was stopped in February 2004, and a March 2004 release noted that the estrogen-only arm had been stopped due to the finding of an increased risk for stroke among participants as well as the failure to identify any cardioprotective properties.

The US Preventive Services Task Force recommends against using HRT for chronic illnesses such as osteoporosis.[14] If a woman and her health care provider feel that HRT is appropriate to treat menopausal symptoms, it should be prescribed at the lowest dose for the shortest duration. The risks and benefits of HRT should be clearly discussed before initiating therapy.

The concern surrounding prescribing HRT for premenopausal breast cancer survivors remains a problematic issue for clinicians. The number of survivors has increased steadily and includes a growing population of women who are "forced" into menopause through chemotherapeutic agents. The premenopausal women who experience an acute, early menopause seem to report more severe symptoms than premenopausal women who experience gradual, natural hormonal decreases over time. Although a majority of these women will enjoy disease-free survival (DFS), their quality of life may be compromised by somatic complaints caused by the dramatic drop in estrogen levels (eg, hot flashes, dyspareunia, and labile mood swings) and physical manifestations (eg, osteoporosis and possible heart disease). Observational studies have demonstrated that HRT may remedy or reduce osteoporosis, ischemic heart disease, vasomotor symptoms, and urogenital atrophy in these young women, but healthcare providers remain reluctant to prescribe it. Giving breast cancer survivors' estrogen therapy is a controversial issue, as the current standard of practice generally precludes prescribing these hormonal agents and the WHI results will likely give added credence to existing practice.[15,16]

Oral contraceptives have also been studied as a possible risk factor for the development of breast cancer. Women who have not taken oral contraceptives for more than 10 years are at no greater risk than women who have never taken oral contraceptives. However, there is an increased risk for breast cancer among women who have taken oral contraceptives for prolonged (> 10 years) periods of time.[11]

## FAMILY HISTORY

Approximately 70% of women who develop breast cancer have no known risk factors. Their disease is considered sporadic (no history of breast cancer through 2 generations). However, women with a family history of breast cancer, especially in first-degree relatives (mother, sister, and daughter), are at increased risk for developing the disease. The risk increases further if more than one first-degree relative has breast cancer or was young (<40 years) at the time of diagnosis. Familial breast cancer is thought to result from an interaction of common lifestyles among families and underlying genetic susceptibility.[16]

Approximately 5% to 10% of breast cancers are thought to be hereditary. Hereditary or genetic breast cancer is defined as a positive family history, often with related cancers (eg, ovarian), consistent with an autosomal dominant factor that includes onset at an early age (average 45), an excess of bilaterality, male breast cancer, and other multiple cancers.[17] Two autosomal dominant gene mutations have been isolated—one on chromosome 17q and another on chromosome 13q that can inactivate tumor suppressor genes.[18,19] Two breast/ovarian cancer susceptibility gene mutations (*BRCA1* and *BRCA2*) have been mapped and cloned. The first mutation identified *BRCA1* (BReast CAncer 1), lies on the long arm of chromosome 17 (17q12–21); *BRCA2* is located on the long arm of chromosome 13 (13q12–13).[19,20]

Inheritance of the *BRCA1* and *BRCA2* susceptibility genes is often associated with a high penetrance (likelihood that the effect of the mutation will result in the disease) for families with multiple breast and ovarian cancers. These gene mutations follow an autosomal dominant pattern, meaning that the mutation can be passed from either parent to a child and that each child (male or female) has a 50% likelihood of inheritance. Given that the science of genetics is constantly evolving, risk estimates can vary depending on the locus of the mutation or ethnicity and should be interpreted with care. These breast cancer susceptibility genes are present in less than 1% of the general population, but the risk for developing invasive breast cancer for their carriers is 41% to 90%.[21] Women who have inherited a mutation on *BRCA1* or *BRCA2* may have up to an 85% risk of developing breast cancer by age 70. The risk for developing ovarian cancer varies from 26% to 54% for *BRCA1* to approximately 27% for *BRCA2*.[22,23] Mutation carriers diagnosed with breast or ovarian cancer have additional risks of developing a second cancer (ovarian, contralateral breast, or primary breast cancer). They also have an increased risk for male breast cancer, prostate, pancreatic, and fallopian tube cancers.[24] The search continues for other genes that confer breast cancer susceptibility, but no probable candidate has been confirmed at this time.[25,26]

The *BRCA1* and *BRCA2* gene mutations are more common among people with an eastern European (Ashkenazi Jewish) background. Three mutations have been identified that are linked with Ashkenazi Jewish heredity, 2 on *BRCA1* and 1 on *BRCA2*. The mutation occurs in 1 in 200 women in the general population and in 1 in 40 women of eastern European descent.[27] The risk of developing breast cancer for this group was initially estimated to be 56% by age 70, and the risk for ovarian cancer is estimated to be 16%.[28] These figures are considerably lower than those for more heterogenous populations. A report from King and colleagues examined 1,008 index cases and reported that the lifetime risk for Ashkenazi women is 82% for breast cancer and 54% for ovarian cancer.[24]

Current information indicates that *BRCA1* and *BRCA2* are responsible for most or all hereditary ovarian cancers but not all hereditary breast cancers.[28] Other, presumably low-penetrance gene variants are thought to be responsible for moderate increases in breast cancer risk. Among these are mutations in *ATM* (ataxia telangiectasia mutated), *Chk2* (checkpoint kinase 2), *p53* (associated with Li-Fraumeni syndrome), and *PTEN* (associated with Cowden disease). *BRCA1* is phosphorylated by *ATM* and *Chk2* in response to DNA damage. All of these genes are components of the cell cycle repair pathway affecting *BRCA1* and *BRCA2*.[29–31]

For the woman who has breast cancer, there is a 0.7% to 0.8% per year risk of developing a second primary breast cancer.[32] Variables that may alter the risk of developing a contralateral breast cancer include a personal early age of onset, having a first-degree relative with early-onset or bilateral disease, or a genetic mutation. Treatment with chemotherapy and/or hormones for breast cancer may reduce the development of a second breast cancer.

Some of the inherited breast cancer mutations are identifiable by molecular testing. However, these tests are expensive and not always covered by medical insurance, and their interpretation is complicated and can be emotionally charged. Many university settings or large community hospitals with dedicated breast cancer centers offer programs for women at high risk for developing breast cancer. These programs are usually staffed by medical and surgical oncologists, genetic counselors, specially trained advanced practice nurses (APNs), and gynecologic oncologists who can guide patients through the process of testing and appropriate interventions that may include prophylactic mastectomy or oophorectomy. The American Cancer Society (ACS) and the American Society for Clinical Oncology strongly urge people who believe they are at high risk to seek the guidance of such programs.[4]

## LIFESTYLE FACTORS

There is convincing evidence that obesity, alcohol consumption, and sedentary lifestyle are risk factors for developing breast cancer.[7] Historically, because countries with high-fat diets have higher breast cancer rates than countries with low-fat diets, high-fat diets were thought to be a risk factor for breast cancer. However, studies have shown that there is no association between fat intake and risk for breast cancer.[33]

Obesity has been shown to increase the risk for breast cancer, particularly in postmenopausal women. The International Agency for Research estimates that obesity and a sedentary lifestyle are linked to 25% of breast cancer cases worldwide.[34] In a study completed in 2002, a weight gain of 55 pounds or more after the age of 18 was found to increase the risk of breast cancer by 18%. A 22 pound weight loss after menopause was associated with a 57% reduction in breast cancer risk.[35] Results from the Women's Health Initiative observational study and the Nurses' Health Study both show that obese postmenopausal women (BMI > 31.1) have a significantly increased risk for developing breast cancer.[36] The mechanism for this increased risk is thought to be related to estrogen production. In postmenopausal women, androgens are converted to estrogen in adipose tissue. It is likely that more of this conversion occurs in obese women.[37] Obesity is a modifiable risk factor. Nurses are instrumental in providing education, support, and encouragement to assist women with weight-reduction programs. Many versions of diet and exercise programs exist that can meet the particular needs of most women who are motivated to reduce their risk of breast cancer as well as improve cardiovascular status.

Conversely, there is mounting evidence that exercise reduces the risk of breast cancer.[38,39] The risk reduction ranged from 10% to 70% for women who exercised most vigorously. The average reduction in risk was 30% to 40% for women who exercised 3 to 4 hours per week. Menopausal status was not a factor in the risk reduction. The mechanism for the relationship between physical activity and reduced breast cancer risk is not clearly understood at this time but is believed to be related to hormones and energy balance.[34,40]

Recent studies indicate that alcohol consumption (more than 2 drinks or 24 g of alcohol per day) is associated with a 21% increased risk of developing breast cancer. The risk is dose dependent but independent of the type of alcohol consumed.[41,42] Alcohol is thought to be a component in the metabolic pathway of estrogen production. Thus, by increasing circulating estrogen levels, alcohol can increase the risk of breast cancer.[43] Women who consume alcohol should be counseled regarding the potential cancer risks. There are no studies that suggest a relationship between cigarette smoking and increased risk for breast cancer.[44]

## RACE, ETHNICITY, AND SOCIOECONOMIC STATUS

Race, ethnicity, and socioeconomic status have emerged as factors that can influence the risk and severity of breast cancer. In 2004, 8% of Caucasian American women, 24% of African American women, 22% of Latino women, 27% of American Indian or Alaskan native women, and 10% of Asian American women lived at a poverty level income. At that time, 11% of Caucasian American women, 19% of African American women, 33% of Latino women, 28% of American Indian or Alaskan natives, and 18% of Asian

American women had no health insurance. The combination of poverty and lack of health insurance negatively impacts access to screening, treatment options, delivery of care, and access to clinical trials. For example, from 1991 to 2004, the mammography prevalence of all women over 40 was 60%. For women with less than a high school education, the prevalence was 40%. For women with no health insurance, the prevalence of mammograms was 30%.[45] The lack of health insurance is also associated with advanced stage of breast cancer at diagnosis.[46] The 5-year survival rate for patients with lower incomes is consistently lower than patients with higher incomes at every stage of the disease.[47,48] In addition to access to care, race, ethnicity, and socioeconomic status are associated with a higher incidence of comorbidities and aggressive tumor characteristics, especially among African American women.[49,50]

## RADIATION

The carcinogenic effects of both low-dose and high-dose ionizing radiation have been well documented. Exposure to ionizing radiation from nuclear accidents or medical procedures increases the risk of breast cancer, especially if the exposure occurred before the age of 40.[51] Women who received mantle radiation for the treatment of Hodgkin's disease, especially if they were younger than 15 when treated, are at a markedly higher risk for developing breast cancer.[52] They should be made aware of this high risk and followed closely by health care professionals with a stringent screening schedule.

The concern about the effects of radiation has generated some apprehension regarding the potential harm of repeated mammograms and chest radiographs. A cumulative exposure greater than 100 cGy is associated with an increase in risk. The doses for these procedures are extremely small, and the potential benefit far outweighs the risk. A mammogram emits a dose of 0.2 to 0.4 cGy per study, and a chest film generates approximately 0.002 cGy to each breast.[53,54]

## CLINICAL FEATURES OF THE BREAST

Clinical features of the breast that increase the risk of breast cancer include breast density and benign breast abnormalities. High breast tissue density (a mammographic finding that compares the amount of glandular tissue to fatty tissue in the breast) was associated with a 4-fold to 6-fold increase in the risk of developing breast cancer in several studies.[55,56] Results from a recent study show that premenopausal women or women younger than 50 who tend to have dense breasts may benefit from digital rather than film mammograms.[57]

Benign breast abnormalities can be separated into 2 groups: nonproliferative lesions and proliferative lesions. Nonproliferative lesions, such as simple cysts, are not a risk factor for breast cancer. Proliferative lesions are further categorized as those without atypia and those with atypia. Proliferative lesions without atypia, such as fibroadenoma exhibit excessive growth of normal ductal or lobular cells and increase the risk of developing breast cancer 1.5-fold to 2-fold. Proliferative lesions with atypia show excessive growth of cells that are abnormal and increase the risk of breast cancer 4 to 5 times. Atypical ductal hyperplasia (ADH) and atypical lobular hyperplasia (ALH) are included in this category. A woman with ADH or ALH and a family history of breast cancer has higher risk for developing breast cancer.[58,59]

Lobular carcinoma in situ (LCIS) is another abnormality that is considered to be a risk factor for breast cancer. Lobular carcinoma in situ lesions are associated with increased risk within both breasts but this abnormality is not considered a premalignant condition.[60] LCIS is characterized by a proliferation of cells that remain in the breast lobules and confers an increased risk of 1% per year for developing breast cancer.[61] This uncommon finding occurs predominately in premenopausal women, with an average age at diagnosis of 44 to 47 years.[62] LCIS is usually not detected by palpation or mammography, but rather is most often an incidental microscopic finding when breast tissue is removed for another reason. Current evidence suggests that LCIS functions as a marker of increased risk for developing an invasive ductal (more common) or lobular (less common) cancer.[63] Mastectomy for LCIS should be considered a prophylactic procedure rather than therapeutic.[61,64] Because many observations have concluded that most women with LCIS do not develop breast cancer, clinicians increasingly believe that LCIS may be treated with local excision and close follow up that employs mammograms twice a year and clinical exam every 3 to 4 months. Improvements in mammography sensitivity have made this approach more feasible. Women who are unable or unwilling to comply with frequent monitoring may opt for a unilateral or bilateral mastectomy with or without reconstruction.

## RISK ASSESSMENT TOOLS

There are several assessment tools that can be used to measure the risk of developing invasive breast cancer. The Breast Cancer Risk Assessment Tool is an interactive tool available on the internet (http://www.cancer.gov/bcrisktool/) that was developed by the National Cancer Institute (NCI) and the National Surgical Adjuvant Breast and Bowel Project (NSABP). This tool is based on the Gail model and covers the areas of personal history of breast cancer, age, age at menarche, age at first live birth, family history of breast cancer, number of breast biopsies, and race/ethnicity. This model estimates a woman's risk of developing breast cancer in the next 5 years and up to age 90 (lifetime risk). The tool has been found to be accurate for estimating a woman's lifetime risk for developing breast cancer but it cannot predict which women will actually develop the disease.[65]

The Gail model is an assessment tool that calculates the risk of invasive breast cancer within a specific time frame. The risk factor data were initially extrapolated from the Breast Cancer Detection Demonstration project and modified for the National Surgical Breast and Bowel Program prevention trial (NSABP P-1). The Gail model has been validated for Caucasian women and has been tested in the Women's Health Initiative for African American women. It is believed to slightly underestimate risk for African American women and has not yet been validated for Hispanic or Asian women. The Gail model is used as a screening tool, but neither the Gail nor the NCI model captures several elements of potential risk—namely, age of relatives' diagnosis, history of bilateral cancer, breast cancer in second-degree relatives, and history of ovarian cancer.[66,67]

The Claus model for breast cancer risk was developed to address some of these deficits.[68] Using data from the Cancer and Steroid Hormone Study, this model gives the age-specific risk for a woman with a family history of one or more relatives. Neither the NCI model that is based on the Gail model nor the Claus model is appropriate for breast cancer mutation carriers. The Myriad tables and the BRCAPRO tool, both of which evaluate mutations, can be used to assess high-risk individuals. The BRCAPRO tool is a statistical model used to calculate the probability of a genetic mutation based on family history that includes second-degree relatives, bilateral breast cancer, and ovarian cancer.[69] The NCI-Gail model and the Claus model are based on the assumption that women are receiving breast exams and screening mammograms and should be used only as part of the discussion about risk.

### NURSING IMPLICATIONS

Timely and appropriate nursing interventions have the potential to lower the risk of breast cancer. Those individuals with nonmodifiable risk factors, such as age, female gender, and positive family history, can be identified and educated regarding their increased risk. They can also be encouraged to follow the appropriate screening schedule and possible genetic testing.

Modifiable risk factors provide many opportunities for nursing interventions. Nurses can identify risk factors among individuals and then educate regarding healthy life styles, including weight reduction for obese patients, the role of exercise in preventing cancer, and moderation in alcohol use. Nurses can educate perimenopausal patients about the recently established link between prolonged HRT and increased risk for breast cancer, and counsel these patients about possible alternatives for managing menopausal symptoms.

In spite of the well-established efficacy of mammograms in detecting breast cancer, the prevalence of this imaging modality has slightly decreased recently among all women, as discussed above. Women of lower socioeconomic status and women from minorities have historically had lower rates of mammograms. In addition, these women, particularly African American women, are diagnosed at a later stage and have lower survival rates than Caucasian women. These trends underscore the need for ongoing education and facilitation for proper screening among all populations.

## PREVENTION, SCREENING, AND EARLY DETECTION

Breast cancer is known to be a slow-growing malignancy caused by the interaction of hormonal, genetic, lifestyle, and environmental factors. Approximately 65% of women with breast cancer have no known risk factors and 85% have no family history of the disease.[70] Guidelines for prevention, screening, and early detection have been established in an effort to prevent or detect breast cancer at an early stage. Recommendations for women at high risk for the development of breast cancer who have genetic or hereditary predisposition include chemoprevention, prophylactic surgery, and genetic counseling. Chemoprevention or prophylactic surgery is also recommended for women at high risk due to family or personal history of breast cancer. Lifestyle modifications and appropriate surveillance are recommended for all women, including those with low to average risk for the development of breast cancer.

### PREVENTION

#### Chemoprevention

Chemoprevention is the use of a chemical agent to prevent or alter the development of cancer. The development of a chemoprevention agent should be based on a disease model that identifies progressive development over several years and involves multiple factors that can be reversed. These interventions must be based on a biological rationale and have minimal toxic effects. Chemoprevention of breast cancer is directed at decreasing the exposure of breast tissue to ovarian hormones. Studies suggest that more than 2 million women in the US could benefit from chemoprevention.[71]

Tamoxifen is the first drug that was approved for the prevention of breast cancer. It is a selective estrogen receptor modulator (SERM) that binds to ERs in the breast, thus inhibiting uptake. It is an oral medication that is to be taken daily in a 20 mg dose. Tamoxifen was originally launched as a treatment for advanced breast cancer in postmenopausal women. Since then, tamoxifen has been found to be effective in the treatment of premenopausal women with advanced disease.[72–74] Tamoxifen has also been found to increase DFS in node-negative, ER positive disease[75] as well as node-positive disease.[72,76] Women taking tamoxifen for primary breast cancer have experienced a reduction in the expected incidence of contralateral breast cancer. This finding strengthened the belief in tamoxifen's chemoprotective effect, and led to its use in a large U.S. prevention trial through the National Surgical Adjuvant Breast and Bowel Program (NSABP).

Tamoxifen was studied as a chemopreventive agent in the NSABP P-1 trial from 1992 to 1997. More than 13,000 high-risk women who were 35 years or older were randomized to 5 years of tamoxifen or a placebo. After a 7 year follow-up period, the rate of invasive breast cancer for those women on the tamoxifen arm was reduced by 49% to 50%, with a similar risk reduction in premenopausal and postmenopausal women. Data regarding efficacy of tamoxifen among *BRCA* mutation carriers are conflicting, but it is commonly prescribed for carriers who have not undergone prophylactic mastectomies.[77]

The major toxicities of tamoxifen are increased risk of endometrial cancer and thromboembolic events, especially among women older than 50 years of age. Other side effects include accelerated cataract formation, amenorrhea or oligomennorhea, and menopausal symptoms such as hot flashes. A beneficial effect of tamoxifen is a decrease in hip, radius, and spine fractures.[78]

Raloxifene (Evista) is the second drug approved by the FDA for the prevention of invasive breast cancer. Like tamoxifen, it is an SERM. While studying raloxifene for the prevention and treatment of osteoporosis in postmenopausal women, researchers noted that it seemed to lower the incidence of invasive breast cancer in this group.[79] The second breast cancer prevention trial, NSABP P-2 or the Study of Tamoxifen and Raloxifene (STAR) opened in 1999. More than 19,000 women who were postmenopausal and had a high risk of breast cancer (>1.67 Gail risk model) participated. Early results indicated that raloxifene, like tamoxifen, reduced the risk of invasive breast cancer by 50%. However, raloxifene does not lower the risk for noninvasive breast cancer or LCIS. It was approved by the FDA in September, 2007 for the prevention of invasive breast cancer among postmenopausal women at high risk.[80] Unlike tamoxifen, it is not indicated for the treatment of breast cancer. It is also a daily oral medication taken in a 50 mg dose. Side effects are similar to tamoxifen, but there is a lower risk of endometrial cancer and a higher risk of thromboembolic events.

Aromatase inhibitors (AIs) are another class of hormones that are being studied as chemopreventive agents. Aromatase is an enzyme that is active in the pathway of converting adrenal androgens and testosterone to estrogen. This conversion or aromatization occurs in adipose tissue, muscle, and the liver. Aromatase is also found in breast tissue and can synthesize estrogen in situ in that location. AIs block the synthesis of estrogen throughout the body. There are 2 classes of AIs: steroidal and nonsteroidal. The steroidal AI is exemestane (Aromasin). Anastrozole (Arimidex) and letrozole (Femara) are nonsteroidal. AIs are used only for postmenopausal women because in premenopausal women they can cause a gonadotropin surge resulting in increased estrogen levels.[81,82]

Aromatase inhibitors are currently used to treat breast cancer in the adjuvant and metastatic settings. Results from a large double-blind randomized trial (Anastrozole, Tamoxifen Alone and in Combination or the ATAC Trial) involving more than 9000 postmenopausal women with early stage breast cancer showed that the incidence of primary invasive breast cancer in the contralateral breast was 58% lower in the anastrozole alone arm.[83] In the MA-17 mammary gland trial, women with early stage breast cancer were given either letrozole or a placebo after 5 years of tamoxifen. There was a 39% reduction in the incidence of contralateral breast cancer in the letrozole arm.[84] Observations from the adjuvant trials have led to 2 large chemoprevention studies. In the MAP-3 (mammary glands prevention) trial, high-risk postmenopausal women are randomized to 5 years of exemestane or a placebo instead of tamoxifen. In the IBISII trial, anastrozole and a placebo are used. AIs are oral medications that are taken daily. Side effects include diffuse arthralgias and mylagias and mild menopausal symptoms. The incidence of endometrial cancer and thromboembolic events is less than that with tamoxifen, but AIs do not confer the same protection against osteoporosis.[85] Presently, tamoxifen is recommended for the prevention of breast cancer among premenopausal women and raloxifene for postmenopausal women.

## Prophylactic surgery

Prophylactic mastectomy is an effective prevention strategy for women at high risk for breast cancer. In the often cited study by Hartmann et al in 1999, there was a 90% risk reduction in the incidence of breast cancer among high-risk women with a family history who underwent bilateral prophylactic mastectomies.[86] Breast cancer has been known to occur in the chest wall or axillary region. It is therefore important for a woman to recognize that some risk of developing breast cancer exists after a prophylactic mastectomy, as breast cancer cells may extend to the clavicle, the latissimus, or the abdomen, and are not included in the mastectomy.[87] The control group in this study was composed of sisters of the women who underwent mastectomies. In a subsequent study, the *BRCA* status of the high-risk women was determined. The benefit of prophylactic mastectomies was confirmed among the mutation carriers as well.[86]

Results from several studies have shown that bilateral prophylactic mastectomy and salpingo-oophorectomy reduce the risk of both ovarian and breast cancers among

*BRCA* mutation carriers.[85,87–90] In addition to reducing the risk of these cancers, the surgery enables earlier diagnosis of ovarian cancer.

The patient must be presented with a clear, in-depth evaluation of her current and potential risk, stressing that although she may have a dramatically increased risk of breast cancer, there is no guarantee that she will develop disease in her lifetime. It is important for women to take adequate time in weighing the risks vs benefits of these procedures. The complications of prophylactic mastectomies are similar to those for other mastectomies. However, if reconstruction is added to this procedure, capsular contracture is another possibility. Additionally, the woman should be evaluated by a gynecological oncologist if she is considering an oophorectomy. As discussed above, a healthy lifestyle, including regular exercise, weight control or weight reduction, and decreased alcohol consumption, and avoiding prolonged use of HRT can all reduce the risk of developing breast cancer.

## SCREENING AND EARLY DETECTION

The goal of screening for breast cancer is to detect the disease at an early stage in asymptomatic individuals. For average-risk, asymptomatic women, the ACS recommends clinical breast exam (CBE) every 3 years from age 20 to 39, then annually, and annual mammograms starting at age 40.[91] Women with dense breasts, identified on conventional mammography, may benefit from digital mammograms. There is no age recommendation for stopping screening mammograms. This decision should be individualized and based on a risk-benefit analysis.[92] The position of the ACS is that breast self-exam (BSE) is optional, but that breast self-awareness can be more effective in detecting abnormalities than BSE. Women should be aware of the baseline appearance and nature of their breasts. They should report any changes to health care professionals, even if a mammogram was recently performed.

Currently, the ACS does not recommend the routine use of breast magnetic resonance imaging (MRI) as a screening tool for breast cancer. The ACS advises women with moderate risk (those with a history of LCIS, ductal carcinoma in situ (DCIS), ADH, or ALH, or dense breasts) to discuss the benefits of adding annual MRIs to their screening program. The ACS recommends the addition of annual breast MRIs to mammography for those women with a high risk for breast cancer (those with known *BRCA* mutations or a first-degree relative with a mutation, a history of radiation therapy (RT) to the chest between the ages of 10 and 30 years, or a personal or family history of Li-Fraumeni or Cowden syndrome).[93]

More than 95% of breast malignancies arise from cells that line the milk ducts. Ductal lavage is a technique that allows cells from milk ducts to be removed via a small catheter inserted through the nipple. Needle aspiration involves gentle suction applied to the nipple to obtain cells. Both of these techniques should ideally provide readily available samples for cytological evaluation with a minimum of discomfort to patients. However, these promising techniques have yielded disappointing results. Samples obtained often produce cellular material that is not adequate for cytological examination, and patients report discomfort from the procedures.[94,95]

## NURSING IMPLICATIONS

Oncology nurses, possibly more than any other members of the health care team, can educate and advocate for patients to receive appropriate screening, prevention, and treatment for breast cancer. Because of the high incidence and mortality and morbidity of breast cancer in this country, prevention and early detection of the disease should be a high priority among nurses.

Mammography has been identified as the most sensitive screening method for detecting early stage breast cancer, possibly years before the malignancy becomes symptomatic. As mentioned above, however, the prevalence of mammography has decreased in recent years, and it has always been lower in non-Caucasian and lower socioeconomic groups. Oncology nurses are in an excellent position to educate and encourage their patients to adhere to the appropriate screening schedule and to promote access to mammograms for patients of lower socioeconomic status. As their role unfolds, patient navigators may have a positive impact on the outcomes for these populations.[96]

Women at moderate or high risk for developing breast cancer should be advised of the more stringent screening schedules recommended for them. In addition to being educated about the implications of their risk, these patients may need to be referred for genetic testing and sent to a high-risk breast cancer center. Nurses may need to advocate for these patients to get insurance approval for additional testing and imaging. Women at risk are often anxious and require early intervention to learn to cope with the lifelong possibility of developing breast cancer.

Women who choose chemoprevention should be made aware of the side effects and risks of endocrine therapy. In addition to teaching patients about side effects, oncology nurses should manage the symptoms, such as hot flashes, and should make patients aware of symptoms to report such vaginal bleeding or limb swelling. Patients receiving AIs should be taught to adhere to appropriate osteoporosis screening and management. Patients of lower socioeconomic status may need assistance from their nurses in obtaining these medications.

Women at high risk for developing breast cancer, especially the *BRCA* mutation carriers, may choose prophylactic surgery. They need to be informed of their surgical options, including reconstruction possibilities, and possible complications such as bleeding, infection, decreased breast and nipple sensation and possible poor cosmetic outcomes. Also, prophylactic mastectomy does not confer complete protection against breast cancer since not all of the breast tissue can be surgically removed. Women who undergo prophylactic salpingo-oophorectomy face the same postoperative risks as well as early menopause. All of these women are at risk for psychological trauma and can benefit from the care of a well-informed, compassionate nurse.

It is important for patients to increase the self-awareness of their breasts, emphasizing that cyclical nodularity and tenderness are normal. Some women may choose to perform BSE. Oncology nurses can teach these patients the correct technique and schedule and can encourage these women to report changes in their breasts to health care professionals.

An additional intervention that oncology nurses can implement is to encourage a healthy lifestyle. As mentioned above, exercise has been shown to reduce the risk of breast cancer. Obesity, a sedentary lifestyle and excessive alcohol intake increase breast cancer risk. While smoking has not been implicated as a risk for breast cancer, smoking cessation and avoiding exposure to tobacco has many health benefits.[44] Perhaps most importantly, by providing the above education, advocacy and support, we can empower our patients with strategies they can use to combat the pervasive threat of breast cancer.

## GENETIC COUNSELING PROGRAMS

About 5% to 6% of all breast cancers are associated with an inherited genetic mutation.[97] The majority of these cases involve the autosomal-dominant *BRCA1* and *BRCA2* genes.[22,98] However, these mutations are rare and affect 1% to 8% of the general population.[21,98] In contrast, 12% to 30% of breast cancers in women of Ashkenazi Jewish descent can be attributed to a *BRCA* mutation.[99,100] As science and biotechnology continue to identify chromosomal abnormalities that confer a high probability for developing breast cancer, the need to provide more comprehensive risk assessment for families as well as genetic counseling and testing will direct practitioners and the public to seek genetic counseling programs. The primary physician will often be responsible for referring a patient for further evaluation and, therefore, must possess a basic working knowledge of the personal and familial histories that may suggest a genetic link. According to Stopfer,[101] genetic counseling should assist the patient and family in understanding the medical information pertinent to the disease(s), comprehending how heredity causes or predisposes one to disease and the personal risk of developing a condition, and creating a plan for follow-up that may include several treatment modalities.[102] Another important consideration is the psychological impact of genetic counseling and testing. A study addressed this issue and found no increase in psychological distress from such counseling.[103] Additionally, Braithwaite and colleagues reviewed controlled trials and prospective studies evaluating the psychological impact of genetic testing and reported no apparent adverse effect on cancer-specific worry or anxiety.[104]

The creation and implementation of a breast cancer genetic counseling program must include the following elements: a database and an assessment model based on known and accepted risk factors; genetic counselors who carefully interview, screen, and educate patients and families; psychosocial support staff to address the emotional and physical consequences of the counseling and testing process; and clinicians, nurses, and researchers who share clinical responsibilities and actively participate in treatment protocols and prevention trials for breast cancer. Confidentiality, informed consent, and insurance issues should be carefully addressed by the counseling program staff. Once risk has been established, the patient and family members should also receive specific recommendations tailored to the needs of the individual (see Table 48-2 for Screening Guidelines for *BRCA1*/*BRCA2* Mutation Carriers).

The American Society of Clinical Oncology (ASCO) issued a revised position paper regarding genetic testing for cancer susceptibility.[105] The ASCO paper recognizes that identifying those individuals with the highest risk will certainly increase early detection and may ultimately lead to the prevention of many cancers. However, ASCO also cites the importance of addressing the actual and potential risks of testing in a setting that offers extensive patient/family counseling and education. Additionally, ASCO endorses pre-test and post-test counseling and testing within a research protocol format that includes a national registry, long-term outcomes, and psychological ramifications.

The Internet has become a valuable source of information for both professionals and patients. Patients may inquire about Web sites that provide basic genetic information, and care must be taken to review any site before making a recommendation. A search engine designed to assist health professionals and the public with genetic information is http://ghr.nlm.nih.gov. Some other appropriate sites for patients and families are http://www.cdc.gov/genomics/, listing information about genetic testing and testing centers as well as links to similar sites; the National Center for Biotechnology Information, http://www.ncbi.nlm.nih.gov, which offers a primer about the biology of genetics and links to the Human Genome Project; and the National Human Genome Institute's Spanish-language talking glossary, http://www.genome.gov/sglossary.cfm. A peer support hotline has been established at the University of Pennsylvania; it is staffed by volunteers located across the country who have undergone genetic testing and can be reached at 866–824-RISK (866–824-7475). Nurses may wish to access other sites of interest: http://www.geneclinics.org has a directory of genetic abnormalities

**TABLE 48-2**

**Screening Guidelines for *BRCA1/BRCA2* Mutation Carriers**

| Type of Cancer | Screening Procedure | Starting Age | Frequency |
|---|---|---|---|
| **Screening for Women With Mutations in *BRCA1* or *BRCA2*** | | | |
| Breast | Mammograms | 25 years | Every 12 months |
| | Physician breast exam | 25 years | Every 6 months |
| | Breast self-exam | 20 years | Once every month |
| | Breast MRI | 25 years | Every 12 months |
| Ovarian | CA125 blood test<br>Ovarian ultrasound<br>*(Note: these tests have never been proven to reduce the risk of dying from ovarian cancer.)* | 25 years, until childbearing complete, then removal of ovaries (prophylactic oophorectomy) | Every 6–12 months |
| Colon | Colonoscopy | 50 years | Every 3–5 years |
| Uterine/Cervical | Pelvic exam/Pap smear | 18 years | Every 12 months |
| **Screening for Men With Mutations in *BRCA1* or *BRCA2*** | | | |
| Breast | Physician breast exam | 50 years | Once every year |
| Prostate | Prostate exam and PSA | 45 years | Once every year |
| Colon | Colonoscopy | 50 years | Every 3–5 years |

*Abbreviations*: *BRCA1*, BReast CAncer 1; *BRCA2*, BReast CAncer 2; MRI, magnetic resonance imaging; PSA, prostate specific antigen.

*Source*: Reprinted with permission from: Cancer Risk Evaluation Program, University of Pennsylvania Cancer Center. These guidelines may change as new data become available and must be individualized.

and testing sites. The International Society of Nurses in Genetics (ISONG) site, http://www.isong.com, lists education, nursing, and genetics resources and standards of practice. Additional sites include http://www.geneticnurse.org; http://www.nchpeg.org, the web site of the National Coalition for Health Education in Genetics; and http://www.geneticalliance.org.

An oncology nurse who receives additional education in the field of genetics will provide a wealth of information for the patient and family. All individuals who seek genetic counseling for breast cancer may not necessarily be at high risk. It is important for the staff to educate the patient and family as well as the referring physician regarding family and personal history assessments.

## PATHOPHYSIOLOGY

### CELLULAR CHARACTERISTICS

The majority of primary breast cancers are adenocarcinomas located in the upper outer quadrant of the breast (Figure 48-1). The most common histological types of breast tumors are summarized in Table 48-3.[106]

*Invasive (infiltrating) ductal* carcinoma is the most common type of breast cancer, accounting for 70% to 80% of all invasive breast tumors. Clinically, these lesions often present as hard, palpable masses or mammographic abnormalities. Invasive ductal carcinomas are divided into 3 histological grades based on a combination of features: tubule formation, mitotic rate, and nuclear grade.[107] Well-differentiated (Grade 1) cancers have little or no mitotic activity, relatively uniform nuclei, and are arranged in small tubules. Moderately-differentiated tumors have more variation in nuclear size and shape, moderate mitotic activity, and less tubule formation. Poorly differentiated (Grade 3) tumors have marked nuclear pleomorphism, considerable mitotic activity, and little tubule formation. These tumors have the tendency to grow and spread more aggressively. Invasive ductal carcinomas have the poorest prognosis of all invasive breast cancers and have the tendency to metastasize via the lymphatics.

*Invasive (infiltrating) lobular* carcinomas are the second most common type and account for 5% to 10% of all breast cancers. The incidence rates for this type of breast cancer are rising and may in part be related to the use of postmenopausal HRT.[108] Invasive lobular cancer can present as a mammographic abnormality or a palpable mass. However, many have a more subtle appearance on mammogram and may feel like a vague thickening on examination. Thus, invasive lobular carcinomas may be significantly greater in size than that measured on physical examination or mammography. Lobular carcinomas have an increased

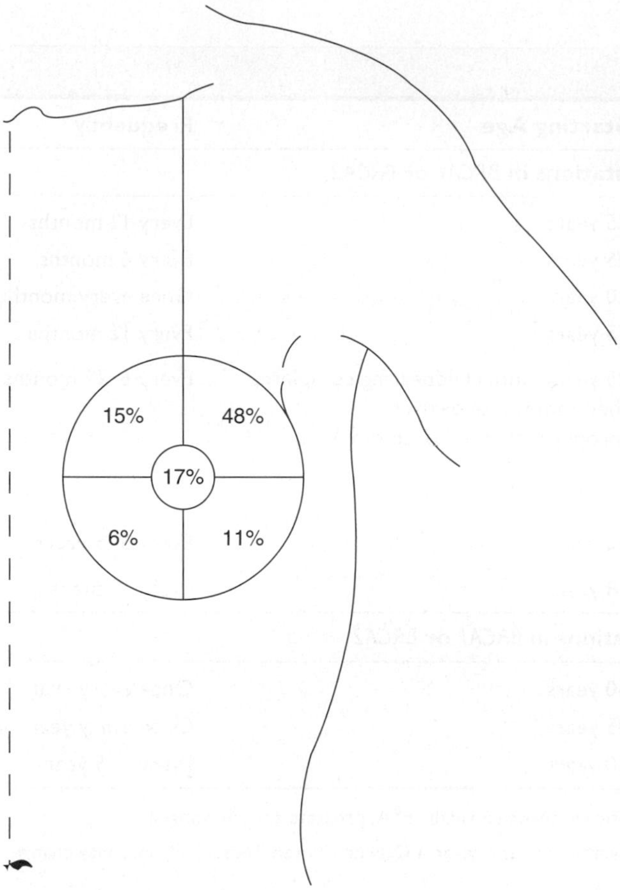


**FIGURE 48-1**

Incidence of breast cancer according to location.

incidence of bilateral breast cancer. The prognosis of these breast cancers is similar to invasive ductal carcinoma.

*Tubular* carcinoma is fairly uncommon and represents a well-differentiated adenocarcinoma of the breast. These cancers typically occur in women age 60 and older. They are characterized by a proliferation of well-formed tubular or glandular structures facilitating early mammographic discovery. Nodal and distant metastases are rare and they have an excellent prognosis.

*Medullary* carcinomas account for 5% to 7% of malignant breast tumors, occurring most commonly in women aged 55 to 65.[109] These tumors often present as palpable, moderately defined masses that are poorly differentiated. Despite an aggressive histological appearance, these cancers are felt to have a favorable prognosis. However, the variable classification systems employed in diagnosing medullary carcinoma make a definitive diagnosis and prognosis uncertain.

*Mucinous* (colloid) carcinoma is uncommon, typically occurring in 2% to 3% of invasive breast cancer and is mostly seen in women aged 70 to 80. This tumor type is characterized by the presence of large pools of mucin interspersed with small islands of tumor cells. These cancers tend to be well circumscribed with a soft, gelatinous consistency. Metastasis to axillary lymph nodes occurs in about 15% of patients. Although metastases are infrequent, late recurrences are seen. Mucinous carcinoma has a very good prognosis.

*Inflammatory* breast cancer occurs infrequently and accounts for less than 4% of breast cancers. This type of cancer often presents with skin edema, erythema, warmth, and induration of the underlying tissue and may be mistaken for cellulitis. Even though it appears to be localized, it is associated with a poor prognosis.

Other malignant tumors of the breast include invasive papillary carcinoma, invasive apocrine carcinoma, invasive cribiform carcinoma, metaplastic carcinoma and Paget's disease.[110]

## PATTERNS OF METASTASIS

Breast cancer is a heterogenous, highly variable disease. Even among individuals with the same histological type, clinical stage, and treatment, some will be cured while others develop metastatic disease within 6 months of therapy. The development of aberrant cell clones, with diverse growth rates and metastatic potential, may in part account for the differences seen in clinical behavior. While the process of metastasis is a complex and poorly understood phenomenon, a growing body of evidence suggests that angiogenesis (neovascularization) of the tumor plays an important role in the biological aggressiveness of breast cancer.[111–113]

Breast cancer metastasizes widely and to almost all organs of the body, but primarily to the skin, bone, lungs, lymph nodes, liver, and brain. Patients with metastatic disease may present with symptoms specific to that organ. For instance, women with metastatic disease to bone often complain of bone pain. Those with liver metastases may report anorexia, weight loss, malaise, and occasionally right upper quadrant pain. Central nervous system metastases may present with specific neurological symptoms such as headache that is more severe in the morning or is accompanied by nausea, or relate to specific neurological damage such as cranial nerve palsies (double vision), motor dysfunction, or spinal cord symptoms. Invasive ductal carcinomas metastasize more commonly to the lungs, liver, and brain.[114] In contrast, invasive lobular carcinomas are more likely to spread to the leptomeninges, retroperitoneum, gastrointestinal tract, and reproductive organs.[114] Metastatic breast cancer is not curable but there are long-term survivors.

# ASSESSMENT

## HISTORY

When evaluating a patient for breast cancer, it is important to take a thorough history. Risk factors including age,

**TABLE 48-3**

**Histological Types of Invasive Breast Cancers**

| Histological Type | Percentage of Occurrence | Clinical Features | Metastatic Pattern | Prognosis |
|---|---|---|---|---|
| Infiltrating ductal carcinoma | 70 | Stony hardness to palpation<br>Prominent lump<br>Malignant cells have invaded through the walls of the duct<br>May have a spiculated appearance on mammogram | Axillary lymph nodes (common)<br>Bone<br>Lung<br>Liver<br>Brain | Poor |
| Infiltrating lobular carcinoma | 10–15 | Diffuse, ill-defined thickness<br>Multicentric<br>Bilaterality (30%) | Axillary lymph nodes (common)<br>Occult lymph node micrometastasis may occur | Poor |
| Tubular | 2 | May be quite large | Axillary lymph nodes (uncommon)<br>Distant metastases uncommon | Favorable |
| Medullary | 5–7 | Well circumscribed<br>Rapid growth rate<br>Bilaterality | Approximately 40% of cases demonstrate lymph node involvement at diagnosis | Favorable |
| Mucinous (colloid) | 3 | Slow growing, bulky | Axillary lymph node involvement in less than one-third of cases at diagnosis | Favorable |

*Source*: Data from Schnitt and Guidi.[106]

gender, genetics, personal history of cancer, radiation exposure, use of exogenous hormones, reproductive history, and family history of cancer should be assessed. The patient should be asked about prior cysts or breast biopsies and any palpable abnormalities. The history of a breast mass includes the length of time it has been present, whether it has changed in size, and any associated tenderness.

## PHYSICAL EXAMINATION

Physical examination of the breasts includes an evaluation of the skin, nipples, breast tissue, and axillary and supraclavicular lymph nodes. Clinical manifestations that are more suspicious of cancer include nipple retraction or elevation, which may be due to tumor fixation or infiltration into the underlying tissues. Nipple discharge or erosion are other concerning findings. Skin dimpling or retraction also may be present and is possibly due to invasion of the suspensory ligaments and fixation to the chest wall. Heat and erythema of the breast skin may be related to inflammation, but they are also signs of inflammatory breast carcinoma. Skin edema, or peau d'orange, the French term for "skin of the orange" (Figure 48-2), is characteristic of malignant disease. The edema is thought to be due to the invasion and obstruction of dermal lymphatics by tumor. Palpable lesions may range from well-circumscribed, discrete masses to ill-defined skin thickening. Malignant breast lesions are rarely tender. It is important to remember that most breast cancers present as a palpable mass without other physical findings.

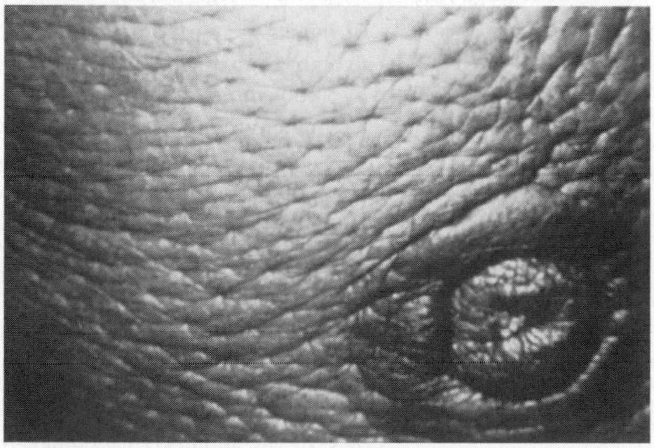

**FIGURE 48-2**

Peau d'orange; characteristic of lymphatic and dermal invasion by adenocarcinoma (inflammatory carcinoma).

## DIAGNOSTIC STUDIES

Routine mammography may reveal a large spectrum of breast pathology, ranging from equivocal benign conditions to those that are considered malignant until proven otherwise. The appearance of these lesions is often a coincidental finding on a screening mammogram of an asymptomatic woman. However, if a palpable abnormality is present, additional diagnostic tools will be utilized to isolate the abnormality and provide more specific information for the clinician.

The diagnostic evaluation of breast lesions may be a simple one-step procedure or may progress to a multilevel process. Several noninvasive and minimally invasive diagnostic tools may aid the clinician in identifying lesions within the breast. The standard "triple test" approach to a reliable diagnosis of a breast abnormality calls for correlating the clinical, imaging, and cytological findings, resulting in a sensitivity and specificity greater than 97% for diagnosing breast cancer. Of the 3 modalities, the 2 that combine to be most reliable are imaging and cytology.[115]

### Mammography

The consensus recommendation is that screening mammography should begin at age 40[116–118] (Table 48-4). Mammograms are successful in detecting breast cancer 90% of the time whereas 10% of cancers are detected solely by physical examination. The goal of screening mammography is to find a cancer before it becomes clinically apparent. A woman who adheres to the screening mammography and clinical breast examination recommendation increases the likelihood that any cancer noted on mammogram will be a smaller size and an earlier stage with a higher survival rate.

Mammographic findings are summarized using the American College of Radiology (ACR) Breast Imaging Reporting and Data System (BIRADS) assessment categories. This is a quality control system where radiologists assign numerical codes after interpreting a mammogram. Across providers and institutions, theses categories standardize the reporting of findings and the recommendations for further management. The BIRADS categories are as follows:[119]

Category 0: Incomplete; need further images or previous mammograms for comparison
Category 1: Negative; routine follow-up recommended
Category 2: Benign finding; routine follow-up recommended
Category 3: Probable benign finding; short interval follow-up recommended
Category 4: Suspicious abnormality; biopsy should be considered
Category 5: Highly suggestive of malignancy; appropriate action should be taken
Category 6: Known, biopsy proven malignancy; appropriate action should be taken

The BIRADS categories were originally developed for mammography findings but have since been adapted for findings related to MRI and ultrasound.

### Screening mammography

Screening mammograms are used for routine breast surveillance for the asymptomatic patient. The screening

**TABLE 48-4**

**American Cancer Society Guidelines for Breast Cancer Detection**

| | |
|---|---|
| Women at average risk | Begin mammography at 40 with a yearly clinical breast examination.<br>Beginning at approximately age 20, women should be told about the benefits and limitations of BSE. Prompt reporting of any new breast symptom to a healthcare professional should be emphasized. Women who choose to perform BSE should have the technique reviewed during a periodic health examination. It is acceptable for women to choose not to do BSE or to do BSE irregularly.<br>Women should have an opportunity to become informed about the benefits, limitations, and potential harms associated with regular screening. |
| Older women | Screening considerations in older women should be individualized by considering the potential risks and benefits of mammography in the context of current health status and estimated life expectancy. As long as a woman is in reasonably good health and would be a candidate for treatment, she should continue to be screened with mammography. |
| Women at increased risk | Women at increased risk of breast cancer might benefit from additional screening strategies beyond those offered to women at average risk, such as earlier initiation of screening, shorter screening intervals, or the addition of screening modalities other than mammography and physical examination such as ultrasound or magnetic resonance imaging. However, the evidence currently available is insufficient to justify recommendations for any of these screening approaches. |

*Abbreviation*: BSE, breast self-examination.

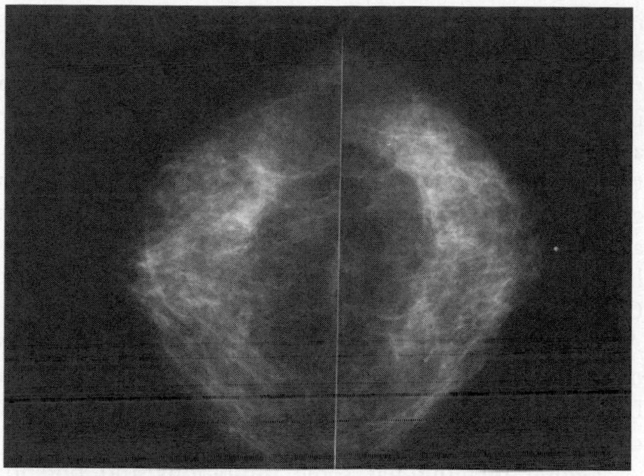

**FIGURE 48-3**

Screening mammography of an asymptomatic breast from above (craniocaudal view).

mammogram usually consists of 4 views, 2 per breast (Figures 48-3 and 48-4). A mediolateral oblique view and a craniocaudal view of each breast enable the technologist to image as much breast as possible (ie, the axillary tail and pectoralis muscle).

Screening mammograms provide a high-sensitivity study at the lowest possible cost and allow for a high-quality image with minimum radiation exposure. They permit the radiologist to detect characteristic benign and malignant masses. Benign masses include cysts, fibroadenomas, and inframammary lymph nodes, all of which have defined borders. Malignant lesions may present as spiculated or ill-defined masses, architectural distortion, asymmetric densities, and microcalcifications (Figures 48-5 and 48-6). Additionally, subtle abnormalities may be noted by the radiologist that requires further studies to determine whether pathology exists.[120]

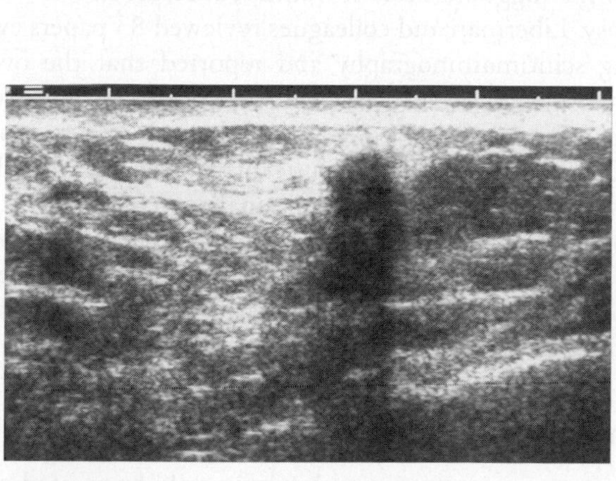

**FIGURE 48-4**

Screening mammography of an asymptomatic breast from the side (mediolateral view).

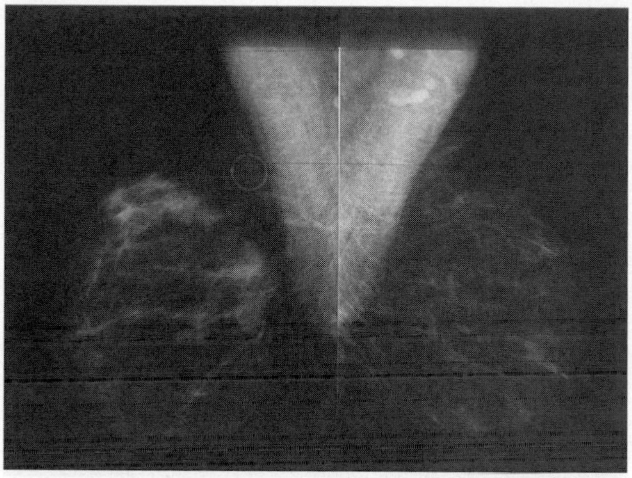

**FIGURE 48-5**

The mediolateral views show the appearance of an asymmetric density.

## Diagnostic mammography

A diagnostic mammogram is performed when the patient reports specific symptoms, suspicious clinical findings exist, or an abnormality has been found on a screening mammogram. A diagnostic film uses additional views of the affected breast as well as the possibility of localized compression and magnification views to increase the specificity when trying to identify the abnormality. The area in question is locally compressed and/or magnified, which enables the radiologist to comment more accurately on the lesion (Figure 48-7). The radiologist should be present during the diagnostic study. The ongoing evaluation of the additional films is crucial for rendering a diagnosis or recommending a plan of care.

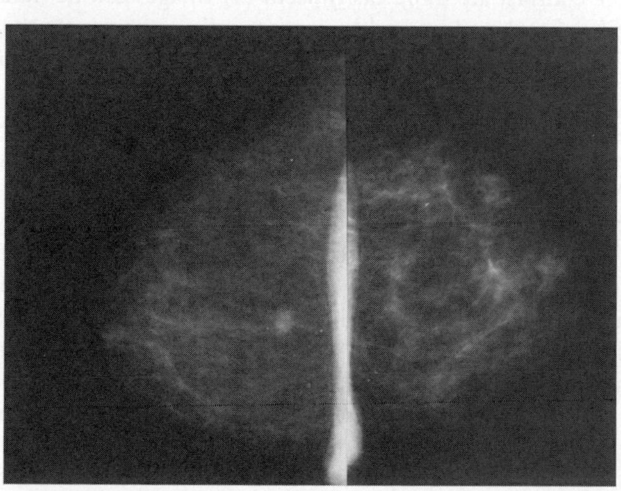

**FIGURE 48-6**

A craniocaudal view demonstrates the presence of spiculated nodules.

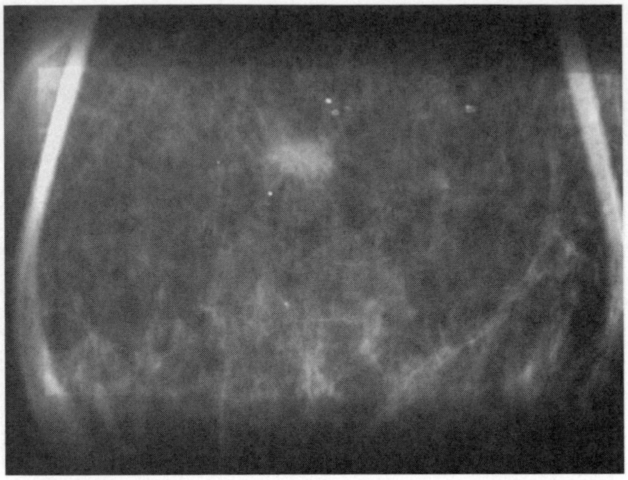

**FIGURE 48-7**

Magnification of the nodule provides a more accurate picture of the irregular border noted on screening mammogram. Note that the border is not clearly defined, but appears fuzzy or hazy, which is especially demonstrated on the left side. The irregular appearance and spiculations make this nodule suspicious for cancer.

## Digital mammography

Digital mammography records the radiographic image in a digital format that can be stored in a computer. This image can be played on a monitor or transferred onto film. Adler and Wahl[121] and Schmidt and Nishikawa[122] listed the advantages of digital technology over film mammography in an early study: (1) Digital technology allows for more variations in exposure. (2) The radiologist's performance is increased by virtue of a second look. (3) Differences in tissue contrast are more easily seen. (4) Images can be transmitted and easily stored.

A comparison of film and digital mammography by Lewin and colleagues reported no statistical difference in detecting cancers, but there was a lower recall rate with digital mammography.[123] Preliminary results from the Digital Mammographic Imaging Screening Trial (DMIST), a clinical trial of digital vs film mammography, showed no difference in detecting breast cancer for the general population of women.[57] However, those with dense breasts, who are premenopausal or perimenopausal or who are younger than age 50, may benefit from having a digital rather than a film mammogram.[57]

Computer-assisted detection (CAD) utilizes a software program to recognize digitalized mammographic patterns and to target potentially suspicious lesions for the radiologist to review and interpret. Recent reports have demonstrated improved detection using computer-aided detection systems,[124–126] but one large study noted no such improvement in detection, suggesting that more studies need to be conducted.[127] Several promising outcomes may result from this method of imaging. The specificity of the image is enhanced by real-time evaluation on a screen, allowing for manipulation of contrast that enhances detection and permits more rapid interventional procedures. The goal of CAD is to reduce the number of false positive results and unnecessary biopsies. Given that specialist radiologists have higher cancer detection rates and lower recall rates, CAD may prove most useful for general radiologists.[120] Additionally, this real-time evaluation will enhance the use of mobile systems in remote areas. Expert consultation may be immediately accessed via satellite, while the unit is still on site.[128]

Digital imaging has some limitations and potential problems. Whole-breast images equal to the quality of film mammography are only recently available for large-breasted women, and it is difficult to do an adequate comparison of previous film-screen studies with the digital images. A limitation of digital mammography is that the spatial resolution is less than what is available with film mammography. However, greater contrast resolution is seen with digital mammography. Cost is another limiting factor for digital imaging and CAD. Additional expense will be incurred as accessory equipment is acquired to fully utilize the capabilities of digital imaging.

## Scintimammography

Scintimammography uses a variety of radioisotopes to scan the axilla and supraclavicular area while imaging the breast,[129] but the most commonly used radiopharmaceutical tracer is technetium-99M sestamibi (MIBI). The tracer is injected intravenously and the rate of tissue absorption is then calculated, with higher rates being suspicious for malignancy. Scintimammography was introduced as a tool with superior specificity compared to mammography, with the suggestion that it would reduce the rate of benign biopsy. Liberman and colleagues reviewed 83 papers evaluating scintimammography and reported that the overall sensitivity and specificity was significantly higher than with mammography (>85%), but the rate of detection of nonpalpable masses was significantly lower (67%) and the sensitivity for detecting cancers smaller than 1 cm was also poorer.[130] Scintimammography could eventually improve the accuracy of breast cancer diagnosis and decrease the number of unnecessary biopsies performed when used as an adjunct to mammography.

## Sonogram

A sonogram or ultrasound has primarily been used as an adjunct to mammography to determine whether a lesion is solid or cystic.[131] However, its sensitivity and specificity are

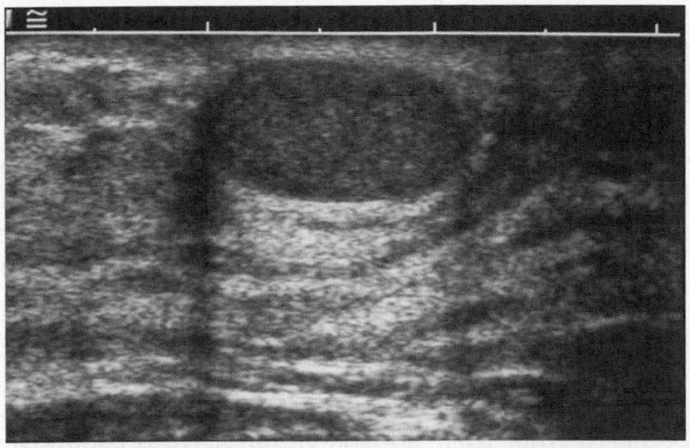

**FIGURE 48-8**

An ultrasound of a palpable mass reveals the characteristics of a fibroadenoma, which is a benign nodule.

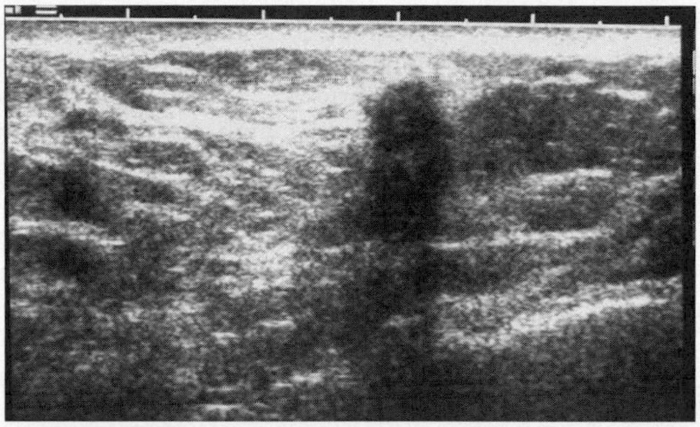

**FIGURE 48-9**

This ultrasound demonstrates 2 characteristics of a suspicious mass: (1) irregular shape and (2) ill-defined borders and spiculations.

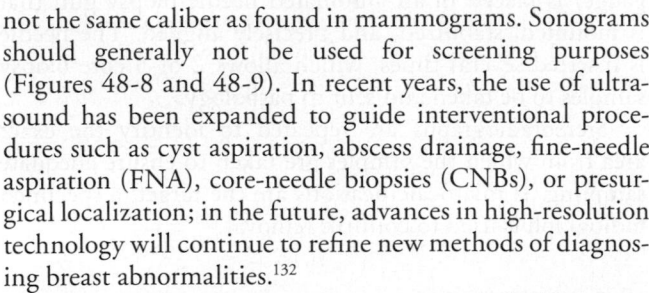

not the same caliber as found in mammograms. Sonograms should generally not be used for screening purposes (Figures 48-8 and 48-9). In recent years, the use of ultrasound has been expanded to guide interventional procedures such as cyst aspiration, abscess drainage, fine-needle aspiration (FNA), core-needle biopsies (CNBs), or presurgical localization; in the future, advances in high-resolution technology will continue to refine new methods of diagnosing breast abnormalities.[132]

Ultrasound is appropriate to investigate palpable lesions in young women whose breasts have dense fibroglandular tissue that may obscure a lesion in the breast or to evaluate suspected implant rupture. It is also useful in pregnant women, who need to be spared radiation when an abscess or galactocele is suspected, or in recently lactating women, whose breasts are extremely dense.

### Magnetic resonance imaging

Magnetic resonance imaging (MRI) uses magnetic fields to produce cross-sectional images of breast tissue. A contrast agent like gadolinium is often administered intravenously to enhance detection of cancerous lesions. MRI evaluates the rate at which the contrast initially enters the breast tissue and the intensity of enhancement. Malignant lesions tend to exhibit an increased enhancement within the first 2 minutes. Absence of uptake and areas of slow enhancement are considered negative findings.[133] Reports have shown that contrast enhanced MRI has a high sensitivity for detecting breast cancer and is not hampered by breast density.[134–136] MRI of the breast is also gaining popularity due to advances in imaging techniques, uniformity in interpretation guidelines, and increased accessibility. However, MRI has been shown to have variable specificity due to the enhancement of benign breast tissue and due to false negative rates ranging from 4% to 12%.[136–138] In addition, it has a high cost and some individuals may not be able to complete the study due to claustrophobia or indwelling metal devices.[132] As a diagnostic and screening tool, MRI can be a useful adjunct to mammograms and sonograms when there are equivocal images or exam findings. Though gaining in popularity, the role of MRI in breast cancer staging has yet to be defined.

In 2006, the ACS convened an expert panel to review the breast MRI screening literature. On the basis of this review, the ACS now recommends breast MRI screening as an adjunct to mammography for women with a *BRCA* mutation, for women with a first-degree relative who is a *BRCA* carrier, or for women with an approximately 20% to 25% or greater lifetime risk of breast cancer.[93] There are several groups for which the evidence was felt to be insufficient to recommend for or against screening, including women with a personal history of breast cancer, LCIS, ADH, and extremely dense breasts on mammography.[93]

### Positron emission tomography

Positron emission tomography (PET) with fluorine-18 fluorodeoxyglucose (FDG) is a radiotracer imaging method that employs metabolic activity to image the breast tissue. It quantifies the overconsumption of glucose by a tumor cell and emits a foci of increased metabolic uptake.[139,140]

Positron emission tomography may be used to locate primary, regional, and systemic metastases.[140] The clinical benefit of PET scanning in the diagnostic and staging evaluation of locoregional disease or in the detection of distant metastases is uncertain. In both instances, it does not appear to contribute more significant information than other imaging modalities.[141–145] The major limitations of this technology are the high cost of the scanners and the half-life of the radiopharmaceuticals, which may not be long enough to sufficiently trace biochemical reactions. PET will not be accepted as a routine screening or diagnostic tool until more definitive data become available.[140]

### Fine-needle aspiration

Fine-needle aspiration (FNA) is employed to evaluate a palpable breast mass. It is a simple and quick office procedure that can be performed with minimal local anesthesia using a small 21-gauge or 23-gauge needle.[146,147] An ultrasound-guided FNA is sometimes done to ensure proper needle placement. The aspirated contents are then sent to cytology for review. In skilled hands, FNA has a high sensitivity and specificity rate.[148] However, further evaluation of a suspicious lesion may be warranted if the result is negative. Although it can lead to the diagnosis of carcinoma, FNA cannot distinguish between an in situ or an invasive cancer.

### Core-needle biopsy

Core-needle biopsy (CNB) is generally used for palpable masses that have some suspicion for cancer. Such biopsies are performed manually or with a spring action "gun," which automatically advances the needle to the lesion and obtains a specimen. The needle gauge is larger than in FNA, 14 or 16 gauge, thereby producing a larger sample of tissue. An ultrasound guided CNB can be used on nonpalpable lesions to confirm needle placement and on palpable lesions that are small, moveable, deep, or barely palpable. CNB is felt to be superior to FNA for several reasons: The diagnosis is based on histological rather than cytological evaluation; a definitive diagnosis is usually rendered; and in situ carcinomas can be distinguished from invasive cancers, although some in situ cancers with microinvasion or small foci of invasion may be missed.[132] With CNB the specimen is also large enough for estrogen receptor (ER), progesterone receptor (PR), and *HER2/neu* testing to be performed.

### Stereotactic core-needle biopsy

The stereotactic CNB is mainly used to target and identify mammographically detected nonpalpable lesions in the breast and is most often employed to identify the morphology of microcalcifications. It is appropriate for sampling most nonpalpable lesions, but is less suitable for very small lesions, lesions close to the chest wall or skin, or those on the extreme medial or lateral area of the breast.[149] This procedure is contraindicated for obese individuals, those on anticoagulant therapy that cannot be held, and for individuals who may not be able to tolerate the positioning required for the biopsy.[150] The stereotactic biopsy permits diagnosis of benign disease without the trauma or scarring of an open biopsy. This procedure has been improved over time and now yields sufficient tissue for diagnosis more than 97% of the time when performed by an experienced practitioner. It also results in a cost savings over excisional biopsy.[151]

The basic principle of stereotactic CNB is to immobilize the breast from fixed horizontal and vertical coordinates so as to calculate the exact position of the lesion within a three-dimensional field.[152] The patient is usually positioned prone, and the breast is suspended through an opening in the examination table. (See Figure 48-10.)

The breast is then compressed, proper placement is confirmed by stereoradiographs or digital mammograms, and the breast is locally anesthetized. A biopsy needle (14–20 gauge) is placed in an automated needle biopsy gun that is mounted, stabilized, and precisely aligned. The needle is inserted several times, which allows 2 or 3 core biopsy samples to be taken and sent to pathology.

Stereoradiographs are repeated to identify the exact area from which the samples are taken to ensure adequate sampling. If microcalcifications are the target, a specimen radiograph is used to confirm removal.[150]

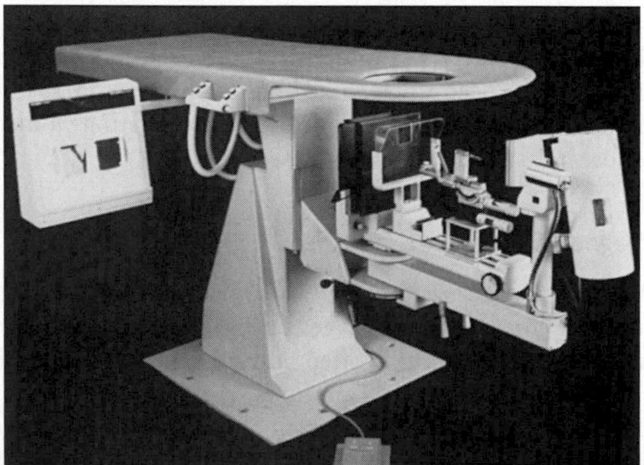

**FIGURE 48-10**

The stereotactic table allows for localization of the nonpalpable lesion between the Plexiglas plates below the opening from which the breast hangs down. Some machines allow for the procedure to be done in a sitting position, which is less favorable due to the possibility of syncope.

*Source*: Photo courtesy of Fischer Imaging, Denver, Colorado.

After the procedure, pressure with or without an ice pack is applied for 5 minutes. The area is then cleaned and a sterile bandage is applied. The patient may shower the next day, but should avoid bathing for 2 days. The patient is also given instructions regarding notification of results.

### Wire localization biopsy

The aim of wire localization biopsy is to radiographically assist the surgeon in locating a nonpalpable lesion for the purpose of excisional biopsy and to minimize the volume of tissue removed to avoid unnecessary deformity.[146] The character of the abnormality is identified after biopsy. (See Figure 48-11.) A histological diagnosis can be made and a highly suspicious abnormality or biopsy-proven lesion can be fully excised.

The needle-localized biopsy requires that the radiologist targets the area via mammography. Once the area is anesthetized, a small wire with a hook on the end or a needle is inserted into the lesion. Multiple lesions may be localized at one time using several wires. A set of repeat mammograms is then taken to ensure proper placement (Figure 48-12). This wire is then taped to the skin of the breast to prevent dislodgement. The patient is sent to the operating room with the mammograms that note the area to be excised.[153] After the biopsy is complete, the specimen is examined microscopically and radiographs are done to ensure that the abnormality has been removed.

### Excisional biopsy/lumpectomy

The excisional biopsy is the most invasive diagnostic procedure. There are several reasons for recommending an excisional biopsy:

1. Sonogram findings show the lesion to be solid and indeterminate.
2. The cytology and/or histology results are insufficient.
3. The clinical or mammographic findings are suspicious.

The objective of this biopsy is to remove the lump or area identified, along with a small margin of surrounding normal tissue. The potential for breast conservation should be considered during the planning for the biopsy. This is done by placing the incision above the lesion, using

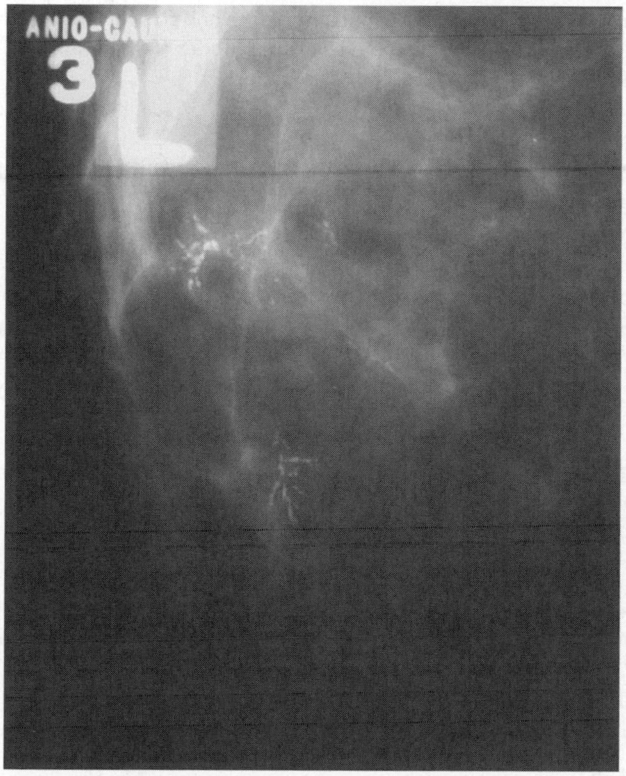


**FIGURE 48-11**

Magnification view of 2 areas of suspicious microcalcifications.

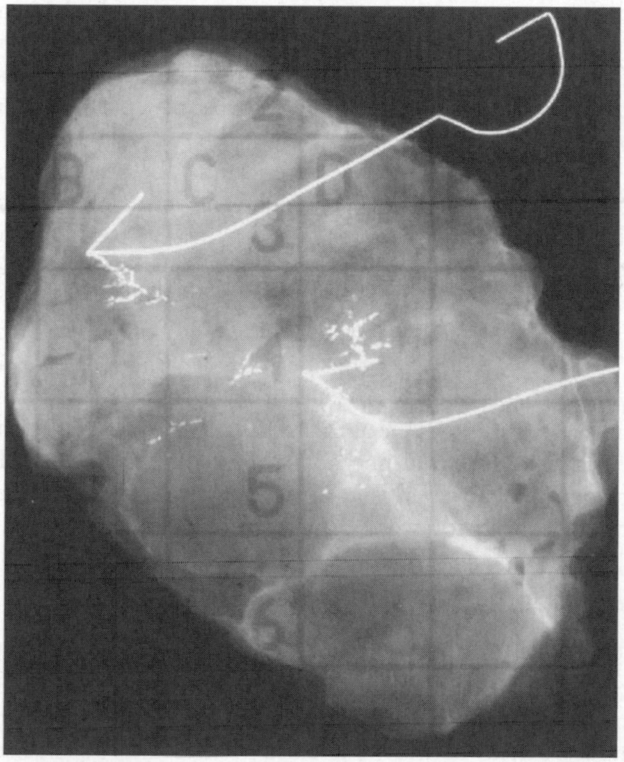

**FIGURE 48-12**

Specimen mammogram: Hook-wires were placed in each area of calcification. They were removed with good margins of surrounding tissue.

the most appropriate incision to follow the lines of tension, and avoiding tunneling. After the tumor is removed, the skin is closed without approximating breast tissue or fat. This method results in less deformity at the biopsy site. The excised tissue is identified and sent to the pathology lab for histopathological diagnosis.

Though rarely done, an incisional biopsy is usually performed on a large mass and removes only part of the lesion for diagnosis. Major surgery would be required to completely remove the lump. If the tumor is very large and a diagnosis and/or additional tumor markers are needed, CNB is usually sufficient and an incisional biopsy is not necessary.

## PROGNOSTIC INDICATORS

When breast cancer is diagnosed and found to be localized without evidence of metastatic spread, it is critical to identify patients who are at a substantial risk of recurrence, either locally or systemically. Identification of variables that are associated with disease recurrence may make it possible to design the most appropriate treatment for the individual based on the biological aggressiveness of the cancer. The identification of various prognostic indicators helps to define the natural history of breast cancer, establish prognosis with increasing accuracy, and, most important, identify those subsets of women who may be cured by local therapy alone vs those who would most benefit from adjuvant systemic therapies.[154]

Valuable parameters for determining the prognosis for patients with breast cancer include the status of the axillary lymph nodes, size of the tumor, invasive nature of the neoplasm, nuclear grade, hormone receptor status, *HER2/neu* overexpression, and histological type. Cell proliferative indices, DNA ploidy, and vascular endothelial growth factor (VEGF) protein are considered to be of high prognostic value in breast cancer, especially for women who have node-negative disease.[155] Age at diagnosis and menopausal status remain controversial prognostic indicators. It is generally recognized, however, that breast cancer patients younger than age 35 have a worse prognosis than older patients.[155]

### Axillary lymph node status

The involvement of axillary nodes by tumor is the single most important factor in determining prognosis in breast cancer (Figure 48-13). Clinical assessment of the axillary nodes carries both a 30% false-positive and 30% false-negative rate. Hence, pathological staging of the lymph nodes is mandatory, including examination for microscopic metastases to the nodes.[156] Once involvement is determined, important issues are the number of nodes involved, the levels of involvement, and whether the lymph node capsule has been invaded. Recovery of a small number of negative lymph nodes during a traditional axillary node dissection may understage disease and lead to an increased rate of regional relapse and poorer survival.[157]

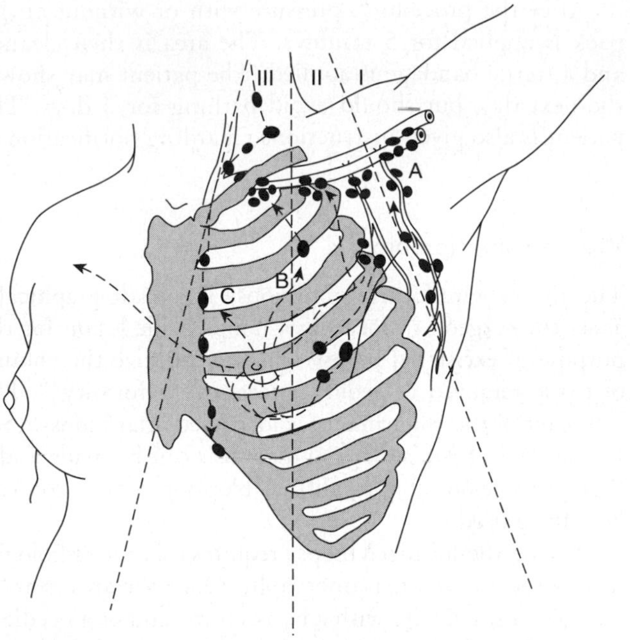


**FIGURE 48-13**

Lymphatics of the breast leading to (A) axillary nodes, which are distributed over a large area from the lateral aspects of the breast proper to the axillary vessels; (B) interpectoral chain leading to interpectoral node (circle detail) and to high nodes in the axilla; and (C) chain of the internal mammary leading frequently to nodes in second interspace and to supraclavicular and cervical nodes. The levels of lymph nodes (I, II, III) are defined by the pectoralis minor muscle.

Women with no evidence of lymph node involvement have a higher survival rate than women with lymph node involvement.[158] Table 48-5 demonstrates the correlation between survival and number of involved nodes in a large population of women.[159] Metastases to the internal

**TABLE 48-5**

**Recurrence Rates in 20,547 Women With Breast Cancer According to the Number of Histologically Involved Axillary Nodes**

| Number of Positive Nodes | Recurrence at 5 Years (%) |
|---|---|
| 0 | 25 |
| 1–3 | 40 |
| 4–6 | 49 |
| 7–9 | 58 |
| 10+ | 78 |

*Source*: Data from Nemoto et al.[159]

mammary nodes have the same significance as metastases to the axillary nodes. Internal mammary node metastasis occurs more readily in patients who have medial lesions. Although internal mammary nodes are not commonly sampled, they are invaded in 10% of patients when axillary nodes are negative. This phenomenon may help to explain the recurrence patterns in some axillary node-negative women.[160]

### Tumor size

Second to nodal status, tumor size of an invasive breast cancer is a very important factor in predicting lymph node involvement and clinical outcomes. Studies have shown that an increase in tumor size is related to an increased risk of recurrence.[161–164] Women with node-negative breast cancer and tumors smaller than 1 cm in diameter have a relative overall 5-year survival rate of nearly 99%.[161] Patients with tumors measuring 1 to 3 cm have a relative 5-year survival rate of approximately 91%, while those with tumors measuring more than 3 cm have a 5-year survival rate of 85%.[160–164] The significance of tumor size is independent of lymph node status.

One unresolved issue for providers is how to assess multifocal, invasive breast cancer. It is not known whether prognosis is related to the largest focus of invasive cancer or to the cumulative size of all the foci of invasive cancer. As additional research is needed, pathologists continue to report their individual sizes rather than their sum.

### Hormone receptor status

Normal breast epithelium contains hormone receptors and responds specifically to the stimulatory effects of estrogen and progesterone. A majority of breast cancers have an overexpression of estrogen and progesterone receptors. These receptors bind to circulating hormones and promote cell growth and division. Upon their removal, invasive and noninvasive breast cancer cells undergo immunohistochemical analysis to quantify ER and PR. The major benefit to knowing a woman's ER and PR status concerns its value in predicting which patients will respond to hormone manipulation. Postmenopausal women tend to be ER positive, while premenopausal women tend to be ER negative.[165]

The prognostic importance of ER and PR status is equivocal. Some studies report an increase in DFS for hormone receptor positive individuals the first 5 to 10 years after treatment.[166,167] Other studies report that over time the prognosis for ER and PR negative patients rivals those with positive receptors.[168]

### Cell proliferative indices and DNA ploidy

Cell proliferative potential has important prognostic significance, especially in node-negative breast cancer. Using flow cytometry, it is possible to measure the DNA content and proliferative activity (S-phase fraction) of a tumor. Patients whose tumors have an abnormal amount of DNA are aneuploid; those with normal DNA are diploid.[155] A high S-phase fraction predicts a poorer prognosis and a greater risk of recurrence compared to a low S-phase calculation.[155] Tumors that are ER negative tend to have a high S-phase fraction, reflecting a more aggressive metastatic potential.[155]

### Histological grade

Tumor grade is an important prognostic variable. Tumors are generally classified according to their histological grade, which takes into account the nuclear pattern, tubule formation, and mitotic activity. Tumors that are well differentiated (Grade 1) have a better prognosis and a lower rate of distant metastases than those that are poorly differentiated (Grade 3).[169–173]

### Molecular and biological factors

A variety of molecular markers have been studied in breast cancer to determine whether pretreatment clinical features and molecular markers can predict treatment response and survival in patients with primary breast cancer.[174]

Under normal circumstances, *p53* is a tumor suppressor gene that codes for a nuclear transcription factor that is involved with cell-cycle regulation and programmed cell death. The loss of functioning of this tumor suppressor gene may be associated with increased aggressive tumor behavior. Mutation of the *p53* gene appears to be an independent prognostic marker of early relapse and could be an important factor in identifying node-negative patients who have a poor prognosis and would therefore benefit from adjuvant systemic therapy.[175,176]

The *HER2/neu* proto-oncogene encodes for a transmembrane protein that appears to be a receptor for a peptide growth factor. Amplification of this gene occurs in approximately 30% of women with breast cancer, resulting in overexpression of the gene product. It appears that overexpression of *HER2/neu* is associated with more aggressive cancers and worse disease-free and overall survival (OS), especially for those patients with node-positive disease. Further, in women with metastatic breast cancer, *HER2/neu* overexpression is correlated with poor response to endocrine therapy and favorable response to chemotherapy—especially cisplatin, doxorubicin and paclitaxel.[154,177]

Vascular endothelial growth factor (VEGF) is an angiogenic factor that stimulates proliferation of vascular endothelial cells. Overexpression of VEGF is thought to be involved in tumorigenesis and metastasis in primary breast cancer. Chemical signals (cytokines) from tumor cells are thought to stimulate resting vascular endothelial cells to begin a rapid growth phase, thereby supporting the growth and spread of the tumor. Increased expression of this growth factor is associated with decreased OS in women with node-negative and node-positive breast cancer.[178–180]

### Gene expression profiling

The 21-gene recurrence score assay (Oncotype DX) is used to assess gene expression. This test analyzes formalin-fixed, paraffin-embedded tissue using the reverse-transcriptase polymerase chain reaction (RT-PCR) method. The recurrence score can be used as a prognostic and predictive indicator for women with newly diagnosed, node-negative, ER positive breast cancer.[181,182] Patients are given a recurrence score and divided into low-risk, intermediate-risk, or high-risk categories based on the expression of a panel of 21 genes. Those with a low recurrence score are likely to benefit from hormonal therapy like tamoxifen and may not require adjuvant chemotherapy. In contrast, those with a high recurrence score would likely benefit from adjuvant chemotherapy more than from hormonal therapy alone.

## CLASSIFICATION AND STAGING

Once breast cancer has been diagnosed, a complete evaluation of the disease is initiated to establish the stage of disease and the most appropriate approach to treatment. The initial staging evaluation typically begins with a thorough history and physical examination, complete blood count, liver function tests, and a complete metabolic profile. Evaluation of a patient's bones, brain, chest, and liver are performed based on their symptoms.[183] For example, to rule out liver metastases a computed tomography (CT) scan of the abdomen or liver may be done if liver enzymes are elevated or hepatomegaly is noted. A bone scan may be warranted if there are complaints of pain or there is an elevated serum calcium level. For those with stage III disease, a bone scan and a CT scan of the chest, abdomen, and pelvis are often done to rule out metastatic disease. If distant metastases are discovered upon initial diagnosis, extensive breast surgery is usually suspended.

Clinical staging is based on the characteristics of the primary tumor, the physical examination of the axillary nodes, and the presence or absence of distant metastases. The clinical evaluation is less reliable than the pathological evaluation. Because of the prognostic significance of axillary node involvement and tumor size, a pathological staging system for breast cancer is necessary. The pathological staging recommended by the American Joint Committee on Cancer (AJCC)[184,185] is presented in Table 48-6.

The 2003 updates to the 2002 staging system take into account the latest cancer research and changes in clinical practice. Recent modifications include reclassification for the number of involved axillary lymph nodes, reclassification for internal mammary and supraclavicular nodal involvement, and discrimination between micrometastases and isolated tumor cells. Stage classification changes using the new AJCC system for breast cancer will result in significant adjustments in reported outcomes by stage.[186] This system is somewhat complicated and can be simplified in terms of the most critical components—tumor size, whether nodes are involved and whether distant metastases are present:

| | |
|---|---|
| Stage I | Tumor 0 to 2 cm in size; negative lymph nodes and no evidence of metastasis |
| Stage II | Tumor size > 2 cm; positive but ipsilateral and mobile lymph nodes; node-negative tumor > 5 cm |
| Stage III | Node-positive tumor > 5 cm; extensive axillary lymph node involvement; supraclavicular lymph node involvement; direct tumor extension to chest wall or skin; inflammatory breast cancer |
| Stage IV | Distant metastases are known to be present.[184–186] |

## THERAPEUTIC APPROACHES AND NURSING CARE

While a breast cancer diagnosis causes significant emotional, social, and economic/vocational upheaval, such distress generally eases over time as therapy is planned and carried out. Most patients actively participate in the decision-making process and are able to articulate their need for information throughout treatment planning and months of therapy. To be a supportive advocate for the patient and their family, the nurse must be knowledgeable concerning the options for therapy, the goals of therapy, the measures to minimize complications of treatment, and the various resources that may needed throughout the treatment period and beyond.

A patient's psychological and social adjustment to the diagnosis and treatment of breast cancer will depend on their previous coping strategies and emotional stability. In addition, social support has consistently been found to influence a woman's adjustment through treatment.[187] The threat to emotional, social, sexual, and physical well-being is multifaceted, and the relative impact of these factors on adjustment varies from patient to patient and assumes varying degrees of importance at different stages of treatment.[188]

A strong source of social support will be extremely valuable throughout all phases of treatment. While the most important sources of social support are the patient's spouse or significant other, family, and friends, other sources of support may be needed to maintain a strong social network. The roles of the psycho-oncologist, the social worker, and various support groups are important resources for patients and their families.

The patient's need for information will vary considerably throughout each phase of treatment. It is not uncommon for the treatment plan to include surgery, radiation, chemotherapy, targeted therapy, and endocrine therapy. For many

**TABLE 48-6**

**American Joint Committee on Cancer Staging for Breast Cancer Tumor-Node-Metastasis (TNM) Classifications**

| **Primary Tumor (T)** | | **Regional Lymph Nodes (N)** | |
|---|---|---|---|
| T0 | No tumor evident | N0 | No regional lymph node metastasis |
| T1s | Carcinoma in situ | pN1 | Metastasis to 1–3 axillary lymph nodes and/or internal mammary nodes identified by sentinel node biopsy |
| T1mic | Less than 1 mm in greatest dimension | pN2 | Metastasis to 4–9 ipsilateral axillary lymph nodes or clinically apparent internal mammary nodes |
| T1a | 1–5 mm | pN2 | Metastasis to 10 or more ipsilateral axillary nodes; clinically apparent internal mammary nodes and 1 or more axillary nodes; or ipsilateral supraclavicular lymph nodes |
| T1b | 6–10 mm | NX | Regional lymph nodes cannot be assessed |
| T1c | 11–20 mm | | Node staging modified by presence of disease identified by immunohistochemistry or molecular studies: see AJCC Staging manual for full details |
| T2 | 21–50 mm (2–5 cm) | **Distant Metastases** | |
| T3 | Larger than 50 mm (> 5 cm) | M0 | No distant metastases |
| T4 | Tumor of any size with direct extension to chest wall or skin | M1 | Distant metastases |
| T4a | Extension to chest wall | MX | Distant metastases cannot be assessed |
| T4b | Edema or ulceration of the skin of the breast or satellite skin nodules on the same breast | | |
| T4c | Both T4a + T4b | | |
| T4d | Inflammatory carcinoma | | |
| TX | Primary tumor cannot be assessed | | |

| **Stage** | **TNM** | **10-Year Overall Survival (%)** |
|---|---|---|
| 0 | Tis N0 M0 | 95 |
| I | T1 N0 M0 | 88 |
| IIA | T0 N1 M0 | 62 |
| | T1 N1 M0 | |
| | T2 N0 M0 | |
| IIB | T2 N1 M0 | 62 |
| | T3 N0 M0 | |
| IIIA | T0 N2 M0 | 29 |
| | T1 N2 M0 | |
| | T2 N2 M0 | |
| | T3 N1 M0 | |
| | T3 N3 M0 | |
| IIIB | T4 N0 M0 | 29 |
| | T4 N1 M0 | |
| | T4 N2 M0 | |
| IIIC | Any T N3 M0 | 29 |
| IV | Any T, Any N, M1 | 7 |

*Source*: Data from the American Joint Committee on Cancer (AJCC).[184]

patients, the time of active treatment lasts at least 6 months to a year. Most patients with breast cancer, also do not realize that they may not feel "back to their normal self" for a year following completion of their treatment. If reconstruction is planned, this rehabilitation phase will be extended. In addition, if patients are on endocrine therapy, they may remain on therapy for 5 to 10 years. Patient-centered nursing care is crucial at each point in the breast cancer trajectory, from diagnosis through survivorship and/or death, to optimize adaptation and well-being.

## PRIMARY BREAST CANCER

The treatment of primary breast cancer is encompassed by complementary but different approaches. One approach is treating the breast and lymph nodes itself, or local–regional treatment. The goal of this is to treat the breast and lymph node itself. This is done by surgery and/or radiation. The other approach is the systemic approach of treating the whole body. The goal of systemic therapy is to eliminate any presumed micrometastatic disease risk of recurrence and death. This is done through chemotherapy, endocrine therapy, and/or targeted therapy. A patient may receive all or only some of these treatments. A central component guiding breast cancer therapy is the full knowledge of the disease extent and its biological features.[189] To properly treat the cancer, it is important to understand the cancer's pathological characteristics that serve as prognostic factors, in addition to the size of the tumor and the number of positive lymph nodes, which are the most predictive.

### Local–regional therapy

While it is true that nearly 60% of women diagnosed with breast cancer today will have localized, node-negative breast cancer and a high chance of cure, many women with early stage breast cancer, stages I to II, will develop metastatic disease from which they will die, regardless of local or systemic treatment. Furthermore, numerous clinical trials have demonstrated that breast-conserving treatment, consisting of removal of the primary tumor by lumpectomy plus breast radiation, results in a survival rate that is equal to that associated with more extensive local therapy, such as mastectomy or modified radical mastectomy.[190–193] Currently, more than one-third of women with breast cancer in the US are managed by lumpectomy and radiation therapy (RT).

## BREAST SURGERY

### Breast-conserving surgery

The goal of breast-conserving surgery is to minimize the risk of local recurrence while leaving the patient with a cosmetically acceptable breast.[194] Breast-conserving therapy is often referred to as a lumpectomy, segmental mastectomy, partial mastectomy, quadrantectomy, wide local excision, and tylectomy, and is used to describe the removal of the breast cancer and various amounts of surrounding normal tissue.[194]

Selection of the most appropriate surgical procedure is critical to local control of the primary cancer so as to reduce the risk of local failure and systemic disease. Most women view breast-conserving surgery as an acceptable surgery, and body image is often able to be maintained. Scar tissue may form and cause some contracture over time, but even with a decrease in breast size, most patients find the cosmetic result acceptable, especially when wearing a bra. Complications following breast-conserving surgery include arm edema, seroma formation, wound infection, shoulder dysfunction, upper extremity weakness, fatigue, and limitations in mobility. Some women may prefer mastectomy or may need to undergo a mastectomy because of contraindications to breast-conserving surgery. Breast-conserving surgery may not be appropriate for women with larger tumors greater than 5 cm, tumors involving the nipple–areola complex, tumors with extensive intraductal disease, tumors that appear to be multicentric or tumors that encompass or grow in all quadrants of the breast. Another contraindication to breast-conserving surgery includes active connective tissue disease such as scleroderma, especially when there is skin involvement, and lupus, because of the inability to receive radiotherapy.[189]

### Mastectomy

A modified radical mastectomy involves the removal of all breast tissue and the nipple–areola complex, plus level I and II axillary node dissection (see Figure 48-13). The pectoralis muscle is preserved. Modified radical mastectomy is indicated for larger, and/or multicentric disease or where cosmesis could not be achieved with conservative surgery. Modified radical mastectomy may be employed as definitive treatment following local recurrence in patients who initially fail conservative surgery and radiation. In general, patients with noninvasive or locally invasive tumors have excellent prognoses following salvage mastectomy. However, patients with predominantly invasive recurrent tumors are at significant risk for further relapse.

Postoperative complications following mastectomy include wound infection, flap necrosis if tissue reconstruction is performed, and seroma formation (a lump or swelling caused by accumulation of serum within a tissue organ). Seromas occur in approximately 10% of patients and generally resolve following aspiration. Antibiotics may be indicated if infection occurs.

Nursing care of the post mastectomy patient centers on wound care, with special attention being paid to maintaining functioning wound drains. If drains become blocked, the wound is more likely to develop a seroma/hematoma, leading to infection and possibly flap necrosis. To maintain suction and an adherent flap, drains may be "milked" to remove small clots. Drains are usually removed within 2 to 4 days following surgery. Patients may be discharged with drains intact.

Post mastectomy exercises to maintain shoulder and arm mobility may begin as early as 24 hours after surgery. The patient is instructed to maintain the affected arm in the adducted position but to perform limited exercises involving the wrist and elbow. Flexing fingers and touching the hand to the shoulder are encouraged. Squeezing a ball is discouraged, as it increases blood flow and, if done too vigorously, leads to swelling in the early postoperative period. Tables 48-7 and 48-8 provide information about hand and arm precautions post mastectomy and exercises that the patient can do after surgery.

Prior to discharge, the patient should have clear instructions regarding wound care, drain management, and care of the axilla. Initial care of the wound involves maintaining a clean incision with dressing changes daily if indicated. Care should also include avoiding the use of creams, deodorants, and shaving under the underarm for 2 weeks after surgery. A return appointment is made to assess the wound and, if necessary, remove stitches. At that time, the patient should receive specific instructions regarding post mastectomy exercises. An analgesic may be indicated to promote arm mobility during exercises and to prevent shoulder dysfunction.

Shoulder stiffness and decreased arm range of motion (ROM) are common and due primarily to postoperative immobility. It is not uncommon for a tightness to develop under the axilla extending to the elbow. This cord-like substance is thought to comprise sclerosed lymphatics that gradually dissipate 2 to 3 months after surgery. ROM exercises and massage therapy are beneficial.

Instructions regarding breast self-care and follow-up are usually given during the first outpatient visit after surgery. Introducing the patient to various prostheses and mastectomy bras can occur in the hospital or after hospitalization. Most patients are advised not to wear a prosthesis until the wound has healed completely, normally within 6 to 10 weeks. Many different kinds of prostheses exist: some are foam filled, others are liquid silicone filled, or still others are of a self-adhering variety. It is important that the prosthesis fit properly and that the weight be similar to the remaining breast. Insurance may pay for prostheses. A prescription or letter demonstrating medical necessity is usually required for insurance reimbursement.

## Axillary and sentinel lymph node dissection

Lymph node status is one of the single most important variables in determining breast cancer prognosis; therefore it is important to evaluate the status of the affected axilla through sentinel lymph node and/or axillary lymph node dissection.[195] The principal reason to perform this procedure is to help determine prognosis and risk for recurrence. Because lymph node dissection is responsible for significant morbidity associated with breast surgery, there has been increasing interest in finding alternative methods to obtain prognostic information.

The sentinel lymph node mapping and resection, the least invasive approach to staging the axilla, is now recommended by the NCCN 2009 panel guidelines as the preferred method to assess the pathological status of the axillary lymph nodes for patients with Stage I or II breast

**TABLE 48-7**

**Patient Information: Hand and Arm Precautions for Patients who have Undergone Breast Surgery**

- Do not permit injections (eg, chemotherapy, blood samples, or vaccinations) to be done on your affected arm unless approved by your physician.
- When trimming cuticles, take extra care not to tear hangnails. Professional manicures are recommended.
- Wear heavy gloves when gardening and digging or handling thorny plants.
- Always use a thimble when sewing to avoid pinpricks, and wear rubber gloves while washing dishes.
- Protect your arm from burns, especially from small appliances such as irons or frying pans, and from the sun.
- Be sure your hand and arm are well protected with an elbow-length mitt when reaching into a hot oven.
- Always have blood pressure measurements taken on the opposite arm. Avoid arm constriction from tight elastic sleeves, or jewelry.
- Do not carry a heavy purse or other objects—especially grocery bags or luggage—with your affected arm.
- Avoid strenuous upper body aerobics unless arm is supported by a properly fitted anti-lymphedema compression sleeve. Lifting weights of any kind is not recommended.
- Apply a good lanolin cream several times daily if your skin appears dry.
- Treat cuts and scratches by washing the area well and applying an antiseptic. Contact your physician if signs of infection, redness, warmth, or swelling occur.

**TABLE 48-8**

**Post mastectomy Exercises**

| When to Begin | Purpose | Exercises: Perform Exercises 5–10 Times Each, 3 Times a Day |
|---|---|---|
| Postoperatively days 1–5 | Prevent and/or reduce swelling | • Position arm against your side in a relaxed position.<br>• Elbow should be level with your heart, and the wrist just above the elbow when resting.<br>• Rotate wrist in a circular fashion.<br>• Touch fingers to shoulder and extend arm fully. |
| After drains are removed | Promote muscle movement without stretching | • While standing, brace yourself with your other arm and bend over slightly, allowing your affected arm to hang freely. Swing the arm in small circles and gradually increase in size. Make 10 circles—rest—repeat in the opposite direction.<br>• Swing arm forward and back as far as you can without pulling on the incision.<br>• While standing, bend over slightly and swing arms across the chest in each direction.<br>• While sitting in a chair, rest both arms at your side. Shrug both shoulders, then relax.<br>• While sitting or standing, pull shoulders back, bring the shoulder blades together. |
| After sutures are removed | Stretch and regain full range of motion; to gain mobility of your shoulder, you must move it in all directions, several times a day | • While lying in bed with arm extended, raise arm over your head and extend backward.<br>• While lying in bed, grasp a cane or short pole with both hands across your lap.<br>• Extend arms straight up and over your head and return.<br>• Repeat, rotating the cane clockwise and then counter clockwise while over your head.<br>• While standing, extend arm straight over your head and down.<br>• Extend your elbow out from your side at a 90° angle—hold it for 10 seconds—relax.<br>• Extend your arm straight out from your side even with your shoulder—extend arm straight up toward the ceiling.<br>• Stand at arm's length facing a wall. Extend arms so your fingertips touch the wall. Creep fingers up the side of the wall, stepping forward as necessary. Repeat the procedure going down the wall—keep arms extended.<br>• Stand sideways to the wall. Extend arm out so fingers touch the wall. Creep up the wall a little more each day.<br>• Use hand and arm normally (see Table 48-7). |
| After 6 weeks | Strengthen arm and shoulder and regain total use of arm and shoulder | • Begin water aerobics.<br>• Begin overall fitness program.<br>• Begin aerobics, Jazzercise, or other resistive exercises.<br>• Avoid using weights as these may increase arm edema and subsequent swelling. |

cancer.[189,196–203] The sentinel lymph node is the first node in the lymphatic basin that receives primary lymphatic flow from the tumor. The histological characteristic of the sentinel lymph node has been found to predict the histological characteristics of the remaining lymph nodes in the axilla. Sentinel lymph node mapping involves the injection of a radioactive substance or blue dye into the area around the tumor, which then drains into the ipsilateral axilla. The axilla is explored through a small incision, and the lymph node that takes up the blue dye or technetium-labeled sulfur colloid is the sentinel node, which is then excised. If the sentinel node is positive for tumor, then the patient undergoes an axillary dissection, but only if doing so will contribute to decisions regarding therapy. If the sentinel node is negative, the remaining axilla is negative 92% to 95% of the time.[204] Debate continues over whether finding micrometastases in the sentinel node dictates proceeding with a full axillary dissection.

Axillary lymph node dissection is reserved for patients who have a positive sentinel lymph node, larger primary tumors, and palpable axillary lymph nodes. Lymphatic drainage generally follows an orderly sequential pattern from level I and II nodes, rarely to level III.[205] Because the axilla receives 75% to 85% of lymphatic drainage from the breast, an axillary lymph node dissection includes dissection of level I and II axillary lymph nodes.[205–208] The surgeon will extract the level I and level II lymph nodes, extending from the latissimus dorsi muscle laterally, the axillary vein superiorly, and the medial border of the pectoralis minor muscle medially.[195] Multiple vessels, nerves and structures will need to be preserved for optimal function and to minimize tissue damage.[195] Risks of axillary lymph node dissection include pain, numbness, swelling, weakness and stiffness, lymphedema, and a decreased quality of life.

## RADIATION THERAPY

The role of radiation in the management of localized breast cancer has evolved over the years to the point where such therapy is now considered standard treatment for a variety of tumors. In fact, with an equivalent survival rate and preservation of the breast, breast-conserving surgery plus radiation is considered preferable to mastectomy for the majority of women with early stage breast cancer. As discussed earlier, the major criteria for selecting patients for breast-conserving surgery and RT are (1) the size of the tumor and the feasibility of resecting the primary tumor without causing major cosmetic deformity, and (2) the likelihood of tumor recurrence in the breast.[209] Local failure following breast-conserving surgery and radiation occurs in 13% of patients at 10 years.[209] Every effort should be made to decrease the local failure rate, mainly by obtaining clear surgical margins and possibly by adding systemic therapy.

Radiation is also used in some cases post mastectomy. For women who are at high risk for local or regional recurrence, radiation and systemic therapy are indicated post mastectomy. These patients include those with large tumors greater than 5 cm, tumors that invade the skin of the breast or the chest wall, or those with more than 4 positive axillary nodes. There is some question on both the role of radiation post mastectomy and left-sided breast cancers. It is less well-established due to the risks associated with radiation to the chest wall. There appears to be a higher risk for fatal myocardial infarction 10 to 15 years later in left-sided breast cancers compared with adjuvant radiation for right-sided breast cancer,[210] although a retrospective study by Vallis and colleagues found no evidence of excess morbidity and mortality from coronary artery disease among women treated with RT to the left breast at 10.2 years of follow up.[211] If a patient requires chemotherapy and radiation, the patient can receive either treatment mode first. It has become the standard approach to receive chemotherapy followed by radiation.[209] If radiation follows chemotherapy, generally it begins within 3 to 4 weeks following chemotherapy.

Radiation doses to the breast are delivered using super voltage equipment and tangential fields to minimize lung and heart exposure. The whole-breast dose ranges from 45 to 50 cGy delivered over 5 to 6 weeks. Whether a radiation boost is given depends on the type of local excision and risk for local recurrence. A boost is an extra 10 to 16 cGy to the tumor bed.[209] The morbidity associated with a boost of moderate size and dose delivered either by electron beam or interstitial implantation is small.[211,212] The cosmetic result following partial mastectomy and RT is generally considered to be good.

The major acute side effects of external beam RT are skin changes; including itching, dryness, scaling, redness, tenderness, burning, skin discoloration. Breast swelling, arm swelling, and pain may occur, but usually later on. The breast may feel sore and warm to touch during radiation treatment. Patients are instructed not to use soap when washing the area and to pat it dry. Dry desquamation can progress to a moist desquamation with infection. It is important to look for any signs or symptoms of infection. Other side effects include fatigue, anemia, and nausea. Later effects include telangiectasia, which are visibly small blood vessels and seen less often, and arm edema, which usually results from radiating the axilla for multiple positive nodes. Breast edema is unique to patients undergoing breast-conserving surgery and radiation. It usually appears during or within the first 6 months after treatment. Breast edema is more common in women who have had an axillary dissection with more than 11 nodes removed and in patients receiving adjuvant chemotherapy. Lymphedema can also occur in patients who have axillary dissection followed by RT to the axilla.

Rare side effects include symptomatic pneumonitis and brachial plexopathy. Radiation pneumonitis is characterized by a dry cough and low-grade fever. It can appear 2 to 3 months after the completion of therapy and occurs in 1% to 3% of patients. Brachial plexopathy manifesting as paresthesias, with or without arm and hand weakness, may be transient or permanent. Rib fractures and cardiac complications are also rare and may be related to dose and treatment with concurrent chemotherapy.

An alternative to external beam therapy for early-stage breast cancer is high dose rate (HDR) brachytherapy. It can be delivered in 2 ways: through the intraoperative placement of a balloon catheter in the lumpectomy site, or via rod placement in the lumpectomy site after completion of adjuvant chemotherapy. In both regimens, fractionated therapy is given twice daily for 5 days, after which the rods or balloon catheter is removed.[213,214] The patient undergoing brachytherapy may find it more convenient to stay in the hospital for the duration of treatment. The radioactive material is removed after each fraction and reinserted for the next fraction. Early single-institution trials have found that HDR partial-breast irradiation has similar outcomes to standard whole-breast external beam therapy.[215,216] If HDR brachytherapy is to follow adjuvant chemotherapy containing an anthracycline, the start of the brachytherapy should be delayed for approximately 6 weeks to avoid radiation recall, or repeat warmth and redness of the previous irradiated skin.

## BREAST RECONSTRUCTION

Mastectomy is indicated for a number of reasons: large or diffuse tumors, multifocal or multicentric tumors, a disparity in tumor size vs breast size, contraindications to radiation, or patient preference. Women who do undergo mastectomy for breast cancer have an increasing number of choices for reconstructive surgery. Breast reconstruction is an option for most women with breast cancer,[217] but it remains a personal decision. The goals of reconstructive surgery are good cosmetic effect and preserving the ability to perform normal activities. In addition, women have an enhanced self-image after reconstruction. Considerations for the suitability of breast reconstruction include the possible need and timing of adjuvant therapies, the patient's general health and habitus, previous breast surgery or radiation, and the condition of possible autologous skin donor sites and the contralateral breast.[218]

Patients who are considering breast reconstruction have a number of decisions to make. The first decision is whether the reconstruction should be immediate or delayed. There is consensus that immediate reconstruction does not delay adjuvant therapy, and it is performed in a majority of procedures today. A significant advantage of immediate reconstruction is that there is one surgical procedure, so the morbidity and overall cost are lower. Immediate reconstruction promotes a positive body image and may enhance psychological and emotional adjustment to all aspects of breast cancer. Also, the development of a skin-sparing mastectomy enables the surgeon to use more breast skin, which greatly improves the outcome of immediate reconstruction.[219]

Delayed reconstruction is indicated when a patient is unable to make a decision about this surgery, possibly because of the emotional trauma of a cancer diagnosis, or because the need for adjuvant chemotherapy is unclear and more time is needed to develop a treatment plan. Also, patients with fixed chest wall masses or involvement of the pectoralis major are not good candidates for immediate reconstruction.[219] Breast reconstruction can occur weeks to years after a mastectomy. There are no differences in recurrence or survival rates noted between immediate or delayed reconstruction.[218] Once the decision regarding timing of surgery has been made, breast reconstruction options fall into 2 broad categories: implant reconstruction and autogenous reconstruction. See Table 48-9 for a comparison of reconstructive procedures.[220]

### Breast implant reconstruction

Tissue expansion followed by breast implant reconstruction is the simplest option with the shortest recovery since there is no use of donor tissue. It is the most common breast reconstruction performed in the US and is recommended for women with small to moderate-sized breasts with little or no ptosis, or tissue drooping. Contraindications to this procedure include the lack of available skin flap to close over the implant, preoperative or postoperative RT or previous RT to the breast area, obesity, and a smoking history.[219] Tissue expansion with permanent breast implant placement is the simplest type of reconstruction, but it is a multistep process and requires a commitment to completing numerous procedures over a period of several months.

Initially, the surgeon creates a subpectoral/subserratus pocket in the breast that is filled with an empty tissue expander. The expander is filled with varying amounts of saline, and the wound is closed. This procedure takes approximately 1 hour, after the mastectomy is performed. Patients usually stay in the hospital 24 to 48 hours. Approximately 2 weeks after the initial procedure, patients begin a series of expansions in the outpatient setting. The expansions involve weekly or biweekly percutaneous injections of saline through ports built into the expanders. Patients report that the expansion process is moderately but briefly uncomfortable. The process usually takes 6 to 8 weeks.[219]

Approximately 3 months after the initial surgery, a second procedure is performed. The tissue expander is surgically removed and replaced with a permanent implant. The FDA approved silicone gel-filled breast implants for breast reconstruction in 2006. There are now a variety of silicone gel and saline permanent breast implants available. The choice for the specific type of implant is made by the patient and her surgeon on the basis of breast size, shape, and contour. Silicone gel implants tend to be softer and feel more like natural breast tissue than the saline implants. Complications associated with tissue expansion and breast implants include postoperative infection, mastectomy flap necrosis, contracture of the implant capsule or wrinkling at the incision line, and migration or deflation of the implant. Complications of the expander/implant technique are less than 10%, in patients who do not receive RT to the breast.[218] Breast implants need to be replaced every 10 to 12 years to minimize rupture. This procedure can be done on an out-patient basis.

Patients who select tissue expansion with permanent implant reconstruction have the option of undergoing mastopexy or augmentation of the contralateral breast to achieve symmetry. This type of reconstructive surgery is favorable for bilateral mastectomies because symmetry is more easily achieved, and donor site adequacy and morbidity are not issues.[219]

### Autogenous breast reconstruction

Autogenous (autologous) tissue reconstruction involves the use of the patient's tissue from donor sites to reconstruct the breast mound after mastectomy. Autogenous reconstruction can be further divided into 2 categories: pedicle flaps and free flaps. Pedicle flap reconstruction procedures include the transverse rectus abdominus myocutaneous (TRAM) flap procedure and the latissimus dorsi

**TABLE 48-9**

**Comparison of Reconstruction Procedures**

| Surgical Procedure | Anesthesia | OR Time | Days in Hospital | Shape and Consistency | Scars |
|---|---|---|---|---|---|
| Insertion of tissue expander | General | 1 hour | 2–3 with mastectomy, ambulatory if delayed | No natural ptosis, firm (temporary stretching device only) | Through mastectomy scar (no new scar) |
| Exchange of tissue expander for permanent implant[a] | General | 1 hour | 0 | Softer than expander; shape and ptosis closer to that of natural breast | Through mastectomy scar (no new scar) |
| Latissimus dorsi flap | General | 3–4 hours | 2–4 | Natural shape, soft | Donor-site scar on back |
| Pedicle TRAM flap | General | 4–5 hours | 4–5 | Natural shape, soft | Donor-site scar on abdomen |
| Free TRAM flap | General | 5–6 hours | 5–7 | Natural shape, soft | Donor-site scar on abdomen |
| Gluteal free flap | General | 6–8 hours | 7–10 | Natural shape, soft | Donor-site scar on gluteus (buttock) |
| Nipple/areolar reconstruction using a skin graft[a] | Local with IV sedation | 1.5 hours | 0 | Reconstructed nipple will have tactile but not erectile sensation | Donor-site scar at inner upper thigh fold (groin fold) |
| Nipple/areolar reconstruction using micropigmentation (tattooing)[a] | Local anesthesia in doctor's office | Procedure time: 20 minutes (approximately) | NA | Gives illusion of the nipple/ areolar | NA |

[a]These procedures are done following initial breast reconstruction.

*Abbreviation*: IV, intravenous; NA, not applicable; OR, operating room; TRAM, transverse rectus abdominus myocutaneous.

*Source*: Data from Baron and Vaziri.[220]

procedure. Free flap reconstruction procedures involve microsurgery and include the TRAM, the deep inferior epigastric perforator (DIEP) flap, the superficial inferior epigastric artery (SIEA) flap, and the superior and inferior gluteal artery flaps.[219]

*Pedicle flaps.* The most widely used autogenous breast reconstruction procedure is the TRAM flap in which skin and fatty tissue from the lower abdomen is used to replace breast tissue removed by a mastectomy. Perfusion of the donor tissue is maintained through the vasculature of the rectus abdominus muscle. Either one rectus muscle (unipedicle flap) or both muscles (bipedicle flap) can be used, depending on surgeon preference. This surgery takes approximately 4 to 5 hours with a 4 to 5 week recovery period after which patients can usually stand upright, walk comfortably, and resume normal activities.[219,221]

Advantages of the TRAM flap include a reconstructed breast that appears natural. A portion of abdominal skin can be used to reconstruct the areola and nipple. Since fat is removed from the abdomen, the abdominal contour is improved (the so-called "tummy tuck" benefit). TRAM flap reconstruction can be performed immediately after a skin-sparing mastectomy, resulting in fewer complications and improved cosmetic results.[218] Disadvantages to this procedure include the prolonged recovery period and abdominal wall weakness. Reconstruction of the abdominal wall with mesh during the surgery can reduce the problems with weakness of the abdominal wall.

Complications of the TRAM flap reconstruction include infection, fat necrosis, and partial or complete flap loss. Contraindications to TRAM flap reconstruction are factors that compromise wound healing and blood supply to the transferred tissue such as prior abdominal surgery or radiation, smoking, obesity, collagen disorders, and insufficient donor tissue. It is the procedure of choice for unilateral breast reconstruction for the appropriate patient.[218,219]

The latissimus dorsi flap (with or without implant) is a viable reconstruction option for women who have inadequate abdominal tissue or prior abdominal surgery or scarring. The procedure involves the rotation of the latissimus muscle with a skin paddle through the axilla to the mastectomy site. The latissimus is sewn to the chest wall and the pectoralis muscle, creating a pocket in which the implant can be placed. The implant may be required to ensure breast symmetry. The vascular supply to this flap is maintained by the thoracodorsal artery and vein. The skin paddle is used to reconstruct the areola and nipple. This surgery also requires 4 hours to complete and requires several intraoperative patient position changes. Like the TRAM flap reconstruction, the latissimus dorsi flap can be performed immediately after mastectomy with all the advantages of a single stage surgical plan. The latissimus dorsi procedure requires a shorter recovery period than the TRAM and is associated with less fat necrosis and flap failure. Cosmesis is reported as excellent. (See Figures 48-14 and 48-15.) Complications include prolonged donor site seroma formation (15% incidence) that may require repeated aspirations, infection, and capsular contracture. Capsular contracture occurs more often among patients who have postoperative radiation. Also, a full lymph node dissection may injure the blood supply of the latissimus flap. A sentinal lymph node biopsy performed prior to reconstruction would provide information regarding the need for axillary dissection.[218,219]

*Free flap.* The free flap represents the newest technique in breast reconstructive surgery. This procedure entails removing a portion of skin and fat from the lower abdomen that may also include a portion of muscle, and grafting it to the mastectomy site with microvascular anastomoses. The free flap has been reported to reduce complications, require shorter hospitalizations, and enhance the cosmetic outcome over pedicled tissue.[222]

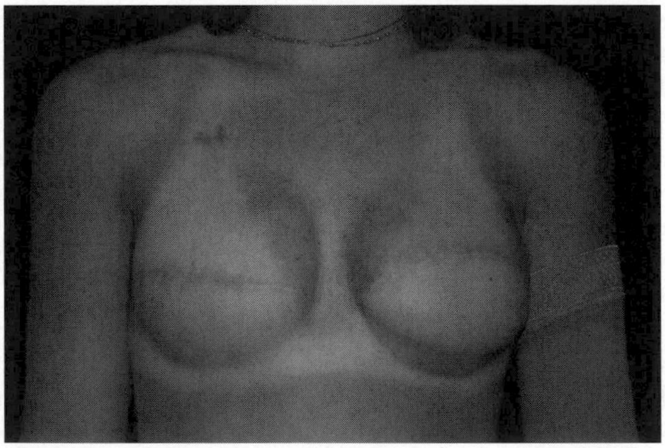

**FIGURE 48-14**

Latissimus flap with implant reconstruction on left in radiated field.

*Source*: Courtesy of Joseph Serletti, MD. Department of Plastic Surgery, Hospital of the University of Pennsylvania.

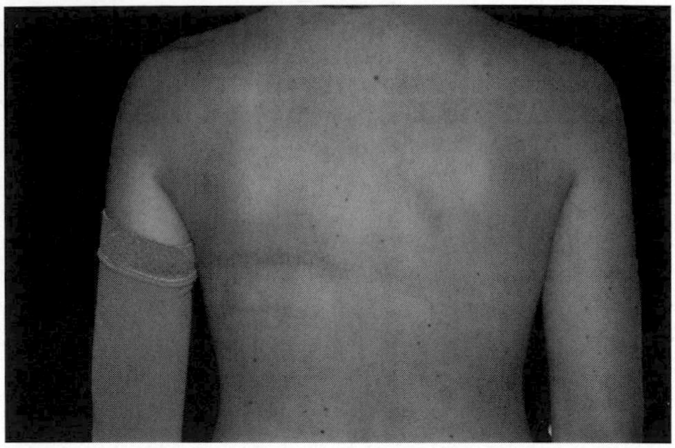

**FIGURE 48-15**

Donor site latissimus dorsi flap.

*Source*: Courtesy of Joseph Serletti, MD. Department of Plastic Surgery, Hospital of the University of Pennsylvania.

In the TRAM free flap procedure, skin, fat fascia, muscle, and vessels are removed from the abdomen and transplanted at the mastectomy site. Deep inferior epigastric perforator (DIEP) and superficial inferior epigastric artery (SIEA) are muscle-sparing procedures in which only abdominal skin, fat, and vessels are removed and transplanted. For patients who are not candidates for abdominal or latissimus dorsi flaps, either by medical history or choice, the superior or inferior gluteal artery flap, the deep circumflex iliac artery flap, of the anterolateral thigh flap can be performed. These procedures may or may not be muscle-sparing, depending on the size and integrity of the vessels involved. There is an increased donor site morbidity and limited amount of donor tissue associated with these procedures. Free flap surgeries are longer than the pedicle procedures, but recovery is shorter because less tissue is dissected. Complications include infection, flap failure, fat necrosis, bleeding, and thrombosis. Free flap reconstruction is an option for certain high-risk patients such as smokers and the obese.[218] (See Figures 48-16 and 48-17.)

## NIPPLE–AREOLAR CONSTRUCTION

Construction of the nipple–areolar complex is the final phase of the breast reconstruction process. The symmetry and cosmetic result of the breast mound should be satisfactory before this procedure is performed. Nipple–areolar reconstruction can be performed after the completion of

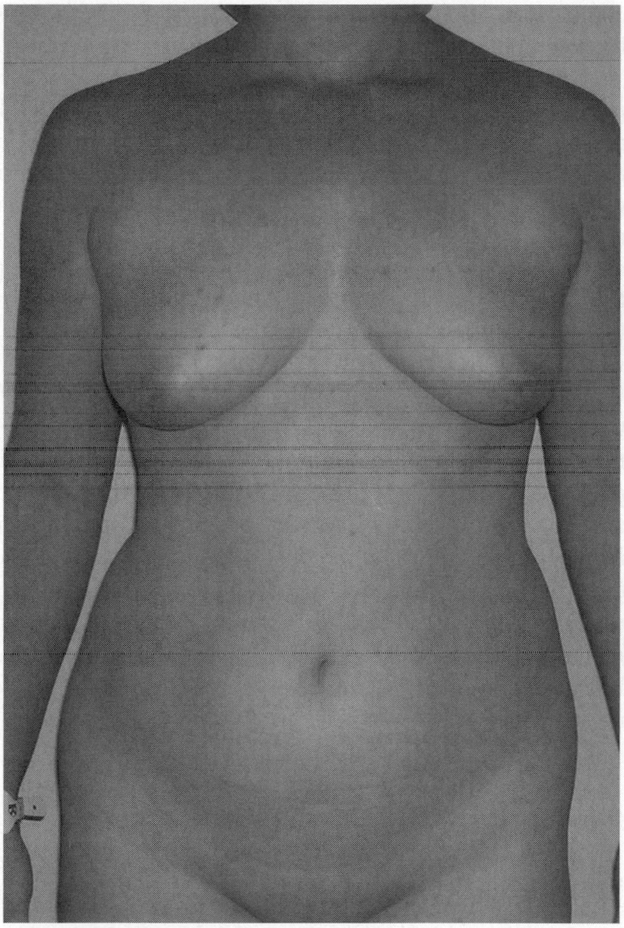

**FIGURE 48-16**

Pre-surgery reconstruction.

*Source*: Courtesy of Joseph Serletti, MD. Department of Plastic Surgery, Hospital of the University of Pennsylvania.

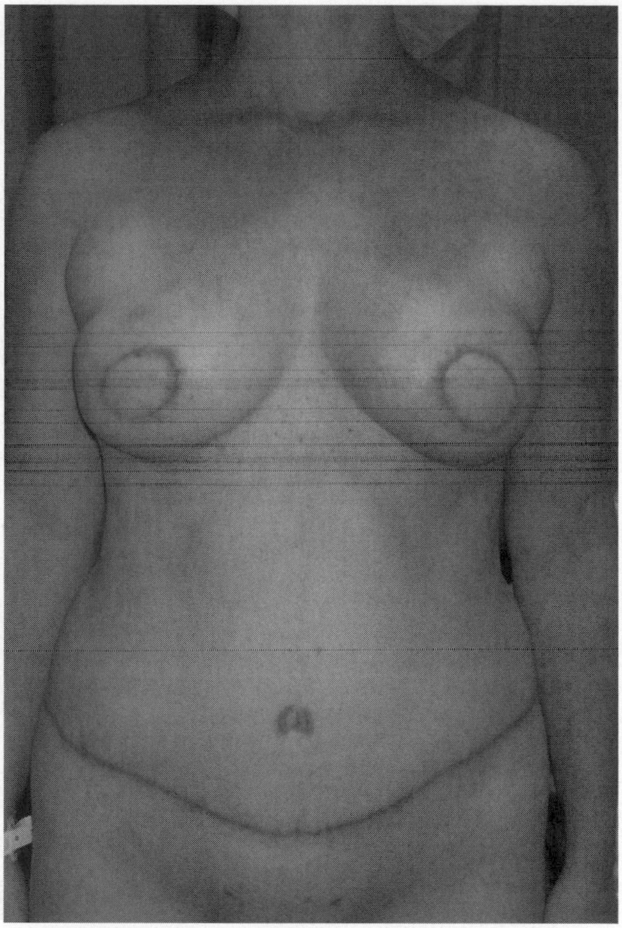

**FIGURE 48-17**

Bilateral free flap reconstruction.

*Source*: Courtesy of Joseph Serletti, MD. Department of Plastic Surgery, Hospital of the University of Pennsylvania.

adjuvant therapy. The nipple should closely match the opposite side in size and pigment.

Tissue may be taken from the opposite breast if an adequate supply is available or if mastopexy has been performed. Tissue can also be harvested from the groin or from excess skin from a TRAM flap. Previously, the nipple was often "banked" to the patient's thigh or groin to be used later. This method has fallen out of favor due to the risk of introducing potentially malignant tissue to the disease-free breast.

Tattooing is the primary method for creating the darker pigment of the areola. Another option is a skin graft from the inner thigh. However, grafts are uncomfortable and can fade, requiring tattooing, so most women prefer to forgo this surgery and have the area tattooed.[223]

Maintaining projection is a challenge that has been met by construction of pedicle flaps. These techniques fold the skin to achieve a slightly protuberant nipple. The most popular methods are the skate flap and the c-v flap technique, in which the skin is raised and folded to achieve a natural nipple profile. Complications are rare with nipple–areolar reconstruction, but may include failure to maintain suitable projection of the nipple, graft failure, and fading of the pigmented areas.[224] (See Figure 48-18.)

## NURSING IMPLICATIONS

Oncology nurses have the opportunity to deliver many levels of care to patients with breast cancer undergoing reconstructive surgery. This care requires quality teaching, assessment, and clinical skills and the ability to attend to the psychological/emotional needs of this population.

Women who are recently diagnosed with breast cancer are uniquely vulnerable. They are given a potentially devastating diagnosis and are then asked to make decisions regarding chemotherapy and/or RT, surgery and possible breast reconstruction. The timing and sequencing of the

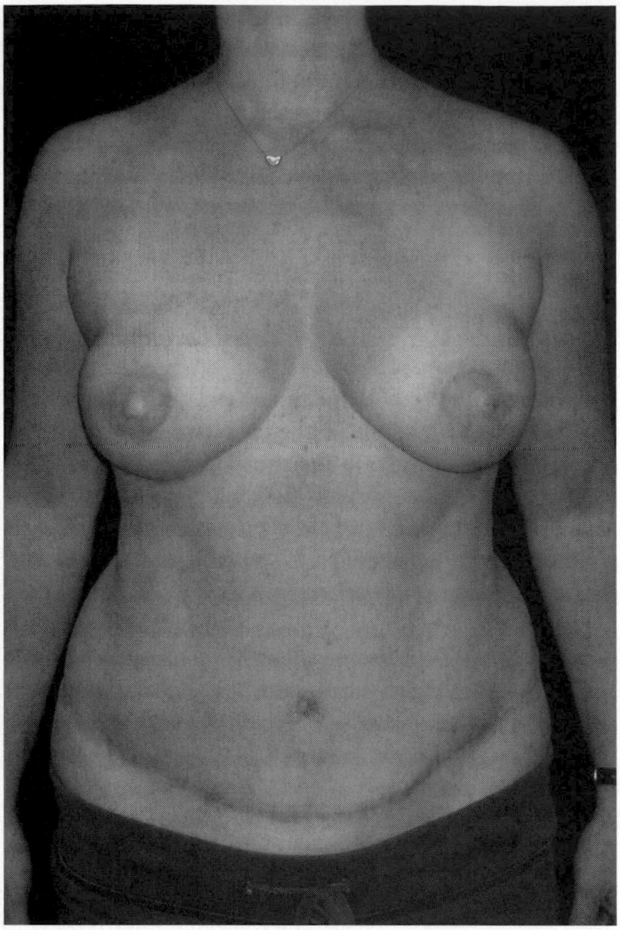

**FIGURE 48-18**

Nipple/areolar reconstruction and tattooing.

*Source*: Courtesy of Joseph Serletti, MD. Department of Plastic Surgery, Hospital of the University of Pennsylvania.

treatment modalities are interdependent. For full efficacy of the treatments, decisions have to be made in a timely fashion. Consequently, many women are overwhelmed by the deluge of information and choices that they must make. It is imperative for oncology nurses to provide emotional support to these patients and their families, offering counseling and social work support when appropriate. Also, adequate patient teaching is of paramount importance so that patients can give their informed consent.

Some teaching points regarding breast reconstruction are that more than one surgeon is involved in the procedure. Usually both an oncologic surgeon and a plastic surgeon participate, and scheduling of the surgery has to be coordinated with both practices. Occasionally, multiple minor surgical procedures are required after reconstruction to achieve optimal cosmesis. Patients need to be aware of the extended time and emotional commitment involved. Patients cannot undergo MRIs while saline expanders are in place because of the metal port. See Table 48-9 for a comparison of reconstruction procedures and Table 48-10 for a comprehensive list of preoperative teaching.[220]

Postoperative nursing care includes monitoring the patient for adequate pain control and wound healing. To prevent failure, flaps should be assessed frequently for color, temperature, circulation, edema, and temperature. Prior to discharge, patients should be taught to monitor for and report signs of infection or poor wound healing as well as drain and wound care. Referral for visiting nurses is helpful. Range of motion exercises should be taught. Arranging for physical therapy is frequently indicated after initial wound healing.[225]

Women with breast cancer who have undergone a mastectomy and reconstruction, regardless of the timing, need effective emotional support from their nurses. The patients can experience fear, loss, body image disturbances, and depression. They can also experience disappointment if the cosmetic results of reconstruction are not what they expected. Their emotional needs can continue long after the incisions have healed. Competent emotional support, including referrals for counseling or support groups when indicated, is an important component of nursing care for these patients.

## SYSTEMIC ADJUVANT THERAPY

### Local–regional breast cancer

Much of the research in breast cancer has concentrated on finding optimal regimens of systemic therapy that have the potential to destroy circulating tumor cells. The need for such research is paramount, given that nearly 90% of women newly diagnosed with breast cancer are potentially curable. Of that group, nearly 60% will have node-negative disease. The results of prospective clinical trials suggest that the rate of disease recurrence in patients with node-negative breast cancer can be reduced 20% to 50% by administration of adjuvant therapy.[226] This led to the conclusion at the NIH Consensus Development Conference on Early Stage Breast Cancer that, although the majority of patients with node-negative breast cancer are cured by breast-conserving treatment or total mastectomy and axillary node dissection, the rate of local and distant relapse following local therapy for node-negative breast cancer is decreased both by combination chemotherapy and by tamoxifen.[227]

*Adjuvant therapy.* Upon completion of surgery and before radiation begins, if indicated, it is important to discuss the role of systemic adjuvant therapy. Systemic therapy includes endocrine therapy, chemotherapy, and/or targeted therapy. The decision to use systemic therapy involves examining the risks vs the benefits of the therapy. The major goal of adjuvant therapy in breast cancer is to decrease the chance of recurrence and improve survival. The benefit of adjuvant

**TABLE 48-10**

**General Preoperative Teaching**

| Preoperative Teaching Topics | Teaching Points |
|---|---|
| Things to expect after surgery | Patients undergoing a flap procedure will have an incision drain(s) at the reconstructed breast site and at the donor site. |
| | Postoperative swelling is normal and may last for a couple of weeks. |
| | There may be temporary skin-color change at the reconstructed site (bruising, pinkish skin). These changes improve with time. |
| | Patients undergoing a flap procedure will experience temporary tightness at the reconstructed site at the donor site. |
| | Any patient having a flap procedure will have a Foley catheter for 2–3 days postoperatively. |
| | Patients having TRAM or gluteal flap procedure are asked to donate 1–2 units of packed red blood cells in case it is needed during or after surgery. |
| | Patients are taught breathing and leg exercises to prevent pneumonia and DVT, respectively. |
| Change in sensation in the reconstructed breast | Patients may experience temporary changes in sensation such as sensitivity to touch, numbness, and tingling (caused by nerve damage during mastectomy). |
| | Some degree of numbness and change of sensation may be permanent. |
| Pain management | Pain medication may include PCA pumps, IM or PO narcotics depending on level of pain . |
| Range-of-motion exercises | Exercises generally begin the day after surgery with appropriate modifications for individual procedures |
| Home care needs | Patients having TRAM flap or gluteal flap will need help at home for at least 1 week following discharge. |
| Time away from work | Approximately 4–6 weeks after implant reconstruction; |
| | 6–8 weeks after latissimus dorsi flap; |
| | 6–12 weeks after TRAM flap and gluteal flap. |

*Abbreviations*: DVT, deep vein thrombosis; IM, intramuscular; PCA, patient-controlled analgesia; PO, oral; TRAM, transverse rectus abdominus myocutaneous.

*Source*: Data from Baron and Vaziri.[220]

chemotherapy or endocrine therapy is in proportion to the risk of breast cancer recurrence.[227] A patient's prognostic and predictive factors play a key role in making a decision in systemic therapy. These factors include age, tumor size, menopausal status, lymph node involvement, comorbidities, ER and PR status, and *HER2/neu* status. In the last 5 to 10 years, research has shown that most individuals will benefit from some combination of endocrine therapy, targeted therapy or chemotherapy

A large statistical analysis demonstrated that optimal use of adjuvant therapy can significantly improve long-term survival in women with stage I and II breast cancer. In women younger than age 50, adjuvant chemotherapy alone reduces the annual odds of recurrence by 35% and the annual odds of death by 27%. Adjuvant chemotherapy is less effective in postmenopausal women older than age 50. Treatment for this group reduces the annual odds of recurrence by 20% and the annual odds of death by 11%.[228]

Typically, for patients with tumors smaller than 1 cm in diameter and negative nodes, the chance of recurrence is less than 10% at 10 years if no chemotherapy is given. It may be reasonable not to offer these patients adjuvant chemotherapy. Chemotherapy can cause may short-term and long-term side effects. However, for some women with node-negative breast cancer, such as ER, PR, and *HER2/neu* negative breast cancer, the incidence of metastatic disease is higher and approaches 50%.[229] Combination chemotherapy can effectively reduce the annual odds of recurrence by at least 30% in this population but to achieve this rate, 70% of patients will receive therapy unnecessarily because they would have been cured by surgery alone. When managing early stage breast cancer, it is important to optimize adjuvant systemic therapy, in order to improve long-term survival and minimize toxicity.[230] Some tools have been developed in the last 10 years to help this decision. Some oncologists are using Adjuvant! Online, an online program that analyzes a patient's breast cancer features to calculate the risk of relapse and mortality. It can also help to predict the benefit of hormonal therapy and chemotherapy.[231] Mammoprint is another assay developed recently to assist oncologists making decisions about adjuvant chemotherapy. It is a scoring system in which a 70 gene assay is performed on fresh breast cancer tissue to predict recurrence.[231] Also, trials in the field of genomics conducted with NSABP have led to approval of a DNA microarray (OncotypeDX Breast Cancer Assay, Genomic Health, Inc, Redwood City, California) that uses a scoring system to assign a numeric risk to individual women based on the particular genetic profile of their breast cancer. This is currently approved for use in breast cancer patients with estrogen positive, node-negative disease. Use of this test along with assessment of existing risk factors for recurrence may allow oncologists to prospectively determine who may require chemotherapy and who may not.[232]

Although prognostic indicators such as cellular ploidy status, proliferative indices, and tumor grade may help to determine a woman's risk of recurrence, no one parameter is completely predictive of recurrence. Most clinicians agree that many women with node-negative breast cancer should receive adjuvant chemotherapy, especially those with larger tumors. Women with the lowest risk of recurrence are those with tumors smaller than 1 cm, a low-grade malignancy, positive ER/PRs, negative *HER2/neu* status, and a low proliferative rate. In contrast, those with tumors larger than 2 cm, a high-grade malignancy, negative ER/PRs, positive *HER2/neu* status, triple negative receptor status (ER, PR, and *HER2/neu* negative), and a high rate of proliferation are at highest risk for tumor recurrence.

### *Adjuvant endocrine therapy*

***Tamoxifen.*** Tamoxifen is a nonsteroidal antiestrogen drug that binds estrogen and modulates the functions mediated by this receptor system. Tamoxifen binds competitively to ER present in tumor cells. By blocking the binding of estrogen, it blocks cell cycle transit in the Gap 1 phase and inhibits tumor growth.

Adjuvant tamoxifen significantly reduces the risks of recurrence and death from breast cancer in women in all age groups who have hormone receptor positive breast cancer. It can be used in premenopausal and post menopausal patients. In women with ER positive breast cancer, adjuvant tamoxifen is the standard of care for endocrine therapy for premenopausal women. It decreases the annual odds of recurrence by 39% and the annual odds of death by 31% irrespective of the use of chemotherapy, patient age, menopausal status, or axillary lymph node status.[166,187] The benefit is greatest when tamoxifen is administered for 5 years and when it is given to women with ER positive tumors. It is also a viable choice in women who present with advanced tumors when chemotherapy is contraindicated. (See Figure 48-19.) Tamoxifen has been shown to significantly reduce the incidence of contralateral breast cancer in women whose primary breast cancer was hormone receptor positive. It may be contraindicated in patients with clotting disorders, immobility, history of uterine dysplasia, or psychiatric disorders, such as depression.

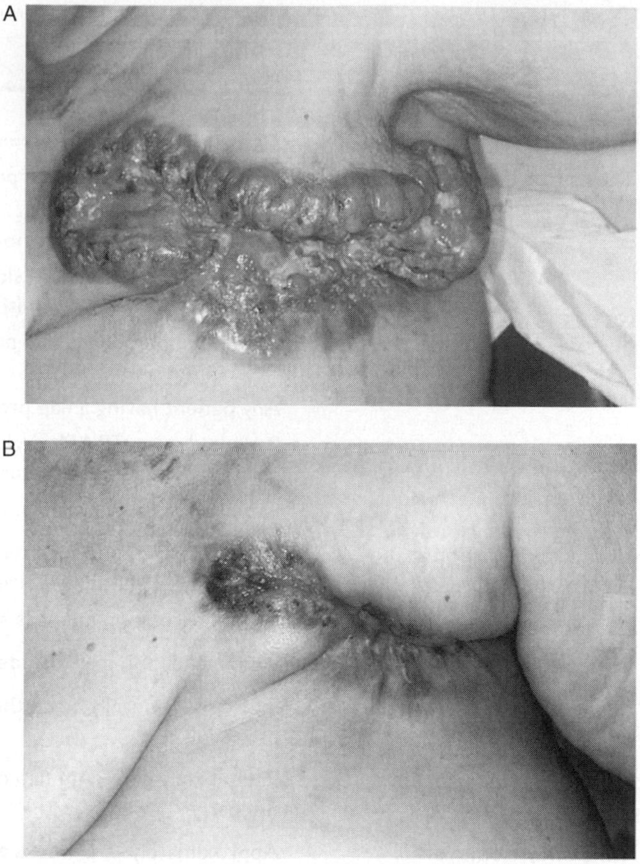


**FIGURE 48-19**

Two pictures depict (A) a patient with a long-neglected breast cancer who was placed on tamoxifen 20 mg per day and (B) the improvement after 6 months of therapy.

Tamoxifen has several side effects. Common side effects include hot flashes, night sweats, vaginal discharge, vaginal dryness, mood swings, leg cramps, weight gain, bloating and swelling. Blood clots, both deep vein thrombosis and pulmonary embolism, and uterine cancer are among the more life threatening side effects of tamoxifen. Undesirable consequences of the estrogen-like effects of SERMs include stimulation of the endometrium. Although tamoxifen may promote endometrial cancer due to its estrogen agonist effects, the benefits of preventing disease recurrence or progression usually outweigh the risk of developing endometrial cancer. The risk of endometrial cancer is greater in postmenopausal women than in those still experiencing regular menses.[229,233–235] Another side effect of tamoxifen is ocular toxicity (retinopathy or keratophy). It is not a clinically significant danger of tamoxifen therapy.[236] After tamoxifen withdrawal, ocular abnormalities are usually found to be reversible. Currently, the recommendation is to continue treatment unless visual symptoms are present. Patients might benefit from routine eye examination, especially those with preexisting ophthalmologic conditions.[236–238]

*Aromatase inhibitors.* Aromatase inhibitors (AIs) function differently from tamoxifen and are now considered to be the optimal endocrine therapy for postmenopausal female hormone positive breast cancer. The conversion of adrenal androgens to estrogens occurs primarily in adipose, muscle, ovarian, brain, and liver tissue, and constitutes the primary source of estrogen in postmenopausal estrogen-dependent breast cancer. AIs reversibly bind to the aromatase enzyme that is responsible for the conversion of androstenedione to estrone. AIs also prevent the peripheral aromatization of other steroids to estrogen, primarily in body fat. The aromatase enzyme acts at the last step in the estrogen-synthesis pathway, catalyzing the conversion of androgens to estrogens. Nonsteroidal AIs, such as letrozole and anastrozole, work by reversible inhibition of aromatase and subsequent reduction of estrogen synthesis.[239] Steroidal AI or exemestane, which is a steroidal aromatase inactivator, has also been studied in the adjuvant setting. It works by irreversibly binding to and inactivating aromatase, therefore inhibiting estrogen production. AIs are not active in women with functioning ovaries and should only be used in postmenopausal women.[189]

In the last several years there have been multiple studies evaluating AIs in the adjuvant breast cancer setting. These trials have examined using AIs in 3 different ways: as initial adjuvant endocrine treatment for 5 years; in patients treated with adjuvant tamoxifen switching after 2 to 3 years and receiving an AI for a total of 5 years of adjuvant endocrine therapy; and in patients who have completed 5 years of adjuvant tamoxifen and will receive 5 years of an AI. All of these studies demonstrated an increased OS with the use of AIs compared to tamoxifen or placebo in the adjuvant setting.[189,195,240–242] Three of these pivotal trials include the ATAC (Anastrozole or Tamoxifen Alone or in Combination), the BIG (Breast International Group) 1–98 trial, and the MA.17 trial. The ATAC trial was a large, randomized clinical trial investigating the use of anastrozole or tamoxifen alone or in combination in the adjuvant setting. ATAC showed anastrozole to be superior to tamoxifen and was a well-tolerated endocrine option in early breast cancer.[243] The BIG 1–98 was a randomized trial testing the use of tamoxifen alone for 5 years, letrozole alone for 5 years, tamoxifen for 2 years followed sequentially by letrozole for 3 years, or letrozole for 2 years followed sequentially by tamoxifen for 3 years.[189] With 8,010 women included with the analysis, DFS was superior in the women treated with up front letrozol for 5 years.[189,244] The MA-17 trial looked at patients who received 4.5 to 6 years of tamoxifen, then within 3 months of stopping endocrine therapy were randomized to received either letrozole or placebo.[245] This trial demonstrated that extended therapy with letrozol provides additional benefit in post menopausal women with hormone positive breast cancer.[189,245,246] A separate, additional analysis of this trial also found significant improvements in both DFS and distant DFS with women who started letrozole after having no endocrine therapy for an extended period.[189,247] Because of these trials, AIs are now the preferred endocrine therapy over tamoxifen in postmenopausal females, although tamoxifen can still be considered in females with relative and absolute contraindications to AIs.

The side effects most commonly reported with AIs include joint aches, joint stiffness, hot flashes and bone loss. Bone loss appears to increase during the first 2 years of therapy, with declining loss thereafter. Also, in a phase III study of letrozole vs megestrol acetate by Buzdar and colleagues, hair thinning, headache, nausea, and diarrhea were reported more frequently in the letrozole arm.[248]

*Adjuvant chemotherapy.* Adjuvant chemotherapy for breast cancer treatment has changed in the last 5 to 10 years. Recent advances in adjuvant chemotherapy for breast cancer includes new standards in adjuvant chemotherapy, the addition of taxane chemotherapy drugs in the adjuvant setting, the need for anthracycline chemotherapy in the adjuvant setting being called into question, and the demonstrated benefit of adding *HER2/neu* targeted therapy to chemotherapy in the adjuvant setting.[230]

Several combination chemotherapy regimens are currently being used to treat local–regional breast cancer. Drugs that are generally used in the adjuvant breast cancer setting include doxorubicin, cyclophosphamide, paclitaxel, doxetaxel, and less frequently fluorouracil, and methotrexate. According to the National Comprehensive Cancer Network consensus based guidelines published in 2009, the preferred adjuvant breast cancer regimens include: (1) docetaxel, doxorubicin, and cyclophosphamide (TAC); (2) doxorubicin and cyclophosphamide (AC); (3) doxorubicin and cyclophosphamide dose dense or every 2 weeks followed by paclitaxel dose dense; (4) doxorubicin and cyclophosphamide followed by weekly paclitaxel; (5) docetaxel plus cyclophosphamide (TC).[189] Doxorubicin based regimens currently have been found in randomized trials to be superior to cyclophosphamide, 5-fluorouracil, and methotrexate (CMF) in relapse-free and overall survival.[189,249,250] CMF is no longer the treatment of choice. If it is used today, all 3 drugs are given intravenously and this regimen is never used concurrently with RT due to the risk of radiation recall of the irradiated skin sites.

In the past decade, the role of paclitaxel or docetaxel in the adjuvant setting has been extensively studied. The addition or substitution of a taxane to adjuvant anthracycline-based chemotherapy improves DFS and OS in women with early stage breast cancer, irrespective of age, menopausal status, hormonal receptor status, and lymph node involvement.[230,251–253] Results available from 16 randomized trials comprising >30,000 women with early-stage breast cancer in which taxane and non-taxane containing regimens were compared in 3 meta-analyses each showing that the addition of taxanes in the adjuvant setting for breast cancer provides benefit.[230] Research is still needed to determine when taxanes are most appropriate. Based upon existing evidence, the role of a taxane appears most appropriate in women who have a high risk of relapse and have no endocrine sensitivity, multiple positive nodes, and *HER2/neu* positive breast cancers.[230] Triple negative patients are another high-risk group who are thought to benefit from an anthracycline plus taxane based regimen.[254]

In recent years researchers have questioned the safety of using anthracyclines as part of adjuvant breast cancer therapy. The experience from clinical trials suggests that the excess risk of cardiac morbidity related to anthracyclines-based therapies is small.[166,230] Many researchers have questioned long-term cardiac side effects and safety, especially in older women and early stage breast cancer.[255,256] In 2000 the Early Breast Cancer Trialists' Collaborative Group (EBCTCG) overview of anthracycline-based regimens were associated with an annual risk of cardiac mortality of 0.08%/year compared to 0.06%/year in patients with non-anthracycline-based regimens.[166,230] In part due to this concern, a recent trial randomized women to 4 cycles of docetaxel-cyclosphosphamide (TC) regimen or 4 cycles of adriamycin-cyclophosphamide (AC) and results were updated in 2007.[230,257] The trial initially demonstrated an improvement in 5-year DFS for TC over AC after a median follow up of 5.5 years and at 7 years median follow up, treatment with TC was associated with a statistically significant improvement in OS (6-year OS 88% for TC vs 84% for AC, hazard ratio = 0.73, $P = 0.045$).[230,258] This trial provided a reasonable option for women with low-intermediate risk disease, especially those at risk for anthracycline-induced cardiomyopathy.[230] It also raised the question of whether or not anthracyclines are needed in adjuvant breast cancer treatment.

Chemotherapy has many side effects, and these depend on the particular regimen used. In general, the side effects seen in adjuvant breast cancer treatment include, but are not limited to, nausea, vomiting, neutropenia, anemia, peripheral neuropathy, arthragias and myalgias. Rare side effects include myelodysplastic syndrome, leukemia, cardiomyopathy, and bladder cystitis.

***Adjuvant targeted-trastuzumab therapy.*** Trastuzumab in the adjuvant setting for breast cancer has given *HER2/neu* positive patients new hope for survivorship. Trastuzumab is a humanized, monoclonal antibody that targets the extra cellular domain of *HER2/neu*.[189,259,260] *HER2/neu* belongs to a family of 4 transmembrane receptor tyrosine kinases that mediate the growth, differentiation, and survival of cells.[260–262] Overexpression of HER2/neu protein, amplification of the *HER2/neu* gene, or both occur in approximately 15% to 25% of breast cancers and this is generally thought of as a negative prognostic factor.[260,263,264] Only those patients with *HER2/neu* positive breast cancer are candidates of trastuzumab therapy.[265]

Recent large phase III trials demonstrated the benefit of trastuzumab in the adjuvant setting. In the NSABP B-31 trial, patients with *HER2/neu* positive, node positive, breast cancer were randomized to 4 cycles of AC every 3 weeks followed by 4 cycles of paclitaxel every 3 weeks, or the same regimen with trastuzumab for 52 weeks following the completion of the paclitaxel.[189] In the North Central Cancer Treatment Group (NCCTG) N9831 trial, patients with *HER2/neu* positive, node positive breast cancer; or if node negative, with primary tumors greater than 1 cm, if ER negative and PR negative, or greater than 2 cm in size if ER or PR positive were similarly randomized, except that paclitaxel was given at a low dose weekly schedule for 12 weeks and a third arm delayed trastuzumab until the completion of paclitaxel.[189] These 2 trials were analyzed together. They show that after a median 4-year follow up, a 52% reduction in the risk of breast cancer recurrence and a 35% decrease in the risk of death in the patients who received trastuzumab.[266] A third important trial showing the benefit of trastuzumab was the Herceptin Adjuvant Trail, HERA trial. This trial tested trastuzumab for 1 or 2 years compared to no therapy after varying standard chemotherapy regimens chosen by the treating MD in patients with node-positive or node-negative disease with tumors larger than 1 cm.[189,260] They found that after a 1-year median follow-up receiving 1 year of trastuzumab, resulted in a 46% reduction in the risk for recurrence compared with those patients who did not have trastuzumab, no difference in OS, and acceptable cardiac toxicity.[189] The 2-year data indicated that 1 year of trastuzumab therapy is associated with an OS benefit when compared with observation.[267] Lastly, the Breast Cancer International Research Group (BCIRG) 006 study randomized 3,222 women with *HER2/neu* negative, node positive, or high-risk node-negative breast cancer to AC followed by docetaxel, AC followed by docetaxel plus trastuzumab for 1 year (AC-TH), or carboplatin and docetaxel plus trastuzumab (TCH) for 1 year.[189,268] This study showed that OS advantage in patients in both trastuzumab arms.[189,268] A novel finding was that cardiac toxicity in the TCH arm was significantly lower than the patients who received AC-TH.[189,268]

Side effects related to trastuzumab include hypersensitivity reactions, or cytokine release syndrome generally seen with the first dose, and cardiotoxicity inducing congestive heart failure.[260] With the use of trastuzumab as a single agent in the metastatic setting, CHF or cardiac death was reported in 1.4% of women.[260,269,270] When combined with chemotherapy drugs, especially an anthracycline, there is a greater risk of cardiotoxicity. In fact, the risk is so high that concurrent use of trastuzumab and an anthracycline is contraindicated. Therefore, it is important to maintain strict cardiac monitoring when trastuzumab is given with chemotherapy. A MUGA or ECHO is often done every 3 months or more to follow patients' cardiac status. Also, when deciding on treatment for *HER2/neu* positive breast patients, it is important to weigh the benefits and risks of those with cardiac disease, especially in older adults.

## LOCALLY ADVANCED BREAST CANCER

Efforts to improve outcomes in patients with more advanced stage, node-positive cancer have focused on the development and application of new drugs and regimens, including targeted molecular therapeutics, in combination with systemic therapy. Dose dense regimens, in which treatment with myelosuppressive agents is given every 2 weeks rather than every 3 weeks, also improve outcomes, likely by increasing intracellular drug concentration. The addition of colony-stimulating factors ameliorates the dose-limiting toxicity of myelosuppression in these dose dense regimens, usually preventing the need for dose reductions or treatment delays. Giving optimal doses at regular, frequent intervals is an important strategy in preventing resistance and ultimate recurrence of disease. An intergroup clinical trial that evaluated dose dense vs standard AC followed by paclitaxel showed that, after a median follow up of 36 months, there was a 26% relative risk reduction in the odds of recurrence. Four-year DFS was 82% for the dose dense treatment vs 75% for the standard, every 3-week regimen. Dose dense treatment was associated with a 31% proportional reduction in mortality.[271,272]

Locally advanced breast cancer is associated with a high risk of developing distant metastases. The larger the size of the primary tumor, and the greater the number of histologically positive lymph nodes, the greater the risk of metastasis and death. Clinical characteristics of locally advanced disease include large (>5 cm) or unresectable primary tumors, fixed axillary nodes, and the classic inflammatory carcinoma. The classic inflammatory cancer diagnosis is based upon a clinical diagnosis and skin biopsy. While distant metastases are presumed to be present, they are not clinically apparent at staging.

If the tumor is fixed to the chest wall, inflammatory carcinoma is present, significant ulceration exists, or the axillary nodes are fixed to one another or other structures, the situation is generally considered inoperable and almost certain risk of recurrence. The presence of positive supraclavicular lymph nodes is also considered locally advanced breast cancer.[184]

The prognosis of patients with locally advanced disease is rarely improved by local therapy alone. Results are superior when chemotherapy and radiation are included in the treatment plan.[273] The use of neoadjuvant chemotherapy may result in significant tumor regression in 60% to 90% of women with locally advanced disease.[274] The advantage of using neoadjuvant therapy includes in vivo assessment of response. Significant tumor shrinkage may permit resection in previously unresectable disease, allowing for less extensive surgical procedures. In addition, neoadjuvant chemotherapy provides immediate treatment to possible micrometastasis that would otherwise be delayed by local therapy. In terms of survival, there is no apparent advantage to preoperative chemotherapy as compared with postoperative chemotherapy.[275] Combined modality therapy employing chemotherapy, surgery, and radiation may result in complete disappearance of disease in many patients, including those with inflammatory cancer.[275,276]

## METASTATIC BREAST CANCER

Despite improved screening techniques and increased awareness of breast cancer as a major health threat, approximately 10% of women diagnosed with breast cancer have metastatic disease at clinical presentation. Furthermore, approximately 30% of women diagnosed with early stage, node-negative disease and roughly 60% with node-positive disease will relapse despite adjuvant therapy. The majority of patients who relapse (80%) do so within 2 years of the diagnosis. Excessive physical examination and testing (x-ray, CT, MRI) to identify disease recurrences and metastases in an effort to institute earlier aggressive treatment have not altered the clinical course of women with metastatic breast cancer and therefore these interventions are not performed unless specific symptoms warrant investigation.[277–279]

Most recurrences or metastases are diagnosed on the basis of symptoms and physical findings. Instead of an obvious physical finding, a patient may complain of a cough that does not go away, an annoying and persistent back or hip pain that may only occur with movement, loss of appetite, mild nausea, or a slightly swollen abdomen. Subsequent diagnostic scans may reveal pulmonary or liver metastasis. An assessment of the extent of disease is carried out, first to document the recurrence of disease and second to determine the most appropriate therapeutic approach. Typically, a chest x-ray, bone scan, CT scan of the chest and liver, and serum chemistries are done at the time of known or suspected recurrence to identify any abnormalities and the need for further investigation of extent of disease. Tumor markers may be done as a baseline, as they may parallel the clinical course. Tumor markers are often normal when there is metastatic disease present, so are not always predictive, but if elevated at the time of metastatic disease diagnosis, they may be useful in following the disease. If disease is suspected, often tissue biopsies are typically performed to document disease and test for predictive factors such ER/PR and are analyzed for *HER2/neu* gene amplification.

The median survival time for stage IV disease is 2 to 3 years; however, reports of 5-year survival range from 12% to 35% and 10-year survival from 5% to 22%.[280] The goal of treatment for metastatic breast cancer is to extend survival and to control symptoms and provide the best quality of life possible given the fact that metastatic breast cancer is currently not curable.

## SITES OF BREAST CANCER METASTASIS

Breast cancer most commonly metastasizes to bone (more than 50% of patients), specifically, the spine, ribs, and proximal long bones. Affected patients may complain of localized, deep-seated, unrelenting pain. Pathological fracture of the proximal femur may occur spontaneously despite efforts to protect the weakened bone. Likewise, persistent back pain may herald a compression fracture and possible neurological impairment. Hypercalcemia may reflect bone resorption due to tumor growth and resultant osteoclastic stimulation. Bone marrow metastasis occurs frequently in patients with extensive multifocal bone disease, generally presenting as either pancytopenia or nocturnal pain. Pancytopenia in patients with a history of breast cancer should be evaluated by bone marrow aspiration and biopsy to rule out bone marrow infiltration by breast cancer cells, myelodysplastic disease, or acute leukemia.

Loss of appetite, abnormal liver function tests, mild nausea and mild right upper quadrant pain may be early symptoms of liver involvement. Late symptoms include right upper quadrant pain, referred right shoulder pain, abdominal distention, nausea, vomiting, periodic fever, jaundice, generalized weakness, and possibly confusion. Pulmonary involvement may begin as a subtle, nonproductive cough or shortness of breath. Lymphangitic pulmonary spread is an ominous sign of rapidly progressive disease. Pleural effusions can progress slowly over time but may respond temporarily to drainage and sclerosing. Renal involvement is extremely rare and generally presents as oliguria or uremia in a woman with deteriorating mental status. Brain metastasis usually occurs in the supratentorial region, in multiple sites, or as carcinomatous meningitis presenting as cranial nerve palsies, altered mentation, seizures, or focal paresis.

Cancer that has spread to the chest wall usually presents as a painless subcutaneous nodule along the mastectomy scar and adjacent chest wall areas. These lesions may respond well to local therapy, but distant disease is presumed to be present.[281] If the disease recurs locally after breast-conserving surgery plus radiation, mastectomy may be indicated, provided that the cancer is present only in the breast tissue and not in the skin or distant sites. Evidence of disease in a supraclavicular node or recurrence in the scar or chest wall after mastectomy generally indicates metastatic spread beyond the breast, warranting systemic therapy.

The management of patients with metastatic breast cancer is aimed at judicious use of local and systemic measures that control and/or palliate symptoms and improve quality of life while extending survival, but is not curative. The initial choice of therapy is generally the one that is the least toxic and carries with it the highest response rate. (See Figure 48-20.) The basic strategy is to achieve optimal control of the disease for as long as possible by sequential administration of appropriate systemic treatments, whether it includes endocrine therapy, chemotherapy, or targeted therapy. Several factors may affect treatment choice, including a patient's performance status, physician and patient preferences, adherence to therapy, drug administration route, comorbidities, drug toxicities, tumor characteristics, hormonal status, efficacy, and prior exposure to a certain class of drugs.[282] Local therapies are added periodically as needed to enhance systemic treatment. For many women, especially those with hormone receptor-positive disease, this can mean many years with better quality of life. Clinical trials of investigational agents should be considered for women with progressive metastatic breast cancer.

## ENDOCRINE THERAPY

### Antiestrogens and aromatase inhibitors

Women who have ER positive breast cancer demonstrate a consistently superior survival after recurrence compared to women who have ER negative disease. It is generally accepted that the greater the ER positivity, the greater the response rate to endocrine therapy. Similarly, the presence of both the ER and the PR on the tumor confers a higher response rate than the presence of only the ER.

When possible, tissue from the recurrent tumor should be tested for hormone receptors. Loss of the ER at relapse is a highly significant predictor of poor response to second-line endocrine therapy. For the patient who has not experienced prior hormonal manipulation, the use of tamoxifen, a selective estrogen receptor modulator (SERM), currently represents the standard of care for premenopausal females.[283] The SERM drugs bind the ER and modulate the functions mediated by this receptor. A new antiestrogen, fulvestrant, degrades and down-regulates the ER but does not bind to DNA; as a result, it has no estrogenic activity. Side effects are minimal. Fulvestrant is indicated when disease has progressed despite tamoxifen therapy.[284]

Aromatase inhibitors including anastrozole, letrozole, and exemestane, have been shown to improve progression-free and OS compared with tamoxifen in postmenopausal patients with advanced, hormone receptive positive breast cancer by approximately 11% across studies.[285,286] AIs show strong evidence of benefit over tamoxifen in the first-line metastatic setting for postmenopausal patients and are generally used first, although tamoxifen is often used through the course of treatment.[283,285] Approximately 40% to 50% of patients who relapse after an initial response to tamoxifen therapy respond to second-line endocrine therapy.[287]

### Androgens

Androgens are most effective in women who are 5 or more years postmenopause. The overall response rate to these agents is low. Androgens block pituitary gonadotropin secretion, thereby opposing endogenous estrogens. These

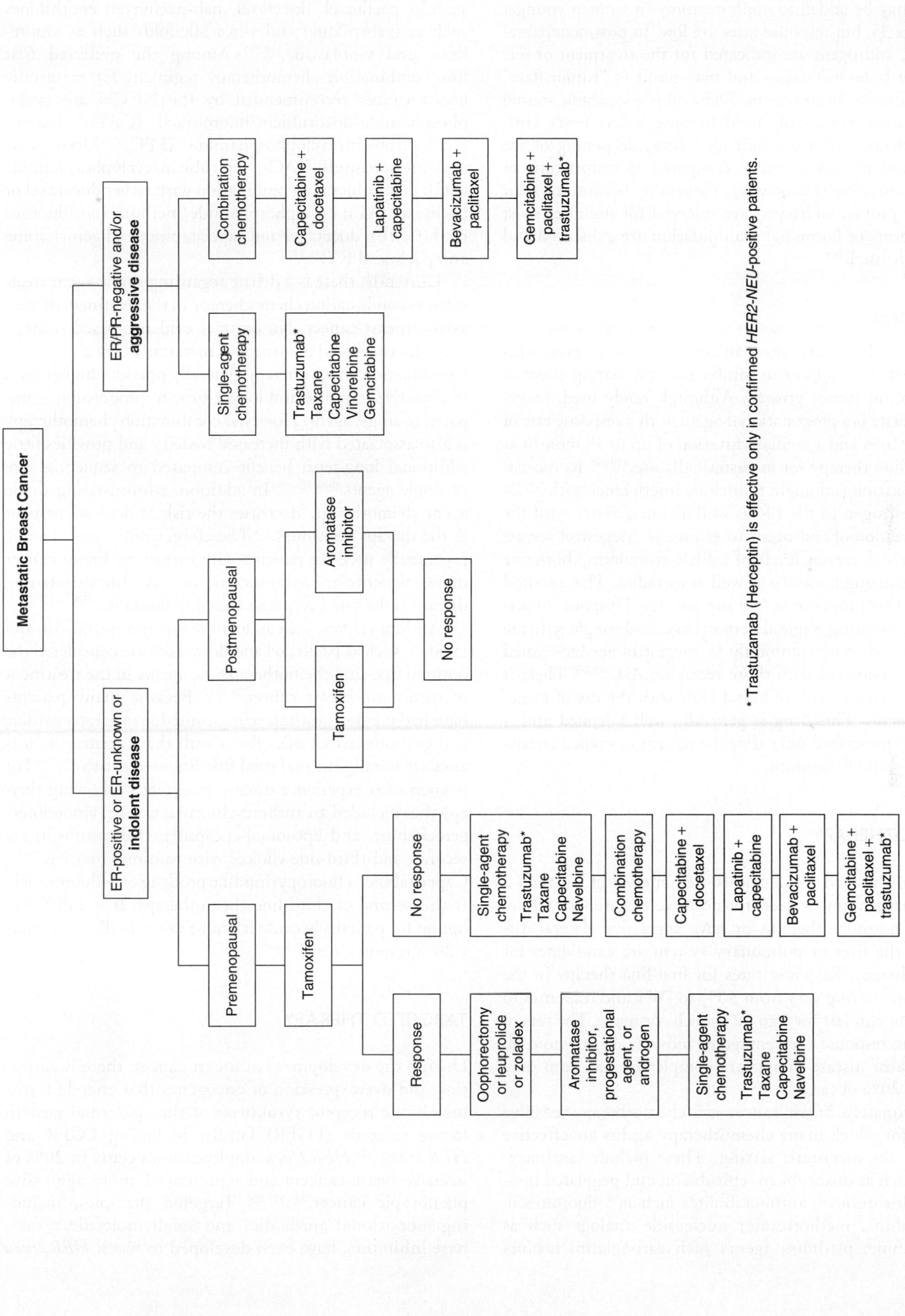


**FIGURE 48-20**

Metastatic breast cancer: systemic approaches to management.

*Abbreviations:* ER, estrogen receptor; PR, progesterone receptor.

drugs may be added to oophorectomy in women younger than age 35, but response rates are low. In postmenopausal women, androgens are indicated for the treatment of soft tissue or bone metastases and may result in "tumor flare" with initiation of treatment. Danazol is a synthetic steroid and is more commonly used because it has fewer virilizing effects (hirsutism, hair loss, acne, deepening of the voice, and increased libido) compared to testosterone or fluoxymesterone (Halotestin). Generally, because of their toxicity profile, androgens are reserved for use after most other forms of hormonal manipulation are exhausted and are rarely used.[288]

### Progestins

Although the precise mechanism of action of progestins is unclear, they appear to inhibit the stimulating effect of estradiol on tumor growth. Although rarely used, megestrol acetate is a progestational agent with a response rate of 12% to 16% and a median duration of up to 18 months as second-line therapy for metastatic disease.[239,248] Its mechanism of action is thought to include interference with binding of estrogen to the ER as well as interference with the aromatization of androgens to estrogens. Megestrol acetate effectively decreases levels of follicle-stimulating hormone and luteinizing hormone as well as estradiol. The standard dose of this progestin is 160 mg per day. Dyspnea, hypertension, sweating, vaginal hemorrhage, and weight gain are all observed more commonly in megestrol acetate-treated patients compared with those receiving AIs.[239,248] There is also an increased risk of blood clots with the use of megestrol acetate. This drug is generally well tolerated and is typically prescribed only after the patient has failed tamoxifen, AIs, and fulvestrant.

## CHEMOTHERAPY

Women who have had a disease-free interval of less than 2 years, have hormone receptor-negative disease, are refractory to hormone therapy, or have aggressive visceral disease in the liver or pulmonary system are candidates for chemotherapy. Response rates for first-line therapy in the metastatic setting vary from 30% to 70% and responses to treatment can last for 9 to 12 months or more. The rate of complete response (percentage of individuals in whom all evidence of disease disappears completely) has been only 10% to 20% of cases.[289–292]

Fortunately, breast cancer is a chemotherapy-sensitive cancer for which many chemotherapy agents are effective even in the metastatic setting. These include: anthracyclines such as doxorubicin, epirubicin, and pegylated liposomal doxorubicin; antimetabolites such as 5-fluorouracil, capecitabine, methotrexate; nucleoside analogs such as gemcitabine; platinum agents such carboplatin; taxanes such as paciltaxel, docetaxel, nab-paclitaxel; epothilones such as ixabepilone; and vinca alkaloids such as vinorelbine and vinblastine.[189,285] Among the preferred first line combination chemotherapy regimens for metastatic breast cancer recommended by the NCCN are cyclophosphamide/doxorubicin/fluorouracil (CAF); fluorouracil/epirubicin/cyclophosphamide (FEC); adriamycin/cyclophosphamide (AC); epirubicin/cyclophosphamide (EC); doxorubicin in combination with either docetaxel or paclitaxel (AT); cyclophosphamide/methotrexate/fluorouracil (CMF); docetaxel and capecitabine; and gemcitabine and paclitaxel (GT).[189]

Currently, there is a debate regarding single agent treatment vs combination chemotherapy in the treatment of metastatic breast cancer. No optimal evidence-based strategy exists for the initial treatment of metastatic breast cancer.[285] Combination chemotherapy generally provides higher rates of objective response and longer time to progression, compared to single agent. However, combination chemotherapy is also associated with increased toxicity and provides little additional long-term benefit compared to sequential use of single agents.[189,293–296] In addition, administering single agent chemotherapy decreases the risk of dose adjustment as the therapy continues.[189] Therefore, single agent therapy is generally used for patients with metastatic breast cancer unless patients are symptomatic or have life-threatening disease and a rapid response is highly desirable.[285]

Anthracyclines, such as doxorubicin and epirubicin, and taxanes, such as paclitaxel and docetaxel, are considered the optimal first-line chemotherapeutic agents in the treatment of metastatic breast cancer.[285,297] Because many patients have had previous anthracyclines, and due to greater cardiac and gastrointestinal side effects with these agents, the taxanes are usually the preferred first-line treatments.[285,298] For women who experience disease recurrence following therapy that included an anthracycline or a taxane, vinorelbine, gemcitabine, and liposomal-encapsulated doxorubicin are second- and third-line choices with minimal toxicity.[290,291] Capecitabine, a fluoropyrimidine prodrug of 5-fluorouracil, is also second or third-line chemotherapy. It is a different option for patients because it can be taken orally, and offers a 20% response rate.[299,300]

## TARGETED THERAPY

During the development of breast cancer, there is activation and overexpression of oncogenes that encode transmembrane receptor tyrokinase of the epidermal growth factor receptor (EGFR) family, including EGFR and *HER2/neu*.[296] *HER2/neu* amplification occurs in 20% of invasive beast cancers and represents a more aggressive phenotypic cancer.[263,301,302] Targeted therapies, including monoclonal antibodies and small molecule tyrokinase inhibitors, have been developed to block *HER2/neu* signaling pathways in breast cancer.[301] Trastuzumab is a recombinant humanized monoclonal antibody that binds to the extracellular domain of the HER2/neu protein.[301] All women who overexpress the *HER2/neu* oncogene should be given trastuzumab at the time of recurrence, either as a single agent or in combination with a cytotoxic chemotherapy. As in the adjuvant setting, cardiac toxicity is the most significant side effect with trastuzumab. Therefore, a patient's cardiac status is serially monitored with MUGA scans or ECHOs. Those patients with significant cardiac disease or some elderly patients with multiple comorbidities may not be good candidates for trastuzumab therapy.

Two other targeted therapies have now been approved for the treatment of metastatic breast cancer, including lapatinib (Tykerb) and bevacizumab (Avastin). Lapatinib is a small molecule inhibitor of the intercellular tyrosine kinase domain of both EGFR and *HER2/neu* receptors.[301] Initial results of a phase III trial demonstrated that lapatinib plus capecitabine is superior to capecitabine alone and should be incorporated as first-line therapy in metastatic breast cancer management.[285,297,301] Side effects of lapatinib include rash, mostly acne-like on the face and upper chest and back, and diarrhea. As with trastuzumab, although it appears to be less frequent, side effects of lapatinib include cardiomyopathy, which warrants close cardiac monitoring.

Bevacizumab is monoclonal antibody that targets VEGF and was approved for the upfront treatment of *HER2/neu* negative metastatic breast cancer in February 2008.[303] It binds to VEGF and prevents the interaction of VEGF to its receptor cell.[303] Patients with breast cancer have elevated serum levels of VEGF; in addition, breast cancer cells have higher levels of VEGF expression than normal cells.[303,304] VEGF inhibition is thought to prevent the development of new tumor growth by blocking new blood vessel development, causing regression of existing tumor blood vessels, causing some direct tumor cell-kill effects, and decreasing intratumoral fluid pressure, which may help chemotherapy to penetrate the tumor.[303,305] The phase III E2100 trial compared bevacizumab plus paclitaxel to paclitaxel alone in patients with metastatic breast cancer who had not received prior chemotherapy. Adding bevacizumab to paclitaxel significantly increased PFS over paclitaxel alone, as well as the response rate, but OS was not superior.[303,306] Currently bevacizumab is also being studied with chemotherapies such as capecitabine, doxorubicin, and albumin-bound paclitaxel. Side effects of bevacizumab include hypertension, proteinuria, cerebrovascular ischemia, fatigue, and infection. Bevacizumab can also impair wound healing, cause bleeding and induce thrombosis.[303,306] All patients should have brain scans to rule out any metastatic disease to the brain. Brain lesions can be vascular and have a high risk of bleeding. Thus, patients with metastatic brain lesions should not receive bevacizumab.

### BISPHOSPHONATE THERAPY

Women with metastases to bone should be placed on a bisphosphonate therapy to slow disease progression, decrease the rate of bone loss, and protect against pathological fracture. Women with bone metastases who are hormone receptor-positive should also receive appropriate endocrine therapy. The bisphosphonate therapy should continue for life, regardless of progression or change in other therapies.

Women with visceral metastases as well as those with bony involvement will also respond to bisphosphonate therapy. Although radiological evidence of bone healing related to bisphosphonate therapy may take as long as 6 months to appear, subjective improvement occurs within a shorter time. For women who have lytic bony disease, zoledronic acid given as an infusion over 15 to 30 minutes once a month has proven useful to promote bone healing, prevent new disease in bone, decrease the fracture rate, decrease the need for palliative radiation, and decrease the use of narcotic analgesics in patients with metastatic disease.[307] Pamidronate, an alternative to zoledronic acid, is given as an infusion over 2 hours once a month. Renal function should be monitored monthly for patients receiving zoledronic acid or pamidronate, given that renal insufficiency has been known to occur in patients receiving long-term intravenous bisphosphonate therapy.[308–310]

## BREAST CANCER IN SPECIAL POPULATIONS

### MALES

There were 1990 new cases of breast cancer diagnosed in men in 2008 and 450 died of their disease.[311] Male breast cancer accounts for less than 1% of all breast cancer cases and 0.2% of all malignancies in men.[312] The anatomical structures of the male breast are the same as those of the female breast. It is the hormonal stimulation present in the female breast but absent in the male that accounts for the developmental and physiological differences between the male and female breast. This lack of hormonal stimulation also may explain the comparatively low incidence of male breast cancer. Nevertheless, the disease is similar in both sexes in terms of epidemiology, natural history, and response to therapy.

The strongest risk factor for male breast cancer is Klinefelter's syndrome, in which the male has inherited an additional X chromosome (47, XXY karyotype). Gynecomastia, atrophic testis, high levels of gonadotropins, and low testosterone levels are characteristic of Klinefelter's syndrome. The risk of breast cancer in males with Klinefelter's syndrome is as much as 50 times that of males in the general population.[313] Other risk factors for the development of breast cancer in men include chronic liver disorders, administration of exogenous estrogen to treat prostate cancer[314] or to maintain female characteristics in transsexuals, obesity, *BRCA2* mutations, and a family history of breast cancer in female relatives.[312,315]

Breast cancer occurs most frequently in men after age 60, with the peak incidence noted between 60 and 69 years. The majority of male breast cancers (81%) are ER positive; however, receptor positivity does not increase with advancing age as it does in women.[313] Male breast cancer typically arises from ductal elements and generally present as infiltrating ductal carcinoma (Table 48-11).[313] Analysis of tumor cells for overexpression of *HER2/neu* by fluorescence in situ hybridization suggests that breast cancer in males has a very low rate (<1%) of protein overexpression.[316] The remaining prognostic factors are the same as in female breast cancer.

A moderately tender, centrally located subareolar mass is usually the first symptom that brings the man to seek medical attention. Pectoral fixation, involvement of skin, nipple changes, bleeding and discharge are commonly present, often because of delay in seeking medical attention. These factors may account for the increased frequency with which advanced disease and early invasion of local and regional lymphatics are diagnosed in men. Ulceration may occur early in the course of the disease and carries a relatively poor prognosis. Because of its relatively central location, male breast cancer can be expected to metastasize to the internal mammary nodes. The lungs and bony skeleton are the most common metastatic sites.

Because of the low incidence of male breast cancer and relatively small number of male patients, it is difficult to conduct controlled clinical trials to aid in establishing appropriate therapy. Giordano and colleagues conducted a population-based sample of 2524 men with breast cancer in an attempt to characterize the disease.[317] Men were found to be significantly older at diagnosis, more likely to present with later-stage disease, more likely to have larger tumors, and more likely to have nodal involvement, ductal histology, and ER positive tumors than women.[317]

The treatment of male breast cancer is based on the treatment of female breast cancer. The modified radical mastectomy has been the mainstay of therapy. Because male breast cancer is often diagnosed at a later stage, the skin and underlying fascia are frequently involved. Skin grafting may be required to adequately close the surgical wound. Adjuvant radiotherapy, hormonal manipulation using SERMs or AIs, and chemotherapy are also part of the approach to treatment.[312,318,319]

Orchiectomy appears to remove the source of estrogen and androgen in recurrent male breast cancer and can result in a prompt remission. With recurrent disease, further hormonal manipulation using tamoxifen, anastrozole, and progestin may be helpful. Anastrozole, tamoxifen, and other forms of hormone manipulation are relatively ineffective without orchiectomy. However, goserelin acetate effectively reduces testosterone to castration levels and may be an important alternative for men who refuse orchiectomy.

**TABLE 48-11**

**Histological Subtypes of Male Breast Cancer**

| Type | Incidence (%) |
|---|---|
| Infiltrating ductal carcinoma | > 80 |
| Papillary carcinoma | 5 |
| Lobular carcinoma | 1 |
| Inflammatory carcinoma | 1 |
| Paget's disease | 1 |
| Medullary, tubular, mucinous | < 1 |

*Source*: Data from Giordano et al.[313]

## YOUNG WOMEN

Breast cancer is a rare occurrence in young women under the age of 45. The incidence of breast cancer from 2002 to 2006 for women under the age of 20 was 0.0%; the incidence increased for women between the ages of 20 and 34 and was 1.9%; and women between 35 and 44 the incidence was 10.5%.[320] When breast cancer occurs in young women it is generally more aggressive biologically and has an unfavorable prognosis compared with older, postmenopausal patients. Tumors in young women tend to present with a higher grade, higher proliferative fraction, and more vascularization than in older women.[321] Younger women are more likely to present with more advanced disease at diagnosis, and the risk of death from breast cancer is highest among the youngest and oldest cohorts as compared with women of intermediate age.[72]

Adjuvant chemotherapy is a nearly universal recommendation for younger women diagnosed with invasive breast cancer. Ovarian suppression in the management of localized breast cancer in premenopausal women has been a controversial issue for some time. In premenopausal women, evidence appears to support a dual mechanism of action of chemotherapy, involving both direct cytotoxicity and ovarian suppression resulting from chemotherapy-induced ovarian failure. Early studies of ovarian suppression indicate that it is a viable treatment with tamoxifen for premenopausal women with ER positive breast cancer.[322]

Treatment questions appropriate for women with breast cancer in regards to the use of endocrine therapy in premenopausal women, ovarian function suppression, and duration and intensity of chemotherapy remain to be answered. The majority of clinical trials upon which treatment decisions are based report data for women age 40 and older. There is a need for clinical investigations of the younger population given that chemotherapy is invariably recommended for these high-risk patients.[323]

In addition to issues related to the poor prognosis and appropriate medical management of young patients with breast cancer, issues of early menopause, sexual functioning, childbearing, and dealing with the young family require support from the physician, nurse, and psychosocial staff. The possibility of pregnancy after treatment for breast cancer remains controversial. Most studies have utilized case-control designs and have shown that pregnancy following breast cancer is not detrimental to survival and, in fact, is often linked to an improvement in survival.[324] Most experts recommend waiting until 2 years postsurgery before attempting conception, but this recommendation is based on limited data from a small and selectively obtained group of patients. Based on available data gleaned largely from retrospective case-control studies, no definitive recommendations can be made with regard to local recurrence, risk of distant metastasis, or OS.

Cancer is generally viewed to be a disease of aging, and the diagnosis of breast cancer in a young woman can be devastating to the woman, her partner, and her family. Many breast cancer support groups, such as Y-ME and Gilda's Club, now include groups specifically geared toward young breast cancer survivors.

## ELDERS

Cancer is largely a disease of aging; that is, the incidence and mortality rates of breast cancer increase with age. The size of the geriatric population (those over the age of 65) is increasing annually. Barring any unforeseen breakthrough in cancer prevention, the number of breast cancer cases will increase exponentially.

A common question raised during the physical assessment of the healthy older woman is how long to continue annual mammographic screening for breast cancer. Breast cancer is a leading cause of cancer death in women older than 65 years of age. Unfortunately, mammographic screening is underutilized in elderly women in the US, with only one-third of women in the 65 to 69 age groups undergoing routine screening mammography.[325] Life expectancy in the US is approximately 83 years for women; therefore, a 65-year-old woman can expect to live another 18 years. Women who are otherwise healthy and would choose to treat breast cancer if it were found should continue mammographic screening and annual breast exams.[326,327] Women whose life expectancy due to comorbid conditions or advancing age is less than 5 years would probably not realize a survival benefit from early diagnosis of breast cancer and therefore should stop screening.[326]

Postmenopausal women are generally diagnosed with stage I or II, hormone receptor-positive, infiltrating ductal carcinoma. Breast cancer in the older woman is associated with more favorable tumor biology, and survival rates for older women are similar to survival rates for the general population.[328] Small tumor size and negative nodes mean that treatment can be effectively confined to local–regional therapy (including surgery and radiation) and endocrine therapy (including SERMs and AIs), both of which are generally well tolerated by elders.[329] Treatment issues arise when the prognosis is poor and recurrence seems likely due to a large tumor or positive axillary nodes or when the tumor is hormone receptor negative or is positive for *HER2/neu*. Evidence from a phase III study indicates that the use of an AI may be more effective than tamoxifen in women who overexpress *HER2/neu*.[330] When chemotherapy is indicated, an accurate assessment of the older patient's comorbidities, tumor biology, functional status, and support systems is necessary. It is difficult to determine optimal treatment regimens for older patients as few clinical trials in the past have included a sizable number of older patients.

Chronic comorbidities increase with aging, and patients with breast cancer are no less likely than the general population to have one or more comorbid conditions. Evaluating the status of the comorbid conditions, the effect of chemotherapy, and the availability of supportive care is necessary before making treatment decisions.[331] Chemotherapy doses may require modification for the appearance of side effects; the side effects may be more or less pronounced in elders or may be masked by symptoms from preexisting conditions. Most chemotherapy dosage adjustments relate only to decreases in creatinine clearance; renal function should be monitored in all older patients receiving chemotherapy.[331] Table 48-12 lists issues to be considered when contemplating chemotherapy in elders.

Many older patients potentially lack sufficient social support systems, and providing the necessary support may become a trying issue for the nurse and family alike. Family caregivers usually play an essential role in caring for patients with cancer. Lack of financial support and physical access to treatment facilities may represent barriers for many older women. Referral to a community-based senior center or psychologist may provide support not otherwise available for the family in an effort to offset the negative aspects of caregiving.[332] Many women, especially older women, are overwhelmed by the prospect of several surgical procedures to obtain a full diagnosis, chemotherapy, RT, and continuing follow-up care. All women, in addition to the elderly, may benefit from the presence of a nurse case manager or patient navigator to assist in directing and obtaining care.[333]

## AFRICAN AMERICAN WOMEN

For many years, the disparities in cancer incidence and survival between African Americans and Caucasians have been the subject of study and controversy. African American women are more likely to die of breast cancer,

**TABLE 48-12**

**Chemotherapy Considerations in Older Breast Cancer Patients**

| Agent or Regimen | Side Effects of Concern | Considerations | Comorbid Condition Alert |
|---|---|---|---|
| Anthracyclines | Cardiotoxicity | Obtain MUGA prior to treatment<br>Avoid use with history of cardiac disease | Congestive heart failure<br>Coronary artery disease<br>History myocardial infarction |
| | Nausea/vomiting | Fluid loss/dehydration | |
| | Myelosuppression | Consider use of growth factor support | |
| Cyclophosphamide | Nephrotoxicity | Monitor urinary function | Renal insufficiency |
| | Nausea/vomiting | Fluid loss/dehydration | |
| Taxanes | Peripheral neuropathy | Monitor motor/sensory function | Diabetes mellitus |
| | Peripheral edema | Monitor fluid retention (docetaxel) | Congestive heart failure |
| | Hand–foot syndrome | Monitor skin changes (docetaxel) | Psoriasis; eczema |
| Vinorelbine | Constipation | Prophylactic bowel regimen | |
| Capecitabine | Hand–foot syndrome | Monitor skin changes | Psoriasis; eczema |
| | Nausea/diarrhea | Fluid loss/dehydration | |

*Abbreviation*: MUGA, multiple gated acquisition.

even though they are less likely to be diagnosed with breast cancer. Whether African American women have biologically more aggressive breast cancer than Caucasian women and whether race acts as a significant independent prognostic factor for survival have not been determined by any large-scale clinical trial. A meta-analysis of articles reporting on OS for African American and Caucasian patients treated similarly for cancer reported only modest cancer-specific survival differences, highlighting the need for further research into differences in treatment, presentation stage, and mortality from other diseases.[334]

Some researchers believe that biology may be responsible for the higher mortality rates among African American patients with breast cancer. One-third of African American women with breast cancer are diagnosed premenopausally (before age 50) compared to 23% of Caucasian women. Estrogen receptor-negative breast cancer is also more common among African American women (40%) compared to Caucasian women (23%).[335] These 2 factors, however, are linked for all women: Premenopausal women of all races tend to have hormone receptor-negative breast cancers.

Continuing genomic research seeking a biological variable that may account for these survival differences recently identified a gene, *BP1*, that may be responsible for the differing survival outcomes between African American and Caucasian women treated for breast cancer. The expression of *BP1* in tissue was closely correlated with both ER negative tumors and race: 89% of tumors from African American women were *BP1* positive, whereas only 57% of tumors from Caucasian women expressed *BP1*. *BP1* could provide a useful target for therapy or early diagnosis, if activation of *BP1* proves to be an early event in carcinogenesis.[336]

Other researchers support the theory that socioeconomic status replaces race as a predictor of poorer outcome after women are diagnosed with breast cancer.[337] Socioeconomic status has been correlated with increased risk of disease and poorer health outcomes. Poorer populations have higher incidence and mortality from all kinds of disease, but especially a number of cancers. African American women with breast cancer have disproportionately more high-grade disease at diagnosis as compared with Caucasian women. It is conceivable that genetic causes of certain cancers may be more prevalent in populations whose members originate from certain geographic areas, such as Africa,[338] but most likely any genetic causes are due to a combination of factors, including genetic makeup.[338]

Whatever the cause, nurses need to be aware that survival of breast cancer is less likely for African American women than for Caucasian women. African American women generally present with later-stage disease. The incidence of small tumors and localized disease is consistently higher in Caucasian women; the incidence of tumors larger than 5 cm and distant-stage disease is higher among African American women.[339] Higher relative survival rates and greater improvement in survival over time are observed in Caucasian women more than in African American women.[280,325]

Access to adequate, high-quality mammographic screening and CBE remains the goal for early detection of breast cancer in all women including African American women. Although federally funded programs for mammographic screening have been available for many years, adequate funding to treat women diagnosed through these screening programs had been lacking. Passage of the Breast and Cervical Cancer Prevention Act of 2000 provides medical assistance through federally funded, state-run Medicaid programs to eligible women who were screened through the Centers for Disease Control and Prevention's National Breast and Cervical Cancer Early Detection Program.[340] African American women who are diagnosed with breast cancer should be evaluated for participation in clinical trials that may provide access to state-of-the-art cancer care that might otherwise be unavailable to them.

## SYMPTOM MANAGEMENT AND SUPPORTIVE CARE

Advances in early detection and adjuvant treatment have improved the OS rates for women with breast cancer, but the natural history of the disease is basically unchanged. Approximately 20%to 30% of patients with breast cancer will develop systemic recurrence, and approximately 10% of patients present with metastatic disease at the time of diagnosis. Once the disease has become metastatic, it is no longer considered to be curable. Only half of these patients will live more than 2 years.[341]

Breast cancer can spread to bone, soft tissue (lymph nodes or scar skin at incision site), liver, lung, and brain. Patients with metastatic breast cancer experience symptoms similar to those associated with other metastatic disease including visceral and neuropathic pain, nausea, dyspnea, fatigue, anorexia/cachexia, and mental status changes. These symptoms require comprehensive management that is covered thoroughly in other chapters of this text.

Many patients with breast cancer experience lymphedema, either as a side effect of surgery and/or radiation or as disease progression. Lymphedema is a chronic condition that occurs when the flow of lymph fluid through lymphatic vessels is impaired and the fluid accumulates in surrounding dependent tissue. Approximately 25% of women with breast cancer develop lymphedema, but the frequency ranges from 6% for women who have undergone lumpectomy only to 68% for women who have had full axillary node dissections. The acceptance of SLNB as the standard approach for initial surgical evaluation of the axilla has decreased the risk of lymphedema. Factors that increase the risk of lymphedema, in addition to axillary surgery, are radiation, high-risk breast cancers (large tumors with positive nodes and lympho-vascular invasion), and obesity.[342,343] Lymphedema is an irreversible condition that progresses without treatment.[343] Its presence is a constant visible reminder that breast cancer has occurred. It can cause body image disturbance, anxiety, depression, physical discomfort, and functional deficits long after adjuvant treatment is completed.

The epidemiology of lymphedema is changing, largely due to lymphatic-sparing surgical techniques and improved treatments. The incidence of lymphedema among early stage breast cancer patients is decreasing while the incidence among patients with stage IV disease is increasing. The latter group is at higher risk for developing lymphedema and they are living longer with advanced disease. The increased morbidity of breast cancer seen among the elderly and women of lower socioeconomic status is mirrored in lymphedema. Women in both groups tend to have more comorbidities and less access to lymphedema treatment.[344] Lymphedema screening, prevention, and treatment should be available to all patients with cancer.

The risk for lymphedema is life-long and should be considered for any patients with breast cancer who have undergone axillary surgery or RT. Early symptoms of lymphedema include swelling of the ipsilateral breast or arm, and a sensation of heaviness, aching, tingling or fatigue in the limb. The area of concern should be inspected for asymmetry, loss of anatomical landmarks, warmth, and erythema. Infection, disease recurrence or progression, and thrombophlebitis should be ruled out. The patient should then be referred to a physical therapist, preferably a lymphedema specialist.[343]

The most effective treatment for lymphedema is prevention. Women at risk should be counseled to avoid injury, needle sticks, and constriction from clothing, jewelry, or blood pressure cuffs, and manicures to the affected limb. The use of a compression garment (sleeve) for air travel is controversial. Women who are at risk for developing lymphedema should make the decision about compression garments based on the extent of their risk. Women who have lymphedema should always wear the garment for air travel. The sleeve should always be worn with a glove to prevent edema of the hand. The sleeve should be provided by a professional fitter. Women should be counseled to monitor for and report rashes or signs of infection in the affected areas. Evidence suggests that exercise and avoiding obesity can protect against lymphedema.[343] Arming patients with lymphedema prevention behaviors may decrease their anxiety and improve their overall sense of control regarding breast cancer. See Table 48-7 for information about hand and arm precautions in patients who have undergone surgery for the management of breast cancer.

Complex or complete decongestive therapy (CDT) was formalized as the standard of care for lymphedema by the International Society of Lymphology in 2001.[345] CDT is a 2-phase system that includes manual lymphatic drainage (MLD), multilayer short-stretch compressive bandaging, skin care, therapeutic exercise, and compression garments. MLD is a specialized form of massage that promotes decongestion of lymphedematous areas by sequestering and rechanneling lymph fluid through functioning lymph vessels. MLD is a gentle, rhythmic massage performed 30 to 60 minutes daily. After MLD, short-stretch bandages that apply pressure during movement but not at rest are applied in layers. If needed for comfort, padding can be applied under the bandages. Therapeutic exercises are performed several times throughout the day with the bandages in place. Rhythmic muscle contraction and relaxation with the compression garments promote an internal pumping mechanism that allows lymph to flow in open channels. Cellulitis is common in lymphedematous areas. The goal of skin and nail care is to avoid infections. The care consists of inspecting the affected area daily, cleansing with mineral based soap and applying moisturizer under the bandages.[343,345]

Phase I of CDT is focused on reducing limb fluid volume and is composed of 45 minutes of MLD followed by the application of bandages and exercise. Ideally, the treatment is performed 7 days per week, with caregivers instructed to rebandage over the weekends. The compressive bandages are left in place for 21 to 24 hours for maximum efficacy.[343] Phase I of CDT usually lasts for 2 to 4 weeks, depending on response to treatment. Patients are gradually transitioned to phase II of the maintenance phase that consists of MLD, compression bandaging, therapeutic exercise, and skin and nail care. Phase II is considered to be lifelong therapy.[344] CDT require commitment on the part of the patient and caregiver. Patients may ask about the benefit of pumps and other compression devices that are less labor-intense, but current recommendations advise against the use of external pumps to treat lymphedema.[343]

Relative contraindications for CDT include hypertension, diabetes, asthma, and paralysis (flaccid limb). Absolute contraindications include infection of the affected area, CHF, and thrombophlebitis. There is conflicting evidence regarding CDT and the potential spread of metastatic disease, but the consensus is that CDT can improve the quality of life of patients with lymphedema.[344,346] See Table 48-13 for a list of lymphedema support groups.

Frequently, woman with cancer experience menopausal symptoms, including hot flashes, fatigue, weight gain, and irregular or absent menses. The exact etiology of these symptoms is unknown but is thought to be related to the disease itself, to treatment (chemotherapy and/or endocrine therapy), or the aging process. A variety of pharmacologic and nonpharmacologic treatments are available, but they may not be effective for all individuals.[347] Careful assessment and ongoing research are needed to successfully manage this cluster of symptoms.

**TABLE 48-13**

| Nonprofit Lymphedema Information Resources |
|---|
| Online information is available from several nonprofit lymphedema information resources: |
| American Cancer Society: http://www.cancer.org |
| Circle of Hope Lymphedema Foundation Inc.: http://www.lymphademacircleofhope.org |
| Lymphedema Research Foundation (LRF): http://www.lymphaticresearch.org |
| Lymphology Association of North America (LANA): http://www.clt-lana.org |
| National Cancer Institute (NCI): http://www.cancer.gov/cancertopics/pdq/supportivecare/lymphedema |
| National Lymphedema Network (NLN): http://www.lymphnet.org |

*Source*: Reproduced with permission from John Wiley & Sons, Inc.[345]

## FUTURE TRENDS

Breast cancer is not one disease but rather an amalgam of many heterogeneous manifestations of disease. It is a challenge to fight this disease, yet scientists and researchers have made great strides in the last 10 to 20 years. It is challenging to isolate suitable targets for preventing the initial steps that cause a normal cell to avoid immune surveillance and apoptosis and become malignant. Toward this goal, scientists use DNA microarrays which allow simultaneous analysis of tens of thousands of genes in a single experiment, in attempts to identify single genes as prognostic indicators or as therapeutic targets. Once it has been established that these molecular targets are valid therapeutic targets, then these molecular targets may be used to screen women deemed at high risk for development of breast cancer. Identification of a target gene may open the door to drugs that will disable the gene and serve as true chemoprevention. In addition, therapies that take advantage of these molecular targets will hopefully continue to advance the success of breast cancer therapy.

Monoclonal antibodies are rapidly becoming an indispensible part of therapy for women with metastatic breast cancer and are currently under investigation as treatment in the adjuvant setting. Bevacizumab is currently being studied in the adjuvant setting. Also, targeted therapies specifically directed at different parts or all of the *HER2/neu* family continue to be investigated for their use in metastatic breast cancer and their potential for improving outcomes in the adjuvant setting. As microarray analysis become a larger part of the diagnostic work-up for patients with breast cancer, researchers will strive to find treatments targeting the variety of genes that appear to play a part in breast cancer. It is not unreasonable to anticipate monoclonal antibody treatments custom-designed for each newly diagnosed patient with breast cancer based on the molecular profile of the individual's particular tumor.

Progress in the treatment of breast cancer has dramatically improved survival rates, but until breast cancer is eradicated, more advanced surgical techniques, diagnostic tools, and evaluation strategies will be proposed. Imaging technologies that will predict even earlier detection of breast cancer, allow image-guided ablation of malignant tumors, provide presurgical evaluation of regional or distant disease, and assess response to therapy are currently being investigated.

Women with dense breasts pose a challenge for mammographers. Breast density is noted predominantly in younger women, but breast density may persist into old age in some women. Higher density has the potential to obscure potential pathological areas. MRI is being studied as a screening tool, and recently is being utilized more in practice. MRI is a better imaging modality, but it continues to be a costly screening tool compared to mammography and insurers are unlikely to reimburse for MRI as a screening tool.

Patients with locally advanced breast cancer often select neoadjuvant chemotherapy to reduce the size of the tumor and allow for a better surgical outcome. Evaluating the response to treatment has been limited to imaging studies assessing for reduction in tumor bulk. Scientists continue to look for additional methods to determine tumor characteristics and response to therapy. Mankoff and colleagues evaluated the blood flow of tumors in women with locally advanced breast cancer before and during treatment, comparing (Tc-99m)-sestamibi uptake with (0–15)-water PET serial imaging.[348] Based on these preliminary findings, the authors created a model of the MIBI kinetics of breast tumors to be used to further assess tumor characteristics.[348] Others are using MRI imaging techniques to examine response to specific chemotherapeutic drugs. Neoadjuvant treatment remains a place where further research needs to be completed. Due to the screening methods that allow for early diagnosis of breast cancer and the recent treatment advances, most patients with breast cancer will survive their cancer for 5 years and beyond.[349] After years of follow-up care with their primary oncologists, many patients and providers struggle with the next step in their care. Many believe patients with breast cancer are a unique population that would benefit from a survivorship clinic that includes their own personal treatment summaries and care plans. With the development of survivor initiatives in cancer programs across the country, survivorship care is being recognized as a distinct phase of the cancer trajectory.[350] This is an excellent opportunity for APNs to practice independently and to provide education on an important part of breast cancer and survivorship treatment.[350] Multiple cancer centers throughout the country are now providing survivorship clinics and these clinics continue to expand as the number of breast cancer survivors continues to grow.

The diagnosis and treatment of breast cancer is no longer based on a traditional hierarchical model, but has become a complex plan designed by the multidisciplinary team. The continuing influx of innovative diagnostic tools and therapies will continue to challenge the knowledge base of all healthcare providers. It is imperative that nurses belong to professional organizations and participate in continuing education courses addressing breast cancer management including novel therapies and techniques. Understanding the basic scientific principles of these new tools and therapies will enable nurses to remain integral members of the team that actively participates in the education, treatment, and support of the patient and family.

## CONCLUSION

Ongoing advances in prevention, detection, and treatment offer patients with breast cancer new hope. Breast cancer, like other cancers is becoming a chronic illness with periods of disease-free status. These developments provide a dual challenge for oncology nurses. Women who have breast cancer or who are at risk for the disease are presented with a myriad of choices and decisions to make. If treatment is indicated, some of these choices have to be made shortly after the diagnosis when the patient and her supporters are particularly vulnerable. At the opposite end of the disease trajectory, with metastatic breast cancer, more difficult decisions may have to be made. In addition to providing comprehensive physical care and symptom management, nurses are called upon to provide support and education along the disease trajectory. The second part of the challenge includes restoring patients to normalcy, helping them to reclaim their lives when treatment is completed. These patients need to be encouraged and enabled to obtain appropriate follow-up care. Also, they need continuing encouragement and support so that anxiety about disease recurrence does not become more malignant than the disease itself.

## REFERENCES

1. Jemal A, Siegel R, Ward E, Hao Y, Xu J, Thun M. Cancer statistics. *CA: Cancer J Clin.* 2009;59:225–249.
2. Jemal A, Siegel R, Ward E, et al. Cancer statistics. *CA: Cancer J Clin.* 2008;58:73–83.
3. Jemal A, Ward E, Thun MJ. Recent trends in breast cancer incidence rates by age and tumor characteristics among US women. *Breast Cancer Res.* 2007;9:R28.
4. American Cancer Society. *Breast Cancer Facts and Figures 2007–2008.* Atlanta: American Cancer Society; 2008:9–11.
5. Ries LAG, Melbert D, Krapcho M, et al, eds. *SEER Cancer Statistics Review, 1975–2004.* Bethesda, MD: National cancer Institute. http://seer.cancer.gov/csr/1975_2004, based on November 2006 SEER data submisson, posted to the SEER Web site, 2007. Accessed January 28, 2010.
6. Breen N, CroninK, Meissner HI, et al. Reported drop in mammography: is this cause for concern? *Cancer.* 2007;109:2405–2409.
7. Wood W, Muss H, Solin L, et al. Malignant tumors of the breast. In: DeVita V, Hellman S, Rosenbery S, eds. *Cancer Principles and Practice of Oncology.* 7th ed. Philadelphia, PA: Lippincott, Williams & Wilkins; 2000:1415–1418.

8. Hulka BS, Moorman PG. Breast cancer: hormones and other risk factors. *Maturitas.* 2001;38:103–113; discussion 113–116.
9. Osteen R. Breast cancer. In: Lenhard RE, Osteen RT, Gansler T, eds. *Clinical Oncology.* Atlanta, GA: American Cancer Society; 2001:2251–2268.
10. Glass A, Lacey J, Carreon D, et al. Breast cancer incidence, 1980–2006: combined roles of menopausal hormone therapy, screening mammography, and estrogen receptor status. *J Natl Cancer Inst.* 2007;99:1152–1161.
11. Willett W, Rockhill B, Hankinson S, et al. Nongenetic factors in the causation of breast cancer. In: Harris J, Lippman M, Morrow M, et al, eds. *Diseases of the Breast.* 3rd ed. Philadelphia, PA: Lippincott, Williams & Wilkins; 2004:228–240.
12. Writing group for the Women's Health Initiative Randomized Controlled Trial: risks and benefits of estrogen plus progestin in healthy postmenopausal women: principal results from the Women's Health Initiative randomized controlled trial. *JAMA.* 2002;288:321–333.
13. Kim C, Kwok YS. Decision analysis of hormone replacement therapy after the Women's Health Initiative. *Am J Obstet Gynecol.* 2003;189:1228–1233.
14. US Preventive Services Task Force. Postmenopausal hormone replacement therapy for primary prevention of chronic conditions: recommendations and rationale. *Ann Intern Med.* 2002;137:834–839.
15. Col NF, Hirota LK, Orr RK, et al. Hormone replacement therapy after breast cancer: a systematic review and quantitative assessment of risk. *J Clin Oncol.* 2001;19:2357–2363.
16. Collaborative Group on Hormonal Factors in Breast Cancer. Familial breast cancer: collaborative reanalysis of individual datat from 52 epidemiological studies including 58,209 women with breast cancer and 101,986 women without the disease. *Lancet.* 2001;358:1389–1399.
17. DeMichele A, Weber B. Inherited genetic factors. In: Harris JR, Lippman ME, Morrow M, et al, eds. *Diseases of the Breast*, 2nd ed. Philadelphia: Lippincott, Williams and Wilkins; 2000:221–236.
18. Wooster R, Bignell G, Lancaster J, et al. Identification of the breast cancer susceptibility gene BRCA2 [see comment] [erratum appears in *Nature.* 1996;379:749]. *Nature.* 1995;378:789–792.
19. Miki Y, Swensen J, Shattuck-Eidens D, et al. A strong candidate for the breast and ovarian cancer susceptibility gene BRCA1. *Science.* 1994;266:66–71.
20. Collins N, McManus R, Wooster R, et al. Consistent loss of the wild type allele in breast cancers from a family linked to the BRCA2 gene on chromosome 13q12–13. *Oncogene.* 1995;10:1673–1675.
21. Risch HA, McLaughlin JR, Cole DE, et al. Population BRCA1 and BRCA2 mutation frequencies and cancer penetrances: a kin-cohort study on Ontario, Canada. *J Natl Cancer Inst.* 2006;98:1694–1706.
22. Ford D, Easton DF, Stratton M, et al. Genetic heterogeneity and penetrance analysis of the BRCA1 and BRCA2 genes in breast cancer families. The Breast Cancer Linkage Consortium. *Am J Hum Genet.* 1998;62:676–689.
23. King MC, Marks JH, Mandell JB, et al. Breast and ovarian cancer risks due to inherited mutations in BRCA1 and BRCA2 [see comment]. *Science.* 2003;302:643–646.
24. The Breast Cancer Linkage Consortium. Cancer risks in BRCA2 mutation carriers. *J Natl Cancer Inst.* 1999;91:1310–1316.
25. Gayther SA, Russell P, Harrington P, et al. The contribution of germline BRCA1 and BRCA2 mutations to familial ovarian cancer: no evidence for other ovarian cancer-susceptibility genes. *Am J Hum Genet.* 1999;65:1021–1029.
26. Thompson D, Szabo CI, Mangion J, et al. Evaluation of linkage of breast cancer to the putative BRCA3 locus on chromosome 13q21 in 128 multiple case families from the Breast Cancer Linkage Consortium. *Proc Natl Acad Sci USA.* 2002;99:827–831.
27. Domchek S, Weber B. Inherited genetic factors and breast cancer. In: Harris J, Lippman M, Morrow M, et al, eds. *Diseases of the Breast.* 3rd ed. Philadelphia, PA: Lippincott, Williams & Wilkins; 2004:277–302.
28. Rahman N, Stratton MR. The genetics of breast cancer susceptibility. *Ann Rev Genet.* 1998;32:95–121.
29. Marsh D, Dahia P, Caron S, et al. Germline PTEN mutations in Cowden syndrome-like families. *J Med Genet.* 1998;35:881–885.
30. Varley J, Haber D. Familial breast cancer and the Hchk2 1100delc mutation: assessing cancer risk. *Breast Cancer Res.* 2003;5:123–125.
31. Chenevix-Trench G, Spurdle AB, Gatei M, et al. Dominant negative ATM mutations in breast cancer families. *J Natl Cancer Inst.* 2002;94.205–215.
32. Samant RS, Olivotto IA, Jackson JS, et al. Diagnosis of metachronous contralateral breast cancer. *Breast J.* 2001;7:405–410.
33. Clark GM. Nongenetic risk factors and inherited predisposition. In: Hassey-Dow K, ed. *Pocket Guide to Breast Cancer.* 3rd ed. Sudbury, MA: Jones and Bartlett; 2006:10.
34. International Agency for Cancer Research (IARC). *IARC Handbook of Cancer Prevention. Vol. 6: Weight Control and Physical Activity.* Lyon: IARC Press; 2002.
35. Eliases AH, Colditz GA, Rosner B, et al. Adult weight change and risk of postmenopausal breast cancer. *JAMA.* 2006;296:193–201.
36. Morimoto LM, White E, Chen Z, et al. Obesity, body size, and risk of postmenopausal breast cancer: The Women's Health Initiative (United States). *Cancer Causes Control.* 2002;13:741.
37. Hankinson SE, Willett WC, Colditz GA, et al. Circulating concentrations of insulin-like growth factors and risk of breast cancer. *Lancet.* 1998;351:810.
38. Thune I, Furberg AS. Physical activity and cancer risk: dose–response and cancer, all sites and site-specific. *Med Sci Sports Exerc.* 2001;33:8530.
39. Holmes MD, Chen WY, Feskanich D, et al. Physical activity and survival after breast cancer diagnosis. *JAMA.* 2005;293:2479–2486.
40. Friedenreich CM. Physical activity and cancer prevention: from observational to intervention research. *Cancer Epidemiol Biomarkers Prev.* 2001;10:287–301.
41. Fentiman IS. Fixed and modifiable risk factors for breast cancer. *Int J Clin Pract.* 2001;55:527–530.
42. Terry MB, Zhang FF, Kabat G, et al. Lifetime alcohol intake and breast cancer risk. *Ann Epidemiol.* 2006;16:230–240.
43. Zhang SM, Lee IM, Manson JE, et al. Alcohol consumption and breast cancer risk in the women's health study. *Am J Epidemiol.* 2007;165:676–676.
44. International Agency for Research on Cancer (IARC) monographs on the evaluation of carcinogenic risks to humans. *Tobacco Smoke and Involuntary Smoking.* Lyon: IARC Press; 2004.
45. Ward E, Jemal A, Cokkinides V, et al. Cancer disparities by race/ethnicity and socioeconomic status. *CA: Cancer J Clin.* 2004:54:78–93.
46. Halpern MT, Bian J, Ward EM, et al. Insurance status and stage of cancer at diagnosis among women with breast cancer. *Cancer.* 2007;110:395–402.
47. Baquet CR, Commiskey P. Socioeconomic factors and breast carcinoma in multicultural women. *Cancer.* 2000;88:1256–1264.
48. Bradlet CJ, Given CW, Roberts C. Disparities in cancer diagnosis and survival. *Cancer.* 2001;91:178–188.
49. Newman LA, Griffith KA, Jatoi I, et al. Meta-analysis of survival in African American and white American patients with breast cancer: ethnicity compared with socioeconomic status. *J Clin Oncol.* 2006;24:1342–1349.
50. Chlebowske RT, Chen Z, Anderson GL, et al. Ethnicity and breast cancer: factors influencing differences in incidence and outcome. *J Natl Cancer Inst.* 2005;97:439–448.
51. van Leeuwen FE, Klotman WJ, Stovall M, Dahler EC, van't Veer EM, et al. Roles of radiation dose, chemotherapy, and hormonal factors in breast cancer following Hodgkin's disease. *J Natl Cancer Inst.* 2003;95:97–100.
52. Bhatia S, Yasui Y, Robinson LL, et al. High risk of subsequent neoplasms continues with extended follow-up of childhood Hodgkin's disease: report from the Late Effects Study group. *J Clin Oncol.* 2003;21:4386.
53. Osuch JR. Breast health and disease over a lifetime. *Clin Obstet Gynecol.* 2002;45:1140–1161.

54. Kruger RL, Schueler BA. A survey of clinical factors and patient dose in mammography. *Med Phys.* 2001;28:1449–1454.
55. Vacek PM, Geller BM. A prospective study of breast cacner risk using routine mammographic breast density measurements. *Cancer Epidemiol Biomarkers Prev.* 2004;13:715–722.
56. Boyd NF, Guo H, Marting IJ, et al. Mammographic density and the risk and detection of breast cancer. *N Engl J Med.* 2007;356:227–236.
57. Pisano ED, Gatsonis C, Hendrick E, et al. Diagnostic performance of digital versus film mammography for breast cancer screening. *N Engl J Med.* 2005;353:1773–1783.
58. Hartmann LC, Sellers TA, Frost MH, et al. Benign breast disease and the risk of breast cancer. *N Engl J Med.* 2005;353:229–237.
59. Collins LC, Baer HJ, Tamimi RM, et al. Magnitude and laterality of breast cancer risk according to histologic type of atypical hyperplasia: results from the Nurses' Health Study. *Cancer.* 2007;109:180–187.
60. Singletary ES. Radiofrequency ablation of breast cancer. *Am Surgeon.* 2003;69:37–40.
61. Lakhani SR. In-situ lobular neoplasia: time for an awakening. *Lancet.* 2003;361:96.
62. Camus MG, Joshi MG, Mackarem G, et al. Ductal carcinoma in situ of the male breast. *Cancer.* 1994;74:1289–1293.
63. Morrow M, Harris JR. Local management of invasive breast cancer In: Harris JR, Lippman ME, Morrow M, et al, eds. *Diseases of the Breast,* 2nd ed. Philadelphia: Lippincott, Williams and Wilkins; 2000: 515–560.
64. Fisher ER, Land SR, Fisher B, et al. Pathologic findings from the National Surgical Adjuvant Breast and Bowel Project: twelve-year observations concerning lobular carcinoma in situ. *Cancer.* 2004;100:238–251.
65. National Cancer Institute. *Breast Cancer Risk Assessment Tool.* http://www.cancer.gov/bcrisktool/. Accessed January 28, 2010.
66. Gail MH, Brinton LA, Byar DP, et al. Projecting individualized probabilities of developing breast cancer for white females who are being examined annually. *J Natl Cancer Inst.* 1989;81:1879–1886.
67. Gail MH, Constantino JP. Validating and improving models for projecting the absolute risk of breast cancer. *J Natl Cancer Inst.* 2001;93:334–335.
68. Claus EB, Risch N, Thompson WD. Autosomal dominant inheritance of early-onset breast cancer: implications for risk prediction. *Cancer.* 1994;73:643–651.
69. Berry D, Parmigiani G, Sanchez J, et al. Probability of carrying a mutation of breast–ovarian cancer gene BRCA1 based on family history. *J Natl Cancer Inst.* 1989;81:1879–1886.
70. National Cancer Institute. *Genetics of Breast and Ovarian Cancer (PDQ).* http://www.cancer.gov/cancertopics/pdq/genetics/breast-and-ovarian/healthprofessional. Accessed January 28, 2010.
71. Silva OE, Zurrida S. *Breast Cancer: A Practical Guide.* 3rd ed. New York: Elsevier; 2005.
72. Hortobagyi GN. Progress in systemic chemotherapy of primary breast cancer: an overview. *J Natl Cancer Inst Monogr.* 2001;30:72–79.
73. Miyoshi Y, Taguchi T, Tamaki Y, et al. Current status of endocrine therapy for breast cancer. *Breast Cancer.* 2003;10:105–111.
74. Cummings FJ. Evolving uses of hormonal agents for breast cancer therapy. *Clin Ther* (suppl). 2002;24:C3-C25.
75. Anonymous. Tamoxifen for early breast cancer: an overview of the randomised trials. Early Breast Cancer Trialists' Collaborative Group. *Lancet.* 1998;351:1451–1467.
76. Gradishar WJ, Jordan VC. The evolving role of endocrine therapy for the treatment and prevention of breast cancer. *Cancer Chemother Biol Response Modif.* 2002;20:227–238.
77. Freedman AN, Granbard BI, Rao SR, et al. Estimates of the number of US women who could benefit from tamoxifen for breast cancer chemoprevention. *J Natl Cancer Inst.* 2003;95:526–532.
78. Fisher B, Constantino JP, Wickerham DI, et al. Tamoxifen for prevention of breast cancer: report of the National Surgical Adjuvant Breast and Bowel Project P-1 Study. *J Natl Cancer Inst.* 1998;90:1371–1388.
79. Dienger M. Hormonal therapy in advanced metastatic disease. In: Hassey-Dow K, ed. *Contemporary Issues in Breast Cancer, a Nursing Perspective.* 2nd ed. Sudbury, MA: Jones and Bartlett Publishers; 2004:38.
80. Cauley JA, Norton L, Lippman ME, et al. Continued breast cancer risk reduction in postmenopausal women treated with raloxifene: 4-year results from the MORE trial. Multiple outcomes of raloxifene evaluation. *Breast Cancer Res Treat.* 2001;65:125–134.
81. National Surgical Adjuvant Breast & Bowel Project (NSABP). *Study of Tamoxifen and Raloxifene.* 2004b. http://www.nsabp.pitt.edu/STAR/Index.html. Accessed October 1, 2009.
82. Goss P, Strasser K. Aromataser inhibitors in the treatment and prevention of breast cancer. *J Clin Oncol.* 2001;19:881–894.
83. Ravdin P. Aromatase inhibitors for the endocrine adjuvant treatment of breast cancer. *Lancet.* 2002;359:2126–2127.
84. ATAC Trialists' Group. Anastrazole-alone or in combination with tamoxifen versus tamoxifen alone for adjuvant treatment of postmenopausal women with early breast cancer: first results of the ATAC randomized trial. *Lancet.* 2002;359:2131–2139.
85. Kauff ND, Satagopan JM, Robson ME, et al. Risk-reducing salpingo-oophorectomy in women with a BRCA1 or BRCA2 mutation. *N Engl J Med.* 2002;346:1609–1615.
86. Hartmann LC, Schaid DJ, Woods JE, et al. Efficacy of bilateral prophylactic mastectomy in women with a family history of breast cancer. *N Engl J Med.* 1999;340:77–84.
87. Bland KI, Chang HR, Chandler GS, et al. Modified radical and total (simple) mastectomy. In: Bland KI, Copeland EM, eds. *The Breast: Comprehensive Management of Benign and Malignant Disorders.* 3rd ed. St. Louis: Saunders; 2004:865–884.
88. Hartmann LC, Sellers TA, Schaid DY, et al. Efficacy of bilateral prophylactic mastectomy in BRCA1 and BRCA2 gene mutation carriers. *J Natl Cancer Inst.* 2001;93:1633–1637.
89. Rebbeck TR, Lynch HT, Neuhausen SI, et al. Prophylactic oophorectomy in carriers of BRCA1 or BRCA2 mutation. *N Engl J Med.* 2002;346:1616–1622.
90. Eisen A, Lubinski J, Klijn J, et al. Breast cancer risk following bilateral oophorectomy in BRCA1 and BRCA2 mutation carriers: an international case-control study. *J Clin Oncol.* 2005;23:7491–7496.
91. Smith RA, CokkinidesV, Eyre HJ. Cancer screening in the United States 2007: a review of current guidelines, practices, and prospects. *CA: Cancer J Clin.* 2007;57:90–104.
92. Walter LC, Covinsky KE. Cancer screening in elderly patients: a framework for individualized decision making. *JAMA.* 2001;285:2750–2756.
93. Saslow D, Boetes C, Burke W, et al. American Cancer Society guidelines for breast screening with MRI as an adjunct to mammography. *CA: Cancer J Clin.* 2007;57:75–89.
94. Danforth DN, Abati A, Filie A, et al. Combined breast ductal lavage and ductal endoscopy for the evaluation of the high-risk breast: a feasibility study. *J Surg Oncol.* 2006;94:555–564.
95. Visvanathan K, Santor D, Ali SZ, et al. The reliability of nipple aspirate and ductal lavage in women at increased risk for breast cancer—a potential tool for breast cancer risk assessment and biomarker evaluation. *Cancer Epidemiol Biomarkers Prev.* 2007;16:950–955.
96. Wells K, Battaglia T, Dudley D, et al. Patient navigation: state of the art or is it science? *Cancer.* 2008;113:1999–2010.
97. Malone KE, Daling JR, Thompson JD, et al. BRCA1 mutations and breast cancer in the general population: analyses in women before age 35 and in women before age 45 years with first-degree family history. *JAMA.* 1998;279:922.
98. Ford D, Easton DF, Peto J. Estimates of the gene frequency of BRCA1 and its contribution to breast and ovarian cancer incidence. *Am J Hum Genet.* 1995;57:1457.
99. Warner E, Foulkes W, Goodwin P, et al. Prevalence and penetrance of BRCA1 and BRCA2 gene mutations in unselected Ashkenazi Jewish women with breast cancer. *J Natl Cancer Inst.* 1999;91:1241.
100. Abeliovich D, Kaduri L, Lerer I, et al. The founder mutations 185delAG and 5382insC in BRCA1 and 6174delT in BRCA2 appear

in 60 percent of ovarian cancer and 30 percent of early-onset breast cancer patients among Ashkenazi Jewish women. *Am J Hum Genet.* 1997;60:505.

101. Stopfer JE. Genetic counseling and clinical cancer genetics services. *Semin Surg Oncol.* 2000;18:347–357.
102. Croyle RT, Lerman C. Risk communication in genetic testing for cancer susceptibility. *J Natl Cancer Inst Monogr.* 1999;30:59–66.
103. Schwartz MD, Peshkin BN, Hughes C, et al. Impact of *BRCA1/BRCA2* mutation testing on psychological distress in a clinic-based sample. *J Clin Oncol.* 2002;20:514–520.
104. Braithwaite D, Emery J, Walter F, et al. Psychological impact of genetic counseling for familial cancer: a systematic review and meta-analysis. *J Natl Cancer Inst.* 2004;96:122–133.
105. Anonymous. American Society of Clinical Oncology policy statement update: genetic testing for cancer susceptibility. *J Clin Oncol.* 2003;21:2397–2406.
106. Schnitt SJ, Guidi AJ. Pathology of invasive breast cancer. In: Harris JR, Lippman ME, Morrow M, et al, eds. *Diseases of the Breast.* 2nd ed. *Philadelphia, Lippincott, Williams and Wilkins*; 2000:425–470.
107. Elston CW, Ellis IO. Pathological prognostic factors in breast cancer I. The value of histological grade in breast cancer: experience from a large study with long-term follow-up. *Histopathology.* 1991;19:403.
108. Chen CL, Weiss NS, Newcomb P, et al. Hormone replacement therapy in relation to breast cancer. *JAMA.* 2002;287:734–741.
109. Rosen PP, Lesser ML, Senie RT, et al. Epidemiology of breast carcinoma IV: age and histologic tumor type. *J Surg Oncol.* 1982;19:44–51.
110. Schnitt SJ, Guidi AJ. Pathology of invasive breast cancer. In: Harris JR, Lippman ME, Morrow M, et al, eds. *Diseases of the Breast.* 3rd ed. Philadelphia, PA: Lippincott, Williams & Wilkins; 2004:541–584.
111. Folkman J. Angiogenesis in breast cancer. In: Bland KI, Copeland EM, eds. *The Breas: Comprehensive Management of Benigh and Malignant Disorderst.* 3rd ed. Philadelphia, PA: W. B. Saunders; 2004:563.
112. Fox SB, Harris AL. Biology of breast tumor angiogenesis. In: Harris JR, Lippman ME, Morrow M, et al, eds. *Diseases of the Breast.* 3rd ed. Philadelphia, PA: Lippincott, Williams & Wilkins; 2004:441–458.
113. Elkin M, Orgel A, Kleinman HK. An angiogenic switch in breast cancer involves estrogen and soluble vascular endothelial growth factor receptor 1. *J Natl Cancer Inst.* 2004;96:875–878.
114. Dixon AR, Ellis IO, Elston CW, et al. A comparison of the clinical metastatic patterns of invasive lobular and ductal carcinomas of the breast. *Br J Cancer.* 1991;63:634–635.
115. Anonymous. The uniform approach to breast fine-needle aspiration biopsy. NIH consensus development conference [see comment]. *Am J Surg.* 1997;174:371–385.
116. Smith RE. A review of selective estrogen receptor modulators and National Surgical Adjuvant Breast and Bowel Project clinical trials. *Semin Oncol.* 2003;30:4–13.
117. Anonymous. Screening for breast cancer: recommendations and rationale. U.S. Preventative Services Task Force. *Arch Intern Med.* 2002;137:344–346.
118. Smith RA, Saslow D, Andrews Sawyer K, et al. American Cancer Society guidelines for breast cancer screening: update 2003. *CA: Cancer J Clin.* 2003;53:141–169.
119. *Breast Imaging Reporting and Data System (BI-RADS) Atlas.* 4th ed. Reston, VA: American College of Radiology; 2003.
120. Sickels EA, Wolverton DE, Dee KE. Performance parameters for screening and diagnostic mammography: specialist and general radiologists. *Radiology.* 2002;224:861–869.
121. Adler DD, Wahl RL. New methods for imaging the breast: techniques, findings, and potential. *AJR Am J Roentgenol.* 1995;164:19–30.
122. Schmidt RA, Nishikawa RM. Clinical use of digital mammography: the present and the prospects. *J Digital Imag.* 1995;8:74–79.
123. Lewin JM, Hendrick RE, D'Orsi CJ, et al. Comparison of full-field digital mammography with screen-film mammography for cancer detection: results of 4,945 paired examinations. *Radiology.* 2001;218:873–880.
124. The JS, Schilling KJ, Hoffmeister JW, et al. Detection of breast cancer with full-field digital mammography and computer-aided detection. *AJR Am J Roentgenol* 2009;192:337.
125. Brem RF, Baum J, Lechner M, et al. Improvement in sensitivity of screening mammography with computer-aided detection: a multiinstitutional trial. *AJR Am J Roentgenol.* 2003;181:687–693.
126. Fenton JJ, Taplin SH, Carney PA, et al. Influence of computer-aided detection on performance of screening mammography. *N Engl J Med.* 2007;356:1399.
127. Gur D, Sumkin JH, Rockett H, et al. Changes in breast cancer detection and mammography recall rates after the introduction of a computer-aided detection system. *J Natl Cancer Inst.* 2004;96:185–190.
128. Newman L. Developing technologies for early detection of breast cancer: a public workshop summary. In: Institute of Medicine, ed. *Early Detection of Breast Cancer.* Washington, DC: National Academy Press; 2000:1–24.
129. Chen J, Wu H, Zhou J, et al. Using TC-99m MIBI scintimammography to differentiate nodular lesions in breast and detect axillary lymph node metastases from breast cancer. *Chin Med J.* 2003;116:620–624.
130. Liberman M, Sampalis F, Mulder DS, et al. Breast cancer diagnosis by scintimammography: a meta-analysis and review of the literature. *Breast Cancer Res Treat.* 2003;80:115–126.
131. Flobbe K, Bosch AM, Kessels AG, et al. The additional diagnostic value of ultrasonography in the diagnosis of breast cancer. *Arch Intern Med.* 2003;163:1194–1199.
132. Bassett LW, Shiroishi M. Breast imaging. In: Bland KI, Copeland EM, III, eds. *The Breast: Comprehensive Management of Benign and Malignant Disorders.* 3rd ed. St. Louis, MO: Saunders; 2004:611–665.
133. Teifke A, Lehr HA, Vomweg TW, et al. Outcome analysis and rational management of enhancing lesions incidentally detected on contrast-enhanced MRI of the breast. *AJR Am J Roentgenol.* 2003;181:655–662.
134. Orel SG, Schnall MD. MR imaging of the breast for the detection, diagnosis, and staging of breast cancer. *Radiology.* 2001;220:13–30.
135. Harms SE, Flamig DP, Hesley KL, et al. MR imaging of the breast with rotating delivery of excitation off resonance: clinical experience with pathologic correlation. *Radiology.* 1993;187:493–501.
136. Bluemke DA, Gatsonis CA, Chen MH, et al. Magnetic resonance imaging of the breast prior to biopsy. *JAMA.* 2004;292:2735.
137. Boetes C, Strijk SP, Holland R, et al. False-negative MR imaging of malignant breast tumors. *Eur Radiol.* 1997;7:1231–1234.
138. Ghai S, Muradali D, Bukhanor K, et al. Nonenhancing breast malignancies on MRI: sonographic and pathologic correlation. *AJR Am J Roentgenol.* 2005;185:481–487.
139. Lobrano MB, Singha P. Positron emission tomography in oncology. *Clin J Oncol Nurs.* 2003;7:379–385.
140. Haberkorn U. The role of diagnostic PET in treatment planning before tumor surgery. *Chirurg.* 2001;72:1010–1019.
141. Adler LP, Faulhaber PF, Schnur KC, et al. Axillary lymph node metastases: screening with [F-18] 2-deoxy-2-fluoro-D-glucose (FDG) PET. *Radiology.* 1997;203:323.
142. Avril N, Rose CA, Schelling M, et al. Breast imaging with positron emission tomography and fluorine-18 fluorodeoxyglucose: use and limitations. *J Clin Oncol.* 2000;18:3495.
143. Quon A, Gambhir SS. FDG-PET and beyond: molecular breast imaging. *J Clin Oncol.* 2005;23:1664.
144. Landheer ML, Steffens MG, Klinkenbijl JH, et al. Value of fluorodeoxyglucose positron emission tomography in women with breast cancer. *Br J Surg.* 2005;92:1363.
145. Weir L, Worsley D, Bernstein V. The value of FDG positron emission tomography in the management of patients with breast cancer. *Breast J.* 2005;11:204.
146. Sakorafas GH. Breast cancer surgery—historical evolution, current status and future perspectives. *Acta Oncol.* 2001;40:5–18.
147. Daltrey IR, Lewis CE, McKee GT, et al. The effect of needle gauge and local anaesthetic on the diagnostic accuracy of breast fine-needle aspiration cytology. *Eur J Surg Oncol.* 1999;25:30–33.

148. Ljung BM, Drejet A, Chiampi N, et al. Diagnostic accuracy of fine-needle aspiration biopsy is determined by physician training in sampling technique. *Cancer.* 2001;93:263.
149. King TA, Fuhrman GM. Image-guided breast biopsy. *Semin Surg Oncol.* 2001;20:197–204.
150. Robinson DS, Sundaram M. Stereotactic imaging and breast biopsy. In: Bland KI, Copeland EM, III, eds. *The Breast: Comprehensive Managemant of Benign and Malignant Disorders.* St. Louis, MO: Saunders; 2004:685–697.
151. Bold RJ. Surgical management of breast cancer: today and tomorrow. *Cancer Biother Radiopharm.* 2002;17:1–9.
152. Liberman L. Percutaneous image-guided core breast biopsy. *Radiol Clin North Am.* 2002;40:483–500, vi.
153. Chung K, Velanovich V. Patient-perceived cosmesis after biopsy: comparison of stereotactic incisional, excisional, and wirelocalized biopsy testniques. *Surgery.* 2002;131:497–501.
154. Clark GM. Interpreting and integrating risk factors for patients with primary breast cancer. *J Natl Cancer Inst Monogr.* 2001;30:17–21.
155. Chang JC, Hilsenbeck, SG. Prognostic and predictive factors. In: Harris JR, Lippman ME, Morrow M, et al, eds. *Diseases of the Breast.* 3rd ed. Philadelphia, PA: Lippincott, Williams & Wilkins; 2004:675–696.
156. Baker M, Gillanders WE, Mikhitarian K, et al. The molecular detection of micrometastatic breast cancer. *Am J Surg.* 2003;186:351–358.
157. Weir L, Speers C, D'yachkova Y, et al. Diagnostic significance of the number of axillary lymph nodes removed in patients with node-negative breast cancer. *J Clin Oncol.* 2002;20:1793–1799.
158. Greenlee R, Murray T, Bolden S, Wingo P. Cancer statistics, 2000. *CA: Cancer J Clin.* 2000;50:7.
159. Nemoto T, Vana J, Bedwani RN. Management and survival of female breast cancer: results of a national survey by the American College of Surgeons. *Cancer.* 1980;45:2917–2924.
160. Hellman S, Harris JR. Natural history of breast cancer. In: Harris JR, Lippman ME, Morrow M, et al, eds. *Diseases of the Breast.* 2nd ed. Philadelphia, PA: Lippincott, Williams & Wilkins; 2000:407–423.
161. Carter C, Allen C, Henson D. Relation of tumor size, lymph node status and survival in 24,740 breast cancer cases. *Cancer.* 1989;63:181–186.
162. Fisher B, Slack NH, Bross IDJ, et al. Cancer of the breast: size of neoplasm and prognosis. *Cancer* 1968; 24:1071–1080.
163. Chia SK, Speers CH, Bryce, CJ, et al. Ten-year outcomes in a population-based cohort of node-negative, lymphatic, and vascular invasion-negative early breast cancers without adjuvant systemic therapies. *J Clin Oncol*, 2004; 22:1630–1637.
164. Rosen PP, Groshen S, Kinne DW, et al. Factors influencing prognosis in node negative breast carcinoma: analysis of 767 T1N0M0/T2N0M0 patients with long term follow-up. *J Clin Oncol.* 1993;11:2090–2100.
165. Elledge RM, Allred DC. Clinical aspects of estrogen and progesterone receptors. In: Harris JR, Lippman ME, Morrow M, et al, eds. *Diseases of the Breast.* 3rd ed. Philadelphia, PA: Lippincott, Williams & Wilkins; 2004:603–617.
166. Early Breast Cancer Trialists Collaborative Group (EBCTCG). Effects of chemotherapy and hormonal therapy for early breast cancer on recurrence and 15-year survival: an overview of the randomised trials. *Lancet.* 2005;365:1687.
167. Grann VR, Troxel AB, Zojwalla NJ, et al. Hormone receptor status and survival in a population-based cohort of patients with breast carcinoma. *Cancer.* 2005;103:2241.
168. Berry DA, Cirrincione C, Henderson IC, et al. Estrogen-receptor status and outcomes of modern chemotherapy for patients with node-positive breast cancer. *JAMA.* 2006;295:1658.
169. Henson DE, Ries L, Freedman LS, et al. Relationship among outcome, stage of disease, and histologic grade for 22,616 cases of breast cancer: the basis for a prognostic index. *Cancer.* 1991;68:2142–2149.
170. Mansour EG, Ravdin PM, Dressler L. Prognostic factors in early breast carcinoma. *Cancer.* 1994;74:381–400.
171. Donegan WL. Tumor-related prognostic factors for breast cancer. *CA: Cancer J Clin.* 1997;47:28–51.
172. Roberti NE. The role of histologic grading in the prognosis of patients with carcinoma of the breast: is this a neglected opportunity? *Cancer.* 1997;80:1708–1716.
173. Page DL, Gray R, Allred DC, et al. Prediction of node-negative breast cancer outcomes by histologic grading and S-phase analysis by flow cytometry: an Eastern Cooperative Oncology Group Study (2192). *Am J Clin Oncol.* 2001;24:10–18.
174. Chang J, Powles TJ, Allred DC, et al. Biologic markers as predictors of clinical outcome from systemic therapy for primary operable breast cancer. *J Clin Oncol.* 1999;17:3058–3063.
175. Jerry DJ, Minter LM, Becker KA, et al. Hormonal control of p53 and chemoprevention. *Breast Cancer Res.* 2002;4:91–94.
176. Marchetti P, Cannita K, Ricevuto E, et al. Prognostic value of p53 molecular status in high-risk primary breast cancer. *Ann Oncol.* 2003;14:704–708.
177. Tan-Chiu E, Piccart M. Moving forward: herceptin in the adjuvant setting. *Oncology.* 2002;63:57–63.
178. Eppenberger U, Kueng W, Schlaeppi JM, et al. Markers of tumor angiogenesis and proteolysis independently define high- and low-risk subsets of node-negative breast cancer patients. *J Clin Oncol.* 1998;16:3129.
179. Linderholm B, Grankvist K, Wilking N, et al. Correlation of vascular endothelial growth factor content with recurrences, survival, and first relapse site in primary node-positive breast carcinoma after adjuvant treatment. *J Clin Oncol.* 2000;18:1423.
180. Linderholm B, Tavelin B, Grankvist K, Henriksson R. Does vascular endothelial growth factor (VEGF) predict local relapse and survival in radiotherapy-treated node-negative breast cancer? *Br J Cancer.* 1999;81:727.
181. Paik S, Shak S, Tang G, et al. A multigene assay to predict recurrence of tamoxifen-treated, node-negative breast cancer. *N Engl J Med.* 2004;351:2817.
182. Harris L, Fritsche H, Mennel R, et al. American Society of Clinical Oncology 2007 update of recommendations for the use of tumor markers in breast cancer. *J Clin Oncol.* 2007;25:5287.
183. Basset L. Breast imaging. In: Bland K, Copeland E, eds. *The Breast: Comprehensive Management of Benign and Malignant Diseases.* 2nd ed. Philadelphia, PA: Saunders; 1998:648.
184. Greene FL, Page DL, Fleming ID, et al, eds. *AJCC Cancer Staging Handbook.* 6th ed. New York: Springer, 2002.
185. Singletary SE, Allred C, Ashley P, et al. Revision of the American Joint Committee on Cancer staging system for breast cancer. *J Clin Oncol.* 2002;20:3628–3636.
186. Woodward WA, Strom EA, Tucker SL, et al. Changes in the 2003 American Joint Commission on Cancer staging for breast cancer dramatically affect stage-specific survival. *J Clin Oncol.* 2003;21:3244–3248.
187. Sammarco A. Psychosocial stages and quality of life of women with breast cancer. *Cancer Nurs.* 2001;24:272–277.
188. Rowland JH, Massie MJ. Psychosocial issues and interventions. In: Harris JR, Lippman ME, Morrow M, et al, eds. *Diseases of the Breast.* 2nd ed. Philadelphia, PA: Lippincott, Williams & Wilkins; 2000:1009–1031.
189. Carlson RW, Allred DC, Anderson BO, et al. Breast cancer: clinical practice guidelines in oncology. *J Natl Compr Canc Netw.* 2009;7:122–191.
190. Kricke A, Armstrong B. Surgery and outcomes of ductal carcinoma in situ of the breast: a population based study in Australia. *Eru J Cancer.* 2004;40:2396–2402.
191. Fisher B, Anderson S, Bryant J, et al. Twenty-year follow-up of a randomized trial comparing total mastectomy, lumpectomy, and lumpectomy plus irradiation for the treatment of invasive breast cancer. *N Engl J Med.* 2002;347:1233–1241.
192. Poggi MM, Danforth DN, Sciuto LC, et al. Eighteen-year results in the treatment of early breast carcinoma with mastectomy versus breast conservation therapy. *Cancer.* 2003;98:697–702.
193. Veronesi U, Cascinelli N, Mariani L, et al. Twenty-year followup of a randomized study comparing breast-conserving

surgery with radical mastectomy for early breast cancer. *N Engl J Med.* 2002;347:1227–1232.

194. Morrow M. Techniques in surgery: lumpectomy for palpable and nonpalpable cancer. In: Harris JR, Lippman ME, Morrow M, et al, eds. *Diseases of the Breast.* 3rd ed. Philadelphia, PA: Lippincott, Williams & Wilkins; 2004:819–834.
195. Cunningham RS. Breast cancer. In: Hassey Dow K, ed. *Nursing Care of Women with Caner.* St. Louis, MO: Mosby, Elsevier; 2006:48–80.
196. Lyman GH, Giuliano AE, Somerfield MR, et al. American Society of Clinical Oncology guideline recommendations for sentinel lymph node biopsy in early stage breast cancer. *J Clin Oncol.* 2005;23:7703–7720.
197. Bass SS, Lyman GH, McCann CR, et al. Lymphatic mapping and sentinel lymph node biopsy. *Breast J.* 1999;5:288–295.
198. Cox CE. Lymphatic mapping in breast cancer: combination technique. *Ann Surg Oncol.* 2001;8:67S-70S.
199. Krag D, Weaver D, Ashikaga T, et al. The sentinel lymph node in breast cancer—a multicenter validation study. *N Engl J Med.* 1998;339:941–946.
200. McMasters KM, Giuliano AE, Ross MI, et al. Sentinel-lymph-node biopsy for breast cancer—not yet the standard of care. *N Engl J Med.* 1998;339:990–995.
201. O'Hea BJ, Hill AD, El-Shirbiny AM, et al. Sentinel lymph node biopsy in breast cancer: initial experience a Memorial Sloan-Kettering Cancer Center. *J Am Coll Surg.* 1998;186:423–427.
202. Veronesi U, Paganelli G, Viale G, et al. A randomized comparison of sentinel-node biopsy with routine axillary dissection in breast cancer. *N Engl J Med.* 2003;349:546–553.
203. Kuehn T, Vogel FD, Helms G, et al. Sentinel-node biopsy for axillary staging in breast cancer: results from a large prospective German multi-institutional trial. *Eur J Surg Oncol.* 2004;30:252–259.
204. Bonnema J, van de Velde CJH. Sentinel lymph node biopsy in breast cancer. *Ann Oncol.* 2002;13:1531–1537.
205. Grube BJ, Rose CM, Guiliano AE. Local management of invasive breast: axilla. In: Harris JR, Lippman ME, Morrow M, et al, eds. *Disease of the Breast.* 3rd ed. Philadelphia, PA: Lippincott, Williams & Wilkins; 2004:745–784.
206. Haagensen C. Anatomy of the mammary glands. In: Haagensen C, ed. *Disease of the Breast.* Philadelphia, PA: WB Saunders; 1986:1–46.
207. Turner-Warkivek R. Lypmphatics in the breast. *Breast J Surg.* 1959;46:574–582.
208. Lacour J, Lee M, Hill C, et al. Is it useful to remove internal mammary nodes in operable breast cancers? *Eur J Surg Oncol.* 1987;13:309–314.
209. Morrow M, Harris JR. Local management of invasive breast cancer. In: Harris JR, Lippman ME, Morrow M, et al, eds. *Diseases of the Breast.* 3rd ed. Philadelphia, PA: Lippincott, Williams & Wilkins; 2004:720–744.
210. Paszat LF, Mackillop WJ, Groome PA, et al. Mortality from myocardial infarction after adjuvant radiotherapy for breast cancer in the surveillance, epidemiology, and end-results cancer registries. *J Clin Oncol.* 1998;16:2625–2631.
211. Vallis KA, Pintilie M, Chong N, et al. Assessment of coronary heart disease morbidity and mortality after radiation therapy for early breast cancer. *J Clin Oncol.* 2002;20:1036–1042.
212. Bartelink H, Horiot JC, Poortmans P. Recurrence rates after treatment of breast cancer with standard radiotherapy with or without additional radiation. *N Engl J Med.* 2001;345:1378–1387.
213. Hevezi JM. Emergeing technology in cancer treatment: radiotherapy modalities. *Oncology.* 2003;17:1445–1456.
214. Truong MT, Hirsch AE, Formenti SC. Novel approaches to postoperative radiation therapy as part of breast-conserving therapy for early-stage breast cancer. *Clin Breast Cancer.* 2003;4:253–263.
215. Kuske RRJ. Breast brachytherapy. *Hematol Oncol Clin North Am.* 1999;13:543–558.
216. Gordils-Perez J, Rawlins-Duell R, Kelvin JF. Advances in radiation treatment of patients with breast cancer. *Clin J Oncol Nurs.* 2003;7:629–636.
217. American Society of Plastic and Reconstructive Surgeons (ASPRS) Socioeconomic Committee. *Position Paper: Breast Reconstruction.* Arlington Heights, IL: American Society of Plastic and Reconstructive Surgeons; 1994.
218. Fine N, Mustoe T. Breast reconstruction. In: Harris J, Lippman M, Morrow M, et al, eds. *Diseases of the Breast.* 3rd ed. Philadelphia, PA: Lippincott, Williams & Wilkins; 2004:801–818.
219. Bucky L, Tuma G. Breast reconstruction. In: Torosian M, ed. *Breast Cancer: A Guide to Detection and Multidisciplinary Therapy.* Totowa, NJ: Humana Press; 2002:111.
220. Baron R, Vaziri N. Reconstructive surgery. In: Hassey-Dow K, ed. Pocket Guide to Breast Cancer. 3rd ed. Sudbury, MA: Jones and Bartlett; 2006:87–96.
221. Shenan S, Kim J, Bienstock A, Yuksei, E. Plastic and reconstructive surgery. In: Bruncardi F, Anderson D, Billiar T, et al, eds. *Schwartz's Principles of Surgery.* 8th ed. New York: McGraw Hill Company, Inc.; 2005:441–448.
222. Sandau KE. Free TRAM flap breast reconstruction. *Am J Nurs.* 2002;102:36–43, quiz 44.
223. Jabor MA, Shayani P, Collins DR, Jr, et al. Nipple–areola reconstruction: satisfaction and clinical determinants. *Plast Reconstruct Surg.* 2002;110:457–463, discussion 464–455.
224. Losken A, Mackay GJ, Bostwick JI. Nipple reconstruction using the c-v flap technique: a long term evaluation. *Plast Reconstruct Surg.* 2001;108:361–369.
225. Baron R, Vaziri N. Reconstructive surgery. In: Hassey-Dow K, ed. *Contemporary Issues in Breast Cancer, A Nursing Perspective.* 2nd ed. Sudbury, MA: Jones and Bartlett Publishers; 2004:90–108.
226. Carlson RW, Edge SB, Theriault RL, et al. NCCN: breast cancer. *Cancer Control.* 2001;8:54–61.
227. Goldhirsh A, Glick JH, Gelber KD, et al. Meeting highlights: International Expert Consensus on the Primary Therapy of Early Breast Cancer. *Ann Oncol.* 2005;16:1569–1583.
228. Group EBCTC. Polychemotherapy for early breast cancer: an overview of the randomized trials. *Lancet.* 1998;352:930–942.
229. Fisher B, Jeong JH, Dignam J, et al. Findings from recent National Surgical Adjuvant Breast and Bowel Project adjuvant studies in stage I breast cancer. *J Natl Cancer Inst Monogr.* 2001;30:62–66.
230. Bedard PL, Cardoso F. Recent advances in adjuvant systemic therapy for early-stage breast cancer. *Ann Oncol.* 2008;19(Suppl. 5): v122-v127.
231. Dobbe E, Gurney K, Kiekow S, et al. Gene-expression assay: new tools to individualize treatment of early stage breast cancer. *Am J Health Syst Pharm.* 2008;65:23–28.
232. Paik S, Shak S, Kim C, et al. Multi-gene RT-PCR Assay for Predicting Recurrence in Node Negative Breast Cancer Patients—NSABP studies B-20 and B-14. San Antonio TX: San Antonio Breast Cancer Symposium; 2003 (abstr 16).
233. Gail MH. The estimation and use of absolute risk for weighing the risks and benefits of selective estrogen receptor modulators for preventing breast cancer. *Ann NY Acad Sci.* 2001;949:286–291.
234. Osborne CK, Zhao H, Fuqua SA. Selective estrogen receptor modulators: structure, function, and clinical use. *J Clin Oncol.* 2000;18:3172–3186.
235. Roe EB, Chiu KM, Arnaud CD. Selective estrogen receptor modulators and postmenopausal health. *Adv Intern Med.* 2000;45:259–278.
236. Sadowski B, Kriegbaum C, Apfelstedt-Sylla E. Tamoxifen side effects, age-related macular degeneration (AMD) or cancer associated retinopathy (CAR)? *Eur J Ophthalmol.* 2001;11:309–312.
237. Noureddin BN, Seoud M, Bashshur Z, et al. Ocular toxicity in low-dose tamoxifen: a prospective study. *Eye.* 1999;13:729–733.
238. Alwitry A, Gardner I. Tamoxifen maculopathy. *Arch Ophthalmol.* 2002;120:1402.
239. Rose C. A comparison of the efficacy of aromatase inhibitors in second-line treatment of metastatic breast cancer. *Am J Clin Oncol.* 2003;26:S9-S16.

240. Cuzick J. Aromastase inhibitors for breast cancer prevention. *J Clin Oncol.* 2005;23:1636–1643.
241. Strasser-Weippl K, Gross PE. Advances in adjuvant hormonal therapy for postmenopausal women. *J Clin Oncol.* 2005;23:1751–1758.
242. Winer EP, Hudis C, Burstein HJ, et al. American Society of Clinical Oncology technology assessment on the use of aromatase inhibitors as adjuvant therapy for postmenopausal women with hormone receptor-positive breast cancer: status report 2004. *J Clin Oncol.* 2005;23:610–629.
243. Buzdar AU. Role of anastrozole in adjuvant therapy for postmenopausal patients. *Semin Oncol.* 2003;30:21–29.
244. Thurlimann B, Keshaviah A, Coates AS, et al. A comparison of letrozole and tamoxifen in postmenopausal women with early breast cancer. *N Engl J Med.* 2005;353:2747–2757.
245. Goss PE, Ingle JN, Martino S, et al. A randomized trial of letrozole in postmenopausal women after 5 years of tamoxifen therapy for early-stage breast cancer. *N Engl J Med.* 2003;349:1793.
246. Goss PE, Ingle JN, Martino S, et al. Randomized trial of letrozole following tamoxifen as extended adjuvant therapy in receptor-positive breast cancer: update and findings from NCIC CTC MA.17. *J Natl Cancer Inst.* 2005;97:1262–1271.
247. Goss PE, Ingle JN, Pater JL, et al. Late extended adjuvant treatment with letrozole improves outcomes in women with early-stage breast cancer who complete 5 years of tamoxifen. *J Clin Oncol.* 2008;26:1948–1955.
248. Buzdar A, Douma J, Davidson N, et al. Phase III, multicenter, double-blind, randomized study of letrozole, an aromatase inhibitor, for advanced breast cancer versus megestrol acetate. *J Clin Oncol.* 2001;19:3357–3366.
249. Fisher B, Anderson S, Wickerham DL, et al. Increased intensification and total dose cyclophosphamide in a doxorubicin–cyclophosphamide regimen for the treatment of primary breast cancer: findings from the National Surgical Adjuvant Breast and Bowel Project B-22. *J Clin Oncol.* 1997;15:1858–1869.
250. Henderson IC, Berry DA, Demetri GD, et al. Improved outcomes from adding sequential paclitaxel but not from escalating doxorubicin dose in an adjuvant chemotherapy regimen for patients with node-positive primary breast cancer. *J Clin Oncol.* 2003;21:976–983.
251. Bria E, Nistico C, Cuppone F, et al. Benefit of taxanes as adjuvant chemotherapy for early breast cacner. *Cancer.* 2006;106:2337–2344.
252. De Laurentiis M, Cancello G, D'Agostino D, et al. Taxane-based combinations as adjuvant chemotherapy for early breast cancer: a meta analysis of randomized trials. *J Clin Oncol.* 2008;26:44–53.
253. Ferguson T, Wilcken N, Vagg R, et al. Taxanes for adjuvant treatment of early breast cancer. *Cocchrane Database Syst Rev.* 2007, Issue 4. Art. No: CD004421. DOI: 10.1002/14651858.CD00421.pub2. Accessed March 9, 2010.
254. Goldhirsh A, Ingle JN, Gelber RD, et al. Thersholds for therapies: highlights of the St. Gallen International Expert concensus on the primary therapy for early breast cancer. *Ann Oncol.* 2009;20:1319–1329; doi:10.1093/annonc/mdp322. Accessed March 9, 2010.
255. Doyle JJ, Neugut Al, Jacobson JS, et al. Chemotherapy and toxicity in older breast cancer patients: a population based study. *J Clin Oncol.* 2005;23:8597–8605.
256. Giordano SH, Duan Z, Kuo Y-F, et al. Use and outcomes of adjuvant chemotherapy in older women with breast cancer. *J Clin Oncol.* 2006;24:2750–2756.
257. Jones S, Holmes F, O'Saughnessy J, et al. Extended follow up and anaylsis by age of the US Oncology Adjuvant trial 9735: docetaxel/cyclosphosphamide is associated with an OS benefit compared to doxorubicin/cyclophosphamide and is well-tolerated in women 65 and older. San Antonio Breast Cancer Symposium Abstr 12, 2007.
258. Jones SE, Savin MA, Holmes FA, et al. Phase III trial comparing doxorubicin plus cyclophosphamide with docetaxel plus cyclophophaside as adjuvant therapy for operable breast cancer. *J Clin Oncol.* 2006;24:5381–5387.
259. Burstein HJ. The distinctive nature of Her2-positive breast cancers. *N Engl J Med.* 2005;353:1652–1654.
260. Piccart-Gerhart MJ, Procter M, Leyland-Jones B, et al. Trastuzumab after adjuvant chemotherapy in Her2-positive breast cancer. *N Engl J Med.* 2005;353:1659–1672.
261. Yarden Y, Sliwkowski M. Untangling the ErbB signaling network. *Nat Rev Mol Cell Biol.* 2001;2:127–137.
262. Gschwind A, Fischer OM, Ullrich A. The discovery of tyrosine kinases: targets for cancer therapy. *Nat Rev Cancer.* 2004;4:361–370.
263. Slamon DJ, Clark GM, Wong SG, et al. Human breast cancer: correlation of relapse and survival with amplification of the Her-2/neu oncogene. *Science.* 1987;235:177–182.
264. Slamon DJ, Godolphin W, Jones LA, et al. Studies of the Her-2/neu proto-oncogene in the human breast and ovarian cancer. *Science.* 1989;244:707–712.
265. Yamauchi H, Stearns V, Hayes DF. When is a tumor marker ready for prime time? A case study of c-erb-2 as a predictive factor in breast cancer. *J Clin Oncol.* 2001;19:2334–2356.
266. Perez EA, Romond EH, Suman VJ, et al. Updated results of the combined analysis of the NCCTG N9831 and NSABP B31 adjuvant chemotherapy with/without trastuzumab in patients with Her2-positive breast cancer [abstract]. *J Clin Oncol.* 2007;25(Suppl. 1): Abstract 512.
267. Smith I, Procter M, Gelber RD, et al. 2-Year follow-up of trastuzmab after adjuvant chemotherapy in HER2-postive breast cancer: a randomized controlled trial. *Lancet.* 2007;369:29–36.
268. Slamon D, Eiermann W, Robert N, et al. Phase III trial comparing AC-T with AC-TH and with TCH in the adjuvant treatment of Her2 positive early breast cancer patients: second interim efficacy analysis [abstract]. Present at the San Antonio Breast Cancer Symposium, San Antonio, TX; December 10–14, 2006, Abstract 52.
269. Vogel CL, Cobleigh MA, Tripathy D, et al. Efficacy and safety of trastuzumab as a single agent in first line treatment of Her2-overexpressing metastatic breast cancer. *J Clin Oncol.* 2002;20:719–726.
270. Baselga J, Carbonell X, Castaneda-Soto NJ, et al. Phase II study of efficacy, safety, and pharmacokinetics of trastuzumab monotherapy administered on a 3 weekly schedule. *J Clin Oncol.* 2005;23:2162–2171.
271. Citron ML, Berry DA, Cirrincione C, et al. Randomized trial of dose-dense versus conventionally scheduled and sequential versus concurrent combination chemotherapy as postoperative adjuvant treatment of node-positive primary breast cancer: first report of Intergroup Trial C9741/Cancer and Leukemia Group B trial 9741. *J Clin Oncol.* 2003;21:1431–1439.
272. Hudis C. Dose-dense chemotherapy for breast cancer: the story so far. *Br J Cancer.* 2000;82:1897–1899.
273. Baum M. The changing face of breast cancer—past, present and future perspectives. *Breast Cancer Res Treat.* 2002;75:S1-S5; discussion S33-S35.
274. Ikeda T, Jinno H, Matsu A, et al. The role of neoadjuvant chemotherapy for breast cancer treatment. *Breast Cancer.* 2002;9:8–14.
275. Buchholz TA, Hunt KK, Whitman GJ, et al. Neoadjuvant chemotherapy for breast carcinoma: multidisciplinary considerations of benefits and risks. *Cancer.* 2003;98:1150–1160.
276. Recht A, Edge SB. Evidence-based indications for postmastectomy irradiation. *Surg Clin North Am.* 2003;83:995–1013.
277. Bast RC, Jr, Ravdin P, Hayes DF, et al. 2000 update of recommendations for the use of tumor markers in breast and colorectectal cancer: clinical practice guidelines of the American Cancer Society of Clinical Oncology. *J Clin Oncol.* 2001;19:1865–1878.
278. Loprinzi CL, Hayes D, Smith T. Doc, shouldn't we be getting some tests? *J Clin Oncol.* 2000;18:2345–2348.
279. Hayes DF. Evaluation of patients after primary therapy. In: Harris JR, Lippman ME, Morrow M, et al, eds. *Diseases of the Breast.* 2nd ed. Philadelphia, PA: Lippincott, Williams & Wilkins; 2000:709–773.
280. Ries LA, Eisner MP, Kosary CL, et al. *SEER Cancer Statistics Review, 1975–2000.* Bethesda, MD: National Cancer Institute; 2003.
281. Moore S. Cutaneous metastatic breast cancer. *Clin J Oncol Nurs.* 2002;6:255–260.

282. Mahon SM. Introduction: the status of metastatic breast cancer management. *Clin J Oncol Nurs.* 2009;13:2–3.
283. Ingle JN. Sequencing of hormonal therapy in breast cancer. *Breast J.* 2002;8:332–337.
284. Jones SE. Fulvestrant: an estrogen receptor antagonist that downregulates the estrogen receptor. *Semin Oncol.* 2003;30:14–20.
285. Palmieri FM, Fry DK, Mahon SM. Current clinical issues in systemic therapy for metastatic breast cancer. *Clin J Oncol Nurs.* 2009;13:4–10.
286. Mauri D, Pavlidis N, Polyzos NP, et al. Survival with aromatase inhibitors and inactivators versus standard hormonal therapy in advanced breast cancer: meta-analysis. *J Natl Cancer Inst.* 2006;98: 1285–1291.
287. Johnston SR, Smith IE, Dowsett M. Place of aromatase inhibitors in the endocrine therapy of breast cancer. In: Miller WR, Santen RJ, eds. *Aromatase Inhibition and Breast Cancer.* New York: Marcel Dekker; 2001:29–49.
288. Kimmick GG, Muss HB. Endocrine therapy in metastatic breast cancer. *Cancer Treat Res.* 1998;94:231–254.
289. Danova M, Porta C, Ferrari S, et al. Strategies of medical treatment for metastatic breast cancer. *Int J Oncol.* 2001;19:733–739.
290. Ellis MJ, Hayes DF, Lippman ME. Treatment of metastatic breast cancer. In: Harris JR, Lippman ME, Morrow M, et al, eds. *Diseases of the Breast.* 2nd ed. Philadelphia, PA: Lippincott, Williams & Wilkins; 2000:749–797.
291. Nabholtz JM, Reese DM, Lindsay MA, et al. Combination chemotherapy for metastatic breast cancer. *Exp Rev Anticancer Therap.* 2002;2:169–180.
292. Perez EA. Update on metastatic breast cancer. *Curr Oncol Rep.* 1999;1:11–15.
293. Carrick S, Parker s, Wilcken N, et al. Single agent versus combination chemotherapy for metastatic breast cancer. *Cochrane Database syst Rev.* 2005;2:CD003372.
294. Sledge GW, Neuberg D, Bernardo P, et al. Phase III trial of doxorubicin, paclitaxel, and combination of doxorubicin and paclitaxel as front-line chemotherapy for metastatic breast cancer: an intergroup trial (E1193). *J Clin Oncol.* 2003;21:588–592.
295. O'Shaughnessy J, Miles D, Vukelja S, et al. Superior survival with capectabine plus doxetaxel combination chemotherapy in anthracycline-pretreated patients with advanced breast cancer: phase III trial results. *J Clin Oncol.* 2002;20:2812–2823.
296. Albain K, Nag S, Calderillo-Ruiz J, et al. Global phase III study of gemcitabine plus paclitaxel (GT) vs, paclitaxel (T) as frontline therapy for metastatic breast cancer. (MBC): first report of overall survival [abstract 510]. *J Clin Oncol.* 2004;22:14s(Suppl. 1).
297. National Comprehensive Cancer Network. (2008) *NCCN Clinical Practical Guidelines in Oncology: Breast cancer[v.2.2008].* http://www.nccn.org/professionals/physician_gls/PDF/breast.pdf. Accessed June 27, 2009.
298. Verma S, Clemons M. First-line treatment options for patients with Her2-negative metastatic breast cancer. The impact of modern adjuvant chemotherapy. *Oncologist.* 2007;12:785–797.
299. O'Shaughnessy J. Clinical experience of capecitabine in metastatic breast cancer. *Eur J Cancer.* 2002;38:10–14.
300. Gerbrecht BM. Current Canadian experience with capecitabine: partnering with patients to optimize therapy. *Cancer Nurs.* 2003;26:161–167.
301. Cameron D, Casey M, Press, M et al. A phase III randomized comparison of lapatinib plus capectabine versus capecitabine alone in women with advanced breast cancer that progressed on trastuzumab: update efficacy and biomarker analyses. *Breast Can Res Treat.* 2008;112:533–543.
302. Press MF, Slamon DJ, Flom KJ, et al. Evaluation of Her-2/Neu gene amplication and over expression: comparison of frequently used assay methods in a molecularly characterized cohort of breast cancer specimens. *J Clin Oncol.* 2002;20:3095–3105.
303. Frye DK, Mahon SM, Palmieri FM. New options for metastatic breast cancer. *Clin J Oncol Nurs.* 2009;13:11–18.
304. Heer K, Kumar H, Read JR, et al. Serum vascular endothelial growth factor in breast cancer: its relation with cancer type and estrogen receptor status. *Clin Cancer Res.* 2001;7:3491–3494.
305. Dvorak HF. Vascular permeability factor/vascular endothelial growth factor: a critical cytokine in tumor angiogenesis and a potential target for diagnosis and therapy. *J Clin Oncol.* 2002;20:4368–4380.
306. Miller K, Wang M, Gralow J, et al. Paclitaxel plus bevacizumab versus paclitaxel alone for metastatic breast cancer. *N Eng J Med.* 2007;357:2666–2676.
307. Rosen LS, Gordon DH, Dugan WJ, et al. Zoledronic acid is superior to pamidronate for the treatment of bone metastases in breast carcinoma patients with at least one osteolytic lesion. *Cancer.* 2003;100:36–43.
308. Rosen LS, Gordon D, Tchekmedyian S, et al. Zoledronic acid versus placebo in the treatment of skeletal metastases in patients with lung cancer and other solid tumors: a phase III, double-blind, randomized trial—the Zoledronic Acid Lung Cancer and Other Solid Tumors Study Group. *J Clin Oncol.* 2003;21:3150–3157.
309. Ali SM, Esteva FJ, Hortobagyi G, et al. Safety and efficacy of bisphosphonates beyond 24 months in cancer patients. *J Clin Oncol.* 2001;19:3434–3437.
310. Hillner BE, Ingle JN, Chlebowski RT, et al. American Society of Clinical Oncology 2003 update on the role of bisphosphonates and bone health issues in women with breast cancer. *J Clin Oncol.* 2003;21:4042–4057.
311. American Cancer Society. *Cancer Facts and Figures 2007–2008.* Atlanta: American Cancer Society, Inc.
312. Buzdar AU. Breast cancer in men. *Oncology.* 2003;17:1361–1364.
313. Giordano SH, Buzdar AU, Hortobagyi GN. Breast cancer in men. *Ann Intern Med.* 2002;137:678–687.
314. Thellenberg C, Malmer B, Tavelin B, et al. Second primary cancers in men with prostate cancer: an increased risk of male breast cancer. *J Urol.* 2003;169:1345–1348.
315. English JC, III, Middleton C, Patterson JW, et al. Cancer of the male breast. *Int J Dermatol.* 2000;39:881–886.
316. Bloom K, Reddy V, Green L, et al. Male breast carcinomas do not show amplification of the *HER-2/neu* gene. *Breast Cancer Res Treat.* 2000;64:127.
317. Giordano SH, Cohen DS, Buzdar AU, et al. Breast carcinoma in men: a population-based study. *Cancer.* 2004;101:51–57.
318. Giordano SH, Valero V, Buzdar AU, et al. Efficacy of anastrozole in male breast cancer. *Am J Clin Oncol.* 2002;25:235–237.
319. Peate I. Caring for men with breast cancer: causes, symptoms and treatment. *Br J Nurs.* 2001;10:975–981.
320. Horner, MJ, Ries LAG, Krapcho M, et al, eds. *SEER Cancer Statistics Review, 1975–2006*, National Cancer Institute. Bethesda, MD. http://seer.cancer.gov/csr/1975_2006/, based on November 2008 SEER data submission, posted to the SEER Web site, 2009. Accessed January 28, 2010.
321. Mintzer D, Glassburn J, Mason B, et al. Breast cancer in the very young patient: a multidisciplinary case presentation. *Oncologist.* 2002;7:547–554.
322. IBCSG. Adjuvant chemotherapy followed by goserelin versus either modality alone for premenopausal lymph node-negative breast cancer: a randomized trial. *J Natl Cancer Inst.* 2003;95:1833–1845.
323. Goldhirsch A, Gelber RD, Yothers G, et al. Adjuvant therapy for very young women with breast cancer: need for tailored treatments. *J Natl Cancer Inst Monogr.* 2001;30:44–51.
324. Upponi SS, Ahmad F, Whitaker IS, et al. Pregnancy after breast cancer. *Eur J Cancer.* 2003;39:736–741.
325. Field LR, Wilson TE, Strawderman M, et al. Mammographic screening in women more than 64 years old: a comparison of 1and 2-year intervals. *Am J Radiol.* 1998;170:961–965.
326. Kimmick GG, Balducci L. Breast cancer and aging. Clinical interactions. *Hematol Oncol Clin North Am.* 2000;14:213–234.

327. Holmes CE, Muss HB. Diagnosis and treatment of breast cancer in the elderly. *CA: Cancer J Clin.* 2003;53:227–244.
328. Diab SG, Elledge RM, Clark GM. Tumor characteristics and clinical outcome of elderly women with breast cancer. *J Natl Cancer Inst.* 2000;92:550–556.
329. Muss HB. Factors used to select adjuvant therapy of breast cancer in the United States: an overview of age, race, and socioeconomic status. *J Natl Cancer Inst Monogr.* 2001;30:52–55.
330. Ellis MJ, Coop A, Singh B, et al. Letrozole is more effective neoadjuvant endocrine therapy than tamoxifen for ErbB-1and/or ErbB-2-positive, estrogen-receptor positive primary breast cancer: evidence from a phase III randomized trial. *J Clin Oncol.* 2001;19:3808–3816.
331. Aapro MS. Progress in the treatment of breast cancer in the elderly. *Ann Oncol.* 2002;13:207–210.
332. Haley WE. Family caregivers of elderly patients with cancer: understanding and minimizing the burden of care. *J Support Oncol.* 2003;1:25–29.
333. Goodwin JS, Satish S, Anderson ET, et al. Effect of nurse case management on the treatment of older women with breast cancer. *J Am Geriatr Soc.* 2003;51:1252–1259.
334. Bach PB, Schrag D, Brawley OW, et al. Survival of blacks and whites after a cancer diagnosis. *JAMA.* 2002;287:2106–2113.
335. Joslyn SA, West MM. Racial differences in breast carcinoma survival. *Cancer.* 2000;88:114–123.
336. Fu SW, Schwartz A, Stevenson J, et al. Correlation of expression of BP1, a homeobox gene, with estrogen receptor status in breast cancer. *Breast Cancer Res.* 2003;5:R82-R87.
337. Cross CK, Harris J, Recht A. Race, socioeconomic status, and breast carcinoma in the U.S. *Cancer.* 2002;95:1988–1999.
338. Brawley OW. Some perspective on black–white cancer statistics. *CA: Cancer J Clin.* 2002;52:322–325.
339. Ghafoor A, Jemel A, Cokkinides V, et al. Cancer statistics for African American. *CA: Cancer J Clin.* 2002;52:326–341.
340. Cancer Prevention and Control. Guidance and Summary of Actions on the Breast and Cervical Cancer Prevention and Treatment Act of 2000. Atlanta, GA: CDC: 2003.
341. Ellis M, Hayes D, Lippman M. Treatment of metastatic breast cancer. In: Harris J, Lippman M, Morrow M, et al, eds. *Diseases of the Breast.* 3rd ed. Philadelphia, PA: Lippincott, Williams & Wilkins; 2004:801–818.
342. Borup Christennson S, Lundgren E. Sequelae of axillary dissection vs. axillary sampling with or without irradiation for breast cancer. A randomized trial. *Acta Chir Scand.* 1989;155:515–519.
343. Cheville A. Current and future trends in lymphedema management: implications for women's health. *Phys Med Rehabil Clin North Am.* 2007;18:540–543.
344. Bernas MJ, Witte CL, Witte MH. The diagnosis and treatment of peripheral lymphedema: draft revision of the 1995 Consensus Document of the International Society of Lymphology Executive Committee for Discussion at the September 3–7, 2001, XVIII International Congress of Lymphology in Genoa, Italy. *Lymphology.* 2001;34:84–91.
345. Lawenda B, Mondry T, Johnstone P. Lymphedema: a primer on the identification and management of a chronic condition in oncologic treatment. *CA: Cancer J Clin.* 2009;59:1–11.
346. Pinell XA, Kirkpatrick SH, Hawkins K, et al. Manipulative therapy of secondary lymphedema in the presence of locoregional tumors. *Cancer.* 2008;112:950–954.
347. Carpenter J. State of the science: hot flashes and cancer, part 2: management and future direstions. *Oncol Nurs Forum.* 2005;32:969–978.
348. Mankoff DA, Dunnwald LK, Gralow JR, et al. [Tc-99m]-sestamibi uptake and washout in locally advanced breast cancer are correlated with tumor blood flow. *Nucl Med Biol.* 2002;29:719–727.
349. Mao JJ, Bowman MA, Stricker CT, et al. Delivery of survivorship care by primary care physicians: the perspective of breast cancer patients. *J Clin Oncol.* 2009;27:933–938.
350. Cunningham RS. Nurses to fill gaps in screening recommendations. *Oncol Nurs News.* 2009;3:1.

CHAPTER 49

*Terri Armstrong, PhD, ANP-BC, FAAN*

# Central Nervous System Cancers

## INTRODUCTION

Cancer of the central nervous system (CNS) includes tumors of the brain and spinal cord that originate in the CNS (primary) and those that metastasize from systemic cancer (secondary or metastatic). Central nervous system cancers are relatively uncommon, but are unique in the associated neurologic symptoms that occur in these patients. Whether benign or malignant, primary or secondary, CNS tumors can be associated with significant morbidity and mortality, having a drastic affect on the patients' functional ability and cognition. Knowledge of the various tumor types and their differences, associated neuroanatomy and neurophysiology, and the many issues related to symptoms associated with both the tumor and its treatment is essential to provide accurate assessment, ongoing intervention, and supportive management for these individuals.

# BRAIN TUMORS

## EPIDEMIOLOGY

Central nervous system cancers can be primary or metastatic. The most prevalent CNS malignancy is the metastatic brain tumor, which occurs ten times more often than primary brain tumors. Brain metastasis is the most common neurological complication of systemic cancer. In the United States, it is estimated that over 170,000 patients will develop brain metastases annually, occurring in 10% to 30% of cancer patients. Prevalence has been increasing and is related to improved survival of cancer patients, the aging of the US population, and enhanced detection with magnetic resonance imaging (MRI).[1] The most common systemic cancers associated with CNS metastases are lung cancer (50%), breast cancer (15%–20%), and melanoma (10%).[1]

Primary CNS cancers represent approximately 2% of all reported malignancies. Approximately 51,410 new cases of primary malignant and nonmalignant CNS tumors were diagnosed in the United States in 2007[2] with 22,070 new cases of malignant primary brain tumors expected to be diagnosed in the United States in 2009.[3] However, any intracranial tumor, regardless of its histological behavior, can potentially invade and displace critical areas of the brain, causing devastating effects. The incidence is slightly higher in men than in women with the exception of meningiomas, which occur more often in women.[4] In children, an estimated 3750 new cases of childhood primary nonmalignant and malignant brain and central nervous system tumors are expected to be diagnosed in the United States in 2007.[2] Brain cancer is the second most common cancer diagnosed in children, second only to leukemia.

Primary malignant CNS tumors are responsible for approximately 2.5% of all cancer-related deaths. In the United States, an estimated 12,920 deaths in 2009 were attributable to primary brain tumors.[3] The 5-year relative survival rate following diagnosis of a primary CNS tumor is 28.8% for males and 31.6% for females.[2] Survival is dependent on tumor type and the degree of malignancy. Median survival for those with the highly malignant glioblastoma (GBM) is only 12 to 15 months.[5]

Over the past three decades, the incidence of primary brain tumors appears to have increased, primarily in the elderly.[6] The increasing incidence of brain tumors is probably due to newer neruoimaging techniques, as well as environmental carcinogens found in industrialized nations, better access to specialized care, changing attitudes toward the care of the elderly, medical support programs, and the increasing size of the elderly population.[5] Historically, the overall number of CNS tumors in the United States may have been substantially underestimated, as a consequence of nonmalignat tumors not being included in tumor registries. The most common primary brain tumor is the malignant glioma, accounting for more than 70% of all malignant CNS cancers.[2]

## ETIOLOGY

### GENETIC FACTORS

Specific causes and risk factors for the majority of CNS tumors have not been identified. Fewer than 5% of CNS tumors are associated with specific genetic disorders. Individuals with specific autosomal dominant disorders (ie, neurofibromatosis, tuberous sclerosis, LiFraumeni syndrome, Turcot syndrome, and von Hippel-Lindau disease) have a higher incidence of brain tumors than the general population.

Neurofibromatosis type 1 (NF-1), also called von Recklinghausen's disease, occurs in 1 out of 3000 individuals.[7] The most common brain tumors associated with NF-1 are optic nerve gliomas, astrocytomas, ependymomas, meningiomas, and neurofibromas.[7,8] Neurofibromatosis type 2 (NF-2) occurs less frequently and is characterized by an increased incidence of schwannomas, meningiomas, ependymomas, and astrocytomas.[9] Tuberous sclerosis, or Bourneville disease, has a reported incidence ranging from 1 in 10,000 to 1 in 50,000. Approximately one-half of individuals with this disorder develop subependymal giant cell astrocytomas.[9] The Li-Fraumeni syndrome is associated with an increased incidence of many different types of cancer, including astrocytomas and primitive neuroectodermal tumors (PNETs). Gliomas, medulloblastomas, and pituitary adenomas have been observed in individuals with Turcot syndrome, a syndrome of CNS tumors in individuals with adenomatous polyposis coli (APC). Approximately 5% of families with APC have this syndrome.[7] Finally, those with von Hippel-Lindau disease are at risk for developing cerebellar hemangioblastomas.[10]

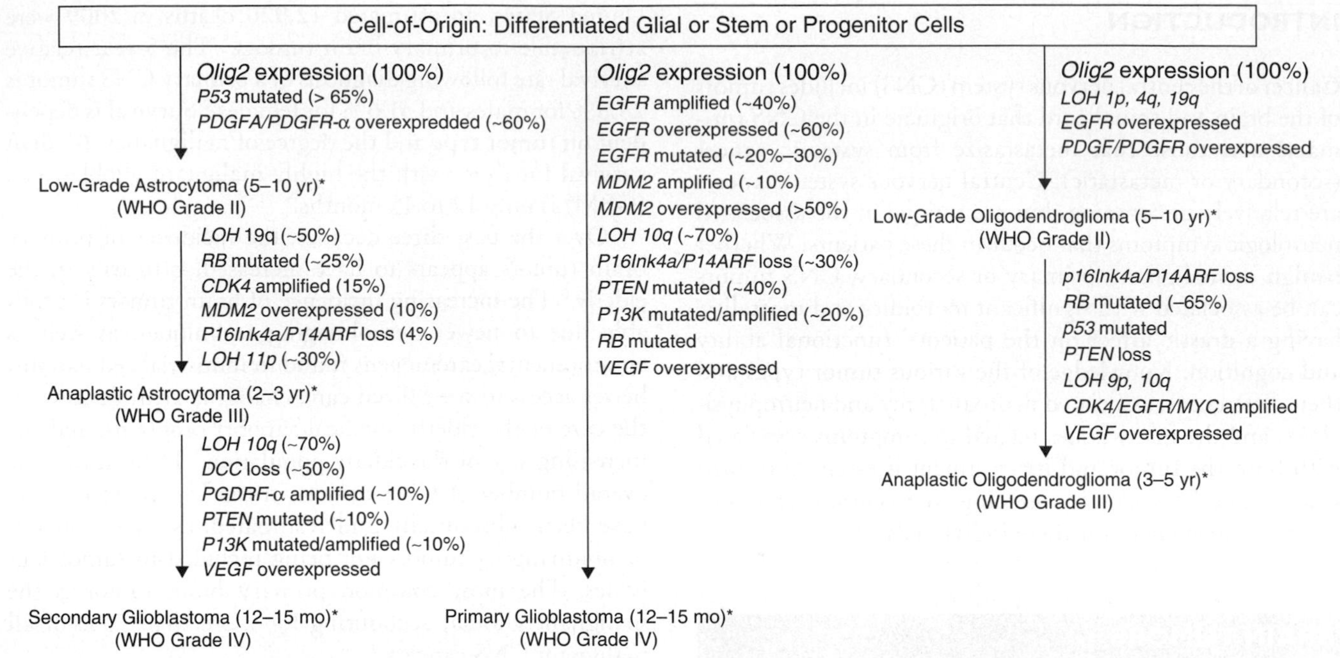


**FIGURE 49-1**

Pathways in the development of malignant gliomas.

*Source*: Reprinted with permission from Wen & Kesari (2008).[5]

As with other cancers, CNS tumor pathogenesis is a multistep process in which tumor suppressor gene inactivation and oncogene activation and overexpression play a part, along with alterations in cell cycle progression, abnormalities in signal transduction pathways, glial cell invasion, and angiogenesis. Malignant transformation in gliomas results from a sequential accumulation of genetic aberrations and disregulation of growth-factor signaling pathways[5,11] and are outlined in Figure 49-1. Recently it has been identified that glioblastoma can be separated into two main suptypes based on these changes: primary GBM and secondary GBM. Primary or de novo GBM is characterized by epidermal growth factor receptor amplification and mutations, loss of heterozygosity of chromosome 10q, deletion of the phosphatase and tensin homologue on chromomsome 10 (PTEN), and p16 deletion. Secondary GBM occur more often in younger patients and are characterized by overexpression of the platelet derived growth factor receptor (PDGR), abnormalities in the p16 and retinoblastoma (Rb) pathways, loss of heterozygosity of chromosome 10q, and mutations in the *p53* tumor suppressor gene.[12] These tumors are morphologically indistinguishable but may respond differently to targeted molecular therapies.[5] Similarly, progression from low-grade to anaplastic oligodendroglioma has been found to be associated with defects in PTEN, Rb, *p53*, and cell cycle pathways.[5,13]

The genetic and signaling pathways noted above have been well characterized, but the exact cellular origin of CNS tumors is not known. There is increasing evidence that neural stem cells or other related progenitor cells can be transformed into cancer stem cells and give rise to CNS tumors.[14] Current laboratory investigations are further defining the role and biologic difference between these cancer stem cells and identified pathways involved in malignant transformation in order to develop selective therapies.

## RADIATION

Ionizing radiation is the only definitive risk factor related to the development of CNS cancers.[6,15] Scalp irradiation, once used for the treatment of tinea capitus, has led to an increase in meningiomas,[16] gliomas, and nerve sheath tumors.[17] Brain irradiation, used in the treatment of pituitary tumors,[18,19] head and neck cancers, and leukemia, has led to an increase in gliomas, meningiomas, and sarcomas.[20]

## IMMUNOSUPPRESSION AND VIRAL FACTORS

Evidence for an etiologic role of allergies and immune function and infectious agents in the development of brain tumors is growing.[21] There is an inverse association between self-reported allergic conditions and for adult gliomas that are not present in meningiomas.[22] Acquired immunosuppression, that results from human immunodeficiency virus

(HIV) infection and the use of immunosuppressive agents after organ transplant, has led to an increased incidence of primary central nervous system lymphoma (PCNSL).[23,24]

## CHEMICAL AND ENVIRONMENTAL FACTORS

Although many chemicals are carcinogenic in animals and produce brain tumors, the possible association of chemical exposure and brain tumors has not truly been established. There may be a relationship between brain tumors and such industries as synthetic rubber, petrochemical, aeronautics, drug manufacturing, nuclear energy, health professionals, and those associated with precision metal work. However the exact neurocarcinogen exposure associated with these occupations has not been defined.[21] Substances that have been investigated include polyvinyl chloride, pesticides, herbicides, fertilizers, organic solvents, phenols, formalin, polycyclic aromatic hydrocarbons, hair dyes, and *N*-nitroso compounds.

## ELECTROMAGNETIC FIELDS

Concern has existed over the possible association between extremely low-frequency electromagnetic fields (ELF-EMFs) and the development of brain tumors, particularly exposure from cellular telephones. Exposure to ELF-EMFs is almost universal today in industrialized nations. In addition to cellular telephones, other sources of ELF-EMF include residential heating, electrical appliances, hand-held radios, electric power lines, transformers, and computer terminals. Some studies have reported a higher than expected incidence of brain tumors, particularly gliomas,[25] among electricians, electronics and communications workers,[26,27] railway workers, and welders.[28] At this point, most of the current research fails to support ELF-EMF from levels experienced in the home environment as a risk factor for brain tumors.[20] Current data on the risk of first generation cellular telephones does not suggest an increased risk of gliomas, meningioma, or acoustic neuromas with short term cell phone use.[29–31]

# PATHOPHYSIOLOGY

## ANATOMY AND PHYSIOLOGY

The nervous system contains two types of cells: neurons and supportive cells referred to as glial cells. The neurons are the basic anatomical and functional unit of the nervous system. The glial cells provide structural support, nourishment, and protection for the neurons. In the CNS, glial cells are subdivided into four main types: astrocytes, oligodendrocytes, ependymal cells, and microglia. Unlike neurons, glial cells in the adult nervous system retain their capacity to divide. They can undergo anaplasia and are the major source of primary tumors of the CNS. The specific tumor type is named for the glial cell of origin. For example, astrocytomas arise from astrocytes, and ependymomas arise from ependymal cells.

The brain is divided into three main areas: the cerebrum, the brain stem, and the cerebellum. The cerebrum contains the two cerebral hemispheres and the diencephalon. The cerebral hemispheres are connected by a large area of white matter, the corpus callosum, which allows each portion of one hemisphere to connect with the corresponding portion of the other hemisphere. It essentially allows communication between the two hemispheres. Each cerebral hemisphere is divided into four lobes: frontal, parietal, temporal, and occipital (Figure 49-2). The diencephalon is composed of the thalamus, hypothalamus, and basal ganglia. The pituitary gland is connected to the hypothalamus. The brain stem is made up of the midbrain, pons, and medulla. The cerebellum has two hemispheres and is connected to the brain stem by the cerebellar peduncles. The functions of these areas are listed in Table 49-1.[32]

### Cranial nerves

The 12 pairs of cranial nerves (CNs) are part of the peripheral nervous system (PNS), but the nuclei or synapses are located in the brain stem with e fiber pathways (axons) exiting the brain. Cranial nerves I and II are located beneath the cerebral hemispheres, the nuclei for cranial nerves III and IV in the midbrain, cranial nerves V to VIII in the pons, and cranial nerves IX to XII in the medulla (Figure 49-3). Their functions are listed in Table 49-2. Symptoms of cranial nerve dysfunction (cranial nerve palsy) can provide valuable information for localizing an intracranial tumor.

### Meninges

The meninges are the membranes covering the brain and spinal cord. There are three layers of meninges: the dura

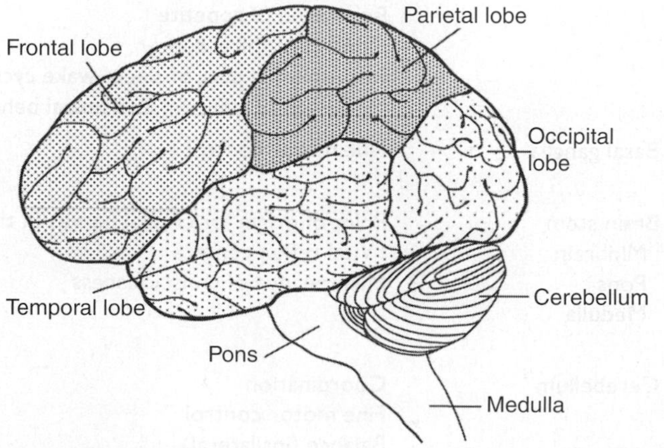


**FIGURE 49-2**

Lobes of the cerebral hemispheres.

**TABLE 49-1**

**Clinical Manifestations of Intracranical Tumors**

| Location | Function | Abnormality |
| --- | --- | --- |
| Frontal lobes | Intellect<br>Personality<br>Judgment<br>Abstract thinking<br>Mood and affect<br>Long-term memory<br>Voluntary motor activity (contralateral)<br>Secondary urinary control<br>Language expression (dominant side) | Intellectual deterioration<br>Personality changes<br>Impaired judgment<br>Emotional lability, flat affect<br>Memory loss<br>Muscle weakness or paralysis<br>Babinski sign, increased deep-tendon reflexes<br>Incontinence<br>Expressive aphasia (Broca's aphasia)<br>Seizures |
| Parietal lobes | Sensory integration (contralateral)<br>Sensory interpretation (contralateral)<br>Ability to carry out and understand special constructs | Decrease or loss of sensation (pain, temperature, pinprick, light touch, proprioception, vibration, two-point discrimination, stereognosis, graphesthesia)<br>Inability to write, calculate<br>Construction apraxia<br>Seizures |
| Temporal lobes | Hearing<br>Short-term memory<br>Language comprehension (dominant side)<br>Intellectual impairment<br>Interpretation of memory<br>Emotion | Hearing changes, hallucinations<br>Memory loss<br>Receptive aphasia (Wemicke's aphasia)<br>Emotional lability<br>Seizures |
| Occipital lobes | Vision<br>Visual interpretation<br>Inability to identify objects or symbols or meaning of written words | Visual field defects (contralateral homonymous hemianopsia), blindness<br>Hallucinations<br>Seizures |
| Thalamus | Sensory relay station<br>Conscious awareness of pain<br>Sleep–wake cycle<br>Focusing of attention<br>Emotion | Sensory abnormality<br>Neuropathic pain<br>Inattentiveness<br>Emotional lability<br>Hydrocephalus, increased ICP |
| Hypothalamus | Coordination of autonomic nervous system function<br>Temperature regulation<br>Regulation of water metabolism<br>Regulation of hormone secretions<br>Regulation of appetite<br>Control of thirst center<br>Regulation of part of sleep–wake cycle<br>Mediation of affective and sexual behavior | Abnormalities in sweating, vasodilation, hypotonia, pulse<br>Hypothermia or hyperthermia<br>Abnormalities in absorption of free water<br>Endocrine dysfunction<br>Increase or decrease appetite<br>Increase or decrease thirst<br>Flat affect<br>Emotional lability |
| Basal ganglia | Fine motor control | Weakness or paralysis<br>Intention tremors, Parkinsonism |
| Brain stem<br>Midbrain<br>Pons<br>Medulla | Point of origin for cranial nerves III through XII<br>Vital reflex centers<br>Maintenance of consciousness | Cranial nerve dysfunction<br>Abnormalities of reflex activities (heart rate, respirations, blood pressure, coughing, sneezing, swallowing, vomiting)<br>Change in level of consciousness |
| Cerebellum | Coordination<br>Fine motor control<br>Balance (ipsilateral) | Ataxia, dysarthria<br>Action tremor, nystagmus,<br>Loss of balance, wide-based gait<br>Hydrocephalus |

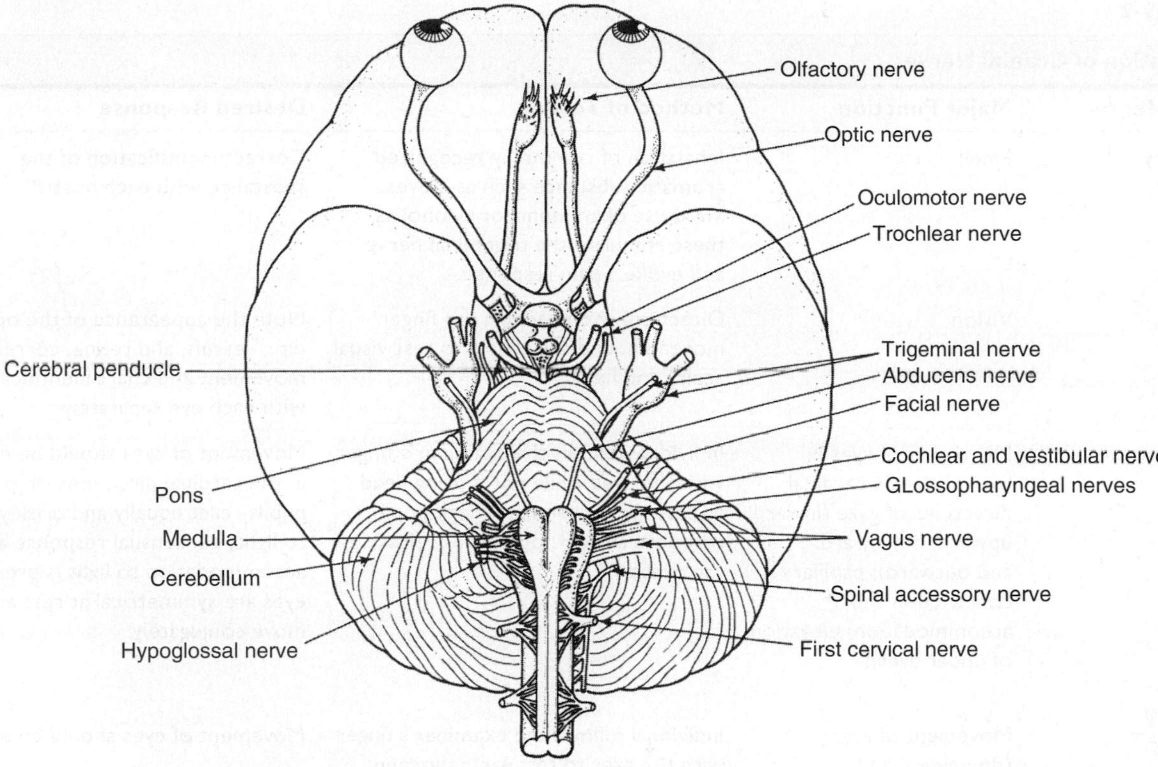


**FIGURE 49-3**

Cranial nerves from the base of the brain.

mater, arachnoid, and pia mater. The outermost layer, the dura mater, lines the interior of the skull. The outer layer of the dura is the periosteum of the cranial bone.[33] There is a potential space between the dura and the skull called the *epidural space.* The inner dural layer extends throughout the skull and folds in on itself to create anatomical compartments. The falx cerebri, the tentorium cerebelli, and the falx cerebelli are three such dural folds. The falx cerebri descends vertically between the two cerebral hemispheres to partially separate the two hemispheres. The tentorium cerebelli divides the skull into the supratentorial space and the infratentorial space. Structures and tumors that lie above the tentorium (cerebral hemispheres, diencephalon, and basal ganglia) are located in the supratentorial compartment; those lying below the tentorium (cerebellum and brain stem) are in the infratentorial compartment, also known as the posterior fossa. An opening in the tentorium—the tentorial notch—allows the brain stem, blood vessels, and nerves to pass through the tentorium. A third fold of dura, the falx cerebelli, separates the two lobes of the cerebellum.

The middle meningeal layer, the arachnoid, is a thin, delicate, transparent membrane that loosely surrounds the brain. There is a potential space between the dura and the arachnoid—the subdural space—which is a common site of hematomas. The pia mater is the innermost meningeal layer. The meshlike, vascular membrane adheres directly to the surface of the brain, dipping down between the convolutions of the brain surface. The pia mater and the arachnoid together are referred to as the *leptomeninges.* The space between the arachnoid and the pia mater, the sub arachnoid space, is where cerebrospinal fluid (CSF) circulates.

## Ventricular system

The ventricular system consists of a series of interconnected chambers and pathways responsible for the production and circulation of CSF around the brain and spinal cord (Figure 49-4). The majority of CSF is formed in the choroid plexuses. Approximately 20 to 25 mL of CSF is produced hourly, and the volume of CSF found in the ventricular system at any one time is 125 to 150 mL. In addition, CSF may be aspirated in expanded areas of the subarachnoid space called *cisterns.* The major cisterns are the cisterna magna, located between the medulla and the cerebellar region, and the lumbar cistern, between vertebrae L2 and S2.[33]

## Cerebrovascular circulation

The cerebral arterial circulation is the body's most complex vascular network. The brain receives approximately 20%

**TABLE 49-2**

**Examination of Cranial Nerves**

| Cranial Nerve | Major Function | Method of Testing | Desired Response |
|---|---|---|---|
| I. Olfactory | Smell | Inhalation of commonly recognized aromatic substance such as cloves; avoid use of ammonia or alcohol as these stimulate the trigeminal nerve and evoke a pain response | Correct identification of the substance with each nostril |
| II. Optic | Vision | Direct ophthalmoscopy; use finger movement and eye charts to test visual acuity and fields | Note the appearance of the optic disc, vessels, and retina; correct eye movement and chart identification with each eye sepatately |
| III. Oculomotor | Movement of eyes in four of the six cardinal directions of gaze (inward, upward, downward, and outward); papillary constriction and accommodation; elevation of upper eyelid | Individual follows the examiner's finger with the eyes while not moving head to test eye movement; check pupil response to light; observe for ptosis of the eyelid | Movement of eyes should be equal in the cardinal directions of gaze; pupils react equally and briskly to light; consensual response and accommodation to light is present; eyes are symmetrical at rest and move conjugately |
| IV. Trochlear | Movement of eyes (downward and inward) | Individual follows the examiner's finger with the eyes to test eye movement | Movement of eyes should be equal |
| V. Trigeminal | Muscles of mastication and eardrum tension; general sensations from anterior half of head including face, nose, mouth | Individual clamps the jaw, opens the mouth against resistance and masticates to check motor division of the nerve; touch both sides of the person's face, checking for pain, touch, and temperature response; gently touch the person's cornea with a cotton wisp to check the cornea reflex | Jaw movement is strong and symmetrical; correct identification of sensations; rapid blinking |
| VI. Abducens | Lateral movement of eyes | Individual follows the examiner's finger to test eye movement (oculomotor, trochlear; and abducens are tested together) | Movement of eyes should be equal |
| VII. Facial | Muscles of facial expression and tension on ear bones; lacrimation and salivation; taste to anterior two-thirds of tongue | Observe for facial symmetry and the individual's ability to contract muscles to check motor division; individual tastes sweet, sour, salty, and acidic flavor | Individual smiles, frowns, wrinkles nose and brow, closes eyes tightly with symmetry; correct identification of tastes |
| VIII. Acoustic (cochlear and vestibular) | Hearing, balance and equilibrium | Test hearing ability with the use of whispered voice and tuning fork at various distances from the ear to check the cochlear nerve; check the vestibular nerve by having the individual stand on one foot with eyes closed | Recognition of sound; maintenance of balance |
| IX. Glossopharyngeal | Gag and swallowing, salivation, taste to posterior third of tongue | Have individual say "ah"; check the gag reflex by touching the pharynx with a tongue depressor, have individual taste different flavors | Soft palate and uvula elevate in the midline; gag response is present, correct identification of tastes |

*(Continued)*

**TABLE 49-2**

**Examination of Cranial Nerves (*Continued*)**

| Cranial Nerve | Major Function | Method of Testing | Desired Response |
|---|---|---|---|
| X. Vagus | Gag and swallowing, laryngeal control, parasympathetic to thoracic and abdominal viscera | Check the individual's swallowing ability, ask individual to cough and speak; glossopharygeal and vagus nerves are examined together because of overlapping innervation of the pharynx | No dysphagia present, speak without hoarseness or weakness |
| XI. Spinal accessory | Movement of head and shoulders | Ask the individual to elevate the shoulders, turn the head, and resist the examlner's attempts to pull the chin back to midline; check the symmetry of the trapezius and sternocleidomastoid muscles | Equal bilateral strength; atrophy may indicate nerve dysfunction |
| XII. Hypoglossal | Movement of tongue | Ask the individual to protrude the tongue and move from side to side and up and down | Absence of deviations, atrophy, or tremors |

of the body's resting cardiac output. This large amount of blood flow reflects the brain's tremendous metabolic requirements, particularly for oxygen and glucose. An adequate cerebral blood flow (CBF) is necessary to deliver oxygen, glucose, and other nutrients to the brain, and to remove carbon dioxide and other metabolic products from the brain. The CBF must remain relatively constant because the CNS has little ability to store oxygen and glucose in its tissue. Even brief circulation failure may result in temporary or permanent loss of neurological function.

Arterial blood flow to the anterior brain is supplied by the two internal carotid arteries and to the posterior brain by the two vertebral arteries. The cerebral venous circulation consists of veins located on the surface of the brain and vascular channels or sinuses located between the two dural layers. The superior sagital sinus is one of the dural venous

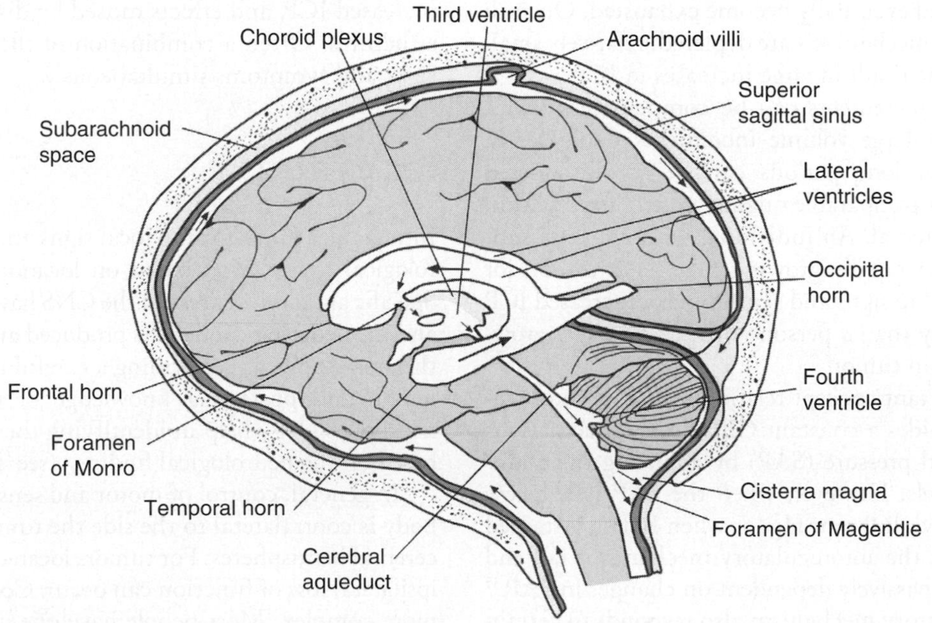


**FIGURE 49-4**

Circulation of cerebrospinal fluid.

sinuses and is a major site of CSF reabsorption. The cerebral veins drain into the cerebral sinuses, empty into the jugular veins, and return blood to the heart. Obstruction of venous outflow can result in increased intracranial pressure (ICP).

## PHYSIOLOGY OF INTRACRANIAL PRESSURE

Intracranial pressure is exerted within the skull and meninges by brain tissue, CSF, and cerebral blood volume (CBV). The skull and meninges form a rigid compartment holding these three major components: brain tissue (representing 80% of the total volume), CSF (constituting 10%), and the blood volume (accounting for the remaining 10%). According to the Monro-Kellie hypothesis, the rigid vault formed by the skull and meninges is filled to capacity with essentially noncompressible contents, which remain relatively constant, and therefore is unyielding to any increases in volume. If any one component increases in volume, a concomitant decrease in the volume of one or both of the remaining components must occur to maintain normal ICP. If the reciprocal compensation does not occur, ICP rises. The normal ICP is 0 to 15 mm Hg (80–180 cm $H_2O$). The mechanism by which this secondary decrease in volume occurs is called *compensation*. Brain tumors increase the brain mass, and the often-accompanying edema can further increase the volume to the point where compensation does not occur resulting in elevated ICP.[34,35]

To maintain a normal ICP, the compensatory mechanisms reduce the amount of CSF, blood volume, or both. The volume of CSF is decreased by increasing absorption or reducing production. These compensatory mechanisms are finite, however, and eventually become exhausted. Once all the compensatory mechanisms are depleted, relatively small increases in volume result in large increases in ICP.

Small volume increments can be compensated for far more readily than large volume increments. Increases in volume made over long periods can be accommodated more easily than a comparable quantity introduced within a much shorter interval. An individual with an acute subdural hematoma or rapidly growing malignant tumor, for example, will develop signs and symptoms of increased ICP much more rapidly than a person with a large, slow growing, low-grade brain tumor.

Another important concept relating to ICP is autoregulation, which provides a constant CBF despite fluctuations in systemic arterial pressure (SAP) by adjusting the diameter of blood vessels. However, when the SAP falls below 60 mm Hg or above 160 mm Hg, or when ICP is sustained above 30 mm Hg, the autoregulatory mechanisms fail and the CBF becomes passively dependent on changes in SAP.[35]

The autoregulatory mechanism also responds to certain metabolic factors. The cerebral blood vessels vasodilate in response to increased $PaCO_2$ and decreased pH, leading to an increased CBF and CBV. Decreased $PaCO_2$ and increased pH lead to constriction of cerebral blood vessels, resulting in decreased CBF and CBV. The cerebral blood vessels are less sensitive to changes in the $PaO_2$. Vasodilation leading to increased CBF and CBV generally does not occur until the $PaO_2$ falls to the hypoxic range.

Another consideration relating to ICP is the cerebral venous system. The cerebral veins do not have valves as do other venous vessels in the body. Any condition that obstructs or compromises the venous outflow may also increase CBV because more blood is backed up in the intracranial cavity.[35] Activities such as coughing, sneezing, or performing the valsalva maneuver increase intrathoracic and intraabdominal pressures that increase ICP by decreasing cerebral venous outflow via the jugular veins. Rotation and extreme flexion or extension of the neck may also obstruct venous outflow and arterial inflow. Positive endexpiratory pressure (PEEP) treatments, hip flexion, and lying on the abdomen also increase thoracic and abdominal cavity pressures.[36] Elevating the head of the bed facilitates venous drainage.

## CLINICAL MANIFESTATIONS

The clinical manifestations of a brain tumor can vary tremendously from one individual to another and among different types of tumors. The particular signs and symptoms with which an individual presents depend on the location within the CNS, size and associated edema of the surrounding brain, method of expansion, and rate of tumor growth. The clinical manifestations can be divided into three major categories: focal effects, generalized effects of increased ICP, and effects caused by displacement of brain structures. Often a combination of these effects produces signs and symptoms simultaneously.

### FOCAL EFFECTS

Intracranial tumors cause focal signs and symptoms of neurological dysfunction based on location within the CNS. Specific anatomical areas in the CNS have unique functions, and the neurological deficits produced are directly related to the area involved. Performing a careful neurological examination and possessing knowledge of neuroanatomy and neurophysiology help in identifying the location of a lesion based on the neurological findings (see Table 49-1).

In general, control of motor and sensory function of the body is contralateral to the side the tumor is located in the cerebral hemispheres. For tumors located in the cerebellum, ipsilateral loss of function can occur. Control of language is more complex. Most people have one cerebral hemisphere that is more developed or dominant than the other with respect to language. In right-handed and most left-handed individuals, the dominant hemisphere is the left. This is important to distinguish because the dominant hemisphere controls language, and for most people this is the left hemisphere. The right hemisphere is the nonverbal or perceptual hemisphere, which processes temporospatial information. Although 95% of right-handed people have left-hemisphere language function, only 18.8% of left-handed people have right-hemisphere language function. Additionally, 19.8% of the left-handed have bilateral language functions.[37]

Seizures occur in patients with both primary and metastatic supratentorial brain tumors. The incidence of seizures is highest in patients with primary low-grade brain tumors, with over 80% of patients experiencing a seizure.[38] Seizures are reported to occur in 30% to 60% of patients with high-grade gliomas, 40% of patients with meningiomas, and approximately 20% of patients with primary CNS lymphoma.[38] Seziures may be the initial presenting symptom in a number of patients, sometimes occurring months to years before the clinical diagnosis is made. Focal or partial seizures involve a particular area of the brain, whereas generalized seizures involve both cerebral hemispheres. In patients wtih brain tumors, seizures usually start locally and then generalize.[39] Focal seizures can aid in localizing the tumor, depending on the pattern of seizure activity.

Tumors of the frontal lobe can lead to inability to concentrate, inattentiveness, difficulty with abstraction, impaired memory, personality changes, quiet flat affect, inappropriate behavior, lack of social control, indifference, emotional lability, and loss of initiative. To complicate the situation, the individual may be unaware that his or her behavior has changed or is inappropriate.[40] Tumors in the posterior portion of the frontal lobe can result in hemiparesis or hemiplegia on the contralateral side of the tumor. Deep-tendon reflexes increase on the paretic side, and a positive Babinski sign is present. Broca's area is located in the frontal lobe (on the left in most people). Damage to this area in the dominant hemisphere results in the inability to express oneself in words even though the individual may comprehend speech and language. Broca's aphasia has been referred to as *expressive aphasia* and can be extremely frustrating for individuals.

Parietal lobe tumors affect sensory and perceptual functions more than motor function, although mild hemiparesis is sometimes seen with these tumors.[41] Common symptoms include impaired sensation, paresthesias, loss of two-point discrimination, and inability to recognize an object by feeling its size and shape (astereognosis) on the side of the body opposite the lesion. In addition they may expereince inability to locate or recognize parts of the body (autotopagnosia), loss of awareness or denial of a motor or sensory defect in the affected body part (anosognosia), inability to write (agraphia) or to calculate numbers (acalculia), and inability to execute learned movements in the absence of weakness or paralysis (apraxia).

Tumors of the temporal lobe can cause impairment of recent memory, aggressive behavior, and psychomotor seizures. Involvement of the dominant side can lead to an inability to recall names (dysnomia), impaired perception of verbal commands, and Wernicke's or receptive aphasia. In this type of aphasia, the patient speaks easily, appears to be making an effort to communicate, and is easily engaged in conversation. However, little meaning is conveyed. The individual does not understand what is being said. He or she may speak in phrases or complete sentences, but the listener is usually unable to make sense of the content. *Receptive aphasia* can make patient teaching extremely difficult.

The meeting point of the temporal, occipital, and parietal lobes is called the *interpretive area*. Lesions in this location can cause a global aphasia, resulting in the inability to express oneself or understand what is being said. Cognitive function will be significantly altered by damage to this area in the dominant hemisphere.[40]

Occipital lobe tumors produce visual symptoms, including homonymous hemianopsia (visual loss in half of each visual field on the contralateral side of the lesion) and visual hallucinations. Tumors located in this area can also interfere with the ability to interpret what is seen. Tumors located in or near the thalamus can lead to hydrocephalus, sensory disturbances, paresthesias, neuropathic pain, emotional lability, and sleep pattern disturbances. Hypothalamic tumors lead to endocrine dysfunction. These tumors can also affect water metabolism, appetite, sexual behavior, and regulation of body temperature, the sleep–wake cycle, and the autonomic nervous system.

Brain stem tumors can produce dire consequences, because the centers that control consciousness, respiration and heart rate are located here. The points of origin of cranial nerves III through XII are also located here, and dysfunction is common. Multiple nerve fiber tracts in the brain stem allow transmission of nerve impulses between the cerebral hemispheres and the spinal cord, including motor and sensory function. Brainstem dysfunction can occur as a direct result of tumor located here or because of compression as intracranial pressure rises.

Tumors located in the cerebellum impair coordination of voluntary movements, control of balance, and fine motor activities ipsilateral to the lesion.. Individuals may have a wide-based ataxic gait, may have difficulty in maintaining balance or performing tasks, a dysarthric speech pattern, tremors and nystagmus. Symptoms of increased ICP are often present because of the location near the base of the brain and compression of the fourth ventricle.

## GENERALIZED EFFECTS OF INCREASED INTRACRANIAL PRESSURE

Brain tumors increase ICP by their size, cerebral edema, or obstruction of CSF pathways. The presence of increased ICP and the speed at which it develops can vary. In some locations of the brain, a very small tumor can lead to marked elevations of ICP. In other areas of the brain, by contrast, large, extensive tumors may not initially cause ICP to rise. A rapidly developing tumor with extensive edema will raise ICP sooner than a slower-growing lesion with little edema.

Signs and symptoms result from the effects of increasing pressure on nerve cells, blood vessels, and the dura. Sustained increases in ICP ultimately cause nerve cell damage and cell death. An expanding tumor (or other space-occupying lesion) can create a vicious cycle of intracranial hypertension (Figure 49-5). After the brain's normal compensatory mechanisms have been exhausted, the increased ICP results in a decreased CBF. A reduction in the brain's blood supply leads to tissue hypoxia because the brain does not receive sufficient oxygen. The diminished blood supply also interferes with the removal of $CO_2$ and lactic acid. These metabolic by-products act as potent vasodilators. Vasodilation of the cerebral blood vessels leads to further edema. As a result, the total volume within the cranium increases, ICP rises further, and the cycle repeats itself.[32]

The signs and symptoms of increased ICP include change in the level of consciousness or cognition, headache, motor and sensory deficits, pupillary changes and papilledema, vomiting, seizures, and changes in vital signs.

Level of consciousness is an index of neurological status and ranges from alert and oriented, restless, confused, unable to follow simple commands, lethargic, to comatose. An individual may have short-term memory loss, impaired judgment, difficulty concentrating, or be forgetful. Drowsiness, personality changes or diminished cognitive ability may occur. Sleeping more is the most commonly reported early sign of the tumor. Many of the initial changes have a gradual onset and can be so subtle that they are

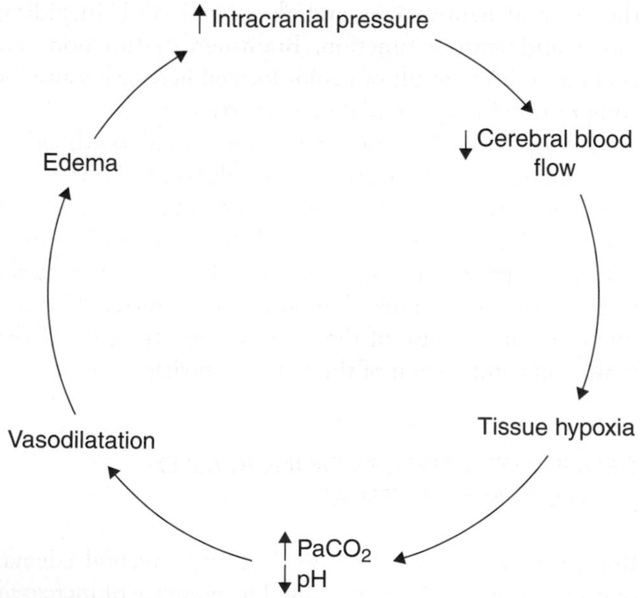


**FIGURE 49-5**

Cycle of intracranial hypertension.

evident only to the family or a skilled observer.[32] Families report that the individual just is not himself or herself.

Headache is a common presenting symptom. The location and characteristics of the headaches must be evaluated to distinguish them from other common types of headaches. The headache is usually bilateral in the frontal, temporal, or retroorbital areas. Typically, the pain occurs during the night or in the early morning, subsides after arising, and recurs the following morning. The pain can be described as dull, sharp, or throbbing. Some individuals complain of an uncomfortable feeling in the head rather than a headache. Bending over, coughing, or performing a valsalva maneuver often aggravates or initiates the pain. The headaches gradually increase in frequency, duration, and severity until, in the later stages, they are almost constant.

Motor signs of increased ICP may include hemiparesis or hemiplegia on the contralateral (opposite) side of the tumor, diminished reflexes, or development of pathological reflexes. Decorticate and decerebrate posturing can occur in the late stages of increased ICP when the diencephalon and brain stem become compressed. Decorticate posturing is an abnormal flexion of the arms with extension of the legs. Decerebrate posturing is an abnormal extension of the arms and legs. Sensory symptoms consist of impaired sensation, inability to interpret sensory information, or both.

Papilledema is considered a cardinal sign of increased ICP, but it may be a late finding. The edema of the optic disk results from compression around the optic nerve impeding the outflow of venous blood. A trained individual using an ophthalmoscope should assess for the presence of papilledema. Other visual signs and symptoms can occur including blurry vision, visual field deficits, and changes in pupillary size and reaction to light.

Vomiting as a sign of increased ICP occurs more commonly in children and in those with infratentorial tumors.[41] It may be preceded by nausea, or it may be sudden, unexpected, and projectile. Vomiting is not related to eating. Increased pressure on the medulla is believed to precipitate this symptom.[32]

Changes in vital signs occur late in the course of increased ICP. They result from increased pressure on the medulla. Systolic blood pressure (SBP) rises and diastolic blood pressure (DBP) drops, widening the pulse pressure. Bradycardia and an abnormal respiratory pattern (usually slowed and irregular respirations) develop. This combination of hypertension, bradycardia, and abnormal respirations, referred to as *Cushing's triad*, is a very late sign of increased ICP. By the time Cushing's triad is identified, the patient is usually already comatose.

## DISPLACEMENT OF BRAIN STRUCTURES

Pressure is normally distributed equally between the supratentorial and infratentorial compartments. A growing tumor mass and the associated edema cause pressure to increase within the compartment. Once the brain's compensatory mechanisms are exhausted, the increased pressure can cause the brain tissue in the high-pressure compartment to protrude into the lower-pressure compartment. This process, called *herniation*, is a life-threatening neurological emergency.[32]

The shifting brain tissue compresses other neural tissue and structures, further increases the edema, causes ischemia from damage to blood vessels, and can obstruct CSF pathways, leading to hydrocephalus. These compressive, ischemic, vascular, and obstructive changes all add to and aggravate the original problem of increased ICP.

Abnormal clinical signs usually follow an orderly progression. Careful neurological assessment in patients at risk for herniation may facilitate early identification of this potentially life-threatening complication. However, herniation can occur with little warning. A sudden change in the ICP or contents (as in an acute hemorrhage or the performance of an LP) will rapidly lead to brain stem compression.

There are two major classifications of herniation: supratentorial and infratentorial. Supratentorial tumors can lead to cingulate, uncal, or central transtentorial herniation. Herniation of the cingulate gyrus under the falx cerebri compresses the contralateral frontal lobe and the anterior cerebral arteries. Such herniation can cause bilateral frontal lobe ischemia, urinary incontinence, leg weakness, and mental status changes. The diencephalon is shifted to the contralateral side, compresses itself and the third ventricle, and leads to diminished consciousness.[42]

Uncal herniation, usually occurring with expanding temporal lobe tumors, forces the temporal lobe (the uncus) into the tentorial notch. The midbrain is compressed laterally. The third cranial nerve, the posterior cerebral artery, and the diencephalon are compressed. Compression of the third cranial nerve, the oculomotor nerve, initially causes the ipsilateral pupil to sluggishly react to light. With further compression, the pupil dilates and becomes unreactive. With midbrain compression, the motor pathways of the cerebral peduncle produce a contralateral hemiparesis. A positive Babinski sign may be seen with the hemiparesis. The enlarging mass also shifts the diencephalon, leading to a progressive loss of consciousness beginning with drowsiness and proceeding to stupor and finally to coma.[42] Compression of the posterior cerebral artery can cause ischemia or infarction of the ipsilateral occipital lobe. Later findings in uncal herniation include decorticate followed by decerebrate posturing, and impaired oculocephalic and oculovestibular reflexes. Oculocephalic reflexes are tested by holding the patient's eyelids open and briskly rotating the head from side to side or by briskly flexing and extending the neck (doll's eyes phenomenon). Oculovestibular reflexes are tested by injecting ice water into the external ear canal. In the comatose patient, testing these reflexes assesses for the presence of brain stem function.

Central or transtentorial herniation results from the downward displacement of the cerebral hemispheres and basal ganglia onto the diencephalon and midbrain, which are then forced through the tentorial notch. Initially, there will be a change in the level of consciousness or behavior. The person becomes drowsy, inattentive, or agitated. Pupil size is reduced. There may be deep sighing or yawning with respirations. As the tumor continues to displace tissue downward, the individual becomes stuporous and eventually comatose. Pupils become nonreactive, eye movements disconjugate, and, as the brain stem becomes compressed, decorticate posturing deteriorates to decerebrate in response to noxious stimuli. Oculocephalic and oculovestibular reflexes may be absent.

Both central and uncal herniations cause changes in the respiratory pattern. Irregular depth and rhythm often are more significant than changes in respiratory rate alone. Initially, respirations may be irregular with occasional pauses, sighs, or gasps. Later respiratory pattern changes include Cheyne-Stokes breathing, sustained hyperventilation, ataxic breathing, apnea, and finally respiratory arrest.[32] The classic vital sign changes of Cushing's triad are seen during the terminal phase of herniation.

Infratentorial herniation results from tumors of the posterior fossa, leading to displacement of the cerebellum either upward through the opening in the tentorium cerebelli or downward through the foramen magnum. In upward transtentorial herniation, the cerebellum compresses the midbrain. Obstruction and blockage of CSF pathways may occur. The individual may lose consciousness immediately. This event may be accompanied by hyperventilation; pinpoint, fixed, and unequal pupils; upward-gaze paralysis; vomiting; and decerebration.

Downward cerebellar tonsillar herniation is more common and results in the downward protrusion of the cerebellar tonsils through the foramen magnum. The lower brain stem is compressed; when the compression is acute, it can cause sudden loss of consciousness followed by respiratory arrest. This may be precipitated by events causing a sudden rise in ICP such as sneezing, coughing, or performing a valsalva maneuver. The outflow of CSF from the fourth ventricle becomes blocked, leading to obstructive hydrocephalus. Other signs include lower cranial nerve dysfunction, suboccipital headache, vomiting, and neck pain. Altered consciousness with resulting coma may be an early sign. Later signs of medullary compression include abnormal respiratory patterns, fluctuating blood pressure and heart rate, and cardiac dysrhythmias. In both types of infratentorial herniation, respiratory arrest, cardiac arrest, or both will occur if the condition goes untreated. Figure 49-6 illustrates the herniation syndromes.

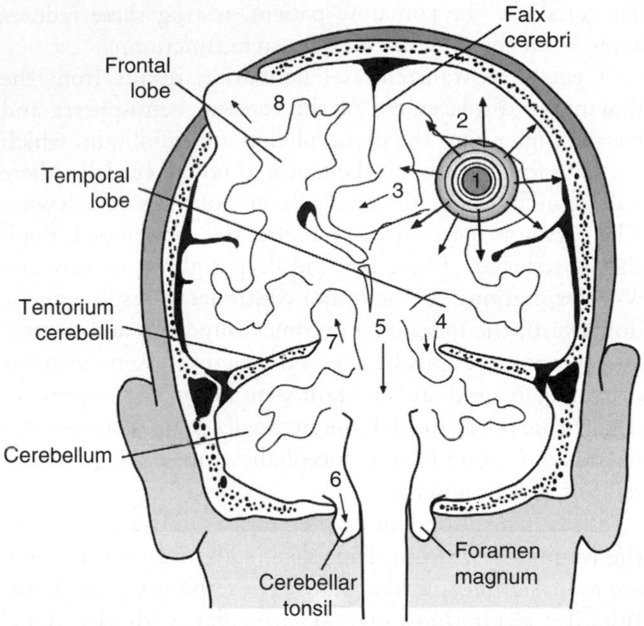


**FIGURE 49-6**

Herniation syndromes. (1) Tumor. (2) Edema. (3) Cingulate herniation. (4) Uncal herniation. (5) Central transtentorial herniation. (6) Downward cerebellar tonsillar herniation. (7) Upward herniation of the cerebellum. (8) Herniation through a cranial defect.

### PATTERN OF SPREAD

The pattern of spread noted with brain tumors differs from that found with other cancers. While brain tumors may spread to other parts of the CNS, metastases outside the brain and spinal cord are rare. Metastases outside the CNS may occur when tumor cells are transferred to the scalp, cerebral blood vessels, or dural sinus during an operative procedure. The spread of glial tumor cells through ventriculopleural and VP shunts has also been reported.

Brain tumors grow by expansion, infiltration, or both. Although gliomas invade locally, cells can sometimes be found at intracranial sites distant from the main tumor, termed multifocal disease. Brain tumors may seed the CSF and spread through the subarachnoid space. Seeding occurs along the surface of the brain and spinal cord, and "drop metastases" can occur. Some tumors, including PCNSLs, ependymomas, and medulloblastomas, seed the CSF more often than others.

Most metastatic brain tumors are theorized to develop from hematogenous spread of tumor cells, usually through the arterial circulation. The grey-white junction in the cerebrum is the most common area for tumors to occur, with two-thirds of brain metastases reported to occur in this area. Tumors in the posterior fossa are thought to occur through Batson's Plexus.[43]

## ASSESSMENT

### PATIENT AND FAMILY HISTORY

Assessment of the individual with a known or suspected brain tumor begins by obtaining the individual's medical history. The description and duration of symptoms, when they occur, the presence of exacerbating or relieving factors, and the order of their appearance are assessed. This assessment is followed by a complete neurological examination.

### PHYSICAL EXAM

An initial neurological assessment is essential because it provides baseline knowledge of the individual's neurological function. Future assessments will be evaluated in comparison with the initial examination, allowing the detection of any changes or abnormalities.

Standard generalized assessment, including vital signs (blood pressure, temperature, pulse and respirations), assessment of cardiac and pulmonary function should be performed. The neurological exam begins with an assessment of the patient's level of consciousness and mental status. The individual whose level of consciousness is impaired must be sufficiently stimulated to be able to appropriately describe the degree of alteration. Levels of alteration ranging from full consciousness to deep coma may occur. Common descriptions include alert and oriented, confused, lethargic, stuporous, obtunded, semicomatose, and comatose. Many institutions have included components of the Glasgow Coma Scale, a tool that assesses neurological function in comatose patients, as part of their neurological assessment form.

Conversing with and observing the individual evaluates mental status and cognitive ability. One should note the person's behavior, appearance, mood, and affect. Observation of actions, posture, facial expressions, and responses to the conversation and environment provide information regarding general cerebral function. Orientation, general knowledge, recent and remote memory, attention span, immediate recall, abstract reasoning, and judgment are also part of the assessment of cognitive function. Standardized assessment scales, such as the Mini Mental Status Exam (MMSE) can often be used as a guide. Language is evaluated for content, flow of speech, speech patterns, and comprehension. The presence of aphasia (the inability to understand or express one's own language), agnosia (the inability to recognize common objects through the senses of sight, touch, and sound), and apraxia (the inability to perform a skilled motor act in the absence of weakness or paralysis) is noted. Mental status changes often go unnoticed by patients. For this reason, family members, significant others, or work colleagues may initially identify a problem. They can often provide valuable information regarding the onset and progression of symptoms. In addition, formal evaluation with neuropsychological testing can often identify components of dysfunction not found on exam or by patient or caregiver report.

Motor and sensory functions are also evaluated. As noted previously, supratentorial lesions often cause deficits on the side of the body opposite the lesion. For infratentorial lesions, deficits occur ipsilaterally. A motor exam assesses whether the individual moves normally or abnormally, what the level of response is, and how strong both the upper and lower extremities are against gravity and resistance. This exam also tests gait, posture, and reflexes. Sensation is assessed by introducing various stimuli to different parts of the body with the eyes closed. Light touch, pain, temperature, and position sense are evaluated bilaterally.

Assessment of cerebellar function focuses on the ability to coordinate movement and to maintain normal muscle tone and equilibrium. The person is asked to perform the finger-to-finger, finger-to-nose, hand patting, Romberg, and tandem walking tests. In addition, assessment for nystagmus and dysarthric speech should be performed.

Testing of cranial nerve function can be the most intimidating portion of the neurological assessment. The 12 pairs of cranial nerves, their function, method of testing, and desired response are listed in Table 49-2.

The performance of the initial assessment is equally important for the person with recurrent or progressive disease. Changes in the neurological assessment, the development of new symptoms, or both can indicate increased ICP, recurrent disease, or side effects of treatment. Any change in symptom characteristics should be identified, along with possible exacerbating or relieving factors. Seizures are another area that warrants investigation. The nurse determines whether the individual has experienced seizures, what the frequency and pattern of occurrence are, and whether the person experiences an aura before the seizure.

## DIAGNOSTIC STUDIES

Developments in neuroimaging have dramatically improved the ability to diagnose, localize, and treat individuals with brain tumors. MRI, administered with and without contrast is the standard imaging technique. Positron emission tomography (PET) and specialized MRI techniques, including perfusion-weighted imaging, diffusion-weighted imaging, proton MR spectroscopy, functional MRI, and multiparametric analysis when multiple MR techniques are evaluated in total are increasingly being utilized to distinguish tumor from radiation necrosis and to increase the understanding of the metabolism and extent of tumors.[44,45]

### Computerized tomography

CT scan allows differentiation between bone, brain tissue, and CSF.[46] It is highly sensitive to blood within the brain and is the technique of choice for evaluating the presence of acute hemorrhage. A CT scan can be used to evaluate skull metastases and other bony pathology,[44] because bony structures are extremely well visualized on CT. This type of study can be performed more rapidly than MRI, an important consideration in emergency situations or when sedation may be contraindicated.[45]

### Magnetic resonance imaging

MRI with and without contrast is the more definitive and preferred imaging study for the individual with a brain tumor.[44] It provides much better resolution than a CT scan and more clearly differentiates between solid tumor, edema, and fluid collection. MRI provides superior definition of the borders of a brain tumor, and the extent of the tumor and its invasiveness can be better demonstrated by MRI. The use of paramagnetic agents such as gadolinium-DTPA allows for contrast scanning with minimal risk of allergic complications. Initially thought to not be associated with risk of renal toxicity, gadolinium exposure during MRI has recently been shown to be associated with nephrogenic systemic fibrosis, resulting in the need for evaluation prior to exposure for those at risk.[47,48]

MRI also demonstrates an increased sensitivity for small (<1 cm) lesions[32] and can detect CT-occult tumors. Such a study may show multiple metastatic lesions that the CT demonstrated as a single one. MRI is also superior to CT scan in imaging the posterior fossa, because bone artifact is not present in MRI. Likewise, it can more readily identify leptomeningeal metastases.

### Diffusion and perfusion-weighted MR imaging

Perfusion-weighted imaging measures the degree of tumor angiogenesis and capillary permeability using methods such as dynamic susceptibility contrast (DSC), dynamic contrast-enhanced (DCE), and arterial spin labeling (ASL).[49] The quantitative variable obtained from this imaging is the relative cerebral blood volume (rCBV), which has been shown to increase with the malignancy of astroyctic tumors. Another measure term $K^{trans}$ is an indicator of endothelial permeability of vessels. It is generated from DCE imaging and has also been shown to determine glioma grade and treatment response.[50]

Diffusion-weighted imaging (DWI) is a technique in which random water motion is measured in terms of an apparent diffusion coefficient (ADC) and directionality by fractional anisotropy (FA).[49] This imaging has been used to distinguish normal brain from necrosis, edema, and tumor. It has also been shown to be a reliable indicator of early stroke.

Diffusion tensor imaging (DTI), also referred to as white matter tractography is different from DWI in that it is sensitive to the direction that water is traveling. In brain tumor patients, this allows visualization of specific fiber bundles and how they are affected by tumor.[51]

### MR spectroscopy

Magnetic resonance spectroscopy is imaging that is utilized to assess the metabolic activity of abnormal versus normal tissue by detecting the levels of metabolities. In neurooncology, this type of imaging is used to distinquish necrosis from active tumor and for planning for biopsy.[44] For malignant tumors, the area of active tumor typically shows an increase in the choline peak compared to creatine and a decrease in the *N*-acetyl aspartate peak.[49]

### Functional magnetic resonance imaging

Specific areas of brain function can be identified using functional MRI (fMRI). This type of study identifies focal changes in cerebral blood flow (termed blood oxygenation level-dependent or BOLD effect) in response to repetition of specific tasks so as to accurately localize specific areas of the brain in relation to the tumor. The changes result in an increased signal intensity on MRI.[49] This technique is helpful for presurgical planning to enable maximal tumor resection while avoiding areas of critical neurological function such as language, motor, and sensory areas.

### Multiparametric analysis

Current efforts are underway to combine the techniques noted above to better define the extent of tumor, reflect changes in tumor vacularity, improve diagnosis of necrosis versus tumor, and for planning of surgery and radiation therapy. The impact of the use of multiple techniques is still to be determined.

### Positron emission tomography

PET is a functional imaging technique that may also be used in individuals with brain tumors. This technique provides dynamic information on CBF and metabolism rather than the precise anatomical localization seen in MRI. PET combines the properties of nuclear scanning with physical characteristics of positron-emitting isotopes of naturally occurring atoms.[52,53] Radioactive isotopes produced in a cyclotron are incorporated into a chosen brain metabolite and injected intravenously. These isotopes disintegrate and form a positively charged electron (a positron). The positron travels until it comes together with an electron; the pair are then converted to a pair of photons traveling in opposite directions. A ring of collimators surrounding the individual's head records these events, computers calculate measurements, and a reconstruction algorithm produces an axial view of brain uptake. Also, by monitoring the arterial concentration of radioactivity via an arterial line, the absolute metabolic rate of areas in the brain can be calculated.

Most PET studies have used $^{18}$F-fluorodeoxyglucose (FDG), a fluorinated glucose analog, to measure glucose metabolism, which is increased in tumor cells.[52] The amount of FDG uptake correlates with the degree of malignancy—ie, low-grade gliomas tend to have lower uptake (hypometabolic) and malignant gliomas have higher uptake (hypermetabolic). In addition to determining tumor grade, this technique is also used to identify optimal site for biopsy, detect recurrent tumor and distinguish between tumor recurrence and radiation necrosis. However, specificity and sensitivity are not ideal, with reports ranging from 73% to 86% and 22% to 56% respectively.[52] Therefore, wide spread use has not occurred.

### Single-emission photon computed tomography

Single-emission photon computed tomography, another functional imaging technique, is used to differentiate high-grade from low-grade tumors and malignant from non-malignant brain lesions.[53] This technique involves the IV administration of isotopes taken up by the brain and tumor cells. These isotopes emit photons, which are then detected by a rotating gamma camera. Regions of intense thallium uptake usually represent active solid tumor recurrence, whereas low thallium uptake generally indicates the presence of radiation necrosis. This technique has also been shown to be effective in distinguishing the presence of infiltrating tumor from solid tumor and in differentiating between tumor and infection in HIV-positive individuals.[54]

### Angiography

Cerebral angiography may be used to confirm that the lesion in question is a vascular malformation or an aneurysm rather than a neoplasm. In other situations (eg, with large meningiomas), angiography may be useful before surgery to determine the blood supply so that it can be embolized during the angiography procedure, obliterated during the surgical procedure, or both.[41] Cerebral angiography involves percutaneous puncture of the femoral artery with injection of radiopaque medium to visualize the cerebral vasculature. Magnetic resonance angiography (MRA) has largely replaced invasive intraarterial angiography.

### Lumbar puncture

CSF is often examined for malignant cells in individuals with tumors such as medulloblastomas, ependymomas, and PCNSLs, all of which have the propensity to seed the subarachnoid space and spread throughout the CSF pathways. Such studies are also evaluated in individuals with known or suspected leptomeningeal disease (LMD) from systemic cancers. An LP should be performed after neuroimaging studies such as MRI and CT scan, especially in an individual with a suspected tumor, because of the risk of herniation.[55] Other studies on the CSF, which help in the diagnosis, is evaluation of CSF cell count, glucose, and protein, and biologic markers associated with the specific cancer.[56] Often several lumbar taps are necessary to obtain positive cytology

## PROGNOSTIC INDICATORS

The prognosis for an individual with a brain tumor varies considerably depending on the specific type and location of the tumor. Those with a higher histological grade, have a poorer prognosis, with median survival for the patient with GBM 12 to14 months. Several important prognostic factors have been identified that may affect the eventual outcome. For patients with malignant gliomas, advanced age, histologic features of glioblastoma, poor performance and neurologic status and unresectable tumors are the most important prognostic factors.[57,58] Histologic grade continues to be an important factor in prognosis. Individuals with anaplastic astrocytoma have a significantly better prognosis than those with GBM, with median survival reported to be 2 to 3 years. Patients with astrocytoma, have median survival of 5 to 7 years. Patients with oligodendrogliomas have a better prognosis then those patients with purely astrocytic tumors, and the tumors are more responsive to therapy. The prognosis of individuals with high-grade gliomas, as with most of the CNS tumors, decreases as their functional status decreases. Those who have severe neurological deficits or are debilitated generally do not tolerate treatment as well as those with a higher performance status. They are also more susceptible to complications.

The extent of surgical resection has been accepted as an important prognostic factor for patients with malignant gliomas,[59] low-grade gliomas,[60] in addition to meningiomas and acoustic neuromas. In terms of recurrence rates and survival efforts are ongoing to identify biologic and genetic alterations in tumors that will provide prognostic information as well as guide optimal therapy.[5] Brain metastases are generally associated with a poor prognosis. However, more favorable outcomes are associated with a KPS >70, age less than 65 years, controlled systemic disease, and metastases to the brain only.[61]

## CLASSIFICATION AND STAGING

Central nervous system neoplasms represent a diverse heterogeneous group of primary and metastatic tumors of the brain and spinal cord. The classification of primary CNS tumors is based on the premise that each type of tumor results from the abnormal growth of a specific cell type. The consistent naming and grouping of similar tumor types are extremely important when gathering information and statistics on the incidence, etiology, effectiveness of treatment, and prognosis of CNS tumors. Figure 49-7 from the Central Brain Tumor Registry of the United Status lists the perentage of all primary CNS tumors by histology.

The most critical feature in the classification of CNS tumors is histopathology. The World Health Organization (WHO) first characterizes a CNS tumor histologically by its cell of origin and then designates a grade based on its similarity to normal cells. Grading assesses the degree of malignancy or aggressiveness of the tumor cells by comparing the cellular anaplasia, differentiation, and mitotic activity with those of the cells' normal counterparts.Tumor classification has clinical implications, dictates the choice of therapy, and predicts prognosis.

The WHO criteria were revised in 2003 and updated in 2007. Central nervous system tumors are classified into the following groups: tumors of neuroepithelial tissue; germ cell tumors; tumors of cranial and paraspinal nerves; tumors of the meninges; lymphomas and hematopoietic neoplasms; tumors of the sellar region; and metastatic tumors. Following is a review of specific subtypes of tumors within these groups.

## GLIOMAS

Gliomas are the most common primary brain tumor in adults. They belong to the group of tumors called tumors of neuroepitheliam tissue and include the astrocytomas, oligodendrogliomas, ependymomas, mixed gliomas, malignant gliomas not otherwise specified, and neuroepithelial

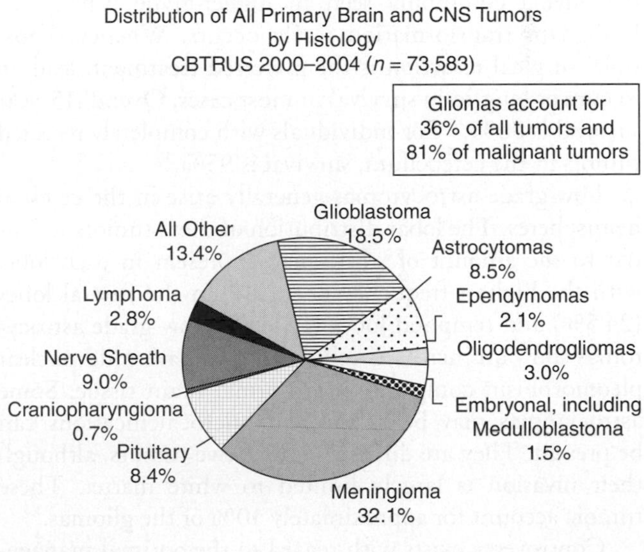


**FIGURE 49-7**

**Statistical report: primary brain tumors in the United States, 2000–2004. Reprinted with permission from CBTRUS (2008).[2] Published by the Central Brain Tumor Registry of the United States.**

tumors The broad category of glioma accounts for 36% of all primary CNS tumors and 81% of malignant tumors.[2]

## Astrocytomas

The majority of gliomas are astrocytomas. These tumors are graded to describe their degree of malignancy. Grade is based on the tumor's microscopic appearance and indicates its similarity to normal cells, its tendency to spread, and its growth rate. A 4-grade system describes these tumors as grades I through IV: pilocytic astrocytoma (grade I), low-grade astrocytoma (grade II), anaplastic astrocytoma (grade III), and glioblastoma multiforme (grade IV). In this system, grade I tumors tend to be benign and grade IV tumors are the most malignant.

Increasing grades of malignancy within the astrocytoma group are often associated with increasing patient age. Approximately 75% of pilocytic astrocytomas occur in individuals younger than age 20.[62] The mean age at diagnosis of a low-grade astrocytoma is 34 years, an anaplastic astrocytoma 40 years, and a GBM is 53 years.[63] Low-grade astrocytomas rarely occur in those older than 50, whereas glioblastomas can occur in younger individuals and children. There is a slightly higher incidence of astrocytomas in males than in females.

Pilocytic astrocytomas represent 5% of the gliomas. Although typically pediatric tumors, 25% occur in individuals older than 18 years.[63] These tumors are usually found in the cerebellum, optic tracts, and diencephalon, but can occur in the cerebral hemispheres and brain stem. On imaging, they are well circumscribed, often cystic, are enhanced with contrast, and usually lack the surrounding edema commonly seen in higher-grade tumors.[62,64] Malignant transformation rarely occurs. Whenever possible, surgical resection is the preferred treatment, leading to cure or long-term survival in most cases. Overall 15-year survival is 80%.[65] For individuals with completely resected tumors in the cerebellum, survival is 95%.[54]

Low-grade astrocytomas generally arise in the cerebral hemispheres. The lobar distribution of these tumors is similar to the amount of white matter present in each lobe, with the highest frequency occurring in the frontal lobes (24.5%) and temporal lobes (19.6%).[2] Low-grade astrocytomas show an increased cellularity and have mild nuclear pleomorphism compared with normal brain tissue. Some astrocytomas may be cystic, and microcalcifications can be present. They are diffusely infiltrative tumors, although their invasion is largely limited to white matter. These tumors account for approximately 10% of the gliomas.[2]

Controversy exists with regard to the optimal management of low-grade astrocytomas.[66] Because much of the available retrospective literature suggests a survival benefit with aggressive surgical resection, the general recommendation is to have as complete an excision of tumor as possible without compromising function.[66] Some low-grade astrocytomas present with well-controlled seizures and are relatively small, asymptomatic, and indolent lesions. Many individuals with these tumors can be safely observed and closely monitored without surgery or other treatment. Intervention would be indicated if the tumor progressed, the radiographic appearance changed (such as the development of new contrast enhancement), or the individual developed new or uncontrolled symptoms.[67] Delayed treatment postpones the risks of surgery and the side effects of radiation therapy (RT). Most individuals with low-grade astrocytomas are prescribed RT, although the timing of treatment is still debated.[66] A prospective randomized study evaluating the prognostic effect of RT in low-grade gliomas showed an improved progression-free survival for patients who received early postoperative RT compared to those who received RT at tumor recurrence.[68] However, overall survival was similar for both groups. Radiation treatment options include RT immediately after surgery, for only incompletely resected tumors, and at the time of tumor recurrence or progression. Currently, there is no established role for chemotherapy in the standard treatment of these tumors, but studies are currently evaluating the use of chemotherapy in this patient population.

Low-grade astrocytomas are rarely cured because they cannot be completely excised as a consequence of the infiltrative nature of the disease. In addition, a large percentage of these tumors undergo malignant transformation to a higher tumor grade over time. Some individuals with low-grade astrocytomas may survive for many years, whereas others experience a malignant course with short survival time. No specific therapy has been identified that can reliably prevent malignant transformation of a low-grade astrocytoma. The median survival for individuals with low-grade astrocytoma is 5 to 8 years with 15% to 20% surviving for 10 years.[62]

Anaplastic astrocytoma and GBM are some times referred to as malignant gliomas or high-grade gliomas. This designation indicates the more malignant nature and worse prognosis associated with these tumors. Also included in this group are tumors referred to as gliomatosis cerebri, which diffusely infiltrates all or much of the brain without necessarily forming a mass lesion. Anaplastic astrocytomas represent 7.5%of all gliomas, whereas GBM is the most common adult primary brain tumor and accounts for more than 50% of all gliomas.[2] The histological features of anaplastic astrocytoma include those seen in low-grade astryctoma, but also include mitotic activity. Glioblastoma multiforme has these characteristics plus either necrosis, vascular proliferation, or both. Like most primary CNS tumors, malignant gliomas tend to recur locally, with 90% recurring at the original tumor site. They can infiltrate the brain and spread throughout the neuroaxis. However, they rarely spread to distant locations outside of the CNS.

Individuals with anaplastic astrocytoma have a better prognosis than those with glioblastoma. With conventional therapy, median survival for anaplastic astrocytoma is approximately 2 to 3 years, with 29.4% of individuals surviving 5 years. A recently published analysis of the 2-year and 5-year survival data in GBM confirms an improvement in overall survival for those whose tumors demonstrate methylated MGMT, a DNA repair enzyme which when the promoter region is methylated, the tumor is less likely to repair damage by chemotherapy (2-year survival of 27.2% versus 10.9% and 9.8% versus 1.9% at 5 years (hazard ratio 0.6, 95% CI 0.5–0.7: $p < 0.0001$).[69]

Conventional treatment for these high-grade gliomas is evolving and includes a combination of surgery, RT, and chemotherapy.[5] Malignat gliomas cannot be completely removed with surgery as a result of the infiltrative nature. However, patients who undergo an extensive resection may have a modest survival advantage.[5,70,72] Radiation is the mainstay of treatment for malignant gliomas and consists of 60 Gy of partial-field external-beam radiation delivered 5 days per week in fractions of 1.8 to 2.0 gy.[5]

The use of chemotherapy, particularly in anaplastic astrocytoma is more controversial. Earlier trials evaluating chemotherapy, have included patients with both anaplastic astrotcytoma and GBM, making clear indication for chemotherapy difficult. Evidence-based management of patients with anaplastic astrocytoma supports the use of maximum resection and radiation therapy, and reserves the use of temozolomide chemotherapy for recurrent disease.[73] For patients with GBM, level I evidence exists that treatment of newly diagnosed GBM with concomitant temozolomide with radiation therapy followed by adjuvant temozolomide increases median survival and significantly improves the two year survival rate.[74] There is no standard of care for treatment at recurrence. Bevacizumab was granted accelerated approval in 2009 based on response in recurrent GBM of 19% to 26% of patients for a medium time of 3.9 to 4.2 months.[75]

## Oligodendrogliomas

Oligodendrogial tumors are being increasingly recognized and account for 3% of primary CNS tumors and 8.4% of all gliomas.[2] Reports suggest that the incidence of oligodendrogliomas has been largely underestimated in the past.[62] Oligodendrogliomas arise from oligodendrocyte cells, which are responsible for the development and maintenance of the myelin sheath. Many of these tumors contain oligodendrocytes, astrocytes, and ependymal cells and are referred to as *mixed gliomas*. Oligodendrogliomas frequently arise in young individuals, with a peak incidence occurring at age 30.[62]

These tumors are usually located in the frontal or temporal lobes of the cerebral hemispheres. Many oligodendrogliomas have calcifications within the tumor and adjacent brain tissue and have a cystic component.[41] The classification of oligodendrogliomas distinguishes between two grades. Low-grade tumors are well-differentiated and have cells that appear to be only slightly abnormal. They tend to be slow growing and may be present for many years before diagnosis. Anaplastic oligodendrogliomas have highly abnormal-looking cells and usually grow more quickly. Anaplastic features include high cellularity, nuclear pleomorphism, frequent mitosis, areas of necrosis, and proliferation of blood vessels. Clinically, these tumors present in the same fashion as other similarly located tumors. However, two features separate the oligodendrogliomas: the antecedent (prodromal) history, averaging 7 to 8 years, tends to be longer, and seizures are more common, occurring in 70% to 90% of patients by the time of diagnosis.[40,41] Oligodengrogliomas and anaplastic oligodendrogliomas have been found to be chemosensitive tumors with dramatic and prolonged responses to chemotherapy seen in tumors whose genetic analysis has shown a loss of heterozygosity on the long arm of chromosome 19 and the short arm of chromosome 1.[76–78] The standard treatment for low-grade oligodendrogliomas has been surgery, when a good neurological outcome is possible. For patients with maximal resection, further treatment is determined by age. For patients ≤ 45, observation with follow-up MRI is typically recommended.[78] For those > 45, external beam RT or chemotherapy for those with demonstrated 1P and 19Q loss can be undertaken. For patients in whom biopsy or partial resection is completed, radiation or chemotherapy with a nitrosurea or temzolomide is recommended.[79]

For patients with anaplastic oligodendrogliomas, treatment may eventually be tailored according to the genetic profile, as anaplastic oligodendrogliomas appear to not be a homogeneous group of tumors. The PCV (procarbazine, lomustine [CCNU], and vincristine) regimen has produced the longest and most reliable response to date with level 1 evidence of effectiveness.[80] In clinical practice, temozolomide is often used as a result of improved tolerability and less toxicity. Studies are underway evaluating the impact of combination therapy with radiation and temozolomide chemotherapy verus temozolomide alone in patients with anaplastic oligodendroglioma who are treated according to chromosomal status.

## Ependymomas

Ependymomas represent approximately 2% of all adult CNS tumors and 6% of gliomas.[2] They occur in all age groups but are most often seen in young adults and children. Ependymomas arise from the ependymal cells, which form the lining of the ventricles and the central canal of the spinal cord. Recent efforts have suggested that radial glial cells are the progenitor cells leading to formation of ependymomas.[81]

Ependymomas may be differentiated and low-grade or anaplastic and high-grade. The characteristic histological pattern of low-grade ependymomas consists of epithelial-like arrangements of cells around an irregular open space or a radiating, tapering process of tumor cells surrounding a blood vessel. In addition to the typical pattern of low-grade tumors, anaplastic ependymomas also have cellular pleomorphism, necrosis, mitoses, and multinucleation. Low-grade tumors are more common, and tend to occur most often in the spine. Anaplastic tumors most commonly occur in the cerebral hemispheres.[82] Standard treatment of ependymomas is maximal safe surgical resection for low-grade tumors and surgery followed by radiation therapy for incompletely resected low-grade and anaplastic tumors.[83] Individuals with totally resected tumors have the best prognosis. Craniospinal radiation is reserved for those individuals with either radiographic or pathologic evidence of craniospinal seeding. The use of chemotherapy is evolving, with limited studies to date exploring the use in adult patients due to the relative rarity of the diagnosis. Overall survival for ependymomas are approximately an 80% two year survival rate and 65% 10-year survival rate.[2] However, tumors involving the spine tend to be low-grade and often do not recur. Tumors involving the brain can recur, with an overall 10-year relapse free survival of 46%, with worse prognosis seen in adults with anaplastic tumors.[84]

## MENINGIOMAS

Meningiomas, the most common benign brain tumor, account for 32% of all adult intracranial tumors.[2] They arise from the meninges and are often located near major venous sinuses, large cerebral blood vessels, and the skull base. They may occur as single or multiple lesions. Meningiomas occur twice as often in women as in men and tend to occur in those aged 50 to 80 years, with the median age of diagnosis being 64.[85]

Most meningiomas are differentiated with low proliferative capacity, limited invasiveness, and well-defined borders. The traditional classification divides meningiomas into three grades including low-grade (grade I) or grade II and III, which are considered more malignant.[86] Grade II and III tumors contain abundant mitoses, nuclear pleomorphism, necrosis, high nuclear-to-cytoplasmic ratio, loss of normal architecture, and invasion of surrounding brain tissue.[87] Malignant meningiomas account for less than 10% of all meningiomas, occur more often in men, are frequently multifocal, cause systemic metastases, and generally have a high recurrence rate.[88] As these tumors tend to not invade the brain, symptoms are produced by compression of surrounding brain tissue. The precise clinical features vary depending on the exact location of the tumor. It has recently been recognized that despite the noninfiltrating nature, grade I meningiomas can be associated with neurocognitive dysfunction and late sequelae based on lesion location and use of anticonvulsants.[89]

The primary treatment modality for meningiomas is surgery, with the extent of surgical resection being the primary factor that influences the recurrence rate. Factors that may prevent complete resection include tumor location, size, consistency, vascular and cranial nerve involvement, and, in the case of recurrence, prior surgery, radiotherapy, or both. The risk of recurrence for completely resected benign meningiomas is small, and postoperative radiation is usually not recommended Recurrence rates for completely resected meningiomas are approximately 3% at 5 years and 20% at 20 years.[54]

Recent efforts have also demonstrated equivalent survival of patients treated with radiosurgey compared to those treated with surgical resection as initial treatment and for recurrence.[77] Radiation is also indicated for individuals with inoperable, partially resected, anaplastic and recurrent meningiomas. Postoperative radiation prolongs the interval to recurrence, prevents tumor regrowth, and improves the survival of some individuals with incompletely resected tumors.[41] Those with malignant meningiomas should receive adjuvant radiation regardless of the extent of resection.[85,90,91] Although chemotherapy and hormonal therapies have played only a limited and investigational role in the management of meningiomas, there have been some responses to alfa-interferon[92] and hydroxyurea.[93]

## VESTIBULAR SCHWANNOMAS (ACOUSTIC NEUROMAS)

Vestibular schwannomas, traditionally called *acoustic neuromas*, are benign tumors arising from the Schwann cells at the vestibular portion of the eighth cranial nerve (vestibulocochlear or acoustic nerve). They account for approximately 9% of all intracranial tumors, occur twice as often in woman, and are found more often in individuals aged 30 to 60.[2] With these very slow-growing tumors, symptoms are related to compression and stretching of cranial nerves, causing interference with their function.[94] As the tumor expands from its origin on the vestibular nerve, it extends into the area between the cerebellum, pons, and medulla known as the *cerebellopontine angle*. The cochlear, trigeminal, and facial nerves are compressed. As the tumor continues to grow, it ultimately compresses the cerebellar peduncles, cerebellum, brain stem, and cranial nerves IX, X, and XI (glossopharyngeal, vagus, and spinal accessory nerves).[95] The most common presenting symptom is a unilateral sensorineural hearing loss. Other initial symptoms are tinnitus, vertigo, and disequilibrium. Late clinical features are facial palsy, facial numbness, headache, ataxia, diplopia, dysphagia, and hydrocephalus.[87,95]

Diagnostic tests include audiometry and brain stem auditory evoked potentials followed by magnetic resonance imaging (MRI) with gadolinium. Surgery and radiosurgery are the primary treatment modalities for most individuals with vestibular schwannomas. The goal of surgery is to completely remove the tumor while preserving facial nerve function and hearing. Factors that predict the success of postoperative hearing preservation are preoperative hearing level and tumor size.[96] Surgical management of these lesions allows a cure rate in 92% to 100% of patients undergoing a complete resection.[85] Radiosurgery has also been shown to be equally effective, without the risk of surgery. As a result, more patients are undergoing radiosurgery as primary treatment.[97]

## PRIMARY CENTRAL NERVOUS SYSTEM LYMPHOMAS

A primary central nervous system lymphoma (PCNSL) is an aggressive non-Hodgkin's lymphoma that arises within and is confined to the CNS. PCNSL is a rare tumor, accounting for almost 3% of all intracranial cancers.[2] Primary central nervous system lymphoma is often associated with acquired or congenital immunosuppression. Its incidence is increasing in both immunocompetent and immunosuppressed individuals, as a consequence of the association with HIV infection, newer imaging modalities, and an increase in organ transplantation.[98,99] Primary central nervous system lymphoma is the second most common brain lesion and the fourth most common cause of death in AIDS patients. Other populations at risk include organ transplant recipients, individuals with collagen vascular diseases, those with congenital immunodeficiencies, and patients with a previous history of cancer.[98]

Primary central nervous system lymphoma is almost always disseminated within the CNS. The sites involved may include the brain, leptomeninges, eyes, and (rarely) the spinal cord. About 95% of patients diagnosed with PCNSL have a brain lesion, and 50% of these lesions are multifocal. The lesions are often periventricular and involve the leptomeninges. As a result, seeding within the CSF often occurs. Positive cytology is found in approximately 30% of patients at diagnosis, and an additional one-third have a suspicious cytology. The eyes are a direct extension of the nervous system and are involved in as many as 20% of patients at diagnosis. PCNSL may develop in the eye only. Eventually 60% to 80% of these patients will go on to develop PCNSL in the brain.[100]

These lymphomas are primarily of B-cell origin and are of the intermediate- to high-grade type. PCNSL is a stage IE lymphoma; that is confined to a single extranodal site. Affected patients show no evidence of a systemic lymphoma, and in fact, systemic lymphoma should be ruled out. Diagnostic work-up includes MRI, CSF analysis, ophthalmologic exam, and a work-up to rule out systemic lymphoma. The lesions are usually multifocal, are uniformly enhanced with contrast, and are located near the ventricles, basal ganglia, and corpus callosum. There is no known survival benefit to debulking surgery, unless surgery is needed for impending herniation. Biopsy is usually performed to obtain tissue for diagnosis. Steroids should be avoided in suspected PCNSL because they can lead to complete remission of contrast-enhancing lesions and reduce the likelihood of a diagnostic specimen being obtained.[98] Radiation therapy is the standard treatment approach for patients with PCNSL. Standard treatment is 45 Gy whole brain radiation therapy (WBRT) with no boost.[98] Some advocate deferring radiation therapy in patients older than 60 years of age to reduce neurotoxicity.[101]

Primary central nervous system lymphoma is chemosensitive, and tumor response and patient survival are improved with the use of high-dose methotrexate (HD-MTX), with a median progression-free survival of 12.8 months with chemotherapy alone and up to 60 months with combination MTX therapy and WBRT.[98] Other treatments include intensifying the dose or delivery of chemotherapy, use of a variety of high-dose methotrexate-based regimens, and blood-brain barrier (BBB) disruption with mannitol followed by intraarterial and systemic chemotherapy without RT.[102]

## BRAIN METASTASES

Brain metastases occur in 20% to 40% of individuals with cancer. The incidence of brain metastases is increasing as patients are living longer, better control of systemic cancer becomes possible, and the incidence of cancers that commonly metastasize to the brain (eg, lung and breast) continues to rise. Other factors contributing to this phenomenon are advances in neuroimaging, use of routine staging tests that assess the CNS, and perhaps the sanctuary effect provided by the BBB, which may isolate the nervous system tissue from the antitumor effects of systemic chemotherapy. Brain metastases occur at three sites: the brain parenchyma itself, the skull and dura, and the leptomeninges, with parenchymal brain metastases found most frequently. Approximately 170,000 new cases will be diagnosed annually.[103] The majority of brain metastases are theorized to result from hematogenous spread from the primary tumor. Although most cancers can metastasize to the brain, melanoma and cancers of the lung, breast, kidney, colon, and thyroid have a particular propensity to do so. The lung is the most common site of origin. Breast and lung cancers are prevalent in the population, whereas melanoma accounts for only 1% of all cancers diagnosed. Nevertheless, melanoma has the highest propensity of all systemic cancers to metastasize to the brain. Almost 40% of patients with melanoma develop brain metastases,[104] making it—despite the rarity of melanoma as a primary tumor—the third most frequent cause of brain metastases.

When neurological symptoms of brain metastases develop, the individual often has widespread systemic disease. Brain metastases are characterized by severe peritumoral edema, which contributes to the neurological symptoms. The presenting signs and symptoms of metastatic brain disease are dependent upon the lesion's location in the brain and can be identical to those of other space-occupying lesions.

The majority of metastatic brain lesions occur in the cerebral hemispheres (80%), with 15% being found in the cerebellum and 5% in the brain stem. Between 50% and 70% of individuals with brain metastases have multiple lesions.[42] Multiple metastatic lesions are often found in melanoma and lung cancer, whereas single lesions tend to occur in colon, breast, and renal cell cancers.[42,105] With early diagnosis and management, brain metastases may respond to therapy. Most individuals benefit from palliative treatment, and an increasing number of patients experience a prolonged remission. Neurological function may be preserved and quality of life maintained. Thus, systemic cancer, rather than neurological disease, usually limits life expectancy.

Treatment of brain metastases depends on the number and location of the lesions, the particular type of primary tumor, patient age and functional status, and the extent of systemic disease present. Surgery is often considered as initial therapy if there is a need for tissue diagnosis, for large lesions or in the setting of impending herniation, or hemorrhage.[104] Two randomized studies have established the efficacy of surgery in addition to radiotherapy alone in preventing recurrence and prolonging survival in patients with solitary brain metastases.[106,107] Patients with multiple (2–4) lesions may also be considered for surgery. Bindel and colleagues compared a group of individuals who had multiple lesions resected to a group who had some lesions left unresected, and found improved survival for those who had lesions resected.[108] Surgery should be considered if one lesion is causing a life-threatening herniation, hemorrhage, or hydrocephalus. Unfortunately, nearly 50% of patients are not candidates for surgery because of the inaccessibility of the tumor(s), extensive systemic disease, or other factors.[108]

Whole brain radiation therapy (WBRT) is the standard treatment approach for those with >3 metastases[104] and is used for most brain tumor patients. For many years, WBRT had been the standard treatment for both single and multiple brain metastases. But today, controversy exists for the use of WBRT for those who are able to undergo surgery or stereotactic radiosurgery (SRS) treatment.[104] Rationale to withhold WBRT after initial treatment includes the amount of time it takes to perform WBRT in patients with limited lifespan, that most patients will not develop distant recurrence, and the potential for neurocognitive effects of WBRT. Radiosurgery is often used as sole initial treatment or in conjunction with fractionated radiotherapy.[109] Retrospective comparisons suggest that survival is comparable for individuals treated with radiosurgery and those who receive the combination of surgery and WBRT,[103,110,111] Combining SRS, WBRT and surgery has not been shown to improve survival in patients with multiple metastases. One study evaluated the addition of SRS to WBRT for improved local control of brain metastases and showed that the response rate was improved in the SRS group, and survival was improved for those with single metastases but not for multiple metastases.[112] At the time of recurrence, WBRT radiosurgery, or chemotherapy may be indicated as a palliative measure.[103,106,112]

Chemotherapy is rarely used as primary therapy for brain metastases. Many tumors that metastasize to the brain, such as nonsmall cell lung cancer, melanoma, and unknown primary cancer, are often resistant to chemotherapy.[105] Adjuvant chemotherapy may be considered for individuals with more chemosensitive tumors (eg, germ cell, breast, and small cell lung cancers). Chemotherapy has been combined with WBRT in an attempt to improve the outcome compared with either modality alone. Survival was longer in patients with brain metastases from small cell lung cancer treated with teniposide and WBRT compared to WBRT alone,[113] and in patients treated with temozolomide and WBRT compared to temozolomide alone.[114] The use of targeted therapies in addition to WBRT or at recurrence are being evaluated for the impact on survival and response.[105]

Systemic cancer can also metastasize to the skull or spread into the CSF. Tumors that metastasize to bone—particularly metastatic tumors of the breast, prostate, and lung, may infiltrate the skull or dura by direct extension and compress the venous sinuses or underlying brain tissue. Treatment may consist of RT, surgical resection, or both. Leptomeningeal metastasis, once thought to be a rare complication of cancer, is increasing in frequency. Also known as meningeal carcinomatosis, it entails a diffuse or multifocal seeding of cancer cells throughout the meninges and CSF. The seeding pattern of growth covers the surface of the brain and spinal cord. Leptomeningeal metastasis is usually an indication of progressive systemic cancer. Presentation consists of multiple symptoms related to the areas of the CNS involved. Symptoms may include cranial nerve abnormalities, spinal nerve root impingement leading to weakness, altered sensation in the legs, or alterations in bowel and bladder control, as well as focal symptoms associated with location in the brain parenchyma.[115]

Although the exact incidence of leptomeningeal metastasis is difficult to determine, it has been reported to have an an overall incidence as high as 8%.[42] While any systemic cancer can seed the meninges, the cancers most commonly leading to meningeal carcinomatosis are leukemia, lymphoma, melanoma, and breast, lung, and gastrointestinal (GI) cancers.[116] The incidence of meningeal involvement from leukemia has decreased, while the incidence of leptomeningeal metastasis from breast and lung cancer is increasing. Diagnosis is established by close examination of the CSF and MRI of the brain and spinal cord. Cerebrospinal fluid analysis is often abnormal, but repeated lumbar punctures (LPs) are often required to identify malignant cells in the CSF. Radionuclide CSF flow studies are performed to detect CSF compartmentalization and are useful in establishing placement of ommaya reservoirs and for treatment planning.

Treatment includes radiation to symptomatic areas or areas of CSF block only, because radiation to the entire neuroaxis leads to bone marrow depression. This RT is followed by chemotherapy administered directly into the CSF. If chemotherapy is given concurrently with WBRT, significant cognitive decline can occur. Chemotherapy can be injected directly into the lateral ventricle of the brain by using an Ommaya reservoir, thereby ensuring optimal consistent CSF levels. Common chemotherapeutic agents include methotrexate, cytarabine, lipsoma cytarabine (Depocyte) and thiotepa. Median survival ranges from 7 to 24 weeks.[42] Clinical trials are underway to evaluate new biological or cytotoxic compounds.[117]

## THERAPEUTIC APPROACHES AND NURSING CARE

Conventional treatment of the high-grade gliomas is usually a combination of surgery, RT, and chemotherapy. The therapy for recurrent tumors is based on the types of therapy that the individual has already received. Each modality has associated side effects and may worsen existing deficits. At the time of first or second recurrence, clinical trials are often available and provide new avenues of treatment for patients.[77]

### SURGERY

Surgery remains the initial treatment for the majority of individuals with brain tumors. Recent technical advances in neuroanesthesia, neuroimaging, and instrumentation have made the surgical treatment of brain tumors safer and more effective. The goal of surgery is often multipurpose: to establish a diagnosis by providing tissue for histological examination; to provide relief of symptoms by quickly reducing the tumor bulk; and to alleviate ICP and the mass effect caused by compression or infiltration of brain tissue. As a result of the decreased mass effect, patients may tolerate RT better and experience fewer side effects.[118] Decreasing the tumor burden may also increase the effectiveness of adjuvant therapies by decreasing the number of tumor cells that must be treated, altering cell kinetics, removing radioresistant hypoxic cells, and removing areas of the tumor inaccessible to chemotherapy.[119]

When evaluating an individual for surgery, many factors must be considered: size and location of the tumor, relationship of the tumor to functional brain regions, presence of widespread or multiple sites of disease, and the individual's age and neurological status. For example, a tumor with well-defined margins or one that is encapsulated in the nondominant hemisphere lends itself to an extensive resection. A rapidly growing infiltrative tumor that extends across the midline and is located in a deep vital structure or within the motor or sensory cortex may not be completely excised. In such a case, a biopsy or partial resection may be a safer option than a radical procedure. PCNSL, a tumor often widely disseminated throughout the CNS, is not usually surgically resected. In addition, tumors involving eloquent areas of the brain, such as the brainstem or motor strip, may not be removed because of the associated risk of significant deficits.

#### Biopsy

The goal of biopsy is to provide the neuropathologist with a representative sampling of the lesion with which to establish a histological diagnosis. Stereotactic biopsy precisely locates areas in the brain using 3-dimensional coordinates without direct visual access. Using a stereotactic frame the patient's head is secured to the head ring, with four percutaneous skull pins to provide rigid skull fixation. A localizing cage composed of vertical and diagonal graphite rods is secured in the head ring, and a CT or MRI is performed. The lesion is referenced to the nine *x*- and *y*-coordinates of the localizing cage, and these points are transformed to create a 3-dimensional space. The localizing cage is removed, and in the operating room a sterile arc guidance system is fixed to the head ring. The center of the arc depicts the target lesion, which can be approached from any angle or point on the arc quadrant. The biopsy probe or needle is accurately directed to within 1 to 2 mm of the target.[54,121] In this way, the needle or probe can be guided to the target along the safest pathway (ie, one that avoids major vascular and functional structures).

Stereotactic biopsy has a diagnostic accuracy of greater than 95%, an overall morbidity rate of 3.2%, and a mortality rate of 0.6%.[122] However, concern exists about the diagnostic accuracy of biopsy for gliomas, as a consequence of the heterogeneous nature of the tumor. Potential complications after a brain biopsy include hemorrhage at the biopsy site, exacerbation of cerebral edema, development of a new neurological deficit, seizures, and infection.

Because they report discomfort with the head frame during placement, patients usually require premedication. In adults, stereotactic biopsy is generally performed under local anesthesia. This approach may decrease complications associated with general anesthesia but requires patient cooperation to perform the procedure. The need for patient cooperation with these systems discourages their use in pediatric patients and patients with dementia,[123] who typically require general anesthesia. Associated mortality and morbidity may be decreased with stereotactic procedures and hospital stays may be shorter.

#### Craniotomy

The goal of brain tumor surgery is to remove the tumor completely while preserving neurological function.[124] Surgical cure is often not possible, because of the infiltrative nature of most CNS tumors, expecially gliomas. Many tumors traditionally considered unapproachable are now being completely removed with success. The advances that make these successes possible include intraoperative monitoring; interactive, image-guided, frameless stereotactic systems; functional imaging with awake craniotomies and intraoperative MRI.[118] Major neurological morbidity has been reduced to 8.5% and mortality to 1.7% for patients undergoing craniotomy for tumor removal.[125]

Intraoperative monitoring includes intraoperative ultrasound (IOUS) and brain mapping techniques. With IOUS, the surgeon receives immediate feedback during the craniotomy and views images that assist in the maximal resection of the tumor. A major advantage of ultrasound is its ability to portray an image of the tumor and operating field in real time, allowing visual tracking of changes in the tumor and shifts in the surrounding brain during the operation. IOUS helps to define the tumor's borders by delineating both the tumor and its transition toward normal tissue and by differentiating edema from solid tumor and normal brain.[119,126] In addition, IOUS is useful in planning the route or approach through normal tissue to reach the tumor.

Preoperative functional MRI imaging and intraoperative brain mapping is useful in surgery in the dominant hemisphere, the motor and sensory regions, and the speech centers. Functional MRI is used to identify eloquent areas of the brain and assists with assessing the feasibility of surgical resection, for surgical planning, and for selecting patients for invasive functional mapping procedures.[127] Brain mapping techniques use either direct stimulation of the cerebral cortex or sensory evoked potentials (SEPs). In direct cortical stimulation, the dura is opened and electrodes are placed on the surface of the brain. The patient is then awakened and, by stimulating the electrodes and having the patient perform repetitive motor or language tasks the eloquent cortex can be located and avoided during surgery. During SEP monitoring, sensory structures are stimulated and the electrical responses of the areas are analyzed on a monitor.[118] This technique permits mapping of the somatosensory, auditory, and visual cortex. Use of these techniques has been reported to facilitate tumor resection in functioning brain regions and allowing for neurologic recovery.[128] However, a randomized trial comparing outcome has not been completed.

Interactive, image-guided, frameless stereotactic systems provide neurosurgeons with precise preoperative and intraoperative patient information. They can improve the accuracy of localizing lesions and aid in defining tumor margins. This allows the surgeon to perform a safe, more effective, and less invasive tumor excision. Before surgery, the patient undergoes a CT or MRI and markers or fiducials, which will be visible on the images, are applied to the patient's head. Some systems do not require markers to be placed but instead use previously referenced surface points on the patient's head. A computer transforms the data into a three-dimensional image for use in the operating room. Before the surgery, the surgeon can plan each step of the procedure and the ideal access to the tumor via the three-dimensional image on the computer screen. The tumor and its surroundings can be viewed from different angles and in relation to land-mark structures. Once in the operating room, the patient's fiducials or coordinates are integrated to the image. A pointing device, such as the viewing wand, is used to quickly communicate surgical locations to the computer system.[123] Some systems use a mechanically linked arm; others communicate through sonic, optical, or magnetic digitizers.[129] At any time during the surgery, the surgeon can place the probe on a structure and, by viewing the screen, determine its location in relation to surrounding structures within 1 to 2 mm.[119] The main limitation of such a system is its reliance on preoperative images. During the surgery, anatomical changes occur. These changes may be related to CSF, edema, or the resection itself. Their occurrence can make the data derived from preoperative images somewhat outdated. Only intraoperative imaging can provide the updated information required to maintain accurate navigation during surgery.[124]

Intraoperative imaging was developed to overcome the limitations of using navigation systems that are based on preoperative images and to provide updated images during the actual procedure. With updated intraoperative images, the course of the surgery may be affected. For example, unrecognized tumor that otherwise would have been seen only on a postoperative MRI done outside the operating room can be removed, allowing for a more complete tumor resection. Unnecessary further dissection may be avoided, thereby decreasing the risk of neurological injury.[124] In addition, once the procedure is complete, a final image may be obtained to evaluate for a hematoma or other complication. Intraoperative MRI (iMRI) designs range from dedicated units requiring the construction of a special operating room, to MRI suites that can be transformed into sterile surgical areas,[130] to iMRI devices designed specifically to work in neurosurgical operating rooms.[131] Comparative trials evaluating outcome for those patients undergoing craniotomy with interoperative imaging versus those who have not have not been completed.

Surgery also provides access for other adjuvant therapies. A stereotactic surgical procedure may be used to place radioactive sources within the tumor or the gliasite balloon. Chemotherapy wafers may be implanted surgically within a tumor cavity and then slowly and continuously release chemotherapy directly into the brain. Ommaya reservoirs may be placed to deliver chemotherapy directly into the CSF.

## Nursing care

Nursing interventions for patients undergoing neurosurgical procedures begin preoperatively in the outpatient setting. A baseline neurological examination is essential. Preoperative teaching consists of education in the planned surgical procedure, postoperative routines, measures to prevent complications, and medications that will be administered. Patients must be instructed to refrain from taking aspirin, aspirin-containing products, anticoagulants and nonsteroidal anti-inflammatory drugs (NSAIDs) preoperatively. Patients scheduled to undergo an awake procedure may have additional emotional issues, including fear, anxiety, and concern for their own responsibility for the outcome.[132]

Postoperative recovery practices vary among institutions. Neurological assessment is conducted on an ongoing basis to identify any variations that may signify potential complications. If no complications occur, patients undergoing craniotomy are usually hospitalized for 3 to 5 days, while those having a stereotactic biopsy require a 24- to 48-hour hospital stay. Some patients will initially be cared for in a postoperative step-down or an intensive care unit. Others will not require intensive monitoring beyond the postanesthesia care unit.

Postoperatively, patients may have new or worsened neurological deficits. The plan of care must be individualized, reflecting the specific deficits encountered. Intensive inpatient rehabilitation may be appropriate for patients with functional deficits, and improved function has been demonstrated as a result of therapy.[133] Safety measures assume the utmost importance for all personnel involved in the patient's care. Family members may not truly understand the severity of the potential risks related to deficits such as impaired judgment, memory loss, weakness or paralysis, and visual field disturbances, and will require frequent reinforcement.

### Postoperative complications

Complications after neurosurgery may include intracranial bleeding, cerebral edema, further neurological impairment, electrolyte imbalance, infection, seizures, venous thromboembolism, and hydrocephalus. Hemorrhage at the operative site can occur within hours after surgery. Bleeding may also occur from traction on the bridging veins between the brain and the dura, leading to a subdural hematoma.[32] Additional areas where bleeding may occur are the epidural space, the subarachnoid space, or within the ventricles. Patients usually present with a new or worsening of a preoperative neurological deficit or seizures and often require surgery to evacuate the hematoma.

Postoperative cerebral edema is especially severe when residual tumor is present, but it occurs even after complete tumor removal. This complication results from the surgical manipulation of the surrounding brain tissue, changes in regional blood flow, or brain injury caused by excessive retraction.[119] The amount of edema varies in each individual but generally reaches its maximum peak at 48 to 72 hours postoperatively. Cerebral edema is treated with corticosteroids, usually dexamethasone; careful fluid management; and osmotherapy when necessary. Other techniques for controlling ICP include hyperventilation, CSF drainage, and the use of anesthetic agents. Activities that can exacerbate ICP should be avoided. The head of the bed is generally elevated 30°.

Electrolyte imbalance—namely, hyponatremia—can occur and may be treated with fluid restriction. Some patients require fluid restriction, although most are kept euvolemic. Hyponatremia can decrease the seizure threshold, exacerbate cerebral edema, and increase neurological deficits. Infection is often prevented by the prophylactic use of antibiotics for 24 to 48 hours postoperatively.

Seizures are managed with prophylactic anticonvulsants and maintenance of therapeutic serum levels. Controversy persists concerning the use of prophylactic anticonvulsants in individuals who have not previously had a seizure.[62] Phenytoin (dilantin) is the most commonly used agent, although other agents including levetiracetam are being used with increasing frequency due to efficacy and improved tolerability.[134] A CT scan may be indicated after a postoperative seizure to rule out hematoma, increased cerebral edema, or pneumocephalus.

Venous thromboembolism is a particular concern in neurosurgery patients because of the length of surgery, immobility of some postoperative patients, hemiparesis, and tumor-related hypercoagulable states.[119] Early ambulation is encouraged whenever possible. The risk of venous thromboembolism is reduced by the use of pneumatic compression devices and prophylactic anticoagulation. This complication may occur early or late in the postoperative period.

Postoperative hydrocephalus may be caused by tumor, periventricular swelling, or intraventricular blood. When severe, it is usually treated with ventriculostomy or VP shunting.

## RADIATION THERAPY

Radiation therapy plays a central role in the treatment of adult brain tumors. Early randomized studies by the Brain Tumor Cooperative Group (BTCG) firmly established the role of postoperative RT in patients with malignant gliomas. Individuals who received postoperative RT had a significantly prolonged survival compared with those who received only postoperative supportive care.[135] These studies were so convincing that subsequent clinical trials evaluating adjuvant therapy for malignant brain tumors have included RT in all treatment arms.[5,136] Likewise, RT plays an important role in the treatment of patients with low-grade gliomas; inoperable, partially resected, or recurrent benign brain tumors; and metastatic brain tumors.

### Conventional radiotherapy

Radiotherapy for malignant gliomas historically was delivered to the whole brain. Neuroimaging studies have shown that the majority of tumors recur within 1 to 2 cm of their original location. In addition, many individuals who survive for extended periods after WBRT develop significant treatment-related morbidity. Therefore, partial brain irradiation or local-field radiotherapy (LFRT) is now accepted as the standard treatment approach. With this approach, radiation is delivered to the tumor and a 3-cm margin of tissue surrounding the perimeter[137] in divided doses (fractions), generally once daily over 5 to 6 weeks, to deliver 60 Gy to the involved field. WBRT is usually reserved for multifocal disease. Intensity-modulated radiation therapy (IMRT) is a term applied to technology that uses nonuniform radiation beams to achieve conformal dose distributions. The theoretical benefit is less exposure to normal brain structures and improved planning for complex lesions.[138] Proton beam radiation therapy is another technique currently being explored in the treatment of CNS tumors. Proton beam uses charged particles, not x-rays to treat the tumor. Theorized benefits include improved dose distributions and the absence of an exit dose reducing injury to critical adjacent structures.[139]

Attempts to improve responses to conventional RT while preserving normal tissue have included further manipulation of the dose and schedule of RT by hyperfractionation and accelerated treatment schedules and the use of radiosensitizers. However, these attempts have not improved the outcome and in some cases have led to increased toxicity.[140]

Other primary brain tumors may be treated with RT. In benign brain tumors such as meningiomas and pituitary adenomas that cannot be completely excised or that recur despite aggressive resection, RT is an important adjuvant therapy. A dose of 54 Gy is recommended for benign tumors. Individuals with malignant meningiomas generally receive postoperative RT, regardless of the extent of resection, and the dose is increased to 60 Gy.[41]

### Three-dimensional conformal radiation therapy

In most centers, the RT plan for primary brain tumor patients uses 3-dimensional treatment planning (3D-CRT). This method of high-precision RT utilizes MRI, CT information, or both, plus powerful computer technology, to plan and deliver external beam radiation treatments that shape the prescription dose distribution to conform to the anatomical boundaries of the tumor in its entire three-dimensional configuration while minimizing the dose to the surrounding tissue. It requires reproducible and precise head immobilization. Comparative two-dimensional and three-dimensional treatment planning studies in brain tumor patients have demonstrated a 30% reduction in the amount of normal brain irradiated when the 3DCRT method is used.[141] In addition, 3D-CRT may allow higher than traditional doses to be safely administered to selected individuals.[62]

Intensity-modulated RT (IMRT) is an advanced form of 3D-CRT that offers an additional refinement of the dose configuration. Dose distributions in this method conform to the shape of the target volume and sculpt around adjacent critical structures.[62]

### Stereotactic radiosurgery

Stereotactic radiosurgery (SRS) uses an imaging-compatible stereotactic device to precisely localize an intracranial target and provides a high radiation dose in a single session without delivering significant radiation to the surrounding normal brain tissue. This technique is performed using a modified linear accelerator or gamma knife unit. A noninvasive, single-day procedure, SRS is usually performed in an outpatient setting. It was initially used for small arteriovenous malformations (AVMs), benign brain tumors, and brain metastases. Malignant tumors were not considered appropriate for SRS because of their invasiveness and large size. However, the use of SRS in the treatment of primary and recurrent malignant brain tumors has increased. Shrieve and associates reported on a group of individuals with recurrent GBM treated with SRS.[137] The median survival was 10.2 months, with a 19% two-year survival. The American Society for Therapeutic Radiology and Oncology (ASTRO) conducted an evidence-based review of the role of radiosurgery for malignant gliomas, and reported that radiosurgery does not have added benefit to external beam radiotherapy along in terms of overall survival, local brain control, or quality of life.[142] Unfortunately, the majority of individuals with malignant gliomas are not eligible for this type of therapy because of the size or shape of their tumors. Tumors larger than 4 cm cannot be treated with SRS, for example. Patients with previously irradiated small lesions have been safely treated with SRS.[143]

### Stereotactic radiotherapy

Stereotactic radiotherapy uses the planning technology and precision of SRS but delivers the treatment using standard fraction ation doses, combining the focal advantages of SRS with the radiobiological advantage of fractionation.[62] SRS hardware, software, and head frames can be relocalized daily in a nontraumatic and reproducible fashion. Standard fractionation avoids the toxicities associated with large single doses, and tumors located near critical structures may be more successfully treated with the precision of the stereotactic technique. This approach is being used for some benign tumors and gliomas.

### Interstitial brachytherapy

Brachytherapy involves the temporary high-activity or permanent low-activity implantation of radioactive sources directly into the brain tumor. Traditionally, catheters are placed into the tumor using stereotactic surgical techniques, and the radiation seeds or pellets are then inserted in the catheters. The implants are removed either after a few days or several months, or are left in permanently, depending on the source used. Iodine-125 ($^{125}I$) and iridium-192 ($^{192}I$) are the most commonly used sources for both temporary and permanent implants. Newer delivery techniques include the development of an inflatable balloon which is filled with liquid radioisotopes and the use of radioimmunotherapy.[144] The technique is limited in that it is estimated that only 30% of patients are eligible for the technique which requires a surgically accessible lesion.[144]

Initial single institution studies reported promising results; however, two prospective randomized studies evaluating traditional bracytherapy for treatment of malignant gliomas failed to show a survival advantage.[145,146] The impact of newer techniques is still being explored.

## Brain metastases

Treatment for patients with brain metastases is determined by number of metastases, location of metastases, status of systemic disease, and patient functional status. The objectives of surgery may include obtaining a tissue diagnosis, removal of mass effect, resolution of edema, definitative therapy for local lesions, and improvement in overall survival when combined with radiation therapy.[105] Radiation is standard treatment for metastatic brain tumors, employing either WBRT, radiosurgery or hypofractionated stereotactic radiosurgery.[147] These individuals and those with multiple metastases typically undergoWBRT. Patients who undergo surgery may receive postoperative WBRT. Studies reported a prolonged survival in which patients who received postoperative WBRT maintained a higher performance status and had fewer intracranial recurrences.[107,142] Traditionally WBRT has been preferred over partial-field RT because multiple metastases may be present even if some are too small to be detected on imaging studies. Typical radiation treatment schedules for metastatic brain tumors consist of a total dose of 30 Gy delivered over 10 fractions.[105] Lower daily fractions and a more protracted course may be indicated in individuals with a better prognosis.[42] As with primary tumors, response rates vary with the histological characteristics of the primary tumor. For example, metastases from breast and small cell lung cancers respond better to RT than do metastases from melanoma, renal, or colon cancers.[32,42]

The use of prophylactic cranial irradiation (PCI) has been investigated for patients at high risk of developing brain metastases, such as those with small cell lung cancer (SCLC). Meta-analyses have shown that use of PCI results in a statistically significant increase in overall survival (5%-6%) over 3 years, leading to this being the standard of care for patients with SCLC.[148,149]

Many metastatic brain lesions are now being treated with SRS. Unlike with surgery, few lesions are inaccessible to SRS because of their location in the brain. Because metastatic tumors are generally small in size and tend not to invade adjacent brain tissue, the individual with brain metastases is an ideal candidate for radiosurgery. Factors favoring surgery over SRS include the need for tissue diagnosis, uncontrolled primary disease, uncontrolled or progressing nonbrain metastases, tumors larger than 3 cm, tumors associated with significant mass effect and neurological symptoms, steroid-dependence, and presence of an intratumoral bleed.[105] Median survival for patients with brain metastases treated with SRS has generally been reported at 7 to 10 months, although Young and colleagues found more than 30% of patients surviving beyond one year and 15% to 20% beyond two years.[150] SRS may be used alone, may be used with WBRT, or may be used to treat recurrent or new metastases after prior WBRT or SRS.[142] An exact algorithm on whether to use SRS alone or inconjunction with WBRT does not exist, and multiple factors (as discussed previously) must be considered.[105] The disadvantages of radiosurgery relate to its high cost, increased risk of radiation necrosis, and failure to control micrometastases elsewhere in the brain.[150,151]

## Side effects

Side effects of RT can be classified as acute, subacute, or delayed. Acute reactions occur during the course of treatment and are temporary. They are manifested as signs of increased ICP or worsening of neurological deficits. These effects result from an increase in cerebral edema; the administration of corticosteroids usually decreases or alleviates symptoms. Steroids are generally administered during the initiation of therapy and can often be tapered to a lower dose or discontinued as therapy progresses. Fatigue is a common occurrence. Other acute adverse effects include nausea, vomiting, anorexia, alopecia, and skin irritation. Alopecia lasting several months occurs after 54 Gy; it may be permanent after 60 Gy or in the area of boost. Acute reactions have been reported to occur in one-third of patients undergoing stereotactic radiosurgery and include headaches, nausea, vomiting, dizziness and vertigo (more commonly with acoustic neuromas), worsening neurological deficit, and seizures.[152]

Subacute reactions generally develop 1 to 3 months after completion of therapy. These, too, are of a temporary nature. Symptoms include anorexia, sleepiness, lethargy, and an increase in neurological deficits. Delayed effects of RT usually occur 6 to 24 months after completion of treatment. These effects are irreversible and often progressive. They result from direct injury to brain tissue and blood vessels. Leukoencephalopathy—that is, degeneration of the white matter—occurs at the tumor site and surrounding irradiated brain. The risk of developing leukoencephalopathy increases with a higher total dose, higher dose per fraction, and concomitant use of neurotoxic chemotherapeutic agents, particularly methotrexate. The clinical manifestations range from mild cognitive neurological impairment to dementia to death. The onset and progression can be quite variable. Radiation necrosis occurs more commonly after brachytherapy and radiosurgery but can occur after conventional RT as well. Individuals at increased risk for long-term radiation effects include children younger than age 2 and adults older than 60. Long-term effects can be initially managed to some degree with corticosteroids and surgery to remove necrotic tissue. Other long-term effects include loss of vision, development of secondary malignancies, and endocrine disturbances. The major complication of both brachytherapy and radiosurgery is the development of symptomatic radiation necrosis requiring prolonged administration of steroids and reoperation. The rate of reoperation is 30% to 40%, usually within 6 months.

### Nursing care

Nursing management of the individual receiving RT includes neurological assessment and evaluation of side effects, and patient and family education regarding treatment schedules, routines, possible side effects, and management of these effects. Additional interventions focus on the specific irradiation method used. The most common method, conventional external beam, is usually administered on an outpatient basis. Assistance may be necessary for transportation arrangements. Most patients will be on steroids to reduce the cerebral edema that occurs during brain irradiation. Education is necessary regarding these agents' many adverse effects. Brain irradiation causes the skin to become dry and peel, and moist desquamation may occur, most often behind the ears.[153] Individuals should be instructed on appropriate skin care, avoidance of over the counter creams containing perfumes, and they must avoid sun exposure. Extreme fatigue occurs during and after treatment, and patients require support and encouragement to manage this distressing symptom. Standard approaches to the management of fatigue should be undertaken, including the use of frequent rest periods and planned activities. Use of adjunctive agents, such as psychostimulants has not shown to be of benefit during radiation therapy.[154]

## CHEMOTHERAPY

Chemotherapy plays an important adjuvant role in the treatment of adult primary brain tumors. The most widely studied group of tumors has been the malignant glioma because it is the most common adult primary brain tumor and accounts for the majority of deaths in individuals with brain tumors. Many studies have evaluated a variety of single chemotherapeutic agents and multiple-drug regimens. BCNU; the combination of procarbazine, procarbazine, and vincristine (PCV); and the most recently approved agent, temozolomide,[54] remain the most commonly used agents for both newly diagnosed and recurrent malignant gliomas.

The delivery of adequate concentrations of intravenous chemotherapy to tumors within the CNS is limited by the presence of the BBB. The BBB is made of a continuous lining of endothelial cells that are connected by tight junctions.[32] Large, water-soluble, charged particles and compounds bound to plasma proteins are unable to penetrate the BBB. This vascular barrier normally protects the brain by limiting the entry of potentially toxic substances into brain tissue. Unfortunately, it also prevents the majority of chemotherapeutic agents from entering brain tissue.

Although the BBB can be a potential obstacle to the delivery of chemotherapy, the most malignant brain tumors are often associated with marked BBB disruption. Water-soluble contrast agents administered with CT or MRI are able to cross the normally impermeable BBB and enter the brain in the region of the tumor. The surrounding normal brain, however, continues to exclude the contrast material because its BBB remains intact. Thus, the enhancing masses seen on CT and MRI represent regions of tumor with a substantially disrupted BBB. Malignant cells, however, often infiltrate adjacent tissue and spread to distant sites. Contrast enhancement usually does not occur in the surrounding normal brain that typically contains micrometastatic disease.[140] The BBB is, therefore, at least partially intact in many brain tumors, particularly in the periphery of the tumor and around infiltrating tumor cells.

After years of study and many trials, alkylating agents such as temozolomide and nitrosoureas (BCNU and CCNU, which is often given in combination with procarbazine and vincristine) have been shown to be the most effective agents for the treatment of malignant gliomas. The nitrosoureas (BCNU and CCNU) cause delayed and cumulative myelosuppression, pulmonary fibrosis, nausea, vomiting and, during administration of BCNU, facial flushing and pain and burning along the IV site. Side effects of procarbazine include rash, myelosuppression, encephalopathy, peripheral neuropathy, hepatotoxicity, and hypertensive crisis with consumption of foods containing tyramine. Side effects of vincristine include peripheral neuropathies, constipation, myelosuppression, alopecia, nausea, and vomiting. Temozolomide, an oral alkylating agent, has mild toxicities including nausea, vomiting, and noncumulative myelosuppression, making this agent an attractive alternative for glioma treatment.

Recently, the use of irinotecan and bevacizumab has been reported to result in tumor shrinkage and improved time to progression for patients with GBM.[155] This treatment is currently undergoing further validation. Other agents that have been shown to have some activity include carboplatin, etopisode, and tamoxifen. Anaplastic oligodendrogliomas have been found to be chemosensitive tumors. The PCV combination has been the most widely studied regimen for these tumors, and positive results have been obtained in both newly diagnosed and recurrent tumors. This regimen is now standard therapy.[156] Mixed gliomas[157,158] and nonanaplastic oligodendrogliomas[159] also appear to respond to these agents. In the clinical setting, temozolomide is often prescribed as a consequence of improved tolerability.[140]

Chemotherapy has not been considered to have a major role in the treatment of brain metastases. There are a paucity of randomized trials exploring this issue.[147] However, studies have been completed showing minimal response in patients with brain metastases from SCLC and germ cell tumors.[160,161] As a consequence, chemotherapy treatment may be given as initial treatment in these patients or adjuvantly with radiation therapy.[147] Response has also been reported in other tumors types, including non-small cell lung cancer (NSCLC and breast cancer. However, radiation therapy remains the standard treatment approach for these and other metastases.

New approaches have been explored in an attempt to increase the efficacy of the currently available chemotherapeutic agents. These options include gene therapy and targeted therapies including antiangiogenic and small molecules.[74]

### Interstitial

Interstitial chemotherapy—the use of biodegradable polymers impregnated with chemotherapeutic agents—is a promising approach in chemotherapy delivery for brain tumors. These polymers are placed intraoperatively in the walls of the tumor cavity after resection and continuously release high local concentrations of chemotherapeutic agents. Chemotherapy delivered directly to the tumor bypasses the variably disrupted BBB, results in high local drug concentrations, and minimizes systemic toxicity. Implantation of BCNU wafers was found to prolong median survival in patients with recurrent high-grade gliomas.[162–165] This route of administration may facilitate the use of new and established chemotherapeutic agents that previously could not be efficiently, safely, or effectively delivered to the brain.

## BIOTHERAPY

To date, biotherapy has had little success in the treatment of malignant brain tumors, but is increasingly the focus of research. Methods investigated include the use of targeted molecular therapies and antiangiogenic agents.[5]

### Targeted molecular therapies

The primary targeted agents currently under investigation include the receptor tyrosine kinases such as PDGFR, VEGFR, and EGFR, in addition to signal-transduction inhibitors including farnesyltransferase, P13K, and mTOR.[5,166–169] Use of single agents has had modest response and no prolongation of 6-month progression free survival.[170,171] This is theorized to result from the fact that malignant gliomas have coactivation as well as redundancy in signaling pathways. Targeting one pathway is therefore ineffective. Current experimental strategies include identifying molecular features of the individual tumor and selecting agents which target these pathways, administration of multiple targeting agents, and adding targeted agents combined with radiation therapy and chemotherapy.

### Antiangiogenesis

Angiogenesis is the growth of new blood vessels. Tumor growth is dependent on the development of a new vascular supply, and endothelial proliferation is a characteristic feature of astrocytomas. Malignant gliomas are among the most vascular of all tumors. The inhibition of tumor-associated new-vessel growth (antiangiogenesis) could retard tumor growth and become a potentially useful treatment modality. Clinical trials report improved response rates when patients are treated with bevacizumab and irinotecan[155,172,173]. As a consequence, there is increased focus on the use of bevacizumab and other antiangiogenic agents in the newly diagnosed and recurrent setting. Recently, it has been identified that some of the decrease in enhancement seen on MRI may be a consequence of a decrease in VEGF. In addition, a change in the pattern of progression, from an enlarging enhancing mass, to a more infiltrative pattern has been identified.[155,172,173] The implications for evaluation of response and impact on long term outcome are still to be determined.

### Nursing care

Nursing management of the individual receiving chemotherapy and biotherapy depends on the method of chemotherapy administration and the specific agents used. It includes assessment and evaluation of side effects; patient and family education regarding treatment schedules, routines, and possible side effects; and interventions to enhance tolerance and maintain functional ability. The use of targeted molecular therapy and antiangiogenic agents has led to additional side effects, such as rash, hypertension, and pancreatitis, that were not previously seen with standard treatment approaches. In addition, alterations in the appearance of tumor on standard imaging have changed response criteria. Understanding the potential side effects and impact on follow-up is a key part of nursing care of the patient receiving investigational agents.

# SPINAL CORD TUMORS

## EPIDEMIOLOGY

Primary spinal cord tumors occur less frequently than primary brain tumors, accounting for only 4% of all primary

CNS tumors.[2] Approximately 2700 of these tumors are diagnosed each year. They occur most often in individuals aged 20 to 60 years. With the exception of meningiomas, which occur more often in women, spinal cord tumors are found with equal frequency in men and women. Metastatic tumors are much more common than primary spinal cord tumors, reportedly afflicting 5% to 10% of individuals with systemic cancer.

## ETIOLOGY

The etiology of the majority of primary spinal cord tumors is unknown. Individuals with NF-1 may develop neurofibromas and astrocytomas of the spinal cord.[174] Spinal nerve root tumors (schwannomas) and ependymomas may be present in patients with NF-2, and individuals with von Hippel-Lindau disease are at risk for developing spinal hemangioblastomas.[174]

## PATHOPHYSIOLOGY

### ANATOMY AND PHYSIOLOGY

The spine is a flexible column formed by a series of vertebrae, each stacked one upon another to support the head and trunk. The vertebral column shown in Figure 49-8 consists of 33 vertebrae: 7 cervical, 12 thoracic, 5 lumbar, 5 sacral, and 4 coccygeal. The five sacral vertebrae fuse to form the sacrum, and the four coccygeal vertebrae fuse to form the coccyx.

The spinal cord, housed within the vertebral column, is an elongated mass of nerve tissue less than 1 inch in diameter and approximately 17 to 18 inches in length. It arises from the medulla oblongata, beginning at the top of the first cervical vertebra, and extends down to the lower border of the first lumbar vertebra, where it ends in a tapered, conelike structure called the *conus medullaris*. The spinal cord is about 10 inches shorter than the vertebral column, and the lower segments of the spinal cord, therefore, are not aligned opposite corresponding vertebrae. Thus, the lumbar and sacral spinal nerves have very long roots. These roots descend in a bundle from the conus, and because of its resemblance to the tail of a horse, this formation is called the *cauda equina*.[175]

There are 31 pairs of spinal nerves exiting from the spinal cord through the intervertebral foramina: 8 cervical, 12 thoracic, 5 lumbar, 5 sacral, and 1 coccygeal. The intervertebral foramina are narrow, and the nerves may easily be compressed at this site by a protruding disk or arthritic spurring. Each spinal nerve has a dorsal root by which afferent (sensory) impulses enter the cord and a ventral root by which efferent (motor) impulses leave the spinal cord. The dorsal roots convey sensory input from skin segments that

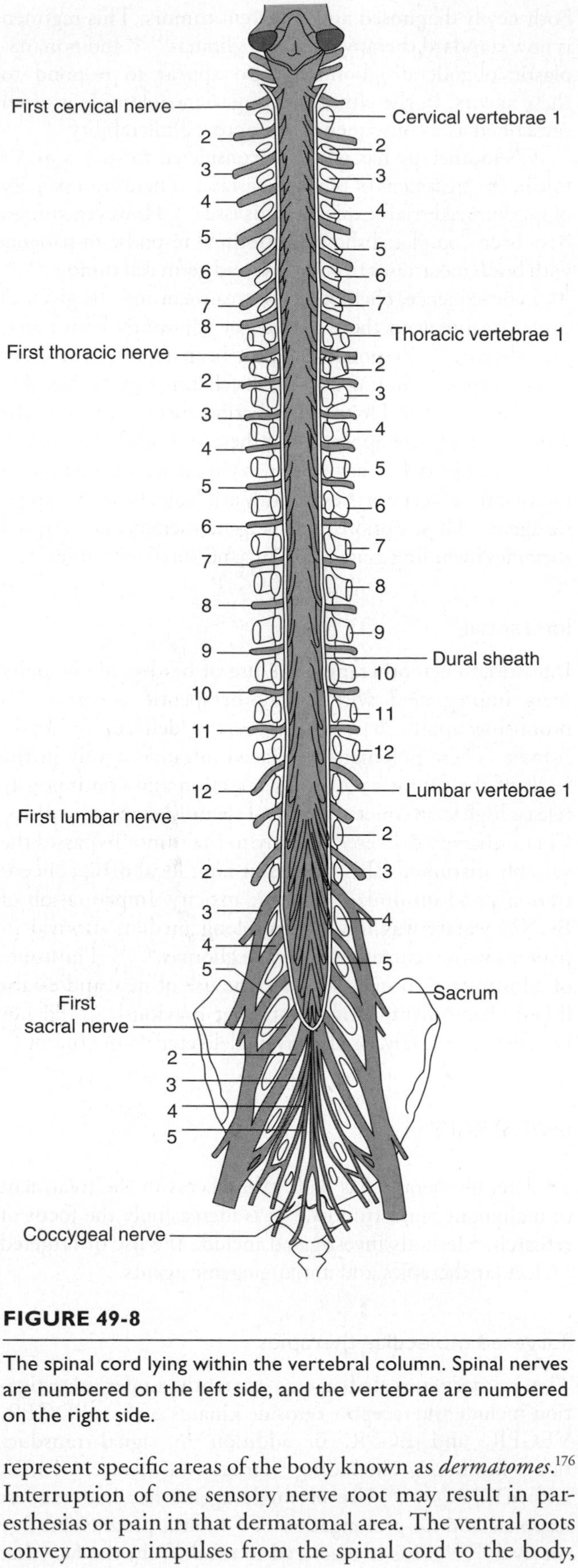


**FIGURE 49-8**

The spinal cord lying within the vertebral column. Spinal nerves are numbered on the left side, and the vertebrae are numbered on the right side.

represent specific areas of the body known as *dermatomes*.[176] Interruption of one sensory nerve root may result in paresthesias or pain in that dermatomal area. The ventral roots convey motor impulses from the spinal cord to the body,

**TABLE 49-3**

**Motor Nerve Roots (Myotomes) and Areas They Innervate Spinal Cord**

| Segment | Muscle Action |
|---|---|
| C-1 to C-4 | Flexion, lateral flexion, extension, and rotation of neck |
| C-3 to C-5 | Diaphagm (inspiration); elevation of upper thorax and scapula |
| C-5 to C-6 | Shoulder movement; flexion of elbow |
| C-5 to C-7 | Forward thrust of shoulder |
| C-5 to C-8 | Adduction of arm from front to back |
| C-6 to C-8 | Extension of forearm and wrist |
| C-6 to T-1 | Thumb and index finger (C-6), middle finger (C-7), ring finger (C-8), and pinky finger (T-1) |
| C-7 to T-1 | Flexion of wrist |
| T-1 to T-12 | Control of thoracic, abdominal, and back muscles |
| L-1 to L-3 | Flexion of hip |
| L-2 to L-4 | Extension of leg; adduction of thigh |
| L-4 to S-2 | Flexion, abduction, and rotation of thigh; flexion of lower leg; extension, flexing, and spreading of toes |
| L-4 to L-5 | Dorsal flexion of foot |
| L-5 to S-2 | Plantar flexion of foot |
| S-2 to S-4 | Perinum and sphincters |

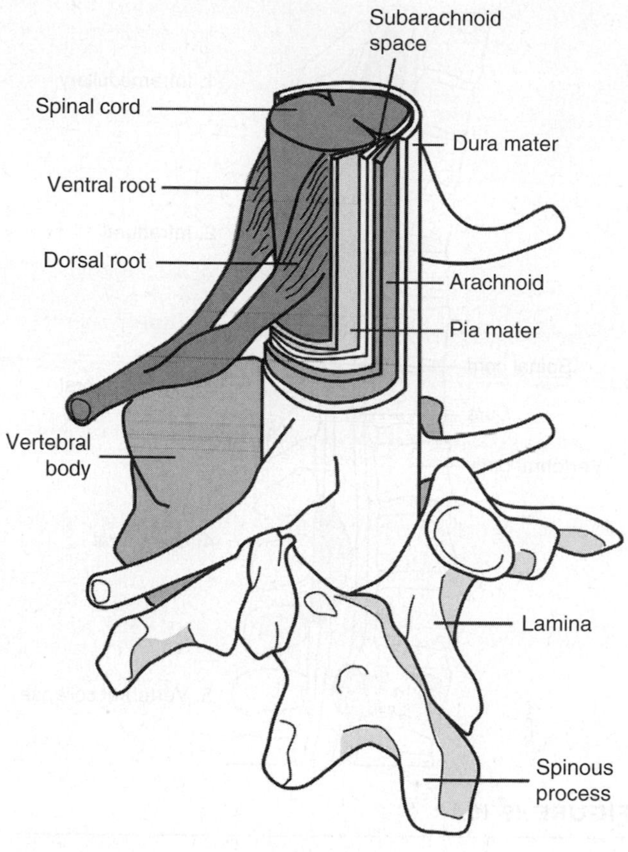


**FIGURE 49-9**

Spinal meninges.

innervating specific areas of muscle groups called *myotomes* (Table 49-3).

The cranial meninges are contiguous within the spinal canal to support and protect the spinal cord. The spinal dura is a continuation of the inner layer of the cerebral dura. The outer dural layer ends at the foramen magnum, being replaced by the periosteal lining of the vertebral canal. The spinal dura encloses the spinal nerves and terminates at the level of the sacrum. The arachnoid layer of the spinal meninges is a continuation of the cerebral arachnoid. The pia mater in the spinal cord is thicker, firmer, and less vascular than that of the brain.[33] The spinal meninges are illustrated in Figure 49-9.

A cross section of the spinal cord shows that it is arranged as a butterfly-shaped area of gray matter surrounded by white matter. The gray matter consists of cell bodies, axon, and dendrites. The white matter consists of longitudinally running fiber tracts. The white matter in each half of the cord is divided into columns. These columns are further divided into tracts, which are the sensory and motor pathways of the spinal cord. Impulses are conducted up the spinal cord via ascending tracts (sensory) to the brain, and the descending tracts conduct impulses from the brain down to the spinal cord (motor). The specific motor and sensory symptoms seen in spinal cord tumors depend on the tumor's involvement of these specific tracts. Knowledge of the specific level of involvement is helpful in understanding the signs and symptoms in relation to the specific dermatomes and myotomes involved.

Tumors are often classified by the cell of original and location in relation to the spinal cord and dura (Figure 49-10). Extradural tumors are located outside of the spinal cord, intradural-extramedullary tumors are within the dura but not within the body of the spinal cord, and intramedullary tumors occur within the spinal cord.[177]

## EXTRADURAL TUMORS

Extradural tumors lie outside the dura and are the most common spinal tumor, accounting for 60% of all cases. Most of these tumors are caused by metastatic cancer to the vertebral column, a common site of bone metastasis. Epidural metastatic tumor causing spinal cord compression is a common complication of cancer and should be considered a neurologic emergency. Often the degree of deficits and recovery are better if the tumor is found early.

Metastases can occur in multiple contiguous vertebrae and in multiple sites of the vertebral column. Metastatic

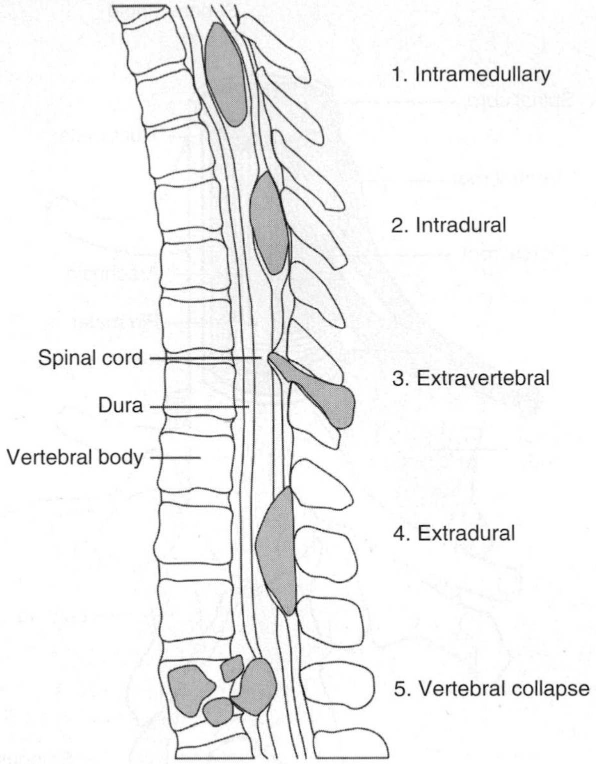


**FIGURE 49-10**

Anatomical location of spinal cord

spinal cord tumors most often originate from cancers of the breast, lung, prostate, and kidney and from multiple myeloma.[178] Less common are cancers of the GI tract, thyroid, lymphoma, sarcoma ,and melanoma. The neurological symptoms seen with extradural tumors often result from compression rather than invasion of the spinal cord. The spinal cord is usually compressed anteriorly, which leads to edema and ischemia of the spinal cord and mechanically distorts and damages the nervous tissue. Spinal cord compression (SCC) occurs either by direct extension of the tumor into the epidural space, by vertebral collapse and displacement of bone into the epidural space, or by direct extension through the intervertebral foramina. The thoracic spine is the most frequent location of epidural SCC (70% of cases), followed by the lumbosacral (20%) and cervical spine (10%).[179] In 30% of cases, multiple levels are involved. Lung and breast cancer most often cause thoracic compression, whereas prostate, renal, and GI tumors are more likely to affect the lower thoracic or lumbosacral vertebrae.

Lymphomas may be a cause of SCC because they can extend directly through the intervertebral foramina. Other tumors such as sarcoma and chordoma may arise as primary extradural tumors. The chordoma is a slow-growing but highly invasive tumor. It often occurs in the sacrum but can also be found in the cervical spine and intracranially at the base of the skull. This tumor erodes bone and soft tissue extensively; even though it is histologically benign, it is difficult to remove in its entirety.

## INTRADURAL TUMORS

Intradural tumors arise from the nerve roots or coverings of the spinal cord (intradural, extramedullary) or develop in the spinal cord itself (intradural, intramedullary). Intradural, extramedullary tumors account for almost 90% of primary spinal cord tumors and 30% of all spine tumors, with meningiomas and nerve sheath tumors (neurofibromas and schwannomas) being the most common.[177] Schwannomas are often located in the lumbar spine on one of the many nerve roots of the cauda equina. Meningiomas commonly arise in the thoracic spine (80% of cases). Both spinal schwannomas and meningiomas can often be completely removed by surgery, and recurrence is rare with complete resection. Sarcomas can also arise as extramedullary tumors. Other less common intradural extramedullary tumors are vascular tumors, chordomas, and epidermoids.[41]

Intradural, intramedullary tumors arise from the same cell as their intracranial counterparts; however, the grade of malignancy is often lower, making the majority of primary spinal cord tumors benign. The majority of intramedullary tumors are ependymomas (60%),[180] followed by astrocytomas (30%).[177,181] Less common histologies include hemangioblastomas and various hemangiomas, oligodendrogliomas, gangliogliomas, and medulloblastomas.[41] Most ependymomas are located in the lumbosacral area. Treatment usually includes maximal surgical resection and RT if incomplete resection or higher grade tumor. Ependymomas that involve the CSF are treated with craniospinal RT. Chemotherapy is usually reserved for recurrent tumors.[180] Astrocytomas are more commonly located in the cervical and thoracic spinal cord. As treatment for them, surgical resection is often attempted followed by RT. As many as 20% of spinal cord astrocytomas are malignant; such high-grade tumors are generally treated only with RT. Hemangioblastomas are vascular tumors evenly distributed throughout the spinal cord except for those associated with von Hippel-Lindau syndrome, in which they are predominantly located in the cervical cord.

## PATTERN OF SPREAD

The most common mechanism of spread for extradural spinal metastases is thought to involve hematogenous arterial spread. A second mechanism is direct invasion through the intervertebral foramina by a paravertebral mass. Another possible mechanism of metastatic epidural spinal cord metastases is retrograde venous spread from the primary site by way of Batson's plexus.[178] Intradural, intramedullary metastases may occur through CSF pathways. In contrast, primary spinal cord tumors rarely metastasize outside the CNS.

## CLINICAL MANIFESTATIONS

The clinical manifestations associated with spinal cord tumors result from compression and, much less frequently, invasion of the spinal cord. Extramedullary tumors affect the cord by compression, causing traction on or irritation of the spinal nerve roots, displacement of the spinal cord itself, interference with the spinal blood supply, or obstruction of CSF circulation.[182] Intramedullary tumors invade and destroy the spinal cord itself. When spinal cord compression occurs, the normal physiology involved in providing an adequate blood supply, maintaining stable cellular membranes, and facilitating afferent and efferent impulses for specific sensory, motor, and reflex functions of the spinal cord and related spinal nerves is altered.[183] Edema results, causing additional deficits.

The clinical manifestations seen with spinal cord tumors depend on the tumor's rate of growth and the level of the spinal cord affected. Symptom duration prior to diagnosis is often in the range of 3 to 4 years for primary spinal cord tumors.[184] A slow-growing, benign tumor better allows the cord to accommodate the mass. Tumors can compress the cord into a thin, ribbonlike structure without causing significant neurological deficits. By contrast, the spinal cord cannot accommodate a sudden mass or rapidly growing lesion such as a hematoma or a metastatic tumor. It has little ability to compensate for such lesions, which increase pressure and create extensive edema causing sudden neurological dysfunction. The signs and symptoms of spinal cord tumors include pain, motor weakness, sensory impairment, and autonomic dysfunction involving bowel and bladder function.

Pain is the most common presenting symptom of a spinal cord tumor. In epidural metastases, back or neck pain may be present for weeks or months, and intradural tumors can cause pain for years before the correct diagnosis is established. Often the pain is initially dismissed as arthritis, back strain, or disc disease, and until other more obvious neurological manifestations appear, the diagnosis of a spinal cord tumor is usually not considered. Back or neck pain in cancer patients, especially those with tumor types that commonly metastasize to bone, should be evaluated for spinal metastases.

The pain may be localized or radicular. Localized pain and tenderness are common over the involved area, particularly with epidural metastases. Radicular pain may be described as bandlike and follows the distribution of the spinal nerve roots (dermatomes). The pain can vary from mild to severe and from dull to sharp or burning, and almost always becomes more severe with time. Pain may be worse at night; a recumbent position often aggravates it. Pain that is aggravated by movement and relieved with immobility may indicate spinal instability. Activities that produce a valsalva maneuver, such as sneezing, coughing, and straining, increase the spinal pressure and cause intensification of pain.

Weakness is the most readily identified objective finding and may follow the appearance of sensory symptoms. It is reported to occur in 35% to 75% of patients.[182] The level of impairment determines the muscle groups involved (myotomes). The weakness is often associated with hyperreflexia, spasticity, and a positive Babinski sign. It will eventually progress to complete paraplegia unless treatment is initiated. Fifty percent to 68% of patients are unable to walk when they are first diagnosed with epidural spinal cord compression.[182,185] Specific motor symptoms will vary depending on where the tumor is located on a cross section of the spinal cord. A lateral tumor will affect voluntary movement in the arms and legs, muscle tone, coordination, and posture. Tumors in the anterior cord will affect voluntary movement of the trunk muscles, equilibrium, and posture.

Sensory deficits are reported to occur in 50% to 70% of patients at diagnosis, and 60% have bowel and bladder symptoms. Specific sensory deficits will depend on where the tumor is located on a cross section of the spinal cord. A lateral tumor will affect pain and temperature, causing symptoms of coldness, numbness, and tingling. Awareness of vibration and proprioception of body parts are affected if the posterior aspect is involved. Touch and pressure on the opposite side of the body will be affected if the tumor is anterior. Compression affects function below the lesion; therefore, it is important to determine the highest functional level. A sensory assessment begins at the toes and moves upward to determine the level at which function remains, which is generally the level of the tumor. However, there may be a discrepancy between the level of remaining function and apparent tumor location. The lesion may be one or two vertebrae above the level of compression. A narrow band of hyperesthesia directly above often accompanies the tumor level.[183]

The effects may be symmetrical and bilateral, asymmetrical, and even unilateral. A combination of sensory and motor deficits may also be seen. A loss of touch, vibration, position sense, and motor ability on the same side as the lesion with contralateral loss of pain and temperature is called the Brown–Séquard syndrome. This syndrome occurs in approximately 20% of patients with spinal cord tumors.[41]

## ASSESSMENT

Assessment of the individual with a known or suspected spinal cord tumor begins by obtaining a history. The description and duration of symptoms, the presence of exacerbating or relieving factors, and the order of their appearance must be established. A neurological examination, especially of motor and sensory function, gait, and reflexes, is performed. In addition, the possible presence of bowel or bladder dysfunction must be established, and a pain assessment is performed. This initial assessment provides a baseline from which all future assessments will be compared. This neurological assessment should attempt to determine where the tumor is likely to be located (cervical, thoracic, or lumbar).

### DIAGNOSTIC STUDIES

The diagnostic procedure of choice for the evaluation of both intramedullary and extramedullary spinal cord tumors is MRI performed with and without contrast. It provides superb anatomical detail of the spinal cord, is noninvasive, and carries fewer risks than myelography. Use of contrast is standard when evaluating spinal cord tumors, as the majority of intramedullary tumors demonstrate enhancement despite the histologic grade.[177] MRI is also helpful for planning radiation therapy and surgery.

Computed tomography myelography may be performed if there is concern of CSF involvement or a block of CSF flow. In CT myelography, contrast medium is injected into the subarachnoid space, usually by means of a lumbar puncture, and CT images of the spinal cord and vertebral column are taken to determine whether a partial or a complete obstruction is present. After a CT myelogram has been performed, the individual must be assessed for any neurological changes and positioned appropriately (usually supine, with the head of the bed elevated at a prescribed level). Possible complications include allergic reaction to the contrast agent, meningeal irritation, headache, nausea, vomiting, infection, and seizure.

Spine x-rays may be performed in individuals suspected of epidural metastases. It is estimated, however, that 30% to 50% of the vertebral body must be destroyed before changes are seen on a plain radiograph.[42] Bone scans are sensitive in identifying vertebral disease, but they are not always specific and may identify pathology other than cancer.

### PROGNOSTIC INDICATORS

The majority of extradural spinal tumors result from metastatic disease, which generally carries a poorer prognosis because of the more advanced stage of disease. Many patients with metastases survive 3 to 6 months.[186] Factors associated with improved survival include the ability to walk before and after treatment, radiosensitive tumor histologies, no visceral or brain metastases, and a single site of cord compression.[186]

The severity of weakness is the most significant prognostic factor for neurological recovery. Eighty percent of those patients who are ambulatory at the time of diagnosis remain so after treatment. As the neurological dysfunction increases, the likelihood of recovery diminishes. Only 30% to 45% of patients who are initially paraparetic and nonambulatory become ambulatory, and those who are paraplegic at diagnosis are likely to remain so, with only 5% regaining the ability to walk. The second most common factor is the rapidity that symptoms develop, with those who develop deficits slowly having a higher likelihood of recovery.

Favorable prognostic factors for intradural tumors include extent of surgical resection, histological grade, performance status, age, and, as in extradural tumors, slow onset of neurological dysfunction. Schwannomas, meningiomas, and ependymomas have a low recurrence rate if completely resected. The same cannot be said for astrocytomas, where the available literature has failed to demonstrate a significant correlation between prognosis and degree of surgical resection.[187,188] A patient's preoperative level of neurological function is the strongest prognostic indicator of postoperative functional outcome.

## CLASSIFICATION AND STAGING

Primary spinal tumors are classified by their cell of origin and their anatomical location. The types of spinal cord tumors are similar to those tumors found in the brain. Histologically, however, they tend to be less malignant. The major anatomical consideration with spinal cord tumors relates to the tumor's location in relation to the spinal dura mater, as described previously.

## THERAPEUTIC APPROACHES AND NURSING CARE

### SURGERY

The first line of treatment, prior to surgery, for most patients is the use of corticosteroids, which is discussed in the section on chemotherapy. In the treatment of spinal cord tumors, the goals of surgery include provision of a diagnosis and partial or complete removal of the tumor. For most intradural, extramedullary tumors, surgery is the primary treatment. Schwannomas and meningiomas can often be completely resected with modern microsurgical techniques and neurosurgical instruments. As in brain tumor surgery, intraoperative monitoring assists the surgeon in maximizing the resection while protecting the spinal cord. In most cases, these tumors can be removed through a posterior (laminectomy) approach. The risk of recurrence is estimated at 10% for complete resections, while recurrence rates increase to 20% for incompletely resected tumors.[185,186] When possible, recurrences are generally treated with repeat surgical resection.

Surgery is the initial treatment for intramedullary tumors (ependymomas and astrocytomas) with the exception of the malignant astrocytomas. The determining factor in the successful surgical treatment of these tumors is the degree of tumor infiltration of the surrounding spinal cord. As with intracranial glial tumors, indistinct tumor margins and microscopic infiltration can prevent complete tumor removal. Attempts at complete removal often risk loss of neurological function. Astrocytomas are less clearly demarcated from the surrounding spinal cord tissue than ependymomas. Some astrocytomas are treated with biopsy only, followed by RT. For well-delineated astrocytomas, surgical removal can provide long-term tumor control, and sometimes, cure. Ependymomas of the spinal cord have a longer natural history than astrocytomas. Recurrence of ependymomas may be delayed up to 12 years, whereas astrocytomas that recur generally do so within 3 years.[177,189]

A randomized trial showed improved ambulatory status and overall survival for patients with extradural tumors who underwent direct decompressive surgery and postoperative radiation therapy as compared to those who received radiation alone.[190] Surgery is also indicated in cases where the cause of SCC is unknown, there is spinal instability or bone collapse into the spinal canal, a recurrence cannot be retreated with additional RT, the tumor is known to be radioresistant, or the individual is rapidly deteriorating neurologically, perhaps during the course of RT. Complications related to surgical intervention include the standard surgical risks as well as the development of neurological deficits, CSF leak, and wound dehiscence. The individual with significant or long-standing preoperative neurological deficits is likely to show no improvement or even progression after surgery. The most significant complication requiring treatment is a new neurological deficit in which the neurological function often may not return. The onset of a new deficit is typically related to vascular insult of or manipulation of the spinal cord during surgery.[189] A CSF leak may develop because the dura is not completely sealed or a tear was not repaired. Such a leak is usually treated with lumbar drainage for several days. If the leakage continues, surgery may be required to repair it.

## RADIATION THERAPY

Radiation therapy is generally not recommended for completely resected intradural low-grade (intramedullary and extramedullary) spinal cord tumors. Both intramedullary and extramedullary tumors may be treated with RT if incompletely resected or on recurrence if repeat surgical resection is not feasible. Doses of 50 to 55 Gy are generally used.[186,189] Ependymomas are radiosensitive tumors. In patients with ependymomas who received adjuvant RT, 5- and 10-year survival rates are 60% to 100% and 68% to 95%, respectively.[82] The 5- and 10-year survival rates for low-grade astrocytomas who received RT are 60% to 90% and 40% to 90% respectively.[188] For individuals with high-grade astrocytomas, RT is the standard treatment approach; even with RT, the prognosis is poor. Survival in such cases is 6 to 8 months.[189]

Radiation therapy and steroids are the most widely used therapies for extradural tumors. The usual dose of radiation administered is 30 Gy in 300 cGy fractions.[42,186] Often, higher doses are administered for the initial treatments, especially if evidence of neurological dysfunction is present.

Spinal RT does not cause acute clinical symptoms. The major complication of spinal cord radiation—radiation myelopathy—results from demyelination and white matter necrosis or intramedullary microvascular injury. Radiation myelopathy may present as a subacute or more severe delayed reaction. A transient subacute myelopathy is clinically manifested by momentary electrical shock-like paresthesias or numbness radiating from the neck down to the extremities, and it is precipitated by flexing the neck (Lhermitte's sign). This syndrome develops after an average of 3 to 4 months following treatment and resolves within 3 to 6 months without the need for intervention.[41]

The more severe delayed radiation myelopathy generally occurs 12 to 28 months following RT, but can take up to 4 years to appear. The clinical manifestations are irreversible; they begin with weakness and can progress to a complete functional loss from the level of the radiation portal down. It is estimated that for doses in the range of 57 to 61 Gy with conventionally fractionated RT, the incidence of myelopathy is 5%.[190] Risk factors for myelopathy include both the total dose and the dose per fraction.

## CHEMOTHERAPY

Corticosteroids are often the first line of treatment. Benefits include the reduction of edema and a tumoricidal effect on lymphomas and in some breast cancer patients. The optimum loading and maintenance dose of corticosteroids have not been determined. Because spinal cord damage becomes irreversible if the compression is not relieved, clinicians often will prescribe high-dose dexamethasone in patients with rapidly progressive symptoms or in those who cannot walk, and then taper during the course of treatment. Patients with minimal symptoms may require lower doses or be able to tolerate therapy without neurologic compromise without corticosteroids.[182]

Chemotherapy is used for epidural tumors that are chemosensitive and in patients with recurrent tumor who have received radiation therapy. Although there have been no trials of chemotherapy for primary spinal cord tumors, drugs active against intracranial gliomas might potentially be effective against these same histologies in the spinal cord. Anecdotal evidence indicates that patients have been treated with nitrosourea-based regimens.[188]

## SYMPTOM MANAGEMENT AND SUPPORTIVE CARE

Individuals with CNS tumors frequently suffer from disabling symptoms that dramatically affect their ability to function. Many of these symptoms are directly related to the tumor, but other symptoms are only indirectly related to the cancer—for example, side effects of medications used for symptom relief, such as corticosteroids and anticonvulsants, and the psychological symptoms resulting from the devastating effects of the nervous system tumor itself (eg, aphasia, paralysis, incontinence, cognitive dysfunction).[191,192] The care of these patients continues to shift to the home and community, regardless of prognosis. Supportive nursing measures assume importance in all areas of patient care. Table 49-4 describes common nursing diagnoses, suggests causes of the problems, and offers some of the associated nursing interventions for the care of these individuals.

Cerebral edema is often managed with corticosteroids such as dexamethasone. Dramatic improvements in neurological function are often seen along with reduction in ICP within hours to days following the initiation of steroids, particularly in those individuals with tumors producing substantial edema.[35,36] In situations where ICP is acutely elevated, steroids alone are insufficient and osmotic diuretics, also referred to as *hyperosmolar agents*, are required. The high concentration of the drug causes water to be drawn from the normal tissue. Diuresis occurs within one to three hours and lasts up to approximately eight hours. An indwelling urinary catheter, strict recording of intake and output, and monitoring of electrolytes are necessary. Other methods to help control increased ICP include fluid restriction, hyperventilation, sedation, and temperature control. Valsalva maneuvers, isometric muscle contractions, coughing, sneezing, straining, and the use of positive-end expiratory pressure (PEEP) should be avoided, as they can further aggravate increased ICP. A decrease in venous outflow will increase the total blood volume within the intracranial space, leading to elevated ICP. Head and neck positions that impair venous outflow include jugular compression, head rotation, neck flexion, and neck extension. The head of the bed should be elevated to promote venous drainage. Lying prone and flexing the hips should be avoided because these positions increase intraabdominal and intrathoracic pressures, also leading to elevations in ICP. When turning or positioning in bed, the head and neck should be maintained in a neutral position. Alert individuals should be instructed not to turn themselves. Many patients unintentionally perform a valsalva maneuver or grab the side rails tightly (isometric muscle contraction) when turning.[36]

Unfortunately, many nursing interventions, although necessary, can aggravate the already increased ICP. Although many of these activities cannot be avoided, they can be better spaced over time. It is a common practice to group these activities together. For example, when a patient is bathed, he or she is turned several times, receives range-of-motion exercises and pulmonary toileting, and is repositioned. The patient is probably suctioned, is medicated, and may have a dressing or two changed before the nurse leaves the room to attend to other patients or responsibilities. While this practice is often considered necessary to manage the nurse's time and remain efficient and organized, it is not always in the best interest of the patient with increased ICP. Spacing out these activities and care can decrease sustained elevations of increased ICP.

Blocked CSF pathways may lead to hydrocephalus. In such cases, a VP shunt or temporary ventriculostomy may be required. A ventriculostomy is indicated when the etiology of the hydrocephalus is believed to be of a temporary nature. Patients with a ventriculostomy require correct head positioning in relation to the level of the drainage system. The drainage system drip chamber level is ordered by the physician and is usually positioned level with the external auditory meatus. The level is changed based on the patient's clinical condition and the amount of CSF drainage. The procedure of leveling the drip chamber at, above, or below the external auditory meatus minimizes the risk of both excessive CSF drainage leading to collapse of the ventricles and insufficient CSF drainage leading to hydrocephalus. The level of the drip chamber is continuously monitored, the amount and consistency of CSF are assessed hourly, and the patient is evaluated for any neurological changes and signs of infection.

Individuals with spinal cord tumors also receive steroids, especially when SCC has developed. Once the condition is determined or even clinically suspected, steroids are initiated immediately. Steroids decrease the edema of the spinal cord and rapidly relieve back pain in many patients. More than 95% of individuals with SCC report having pain. While the administration of steroids provides pain relief for many individuals, others require additional analgesics. Effective analgesia needs to be established early on and dosages adjusted as the steroids and treatmentfurther reduce the pain.

The goal of treatment is to preserve and maintain existing neurological function. Patient assessment is therefore crucial throughout this period to evaluate neurological status. Changes in the neurological exam or the development of new deficits must be followed up immediately.

Glucocorticoid hormones are commonly used in neurooncology. Unfortunately, they have many unwanted side effects. Some of the common side effects, while distressing to the individual, are considered mild: insomnia, fatigue, increased appetite, hiccups, blurry vision, behavioral changes, acne, edema, abdominal bloating, and the

**TABLE 49-4**

**Nursing Management of an Individual With a CNS Tumor**

| Nursing Diagnosis | Possible Cause | Nursing Interventions |
|---|---|---|
| Altered cerebral tissue perfusion | Tumor size<br>Cerebral edema<br>Obstruction of CSF pathways<br>Decreased cranial venous outflow<br>Increased intraabdominal and intrathoracic pressure<br>Increased systemic arterial blood pressure | Neurological assessment<br>Corticosteroid administration<br>ICP monitoring<br>Avoid cumulative activities<br>Ventriculostomy<br>Elevate head of bed<br>Avoid head rotation, neck flexion, and extension<br>Avoid hip flexion and prone position<br>Avoid valsalva maneuvers, isometric muscle contraction, coughing emotional arousal |
| High risk for seizures | Disturbance of intracranial contents<br>Electrolyte abnormality | Prophylactic anticonvulsants<br>Institute seizure precautions<br>Maintain safe environment<br>Be aware of concurrent medications that interfere with anticonvulsant action, absorption, or both<br>Correct electrolyte abnormalities |
| Impaired cognition<br>Memory<br>Judgment<br>Thought processes | Frontal tumor<br>Cerebral edema<br>Hydrocephalus<br>Radiation therapy<br>Medication effects | Maintain as close to normal function as possible<br>Reorient individual<br>Utilize calendars, clocks, labels, photographs, etc., as visual cues or reminders<br>Maintain as close to normal function as possible<br>Encourage social activities<br>Instruct family members<br>Provide written instructions |
| Impaired physical mobility<br>Hemiparesis<br>Hemiplegia<br>Paraparesis<br>Paraplegia<br>Ataxic gait<br>Level of consciousness | Frontal tumor<br>Parietal tumor<br>Spinal tumor<br>Spinal RT<br>Steroids | Maintain maximal activity level<br>Provide assistance as necessary for ambulation, transfer, ADLs<br>Encourage proper footwear (nonskid soles that enclose the foot)<br>Maintain safe environment<br>Keep needed objects close at hand<br>Physical and occupational therapy<br>Range-of-motion exercises<br>Teach proper use of assistive devices (brace, cane, walker)<br>Institute measures to prevent complications such as DVT, pressure ulcer, foot drop, pneumonia<br>Develop specific interventions to compensate for deficits<br>Instruct patient and family in safety measures and above techniques<br>When preparing for discharge, obtain necessary equipment for home (wheel-chair, bed, commode, walker, guardrail for bathroom, stool for shower)<br>Assess home for physical setup and safety (stairs, rugs) |
| Alteration in sensory/ perceptual ability | Occipital tumor<br>Parietal tumor<br>Frontal tumor<br>Spinal cord tumor<br>Peripheral neuropathy | Monitor sensory function<br>Identify highest level of intact sensory function<br>Instruct patient and family on methods of compensation (checking position of involved areas visually, turning head completely to scan area)<br>Occupational therapy for assistive devices<br>Instruct patient and family in safety measures, proper clothing, and foot wear |
| Knowledge deficit<br>Disease<br>Treatment<br>Medications<br>Discharge | New diagnosis<br>Anxiety | Provide education to patient and family appropriately<br>Encourage questions<br>Clarify misconceptions<br>Refer to resources as needed<br>Provide written materials and written instructions |

*(Continued)*

**TABLE 49-4**

**Nursing Management of an Individual With a CNS Tumor (*Continued*)**

| Nursing Diagnosis | Possible Cause | Nursing Interventions |
|---|---|---|
| Alteration in comfort<br>Headache<br>Back pain | Intracranial tumor<br>Increased ICP<br>Spinal cord compression<br>Steroid withdrawal | Assess for verbal and nonverbal indicators of pain<br>Have patient rate pain using 0-10 scale, if possible<br>Administer analgesics, steroids, or other non-narcotic agents and evaluate effectiveness<br>Encourage relaxation techniques or meditation<br>Encourage diversional activities |
| High risk for impaired skin integrity | Immobility<br>Sensory changes<br>Poor nutrition | Assess skin condition frequently<br>Frequent, thorough skin care<br>Use of pressure-relieving devices<br>Maximize nutrition<br>Instruct patient and family on measures to prevent skin breakdown (proper positioning techniques, lotion, massage, bathing, nutritious snacks, and meals) |

characteristic moon face. Other effects can be more serious: GI bleeding, bowel perforation, hyperglycemia, hallucinations, psychosis, myopathy manifested by proximal leg weakness, osteoporosis, and acute adrenal insufficiency resulting from steroid withdrawal. Immunosuppression caused by prolonged steroid administration can lead to opportunistic infections, particularly *Pneumocystis carinii* pneumonia (PCP). In some cases, individuals on prolonged steroid therapy may also receive PCP prophylaxis. Common options for prophylaxis and treatment include trimethoprim and sulfamethoxazole (Bactrim), pentamidine, or dapsone.[193] Ongoing assessment is necessary because neurooncology patients often receive steroids for prolonged and repeated periods of time. Patients and families need to be educated regarding the medications, including the side effects to observe for and interventions to take, indications to call their physician, and the absolute necessity of taking the prescribed dose. Sudden withdrawal of steroids can lead to adrenal insufficiency. Symptoms of this condition include fatigue, muscular weakness, joint pain, fever, anorexia, nausea, and orthostatic hypotension.[32] Steroid dosages are tapered slowly to prevent these symptoms of withdrawal. Patients should be given written instructions about the schedule of the steroid taper and should be monitored for increased neurological symptoms as the dose is decreased. Some individuals may become steroid-dependent and do not tolerate even a slow taper. It is also important to be familiar with the drug interactions of steroids and other medications that the individual may be taking. Drugs such as dilantin, phenobarbital, and perhaps carbamazepine increase the metabolic clearance of steroids and may decrease their therapeutic effect.

Anticonvulsants are commonly used to treat and prevent seizures in individuals with primary and metastatic brain tumors. These agents are not without side effects, and many of these agents cause drowsiness and cognitive dysfunction. Worsening neurological symptoms occur at toxic therapeutic levels and can add to existing neurological dysfunction. Patients on anticonvulsatns require monitoring of drug levels, if appropriate, and for signs of toxicity. Individuals should be encouraged to obtain and wear a medic alert bracelet.

Many individuals with CNS cancers experience anxiety and depression. The psychological impact of the diagnosis, with its relatively poor prognosis, can be devastating. While considered natural responses to the illness with its disabling neurological deficits, anxiety and depression are sometimes overlooked. Antidepressants and antianxiolytics may help improve the psychological symptoms. Counseling can be of benefit to both the individual and his or her family who are grieving the loss of the "person they once knew." The debilitating effects of CNS cancers are not limited to obvious neurological deficits; perhaps more devastating are the effects on the "persona." The personality of the individual is often permanently changed due to the disease, treatment, or both.

## CONCLUSION

Malignancies of the CNS present tremendous challenges for individuals, families, and caregivers. Because the clinical manifestations, course of treatment, and complications vary with the type and site of tumors, individuals with CNS cancers require highly individualized plans of care. Supportive care takes on a role of utmost importance and encompasses the entire course of illness from diagnosis through the terminal phase of disease. Even with advances in overall therapeutic modalities, successful treatment of CNS cancers remains elusive. Outcomes can range from cure to permanent disability to life prolonged by a few days, weeks, or months. The ongoing physical and emotional support necessary for both the individual and the family create a challenging role for oncology nurses.[194] The neurological symptoms and complications produced by CNS cancers are, unfortunately, profoundly disabling and severely affect quality of life. Assisting the individual to manage problems of daily living, maintain normal function to the best of his or her ability, and attain quality of life are nurses' ultimate goals.

## REFERENCES


1. Norden, AD, Wen PY, Desari, S. Brain Metastases. *Curr Opin Neurol.* 2005;18:654–661.
2. CBTRUS. *Statistical Report: Primary Brain Tumors in the United States, 2000–2004.* Published by the Central Brain Tumor Registry of the United States; 2008.
3. American Cancer Society. *Cancer Facts and Figures 2009.* Atlanta: American Cancer Society; 2009.
4. Ries LAG, Melbert D, Krapcho M, et al., eds. *SEER Cancer Statistics Review, 1975–2004.* Bethesda, MD: National Cancer Institute. http://seer.cancer.gov/csr/1975_2004, poster 2007 obtained July 2008.
5. Wen PY, Kesari S. Malignant gliomas in adults. *N Engl J Med.* 2008;359:492–507.
6. Fisher JL, Schwartzbaum JA, Wrensch M, Wiemels, JL. Epidemiology of brain tumors. *Neurol Clin.* 2007;25:867–890.
7. Bohnen NI, Radhakrishnan K, O'Neill BP, et al. Descriptive and analytic epidemiology of brain tumors. In: Black PM, Loeffler JS, eds. *Cancer of the Nervous System.* Cambridge, Blackwell Science; 1997:3–24.
8. Friedman JM. Neurofibromatosis 1: clinical manifestations and diagnostic criteria. *J Child Neurol.* 2002;17:548–554.
9. National Brain Tumor Foundation (NBTF): *Brain Tumors: A Guide.* Oakland, CA: National Brain Tumor Foundation; 2007.
10. Martz CH. von Hippel-Lindau disease: a genetically transmitted multisystem neoplastic disorder. *Semin Oncol Nurs.* 1992;8:281–287.
11. Furnari FB, Fenton T, Bachoo RM, et al. Malignant astrocytic glioma: genetics, biology, and paths to treatment. *Genes Dev.* 2007;21: 2683–2710.
12. Ohgako H, Kleihues, P. Genetic pathways to primary and secondary glioblastoma. *Am J Pathol.* 2007;170:1445–1453.
13. Louis DN, Ohgaki H, Wiestler OD, et al. *The 2007 WHO Classification of Tumors of the Central Nervous System.* Lyon, France: IARC Press; 2007.
14. Sanai N, Alvarez-Buylla, A. Berger, MS. Neural stem cells and the origin of gliomas. *N Engl J Med.* 2005;353:811–822.
15. Bondy ML, Scheurer ME, Malmer B, et al. Brain tumor epidemiology: consensus from the Brain Tumor Epidemiology Consortium. *Cancer.* 2008;113(suppl):1953–1968.
16. Sadetzki S, Modan B, Chetrit A, et al. An iatrogenic epidemic of benign meningioma. *Am J Epidemiol.* 2000;151:266–272.
17. Ron E, Modan B, Boice JD, et al. Tumors of the brain and nervous system after radiotherapy in childhood. *N Engl J Med.* 1988;319:1033–1039.
18. Tsang RW, Laperriere NJ, Simpson WJ, et al. Glioma arising after radiation therapy for pituitary adenoma. *Cancer.* 1993;72:2227–2233.
19. Alexander MJ, DeSalles AA, Tomiyasu U. Multiple radiation-induced intracranial lesions after treatment for pituitary adenoma. *J Neurosurg.* 1998;88:111–115.
20. Walter AW, Hancock ML, Pui CH, et al. Secondary brain tumors in children treated for acute lymphoblastic leukemia at St. Jude Children's Research Hospital. *J Clin Oncol.* 1998;16:3761–3767.
21. Davis FS. Epidemiology of brain tumors. *Expert Rev Anticancer Ther.* 2007;7(suppl):S3–S6.
22. Schwartzbaum J, Johsson F, Ahlbom A, et al. Cohort studies of association between self-reported allergic conditions, immune-related diagnoses and glioma and meningioma risk. *Int J Cancer.* 2003;106:423–428.
23. Schiff D, Suman VJ, Yang P, et al. Risk factors for primary central nervous system lymphoma. *Cancer.* 1998;82:975–982.
24. Schabel M. Epidemiology of primary CNS lymphoma. *J Neurooncol.* 1999;43:199–201.
25. Heath CW. Electromagnetic field exposure and cancer: a review of epidemiologic evidence. *CA Cancer J Clin.* 1996;46:29–44.
26. Berleur MP, Cordier S. The role of chemical, physical, or viral exposures and health factors in neurocarcinogenesis: implications for epidemiologic studies of brain tumors. *Cancer Causes Control.* 1995;6: 240–256.
27. Sahl JD, Kelsh MA, Greenland S. Cohort and nested case-control studies of hematopoietic cancers and brain cancers among electric utility workers. *Epidemiology.* 1993;4:104–114.
28. Floderus B, Persson T, Stenkind C, et al. Occupational exposure to electromagnetic fields in relation to leukemia and brain tumors: a case-control study in Sweden. *Cancer Causes Control.* 1993;4:465–476.
29. Shoemaker M, Swerdlow A, Ahlbom A, et al. Mobile phone use and risk of acoustic neuroma: results of the Interphone case-control study in five North European countries. *Br J Cancer.* 2005;93:842–848.
30. Kan P, Simonsen SE, Lyon JL, Kestle JR. Cellular phone use and brain tumor: a meta-analysis. *J Neurooncol.* 2008;86:71–78.
31. Lahkola A, Auvinen A, Raitanen J, et al. Mobile phone use and risk of glioma in 5 North European countries. *Int J Cancer.* 2007;120: 1769–1775.
32. Chaffee EE, Lytle IM. *Basic Physiology and Anatomy.* Philadelphia: Lippincott; 1980.
33. Belford K:. Central nervous system cancers. In: Yarbro CH, Frogge MH, Goodman M, eds. *Cancer Nursing: Principles and Practice.* 6th ed. Sudbury, MA: Jones and Bartlett; 2005:1089–1136.
34. Hickey JV. Overview of neuroanatomy and neurophysiology. In Hickey JV, ed. *The Clinical Practice of Neurological and Neurosurgical Nursing.* 5th ed. Philadelphia: Lippincott; 2002:45–93.
35. Lee, Eva Lu T, Armstrong TS. Increased intracranial pressure. *Clin J Oncol Nurs.* 2008;12:1–4.
36. Hickey JV. Intracranial pressure theory and management of increased intracranial pressure. In: Hickey JV, ed. *The Clinical Practice of Neurological and Neurosurgical Nursing.* 5th ed. Philadelphia: Lippincott; 2002:285–319.
37. Taylor I, Taylor MM. *Psycholinguistics: Learning and Using Language.* Englewood Cliffs, NJ: Prentice Hall; 1990:362.
38. Hildebrand J, Lecaille C, Perennes J, Delattre, JY. Epileptic seizures during follow-up of patients treated for primary brain tumors. *Neurology.* 2005;65:212–215.
39. Westcarth L, Armstrong T. Seizures in people with cancer. *Clin J Oncol* Nurs. 2007;11:33–37.
40. Armstrong TS, Kanusky J, Gilbert MR. Seizure the moment to learn about epilepsy in the person with cancer. *Clin J Oncol Nurs.* 2003;7:163–169.
40. Lovely MP. Symptom Management of brain tumor patients. *Semin Oncol Nurs.* 2004;20:273–283.
41. Levin VA, Leibel SA, Gutin PH. Neoplasms of the central nervous system. In: Devita VT Jr, Hellman S, Rosenberg SA, eds. *Cancer: Principles and Practice of Oncology.* 6th ed. Philadelphia: Lippincott, Williams and Wilkins; 2001:2100–2160.
42. Posner JB. *Neurologic Complications of Cancer.* Philadelphia: Davis; 1995.
43. Armstrong TS, Gilbert MR. Metastatic brian tumors: diagnosis, treatment, and nursing interventions. *Clin J Oncol Nurs.* 2000;4:217–225.
44. Armstrong TS, Cohen MZ, Weinberg J, Gilbert MR. Neuroimaging in neuro-oncology. *Semin Oncol Nurs.* 2004;20:231–239.
45. Newton HB, Ray-Chaudhury A, Cavaliere R. Brain tumor imaging and cancer management: the neuro-oncologists perspective. *Top Magn Reson Imaging.* 2006;17:127–136.
46. Hickey JV. Diagnostic procedures and laboratory tests for neuroscience patients. In: Hickey JV, ed. *The Clinical Practice of Neurological and Neurosurgical Nursing.* 5th ed. Philadelphia: Lippincott; 2002:93–117.

47. Grobner T, Prischl FC. Patient characteristics and risk factors for nephrogenic systemic fibrosis following gadolinium exposure. *Semin Dial.* 2008;21:135–139.
48. Wiginton CD, Kelly B, Oto A, Jesse M, Aristimuno P. Gadolinium-based contrast exposure, nephrogenic systemic fibrosis, and gadolinium detection in tissue. *AJR.* 2008;190I:1060–1068.
49. Chawla S, Poptani H, Melhen, ER. Anatomic, physiologic, and metabolic imaging in neuro-oncology. *Cancer Treat Res.* 2008;143:3–42.
50. Roberts HC, Roberts TP, Brasch RC, Dillon, WP. Quantitative measurement of microvascular permeability in human brain tumors achieved using dynamic contrast-enhanced MRI: correlation with histology grade. *AJNR.* 2000;21:891–899.
51. Yu Cs, Li KC, Xuaa Y, Ji XM, Qin W. Diffusion tensor tractography in patients with cerebral tumors: a helpful technique for neurosurgical planning and postoperative assessment. *Eur J Radiol.* 2005;56:197–204.
52. Fischman AJ. PET imaging fo brain tumors. *Cancer Treatm Res.* 2008; 143:67–92.
53. Hoffman JM. New advances in brain tumor imaging. *Curr Opin Oncol.* 2001;13:148–153.
54. Abrey LE, Mason WP, eds. *Brain Tumors: Fast Facts Indispensable Guides to Clinical Practice.* Oxford: Health Press; 2003.
55. Van den Bent MJ. The role of chemotherapy in brain metastases. *Eur J Cancer.* 2003;39:2114–2120.
56. Gleissner B, Chamberlain MC. Neoplastic meningitis. *Lancet Neurol.* 2006;5:443–452.
57. Lamborn KR, Chang SM, Prados MD. Prognostic factors for survival of patients with glioblastoma: recursive partitioning analysis. *Neuro-oncology.* 2004;6:227–235.
58. Martinez R, Volter C, Behr R. Parameters assessing neurologic status in malignant glioma patients: prognostic value for survival and relapse-free time. *Br J Neurosurg.* 2008;6:1–6.
59. Berger MS. Malignant astrocytomas: surgical aspects. *Semin Oncol.* 1994;21:172–185.
60. Berger MS, Rostomily RC. Low-grade gliomas: functional mapping resection strategies, extent of resection, and outcome. *J Neurooncol.* 1997;34:85–101.
61. Gaspar L, Scott C, Rotman M. Recursive partitioning analysis (RPA) of prognostic factos in three Radiation Oncology Group (RTOG) brain metastases trials. *Int J Radiat Oncol Biol Phys.* 1997;37:745–751.
62. DeAngelis LM, Gutin PH, Leibel SA, Posner JB, eds. *Intracranial Tumors Diagnosis and Treatment.* London: Martin Dunitz; 2002.
63. Shafqat S, Hedley-Whyte TE, Henson JW. Age-dependent rate of anaplastic transformation in low-grade astrocytoma. *Neurology.* 1999;52:867–869.
64. Behin A, Hoang-Xuan K, Carpentier AF, et al. Primary brain tumors in adults. *Lancet.* 2003;361:323–331.
65. Shaw EG, Scheithauer BW, O'Fallon JR. Supratentorial gliomas: a comparative study by grade and histologic type. *J Neurooncol.* 1997;31:273–278.
66. Brown PD. Low-grade gliomas: the debate continues. *Curr Oncol Rep.* 2006;8:71–77.
67. Macdonald DR. Low-grade gliomas, mixed gliomas, and oligodendrogliomas. *Semin Oncol.* 1994;21:236–248.
68. Karim ABMF, Afra D, Cornu P, et al. Randomized trial on the efficacy of radiotherapy for cerebral low-grade glioma in the adult: European Organization for Research and Treatment of Cancer Study 22845 with the Medical Research Council Study BR04: an interim analysis. *Int J Radiat Oncol Biol Phys.* 2002;52:316–324.
69. Stupp R, Hegi ME, Mason WP, et al. Effects of radiotherapy with concomitant and adjuvant temozolomide versus radiotherapy alone on survival in glioblastoma in a randomised phase III study: 5-year analysis of the EORTC-NCIC trial. *Lancet Oncol.* 2009;10:459–466.
70. Asthagiri AR, Pouratian N, Sherman J, Ahmed G, Shaffrey ME. Advances in brain tumor surgery. *Neurol Clin.* 2007;25:975–1003.
71. Lacroix M, Abi-Said D, Fourney D, et al. A multivariate analysis of 216 patients with glioblastoma multiforme: prognosis, extent of resection, and survival. *J Neurosurgery.* 2001;95:190–198.
72. Sanai N, Berger MS. Glioma extent of resection and its impact on patient outcome. *Neurosurgery.* 2008;62:753–764.
73. Chamberlain MC, Chowdhary SA, Glantz MJ. Anaplastic astrocytomas: biology and treatment. *Expert Rev Neurother.* 2008;8:575–586.
74. Stupp R, Mason WP, van den Bent MJ, et al. Radiotheapy plus concomitant and adjunvant temozolomide for glioblastoma. *N Engl J Med.* 2005;352:987–996.
75. Cohen MH, Shen YL, Keegan P, Pazdur R. FDA drug approval summary: bevacizumab (Avastin) as treatment of recurrent glioblastoma multiforme. *Oncologist,* 2009;14:1131–1138.
76. Cairncross JG, Ueki K, Zlatescu MC, et al. Specific genetic predictors of chemotherapeutic response and survival in patients with anaplastic oligodendroglioma. *J Natl Cancer Inst.* 1998;90:1473–1479.
77. Bigner SH, Rasheed K, Wiltshire RN, et al. Morphologic and molecular genetic aspects of oligodendroglial neoplasms. *Neurooncology.* 1999;1:52–60.
78. Ino Y, Betensky RA, Zlatescu MC, et al. Molecular subtypes of anaplastic oligodendroglioma: implications for patient management at diagnosis. *Clin Cancer Res.* 2001;7:839–845.
79. National Comprehensive Cancer network. *NCCN Practice Guildeines Central Nervous system Cancers.* Jenkintown, PA: National Comprehensive Cancer network; 2008.
80. Cairncross G, Berkey B, Shaw E, et al. Phase III trial of chemotherapy plus radiotherapy compared with radiotherapy alone for pure and mixed anaplastic oligodendroglioma: Intergroup Radiation Therapy Oncology Group Trial 9402. *J Clin Oncol.* 2006;24:2707–2714.
81. Taylor MD, Poppleton H, Fuller C, et al. Radial glia cells are candidate stem cells of ependymoma. *Cancer Cell.* 2005;8:323–334.
82. Metellus P, Barrie M, Figarella-Branger D, et al. Multicentric french study on adult intracranial ependymomas: prognostic factors analysis and therapeutic considerations from a cohort of 152 patients. *Brain.* 2007;130:1338–1349.
83. Reni M, Brandes A, Vavassori V, et al. A multicenter study of the prognosis and treatment of adult brain ependymal tumors. *Cancer.* 2004;100:1221–1229.
84. McLaughlin MP, Marcu RB, Buatti JM, et al. Ependymoma: result, prognostic factos and treatment recommendations. *Int J Radiat Oncol Biol Phys.* 1998;40:845–850.
85. Asthagiri AR, Helm GA, Sheehan JP. Current concepts in management of meningiomas and schwannomas. *Neurol Clin.* 2007;25: 1209–1230.
86. Kleihues P, Cavenee WB, eds. World Health Organization Classification of Tumors: Pathology and Genetics: Tumors of the nervous system. Lyon, France: IARC Press; 2000:2.
87. Black PM. Brain tumors. N Engl J Med. 1991;324:1555–1564.
88. Younis GA, Sawaya R, DeMonte F, et al. Aggressive meningeal tumors: review of a series. *J Neurosurg.* 1995;82:17–27.
89. Dijkstra M, van Nieuwenhuizen D, Stalpers LJ, et al. Late neurocognitive sequelae in WHO grade I meningioma patients. *J Neurol Neurosurg Psychiatr.* 2009;80:910–915.
90. Wilson CB. Meningiomas: genetics, malignancy, and the role of radiation in induction and treatment. *J Neurosurg.* 1994;81:666–674.
91. Hug EB, DeVries A, Thornton AF, et al. Management of atypical and malignant meningiomas: role of high-dose, 3D-conformal radiation therapy. *J Neurooncol.* 2000;48:151–160.
92. Kaba SE, DeMonte F, Bruner JM, et al. The treatment of recurrent unresectable and malignant meningiomas with interferon alpha-2B. *Neurosurgery.* 1997;40:271–275.
93. Mason WP, Gentili F, Macdonald DR, et al. Stabilization of disease progression by hydroxyurea in patients with recurrent or unresectable meningioma. *J Neurosurg.* 2002;97:341–346.
94. Campbell C. Acoustic neuroma: nursing implications related to surgical management. *J Neurosci Nurs.* 1991;23:50–60.
95. Black PM. Benign brain tumors. In: Wen PY, Black PM, eds. *Neurologic Clinics: Brain Tumors in Adults.* Philadelphia: Saunders; 1995: 927–954.

96. Koos WT, Day JD, Matula C, et al. Neurotopographic considerations in the microsurgical treatment of small acoustic neurinomas. *J Neurosurg.* 1998;88:506–512.
97. Flickinger JC, Kondziolka D, Niranjan A, et al. Results of acoustic neuroma radiosurgery: an analysis of 5 years' experience using current methods. *J Neurosurg.* 2001;94:1–6.
98. Mohile NA, Abrey LE. Primary central nervous system lymphoma. *Neurol Clin.* 2007;25:1193–1207.
99. Kadan-Lottick NS, Skluzacek MC, Burney JG. Decreasing incidence rates of primary central nervous system lymphoma. *Cancer.* 2002;95:193–202.
100. DeAngelis LM. Current management of primary central nervous system lymphoma. *Oncology.* 1995;9:63–71.
101. Gavrilovic IT, Hormigo A, Yahalom J. Long-term follow-up of high-dose methotrexate-based therapy with and without whole brain irradiation for newly diagnosed primary CNS lymphoma. *J Clin Oncol.* 2006;24:4570–4574.
102. Dahlborg SA, Braziel R, Crossen JR, et al. Non-AIDS primary CNS lymphoma: first example of a durable response in a primary brain tumor using enhanced chemotherapy delivery without cognitive loss and without radiotherapy. *Cancer J Sci Am.* 1996;2:166–174.
103. Young RF. Radiosurgery for the treatment of brain metastases. *Semin Surg Oncol.* 1998;14:70–78.
104. Ewend MG, Morris DE, Carey LA, Ladha AM, Brem S. Guidelines for the initial management of metastatic brain tumors: role of surgery, radiosurgery, and radiation therapy. *J Natl Compr Cancer Netw.* 2008;6:505–513.
105. Sitton E. Central nervous system metastases. *Semin Oncol Nurs.* 1998;14:210–219.
106. Patchell RA, Tibbs PA, Walsh JW, et al. A randomized trial of surgery in the treatment of single metastases to the brain. *N Engl J Med.* 1990;322:494–500.
107. Vecht CJ, Haaxma-Reiche H, Noordijk EM, et al. Treatment of single brain metastasis: radiotherapy alone or combined with neurosurgery? *Ann Neurol.* 1993;33:583–590.
108. Bindel RK, Sawaya R, Leavens ME, et al. Surgical treatment of multiple brain metastases. *J Neurosurg.* 1993;79:210–216.
109. Mehta MP, Tsao MN, Whelan TJ, et al. The American Society for Therapeutic Radiology and Oncology (ASTRO) evidence-based review of the role of radiosurgery for brain metastases. *Int J Radiat Oncol Biol Phys.* 2005;63:37–46.
110. Oben A, Moriarty TM, Loeffler JS. Radiosurgery for metastases. *J Neurooncol.* 1996;27:279–285.
111. Muacevic A, Kreth FW, Horstmann GA, et al. Surgery and radiotherapy compared with gamma knife radiosurgery in the treatment of solitary cerebral metastases of small diameter. *J Neurosurg.* 1999;91:35–43.
112. Aoyama H, Shirato H, Tago M, et al. Stereotactic radiosurgery plus whole-brain radiation therapy vs stereotactic radiosurgery alone for treatment of brain metastases: a randomized controlled trials. *JAMA.* 2006;281:2483–2491.
113. Postmus PE, Haaxma-Reiche H, Smit EF, et al. Treatment of brain metastases of small-cell lung cancer: comparing teniposide and teniposide with whole-brain radiotherapy—a phase III study of the European Organization for the Research and Treatment of Cancer Lung Cancer Cooperative Group. *J Clin Oncol.* 2000;18:3400–3408.
114. Antonadou D, Paraskevaidis G, Sarris N, et al. Phase II randomized trial of temozolomide and concurrent radiotherapy in patients with brain metastases. *J Clin Oncol.* 2002;20:3644–3650.
115. Gordon BM, Myers JS. Leptomeningeal metastases. *Clin J Oncol Nurs.* 2003;7:151–155.
116. Taillibert S, Laigle-Donadey F, Chodkiewicz C, Sanson M, Hoang-Xuan K, Delattre JY. Leptomeningeal metastases from solid malignancy: a review. *J Neurooncol.* 2005;75:85–99.
117. Jaeckle KA. Improving the outcome of patients with leptomeningeal cancer: new clinical trials and experimental therapies. *Cancer Treat Res.* 2005;125:181–193.
118. Bohan E, Glass-Macenka D. Surgical management of patients with primary brain tumors. *Semin Oncol Nurs.* 2004;20:240–252.
119. Sawaya R, Rambo WM, Hammond MA, et al. Advances in surgery for brain tumors. In Wen PY, Black PM, eds. *Neurologic Clinics: Brain Tumors in Adults.* Philadelphia: Saunders; 1995:757–771.
120. Heilbrun MP, Roberts TS, Apuzzo MLJ, et al. Preliminary experience with Brown-Roberts-Wells (BRW) computerized tomography stereotaxic guidance system. *J Neurosurg.* 1983;59:217–222.
121. Arbour RA: Stereotactic localization and resection of intracranial tumors. *J Neurosci Nurs.* 1993;25:14–21.
122. Krieger MD, Chandrasoma PT, Zee CS, et al. Role of stereotactic biopsy in the diagnosis and management of brain tumors. *Semin Surg Oncol.* 1998;14:13–25.
123. League D. Interactive, image-guided, stereotactic neurosurgery systems. *AORN J.* 1995;61:360–370.
124. Schulder M, Carmel PW. Intraoperative magnetic resonance imaging: impact on brain tumor surgery. *Cancer Control.* 2003;10:115–124.
125. Hentschel SJ, Sawaya R. Optimizing outcomes with maximal surgical resection of malignant gliomas. *Cancer Control.* 2003;10:109–114.
126. Gooding GA, Edwards MS, Rabskin AE, et al. Intraoperative real-time ultrasound in the localization of intracranial neoplasms. *Radiology.* 1983;146:459–461.
127. Lee CC, Ward HA, Sharbrough FW, et al. Assessment of functional MRI imaging in neurosurgical planning. *AJNR Am J Neuroradiol.* 1999;20:1511–1519.
128. Meyer FB, Bates LM, Goerss SJ, et al. Awake craniotomy for aggressive resection of primary gliomas located in eloquent brain. *Mayo Clin Proc.* 2001;76:677–687.
129. Chen TC, Apuzzo MLJ. Principles of stereotactic neurosurgery. In: Black PM, Loeffler JS, eds. *Cancer of the Nervous System.* Boston: Blackwell Science; 1997:156–177.
130. Hall W, Liu H, Martin AJ, et al. Safety, efficacy, and functionality of high-field strength interventional magnetic resonance imaging for neurosurgery. *Neurosurgery.* 2000;46:632–642.
131. Sutherland GR, Kaibara T, Louw D, et al. A mobile high-field magnetic resonance system for neurosurgery. *J Neurosurg.* 1999;91:804–813.
132. Palese A, Skrap M, Fachin M, Visioli S, Zannini L. The experience of patients undergoing awake craniotomy: in the patients' own words. A qualitative study. *Cancer Nurs.* 2008;31:166–172.
133. Greenberg E, Treger I, Ring H. Rehabilitation outcomes in patients with brian tumors and acute stroke: comparative study of inpatient rehabilitation. *Am J Phys Med Rehabil.* 2006;85:568–573.
134. Newton HB., Goldlust SA, Pearl D. Retrospective analysis of the efficacy and tolerability of levetiracetam in brain tumor patients. *J Neurooncol.* 2006;78:99–102.
135. Walker MD, Alexander E, Hunt WE, et al. Evaluation of BCNU and/or radiotherapy in the treatment of anaplastic gliomas. *J Neurosurg.* 1978;49:333–343.
136. Fine HA, Dear KB, Loeffler JS, et al. Meta-analysis of radiation therapy with and without adjuvant chemotherapy for malignant gliomas in adults. *Cancer.* 1993;71:2585–2597.
137. Shrieve DC, Alexander E, III, Wen PY, et al. Comparison of stereotactic radiosurgery and brachytherapy in the treatment of recurrent glioblastoma multiforme. *Neurosurgery.* 1995;36:275–284.
138. Grant W, Woo SY. Clinical and financial issues for intensity-modulated radiation therapy delivery. *Semin Radiat Oncol.* 1999;9:99–107.
139. Levin WP, Kooy H, Loeffler JS, DeLaney, TF. Proton beam therapy. *Br J Cancer.* 2005;17:849–854.
140. Gonzalez J, Gilbert MR. Treatment of astrocytomas. *Curr Opin Neurol.* 2005;18:632–638.
141. Thorton AF, Hegarty TJ, Ten Haken RK, et al. Three-dimensional treatment planning of astrocytomas, a dosimetric study of cerebral irradiation. *Int J Radiat Oncol Biol Phys.* 1991;20:1309–1315.

142. Tsao MN, Lloyd NS, Wong RK, Rakovitch E, Chow E, Laperriere N. Radiotherapeutic management of brain metastases: a systematic review and meta-analysis. *Cancer Treat Rev.* 2005;31:256–273.
143. Bhatnagar A, Heron DE, Kondziolka D, et al. Analysis of repeat stereotactic radiosurgery for progressive primary and metastatic CNS tumors. *Int J Radiat Oncol Biol Phys.* 2002;53:527–532.
144. Vitaz TW, Warnke PC, Tabar V, Gutin PH. Brachytherapy for brain tumors. *J Neurooncol.* 2005;73:71–86.
145. Laperriere N, Leung P, McKenzie S, Milosevic M, Wong S, Glen J. Randomized study of brachytherapy in the initial management of patients with malignant astrocytoma. *Int J Radiat Oncol Biol Phys.* 1998;41:1005–1011.
146. Selker RG, Shapiro WR, Burger PC, et al. Brain tumor cooperative group: the brain tumor cooperative group NIH trial 87–01: a randomized comparison of surgery, external radiotherapy, and carmustine versus,surgery, interstitial radiotherapy boost, external radiation therapy, and carmustine. *Neurosurgery.* 2002;51:343–355.
147. Soffietti R, Costanza A, Laguzzi E, Nobile M, Ruda R. Radiotherapy and chemotherapy of brain metastases. J Neurooncol. 2005;75:31–42.
148. Vines EF, Le Pechoux C, Arriagada R. Prophylactic cranial irradiation in small-cell lung cancer. *Semin Oncol.* 2003;30:38–46.
149. Meert AP, Paesmans M, Berghmans T, et al. Prophylactic cranial irradiation in small-cell lung cancer: a systematic review of the literature with meta-analysis. *BMC Cancer.* 2001;1:5.
150. Young RF, Jacques DB, Duma C, et al. Gamma knife radiosurgery for treatment of multiple brain metastases: a comparison of patients with single versus multiple lesions. *Radiosurgery.* 1995;1:92–101.
151. Sneed PK, Lamborn KR, Forstner JM, et al. Radiosurgery for brain metastases: is whole brain radiotherapy necessary? *Int J Radiat Oncol Biol Phys.* 1999;43:549–558.
152. Werner-Wasik M, Rudoler S, Preston PE, et al. Immediate side effects of stereotactic radiotherapy and radiosurgery. *Int J Radiat Oncol Biol Phys.* 1999;43:299–304.
153. Hancock CM, Burrow MA. The role of radiation therapy in the treatment of central nervous system tumors. *Semin Oncol Nurs.* 2004;20:253–259.
154. Butler JM, Case LD, Atkins J, et al. A phase II, double-blind, placebo-controlled prospective randomized clinical trial of d-threo-methylphenidate HCL in brain tumor patients receiving radiation therapy. *Int J Radiat Oncol Biol Phys.* 2007;69:1496–1501.
155. Vredenburgh JJ, Desjardins A, Herndon JE, et al. Phase II trial of bevacizumab and irinotecan in recurrent malignant glioma. *Clin Cancer Res.* 2007;13:1253–1259.
156. Conrad CA, Milosavljevic VP, Yung WK. Advances in chemotherapy for brain tumors. In Wen PY, Black PM, eds. *Neurologic Clinics: Brain Tumors in Adults.* Philadelphia: Saunders; 1995:795–812.
157. Glass J, Hochberg FH, Gruber ML, et al. The treatment of oligodendrogliomas and mixed oligodendrogliomas-astrocytomas with PCV chemotherapy. *J Neurosurg.* 1992;76:741–745.
158. Kyritsis AP, Yung WKA, Bruner J, et al. The treatment of anaplastic oligodendrogliomas and mixed gliomas. *Neurosurgery.* 1993;32:365–371.
159. Mason WP, DeAngelis LM. Procarbazine, CCNU, vincristine (PCV) chemotherapy (CT) for benign oligodendroglioma. *Neurology.* 1994;44:A262–A263.
160. Fossa SD, Bokemeyer C, Gerl A, et al. Treatment outcome of patients with brain metastases from malignant germ cell tumors. *Cancer.* 1999;85:988–997.
161. Grossi F, Scolaro T, Tixi L, Loprevite M, Ardizzoni A. The role of systemic chemotherapy in the treatment of brain metastases from small-cell lung cancer. *Crit Rev Oncol Hematol.* 2001;37:61–67.
162. Olivi A, Brem H. Interstitial chemotherapy with sustained release polymer systems for the treatment of malignant gliomas. *Recent Results Cancer Res.* 1994;135:149–154.
163. Brem H, Piantadosi S, Burger PC, et al. Intraoperative controlled delivery of chemotherapy by biodegradable polymers: safety and effectiveness for recurrent gliomas evaluated by a prospective multi-institutional placebo-controlled clinical trial. *Lancet.* 1995;345:1008–1012.
164. Westphal M, Hilt DC, Bortey E, et al. A phase III trial of local chemotherapy with biodegradable carmustine (BCNU) wafers (Gliadel wafers) in patients with primary malignant glioma. *Neuro-oncology.* 2003;5:79–88.
165. Giese A, Kucinski T, Knopp U, et al. Pattern of recurrence following local chemotherapy with biodegradable carmustine (BCNU) implants in patients with glioblastoma. *J Neurooncol.* 2004;66:351–360.
166. Rich JN, Reardon DA, Peery T, et al. Phase II trial of gefitinib in recurrent glioblastoma. *J Clin Oncol.* 2004;22:133–142.
167. Wen PY, Yung WK, Lamborn KR, et al. Phase I/II study of imatinib mesylate for recurrent malignant gliomas: North American Brain Tumor Consortium Study 99–08. *Clin Cancer Res.* 2006;12:4899–4907.
168. Batchelor TT, Sorensen AG, di Tomaso E, et al. AZD2171, a pan-VEGF receptor tyrosine kinase inhibitor, normalizes tumor vasculature and alleviates edema in glioblastoma patients. *Cancer Cell.* 2007;11:83–95.
169. Chang SM, Wen P, Cloughesy T, et al. Phase II study of CCI-779 in patients with recurrent glioblastoma. *Invest New Drugs.* 2005;23:357–361.
170. Chi AS, Wen PY. Inhibiting kinases in malignant gliomas. *Expert Opin Ther Targets.* 2007;11:473–496.
171. Sathornsumetee S, Reasrdon DA, Desjardins A, Quinn JA, Vrendenburgh JJ, Rich JN. Molecularly targeted therapy for malignant glioma. *Cancer.* 2007;110:13–24.
172. Vredenburgh JJ, Desjardins A, Herndon HE, et al. Bevacizumab plus irinotecan in recurrent gliomblastoma multiforme. *J Clin Oncol.* 2007;25:4722–4729.
173. Chi A, Norden AN, Wen PY. Inhibition of angiogenesis and invasion in malignant gliomas. *Expert Rev Anticancer Ther.* 2007;7:1537–1560.
174. Parsa AT, Fiore AJ, McCormick PC, et al. Genetic basis of intramedullary spinal cord tumors and therapeutic implications. *J Neurooncol.* 2000;47:239–251.
175. Gilman S, Newman SW. *Manter and Gatz's Essentials of Clinical Neuroanatomy and Neurophysiology.* 10th ed. Philadelphia: Davis; 2003.
176. Barr ML, Kiernan JA. *The Human Nervous System.* 8th ed. Philadelphia: Lippincott; 2005.
177. Van Goethen JWM, van den Hauwe L, Ozsarlak O, De Schepper, AMA, Parizel PM. Spinal tumors. *Eur J Radiol.* 2004;50:159–176.
178. Penas-Prado M, Loghin ME. Spinal cord compression in cancer patients: review of diagnosis and treatment. *Curr Oncol Rep.* 2008;10:78–85.
179. Marrs JA. Nurse, my back hurts: understanding malignant spinal cord compression. *Clin J Oncol Nurs.* 2006;10:114–116.
180. Schild SE, Nisi K, Scheithauer BW, et al. The results of radiotherapy for ependymomas: the Mayo Clinic experience. *Int J Radiat Oncol Biol Phys.* 1998;42:953–958.
181. Houten JK, Cooper PR. Spinal cord astrocytomas: presentation, management and outcome. *J Neurooncol.* 2000;47:219–224.
182. Cole JS, Patchell RA. Metastatic epidural spinal cord compression. *Lancet Neurol.* 2008;7:459–466.
183. Hickey JV, Armstrong TS. Spinal cord tumors. In: Hickey JV, ed. *The Clinical Practice of Neurological and Neurosurgical Nursing.* 5th ed Philadelphia: Lippincott; 1997:509–521.
184. Schwartz TH, McCormick PC. Intramedullary ependymomas: clinical presentation, surgical treatment strategies and prognosis. *J Neurooncol.* 2000;47:211–218.
185. Helweg-Larsen S, Sorenson PS. Symptoms and signs in metastatic spinal cord compression: a study of progression from ffirst symptoms until diagnosis in 153 patients. *Eur J Cancer.* 1994;30A:396–398.
186. Rades D, Fehlauer F, Schulte R, et al. Prognostic factors for local control and survival after radiotherapy of metastatic spinal cord comprlession. *J Clin Oncol.* 2006;24:3388–3393.
187. Abernathey CD. Spinal intradural extramedullary tumors. In: Rengachary SS, Wilkins RH, eds. *Principles of Neurosurgery.* London: Wolfe; 1994:38–1-38–8.

188. Minehan KJ, Shaw EG, Scheithauer BW, et al. Spinal cord astrocytoma: pathological and treatment considerations. *J Neuro Surg.* 1995; 83:590–595.
189. Linstadt DE, Wara WM, Leibel SA, et al. Postoperative radiotherapy of primary spinal cord tumors. *Int J Radiat Oncol Biol Phys.* 1989;16:1397–1403.
190. Patchell RA, Tibbs PA, Regine WF, et al. Direct decompressive surgical resection in the treatment of spinal cord compression caused by metastatic cancer: a randomized trial. *Lancet.* 2005;366:643–648.
191. Daly FN, Schiff D. Supportive management of patients with brain tumors. *Expert Rev Neuropather.* 2007;7:1327–1336.
192. Drapatz J, Schiff D, Desari S, Norden AD, Wen PY. Medical management of brain tumor patients. *Neurol Clin.* 2007;25:1035–1071.
193. D'Avignon LC, Schofield CM, Hospenthal DR. Pneumocystis pneumonia. *Semin Respir Crit Care Med.* 2008;29:132–140.
194. Jamda M, Steginga S, Dunn J, Langbecker D, Walker D, Easkin E. Unmet supportive care needs and interest in services among patients with a brain tumour and their careers. *Patient Educ Couns.* 2008;71:251–258.

CHAPTER

50

Virginia R. Martin, MSN, RN, AOCN®, Susan Vogt Temple, RN, MSN, AOCN®

# Cervical Cancer

## INTRODUCTION

Cervical cancer is the second most common cancer in women worldwide. Persistent infection with oncogenic human papillomavirus (HPV), most frequently contracted through genital skin to skin contact/vaginal intercourse, is necessary for the development of cervical cancer and high-grade precursor lesions. Virtually all cases of invasive cervical cancer harbor HPV DNA sequences. Fortunately, most sexually active women in the US have transient HPV infections and clear the virus to undetectable or negligible levels within 1 to 2 years following exposure. In the US, the majority of cervical lesions are diagnosed in the preinvasive stages of intraepithelial neoplasia, when the disease is curable. Like many other cancers, cervical cancer can be cured when it is diagnosed in early stages. However, in developing nations and among older women, ethnic minorities, and the medically underserved in the US, cervical cancer screening is unavailable or inaccessible.

## EPIDEMIOLOGY

Cervical cancer remains a significant source of morbidity and mortality for women worldwide, with more than 500,000 women being diagnosed with invasive disease. Approximately 300,000 deaths are attributed to progressive disease and concomitant complications yearly.[1] Globally, cervical cancer ranks as the second most common cancer in women and is one of the leading causes of cancer-related deaths for women in developing nations. The highest incidence of invasive cervical cancer is reported in sub-Saharan Africa, the Caribbean, Central and South America, and southern Asia.[1] A disproportionate share (more than 80%) of cervical cancer deaths occur in those nations that lack the necessary resources and infrastructure for ongoing screening, surveillance, and treatment of preinvasive and invasive lesions.[2]

According to the American Cancer Society, 11,270 new cases of invasive cervical cancer will have been diagnosed in the US in 2009, and 4,070 women will die of the disease. Deaths from invasive cervical cancer decreased by 74% between 1955 and 1992, and they continue to decline by about 2% per year.[2,3] This dramatic decline can be attributed, in part, to increased utilization of the Pap test, which can identify premalignant changes in cervical cytology.[2,4] Cervical cancer rarely affects women younger than age 25.[2,5] Half of all women diagnosed with cervical cancer are between the ages of 35 and 55.[2] Nevertheless, invasive cervical cancer remains a significant health problem in women who are less likely to undergo regular screening and are at increased risk for cervical cancer, including women age 65 and older, minority populations including African American and Hispanic women, and those who are medically underserved.[2,4,5–7]

Although the incidence of invasive cervical cancer has decreased dramatically, the incidence of noninvasive disease or carcinoma in situ (CIS) in the US has climbed since 1945; this type of cancer is currently about 4 times more common than invasive disease. The increased incidence is due, in part, to early detection of preinvasive disease through screening and surveillance. Women with premalignant/CIS lesions are usually 10 to 15 years younger, on average, than women with invasive cervical cancer. This prolonged natural history, representing progression from preinvasive disease or intraepithelial carcinoma to clinically invasive disease, can allow for effective screening and early intervention.[5,8,9]

## ETIOLOGY

Epidemiological studies have produced substantial evidence indicating that *persistent infection with oncogenic HPVs* is the most significant risk factor for the development of preinvasive or invasive cervical cancer.[8–11] HPV is the most prevalent sexually transmitted disease; more than 100 distinct types of HPV have been identified and more than 40 types of HPVs can be sexually transmitted.[12,13] Low-risk forms of HPV (lrHPV), primarily HPV 6 and 11, are implicated in the etiology of genital warts (condylomata acuminata) and rarely lead to carcinogenesis, whereas oncogenic HPVs are referred to as "high-risk" viruses (hrHPV).[12–15]

Sexually transmitted high-risk HPVs induce cellular hyperproliferation and are integrated into the host genome in carcinomas. In HPV infections, the E2 protein binds to numerous sites in the nucleus, blocks gene transcription, and regulates cell growth indirectly through down-regulation of the *E6* and *E7* oncogenes. The E6 and E7 viral oncoproteins from oncogenic types of HPV inactivate the cell cycle regulators *p53* and retinoblastoma, providing the initiating event in abnormal cellular proliferation and carcinogenesis.[13,14,16,17] High-risk HPVs include types 16, 18, 31, 33, 35, 39, 45, 51, 52, 56, 58, 59, 66, 68, and 73.[13,14] In particular, HPV 16, 18, 31, 33, and 51 have been recovered from more than 95% of all invasive cervical neoplasms.[13,14] One 1999 study estimated that 99% of cervical cancers worldwide contain HPV DNA sequences.[9] Based on available data, the World Health Organization's International Agency for Research on Cancer has classified HPV 16 and 18 as carcinogenic in humans.[13,14] HPV 18 is associated with 15% to 50% of invasive cervical cancer lesions and is the most common papillomavirus found in women with adenocarcinoma of the cervix. HPV 16 is more commonly associated with squamous cell carcinomas.[5,16]

All sexually active women are at risk for HPV infection.[11] The list of risk factors for cervical cancer includes behaviors that increase the potential for exposure to oncogenic HPV (Table 50-1) as well as demographic and gynecologic factors. An estimated 20 million people in the US are infected with HPV, yet few of the women who have been exposed actually develop invasive cervical cancer.[17,18]

**TABLE 50-1**

| Risk Factors for Oncogenic HPV Exposure, Cervical Cancer Precursors, and Cervical Cancer |
|---|
| Infection with oncogenic forms of HPV |
| Cigarette smoking |
| Large number of sexual partners |
| Immunosuppression |
| Unavailability/lack of screening |
| Ethnic minority |
| Older age |
| Long-term oral contraceptive use |
| History of sexually transmitted diseases |
| Early age at first coitus |
| Partner sexual behaviors/number of sexual encounters |
| Partner whose partner/first wife was diagnosed with cervical cancer |
| DES exposure in utero |
| Diet low in folate, carotene, and vitamin C |
| Multiparity |

*Abbreviations*: DES, diethylstilbestrol; HPV, human papillomavirus.

HPV infection is suppressed or cleared in the majority of cases; only a minority of women exposed to high-risk forms of HPV develop a latent or persistent infection.[12–14,19]

Data indicate that oncogenic HPV infection by itself is a necessary but insufficient factor for the development of cervical neoplasia.[9,10] Other host and environmental cofactors have yet to be fully elucidated. Cofactors that may play a role in carcinogenesis include immunosuppression (HIV/AIDS and transplant-related immunosuppression)[12,20]; age; smoking/exposure to tobacco products[21–23]; and multiparity, long-term use of oral contraceptives, and the presence of other sexually transmitted diseases.[24] Cigarette smoking and tobacco use have been identified as cofactors for squamous cell cervical cancer development, as nicotine and the tobacco-specific carcinogen, cotinine, have been isolated from the cervical mucus and genital tracts of both women who use tobacco products and women who are passively exposed to cigarette smoke.[21–23]

Squamous cervical carcinoma is rare in women who are nulliparous, as well as in those who are lifetime celibates or in lifetime monogamous relationships. Females exposed to diethylstilbestrol (DES) in utero have a higher incidence of clear-cell adenocarcinoma of the cervix and vagina.[5]

Since 1993, cervical cancer has been designated as an AIDS-defining illness by the Centers for Disease Control and Prevention, and cervical intraepithelial neoplasia (CIN) has been designated as a human immunodeficiency virus (HIV)-related condition. Women with HIV infection are at higher risk for developing high-grade squamous intraepithelial lesions (HSIL) of the cervix; the increased risk may be due to an inability to effectively clear the virus. In HIV-infected females, cervical cancer may manifest itself in unusual ways, be more aggressive, and run a more fulminant course.

## PREVENTION, SCREENING, AND EARLY DETECTION

Prevention of cervical cancer centers on modifying sexual behavior, thereby limiting a woman's exposure to oncogenic HPV. Risk-reducing behaviors include limiting the number of lifetime sexual partners, maintenance of a lifetime monogamous relationship by both sexual partners, limiting sexual activity in the teenage years, use of barrier contraceptives to reduce exposure to other sexually transmitted diseases, and an increased understanding and practice of safe sexual behavior. In addition, screening (Pap test) at appropriate intervals and prompt treatment of cervical cancer precursors are integral to prevention and early detection. Women should also be encouraged to stop smoking and to avoid tobacco use.[25]

The Pap test is an effective and economical screening technique to detect cervical neoplasia. In the traditional Pap test, an Ayres spatula and cytobrush are used to collect squamous and endocervical cells. The collection/sample is then smeared on a glass slide, with the spatula used first, followed by the endocervical brush; the slide is then sprayed with a fixative. Accuracy of the Pap smear results depends on the sampling method, staining, and microscopic examination.[26–29] In 1999, the Agency for Health Care Policy and Research reported the results of a meta-analysis of 84 robust studies, which found that conventional Pap smears have a specificity of 98% and a sensitivity of 51%.[26]

Liquid-based cytology was developed to respond to 5 major limitations of conventional Pap tests: failure to capture the complete specimen; inadequate fixation/drying artifact; presence of elements that obscure evaluation; random distribution of abnormal cells; and technical variance in smear quality. When using liquid-based cytology, the cellular collection is not smeared on a slide but rather is transferred to a vial containing a liquid medium. Cells are separated from mucus and blood and placed in a single layer, which is then reviewed. Liquid-based cytology is more expensive than standard Pap tests but offers the advantages of greater accuracy and possibility of reflex HPV testing. "Reflex" testing refers to testing either the original liquid-based cytology residual specimen or a separate sample collected at the time of the initial screening visit for HPV testing. The increased accuracy of the test, when adjunctive HPV testing is done, reduces the need for repeat Pap tests and colposcopic evaluation. HPV testing is often used to triage equivocal Pap test results in the US and is also approved in primary screening in women 30 years and older.[30]

Automated interpreters can be useful in the detection of cervical abnormalities and can lower false-negative rates. High-resolution video scanners are able to distinguish between normal and abnormal cytologic specimens and can decrease mistakes due to human error.[5,31]

The National Cancer Institute (NCI), the Society of Gynecologic Oncologists, and the Society of Gynecologic Nurse Oncologists support recently revised guidelines on screening for cervical cancer and precursor lesions. The American Cancer Society[32] released its revised guidelines in November 2002 and currently is in the process of reviewing these guidelines again; the US Preventive Services Task Force published its recommendations in January 2003.[33] Summary points include the following:

- All women who are or have been sexually active should begin having Pap tests 3 years following initiation of vaginal intercourse but no later than at 21 years old.
- Screening should be done every year with the conventional Pap test or every 2 years when using the newer liquid-based Pap test.
- Beginning at age 30, women who have had 3 or more consecutive normal Pap tests in a row may be screened every 2 to 3 years with the conventional Pap test or liquid-based Pap test.
- Women with specific risk factors (eg, immunosuppression, exposure to DES in utero) may need to be screened more frequently.
- Women 70 years of age or older who have had 3 or more normal Pap tests in a row and no abnormal Pap tests in the last 10 years may opt to stop cervical cancer screening. Women with a history of cervical cancer, DES exposure in utero, HIV infection, or immunosuppression should continue to be screened.
- Women who have had a total hysterectomy (including removal of the cervix) may choose to stop cervical cancer screening unless the surgery was done for cervical cancer or precursor lesions. Women who have a cervix should screen according to the preceding guidelines.

In November 2009, the American College of Obstetricians and Gynecologists (ACOG) revised cervical cancer screening guidelines to recommend women begin cervical cancer screening at age 21, instead of 3 years after the onset of sexual activity. Additionally ACOG has recommended that women 30 years or older should be screened by conventional or liquid Pap test once every two years (http://www.acog.org/publications/educational_bulletins/pb109.cfm).

## PREINVASIVE DISEASE

### SQUAMOUS INTRAEPITHELIAL LESIONS

The cervix—the lower part of the uterus—extends from the isthmus into the vagina and is divided into 2 major parts: the endocervix and the exocervix. The endocervix is contiguous to the exocervix, which includes the external os and extends to the vaginal fornix. Squamous epithelial cells line the outside surface of the cervix and the vagina, while columnar epithelial cells line the rest of the cervix and the uterus. The *squamocolumnar junction* (often identified as the transformation zone) refers to the area where the columnar epithelium of the endocervix joins the squamous epithelium of the exocervix at the os (Figure 50-1). The position of the transformation zone changes over time, moving up and into the endocervical canal as stratified squamous epithelium replaces the glandular epithelium.[34] Cancer of the cervix is a culmination of a progressive disease that begins as a series of events that occurs in the squamocolumnar junction—HPV infection, persistence, progression into precursor lesions, and invasive cancer.[34] Over time, precursor lesions, termed high-grade cervical intraepithelial neoplasia (CIN2 or CIN3), can progress to involve the full thickness of the epithelium and invade the stromal tissue of the cervix.[5,31]

#### Assessment

Despite the presence of CIN, no gross lesions or abnormality may be observed during the visual inspection of the cervix. Visual inspections are limited because only a portion of the cervix is visible for assessment.

The Pap smear is an effective and economical screening and assessment tool. There have been many refinements made in this technology. The terminology used to describe cervical cytology has changed since the original Papanicolaou numeric system was introduced. Originally, Pap smear findings were divided into 5 classes (I to V) that described atypical changes in cervical cells. In 1988,

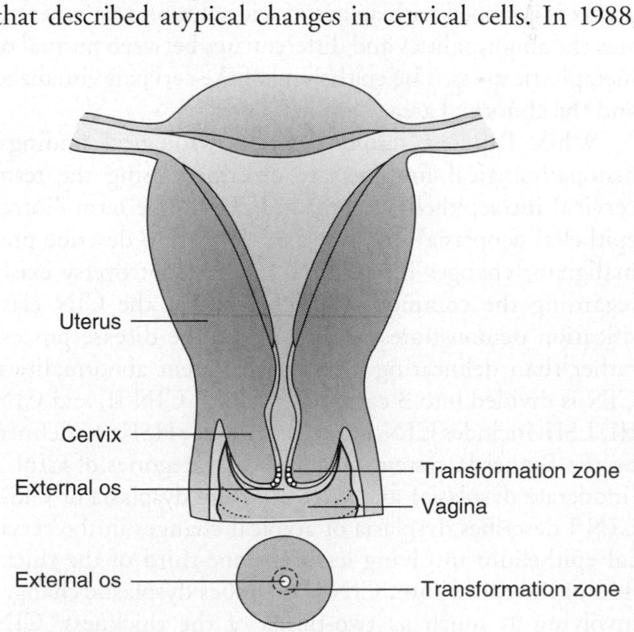


**FIGURE 50-1**

Cervical transformation zone.

a workshop sponsored by the NCI was held in Bethesda, Maryland, to address problems inherent in the Papanicolaou system. The goal was to review existing terminology and to make recommendations for a more effective method of reporting. The outcome of this conference was the Bethesda system (TBS).[25,31,35,36]

The Bethesda system, proposed in 1988, updated in 1991, and revised in 2001, describes the type and adequacy of the specimen submitted, indicates the testing performed, and gives an interpretation of the results.[25,35–37] Under the 2001 Bethesda guidelines, the Pap test can be "negative for intraepithelial lesion" or it can evidence "epithelial cell abnormalities." Epithelial cell abnormalities are divided into squamous cell or glandular cell abnormalities. Squamous cell abnormalities include *atypical squamous cells of undetermined significance* (ASC-US), *atypical squamous cells—cannot exclude high-grade squamous intraepithelial abnormality* (ASC-H), *low-grade squamous intraepithelial lesion* (LSIL), HSIL, and *squamous cell carcinoma*. Glandular cell abnormalities include *atypical glandular cells* (AGC), with qualifying statements being added to indicate the cellular origin of the atypical cells (endometrial, glandular, or endocervical). AGCs detected on cervical Pap tests may indicate significant cervical or endometrial pathology, and additional testing is required in certain situations.[25,35–37]

When the Pap test report shows ASC-H or SIL, or if the patient is considered to be at high risk for cervical cancer, referral for colposcopic examination with endocervical assessment, biopsy, and/or treatment is indicated. Colposcopy is performed on an outpatient basis, using a stereoscopic, binocular microscope that illuminates and magnifies the view of the cervix. During this procedure, the cervix is swabbed with an acetic acid solution that accentuates the abnormalities and differentiates between normal or metaplastic areas. The epithelium of the cervix is visualized and the abnormal areas biopsied.[5,25,31,35,37]

While Pap test results describe cytological findings, histopathological findings are described using the term cervical intraepithelial neoplasia (CIN). The term "intraepithelial neoplasia" or "dysplasia" is used to describe premalignant changes in epithelial tissue. Controversy exists regarding the commonly held belief that the CIN classification demonstrates progression of the disease process rather than delineating distinctly different abnormalities. CIN is divided into 3 categories: CIN I, CIN II, and CIN III. LSIL includes CIN 1 and condyloma; HSIL, as defined by the Bethesda system, includes the categories of CIN 2 (moderate dysplasia) and CIN 3 (severe dysplasia or CIS). CIN I describes dysplasia or atypical changes in the cervical epithelium involving less than one-third of the thickness of the epithelium. CIN II describes dysplastic changes involving as much as two-thirds of the thickness. CIN III, also known as severe dysplasia or CIS, involves two-thirds to full thickness involvement of the epithelium with no areas of stromal invasion or metastases (Figure 50-2).

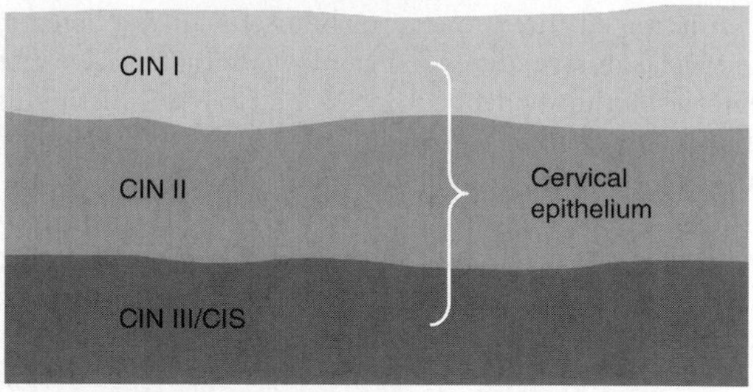


**FIGURE 50-2**

Atypical changes in the cervix.

Once the disease progresses beyond the basement membrane and invades the cervical stroma, it is considered invasive.[5,25,31,35,37]

In 2006 a group of 146 experts met to develop consensus guidelines for the management of women with abnormal cervical cancer screening test results. The results published included some additional information and direction for the management of women with cytologic abnormalities in 2007.[30] Many of the recommendations listed previously remain unchanged but a few additional clarifications were developed to help guide practitioners. Managing ASC-US or LSIL is unchanged except adolescents with these results are now recommended to have cytological follow-up for 2 years. The management of HSIL and AGC has more emphasis on immediate screening and treatment for HSIL. HPV testing is incorporated in to the management of AGC after initial evaluation with colposcopy and endometrial sampling. In addition, the 2004 HPV guidance for testing was adopted, which outlines HPV testing as an adjunct to cervical cytology screening for women 30 years and older.

An international study published this year may change testing for women in developing countries. The study compared HPV testing vs cytological testing, vs visual inspection of the cervix with acetic acid, vs standard care to 131,746 healthy women in 52 village clusters in India. The results found that single round HPV testing was associated with a significant decline in the rate of advanced cervical cancers and associated deaths compared to the unscreened group.[38] In addition, there was no significant reduction in the rate of death in either the cytological testing group or the visual inspection group as compared with the control group.[38] The authors conclude that the higher sensitivity of HPV testing to detect lesions with a higher potential for malignant transformation resulted in the reduction of incidence of advanced cancer and death.

## THERAPEUTIC APPROACHES AND NURSING CARE

Each type of SIL lesion can regress, persist, or become invasive. High-grade SIL (CIN 3) is more likely to progress than the milder forms, which may regress spontaneously to normal. The rate of progression from LSIL to HSIL is less than 20%. Unlike LSIL, however, HSIL (CIN 2 and 3) has a greater potential to progress to invasive cervical cancer if left untreated. Because there is no way to predict which lesions will become invasive and which will not, patients with low-grade lesions are followed and high-grade lesions are treated when they are discovered.[5,18,19,31,35,37,39–41]

It is critical that the extent of the lesion be determined as accurately as possible before treatment begins. The Pap test, colposcopy, and colposcopically directed biopsies may determine the extent, depth, and severity of the cervical lesion, differentiating between SIL, CIS, and invasive carcinoma of the cervix. Treatment for SIL includes a diagnostic excisional procedure such as a direct cervical biopsy, cryotherapy, laser surgery, electrosurgery, cone biopsy, or hysterectomy. The selection of therapy is based on the extent of the disease, patient compliance with follow-up, the patient's wishes to preserve ovarian and reproductive function, and the physician's recommendation. In general, complications of excisional therapies are related to the amount of endocervix that is removed.[5,25,31,35,37,41]

Cryotherapy has been used for more than 50 years and is an effective option for the treatment of CIN in selected patients. This technique uses liquid nitrogen to induce freezing of cervical tissue. A portable probe is placed on the lesion; the probe is then activated to initiate freezing, which in turn leads to tissue necrosis. Cryotherapy is a cost-effective and relatively painless treatment with low morbidity that can be performed on an outpatient basis. Patients most often complain of a watery discharge for 2 to 4 weeks after treatment. Reepithelialization is complete within 3 months of therapy. Serious complications secondary to cryotherapy are rare.[5,25,35,37,41]

Laser technology can also be used to eradicate SIL. The laser is mounted on the colposcope, and the beam is directed under colposcopic control. The advantage of using a laser is that significantly less disease-free tissue is removed with the entire lesion. Patients may experience a little more discomfort than with cryosurgery, but there is usually less vaginal discharge, and complete healing occurs in about 2 weeks. A primary disadvantage of laser treatment is that it may cause thermal damage to the tissue specimen, making it difficult for the pathologist to rule out invasive cancer.[5,25,31,35,37,41]

The most widespread excisional technique used in the treatment of SIL is the loop electrosurgical excision procedure (LEEP) or large loop diathermy excision of the transformation zone (LLETZ). LEEP uses a thin wire loop and a low level of electricity to excise affected cervical tissue with minimal ablation. Because very thin wires are used, greater control can be exercised over the amount of tissue removed; additionally, the excised tissue contains minimal thermal artifact that might hinder the histopathological evaluation. The patient can expect a heavy, brown, and sometimes malodorous discharge for 2 to 3 weeks following the LEEP. Patients should avoid heavy lifting or strenuous activity for several weeks after the procedure and should not insert anything into the vagina for 4 weeks. Complications of loop excision therapy occur in 1% to 2% of patients and include infection and heavy bleeding. Later complications may include delayed bleeding and cervical stenosis. In selected patients, use of LEEP may allow for diagnosis and treatment of SIL during one outpatient visit. The "see and treat" office visit avoids the usual 2 sessions (diagnosis at initial visit and biopsy during the second) and is particularly advantageous in situations where patient follow-up is episodic or inconsistent.[5,25,31,35,37,41,42]

Cold knife conization involves removal of a cone-shaped piece of tissue from the exocervix and the endocervix. Performed under general anesthesia on an outpatient basis, conization can be used in 4 situations as follows:

1. For diagnosis, if no lesion of the cervix is noted and an endocervical tumor is suspected
2. To determine the extent of the lesion if microinvasion is diagnosed on biopsy; or if the entire lesion cannot be seen with the colposcope;
3. If there are discrepancies between the cytological report (Pap test) and the histological appearance of the lesions on biopsy;
4. When the patient cannot be relied upon for long-term follow-up.

Major immediate complications of conization may include hemorrhage, uterine perforation, and complications of anesthesia. Delayed complications may include bleeding, cervical stenosis, infertility, cervical incompetence, and increased chances of preterm (low-birth-weight) delivery.[5,25,35,37,41,43]

Total vaginal hysterectomy (TVH) may be employed for treatment of individuals with HSIL (CIN III). This option is appropriate for individuals with HSIL who have completed childbearing. These individuals must be followed as closely for recurrence as those patients who are treated with more conservative measures.[5,25,41,43]

The primary nursing responsibilities for women with SIL relate to education. This educational process includes defining the disease, explaining the treatment, teaching the importance of close follow-up, and modifying high-risk behaviors.[25,37,41]

If the biopsy indicates the presence of SIL, the woman may erroneously think that she has invasive cancer. She may also blame herself, her past sexual behavior, and her sexual partners for exposure to oncogenic HPV and subsequent development of SIL. The nurse must assure the patient that she does not have cancer and that SIL is an easily treated premalignant condition. In women treated for SIL, self-esteem may drop and anxiety may increase during the initial and postsurgical visits. In addition, women may fear losing fertility and sexual function. The nurse should help the woman understand the type of treatment recommended, explain the nature and purpose of treatment, and describe the side effects of the therapy.[25,31,37]

Following treatment, the nurse instructs the woman on how to care for herself at home. Douching, tampons, and sexual intercourse are prohibited for at least 2 to 4 weeks, depending on the treatment. A return visit must be scheduled for 2 to 4 weeks, then every 3 months for a year, and every 6 months thereafter. The importance of this follow-up must be stressed, because there is a possibility of treatment failure or recurrence of the SIL. Minimal bleeding and vaginal discharge may be present for a week or longer after biopsy, cryosurgery, LEEP, or laser and for several weeks following conization.[25,31,37]

Information concerning sexual functioning and fertility should be discussed with women undergoing treatment for SIL, although electrocautery, cryosurgery, laser therapy, and conization rarely cause physiological sexual dysfunction. Most women report no change in libido, orgasm, coital frequency, or overall satisfaction with their sex life. Fertility is usually maintained, but difficulty with conception may occur. Nurses should take time to educate women about reducing risk factors (eg, HIV and multiple sexual partners) and preventive measures (eg, smoking reduction, minimizing the number of sexual partners, and barrier protection) related to preinvasive disease. Table 50-2 summarizes issues specifically related to nursing management of patients with preinvasive disease.[25,31,37]

Although mortality rates for cervical cancer have decreased over the past 40 years, the rates among ethnic minorities, poor women, and elderly women of all races are higher due to decreased utilization of screening methods in these populations. Access to cervical cancer screening for African Americans, Hispanics, older women, and those who are economically disadvantaged should be a priority for healthcare professionals. Barriers that discourage women from taking advantage of cervical screening include embarrassment, discomfort, financial burden, fatalism, lack of access, lack of transportation, population mobility, opposition by partners, lack of education, lack of health insurance, and age.[4–7,25] Researchers have employed some creative approaches to increase cervical cancer screening and follow-up for underserved groups, including a screening program in a public hospital emergency room, Pap smear screening offered in an inpatient setting, the use of lay educators, the use of nurse practitioners for cervical screening in medically underserved areas, culturally based educational programs, and interventions based on socioeconomic status.[4–7,25]

## INVASIVE DISEASE

### PATHOPHYSIOLOGY

#### Cellular characteristics

Invasive cervical cancer types are divided into 3 major categories: squamous carcinoma, adenocarcinoma, and other types. Histologically, 80% to 90% of cervical tumors are squamous cell carcinomas; 10% to 20% are adenocarcinomas. A very small number of epithelial cervical cancers include adenosquamous and glassy cell carcinomas, and neuroendocrine variants including carcinoid, large cell neuroendocrine, and small cell cancers of the cervix. Squamous carcinomas originate in the squamocolumnar junction and are often associated with CIS, microinvasive disease, and invasive carcinoma. They are assigned 1 of 4 grades: well differentiated (G1), moderately differentiated (G2), poorly differentiated (G3), or undifferentiated (G4).[43]

Adenocarcinomas generally occur in younger women and carry a greater risk, because the tumor arises within the endocervical mucus-producing gland cells. The tumor can become quite bulky before it becomes clinically evident. The bulkiness makes the tumor harder to treat, so this type of cancer has a high rate of local recurrence. Adenocarcinomas appear to be increasing in prevalence and are more difficult to detect than squamous carcinomas. There is no consistent definition of this histological type, no uniform reporting method, and no clear-cut histological pattern for correlation of cytological features.[43,44] Oral contraceptives may be associated with higher rates of adenocarcinoma in younger women, especially if oral contraceptives are used during adolescence when the cervix has not fully matured.[5,43]

Primary sarcomas and lymphomas of the cervix have been described in the literature. The incidence of primary or secondary sarcomas and lymphomas is very rare.[5,43]

#### Progression of disease

Initially, the invasive malignant process breaks through the basement membrane to invade the cervical stroma. The lesion may infiltrate the endocervix, be exophytic and extend into the exocervix, or be visible as a superficial ulceration. The lesion may then spread in any direction by direct extension. For example, it may begin on the endocervix and spread through cervix, into the parametrial tissue, and through the vesicovaginal and rectovaginal septae into the bladder and rectum. The upper vagina and corpus of the uterus may also become involved.[5,43,45]

Involvement of the lymph nodes in the spread of cervical cancer is fairly predictable and includes paracervical and parametrial lymphatics. Obturator, hypogastric, and other external iliac nodes may be involved; the tumor may also metastasize to the common iliac or para-aortic lymph nodes. Parametrial lymph node metastasis occurs and may be correlated with involvement of iliac lymph nodes.[5,43]

Hematogenous spread through the venous plexus and the paracervical veins occurs less frequently than lymphatic spread but is relatively common in the more advanced stages of disease. The most common sites of distant metastasis are the mediastinal and supraclavicular nodes, lungs, liver, and bone.[5,43]

**Treatment Modalities and Nursing Management of the Woman With Cervical Preinvasive or Invasive Disease**

| Treatment Modalities | Nursing Management |
|---|---|
| Local therapies (eg, laser cryosurgery, electrocautery) for preinvasive (SIL, CIN) disease | Explain the disease. Assure patient that SIL (CIN) is not cancer.<br>Explain treatment and possible complications of treatment.<br>Discuss possibility of treatment failure.<br>Instruct in self-care after treatment (no douching, tampons, sexual intercourse for 2–4 weeks).<br>Stress importance of follow-up care (next appointment, call physician if fever, bleeding develops).<br>Assess concerns related to sexual function (changes in libido, orgasm, coital frequency, fertility).<br>Assess for anxiety, depression, changes in body, self-image.<br>Assess for psychological issues associated with sexually transmitted disease (guilt, blame, mistrust). |
| Surgery | Instruct patient preoperatively in use of incentive spirometer, importance of turning, coughing, deep breathing, abdominal splinting, early ambulation, and use of antiemboletic stockings. Have patient do return demonstration as indicated.<br>Review bowel preparation procedure.<br>Review need for IV, urinary catheter, colostomy, ileal conduit as indicated.<br>Begin ostomy teaching preoperatively as indicated.<br>Stress availability of pain medication.<br>Review use of patient-controlled analgesia as indicated.<br>Explore nonpharmacologic pain relief measures with patient.<br>Provide postoperative wound care.<br>Encourage patient to participate in wound care as indicated.<br>Assess concerns related to sexual function (changes in libido, orgasm, coital frequency, fertility).<br>Assess cultural beliefs as they relate to treatment (blood transfusions, avoidance of drugs, dietary restrictions).<br>Assess spiritual needs/concerns.<br>Assess vital signs, body systems, lab values postoperatively.<br>Assess for deep-vein thrombosis.<br>Assess nutritional status, lymphedema, skin integrity hazards of immobility, alteration in sleep/rest patterns.<br>Assess psychosocial functioning. |
| Radiotherapy | Review treatment procedure (eg, external beam, intracavitary).<br>Review side effects of therapy (eg, to skin, effect on blood values, vaginal stenosis as indicated).<br>Explain mobility restrictions with intracavity, interstitial radiotherapy as indicated.<br>Assess for deep-vein thrombosis.<br>Encourage diversional activities to relieve boredom.<br>Emphasize availability of pain relief measures.<br>Explore nonpharmacologic pain relief measures with patient.<br>Assess concerns related to sexual function (changes in libido, orgasm, coital frequency, fertility).<br>Assess cultural beliefs as they relate to treatment (blood transfusions, avoidance of drugs, dietary restrictions).<br>Assess spiritual needs/concerns. |
| Chemotherapy | Explain treatment (rationale for chemotherapy, name of chemotherapy agents, nadir, method of administration, side effects).<br>Assess psychological status of patient.<br>Assess for anxiety, depression, changes in body, self-image.<br>Assess effects of treatment on quality of life.<br>Assess concerns related to sexual function.<br>Assess cultural beliefs as they relate to treatment (blood transfusions, avoidance of drugs, dietary restrictions).<br>Assess spiritual needs/concerns. |
| Clinical trials | Review information related to clinical trials if indicated. |

### Clinical manifestations

Cervical cancer is usually asymptomatic in its preinvasive and early stages, although women may notice a watery or mucoid vaginal discharge. In the majority of cases, the disease is discovered by Pap test during routine examination. Later symptoms that often prompt the woman to seek medical attention in cervical cancer include postcoital bleeding, intermenstrual bleeding, or heavy menstrual flow. If this bleeding is chronic, the woman may complain of symptoms related to anemia. A common complaint in advanced cervical malignancy is that of a foul-smelling, serosanguineous, or yellowish vaginal discharge.[5,43,45]

Other late symptoms, which are indicative of advanced disease, include pain in the pelvis, hypogastrium, lumbosacral or gluteal area, flank, or leg. This pain occurs secondary to involvement of the pelvic wall, ureters, lymph nodes, or sciatic nerve roots. Urinary and rectal symptoms may indicate invasion of these structures by tumor. End-stage disease may be characterized by edema of the lower extremities due to lymphatic and venous obstruction. Massive vaginal hemorrhage and development of renal failure may result from local invasion of blood vessels and bilateral ureteral obstruction by tumor.[5,43,45]

## ASSESSMENT

### Physical examination

The most frequent physical finding for invasive cervical cancer is a lesion on the cervix. Suspicious lesions should be biopsied to an adequate depth to confirm the diagnosis of invasive carcinoma. Lesions that extend into the exocervix are termed exophytic; lesions may also be ulcerative or plaque-like. Cervical cancer is staged clinically by bimanual pelvic and rectovaginal examination, with careful attention being paid to the size of the lesion and free space between the tumor and the pelvic sidewall. The tumor may extend into the adjacent vaginal fornices or to the paracervical and parametrial tissues; if untreated, it may invade the bladder, rectum, or both.[5,43,45]

Surgical staging to ascertain pelvic and para-aortic lymph nodes status before treatment has been evaluated in several clinical trials. Although surgical findings do not change the clinical stage, information obtained via surgery may influence therapeutic interventions.[5,43,45]

### Diagnostic studies

Diagnostic testing may include chest and computerized tomography (CT) scans, complete blood count (CBC), and blood chemistries. Computerized axial tomograms may be used to determine the extent of pelvic disease, to define radiotherapy portals, and to evaluate lymph node status. However, CT and magnetic resonance imaging (MRI) are not effective in detecting small metastases. The main use of CT is to help identify enlarged lymph nodes in the pelvis and para-aortic areas. MRI offers no advantage over CT in evaluating lymph node metastasis or assessing the parametrium. Researchers have found, however, that MRI provides improved evaluation of tumor size, stromal invasion, and extent of disease as compared to CT.[46] Both CT and MRI are generally able to evaluate lymph node metastasis (86% each). Although MRI has been used to assess the response of cervical cancer to neoadjuvant chemotherapy, it is not as precise as surgical staging. Verification of tumor volume (the most important prognostic factor for survival of the patient with cervical cancer) by MRI may help the physician to determine the best treatment modality. Positron emission tomography (PET) may be able to detect disease not seen on CT or MRI. In addition, PET, if used in conjunction with CT and MRI, may be better able to determine the extent of local disease and nodal involvement.[5,43,45]

Ureteral obstruction has been found in 30% of patients with stage III disease and as many as 50% of women with stage IV disease; these patients will present with hydronephrosis on the affected side and require insertion of ureteral stents. Cystoscopy and rectosigmoidoscopy, often done under anesthesia (EUA), are indicated in patients with advanced-stage disease.[5,43,45]

A supraclavicular node biopsy is performed if one of these nodes is palpable or if para-aortic nodes are positive. The left node is most often positive—it is where the thoracic duct enters into the subclavian vein. Positive supraclavicular nodes are often associated with a positive aortic node. In such cases, a blind scalene node biopsy is recommended. If this biopsy is positive, systemic therapy is necessary. Following a thorough evaluation, the clinical stage is determined.[5,43,45]

### Prognostic indicators

Factors that influence prognosis include stage, tumor volume, tumor histology and grade, lymph node and endometrial involvement, and presence of lymphovascular space invasion in the pathological specimen.[5,43,45,47,48] Coexpression of epidermal growth factor receptors (EGFRs) and cyclooxygenase-2 portends a poorer prognosis in patients with stage IIB disease. Performance status and patient age are also significant in more advanced stages.[49] Both squamous cell antigens and tumor markers have been evaluated for their clinical significance; however, application of the information gleaned from these data has been limited to clinical studies. These measures are not readily available for screening or for ongoing clinical evaluation.[45]

## CLASSIFICATION AND STAGING

Cervical cancer is staged clinically by physical exam, with confirmation being obtained from bimanual pelvic and rectovaginal examinations completed with the patient under anesthesia. Research in the direction of surgical staging is encouraged.[50] The exam under anesthesia approach allows for more accurate staging, including visualization of the upper vagina and palpation of parametrial and lateral side wall tissues. Evaluation under anesthesia (EUA) usually occurs at the same time as the planned surgical intervention or when radiation implants are inserted.[43,45,51,52] The clinical stage is not changed if disease recurs.

The most commonly used staging system used today is the International Federation of Gynecology and Obstetrics (FIGO) system (Table 50-3). This system was most recently revised in 2009. The American Joint Committee on Cancer staging system may also be used; both staging systems are applicable to all histological types. The identifier microinvasion, however, is used only with squamous cell carcinoma.[43,45,51]

Disease that is confined to the cervix is defined as stage I. Stratification into particular substages is based on depth and breadth of invasion. Stage IA lesions are considered microinvasive, and risk of lymph node metastases and recurrent disease is low. Stage II disease includes lesions in which the tumor has extended beyond the cervix but has not extended to the pelvic wall. The tumor has extended to the pelvic wall in stage III disease. Tumors that involve the lower one-third of the vagina and all cases with hydronephrosis or nonfunctioning kidney are considered to be stage III (unless they are due to other comorbid conditions). Spread to adjacent organs or a distant site is included in stage IV.[43,45,51]

## THERAPEUTIC APPROACHES AND NURSING CARE

Once invasive cervical cancer is diagnosed and the clinical stage is established, treatment is based on the woman's age, general medical condition including comorbidities, extent of the cancer, and the presence of any complicating abnormalities. Either surgery or radiation therapy can be used with equal efficacy for patients with early-stage disease; surgical procedures may be accomplished using a laparotomy

**TABLE 50-3**

**Revised Federation of Gynecology and Obstetrics (FIGO) Staging for Carinoma of the Cervix**

| Stage | Description |
|---|---|
| 0 | Carcinoma in situ, intraepithelial carcinoma. |
| I | The carcinoma is strictly confined to the cervix. |
| IA | Invasive cancer identified only microscopically. All gross lesions even with superficial invasion are stage IB cancers. Invasion is limited to measured stromal invasion with maximum depth of 5 mm and no wider than 7 mm. |
| IA1 | Measured invasion of stroma no greater than 3 mm in depth and no wider than 7 mm. |
| IA2 | Measured invasion of stroma greater than 3 mm and no greater than 5 mm in depth, and no wider than 7 mm. |
| IB | Clinical lesions confined to the cervix or preclinical lesions greater than stage IA. |
| IB1 | Clinical lesions no greater than 4 cm in size. |
| IB2 | Clinical lesions greater than 4 cm in size. |
| II | The carcinoma extends beyond the cervix but has not extended to the pelvic wall. The carcinoma involves the vagina but not as far as the lower third. |
| IIA1 | Tumor size of less than or equal to 4 cm. with involvement of less than the upper two-thirds of the vagina. |
| IIB2 | Tumor size of more than 4 cm. with involvement of less than the upper two-thirds of the vagina. |
| III | The carcinoma has extended to the pelvic wall. On rectal examination, there is no cancer-fee space between the tumor and the pelvic wall. The tumor involves the lower third of the vagina. All cases with hydronephrosis or nonfunctioning kidney are included unless they are known to be due to other causes. |
| IIIA | No extension to the pelvic wall. |
| IIIB | Extension to the pelvic wall and/or hydronephrosis of nonfunctioning kidney. |
| IV | The carcinoma has extended beyond the true pelvis or has clinically involved the mucosa of the bladder or rectum. A bullous edema as such does not permit a case to be allotted to stage IV. |
| IVA | Spread of the growth to adjacent organs. |
| IVB | Spread to distant organs. |

*Source*: Data from Pecorelli et al.[50]

incision or using minimally invasive techniques.[43,45] With either radiation therapy or surgery, the 5-year survival rate for early-stage cervical cancer is 85%.[5,43] In the past 20 years, outcomes for locally advanced disease have improved with radiation therapy. This trend reflects more adequate placement of intracavitary brachytherapy, higher paracentral doses, and reduction of overall treatment time. Radiation therapy can be used for all individuals, whereas surgery is indicated only for women who are considered good surgical candidates. In general, patients with more advanced disease (stages IIb to IV) are treated with radiation therapy.[5,43,53–55]

Several randomized trials have shown a survival advantage for cisplatin-based chemotherapy given concurrently with radiation therapy.[53–61] The positive trials vary in terms of disease stage, radiation dose, and schedule of chemotherapy/radiation therapy, yet all demonstrate a significant benefit of concurrent therapy. The risk of death from cervical cancer is reduced by 30% to 50%, suggesting that cisplatin-based chemotherapy should be given to women who require radiation therapy for the treatment of cervical cancer.[53–61]

## STAGES IA1, IA2, AND IB1

Stage IA disease (microinvasive carcinoma) has been subdivided into 2 stages, IA1 and IA2. Stage IA1 (≤3 mm depth of invasion, horizontal dimension < 7 mm, no lymphatic or vascular space involvement) should be treated by total abdominal hysterectomy (TAH) or TVH if the patient is healthy and does not desire further childbearing. Conization can be done for those women who are poor surgical risks or who wish to preserve fertility, as long as the biopsy margins are free of disease and the patient is followed closely. Intracavitary radiation may also be utilized to treat cervical cancer in this stage.[5,43,45,48]

Stage IA2 disease is treated by TAH or TVH if invasion is less than 3 mm and there is no lymphovascular involvement. If the invasion is greater than 3 mm or lymphovascular invasion has occurred, the disease is managed the same way as stage IB disease. Five-year survival in patients with properly staged IA cervical cancer is close to 100%. Conservative measures are recommended to treat stage IA1 cervical cancer, whereas more aggressive measures (radical or modified radical hysterectomy with pelvic lymph node dissection) are indicated for stage IA2 because of the higher risk of lymphovascular involvement.[5,43,45]

Some patients who desire a fertility sparing procedure may be candidates for radical vaginal or abdominal trachelectomy. Young women with stage IAI, IA2, and IBI can be considered for radical trachelectomy; this procedure is a conservative, yet radical approach in which the corpus uteri is left intact and fertility potential may be maintained. The cervix, parametrium, and vaginal cuff are excised; lymphadenectomy is accomplished laproscopically.[62–65]

## STAGES IB2 AND IIA

In 1995, FIGO subdivided stage IB into stage IB1 (lesions ≤ 4 cm in size) and stage IB2 (lesions > 4 cm in size), also called bulky disease. The choice of therapy for patients with stage IB2 and IIA disease remains controversial. There are 3 directions for treatment of women with bulky disease: primary chemoradiotherapy; neoadjuvant chemotherapy followed by radical hysterectomy and subsequent chemoradiotherapy; or primary radical hysterectomy and lymphadenectomy followed by tailored radiotherapy with concomitant radiotherapy.[66]

Some gynecologic oncologists prefer surgery to radiotherapy because ovarian function may be preserved with the former approach. Radical hysterectomy involves removal of the uterus, upper third of the vagina, entire uterosacral and uterovesical ligaments, all of the parametria, and pelvic node lymphadenectomy. It is a complex procedure because the organs removed are proximal to many vital body structures—the bladder, ureters, rectum, and great vessels of the pelvis. The major complications of radical hysterectomy include ureteral fistulas, bladder dysfunction, pulmonary embolus, lymphocysts, pelvic infection, bowel obstruction, rectovaginal fistulas, and hemorrhage. The vagina usually remains more pliable after surgery than with radiation, the overall treatment time is shorter, and long-term radiation complications to pelvic tissue can be avoided. Postoperative bladder dysfunction is manifested by the loss of the sense to void and inability to empty the bladder. A suprapubic catheter is placed intraoperatively, and the patient is taught bladder training before discharge. Alternatively, the patient may be taught intermittent self-catheterization. Postoperatively, potential complications include bleeding, infection, pneumonia, pulmonary embolus, myocardial infarction, and deep-vein thrombosis. Patients should be ambulatory on the first postoperative day.

The upper portion of the vagina is removed in a radical hysterectomy; the vagina may be shorter but remains distensible. Psychosexual sequelae following radical hysterectomy include sexual dysfunction and infertility.[5,43,45]

Radiation therapy has the advantages of avoiding major intraoperative and postoperative complications and allowing the patient to receive the therapy as an outpatient. Acute and chronic complications following radiation therapy include diarrhea, abdominal cramping, desquamation of the skin, anemia, sexual dysfunction and infertility, fistulas, bowel obstructions, and vaginal stenosis. Patients should be instructed to engage in vaginal intercourse or use a vaginal dilator 3 times a week in an effort to delimit vaginal stenosis.[45,47]

Patients with bulky disease (barrel-shaped cervix) have a higher incidence of central recurrence, pelvic and para-aortic lymph node metastases, and distant dissemination. An increased dose of radiation to the central pelvis followed 6 weeks later by radical hysterectomy, or both, have been advocated in patients with bulky disease. Radical surgery followed by radiation therapy remains controversial because the patient faces the prospect of complications associated with each treatment modality and the potential for concomitant toxicity from combination therapy.[5,43,45]

The clinical trials in locally advanced cervical cancer have provided the data that the use of cisplatin with radiotherapy is more beneficial than radiotherapy alone. More recently, a Gynecology Oncology Group (GOG) trial in women with earlier stage disease showed radiation treatment with randomization to with or without cisplatin resulted in a 50% reduction in risk of recurrent disease in the chemotherapy arm and improved survival.[46,59,66,67]

Since cervical cancer is a chemosensitive disease, studies have suggested that neoadjuvant therapy may improve the resectability of bulky lesions. A prospective trial compared surgery with or without neoadjuvant chemotherapy in 205 women with stage IB disease > 2 cm. The women were randomly assigned to surgery followed by radiotherapy or neoadjuvant chemotherapy with cisplatin, vincristine, and bleomycin for 3 courses followed by surgery and postoperative radiotherapy. The results showed only a small trend toward better survival in the neoadjuvant group (82% vs 77%).[66,68] The neoadjuvant group did however show improved long-term survival even though postoperative therapy was radiotherapy alone and as stated above this approach is now known to be inferior to concomitant chemoradiotherapy. Thus, neoadjuvant therapy continues to be investigated and a trial is underway in Europe that compares chemoradiotherapy to neoadjuvant chemotherapy followed by surgery.

## STAGES IIB, III, AND IVA—LOCALLY ADVANCED DISEASE

Women with stage IIB, III, or IV cervical cancer are treated with high doses of external pelvic radiation followed by high dose rate (HDR) or low dose rate (LDR) brachytherapy and concomitant chemotherapy. Randomized trials and meta-analysis reported a 30% to 50% reduction in the risk of death from cervical cancer for women with locally advanced disease undergoing radiotherapy and concomitant cisplatin-based chemotherapy compared to radiotherapy alone, which has resulted in a new standard of care.[56–59,66,69–71] The Cochrane meta-analysis summary showed that the combination of chemoradiotherapy had a 31% reduction in the risk of death, 34% improval in progression free survival, and a significant decrease in both local and distant recurrence rates.[70] The recommended treatment schedule is a weekly dose of cisplatin of 40 $mg/m^2$ to a cumulative dose of 200 $mg/m^2$ during radiotherapy.

The initial dose of external radiation may help reduce tumor load and facilitate placement of vaginal applicators to enhance the effects of brachytherapy. HDR technique allows the patient to be treated on an outpatient basis; treatment is quicker and enables the patient to be ambulatory. Treatment is usually completed in approximately 8 weeks. Cumulative tumor doses of 75 to 85 Gy for nonbulky disease and 85 to 90 Gy for bulky disease is necessary for local tumor control.[72,73] The 5-year survival rate of patients with stage IIB cancer is 60% to 79%, while those with stage III disease is 25% to 50%, and those with stage IVA disease is 18% to 34%. The advantages of radiation over surgery for advanced disease are that radiation can be given on an outpatient basis, it avoids surgery, and it is suitable for women who are poor surgical candidates.[5,43,45]

Morbidity resulting from properly administered radiotherapy in cervical cancer is usually manageable. Adverse reactions have been reported when poor technique is used, but these reactions occur infrequently in properly treated women. The higher the dose of radiation, the higher the rate of complications. Some morbidity attributed to radiation is secondary to uncontrolled tumor growth or the compounded effects of multiple therapies and is not a direct result of the radiation therapy. Major complication rates range from 3% to 5% for stage I and IIA disease and from 10% to 15% for stage IIB and III disease.[5,43,45]

The major complications related to radiotherapy include vaginal stenosis, fistula formation, sigmoid perforation or stricture, uterine perforation, rectal ulcer or proctitis, intestinal obstruction, fistulas, ureteral stricture, severe cystitis, pelvic hemorrhage, and pelvic abscess. Other problems related to radiation therapy include nausea, vomiting, diarrhea, and, rarely, radiation myelitis.[5,43,45]

Sexual dysfunction secondary to vaginal atrophy, stenosis, and lack of lubrication is a known effect of the radiation therapy. Radiation causes thinning of the vaginal epithelium, and the vagina may become shortened, less flexible, and partially obliterated. Vaginal intercourse may cause dyspareunia and bleeding. Women who are not sexually active experience a higher incidence of atrophy and stenosis than do sexually active women. The use of vaginal dilators and water-soluble lubricants can minimize the effects of radiation. Patients should be instructed to engage in vaginal intercourse and/or use a vaginal dilator 3 times a week in an effort to delimit vaginal stenosis.[5,43,45]

Surgical staging of advanced disease before initiating treatment is advocated in an attempt to gain a more precise evaluation of the extent of the disease. Arguments in favor of pretreatment laparotomy are that (1) the extent of the disease can be ascertained, (2) patients who have disease not curable by radiation may be offered palliative therapy, and (3) those patients most likely to benefit from extended-field radiation are identified. Arguments against pretreatment laparotomy are that (1) surgical staging can cause morbidity and mortality, (2) many patients with para-aortic nodal metastases also have systemic disease not detected by surgery, (3) there is only minimal improvement in net survival, and (4) surviving patients have high morbidity.

Currently, surgeons choose to use alternative extraperitoneal staging methods to determine the extent of disease. One approach involves making a small incision near the umbilicus and outside the proposed radiation field. This strategy allows sampling of the aortic and/or common iliac nodes, collection of peritoneal fluids for cytology, and palpation of pelvic structures.[5,43]

## RECURRENT OR PERSISTENT DISEASE

Approximately 35% of women with invasive cervical cancer will have recurrent or persistent disease. Therefore, thorough, regular follow-ups after treatment are mandatory. Recurrent cervical cancer is difficult to diagnose. Clinical and cytological evaluation of an irradiated cervix is problematic because the cells and configuration of the cervix are distorted from the radiation. Therefore, histological confirmation of recurrence is essential.[5,43]

Favorable prognostic indicators in recurrent disease include: a localized, central pelvic recurrence; a disease-free interval greater than 6 months; the size of recurrence is less than 3 cm in diameter; and no side wall fixation.[74,75] Almost 80% of recurrences become manifest within 2 years after therapy.[75] The signs and symptoms may be subtle and varied, including unintentional weight loss; unilateral leg edema; pain in the buttock, pelvis, or thigh; serosanguinous vaginal discharge; ureteral obstruction; supraclavicular lymph node enlargement (usually of the left side); cough; hemoptysis; and chest pain. The triad of sciatic pain, hydronephrosis, and leg edema is particularly ominous. Evaluation following histological confirmation generally includes a chest x-ray, intravenous pyelogram (IVP), CBC, and blood chemistries. A PET scan, CT scan, lymphangiography, or fluoroscopically directed needle biopsies to evaluate the status of the regional lymph nodes, liver, and kidneys may be performed. These procedures have replaced more elaborate operative procedures to provide histological confirmation of recurrence, which may save the woman from unnecessary surgery. In general, the prognosis for women who have central recurrence of disease is better than for those who experience recurrence in the pelvic wall.

Following surgery or radiotherapy as primary treatment for patients with cervical cancer, approximately half of all recurrences are local (cervix, uterus, vagina, parametrium, and regional lymph nodes). The remaining cases involve distant metastases to the lung, liver, bone, mediastinal, or supraclavicular lymph nodes.[5,43]

The prognosis for patients with persistent or recurrent carcinoma of the cervix is dismal. One-year survival rates are 10% to 15%. Survival averages 6 to 10 months once recurrent cervical cancer is diagnosed. The aim of treatment in recurrent disease is palliation because control or cure is rare.[5,43]

### Surgery

Pelvic exenteration entails en bloc removal of the pelvic organs and is limited to those patients with a central recurrence of their disease. A total pelvic exenteration includes a radical hysterectomy, pelvic lymph node dissection, and removal of the bladder and rectosigmoid colon. The surgical procedure is aborted if the patient is found to have recurrent disease outside the pelvis, positive lymph nodes, or disease fixed to the pelvic side wall. Occasionally, a posterior exenteration (which preserves the bladder) or anterior exenteration (which preserves the rectum) can be performed. The number of total pelvic exenterations has decreased dramatically in the past 20 years, and today this procedure is performed only in a selected group of patients. It is important to ensure that patients will be psychologically able to adjust to the changes in body function and body image. Unfortunately, inoperable disease is found about 60% of the time in candidates for pelvic exenteration.[5,43]

Extensive preoperative evaluation must be done to ensure that no disease exists outside the pelvis and that renal function is adequate. Studies usually performed include chest x-ray, IVP, blood chemistries, creatinine clearance, CT scan, bone scan, and liver-spleen scan. Some clinicians also order lymphangiography as well as an abdominal CT scan to evaluate the regional lymph nodes. If lymphadenopathy is present, a needle aspiration of the nodes may be done. If the aspirate is positive for malignancy, the woman may be spared an unnecessary laparotomy. A blind scalene node biopsy may be recommended to complete the evaluation. Preoperative evaluation of nutritional status is also important in this population. As many as 60% of cancer patients may exhibit laboratory or clinical evidence of malnutrition.[5,43]

At laparotomy, the entire abdomen and pelvis are explored in search of metastases. A selective para-aortic lymphadenectomy, bilateral pelvic lymphadenectomy, and biopsies of the pelvic side walls are done and sent for frozen section. If any of these samples test positive, or if the patient has positive intraoperative washings for disease, the exenteration is abandoned as the disease is considered incurable.[5,43]

The use of the end-to-end anastomotic (EEA) stapling device has resulted in patients' not requiring a permanent colostomy after pelvic exenteration; the creation of a continent conduit may be a surgical alternative to a more traditional urinary diversion. The EEA reduces the risk of anastomotic leaks, fistula formation, and late strictures, and it decreases operative time. Permanent colostomy can also be avoided by using a segment of sigmoid colon as a rectal substitute.[5,43]

Immediate postoperative problems include pulmonary embolism, pulmonary edema, cerebrovascular accident, hemorrhage, myocardial infarction, sepsis, and small-bowel obstruction. Long-term problems include fistula formation, urinary obstruction, infection, and sepsis. The use of pelvic exenteration has been limited to a very narrowly defined group of candidates, because reports indicate a 5-year survival rate of 23% to 50% and an operative mortality rate of approximately 9.8%. Women younger than age 35 have a better prognosis as compared with those older than age 35. Psychosexual and social rehabilitation of surviving patients is a major challenge. Vaginal reconstruction at the time of exenteration and psychological support in the postoperative period can help patients adjust. Survival statistics are worse for women who have recurrent disease greater than 3 mm, bladder involvement, positive pelvic lymph nodes, and recurrence less than a year after previous treatment.[5,43,45]

### Radiation therapy

In previously irradiated individuals, metastatic disease outside the initial radiation field may be treated cautiously with radiation to provide local control and relieve symptoms. In selected cases, radiation within previously treated areas may be used. For women treated initially with surgery, full-dose radiotherapy using a combination of external and intracavitary implants may afford excellent palliation or even cure.[5,43]

### Chemotherapy

In general, surgery or radiation will not be curative for most women who have recurrent cervical cancer. Previous radiation therapy to the pelvis alters the vascular supply, which limits potential drug delivery to tumor sites located in previously irradiated fields. Additional challenges are that the therapeutic doses of radiation therapy to the pelvis will compromise bone marrow reserve, and poor renal function secondary to previous radiation or surgery and ureteral obstruction from tumor or scarring may necessitate or delimit chemotherapeutic options.[45,47]

Response rates for patients with recurrent cervical cancer treated with single agent and investigational chemotherapy range from 0% to 48%, with most studies reporting a response rate less than 20%. In general, there is no long-term benefit from chemotherapy, as responses last less than 9 months with variable lengths of survival. Response rates are higher in patients who have received no prior radiation therapy or chemotherapy and new challenges have been presented since the 1999 NCI clinical announcement and new treatment paradigm for locally advanced cervical cancer.[5,43,45,71]

Activity has been documented for a number of single agents, including cisplatin, ifosfamide, paclitaxel, vinorelbine, topotecan, and irinotecan.[76–87] Other agents with demonstrated activity include cyclophosphamide, chlorambucil, melphalan, doxorubicin, carboplatin, 5-fluorouracil, methotrexate, vincristine, vindesine, and hexamethylmelamine.[5,43] Recently, gemcitabine has exhibited antitumor activity against cervical cancer in phase II clinical trials.[88] Topotecan has also shown efficacy against cervical cancer in phase II trials.[87] Of the single agents, cisplatin remains the drug with the greatest antineoplastic activity, although carboplatin may be used as first-line treatment as well. Even so, objective response rates with cisplatin only range between 17% and 30%, and the drug does not provide any increase in survival time for patients.[5,43]

Combination chemotherapy regimens have been compared with single agents and benefit has been proven. Early trials showed a modest benefit but greater toxicity, which led to trials with quality of life components for better comparison. The GOG 169 trial compared cisplatin alone with cisplatin plus paclitaxel. The objective response was 19% for cisplatin alone vs 36% for cisplatin plus paclitaxel ($P = 0.002$).[89,90] Median progression free survival was also improved but not overall survival. Myelosuppression was more significant in the paclitaxel arm, but it did not worsen quality of life.

A subsequent GOG trial compared cisplatin alone vs cisplatin plus topotecan and reported objective response rates of 13% vs 26%, respectively.[91] The median survival was 6.5 months vs 9.4 months, and despite increased toxicity, it did not reduce reported patient quality of life.

A recently closed study, GOG 204, compared cisplatin plus 1 of 4 agents: paclitaxel, topotecan, vinorelbine, or gemcitabine. After 513 patients were evaluated, the study was closed as an interim analysis indicated no superior efficacy of any of the experimental arms over cisplatin plus paclitaxel.[92]

Future directions of treatment are being pursued as the goal of a highly active or curative therapy for advanced or recurrent cervical cancer is still elusive. Bevacizumab has been studied in cervical cancer as angiogenesis plays a role in cervical cancer. A phase II trial with bevacizumab at 15 mg/kg given every 21 days was administered to 46 patients and was well tolerated, and it demonstrated modest activity in second and third line treatment for recurrent cervical cancer.[73]

A planned phase III trial to investigate the impact of bevacizumab with combination chemotherapy is underdevelopment. Also, cervical cancer has a high overexpression of EGFR; thus, EGFR is another attractive target for future therapy.[92]

Complications of chemotherapy may manifest themselves in any organ system and depend on the agent, dose, and route utilized. In addition, chemotherapy may adversely affect psychological, emotional, and psychosocial aspects of the cancer patient's life. Side effects associated with cisplatin include nausea and vomiting, renal dysfunction, peripheral neuropathy, anemia, neutropenia, hypomagnesemia, and ototoxicity.[5,43,45]

## SYMPTOM MANAGEMENT AND SUPPORTIVE CARE

Symptoms seen in patients with progressive cervical cancer include the development of ureteral obstruction, pain, cachexia, bleeding and anemia, and lymphedema. Patients with recurrent cervical cancer to the lung may complain of hemoptysis, cough, shortness of breath, and chest pain. Patients may have bony or brain metastases with the expected symptomatology associated with these lesions. Urinary diversion may be considered and is palliative in those patients with ureteral obstruction; embolization or additional radiation may be used for vaginal bleeding or hemorrhage. Spot radiation may be an option for metastatic lesions or areas of pain.

Patients who are cured are seen every 3 months for the first 2 to 3 years with gradual lengthening of posttherapy evaluations. Those individuals receiving definitive radiation therapy should be instructed to engage in vaginal intercourse or use a vaginal dilator at least 3 times a week. Significant vaginal stenosis precludes optimal posttherapy follow-up and evaluation.

## CONCLUSION

The burden of cervical cancer incidence, morbidity, and mortality is felt primarily in developing nations. Cancer prevention efforts worldwide have focused on screening women using the Pap smear/test and treating precursor lesions before the development of a malignancy. Unfortunately, developing nations often do not have the necessary infrastructure to provide access to screening, educational programs to create awareness, or availability to provide Pap smear screening services and follow-up. Currently, screening efforts in areas with limited resources continue to focus on intermittent visual inspections of the cervix. The cervix is swabbed with an acetic acid solution, which highlights differences in cell structure. Healthcare practitioners then visually inspect for evidence of cervical lesions. Clinical trials using magnification with visual inspections may be useful in identifying moderate to severe cervical lesions.[31]

Cervical cancer is preventable, as the vast majority of cases are caused, in part, by persistent infection with oncogenic HPVs. Primary prevention efforts have focused on the development of HPV vaccines to prophylax/prevent oncogenic HPV infection. Studies on HPV prophylaxis and prevention have been conducted and are currently under way in both the US and developing nations.[93–97]

Cervical cancer accounts for significant morbidity and mortality worldwide. Of the gynecological malignancies, only cervical cancer has an effective screening method for early detection. The potential for cure is enhanced when the disease is diagnosed in early stages. Treatment modalities for women with invasive disease can be very aggressive and may result in a variety of illness-related demands on the woman and her family. In addition, when recurrences appear, expectations for cure may be unrealistic and effective palliation remains to be discovered. Risk factors in the development of preinvasive and invasive disease are well known, but it may take many years for invasive disease to develop. Additional research should target the goal of improving the percentage of women who receive regular screening in an effort to diagnose the disease in its earliest stages.

## REFERENCES


1. American Cancer Society. *Global Cancer Facts and Figures, 2007.* http://caonline.amcancersoc.org/cgi/content-nw/full/56/2/106/TBL16. Accessed October 1, 2009.
2. American Cancer Society. *2009 Facts and Figures.* http://www.cancer.org/statistics/selectcancers.htm/#cervix. Accessed October 1, 2009.
3. Jemal A, Siegel R, Ward E, Hao Y, Xu J, Thun M. Cancer Statistics 2009. *CA: Cancer J Clin.* 2009;59:225–249.
4. Symonds RP. Screening for cervical cancer: different problems in the developing and developed world. *Eur J Cancer Care.* 1997;6:275–279.
5. DiSaia PJ, Creasman WT. *Clinical Gynecologic Oncology.* 6th ed. St. Louis, MO: Mosby; 2002.
6. Borrayo EA, Thomas JJ, Lawsin C. Cervical cancer screening among Latinas: the importance of referral and participation in parallel cancer screening behaviors. *Women Health.* 2004;39:13–29.
7. Reynolds D. Cervical cancer in Hispanic/Latino women. *Clin J Oncol Nurs.* 2004;8:146–150.
8. Bosch FX, Manos MM, Munoz N, et al. Prevalence of human papillomavirus in cervical cancer: a worldwide perspective. International Biological Study on Cervical Cancer (IBSCC) study group. *J Natl Cancer Inst.* 1995;87:796–802.
9. Wallboomers JM, Jacobs MV, Manos MM, et al. Human papillomavirus is a necessary cause of invasive cervical cancer worldwide. *J Pathol.* 1999;189:12–19.
10. National Institute of Health. *Consensus Statement on Cervical Cancer.* Bethesda, MD: National Institute of Health; April 1–3, 1996.
11. Wolf JK, Franco EL, Arbeit JM, et al. Innovations in understanding the biology of cervical cancer. *Cancer.* 2003;98:2064–2069.
12. Viscidi R. Epidemiology of genital tract human papillomavirus infections. In: Apgar B, Brotzman G, Spitzer M, eds. *Colposcopy: Principles and Practice.* Philadelphia, PA: W.B. Saunders; 2002:1–2.
13. Schlossser BJ, Howett MK. Human papillomaviruses: molecular aspects of the viral life cycle and pathogenesis. In: Apgar B, Brotzman G, Spitzer M, eds. *Colposcopy: Principles and Practice.* Philadelphia, PA: W.B. Saunders; 2002:23–39.
14. Munoz N, Bosch FX, de Sanjose S, et al. Epidemiologic classification of human papillomavirus types associated with cervical cancer. *N Engl J Med.* 2003;348:518–527.
15. Trottier H, Granco EL. The epidemiology of genital human papillomavirus infection. *Vaccine.* 2006;24(suppl 1):S1/4–S1/15.
16. Burk RD, Terai M, Gravitt PE, et al. Distribution of human papillomavirus types 16 and 18 variants in squamous cell carcinomas and adenocarcinomas of the cervix. *Cancer Res.* 2003;63:7215–7220.
17. Ostor AG. Natural history of cervical intraepithelial neoplasia: a critical review. *Int J Gynecol Pathol.* 1993;12:186–192.
18. Melnikow J, Nuovo J, Willan AR, et al. Natural history of cervical squamous intraepithelial lesions: a metaanalysis. *Obstet Gynecol.* 1998;92:727–735.
19. Franco EL, Villa LL, Sobrinho JP, et al. Epidemiology of acquisition and clearance of cervical human papillomavirus infection in women from a high risk area for cervical cancer. *J Infect Dis.* 1999;180:1415–1423.

20. Maiman M, Fruchter RG, Clark M, et al. Cervical cancer as an AIDS-defining illness. *Obstet Gynecol.* 1997;89:76–80.
21. Castellsague X, Munoz N. Cofactors in human papillomavirus carcinogenesis—role of parity, oral contraceptives, and tobacco smoking. *J Natl Cancer Inst Monogr.* 2003;31:20–28.
22. Harris TG, Kulasingam SL, Kiviat NB, et al. Cigarette smoking, oncogenic human papillomavirus, Ki-67 antigen, and cervical intraepithelial neoplasia. *Am J Epidemiol.* 2004;159:834–842.
23. Plummer M, Herrero R, Franceschi S, et al. Smoking and cervical cancer: pooled analysis of the IARC multi-centric case-control study. *Cancer Causes Control.* 2003;14:805–814.
24. Munoz N, Castellsague Z, de Gonzalez AB, Gissmann L. HPV in the etiology of human cancer. *Vaccine.* 2006;24(suppl 3):s3/1–10.
25. Spinelli A. Preinvasive diseases of the cervix, vulva, and vagina. *Semin Oncol Nurs.* 2002;18:184–192.
26. Agency for Healthcare Policy and Research. *Evidence Report/Technology Assessment, Number 5. Evaluation of Cervical Cytology.* Bethesda, MD: AHCPR Publication No. 99-E010; 1999.
27. Cox JT. Advances in cervical cancer screening: Pap testing. *Contemp Obstet Gynecol.* 2001;46(suppl):3–18.
28. Bernstein SJ, Sanchez-Ramos L, Ndubisi B. Liquid-based cervical cytologic smear and conventional Papanicolaou smears: a metaanalysis of prospective studies comparing cytologic diagnosis and sample adequacy. *Am J Obstet Gynecol.* 2001;185:308–317.
29. Sptizer M, Johnson C. Terminology in cervical cytology: B. conventional cytology. In: Apgar B, Brotzman G, Spitzer M, eds. *Colposcopy: Principles and Practice.* Philadelphia, PA: W.B. Saunders; 2002:52–56.
30. Wright TC, Massad S, Dunton CJ, Spitzer M, Wilkinson EJ, Solomon D. 2006 consensus guidelines for the management of women with abnormal cervical cancer screening tests. *Am J Obstet Gynecol.* 2007;197: 346–355.
31. Wright T Jr. Pathogenesis and diagnosis of preinvasive lesions of the lower genital tract. In: Hoskins WJ, Perez CA, Young RC, eds. *Principles and Practice of Gynecologic Oncology.* 3rd ed. Philadelphia, PA: Lippincott, Williams & Wilkins; 2000:735–774.
32. Saslovar D, Runowicz CD, Solomon D, et al. American Cancer Society guideline for the early detection of cervical neoplasia and cancer. *CA: Cancer J Clin.* 2002;52:342–362.
33. US Preventive Services Task Force. Recommendations and Rationale: Screening for Cervical Cancer. http://www.ahrq.gov/clinic/uspstf/uspscerv.htm. Accessed October 1, 2009.
34. Schiffman M, Castle PE, Jeronimo J, Rodriguez AC, Wacholder S. Human papillomavirus and cervical cancer. *Lancet.* 2007;370:890–907.
35. Wright TC Jr, Cox JT, Massad LS, et al. 2001 consensus guidelines for the management of women with cervical cytological abnormalities. *JAMA.* 2002;287:2120–2129.
36. Sptizer M, Johnson C. Terminology in cervical cytology: A. the Bethesda system. In: Apgar B, Brotzman G, Spitzer M, eds. *Colposcopy: Principles and Practice.* Philadelphia, PA: W.B. Saunders; 2002: 41–52.
37. Apgar B, Brotzman G. High grade squamous intraepithelial lesion. In: Apgar B, Brotzman G, Spitzer M, eds. *Colposcopy: Principles and Practice.* Philadelphia, PA: W.B. Saunders; 2002:249–263.
38. Sankaranarayanan R, Nene BM, Shastri SS, et al. HPV screening for cervical cancer in rural India. *N Eng J Med.* 2009;360:1385–1394.
39. Schlecht NF, Platt RW, Duarte-Franco E, et al. Human papillomavirus infection and time to progression and regression of cervical intraepithelial neoplasia. *J Natl Cancer Inst.* 2003;95:1336–1343.
40. The Atypical Squamous Cells of Undetermined Significance/Low-Grade Squamous Intraepithelial Lesions Triage Study (ALTS) Group. Human papillomavirus testing for triage of women with cytologic evidence of low-grade squamous epithelial lesions: baseline data from a randomized trial. *J Natl Cancer Inst.* 2000;92:397–402.
41. Cox JT. Management of precursor lesions of cervical carcinoma: history, host defense, and a survey of modalities. *Obstet Gynecol Clin North Am.* 2002;29:751–785.
42. Wright TC Jr, Gagnon S, Richart RM, et al. Treatment of cervical intraepithelial neoplasia using the loop electrosurgical excision procedure. *Obstet Gynecol.* 1992;79:173–178.
43. Stehman FB, Perez CA, Kurman RJ, et al. Uterine cervix. In: Hoskins WJ, Perez CA, Young RC, eds. *Principles and Practice of Gynecologic Oncology.* 3rd ed. Philadelphia, PA: Lippincott, Williams & Wilkins; 2000:841–918.
44. Widrich T, Kennedy AW, Myers TM, et al. Adenocarcinoma in situ of the uterine cervix: management and outcome. *Gynecol Oncol.* 1996;61:304–308.
45. Fischer M. Cancer of the cervix. *Semin Oncol Nurs.* 2002;18:193–199.
46. Mitchell DG, Snyder B, Coakley F, et al. Early invasive cervical cancer: tumor delineation by magnetic resonance imaging and computed tomography, and clinical examination verified by pathologic results, in the ACRIN 6651/GOG183 Intergroup Study. *J Clin Oncol.* 2006;24:5687–5694.
47. Stanley MA. Prognostic factors and new therapeutic approaches to cervical cancer. *Virus Res.* 2002;89:241–248.
48. Creasman WT, Zaino RJ, Major FJ, et al. Early invasive carcinoma of the cervix (3 to 5 mm invasion): risk factors and prognosis. A Gynecology Oncology Group study. *Am J Obstet Gynecol.* 1998;178:62–65.
49. Kim GE, Kim YB, Cho NH, et al. Synchronous coexpression of epidermal growth factor receptor and cyclooxygenase-2 in carcinomas of the uterine cervix: a potential predictor of poor survival. *Clin Cancer Res.* 2004;10:1366–1374.
50. Pecorelli S, Zigliani L, Odicino F. Revised FIGO staging for carcinoma of the cervix. *Int J Gynecol Obstet.* 2009;105:107–108.
51. AJCC. Cervix uteri. In: Greene FL, Page DL, Fleming ID, et al, eds. *American Joint Committee on Cancer: AJCC Cancer Staging Manual.* 6th ed. New York: Springer; 2000:260.
52. Hoffman MS, Cardosi RJ, Roberts WS, et al. Accuracy of pelvic examination in the assessment of patients with operable cervical cancer. *Am J Obstet Gynecol.* 2004;190:986–993.
53. Thomas GM. Improved treatment for cervical cancer—concurrent chemotherapy and radiotherapy. *N Engl J Med.* 1999;340:1198.
54. Thomas GM. Concurrent chemotherapy and radiation for locally advanced cervical cancer: the new standard of care. *Semin Radiat Oncol.* 2000;10:44–50.
55. Rose PG, Bundy BN. Chemoradiation for locally advanced cervical cancer: does it help? *J Clin Oncol.* 2002;20:891.
56. Pearcey R, Brundage M, Drouin P, et al. Phase III trial comparing radical radiotherapy with and without cisplatin chemotherapy in patients with advanced squamous cell carcinoma of the cervix. *J Clin Oncol.* 2002;20:966–972.
57. Whitney CS, Sause W, Bundy BN, et al. Randomized comparison of fluoruracil plus cisplatin vs hydroxyurea as an adjunct to radiation therapy in stage IIB—IVA carcinoma of the cervix with negative para-aortic lymph nodes: a Gynecology Oncology Group and Southwest Oncology Group study. *J Clin Oncol.* 1999;17:1339–1348.
58. Morris M, Eifel PJ, Lu J, et al. Pelvic radiation with concurrent chemotherapy compared with pelvic and para-aortic radiation for high-risk cervical cancer. *N Engl J Med.* 1999;340:1137–1143.
59. Rose PG, Bundy BN, Watkins EB, et al. Concurrent cisplatin based radiotherapy and chemotherapy for locally advanced cervical cancer. *N Engl J Med.* 1999;340:1144–1153.
60. Keys HM, Bundy BN, Stehman FB, et al. Cisplatin, radiation, and adjuvant hysterectomy compared with radiation and adjuvant hysterectomy for bulky stage I cervical carcinoma. *N Engl J Med.* 1999;340:1154–1161.
61. Peters WA III, Liu PY, Barrett RJ II, et al. Concurrent chemotherapy and pelvic radiation therapy compared with pelvic radiation therapy alone as adjuvant therapy after radical surgery in high-risk, early stage cancer of the cervix. *J Clin Oncol.* 2000;18:1606–1613.
62. Schlaerth JB, Spirtos N, Schlaerth AC. Radical trachelectomy and pelvic lymphadenectomy with uterine preservation in the treatment of cervical cancer. *Am J Obstet Gynecol.* 2003;188:29–34.

63. Koiopoulos G, Sotiriadis A, Kyrgiou M, et al. Conservative surgical methods for FIGO stage IA2 squamous cervical carcinoma and their role in preserving women's fertility. *Gynecol Oncol.* 2003;93:469–473.
64. Abu-Rustum NR, Sonoda Y. Fertility-sparing radical abdominal trachelectomy for cervical carcinoma. *Gynecol Oncol.* 2007;104:s56–s59.
65. Carter J, Sonoda Y, Chi DS, Raviv L, Abu-Rustum NR. Radical trachelectomy for cervical cancer: postoperative physical and emotional concerns. *Gynecol Oncol.* 2008;111:151–157.
66. Holschneider CH, DeLosSantos JF. Invasive cervical cancer: management of stages IB2, bulky IIA, and locally advanced disease. UpToDate, version 17.1, January 15, 2009.
67. Stehman FB, Ali S, Keys HM, et al. Radiation therapy with or without weekly cisplatin for bulky stage IB cervical carcinoma: follow up of a Gynecologic Oncology Group trial. *Am J Obstet Gynecol.*2007;197:503,e1–6.
68. Sardi JE, Giaroli A, Sananes C, et al. Long-term follow-up of the first randomized trial using neoadjuvant chemotherapy in stage IB squamous carcinoma of the cervix: the final results. *Gynecol Oncol.* 1997;67:61–69.
69. Eifel PJ, Winter K, Morris M, et al. Pelvic irradiation with concurrent chemotherapy versus pelvic and para-aortic irradiation for high-risk cervical cancer: an update of radiation therapy oncology group trial (RTOG) 90–01. *J Clin Oncol.* 2004;22:872–880.
70. Green J, Kirwan J, Tierney J, et al. Concomitant chemotherapy and radiation therapy for cancer of the uterine cervix. Cochrane Database Syst Rev 2005;20(3):CD002225.
71. National Cancer Institute. Concurrent chemoradiaiton for cervical cancer. Clinical announcement, Washington, DC, February 22, 1999.
72. Stewart A, Viswanathan A. Current controversies in high-dose rate versus low-dose rate brachytherapy for cervical cancer. *Cancer.* 2006;107:908–915.
73. Monk BJ, Tewari KS, Kow WJ. Multimodality therapy for locally advanced cervical carcinoma: state of the art and future directions. *J Clin Oncol.* 2007;27:2952–2965.
74. Friedlander M. Guidelines for the treatment of recurrent and metastatic cervical cancer. *Oncologist.* 2002;7:342–347.
75. Holschneider CH. Management of diseeminated or recurrent cervical cancer. http://www.UpToDate.com. January 8, 2009.
76. Alberts DS, Kronmal R, Baker LH, et al. Phase II randomized trial of cisplatin chemotherapy regimens in the treatment of recurrent or metastatic squamous cell cancer of the cervix: a Southwest Oncology Group Study. *J Clin Oncol.* 1987;5:1791–1795.
77. Thigpen JT, Blessing JA, DiSaia PJ, et al. A randomized comparison of a rapid versus prolonged (24 hr) infusion of cisplatin in therapy of squamous cell carcinoma of the uterine cervix: a Gynecologic Oncology Group study. *Gynecol Oncol.* 1989;32:198–202.
78. Coleman RE, Harper PG, Gallagher C, et al. A phase II study of ifosfamide in advanced and relapsed carcinoma of the cervix. *Cancer Chemother Pharmacol.* 1986;18:280–283.
79. Kudelka AP, Winn R, Edwards CL, et al. An update of a phase II study of paclitaxel in advanced or recurrent squamous cell cancer of the cervix. *Anticancer Drugs.* 1997;8:657–661.
80. Thigpen JT, Vance RB, Khansur T. The platinum compounds and paclitaxel in the management of carcinomas of the endometrium and uterine cervix. *Semin Oncol.* 1995;22(suppl 12):67–75.
81. McGuire WP, Blessing JA, Moore D, et al. Paclitaxel has moderate activity in squamous cervix cancer: a Gynecologic Oncology Group study. *J Clin Oncol.* 1996;14:792–795.
82. Morris M, Brader K, Levenback C, et al. Phase II study of vinorelbine in advanced and recurrent squamous cell carcinoma of the cervix. *J Clin Oncol.* 1998;16:1094–1098.
83. Lacava JA, Leone BA, Machiavelli M, et al. Vinorelbine as neoadjuvant chemotherapy in advanced cervical carcinoma. *J Clin Oncol.* 1997;15:604–609.
84. Coleman RL, Miller DS. Topotecan in the treatment of gynecologic cancer. *Semin Oncol.* 1977;24(suppl):S20–S55.
85. Buxton EJ, Meanwell CA, Hilton C, et al. Combination bleomycin, ifosfamide, and cisplatin chemotherapy in cervical cancer. *J Natl Cancer Inst.* 1989;81:359–361.
86. Verschraegen CF, Levy T, Kudelka AP, et al. Phase II study of irinotecan in prior chemotherapy-treated squamous cell carcinoma of the cervix. *J Clin Oncol.* 1997;15:625–631.
87. Look KY, Blessing JA, Levenback CA, et al. A phase II trial of CPT-11 in recurrent squamous cell carcinoma of the cervix: a Gynecologic Oncology Group study. *Gynecol Oncol.* 1998;70:334–338.
88. Carmichael J. The role of gemcitabine in the treatment of other tumors. *Br J Cancer.* 1998;78:21–25.
89. Moore DH, Blessing JA, McQuellon RP, et al. Phase III study of cisplatin with or without paclitaxel in stage IVB, recurrent or persistent squamous cell carcinoma of the cervix: a Gynecologic Oncology Group study. *J Clin Oncol.* 2004;22:3113–3119.
90. Moore DH. Chemotherapy for advanced, recurrent, and metastatic cervical cancer. *J Natl Compr Canc Netw.* 2008;6:53–57.
91. Monk BJ, Huang HQ, Cella D, Long HJ. Quality of life outcomes from a randomized phase III trial of cisplatin with or without topotecan in advanced carcinoma of the cervix: a Gynecologic Oncology Group study. *J Clin Oncol.* 2005;23:4626–4633.
92. Tewari KS, Monk BJ. Recent achievements and future developments in advanced and recurrent cervical cancer: trials of the Gynecologic Oncology Group. *Semin Oncol.* 2009;36:170–180.
93. Chu NR. Therapeutic vaccination for the treatment of mucosotropic human papillomavirus-associated disease. *Expert Opin Biol Ther.* 2003;3:477–486.
94. Koutsky LA, Ault KA, Wheeler CM, et al. A controlled trial of human papillomavirus type 16 vaccine. *N Engl J Med.* 2002;347:1645–1651.
95. National Cancer Institute. Future directions in epidemiologic and preventive research on human papillomavirus and cancer. *J Natl Cancer Inst Monogr.* 2003;31:1–130.
96. Mandic A, Vujkov T. Human papillomavirus vaccine as a new way of preventing cervical cancer: a dream or the future? *Ann Oncol.* 2004;15:197–200.
97. Goldie SJ, Kohli M, Grima D, et al. Projected clinical benefits and cost-effectiveness of a human papillomavirus 16/18 vaccine. *J Natl Cancer Inst.* 2004;96:604–615.

CHAPTER

51

Gail M. Wilkes, MS, RN, ANP-BC, AOCN®

# Colon, Rectal, and Anal Cancers

## Colon Cancer

### INTRODUCTION

Colon and rectal cancers are combined in the term "colorectal cancer," and most available statistics on these cancers are also combined. Colorectal cancer is the third leading cause of cancer in both men and women and is the leading cause of death from cancer in men and women combined. If women and men are considered separately, it is still the third leading cause of cancer deaths led by lung and breast cancer in women and lung and prostate cancer in men. In 2009, the American Cancer Society (ACS) estimated that 106,100 people developed colon cancer (52,010 men and 54,090 women), and 40,870 developed rectal cancer (23,580 men and 17,290 women). The ACS expected 49,920 people to die of colon and rectal cancers in 2009: 25,240 men and 24,680 women.[1] Colorectal cancer represents 9% of all cancer deaths, but fortunately, there has been a steady decrease in incidence over the last 20 years. However, colon and rectal cancers combined are a major public health problem. In terms of incidence, colon cancer is 2.5 times more common than rectal cancer, and anal cancers account for fewer than 4% of all lower gastrointestinal (GI) cancers.[2]

Despite the fact that colon and rectal cancers may share a similar cellular path of carcinogenesis, they are two separate diseases. In this chapter, they will be discussed together and differences pointed out in their epidemiology, as many of the studies and statistics discuss both cancers concurrently. The chapter will then discuss them separately in terms of treatment. Anal cancer is histologically different and is discussed in a separate subsection.

Colon cancer is, in most cases, a *preventable and curable disease*, which is known to be influenced by genetic as well as environmental factors such as micronutrients, exercise, and obesity. Strong evidence of these relationships is emerging, and counseling about exercise and elimination of obesity is included in prevention regimens. For both colon and rectal cancers, 90% of disease occurs in individuals who are age 50 and older. Many reasons explain the high incidence and mortality figures, ranging from cultural aversions to discussion of bowel function, primary care providers' lack of compliance with standard recommended screening, lack of access to standard care among socioeconomically disadvantaged populations, as well as a more aggressive biology of disease in patients younger than 50 years old. Screening and early detection activities are critical for all individuals aged 50 years or older, and for younger individuals who are at risk for the development of colon cancer. As the twenty-first century unfolds, it will bring a better genetic understanding of cancer with the deciphering of the human genome. It is therefore imperative that we understand the changes that occur in the malignant transformation in colon and rectal cancers.

Colon cancer is the most extensively studied of the GI malignancies, particularly in terms of its genetic, molecular, biological, environmental, and dietary aspects. Because this cancer may be silent until it reaches an advanced stage, screening and early detection have become the primary methods for reducing morbidity and mortality. Advances in endoscopy, specialty radiology, and surgical resection for primary as well as metastatic disease, together with improvements in chemotherapy, biotherapy, and radiation therapy over the last decade, have helped to diminish the mortality and morbidity of colon cancer. Nurses, physicians in primary care, and members of the healthcare team can help increase awareness that screening is available and that prevention methods are effective and valuable. More than 30,000 lives could be saved each year if the general public, primary care physicians, and managed care companies were more aware of and promoted methods of early detection and treatment.[3] State-of-the-art treatment and care can be provided by healthcare professionals as genetic mapping, clinical trials, advancements in the management of side effects, and alternative methods of treatment and support are developed.

### EPIDEMIOLOGY AND ETIOLOGY

Approximately 6% of the US population will at some point develop colorectal cancer.[1] Colon and rectal cancers combined are one of the leading causes of cancer-related deaths in the Western world. They account for approximately two-thirds of all cancers arising in the GI tract. Their peak incidence occurs in the sixth and seventh decades of life. More women than men develop colon cancer, but more men than women develop rectal cancer.[1] Adenocarcinomas of the colon can be hereditary or sporadic. Inherited colon cancers account for about 5% of colon cancers and include either familial adenomatous polyposis (FAP) or hereditary nonpolyposis colorectal cancer (HNPCC). Of the sporadic colon cancers, 15% to 30% arise in individuals at risk for developing colon cancer due to a personal or family history of colon cancer: having had colon cancer or adenomatous polyps, or having a first degree relative who had colon cancer or adenomatous polyps before the age of 60.[4]

Colon cancer develops as the result of an accumulation of genetic mutations. With or without familial risk, colon cancers seem to develop from mutations in similar genes, although the progression of accumulated mutations may differ.[5] Advances in microarray technology will help establish the pathways via distinct mutational gene signatures, and in the future, enable individualized care.[6] The most commonly mutated genes in colon cancer are the adenomatous polyposis coli (*APC*) genes, which are tumor suppressor genes, the *K-ras* oncogene, the *p53* tumor suppressor gene, the *deleted-in-colon-cancer* tumor suppressor gene, and the *DNA mismatched pair* genes. Other molecular characteristics that are associated with an aggressive phenotype are mutation in p27, a cyclin-dependent kinase inhibitor that helps balance active cell division with no cell division based on the body's needs; epidermal growth factor receptor (EGFR) overexpression, which inhibits apoptosis (programmed cell death) and leads to the formation of new blood vessels (angiogenesis) and metastatic spread; and DNA aneuploidy (an incorrect number of chromosomes), which is associated with colon cancer recurrence and poor outcomes. In this patient group representing about 85% of patients with colorectal cancer, the pathway is one of chromosomal instability (CIN).

Alternatively, 15% of patients with colorectal cancer have microsatellite instability (MSI), related to errors in DNA replication. Hereditary nonpolyposis colorectal cancer arises from mutations in one of the four genes that participate in mismatch repair, or the repair of defective DNA strands. When mismatch repair does not function, mutations occur in one or more of the genes that are important to the control of cell growth, and the mutations are perpetuated in subsequent generations of colon mucosal epithelial cells.[5] The mutated genes in cancer syndromes have been identified, and genetic testing is available for patients and their first-degree relatives.

About 95% or more of colon cancers occur in individuals without obvious genetic syndromes and are referred to as *sporadic* or *common* cancers. About 10% of adults in Western countries have a first-degree relative who is affected by colon cancer. These persons have a twofold to threefold increased risk of acquiring the disease. Having multiple relatives with colon cancer or relatives with a diagnosis at a younger age further increases the risk.[7] Colon cancers are generally known to evolve through a multistep process involving a benign adenomatous polyp that eventually becomes cancerous. This entire process can take approximately 10 years. Early colon and rectal carcinomas confined to the mucosa or submucosa usually produce a polypoid mass. There is generally no risk of invasive malignancy in polyps smaller than 5 mm, which are commonly hyperplastic. In contrast, adenomas > 1 cm in size have a 15% likelihood of becoming malignant in 10 years.[4] Incidence and mortality rates among racial and ethnic groups differ, perhaps as the result of differences in socioeconomic status, especially in terms of access to standard health care where regular screening may occur less commonly in socioeconomically disadvantaged individuals, compared to that of Caucasians. In addition, the purchase of fresh fruit and vegetables and eating a healthy diet are often less possible for the socioeconomically disadvantaged.[8] Among African Americans, the incidence of colorectal cancer is 15% higher than in Caucasians, and mortality is about 40% higher.[8] According to ACS statistics for the period 2000 to 2004, the incidence rate (per 100,000) among African American males was 72.6 compared to 60.4 in Caucasian males and 55.0 for African American females vs 44.0 for Caucasian females. Death rates (per 100,000) are also higher: 32.7 for African Americans men vs 22.9 for Caucasian men, and 22.9% for African American women compared to 15.9 in Caucasian women.[9] The incidence and death rates of colon and rectal cancers for the same period among Asians/Pacific Islanders, American Indians/Alaskan Natives, and Hispanics/Latinos (although not mutually exclusive from all others such as Caucasian) are lower than those among Caucasians.[9]

The higher incidence and mortality rates in African Americans are believed to be due to reduced access to regular screening and, in some cases, due to poorer access to timely, high-quality treatments.[1] For example, ACS statistics show that 38% of Caucasian patients present with localized colon and rectal cancers, while only 34% of African Americans present with localized disease; 19% of Caucasians present with distant disease compared to 24% of African Americans. The question of whether colon and rectal cancers have a more aggressive biology in African Americans has been raised, but a study by McCollum and colleagues showed that with equal staging (high-risk stage II and stage III colon cancer) and similar access to healthcare resources and treatment with adjuvant chemotherapy, Caucasians and African Americans with colon cancer have similar 5-year survival and overall survival rates.[10] In addition, health beliefs of patients of lower socioeconomic means pose challenges. For example, many African Americans use emergency rooms for evaluation of health problems, rather than prevention; they may have a sense of fatalism with the belief that cancer means death, together with an aversion to discussion of any aspects of bowel elimination; and inability to buy healthy foods so that they eat canned foods and high-fat foods, resulting in obesity. Interestingly, the absolute difference in death rates between less educated and more educated individuals in general cancer situations was greater than the difference in death rates between African Americans and Caucasians.[1]

The incidence of colorectal cancer has been decreasing over the last 20 years, with a steeper decrease of 2.3% per year from 1998 to 2004, a trend believed to be partially related to improved screening,[9] and possibly to the increased use of hormone replacement therapy and non-steroidal anti-inflammatory drugs during this time.[8] American Cancer Society statistics reveal that mortality rates are also decreasing in both men and women, more steeply over the last few years (1.8% per year decrease from 1985–2002, and 4.7% from 2002–2004) [9] In addition there have been increases in 5-year survival rates.

Only about 39% of individuals who have colon and rectal cancers present with localized disease with the promise of a 90% 5-year survival; the remaining 61% have regional disease (lymph node involvement or involvement of adjacent organs) or advanced disease at diagnosis[9] Regional spread to lymph nodes or adjacent organs reduces the 5-year survival rate to approximately 67%. If the cancer has spread to distant sites the 5-year survival is 10% or less.[8]

While colon cancer has always been considered a primary disease of the left colon, there is a documented increase in the incidence of right sided (proximal) lesions while that in the left colon (distal) is decreasing.[4] Possible reasons include increased longevity, possible differences in response to carcinogens in the proximal and distal colon, and genetic differences where tumors in the right (proximal) colon tend to be microsatellite unstable (MSI) while those in the distal colon are chromosomally unstable (CIN).[4,11] Of critical importance is that proximal lesions are missed by flexible sigmoidoscopy.[12] The incidence of colon and rectal cancers is high in industrialized regions like North America, northwestern Europe, and Australia. Incidence is low in less developed regions such as Asia, Africa, and South America. Residents of high-risk countries typically consume diets that are high in total fat, animal fat, and protein, and that are relatively low in fruits, vegetables, and fiber. Individuals moving from a low-risk country to a high-risk one assume the higher risk of their new country within one generation. In addition to diet, many lifestyle habits are related to a higher risk of colorectal cancer.[8]

The incidence of colon cancer increases with age. Factors that have been identified as contributing to the development of colon cancers over a person's lifetime include diet, fecal carcinogens, bile acids, lifestyle, alcohol intake, inflammatory bowel conditions, cholecystectomy, and familial and genetic factors.[11] The most important factors are age, obesity, familial/genetic factors, activity level, and diet (micronutrient deficiency, and factors that slow bowel transit time). Meyerhardt et al, in an observational study, found that a diet high in red and processed meats, concentrated carbohydrates such as sweets (eg, candy), desserts, french fries, and refined grains appeared to increase the risk of colon cancer recurrence and decrease survival in individuals who had undergone surgical resection for stage III colon cancer followed by adjuvant chemotherapy.[13]

## FAMILIAL/GENETIC AND LIFESTYLE FACTORS

Table 51-1 summarizes primary prevention strategies. Lieberman and colleagues studied 3121 asymptomatic patients aged 50 to 75 years from 13 Veterans Affairs medical centers over the period 1994 to 1997, all of whom had an adenoma greater than 10 mm in diameter, villous adenoma, an adenoma with high-grade dysplasia, or invasive cancer.[14] They found positive associations for history of a first-degree relative with colorectal cancer, current smoking, and current moderate or heavy alcohol use. Inverse or protective associations were found for cereal fiber intake (more than 4.2 g per day), vitamin D intake (greater than 645 IU per day), and daily use of nonsteroidal anti-inflammatory drugs (NSAIDS). The authors reported that slightly protective factors were physical activity, daily multivitamin use, intake of calcium, and low consumption of fat derived from red meat. No association was found with body mass index (BMI) or prior cholecystectomy. In patients for whom hyperplastic polyps were the only finding at colonoscopy, risk was similar to that of patients with no polyps, except that current or past smoking increased the risk for hyperplastic polyps.

A decrease in physical activity or sedentary lifestyle leads to a decrease in intestinal tract transit time and allows potential carcinogens to have longer contact with gut mucosa. Vigorous exercise is associated with a decreased risk of colon cancer. Meyerhardt et al, found that recreational activity after the diagnosis of stages I to III colon cancer appeared to reduce both specific and overall risk of colorectal cancer mortality.[29] There is a noted association between obesity, as well as increased caloric intake in excess of energy expenditure, and an increased risk for colon cancer.[2] Diets high in fat increase the production of bile salts and change their composition. Altered bile salts are converted into potential carcinogens by intestinal flora.

Through a complex relationship, cyclooxygenase (COX) exerts an inflammatory effect systemically within the body, and this sets the stage for malignant transformation. Colorectal cancers often express COX-2, and this expression correlates with tumor angiogenesis, more invasive tumor phenotype, resistance to apoptosis, and systemic immunosuppression.[34] COX-2 inhibitors can reduce the growth of colorectal polyps. For this reason, the drug celecoxib (Celebrex) is indicated for the prevention of FAP in high-risk individuals.[35]

Studies have produced conflicting results regarding the role of dietary fiber in reducing risk. The protective mechanism of dietary fiber is through increasing fecal bulk, which changes the bacterial composition of the feces and accelerates the transit time in the intestinal tract.

Heavy alcohol consumption is a factor in the development of colon and rectal cancers.[36] Su and Arab reported the follow-up results of the national Health and Nutrition Examination Survey I, which demonstrated a significant

**TABLE 51-1**

**Primary Prevention Strategies**

| Prevention Strategy | Study, Findings, or Article | Reference |
|---|---|---|
| Cereal fiber, vitamin D, daily use of NSAIDs | Inverse or protective association for cereal fiber intake (> 4.2 g/day), vitamin D intake greater than 645 IU/day, and daily use of NSAIDs. | Lieberman et al[14] |
| Dietary fiber | Prospective study of 88,757 women aged 34–59 years without a history of cancer or colon cancer risk factors, who were followed for 16 years. No association was found between the intake of dietary fiber and development of adenoma or risk of colon or rectal cancer. | Fuchs et al[15] |
| Diet high in vegetables, fruits, grains | Increased risk in men for the development of colorectal adenoma from a diet high in saturated fat and low in fiber. Diet of chicken and fish instead of red meat, and increased intake of vegetables, fruits, and grains are protective against CRC in men. | Giovonnucci et al[16] |
| Dietary fiber | RCT of 33,971 subjects [Prostate, Lung, Colorectal, and Ovarian (PLCO) Cancer Screening Trial]: high intake of dietary fiber was associated with a lower risk of colon and rectal adenomas. Individuals ingesting the highest amounts of fiber had a 27% lower risk of distal colonic adenoma as compared to the lower quintile with fiber from grains, cereals, and fruits conferring the most protection; no reduction in risk for rectal adenomas. | Peters et al[17] |
| Dietary fiber | Large prospective study (*N* = 519,978) of the association between dietary fiber intake and the incidence of CRC. Highest intake group (fiber 35 g/day) had a 27% lower incidence of adenoma (*P* = 0.002) after an average follow-up of 4.5 years. Dietary fiber intake as inversely proportional to the incidence of colon cancer, and the protective effect was greatest for left-sided colon cancers and least for rectal cancer. | Bingham et al[18] |
| Fruit and vegetables | Inverse relationship between the amount of fruit and vegetables consumed and the risk of CRC | Terry et al[19] |
| Red meat | Diets high in animal fats and red meat were associated with an increased risk of colonic adenomas in women and colon cancer in men | Willett et al[20] |
| Red meat | Meta-analysis of articles published 1973–1999 showed that high intake of red meat, especially processed meat, was associated with a moderate but significant increase in CRC risk. Total meat intake was not significantly associated with CRC risk. | Norat et al[21] |
| Micronutrients | Nurses' Health Study data from 88,756 women showed that women who had taken multivitamins containing folic acid for at least 15 years had a significant reduction in the risk of developing colon cancer but not of developing rectal cancer. | Giovannucci et al[22] |
| Folate | DNA in adenomas was hypomethylated compared to controls that did not have adenomas, and patients with CRC had a significantly lower folate status than controls. Patients who had a high folate status as determined by dietary intake, plasma, and erythrocyte folate concentrations had significantly reduced risk of developing colon cancer. | Pufulete et al[23] |
| Calcium | Nurses' Health Study and Health Professionals' Follow-Up Study: higher calcium intake was associated with a significantly lower risk of cancer in the distal colon but not the proximal colon. | Wu et al[24] |
| Calcium | In a prospective study of 803 patients with a history of colorectal adenomas, calcium supplementation statistically reduced the risk of adenoma recurrence in those patients who had adequate vitamin D levels (29.1 ng/mL). | Grau et al[25] |
| Exercise | Harvard University alumni studied. Those who were highly active (energy expenditure of 2500 kilocalories per week) had 50% the risk of developing colon cancer compared to those who were physically inactive (< 1000 kilocalories per week). | Lee et al[26] |

(Continued)

**TABLE 51-1**

**Primary Prevention Strategies (Continued)**

| Prevention Strategy | Study, Findings, or Article | Reference |
|---|---|---|
| Exercise | Nurses' Health Study data showed vigorous exercise reduced the risk for developing colon adenoma and cancer in both men and women. Women with the highest energy expenditure quintile had 57% of the risk of developing large adenoma of sedentary women. | Giovannucci et al[27] |
| Exercise | Review of literature showing a relationship between exercise and reduced risk of colon cancer: 50% reduction in incidence of colon cancer in individuals with the highest level of activity, which persisted when controlled for diet and other factors that might reduce or increase risk of colon cancer. | Colditz et al[28] |
| Exercise | Prospective observational study of 573 women with stage I-III CRC showed that increasing levels of exercise after diagnosis of nonmetastatic CRC reduced cancer-specific mortality and overall mortality. | Meyerhardt et al[29] |
| Aspirin and NSAIDs | Reduces incidence of premalignant adenomas and colon cancer | Muscat et al[30] |
| Selective COX inhibitors | Reduction in mean number of polyps by 28% in patients with familial adenomatous polyposis | Gwyn and Sinicrope[31] |
| Aspirin 325 mg daily | Prospective study of 635 patients with a history of colon cancer who were randomized into groups taking 325 mg daily or placebo. The aspirin group had significantly fewer adenomas than did the placebo group, and a longer time to adenoma detection as compared to the placebo group. | Sandler et al[32] |
| Aspirin 81 mg vs 325 mg daily | Placebo-controlled trial of 1121 patients with a history of adenoma, who were randomized into one of three groups: aspirin 81 mg daily, aspirin 325 mg daily, or placebo. Only the group receiving aspirin 81 mg daily had a significantly reduced risk of developing adenomas as compared to placebo. While 7 patients in the aspirin group had a stroke, the number was not statistically significant. | Baron et al[33] |

*Abbreviations*: COX, cyclooxygenase; CRC, colorectal cancer; IU, international unit; NSAID, nonsteroidal anti-inflammatory drug; RCT, randomized controlled trial.

association between alcohol consumption and the development of colon and rectal cancers. Individuals with a greater than 34 year history of alcohol ingestion had a 70% increased risk of the development of colon and rectal cancer, compared to nondrinkers.[36] Alcohol is thought to stimulate gastrointestinal cell proliferation and promote carcinogenesis secondary to an excess of unabsorbed carcinogens such as the nitrosamines found in beer and whiskey.[36] The body's demand for folate increases with alcohol consumption, and low folate levels may actually confer the risk for the development of these cancers. Larsson et al found in a large Swedish mammography study, that vitamin B6 ingestion conferred protection from colorectal cancer in women who drank alcohol.[37]

Women with a history of endometrial, ovarian, or breast cancer have an increased chance of developing colorectal cancer.[2] Persons with a history of colorectal carcinoma are also at increased risk of developing a second primary colon cancer. Patients who have undergone a cholecystectomy have also been noted to have a higher incidence of colon cancers, but studies conflict as to the exact level of risk.[2]

The National Cancer Institute (NCI) has developed colorectal cancer mortality projections, based on large, older prospective epidemiological studies, and simulated the risk for individuals to develop CRC if they continued high risk lifestyle patterns. The calculated relative risk for developing CRC as compared to those who do not develop CRC (who have a risk of 1.0), is 1.64 for smoking, 1.11 for obesity (BMI>30), and 1.07 for eating red meat 2 times a week as a main meal. Protective effects reduce the relative risk of developing CRC: exercise (20+ met-hours/week) to 0.87, high vegetable consumption (5+ servings/day 0.99), multivitamin daily intake 0.54, aspirin use (2+ tablets/week), and hormonal replacement therapy in post-menopausal women 0.68.[38]

Inflammatory bowel disease (IBD) increases the risk of colon cancer.[39] In general, cancer that develops in individuals with IBD begins with dysplastic changes in the intestinal mucosa and occurs at site of active disease. The relative risk of colon cancer increases with the duration of IBD, as well as severity of disease and concurrent primary sclerosing cholangiitis. Over the last two decades, mortality rates for colorectal cancer in many developed countries have declined in women but not in men. A possible explanation for the decrease in women is the use of oral contraceptives and hormone replacement therapy. A 20% to 40% risk reduction is reported among users of hormone replacement therapy. The apparent protection is related to estrogen, and tended to be stronger among recent users.[2]

Risk factors for colorectal cancer can be broadly classified as environmental and genetic. Environmental factors include diet, lifestyle, and nonsteroidal inflammatory drugs while environmental risk factors include occupational exposure to asbestos, acrylonitrile, ethyl acrylate, synthetic fibers, halogens, printing materials, and fuel oils. Genetic risk factors are related to inherited germ-line mutations (such as familial adenomatous polyposis (FAP) with a mutation in the adenomatous polyposis coloni *(APC)* gene or hereditary nonpolyposis colon cancer (HNPCC), related to mutation in the *MMR* gene), or inherited risk conferred by a first-degree relative having colon cancer. Several genetic polyposis syndromes are associated with a high risk of colon and rectal cancers. FAP is an inherited autosomal dominant trait that results in the development of multiple polyps throughout the colon and rectum. This process generally starts in late adolescence. Persons with this syndrome have a 100% lifetime risk of developing colorectal cancer.[4] Hereditary nonpolyposis colorectal cancer (HNPCC) is an inherited autosomal dominant condition characterized by the occurrence of colorectal cancer at an average age of 45 years. An individual with HNPCC has a 80% lifetime risk of developing colorectal cancer, and for women, a 40% lifetime risk for developing endometrial cancer.[4] Hereditary nonpolyposis colon cancer occurs as type A (Lynch type I) or type B (Lynch type II). Type A is familial, site-specific, nonpolyposis colon cancer. Type B is also nonpolyposis colon cancer but is found in association with other forms of cancer such as breast, endometrial, gastric, and ovarian cancer. Once an individual at risk for HNPCC develops cancer, a subtotal colectomy should be performed. Prophylactic hysterectomy and/or bilateral salpingoophorectomy should be considered for women with HNPCC who are diagnosed with cancer or who are genetic carriers of this disease.

A variant of FAP consists of multiple, flat adenomas that have an increased risk of becoming cancerous. Other genetic premalignant polyposis syndromes associated with a high risk of colorectal cancer include hamartomatous polyposis syndromes (Peutz-Jeghers, juvenile polyposis, Cowden's disease (multiple hamartoma syndrome), and neurofibromatosis) and types of adenomatous polyposis (Gardener's syndrome and Turcot's syndrome).[4]

Inherited risk conferred by a first-degree and second-degree family member with colorectal cancer has been established by earlier, large, prospective epidemiological studies. These patients represent about 20% to 25% of patients with CRC. Relative risk increases to 1.8 (1.0 being normal risk) if a sibling or parent has adenomatous polyps. Risk is increased to three times normal if one or two first-degree relatives aged <50 years old develops colon cancer, and is increased two times if a second degree relative has colon cancer.[4] Selected studies on primary prevention are summarized in Table 51-1. There is still controversy about which factors directly or indirectly cause colon cancer. At this time, it is known that the following factors definitely increase risk and play a role in the development of colon cancer: familial/genetic factors, obesity, inflammatory bowel disease (IBD), inactivity, and micronutrient deficiency.

## PREVENTION, SCREENING, AND EARLY DETECTION

While family history or history of colon adenomas or colon cancer cannot be changed, much can be done to reduce an individual's risk. Two types of prevention are recognized for colorectal cancer: primary and secondary. *Primary prevention* involves minimizing external risk factors such as obesity and improving areas that are likely to be protective such as, diet,[14–21] micronutrients,[22–25] exercise,[26–29] and factors that may minimize polyp formation such as aspirin (if the benefit outweighs risk of side effects).[31–33] Table 51-1 describes studies in these areas, their findings, and references for further reading. It is estimated that as many as 80% of colon cancers can be prevented by dietary change. *Secondary prevention*, or the identification and modification of risk factors following the development of a colonic polyp, involves surgical removal of suspicious adenomatous or malignant polyps to prevent the development of colon cancer.

### PRIMARY PREVENTION

The data shown in Table 51-1 continue to underscore the importance of diet. It is hypothesized that obesity and lack of exercise together may be responsible for altering the metabolism of insulin and insulin-like growth factors.[40] Insulin regulates energy metabolism and anabolic signals related to hyperinsulinemia can promote tumorigenesis (stimulating cell proliferation and inhibiting apoptosis).[41] Dietary fiber has long been touted as a way to protect the colonic and rectal carcinogens through increasing the transit rate of fecal material containing carcinogens. General daily dietary recommendations for fiber intake are 20 to 30 grams per day or more, especially wheat bran[1] and eating at least 5 fruits and vegetables each day. Exercise appears to be an important preventive factor, and many studies have consistently shown a decreased risk for development of adenoma in individuals who exercised vigorously as measured in energy expenditure, after controlling for other factors such as diet and body mass index. Today, the most important primary prevention strategies are weight reduction to appropriate weight for height; regular exercise; eating 5 or more fruits and vegetables per day; including micronutrients such as folate, calcium, and vitamin D in the diet; and taking a baby aspirin or NSAIDs daily if at risk and appropriate.

## SECONDARY PREVENTION AND SCREENING

It is well known that certain polyps are precursors to colon and rectal cancers. Secondary prevention involves removing premalignant polyps, thereby preventing the evolution of colon cancer in most cases. Polyps commonly form in the colon and rectum as an individual ages, with risk increasing beyond 50 years of age. A primary screening goal is to identify polyps before they become malignant. Often polyps bleed as they enlarge, and bleeding can be identified by use of the fecal occult blood test (FOBT). It was estimated that deaths from colon and rectal cancer could have been reduced by 50% or more if Americans age 50 to 80 years had followed the American Cancer Society Guidelines prior to 2008 (FOBT annually, sigmoidoscopy every 5 years, or colonoscopy every 10 years or double contrast barium enema every 5 years).[42] Based on reports by the Congressional Office of Technology Assessment and the National Cancer Institute, the cost per year of lives saved by colon and rectal cancer screening renders the mass screening cost-effective and could save as many as 30,000 lives per year.[3]

Unfortunately, despite the fact that adherence to colorectal cancer screening recommendations is improving, 2005 screening data for adults aged 50 to 64 years showed that 44.2% had had a recent screening (an increase from 37.6%) and 56.4% (from 48.7%) of persons aged 65 or older had undergone a recent screening.[42] The prevalence of colonoscopy increased to 39.2% from 20%.[42] As a result of this, as well as the fact that the screening options were complex, a consensus group was organized composed of the American Cancer Society, the US Multi-Society Task Force on Colorectal Cancer (USMSTF), made up of representatives from the American College of Gastroenterology, American Gastroenterological Association, and the American Society for Gastrointestinal Endoscopy, and the American College of Radiology. The group published consensus guidelines for asymptomatic, average-risk individuals, which recommended tests that either detect adenomatous polyps and cancer, and those which primarily detect cancer, based on the individual's willingness and ability to adhere to the recommended testing.[43] See Tables 51-2 and 51-3.

Ideally, the patient will consider the tests that find both polyps and cancer early (eg, either colonoscopy every 10 years, double contrast barium enema (DCBE) every 5 years, flexible sigmoidoscopy (FSIG) every 5 years, or CT colonography (virtual colonoscopy, CTC) every 5 years). However, the test must be available (both physically and affordable) and the patient must be willing to do the follow-up (eg, if examination is positive, a colonoscopy will be required for FSIG, DCBE, or CTC if polyps are ≥ 6 mm). If patients are unwilling or unable to have an invasive test requiring bowel preparation, then tests that primarily detect cancer are recommended, such as guaiac FOBT annually, fecal immunochemical test (FIT) annually, or a stool DNA test (sDNA) frequency unknown. Again, the patient should understand that these tests are less likely to prevent cancer, and be willing to adhere to having the test regularly, and to comply with the follow-up recommendations. Having access to health screening is very important, as is the recommendation of the clinician. The National Health Interview Survey (NHIS, the Center for Disease Control, or CDC's, principal source of health information about civilian, non-institutionalized Americans) and the Behavioral Risk Factor Surveillance Survey (BRFSS) both show that uninsured individuals have lower levels of colorectal cancer screening than those with health insurance.[9] In addition, the 2005 NHIS survey showed that for men and women aged 50 to 64 who had private insurance, 48.3% had screening recommended by their healthcare provider within the prior 10 years, 39.6% who had Medicaid insurance, and 18.8% who were uninsured. Health insurance was shown to be an important predictor of screening across racial and ethnic groups. In addition, at all levels of education, individuals with health insurance were twice as likely to have colorectal cancer screening as those without health insurance.[9]

While controversy remains regarding the equivalence of double-contrast barium enema plus flexible sigmoidoscopy or colonoscopy, it is quite clear that if an individual has any increased risk for the development of colon cancer, then a colonoscopy should be performed (see Table 51-2 and 51-3). In addition, if there is any suggestion that a tumor may be on the right (proximal) side, such as with obese women or African American men, or if distal adenomas are found at sigmoidoscopy, a colonoscopy must be performed.

Persons with an inherited risk for colorectal cancer, such as family history of FAP, should begin screening by colonoscopy between the ages of 10 and 12. Individuals with 1 or more first-degree relatives who developed colon cancer before the age of 55 should have an annual fecal occult blood test and a colonoscopy or double-contrast barium enema every 5 years starting 10 years before the age of onset in the relative. Persons with lower levels of risk (one relative with colorectal cancer diagnosed at an age more than 60 years) should have standard screening starting at age 50. The Society of Gastroenterology Nurses and Associates supports routine screening using flexible sigmoidoscopy performed by trained nurses as a way to increase access to screening.[44]

The FOBT and periodic flexible sigmoidoscopy are two easy methods of screening. Most studies, including

**TABLE 51-2**

**2008 Consensus Guidelines for Colorectal Cancer Screening: Average-Risk Individuals Age 50 and Over**

| Test | Discussion Points With Patients to Help Select Test |
|---|---|
| ***A. Tests to prevent cancer through detection of adenomatous polyps and early cancer (preferred)*** | |
| Flexible sigmoidoscopy | Performed every 5 years; only examines up to the splenic flexure (40 cm); will need colonoscopy if positive findings; requires bowel preparation |
| Colonoscopy | Performed every 10 years; examines full colon and rectum, including proximal colon and permits biopsy and excision of polyps; full bowel prep required; conscious sedation is used and must have someone to bring the person home; risks include perforation (3%) and bleeding after polypectomy |
| Double contrast barium | Performed every 5 years; examines full colon and rectum but colonoscopy requiring another full bowel prep must be done if polyp(s) ≥6 mm in size are found; cannot biopsy or remove polyps; minimal risk for complications |
| Virtual colonoscopy (computerized tomography colonography, CTC) | Performed every 5 years; examines full colon and rectum with state-of-the art equipment by a skilled physician; requires full bowel prep; colonoscopy required if polyp(s) ≥6 mm in size are found; may find extracolonic abnormalities; rare complications; may be uncomfortable as no sedation and gas distends the bowel |
| ***B. Tests to detect cancer*** | |
| Guaiac fecal occult blood test (gFOBT) | Performed annually; strict preparation (diet, avoidance of aspirin, NSAIDs); 2–3 sequential stool samples obtained at home, and must be returned to be read; follow-up including colonoscopy is necessary if blood is found |
| Fecal immunochemical test (FIT) | Performed annually; expensive; follow-up including colonoscopy is necessary if blood is found |
| Stool DNA test (sDNA) | Frequency is unknown; expensive; must follow directions (eg, adequate sample, preservative, shipping to laboratory); technology is changing; follow-up including colonoscopy is necessary if blood is found |

*Note*: One test is selected, and screening for prevention is preferred. Individual must be willing and able to participate in necessary follow-up if the test reveals positive findings.

*Source*: Data from Levin et al.[43]

randomized trials, show that periodic FOBT reduces the risk of death from colon and rectal cancer by 15% to 33%.[45] Mandel and colleagues[46] studied the effect of FOBT screening on the incidence of colorectal cancer. They found that (1) the number of positive FOBT slides was associated with a positive predictive value for both colorectal cancer and adenomatous polyps at least 1 cm in diameter and (2) use of either annual or biennial FOBT significantly reduced the incidence of colorectal cancer. In screening general populations, it is estimated that 1% to 16% of patients have positive FOBT, depending on age, whether the sample is rehydrated, and the purpose of the test. Following colonic evaluation, the rate of finding colon or rectal cancer is only 2% to 17%, and the rate of finding early colon or rectal cancer is 2% to 14%.[45] However, once a positive FOBT is found, there must be adequate evaluation of the colon and follow-up. The sensitivity and specificity of guaiac FOBT is variable, and depends on the manufacturer, collection technique, number of samples tested, whether the sample is hydrated, and compliance to the preparation (avoidance of aspirin, nonsteroidal anti-inflammatory drugs, vitamin C, red meat, poultry, fish, and raw cruciferous vegetables).[45]

The fecal immunochemistry test (FIT) is more expensive than the guaiac FOBT: it detects human globulin (from hemoglobin) but is more specific for human blood (in the lower GI tract) and does not give a false-positive when combined with vitamin C. The test does not require restrictions or the complex 3 sequential stool tests as with guaiac FOBT. A study comparing guaiac FOBT and FIT testing showed that the sensitivity for colorectal cancer was 81.8% for the FIT compared to 64.3% of the guaiac FOBT; however, the guaiac FOBT was more sensitive to identify advanced adenomas (41.3%) compared to the FIT (29.5%).[47]

DNA stool testing is based on the fact that adenoma or carcinoma cells containing mutated DNA are shed continuously into the stool from the intestinal mucosa, and can be detected by a multi-targeted stool assay.[48] Mutations identified include those in *K-ras, APC, p53* genes as well as markers for microsatellite instability (BAT-26) and DNA integrity. Sensitivity for colorectal cancer ranged from 52% to 91%, and specificity 93% to 97%, and although less sensitive for advanced adenomas, it was still superior to guaiac FOBT.[48] The consensus guidelines state that although the

**TABLE 51-3**

**2008 Consensus Guidelines for CRC Screening: Increased or High-Risk Individuals**

| Risk Etiology | Recommendations |
|---|---|
| ***Polyps found at colonoscopy*** | |
| Hyperplastic | Colonoscopy interval for average-risk individuals |
| 1–2 tubular adenomas, low-grade dysplasia | Colonoscopy 5–10 years after initial polypectomy |
| 3–10 adenomas, or > 1 cm, or villous features, or high-grade dysplasia | Colonoscopy 3 years after initial polypectomy |
| > 10 adenomas on examination | < 3 years after initial polypectomy |
| Sessile adenoma, fragmented excision | Colonoscopy 2–5 months after removal |
| ***Personal history of CRC*** | |
| Following resection for cure | 1 year after resection; if WNL, repeat in 3 years, then 5 years |
| Synchronous tumors | 3–6 months after resection |
| Obstructing colon cancer | Virtual colonoscopy with IV contrast or DCBE |
| ***Family history of CRC*** | |
| First degree relative before age 60 years with CRC or adenomatous polyp, or in ≥ 2 first degree relatives at any age | Colonoscopy at age 40, or 10 years before youngest case in immediate family, and repeat every 5 years |
| First degree relative age ≥ 60 years with CRC or adenomatous polyps, or in 2 second degree relatives with CRC | Begin screening at age 40 with testing for average-risk individuals |
| ***Genetic disease risk, or IBD*** | |
| Diagnosis of FAP or suspected without genetic test results | Begin annual flexible sigmoidoscopy at age 10–12 years to determine if genetic abnormality expressed; genetic testing with counseling if not already done |
| Genetic or clinical diagnosis of HNPCC or at risk for HNPCC | Colonoscopy every 1–2 years, beginning at age 20–25 years, or 10 years before the youngest case in the immediate family; genetic testing with counseling |
| IBD, chronic ulcerative colitis, or Crohn's colitis | Colonoscopy with biopsies for dysplasia q 1–2 years, by experienced endoscopists familiar with IBD |

*Abbreviations*: CRC, colorectal cancer; DCBE, double contrast barium enema; FAP, familial adenomatous polyposis; HNPCC, hereditary nonpolyposis colon cancer; IBD, inflammatory bowel disease; IV, intravenous; WNL, within normal limits.
*Source*: Data from Levin et al.[43]

technology is still evolving, there is sufficient data to recommend this test for asymptomatic, average risk individuals, as patient satisfaction is high. The frequency of performing this test is unclear presently.[43]

Digital rectal examinations are simple but can detect abnormalities only up to 7 cm from the anal verge. Thus they are not useful for colon cancer screening. FOBT should not be obtained via a digital rectal exam.

Sigmoidoscopy using a flexible, fiber-optic sigmoidoscope is easy to perform, requires no sedation, and detects as many as 65% of colorectal tumors within 60 cm from the anal verge.[49] If adenomas are found in the distal colon, then colonoscopy is usually performed to examine the proximal colon. Advanced proximal lesions are more likely if the individual is older than age 65, and if villous or tubulovillous distal adenomas were found, or there is a family history of colon or rectal cancer or multiple distal polyps,[11] or as mentioned previously, in obese women or African American men. If adenomas can be found and removed early, colon cancer can be prevented. Schoen and colleagues[49] reported on data from the Prostate, Lung, Colorectal and Ovarian (PLCO) Cancer Screening trial showing that a repeat sigmoidoscopy 3 years following a negative sigmoidoscopy found a polyp or lesion in the rectum or distal sigmoid in 13.9% of patients (1292 out of 9317 subjects). Most of the polyps were benign, but 2.3% of subjects (214 out of 9317) had adenomas that were not advanced, and 0.8% (78 out of 9317) had advanced adenoma or cancer. Of patients with advanced adenoma or malignancy, 80% had a thorough examination 3 years earlier. The PLCO is a large, randomized, prospective study that will continue to accrue patients through 2015.

According to Gatto and colleagues,[50] there is a risk of perforation during sigmoidoscopy (incidence = 0.88/1000 procedures), especially in elderly patients with two or more co-morbidities. The risk is less than that of colonoscopy, although the risk of perforation with colonoscopy is decreasing.

Most sigmoidoscopies are performed by physicians, but evidence indicates that nurse endoscopists are equally able to do effective examinations. As early as 1994, Maule[51] described a comparative study of nurse performance of sigmoidoscopy compared to physicians: Nurses performed 1881 independent exams compared to 730 by physicians. The mean depth of insertion of the sigmoidoscope was significantly greater by physicians (48 cm vs 46 cm in men, and 41 cm vs 38 cm in women). There was no significant difference in the number of adenomas or cancer found or in the complications (none) between nurses and physicians. There was however, a highly significant difference between the number of patients who returned for follow-up sigmoidoscopy: more patients examined by nurses returned as compared to those examined by physicians ($P = 0.001$). More recently, Kelly et al described the experiences of a nurse specialist-led flexible sigmoidoscopy practice in an outpatient setting in the United Kingdom from 1999 to 2004, demonstrating efficient and safe screening and evaluation of colorectal symptoms.[52] In the US, the Society of Gastroenterology Nurses and Associates has developed standards and guidelines for performance of flexible sigmoidoscopy by registered nurses for the purpose of colorectal cancer screening.[53]

Combining FOBT and flexible sigmoidoscopy should increase early detection of advanced adenomas or early-stage cancers, but two studies showed no significant difference between both modalities compared to sigmoidoscopy (or colonoscopy as a surrogate) alone.[54,55] Winawer and colleagues[56] compared colonoscopy and double-contrast barium enema for surveillance after polypectomy as part of the National Polyp Study Work Group, and found that colonoscopy was a more effective method of surveillance than double-contrast barium enema. Colonoscopy is a more sensitive tool for detecting tumors throughout the entire colon. Biopsy specimens can be obtained and polyps removed during the actual procedure. The accuracy of the colonoscopy examination depends on the ability of the endoscopist to reach the cecum and to negotiate blind corners and mucosal folds. To achieve a satisfactory examination, patient teaching for preparation and support during the procedure itself are crucial. In addition, the rate for missing large adenomas (10 mm) is 6% to 12%, while that for cancer is 5% with colonoscopy.[57]

Lieberman and colleagues[58] studied 3121 veterans and found that patients with distal polyps were also more likely to have proximal polyps. However, Imperiale and colleagues[59] showed that all patients with proximal neoplastic lesions do not have distal polyps; hence, if colonoscopy was reserved only for high-risk patients or those with distal polyps, then 46% or more of patients with proximal lesions will be missed. The authors concluded that the risk of perforation from colonoscopy is double that of sigmoidoscopy, but the difference between the two modalities is decreasing. Colonoscopy acceptance by patients has increased since the publicity of major figures made it socially acceptable to discuss. However, a number of patients are still dissatisfied with the 1 to 2 days of bowel preparation, the fact that the procedure requires IV conscious sedation, and someone to drive the person home.

## Virtual colonoscopy or colonography

Recently, much attention has been focused on virtual colonoscopy or colonography as a means to examine the colon. Virtual colonoscopy uses computer-generated images from abdominal computed tomography (CT) or magnetic resonance imaging (MRI) to simulate colonoscopic examination. There have been advances in CT technology that produce thin sliced images of the entire bowel wall, along with integrated 3D graphics. The preparation and procedure may be as uncomfortable for the patient as colonoscopy, as the bowel must be adequately prepared, and the bowel distended with gas to permit visualization. In addition, it is unclear whether virtual colonoscopy provides the same accuracy in identifying polyps, especially if they are smaller than 1 cm, or if it can provide the same reliability when used for follow-up of lesions as does conventional colonoscopy.

A number of important studies have examined this technology, and as a screening modality, virtual colonoscopy has been included in the consensus guidelines. Summers et al reported a National Institutes of Health study of 1186 patients using virtual colonoscopy combined with a computer-aided polyp detector (CAD). The findings showed that this technique is comparable to optical colonoscopy, as CAD was able to detect 83% of polyps that were 10 mm (1 cm) or larger, 81% of polyps that were 8 mm or larger, and 61% of polyps that were 6 mm or larger. Missed polyps were hidden under fluid, or on a fold. The false positive rate per patient was: two false positives (10+ mm), seven false positives (8+ mm), and eight false positives (6+ mm).[60]

Unfortunately, virtual colonoscopy does not permit excision of polyps once found; patients still need to have a conventional colonoscopy for polypectomy. The consensus guidelines recommend that all patients with 1 or more polyps $\geq 10$ mm or 3 or more polyps $\geq 6$ mm should have a colonoscopy.[43] The consensus guidelines state that CTC is equivalent to optical colonoscopy for the detection of cancer and significantly sized polyps, when state-of-the-art techniques are used.[43] Further study will help establish criteria for CTC reporting, as well as define the interval testing time when the test results are normal.

## Other screening technologies

Laboratory tests for gene mutations are now available, thus making it possible to screen individuals at increased risk for developing colorectal cancer as a result of inherited mutations. Genetic analysis of populations at risk could result in more specific measures to reduce risk and earlier identification of the colorectal malignancy. Unfortunately, persons at high risk who should be genetically tested are potentially more likely to lose their insurance coverage. The role of the nurse and/or the genetic counselor in this situation is to provide the necessary information needed for the patient to be able to make an informed decision. In the past, many patients pay out of pocket for genetic testing to avoid insurance cancellation or loss of employment. The Genetic Information Nondiscrimination Act (GINA) now protects individuals against discrimination based on their genetic history, in terms of employment or health insurance.[61] Genetic testing and clinical screening usually should not be undertaken until 10 to 12 years of age.[3] Table 51-3 outlines the consensus guidelines for screening and surveillance for the early detection of colorectal adenomas and cancer in individuals at increased risk or high risk.[43]

## PATHOPHYSIOLOGY

### CELLULAR CHARACTERISTICS

In colorectal cancers, a series of mutations occurs in the epithelial cells of the colonic and rectal mucosa. Carcinogens that stimulate these changes include fecal mutagens, meat intake, bile acids, altered vitamin and mineral intake, and fecal pH.[11] These mutations affect the genes of *somatic* cells of the body (but not the reproductive cells), and involve both proto-oncogenes (genes that encourage the cell to go through active division) and suppressor genes (genes that discourage the cell from going into active division). These changes are not passed from parent to offspring. In contrast, in a small percentage of individuals, similar mutations occur in the *germ-line* (reproductive) proto-oncogenes and some germ-line tumor suppressor genes. These mutations are passed from parent to child, and affect all cells that arise from the inherited cells with mutations. This genetic predisposition accounts for only 7% to 8% of patients with colon or rectal cancer.[62]

Kinzler and Vogelstein[62] were able to trace the genetic mutations in patients with HNPCC from the time that the initial mutation occurred in the colonic mucosa, to the formation of an adenoma on the mucosal surface, and continuing to an adenocarcinoma during the period of 10 to 20 years it took for an invasive adenocarcinoma to develop. Carcinogens cause mutations, but normally the cells are able to repair themselves using functional DNA repair genes. At some point, a mutation occurs in the *APC* gene, which acts as a tumor suppressor gene. When the mutation in the *APC* gene is not corrected, the mutation is carried through the cell division cycle, and the DNA mutation passes into each of the two daughter cells. This mutation results in the loss of a portion of the *APC* gene (5q21, long arm of chromosome 5). Loss of a portion of a chromosome is called loss of heterozygosity (LOH). This initial genetic mutation occurs in somatic cells in 80% of the sporadic cancers, and is the inherited (germ-line) mutation in individuals with FAP and HNPCC. There are two alleles for this gene. One is passed from parent to child. When the other copy of the gene is inactivated through exposure to carcinogens, and both are mutated, the gene is inactivated. This removes the tumor suppressor function, so that no force opposes the continual cell division. In addition, the *APC* gene makes a protein that regulates cell-cell adhesion, cell migration, and influences apoptosis. Genetic analysis shows that both *APC* alleles are inactivated in most colon and rectal adenomas, and in inherited as well as 80% of sporadic colon and rectal adenocarcinomas.[4] Another gene that is mutated and often associated with the mutation in the *APC* gene is beta-catenin, which keeps cells attached to the cytoskeleton. Adenomatous polyposis coli (APC) is a major binding partner and regulator of the beta-catenin protein, so when both *APC* alleles are mutated, beta-catenin is not degraded, and continues to activate the Wnt signaling pathway leading to cell proliferation and migration.[4] (Wnt signaling is a signal transduction pathway involved in embryogenesis that keeps stem cells in an undifferentiated state. It is mutated in many cancers, and is implicated in about 90% of CRCs.) In the small number of tumors where the *APC* gene is not mutated, beta-catenin is mutated, again leading to activated Wnt signaling.[2] The mutation occurs on the short arm of chromosome 3 (3p21), which is an area often mutated in many cancers. The mutation removes the regulation of the cell adhering to the cytoskeleton, so that cells can over time, grow away from the cytoskeleton and migrate, which normally cause them to die (automatically go into programmed cell death). In malignant cells, this phenomenon allows the cell to become invasive and to metastasize. There appear to be at least three pathways resulting in CRC.[4] In the first pathway, a normal cell undergoes inactivation of the *APC* gene (5q loss) forming a dysplastic crypt. Then there is mutation of the *K-Ras* proto-oncogene, forming an oncogene. This leads to an adenoma with chromosomal abnormalities (CIN). Over time, the next genes that become mutated are tumor suppressor genes, the *deleted-in-colon-cancer* (DCC), as well as *DPC4* gene (17p loss). As there is no opposition to the activated oncogene, cell division continues and results in the formation of a late adenoma. The tumor suppressor gene, *p53*, "the brakes of the cell cycle," is then mutated and becomes inactive. This mutation removes the final opposing force to uncontrolled cell division and moves the late adenoma into malignant transformation.

In the second and third pathways, the first step leads to inactivation of one or more mismatch repair genes. In HNPCC, this is the familial MSI-H (microsatellite instability-high) pathway, followed by mutation of *APC*, beta-catenin, and *Axin* 2 (a tumor suppressor gene that helps to regulate beta-catenin expression). This is followed by mutation and formation of the *K-Ras* oncogene, leading to an adenoma, then over time, there are more mutations of genes with microsatellites, *p53*, and a carcinoma forms. The third pathway starts with inactivation of mismatch repair gene *MLH1* via epigenetic causes (inheritable changes in DNA function not caused by changes in DNA sequence; often caused by DNA methylation in this case, hypermethylation of the *MLH1* promoter). The next step is similar to the second pathway, where *APC*, beta-catenin, and *Axin* 2 are mutated, but here these are followed by a genetic mutations in *B-Raf*, as well as *K-Ras* leading to the formation of a serrated adenoma. Then, similar to the second pathway, there are mutations in genes with microsatellites leading to their inactivation, and malignant transformation.[4]

This information has helped to divide colon tumors into two general classes: those with chromosomal instability (CIN) and those with microsatellite instability (MSI). About 85% of sporadic colon cancers have CIN and 15% have MSI. Characteristics of CIN include nonrandom chromosome losses (long or short arms of chromosomes 5q, 12p, 18q, 17p in *APC*, beta-catenin, *K-ras*, and *DCC* genes). Microsatellite instability (MSI) characteristics are related to defects in mismatched repair (*MMR*) genes; are common in HNPCC; have an increased mutation rate in *APC*, beta-catenin, and *K-ras* genes due to defects in *MMR* genes so the cell cannot correct the DNA mistakes; and produce replication errors in transforming growth factor-beta (TGF-β) and *BAT-26* gene loci.

Interestingly, patients with MSI tumors have an increased response to chemotherapy. MSI often involves *MLH1* (one of the DNA mismatch repair genes that when mutated prevents certain types of DNA repair). In HNPCC, *MLH1* is an inherited mutation; in the sporadic cancers, it is brought about by epigenetic (involving a mutation or change in the chromatin structure in the gene) silencing by *hypermethylation* of the promoter region. Both avenues result in the same MSI phenotype.[63] DNA methylation is a normal process that allows the cell to shut off or silence gene expression, so that the gene no longer is transcribed to make a specific protein that the body no longer needs. For example, during embryogenesis, the embryo cells must differentiate into specific body tissues; once the fetus is formed, the responsible genes are silenced or shut off. As the colon and rectal mucosa ages, methylation of the DNA slowly occurs. Although a small amount of gene methylation is found in normally aging colorectal mucosal epithelial cells, age-related hypermethylation may result in the silencing of tumor suppressor genes, leading to malignant transformation.[62] It is believed that abnormal DNA methylation occurs early in the formation of an adenoma, especially villous adenomas.

### Inherited colon cancer

***Familial adenomatous polyposis.*** Familial adenomatous polyposis (FAP) involves a mutation in the *APC* tumor suppressor gene. Normally, this gene brings about death of the colonic cells once their usefulness is complete. It also helps to keep the protein beta-catenin in check. If the protein beta-catenin is allowed to accumulate in the cell, it stimulates genes that turn on cell division. The *APC* gene is an autosomal dominant gene: the *APC* gene on one of the nonsex chromosomes is always expressed or turned on, even if only one copy of the gene or allele is present. The mutation renders the gene inactive. The chance of passing the gene to offspring is 50% for each pregnancy. Every cell in the affected person's colonic and rectal mucosa has one normal copy of the gene and one mutated copy of the gene that was inherited (it is a germ-line mutation). A second mutation in the normal allele will inactivate the tumor suppressor function, leading to development of an adenomatous polyp. The more frequently the cells divide, the more likely another mutation will occur, thereby initiating the process of malignant transformation. The mutation of the *APC* gene is highly penetrant: If a person inherits the gene, the likelihood of developing colon or rectal cancer over the individual's lifetime is 100%. Familial adenomatous polyposis affects about 1 in 8000 individuals, with polyps usually beginning at age 16, and malignant transformation usually occurring between the ages of 30 and 40 years. Familial adenomatous polyposis represents 0.5% of all colon and rectal cancers. The affected individual develops hundreds to thousands of polyps in the colon and rectum. Thus, screening begins at puberty and genetic counseling is important to prevent or detect at an early stage any malignant transformation so that curative resection can occur. Prophylactic total colectomy may be offered, or celecoxib may be indicated for the prevention of polyp formation in individuals with FAP.[64] Unfortunately, celecoxib is associated with rare but increased risk of cardiovascular events so benefit should outweigh risk. A study by Bertagnolli et al demonstrated that celecoxib is associated with a significant decrease in polyp formation (60.7% incidence in group receiving placebo, compared to 43.2% (celecoxib 200 mg PO twice daily) and 37.5% (celecoxib 400 mg PO twice daily). Adverse events were significantly higher in patients treated with celecoxib, although by a small amount: 18.8% in the placebo group compared to 20.4% (low dose celecoxib) and 23% (high dose group); and risk ratio for cardiovascular events in the celecoxib arms compared to placebo was 2.6 (low dose) and 3.4 (high dose).[64] The authors caution that while celecoxib is effective, it cannot be routinely recommended given the potential cardiovascular risks.

***Hereditary nonpolyposis colorectal cancer.*** Hereditary nonpolyposis colorectal cancer (HNPCC) is also known as Lynch I syndrome. In contrast to patients with FAP, individuals with HNPCC do not present with multiple polyps. These genetic mutations are also autosomal dominant, but the penetrance is incomplete, so only 80% of individuals with the genetic mutations develop the colon or rectal cancer. Hereditary nonpolyposis colorectal cancer affects about 1 in 1000 individuals, and 1 in 100 individuals with colon or rectal cancer. This disease accounts for about 7% of all colorectal cancers.[65]

The germ-line genetic mutations (passed on in the reproductive cells of the parent), appear in one of the 5 DNA mismatch repair genes (proofreading molecules on DNA—*MSH2, MLH1, PMS1, PMS2,* and *MSH6*).[66] The mismatch repair genes ensure that the cell's genes are identical to the parent cells' genes (genomic fidelity). The mismatch repair genes repair base-base mismatches, insertion-deletion loops, and mistakes that occur during DNA replication and recombination, as well as activation of cell-cycle checkpoint function and induction of apoptosis if the DNA mutation cannot be repaired.[66] These cancers tend to be MSI and occur in the right, proximal colon. The current standard for diagnosis of this syndrome is known as the revised Bethesda criteria (see Table 51-4). There appear to be some racial and ethnic variations in HNPCC, and other countries such as Japan and China have slightly different criteria. In the US, Lynch and colleagues[65,67] suggest that when an individual undergoes genetic testing for HNPCC, the primary DNA sequence of the *MSH2* gene should be tested first; if it is positive for a mutation, then the rest of the genes should be tested as the individual most likely has HNPCC.

**TABLE 51-4**

**Revised Bethesda Criteria for HNPCC Diagnosis, 2003**

- Diagnosed with CRC before the age of 50 years old.
- Synchronous or metachronous colorectal or other HNPCC-related tumors, including stomach, bladder, ureter, renal pelvis, biliary tract, brain (glioblastoma), sebaceous gland adenomas, keratoacanthomas, and carcinoma of the small bowel, regardless of age.
- CRC with high MSI morphology that was diagnosed before the age of 60 years.
- CRC with one or more first-degree relatives with CRC or other HNPCC-related tumors. One of the cancers must have been diagnosed before the age of 50 years, including adenoma, which must have been diagnosed before the age of 40 years.
- CRC with two or more relatives with CRC or other HNPCC-related tumors, regardless of age.

*Note*: Only one criteria needs to be met.
Abbreviations: CRC, colorectal cancer; HNPCC, hereditary nonpolyposis colorectal cancer; MSI, microsatellite instability.
*Source*: Data from Umar et al.[66]

Lynch II syndrome refers to the development of extracolonic cancers such as ovarian, endometrial, breast, and biliary cancers. A woman with HNPCC has a 60% lifetime risk of developing endometrial cancer.

## PROGRESSION OF DISEASE AND PATTERNS OF SPREAD

The colon is made up of four layers: the mucosa, the submucosa, the muscularis, and the serosa. The mucosa and submucosa are divided by the muscularis. Reproduction of cells in the colon takes place in the crypts of Lieberkuhn, which are located in the mucosal layer. As new cells are produced, old cells mature, migrate out of the crypt, and are shed. Damage to the crypts will affect reproducing cells and cause the crypts to become prone to errors and to the formation of early adenomas.[11]

The large intestine consists of the cecum, ascending colon, transverse colon, descending colon, sigmoid colon, and rectum, as shown in Figure 51-1. The ascending colon and descending colon are considered extraperitoneal organs because they lie in the anterior pararenal space and are covered by a single layer of the posterior peritoneum. The transverse and sigmoid colon are suspended in the peritoneal cavity by the mesocolon that is formed by two layers of peritoneal linings. The cecum is attached to the ileocolic mesentery in the right iliac fossa. The arterial supply to the cecum, ascending colon, and transverse colon derives from the superior mesenteric artery. The blood supply to the sigmoid colon and descending colon comes from the inferior mesenteric artery. The superior mesenteric vein drains the cecum, ascending colon, and transverse colon. The artery and vein supplying and draining each segment of the colon accompany each other in the mesocolon. The venous system of the colon drains into the portal circulation.

Nodal spread from each segment of the colon follows the blood vessels in the mesocolon.[11] Invasion of the venous system yields a poor prognosis. Once tumor cells invade the vascular system, widespread dissemination of the disease follows; it is not amenable to surgical resection, and chemotherapy and radiation therapy have only limited effects. Local invasion into the neighboring structures is more common in the cecum and rectosigmoid areas. The liver is the most frequent site of metastatic involvement. Solitary pulmonary metastasis is rare. Other areas of metastasis include the brain (cerebellum), bones, kidneys, and adrenals.[11] By the time of diagnosis, approximately 25% of colon cancers will have extended through the bowel wall.[2] Implantation of tumor cells at other sites can occur as a result of surgical manipulation of the tumor, intraluminal spread, or shedding of tumor cells into the peritoneum. Intraperitoneal seeding and carcinomatosis may occur even without lymphatic or visceral spread.

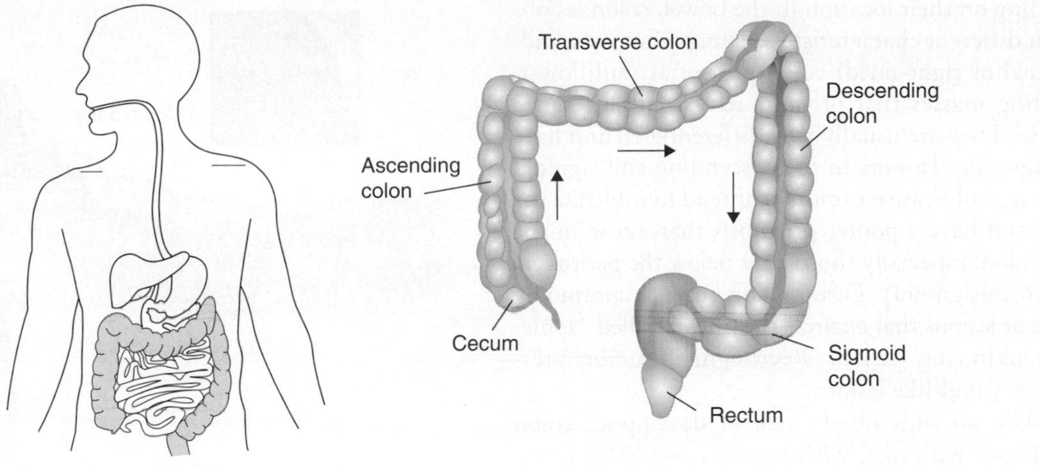


**FIGURE 51-1**

Anatomy of the colon.

*Source*: Data from National Institute of Diabetes and Digestive and Kidney Diseases.[68]

## Histology

The most common histological type of colon cancer is adenocarcinoma. The degree of differentiation of the tumor is based on the appearance of well-formed glands, and poorly differentiated tumors do not show well-defined glandular structures.[69] Most adenocarcinomas are moderately well differentiated. If cells are poorly differentiated or high grade, the cancer is more aggressive and often associated with lymphatic or vascular invasion. Many tumors produce mucin, which either stays inside the cells or is secreted. Secreted mucin helps the cells move away into neighboring cells. If more than 50% of the tumor mass is made up of extracellular mucin, it is called a mucinous carcinoma. These are found principally in the sigmoid (descending) colon and rectum, account for 11% to 17% of colon and rectal cancers, and often are diagnosed at a more advanced stage of disease.[69] If mucin stays inside the cell in more than 50% of the tumor mass, it is called a signet ring carcinoma. These cancers are rare, accounting for 1% to 2% of colon and rectal cancers, but are very aggressive. In one study, more than 93% of patients with signet ring carcinoma presented with stage III or IV disease at diagnosis, and 64% of patients had peritoneal spread.[70] Some distal colon cancers may include areas of squamous cells, so the cancers are called adenosquamous carcinomas.[71] Rarely, there may be small areas of neuroendocrine cells, especially in poorly differentiated tumors. When these are present in larger amounts in non-glandforming tumors, they are called small cell carcinomas and have a poor prognosis.[69] Lastly, medullary carcinoma is a type of non-gland-forming colon cancer that is characterized by tumor-infiltrating lymphocytes, microsatellite instability, and HNPCC.[69]

Other tumors may involve the colon rarely, such as Kaposi's sarcoma, primary non-Hodgkin's lymphoma (cecum, right colon, or rectum), and carcinoid (cecum or rectum). Sometimes the primary tumor is unclear. Adenocarcinomas of colorectal origin are almost always cytokeratin 20 positive and cytokeratin 7 negative by immunohistochemistry.[72] While molecular diagnosis is still being clinically explored, eventually microarray gene profiling may permit rapid diagnosis and treatment planning.

Previously the most common sites of colon cancers were the sigmoid and descending colon, but the proximal colon is now the site of highest incidence at 54.7%.[11] Evidence indicates that sporadic left colon tumors differ genetically from right-sided or proximal tumors. Olesen and colleagues[73] found 44 different abnormal gene expressions between right and left-sided colon cancer lesions when genes were analyzed using microarray technology. These differences in gene expression were not based on microsatellite instability. The researchers also found both right and left-sided cancers share 30 genes that are not present in normal colonic mucosa, which can be used as tumor markers. Therefore, in developing molecular-targeted therapy against colon cancer using gene expression as a guide, separate strategies will be needed for targeting right-vs left-sided colon adenocarcinomas.

Adenocarcinomas of the colon and rectum develop initially in the mucosa. The tumor then locally invades into the lumen of the bowel wall. When it has traversed the muscularis mucosa and infiltrated the serosa, it is termed *invasive*. Further infiltration by way of the lymph and vascular system occurs next, and direct extension may occur into the peritoneal surfaces as well.

Depending on their location in the bowel, colon lesions may exhibit different characteristics. Tumors in the ascending (proximal or right-sided) colon present as cauliflower-like fungating masses that progress to become ulcerative and necrotic. They are usually well differentiated and have a better prognosis. Tumors in the descending and sigmoid colon present as ulcerative tumors that tend to infiltrate the bowel wall and have a poorer prognosis than those in the ascending colon, especially those at or below the peritoneal reflection (rectosigmoid). Distal colon tumors commonly are annular or lesions that encircle the bowel, called "apple-core" or "napkin ring" lesions. Rectosigmoid tumors present as villous, frond-like lesions.

In the US, an individual's risk of developing colon cancer increases with age, with most cases (90%) being diagnosed in individuals older than 50 years of age.[11] At age 60, about 50% of individuals will have at least one polyp. Initially, polyps form when the intestinal glandular epithelium undergoes mutation. Most polyps are adenomatous polyps or adenomas. About 75% of all polyps are adenomas. Other types of polyps are always benign: hyperplastic, inflammatory, and hamartomatous polyps. Adenomatous polyps or adenomas have the ability to become malignant. Two factors influence the likelihood that an adenoma will become malignant: histology and size. Histologically, adenomas can be tubular (shaped like a tube), villous (tiny projections), or tubulo-villous (tubes and fingerlike projections). Most adenomas are tubular polyps, which represent 70% of adenomas. Villous adenomas confer the highest risk, and tubular adenomas have the lowest risk of transformation. As the polyp becomes larger, the risk of malignant transformation increases. When a polyp reaches 2 cm or larger, the risk of malignant transformation is 20%. This relationship between size and malignancy underscores the importance or removing polyps when they are small. The time from polyp formation to malignant transformation can be as long as 10 years. At age 50, the incidence of adenomas is 25%; by age 70, the risk increases to 50%.[74] Further, inflammatory conditions near the polyp increase the risk of malignant transformation. As previously discussed, ulcerative colitis (UC) increases the risk of colorectal cancer due to the chronic cycles of mucosal injury, with subsequent regrowth resulting in dysplasia. Polyps are either pedunculated (stalk-like) or sessile (flat). Sessile polyps are closer to the bowel wall, so as they enlarge, they can more easily invade the bowel mucosa as compared to pedunculated polyps. Sessile polyps are also more difficult to remove. Sometimes they are flat, plaque-like polyps that are difficult to visualize except on colonoscopy, as they may lie slightly below the surface of the bowel mucosa. Figure 51-2 shows a pedunculated polyp.[75]

Polyps are removed at colonoscopy, with the site marked. Superficial adenomatous polyps with malignant transformation are simply removed with close follow-up. If they have deep invasion into the stalk, are high grade (poorly differentiated (grade 3) or undifferentiated (grade 4)), or show lymphatic invasion, or if the surgical margins show residual tumor, then a colectomy with en bloc removal of the regional lymph nodes is performed.[76]

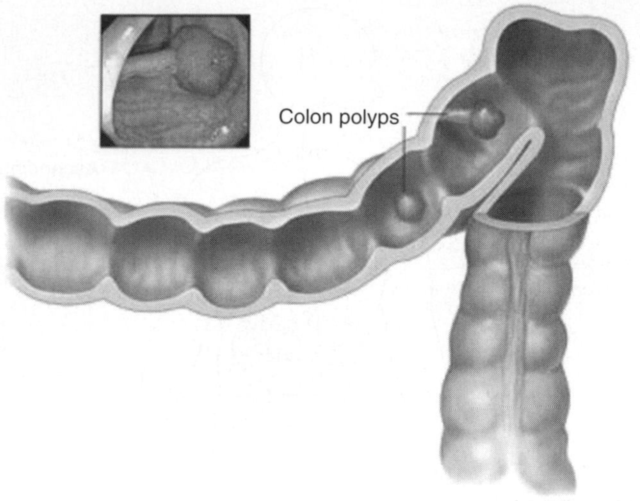


**FIGURE 51-2**

Pedunculated polyp.

*Source*: Data from National Cancer Institute.[75]

If the polyp is a villous adenoma or villoglandular adenoma during colonoscopy the polyp is removed and the site marked. An in situ malignancy with negative margins is removed, and the patient closely followed. If the tumor specimen is fragmented, is high grade, or has penetrated to the submucosa or deeper, or if the margins are involved with tumor, then a colectomy with en bloc removal of the regional lymph nodes is performed.[76]

Patients with a history of colorectal cancer are at increased risk of developing a second primary colon cancer or other malignancy, especially at the site where an anastomotic connection was made by the previous surgery. Patients with UC are also at increased risk of developing colorectal cancer, depending on the extent of colitis, the development of mucosal dysplasia, and the duration of symptoms. Colorectal cancer risk is also higher than normal in patients with Crohn's disease, an inflammatory disease usually involving all layers of the intestinal mucosa.

## CLINICAL MANIFESTATIONS

General signs and symptoms of colon cancer are listed in Table 51-5. Clinical manifestations of tumors in the colon vary depending on location. Tumors in the *cecum and ascending or right colon* occur in 54% of patients, and may be large and bulky if not detected early. As digested food moves down the gastrointestinal tract, liquid or semi-liquid

**TABLE 51-5**

| Clinical Manifestations of Colon Cancer |
|---|
| • Progressive fatigue |
| • Black tarry stools with or without mucus or bright red blood in the stool |
| • A feeling of incomplete stooling |
| • Change in bowel habits, such as constipation, diarrhea, or one alternating with the other |
| • Change in size or shape of the stool, such as pencil or ribbon-like |
| • Cramping, pain, or discomfort in the stomach or abdomen |
| • Abdominal distention or bloating |
| • Jaundice |

material enters the ascending colon. Thus, there is no change in bowel habits as a presenting sign. However, there can be intermittent or chronic bleeding, which over time, leads to iron-deficiency anemia. Symptoms generally include those of anemia (fatigue, weakness, shortness of breath, and exercise intolerance), melena, anorexia, and vague, dull pain or aching. Signs include a palpable mass in the right lower quadrant on physical exam and weight loss. There is an increasing incidence of proximal or right-sided colon cancers, especially in the cecum.

The *transverse colon* is the site of water absorption, where the fecal material begins to become formed and firm. About 10% of colon cancers appear here. Signs and symptoms of a malignant lesion in the transverse colon include gas, a change in bowel habits, abdominal cramping, partial or complete obstruction, possible perforation of the bowel, and blood in the stool. Signs and symptoms of anemia may also occur.

About 36% of colon cancers are found in the *descending and sigmoid colon*. Here, a lesion may partially occlude the lumen, causing a change in bowel habits as well as a change in caliber of the stool, so the stool may be pencil-like or ribbon-like and narrow. Partial obstruction of the bowel lumen can cause cramps, flatulence, constipation alternating with diarrhea, abdominal pain, bright red blood on stooling, a feeling of incomplete stooling, and obstructive symptoms such as nausea and vomiting; melena may occur, as may bowel perforation. In 3% to 5% of patients, synchronous lesions will appear in two different places in the colon, and the clinical manifestations will reflect the locations of both tumors.

Early in the course of malignancy, the individual may be asymptomatic. Early signs and symptoms may include vague abdominal pain, flatulence, and minor changes in bowel movements with or without (rectal) bleeding. This is in contrast to signs and symptoms of late cancer, which include severe pain, anorexia and weight loss, sacral or sciatic pain, jaundice, pruritus, ascites, hepatomegaly, and renal impairment.[2] Carcinoma of the colon or rectum during pregnancy is rare, but has been noted. Early diagnosis is difficult because symptoms are similar to those of pregnancy.[77]

## ASSESSMENT

### PATIENT AND FAMILY HISTORY

Assessment includes a thorough history, as well as a full review of systems and family history, and physical exam. Specifically, the history should include a symptom analysis focusing on presenting signs and symptoms: recent weight loss or gain; changes in appetite; changes in the size, shape, caliber, or color of stools; difficulty passing stool; nausea and/or vomiting; blood in the stools; abdominal pain; bloating; fatigue; palpitations; skin color changes; and unusual itching. Social history should include lifestyle factors such as diet, smoking and alcohol intake, occupational history, exposure to chemicals or radiation, and prior medical and surgical procedures. Medical history should include history of inflammatory bowel disease, adenoma or cancer in the colon, any other malignancy such as those associated with HNPCC (colon or rectum, uterus, ovary, ureter, bladder), and hemorrhoids. The family history should be as complete as possible, including first-degree relatives for two generations and the age at onset of cancer in each family member who has had colon or rectal cancer. The review of systems will elicit symptoms or changes in function outside the gastrointestinal system and help to give a full picture of the extent of disease.

### PHYSICAL EXAMINATION

The physical examination focuses on the abdomen, breasts, rectum, and lymph nodes to identify any abnormalities that reflect the status of primary or metastatic colon cancer. Initially, general features are assessed such as weight, vital signs, and functional and mental ability, as well as overall nutritional status of facial muscles (wasting of the temporal or masseter muscles), which may signify advanced disease.

Auscultation of the abdomen reveals bowel status: high-pitched bowel sounds reflect hypermotility and possible partial bowel obstruction, while faint-pitched or absent bowel sounds suggest complete bowel obstruction. Observe the abdomen for distention and any abnormalities.

Palpation is useful in identifying masses, especially of right-sided or proximal lesions; areas of tenderness; ascites; and rebound tenderness that may signal bowel perforation. Bowel perforation may be acute or chronic. Acute perforation is accompanied by pain, fever, and a palpable mass, and the differential diagnosis will include appendicitis or diverticulitis depending on the patient's history. In chronic perforation, acute signs are absent and fistulae may form, with resulting signs and symptoms. If a sigmoid cancer develops a fistula into the bladder, the patient will develop symptoms of chronic urinary tract infection and hematuria. Percussing and palpating the right upper quadrant will give information about possible liver metastases, the most common metastatic site of colon cancer. Approximately 10% to 15% of patients will have liver metastases at presentation. To augment assessment of liver metastases, inspect the eye sclera for icterus, which precedes jaundice related to biliary obstruction. In addition, if the history elicited shoulder pain unrelated to injury, which suggests referred pain from liver metastases, assess shoulder range of motion and whether pain increases during movement. If pain increases it is unlikely to be referred pain.

Systematically assess the lymph nodes. If a female patient has pelvic pain, a pelvic exam should be done to identify metastases to the ovary or cul-de-sac. The neurological exam gives information about possible brain metastases or metastases to the spinal cord with spinal cord compression. Rarely, patients may present with paraneoplastic symptoms, such as superficial or deep-vein thrombosis related to hypercoagulability. Patients with advanced disease are most likely to have a history of right upper quadrant pain, abdominal distention, early satiety, and palpable supraclavicular or umbilical/periumbilical nodules.

## DIAGNOSTIC STUDIES

A definitive biopsy confirms the diagnosis, often done via colonoscopy. Complete blood count, electrolytes, renal and liver function studies, and coagulation assays are done. A baseline carcinoembryonic antigen (CEA) level is drawn once a diagnosis of colon cancer is made. Computerized tomography (CT) scans of the chest, abdomen, and pelvis are performed to evaluate metastases in the lungs, liver, and extracolonic tissue.[76] Magnetic resonance imaging (MRI) is used to further explore questionable areas found on CT or to evaluate recurrence. Positron emission tomography (PET) scans provide whole-body evaluation and highlight active tumors within the body. Malignant tumors have an increased rate of glycolysis, shown by an increased uptake of a glucose analog tracer, which is then trapped in the tumor cells. Positron emission tomography scan is not the standard diagnostic test at this time for initial diagnosis and staging, but is performed if the patient has potentially resectable metastases in the liver and/or lung.[76] A bone scan should be done to identify bony metastases, as their presence will affect the treatment plan. If the patient is young and has a profile suggestive of FAP or HNPCC, genetic testing should be offered. If positive, then genetic counseling should be offered to siblings and children.

In addition to the previously mentioned diagnostic tests, patients with recurrent or metastatic disease may have other tests to evaluate the extent of disease. In patients with occult cancer, combining a CEA scan with conventional imaging techniques significantly increases diagnostic accuracy.[2] Magnetic resonance imaging may also be performed for patients with potentially resectable metastases, or who are allergic to CT contrast material. Fine-needle aspiration, with or without other diagnostic tests, is generally indicated to confirm the recurrence of disease.

## PROGNOSTIC INDICATORS

Stage of disease at presentation is the most important prognostic factor in colon cancer. Patients who are symptomatic at diagnosis have a worse prognosis.[11] The prognosis is dependent on depth of invasion or penetration through the wall of the colon, involvement of local and regional lymph nodes, and presence of disease in distant sites. Another factor that affects prognosis is whether the lesion causes obstruction or perforation in patients with stage II and III colon cancers. Many years ago, the National Surgical Adjuvant Breast and Bowel Project (NSABP) showed that disease-free survival was negatively associated with obstruction and bowel perforation in Duke's B2 and C, or stage II and III, colon cancer.[78] Location of tumor—either right, left, or rectosigmoid—did not correlate with survival or disease-free survival. This study was replicated by Steinberg and colleagues[79] as part of the Gastrointestinal Tumor Study Group, with similar findings. Other studies have found a difference in survival related to right or left colon cancer location. Halvorsen and Johannesen[80] found that for each stage of disease, those patients with lesions located at or below the peritoneal reflection (rectosigmoid and rectum) had a shorter survival compared to patients with a more proximal lesion. Another prognostic factor is pretreatment level of CEA, where a high CEA level confers a poor prognosis.[76]

Following the development of microarray technology and further elucidation of the sequence of genetic mutations in colon cancer, many molecular markers have been identified as prognostic indicators. Microsatellite instability (MSI) is associated with improved survival, as well as the presence of tumor-infiltrating lymphocytes.[81] MSI means there are a high number of mistakes in DNA replication and instability of 30 or more microsatellite loci that result in expansion or contraction of short, repeated DNA sequences caused by insertion or deletion of repeated units.[82,83] Even though tumors with MSI are often poorly differentiated, patients are more likely to respond to chemotherapy and have longer survival.

Loss of heterozygosity (LOH) confers a poor prognosis. It refers to the loss of an allele or copy of chromosome. Of interest is the long arm of chromosome 18 (18q), which contains a number of tumor suppressor genes, and when lost, is involved in tumorigenesis. The *DDC* gene is located on this arm of this chromosome. When this tumor suppressor gene is mutated, it takes the brakes off uncontrolled cell division. In one study, patients with stage II colon cancer who had LOH 18q had the same risk as patients with stage III disease.[84] Other interesting factors that have not been adequately studied to date include DNA content (aneuploidy or abnormal DNA content in cells is associated with a poor prognosis); molecular markers such as LOH in tumor suppressor genes; the oncogenes *K-ras, c-myc; bcl-2*, and *BAX*; DNA synthesis-related genes; growth factors and growth factor receptor genes; cell cycle regulator genes *p27* and *p21*; and angiogenesis-related genes for vascular endothelial growth factor (VEGF), among others.[85]

## CLASSIFICATION AND STAGING

The prognosis for persons with colon cancer is directly related to the stage of the disease at the time of diagnosis. Stage is determined by the depth of penetration of the tumor into and through the intestinal wall, involvement of contiguous organs, the number of regional lymph nodes involved, and the presence or absence of distant metastases.

There are three staging systems available, but most clinicians use the American Joint Committee on Cancer (AJCC) staging system. Colon cancer stage is determined by the T (tumor depth of invasion), N (lymph node involvement), and M (metastastic spread to distant organs) system (Table 51-6).[86] Lymph nodes are extensive over the large bowel and are the first barrier that malignant cells traverse after leaving the colon. The more lymph nodes removed at colon cancer surgery, the more accurate the nodal staging, and the more appropriate the treatment plan. The portal venous system brings embolized colon malignant cells to the liver, and cells can be disseminated by tumors that penetrate through the full thickness of the bowel wall and onto the periotoneal surface. The recognition of this phenomenon has led to improved staging classification of T3 and T4 tumors (stage II) as well as subdivisions in stage III, as there are significant differences in survival based on the stratification. With the revised staging, the 5-year survival rate for patients with stage I is 93.2%, stage IIA is 84.7%, stage IIB is 72.2%, stage IIIA is 83.4%, IIIB is 64.1%, and IIIC is 44.3%, and stage IV is 8.1%.[86] The sixth edition of the *AJCC Cancer Staging Manual* contains a number of additions[86]:

1. Smooth metastatic nodules in the pericolic fat are considered lymph node metastases (N).
2. Irregularly shaped metastatic nodules in the peritumoral fat are considered vascular invasion.
3. Stage II is subdivided into IIA (T3 lesions) and IIB (T4 lesions).
4. Stage III is subdivided into IIIA (T1-2, N1, M0), IIIB (T3-4, N1, M0), and IIIC (any T, N2, M0).

**TABLE 51-6**

**Tumor, Node, and Metastases Staging of Colon Cancer**

**Staging Groups**

| *Stage* | *T* | *N* | *M* |
|---|---|---|---|
| 0 | Tis | N0 | M0 |
| IA | T1 | N0 | M0 |
| IB | T2 | N0 | M0 |
| IIA | T3 | N0 | M0 |
| IIB | T4 | N0 | M0 |
| IIIA | T1–T2 | N0 | M0 |
| IIIB | T3–T4 | N1 | M0 |
| IIIC | Any T | N1 | M0 |
| IV | Any T | Any N | M1 |

*Staging definitions*

| | |
|---|---|
| T0 | No evidence of primary tumor |
| Tis | Carcinoma in situ: intraepithelial or invasion of lamina propria |
| T1 | Tumor invades submucosa |
| T2 | Tumor invades muscularis propria |
| T3 | Tumor invades through the muscularis propria into the subserosa, or the nonperitonealized pericolic or perirectal tissues; V and L substaging are used to identify the presence or absence of vascular or invasion |
| T4 | Tumor directly invades other organs or structures, and/or perforates visceral peritoneum; V and L substaging are used to identify presence or absence of vascular or lymphatic invasion |
| N1 | Metastases in 1–3 regional lymph nodes |
| N2 | Metastases in 4 or more regional lymph nodes |
| M1 | Distant metastases |

*Histological grade*

| | |
|---|---|
| G1 | Well differentiated |
| G2 | Moderately differentiated |
| G3 | Poorly differentiated |
| G4 | Undifferentiated |

*Source*: Data from Greene et al.[86]

5. The surgeon should mark the specimen where the tumor penetration is the deepest so the radial margin can be evaluated, and also should indicate whether the tumor was completely resected with negative margins (R0), incompletely resected with microscopic margins (R1), or incompletely resected with gross residual tumor (R2).

Following surgical resection of colorectal tumors, pathological stage is the single most important prognostic factor. The prognosis for stage I and II disease is more favorable, whereas stage III and IV disease have a poorer prognosis. In the TNM classification, each of the three subsets of tumor, nodal, and metastatic categories does not make any assumptions about the status in another part of the system. Two areas in staging are of particular concern: (1) lymph node sampling to determine accurate staging must be adequate, and (2) T4 tumors (stage IIB) have biological characteristics that allow them to invade through the bowel wall and into contiguous tissues.

In past practice, the number of lymph nodes sampled during standard colectomy for colon cancer varied, with the average being 8 lymph nodes. Esser and colleagues[87] estimated that to correctly classify lymph node status with 95% confidence, the surgeon needed to sample 20 lymph nodes for T1 lesions, 17 nodes for T2 lesions, and 15 nodes for T3 lesions. They found that patients with stage I disease who had fewer than 10 lymph nodes sampled had shorter survival than patients who had 10 or more lymph nodes evaluated ($P < 0.01$). Thus, a number of patients have been incorrectly staged because insufficient lymph nodes were sampled, and the patient's stage was therefore underestimated. Le Voyer and colleagues[88] performed a secondary analysis and found that survival decreased with increasing numbers of lymph nodes involved with tumor, and survival increased as more lymph nodes were removed and analyzed. The current standard is that a minimum of 12 lymph nodes should be examined to identify a T3 colon cancer lesion as node negative. If less than 12 lymph nodes are examined, the patient is at risk for understaging and should be offered adjuvant chemotherapy following surgical resection.[76]

Lennon and colleagues[89] studied patients with stage II disease after excluding those with perforation or tumor involving adjacent organs at the time of surgery. They found that the peritoneal space contained tumor cells in 13.6% of patients and that these patients had high rates of lymphovascular invasion and neural invasion (69% and 44%, respectively). Of this group of patients, 60% died of recurrent disease within three years of initial surgery. The AJCC's Prognostic Factors Group has recommended that T4 lesions be subgrouped into T4a (tumor invading adjacent structures or organs) and T4b (tumor involves the visceral peritoneum).[90] It is well recognized that patients with stage II colon cancer who have obstruction, perforation, or ulceration have a poorer prognosis than patients without these complications. For this reason, patients, with obstruction, perforation, or ulceration are encouraged to consider adjuvant chemotherapy or entry into a clinical trial.

## THERAPEUTIC APPROACHES AND NURSING CARE

### SURGERY

The National Comprehensive Cancer Network (NCCN) has developed practice guidelines for the management of advanced adenomas and colon cancer.[76] Surgery is the primary treatment for colon cancer. The goal of surgery is to eliminate disease in the colon, nodal basins, and contiguous organs. The tumor location, blood supply, and lymph node pattern in the involved region will define the extent of surgical resection.

The procedure of choice for resectable colon cancer is a colectomy with en bloc removal of regional lymph nodes.[11] Laparoscopic colectomy has been studied, and a number of studies and meta-analyses have shown equivalence to open colectomy.[91–95] A laparoscopic colectomy may be considered if the surgeon has experience doing this procedure, the patient has no disease in the rectum, has no significant adhesions, no advanced local or metastatic disease, no cancer-related acute bowel obstruction or perforation, and a thorough abdominal exploration must be possible.[76] The various surgical options as well as their indications and major morbidities are briefly discussed below and illustrated in Figure 51-3. With these procedures, the lymphadenectomy

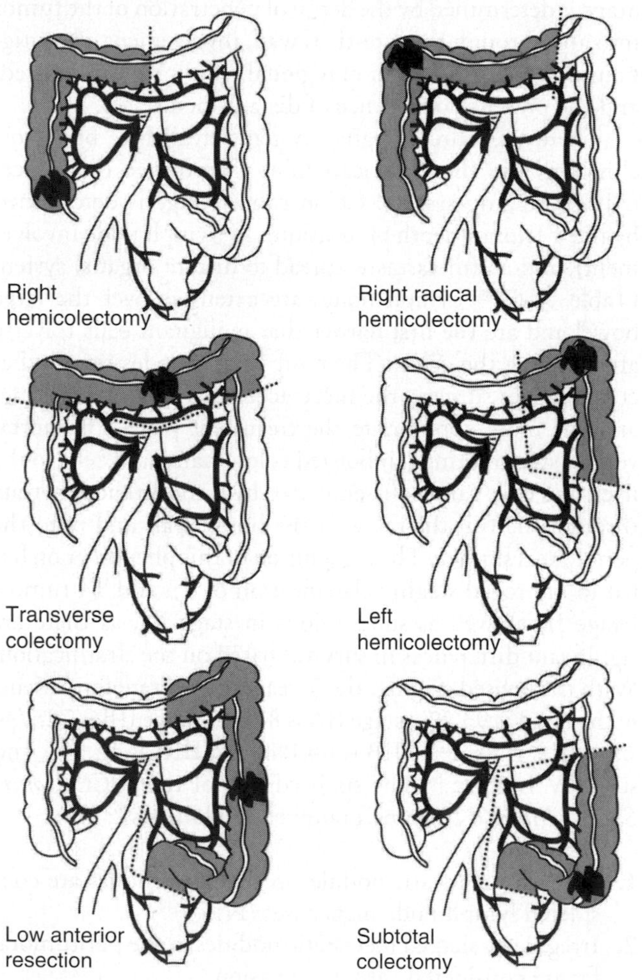


**FIGURE 51-3**

The procedure selected relates to the location and extent of the tumor.

should include: identification of lymph nodes at the origin of feeding vessels and collection for pathological examination, biopsy or removal of suspicious lymph nodes outside the resection field, at least 12 lymph nodes to establish stage II colon cancer, and removal of as many lymph nodes as possible for stage III colon cancer, as this correlates with survival.[76] If lymph nodes are left behind, this indicates an incomplete resection (R2).

*Right hemicolectomy* involves removal of the distal 5 to 8 cm of the ileum, right ascending colon, hepatic flexure, and transverse colon proximal to the middle colic artery. This procedure is indicated for cecal, ascending colon, and hepatic flexure lesions. Major morbidities include ureteral injury, duodenal injury, and bile acid deficiency. Bile acid deficiency is rarely seen and only with extensive resection of the terminal ileum.

*Right radical hemicolectomy* involves the removal of the transverse colon (including resection of the middle colic artery at its origin) in addition to structures removed in the right hemicolectomy. Indications for this procedure are lesions of the hepatic flexure or transverse colon. In addition to the complications associated with right hemicolectomy, morbidities include anastomotic dehiscence and diarrhea.

*Transverse colectomy* is the segmental resection of the transverse colon. This procedure is indicated for midtransverse colon lesions. The major morbidity is anastomotic dehiscence. This procedure is rarely performed because of the difficulty of achieving a tension-free anastomosis with adequate blood supply, as the marginal artery of Drummond is sacrificed. Surgeons prefer to perform an extended right radical hemicolectomy with an ileosigmoid anastomosis.[11]

*Left hemicolectomy* includes the removal of the transverse colon distal to the right branch of the middle colic artery and the descending colon up to, but not including, the rectum, plus division and ligation of the inferior mesenteric artery (IMA). Indications for this procedure are left colon lesions. Anastomotic dehiscence is the major morbidity.

*Low anterior resection* involves the removal of the descending colon distal to the splenic flexure, sigmoid colon, upper two-thirds of the rectum, and ligation of IMA and inferior mesenteric vein either at the origin or just distal to the origin of the left colic artery. This procedure is indicated for lesions of the sigmoid colon and proximal rectum. Morbidities include anastomotic dehiscence and bowel ischemia secondary to inadequate flow through the marginal artery of Drummond.

*Subtotal colectomy* is the removal of the right, transverse, descending, and sigmoid colon with ileorectal anastomosis. This procedure is indicated for multiple synchronous colon tumors and distal transverse colon lesions particularly in a patient with a clotted IMA. Morbidities include diarrhea, perineal excoriation, and anastomotic dehiscence.[96] If the patient is obstructed by tumor (actual or imminent), if the colon cannot be resected, a diverting colostomy, bypass of impending obstruction, or stent placement is performed.[96] Table 51-7 identifies potential complications of colorectal cancer surgery.

The role of sentinel lymph node (SLN) mapping and biopsy in staging remains under investigation. Sentinel lymph node mapping follows the template established for melanoma and breast cancer. Sentinel lymph nodes that are the first lymph nodes to be reached by malignant cells are identified by dye or labeling, and then biopsied to see if they contain tumor. If tumor is found, then it is likely more lymph nodes are involved. If the biopsy is negative, then it is likely that none of the remaining lymph nodes are involved. Dye is injected around the tumor, and the sentinel lymph nodes are identified by their uptake of the dye. Saha and colleagues[97] described their multi-institutional study of 203 patients and found that SLN mapping (1–4 lymph nodes) was 98% successful. In this study, 14% of patients had micrometastases and were upstaged from stage I/II to stage III. Skipped metastases were found in 0.03% of patients. The authors concluded that SLN was simple and cost-effective. More recently, Redston et al reported the results of Cancer and Leukemia Group B (CALGB) trial 80001 that aimed to determine if sentinel lymph node (SLN) sampling could reduce the number of lymph nodes required to characterize micrometastatic disease in patients with potentially curable colon cancer.[98] They found that sentinel lymph nodes did not accurately predict the presence of lymph nodes or micrometastatic

**TABLE 51-7**

**Potential Complications of Colorectal Surgery**

| Complication | Signs and Symptoms |
|---|---|
| Anastomotic leak | Abdominal pain, postoperative fever, ileus, elevated WBC count |
| Intra-abdominal abscess | Persistent, recurring postoperative fever; elevated WBC count |
| Bowel obstruction | Abdominal distention and pain, constipation, nausea/vomiting, high pitched (partial) to absent (complete) bowel sounds |
| Alternations in bowel elimination pattern | Irregular bowel elimination, constipation; diarrhea, fecal incontinence (uncommon); temporary or permanent stoma |
| Alteration in urinary elimination | Urgency; bladder dysfunction, with injury to bladder or ureters, urine can leak through incision; oliguria |
| Sexual dysfunction | Impotence, difficulty with ejaculation; short-or long-term problems depend upon nerve preservation |
| Stoma dysfunction | Skin breakdown, stomal prolapse, hernia, injection of peristomal skin, bleeding |

*Abbreviation*: WBC, white blood cell.

disease. Sentinel lymph node mapping has brought benefits of improving the accuracy of lymph node evaluation in lymph node-negative patients, as approximately one-third of patients with lymph node-negative cancer develop recurrent disease. Bilchik and colleagues[99] studied lymphatic mapping followed by focused analysis of sentinel nodes using molecular profiling. They found that 8 of 31 patients with lymph node-negative disease had micrometastases using molecular profiling, and were upstaged to stage III. This change in stage has important implications, as these patients would otherwise not have received adjuvant chemotherapy.

Feig and colleagues[100] cautioned surgeons about the value of SLN mapping in colon and rectal cancer. They reported that they were successful in finding sentinel lymph nodes in 98% of patients. They found a false-negative rate of 38%, however, and recommended large prospective studies to evaluate the accuracy and potential of SLN mapping in colon cancer.

In reviewing the literature, Haas et al found that accuracy rates were between 78% to 100%, sensitivity rates between 25% to 100%, and true upstaging rates between 0 and 26%.[101] Finally, the NCCN states that the use of sentinel lymph nodes and detection of cancer cells by immunohistochemistry alone should be considered investigational, and the results used with caution in managing patients.[76]

### Liver metastases

An estimated 20% of patients will present with liver metastases, another 20% to 30% will develop liver metastases as a site of recurrence following primary treatment, and as many as 70% of patients who are not cured will ultimately develop liver metastases.[76] For some patients, however, resection of isolated metastases can result in cure. Figueras et al demonstrated a 53% 5-year overall survival,[102] Choti et al demonstrated a 58% 5-year survival,[103] and Abdella et al demonstrated a 58% 5-year survival.[104]

The NCCN identifies the following requirements for resectable metastases: first, it must be surgically feasible to completely resect the lesion (R0) based on the anatomy and extent of disease, and second, there must be adequate hepatic reserve after resection (adequate liver remnant).[76] In addition, the primary tumor must have been resected (R0) for cure, and there should be no unresectable extrahepatic sites of disease. Some patients may be initially unresectable, but following neoadjuvant antineoplastic therapy, may be reconsidered if their disease is now resectable. Solitary lesions have a better prognosis than multiple metastases in the liver. If the patient develops recurrent disease after metastectomy, re-resection may be considered in selected patients. Finally, intra-arterial embolization should not be routinely used outside of a clinical trial.

Fong and colleagues found that seven factors were significant and independent predictors of poor long-term outcome: positive surgical margins, extrahepatic disease, node-positive primary tumor, disease-free interval from primary tumor to metastases less than 12 months, more than one hepatic tumor, largest hepatic tumor more than 5 cm, and CEA level greater than 200 ng/mL.[105] The authors recommended that if a patient has two or fewer of the factors, there is a favorable outcome; however, if the patient has three or more factors, the individual should consider experimental adjuvant trials following resection. Of patients who undergo hepatic resection, 50% are alive at 5 years.[76,106]

To be able to effectively resect metastases in the liver, the patient must be thoroughly evaluated immediately during the diagnostic workup, and the multi-disciplinary team mobilized. First, the patient has a PET scan to determine the extent of metastatic disease, and sites of extrahepatic disease. Sometimes, it is feasible to perform a synchronous resection, or plan a staged resection of the primary as well as the metastatic site.

If the patient has resectable liver metastases, and has not received prior chemotherapy, they may receive initial resection followed by chemotherapy, or neoadjuvant chemotherapy followed by resection, and additional post-operative chemotherapy. If the patient has had prior adjuvant chemotherapy within the prior 12 months, then the patient should have an alternative, active chemotherapy for metastatic disease.[76]

If the tumor and/or the metastatic disease is not resectable, neoadjuvant therapy with the 5-fluorouracil (5-FU) and leucovorin (LV) based regimen FOLFIRI (with irinotecan), FOLFOX (with oxaliplatin), or capecitabine (5-FU prodrug, which mimics a 5-FU continuous infusion) together with oxaliplatin (CapeOx), with or without bevacizumab is recommended for 2 to 3 months. Bevacizumab, an anti-angiogenesis agent, should be stopped 4 to 6 weeks prior to surgery to enhance surgical healing. Then either a synchronous or staged colectomy and resection of metastatic disease can be performed, or the patient may have colectomy, followed by the above neoadjuvant chemotherapy, with a staged resection of the metastatic disease.

The NCCN recommends adjuvant chemotherapy for 6 months following potentially curable hepatic resection; if neoadjuvant chemotherapy was given, then adjuvant therapy is given for 3 to 4 months.[76] Options include active combination regimens discussed above, or hepatic artery infusion (HAI) therapy with or without systemic 5-FU/LV. Kemeny and colleagues[107] presented Cancer and Leukemia Group B (CALGB) data showing superior response (48% vs 25%, $P = 0.009$) and survival (22.7 months vs 19.8 months, $P = 0.027$) of patients with liver-only metastases from colon and rectal cancer receiving HAI fluoxouridine, leucovorin, and dexamethasone as compared to patients receiving 5-FU and leucovorin (5-day Mayo regimen). Median time to progression was not significantly different. Quality of life as measured by physical functioning was similar at 9 months, but poorer at 12 months in the group receiving systemic chemotherapy. Of interest, the patients who did best had lower gene expression of thymidylate synthase and *p21* (cyclin-dependent kinase inhibitor). Finally, in the cost-benefit analysis, the lifetime cost for HAI was $157,800 compared to $97,600 for systemic therapy; some of the greater cost for HAI was related to patients surviving longer and receiving more drug.

Radiofrequency ablation is an option for patients who are not eligible for resection of liver metastases. It uses ultrasound guidance to deliver high temperatures to the hepatic tumor and provides long-term control for some patients. Another treatment technique is chemo-embolization, in which drug is directly injected into the tumor, and then the vessel is embolized to keep the drug in that specific location. This technique is being studied to try to increase hepatic reserve for patients who are otherwise resectable. Cryotherapy is also used to freeze the hepatic lesions, thereby killing the tumor cells. Both radiofrequency and cryotherapy ablation techniques are being studied with combination intrahepatic artery and systemic chemotherapy. These techniques are not options in patients with widespread liver metastases or other systemic disease.

### Peritoneal metastases

Peritoneal carcinomatosis may occur in patients with colon cancer. Studies have defined the lymphatic and portal dissemination of malignant cells, where the cells may or may not successfully become implanted and begin to divide and establish a blood supply of their own as a metastatic site (metastatic inefficiency).[76] In contrast, colon cancer cells that are disseminated into the peritoneum metastasize efficiently and are able to implant successfully. Unfortunately, positive peritoneal washings in such cases confer a uniformly dismal prognosis. Malignant cells reach the peritoneum through invasion through the bowel wall (T3 and T4 lesions) as well as a possible iatrogenic introduction via surgery itself. If tumor contaminates the surgical site, the healing process, including angiogenesis, enhances tumor growth and metastatic efficiency.[108]

The recommended treatment options are limited colon resection for nonobstructing abdominal/peritoneal metastases; or for impending obstruction, limited resection, diverting colostomy, or bypass of the impending obstruction followed by salvage chemotherapy are treatment options.[76]

In an effort to minimize the growth of metastatic cells in the peritoneum, new combination techniques using peritonectomy plus intraperitoneal chemotherapy are being studied. All visible tumor is removed at surgery, and heated intraoperative intraperitoneal chemotherapy is used to kill the remaining tumor cells. The heated intraperitoneal chemotherapy may be repeated if well tolerated during the first 5 postoperative days.[109–111] Chemotherapy drugs used are fluorouracil, mitomycin C, doxorubicin, cisplain, paclitaxel, gemcitabine, and oxaliplatin. The NCCN does not recommend this treatment outside of a clinical trial.[76]

### Pulmonary metastases

While endobronchial metastases are rare, colorectal carcinoma is one of the most common primary tumors with pulmonary metastases.[11] Colorectal tumors that metastasize to the lungs may present as solitary masses or multiple nodules. Individuals who experience pulmonary metastases from a colorectal primary tumor may present with symptoms of dyspnea, but it has been estimated that 85% of such patients are asymptomatic for pulmonary problems.[11] Most colorectal metastases to the lungs are detected by routine chest x-ray. More definitive evaluation can be accomplished by a CT scan of the chest, which further defines the number and location of the lesions. In evaluation of metastectomy, a PET scan should be performed to identify extent of disease, including any extra-pulmonary disease. The primary, pulmonary lesion, and any extrapulmonary disease must be able to be resected completely (R0) with negative surgical margins. There must be adequate pulmonary reserve and function remaining.[76]

Pulmonary resection of the metastatic area provides the best long-term survival, with patients achieving 63.7% 5-year survival in one study.[112] With aggressive patient follow-up, small lesions measuring 1 cm or less can be seen on CT. However, the primary lesion as well as any other metastatic sites must be controlled. In this study, patients with four or fewer pulmonary metastases and adequate pulmonary reserve underwent lobectomy; if the metastases were >3 cm in size, lymph node dissection was added. Patients that benefited most in this trial had tumors with well-differentiated adenocarcinoma histology, a solitary metastatic nodule, and had a disease-free interval of at least 2 years following initial surgery.[112]

### Complications of colorectal surgery

Some of the options for colon surgery are shown in Figure 51-3. The primary surgical procedure may produce both anatomical and functional alterations. If the patient requires a diverting colostomy, he or she will require preoperative teaching and a visit by the Certified Wound, Ostomy, Continence Nurse (CWOCN; also known as an enterostomal therapist or ET nurse), as well as postoperative teaching and follow-up. Emotional as well as physical self-care strategies will need to be supported so the patient will be able to function as independently as possible.

## RADIATION THERAPY

Radiation poses significant toxicity potential to the cells of the gut due to the rapid turnover of mucosal cells. However, in some studies postoperative radiation combined with chemotherapy improves survival in patients with bulky, locally advanced disease (T4, N0, M0; T4, N1-2, M0;

or T3, N0, M0 disease with perforation, close indeterminate resection margins, or positive resection margins).[113,76] Radiation provides local and regional control, while systemic chemotherapy theoretically attacks metastatic cells that have embolized. The NCCN recommends consideration of radiotherapy for patients with T4 lesions that are fixed to contiguous organ(s), or locally recurrent disease.[76] Potential side effects of radiation for locoregional control include enteritis, diarrhea (small bowel), nausea and vomiting (stomach, liver), and flank pain (kidneys). Side effects are minimized by intensity modulated radiation therapy (IMRT) and pre-operative radiological imaging or surgical clips. As another option, a clinical trial or observation could be selected as a treatment choice.[76]

Concurrent chemotherapy, usually a continuous infusion of 5-FU or a prodrug (capecitabine) which mimics a continuous 5-FU infusion, during radiation increases the cells' sensitivity to radiation damage, called radiosensitization. Efficacy in local-regional control, especially for patients with T4 lesions, and no lymph node or metastatic involvement, where patients achieved a 80% disease free survival; patients with lymph node involvement had a 53% disease free survival, compared to historical controls.[113] This and other seminal studies have provided the evidence for the NCCN recommendation.[76] The dose-limiting toxicities of continuous 5-FU infusion are mucositis and diarrhea. Palmar–plantar erythrodysesthesia (hand-foot syndrome) has also been noted with protracted infusions of 5-FU.[2]

## CHEMOTHERAPY

### Adjuvant

Chemotherapy plays a significant role in the management of colon cancer. While patients with stage I disease are considered cured with surgery alone, one-third of patients with stage II disease will have recurrence following surgery. Patients with stage III disease, with lymph node involvement, are at highest risk for recurrence. For this reason, chemotherapy is recommended for all patients with stage III colon cancer, and to be considered for patients with high-risk stage II disease. High-risk features are high-grade tumor (3/4), lymphatic/vascular invasion, bowel obstruction, < 12 lymph nodes examined, localized perforation, or close indeterminate or positive margins), or T4 tumor. Thus, for patients with stage IIA with high-risk features, or patients with stage IIB, adjuvant chemotherapy or entry into a clinical trial is recommended.[75]

Survival in patients with stage III disease (lymph node involvement) is significantly improved with adjuvant chemotherapy. Chemotherapy regimens are presented in greater detail in Table 51-8, and selected toxicities in Table 51-9. At one time, the standard adjuvant therapy for stage III colon cancer was 5-FU plus levamisole. In 1988, studies that added leucovorin (LV) to 5-FU demonstrated stabilization of the 5-FU-thymidylate-synthase complex, thereby increasing the period of tumor inhibition. While overall survival was not increased with leucovorin and 5-FU therapy, the response rate was increased significantly. Studies also showed that 12 months of adjuvant therapy was not superior to 6 months of therapy.[76] Thus, the standard is now 6 months of adjuvant chemotherapy with either 5-FU/LV, capecitabine alone, which mimics a continuous infusion of 5-FU, or the combination folinic acid, bolus followed by infusional 5-FU, oxaliplatin (FOLFOX). The MOSAIC study, a large multi-centered randomized controlled trial (RCT) showed at 6 years, had a 20% reduction in the risk of dying from colon cancer, compared to patients receiving 5FU/LV.[114]

Toxicities included neutropenia in almost 80% of patients (neutropenic fever/infection was 1.8%), peripheral sensory neuropathy in 91% of patients, which was reversible, nausea (73%), diarrhea (56%), and vomiting (47%).

A similar trial, the NSABP C07, also a large RCT, compared bolus 5-FU/LV with bolus 5-FU/LV plus oxaliplatin (FLOX) and found at 4 years almost identical results as the MOSAIC trial. Toxicities differed in that the patients in the FLOX arm had more grade 3/4 diarrhea and dehydration related to bowel wall thickening. The incidence of grade 3/4 peripheral neuropathy was less in the FLOX group compared to FOLFOX4, as the total cumulative dose of oxaliplatin was less.[115]

Capecitabine, an oral prodrug of 5-FU, was shown in the metastatic setting to be at least as effective as bolus 5-FU/LV, so it was tested in the adjuvant setting. The X-ACT trial was a phase III RCT of 1870 patients with stage III colon cancer randomized patients to receive either capecitabine, or IV bolus 5-FU/LV (Mayo regimen). This non-inferiority study showed that capecitabine was as effective as bolus 5-FU/LV.[116] Interestingly, patients who developed grades 1 to 3 hand–foot syndrome (HFS) had a 5-year OS of 73.78% compared to patients who did not develop HFS and had an OS of 66.25%. In addition, there were less grade 3/4 toxicity events in the capecitabine arm compared to the 5-FU/LV arm. Adjuvant clinical trials are evaluating the benefit of the addition of either or both of the biological agents bevacizumab (Avastin, an antiangiogeneic agent), and cetuximab (Erbitux, an Epidermal Growth Factor Receptor (EGFR) inhibitor) to 5-FU and/or FOLFOX.

For patients with stage II colon cancer, the answers are not as clear. The 5-year survival rate without chemotherapy for stage II colon cancer is 75% to 80%. Advances have been made in identifying genetic mutational sequences that predict recurrence in small studies of patients but these need to be validated in larger, prospective trials so that one day adjuvant chemotherapy can be individually tailored to each patient. For example, Johnston et al reported the identification and testing of a 48-gene signature that predicted recurrence of patients with stage II colon cancer 100% of the

**TABLE 51-8**

**Chemotherapeutic Regimens for Colon Cancer: Adjuvant Therapy and Treatment of Advanced Colorectal Cancer**

| Regimen Name | Regimen Dosage | Reference |
|---|---|---|
| 5-FU/LV Roswell Park (high dose) | Day 1: 5-FU 500 mg/m$^2$ IV weekly ×6 administered midway through LV;<br>Day 1: LV 500 mg/m$^2$ IV over 2 hours weekly ×6;<br>Repeat every 8 weeks ×4 cycles | Wolmark et al[119] |
| LV/5-FU2 | Days 1 and 2: LV 200 mg/m$^2$ IV over 2 hours, then 5-FU 400 mg/m$^2$ IVP, then 5-FU infusion over 22 hours | de Gramont et al[114] |
| Simplified LV/5-FU2 | Day 1: LV 400 mg/m$^2$ IV over 2 hours; then<br>Day 1: 5-FU 400 mg/m$^2$ IVP; then<br>Days 1 and 2: 5-FU infusion 1200 mg/m$^2$ IV continuous infusion ×2 days (total dose 2400 mg/m$^2$) over 46–48 hours;<br>Repeat every 2 weeks × 6 months | de Gramont et al[114] |
| FOLFOX4 | Day 1: Oxaliplatin 85 mg/m$^2$ IV over 2 hours;<br>Days 1 and 2: Leucovorin 200 mg/m$^2$ IV over 2 hours;<br>Days 1 and 2: 5-FU 400 mg/m$^2$ IVB; then<br>Days 1 and 2: 5-FU 600 mg/m$^2$ IV over 22 hours;<br>Repeat every 2 weeks | de Gramont et al[114] |
| FLOX | Day 1 of each week: 5-FU 500 mg/m$^2$ IVB weekly ×6; with<br>Day 1 of each week: Leucovorin 500 mg/m$^2$ IV weekly ×6, each 8-week cycle ×3; with<br>Weeks 1, 3, and 5: Oxaliplatin 85 mg/m$^2$ IV over 2 hours, each 8-week cycle ×3 | Wolmark et al[119] |
| mFOLFOX6 | Day 1: Oxaliplatin 85 mg/m$^2$ IV over 2 hours;<br>Day 1: Leucovorin 400 mg/m$^2$ IV over 2 hours;<br>Day 1: 5-FU 400 mg/m$^2$ IVB then 1200 mg/m$^2$/day ×2 days (total 2400 mg/m$^2$ over 46–48 hours) continuous infusion;<br>Repeat every 2 weeks | Hochster et al[121] |
| Capecitabine | Days 1–14: 1250 mg/m$^2$ PO BID, repeat q 21 days, ×6 months | Twelves et al[116];<br>Cassidy et al[120] |
| **Metastatic Treatment** | | |
| Bevacizumab and 5-FU containing regimens | Day 1: Bevacizumab 5 mg/kg IV every 2 weeks + 5-FU and leucovorin or FOLFIRI or 10 mg/kg IV every 2 weeks with FOLFOX<br>Or<br>Day 1: Bevacizumab 7.5 mg/kg IV every 3 weeks with CapeOx | Hochster et al[121];<br>Hurwitz et al[122] |
| Bevacizumab + FOLFOX4 | Day 1: Bevacizumab 10 mg/kg IV;<br>Day 1: Oxaliplatin 85 mg/m$^2$ IV over 2 hours;<br>Days 1 and 2: Leucovorin 200 mg/m$^2$ IV over 2 hours;<br>Days 1 and 2: 5-FU 400 mg/m$^2$ IVB, then 600 mg/m$^2$ IV over 22 hours;<br>Repeat every 2 weeks | Giantonio et al[128] |
| Capecitabine | Days 1–14: Capecitabine 1250 mg/m$^2$ PO BID repeated every 21 days (variations include dose of 1000 mg/m$^2$ PO BID days 1–14) | Hoff et al[123] |
| CapeOx | Day 1: Oxaliplatin 130 mg/m$^2$ IV over 2 hours, capecitabine 850 mg/m$^2$ PO BID days 1–14, repeat cycle every 21 days | Hochster et al[121] |
| Cetuximab | Day 1: 400 mg/m$^2$ IV over 2 hours weekly, then 250 mg/m$^2$ IV over 1 hours weekly<br>In combination with irinotecan containing regimen, or alone if unable to tolerate irinotecan | Cunningham et al[124];<br>Jonker et al[125] |

*(Continued)*

**TABLE 51-8**

**Chemotherapeutic Regimens for Colon Cancer: Adjuvant Therapy and Treatment of Advanced Colorectal Cancer (*Continued*)**

| Regimen Name | Regimen Dosage | Reference |
|---|---|---|
| Cetuximab ± irinotecan | Day 1: Cetuximab 400 mg/m² IV over 2 hours, then 250 mg/m² IV weekly over 1 hour<br>Or<br>Cetuximab 500 mg/m² IV every 2 weeks ± irinotecan 300–350 mg/m² IV every 3 weeks<br>Or<br>180 mg/m² IV every 2 weeks<br>Or<br>125 mg/m² IV every week ×4<br>Repeat every 6 weeks | Cunningham et al[124] |
| Douillard | Day 1: Irinotecan 180 mg/m² IV over 90 minutes;<br>Days 1 and 2: Leucovorin 200 mg/m² IV over 2 hours;<br>Days 1 and 2: 5-FU 400 mg/m² IVB;<br>Days 1 and 2: 5-FU 600 mg/m² IV over 22 hours (as continuous infusion);<br>Repeat every 2 weeks | Douillard et al[126] |
| FOLFIRI | Day 1: Irinotecan 180 mg/m² IV over 90 min;<br>Day 1: Leucovorin 400 mg/m² IV over 2 hours;<br>Day 1: 5-FU 400 mg/m² IVB;<br>Days 1 and 2: 5-FU (total dose 2400–3000 mg/m² IV over 46–48 hours as continuous infusion)<br>Repeat every 2 weeks | Tournigand et al[127] |
| FOLFOX4 | Day 1: Oxaliplatin 85 mg/m² IV over 2 hours;<br>Days 1 and 2: Leucovorin 200 mg/m² IV over 2 hours;<br>Days 1 and 2: 5-FU 400 mg/m² IVB, then 600 mg/m² IV over 22 hours;<br>Repeat every 2 weeks | Giantonio et al[128] |
| mFOLFOX6 | Day 1: Oxaliplatin 85 mg/m² IV over 2 hours;<br>Day 1: Leucovorin 400 mg/m² IV over 2 hours;<br>Days 1 and 2: 5-FU 400 mg/m² IVB, then 1200 mg/m²/day ×2 days (total 2400 mg/m² over 46–48 hours) continuous infusion;<br>Repeat every 2 weeks | Giantonio et al[128] |
| FOLFOX6 | Day 1: Oxaliplatin 100 mg/m² IV over 2 hours; at same time as<br>Day 1: Leucovorin 400 mg/m² IV over 2 hours;<br>Day 1: 5-FU 400 mg/m² IVB<br>Days 1 and 2: 5-FU 1200–1500 mg/m² ×2 days (total 2400–3000 mg/m² IV over 46–48 hours) continuous infusion;<br>Repeat every 2 weeks | Tournigand et al[127] |
| FOLFOX7 | Day 1: Oxaliplatin 130 mg/m² IV over 2 hours through arm of Y-set;<br>Day 2: Leucovorin 400 mg IV through second arm of Y-set, over 2 hours, flush with D5W;<br>Days 1 and 2: 5-FU 1.2 g/m² ×2 days (2.4 g/m² IV infusion over 46 hours);<br>Repeat every 2 weeks | Tournigand et al[129] |
| Simplified 5-FU/LV biweekly infusional sLV5FU2 | Day 1: Leucovorin 400 mg/m² IV over 2 hours; followed by<br>Day 1: 5-FU 400mg/m² IVB; and then<br>Days 1 and 2: 5-FU 1200 mg/m²/day ×2 days (total 2400 mg/m² over 46–48 hours) continuous infusion;<br>Repeat every 2 weeks | de Gramont et al[114] |
| Panitumumab | 6 mg/kg IV over 1 hour every 2 weeks | Van Cutsem et al[130] |
| XELOX | Day 1: Oxaliplatin 130 mg/m² IV over 2 hours;<br>Days 1–14: Capectiabine 1000 mg/m² PO BID, evening day 1 through morning day 15;<br>Repeat every 3 weeks | Cassidy et al[131]; Saltz et al[132] |

*Abbrevations*: 5-FU, 5-flurouracil; IV, intravenous; IVB, intravenous bolus; IVP, intravenous piggback; LV, leucovorin.

**TABLE 51-9**

**Toxicities of Major Agents Used in the Treatment of Colon and Rectal Cancers**

| Drug | Major toxicities |
|---|---|
| 5-FU/LV | Bone marrow suppression, nadir days 10–14; mucositis, diarrhea, dry skin and photosensitivity, nausea, blepharitis (tear duct stenosis), hand-foot syndrome (palmar-plantar erythrodysesthesia), rare cerebellar toxicity and angina |
| Irinotecan | Diarrhea (acute and late), bone marrow suppression especially febrile neutropenia, mucositis, mild alopecia, asthenia, fever, vascular syndrome |
| Oxaliplatin | Rare hypersensitivity reactions; acute and chronic/persistent neuropathy, mild bone marrow suppression, nausea and vomiting, diarrhea |
| Bevacuzimab | Uncommon: hemorrhage, gastrointestinal perforation, delayed wound healing (delay until ≥ 21 days from or before surgery)<br>More common: asthenia, pain, abdominal pain, headache, hypertension, diarrhea, nausea, vomiting, anorexia, stomatitis, constipation, upper respiratory infection, epistaxis, dyspnea, exfoliative dermatitis, proteinuria |
| Cetuximab | Rare: severe infusion reaction and pulmonary toxicity<br>More common: acne-like rash, diarrhea, pain, fever, nausea, vomiting, anorexia, constipation, headache |

*Abbrevations*: 5-FU, 5 fluorouracil; LV, leucovorin

time.[117] In the meanwhile, controversy continues as to the absolute benefit of adjuvant therapy for patients with stage II colon cancer due to lack of sufficiently powered clinical trials and data. At most, adjuvant therapy would offer a 5% survival advantage[118] Currently, various online models can assist with decision making regarding what adjuvant treatment a patient with stage II colon cancer should receive, such as Adjuvant Online (http://www.adjuvantonline.com) and the Mayo Clinic Calculator (http://www.mayoclinic.com/calcs). Table 51-8 describes adjuvant therapy and treatment options for patients with advanced colon and rectal cancers.

## ADVANCED OR METASTATIC DISEASE CHEMOTHERAPY AND TARGETED THERAPY

Within the last decade, significant advances have occurred in the management of metastatic colorectal cancer. In review, the combination of 5-FU/LV results in a response rate of 20% to 25%, with an overall median survival of 11 to 12 months[114] Capecitabine (Xeloda) was shown to be equivalent in effectiveness to 5-FU and LV, so the drug is FDA approved for this first-line indication as well, when fluoropyrimidines alone are preferred. In Europe, the de Gramont regimen of infusional 5-FU/LV demonstrated an increased response, but equivalent overall survival with significantly reduced toxicity using infusional 5-FU compared with bolus LV.[133] Irinotecan (Camptosar) when given with infusional 5-FU, is known as FOLFIRI; when given as a bolus, it is known as IFL. IFL is no longer recommended as it was shown inferior to FOLFIRI and is more toxic.[134]

Evidence suggests that patients who survive the longest have had the opportunity to receive three available drugs: 5-FU/LV, oxaliplatin, irinotecan.[135] Following this, the advent of the antiangiogenic agent bevacizumab increased survival, so that now patients diagnosed with advanced colorectal cancer have a median survival of greater than 21 months, approaching 25 months with the use of bevacizumab.[122] The NCCN recommends that patients who can tolerate intensive therapy begin with FOLFOX or Capecitabine (Cape) Oxaliplatin (Ox) called CapeOx, or Folinic acid (FOL) 5-FU (F) Irinotecan (IRI) called FOLFIRI, or 5-FU/LV alone, plus bevacizumab.[76] If the patient had received FOLFOX as adjuvant chemotherapy within 12 months, then the recommended initial regimen would be FOLFIRI. Upon progression, the patient would change to an alternate regimen. It is unclear whether bevacizumab should be continued and the chemotherapy agents changed, or stopped with the change to different chemotherapy. Grothey et al found that continuing bevacizumab after disease progression, as well as second line chemotherapy, were each independently associated with increased overall survival (OS).[136]

Oxaliplatin in combination with 5-FU/LV is known as FOLFOX. The acronym is derived from Folinic acid (leucovorin), F (fluorouracil or 5-FU), and OX (oxaliplatin). FOLFOX 4 was shown to increase overall response rate to 45% compared to IFL (31%), and overall survival of 19.5 months compared to IFL (15.0 months).[137] FOLFOX has a number of iterations, and is most commonly prescribed as modified or m-FOLFOX6. See Table 51-8.

Although cure is possible for some patients with resectable metastases, it is not possible for those who have progressive disease or are unresectable. For these patients, quality of life is a critical benefit. In an effort to see if chemotherapy could be interrupted, or changed to maintenance chemotherapy, investigators conducted the OPTIMOX 1 (oxaliplatin in a "stop-and-go" approach) and 2 trials. OPTIMOX1 trial randomized patients to receive either FOLFOX4 every other week until disease progression, or FOLFOX 7 for 6 cycles followed by 12 cycles of infusional 5-FU/LV, unless progression came first, and then resumption with the oxaliplatin containing regimen. Patients in both groups had similar time to progression (TTP, 10.3 months and 12.3 months) and grades 3/4 neutropenia and neurotoxicity were significantly less in the arm using maintenance 5-FU/LV.[129] The

OPTIMOX2 trial attempted to halt chemotherapy entirely, but this resulted in inferior progression free survival (PFS) times so this is not recommended.[138]

## Chemotherapy and molecular targeted therapy

Two major molecular targeted therapies have been approved for use in advanced colon and rectal cancers: bevacuzimab and cetuximab, both monoclonal antibodies, which have been discussed in combination with chemotherapy. Significant advances have been made in the management of colon cancer. The current treatment options are summarized in Table 51-10.

Bevacuzimab, a monoclonal antibody against vascular endothelial growth factor (VEGF), prevents the proliferation and migration of endothelial cells to form new blood

**TABLE 51-10**

**Management of Colon Cancer**

| Pathology and Extent of Disease | Surgical Management | Follow-Up and Adjuvant Therapy |
|---|---|---|
| ***Polyps*** | | |
| Pedunculated polyp with invasive cancer:<br>• Adenoma with deep invasion into stalk<br>• Adenoma with margins that cannot be assessed, high-grade lesion (3–4), vascular or lymphatic invasion, positive margins | Colectomy with excision of regional lymph nodes (en bloc) | Superficial, completely removed polyps: no further surgery<br>Follow-up depends on pathological stage |
| Sessile adenomatous polyp, villous adenoma, or villoglandular adenoma with invasive cancer with high risk for recurrence:<br>• Fragmented specimen, tissue margins that cannot be assessed, or adverse pathology)<br>• ≥ T1 or positive margins | Colectomy with excision of regional lymph nodes (en bloc) | Single specimen,Tis, with negative margins, completely removed: no further surgery<br>Follow-up depends upon pathological stage |
| ***Colon Cancer*** | | |
| Nonobstructing lesion | Colectomy with excision of regional lymph nodes (en bloc) | Adjuvant chemotherapy based on stage:<br>Stage I: none |
| Resectable, obstructing lesion (unprepped) | Colectomy with excision of regional lymph nodes (en bloc) if possible; otherwise resection with diversion or stent | Stage IIA (T3): clinical trial or observation, or 5-FU/LV, FOLFOX, capecitabine if high risk for recurrence (high grade, LVI, vascular invasion, bowel obstruction)<br>Stage IIB (T4) or T3 with high risk of recurrence (positive margins, perforation): 5-FU/LV with or without XRT, FOLFOX or capecitabine chemotherapy;clinical trial, or observation<br>Stage III: FOLFOX, 5-FU/LV, or capecitabine;consider addition of XRT for T4 lesion if high risk |
| Unresectable lesion | Palliative resection, diversion or stent | Salvage chemotherapy: First line: FOLFOX, FOLFIRI, bevacizumab + 5-FU–based regimen *if patient can tolerate intensive therapy*; if not, capecitabine, 5-FU/LV, or 5-FU CI Second line: FOLFOX or FOLFIRI (depending on first line chemotherapy), irinotecan ± cetuximab |

*(Continued)*

**TABLE 51-10**

**Management of Colon Cancer (*Continued*)**

| Pathology and Extent of Disease | Surgical Management | Follow-Up and Adjuvant Therapy |
|---|---|---|
| ***Metastatic Disease*** | | |
| ***Liver metastases*** | | |
| • Isolated, resectable | Resection of primary lesion, excision of regional lymph nodes (en bloc), with liver resection or later, staged liver resection; neoadjuvant chemotherapy as needed to make resection possible with FOLFOX or FOLFIRI or CapeOX ± bevacizumab | 6 months of adjuvant chemotherapy using 5-FU/LV (bolus or CI), capecitabine, FOLFOX, FOLFIRI, hepatic artery infusion ± 5-FU/LV (bolus or CI), or FU CI, or observation |
| • Unresectable | Palliative colectomy if at high risk for obstruction | Salvage chemotherapy: First line: FOLFOX, FOLFIRI, bevacizumab + 5-FU–based regimen *if patient can tolerate intensive therapy*; if not, capecitabine, 5-FU/LV, or 5-FU CI Second line: FOLFOX or FOLFIRI (depending on first line chemotherapy), irinotecan ± cetuximab |
| ***Lung metastases*** | | |
| • 1–3 nodules, resectable | Resection of primary tumor with excision of regional lymph nodes (en bloc), then resection of pulmonary lesions | 6 months of adjuvant chemotherapy using 5-FU/LV (bolus or CI), capecitabine, FOLFOX, FOLFIRI, hepatic artery infusion ± 5-FU/LV (bolus or CI), or FU CI or observation |
| • Multiple nodules, unresectable | Palliative resection of primary tumor is an option | Salvage chemotherapy:<br>First line: FOLFOX, FOLFIRI, bevacizumab + 5-FU–based regimen *if patient can tolerate aggressive therapy*; if not, capecitabine, 5-FU/LV, or 5-FU CI<br>Second line: FOLFOX or FOLFIRI (depending upon first line chemotherapy), irinotecan ± cetuximab. |
| ***Abdominal/peritoneal metastases*** | Option of limited resection of primary tumor, diverting colostomy or bypass if impending obstruction | Salvage chemotherapy:<br>First line: FOLFOX, FOLFIRI, bevacizumab + 5-FU-based regimen *if patient can tolerate intensive therapy*; if not, capecitabine, 5-FU/LV, or 5-FU CI<br>Second line: FOLFOX or FOLFIRI (depending upon first line chemotherapy), irinotecan ± cetuximab. |
| ***Local recurrence*** | | |
| • Resectable | PET scan shows no further metastatic disease so resection | Adjuvant therapy for 6 months if not already received |
| • Unresectable or multiple lesions | Treatment plan based on performance status | Salvage chemotherapy or best supportive care based on performance status |

*Abbreviations*: 5-FU, 5-fluorouracil; FOLFIRI, 5-FU + irinotecan + leucovorin; FOLFOX, 5FU + oxaliplaton + leucovorin; Cape Ox, capecitabine + oxaliplatin; CI, continuous infusion; LV, leucovorin; LVI, lymphatic and/or vascular invasion; PET, positron emission tomography; TIS, tumor in situ; XRT, radiation therapy.

*Source*: Data from National Comprehensive Cancer Network[76]; Choti[103]; Kemeny et al[107]; de Gramont et al[114,133,137]; Hochster et al[121]; and Hurwitz et al.[122]

vessels for the developing malignancy. The addition of bevacizumab to IFL increased the objective response rate in newly diagnosed patients with metastatic colon cancer to 45% (compared to 35% with IFL) and median survival of 20.3 months (compared to 15.6 with IFL).[120] Bevacizumab (Avastin) is the first antiangiogeneis agent approved by the FDA. It is indicated for first-line treatment of advanced colon and rectal cancers in combination with a 5-FU-based regimen.

Colon and rectal cancers overexpress the EGFR, prompting cells to continually divide, become invasive, block apoptosis (programmed cell death), and make new blood vessels. Cetuximab (Erbitux), a monoclonal antibody directed against EGFR, when given in combination with irinotecan resulted in an improved response in previously treated, refractory patients with advanced colon and rectal cancers. Patients must test positive to receive the drug, but the NCCN Guidelines state that no patient should be denied the drug based on EGFR testing and a K-Ras wildtype genotype. This is because mutated K-Ras continues to stimulate cell proliferation even when EGFR is blocked[76] The overall response rate in the cetuximab-treated arm of one study was 22.9% compared to 10.8% in the irinotecan monotherapy arm, and overall survival was 8.6 months compared to 6.9 months in the single-agent irinotecan arm.[124] As a single agent, cetuximab was compared to best supportive care (BSC), and resulted in a significant increase in median overall survival of 6.1 month compared to 4.6 months in the BSC group.[125] Patients who experienced a grade 2 or higher rash were more likely to have increased survival ($P = 0.001$). Studies have shown that cetuximab is ineffective in patients with a mutation in the *K-ras* gene.[139] Cetuximab is being studied in other combinations.

Panitumumab, the newest monoclonal antibody directed against the EGFR, is FDA-approved as a single agent. When compared to BSC, patients receiving panitumumab had a significantly longer PFS (8 week vs 7.3 week) but there was no difference in overall survival.[130] In preclinical studies, panitumumab was active in combination with chemotherapy. The Panitumumab Advanced Colorectal Cancer Evaluation (PACCE) trial was an open-label, phase III study that randomized 1000 patients to receive either panitumumab plus bevacizumab or bevacizumab alone in combination with investigator-selected chemotherapy (oxaliplatin or irinotecan based). The study was terminated early when an interim analysis showed that PFS and OS were superior in the control arm (bevacizumab alone) and there was an increased incidence of grade 3/4 diarrhea, dehydration and infection in the panitumumab containing arm.[140] However, similar to cetuximab, panitumumab shows efficacy only in wild type or non-mutated *K-ras* tumors,[141] and response correlates with rash.

Finally, there is no predictive value in EGFR testing in colon cancer, so routine EGFR testing is not recommended by NCCN, and no patient should be restricted from cetuximab or panitumumab therapy based on EGFR testing.[76]

### Side effects of chemotherapy

Side effects from chemotherapy can be severe. The nurse's role is critical in safely administering the drug(s), as well as providing education about potential side effects, self-assessment, and self-care measures to minimize toxicity and maximize quality of life. The Oncology Nursing Society (ONS) standards help to ensure that the patient's physical, psychosocial, and educational needs are being addressed, and the evidence based symptom management recommendations (Putting Evidence into Practice, or PEP, resources) provide a foundation. Educating patients about adverse treatment effects helps them to manage symptoms and helps alleviate the serious or life-threatening treatment complications. Irinotecan combinations are perhaps the most challenging. During one clinical trial, the arm containing irinotecan was stopped pending further investigation. Although it was found that the mortality rate was not significantly higher, clinicians were reminded that patients receiving IFL require close monitoring for febrile neutropenia and late onset of diarrhea. This is one of the reasons IFL is no longer recommended.[142] Diarrhea can be severe, and a suggested approach to its management is a 4 mg loading dose of loperamide at the first sign of diarrhea, then 2 mg doses every 2 hours until diarrhea abates, for at least 12 hours. Potential side effects from the combination of 5-FU and leucovorin include nausea, vomiting, diarrhea, mucositis, fever, leukopenia, thrombocytopenia, and hypotension. The major toxicities of each drug are shown in Table 51-9. The dose-limiting toxicities for irinotecan are diarrhea and neutropenia; and for oxaliplatin, persistent neurotoxicity.

### Side effects of molecular targeted therapy

The dose-limiting toxicities for bevacizumab are hemorrhage and hypertension; and for cetuximab and panitumumab, severe acne-like rash and diarrhea. Cetuximab can also rarely cause anaphylaxis. Oncology nurses play a critical role in assessing and managing patients who are receiving chemotherapy, together with biotherapy, as well as teaching them self-care measures as the patient moves along the disease continuum.

## PATIENT MANAGEMENT AND SUPPORTIVE CARE

Many patients have uncomplicated, curative surgery for colon cancer. Table 51-11 describes post treatment follow-up. For others, their course may be complicated by several expected and unexpected developments. Symptoms produced by disease and progression can affect quality of life, self-care and symptom management needs, and educational needs for self care. Bowel obstruction and fistula formation require supportive care and symptom management, as does palliative care for patients with progressive disease.

### BOWEL OBSTRUCTION

Bowel obstruction is a common complication in patients with abdominal or pelvic cancers, such as those arising in

**TABLE 51-11**

**Post-Treatment Surveillance for Colon Cancer**

| | |
|---|---|
| Curative resection and NED | H&P q 3 months ×2 years, then q 6 months for the next 5 years. Colonoscopy within 1 years of resection or 3–6 months postoperatively; repeat annually if malignant polyp(s) found; otherwise repeat colonoscopy at least every 3 years. |
| ≥T2 lesions | CEA blood test baseline then q 3 months ×2 years, then q 6 months for the next 2–5 years if curative. Aggressive surgery for detected recurrence is feasible. Colonoscopy within 1 years of resection or 3–6 months postoperatively; repeat q year if neoplastic polyps found; otherwise at least every 3 years. |
| Increasing CEA level after resection | Colonoscopy; CT (chest, abdominal, pelvic), H&P. If scans are WNL despite increasing CEA, repeat scans every 3 months if symptoms occur. PET scan may be helpful in identifying isolated metastases, and should be done to establish whether recurrence is respectable. |

*Abbreviations*: CEA, carcinoembryonic antigen; CT, computerized tomography; H&P, history and physical exam; NED, no evidence of disease; PET, positron emission tomography; WNL, within normal limits.
*Source*: Data from the National Comprehensive Cancer Network.[76]

the colon, ovary, and stomach. Although bowel obstruction may develop at any time, it is more common and may evolve more rapidly in patients with advanced disease. If the patient presents with an obstructing lesion, and the bowel cannot be adequately prepped for resection, a flexible stent may be placed temporarily, or it may be placed for palliation.[76]

Bowel obstruction secondary to advanced colon or rectal carcinoma may be extrinsic or intrinsic. Extrinsic compression of the bowel may occur as a result of abdominal carcinomatosis or tumor studding along the bowel wall. Intrinsic compression of the bowel can result from growth and progression of the tumor within the lumen of the bowel itself. Signs and symptoms of bowel obstruction include nausea and vomiting, abdominal pain, progressive constipation, and the absence of bowel sounds over the affected area. Initially, there is sporadic vomiting, but it increases progressively until it occurs 68% to 100% of the time. Vomiting can remain intermittent or become continuous. It develops early and in large amounts with obstruction of the gastric outlet or small intestine, but develops later in large bowel obstruction.[143] Biliary vomiting is almost odorless and indicates an obstruction in the upper part of the abdomen. The presence of foul-smelling, fecaloid vomiting can be the first sign of an ileal or colonic obstruction.

Diagnosis of a bowel obstruction is made via radiologic assessment. An abdominal x-ray is taken in a supine or standing position to document dilated loops of bowel, air-fluid interfaces, or both. An x-ray following the ingestion of contrast dye can distinguish obstruction from metastases, radiation injury, or adhesions. A more definitive examination can be done with colosigmoidoscopy.[143]

The usual treatment for symptom control is nasogastric suction and administration of parenteral fluids. This inpatient treatment decompresses the stomach and/or intestine and corrects fluid and electrolyte imbalances before surgery or while the decision for surgery is being made. To prevent the tube from becoming occluded, periodic flushing or replacement is needed.

If the obstruction continues for more than a few days, a gastrostomy tube is a much more acceptable and well-tolerated route for decompression than nasogastric intubation.[144] Intermittent venting of the gastrostomy tube allows the patient to continue oral intake and maintain an active lifestyle without the inconvenience of a nasogastric tube. The two options currently available are surgically placed gastrostomy and percutaneous endoscopic gastrostomy (PEG). A gastrostomy tube placed at the time of surgical exploration is the traditional method of long-term gastric decompression. It should be done whenever the surgeon's intraoperative impression is that complete bowel obstruction is imminent or may be prolonged or imminent. PEG entails the insertion of a tube into the stomach through the abdominal wall under fluoroscopic or endoscopic guidance. It can be performed safely as a venting procedure for patients with advanced cancer who are suffering from nausea and vomiting due to bowel obstruction.

Colicky pain occurs in 72% to 76% of patients, and continuous abdominal pain is present in more than 90% of cancer patients with bowel obstruction.[143] Pain may be due to abdominal distention, tumor mass, or hepatomegaly, as well as the obstruction itself.

Initially described 14 years ago, the pharmacological management of bowel obstruction due to advanced cancer focuses on the treatment of pain, nausea, vomiting, and other symptoms without the use of nasogastric tube or intravenous hydration. Palliative care units worldwide now use this approach. Somatostatin or octreotide can be used to minimize intestinal secretions. Antiemetic and pain regimens are well established.[144] The average survival of patients who have inoperable bowel obstruction and are treated with drugs ranges from 2 to 50 days.[144]

## FISTULA

Solid tumors may extend into the bowel from adjacent organs or may spread from the bowel to create fistulous openings to the skin, the vagina, or other organs. Fistulas also may occur as a result of anastomotic breakdown following a surgical procedure on the bowel or as a complication of radiation therapy.

Initial interventions for the patient with a fistula involving the intestinal tract include fluid and electrolyte stabilization and control of infection.[143] Specific fluid and electrolyte needs depend on the type and volume of fistula output; for example, small bowel fistulas usually produce high volumes of effluent containing significant amounts of sodium, potassium, and bicarbonate.[145] The patient with high-output fistula requires close monitoring of fluid-electrolyte balance, with replacement titrated in response to the type and volume of output and laboratory indices. Initial management also involves careful evaluation for any intra-abdominal infectious process. Abscesses are drained via open surgical exploration and irrigation or via percutaneous catheter placement.[145]

Fistula closure is typically achieved either through medical management promoting spontaneous closure or through surgical resection or bypass of the fistulous tract. Usually, conservative medical management is tried first, assuming no intra-abdominal infection is present and the distal bowel is patent. This conservative medical approach is based on studies indicating that in the absence of distal obstruction about 50% of fistulas will close spontaneously within four to six weeks and that surgical closure is frequently ineffective until the underlying factors contributing to fistula development have been corrected.[145] The two major principles on which conservative management is based are (1) provision of nutritional support and (2) bowel rest for the involved segment of the intestine.

Recently, a number of studies have demonstrated a significant reduction in fistula output and in the time required for spontaneous fistula closure with the administration of somatostatin or its analog, octreotide acetate. Somatostatin is a naturally occurring intestinal hormone that reduces the volume of intestinal secretions.[145] A major component of effective fistula management is the containment of the effluent and odor and the protection of the surrounding skin, as these aspects of care have a profound impact on the patient's quality of life. Many products and techniques are now available for achieving and maintaining these goals.

## PROGRESSIVE DISEASE

Symptoms of progressive disease relate to the areas of metastases. The most common metastatic sites in colon cancer are the lymph nodes, liver, and lungs, with metastases to the brain and bone occurring less commonly. The liver is a large organ and can accommodate many metastatic tumors before the patient experiences signs and symptoms of an obstructed liver. As the liver becomes replaced with tumor, liver function tests start to become abnormal. Patients develop nausea, anorexia, cachexia, and ascites as the serum albumin falls, decreasing the colloidal osmotic pressure in the blood vessels. Fluid shifts into the third space, with pedal edema that becomes pitting, which may progress up the calf and thigh. Dyspnea on exertion occurs as the peritoneal fluid pushes up the diaphragm, shrinking the area of lung expansion. Nurses work with the patient and family to minimize, manage, or prevent complications.

The challenging anorexia-cachexia syndrome often requires the assistance of the dietitian, but focuses on helping the patient eat small, frequent feedings of foods and fluids that are pleasing and calorie dense, because the stomach fills quickly. Loss of appetite can be distressing to patients. Despite the fact that this loss does not affect survival, it may affect quality of life. As a consequence, appetite stimulants may be prescribed, such as megestrol acetate. It is important to avoid using total parenteral nutrition for the patient with progressive disease unless there is a chance of reversing the disease with aggressive therapy. Antiemetic control is also critical with progressive disease.

Dyspnea can be distressing, so the nurse focuses on teaching the patient positioning to help the diaphragm descend and increase space for lung expansion, such as using 2 to 3 pillows, a high Fowler's position, or a cardiac recliner. Although the administration of salt-poor albumin should theoretically reverse the colloidal osmotic pressure in the blood vessels, or paracentesis should reduce ascites, unfortunately the fluid often quickly reaccumulates following these measures, thus they are not the standard of care. A trial of diuretic therapy may be effective in reducing painful peripheral edema, together with elevation of the lower extremities. Nurses teach self-administration of diuretics, evaluate responses, and teach other self-care activities to prevent skin breakdown.

Patients may have visceral pain, requiring opioid analgesics. The nurse works closely with both the patient and family to achieve established pain management goals, with care to prevent constipation or other opioid-induced complications. As the disease advances, talking with the patient, about advanced directives can be challenging, but rewarding as the patient makes important decisions, such as making a will while still feeling well enough. Many patients wish to die at home surrounded by their family, so involving the hospice team can be critical to ensure that symptoms are managed, and that the patient maintains the highest quality of life until death. The nurse is a catalyst, stimulating the healthcare team to continue to strive for management and control of symptoms, and an advocate, ensuring that, given the particular set of circumstances, the highest quality of life for each patient is achieved. For information on palliative care measures, see chapters Chapters 74 and 75.

## LONG-TERM MONITORING AND FOLLOW-UP

In today's healthcare environment, the delivery of care takes place in an accelerated fashion. The time span between presentation, work-up, diagnosis, acute intervention, and follow-up treatment can be compressed into a month. Often a multitude of healthcare professionals are involved in the individual's care, which makes communication and coordination of the treatment plan paramount. It has been estimated that 62% of Caucasians and 53% of African Americans diagnosed with colon cancer will attain the 5-year survival rate.[1] Continuity of care during the disease trajectory is critical to assure regular follow-up and intervention as needed.

The average length of stay for someone who has undergone a surgical resection secondary to colorectal carcinoma is less than 5 days. At the time of admission, the appropriate referrals need to be made. Should the individual need a colostomy, and the institution employs, a wound and enterostomal nurse (CWOCN) needs to be involved. A registered dietitian lends support for caloric calculations, hyperalimentation guidelines, and dietary specifics. Social service may be needed as dictated by the individual's home and support situation. Home care is also a consideration to meet specific healthcare needs once the individual is discharged.

At discharge, the individual needs to know when to call their healthcare provider for problems such as fever, chills, shortness of breath, or hemoptysis. Should any change occur with the incision, such as erythema, drainage, or wound separation, the surgeon also needs to be notified. Information about discharge medications and resuming previous medications must be reviewed and clarified.

Upon the patient's return for the postoperative check, an overall physical assessment takes place and the final pathology is shared with the individual and family if the tissue diagnosis was not available at the time of discharge. The general plan for follow-up treatment can be discussed. While additional adjunctive therapy may not begin for another few weeks, the appropriate referrals to the radiation oncologist or medical oncologist need to be made in a timely fashion. Post-treatment surveillance is important and a schema is shown in Table 51-11. Some controversy exists regarding the exact sequence and measures, however, and outcome studies are being conducted.

If the disease is advanced, palliation of symptoms is part of the spectrum of care. The individual and family should be educated regarding the gradual progression of the disease and options available for the treatment of these symptoms. The individual and family can be offered the services and support of hospice. Discussion about advanced directives should occur in a supportive environment. Options for interventions need to be explored so that an informed decision can be made. Most symptoms can be handled within the comfort of the individual's home if so desired. Should a hospital admission become necessary, however, decisions regarding life-support measures need to be explored with the individual and family prior to the hospitalization.

## CONCLUSION

The last decade has seen an awakening realization of the importance of prevention and early detection of colon cancer. However, much work remains to be done to ensure that basic screening tests are offered and made accessible to Americans, especially those age 50 years or older. Although public education efforts in primary prevention have increased, obesity—a known risk factor for colon cancer—remains an enormous problem in the US. Great strides have been made in the management of advanced colon cancer, especially in terms of chemotherapy and biotherapy, and similar advances need to be made in adjuvant therapy so that patients with colon cancer can, indeed, be cured.

# RECTAL CANCER

## INTRODUCTION

In 2009, the ACS estimates that 40,870 people will develop rectal cancer (23,580 men and 17,290 women).[1] In addition, the ACS estimates that 49,920 people will die from colon and rectal cancers combined in 2009 (25,240 men and 24,680 women).[1] Similar to colon cancer, rectal polyps can be found early and removed so that rectal cancer in most cases can be prevented, or detected early so it can be cured through regular, routine screening. For both colon and rectal cancers, 90% of disease occurs in individuals who are age 50 or older.

## EPIDEMIOLOGY AND ETIOLOGY

Rectal cancer is seen more frequently in men than in women.[2] The mortality from rectal cancer has decreased during the last 30 years.[146] Risk factors for rectal cancer are age (risk increases with age more than 50 years old), genetic history of FAP, family history (first-degree relative with adenomas or invasive rectal carcinoma), smoking history in some studies, and history of ulcerative colitis.

## PREVENTION, SCREENING, AND EARLY DETECTION

Peters and colleagues[17] studied 33,971 subjects in the randomized Prostate, Lung, Colorectal and Ovarian (PLCO) cancer screening trial, and found that a high intake of dietary fiber was associated with a lower risk of colon but not rectal adenomas. Individuals ingesting the highest amounts of fiber had a 27% lower risk of distal colonic adenoma as compared to the lowest quintile, with fiber from grains, cereals, and fruits conferring the most protection. The researchers did not find a reduction in risk for rectal adenoma.[17] Giovannucci and colleagues[22] reviewed the Nurses' Health Study data from 88,756 women, and found that women who had taken multivitamins containing folic acid for at least 15 years had a significant reduction in the risk of developing colon cancer, but not the risk of developing rectal cancer. Tsong et al[147] found a significant increase in rectal cancer in Asian patients who smoked heavily and drank alcohol. Exercise does not appear to reduce the risk of rectal cancer.[27]

Digital rectal examination allows exploration of the rectum as far as 7 cm from the anal verge. Herrinton and colleagues[148] used a case-controlled study to show that routine digital rectal exam did not significantly reduce mortality from rectal cancer. Thus, patients age 50 or older should be screened using the same standard as those with colon cancer, shown in Table 51-2.

Bleeding from the anus is often an early sign of rectal cancer, and leads to prompt intervention and likelihood of cure. This underscores the need for colon and rectal cancer screening as part of the annual physical exam in all individuals age 50 or older, and starting at age 40 for individuals at risk as discussed previously. Later symptoms occur when large polyps or lesions bleed or cause tenesmus or incomplete evacuation of stool, cramping, abdominal pain, and obstructive symptoms. These cases have a lower chance of cure.

## PATHOPHYSIOLOGY

The rectum is divided into three sections:

- Lower rectum, 3 to 6 cm from the anal verge; extraperitoneal
- Midrectum, 6 to 10 cm from anal verge; extraperitoneal
- Upper rectum, 10 to 15 cm above the anal verge but with the upper limit of the rectum approximately 12 cm from the anal verge; surrounded by peritoneum on its anterior and lateral surfaces

The rectum temporarily stores fecal waste from which water, electrolytes, and nutrients have been removed as it travels down the intestines. When stimulated, it propels the waste into the anus for evacuation. The rectal mucosa secretes mucus that helps move the waste to the anus. The rectum, together with the muscles in the pelvic floor, help maintain continence. As the rectum fills with fecal waste, sensory nerves stimulate conscious or unconscious tightening of the external anal sphincter until it is appropriate to evacuate the stool, when the sphincter is relaxed. See Figure 51-4.

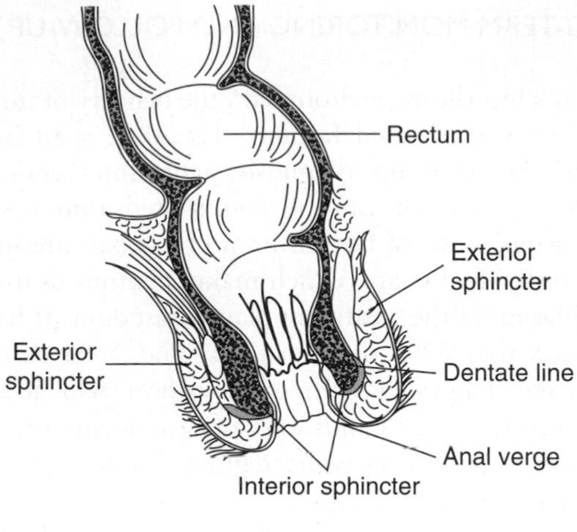


**FIGURE 51-4**

Anatomy of the rectum.

*Source*: Data from National Digestive Diseases Information Clearinghouse.[149]

The rectum has a number of lymphatic channels, and most of the lymphatic drainage follows the hemorrhoidal artery toward the mesenteric artery, as does the drainage from the perirectal lymph nodes that lie mid-rectum and above.[150] The lower perirectal lymph nodes drain laterally, and the hypogastric and iliac lymph node drainage is carried along the aorta. The autonomic nervous system innervates most of the pelvic organs and is important to sexual and bladder function. The sympathetic nerves form the hypogastric plexus; the nerve trunks lie under the pelvic peritoneum, lateral to the mesorectum (the fold of mesentery or peritoneum that is attached to the rectum). These nerve fibers lie close to the arteries supplying the pelvic organs. Parasympathetic fibers leave the 2 to 4 sacral nerve roots to innervate the pelvic viscera, and join the sympathetic fibers at the pelvic plexus. It is critical that the autonomic nerves be preserved during resection of the mesorectum so as to preserve sexual and bladder function.[151]

The location of a rectal tumor is identified by the distance from the lower edge of the tumor to the anal verge (distance from the end of the anal canal where it meets perianal skin), dentate line (line of tissue on the top of the anal canal, separating rectum from anus), or anorectal ring (upper border of the rectal sphincter). Progress in surgical technique has led to the selection of patients for whom sphincter-sparing resection of the rectum is a viable option. This choice is discussed in greater detail in the "Therapeutic Approaches and Nursing Care" section.

### CELLULAR CHARACTERISTICS

Rectal and colon cancers appear to share similar mutations, which results first in adenomatous polyp formation, followed by malignant transformation. Most cancers of the rectum are adenocarcinomas, or carcinomas arising in glandular cells in the mucosa. Adenocarcinomas can be either mucinous (colloid) or signet ring types. Other histological types are scirrhous, neuroendocrine (which confers a poorer prognosis than pure adenocarcinoma), and carcinoid tumors. Squamous cell carcinomas and adenosquamous and undifferentiated carcinomas have been found in the rectum as well.[2] Rarely, carcinoid tumors may arise in the rectum, often appearing as submucosal nodules, and may be indolent; in contrast colonic carcinoid tumors are aggressive and metastasize.[152] Uncommonly, small cell histologies have been described in the rectum, in some cases associated with ulcerative colitis.[153]

Adenocarcinomas of the rectum develop initially in the mucosa, and then locally invade into the lumen of the bowel wall. When the tumor has traversed the muscularis mucosa and infiltrated the submucosa, it is termed *invasive*. Further infiltration by way of the lymph and vascular systems occurs next, and direct extension may occur onto the peritoneal surfaces as well. If the tumor secretes large amounts of mucin (more than 50% of the tumor mass is made up of extracellular mucin), it is called a mucinous carcinoma.

### PROGRESSION OF DISEASE AND PATTERNS OF SPREAD

The large intestine consists of the cecum, ascending colon, transverse colon, descending colon, sigmoid colon, and rectum. The rectum is surrounded by extraperitoneal perirectal fat in the pelvis. The blood supply to the sigmoid colon, descending colon, and upper rectum comes from the inferior mesenteric artery. The lower rectum is supplied by the internal iliac arteries. The rectum is drained by two routes: the superior hemorrhoidal veins, which empty into the portal venous system, and the middle and inferior hemorrhoidal veins, which empty into the inferior vena cava.[18]

By the time of their diagnosis, rectal cancers will have penetrated through the wall in 50% to 77% of patients and will have metastasized to lymph nodes in 50% to 60% of cases.[2] Implantation of tumor cells at other sites can occur as a result of surgical manipulation of the tumor, intraluminal spread, or shedding of tumor cells into the peritoneum. Intraperitoneal seeding and carcinomatosis may occur even without lymphatic or visceral spread. The most common sites of distant metastases for rectal cancer are the liver and lung. Solitary pulmonary metastasis is rare, but may occur with distal rectal cancers.[2] Other areas of metastasis include the brain (cerebellum), bones, kidneys, and adrenals.[153]

The most common sites of rectal cancer recurrence are (1) anterior local recurrence—anastomotic site, prostate and seminal vesicles in men, and vagina, uterus, or bladder in women; and (2) posterior local recurrence—sacrum, pyriformis muscle, sciatic nerve, and pelvic sidewalls.[150]

## CLINICAL MANIFESTATIONS

Signs and symptoms of rectal cancer relate to the location of the tumor near the end of the descending (sigmoid) colon in the rectum. As the malignancy increases in size, signs and symptoms reflect the degree of obstruction in the rectum, such as changes in bowel elimination patterns. In contrast to right-sided colon cancers, which may cause anemia, left-sided colon cancers and rectal cancers have a higher incidence of bright red bleeding.[148] Early signs are bleeding from the anus and painful defecation. Other symptoms include a change in bowel habits such as new onset of constipation or diarrhea, or constipation with diarrhea where diarrhea occurs due to the partial obstruction created by the tumor; changes in the caliber of stool; increased pain on defecation; and a feeling of incomplete stooling or fullness after defecation.

Late signs of rectal cancer are tenesmus, or urgent feeling of having to defecate, but inability to empty the rectum because of circumferential growth and transmural penetration by the rectal tumor[2]; abdominal pain; jaundice; malaise; pelvic pain; anorexia; weight loss; pruritus; ascites; and hepatomegaly. In cases where bleeding from the rectum has continued for a long period of time the signs and symptoms of anemia (fatigue, shortness of breath) can occur. If the tumor locally invades neighboring organs, such as the prostate, bladder, or high sacral nerve roots, the patient will have dysuria, hematuria, or other urinary symptoms. If the tumor locally invades posteriorly, the patient will complain of buttock or perineal pain.[2] Very late signs are urinary signs related to local invasion of neighboring organs such as the prostate or bladder, and destruction of sacral nerve roots causing sacral or sciatic pain, and buttock or perineal pain.[2]

The sensation of a mass in the rectum is often mistakenly attributed to hemorrhoids or anal fissures and may require a rectal examination and biopsy for accurate diagnosis. A proctosigmoidoscopy will provide an adequate examination to secure biopsy and provide a baseline for surgical assessment. Instructing the patient, assisting with the examination, and providing support and privacy for the patient during the procedure are crucial to a successful examination.

## ASSESSMENT

### PATIENT AND FAMILY HISTORY

The history should include patient and family history, with attention being paid to a personal history of FAP or

HNPCC; rectal or colon adenomas; rectal, colon, uterine, ovarian, bladder, or other cancers; and a history of inflammatory bowel diseases. Family history of adenomas or rectal, colon, or other cancers, and their age at onset, should be elucidated. Social history of smoking or alcohol consumption should be queried. In addition, a systems review should be done, with a careful exploration of bowel habits, changes, rectal sensation of fullness or incomplete stooling, bleeding, and hemorrhoids.

## PHYSICAL EXAMINATION

Key features of the physical examination are assessment of the abdomen, breasts, rectum, and lymph nodes to identify any abnormalities that reflect the status of primary or metastatic rectal cancer. Initially, general features are assessed, such as weight, functional and mental ability, and nutritional status, with a focus on wasting of the temporal or masseter muscles. If the rectal cancer invades the bladder or develops a fistula into the bladder, the patient will develop symptoms of chronic urinary tract infection and hematuria. Percussing and palpating the right upper quadrant will give information about possible liver metastases, the most common metastatic site of rectal cancer. To augment assessment of liver metastases, assess the eye sclera for icterus, which precedes jaundice related to biliary obstruction. A digital rectal exam should be performed to locate masses and identify tenderness. In men, assessment for rectal cancer should include a prostate exam and in women a bimanual vaginal exam should be performed.

## DIAGNOSTIC STUDIES

Diagnostic studies include proctoscopy with biopsy of the suspicious lesion with pathological analysis of depth of invasion of the muscularis mucosa as well as marking the tumor; chest, abdominal, and pelvic CT; serum CEA level, CBC, electrolytes, and liver function tests[146]; and endorectal ultrasound (EUS) or endorectal or pelvic MRI, which provides information about depth of invasion and lymph node status.[154] Colonoscopy is recommended to rule out any synchronous polyps or tumors in the colon. These studies provide adequate information to identify clinical stage and treatment of choice. EUS helps to clarify surgical options and contributes to choosing a sphincter-saving procedure. EUS is superior to CT scan in evaluating the depth of wall invasion and the involvement of adjacent soft tissues, but it may not be sensitive enough to detect microinvasion of the submucosa. In a meta-analysis, EUS had a high, similar sensitivity to MRI, but was more specific (86% vs 69%) in identifying depth of tumor invasion.[154] When MRI is used in preoperative staging, it can detect pelvic sidewall and ascral involvement, so it complements the information gained from EUS.[154] If synchronous liver metastases (single or potentially resectable) are identified, PET/CT or contrast-enhanced CT is recommended to evaluate resectability and to establish a baseline for posthepatectomy follow-up.[146]

Magnetic resonance imaging is also useful in diagnosing advanced disease and can detect recurrent rectal cancer or tumors too small to be evaluated on CT scan. Magnetic resonance imaging may also be done for patients who are unable to tolerate the CT scanner or who are allergic to the contrast material. Fine-needle aspiration, with or without the above diagnostic tests, is generally indicated to confirm the recurrence of disease.

## PROGNOSTIC INDICATORS

In rectal cancer, as in colon cancer, staging of the tumor is based on depth of invasion rather than size of the tumor because depth of tumor penetration has been shown to independently influence survival.[153] The most important predictors of long-term survival of patients with rectal cancer are pathological stage at diagnosis, presence of distant metastases, extent of local tumor, number of positive lymph nodes, and residual disease after definitive therapy. As the molecular basis of carcinogenesis has become better understood, other biological, genetic, molecular, and tissue factors have been identified, in addition to TNM staging, that influence survival for the patient with rectal cancer. Seven prognostic indicators are supported by multiple, statistically robust clinical trials[153]:

1. Local extent of tumor defined as depth of tumor penetration
2. Serosal involvement by tumor
3. Regional lymph node involvement
4. Nodal micrometastases, where lymph nodes that contain a tumor measuring 3 mm or larger in diameter are considered positive, while those containing tumor measuring 0.2 mm or smaller or identified by nonhistological means such as polymerase chain reaction or immunostaining are considered micrometastases
5. Lymphatic or vascular invasion (LVI), which predicts local or regional recurrence regardless of tumor status
6. Residual tumor following definitive therapy
7. Elevated preoperative serum level of CEA ≥ 5.0 ng/mL, which predicts reduced survival

# CLASSIFICATION AND STAGING

Tumor, Node, Metastases (TNM) staging is the most widely accepted form of staging for rectal cancer (see Table 51-12). The most important predictor of survival is stage at presentation. Five-year survival rates by stage are

**TABLE 51-12**

**Staging for Rectal Cancer**

| Stage | Tumor | Nodal Status | Metastases | Duke's Stage |
|---|---|---|---|---|
| 0 | Tis (in situ intraepithelial or invades lamina propria) | N0 (no metastasis in the lymph nodes) | M0 (no distance metastasis) | – |
| I | T1 (invades submucosa) | N0 | M0 | A |
| | T2 (invades muscularis propria) | N0 | M0 | A |
| IIA | T3 (through muscularis into subserosa or into nonperitonealized pericolic or perirectal tissue) | N0 | M0 | B |
| IIB | T4 (directly invades other organs or structures, and/or perforates visceral peritoneum) | N0 | M0 | B |
| IIIA | T1–T2 | N1(metastasis to 1–3 regional lymph nodes) | M0 | C |
| IIIB | T3–T4 | N1 | M0 | C |
| IIIC | Any T | N2 (metastasis to 4 or more regional lymph nodes) | M0 | C |
| IV | Any T | Any N | M1 (distant metastasis) | D |

*Source*: Data from Greene et al.[85]

as follows: stage I, 79%; stage II, 52%; stage III, 37%; and stage IV, 4%. Each stage has a lower 5-year survival rate than the comparable stage of colon cancer.[153] Stage III rectal cancer patients are now stratified into three subsets, each with a different prognosis.[153] Stage IIIA patients with T1-2, N1 lesions have a 5-year survival rate of 39% when treated with surgery alone, compared to 55.1% (relative survival, 67.2%) when surgery is followed by adjuvant chemotherapy and radiation therapy. Stage IIIB patients with T3-4, N1 lesions have a 5-year survival rate of 21.7% when treated with surgery alone, compared to 40.9% with surgery plus adjuvant therapy. Stage IIIC patients have any T, N2 disease and a 12.2% 5-year survival rate, which increases to 28.9% when treated with surgery combined with chemotherapy and radiation. Staging is done preoperatively as clinical staging ("c" prefix) and postoperatively by the pathologist (indicated with a "p" prefix). If neoadjuvant therapy is given, such as preoperative chemotherapy, a "y" prefix is used, and an "r" prefix signifies cancers that have recurred.[152]

## THERAPEUTIC APPROACHES AND NURSING CARE

Table 51-13 details strategies developed by leading experts for the management of rectal cancer.[146] The approaches have become widely adopted as the standard of care. If neoadjuvant chemoradiation is given prior to surgery, to downstage the tumor, surgery is delayed for 5 to 10 weeks to ensure healing.[146]

### SURGERY

The successful management of rectal cancer has 5 goals: cure, local control, restoration of intestinal continuity, preservation of anorectal sphincter function, and preservation of the patient's sexual and urinary function. The initial treatment planning is complex and balances the goal/intent (cure or palliation) and function with the preservation of normal bowel function if possible.[146] Because of the anatomical constraints of the bony pelvis, it may be difficult in some cases to achieve adequate sphincter, sexual, and urinary function without compromising cure and local control.

Local control is an extremely important aspect of treatment. As many as 25% of the patients who die of rectal cancer will have local recurrence only; another 50% will have local recurrence in addition to distant disease. For patients with local recurrence after initial treatment for rectal cancer, additional surgery rarely has advantages. Many of these patients with advanced disease experience significant problems with bone and nerve pain, hemorrhage, pelvic sepsis, and bowel and urinary obstruction.

The surgical procedure employed for rectal cancer depends on the stage and depth of tumor invasion of the mucosa. Total mesorectal excision is the standard, in which

**TABLE 51-13**

**Management of Rectal Cancer**

| Stage of Disease | Primary Treatment | Adjuvant Treatment |
|---|---|---|
| **T1–2, N0** | | |
| • T1-2, N0, M0 | Abdominoperineal resection, low anterior resection, or coloanal anastomosis (total mesorectal excision) | Observe |
| • pT3, N0, M0 or T1-3, N1-2 | Abdominoperineal resection, low anterior resection | 5-FU ± LV or FOLFOX or capecitabine then CI 5-FU/RT or 5-FU/LV/RT or capecitabine/RT, then 5-FU ± LV or FOLFOX or capecitabine |
| • T1, NX, negative margins after primary treatment | Transanal excision (if tumor < 30% of bowel circumference, < 3 cm in size, clear margins, mobile, within 8 cm of anal verge, no LVI, well- to moderately well differentiated, grade 1–2. | Observe |
| • T1-2, NX, positive margins, LVI, grade 3–4 after primary treatment | Abdominoperineal resection, low anterior resection, or coloanal anastomosis (total mesorectal excision) | If pathological (p) T1-2, N0, M0 observe;<br>If pT3, N0, M0, or pT1-3, N1-2: 5-FU ± LV or FOLFOX or capecitabine then CI 5-FU/RT or bolus 5-FU/LV/RT or capecitabine/RT; then 5-FU ± LV or FOLFOX or capecitabine |
| • T2, NX, margins clear | Abdominoperineal resection, low anterior resection, or coloanal anastomosis (total mesorectal excision) or 5-FU/XRT | Consider systemic chemotherapy |
| **T3, N0 or T any, N1N2** | Preoperative CI 5-FU/XRTfor lymph node–positive disease, or bolus 5-FU/LV/RT or capecitabine/RT; then abdominoperineal resection, low anterior resection, or coloanal anastomosis (total mesorectal excision).<br>For patients unable to tolerate combined modality therapy: Abdominoperineal resection, low anterior resection, or coloanal anastomosis using mesorectal excision alone. | 5-FU ± LV or FOLFOX or capecitabine<br>pT3, N0, M0, or pT1-3, N1-2: Reconsider: 5-FU ± LV or FOLFOX or capecitabine; then CI 5-FU/RT or bolus 5-FU/LV/RT or capecitabine/RT; then 5-FU ± LV or capecitabine |
| **T4** | CI 5-FU/RT or bolus 5-FU/LV/RT or capecitabine/RT, followed by resection if possible | 5-FU ± LV or FOLFOX or capecitabine |
| **T any, N any, M1 resectable** | FOLFOX ± bevacizumab or FOLFIRI ± bevacizumab or CapeOX ± bevacizumab, followed by staged or synchronous resection of rectal primary and metastases<br>Or<br>Staged or synchronous resection of rectal primary and metastases<br>Or<br>CI 5-FU/pelvic RT or bolus 5-FU/LV/RT or capecitabine/RT, followed by synchronous resection of rectal primary and metastases. | CI 5-FU/pelvic RT or bolus 5-FU/LV/pelvic RT or capecitabine/RT<br>If T1-2, N0, M1: 5-FU ± LV ×6 months or FOLFOX ± bevacizumab ×4–6 months, or FOLFIRI ± bevacizumab × 4–6 months, or Cape Ox ± bevacizumab<br>If pT3-4, any N, or any T, N1-2: 5-FU ± LV or FOLFOX or capecitabine; then CI 5-FU/RT or bolus 5-FU/LV/RT or capecitabine/RT; then<br>5-FU ± LV or FOLFOX or capecitabine<br>5-FU ± LV or FOLFOX ± bevacizumab or FOLFIRI ± bevacizumab or CapeOx ± bevacizumab<br>Optional 5-FU/pelvic XRT T1-2, N0, M1: 5-FU ± LV or FOLFOX or FOLFIRI for 4–6 months<br>T3-4, any N, or any T, N1-2: 5-FU ± LV or FOLFOX, then CI 5-FU/XRT or capecitabine/XRT, then 5-FU ± LV |
| **Any T, any N, M1 unresectable** | Options include resection of tumor, diverting colostomy, stenting, laser photocoagulation, 5-FU/RT or capecitabine/RT, single-modality chemotherapy | Chemotherapy regimens: First line: FOLFOX, FOLFIRI, bevacizumab<br>+ 5-FU–based regimen *if patient can tolerate intensive therapy*; if not, capecitabine, 5-FU/LV, or 5-FU CI<br>Second line: FOLFOX or FOLFIRI (depending on firstline chemotherapy), irinotecan ± cetuximab |

*Abbreviations*: 5-FU, 5-fluorouracil; CI, continuous infusion; LV, leucovorin; LVI, lymphovascular invasion; NX, nodal status unknown; pTNM, pathological tumor node metastases staging; XRT, radiation therapy.

*Source*: Data from Libutti et al[11]; National Comprehensive Cancer Network[146]; and Libutti et al.[150]

the tumor, blood vessels, and lymphatics are removed to decrease the risk of locoregional recurrence, since lymphatic spread from rectal cancers occurs upward, lateral, and distal. Criteria for a local, transanal excision are that the tumor is less than 30% of the bowel circumference, smaller than 3 cm in size, resectable with clear margins (T1 lesion), mobile, within 8 cm of the anal verge, without lymphatic or vascular invasion (LVI); well to moderately well differentiated; and Grade 1 to 2.[146] A low anterior resection (LAR) or coloanal anastomosis (CAA) is appropriate for uncomplicated lesions in the mid and upper rectum.[2] Either procedure will preserve the sympathetic and parasympathetic nerves as long as there is adequate blood supply, sphincter muscle function, and no tension at the anastamosis.[150]

If the sphincter muscles are involved or the tumor extends to within 2 cm of the dentate line, abdominoperineal resection (APR) with sacrifice of the sphincter is necessary. This radical surgical approach involves transabdominal resection of the rectum and mesorectum from the level of the inferior mesenteric vessels to the levator muscles, in combination with transperineal excision of the anus and distal rectum.[150] Although a neosphincter has been FDA approved, it requires careful anorectal reconstruction and prosthesis implantation, The NCT00059891 study is currently exploring the risks and complications of the neosphincter, ease of use, efficacy, and quality of life of patients compared to APR,[155] Abdominoperineal resection is currently indicated for tumors of the distal third of the rectum within 3 cm of the anal verge, tumors involving the anal-sphincter musculature, tumors of the rectovaginal septum, patients with poor continence preoperatively, and patients with diarrheal disorders.[146]

In recent years, the use of adjuvant therapy, the introduction of circular stapling devices, and the demonstrated adequacy of 2 cm distal margins have allowed safe use of sphincter-preserving surgery for resection of midrectal and some distal rectal cancers.[150] In low anterior resection, as described earlier, the dissection and anastomosis are performed below the peritoneal reflection.

A coloanal anastomosis preserves the sphincter mechanism in patients with low-lying rectal tumors whose negative distal margin of resection is up to, but does not include, the anal-sphincter musculature. The operative dissection is similar to that of LAR and APR, with transection of the distal margin at the level of the levator ani muscles within the abdomen. Through a perineal approach, the remaining anal mucosa is stripped and an anastomosis is made between the colon and the anus to restore intestinal continuity.[146] To provide adequate bowel length and a tension-free anastomosis, the splenic flexure of the colon is completely mobilized. The vascular supply of the left colon is then based on the middle colic artery. The surgeon will perform a protective diverting ileostomy in all patients who have coloanal anastomosis. Contraindications for an LAR or coloanal anastomosis include tumors involving the anal-sphincter musculature, tumors involving the rectovaginal septum, patients with poor continence preoperatively, patients with diarrhea disorders, and unfavorable anatomical constraints (eg, obesity, narrow pelvis).

The success and options presented to patients for surgical management of rectal cancers depend on the skill of the surgeon. Meyerhardt and colleagues[156] studied the impact of hospital procedure volume on surgical operations and long-term outcomes in high-risk (stage II and III), curatively resected patients with rectal cancer. They found a significant difference in the rates of APR as a function of hospital procedure volume: a 46% rate in low-volume hospitals compared to a 31.8% rate in high-volume hospitals. However, overall, they found there was no significant difference in rectal cancer recurrence or survival when patients completed standard adjuvant therapy.

## RADIATION THERAPY

Combined modality therapy with chemotherapy and radiation therapy has a significant role in the management of patients with rectal cancer (below the peritoneal reflection). Loco-regional failure with surgical therapy alone in the treatment of patients with stage II and III rectal cancer approaches 50%. Randomized clinical trials have shown that adjuvant chemotherapy combined with radiation therapy improves survival for patients with stage II and III rectal cancer, so most patients with stage II (tumor penetration through the muscle wall) and III (positive lymph nodes) receive surgery, radiation and chemotherapy.[150] Three-dimensional, conformal radiation treatment planning is used in many centers for more precise targeting of radiation, because it yields an improved ability to plan and localize the target and normal tissues of treatment volume as compared to traditional radiation therapy.

When considering preoperative radiation, it is important to note that tumor cells are often well-oxygenated because the blood supply to the tumor has not been surgically manipulated. Well-oxygenated cells are believed to have increased radiosensitivity; as a consequence, tumor cell killing by radiotherapy may be increased.[146] Despite these radiobiological advantages, preoperative radiation alone has not affected overall rates of survival, distant recurrence, or cure rates.[146] However, locoregional tumor control rates have improved with preoperative radiation. Randomized studies have shown a significant decrease in local recurrence rates when preoperative doses of radiotherapy were higher than 34.5 Gy.[146] In addition, the sphincter preservation rate for patients with T3 and T4 lesions treated with preoperative radiotherapy is increased.[146] Preoperative chemoradiation may be more effective than postoperative adjuvant treatment, especially in patients with T3 or T4 lesions. Such treatment may improve resectability and produce fewer complications compared to the postoperative treatment. Radiation doses of 45 to 55 Gy are recommended in combination with 5-FU-based chemotherapy.[2] Patients receiving pre-operative chemoradiation should wait 5 to 10 weeks after treatment is completed before undergoing surgery. Following surgery, the patient should receive adjuvant chemotherapy for 6 months.[146]

Unresectable rectal tumors may be treated with palliative radiation, and radiation therapy is used for palliation of advanced rectal cancer symptoms. The pain from the local recurrence of rectal cancer is very difficult to control, and radiation may reduce pain.

### Radiation side effects

Injury to the bowel may occur as a result of radiation therapy. Some side effects of radiation may require surgical intervention, but most side effects subside when radiation therapy is stopped. Chronic radiation enteritis can lead to bowel mucosal thinning and inflammation, eventually resulting in ulceration.

### CHEMOTHERAPY

Adjuvant chemotherapy is recommended for patients with tumors having positive circumferential or radial margins (CRM), defined as a tumor within 1 mm of the tumor margin. See Table 51-13 for the chemotherapy regimens available, in combination with radiation therapy. Because of the bony pelvis limitation, surgeons may find it difficult to achieve wide resection margins. A positive margin is one of the most important predictive factors for both local and distant recurrence. In addition, patients with stage II and III rectal cancers are at high risk of recurrence. Thus, aggressive adjuvant chemotherapy combined with radiotherapy is used to reduce local recurrence and increase overall survival.

For patients with metastatic rectal cancer, the NCCN guidelines suggest that single, isolated metastases may be resected together with the primary rectal lesion, followed by adjuvant chemotherapy and radiotherapy to the pelvis.[146] For patients with unresectable metastases, FOLFOX 4 together with bevacizumab, is one of several treatment options that is effective as palliative therapy. The chemotherapy regimens used in the treatment of patients with rectal cancer are similar to those used in the treatment of colon cancer. Please refer to Tables 51-8 and 51-13 for descriptions of these regimens. In addition, the discussion of chemotherapy side effects and management are discussed in the colon cancer section. See the discussion for colon cancer on bevacizumab and cetuximab, both of which are indicated in combination with chemotherapy for the treatment of advanced rectal cancer.

## SYMPTOM MANAGEMENT AND SUPPORTIVE CARE

Patients who have an APR will have a permanent sigmoid or descending colostomy; those who undergo a LAR or CAA, may have a temporary ileostomy. All of these patients will benefit from consultation with a CWOCN from the first visit when they are told the diagnosis through the preoperative and postoperative phases. Nursing management focuses on early recognition of potential problems.

Postoperative care is focused on facilitating an uncomplicated recovery with healing of the operative site and recovery of baseline function and patterns. If the patient has a stoma, another goal is to empower the individual to effectively care for it. Nurses play a critical role in providing patient education, emotional support, and coordination of care across care boundaries.

### PERINEAL WOUND HEALING

The perineal wound or incisional site may be closed immediately following the removal of the rectum, anus, muscle, and fatty tissue, or it may be left open to heal by secondary intention. Primary closure of the perineal wound site at the time of surgery is the preferred technique, because it is more comfortable for the patient and requires much less care. Closed suction drains are inserted at the time of surgery and exit either through the incisional area or through a separate stab wound in the buttocks. The drains are removed on the third or fifth postoperative day. Primary closure is contraindicated when fecal spillage occurs, the bowel is perforated, an infected hematoma is present, or there is perineal disease such as abscess or fistula.[145]

Perineal wound healing by secondary intention prolongs the healing process, which may take as long as four months. The wound requires packing and meticulous care to promote granulation and to avoid infection. Irrigations and sitz baths facilitate wound healing. The drainage and healing process must be carefully monitored by the nurse, and any untoward signs and symptoms of infection must be reported. Nursing care can range from complex dressing changes to washing the area with soap and water, monitoring intake and output, and checking for patency of drainage tubes.

### STOMA AND COLOSTOMY MANAGEMENT

Careful selection of the stoma site is an important step toward ensuring the patient's quality of life after surgery. By assessing the patient's abdomen in lying, sitting, and standing positions, the healthcare provider can ensure that the selected stoma site is within the rectus muscle and is in an area that can physically support ostomy equipment. It is important that the patient is able to visualize the proposed stoma site so that self-care will be easier.[143] Scars, folds, bony prominences, belt and waistlines, and the umbilicus need to be avoided to ensure proper fit of the ostomy equipment. The anatomical location of the stoma influences the abdominal quadrant placement as well as the surgical technique employed.

The stoma must be evaluated for viability, condition, size, and shape, and it must be determined whether all sutures are holding the everted stoma onto the abdomen. A red, shiny, moist, budded, or flush stoma with all sutures and peristomal skin intact is the desired outcome. Deviations from this finding should be reported to the surgeon, as they may indicate early problems and require immediate surgical intervention.[143]

Psychological support of the patient begins preoperatively with an explanation of the surgery to be performed and introduction to the pouching system and equipment. After surgery, support shifts to coping and adaptation, particularly when the patient first looks at his or her stoma, which can be very upsetting. The initial size of the stoma will depend on the portion of the bowel segment involved and any bowel obstruction that existed prior to surgery. The initial bowel edema gradually subsides following surgery, and the actual stoma size is established in six to eight weeks.[143] This is an important variable to remember when preparing the pouch opening to ensure proper sizing.

Initially the patient will have serosanguineous fluid in the pouch. The time at which the stoma begins to function depends on the preoperative cleansing and prior obstruction. If this was an emergent surgery or poor cleansing was performed, stool will be present almost immediately. Once peristalsis returns and flatus is passed, food is introduced. Stool will soon be expelled from the stoma. Usually, the more proximal a stoma is in the bowel, the sooner it functions and the more liquid the stool content.

The key principles in stoma management include the containment of the effluent and odor and the protection of the peristomal skin. The degree of skin protection required is dictated by the characteristics of the effluent. Effluent that is proteolytic, highly acidic, or highly alkaline (ileostomy, cecostomy, ascending colostomy) requires meticulous protection of peristomal skin. Nonenzymatic effluent with a pH that is essentially neutral primarily requires protection against pooling of drainage that can macerate the skin (descending/sigmoid colostomies).

Equipment costs vary but are reimbursable to some degree by Medicare and most private insurers. Certain agencies help with the costs for those individuals who have particular needs; however, these groups differ across the country. Patient teaching proceeds in a stepwise fashion from the simple to the complex. Asking the patient what he or she wants to learn first may relieve some of the patient's anxiety. With a family member or significant other present to serve as a backup caregiver when the patient is at home, the teaching usually proceeds from removing or applying the pouch closure clamp, to looking at and cleansing the stoma, to applying and emptying the pouch. The goal is for the patient to independently manage the pouch changing and stoma care prior to discharge.

Case managers coordinating the discharge plan for the patient should be encouraged to recommend home health agencies with CWOCN consultants to ensure continuity of care and management of any peristomal complications. Many hospital-based CWOCN consultants will also see outpatients for post-discharge care and instruction. Individualized patient education materials, mail-order catalogs and a list of the supplies, names of community vendors, and support groups at the United Ostomy Association or the American Cancer Society are available to facilitate patients' self-care.

## SEXUAL DYSFUNCTION

Early-stage rectal cancer treated with resection of the rectal lesion may interfere with an individual's potential for orgasm, although erectile dysfunction is less common. In contrast, patients who undergo more extensive surgery have a far higher incidence of sexual dysfunction, especially males. In 1999, a study of 60 men who were sexually active prior to pretreatment and who received either high anterior resection, low anterior resection, or abdominoperineal resection demonstrated that patients in the APR arm had the highest percentage of sexual problems. About 65% became sexually inactive, 50% were unable to ejaculate, and 45% reported erectile dysfunction.[157] More recently in 2005, a study by Hendren et al[158] measured sexual function and quality of life after rectal cancer treatment. They found that of the 32% of women and 50% of men who were sexually active, 29% of the women and 45% of the men said their sex lives were worse following the surgery. More concerning, the patients rarely remembered discussing the sexual risks preoperatively, or treatment for their sexual dysfunction. Despite this, global quality of life scores were high. Thus, early multi-disciplinary treatment planning, including neoadjuvant therapy as appropriate to avoid APR, is necessary. In addition, patient assessment of patients' sexuality should occur prior to treatment, and after, with care planning to include patient education, therapy, and referral as needed to minimize sexual dysfunction following therapy.[159]

Patients with ostomies can become concerned with their body image as they worry about stoma appearance, stool collecting in the pouch, pouch leakage, sounds, and odors. These can all cause the person to feel unattractive and to have a diminished libido. Fear of rejection by one's significant other can cause stress in the relationship and have a negative impact on the patient's self-concept.

Support for the patient and significant other includes the following[160,161]:

1. *Depression or anxiety.* Antidepressants may be useful but some drugs can interfere with erectile function; those who prescribe should consult with a pharmacist.
2. *Fatigue.* Napping prior to sexual activity as well as avoiding heavy meals and alcohol can be helpful. Trying different positions during sexual activity that require minimal effort, such as the side-lying position, may be helpful.
3. *Pain.* Timing of medication is important to provide pain control without drowsiness. Relaxation techniques, warm baths or soaks, and massage may decrease pain and can be an opportunity for sexual foreplay when done as a couple.
4. *Nausea.* Medicating with antiemetics prior to sexual activity is often suggested. A light meal or crackers prior to activity may also be helpful. Usual accoutrements of sexual activity, such as perfumes, colognes, and scented candles, may have to be avoided if smells cause nausea.
5. *Odors.* Elimination ostomies should be emptied prior to sexual activity. Deodorizers or odor eliminators are available if odors are a concern. Pouch covers are also available to shield the pouch contents.

### URETERAL OBSTRUCTION

With advanced rectal cancer, bilateral ureteral obstruction can occur as a result of direct tumor compression of the ureters. Individuals with ureteral obstruction present with oliguria and elevated serum creatinine. A cystoscopy and bilateral retrograde pyelogram are the most reliable diagnostic tools for determining ureteral obstruction. These exams also determine whether the obstruction is intrinsic to the ureter or extrinsic, as would be seen with an advancing colorectal lesion.

Treatment of ureteral obstruction may be accomplished at the time of the retrograde pyelogram. Urinary stents can be inserted into the ureters to establish patency and prevent further compression by the tumor. Stents can circumvent the need for a surgical procedure. If the ureteral stents become occluded, they can be usually changed via cystoscopy. In some situations, however, urinary stents cannot be utilized because of ureteral strictures or inability to visualize the ureters. In such cases, percutaneous nephrostomy tubes can be used to treat the obstruction. Nephrostomy tubes placed directly into the kidney via a percutaneous approach allow adequate urinary drainage from the renal pelvis.

### LIVER METASTASES

Initial evaluation of a patient with liver metastases should include whether the liver lesion(s) are resectable. If so, then the primary tumor and metastatic site can be resected synchronously, or as a staged plan. If the tumor does not appear resectable, neoadjuvant therapy may be planned and then the patient re-evaluated. See previous discussion for the patient with metastatic colon cancer.

In addition to the symptoms experienced by a patient with advanced colon cancer a patients with advanced rectal cancer may experience symptoms of intermittent obstruction, as well as pain and dysfunction depending on the organs involved by local invasion. Nursing care is directed toward support and symptom management to help the patient maximize the quality of life for the time remaining. Community resources such as hospice should be consulted early in the period of advanced disease so that relationships can be established, and a symptom management plan can be instituted when needed.

### FOLLOW-UP

The National Comprehensive Cancer Network (NCCN) identifies recommended follow-up based on stage of disease and treatment.[146] Patients should have a history and physical every 3 months for 2 years, then every 6 months for a total of 5 years. Carcinoembryonic antigen measurements should generally be repeated every 3 months for 2 years; for patients with T2 or greater lesions, they should be repeated every 6 months for 2 to 5 years. Colonoscopy should be performed in 1 year following treatment, then repeated in 1 year if abnormal or at least every 2 to 3 years if negative for polyps. If the patient did not have a preoperative colonoscopy due to obstruction, then it should be performed 3 to 6 months after initial treatment.

## CONCLUSION

Screening and early detection strategies must be perfected so that patients will be diagnosed earlier, especially in minority communities. Adenomatous polyps can be removed to prevent rectal cancer. If a tumor is not prevented, it can be cured when diagnosed early and removed by endoscopy. Continued improvements in combination chemotherapy, radiation therapy, and molecular targeted therapy will offer improved control in both the adjuvant and the metastatic settings.

# ANAL CANCER

## INTRODUCTION

Anal cancer is comprised of cancers of the anal canal and anal margin (perianal skin). Anal canal cancer is an uncommon yet potentially curable cancer. Several subcategories of disease with different risks and etiologies exist. In HIV-positive men and women who have receptive anal intercourse, cancer results from sexually transmitted human papillomavirus (HPV) infection. The incidence of this disease increased markedly in the 1980s in relation to HIV infection, and it appears to be increasing with the prolongation of longevity in HIV-positive men who have sex with men. The incidence of anal canal cancer is increasing and major risk factors are (1) infection with human papillomavirus (HPV)-16, and to a lesser extent -18, 31, 33, 35; (2) immunosuppression; and (3) tobacco smoking.[162] Most cancers are squamous histology, and effective combination chemotherapy and radiation treatment results in an 80% 5-year survival rate with sphincter preservation.[163] Radical surgery is reserved for salvage, and for patients with recurrence or progression, APR may result in cure.[164]

## EPIDEMIOLOGY AND ETIOLOGY

Anal cancer represents less than 4% of all gastrointestinal cancers, but its incidence is increasing. The ACS estimated that 5290 people would develop the disease, and 710 people would die in 2009.[1] More women (17%) die of anal cancer than men (11%).[1] About 80% of anal cancers are diagnosed in patients age 60 or older, but in patients younger than age 35, men are more frequently affected than women.[164]

Three main risk factors have been identified: infection by HPV-16, immunosuppression, and tobacco smoking, but the major risk factor appears to be persistent infection with HPV-16. Anal cancer in HIV-infected men and women appears to be related to the sexual transmission of HPV-16 by receptive anal intercourse, resulting in the initial mutational event. The incidence of anal cancer among single men is said to be six times higher than that among married men.[2] A history of genital warts (condylomata) is also associated with anal cancer, again suggesting that HPV may be a causative factor. Pfister and Fuchs[165] showed that HPV-16 infection is associated with high-grade anal intraepithelial neoplasia (AIN) and risk of anal cancer, but many patients with HPV-16-positive cytologies do not develop anal cancers. Other sexually transmitted diseases besides genital warts have been linked to increased risk for anal cancer, including a history of cervical cancer.[162] Smoking tobacco has been identified as another risk factor, independent of sexual behavior.[166] Immunosuppression is a major risk factor, and there is an increased risk of anal canal cancer in patients who are immunosuppressed after solid organ transplantation, infected by human immunodeficiency virus, or who have a history of vulvar or vaginal cancer.[162] Patients who have undergone renal transplant have 100-fold higher risk. Patients with HIV infection have a 15 to 30 times higher risk, with risk increasing as CD4 levels fall below 200/μL.[1] Another study showed that homosexual men who were HIV positive had a 13.9 relative risk, which jumped to 84.1 when the infection evolved into AIDS.[167]

## PREVENTION, SCREENING, AND EARLY DETECTION

Prevention strategies are based on known etiology. Because the greatest risk for anal cancer appears to be persistent HPV-16 infection, and this is magnified in individuals who are immunosuppressed, such as with HIV-infection. Thus, teaching HIV-infected patients who have receptive anal intercourse protective sexual practices, and encouraging screening should be encouraged. Women who have high numbers of life-time sexual partners are at risk for HPV-16 infection. In one study involving female subjects, Friis and colleagues[166] found that (1) women with more than 10 lifetime sexual partners had a 5 times greater risk for anal cancer compared to women with one lifetime partner; (2) women who had more than four partners before the age of 20 had a three times higher risk than women who had not had intercourse before age 20; and (3) women with anal warts had a tenfold increased risk, while women with a prior history of sexually transmitted diseases or cervical neoplasia also had increased risk. All individuals who are sexually active should be encouraged to use condoms during sexual activity. Indeed, for those who engage in receptive anal intercourse, condoms are critical.

For those individuals at risk (ie, those with immunosuppression and the possibility of HPV-16 infection), screening for anal cancer should be considered as soon as the risk is identified. The standard for screening is an anal Pap smear followed by high-resolution anoscopy. However, the sensitivity and specificity of anal cytology is poor. The value of screening for anal intraepithelial neoplasia (AIN) in homosexual and bisexual HIV-infected individuals has been shown in one study to be cost-effective and resulted in improved survival. Salit and colleagues[168] reported data for an anal cancer screening program in HIV-positive men. Out of a total of 680, 75 men with HIV-positive were screened using anal Pap smears, HPV detection, and high-resolution anoscopy. High-risk oncogenic HPV was found in 80% of patients; Pap smears were abnormal in 70% of the patients, with high-grade changes (high-grade squamous intraepithelial lesions, HSIL) in 17% and low-grade changes (low-grade squamous intraepithelial lesions, LSIL) in 38%; anal biopsies were abnormal in 56% of the patients, with a distribution of 25% LSIL, 28% HSIL, and 1% anal cancer. More recently, it appears that among HIV-infected patients, high-grade squamous intraepithelial lesions are not more prevalent in patients on highly active antiretroviral therapy. Research is necessary to identify the subgroups of HIV-infected patients, of men who have sex with men who would benefit from screening, and intensive follow-up using high resolution anoscopy.[169,170] Additional data sources may include HPV viral loads, adjuncts to cytology such as *p16ink4a* (gene for cyclin-dependent kinase inhibitor 2A) staining.[169] Often symptoms of anal cancer, such as bleeding, pain, and a sensation of fullness, are attributed to hemorrhoids or anal fissure, with resulting delay in evaluation and diagnosis.

## PATHOPHYSIOLOGY

The anus is the terminal 4 to 6 cm of the gastrointestinal tract, and the anal canal connects the rectum to the perianal skin (see Figure 51-4). It is lined by an epithelial mucous membrane that covers the internal sphincter[163] and is responsible for maintaining continence. The anal canal is that region extending from the anal verge to the rectal mucosa. Another way of describing this area is the area between the anal verge and the anorectal ring. The anorectal ring is easily palpable and corresponds to the junction of a portion of the levator muscle with the external anal sphincter. The dentate line is located at the transition zone, where the columnar epithelium of the proximal canal meets the stratified squamous epithelium of the lower canal. The anal glands empty here.[163] Squamous cell tumors may develop in the anal canal or the anal margin. Cloacogenic carcinomas develop above the dentate line. Adnocarcinomas arise from the glands located at the dentate line. Anal margin tumors may consist of squamous cell, basal cell, Bowen or Paget's disease, verrucous carcinoma, or Kaposi's sarcoma. Melanomas tend to develop below the dentate line.[163]

The arteries supplying the distal rectum and anal canal are the superior, middle, and inferior hemorrhoidal arteries; venous drainage parallels the arteries. Sympathetic nerves innervate the internal rectal sphincter muscles, while parasympathetic fibers in sacrum sense distention of the rectum and anus. Lymphatic vessels drain the anal canal via the inguinal, pelvic visceral, and hypogastric nodes, which are interconnected, and ultimately empty into the para-aortic nodes.[163]

### CELLULAR CHARACTERISTICS

Most anal cancers are squamous cell (epidermoid) carcinomas. Less common cell types are cloacogenic, basaloid, transitional, and mucoepidermoid carcinomas.[2] Unusual tumors arising in the anal canal include small cell carcinomas, melanomas, and adenocarcinomas. Small cell carcinomas of the anal canal are aggressive and signal early distant metastases; adenocarcinomas carry a poor prognosis and should be managed aggressively with multimodality treatment.[163] Nononcogenic HPV types 6 and 11 are implicated in the formation of genital warts, in contrast to the oncogenic HPV-16, which is associated with both cervical and anal cancers. The malignant transformation may be related to the two viral proteins E7 and E6 which bind to the tumor suppressor gene products *Rb* and *p53* in the anal epithelial mucosal cells. The proteins E7 and E6 help the virus divide and infect the epithelial cell DNA. Likewise, *Rb* and *p53* protect against uncontrolled cell growth and the inclusion of mutated DNA into the cell's DNA. Once the viral genetic material is incorporated into the anal mucosal cells' DNA, cell division results in E6 and E7 proteins being transcribed, causing the cell to move from premalignant to malignant. HPV genetic material is commonly found in the DNA of anal cancer cells.[171] HIV apparently enhances the malignant transformation, a result that is believed to be due to the HIV tat protein, which helps to produce more E6 and E7.[171]

The first changes seen clinically are similar to those found in HPV-induced cervical cancer. HPV first causes dysplasia in the epithelial mucosal cells: low-grade squamous intraepithelial lesions are called LSIL while high-grade intraepithelial lesions are called HSIL (which includes moderate and severe dysplasia, as well as carcinoma in situ). HIV infection, history of receptive anal intercourse, and lower CD4 levels are associated with HSIL. There is hyperplasia, angiogenesis, and loss of apoptosis (programmed cell death).[163] As in cervical cancer, the Pap smear in the anal canal is performed at the transition zone.

The risk for developing anal cancer in HIV-positive men doubles from 15 to 30 times as the CD4 levels falls, and is increased even further if the patient is also infected with other oncogenic strains of HPV. It is unknown how rapidly the progression from HSIL occurs, if it occurs at all. Nevertheless, it appears that for HIV-infected patients, as their survival increases due to HAART therapy, patients with unknown HSIL will progress to invasive squamous cell cancer.[162] Use of the Pap test in screening may identify dysplastic changes in the anal epithelial cells.

### PROGRESSION OF DISEASE

The distribution of anal and perianal cancers can be predicted based on the anatomy because the tumor usually spreads by direct extension, through the lymphatic system, more commonly than via the bloodstream. The primary tumor grows along the length and circumference of the anal canal, and can invade the sphincter muscles and connective tissue early.[162] Proximal tumors may spread upward for 5 to 6 cm before ulcerating into the rectum; extension beyond the canal into the rectum or perianal skin occurs in up to half of patients.[162] Tumors extending locally rarely invade the bladder, sacrum, prostate, or vagina. While tumors in the anal margin are unlikely to metastasize, those in the anal canal may. Tumors developing on or above the dentate line tend to metastasize by the venous route into the portal system, with the ensuing development of liver, lung, or bone metastases in a small number of patients. Lymph node metastases are more common, with inguinal lymph node involvement in 15% to 63% of patients, with highest incidence in patients with distal anal cancers.[167] Lymphatic drainage for anal cancer above the dentate line goes into the perirectal and paravertebral nodes similar to rectal adenocarcinoma, while tumors below this line drain into the inguinal and femoral lymph nodes.[162] Proximal lesions above the dentate line are more likely to involve the mesenteric nodes than distal lesions.

## CLINICAL MANIFESTATIONS

Many of the signs and symptoms of anal cancer are attributed to benign conditions such as hemorrhoids, even by primary care physicians. Common signs and symptoms are change in bowel elimination patterns, bleeding, anal discharge or itching, anal mass, tenesmus, tenderness on palpation, pain on defecation, pruritus, and rarely inguinal lymph node swelling. Pain or the sensation of a rectal mass occurs in 30% of patients as a presenting symptom.[167]

## ASSESSMENT

### PATIENT AND FAMILY HISTORY

A systematic history is taken, beginning with patient factors including present and past medical history, social history including sexual practices, history of sexually transmitted diseases (STDs), benign anal diseases such as fissure, and perineal condylomata. A complete symptom analysis should be performed of the presenting symptoms, asking about anal pruritus, bleeding, tenesmus, changes in bowel habits, anal discharge, and pain. In women, signs and symptoms should be elicited that would suggest tumor infiltration of the vagina. A detailed review of systems should follow.

### PHYSICAL EXAMINATION

Physical examination includes a full examination, including digital rectal exam palpating for any lesions, and in women, a gynecological exam including cervical screening.[163] An intraluminal mass should be described in terms of location, size, extent, and relationship to dentate line. Most tumors are hard, indurated, and, as they enlarge, become fixed. Palpation for lymph nodes should be performed, especially the inguinal area. If lymph nodes are enlarged, a biopsy or fine needle aspiration should be done.[167]

### DIAGNOSTIC STUDIES

The NCCN recommends that anoscopy as well as abdominal/pelvic CT scan or MRI be performed as part of the workup for evaluation of anal canal cancers.[162] Pelvic CT or MRI may help determine whether pelvic or inguinal lymph nodes, as well as the liver, are involved with tumor. A PET scan should be considered as well, although not for anal margin cancers. Transrectal ultrasound may prove helpful in defining depth of invasion and involvement of adjacent organs.[162] Anal lesions often appear flat or slightly raised with indurated borders and should be biopsied.[167] HIV testing should be performed, and, if positive, CD4 should be assessed.

### PROGNOSTIC INDICATORS

The most important prognostic factors in anal canal cancer are the size of the primary tumor and the extent of lymph node involvement.[2] If the tumor is 2 cm or smaller, the patient has a 80% likelihood of cure; by comparison, a patient with a tumor larger than 5 cm has a 50% chance of cure. However, if metastasis is present, then these factors no longer are important. Patients with T3 and T4 tumors (larger than 5 cm) have a 50% likelihood of recurrence even after combined modality therapy.[162] Anal margin cancers behave much like skin cancers and rarely metastasize.

## CLASSIFICATION AND STAGING

Most anal cancers are squamous cell cancers and are treated with combined modality therapy, which is reflected in the staging. Table 51-14 depicts the AJCC staging for anal canal cancers.

## THERAPEUTIC APPROACHES AND NURSING CARE

The most common approaches to the management of anal cancer are reviewed in Table 51-15.[162,167,172–175] Early, in situ lesions may be curable by surgery alone, but most require multimodality therapy. Patients with stage IIIB anal canal cancer with positive inguinal nodes have a poor prognosis, although some may be cured. Available clinical trials should be discussed with these patients.

### SURGERY

Surgical resection alone is indicated only for small, in situ lesions that do not involve the anal sphincter and

**TABLE 51-14**

**Staging of Anal Canal Cancer**

| Stage | Tumor | Nodal Status | Metastases |
|---|---|---|---|
| 0 | Tis (carcinoma in situ) | N0 (no metastasis in the lymph nodes) | M0 (no distant metastasis) |
| I | T1 (tumor ≤2 cm in greatest dimension) | N0 | M0 |
| II | T2 (tumor >2 cm and <5 cm in greatest dimension) | N0 | M0 |
| | T3 (tumor >5 cm in greatest dimension) | N0 | M0 |
| IIIA | T1 | N1 (metastasis in perirectal lymph nodes) | M0 |
| | T2 | N1 (metastasis in perirectal lymph nodes) | M0 |
| | T3 | N1 (metastasis in perirectal lymph nodes) | |
| | T4 (tumor of any size invades adjacent organ(s), such as vagina, urethra, or bladder) | N0 | M0 |
| IIIB | T4 | N1 (metastasis in perirectal lymph nodes) | M0 |
| | Any T | N2 (metastasis in unilateral internal iliac and/or inguinal lymph nodes) | M0 |
| | Any T | N3 (metastasis in perirectal and inguinal lymph nodes and/or bilateral internal iliac and/or inguinal lymph nodes) | M0 |
| IV | Any T | Any N | M1 |

*Source*: Data from Greene et al.[86]

when it is expected that adequate surgical margins can be obtained. Unfortunately, most anal canal cancers are not detected at this early stage.[162] In the past, APR for anal canal tumors was considered the treatment of choice for stage I and II lesions, and resulted in a 5-year survival rate of approximately 70%. Currently survival is at least as likely using lower-dose radiation and chemotherapy with sphincter preservation.[162,163] Surgical resection is indicated for the treatment of residual or recurrent anal canal cancer following nonsurgical primary therapy.[163] Palliative surgery may be indicated for stage IV anal canal cancer.

**TABLE 51-15**

**Management of Anal Canal Cancer**

| Stage | Primary Treatment | Comments |
|---|---|---|
| Tis | Local excision | Re-excision if inadequate margins or local XRT ± 5-FU based chemotherapy |
| T1, N0 | Mitomycin/5-FU plus XRT | PE including DRE at 8–12 weeks post-therapy; biopsy if suspicious lesion or signs/symptoms of progress disease.<br>– If recurrence, APR ± preceded by 5-FU/cisplatin chemotherapy |
| T2–4, N0, or N+ | Mitomycin/5-FU plus XRT (45–59 Gy) | PE including DRE at 8–12 weeks post-therapy; biopsy if suspicious lesion or signs/symptoms of progress disease.<br>– If recurrence, APR ± preceded by 5-FU/cisplatin chemotherapy; if LN+ on groin dissection, XRT if not previously given<br>– If distant metastasis, platinum-containing chemotherapy regimen |

*Abbreviations*: 5-FU, 5-fluorourcil; APR, abdominoperineal resection; CI, continuous infusion; DRE, digital rectal exam; LN, lymph node; LV, leucovorin; LVI, lymphovascular invasion; NX, nodal status unknown; PE, physical exam; pTNM, pathological TNM staging; XRT, radiation therapy.

*Source*: Data from Allal et al[172]; Ellenhorn et al[173]; Flam et al[174]; Hung et al[175]; the National Comprehensive Cancer Network[163]; and Ryan et al.[167]

In the care of HIV-infected patients with HSIL, Chang and colleagues[176] reported their prospective study of surgical treatment (excision and cautery) using high-resolution anoscopy. The procedure was effective in eliminating HSIL in HIV-negative patients, but the HIV-positive group showed a high degree of HSIL persistence and recurrence.

### RADIATION THERAPY

Chemoradiation is the preferred treatment for anal cancers. Approximately 80% to 90% of patients will achieve a complete response with combination therapy. Stage I, II, and III anal canal cancers are treated with mitomycin-c/5-FU infusional therapy plus external beam radiotherapy as definitive therapy. A major clinical trial involving the Eastern Cooperative Oncology Group (ECOG) and the Radiation Therapy Oncology Group (RTOG) demonstrated that the addition of chemotherapy to radiation alone increased the disease-free survival rate from 51% to 73% ($P = 0.0003$) and resulted in a lower colostomy rate (9% compared to 22%, $P = 0.002$).[174] Patients with large squamous cell tumors (T3 and T4) and lymph node involvement (bulky N2 or N3) have a poor prognosis. Meropol, et al reported the findings of a large CALGB trial that established the safety and efficacy of induction chemotherapy with infusional 5-FU plus cisplatin followed by 5-FU plus mitomycin C with concurrent radiation.[177] At 4 years of follow-up, 68% of patients are alive, 61% disease free, and 50% colostomy free. Residual masses may take a few months to regress fully, and any suspicious residual areas should be biopsied.[163] Palliative radiotherapy may be indicated alone, or in combination with chemotherapy, for treatment of stage IV anal canal cancer.

### CHEMOTHERAPY

Flam and colleagues[174] demonstrated the efficacy of mitomycin-c together with 5-FU continuous infusion for anal canal cancer, in combination with external beam radiotherapy. However, mitomycin-c has potentially severe side effects. Its principal toxicities are delayed myelosuppression with cumulative neutropenia and thrombocytopenia, nausea and vomiting, anorexia, fatigue, and mucositis. The drug can also cause hemolytic-uremic syndrome that may be fatal as well as interstitial pneumonitis. Hung and colleagues demonstrated in a phase II study that cisplatin in combination with 5-FU produced equivalent results with less toxicity.[175] However, more recently, the question as to whether cisplatin-based therapy with radiation would improve survival compared to mitomycin-c/5-FU with radiation was tested in the RTOG 98–11 clinical trial and at a median follow-up of 2.51 years, showed no significant difference.[178] The results showed there was no difference in disease-free survival between the groups. However, patients in the mitomycin-c containing group had significantly more hematological toxicity while patients in the cisplatin containing group had significantly more colostomies. Chemotherapy regimens are described in Table 51-16.

### MOLECULAR TARGETED THERAPY

Biotherapeutic approaches are being investigated in the treatment of anal canal cancer. Studies are exploring the use of HPV vaccines for the treatment of anal canal cancer. With the success of HPV vaccine in the prevention of cervical cancer, investigators are exploring whether this vaccine can be effective in high risk individuals in preventing anal cancer. Joura, et al found that women in their study of the HPV vaccine had a significant reduction in premalignant lesions in the anus, as well as in the vulva and cervix.[179]

In a study by Sobhani and colleagues,[180] the authors found that HPV infection increased the number of dendritic cells in the anal mucosa of HIV-negative patients that was associated with anal condylomata. Human immunodeficiency virus-infected patients have significantly fewer dendritic cells, which may contribute to the development of invasive anal canal cancer. Dendritic cells are special, powerful immune cells that are antigen-presenting cells, responsible for activating T lymphocytes. Dendritic cell vaccines are being studied in melanoma and renal cell cancer and have a promising future in the treatment of cancers with identifiable, specific antigens. Unfortunately, there are no known specific antigens on anal cancer cells.

As molecular profiling is applied to anal canal cancer, the specific mutations and intracellular flaws may become the focus of molecularly targeted therapy. Squamous cell cancers often overexpress the epidermal growth factor (EGFR), and this appears true of anal canal cancer.[181] Often tumors that overexpress EGFR are resistant to radiotherapy.[182] The ECOG E3205 clinical trial is studying the value of the addition of cetuximab, an EGFR inhibitor, to cisplatin, 5-FU and radiation therapy in the treatment of immunocompetent patients with stage I-IIIB invasive anal carcinoma.[183]

## SYMPTOM MANAGEMENT AND SUPPORTIVE CARE

Nurses play an important role in the care of patients at risk for anal canal cancer. HIV-infected individuals, as well as other individuals who practice anal receptive intercourse; have a history of cervical, vaginal or vulvar cancer; or who are immunosuppressed, are at higher risk for this cancer. Nurses help teach patients and their partners about risk, protective precautions, and screening methods. Once HSIL

**TABLE 51-16**

**Chemotherapy Regimens Used in the Treatment of Anal Canal Cancer**

| Therapy | | Reference |
|---|---|---|
| *Wayne State 5FU/Mitomycin/Radiation* | | |
| 5-Fluorouracil | 1000 mg/m²/day IV CI, days 1–4, 29–32 | Nigro et al[184] |
| Mitomycin C | 15 mg/m² IV, day 1 | |
| Radiation therapy | 200 cGy/day, days 1–5, 8–12, and 5–19 | |
| *EORTC 5FU/Mitomycin/Radiation* | | |
| 5-Fluorouracil | 750 mg/m²/day IV CI, days 1–5, 29–33 | Bartelink et al[185] |
| Mitomycin C | 15 mg/m² IV, day 1 | |
| Radiation therapy | 180 cGy/day over 5 weeks<br>Total dose 4500 cGy | |
| *Chemotherapy Given Concurrently with Radiation Therapy* | | |
| Lf PR or CR, radiation boost | 1500–2000 cGy | |
| *M.D. Anderson 5FU/Cisplatin/Radiation* | | |
| 5-Fluorouracil | 250 mg/m²/day IV CI, days 1–5, each week of radiation | Hung et al[175] |
| Cisplatin | 4 mg/m²/day IV CI, days 1–5 each week of radiation | |
| Radiation therapy | 180 cGy/day over 6 weeks+<br>Total dose 5500 cGy | |
| Chemotherapy given concurrently with radiation therapy. | | |
| *Metastatic/Salvage 5FU and Cisplatin* | | |
| 5-Fluorouracil | 1000 mg/m²/day IV CI, days 1–5, repeat every 21–28 days | Flam et al[174] |
| Cisplatin | 100 mg/m² IV on day 2 | |

*Abbreviations*: 5-FU, 5-fluorouracil; CI, continuous infusion; EORTC, European Organization on Research and Treatment of Cancer; IcGy, 1/100 Gy, the international system unit of absorbed dose of radiation; IV, intravenous; 1 Gy, 100 rad.

is diagnosed, the patient requires definitive treatment and close follow-up.

Once a patient has developed anal canal cancer, symptoms relate to bowel elimination. The nurse provides support and teaching prior to definitive treatment. Ideally, symptoms will resolve with combined chemotherapy and radiotherapy. New approaches are reducing the number of patients requiring a colostomy for patients with residual or recurrent disease.

Symptoms of progressive disease relate to metastases in the liver, lung, and bone. Symptom management and care of patients with lung or liver metastases from anal cancer is the same as that for colon cancer metastases.

## LONG-TERM MONITORING AND FOLLOW-UP

For many patients, anal canal cancer is a curable cancer. Unfortunately, some patients—especially those with large, bulky tumors—may develop local recurrence, which can be effectively treated by resection and salvage therapy. Following definitive therapy, anal cancer will continue to regress for as long as 3 months or more. A biopsy should be done of the tumor site at least 3 months following completion of combined treatment, and repeated until either a complete response is achieved, or there is a persistent residual mass requiring further therapy. Recurrence usually occurs within the first 3 years.[163] According to the NCCN guidelines, follow-up and long-term monitoring should included examinations every 3 months for 2 years, with a digital rectal exam, anoscopy, and inguinal node palpation.[163] If post-definitive treatment biopsy shows persistent disease, or if the patient recurs, an APR is effective in providing long-term control and survival in 40% to 50% of patients.[162]

## CONCLUSION

Clinical trials are exploring advances in screening and early detection for anal cancer in HIV-infected patients and in immunologically suppressed patient populations. Given that the majority of anal canal cancers are virally induced, vaccines could potentially prevent malignant transformation. Research into the molecular flaws leading to malignant transformation is needed to help new therapies target anal canal malignancy and to improve treatment of large, bulky tumors. Improved therapeutic regimens with greater efficacy in achieving a complete response for patients with larger tumors as well as those with lymph node-positive disease are needed as well.[163]

In the past 30 years, there has been a downward trend in the incidence, morbidity, and mortality associated with colon and rectal cancers. Current screening mechanisms, diagnostic techniques, surgical interventions, and adjuvant therapy regimens have enabled individuals diagnosed with such malignancies to experience improved long-term survival and enhanced quality of life. However, despite the fact that colon and rectal cancers are preventable in most situations through removal of polyps, and otherwise highly curable if found early, colon and rectal cancers combined remain the third leading cause of incidence and mortality from cancer. Anal cancer, although uncommon, has shown an increase in incidence that appears to correlate with HPV infection and high-risk sexual behaviors. Although highly curable when found early, many patients delay seeking a diagnosis due to assumptions that symptoms relate to benign anal conditions such as hemorrhoids.

Factors that contribute to the pathogenesis of colon and rectal cancers are multifactorial. Age, diet, genetics, alcohol use, environment, inflammatory bowel conditions, and prior radiation therapy are all risk factors for the development of colorectal cancer. The understanding of gene mutational sequence for colon and rectal cancers is providing direction in the development of novel screening and early detection strategies.

Surgery continues to be the mainstay of therapy for adenocarcinoma of the colon and rectum. To accurately stage these malignancies, sufficient numbers of lymph nodes must be sampled, so that appropriate adjuvant therapy can be delivered. Chemotherapy, radiation therapy, and molecularly targeted therapy are utilized preoperatively, intraoperatively, postoperatively, and in patients with advanced disease to achieve better long-term survival. In instances when APR is indicated for optimal treatment, nurses contribute much to the patient preparation, supportive management, and prevention of complications for patients who require an ostomy.

Today's healthcare environment continues to change rapidly; more is accomplished on an outpatient basis and hospital lengths of stay continue to dwindle. A multitude of specialized nurses and physicians will care for the individual with colon, rectal, or anal carcinoma. The coordination and quality of care delivered is paramount as we move toward earlier diagnosis and better long-term survival for this disease.

## REFERENCES


1. Jemal A, Siegel R, Ward E, Hao Y, Xu J, Thun MJ. *CA: Cancer J Clin.* 2009;59:225–249.
2. Ellerhorn JDI, Cullinane CA, Coia LR, Alberts SR. Colon, rectal and anal cancers. In: Pazdur R, Coia LR, Hoskins WJ, Wagman LD, eds. *Cancer Management: A Multidisciplinary Approach.* 10th ed. San Francisco, CA: Oncology Publishing Group; 2006:350–375. http://www.cancernetwork.com/cancer-management/chapter16/article/10165/1171391. Accessed September 29, 2009.
3. Levin B, Smith RA, Feldman GE, et al. Promoting early detection tests for colorectal carcinoma and adenomatous polyps. *Cancer.* 2002; 95:1618–1628.
4. Fearon ER, Bommer GT. Molecular biology of colorectal cancer. In: DeVita VT, Lawrence TS, Rosenberg SA, eds. *Cancer: Principles and Practice on Oncology.* 8th ed. Philadelphia, PA: Lippincott, Williams & Wilkins; 2008:1219–1231.
5. Alberici P, Fodde R. The role of the APC tumor suppressor in chromosomal instability. *Genome Dis.* 2006;1:149–170.
6. Sjoblom T, Jones S, Wood LD, et al. The consensus coding sequences of human breast and colorectal cancers. *Science.* 2006;314:268–274.
7. Boardman LA, Morlan BW, Rabi KG, et al. Colorectal cancer risks in relatives of young-onset cases: is risk the same across all first-degree relatives? *Clin Gastroenterol Hepatol.* 2007;5:1195–1198.
8. American Cancer Society. *Colorectal Cancer Facts and Figures: Special Edition 2005.* Atlanta, GA: American Cancer Society; 2005.
9. American Cancer Society. *Cancer Facts and Figures, 2008.* Atlanta, GA: American Cancer Society; 2008.
10. McCollum AD, Catalano PJ, Haller DG, et al. Outcomes and toxicities in African-American and Caucasian patients in a randomized adjuvant chemotherapy trial for colon cancer. *J Natl Cancer Inst.* 2002;94:1160–1167.
11. Libutti SK, Saltz LB, Tepper JE. Cancer of the colon. In: DeVita VT, Lawrence TS, Rosenberg SA, eds. *Cancer: Principles and Practice of Oncology.* 8th ed. Philadelphia, PA: Lippincott, Williams & Wilkins; 2008;1232–1285.
12. Singh V, Das A. Racial variability in secular trends in the incidence of proximal colon cancer: results from a national cancer registry. [Abstract 100] *Gastrointest Endosc.* 2007;65.
13. Meyerhardt JA, Niedzwiecki D, Hollis D, et al. Association of dietary patterns with cancer recurrence and survival in patients with stage III colon cancer. *JAMA.* 2007;298:754–764.
14. Lieberman DA, Prindiville S, Weiss DG, et al. Risk factors for advanced neoplasia and hyperlastic polyps in asymptomatic individuals. *JAMA.* 2003;290:2959–2967.
15. Fuchs CS, Giavonnucci EL, Colditz GA, et al. Dietary fiber and decreased risk of colorectal cancer and adenoma in women. *N Engl J Med.* 1999;340:169–176.
16. Giavonnucci E, Stampfer MJ, Colditz GA, et al. Relationship of diet to risk of colorectal adenoma in men. *J Natl Cancer Inst.* 1992;84:91–98.
17. Peters U, Sinha R, Chatterjee N, et al. Dietary fibre and colorectal adenoma in a colorectal cancer early detection programme. *Lancet.* 2003;361:1491–1495.
18. Bingham SA, Day NE, Luben R, et al. Dietary fibre in food and protection against colorectal cancer in the European Prospective Investigation into Cancer and Nutrition (EPIC): an observational study [erratum in *Lancet.* 2003;362:1000]. *Lancet.* 2003;361:1496–1501.
19. Terry P, Giovannucci E, Michels KB, et al. Fruit, vegetables, dietary fiber, and risk of colorectal cancer. *J Natl Cancer Inst.* 2001;93:525–533.
20. Willett WC, Stampfer MJ, Colditz GA, et al. Relation of meat, fat, and fiber intake to the risk of colon cancer in a prospective study among women. *N Engl J Med.* 1990;323:1664–1672.
21. Norat T, Lukanova A, Ferrari P, et al. Meat consumption and colorectal cancer risk: dose-response meta-analysis of epidemiological studies. *Int J Cancer.* 2002;98:241–256.
22. Giovannucci E, Stampfer MJ, Colditz GA, et al. Multivitamin use, folate, and colon cancer in women in the Nurses' Health Study. *Ann Intern Med.* 1998;129:517–524.
23. Pufulete M, Alghnaniem R, Leather AJ, et al. Folate status, genomic DNA hypomethylation, and risk of colorectal adenoma and cancer: a case control study. *Gastroenterology.* 2003;124:1240–1248.
24. Wu K, Willett WC, Fuchs CS, et al. Calcium intake and risk of colon cancer in women and men. *J Natl Cancer Inst.* 2002;94:437–446.
25. Grau MV, Baron JA, Sandler RS, et al. Prolonged effect of calcium supplementation on risk of colorectal adenomas in a randomized trial. *J Natl Cancer Inst.* 2007;99:129–136.

26. Lee IM, Paffenbarger RS Jr, Hsieh C. Physical activity and the risk of developing colorectal cancer among college alumni. *J Natl Cancer Inst.* 1991;83:1324–1329.
27. Giovannucci E, Ascherio A, Rimm EB, et al. Physical activity, obesity, and risk for colon cancer and adenoma in men. *Ann Intern Med.* 1995;122:227–263.
28. Colditz GA, Cannuscio CC, Frazier AL. Physical activity and reduced risk of colon cancer: implications for prevention. *Cancer Causes Control.* 1997;8:649–667.
29. Meyerhardt JA, Giovannucci EL, Holmes MD, et al. Physical activity and survival after colorectal cancer diagnosis. *J Clin Oncol.* 2006;24:3527–3534.
30. Muscat JE, Stellman SD, Wynder EL. Nonsteroidal anti-inflammatory drugs and colorectal cancer. *Cancer.* 1994;74:1847–1854.
31. Gwyn K, Sinicrope FA. Chemoprevention of colorectal cancer. *Am J Gastroenterol.* 2002;97:13–21.
32. Sandler RS, Halabi S, Baron JA, et al. A randomized trial of aspirin to prevent colorectal adenomas in patients with previous colorectal cancer. *N Engl J Med.* 2003;348:883–890.
33. Baron JA, Cole BF, Sandler RS, et al. A randomized trial of aspirin to prevent colorectal adenomas. *N Engl J Med.* 2003;348:891–899.
34. Blanke CD, Benson AB, Dragovich T, et al. A phase II trial of celecoxib (CX), irinotecan (I), 5-fluorouracil (5FU), and leucovorin (LCV) in patients with unresectable or metastatic colorectal cancer (CRC). [Abstract 505] *Proc Am Soc Clin Oncol.* 2002;38.
35. Celebrex package insert. New York, NY: Pfizer; Jan 2008.
36. Su LJ, Arab L. Alcohol consumption and risk of colon cancer: evidence from the national health and nutrition examination survey I epidemiologic follow-up study. *Nutr Cancer.* 2004;50:111–119.
37. Larsson SC, Giovannucci E, Wolk A. Vitamin B intake, alcohol consumption, and colorectal cancer: a longitudinal population-based cohort of women. *Gastoenterology.* 2005;128:1830–1837.
38. National Cancer Institute. Colorectal cancer mortality projections. http://cisnet.cancer.gov/projections/colorectal/risk.php. Accessed September 28, 2009.
39. Jess T, Loftus EV, Velayos FS, et al. Risk factors for colorectal neoplasia in inflammatory bowel disease: a nested, case-controlled study from Copenhagen County, Denmark and Olmsted County, Minnesota. *Am J Gastroenterol.* 2007;102:829–836.
40. Schoen RE, Weissfeld JL, Kuller LH, et al. Insulin-like growth factor-1 and insulin are associated with the presence and advancement of adenomatous polyps. *Gastroenterology.* 2005;129:464–475.
41. Kaaks R, Lukanova A. Energy balance and cancer: the role of insulin and insulin-like growth factor. *Proc Nutr Soc.* 2001;60:91–98.
42. Smith RA, Cokkinides V, Brawley OW. Cancer screening in the United States, 2008: a review of current American Cancer Society guidelines and cancer screening issues. *CA: Cancer J Clin.* 2008;58:161–179.
43. Levin B, Lieberman DA, McFarland B, et al. Screening and surveillance for the early detection of colorectal cancer and adenomatous polyps, 2008: a joint guideline from the American Cancer Society, the US Multi-Society Task Force on Colorectal Cancer, and the American College of Radiology. *CA: Cancer J Clin.* 2008;58:130–160.
44. American Gastroenterology Nurses and Associates. *Standards and Guidelines for the Performance of Flexible Sigmoidoscopy by Registered Nurses for the Purpose of Colorectal Cancer Screening.* Chicago, IL: Society of Gastroenterology Nurses and Associates; 2003.
45. Allison JE, Sakoda LC, Levin TR, et al. Screening for colorectal neoplasms with new fecal occult blood tests: update on performance characteristics. *J Natl Cancer Inst.* 2007;99:1462–1470.
46. Mandel JS, Church TR, Bond JH, et al. The effect of fecal occult-blood screening on the incidence of colorectal cancer. *N Engl J Med.* 2000;343:1603–1607.
47. Whitlock EP, Lin JS, Liles E, Beil TL, Fu R. Screening for colorectal cancer: a targeted, updated systematic review for the US Preventive Services Task Force. *Ann Intern Med.* 2008;149:638–658.
48. Ahlquist DA, Sargent DJ, Loprinzi CL, et al. Stool DNA and occult blood testing for screen detection of colorectal neoplasia. *Ann Intern Med.* 2008;149:441–450.
49. Schoen RE, Pinsky PF, Weissfeld JL, et al. Results of repeat sigmoidoscopy 3 years after a negative examination. *JAMA.* 2003;290:41–50.
50. Gatto NM, Frucht H, Sundararajan V, et al. Risk of perforation after colonoscopy and sigmoidoscopy: a population-based study. *J Natl Cancer Inst.* 2003;95:230–236.
51. Maule WF. Screening for colorectal cancer by nurse endoscopists. *N Engl J Med.* 1994;330:183–187.
52. Kelly SB, Murphy J, Smith A, et al. Nurse specialist led flexible sigmoidoscopy in an outpatient setting. *Colorectal Dis.* 2007;10:390–393.
53. Ball M, Bohlander SL, Huber D, et al. Standards and guidelines: performance of flexible sigmoidoscopy by registered nurses for the purpose of colorectal cancer screening. Chicago, IL: Society of Gastroenterology Nurses and Associates; 2003.
54. Lieberman DA, Weiss DG. Veterans Affairs Cooperative Study Group 380: one time screening for colorectal cancer with combined fecal occult-blood testing and examination of the distal colon. *N Engl J Med.* 2001;345:550–560.
55. Gondal G, Grotmol T, Hofstad B, et al. The Norwegian Colorectal Cancer Prevention (NORCAPP) screening study: baseline findings and implementations for clinical work-up in age groups 50–64 years. *Scand J Gastroenterol.* 2003;38:635–644.
56. Winawer SJ, Stewart ET, Zauber AG, et al. A comparison of colonoscopy and double-contrast barium enema for surveillance after polypectomy. National Polyp Study Work Group. *N Engl J Med.* 2000;342: 1766–1772.
57. Pickhardt PJ, Nugent PA, Mysliwiec PA, et al. Location of adenomas missed by optical colonoscopy. *Ann Intern Med.* 2004;141:352–359.
58. Lieberman DA, Weiss DG, Bond JH, et al. Use of colonoscopy to screen asymptomatic adults for colorectal cancer. Veterans Affairs Cooperative Study Group 380. *N Engl J Med.* 2000;343:162–168.
59. Imperiale TF, Wagner DR, Lin CY, et al. Using risk for advanced proximal colonic neoplasia to tailor endoscopic screening for colorectal cancer. *Ann Intern Med.* 2003;139:959–965.
60. Summers RM, Yao J, Pickhardt PJ, et al. Computed tomographic virtual colonoscopy computer-aided polyp detection in a screening population. *Gastroenterology.* 2005;129:1832–1844.
61. National Human Genome Research Institute. Genetic Information Nondiscrimination Act: 2007–2008. http://www.genome.gov/24519851. Accessed September 28, 2009.
62. Kinzler K, Vogelstein B. Lessons from hereditary colorectal cancer. *Cell.* 1996;87:159–170.
63. Niv Y. Microsatellite instability and MLH1 promoter hypermethylation in colorectal cancer. *World J Gastroenterol.* 2007;13:1767–1769.
64. Bertagnolli MM, Eagle CJ, Zauber AG, et al. Celecoxib for the prevention of sporadic colorectal adenomas. *N Engl J Med.* 2006;355:873–884.
65. Lynch HT, Coronel SM, Okimoto R, et al. A founder mutation of the *MSH2* gene and hereditary nonpolyposis colorectal cancer in the United States. *JAMA.* 2004;291:718–724.
66. Umar A, Boland CR, Terdiman JP, et al. Revised Bethesda Guidelines for hereditary nonpolyposis colorectal cancer (Lynch syndrome) and microsatellite instability. *J Natl Cancer Inst.* 2004;96:261–268.
67. Cortellino S, Turner D, Masciullo V, et al. The base excision repair enzyme MED1 mediates DNA damage response to antitumor drugs and is associated with mismatch repair system integrity. *Proc Natl Acad Sci USA.* 2003;100:15071–15076.
68. National Institute of Diabetes and Digestive and Kidney Diseases. Anatomic problems of the colon. Bethesda, MD: National Digestive Diseases Clearinghouse; 2005. Accessed September 28, 2009. http://digestive.niddk.nih.gov/ddiseases/pubs/anatomiccolon.
69. Compton CC, Fielding LP, Burgart LJ. Prognostic factors in colorectal cancer. College of American Pathologists consensus statement 1999. *Arch Pathol Lab Med.* 2000;124:979–994.

70. Frizelle FA, Hobday KS, Batts KP, et al. Adenosquamous and squamous carcinoma of the colon and upper rectum: a clinical and histopathologic study. *Dis Colon Rectum*. 2001;44:341–346.
71. Chu P, Wu E, Weiss LM. Cytokeratin 7 and cytokeratin 20 expression in epithelial neoplasms: a survey of 435 cases. *Mod Pathol*. 2000; 13:962–972.
72. Birkenkamp-Demtroder K, Olesen SH, Sorensen FB, et al. Differential gene expression in colon cancer of the caecum, sigmoid and rectosigmoid. *Gut*. 2005;54:374–384.
73. Olesen SH, Frederiksen CM, Sorensen FB, et al. Differential Gene Expression in Right and Left Sided Colon Cancers Identified by Microarray Analysis. In: 94th Annual Meeting, July 11–14, 2003. [Abstract 1481] Washington, DC: American Association for Cancer Research.
74. Winawer S, Fletcher R, Rex D, et al. Colorectal cancer screening. *Gastroenterology*. 2003;124:544–548.
75. National Cancer Institute. Colon cancer: treatment—patient information [NCI PDQ]. http://www.peacehealth.org/kbase/nci/ncicdr0000062954.htm. Accessed September 28, 2009.
76. National Comprehensive Cancer Network. *Practice Guidelines in Oncology: Colon Cancer, v.4.2009*. Jenkintown, PA: National Compre-hensive Cancer Network. http://www.nccn.org/professionals/physician_gls/f_guidelines.asp. Accessed September 28, 2009.
77. Minter A, Malik R, Ledbetter L, et al. Colon cancer in pregnancy. *Cancer Control*. 2005;12:196–202.
78. Wolmark N, Wieand HS, Rockette HE, Fisher B. The prognostic significance of tumor location and bowel obstruction in Dukes B and C colorectal cancer. Findings from the NSABP clinical trials. *Ann Surg*. 1983;198:743–748.
79. Steinberg SM, Barkin JS, Kaplan RS, et al. Prognostic indicators of colon tumors. The Gastrointestinal Tumor Study Group experience. *Cancer*. 1986;57:1866–1870.
80. Halvorsen TB, Johannesen E. DNA ploidy, tumor site, and prognosis in colorectal cancer. *Scand J Gastroenterol*. 1990;25:141–146.
81. Locker GY, Hamilton S, Harris J, et al. ASCO 2006 update of recommendations for the use of tumor markers in gastrointestinal cancer. *J Clin Oncol*. 2006;24:5313–5327.
82. Zlobec I, Baker K, Terracciano LM, Lugli A. RHAMM p21 combined phenotype identifies microsatellite instability-high colorectal cancers with a highly adverse prognosis. *Clin Cancer Res*. 2008;14:3798–3806.
83. Kim GP, Colangelo LH, Paik S, et al. Predictive value of microsatellite instability high remains controversial. *J Clin Oncol*. 2008;25: 4857–4867.
84. Schepeler T, Reinert JT, Ostenfeld MS, et al. Diagnostic and prognostic microRNAs in stage II colon cancer. *Cancer Res*. 2008;68:6416–6424.
85. Ogino S, Goel A. Molecular classification and correlates in colorectal cancer. *J Mol Diagnostics*. 2008;10:13–27.
86. Greene FL, Page DS, Fleming ID, et al. *American Joint Committee on Cancer. AJCC Cancer Staging Manual*. 6th ed. New York, NY: Springer-Verlag; 2002.
87. Esser S, Reilly WT, Riley LB, et al. The role of sentinel lymph node mapping in staging of colon and rectal cancer. *Dis Colon Rectum*. 2001; 44:850–854.
88. Le Voyer TE, Sigurdson ER, Hanlon AL, et al. Colon cancer survival is associated with increasing number of lymph nodes analyzed: a secondary survey of intergroup trial INT-0089. *J Clin Oncol*. 2003;21:2912–2919.
89. Lennon AM, Mulcahy HE, Hyland JMP. Peritoneal involvement in stage II colon cancer. *Am J Clin Pathol*. 2003;119:108–113.
90. Compton C, Fenoglio-Preiser CM, Pettigrew N, et al. American joint committee on cancer prognostic factors consensus conference: colorectal working group. *Cancer*. 2000;88:1739–1757.
91. Lacy AM, Garcia-Valdecasa JC, Delgado S, et al. Laparoscopy assisted colectomy versus open colectomy for treatment of non-metastatic colon cancer: a randomized trial. *Lancet*. 2002;359:2224–2229.
92. Jayne DG, Guillou PJ, Thorpe H, et al. Randomized trial of laparoscopic-assisted resection of colorectal carcinoma: 3-year results of the UK MRC CLASICC trial Group. *J Clin Oncol*. 2007;25:3061–3068.
93. The Clinical Outcomes of Surgical Therapy Study Group. A comparison of laparoscopically assisted and open colectomy for colon cancer. *N Engl J Med*. 2004;350:2050–2059.
94. Bonjer HJ, Hop WC, Nelson H, et al. Laparoscopically assisted vs open colectomy for colon cancer: a meta-analysis. *Arch Surg*. 2007; 142:298–303.
95. Jackson TD, Kaplan GG, Arena G, et al. Laparoscopic versus open resection for colorectal cancer: a meta-analysis of oncologic outcomes. *J Am Coll Surg*. 2007;204:439–446.
96. Schwartzentruber DJ, Lublin M, Hostletter RB. Bowel obstruction. In: Berger AM, Shuster JL, Von Roenn JH, eds. *Principles and Practice of Palliative Care and Supportive Oncology*. 3rd ed. Philadelphia, PA: Lippincott, Williams & Wilkins; 2006:181.
97. Saha S, Bilchik A, Wiese D, et al. Ultrastaging of colorectal cancer by sentinel lymph node mapping technique—a multicenter trial. *Ann Surg Oncol*. 2001;8(suppl):94S–98S.
98. Redston M, Compton CC, Miedema BW, et al. Analysis of micrometastatic disease in sentinel lymph nodes from respectable colon cancer: results of Cancer and Leukemia Group B trial 80001. *J Clin Oncol*. 2006;24:878–883.
99. Bilchik AJ, Nora DT, Saha S, et al. The use of molecular profiling of early colorectal cancer to predict micrometastases. *Arch Surg*. 2002;137:1377–1383.
100. Feig BW, Curley S, Lucci A, et al. A caution regarding lymphatic mapping in patients with colon cancer. *Am J Surg*. 2001;182:707–712.
101. Haas R, Wicherts D, Hobbelink M, et al. Sentinel lymph node mapping in colon cancer: current status. *Ann Surg Oncol*. 2006;14:1070–1080.
102. Figueras J, Valls C, Rafecas A, et al. Resection rate and effect of postoperative chemotherapy on survival after surgery for colorectal liver metastases. *Br J Surg*. 2001;88:980–985.
103. Choti MA, Sitzmann JV, Tiburi MF, et al. Trends in long-term survival following liver resection for hepatic colorectal metastases. *Ann Surg*. 2002;235;759–766.
104. Abdalla EK, Vauthey JN, Ellis LM, et al. Recurrence and outcomes following hepatic resection, radiofrequency ablation, and combined resection/ablation for colorectal liver metastases. *Ann Surg*. 2004;239: 815–825.
105. Fong Y, Fortner J, Sun RL, et al. Clinical score for predicting recurrence after hepatic resection for metastatic colorectal cancer: analysis of 1001 consecutive cases. *Ann Surg*. 1999;230:309–318; discussion 318–321.
106. Pawlik TM, Scoggins CR, Zorzi D, et al. Effect of surgical margin status on survival and site of recurrence after hepatic resection for colorectal metastases. *Ann Surg*. 2005;241:715–722.
107. Kemeny NE, Niedzwiecki D, Hollis DR, et al. Hepatic arterial infusion (HAI) vs systemic therapy for hepatic metastases from colorectal cancer: a CALGB randomized trial of efficacy, quality of life (QOL), cost effectiveness, and molecular markers [abstr 1010]. *Proc Am Soc Clin Oncol*. 2003;22:252.
108. Sugarbaker PH. Managing the peritoneal surface component of gastrointestinal cancer. Part I. Patterns of dissemination and treatment options. *Oncology*. 2004;18:51–59.
109. Glehen O, Kwiatkowski F, Sugarbaker PH, et al. Cytoreductive surgery combines with perioperative intraperitoneal chemotherapy for the management of peritoneal carcinomatosis from colorectal cancer: a multi-institutional study. *J Clin Oncol*. 2004;22:3284–3292.
110. Verwaal VJ, van Ruth S, de Bree E, et al. Randomized trial of cytoreduction and hyperthermic intraperitoneal chemotherapy vs systemic chemotherapy and palliative surgery in patients with peritoneal carcinomatosis of colorectal cancer. *J Clin Oncol*. 2003;21: 3737–3743.

111. da Silva RG, Sugarbaker PH. Analysis of prognostic factors in seventy patients having a complete cytoreduction plus perioperative intraperitoneal chemotherapy for carcinomatosis from colorectal cancer. *J Am Coll Surg.* 2006;203:878–886.
112. Ike H, Shimada H, Ohki S, et al. Results of aggressive resection of lung metastases from colorectal carcinoma detected by intensive follow-up. *Dis Colon Rectum.* 2002;45:468–473.
113. Willett CG, Goldberg S, Shellito PC, et al. Does postoperative irradiation play a role in the adjuvant therapy of stage T4 colon cancer? *Cancer J Sci Am.* 1999;5:242–247.
114. de Gramont A, Boni C, Navarro M, et al. Oxaliplatin/5FU/LV in adjuvant colon cancer: updated efficacy results of the MOSAIC trial, including survival, with a median follow-up of six years. *J Clin Oncol.* 2007;25:4007.
115. Wolmark N, Wieand HS, Kuebler JP, et al. A phase III trial comparing FULV to FULV + oxaliplatin in stage II or III carcinoma of the colon: results of NSABP Protocol C-07. ASCO Annual Meeting Proceedings. *J Clin Oncol.* 2005;23:3500.
116. Twelves C, Scheithauer W, McKendrick J, et al. Capecitabine vs 5-FU/LV in stage III colon cancer: updated 5-year efficacy data from X-ACT trial and preliminary analysis of relationship between hand-foot syndrome (HFS) and efficacy. In: *2008 Gastrointestinal Cancers Symposium.* Orlando, FL: American Society of Clinical Oncology; [Abstract 274].
117. Johnston G, Mulligan K, Kay E, et al. A genetic signature of relapse in stage II colorectal cancer derived from formalin fixed paraffin embedded tissue (FFPE) tissue using a unique disease specific colorectal array [abstr 3519]. *J Clin Oncol.* 2006;24(suppl):150s.
118. Kopetz S, Freitas D, Calabrich AFC, Hoff PM. Adjuvant chemotherapy for stage II colon cancer. *Oncology.* 2008;22:260–270.
119. Wolmark N, Rockette H, Fisher B, et al. The benefit of leucovorin-modulated fluorouracil as postoperative adjuvant therapy for primary colon cancer: results from National Surgical Adjuvant Breast and Bowel Project Protocol C-03. *J Clin Oncol.* 1993;11:1879–1887.
120. Cassidy J, Scheithauer J, McKendrick H, et al. Capecitabine (X) vs. bolus 5-FU/leucovorin (LV) as adjuvant therapy for colon cancer (the X-ACT study): efficacy results of a phase III trial. *J Clin Oncol.* 2004;22:3509.
121. Hochster HS, Hart LL, Ramanathan RK, et al. Regimens with or without bevacizumab as first-line treatment of metastatic colorectal cancer: results of the TREE study. *J Clin Oncol.* 2008;21: 3523–3529.
122. Hurwitz H, Fehrenbacher L, Novotny W, et al. Bevacizumab plus irinotecan, fluorouracil, and leucovorin for metastatic colorectal cancer. *N Engl J Med.* 2004;350:2335–2342.
123. Hoff PM, Ansari R, Batist G, et al. Comparison of oral capecitabine vs intravenous fluorouracil plus leucovorin as firstline treatment in 605 patients with metastatic colorectal cancer: results of a randomized phase III study. *J Clin Oncol.* 2001;19:2282–2292.
124. Cunningham D, Humblet Y, Siena S, et al. Cetuximab monotherapy and cetuximab plus irinotecan in irinotecan-refractory metastatic colorectal cancer *N Engl J Med.* 2004;351:337–345.
125. Jonker DJ, O'Callaghan CJ, Karapetis CS, et al. Cetuximab for the treatment of colorectal cancer. *N Engl J Med.* 2007;357:2040–2048.
126. Douillard JY, Cunningham D, Roth AD, et al. Irinotecan combined with fluorouracil compared with fluorouracil alone as first-line treatment for metastatic colorectal cancer: a multicentre randomized trial. *Lancet.* 2000;355:1041–1047.
127. Tournigand C, Andre T, Achilee E, et al. FOLFIRI followed by FOLFOX6 or the reverse sequence in advanced colorectal cancer: a randomized GERCOR study. *J Clin Oncol.* 2004;22:229–237.
128. Giantonio BJ, Catalano PJ, Meropol NJ, et al. Eastern Cooperative Oncology Group Study E3200. Bevacizumab in combination with oxaliplatin, fluorouracil, and leucovorin (FOLFOX4) for previously treated metastatic colorectal cancer: results from the Eastern Cooperative Oncology Group Study E3200. *J Clin Oncol.* 2007;25:1539–1544.
129. Tournigand C, Cervantes A, Figer A, et al. Optimox 1: a randomized study of FOLFOX4 or FOLFOX7 with oxaliplatin in a stop-and-go fashion in advanced colorectal cancer-A GERCOR study. *J Clin Oncol.* 2006;24:394–400.
130. Van Cutsem E, Peeters M, Siena S, et al. Open-label phase III trial of panitumumab plus best supportive care compared with best supportive care aolone in patients with chemotherapy-refractory metastatic colorectal cancer. *J Clin Oncol.* 2007;25:1658–1664.
131. Cassidy J, Clarke S, Díaz-Rubio E, et al. Randomized phase III study of capecitabine plus oxaliplatin compared with fluorouracil/folinic acid plus oxaliplatin as first-line therapy for metastatic colorectal cancer. *J Clin Oncol.* 2008;26:2006–2012.
132. Saltz LB, Clarke S, Díaz-Rubio E, et al. Bevacizumab in combination with oxaliplatin-based chemotherapy as first-line therapy in metastatic colorectal cancer: a randomized phase III study. *J Clin Oncol.* 2008; 26:2013–2019.
133. de Gramont A, Bossett JF, Milan C, et al. Randomized trial comparing monthly low-dose leucovorin and fluorouracil bolus with bimonthly high-dose leucovorin and fluorouracil bolus plus continuous infusion for advanced colorectal cancer: a French intergroup study. *J Clin Oncol.* 1997;15:808–815.
134. Sargent DJ, Niedzwiecki D, O'Connell MJ, et al. Recommendation for caution with irinotecan, fluorouracil and leucovorin for colorectal cancer. *N Engl J Med.* 2001;345:144–146.
135. Goldberg RM, Sargent DJ, Morton RF, et al. A randomized controlled trial of fluorouracil plus leucovorin, irinotecan, and oxaliplatin combinations in patients with previously untreated metastatic colorectal cancer. *J Clin Oncol.* 2004;22:23–30.
136. Grothey A, Sugrue MM, Purdie DM, et al. Bevacizumab beyond first progression is associated with prolonged overall survival in metastatic colorectal cancer: results from a large observational cohort study (BRiTE). *J Clin Oncol.* 2008;26:5326–5334.
137. de Gramont A, Figer A, Seymour M, et al. Leucovorin and fluorouracil with and without oxaliplatin as first-line treatment in advanced colorectal cancer. *J Clin Oncol.* 2000;18:2938–2947.
138. Maindrault-Goebel F, Lledo G, Chibaudel B, et al. Final results of OPTIMOX2, a large randomized phase II study of maintenance therapy or chemotherapy-free intervals (CFI) after FOLFOX in patients with metastatic colorectal cancer (MCRC): a GERCOR study. ASCO Annual Meeting Proceedings Part I, 2007. *J Clin Oncol.* 2007;25:4013.
139. Khambata-Ford S, Garrett CR, Meropol NJ, et al. Expression of epiregulin and amphiregulin and K-ras mutation status predict disease control in metastatic colorectal cancer patients treated with cetuximab. *J Clin Oncol.* 2007;25:3230–3237.
140. Hecht JR, Mitchell E, Chidiac T, et al. Interim results from PACCE: irinotecan (Iri)/bevacizumab (bev) +/− panitumumab (pmab) as first-line treatment (tx) for metastatic colorectal cancer (mCRC). In: *Gastro-intestinal Cancers Symposium.* American Society of Clinical Oncology; Presented January 25–27, 2008; Orlando, FL. [Abstract 273, 279].
141. Amado RG, Wolf M, Peeters M, et al. Wild-type K-RAS is required for panitumumab efficacy in patients with metastatic colorectal cancer: results from a phase IIII trial of panitumumab compared to best supportive care. *J Clin Oncol.* 2008;26:1626–1634.
142. Rothenberg ML, Meropol NJ, Poplin EA, et al. Mortality associated with irinotecan plus bolus fluorouracil/leucovorin: summary findings of an independent panel. *J Clin Oncol.* 2001;19:3801–3807.
143. Schmelser L. Nursing management of lower intestinal problems. In: Lewis SM, Heitkemper MM, Dirkson SR, O'Brien P, Bucher L, eds. 7th ed. *Medical Surgical Nursing: Assessment and Management of Clinical Problems.* St. Louis, MO: Mosby-Elsevier; 2007:200–275.
144. National Comprehensive Cancer Network. *Practice Guidelines in Oncology: Palliative Care, v.1.2009.* Jenkintown, PA: National Comprehensive Cancer Network. http://www.nccn.org/professionals/physician_gls/f_guidelines.asp. Accessed September 28, 2009.

145. Pontieri-Lewis V. Management of gastrointestinal fistulas. *Med Surg Nurs*. 2005;14:68–72.
146. National Comprehensive Cancer Network. *Practice Guidelines in Oncology: Rectal Cancer, v.4.2008*. Jenkintown, PA: National Comprehensive Cancer Network. http://www.nccn.org/professionals/physician_gls/f_guidelines.asp. Accessed September 28, 2009.
147. Tsong WH, Koh W-P, Yuan J-M, et al. Cigarettes and alcohol in relation to colorectal cancer: the Singapore Chinese health study. *Br J Cancer*. 2007;96:821–827.
148. Herrinton LJ, Selby JV, Friedman GD, et al. Case-control study of digital-rectal screening in relation to mortality from cancer of the rectum. *Am J Epidemiol*. 1995;142:961–964.
149. National Institute of Diabetes and Digestive and Kidney Diseases. Fecal incontinence. Bethesda, MD: National Digestive Diseases Information Clearinghouse; 2007. http://digestive.niddk.nih.gov/ddiseases/pubs/fecalincontinence. Accessed September 28, 2009.
150. Libutti SK, Tepper JE, Saltz LB. Rectal cancer. In: DeVita VT, Lawrence TS, Rosenberg SA, eds. *Cancer: Principles and Practice in Oncology*, 8th ed. Philadelphia PA: Lippincott, Williams & Wilkins; 2008:1285–1301.
151. Ono A, Fujii T, Saito Y, et al. Endoscopic submucosal resection of rectal carcinoid tumors with a ligation device. *Gastrointest Endosco*. 2003; 57:583–587.
152. Compton CC, Greene FL. The staging of colorectal cancer: 2004 and beyond. *CA: Cancer J Clin*. 2004;54:295–308.
153. Compton CC. Colorectal carcinoma: diagnostic, prognostic and molecular features. *Mod Pathol*. 2003;16:376–388.
154. Bipat S, Glas AS, Slors FJ, et al. Rectal cancer: local staging and assessment of lymph node involvement with endoluminal US, CT, and MR imaging—a meta-analysis. *Radiology*. 2004;232:773–783.
155. Anal sphincter prosthesis in treating patients who are undergoing surgery for anal or rectal cancer. http://clinicaltrials.gov/ct2/show/NCT00059891. Accessed September 28, 2009.
156. Meyerhardt JA, Tepper JE, Niedzwiecki D, et al. Impact of hospital procedure volume on surgical operation and long-term outcomes in high-risk curatively resected rectal cancer: findings from the Intergroup 0114 study. *J Clin Oncol*. 2003;22:166–174.
157. Koukouras D, Spiliotis J, Scopa C, et al. Radical consequences in the sexuality of male patients operated for colorectal carcinoma. *Eur J Surg Oncol*. 1991;17:285–288.
158. Hendren SK, O'Connor BI, Liu M, et al. Prevalence of male and female sexual dysfunction is high following surgery for rectal cancer. *Ann Surg*. 2005;242:212–223.
159. Hassan I, Cima RR. Quality of life after rectal resection and multimodality therapy. *J Surg Oncol*. 2007;96:684–692.
160. Barton-Burke M, Gustason CJ. Sexuality in women with cancer. *Nurs Clin North Am*. 2007;42:531–554.
160. Manderson L. Boundary breaches: the body, sex and sexuality after stoma surgery. *Soc Sci Med*. 2005;61:405–415.
162. Cummings BJ, Swallow CJ, Ajani JA. Cancer of the anal region. In: DeVita VT, Lawrence TS, Rosenberg SA, eds. *Cancer: Principles and Practice in Oncology*. 8th ed. Philadelphia, PA: Lippincott, Williams & Wilkins; 2008:1301–1313.
163. National Comprehensive Cancer Network. *Practice Guidelines in Oncology: Anal Canal Cancer, v.2.2008*. Jenkintown, PA: National Comprehensive Cancer Network; 2008.
164. Johnson LG, Madeleine MM, Newcomer LM, et al. Anal cancer incidence and survival: the surveillance, epidemiology, and end results experience, 1973–2000. *Cancer*. 2004;101:281–288.
165. Pfister H, Fuchs PG. Relation of papillomaviruses to anogenital cancer. *Dermatol Clin*. 1991;9:267–270.
166. Friis S, Kjaer SK, Frisch M, et al. Cervical intraepithelial neoplasia, anogenital cancer, and other cancer types in women after hospitalization for condyloma acuminata. *J Infect Dis*. 1997;175:743–748.
167. Ryan DP, Compton CC, Mayer RJ. Carcinoma of the anal canal. *N Engl J Med*. 2000;342:792–800.
168. Salit IE, Tinmouth J, Lytwyn A, et al. Screening for anal cancer. In: Community Alliance for Health Research; 2004; Ottawa, Ontario: Canadian Institutes of Health Research. Abstract 158.
169. Fox P. Anal cancer screening in men who have sex with men. *Curr Opin HIV AIDS*. 2009;4:64–67.
170. Chiao EY, Giordano TP, Palefsky JM, Turing S, El Serag H. Screening HIV-infected individuals for anal cancer precursor lesions: a systematic review. *Clin Infect Dis*. 2006;43:223–233.
171. Vernon SD, Hart CE, Reeves WC, et al. The HIV-1 tat protein enhances E-2 dependent human papillomavirus 16 transcription. *Virus Res*. 1993;27:133–135.
172. Allal AS, Laurencet FM, Reymond MA, et al. Effectiveness of surgical salvage therapy for patients with locally uncontrolled anal carcinoma after sphincter-conserving treatment. *Cancer*. 1999;86:405–409.
173. Ellerhorn JD, Enker WE, Quan SH. Salvage abdominoperineal resection following combined chemotherapy and radiotherapy for epidermoid carcinoma of the anus. *Ann Surg Oncol*. 1994;1:105–110.
174. Flam M, John M, Pajak TF, et al. Role of mitomycin in combination with fluorouracil and radiotherapy, and of salvage chemoradiation in the definitive nonsurgical treatment of epidermoid carcinoma of the anal canal: results of a phase III randomized intergroup study. *J Clin Oncol*. 1996;14:2527–2539.
175. Hung A, Crane C, Delclos M, et al. Cisplatin-based combination modality therapy for anal carcinoma: a wider therapeutic index. *Cancer*. 2003;97:1195–1202.
176. Chang GJ, Berry JM, Jay N, et al. Surgical treatment of high-grade anal squamous intraepithelial lesions: a prospective study. *Dis Colon Rectum*. 2002;45:453–458.
177. Meropol NJ, Niedzwiecki D, Shank B, et al. Induction therapy for poor-prognosis anal canal carcinoma: a phase II study of the Cancer and Leukemia Group B (CALGB 9281). *J Clin Oncol*. 2008;26: 3229–3234.
178. Ajani JA, Winter KA, Gunderson LL, et al. Fluorouracil, mitomycin, and radiotherapy vs fluorouracil, cisplatin, and radiotherapy for carcinoma of the anal canal: a randomized controlled trial. *JAMA*. 2008;299:1914–1921.
179. Joura EA, Leodolter S, Hernandez-Avila M, et al. Efficacy of a quadrivalent prophylactic human papillomavirus (types 6,1,16,18) L1 virus-like-particle vaccine against high grade vulval and vaginal lesions: a combined analysis of three randomized clinical trials. *Lancet*. 2007;12:524–534.
180. Sobhani I, Walker F, Aparicio T, et al. Effect of anal epidermoid cancer-related viruses on the dendritic (Langerhans') cells of the human anal mucosa. *Clin Cancer Res*. 2002;8:2862–2869.
181. Le LH, Chetty R, Moore MJ. Epidermal growth factor receptor expression in anal canal carcinoma. *Am J Clin Pathol*. 2005;124:20–23.
182. Gee JMW, Nicholson RI. Expanding the therapeutic repertoire of epidermal growth factor receptor blockade: radiosensitization. *Br Can Res*. 2003;5:126–129.
183. National Cancer Institute Clinical Trials (PDQ). Phase II study of cetuximab, cisplatin, fluorouracil, and radiotherapy in immunocompetent patients with stage I-IIIB invasive anal carcinoma. http://www.cancer.gov/clinicaltrials/ECOG-E3205. Accessed September 28, 2009.
184. Nigro ND, Seydel HG, Considine B, et al. Combined preoperative radiation and chemotherapy for squamous cell carcinoma of the anal canal. *Cancer*. 1983;51:1826–1829.
185. Bartelink H, Roelofsen F, Eschwege F, et al. Concommitant radiotherapy and chemotherapy is superior to radiotherapy alone in the treatment of locally advanced anal cancer: results of a phase III randomized trial of the European Organization for Research and Gastrointestinal Cooperative Groups. *J Clin Oncol*. 1997;15:2040–2049.

CHAPTER 52

Colleen O'Leary, RN, MSN, AOCNS®

# Endocrine Malignancies

## INTRODUCTION

Endocrine system cancers are malignant neoplasms that occur in the glands responsible for producing and secreting hormones that coordinate activities throughout the body. When a malignancy occurs in the endocrine system, it causes the gland to produce too little or too much of the hormone that is normally produced. This abnormal hormone production is what is responsible for the symptoms associated with each endocrine cancer and is often the only sign of cancer in these individuals. Other than thyroid cancer, the incidence of endocrine cancers is relatively rare accounting for only 2% of all cancers.[1] There were an estimated 39,330 new cases of endocrine cancers in the US in 2009.[1] Because of a high rate of cure for most endocrine cancers, the estimated death rate for these cancers in 2009 was approximately 2470. Thyroid cancer is the most common of the endocrine cancers accounting for 95% of all endocrine cancers and 6% of the deaths from endocrine cancers.[1] Other glands that are commonly discussed with the endocrine cancers include the parathyroids, pituitary, and adrenals. In addition, this chapter will cover pheochromocytomas and multiple endocrine neoplasia (MEN) syndromes.

## THYROID TUMORS

The thyroid is a gland at the front of the neck beneath the larynx. A healthy thyroid is usually about the size of a quarter and cannot be felt through the skin without manipulation of the larynx. Tightly packed follicular epithelial cells interspersed with parafollicular or C cells make up the 2 lobes of the thyroid that are separated by a thin piece of tissue, the isthmus. The follicular cells use iodine from the body to produce thyroid hormone. Thyroid hormone affects the weight, heart rate, blood pressure, and body temperature. Hyperthyroidism can cause hunger, trouble sleeping, nervousness, weight loss, rapid or irregular heartbeat, and a feeling of being too warm. Hypothyroidism causes a person to slow down, feel tired, and gain weight. The amount of thyroid hormone released from the thyroid is regulated by the pituitary gland at the base of the brain through the release of thyroid-stimulating hormone (TSH). The C cells make calcitonin, which plays a small role in regulating calcium levels in the body.

### EPIDEMIOLOGY

Thyroid cancer is the most common of the endocrine cancers. Although the incidence of most head and neck cancers in the US is decreasing, a number of registries have reported that the incidence of thyroid cancer is increasing.[1–4] The annual incidence of thyroid cancer has risen nearly 50% since 1975 affecting 37,200 people in 2009.[1,3] More than 70% of the cases of thyroid cancer will occur in women, and unlike many adult cancers, it is found more often in younger people between the ages of 20 and 55 with the majority occurring after age 45.[1,3]

Thyroid cancer is one of the most curable cancers. The 5-year survival rate for all types of thyroid cancer is 97% with a 10-year survival of 85% to 93%.[1,3,5] Age is an important determinant of prognosis with patients younger than age 45 years doing much better as compared with those older than 45 years. Thyroid cancer is the only cancer that includes age in the staging system by the American Joint Committee on Cancer (AJCC).[6] (See Table 52-1.) Also notable within this staging system is the fact that the presence of nodal metastasis has no bearing on prognosis.[6] Forty-year recurrence rates are about 35%, two thirds of which occur in the first decade after initial therapy. Local disease comprises 68% of the recurrence with distant metastasis, mostly to the lung, comprising 32% of the recurrence.[4] All recurrences, whether local or distant, occur more frequently under age 20 years and over age 60.[4]

### ETIOLOGY

Ionizing radiation is the only known environmental cause for thyroid carcinoma, usually causing papillary thyroid cancer (PTC). This is especially true in children whose thyroid gland has one of the highest risks of developing cancer than any other organ.[3] After the Chernobyl nuclear reactor accident in 1986 many children developed PTC after being exposed to radioiodine fallout. It became clear that $^{131}$Iodine ($^{131}$I) and other short-lived radioiodines were potent thyroid carcinogens in children. In addition, the risk of radiation-induced thyroid cancer is higher in women, in certain Jewish populations, and in patients with a family history of thyroid cancer. This has led to the increasing knowledge of genetic mutations related to thyroid cancer.

Oncogenes are genes involved in the development of cancer that affect the DNA's ability for maintenance and repair. Tumor suppressor genes slow down cell division or induce apoptosis at appropriate times. Thyroid cancer harbors several highly prevalent genetic alterations. Classical gene alterations commonly seen in thyroid cancer include *K-Ras* mutations, *p53* mutations, and rearranged during transfection (*RET*) mutations. Rearrangement of the *RET* gene, also known as *RET/PTC* rearrangement, is the most common genetic alteration identified to date in thyroid cancer.[7] The prevalence of *RET/PTC* in papillary cancers is 10% to 30%.[7,8] The *RET* mutations are usually acquired over a person's life time rather than being inherited. However, since every person has 2 *RET* genes, the possibility of passing a mutation on to offspring is 50%.[7]

**TABLE 52-1**

**TNM Classification System for Differentiated Thyroid Cancer**

| **Definition** | | |
|---|---|---|
| TI | Tumor diameter 2 cm or smaller | |
| T2 | Primary tumor diameter > 2 cm to 4 cm | |
| T3 | Primary tumor diameter > 4 cm | |
| T4a | Tumor of any size extending beyond the thyroid capsule to invade subcutaneous soft tissues, larynx, trachea, esophagus, or recurrent laryngeal nerve | |
| T4b | Tumor invades prevertebral fascia or encases carotid artery or mediastinal vessels | |
| TX | Primary tumor size unknown, but without extrathyroidal invasion | |
| NO | No metastatic nodes | |
| NIa | Metastases to level VI (pretracheal, paratracheal, and prelaryngeal/Delphian lymph nodes) | |
| NIb | Metastasis to unilateral, bilateral, contralateral cervical or superior mediastinal node metastases | |
| NX | Nodes not assessed at surgery | |
| M0 | No distant metastases | |
| MI | Distant metastases | |
| MX | Distant metastases not assessed | |
| | **Stages** | |
| | **Patient age < 45** | **Patient aged 45 years or older** |
| Stage I | Any T, any N, M0 | TI, N0, M0 |
| Sage II | Any T, any N, MI | T2, N0, M0 |
| Stage III | | T3, N0, M0 |
| | | TI, NIa M0 |
| | | T2, NIa M0 |
| | | T3, NIa M0 |
| Stage IVA | | T4a, N0, M0 |
| | | T4a, NIa, M0 |
| | | TI, NIb, M0 |
| | | T2, NIb, M0 |
| | | T3, NIb, M0 |
| | | T4a, NIb, M0 |
| | | TI, NIb, M0 |
| Stage IVB | | T4b, Any N, M0 |
| Stage IVC | | Any T, Any M, MI |

*Source*: Data from Greene.[6]

Scientists have recently identified that a mutation in the *B-type Raf kinase* (*BRAF*) gene is present in 30% to 70% of PTCs.[6,7] The *BRAF* mutation is less likely to be present in children and is uncommon in those whose cancer is thought to arise from radioactive materials. Both *BRAF* and *RET/PTC* mutations are thought to be oncogenes rather than tumor suppressor genes. It is uncommon to have both the *BRAF* and the *RET/PTC* mutation simultaneously. Those with the *BRAF* mutation tend to have a more aggressive growth and higher incidence of metastasis.

Various activating *Ras* mutations, considered oncogeneic and widely seen in other cancers as well, occur mainly in follicular thyroid cancer (FTC).[7,8] Mutations in the tumor suppressor *p53* gene are also seen in follicular anaplastic thyroid cancer (ATC).[7,8] Individuals with medullary thyroid cancer (MTC) also have a mutation of the *RET* gene, but it is found on a different point on the gene than those seen in PTC. Nearly all of the individuals with the inherited form of MTC and 1 out of 5 with sporadic MTC have a mutation in the *RET* gene. In those who have the sporadic MTC, the genetic mutation is only found in the cancer cells whereas those with inherited MTC express the mutation in all of their cells.

## PATHOPHYSIOLOGY

There are 4 main histological types of thyroid cancer: follicular thyroid cancer, pituitary thyroid cancer, anaplastic thyroid cancer, and medullary thyroid cancer. Pituitary thyroid cancers and follicular thyroid cancers, often referred to together as differentiated thyroid cancer (DTC), account for 95% of all thyroid cancers with 80% of those being PTC.[5,9]

Differentiated thyroid cancer begins in the follicular cells and grows slowly. Medullary thyroid cancer accounts for about 3% of thyroid cancers and arises in the C cells of the thyroid.[5,9] Medullary thyroid cancer grows slowly and can be easier to control if found early before it metastasizes to other parts of the body. Anaplastic thyroid cancer accounts for the remaining 2% of thyroid cancers. It also arises in the follicular cells but grows very quickly.[5,9] It is the most difficult type of thyroid cancer to control. Prognosis and treatment are mainly related to grading and staging of the tumor as well as the patient's age and performance status.[10]

### Papillary and follicular tumors

Papillary thyroid tumors arise from both papillary and follicular cells in the thyroid and grow in finger-like projections. It grows slowly, is more common in women than men, and often occurs before age 45. Papillary thyroid cancer is the most common type of thyroid cancer.[9] Papillary thyroid tumors are usually multifocal and infiltrate local tissue. Differentiated thyroid cancer is one of the most curable cancers and is associated with a favorable prognosis. Differentiated thyroid cancer occurs more frequently in women than in men with most cases being found in people between the ages of 20 and 60. Papillary and follicular thyroid carcinomas carry 10-year overall survival rates of 93% and 85%, respectively.[5] The mortality for DTC is similar in patients of comparable age and disease stage. Both have an excellent prognosis if the tumors are confined to the thyroid. Vascular invasion and metastasis to a distant site, such as bone and lung, are more common in papillary tumors than in follicular tumors.[11]

Distant metastasis in DTC can be divided into 2 categories: occurring as the initial presenting diagnosis and distant metastasis after initial treatment of thyroid cancer. The incidence of distant metastasis after initial treatment of DTC is between 7% and 23%.[5] The frequency of individuals diagnosed with DTC presenting initially with distant metastasis ranges from 1% to 9%.[5]

Follicular thyroid cancer arises in the follicular cells, grows slowly, and has a high cure rate. Follicular tumors are typically a single encapsulated tumor that tends to be more aggressive than papillary tumors. Follicular thyroid cancers are more common in areas of the world in which people's diets are low in iodine. This is an uncommon finding in the US due to the addition of iodine to table salt. However, a diet low in iodine may increase a person's risk of PTC especially if the person is also exposed to radiation.[9]

Exposure to radiation is a proven risk factor for the development of thyroid cancer. Sources of radiation exposure include medical treatments as well as radiation fallout from power plants or nuclear weapons. Having a history of radiation for head and neck cancer increases a person's risk for thyroid cancer as well.

### Medullary tumors

Medullary thyroid cancer makes up about 3% of all thyroid cancers[9] and begins in the neuroendocrine C cells of the thyroid. MTC occurs equally in men and women and usually occurs after age 50. About 1 out of 5 MTCs result from an inherited gene mutation.[8] These cases are known as familial medullary thyroid cancer (FMTC). FMTC can occur alone or in combination with other cancers. The combination of FMTC with tumors of other endocrine glands is known as multiple endocrine neoplasia syndrome, which is discussed later in this chapter. Many patients with MTC have tumor spread to their cervical lymph nodes at the time of diagnosis. Regional lymph node spread indicates a poor prognostic sign with the 10-year survival rate being only 42%.

### Anaplastic tumors

Anaplastic thyroid cancer makes up about 2% of all thyroid cancers.[9] It arises in the follicular cells of the thyroid. Unlike other thyroid cancers, ATC grows and spreads rapidly and is hard to control. Men are more likely than women to have ATC and most are over the age of 60. Potential risk factors include having a long standing benign thyroid nodule, goiter, or other thyroid lesion. ATC arises from these long standing nodules in the thyroid. The patient often experiences rapid and marked enlargement of the lesion. Because of the rapid growth and spread of ATC, most patients live for only 4 to 12 months following diagnosis. The most common areas of metastasis that are seen at the time of diagnosis include lung, pleura, bone, and brain. Neither radiation nor chemotherapy has shown to significantly reduce survival rates.

## CLINICAL MANIFESTATIONS

Thyroid malignancies are usually asymptomatic for long periods of time and commonly present as a solitary thyroid nodule. Both benign and malignant nodules are often asymptomatic giving no clinical clue to their diagnosis. About 50% of malignant nodules are discovered during a routine physical examination, on imaging studies, or during surgery for benign disease.[3,4] The other 50% are noticed by the patient as an asymptomatic nodule. Some common symptoms that patients experience as a nodule develops include a lump in the front of the neck, hoarseness or voice changes, swollen lymph nodes in the neck, trouble swallowing or breathing, or pain in the throat or neck that does not go away. Most often these symptoms are not due to cancer but a benign thyroid nodule or other condition. However, evaluating all nodules for malignancy is difficult given the fact that benign nodules are so prevalent and thyroid cancer, by contrast, is so uncommon.

## ASSESSMENT

Diagnostic procedures for determining thyroid malignancies include physical examination, including personal and family history, laboratory tests, and imaging procedures followed by biopsy to confirm diagnosis. Prompt diagnosis has a bearing on outcome; however, a delay of 12 months or more was found in almost 30% of the patients managed by primary care physicians in one study.[4]

Since 50% of thyroid malignancies are found on routine physical examination, this is an important tool in clinical diagnosis. In addition to palpation of the thyroid and neck structures, patients should be assessed for any symptoms of potential malignancy. According to guidelines developed by the American Association of Clinical Endocrinologists (AACE) and the Associazione Medici Endocrinologi (AME), the Italian Endocrinology Medical Association, when assessing for thyroid malignancies a patient history and physical examination should include family history of thyroid disease, previous neck disease or treatment, growth of a neck mass, hoarseness, dysphonia, dysphagia or dyspnea, location, consistency, and size of the nodule, neck tenderness or pain, cervical adenopathy, and symptoms of hyperthyroidism or hypothyroidism.[12] Factors suggesting increased risk of malignant disease potential include male gender, fixed nodule, cervical adenopathy, disease age < 20 or > 70 years, persistent hoarseness, dysphonia, dysphagia or dyspnea, growing nodule, firm or hard consistency, history of head and neck irradiation, and family history of MTC or multiple endocrine neoplasia 2 (MEN2).[3,12]

Although no laboratory test can determine whether a thyroid nodule is malignant, measurement of serum thyrotropin (TSH) concentration is the single most useful laboratory test in the initial evaluation of thyroid nodules because of the high sensitivity of the TSH assay in detecting even subtle thyroid dysfunction.[3,9,12] Calcitonin testing is imperative in those patients with a history of familial MTC or MEN2, but routine testing of serum calcitonin in all patients with unselected thyroid nodules does not seem to be cost-effective. In addition, the risk of false-positive results should be considered since high levels of serum calcitonin can be present in patients with other conditions such as C-cell hyperplasia, pulmonary and pancreatic tumors, and kidney failure as well as systemic inflammatory response syndrome and sepsis. Therefore, routine use of serum calcitonin levels is not recommended.[3,9,12]

Imaging studies useful in the diagnosis of thyroid malignancies consist of ultrasound and nuclear medicine scans including radioiodine scans and positron emission tomography (PET). High-resolution ultrasound is the most sensitive test available to detect thyroid lesions, measure their dimensions accurately, identify their structure, and evaluate diffuse changes in the thyroid gland. Ultrasound is helpful in determining if a nodule is solid or filled with fluid and can be used to determine the number and size of nodules. Ultrasound should be performed in all patients with a history of familial thyroid cancer, MEN2, or childhood cervical irradiation even if palpation yields normal findings.[12]

The most common nuclear medicine scan used in the diagnosis of thyroid malignancies is the radioiodine thyroid scintigraphy scan, more commonly known as a thyroid scan. A thyroid scan is the only technique that allows for assessment of thyroid regional function and detection of functional tissue. On the basis of amount of the radioisotope taken up by the tissue, it may be classified as hyperfunctioning ("hot") or hypofunctioning ("cold"). Hot nodules almost never represent clinically significant malignant lesions, whereas cold nodules have a reported malignant risk of about 5% to 8%.[3,12] Radioiodine scans work best in patients with a high level of TSH and because iodine in the body can interfere with the results of the test, patients are generally told not to ingest foods or medicines that increase iodine for 1 day prior to the examination.

Biopsy is the only definitive way to diagnose a thyroid malignancy. Fine-needle aspiration (FNA) has become a reliable, safe, and cost-effective method for evaluating thyroid nodules. Traditionally, FNA biopsy results are divided into 4 categories: nondiagnostic, malignant, indeterminate, or suspicious for neoplasm and benign. About 70% of FNA specimens are classified as benign, 5% are malignant, 10% are suspicious, and 10% to 20% are nondiagnostic or unsatisfactory.[3,11,12] The results are important in determining whether to treat the patient medically or surgically. If a diagnosis cannot be made from FNA, a surgeon removes the whole nodule. In addition, if FTC is suspected complete surgical excision may be needed for diagnosis.

## CLASSIFICATION AND STAGING

Histological diagnosis and age are the 2 most important determinants to staging and prognosis for thyroid malignancies. There are several staging and clinical prognostic scoring strategies that use patient age older than 45 years as a major feature to identify cancer mortality from thyroid malignancies.[3] However, as noted earlier, both histology and age are incorporated into the AJCC staging system, which is the preferred staging system for thyroid malignancies (see Table 52-1).

## THERAPEUTIC APPROACHES AND NURSING CARE

### Surgery

Surgery is the primary treatment for thyroid cancer and is used in nearly every case, except perhaps ATCs. Once results of the FNA indicate thyroid cancer, surgery to remove the tumor and all or part of the remaining thyroid gland is recommended.[3,4,11] Thyroidectomy is used for all types of thyroid malignancies. Near-total or total thyroidectomy is recommended if any of the following are present: the primary thyroid carcinoma is more than 1 to 1.5 cm, contralateral thyroid nodules, regional or distant metastases, patient has a personal history of radiation therapy to the head and neck, or a first-degree family history of DTC.[12] Older age (>45 years) may also be a criterion for recommending near-total or total thyroidectomy because of higher recurrence rates in this age group. These recommendations also apply to children and young adults because 60% to 80% have regional lymph node involvement and 10% to 20% have distant metastases.[4] If all of the thyroid tissue cannot be removed, remaining tissue may be destroyed using radioactive iodine at a later date.

Some patients with follicular or PTC may have a lobectomy rather than thyroidectomy. One lobe and the isthmus are removed. At times a second surgery is needed to remove the remaining lobe, but more frequently radioactive iodine or radiation therapy may be used to destroy remaining tissue. Performing a lobectomy alone may result in a 5% to 10% recurrence rate in the opposite thyroid lobe, a high tumor recurrence rate, and a high (11%) incidence of subsequent pulmonary metastases.[4] The thyroid tissue removed contains the cells that produce thyroid hormone. Daily thyroid hormone replacement therapy will need to be initiated on all patients who have their thyroid removed.

Postoperative complications of thyroid surgery include temporary or permanent hoarseness or loss of voice, damage to the parathyroid glands, excessive bleeding or formation of hematoma, recurrent laryngeal nerve paralysis, vocal cord paralysis, thyroid storm, and wound infection.[8,9,11] Damage to the parathyroid glands can cause hypoparathyroidism that can lead to low serum calcium levels causing muscle spasms and peripheral neuropathies. Thyroid storm, or thyrotoxic crisis, is an acute episode of thyroid overactivity that is characterized by high fever, tachycardia, delirium, dehydration, and extreme excitability.

Nursing management of the surgical patient demands keen assessment for signs and symptoms of bleeding, infection, tetany, hypocalcemia, vocal cord paralysis, and thyrotoxic crisis. Assessing respiratory status every hour for 12 hours is recommended in the immediate postoperative period.[11] The respiratory assessment should include vital signs every 4 hours, inability to speak, retraction of neck muscles, crowing respirations, dyspnea, and cyanosis. The nurse should also observe for hematoma, hoarseness, and vocal cord paralysis. Nursing interventions include keeping the head of the bed elevated to >45° at all times, maintaining neck support by placing the hands behind the neck with elbows raised when moving or sitting, and having the patient turn, cough, and deep breath every 2 hours.

Calcium levels are monitored daily due to the fact that 1% of patients undergoing near-total thyroidectomy and 6% to 8% of patients undergoing total thyroidectomy will experience temporary or permanent hypoparathyroidism. Hypoparathyroidism occurs at a rate as high as 10% in adults and may be twice as high in children.[4] Hypoparathyroidism results in hypocalcemia. The symptoms of hypocalcemia include numbness, tingling or cramps in the extremities, numbness and tingling around the mouth, stiffness, twitching or spasms in the hands or feet, positive Chvostek's sign, and positive Trousseau sign. A positive Chvostek's sign refers to an abnormal reaction to the stimulation of the facial nerve. When the facial nerve is tapped at the angle of the jaw, the facial muscles on the same side of the face will contract momentarily. To elicit a Trousseau sign, a blood pressure cuff is inflated to occlude the brachial artery for several minutes. Carpopedal spasms will be seen that include flexion at the wrist, flexion at the metacarpophalangeal joints, extension of the interphalangeal joints, and adduction of the thumbs and fingers. Patient may be required to take calcium gluconate to avoid hypocalcemia. Patient education should include avoiding foods that suppress calcium absorption such as spinach, Swiss cheese, beets, bran, and whole-grain cereals.

## Radiation therapy

Radioactive iodine therapy (RAI) using $^{131}I$ has been shown to improve the survival rate of patients with metastatic papillary or FTC, and this treatment is now standard practice in such cases.[12] But, the benefits of RAI therapy are less clear for patients with nonmetastatic cancers of the thyroid gland that are relatively small in size. In addition, for 4 to 6 weeks following surgery, RAI is administered to ablate any remaining functioning thyroid tissue as well as residual local and metastatic tumor. RAI is not used to treat anaplastic and medullary thyroid carcinomas because these types of cancer do not take up iodine.

Short-term side effects of RAI include neck tenderness, nausea, swelling and tenderness of the salivary glands, dry mouth, taste changes, fatigue, headache, bone marrow suppression, and pain.[3,4,9] Men who receive large total doses with RAI may become infertile or have lower sperm counts. Radioactive iodine may also affect a woman's ovarian function, and some women may have irregular periods for up to a year after treatment. Some physicians recommend that women avoid becoming pregnant for 6 months to a year after treatment. Both men and women who have had RAI therapy may have a slightly increased risk of developing leukemia in the future. There is disagreement on exactly how much this risk is increased, but most of the largest studies have found that this is an extremely rare complication and some research even suggests the risk of leukemia may not be significantly increased.[8,9]

Nursing care focuses on symptom management and patient education. The nurse should begin by reviewing the purpose and administration of the RAI with the patient ensuring that they understand that the treatment will occur in the hospital and not on an outpatient basis. The patient will be instructed that they will drink the RAI from a special container that will be given to them. They should be instructed not to bring any articles from home. In addition, it is the nurse who may help to minimize a patient's sense of isolation during treatment as well as providing radiation safety instructions for patients and visitors. The nurse should be sure that the patient is aware that visitors will only be able to stay for 30 minutes at a time and that no pregnant women should visit. Education regarding side effects including nausea, vomiting, tiredness, headache, mucositis, and neutropenia should be reviewed assuring the patient that these side effects can be managed with a variety of interventions. Education and clarification of misconceptions regarding RAI is an important nursing intervention.[11] Discharge instructions should include the fact that the patient will still be radioactive for a few days and, thus, should sleep alone and not hold children close to them for a period of 3 days after discharge. In addition, precautions should be taken to always sit on the toilet when urinating and to flush the toilet 3 times after voiding. Instructing the patient to drink at least 2 quarts of fluid for several days will help the body to rid itself of the RAI. (See Figure 52-1.)

External beam radiation therapy (EBRT) may be used for anaplastic tumors that do not take up RAI, for tumors that recur after standard treatment, or to treat bone pain resulting from metastasis. The timing, dose, and mode of delivery of EBRT remain controversial. The goal of EBRT is achieving local control. However, EBRT has considerable toxicities associated with it and often does not achieve the goal. The 5-year survival rate being approximately 5% with any currently available treatment has led to the development of a variety of fractionation regimens and concurrent radiation-chemotherapy and surgical resection.[13] Despite the fact that all of the regimens studied showed local control from 41% to 68%, the significant toxicities have shown them to be unacceptable. Careful patient selection should be exercised when choosing EBRT regimens. For patients with a good performance status and no metastasis, a reasonable regimen is to use standard fractionation to total doses of 50 to 60 Gy or accelerated hyperfractionated EBRT without chemotherapy, 60 Gy in 40 fractions (1.5 Gy/fraction given twice a day) over 4 weeks.[13] With any regimen, the efficacy of EBRT needs to be balanced with its toxicity. Toxicity depends on the amount of radiation received and what part of the body is irradiated. Radiation to the neck may cause xerostomia and mucositis severe enough to necessitate use of intravenous fluids or enteral tube feedings. Local irritation of skin is progressive and can range from redness to moist desquamation. Fatigue is also a significant side effect that most patients experience during treatment.

**What is $^{131}$I?**
$^{131}$I is radioactive iodine that goes to the thyroid gland and thyroid cancer cells. It is toxic to these cells, and the aim of treatment is to kill cancer cells. It will also kill normal thyroid cells.

**Where will I go to get the $^{131}$I treatment?**
You will have to go to the hospital to get this treatment. While in the hospital, you will wear only hospital gowns, robe, and slippers. Do not bring things from home.

**How will I take the $^{131}$I?**
You will be given a special container of $^{131}$I, and you will drink it through a straw.

**Will I be able to have visitors while I am in the hospital?**
You may have adult visitors while you are in the hospital, but because you will be radioactive there are some rules:

1. No pregnant women can visit.
2. Visitors will only be able to stay for 30 minutes or less for the first 48 hours.

**Will I have any side effects from $^{131}$I?**
Possible side effects may include nausea and vomiting, tiredness, headache, a sore mouth, and a lowered white blood count after you get the treatment. Your nurse will give you medicine for the nausea or the headache if you have them, and your doctor may want you to get a blood test after you go home. You may also have a metallic taste in your mouth for several days after taking $^{131}$I.

**Will I still be radioactive when I go home?**
Yes, you will be radioactive for a few days. For 3 days after you go home you should:

1. Sleep alone.
2. Not hold children close to you.

**How can I help my body to get rid of the $^{131}$I?**
You need to drink as much fluid as you can (at least 2 quarts) for several days after getting the $^{131}$I. This can include water, juices, sodas and so forth. The $^{131}$I will pass out of your body in your urine, so when you go to the bathroom you should:

1. Sit on the toilet to urinate so urine does not splash anywhere.
2. Flush the toilet 3 times after you pass urine.

**How will my doctor know if the thyroid cancer is gone?**
Your doctor will schedule you for a body scan in about 3 to 6 months. If the scan shows that there aren't any more thyroid cancer cells, you will not need any more $^{131}$I. If there are any thyroid cancer cells that show up on the scan, you will get another $^{131}$I treatment.

**If you have any other questions, please write them down so you remember to ask your doctor or your nurse.**

**FIGURE 52-1**

Teaching sheet for the patient receiving $^{131}$I treatment

## Chemotherapy

There are no data to support the use of adjuvant chemotherapy in the management of DTC.[3,14] Doxorubicin may act as a radiation sensitizer in some tumors of the thyroid origin and so has been considered for patients with locally advanced disease undergoing external beam radiation. Anaplastic thyroid cancers, which are not receptive to RAI, have shown partial remissions with the use of chemotherapy in some patients. Although doxorubicin is the most commonly used chemotherapeutic agent for thyroid cancer, the results of monotherapy with doxorubicin have been poor with only about 17% of patients achieving a partial remission.[15] However, the combination of doxorubicin (60 mg/m$^2$) plus cisplatin (40 mg/m$^2$) appears to be more active than doxorubicin alone and has been reported to produce more complete responses with 30% of patients responding to treatment.[15]

A current phase II and III clinical trial uses a combination of combrestastatin with paclitaxel/carboplatin for ATC. No current results are available. Another active clinical trial for children ages 5 to 18 is studying the side effects and best dose of vandetanib to establish effectiveness in treating patients with MTC.[9]

## PARATHYROID TUMORS

The parathyroid glands are 4 pea-sized organs found in the neck near the thyroid gland. The parathyroid glands make parathyroid hormone (PTH or parathormone). PTH helps the body use and store calcium to keep serum calcium levels normal. When the parathyroid gland becomes overactive, it makes too much PTH causing hyperparathyroidism. The result of hyperparathyroidism is hypercalcemia. The hypercalcemia caused by hyperparathyroidism is more serious and life threatening than parathyroid cancer itself, and treating hypercalcemia is as important as treating the cancer.

## EPIDEMIOLOGY

Parathyroid cancer is a rare neoplasm that reportedly account for <1% of the cases of hyperparathyroidism.[16] Parathyroid carcinomas tend to be localized in the inferior parathyroid glands. Several oncogenes and tumor suppressor genes have been linked to parathyroid carcinoma. The loss of a region on chromosome 13 associated with parathyroid cancer has been reported.[16]

A more recently described tumor suppressor is the *hyperparathyroidism-2* (*HRPT2*) gene, which is associated with the hyperparathyroidism-jaw tumor (HPT-JT) syndrome.[16] The inactivation of *HRPT2* is involved directly in predisposition to HPT-JT and in the development of some sporadic parathyroid tumors. It has been proposed that *HRPT2* mutations constitute an early event that may lead to parathyroid cancers, and may be a marker of malignant potential in both familial and sporadic parathyroid tumors. It has been shown that the *cyclin dependent 1* (*CCND1*) or *parathyroid adenoma 1* (*PRAD1*) oncogene is overexpressed frequently in parathyroid cancer, and it has been proposed that *PRAD1* plays an important role in the malignant transformation of parathyroid cancers.[16]

## ETIOLOGY

There are no definitive risk factors that have been identified for parathyroid carcinoma. However, it has been suggested that having familial isolated hyperparathyroidsim (FIHP) or multiple endocrine neoplasia type 1 (MEN1) may increase a person's risk of developing parathyroid cancer,[17] both of which are rare hereditary disorders. There has been found to be some association between patients with chronic renal failure and dialysis with the development of parathyroid cancer also. One explanation focuses on the relationship between parathyroidism and chronic hypocalcemia caused by renal insufficiency, hypovitaminosis D, malabsorption of calcium in the gut, or PTH resistance.[11]

## PATHOPHYSIOLOGY

The cells involved with parathyroid tumors appear to be histologically similar to parathyroid adenomas, making it difficult to establish that a tumor is benign or malignant. However, whereas parathyroid adenomas tend to be soft and oval, parathyroid cancers tend to be larger in size, often > 3 cm, firm, lobulated, and have a dense, fibrous capsule.[16] Adenomas usually involve only one parathyroid gland and are surrounded by a rim of normal parathyroid tissue. Cancers of the parathyroid tend to have more mitosis and may be surrounded by a thick irregular capsule.[17]

Parathyroid cancers tend to be indolent, so diagnosis may occur late. The recurrence of hypercalcemia or elevated PTH following surgery to remove a tumor previously deemed benign may be a good indication that the tumor was malignant and has since recurred. Because of the low incidence of parathyroid cancer, an AJCC staging has not been formulated. In addition, neither lymph node status nor tumor size seems to be prognostic markers for parathyroid cancer. Patients are considered to have either localized or metastatic disease. Parathyroid cancers generally metastasize to regional lymph nodes and lungs and may involve other distant sites such as the liver, bone, pleura, and pancreas.[16]

## CLINICAL MANIFESTATIONS

Most of the symptoms related to parathyroid cancer are caused by the hypercalcemia that develops. These symptoms may include weakness, fatigue, nausea and vomiting, loss of appetite, unexplained weight loss, polydipsia, polyuria, constipation, and confusion. Typically a patient with parathyroid cancer has serum calcium levels that exceed 14 mg/dL. The effects of prolonged hypercalcemia include rheumatoid symptoms, renal calculi, and calcifications of the cornea and other soft tissues. Symptoms that include chronic hoarseness and recurrent laryngeal nerve palsy in a patient with primary hyperparathyroidism who has not had previous neck surgery are suggestive of parathyroid carcinoma.

## ASSESSMENT

Once hyperparathyroidism has been diagnosed, imaging tests may be done to determine which parathyroid glad is overactive. However, because of the difficult distinction between benign and malignant tumors, as previously discussed, the patient's symptoms, serum calcium levels, and serum PTH levels are used to make a diagnosis.

Physical examination should include checking for general signs of health as well as any signs of lumps or nodules. A history of the patient's general health habits, and past illnesses and treatments should be taken. With hypercalcemia that is otherwise unexplained, an immunoassay for parathyroid hormone (iPTH) is completed. With parathyroid tumors, the iPTH level is markedly increased. Because the majority of parathyroid tumors are nonpalpable, the use of imaging procedures including magnetic resonance imaging (MRI) and computerized tomography (CT) can be helpful. MRI and CT may be used to locate and identify tumors as well as evaluate tumor mass following surgery. A type of radionuclide scan, the sestamibi scan, uses 99m-technetium sestamibi to locate an overactive parathyroid gland and determine whether the disease is confined to one or more glands.[17] Radiographs may also be useful to confirm bone or lung metastasis. Prognostic factors related to parathyroid cancer include the ability to control hypercalcemia, local or metastatic disease, the ability to completely remove the tumor and the capsule enclosing it, and the patient's general state of health.

## THERAPEUTIC APPROACHES AND NURSING CARE

### Medical management

The morbidity and mortality associated with parathyroid cancer generally are due to PTH secretion and hypercalcemia rather than the tumor burden itself. Treatment modalities for hypercalcemia, especially in patients with unresectable disease or without measurable disease, become paramount. Conventional treatment to help control or ameliorate the hypercalcemia includes intravenous fluids and diuretics to help flush out excess calcium, and antiresorptive agents such as bisphosphonates, gallium, or mithramycin to decrease the amount of calcium in the bloodstream.

### Surgery

Surgery is the recommended treatment for both localized and metastatic parathyroid cancer. Initially, surgery should include an en bloc resection of the tumor that takes care to avoid rupture of the tumor capsule and to ensure that the margins are free of tumor. This procedure will involve a parathyroidectomy, typically an ipsilateral thyroidectomy (thyroid lobectomy), and possibly resection of adjacent cervical muscles, paratracheal tissues, and the recurrent laryngeal nerve, if involved.[11,16–18] Lymphadenectomy, beyond that necessary to achieve an en bloc excision of the primary malignancy, is not indicated unless there is presence of enlarged or firm nodes. Local recurrence may be minimized by an en bloc resection approach. Preoperative medical management to lower elevated calcium levels and to correct other metabolic disturbances that are due to hyperparathyroidism is critical. Metastatic disease can appear shortly after the initial diagnosis and surgery or for up to 20 years later. Because of the difficulty in making a histological diagnosis, the appearance of recurrent or metastatic disease in a patient previously treated surgically for hypercalcemia can be the first indicator that the tumor was malignant. Approximately 50% of the patients who experience recurrence will have distant metastases.[17] The most common site of distant metastasis is the lung.[16,17] Some patients experience years of survival even after the diagnosis of distant metastases.[16] Aggressive surgical resection has been associated with a 49% 10-year survival rate according to data from the US National Cancer Database.[19]

The focus of postoperative nursing care is to monitor for signs of infection and hemorrhage, monitor serum calcium levels and provide patient and family education. A syndrome commonly referred to as hungry bone syndrome may occur as calcium and phosphorus are deposited into the skeleton causing symptomatic hypocalcemia. Occurrence of hungry bone syndrome indicates successful tumor removal. The patient will require intravenous calcium and calcitrol until the remaining parathyroid glands recover. It is common to monitor serum calcium and PTH levels every 3 months for elevation, which could indicate recurrent local or metastatic disease.

### Radiation therapy

In selected patients, adjuvant radiation therapy appears to decrease the local recurrence rate effectively.[16] Especially in high-risk patients, radiation therapy appears to improve the disease free interval. In addition, local recurrence rates are lower if adjuvant radiation is applied after initial surgery regardless of the type of surgery or disease stage.

### Chemotherapy

Overall, chemotherapy has been judged ineffective for treatment of parathyroid cancer. Because parathyroid cancers are so rare there are no reported chemotherapy studies. However, anecdotal reports show that short-term remissions with chemotherapy are possible.[16,17] In these reports, combination regimens including fluorouracil, cyclophosphamide, and paclitaxel have been used.

### Palliative care

Supportive care for hypercalcemia is often the focus in patients with parathyroid cancer. Control of hypercalcemia is difficult because it is caused by tumor recurrence. When additional surgery is not possible, recurrent hypercalcemia is treated with the same drugs used to treat other instances of hypercalcemia. Even with the use of calcitonin, bisphosphonates, or other antiresorptive therapies, calcium levels may remain persistently elevated. Chronic uncontrolled hypercalcemia that causes intractable nausea, vomiting, and dehydration, remains the cause of death for most patients with parathyroid tumors.

## PITUITARY TUMORS

Pituitary tumors represent from 10% to 25% of all intracranial cancers. Pituitary tumors can be classified into 3 groups according to their biological behavior: benign, invasive adenoma, and carcinoma. Adenomas comprise the largest portion of pituitary tumors with an overall estimated prevalence of approximately 17%.[20] Only a minority of adenomas are symptomatic. Invasive adenomas, which account for approximately 35% of all pituitary neoplasms, may invade the dura mater, cranial bone, or sphenoid sinus.[20] Cancers account for 0.1% to 0.2% of all pituitary tumors.[20]

The pituitary gland is found inside the skull just above the nasal passages. It sits in a tiny bony space called the sella turcica. This small gland is connected directly to the hypothalamus. This connection to the hypothalamus provides a key link between brain activity and the endocrine system. The pituitary gland has 2 parts—the posterior pituitary and the anterior pituitary—each with distinct functions. The smaller posterior pituitary is really an extension of brain tissue. The posterior pituitary is where the hormones vasopressin, also called antidiuretic hormone, and oxytocin are made and secreted. Vasopressin causes the kidney to retain water and not excrete it in the urine. Without vasopressin, a person would develop diabetes insipidus (DI) by excreting too much urine. Vasopressin also can raise blood pressure by constricting blood vessels. The hormone oxytocin is primarily a hormone of pregnancy causing the uterus to contract during childbirth and the breasts to release milk when nursing. Tumors rarely develop in the posterior pituitary gland.

Most pituitary tumors begin in the larger anterior pituitary gland, which is not brain tissue. It is a true gland. It produces several hormones that control other endocrine glands. Growth hormone (GH), also known as somatotropin, promotes body growth during childhood. Adults make only small amounts of GH. If an adult continues to make GH, acromegaly develops. Thyroid-stimulating hormone (TSH), also known as thyrotropin, stimulates growth of the thyroid gland and the release of thyroid hormone. Adrenocorticotropic hormone (ACTH), also known as corticotropin, causes adrenal gland growth and production of steroid hormones by the adrenal glands. Too much of this hormone from the pituitary gland produces Cushing's syndrome. The gonadotropins luteinizing hormone (LH) and follicle-stimulating hormone (FSH) regulate the cycle of ovulation and menstruation in women. In men, LH and FSH control testosterone and sperm production in the testicles. Prolactin (PRL), another pituitary hormone, causes milk production in the female breast. Its function in men is not known.

## EPIDEMIOLOGY

Although approximately 10% of brain tumors are pituitary tumors, these tumors generally remain small and silent.[11] An estimated 11% of pituitary cancers are discovered either on autopsy or via MRI or CT done for other reasons. The role of gender is dependent upon the hormone produced in each tumor type. Women are 4 times more likely to develop prolactinoma and 3 times more likely to develop Cushing's syndrome (CS). The majority of pituitary cancers occur between the ages of 30 to 50 years, but they can also develop in children and teenagers.

## ETIOLOGY

There has been no unequivocal histological pathogenesis identified thus far for pituitary cancers. Most scientists believe that pituitary tumors arise from repeated mutations of a single cell thus making them monoclonal in origin. One gene that is thought to play a part in the pathogenesis of pituitary tumors is *pituitary tumor-transforming gene* (*PTTG*). *PTTG* has been found in all types of pituitary tumors as well as normal pituitary tissue. However, research has shown that the amount of *PTTG* in pituitary tumors can be as much as 80% higher than that in normal pituitary tissue.[21] Because of this *PTTG* has been used as a molecular marker for pituitary tumor invasiveness and aggressiveness.

Scientists are also studying the relationship between the genetic mutations found in people with MEN1 and pituitary tumor formation. Even though hereditary pituitary tumors account for only about 3% of all pituitary tumors, MEN1 is responsible for the vast majority of hereditary pituitary tumors.[21] In patients with MEN1, pituitary tumors are generally not seen until adulthood. Much less is known about the causes of nonhereditary pituitary tumors, although recent studies indicate that about 40% of GH-secreting adenomas have an acquired mutation in a specific protein called Gs alpha.[21] Gs alpha mutations are much less common in other types of pituitary adenomas.

Several other genetic abnormalities have been found in other types of pituitary adenomas, but it is not clear whether abnormal genes are essential for pituitary tumor formation. What is known is that there is a loss of the normal regulatory mechanism that keeps the glandular cells from overproducing their hormone and growing. This is probably the result of the gene alterations.

## PATHOPHYSIOLOGY

Because no unequivocal histopathological features of cancer exist in pituitary cancer, the diagnosis of malignancy is reserved for pituitary cancers that have metastasized to remote areas of the central nervous system (CNS) or outside of the CNS.[20] In a review of 95 cases of pituitary cancer, 68% of the cases were found to be hormone-producing; PRL (26%) and ACTH (25%) being the most common hormonal subtypes.[20] Pituitary cancers producing GH were the second most common of the hormonal subtypes, and FSH/LH-producing and TSH-producing cancers are even more rarely reported. Other reports indicate that as many as 88% of pituitary cancers are hormone producing, with ACTH-secreting tumors being the most common.[21] In a series of 15 cases, cancers showed a greater tendency toward systemic metastasis than craniospinal metastasis; the rate of systemic metastasis was 71% for PRL-producing cell tumors and 57% for ACTH-producing tumors.[20]

## CLINICAL MANIFESTATIONS

The signs and symptoms associated with pituitary tumors are directly related to the hormone that is being hypersecreted. Most of the tumors that make LH and FSH do not make enough hormones to cause symptoms. These are referred to as nonfunctioning tumors. However, when a functioning tumor over secretes a hormone, the ensuing signs and symptoms depend on that hormone. The most frequently seen functional tumor over-secretes prolactin. Sign and symptoms include headache, oligomenorrhea, amenorrhea, galactorrhea, infertility, and impotence in men. Commonly seen symptoms regardless of the hormone being secreted include headache, seen in 40% to 60% of patients, and visual changes including blurred vision, double vision or loss of peripheral vision, seen in 60% of patients with pituitary cancer.[20]

### Hormone effects

*Prolactinomas.* Forty percent of all pituitary tumors are prolactinomas causing hyperprolactinemia and its clinical sequelae.[20] Women are more likely to have small microadenomas whereas larger macroadenomas are seen more frequently in men. The most common side effects seen in women are galactorrhea or other menstrual irregularities including oligomenorrhea, amenorrhea, or infertility. Men with hyperprolactinemia exhibit decreased libido or impotence and galactorrhea in some cases.

*Growth hormone-secreting tumors.* Almost 95% of all GH-secreting tumors arise in the pituitary gland.[22] These tumors produce acromegaly in adults and gigantism in prepubescent children. Acromegaly is a chronic disease that because of its slowly progressive, and insidious nature, often remains undetected for up to 10 years before formal diagnosis. The delay in diagnosis may exaggerate the complications due to GH hypersecretion. The classic clinical findings in a patient with advanced acromegaly include frontal bossing, which is an unusually prominent forehead, sometimes associated with a heavier than normal brow ridge, coarse facial features, wide nasal bridge, thick lips, protruding jaw with widely spaced teeth, and large hands and feet. Patients with acromegaly often complain of headaches and fatigue. Hypertension is present in approximately 30% of cases of acromegaly.[22] Musculoskeletal complications include enlargement of the synovial tissue and cartilage, causing hypertrophic arthropathy. The arthropathy, primarily of the weight-bearing joints, can lead to degenerative changes and the need for surgical replacement of joints. Individuals with acromegaly are at increased risk for premalignant colonic polyps, which are present in up to 30% of such individuals. A retrospective study has suggested an increased risk of colon cancer in patients with acromegaly.[22] The mortality rate of patients with acromegaly is 2 to 4 times higher than the general population, primarily attributable to cardiovascular disease.

Over secretion of ACTH is the most frequent cause of CS causing 80% to 85% of all cases.[23] The suspicion of CS in an individual arises from the presence of acne, hirsutism, fatigue, thinned skin, purple striae, high blood pressure, glucose intolerance, menstrual irregularity, a cervical fat pad, proximal muscle weakness, the characteristic moon face, and central obesity with supraclavicular fat accumulation. Neuropsychological disturbances including depression, emotional irritability, sleep disturbances, and cognitive deficits are also frequently observed. Muscular atrophy and purple striae are particularly helpful stigmata in adults, whereas in children growth retardation is frequently present. Because the symptoms of CS are often subtle, patients often are not diagnosed until long after symptoms are first seen. Patients are generally treated for individual symptoms until a definitive diagnosis of CS is eventually made. Mortality is as high as 50% within 5 years of diagnosis with causes including cardiovascular disease, infection, and suicide secondary to depression.[23]

## ASSESSMENT

Definitive diagnosis of pituitary tumors involves a series of assessments including history and physical examination, endocrinology testing, radiologic testing, and histopathological findings. Since many pituitary tumors progress slowly, a thorough history and physical examination to identify subtle changes is important. An eye examination to test the patient's overall eye health as well as visual field examination should be completed. In addition, a neurological examination to test for muscle strength and coordination can offer important information. Important information from the patient's history includes a family history of pituitary gland tumors, hyperparathyroidism, multiple kidney stones, hypoglycemia, or adrenal gland tumors. These may all be indicative of MEN1. Once a suspicion of pituitary tumor arises, endocrinology testing will follow to test the serum hormone levels. If serum hormone levels are increased in the absence of other causes, a pituitary tumor is suspected. In some cases, additional testing may be required for stimulation or suppression of pituitary hormones.

Radiological testing may be done to confirm abnormalities. Although CT scans can find a pituitary tumor if it is large enough, MRI is the preferred diagnostic tool. MRI is the best imaging test to identify pituitary tumors of all types. MRI can identify a macroadenoma of the pituitary gland, as well as most microadenomas. But the MRI may not be able to detect microadenomas that are smaller than 3 mm (about 1/8 in).[22]

## CLASSIFICATION AND STAGING

Pituitary tumors are classified according to hormone secretion, secretory ability, size, and invasiveness. Most tumors are functioning, meaning that they are secreting a hormone and cause the ensuing clinical sequelae of the hormone secreted. Other tumors either do not secrete hormones or secrete them in such small amounts that no clinical manifestations are seen. Prolactinomas are the most common accounting for 40% of all functioning pituitary tumors. GH-secreting tumors resulting in acromegaly occur in approximately 20% of the cases, and ACTH-secreting tumors resulting in CS are found in approximately 10% of the tumors.[20]

Pituitary tumors are also classified according to size and divided into microadenomas with the greatest diameter being <10 mm and macroadenomas with the greatest diameter being ≥10 mm.[20] Most pituitary adenomas are microadenomas. Tumors are also characterized as intrasellar or extrasellar, depending on their ability to expand outside the sella turcica. In addition, depending on whether they can infiltrate into the dural and osseous walls, these tumors will be deemed invasive or noninvasive.[20] (See Table 52-2 for the staging of pituitary tumors).[24]

**TABLE 52-2**

**Staging of Pituitary Tumors**

The radiographical classification for pituitary adenomas

0. Normal pituitary appearance
I. Enclosed within the sella turcica, microadenoma, smaller than 10 mm
II. Enclosed within the sella turcica, macroadenoma, 10 mm or larger
III. Invasive, locally, into the sella
IV. Invasive, diffusely, into the sella

The grading schema for suprasellar extensions

1. 0 to 10 mm suprasellar extension occupying the suprasellar cistern
2. 10 to 20 mm extension and elevation of the third ventricle.
3. 20 to 30 mm extension occupying the anterior of the third ventricle
4. A larger than 30 mm extension, beyond the foramen of Monro, or Grade C with lateral extensions

*Source*: Data from National Cancer Institute.[24]

## THERAPEUTIC APPROACHES AND NURSING CARE

The goals of treatment for pituitary tumors include normalization of hormonal secretion and resolution or cessation of the progression of neurological defects. Interventions may include surgery, medical therapy, radiation therapy, or a combination of these modalities. The treatment of choice must be individualized and is dictated by the type of tumor, the nature of the excessive hormonal expression, and whether or not the tumor extends into the brain around the pituitary gland.

### Surgery

Surgery is the treatment of choice for most pituitary tumors. The exception is prolactinomas, which are generally managed medically. The transsphenoidal microsurgical approach to a pituitary lesion is the most widely employed surgical approach to pituitary lesions and represents a major development in the safe surgical treatment of both hormonally active and nonfunctioning tumors. See Figure 52-2. This approach is often successful in debulking tumors, even those that have a significant suprasellar extension. First the surgeon makes a small incision under the upper lip or along the nasal septum. The incision is then advanced along the septum back toward the sphenoid sinus. The boney walls of the sphenoid sinus are opened to reach the pituitary. The advantages of this approach are that no other part of the brain is touched, the neurological complication rate is very low, and there is no visible scar. The disadvantage of this technique is that it is difficult to remove large tumors. If the tumor is a microadenoma, then the cure rates are greater than 80%, if surgery is done by an experienced neurosurgeon.[21] If the tumor is large or has invaded the nearby nerves, brain tissue or its coverings, the chances for a cure by surgery are lower.

A contraindication to this approach includes tumors with a significant suprasellar extension with an hourglass-shaped narrowing between the intrasellar and suprasellar component causing blind attempts to reach the suprasellar tumor, which may lead to cerebral damage. In addition, an infection in the sphenoid sinus is potentially a contraindication to the transsphenoidal approach. In such cases, craniotomies via a pterional or subfrontal approach may be performed.[20] Rapid deterioration of vision is an immediate indication for surgery to relieve pressure produced by an expanding tumor mass, except in the case of macroprolactinomas where intensive observation with a patient on dopaminergic agonists may be an acceptable alternative.

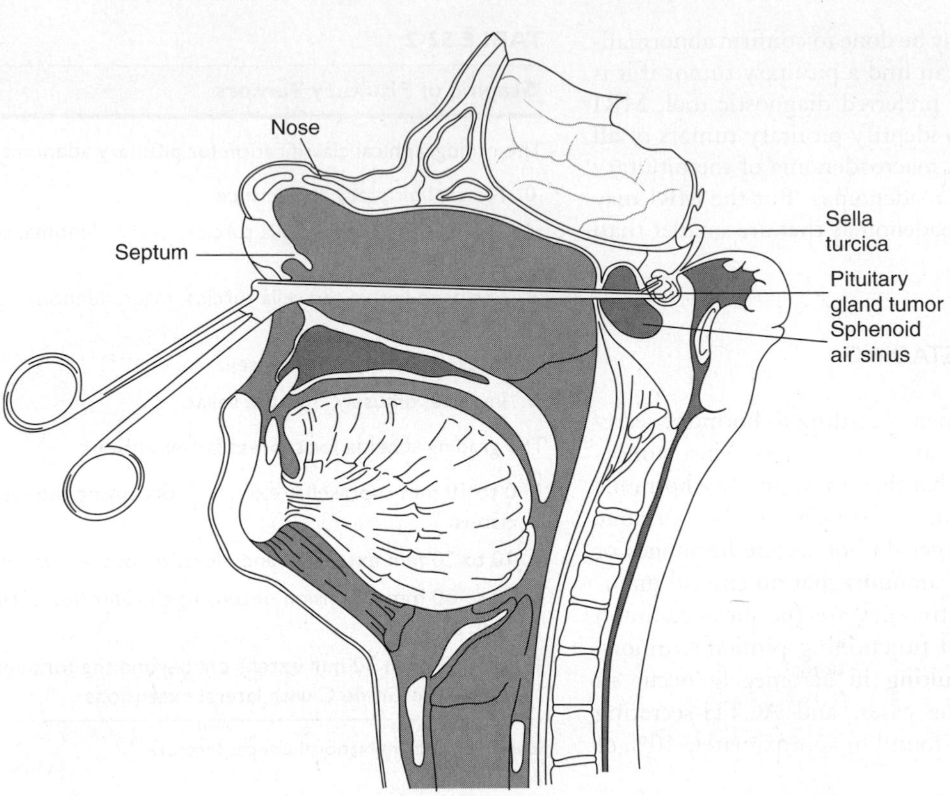


**FIGURE 52-2**

Transsphenoidal surgical resection of a pituitary tumor. The upper lip is retracted and an incision is made in the gingival mucosa. After displacing the septal cartilage, the surgeon removes the anterior wall of the sphenoid sinus and the floor of the sella turcica. The pituitary tumor is removed using the microsurgery technique in an attempt to preserve normal pituitary structure and function.

Progressive deterioration of visual fields is often the primary neurological criterion on which surgical management decisions are based.

Recently, surgeons have been using endoscopic surgery. The surgeon passes instruments through the nasal passages and opens the sphenoid sinus to reach the pituitary gland and remove the tumor. This procedure may take less time than the usual one and causes fewer complications, but its use is limited by the tumor size and position, and the character of the sphenoid sinus.[20]

## Radiation therapy

Conventional radiation therapy is an effective adjunct to the treatment of pituitary tumors. The advantages of radiation therapy are that it is noninvasive and suitable for surgically high-risk patients. The clinical and biochemical response, however, is slow and may require from 2 to 10 years to determine a complete and sustained remission. In addition, radiation therapy carries a substantial risk of hypopituitarism, approximately 30% at 10 years.[20] Stereotactic radiation surgery by gamma knife may be a treatment option for patients with recurrent or residual adenomas. In these tumors, this approach aims to obtain the arrest of cell proliferation and hormone hypersecretion using a single, precise, high dose of ionizing radiation, thereby sparing surrounding structures.[11]

## Drug therapy

Unlike other pituitary tumors, surgery is usually not the first treatment for prolactin-secreting adenomas. Dopamine agonists, bromocriptine (Parlodel) and cabergoline (Dostinex) are drugs that are effective in both blocking prolactin production by these adenomas and preventing growth of these tumors so that surgery is usually not necessary. Cabergoline has an advantage of lasting longer, so it does not need to be taken as often. Side effects may also be fewer with cabergoline. About 80% to 90% of patients are able to control their prolactin levels with medication.[20] The drugs are very effective in reducing the size of prolactin-secreting macroadenomas. About 60% of these tumors shrink to less than half of their original size after medical treatment. Only about 15% to 20% of the tumors show no decrease in size after treatment. In addition, these drugs usually prevent prolactinomas from growing larger.[19] If successful, the drug treatment may be continued for life. Within 3 months of starting treatment, the blood prolactin level is measured again and the MRI scan is repeated to check whether the medication has been effective. If the response has not been good after 6 months or if serious side effects occur, then surgery may be considered. Possible side effects of these drugs include drowsiness, dizziness, nausea, vomiting, diarrhea or constipation, confusion, and depression.

If surgery is ineffective for GH-secreting tumors, medication management may be attempted. Drugs such as bromocriptine or cabergoline may reduce GH levels in about 20% of patients. Unfortunately, the high doses often needed to be effective are not well tolerated by some patients. Since higher doses are often used in treating GH-secreting adenomas, the side effects for these patients may be worse and occur more often. The advantage of these drugs is that they are taken orally.

Octreotide is a modified form of the natural hormone somatostatin. Somatostatin is made in the pituitary and other glands and was named for its ability to inhibit GH (somatotropin) secretion. Octreotide blocks GH production by adenomas and returns insulin-like growth factor-I (IGF-I) to normal levels in about 65% of patients. It is first given 50 to 100 μg as a subcutaneous injection 2 to 3 times per day. The dosage is then increased according to individual biochemical responses to a maximum level of 500 μg 3 times per day. A newer drug, lanreotide, has been effective in suppressing GH secretion and is given as an injection every 1 to 2 weeks or every month.[21] Both these drugs have minor side effects such as nausea, vomiting, diarrhea, stomach pain, dizziness, headache, and pain at the site of injection. Because these newer, long-acting preparations are convenient and effective, practitioners are beginning to question whether surgery should always be the first treatment for people with GH-secreting adenomas. In those who might have difficulty with surgery, such as frail elderly people, drug treatment might be a good choice as the first treatment.

## Nursing care

Patient teaching and monitoring is a crucial part of care provided by nurses to patients with pituitary tumors. From the time of diagnosis through treatment, observation and monitoring of subtle changes in neurological, visual, and physical status may indicate tumor growth or progression. Adequate teaching regarding diagnostic testing and significance of results is imperative in order for the patient and family to effectively manage diagnosis and treatment.

Postsurgical monitoring is one of the most important roles of the nurse in the care of the patient with a pituitary tumor. Patients are cared for in either an intensive care or neurological intensive care area immediately following surgery. Nurses monitor for postoperative complications that are usually transient but may have some long lasting effects. The most common of these complications is surgical trauma-related swelling of the pituitary and pressure on the pituitary stalk or posterior pituitary. If untreated, this may cause temporary DI that result in secretion of large volumes of dilute urine and sodium retention. If DI occurs, fluid losses are replaced, on a milliliter per milliliter basis each hour, until DI improves. Mild DI is usually managed with isotonic intravenous fluids. Vasopressin is administered in more severe cases, with the usual dose being 5 units subcutaneously every 4 to 6 hours until urine volume becomes normal.

Another complication of transsphenoidal surgery is a cerebrospinal fluid (CSF) fistula and leak that can lead to meningitis or tension pneumocephalus. The nurse must monitor the patient for signs and symptoms of meningitis, and check the dressing for glucose in any drainage, which would indicate CSF fluid. CSF leak presents as a persistent postnasal drip. Patients need to be educated to alert their health care professional if they experience a salty taste in their mouth, frequent swallowing or increased drainage when bending over. If CSF leak is confirmed, elevating the head of the bed and maintaining bed rest to decrease pressure are indicated. Other complications of surgery occur due to the proximity of the pituitary gland to other structures and includes vascular injury to the carotid artery, damage to cranial nerves III, IV, V, and VI, optic nerve or optic chiasm damage, anterior pituitary insufficiency and death.

Patients who undergo transsphenoidal surgery may be discharged from the hospital in as few as 3 days. Clear postoperative education is imperative. Patients are instructed regarding signs and symptoms of infection, medications to be taken, and diet and activity restrictions. They should be instructed to notify the surgeon for any fever greater than 101° F, any symptoms of meningitis including headache and stiff neck, persistent clear nasal drainage, persistent headache, visual changes and excessive thirst. Nurses are the key in reinforcing the need for follow-up both in the immediate postsurgical period and at regular intervals thereafter. Complications of therapy including hypopituitarism and tumor recurrence can occur as late as 30 years after treatment.

# ADRENAL TUMORS

The adrenals are triangular shaped glands that sit atop each kidney. They influence or regulate the body's metabolism, salt and water balance, and response to stress by secreting a variety of hormones.[25] The adrenal glands measure about one-half inch in height and 3 inches in length. Each gland consists of a medulla, the center of the gland, which is surrounded by the cortex. The adrenal cortex comprises about 90% of the adrenal gland. It synthesizes several corticosteroids essential for life in response to signals from the pituitary gland and other systems. The most important corticosteroids of the adrenal cortex are the glucocorticoid cortisol (hydrocortisone) and the mineralocorticoid aldosterone. In addition, the adrenal glands synthesize small amounts of androgens including testosterone and estradiol. Corticosteroids play an important role in the regulation of body systems and homeostasis including glucose, protein and lipid metabolism as well as wound healing, myocardial contractility and arteriolar tone. Corticosteroids also reduce the formation of inflammatory mediators such as prostaglandins, leukotrienes and histamine causing an overall general immunosuppression. Mineralocorticoids are critical to maintaining normal serum sodium balance and, to some degree, potassium balance. The primary stimulation for the synthesis of aldosterone is fluid loss with the pituitary playing a small part. Aldosterone causes the kidneys to secrete renin and continue production of angiotensin. Even though adrenal cortical hormones are released slowly, their actions are long lasting.

In the inner adrenal medulla the chromaffin cell is the principle cell type. The medulla is richly innervated by preganglionic sympathetic fibers and is, in essence, an extension of the sympathetic nervous system. It is a source of the catecholamines epinephrine and norepinephrine. Once these hormones are released into blood they bind adrenergic receptors on target cells, where they induce essentially the same effects as direct sympathetic nervous stimulation, although their effect is longer lasting. The physiological consequences of medullary catecholamine release are framed as responses that aid in dealing with stress. Some major effects mediated by epinephrine and norepinephrine are increased rate and force of contraction of the heart muscle, constriction of blood vessels, resulting in increased resistance and hence arterial blood pressure, dilation of bronchioles, stimulation of lipolysis in fat cells providing fatty acids for energy production, increased metabolic rate, and inhibition of certain "nonessential" processes such as gastrointestinal secretion and motor activity.[26]

Adrenal masses are among the most common tumors in humans, and although most cause no symptoms or health problems, a small proportion can lead to serious diseases. Approximately 1 out of every 4,000 adrenal masses is cancerous.[25] Several types of adrenocortical tumors arise from the cortex and pheochromocytomas arise from the medulla.

## ADRENOCORTICAL TUMORS

### Epidemiology

Adrenal cortical tumors, mostly benign adenomas, are frequent in the general population and most often found incidentally.[25] By contrast, adrenal cortical cancer (ACC) is rare with an estimated prevalence between 4 and 12 per million in adults.[26] In children, the incidence is approximately 10 times lower. In addition, ACC occurs more often in females. Although adrenal cancer is potentially curable at early stages, only 30% of these malignancies are confined to the adrenal gland at the time of diagnosis.[26]

### Etiology

There have been no absolute risk factors identified for the development of adrenal cortical tumors. Chromosomal alterations are observed in 28% of benign adrenocortical tumors.[26] Most of the changes observed concern losses on chromosomes 2, 11q, and 17p and gains on chromosomes 4 and 5. Over the past several years there has also been progress in understanding how certain genetic changes cause cells in the adrenal gland to become cancerous. The *insulin like growth factor-II* (*IGF-II*) gene is involved in the development of the adrenal cortex and its role has been documented in adrenocortical tumors.[26] *IGF-II* is strongly overexpressed in malignant adrenocortical tumors, with such overexpression observed in approximately 90% of ACC.[26] Germline mutations in the *tumor protein p-53* (*TP53*) gene are identified in 70% of families with Li-Fraummeni syndrome (LFS). LFS results in a very high risk of developing one or more types of cancer including ACC. Only small numbers of ACC are due to this syndrome, however, many other ACCs have also been found to have abnormal *p53* genes. Another genetic mutation linked with ACC is the *MEN1* gene. Adrenocortical tumors are observed in 25% to 40% of MEN1 patients.[26] The angiogenic status of a tumor can be assessed by the study of vascular endothelial growth factor (VEGF) expression. In ACC, an overexpression of VEGF by comparison with adrenal adenomas has been observed. Serum VEGF levels were significantly higher in patients with ACC than in patients with adrenal adenomas and normal subjects.[26]

### Pathophysiology

Adrenocortical cancer can be classified as differentiated, anaplastic or hormonal. Functioning tumors are usually differentiated. Production of hormones by anaplastic tumors is rare. Approximately 60% of adrenocortical cancers produce hormones. The associated clinical syndromes include the following; CS, adrenogenital syndrome, virilization, feminization, precocious puberty, hyperaldosteronism, and primary hyperaldosteronism (Conn's syndrome).

### Clinical Manifestations

In about half of the people with ACC, symptoms are caused by the hormones the tumor secretes. In the other half, symptoms occur because the tumor has grown so large that it invades nearby organs. In children symptoms are most often caused by androgens that the tumor secretes. The most common symptoms are excessive growth of facial, pubic and axillary hair, and enlargement of the penis in boys or the clitoris in girls. If the tumor secretes estrogens, however, the symptoms would include early puberty in girls, with breast enlargement and the beginning of menses. Breast enlargement may also be seen in boys. In adults with androgen or estrogen secreting tumors, the symptoms are less noticeable since their primary sexual characteristics are more fully developed. However, men with estrogen secreting tumors may have slight breast tenderness and enlargement. They may also experience impotence and decreased libido. Women with androgen secreting tumors may experience virilization including progressive hirsutism, acne, clitoral hypertrophy, menstrual abnormalities, deepening of the voice, frontal baldness and increased libido.

Benign or malignant adrenal cortical tumors are the cause of 20% to 25% of all cases of CS and result in symptoms in multiple body systems.[23] Patients with aldosterone secreting tumors present with symptoms of Conn's syndrome. These symptoms include hypertension, hypokalemia with serum potassium usually less than 3.5 mEq/L, hypernatremia and suppressed rennin effects. The hypokalemia may cause the most serious and life threatening symptoms including cardiac arrhythmias, abnormal electrocardiogram (ECG) changes, digitalis toxicity, weakness, polydipsia, and visual disturbances.

## Assessment

Often the diagnosis of adrenocortical tumors is delayed because the clinical manifestations are nonspecific. In addition, given the fact that ACC is so rare, most clinicians would not initially include this as a differential diagnosis with the presenting symptoms. Once ACC is suspected, confirmation is completed by correlating physical findings with laboratory findings and imaging studies. A 24 hour urine test is most often completed on patients with symptoms of high cortisol levels. This urine test will measure levels of cortisol and 17-hydroxy steroids in the urine. If a cortisol-producing tumor is present, levels will be abnormally high. Dexamethasone suppression tests may be added to the 24 hour urine or completed on serial serum samples. After administration of dexamethasone the urine or serum is tested for cortisol. The dexamethasone will decrease production of cortisol in people who do not have adrenal tumors. Therefore, if the cortisol level remains high, a cortisol secreting tumor is likely. Complete serum evaluation including complete blood counts, comprehensive chemistry and serum hormone levels will be completed for those patients suspected of having aldosterone, androgen or estrogen secreting hormones. Serum levels of these hormones will initially be evaluated. Patients with aldosterone secreting tumors will also have lower serum potassium, increased serum aldosterone and decreased serum rennin. For those patients with androgen or estrogen secreting tumors, there will be an increase in serum androgen or estrogen as well as an increase in urine 17-ketosteroids and 17-hydroxysteroids.[25,26] Serum FSH may also be measured with an elevation indicating an adrenocortical tumor.[25,26]

Imaging studies commonly used to assist in the diagnosis of ACC include ultrasound, CT, PET, and MRI. Ultrasound can be used to determine if there is a mass in the adrenal gland. CT shows the adrenal glands clearly and can often confirm the location of the tumor. An updated type of PET has been developed that uses a radioactive form of metomidate. This substance concentrates in adrenal cortical tissue, particularly adenomas and carcinomas.[27] MRI may sometimes provide more information than CT because it can better distinguish adrenal carcinoma from adenomas and may be able to confirm whether a tumor is invading into blood vessels.

## Classification and Staging

It is often difficult to histopathologically differentiate adrenocortical adenomas and carcinomas. Tumors do not synthesize hormones as efficiently as normal adrenal glands and tend to become large by the time they cause symptoms and are detected. Generally, adrenal tumors with malignant potential grow faster than those with a benign phenotype. But it has been noted that even adrenal tumors smaller than 2 cm at detection have already been metastatic.[11] Analysis has shown that ACC consists of monoclonal populations of cells indicating that tumor progression is the end result of an intrinsic genetic mutation, whereas benign tumors might be monoclonal as well as polyclonal.

A modified MacFarlane staging system in conjunction with traditional TNM staging is widely accepted in staging adrenocortical cancer.[23,28] Four different stages are differentiated with this staging system.[28] (See Table 52-3.) Stage I and II tumors are localized to the adrenal cortex and present a maximum diameter below or above 5 cm respectively.

**TABLE 52-3**

**Adrenal Cortical Cancer Staging Groups**

| Stage | Tumor Size | Local Metastasis | Distant Metastasis |
|---|---|---|---|
| I | Smaller than 5 cm (2 inches) | None | None |
| II | Larger than 5 cm (2 inches) | None | None |
| III | Any size | Yes | None |
| IV | Any size | Yes or No | Yes |

*Source*: Data from National Cancer Institute.[26]

Locally invasive tumors or tumors with regional lymph node metastases are classified as stage III, whereas stage IV consists of tumors invading adjacent organs or presenting with distant metastases. Stage I tumors have the best prognosis with 5-year survival rates for patients with stage I and II disease at about 50% to 60%.[28] Patients with stage III disease have a 5-year survival rate of about 20% with a corresponding rate of 10% for those with stage IV disease.[27] A better survival is usually reported in younger patients. Cortisol secreting tumors are associated with a worse prognosis. This could be due to the morbidity associated with CS.

### Therapeutic Approaches and Nursing Care

*Surgery.* Surgery of the adrenocortiol tumor is the major treatment of stage I, II and III ACC. Only complete tumor removal can lead to long-term remission. Open adrenalectomy is currently recommended as laparoscopic removal of malignant adrenocortical tumors could be associated with a high risk of peritoneal dissemination.[26] Substitutive glucocorticoid therapy should be started after surgery of cortisol secreting tumors to avoid adrenal deficiency. In stage IV patients, with distant metastases, tumor debulking with removal of the primary adrenal tumor may be used in order to improve both prognosis and reduce steroid excess.

*Radiation therapy.* Radiation therapy is usually considered not very effective to control tumor growth. However, it has been suggested in a recent study that tumor bed radiation therapy is effective in preventing local recurrence after surgical removal.[28]

*Chemotherapy.* When complete tumor removal is not possible, or in the case of recurrence, treatment with mitotane is recommended. Mitotane has both an anticortisolic action and inhibits steroid synthesis specific to the adrenal cortex. One review suggests that an objective tumor regression was observed in 25% of cases where mitotane was used.[29] In addition, a retrospective study on patients with cortisol-secreting ACC showed a better survival rate when starting treatment with mitotane 3 months following the surgery of adrenal tumor.[30] There are significant side effects associated with mitotane, mainly digestive and neurological, which often limit the ability to reach optimal blood levels. Toxicities include anorexia, nausea and vomiting, diarrhea, depression, somnolence, vertigo and peripheral neuropathy.

Several cytotoxic chemotherapy regimens have been used in ACC. They are usually considered in patients with tumor progression who have been treated with mitotane therapy. The current recommendations include a combined treatment with cisplatin, etoposide, and doxorubicin (EDP) along with mitotane or streptozotocin along with mitotane.[31] An international trial, the first international randomized trial in locally advanced and metastatic adrenocortical carcinoma treatment (FIRM-ACT) is currently being completed to investigate the efficacy of these 2 treatments.[26]

*Symptom management and supportive care.* Many patients with adrenal tumors have progressive disease at presentation due to delays in diagnosis. Because of the late stage of their disease, many do not respond to treatment. Palliative treatment is important for these patients in order to reduce the symptoms produced by excess hormone secretions. Patients with CS may be treated with drugs to block steroid synthesis that include aminoglutethimide, metyrapone and ketoconazole. Other drugs, such as mefiristone, block steroid actions in target organs. These drugs may all control symptoms but not tumor growth. Those patients with Conn's syndrome are treated with spironolactone, a potassium sparing diuretic, which is often administered to correct tumor induced hypokalemia. Nursing interventions aimed at identifying and treating side effects of hormone hypersecretion is crucial in the effective treatment of patients with adrenal tumors.

## PHEOCHROMOCYTOMA

### Epidemiology

Pheochromocytoma is a rare tumor of chromaffin cells most commonly arising from the adrenal medulla. An estimated 800 cases are diagnosed yearly in the US.[31] The peak incidence is in patients in their 20s, 30s, and 40s and occurs with equal frequency in males and females.[33,34] Bilateral disease is present in approximately 10% of patients. Bilaterality is much more common in familial pheochromocytoma and is often found in association with the familial multiple endocrine neoplasia syndromes (MEN, types 2A and 2B). Extra-adrenal pheochromocytoma or functional paraganglioma occurs in approximately 10% to 15% of cases and may arise from any extra-adrenal chromaffin tissue in the body associated with sympathetic ganglia. Extra-adrenal pheochromocytoma is most often located within the abdomen and may have greater malignant potential than adrenal pheochromocytomas. Extra-adrenal tumors usually have a poorer prognosis than adrenal tumors. Because of the production and release of catecholamines, pheochromocytomas cause hypertension. Only 0.1% to 2% of all patients with hypertension, however, will be found to have a pheochromocytoma.[35] The importance of the recognition of this disease is that more than 90% of patients properly diagnosed and treated are curable.[32]

## Etiology

Approximately 90% of pheochromocytoma tumors occur sporadically and the remainder occurs as part of MEN2A, MEN2B or other neuroectodermal syndromes. Other syndromes associated with pheochromocytoma include neurofibromatosis, von Hippel-Lindau disease, cerebellar hemangioblastoma, Sturge-Weber syndrome, and tuberous sclerosis. In a series of 82 unselected patients with pheochromocytoma, 23% were found to be carriers of associated familial disorders.[32] Therefore, all patients with pheochromocytomas should be screened for MEN2 and von Hippel-Lindau disease to avert further morbidity and mortality in the patients and their families.

## Pathophysiology

Histologically, pheochromocytoma is composed of large pleomorphic chromaffin cells. Approximately 10% of pheochromocytomas are considered to be malignant. No histological features exist that distinguish benign from malignant tumors. Microscopic evidence for local invasion of tissue or blood vessels, however, suggests malignancy. Criteria based on tumor size, mitotic index, and DNA ploidy have been reported to be helpful in some series, though they are not always reliable predictors of biological behavior.[32] Because the distinction between benign and malignant tumors cannot be made with certainty, careful surveillance is needed for a prolonged period after the initial surgical resection. Malignant tumors can metastasize to lymph nodes, bone, lung, liver, brain and omentum.

## Clinical Manifestations

The release of catecholamine is what causes the typical manifestation of pheochromocytomas: hypertension. Tumors that also produce large amounts of epinephrine can cause many symptoms in all organ systems. The hypertension caused by pheochromocytoma may be sustained or paroxysmal and is often severe with occasional malignant features of encephalopathy, retinopathy, and proteinuria and is experienced by 82% of patients.[11] Other clinical features of pheochromocytoma include headache, sweating, palpitation, tachycardia, and severe anxiety along with epigastric or chest pain. Perfuse sweating, palpitations, and headache are known as the "classic triad" and are often the presenting symptoms of someone with an undiagnosed pheochromoctytoma, although one review noted that this triad is appearing less often than was previously thought.[33] Orthostatic hypotension is frequently present and is probably caused by reduced intravascular volume following chronic adrenergic stimulation. Symptoms usually occur during a life-threatening crisis when excessive catecholamines are released into the bloodstream. However, excessive catecholamine release can also be spontaneously triggered by changes in position, increased abdominal pressure, exercise, micturation, intercourse, pain, labor, anesthesia, surgery or chemotherapy. Anticholinergic drugs may also cause catastrophic tachycardias, and other drugs including dopamine antagonists, tricyclic antidepressants, and naloxone may precipitate extreme hypertension.

The most severe complication is pheochromocytomas crisis, which may lead to encephalopathy that can progress to coma, shock, disseminated intravascular coagulation and multiple organ system failure.[32] Crisis episodes can vary from several minutes to an hour and can occur daily or sporadically. After a crisis episode the patient may have tremors and feel short of breath, weak or exhausted.

## Assessment

The diagnosis of pheochromocytomas is often delayed because hypertension is much more likely to be caused by other factors. Diagnosis is confirmed by correlating physical findings with laboratory results and localization procedures. The diagnosis of pheochromocytoma is established by the demonstration of elevated 24-hour urinary excretion of free catecholamines (norepinephrine and epinephrine) or catecholamine metabolites (vanillylmandelic acid and total metanephrines). The measurement of plasma catecholamines can also be of value in the diagnosis of pheochromocytoma. The measurement of plasma catecholamines, however, has limited sensitivity and specificity. Plasma metanephrines have been reported to be more sensitive than plasma catecholamines.[32] When 52 patients with pheochromocytoma were studied, every patient was found to have elevated plasma levels of metanephrines, but 8 of the patients had normal levels of plasma catecholamines.[32]

Once the diagnosis is confirmed by biochemical determinations, the localization and extent of disease should be determined. Ninety-seven percent of the tumors are found in the abdomen, 2% to 3% are found in the thorax, and 1% are found in the neck.[32] CT has a 93% to 100% sensitivity for detecting intra-adrenal pheochromocytomas of approximately 0.5 cm in diameter. The sensitivity of CT is slightly lower at 90% for localizing extra-adrenal disease of approximately 1 cm in size.[36] MRI offers slightly better sensitivity.

$^{131}$I metaiodobenzylguanidine (MIBG) has been found to be useful as a scintigraphic localization agent. If the tumor is not adequately localized by these methods, then MRI, or rarely, vena cava catheterization with selective venous sampling for catecholamines may be indicated. MIBG scanning has a lower sensitivity of only 80% but a specificity of 100%.[32] If extra-adrenal or metastatic disease is suspected, additional studies such as bone scan, liver-spleen scan, chest CT scan, or ultrasound may aid in determining the extent of disease.

## Classification and Staging

Most pheochromocytomas are benign and the presence of metastasis is the only reliable indicator of malignancy. There is no accepted staging system for pheochromocytoma. Data suggest that for patients with resectable, benign pheochromocytoma, the overall survival is equal to that of the age-matched normal population. Data reported from a systematic review suggest that the 5-year survival rate for patients with metastatic, malignant pheochromocytoma is approximately 40%.[32] In 3 retrospective studies of patients with either metastatic or recurrent pheochromocytoma, the 5-year survival ranged from 32% to 60%.[32] Patients with benign or malignant tumors may succumb from complications related to excessive catecholamine effects on normal systems, such as cardiovascular disease, cerebral vascular accident, renal disease or diabetes mellitus.

## Therapeutic Approaches and Nursing Care

*Surgery.* Surgery is the treatment of choice for pheochromocytomas that are benign, localized, or regional and may cure resectable disease. Surgery is also indicated to resect or debulk recurrent disease and metastases. The standard anterior approach to the adrenal gland is used, and the entire gland is removed; simple tumor excision should not be attempted.[31] The abdomen and retroperitoneum are examined thoroughly for the presence of extra-adrenal disease. After 1 week or more following surgery, repeated biochemical assays for catecholamines and/or metabolites are performed to confirm that all functioning pheochromocytoma has been removed. Preoperative medical management of the effect of excessive adrenergic stimulation is necessary. Preoperative nursing care focuses on ensuring adequate hydration, monitoring blood pressure and patient teaching. Patient teaching includes avoidance of straining and rapid changes in position. Intraoperatively, blood pressure is controlled by titration of small doses of phentolamine or nitroprusside, and cardiac arrhythmias may be treated with propranolol or lidocaine.[11] Postoperative monitoring of vital signs, hemodynamic status, fluid and electrolyte status and urinary output are crucial. Hypotension is common and should be treated with volume expansion. Postoperative hypertension is best treated with diuretics. The nurse also monitors for other postoperative complications including pain, bleeding, and infection.

*Radiation therapy.* Radiation therapy may be palliative for symptoms or for the morbidity resulting from local invasion by tumor. Treatment with targeted radiation therapy using $^{131}$I metaiodobenzylguanidine ($^{131}$I MIBG) has met with limited success. In approximately 35% of the patients screened, the tumor has sufficient uptake of the radioisotope to allow for a therapeutic dose.[32,37] In a group of 28 patients shown to have sufficient uptake of $^{131}$I MIBG, objective partial responses were observed in 29% of the patients, and biochemical improvement was noted in 43% of the patients.[32] In addition, radiation therapy can be effective for palliation of symptoms associated with bone metastases.

*Chemotherapy* Chemotherapy has been considered ineffective for pheochromocytoma. Several single agents and drug combinations have been evaluated in a limited number of patients with variable results. The most active chemotherapy regimen appears to be the combination of cyclophosphamide, vincristine, and dacarbazine (CVD).[32] CVD has been shown to produce partial remissions of moderate duration in symptomatic patients. Analysis of 23 patients treated with CVD showed 61% of the patients had objective evidence of tumor regression, and 74% of the patients had evidence of biochemical response.[37] In addition, improved control of hypertension, reduced need for antihypertensive medications, and improvement in overall performance status was observed.[32,37] Since hypertensive episodes have been reported following chemotherapy, patients need to be prepared with adrenergic blockers prior to treatment. No evidence exists that chemotherapy contributes to improved patient survival. Chemotherapy should be used only for palliation in symptomatic patients.

*Symptom management and supportive care* Patients with unresectable metastatic disease may experience recurrent hypertension that is normally managed with phenoxybenzamine, propanolol or labetolol.[32] It is important to point out that phenoxybenzamine, an irreversible, long-acting alpha-adrenergic antagonist, has several adverse effects including postural hypotension, tachycardia, miosis, nasal congestion, inhibited ejaculation, diarrhea and fatigue. This agent is initially administered at low doses and gradually increased. Another drug that patients may receive is metyrosine, which prevents the conversion of catecholamine precursors to catecholamines. The benefit of metyrosine is that it allows the use of lower doses of alpha-adrenergic blockers, which in turn, minimizes the potential side effects of those agents.

# MULTIPLE ENDOCRINE NEOPLASIA

Multiple endocrine neoplasia syndromes are rare, inherited conditions in which several endocrine glands simultaneously develop benign or malignant tumors or grow excessively without forming tumors. Symptoms vary depending on which glands are affected. (See Table 52-4.) MEN syndrome can appear in infants or in individuals as old as age 70.

**TABLE 52-4**

**Multiple Endocrine Neoplasia Syndromes**

| Syndrome | Major Organ Tumors | Presenting Symptoms/Comments |
|---|---|---|
| MEN1 | Parathyroid (hyperplasia), 80%–100%<br>Pancreas (insulinoma), 40%–85%<br>Duodenum (gastrinoma, VIPoma), 25%<br>Pituitary (prolactinoma, growth hormone-secreting adenoma), 30%–65%<br>Neuroendocrine (carcinoids), other sites, 5%–9% | • Presenting symptoms depend on organs involved and whether tumor secretes hormone. May include:<br>Hypercalcemia, urolithiasis<br>Hypoglycemia<br>Peptic ulcer, diarrhea<br>Galactorrhea, acromegaly<br>• Other, less common tumors: thymus, stomach, carcinoid, lipoma, spinal cord ependymoma<br>• Prediagnostic manifestations: 50% of patients have cutaneous manifestations, including angiofibromas, café-au-lait spots, confetti-like hypopigmented macules, multiple gingival papules |
| MEN2 | | |
| MEN2A | Thyroid (MTC), 70%<br>Adrenal medulla (pheochromocytoma), >50%<br>Parathyroid (adenoma), 15%–30% | • Presenting symptoms depend on organs involved and whether tumor secretes hormone. May include:<br>Diarrhea<br>Hypertension, palpitations<br>Hypercalcemia, urolithiasis |
| MEN2B | Thyroid (MTC), 100%<br>Adrenal medulla (pheochromocytoma) | • Onset of MTC is 10 years earlier than MEN2A, most aggressive<br>• Developmental abnormalities accompany syndrome: typical facies, marfanoid appearance, oral mucosa, conjunctiva, intestinal mucosa<br>• Ganglioneuromas may cause difficult swallowing, vomiting, constipation, diarrhea<br>• Parathyroid adenomas are noted to be rare to absent |
| Familial MTC | | • Hypercalcemia, urolithiasis<br>• More benign than MEN2A, good prognosis |

*Abbreviations*: MEN, multiple endocrine neoplasia; MTC, medullary thyroid cancer, VIP, vasoactive intestinal peptide.

*Source*: Data from Yip et al[37]; Komminoth et al[38]; Marx[39]; Gibril et al[40]; and Hermans et al.[41]

MEN syndromes occur in 3 patterns, types 1, 2A, and 2B, although the types occasionally overlap.[43] (See Table 52-5.) The tumors and the abnormally large glands often produce excess hormones. Although tumors or abnormal growth may occur in more than 1 gland at the same time, changes often take place over time. MEN syndromes are caused by inherited genetic mutations. A single gene responsible for type 1 disease has been identified. Abnormalities in a different gene have been identified in people with types 2A and 2B disease.

## MULTIPLE ENDOCRINE NEOPLASIA 1

Multiple endocrine neoplasia 1 includes a varying combination of more than 20 endocrine and nonendocrine tumors. The most frequent endocrine tumors associated with MEN1 include parathyroid tumors, anterior pituitary tumors, and endocrine tumors of the gastro-entero-pancreatic tract. Patients may have tumors in one or more of these sites simultaneously. Parathyroid tumors are seen in 80% to 100% of all patients with MEN1 at a mean age of 19, whereas 30% to 65% of patients develop an additional single, pituitary adenoma.[43] Less frequently, patients may develop thyroid tumors, carcinoid tumors or adrenocortical tumors. Nonendocrine tumors associated with MEN1 include facial angiofibromas, collagenomas, lipomas, menigiomas, ependymomas and leiomyomas. MEN1 is quite rare, occurring in about 3 to 20 persons out of 100,000. It affects both genders equally and shows no geographical, racial or ethnic preferences.

### Etiology

Multiple endocrine neoplasia 1 is inherited in an autosomal-dominant manner. Approximately 10% of cases are caused by de novo mutations. Each child of an individual

**TABLE 52-5**

**Conditions That Occur With Multiple Endocrine Neoplasia (MEN)**

| Condition | MEN1 | MEN2A | MEN2B |
|---|---|---|---|
| Parathyroid gland tumors | ≥ 90% | 10–20% | – |
| Pancreatic tumors | 60%–70% | – | – |
| Pituitary gland tumors | 15%–42% | – | – |
| Thyroid gland tumors (specifically medullary carcinoma) | – | > 90% | >90% |
| Pheochromocytoma (tumor of the adrenal glands) | – | 50% | 60% |
| Neuromas on mucous membranes | – | – | ≅ 100% |
| Bodily changes similar to those in people with Marfan syndrome | – | – | ≅ 100% |

*Source*: Used with permission from Porter.[42] Copyright © 2008 by Merck & Co, Inc.

*Abbreviation*: MEN, multiple endocrine neoplasia.

with MEN1 has a 50% chance of inheriting the mutation. Multiple endocrine neoplasia is the only gene known to be associated with MEN1 syndrome. It is found on the long arm of chromosome 11, and has been confirmed to lie at 11q13. The function of the *MEN1* gene is unknown and at least 12 mutations have been identified. Multiple endocrine neoplasia germline mutations are identified in about 80% to 90% of patients with familial MEN1 syndrome and in 65% of individuals with nonfamilial MEN1 syndrome.[44,45] Approximately one half of the mutations involve chromosomal deletions while only about 15% involve insertions.[45] Tumors occur because of a second mutation in the normal allele that results in the loss of that allele, suggesting that *MEN1* is a tumor suppressor gene.[45]

## MULTIPLE ENDOCRINE NEOPLASIA 2

Approximately 1 out of 500,000 individuals will develop MEN2. Individuals with MEN2 develop hyperplasia or tumors of the thyroid, parathyroid and adrenal glands. The MEN2A subcategory is more common and accounts for 90% of cases whereas 5% of cases are attributed to MEN2B.[43]

### Multiple endocrine neoplasia 2A (MEN2A)

The most common and classic sign of MEN2A is hyperplasia of thyroid C cells that progress to MTC. The *RET* gene is most commonly associated MEN2A. The majority of carriers, 70%, develop tumors by age 70 years and more than 95% develop MTC. Prognosis depends on successful treatment of MTC. About 50% of patients with MEN2A also develop pheochromocytomas. Most of these tumors are benign and manifest with severe and often prolonged hypertension. Parathyroid adenomas occur less frequently affecting 15% to 30% of patients with development of the tumor occurring much later than those with MEN1.

### Multiple endocrine neoplasia 2B (MEN2B)

Multiple endocrine neoplasia2B can consist of MTC, pheochromocytomas, and neuromas. Some individuals with MEN2B disease have no family history and only de novo gene mutations. The MTC that occurs in MEN2B disease tends to develop at an early age and has been found in infants as young as 3 months of age. The medullary thyroid tumors in MEN2B disease grow faster and spread more rapidly than those in MEN2A disease. Most people with MEN2B disease develop neuromas in their mucous membranes. The neuromas appear as glistening bumps around the lips, tongue, and lining of the mouth. Neuromas may also occur on the eyelids and glistening surfaces of the eyes, including the conjunctiva and cornea. The eyelids and lips may thicken. Digestive tract abnormalities cause constipation and diarrhea. Occasionally, a megacolon develops. These abnormalities probably result from neuromas growing on the intestinal nerves. Individuals with MEN2B disease often develop spinal abnormalities, especially kyphosis, scoliosis and lordosis. They may also have abnormalities of the bones of the feet and thighs. Many people have long limbs and loose joints. Puberty is delayed in patients with MEN2B, and their reproductive rates are low secondary to mortality, impotence, and infertility.

### Etiology

Rearranged during transfection, a proto-oncogene located on the long arm of chromosome 10 has been confirmed to be responsible for MEN2. A number of different mutations can lead to MEN2A, but only one specific genetic alteration leads to MEN2B. *RET* is a dominant transforming gene for cancer and a mutation results in a permanently activated mutant receptor that responds to its intrinsic tyrosine kinase enzyme activity. A mutation in only one copy of the *RET* gene is sufficient to cause disease. More than 92% of patients in MEN2 families have mutations in the *RET* gene.[11]

## ASSESSMENT AND SCREENING

Because about one half of the children of individuals with MEN syndromes inherit the disease, baseline and ongoing screening for these individuals is the focus of management. There are no standard recommendations for screening because of the differences in availability of genetic screening and treatment options. However, annual screening may focus on laboratory evidence of the overexpression of hormones from hypersecreting tumors. Classical diagnosis of MEN is based on clinical features and on testing for elevated hormone levels. For MEN1, the relevant hormone is PTH. For both types of MEN2, the greatest concern is development of MTC. It can be detected by measuring levels of the thyroid hormone, calcitonin. Numerous other hormone levels can be measured to assess the involvement of the various other endocrine glands. Diagnosis of MEN2B can be made by physical examination alone. However, MEN2A shows no distinct physical features and must be identified by measuring hormone levels or by finding endocrine tumors.

Multiple endocrine neoplasia 1 is most commonly diagnosed when patients are in their forties, but can be diagnosed in the teens or twenties if stringent monitoring of serum hormone levels is completed. It is recommended that annual testing begin between the ages of 8 and 15. If an individual does not show evidence of disease by age 30, the risk of being a gene carrier is decreased to 10%.[46] However, testing should continue since the maximal age for conversion is unknown.

Genetic testing for *RET* mutations in family members with a known risk for MEN2A and MEN2B is the diagnostic method of choice.[43] In more than 90% of cases a *RET* mutation can be determined. Individuals who are identified as carriers of the *RET* gene can be offered total thyroidectomy on a prophylactic basis to prevent the development of MTC.

Annual screening for MEN2A gene mutation carriers is recommended to start by age 4 or 5 and continue to age 20. This screening includes laboratory testing for plasma calcitonin after intravenous pentagastrin or calcium stimulation, urinary or serum catecholamines, and serum calcium, and monitoring of blood pressure. Imaging of the adrenal glands may also be employed. Testing for calcitonin involves the injection of pentagastrin or calcium and the measurement of serum calcitonin at baseline, 2 to 3 minutes post-injection, and 5 to 10 minutes post-injection. Reproducible serum calcium elevations above normal indicate the need to proceed to total thryroidectomy. Patients whose calcitonin levels are borderline are retested in 3 to 6 months. Unfortunately, these calcitonin provocation tests may result in false-negative and false-positive results.[43]

## THERAPEUTIC APPROACHES AND NURSING CARE

Physicians, nurses, genetic counselors and psychologists that are knowledgeable in inherited cancer syndromes are imperative for effective treatment of patients with MEN syndromes. Skill in gathering a family history that includes a pedigree is most beneficial in the interpretation of risk and identification for further diagnostic testing. Nurses should be knowledgeable in the issues surrounding genetic testing and offer education and support to the patient and family.

There is no known cure for any of the multiple endocrine neoplasia syndromes. Changes in each gland are treated individually. Tumors are treated by surgical removal when possible. Drugs to correct the hormone imbalance caused by gland overactivity are also administered. Because MTC is ultimately fatal if untreated, prophylactic surgical removal of the thyroid gland if genetic testing has revealed evidence of type 2A or type 2B disease, even if the diagnosis of MTC has not been made is recommended. Once the thyroid is removed, individuals must take thyroid hormone for the rest of their life.

## CONCLUSION

Most of the endocrine tumors that occur are rare and benign. However, when they do occur, both benign and malignant tumors may cause significant morbidity, mortality and decreased quality of life. Because of the rarity of these cancers and the seemingly common clinical manifestations accompanying them, diagnosis is often delayed to a point beyond curative treatment. Because of the delay in diagnosis, the continued hypersecretion of hormones can be devastating to normal physiological functions. Nursing care for patients with endocrine tumors requires knowledge of hormone secretion and their effects on body systems. Monitoring of these hormonal effects and administration of recommended therapies often falls in the hands of the nurse. With knowledge of the genetic etiology of many of these tumors including hereditary and non hereditary causes, the nurse can help to identify risk and decrease the time to diagnosis. Symptom assessment and management is often the focus of nursing, particularly when dealing with individuals with endocrine tumors.

## REFERENCES

1. Jemal A, Siegel R, Ward E, Hao Y, Xu J, Thun MJ. Cancer Statistics, 2009. *CA: Cancer J Clin.* 2009;59:225–249.
2. Burke JP, Hay ID, Dagan F, et al. Long term trends in thyroid carcinoma: a population based study in Olmsted County, Minnesota, 1935–1999. *Mayo Clinic Proc.* 2005;80:753–758.
3. Davies L, Welch HG. Increasing incidence of thyroid cancer in the United States, 1973–2002. *JAMA.* 2006;295:2164–2167.

4. Mazzaferri EL, Kloos RT. Clinical review 128: current approaches to primary therapy for papillary and follicular thyroid cancer. *J Clin Endocrinol Metab.* 2001;86:1447–1463.
5. Sampson E, Brierley JD, Le LW, et al. Clinical management and outcome of papillary and follicular (differentiated) thyroid cancer presenting with distant metastasis at diagnosis. *Cancer.* 2007;110:1451–1456.
6. Greene FL, Page DL, Fleming ID, et al. *AJCC Cancer Staging Manual,* 6th ed. New York: Springer; 2002.
7. Xing M. BRAF mutation in thyroid cancer. *Endocrine-Related Cancer.* 2005;12:245–262.
8. Fragin JA. Challenging dogma in thyroid cancer molecular genetics—role of RET/PTC and BRAF in tumor initiation. *J Clin Endocrinol Metab.* 2004;89:4280–4284.
9. Sherman SI. Thyroid carcinoma. *The Lancet.* 2003;361:501–511.
10. Sywak M, Pasieka JL, Ogilvie T. A review of thyroid cancer with intermediate differentiation. *J Surg Oncol.* 2004;86:44–54.
11. Goodman M, Wickham R. Endocrine malignancies. In: Yarbro CH, Frogge MH, Goodman M, eds. *Cancer Nursing Principles and Practice.* 6th ed. Sudbury, MA: Jones and Bartlett; 2005:1215–1243.
12. American Association of Clinical Endocrinologists and Associazione Medici Endocrinologi. American association of clinical endocrinologists and assiciazione medici endocrinology medical guidelines for clinical practice for the diagnosis and management of thyroid nodules. *Endocr Pract.* 2006;12:63–102.
13. Brierley JD, Tsang RW. External beam radiation therapy for thyroid cancer. *Endocrinol Metab Clin.* 2008;37:497–509.
14. Cooper DS, Doherty GM, Haugen BR, et al. Management guidelines for patients with thyroid nodules and differentiated thyroid cancer. *Thyroid.* 2006;16:109–143.
15. Carling T, Udelsman R. Thyroid tumors. In: DeVita VT Jr, Hellman S, Rosenberg SA, eds. *Cancer: Principles and Practice of Oncology.* 7th ed. Philadelphia: Lippincott, Williams & Wilkins; 2005:1502–1519.
16. Clayman GL, Gonzalez HE, El-Naggar A, et al. Parathyroid carcinoma: evaluation and interdisciplinary management. *Cancer.* 2004;100:900–905.
17. Shane E. Clinical review 122: parathyroid carcinoma. *J Clin Endocrinol Metab.* 2001;86:485–493.
18. Fraker DL. Parathyroid Tumors .In: DeVita VT Jr, Hellman S, Rosenberg SA, eds. *Cancer: Principles and Practice of Oncology.* 7th ed. Philadelphia: Lippincott, Williams & Wilkins; 2005:1521–1527.
19. Messerer CL, Bugis SP, Baleski C, et al. Normocalcemic parathyroid carcinoma: an unusual clinical presentation. *World J Surg Oncol.* 2006;4:10–15.
20. Chanson P, Salenave S. Diagnosis and treatment of pituitary adenomas. *Minerva Endocrinol.* 2004;29:241–275.
21. Ghandi CD, Post KD. Neoplasms of the endocrine glands: pituitary neoplasms. In: Kufe DW, Pollock RE, Weichselbaum RR, et al, eds. *Cancer Medicine,* 6th ed. Hamilton, Ontario: BC Decker; 2003:1251–1258.
22. Cook DM, Ezzat S, Katznelson, et al. American Association of Clinical Endocrinologists (AACE) medical guidelines for clinical practice for the diagnosis and treatment of acromegaly. *Endocr Pract.* 2004;10:213–225.
23. Arnaldi T, Angeli A, Atkinson AB, et al. Diagnosis and complications of Cushing's syndrome: a consensus statement. *J Clin Endocrinol Metab.* 2003;88:5593–5603.
24. National Cancer Institute: Pituitary Tumors. http://www.cancer.gov/cancertopics/pdq/treatment/pituatry/healthprofessional. Accessed December 28, 2009.
25. Grumbach MM, Biller BMK, Braunstein GD, et al. Management of clinically inapparent adrenal mass ("Incedentiloma") NIH Conference. *Ann Intern Med.* 2004;138:424–429.
26. Libe R, Fratticci A, Berthearat J. Adrenocortical cancer: pathophysiology and clinical management. *Endocrine-Related Cancer.* 2007;14:13–28.
27. National Cancer Institute. *Adrenocortical Carcinoma Treatment.* http://www.cancer.gov/cancertopics/pdq/treatment/adrenocortical/HealthProfessional. Accessed January 1, 2010.
28. Norton JA. Adrenal tumors. In: DeVita VT Jr, Hellman S, Rosenberg SA, eds. *Cancer: Principles and Practice of Oncology.* 7th ed. Philadelphia, PA: Lippincott, Williams & Wilkins:; 2005:1528–1539.
29. Allolio B, Fassnacht M. Adrenocortical carcinoma: clinical update. *J Clin Endocrinol Metab.* 2006;91:2650.
30. Abvien G, Coste J, Groussin L, et al. Bioclinical features in the prognosis of adrenocortical cancer: poor outcome of cortisol-secreting tumors from a series of 202 consecutive patients. *J Clin Endocrinol Metab.* 2006;91:2650–2655.
31. Fassnacht M, Hahner S, Polat B, et al. Efficacy of adjuvant radiotherapy of the tumor bed on local recurrence of adrenocortical carcinoma. *J Clin Endocrinol Metab.* 2006;91:4501–4504.
32. Petri BJ, vanEijck CHJ, deHerderer WW, Wagner A, Krijger RR Pheochromocytomas and sympathetic paragangliomas. *Br J Surg,* 2009; 96:1381–1392.
33. Reisch N, Peczkowska M, Januszewicz A, et al. Pheochromocytoma: presentation, diagnosis, and treatment. *J Hypertension.* 2006;24: 2341–2143.
34. Cook LK. Emergency: pheochromocytoma. *Am J Nurs.* 2009;109: 50–53.
35. Calhoun DA, Jones D, Textor S, et al. Resistant hypertension: diagnosis, evaluation, and treatment: a scientific statement from the American Heart Association Professional Education Committee of the Council for High Blood Pressure Research. *Circulation.* 2008;117:e510-e526.
36. Ilias I, Pacak K. A clinical overview of pheochromocytomas/paragangliomas and carcinoid tumors. *Nucl Med Biol.* 2008;35(suppl 1): S27-S34.
37. Huang H, Abraham J, Hung E, et al. Treatment of malignant pheochromocytoma/paraganglioma with cyclophosphamide, vincristine, and dacarbazine: recommendation from a 22-year follow-up of 18 patients. *Cancer.* 2008;113:2020–2028.
38. Yip L, Gilbert JC, Shapiro SE, et al. Multiple endocrine neoplasia type 2: evaluation of the genotype-phenotype relationship. *Arch Surg.* 2003;138:409–416.
39. Lomminoth P, Heitz PU, Kloppel G. Pathology of MEN-1: morphology, clinicopathologic correlations and tumor development. *J Intern Med.* 1998;243:455–464.
40. Marx SJ. Multiple endocrine neoplasia type 1. In: Vogelstein B, Kinzler KW, eds. *The Genetic Basis of Human Cancer.* New York, McGraw-Hill; 1998:489–506.
41. Gibril F, Schumann M, Pace A, et al. Multiple endocrine neoplasia type 1 and Zollinger-Ellison syndrome: a prospective study of 107 cases and comparison with 1009 cases from the literature. *Medicine.* 2004;83:43–83.
42. Hermans MMH, Lips CJM, Bravenboer B. Growth hormone overproduction in a patient with multiple endocrine neoplasia type 1. *J Intern Med.* 2000;248:525–530.
43. Porter RS, ed. Conditions that occur with multiple endocrine neoplasia. *The Merck Manual of Medical Information,* 2nd ed. Whitehouse Station, NJ: Merck & Co, Inc. http://www.merck.com/mmhe. Accessed October 1, 2009.
44. Skogseid B. Multiple endocrine neoplasia type 1. *Br J Surg.* 2003;90:383–385.
45. National Endocrine and Metabolic Diseases Information Service. *Multiple Endocrine Neoplasia Type 1.* http://www.endocrine.niddk.nih.gov/pubs/men1/men1.htm. Accessed October 1, 2009.
46. Lairmore TC, Piersall LD, DeBenedetti MK, et al. Clinical genetic testing and early surgical intervention in patients with multiple endocrine neoplasia type 1 (MEN1). *Ann Surg.* 2004;239:637–647.

CHAPTER

53

Lois Almadrones Cassidy, RN, MS, FNP, MPA

# Endometrial Cancer

## INTRODUCTION

Endometrial cancer is the fourth leading cause of cancer in women in the US where it is the predominant cancer of the female genital tract (see Table 53-1).[1] Globally, it is the seventh leading cancer in females and follows with cervical cancer.[2] Endometrial cancer has 10 times the incidence in North America and Europe than in the developing countries and is rising as life expectancy increases.[3] It may be the most curable cancer when diagnosed early. Endometrial carcinomas make up 97% of all cancers of the corpus uteri and are the subject of this chapter. The remaining 3% are uterine sarcomas.[4]

## EPIDEMIOLOGY

In 2009, an estimated 42,160 new cases of endometrial cancer were diagnosed in the United States, and an estimated 7780 women died of the disease.[1] Although incidence rates have been relatively stable, the number of deaths has more than doubled since the 1980s.[1,5] A woman's lifetime risk of developing endometrial cancer is 2.48 or 1 in 40.[1] The Federation of Gynecological Oncologists (FIGO) and the National Cancer Institute's Surveillance, Epidemiology, and End Results (SEER) data suggest that approximately 83% of endometrial cancers are diagnosed locally or in early stages I or II and survival rates range from 81% to 96%.[6,7] Although the age-adjusted incidence is 31% lower among African American women than Caucasian women, the age-adjusted mortality among African American women is 84% higher. This disparity is one of the largest observed in the SEER Program.[8]

The racial disparity with regard to incidence and mortality rates has been of great concern and the focus of several epidemiological studies. Ueda et al's[5] multivariate analysis of SEER data from 1988 to 2001 suggest that older age, African American race, lack of primary staging procedures, advanced stage, high grade, and nonendometriod histology were independent prognostic factors for worse survival rate.

**TABLE 53-1**

**Leading Sites of Cancer in US Women in 2009**

| Site | Incidence |
|---|---|
| Breast | 192,370 |
| Lung and bronchus | 103,350 |
| Colon and rectum | 71,380 |
| Endometrium | 42,160 |
| Non-Hodgkin's lymphoma | 29,900 |

Source: Data from Jemal et al.[1]

Madison et al[9] in a population-based study multivariate analysis suggest that the advanced stage of the disease at diagnosis was associated with race/ethnicity or income, but not both. Mortality was found to be statistically associated with African American ethnicity, increased age, aggressive histology, poor tumor grade, and advanced stage of the disease. Higher income and hysterectomy were associated with a decreased risk for death.[9]

Endometrial cancer is primarily a disease of postmenopausal women. The median age at diagnosis is 61 years. Approximately 5% of women will be diagnosed with the disease before the age of 40, and 20% to 25% will be premenopausal when diagnosed.[10]

## ETIOLOGY

Endometrial cancer has been classified as 2 types (I and II) and each type has different risk factors.[11] Type I is more common and is associated with hyperestrogenism. Type II, which does not appear to be related to hyperestrogenism, arises in atrophic endometrium of older women, has a more aggressive histology and less favorable prognosis.[12] Risk factors for the development of type II are less known than those for type I, but seem to be associated with the histological precursor of endometrial intraepithelial carcinoma (EIC).[13] The hyperestrogenism associated with type I can be attributed to obesity, anovulation, or exposure to excessive estrogen.[3] Endometrial cancer is therefore primarily related to postmenopausal status, obesity, nulliparity, late menopause, diabetes mellitus, polycystic ovarian syndrome, or the use of either tamoxifen or unopposed estrogen. Among these risk factors, obesity has the highest associated risk ratio.[14] The risk of dying from endometrial cancer is 6.25-fold higher in women with a body mass index (BMI) > 40 kg/m$^2$ than in women of normal weight.[15]

Obesity is defined as BMI (calculated as the weight in kilograms divided by the height in square meters) of 30 kg/m$^2$ or more.[16] The term overweight is defined as a BMI equal or greater than 25 kg/m$^2$. Obesity has increased to epidemic proportions in the United States, with the prevalence of age-adjusted obesity rising from 22.9% in 1988–1994 to 30.5% in 1999–2000 among US adults.[17–19] Among races and ethnic differences, African American women have the highest prevalence of obesity (33.2%) nearly twice as that of Caucasian women (17.3%) and 5 times more than Asian/Pacific Islander women (5.9%).[16] Obesity at the time of diagnosis (but not at younger ages) has been associated with the risk for endometrial cancer.[20] A prospective study in Sweden found that the relative risk (RR) for endometrial cancer in obese women vs the general population was 2.9, consistent with the literature in the United States (which finds an RR ranging from 2 to 4).[21] Saltzman et al[22] evaluated the risk in diabetic women and suggests that obesity is only a partial mechanism linking diabetes to endometrial cancer. The authors observed that the risk of endometrial cancer is particularly high in women with a recent diagnosis of diabetes. Two reasons are hypothesized: (1) women in the prediabetic and early diabetic states have elevated levels of circulating insulin and (2) like other hormones, eg, estrogen, insulin can influence endometrial cancer risk relatively quickly. Research by Lukanova et al[23] suggests women in the highest fifth of C-peptide levels (a marker of pancreatic insulin production whose production mirrors those of circulating insulin) after adjusting for BMI still had a 4.4-fold increase in endometrial cancer compared to women in the lowest fifth.[23] Diabetes and previously diagnosed hypertension are also strongly associated with the risk of endometrial cancer but the exact mechanism of action is not known.[22]

Excessive endogenous estrogen metabolism or production or inadequate progesterone levels have also been associated with the development of endometrial cancer. Several hormonal aberrations can be linked to obesity. Increased body size plays a role in androgen conversion to estrogen.[4,24] Women who are more than 50 pounds overweight would face a 10-fold increased risk of developing endometrial cancer.[4] In addition, body fat distribution may be an independent risk factor with the highest risk being in women who carry weight abdominally rather than peripherally.[13] Fat cells are an excellent storage depot for estrogen, and the chronic slow release of estrogen from these cells may account for the increased risk. In obese, postmenopausal women, secretion of serum sex-hormone-binding globulin (SHBG) is depressed, leaving higher concentrations of free estradiol in the blood. Obese women tend to have endocrine malfunctions, such as inadequate progesterone levels that cause anovulatory cycles with irregular menses. Chronic anovulation, such as in polycystic ovarian disease, results in the failure of progesterone to oppose chronic estrogen effects on the endometrium. Another source of endogenous estrogen can be feminizing ovarian tumors (eg, granulosa cell tumors).[4]

The use of unopposed estrogen therapy has been linked to an increased incidence of endometrial cancer. This problem can be virtually eliminated by cycling or combining estrogen and progesterone. Progesterone should be administered a minimum of 10 days per month.[25,26] Results of the Women's Health Initiative (WHI) study reported that women who took 0.625 mg of conjugated equine estrogen and 2.5 mg of medroxyprogesterone acetate daily were less likely to develop endometrial cancer than placebo group patients who did not take hormones (hazard ratio (HR) 0.81). However, there was an increased risk of ovarian cancer (HR 1.58), and more endometrial biopsies to assess vaginal bleeding were required in the estrogen with progesterone group. Therefore, the authors suggest caution in the use of continuous combined hormones.[27]

Tamoxifen, which acts as an antiestrogen on breast tissue, has a weak estrogenic effect on endometrial tissue and has been associated with thickening of the endometrium and changes from polyps to hyperplasia and cancer.[28–30] As early as 1989, Fornander and colleagues reported a 6.4-fold increase in women with breast cancer, receiving tamoxifen 40 mg daily vs the placebo group.[29] Data from the National Surgical Adjuvant Breast and Bowel Project (NSABP) in breast cancer prevention demonstrated a 2.53% increase in risk for endometrial cancer in women taking tamoxifen (95% confidence interval = 1.35–4.97). The greatest risk was in women over the age of 50. All endometrial cancers among the study group were diagnosed as stage I.[31] A genetic link also exists for a predisposition to develop endometrial cancer, particularly if the disease in family members is diagnosed at a young age.[11] Lynch II or hereditary nonpolyposis colorectal cancer (HNPCC) syndrome is associated with a lifetime risk of 40% to 60% for the development of endometrial cancer.[32,33] A woman should be referred to genetic counseling if she meets the modified Amsterdam criteria for this syndrome, which is defined as follows: three family members who have had an HNPCC-associated cancer—one being a first-degree relative and one of the other two having been diagnosed before the age of 50—in at least two successive generations.[11] Lu et al[34] concluded, after reviewing 223 families (who met the modified Amsterdam criteria), that women are at equal or higher risk of developing endometrial cancer than colon cancer, and that endometrial cancer as well as ovarian and colon cancer may be the initial cancer diagnosis.

## PREVENTION, SCREENING, AND EARLY DETECTION

The 2 most important factors that appear to have a protective effect against the development of endometrial cancer are oral contraceptives and cigarette smoking. Both of these factors are protective because they reduce the estrogenic stimulation on the endometrium known to be the causative factor in type I endometrial cancer.[11] Use of oral contraceptives, which since the 1970s have consisted mostly of progesterone, decreases a woman's risk of developing endometrial cancer for at least 12 months; this protection seems to persist for up to 15 years in nulliparous women. Similarly, smoking has been correlated with a reduction in risk, especially in women over the age of 50 due to the antiestrogenic effect of cigarette smoking on circulating estrogen concentrations, a reduction of body weight, and an earlier age of menopause among cigarette smokers. However, the risks of developing lung cancer and other health problems well outweigh any protection gained against endometrial cancer.[10,35] Pregnancy also reduces the risk of endometrial cancer because of the protective effect of high progesterone levels during pregnancy. Nulliparous women are twice as likely to develop endometrial cancer as women who have delivered a child.[11] The effect of physical activity on endometrial cancer has been studied but results vary. Friedenreich et al[36] reported in a cohort study of over 250,000 women in 9 European countries that no protective benefit was found in all women studied but some benefit was observed in the cohort of premenopausal women who reported either active or moderately active physical activity compared to inactive. Important risk reducing strategies that most women can control themselves are weight management and physical activity. Prevention of obesity through dietary intake that includes less animal fat and more fruits and vegetables as well as regular physical activity can contribute to the reduction of endometrial cancer.[12,37] A review of the evidence-based policy recommendations on cancer screening and prevention in both Canada and the United States found the following recommendations for preventing endometrial cancer: using progesterones to prevent cancer associated with estrogen replacement; using combination oral contraceptives; avoiding tamoxifen; controlling obesity, diabetes, and hypertension; avoiding a high-fat diet; and increasing breast feeding and physical activity.[38]

Endometrial atypical hyperplasia has a risk of progression to carcinoma of approximately 25%, and the standard treatment recommendation is hysterectomy. Although the incidence of endometrial cancer is 3% to 5% in women under 40 years of age, fertility preservation may be desired in the younger patient population.[39] Studies indicate that women with either atypical hyperplasia or well-differentiated adenocarcinoma confined to the endometrium who wish to maintain fertility may be offered the option of progesterone therapy with successful regression of their hyperplasia or early endometrial cancers in up to 75% of cases, with subsequent pregnancies reported.[40,41] There is no consensus on the ideal progestational agent, dosage, duration of treatment, or schedule for long-term surveillance.[42] The use of progestin-containing intrauterine devices (IUD) have also been successfully used to treat this population with grade 1 endometrial cancer and no evidence of extrauterine disease.[43] For these young women, who are compliant with treatment and undergo careful monitoring, including repeat endometrial biopsies usually every 3 to 6 months, to evaluate response, a benefit may be offered from this experimental option.[42]

Unfortunately, there is no sensitive and specific screening test for endometrial cancer. The Papanicolaou (Pap) smear will only occasionally detect an endometrial cancer. Although endometrial biopsy is 90% effective in detecting a cancer and can be accomplished in the outpatient setting, the procedure is not without morbidity and cost and is not recommended at this time as a screening procedure for the general population. The American Cancer Society currently recommends that women with an average or increased risk should be informed about the risks and symptoms of endometrial cancer at the onset of menopause and should be strongly encouraged to report any unexpected vaginal bleeding or spotting to their physicians. Women with a genetic risk belonging to an HNPCC kindred have a lifetime risk of 42% to 60% of developing endometrial cancer are advised to begin annual screenings at age 35, although this recommendation is based on expert opinion without definitive scientific evidence.[44] Special screenings of asymptomatic women on tamoxifen with either periodic endometrial biopsies or pelvic ultrasounds have shown no proven benefit.[45–47] Annual gynecological examinations are recommended for these women, as well as for the population at large.[12,31] Other screening techniques, such as transvaginal ultrasonography and endometrial biopsy, have been investigated but are not currently recommended as appropriate for screening in asymptomatic women.[11]

## PATHOPHYSIOLOGY

### CELLULAR CHARACTERISTICS

The uterine corpus is a muscular, hollow, pear-shaped organ with an endometrial lining composed of ciliated epithelial cells. Throughout the epithelium are small, tubular glands that extend to the myometrium, or muscle wall of the corpus. Endometrial cancer develops in the tubular glands of the epithelial layer. Tumors that arise in the lower uterine segment involve the cervix sooner and have a higher incidence of pelvic and para-aortic lymph node involvement than do tumors that arise higher in the fundus or other locations in the uterus. Similarly, tumors that have deep myometrial invasion tend to be more aggressive and those affected have a poorer survival rate.[10,48] Endometrial hyperplasia, primarily the atypical type, is a premalignant or precursor cytologic change that can progress to malignancy. However, simple or complex hyperplasia without atypia rarely progresses to cancer.[39] Newer terminology being discussed by the World Health Organization for these precursor lesions further distinguishes each into the precursor lesions associated with type I or type II endometrial cancer. The term endometrial intraepithelial neoplasia (EIN) represents the histopathological presentation of a monoclonal endometrial preinvasive glandular proliferation that is the immediate precursor to type I endometrial adenocarcinoma. The proposed term for the precursor lesion of type II endometrial cancer is EIC.[49]

The majority of endometrial cancers are adenocarcinomas. Three types of adenocarcinomas account for more than 80% of histological patterns—pure endometrioid adenocarcinoma, adenocarcinoma with a squamous metaplasia (formerly adenoacanthoma), and adenocarcinoma with squamous differentiation (formerly adenosquamous). The less frequent patterns include clear cell (mesonephroid) carcinomas, undifferentiated carcinomas, and papillary serous carcinomas. The clear cell and serous patterns are more aggressive than the other carcinomas.[10]

## PROGRESSION OF DISEASE AND PATTERNS OF SPREAD

Multiple factors affect the natural history and prognosis of endometrial cancer (see Table 53-2). These include histological type and differentiation (grade), stage of disease, myometrial invasion, peritoneal cytology, isthmus-cervix extension, pelvic and aortic lymph node metastasis, intraperitoneal spread, and adnexal metastasis.[10]

Endometrial cancer usually starts in the fundus and can spread to involve the entire endometrium. Through direct extension and infiltration, the cancer spreads to the myometrium, endocervix, cervix, fallopian tubes, and ovaries. In a landmark Gynecologic Oncology Group (GOG) study of patterns of disease spread, it was found that 22% of patients with seemingly uterine confined disease were found to have extrauterine spread, 11% had pelvic and/or para-aortic metastasis, 12% had positive peritoneal cytology, 5% had adnexal involvement, and 6% had gross intraperitoneal spread. Nodal metastases were related to tumor grade and depth of myometrial invasion, and patients with positive cytology, adnexal, or intraperitoneal spread also had increased frequency of nodal disease.[50] Recurrence appears in 38% of women with adnexal spread compared to 11% in women without such involvement.[50]

Metastatic spread is usually to the pelvic and para-aortic lymph nodes and has been positively correlated with tumor differentiation, stage of disease, and amount of myometrial invasion. Pelvic and para-aortic lymph node metastases can be present even in women with stage I disease, among which approximately 10% will have positive pelvic nodes, and stage II disease with positive pelvic nodes will have 30% to 40% positive para-aortic nodes.[48] Less common sites of metastases include the vagina, peritoneal cavity, omentum, and inguinal lymph nodes. Hematogenous spread often involves the lung, liver, bone, and brain. The size of the uterus, measured by uterine sound, has been used as an indicator of survival. However, because large uterine size can be secondary to concomitant disease, such as fibroids, uterine size is no longer included in the staging and prognosis of endometrial cancer.[10,48,50]

Histological differentiation is one of the most sensitive indicators of metastases and prognosis.[48] The less differentiated the tumor, the poorer the prognosis. grade 1 tumors are highly differentiated, grade 2 tumors are moderately differentiated, and grade 3 tumors are mostly solid or undifferentiated carcinomas.[48] Overall 5-year survival rates are 99.2% for patients with grade 1 tumors, 90.8% for those with grade 2 tumors, and 64.9% for those with grade 3 tumors and 54.9% for those with anaplastic tumors (Figure 53-1).[51]

The degree of myometrial invasion, another prognostic indicator, is generally classified as none (localized to the endometrium), superficial (invasion that is less than 50%), or deep (greater than 50%).[10,48] The greater the invasion, the poorer the prognosis. In addition, the less differentiated the tumor, the greater the chance of myometrial invasion. Thus, the grade of the tumor is combined with the degree of myometrial invasion to estimate survival.

During surgery, in addition to biopsies or resection, samples of peritoneal fluid or washings of the peritoneal cavity are obtained for staging purposes. Women with positive peritoneal washings associated with extrauterine disease usually have a more aggressive disease and a worse prognosis.[48,52]

**TABLE 53-2**

**Prognostic Indicators for Endometrial Cancer**

| Indicator | Good Prognosis | Poor Prognosis |
|---|---|---|
| Stage of disease | I | II, III, IV |
| Histology | Adenocarcinomas: nonserous, non-clear cell | Serous or clear cell |
| Tumor differentiation | Grade I | Grades 2, 3 |
| Myometrial invasion | Superficial or none | Deep (> 50%) |
| Nodal metastasis | None | Present |
| Peritoneal cytology | Negative | Positive |

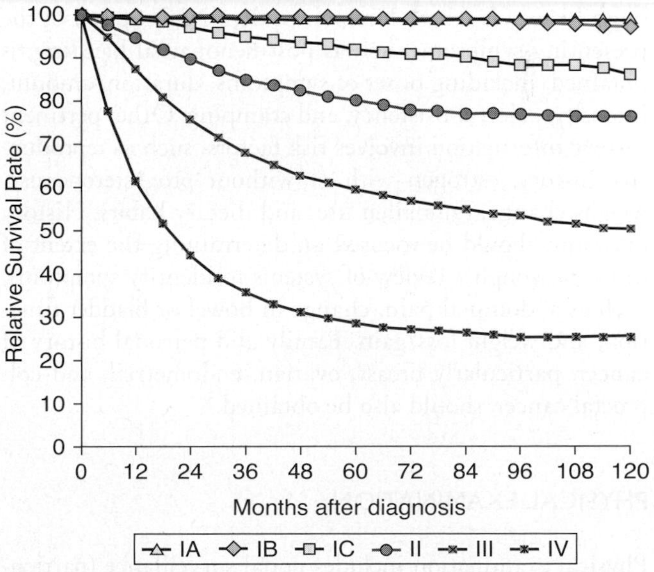


**FIGURE 53-1**

Adenocarcinoma of the corpus uteri: relative survival rate (%) by AJCC stage (SEER modified 3rd edition). Ages 20+, 12 SEER Areas, 1988–2001.

*Source*: Data from Kosary.[51]

Endometrial cancer tends to recur within the first 3 years following surgery. It can recur locally in the pelvis, regionally in the abdomen, or at distant sites outside the abdominal–peritoneal cavity. Patients whose tumors have good prognostic indicators rarely have distant metastases, while women with poorer prognoses more frequently have distant metastases.[48]

## CLINICAL MANIFESTATIONS

Abnormal vaginal bleeding, an early symptom associated with endometrial cancer, usually prompts women to seek medical attention. Postmenopausal bleeding should always be evaluated, even though only 20% of women with this symptom will have cancer. Any serosanguinous vaginal discharge or new heavy bleeding should also be evaluated. Premenopausal onset of irregular or heavy menstrual flow may be significant, especially if the patient is infertile with anovulatory cycles. Other less frequent symptoms include pyometria and hematometria, particularly in older women; and abdominal distension, lumbosacral, hypogastric, and pelvic pain in women may indicate more advanced disease.[48,53]

## ASSESSMENT

### PATIENT AND FAMILY HISTORY

In women suspected of having endometrial cancer, a thorough history is taken. First, an in-depth description of the presenting symptom, such as postmenopausal bleeding, is obtained, including onset of symptoms, duration, amount, intensity, color, consistency, and cramping. Other pertinent history information involves risk factors, such as reproductive history, estrogen with or without progesterone use, weight change, tamoxifen use, and dietary habits. History questions should be focused on determining the extent of disease through a review of systems to identify symptoms, such as abdominal pain, change in bowel or bladder function, and weight loss/gain. Family and personal history of cancer, particularly breast, ovarian, endometrial, and colorectal cancer, should also be obtained.[54]

### PHYSICAL EXAMINATION

Physical examination includes nodal surveillance (particularly supraclavicular and inguinal lymph nodes), lungs, abdomen for evidence of disease and organomegaly, and a complete pelvic examination (external genitalia, vagina, cervix, uterine size, adnexa, and rectovaginal bimanual examination) to evaluate the parametria and rectovaginal area.[54]

### DIAGNOSTIC STUDIES

A Pap smear will only occasionally detect an endometrial cancer. A more reliable diagnostic technique is endometrial biopsy, which allows histological rather than cytological examination. Endometrial biopsy, endocervical curettage, or Pap smears done in the outpatient setting have shown a 99% rate of detection of cancer in postmenopausal women. If the endometrial biopsy is negative and symptoms persist, a fractional dilatation and curettage (D&C) should be performed to obtain a differential diagnosis.[53,55]

Other diagnostic tests include transvaginal ultrasound, chest x-ray, stool guaiac, complete blood count (CBC), and blood chemistry profiles, including liver function studies. Cystoscopy, barium enema, and proctoscopy may be performed if bladder or rectal involvement is suspected. Though not routinely recommended, other studies that may be used to evaluate the status of pelvic, abdominal, and nodal disease include hysterography, hysteroscopy, lymphangiography, magnetic resonance imaging (MRI), and computerized axial tomogram scan.[48] A CA-125 level may be drawn and, if elevated, may indicate the presence of advanced or metastatic disease.[56] Although an MRI cannot distinguish benign from malignant neoplasms, it is effective in detecting the degree of myometrial invasion.[57] An MRI that shows no myometrial invasion may be of value in the decision to recommend progesterone therapy for women with early-stage endometrial cancer or atypical endometrial hyperplasia who desire to preserve fertility.[58]

### PROGNOSTIC INDICATORS

Prognostic indicators in endometrial cancer are obtained through surgical staging and pathological information. Good prognostic indicators include having risk factors that relate to endogenous or exogenous estrogen levels, such as obesity, estrogen use without progesterone, nulliparity, and late menopause; estrogen-related risk factors; histological grade 1 or 2; superficial myometrial invasion; no nodal metastasis; and stage I disease. In contrast, a poor prognosis involves histological grade 3, deep myometrial invasion, nodal metastasis, high stage, and aggressive histological behavior (usually clear cell or papillary serous).[48]

## CLASSIFICATION AND STAGING

Endometrial cancer is staged surgically (see Table 53-3),[59] if medical conditions and intra-abdominal disease permit the woman to be a candidate for surgery. Staging helps to define primary tumor size, location, and the extent of spread beyond the uterus. According to SEER data, approximately 70% of tumors are diagnosed in stage I, 9% in stage II, 6.8% in stage III, 9% in stage IV, and 4.8% unknown stage.[51]

**TABLE 53-3**

**FIGO Staging Classification: Corpus Uteri**

| | |
|---|---|
| I | Tumor confined to corpus uteri |
| IA | Tumor limited to endometrium |
| IB | Tumor invades up to or less than one-half of the myometrium |
| IC | Tumor invades more than one-half of the myometrium |
| II | Tumor invades cervix but does not extend beyond uterus |
| IIA | Endocervical glandular involvement only |
| IIB | Cervical stromal invasion |
| III | Local and/or regional spread |
| IIIA | Tumor involves serosa and/or adnexa (direct extension or metastasis) and/or cancer cells in ascites or peritoneal washings |
| IIIB | Vaginal involvement (direct extension or metastasis) |
| IIIC | Metastasis to pelvic and/or para-aortic lymph nodes |
| IV | |
| IVA | Tumor invades bladder mucosa and/or bowel mucosa |
| IVB | Distant metastasis (excluding metastasis to vagina, pelvic serosa, or adnexa, and including metastasis to intra-abdominal and/or inguinal lymph nodes) |

*Source*: Reprinted from the International Federation of Gynecology and Obstetrics (FIGO).[59]

The standard surgical staging and treatment of endometrial cancer includes bimanual examination under anesthesia, laparotomy through an adequate abdominal incision (usually vertical), exploration of the peritoneal cavity, peritoneal cytology, biopsies of suspicious areas, selective pelvic and para-aortic lymphadenectomy, total abdominal hysterectomy (TAH), bilateral salpingo-oophorectomy (BSO), and possible omentectomy and resection of tumor implants.[48,60] The best-trained physician to treat any gynecological cancer is a gynecologic oncologist. The Society of Gynecologic Oncologists recommends referral of women with known or suspected endometrial cancer to a gynecologic oncologist for surgery and subsequent surveillance.[61]

## THERAPEUTIC APPROACHES AND NURSING CARE

### EARLY-STAGE DISEASE

The goals of treatment in stage I and II disease are for cure and long-term survival; thus, nursing care must focus on managing the side effects of treatment and promoting health maintenance behaviors.

#### Surgery

Treatment of endometrial cancer includes surgical staging, TAH, BSO, pelvic and para-aortic lymphadenectomy, and peritoneal washings. Surgical staging is initially done on all women who are surgical candidates so that adjuvant radiation, if needed, can be tailored to the individual's extent of disease. Many women with early-stage disease will not need additional therapy beyond the initial surgery, thus avoiding the time, effort, and morbidity associated with adjuvant radiation therapy. A second reason for initial surgical staging is because the pathologist is better able to evaluate untreated tissue for the histological indicators of prognosis (histological type, grade, and myometrial invasion).[60,62]

An alternative method for surgical staging of endometrial cancer that has gained popularity is minimally invasive surgery (see Figure 53-2).[63] Childers and associates first reported successful laparoscopically assisted vaginal hysterectomies (LAVHs) in women with early-stage endometrial cancer.[64] Laparoscopy is associated with few complications, shorter hospital stays and recovery time, cosmetically better outcomes, and lower overall hospital charges. Women also report a higher level of satisfaction with laparoscopy compared to women treated with laparotomy.[63,65] Barakat and associates reported that the median number of lymph nodes sampled during surgery increased with laparoscopy, which led to fewer women requiring whole abdominal radiation postoperatively. This change in the treatment paradigm also seems to decrease morbidity with no significant difference in overall survival.[66] LAVH must be done by a physician who is well trained in this technique, including laparoscopic lymph node dissections. One contraindication

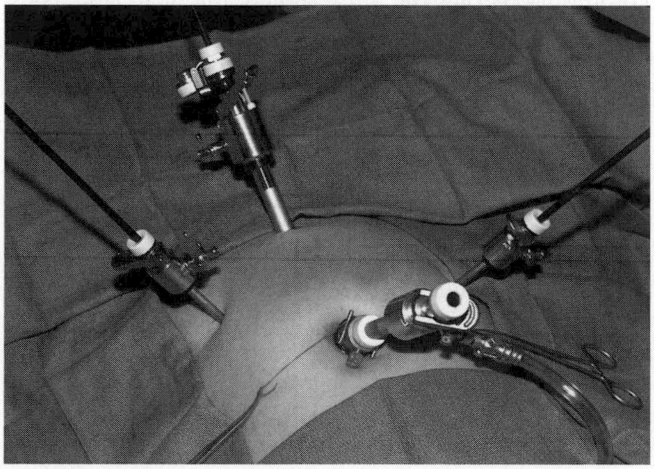

**FIGURE 53-2**

Minimally invasive surgical staging procedure using reusable or disposable trocars.

*Source*: Reprinted from Sonoda,[63] courtesy of Levine et al.

for laparoscopic surgery may be the obese patient, with a BMI greater than 28—a relative weight greater than 120% of the desirable weight.[67] The GOG is currently analyzing results of a randomized phase III (GOG-LAP2) trial comparing LAVH to the standard laparotomy to determine equivalency in cancer outcomes and quality of life.[68] National Comprehensive Cancer Network (NCCN) guidelines recommend that LAVH with pelvic and para-aortic dissection patients should be followed over a long term to compare their outcomes with those women who have traditional laparotomy.[60]

Prior to undergoing surgery for endometrial cancer, women must be thoroughly informed about surgical procedures, recovery, and self-care issues (see Table 53-4). Postoperative care includes fluid and electrolyte monitoring, progressive ambulation, and cardiopulmonary monitoring and intervention. Since many of these women may be overweight or obese and over the age of 60, they may have concurrent medical problems, such as hypertension, diabetes, or renal compromise, that will require careful assessment and monitoring. Due to shortened hospital stays, discharge planning must begin early, even in the preoperative period. Assessment includes identifying the need for home care, ongoing monitoring, and follow-up care. Because hysterectomy is still associated with a loss of femininity and sexuality, psychosocial support is an important part of follow-up care. Sexual alterations may be particularly important when the woman is still of childbearing age and premenopausal, since the surgery itself will render her sterile and place her abruptly into menopause. Mobilization of support resources, such as family, friends, social workers, spiritual counselors, and home-care nurses, may assist the woman in coping with these changes. Some of the most common postoperative complications that the nurse should anticipate and assess include bleeding, wound infection, deep venous thrombosis, pulmonary atelectasis, and pneumonia. Long-term complications may include lower extremity lymphedema and symptomatic lymphocysts related to the more thorough pelvic lymphadenectomy.[66]

## Radiation

The need for adjuvant radiation therapy for endometrial cancer is determined by stage and pathological risk factors (see Table 53-2).[9] Women with stage IA, grade 1 or 2 disease and no myometrial invasion are considered at low risk for recurrence and require no further treatment.[60] The vagina is the most common site of local recurrence; therefore, adjuvant intravaginal brachytherapy may be recommended for women with intermediate risk—less than 50% myometrial invasion.[69] Intravaginal brachytherapy is administered in the outpatient setting in 3 divided fractions delivered every 2 weeks.[69,70] Morbidity is minimal and consists of mild gastrointestinal and urinary symptoms and vaginal dryness.[69,70] The role of external pelvic radiation added to intravaginal brachytherapy remains controversial in women with adequate surgical staging and no extrauterine disease because it adds to morbidity and cost. It has also been demonstrated that women can be treated at the time of recurrence with no negative effect on overall survival.[70,71]

Indications for pelvic external-beam radiation therapy (which allows treatment of all pelvic tissue, including nodes and lymphatics) usually include disease localized to the pelvis, a high-grade tumor, and greater than 50% myometrial invasion. Women with stage IC or IIA disease are recommended, based on risk factors, to receive either observation, intravaginal brachytherapy, or whole pelvic radiation; stage IIB treatment recommendations include intravaginal and whole pelvic radiation; stage III therapy varies but NCCN guidelines recommend chemotherapy with or without tumor-directed radiation to the whole pelvis, or abdominopelvic with or without chemotherapy; and stage IV treatment may include pelvic and abdominal radiation, and/or intracavitary, as well as chemotherapy.[60] Finally, in women who are poor surgical candidates, eg, comorbidity, obesity, radiation is a justifiable option.[72]

Women who have been incompletely surgically staged may be offered surgical restaging procedures if radiologic imaging indicate extrauterine disease and then appropriate radiation therapy. However, older women treated with high-risk locally advanced endometrial cancer have a poorer survival and greater risk of recurrence following postoperative radiation therapy, independent of other prognostic factors. These women may benefit from other modalities of treatment.[72]

Before receiving radiation therapy women should be educated about the treatment plan, side effects, monitoring, self-care, and quality-of-life issues. During therapy, the patient is monitored closely for side effects of the treatment so that timely intervention can occur. These side effects of pelvic and abdominal radiation will be directly related to the organs or systems included in the radiation port. Potential side effects include nausea, diarrhea, urinary urgency or burning, myelosuppression, and skin changes, such as erythema, dryness, itching, burning, and desquamation. Vaginal atrophy and stenosis resulting from radiation therapy can lead to sexual dysfunction, which may have a negative effect on self-image and self-esteem and diminish quality of life. The nurse should incorporate a sexual assessment at every visit and address the women's specific needs related to sexuality. Some suggestions may be the liberal and adequate use of vaginal lubricants to help minimize dryness and painful intercourse. Other suggestions may include longer time for foreplay and more comfortable positions for intercourse. If the woman is not sexually active, the use of vaginal dilators with lubricants may help prevent vaginal stenosis.[73,74] For specific radiation therapy issues and nursing care, see Chapters 13 and 14.

**TABLE 53-4**

**Information Needs Related to Endometrial Cancer**

| Topic | Information |
|---|---|
| **Health maintenance issues that affect risk** | |
| Estrogen replacement therapy (ERT) | Indications:<br>Vaginal atrophy with infection or sexual dysfunction<br>Loss of pelvic support with incontinence<br>Perimenopausal emotional lability<br>Early surgical and radiation castration<br>Vasomotor instability<br>Estrogen cycled with progesterone<br>Annual pelvic exam<br>Annual mammogram<br>Seek medical attention if any abnormal vaginal bleeding occurs, including postmenopausal bleeding (PMB) |
| Breast self-examination (BSE) | Importance of BSE in conjunction with ERT<br>Determine schedule to aid in compliance<br>Technique for performing BSE and demonstration of skill |
| Diet and weight control | Low-fat calcium-rich diet, calcium supplements, diphosphonate therapy for osteopenia<br>Maintain weight within normal range<br>Large amounts of caffeine and fiber may decrease calcium absorption<br>Weight-bearing exercises to decrease bone loss (eg, walking) |
| Abnormal vaginal bleeding | Seek medical attention for new onset of abnormal bleeding, including intramenstrual and PMB<br>PMB and abnormal bleeding in the infertile patient with anovulatory cycles must be evaluated, even though only 20% of PMB is associated with malignancy<br>Evaluation of abnormal bleeding included pelvic exam and endometrial biopsy |
| **Therapeutic interventions** | |
| Surgery | Types of surgery planned, what will be removed, change in anatomy and function anticipated<br>Clarify, reinforce informed consent<br>Role in postoperative care to facilitate recovery, eg, progressive ambulation respiratory care<br>Discharge planning related to self-care issues, need for assistance, and appointment for postoperative follow-up |
| Radiation | Type of therapy planned<br>Associated morbidity, eg, GI, GU<br>Appointments for follow-up |
| Hormonal | Schedule for medications<br>Expected side effects |
| Chemotherapy | Types of drugs and regimen planned<br>Side effects and toxicities of drugs<br>Inpatient vs outpatient vs home chemotherapy<br>Duration of therapy<br>Need for venous access device<br>Regular appointments to monitor response |
| **Psychosexual concerns** | |
| Role functioning | Dispel myths related to perceived loss of feminity due to removal of uterus, tubes, and ovaries, eg, weight gain, loss of sexual interest/enjoyment, aging, mental deterioration<br>Help redefine self in terms of other than reproduction |
| Sexual functioning | Review anatomy, physiology, and sexual functioning preoperatively<br>Complete sexual assessment<br>Alteration in sexual response secondary to hysterectomy:<br>Cervix contributes, but is not essential for orgasm<br>Uterus elevates during excitement phase and contracts rhythmically during orgasm |

*(Continued)*

**TABLE 53-4**

**Information Needs Related to Endometrial Cancer (*Continued*)**

| Topic | Information |
|---|---|
| **Psychosexual concerns (*Continued*)** | |
| | Alteration in sexual functioning secondary to radiation: |
| | Vaginal dryness and stenosis may result in patient who is not sexually active, unless vaginal dilators and lubricants are employed |
| | Use of water-soluble lubricants during intercourse, such as Astroglide or nonhormonal moisturizers used 3 times a week, such as Replens |
| | Use of low-dose estrogen vaginal pellets (Vagifem) or ring device (Estring) that release minimal systemic estrogen |
| | Nonhormonal therapy for menopausal symptoms: |
| | Low-dose antidepressants—vasomotor instability |
| | Layered cotton, light wool clothing |
| | Paced respirations/relaxation techniques |
| | Cool environment |
| | Avoid hot baths, hot tubs, hot food before bedtime |
| | Regular exercise |

## ADVANCED OR RECURRENT DISEASE

Treatment goals for stage III or IV or for recurrent disease include controlling the disease and associated symptoms. Responses to treatment are usually partial and last for 3 to 6 months with median survival lasting only 7 to 10 months.[75] Palliation and supportive care are important nursing management goals in order to maximize the patient's quality of life.

### Surgery and radiation

Endometrial cancer is difficult to treat if it has metastasized or recurred. Women with isolated vaginal recurrences can be treated curatively with radiation therapy.[75] However, women with recurrences outside the upper vagina (pelvis or distant) require multimodal therapy, and the 5-year progression-free survival is only approximately 20%.[53] Radical surgery with pelvic exenteration has been attempted in women with central pelvic recurrences after radiation, but morbidity is high and overall long-term survival is approximately 20% to 45%.[76] Another approach to central recurrence is the combination of exenteration (total, anterior, or posterior) with intraoperative radiation therapy delivered directly to the site with the highest risk of local failure. Although morbidity is high with this combined therapy, local control and salvage are possible in patients who would otherwise be offered only palliative treatment.[77] Palliative radiation can be used to control heavy vaginal bleeding in patients with advanced, incurable disease.

### Hormonal therapy

The most commonly used systemic therapy for recurrent endometrial cancer has been synthetic progestational agents although aromatase inhibitors are also being used. National Comprehensive Cancer Network guidelines do not recommend any particular hormone drug, dose, or schedule.[60] A GOG study reported that estrogen receptor alpha (ER-$\alpha$) measured in metastatic endometrial carcinoma tissue prior to hormonal therapy was statistically significantly related to clinical response to daily tamoxifen and intermittent medroxyprogesterone acetate. No correlation with progesterone receptors and response was found in this group of patients.[78]

Single-agent tamoxifen has also been studied; the overall response is only 10%, but when combined with megestrol acetate responses increased to 27%.[79,80] Oral preparations of megestrol acetate or intramuscular medroxyprogesterone acetate are effective agents against endometrial cancer and are continued until the disease progresses. At that time, chemotherapy is considered. Other selective estrogen-receptor modulators (SERMs), eg, anastrozole, are currently under investigation.[48] Arzoxifene was studied and found to have a response rate of 31% in patients with recurrent or advanced endometrial cancer with a median duration of response of 13.9 months.[81]

Patient education, close assessment, and monitoring for side effects of the progestational agents are important components of care. The side effects include fluid retention, phlebitis, and thrombosis. Feelings of well-being, as well as weight gain, while taking progesterones are also possible. Side effects are usually minimal, unless high doses are employed.

### Chemotherapy

Cytotoxic agents historically have had a limited role in the treatment of advanced-stage endometrial cancer and were reserved for palliative treatment after failure of hormonal therapy. The most active chemotherapeutic agents in patients with no prior chemotherapy are platinum agents, taxanes, and anthracyclines with response rates ranging from 20% to 30%.[12] Two phase III studies by the GOG and the European Oncology Research Trial Cooperative (EORTC) both showed a modest survival benefit (9 months vs 7 months) with combination therapy cisplatin and doxorubicin vs doxorubicin alone, albeit worse hematologic and nausea/vomiting. These regimens are currently the standard of care.[82,83]

Another GOG study incorporating the standard therapy of cisplatin and doxorubicin plus paclitaxel and filgrastin (for bone marrow support) showed a better response rate (57%) but only a small improvement in overall survival.[84]

Serous or clear cell carcinomas of the endometrium act more like ovarian cancer in patterns of spread and aggressive clinical behavior. Women diagnosed with these types cancers are often treated similarly to ovarian cancer with surgical debulking followed by paclitaxel and carboplatin and appropriate radiation therapy.[48]

Initially, the woman will need intensive education regarding the chemotherapy regimen, schedule, and side effects of the drugs. Once treatment has been started, ongoing assessment and monitoring for side effects will permit early recognition of problems and prompt intervention. Continuous psychosocial support is needed to assist the woman and her family in coping with the side effects of treatment, such as nausea, vomiting, hair loss, myelosuppression, and peripheral neuropathy. For specific issues and side effects of chemotherapy, refer to Chapters 15, 16, and 17.

## SYMPTOM MANAGEMENT AND SUPPORTIVE CARE

The woman with early-stage endometrial cancer can expect long-term, disease-free survival. Since the majority of women with endometrial cancer fall into this favorable category, health maintenance will be a major focus of their ongoing care. It is important to note that this population of women will live their remaining lives without the potential health benefits of endogenous estrogen because of surgical hormonal ablation, and they may experience uncomfortable menopausal symptoms.

Estrogen replacement therapy (ERT) without progesterone is often discussed as an important factor for quality of life and relief of menopausal symptoms, but the issue is controversial, especially after the results of the WHI showed no added cardiac benefit and an increase in both breast and ovarian cancers in women who took hormones.[27] A randomized study was done by the GOG to evaluate the effect of ERT on recurrence-free survival and overall survival in women with stage I or II endometrial cancer. Unfortunately, the study was closed early due to decreased enrollment after publication of the WHI. Although the number of participants in the study before it closed reached only 1240 of the proposed 2107 patients needed for statistical validity, reported results suggested that ERT in stage I/II endometrial cancer patients did not increase either recurrence of their endometrial cancer or new malignancy.[85] A subgroup retrospective analysis done on African American women in the GOG study showed that even controlling for all risk factors for recurrence, rates of recurrence-free survival in early-stage African American women who took ERT was statistically higher than in Caucasian women who took ERT ($P \geq 0.0005$).[86]

The NCCN guidelines agree that ERT is a reasonable option in women who are at low risk for recurrence but this should only be initiated after discussion between the patient and physician. If a patient receives adjuvant therapy NCCN recommends a 6 to 12 month waiting period before initiation of hormone replacement therapy.[60]

In addition, as younger women develop endometrial cancer, conservative fertility-sparing therapy for early-stage, low-grade disease has demonstrated efficacy, but long-term outcomes are still unknown. Another major area for assessment and intervention is knowledge related to health-maintenance behaviors, therapeutic interventions, and psychosocial concerns.

For those women who present with an advanced-stage disease, an aggressive histological cell type like serous or clear cell carcinoma type or who have a recurrence, the challenges of care will vary according to the location and extent of disease. Women with local, pelvic recurrence will have symptoms related to the structures that are involved, such as hematuria (if the bladder is involved), fecal incontinence (if a rectovaginal fistula is present), or pain (if nerves are involved). Regional recurrence in the abdominal cavity can include ascites, a change in bowel habits due to compression or involvement of the bowel, or right upper quadrant pain from liver involvement. Finally, distant recurrence can involve respiratory compromise with lung metastases/effusions or central nervous system morbidity with brain metastases. The type of therapy used will depend on the specific recurrence. Although surgery or radiation may be used in selected situations, such as when removing an isolated mass or treating an area that did not previously receive any radiation, chemotherapy is usually offered. Important considerations include the side effects of therapy and how to manage them; self-care issues, such as care of a venous access device, nutritional intake, and pain control; and community resources for assistance, including home-care resources, support groups, and counseling. Quality of life is also an important issue to discuss with the woman and her family, particularly focusing on physical changes and functional status, psychosocial concerns (such as changes in roles within the family), economic concerns, and spiritual and religious concerns. When the goal of treatment is supportive care, hospice care and bereavement counseling are the focus.

For the vast majority of women with endometrial cancer, the major nursing challenges relate to compliance and regular follow-up. Since most patients will be cured with their primary surgery, regular follow-up will be the focus of their care. Follow-up usually involves regular pelvic examinations, at least quarterly in the initial years after diagnosis. Other tests and scans are performed as clinically indicated. Education about the importance of follow-up, as well as of a healthy lifestyle, must be stressed. A healthy lifestyle includes weight reduction, if appropriate, a diet low in fat, regular exercise, and regular screening for other cancers, including mammography, Pap smears, and colonoscopy.

For women who have advanced disease, mobilization of resources will be important in order to maximize care and quality of life. Coordination of care or case management is important to ensure that all physical and psychosocial needs are being addressed, either at the time of discharge from the hospital or when care requirements change. Local ambulatory and home care resources, including nursing, social work, support groups, and spiritual counseling, can help the woman remain at home during ongoing care for advanced-stage disease, whether the goal is cure, palliation, or comfort measures.

Although the majority of women are diagnosed with early-stage endometrial cancer, women still die from recurrent or advanced-stage disease. Ongoing efforts strive to define appropriate screening techniques, adjuvant therapy, and new cytotoxic agents and regimens to improve survival. Comprehensive, holistic nursing management will assist the woman and her family to achieve optimal health and quality of life.

## CONCLUSION

One of the biggest challenges faced by healthcare providers is educating women about the correlation between obesity and endometrial cancer. Obesity is a growing epidemic, especially in the United States, and can be prevented with a healthy diet and exercise. Nurses can have a significant role in educating and empowering women about the benefits of good nutritional habits, which may help to prevent many medical conditions, including endometrial cancer.

Economics and reimbursement issues continue to influence the delivery of health care. Laparoscopic surgery reduces the length of hospital stays; therefore, the results of the GOG randomized trial of laparoscopy vs standard laparotomy for the initial treatment of early-stage endometrial cancer are eagerly awaited. If laparoscopy is shown to be equivalent to laparotomy in clinical outcomes and improves a woman's quality of life, it may become a new standard surgical approach for this disease. Robotic surgery is also being evaluated for treatment of endometrial cancer.[87]

The role of genetics in endometrial cancer will continue to be explored and may lead to the discovery of a gene linked to endometrial cancer. A gene would identify women at higher risk for this form of cancer, which may lead to early intervention.

Investigational agents being studied include specific molecular pathway targeting agents like mTOR inhibitors, c-Kit, Abl, and platelet-derived growth factor inhibitors, EGF, HER-2/*neu*, and VEGF-targeted agents, all of which may have a role in future treatment regimens.[48]

## REFERENCES


1. Jemal A, Siegel R, Ward E, Yongping H, Jiaquan X, Thun M. Cancer Statistics, 2009. *CA: Cancer J Clin.* 2009;59:225–249.
2. Parkin D, Bray F, Ferlay J, Pisani P. Global Cancer Statistics, 2002. *CA Cancer J Clin.* 2005;55:74–108. http://caonline.amcancersoc.org/cgi/content/full/55/2/74. Accessed September 28, 2009.
3. Amant F, Moerman P, Neven P, Timmerman D, Van Limbergen, Vergote I. Endometrial cancer. *Lancet.* 2005;366:491–505.
4. Rose P. Endometrial carcinoma. *N Engl J Med.* 1996;335:640–649.
5. Ueda SM, Kapp DS, Cheung MK, et al. Trends in demographic and clinical characteristics in women diagnosed with corpus cancer and their potential impact on the increasing number of deaths. *Am J Obstetrics Gynecol.* 2008;198:218.e1–218.e6.
6. Trimble EL, Harlan LC, Clegg L, Stevens JL. Pre-operative imaging, surgery, and adjuvant therapy for women diagnosed with cancer of the corpus uteri in community practice in the US. *Gynecol Oncol.* 2005;96: 741–748.
7. Creasman WT, Odicino F, Maisonneuve P, et al. Carcinoma of the corpus uteri: FIGO 6th Annual report on the results of treatment in gynaecological cancer. *Int J Gynaecol Obstet.* 2006;95(suppl):S105–S143.
8. Ries LAG, Eisner MP, Kosary CL, et al, eds. *SEER Cancer Statistics Review, 1975–1998. SEER Cancer Statistics Review, 1973–1998.* Bethesda, MD: National Cancer Institute; 2001.
9. Madison T, Schottenfeld D, James S, Schwartz A, Gruber S. Endometrial cancer: socioeconomic status and racial/ethnic differences in stage at diagnosis, treatment and survival. *Am J Public Health.* 2004;94:2104–2111.
10. DiSaia PJ, Creasman WT. *Clinical Gynecologic Oncology.* 6th ed. St. Louis, MO: Mosby; 2002.
11. Sonoda Y, Barakat R. Sreening and the prevention of gynaecologic cancer: endometrial cancer. *Best Pract Res Clin Obstet Gynaecol.* 2006;20: 363–377.
12. Bakkum-Gamez JN, Gonzales-Bosquet J, Laack NN, Mariani A, Dowdy SC. Current issues in the management of endometrial cancer. *Mayo Clin Proc.* 2008;83:97–112.
13. Ambros R, Sherman M, Zahn C, Bitterman P, Kurman R. Endometrial intraepithelial carcinomas: a distinctive lesion specifically associated with tumors displaying serous differentiation. *Hum Pathol.* 1995;26: 1260–1267.
14. Soliman PT, Oh JC, Schmeler KM, et al. Risk factors for young premenopausal women with endometrial cancer. *Obstet Gynecol.* 2005;105: 575–580.

15. Calle E, Rodriguez C, Walker-Thurmond K, Thun M. Overweight, obesity and mortality from cancer in a prospectively studied cohort of US adults. *N Engl J Med.* 2003;348:1625–1638.
16. Prevalence of overweight and obesity among adults in the United States. http://www.cdc.gov/nchs/products/pubs/pubd/hestats/obese/obse99.htm. Accessed September 28, 2009.
17. Mokdad AH, Bowman BA, Ford ES, et al. The continuing epidemics of obesity and diabetes in the United States. *JAMA.* 2001;286:1195–1200.
18. Flegal KM, Carroll MD, Ogden CL, et al. Prevalence and trends in obesity among US adults 1999–2000. *JAMA.* 2002;288:1723–1727.
19. Polednak AP. Trends in incidence rates for obesity-associated cancers in the US. *Cancer Detect Prev.* 2003;27:415–421.
20. Persson I, Adami HO. Endometrial cancer. In: Adami HO, Hunter D, Trichopulos D, eds. *Textbook of Cancer Epidemiology.* New York: Oxford University Press; 2002:359–377.
21. Wolk A, Gridley G, Svensson M, et al. A prospective study of obesity and cancer risk in Sweden. *Cancer Causes Control.* 2001;12:13–21.
22. Saltzman BS, Doherty JA, Hill DA, et al. Diabetes and endometrial cancer: an evaluation of the modifying effects of other known risk factors. *Am J Epidemiol.* 2008;167:607–614.
23. Lukanova A, Zeleniuch-jacquotte A, Lundin E, et al. Pre-diagnostic levels of C-peptide, IGF-I, IFBP-1,-2 and -3 and risk of endometrial cancer. *Int J Cancer.* 2004;108:262–268.
24. Goodman MT, Hankin JH, Wilkens LR, et al. Diet, body size, physical activity, and the risk of endometrial cancer. *Cancer Res.* 1997;57:5077–5085.
25. Archer D. The effect of the duration of progestin use on the occurrence of endometrial cancer in postmenopausal women. *J North Am Menopause Soc.* 2001;8:245–251.
26. Pike M, Peters R, Cozen W, et al. Estrogen-progestin replacement therapy and endometrial cancer. *J Natl Cancer Inst.* 1997;89:1110.
27. Anderson GL, Judd HL, Kaunitz AM, et al. Effects of estrogen plus progesterone on gynecologic cancers and associated diagnostic procedures: the Women's Health Initiative randomized trial. *JAMA.* 2003;290:1739–1748.
28. Fisher B, Costantino JP, Redmond CK, et al. Endometrial cancer in tamoxifen-treated breast cancer patients: findings from the National Surgical Adjuvant Breast and Bowel Project (NSABPP) B-14. *J Natl Cancer Inst.* 1994;86:527–537.
29. Fornander T, Rutquist LE, Cedarmark B, et al. Adjuvant tamoxifen in early breast cancer: occurrence of new primary cancers. *Lancet.* 1989;1:117–129.
30. Cuzick J, Powles T, Veronesi U, et al. Overview of the main outcomes in breast cancer prevention trials. *Lancet.* 2003;361:296–300.
31. Fisher B, Costantino JP, Wickerham DL, et al. Tamoxifen for prevention of breast cancer: report of the National Surgical Adjuvant Breast and Bowel Project P-1 study. *J Natl Cancer Inst.* 1998;90:1371–1388.
32. Aarnio M, Sankila R, Pakkala E, et al. Cancer risk in mutation carriers of DNA mismatch-repair genes. *Int J Cancer.* 1999;81:214–218.
33. Watson P, Lynch H. Cancer risk in mismatch repair gene mutation carriers. *Fam Cancer.* 2001;1:57–60.
34. Lu K, Dinh M, Kohlmann W, et al. Gynecologic cancer as a "sentinal cancer" for women with hereditary nonpolyposis colorectal cancer syndrome. *Obstet Gynecol.* 2005;105:569–574.
35. Terry PD, Rohan TE, Franceschi S, et al. Cigarette smoking and the risk of endometrial cancer. *Lancet.* 2002;3:470–480.
36. Freidenreich C, Cust A, Lahmann P, et al. Physical activity and risk of endometrial cancer: the European prospective investigation into cancer and nutrition. *Int J Cancer.* 2007;121:347–355.
37. McTiernan A, Tworoger S, Ulrich C, et al. Effect of exercise on serum estrogens in postmenopausal women: a 12-month randomized clinical trial. *Cancer Res.* 2004;64:2923–2928.
38. Franco EL, Duarte-Franco E, Rohan TE. Evidence-based policy recommendations on cancer prevention and screening. *Cancer Detect Prev.* 2002;26:350–361.
39. Kurman RJ, Kaminski PE, Norris HJ. The behavior of endometrial hyperplasia: a long term study of untreated hyperplasia in 170 patients. *Cancer.* 1985;56:403–412.
40. Kaku T, Yoshikawa H, Tsuda H, et al. Conservative therapy for adenocarcinoma and atypical endometrial hyperplasia of the endometrium in young women: central pathologic review and treatment outcome. *Cancer Lett.* 2001;167:39–48.
41. Lowe M, Cooper B, Sood A. Implementation of assisted reproductive technologies following conservative management of FIGO grade 1 endometrial adenocarcinoma and/or complex hyperplasia with atypia. *Gynecol Oncol.* 2003;9:569–572.
42. Rackow B, Arici A. Endometrial cancer and fertility. *Curr Opin Obstet Gynecol.* 2006;18:245–252.
43. Montz F, Bristow R, Bovicelli A, et al. Intrauterine progesterone treatment of early endometrial cancer. *Am J Obstet Gynecol.* 2002;186:651–657.
44. Smith RA, Cokkinides V, Eyre H. American Cancer Society guidelines for the early detection of cancer, 2005. *CA: Cancer J Clin.* 2005;55:31–44.
45. Barakat RR, Gilewski A, Almadrones LA, et al. Effect of adjuvant tamoxifen on the endometrium in women with breast cancer: a prospective study using office endometrial biopsy. *J Clin Oncol.* 2000;18:3459–3463.
46. Burgmann S, Goodman A. Surveillance for endometrial cancer in women receiving tamoxifen. *Ann Int Med.* 1999;131:137–135.
47. Gerber B, Krause A, Muller H, et al. Effects of adjuvant tamoxifen on the endometrium in postmenopausal women with breast cancer: a prospective long-term study using transvaginal ultrasound. *J Clin Oncol.* 2000;18:3464–3470.
48. McMeekin DS, Alektiar KM, Sabbatini P, Zaino RJ. Corpus: epithelial tumors. In: Barakat RR, Markman M, Randall ME, eds. *Principles and Practice of Gynecologic Oncology.* 5th ed. Baltimore, MD: Lippincott, Williams, & Wilkins; 2009:683–732.
49. Horn LC, Meinel A, Handzel R, Einenkel J. Histopathology of endometrial hyperplasia and endometrial carcinoma. *Ann Diagn Pathol.* 2007;11:297–311.
50. Creasman WT, Morrow CP, Bundy BN, et al. Surgical pathologic spread patterns of endometrial cancer: a Gynecologic Oncology Group study. *Cancer.* 1987;60:2035–2041.
51. Kosary CL. Cancer of the corpus uteri. *SEER survival monograph.* 123–132. http://seer.cancer.gov/publications/survival/surv_corpus_uteri.pdf. Accessed September 28, 2009.
52. Hirai Y, Takeshima N, Kato T, Hasumi K. Malignant potential of positive peritoneal cytology in endometrial cancer. *Obstet Gynecol.* 2001;97:725–728.
53. Sonoda Y. Optimal therapy and management of endometrial cancer. *Expert Rev Anticancer Ther.* 2003;3:37–47.
54. Greven KM, Corn BW. Endometrial cancer. *Curr Probl Cancer.* 1997;21:72–127.
55. Dijkhuizen FP, Mol BW, Brolmann HA, et al. The accuracy of endometrial sampling in the diagnosis of patients with endometrial carcinoma and hyperplasia: a meta-analysis. *Cancer.* 2000;89:1765–1772.
56. Sood AK, Buller RE, Burger RA, et al. Value of preoperative CA 125 level in the management of uterine cancer and prediction of clinical outcome. *Obstet Gynecol.* 1997;90:441–447.
57. Barakat RR, Hricak H. What do we expect from imaging? *Radiol Clin North Am.* 2002;40:521–526.
58. Ben-Shacher I, Vitelles K, Cohn D. The role of MRI n the conservative management of endometrial cancer. *Gynecol Oncol.* 2004;93:233–237.
59. International Federation of Gynecology and Obstetrics (FIGO). Pecorelli S, Ngan HYS, Hacker NF, eds. *Staging Classifications and Clinical Practice Guidelines for Gynaecological Cancers. A Collaboration Between FIGO and IGCS.* 3rd ed. London: Author; 2006.
60. Greer BE, Koh WJ, Abu-Rustum N, et al. Uterine Neoplasms. *The NCCN Practice Guidelines in Oncology.* Version 2.2009. National Comprehensive Cancer Network. http://www.nccn.org. Accessed September 28, 2009.

61. Society of Gynecologic Oncologists. Referral guidelines in gynecologic oncology. *Gynecol Oncol.* 2000;78:S1–S13.
62. American College of Obstetricians and gynecologists. ACOG practice bulletin, clinical management guidelines for obstetricians-gynecologists, #65, August 2005: management of endometrial cancer. *Obstet Gynecol.* 2005;106:413–425.
63. Sonoda Y. Laparoscopic staging procedures. In: Levine DA, Barakat RR, Hoskins WJ, eds. *Atlas of Procedures in Gynecologic Oncology.* London: Martin Dunitz; 2003:105.
64. Childers JM, Brzechffa PR, Hatch KD, et al. Laparoscopically assisted surgical staging of endometrial cancer. *Gynecol Oncol.* 1993;51:33–38.
65. Gemignani ML, Curtin JP, Zelmanovich J, Patel DA, Venkatraman E, Barakat RR. Laparoscopic-assisted vaginal hysterectomy for endometrial cancer: clinical outcomes and hospital charges. *Gynecol Oncol.* 1999;73:5–11.
66. Barakat RR, Lev G, Hummer AJ, et al. Twelve-year experience in the management of endometrial cancer: a change in surgical and postoperative radiation approaches. *Gynecol Oncol.* 2007;105:150–156.
67. Eltabbakh GH, Sahmonki MI, Moody JM, et al. Hysterectomy for obese women with endometrial cancer: laparoscopy or laparotomy? *Gynecol Oncol.* 2000;78:329–335.
68. Walker J, Mannel R, Piedmonte M, et al. Phase III trial of laparoscopy versus laparotomy for surgical resection and comprehensive surgical staging of uterine cancer: a Gynecologic Oncology group study funded by the National Cancer Institute [abstract]. *Gyencol Oncol.* 2006;101:S11.
69. Chadha MP, Nanavati PJ, Liu P, et al. Patterns of failure in endometrial carcinoma Stage IB, grade 3 and IC patients treated with postoperative vaginal vault brachytherapy. *Gynecol Oncol.* 1999;75:103–107.
70. Sabbatini P, Alektiar KM, Barakat RR. Endometrial cancer. In: Barakat RR, Bevers MN, Gershenson DM, et al, eds. *Handbook of Gynecologic Oncology.* London: Martin Dunitz; 2000:265–278.
71. Creutzberg CL, van Putten WL, Koper PC, et al. Surgery and postoperative radiotherapy versus surgery alone for patients with Stage I endometrial carcinoma: multicenter randomized trial. PORTEC Study Group: Post Operative Radiation Therapy in Endometrial Carcinoma. *Lancet.* 2000;355:1405–1411.
72. Jolly S, Vargas CE, Kumar T, et al. The impact of age on long-term outcome in patients with endometrial cancer treated with postoperative radiation. *Gynecol Oncol.* 2006;103:87–93.
73. Mick J. Sexuality Assessment: 10 strategies for improvement. *Clin J Oncol Nurs.* 2007;11:671–675.
74. Stilos K, Doyle C, Daines P. Addressing the sexual health needs of patients with gynecologic cancers. *Clin J Oncol Nurs.* 2008;12:457–463.
75. Amant F, Moreman P, Neven P, Timmerman D, Van Limbergen E, Vergote I. Treatment modalities in endometrial cancer. *Curr Opin Oncol.* 2005;19:479–485.
76. Barakat RR, Goldman NA, Patel DA, et al. Pelvic exenteration for recurrent endometrial cancer. *Gynecol Oncol.* 1999;75:99–102.
77. Gemignani ML, Alektiar KM, Leitao M, et al. Radical surgical resection and high-dose intraoperative radiation therapy in patients with recurrent gynecologic cancers. *Int J Radiat Oncol Biol Phys.* 2001;3:687–694.
78. Singh M, Zaino RJ, Filiaci VJ, Leslie KK. Relationship of estrogen and progesterone receptors to clinical outcome in metastatic endometrial carcinoma: a Gynecologic Oncology Group Study. *Gynecol Oncol.* 2007;105:59–65.
79. Thigpen JT, Brady MF, Alvarez RD, et al. Oral medroxyprogesterone acetate in the treatment of advanced or recurrent endometrial carcinoma: a dose-response study by the Gynecologic Oncology Group. *J Clin Oncol.* 1999;17:1736–1744.
80. Thigpen T, Brady MF, Homesley HD, et al. Tamoxifen in the treatment of advanced or recurrent endometrial carcinoma: a Gynecologic Oncology Group study. *J Clin Oncol.* 2001;19:364–367.
81. McMeekin DS, Gordon A, Fowler J, et al. A phase II trial of arzoxifene, a selective estrogen response modulator, in patients with recurrent or advanced endometrial cancer. *Gynecol Oncol.* 2003;90:64–69.
82. Aapro M, van Wijk F, Bolis G, et al. European Organization for Research and Treatment of Cancer (EORTC) Gynecological Cancer Group. Doxorubicin versus doxorubicin and cisplatin in endometrial carcinoma: definitive results of a randomized study (55872) by the EORTC Gynaecological Cancer Group. *Ann Oncol.* 2003;14:441–448.
83. Thigpen JT, Brady MF, Homesley HD, et al. Phase III trial of doxorubicin with or without cisplatin in advanced endometrial carcinoma: a Gynecologic Oncology Group study. *J Clin Oncol.* 2004; 22:3902–3908.
84. Fleming G, Brunetto V, Cella D, et al. Phase II trial of doxorubicin plus cisplatin with or without paclitaxel plus filgrastim in advance endometrial carcinoma: a Gynecologic Oncology Group (GOG) study. *J Clin Oncol.* 2004;22:2159–2166.
85. Barakat RR, Bundy B, Spiritos N, Bell J, Mannel R. Randomized double-blind trial of estrogen replacement therapy versus placebo in women with Stage I or II endometrial cancer: a Gynecologic Oncology Group (GOG) study. *Br J Clin Pharmacol.* 2006;62:56–70.
86. Maxwell GL, Tian C, Risinger JI, Hamilton CA, Barakat RR. for the Gynecologic Oncology Group Study. Racial disparities in recur-rence among patients with early-stage endometrial cancer: is recurrence increased in black patients who receive estrogen replacement therapy? *Gynecol Oncol.* 2007;106:325–333.
87. Bandera CA, Magina JF, Robotic surgery in gynecologic oncology. *Curr Opin Obstet Gynecol.* 2009;21:25–30.

CHAPTER 54

*Nancy D. Tsottles, RN, BSN, H. Piersol Byrnes, RN, BSN, OCN®*

# Esophageal Cancer

## INTRODUCTION

The esophagus is a tube that extends from the pharynx at the area of the cervical spine and ends at the junction connecting it to the stomach. It lies posterior to the trachea and is divided into the cervical (proximal) esophagus and the thoracic (mid and distal) esophagus (see Figure 54-1).[1] Its function is to facilitate the swallowing process by peristaltic movements so that food and liquid can pass from the mouth to the stomach. The esophagus is made up of 4 layers; from innermost to outermost, they are the (1) mucosal, (2) submucosal, (3) muscularis propria, and (4) adventitia layers.[2] The mucosal layer is convoluted, is lined with epithelial tissue, and secretes mucus and other substances to keep the surface moist and flexible—features necessary for swallowing. Beneath the epithelium are the lamina propria, where the exocrine glands are located, and the muscularis mucosa, which is a thin layer of muscular tissue. Between the mucosa and submucosa are located the major blood and lymphatic vessels. The submucosa, the second layer, consists of the submucus nerve plexus, an area rich in nerve fibers. The third layer, the muscularis propria, consists of both circular and longitudinal muscles as well as nerve tissue. The adventitia is the fourth and outer layer. There is no serosal layer in the esophagus.

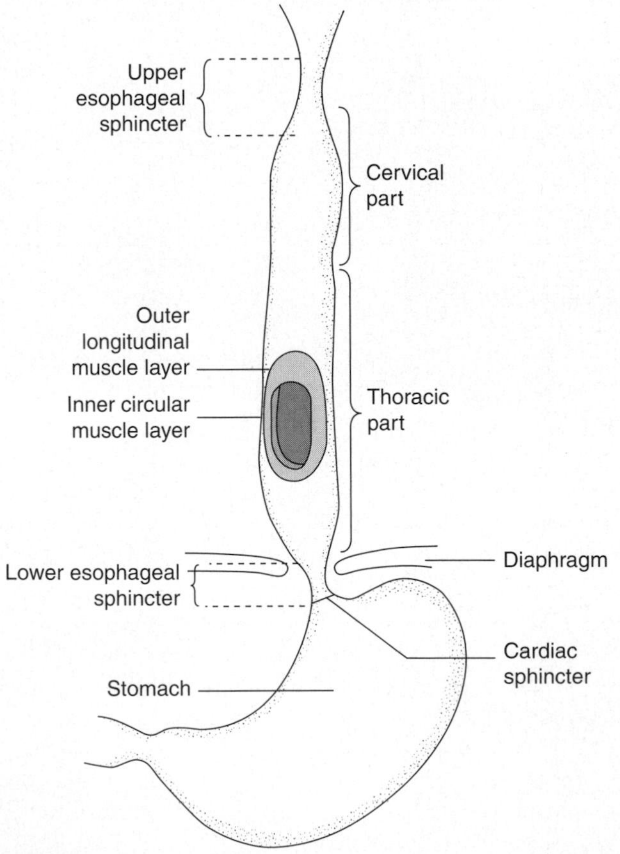


**FIGURE 54-1**

Normal anatomy of the esophagus with cutaway to show muscle layer.

Because of its location and function, the esophagus is subject to both internal and external factors that may affect its health. For example, the type and temperature of foods consumed, overflow of substances inhaled into the trachea, and acid refluxed from the stomach are all factors that are potentially harmful and damaging to the cells of the esophagus. One of the possible adverse outcomes of this cellular damage is the development of cancer of the esophagus.

## EPIDEMIOLOGY

In the United States, an estimated 16,470 new cases of esophageal cancer and 14,280 deaths were expected in 2008.[3] This accounts for approximately 1% of all cancers diagnosed in the United States.[4] Worldwide, esophageal cancer is ranked as the eighth most common malignancy[4] and the sixth leading cause of death from cancer.[5] Regions noted to have a high incidence of esophageal cancer include Asia, southern and eastern Africa, and northern France.[4] In the United States, the incidence of esophageal cancer is higher in the eastern part of the country and in major urban centers.[6] Cancer of the esophagus is more prevalent in men than in women and occurs more frequently in those over age 50. There are 2 major histologic types of esophageal cancer: squamous cell carcinoma (SCC) and adenocarcinoma (AC). Squamous cell carcinomas are most often found in the proximal and mid-esophagus, whereas ACs are most often found in the distal esophagus and gastroesophageal (GE) junction.[6] Squamous cell carcinoma is more prevalent among Asians and African Americans,[7] while AC is more prevalent among Caucasians.[4,6] Squamous cell carcinoma is the leading type of esophageal cancer in countries such as Japan, China, and Iran. Adenocarcinoma is more common in North America and many western European countries.[4] In Western countries like the United States, the incidence of AC has increased by 350% between 1976 and 1994.[8,9] Thus AC of the esophagus is one of the most rapidly increasing types of cancer today. Currently, approximately 60% to 70% of new cases of esophageal cancer are ACs.[10] The reason for this increase is not clear. It may be linked to the increasing prevalence of obesity and gastroesophageal reflux disease (GERD), and the decreasing prevalence of *Helicobacter pylori* infection in the population.[8,9,11] Obesity is felt to increase intra-abdominal pressure and GERD[5] and may be associated with a 4-fold increase in the risk of AC.[8] *Helicobacter pylori* infection may provide protection against the development of AC,[5] as it can lead to the development of chronic atrophic gastritis and a decrease in gastric acid secretion, potentially negating the effects of chronic reflux.[8,12] In the United States, the decrease in SCC of the esophagus may be linked to the decline in smoking, especially among men.[8]

## ETIOLOGY

The cause of esophageal cancer is not completely known but is probably multifactorial. The major risk factors associated with the development of SCC are cigarette smoking and alcohol consumption (drinking more than 1 alcoholic beverage per day).[12] Alcohol acts as a mechanical irritant, promotes dietary deficiency, and may contribute to susceptibility to other carcinogens.[12] A recent study conducted in Australia found that the highest risks for SCC were observed among current drinkers with alcohol intakes greater than 170 g/week, which is above levels of intake recommended by US dietary guidelines (up to 140 g/week).[13] Smoking cessation has been found to significantly decrease the risk of the development of SCC.[4] Low socioeconomic status,[12] caustic injury to the esophagus, prior radiation to the chest, and a prior diagnosis of head and neck cancer are other risk factors in the development of SCC of the esophagus.[5] The most noted risk factors for AC are GERD and Barrett's esophagus.[4] GERD is associated with obesity and affects up to 30% of the Western population.[4] Barrett's esophagus is a condition caused by injury from chronic reflux of gastric contents into the esophagus, resulting in the squamous epithelium in the distal esophagus being replaced by columnar epithelium. Evidence of Barrett's esophagus exists in approximately 62% of cases of esophageal cancer.[4] Other risk factors for AC of the esophagus may be smoking, obesity, and a diet lacking fruits and vegetables that contain vitamins A, C, E, selenium, carotenoids, and fiber.[12] Hiatal hernia has also been shown to be an independent risk factor and, when found in combination with reflux symptoms, can lead to an 8-fold increase in the risk of AC of the esophagus.[14] Medications such as beta-blockers, aminophyllines, and anticholinergic agents that may decrease lower esophageal sphincter (LES) pressure, possibly increasing reflux, have also been associated with AC of the esophagus.[5,15]

Dietary links may play a role in the development of both types of esophageal cancer. Diets low in fruits and vegetables[12] and foods high in nitrosamine concentrations such as pickled and fermented foods may increase the risk. An increased risk has also been associated with diets high in vitamin B12, animal protein, total fat, saturated fat, and cholesterol.[8] In contrast, diets high in vitamins C, B6, and E, folate, beta carotene, and fiber are associated with a reduced risk.[8] Silvera et al[16] found an increased risk of AC of the esophagus with high intake of meats (particularly red meats), refined grains, high-fat dairy foods, and low intake of vegetables in a population-based case-control study. Intake of noncitrus fruits, deep yellow, dark green, and raw vegetables decreased the risk of AC of the esophagus.[16] High-fat dairy intake and low fruit and vegetable intake were associated with an increased risk of SCC, while meat alternates (eggs, nuts, and beans) were associated with a decreased risk of the development of SCC of the esophagus.[16]

Another possible risk factor for developing esophageal cancer is viral infection. Recent data suggest that human papilloma virus (HPV) may contribute to the development of SCC of the esophagus in high-incidence regions such as Asia and South Africa.[7,12] Human papilloma virus is an oncogenic virus that encodes 2 proteins (E6 and E7), which sequester the retinoblastoma (Rb) protein and *p53* tumor suppressor gene products leading to tumor growth.[12] There may also, in fact, be genetic components that contribute to the development of esophageal cancer. Genetic alterations can modify the cell cycle causing unchecked growth and proliferation and avoidance of programmed cell death.[12] Both tumor suppressor genes, such as *p53*, *p16*, and the adenomatous polyposis coli *(APC)* gene and proto-oncogenes including the epidermal growth factor receptor (EGFR) and *ERB-2* may be involved. Epidermal growth factor receptor overexpression has been found in Barrett's esophagus related AC and SCC and may predict a poor response to chemoradiotherapy.[12] The *p53* gene mutations are found with increasing frequency in the progression from Barrett's esophagus, to dysplasia, to AC.[12] *p53* inactivation may be an early step in carcinogenesis and has been found in approximately 50% to 90% of esophageal AC.[17] Cyclin D1 is an oncogene that may play an early role in carcinogenesis and overexpression has been linked to the development of AC and SCC.[12,17] Cyclin D1 overexpression has been correlated with regional and distant metastases, advanced tumor grade and stage, poor response to chemotherapy, and decreased overall survival and thus is a predictor of poor outcome.[12]

## PREVENTION, SCREENING, AND EARLY DETECTION

Flexible upper endoscopy is the most reliable screening tool for detecting esophageal cancers, since it allows direct visualization of the esophagus and the GE junction.[18] However, this procedure is generally done under conscious intravenous sedation, is costly, and it is not practical to use to screen large populations. Recently, transnasal endoscopy has been introduced and may be more useful for population screening in the future. This method does not require sedation, can be done in an office, requires less time, and is reportedly equally tolerable and effective for patients.[18]

There are no current recommendations in the United States for screening and early detection programs for esophageal cancer in the general population. The relatively small number of patients diagnosed with esophageal cancer each year may make developing and using a mass-screening program impractical. Screening programs used in clinical practice usually concentrate on high-risk candidates with tobacco and alcohol use, poor dietary habits, history of GERD, and family history of Barrett's esophagus or esophageal cancer. Individuals should be educated about the role of tobacco, alcohol, and diet in the potential development of esophageal cancer.

The presence of risk factors such as long-standing, frequent symptoms of gastroesophageal (GE) reflux, obesity, and male gender may identify individuals who should undergo screening for Barrett's esophagus. Patients diagnosed with Barrett's esophagus have a 40- to 125-fold higher risk of progressing to AC of the esophagus than the general population.[12] Unfortunately, screening does not reduce the rate of progression of Barrett's esophagus to AC[18] nor does it decrease cancer mortality.[19] It has not been proven that screening patients with GERD reliably identifies individuals at high risk for AC, as up to 40% of patients with AC have no history of GERD symptoms.[17]

Once cellular changes associated with Barrett's esophagus are detected, it is recommended that regular endoscopic surveillance with biopsy sampling be conducted. The National Comprehensive Cancer Network (NCCN) Esophageal Cancer Guidelines recommend endoscopic screening with 4-quadrant biopsy every 1 to 3 years with the screening interval decreased to 6 to 12 months, if low-grade dysplasia is found.[4] If high-grade dysplasia is found, this should be confirmed by a second pathologist, as cancer is actually present in up to 50% of these patients.[4] Studies suggest that individuals with Barrett's esophagus who have regular endoscopic surveillance may present with smaller, lower-grade tumors at an earlier stage than individuals who do not receive surveillance and who usually present with tumor-related symptoms of more advanced disease, such as dysphagia and weight loss.[18,19] Therefore, for those with Barrett's esophagus that eventually develops into esophageal cancer, the 5-year survival rate is close to 60% if they had ongoing surveillance for Barrett's esophagus vs 20% or less for individuals without previously documented Barrett's esophagus.[18,20]

A person who reports frequent, chronic gastric reflux symptoms should be evaluated for the presence of Barrett's esophagus and should be medically managed with antireflux therapy, specifically proton pump inhibitors (PPIs). Studies have shown that patients with Barrett's treated with PPIs developed dysplasia less often than those treated with histamine H2-receptor antagonists.[17] Souza and Spechler[17] recommend that patients with Barrett's esophagus be treated with PPIs at a dose that eliminates the symptoms and endoscopic signs of GERD. Even though antireflux medications are highly effective in controlling the symptoms of GERD, they are not proven to reduce the risk of AC.[21] Anti-reflux surgery, fundoplication, has also been used in trying to prevent cancer in patients with Barrett's esophagus.[17] However, no medical or surgical treatment thus far has been proven to decrease the risk of AC in Barrett's esophagus.[17]

Prevention of esophageal cancer must focus on reducing the risk factors associated with developing the disease. The risk of SCC may be reduced by eliminating smoking, limiting alcohol intake, limiting intake of high-fat dairy products, and increasing intake of fruits and vegetables, and meat alternates.[5,16,22] The risk of AC may be reduced by eliminating smoking, reducing obesity, limiting intake of red meats, refined grains, and high-fat dairy, increasing intake of fruits and vegetables (particularly deep yellow, dark green, and raw vegetables), and reducing GERD.[16,22] Nurses can play a key role in educating patients and the public regarding ways to reduce risk factors.

## PATHOPHYSIOLOGY

### CELLULAR CHARACTERISTICS

The esophagus is lined in a continuous manner with squamous epithelium until the GE junction, where it is lined with columnar tissue. Although a range of cellular differentiation is found in esophageal tumors, SCCs are generally more differentiated at diagnosis than ACs.[23] Squamous cell carcinomas are most frequently found in the proximal esophagus or mid-esophagus. Cellular atypia usually precedes the development of SCC and is found more often in smokers than nonsmokers.[5] Squamous cell carcinoma of the esophagus can be classified as polypoid, ulcerative, or infiltrative.[24] Tumor growth in the esophagus that is infiltrative in nature thickens the wall and leads to luminal narrowing. Frequently, the tumor is a polypoid mass that projects into the lumen of the esophagus. If not detected and removed, the tumor will grow until the esophagus is completely obstructed. Tumors that are ulcerative in nature are elevated with irregular, nodular edges. These ulcerative tumors expand into the submucosa and can be elevated to the point of obstruction. Some of these tumors will remain localized, while others will extend throughout large areas of the esophagus.

Adenocarcinomas frequently arise from the columnar epithelium of the distal esophagus or GE junction. The cellular changes in the columnar epithelium are most often attributed to Barrett's esophagus, discussed in detail later in this chapter. These tumors may be fungating or stenotic in appearance.[12]

### PROGRESSION OF DISEASE

Because the esophagus does not have a serosal outer layer, it is easy for tumors to spread into adjacent tissues early in the disease. Frequently, the disease has spread to adjacent tissue and/or regional lymph nodes before it is detected. More than 50% of patients have either metastatic disease or unresectable tumors at the time of diagnosis.[5] Tumors of the cervical esophagus can involve the left main stem bronchus, thoracic duct, aortic arch, or pleura. Tumors of the more distal areas of the esophagus can penetrate into the pericardium, pleura, descending aorta, and diaphragm.

Invasion into these adjacent structures can make the tumor unresectable. The presence of a rich lymphatic system makes it easy for the tumor to metastasize to distant sites, and such tumors are incurable. Evidence suggests that occult micrometastases are often present at the time of initial diagnosis, even when distant disease is not clinically evident.[12] Therefore, some clinicians consider this to be a systemic disease at diagnosis.[25]

### PATTERNS OF SPREAD

The area surrounding the esophagus is rich in lymph nodes and vessels. These lymph nodes begin at the cervical esophagus and include the scalene, internal jugular, upper cervical, periesophageal, supraclavicular, and cervical nodes. Biopsy-proven, positive nodes in these areas are considered to be localized disease for cervical esophageal tumors but are considered distant disease for more distal tumors of the esophagus.

More distally located nodes surrounding the esophagus include the tracheobronchial, superior mediastinal, peritracheal, carinal, hilar, periesophageal, perigastric, pericardial, and mediastinal nodes. Positive nodes in these areas are considered localized disease for tumors of the thoracic esophagus but distant disease for tumors of the proximal esophagus.

The most distal nodes are the celiac axis nodes. When the celiac axis nodes are positive, it is considered localized disease for tumors of the distal esophagus and gastroesophageal junction but distant disease for tumors of the proximal and mid-esophagus.

Common metastatic sites beyond the esophageal area are the liver, lungs, pleura, and bone.[6] Other metastatic sites include the adrenals, kidney, peritoneum, and brain.[6,26] The depth of tumor invasion and presence of involved lymph nodes are predictors of distant tumor spread.[12] Tumor location and histology may influence the pattern of recurrence postesophagectomy.[12] Squamous cell carcinoma generally found in the upper- and middle-third of the esophagus tends to recur locoregionally following treatment.[12] Adenocarcinoma found most often in the lower third or GE junction tends to recur in abdominal nodes and distant organ sites.[12,26] Observations such as these have lead to the belief that SCC and AC of the esophagus are distinct clinical entities and may respond differently to treatments.[27,28]

## CLINICAL MANIFESTATIONS

Weight loss and dysphagia are the most common presenting symptoms of esophageal cancer.[6,10,29] The dysphagia is gradually progressive with difficulty initially in swallowing solids, then liquids.[12,29] Dysphagia may be described as foods "sticking" or getting caught, throat fullness, chest discomfort, or a feeling of obstruction.[6] Dysphagia with significant weight loss is seen in approximately 90% of patients with SCC.[12] Loss of appetite, malaise, regurgitation, and painful swallowing (odynophagia) may also be present. An individual may be unable to swallow or clear salivary secretions if the esophagus is obstructed. There may also be pain if a bone metastasis is present, or the person may have elevated liver enzymes if a liver metastasis is present. Other presenting symptoms may include cough or hoarseness secondary to paratracheal nodal or recurrent laryngeal nerve involvement, dull retrosternal pain due to invasion of mediastinal structures,[12,30] and anemia from a chronic gastrointestinal (GI) bleed from the mucosal lesion.[28] Manifestations of late-stage disease may include persistent hiccups due to diaphragmatic involvement, halitosis, Horner's syndrome (miosis, ptosis, absence of sweating in ipsilateral face and neck), supraclavicular adenopathy, and tracheoesophageal fistula.[30]

## ASSESSMENT

It is important to accurately determine the extent of the disease and the overall health status of the individual in order to provide the proper therapy. The first step in this assessment process is an extensive history and physical examination. Diagnostic studies and prognostic indicators, all contribute to a comprehensive assessment for esophageal cancer. Exploring the individuals' socioeconomic status, insurance coverage, educational background, and cultural and religious practices can elicit important information and factors to consider when planning and individualizing care.[31] A multidisciplinary assessment by an experienced team is beneficial, since the management and treatment of esophageal cancer requires the involvement of many disciplines. Evaluation by medical oncology, radiation oncology, thoracic surgery, endoscopy, nutrition, nursing, and social work may all be a part of the assessment process.[26]

### PATIENT AND FAMILY HISTORY

The history should include information on any tobacco and alcohol use; diet; weight loss and over what period of time this loss has occurred; presence of dysphagia; pain, especially with swallowing; heartburn; or gastric reflux, as well as the presence of comorbid conditions such as heart disease, pulmonary disease, and diabetes. Any history of prior upper aerodigestive tract cancer, such as lung or oropharyngeal, should be noted, as these patients can develop secondary primary cancers at a rate of approximately 4% per year.[12] Nearly 10% of these secondary malignancies arise in the esophagus.[12] Any family history of cancer is also obtained.

There is some evidence of familial tendency toward reflux, Barrett's esophagus, and AC of the esophagus.[32] In a study by Chak et al,[33] familial Barrett's esophagus was found in 7.3% of persons presenting with Barrett's esophagus, or AC of the esophagus or GE junction. The presence of familial Barrett's esophagus may be related to shared environmental factors or to inheritance of common susceptibility gene(s).[33] However, larger studies are needed to identify the gene(s) that confer an inherited susceptibility to the development of Barrett's esophagus and Barrett's-related AC.[33] Performance status is a reliable indicator of general condition. Performance status usually correlates with the length of time the individual has experienced dysphagia, weight loss, and other symptoms. It is also important to determine what medications the individual is taking as well as the presence of any allergies. Since alternative therapies are becoming more common, the use of any natural remedies to treat the disease or control symptoms should be included in the general history.

## PHYSICAL EXAMINATION

Physical examination alone may not be particularly helpful in detecting esophageal cancer. However, the overall assessment of the person's condition is useful to determine the ability to tolerate treatment. A thin, emaciated appearance could indicate more advanced disease. Weight loss in excess of 10% of body mass is indicative of a poor prognosis.[5] Other foci of the physical examination might include assessment for the presence of lymph nodes in the cervical and supraclavicular areas, focal tenderness, abdominal masses, or an enlarged or nodular liver.

## DIAGNOSTIC STUDIES

Endoscopy with biopsy is the only definitive method for diagnosing the presence of esophageal cancer. Endoscopic biopsies and cytologic brushings will provide a diagnosis in 90% of patients.[28] Histologic examination of biopsied tissue will also determine cellular differentiation. Cancer cells are classified as well differentiated, moderately differentiated, poorly differentiated, or undifferentiated.

Evaluation to determine extent of the disease should include a computerized tomography (CT) scan of the chest and complete abdomen. This will provide information regarding potential metastases of the lung, liver, and celiac axis. The endoscopic ultrasound (EUS) and EUS-guided fine-needle aspiration (FNA) are regarded as invaluable tools for accurate pre-treatment staging. The EUS is able to clearly delineate the multiple layers of the esophageal wall, thus allowing for accurate determination of both the tumor (T) and nodal (N) stage of the cancer. Studies have shown that the EUS is superior to the CT scan in both tumor and nodal staging, with an overall accuracy of approximately 85% for tumor staging, and 75% for the nodal stage.[12] The EUS is also helpful in identifying aortic invasion, although CT scans are more accurate in determining distant metastases to the lung, liver, and peritoneum. Endoscopic ultrasound can also be used to determine response to neoadjuvant therapy. In a study by Chak and colleagues,[34] measurement of reduction in tumor size by EUS, following neoadjuvant therapy, helped identify patients who had achieved a pathological response. The authors then compared survival time of patients classified as responders vs those classified as nonresponders by EUS. This prospective study found that the overall survival rate of responders was 17.6 months as compared to 14.5 months for nonresponders. Furthermore, it was discovered that the survival time of the subset of responders who then went on for surgical resection was also significantly higher than the nonresponders who underwent resection. The study thus concluded that EUS was the only clinical variable associated with survival time.[34]

Positron emission tomography (PET) is a newer technology that uses the uptake of a radiolabeled glucose analogue by tumors to detect the presence and extent of disease. Unlike CT scans, which have a structural-based technology, PET has a metabolism-based technology. While the accuracy of the fludoxyglucose positron emission tomography (FDG-PET) in assessing regional lymph nodes falls somewhere between the low accuracy of a CT scan and the high accuracy of the EUS,[35] numerous studies confirm that the FDG-PET is superior to the CT scan in the detection of distant metastases with a sensitivity, specificity, and accuracy of 80% to 90%.[12,35] This ability of the PET scan to identify metastatic disease in patients who might otherwise receive inappropriate definitive local therapy has rendered it a standard staging test. A prospective study found an overall accuracy of 82% of the PET in identifying stage IV disease, vs 64% accuracy of the CT scan and EUS combined. In this same study, the addition of the PET to the CT scan and EUS revealed a change in staging that altered the treatment plan in 22% of the patients studied.[28,36] The PET also appears to have increased benefit in evaluating the response to chemotherapy and radiation.[12,37]

Another method for determining the presence or absence of metastatic disease is the exploratory laparoscopy. Through small abdominal incisions, the area is visually explored for the presence of nodes or tissue that appears suspicious. If something suspicious is observed, a biopsy is taken so a definitive diagnosis can be made. Intraperitoneal metastases and/or small liver metastases that may not have previously been identified by imaging studies may be detected during laparoscopy.

When the tumor involves the upper two-thirds of the esophagus, bronchoscopy is performed to rule out invasion into the trachea or formation of a tracheoesophageal fistula.[10] These findings may preclude the patient from having esophageal surgery.

Thorough staging involves the combination of all these diagnostic procedures to ensure the most accurate staging of the disease. This extensive assessment is extremely important in order to determine the best treatment approach.

### PROGNOSTIC INDICATORS

The prognosis for patients with esophageal cancer is poor. This is partly due to the absence of a serosal layer in the esophagus that makes it easier for a tumor to extend beyond the esophageal wall. Also, the rich lymphatic system in the esophageal area lends itself to early metastasis of the disease. At presentation, more than 50% of patients with esophageal cancer have unresectable or metastatic disease.[5] In the US, the overall 5-year survival rate for all stages of esophageal cancer remains at 16%.[3]

Prognostic factors include stage, sex, age, performance status, anatomic location of the tumor, degree of weight loss, depth of tumor invasion, and involvement of lymph nodes.[5,26] Two key prognostic indicators for esophageal cancer are the depth of tumor invasion into or through the esophageal wall (T3 or T4) and the presence or absence of abdominal metastasis (M1).[38] Patients with T3N0 (stage IIA) disease have a 30% to 40% 5-year survival rate post-surgical resection.[5,6] The 5-year survival rate drops to less than 20% for T3N1 (stage III) disease.[5,6] The median survival is less than 1 year for patients with metastatic disease treated with chemotherapy.[5]

There are no serum tumor markers that have a proven role in the evaluation of esophageal cancer.[25] The pathological stage of the resected esophagus has been found to be a predictor of survival.[4,28] When no residual tumor is found in the resected esophagus and lymph nodes, this is classified as a pathological complete response (pCR). Results of phase II and III preoperative chemoradiation trials demonstrate that at the time of surgery, patients with a pCR or minimal residual tumor (stage I) have the best prognosis, with overall survival rates of 60% to 70% at 5 years.[28] This information may be useful in advising patients and selecting high-risk patients for trials of novel adjuvant therapies in an effort to improve survival.[28]

## CLASSIFICATION AND STAGING

Staging for esophageal cancer involves both clinical and pathological staging of the disease. Clinical staging, conducted prior to treatment, involves disease that can be examined objectively. Included are history, physical examination, biopsy of the tumor, laboratory results, endoscopic examination, and radiologic imaging.[38]

Pathological staging is based on surgical exploration, such as exploratory laparoscopy, and the examination of the surgically resected tissue and associated lymph nodes. Involvement of adjacent structures and detection of any distant metastatic sites must be documented in order to treat the disease appropriately.

Staging of the disease (Table 54-1) is based on the American Joint Committee on Cancer (AJCC) TNM system and includes the depth of invasion of the primary tumor, invasion into surrounding tissue, nodal involvement, and the presence or absence of metastasis.[38] The letter "T" indicates the presence and depth of invasion of the primary tumor, "N" indicates the presence of positive lymph nodes, and "M" indicates the presence of metastatic disease. The majority of people with esophageal cancer present with stage III disease and are classified as either T3N1 (invasion of the adventitia and spread to regional nodes) or T4 (penetration into adjacent structures).[5]

## THERAPEUTIC APPROACHES AND NURSING CARE

Treatment for esophageal cancer is varied and depends on the stage of the disease and upon the general health status of the patient. For instance, tumor invasion into the aorta, vena cava, pericardium, or tracheobronchial tree or T4 classification makes the tumor unresectable.[26] The presence of metastatic disease eliminates surgery (except for palliation) as an option. Presence of comorbid conditions may also preclude certain treatments. It is therefore important to have thorough staging and evaluation of the individual's condition, and to make sure that he or she understands the risks and benefits of the various therapies before proceeding.

Nursing care for an individual with esophageal cancer is complex and sometimes difficult. Aggressive measures for symptom control and support of the patient and family throughout treatment need to be coordinated and implemented. Because treatment may cross many settings—inpatient, outpatient, home care, and hospice—and requires the use of many resources, coordination is a critical component of care. The number and severity of side effects of treatment and the nursing care to manage these side effects depends on the extent of disease and the treatment given.

### BARRETT'S ESOPHAGUS

Barrett's esophagus is a premalignant condition resulting from GERD that may be exacerbated by obesity or hiatal hernia.[26] Barrett's esophagus develops in 5% to 20% of patients with chronic GERD.[20] Symptoms associated with GERD can include heartburn, regurgitation, chest pain, hoarseness, sore throat, and asthma/cough.[39] An endoscopy with esophageal biopsy is needed to diagnose Barrett's esophagus.[19] Normal squamous lining is pale and glossy in appearance, whereas the characteristic lining of Barrett's esophagus is dull and reddish in color.[19] If the area

**TABLE 54-1**

**AJCC TNM Staging for Esophageal Cancer**

| | | | |
|---|---|---|---|
| **Primary Tumor (T)** | | | |
| TX | Primary tumor cannot be assessed | | |
| T0 | No evidence of primary tumor | | |
| Tis | Carcinoma *in situ* | | |
| T1 | Tumor invades lamina propria or submucosa | | |
| T2 | Tumor invades muscularis propria | | |
| T3 | Tumor invades adventitia | | |
| T4 | Tumor invades adjacent structures | | |
| **Regional Lymph Nodes (N)** | | | |
| NX | Regional lymph nodes cannot be assessed | | |
| N0 | No regional lymph node metastasis | | |
| N1 | Regional lymph node metastasis | | |
| **Distant Metastasis (M)** | | | |
| MX | Distant metastasis cannot be assessed | | |
| M0 | No distant metastasis | | |
| M1 | Distant metastasis | | |
| **Tumors of the Lower Thoracic Esophagus** | | | |
| M1a | Metastasis in celiac lymph nodes | | |
| M1b | Other distant metastasis | | |
| **Tumors of the Midthoracic Esophagus** | | | |
| M1a | Not applicable | | |
| M1b | nonregional lymph nodes and/or other distant metastasis | | |
| **Tumors of the Upper Thoracic Esophagus** | | | |
| M1a | Metastasis in cervical nodes | | |
| M1b | Other distant metastastis | | |
| **Stage Grouping** | | | |
| Stage 0 | Tis | N0 | M0 |
| Stage I | T1 | N0 | M0 |
| Stage IIA | T2 | N0 | M0 |
| | T3 | N0 | M0 |
| Stage IIB | T1 | N1 | M0 |
| | T2 | N1 | M0 |
| Stage III | T3 | N1 | M0 |
| | T4 | Any N | M0 |
| Stage IV | Any T | Any N | M1 |
| Stage IVA | Any T | Any N | M1a |
| Stage IVB | Any T | Any N | M1b |

of abnormal columnar epithelium is less than 3 cm, it is characterized as short-segment Barrett's esophagus, and if the area is 3 cm or larger, it is characterized as long-segment Barrett's esophagus.[19,20] However, no length of columnar lined epithelium is considered normal.[28] Short-segment Barrett's esophagus is also susceptible to the development of dysplasia and AC.[28] Varying degrees of cellular dysplasia are associated with Barrett's esophagus, and thus varying approaches are taken to its treatment. Cellular dysplasia is classified as low, intermediate, and high grade. Dysplasia in Barrett's esophagus is thought to precede the development of invasive AC.[28] Low-grade dysplasia is felt to be potentially reversible.[28] Barrett's esophagus with low-grade dysplasia may be treated with intensive (twice-daily treatment with a PPI) medical antireflux therapy for 8 to 12 weeks and repeated endoscopic examination.[21] Endoscopy should be repeated after 6 and 12 months, followed by yearly endoscopy, if there is no progression.[21] Some studies suggest that nonsteroidal anti-inflammatory drugs (NSAIDs) including aspirin may help to alter the rate of neoplastic progression in patients with Barrett's esophagus.[17] However, further studies are needed to establish efficacy.[17]

The duration of the surveillance interval remains controversial due to the lack of data from randomized trials. Gopal and colleagues[20] report patient age and the segment length of involved Barrett's esophagus as risk factors for the development of dysplasia. The authors note an increase in the risk of dysplasia by 3.3% per year in persons over 40 years of age and a 14% increase in risk per 1 cm increase in the segment length of involved Barrett's esophagus.[20] The American College of Gastroenterology recommends that patients with Barrett's esophagus have regular surveillance endoscopy with biopsies to detect dysplasia every 3 years for patients who have had 2 consecutive endoscopies without evidence of dysplasia.[19] For patients found to have low-grade dysplasia, endoscopy every 6 to 12 months is recommended.[4,19] Patients with high-grade dysplasia should have repeat endoscopy with multiple biopsies to rule out invasive cancer. If the high-grade dysplasia is focal or limited, the condition should be monitored at 3-month intervals with endoscopic surveillance.[19] For patients with multifocal high-grade dysplasia, surgical resection may be considered.[22] It is estimated that patients with Barrett's esophagus have an annual cancer incidence ranging from 0.1% to 0.5%.[5,19,20]

The treatment for Barrett's esophagus with high-grade dysplasia is more controversial and involves 3 options: esophagectomy, endoscopic ablative therapy with continued surveillance, or an intensive endoscopic biopsy surveillance program every 2 to 3 months.[19,21,28] An important rationale supporting surgical resection is the prevalence of AC in 45% to 50% of specimens surgically removed from people with high-grade dysplasia.[28] Esophagectomy is the only treatment that can definitively prevent the progression from dysplasia to cancer and thus is the treatment of choice.[4,12,19,21] Several nonsurgical treatment options have been developed for patients who are not surgical candidates. Mucosal ablative techniques including photodynamic therapy (PDT), laser ablation, and argon plasma coagulation, all provide destruction of the mucosal layer.[12] The premise of these therapies is that mucosal injury in an acid-controlled environment eliminates the premalignant mucosa and resurfaces the esophageal lining with regenerated squamous epithelium.[12] Endoscopic laser therapy in combination with a PPI is a nonsurgical option for patients with high-grade dysplasia or early AC.[18] Proton pump inhibitors such as omeprazole, lansoprazole, rabeprazole, pantoprazole, and esomeprazole are potent acid-suppressive drugs.[39] In some patients with Barrett's esophagus, the combination of administering a PPI and endoscopic ablation may result in the abnormal mucosa returning to normal squamous mucosa.[5] Esophageal perforation is the main risk of thermal ablation therapy.[12] However, no study has shown that ablative therapy decreases the long-term risk for developing cancer in the presence of Barrett's esophagus.[19]

Endoscopic mucosal resection (EMR) can be used to treat high-grade dysplasia or superficial cancers found by endoscopy.[12,18,28] Endoscopic mucosal resection involves the submucosal injection of fluid to lift and separate the lesion from the underlying mucosal layer, allowing full resection, and retrieval of tissue for histologic examination.[12] Photodynamic therapy has also been studied for the treatment of Barrett's esophagus with high-grade dysplasia, and is felt to be superior for ablation of metaplastic and dysplastic epithelium.[4] Resolution of high-grade dysplasia has been found in 78% of patients treated with PDT, over a 5-year follow-up.[28,40] Complications of PDT include photosensitivity and formation of strictures.[12] Lifelong endoscopic surveillance with biopsies is still required for patients with high-grade dysplasia following treatment with PDT or EMR.[4] Another option is a more conservative treatment similar to that for lower grades of dysplasia as described earlier, with intense endoscopic biopsy surveillance at 3-month intervals. However, limited data exist on the safety and efficacy of this approach.[21] Invasive carcinoma may develop within 3 years in up to 50% of patients with untreated high-grade dysplasia.[5]

Nursing care for people with Barrett's esophagus is focused on education about the disease process and the risk of the disease progressing to AC. The person must understand the importance of scheduled follow-up evaluations and appropriate treatment with antireflux medications, preferably PPIs.[17] For many individuals, reflux symptoms may have been present for lengths of time varying from months to years prior to the diagnosis of Barrett's esophagus or esophageal cancer. Reflux symptoms may also recur following esophagectomy surgery. In addition to using medications, patients need to be taught lifestyle modifications to assist in controlling reflux symptoms. They need to be aware of foods that may increase reflux, such as coffee, alcohol, chocolate, fat, onions, citrus, and tomato products, and should limit their intake of these foods.[19,39] Avoiding meals for 3 hours prior to bedtime, elevating the head of the bed, and sleeping on the left side can improve clearance of esophageal acid and reduce night time exposure.[39] Loose-fitting clothing should be worn, since tight clothing may increase intragastric pressure.[39] Obesity should be avoided, as it has been shown to correlate with reflux and decreased lower esophageal sphincter pressures.[39] Smoking should also be avoided, as it has been documented to increase esophageal acid exposure.[39] The care of the individual with a surgically resected esophagus is discussed in the following section.

## LOCAL AND LOCOREGIONAL ESOPHAGEAL CANCER

### Surgery alone

Surgical resection of the esophagus is the primary treatment for local and locoregional cancer for people with resectable disease whose comorbid conditions do not prohibit surgical treatment. This has been the standard treatment, particularly in settings where clinical trials are not available. Numerous studies have demonstrated a statistically significant association between surgery performed in hospitals designated as high-volume esophagectomy institutions and lower complication and mortality rates.[12,30,41] Therefore, it is recommended that esophagectomy surgery be performed in centers with experience in this surgery.[4] Several different resection approaches have been developed. The approach selected depends on the location of the tumor and the preference and expertise of the surgical team. The different approaches are radical en bloc esophagectomy, left thoracoabdominal approach, combined abdominal and right thoracotomy approach (Ivor-Lewis), and transhiatal approach.[10,28] No survival advantage related to the surgical approach used has been demonstrated in prospective studies.[28]

The radical en bloc approach advocates a 2- or 3-field lymphadenectomy in conjunction with an esophageal resection and replacement. It involves a complete resection of the esophagus 10 cm above and below the tumor, with resection of adjacent structures including arterial and venous supplies of the tumor as well as selected tissues. This particular surgical approach is a much more complex surgery than standard techniques, which is reflected in morbidity rates as high as 58%.[28] The combined abdominal and right thoracotomy approach is used for cancers of the upper esophagus and mid-esophagus because it allows for better visualization of the involved area. The left thoracoabdominal and transhiatal approaches are typically used for cancers of the distal esophagus and GE junction or for resection of Barrett's esophagus. The thoracoabdominal approach involves making an incision across the left abdomen and thorax and then resecting the distal esophagus and the proximal stomach. The remaining stomach is prepared as a conduit and attached to the esophageal stump with an intrathoracic or cervical anastomosis.[4,28]

The transhiatal esophagectomy (THE) (Figure 54-2)[42] has become more extensively used in recent years. In this procedure, the intrathoracic esophagus is removed, the stomach is repositioned in the posterior mediastinum where the esophagus was located, and the gastric fundus is anastomosed to the cervical esophagus above the level of the clavicles. The advantages of this approach include the ability to avoid a thoracotomy, with its attendant complications, such as pain leading to ineffective breathing and atelectasis. Wide proximal esophageal margins ensure complete resection of the tumor and Barrett's mucosa.[28,29] Since the anastomosis site is in the neck as opposed to the chest, consequences of anastomotic leak are minimized.[29] The esophageal reconstruction also results in an excellent quality of swallowing. Disadvantages of the THE include limited visualization of

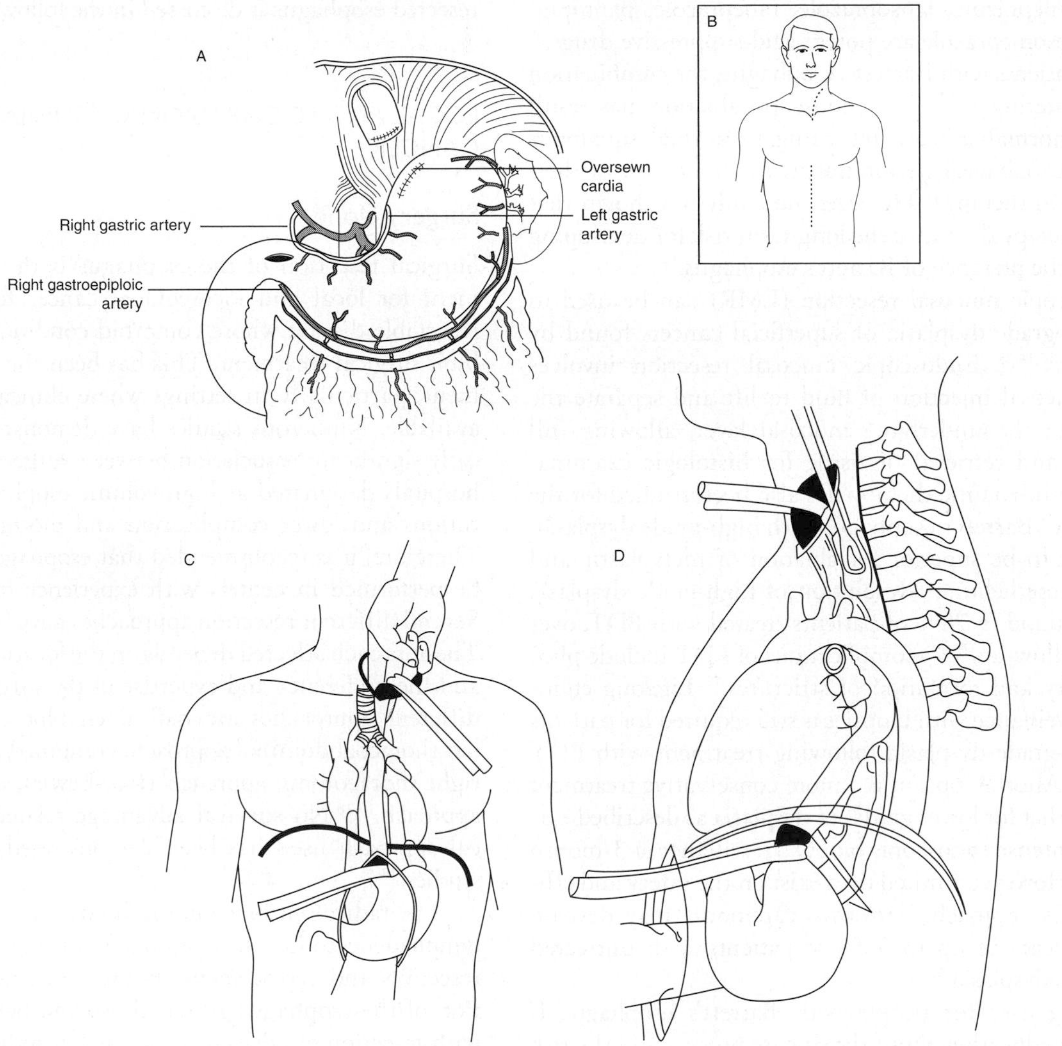


**FIGURE 54-2**

(**A**) Standard mobilization of the stomach for esophageal replacement either in the posterior mediastinal or substernal position. The left gastric artery and left gastroepiploic vessels have been divided. The mobilized stomach is based on the remaining right gastric and right gastroepiploic arteries that are preserved. A pyloromyotomy and generous Kocher maneuver are performed. (**B**) Left cervical incision and upper midline abdominal incision used for transhiatal esophagectomy and esophageal replacement with stomach in the posterior mediastinum. (**C**) Transhiatal mobilization of the thoracic esophagus from the posterior mediastinum using blunt dissection and traction on rubber drains placed around the esophagogastric junction and the cervical esophagus. The volar aspects of the fingers are kept against the esophagus to reduce the risk of injury to adjacent structures. (**D**) Lateral view showing transhiatal mobilization of the esophagus away from the prevertebral fascia using a half sponge on a stick inserted through the cervical incision and advanced until it makes contact with the hand inserted from below through the diaphragmatic hiatus. Arterial pressure is monitored as the heart is displaced forward by the hand in the posterior mediastinum.

*Source*: Reprinted with permission from Orringer.[42]

middle or proximal third tumors, the inability to complete an intrathoracic regional lymphadenectomy, the potential for injury to intrathoracic structures, and the need for long-segment esophageal replacement.[28,43]

Recently, minimally invasive techniques for esophagectomy have been developed and are under investigation. These techniques include laparoscopic, thoracoscopic, combined laparoscopic and thoracoscopic, and hand-assisted techniques.[12] Minimally invasive esophagectomy is associated with decreased morbidity, and shorter recovery time leading to reduced hospital stay when compared to open esophagectomy.[4,12,41] These techniques may be useful for older patients and those patients with early-stage disease.[4] However, no randomized trials have assessed whether the minimally invasive techniques improve survival when compared to open esophagectomy.[4]

Complications of surgery include respiratory compromise, wound infection, and leak at the anastomosis site. Following surgery, patients should be turned frequently, instructed to cough and deep breathe and to use an incentive spirometer at regular intervals throughout the day. Fluid balance should be monitored closely, as over-hydration can lead to respiratory compromise. All wounds and tubes should be observed for signs of infection or bleeding.[31] People who have undergone esophagectomy have an altered gastric passageway that changes the way they swallow and digest. Rapid passage of food through the GI tract that now lacks an esophagus can lead to gastric stasis, steatorrhea, diarrhea, early satiety, regurgitation, and dumping syndrome.[31] Nutrition is a significant concern for any patient who has undergone esophageal surgery, so a nutritionist should be consulted early in the process. Initially, people are fed by tube feedings or parenterally following esophagectomy. After performing a swallowing test to determine whether there is leakage, the individual is advanced from a liquid to a soft diet to a regular diet as tolerated. Because the stomach is small as a result of the partial gastrectomy, the person must eat frequent small meals. This is quite often a struggle for people, and they commonly lose weight after surgery until they are able to take in enough calories to maintain nutritional requirements. It is usually a trial-and-error process for the person to find the foods that can be eaten and tolerated best. Eventually, the individual is able to eat in a more normal way and maintain or even regain some weight. However, stenosis caused by scar tissue can occur at the surgical site, which may require mechanical dilatation at intervals following surgery. This stenosis and dilatation process can be very frustrating for the person who expected to be free of swallowing problems once recovered from surgery. In addition, patients may fear that difficulty in swallowing is indicative of a recurrence of cancer.

Nursing care involves educating the person about what to expect following surgery. Expectations play a major role in how the patient and family view postsurgical status and progress. Following surgery, the patient will recover in an Intensive Care Unit for up to 2 days, and will then be transferred to a medical/surgical unit for an additional 5 to 10 days.[2] The patient will likely have chest tubes, a nasogastric (NG) tube, enteral or parenteral nutrition, patient-controlled analgesia (IV or epidural), an indwelling urinary catheter, and possibly supplemental oxygen. The NG tube will remain in place 5 to 7 days after surgery, and is used for decompression to facilitate healing of the anastomosis between the stomach and the esophagus. A barium swallow test will likely be performed to evaluate for leakage at the anastomosis site. Once it has been determined that the anastomosis has healed, and once the patient has regained normal bowel function, the NG tube will be removed, and oral feedings started. Oral feedings are advanced slowly from clear liquids to an esophagectomy diet, as tolerated (see Table 54-2).[44]

Depending on the procedure, one or more chest tubes may be placed. While present, the patient should be monitored for fever, tachycardia, shortness of breath, chest pain, and increased chest tube drainage or color change in the drainage, all of which may be signs of pulmonary embolism or esophageal anastomosis leak.[2]

Aggressively evaluating weight and fluid balance post-surgery is important. Cardiac assessment is important following the surgical procedure, since atrial fibrillation due to irritation of the vagus nerve during surgery may occur early in the postoperative period. It may be necessary to administer medications to control this dysrhythmia. Pulmonary assessment is also important to detect postsurgical fluid overload and the development of pneumonia. Once the patient is extubated, usually 24 hours postsurgery, aggressive pulmonary management is needed.[31] After discharge from intensive care, physical therapy is initiated to gradually increase mobility. Pulmonary complications are less likely with the transhiatal esophageal approach, since a thoracotomy is not performed. Drainage tubes need to be maintained for patency and the drainage assessed for signs of bleeding, infection, or anastomotic leak. Surgical wounds need to be monitored for signs and symptoms of infection. Once oral intake is initiated, assessment of the ability to swallow is important, since the person may need encouragement to try different positions and approaches to swallowing. Initiating a nutritional consult to further educate the individual regarding dietary needs and possible supplements is essential. The individual needs assurance that there will be gradual improvement in his or her ability to tolerate varied and larger quantities of food.

The patient may experience a dumping syndrome following surgery, which results from the unusually rapid passage of food from the mouth to the intestine due to removal of the esophagus. Symptoms associated with dumping syndrome are nausea, vomiting, diarrhea, abdominal pain, bloating, dizziness, flushing, and palpitations with onset within 15 to 60 minutes after a meal.[31,30] This syndrome improves with dietary correction, including the amount

**TABLE 54-2**

**Special Considerations for Nutrition for Patients Who Have Had an Esophagectomy**

| Treatment | Diet Upgrade in Hospital | Diet Upgrade After Discharge |
|---|---|---|
| Esophagectomy | • Usually nothing by mouth until postoperative day 4<br>• On day 4, a clear liquid diet, as well as an isotonic feeding is started.<br>• Tube feedings are cycled to night feedings to free the patient through the day and to encourage increased oral intake. The patient may be on tube feedings from 2 to 4 weeks.<br>• By postoperative day 7 or 8, the patient's diet is increased to a full liquid diet.<br>• By 2 to 4 weeks after surgery, tube feeds will be decreased as soft foods are tolerated. | • Suggest 2 ounces of clear liquids. every 2 hours, and increase until the patient is able to tolerate 6 ounces every 4 hours. Continue this schedule as the patient goes to full liquids.<br>• Encourage the patient to avoid carbonated soft drinks the first 6 to 8 weeks after surgery.<br>• Encourage the patient to drink nutritional supplements several times per day if unable to eat enough regular foods to meet his or her nutritional needs.<br>• Avoid dairy products such as milk, cottage cheese, and pudding, as these may cause diarrhea.<br>• Encourage small, frequent meals throughout the day.<br>• Recommend that the patient sit up straight for one to 2 hours after each meal.<br>• Tell the patient to avoid sweets such as pies, cookies, and pastries that may cause diarrhea or dumping syndrome.<br>• Avoid foods that are spicy and gas forming to eliminate gastrointestinal distress. |

*Source:* Reprinted with permission from Churma SA, Horrell CJ. Esophageal and gastric cancers. In: Kogut VJ, Luthringer SL, eds. *Nutritional Issues in Cancer Care*. Pittsburgh, PA: Oncology Nursing Society; 2005:45–63.[44]

eaten and the frequency of meals. Smaller meals eaten more frequently, such as 6 small meals daily, are usually better tolerated. Dietary supplements such as Ensure that may have been helpful prior to surgery often exacerbate the dumping syndrome postsurgery. Antidiarrheal drugs may also be useful. Other symptoms include fatigue and anxiety.[45] People should be encouraged to keep their follow-up appointments and to call the surgeon if there are problems after discharge.

Unfortunately, the prognosis following surgical treatment alone is poor. Most people die of distant metastasis within 2 years. Following surgical resection, even with improvements in surgical technique and postoperative care, current studies with a comparative arm of surgery alone show an average 5-year survival rate of 14% to 22% as opposed to surgery following neoadjuvant treatment.[46–48]

## Combined therapy

Since the late 1970s, in an attempt to improve both local and systemic control of esophageal cancer, multimodality treatment approaches have been investigated. These early trials led to the development of 4 multimodality approaches to treat locally advanced esophageal cancer: chemoradiotherapy without surgery, neoadjuvant chemotherapy followed by surgery, neoadjuvant chemoradiotherapy followed by surgery, and surgery with pre- or postoperative radiation[27](see Table 54-3).[28]

*Combined chemoradiotherapy without surgery.* Combined chemoradiotherapy alone can be utilized for patients who have localized, potentially curable disease and either decline surgery or have comorbid conditions that preclude them from surgery. It is also the preferred treatment for cancers located in the cervical esophagus, thereby avoiding an extensive surgical procedure.[26] Combined chemoradiotherapy for the treatment of esophageal cancer has been shown to be more effective than radiation alone. The landmark Intergroup Radiation Therapy Oncology Group (RTOG 85–01) study reported by Herskovic and colleagues proved that radiation therapy alone was not curative and established chemoradiotherapy as a curative option.[49,50] Patients were randomized to receive either radiation alone (64 Gy at 2 Gy/day) or 4 cycles of fluorouracil (5-FU) 1000 mg/m$^2$/day for 4 days and cisplatin 75 mg/m$^2$ on day 1 given in weeks 1, 5, 8, and 11 with radiation (50 Gy at 2 Gy/day).[49,50] Five-year survival was 0% in the patients receiving radiation alone and 27% in those receiving combined modality therapy.[49,50] Successive trials have looked at escalating systemic therapy by increasing the dose of each drug, total number of cycles, and total dose of radiation. This approach was eventually abandoned, as the majority of patients failed to complete the entire course due

**TABLE 54-3**

**Options in the Therapy of Esophageal Carcinoma**

| Treatment | Recommendation |
|---|---|
| **Single Modality** | |
| Surgery | • Accepted standard for resectable AC and SCC |
| Radiotherapy | • Recommended for high-grade dysplasia and stage I carcinoma<br>• Definitive treatment of inoperable patients unsuitable for chemoradiation<br>• Palliation of obstructive symptoms |
| **Combined Modality** | |
| Definitive chemoradiation | • Inoperable SCC and selected resectable SCC |
| Preoperative chemotherapy | • Inoperable AC |
| Preoperative chemoradiation | • Investigational<br>• Preferred approach for resectable SCC and AC |
| **Postoperative Adjuvant Therapy** | |
| Following preoperative chemotherapy or chemoradiation | • No demonstrated benefit |
| Following surgery alone | • RO resection: no demonstrated benefit for adjuvant radiotherapy, chemotherapy, or chemoradiation for SCC; potential benefit for AC based on gastric trial data<br>• Microscopic or gross residual tumor: consider chemoradiation in good performance status patients or radiation indicated |

*Abbreviations*: AC, adenocarcinoma of the distal esophagus and gastroesophageal junction; SCC, squamous cell carcinoma.
*Source*: Reprinted with permission from Kleinberg L, Gibson MK, Forastiere AA. Chemoradiotherapy for localized esophageal cancer: regimen selection and molecular mechanisms of radiosensitization. *Nat Clin Pract Oncol*. 2007;4:282–294.[28]

to toxicities, and there was no suggestion of improved efficacy.[46] Another trial (RTOG 9405) looked at intensifying the radiation dose while keeping the same dose of cisplatin (75 mg/m² day 1) with continuous 5-FU 1000 mg/m²/day × 96 hours, repeated every 21 days. This study revealed no improvement in median survival (13.0 months vs 18.1 months) or 2-year survival (31% vs 40%) as well as no beneficial effect on locoregional control.[51] Thus, the current standard of care for chemoradiotherapy remains the same as that published in 1992 from RTOG 85–01.[28,52] Long-term survival remains at 27% at 5 years, with a median of 12.5 months in patients treated with combined chemoradiotherapy utilizing cisplatin and fluorouracil-based regimens.[5,28]

*Neoadjuvant therapy prior to surgery.* Neoadjuvant therapy is used to debulk or downstage the tumor, thus facilitating surgical resection. This approach provides local and systemic therapy. The use of combined chemoradiotherapy prior to surgery has been investigated for the past 2 decades, with a goal of improving survival. This is based on the premise that to enhance local control, neoadjuvant chemoradiotherapy followed by surgery, allows for the down-staging of the tumor to microscopic disease, leaving only residual disease for surgery, and thus optimizing the potential for cure.[46] Although to date, there has not been an adequately powered prospective randomized trial that satisfactorily demonstrates a survival benefit with this option, the neoadjuvant chemoradiotherapy approach has been integrated into the standard treatment of patients with locally advanced, operable esophageal cancer.[27] Because the combination of cisplatin and 5-FU demonstrated significant benefit when added to radiation in RTOG 85–01, these 2 chemotherapy agents have become the backbone of many studies and remain a commonly used combination with concurrent radiation.[27] A series of randomized trials have looked at preoperative cisplatin, 5-FU with concurrent radiation vs surgery alone, and the results are conflicting. Two trials by Walsh and Urba's groups demonstrated a survival benefit,[23,53] while 2 studies by Bosset and LePrise's groups did not.[54,55] What all of these trials have demonstrated is that locoregional failure was significantly less in the chemoradiotherapy group (42% vs 19%) and the percentage of patients with distant metastases did not differ (65% vs 60%).[23,53–55]

In clinical trials at Johns Hopkins, it was found that patients who had undergone combined chemoradiotherapy and had no residual tumor (a pathologic complete response [pCR]) at surgical resection had the best prognosis.[56] Two sequential protocols utilizing cisplatin, protracted infusion 5-FU, and 44 Gy of radiation therapy followed by transhiatal esophagectomy resulted in a pCR rate of 33%.[56] The 5-year survival rate was 67% for patients with a pCR and 27% for the remainder of the patients.[56]

Recent studies have looked at alternative regimens to cisplatin/5-FU. A randomized phase II study through the Eastern Cooperative Oncology Group, ECOG 1201, addressed the question of whether outcome could be improved using alternative regimens, with a pCR rate as the primary endpoint.[57] This trial was limited to patients with AC of the GE junction, distal esophagus, and cardia (upper part of the stomach just below the GE junction). Patients were randomized to receive either cisplatin 30 $mg/m^2$ plus irinotecan 65 $mg/m^2$ on days 1, 8, 22, and 29 with concurrent radiation at 45 Gy (given as 1.8 Gy per day 5 days per week for 5 weeks); or cisplatin 30 $mg/m^2$ and paclitaxel 50 $mg/m^2$ as a 1 hour infusion on days 1, 8, 15, 22, and 29 with radiation therapy (RT) at 45 Gy (given as 1.8 Gy per day 5 days per week for 5 weeks). Of these patients, 83% of those receiving the cisplatin/irinotecan arm had a complete resection with negative margins and 15% had a pCR.[28,57] Of those receiving the cisplatin/paclitaxel arm, 70% had a complete resection with negative margins, and 16% achieved a pCR.[28,57] These results were not superior to those expected with standard neoadjuvant cisplatin/5-FU/RT, but as this study is recent, survival outcome is not yet available.[28,52,57] Additional phase II trials have looked at other platinum-based regimens containing paclitaxel, docetaxel, oxaliplatin, or irinotecan; pCR rates, preliminary survival outcome, and toxicity do not appear to be improved over those of cisplatin/5-FU.[28]

As current chemoradiotherapy regimens appear to have reached the limits of toxicity, areas of future investigation are looking to incorporate molecularly targeted therapies into combined modality treatment paradigms. Cetuximab is a monoclonal antibody that targets the EGFR. It is currently being used as a radiation sensitizer in combination with chemotherapy in head and neck cancer. As of this writing, there is a new ECOG preoperative trial (E2205) that combines 5-FU, oxaliplatin, and cetuximab with radiation for the management of esophageal cancer.[46] There is an ongoing trial at the Johns Hopkins University looking at the pCR in response to neoadjuvant paclitaxel, cisplatin, and radiation combined with gefitinib.[27] While studies show that multimodality approaches are clearly superior to single modality surgery or radiation alone, most patients present with disease that has already spread to regional nodes, and thus will die with distant metastases.[46] Clearly, improved strategies for treatment are needed, and the challenge will be to design therapies that are not only efficacious but tolerable for the patient.

Although the combined approach may result in a better tumor response and longer survival, it also has more associated toxicities, and thus more complex nursing care is required. There are the postesophagectomy complications discussed earlier, plus the toxicities associated with chemotherapy and radiation therapy administered prior to surgery (see Table 54-4).[44] One of the more serious complications of chemotherapy includes myelosuppression, resulting in decreased levels of white blood cells (WBCs), red blood cells (RBCs), and platelets. Routine monitoring of blood counts is required so that the specific type of deficiency can be treated appropriately. Individuals may need transfusions of RBCs and platelets during the course of treatment. Colony-stimulating factors, such as erythropoietin to stimulate RBC growth and filgrastim to stimulate WBC growth, may also be used in some clinical situations. The American Society of Clinical Oncology (ASCO) and the American Society of Hematology (ASH) have developed clinical practice guidelines to follow when using hematopoietic colony-stimulating factors.[58] The 2007, ASCO/ASH guidelines recommend initiating an erythropoiesis-stimulating agent (ESA) once hemoglobin (Hgb) reaches, or falls below 10 g/dL. An ASCO/ASH Update Committee found no conclusive evidence that initiating ESAs at Hgb levels greater than 10 g/dL would prevent the need for transfusions or substantially improve of life.[58] Sufficient iron stores must be available for the stimulation of RBCs to be effective. Growth-stimulating factors are given on varying schedules from daily to every other week, depending on the medication being used. They are given by subcutaneous injection, either during a clinic visit or at home by the patient or a family member who has been trained. Prior to initiating ESA therapy, ASCO/ASH guidelines recommend that clinicians evaluate patients for other correctable causes of anemia. A thorough history and physical should be performed and relevant diagnostic tests ordered.[58] The patient may need to be started on prophylactic antibiotics should neutropenia develop (usually when the absolute neutrophil count (ANC) drops to less than 1000/$mm^3$). The patient will also need to monitor his or her temperature and should be advised to call if a fever of 100.5°F (38.3°C) or greater develops. Combining the use of growth factors and prophylactic antibiotics may enable the patient who has previously experienced a neutropenic fever to tolerate chemotherapy treatments at higher and more effective doses. Growth-stimulating factors are expensive, and the patient's insurance benefits and financial status need to be taken into consideration before initiating treatments with these medications.

Gastrointestinal complications are another serious and common side effect of chemotherapy and RT. Prior to any treatment, people with esophageal cancer typically experience dysphagia and weight loss. In order to provide adequate nutritional support through treatment, it is often necessary to place a gastrostomy or jejunostomy feeding tube for aggressive supplementation. A nutritional consult will be needed once the tube is placed and the person educated as to the amount and type of feeding to be used. Caloric requirements are increased during treatment, and often a daily intake of 2000 calories or more is necessary

**TABLE 54-4**

**Common Side Effects of Esophageal Cancer Treatment, Causes, and Management**

| Side Effect | Possible Causes | Management |
|---|---|---|
| Difficulty or painful swallowing | Tumor location<br>Inflammation/pain in esophagus because of endoscopic surgery, radiation, or chemotherapy<br>Anastomotic stricture after esophagectomy<br>Tumor recurrence<br>Tumor ingrowth in stent | Encourage small, frequent, soft, moist meals, and snacks<br>Encourage patient to drink high-calorie liquid nutritional supplements several times per day if patient is unable to eat enough regular foods to meet his or her nutritional needs<br>Insert feeding tube if patient is unable to drink and eat sufficient calories to maintain his or her weight |
| Early satiety, anorexia, and weight loss | Tumor location, surgical treatment, chemotherapy, and radiation | Encourage small, frequent meals<br>Encourage patient to consume high-calorie foods such as ice cream, puddings, cheeses, milkshakes, cream soups, eggs, and lunch-meats and spreads, such as tuna and chicken<br>Limit fluids with meals, but encourage patient to sip fluids throughout the day to meet fluid intake needs<br>Augment meals with liquid supplements<br>Patients who have had an esophagectomy must drink slowly to decrease chance of dumping syndrome<br>Provide appetite stimulants<br>Cycle or decrease tube feeds to help to increase oral intake |
| Gas, bloating | Altered anatomy | Use anti-flatulence medication, such as simethicone<br>Encourage small, frequent meals |
| Reflux, regurgitation, and esophagitis | Removal of distal esophageal sphincter with esophagectomy<br>Stents and lasers placed at the gastroesophageal junction<br>Increased incidence of heartburn | Follow anti-reflux diet (ie, no citrus, tomato, fatty foods, coffee, or chocolate)<br>Encourage small, frequent meals<br>Encourage patient to stand up or walk after eating<br>Elevate head of bed 30°-45° during times of rest or bedtime, especially if patient is receiving tube feedings<br>Use anti-reflux medications if needed<br>Try aloe vera liquid before meals |
| Dumping syndrome and diarrhea | Occurs in patients who have had an esophagectomy secondary to removal of the distal esophageal sphincter<br>Symptoms that may occur 15–60 minutes after a meal include nausea, vomiting, diarrhea, dizziness, and palpitations<br>Tube feeding intolerance<br>Infectious diarrhea | Encourage small, frequent meals<br>Avoid lactose in diet<br>Avoid large amounts of concentrated sweets<br>Eat dry meals with fluids consumed 30 minutes after meals<br>Change tube feeding formula if not tolerated<br>Begin standard antidiarrheal medications<br>Use medication if infectious diarrhea is present<br>Try probiotics, such as Lactinex, or yogurt<br>Encourage patient to eat a low-fat and low-roughage diet<br>Encourage increased fluid intake; patient may need IV hydration |
| Constipation | Both pain and antinausea medications have a constipating effect<br>Changes in eating habits or eating a decreased amount<br>Decreased physical activity<br>Decreased fluid intake | Encourage patient to use laxatives and stool softeners as directed<br>Encourage patient to eat at the same times every day<br>Encourage patient to drink 8–10 cups of liquid each day, including water, prune juice, and warm liquids<br>Encourage patient to eat more high-fiber foods<br>Begin bowel program with stool softeners and laxatives, as needed |

(Continued)

**TABLE 54-4**

**Common Side Effects of Esophageal Cancer Treatment, Causes, and Management (*Continued*)**

| Side Effect | Possible Causes | Management |
|---|---|---|
| Chyle leak | Thoracic duct is accidentally nicked during surgery | Try a very low-fat diet (less than 10 grams) to include flat soft drinks, juices, and broths<br>Use tube feedings that are semi-elemental and high in MCT oils<br>Use total parenteral nutrition if drainage persists with the above recommendations<br>Somatostatin may be of benefit once leak is determined |

*Source*: Reprinted with permission from Churma SA, Horrell CJ. Esophageal and gastric cancers. In: Kogut VJ, Luthringer SL, eds. *Nutritional Issues in Cancer Care*. Pittsburgh, PA: Oncology Nursing Society; 2005:45–63.[44]

to maintain weight. Home nursing visits may need to be initiated once the tube is placed to educate the individual and family regarding the care of the tube as well as how to deliver the feedings. Chemotherapy, particularly cisplatin-based regimens, can cause nausea, vomiting, diarrhea, constipation, taste changes, mucositis, and loss of appetite. All of these side effects make it difficult to manage a patient's nutritional and fluid status. Antiemetics are utilized to prevent and control nausea and vomiting. Over the years antiemetic regimens have been refined and improved. The use of the 5-hydroxytryptamine receptor antagonist (5-HT3) blockers such as granisetron, dolasetron, and ondansetron are standard for patients receiving highly emetogenic chemotherapies such as cisplatin. The combination of Aprepitant, a new neurokinin 1 (NK1) receptor antagonist, and a 5-HT3 blocker targets both key pathways involved in cisplatin-induced nausea and vomiting. For highly emetogenic regimens, the Oncology Nursing Society (ONS) and the NCCN guidelines recommend combining a 5-HT3 blocker (granisetron, ondansetron, dolasetron, or palonosetron) on day 1, aprepitant 125 mg day 1, 80 mg days 2 and 3, and dexamethasone 12 mg day 1, 8 mg days 2 to 4.[59–61] It is important to counsel patients to take these medications as prescribed regardless of whether or not they are feeling nauseated. In the event of breakthrough nausea, additional medications such as prochlorperazine, promethazine, metoclopramide, and lorazepam can be used on an as-needed basis. Diarrhea and constipation are also common side effects. Diarrhea can be caused by dumping syndrome, enteral nutrition, or the chemotherapy itself. It is typically managed with medications and fluid intake. Irinotecan, in particular, is known for causing both acute and delayed diarrhea, and can be severe. Patients receiving irinotecan should be counseled on aggressive use of loperamide, and should be instructed to call their healthcare provider should the diarrhea fail to be controlled with loperamide. Patients may also experience constipation, especially those patients receiving analgesics for esophagitis. Patients should be educated about the appropriate use of stool softeners and laxatives to prevent severe constipation.

Loss of taste and appetite are some of the more common side effects of chemoradiotherapy. Patients often find that food does not taste "right" or even taste at all, and thus are less inclined to eat as much food as they should for their required caloric intake. Foods served at room temperature are often better tolerated than heated foods and have fewer odors that people undergoing chemotherapy may find intolerable. Adding spices such as cinnamon or ginger may help improve the taste of foods. Patients should be advised to eat smaller meals at more frequent intervals. Tobacco and alcohol use should be avoided, since they further irritate the GI lining.

Espohagitis is a common early side effect of radiation, usually occurring 2 to 3 weeks after the start of radiation and resolving within several weeks of the conclusion of therapy.[28] Analgesics, which are usually required at some point in treatment, are generally more easily given transdermally or through a feeding tube, since the patient may have difficulty swallowing. Patients and their families are educated about the use and side effects of analgesic medications and how to apply the transdermal medications or give medications through the feeding tube. Topical anesthetics such as viscous lidocaine may also be used to control discomfort during eating. Other less common early side effects of radiation include skin reactions, laryngeal toxicity (if in the treatment field), and pneumonitis.[28] The most common serious late complication of radiation is benign stricture, seen in 12% to 30% of curatively treated patients.[28] Dilation of the esophagus is generally effective in treating benign strictures.

Fatigue is cited as a common side effect experienced by patients with cancer; and is often experienced by those with esophageal cancer who are receiving chemoradiotherapy.[2] A survey conducted by the Fatigue Coalition (a multidisciplinary group of medical practitioners, researchers, and patient advocates) identified a fatigue prevalence rate of 76% in patients with cancer treated with chemotherapy alone or with radiotherapy.[62] It is often distressing to patients and their families because they may perceive that fatigue is an indicator of their disease status, and because fatigue interferes with the routines of daily life. This type of treatment-induced fatigue may not be relieved by rest, and people need to learn new ways to manage it. There is a high level of evidence supporting the benefit of exercise in the management of fatigue during and following cancer treatment.[61,63] It is important to maintain a balance between activity and rest. For example, daily walks and afternoon naps help establish a routine that can be managed by most people staying at home. Daily fatigue diaries can help identify times during the day when the person is most fatigued so that the day's activities can be adjusted accordingly. Priorities may need to be set and limits established, since patients often do not feel up to their pretreatment activity level.

Anxiety, fear, worry, and depression are understandable and expected reactions to the diagnosis and treatment of esophageal cancer. Patients and their families may need counselling to help them cope with the challenges of therapy and outcomes of the disease. A social work or psychological consult may be necessary. Financial burdens brought on by the cost of treatment or the inability to work may be a major source of stress. A social work consult may be helpful in assisting the individual and family to apply for disability benefits or other areas of financial assistance. Patients may find it beneficial to utilize self-care approaches such as massage therapy or other relaxation techniques to manage anxiety and stress. Patients and their families may also benefit from talking to others who have successfully undergone similar treatments for esophageal cancer.

Other side effects of chemotherapy include cardiac toxicity manifested by irregular cardiac rhythms, particularly with the taxanes. Hepatic toxicity is evidenced by an increase in liver enzyme levels. Nephrotoxicity and ototoxicity can occur with cisplatin. Peripheral neuropathy is a side effect associated with cisplatin and the taxanes that is initially manifested by numbness and tingling of the fingers and toes. Fluorouracil can produce a "hand/foot" syndrome, which is a redness and peeling of the skin that will resolve over time. The use of lotions and protection from the elements are usually adequate treatments. Alopecia, rashes, and dry skin are other common side effects associated with chemotherapy. Wigs, hats, or turbans may be used depending on cost and personal preference. Patients should be educated regarding which side effects to expect with their particular chemotherapy regimen and how to assess themselves for early signs of complications throughout treatment.

Educating the individual and family about the disease process and side effects of treatments can involve verbal instruction, written information, and audiovisual material to help the patient and family assimilate the information. Frequent review of the educational information is necessary, since high stress levels may make it difficult for the patient and family to remember much of the information initially provided. Often, talking to someone else who has had the disease and experienced similar treatments may be helpful. Support groups where people can talk about their experiences and share with others can also be helpful. Many patients find using the Internet helpful when looking for information. The National Cancer Institute (NCI) web sites http://www.nci.nih.gov and http://cancertrials.nci.nih.gov contain information about the NCI and its programs and information on clinical trials. Other web sites patients and families may find useful are as follows: http://cancernet.nci.nih.gov, http://rex.nci.nih.gov, and http://chid.nih.gov/ncichid, to name a few.

Follow-up for patients who have undergone treatment for locoregional disease includes a complete history and physical examination, with labs and radiological evaluations as clinically indicated, every 3 to 4 months for 1 year, then every 6 months for 2 years, and yearly thereafter.[4]

## NONRESECTABLE OR METASTATIC DISEASE

Tumors may be considered to be nonresectable for various reasons. Patients may have comorbid conditions that preclude surgical resection. The location of the tumor may be such that resection is not feasible. This is often the case with tumors located in the proximal cervical esophagus, as they require an extensive surgical procedure, which may include a total laryngectomy. Nonresectable tumors may include those that involve the heart, great vessels, trachea, or adjacent organs including the liver, pancreas, lung, and spleen.[4] Nonresectable tumors are often treated with radiation alone or with radiation combined with chemotherapy. This combination has been shown to be more effective than radiation therapy alone.[5,26] It is the treatment of choice in people with localized disease that is considered nonresectable either because of comorbid conditions or the location of the tumor. The current standard of care regimen for definitive chemoradiotherapy is cisplatin plus 5-FU, as per the RTOG 85–01 study published in 1992.[28] Fluoropyrimidines such as 5-FU and capecitabine are the most established radiosensitizers.[27] Other regimens used for definitive chemoradiation include cisplatin plus paclitaxel or irinotecan, oxaliplatin plus 5-FU or capecitabine, and docetaxel or paclitaxel plus 5-FU or capecitabine.[4] Currently, a phase III trial is being conducted comparing FOLFOX4 to cisplatin plus 5-FU.[4,64] It is not clear whether any of these regiments improve survival compared to best supportive care, nor is it known whether any 1 regimen is superior in terms of response, survival, or palliation of symptoms.[28]

The presence of metastatic disease eliminates the option of surgery except as a palliative procedure. Treatment approaches utilized in patients with metastatic disease are palliative in intent and include best supportive care alone or together with chemotherapy.[4] The major goals of therapy should be palliation of symptoms and improvement in quality of life (QOL).[28] The patient's performance status should guide the type of therapy offered. Patients with an ECOG performance status of 3 (capable of only limited self-care, confined to bed or chair 50% or more of waking hours) or 4 (completely disabled, cannot carry on any self-care, totally confined to bed or chair) should be offered only best supportive care.[4] Patients with a performance status of ECOG 2 (ambulatory and capable of all self-care but unable to carry out work activities, up and about more than 50% of waking hours) or better may be offered chemotherapy.[4] Chemotherapy is utilized to decrease the size of the tumor in order to provide symptom relief. Although SCC and AC are both responsive to chemotherapy, the duration of response is usually short, lasting only a few months.[5] Tumor shrinkage may occur in 35% to 55% of patients with metastatic disease.[5,28] Combinations of usually 2 chemotherapy drugs that may include cisplatin, 5-FU, a taxane, or irinotecan are used.[5] Capecitabine may also be used as a single agent for patients with a reduced performance status or an inability to tolerate combination chemotherapy.[26] The use of capecitabine combined with agents such as docetaxel, cisplatin, or oxaliplatin is also being studied. Clinical trials are ongoing to evaluate these and other drug combination regimens in the metastatic setting. The cooperative groups ECOG and Cancer and Leukemia Group B (CALGB) are currently enrolling patients on a joint randomized phase II study comparing 3 treatment arms consisting of ECF-C (epirubicin, cisplatin, continuous infusion 5-FU, and cetuximab), IC-C (irinotecan, cisplatin, and cetuximab), and FOLFOX-C (5-FU, oxaliplatin, leucovorin, and cetuximab) for patients with metastatic esophageal and GE junction cancer. It is not clear whether any of these regimens improve survival compared to best supportive care, nor is it known whether any 1 regimen is superior in terms of response, survival, or palliation of symptoms.[28]

The components of best supportive care are dependent on the patient's symptoms. Stent placement, laser therapy, PDT, radiotherapy (external or brachytherapy), or a combination of these may be used for the patient with esophageal obstruction.[4] Esophageal dilatation may also be helpful. Medications and/or radiotherapy may be used to achieve pain control.[4] Enteral feedings may be required to provide nutritional support. Patients with bleeding from the tumor may need surgery, radiotherapy, and/or endoscopic therapy to achieve control of the bleeding.[4]

In the setting of metastatic disease, radiation may be used to relieve dysphagia or to relieve symptoms associated with conditions such as lytic bone lesions and brain metastases. Brachytherapy, alone or in combination with external beam radiation, is one treatment option for patients with nonresectable tumors or metastatic disease. Brachytherapy has been shown to improve dysphagia due to obstruction by the tumor. An advantage of brachytherapy is the ability to directly treat the nonresectable tumor while limiting exposure to surrounding tissue. Side effects of brachytherapy to the esophagus include ulceration, stricture, and fistula formation. Endoscopic esophageal dilatation with surgical instruments can also help alleviate dysphagia but must be repeated frequently or performed in conjunction with other treatments such as radiation. Serious side effects include bleeding and perforation and occur in about 0.5% of all esophageal dilation procedures.[19] It is also possible to place an esophageal stent during an endoscopic procedure that can be performed during an outpatient visit or overnight stay, which usually provides relief longer than dilatation. Swallowing is improved with placement of an esophageal stent in 88% to 100% of patients with malignant dysphagia.[12,28] Stent placement is associated with less risk of perforation and bleeding than dilatation. A barium swallow may be performed after stent placement to assess for perforation. Newer self-expanding metallic stents (SEMS) are covered with polyethylene, polyurethane, or silicone sheaths that may delay or prevent tumor ingrowth, and subsequent esophageal obstruction.[12,28] Self-expanding metallic stents require less tumor dilatation for insertion and expand to greater luminal diameter and have thinner walls to minimize erosion and hemorrhage than rigid stents.[28] They may be stacked on top of another to manage tumor overgrowth over the top of a previously placed stent.[28] However, stent placement traversing the GE junction may cause severe acid reflux.[5,12,28] Other complications of stent placement include pain, perforation, food impaction, reflux, and stent migration requiring removal.[28]

Laser therapy is another treatment option for people with tumors in locations amenable to laser therapy and for those who have a completely obstructed esophagus. Neodymium yttrium aluminum garnet (Nd:YAG) laser therapy vaporizes tumor tissue by delivering high-energy beams through an endoscopically introduced fiber.[7,12] Tumors in the midesophagus are most amenable to this therapy.[12] The complication rate of the laser procedure is low, with perforation and bleeding being the most common complications. Photodynamic therapy is a more recent treatment option and can be used to treat total or partial obstructed esophageal lesions. A chemical sensitizer, Photofrin, is given intravenously and is selectively taken up by the tumor. Through endoscopy, the chemical sensitizer is activated in the presence of molecular oxygen by a laser light source using a specific wavelength that damages the tumor. The PDT process can be repeated as often as needed to open the obstructed esophagus. Complications of PDT include esophagitis, fistula and stricture formation, and photosensitivity that can last 4 to 6 weeks and may be mild to severe in nature. Photosensitivity to visible light begins immediately after the patient is injected with Photofrin, requiring implementation of photosensitivity precautions.[65] Patients need to be taught that sunscreen is ineffective, as it blocks only the invisible ultraviolet rays. It is important for the patient to wear clothes that fully cover their body when outdoors during daylight hours.[65] Body cover needs to include the use of a ski mask, gloves, long-sleeved shirts, long pants, and sunglasses. Sunglasses may also be needed at night because bright lights, such as car headlights, may cause ocular pain. When possible, fluorescent lights should be used when indoors. Other lights that are considered safe are light from the television, computer, or movie screen.[65] Inflammation and cell death begin 8 to 10 hours following PDT.[65] Once this occurs, patients may experience symptoms such as anorexia, nausea, vomiting, hiccoughs, burping, discomfort with swallowing, and pain in the mid-chest.[65] Patients may require antiemetics, pain medications, and intake of a liquid or soft diet to control symptoms. One patient satisfaction study reported that odynophagia and dysphagia were the patients' most significant reported problems following PDT.[66] This may result in a decrease in nutritional and fluid status, which will need to be managed. Most patients with obstruction due to an unresectable tumor can be palliated with PDT and/or placement of a SEMS.

Nursing care of the patient with advanced disease involves the management of physiological side effects of treatment as well as the psychosocial issues that are most often present. The patient and family must make difficult decisions about whether to undergo a particular treatment, when to stop treatment, financial matters associated with treatment, and how they wish the dying process to occur. Support through social work consult, open discussions with individuals and families, and referral to hospice care are all appropriate approaches that depend on personal preference, cultural differences, and social supports. Pain control and nutritional support are ongoing care needs.

## SYMPTOM MANAGEMENT AND SUPPORTIVE CARE

Dysphagia and weight loss are the most common clinical symptoms associated with esophageal cancer.[6,10] Therefore, nutritional needs are often the most pressing initial problems to address. Assessment of swallowing capabilities of the individual and nutritional consults should be made. Patients who are able to swallow soft and liquid foods may be able to supplement their diet with high-calorie liquids such as Boost, Ensure, Ensure Plus, or Scandi Shakes. If the patient is unable to swallow adequately and maintain nutritional requirements, feeding tubes can be placed and the individual started on tube feedings as a means of achieving complete nutrition. Nutrition can also be provided by parenteral infusions if alternative strategies fail. The patient may also be dehydrated, so fluid requirements must be taken into account.

Patients who have problems with nutritional intake and are fed through tubes often have other GI complications such as diarrhea or constipation. Often the type and amount of enteral solution and fluids will need to be adjusted. Patients may need to take medications to control diarrhea or constipation. Those persons with jejunostomy tubes may experience the dumping syndrome, and the types, amounts, and frequency of feedings may need to be adjusted. Patients will need to be followed closely for weight changes and dehydration until tube feedings are adequately adjusted.

Individuals who have tumors that occlude the esophagus are not able to adequately clear their secretions. Consequently, they expectorate frequently. This is often frustrating and embarrassing for them. They may also be fearful of choking on the secretions, especially at night while sleeping. It may be helpful for the person to sleep with the head of the bed elevated so the risk of aspiration is decreased. Individuals with obstructing esophageal tumors need to have palliative treatment such as stent placement or dilatation as soon as possible to open up the area so secretions can be cleared adequately.

Tumors that are extensive can erode into surrounding tissue and vasculature, causing hemorrhage. Emergency surgery may be required. Esophagothoracic fistulas may form, especially after radiation to the site of the primary tumor. Esophageal tumors can also invade surrounding organs or structures such as the lung and mediastinum, causing pain and respiratory complications.

Distant metastatic disease can result in impairment of organ function such as hepatic failure. Elevated liver enzymes can lead to impaired mental function. The person with advanced esophageal cancer may also experience pain associated with bone metastasis. Supportive care includes home nursing, pain and nutritional management, respite care for the family, and hospice care.

It has been shown that increased symptoms are associated with a decreased QOL.[67] Therefore, symptom management should be directed toward symptoms that interfere with the patient's QOL.[67] Postesophagectomy, symptoms such as early satiety, dysphagia, diarrhea, vomiting, reflux, postprandial sweating, and weight loss have been reported.[67] Patient education presurgery should include discussion regarding possible postoperative symptoms and treatments. Patient assessment and intervention are important aspects of nursing, in order to manage symptoms and optimize the patient's QOL.[67]

Complications of esophageal cancer as well as of the treatments delivered are multifaceted, and the nursing care required to manage them is complex. Thorough physical and psychosocial assessments must be made in order to develop a plan of care optimal for the patient and family. Symptom management is necessary in order to help the individual tolerate treatment. Coordination of various resources to provide care across the continuum and at the various stages of the disease is essential in addressing the needs of this population. Educating and supporting the individual and family so they can make informed decisions about treatments and life issues helps them to maintain some measure of control at one of the most difficult times in their lives.

## CONCLUSION

Although the incidence of esophageal cancer is relatively low, it is one of the more rapidly increasing types of cancer today. The prognosis for esophageal cancer is generally poor; however, if the disease is diagnosed early there are options for treatment that may increase the likelihood for survival. While management of Barrett's esophagus is controversial, there is reason to consider prophylactic surgery for people with high-grade dysplasia in order to prevent the development of AC. For people with locally advanced, operable disease, a combined approach using neoadjuvant chemoradiotherapy followed by esophagectomy has been integrated into the standard treatment. For people with unresectable disease, various options are available, but the combination of radiation and chemotherapy seems to be superior. The person with metastatic disease also has several options for treatment and palliation, depending on such factors as complications the person is experiencing, performance status, and personal preferences.

Prevention and early detection of esophageal cancer may be key factors in reducing the incidence and mortality of this devastating disease. Public education regarding known risk factors and efforts to reduce these factors may affect the increasing incidence. Improved screening for persons at risk for developing cancer and standardized surveillance programs for persons with Barrett's esophagus may lead to earlier diagnosis of the disease and improved survival. New chemotherapeutic agents including antiangiogenic agents, gene therapy, vaccines, and antireceptor agents may lead to future advances in treatment and thereby affect survival.[4] Incorporating targeted therapies with chemotherapy regimens, particularly those that target EGFRs or cyclooxygenase-2 inhibitors warrant further study.[5] Identifying and using biological markers to predict response to therapy may allow for adjusting therapies to the individual patient's tumor in the future.[68] It is clear that much progress is needed to improve patient survival for this often lethal disease.

## REFERENCES


1. Given BA, Simmons SJ. *Gastroenterology in Clinical Nursing.* St Louis, MO: Mosby; 1979:942.
2. Edmondson D, Schiech L. Esophageal cancer—a tough pill to swallow. *Nursing.* 2008;2008:44–50.
3. Jemal A, Siegel R, Ward E, et al. Cancer statistics, 2008. *CA: Cancer J Clin.* 2008;58:71–96.
4. National Comprehensive Cancer Network. Esophageal cancer. Clinical practice guidelines in oncology. version 1, 2008. http://www.nccn.org. Accessed November 1, 2009.
5. Enzinger PC, Mayer RJ. Esophageal cancer. *N Engl J Med.* 2003;349: 2241–2252.
6. Brooks-Brunn JA. Esophageal cancer: an overview. *Medsurg Nurs.* 2000; 9:248–254.
7. O'Dea DG, Macdonald JS. Esophageal and gastric cancers. In: Griffin-Sobel JP, ed. *Site-Specific Cancer Series: Gastrointestinal Cancers.* Pittsburgh, PA: Oncology Nursing Society (ONS); 2007:31–42.
8. Mayne ST, Navarro SA. Diet, obesity and reflux in the etiology of adenocarcinomas of the esophagus and gastric cardia in humans. *J Nutr.* 2002;132(suppl 11):3467–3470.
9. Brown LM, Devesa SS. Epidemiologic trends in esophageal and gastric cancer in the United States [abstract]. *Surg Oncol Clin North Am.* 2002;11:235–256.
10. Leonard GD, Kelsen DP, Allegra CJ. Esophageal cancer. In: Abraham J, Allegra C, Gulley J, eds. *Bethesda Handbook of Clinical Oncology.* 2nd ed. Philadelphia, PA: Lippincott, Williams, and Wilkins; 2005:61–71.
11. Holtmann G. Reflux disease: the disorder of the third millennium. *Eur J Gastroenterol Hepatol.* 2001;1(13 suppl):S5-S11.
12. Posner MC, Forastiere AA, Minsky BD. Cancers of the gastrointestinal tract. In: DeVita VT, Hellman S, Rosenberg S, eds. *Cancer: Principles and Practice of Oncology.* 7th ed. Philadelphia, PA: Lippincott Williams and Wilkins; 2005:861–909.
13. Pandeya N, Williams G, Green A, et al. Alcohol consumption and the risks of adenocarcinoma and squamous cell carcinoma of the esophagus. *Gastroenterology.* 2009;136:1215–1224.
14. Wu AH, Tseng CC, Bernstein L. Hiatal hernia, reflux symptoms, body size, and risk of esophageal and gastric adenocarcinoma [abstract]. *Cancer.* 2003;98:940–948.
15. Corley DA, Buffler PA. Oesophageal and gastric cardia adenocarcinomas: analysis of regional variation using the Cancer Incidence in Five Continents database. *Int J Epidemiol.* 2001;30:1415–1425.
16. Silvera SAN, Mayne ST, Risch H, et al. Food group intake and risk of subtypes of esophageal and gastric cancer. *Int J Cancer.* 2008;123:852–860.
17. Souza RF, Spechler SJ. Concepts in the prevention of adenocarcinoma of the distal esophagus and proximal stomach. *CA: Cancer J Clin.* 2005;55:334–351.
18. Gerson LB, Triadafilopoulos G. Screening for esophageal adenocarcinoma: an evidence-based approach. *Am J Med.* 2002;113:499–505.
19. Spechler SJ. Clinical manifestations and esophageal complications of GERD. *Am J Med Sci.* 2003;326:279–284.
20. Gopal DV, Lieberman DA, Margaret N, et al. Risk factors for dysplasia in patients with Barrett's esophagus (BE): results from a multicenter consortium. *Dig Dis Sci.* 2003;48:1537–1541.
21. Spechler SJ. Barrett's esophagus. *N Engl J Med.* 2002;346:836–842.
22. Engel LS, Chow WH, Vaughan TL, et al. Population attributable risks of esophageal and gastric cancers. *J Natl Cancer Inst.* 2003;95:1404–1413.
23. Walsh TN, Noonan N, Hollywood D, et al. A comparison of multimodal therapy and surgery for esophageal adenocarcinoma. *N Engl J Med.* 1996;335:462–467.
24. Livinstone EM, Skinner DB. Tumors of the esophagus. In: Berk JE, ed. *Gastroenterology.* Philadelphia, PA: Saunders; 1985:818–840.
25. Khushalani N. Symposium on solid tumors. Cancer of the esophagus and stomach. *Mayo Clin Proc.* 2008;83:712–722.
26. Gibson MK, Forastiere AA. Cancer of the esophagus. In: Bayless T, ed. *Advanced Therapy of Gastroenterology and Liver Disease.* Toronto, ON: BC Decker; 2004:5–68.
27. Kleinberg L, Gibson MK, Forastiere AA. Chemoradiotherapy for localized esophageal cancer: regimen selection and molecular mechanisms of radiosensitization. *Nat Clin Pract Oncol.* 2007;4:282–294.
28. Kleinberg L, Brock MV, Jagannath SB, et al. Cancer of the esophagus. In: Abeloff MD, Armitage JO, Niederhuber JE, eds. *Abeloff's Clinical Oncology.* 4th ed. Philadelphia, PA: Churchill Livingstone; 2008:1399–1423.
29. Mackenzie DJ, Popplewell PK, Billingsley KG. Care of patients after esophagectomy. *Critical Care Nurse.* 2004;24:16–29.
30. Sweed MR, Edmonson D, Cohen SJ. Tumors of the esophagus, gastroesophageal junction, and stomach. *Semin Oncol Nurs.* 2009;25:61–75.
31. Griffen-Sobel JP. Nursing care of patients with gastrointestinal cancers. In: Griffen-Sobel JP, ed. *Site-Specific Cancer Series: Gastrointestinal Cancers.* Pittsburgh, PA: Oncology Nursing Society (ONS); 2007:59–73.

32. Wild CP, Hardie LJ. Reflux, Barrett's oesophagus and adenocarcinoma: burning questions. *Nature.* 2003;3:676–684.
33. Chak A, Ochs-Balcom H, Falk G, et al. Familiality in Barrett's esophagus, adenocarcinoma of the esophagus, and adenocarcinoma of the gastroesophageal junction. *Cancer Epidemiol Biomarkers Prev.* 2006;15:1668–1673.
34. Chak A, Canto MI, Cooper GS, et al. Endosonographic assessment of multimodality therapy predicts survival of esophageal carcinoma patients [abtract]. *Cancer.* 2000;88:1788–1795.
35. Luketich JD, Schauer PR, Meltzer CC, et al. Role of positron emission tomography in staging esophageal cancer. *Ann Thorac Surg.* 1997;64:765–769.
36. Flamen P, Lerut A, Van Cutsem E, et al. Utility of positron emission tomography for the staging of patients with potentially operable esophageal carcinoma. *J Clin Oncol.* 2000;18:3202–3210.
37. Weber WA, Ott K, Becker K, et al. Prediction of response to preoperative chemotherapy in adenocarcinomas of the esophagogastric junction by metabolic imaging. *J Clin Oncol.* 2001;19:3058.
38. Greene FL, Page DL, Fleming ID, et al. *AJCC Cancer Staging Handbook.* 6th ed. New York: Springer-Verlag; 2002:101–109.
39. Tutuian R, Castell DO. Management of gastroesophageal reflux disease. *Am J Med Sci.* 2003;326:309–318.
40. Overholt BF, Wang KK, Burdick JS, et al. Five-year efficacy and safety of photodynamic therapy with Photofrin in Barrett's high-grade dysplasia. *Gastroentest Endosc.* 2007;66:460–468.
41. Luketich JD, Alvelo-Rivera M, Buenaventura PO, et al. Minimally invasive esophagectomy: outcomes in 222 patients. *Ann Surg.* 2003;238:486–494; discussion 494–495.
42. Orringer MB. Tumors, injuries, and miscellaneous conditions of the esophagus. In: Greenfield LJ, Mulholland M, Oldham KT, et al. eds. *Surgery: Scientific Principles and Practice.* 2nd ed. Philadelphia, PA: Lippincott-Raven; 1997:694–735.
43. Orringer MB, Marshall B, Chang AC, et al. Two thousand transhiatal esophagectomies: changing trends, lessons learned. *Ann Surg.* 2007;246:363–372; discussion 372–374.
44. Churma SA, Horrell CJ. Esophageal and gastric cancers. In: Kogut VJ, Luthringer SL, eds. *Nutritional Issues in Cancer Care.* Pittsburgh, PA: Oncology Nursing Society; 2005:45–63.
45. Brooks JA, Kesler KA, Johnson CS, et al. Prospective analysis of quality of life after surgical resection for esophageal cancer: preliminary results. *J Surg Oncol.* 2002;81:185–194.
46. Juergens RA, Forastiere A. Combined modality therapy of esophageal cancer. *J Natl Comprehens Cancer Netw.* 2008;6:851–860.
47. Burmeister BH, Smithers BM, Gebski V, et al. Surgery alone versus chemoradiotherapy followed by surgery for resectable cancer of the oesophagus a randomised controlled phase III trial. *Lancet Oncol.* 2005;6:659–668.
48. Kelsen DP, Ginsberg R, Pajak TF, et al. Chemotherapy followed by surgery compared with surgery alone for localized esophageal cancer. *N Engl J Med.* 1998;339:1979–1984.
49. Herskovic A, Martz K, Al-Sarraf M, et al. Combined chemotherapy and radiotherapy compared with radiotherapy alone in patients with cancer of the esophagus. *N Engl J Med.* 1992;326:1593–1598.
50. Cooper JS, Guo MD, Herskovic A, et al. Chemoradiotherapy of locally advanced esophageal cancer: long-term follow-up of a prospective randomized trial (RTOG 85–01). Radiation Therapy Oncology Group. *JAMA.* 1999;281:1623–1627.
51. Minsky BD, Pajak TF, Ginsberg RJ, et al. INT 0123 (Radiation Therapy Oncology Group 94–05) phase III trial of combined-modality therapy for esophageal cancer: high-dose versus standard-dose radiation therapy. *J Clin Oncol.* 2002;20:1167–1174.
52. Kleinberg L, Forastiere A. Chemoradiation in the management of esophageal cancer. *J Clin Oncol.* 2007;25:4110–4117.
53. Urba SG, Orringer MB, Turrisi A, et al. Randomized trial of preoperative chemoradiation versus surgery alone in patients with locoregional esophageal carcinoma. *J Clin Oncol.* 2001;19:305–313.
54. Bosset JF, Gignoux M, Triboulet JP, et al. Chemoradiotherapy followed by surgery compared with surgery alone in squamous-cell cancer of the esophagus. *N Engl J Med.* 1997;337:161–167.
55. LePrise E, Etienne PL, Meunier B, et al. A randomized study of chemotherapy, radiation therapy, and surgery versus surgery for localized squamous cell carcinoma of the esophagus. *Cancer.* 1994;73:1179–1784.
56. Kleinberg L, Knisely J, Heitmiller R, et al. Mature survival results with preoperative cisplatin, protracted infusion 5-fluorouracil, and 44-Gy radiotherapy for esophageal cancer. *Int J Radiat Oncol Biol Phys.* 2003;56:328–334.
57. Kleinberg L, Powell ME, Forastiere A, et al. E1201: an Eastern Cooperative Oncology Group (ECOG) randomized phase II trial of neoadjuvant preoperative paclitaxel/cisplatin/RT or irinotecan/cisplatin/RT in endoscopy with ultrasound (EUS) staged adenocarcinoma of the esophagus [Post meeting edition]. *Proc Am Soc Clin Oncol.* 2007;25.
58. Rizzo D, Somerfield MR, Hagerty KL, et al. The use of epoetin and darbepoetin in patients with cancer: 2007 American Society of Clinical Oncology/American Society of Hematology Clinical Practice Guideline Update. *J Oncol Prac.* 2008;4:48–52.
59. Tipton J, McDaniel R, Barbour L, et al. *Chemotherapy-Induced Nausea and Vomiting. ONS PEP CARD.* Pittsburgh, PA: Oncology Nursing Society (ONS); 2006.
60. National Comprehensive Cancer Network. Antiemesis. Clinical practice guidelines in oncology, version 3, 2009. http://www.nccn.org. Accessed November 1, 2009.
61. Eaton LH, Tipton JM, eds. *Putting Evidence into Practice: Improving Oncology Patient Outcomes.* Pittsburgh, PA: Oncology Nursing Society (ONS); 2009.
62. Curt GA, Breitbart W, Cella D, et al. Impact of cancer-related fatigue on the lives of patients: new findings from the fatigue coalition. *Oncologist.* 2000;5:353–360.
63. Mitchell S, Beck S, Hood L, et al. *Fatigue. ONS PEP CARD.* Pittsburgh, PA: Oncology Nursing Society (ONS); 2006.
64. Conroy T, Yataghene Y, Etienne PL, et al. Definitive chemoradiotherapy (CRT) with FOLFOX 4 or 5-FU-cisplatin as first line treatment for patients (pts) with inoperable esophageal cancer (IEC): final results of a randomized phase II study [Abstract 4532]. *J Clin Oncol.* 2007;25(18 suppl):4532.
65. Phan M, Dyke S, Whittaker MA, et al. An educational tool for photodynamic therapy of Barrett esophagus with high-grade dysplasia: from screening through follow-up. *Gastroenterol Nurs.* 2005;28:413–419.
66. Hemminger LL, Wolfsen HC. Photodynamic therapy for Barrett's esophagus and high grade dysplasia: results of a patient satisfaction survey. *Gastroenterol Nurs.* 2002;25:139–141.
67. Sweed MR, Schiech L, Barsevick A, et al. Quality of life after Esophagectomy for cancer. *Oncol Nurs Forum.* 2002;29:1127–1131.
68. Refaely Y, Krasna MJ. Multimodality therapy for esophageal cancer [abstract]. *Surg Clin North Am.* 2002;82:729–746.

CHAPTER 55

Mary B. Hodgin, MS, CMSRN

# Gallbladder and Bile Duct Cancer

## GALLBLADDER CANCER

### INTRODUCTION

The two most common malignancies of the biliary tree are adenocarcinoma of the gallbladder and of the bile duct (cholangiocarcinoma). Although there is some overlap in the diagnosis and treatment of these two cancers, they are distinct enough to require separate discussions. Carcinoma of the gallbladder, which we consider first, is a rare form of cancer and as such has a distinct etiology, pathophysiology, clinical presentation, and treatment. In most patients, the disease is not suspected clinically and is found at an advanced stage, often during surgery for cholelithiasis.

### EPIDEMIOLOGY

Although gallbladder cancer is a rare form of cancer, it is the most common malignancy of the biliary tract and the fifth most common cancer of the gastrointestinal (GI) tract.[1] Approximately 9500 cases are diagnosed in the United States each year. The incidence of gallbladder cancer in the United States is 2.5 per 100,000 residents.[2] Wide variations in incidence exist throughout the world and in different regions of the United States. In the United States, the incidence is highest in the Southwest, where the occurrence is most common among Native Americans and Hispanic Americans.[3,4] Other countries with high rates of gallbladder cancer include India, Pakistan, the Andean areas of Ecuador, Bolivia, Chile, and northern Japan. European countries include Poland, the Czech republic, and Slovakia.[3,4] In contrast, gallbladder cancer rates are low in most northern European countries, Nigeria, Singapore, the United States, and Canada.[4]

Women develop gallbladder cancer 5 times more often than men, similar to the incidence of gallstones.[3,5] Studies have also shown that female sex, age, postmenopausal status, and cigarette smoking are risk factors. Other studies have identified overweight and obesity as significant risk factors.[3,6] Gallbladder cancer is rare in individuals under age 50, with most cases occurring among those in their late 60s and early 70s.[7]

### ETIOLOGY

Several factors are associated with an increased risk for gallbladder cancer (see Table 55–1). Gallstones are the most common etiologic factor, probably due to their high prevalence in the general population. More than 90% of individuals with gallbladder cancer have coexistent chronic cholecystitis (inflamed gallbladder) and cholelithiasis (gallstones). Gallbladder cancer is more likely to occur in individuals with a single large gallstone than in those with multiple smaller stones. Patients having gallstones greater than 3 cm have 10 times greater risk of developing gallbladder cancer.[6,8] It is presumed that the large gallstones have been present for a long period of time, causing chronic irritation of the gallbladder wall and thus predisposing it to the development of carcinoma.[8]

**TABLE 55-1**

| Risk Factors for Gallbladder Cancer |
|---|
| Gallstones (single gallstone usually larger than 3 cm) |
| Choledochal cyst |
| Anomalous pancreatobiliary duct junction |
| Carcinogens |
| Rubber plant workers |
| Azotoluene |
| Nitrosamines |
| Obesity |
| Estrogens |
| Typhoid carriers |
| Porcelain gallbladder (calcification of the gallbladder wall) |
| Gallbladder polyps |

Individuals with a choledochal cyst may develop carcinoma throughout the biliary tree, but most tumors arise in the gallbladder. The chance of developing an associated gallbladder or bile duct cancer increases for women beginning at age 40. In their 70s and 80s the ratio of incidence for men to women is about 1 to 3.[9] Recent studies have suggested that an anomalous pancreatobiliary duct junction (APBDJ) is associated with an increased incidence of gallbladder cancer in individuals with a choledochal cyst, a congenital cystic dilation of the biliary tree.[7,8,10] This common channel abnormality between the common bile duct and pancreatic duct allows reflux of pancreatic juice into the biliary tree. The question still remains whether it is the regurgitation of pancreatic juice or the relationship of the abnormal junction to bile stasis and the subsequent retention of carcinogens within the biliary tree that causes gallbladder cancer.[5,8,11] Further, animal studies have suggested that azotoluene and nitrosamines can cause gallbladder cancer, and an association between gallbladder cancer and obesity and estrogens has been suggested in epidemiological studies.[1, 3, ,] Recent studies, however, have failed to validate the previously held concept that certain industrial carcinogens are linked to gallbladder cancer.[8,12]

Typhoid carriers have an increased risk of gallbladder and bile duct cancer. The higher incidence of gallbladder cancer in chronic typhoid carriers is also thought to result from chronic irritation and degradation of bile acids.[6,13] Calcification of the gallbladder wall, the so-called porcelain gallbladder, is associated with sustained chronic cholecystitis and gallbladder cancer.[4] Gallbladder polyps are also a risk factor for cancer. Polyps larger than 1 cm are most likely to become malignant and are an indication for cholecystectomy.[4,6]

## PREVENTION, SCREENING, AND EARLY DETECTION

At present there is no effective screening method for gallbladder cancer, as it is a rare tumor that is often confused with other biliary cancers. The presenting symptoms of gallbladder cancer usually occur with advanced disease, making early detection almost impossible. Effective ways to eliminate the formation of gallstones in the general population, and especially in high-risk individuals, would be beneficial for many reasons, one of which is decreased gallbladder cancer. Consideration may be given to more aggressive screening of high-risk individuals and early resection of the gallbladder with any findings suggestive of gallbladder cancer.[14] Heightened awareness of the incidence of gallbladder cancer through education of high-risk individuals may lead to routine surveillance and early detection. Wide geographical, ethnic, and cultural variations exist in the incidence of gallbladder cancer, which suggests that there are major genetic and environmental influences on the development of the disease, including diet and lifestyle. Identifying and eliminating these factors could lead to prevention and control of gallbladder cancer.

Carcinoembryonic antigen (CEA), alpha-fetoprotein (AFP), and carbohydrate antigen 19–9 (CA 19–9) are serum markers that may raise suspicion of malignancy associated with gallbladder carcinoma, but more recent studies have shown no diagnostic or prognostic significance for this cancer. These markers may have greater significance when used in combination.[15,16] Novel tumor markers are being investigated to determine whether they are expressed in gallbladder and biliary cancers. The existence of such markers would be useful in developing diagnostic tests and treatment paradigms for these tumors.[17]

## PATHOPHYSIOLOGY

### Cellular characteristics

The vast majority of gallbladder cancers are adenocarcinomas, which occur in 85% of patients, followed in frequency by papillary carcinoma and mucinous adenocarcinoma. Cancers of the gallbladder can be one of several histologic types, including papillary, nodular, tubular, and combinations. Histologic grades of gallbladder carcinoma include well differentiated, moderately differentiated, poorly differentiated, and undifferentiated.[18]

### Progression of disease

Since most individuals with cancer of the gallbladder present with disease at an advanced stage, it is difficult to know the exact progression of the disease. Gallbladder cancer is a locally invasive tumor that can extend directly into the gallbladder bed of the liver, extrahepatic bile ducts, duodenum or transverse colon, portal vein, hepatic artery, or pancreas. A tumor may originate anywhere in the gallbladder, with the most common site being the fundus, although the site of origin may be difficult to determine because most gallbladder cancers have grown beyond the limits of resectability before they are discovered.[18,19]

The patterns of spread predictably follow lymphatic and venous drainage of the gallbladder and peritoneal "drop" metastases. Venous drainage of the gallbladder is directly into the adjacent liver, and the most common pattern of spread of gallbladder cancer is through direct extension into the liver. The lymphatic drainage of the gallbladder is to the cystic duct lymph nodes and periportal lymph nodes, and then to the celiac and superior mesenteric lymph nodes. These tumors can spread into and around the cystic duct and can extend into the common bile duct, causing biliary obstruction (Figure 55-1).[20] Thus, jaundice may be the first clinical manifestation of a problem. Diffuse peritoneal seeding and distant metastasis are less common and occur late in the course of the disease.[4,19]

## CLINICAL MANIFESTATIONS

In its early stages, carcinoma of the gallbladder is usually asymptomatic. This fact contributes to the low curability rate of gallbladder carcinoma, since the lack of symptoms precludes the early diagnosis of the disease.

When signs and symptoms of gallbladder cancer manifest, they usually resemble those of benign gallbladder disease. Common symptoms are pain in the right upper abdominal quadrant, nausea, vomiting, an intolerance of fatty food, chills, and fever. Advanced age should raise the index of suspicion.[21] Individuals with gallbladder cancer commonly have advanced disease and present with nonspecific signs of malaise, anorexia, weight loss, abdominal distention, jaundice, and pruritus. Most individuals have multiple symptoms. Almost half of individuals with gallbladder cancer will present with jaundice, in addition to the clinical symptoms suggestive of biliary tract disease. This usually denotes advanced disease. Tumor invasion of the cystic duct can cause cystic duct obstruction, resulting in the development of acute cholecystitis. In advanced stages of the disease, individuals may present with a palpable mass in the right upper quadrant resulting from obstruction and distention of the gallbladder. Hepatomegaly, jaundice, cachexia, fever, and ascites may also be present as evidence of progressive disease and liver failure. Definitive diagnosis often is made at the time of surgery for jaundice or acute cholecystitis.[4]

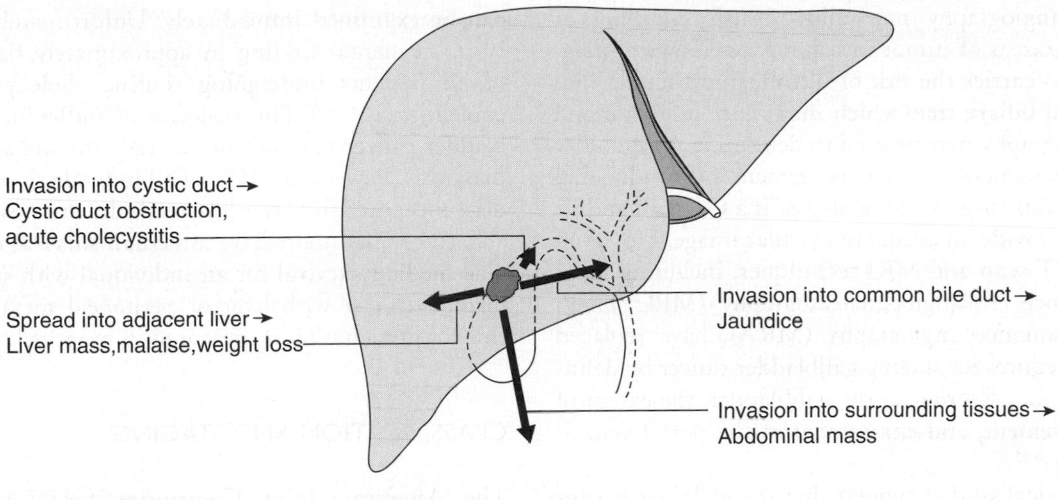


**FIGURE 55-1**

Tumor spread and presenting signs in gallbladder cancer. Gallbladder cancer commonly spreads by direct extension into surrounding tissues. This tumor extension results in the clinical presentations of jaundice, acute cholecystitis, abdominal mass, and weight loss. *Source*: Adapted with permission from Norwold DL, Dawes LG. Biliary neoplasms. In: Greenfield LJ, et al, eds. *Surgery: Scientific Principles and Practice*. 2nd ed. Philadelphia, PA: Lippincott-Raven; 1997:1056–1067.[20]

## ASSESSMENT

### Patient and family history

The individual may have had no previous symptoms or may have vague, chronic complaints of right upper quadrant pain. A change in the character of the symptoms may prompt the person to seek medical attention. Any individual who is at high risk for gallbladder cancer or who has a family history of the disease should receive a thorough evaluation.

### Physical examination

Jaundice with pruritus may be evident in individuals with an obstructing gallbladder cancer. In advanced carcinoma of the gallbladder, an individual with severe weight loss may have a visibly palpable gallbladder when supine.

### Diagnostic studies

With the exception of jaundice, no specific laboratory abnormalities may be seen. Some individuals present with acute cholecystitis manifested by fever and leukocytosis on complete blood count (CBC). Other laboratory findings may include anemia, elevated sedimentation rate, and reduced serum albumin. In more advanced cases, elevated transaminase and coagulation abnormalities may reflect liver failure.

Radiographic imaging is used to determine the extent of liver invasion, invasion of adjacent organs, vascular involvement, extent of biliary involvement, presence of nodal metastases, and presence of peritoneal metastases. The finding of a nonuniform mass replacing all or part of the gallbladder is most suspicious for a gallbladder cancer.[23]

Ultrasonography (US), computerized tomography (CT) scan, magnetic resonance imaging (MRI), cholangiography, and angiography may all be helpful in evaluating individuals with suspected gallbladder cancer.[4,22] Ultrasonography is used to identify a thickened gallbladder wall or a mass protruding into the gallbladder, either filling or replacing the gallbladder. It also may show tumor invasion of the liver or porta hepatis and may visualize adjacent adenopathy. A dilated biliary tree and hepatic metastasis may also be evaluated by ultrasound.[16] Studies suggest that US underestimates lymph node involvement and often fails to differentiate between gallbladder cancer and chronic cholecystitis.[18,23] A CT scan can demonstrate a gallbladder cancer as an intraluminal mass, a mass replacing the gallbladder, or a mass extending from the gallbladder. Computed tomography scans also allow accurate assessment of the spread of the disease. Direct invasion of the liver or porta hepatis, involvement of adjacent lymph nodes, liver metastases, and invasion of adjacent structures can also be evaluated by CT scans.[16]

New magnetic resonance cholangiography and vascular enhancement techniques make it possible to visualize biliary obstruction, encasement of the portal vein, and hepatic involvement.[8,16] Cholangiography can be useful for diagnosing gallbladder cancer in an individual with jaundice. Percutaneous transhepatic cholangiography (PTC) or endoscopic retrograde cholangiopancreatography (ERCP) may both be beneficial. The typical finding with either study is a long stricture of the common hepatic duct.[24]

Direct cholangiography may allow brush sampling or biopsy of the areas of tumor invasion for cytological diagnosis but also carries the risk of introducing bacteria into an obstructed biliary tree, which may cause infection and sepsis. Angiography may be used to determine resectability through assessment of vascular encasement if the individual has had previous surgery in the area or if a CT scan and/or MRI fail to provide an adequate vascular image. However, new spiral CT scan and MRI techniques, including magnetic resonance cholangiopancreatography (MRCP) and magnetic resonance angiography (MRA), have replaced invasive procedures for staging gallbladder cancer by defining the presence of tumor in the gallbladder, the extent of biliary involvement, and encasement of the portal vein or hepatic artery.[8,25]

If radiological studies suggest that the gallbladder cancer may be resectable or if palliative surgery is considered, tissue diagnosis is not required before surgery. However, if resection is deemed not possible due to extensive liver invasion, liver or peritoneal metastases, or encasement of the main portal vein, a biopsy of the tumor is necessary to help establish a diagnosis and confirm the stage of tumor. A percutaneous fine needle biopsy with US or CT scan guidance can assist in establishing the diagnosis.[24] The advent of endoscopic ultrasound (EUS) has become another means of obtaining tissue diagnosis.[18,24] Brushings of obstructed bile ducts or bile cytology via PTC or ERCP have a low yield of samples for diagnosis.[16] Laparoscopy may also be used to obtain a biopsy of the liver, peritoneum, or tissue around the gallbladder.[4,6,26]

### Prognostic indicators

The histologic grade of gallbladder cancer has significant prognostic implications. The presence or absence of metaplasia is an important prognostic factor. Individuals with metaplasia have a better prognosis than those with dysplasia. This period of histologic change generally occurs over a 3-year period.[27] Poorly differentiated infiltrating tumors have a strong association with gallstones, lymph node metastases, and direct extension into the liver. Papillary cell tumors are less likely to invade the liver directly and have a lower incidence of lymph node metastasis. They are also less likely to have associated gallstones. Nodular forms of tumor are more likely to infiltrate early, to invade the liver, and to have lymph node metastases along with a higher incidence of gallstones. Tubular tumors are in the midrange with respect to their aggressive metastatic behavior.[4,28]

The degree of invasion by the tumor is predictive of survival. Tumors with the best prognosis are those found incidentally at the time of cholecystectomy for symptomatic gallstone disease. This serendipitous finding emphasizes the importance of surgically opening the gallbladder at the time of cholecystectomy so that any suspicious lesion can be examined immediately. Unfortunately, carcinoma is an incidental finding in approximately 0.3% to 1.5% of all patients undergoing routine cholecystectomy for cholelithiasis.[4,19,29] The majority of individuals with gallbladder cancer have advanced stage tumors at the time of diagnosis. Fewer than 15% of all individuals with gallbladder cancer are alive after 5 years. Individuals with unresectable stage III tumors have a median survival of 6 months. The median survival for an individual with stage IV gallbladder cancer with liver or peritoneal metastases at the time of presentation is measured in months.[4]

## CLASSIFICATION AND STAGING

The American Joint Committee for Cancer Staging (AJCC) has established the TNM classification presented in Table 55–2.[30] Alternative classification schemes are currently used in Europe and Japan. Histologic grading on the basis of differentiation and the degree of invasion of the tumor are both important factors in staging gallbladder cancer and determining survival. Almost all known survivors of gallbladder cancer have had well-differentiated tumors. The higher the histologic grade, greater is the association with advanced stage and rapid disease progression. No ideal staging system exists that adequately correlates all aspects of gross and histologic pathology of cancer of the gallbladder.

## THERAPEUTIC APPROACHES AND NURSING CARE

The individual and the stage of the tumor must be considered when deciding on the appropriate treatment for gallbladder cancer. An individual's general medical condition is more important than the chronological age of the patient. When surgery is contemplated, several factors must be considered. Special attention must be given to any liver problems, as cirrhosis and portal hypertension will increase surgical risk. Obstructive jaundice may alter organ and immune function and should be treated preoperatively if liver resection is being considered. Altered renal function, poor nutritional status, and sepsis are other parameters that increase the risk for a poor surgical outcome in individuals who are jaundiced. The majority of patients undergoing treatment for gallbladder cancer is in their seventh decade of life and may be at increased risk for major surgery as a consequence of concomitant medical problems.

Local invasion of the liver is a common finding that can sometimes be managed with a wedge resection of the liver. More extensive liver involvement may require a larger liver resection. Extension of the tumor into the colon may require a colon resection. Progression of tumor into the

**TABLE 55-2**

**AJCC TMN Staging for Gallbladder Cancer**

| | | | |
|---|---|---|---|
| **Primary Tumor (T)** | | | |
| TX | Primary tumor cannot be assessed | | |
| T0 | No evidence of primary tumor | | |
| Tis | Carcinoma in situ | | |
| TI | Tumor invades lamina propria or muscle layer | | |
| TIa | Tumor invades lamina propria | | |
| TIb | Tumor invades muscle layer | | |
| T2 | Tumor invades perimuscular connective tissue; no extension beyond serosa or into liver | | |
| T3 | Tumor perforates the serosa (visceral peritoneum) and/or directly invades the liver and/or one other adjacent organ or structure, such as stomach, duodenum, colon, or pancreas, omentum or extrahepatic bile ducts | | |
| T4 | Tumor invades main portal vein or hepatic artery or invades multiple extrahepatic organs or structures | | |
| **Regional Lymph Nodes (N)** | | | |
| NX | Regional lymph nodes cannot be assessed | | |
| N0 | No regional lymph node metastasis | | |
| NI | Regional lymph node metastasis | | |
| **Distant Metastasis (M)** | | | |
| MX | Distant metastasis cannot be assessed | | |
| M0 | No distant metastasis | | |
| M2 | Distant metastasis | | |
| **Stage Grouping** | | | |
| Stage 0 | Tis | N0 | M0 |
| Stage IA | TI | N0 | M0 |
| Stage IB | T2 | N0 | M0 |
| Stage IIA | T3 | N0 | M0 |
| Stage IIB | TI | NI | M0 |
| | T2 | NI | M0 |
| | T3 | NI | M0 |
| Stage III | T4 | Any N | M0 |
| Stage IV | Any T | Any N | MI |

*Source*: Data from Greene et al.[30]

duodenum or pancreatic head can be resected with a pancreaticoduodenectomy. Multiple metastases in both lobes of the liver or peritoneum or distant metastases are considered contraindications to resection of the primary gallbladder tumor.

## Surgery

Although fewer than 50% of cancers of the gallbladder are resectable, the most effective treatment for this form of cancer is resection of the primary tumor and areas where it has locally invaded.[19] With improving safety of liver resections and biliary reconstructions, major resections are being performed and have shown a curative potential even for advanced disease.[29]

Cholecystectomy is the primary treatment for stage I gallbladder carcinoma. Many gallbladder cancers are found incidentally at the time of elective cholecystectomy. Reexploration to perform an extended resection may then be recommended within a few weeks of the original cholecystectomy.[4,6,8,24]

The treatment approach also depends on the depth of invasion of the gallbladder wall. If the tumor is limited to the mucosa, a simple cholecystectomy is sufficient therapy and has a very good prognosis. If the tumor penetrates the serosa, however, a simple cholecystectomy is not adequate. The position of the tumor within the gallbladder wall may also dictate further therapy. If the tumor is next to the liver bed, with minimal invasion, the recurrence rate may be high. Likewise, if the tumor is superficial and away from the liver, cholecystectomy may be an adequate operation.[6,18]

Laparoscopic removal of known gallbladder cancer is not recommended. Tumor implantation at the port sites has been found when gallbladder cancer was removed laparoscopically. Laparoscopic manipulation of the tumor could also lead to tumor dissemination in the abdomen.[6,18]

When the cancer involves deeper layers of the gallbladder wall, the prognosis is grim. A radical or extended cholecystectomy has been recommended in the hopes of improving survival. The extended procedure consists of a cholecystectomy with a wide resection of the liver around the gallbladder bed and a major lymph node dissection[19] (Figure 55-2). If the tumor is near the cystic duct or if the bile duct is involved with the tumor, a bile duct resection may be performed at the time of the extended cholecystectomy. Studies have shown an improved 5-year survival as high as 35% with this extended cholecystectomy approach.[19,24] Even when the serosa is involved, extended cholecystectomy provides a better survival advantage over simple cholecystectomy. This extensive resection should be considered the therapy of choice for preoperatively recognized and potentially resectable gallbladder cancer.[4,19,24] More extensive resections that include both the liver and the duodenum or pancreas have been advocated by some researchers. In recent years, the morbidity and mortality have been significantly reduced particularly when this surgery is performed at a high volume hepatobiliary center.[19,24,31] Survival after surgical resection depends on tumor stage and the operation performed. For stage I tumors, the 5-year survival after routine cholecystectomy is greater than 85%. For stage II, III, and IV tumors, 5-year survival is approximately

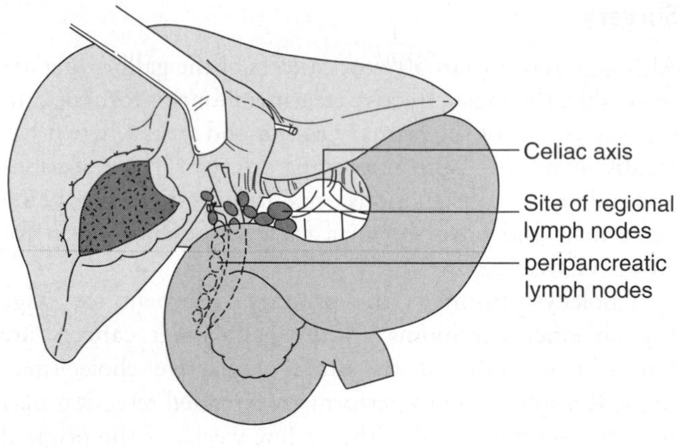


**FIGURE 55-2**

Treatment for invasive gallbladder cancer is cholecystectomy and a wedge resection of the liver along with a regional lymphadenectomy. The wedge resection of the liver is illustrated along with the lymph node regions that drain the gallbladder and that should be removed during the operation for gallbladder cancer.

*Source*: Adapted with permission from Norwold DL, Dawes LG. Biliary neoplasms. In: Greenfield LJ, et al, eds. *Surgery: Scientific Principles and Practice*. 2nd ed. Philadelphia, PA: Lippincott-Raven; 1997:1056–1067.[20]

25%, 10%, and 2%, respectively. Individuals with stage II tumors treated with an extended cholecystectomy may be expected to have a 5-year survival of better than 78%.[23] The best survival for individuals with advanced tumors has been attained in Japan with more radical surgery, including removal of adjacent liver, lymph nodes, and/or involved adjacent viscera.[8] Results from major hepatobiliary centers in the United States are revealing improved survival with reoperation after an incidental finding of gallbladder cancer during cholecystectomy and radical resection in patients with advanced disease.[8,24,26]

*Postoperative care.* Routine postoperative care is necessary for an individual having a simple cholecystectomy. The surgery may be done on an outpatient basis or with a hospitalization of only a few days. For an extensive surgery involving the removal of any part of the liver or surrounding tissues, more intensive monitoring and assessment are needed. The nursing care for these individuals is the same as for anyone having a major liver resection. The main concerns in the care of an individual following hepatic surgery are control of hemorrhage, replacement of blood loss, prevention of infection and pneumonia, and appropriate supportive care. Postoperative complications include hemorrhage, biliary fistula, infection, transient metabolic consequences, subphrenic abscess, pneumonia, atelectasis, portal hypertension, and clotting defects. Careful attention to any wound, tubes, and drains, along with critical analyses of the appearance of drainage, is also vital. Knowledge of the potential complications, expected reactions, and anticipatory nursing care will aid greatly in the postoperative period.

Adjuvant treatment modalities are limited. It can be disconcerting to the individual to learn that there is little treatment to offer with any proven benefit for advanced cancer of the gallbladder. The nurse should review and explain postoperative treatment. Listening and supporting patients during their perioperative care help them and their families during a stressful time. While hospitalization is often minimal after surgery, patients are faced not only with attempting to recover from a physical insult but also with the psychological impact of a cancer with a grim prognosis.

## Palliative therapy

Most therapies for gallbladder cancer are palliative. Palliative management for gallbladder cancer is directed at the relief of jaundice, treatment of sepsis, and palliation of pain. The majority of gallbladder tumors are unable to be resected with negative margins. If a tissue diagnosis can be obtained through percutaneous liver biopsy or by laparoscopy, nonoperative palliation should be considered.

*Nonoperative management.* Many individuals with gallbladder cancer will have obstructive jaundice, which can be relieved and managed with an endoscopic biliary stent or percutaneous transhepatic biliary stent.[4] If metastatic disease is found, the jaundice may be relieved with a percutaneous transhepatic biliary stent, which may be left in place or changed to an internal stent. Patients with a percutaneous transhepatic biliary stent may develop acute cholecystitis, which subsequently may require percutaneous drainage of the gallbladder and intravenous antibiotics.[32] Recurrent jaundice and cholangitis are problems that may recur during the course of the disease due to tumor obstruction of the biliary tree or biliary stent. However, when a patient has a biliary stent placed that resolves jaundice and pruritus, an improvement in appetite, nausea, and quality of life also occur.[33]

Unfortunately, individuals who require nonoperative palliation usually do not survive more than 3 months. Pain should be treated aggressively to improve the individual's quality of life. Opiates are given as indicated. Radiation therapy may help to reduce the pain. Percutaneous celiac nerve block may also be helpful for this purpose.

*Operative palliation.* Surgery may be performed to obtain a tissue diagnosis, remove the gallbladder to prevent acute cholecystitis, relieve or prevent pain, and treat or prevent gastric outlet obstruction. A gastrojejunostomy bypass may be performed to relieve or prevent gastric outlet obstruction.

For a tumor that is locally unresectable without extension to adjacent organs (duodenum or pancreas), a Roux-en-Y choledochojejunostomy (anastomosis of a loop of jejunum to the common bile duct proximal to the obstruction) may be performed. At the time of exploration, the tumor margins should be marked with radiopaque clips if external beam radiotherapy is being considered. Nursing care is the same as for any abdominal surgery.

The addition of an internal–external percutaneous transhepatic biliary stent depends on the extent of the disease and the choice of the physician in treating jaundice. The individual and the family will need to be taught how to care for and flush the stent, as it may be left in place for the rest of the person's life. The stent is usually flushed twice a day with sterile normal saline solution. Daily cleansing of the stent site is required. A patient may require right and left biliary stents to drain both lobes of the liver if the tumor is obstructing the bifurcation of the biliary tree into the liver. Signs and symptoms of complications related to the stent must be reviewed to enable the individual and family to notify the clinician promptly to avoid problems and unnecessary hospitalization. The use of an internal self-expandable metallic stent to palliate obstructive jaundice is now favored for individuals with only a few months to live.[34] The stent may be placed by an interventional radiologist or endoscopist.

The majority of individuals with gallbladder cancer have advanced stage tumors at the time of diagnosis. Fewer than 15% of all individuals with gallbladder cancer are alive after 5 years. Individuals with unresectable stage III tumors have a median survival of 5 months.[35] The median survival for an individual with stage IV gallbladder cancer with liver or peritoneal metastases at the time of presentation is only 1 to 3 months.[35]

### Radiation therapy

Radiation therapy has been used to treat individuals with resected gallbladder cancer as well as those with unresectable tumors. There has been no proven, survival advantage with external beam radiation, alone or after surgery. In unresectable cancer, external beam radiation has been used to help relieve pain or to relieve biliary obstruction. Intraoperative radiation has also been used, but the advantage of this technique combined with resection and/or external beam radiotherapy has not been proven, and further trials regarding this modality are necessary.[4,36] Likewise, the role of radiation sensitizers, such as fluorouracil (5 FU), and the addition of leucovorin to intraoperative or external beam radiation therapy has yet to be conclusively studied in individuals with gallbladder cancer.[37] Overall, the data in support of using radiotherapy are meager but hopeful, supporting the need for additional research.[8] The curative potential of an operation may be enhanced by postoperative radiotherapy. Palliation, including relief from obstruction, may be achieved for a period in patients with advanced disease.[8,31]

### Chemotherapy

Chemotherapy agents for the treatment of gallbladder cancer have been limited due to poor tumor response. Mitomycin C and 5 FU have been most commonly used. Gemcitabine has shown promise for treatment of advanced gallbladder carcinoma, in a number of small studies with reported response rates between 8% and 60%.[31] In individuals suspected of having microscopic disease after resection, chemotherapy may be considered as adjuvant therapy, but its effectiveness has been difficult to document. Intra-arterial and intraperitoneal delivery of chemotherapeutic agents has been tried, with varying results. Molecular biology provides some new and hopeful treatment options. Cytokines, tumor necrosis factor, and epidermal growth factor are examples of concepts being used in the development of new therapeutics.[38] These biological agents target specific cell locations to interrupt the progression of disease based on the specific molecular expression of the disease.[38] Chemotherapy combined with radiation therapy may have value postoperatively for patients who have had resection for advanced disease[6,23]

The rarity of gallbladder cancer limits the ability to perform prospective, randomized studies of therapy, as the majority of cases present at an advanced stage. Since there is no standard therapy for advanced gallbladder cancer, individuals should be offered the opportunity to participate in controlled clinical trials.

## SYMPTOM MANAGEMENT AND SUPPORTIVE CARE

Individuals with advanced cancer of the gallbladder usually have disease involving the liver and biliary tree. Obstructive jaundice, liver abscess, and liver failure are potential complications. The patient and family must be taught how to manage any drain or percutaneous transhepatic biliary stent. Teaching them the signs and symptoms of potential problems resulting from the tumor or any tubes and drains may allow for earlier intervention and less need for hospitalization. Persistent pain, fever, chills, and recurrent jaundice may be symptoms of a liver abscess caused by obstructed bile ducts, or of a malfunctioning endoscopic or percutaneous biliary stent.

With progressive liver failure, ascites and increased abdominal girth may cause pain, discomfort, and dyspnea. Supportive measures include aggressive pain management and proper body positioning. Ascites can be controlled by fluid and sodium restriction along with diuretic therapy. A peritoneal tap may be necessary to relieve abdominal distention and provide comfort and easier breathing.

Intra-abdominal spread of tumor can cause pain and palpable or visible tumor.

Nutritional intake is poor in the individual with gallbladder cancer and jaundice. Elevated bilirubin levels cause changes in taste, leading to a decrease in appetite and weight loss. Cold foods may be better tolerated. Food prepared with spices that enhance taste can be tried. Plastic silverware can be used if the individual complains of a metallic taste in the mouth. Small, frequent snacks and a change in the environment may be helpful. Nausea, vomiting, and anorexia can also hinder nutrition. Antiemetics prior to eating may assist in controlling nausea and vomiting. Megestrol acetate and cannabinoids may help to manage anorexia.

Liver failure usually develops as the disease progresses and follows a progression of lethargy and weakness to encephalopathy and hepatic coma. Renal failure is also common at this time. The nurse can assist the family by explaining what to expect as the symptoms develop. Individual and family support is the major goal of nursing care.

Most individuals with gallbladder cancer present with advanced disease and rapid decline. Palliative care should be initiated early with transition to hospice care. Communication from the inpatient or outpatient nurse to home care, palliative care, and hospice nurses can be invaluable in providing quality care to an individual with a rapidly changing condition. Attention to individual and family needs is made easier when the nurses who know the most about the individual share information. The burden to the family and their experience with cancer can be greatly eased by anticipatory management and supportive care.

### FUTURE TRENDS

Advances in the understanding of the genetics of gallbladder cancer may help in diagnosing this form of cancer, screening patients at risk, and developing new therapies. The use of noninvasive radiographic imaging will continue to enhance the diagnosis of carcinoma of the gallbladder. Surgical innovations for gallbladder cancer will continue to be a challenge for the surgeon and nurses caring for these patients. Multi-institutional clinical trials are needed before routine use of any neoadjuvant or adjuvant chemotherapy and/or radiation therapy for gallbladder cancer can be recommended.

## BILE DUCT CANCER

### INTRODUCTION

Adenocarcinoma of the bile duct is also referred to as *cholangiocarcinoma.* It is a rare malignancy that can occur anywhere in the biliary tree. The spectrum of cholangiocarcinoma is best classified into 3 anatomic groups: (1) perihilar, (2) distal, and (3) intrahepatic. Perihilar lesions are the most common, accounting for approximately 50% of these tumors. Distal tumors are the second most common and intrahepatic cholangiocarcinomas occur in 5% to 10% of cases (Figure 55-3).[8,39] Cholangiocarcinoma occurs with conditions in which bile is stagnant, infected, or both, and with the formation of bile duct stones. A diagnosis of cholangiocarcinoma should be considered in every case of obstructive jaundice. Diagnosis and management of cholangiocarcinoma are often challenging and complex. Ideally, diagnosis of an early cholangiocarcinoma may reveal a small, localized tumor that may be amenable to an aggressive multidisciplinary approach.

### EPIDEMIOLOGY

Approximately 21,000 new cases of liver and intrahepatic bile duct cancer are diagnosed annually in the United States.[2] Intrahepatic cholangiocarcinoma is much less common than liver cancer and also occurs less frequently than extrahepatic cholangiocarcinoma. A recent study reports between 2500 and 4000 new cases of extrahepatic cholangiocarcinoma in the United States annually.[8] The US incidence approaches 2 per 100,000 people each year, with a higher incidence in specific groups at high risk for the disease.[40] The incidence of cholangiocarcinoma increases with age, with the mean age at presentation being over 65 years. These tumors occur with similar frequency in

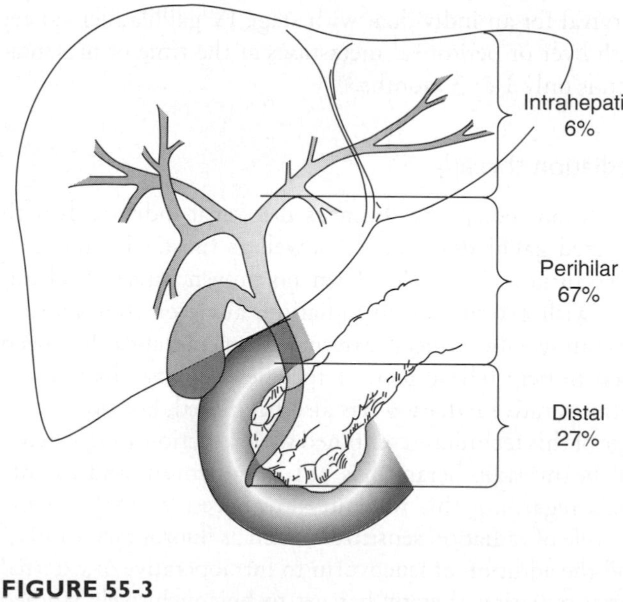


**FIGURE 55-3**

Distribution of 294 cholangiocarcinomas into intrahepatic, perihilar, and distal subgroups.

*Source:* Used with permission from Nakeeb A, Pitt HA, Sohn TA, et al. Cholangiocarcinomas: a spectrum of intrahepatic, perihilar, and distal tumors. *Ann Surg.* 1996;224:463–475.[39]

men and women.[41,42] Increased frequency of cancers of the biliary tract have been reported in Southeast Asia, Japan, Eastern Europe, Central and South America, and among American Indians and Hispanic Americans.[41]

## ETIOLOGY

Several risk factors have been linked to cholangiocarcinoma (Table 55–3). Factors common to a number of these etiological parameters include biliary stasis and infection with and without intrahepatic or common bile duct stones. Only a small proportion of individuals with cholangiocarcinoma typically have these risk factors.

Strong associations have been seen in individuals with cystic dilatation of the bile duct, including both choledochal cyst disease and Caroli's disease (congenital dilatation of the intrahepatic bile ducts). Individuals with cholangiocarcinoma associated with choledochal cysts are usually diagnosed at a median age of 34.[8] The origin of choledochal cysts and subsequent formation of cholangiocarcinoma has been explained by an APBDJ, where there is a high entry of the pancreatic duct into the extrahepatic biliary tree. This finding suggests that reflux of pancreatic exocrine secretions into the bile duct may lead to malignant transformation of the biliary epithelium. Other factors that may lead to malignant transformation in choledochal cysts include bile stasis within the cyst, stone formation, chronic inflammation, and bacterial infection.[8,43] These same factors may play a role in the high incidence of cholangiocarcinoma in individuals with Caroli's disease.[41]

In East Asia, a clear association has been recognized between cholangiocarcinoma and infection with the liver fluke *Clonorchis sinensis*. This infection results from consuming infected raw fish. The parasite usually occupies the intrahepatic bile ducts, obstructing the flow of bile. Another liver fluke, *Opisthorchis viverrini*, is endemic to Thailand and is also associated with cholangiocarcinoma.[43,44] The combination of liver fluke infestation and a diet high in nitrosamines may explain the high incidence of cholangiocarcinoma in this region.[45] It has been suggested that the presence of *Opisthorchis viverrini* may induce DNA damage and mutation in the intrahepatic biliary epithelium.[43]

**TABLE 55-3**

**Risk Factors for Bile Duct Cancer**

| High Risk | Possible Increased Risk |
|---|---|
| Cystic dilation of bile duct | Asbestos |
| Choledochal cyst | Dioxin (Agent Orange) |
| Caroli's disease | Isoniazid |
| Clonorchis | Methyldopa |
| Hepatolithiasis | Nitrosamines |
| Sclerosing cholangitis | Opisthorchiasis |
| Thorium dioxide (Thorotrast) | Oral contraceptives |
| Ulcerative colitis | Polychlorinated biphenyls |

The cause and effect relationship between cholelithiasis and cholangiocarcinoma has not been established. Yet a recent study showed that the risk of biliary tract cancer among women was significantly associated with a history of cholelithiasis and postmenopausal status.[46,47]

Individuals with hepatolithiasis, which is commonly found in Southeast Asia, have a 5% to 10% risk of developing cholangiocarcinoma during their lifetime. Bile stasis, infected bile, and cystic dilatation of the intrahepatic biliary tree may all be risk factors for the development of bile duct cancer.[41,45]

Individuals with sclerosing cholangitis are also at increased risk for developing cholangiocarcinoma. Primary sclerosing cholangitis (PSC) is an idiopathic disease characterized by multiple intrahepatic and extrahepatic inflammatory bile duct strictures that cannot be attributed to specific causes.[48] Cholangiocarcinoma that develops in individuals with sclerosing cholangitis is often manifested by rapid clinical deterioration and progressive jaundice.[49] The majority of individuals with sclerosing cholangitis have coexisting ulcerative colitis. The prevalence of cholangiocarcinoma in individuals with ulcerative colitis is significantly greater than the risk for the general population.[45,51] Ulcerative colitis is often quiescent in individuals who develop sclerosing cholangitis, and can go unrecognized. The colitis precedes the cholangiocarcinoma by an average of 5 years. Individuals with sclerosing cholangitis or ulcerative colitis who develop bile duct cancer are usually in their fifth decade, approximately 20 years younger than individuals without these risk factors.[51]

The radiocontrast agent thorium dioxide (Thorotrast) has also been shown to cause hepatic and bile duct malignancies. Thorotrast was used as a contrast agent for radiography from the late 1920s until the 1940s. It emits energy as alpha particles and, when injected intravenously, is retained in the reticuloendothelial system for life. Cholangiocarcinomas have been diagnosed in individuals on an average of 35 years after exposure.[52] A number of chemicals and several other drugs have been associated with cholangiocarcinoma, including asbestos, dioxin (Agent Orange), isoniazid, and methyldopa.[42] Dietary nitrosamines, which are present in cured meats, have also been suspected.[42] A clustering of persons with cholangiocarcinoma has been reported in certain geographical areas of the United States, underscoring the importance of environmental factors in the pathogenesis of cholangiocarcinoma.[53,54] Exposure to chemicals used in the rubber, automobile, wood finishing, and metal fabricating industries has been associated with an increased risk of gallbladder carcinoma.[8,43]

## PREVENTION, SCREENING, AND EARLY DETECTION

At present there is no effective screening for cancer of the biliary tree. Studies are needed to develop a serum or a bile marker for early detection of cholangiocarcinoma in high-risk individuals with hepatolithiasis, choledochal cysts, sclerosing cholangitis, or ulcerative colitis. Further genetic, dietary, occupational, and environmental analysis of clusters of people with cholangiocarcinoma may provide additional clues to the pathogenesis of these rare tumors.

The role of prevention is important, as there is limited benefit from surgery in these patients, and other therapies are even less effective. Early detection with timely resection is necessary to improve the survival rate of persons with biliary carcinoma. Screening and removal of stone-containing gallbladders may gain acceptance with the advent of innovative surgical techniques.

## PATHOPHYSIOLOGY

### Cellular characteristics

Cholangiocarcinomas arise from the epithelium of the intrahepatic and extrahepatic bile ducts. They appear as firm, gray-white tumors. Central necrosis may be observed. The majority of bile duct cancers are adenocarcinomas, with papillary adenocarcinoma and mucinous and mucin-producing adenocarcinomas, the next largest groups. Extrahepatic bile duct papillary adenocarcinomas have the best prognosis, while mucinous adenocarcinomas have the poorest outcome.[55]

The tumors range from well-differentiated to poorly differentiated varieties that exhibit glandular or acinar structures. Mucin is almost always found within the cytoplasm of the cells. Cells tend to be cuboidal or low columnar and resemble biliary epithelium, though bile production is not usually seen.[28]

Other histologic types of bile duct cancers include squamous, mucoepidermoid, leiomyosarcoma, rhabdomyosarcoma, cystadenocarcinoma, carcinoid, and granular cell carcinoma.[28] The pathological determination of malignancy may be difficult, especially if there is cholangitis, hepatolithiasis, biliary obstruction, and stents. The pathological diagnosis is supported by any additional finding of (1) a positive reaction to CEA, (2) nuclear size variation, (3) distended intracytoplasmic lumina, or (4) neural invasion. Most cholangiocarcinomas will stain positively for CEA as well as for the carbohydrate antigens CA 125 and CA 19–9.[41] New digital imaging techniques such as fluorescence in situ hybridization (FISH) analyze cell contents to identify aneuploidy. By comparing digital renderings, variants of normal can then be correlated to cytology with a high degree of accuracy for cholangiocarcinoma.[41,45,56]

### Progression of disease

Cholangiocarcinoma originating within the hepatic parenchyma is usually a solitary and large mass. Tumor invasion of the large portal or hepatic veins may occur. Intrahepatic tumors tend to present as solitary masses. Perihilar cholangiocarcinoma may present as an infiltrative mass that extends from the hilum into the parenchyma of the liver as a sclerotic mass that encircles a large bile duct, or as a polypoid tumor that invades the lumen of a large bile duct. Distal bile duct cancers tend to infiltrate locally.[51]

In both the gallbladder and extrahepatic bile ducts, areas of dysplasia and carcinoma in situ may be found adjacent to invasive carcinoma, suggesting such a sequence in the development of these tumors.[51]

Extrahepatic metastases occur more frequently through the lymphatic system than through the hematogenous route. Peripancreatic and hilar lymph nodes are involved in approximately half of the cases. Metastases to the liver or peritoneal cavity are common in cholangiocarcinoma. Perineural and periductal spaces and portal tracts tend to be invaded by tumor. Lung, bone, and other sites are much less likely to be involved. When the tumor causes chronic biliary obstruction, the liver may develop secondary biliary cirrhosis.[28]

## CLINICAL MANIFESTATIONS

The majority (more than 90%) of individuals with cholangiocarcinoma present with jaundice. Pruritus, mild abdominal pain, fatigue, anorexia, and weight loss occur less frequently. Cholangitis is rarely a presenting symptom but commonly occurs following endoscopic or percutaneous biliary tract manipulation. Except for jaundice and multiple excoriations of the skin from pruritus, the physical examination is usually normal. A mass may be palpable or the liver may be enlarged with intrahepatic biliary tumors. A person with perihilar cholangiocarcinoma typically presents with mild upper abdominal pain and unilobular hepatic enlargement, as the tumor may be obstructing the intrahepatic biliary tree in either the right or left lobe of the liver.[28]

An individual who presents with upper abdominal symptoms or abnormal hepatic function without jaundice will require diagnostic studies to assist in the early diagnosis of possible bile duct carcinoma. Bile duct carcinoma without jaundice can be regarded as being in a relatively early stage and is likely to have a more favorable outcome than most bile duct carcinomas with jaundice.[25,57]

## ASSESSMENT

### Patient and family history

The individual diagnosed with cholangiocarcinoma may have had subtle weight loss, malaise, indigestion, and vague abdominal pain; or there may have been no previous symptoms. Pruritus along with the appearance of tea-colored urine and clay-colored (acholic) stools may be noticed before jaundice is evident.

Cholangiocarcinoma is difficult to diagnose in the presence of PSC. Rapid elevation of bilirubin associated with weight loss and abdominal discomfort in an otherwise stable person with PSC should alert the clinician to the possibility of cholangiocarcinoma.[42,50] Individuals should be questioned regarding any conditions that predispose them to cholangiocarcinoma.

### Physical examination

Apart from jaundice, the physical examination is usually normal in individuals with perihilar tumors. A mass may be palpable or the liver may be enlarged with an intrahepatic bile duct tumor. In an individual with a distal bile duct tumor, a distended, nontender gallbladder may be palpable.

### Diagnostic studies

*Laboratory data.* Laboratory evaluation reveals elevation of total serum bilirubin (greater than 10 mg/dL) in most individuals with cholangiocarcinoma at the time of presentation. Marked elevations of alkaline phosphatase and gamma-glutamyl transferase levels reflect bile duct epithelial cell injury. Markers of hepatocyte injury such as alanine amino transferase and aspartate amino transferase may be only slightly elevated. Individuals with chronic biliary obstruction may have laboratory evidence of depressed hepatocyte function, such as low albumin or prolonged prothrombin time.[28]

Serum tumor markers such as CEA and AFP are usually normal. Serum CA 19–9 and CA 50 may be elevated in individuals with cholangiocarcinoma, and they may be useful in screening those individuals at high risk of developing cholangiocarcinoma. The use of serum and bile tumor markers has been shown to improve the early detection of cholangiocarcinoma in persons with PSC.[42] Other serum tumor markers are being investigated. High levels of interleukin 6 (IL-6) have been found in individuals with cholangiocarcinoma and correlate with tumor burden. In association with other tumor markers such as AFP, CEA, and CA 19–9, IL-6 may be useful in distinguishing among hepatic neoplasms.[58] Currently, no accurate serum or bile screening test for bile duct cancer exists.

*Radiological evaluation.* The goal of radiological evaluation for individuals with cholangiocarcinoma is delineation of the extent of the tumor, including involvement of the bile ducts, liver, portal vessels, and distant metastases. An ordered sequence of studies will achieve this goal. Cholangiocarcinoma is suspected on the basis of an abnormal US or CT scan. An intrahepatic tumor is visualized as a liver mass, with or without peripherally dilated bile ducts. A perihilar cholangiocarcinoma produces a picture of dilated intrahepatic bile ducts, a normal or collapsed gallbladder, and a normal pancreas. A distal cholangiocarcinoma causes dilation of intrahepatic and extrahepatic bile ducts as well as of the gallbladder, with or without a mass in the head of the pancreas.

Ultrasonography and CT scans have comparable accuracy in depicting the level of biliary obstruction.[22,55] CT is more useful than US for determining resectability because of its greater sensitivity in depicting the actual tumor mass, vascular invasion, spread to adjacent organs, and distant metastases.[59] However, a primary tumor mass often does not visualize on a standard CT scan or US. The newer helical 3-dimensional CT techniques and even MRI are better at detecting the parenchymal extent of the tumor. Magnetic resonance cholangiopancreatography is a noninvasive method for detecting the existence and extent of a bile duct tumor, and MRA is effective in assessing vascular invasion by a tumor.[42,60]

In some institutions, after documentation of bile duct dilation, biliary anatomy may be better defined cholangiographically through either the percutaneous transhepatic or endoscopic retrograde route. The proximal extent of the tumor is the most important feature in determining resectability. In tumors of the perihilar region/hepatic hilum, PTC is favored because it best defines the proximal (uppermost) extent of tumor involvement. This approach also allows the preoperative placement of percutaneous transhepatic biliary stents to drain the obstructed biliary tree for partial or complete relief of jaundice. For neoplasms involving the proximal common hepatic duct or the bifurcation of the bile duct, both the left and right hepatic ducts may be intubated with transhepatic biliary stents to drain both lobes of the liver.[61] A noninvasive approach is now favored in the diagnosis of bile duct cancer, as it prevents biliary instrumentation and infection associated with preoperative morbidity.

For tumors of the distal common bile duct, the use of ERCP may allow visualization of both the proximal and distal extent of the tumor within the extrahepatic biliary tree. Decompression of the obstructed biliary tree can be performed by the placement of a biliary endoprosthesis.[56,61]

*Biopsy/cytology.* Brush or scrape biopsy, or cytological examination of bile may determine a tissue diagnosis.[56] Percutaneous needle aspiration biopsy is not recommended because of the possibility of tumor seeding.[45] The use of needle biopsy to establish a diagnosis may be required only when the tumor is deemed unresectable. In this setting, punch biopsies from the lumen of the bile duct before placement of transhepatic biliary stents may yield the best diagnostic information.[28] These techniques are not performed in persons with presumed bile duct cancer to confirm diagnosis, as those individuals will ultimately be explored for resection or palliation.

## CLASSIFICATION AND STAGING

In the United States, cholangiocarcinoma is staged by the TMN classification developed by the AJCC (Table 55-4).[62] In this system, stage I tumors are confined to the bile duct mucosa or muscular layer, whereas stage II tumors invade periductal tissues. Stage III tumors have spread to regional lymph nodes and stage IV tumors either invade adjacent structures or have distant metastases. In Europe, the International Union Against Cancer classifies cholangiocarcinomas in a similar fashion. In Japan, a more complex system devised by the Japanese Cancer Society takes into account invasion of specific adjacent organs or blood vessels.

A combination of CT scan, MRI, and endoscopy may be used to stage cholangiocarcinoma. CT scan findings of bilobar peripheral hepatic metastases or extrahepatic disease preclude curative resection. Atrophy of the lobe containing the tumor with hypertrophy of the other lobe is also a sign that resection may not be possible. Cholangiography findings of extensive bilobar intrahepatic duct involvement are another indicator of unresectability. Radiographic evidence of encasement or occlusion of the common hepatic artery or main portal vein by tumor is also indicative of unresectability.[42]

As imaging technology improves, more patients with unresectable disease will be identified avoiding the need for laparotomy. The importance of staging laparoscopy in abdominal malignancies has been increasingly recognized.

## THERAPEUTIC APPROACHES AND NURSING CARE

### Surgery

Surgical resection is the most effective therapy for cancer of the bile duct. It is the appropriate option for prolonged survival and potential cure. Diagnostic imaging may not provide enough accuracy for a definitive decision regarding resectability. Obtaining a histologically proven diagnosis of malignancy may not be possible. Laparoscopy is becoming a major tool for better predicting the resectability of hepatobiliary malignancies. A staging laparoscopy may correctly identify unresectable disease and prevent unnecessary laparotomy.[56,63]

The type of surgical resection performed depends on the anatomic location of the tumor. A pancreaticoduodenectomy, or Whipple procedure, is usually the surgical operation for a distal bile duct carcinoma (see Chapter 63). The median survival rate has been reported to be 22 months. Intrahepatic cholangiocarcinoma is managed optimally with hepatic resection (see Chapter 56).[64] The prognosis for resectable intrahepatic cholangiocarcinoma is more favorable than that for perihilar cholangiocarcinoma, with a median survival rate of 9 to 30 months.[53] Incidental bile duct carcinomas may be found at the time of liver transplantation performed for PSC.[53]

Although controversial, percutaneous transhepatic biliary drains (PTBD) may be inserted preoperatively in individuals undergoing surgical exploration for perihilar

**TABLE 55-4**

**AJCC TNM Staging for Extrahepatic Bile Duct Tumors**

| | | | |
|---|---|---|---|
| **Primary Tumor (T)** | | | |
| TX | Primary tumor cannot be assessed | | |
| T0 | No evidence of primary tumor | | |
| Tis | Carcinoma in situ | | |
| T1 | Tumor confined to the bile duct histologically | | |
| T2 | Tumor invades beyond the wall of the bile duct | | |
| T3 | Tumor invades the liver, gallbladder, pancreas, and/or unilateral branches of the portal vein (right or left) or hepatic artery (right or left) | | |
| T4 | Tumor invades any of the following: main portal vein or its branches bilaterally, common hepatic artery, or other adjacent structures, such as colon, stomach, duodenum, or abdominal wall | | |
| **Regional Lymph Nodes (N)** | | | |
| NX | Regional lymph nodes cannot be assessed | | |
| N0 | No regional lymph nodes metastasis | | |
| N1 | Regional lymph node metastasis | | |
| **Distant Metastasis (M)** | | | |
| MX | Distant metastasis cannot be assessed | | |
| M0 | No distant metastasis | | |
| M1 | Distant metastasis | | |
| **Stage Grouping** | | | |
| Stage 0 | Tis | N0 | M0 |
| Stage IA | T1 | N0 | M0 |
| Stage IB | T2 | N0 | M0 |
| Stage IIA | T3 | N0 | M0 |
| Stage IIB | T1 | N1 | M0 |
| | T2 | N1 | M0 |
| | T3 | N1 | M0 |
| Stage III | T4 | Any N | M0 |
| Stage IV | Any T | Any N | M1 |

*Source*: Data from Greene et al.[30]

cholangiocarcinoma. These drains (biliary stents) provide decompression of the biliary tree and palliation of symptomatic jaundice.[57,65] The stents assist in the technical aspects of hilar dissection by allowing palpation of the catheter within the biliary tree to identify and dissect the hepatic duct bifurcation at the time of exploration.[66]

Stents may also be placed endoscopically. Endoscopic biliary drainage (EBD) is less invasive but often needs to be converted to percutaneous drainage when decompression is needed for a prolonged period.[60,67] Controversy still exists whether a single lobe of the liver or total hepatic drainage should be performed even though only 25% to 30% of the liver needs to be drained to ameliorate jaundice.[68] The overall impact of these procedures on morbidity and mortality remains unclear. Research is ongoing.[68]

Perihilar bile duct carcinomas may be removed with a hilar resection at the hepatic duct bifurcation combined with a hepaticojejunostomy (biliary enteric anastomosis).[54]

Perihilar cholangiocarcinoma may extend along either the right or left hepatic duct into the hepatic parenchyma. A hepatic lobectomy may be considered in addition to the hilar resection.[22,57] The role of total hepatectomy and liver transplantation in treating intrahepatic cholangiocarcinoma remains a viable option although there is a scarcity of available donor organs. Patients with unresectable disease but with otherwise normal biliary and hepatic structure and function may benefit from liver transplantation.[45] Patients with PSC are also candidates for liver transplantation. For this reason it is important to maintain surveillance of their condition, so that transplant can occur before progression to advanced disease.[50] Combination of neoadjuvant chemotherapy and radiation may further improve results after liver transplantation.[22]

Factors shown to be predictors of survival in patients with resection for bile duct carcinomas include negative margin status, preoperative albumin level, postoperative sepsis, serum bilirubin concentration, preoperative jaundice, lymph node involvement and tumor grade. Nutritional status may also play an important role in the eventual outcome.[69–71]

The care of the patient after surgery for bile duct cancer is the same as for any major abdominal procedure. Expert nursing care is essential in managing stents and potential complications. Patients and their families are helped throughout the perioperative period by education and support provided by the nurse.

## Palliative therapy

Although much progress has been made in the diagnosis and management of perihilar cholangiocarcinoma, complete surgical resection is usually impossible because of local tumor invasion. Most patients can be managed only by palliative drainage.

Palliative therapy in patients with cholangiocarcinoma can include both nonoperative and operative procedures. Patients who need nonoperative palliation may have biliary decompression performed using stents placed by either the percutaneous or endoscopic route.[40,57] Most patients with unresectable perihilar tumors are not candidates for endoscopic biliary stents. The placement of percutaneous transhepatic biliary stents and subsequent placement of self-expandable metallic stents is the palliative procedure of choice for these patients. Percutaneous transhepatic biliary stents are left in place and may be exchanged for larger diameter, softer silastic transhepatic stents by interventional radiology (Figure 55-4).[42,72] Transhepatic biliary stents may also be placed to facilitate the delivery of high doses of local radiation (brachytherapy). Radioactive seeds on long guidewires are placed directly adjacent to the site of the tumor through the transhepatic stent (Figure 55-5).

A patient who is found at laparotomy to have a widespread intraperitoneal tumor will have his or her gallbladder removed to prevent the subsequent development of acute cholecystitis, which may result from the preoperative placement of percutaneous transhepatic biliary stents causing obstruction of the cystic duct.

A patient with a locally advanced unresectable perihilar tumor may have a Roux-en-Y choledochojejunostomy with intraoperative placement of larger silastic transhepatic stents. A segment III bypass to the left intrahepatic ducts may be performed for biliary decompression.[73] For distal bile duct tumors, a double bowel bypass, choledochojejunostomy, and gastrojejunostomy are usually the procedures of choice (see Chapter 63).

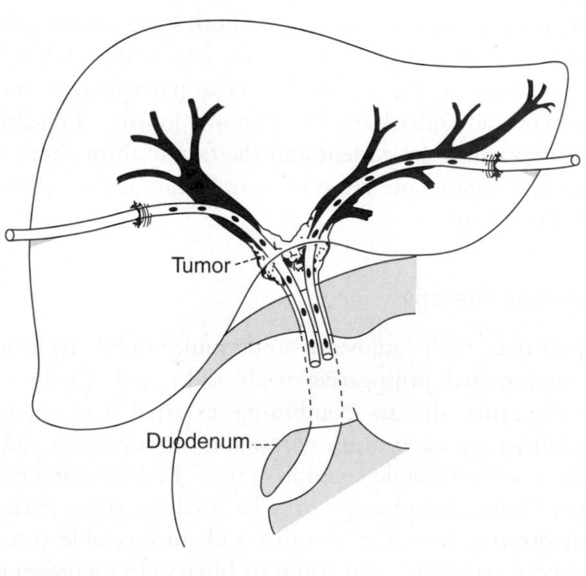


**FIGURE 55-4**

Transhepatic stents are placed in both the right and left hepatic ductal system for palliation of an obstructing proximal tumor. The internal ends of the tubes are left in the distal common bile duct.

*Source:* Used with permission from Rossi et al.[72]

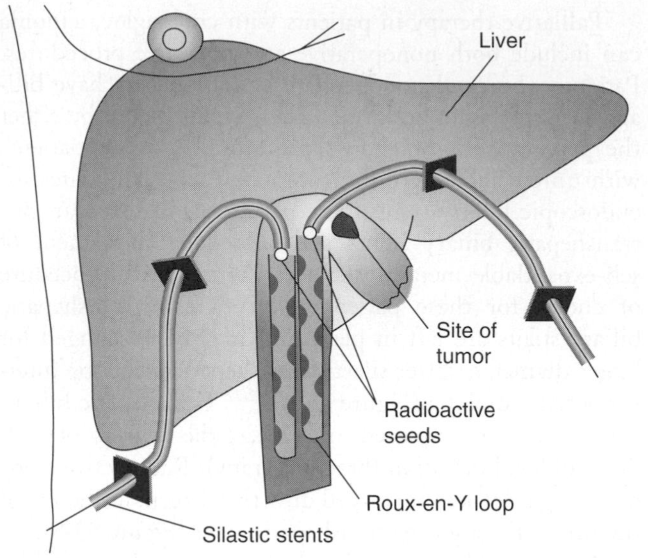


**FIGURE 55-5**

Transhepatic silastic stents can be used as conduits for delivering radioactive $^{192}$Ir seeds to the site of tumor.
*Source*: Used with permission from Rossi et al.[73]

Newer therapies such as photodynamic therapy, transarterial embolization, and intraluminal brachytherapy have also been employed in the treatment of patients with unresectable perihilar bile duct cancer.[40,56,60] Preoperative portal vein embolization has been used to provide safer liver surgery and to make these difficult perihilar tumors more resectable.[60]

Chemotherapy or radiation or both have offered generally poor results as palliative therapy for unresectable bile duct carcinoma. Patients may elect to participate in novel therapies and embark on an unknown journey. Educating and supporting the patient and the family throughout the diagnosis, treatment, and disease trajectory is the hallmark of nursing care.

### Radiation therapy

Experience with adjuvant and multimodal treatment in randomized prospective trials is limited. Reports in the literature discuss combining external and internal brachytherapy via iridium wires, and intraoperative radiotherapy with systemic chemotherapy.[57] Radiotherapy combined with chemotherapy may be used for those patients with positive resection margins and unresectable tumors to relieve pain and contribute to biliary decompression.[73] Neoadjuvant radiation and chemoradiation in combination with other modalities such as photodynamic therapy have also been investigated. These studies show no clear benefit and neoadjuvant therapies are not included in the standard of care.[40,60]

Retrospective studies suggest that patients who receive external beam radiation therapy combined with self-expanding metallic stents have improved survival and stent patency compared with patients receiving stenting alone.[74] A recent retrospective analysis of over 3800 patients suggests that adjuvant radiation improves overall survival with little impact on cure rates.[73]

### Chemotherapy

The use of chemotherapy alone, using 5 FU and multiple other chemotherapeutic drugs, has not been shown to improve survival in patients with either resected or unresected bile duct carcinoma. 5 FU and cisplatin or 5 FU and gemcitabine may be promising regimens in the palliative treatment of unresectable bile duct cancer. Other drugs—including hormones, antiestrogens, cholecystokinin, somatostatin, and antibiotics used as cytotoxic agents—have been tried as novel approaches.[28] There is interest in therapy related to HER-1 and HER-2 receptors as well as anti-VEGF targeted therapies. Although promising, at this time no definitive data is available.[40,41] Some studies show that photodynamic therapy may provide some benefit.[42,55] Controlled human trials are necessary to determine whether any of these have an impact on this type of tumor.

## SYMPTOM MANAGEMENT AND SUPPORTIVE CARE

The symptom management of individuals with advanced bile duct cancer parallels that of individuals with gallbladder cancer. Palliation of obstructive jaundice by endoscopic or percutaneous stents may be a primary objective. Internal metallic, expandable stents placed in the biliary ducts to maintain lumen patency may be the optimal intervention for patients with only a couple of months to live. Liver abscess due to obstruction of the biliary ducts, as well as liver failure are potential complications. The symptoms of persistent pain, fever, chills, and recurrent jaundice may indicate a liver abscess, which can be treated by percutaneous drainage and antibiotics. Malfunctioning endoscopic or percutaneous biliary stents can also present as fever, chills, and recurrent jaundice. Internal, metallic expandable stents may become occluded with debris or tumor. A percutaneous transhepatic biliary stent may need to be placed to relieve the obstruction from a metallic stent.

Erosion of tumor into a major blood vessel, such as the portal vein or hepatic artery, is another potential problem that can cause a massive bleed and death. Support for the family is important, as the individual may unexpectedly meet a rapid demise. The nurse can assist the patient and family by explaining what to expect as symptoms develop.

Maintenance of nutrition is a challenge, as individuals with obstructive jaundice have major interference of their taste buds and decreased appetite due to lack of bile in the

GI system. Different food preparations or appetite stimulants can be tried to help bolster an individual's intake.

Individuals who succumb to progressive liver failure usually lapse into hepatic coma. Progressive liver failure must be recognized and supportive nursing care rendered. The major goals of nursing care in individuals with carcinoma of the biliary tree are recognition of overt as well as subtle symptoms and their impact as the disease progresses. Comfort measures are paramount in these patients. Family support is also important to help them cope with the inevitable loss of a loved one.

Most individuals with bile duct cancer present at an advanced stage and rapidly decline. For those individuals who have surgical intervention, and whose length of survival may be extended, the outcome of the disease is the same. The nurse must be aware of how the individual and the family are coping. Not only the physical status of the patient, but also the psychosocial welfare must be considered. Whatever treatment modality the patient embarks upon, there is always a reason to provide hope and encouragement. When the patient truly declines and enters the terminal stage of the disease, palliative care with emphasis on quality of life becomes paramount.

### FUTURE TRENDS

Therapy for cholangiocarcinoma is limited. Surgery remains the principal treatment modality and the only potential for cure. Laparoscopy is an increasingly important modality in determining the resectability of these tumors. The role of chemotherapy and radiation remains controversial, as there are no data supporting a survival advantage for patients. As most patients present with advanced disease, relief of biliary obstruction via biliary stents, with or without photodynamic therapy, constitute the only palliative options. The continued investigation into newer agents and novel therapies may hold promise in the treatment of these difficult malignancies. Any further advances in the therapy of cholangiocarcinoma will most likely be based on a molecular understanding of the disease.

## CONCLUSION

Significant advances in the pathogenesis, diagnosis, and treatment of malignancies of the biliary tract have been made in recent years. Most patients with carcinoma of the gallbladder and bile duct, however, continue to have a poor prognosis. Identification of the gene responsible for biliary anomalies and the development of serum or bile tumor markers may make early detection and prevention of these cancers possible for persons at risk. Dietary, occupational, environmental, and further genetic analysis of clusters of patients may provide more clues to the pathogenesis of these rare tumors.

Advances in technology will allow less-invasive imaging diagnostic studies. Quality of life and length of survival will continue to be assessed in both palliated and aggressively surgically resected patients. New chemotherapeutic agents and novel therapies need to be tested. Advances in our understanding of the genetics of the disease will help in diagnosing bile duct cancer, as well as in screening patients at risk and developing new therapies. Safer surgeries and more effective adjuvant therapy are needed to improve the outlook for future patients with malignancies of the gallbladder and biliary tract. Further innovations will require multidisciplinary collaboration to treat these patients based on the foundation of nursing care.

## REFERENCES


1. Lai CH, Lau WY. Gallbladder cancer—a comprehensive review. *Surgeon.* 2008;2:101–110.
2. American Cancer Society. *Cancer Facts and Figures, 2008.* Atlanta, GA: American Cancer Society; 2008.
3. Randi G, Franceschi S, LaVecchia C. Gallbladder cancer worldwide: geographical distribution and risk factors. *Int J Cancer.* 2006;118:1591–1602.
4. Gourgiotis S, Kocher HM, Solaini L, Yarollahi A, Tsiambas E, Salemix NS. Gallbladder cancer. *Am J Surg.* 2008;196:252–264.
5. Wistuba II, Gazdar AF. Gallbladder cancer: lessons from a rare tumor. *Nat Rev Cancer.* 2004;4:695–706.
6. Miller G, Jarnagin WR. Gallbladder carcinoma. *J Cancer Surg.* 2008;34:306–312.
7. Khan ZR, Neugut AI, Chabot JA. Risk factors for biliary tract cancers. *Am J Gastroenterol.* 1999;94:149–152.
8. Cleary SP, Dawson LA, Knox JJ, Gallinger S. Cancer of the gallbladder and extrahepatic bile ducts. *Curr Probl Surg.* 2007;44:396–482.
9. Kumar JR, Tewari M, Rai A, Sinha R, Mohapatra SC, Shukla H. An objective assessment of demography of gallbladder cancer. *J Surg Oncol.* 2006;93:610–614.
10. Bismuth H, Krissat J. Choledochal cystic malignancies. *Ann Oncol.* 1999;10(suppl 4):94–98.
11. Roiukounakis N, Moanlakopoulos S, Tzourmakliotis D, Bethanis S, McCarty TM, Cuhn J. Biliary tract malignancy and abnormal pancreaticobiliary junction in a western population. *J Gastroenterol Hepatol.* 2007;22:1949–1952.
12. Pandey M. Environmental pollutants in gallbladder carcinogenesis. *J Surg Oncol.* 2006;93:640–643.
13. Kumar S., Kumar S, Kumar S. Infection as a risk for gallbladder cancer. *J Surg Oncol.* 2006;93:633–639.
14. Misra S, Chaturvedi A, Misra NC, et al. Carcinoma of the gallbladder. *Lancet Oncol.* 2003;4:167–175.
15. Shukla VK, Gurubachan, Sharma D, Dixit VK, Usha. Diagnostic value of serum CA 242, CA 19–9, CA 15–3 and CA 125 in patients with carcinoma of the gallbladder. *Trop Gastroenterol.* 2006;27:1–165.
16. Tsukada K, Takada T, Miyazaki M, et al. Diagnosis of biliary tract and ampullary carcinomas. *J Hepatobiliary Pancreat Surg.* 2008;15:31–40.
17. Swierczynski SL, Maitra A, Abraham SC, et al. Analysis of novel tumor markers in pancreatic and biliary carcinomas using tissue microarrays. *Hum Pathol.* 2004;35:357–366.
18. Reid KM, Ramos-De la Medina A, Donohue JH. Diagnosis and surgical management of gallbladder cancer: a review. *J Gastrointest Surg.* 2007;11:671–681.
19. Mekeel KL, Hemming AW. Surgical management of gallbladder carcinoma: a review. *J Gastrointest Surg.* 2007;11:1188–1193.

20. Norwold DL, Dawes LG. Biliary neoplasms. In: Greenfield LJ, et al., eds. *Surgery: Scientific Principles and Practice*. 2nd ed. Philadelphia, PA: Lippincott-Raven; 1997:1056–1067
21. Kwon A-H, Matsui Y. Laparoscopic cholecystectomy in patients aged 80 years and over. *World J Surg.* 2006;30:1204–1210.
22. Bridgewater J, Imber C. New advances in the management of biliary tract cancer. *HPB.* 2007;9:104–111.
23. Malik IA. Gallbladder cancer: current status. *Expert Opin Pharmacother.* 2004;5:1271–1277.
24. Pitt HA, Nakeeb A. Operative approach to gallbladder cancer. *Curr Gastroenterol Rep.* 2006;8:161–167.
25. Gore RM, Shelhamer RP. Biliary tract neoplasms: diagnosis and staging. *Cancer Imaging.* 2007;7:S15–S23.
26. Lai CH, Lau WY. Gallbladder cancer—a comprehensive review. *Surgeon.* 2008;6:101–110.
27. Mukhopadhyay S, Landas SK. Putative precursors of gallbladder dysplasia: a review of 400 routinely resected specimens. *Arch Pathol Lab Med.* 2005;129:386–390.
28. Levin B. Gallbladder carcinoma. *Ann Oncol.* 1999;10(suppl 4): 129–130.
29. Chan SY, Poon RT, Lo CM, Ng KK, Fan ST. Management of carcinoma of the gallbladder: a single-institution experience in 16 years. *J Surg Oncol.* 2008;97:156–164.
30. Greene FL, Page DL, Fleming ID, et al. *AJCC Cancer Staging Manual.* 6th ed. New York, NY: Springer Verlag;2002:139–144.
31. Misra S, Chaturvedi A. Misra NC. Gallbladder cancer. *Curr Treat Options Gastroenterol.* 2006;9:95–106.
32. Tsuyuguchi T, Takada T, Miyazaki M, et al. Stenting and interventional radiology for obstructive jaundice in patients with unresectable biliary tract carcinomas. *J Hepatobiliary Pancreat Surg.* 2008;15: 69–73.
33. Makino T, Fujitani K, Tsujinaka T, et al. Role of percutaneous transhepatic biliary drainage in patients with obstructive jaundice caused by local recurrence of gastric cancer. *Hepatogastroenterology.* 2008;81:54–57.
34. Yoshida H, Mamada Y, Taniai N, et al. One-step palliative treatment method for obstructive jaundice caused by unresectable malignancies by percutaneous transhepatic insertion of an expandable metallic stent. *World J Gastroenterol.* 2006;12:2423–2426.
35. Kiran RP, Pokala N, Dudrick SJ. Incidence pattern and survival for gallbladder cancer over three decades: an analysis of 10,301 patients. *Ann Surg Oncol.* 2006;14:827–832.
36. Reddy SK, Clary BM. Surgical management of gall bladder cancer. *Surg Oncol Clin North Am.* 2009;18:307–324.
37. Kresl JJ, Schild SE, Henning GT, et al. Adjuvant external beam radiation therapy with concurrent chemotherapy in the management of gallbladder carcinoma. *Int J Radiat Oncol Biol Phys.* 2002;52: 167–175.
38. Thomas MB. Targeted therapies for cancer of the gallbladder. *Current Opin Gastroenterol.* 2008;24:372–376.
39. Nakeeb A, Pitt HA, Sohn TA, et al. Cholangiocarcinomas: a spectrum of intrahepatic, perihilar, and distal tumors. *Ann Surg.* 1996:224: 463–475.
40. Demols A, Marechal R, Deviere J, VanLaehtem J. Biliary tract cancers: from pathogenesis to endoscopic treatment. *Best Pract Res Clin Gastroenterol.* 2007;21:1015–1029.
41. Blechasz BRA, Gores GJ. Cholangiocarcinoma. *Clin Liver Dis.* 2008;12:131–150.
42. Khan SA, Thomas HC, Davidson BR, Taylor-Robinson SD. Cholangiocarcinoma. *Lancet.* 2005;366:1303–1314.
43. Shaib Y, El-Serag HB. The epidemiology of cholangiocarcinoma. *Semin Liver Dis.* 2004;24:115–125.
44. Sripa B, Kaewkes S, Sithithaworn P, et al. Liver fluke induces cholangiocarcinoma. *PLoS Med.* 2007;4:1148–1155.
45. Mahli H, Gores GJ. Cholangiocarcinoma: modern advances in understanding a deadly old disease. *J Hepatol.* 2006;45:856–867.
46. Okuda K, Nakanuma Y, Miyazaki M. Cholangiocarcinoma: recent progress, part I: epidemiology and etiology. *J Gastroenterol Hepatol.* 2002;17:1049–1055.
47. Khan ZR, Neugut AI, Ahsan H, et al. Risk factors for biliary tract cancers. *Am J Gastroenterol.* 1999;94:149–152.
48. Oldakowksa-Jedynak U, Nowak M, Mucha K, Foroncewicz B, Nyckowski P, Zieniewicz K, et al. Recurrence of primary sclerosing cholangitis in patients after liver transplantation. *Tansplantation Proc.* 2006;38:240–243.
49. Stiehl A. Primary sclerosing cholangitis: neoplastic potential in bile ducts and the pancreas? *J Hepatol.* 2002;36:433–435.
50. Yachimski P, Pratt DS. Cholangiocarcinoma: natural history treatment, and strategies for surveillance in high-risk patients. *J Clin Gastroenterol.* 2008;42:178–190.
51. Molmenti EP, Marsh JW, Dvorchik I, et al. Hepatobiliary malignancies: primary hepatic malignant neoplasms. *Surg Clin North Am.* 1999;79:43–57.
52. Lipshutz GS, Brennan TV, Warren RS. Thorotrast-induced liver neoplasia: a collective review. *J Am Coll Surg.* 2002;195:713–718.
53. Gores GJ. Cholangiocarcinoma: current concepts and insights. *Hepatology.* 2003;37:961–969.
54. Ahrendt SA, Nakeeb A, Pitt HA. Cholangiocarcinoma. *Clin Liver Dis.* 2001;5:191–218.
55. Lim JH. Cholangiocarcinoma: morphologic classification according to growth pattern and imaging findings. *AJR Am J Roentgenol.* 2003;181:819–827.
56. Patel T, Singh P. Cholangiocarcinoma: emerging challenges to a challenging cancer. *Curr Opin Gastroenterol.* 2007;23:317–323.
57. Sandhu DS, Roberts LR. Diagnosis and management of cholangiocarcinoma. *Curr Gastroenterol Rep.* 2008;10:43–52.
58. Cheon YK, Cho YD, Moon JH, et al. Diagnostic utility of interleukin-6 (IL-6) for primary bile duct cancer and changes in serum IL-6 levels following photodynamic therapy. *Am J Gastroenterol.* 2007;102: 2164–2170.
59. Mortele KJ, Ji H, Ros PR. CT and magnetic resonance imaging in pancreatic and biliary tract malignancies. *Gastrointest Endosc.* 2002;56(suppl 6):S206-S212.
60. Tajiri T, Yoshida H, Mamada Y, Taniai N, Yokomuro S, Mizuguchi Y. Diagnosis and initial management of cholangiocarcinoma with obstructive jaundice. *World J Gastroenterol.* 2008;14:3000–3005.
61. Stern N, Sturgess R. Endoscopic therapy in the management of malignant biliary obstruction. *EJSO.* 2007;34:313–317.
62. Szklaruk J, Tamm E, Charnsangavej C. Preoperative imaging of biliary tract cancers. *Surg Oncol Clin North Am.* 2002;11:865–876.
63. Corvera CU, Weber SM, Jarnagin WR. Role of laparoscopy in the evaluation of biliary tract cancer. *Surg Oncol Clin North Am.* 2002;11: 877–891.
64. Martin R, Jarnagin W. Intrahepatic cholangiocarcinoma: current management. *Minerva Chir.* 2003;58:469–478.
65. Paik WH, Park YS, Hwang JH, et al. Palliative treatment with self-expandable metallic stents in patients with advanced type III if IV hilar cholangiocarcinoma: a percutaneous versus endoscopic approach. *Gastrointest Endosc.* 2009;69:55–62.
66. Ahrendt SA, Pitt HA. Biliary tract. In: Townsend CM, ed. *Sabiston Textbook of Surgery: The Biological Basis of Modern Surgical Practice.* 16th ed. Philadelphia, PA: WB Saunders; 2001:1076–1111.
67. Guglielmi A, Ruzzenente A, Iacono C, eds. Surgical treatment of hilar and intrahepatic cholangiocarcinoma. *Preoperative Biliary Drainage.* Milan, Italy: Springer; 2008:57–65.
68. Larghi A, Tringali A, Lecca PG, Giordano M, Caostamagna G. Management of hilar biliary strictures. *Am J Gastroenterol.* 2008;103: 458–473.
69. Anderson CD, Pinson CW, Berlin J, Chari RS. Diagnosis and treatment of cholangiocarcinoma. *Oncologist.* 2004;9:43–57.
70. Ustundag, Y. Cholangiocarcinoma: a compact review of the literature. *World J Gastroenterol.* 2008;14:6458–6466.

71. Kloek JJ, Ten Kate FJ, Busch RC, Gouma DJ, Van Gulik TM. Surgery for extrahepatic cholangiocarcinoma: predictors of survival. *HPB.* 2008;10:190–195.
72. Rossi RL, Gordon M, Braasch JW. Intubation techniques in biliary tract surgery. *Surg Clin North Am.* 1980;60:297–312.
73. Shinohara ET, Mitra N, Guo M, Metz JM. Radiation therapy is associated with improved survival in the adjuvant and definitive treatment of intrahepatic cholangiocarcinoma. *Int J Radiat Oncol Biol Phys.* 2008;72:1495–1501.
74. Yoon JH, Gores GJ. Diagnosis, staging, and treatment of cholangiocarcinoma. *Curr Treat Options Gastroenterol.* 2003;6:105–112.

CHAPTER 56

*Ellen Carr, RN, MSN, AOCN®*

# Head and Neck Malignancies

## INTRODUCTION

For many years, the standard treatment for head and neck cancers has consisted of a combination of treatment modalities—surgery, radiation, and chemotherapy. With the addition of targeted therapies to the arsenal of treatment modalities, patients with head and neck cancer have more treatment options. A multidisciplinary focus of treatment and system management remains the standard of care for these patients. This chapter provides an overview of head and neck cancers—their etiology, treatment modalities, and the many components of rehabilitation that these patients can face.

Head and neck cancers include cancers that begin in the cells that line the mucosal surfaces in the head and neck area, eg, mouth, nose, and throat. Specifically head and neck cancers include cancers of the oral cavity, salivary glands, paranasal sinuses and nasal cavity, pharynx, nasopharynx, oropharynx, hypopharynx, larynx, and lymph nodes in the upper part of the neck. When tumor cells are found in the cervical lymph nodes and no evidence of cancer is in other parts of the head and neck, the cancer is called *unknown (occult) primary*.[1,2]

## EPIDEMIOLOGY

Head and neck cancers account for approximately 5% of all cancers.[3] In 2009, an estimated 83,730 Americans developed cancer of the head and neck, and nearly 18,860 died from their disease.[3,4] Most of these tumors were preventable. The majority of head and neck tumors occur in the oral cavity, larynx, and oropharynx.[3]

For all head and neck cancer sites, the overall survival rate 3 years from time of diagnosis is 64.4%. This was an increase in observed survival from 47.8% over the 25-year period of 1973 to 1998, including patients still alive in 2003.[4,5]

Tobacco is the most preventable cause of death from head and neck cancer. In the United States in 2008, as many as 170,000 people die each year from tobacco use.[3,6] The rate at which new cases of head and neck cancers are diagnosed has increased in recent years. According to the American Cancer Society (ACS), oral cancer accounts for 3% of all cancers in the United States, or the tenth most common cancer. In 2009, the incidence rate was an estimated 35,720 with 7600 deaths. More than 25% of those diagnosed die of oral cancer.[7,8] From 1979 to 2006, the death rate from oral cancers has slightly decreased.[4,9] According to the American Dental Association (ADA), approximately 75% of patients diagnosed with oral cancer have been smokers.[10]

New cases of oral cancer are 2.5 times as common in men as in women. In men, 3% of all cancer cases are oral cancers. About 90% of oral cancers occur in patients aged 45 years or older.[3] According to the ADA, on an average, only half of those diagnosed with the disease will survive more than 5 years.[10] African Americans are especially vulnerable; the incidence rate is one-third higher than whites and the mortality rate is almost twice as high.[3]

For the period 1996 to 2003, for patients with oral cavity or pharyngeal malignancies, the overall 1-year survival in the United States was 82%. The 5-year survival rate for this group of patients was 59.1% and the 10-year survival rate was 48%.[3,4] For tumors that were localized at the time of diagnosis, the 5-year survival rate was 81.8%. For tumors spreading regionally, the 5-year survival rate was 42.1%. For distant tumors at diagnosis, the survival rate was 26.5%.[3]

In 2009 in the United States, new incidence of cancer of the larynx accounted for new cases. In the United States, the median average age of a patient diagnosed with cancer of the larynx is 69 years. The overall 5-year survival rate for laryngeal cancer is 62.5%.[11]

Cancer of the hypopharynx is uncommon. Approximately 2500 new cases are diagnosed in the US each year, with peak incidence occurring in those 60 years or older. More men than women are diagnosed with hypopharyngeal cancer. In the United States, 65% to 85% of hypopharyngeal cancers involve the pyriform sinuses.[12]

## ANATOMY

### NASAL FOSSA AND PARANASAL SINUSES

The nasal cavity (Figure 56-1) is supported by the hard palate and soft palate (floor), divided by the septum, and topped by the ethmoid bone, which separates the superior aspect of the nasal fossa from the cranial cavity. Three

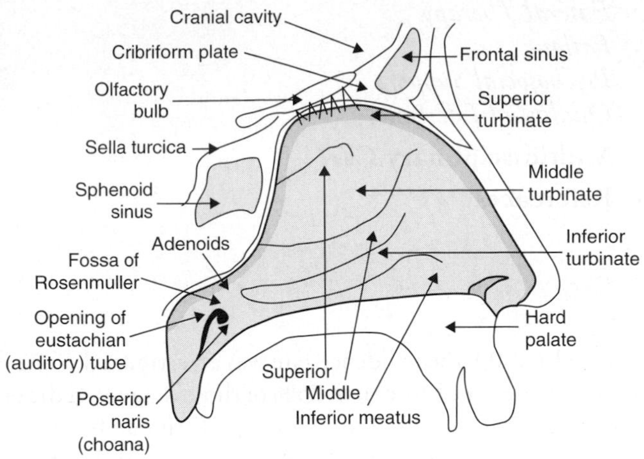


**FIGURE 56-1**

Structures of the nose and nasopharynx.

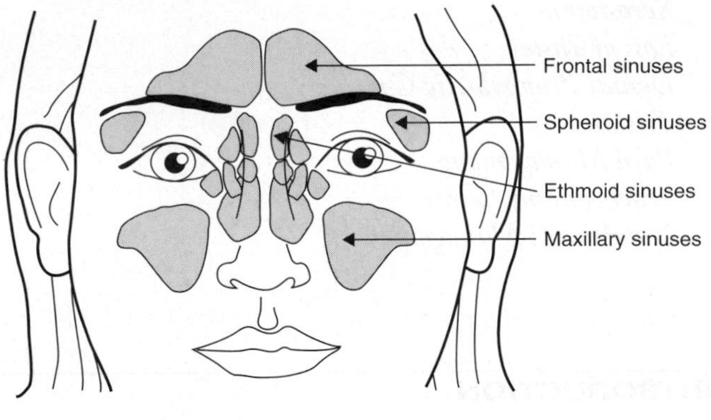


**FIGURE 56-2**

The paranasal sinuses.

curving, scroll-like bones form the lateral walls of the nasal cavity. These bones are the superior turbinate, middle turbinate, and inferior turbinate. Each of these bones has a tiny meatus (opening) for drainage to specific sinus regions. The masolacrimal duct drains into the inferior meatus. The middle turbinate meatus drains the maxillary, anterior ethmoid, and frontal sinuses (Figure 56-2). The superior turbinate drains the posterior ethmoid and sphenoid sinuses. The four paired, paranasal sinuses are the maxillary, ethmoid, frontal, and sphenoid sinuses. Each pair of sinuses is named according to the skull bone housing it. The majority of sinus malignancies occur in the maxillary sinuses.

## SKULL BASE

The skull base is divided into three regions—anterior, middle, and posterior. The anterior region includes the ethmoid sinuses, frontal sinuses, and superior hemispheres of the orbits. The middle region includes the greater and lesser wings of the sphenoid bone, infratemporal bone, infratemporal fossa, optic apex, and optic chiasm. The posterior skull base region contains the clivis, posterior fossa, jugular foramen, and interior auditory canal. Tumors can originate intracranially and extend into head and neck sites. Malignancies also can spread from the nasal fossa, paranasal sinuses, nasopharynx, or infratemporal fossa.

## NASOPHARYNX

The nasopharynx is bordered anteriorly by the posterior naris/choana and posteriorly by the adenoids, body of the sphenoid, and basilar process of the occipital bones (Figure 56-2). Interiorly, the nasal passage merges with the oropharynx at the level of the soft palate. The eustachian tube orifice is just anterior to the fossa of Rosenmuller, which is also called the pharyngeal recess. The majority of nasopharyngeal malignancies occur in the fossa of Rosenmuller. Anterior to the fossa of Rosenmuller are the adenoids (pharyngeal tonsils).

Lymphatic drainage is abundant, with spread going to ipsilateral and contralateral retropharyngeal nodes. Regional spread usually occurs early as nasopharyngeal cancer progresses. Due to the abundant capillary lymphatic system, spread initially involves the cervical triangle, upper/middle/lower jugular chains, or supraclavicular nodes. The common carotid provides the blood supply.

## ORAL CAVITY

The boundaries of the oral cavity are the upper and lower alveolar processes. The oral cavity extends from the anterior vermilion border of the lips superiorly to the posterior border of the hard palate and superior maxillary bone. Inferiorly, the oral cavity extends to the circumvallate papillae of the base of the tongue (BOT) and the floor of mouth (FOM) muscle. Lateral boundaries are the palatine arches or cheeks and include the muscle of the cheek. The oral cavity includes the lips, tongue, salivary glands, FOM, mesopharynx, and hypopharynx. The most commonly encountered tumors involve the lips, tongue, and FOM (Figure 56-3). Of the head and neck cancers, oral cancers are the least likely to spread to the cervical lymph nodes.

## OROPHARYNX

The oropharyngeal region borders the facial arch, which includes the inferior surface of the soft palate, the uvula, and the anterior border of the tonsillar pillar as well as the lingual tonsils, also called the pharyngeal tonsils; posterior one-third of the tongue; and the adjacent pharyngeal wall

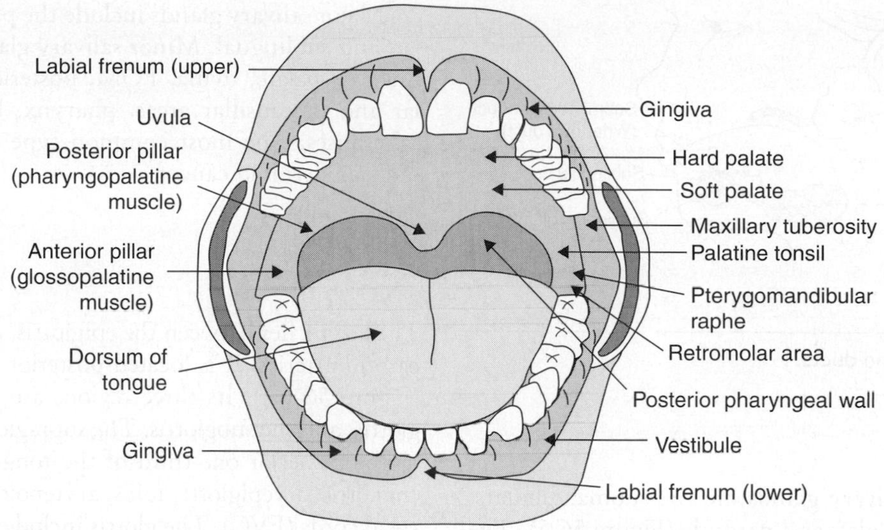


**FIGURE 56-3**

The oral cavity.

(Figure 56-4). All structures of the oropharynx contribute to aerodigestion, including mastication, deglutition, phonation, and respiration. Malignancies of the oropharynx are infrequent and difficult to diagnose because they tend to be hidden. Carcinoma of the tonsil (tonsillar fossa or pillars) is the most common oropharyngeal malignancy. These tumors usually begin in the tonsil, soft palate, or tonsil-like tissue of the tongue base.

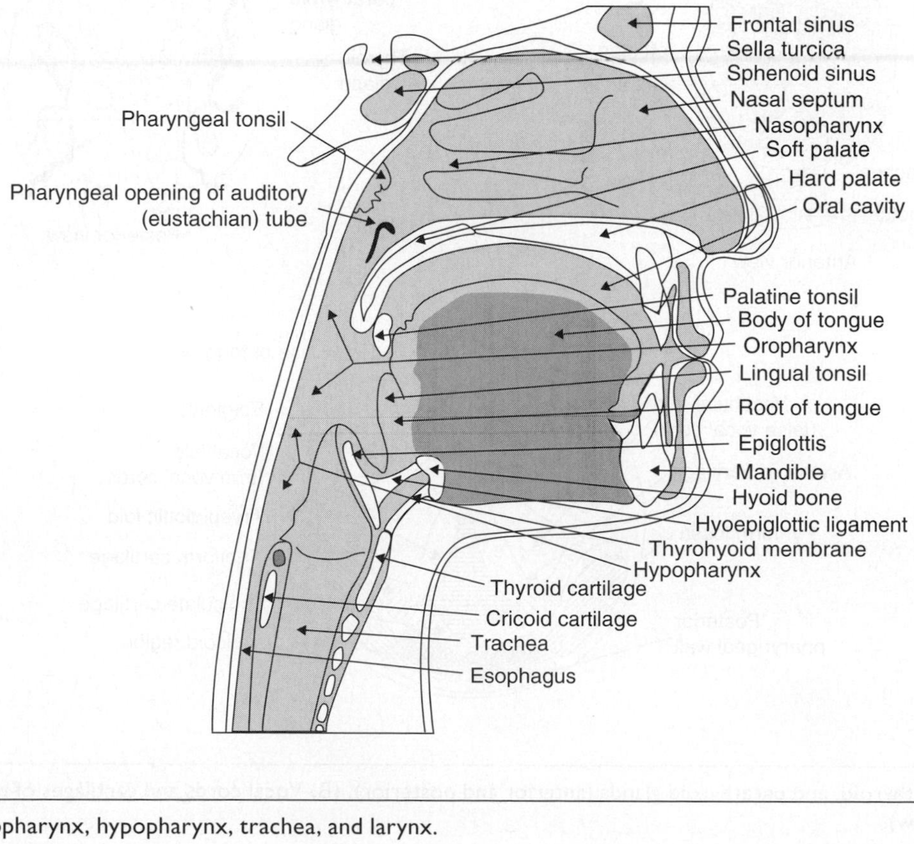


**FIGURE 56-4**

Structures of the oropharynx, hypopharynx, trachea, and larynx.

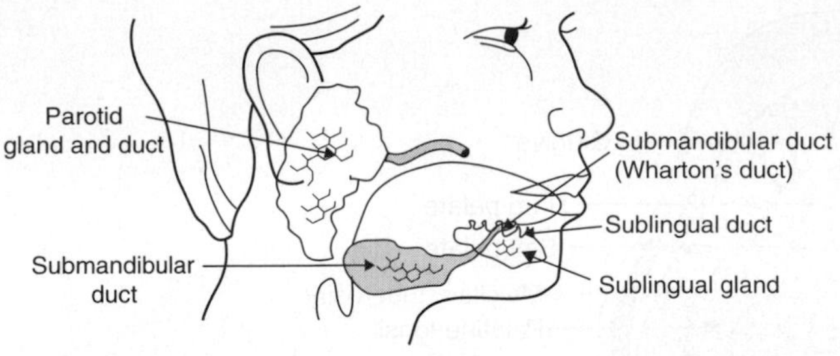


**FIGURE 56-5**

Major salivary glands and ducts.

## SALIVARY GLAND

The three paired salivary glands are the submandibulars, sublinguals (submentals), and parotids (Figure 56-5). The parotids are in the preauricular areas, the sublinguals are within the FOM, and the submandibulars are deep and inferior to the mandible.

Major salivary glands include the parotid, submandibular, and sublingual. Minor salivary glands include the oral mucosa, palate, uvula, FOM, posterior tongue, retromolar and pretonsillar areas, pharynx, larynx, and paranasal sinuses. The most common type of salivary tumor is mucoepidermoid cancer.

## LARYNX

The larynx lies between the epiglottis, cricoid cartilage, and carotid arteries. It is located posterior to the thyroid gland (Figure 56-6A). Its three regions are the supraglottic, the glottis, and the subglottis. The supraglottic region is inferior to the posterior one-third of the tongue, and includes the epiglottis, aryepiglottic folds, arytenoid cartilages, and false vocal cords (FVC). The glottis includes the true vocal cords (TVC), rima glottis, and glottic slit, which separates the TVC (Figure 56-6B). The subglottis extends 1 cm below the TVC to the cricoid cartilage or first tracheal ring. Recurrent

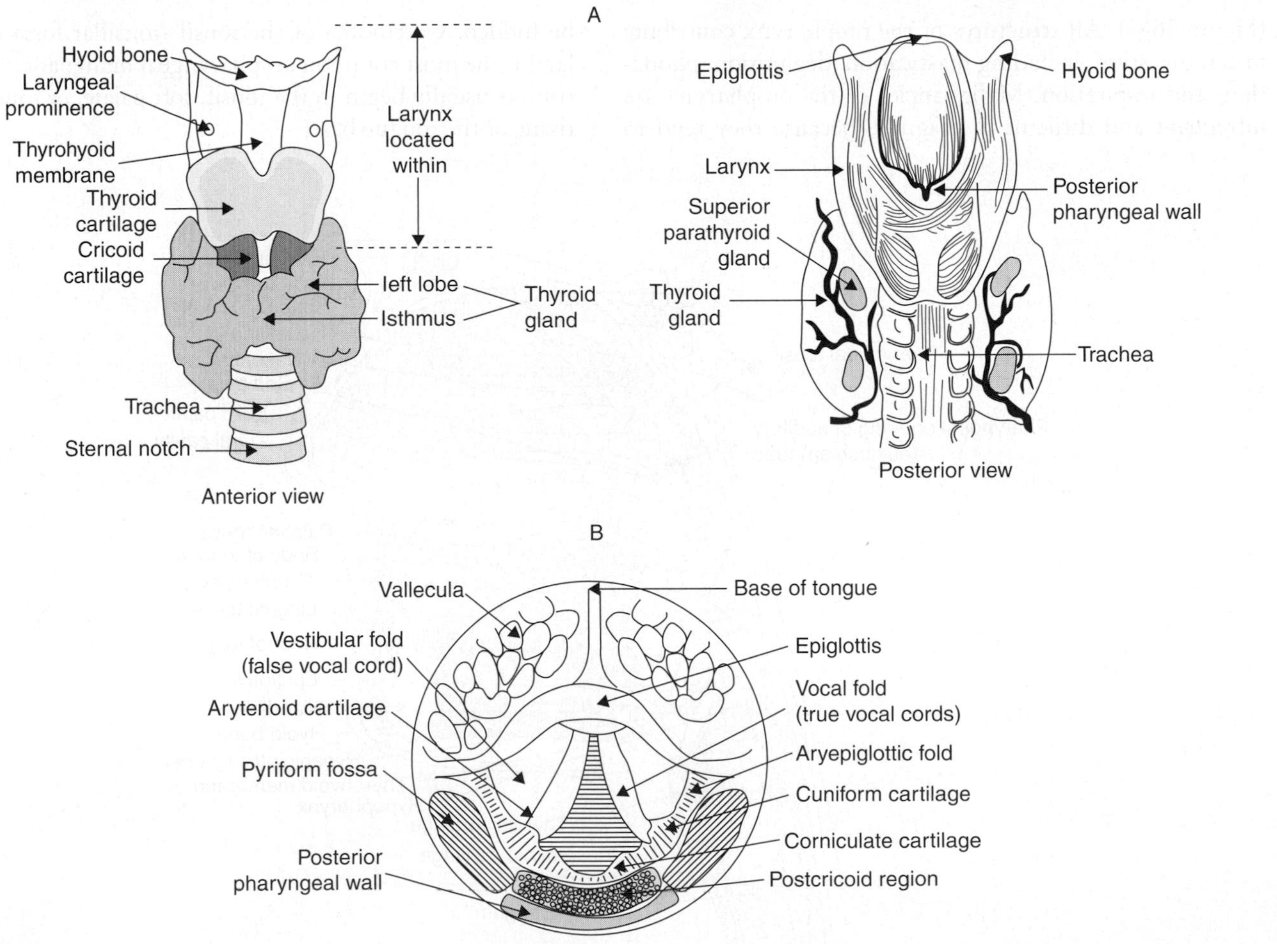


**FIGURE 56-6**

(A) Larynx, trachea, thyroid, and parathyroid glands (anterior and posterior). (B) Vocal cords and cartilages of the larynx and epiglottis (mirror view).

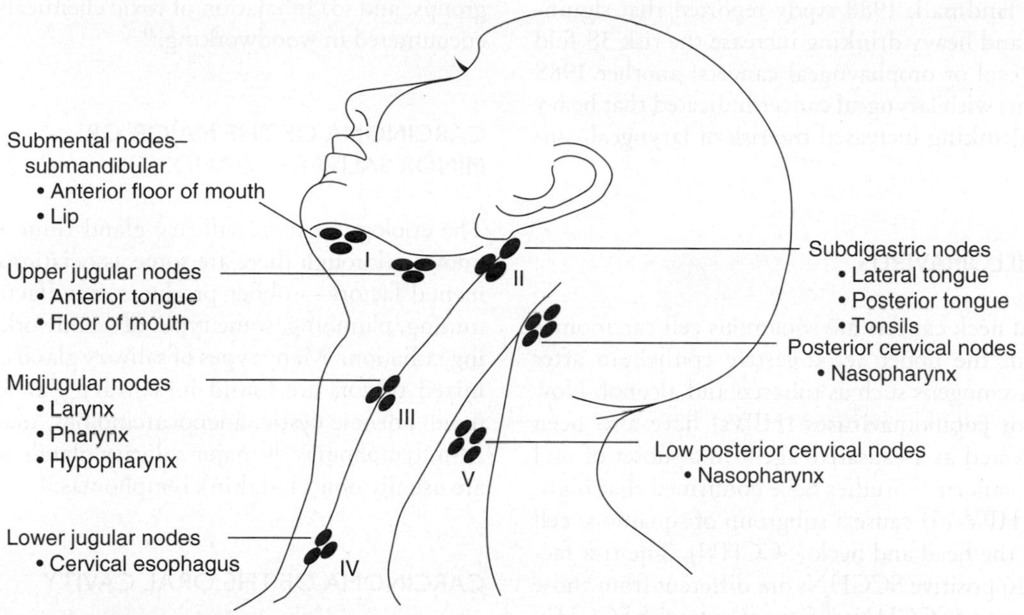


**FIGURE 56-7**

Lymphadenopathy of the head and neck area provides important clues to the location of the primary site.

and superior laryngeal nerves innervate the area; they are branches of the vagus nerve (Cranial nerve [CN] X). Glottic carcinoma is the most common laryngeal malignancy. The subglottic site is the least common location for cancer.

### HYPOPHARYNX AND NECK

The hypopharynx (Figure 56-4), also called the laryngopharynx, connects the oropharynx from the hyoid bone to the esophageal introitus. The lower end is at the level of the sixth cervical vertebra. The hypopharynx is divided into three regions: (1) the paired pyriform sinuses, (2) the posterior pharyngeal walls, and (3) the postcricoid area (lower pharyngeal wall). The majority of hypopharyngeal lesions start in one of the pyriform sinuses. Once cancer cells have penetrated the mucosa of the pharynx, they can easily spread regionally. The neck nodes (Figure 56-7) provide avenues for lymphatic drainage from the base of skull to the clavicle. The level of lymph node involvement is indicative of the location of the primary tumor.

## ETIOLOGY AND RISK FACTORS

### TOBACCO

Tobacco abuse has been implicated as a risk factor for all head and neck tumor sites. Cigarettes, pipes, cigars, smokeless tobacco, and habitual use of marijuana are all considered to be physical carcinogens. Tobacco use increases the risk of developing head and neck cancer more than 25-fold.[6] When a patient with cancer continues to smoke and use alcohol, the cure rate—regardless of treatment plan—diminishes. The risk of oral cancer can be halved within 5 years of cessation of smoking.[6]

Every type of tobacco has been connected to dysplastic injuries and carcinogenic changes in all head and neck primary malignancy sites. Smokers who quit smoking before the age of 50 reduce their risk of dying within 15 years compared with people who continue to smoke; the risk of dying is reduced substantially even among persons who stop smoking after the age of 70.[6]

### TOBACCO AND ALCOHOL

At least 75% of head and neck cancers are attributed to a combination of cigarette smoking and alcohol drinking.[13] Among those who have never used tobacco, alcohol consumption is associated with an increased risk of head and neck cancer only when alcohol was consumed at high frequency. The association with high-frequency alcohol intake is most notable in cancers of the oropharynx/hypopharynx and larynx.[13] Upper hypopharyngeal cancer is associated with heavy drinking and smoking.[12] Risk also increases with the amount smoked per day.[7]

The strongest link between alcohol and cancer is evident with cancers of the oral cavity, esophagus, larynx, pharynx, and liver.[6,7] A landmark 1988 study reported that significant smoking and heavy drinking increase the risk 38-fold of developing oral or orophayngeal cancers; another 1988 study of patients with laryngeal cancer indicated that heavy smoking and drinking increased the risk of laryngeal cancer 42-fold.[14]

## HUMAN PAPILLOMAVIRUS

Most head and neck cancers are squamous cell carcinomas that develop in the upper aerodigestive epithelium after exposure to carcinogens such as tobacco and alcohol. Now selected human papillomaviruses (HPVs) have also been strongly implicated as a causative agent in a subset of oral squamous cell cancers.[15] Studies have confirmed that high-risk HPV (ie, HPV-16) cause a subgroup of squamous cell carcinomas of the head and neck (SCCHN). The risk factors for HPV-16 positive SCCHNs are different from those for HPV-16 negative SCCHNs.[16] For patients with SCCHN of the oropharynx, tumor HPV status is strongly associated with treatment response and survival.[17,18] Therefore, further identification of selected HPV in head and neck cancers will open up more avenues for diagnosis, therapy, screening, and prevention.

Oral cancer has also been linked to HPV, and precancerous oral lesions, called leukoplakia.[19] The body of knowledge about etiological factors is growing, especially relating to genetics. Studies have shown that oral cancer tumors have missing chromosome arms—specifically, 3, 17, and 19. Future treatments will likely focus on the genetic basis for these tumors, expanding our knowledge of gene suppressor proteins.[20]

## CARCINOMA OF THE NASAL CAVITY AND PARANASAL SINUSES

Exposure to tobacco, alcohol, chemicals (such as nickel), and chemical inhalants (such as those found in furniture making, shoe leather working, and textile work) have been associated with increased incidence of cancers of the nasal cavity and paranasal sinuses. In addition, chronic sinusitis has been linked with carcinoma of the maxillary sinus.

## CARCINOMA OF THE NASOPHARYNX

Nasopharyngeal carcinoma risk factors—unlike risk factors for other head and neck cancers—are not primarily linked to tobacco and alcohol. They include (1) infection by the Epstein-Barr virus (EBV), which is applicable for all ethnic cultures; (2) routine inhalation of the nitrosamines in salt-cured, steamy foods such as meats, fish, eggs, and leafy vegetables, especially for Chinese and other Asian cultural groups; and (3) inhalation of toxic chemicals, such as those encountered in woodworking.[21]

## CARCINOMA OF THE MAJOR OR MINOR SALIVARY GLANDS

The etiology of most salivary gland tumors is not clearly known, although there are some associations with environmental factors—rubber products manufacturing, asbestos mining, plumbing, some types of woodworking, and ionizing radiation.[7] Many types of salivary gland carcinomas and mixed tumors are found in salivary glands: mucoepidermoid, adenoic cystic, adenocarcinomas, malignant mixed. Also, lymphomas of major salivary glands can occur; they are usually non-Hodgkin's lymphomas.[14]

## CARCINOMA OF THE ORAL CAVITY

Tobacco use is responsible for 90% of oral cancers in men and 60% of cases in women.[7,10] Although the use of tobacco and alcohol are risk factors in developing oral cancer, approximately 25% of patients with oral cancer have no known risk factors. There has been nearly a 5-fold increase in incidence in patients with oral cancer under age 40, many with no known risk factors.[10]

The incidence of oral cancer in women has increased significantly, largely due to an increase in women smoking. In 1950, the male-to-female ratio of smokers was 6:1; by 2002, for every 2 male smokers, there is 1 female smoker.[10] The risk of oral cancer decreases by as much as 50% within 3 to 5 years after a person stops smoking. It returns to a normal level within 10 years of stopping smoking. Heavy cigar smoking is particularly closely associated with oral cancer.[7]

The synergistic effects of tobacco use and alcohol consumption increase the risk for developing oral cancer, compared to exposure to either risk factor alone.[7] The risk of developing cancer with tobacco use increases when the person drinks and continues to smoke or chew tobacco.[6] Approximately 75% to 80% of patients with oral cancer drink alcohol frequently, and as many as 90% of patients with oral cancer have a history of tobacco use.[7,10] For oral cancer, additional risk factors include poor oral hygiene, mechanical irritation, and Plummer–Vinson syndrome.

## CARCINOMA OF THE LIP

Prolonged exposure to sunlight is linked with cancer of the lip and is an established major cause of skin cancer[7] (see Chapter 66, Skin Cancer). SCC and basal cell carcinoma are the major nonmelanomatous skin cancers of the head and neck area. Lip malignancies occur most frequently on the lower lip. The carcinogenic effect on the skin is compounded if the individual is fair-skinned.

## CARCINOMA OF THE LARYNX

The majority of individuals who develop laryngeal cancer have a long history of habitual tobacco use and alcohol abuse. Other etiological factors may include constant irritation of the vocal cords due to chronic laryngitis or an overprojection of the voice, sometimes called voice abuse.[12]

## CARCINOMA OF THE HYPOPHARYNX

Upper hypopharyngeal cancer is associated with heavy drinking and smoking. Hypopharyngeal cancer has not been associated with any specific chromosomal or genetic abnormalities. However, loss of chromosome 18 was observed in 57% of hypopharyngeal tumors in one study. Other studies have emphasized the importance of chromosome 11q13 amplification, which may be related to nodal metastases, local tumor aggressiveness, and a higher incidence of tumor recurrence.[12]

## CLINICAL MANIFESTATIONS

Cancer of the head and neck is curable if detected early. Many of these malignancies are associated with early symptoms, which have been present for a while before the patient sees a physician for evaluation (Table 56-1). Unfortunately, the majority of head and neck cancers are diagnosed at more advanced stages.[1]

The symptoms of the various head and neck cancers correspond to changes in function caused by tissue injury to the specific anatomical site. Common symptoms for all sites include weight loss and a persistent unilateral lump or mass. A neck mass is highly suspicious of regional spread of the carcinoma.

Other general symptoms of tumor growth include the following:

- *Expectorating blood.* This symptom is often caused by something other than cancer. However, tumors in the nose, mouth, throat, or lungs can cause bleeding. Individuals who have blood in their saliva or phlegm for more than a few days should see a physician.[1]
- *Swallowing problems.* Cancer of the throat or esophagus may make swallowing solid foods difficult.
- *Persistent earache.* Constant pain in or around the ear when swallowing can be a sign of infection or tumor growth in the throat.
- *A lump in the neck.* When the lump lasts more than 2 weeks, the person should be seen by a physician as soon as possible. Not all lumps are cancer, but a lump in the neck can be the first sign of cancer of the mouth, throat, larynx, or thyroid gland, or of certain lymphomas or leukemias. Most masses are painless and enlarged on physical exam.

**TABLE 56-1**

**Symptoms of Head and Neck Malignancies**

| Tumor Site | Symptoms |
|---|---|
| Oral cavity (including lip, floor of mouth, tongue, hard palate) | Nonhealing white, red, or white/red patch on gums, tongue, tonsil, or lining of the mouth; pain; loosening teeth, ill-fitting dentures; gingival swelling; hyperplasia; dysplasia; difficulty chewing or moving the tongue; sore throat (feels that something is caught) |
| Nose and paranasal sinuses | Unilateral obstruction of naris; nonhealing ulcer; intermittent epistaxis |
| Nasopharynx | Nasal obstruction; pain; may present without mucosal changes; painless, enlarged lymph node(s) in neck; recurrent otitis media |
| Oropharynx (base of tongue, tonsil, soft palate) | Asymmetry; dull ache; pain; dysphagia; superficial diffuse erythroplakia; referred otalgia; trismus; muffled voice; neck mass |
| Trachea | Not a primary tumor site (distant spread from larynx, lung, or esophagus) |
| Larynx, hypopharynx | Voice changes (early stage when lesion is on vocal cord); leukoplakia or erythroplakia; stridor or dyspnea; skip lesions |
| Supraglottic | Dysphagia; sore throat; aspiration; referred ear pain; tickling sensation in throat; change in vocal quality; hoarseness; enlarged neck nodes |
| Glottic | In addition, stridor with large tumors |
| Subglottic | In addition, hemoptysis |
| Salivary gland | Unilateral symptoms; impaired jaw mobility; neurological changes (numb lower lip); face numbness or persistent facial pain; painless gland swelling |

## SKULL BASE MALIGNANCIES

Epidermoid, mucoepidermoid, and adenoid cystic adenocarcinoma skull base tumors are rare. Presenting symptoms include otalgia, facial pain, epistaxis, headaches, changes in vision or hearing, and recurrent sinus infections.

Abnormalities commonly correlate with cranial nerve (CN) involvement.

## NASAL CAVITY, PARANASAL SINUSES, AND NASOPHARYNGEAL MALIGNANCIES

In the US, nasal cavity SCC occurs rarely, and the majority of nasal tumors are of a low grade at diagnosis. The most common paranasal sinus malignancies involve the maxillary sinus. Symptoms of a malignancy of the nasal cavity or paranasal sinus may include nasal obstruction, epistaxis, localized pain, facial swelling, trismus, loosened teeth, localized mass, and facial nerve (CN VII) dysfunction. Malignant changes of the nasopharynx may present with symptoms similar to those noted with cancer of the nasal cavity, such as epistaxis, nasal obstruction, and impaired CN VII function. Additional signs are enlarged but pain-free lymph nodes of the neck, tinnitus, recurrent otitis media, headache, and other symptoms associated with CN compression (see Table 56-2). Sinus cancers are associated with a poor prognosis due to early perineural and skull base invasion.

**TABLE 56-2**

**Examination Techniques by Cranial Nerve Distribution**

| Region | Evaluates | Assessment |
|---|---|---|
| Head | CN V–Trigeminal | |
| | Sensory: maxillary sinus, teeth | Place hands on temporal muscles and then masseter muscles to palpate muscle contractions for symmetry |
| | Motor: chewing action | |
| | CN VII–Facial | |
| | Motor: assess symmetry | Ask patient to lift both eyebrows, tightly close eyes, make exaggerated frown and then wide smile, puff cheeks |
| | Sensory: taste | Taste test |
| Auditory | CN VIII–Acoustic | |
| | Sensory: hearing | Refer to audiologist to evaluate unilateral changes in hearing |
| | CN IX–Glossopharyngeal | |
| | Sensory: middle ear | |
| Nose and paranasal sinuses | CN I–Olfactory | |
| | Sensory: smell | Test smell with scratch card if possible, alcohol swab may be used |
| | Nasal structure | Inspect with headlight and nasal speculum |
| | Frontal sinuses<br>Maxillary sinuses<br>Ethmoid sinuses | Palpate sinuses bilaterally for lumps, tenderness; transilluminate sinuses |
| Mouth and pharynx | Parotid | Palpate for unilateral mass |
| | Mucosa | Inspect oral cavity for leukoplakia, erythroplakia, ulcer, mass |
| | CN IX–Glossopharyngeal | Test on both sides of back of tongue with tongue blade for gag reflex |
| | CN X–Vagus | Watch for rise of uvula/soft palate when patient says "ah" |
| | Mucosal changes | |
| Hypopharynx and larynx | CN X–Vagus | Apply local anesthetic spray to oropharynx, ask to breathe through mouth, stick out tongue, and repeat vowels "a" and "e" while examining, using laryngeal mirror and headlight or fiber-optic equipment |
| Neck | CN XI–Accessory | Palpate for masses, tenderness or pain, swelling along the cervical lymph node chains |
| | | Gently hold neck and have patient turn head from side to side against resistance |
| | | Direct patient to shrug shoulders against resistance |

## ORAL CAVITY AND OROPHARYNX MALIGNANCIES

Structures of the oral cavity that may be affected by malignant changes include the lip, upper and lower buccal mucoses, upper and lower alveolar ridges, retromolar trigone, hard palate, anterior two-thirds of the tongue, and FOM.

Abnormalities of any of these structures may include a nonhealing ulcer vs a painless, firm mass, and they may involve either leukoplakia or erythroplakia. The individual's first symptom may be that dentures no longer fit comfortably. Malignancies of the oropharynx are difficult to diagnose, as the same symptoms can readily be ascribed to nonmalignant conditions. Generalized symptoms may include mild but persistent dull ache and sore throat, referred otalgia, dysphagia with ongoing weight loss, and worsening airway obstruction.

Most cancers of the mouth or tongue cause a sore or swelling that does not go away. These sores and swellings may be painless unless they become infected. Bleeding may occur, but often not until late in the disease. If an ulcer or swelling is accompanied by lumps in the neck it is considered a particularly ominous sign.

## LARYNGEAL MALIGNANCIES

Most cancers of the larynx cause some change in voice. Any hoarseness or other voice change lasting more than 2 weeks is significant.

Symptoms of laryngeal carcinomas are associated with the region of the larynx where the tumor originated. The larynx is divided into three areas: supraglottic, glottic, and subglottic. Early on, presenting symptoms can be masked due to the persistent irritation that the person has experienced over many years of habitual tobacco use or occupational exposure to irritants such as petroleum products or wood dust. The presence of a neck mass indicates regional lymph node spread. Presenting symptoms will be determined by the anatomical structures involved.

## HYPOPHARYNGEAL MALIGNANCIES

Because of the anatomical location of the hypopharynx, tumors in this area are often detected late, after they have invaded muscle and adjacent structures. As with laryngeal carcinomas, early symptoms are often masked by years of chronic irritation from tobacco and alcohol use. Pyriform sinus lesions may present with otalgia, which is usually described as dull ear pain. Voice changes and dysphagia tend to occur late, when advanced disease is present. Posterior pharyngeal wall lesions may present as a sore throat or with a feeling of mucous retention after swallowing.

# PATHOPHYSIOLOGY

## CELLULAR CHARACTERISTICS

More than 90% of head and neck tumors are SCC in origin. These tumors arise from the epithelium. Those that do not originate in squamous cells arise in white blood cells (lymphoma) or glandular cells (adenocarcinoma).[22]

An invasive carcinoma will be well differentiated, moderately well differentiated, poorly differentiated, or undifferentiated. Other categories used include infiltrative (originating within the epithelium), exophytic (originating on the surface of the epithelium), and verrucous (wart-like) carcinomas. Microscopic variants of SCCs are further classified as keratinizing (well-differentiated and moderately well-differentiated changes) or nonkeratinizing (anaplastic). Nonkeratinizing cells include the less common lymphoepithelioma, transitional cell, and spindle cell SCCs of the head and neck.

Adenocarcinomas of the major and minor salivary glands include poorly differentiated, high- or low-grade mucoepidermoid, adenoid cystic, acenic cell, and malignant mixed adenocarcinomas (which include more than one of the adenocarcinoma tumor types). Thyroid cancer, a head and neck malignancy, is discussed with endocrine conditions (see Chapter 52, Endocrine Malignancies).

When the carcinoma is noninvasive, it is called "carcinoma in situ." In oral cancer, "leukoplakia" is a clinically descriptive term indicating a white patch that does not rub off. The significance of leukoplakia is based on its histology. Leukoplakia can range from hyperkeratosis to early invasive carcinoma, or it may merely represent a fungal infection, lichen planus, or other benign oral disease.[14]

## PROGRESSION OF DISEASE

Head and neck tumors tend to recur locally. The basement membrane, which underlies the squamous epithelium, provides an important natural barrier to local tumor cell invasion. However, primary head and neck lesions are locally invasive because specific neoplastic receptors can advance tumor growth into the basement membrane.

In establishing a treatment plan, the intensity of therapy takes into account several prognostic factors. Among these prognostic parameters are the tumor (T), node (N), and metastatic (M) stage; the presence of extranodal growth (extracapsular spread); tumor volume; lymph node burden; extent of tumor necrosis; and histological grading.

The incidence of spread to regional lymph nodes at diagnosis is high. Based on the tumor's location, there may be either early or late spread to one or more of the adjacent superficial or deep cervical lymph node chains (Figure 56-7). Lymph node involvement is predictable and based on the anatomical location of the tumor. When there is involvement of distant lymph nodes, such as mediastinal nodes, the cancer is considered metastatic.

Lymph node metastasis is an important factor in head and neck cancer prognosis. Lymph node involvement is staged as stage III or IV disease.[22] The most common area of lymph node spread is bilaterally along the internal jugular vein underneath the sternocleidomastoid muscle, especially along the angle of the jaw. The risk of distant metastasis is increased if the tumor has spread to the neck lymph nodes and multiple lymph nodes are involved. Lymph node involvement in the lower neck is more ominous than involvement of lymph nodes in the upper neck. As a general rule, as tumor cells proceed from the lips posterior to the hypopharynx, prognosis worsens. Tumor thickness correlates with lymph node spread and poor survival rates. At the time of diagnosis, most patients with head and neck cancer have metastatic disease (43% nodal involvement; 10% distant metastasis).[23] Patients with head and neck cancer often develop a second primary tumor, usually of the upper aerodigestive tract or lung.[23]

In oral cancers, a positive margin or tumor depth greater than 5 mm increases the risk of local recurrence in oral/lip cancer. No statistically significant correlation between degree of differentiation and the biological behavior of the cancer exists; however, vascular invasion is a negative prognostic factor.[8]

For salivary tumors, the etiology of these tumors is not clear. Exposure to low dose radiation or cumulative exposure to radiation has been identified as contributing to the development of these tumors. Unlike other head and neck cancers, exposure to tobacco and alcohol are not contributors to salivary tumors.[14]

The prognosis for small laryngeal cancers that have not spread to lymph nodes is good. Cure rates range from 75% to 90%, depending on tumor size, site, and degree of infiltration. In laryngeal cancer, 25% to 50% patients present with involved lymph nodes.[11] Locally advanced lesions are difficult to treat and distant metastases are common, even if primary laryngeal cancer is controlled. For laryngeal cancer, the most adverse prognostic factor is higher T and N stage. Other prognostic factors include sex, age, performance status, and pathology. Patients with laryngeal cancer are at highest risk of recurrence after treatment in their first 2 to 3 years after diagnosis. Recurrences after 5 years are rare. If cancer is found in and around the larynx 5 years after treatment, it is generally considered a new primary.[11]

For patients with hypopharyngeal tumors, 50% present with cervical lymph node involvement and one-fourth have a second primary tumor. Hypopharyngeal tumors tend to spread within the mucosa, beneath intact epithelium, and can skip metastasis, resurfacing at various remote locations. When diagnosed, these tumors are at an advanced stage.[12] The most important features determining prognosis are the size and extent of local spread of the primary carcinoma and the extent of involvement of regional lymph nodes. These tumors have a relatively high incidence of delayed regional spread (2 or more years after completing primary therapy) and distant metastasis.[12]

Nasopharyngeal cancer prognosis is associated with the size of the tumor, stage, and neck node involvement. Other factors include the patient's age, diminished immune function at diagnosis, and incomplete excision of the initial tumor.[21]

## ASSESSMENT

Once a clinical evaluation is suspicious for a malignancy, further diagnostic testing follows. For many head and neck evaluations, more sophisticated scoping is possible with a flexible fiber-optic laryngoscope, which is an office-based examination. This examination allows the physician to see the patient's nasal cavity, nasopharynx, oropharynx, and larynx. Before the exam, the patient's nasal area is sprayed with a topical anesthetic. The patient remains able to respond to verbal requests during the exam, such as making the sound "a" or "e" to see movement of the vocal cords. After being scoped, the patient is advised to avoid eating or drinking for 30 minutes until the gag reflex returns.

To stage the tumor, tissue is biopsied (incisional, excisional, needle biopsy) to establish a histopathic diagnosis. Pathological review of biopsied tissue is the only way to establish a definitive diagnosis.[24] Some biopsies can be performed in the clinic office with the biopsy area anesthetized locally. A fine-needle aspiration (FNA) can be attempted in the clinic in an effort to evaluate a gland or neck mass.

If the suspected tumor in the oral cavity or pharynx cannot be viewed easily with the fiber-optic laryngoscope, then the physician will view the area with an esophagoscope. The patient is under general anesthesia during the procedure. A direct laryngoscopy (DL) is also called a *panendoscopy*. During the procedure, the surgeon will take excisional samples for a biopsy, then send them to the pathology laboratory for histological evaluation.

Radiological studies are crucial in the evaluation of tumor size, invasion, and lymph node spread so that the best treatment option can be determined.[25]

## IMAGING

Imaging contributes to decisions as to how to treat the cancer initially and in follow-up during treatment and after treatment ends. In addition to the diagnostic value of imaging, studies have shown that imaging studies can have predictive value for patient outcomes, independent from standard TNM classifications for staging and treatment.[26]

## MAGNETIC RESONANCE IMAGING

Magnetic resonance imaging (MRI) is considered superior to computed tomography (CT) for showing the depth of primary tumor invasion in soft tissues and fatty areas. It shows malignant changes from inflammation and better illuminates metastasis to the lymph nodes.[25] MRI is the preferred diagnostic film for tumors of the parotid, parapharyngeal, retropharyngeal, and prevertebral spaces, since it shows greater contrast resolution. It also provides better soft tissue contrast in images of the tongue, oropharynx, and tonsil.[25]

For most head and neck tumors, MRI is better than CT when identifying mature scarring, bony involvement, tumor recurrence, and postradiation complications. For nasopharyngeal cancer, CT is widely used because it offers greater availability, is less expensive, and is less time-consuming. However in most cases, MRI is the preferred imaging modality in head and neck cancers. For example, in some nasopharyngeal cancer cases, MRI cannot reliably demonstrate mucosal recurrence or differentiate tumor recurrence from postradiation tissue changes.[25]

## COMPUTED TOMOGRAPHY

For malignancies of the pharynx (nasopharynx, oropharynx, and hypopharynx) as well as the sinuses, CT is superior to x-rays in distinguishing inflammation from tumor. It also can show cartilage invasion, bony destruction or erosion, and the extent of disease for most of the head and neck malignancies.[25] Tumors of the oropharynx, larynx, and hypopharynx can be imaged with CT, which is less affected by breathing and swallowing artifacts that accompany MRI. There is no clear advantage of CT or MRI for evaluation of nodal disease.[25]

## POSITRON EMISSION TOMOGRAPHY

Positron emission tomography, or a PET scan, is a diagnostic examination that shows physiological images of the entire body based on the detection of biochemical changes. The value of a PET scan is enhanced when it is part of a larger diagnostic workup with CT or MRI. PET scanning has become a major advancement in clinical oncology when determining whether disease has spread from the locoregional area to sites of distant metastasis.[27]

A PET scan is indicated in patients with head and neck cancer (1) to guide biopsy or local resection at the initial stage of an unknown primary; (2) to prevent unnecessary further treatment in high-risk patients; (3) to monitor tumor response before full-dose irradiation; (4) to detect residual, recurrent, or secondary neoplasms after definitive radiotherapy; (5) in patients with no known nodal disease, to evaluate the necessity of neck treatment; and (6) in cases when laryngeal cancer recurrence is suspected with no objective findings, to determine whether a biopsy is warranted.[27]

## POSITRON EMISSION TOMOGRAPHY/COMPUTED TOMOGRAPHY

The integration of functional imaging with CT anatomical imaging (PET/CT) has dramatically increased the clinical applicability of PET alone.[27] Positron emission tomography/computed tomography is a means to noninvasively stage many head and neck cancers, providing a functional assay of tumor metabolic activity. It is used with physical examination and other imaging to determine the levels of nodal metastases as well to identify the site of head and neck involvement. For most patients evaluated with PET/CT, tumors on PET/CT are either larger or smaller than tumors outlined on CT scan only.[28]

Positron emission tomographies/computed tomographies continue to be a diagnostic tool to evaluate tumor occurrence or growth after treatment. PET/CT is also being considered a method to plan radiation treatment and to better manage further treatment decisions of previously untreated patients with head and neck cancer.[29,30]

## OTHER IMAGING STUDIES

For T1 to T2 laryngeal tumors, videostroboscopy is used for early detection. Videolaryngoscopy permits assessment of larger lesions. If the individual has a hypopharyngeal or pyriform sinus malignancy, a barium sulfate cinefluoroscopy of the upper gastrointestinal (GI) tract is ordered to assess tracheoesophageal function and to detect a second primary tumor.

Angiography is another radiological test that can define collateralization, especially when the tumor is adjacent to or invading the carotid artery. Following the angiogram, the patient will undergo frequent neurological checks. When resection of the carotid artery is anticipated, cerebral contralateral blood flow is evaluated using a balloon test occlusion (BTO) with single-photon emission computerized tomography (SPECT).

# CLASSIFICATION AND STAGING

Staging of head and neck cancers is key to treatment decisions, providing a baseline for the evaluation of treatment outcomes and prognosis.

The American Joint Committee on Cancer (AJCC) has established a staging criteria for lip and oral, nasal cavity and paranasal, nasopharynx, major salivary, hypopharynx, and laryngeal cancers.[31] Table 56-3 provides the criteria for lip and oral cancers.[32]

**TABLE 56-3**

**Lip and Oral Cavity Staging**

**TNM Definitions**

**Primary tumor (T)**

| | |
|---|---|
| TX | Primary tumor cannot be assessed |
| T0 | No evidence of primary tumor tissue: Carcinoma in situ |
| T1 | Tumor 2 cm or less in greatest dimension |
| T2 | Tumor more than 2 cm but not more than 4 cm in greatest dimension |
| T3 | Tumor more than 4 cm in greatest dimension |
| T4 | (lip) Tumor invades through cortical bone, inferior alveolar nerve, floor of mouth, or skin of face (ie, chin or nose) |
| T4a | (oral cavity) Tumor invades adjacent structures (eg, through cortical bone, into deep [extrinsic] muscle of tongue [genioglossus, hyoglossus, palatoglossus, and styloglossus], maxillary sinus, skin of face) |
| T4b | Tumor invades masticator space, pterygoid plates, or skull base and/or encases internal carotid artery (*Note:* Superficial erosion alone of bone/tooth socket by gingival primary is not sufficient to classify a tumor as T4.) |

**Regional lymph nodes (N)**

| | |
|---|---|
| NX | Regional lymph nodes cannot be assessed |
| N0 | No regional lymph node metastasis |
| N1 | Metastasis in a single ipsilateral lymph node, 3 cm or less in greatest dimension |
| N2 | Metastasis in a single ipsilateral lymph node, more than 3 cm but not more than 6 cm in greatest dimension; or in multiple ipsilateral lymph nodes, none more than 6 cm in greatest dimension; or in bilateral or contralateral lymph nodes, none more than 6 cm in greatest dimension |
| N2a | Metastasis in a single ipsilateral lymph node more than 3 cm but not more than 6 cm in dimension |
| N2b | Metastasis in multiple ipsilateral lymph nodes, none more than 6 cm in greatest dimension |
| N2c | Metastasis in bilateral or contralateral lymph nodes, none more than 6 cm in greatest dimension |
| N3 | Metastasis in a lymph node more than 6 cm in greatest dimension |

In clinical evaluation, the actual size of the nodal mass should be measured and allowance should be made for intervening soft tissues. Most masses larger than 3 cm in diameter are not single nodes but are confluent nodes or tumors in soft tissues of the neck. There are 3 stages of clinically positive nodes: N1, N2, and N3. The use of subgroups a, b, and c is not required but recommended. Midline nodes are considered homolateral nodes

**Distant metastasis (M)**

| | |
|---|---|
| MX | Distant metastasis cannot be assessed |
| M0 | No distant metastasis |
| M1 | Distant metastasis |

**AJCC Stage Groupings**

| | |
|---|---|
| Stage 0 | Tis, N0, M0 |
| Stage I | T1, N0, M0 |
| Stage II | T2, N0, M0 |
| Stage III | T3, N0, M0 |
| | T1, N1, M0 |
| | T2, N1, M0 |
| | T3, N1, M0 |
| Stage IVA | T4a, N0, M0 |
| | T4a, N1, M0 |
| | T1, N2, M0 |
| | T2, N2, M0 |
| | T3, N2, M0 |
| | T4a, N2, M0 |
| Stage IVB | Any T, N3, M0 |
| | T4b, any N, M0 |
| Stage IVC | Any T, any N, M1 |

*Source*: Data from American Joint Committee on Cancer.[32]

The latest revision of the AJCC staging criteria[31,32] takes into account detailed local anatomical features, recognizing that the degree of locoregional tumor involvement of these structures may be as important as distant metastasis. The latest revision includes criteria of more advanced cases (T4 categories and stage IV disease), which better clarify the goal of cure or palliation.[33]

## THERAPEUTIC APPROACHES

In most cases, treatments for head and neck cancer include a combined modality approach, which can include one or more of the following: surgery, radiation therapy (RT), chemotherapy, and targeted therapies.[34–36]

### SURGERY

For early-stage disease, surgery alone is the standard of care for most patients with SCCHN. For stage I and stage II disease, when no cervical nodes are involved, surgical resection can remove the tumor with clear margins. (Note: Radiation therapy alone is another treatment option for certain stage I and II malignancies and is also a standard of care for early disease.)[37] Negative margins predict high probability of tumor control at stage I or II.

With stage III and IV malignancies, the tumor is surgically removed. Then adjuvant treatment is given—chemotherapy and/or radiation treatment or chemotherapy/targeted therapy and/or RT.[37]

Surgery typically precedes other modality treatments. Surgery after RT has been shown to benefit selected patients with regional advanced disease. When straightforward surgical excisions and resections are not adequate because of cervical lymph node involvement, the surgeon can perform a radical neck dissection (RND) or a modified neck dissection (MND).[38]

When definitive staging based on imaging is not clear, elective neck dissections (unilateral or bilateral, radical or selective, as appropriate) are performed. This is the case when occult nodal metastases are suspected even if patient has a relatively small T1 or T2 tumor.

#### Surgery of the neck

Preoperative teaching present concepts and skills that will eventually be the responsibility of the patient: short- and long-term airway management, nutritional support, wound care, pain management, and communication. Depending on the procedure, some patients will undergo placement of both a temporary tracheostomy tube and a temporary gastric tube.

After surgery, attentive tracheostomy suctioning and care will help promote tissue oxygenation as well as improve pulmonary functioning. With a total laryngectomy plus neck dissection, postoperative complication risks increase, such as fistula formation, carotid rupture, wound infection, and pharyngeal stenosis. These risks are especially of concern when the tumor is recurrent and the individual has received prior radiation treatments to the tumor site. The healing of a fistula to the laryngeal region requires meticulous management of fistula drainage, with scheduled irrigations and packing of the wound.[39]

Salivary drainage from a fistula, when there is insufficient tissue coverage of the carotid, can create a critical complication—carotid artery rupture. If the patient is at risk for this condition, carotid artery blowout precautions are instituted. For carotid blowout, supplies kept at the bedside include gloves, a cuffed tracheostomy tube of the correct size, sterile saline, and towels for padding.[39]

Should a carotid rupture occur, the patient's care team should follow standard procedures to promptly secure the airway with the inflation of the cuffed tracheostomy tube, start suctioning, and applying pressure to the site (using saline-soaked gauze for intraoral bleeding and padding to the neck for an external rupture). Later laryngeal complications, which can require surgical repair, include tracheostomal stenosis and hypopharyngeal stricture.[38]

#### Paranasal surgery

At one month post-resection, patients are taught to loosen crusting by using a 50% solution of 3% hydrogen peroxide and water. To further clean the cavity, use a sponge-tipped applicator to gently scrub the skin graft, then rinse the cavity with a salt-and-soda solution. These patients are at risk for infection; postoperative tissue changes decrease the blood supply. Therefore, patients are advised to change their irrigation solution daily and clean equipment regularly with soap and water.[39]

If the sinus tumor has invaded the patient's orbit, treatment is a radical maxillectomy with orbital exteneration. Following this procedure, check the oral cavity for displaced packing and replace it if necessary. Elevate the patient's bed to promote nasal drainage, minimize edema, and improve nasal breathing. Support the patient with accommodations to offset the loss of vision in one eye. The patient is at increased risk for falls during the postoperative phase. Prior to discharge, patient teaching includes oral irrigation and hygiene skills and care of the prosthetic device.

#### Salivary gland surgery

When surgery affects the facial nerve and its control of eye blinking, the cornea needs protection from eye abrasions. Eye drops and ophthalmic ointments provide moisture to the cornea. If facial numbness occurs, protect the skin from sun, wind, and cold exposure.

### Postoperative care: care of flaps and grafts

Skin grafts (SG) and flaps to replace or augment the surgically removed area allow blood flow to and from the affected area, allowing nutritional support, oxygenation, thermoregulation, and transport of metabolic waste. To ensure proper healing, the donor and recipient sites are frequently assessed and the conditions documented.

Full-thickness skin graft (FTSG) and split-thickness skin graft (STSG) are secured by suturing the graft into the recipient defect. Full-thickness grafts usually are harvested from areas of the body which have natural creases, such as the preauricular, supraclavicular, or lower lateral regions of the neck. Split-thickness skin grafts may also be taken from the lateral thigh.[38]

When the recipient site is the FOM, the area is bolstered in the operating room with gauze saturated with bismuth tribromophenate (XeroForm). This bolus packing is not disturbed until removal approximately 5 days postsurgery. While the dressing remains in place, the patient's oral cavity is assessed frequently for drainage, odor, and infection. Regular oral care starts when the bolus dressing is removed and the patient can resume oral hygiene.[39]

In the operating room, donor sites for skin grafts are often covered with a transparent adhesive film product that is occlusive to liquids and bacteria. The film product provides a moist environment that promotes healing (and limits scarring), allowing for observation and assessment. The transparent dressing conforms to the patient's wound and may stay in place, undisturbed, for as long as 7 days. Once the dressing is ready to be removed, it causes less discomfort to the patient.

If the surgeon uses a dry dressing, generally it is padded with a circular gauze dressing and stays in place for several days after surgery. Sterile technique is used when changing the dressing. If it becomes dry and adheres to the wound, saline-soaked gauze is applied to the area for several minutes to release it. Gentle manipulation is used when removing the dressing to prevent damage to viable tissue and bleeding which delays healing.[39]

The patient is more likely to report pain at the donor site than at the recipient defect site. Administer analgesics every 3 to 4 hours. During the early postsurgery days, friction on the donor graft can increase the individual's discomfort. With flaps, avoid placing pressure on the flap from tracheostomy ties or dressings to promote blood flow to the flap.

If ischemia of the graft occurs, there is decreased perfusion pressure and lowered platelet activation followed by thrombus development at the level of the anastomoses. If lymphatic drainage is obstructed, then interstitial pressure may increase, causing edema.[39]

When myocutaneous flaps are used, follow protocols as to how to maintain proper positioning to and prevent tension or entanglement of the pedicle of the graft. The incision sites are to be kept clean, typically by using a 50% hydrogen peroxide and 50% normal saline solution, 3 or 4 times per day. Keep attention to the suture line since fibrin build-up there interferes with granulation and provides an avenue for infection.[38,39]

### Surgical restoration: reconstruction

Microvascular free tissue transfer (reconstruction flaps) are used to reconstruct post oncologic surgical defects in the head and neck region.[38]

With a wide resection, reconstruction involves pedicle flaps and grafts to close defects.[38] Recent advances in reconstructive surgical techniques include neovascularization, microvascular soft tissue transfer, and delivery of sufficient blood flow through the flap or graft. Full-thickness skin grafts (epidermis and dermis) may cover large defects. Such grafts to cover facial defects (nasal tip, eyelid, or auricle) are harvested from preauricular or postauricular areas.

Split-thickness skin grafts (STSG) are nearly transparent, with a thickness between 0.006 and 0.02 inch. They have been shown to provide good functional outcomes.[38] The lateral thigh is a common site for the STSG harvest. This type of graft has limited use in facial reconstruction, because the thin graft can shrink or shift as it contracts and wrinkles following RT.[38] Post-graft surgery, complications are associated with the type of graft; revascularized flaps have been shown to have fewer complications.[38]

## RADIATION THERAPY

The treatment of locally advanced or recurrent head and neck cancers has improved from single modality interventions of surgery and RT alone to include combined modality therapy—surgery, chemotherapy, and radiation. Combined therapy has led to improved local control and disease-free survival.[40]

Developments to improve the delivery, dosing, and effectiveness of RT include altered fractionation, three-dimensional conformal radiotherapy, intensity-modulated radiation treatment (IMRT), stereotactic radiosurgery, fractionated stereotactic radiotherapy, charged-particle radiotherapy, neutron-beam radiotherapy, and brachytherapy.[40–43]

### Early-stage treatment

Early-stage cancer of the head and neck can be treated with RT or surgery. Radiation has been used successfully alone for early-stage tumors (T1, T2) and for cases when resection is not advisable (ie, neck dissection is not feasible based on the extent of the tumor, the patient's general medical condition, or an anticipated unacceptable deficit).[44]

### Adjuvant radiation treatment

Postoperative or adjuvant RT reduces the risk of local–regional failure and probably improves survival. Patients who are at high risk for recurrence after surgery may benefit from more aggressive dose-fractionation schedules that may include altered fractionation to decrease the overall time from surgery to the completion of RT. Adjuvant chemotherapy also appears to improve the probability of cure in high-risk patients.[44,45]

For locally advanced tumors (T3, T4) and for patients at high risk of local recurrence, RT follows surgery as the combined treatment of choice. High-risk cases include T4 tumors, close or positive margins, perineural/perilymphatic/vascular invasion of the same tumor, multiple positive nodes, and extracapsular invasion. Studies have established a dose of up to 60 Gy (200 cGy/day) in 5 to 6 weeks as standard adjuvant treatment for locally advanced cancers of the mouth and throat.

In ongoing efforts to establish a consensus about treatment regimens for locoregional control and advanced disease, hundreds of clinical trials are in effect. Studies continue to look at patient selection for altered fractionation regimens, type of chemoradiotherapy association, radiation or chemotherapy dose schedule.[46]

In a 2007 study of more than 5000 head and neck patients, adjuvant radiotherapy was evaluated for node-positive head and neck squamous cell carcinoma treated with primary surgery. The median follow-up period was 4.4 years. Adjuvant RT significantly improved 5-year overall survival by more than 10% from surgery alone compared to surgery and adjuvant RT.[47]

Efforts to minimize radiation toxicity have involved advances in radiation physics and development of pharmacological agents. Radiation techniques include conformal and IMRT, which minimizes dose to normal tissues while delivering high doses to tumor targets.[48]

Advanced treatment techniques such as altered fractionation, reduction of overall treatment time, and combined postoperative RT, and chemotherapy can minimize adverse effects.[41]

### Intensity-modulated radiation treatment

Intensity-modulated radiation treatment is proving to provide comparable outcomes to external radiation but with less debilitating complications of mucositis and xerostomia.[49–54]

In many studies, IMRT treatments have been encouraging, providing locoregional control of advanced laryngeal and hypopharyngeal carcinomas. After IMRT, xerostomia has been shown to improve over time. Pharyngoesophageal stricture—limiting oral intake (and requiring the patient to receive nutrition from a percutaneous gastrostomy tube)—remains a problem. This is true, particularly for patients with hypopharyngeal carcinoma and, to a lesser extent, those with laryngeal cancer.[49]

Intensity-modulated radiation treatment is the latest evolutionary step for three-dimensional conformal radiotherapy (3-DCRT). IMRT plans are generated with computer-optimized nonuniform radiation beam focused on a narrowly defined target or field. The technique better regulates and controls the dosage given by fractionation so that higher doses are possible without more intense side effects. The tumor receives higher doses; lower doses go to areas of subclinical disease.

Intensity-modulated radiation treatment has been compared with conventional RT, looking at quality-of-life (QOL) indicators of head and neck cancer survivors. In a 2007 study, two comparable groups (67 pairs) of head and neck patients were evaluated. The IMRT group reported less distress from mucositis, especially for dry mouth and sticky saliva. These QOL data suggest a clear benefit from IMRT, particularly in the areas of salivary dysfunction and oral pain.[54]

### Brachytherapy

Brachytherapy is a retreatment alternative to external beam radiation therapy (EBRT). Successful brachytherapy treatment of head and neck tumors uses low-dose rate brachytherapy.[55] In selected oropharyngeal tumors, combined external beam and brachytherapy protocols have been effective.[56]

Brachytherapy for head and neck tumors places radioactive material in close proximity to or directly into the tumor on a temporary basis. The treatment is generally well tolerated. A commonly used radioisotope for this treatment is cesium-137, which is used for both intercavitary and interstitial implants. Other radioisotopes used for head and neck tumors include iridium-192 and gold-198. The determination of a specific radionuclide for brachytherapy is based on its half-life. For example, the half-life of cesium-137 is 30 years, while iridium-192 has a half-life of 74 days.

Implants are most often placed in the operating room, under general anesthesia. When surgery is not an option, brachytherapy may be combined with external beam therapy to boost the total dose of radiation to the tumor.

Primary tumor sites that are more often treated with implants are the tongue, lip, FOM, skin, nasal vestibule, and buccal mucosa. Implants are generally uncomfortable. Base of the tongue lesions, for example, may be treated with needles placed into the dorsum and through the tongue to the BOT region. Pain must be managed and nutritional status monitored. Oral intake may be too uncomfortable for the patient. Also, brachytherapy may adversely affect the individual's ability to speak and enunciate. Only limited experiences exist with high-dose rate brachytherapy (HDRBT) in patients with head and neck cancers.[57]

### Chemoradiation

Since the 1990s, many studies have shown that combining simultaneous chemotherapy and RT are effective in advanced SCCHN. Concurrent chemoradiotherapy is more efficacious than chemotherapy or radiotherapy alone as a locoregional treatment for high-risk patients (stage III/IV, recurrent or second primary tumors) with SCCHN.[58] These chemoradiation protocols have improved response rates as primary treatments or in the adjuvant setting, as well as better controlling treatment side effects.[58,59]

A typical chemoradiation protocol is daily radiation to 70 Gy over 7 weeks with concurrent cisplatin-based chemotherapy protocols (20 mg/m$^2$ during days 1 to 4 of weeks 1 and 5). Cisplatin chemotherapy given concurrently with radiotherapy is the best studied platform, but cisplatin-related toxicities and evidence of higher survival have lead to the increasing adoption of multiagent-based chemoradiotherapy platforms.[58]

## RADPLAT

Organ preservation with concurrent chemoradiotherapy was first established in laryngeal carcinoma post surgery.[34] The RADPLAT protocol was developed in the late 1990s to provide more durable survival rates while preserving organ function. RADPLAT involved weekly administration of high-dose cisplatin directly to the tumor site (150 mg/m$^2$) with simultaneous intravenous thiosulfate (9 g/m$^2$). Radiation therapy was also given during the treatment period.[60]

Patients receiving treatment under the RADPLAT protocol had better survival rates with organ preservation. A study published in 2001 reported on 213 patients with stage III/IV head and neck cancer who were treated with the RADPLAT protocol. In the study, 80% of the patients had a complete response in the primary site of tumor and 62% had a complete response in the regional site. Coupled with neck dissection, 98% of the patients showed no regional disease. The recurrence rate was 26%, and the 5-year survival rates were calculated at 38.8% overall and 53.6% cancer related.[61] Although providing excellent treatment of locoregional disease, RADPLAT has shown to have limited effectiveness for patients with subclinical metastases or micrometastases at distant sites.[61]

Since the initial promising reports of RADPLAT as a concurrent chemoradiation, clinicians have developed variations of salvage protocols for local and regionally advanced SCCHN. Because the intraarterial scheduling of RADPLAT has proved to be operationally difficult, chemoradiation schedules—with chemotherapy delivery through regular intravenous and oral routes—are more prevalent.

Now chemoradiation as a treatment is showing benefit in many head and neck cancers, as measured by selection criteria and treatment outcomes, risk levels, and patient side effects.[62,63] Additional chemoradiation trials are adding or substituting various chemotherapies: capecitabine,[64] carboplatin,[65] docetaxel,[66,67] epirubicine,[68] or trying various chemotherapy or radiation schedules.[69,70]

### Radiation and targeted therapies

Anti-EGFR based chemoradiotherapy is efficacious and well tolerated, but no comparative data with standard chemoradiotherapy exist. Its use is recommended only for elderly patients and patients with poor performance status until additional data become available.[58]

## CHEMOTHERAPY

Chemotherapy alone is rarely the treatment for SCCHN. Nearly all patients with locally advanced head and neck cancer receive chemotherapy as part of initial multimodality curative treatment. Three decades of collaborative research have integrated platinum-based chemotherapy (with accompanying RT) into the curative management of laryngeal, oropharyngeal, and nasopharyngeal cancers and patients with head and neck cancer with unresectable disease or high risk of recurrence.

These multimodality treatments (which include chemotherapy) have improved local–regional control, organ preservation, and survival endpoints.[71] For patients with unresectable disease, the use of platinum-based chemoradiotherapy has improved the 3-year survival rate from 15%-20% to 35%-50%.[72]

Chemotherapy induction protocols began as cisplatin based. A typical induction regimen has been cisplatin 100 mg/m$^2$ IV on day 1 with 5-fluorouracil (5-FU), 1000 mg/m$^2$ per day as continuous infusion for 5 consecutive days, repeating every 3 weeks. Now protocols have expanded to include other chemotherapies such as taxanes.[72]

Phase II studies have suggested that the standard regimen of cisplatin and fluorouracil (PF) plus docetaxel (TPF) improve progression-free and overall survival outcomes in SCCHN.[67,73,74] Studies are looking at several optimal three drug induction chemotherapy protocols. Chemoinduction is then followed by concurrent chemoradiation to improve outcomes.[75,76]

Phase II studies using paclitaxel and capecitabine have also shown comparable outcomes to standard cisplatin/5-FU regimens.[77] Yet the combination of paclitaxel, cisplatin, and 5-FU had efficacy similar to that of standard treatment regimens in patients with advanced or recurrent SCCHN but with increased toxicity.[78] Other studies are evaluating survival or side effect benefits with the addition of gemcitabine to protocols.[79]

## TARGETED THERAPIES

Although combination treatment modalities involving surgery, RT, and chemotherapy have improved the therapies available for SCCHN, the addition of targeted therapies to regimens hold great promise and shifts the paradigm of treatment strategies.[80] These so-called novel or targeted therapies, with highly targeted mechanisms of action and synergistic effects with current therapies, are being evaluated to improve the treatment failure endpoints of tumor recurrence, secondary tumors, and comorbidities. They also may improve treatment approaches often limited by toxicities.[81,82]

Epidermal growth factor receptor has been identified as a factor in the development and progression of squamous cell cancer of the head and neck and is associated with a poor prognosis.[83,84] The anti-EGFR monoclonal antibody (MoAb) cetuximab (Erbitux) is the first targeted therapy to be developed for SCCHN. Anti-EGFR agents prevent ligand binding, interrupting the signal cascade, subsequently, inhibit tumor growth and metastasis.[81,82,85] More approved targeted therapies are on the horizon.

Cetuximab plus 7-week RT in patients with locally advanced SCCHN has increased survival and improved locoregional control of SCCHN.[67,86] This is the first phase III trial to confirm a survival advantage with the addition of a molecular-targeted agent to radiation.[86] Studies have indicated a 13% overall objective response rate in platinum-refractory patients with SCCHN.[82] Moreover, the addition of cetuximab to RT treatment regimen did not adversely affecting QOL.[87]

Single-agent cetuximab conferred clinical benefits for patients with platinum-refractory metastatic disease. A phase III trial demonstrated a survival benefit with cetuximab and standard platinum-based therapy in the front-line treatment of recurrent/metastatic disease.[81] Further studies will establish the optimal way of integrating EGFR-directed therapies into standard chemoradiation protocols.[88] The side effects from cetuximab therapy have been reported as milder than that of standard chemotherapy and chemoradiation therapy treatments; cetuximab therapy appears to not exacerbate RT toxicity.[80,81]

Although oral toxicities common to chemoradiation protocols are less with cetuximab, adverse cutaneous reactions appear to be a marker for response.[82,89] Studies have reported that the acneiform rash occurred in 70% to 80% of patients treated with cetuximab.[90] Presence of the characteristic rash is significantly associated with response and/or survival. Therefore, patient education about this rash is an important component to multidisciplinary patient care.[91] Ongoing head-to-head comparative trials comparing cetuximab with other biological agents are ongoing.[82,92,93]

Other targeted therapies in clinical trials for SCCHN are small-molecule EGFR-tyrosine kinase inhibitors in combination with chemoradiotherapy or as single agents, and antiangiogenesis agents.[81,88,89,92,94]

## FUTURE TREATMENT AND MANAGEMENT STRATEGIES

For the next few years, targeted and novel therapies will be among the main clinical environments to develop or perfect treatments for SCCHN. Studies will offer a better understanding of the molecular and genetic foundation of disease, cell mechanisms, as well as clinical strategies.

Additional studies will look at the efficacy of anti-EGFR agents. Erlotinib, an EGFR tyrosine kinase inhibitor, has shown favorable results in phase II trials as monotherapy and in combination with chemotherapy. Gefitinib, another EGFR tyrosine kinase inhibitor, has shown efficacy as monotherapy, in combination with chemotherapy, and with chemoradiotherapy.[95] The intent of these approaches is that more low-toxicity, tumor-specific targeting strategies will be available for patients with SCCHN.

An additional challenge in treatment will be to establish assays to determine which patients are most likely to benefit from these agents.[95] Identification of predictive biomarkers of resistance or sensitivity to these therapies remains the main challenge; selecting of patients most likely to benefit.[89,96,97]

As our understanding of the inherited genetic factors for head and neck cancers grows, agents target those tumors that show genetic susceptibility. Gene expression patterns of individual tumors have shown promise to improve discovery of biomarkers for (1) progression of premalignant lesions, (2) disease presence or absence, (3) prediction of clinical outcome, and (4) identification of targets for therapy.[98]

Human papillomavirus will continue to be a focus of study since it has been found to be associated with SCCHN. Vaccines are in development to stimulate HPV-specific immune responses. Two HPV oncogenic proteins, E6 and E7, have been targeted in experimental vaccine systems.[99]

Alteration of the *p53* tumor suppressor gene has been shown to be associated with a high risk of developing SCCHN.[100] Thus, *p53* appears to play an important role in the pathogenesis and progression of head and neck cancers. Further understanding of the role of *p53* gene mutations might clarify the diagnosis, prognosis, and treatment of high-risk patients.[101,102] For example, local recurrence is the most common cause of mortality after SCCHN surgery; *p53* gene mutations have been observed in tissue adjacent to the tumor, and constitute a good prognostic marker of tumor recurrence. Resected tumors with negative margins have been shown to have residual tumor cells with persistent *p53* mutations at the margins.

Given that the mutation of *p53* is one of the most frequent genetic changes found in human cancer, gene therapy that capitalizes on the effects of *p53* has been targeted in radiotherapy and thermotherapy treatments. Using *p53* as a foundation, clinical trials continue—looking at adenoviruses engineered to function as vectors for delivering therapeutic genes for gene therapy. One of these adenoviruses targeted to head and neck cancers is ONYX-015.[102]

## HEAD AND NECK SPECIALIZED PROGRAMS OF RESEARCH EXCELLENCE

The Head and Neck Cancer Specialized Programs of Research Excellence (SPOREs) are research programs, sponsored by grants from National Cancer Institute (NCI). SPOREs projects are interdisciplinary, championing collaboration among project teams at each institution and among SPOREs-funded institutions. SPOREs projects are involved with new treatment and prevention strategies and with investigating molecular mechanisms and innovative therapies. SPOREs programs also partner with other NCI/NIH programs, industry involved public–private partnerships, nonprofit organizations, patient advocates, and international investigators in Europe, Canada, Asia, and Mexico.[103]

Begun in 2002, a main focus of SPORE research is translational head and neck cancer research. As of 2008, the institutions involved in SPORE research are Emory University, the University of Michigan Health System, The University of Texas MD Anderson Cancer Center, Johns Hopkins University, and University of Pittsburgh.[103]

For example, at the University of Michigan, five major projects have been developed that will study the molecular structure of cancer cells, explore the possibility of their use as a predictive measures of response to chemotherapy and radiation treatment options, and predict the risk of spread of cancer or cancer recurrence.[104]

At Johns Hopkins, SPOREs research initiatives include the study of HPV in cancer development and how the virus is transmitted to the upper airway. Scientists at the Johns Hopkins Kimmel Cancer Center were the first to discover that HPV also is a likely cause of certain cancers of the head and neck and is an indicator of improved survival.[105]

## TREATMENT STRATEGIES FOR SPECIFIC HEAD AND NECK CANCERS

As a standard of care, a multidisciplinary treatment plan is established for all patients diagnosed with head and neck cancer.[106] In general, early-stage head and neck cancers can be treated with surgery and/or RT. For advanced resectable tumors (laryngeal and hypopharyngeal), standard treatment after surgery includes neoadjuvant chemotherapy regimens (platinum) and RT. Unresectable tumors are treated with chemoradiation, either concurrently or concomitantly.[37,106]

### Nasal fossa and paranasal sinuses

Small tumors can be treated by either surgery or RT. Surgery and postoperative RT may result in improved local control and survival with no evidence of disease recurrence, but complications are more severe when compared with RT alone.[107] Elective neck irradiation has been seen as unnecessary for patients with early-stage disease.

Tumor spread commonly occurs along the lateral walls of the nasal cavity. Local spread is to the maxillary sinus or nasopharynx and may be present upon initial diagnosis. Concomitant or sequential multimodal treatment can provide improved local and regional control.

For maxillary sinus lesions, when the tumor is confined to the sinus, a maxillectomy will usually be performed. Prior to surgery, a consultation with the maxillofacial prosthodontist will be scheduled. The prosthodontist will make impressions of the hard and soft palates and then create an obturator that will be used to fill the surgical defect. Following resection of the cancer, a skin graft may be required to cover the surgical defect. The graft also counters contraction of the tissue, which is a normal part of the healing process. The obturator will be wired into place in the operating room following resection, after the defect is packed with petroleum-based gauze or nonadhering intermediate reline resin.

The ability to speak and to complete the oral phases of swallowing are restored for the patient with placement of the obturator, so there may be no need for a nasogastric tube postoperatively. After about 5 days, the surgeon removes the obturator and gauze and examines the surgical site. A removable obturator is designed by the prosthodontist. The patient is taught how to remove, clean, and replace the obturator. It can take as many as 6 months of revisions before the fit of the obturator is satisfactory, depending on the size of the defect and the healing necessary following chemotherapy and radiation. The patient is taught to remove the obturator after every meal and at bedtime. The patient then irrigates the cavity with a solution of normal saline and baking soda, which cleanses the area without causing irritation.

### Skull base

Large lesions are treated with a combination of surgery and chemotherapy, while small tumors can be treated with RT alone. Surgery can involve the head and neck surgeon, neurosurgeon, microvascular surgeon, and plastic surgeon. For patients with stage III or IV tumors, chemotherapy is combined with RT.

In addition to the risk of standard complications following surgery (aspiration pneumonia, pulmonary edema, congestive heart failure, myocardial infarction, and sepsis), postsurgical complications may include cerebrospinal fluid (CSF) leak, increased intracranial pressure (cerebral edema), artery thrombosis, seizure, and stroke.

Close monitoring of intracranial pressure (ICP) assists in detecting subtle changes requiring immediate interventions to correct bleeding or promote adequate ventilation. Headache is an early sign of increasing ICP. Fluid balance can be erratic. Wide fluctuations in blood pressure can occur postoperatively as a result of vasoconstriction and insufficient cerebral perfusion.

As the patient recovers from treatment, he or she may need rehabilitation for impaired vision and for defects in swallowing, hearing, mobility, and balance.

### Nasopharynx

Treatment of small nasopharyngeal cancers with radiation is the treatment of choice and yields 80% to 90% survival rates.[12] Surgery is generally not recommended due to the difficulty in accessing this location.

For nasopharyngeal RT, both sides of the patient's neck are usually treated, even when there is no current evidence of lymph node spread. This is because the risk is high for undetectable neck disease. The delivery of RT to this site is complex, with critical attention being paid to the protection of the spinal cord from injury.

Serous otitis media, with obstruction of the eustachian tube, is associated with treatment of nasopharyngeal malignancies. Prior to any RT, in anticipation of serous drainage during treatment, the surgeon may perform a myringotomy with ventilation tube insertion.

For locoregional control of advanced disease (T3, T4), chemotherapy is given in conjunction with RT. One effective regimen combines epirubicin, cisplatin, and infusional 5-FU chemotherapy followed by radiation with concurrent cisplatin.[71]

### Oral cavity

Early-stage cancers (stages I and II) of the lip and oral cavity are highly curable by surgery or by RT. For early-stage oral cancer, EBRT and brachytherapy have been used successfully. The presence of a positive margin or a tumor depth greater than 5 mm significantly increases the risk of local recurrence and suggests the need for combined modality treatment.

With oral cavity tumors, depending on the clinical stage, a continuous or discontinuous ipsilateral neck dissection is performed to prevent regional spread, followed by adjuvant RT.[7] Chemoradiation protocols are used for patients with advanced, recurrent, and metastatic head and neck cancer.[49]

Intensity-modulated radiation treatment has been shown to benefit patients by allowing the option of reradiating fields when locoregional relapses occur. IMRT may reduce the toxicities associated with standard RT.[108]

### Oropharynx

Stage I and II tumors of the oropharynx are managed similarly to early-stage oral cavity malignancies.

Early carcinoma of the tonsil can effectively be treated using single modality therapy. Local regional control and survival are similar following surgery or radiotherapy. Radiation therapy is used for recurrent disease. Advanced disease warrants multimodality therapy.[109] Tumors of the pharynx (oropharynx or hypopharynx) are treated primarily with combined chemoradiation. Base of the tongue cancers can be treated with surgery and postoperative radiation. These strategies offer patients a high probability of locoregional control, survival, and good QOL.[110]

A surgical resection of the BOT carcinoma is the most difficult site of the oropharynx to manage postoperatively. Therefore, primary high-dose irradiation, often with brachytherapy, is added. A higher level of tumor control may be achieved with a local surgical resection plus a neck dissection.

For advanced (T4) BOT tumors, treatment is usually a total laryngectomy in conjunction with total resection of the tongue base. A laryngectomy is necessary when the adjacent preepiglottic space, which is separated by only a thin membrane from the tongue base, has tumor invasion. A total laryngectomy removes the entire tumor. Laryngeal cancers are also treated with chemoradiation if the larynx is functional. However, if the tumor has destroyed the laryngeal skeleton, surgery (generally total laryngectomy) may be required to restore an adequate airway and maintain swallowing.

With the recent advances in combination therapy, however, tumor control may be accomplished without the need for a laryngectomy. This organ-sparing treatment involves a hyperfractionated (twice daily) schedule of RT and may include brachytherapy as part of the treatment plan.

Adjuvant chemotherapy can maintain local tumor control.[109] For advanced oropharyngeal tumors, concomitant chemotherapy with RT has been shown to be more effective than RT alone in terms of disease-free survival. Nevertheless, overall survival has not been shown to improve.[52,109]

### Salivary gland

For patients with parotid tumors, the standard treatment is a superficial parotidectomy with facial nerve dissection. This procedure may be both diagnostic (with the biopsy confirming the histology) and therapeutic (removal of the tumor).

Distant metastasis is the most common cause of treatment failure. Total parotidectomy with neck dissection and adjunctive RT remains the preferred treatment for local and regional control of disease.[38]

Radiation may be a treatment option for inoperable locoregional disease. Surgery, radiation, and repeat radiation are treatment options for local relapse, whereas RND is indicated for regional relapses. Metastatic disease may be either treated with radiotherapy or palliative chemotherapy, depending on the site of metastasis.[52]

### Glottis and larynx

Unlike supraglottic tumors, glottic carcinomas initially remain localized. Lymphatic supply is limited in this region, resulting in a lower percentage of early spread to the cervical neck nodes. Glottic tumors are also more likely to be detected early because the individual promptly develops symptoms of hoarseness.

In situ tumors can be treated with laser vaporization, microexcision, or RT.[111] The advantage of laser excision and irradiation to the glottis over surgical treatment is the retention of a near-normal voice. With microexcision surgery, the voice changes the least.

Patients with T2 glottic carcinomas with fixed, immobile vocal cords may be treated with irradiation alone or by a vertical hemilaryngectomy. For the vertical hemilaryngectomy, the surgeon removes a part or all of the TVC and FVC, as well as the associated half of the thyroid cartilage. If the vocal cord is fixed and evidence of tumor extension or invasion is found, generally a total laryngectomy will be necessary.

For early-stage laryngeal cancer, both surgery and radiotherapy are effective treatment modalities, offering a high rate of local control.[112] RT as a choice for treatment is based on the locoregional extent of the malignancy, efforts to maintain the patient's functioning vocal cords, and expected disease free and survival outcomes of disease.[52]

## SYMPTOM MANAGEMENT AND SUPPORTIVE CARE

Standard of care for head and neck cancer requires multimodality treatment strategies to improve outcomes. Accompanying those treatments can be a myriad of acute and late adverse effects.[113] These effects can impact the patient physically and emotionally.

More studies are looking at symptom burden and control, with evaluation based on valid and reliable instruments.[114,115] These studies show that accompanying side effects to treatment cause patients' distress and effect their QOL.[114] Therefore, not only do side effects need to be addressed but they also require their own foundation of evidence-based practice, establishing thresholds for acceptable or positive outcomes.[116]

### SWALLOWING

Preservation and/or restoration of swallowing is a primary rehabilitation goal after most initial head and neck cancer treatments and through the palliative phase of treatment.[117] Collaboration among different specialists (physicians, speech pathologist, dietitian, and psychologists) remains key to a desirable outcome.[118] Fortunately, with modifications in treatment delivery (IMRT sparing protocols, dose reduction, brachytherapy), the extent of dysphagia is less.[119]

A speech pathologist in partnership with a radiologist helps evaluate and treat patients who have diminished or no swallowing function (dysphagia) due to their disease or treatment.

Patients with long-term dysphagia after treatment for head and neck cancer are at risk of aspiration.[120] After treatment, swallowing function for patients—especially pharyngeal and laryngeal cancer, who have received RT—can continue to deteriorate over time, even many years after RT has ended.[121]

Before a patient takes food or fluid orally, swallowing function is evaluated and rehabilitation efforts are put in place. For example, a patient who has had a tongue resection will need to learn how to use the remainder of the tongue to propel a bolus of food back to and through the anterior faucial arches as the first phase of swallowing. The swallow trigger is affected when the CNs have been impaired or damaged by disease or treatment. Cranial nerves that can be affected are the trigeminal (V), facial (VII), glossopharyngeal (IX), vagus (X), spinal accessory (XI), or hypoglossal (XII) nerves (Table 56-2).

To assess an individual's degree of dysphagia, it is important to determine the presence or absence of aspiration, any voice impairment, ease of movement of the larynx, any evidence of gurgling with respiration, and the degree of fatigue. Further assessment by video-fluoroscopy or modified barium swallow shows how liquid or food travels. Evaluation includes the presence or absence of aspiration, the amount of pharyngeal residue postswallow, and the amount of time it takes to complete all three phases of swallowing.

### SWALLOW THERAPY

The action of swallowing requires mobility of pharyngeal structures, which allow liquid or food boluses to move through the patient's oral cavity, fauces, pharynx, and esophagus, and into the stomach. For example, a supraglottic laryngectomy affects the pharyngeal phase of swallowing, decreasing protection of the glottis. Until swallowing techniques are learned, the patient is at risk of aspiration.[121] When structures in the oral cavity and oropharynx undergo extensive resections (requiring flap reconstruction), swallowing phases change, creating difficulties such as drooling of saliva, decreased mastication, aspiration, and pooling of food and fluids. In addition, RT to this area causes xerostomia, with loss of lubrication of the food bolus and taste changes.

The speech therapist works with patients in anticipation of the first oral intake, Normally, aspiration is prevented during the pharyngeal phase of swallowing by spontaneous, sequential actions: (1) the epiglottis closes to protect the laryngeal inlet; (2) the TVC come together; (3) the larynx rises and moves forward; (4) the cricopharyngeus opens in response to the laryngeal pull; and (5) the bolus travels above the larynx to the open cricopharyngeus and on to the esophagus.

Supraglottic swallowing is a technique that protects the airway from aspiration. It includes the following steps:

- Prepare the bolus of food in the oral preparatory phase.
- Before initiating the swallow, hold one's breath to close the vocal cords.
- Swallow while still holding one's breath.
- Cough while exhaling after the swallow to expectorate remaining food or fluids on top of vocal cords, thereby preventing aspiration.

Additional compensatory strategies that the speech pathologist may recommend include postural changes that facilitate passage of food into the oral cavity and pharynx (head elevated); changes in food consistency (ie, thin vs thick fluids, semi-solid vs pureed foods—Jello, applesauce, or mashed potatoes); indirect swallowing therapy—jaw and tongue range of motion exercises; and adduction of tongue exercises; to improve laryngeal closure.

Table 56-4 provides an example of a plan of care for dysphagia, which a speech therapist might follow during the patient's rehabilitation.

**TABLE 56-4**

**Dysphagia in Head and Neck Cancer Patients: Exercises and Compensatory Swallow Techniques**

| Problem | Technique |
|---|---|
| **Oral Preparatory Phase Problems** | |
| Decreased lip closure | Labial strength/ROM |
| Decreased mandibular ROM | ROM exercises |
| Decreased tongue ROM | ROM exercises/head tilt |
| | Palatal augmentation prosthesis |
| | Effortful swallow |
| | Reduce each bolus volume |
| | Head back position |
| **Pharyngeal Phase Problems** | Alternate liquids/solids |
| | Limit diet to liquids/pureed foods |
| | Multiple swallows per bolus |
| | Turn head toward affected side |
| | Tilt head toward stronger side |
| **Laryngeal Protection Problems** | Mendelsohn maneuver |
| | Supraglottic swallow |
| | Chin tuck maneuver |
| | Laryngeal adduction exercises |

*Abbreviation*: ROM, range of motion.

*Source*: Data from Stephen Goldman MACC, Speech Pathology Associates, San Diego, CA; 2004 (*personal communication*).

## SPEECH

Rehabilitation efforts that concentrate on improving or restoring the patient's ability to speak are key to a patient's continued progress in recovery and beyond. Studies indicate that the communication needs, communication methods, and perception of voice quality among patients with head and neck cancer are key QOL issues for patients.[114] Patients with nonlaryngeal head and neck cancer report significant objective and subjective changes in vocal function (articulation and phonation) long after treatment ends.[122]

To offset the limitations affecting communication ability post-treatment, standards have been established for rehabilitation of individuals who use laryngeal speech.[123] These standards include support and plans of care that prescribe speech therapy. As part of these care plans, speech pathologists recommend exercises to increase strength, range of motion, coordination, and accuracy of tongue movement. In addition, these plans support the use of oral prostheses to compensate for tissue loss and allow for greater contact of the tongue with the palate, thereby creating more intelligible speech.

Before therapy begins for patients with laryngeal cancer whose voice if compromised due to disease or treatment, the patient needs to establish ways to communicate. These methods will sustain him or her after treatment starts. Simple means to continue communication include pads of paper and pens or pencils, a computer or other electronic device, an erasable whiteboard, or a picture book, which shows commonly used phrases or items.

In esophageal speech, air that is swallowed becomes trapped in the esophagus, then is released. This technique allows air to vibrate against the walls of the esophagus. The puff of air is like a burp. It vibrates the walls of the throat, making sound for the new voice. The tongue, lips, and teeth form words as the sound passes through the mouth. This type of speech sounds low pitched and gruff, but it usually more closely resembles a natural voice than speech made by a mechanical larynx.[123,124]

A tracheoesophageal prosthesis or puncture (TEP) uses an opening created by the surgeon, called a tracheoesophageal fistula. A small plastic or silicone valve fits into this opening. The valve keeps food out of the trachea. After a TEP, patients can cover their stoma with a finger and force air into the esophagus through the valve. The air produces sound by making the walls of the throat vibrate. Sound is formed by air from the lungs, creating a better quality of esophageal speech.[123–125]

Mechanical speech using a handheld, battery-operated electrolarynx or pneumatic larynx transmits the vibration of sound when the patient holds the device to his or her neck or near the mouth. A pneumatic larynx is held over the stoma and uses air from the lungs instead of batteries to make it vibrate.

Voice function decline is well documented after RT.[118,120] Nevertheless, because voice function has been shown to decline with age, the additional impact of postradiation therapy changes can be equal to dystonia that comes with age.[126]

## MUCOSITIS

Oral mucositis remains the most common complication among patients with head and neck cancer.[127] Radiation and/or chemotherapies can destroy the rapidly regenerating epithelial cells on the mucous membrane. With this damage comes oral mucositis, an inflammation that is both progressive and painful.[128]

Tissues that are at risk of mucositis include the buccal mucosa, soft palate, tonsillar pillars, lateral tongue, pharyngeal walls, and larynx. Mucositis can appear as early as the first week of RT, and its severity can increase over time.[129] Clinical reports indicate that mucositis can be more severe with altered fractionation of RT.[127,130] This trend may be associated with late effects of radiotherapy, characterized by a decreased number of blood vessels and by significantly different expression patterns of the adhesion and of integrins and macrophage subpopulations.[128]

Patients report that pain is the worst part of their treatment experience and that the mucositis accompanying a sore throat is more than just a sore mouth.[129,130] Mucositis affects the patient's ability to eat and enjoy a full QOL.[131] When eating is difficult (no taste, dry mouth), patients report that their QOL is significantly compromised. They need additional emotional and psychosocial support because the sequelae from mucositis may extend beyond physical or pharmaceutical treatment of the mucositis.[132]

Table 56-5 [133] describes a scoring system that takes into account mucositis as well as xerostomia.

## ORAL CARE

Oral care is key to management of mucositis. Therapies have been designed to interfere with the causative factors of mucositis, thereby protecting normal mucosa either through direct radioprotection or by manipulation of growth factors and cytokines that are involved in mucosal repopulation. Other therapies have tried to counter inflammation or infection.[134,135] Weak evidence suggests that local antibiotics have a clinically significant ability to prevent acute radiotherapy side effects. There is insufficient evidence that radioprotective agents offer clinically significant protection of parotid glands.[129,130,135]

Patients are cautioned to use only the recommended mouth rinses and to avoid using solutions containing alcohol. Individuals also should be taught to avoid spicy and acid-containing fruits, vegetables, and juices (eg, oranges, grapefruits, lemons, and tomatoes). Both hot and cold foods can induce pain. Systemic analgesics such as hydrocodone or acetaminophen alone or with codeine may be necessary on a round-the-clock schedule or as needed.

Although a number of strategies and products are being investigated for oral care of patients with head and neck cancer, none are clearly superior to traditional regimens.[135,136] Most treatment protocols to prevent mucositis are based on clinical experience, but alternatives based on fundamental basic and clinical research are becoming more widely available.[137]

The results of studies that have evaluated prophylactic and ongoing treatment for oral mucositis are summarized in Table 56-6. Agents that have shown some positive benefits include benzydamine oral rinse and fluconazole for candida mucositis, allopurinal, and vitamin E.[135,136] In a review of interventions for treating oral mucositis, several agents—benzydamine HCl, tetrachlorodecaoxide, chlorhexidine, and "magic" (lidocaine solution, diphenhydramine hydrochloride, and aluminum hydroxide suspension)—had mixed records of effectiveness.[138]

The most effective way to treat radiation-induced mucositis in patients with head and neck cancer remains frequent oral rinsing with a bland mouthwash, such as saline or a sodium bicarbonate rinse, to reduce the amount of oral microbial flora. Dental care, consistent oral assessments, and the initiation of a standardized oral hygiene protocol before cancer treatment begins are the most effective approaches for oral mucositis.[135,136,139]

Patients benefit most when they cleanse the oral cavity every 3 to 4 hours during the day and at night, if possible. Cleansing the oral cavity with a soft bristle brush, using toothpaste with baking soda or saline/soda rinses, and flossing regularly are important components of oral care.[134–136] Despite such rigorous oral hygiene, white or yellow patches may appear. By the fourth to fifth week of treatment, the discomfort has been building and the tissue is vividly erythemic.

After treatment ends, late complications are common, especially in elderly patients. Repeat irradiation may induce serious complications (additional mucositis, xerostomia, malnutrition, pain) because of overdosage to previously irradiated areas. There are reports of severe late complications developing 3 to 10 months after reirradiation.[134,135]

Pain can be managed topically by a pharmaceutical mixture of anesthetic and anti-inflammatory medications along with an antacid, which provides a coating action to promote its adherence to tissues. Patients are taught to swish this mixture for 2 to 3 minutes, then expectorate or swallow (if allowed) 4 times a day (eg, after meals and at bedtime). Coating agents may also be topically applied in the event of breakthrough discomfort.

**TABLE 56-5**

**RTOG Scoring for Skin, Mucosal, and Tongue Reactions**

| | 1 | 2 | 3 | 4 |
|---|---|---|---|---|
| Acute skin reaction | Follicular, faint or dull erythema, epilation, dry desquamation, decreased sweating | Tender or bright erythema, patchy moist desquamation, moderate edema | Confluence, moist desquamation other than skin folds, pitting edema | Ulceration, hemorrhage, or necrosis |
| Acute mucous membrane reaction | Inflammation, may experience mild pain not requiring analgesic | Patchy mucositis that may produce an inflammatory serosanguineous discharge, may experience moderate pain requiring analgesics | Confluent fibrinous mucositis, may include severe pain requiring narcotic | Ulceration, hemorrhage, or necrosis |
| Acute salivary gland reaction | Mild mouth dryness, slightly thickened saliva may have slightly altered taste such as metallic taste, these changes not reflected in baseline feeding behavior, such as increased liquid with meals | Moderate mouth dryness, thick sticky saliva, markedly altered taste | Complete mouth dryness, markedly altered taste or absence of taste | Acute salivary gland necrosis |
| Acute pharynx reaction | Mild dysphagia or odynophagia, may require topical anesthetic or non-narcotic analgesics, may require soft diet | Moderate dysphagia or odynophagia, may require narcotic analgesics, may require soft or liquid diet | Severe dysphagia or odynophagia with dehydration or weight loss (>15% from pretreatment baseline) requiring NG feeding tube, IV fluids, or hyperalimentation | Complete obstruction, ulceration, perforation, fistula |
| Acute larynx reaction | Mild or intermittent hoarseness, cough not requiring antitussive, erythema of mucosa | Persistent hoarseness but able to vocalize, referred ear pain, sore throat, patchy fibrinous exudate or mild arytenoids, edema not requiring narcotic, cough requiring antitussive | Whispered speech, throat pain or referred ear pain requiring narcotic, confluent fibrinous exudate, marked arytenoids edema | Marked dyspnea, stridor or hemoptysis with tracheostomy or intubation necessary |
| Acute tongue reaction | Mild erythema, may have slightly altered taste not affecting nutritional intake | Tender, bright erythema, coated, loss of papillae with shiny appearance, markedly altered taste, moderate pain requiring analgesia | Blistered, cracked appearance, markedly altered taste or absence of taste, severe pain requiring narcotic | Ulceration, hemorrhage, or necrosis |

*Source*: Data from Radiation Therapy Oncology Group.[133]

Because mucositis represents the dose-limiting acute toxicity and xerostomia ranks as the most common long-term QOL complaint, a reduction of the external beam RT dose may provide an important benefit in reducing toxicity. IMRT regimens have been shown to be less toxic for the side effects of mucositis and xerostomia.[48,49]

## XEROSTOMIA

Radiation injury can cause permanent, noncorrectable xerostomia or the lack of saliva. Because RT can damage the salivary glands, the patient's production of saliva may decrease by as much as 50% during the first 1 to 2 weeks of treatment. As treatment progresses, the saliva becomes thick, tenacious, ropey, or even nonexistent. Without saliva, the patient experiences burning sensations or ulcerations, difficulty in swallowing, and oral friction that is associated with tongue adherence to the palate or buccal mucosa. Various studies have reported that xerostomia is one of the major patient-reported distresses from therapy.[127,129]

Xerostomia is commonly measured and graded using objective measures of major salivary gland output and

**TABLE 56-6**

**Treatment for Oral Mucositis**

| Category | Agent | Efficacy | Comments |
|---|---|---|---|
| Saliva stimulant | Pilocarpine | Mixed results, may be more efficacious for nonradiation-induced xerostomia | Can take up to 12 weeks for effect in radiotherapy patients; can cause sweating, headache, urinary frequency |
| | Artificial saliva (mucin or carboxymethylcellulose based) | Short duration | Mucin (porcine derivative) unsuitable for Muslims, religious Jews, other groups |
| | Vitamin C | Limited data, subjective findings demonstrate superiority over artificial saliva only | Local irritation, demineralization of teeth make it unsuitable for long-term use in dentate patients |
| | Citric acid | Limited data demonstrating efficacy in non-RT-related xerostomia only | May cause burning sensation, demineralization of teeth |
| Oral rinse, antimicrobial | Chlorhexidine | Overall no significant change in severity or suppression | Reports of rinse-induced discomfort, taste alteration, teeth staining |
| Oral rinse, antiseptic | Hydrogen peroxide | Mixed results in clinical trials | Long-term use discouraged; breaks down granulation tissue, disrupts flora |
| | Providone-iodine | Data indicate possible advantage over hydrogen peroxide in terms of severity and duration | Should be diluted; full-strength formulation damages new granulated tissue |
| | 0.9% Saline solution | No formal evaluation available | Relatively innocuous, economical |
| | Sodium bicarbonate | No formal evaluation available | Creates alkaline environment that promotes bacterial microflora; unpleasant taste; NCI recommended |
| | 0.9% Saline/sodium bicarbonate | No formal evaluation | NCI recommended |
| Coating agent, mucosal protectant | Sucralfate suspension | Most data demonstrate no statistically significant difference in severity, pain intensity scores, and other subjective symptoms (taste alterations, dry mouth) | May offer little or no benefit compared to oral hygiene, symptomatic treatment |
| | Hydroxypropyl cellulose film | Initial studies are mostly open label; some products provide relief for at least 3 hours | Further study needed |
| | Kaolin pectate | Limited data, usually mixed in "cocktail" | NCI recommended |
| | Aluminum hydroxide | Limited data, usually mixed in "cocktail" | Coating may interfere with oral assessment |
| Mucosal protectant cytokine-like agent | Granulocyte-macrophage colony-stimulating factor | Some data indicate reduction in severity, pain | May prove especially beneficial for chemotherapy or radiotherapy patients; with use, patients discontinue due to intolerable side effects: local skin reactions, fever, bone pain, nausea when administered subcutaneously |
| | Granulocyte colony-stimulating factor | Limited data, some indication of significant reductions in bone marrow transplant patients; occurrences less in radiotherapy patients when used as prophylactic | Further study needed |

(Continued)

**TABLE 56-6**

**Treatment for Oral Mucositis (*Continued*)**

| Category | Agent | Efficacy | Comments |
|---|---|---|---|
| Anti-inflammatory, immunity promotion | Immunoglobulin | Limited data, may lessen severity in patients receiving radiation and chemotherapy | Further study needed |
| Topical anesthetic | Viscous lidocaine | Limited data, may provide significant relief of limited duration | Further study needed |
| | Benzocaine sprays/ gels; Dyclonine rinse; Diphenhydramine solution | See viscous lidocaine | See viscous lidocaine |

observer-rated toxicity grading.[140,141] Additional elements of grading have better defined functional deficits.

Although artificial saliva products are available, the soothing effect is costly and only temporary. Xerostomia may be equally relieved with frequent small sips of water. Patients are advised to always carry a water bottle with them. Hard candies and sugarless gum are other ways to moisten the oral mucosa. It is usually recommended that dentures not be worn. The use of either tobacco or alcohol further dries and irritates the mucosa.

Sodium bicarbonate toothpaste and swabs will help to thin the saliva and can partially correct the acidic effect of xerostomia. Zinc sulfate may play a role in the perception of taste by the patient who receives radiation.

The combination of partial salivary gland sparing and radiation protectors/stimulants may provide additive or synergistic gains in reducing the severity of xerostomia.[135] To increase secretions from the remaining portions of the salivary gland, a few medications may help. Pilocarpine may be prescribed either upon beginning or following RT.[142,143] To offset the diaphoresis as a side effect of pilocarpine, patients are encouraged to increase fluid intake.

Along with pilocarpine, anethole trithione promotes saliva secretion. The radioprotectant amifostine has been shown to be effective in reducing mucositis and dysphagia following RT.[144]

## LOSS OF TASTE

Diminished saliva flow results in changes to taste and smell, especially when taste or olfactory cells are in the radiation field. Taste changes are typically first reported by the second week of RT and become most pronounced 2 months after treatment begins. The alterations to the taste of salty and bitter foods are the most pronounced changes, while the taste of sweets is the least affected.[145]

## DENTAL PROPHYLACTIC CARE

A dental evaluation should precede RT, with extractions as necessary. A preradiation oral examination and treatment[146] will identify existing oral disease, the potential risk of oral disease, remove infectious dental/oral areas, and establish an adequate standard of ongoing oral hygiene and care.[146] Among the effects of RT are reduced vascularity and oxygen tension of the oral hard and soft tissues and salivary gland dysfunction. These changes increase the risk of dental decay and oral infections and may lead to reduced healing capacity following oral surgery procedures. An additional severe complication of RT is osteoradionecrosis of the jaw bone.[147] To improve mastication, speech, and saliva control for patients with osteoradionecrosis, the patient can benefit from acrylic/rubber prosthetics.[147] Patients are commonly instructed about appropriate oral hygiene and the use of fluoride trays.

## TRISMUS

Patient treatment involving the oral cavity (eg, surgery or grafts) can affect muscles for mastication and the posterior mandible. When the oral cavity opening is tightly restricted, the condition called trismus results. With trismus, the patient is at risk of developing fibrosis of oral cavity muscles. With time, exercises can stretch the interarch of the oral cavity. An example of such an exercise is increasing the number of stacked tongue blades to stretch the opening. This exercise should be done three or four times a day.

## PAIN MANAGEMENT

Pain is a significant problem for patients with head and neck cancer during treatment as their tumors grow.[113,114] Pain can occur because of surgery. For example, severed superficial nerves may cause numbness in the initial postoperative period. Then pain resumes when numbness subsides. Subsequent edema may cause feelings of pressure. When the jugular vein has been ligated or occluded, the increase in spinal fluid pressure may cause the patient to experience throbbing, pounding, and pressure sensations in the head.

Pain from mucositis and skin erythema, as well as toxicities from radiation and chemotherapy treatment, can build as treatment courses progress. In a study of patients with head and neck nasopharyngeal cancer, the pain from RT can continue to be severe and undertreated, affecting swallowing and talking more than sleeping or other general activities.[114] In a similar study of individuals who had pain post-treatment, 31% of the patients had pain at diagnosis. Later, 74% reported some degree of pain at 6 to 12 months following treatment. With a multidisciplinary approach to care, pain as a significant symptom from treatment becomes all everyone's concern, mobilizing pharmaceutical pain management strategies, as well as resources from nutritionists, speech and swallow therapists, social workers, psychiatrists, and dentists.[148]

A significant number of patients rejected regular pharmacological management and employed a variety of other pain-relieving methods. The authors concluded that this patient population has a unique pain experience and attitudes toward pain management.[148]

## TRACHEOSTOMY CARE

When the airway is compromised by tumor or postoperative edema, the surgeon will perform a tracheostomy. The procedure is needed if an airway obstruction is anticipated or to manage an existing, compromised pulmonary function. The tracheostomy may be temporary or permanent.

As a form of treatment, the surgeon may perform a total laryngectomy (TL). A TL results in a complete separation of the pharynx from the trachea. It removes the cricoid and thyroid cartilage, both arytenoids, both TVCs, both TVCs, the epiglottis, the preepiglottic and paraglottic spaces, and the hyoid bone.

Care for patients with laryngeal cancer includes ongoing attention to tracheostomy care and suctioning. The general recommendations for tracheostomy cleaning include

- Removing the tube and cleaning it in a solution of equal parts hydrogen peroxide and normal saline.
- If the inner cannula is disposable, replace it with a new cannula of the same size.
- Clean the peristomal site at least every 8 to 12 hours with half-strength hydrogen peroxide, rinse with normal saline, and dry.[39]

Individuals with a total laryngectomy will require only a temporary laryngectomy tube, which is short and wide

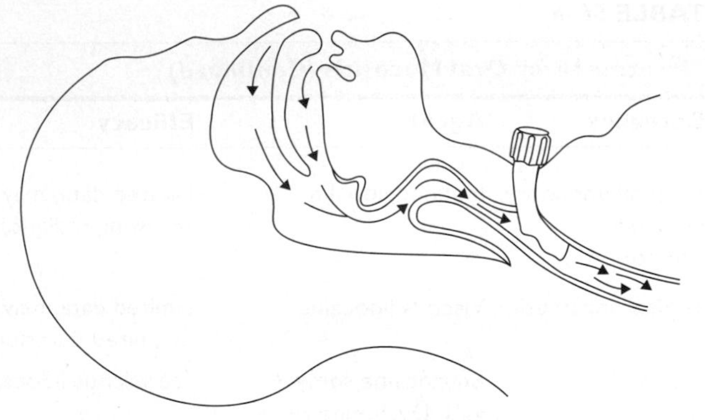

**FIGURE 56-8**

Airway using a fenestrated trache tube.
*Source*: Data from Nelcor Puritan Bennett.[149]

in comparison to the conventional tracheostomy tube. The laryngectomy tube helps to shape the stoma (Figure 56-8.[149]) Table 56-7 lists ways to troubleshoot problems that may arise for individuals with a tracheostomy tube.

Individuals with altered airways have lost their ability to moisten, warm, or filter the air they breathe. This results in thick, tenacious, dry tracheal secretions that are a challenge to clear by coughing. If they cannot be cleared, the secretions may create mucous plugs that obstruct the tracheostomy tube and can block breathing.

To avoid developing these plugs, supplemental humidity is necessary. In the hospital, warm, humidified oxygen should be administered via tracheostomy collar when the patient is at rest. At home, a large (10-gallon) humidifier in the living area and a small bedside humidifier in the sleeping room are useful to provide needed humidity. Patients can apply moistened gauze pads at the trache site and foam or crocheted stoma covers to collect the moisture of exhaled air and optimize humidity. Also, they can instill up to 5 mL of normal saline or spray 4 to 5 puffs of normal saline into the stoma using a nasal atomizer.[39]

## NUTRITIONAL MANAGEMENT

Nutritional support provides the calories for healing after surgical resection and during intensive radiation or chemotherapy treatments. Before their diagnosis, many patients with head and neck cancer already have nutritional deficits. When the malignant process starts or treatment begins, cancer-related weight loss is common because diseases of the head and neck cause impairments in mastication and/or deglutition.[150] Patients can become malnourished after surgery or during treatment, increasing their risk of complications—specifically, infection and delayed wound healing.[150] Loss of appetite and weight contribute to weakness and lethargy and predict a poor prognosis for patients

**TABLE 56-7**

**Tracheostomy Tubes: Solving Problems**

| Symptom | What May Have Happened | What to Do |
|---|---|---|
| Excessive air leak through nose and mouth | Insufficient air in cuff (cuffed tubes only) | Deflate and reinflate the cuff with the proper amount of air |
| | Leak in cuff, inflation line, pilot balloon, or luer valve (cuffed tubes only) | Replace the tube |
| | Tube too small for trachea | Call doctor |
| | Uncuffed vs cuffed tube | Call doctor |
| | Fenestrated inner cannula is in tube (see Figure 56-8) | Remove and replace with nonfenestrated inner cannula |
| Tube comes out of neck opening | Excessive pull or weight at the connector | Readjust tubing to reduce pulling |
| | Trach tube ties are too loose or are tied incorrectly | Retie and secure |
| Difficulty when removing inner cannula for fenestrated tube | Tracheal lining may be pushing through the fenestration | Call doctor |
| | Trach tube alignment has changed | Call doctor |
| Tube or part of tube breaks or does not work | Excessive use or wear on the tube | Replace tube |
| | Trach tube was cleansed using wrong cleaning agents | Replace tube; use recommended cleaning agents |
| | Excessive pulling or weight on connector | Readjust tubing to reduce pulling |
| | Trach tube ties are too loose or are tied incorrectly | Retie and secure |
| Unable or difficult to pass suction catheter through trache tube | Mucous plug | Remove inner cannula and clean it if reusable; replace it if disposable |
| | Catheter is too large for tube size | Replace with correct size |
| | Tube is not properly positioned in the trachea | Reposition the tube |
| | Fenestrated inner cannula is in the tube | Replace with a nonfenestrated inner cannula |

with cancer.[150] In addition, patients with these malignancies may be severely malnourished because of years of tobacco or substance abuse, which can contribute to liver disease.

## ENTERAL THERAPY

If the upper GI tract is compromised or fully obstructed because of disease or treatment, the patient's ability to swallow is impaired. In such cases, enteral feedings may be necessary through a nasogastric feeding tube (NG tube) or a gastrostomy tube (G-tube), which is placed by a surgeon. Placement of the feeding tube before treatment is a prophylactic strategy to offset weight loss inevitably suffered with treatment.[151] Another option is the percutaneous puncture (PEG tube), a gastrostomy tube with a small diameter, which is placed by an interventional radiologist. Before it is used, its placement is checked by x-ray.[152]

Tube feeding can start when the patient has bowel sounds. For either the NG tube or the G-tube, the patient assumes a sitting position or elevates the head of the bed. Generally, feedings start at the slow rate of 25 to 30 mL/hour, increasing to 25 additional mL/hour per day to meet volume and calorie goals.

Tube feedings can occur via gravity or pump (bolus every 4–6 hours or continuous flow). Changes to the nutritionals used or the feeding schedule may be necessary if side effects develop, such as diarrhea. Diarrhea can be caused by certain antibiotics and medications containing sorbital.

## FATIGUE

Fatigue has become a focus of concern in helping patients manage the side effects of cancer treatment. Still its effect on this particular patient population is still not well studied.

In a 2007 study of head and neck patients undergoing RT, fatigue was found to reach its maximum intensity at the sixth week of treatment and then slowly decreases thereafter. Age, thyroid dysfunction, psychological disorders, pre-RT fatigue score, CT, and cortisone use were correlated with RT-related fatigue levels.[153]

A 2005 study of fatigue after RT reported that head and neck patients were among patients who reported severe fatigue. Fatigue was a common adverse effect of RT, reported by more than three-fourths of patients by the third to fifth weeks of treatment.[154]

## PSYCHOSOCIAL SUPPORT

Those diagnosed with head and neck malignancies face many challenges during treatment and its aftermath. Among the main concerns of these patients are dysfunction and disfigurement.[155] Because key components of self-esteem can be affected—including sight, taste, smell, hearing, and sense of touch—the social isolation for these patients can be paralyzing.[155] Patients can best be supported with a variety of interventions. Among them are education about their conditions and accompanying side effects and about coping strategies to help them keep involved in important relationships, activities, and interests.[156]

Because of the challenge of treatment and its accompanying side effects, patients with head and neck cancer are at risk for depression.[157,158] Studies show that patients should be continually assessed for depression with interventions tailored to the patient as needed.[159] But keep in mind, these patients may have been depressed before treatment begins.

Studies show that the lack of psychosocial support can affect survival. A 2006 study of patients with head and neck cancer looked at the coping methods of males, who did not have a partner. The study identified prognostic variables independent of disease-related variables for survival based on age, marital/partner status, and income. According to the study, the apparent disadvantage of unpartnered men was striking related to coping and survival outcomes. The study called for simple supportive interventions to improve outcomes.[160]

Laryngectomy patients have been reported to be at increased risk of psychosocial stressors, depression, and suicide.[161] The patients also report problems with trismus, xerostomia, speech and swallowing disorders, fatigue, and self-image. Supporting these patients by recognizing and addressing their challenges has been shown to help with coping and improved patient-perceived QOL. Conscientious assessment of coping, social situations, risk factors, systematic rehabilitation efforts, ongoing counseling, and support may improve outcomes for patients.[161]

Signs of effective coping immediately after surgery include the patient's attention to self-care and resocialization.[161] For example, after laryngectomy, a patient needs to learn how to take care of what can be a complex set of new skills: dressing changes, tracheostomy care, and suctioning, as well as enteral feeding responsibilities and tasks. Appropriate interventions to help patients and their families will support the patient in his or her skill building, help set boundary limits, and help the patient focus on dealing with current problems. Such interventions support the building and expanding of coping mechanisms.

To boost psychosocial support, a visit by a recovered patient with a similar diagnosis may be requested from the Lost Chord Club, ACS, or another community support group. Such a visit may be well received about 7 days after surgery. Contact with Internet support groups may also benefit the patient (Table 56-8). Nevertheless, it is important to provide continued clinical support and follow-up to augment Internet resources and connections.[161]

## QUALITY-OF-LIFE ISSUES

A 2005 study identified that both psychosocial and physiological factors influence quality of life in patients with head and neck cancer, but many QOL measures are most strongly influenced by psychosocial considerations.[162]

Treatments for head and neck cancer have modestly improved, preserving organ function and extending disease-free periods. Research on QOL with patients with cancer is more prevalent. Yet as important as QOL is for head and

**TABLE 56-8**

**Selected Web-Based Sources of Information and Support for Patients with Head and Neck Cancer**

| |
|---|
| Support for People with Oral and Head and Neck Cancer<br>*http://www.spohnc.org* |
| Let's Face It USA<br>*http://www.faceit.org* |
| National Cancer Institute<br>*http://www.nci.nih.org* |
| International Association of Laryngectomee's<br>*http://www.larynxlink.com* |
| Head and Neck Cancer Community<br>*http://www.headandneckcancer.org* |

neck patients, the factors that contribute to a person's perception of quality of life remain poorly understood.[155] More studies are using well-accepted and valid QOL instruments with this patient population to further clarify the unique issues for these patients, suggesting interventions that are credible and effective with these patients.[155]

Psychological challenges of treatment and survivorship go hand and hand with perceived QOL. Frequently cited problems that patients must address during and following treatment include pain, xerostomia, speech and swallowing disorders, trismus, fatigue, weakness, and weight loss.[163]

Although QOL is multifactorial and subjective, studies show that some improvement may be achieved when healthcare professionals recognize and address symptoms and the challenges of coping during the course of treatment.[164] QOL can also be improved when social and family well-being are addressed, as well as when the healthcare team pays attention to continued smoking behavior and depression.[165]

One of the few larger, longitudinal, case–control studies published that evaluated the effect of a psychosocial support program on QOL in patients with head and neck cancer was undertaken by Petruson et al.[166] A total of 142 newly diagnosed patients with head and neck cancer in Sweden were included in this study. Throughout the first year after diagnosis, 52 participants in the study group were given additional emotional support and information on head and neck cancer, its treatment, and side effects. Patients were evaluated at various milestones. The study and control group's QOL scores initially did not differ significantly. However, at a 1-year follow-up, the control group had a clinically and statistically better global QOL score. At 3-year follow-up, both groups had high levels of depression and treatment-related side effects were also prevalent in both groups.[166]

A 2008 study analyzed the prospectively collected health-related QOL data from head and neck patients. The focus of the study was to assess QOL as an independent prognostic factor for locoregional control and/or overall survival. Study results demonstrated the importance of baseline QOL scores as a significant and independent predictor of the patient's illness.[167]

Further studies have indicated that pain and the functional impairment of chewing and swallowing are the most important parameters before treatment. Immediately after surgical treatment, other variables that are fundamental to QOL are speech intelligibility and mobility disorders in the head, neck, and shoulder regions.[168,169] Yet, studies indicate that no amount of preoperative counseling prepares patients and families for the aftermath of laryngectomy surgery. One study reported that the period for the highest level of stress within families is 6 months after surgery. Then the stress plateaus by 12 months, and reaches a stable level with improved QOL measured at 2 years after treatment.[170]

In a study of post-treatment oropharyngeal patients, when physical, role, emotional, cognitive, and social functioning can be addressed and problem solved, QOL is rated as generally good.[171] Yet head and neck cancer involves very distinct sites. Researchers caution that the specific type of head and neck cancer must be taken into account when assessing QOL. Morton and Izzard found that organ-preservation techniques do not necessarily lead to better QOL outcomes, especially in laryngeal cancer.[172] Moreover, not much is known about the comorbidity of continued alcohol abuse and tobacco use after surgery in laryngectomy patients.[161]

Healthcare providers commonly perceive disfigurement, alternation in function (loss of voice), and disease control as the most relevant issues in the postoperative period. Patients and families give high ratings to management of physical symptoms, social reintegration, participation in enjoyed activities, vocation issues, and communications impairment. Patients may be able to meet rehabilitation goals (talk and eat) but cannot cope with day-to-day living (relationships with family, spouse, finances, work, sexual interest, and performance).[168]

## MULTIDISCIPLINARY CARE

Care of the patient with head and neck cancer is challenging. Barriers to providing care, which requires many disciplines and resources, reside in a healthcare system that is already taxed by many demands. Patients expect optimal care even when insurance coverage is limited. With many patients being underinsured or lacking any insurance, the challenges become even greater.[173]

Many components in the patient's delivery of care are affected by dwindling healthcare resources. Surgical procedures now performed in same-day units limit the opportunity for presurgical and postprocedure teaching. Chemotherapy and RT are usually outpatient procedures. Even if the patient requires a hospital admission, the stay is usually short. Therefore, the opportunity to provide adequate teaching and support is limited. Due to the risk factors that are associated with these patients, their compliance with ongoing and after-care may be shaky.[174] These patients tend to be less health conscious and to have less social support than most other groups of patients with cancer.

Integrating the rehabilitation team in outpatient and after-care is another challenge. Among the multidisciplinary team members who come together for a patient with head and neck cancer are the oncologist, head and neck surgeon, dentist, nurse, dietician, physical therapist, social worker, and, in some instances, plastic surgeon, prosthodontist, and psychologist. Their services need coordination for these patients—specifically, in managing follow-up appointments, supplies and equipment, therapy sessions, dental care, symptom management, and psychosocial support.[175]

Repeated studies, based on evidence-based practice guidelines, show the quality of care for head and neck patients can be greatly improved with a more comprehensive, integrated, and multidisciplinary focus to care delivery.[176]

Studies have also shown that nurses are integral members of the team—if not the leaders of multidisciplinary care teams. Patients consider their connection with the head and neck cancer nurse one of the key relationships they establish, which helps them maintain a sense of continuity and clarity about their care.[177,178]

Many studies are able to show that multidisciplinary teams better address the patient's physical, nutritional, and psychosocial stresses. Patients are better managed, with fewer complications and setbacks and improved staff communication.[175,179–184]

## REFERENCES


1. National Cancer Institute (NCI). Head and neck cancer. http://www.cancer.gov/cancertopics/factsheet/Sites-Types/head-and-neck. Published 2005. Accessed February 26, 2010.
2. National Cancer Institute (NCI). A snapshot of head and neck cancer. http://planning.cancer.gov/disease/Head_and_Neck-Snapshot.pdf. Published 2008. Accessed February 26, 2010.
3. American Cancer Society (ACS). *Cancer Facts and Figures 2009.* Atlanta, GA: American Cancer Society; 2009:16–18.
4. Reis LAG, Melbert D, Krapcho M, et al, eds. *SEER Cancer Statistics Review, 1975–2005.* Bethesda, MD: National Cancer Institute. http://seer.cancer.gov/csr/1975_2005/. Accessed February 24, 2010.
5. Fuller C, Wang S, Thomas C, et al. Conditional survival in head and neck squamous cell carcinoma: results from the SEER dataset 1973–1998. *Cancer.* 2007;109:1331–1343.
6. National Cancer Institute (NCI). Prevention and cessation of cigarette smoking: control of tobacco use (PDQ). http://www.cancer.gov/cancertopics/pdq/prevention/control-of-tobacco-use/healthprofessional. Published 2008. Accessed November 1, 2009.
7. National Cancer Institute (NCI). Oral cancer prevention. http://www.cancer.gov/cancertopics/pdq/prevention/oral/healthprofessional. Published 2008. Accessed November 1, 2009.
8. National Cancer Institute (NCI). Oral cancer screening. http://www.cancer.gov/cancertopics/pdq/screening/oral/healthprofessional. Published 2008. Accessed November 1, 2009.
9. Horner MJ, Ries LAG, Krapcho M, et al, eds. SEER Cancer Statistics Review, 1975–2006. National Cancer Institute. Bethesda, MD. http://seer.cancer.gov/csr/1975_2006. Accessed November 1, 2009.
10. American Dental Association (ADA) Oral Cancer. http://www.ada.org/public/topics/cancer_oral.asp. Published 2007. Accessed November 1, 2009.
11. National Cancer Institute (NCI). Throat (laryngeal and pharyngeal) cancer. http://www.cancer.gov/cancertopics/types/throat. Published 2008. Accessed November 1, 2009.
12. National Cancer Institute (NCI). Hypopharyngeal cancer treatment (PDQ). http://www.cancer.gov/cancertopics/pdq/treatment/hypopharyngeal/healthprofessional. Published 2008e. Accessed November 1, 2009.
13. Hashibe M, Brennan P, Benhamou S, et al. Alcohol drinking in never users of tobacco, cigarette smoking in never drinkers, and the risk of head and neck cancer: pooled analysis in the International Head and Neck Cancer Epidemiology Consortium. *J Natl Cancer Inst.* 2007;99:777–789.
14. Colwill M, Lozio-Stegall HM. Prevention and early detection. In: Clarke LK, Dropkin MJ, eds. *Site-Specific Cancer Series: Head and Neck Cancer.* Pittsburgh, PA: Oncology Nursing Society; 2006:29–34.
15. Argiris A, Karamouzis M, Raben D, et al. Head and neck cancer. *Lancet.* 2008;371:1695–1709.
16. Gillison M, D'Souza G, Westra W, et al. Distinct risk factor profiles for human papillomavirus type 16-positive and human papillomavirus type 16-negative head and neck cancers. *J Natl Cancer Inst.* 2008;100:407–420.
17. Fakhry C, Westra W, Li S, et al. Improved survival of patients with human papillomavirus-positive head and neck squamous cell carcinoma in a prospective clinical trial. *J Natl Cancer Inst.* 2008;100:261–269.
18. Fakhry C, Gillison M. Clinical implications of human papillomavirus in head and neck cancers. *J Clin Oncol.* 2006;24:2606–2611.
19. Ji X, Neumann A, Sturgis E, et al. P52 codon 72 polymorphism associated with risk of human papillomavirus-associated squamous cell carcinoma of the oropharynx in never smokers. *Carcinogenesis.* 2008;29:875–879.
20. Silverman S. *Oral Cancer: American Cancer Society, Atlas of Clinical Oncology.* Ontario, Canada: BC Decker; 2002.
21. National Cancer Institute (NCI). Nasopharyngeal cancer treatment (PDQ). http://www.cancer.gov/cancertopics/pdq/treatment/nasopharyngeal/healthprofessional. Published 2008. Accessed February 26, 2010.
22. Hickey M. Pathophysiology. In: Clarke LK, Dropkin MJ, eds. *Site-Specific Cancer Series: Head and Neck Cancer.* Pittsburgh, PA: Oncology Nursing Society; 2006:17–28.
23. Ridge J, Glisson B, Horwitz E, Meyers M. Head and neck tumors. In: Pazdur R, Coia L, Hoskins W, Wagman L, eds. *Cancer Management: A Multidisciplinary Approach.* 8th ed. Manhassett, NY: CMP Healthcare Media; 2004:39–85.
24. Dawson C. Patient assessment. In: Clarke LK, Dropkin MJ, eds. *Site-Specific Cancer Series: Head and Neck Cancer.* Pittsburgh, PA: Oncology Nursing Society; 2006:35–48.
25. Rumboldt Z, Gordon L, Gordon L, et al. Imaging in head and neck cancer. *Curr Treat Options Oncol.* 2006;7:23–34.
26. Hermans R. Head and neck cancer: how imaging predicts treatment outcome. *Cancer Imaging.* 2006;31;6:S145-S153.
27. Corry J, Rischin D, Hicks R, Peters L. The role of PET-CT in the management of patients with advanced cancer of the head and neck. *Curr Oncol Rep.* 2008:10:149–55.
28. Ahn P, Garg M. Positron emission tomography/computed tomography for target delineation in head and neck cancers. *Semin Nucl Med.* 2008;8:141–148.
29. Corry J, Rischin D, Hicks R, et al. The role of PET-CT in the management of patients with advanced cancer of the head and neck. *Curr Oncol Rep.* 2008;10:149–155.
30. Fleming A, Smith S, Paul C, et al. Impact of [$^{18}$F]-2 fluorodeoxyglucose-positron emission tomography/computed tomography on previously untreated head and neck cancer patients. *Laryngoscope.* 2007;117:1173–1179.
31. American Joint Committee on Cancer (AJCC). *American Joint Committee on Cancer: AJCC Cancer Staging Manual.* 6th ed. New York: Springer; 2002.
32. American Joint Committee on Cancer (AJCC). *Cancer Staging Manual.* 7th ed. New York: Springer; 2010:21–100.
33. O'Sullivan B, Shah J. New TNM staging criteria for head and neck tumors. *Semin Surg Oncol.* 2003;21:30–42.
34. Wirth L, Posner M. Recent advances in combined modality therapy for locally advanced head and neck cancer. *Curr Cancer Drug Targets.* 2007;7:674–680.
35. Bernier J. A multidisciplinary approach to squamous cell carcinomas of the head and neck: an update. *Curr Opin Oncol.* 2008;20:249–255.
36. Licitra L, Bossi P, Locati L. A multidisciplinary approach to squamous cell carcinomas of the head and neck: what is new? *Curr Opin Oncol.* 2006;18:253–257.
37. National Comprehensive Cancer Network (NCCN). Practice Guidelines in Oncology: Head and Neck Cancers v.2.2008. http://www.nccn.org/professionals/physician_gls/PDF/head-and-neck.pdf. Published 2008. Accessed February 26, 2010.

38. Scarpa R, Zevallos J. Surgical management of head and neck malignancies. In: Clarke LK, Dropkin MJ, eds. *Site-Specific Cancer Series: Head and Neck Cancer.* Pittsburgh, PA: Oncology Nursing Society; 2006: 49–61.
39. Sievers A. Postoperative management of the head and neck surgical patient. In: Clarke LK, Dropkin MJ, eds. *Site-Specific Cancer Series: Head and Neck Cancer.* Pittsburgh, PA: Oncology Nursing Society; 2006:85–102.
40. Bangalore M, Matthews S, Suntharalingam M. Recent advances in radiation therapy for head and neck cancer. *ORL J Otorhinolaryngol Relat Spec.* 2007;69:1–12.
41. Marshak G, Popovtzer A. Is there any significant reduction of patients' outcome following delay in commencing postoperative radiotherapy? *Curr Opin Otolaryngol Head Neck Surg.* 2006;14:82–84.
42. Cummings B, Keane T, Pintilie M, et al. Five year results of a randomized trial comparing hyperfractionated to conventional radiotherapy over four weeks in locally advanced head and neck cancer. *Radiother Oncol.* 2007;85:7–16.
43. Bouris J, Overgaard J, Audry H, et al. Hyperfractionated or accelerated radiotherapy in head and neck cancer: a meta-analysis. *Lancet.* 2006;368:843–854.
44. Sheahan P, O'Keane C, Sheahan J, et al. Predictors of survival in early oral cancer. *Otolaryngol Head Neck Surg.* 2003;129:571–576.
45. Popovtzer A, Eisbruch A. Advances in radiation therapy of head and neck cancer. *Expert Rev Anticancer Ther.* 2008;8:633–644.
46. Corvo R. Evidence-based radiation oncology in head and neck squamous cell carcinoma. *Radiother Oncol.* 2007;85:156–170.
47. Kao J, Lavaf A, Teng M, Huang D, Genden E. Adjuvant radiotherapy and survival for patients with node-positive head and neck cancer: an analysis by primary site and nodal stage. *Int J Radiat Oncol Biol Phys.* 2008;71:362–370.
48. Garden A, Lewin J, Chambers M. How to reduce radiation-related toxicity in patients with cancer of the head and neck. *Curr Oncol Rep.* 2006;8:140–145.
49. Lee N, Puri, D, Blanco A, Chao K. Intensity-modulated radiation therapy in head and neck cancers: an update. *Head Neck.* 2007;29:387–400.
50. Lee N, O'Meara W, Chan K, et al. Concurrent chemotherapy and intensity-modulated radiotherapy for locoregionally advanced laryngeal and hypopharyngeal cancer. *Int J Radiat Oncol Biol Phys.* 2007;69: 459–468.
51. Feng M, Eisbruch A. Future issues in highly conformal radiotherapy for head and neck cancer. *J Clin Oncol.* 2007;25:1009–1013.
52. Biagioli M, Harvey M, Roman E, et al. Intensity-modulated radiotherapy with concurrent chemotherapy for previously irradiated, recurrent head and neck cancer. *Int J Radiat Oncol Biol Phys.* 2007;69:1067–1073.
53. Schoenfeld G, Amdur R, Morris C, Li J, Hinerman R, Mendenhall W. Patterns of failure and toxicity after intensity-modulated radiotherapy for head and neck cancer. *Int J Radiat Oncol Biol Phys.* 2008;71:377–385.
54. Graff P, Lapevre M, Desandes E, et al. Impact of intensity-modulated radiotherapy on health-related quality of life for head and neck cancer patients: matched pair comparison with conventional radiotherapy. *Int J Radiat Oncol Biol Phys.* 2007;67:1309–1317.
55. Grimard L, Esche B, Lamothe A, Cygler J, Spaans J. Interstitial low-dose rate brachytherapy in the treatment of recurrent head and neck malignancies. *Head Neck.* 2006;28:888–895.
56. Chen J, Pappas J, Moeller H, Rankin J, Sharma P. Treatment of oropharyngeal squamous cell carcinoma with external beam radiation combined with interstitial brachytherapy. *Head Neck.* 2007;29:362–369.
57. Narayana A, Cohen G, Zier M, et al. High-dose-rate interstitial brachytherapy in recurrent and previously irradiated head and neck-cancers—preliminary results. *Brachytherapy.* 2007;6:157–163.
58. Seiwert T, Salama J, Vokes E. The chemoradiation paradigm-head and neck cancer. *Natl Clin Pract Oncol.* 2007;4:156–171. http://www.medscape.com/viewarticle/553553. Accessed February 26, 2010.
59. Brizel D, Esclamado R. Concurrent chemoradiotherapy for locally advanced, nonmetastatic, squamous carcinoma of the head and neck: consensus, controversy, and conundrum. *J Clin Oncol.* 2006;24: 2612–2617.
60. Argiris A. Update on chemoradiotherapy for head and neck cancer. *Curr Opin Oncol.* 2002;14:323–329.
61. Doweck I, Robbins K, Viera F. Analysis of risk factors predictive of distant failure after targeted chemoradiation for advanced head and neck cancer. *Arch Otolaryngol Head Neck Surg.* 2001;127:1315–1318.
62. Bernier J, Vrielind C. Docetaxel in the management of patients with head and neck squamous cell carcinoma. *Expert Rev Anticancer Ther.* 2008;8:1023–1032.
63. Adelstein D, Saxton J, Rybicki L, et al. Multiagent concurrent chemoradiotherapy for locoregionally advanced squamous cell head and neck cancer: mature results from a single institution. *J Clin Oncol.* 2006; 24:1064–1071.
64. Kim J, Sohn S, Kim D, et al. Phase II study of concurrent chemoradiotherapy with capecitabine and cisplatin in patients with locally advanced squamous cell carcinoma of the head and neck. *Br J Cancer.* 2005;93:1117–1121.
65. Budach W, Hehr T, Budach V, Belka C, Dietz K. A meta-analysis of hyperfractionated and accelerated radiotherapy and combined chemotherapy and radiotherapy regimens in unresected locally advanced squamous cell carcinoma of the head and neck. *BMC Cancer.* 2006;31: 6–28.
66. Tishler R, Posner M, Norris C, et al. Concurrent weekly docetaxel and concomitant boost radiation therapy in the treatment of locally advanced squamous cell cancer of the head and neck. *Int J Radiat Oncol Biol Phys.* 2006;65:1036–1044.
67. Bernier J, Schenider D. Cetuximab combined with radiotherapy: an alternative to chemoradiotherapy for patients with locally advanced squamous cell carcinomas of the head and neck? *Eur J Cancer.* 2007;43:35–45.
68. Karmar S, Esassolak M, Yalman D, et al. Mature results of neoadjuvant chemotherapy followed by radiotherapy in nasopharyngeal cancer: is it really old fashioned? *Med Oncol.* 2008;25:93–99.
69. Salama J, Vokes E, Chmura S, et al. Long-term outcome of concurrent chemotherapy and reirradiation for recurrent and second primary head-and-neck squamous cell carcinoma. *Int J Radiat Oncol Biol Phys.* 2006;64:382–391.
70. Langer C, Harris J, Horwitz E, et al. Phase II study of low-dose paclitaxel and cisplatin in combination with split-course concomitant twice-daily reirradiation in recurrent squamous cell carcinoma of the head and neck: results of Radiation Therapy Oncology Group Protocol 9911. *J Clin Oncol.* 2007;25:4800–4805.
71. Forastiere A. Chemotherapy in the treatment of locally advanced head and neck cancer. *J Surg Oncol.* 2008;97:701–707.
72. Awada A, Ismael G. The challenging integration of platinum compounds, taxanes, and molecular-targeted therapies in the multidisciplinary treatment of squamous cell carcinoma of the head and neck. *Curr Opin Oncol.* 2007;19:177–179.
73. Vermorken J, Remenar E, vanHerpen C, et al. Cisplatin, fluorouracil and docetaxel in unresectable head and neck cancer. *N Engl J Med.* 2007;357:1695–1704.
74. Posner M, Hershock D, Blajman C, et al. Cisplatin and fluorouracil alone or with docetaxel in head and neck cancer. *N Engl J Med.* 2007;357:1705–1715.
75. Adelstein D, Leblanc M. Does induction chemotherapy have a role in the management of locoregionally advanced squamous cell head and neck cancer? *J Clin Oncol.* 2006;24:2624–2628.
76. Haddad R, Tishler R, Wirth L, et al. Rate of pathologic complete responses to docetaxel, cisplatin and fluorouracil induction chemotherapy in patients with squamous cell carcinoma of the head and neck. *Arch Otolaryngol Head Neck Surg.* 2006;132:678–681.
77. Bentzen J, Hansen H. Phase II analysis of paclitaxel and capecitabine in the treatment of recurrent or disseminated squamous cell carcinoma of the head and neck region. *Head Neck.* 2007;29:47–51.
78. Worden F, Moon J, Samlowski W, et al. A phase II evaluation of a 3-hour infusion of paclitaxel, cisplatin and 5-fluorouracil in patients with

advanced or recurrent squamous cell carcinoma of the head and neck: Southwest Oncology Group study 0007. *Cancer.* 2006;107:319–327.
80. Panikkar R, Astsaturov I, Langer C. The emerging role of cetuximab in head and neck cancer: a 2007 perspective. *Cancer Invest.* 2008;26:96–103.
81. Langer C. Targeted therapy in head and neck cancer: state of the art 2007 and review of clinical applications. *Cancer.* 2008;112:2635–2645.
82. Blick S, Scott L. Cetuximab: a review of its use in squamous cell carcinoma of the head and neck and metastatic colorectal cancer. *Drugs.* 2007;67:2585–2607.
84. Hitt R, Echarri MJ. Molecular biology in head and neck cancer. *Clin Transl Oncol.* 2006;8:776–779.
85. Bossi P, Locati L, Licitra L. Biological agents in head and neck cancer. MedScape. http://www.medscape.com/viewarticle/567643. Published 2007. Accessed November 1, 2009.
86. Harari P. Stepwise progress in epidermal growth factor receptor/radiation studies for head and neck cancer. *Int J Radiat Oncol Biol Phys.* 2007;69(suppl 2):S25–S27.
87. Curran D, Giralt J, Harari P, et al. Quality of life in head and neck cancer patients after treatment with high-dose radiotherapy alone or in combination with cetuximab. *J Clin Oncol.* 2007;25:2191–2197.
88. Ahmed S, Cohen E. Treatment of squamous cell carcinoma of the head and neck in the metastatic and refractory settings: advances in chemotherapy and the emergence of small molecule epidermal growth factor receptor kinase inhibitors. *Curr Cancer Drug Targets.* 2007;7:666–673.
89. Le Tourneau C, Siu L. Molecular-targeted therapies in the treatment of squamous cell carcinomas of the head and neck. *Curr Opin Oncol.* 2008;20:256–263.
90. Burtness B. The role of cetuximab in the treatment of squamous cell cancer of the head and neck. *Exp Opin Biol Ther.* 2005;5:1085–1093.
91. Fish-Steagall A, Searcy P, Sipples R. Clinical experience with anti-EGFR therapy. *Semin Oncol Nurs.* 2006;22(suppl 1):10–19.
92. Mehra R, Cohen R, Harari P. EGFT inhibitors for the treatment of squamous cell carcinoma of the head and neck. *Curr Oncol Rep.* 2008;10:176–184.
93. Reuter C, Morgan M, Edkardt A. Targeting EGF-receptor-signalling in squamous cell carcinomas of the head and neck. *Br J Cancer.* 2007;96:408–416.
94. Riesterer O, Milas L, Ang K. Combining molecular therapeutics with radiotherapy for head and neck cancer. *J Surg Oncol.* 2008;97:708–711.
95. Chai R, Grandis J. Advances in molecular diagnostics and therapeutics in head and neck cancer. *Curr Treat Options Oncol.* 2006;7:3–11.
96. Hass H, Schmidt A, Nehls O, Kaiser S. DNA ploidy, proliferative capacity and intratumoral heterogeneity in primary and recurrent head and neck squamous cell carcinomas. (HNSCC)—potential implications for clinical management and treatment decisions. *Oral Oncol.* 2008;44:78–85.
97. Giri U, Ashorn C, Ramdas L, et al. Molecular signatures associated with clinical outcome in patients with high-risk head-and-neck squamous cell carcinoma treated by surgery and radiation. *Int J Radiat Oncol Biol Phys.* 2006;64:670–677.
98. Chung C, Levy S, Yarbrough W. Clinical applications of genomics in head and neck cancer. *Head Neck.* 2006;28:360–368.
99. Devaraj K, Gillison ML, Wu T. Development of HPV vaccines for HPV-associated head and neck squamous cell carcinoma. *Crit Rev Oral Biol Med.* 2003;14:345–362.
100. Psyri A, DiMaio D. Human papillomavirus in cervical and head-and-neck cancer. *Natl Clin Pract Oncol.* 2008;5:24–31.
101. Keum K, Chung E, Koom W, et al. Predictive value of p53 expression for occult neck metastases in patients with clinically node-negative oral tongue cancer. *Otolaryngol Head Neck Surg.* 2006;135:858–864.
102. Vattemi E, Claudio P. Adenoviral gene therapy in head and neck cancer. *Drug News Perspect.* 2006;19:329–337.
103. Specialized Programs of Research Excellence (SPOREs). Head and neck SPOREs. http://spores.nci.nih.gov/current/hn/hn.html. Published 2008. Accessed November 1, 2009.
104. University of Michigan Health System (UMHS). SPORE in head and neck cancer. http://www2.med.umich.edu/cancer/hnspore/index.cfm. Published 2007. Accessed November 1, 2009.
105. Hopkins Medical Center. Excellence in head and neck cancer research: the Johns Hopkins Head and Neck Cancer SPORE. http://www.hopkinskimmelcancercenter.org/kpr/spore_headandneck.cfm. Published 2007. Accessed November 1, 2009.
106. European Society for Medical Oncology (ESMO). Squamous cell carcinoma of the head and neck: ESMO clinical recommendations for diagnosis, treatment and follow-up. *Ann Oncol.* 2007;18(supp 2): ii65–ii66.
107. Katz T, Mendenhall W, Morris C, et al. Malignant tumors of the nasal cavity and paranasal sinuses. *Head Neck.* 2002;24:821–829.
108. National Cancer Institute (NCI). Lip and oral cavity cancer treatment (PDQ). http://www.cancer.gov/cancertopics/pdq/treatment/lip-and-oral-cavity/healthprofessional. Published 2008. Accessed November 1, 2009.
109. National Cancer Institute (NCI). Oropharyngeal cancer treatment (PDQ). http://www.cancer.gov/cancertopics/pdq/treatment/oropharyngeal/healthprofessional. Published 2008. Accessed November 1, 2009.
110. Harrison L, Ferlito A, Shaha A, et al. Current philosophy on the management of cancer of the base of the tongue. *Oral Oncol.* 2003;39: 101–105.
111. Flint P. Minimally invasive techniques for management of early glottic cancer. *Otolaryngol Clin North Am.* 2002;35:vi-vii, 1055–1066.
112. National Cancer Institute (NCI). Laryngeal cancer treatment (PDQ). http://www.cancer.gov/cancertopics/pdq/treatment/laryngeal/healthprofessional. Published 2008. Accessed November 1, 2009.
113. Murphy B, Gilbert J, Cmelak A, Ridner S. Symptom control issues and supportive care of patients with head and neck cancer. *Clin Adv Hematol Oncol.* 2007;5:807–822.
114. Rosenthal D, Mendoza T, Chambers M, et al. Measuring head and neck cancer symptom burned; the development and validation of the M.D. Anderson symptom inventory, head and neck module. *Head Neck.* 2007a;29:923–931.
115. Jones H, Hershock D, Machtay M, et al. Preliminary investigation of symptom distress in head and neck patient population: validation of a measurement instrument. *Am J Clin Oncol.* 2006;29:158–162.
116. Cox L, Davis M. Swallowing dysfunction in patients with head and neck cancer receiving radiation therapy: using performance improvement to enhance practice. *Oncol Nurs Forum.* 2008;35:504. [abstract 2747]
117. Roe J, Leslie P, Drinnan M. Orophayngeal dysphagia: the experience of patients with non-head and neck cancers receiving specialist palliative care. *Palliat Med.* 2007;21:567–574.
118. Nguyen N, Smith J, Sallah S. Evaluation and management of swallowing dysfunction following chemoradiation for head and neck cancer. *Curr Opin Otolaryngol Head Neck Surg.* 2007;15:130–133.
119. Eisbruch A, Levendag P, Feng F, et al. Can IMRT or brachytherapy reduce dysphagia associated with chemoradiotherapy of head and neck cancer? The Michigan and Rotterdam experiences. *Int J Radiat Oncol Biol Phys.* 2007;69(suppl 2):S40-S42.
120. Nguyen N, Moltz C, Frank C, et al. Long-term aspiration following treatment for head and neck cancer. *Oncology.* 2007;74:25–30.
121. Nguyen N, Moltz C, Frank C, et al. Impact of swallowing therapy on aspiration rate following treatment for locally advanced head and neck cancer. *Oral Oncol.* 2007;43:352–357.
122. Perry A, Shaw M, Cotton S. An evaluation of functional outcomes (speech, swallowing) in patients attending speech pathology after head and neck cancer treatments: results and analysis at 12 months post intervention. *J Laryngol Otol.* 2003;117:368–381.
123. National Cancer Institute (NCI). What you need to know about cancer of the larynx. NIH Publication No. 02–1568. http://www.nci.nih.gov/cancerinfo/wyntk/larynx. Published 2003. Accessed November 1, 2009.

124. Eksteen E, Rieger J, Nesbit M, et al. Comparison of voice characteristics following three different methods of treatment for laryngeal cancer. *J Otolaryngol.* 2003;32:250–253.
125. Koch W. Total laryngectomy with tracheoesophageal conduit. *Otolaryngol Clin North Am.* 2002;35:1081–1096.
126. Behrman A, Abramson A, Myssiorek D. A comparison of radiation-induced and presbylaryngeal dysphonia. *Otolaryngol Head Neck Surg.* 2001;125:193–200.
127. Eilers J, Million R. Prevention and management of oral mucositis in patients with cancer. *Semin Oncol Nurs.* 2007;23:201–212.
128. Dodd M. The pathogenesis and characterization of oral mucositis associated with cancer therapy. *Oncol Nurs Forum.* 2007;31(suppl):5–11.
129. Cawley M, Benson L. Current trends in managing oral mucositis. *Clin J Oncol Nurs.* 2005;9:584–592.
130. Davison D. Oral mucositis. *Clin J Oncol Nurs.* 2006;10:283–284.
131. Armstrong J, McCaffrey R. The effects of mucositis on quality of life in patients with head and neck cancer. *Clin J Oncol Nurs.* 2006;10:53–56.
132. Rosenthal D. Consequences of mucositis-induced treatment breaks and dose reductions on head and neck cancer treatment outcomes. *J Support Oncol.* 2007;5(suppl 4):23–31.
133. Radiation Therapy Oncology Group (RTOG). Acute Radiation Morbidity Scoring Criteria. http://www.rtog.org/members/toxicity/acute.html. Published 1995. Accessed November 1, 2009.
134. Harris D, Eilers J, Harriman A, Cashavelly B, Maxwell C. Putting evidence into practice: evidence-based interventions for the management of oral mucositis. *Clin J Oncol Nurs.* 2008;12:141–152.
135. Eilers J. Nursing interventions and supportive care for the prevention and treatment of oral mucositis associated with cancer treatment. *Oncol Nurs Forum.* 2007;31(suppl 4):13–23.
136. Dirix P, Nuyts S, Vanden Bogaert W. Radiation-induced xerostomia in patients with head and neck cancer: a literature review. *Cancer.* 2006;107:2525–2534.
137. Silverman S. Diagnosis and management of oral mucositis. *J Support Oncol.* 2007;5(suppl 1):13–21.
138. Worthington H, Clarkson J, Eden O. Interventions for treating oral mucositis for patients with cancer receiving treatment (Cochrane Review). In: *The Cochrane Library.* Issue 1. Chichester, UK: John Wiley and Sons; 2004.
139. Sonis ST. Mucositis: the impact, biology and therapeutic opportunities of oral mucositis. *Oral Oncol.* 2009; 45: 1015–1020.
140. Jaroneski L. The importance of assessment rating scales for chemotherapy-induced oral mucositis. *Oncol Nurs Forum.* 2006;33:1085–1093.
141. Bruce S. Radiation-induced xerostomia: how dry is your patient? *Clin J Oncol Nurs.* 2004;8:61–67.
142. Nyarady A, Nemeth A, Ban A, et al. A randomized study to assess the effectiveness of orally administered pilocarpine during and after radiotherapy of head and neck cancer. *Anticancer Res.* 2006;26:1557–1562.
143. Scarantino C, LeVeque F, Swann R, et al. Effect of pilocarpine during radiation therapy: results of RTOG 98–09, a phase III randomized study in head and neck cancer patients. *J Support Oncol.* 2006;4:252–258.
144. Wasserman T, Brizel D, Henke M, et al. Influence of intravenous amifostine on xerostomia, tumor control and survival after radiotherapy for head and neck cancer: 2 year follow-up of a prospective, randomized phase III trial. *Int J Radiat Oncol Biol Phys.* 2005;63:985–990.
145. Maes A, Huygh I, Weltens C, et al. De Gustibus: time scale of loss and recovery of tastes caused by radiotherapy. *Radiother Oncol.* 2002;63:195–201.
146. Koga D, Salajoli J, Alves F. Dental extractions and radiotherapy in head and neck oncology: review of the literature. *Oral Dis.* 2008;14:40–44.
147. Ben-David M, Diamante M, Radawski J, et al. Lack of osteoradionecrosis of the mandible after intensity-modulated radiotherapy for head and neck cancer: likely contributions of both dental care and improved dose distributions. *Int J Radiat Oncol Biol Phys.* 2007;68:396–402.
148. Haddad R. Current and future directions in the treatment of squamous cell carcinoma of the head and neck: multidisciplinary symposium on head and neck cancer. *Exp Opin Ther Targets.* 2006;10:333–336.
149. Nellcor Puritan Bennett. *Tracheostomy Tube: Adult Home Care Guide.* Boulder, CO: Covidien-Puritan Bennett; 2004.
150. Cady J. Nutritional support during radiotherapy for head and neck cancer: the role of prophylactic feeding tube placement. *Clin J Oncol Nurs.* 2007;11:1092–1095.
151. Wiggenraad R, Flierman L, Goossens A, et al. Prophylactic gastrostomy placement and early tube feeding may limit loss of weight during chemoradiotherapy for advanced head and neck cancer: a preliminary study. *Clin Otolaryngol.* 2007;32:384–390.
152. Nguyen P, North D, Smith H, et al. Safety and effectiveness of prophylactic gastrostomy tubes for head and neck cancer patients undergoing chemoradiation. *Surg Oncol.* 2006;15:199–203.
153. Jereczek-Fossa B, Santoro L, Alterio D, et al. Fatigue during head and neck radiotherapy: prospective study on 117 consecutive patients. *Int J Radiat Oncol Biol Phys.* 2007;68:403–415.
154. Hickok J, Roscoe J, Morrow G, et al. Frequency, severity, clinical course, and correlates of fatigue in 372 patients during 5 weeks of radiotherapy for cancer. *Cancer.* 2005;104:1772–1778.
155. Semple C, Sullivan K, Dunwoody L, Kernohan G. Psychosocial interventions for patients with head and neck cancer. *Cancer Nurs.* 2004;27:434–441.
156. Cherith J, Sullivan K, Dunwoody L, et al. Psychosocial interventions for patients with head and neck cancer. *Cancer Nurs.* 2004;27:434–441.
157. Coyne J, Pajak T, Harris J, et al. Emotional well-being does not predict survival in head and neck cancer patients: a Radiation Therapy Oncology Group study. *Cancer.* 2007;110:2568–2575.
158. Kelly C, Paleri V, Downs C, et al. Deterioration in quality of life and depressive symptoms during radiation therapy for head and neck cancer. *Otolaryngol Head Neck Surg.* 2007;136:108–111.
159. Haisfield-Wolfe M, McGuire D, Soeken K, et al. Prevalence rates of depression in studies of head and neck cancer patients across the treatment trajectory: How do they inform practice? *Oncol Nurs Forum.* 2008;35:512. [abstract 2799]
160. Konski A, Pajak T, Movsas B, et al. Disadvantage of men living alone participating in Radiation Therapy Oncology Group head and neck trials. *J Clin Oncol.* 2006;24:4177–4183.
161. Cady J. Laryngectomy: beyond loss of voice—caring for the patient as a whole. *Clin J Oncol Nurs.* 2002;6:347–351.
162. Holloway R, Hellewell J, Marbella A. et al. Psychosocial effects in long-term head and neck cancer survivors. *Head Neck.* 2005;27:281–288.
163. Rose-Ped AL, Bellm L, Epstein J, et al. Complications of radiation therapy for head and neck cancers. *Cancer Nurs.* 2002;6:461–467.
164. Talmi Y. Quality of life issues in cancer of the oral cavity. *J Laryngol Otol.* 2002;116:785–790. [Review]
165. Ronis D, Duffy S, Fowler K, et al. Changes in quality of life over 1 year in patients with head and neck cancer. *Arch Otolaryngol Head Neck Surg.* 2008;134:241–248.
166. Petruson K, Silander E, Hammerlid E. Effects of psychosocial intervention on quality of life in patients with head and neck cancer. *Head Neck.* 2003;25:576–584.
167. Siddiqui R, Pajak T, Watkins-Bruner D, et al. Pretreatment quality of life predicts for locoregional control in head and neck cancer patients: a radiation therapy oncology group analysis. *Int J Radiat Oncol Biol Phys.* 2008;70:353–360.
168. Gellrich N, Schimming R, Schramm A, et al. Pain, function, and psychologic outcome before, during, and after intraoral tumor resection. *J Oral Maxillofac Surg.* 2002;60:772–777.
169. Laverick S, Lowe D, Brown J, et al. The impact of neck dissection on health-related quality of life. *Arch Otolaryngol Head Neck Surg.* 2004;130:149–154.

170. de Leeuw J, de Graeff A, Ros W, et al. Prediction of depression 6 months to 3 years after treatment of head and neck cancer. *Head Neck.* 2001;23:892–898.
171. Tschudi D, Stoeckli S, Schmid S. Quality of life after different treatment modalities for carcinoma of the oropharynx. *Laryngoscope.* 2003;113:1949–1954.
172. Morton R, Izzard M. Quality-of-life outcomes in head and neck cancer patients. *World J Surg.* 2003;27:884–889.
173. Mignogna M, Fedele S, Lo Russo L, et al. Costs and effectiveness in the care of patients with oral and pharyngeal cancer: analysis of a paradox. *Eur J Cancer Prev.* 2002;11:205–208.
174. Specht L. Oral complications in the head and neck radiation patient. Introduction and scope of the problem. *Support Care Cancer.* 2002;10:36–39.
175. Gibson M, Forastiere A. Multidisciplinary approaches in the management of advanced head and neck tumors: state of the art. *Curr Opin Oncol.* 2004;16:220–224.
176. Ouwens M, Marres H, Hermens R, et al. Quality of integrated care for patients with head and neck cancer: development and measurement of clinical indicators. *Head Neck.* 2007;29:378–386.
177. Wells M, Donnan P, Sharp L, Ackland C, Fletcher J, Dewar J. A study to evaluate nurse-led on-treatment review for patients undergoing radiotherapy for head and neck cancer. *J Clin Nurs.* 2008;17:1428–1439.
178. Larsson M, Hedelin B, Athlin E. A supportive nursing care clinic: conceptions of patients with head and neck cancer. *Eur J Oncol Nurs.* 2007;11:49–59.
179. Duffy E. Development of a multidisciplinary patient care team: a collaborative approach to optimize care for patients with head and neck cancer. [Abstract] *Oncol Nurs Forum.* 2008;35:2955.
180. Schlech L. Coaching for success: a multidisciplinary approach to preparing a patient for head and neck surgery. Oncology Nursing Society 32nd Annual Congress Podium and Poster Abstracts. *Oncol Nurs Forum.* 2007;34:2060.
181. Wiederholt P, Connor N, Hartig G, Harari P. Bridging gaps in multidisciplinary head and neck cancer care: nursing coordination and case management. *Int J Radiat Oncol Biol Phys.* 2007;69(suppl 2):S88–S91.
182. Cleary J. Integrating palliative care into head and neck oncology. *Int J Radiat Oncol Biol Phys.* 2007;69(suppl 2):S83-S85.
183. Mendenall W, Mancuso A, Hinerman R, et al. Multidisciplinary management of laryngeal carcinoma. *Int J Radiat Oncol Biol Phys.* 2007;69(suppl 2):S12-S14.
184. Funk G, Gosselin-Acomb T. Improving care of the head and neck cancer patient receiving combination chemotherapy and radiation therapy. [Abstract] *Oncol Nurs Forum.* 2006;33:104.

CHAPTER

57

Sandra E. Kurtin, RN, MS, AOCN®, ANP-C

# Leukemia and Myelodysplastic Syndromes

## INTRODUCTION

The leukemias represent a group of heterogeneous clonal myeloid and lymphoid malignancies that originate in the bone marrow due to a stem cell defect with variable clinical presentations, pathological characteristics, prognosis and recommended treatment. The diseases arise from either B or T lymphocytes or myeloid progenitor cells at different stages of maturation. Each is categorized based on the lineage (lymphoid or myeloid), the specific stage of maturation, and the disease trajectory (chronic vs acute). Robust scientific discovery over the last decade has improved selection of therapies based on specific disease attributes, prognostic variables, and individual patient characteristics. Further refinement of morphological, immunophenotypic, cytogenetic, and molecular analysis has established a separate classification system for the myelodysplastic syndromes (MDS), previously included as a myeloid leukemia and now categorized as a distinct disease with specific diagnostic, prognostic, and treatment guidelines.

This chapter will provide an overview of the epidemiology, etiology, pathobiology, classification, clinical presentation, risk stratification, treatment and nursing management of patients with acute leukemia, chronic leukemia, or MDS, including: acute myeloid leukemia (AML), chronic myeloid leukemia (CML), MDS, acute lymphocytic leukemia (ALL), and chronic lymphocytic leukemia (CLL). Most of these diseases are considered incurable, but most are highly treatable. Understanding the unique attributes of each disease, available treatment options, and strategies for clinical management of the patient using a life-span approach is critical to achieving optimal outcomes for the patient.

## EPIDEMIOLOGY

Worldwide there were 330,963 new cases of leukemia with 279,658 deaths reported in 2007.[1] These hematological diseases are not the most common malignancies and no 1 subtype exceeded an incidence rate of 20,000 in the US in 2009. Collectively, the incidence of leukemia in 2009 in the US for both sexes was 44,790 new cases, with CLL being the most common (15,490) and CML being the least common (5050)[2] (Table 57-1[3-4]). All subtypes were found to be slightly more common in men, and most were diagnosed 10 times more frequently in adults than children. The median age at diagnosis varies, with peak incidence in patients over the age of 60 with the exception of ALL, which is more common in children with only 16.2% of cases diagnosed over the age of 45.[3]

Epidemiologic data specific to MDS has only been collected in the US since 2001,[4] thus comparative trends are not available. Prior to 1973, only 143 cases of MDS were reported. Today, there are 10,000 to 15,000 new cases of MDS annually in the US and the prevalence is estimated to be 35,000 to 55,000 cases based on typical life expectancy. There is an increase in the incidence of MDS with advancing age, highest at ages 80 to 84, then decreasing dramatically at age 85.

Clinical advances in the treatment of leukemia and available supportive care measures have improved survival rates for these diseases. Death rates have decreased by approximately 0.8% per year since 1995.[5]. The mortality rate for CML in particular has declined significantly due to characterization of the *BCR-ABL* fusion gene and development of therapies that target this specific molecular abnormality. The annual mortality rate for CML has been reduced from 15% to 20% to 2% and the median survival is expected to exceed 15 to 20 years based on the current rates.[5]

## ETIOLOGY

Many potential risk factors have been identified for each disease, including antecedent hematological disorders (AHD), genetic predisposition, prior treatment for malignancy, chemical exposures, ionizing radiation, and concomitant autoimmune diseases. In most cases no clear etiology is identified, however, there are distinct differences in suspected risk factors for each disorder. There are no known hereditary, familial, geographic, ethnic, infectious, or economic associations identified with the risk of developing CML, therefore CML does not appear to be preventable.[6] CLL has not been associated with ionizing radiation, chemical exposure, viruses, or prior chemotherapy, but does appear to have some familial trends in 5% to 10% of patients, suggesting an underlying genetic predisposition.[7] Older age is a predisposing risk factor for MDS and is thought to be a result of hematopoietic senescence.[8] Secondary MDS may develop after exposure to high doses of radiation, chemotherapy, or industrial toxins such as benzene. Benzene is the best studied and most widely used potentially leukemogenic agent. Inherited genetic predisposition for developing MDS and congenital abnormalities are rare. Chemotherapeutic agents, such as alkylating agents and topoisomerase II inhibitors, have been reported to increase the incidence of AML.[9] Persons exposed to embalming fluids, ethylene oxides, and herbicides also appear to be at increased risk. Tobacco use has been associated with an increased risk of developing AML (particularly of French American British [FAB] subtype M2), especially in those persons aged 60 to 75.[10]

In both ALL and AML specific genetic abnormalities thought to have underlying chromosomal fragility have been associated with development of disease [11,12] Patients with chromosomal abnormalities including Kleinfelter's syndrome (XXY), Fanconi anemia, trisomy 21 (Down syndrome), Bloom syndrome, and ataxia telangiectasia have a higher risk of developing ALL. Similarly, AML has been associated with these same disorders as well as

**TABLE 57-1**

**Recent Epidemiological Trends for Leukemia in the US**

| Disease | New Cases (US, 2009) | Deaths (US, 2009) | Median Age at Diagnosis (years) | 5-Year Relative Survival Rates 1996–2004 (%)[a] |
|---|---|---|---|---|
| All leukemias | 44,790[b] | 21,870 | | 50 |
| Acute myelogenous leukemia | 12,810 | 9000 | 67 | 21.9 |
| Chronic myelogenous leukemia | 5050 | 470 | 66 | 50.2 |
| Acute lymphocytic leukemia | 5760 | 1400 | 13 | 64.7 |
| Chronic lymphocytic leukemia | 15,490 | 4390 | 72 | 75.9 |
| Myelodysplastic syndrome | 9730 | NA | 70 | 45 (3 year survival rate) |

[a]Excludes myelodysplastic syndrome.
[b]Incidence rate and 3-year survival rates based on data obtained from 2001–2004.
*Source*: Data from SEER[3]; and Rollison et al.[4]

Wiskott-Aldrich syndrome, Kostmann syndrome, and Patau (trisomy of chromosome 13).[13] Given the relatively small numbers of patients diagnosed with each disease, further characterization of specific genetic risk factors has been limited. Similar to other lymphoid malignancies, infectious etiologies have been described as possible predisposing factors for the development of ALL including Epstein-Barr virus (EBV), human immunodeficiency virus (HIV), and human T-cell lymphotrophic virus type 1 (HTLV1).[12]

Perhaps the greatest challenge is the clear association between chemical exposure and the development of AML and MDS. Alkylating agents, epipodophyllotoxins, topoisomerase II inhibitors, anthracyclines, mitoxantrone, and radiotherapy have all been associated with treatment-related AML and MDS.[13] Specific agents are associated with either early or late onset of secondary AML and MDS. The peak onset of treatment related AML or MDS is 5 to 10 years after therapy. Given the incurable nature of these disorders, particular attention must be placed on a life span approach to therapy with attention to potential secondary effects and quality of life.

## PREVENTION, SCREENING, AND EARLY DETECTION

Prevention of leukemia and MDS is difficult outside of avoidance of known chemical and environmental exposures. Radiation safety programs, guidelines set by the Occupational Safety and Health Administration (OSHA), and regulation of pesticide use may provide some protection from possible exposures. Smoking cessation programs may also provide benefit as there is growing evidence that tobacco exposure is associated with bone marrow disorders.[10] As the ability to control a variety of cancers over an extended period using continuous and/or intermittent therapies has grown, there has also been an increase in the number of treatment-related bone marrow disorders including AML and MDS. Long-term follow up of patients using epidemiological approaches will be necessary to better characterize any common agents, dosing parameters, and time of onset for these secondary diseases.

There are no proven screening or early detection programs to date. These diseases are often diagnosed incidentally on a general physical exam or emergency room visit. Increasing provider awareness of the presenting symptoms may facilitate diagnosis, which is often critical to initiating therapy early and achieving optimal clinical outcomes. Encouraging regular health maintenance and screening visits will provide the best opportunity for early detection of subtle changes in blood work and physical findings such as cytopenias, adenopathy, or organomegaly. This will also provide useful analysis of trends over time, which is particularly useful in estimating the onset of disease and characterizing the disease trajectory.

## PATHOBIOLOGY

The leukemias represent a group of heterogeneous clonal myeloid and lymphoid malignancies that originate in the bone marrow due to a stem cell defect. The underlying pathobiology for each disease includes abnormalities in the malignant clone itself (intrinsic abnormalities) and in the tumor microenvironment (extrinsic abnormalities). With the exception of CML where there is a distinct clonal abnormality called the Abelson-breakpoint cluster region or *BCR-ABL* fusion gene, much of the pathobiology of these diseases has yet to be fully characterized. There are several morphological, immunophenotypic, cytogenetic, molecular, and physiological attributes that are known to be associated with each disease. Characterization of these attributes is necessary for classification, staging, and risk stratification. This in turn is used to guide treatment decisions and to estimate prognosis.

Diagnosis of each of these hematological disorders is guided by careful analysis of tissue specimens, most often a bone marrow biopsy and aspirate and/or lymphoid specimens (lymph nodes, spleen, or other extramedullary sites of disease). These specimens allow hematopathologists to apply a series of diagnostic criteria that differentiate the disease as being either myeloid or lymphoid in origin and then within each cell line indicate a specific disease entity. Understanding the key principles of pathobiology including intrinsic and extrinsic abnormalities of each disease will assist the oncology nurse in understanding the variability in clinical presentation, diagnostic criteria, treatment selection, evaluation of response, and estimation of prognosis for each disease.

There are many similarities in the pathobiology of leukemia and MDS but there are key differences that define each disease, and in some cases determine specific treatment selection. Leukemia and MDS are thought to originate as a result of complex interactions between malignant progenitor cells (malignant clone), the bone marrow stroma and microenvironment. There are both intrinsic (within the malignant clone itself) and extrinsic factors (bone marrow microenvironment and stroma) thought to play a role in the pathogenesis of each disease.[14] Intrinsic factors include cytogenetic abnormalities, epigenetic DNA changes and gene mutations or disordered gene expression. Cytogenetic abnormalities are common in hematological malignancies and have long been identified as key elements of the diagnostic process for AML and CML.[15–17] More recently, cytogenetic abnormalities have been elucidated as key diagnostic and prognostic elements of the lymphoid leukemias and MDS. Chromosomes can be considered the "blueprint" for production of each cell line. Cytogenetic abnormalities are in effect, a faulty instruction manual for the production of cells. More complex defects imply a decreased probability of normal cell production. Cytogenetic abnormalities are now considered one of the most critical independent risk factors for prognosis in the hematological malignancies.[18] There are rare inherited cytogenetic predispositions to some of these diseases, however in most cases chromosomal abnormalities are a result of acquired insults to the clone. Hematopoietic senescence as a result of aging and mutagenic and genotoxic stresses, including prior chemotherapy or radiation exposure, environmental and occupational exposures to solvents, and tobacco abuse, have been associated with the development of cytogenetic abnormalities.[18]

Epigenetic DNA changes, unlike genetic changes such as mutations or deletions, which are irreversible (with the exception of treatment with an allogeneic stem cell transplant); represent potentially reversible modifications to DNA and chromatin. The interactions between DNA and chromatin contribute to the regulation of transcription, chromosome stability, DNA repair and replication independent of the genetic code.[19] The best known epigenetic marker is DNA methylation. DNA methylation plays critical roles in the control of gene expression and the architecture of the nucleus of the cell. Patients with AML and MDS have CpG islands that are often hypermethylated, resulting in silencing of critical regulatory or suppressor functions (signal transduction pathways) necessary for normal hematopoiesis (differentiation and apoptosis).[20] Of particular interest is the role of DNA hypermethylation in leukemogenesis. Aberrant DNA methylation is suggested as a primary mechanism for progression of MDS to AML.[21] Drugs that inhibit DNA methylation promote expression of previously silenced genes. Gene expression may also be blocked by changes in chromatin structure caused by histone deacetylation. Chromatin is comprised of DNA, RNA, and proteins that collectively make up chromosomes. Histone deacetylase inhibitors remodel the chromatin structure to enable transcription of previously blocked genes. Because the process of hypomethylation can occur only when cells are actively dividing, treatment must be administered for an extended period of time before results may be achieved and prolonged treatment may be necessary because gene expression typically reverses when treatment ceases.[22]

More recent investigations have identified key molecular aberrations that are associated with disease development, prognosis, and in some cases specific targets for therapy. Application of these principles to specific disease types illustrates the evolving science of the hematological malignancies. The most notable molecular fusion gene is *BCR-ABL*, which is found in all patients with CML. The *BCR-ABL* fusion gene represents a reciprocal translocation of the distal material of chromosome 22 (Ph) and chromosome 9 at specific break points (t (9;22)(q34;q11). Fusion of the Abelson (*ABL*) proto-oncogene from chromosome 9 to the breakpoint cluster region (*BCR*) of chromosome 22 results in the *BCR-ABL* fusion gene. This is a tyrosine kinase protein (oncoprotein) thought to trigger intracellular signal transduction pathways resulting in disordered myelopoiesis with accelerated cell growth, decreased apoptosis, and weakening of cellular adhesion. [23] These changes result in the characteristic clinical findings of leukocytosis, thrombocytosis, splenomegaly, and anemia seen in CML. They are also thought to contribute to the development of the more aggressive blast phase of the disease. *BCR-ABL* is present in approximately 30% of adult ALL cases and is associated with a poor prognosis.[24] The administration of tyrosine kinase inhibitors (TKI) targeting the *BCR-ABL* fusion gene, such as imatinib, dasatinib, and nilotinib, has provided significant improvement in the treatment of these disorders, in particular CML.

Additional molecular attributes have been identified in the other hematological malignancies. Acute promyelocytic leukemia (APL) is characterized by the balanced reciprocal translocation between chromosome 15 and 17 (t15;17) that results in the fusion of the promeylocytic gene (*PML*) and the retinoic acid receptor α (*RAR*α) resulting in the *PML-RAR*α oncogene. This fusion gene is associated with transcriptional repression and inhibition of differentiation of promyelocytic blasts. The introduction of all-trans retinoic acid (ATRA) and arsenic trioxide (ATO) that reverse the transcriptional repression and allow normal differentiation of promyelocytes through chromatin modifying proteins has reduced the morbidity associated with APL due to bleeding diatheses and hyperleukocytosis.[18] APL is now considered the most curable acute leukemia.[25]

Another important molecular abnormality occurs in the FMS-like tyrosine kinase (TK) 3 or *Flt-3*, which is a member of class 3 TK receptors. Other members of this class are c-Kit, platelet-derived growth factor receptor (PDGFR), and c-Fms. Flt-3 protein is expressed in early hematopoietic progenitors and has a major role in early stem cell survival and myeloid differentiation. One of the most important mutations in the gene *Flt-3* is the internal tandem duplication (ITD), which results in constitutive activation of the TK activity of *Flt-3*, leading to activation of downstream molecules (STAT5, Ras, Raf, MAP kinases, P13/AKT) that stimulate survival and proliferation signaling pathways.[26] *FLT3* ITD are thought to confer a growth advantage to AML and APL cells and have been associated with a higher risk of relapse, but are not felt to be sufficient to cause these diseases themselves.[17,26–28] There are a number of *FLT-3* inhibitors under investigation in combination with standard therapies in an attempt to target this molecular abnormality.

Similar molecular and cytogenetic abnormalities have been identified in the pathogenesis of lymphoid leukemias and provide diagnostic and prognostic information as well as opportunities for targeted therapies.[12] Refined characterization of the mutational status of *immunoglobulin variable gene* (*IgV*) status and genomic attributes in CLL has provided critical prognostic and treatment information. Four distinct prognostic attributes have been identified including mutational status of the heavy chain variable gene (*VH*) 17p deletion, 11q deletion—all unfavorable, and 13q—favorable.[29,30] The unfavorable attributes are thought to be associated with B-cell receptors and specific antigen-binding pockets that promote clonal expansion of the leukemic cells in response to other cells, cytokines, and chemokines.[30]

Extrinsic factors that play a role in the pathobiology of the leukemias and MDS include medullary angiogenesis, stromal dysregulation, and the balance of apoptosis and proliferation. The primary mediator of medullary angiogenesis is vascular endothelial growth factor (VEGF) that is over-expressed in the bone marrow of patients with myeloid malignancies and plays an important role in the pathogenesis of these diseases. VEGF overexpression is associated with myeloblast self-renewal and release of inflammatory cytokines, resulting in increased survival of the malignant clone. The bone marrow stroma is comprised of fibroblasts, fat cells, adhesion molecules, endothelial cells, osteoclasts, and osteoblasts. A primary difference between acute myeloid leukemia and MDS is the balance of apoptosis and proliferation. Apoptosis of stromal cells may be increased in MDS resulting in altered distribution of cell types in the bone marrow, such as atypical localization of immature precursors (ALIP), which is associated with a poor prognosis and early leukemic transformation. Bone marrow stroma derived from patients with MDS has been found to be ineffective in supporting bone marrow progenitor cells of healthy donors.[31] Large numbers of hematopoietic cells are rapidly proliferating in the bone marrow but are also undergoing apoptosis. Accelerated apoptosis of hematopoietic progenitors leads to ineffective hematopoiesis and eventual bone marrow failure due to premature loss of progenitor cells. Cytokines such as TNF , interleukin-1 , and IL-6 have been shown to mediate apoptosis in hematopoietic cells. Excessive apoptosis is an attractive explanation for how clonal expansion of marrow progenitor cells could result in ineffective hematopoiesis, peripheral cytopenias, and marrow failure despite a hypercellular bone marrow. As the disease progresses toward leukemic transformation, the rate of proliferation exceeds apoptosis and the patient will demonstrate increasing peripheral blasts. Several new agents target 1 or more of these areas to induce improvement in hematopoiesis and represent an attempt to affect the underlying disease.

## CLASSIFICATION AND STAGING

All of the leukemias represent heterogeneous hematological disorders that originate in the myeloid or lymphoid progenitor cells. Two primary classification systems are used to describe AML, ALL, and MDS. These include the French American British Classification System (FAB) and the World Health Organization (WHO) system. Table 57-2[32-39] (AML/ALL) and Table 57-3[40-42] (MDS) provide a review of these classification systems. Both systems assign a specific category of disease based on morphological descriptions of both peripheral blood and bone marrow findings. The FAB classification system was the standard classification system for many decades using morphology, cytochemistry, and immunophenotyping to differentiate myeloid vs lymphoid lineage, blast percentage, and specific point of differentiation for the neoplastic lineage to categorize the specific subtype of leukemia. The FAB classification system classifies the histologic sub-types of AML from M0 through M7. The WHO incorporated more recent molecular and clinical attributes to refine the diagnostic and prognostic relevance of the classification systems.[42] Several limitations exist in the current classification systems, most notably a limited ability

**TABLE 57-2**

**Selected Criteria From the French American British Classification (FAB) and World Health Organization (WHO) Classification for Acute Leukemia**

| FAB Subtype<br>WHO Classification | Bone Marrow Morphology and<br>Common Immunophenotype | Additional Clinical Findings |
|---|---|---|
| | **Acute Myeloid Leukemia (AML)** | |
| FAB: AML-**M0**, undifferentiated AML<br>WHO: AML NOS, without maturation | Blasts are nondescript, difficult to detect without immunophenotyping<br>Auer rods, and positive MPO staining<br>CD13, CD33, CD117 | 5%–10% of AML<br>Molecular findings: Associated with RUNX1-RUNX1T1<br>Poorer prognosis<br>Presentation with high blast count is common<br>Median age is 46 years |
| FAB: AML-**M1**, AML with minimal maturation<br>WHO: AML NOS, with minimal maturation | Sparse cytoplasmic granules, only occasional Auer rods, and positive MPO staining<br>Express early hematopoietic antigens: CD34, CD38, HLA-DR<br>TdT expression in 50% of cases<br>CD7 in 40% of cases | < 5% of AML<br>Inv (3) associated with thrombocytosis<br>Cytogenetic findings: 16%–22% are *FLT3*$^+$<br>Molecular findings: *RUNX1*<br>Poor prognosis in adults<br>Most common in infants or older adults<br>Commonly present with cytopenias and leukocytosis with evidence of bone marrow failure |
| FAB: AML-**M2**, AML with maturation<br>WHO: AML, with recurrent cytogenetic abnormalities | More clearly myeloid in origin, increased cytoplasmic granules, MPO positivity, frequent presence of Auer rods<br>Considered AML regardless of blast count<br>CD34, CD13, CD15, HLA-DR | 5% of AML<br>10% of FAB M2<br>Cytogenetic findings: t(8;21)(core-binding translocation) has a favorable prognosis<br>Molecular findings: Associated with *RUNX1-RUNX1T1*<br>More favorable response and long-term disease free survival to high-dose cytarabine in the consolidation phase<br>More common in younger patients |
| FAB: AML-**M3**, promyelocytic leukemia<br>WHO: AML, with recurrent cytogenetic abnormalities | Intense cytoplasmic granulation that often obscures the nucleus, blasts stain intensely with Sudan black or MPO<br>Considered AML regardless of blast count<br>Low expression or absence of HLA-DR, CD34, CD11a, CD11b, and CD18; high expression of CD33 | 5%–8% of AML<br>Cytogenetic findings: t(15;17)(q22;q23)<br>Molecular findings: *PML/RARα*<br>Best prognosis of all AML subtypes<br>Responsive to differentiation therapy: all-transretinoic acid (ATRA)<br>High risk of disseminated intravascular coagulation (DIC)<br>More common in younger adults |
| AML-**M3v** (variant) | Abnormal promyelocytes lack granules or Auer rods; weaker cytochemical stains<br>Expression of CD56 | Molecular findings: ZBTB16/*RARα* and variants<br>Poor response to ATRA<br>Correlates to expression of CD56 |
| FAB: AML-**M4**, myelomonocytic leukemia<br>WHO: AML NOS | Dysplastic features, such as hypogranular cytoplasm and nuclear hyposegmentation, blasts stain with both MPO and nonspecific esterase<br>Myeloid antigens (CD13, CD33, CD56, CD15) and variable expression of monocytic antigens in the blasts (CD14, CD4, CD11, CD64, CD36), HLA-DR | 5%–10% of AML<br>Cytogenetic findings: +8 Common<br>Evidence of monocytic and granulocytic differentiation<br>Extramedullary involvement can be seen<br>Median age is 50 years<br>More common in men<br>Favorable prognosis |
| FAB: AML-**M4eo**, myelomonocytic leukemia with eosinophilia<br>WHO: AML NOS | Abnormal basophilic eosinophils are seen in the marrow, which is similar to that of M4<br>Immunophenotype as for M4 | 5%–8% of AML<br>Cytogenetic findings: Inv(16)/t(16;16)<br>Molecular findings: *CBFB/MYH11*<br>Intermediate prognosis<br>Extramedullary involvement is often seen<br>Increased risk of central nervous system (CNS) disease/relapse<br>May present with bleeding disorders |

*(Continued)*

**TABLE 57-2**

**Selected Criteria From the French American British Classification (FAB) and World Health Organization (WHO) Classification for Acute Leukemia (*Continued*)**

| FAB Subtype WHO Classification | Bone Marrow Morphology and Common Immunophenotype | Additional Clinical Findings |
|---|---|---|
| FAB: AML-**M5 A**, monocytic leukemia<br>WHO: AML NOS | Blasts with folded nuclei and abundant cytoplasm that stains positively with nonspecific esterase but is MPO negative (CD14, CD4, CD11b, CD11c, CD64, CD36 and lyzozyme⁺)<br>HLA-DR⁺ | Cytogenetic findings: t(11q23)<br>Molecular findings: MLL<br>Poorer prognosis<br>Median age 49 years<br>Extramedullary disease is common<br>Increased risk of CNS disease/relapse |
| FAB: AML-**M5 B**, monocytic leukemia with differentiation<br>WHO: AML NOS | As for M5 A except that < 80% of monocytic lineage are blasts<br>As for M5 A, CD34(–) | Cytogenetic findings: t(8;16)<br>Associated with erythrophagocytosis<br>Intermediate prognosis |
| FAB: AML-**M6**, erythroid leukemia<br>WHO: AML NOS | Acute erythroid leukemia, may be associated with a variable appearance but usually is accompanied by dysplastic erythroid elements<br>Generally lack myeloid markers<br>Similar to M0 and M1 | < 5% of AML<br>Cytogenetic findings: Deletions of 5 and 7 are often seen<br>Poorer prognosis; often preceded by a myelodysplastic syndrome; seen in older patients |
| FAB: AML-**M7**, megakaryoblastic leukemia<br>WHO: AML NOS | Requires that more than 30% of blasts be of the megakaryocytic lineage; blasts often display clumping, multinucleation, and cytoplasmic blebbing<br>Immunophenotyping is usually required to make the diagnosis; expression of platelet glycoproteins (CD41, CD16, CD42) and CD36 | < 5% of AML<br>Cytogenetic findings: Occassional inv(3)<br>Complex karyotypes common in MDS<br>Poor prognosis<br>Antecedent myeloid disorders are common |
| | **Acute Lymphoblastic Leukemia (ALL)** | |
| FAB: ALL-L1<br>WHO: B lymphoblastic leukemia with recurrent genetic abnormalities | Small cells with minimal cytoplasm and no granules; rare nucleoli<br>B-ALL: CD10, CD19, CD20, CD22, CD34, HLA-DR, TdT cytoplasmic Ig; CD25 associated with t(9;22) | 20% of ALL in adults<br>Cytogenetic findings: t(9;22)<br>Molecular findings: *BCR-ABL*<br>Less favorable than B-ALL without *BCR-ABL*<br>More common in adults<br>Treatment with imatinib in addition to chemotherapy is recommended |
| FAB: ALL-L1<br>WHO: T lymphoblastic leukemia | Small cells with minimal cytoplasm and no granules; rare nucleoli; immunophenotyping is required to differentiate from B-ALL<br>T-ALL: CD2, CD5, CD7, CD8, CD34, may be CD10⁺ | 25% of ALL in Adults<br>Variable cytogenetic and molecular findings<br>Most common subtype in children<br>Often present with cytopenias<br>Extramedullary involvement including CNS is common<br>Mediastinal masses are common |
| FAB: ALL-L2, mature B-cell<br>WHO: B lymphoblastic leukemia | Larger cells with moderate amounts of cytoplasm and prominent nucleoli; TdT positive<br>As for ALL-L1 | 50% of ALL in adults<br>Cytogenetic findings: 5% t(8;14)/*c-myc*<br>Molecular findings: IgH in mature B-cell<br>Most common subtype in adults<br>More favorable prognosis |
| FAB: ALL-L3, B-cell or Burkitt's type leukemia<br>WHO: Variable categories based on cytogenetic and molecular findings | Large round cells with deeply basophilic cytoplasm and vacuoles CD10, CD19, CD20, CD21, CD22, surface Ig | 5% of ALL in adults<br>Cytogenetic findings: t(8;14); t(2;8); t(8;22)<br>Poor prognosis with standard ALL treatment regimens |

*Abbreviations*: ALL, acute lymphoblastic leukemia; AML, acute myelogenous leukemia; BCR-ABL, Abelson-breakpoint cluster region; CD, cluster of differentiation; CNS, central nervous system; c-myc, myclocytomatosis viral oncogene; Flt3, FMS-like tyrosine kinase; HLA, human leukocyte antigen; Ig, immunoglobulin; inv, inversion; MLL, mixed lineage leukemia; MPO, myeloperoxidase; NA, not available; NOS, not otherwise specified; PML/RARa, promyelocytic leukemia protein/retinoic acid receptor alpha; RUN, runt-related transcription factor; t, translocations; TdT, terminal deoxynucleotidyl transferase; ZBT B16/RARa, zinc finger and BTB domain containing protein/retinoic acid receptor alpha.

*Source*: Data from Delauney et al[32]; Arber et al[33]; Vardiman et al[34]; Scheinberg et al[35]; Arber et al[36]; Arber et al[37]; Borowitz and Chan[38]; and Borowitz and Chan.[39]

**TABLE 57-3**

**Selected Diagnostic and Prognostic Criteria for Classification of Myelodysplastic Syndromes (MDS)**

| FAB Subtype | WHO Modification | Morphological and Cytogenetic Findings |
|---|---|---|
| RA; < 5% blasts | RA | Unilineage dysplasia; <5% blasts; < 15% RS |
| | RCMD | Dysplasia in ≥ 10% or ≥2 myeloid lineages; no Auer rods; ± 15% RS |
| | MDS-U | Dysplasia in < 10% of 1 or more myeloid lineages; < 5% blasts; evidence of cytogenetic abnormalities common in MDS |
| | MDS with isolated del(5q)–5q syndrome | Normal or increased megakaryocytes; isolated del(5q)abnormality; no Auer rods; < 5% blasts |
| RARS (RA with ≥ 15% RS) | RARS | ≥ 15% RS; erythroid dysplasia only; <5% blasts |
| | RCMD-RS | Dysplasia in ≥ 10% or ≥ 2 myeloid lineages; no Auer rods; > 15% RS |
| RAEB; 5%–20% blasts | RAEB-I (5%–10% blasts) | Unilineage or multilineage dysplasia; 5%–9% blasts; no Auer rods |
| | RAEB-II (11%–20% blasts) | Unilineage or multilineage dysplasia; 10%–19% blasts; Auer rods may be present |
| RAEB-t; 21%–30% blasts | AML | Blasts > 20%; characteristics of AML with antecedent hematological malignancy |

*Abbreviations*: AML, acute myeloid leukemia; del, deletion; FAB, French American British; MDS, myelodysplastic syndromes; MDS-U, unclassified MDS; RA, refractory anemia; RAEB, refractory anemia with excess blasts; RAEB-t, RA with excess blasts in transformation; RARS, refractory anemia with ringed sideroblasts; RCMD, refractory cytopenias with multilineage dysplasia; RS, ringed sideroblasts; WHO, World Health Organization.

*Source*: Data from Brunning et al[40]; Harris et al[41]; and Vardiman et al.[42]

to incorporate the rapidly expanding characterization of disease attributes thought to indicate both favorable and unfavorable disease within a morphological subtype or stage of disease. The FAB classification system for ALL is thought to provide limited clinical benefit with the primary determinants of prognosis characterized by immunophenotype and genomics.[43] However, historical clinical trials are based on the FAB and WHO criteria and continue to require classification for comparative analysis with any recent clinical trials. Similarly, the use of the FAB classification system alone for AML is felt to be inadequate.[44] Consideration of specific genetic abnormalities and differentiation of de novo AML (DN-AML) and myelodysplasia-related AML (MDR-AML) are suggested as more accurate predictors of prognosis.

Identification of key molecular attributes has led to the development of risk stratification tools and refinement of staging criteria for each disease. For example, the International Prognostic Scoring System (IPSS) (Table 57-4[45,46]) was developed to include cytogenetic information and specific disease characteristics associated with either favorable or unfavorable prognosis or risk for leukemic transformation in patients with MDS. The IPSS relies on the number of cytopenias, cytogenetic profile, and the percentage of blasts in the bone marrow to group patients with MDS into 1 of 4 prognostic categories as follows: low risk, intermediate 1 risk, intermediate 2 risk, and high risk.[40] Cytogenetic abnormalities are present in approximately 40% to 50% of de novo MDS patients.[47] The most common abnormalities include deletions of chromosomes 7 (unfavorable), 5, and 20 (favorable), and trisomy of chromosome 8 (intermediate). Patients with lower risk disease (low-intermediate 1) have more favorable survival projections and are less likely to transform to acute leukemia. Treatment goals for the lower risk patients are aimed at improving hematopoiesis. Patients with higher risk disease (intermediate 2 or high) may transform very rapidly to acute leukemia and prognosis is generally poor. Treatment is aimed at survival. Consideration of diagnostic findings that may favor selection of specific therapies is critical to initiating the therapy with the greatest potential benefit early in the course of disease. More recent analysis of prognostic factors has revealed limitations in this system including the clinical importance of severe (life-threatening) thrombocytopenia or neutropenia, refined cytogenetic risk criteria, anemia, and transfusion requirements.[42,48,49] However, the IPSS criteria remain widely used in clinical practice to estimate risk and guide treatment selection. It is likely that the criteria will continue to undergo revision as new data emerges in the diagnosis and treatment of MDS.

The chronic leukemias are classified using disease specific descriptions based either on phase of illness (CML) or disease characteristics (CLL). These systems have been modified since their inception to include key molecular attributes found to have prognostic significance. For instance, several key prognostic factors have been identified for CLL including a rapid lymphocyte doubling time, elevated serum $\beta^2$microglobulin, unmutated immunoglobulin heavy chain (*IgVH*), CD38 expression, ZAP-70 expression, and FISH cytogenetics, including 17p-, 11q-, +12, and 13q.[50,51] As with many of these diseases, the original staging

**TABLE 57-4**

**Risk-Based Stratification of Myelodysplastic Syndromes—International Prognostic Scoring System (IPSS) and Proposed Modifications**

| Score | 0 | 0.5 | 1.0 | 1.5 | 2.0 | Risk Category | Numeric Score |
|---|---|---|---|---|---|---|---|
| Bone marrow myeloblasts | < 5% | 5%–10% | | 11%–20% | 21%–30% (considered AML) | Low<br>Intermediate-1<br>Intermediate-2<br>High | 0<br>0.5–1.0<br>1.5–2.0<br>≥ 2.5 |
| Karyotype | Normal, or del(5q), del(Y), del(20q) as sole abnormalities | Other abnormalities | del(7), 7+ or 3+ abnormalities | Proposed revision:<br>Favorable: del(12p),del(9q),t(15q), del(15q),$21^+$,$X^-$, t(7q), $21^-$<br>Intermediate-1: del(11q), ($8^+$)<br>Intermediate-2: t(11q23), any del3q abnormality,$19^+$, del(7q), exactly 3 abnormalities<br>Unfavorable: > 3 abnormalities and t(5q) | | | |
| Number of cytopenias | 0.1 | 2.3 | Anemia (hemoglobin <10 g/dL), neutropenia (absolute neutrophil count [ANC] < 1800/μL), and/or thrombocytopenia (platelets < 100,000/μL) | | | | Proposed revision:<br>Adverse risk:<br>Thrombocytopenia at presentation<br>High transfusion burden |

*Abbreviations*: AML, acute mylelogenous leukemia; del, deletion; t, translocation

*Source*: Data from Larson and Anastasi[43]; Head and Thompson[44]; Malcovati et al[48]; and Kao et al.[49]

systems were developed prior to the availability of molecular testing and the appreciation of the prognostic value of many of these attributes. For CLL the 2 primary staging systems are the RAI (US) and Binet (Europe). These have similar criteria with the difference in the stages represented as numeric or alphabetical. (Table 57-5[29,52–54]). Similarly, the staging criteria used for CML have evolved over time. The staging for CML reflects phases of illness (chronic phase, accelerated phase and blast phase) rather than an absolute morphological or molecular criteria (Table 57-6[55,56]). The universal diagnostic criteria is the presence of the *BCR-ABL* fusion gene (t9;22).[55,56]

## CLINICAL MANIFESTATIONS

The clinical presentation differs for each disease based on the cell lineage involved, the disease trajectory (acute vs chronic), and the general characteristics of the individual patient. Many of the patients with these diseases are older and commonly present with vague symptoms of fever, fatigue, malaise, night sweats, leukocytosis, lymphocytosis, or unusual bruising associated with underlying cytopenias. Adenopathy, organomegaly, or skin nodules may also be present and are more common in the lymphoid disorders and selected subtypes of AML. Central nervous system symptoms of headache, visual disturbances, ataxia, nausea or vomiting are most common in ALL resulting from meningeal infiltration and increased intracranial pressure.[12] Symptoms may progress slowly over weeks or months for patients with CLL, CML, or MDS. In contrast, clinical presentation may be abrupt and dramatic for patients with ALL or AML.

## ASSESSMENT

A complete family and personal history, medication review, and physical exam are essential to the diagnostic process. Attention to historical episodes of illness is useful in estimating the onset of illness in CLL, CML, and MDS. Careful attention to specific physical findings indicating tissue infiltration, organomegaly, adenopathy, or CNS disease is necessary to identify patients who may be at a higher risk of treatment-related toxicities. Laboratory evaluation should include analysis of the peripheral smear by a hematopathologist, a complete blood count, differential and platelet count, hepatic and renal profiles, hemolysis parameters,

**TABLE 57-5**

**Selected Diagnostic and Prognostic Criteria for Classification of Chronic Lymphocytic Leukemia (CLL)**

| Diagnostic Criteria | RAI Staging | | | | | Binet Staging | | | Clinical Significance |
|---|---|---|---|---|---|---|---|---|---|
| Stage | 0 | I | II | III | IV | A | B | C | All Stages in either RAI or Binet Systems |
| Lymphocytosis (> 15,000/μL) | + | + | + | + | + | + | + | + | Key diagnostic factor to differentiate from other mature B-cell neoplasms |
| Duration of lymphocytosis > 2 years | | | | | | | | | Validation of chronic disease |
| Bone marrow lymphocytes >30% | | | | | | | | | Differentiation from other indolent B-cell neoplasms |
| Lymphadenopathy (> 1 cm) | – | + | +/– | +/– | +/– | | | | More extensive lymphadenopathy |
| Lymphadenopathy (> 3 sites), including hepatosplenomegaly | | | | | | – | + | +/– | Extramedullary sites of disease (liver, spleen) are common, and in the absence of cytopenias or other high-risk features are considered intermediate risk |
| Hepatosplenomegaly | – | – | + | +/– | +/– | – | + | +/– | |
| Anemia (hemoglobin < 11 g/dL) | – | – | – | + | +/– | | | | Cytopenias reflect bone marrow infiltration or failure and are indicative of high risk disease |
| Anemia (hemoglobin < 10 g/dL) | | | | | | – | – | + | |
| Thrombocytopenia (< 100,000/μL) | | | | | + | – | – | + | |
| **High Risk Features for CLL** | | | | | | | | | |
| CD38 expression in > 30% of lymphocytes | | | | | | | | | Presence of large-cell transformation |
| High risk cytogenetics: 14q, 11q, 17p, 12+ | | | | | | | | | Elevated β2 microglobulin |
| Unmutated (germline) *IgVH* gene | | | | | | | | | Doubling time of lymphocyte count <12 months |
| ZAP-70 expression in > 30% of lymphocytes | | | | | | | | | RAI stage 3 or 4, Binet stage C |
| Elevated serum thymidine kinase | | | | | | | | | |

*Abbreviation*: CD, cluster of differentiation; IgVH, immunoglobulin heavy chain variable; ZAP-70, zeta-chain (TCR) associated protein kinase.

*Source*: Data from Seiler et al[29]; Smith and Boldt[52]; Rai et al[53]; and Binet et al.[54]

tumor lysis screen, and coagulation studies in the instance of APL. Additional laboratory parameters may be ordered for specific disease entities as a baseline analysis for potential treatment-related toxicities (Table 57-7[57,58]). Imaging studies are of particular importance in the lymphoid disorders and CML, as adenopathy and organomegaly are more common due to extramedullary clonal expansion. Baseline studies for underlying infections or organ function are also important to exclude concurrent illnesses or antecedent organ dysfunction.

**TABLE 57-6**

**Chronic Myelogenous Leukemia: Phases of Disease**

| Phase | Characteristics |
|---|---|
| Chronic phase | Indolent course, often asymptomatic, and found incidentally on routine physical exam<br>Predominance of mature white blood cells<br>Approximately 90% of patients are diagnosed at this stage<br>Median survival is 4–6 years (pre-tyrosine kinase inhibitor [TKI] therapy) |
| Accelerated phase | Transition generally occurs over a period of 1 year or more; duration is 4–6 months<br>Associated with progressive leukocytosis, thrombocytosis or thrombocytopenia, basophilia, splenomegaly, fever, bone pain, and thrombotic or bleeding complications<br>Clonal evolution is present |
| Blast phase | Lasts only a few months—survival is poor if untreated<br>Associated with increasing blasts (>30%), progressive splenomegaly despite treatment, and clonal evolution |

*Source*: Data from Calabretta and Perotti[55]; and Cortes et al.[56]

**TABLE 57-7**

**Diagnostic Evaluation of Patients With Acute Leukemias, Chronic Leukemias, and Myelodysplastic Syndrome**

| Peripheral Blood Evaluation | Clinical Significance |
|---|---|
| CBC, differential, and platelet count, reticulocyte count with evaluation of the peripheral smear | Evaluate for the presence of leukocytosis, basophilia, thrombocytosis, monocytosis, peripheral blasts, and morphological abnormalities<br>Establish baseline for monitoring of treatment-induced cytopenias |
| LDH, uric acid, PO4, $Ca^{++}$, $K^{+}$ | Evaluation of high cell turnover or tumor burden and increased risk for tumor lysis syndrome |
| Baseline hepatic, renal, and electrolyte profiles | Mild and transient transaminitis and hyperbilirubinemia are common with treatment<br>Renal toxicities are more common in the elderly<br>Many active therapies have potential renal and hepatic toxicities or may be affected by renal or hepatic insufficiencies |
| Human leukocyte antigen typing | For possible bone marrow or stem cell transplant |
| Serum iron, ferritin, TIBC, folic acid, vitamin B12 | Evaluate for other possible causes of anemia |
| LDH, haptoglobin, reticulocyte count, coombs | Evaluate for possible underlying hemolysis |
| Vitamin $B_{12}$ erythropoietin | Baseline evaluation of levels to determine role for growth factors vs active therapies in patient needing treatment for MDS |
| **Other laboratory studies** | **Clinical Significance** |
| Thyroid profile | Immunomodulatory agents may be associated with hypothyroidism<br>Hypothyroidism may contribute to anemia |
| Serum testosterone | Hypogonadism is common in elderly men and may contribute to fatigue |
| Coagulation profile:<br>Fibrinogen, PT, PTT, D-dimer | Presence of DIC: particularly important in APL with induction therapy |
| Lumbar puncture | Evaluate presence of CNS involvement (most common in ALL) |
| **History, Physical, Radiology Examination** | **Clinical Significance** |
| History of present illness | Document onset of suspicious symptoms, acute episodes of illness and prior transfusion history |
| Co-morbid conditions | Co-morbid conditions and effective management may play a critical role in determining potential therapies, including diabetes, hypertension, coronary artery disease, cardiomyopathy, congestive heart failure or pleural effusions, chronic renal disease, hepatitis or hepatic disease |
| Concomitant medications—including drug allergies | Review of medication profile to identify any potential medication-induced cytopenias, drug–drug interactions, QTc prolongation, or organ toxicity<br>There are numerous potential drug interactions with tyrosine kinase inhibitors used in the treatment of CML |
| Physical exam | Organomegaly: splenomegaly or hepatomegaly<br>Lymphadenopathy<br>Cutaneous manifestations and baseline skin evaluation—more common with M4 histological subtype of AML<br>Baseline cardiac and pulmonary evaluation |
| Radiology | Baseline CXR<br>Abdominal ultrasound if further evaluation of splenomegaly is indicated<br>Baseline MUGA scan or echocardiogram for patients with cardiovascular risk factors or for those patients receiving anthracycline therapy<br>CT scan of the chest, abdomen and pelvis for patients with CLL, CML or with adenopathy or organomegaly |

*(Continued)*

**TABLE 57-7**

**Diagnostic Evaluation of Patients With Acute Leukemias, Chronic Leukemias, and Myelodysplastic Syndrome (*Continued*)**

| Bone Marrow or Tissue Biopsy | Clinical Significance |
|---|---|
| Aspirate<br>Should include spicules and be cellular enough to assess at least 500 cells. | Evaluation of morphological abnormalities of hematopoietic precursors to allow FAB/WHO classification (dysplasia, blast percentage, monocytes, ringed sideroblasts, atypical megakaryocytes)<br>Used for flow cytometry, FISH analysis, and cytogenetics |
| Biopsy<br>Should be of adequate size for evaluation: 1–2 cm | Evaluate cellularity, topography, presence of atypical localization of immature precursors (ALIP; considered a poor prognostic finding), exclusion of other bone marrow disorders or bone marrow infiltration by solid tumors |
| Cytogenetics | Evaluate for possible nonrandom chromosomal abnormalities<br>Usually based on evaluation of 20 metaphases; greater than 2 metaphases are considered nonrandom<br>See individual disease overviews for prognostic significance |
| Tissue biopsy | Lymph nodes, cutaneous lesions, pleural effusions, or other focal areas of disease should be sent for cytology, immunophenotyping, and flow cytometry to describe the extent of disease and rule out infectious etiology |

*Abbreviations*: ALIP, atypical localization of immature precursors; ALL, acute lymphocytic leukemia; AML, acute myeloid leukemia; APL, acute promyelocytic leukemia; $Ca^{++}$, calcium; CBC, complete blood count; CNS, central nervous system; COC, complete blood count; CML, chronic myeloid leukemia; CT, computed tomography; CXR, chest x-ray; DIC, disseminated intravascular coagulation; FAB, French American British; FISH, fluorescent in situ hybridization; $K^+$, potassium; LDH, lactate dehydrogenase; MDS, myelodysplastic syndrome; MUGA, multigated acquisition scan; $PO_4$, phosphate; PT, prothrombin time; PTT, partial thromboplastin time; TIBC, total iron-binding capacity; WHO, World Health Organization.

*Source*: Data from Kurtin[57]; and Kurtin.[58]

The diagnostic process differs for each disease, with a focus on the characteristics of the malignant clone, associated symptoms, and any secondary organ affects. A tissue diagnosis is essential to a precise diagnosis and generally includes peripheral blood, bone marrow aspirate and biopsy, and tissue diagnosis in the presence of lymphadenopathy, organomegaly, or other extramedullary sites of disease. Sampling of the cerebrospinal fluid (CSF) is routine in ALL due to the increased potential for meningeal disease. A variety of diagnostic processes are used to determine the specific subtype of the disease including morphology, cytochemistry, immunophenotyping, cytogenetics analysis, and selected molecular testing using either fluorescent in situ hybridization (FISH) or polymer chain reaction (PCR) technologies. An adequate tissue sample is critical at the time of initial diagnosis as treatment is often initiated immediately and exposure to cytotoxic or targeted therapies may obscure key elements of the pathological diagnosis in subsequent samples. The presence of dysplasia, a hallmark of MDS, is often subtle and requires adequate bone marrow sampling to accurately characterize the disease. A recent analysis of 1317 patients with a diagnosis of AML suggests a delay in induction therapy is associated with inferior complete response and overall survival in patients less than 60 years ($P < 0.001$) but did not seem to correlate with these variables in patients greater than 60 years. This may be critical in allowing additional time to completely analyze the risk profile for the older patients with AML who have a poorer response to standard induction and a higher incidence of AHD.[59]

## THERAPEUTIC APPROACHES AND NURSING MANAGEMENT

The primary treatment modality for these hematological diseases requires a systemic treatment approach using chemotherapy, immunotherapy, and more recently targeted therapies. The role of surgery or radiotherapy is limited. Treatment strategies are based on the need to suppress the malignant clone. The goals of therapy include normalization of hematopoiesis with resolution of cytopenias or leukocytosis/lymphocytosis, effective treatment of potential sanctuary sites or extramedullary disease, elimination of minimal residual disease, and suppression of emerging resistant clones. Minimizing treatment related toxicities while maintaining or improving quality of life is critical to effective treatment. Thus, instituting the most effective therapy based on diagnostic and prognostic profiles will provide the best opportunity for a favorable clinical outcome.

The basic principles of induction therapy (initial aggressive treatment to reduce bulky disease and suppress the malignant clone) followed by consolidation (similar agents often given with decreased intensity) and in some cases long-term maintenance therapy are applied for the treatment of AML and ALL. More recently, selected targeted therapies have been added for improved response. The specific agents used, drug sequencing, and duration of therapy are different for AML and ALL. Treatment of CML, CLL, and MDS is dependent on the presenting symptoms and specific molecular and cytogenetic attributes. Active therapies may not be initiated at the time of diagnosis for patients with MDS or CLL in the absence of clinical indications for treatment. Active therapy is started immediately in the case of ALL, AML, and CML. Stem cell transplantation remains the only curative therapy for most of these diseases due to the limited effect of standard therapies on the leukemic stem cell. In many cases, an allogeneic transplant is necessary to effect a cure.[58] The most common treatment toxicities are attributed to the specific agent(s), the underlying disease, and characteristics of the individual patient.

## SPECIAL CONSIDERATIONS FOR THE ELDERLY POPULATION

Managing the hematological diseases is complicated by the generally advanced age of the patients (median age ranges from 65 to 70), presence of nonhematological comorbid conditions, and the potential inability of the older patient to tolerate certain intensive forms of therapy. Elderly patients commonly have multiple medical problems, use medications to manage them, and are more likely to have more than 1 healthcare provider involved in their care thereby increasing the risk for drug interactions and treatment toxicities. Manifestations of common toxicities or illnesses may be more subtle in the elderly due to age associated functional deficits in multiple organ systems.[60] Particularly important to the elderly patient with hematological malignancies is the age related decline in normal bone marrow function, including diminished capacity for response to stressors such as infection or myelosuppressive treatments.[61,62]

Acute myeloid leukemia in the elderly patient is more often associated with unfavorable disease related factors such as AHD, unfavorable cytogenetics, and the common occurrence of the multidrug resistance gene (*MDR*). Elderly patients with AML, generally defined as age > 60 years in the literature, have been found to have inferior rates of complete response and overall survival when compared to patients younger than age 60.[63] Due to the poor outcomes in older patients with AML receiving standard therapies, clinical trials specifically designed to evaluate AML in the elderly have become more common. Several targeted agents have been evaluated in the treatment of the older adult including Anti-CD33 antibodies, MDR inhibitors, farnesyltransferase inhibitors (FTI), novel nucleoside analogues, and FLT-3 inhibitors.[63–67]. Chronological age alone, however, should never exclude treatment.

Integrating geriatric and oncology nursing strategies allow an individualized approach to this unique population. As with many diseases in the elderly, reliance on family members or friends to maintain the prescribed treatments, including travel to appointments, may place additional stressors on the patient and their support network. Careful evaluation of functional status, ability to tolerate treatments, effect of disease progression, and general overall health can provide the best opportunity for nursing support of these patients. Assessment of activities of daily living may detect deficiencies or deficits that require early intervention before they become problematic.

## TREATMENT STRATEGIES FOR ACUTE MYELOGENOUS LEUKEMIA

### General considerations

The clinical presentation of AML, including APL, is generally abrupt and initiation of therapy needs to be immediate. Complete blood count, bone marrow, and radiological testing are essential prior to initiating therapy. Cytogenetic or molecular test results are generally unavailable prior to the administration of induction therapy. Therefore, initial therapy for AML is based on the age of the patient, presenting symptoms, performance status, total white blood cell count, blast count and comorbidities. AML in the older patient has been previously reviewed. The presence of leukocytosis (WBC > 30 $\times 10^9$ cells) is associated with increased treatment-related death (~50% of cases), often as a result of tumor lysis and aggressive disease.[63] Poor performance status, the presence of infection at the time of presentation, and complex or poorly controlled comorbidities are also considered unfavorable findings. Treatment related mortality is associated with increasing age, abnormal organ function, and a poor performance status.[12] Treatment failure is associated with specific karyotypes, AHD, FLT-3 ITD, MDR1, other molecular attributes that are less common, and treatment-induced AML. Table 57-8 provides an overview of AML and APL and their treatment.[25,28,63,68,69])

### Induction therapy

The standard regimen for induction-remission therapy in AML continues to be a regimen known as "7+3", using 7 days of continuous infusion cytarabine with 3 consecutive days of idarubicin or daunorubicin. Alternative anthracyclines and modified doses and schedules of cytarabine may be used in selected patients. Randomized clinical trials to date show no clear superiority with any 1 anthracycline or alternative use of mitoxantrone when used at equivalent doses.[12] Standard induction therapy is indicated for patients with favorable risk profiles and younger patients with intermediate risk disease. Patients with higher risk disease, such

**TABLE 57-8**

**Disease Overview: Acute Myelocytic Leukemia (AML)/Acute Promyelocytic Leukemia (APL)**

| Feature | Key Findings | | |
|---|---|---|---|
| **Epidemiology** | **New Cases in 2008:** 12,810 **Average Age at Diagnosis:** 67 years | | |
| **Etiology** | Genetic instability<br>Chemical exposure | Mutagens<br>Tobacco | |
| **Stem Cell Defect** | Myeloid progenitor cell | | |
| **Prognostic factors: genetics** | **Favorable**<br>Translocation (t)(15;17) (APL), t(8;21), and inversion(16)<br>Nucleophosmin NPM1 mutation, FMS-related tyrosine kinase 3 (FLT3) | **Intermediate**<br>+8, +6, +21, –Y, 12p–, NPM mutation (Flt3+), C/EBPα mutation | **Poor risk**<br>Complex (> 3 abnormalities)<br>Abnormalities of chromosome 5 or 7<br>17p abnormality, t(6;9), t(3;21)<br>11q23 deletion (del) (common in MDR-AML) |
| **Additional prognostic factors** | Age: Older age is associated with a reduced incidence of complete response<br>Antecedent hematological disorder or secondary AML—These subgroups have a lower incidence of complete response and a reduced overall survival | | |
| **Staging** | FAB/WHO (morphology) | | |
| **Clinical Presentation** | Leukocytosis, leukemia cutis (leukemic skin infiltrates), cytopenias, infection, bleeding, bleeding diathesis (APL) | | |
| **Indication to Treat** | Confirmed diagnosis, presentation with leukocytosis, bleeding diathesis, tumor lysis | | |
| **Key Concepts for Effective Treatment** | Induction therapy is aimed at suppression of the malignant clone with induced hypoplasia and resolution of extramedullary sites of disease<br>Consolidation and maintenance therapy are aimed at achieving a durable molecular remission with eradication of minimal residual disease.<br>Allogeneic bone marrow transplantation is the only potentially curative therapy for AML<br>Differentiation agents (eg, all-transretinoic acid) together with anthracyclines can induce cure in up to 95% of APL cases<br>Aggressive management of cytopenias, leukocyte differentiation syndrome and bleeding diathesis is necessary to avoid treatment-related death during induction therapy for APL | | |
| **FDA Approved Therapies** | **AML:**<br>**Induction and Consolidation:**<br>Anthracyclines: Idarubicin, Daunorubicin<br>Mitoxantrone<br>Cytarabine<br>**Relapse:**<br>Gemtuzumab Ozogamicin | **APL: Induction:**<br>Daunorubicin or Idarubicin<br>All-transretinoic Acid (ATRA)<br>**Maintenance:**<br>6-Mercatopurine<br>Methotrexate<br>ATRA<br>**Relapse:**<br>Arsenic Trioxide<br>Gemtuzumab Ozogamicin | |
| **In Clinical Trials or Used Based on Other Approved Indications** | Gemtuzumab Ozogamicin (Anti CD33 Monoclonal Antibodies)<br>PSC833, Zosuquidar (MDR inhibitors)<br>Tipifarnib (FTI)<br>PKC412, CEP701, Sunitinib (FLT3-inhibitors)<br>Clofarabine, Troxacitabine (nucleoside analogs)<br>Valproic Acid, SAHA, MS-275 (HDAC inhibitors)<br>Bcl-2 antisense (anti-apoptotic)<br>Azacitidine, Decitabine (Hypomethylating agents)<br>Cloretazine (Alkylating agent) | | |
| **Key Supportive Care Concerns** | Myelosupression: infection, differentiation syndrome, mucositis, disseminated intravascular coagulation, neurotoxicity, cardiomyopathy | | |

*Abbreviations*: DIC, disseminated intravascular coagulation; HDAC, histone deacetylases; MRD, minimal residual disease; WHO, World Health Organization.

*Source*: Data from Lo-Coco et al[25]; Burnett and Knapper[28]; Estey[63]; NCCN[68]; and Tallman.[69]

as those over the age of 60, should have modified dosing of cytarabine based on the increased risk of cerebellar toxicity and treatment related toxicity. Improved cure rates have been noted in younger patients and those with favorable cytogenetics t(8;12) and inversion 16 when using high dose cytarabine.[70] The goal of induction therapy is to clear the bone marrow of leukemic cells and to induce hypoplasia. A repeat bone marrow biopsy is performed 2 weeks after the initial induction to assess treatment response. The absence of disease (<5% blasts in an aspirate with spicules, no blasts with Auer rods, no persistent extramedullary disease) is considered a favorable finding. As the peripheral blood counts recover, the bone marrow biopsy is repeated. If there continues to be no evidence of disease, the patient is considered to be in a complete remission (CR). Obtaining a CR with the initial induction regimen is the sole outcome measure associated with improved survival in phase III clinical trials [71] Patients who do not achieve a CR with first induction will be rechallenged with a second cycle of induction therapy often using alternative agents or doses.

The most common treatment-related toxicities during induction therapy include cytopenias requiring transfusion support, treatment of infections, renal, hepatic, and cardiac toxicities related to the specific agents used or preexisting conditions, and gastrointestinal toxicities (nausea, vomiting, diarrhea, mucositis). Drug specific toxicities such as neurotoxicity and acral erythema associated with nucleoside analogs are seen less frequently. Patients are at particular risk for infection as a result of immune compromise due to the disease itself and the presence of neutropenia and concurrent mucositis. Atallah et al [72] reviewed records for 1534 patients with AML and found that Grade 3 or 4 neutropenia occurred in 91% of the patients, and febrile episodes were common (94%). Documented infections were noted in 64% of patients, 28% of the patients required admission to the intensive care unit, and respiratory support or dialysis were necessary in 16% of patients demonstrating the potential serious adverse events attributed to induction therapy for AML and the importance of supportive care strategies during this phase of treatment.

### Postremission therapy (consolidation therapy)

The second phase of treatment for AML is consolidation therapy with the goal of maintaining a CR by suppressing any microscopic disease. Treatment consists of a modified induction regimen in most cases. The role of stem cell transplant (SCT) in first CR remains controversial. There are variable outcomes related to SCT based on the age of the patient and the underlying characteristics of the disease.[73] Careful selection criteria with treatment on a clinical trial is recommended to facilitate refinement of the guidelines for transplantation in the older adult with AML. The advantage of an allogeneic transplant is thought to be related to the graft vs leukemia effect. This is thought to be a result of immune modulation and suppression of the malignant clone by immunocompetent donor T-cells. A recent meta-analysis of 3100 subjects with AML demonstrated a survival advantage for allogeneic transplantation for patients with high-risk AML (hazard ratio [HR] 1.39) but did not show a survival advantage in patients with favorable risk cytogenetics (HR 0.9).[74] Patients with secondary AML (treatment-induced or AHD) tend to have resistant disease and should be evaluated for an allogeneic SCT at the time of diagnosis. Patients who fail induction therapy should also be evaluated for an allogeneic SCT. Difficulties in locating a suitable donor prior to disease progression or treatment-related morbidity or mortality make this a particularly high-risk group of patients. Studies have also identified that infusion of donor lymphocytes after the transplant conditioning regimen and an allogeneic hematopoietic stem cell transplant (HSCT), can successfully treat leukemia relapse.[75]

The recent development of molecular testing for minimal residual disease (MRD) has elucidated the molecular pathogenesis of the disease, specifically the presence of a leukemic stem cell.[76] Minimal residual disease is defined by levels of expression for selected molecular attributes of disease that are not detectable by routine morphological or immunohistochemical techniques.[66,77] This is thought to contribute to the common occurrence of relapse despite significant tumor reduction with standard chemotherapy. Relapsed AML is frequently resistant to standard chemotherapy. More recent clinical trials have included agents that target some of the unfavorable cytogenetic and molecular attributes including antibody-based therapy targeting CD33, FLT-3 inhibitors, FTI, c-Kit inhibitors, demethylating agents, and histone deacytylase inhibitors, MDR1 antagonists, and BCl-2 antagonists.[78] Clinical trials participation is critical to fully understanding the role of these newer agents in the suppression of leukemogenesis and improving remission rates in patients who are not candidates for an allogeneic transplant and have poor-risk AML.

## TREATMENT STRATEGIES FOR ACUTE PROMYELOCYTIC LEUKEMIA

### Induction therapy

Acute promyelocytic leukemia (see Table 57-8) is a distinct histological subtype (M3) of AML and is now thought to be a curable disease in the majority of patients who receive molecularly directed therapy. APL is a subtype of AML defined by the presence of t(15;17) and expression of the PML and retinoic acid receptor alpha $\alpha$ (RAR) resulting in the fusion gene *PML-RARα* present in more than 95% of cases, which is detectable by FISH or polymerase chain reaction (PCR).[12] APL represents 10% to 15% of all cases of AML and patients tend to be younger than those with other types of AML. APL typically has a rapid onset with a high risk of treatment-related death during induction therapy due to bleeding diatheses and leukocyte differentiation syndrome (described below). Therefore, identification of this specific subtype of AML is critical at presentation as the treatment is specific to APL and standard therapy for AML is not beneficial. Signs and symptoms that are common in the presentation of APL specifically include mucocutaneous infiltrates with or without hemorrhage, increased coagulation time and elevated fibrinogen levels. Standard therapy for APL consists of a combination of an anthracycline (daunorubicin or idarubicin) and all-transretinoic acid (ATRA) an oral differentiating agent. In patients with APL, ATRA therapy accelerates the terminal differentiation of malignant promyelocytes to mature neutrophils, leading to apoptosis and CR without myelosuppression and bone marrow hypoplasia.[79]

### Postremission therapy

Following induction therapy, 2 additional cycles of anthracycline based therapy are administered with continuation of ATRA. This approach to treatment in patients with molecularly confirmed APL has resulted in molecular remissions and CR rates of 90% to 95%. The role of arsenic trioxide (ATO) in the initial treatment of APL has gained attention due to the selective partial differentiation of APL blast cells.[25] ATO is currently indicated for relapsed or refractory disease. Additional agents, including FLT-3 inhibitors, are in clinical trials. The role of stem cell transplant is limited in APL due to the high rate of complete molecular remissions with current frontline therapy. Following induction and consolidation, maintenance therapy with ATRA for up to 1 year using intermittent dosing is recommended.

The initiation of treatment for APL requires specific monitoring and institution of preventative supportive care measures. Patients who present with elevated WBC counts ($>10\times10^9$/L) are at increased risk for coagulopathies and leukocyte differentiation syndrome.[12] The mechanism for the bleeding diathesis is poorly understood but is known to be associated with fibrinolysis.[80] The bleeding diathesis is most common in the first week of treatment. Initiating treatment with a differentiation agent (ATRA) together with treatment of the coagulopathy with fibrinogen, fresh frozen plasma, and platelet transfusions to keep the fibrinogen level >150 mg/dL and platelets above 30,000 to 50,000/$mm^3$ have reduced treatment related deaths significantly. The leukocyte differentiation syndrome is associated with administration of ATRA. Fever, a rapid increase in WBCs, pulmonary infiltrates and secondary symptoms of shortness of breath and hypoxia are most common and may occur at variable times during the induction therapy. This syndrome is associated with rapid deterioration in pulmonary function, pleural and pericardial effusions. The immediate institution of dexamethasone at the onset of symptoms can effectively reverse these symptoms.

Arsenic trioxide also requires specific monitoring due to the potential for electrolyte abnormalities and QT prolongation. Baseline and weekly evaluation of serum electrolytes (calcium, potassium, and magnesium) with replacement as needed to maintain concentrations of potassium above 4.0 mEq/L and magnesium above 1.8mg/dL together with interval electrocardiograms to evaluate QTc intervals (<500 milliseconds) will effectively reduce the potential for serious cardiac events such as torsades de pointe.

## TREATMENT STRATEGIES FOR ACUTE LYMPHOCYTIC LEUKEMIA

### General considerations

The treatment of ALL is very different than the treatment for AML in a number of ways. (Table 57-9[45,81–87])The goals of therapy include restoring normal hematopoiesis, preventing the emergence of resistant clones, effectively treating sanctuary sites including the CNS, and eliminating MRD. To achieve these goals, treatment includes induction, consolidation, CNS prophylaxis, and long-term maintenance therapy using a variety of drugs in complex sequencing. Specific drug combinations given at defined intervals over an extended treatment course (up to 3 years) provides the most favorable outcome in ALL. Short-term dose intensification, common in AML, is not felt to be beneficial in ALL with the exception of mature B-cell ALL. The absence of MRD (<0.01%) during or following completion of initial induction therapy is associated with high levels of CR (up to 85% in adults).[81] Advanced age, high leukocyte count at presentation, delayed time to achieve a CR (>4–5 weeks), specific immunophenotype and cytogenetic abnormalities are associated with decreased CR rates, shorter remission duration, decreased overall survival (OS), and increased CNS relapse. Age in particular is felt to be critical in adult ALL patients; patients of age less than 30 years have an OS of 34% to 57% and age greater than 30 years have an OS of 15% to 17%.[88] Approximately 20% to 30% of adult ALL patients (as many as 50% of elderly patients) have Philadelphia chromosome positive ($Ph^+$) disease that is associated with unfavorable outcome.[89] The addition of tyrosine kinase inhibitors targeting the Ph chromosome given concurrently with standard chemotherapy offers improved response rates. These patients are primary candidates for allogeneic transplantation.

### Induction therapy

The most common agents used in the induction phase of treatment for ALL include a corticosteroid (prednisone, dexamethasone), vincristine, and an anthracycline (most often danorubicin). There are a number of regimens that include a variety of other agents with variable dosing and sequencing including asparaginase, cyclophosphamide, teniposide, and cytarabine. The induction phase of treatment is most often administered in an inpatient setting as the patient is

**TABLE 57-9**

**Disease Overview: Acute Lymphocytic Leukemia (ALL)**

| Feature | Key Findings | |
|---|---|---|
| **Epidemiology** | **Incidence (per year):** 5,430 **Median Age at Diagnosis:** 13 years | |
| **Etiology** | Genetic | Autoimmune disease |
| **Stem Cell Defect** | Clonal B cells (most common) or T cells (rare) arrested in the various phases of differentiation | |
| **Chromosomal Findings** | **Intermediate risk**<br>Normal karyotype<br>abn 11q, del(6q), del(17p), del(12p), −13/del(13), t(14q32), t(10;14)<br>Others markers are under investigation | **High risk**<br>−7(Ph neg), del(7p), +8, t(1;19), t(17;19)<br>t(9:22)—Ph+<br>t(4;11) with the *MLL-AF4* gene<br>Complex abnormalities (≥5)<br>Other molecular markers are under investigation |
| **Additional Prognostic Factors Indicating High-Risk Disease** | *BCR-ABL* positive disease<br>Undifferentiated leukemia<br>Null ALL<br>$CD10^+$ (CALLA); mature B-cell ALL<br>WBC > $30x10^9$/L at diagnosis<br>Greater than 4–5 wks to achieve a CR (≥ 0.1% residual disease by PCR)<br>Age > 35 years | |
| **Staging** | Based primarily on immunophenotype and WBC at presentation | |
| **Response Criteria** | CR = < 0.1% residual disease by PCR | |
| **Disease Characteristics** | **B cell ALL**<br>Mature B cell less favorable; treated with intense induction followed by Allogeneic SCT | **T cell ALL**<br>More favorable in adults with initial diagnosis; relapse, however, is difficult to treat<br>More commonly involves extra-medullary sites |
| **Clinical Presentation** | Leukocytosis<br>Splenomegaly<br>Hepatomegaly | Infections<br>Tumor lysis<br>CNS Symptoms: Headache, ataxia |
| **Indication to Treat** | Confirmation of diagnosis, leukocytosis, tumor lysis, CNS symptoms | |
| **Key Concepts for Effective Treatment** | Chemotherapy has been effective alone and in combination with other agents<br>New targeted therapies have increased response rates<br>Chromosomal abnormalities have prognostic value<br>Aggressive concurrent management of infection risk is essential to effective therapy<br>CNS prophylaxis is critical to long-term response | |
| **FDA Approved Therapies** | **Induction:** Most common: Daunorubicin, Vincristine, Prednisone, Asparaginase<br>Ph+- add Imatinib<br>CNS treatment if positive at presentation | |
| | **Consolidation:**<br>Cytarabine<br>Etoposide<br>Asparaginase<br>Daunorubicin/Vincristine/Prednisone<br>CNS-Prophylaxis | **Maintenance:**<br>6-Mercaptopurine<br>Methotrexate<br>Vincristine<br>Prednisone<br>Imatinib or Dasatinib if Ph+ |
| **In Clinical Trials or Used Based on Other Approved Indications** | Nelarabine<br>Clofarabine<br>Forodesine<br>MLN518<br>CEP701<br>Tipifarnib | Rituximab<br>Gemtuzumab Ozogamicin<br>SAHA<br>Valproic Acid<br>MS275<br>MK0752 |
| **Key Supportive Care Concerns** | Tumor lysis syndrome, cytopenias, CNS symptoms: acute and chronic, immunosuppression, neurotoxicity, coagulation abnormalities (asparaginase) | |

*Abbreviations*: ALL, acute lymphocytic leukemia; BCR-ABL, abelson break point cluster region; CNS, central nervous system; CR, creatinine; PCR, polymerase chain reaction; Ph+, Philadelphia chromosome positive; SCT, stem cell transplant; t, translocation; WBC, white blood cell.

*Source*: Data from Greenberg et al[45];Pui and Evans[81]; Moorman et al[82]; Pullarkart et al[83]; Huget et al[84]; Larson[85]; Linker et al[86]; and Kantarjan et al.[87]

newly diagnosed and frequent monitoring for treatment toxicities is necessary. Cytopenias and mucositis are common. Treatment of infections with antibiotic support is similar to that used in AML. Monitoring of coagulation parameters, risk for hypersensitivity, hyperglycemia, and hyperbilirubinemia is necessary with the use of asparaginase.

### CNS prophylaxis

Involvement of the central nervous system, a sanctuary site not easily treated with standard systemic therapy, is common over the course of disease with ALL. Although it may be present in fewer than 10% of patients at initial diagnosis, the incidence over the course of disease is as high as 75% at 1 year without specific therapy aimed at treating the CNS.[86] The primary strategy for CNS prophylaxis is the administration of intrathecal methotrexate with serial testing of the cerebral spinal fluid (CSF) for disease. Cranial irradiation, historically a primary modality, is now reserved for selected high-risk patients (positive CSF, high presenting WBC, T-cell phenotype) due to the treatment related long-term effects including neurocognitive deficits and endocrinopathies.[89]

### Postremission therapy (consolidation therapy)

Post-remission consolidation is instituted following hematologic recovery and may include modified repetition of the induction schedule. Use of higher doses of cyclophosphamide and subcutaneous cytarabine are common. Patients with good performance status and support networks can often receive consolidation treatment in an outpatient setting where laboratory testing, transfusion and infusion capabilities are readily available. Late-intensification using a second course of induction therapy administered during the first few months of remission provides improved outcomes for patients of intermediate risk.[86]

Maintenance therapy includes the use of monthly vincristine, pulse doses of prednisone, and daily dosing of 6-Mercaptopurine and methotrexate. All of the drugs except for vincristine are administered orally. This phase of treatment is generally well-tolerated with minimal incidence of cytopenias or mucositis. Transient elevation of transaminase levels is common. Treatment is continued for at least 2 years. Attempts to shorten the maintenance therapy have resulted in inferior outcomes.[81] Patients with Ph+ disease will continue concurrent administration of imatinib throughout the maintenance phase or until they receive an allogeneic HSCT.[90]

## TREATMENT STRATEGIES FOR CHRONIC MYELOGENOUS LEUKEMIA

Scientific discovery and clinical advances in the diagnosis and treatment of CML, including identification of distinct cytogenetic and molecular characteristics, have resulted in the development of targeted therapies that have significantly improved overall prognosis for this disease. (Table 57-10[91-95]) A new class of drugs targeted at the *BCR-ABL* tyrosine kinase, present in all patients with the disease, has improved clinical responses in the chronic phases of the disease to 83% at 5 years.[96] The first TKI was imatinib that earned FDA approval as first-line therapy for CML in 2001. A second TKI agent, dasatinib, earned FDA approval in 2006 for the treatment of CML in patients with resistance or intolerance to imatinib. Nilotinib, the third TKI, was approved in 2007 for the treatment of CML (Table 57-11[97-100]). However, drug resistance to these new agents may develop over time or be present at the time of diagnosis due to molecular mutations. Complete and thorough diagnostic evaluation of the patient at the time of diagnosis and throughout the course of treatment is essential to optimal therapeutic outcomes.

### Chronic phase

Treatment goals have changed with the development of TKI therapies, with a shift from hematological responses and cytogenetic remission to molecular responses (MR). The primary goal is to induce a complete molecular remission (CMR) early in the clinical course of the disease with a tolerable level of toxicity. Reduction of mortality through vigilant monitoring of molecular status to identify suboptimal response, disease progression, or existing or evolving drug resistance is critical to allow selection of the best potential therapy or the need for a change in therapy.

Refinement of the molecular analysis of CML has shifted the definition of treatment response and is critical to identification of patients who will require a change in therapy. Real-time quantitative polymerase chain reaction (RT-PCR) for *BCR-ABL* has become the gold standard for analysis of treatment response and the presence of residual disease. It is performed with peripheral blood and should be monitored consistently at a single institution if possible to minimize any variance. The achievement of a major molecular response (MMR) following 12 months of imatinib therapy was associated with 100% probability of transformation-free survival at 60 months.[98] Increasing *BCR-ABL* levels that are detected by RT-PCR may indicate mutation or progression of disease.

The National Comprehensive Cancer Network (NCCN) recommends hematological, cytogenetic, and molecular measures at baseline and repeated at regular intervals with initiation of therapy.[97] Hematological parameters are monitored regularly to evaluate for response and treatment toxicity. Dose escalation should be considered if there is no evidence of hematological response at 3 months. Cytogenetics are evaluated at 6 and 12 months, if a complete cytogenetic response is noted, the patient should continue the same dose. If a partial cytogenetic response is noted, the dose is increased and

**TABLE 57-10**

**Disease Overview: Chronic Myelogenous Leukemia (CML)**

| Feature | Key Findings | |
|---|---|---|
| **Epidemiology** | **Incidence (per year):** 5050 **Median Age at Diagnosis:** 66 years | |
| **Etiology** | Unknown | |
| **Stem Cell Defect** | **Myeloid progenitor cell** | |
| **Prognostic Findings** | Favorable: Low WBC count, *BCR-ABL* positive<br>Unfavorable: High WBC count, organomegaly, *BCR-ABL* negative disease | |
| **Staging and Classification** | FAB/WHO Classification of limited prognostic value | |
| **Disease Characteristics** | **Chronic Phase**<br>Indolent course, often asymptomatic and found incidentally on routine physical exam<br>Predominance of mature white blood cells<br>Approximately 90% of patients are diagnosed at this stage<br>Median survival is 4–6 years (pre-TKI therapy)<br>**Accelerated Phase**<br>Transition generally occurs over a period of 1 year or more; duration is 4–6 months<br>Associated with progressive leukocytosis, thrombocytosis or thrombocytopenia, basophilia, splenomegaly, fever, bone pain, thrombotic or bleeding complications<br>Clonal evolution is present<br>**Blast Phase**<br>Lasts only a few months—survival is poor if untreated<br>Associated with increasing blasts (> 30%), progressive splenomegaly despite treatment, and clonal evolution | |
| **Response Criteria**<br>*Cytogenetic response is based on analysis of at least 20 metaphases | Complete hematological response | Normal CBC and differential, no extramedullary disease |
| | Minimal cytogenetic response | 65%–95% Ph-positive metaphases (analysis of at least 20 metaphases) |
| | Minor cytogenetic response | 36%–65% Ph-positive metaphases |
| | Partial cytogenetic response | 1%–35% Ph-positive metaphases |
| | Complete cytogenetic response | 0% Ph-positive metaphases |
| | Major molecular response (MMR) | ≥ 3-log reduction of *BCR-ABL mRNA* |
| | Complete molecular remission (CMR) | Negativity by RT-PCR |
| **Clinical Presentation** | Cytopenias or leukocytosis, splenomegaly, fatigue, cutaneous manifestation—less common | |
| **Indication to Treat** | Confirmed diagnosis with *BCR-ABL* by FISH or PCR | |
| **Key Concepts for Effective Treatment** | Therapy is likely to continue indefinitely<br>Evaluation of response using hematologic, cytogenetic and molecular benchmarks is critical to effective therapy and early identification of resistance | |
| **FDA approved therapies** | Imatinib<br>Nilotinib | Dasatinib<br>Hydrea<br>Interferon |
| **In clinical trials** | Bosutinib | Decitabine |
| **Key supportive care concerns** | Myelosuppression, hepatic function abnormalities, congestive heart failure, gastrointestinal toxicities, QT prolongation, drug-drug interactions | |

*Abbreviations*: BCR-ABL, abelson break point cluster region; CBC, complete blood count; FAB, French American British; FISH, fluorescent in situ hybridization; Ph, Philadelphia chromosome; RT-PCR, real-time polymerase chain reaction; TKI, tyrosine kinase inhibitor; WHO, World Health Organization.

*Source*: Data from Deininger[91]; NCCN[92]; Shah[93]; Giles et al[94]; and Talpaz et al.[95]

testing is repeated at 18 months. If there is a minor or minimal cytogenetic response at 12 months, recommendations are to change therapy to dasatinib or nilotinib, consider an HSCT, or a clinical trial. Real time quantitative polymerase chain reaction should be performed every 3 months—indefinitely. If levels are rising the PCR frequency should increase to monthly and testing for *ABL* kinase domain (KD) mutations should be considered. These parameters are being

**TABLE 57-11**

**FDA Approved Therapies for Chronic Myelogenous Leukemia (CML)**

| Agent | Mechanism of Action | Dosing and route of administration | Common Toxicities |
|---|---|---|---|
| Imatinib | *BCR-ABL* selective tyrosine kinase inhibitor | 400 mg po daily<br>Dose escalation to 600–800 mg/day is indicated in accelerated or blast phase or sub-optimal response<br>Available: 100 mg or 400 mg tablets | Myelosuppression<br>Superficial edema<br>Gastrointestinal toxicities: nausea, vomiting, diarrhea<br>Muscle cramping<br>Rash<br>Pulmonary edema, pleural effusions, ascities: rare<br>QT prolongation |
| Dasatinib | Second generation *BCR-ABL* tyrosine kinase inhibitor<br>Indicated for imatinib-resistant disease<br>No benefit with T315I mutation | 70 mg po bid (accelerated or blast phase) or<br>100 mg po q day (chronic phase)<br>Available: 20 mg, 50 mg, 70 mg, and 100 mg tablets | Myelosuppression<br>Superficial edema<br>Gastrointestinal toxicities: diarrhea, nausea, vomiting<br>Headaches<br>Dyspnea or pulmonary edema: most common in blast phase<br>Rash<br>Asthenia<br>Transaminase elevation<br>QT prolongation |
| Nilontinib | Second generation *BCR-ABL* tyrosine kinase inhibitor<br>Indicated for imatinib resistant disease | 400 mg po twice daily<br>Available: 200 mg capsules | Myelosuppression<br>Gastrointestinal: diarrhea, nausea<br>Hyperbilirubinemia<br>Hyperglycemia<br>Headache<br>Hypophosphatemia<br>Elevated serum lipase<br>Rash<br>Pruritus<br>Arthralgias/myalgias<br>QT prolongation |

*Abbreviation*: BCR-ABL, abelson breakpoint cluster region.
*Source*: Data from NCCN[97]; Novartis Pharmaceuticals[98]; Bristol-Myers Squib[99]; and Novartis Pharmaceuticals.[100]

refined as new agents are developed and more patients are evaluated in long-term follow up.

### Terminal phase

In patients with more advanced disease, control of the accelerated phase of the disease with induction of chronic phase and continued therapies to induce MRD should be the goal.

## TREATMENT STRATEGIES FOR CHRONIC LYMPHOCYTIC LEUKEMIA

The overall 5-year survival for patients with newly diagnosed CLL is approximately 60%, depending on disease stage. (Table 57-12[7,29,30,101]) For patients with progressive CLL, treatment with conventional chemotherapy is not curative, although allogeneic HSCT can help prolong disease-free survival. Patients with aggressive CLL typically have bulky disease, B symptoms (fever, night sweats, and unexplained weight loss in the previous 6 months), and RAI stage III or IV disease with a compromised marrow indicating a poor prognosis and decreased survival. Given the rapid development of new treatment options and refinement of risk-based treatment selection, the treatment strategies for CLL have been in flux. Watchful waiting is still considered appropriate for patients with low tumor burden and no adverse risk factors. Patients with high-risk or aggressive disease should initiate therapy to avoid further complications associated with the treatment of bulky disease. The most common agents

**TABLE 57-12**

**Disease Overview: Chronic Lymphocytic Leukemia (CLL)**

| **Feature** | **Key Findings** | | |
|---|---|---|---|
| **Epidemiology** | **Incidence (per/year):** 15,000 **Average Age at Diagnosis:** 72 years | | |
| **Etiology** | Genetic<br>Autoimmune disease | | |
| **Stem Cell Defect** | Clonal B cells arrested in the B-cell differentiation pathway (95%) | | |
| **Chromosomal findings** | Favorable<br>del(13q) as sole abnormality | Neutral<br>+12 | Poor<br>17p-, t(11q;v), 11q- |
| **Additional prognostic factors indicating high-risk disease** | ZAP-70 > 20% (correlates with unmutated Immunoglobulin heavy chain variable gene (*IgVh* status; suggests poor outcome)<br>CD38+ (aggressive disease)<br>*p53+* (poor response to conventional chemotherapy)<br>Elevated LDH<br>CD69 expression (worse survival outcomes exclusive of ZAP-70 status) | | |
| **Staging** | Binet and RAI Systems | | |
| **Response Criteria** | International Working Group (IWG) Response Criteria | | |
| **Disease Characteristics** | **Indolent:**<br>Low tumor burden, normal marrow function | **Progressive:**<br>High tumor burden, impaired marrow function, hypogammaglobulinemia<br>Auto-immune hemolytic anemia | |
| **Clinical Presentation** | Lymphocytosis<br>Splenomegaly<br>Hepatomegaly<br>Asymptomatic-20% | Infections (agranulocytosis and hypogammaglobulinemia)<br>Adenopathy<br>Hemolytic anemia | |
| **Indication to Treat** | Bulky disease (spleen, liver, nodes)<br>Repeated infections<br>Progressive marrow failure | Autoimmune cytopenias<br>Rapid doubling time (< 6 months)<br>Histological transformation | |
| **Key Concepts for Effective Treatment** | Chemotherapy has been effective alone and in combination with other agents<br>New targeted therapies have increased response rates<br>Chromosomal abnormalities have prognostic value<br>Aggressive concurrent management of infection risk is essential to effective therapy | | |
| **FDA Approved Therapies** | Bendamustine<br>Alemtuzumab<br>Melphalan | Ofatumumab | |
| **In Clinical Trials or Used Based on Other Approved Indications** | Flavopiridol<br>Oblimersen<br>Regimens used for indolent lymphomas | Rituximab<br>Lenalidomide | |
| **Key Supportive Care Concerns** | Tumor lysis syndrome<br>Infections<br>Infusion reactions | Hemolytic anemias | |

*Abbreviations*: CD, cluster of differentiation; del, deletion; IgVH, unmutated immunoglobin heavy chain; LDH, lactate dehydrogenase; t, translocation; ZAP, zeta chain (TCR) associated protein kinase 70.

*Source*: Data from Seiler et al[29]; Chiorazzi et al[30]; and NCCN.[101]

used in the initial treatment of CLL include chlorambucil, the combination of cytoxan, vincristine, and prednisone (CVP) with adriamycin added for more aggressive disease (CHOP), and fludarabine that may be used in combination with cytoxan (FC) and rituximab (FCR).

The most recent NCCN guidelines for CLL have been updated to include several agents recently approved for treatment including bendamustine, alemtuzumab, and various chemoimmunotherapy combinations with pentostatin or fludarabine (Table 57-13[51,102–106]). Alemtuzumab is considered the preferred agent for treatment of elderly patients with del(17p) mutation based on clinical response rates.[101] Bendamustine, the most recently approved drug for the treatment of CLL has dual mechanisms of action, both as a DNA-alkylating agent and as an antimetabolite purine analog—2 of the primary class of drugs used to treat CLL. It is bound to plasma proteins and blocks cells from progressing from Gap 1 to the Gap 2 phase in the cell cycle. These dual mechanisms of action appear to promote apoptosis in lymphoma cell lines.[107]

In addition, several new agents have shown promising results in clinical trials for the treatment of CLL. Lenalidomide, an immunomodulatory agent already approved for the treatment of MDS and multiple myeloma, which is discussed elsewhere, has been shown to have activity in CLL, including in patients with relapsing disease and in patients with del(11q) and del(17p), all indicating high-risk disease.[108] Oblimersen, a Bcl-2 antisense agent has been shown to generate long-lasting CRs and nodular partial remissions when combined with chemotherapy.[109] Ofatumumab is a fully humanized anti-CD20 antibody that appears effective in the presence of few antigen sites, a common characteristic in CLL.

Additional trials have studied treatment specifically in the elderly population, adding to the refinement of selecting individualized therapy to maximize therapeutic outcome and minimize toxicity. Individual risk analysis is necessary, as the most common complications of treatment include immunosuppression and recurrent or atypical infections, cytopenias, and tumor lysis syndrome. As previously noted, many of the patients with CLL are older and will be at increased risk for these complications.

## Hairy cell leukemia

Hairy cell leukemia (HCL) is a rare indolent B-cell malignancy that represents less than 2% of the lymphoid leukemias.[110] It is more common in men (male:female ratio—5:1) and the median age at presentation is 50 years.[110] Because it is so rare, with less than 1000 new cases each year, the majority of clinical trials have fewer than 50 patients.[111] The hallmark diagnostic features are hair-like projections noted on the B-cells and a "fried egg" appearance on bone marrow samples. HCL commonly infiltrates the bone marrow, spleen, and liver. Thus hepatomegaly, splenomegaly, and bone marrow fibrosis are common. Patients often present with anemia, fatigue and vague left upper quadrant pain as a result. No distinct chromosomal aberrations are known, although immunophenotyping will reveal high expression of CD45, and antigens common to the B-cell lineage (CD19, CD20, CD22, and CD79). The standard approach to treatment is use of a purine analog such as cladribine and pentostatin.[111] The overall survival of HCL patients treated with purine analogues is >80%-85% at

**TABLE 57-13**

**FDA Approved Therapies for Chronic Lymphocytic Leukemia (CLL)**

| Agent | Mechanism of Action | Dosing and Route of Administration | Common Toxicities |
|---|---|---|---|
| Alemtuzumab | Anti-CD52 monoclonal antibody | 30 mg IV 3 times per week for 4–12 weeks | Infusion reactions<br>Myelosuppression<br>Lymphopenia<br>Hemolytic anemia: rare |
| Bendamustine | Combined alkylating agent and purine analog | 100 mg/m² IV on days 1 and 2 repeated every 28 days | Myelosuppression<br>Mild gastrointestinal upset |
| Chlorambucil | Alkylating agent | Variable dosing<br>Administered orally | Myelosuppression<br>Late effects: secondary malignancies |
| Fludarabine | Purine analog | 25 mg/m² days 1–5 every 28 days as a single agent<br>Variable dosing in combination regimens | Myelosuppression<br>Infections<br>Hemolytic uremic syndrome: rare |
| Pentostatin | Purine analog | Used in combination regimens<br>4 mg/m² IV on day 1, repeated every 28 days | Myelosuppression<br>Infections<br>Lymphopenia |
| Rituximab | Anti-CD20 monoclonal antibody | Split dosing recommended with initial dose: 50 mg/m² day 1, and 325 mg/m² day 2<br>Standard dosing in subsequent cycles of 375 mg/m²<br>Repeated every 28 days | Infusion reactions<br>Reactivation of hepatitis B<br>Rare mucocutaneous reactions |

*Source:* Data from Abbott and Estey[51]; Genzyme Corp[102]; Cephalon Inc[103]; Ben Venue Laboratories[104]; Pentostatin[105]; and Genentech Inc.[106]

>8–10 years of follow up. Resistant cases can be treated with rituximab.

## TREATMENT STRATEGIES FOR MYELODYSPLASTIC SYNDROMES

### General considerations

Supportive care has been the mainstay of treatment for myleodysplastic syndromes (MDS) over the last 20 years. Until recently, no active therapies were available. Supportive care continues to be important in treatment of symptoms associated with the disease or toxicities of newly developed active therapies. Supportive care includes observation, quality of life assessment, growth factors, antibiotics, iron chelation therapies, and transfusion support. However, it is important to recognize that supportive care measures do not change the underlying disease. (Table 57-14[58,59,110])

The goals of therapy for MDS are based on individualized disease characteristics, patient characteristics, and risk category. Current treatment guidelines are no longer based on age and performance status. Transfusion dependence or progressive or symptomatic cytopenias generally indicate the need for active therapy. For low-risk disease the goals are to improve hematopoiesis, improve quality of life, and minimize toxicity. In high-risk disease, the goal is survival. These patients are at high risk for early transformation to acute leukemia and generally require immediate and aggressive therapy. De-novo MDS is associated with a more favorable outcome when compared to treatment-induced MDS, which is associated with poor response to standard therapies. Three agents have been approved by the FDA since May, 2004, for the active treatment of MDS: azacitidine (approved May, 2004) and decitabine (approved May, 2006), both DNA methylation inhibitors, and lenalidomide (approved December, 2005), an oral agent that has several mechanisms of action and is considered an immunomodulatory agent. Complete disease evaluation is necessary to select the best available therapy for the individual patient. Patients with low serum erythropoietin levels and low transfusion requirements may benefit from erythropoietin stimulating proteins. Lenalidomide is the treatment of choice for patient with del 5q.[110] A small subset of patients who are positive for HLA-DR15 may benefit from administration of anti-thymocyte globulin (ATG). Hypomethylating agents are the treatment of choice for patients with intermediate-2 or high-risk disease or in patients with intermediate 1-risk disease not meeting the previous characteristics. Other agents have been used clinically in the treatment of MDS, including thalidomide and ATO. Each agent has been shown to have some activity in the reduction of transfusions and changes in cytogenetic findings. Several other agents are being studied in ongoing clinical trials or in combination with existing agents.

Each agent has specific potential toxicities and nursing implications. (Table 57-15[112-114]) The most common treatment-related toxicity for active therapies for MDS is myelosuppression. Most therapies require a minimum of 3 to 4 months of treatment to fully evaluate efficacy. Therefore, aggressive management of cytopenias is a critical component of effective treatment.

Transfusion independence, cytogenetic remission, and improvement in quality of life have become the desired end points for clinical trials for MDS. Transfusion independence not only improves the quality of life for MDS patients, but decreases secondary organ effects and decreases the economic and clinical burden. Cytogenetic responses have been shown to correlate with improved survival in patients with chromosome 5q deletion.[115] Maturing data have shown improvement in the overall survival of patients receiving azacitidine for high-risk MDS, compared with supportive care alone.[116] Survival was not dependent of a complete response.[117] Transfusion dependence is common in patients with MDS and secondary iron overload is associated with several negative effects. Administration of iron-chelation therapy is a key supportive care strategy and requires specific monitoring for safe administration. Allogeneic HSCT remains the only potentially curative treatment for MDS and may be considered in younger patients who have a suitable donor.[118]

## SYMPTOM MANAGEMENT AND SUPPORTIVE CARE

Supportive care is an integral component of an effective individualized cancer treatment plan that minimizes potential toxicities, maximizes therapeutic outcomes, and maintains optimal quality of life for the patient. Anemia, neutropenia, thrombocytopenia, and mucositis are some of the most common toxicities associated with treatment of the hematologic malignancies. They may result in dose reductions, dose delays, premature discontinuation of therapy, and increases in morbidity and mortality. Other common treatment related toxicities are summarized in Table 57-16.[58-59]

Myelosuppression is the most common adverse event as most therapies require marrow hypoplasia to effectively suppress the malignant clone. The duration and severity of cytopenias vary based on the status of the underlying disease including tumor burden and subtype, history of prior therapies, and agents used for treatment. Recent advances in transfusion medicine, the availability of cytokine therapies for anemia and neutropenia, and improved awareness of risk factors and early signs and symptoms of toxicity have improved clinical outcomes. In many cases, effective management of these toxicities has allowed patients to be treated in an outpatient setting. Thrombocytopenia is another common complication of cancer and cancer treatment and

**TABLE 57-14**

**Disease Overview: Myelodysplastic Syndromes (MDS)**

| Feature | Key Findings | | |
|---|---|---|---|
| **Epidemiology** | **Incidence:** 15,000–20,000 new cases/year, with 35,000–50,000 existing cases<br>**Average Age at Diagnosis**: 70 years | | |
| **Etiology** | Genetic instability<br>Chemical exposure<br>Tobacco | Mutagens<br>Autoimmune disease<br>Unknown in the majority of cases (~80%) | |
| **Stem Cell Defect:**<br>Myeloid progenitor cell | **Intrinsic Factors:**<br>Malignant clone<br>Cytogenetic abnormalities<br>Epigenetic DNA modification | **Extrinsic Factors:**<br>Bone marrow microenvironment<br>Stromal dysregulation<br>Cytokine abnormalities<br>Imbalance of apoptosis and proliferation | |
| **Chromosomal Findings:**<br>Cytogenetic abnormality present in ~50% | **Favorable**<br>-Y, del 5q, -20q | **Intermediate Risk**<br>+8 and other | **Poor Risk**<br>Complex (> 3 abnormalities)<br>Chromosome 7 abnormalities: 7q, -7, del 7p;<br>inv16, t(8:12) implies diagnosis of AML |
| **Additional Prognostic Factors Indicating High-Risk Disease** | Increased blast cells (> 20% implies leukemic transformation)<br>Increased transfusion burden (> 2 units in 4 weeks)<br>CD7 or CD56 expression by flow cytometry<br>Atypical localization of immature precursors (ALIP)<br>Ongoing analysis of more sensitive testing for chromosomal and molecular attributes<br>Severe thrombocytopenia or neutropenia | | |
| **Staging** | FAB/WHO (morphology) and IPSS/WPSS (risk stratification) | | |
| **Response Criteria** | International Working Group (IWG) Criteria 2006 | | |
| **Disease Characteristics**<br>(All are incurable) | **Low-Intermediate 1 Risk**<br>Indolent course<br>Low probability of leukemic transformation | **Intermediate-High 2 Risk**<br>Progressive course with early transformation to acute leukemia | |
| **Clinical Presentation** | Cytopenias: anemia most common, infection, fatigue, bleeding | | |
| **Indication to Treat** | Transfusion dependence, progressive cytopenias, increased blasts | | |
| **Key Concepts for Effective Treatment** | Supportive care alone does not prevent disease progression (no effect on the underlying disease)<br>Active therapies for MDS generally require a minimum of 3–4 months to achieve a response; premature discontinuation may limit the potential for an optimal response<br>Aggressive concurrent management of cytopenias is essential to effective therapy<br>Treatment goals: reduce transfusion requirements, delay time to leukemic transformation and improve quality of life<br>Chromosomal abnormalities have prognostic value | | |
| **FDA Approved Therapies** | Azacitidine<br>Decitabine<br>Lenalidomide | | |
| **In Clinical Trials or Used Based on Other Approved Indications** | TLK199<br>Src family kinase inhibitors<br>Clofarabine | Arsenic trioxide<br>Valproic acid<br>Thalidomide | |
| **Key Supportive Care Concerns** | Iron overload, injection site reactions, cytopenias and infections, gastrointestinal toxicities | | |

*Abbreviations*: CD, cluster of differentiation; del, deletion; inv, inversion; IPSS, International Prognostic Scoring System; WHO, World Health Organization; WPSS, WHO-classification based Prognostic Scoring System.

*Source*: Data from Kurtin[57]; Kurtin.[58]; and Revlimid (lenalidomide) prescribing information.[112]

**TABLE 57-15**

**FDA Approved Therapies for Myelodysplastic Syndromes (MDS)**

| Agent | Mechanism of Action | Dosing and Route of Administration | Common Toxicities |
|---|---|---|---|
| Lenalidomide | Immunomodulatory and antiangiogenic | 10 mg/day continuous or days 1–21 every 28 days | Myelosuppression<br>Pruritus (mild)<br>Safety program for potential teratogenicity: RevAssist<br>Diarrhea (mild) |
| Azacitidine | Demethylating agent | 75 mg/m²/day SC or IV days 1–7 every 28 days for a minimum of 4 cycles or until disease progression<br>Alternative dosing regimens in recent trials | Myelosuppression<br>Injection site erythema<br>Nausea and vomiting<br>Transient elevation of transaminases<br>Low-grade fevers<br>Contraindicated in patients with sensitivity to mannitol or with extensive hepatic disease |
| Decitabine | Demethylating agent | 15 mg/m²/day IV over 3 hours q 8 hours days 1–3 every 6 weeks<br>20mg/m² IV over one hour days 1–5 every 28 days.<br>Alternative dosing regimens in recent trials | Myelosuppression: neutropenia, thrombocytopenia, leukopenia<br>Nausea and vomiting<br>Transient elevation of transaminases<br>Infections<br>Contraindicated in patients with extensive hepatic disease |

*Abbreviations*: IV, intravenous; SC, subcutaneous.

*Source*: Data from Revlimid (lenalidomide) prescribing information[112]; and Pharmion.[113]

increases the risk of bleeding for the patient. Standards for treatment rely primarily on platelet transfusions or changes in therapy to reduce the incidence. Oncology nurses can assist the patient by providing instruction for bleeding precautions, avoidance of medications such as aspirin or alcohol that may precipitate bleeding, and immediate reporting of uncontrolled bleeding or bruising.

Mucositis and gastrointestinal toxicities are also common during therapy for AML and ALL, in large part due to the specific agents and doses used for treatment. Mucositis in the presence of sustained neutropenia is a significant risk factor for systemic bacteremia. Close monitoring for fever or other subtle signs of infection with prompt initiation of antibiotic therapies and other supportive measures will reduce the mortality associated with febrile neutropenia. Most interventions for treatment of mucositis have been focused on pain management, improved nutritional support (enteral and parenteral feedings), and prevention of secondary infections (oral rinses, antibiotics, and antifungals). The recent development of cytoprotective agents provides hope for prevention of severe oral mucositis. However, these agents are not likely to eliminate the need for effective oral hygiene regimens. Patients should be instructed in the use of a mucolytic rinse such as bicarbonate solution, followed by a normal saline rinse throughout the day. Antibacterial, antifungal, antihistamine, and topical anesthetic agents may be used if indicated; however, chronic use of these agents may be associated with adverse secondary effects such as drying of the mucosa.

Tumor lysis syndrome (TLS) is a potentially life-threatening metabolic disorder that develops as a result of cell lysis most commonly seen with bulky disease or aggressive tumors with the initiation of therapy. Intracellular molecules (potassium, nucleic acids, phosphorus) are released into the extracellular fluids with resulting electrolyte imbalances (hyperkalemia, hyperphosphatemia, hyperuricemia, and hypocalcemia), and secondary systemic effects. If untreated, patients can develop acute renal failure and cardiac arrhythmia, with the potential for cardiac arrest. Patients with rapidly dividing or bulky lymphoproliferative disorders, such as CLL, are at particular risk. Baseline laboratory analysis and frequent monitoring during therapy is necessary in the first 48 to 72 hours after treatment to allow effective management. Patients at high risk should be treated in an inpatient setting, where renal dialysis and cardiac support services are readily available. Prophylactic treatment with allopurinol instituted 24 to 48 hours prior to therapy is effective in the majority of patients. Rasburicase, a potent IV uric acid–lowering formulation is indicated for patients with TLS prior to initiating treatment or in those who have rapidly dividing tumors. Intensive management in the

**TABLE 57-16**

**Nursing Management of Common Disease or Treatment Related Toxicities**

| Clinical Findings | Signs and Symptoms | Nursing Considerations |
|---|---|---|
| Anemia | Fatigue, dyspnea, dizziness, tachycardia, palpitations | Transfusion management:<br>Patients with underlying cardiac disease are at increased risk for CHF exacerbation and may require diuresis with transfusions<br>Benefits are temporary and rarely restore hematocrit (Hct) to normal<br>Transfusions should be based on symptoms not general hemoglobin (Hgb) or Hct parameters<br>Monitoring for iron overload in transfusion dependent patients and need for iron chelation therapy (initiate at ferritin >1000 ng/mL)<br>Administration of erythropoietin agents for MDS patients with serum erythropoietin (epo) level < 500 or who require > 4 units of PRBCs every 8 weeks<br>Careful monitoring for safety in administration of erythropoietin agents in patients at risk for thrombotic events<br>Initiate active therapies for transfusion dependent MDS patients with serum epo level > 500 or PRBCs > 2 units/4 weeks<br>Assist the patient in maintaining a flow sheet for lab results and transfusion dates, blood type, and any antibodies. |
| Neutropenia | Fever, cough, dysuria, abdominal pain or diarrhea | Early recognition of infections<br>Patient education for infection precautions and reportable signs and symptoms<br>Patients receiving active therapies may require drug holiday and dose adjustment<br>Monitoring of CBC, differential and platelet count daily for initial treatment of acute leukemia, weekly for the first 8 weeks for active therapies in CML and MDS, and at varied intervals for the treatment of CLL based on the disease and specific treatment<br>Administration of recombinant granulocyte growth factors<br>Should not be administered on the same day of cytotoxic agents<br>Antimicrobial therapy for active infections; prophylactic antibiotics are not generally recommended to avoid resistance |
| Thrombocytopenia | Petechiae, ecchymosis, epistaxis, hemoptysis, hematuria | Platelet transfusions based on risk of bleeding (platelets < 10,000 $mm^3$ or active bleeding)<br>Careful monitoring of concomitant medications with antiplatelet effect<br>Patient education for bleeding precautions, emergency management and reportable signs and symptoms<br>Aminocaproic acid may be used in transfusion refractory patients<br>Thrombopoiesis stimulating proteins currently in clinical trials<br>Patients receiving active therapies may require drug holiday and dose adjustment |
| Iron chelation for hemosiderosis (iron overload) | Elevated hepatic enzymes, fatigue, confusion, CHF, vague abdominal bloating and pain, MRI findings of iron overload of the liver | Institute iron chelation therapy for serum ferritin > 1000 ng/mL<br>Selected patients responding to active therapies may benefit from phlebotomy<br>Safety monitoring for iron chelation therapy; renal toxicity; increase in serum creatinine, rare cases of acute renal failure reported, and intermittent proteinuria<br>Baseline and regular monitoring of renal function<br>Hepatotoxicity: elevated transaminase levels<br>Baseline and regular monitoring of hepatic function<br>Pancytopenia: neutropenia, agranulocytosis, thrombocytopenia reported in MDS patients<br>Baseline and regular monitoring of CBC, differential, and platelet count<br>Auditory: high-frequency hearing loss, decreased hearing<br>Baseline and yearly audiology evaluation<br>Ocular: cataracts, lens opacities, increased pressure, retinal disorders<br>Baseline and yearly slit-eye and fundoscopic exam |

(Continued)

**TABLE 57-16**

**Nursing Management of Common Disease or Treatment Related Toxicities (*Continued*)**

| Clinical Findings | Signs and Symptoms | Nursing Considerations |
|---|---|---|
| Tumor lysis syndrome | Hyperkalemia<br>Hyperphosphatemia<br>Hypocalcemia<br>Hyperuricemia<br>Cardiac arrhythmias<br>Acute renal failure | Monitor: comprehensive metabolic profile, LDH, uric acid, phosphorus<br>Clinical observation: vital signs, weight, edema, intake and output<br>Hydration: begin 24–48 hours pre-therapy, continue 48–72 hours post-therapy if high risk<br>ECG: if hyperkalemia<br>Allopurinol: 300–900 mg/day (renal function)<br>Rasburicase: 50–100 U/kg/day (contraindicated if glucose-6-phosphate dehydrogenase [G-6-PD] deficient)<br>Oral phosphate binders: amphogel<br>Hemodialysis |
| Bleeding diatheses or coagulopathy | Bleeding<br>Mucocutaneous hemorrhage<br>Thrombosis<br>Disseminated intravascular coagulation | Common with initial therapy for APL when using differentiating agents (ATRA, ATO)<br>Baseline coagulation studies including PT, PTT, fibrinogen<br>Administration of coagulation factors and fibrinogen: cryoprecipitate, platelets, and fresh frozen plasma<br>Maintain fibrinogen above 150 mg/dL<br>Maintain platelets above 30,000 $mm^3$ |
| Mucositis<br>Typhlitis | Oral ulceration and pain<br>Rectal pain and ulceration or abscess | Most often associated with higher doses of cytarabine and anthracyclines<br>Cytoprotective agents may be used in the bone marrow transplant setting<br>Oral hygiene regimens using a mucolytic agent (bicarbonate solution) followed by a normal saline rinse can reduce discomfort and secondary infection<br>Medicated rinses may be used for active infection or for pain management<br>Evaluation of rectal pain is necessary to exclude the presence of a rectal abscess in patients treated with high-dose cytarabine |
| Central nervous system toxicities | Ataxia<br>Confusion<br>Impaired hand–eye coordination<br>Sensory deficits | Cerebellar toxicity is a dose-limiting toxicity with high-dose cytarabine and dose reductions are recommended in older patients<br>Daily neurological evaluations should be conducted and treatment should be held in the presence of changes<br>Peripheral neuropathies are uncommon with the exception of long-term treatment with vincristine in ALL |
| Cutaneous toxicities | Painful plantar and palmar erythema<br>Blistering or desquamation if severe | Acral erythema is a possible complication of high-dose cytarabine.<br>Drug-related rashes are common with antibiotics, allopurinol, and selected active therapies; baseline assessment and ongoing monitoring are essential<br>Leukemia cutis may be present at the time of diagnosis<br>Fungal infections may be associated with skin infiltrates; infiltrates should be biopsied to determine the underlying abnormality (disease vs infectious) |
| Cardiotoxicity | Congestive heart failure<br>Cardiomyopathy<br>QT prolongation and torsades de pointe | Baseline cardiac evaluation including an echocardiogram or MUGA scan<br>Baseline ECG and repeated testing at regular intervals is necessary for ATO and TKI therapy to evaluate QTc interval; treatment should be held for QTc > 500 milliseconds<br>Careful medication review is necessary to identify agents that are associated with QT prolongation<br>Evaluate patients at high risk: cumulative anthracycline dose, history of prior radiotherapy to the chest, and underlying cardiovascular disease |
| Ocular toxicities | Keratoconjunctivitis | Prophylactic administration of steroid eye drops when using doses of Cytarabine of > 2 $gm/m^2$<br>Should begin eye drops 24 hours prior to and continue 48 hours beyond the last dose of cytarabine |

*Abbreviations*: ALL, acute lymphocytic leukemia; APL, acute promyelocytic leukemia; ATO, arsenic trioxide; ATRA, all-transretinoic acid; CHF, congestive heart failure; CLL, chronic lymphocytic leukemia; CML, chronic myeloid leukemia; ECG, electrocardiogram; LDH, lactate dehydrogenase; MDS, myelodysplastic syndrome; MRI, magnetic resonance imaging; MUGA, multigated acquisition scan; PRBCs, packed red blood cells; PT, prothrombin time; PTT, partial thromboplastin time; TKI, tyrosine kinase inhibitor.

*Source*: Data from Kurtin[57]; and Kurtin.[58]

first few days following therapy may be necessary. Most patients can be effectively treated with no sustained renal or cardiac abnormalities and will be at a lower risk with subsequent treatments due to decreased tumor burden.

## CONCLUSION

Strategies for the diagnosis, risk stratification and treatment of hematological malignancies, leukemia and MDS, have expanded at an unparalleled rate offering improved response rates, overall survival, and disease control for patients. Numerous clinical trials are ongoing that offer promising therapies for future use either as single agents or in combinations. Refinement of the diagnostic evaluation and application of prognostic criteria for these disorders has shifted the treatment paradigm from general intensive therapy to selective treatment based on the individual disease and the unique attributes of the patient. Several challenges remain as the rate of scientific discovery has outpaced generalized clinical application. Patient enrolment in clinical trials will be critical to refine the application of molecular and genetic factors in risk analysis and treatment selection. The concept of minimal residual disease, which has been verified for CML and APL does not appear to apply to MDS. Therefore the goal of treatment in each disease may be different based on the current understanding of response vs survival and emphasizes the heterogenicity of these disorders. The consistency and quality of tissue and blood specimens, standardized testing for analysis, and development of clinical guidelines for their use will continue to present a challenge for clinical trials, analysis, and treatment application. Treatment guidelines are likely to be modified frequently as new data emerge. Oncology nurses play a critical role in the daily assessment, treatment, and management of patients with hematological diseases. Understanding novel mechanisms of antitumor activity, associated toxicities, and clinical management strategies for these new therapies is critical to safe and effective management of patients receiving them. Concurrent supportive care is critical to allow continuation of effective therapies. Consideration of the unique characteristics of the individual patient using a life span approach will facilitate individualized treatment strategies.

## REFERENCES


1. Global Cancer Facts and Figures. 2007. http://www.cancer.org/docroot/STT/content/STT_1x_Global_Cancer_Facts_and_Figures_2007.aspAccessed January 9, 2010.
2. American Cancer Society Facts & Figures. 2009. http://www.cancer.org/docroot/STT/stt_0_2008.asp?sitearea=STT&level=1. Accessed January 9, 2010.
3. Surveillance, Epidemiology, and End Results (SEER) Program (www.seer.cancer.gov) SEER* Stat Database: Incidence–SEER 9 Regs Limited-Use, Nov 2008 Sub (1973–2006) http://seer.cancer.gov/index.html. Accessed October 1, 2009.
4. Rollison D, Howlander N, Smith M, et al. Epidemiology of myelodysplastic syndromes and chronic myeloproliferative disorders in the United States, 2001–2004, using data from the NAACCR and SEER programs. *Blood*. 2008;112:45–52.
5. Alvarez RH, Kantarjan H, Cortes JE. The biology of chronic myelogenous leukemia: implications for imantinib therapy. *Semin Hematol.* 2007;44:4–14.
6. Quintas-Cardama A, Cortes J. Chronic myeloid leukemia: diagnosis and treatment. *Mayo Clin Proc*. 2006;81:973–988.
7. Yee K, Obrien S. Chronic lymphyocytic leukemia: diagnosis and treatment. *Mayo Clin Proc*. 2006;81:1105–1129.
8. Mufti G, List AF, Gore SD, et al. Myelodysplastic syndrome. *Hematology*. 2003;176–199.
9. Le Beau MM, Albain KS, Larson RA, et al. Clinical and cytogenetic correlations in 63 patients with therapy-related myelodysplastic syndromes and acute nonlymphocytic leukemia: further evidence for characteristic abnormalities of chromosomes no. 5 and 7. *J Clin Oncol.* 1986;4:325–345.
10. Pogoda JM, Preston-Martin S, Nichols PW, Ross RK. Smoking and risk of acute myeloid leukemia: results from a Los Angeles County case–control study. *Am J Epidemiol*. 2002;155:546–553.
11. Pederson-Bjergaard J, Christiansen DH, Andersen MK, Skovby F. Causality of myelodypslasia and acute myeloid leukemia and their genetic abnormalities. *Leukemia*. 2002;16:2177–2184.
12. Jabour E, Estey E, Kantarjan H. Adult acute myeloid leukemia: diagnosis and treatment. *Mayo Clin Proc*. 2006;81:247–260.
13. Deschler B, Lubbert M. Acute myeloid leukemia: epidemiology and etiology. *Cancer*. 2006;107:2099–2107.
14. Corey SJ, Minden MD, Barber DL, Kantarjan H, Wang JC, Schimmer AD. Myelodysplastic syndromes; the complexity of stem cell diseases. *Nat Rev*. 2007;7:118–129.
15. Haase D, Germing U, Schanz J, et al. New insights into the prognostic impact of the karyotype in MDS and correlation with subtypes: evidence from a core dataset of 2124 patients. *Blood*. 2007;110: 4385–4395.
16. Byrd JC, Mrozek K, Dodge RK, et al. Pre-treatment cytogenetic abnormalities are predictive of induction success, cumulative incidence of relapse, and overall survival in adult patients with denovo acute myeloid leukemia: results from Cancer and Leukemia Group B (CALBG 8461) *Blood*. 2002;100:4325–4336.
17. Mrozek K. Cytogenetic, molecular genetic, and clinical characteristics of acute myeloid leukemia with a complex karyotype. *Semin Oncol.* 2008;35:365–437.
18. Frohling S, Dohner H. Chromosomal abnormalities in cancer. *N Engl J Med*. 2008;359:722–734.
19. Plass C, Oakes C, Blum W, Marcucci G. Epigenetics in acute myeloid leukemia. *Semin Oncol*. 2008;35:378–387.
20. Leone G, Teofili L, Voso MT, et al. DNA methylation and demethylating drugs in myelodysplastic syndromes and secondary leukemia's. *Haematologica*. 2002;87:1324–1341.
21. Jiang Y, Dunbar A, Godnek L, Mohan S, et al. Abberrant DNA methylation is a dominant mechanism in MDS progression to AML. *Blood*. 2009;113:1315–1325.
22. Rice KL, Hormaeche I, Licht JD. Epigenetic regulation of normal and malignant hematopoiesis. *Oncogene*. 2007;26:6697–6714.
23. Kantarjan HM, Deisseroth A, Kurzock R, Estrov Z, Talpaz M. Chronic myelogenous leukemia: a concise update. *Blood*. 1993;82:691–703.
24. Lee S, Kim SJ, Min CK, et al. The effect of first-line imatinib interim therapy on the outcome of allogeneic stem cell transplantation in adults with newly diagnosed Philadelphia chromosome-positive acute lymphoblastic leukemia. *Blood*. 2005;105:3449–3457.
25. Lo-Coco F, Ammatuna E, Montesinos P, Sanz MA. Acute pro-myelocytic leukemia: recent advances in diagnosis and management. *Semin Oncol*. 2008;35:401–409.
26. Dohner H. Implication of the molecular characterization of acute myeloid leukemia. *Hematology*. 2007;412–419.

27. Bacher U, Haferlach, Kern W, Haferlach T, Schnittger S. Prognostic relevance of FLT3-TKD mutations in AML: the combination matters—an analysis of 3082 patients. *Blood.* 2008;111:2527–2537.
28. Burnett A, Knapper S. Targeting treatment in AML. *Hematology.* 2007;429–434.
29. Seiler T, Dohner H, Stilgenbauer S. Risk stratification in chronic lymphocytic leukemia. *Semin Oncol.* 2006; 33;186–194.
30. Chiorazzi N, Rai K, Ferrarini M. Chronic lymphocytic leukemia. *N Engl J Med.* 2005;352:804–815.
31. Aizawa S, Nakano M, IwaseO, et al. Bone marrow stroma from refractory anemia of myelodysplastic syndrome is defective in its ability to support normal CD34 positive cell proliferation and differentiation in vitro. *Leuk Res.* 2004;99:239–246.
32. Delauney J, Vey N, Leblanc T, et al. Prognosis of (inv)(IL)/t(16;16) acute leukemia: a survey of 110 cases from the French AML Intergroup. *Blood.* 2003;102:462–469.
33. Arber D, Stein AS, Carter NH, et al. Prognostic impact of acute myeloid leukemia classification. *Am J Clin Pathol.* 2003;119:672–680.
34. Vardiman JW, Brunning RD, Arber DA, et al. Introduction and overview of the classification of the myeloid neoplasms. In: Swerdlow S, Campo E, Harris N, et al, eds. *World Health Organization: World Health Organization Classification of the Tumours of the Hematopoietic and Lymphoid Tissues.* Geneva: World Health Organization; 2008:18–30.
35. Scheinberg D, Masiak P, Weiss M. Management of acute leukemias. In: DeVita VT Jr, Hellman S, Rosenberg SA, eds. *Cancer: Principles and Practice of Oncology.* Philadelphia: Lippincott, Williams & Wilkins; 2005:2088–2120.
36. Arber DA, Brunning RD, LeBeau MM, et al. Acute myeloid leukemia with recurrent genetic abnormalities. In: Swerdlow S, Campo E, Harris N, et al, eds. *World Health Organization: World Health Organization Classification of the Tumours of the Hematopoietic and Lymphoid Tissues.* Geneva: World Health Organization; 2008:110–123.
37. Arber DA, Brunning RD, Orazi A, et al. Acute myeloid leukemia, not otherwise specified. In: Swerdlow S, Campo E, Harris N, et al, eds. *World Health Organization: World Health Organization Classification of the Tumours of the Hematopoietic and Lymphoid Tissues.* Geneva: World Health Organization; 2008:137–141.
38. Borowitz MJ, Chan JKC. B lymphoblastic leukemia/lymphoma with recurrent genetic abnormalities. In: Swerdlow S, Campo E, Harris N, et al, eds. *World Health Organization: World Health Organization Classification of the Tumours of the Hematopoietic and Lymphoid Tissues.* Geneva: World Health Organization; 2008:171–175.
39. Borowitz MJ, Chan JKC. T Lymphoblastic leukemia/lymphoma. In: Swerdlow S, Campo E, Harris N, et al, eds. *World Health Organization: World Health Organization Classification of the Tumours of the Hematopoietic and Lymphoid Tissues.* Geneva: World Health Organization; 2008:176–178.
40. Brunning RD, Razi A, Germing U, et al. Myelodysplastic syndromes/neoplasms, overview. In: Swerdlow S, Campo E, Harris N, et al, eds. *World Health Organization: World Health Organization Classification of the Tumours of the Hematopoietic and Lymphoid Tissues.* Geneva: World Health Organization; 2008:88–93.
41. Harris N, Jaffe E, Diebold J, et al. World Health Organization of neoplastic diseases of the hematopoietic and lymphoid tissues: report of the Clinical Advisory Committee meeting—Airlie House, Virginia, November 1997. *J Clin Oncol.* 1999;17:3835–3849.
42. Vardiman J, Harris N, Brunning RD, et al. The World Health Organization (WHO) classification of the myeloid neoplasms. *Blood.* 2002;100:2292–2302.
43. Larson R, Anastasi J. Acute lymphoblastic leukemia: clinical presentation, diagnosis, and classification. In: Estey E, Faderl S, Kantarjan H, eds. *Hematologic Malignancies: Acute Leukemias.* Berlin Heidelberg, NY: Springer; 2008:109–118.
44. Head D, Thompson MA. Diagnosis and classification of the acute myeloid leukemias (with discussion of the role of the myelodysplastic syndromes in AML pathogensis). In: Estey E, Faderl S, Kantarjan H, eds. *Hematologic Malignancies: Acute Leukemias.* Berlin Heidelberg, NY: Springer; 2008:21–43.
45. Greenberg P, Cox C, LeBeau M, et al. International scoring system for evaluating prognosis in myelodysplastic syndromes. *Blood.* 1997;89:2079.
46. Haase D, Germing U, Schanz J, et al. New insights into the prognostic impact of the karyotype in MDS and correlation with subtypes: evidence from a core dataset of 2124 patients. *Blood.* 2007;110:4385–4395.
47. Nimer S. Myelodysplastic syndromes. *Blood.* 2008;11:4841–4851.
48. Malcovati L, Germing U, Kuendgen A, et al. Time-dependent prognostic scoring system for predicting survival and leukemic evolution in myelodysplastic syndromes. *J Clin Oncol.* 2007;25:3503–3510.
49. Kao J, McMillan A, Greenberg P. International MDS risk analysis workshop (IMRAW)/IPSS reanlalyzed: impact of cytopenias on clinical outcomes in myelodysplastic syndromes. *Am J Hematol.* 2008;83:765–770.
50. Seiler T, Dohner H, Stilgenbauer S. Risk stratification in chronic lymphocytic leukemia. *Semin Oncol.* 2006;33:186–194.
51. Abbott B, Estey E. Management of myelodysplastic syndromes. *Oncology.* 2008;12:1360.
52. Smith M, Boldt D. Hematological malignancies: current perspectives on diagnosis, prognosis, and treatment. *Oncology.* 2008;22:9–31.
53. Rai K, Sawitsky A, Cronkite E, et al. Clinical staging of chronic lymphocytic leukemia. *Blood.* 1975;46:219–234.
54. Binet JL, AuquierA, Dighiero G, et al. A new prognostic classification of chronic lumphocytic leukemia derived from a multivariate survival analysis. *Cancer.* 1981;48:198–206.
55. Calabretta B, Perotti D. The biology of blast crisis. *Blood.* 2004;103:11, 4010–4022.
56. Cortes JE, Talpaz M, Obrien S, et al. Staging of chronic myeloid leukemia in the imantinib era: an evaluation of the World Health Organization Proposal. *Cancer.* 2006;106:1306–1315.
57. Kurtin SE. Myelodysplastic syndromes: diagnosis, treatment planning, and clinical management. *Oncology: Nurse Edition.* 2007;21:41–48. http://cancernetwork.com/oncology/showArticle.jhtmlarticleId=202402608. Accessed January 9, 2010.
58. Kurtin S. Updates and strategies for the management of MDS, CLL, and MM. Meniscus Educational Institute. August 2008. https://www.meniscus.com/mds-cll-mm Accessed October 1, 2009.
59. Sekeres M, Elson P, Kalaycio M, Advani A, et al. Time from diagnosis to treatment initiation predicts survival in younger, but not older, acute myeloid leukemia patients. *Blood.* 2009;113:28–36.
60. Green JM, Hacker ED. Chemotherapy in the geriatric population. *Clin J Oncol Nurs.* 2004;8:591–597.
61. Berger A. Bone marrow function decline with aging. *Oncol Support Care Q.* 2003;2:22–31.
62. Van Cleave J. Supportive care of the elderly patient with cancer. *Oncol Support Care Q.* 2003;2:44–59.
63. Estey E. Acute myeloid leukemia and myelodysplatic syndromes in the older patient. *J Clin Oncol.* 2007;25:1908–1915.
64. Erba H. Prognostic factors in elderly patients with AML and the implications for treatment. *Hematology.* 2007;7:420–428.
65. Stone RM, O'Donnell M, Sekeres M. Acute myeloid leukemia. *Hematology.* 2004;98–117.
66. Applebaum FR, Gundacker H, Head D, Slovak M,Willman C, Godwin J, Petersdorft S. Age and acute leukemia. *Blood.* 2006;107:3481–3485.
67. Laubach J, Rao A. Current and emerging strategies for the management of acute myeloid leukemia in the elderly. *Oncologist.* 2008;13:1097–1108.
68. NCCN practice guidelines in oncology:acute myeloid leukemia v2.2009. http://www.nccn.org/professionals/physician_gls/PDF/aml.pdf. Accessed, January 9, 2010.
69. Tallman S. New strategies in the treatment of acute myeloid leukemia including antibodies and other novel agents. *Hematology.* 2005;143–150.
70. Kern W, Estey EH. High dose cytosine arabinoside in induction treatment of acute myeloid leukemia: meta-analysis of three trials involving 1691 randomized patients [abstract 581]. *Blood.* 2008;pt1:155a.

71. Cheson BD, Bennett J, Kopecky KJ, et al. Revised recommendations of the international working group for diagnosis, standardization of response criteria, treatment outcomes, and reporting standards for therapeutic trials in acute myeloid leukemia. *J Clin Oncol.* 2003;21:4642–4649.
72. Atallah E, Cortes J, Obrien S, et al. Establishment of baseline toxicity expectations with standard frontline chemotherapy in acute myelogenous leukemia. *Blood.* 2007;110:3547–3551.
73. Klepin H, Balducci L. Acute myelogenous leukemia in older adults. *Oncologist.* 2009;14:222–232.
74. Yanada M, Matsuo K, Emi N, Naoe T. Efficacy of allogeneic hematopoietic stem cell transplantation depends on cytogenetic risk for acute myeloid leukemia in first disease remission: a meta-analysis. *Cancer.* 2005;103:1652–1658.
75. Collins RH Jr, Shpilberg O, Drobyski WR, et al. Donor leukocyte infusions in 140 patients with relapsed malignancy after allogeneic bone marrow transplantation. *J Clin Oncol.* 1997;15:433–444.
76. Chan WI, Huntly B. Leukemia stem cells in acute myeloid leukemia. *Semin Oncol.* 2008;35:326–335.
77. Freeman S, Jovanovic J, Grimwalde D. Development of minimal residual disease-directed therapy in acute myeloid leukemia. *Semin Oncol.* 2008;35:388–400.
78. Estey E. Therapy of AML. In: Leukemias. 2008.
79. Wang ZY, Chen Z. Acute promyleocytic leukemia: from highly fatal to highly curable. *Blood.* 2008;111:2505–2515.
80. Barbui T, Finazzi G, Falanga A. The impact of all-trans-retinoic acid on the coagulopathy of acute promyelocytic leukemia. *Blood.* 1998;91: 3093–3102.
81. Pui CH, Evans W. Treatment of acute lymphoblastic leukemia. *N Engl J Med.* 2006;354:166–178.
82. Moorman A, Harrison C, Buck G, Richards S. Karyotype is an independent prognostic factor in adult acute lymphoblastic leukemia (ALL): analysis of cytogenetic data from patients treated on the Medical Research Council (MRC) UKALLII/Eastern Cooperative Oncology Group (ECOG) 2993 trial. *Blood.* 2007;109:3189–3197.
83. Pullarkart V, Slovak M, Kopecky K, Forman S, Appelbaum F. Impact of cytogenetics on the outcome of adult acute lymphoblastic leukemia: results of Southwest Oncology Group 9400 study. *Blood.* 2008;111:2563–2572.
84. Hugnet F, Leguay T, Raffoux et al. Pediatric inspired therapy in adults with Philadelphia chromosome-negative acute lymphoblastic leukemia: the GRAALL-2003 trial. *J Clin Oncol.* 2008:27:911.
85. Larson R. Three new drugs for acute lymphoblastic leukemia: nelarabine, clofarabine, and forodesine. *Semin Oncol.* 2007;34:S13-S20.
86. Linker C, Damon L, Ries C, and Navarro W. Intensified and shortened cyclic chemotherapy for adult lymphoblastic leukemia. *J Clin Oncol.* 2002;20:2464–2471.
87. Kantarjan HM, Walters RS, Smith TL, et al. Identification of risk groups for development of central nervous system leukemia in adults with acute lymphoblastic leukemia. *Blood.* 1998;72:1784–1789.
88. Gokbuget N, Hoelzer D. Treatment of adult acute lymphoblastic leukemia. *Hematology.* 2006;133–141.
89. Rowe J, Goldstone A. How I treat acute lymphocytic leukemia in adults. *Blood.* 2007;110:2268–2275.
90. Pui CH, Cheng C, Leung, et al. Extended follow-up of long-term survivors of acute lymphoblastic leukemia. *N Engl J Med.* 2003;349:640–649.
91. Deininger M. Chronic myeloid leukemia: management of early stage disease. *Hematology.* 2005;174–182.
92. NCCN practice guidelines in oncology: Chronic Myeloid Leukemia, v1, 2009. http://www.nccn.org/professionals/physician_gls/PDF/cml.pdf. Accessed January 9, 2010.
93. Shah N. Medical management of CML. *Hematology.* 2007;371–375.
94. Giles F, DeAngelo D, Baccarani M, et al. Optimizing outcomes for patients with advanced disease in chronic myelogenous leukemia. *Semin Oncol.* 2008;35:S1-S7.
95. Talpaz M, Shah N, Kantarjan H, et al. Dasatinib in imantinib-resistant Philadelphia chromosome-positive leukemias. *N Engl J Med.* 2006;354:2531–2541.
96. Druker BJ, Guiholt F, Obrien S, et al. Five year follow-up of patients receiving imantinib for chronic myelogenous leukemia. *N Engl J Med.* 2006;355:2408–2417.
97. NCCN Practice Guidelines in oncology: Chronic Myelogenous Leukemia. V2, 2009. http://www.nccn.org/professionals/physician_gls/PDF/cml.pdf
98. Novartis Pharmaceuticals. Gleevac (prescribing information). East Hanover, NJ: Novartis Pharmaceuticals; 2007.
99. Bristol-Myers Squib. Sprycel (prescribing information). New York, NY: Bristol-Myers Squib; 2007.
100. Novartis Pharmaceuticals. Tasigna (prescribing information) East Hanover, NJ: Novartis Pharmaceuticals; 2007.
101. NCCN Practice Guidelines: Chronic Lymphocytic Leukemia, v2, 2009. http://www.nccn.org/professionals/physician_gls/PDF/nhl.pdf. Accessed October 1, 2009.
102. Genzyme Corp. Alemtuzumab (prescribing information). Cambridge, MA: Genzyme Corp; 2007.
103. Cephalon Inc. Bendamustine (prescribing information). Frazer, PA: Cephalon Inc; 2008.
104. Ben Venue Laboratories. Fludarabine (prescribing information). Bedford, OH: Ben Venue Laboratories; 2008.
105. Pentostatin (prescribing information). SuperGen Inc; Dublin, Delaware;2007.
106. Genentech Inc. Rituxumab (prescribing information). San Francisco, CA: Genentech Inc; 2008.
107. Knauf WU, Lissichkov T, Aldaoud A, et al. Bendamustine versus chlorambucil in treatment naïve patients with B-cell chronic lymphocytic leukemia (B-CLL): results of an international phase III study [abstract 2043]. *Blood.* 2007;110:609a.
108. Ferrajoli A, Lee BN, Schlette E, et al. Lenalidomide induces complete and partial remissions in patients with relapsed and refractory chronic lymphocytic leukemia. *Blood.* 2008;111:5291–5297.
109. O'brien S, Moore JO, Boyd TE, et al. Randomized phase III trial of fludarabine plus cyclophosphamide with or without oblimersen sodium (Bcl-2 antisense) in patients with relapsed or refractory chronic lymphocytic leukemia. *J Clin Oncol.* 2007;25:1114–1120.
110. Foucar K, Falini B, Catovsky D, Stein H. Hairy cell leukemia. In: Swerdlow S, Campo E, Harris N, et al, eds. *World Health Organization: World Health Organization Classification of the Tumours of the Hematopoietic and Lymphoid Tissues.* Geneva: World Health Organization; 2008:188–190.
111. Tiacci E, Liso A, Piris M, Falini B. Evolving concepts in the pathogenesis of hairy cell leukemia. *Nat Rev.* 2006;6:437–448.
112. Revlimid (lenalidomide) prescribing information. Celgene Corporation, Summit, NJ, 2006. http://www.revlimid.com/pdf/REVLIMID_PI.pdf. Accessed February 14, 2010.
113. Pharmion. Vidaza (azacitidine for injectable suspension): prescribing information. http://www.pharmion.com/CorporateWeb/home.nsf/AttachmentsByTitle/VidazaFullPrescribingInformation.pdf/$FILE/VidazaFullPrescribingInformation.pdf. Accessed October 1, 2009.
114. MGI Pharma Inc. DACOGEN (decitabine) for Injection Prescribing Information. Bloomington, MN: MGI Pharma Inc; http://www.fda.gov/cder/foi/label/2006/021790lbl.pdf. Accessed October 1, 2009.
115. List AF, Wride K, DeWald GW, et al. Cytogenetic response to lenalidomide is associated with improved survival in patients with chromosome 5q deletion. *Leuk Res.* 2007;31(S1):C028,S38.
116. Fenaux P, Mufti GJ, Santini V, et al. Azacitidine (AZA) treatment prolongs survival (OS) in higher risk MDS patients compared with conventional care regimens (CCR): results of the AZA-001 phase III study [abstract 817]. *Blood.* 2007;110–78a.
117. List AF, Fenaux P, Mufti GJ, et al. Effect of azacitadine (AZA) on overall survival in higher-risk myelodysplastic syndromes (MDS) without complete remission [abstract 7006]. *J Clin Oncol.* 2008;26.
118. NCCN Clinical Practice Guidelines in Oncology: Myelodysplastic Syndromes—v.1.2009. http://www.nccn.org/professionals/physician_gls/PDF/mds.pdf. Accessed March 1,2009.

CHAPTER

58

*Nina N. Grenon, MS, ANP-BC, GNP-BC, AOCN®*

# Liver Cancer

## INTRODUCTION

Primary and secondary cancers of the liver constitute a significant challenge to the multidisciplinary oncology team. Worldwide, hepatocellular carcinoma (HCC) is among the most frequent causes of death from malignancy. The liver is the second most commonly involved organ by metastatic disease.

Hepatocellular carcinoma is the most common malignant tumor of the liver and accounts for as many as 500,000 deaths annually worldwide.[1] In some parts of the world, HCC is the most common malignancy and the most common cause of death from cancer. Although HCC is less common in most of the developed Western world, over the past 3 decades its incidence has increased by about 80% in the United States and Western Europe.[2] This increase has been attributed to the high prevalence of chronic infection with hepatitis C virus (HCV) within these populations. Patients usually present with advanced disease, so treatment options are limited, prognosis is poor, and survival is relatively short. The majority of patients with HCC have underlying cirrhosis and hepatic dysfunction, which complicates the administration of systemic chemotherapy and conducting clinical trials with novel agents. Because of the availability of new forms of therapies for early stage HCC, a growing emphasis is being placed on recognition of risk factors, screening programs, and early diagnosis. In addition, efforts are being made to prevent HCC by using antiviral drugs to treat chronic viral hepatitis.

In the United States, a focal liver lesion is more likely to represent metastatic disease than a primary malignancy. The liver may be the site of metastasis from virtually any primary cancer. Common primary sources of metastases to the liver are cancers of the eye, colon, stomach, pancreas, breast, and lung. Colorectal carcinoma (CRC) is the single most common primary malignancy that results in hepatic metastasis. If liver metastases are found early in the course of colon cancer, surgical resection for metastases is more common than for primary liver cancer.

## EPIDEMIOLOGY

### HEPATOCELLULAR CARCINOMA

Hepatocellular carcinoma is the most common cell type among primary malignant tumors of the liver, ranking fifth in incidence among all malignancies in the world. Approximately 90% of all cases of primary liver cancer are HCC.[1] In the United States an estimated 21,370 new cases of liver and intrahepatic bile duct cancer occurred in 2008, with an annual mortality of 15,190 cases, which reflects the rapid course and grave prognosis of the disease.[3]

The incidence of HCC varies considerably in different parts of the world.[4–6] High-incidence regions (more than 15 cases per 100,000 population per year) include sub-Saharan Africa, the People's Republic of China, Hong Kong, and Taiwan. In these areas, causative factors associated with HCC are chronic hepatitis B virus (HBV) infection acquired predominately through perinatal infection and a high incidence of HBV carriers who acquired the virus early in life. North and South America, Europe, Australia, and parts of the Middle East are low-incidence areas, with fewer than 3 cases reported per 100,000 population per year. In the United States, the incidence of HCC has increased over the past 2 decades, probably due to the existence of a large pool of people with a history of chronic HCV.[7] Intermediate-incidence areas include several countries in eastern and western Europe, Thailand, Indonesia, Jamaica, Haiti, New Zealand (Maoris), and Alaska (Eskimos).[1] The extreme differences in distribution of HCC are probably due to regional variations in exposure to HBV, HCV, and environmental pathogens.

Males are 2 to 3 times more likely to develop HCC than females. The differences in sex distribution may reflect variations in chronic hepatitis carriers, exposure to environmental toxins, and the trophic effects of androgens.[8,9] Although cases can be identified in childhood, this disease typically begins to occur in substantial numbers by the third and fourth decades of life.[10] The majority of HCC cases occur in people with chronic liver disease or cirrhosis. Thus, the rates of HCC incidence also increase with age. In countries with the highest rate of occurrence, HCC tends to affect people at an earlier age, almost invariably due to HBV infection, such as occurs in China and southern Africa.[10]

### LIVER METASTASES

The true incidence of liver metastases is unknown because most data are from autopsy series that reflect the end-stage disease. Depending on the site of the primary tumor, 30% to 70% of patients who die of cancer have liver metastasis.[11]

Gastrointestinal malignancies are prone to spread to the liver, facilitated by the portal venous system. Metastases to the liver from primary colorectal cancer are common, with 15% of patients presenting with synchronous metastasis at the time of diagnosis and an additional 60% of patients developing metastasis later in the course of their disease.[12,13] Other tumors metastasize to the liver less often, including breast cancer (4%), lung cancer (15%), and melanoma (25%).[13]

## ETIOLOGY

### HEPATOCELLULAR CARCINOMA

Unlike most cancers, a number of causative factors for the development of HCC have been identified. Common risk factors include chronic viral hepatitis and underlying liver disease in the form of cirrhosis. Other risk factors in the development of HCC include environmental and chemical toxins, hormones, alcohol and smoking, a number of hereditary disorders, nonalcoholic fatty liver disease (NAFLD), and diabetes mellitus (DM). Nevertheless, HCC can occur in individuals without any known risk factors.[10,13,14]

Hepatitis B virus was the first virus identified as causing tumors in humans, and it is currently believed to be—along with tobacco—the most significant carcinogen to which humans are exposed. Worldwide, HBV is the most frequent underlying cause of HCC. A strong positive correlation exists between HCC incidence rates and the prevalence of hepatitis B surface antigen (HBsAg) in the population, especially in regions where the incidence of HCC is very high.[1] In areas of endemic HBV infection, such as Southeast Asia and sub-Saharan Africa, 10% to 20% of the population is seropositive for HBsAg, with a lifetime risk of developing HCC as high as 80%.[15,16] The majority of HBV infections are acquired in the neonatal period and early childhood and then become chronic; the lifetime relative risk of developing HCC is 70% to 90%.[1] As many as 45% of HBV-infected individuals will die from the tumor, from the infection, or from both. Because of neonatal exposure to HBV, the age of onset of HCC in these countries is younger than that found in Europe and North America.[16,17]

Hepatitis B virus infection in Europe and North America is more commonly the result of sexual or parenteral exposure, occurring later in life than in endemic areas. As a result, HCC in Europe and North America is typically diagnosed after the fourth decade of life. Additional risk factors to the development of HCC in individuals with chronic HBV infection are alcohol and tobacco. A synergism occurs between the infection and alcohol; the risk of HCC increases 2-fold in persons with HBV who consume more than 60 g/day of alcohol.[18] In a study of 53,000 Chinese individuals with HBV who smoked more than 20 cigarettes per day the risk of HCC was increased 2-fold compared with nonsmokers.[19] The risk of HCC climbs after several decades of exposure to HBV, typically after cirrhosis has developed.[17]

Hepatitis C virus is the leading cause of HCC in the US, Europe, and Japan. The annual risk of developing HCC increases as the duration of cirrhosis due to HCV increases. The development of HCC in HCV-infected persons has also been linked to several risk factors, such as viral load, age greater than 60 years, histologic grade of HCC, injury to the liver parenchyma from cirrhosis, severity of transaminase elevation, and failure to respond to interferon treatment. Among HCV-infected individuals, a history of alcohol abuse and HBV infection increase the risk of HCC 2-fold.[20] Concomitant infection with both HBV and HCV is associated with a 3 to 5 times greater risk of developing HCC than infection with either virus alone.[17,20]

The mechanism by which chronic viral hepatitis causes HCC is not known. HBV has a DNA genome that can become incorporated within the genomes of host cells. These integration events may lead to the development of cancer.[21] In contrast, HCV has an RNA genome that does not become integrated into host chromosomes. It is believed that HCV infection leads to HCC through the chronic inflammation and regeneration that are commonly encountered with cirrhosis.[10]

In some parts of the world, high levels of dietary aflatoxin intake have been associated with HCC. Aflatoxin is a mycotoxin produced by molds (*Aspergillus flavus* and *Aspergillus parasiticus*) that contaminate stored foodstuffs such as corn, soybeans, and peanuts.[22,23] Mutations of the *p53* tumor suppressor gene have been identified in patients with HCC who have been chronically exposed to aflatoxin.[5,24] The blue-green algal toxin *Microcystin*, which commonly contaminates ponds in rural China, is thought to be a strong promoter of HCC.[25] In this geographic area, there is a higher mortality rate from HCC among people who drink pond ditch water than among those who drink well water (100 deaths vs fewer than 20 deaths per 100,000 population per year).[26]

Chemical carcinogens linked to primary liver cancer include nitrites, hydrocarbons, solvents, organochlorine pesticides, primary metals, and polychlorinated biphenyls.[25] An increased incidence of HCC has been associated with smoking.[27] Alcohol has been to linked to the development of HCC, but the dose and duration are unclear. Both alcohol abuse and the subsequent development of hepatic cirrhosis are predisposing factors for HCC. Alcohol can act as a synergistic carcinogen with other agents such as HBV, HCV, hepatotoxins, and tobacco.[27,28]

It has been suggested that androgenic steroids (in men) and estrogenic steroids (in women) may increase the risk of HCC. However, a meta-analysis of observational epidemiological studies examining the association between oral contraceptives and the risk of HCC found inconclusive evidence to establish a causal relationship.[29]

Some rare hereditary disorders are associated with an increased risk of developing HCC. Hemochromatosis and alpha-1-antitrypsin deficiency usually cause cirrhosis and are believed to be major contributors to the neoplastic transformation into HCC.[30] Likewise, Wilson's disease, primary biliary cirrhosis, type 1 glycogen storage disease, and porphyria are all thought to increase the risk of HCC.[31]

Another risk factor for the development of HCC is membranous obstruction of the inferior vena cava, thought to be either a congenital abnormality or the result of vena cava thrombosis. Hepatocellular carcinoma develops in 46% of South African blacks and 36% of Japanese with this abnormality.[32]

Diabetes mellitus (DM) and obesity have been suggested to be risk factors for HCC. DM has been associated with NAFLD, including the most severe form, nonalcoholic steatohepatitis (NASH),[33] NASH is a chronic necroinflammatory condition that can lead to liver fibrosis, cirrhosis, and subsequently HCC.[34] Whether the development of HCC is related to obesity and diabetes or to underlying NAFLD-related changes is not clear.[35] In a series of patients who underwent surgical resection for cryptogenic liver disease-related HCC, a study revealed that these patients frequently exhibited the same risk factors as those for NAFLD. These results support the contention that NAFLD is also a significant risk for HCC.[36]

Coffee consumption has been implicated as a protective factor in liver cancer. The consumption of 2 or more cups of coffee per day is associated with a 43% reduction in liver cancer, according to a recent meta-analysis. Coffee contains antioxidants, suggesting the possibility of a protective effect. In addition, coffee and caffeine have been linked to reducing aminotransferase levels and the risk of cirrhosis.[37]

### LIVER METASTASES

The liver has a rich blood supply from both the hepatic artery and the portal circulation. As a consequence, metastases can reach the liver from any organ. The direct passage of blood from the gastrointestinal tract to the portal circulation explains the high rate of liver metastases. Differences are seen in the natural history of the liver metastases from gastrointestinal tumors. Liver metastases found in patients with gastric or pancreatic cancer usually indicate widespread metastatic disease. In contrast, a significant number of patients with colorectal cancer may have isolated liver metastases.

## PREVENTION, SCREENING, AND EARLY DETECTION

Primary prevention aims at reduction of the risk of developing a disease by implementing strategies such as lifestyle modifications, chemoprevention, and vaccination. In the case of HCC, primary prevention seeks to prevent viral hepatitis and control disease in those already infected with HBV and HCV. In Taiwan, a vaccination program for HBV was established in the mid-1980s; after 10 years, the percentage of HBsAg-positive children declined from 10% to less than 2%. The incidence of HCC among children between the ages of 6 and 9 was reduced by 80%.[38] Vaccination for HBV will most likely reduce the risk of HCC in the next decade.[15] In the US, the current recommendation is that all newborns be vaccinated against HBV. In contrast, no vaccine for HCV is available, and it may be some time before any such vaccine is developed. However, vigorous screening of blood used for transfusions has greatly reduced the incidence of HCV infection.

In those individuals who are already infected with HBV and HCV, prevention of HCC has focused on using chemoprevention to treat the viral infection. Interferon has been the primary means of chemoprevention. Several reports have demonstrated the ability of interferon-alpha to lower the incidence of HCC.[39] However, these reports have primarily relied on retrospective nonrandomized data, so their results should be interpreted with caution. Recent reports of large, prospective, randomized trials using the combination of interferon and ribavirin in patients with HCV infection show that this regimen can slow the progression of fibrosis, decrease viral load, and lessen histologic and biological markers of inflammation. The impact on the reduction of cirrhosis and HCC remains to be determined. Of interest, these reports indicate that people who do not respond to interferon are at a higher risk for developing HCC.[40–42]

Currently, cyclooxygenase-2 inhibitors (COX-2 inhibitors) are used as chemoprevention agents in patients with documented cirrhosis from viral hepatitis, alcohol abuse, hemochromatosis, or other causes. Cirrhosis represents a premalignant state for HCC, and increased COX-2 expression is noted in both cirrhosis and dysplasias. It is also believed that angiogenesis inhibitors may represent a potential novel strategy to prevent HCC, and COX-2 inhibitors are known to have some antiangiogenic effects. Clinical trials are currently attempting to determine the actual role of COX-2 in human hepatocarcinogenesis and to identify whether COX-2 inhibitors may have a potential role in the primary or secondary (early detection of disease before it is clinically apparent) prevention of HCC.[43] Strategies for the prevention of HCC in nonviral cirrhosis include decreasing iron overload in patients with hemochromatosis by the regular use of phlebotomy, and decreasing exposure to hepatotoxic agents such as alcohol and aflatoxins.[15]

Regular screening of patients at risk for developing HCC remains controversial; data demonstrating a survival advantage are inconsistent.[44,45] Nevertheless, HCC may be diagnosed at an earlier stage in patients who undergo screening at regular intervals. When the disease is caught early, liver resection and transplantation, which offer the best chance for a cure, are more likely to be treatment options.[46] The American Association for the Study of Liver Diseases issued guidelines suggesting surveillance for patients at risk, including ultrasonography every 6 to 12 months. This interval is based primarily on observational data and the expected growth of rates of HCC (Tables 58-1 and 58-2).[47–49]

## PATHOPHYSIOLOGY

### CELLULAR CHARACTERISTICS

Primary liver cancers are commonly adenocarcinomas that arise from epithelial cells.[50] Among the cell types that are

**TABLE 58-1**

**American Association for the Study of Liver Diseases (AASLD) Recommends Surveillance for the Following Groups of Patients**

- Hepatitis B (HBV) carriers who are Asian (Males ≥ 40, Females ≥ 50)
- Cirrhotic HBV carriers
- Those with a family history of hepatocellular carcinoma (HCC)
- Africans over the age of 20

For patients who are not listed above, the risk varies depending upon the severity of the underlying liver disease and current and past hepatic inflammatory activity. Patients with high HBV DNA concentrations and those with ongoing hepatic inflammation remain at risk for HCC.

- Non-hepatitis B cirrhosis from alcohol
- Hepatitis C
- Genetic hemochromatosis
- Primary biliary cirrhosis

Although the following groups have an increased risk of HCC, no recommendations for or against surveillance can be made because a lack of data precludes an assessment of whether surveillance would be beneficial:

- Alpha 1-antitrypsin deficiency
- Non-alcoholic steatohepatitis
- Autoimmune hepatitis

*Source*: Data from Bruix and Sherman.[49]

sources of HCC are hepatocytes, which account for the majority of primary liver cancers. The remainder is cholangiocarcinomas, which arise from the bile duct epithelium. In rare cases, there is a mixed-type pattern that is usually poorly differentiated. Fewer than 3% of primary liver cancers arise from mesenchymal cells; these malignancies include sarcomas, angiosarcomas, epithelioid tumors, and hemangioendotheliomas.[51]

**TABLE 58-2**

**American Association for the Study of Liver Diseases (AASLD) Recommendations Regarding Surveillance**

- Patients at high risk for developing hepatocellular carcinoma (HCC) (see Table 58-1) should be entered into surveillance programs.
- Patients on the transplant waiting list should be screened for HCC because in the US the development of HCC gives increased priority for Orthotopic Liver Transplant (OLT), and because failure to screen for HCC means that patients may develop HCC and progress beyond listing criteria without the physician being aware.
- Alpha fetoprotein alone should not be used for screening unless ultrasound is not available.
- Patients should be screened at 6- to 12-month intervals
- Surveillance interval does not need to be shortened for patients at higher risk of HCC.

*Source*: Data from Bruix and Sherman.[49]

Fibrolamellar carcinoma is an uncommon variant of HCC that generally occurs in young persons in Western countries and presents in the absence of cirrhosis. The tumor is well demarcated and often encapsulated. Also, the alpha-fetoprotein (AFP) level is not usually elevated and is associated with prolonged survival when compared with the typical HCC. This tendency most likely reflects the fact that the tumor is well demarcated and that a wider range of treatment options are available in the absence of cirrhosis.[52]

The gross appearance of HCC can be characterized as a single mass, multiple nodules, or diffuse liver involvement, referred to as *massive, nodular,* and *diffuse* forms, respectively. The carcinomas may range from well-differentiated lesions to highly anaplastic undifferentiated lesions. In well-differentiated and moderately well-differentiated tumors, hepatocystic cells assume a trabecular (the most common histologic variant), acinar, or pseudoglandular pattern (often characterized by bile-filled strictures).[53,54] It is important to determine the differential diagnosis for well-differentiated HCC, which includes liver cell adenomas and dysplastic nodules.[54] In poorly differentiated tumors, cells take on a pleomorphic appearance characterized by numerous anaplastic, giant cells as well as small, completely undifferentiated cells, and sometimes can resemble a spindle cell sarcoma.[53]

Well-differentiated and moderately well-differentiated HCC can be easily diagnosed, while poorly differentiated tumors may need to be distinguished from primary HCC or metastatic disease to the liver. Liver cancer can be distinguished from other metastatic tumors by examining the production of bile and the presence of albumin mRNA. Staining studies for the expression of AFP, biliary glycoprotein 1, and CD10 may also help identify HCC. In 67% of HCCs, the immunostain is positive for AFP.[54]

## PROGRESSION OF DISEASE

The natural course of primary liver cancer can be progressive, with enlargement of the primary mass until it encroaches on hepatic function or metastasizes. Hematogenic tumor spread most commonly occurs to the lungs, followed by the adrenal glands, bones, gastrointestinal tract, gallbladder, and pancreas. Lymphatic metastases can be found in approximately 25% of patients with HCC and usually occur in the hilum or peripancreatic nodes. More distant lymph nodes, such as perigastric and periaortic nodes, can be involved with advanced disease.[54–57] Death from HCC usually occurs less than 12 months after the diagnosis due to cachexia, gastrointestinal or esophageal varices bleeding, liver failure with hepatic coma, or rarely fatal hemorrhage from tumor rupture.[6]

## CLINICAL MANIFESTATIONS

Most patients with liver cancer will be asymptomatic. The most common symptom of HCC is abdominal pain in the right upper quadrant. It is most often felt in the right hypochondrium and epigastrium and sometimes in the back and lower abdomen. The pain is described as a constant dull ache, which may become severe in the advanced stages of the disease. It sometimes radiates through the back or refers to the right shoulder. The pain may cause the patient to become aware of an upper abdominal mass.[56] The patient may present with increased abdominal girth from ascites, which may be the source of pain, although this is a different pain from that generated by liver tumors. Weight loss, anorexia, and early satiety often indicate advanced lesions.[57] Fever may be present without infection; fever may be accompanied by leukocytosis, which may be misleading by suggesting that the patient has an infection. Pyrexia is thought to be the result of pyrogens released into the bloodstream from the malignant necrotic liver cells. Typically, the fever is intermittent and self-limited.[56]

Obstructive jaundice can be caused by compression of the major intrahepatic ducts from the primary tumor, by obstruction of the common bile duct from nodal metastasis in the porta hepatis, by direct invasion of the biliary tree, or rarely as the result of hemobilia (hemorrhage in the biliary tract).[56] Diarrhea can occur and may be severe and intractable, leading to electrolyte and fluid imbalance. Diarrhea may result from the HCC tumor behaving as a carcinoid tumor (see the discussion of paraneoplastic syndromes). Other gastrointestinal symptoms may include nausea, vomiting, indigestion, and constipation. Gastrointestinal bleeding may occur in the later stages of the disease or in patients with known cirrhosis. It is most likely due to portal hypertension causing gastroesophageal varices, and is frequently a terminal event.[56]

Pain can result from bone metastases localized to the ribs, skull, femur, sacrum, or vertebrae. Dyspnea may be related to pleural effusion, a markedly elevated hemidiaphragm, or extensive lung metastasis.

Occasionally, patients with HCC may develop paraneoplastic syndromes. Hypoglycemia can occur in advanced HCC as a result of the tumor's high metabolic need. Although typically the hypoglycemia is mild, in some instances the decrease in serum glucose can be severe, resulting in lethargy and confusion. In a small percentage of patients, hypoglycemia can occur early in the disease when the tumor secretes insulin-like growth factor, which acts as an insulin agonist and causes severe symptomatic hypoglycemia.[56,58,59]

Erythrocytosis in HCC is thought to be due to secretion of erythropoietin by the tumor. Raised serum erythropoietin levels may be found in as many as 23% of patients with HCC, elevations in packed cell volume and hemoglobin concentration are uncommon, and the majority of patients are anemic.[60]

Hypercalcemia can occur as a result of osteolytic metastases, which are uncommon in HCC. Most often, hypercalcemia is due to secretion of parathyroid hormone-related protein.[56,61] The patient with hypercalcemia may be severely symptomatic and require urgent treatment.

Watery diarrhea is significantly more common in patients with cirrhotic HCC. The diarrhea may be severe and intractable. Although the mechanism involved is not well understood, the diarrhea may be caused by the expression of peptides that cause increased intestinal secretions.[62]

Metastatic disease in the liver usually remains asymptomatic. Many patients with liver metastasis from colorectal cancer are diagnosed through routine surveillance laboratory tests, such as elevated CEA or serum alkaline phosphatase. Early symptoms of liver metastases may include fatigue and abdominal pain. If the metastases involve extensive liver tissue, the patient may present with the same symptoms as with primary HCC.

## ASSESSMENT

### PATIENT AND FAMILY HISTORY

To assess for primary liver cancer or metastases, the history should identify any potential risk factors, such as HBV or HCV infection, cirrhosis, or exposure to toxins. The history should also identify possible risk factors for the development of cancer that could prompt metastasis to the liver, such as a history of any genetic syndrome that might increase an individual's risk for the development of primary liver cancer, colorectal cancer, or breast cancer. Other disease states should also be considered—for example, a history of inflammatory bowel disease and the subsequent risk of developing colorectal cancer. Most important, investigating a family history of cancer and recognizing the development of various carcinomas within each generation will provide information regarding a possible genetic mutation. This information may prompt genetic counseling that can recommend screening the individual who is deemed to be at risk of developing other cancers.

### PHYSICAL EXAMINATION

The most frequent finding on physical examination in patients with HCC is an enlarged liver. One or both lobes may be enlarged, and the surface may be nodular. The liver may be hard or just firm. Focal or generalized tenderness may be present on palpation. Often an elevated right hemidiaphragm can be found on the exam due to the enlarged liver. A bruit caused by compression of the aorta over the liver may be occasionally heard.[56,63,64] Ascites is present in more than 50% of patients with HCC and indicates decompensated cirrhosis.[56,57] Splenomegaly is another common finding as a result of chronic portal hypertension from cirrhosis. Often the enlarged spleen is difficult to feel due to tense ascites and an enlarged left lobe of the liver.[56,57] Muscle wasting becomes evident as the disease runs its course and may be evident at presentation with large, rapidly growing tumors. Slight to moderate jaundice may be observed at initial diagnosis. A sudden onset of acute abdominal pain, accompanied by hypovolemic shock, abdominal distention, absent bowel sounds, and diffuse abdominal tenderness, can result from tumor rupture. This is a rare and usually catastrophic event. The rupture is typically confirmed by radiologic exam, which reveals a liver mass and free intraperitoneal blood.[56,65]

Patients with liver metastases will present with a different physical exam from the preceding profile. The liver may be extensively replaced by disease in the advanced state. Although any of the above findings may be present on exam, the most commonly encountered signs and symptoms are liver enlargement, ascites, jaundice, and muscle wasting.

## DIAGNOSTIC STUDIES

### Laboratory studies

In the early stages of liver cancer, laboratory data such as liver function tests (LFTs) may be normal. After a significant volume of the liver parenchyma is involved by tumor, abnormalities in LFTs may be seen. In the setting of cirrhosis, elevated bilirubin and lowered albumin levels are indicative of poor survival. Serum gamma-glutamyl transferase (GGT) is elevated in most cases of HCC, and alkaline phosphatase can be slightly elevated in metastatic disease. Laboratory evaluation should include HBV and HCV titers and serology alpha fetoprotein(AFP).

The serum AFP measurement is helpful in the diagnosis and management of HCC. The AFP level is elevated to greater than 20 ng/mL in more than 70% of patients with HCC. Elevation from 500 to 1000 ng/mL can be seen in patients with viral hepatitis who do not have HCC.[66,67] In patients with known chronic hepatitis, persistently elevated AFP values indicate a higher risk of developing HCC.[67] AFP does not correlate to tumor size or growth rate. The lack of specificity limits the use of the AFP value except in those patients in whom the level is elevated to greater than 400 ng/mL. However, AFP is useful in monitoring response to treatment and detecting recurrence after treatment of HCC if it was elevated before treatment.[66]

Carcinoembryonic antigen (CEA) is widely used in the detection of colorectal cancer recurrences. Mildly elevated levels of CEA can be detected among smokers and in many benign conditions, including peptic ulcer disease, pancreatitis, and prostatitis. In addition, CEA levels can be elevated in a number of malignancies, including colon, breast, pancreas, liver, and gastric cancer. Due to its lack of specificity, CEA cannot be used as a diagnostic or screening test. Nevertheless, CEA levels are monitored after resection of a primary colorectal cancer or resection of liver metastases. A rise in CEA usually predicts recurrence 6 to 8 months before the patient is symptomatic or findings of disease recurrence appear on radiologic tests.[68] One large study revealed that measurement of the CEA level appeared to be more sensitive for hepatic metastases and less sensitive for focal or peritoneal disease. Overall, 75% to 90% of patients with hepatic colorectal metastases have elevated CEA levels.[68]

### Imaging studies

Imaging studies play a key role in the diagnosis of lesions in the liver and can differentiate between a primary liver cancer and metastatic disease to the liver. The imaging tests most commonly used to diagnose HCC are ultrasound (US), computed tomography (CT), magnetic resonance imaging (MRI), and in some rare instances angiography, CT hepatic arteriography, and arterial portography. In metastatic liver disease, CT scans of the abdomen and liver, MRI of the liver, and positron emission tomography (PET) scans can be useful. In addition, a CT scan of the chest is routinely performed with staging to detect pulmonary metastasis.

The HCC lesions detected by US have different echogenicity from the surrounding liver tissue. Small HCC tumors are typically hypoechoic but may be hyperechoic as the lesions enlarge and can be difficult to distinguish from normal surrounding tissue.[66] Visualization of lesions under the right hemidiaphragm, with overlying gas, or in obese patients can be difficult. Although US cannot distinguish HCC from other solid tumors in the liver, it can be used as a screening tool for HCC. An added benefit of US is its use in the assessment of the patency of the hepatic blood supply and the presence of vascular invasion by the tumor in the portal vein. It can also be used intraoperatively to detect small tumor nodules during hepatic resection. However, CT and MRI have largely replaced US in the diagnosis of HCC.

Computed tomography is often performed to evaluate an abnormality of the liver that was detected on US. It can also be used as a primary screening modality for HCC in patients with cirrhosis. Developments in helical CT imaging include spiral scanners that allow rapid imaging of the liver after infusion of intravenous contrast agents, and the adaptation of scanning protocols that delineate the vascularity of the tumors. Hepatocellular carcinoma derives its blood supply primarily from the hepatic artery; the remainder of the liver receives its blood supply from both the arterial and portal veins. On CT exam, liver carcinomas appear enhanced early during the infusion of dye in the arterial phase (the first 20–40 seconds), allowing for detection of hypervascular HCCs as small as 3 mm.[66,69] The liver parenchyma is enhanced during the portal venous phase (50–90 seconds after the infusing contrast). The term *triphasic CT scan* is used to describe the process of enhancement before contrast and during the arterial phase and the portal venous phase.[66] Tumors that isoattenuate (present in the same enhancing pattern) on both arterial and portal phase imaging can be missed, but may be detected in delayed-phase imaging.[69] The sensitivity of helical CT for detecting HCC has been reported to be as high as 90%.[69] Metastases from colorectal cancer are typically hypovascular and are best identified as nonenhancing lesions on portal phase imaging.[70]

Magnetic resonance imaging is another imaging modality that can distinguish HCC from normal liver tissue.[57] Although MRI has a similar sensitivity for the diagnosis of HCC to helical CT, it has better sensitivity and specificity than CT and US in patients with cirrhotic livers.[71] MRI is also superior in distinguishing benign vascular lesions such as hemangioma and focal fatty changes within the liver. Likewise, MRI is the preferred imaging test in patients with renal insufficiency or in those patients with an allergy to contrast media agents.

To improve the detection and characterization of HCC, angiography can be combined with CT and MRI in a technique known as CT hepatic arteriography and arterial portography.[72] Immediately prior to MRI or CT, contrast dye is injected intra-arterially in the superior mesenteric, hepatic, or splenic artery; images are then obtained during the arterial and portal venous phases. This technique can detect HCCs smaller than 1 cm in diameter.[73] Hepatic arteriography delineates the hepatic arterial anatomy and has been used for preoperative evaluation of HCC, chemoembolization, or infusion of antineoplastic drugs directly into the hepatic artery.[57] This diagnostic technique is not commonly used in the United States. The benefit of CT hepatic arteriography and arterial portography over MRI is unclear due to the former's invasiveness without added benefit of accuracy.[73]

Positron emission tomography is the latest advance in imaging techniques. It evaluates cell metabolism using a glucose analog, F-fluorodeoxyglucose (FDG). Tumors typically have higher rates of glucose uptake and metabolism than surrounding tissues. When FDG is given to the patient, the increased uptake of the glucose analog by the tumor can be detected by the PET scanner.[74] This imaging modality can be used to detect recurrent or metastatic disease, and it can be an accurate imaging technique for differentiating hepatic metastasis, although it may not detect lesions smaller than 1 cm.

Future imaging modalities for HCC include a technetium-99m ($^{99m}$Tc)-labeled anti-AFP Fab imaging kit.[75] Gallium scanning was a common imaging technique for the diagnosis of HCC prior to the advent of CT and MRI. It can still play a role in patients where a diagnosis remains unclear after other noninvasive testing and where more aggressive diagnostics may be inappropriate.[76]

### Liver biopsy

Tissue examination is usually recommended and commonly performed in patients with focal liver lesions in which the diagnosis is uncertain. The routine use of needle biopsy in HCC is controversial, especially in patients with HCC who are candidates for resection and transplantation, because the risks of biopsy include bleeding and spreading of tumor cells along the needle track. Some reports suggest local spread of HCC can occur in 1% of patients after a needle biopsy.[66,77,78] A biopsy may not be needed if the diagnosis is obvious, such as in the case of a large mass found in the liver associated with elevated serum AFP.

Several methods are available for biopsy procedures. Fine-needle aspiration (FNA) biopsy can be performed under US or CT radiologic guidance.[79] Directed core biopsy is more useful than FNA because more tissue can be obtained.[79] If the tumor is massive or spread extensively throughout the liver, a blind biopsy is performed by palpating the mass. Open surgical biopsy procedure is usually indicated if the tumor cannot be radiologically located with precision.[66]

## CLASSIFICATION AND STAGING

Staging is essential for the management of HCC. The purpose of staging is to group patients on the basis of the characteristics of their disease to determine the most appropriate treatment.[80] The prognosis for HCC, unlike other cancers, depends on both the functional state of the liver and the extent of tumor growth.[66,81] The functional status of the liver in a patient with cirrhosis is usually assessed by the Child-Pugh classification (Table 58-3).[82] The Child-Pugh classification helps to assess the severity of liver disease according to the degree of ascites, the plasma concentration of bilirubin and albumin, the prothrombin time, and the degree of encephalopathy. Points are assigned to each element so that a total score can be obtained. A total score of 5 to 6 is considered Grade A (well-compensated disease); 7 to 9 is Grade B (significant functional compromise); and 10 to 15 is Grade C (decompensated disease).[83]

The 2 most popular HCC staging systems are the Okuda system and the tumor-node-metastasis (TNM) classification of the International Union Against Cancer. The Okuda staging system takes into account the extent of the tumor; the patient is evaluated on the 4 criteria of ascites, serum albumin, serum bilirubin, and tumor size (largest cross-sectional area of the tumor), then is staged

**TABLE 58-3**

**Child-Pugh Classification of Severity of Liver Disease**

| Parameter | Points Assigned | | |
|---|---|---|---|
| | 1 | 2 | 3 |
| Ascites | Absent | Slight | Moderate |
| Bilirubin (mg/dL) | < 2 | 2–3 | > 3 |
| Albumin (g/dL) | > 3.5 | 2.8–3.5 | < 2.8 |
| Prothrombin time: seconds over control | 1–3 | 4–6 | > 6 |
| INR | < 1.7 | 1.8–2.3 | > 2.3 |
| Encephalopathy | None | Grade 1–2 | Grade 3–4 |

Grade A, 5–6 points; Grade B, 7–9 points; Grade C, 10–15 points.

*Source*: Data from Child, Turcotte.[82]

as I, II, or III (Table 58-4).[84] Survival with no therapy for patients with stage I, II, or III disease is 8.3, 2.0, or 0.7 months, respectively.[84] The TNM staging system classifies patients from stages I through IV solely on the basis of tumor size and number, lobar involvement, and nodal and distant metastasis (Table 58-5).[85] The TNM staging system is based primarily on imaging studies. It is generally felt that this approach leads to the risk of understaging of patients, especially preoperatively.[80]

More recently, the Cancer of the Liver Italian Program (CLIP) group proposed a new prognostic score that includes the Child-Pugh score, tumor morphology, serum AFP levels, the presence or absence of portal vein thrombosis, with an index of severity of cirrhosis to determine a prognostic score ranging from 0 to 6. (Table 58-6).[86] A number of studies from various geographic locations have suggested that the CLIP performed better at predicting survival than the TNM, Okuda or Child-Pugh system, particularly in patients undergoing nonsurgical therapy.[87,88]

**TABLE 58-4**

**Okuda Staging System for Hepatocellular Carninoma**

| Criterion | Positive | Negative |
|---|---|---|
| Tumor size | > 50% | <50% |
| Ascites | Clinically detectable | Clinically undetectable |
| Serum albumin | < 3 g/dL | > 3 g/dL |
| Serum bilirubin | > 3 mg/dL | < 3 mg/dL |
| Stage | | |
| I | No positive | |
| II | One or two positives | |
| III | Three or four positives | |

*Source*: Data from Okuda et al.[84]

**TABLE 58-5**

**TNM for Hepatocellular Carninoma: Stage Grouping**

| | | | |
|---|---|---|---|
| Stage I | T1 | NO | MO |
| Stage II | T2 | NO | MO |
| Stage IIIA | T3 | NO | MO |
| Stage IIIB | T4 | NO | MO |
| Stage IIIC | Any T | N1 | MO |
| Stage IV | Any T | Any N | M2 |

*Source*: Data from Greene et al.[85]

## THERAPEUTIC APPROACHES AND NURSING CARE

### HEPATOCELLULAR CARCINOMA

A number of therapeutic interventions are available for the treatment of primary liver cancer with the goal of either

**TABLE 58-6**

**CLIP Score: Cancer of the Liver Italian Program**

| Variable | Score |
|---|---|
| Child-Pugh stage | |
| A | 0 |
| B | 1 |
| C | 2 |
| Tumor morphology | |
| Uninodular and extension < 50% | 0 |
| Multinodular and extension < 50% | 1 |
| Massive or extension > 50% | 2 |
| Alpha fetoprotein (AFP) | |
| < 400 ng/ml | 0 |
| > 400 ng/ml | 1 |
| Portal vein thrombosis | |
| No | 0 |
| Yes | 1 |

*Source*: Data from Cancer of the Liver Italian Program (CLIP) Investigators.[86]

cure or palliation (Table 58-7).[89] Of the treatment options available, surgical resection with partial hepatectomy or liver transplantation, or both, offers the only potential for a cure. Patients with unresectable HCC have a number of palliative treatment modalities available, including regional therapy, ablative or cytoreductive therapy, external beam radiation, and systemic chemotherapy. All treatment options may affect normal liver parenchyma and, ultimately, liver function. Supportive care includes pain management, nutritional support, control of nausea and vomiting, management of ascites, minimization of the discomfort of jaundice, management of encephalopathy, and attempts to minimize psychosocial distress and disturbances in body image.

Once a diagnosis of HCC is established through a combination of history, physical assessment, imaging studies, and laboratory tests, a decision is made whether to biopsy. Once the disease has been appropriately staged, treatment options will be based on the extent of liver involvement, size of the tumor, portal vein involvement, performance status, comorbid conditions, and patient preference. Figure 58-1 provides a treatment algorithm for HCC.

### Partial hepatectomy

Partial hepatectomy offers the best option for cure in patients with HCC. The ideal candidate for resection will have disease confined to the liver, with a solitary lesion usually smaller than 5 cm and no nodal metastasis. Radiologic evidence should confirm the lack of hepatic vascular involvement, and the patient should have normal LFTs and no ascites, portal hypertension, or coagulopathies.[90–92] Surgical resection is attempted in patients with Child-Pugh stage A, TNM stages I and II, and Okuda stage 1 lesions.[93] Unfortunately, most patients do not fall into this category. In geographic areas with a high incidence of HCC, only 10% to 15% of patients are potentially curable; in low-incidence areas, 15% to 30% of patients may be suitable candidates for resection.[94–96] Resection is associated with a 5-year survival rate of 30%. In patients with no cirrhosis, the mortality rate associated with surgical liver resection is less than 5%.[97]

**TABLE 58-7**

| Treatment Modalities for HCC |
|---|
| Potentially Curative Treatments |
| Hepatic resection |
| Liver transplantation |
| Palliative Treatments |
| Chemoembolization |
| Hepatic artery infusion |
| Percutaneous interstitial ablation |
| Percutaneous ethanol injection |
| Radiofrequency ablation |
| Microwave coagulation therapy |
| Cryosurgery |
| Radiation therapy |
| External beam radiation |
| Internal radiation |
| Systemic chemotherapy |
| Hormonal therapy |
| Immunotherapy |
| Gene therapy |

*Source:* Data from Bruix.[49]

Intraoperative staging via laparoscopy and intraoperative ultrasound (IOUS) can improve the selection of patients who can be potentially cured by resection. Intraoperative ultrasound can accurately determine the size of the primary tumor and identify portal and hepatic vein involvement. In addition, IOUS can be used to identify major intrahepatic vascular structures and can guide segmental and anatomic resection.[98]

For patients with cirrhosis, liver resection is associated with a number of risks, leading to increased morbidity and mortality in this population. Typically, patients with cirrhosis have rigid liver parenchyma with varices, making it difficult to resect. Many of these patients also have thrombocytopenia and coagulation abnormalities that place them at even greater risk for hemorrhage. Postoperative complications may include liver failure due to the liver not being able to regenerate, and exaggeration of portal hypertension, leading to ascites and variceal bleeding.

The type and extent of resection depends on the tumor location. The type of incision used to perform liver resection is usually subcostal; with this approach, the incision can be extended further if the tumor is bulky or invades the diaphragm. Resections can be classified as either minor or major. Major resections include hepatic lobectomy or extended hepatic lobectomy, also referred to as trisegmentectomy. Minor resection includes nonanatomic wedge resection or anatomic resection of a specific segment. An example of a more difficult resection would involve removing a lesion located within the posterior segment of the right lobe, which is complicated by the location of the hepatic veins.

### Liver transplantation

In patients with localized HCC and no distant metastasis, liver transplantation (LT) can offer the best chance for long-term survival, as it can eradicate the cancer as well as the underlying disease (cirrhosis). Studies over the past several years have shown that survival in carefully selected patients with HCC who undergo LT is the same as survival for those patients who undergo LT for nonmalignant causes.[99–101] The criteria used to identify a suitable candidate include size of a single tumor (smaller than 5 cm or

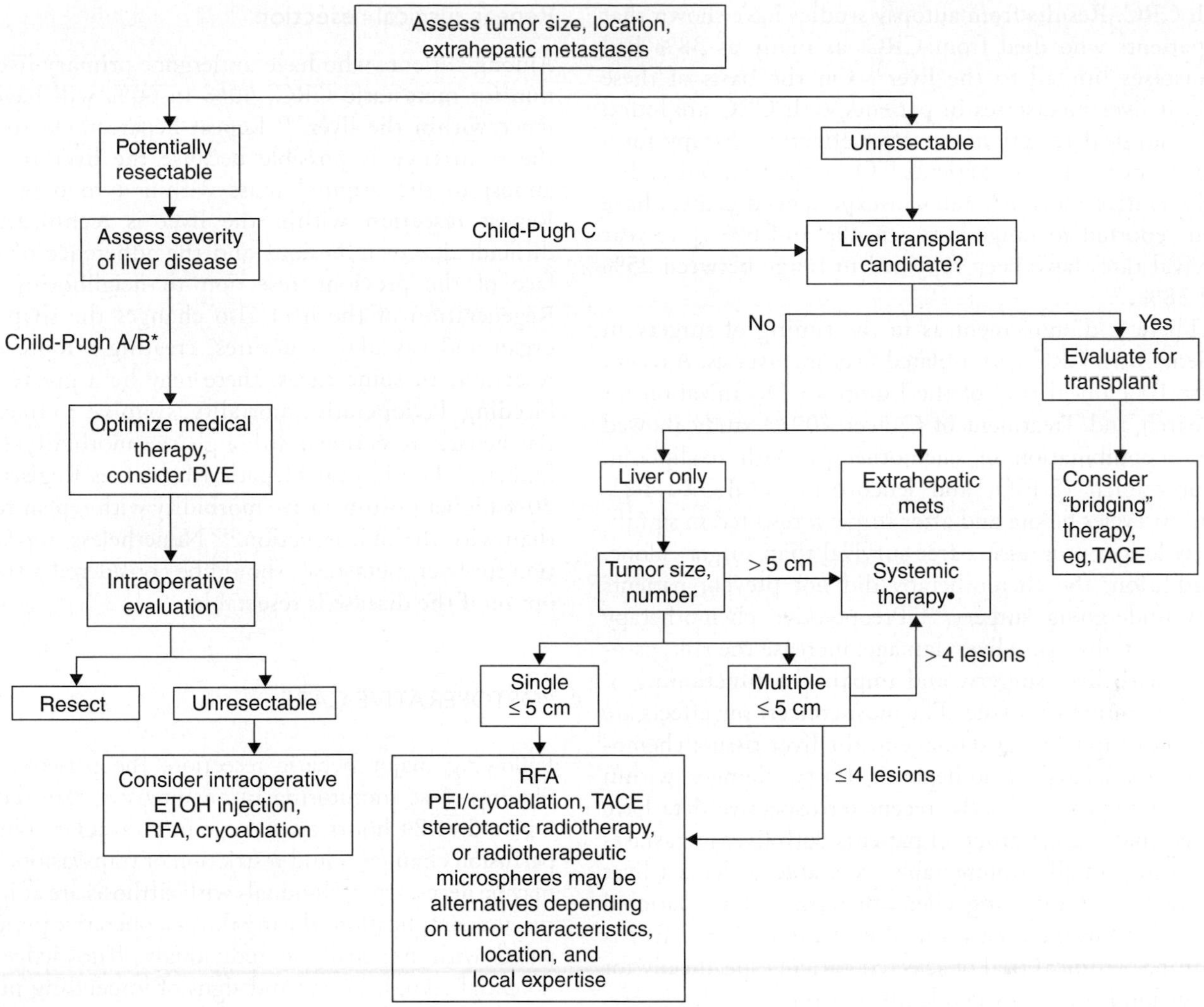


**FIGURE 58-1**

Treatment algorithm for hepatocellular carcinoma.

*Abbrevations*: ETOH, alcohol; PEI, Percutaneous ethanol injection; PVE, Portal vein embolization; RFA, Radiofrequency ablation; TACE, Transcatheter arterial chemoembolization.

*Suitability of patients with Child-Pugh B cirrhosis for surgical resection is highly controversial.

Systemic therapy options include participation in a clinical trial (preferred) or sorafenib.

smaller than 3 cm if there are 1 to 3 tumors), the number of tumor nodules (less than 3), the absence of vascular invasion, and a well-differentiated histology. These criteria are merely guidelines; they are not mandatory. An overall 5-year survival rate of 70% has been reported.[99]

A complicating factor for LT patients with HCC is the waiting period for an available donor. Chemoembolization (also known as transarterial chemoembolization) is a common treatment modality used in patients waiting for LT. Randomized trials of chemoembolization prior to LT have been shown to prolong the survival of unresectable patients with HCC.[102,103] Given the risk of disease progression of patients waiting for LT, adjuvant therapy is currently provided in most centers.

## LIVER METASTASES

### Initial resection

Resection of liver metastases from stomach or pancreatic cancer is not an option due to the aggressive biological nature of these cancers. Occasionally, solitary lesions from breast cancer metastases can be resected with good results. However, resection of liver metastases is done only when strong evidence indicates that the liver is the only site of metastasis. The role of hepatic resection in metastatic neuroendocrine cancers is not known due to the rarity of these tumors. Resection of hepatic metastases is most often appropriate in the management of CRC. The liver may often be the only site of metastases in patients with CRC. Results from autopsy studies have shown that in patients who died from CRC, as many as 38% had metastases limited to the liver.[11] On the basis of these data, if liver metastases in patients with CRC are found early, surgical resection can offer effective therapy for a significant number of patients.[11] Over the past 3 decades, perioperative mortality rates in experienced centers have been reported to range between 4% and 6%. Five-year survival rates have been reported to range between 25% and 38%.[104]

There is disagreement as to the timing of surgery in patients with CRC with isolated liver metastases. A recent phase III clinical trial of the European Organization for Research and Treatment of Cancer 40983 study showed that a combination of chemotherapy with oxaliplatin, 5-fluorouracil (5-FU), and leucovorin (FOLOX4 regimen), 6 cycles before and after surgery, resulted in significantly longer progression-free survival than surgery alone. In addition, the chemotherapy did not prevent patients from undergoing surgery.[105] Preoperative chemotherapy can potentially cause liver damage, increase the risks associated with liver surgery, and impair the functioning of the remaining liver tissue. The most concerning effects are those causing vascular damage to the liver tissue: chemotherapy-associated steatohepatitis (fatty changes within the liver tissue).[106] Finally, recent retrospective data have proven that a select group of patients with liver metastases who were initially unresectable were able to have a liver resection after receiving chemotherapy.[107] The National Surgical Adjuvant Breast and Bowel Project (NSABP) is planning a clinical trial of selected patients specifically for conversion from unresectable disease to resectable disease. This study will use an EGFR inhibitor and patients will be tested for *K-ras* status. Patients with tumors that test for the nonmutant type, such as *K-ras* wild type, will be enrolled in the trial.[108]

Guidelines for resection of liver metastases include the following: there should be no distant metastases or extrahepatic intra-abdominal metastases; if the periportal lymph nodes have metastatic disease present, the resection is typically aborted. The extent of the resection can range from a small nodule to a trisegmentectomy, where as much as 75% of the liver is removed. If a patient has cirrhosis, extensive resection is typically not performed because it is not possible to predict which patients can survive with 75% of the liver removed. Patients with poor performance status are typically not good candidates for liver resection. Age alone is not a contraindication for a patient's eligibility for liver resection.[12]

Resectable synchronous liver lesions can be found at the time of the resection of the primary colorectal tumor. Typically, the liver lesions are biopsied at the time of the colorectal resection, with a plan to resect the metastases at a later date. Intraoperative US is utilized to confirm resectability.

### Repeat surgical resection

Among patients who have undergone primary liver resection for metastatic CRC, 50% to 60% will have recurrence within the liver.[109] Repeat hepatectomy to remove the recurrence is possible because the liver regenerates almost to the original mass within 4 to 6 weeks.[110,111] Repeat resection within the liver is technically more difficult due to adhesions and the adherence of the surface of the previous resection to neighboring organs. Regeneration of the liver also changes the shape of the organ and vascular structures, creating a more difficult resection. In some cases, there may be a greater risk of bleeding. Perioperative mortality is similar to that for initial hepatic resections, although the morbidity rates are higher.[112] The Repeat Hepatic Metastases Registry noted 20% higher postoperative morbidity with repeat resection than with the first resection.[113] Nonetheless, repeat resection for liver metastases should be considered a treatment option if the disease is resectable.

## POSTOPERATIVE CARE

Following major hepatic resection, the patient typically requires close monitoring in an intensive care setting for a period of 24 hours to manage intravascular volume and perfusion changes. Fluid restriction or transfusion, or both, may be necessary. Individuals with cirrhosis are at increased risk for complications during the postoperative period compared with noncirrhotic individuals. Knowledge of the potential complications and signs of impending problems, together with aggressive treatment, are vital in caring for a patient postoperatively.

Monitoring LFTs, phosphate, and glucose frequently is important until a downward trend in transaminase levels is noted. Hypophosphatemia is commonly seen postoperatively, and replacement of phosphate may be necessary. The levels seen in LFTs rise immediately postoperatively but will usually return to normal within 7 to 10 days postoperatively. The degree of elevation depends on the extent of liver resected and intraoperative ischemic time. If LFT results are extraordinarily high in the early postoperative period, they may indicate an injury to vascular inflow or outflow in the retained liver segment. In this case, a Doppler US of the liver should be performed to rule out portal vein thrombosis. In addition, it is important to monitor an individual's glucose level, as it may also be indicative of hepatic failure. Decreased albumin levels are also noted following liver resection, related to protein loss in the abdomen. No benefit from administration of albumin has been noted.[114] The patient's diet is slowly advanced with resolution of a postoperative ileus. Drainage tubes, if placed, are discontinued when the biliary output tapers off and no bile leak is evident.

**TABLE 58-8**

**Postoperative Complications Following Liver Resection**

| | |
|---|---|
| Liver-related complications | |
| | Hemorrhage |
| | Bile fistula |
| | Biloma |
| | Subphrenic abscess |
| | Ascites |
| | Liver failure |
| | Portal hypertension |
| | Coagulopathy |
| Infections | |
| | Wound |
| | Urinary tract |
| | Pneumonia |

If the patient develops ascites, it may interfere with nutritional intake and ventilation. Therefore, it is important to restrict sodium intake to 1000 to 1500 mg per day and fluid intake to 1500 mL per day. Addition of a loop diuretic and spironolactone will likely decrease the patient's weight by 0.5 to 1.0 kg. With this particular intervention, the patient's potassium, blood urea nitrogen (BUN), and creatinine should be monitored closely, with potassium being replaced as necessary. Following hepatic resection, potential complications include hemorrhage, biliary leak or biloma, subphrenic abscess, infection, pneumonia, pleural effusion, transient metabolic consequences, portal hypertension, clotting defects, and hepatic failure (Table 58-8).

### Hemorrhage

The liver is a vascular organ, and with hepatic resection a raw surface area of the liver could produce bleeding in the first 24 hours postoperatively. Bleeding may be indicated by hypotension, tachycardia, and increasing abdominal girth. Intra-abdominal hemorrhage will require immediate exploratory laparotomy to repair the bleeding area. Nursing observations and assessment include frequent monitoring of vital signs and central venous pressure; assessing skin for adequate perfusion; measuring abdominal girth; assessing for bleeding from the incision site; assessing urine and stool; and serial monitoring of hemoglobin and hematocrit. In addition, cirrhotic individuals are at increased risk for bleeding complications and should be evaluated for overt and subclinical signs of bleeding disorders.

### Biliary leak or biloma

Wound drains—typically Jackson-Pratt drains—are placed to prevent bile accumulation. A subhepatic drain is placed, and a small amount of bile may be noted from necrosis on the edge of the liver. When no drains are present or when the bile leak does not resolve following drain placements, a collection of bile, called biloma, may develop. Fever, pain, and a distended abdomen may also indicate a biliary leak or biloma. The drain remains until a leak is no longer noted. If the leak persists, the patient may require further percutaneous drainage.

### Subphrenic abscess

Perihepatic infection or necrosis of the remaining liver may precipitate a subphrenic abscess. Warning signs include sharp, piercing right upper quadrant pain and low-grade fever. Auscultation of the base of the lungs may detect fluid and possible abscess. Given the short length of the typical hospital stay, patients will be at home and need to notify the physician of these symptoms as they appear later in the postoperative course.

### Infection

Individuals with cirrhosis are at increased risk for infection following hepatic resection as a result of decreased protein stores. The mortality rate associated with infection is high.[115] Continued assessment of vital signs, wound healing, and drain patency is crucial. Aggressive intervention is required early.

### Pleural effusion and pneumonia

Pleural effusion is common following liver resection, most often after right hepatectomy. In most cases, patients are asymptomatic and should not be treated for the effusion. Aggressive pulmonary toilet with incentive spirometry and deep breathing can prevent pneumonia. Individuals are often reluctant to perform respiratory exercises due to the pain experienced with a subcostal incision, so they need encouragement. In addition, frequent ambulation and administration of analgesics prior to conducting respiratory exercises are important nursing measures.

### Transient metabolic consequences

A transient elevation in LFTs occurs postoperatively. Concern arises when a persistent upward trend is noted in the bilirubin and LFTs. If this is accompanied by jaundice and signs of hepatic failure, mechanical obstruction and portal vein thrombosis must be ruled out.

### Portal hypertension

Portal hypertension results from the surgical rerouting of the portal venous flow through a small remnant of liver. This leads to sequestration of blood in the splanchnic circulation. Fortunately, the liver has a great potential for increasing blood flow if it has adequate time to compensate.

Central venous pressure monitoring is a reliable indicator of blood volume. Bleeding from a puncture site, wound, or cavity requires immediate attention.

### Clotting defects

A slight rise in the prothrombin time may be noted postoperatively. Severe coagulopathies may develop and need to be treated with fresh frozen plasma. The nurse can detect complications from deficiencies in clotting mechanisms by observing puncture sites for bleeding, monitoring abdominal girth, and testing urine and stool for blood.

### Hepatic failure

Hepatic failure following hepatic resection can occur as a result of portal vein thrombosis or insufficient hepatic parenchyma. Insufficient parenchyma is more frequently the cause of hepatic failure in a cirrhotic individual. A continued rise in bilirubin and LFTs will occur if hepatic failure is developing. In addition, the patient may display mental confusion with an increase in serum ammonia levels. Other systems (eg, renal, neurological, and cardiac systems) may be also compromised. Frequent monitoring of mental status, vital signs, and laboratory studies are important nursing measures.

## POST-TRANSPLANT CARE

Postoperative care following transplantation is similar initially to care following hepatic resection. However, the most important aspect of postoperative care in LT is the administration of immunosuppressive therapy to prevent organ rejection. Ongoing support to patients is critical because they are often overwhelmed with the number of medications that must be taken on a daily basis. Studies of posttransplant improvement in emotional well-being have found that male spouses demonstrate more family cohesion with less conflict, whereas female spouses experience a higher level of stress. At 1 year, patients' and families' overall quality of life is generally improved.[116]

## PALLIATIVE TREATMENTS

### Regional therapy

***Hepatic artery infusion (HAI) for hepatocellular cancer.*** Hepatic artery infusion is a treatment modality used for unresectable HCC confined to the liver. The hepatic artery is the main supply of blood flow to the liver.[93] Chemotherapy with effective first-pass hepatic extraction can be delivered selectively to the tumor via the hepatic artery. Thus, HAI can, in theory, result in a higher concentration of drug to the tumor tissue with fewer systemic side effects.[117] Complications of HAI may include impaired liver function, biliary sclerosis, liver abscess, and dislodgment of the infusion catheter tip. An implantable pump is placed surgically for continuous delivery of the drugs. Chemotherapy agents used for HAI include fluorouracil and floxuridine (FUDR), fluorouracil/cisplatin, floxuridine/mitomycin, doxorubicin, and floxuridine/leucovorin/doxorubicin/platinol (FLAP).[93] Tumor response rates have been reported to be 40%, with a modest survival advantage of a few months.[117]

However, the studies on HAI for the most part have been small, and patients selected for the studies have had less advanced liver disease, good performance status, and the ability to withstand abdominal surgery for pump placement. Potential selection bias needs to be taken into account when interpreting the results of improved survival.[89]

In summary, HAI therapy does not seem to offer a greater survival advantage than systemic therapy. In addition, the risks associated with performing a major surgical procedure for pump placement need to be taken into account. HAI therapy is not to be considered standard therapy for unresectable HCC confined to the liver, but it may be considered in a clinical trial setting.

***HAI for liver metastasis.*** Regional chemotherapy via HAI is a treatment option that is used mostly for unresectable hepatic metastases from colorectal cancer. The principle utilized in the delivery of HAI chemotherapy is that normal hepatic parenchyma derives the majority of its blood supply from the portal system, whereas metastatic lesions in the liver derive most of their afferent blood supply from the hepatic artery.[117,118] Therefore, high doses of chemotherapeutic agents are delivered directly into the hepatic artery, increasing the concentration of drug to which the tumor is exposed, while limiting both normal liver and systemic exposure and toxicity. The systemic toxicities are limited because the chemotherapeutic agents delivered have short half-lives and are extracted by the liver on the first-pass liver metabolism. Most commonly, floxuridine is used for HAI, because of the high percentage of first-pass extraction.

Regional chemotherapy delivers drugs via the hepatic artery with an implantable pump. Preoperative angiography with selective injection of the celiac and superior mesenteric arteries should be performed to assure proper placement of the catheter. The standard anatomy is classified as the common hepatic artery arising from the celiac artery.[119]

The patient then undergoes exploratory laparotomy via right subcostal incision and exploration of the abdomen to rule out extrahepatic metastases. An implantable pump is placed in a subcutaneous pocket in the lower abdominal wall, and the catheter is attached to a subcutaneously implanted port. Fluorescein injection is performed intraoperatively with an ultraviolet lamp to determine adequate perfusion of both lobes of the liver. Cholecystectomy is routinely performed at the time of pump implant to prevent potential complications related to chemotherapy. Postoperatively, a nuclear scan is used to assess the perfusion of the liver. Bilobular flow must be documented and extrahepatic perfusion ruled out.

Surgical expertise is a key factor in the implantation of hepatic arterial pumps, especially when variant anatomy of the liver is present. An inadequate surgical technique can result in both gastroduodenal ulceration and inadequate liver perfusion.[120,121] In addition, medical oncologists must be familiar with the management of HAI chemotherapy in terms of determining the need for decreased dosage vs discontinuation of therapy, because HAI treatment may trigger the beginning of sclerosing cholangitis. Medical management includes close follow-up of biweekly laboratory tests and close attention to rising LFTs, especially bilirubin and alkaline phosphatase. Carcinoembryonic antigen levels are also measured monthly. Fluoropyrimidines (eg, fluorouracil and floxuridine) are utilized to treat hepatic metastases. Regional chemotherapy can be delivered every 2 weeks or weekly on a protracted basis. Therefore, the tumor cells are exposed to the drug throughout the vulnerable phase of their mitotic cycle.[122]

Regional chemotherapy can produce a variety of side effects related to the toxicity of the specific drug. In the early development of hepatic intra-arterial infusion of floxuridine, a high incidence (10%–56%) of gastroduodenal ulceration occurred.[123–125] With increased expertise in surgical technique, this complication has been seen less frequently.

Other complications from HAI chemotherapy can include partial or complete thrombosis of the hepatic artery, occlusion or displacement of the catheter, hemorrhage, infection of the device or catheter, and acalculous cholecystitis.[126]

Another complication of regional chemotherapy with the delivery of floxuridine is "chemical hepatitis," which is demonstrated by a rise in the levels of liver enzymes and bilirubin.[123] Bilirubinemia and strictures of the bile duct may indicate biliary sclerosis.[127] To distinguish this condition from biliary obstruction as a result of nodal metastases in the porta hepatis (transverse fissure of the liver) or stricturing of the bile ducts, a cholangiography should be conducted.

To detect sclerosing cholangitis early, it is important to monitor serum bilirubin frequently. A slight elevation of serum bilirubin should prompt temporary discontinuation of floxuridine treatment. Also, dexamethasone has been given through the hepatic artery to normalize alkaline phosphatase and persistent bilirubin elevation in those patients undergoing hepatic arterial chemotherapy. Patients with extensive liver involvement may experience diarrhea due to impaired fluoropyrimidine hepatic metabolism.[128] Overall, complications of HAI therapy can vary and chemotherapy may need to be discontinued.[129]

Hepatectomy rarely can be performed following intra-arterial chemotherapy unless the tumor volume has been reduced enough to render it surgically resectable.[130] It may be difficult to quantify the size and number of lesions due to the steatosis (fatty degeneration) that can result from intra-arterial therapy. It may also be more difficult to determine whether enough functional hepatic parenchyma remains to prevent postoperative hepatic failure. Technically, it is more difficult to perform hepatectomy because the hepatic artery has been ligated and multiple collateral vessels may have developed.[131] Emerging data from randomized trials suggest a potential benefit of combined regional and systemic chemotherapy following liver resection due to metastatic colorectal cancer.[132]

The use of HAI therapy plus systemic chemotherapy after a hepatic resection has been found to decrease the rate of hepatic recurrence. In addition, it improves 2-year survival rates when compared with systemic chemotherapy alone.[133]

*Embolization/chemoembolization.* Chemoembolization is a local regional treatment option involving drugs or devices to restrict blood flow to certain areas of the liver. The majority of tumors receive blood flow from the hepatic artery, and normal hepatic parenchyma receives its blood supply from the portal vein.[134] It has been shown that chemotherapy given during surgery achieves a 10 times higher intratumoral concentration when it is given through the artery rather than through the portal vein.[135] As a consequence, arterially directed embolization can make the tumor ischemic, while uninvolved liver is spared. Chemoembolization is best for treating hypervascular tumors (eg, HCC and neuroendocrine liver metastases). CRC lesions are hypovascular and limit the ability to deliver adequate chemotherapy and embolic agents. Patient selection criteria required for possible chemoembolization include adequate hematologic and renal function, well-preserved hepatic function, and portal vein patency. On a case-by-case basis, patients with focal tumors with partial portal vein occlusion may still be feasible candidates for chemoembolization.[136,137]

Prior to the chemoembolization procedure, tissue diagnosis should be obtained in addition to CT or MRI to exclude extrahepatic disease. Laboratory studies include complete blood count, LFTs, tumor markers, and partial thromboplastin and prothrombin times. Patient education should focus on side effects related to the postembolization syndrome.

The chemoembolization procedure is performed in the angiography suite with the patient under conscious sedation. A catheter is inserted in the common femoral artery; alternatively, the brachial artery may be used. A diagnostic mesenteric and hepatic arteriography is performed to determine arterial blood supply to the liver and mesentery and to confirm patency of the portal vein. A catheter is then introduced into the right or left hepatic artery depending on which lobe contains the tumor.[138] A coil is introduced into the gastroduodenal artery to protect the stomach and duodenum from potential reflux of the embolic agent.

With the catheter in the appropriate vessel supplying the tumor, the chemotherapy mixture is then injected. Some centers use a single agent, such as doxorubicin, while others add different drugs such as cisplatin, mitomycin, or fluorouracil. Lipiodol (ethiodized oil), a cottonseed oil-based contrast agent, is frequently added to form a chemoemulsion, which suspends droplets of chemotherapeutic agents in an oil matrix. When embolic emulsions are added, this agent increases the response rate. Embolization creates impedance to arterial blood flow and increases the exposure of chemotherapy to the metastatic lesions.

A gelatin sponge, mixed with the chemotherapy, is inserted to block hepatic artery flow that induces ischemic necrosis of bulky tumors. The sponge also retains ethiodized oil for a period of time and maintains a high concentration of chemotherapeutic agents. The drug concentration delivered to the tumor is 10 to 25 times higher than that achieved by systemic infusion.[139] Various centers administer antibiotics before and after the procedure to decrease the risk of infection and abscess formation.[140]

The patient is typically admitted following the chemoembolization procedure, for a period of 24 to 48 hours. Side effects from the treatment are common but self-limited. Most patients will experience postembolization syndrome, characterized by fever, dull right upper quadrant pain, nausea, and vomiting due to transient liver capsule stretching. The symptoms are treated with antipyretics and hydrocortisone, which achieve good control in most cases.[117] Transient elevation in LFTs is common in patients treated with chemoembolization. Rarely, patients may develop bacteremia, pneumonia, ascites, renal dysfunction, pleural effusions, or encephalopathy.[141] More serious but rare complications include liver failure, cerebral hemorrhage, liver abscess, tumor lysis syndrome, gallbladder ischemia, pancreatitis, and gastric and duodenal ulcers.[141]

For an individual with cirrhosis, a rising bilirubin level is a warning sign of potential irreversible liver necrosis. To reduce significant hepatic toxicity, chemoembolization is typically restricted to 1 lobe or major branch of the hepatic artery. The patient is then brought back in 4 weeks, once toxicities and laboratory values return to normal, to complete the procedure in the opposite lobe.

Despite the liver parenchyma's sensitivity to chemotherapy drugs, chemoembolization is safe due the liver's unique vascular supply. The portal vein supplies 70% to 80% of the liver parenchyma, whereas HCC is entirely supplied by the branches of the hepatic artery due to angiogenesis. Hence, repeated chemoembolization procedures are possible without causing significant permanent liver damage.[142]

### Ablative/cytoreductive therapy

*Percutaneous ethanol injection.* Percutaneous ethanol injection (PEI) is an appropriate treatment modality for patients with HCC who have solitary tumors smaller than 2 cm in diameter and who do not have the hepatic reserve to withstand a surgical resection. Because local recurrences are common, PEI is generally not recommended for patients with tumors larger than 5 cm.[143] PEI may also be performed for patients who are transplantation candidates and may be on a long waiting list, as a means of controlling disease while awaiting a transplant.

Injection of 95% ethanol into a tumor induces tumor necrosis and shrinkage. The mechanism of action is cytoplasmic dehydration with subsequent intracellular coagulation, leading to necrosis. Ethanol also affects endothelial cells, causing platelet aggregation, thrombosis, vascular occlusion, and fibrosis—all of which can decrease the blood supply to the tumor.[144]

Percutaneous ethanol injection may be performed as an outpatient procedure for smaller lesions, with multiple separate injections of 1 to 8 mL ethanol being administered twice weekly, for a total of 4 to 12 sessions.[145,146] The survival rates for patients with Child-Pugh stage A cirrhosis (no ascites or encephalopathy, well-preserved liver function) and tumors smaller than 5 cm at 1, 3, and 5 years have been reported to be 98%, 79%, and 47%, respectively.[145,146] Poorer results have been reported in less stringently selected patients.[144–148]

In general, PEI is well tolerated. Common side effects include localized pain due to tumor necrosis and peritoneal irritation due to ethanol leakage. Rare complications occurring in less than 5% of patients may include intraperitoneal hemorrhage, hepatic insufficiency, bile duct or biliary fistula, hepatic infarction, hypotension, and renal failure.[149]

*Cryoablation.* Cryoablation is an ablative therapy for patients with unresectable HCC who have multifocal lesions, typically fewer than 5 total lesions, with each being smaller than 5 cm in diameter. The cryoablation technique involves inserting a cryoprobe then circulating liquid nitrogen to achieve subzero temperature to less than –35°C; it leads to the death of both tumor and normal cells, either immediately or during the subsequent thawing period. Using multiple freeze–thaw cycles increases the percentage of tumor cells killed.[150] To achieve adequate margins, ultrasound guidance is used to direct the site of the freezing procedure. Cryoablation has not been compared prospectively with hepatic resection in noncirrhotic patients. In patients with HCC, survival rates have been reported to approach 20%.[151]

Postoperatively, patients are monitored in the intensive care unit with frequent serial laboratory evaluation, including complete blood count, coagulation profile, electrolytes, BUN, serum creatinine, and myoglobin. Alkaline hydration is administrated until the urine is free of myoglobin.[152–154] Complications arise frequently with cryoablation. They may include cracking of the ice ball, liver surface fracture,[152–154] hypothermia and associated coagulopathy, cardiac arrhythmia, consumptive coagulopathy,[155] thrombocytopenia,[154] biliary fistula,[156] bleeding,[153,156,157] electrolyte disturbance,[151,152] iatrogenic probe injury, cryogenic shock,[152,154] abscess, pleural effusion,[156] myoglobinuria,[153,154,156] and acute renal failure.[157] Due to the relatively high rate of complications associated with cryoablation, radiofrequency ablation is currently favored over cryoablation, as the latter treatment is associated with lower rates of both recurrences and complications.

*Radiofrequency ablation.* Radiofrequency ablation (RFA) is another type of ablative modality used in treating patients with HCC (Figure 58-2), liver metastases from CRC, and neuroendocrine tumors. RFA is typically used in those patients who do not meet the criteria for surgical resection but who are candidates for liver-directed procedures based on the absence of extrahepatic disease. The RFA technique uses high-energy heat greater than 60°F to produce cell destruction and tissue necrosis.[158,159] The RFA procedure may be done percutaneously under US or CT guidance, laparoscopically, or as an open laparotomy procedure. US is used to guide placement of a needle electrode, which is then advanced into the area of the tumor to be treated. The needle electrode is attached to a radiofrequency generator, and the treatment is delivered (Figure 58-3). To obtain a tumor-free margin, the thermal electrode is used to produce a thermal lesion encompassing the entire treated area, including not only the tumor but also nondiseased liver tissue of 1 cm around the tumor.[160] The patient is monitored with CT to determine whether additional therapy is necessary (Figure 58-4).

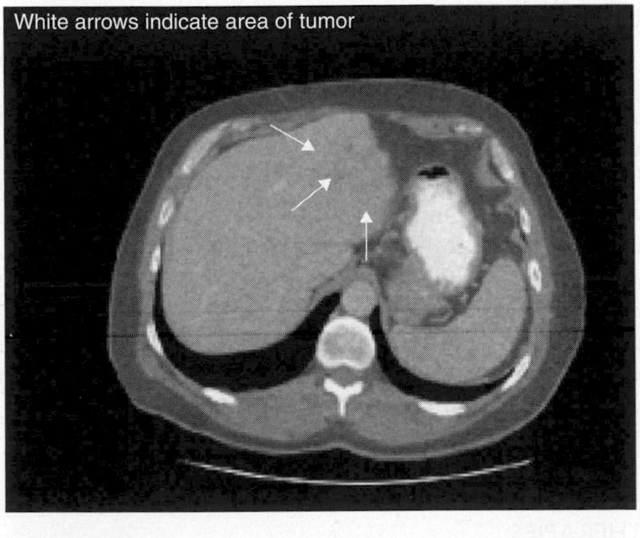


**FIGURE 58-2**

Hepatocellular carcinoma of right medial lobe. Computerized tomography scan before radiofrequency ablation.

*Source*: Photo courtesy of the Massachusetts General Hospital Department of Interventional Radiology.

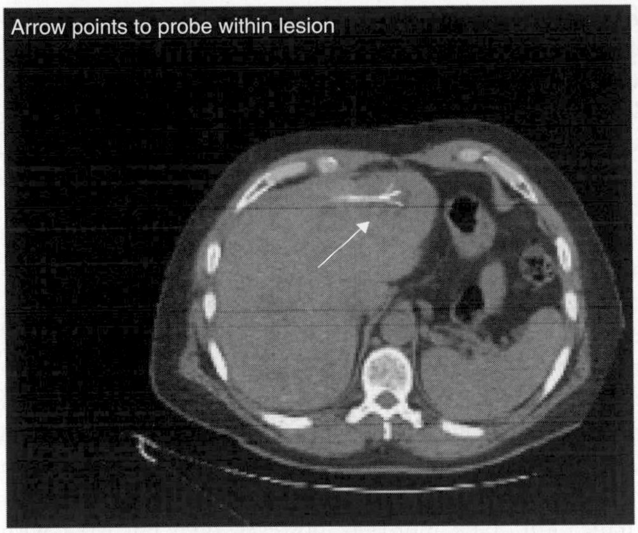


**FIGURE 58-3**

Radiofrequence ablation probe within the lesion.

*Source*: Photo courtesy of the Massachusetts General Hospital Department of Interventional Radiology.

## RADIATION THERAPY

External beam radiotherapy has limited use in the treatment of HCC because normal liver tissue has low tolerance

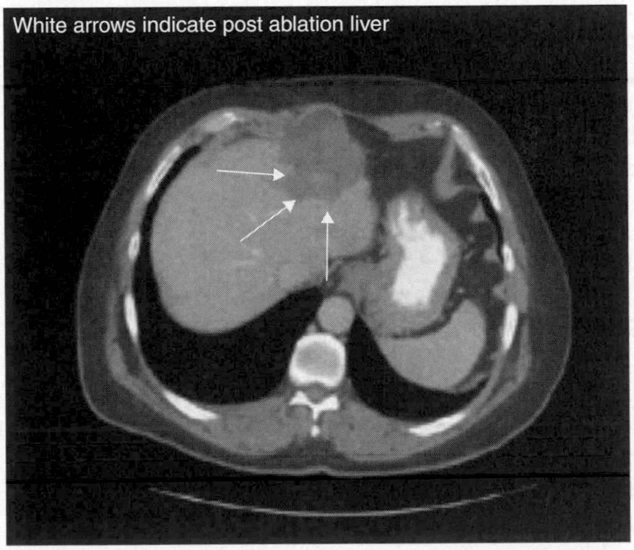


**FIGURE 58-4**

Post-radiofrequency ablation of hepatocellular carcinoma lesion computerized tomography (CT) scan. The goal of treatment with radiofrequency ablation is complete destruction of the tumor and a surrounding margin of hepatic parenchyma. Post-ablation computerized tomography scan (4 weeks) shows lesions larger than original tumor.

*Source*: Photo courtesy of the Massachusetts General Hospital Department of Interventional Radiology.

for radiation. A dosage of greater than 50 Gy has been recommended to kill HCC cells, but this dosage will provoke radiation-induced hepatitis and liver failure.[161] Survival following radiation therapy is short, with most patients dying within 6 months.[162] Conventional radiotherapy in the range of 30 to 35 Gy can be used in patients who require palliation of painful liver lesions.

Larger doses of radiation can be delivered via linear accelerator and proton beam therapy because of the better targeting of the radiation to the tumor. Large doses of radiation are directed at the tumor via 3-dimensional radiation ports. A 50% reduction in tumor size has been reported with minimal side effects and good quality of life.[161] Radiotherapy can be used safely in patients with Child-Pugh stage A cirrhosis and tumors smaller than 8 cm or in patients with Child-Pugh stage B and tumors smaller than 5 cm. This approach, however, does not work with micrometastatic or multifocal disease.[93]

Like many other treatment options, radiation therapy has yet to be defined in regard to unresectable HCC. It can be an option in patients with localized disease who have failed other local therapies, have no extrahepatic disease, and have limited tumor burden and good liver function.

Intra-arterially administered yttrium-90 glass microspheres have also been used in HCC.[162,163] This approach uses drug-eluting beads specifically designed to release chemotherapy, in turn decreasing systemic side effects. Clinical trials of this procedure in the US are ongoing. Early results are promising using this approach as an alternative to chemoembolization.[164] However, published experience is limited. In Europe and Canada, doxorubicin-loaded beads are approved (DC Bead, Biocompatibles International Inc.). In the US, LC beads (Angiodynamics, Inc.)[165] are commercially available in a variety of sizes and approved as a medical device. Doxorubicin can be mixed by a specialized oncology pharmacist using a special mixing technique.

## SYSTEMIC CHEMOTHERAPY

Chemotherapy may be the only potential treatment option for patients with advanced HCC, because the majority of these patients are not candidates for curative resection. To date, many chemotherapy agents have been studied to treat advanced HCC without much success, because several limitations exist in treating the disease. For example, HCC is known to be a chemotherapy-refractory tumor. This tendency could be due to its high rate of expression of drug-resistant genes, and the heterogeneous nature of the tumor.[144,166–168] In addition, patients with advanced HCC who have significant liver dysfunction cannot tolerate systemic chemotherapy.[151] In one study, no objective responses were found in patients with poor performance status, ascites, portal vein thrombus, or serum bilirubin greater than 2 mg/dL.[169]

Single agent and combination chemotherapy have been studied. Doxorubicin is perhaps the most widely used drug as a single agent. A number of small studies have reported partial response rates of less than 20%.[170–172] One small trial suggested a survival benefit compared with best supportive care (median survival of 10.6 months vs 7.5 months).[173,174]

Another agent with a low toxicity profile and broad antitumor activity is fluorouracil. Despite the fact that fluorouracil is extensively metabolized by the liver, adequate doses can be administered in the setting of liver dysfunction. When it is given as a single agent, response rates are low. When it is given in combination with leucovorin, response rates can be as high as 28% for the management of HCC.[173]

Oral agents such as capecitabine[175] or the anti-angiogenic agent thalidomide[176] have been associated with minor objective tumor activity and, in some patients, with stabilization of disease growth. A complete response on radiologic examination has been observed in 1 patient with HCC after receiving capecitabine.[175]

Combination chemotherapy agents have been studied in patients with advanced HCC. These studies have not shown a survival benefit. Of the combination regimens, cisplatin-based regimens have produced higher objective response rates than non-cisplatin-based regimens. Cisplatin-containing regimens include a combination of cisplatin and epirubicin; cisplatin and infusional fluorouracil; sequential low-dose infusional cisplatin plus infusional fluorouracil; and gemcitabine and cisplatin. Median survival in all studies of these agents was 4.4 to 11 months.[177–184]

Interferon-alpha (IFN-α) has been studied as a single agent, with 3 times weekly subcutaneous injections achieving a response rate of 31% and improved median survival benefit when compared with the best supportive care group. Tolerability was good, with fatigue being cited as the major toxicity.[185]

Combination regimens with IFN-α, such as IFN-α and fluorouracil or IFN-α and cisplatin, when compared with best supportive care, have better 1-year survival rates.[186] In addition, the regimen toxicity profile is acceptable. The combination regimen of cisplatin, IFN-α, doxorubicin, and infusional fluorouracil (PIAF) resulted in response rates of approximately 26%, with some patients achieving complete response.[187] However, this regimen is associated with significant toxicity. It may be an appropriate choice in young patients with adequate liver function.[187]

## HEPATOCELLULAR CARCINOMA AND TARGETED THERAPIES

Better understanding of the molecular mechanism of the hepatocarcinogenesis process and the advent of the newly developed molecular targeted agents have provided the opportunity to study some of the novel agents in HCC. It appears that HCC development involves such pathways as angiogenesis, aberrant signal transduction, and dysregulation of cell cycle control. Many of the molecular changes found in HCC are attributed to underlying cirrhosis, and others are found in the dysplastic nodule of the HCC lesions.[188] A number of early clinical studies have examined the efficacy and safety of targeting of some of these pathways in HCC. The expression of epithelial growth factor receptor 1 (EGFR/HER-1) and its ligands EGF and transforming growth factor-alpha have been highlighted in hepatocarcinogenesis.[189] Cetuximab (Erbitux) in combination with gemcitabine and oxaliplatin (GEMOX) suggests activity. In a preliminary report, there were 8 partial responses, and disease control (partial response plus stable disease) was 65%. The treatment is generally well tolerated with Grade 2 and 3 neurotoxicity in 16% and 5%, respectively.[190]

HCCs are known to be vascular tumors; they are also known to express high levels of vascular endothelial growth factor (VEGF).[191] High levels of VEGF expression have also been associated with poor survival.[192] Hence, agents such as bevacizumab (Avastin), an anti-angiogenic agent, a humanized monoclonal antibody that targets VEGF, are believed to benefit patients with HCC.[193] Studies are underway with bevacizumab with and without chemotherapy for the treatment of HCC.

Sorafenib (Nexavar) is the first drug to demonstrate a survival benefit in patients with HCC. Sorafenib is an orally active multitargeted molecule tyrosine kinase inhibitor that inhibits *Ras* kinase and also blocks the intracellular portion of the VEGF receptor.[194] In phase III clinical trials comparing sorafenib to best supportive care, the sorafenib proved survival benefit. Hence, the results of the Sorafenib Hepatocellular Carcinoma Assessment Randomized Protocol (SHARP) trial led to the approval of sorafenib monotherapy as the new reference for standard systemic treatment for HCC in the US.[195]

## GENE THERAPY

Gene therapy represents an exciting and promising approach for the treatment of HCC, although currently it is largely confined to the preclinical and experimental settings. Gene therapy can produce a biological effect by the transfer of foreign genes into the target cells using viral or nonviral vectors.[196] Gene therapies that have been studied for the treatment of HCC include gene replacement therapy with *p53,* a tumor suppressor gene; antisense therapy against the *K-ras* oncogene; drug sensitization with a suicide gene encoding a foreign enzyme that transforms a nontoxic prodrug into a toxic compound in transfected cells; and genetic immunotherapy that seeks to stimulate a more effective response against tumor antigens. Technical problems need to be overcome prior to successful clinical application of gene therapy, including better gene delivery, improved tumor specificity, more stable transgene expressions, and larger therapeutic windows.[197]

## SYMPTOM MANAGEMENT AND SUPPORTIVE CARE

At diagnosis, the clinical course of primary liver cancer and metastatic liver cancer may vary widely. However, as the disease in the liver and the metastatic process progress, their clinical courses will be very similar. Palliative approaches for treating patients with advanced or metastatic liver cancer may rely on systemic chemotherapy, regional therapy, or radiation therapy. Patients may initially present with advanced disease and impaired liver function that is not possible to treat. Regardless of the stage of the disease, comfort measures and management of distressing symptoms should be provided.

Pain can be a common symptom of advanced disease. The etiology of pain in this patient population may include pain caused by abdominal fullness, stretching of the liver capsule, ascites, or intra-abdominal disease metastasis. The 3-step analgesic ladder developed by the World Health Organization should guide pain management therapy.[198] Initially, pain may be controlled with anti-inflammatory drugs and acetaminophen. Due to their gastrointestinal, hepatotoxic, and hematologic side effects, these drugs often have limited long-term use. Transdermal and long-acting oral opioids are used along with short-acting narcotics for breakthrough pain. A bowel regimen should be instituted to avoid or treat constipation. If pain cannot be adequately controlled, external beam radiation with or without chemotherapy may be used to palliate the pain of advanced liver cancer.

As the liver fails and secretes less bile, bilirubin will accumulate in the blood. Clinically, jaundice becomes apparent when bilirubin levels exceed 3 mg/dL. Hemolysis of red blood cells may add to the jaundice. Pruritus can become distressing to the patient. Management of pruritus may include avoiding hot baths and hot drinks that can cause blood vessel dilation; applying local ice pack to areas of most severe itching; taking starch or oatmeal baths; and applying moisturizing agents with topical lotions containing menthol, camphor, phenol, zinc oxide, calamine, doxepin, or corticosteroids. Systemic oral antihistamines may be effective when given in high doses at bedtime. Cholestyramine may be used to remove bile acids if the patient is able to tolerate oral intake.

With advanced disease, ascites can cause pain and dyspnea. Paracentesis can lead to loss of albumin, volume depletion, hypotension, and the risk of peritonitis. Low doses of morphine may help with the dyspnea,[199] and pain management intervention as discussed previously should be instituted. Diuretics, such as furosemide and spironolactone, can be used as needed. Peritoneovenous catheters or shunts are sometimes used for palliation of ascites, depending on the patient's goals.

Nausea, vomiting, and early satiety may be present and should be treated with antiemetics such as prochlorperazine and haloperidol. Allowing the patient to self-regulate oral intake and consume small frequent meals may help.

Psychological distress should be assessed. If present, clinical depression should be treated. There is no particular class of antidepressants that is especially advantageous for this patient population. Selective serotonin reuptake inhibitors (SSRIs) may be a good choice because they have fewer side effects and the potential to improve energy levels. The use of psychostimulants may also be indicated to improve mood, increase appetite, and counter the sedation of opioid treatments. Counseling and a support group for patients and caretakers may benefit these individuals as well.

Generalized debilitation, fatigue, weight loss, and cachexia will be present in advanced disease. Supportive nutritional management initially may include caloric supplementation and oral hydration. Enteral or parental nutrition is usually not preferred in most cases of the anorexia/cachexia syndrome in patients with advanced cancer because it does not yield any prolonged benefit.[200] Appetite stimulants such as megesterol acetate at doses of 200 to 800 mg/day and corticosteroids can be used to treat anorexia.[201–203] Another class of drugs that may be used alone or in conjunction with other agents to stimulate appetite are the cannabinoids. Dronabinol has been proven to improve chemotherapy-induced nausea and vomiting in 65% of cancer patients.[187] It also improves appetite in HIV-associated cachexia. Fatigue is a persistent symptom with many causes, including the disease itself, side effects of treatment, and depression. Fatigue may be reduced by aggressively treating contributing factors such as depression, anxiety, and uncontrolled pain. Anemia may be a contributing factor to fatigue anywhere along the disease trajectory. Once diagnosed, it should be treated with blood transfusion. If appropriate, recombinant human erythropoietin can also be used to promote adequate hemoglobin levels.

Clinical indicators of end-stage liver failure include hepatic encephalopathy, hepatorenal syndrome, recurrent variceal bleeding, ascites, and coagulopathies refractory to indicated therapies. Hepatic encephalopathy is considered an early stage of hepatic coma. Due to the inability of the liver to perform detoxifying functions, ammonia and other substances toxic to the brain will be present in the circulation.

Clinical features of hepatic encephalopathy include drowsiness, confusion, irritability, and characteristic flapping tremors (asterixis). Treatment may include diazepam and haloperidol for agitation and hallucinations. Ammonia levels can be decreased by administering lactulose 30 mL every 8 hours, titrated to produce 2 to 3 stools daily. Likewise, neomycin 1 g daily can be used to decrease ammonia levels.[204]

Anticipatory management of rapidly developing symptoms of the patient and family support are major goals in advanced and end-stage disease. Psychosocial, spiritual, and symptom management are all equally paramount concerns. The person dying from liver failure, whatever its cause, is dying from multisystem failure. For some patients, death may be precipitated by an acute event such as gastrointestinal bleeding, respiratory failure, hypovolemic shock, sepsis, or pneumonia. For others, death may occur quietly, with the patient lapsing into a coma.

## CONCLUSION

Oncology nurses caring for patients with primary liver cancer and metastatic liver disease face a tremendous challenge. Treatment options in patients with HCC are generally limited due to the presence of underlying severe liver disease, advanced tumor stage, and restricted options for transplantation. In the future, improved screening tools and treatment for HCC, as well as the discovery of new treatments such as gene therapy, hold promise for improving survival of patients with HCC. Continued refinements in the surgical management of patients with CRC liver metastasis and regional therapies such as HAI infusion pump and RFA will contribute to improved survival rates.

Preventive strategies will most likely make the greatest impact. As in the case of hepatitis B, vaccination of children in Taiwan resulted in a decline in HCC incidence. In addition, using antiviral therapy in patients with HBV and HCV infection should contribute to the prevention of HCC. Further primary prevention aimed at public health measures to reduce food contamination with aflatoxins and to eliminate excessive alcohol use should also reduce the incidence of liver disease, cirrhosis, and hence HCC.

Oncology nurses can play a key role within the multidisciplinary team caring for patients with HCC and liver metastases. Providing education to patients about disease prevention, screening options for early disease, and treatment options can empower patients and their families in making decisions regarding their treatment and care. In addition, oncology nurses play a key role in providing expert care in the area of symptom assessment and management of pain, nutrition, functional status, and spiritual well-being. In the future, nursing research related to the care of patients with HCC and liver metastases and focused on quality of life, symptom experience from the disease, and treatment can contribute to improving patient outcomes and quality of care.

## REFERENCES

1. Bosch FX, Ribes J, Cleries R, Diaz M. Epidemiology of hepatocellular carcinoma. *Clin Liver Dis.* 2004;9:191–211.

2. El-Serag HB. Hepatocellular carcinoma: recent trends in the United States. *Gastroenterology.* 2004;127:S7-S34.
3. Jemal A, Siegel R, Ward E, et al. Cancer Statistics, 2008. *CA: Cancer J Clin.* 2008;58:71–96.
4. Parkin DM. Global cancer statistics in the year 2000. *Lancet Oncol.* 2001;2:533–543.
5. El-Serag HB. Epidemiology of hepatocellular carcinoma. *Clin Liver Dis.* 2001;5:87–107.
6. Parkin DM, Muir CS, Whelan SL, et al, eds. *Cancer Incidence in Five Continents, vol 6.* Lyon, France: International Agency for Research on Cancer; 1997.
7. Davlla, JA, Morgan RO, Shaib Y, et al. Hepatitis C infection and the increasing incidence of hepatocelllular carcinoma: A population-based study. *Gastroenterology* 2004; 127:1372–1380.
8. Kew MC. Epidemiology of hepatocellular carcinoma. *Toxicology.* 2002;181–182:35–38.
9. Bosch FX. Global epidemiology of hepatocellular carcinoma. In: Okuda K, Tabor E, eds. *Liver Cancer.* New York: Churchill Livingstone; 1997:13–28.
10. DiBisceglie AM. Epidemiology and clinical presentation of hepatocelluar carcinoma. *J Vasc Interv Radiol.* 2002;13:S169-S171.
11. Gilbert HA, Hakagn AR. Metastases: incidence, detection. An evaluation without histologic confirmation. In: Weiss L, ed. *Fundamental Aspects of Metastasis.* Amsterdam: North-Holland; 1976:385–405.
12. Kelvin JF, Scagliola J. Metastases involving the gastrointestinal system. *Semin Oncol Nurs.* 1998;14:187–198.
13. Kemeny N, Kemeny M, Dawson L. Liver Metastases. In Ableoff: *Abeloff's Clinical Oncology.* Armitage JO, Niederhuber JE, Abeloff MD (eds) 4th ed. Orlando: W. B. Saunders Co. 2008:10.
14. Sherman M. Hepatocellular Carcinoma: Epidemiology, Screening and Prevention. In: *Principle and Practice of Gastrointestinal Oncology.* Kelesen D, Daly JM, Kern SE, Levin B, Tepper JE (eds). Philadelphia: Lippincott, Williams and Wilkins, 2007; 395–404.
15. Bralet MP, Regimbeau JM, Pineau P, et al. Hepatocellular carcinoma occurring in nonfibrotic liver: epidemiologic and histopathologic analysis of 80 French cases. *Hepatology.* 2000;32:200–204.
16. Beasley RP, Hwang LY. Epidemiology of hepatocellular carcinoma. In: Vyas GN, Dienstag JL, Hoofnagle JH, eds. *Viral Hepatitis and Liver Disease.* Orlando, FL: Grune and Stratton; 1984:209–244.
17. International Agency for Research on Cancer. Hepatitis virus. *IARC Monogr Eval Carcinog Risks.* 1994;159:66–97.
18. Donato F, Tagger A, Gelatti U, et al. Alcohol and hepatocellular carcinoma: the effect of life time intake and viral hepatitis infection in men and women. *Am J Epidemiol.* 2002;155:323–331.
19. Chen ZM, Liu BQ, Borehamj, et al. Smoking and liver cancer in China: case control comparison of 36,000 liver cancer deaths vs cirrhosis deaths. *Int J Cancer.* 2003;107:106–112.
20. Nissen NN, Martin P. Hepatocellular carcinoma, the high-risk patient. *J Clin Gastroenterol.* 2002;13(Suppl 2):79–85.
21. Monto A, Wright TL. The epidemiology and prevention of hepatocellullar carcinoma. *Semin Oncol.* 2001;28:441–449.
22. Chen CJ, Wang LY, Lu SN, et al. Elevated aflatoxin exposure and increased risk of hepatocellular carcinoma. *Hepatology.* 1996;24:38–42.
23. Wang JS, Huang T, Su J. Hepatocellular carcinoma and aflatoxin exposure in Zhuqing village, Fusui county, People's Republic of China. *Cancer Epidemiol Biomarker Prevent.* 2001;10:143–146.
24. Szymanska K, Hainaut P. TP53 and mutations in human cancer. *Acta Biochimica Polonica.* 2003;50:231–238.
25. Ueno Y, Nagata S, Tsutsumi T, et al. Detection of microcystins, a blue-green algal hepatotoxin, in drinking water sampled in Haimen and Fusui, endemic areas of primary liver cancer in China, by highly sensitive immunoassay. *Carcinogenesis.* 1996;17:1317–1321.
26. Tabor E, DiBisceglie AM. Hepatocellular carcinoma. *Clin Liver Dis.* 1999;3:327–348.
27. Kuper H, Tzonou A, Kaklamani E, et al. Tobacco smoking, alcohol consumption and their interaction in the causation of hepatocellular carcinoma. *Int J Cancer.* 2000;85:498–502.
28. Donato F, Tagger A, Gelatti U, et al. Alcohol and hepatocellular carcinoma: the effect of lifetime intake and hepatitis virus infections in men and women. *Am J Epidemiol.* 2002;155:323–331.
29. Maheshwari S, Sarraj A, Kramer J, et al. Oral contraception and the risk of hepatacellular carcinoma. *J Hepatol.* 2007;47:506–513.
30. Elmberg M, Hultcrantz R, Ekbom A, et al. Cancer risk in patients with hereditary hemochromatosis and in their first degree relatives. *Gastroenterology.* 2003;125:1733–1741.
31. Mandioshona E, MacPhail AP, Gordeuk VK, et al. Dietary iron overload as a risk factor for hepatocellular carcinoma in black Africans. *Hepatology.* 1998;27:1563–1567.
32. Simson IM. Membranous obstruction of the inferior vena cava and hepatocellular carcinoma in South Africa. *Gastroenterology.* 1998;82:171–178.
33. Regimbeau JM, Colombat M, Mognol P, et al. Obesity and diabetes as a risk factor for hepatocellular carcinoma. *Liver Transpl.* 2004;10(Suppl 2):S69-S73.
34. El-serag HB, Tran T, Everhart JE. Diabetes increases the risk of chronic liver disease and hepatocellular carcinoma. *Gastroenterology.* 2004;126:460–468.
35. Yang S, Lin HZ, Hwang H, et al. Hepatic hyperplasia in noncirrhotic fatty livers: obesity steatosis, a premalignant condition? *Cancer Res.* 2001;61:5016–5023.
36. Poonawala A, Nair S, Thuluvath P. Prevalance of obesity and diabetes in patients with cryptogenic cirhhosis: a case control study? *Hepatology.* 2000;32:689–692.
37. Larsson SC, Wolk A. Coffee consumption and risk of liver cancer: a meta-analysis. *Gastroenterology.* 2007;132:1740–1745.
38. Huang K, Lin S. Nationwide vaccination: a success story in Taiwan. *Vaccine.* 2000;1:S35-S38.
39. Camma CM, Giunta P, Andreone P, Craxì A. Interferon and prevention of hepatocellular carcinoma in viral cirrhosis an evidence-based approach. *J Hepatol.* 2001;34:593–602.
40. Marrero CR, Marrero JA. Viral hepatitis and hepatocellullar carcinoma. *Arch Med Res.* 2007;38:612–620.
41. Tanaka H, Tsukuma H, Kasahara A, et al. Effect of interferon therapy on the incidence of hepatocellular carcinoma and mortality of patients with chronic hepatitis C: a retrospective cohort study of 738 patients. *Int J Cancer.* 2000;87:741–749.
42. Hayashi K, Kumada T, Nakano S, et al. Incidence of hepatocellular carcinoma in chronic hepatitis C after interferon therapy. *Hepatogastroenterology.* 2002;49:508–512.
43. Koga H. Hepatocellular carcinoma: is there a potential for chemoprevention using cylooxygenase-2 inhibitors? *Cancer.* 2003;98:661–667.
44. Collier J, Sherman M. Screening for hepatocellular carcinoma. *Hepatology.* 1998;27:273–278.
45. Larcos G, Sorokopud H, Berry G, et al. Sonographic screening for hepatocellular carcinoma in patients with chronic hepatitis or cirrhosis: an evaluation. *AJR Am J Roentgenol.* 1998;171:433–435.
46. Okuda K. Hepatocellular carcinoma. *J Hepatol.* 2000;32(Suppl 1):225–237.
47. Trevisani F, De NS, Rapaccini G, et al. Semi annual and annual surveillance of cirrhotic patients for hepatocellullar carcinoma: effects on cancer stage and patient survival (Italian experience). *Am J Gastroenterol.* 2002;97:734–744.
48. Santagostino E, Colombo M, Rivi M, et al. A 6-month vs a 12-month surveillance for hepatocellular carcinoma in 559 hemophilliacs infected with the hepatitis C virus. *Blood.* 2003;102:78–82.
49. Bruix J, Sherman M. Management of hepatocellular carcinoma. *Hepatology.* 2005;42;1208–1236.
50. Bisgard HC, Thorgeirsson SS. Hepatic regeneration: the role of regeneration in pathogenesis of chronic liver disease. *Clin Lab Med.* 1996;16:325–329.
51. Bartlet DL, Carr BI, Marsh JW. Cancer of the Liver. In: DeVita VT, Hellman S, Rosenberg SA, eds. *Cancer: Principales and Practice.* 7th ed. Philadelphia: Lippincott, Williams & Wilkins; 2005:987–1111.
52. Rolfes DB. Fibrolamellar carcinoma of the liver. In: Okuda K, Shak KG, eds. *Neoplasms of the Liver.* Tokyo: Springer-Verlag; 1987:137–142.

53. Nakanuma Y. Pathology of hepatocellular cancer. In: Rustgi AK, ed. *Gastrointestinal Cancers.* New York: Saunders; 2003:593–604.
54. Crawford JM. The liver and the biliary tract. In: Cotran RS, Kumar V, Collins T, eds. *Robbins Pathologic Basis of Disease.* 6th ed. Philadelphia: W.B. Saunders; 1999:845–901.
55. Katyal S, Oliver JH, Peterson MS, et al. Extrahepatic metastases of hepatocellular carcinoma. *Radiology.* 2000;216:698–703.
56. Kew MC. Clinical aspects of hepatocellular cancer. In: Rustgi AK, ed. *Gastrointestinal Cancers.* New York: Saunders; 2003:564–574.
57. Kew MC. Hepatocellular cancer a century of progress. *Clin Liver Dis.* 2000;4:257–259.
58. Eastman RC, Carson RE, Orloff DG, et al. Glucose utilization in a patient with hepatoma and hypoglycemia. Assessment by a positron emission tomography. *J Clin Invest.* 1992;89:1958–1963.
59. Tietge UJ, Schofl C, Ocran KW, et al. Hepatoma with severe non-islet tumor hypoglycemia. *Am J Gastroenterol.* 1998;93:997–1000.
60. Kew MC, Fisher JW. Serum erythropoietin concentration in patients with hepatocellular carcinoma. *Cancer.* 1986;58:2486–2488.
61. Yen TC, Hwang SJ, Wang CC, et al. Hypercalcemia and parathyroid hormone-related protein in hepatocellular carcinoma. *Liver.* 1993;13:311–315.
62. Bruix J, Castells, Calvet X, et al. Diarrhea as a presenting symptom of hepatocellular carcinoma. *Dig Dis Sci.* 1990;35:681–685.
63. Weber S, Jarnagian W, Duffy A, O'Reilly EM, Abou-Alfa GK, Blumgart L. Liver and bile duct cancer. In: *Abeloff's Clinical Oncology.* Armitage, JO, Niederhuber JE, Abeloff MD, eds. 4th ed. Orlando: W.B. Saunders Co. 2008.
64. Gonzalez KB, Woodall M. Hepatocellular carcinoma: surgical treatment options. *Nurs Clin North Am.* 2001;36:593–603.
65. Yeh CN, Lee WC, Jeng LB. Spontaneous tumour rupture and prognosis in patients with hepatocellular carcinoma. *Br J Surg.* 2002;89:1125–1129.
66. Befeler AS, Di Disceglie AM. Hepatocellular carcinoma: diagnosis and treatment. *Gastroenterology.* 2002;122:1609–1619.
67. Chen DS, Sung JL, Lai MY, et al. Serum alpha-fetoprotein in the early stage of hepatocellular carcinoma. *Gastroenterology.* 1984;86:1404–1409.
68. Moertel CG, Fleming TR, Macdoald JS, et al. An evaluation of the carcinoembryonic antigen (CEA) test for monitoring patients with resected colon cancer. *JAMA.* 1993;270:943–947.
69. Lim JH, Choi D, Kim SH, et al. Detection of hepatocellular carcinoma: value of adding delayed phase imaging to dual-phase helical CT. *AJR Am J Roentgenol.* 2002;179:67–73.
70. Miller FH, Butler RS, Hoff FL, et al. Using triphasic helical CT to detect focal hepatic lesions in patients with neoplasms. *AJR Am J Roentgenol.* 1998;171:643–649.
71. Libbrecht L, Bielen D, Verslype C, et al. Focal lesions in cirrhotic explant livers: pathologic evaluation and accuracy of pretransplantation imaging examinations. *Liver Transpl.* 2002;8:749–761.
72. Yu AS, Kim KW, Lee JT, et al. MR imaging during arterial portography for assessment of hepatocellular carcinoma: comparison with CT during arterial portography. *AJR Am J Roentgenol.* 1998;170:1501–1506.
73. Choi D, Kim S, Lim J, et al. Preoperative detection of hepatocellular carcinoma: ferumoxides-enhanced MR imaging versus combined helical CT during arterial portography and CT hepatic arteriography. *AJR Am J Roentgenol.* 2001;176:475–482.
74. Wudel LJ, Delbeke D, Morris R, et al. The role of [18F] fluorodeoxyglucose positron emission tomoraphy imaging in the evaluation of hepatocellular carcinoma. *Am Sur.* 2003;69:117–124.
75. Dresel S, Kirsch CM, Tatsch K, et al. Detection of hepatocellular carcinoma with a new alpha-fetoprotein antibody imaging kit. *J Clin Oncol.* 1997;15:2683–2690.
76. Serafini AN, Jeffers LJ, Reddy KR, et al. Early recognition of recurrent hepatocellular carcinoma utilizing gallium-67 citrate scintigraphy. *J Nucl Med.* 1998;29:712–716.
77. Takumoru R, Wong LL, Dang C, Wong L, et al. Needle tract implantation from hepatocellular cancer: is needle bipsy of the liver always necessary? *Liver Transpl.* 2000;6:67–72.
78. Durand F, Regimbeau JM, Belghiti J, et al. Assessment of the benefits and risks of percutaneous biopsy before surgical resection of hepatocellular carcinoma. *J Hepatol.* 2001;35:254–258.
79. Kuo FY, Chen WJ, Lu SN, et al. Fine needle aspiration cytodiagnosis of liver tumors. *Acta Cytol.* 2004;48:142–148.
80. Nguyen MH, Keeffe EB. Treatment of hepatocellular cancer. In: Rustgi AK, ed. *Gastrointestinal Cancers.* New York: Saunders; 2003:605–622.
81. Yu AS, Keeffe EB. Management of hepatocellular carcinoma. *Rev Gastroenterol Disord.* 2003;3:8–24.
82. Child CG III, Turcotte JG. Surgery in portal hypertension. In: Child CG III, ed. *The Liver and Portal Hypertension.* Philadelphia: W.B. Saunders; 1964:50.
83. Kadry Z, Furudawa H, Todo S, Clavien AP. Assessment of liver function and mass in cirrhotic and noncirrhotic livers. In: Clavien AP, Fong Y, Lyerly H, Morse MA, Venook AP, eds. *Malignant Liver Tumors: Current and Emerging Therapies*, 2nd ed. Sudbury, MA: Jones and Bartlett; 2004.
84. Okuda K, Ohtuki T, Obata H, et alNatural history of hepatocellular carcinoma and prognosis in relation to treatment: study of 850 patients. *Cancer.* 1985;56:918–928.
85. Greene FL, Page DL, Fleming ID, et al, eds. *AJCC (American Joint Committee on Cancer) Cancer Staging Manual.* 6th ed. New York: Springer-Verlag; 2002:148.
86. Cancer of the Liver Italian Program (CLIP) Investigatros. Prospective validation of the CLIP score: a new prognostic system for patients with cirrhosis and hepatocellular carcinoma. *Hepatology.* 2000;31:840–845.
87. Villa E, Colantoni A, Camma C, et al. Estrogen recepotors for clinical staging for hepatocellullar carcinoma: comparison with clinical staging systems. *J Clin Oncol.* 2003;21:441–446.
88. Cho YK, Chung JW, Kim JK, et al. Comparison of 7 staging systems for patients with heaptocellular carcinoma undergoing transarterial chemoembolization. *Cancer* 2008;112:352–361.
89. Llovet JM, Burroughts A, Bruix J. Hepatocellular carcinoma. Lancet. 2003;362:1907–1917.
90. Duffy JP, Hiatt JR, Busuttill RW. Surgical resection of hepatocellullar carcinoma. *Cancer J.* 2008;14:100–110.
91. Aguayo A, Patt YZ. Liver cancer. *Clin Liver Dis.* 2001;5:479–507.
92. Tung-Ping PR, Fan ST, Wong J. Risk factors, prevention, and management of postoperative recurrence after resection of hepatocellular carcinoma. *Ann Surg.* 2000;232:10–24.
93. Poon RT, Fan ST. Hepatectomy for hepatocellullar carcinoma: patient selection and postoperative outcome. *Liver Transpl.* 2004;10(Suppl 1):S39-S45.
94. Kaibori M, Matsui Y, Kitade H, et al. Hepatic resection for hepatocellular carcinoma in severely cirrhotic livers. *Hepatogastroenterology.* 2003;50:491–496.
95. Llovert JM, Bruix J, Gores GJ. Surgical resection versus transplantation for early hepatocellullar carcinoma: clues for the best strategy. *Hepatology.* 2000;31:1019–1021.
96. Yoo HY, Patt CH, Geshwind JF, et al. The outcome of liver transplantation in patients with hepatocellular carcinoma in the United States between 1988 and 2001: 5-year survival has improved significantly with time. *J Clin Oncol.* 2003;21:4329–4335.
97. Little SA, Fong Y. Hepatocellular carcinoma: current surgical management. *Semin Oncol.* 2001;28:474–486.
98. Lo CM, Lai EC, Liu CL, et al. Laparoscopy and laparoscopic ultrasonography avoid exploratory laparotomy in patients with hepatocellular carcinoma. *Ann Surg.* 1998;227:527–532.
99. Shetty K, Timmins K, Brensinger S, et al. Liver transplantation for hepatocellular carcinoma validation of present selection criteria in predicting outcome. *Liver Transpl.* 2004;10:911–918.

100. Leung JY, Zhu AX, Gordon FD, et al. Liver transplantation outcomes in early-stage heaptocellular carcinoma: results of a multicenter study. *Liver Transpl.* 2004;10:1343–1354.
101. Duffy JP, Vardanian A, Benjamin E, et al. Liver transplantation criteria for heaptocellular carcinoma should be expanded: a 22-year experience with 467 patients at UCLA. *Ann Surg.* 2007;246:502–511.
102. Lo CM, Ngan H, Tso WK, et al. randomized controlled trial of transarterial lipiodol chemoembolization for unresectable heapatocellular carcinoma. *Hepatology.* 2002;35:1164–1171.
103. Llovet JM, Rael MI, Montana X, et al. Arterial embolization or chemoembolization versus symptomatic treatment in patients with unrsectable heapatocelllular carcinoma: a randomized controlled trial. *Lancet.* 2002;359:1734–1739.
104. Fong Y, Cohen AM, Fortner JG, et al. Liver resection for colorectal metastases. *J Clin Oncol.* 1997;15:938–946.
105. Nordlinger B, Sorbye H, Collette L, et al. Final results of the EORTC Intergroup randomized phase III study 40983 [EPOC] evaluating the benefit of peri-operative FOLFOX4 chemotherapy or patients with potentially resectable liver metastases. *J Clin Oncol.* 2007;25(Suppl 18 ):LBA5.
106. Rubbia-Brandt L, Audard V, Sartoretti P, et al. Severe hepatic sinusoidal obstruction associated with oxaliplatin-based chemotherapy in patients with metastatic colorectal cancer. *Ann Oncol.* 2004;15:460–466.
107. Baize N, Gerard B, Bleiberg H, et al. Long-term survival of patients down-staged by oxaliplatin and 5-flurouracil combination followed by rescue surgery for unresectable colorectal liver metastases. *Gastroenterol Clin Biol* 2006; 30: 1349–1353.
108. Alberts SR, Wagman LD. Chemotherapy or colorectal cancer liver metastases. *Oncologist.* 2008;13:1063–1073.
109. Bismuth H, Adam R, Navarro F, et al. Re-resection for colorectal metastases. *Surg Oncol Clin North Am.* 1996;5:353–363.
110. Kin T, Nakajima Y, Kanehiro H, et al. Repeat hepatectomy for recurrent colorectal metastases. *World J Surg.* 1998;24:620–621.
111. Fong Y, Blumgart LH, Cohen A. Repeat hepatic resections for metastatic colorectal cancer. *Ann Surg.* 1994;220:657–662.
112. PetrowskyH, Gonen M, Jarnagin W, et al. Second liver resections are safe and effective treatment for recurrent hepatic metastases for colorectal cancer: a bi-institutional analysis. *Ann Surg.* 2002;235:863–871.
113. Adam R, Bismuth H, Castaing D, et al. Repeat hepatectomy for colorectal liver metastases. *Ann Surg.* 1997;225:51–62.
114. Degremont AC, Ismail M, Arthaud M, et al. Mechanisms of postoperative prolonged plasma volume expansion with low molecular weight hydroxethy (HES 200/0.62, 6%). *Intensive Care Med.* 1995;21:577–583.
115. Vauthey JN, Klimstra D, Franceschi D, et al. Factors affecting longterm outcome after hepatic resection for hepatocellular carcinoma. *Am J Surg.* 1995;169:28–34.
116. Tarter RE. Quality of life following liver transplantation. *Hepatogastroenterology.* 1998;45:1398–1403.
117. Colleoni M, Audisio RA, De Braud F, et al. Practical considerations in the treatment of hepatocellular carcinoma. *Drugs.* 1998;55:367.
118. Watkins E, Khazei AM, Nahra KS. Surgical basis for arterial infusion chemotherapy of disseminated carcinoma of the liver. *Surg Gynecol Obstet.* 1970;130:581–605.
119. Lin G, Lunderquist A, Hagerstrand I, et al. Postmortem examination of the blood supply and vascular pattern of small liver metastases in man. *Surgery.* 1984;96:517–526.
120. Campbell KA, Burns RC, Sitzmann JV, et al. Regional chemotherapy devices: effect of experience and anatomy on complications. *J Clin Oncol.* 1993;11:822–826.
121. Daly J, Kemeny N, Sigurdson E, et al. Regional infusion of colorectal hepatic metastases: a randomized trial comparing the hepatic artery versus the portal vein. *Arch Surg.* 1987;122:1273–1277.
122. Mavlight GM, Patt YZ, Haynie TP, et al. Differential tumor progression in patients with bilobar hepatic metastases and dual arterial supply: evidence supporting the advantage of intra-arterial over intravenous route of drug delivery. *Sel Cancer Ther.* 1989;5:37–45.
123. Hohn DC, Stagg RJ, Price DC, et al. Avoidance of gastroduodenal toxicity in patients receiving hepatic arterial 5-fluoro-2-deoxyuridine. *J Clin Oncol.* 1985;3:1257–1260.
124. Ensminger WD. Intrahepatic arterial infusion of chemotherapy: pharmacologic principles. *Semin Oncol.* 2002;29:119–125.
125. Kemeny N, Daly J, Oderman P, et al. Hepatic artery pump infusion: toxicity and results in patients with metastatic colorectal carcinoma. *J Clin Oncol.* 1984;2:595–600.
126. Lorenz M, Muller HH. Randomized, multicenter trial of fluorouracil plus leucovorin administered either via hepatic arterial or intravenous infusion versus fluorodeoxyuridine administered via hepatic arterial infusion in patients with nonresectable liver metastases from colorectal carcinoma. *J Clin Oncol.* 2000;18:243–254.
127. Kemeny MM, Goldberg DA, Browning S, et al. Experience with continuous regional chemotherapy and hepatic resection as treatment of hepatic metastases. *Cancer.* 1985;55:1265–1270.
128. Kemeny MM, Hogan JM, Goldberg DA, et al. Continuous hepatic artery infusion with an implantable pump: problems with hepatic artery anomalies. *Surgery.* 1986;99:501–504.
129. Kemeny N. Management of liver metastases from colorectal cancer. *Oncology* 2006;20:1161–1176.
130. Kemeny N, Seiter K, Conti JA, et al. Hepatic arterial floxuridine and leucovorin for unresectable liver metastases from colorectal carcinoma. *Cancer.* 1994;73:1132–1142.
131. Elias D, Lasser P, Rougier P, et al. Frequency, technical aspects, results and indications of major hepatectomy after prolonged intra-arterial hepatic chemotherapy for initially unresectable tumors. *J Am Coll Surg.* 1995;180:213–219.
132. Cohen AD, Kemeny NE. An update on hepatic arterial infusion chemotherapy for colorectal cancer. *Oncologist.* 2003;8:553–566.
133. Mocellin S, Pilati P. Lise M, et al Hepatic arterial infusion (HAI) compared to systemic chemotherapy for the treatment of unresectable liver metastases from colorectal carcinoma: a systemic review and meta-analysis of randomized controlled trials. *J Clin Oncol.* 2007;25(18 Suppl):626S.
134. Liapi E, Geschwind JFH. Transcatheter and ablative approaches for solid malignancies. *J Clin Oncol.* 25:978–986.
135. Shankar A, Loizidou M, Taylor I. The vascularity of colorectal liver metastases. *Eur J Surg Oncol.* 1996;22:389–396.
136. Perry LJ, Stuart KE. Hepatic chemoembolization. In: Saini S, Gazelle GS, Mueller PR, eds. *Hepatobiliary and Pancreatic Radiology.* New York: Thieme; 1998:448–469.
137. Stuart K. Chemoembolization in the management of liver tumors. *Oncologist.* 2003;8:425–437.
138. Venook AP, Stagg RJ, Lewis JL, et al. Chemoembolization for hepatocellular carcinoma. *J Clin Oncol.* 1990;8:1108–1114.
139. Konno T. Targeting cancer chemotherapeutic agents by use of lipiodol contrast medium. *Cancer.* 1990;66:1897–1903.
140. Castells A, Ayusu C, Bru C, et al. Transarterial embolization for hepatocellular carcinoma: antibiotic prophylaxis and clinical meaning of postembolization fever. *J Hepatol.* 1995;22:410–415.
141. Venhook AP. Treatment of hepatocellular carcinoma: too many options? *J Clin Oncol.* 1994;12:1323–1334.
142. Georgiades CS, Hong K, Geschwind JF. Radiofrequency ablation and chemoembolization for hepatocelluar carcinoma. *Cancer J.* 2008;14:117–122.
143. Livraghi T, Benedini V, Lazzaroni S. Long-term results of single session percutaneous ethanol injection in patients with large hepatocellular carcinoma. *Cancer.* 1998;83:48–57.
144. Livraghi T, Giorgio A, Marin G, et al. Hepatocellular carcinoma and cirrhosis in 746 patients: long-term results of percutaneous ethanol injection. *Radiology.* 1995;197:101–108.
145. Livraghi T, Bolondi L, Lazzaroni S, et al. Percutaneous ethanol injection in the treatment of hepatocellular carcinoma in cirrhosis. A study of 207 patients. *Cancer.* 1992;69:925–929.

146. Livarghi T, Bolondi L, Buscarini L, et al. No treatment, resection, and ethanol injection in hepatocellular carcinoma: a retrospective analysis of survival in 391 patients with cirrhosis. Italian Cooperative HCC Study Group. *J Hepatol.* 1995;22:522–526.
147. Hasegawa S, Yamaski N, Hiwaki T, et al. Factors that predict intrahepatic recurrence of hepatocellular carcinoma in 81 patients initially treated by percutaneous ethanol injection. *Cancer.* 1999;86:1682–1690.
148. Khan KN, Yatsuhashi H, Yamasaki K, et al. Prospective analysis of risk factors for early intrahepatic recurrence of hepatocellular carcinoma following ethanol injection. *J Hepatol.* 2000;32:269–278.
149. Kurokohchi K, Masaki T, Miyauchi, et al. Percutaneous ethanol and lipiodol injection therapy for hepatocellullar carcinoma. *Int J Oncol.* 2004;24:381–387.
150. Ravikumar TS, Steele GD. Hepatic cryosurgery. *Surg Clin North Am.* 1989;69:433–440.
151. Zhou XD, Tang ZY, Yu YQ, et al. Clinical evaluation of cryosurgery in the treatment of primary liver cancer. Report of 60 cases. *Cancer.* 1988;61:1889–1892.
152. Onik GM, Atkinson D, Zemel R, et al. Cryosurgery of liver cancer. *Semin Surg Oncol.* 1993;9:309–317.
153. Onik G, Rubinsky B, Zemel R, et al. Ultrasound-guided hepatic cryosurgery in the treatment of metastatic colon carcinoma. *Cancer.* 1991;67:901–907.
154. McKinnon JG, Temple WJ, Wiseman DA, et al. Cryosurgery for malignant tumours of the liver. *Can J Surg.* 1996;39:401–406.
155. Morris DL, Ross WB. Australian experience of cryoablation of liver tumors: metastases. *Surg Oncol Clin North Am.* 1996;5:391–397.
156. Weaver ML, Atkinson D, Zemel R. Hepatic cryosurgery in treating colorectal metastases. *Cancer.* 1995;76:210–214.
157. Ross WB, Horton M, Bertolino P, et al. Cryotherapy of liver tumours—a practical guide. *HPB Surg.* 1995;8:167–173.
158. Barnett CC, Curley SA. Ablative techniques for hepatocellular carcinoma. *Semin Oncol.* 2001;28:487–496.
159. McGahan JP, Dodd GD III. Radiofrequency ablation of the liver. *Am J Roentgenol.* 2001;176:3–16.
160. Curley SA. Radiofrequency ablation of malignant liver tumors. *Oncologist.* 2001;6:14–23.
161. Aguayo A, Patt YZ. Nonsurgical treatment of hepatocellular carcinoma. *Semin Oncol.* 2001;28:503–513.
162. Ho S, Lau JW, Leung TW. Intrahepatic (90)Y-microspheres for hepatocellular carcinoma. *J Nucl Med.* 2001;42:1587–1589.
163. Lau W, Ho S, Leung T, et al. What determines survival duration in hepatocellular carcinoma treated with intra-arterial yttrium90 microspheres. *Hepatogastroenterology.* 2001;48:338–340.
164. DelPoggio P, Maddeo A, Zabbialini G, Piti A. Chemoembolization of hepatocellular carcinoma with drug eluting beads. *J Hepatol.* 2007;47:157.
165. Malagari K. Drug-eluting particles in the treatment of HCC: chemoembolization with doxorubicin-loaded DC Bead. *Expert Rev Anticancer Ther* 2008;8:1643–1650.
166. Soini Y, Virkajarvi N, Raunio H, et al. Expression of P-glycoprotein in hepatocellular carcinoma: a potential marker of prognosis. *J Clin Pathol.* 1996;49:470–473.
167. Huang CC, Wu MC, Xu GW, et al. Over-expression of the NDR1 gene and P-glycoprotein in human hepatocellular carcinoma. *J Natl Cancer Inst.* 1992;84:262.
168. Caruso ML, Valentini AM. Overexpression of p53 in a large series of patients with hepatocellular carcinoma: a clinicopathological correlation. *Anticancer Res.* 1999;19:3853–3856.
169. Nagahama H, Okada S, Okusaka T, et al. Predictive factors for tumor response to systemic chemotherapy in patients with hepatocellular carcinoma. *Jpn J Clin Oncol.* 1997;27:321–324.
170. Plweny CL, Toya T, Katongole-Mbidde E, et al. Treatment of hepatocellular carcinoma with adriamycin. Preliminary communication. *Cancer.* 1975;36:1250–1257.
171. Chelbowski RT, Brzechwa-Adjukiewicz A, Cowden A, et al. Doxorubicin (75 mg/m2) for hepatocellullar carcinoma: clinical and pharmacokinetic results. *Cancer Treat Rep.* 1984;68:487–491.
172. Ihde DC, Kane RC, Cohen MH, et al. Adriamycin therapy in American patients with hepatocellular carcinoma. *Cancer Treat Rep.* 1977;61:1385–1387.
173. Nerenstone SR, Ihde DC, Friedman MA. Clinical trials in primary hepatocellular carcinoma: current status and future directions. *Cancer Treat Rev.* 1988;15:1–31.
174. Lai CL, WU PC, Chan GC, et al. Doxorubicin versus no antitumor therapy in inoperable hepatocellular carcinoma. A prospective randomized trial. *Cancer.* 1988;62:479–483.
175. Lozano RD, Patt YZ, Hassan MM, et al. Oral capecitabine for the treatment of hepatobiliary cancers. [Abstr] *Proc Am Soc Clin Oncol.* 2000;19:264a.
176. Patt YZ, Hassan MM, Lozano RD, et al. Phase II trial of thalidomide for treatment of non-resectable hepatocellular carcinoma. [Abstr] *Proc Am Soc Clin Oncol.* 2000;19:266a.
177. Porta C, Moroni M, Nastasi G, et al. 5-Fluorouracil and d, 1-leucovorin calcium are active to treat unresectable hepatocellular carcinoma patients: preliminary results of a phase II study. *Oncology.* 1995;52:487–491.
178. Yang TS, Wang CH, Hsieh RK, et al. Gemcitabine and doxorubicin for the treatment of patients with advanced hepatocellular carcinoma: a phase I-II trial. *Ann Oncol.* 2002;13:1771–1778.
179. Okada S, Okusaka T, Ueno H, et al. Phase II trial of cisplatin, mitoxantrone, and continuous infusion 5-fluorouracil (5-FU) (FMP therapy) for hepatocellular carcinoma (HCC). [Abstr] *Proc Am Soc Clin Oncol.* 1999;18:248a.
180. Ellis PA, Norman A, Hill A, et al. Epirubicin, cisplatin and infusional 5-fluorouracil (5-FU) (ECF) in hepatobiliary tumors. *Eur J Cancer.* 1995;31A:1594–1598.
181. Rai K, Tsuji A, Morita S, et al. Continuous infusion of 5-FU and low-dose consecutive CDDP therapy in advanced hepatocellular carcinoma: a phase II study. [Abstr] *Proc Am Soc Clin Oncol.* 2002;21:164a.
182. Parikh PM, Fuloria J, Babu G, et al. Phase II study of gemcitabine and cisplatin in patients with advanced hepatocellular carcinoma. *Trop Gastroenterol* 2005; 26: 115–118.
183. Chia WK, Ong S, Toh, HC, et al. Phase II trial of gemcitabine in combination with cisplatin in inoperable or advanced hepatocellular carcinoma. *Ann Acad Med Singapore.* 2008;37:554–558.
184. Boucher E, Corbinais S, Brissot P, et al. Treatment of hepatocellular carcinoma (HCC) with systemic chemotherapy combining epirubicin, cisplatinum and infusion 5-fluorouracil (ECF regimen). *Cancer Chemother Pharmacol.* 2002;50:305–308.
185. Llovet JM, Sala M, Castellas L, et al. Randomized controlled trial of interferon treatment for advanced hepatocellular carcinoma. *Hepatology.* 2000;31:54–58.
186. Chung YH, Song IH, Song BC, et al. Combined chemotherapy consisting of intra-arterial cisplatin infusion and systemic interferon-alpha for hepatocellular carcinoma patients with major portal vein thrombosis or distant metastasis. *Cancer.* 2000;88:1986–1991.
187. Leung TW, Tang AM, Zee B, et al. Factors predicting response and survival in 149 patients with unresectable hepatocellular carcinoma treated by combination cisplatin, interferon-alpha, doxorubicin and 5-fluorouracil chemotherapy. *Cancer.* 2002;94:421–427.
188. Zhu AX. Systemic therapy of advanced hepatocellular carcinoma: how hopeful should we be. *Oncologist.* 2006;11:790–800.
189. Harada K, Shiota G, Kawasaki H. Transforming growth factor alpha and epidermal growth factor receptor in chronic liver disease and hepatocellular carcinoma. *Liver.* 1999;19:318–325.
190. Louafi S, Hebbar M, Rosmorduc O, et al. Gemcitabine, oxaliplatin (GEMOX) and cetuximab for treatment of hepatocellular carcinoma (HCC): results of the phase II study ERGO (abstract). *J Clin Oncol.* 2007;25:221s.

191. Yamaguchi R, Yano H, Iemura A, et al. Expression of vascular endothelial growth factor in human hepatocellular carcinoma. *Hepatology.* 1998;28:68–67.
192. Chao Y, Li CP, Chau GY, et al. Prognostic significance of vascular endothelial growth factor, and angiogenin in patients with resectable hepatocellular carcinoma after surgery. *Ann Surg Oncol.* 2003;10:355–362.
193. Schwartz JD, Shwartz M, Sung M, et al. Bevacizumab in unresectable hepatocellular carcinoma for patients without metastasis and without invasion to the portal vein. American Society of Clinical Oncology Gastrointestinal Cancers Symposium, San Francisco, CA, January 26–28, 2006.
194. Liu L, Cao Y, Chen C, et al. Sorafenib blocks the RAF/MEK/ERK pathway, inhibits tumor angiogenesis, and induces tumor cell apoptosis in hepatocellulat carcinoma model PLC/PRF/5. *Cancer Res.* 2006;66:11851–11858.
195. Llovet JM, Ricci S, Mazzaferro V, et al. Sorafenib in Advanced Hepatocellular Carcinoma. *N Engl J Med.* 2008;359:378–390.
196. Qian C, Drozdzik M, Caselmann WH, et al. The potential of gene therapy in the treatment of hepatocellular carcinoma—review. *J Hepatol.* 2000;32:344–351.
197. Sangiro B, Qian C, Schmitz V, et al. Gene therapy of hepatocellular carcinoma and gastrointestinal tumors. *Ann NY Acad Sci.* 2002;963:6–12.
198. Levy M. Pharmacology treatment of cancer pain. *N Engl J Med.* 1996;335:1124–1132.
199. Ben-Aharon, I, Gafter-Gvili A, Paul M, et al. Interventions for alleviating cancer-related dyspnea: a systemic review. *J Clin Oncol.* 2008;26:2396–2404.
200. Loprinzi C. Anorexia and cachexia. In: Loprinzi C, ed. *Cancer Management: A Multidisciplinary Approach.* 6th ed. Melville, NY: Publishers Research and Representation; 2002:831–834.
201. Inui A. Cancer anorexia-cachexia syndrome: current issues in research and management. *CA: Cancer J Clin.* 2002;52:72–91.
202. Gagnon B, Breura E. A review of the drug treatment associated with cancer. *Drugs.* 1998;55:675–688.
203. Jatoi A, Windschitl HE, Loprinzi CL, et al. Dronabinol versus megesterol acetate versus combination therapy for cancer-associated anoraxia: a north central cancer treatment group study. *J Clin Oncol.* 2002;20:567–573.
204. Suh B, Stephens, J and Kunin C. Oral neomycin dosage schedules for suppression of ammonia production by bowel flora. *Antimicrob Agents Chemother.* 1979:16:519–522.

CHAPTER 59

Beth Eaby-Sandy, MSN, CRNP, OCN®

# Lung Cancer

## INTRODUCTION

Lung cancer is the leading cause of cancer deaths in both men and women in the US and worldwide.[1,2] Cigarette smoking continues to be the overwhelming risk factor for developing lung cancer, although there is recent evidence to suggest that more cases of lung cancer may be presenting in minimal or never smokers.[3] Although advances in radiological imaging have yielded earlier detection and improved staging, a screening tool has yet to emerge from clinical trials in lung cancer showing an improvement in mortality.

Despite significant advances in surgery, radiation, and chemotherapy over the past decade, overall 5-year survival rates in lung cancer have improved by only 3% in the past 25 years, as compared with rates for prostate cancer and breast cancer, which have improved by 30% and 14%, respectively, over the past 25 years.[1] Tobacco use prevention and education are vital to improving incidence rates of lung cancer. Newer radiation techniques, chemotherapy, and biological targeted agents have improved cure rates as well as overall survival rates, albeit modestly. Future direction in the treatment of lung cancer will include a personalized approach, as scientists learn to identify gene-specific and disease-specific features that may affect the prognosis and the probability of responding to certain treatments.

## EPIDEMIOLOGY

Deaths from lung cancer saw a sharp rise between 1930 and the 1970s for males and females, and peaked in the 1990s for males (Figure 59-1A) and later for females (Figure 59-1B). The rise likely correlates with the popularity and advertising of cigarettes in the 1920s and 1930s. In 2009, there were an estimated 219,440 new cases of lung cancer, resulting in an estimated 159,390 deaths, 28% of all cancer deaths.[1] Lung cancer is the overall leading cause of cancer deaths, resulting in more deaths than breast, prostate, and colon cancer combined. Five-year survival rates are very low, and have not significantly improved over the past 10 years (Table 59-1).

Lung cancer is also the second most commonly diagnosed cancer next to breast cancer in women and prostate cancer in men. The 2009 reported lifetime risk of developing lung cancer for men was 1 in 13, and for women was 1 in 16.[1] In 2000, the lifetime risk for men was 1 in 12 and for women it was 1 in 18, showing how over the past 9 years, the risk of developing lung cancer has increased in women and decreased in men.[4] Lung cancer rates in women are now approaching a plateau for the first time, after many decades of increase.[1,5] Lung cancer is still a disease of the elderly, with an average diagnosis at 71 years of age and two thirds of all cases diagnosed between the ages of 65 and 84.[5]

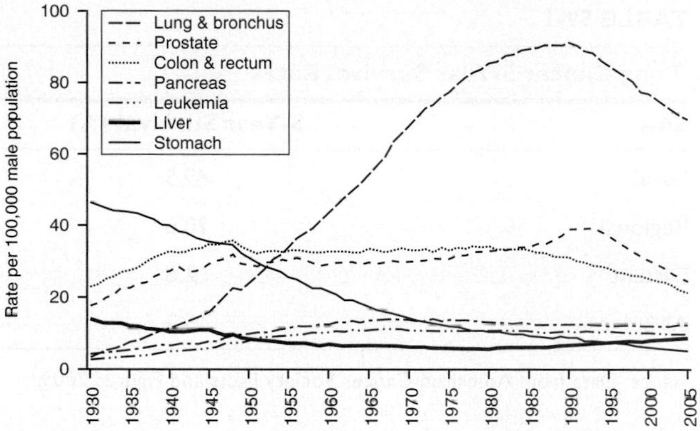


*Per 100,000, age adjusted to the 2000 US standard population

**FIGURE 59-1A**

Age-adjusted cancer death rates per 100,000 males by site in the US, 1930–2005. Data age adjusted to the 2000 US standard population.

*Note*: Due to changes in ICD coding, numerator information has changed over time. Rates for cancer of the liver, lung and bronchus, and colon and rectum are affected by these coding changes. (US Mortality Data, 1960 to 2005, US Mortality Volumes, 1930 to 1959, National Center for Health Statistics, Centers for Disease Control and Prevention, 2009, American Cancer Society.[1])

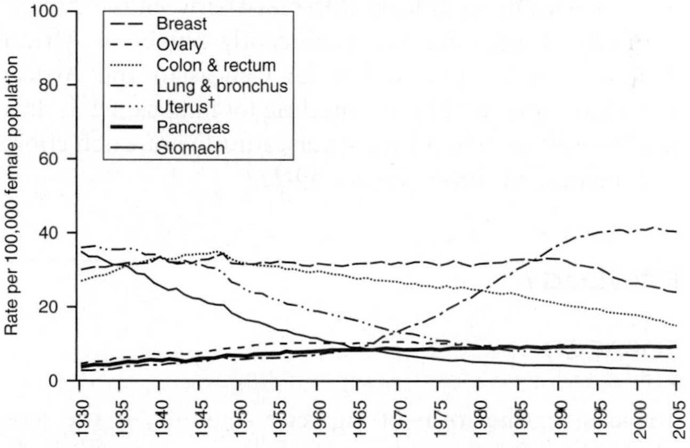


*Per 100,000, age adjusted to the 2000 US standard population †Uterus cancer death rates are for uterine cervix and uterine corpus combined

**FIGURE 59-1B**

Age-adjusted cancer death rates per 100,000 females by site in the US, 1930–2005. Data age adjusted to the 2000 US standard population.

*Note*: Due to changes in ICD coding, numerator information has changed over time. Rates for cancer of the liver, lung and bronchus, and colon and rectum are affected by these coding changes. (US Mortality Data, 1960 to 2005, US Mortality Volumes, 1930 to 1959, National Center for Health Statistics, Centers for Disease Control and Prevention, 2009. American Cancer Society.[1])

**TABLE 59-1**

**Lung Cancer 5-Year Survival Rates**

| Site | 5-Year Survival (%) |
|---|---|
| Local | 49.5 |
| Regional | 20.6 |
| Distant | 2.8 |
| All stages | 15.2 |

*Source*: Data from American Cancer Society Facts and Figures 2009.[1]

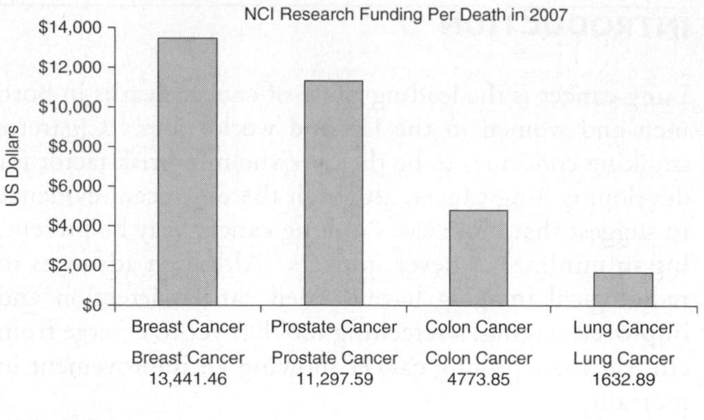


**FIGURE 59-2**

NCI research funding per death in 2007.

Data on never or minimal smokers with lung cancer are limited. The National Cancer Institute (NCI) Surveillance Epidemiology and End Results (SEER) database collects and publishes cancer statistics annually. It is the largest US cancer database; however, smoking status is not captured. Some studies have looked at smoking status and lung cancer with data gathered from long-term general health studies, such as the Nurses Health Study. In the never-smoking population, women are more likely than men to develop lung cancer and there is a suggestion that never-smoking lung cancer cases may be on the rise.[3,6,7]

SEER data report that the age-adjusted incidence of lung cancer is much higher in African American males per 100,000 men than in Caucasian, Asian, Hispanic, and Native American/Alaskan Native males.[5,8] In women, the incidence is highest in Caucasian and African American women, with no significant difference between the 2 races.[5] Similarly, death rates are significantly higher in African American males, but similar for Caucasian and African American women.[5] Finally, funding for lung cancer is drastically lower than in other cancers, stunting research efforts and medical advances (Figure 59-2).[9]

## ETIOLOGY

### TOBACCO

Tobacco, in the form of cigarette smoking, is the most common and preventable cause of all cancers, and is by far the biggest risk factor in lung cancer, accounting for up to 85% to 90% of all lung cancer cases.[1,2] About 43.4 million Americans are current smokers, representing 21% of the total population.[1] Following a 50% decline in smoking from 1965 to 2004, smoking rates have reached a plateau in the past 4 years.[1] Although initially much more popular among men, cigarette smoking prevalence evened out between the genders by the mid-1990s and has remained about 3% greater in Caucasian men than Caucasian women, and 9% more in African American men than African American women.[1]

Cigarette design in the 1950s introduced filtered tobacco, thus allowing cigarette smokers to inhale more deeply.[10] In 1964, the US Surgeon General released the conclusion that cigarette smoking caused lung cancer.[11] Tobacco smoke is the most common and most preventable carcinogen to humans, due to the polycyclic aromatic hydrocarbons and tobacco-specific nitrosamines.[2] The chronic and constant assault of these chemicals on the epithelial cells of the airways causes molecular lesions and decreased repair ability, leading to the development of lung cancer.[2]

The risk of developing lung cancer substantially decreases with the number of years of quitting smoking, even for those who quit well into and after middle age.[12] Those who quit smoking prior to middle age decrease their risk of developing lung cancer by 90%,[12] thus reinforcing how education targeting young audiences can dramatically reduce the incidence of and deaths from lung cancer. The longer the period of smoking, the higher the risk of developing lung cancer; however, even quitting later in life still can have positive effects on decreasing the risk of lung cancer.[12] Therefore, it is never too late to quit smoking to decrease lung cancer risk.

Race and ethnicity also play a factor in the risk of developing lung cancer. Among cigarette smokers, African Americans and Native Hawaiians are at higher risk of developing lung cancer than Caucasian Americans, Japanese Americans, and Latinos.[8,12] However, when smoking exceeds 30 cigarettes in a day, there are no significant differences in risk among different races and ethnic groups.[8] Across ethnic groups, the mean age at smoking initiation and rates of quitting were all similar.[8] However, in regards to quantity, the risk of Caucasian developing lung cancer is significantly lower than the risk for African Americans when smoking 10 or fewer cigarettes per day.[11] Metabolism of nicotine may vary among different ethnic and racial populations. African Americans have higher cotinine levels than Causasian and Hispanic smokers when smoking the same number of cigarettes.[13] There are also reports that African Americans may inhale more nicotine per cigarette, therefore increasing the exposure to tobacco and resulting in a higher incidence of lung cancer when smoking the same number of cigarettes or fewer per day as other racial groups.[14]

Women seem to have an increased susceptibility to tobacco carcinogens; however, they have a lower rate of fatal outcomes than men.[11,15] Women also exhibit more tobacco-related mutations than men, such as mutations of the *TP53* gene, which is common in lung cancer and has been suggested to play a role in carcinogenesis.[16]

## RADON

Radon is a colorless, odorless, inert gas that is produced as a breakdown product from decaying radium or uranium. It is an alkaline earth metal and is considered very radioactive; it is the largest source of natural ionizing radiation. It is usually confined to basements or dwellings underground that are poorly ventilated, but also can be found in hot springs. According to the Environmental Protection Agency (EPA), it is a human carcinogen; it is the second leading cause of lung cancer after cigarette smoking, and the leading cause of lung cancer in nonsmokers.[17] When radon is inhaled, it can be deposited in the bronchial epithelium, exposing these cells to ionizing radiation.[18,19] There is a significant increase of lung cancer risk from exposure to radon, even at lower levels, when combined with cigarette smoking.[18,19] In 1996, after sufficient evidence surfaced of the risk of lung cancer associated with radon exposure, the World Health Organization (WHO) put forth recommendations and guidelines for countries to follow to take action for risk management associated with radon exposure.[20] The current WHO International Radon Project is accruing data from 2005 to 2008 to put forth further guidelines, evaluate current action policies, and estimate global risk for radon exposure and how it relates to the development of lung cancer.[20]

## ENVIRONMENTAL TOBACCO SMOKE

Passive smoke, otherwise known as environmental tobacco smoke (ETS) or secondhand smoke (SHS), can come from various sources and in various quantities, and is smoke inhaled by people who are in close proximity to tobacco smoke. It can be the smoldering smoke of a cigarette or smoke inhaled from the smoke exhaled by another person. Environmental tobacco smoke contains up to 4000 chemicals and is estimated to lead to 3000 nonsmoking deaths from lung cancer per year.[1] SHS is also known to contain most of the same carcinogens as firsthand smoke, although often in lower concentrations. However, SHS can have the same genotoxic and epigenetic effects as mainstream smoke.[21] A meta-analysis in 2002 found a 25% increased risk of lung cancer associated with marriage to a smoker,[22] similar to an earlier meta-analysis showing a 29% increased risk of lung cancer in women whose husbands were smokers.[23]

Secondhand smoke poses an elevated risk of lung cancer for both smokers and never smokers, and represents a worse overall survival when the cancer is diagnosed as early stage non-small cell lung cancer (NSCLC).[24] The most significantly elevated risk is for patients exposed to SHS at work, sometimes classified as "occupational" exposure, as compared with those exposed at home or during leisure activities. The risk associated with SHS was also higher for heavy smokers, compared with light smokers, suggesting that heavier smokers could have already acquired more tobacco-related mutations or are generally sicker. There is also evidence that individuals with SHS exposure before the age of 25 have a higher risk of developing lung cancer than those exposed past the age of 25.[25]

## OCCUPATIONAL HAZARDS

Exposure to occupational human carcinogens accounts for about 9% of lung cancer deaths, with a much higher proportion in men than in women.[26] The risk is sharply increased when combined with cigarette smoking.[27] The risk has improved in developed countries where occupational provisions have been enforced by government agencies.[2] Many less developed countries do not report the statistics, making it difficult to assess occupational risk of lung cancer.[2,26] Many chemicals and metals used worldwide have been identified as human carcinogens related to occupational exposure (Table 59-2).[2]

Asbestos, most commonly associated with malignant mesothelioma, is also a risk factor for lung cancer. It is an insulating fiber used in many industrial, shipping, and heating or cooling occupations, and often the fibers can stick to clothing, causing exposure in family members in close contact. Since the 1950s, regulations have been enforced by government occupational agencies to restrict exposure and provide personal protective equipment to employees who are exposed to asbestos.

## CANNABIS

Cannabis, or marijuana, is likely a risk factor for lung cancer, although the risk has been difficult to study and quantify. Similar carcinogens have been found in cannabis to those found in tobacco. However, variations in methods of smoking, reporting bias because of legality issues, and the often combined tobacco use make it difficult to determine the actual risk associated with smoking cannabis. A meta-analysis reviewing 2 cohort studies and 14 case-controlled studies of cannabis use failed to show adequate data to

**TABLE 59-2**

**Human Carcinogens Primarily From Occupational Exposure**

| Exposure | Target Organ | Main Industry Use |
|---|---|---|
| Arsenic and arsenic compounds | Lung, skin | Glass, metals, pesticides |
| Asbestos | Lung, pleura | Insulation, construction |
| Beryllium, and beryllium compounds | Lung | Aerospace metals |
| Bis(chloromethyl)ether[a] | Lung | Chemical |
| Chloromethyl methyl ether[a] | Lung | Chemical |
| Cadmium and cadmium compounds | Lung | Pigment, battery |
| Chromium (IV) compounds | Nasal cavity, lung | Metal plating, pigment |
| Coal-tar pitches | Skin, lung, bladder | Construction, electrodes |
| Coal-tars | Skin, lung, bladder | Fuel |
| Mustard gas (sulfur mustard)[a] | Pharynx, lung | War gas |
| Radon-222 and its decay products | Lung | Mining |
| Silica, crystalline | Lung | Construction, mining |
| Soots | Skin, lung | Pigment |
| Strong-inorganic-acid mists containing sulfuric acid | Larynx, lung | Chemical |
| Talc-containing asbestiform fibers | Lung | Paper, paint |

[a]Agent mainly of historical interest.
*Source*: Adapted with permission from the World Health Organization, International Agency for Research on Cancer, World Cancer Report 2008.[2]

support an increased risk of cancer.[28] But a more recent study that adjusted for tobacco use and quantity of cannabis consumption showed that smoking cannabis added 8% to any other factors in the risk of developing lung cancer.[29] It equated 1 cannabis joint to 20 to 30 cigarettes. Future study of cannabis use and its relationship to lung cancer risk will need to adjust for concurrent tobacco use and seek methods to measure cannabis use.

## DIETARY FACTORS

Risk of lung cancer associated with dietary nutrients is much less significant than the risk associated with tobacco smoking; however, there are some minor risk increases or decreases with certain foods. Although there has been strong evidence for dietary risk in cancers of the gastrointestinal (GI) tract, fewer data have emerged for lung cancer until very recently. A number of studies have supported the idea that there is a protective anticarcinogenic effect against lung cancer in fruits and vegetables, especially those containing antioxidants or botanicals.[30,31] There are also data showing an inverse relationship between vitamin E (alpha-tocopherol) intake and lung cancer risk, although larger, controlled studies are required to examine this relationship.[32,33]

Conversely, beta-carotene supplementation has a proven detrimental relationship in smokers to the development of lung cancer. This was shown in 2 large randomized clinical trials: the Beta-Carotene and Retinol Efficacy Trial (CARET) and the Alpha-Tocopherol, Beta-Carotene (ATBC) Cancer Prevention Study.[34,35] The conclusion of these studies was that smokers should avoid beta-carotene supplements. That said, foods that are high in carotenoids can be protective for lung cancer risk in dietary intake over long periods, so high-risk populations and smokers need not stop or decrease dietary carotenoid intake.[36]

## OTHER FACTORS

Environmental risk factors, such as exposure to pesticides and air pollution, have also been linked to lung cancer.[37] European studies showed that nonsmokers residing near heavy traffic areas had a small increased risk of lung cancer; however, in the smoking group, there was no associated increased risk.[37,38] There are also increased cases of lung cancer in nonsmokers of Asian ethnicity. One study suggested that exposure to polycyclic aromatic hydrocarbons (PAHs) from using indoor coal cooking methods and then ingesting the PAHs in the food cooked in this manner contributes to the development of lung cancer.[39] Many studies showing increases in lung cancer risk associated with environmental factors have failed to control for tobacco use, so the quality of these data needs to be validated with studies that analyze tobacco use as a confounding risk factor.

Genetic predisposition also plays a role in the development of lung cancer, as evidenced by the wide variations in the number of smokers who actually develop lung cancer. In a study by Bach and colleagues, the risk ranged from 0.8% in former smokers to 15% in lifelong heavy smokers.[40] There are also positive findings of familial risk of lung cancer, especially for those between the ages of 40 and 59 with a history of first-degree relatives with lung cancer.[41] However, it is likely also that a large component of epigenetic changes, such as deficiency in DNA repair genes and differences in tobacco carcinogen metabolism, cause some smokers to be placed at higher risk.[12] Collecting biomarkers for study, such as tissue, blood, and urine samples, can help to further validate these findings and lead to the development of a quality risk assessment model in the future.

A history of alkylating agents and radiation therapy to the chest to treat Hodgkin's disease can cause an increased risk of lung cancer. The risk is dose-dependent and is enhanced when combined with tobacco use.[42]

The presence of acquired lung disease, such as chronic obstructive pulmonary disease (COPD) or emphysema, has also been shown to increase the risk of lung cancer, even when controlling for tobacco use.[43,44] Potential explanations of this could be mucociliary dysfunction, free radical damage to DNA, and chronic inflammation leading to endogenous DNA mutations.[43]

## PREVENTION

### PRIMARY PREVENTION

Risks of lung cancer associated with smoking and environmental tobacco smoke are well documented and understood, making tobacco prevention the most important form of primary prevention. Programs and legislation that protect the general public and educate current smokers are important and essential to reducing mortality from the worldwide lung cancer epidemic. The US Surgeon General first suggested in 1972 that the public may be at risk from ETS, and in 1986 the first report was released of a risk to nonsmokers from involuntary exposure to ETS.[45] Surgeon General C. Everett Koop, in 1986, stated, "the rights of smokers to smoke ends when their behavior affects the health and well-being of others."

In 1989, the California Tobacco Control Program (CTCP) evolved as the first major statewide tobacco control program, with the goal to change the social norm in order to discourage future tobacco users.[46] It was based on 3 main principles: the tobacco companies lie, nicotine is addictive, and secondhand smoke kills.[47] The program sought to promulgate these principles by using the media and toll-free quit-lines to make tobacco less desirable and less acceptable. Restricting smoking in public places and enforcing laws against selling tobacco to youths made tobacco less accessible. During its first decade of existence, the program was associated with 11,000 fewer cases of lung cancer.[48] In addition to reducing lung cancer incidence, the CTCP reduced personal health care costs by $86 billion in its first 15 years, and with the substantial decrease in cigarette sales, cost the tobacco industry $9.2 billion in pretax sales.[47]

The 1998 Master Settlement Agreement was money recovered from the tobacco industry and designated for statewide programs to prevent smoking and promote smoking cessation.[49] This agreement prohibits tobacco advertising to people under 18 years old and provided dollars per capita to each state. However, each state spends much less annually per capita than was allotted under the Master Settlement Agreement.[50] The Centers for Disease Control (CDC) publishes guidelines, most recently in 2007, showing what each state spends per capita, and puts forth recommendations for statewide spending and community programs to promote tobacco use prevention and cessation.[50]

Chemoprevention is the use of natural or chemically synthesized compounds to prevent, inhibit, or reverse the process of carcinogenesis.[51] Primary chemoprevention is prevention in healthy high-risk patients. Although trials with retinoids and alpha-tocopherol (vitamin E) in heavy smokers showed negative results,[34,35] high blood levels of vitamin E in light smokers were associated with a decrease in lung cancer incidence, but this needs to be studied in a prospective fashion.[36] Studies of cyclooxygenase-2 (COX-2) inhibitors and aspirin in smokers suggest a possible inhibition of lung cancer by decreasing the inflammatory response to damaged cells.[52,53] A prospective study of nonsteroidal anti-inflammatory drugs (NSAIDs) suggested a modified lung cancer risk, which was interpreted separately in relation to genotype.[53] Dietary trace metals such as zinc, copper, selenium, iron, and calcium may also play a role in primary chemoprevention of lung cancer by stabilizing DNA repair capacity. These have been studied in retrospective analyses using diet recall questionnaires. These studies have yielded mixed results;[54–56] however, prospective studies in the future may guide possible dietary recommendations to prevent lung cancer.

### SECONDARY PREVENTION

The most effective secondary prevention of lung cancer is smoking cessation. Quitting smoking, even later in life, reduces the risk of lung cancer (Table 59-3).[11] However, an increased risk of lung cancer remains even 30 years after quitting smoking, especially of adenocarcinoma and for heavy smokers.[57] It is important for healthcare providers, at each patient visit, to address smoking status and offer smoking cessation.[58] Smoking cessation strategies in the form of medications or behavior management have been a major advance in decreasing the health risks of smoking.

Nicotine replacement therapy (NRT) is a vehicle that delivers nicotine to the bloodstream to prevent withdrawal symptoms when a patient attempts to quit smoking. NRT is available in different forms, such as gum, transdermal patches, nasal sprays, and inhalers (Table 59-4).[59] All of these preparations are equivalent in efficacy and can double the smoking cessation rate when compared with a placebo.[60,61] Since the patch provides a constant dose, it may be more effective when used as maintenance therapy in the early stages of smoking cessation, and the gum, inhaler, and

**TABLE 59-3**

**It Is Never Too Late to Quit Smoking**

| Age at which quit smoking | Cumulative risk of lung cancer by age 75 in Men |
|---|---|
| Lifelong Nonsmokers | 0.4% |
| 30 | 1.7% |
| 40 | 3.0% |
| 50 | 6.0% |
| 60 | 9.9% |
| 70 | 16.0% |

*Source*: Data from Peto and Doll.[11]

nasal spray may be used as needed for cravings or as an adjunct to the patch.[59]

Bupropion SR (Zyban, GlaxoSmithKline, Research Triangle Park, NC) was the first non-nicotine-containing medication to be approved by the US Food and Drug Administration (FDA) and used for smoking cessation. It contains the same ingredients as Wellbutrin (GlaxoSmithKline, Research Triangle Park, NC), an antidepressant, and therefore carries a black box warning of increased risk of suicidal thinking, suicidal behavior, and major depressive disorder. However, in 3 placebo-controlled studies, bupropion SR in combination with smoking cessation counseling showed an improvement in smoking quit rates.[62] The recommended dose is 150 mg daily for 3 days, then 300 mg/day.

Varenicline (Chantix, Pfizer Inc, Mission, KS) is the newest and most effective smoking cessation aid currently available. In a study of varenicline vs bupropion SR vs placebo, the varenicline showed a significant improvement in continuous abstinence rates from weeks 9 to 12, with smoking abstinence rates of 44% for varenicline, 29.5% for bupropion SR, and 17.7% for placebo.[63] It is also significantly better than placebo at maintaining smoking cessation when given in maintenance dosing from weeks 13 to 24, and even up to week 52 after treatment was completed.[64] Varenicline is prescribed as a starter pack initially, and then builds a patient up to the 1 mg twice a day recommended dose.[65] Following the starter pack, the patient should be treated with the 1 mg twice daily dosing for up to 12 weeks.

Counseling strategies and behavior management techniques have been successful as conjunctive treatment with medical management to improve smoking cessation rates. Many states have offered and advertise toll-free quit-lines that provide advice and support. Quit rates are higher when participants adhere to a phone and Web-based quitting support group.[66] Financial incentives offered by employers have also shown significant increases in smoking cessation rates.[67] A future approach to smoking cessation includes identifying populations who are genetically at risk of smoking addiction and aiming to prevent them from starting smoking or understand why they may have a much harder time quitting than others.

Radon screening and reduction techniques are important for high-risk homes and smokers. A study of radon screening as a public service offering yielded only a very minimal improvement in lung cancer risk; therefore, it may

**TABLE 59-4**

**Nicotine Replacement Therapy**

| Type | Onset (min) | Dose | Advantages | Problems |
|---|---|---|---|---|
| Patch | 50 | < 15 cig/day: 7 to 14 mg/day<br>< 20 cig/day: 15 to 21 mg/day<br>< 40 cig/day: 21 to 35 mg/day<br>> 40 cig/day: 42 mg/day | Constant dose<br>Easy dose | Local skin irritation if used at night<br>Sleep disturbances |
| Gum | 30 | Light smokers—2 mg<br>Heavy smokers—4 mg<br>2 sticks/hr | Quick onset<br>Easy to vary dose | Jaw pain<br>Dental problems<br>Swallowing leads to GI effects |
| Nasal Spray | 10 | 1–2 doses per hours, 8–10 doses/day | Quick onset<br>Easy to vary doses | Nasal symptoms<br>Difficult to use with nasal congestion |
| Inhaler | 30 | 4 mg cartridge, 6–8 cartridges/day | Quick onset | Local irritation<br>Oral stimulation |

*Source*: Reprinted with permission from PMPH-USA. *Lung Cancer.* Ginsberg RJ, editor. PMPH-USA; Shelton, CT, 2002.

not be cost-effective in general, but is important in public buildings prior to construction and schools.[68] Radon is measured as picocuries of radon per liter of air (pCi/L) and is mostly found in high levels in basements and crawl spaces under a house. The EPA recommends actions to fix radon levels if they read 4 pCi/L or higher.[69] Techniques to fix radon levels include soil suction, sealing cracks, and installing exhaust fans; all are best carried out by a contractor specializing in radon mitigation.

Secondary chemoprevention aims to prevent premalignant lesions from forming into lung cancer. The carcinogenesis of lung cancer is a multistep process through which a series of molecular changes progresses into invasive disease. Retinoids have been studied extensively as chemoprevention agents in lung cancer, and results have all been negative.[70] Examples of molecular markers for chemoprevention targets include COX-2, the ras-signaling pathway through farnesyl transferase inhibitors (FTIs), and the tyrosine kinase/epidermal growth factor receptor (EGFR) pathway.[71,72] However, the FDA and the medical community are following a model of first testing these drugs in the adjuvant setting to prevent a recurrence of lung cancer before trialing them in the chemoprevention setting.

### TERTIARY PREVENTION

Tertiary chemoprevention is the use of natural or synthetic agents in patients who have had curative treatment for lung cancer to prevent the development of a recurrence or a second lung cancer. Adjuvant chemotherapy is not considered chemoprevention because it is theoretically treating micrometastatic disease. Currently there are no standard agents used for chemoprevention in this setting. One current trial, Eastern Cooperative Oncology Group (ECOG) 5597, is looking at selenium in preventing second primary lung tumors after surgical resection of early stage NSCLC. Other trials are looking at EGFR inhibitors or FTIs as chemoprevention after resection of early stage NSCLC in specific populations. Also, COX-2 inhibitors are of interest in chemoprevention strategies for lung cancer, and with the confirmation of COX-2 as a molecular target, trials will likely begin to look at these agents for chemoprevention.[73]

## SCREENING AND EARLY DETECTION

### SPUTUM CYTOLOGY

There are abnormal biomarkers that can be found in sputum showing cellular dysplasia, which can identify premalignancy. Genetic aberrations found in sputum, such as tobacco-related *HYAL2* and *FHIT* deletions, have been identified as possible precursors for lung cancer.[74] At this time, there is no standard of care for chemoprevention for premalignant lesions; however, these patients would be eligible for ongoing chemoprevention trials.

### RADIOGRAPHIC IMAGING

Chest x-ray (CXR) is a cost-effective, simple measure to detect lung cancer. Screening trials from 1960 to 1980, including the Mayo Lung Project, the Czech Study on Lung Cancer, the Johns Hopkins Lung Project, and the Memorial Sloan-Kettering Lung Cancer Screening Program, failed to demonstrate a benefit with CXR and sputum cytology in lowering lung cancer mortality.[75] Although these trials have been negative, many clinicians still use CXRs as a surveillance method due to their low cost and safety.

Low-dose spiral chest computed tomography (CT) has been used since the 1990s by imaging 5 to 10-mm horizontal slices down through the body. Studies have shown an improved ability over CXR to detect lung nodules larger than 5 mm, but have not been able to show improvement in survival.[76,77] CT imaging for screening and surveillance has many critics. Often, small nodules in the lung parenchyma are found, causing much worry in patients, but they are too small to biopsy. Many times the nodules or opacities can be related to infection, trauma, or granulomatous disease.

The International Early Lung Cancer Action Program (I-ELCAP) is a large study that randomized high-risk patients to either CXR or chest CT. The study found that with annual CT screening, 85% of patients were diagnosed with stage I lung cancer, and 92% were alive at 10 years.[78] These results were improvements in terms of earlier stage at diagnosis and increased overall survival. However, the I-ELCAP does not show a benefit to CT screening in terms of lives saved. Because of the absence of a reduction in mortality, it is not considered an effective screening tool at this time.[74,79]

In response to the I-ELCAP study, the NCI has launched the National Lung Screening Trial (NLST), which by 2004 had accrued 50,000 patients. Similar to I-ELCAP, this study randomized high-risk patients to either CXR or CT scanning. Currently the study is closed to enrollment, follow-up will conclude in 2009, and results will be analyzed and reported in the near future.[80]

### BRONCHOSCOPIC PROCEDURES

There are currently no approved methods for early detection or screening for lung cancer using bronchoscopic procedures. However, the detection of premalignant lesions or carcinoma in situ in the respiratory tract can be facilitated using different bronchoscopic techniques. Photosensitizers are retained by neoplastic tissues; however, photodynamic techniques have been cumbersome and are associated with side effects, so they are not often used for early detection.[81] White-light bronchoscopy (WLB) is a conventional method using white light, all wavelengths from blue to red, to detect carcinoma in situ. Autofluorescence bronchoscopy (AFB) uses a sophisticated camera, a light source, and computer images to examine the airway and detect early stage malignant changes that are of too low intensity to be seen by the human eye.[81,82] With AFB, normal tissue is illuminated as green, but as the tissue changes or blood supply is increased, there is a progressive decrease in green autofluorescence (Figure 59-3A, B).[81] Studies have shown that using AFB in addition to WLB improved detection of preneoplastic lesions and carcinoma in situ.[83,84] This combination system is often referred to as the Onco-LIFE system. Optical coherence tomography is a promising technique for the future that uses ultrasound imaging with infrared light waves that can detect airway abnormalities as small as 20 μm.[81]

## PATHOPHYSIOLOGY

### CELLULAR CHARACTERISTICS

Tissue diagnosis, otherwise known as pathology, is imperative before starting any type of chemotherapy or radiation treatment for lung cancer. A specific pathological diagnosis will guide therapy and predict prognosis. Lung cancer is generally broken down into 2 major categories: NSCLC, accounting for about 87% of cases, and small cell lung cancer (SCLC), accounting for about 13% of cases.[1] NSCLC is further classified into the histological subtypes adenocarcinoma, squamous cell carcinoma, and large cell carcinoma. The ability to differentiate among histological diagnoses has become important for clinicians to guide which chemotherapeutic agents may give favorable response rates, and also may exclude patients from certain targeted agents due to toxicity concerns.

#### Non-small cell lung cancer

Adenocarcinoma arises from alveolar surface epithelium, and bronchial mucosal glands, and is known to produce mucin.[85] It is currently the most commonly occurring NSCLC in the US, representing 40% of primary tumors, and is the subtype most commonly found in nonsmokers and women.[85,86] Adenocarcinoma is subdivided into 6 categories: acinar, papillary, bronchioloalveolar, solid adenocarcinoma with mucin formation, mixed, and variants. Variants include mucinous, signet ring, and clear cell.[87,88] Bronchoalveolar carcinoma (BAC) is a distinct subtype that spreads along alveolar septae but does not invade lung parenchyma.[86] Tumors of the adenocarcinoma subtype are often located in the periphery of the lung parenchyma, and therefore the patient often presents with fewer symptoms. Changes in smoking behavior, such as filtered cigarettes causing smokers to inhale more deeply, have likely contributed to an increase in adenocarcinoma.[10]

Squamous cell carcinoma (SCC), once the predominant type of NSCLC, now represents 30% to 35% of

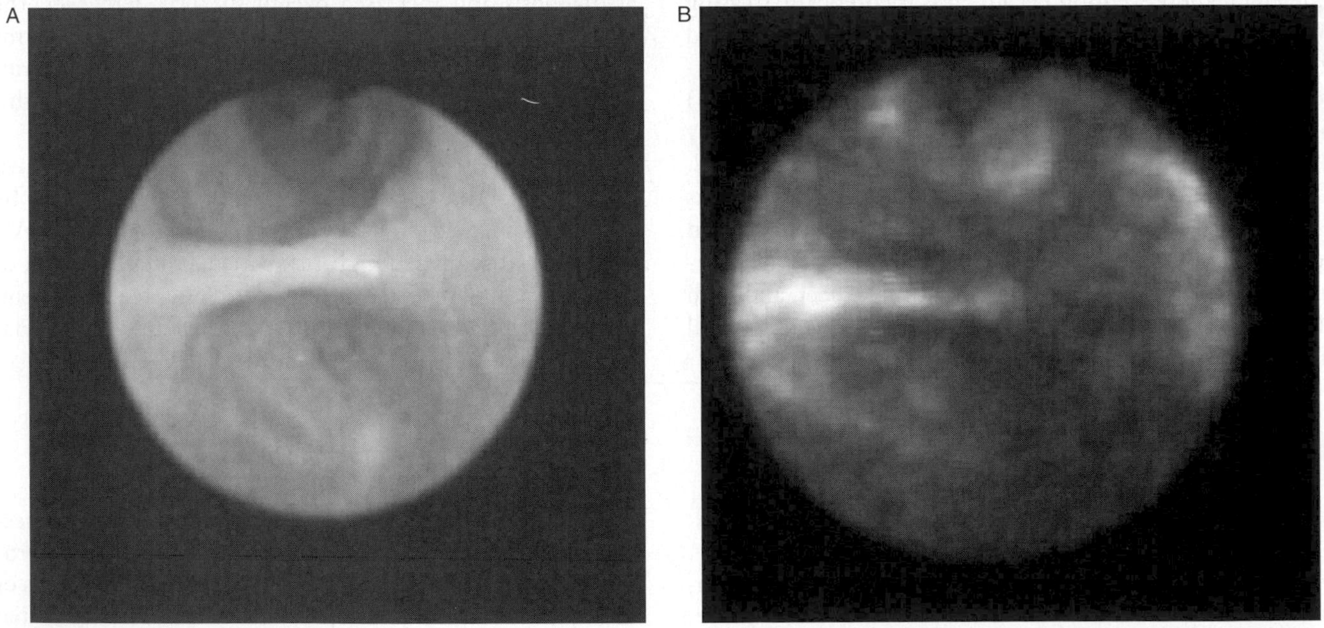


**FIGURE 59-3**

Premalignant lesions as seen on (**A**) white-light bronchoscopy and (**B**) autofluorescence bronchoscopy. (Courtesy Dr. Michael Unger, Fox Chase Cancer Center, Philadelphia, PA.)

cases. It arises from more centrally located areas of the lungs. SCC progresses from noninvasive metaplasia and dysplasia to carcinoma in situ. Once a carcinoma in situ penetrates the basement membrane, involving the lamina propria, it becomes invasive and has the ability to metastasize.[85] It is the subtype most amenable to diagnosis on sputum cytology or bronchial brushes because of its central location.[86] Also due to the central location of these tumors, symptoms such as cough, hemoptysis, and obstructive pneumonia often lead individuals to seek medical attention, which leads to a diagnosis of SCC. Necrosis and cavitation occur in approximately 10% of SCC lung tumors,[85] which, together with the risk of bleeding, can limit options for treatment with biological agents containing vascular endothelial growth factor (VEGF) receptor inhibitors.

Large cell carcinoma represents approximately 15% of all lung cancers. This undifferentiated tumor displays no evidence of squamous or glandular maturation. The diagnosis is made by exclusion. Its incidence has decreased over the years because better histopathological techniques are now available to distinguish those adenocarcinomas and SCC that were previously defined as large cell undifferentiated tumors.[85,86] Large cell tumors frequently contain neuroendocrine features, which are associated with a poorer prognosis.[85]

### Small cell lung cancer

Small cell lung cancer, otherwise known as oat cell lung cancer, is a neuroendocrine tumor. Approximately 98% of cases are associated with cigarette smoking.[89] The incidence of SCLC has declined from a peak of 20% to 25% to a current low of 13%, presumably because of downward trends in cigarette smoking 20 years ago.[1,87] SCLC is an aggressive cancer that usually arises from the large central airways and frequently metastasizes early.[85] Survival in patients with extensive disease without treatment is often measured in weeks. Little is known about the pathogenesis of SCLC, except that there can be hyperplasia of the pulmonary neuroendocrine cells, which function as oxygen sensors.[89] The majority of SCLCs also express the c-KIT oncoprotein; however, there is a lack of c-KIT exon 11 activating mutations in most tumors, explaining why imatinib has been ineffective at treating SCLC.[90]

### Immunostains

Determining whether tumor tissue originates from the lung or another primary site is also very important and directs therapy. For instance, if an adenocarcinoma of the lung displays estrogen receptors, it is important to determine whether it originally came from the breast or the lung. Thyroid transcription factor-1 (TTF-1) is among the most common stains that is specific for a tumor arising from the lung or the thyroid, although in rare instances it can be a metastasis from the colon.[91,92] However, TTF-1 is positive in only about 5% of squamous cell tumors in the lung.[91] Also, most lung cancers that are squamous cell or large cell will stain positive for cytokeratins (CK) 5 or 6, as will acinar adenocarcinomas.[93] The p63 antibody is also commonly used to distinguish between NSCLC and SCLC, as well as adenocarcinoma and squamous cell carcinoma.[94] There are many stains that a pathologist uses to determine an appropriate histological diagnosis; however TTF-1, CK 5 and 6, and p63 are important factors, looked at together, to determine histological cell types for poorly differentiated carcinomas of the lung.[94,95]

## PROGRESSION OF DISEASE

Lung cancer originates in the lung parenchyma and spreads through lymphatic channels in the chest or via direct extension into structures in the chest. From the lymph nodes, the cancer then spreads through either lymphatic channels or the bloodstream to distant sites. The pattern of nodal spread often begins with the adjacent nodes, the hilar lymph nodes, then the mediastinal lymph nodes, and then more distant sites or supraclavicular lymph nodes. Sometimes there will be a malignant pleural effusion, where fluid accumulates in the pleura due to obstruction of lymph node drainage, irritation to the pleura, pleural metastases, or direct extension of tumor into the pleura.

Approximately 50% of lung cancers arise from the central structures in the chest and they can often involve large airways, resulting in hemoptysis, dyspnea, hoarseness, atelectasis, and postobstructive pneumonia.[75] The tumor can directly extend and invade into contiguous structures in the chest, often resulting in metastatic dissemination to distant sites.[96] The brain is also a common site of metastases. In a lung cancer autopsy series, 54% of patients with NSCLCs and 80% with SCLCs had brain metastases at the time of their death.[97] Other common sites of metastases are liver, bone, and adrenal glands.

Mechanisms promoting the spread and growth of lung cancer are currently beginning to be understood and studied. One pathway that has been linked to lung cancer, and other cancers, is the VEGF receptor pathway. A tumor secretes VEGF, which attracts a new blood supply and promotes survival of immature vessels to nourish the cell in a process called angiogenesis.[98] Lung tumors are also known to overexpress and have dysregulation of the EGFR protein.[99] Activation of these receptors on cancer cells promotes invasion, metastasis, inhibition of apoptosis, angiogenesis, proliferation, and survival.[100] There are numerous other growth factor pathways, mutations, and tumor cell receptors involved with lung cancer and its ability to proliferate, including resistance genes that mutate after drug response. There are many agents in phase II and phase III clinical trials currently investigating therapeutic agents targeting these pathways.

## CLINICAL MANIFESTATIONS

### SIGNS AND SYMPTOMS RELATED TO THE PRIMARY TUMOR

Cough is the most common presenting symptom of lung cancer. It can be dry or containing mucus. Many times, the cough is treated conventionally as an upper respiratory infection or a COPD flare. However, when treatment is ineffective and the cough persists, usually a diagnostic work-up ensues. The cough is likely a result of the primary tumor irritating the lung parenchyma, a pleural effusion, or a postobstructive pneumonia.[101] The incidence and prevalence of cough as it relates to presentation of lung cancer varies widely due to the differences in symptom measurement techniques.[102]

Hemoptysis can be a presenting symptom, although it is not nearly as common as cough and shortness of breath. This is most common in SCLC, the squamous cell histology of NSCLC, and tumors that are centrally located. It originates from interference with either the high-pressure bronchial circulation or the low-pressure pulmonary circulation, but up to 90% of the bleeding is from bronchial arteries.[103] Scant hemoptysis refers to flecks of blood in the mucus, and frank hemoptysis describes actual clots of blood in the mucus.

Dyspnea is a result of hypoxemia related to primary tumor obstruction. Usually it is a result of direct involvement in the airways, lung parenchyma, or a pleural effusion.[104] Obstruction can, in turn, produce a pneumonia and atelectasis, complicating dyspnea and causing infection. There can also be a pattern of lymphangitic carcinomatosis, a microspread of the cancer along the lymphatic channels resulting in a diffuse-looking pattern on the CT scan. Phrenic nerve paralysis and an elevated diaphragm from the tumor can also cause shortness of breath.

### SIGNS AND SYMPTOMS RELATED TO INTRATHORACIC EXTRAPULMONARY SPREAD

Chest pain can be a presenting symptom in patients with pleural metastases or direct extension of the tumor into the structures in the chest cavity. Pancoast tumors or superior sulcus tumors, which are tumors located in the lung apex, tend to induce significant pain due to the invasion of the brachial plexus nerves and sometimes the first to third ribs.[105] There can also be upper-extremity paresthesias or Horner's syndrome, which is characterized by ptosis and decreased sweating on the ipsilateral side of the face, from a superior sulcus tumor. Retrosternal chest pain can be related to large mediastinal adenopathy; however, most adenopathy does not produce pain. Pleuritic chest pain can be related to direct extension of the disease; however, it can also indicate a pulmonary embolism.

Pleural effusions are a result of increased fluid production due to tumor implants present in the pleura or from decreased absorption due to lymphatic or bronchial obstruction.[106] They are a common presenting sign of pulmonary malignancy, and are usually coupled with a nagging, dry cough and shortness of breath on exertion. A malignant pleural effusion is usually serosanguineous, with high protein and lactate dehydrogenase (LDH) levels and low glucose levels.[106]

Superior vena cava (SVC) syndrome is most commonly a result of primary lung tumor or mediastinal lymph node encroachment into the SVC and is often considered an oncologic emergency. The SVC drains into the right atrium and is a large, low-pressure vessel that is easily compressible.[107] About 60% to 90% of all SVC cases are caused by cancer, and about 65% are due to lung cancer.[107,108] Almost all patients develop facial and upper-extremity swelling, and some develop dilated collateral veins across the chest, coupled with cough and dyspnea.[108] Less frequent symptoms associated with SVC syndrome are chest pain, syncope, headaches, hoarseness, and dysphagia.[108]

Hoarseness can also be a presenting symptom associated with lung cancer. It is usually a result of aortopulmonary window lymphadenopathy causing impingement on the left recurrent laryngeal nerve, which passes through the aortic arch.[109] Hoarseness is usually not linked with a sore throat or signs of infection. It is an indicator of locally advanced disease and is often a factor that surgeons weigh heavily in the decision to perform surgery due to the complications that it implies.

Pericardial effusion or tamponade, dysphagia, and bronchorrhea are other, rarer but possible symptoms. Lymphadenopathy and lymphangitic spread from primary lung cancers are also conditions seen on radiographic imaging that can cause a myriad of respiratory symptoms to develop.

### SYMPTOMS RELATED TO EXTRAPULMONARY SPREAD

Fatigue is a common symptom seen with metastatic lung cancer. In a pilot study of 20 patients, fatigue was reported as the most troublesome symptom or side effect associated with lung cancer.[102] Often it can be caused by other factors, such as anemia of chronic disease and malnutrition. It can also be exacerbated by general weakness, shortness of breath, and depression. Fatigue is often present even when none of these other factors is present and can be very difficult to treat given the subjective nature and lack of etiology.

Pain can be a presenting and lingering symptom indicative of extrathoracic spread of lung cancer. Most often it is a result of bone metastases and if it is severe or poses a threat of fracture, the patient will need surgery or urgent radiation to the site. Sometimes corticosteroids and narcotics are necessary to alleviate this type of pain. Spine metastases can be the cause of back pain, and a thorough neurological exam is necessary to identify possible signs of spinal cord compression, which is an oncologic emergency. Adrenal metastases are also common as a result of lung cancer and can cause abdominal or back pain.

Brain metastases are a presenting factor in about 10% of patients with lung cancer.[110] Seizures, headaches, a change in mental status, or nausea/vomiting are common complications of brain metastases. These symptoms are often caused by edema surrounding the brain metastasis, and prompt, high-dose steroids are necessary to control the edema. Magnetic resonance imaging (MRI) of the brain with gadolinium is the gold standard for detecting and determining the location and severity of brain metastases. If the patient has a contraindication to MRI, a head CT can be substituted; however, intravenous (IV) contrast is highly recommended to detect brain tumors and edema.

Gastrointestinal symptoms can manifest as a result of the disease in general or from specific metastatic tumors directly involving the GI tract. Anorexia and weight loss are prevalent at presentation, and a loss of even just 5% of the normal body weight at diagnosis can be a poor prognostic indicator.[111] Other symptoms related to the GI tract can be associated with hepatic metastases. Metastases to the stomach and bowel are rare in lung cancer; however, GI obstruction can occur from invasion by local metastatic sites such as liver, adrenals, and any abdominal lymph nodes.

## PARANEOPLASTIC SYNDROMES: SIGNS AND SYMPTOMS INDIRECTLY RELATED TO THE TUMOR

Paraneoplastic syndromes in lung cancer are fairly rare, occurring in about 10% of patients, and are the result of substances such as hormones, growth factors, cytokines, or antibodies secreted by the tumor.[112] They are more common in SCLC and may preclude the diagnosis of cancer, prompting clinicians to seek out a primary tumor. The mechanism of the paraneoplastic syndrome is not well understood, and treatment of the primary tumor is often the best treatment. When linked to a lung cancer diagnosis, paraneoplastic syndromes are often correlated with a poor prognosis.

Endocrine paraneoplastic syndromes include hypercalcemia, syndrome of inappropriate antidiuretic hormone (SIADH), and Cushing's syndrome. Normal calcium levels are from 9 to 11 mg/dL, and hypercalcemia is defined when calcium levels rise above 11 mg/dL. In patients without cancer, it is mostly a result of hyperparathyroidism; however, in lung cancer it is mostly due to bone metastases. Symptoms include a change in mental status, constipation, nausea/vomiting, and in severe cases renal failure, cardiac arrhythmias, or coma. Treatment is centered around hydration in combination with bisphosphonates.

Paraneoplastic adrenocorticotropic hormone syndrome, which causes Cushing's syndrome and SIADH, is most common in patients with SCLC. Patients with Cushing's syndrome typically present with muscle weakness, hypertension, hypokalemia, and glucose intolerance, and in more severe cases metabolic alkalosis.[112] Diagnosis is determined by high cortisol levels in the blood and urine. The most common treatment is oral ketoconazole, metyrapone, and octreotide; however, the development of Cushing's syndrome in a lung cancer patient is a very poor prognostic indicator.[113] SIADH is the abnormal production and secretion of antidiuretic hormone, which causes water reabsorption and hyponatremia. Signs and symptoms of hyponatremia include confusion, nausea/vomiting, diarrhea, increased thirst, decreased urine output, loss of deep tendon reflexes, and in severe cases sodium levels lower than 115 mEq/L, seizures, and coma.[112,114] Fluid restriction of 800 to 1000 ml/day, isotonic or hypertonic IV hydration, and demeclocycline are all used to correct sodium levels, but treatment of the underlying cancer is sometimes also effective.[115]

Neuromuscular paraneoplastic syndromes include Lambert-Eaton myasthenic syndrome (LEMS), encephalitis, and cerebellar degeneration. LEMS has a classic presentation of proximal muscle weakness and muscle fatigue when exercising or getting out of a chair.[112] Other neurological paraneoplastic syndromes include different types of encephalitis, such as limbic encephalitis, brainstem encephalitis, cerebellar degeneration, myelitis, and multifocal encephalomyelitis. They are often associated with a myriad antibodies, and immunotherapy can sometimes be an effective treatment.[116]

Musculoskeletal paraneoplastic syndromes include clubbing and hypertrophic pulmonary osteoarthropathy (HPOA). Clubbing is when the angle of the nail bed changes from the normal 15 degrees between the cuticle and the proximal nail and paronychial soft tissue expansion develops (Figure 59-4).[117] HPOA manifests as painful and sometimes swollen joints and is a clinical diagnosis. The pathogenesis for both conditions is largely unknown. Treatment with nonsteroidal anti-inflammatory agents and narcotics can allay the symptoms; however, treating the cancer often improves HPOA, sometimes without a radiographic tumor response.[117]

Other paraneoplastic syndromes associated with lung cancer are anorexia, cachexia, weight loss and fatigue, many of which come in clusters and indicate a poor prognosis. Dermatologic syndromes can manifest as hyperpigmented skin plaques and seborrheic keratoses, in which no therapy is recommended.[117] Anemia, leukocytosis, and platelet disorders are also evident as part of chronic disease and inflammatory cytokines in lung cancer patients. Thrombosis and thromboembolism, otherwise known as

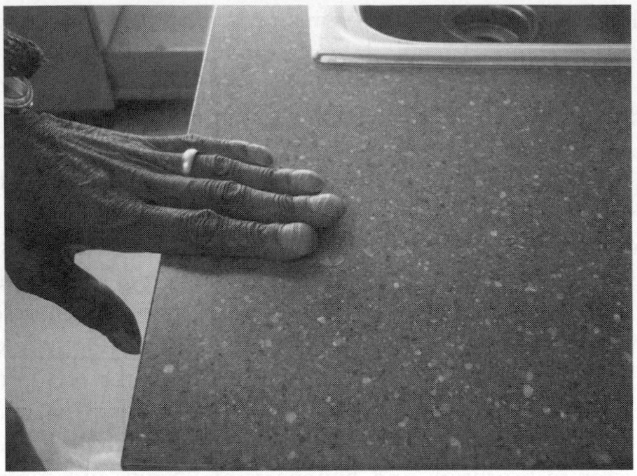

**FIGURE 59-4**

Clubbed fingernails.

Trousseau's syndrome, are also complications common in lung cancer and require aggressive anticoagulation.

## ASSESSMENT

### PATIENT AND FAMILY HISTORY

A detailed history of the patient with lung cancer is essential for both the treatment and future study and understanding of the disease. The patient's history of present illness (HPI), with specific dates of when symptoms occurred, will usually provide a general picture of the trajectory of the disease and can help predict aggressiveness of disease. Data from the HPI and patient demographics can also be entered into an institution's database in order to track and report treatment and survival outcomes.[118] The HPI will also help uncover what studies the patient has completed so far in the work-up and the patient's general understanding of the disease and prognosis before the physician discusses treatment options.

Family, medical, and social histories are also vital to understanding and treating lung cancer. The family history should include the immediate family's medical conditions and history of cancer, indentifying type of cancer(s), whether they were treated and cured, or whether the cancer resulted in death. The medical history of the patient will guide the clinician as to what therapies may be appropriate or contraindicated and generally. Performance status needs to be evaluated as it is important in projecting survival and treatment options in lung cancer patients.[119] Specifically, the interviewer must ask about respiratory conditions, current treatments, and the length of time the patient has suffered from the respiratory illnesses. A surgical history can help identify medical problems, anatomic changes, and how well the patient recuperated. Eliciting a list of prescription and over-the-counter medications will help to identify past or existing medical conditions.

A social history is also quite important for the patient with lung cancer. The smoking history needs to be detailed and the patient needs to be reminded this information is important to make treatment decisions and understand pathology. With instances of undetermined pathology, a nonsmoker would be much less likely to have small cell lung cancer, which is highly linked to cigarette smoking. When taking a smoking history, it is important to identify cigarettes vs cigars, pipes, smokeless tobacco, or marijuana, the age at initiation, the number of packs per day, and the age when the patient quit or whether they have quit. The patient's age at initiation and age at quitting are important because some patients will say they smoked for 20 years, when in reality the gap between starting and quitting is often much longer. A commonly used term in the oncology community is "pack-years." This is a multiplication of number of years of smoking by the number of packs per day. For example, if a patient smoked 1 pack/day for 40 years, this would be called a 40-pack-year history. Another example would be someone who smoked 3 packs/day for 40 years, which would be considered a 120-pack-year history.

Other social history questions of importance, especially in nonsmokers, include occupation and possible exposure to radon. An example of possible radon exposure would be someone who spends a large amount of the day underground, such as living in a basement or working underground or on a floor of a building that is below the ground surface. This is also a good time in the history interview to ask whether the patient is retired, married, and has children. It will open doors of communication with the clinician to explore possible support systems for the patient and physical and emotional barriers, and it often provides an opportunity to offer smoking cessation counseling and health education.

### REVIEW OF SYSTEMS

A full review of systems will add information to the patient's clinical picture. Assessment of each site of pain will uncover possible sites of metastatic disease or other medical conditions. Shortness of breath, cough, and history of hemoptysis are very important to the performance status and treatment options. Weight loss is a significant prognostic factor, and it should be determined how much weight the patient has lost in the past 6 months, and whether this is more than 10% of the patient's usual weight. Other body systems must be reviewed for abnormalities and considered in the diagnostic workup for prognosis and ability to endure different treatment options.

## PHYSICAL EXAMINATION

A full physical exam should be performed on the patient at the initial visit, including special attention to the respiratory, lymphatic, abdominal, and neurological systems, where the clinician could pick up signs of metastases. The respiratory exam should include all 4 techniques of physical exam: inspection, including respiration rate or dyspnea, palpation, percussion, and auscultation.[120] Observation will show signs of retraction upon inspiration, asymmetry, or impaired lung function. Palpation can test for chest expansion and tactile fremitus. Percussion can reveal an area of dullness over a pleural effusion or a lung mass. It is often used to determine the location and size of a pleural effusion prior to thoracentesis. Normal lung tissue should have a sound of resonance on percussion, signifying air in the lungs. Crackles or rales are often heard at the bases and can signify fluid overload from congestive heart failure or a pneumonia. A pleural friction rub can signify an abnormality in the pleura. Wheezes heard in constricted upper airways are consistent with asthma or COPD flares, and sometimes anxiety attacks. Rhonchi are usually loud and coarse, heard any place in the lungs, and are usually a result of loose secretions. Finally, hearing quiet lung sounds implies a mass, pleural effusion, atelectasis, pneumonia, or severe respiratory disease such as COPD.

The remainder of the physical exam focuses on evaluating for sites of metastatic disease. Palpating the abdomen for masses, searching the skin for subcutaneous metastases, and a neurological exam looking for signs of central nervous system metastases are all important findings to report as positive or negative. Also, a thorough lymph node assessment, including submandibular, cervical, supraclavicular, and axillary nodes, can reveal common sites of lung cancer metastases.

## PREOPERATIVE EVALUATION

If the patient presents with early stage disease, he or she may be a candidate for surgical intervention. Numerous issues factor into the decision of whether to perform thoracic surgery on a patient with lung cancer. Lung cancer surgery can leave a patient at risk for permanent pulmonary disability. One risk factor is age, although the fit elderly should be considered: long-term survival in lung cancer patients is improved with patients who are under the age of 70.[121] Also, pulmonary function tests, specifically looking at forced expiratory volume ($FEV_1$) and diffusion capacity, which measures carbon monoxide gas exchange (DLCO), are important. It is suggested that the $FEV_1$ should be 2 L for consideration of pneumonectomy and 1.5 L for lobectomy.[122] However, a predicted postoperative $FEV_1$ may be a more useful tool when an $FEV_1$ is low; surgeons are generally searching for a predicted value of greater than 40%, although that percentage varies in different studies.[123] Carbon monoxide gas exchange is also a predictive value for postoperative complications and morbidity. Generally, studies report that the cutoff for a preoperative DLCO should be between 60% and 70%, and lower values have been associated with postoperative complications.[122]

Measuring exercise tolerance via pulse oximetry and stair climbing also contributes to evaluation of a good surgical candidate. Also, identifying colonized potentially pathogenic microorganisms on bronchoscopy can predict for postoperative infection.[124] The extent of cardiovascular comorbidities and COPD are health problems that are weighed significantly prior to lung surgery. Stage and location of tumor, as well as extent of surgery needed, are major concerns when combined with the other risk factors that influence the decision to perform surgery in the patient with lung cancer.

## DIAGNOSTIC STUDIES

### Diagnostic tissue sampling

Other than surgery, there are many ways to obtain tissue for diagnosis of a suspected lung carcinoma. A pathological diagnosis is of utmost importance and must be obtained prior to cytotoxic treatment. Many times, the goal is to use the most noninvasive, safest approach to gather a pathological and, when possible, a histological diagnosis. Sampling of the mediastinal lymph nodes is also important for determining stage, which guides treatment decisions.

Sputum cytology is a low-risk, noninvasive method to investigate or diagnose lung cancer by collecting or inducing sputum from a patient. The use of sputum to identify premalignant lesions or diagnose lung cancer dates back to the early use of the Papanicolaou (Pap) test.[125] Sputum cytology, if diagnostic, will usually yield squamous cell histology of NSCLCs because these tend to be centrally located tumors in the chest. Often, serial sputum collections are required for verification or diagnosis. In a study comparing conventional prep using the Pap technique with prep using the Thinprep technique, the latter showed an improvement in diagnostic accuracy by reducing the unsatisfactory and false-negative results.[126] Although this is a simple way to detect or diagnose lung cancer, sputum cytology is often associated with false negatives and is not a reliable measure for diagnosis.[127]

Bronchoscopy is among the most common and most reliable methods to diagnose lung cancer. It is performed by a surgeon or pulmonologist; a flexible bronchoscope is passed through the nose or mouth to allow visual access to the airways. Patients are usually given general anesthesia for this procedure. Transbronchial needle aspiration (TBNA) is the technique of passing a needle through the bronchoscope to biopsy suspicious lung masses or gather bronchial washings to assess for malignant cells.[128] Limitations of TBNA are that it is usually a blind pass and often the sample is small and cannot be used to identify a histological subtype. The risks are mostly associated with general anesthesia and aspiration. A similar technique is an endoscopic ultrasound-guided needle aspiration utilizing an esophagoscope with ultrasound to biopsy a mass or lymph nodes.

Transthoracic needle aspiration (TTNA) or fine-needle aspiration (FNA) is also a commonly used technique for diagnosing lung cancer. This is performed by a radiologist aided by CT imaging, and is sometimes referred to as CT-guided needle biopsy. The needle is placed percutaneously through the chest wall while the patient is awake. Risks with this procedure include pneumothorax and hemorrhage. The limitations are geographically difficult lesions such as centralized tumors, which are difficult to reach so that several passes with the needle may be necessary, thus increasing risk of complications.

A malignant pleural effusion can also yield cancer cells. If a patient has a nonloculated pleural effusion in the setting of suspected lung cancer, it is reasonable to drain the fluid from the pleural space via a thoracentesis procedure and send the collection for cytopathological evaluation. Often the patient will need this fluid drained for symptomatic reasons such as pain or shortness of breath, so it is a prime opportunity to acquire cells for diagnosis. Also, if there is enough fluid available, the pathology team can formulate cell blocks to perform molecular pathology testing for more information.

Endobronchial ultrasound with transbronchial needle aspiration (EBUS-TBNA) has emerged as a diagnostic tool that is more sensitive than traditional bronchoscopy because of its ability to detect and biopsy lung masses that are not easily seen or accessed by conventional bronchoscopy.[129,130] However, the goal of tissue biopsy is not only to acquire a diagnosis, but also to determine the stage of disease by biopsying the mediastinal lymph nodes. The EBUS-TBNA technique has been shown to be a reliable tool to stage the mediastinum when obtaining 3 aspirations at each lymph node station.[131] Also, the combination of EBUS-TBNA and EUS-FNA can be used as an alternative method to surgical staging of the mediastinal lymph nodes.[130]

The most accurate way to achieve mediastinal lymph node staging is by performing a cervical mediastinoscopy, where a surgeon makes a small incision above the suprasternal notch and passes a scope down through the mediastinum to biopsy lymph nodes at various stations. Important lymph nodes to biopsy are the left and right high and low paratracheal nodes, pretracheal nodes, and anterior subcarinal nodes. Nodes that cannot be assessed include the posterior subcarinal, inferior mediastinal, and aortopulmonary window nodes (Figure 59-5).[132] If there is a contraindication to the cervical mediastinoscopy, an anterior mediastinotomy (Chamberlain procedure) can be performed. These procedures are performed in the operating room under general anesthesia, or a cervical mediastinoscopy can be performed as an outpatient procedure when it is not being done at the time of surgery. The complication rate is about 1.7% in the experienced thoracic surgeon's hands. Potential complications include pneumothorax, left recurrent laryngeal nerve injury, bleeding, and infection.[133]

## Diagnostic imaging

Chest x-ray is the oldest, easiest, and most cost-effective imaging study to grossly detect a lung mass, pleural effusion, pneumonia, and sometimes adenopathy.[134] However, it is a limited study that shows only a 2-dimensional image of a 3-dimensional person.[118] In a patient with new symptoms prior to diagnosis, it is the first imaging study that can quickly detect a lung mass. However, subcentimeter nodules are difficult to see on CXR and mediastinal lymph nodes are often obscured from view due to the heart and large blood vessels in the center of the chest.

A computed axial tomography (CAT or CT) of the chest is the gold standard for further staging.[135] It is a 3-dimensional scan able to detect small subcentimeter nodules or ground glass opacities that may have been missed on CXR. Spiral CT of the chest, also known as helical CT, is a higher-definition, faster scan in which the patient is constantly moving through the scanner. Administering IV contrast with the CT makes it easier to differentiate mediastinal lymph nodes from the blood vessels and determine whether the nodes are enlarged. Computed tomography imaging of the chest also encompasses the upper abdomen, including the liver, adrenal glands, and kidneys, all sites of possible metastases.

Fluorodeoxyglucose positron emission tomography (FDG-PET) imaging is an important study in evaluating the stage of lung cancer. Positron emission tomography scans are interpreted by evaluating and measuring the maximal standardized uptake values (SUVs). The SUV in NSCLC tumors has been a predictor of stage, nodal status, and survival.[136] PET imaging fused with CT imaging (PET/CT) has become a widely utilized imaging technique to help determine positive CT findings and the probability that they are malignant. Currently, PET scanning is approved in lung cancer for indeterminate lung nodule, staging, or restaging.[137] Its usefulness in evaluating response to chemotherapy and biotherapy is still being evaluated. It has a higher sensitivity and specificity than CT for mediastinal lymph node staging. Combination PET/CT has a high negative predictive value, up to 97%, meaning that if the scan is negative, it is likely that there is no cancer in the mediastinal lymph nodes, and invasive mediastinoscopy can be avoided.[138] However, it does not seem to have as good a positive predictive value, so if there is positivity in the mediastinal nodes on PET imaging, proper mediastinal staging still needs to be completed.[138] The SUVs are measured on a numeric scale. For

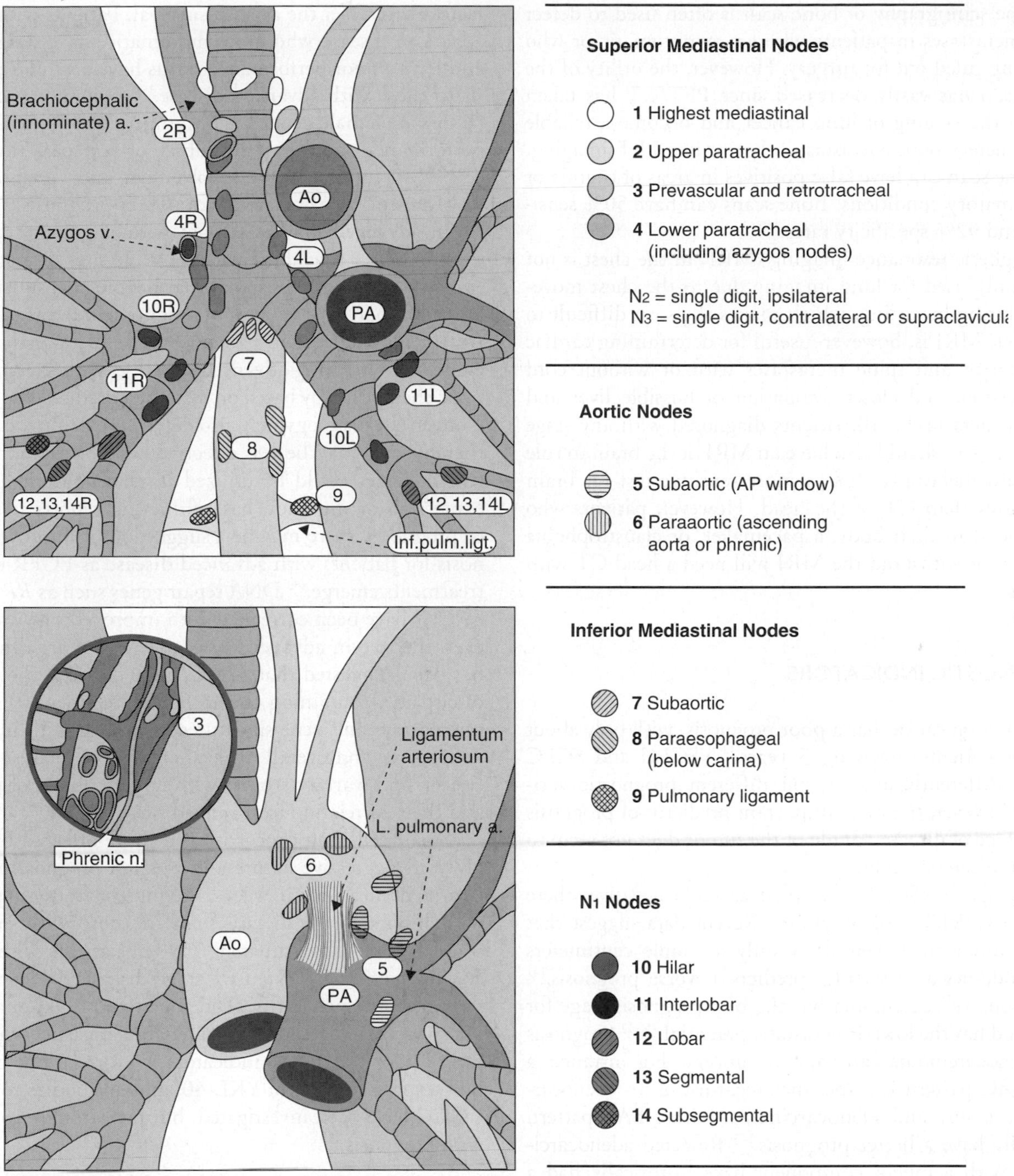


**FIGURE 59-5**

Regional lymph node stations for lung cancer staging.

*Source*: Reprinted from Mountain and Dresler.[132]

an indeterminate lung nodule, when SUV was 0 to 2.5, there was only a 24% chance that it was cancer; however, the higher the SUV, the more likely the mass is cancer.[139] Finally, PET/CT is also a reliable test to detect distant metastases, except for those in the heart, brain, bladder, and sometimes kidneys, which have normal biological uptake of the FDG. PET scans can have false positives due to inflammation, infection, active tuberculosis, and many other inflammatory conditions seen in the lungs or other areas of the body.

Bone scintigraphy or bone scan is often used to detect bone metastases in patients who are symptomatic or who are being ruled out for surgery. However, the utility of the bone scan has vastly decreased since PET/CT has taken over in the staging of lung cancer and become a reliable test to detect bone metastases. Again, like PET imaging, the bone scan can have false positives in areas of trauma or inflammatory conditions. Bone scans can have 50% sensitivity and 92% specificity rates.[140]

Magnetic resonance imaging (MRI) in the chest is not commonly used for lung imaging due to the chest movement during breathing, which makes the scan difficult to interpret. MRI is, however, useful for determining cardiac involvement and spine metastases with or without cord compression, and closer evaluation of possible liver and adrenal metastases. All patients diagnosed with any stage of lung cancer should also have an MRI of the brain to rule out brain metastases. It is a more sensitive test for brain metastases than CT of the head. However, patients who have metal in their body, a pacemaker, or claustrophobia and cannot withstand the MRI will need a head CT with contrast.

### PROGNOSTIC INDICATORS

Overall, lung cancer has a poor prognosis, with only about 15% of patients surviving 5 years.[1] NSCLC and SCLC behave differently and exhibit different prognostic variables. However, the most important predictor of prognosis is the stage of disease. Grade of the tumor does not seem to make a difference in lung cancer.

In stage I NSCLC, classified as node negative, there is much variability of prognosis. Recent data suggest that larger tumor size, even if by only a couple centimeters in a node-negative setting, predicts a worse prognosis.[141] Squamous cell carcinoma has the best prognosis stage for stage and has the lowest metastatic potential.[75,142] Prognosis for adenocarcinoma can vary by subtype. For instance, a pure BAC pattern is sometimes regarded as an adenocarcinoma in situ, and adenocarcinomas with a BAC pattern generally have a better prognosis.[143] Resected adenocarcinomas with a mucin component have historically had a poorer prognosis.[142] Cyclooxygenase-2 and VEGF-C are factors that contribute to lymphatic microvessel density and lymph node invasion, which is associated with poor survival.[144] Thyroid transcription factor 1 is considered a good prognostic factor.[145] Poor performance status, weight loss, and low socioeconomic status are patient characteristics also associated with poor prognosis in early stage patients.[146] Finally, literature on EGFR overexpression has conflicting reports about its effect on survival, with studies showing both better and poorer prognoses.[147–149]

Locally advanced NSCLC has a better prognosis than advanced stage/metastatic disease; however, many factors can affect the average survival. Patients with locally advanced disease who are symptomatic, have weight loss, and have a poor performance status have a similar prognosis to those with advanced disease.[150] Favorable prognostic factors are female gender, age younger than 70, and a good performance status. In the subset of pancoast tumors or T3N0M0 tumors, nerve involvement and vertebral body involvement are associated with poorer prognosis.[150]

In advanced NSCLC, those with oligometastatic disease do better that those with multiple sites of metastases. A recent meta-analysis shows that histological subtypes are also an important predictor of prognosis in terms of clinical treatments available to patients.[151] The meta-analysis concluded that treating advanced NSCLC with specific cytotoxic chemotherapy based on histology predicted outcomes. Conversely, histology may also determine cytotoxic chemotherapy that may be less effective, and other more effective therapies could be utilized instead. Although EGFR expression or mutation has conflicting reports in regards to prognosis, there may be a suggestion of improved prognosis for patients with advanced disease as EGFR-targeted treatments emerge.[152] DNA repair genes such as *RRM1* and *ERCC1* have been correlated with improved survival; however, the role in advanced disease is less clear, although it has been suggested that *ERCC1* may decrease the efficacy of cisplatin-containing chemotherapy regimens.[153,154] Gene microarrays and gene signatures associated with improved relapse-free and overall survival are also of interest in lung cancer, and warrant studies with larger cohorts of patients and their correlation to advanced stage disease.[155,156]

Small cell lung cancer is even more affected by stage, given its aggressive nature and median prognosis without treatment measured in weeks. Prognosis is better in patients with limited stage disease than in those with extensive stage disease. Unfortunately, 75% of patients with SCLC are diagnosed with extensive stage disease.[118] Pleural effusion, performance status, gender, elevated LDH or alkaline phosphatase, low sodium, and paraneoplastic syndromes are all poor prognostic indicators.[157] Correlations between KIT expression, serum YKL-40, and antibodies to HU or VGCC have been investigated, but not strongly correlated with prognosis.[158]

## CLASSIFICATION AND STAGING

### NON-SMALL CELL LUNG CANCER

Treatment of NSCLC depends on the stage of the disease at presentation. Staging for NSCLC applies the T (tumor), N (lymph node), M (metastasis) system that is commonly used for many solid tumors. Until 2009, the American Joint Committee on Cancer set the TNM definitions for lung cancer; however, these definitions have recently undergone intense review and a new staging system with definitions of TNM for lung cancer has been published and was presented at the 2009 World Conference on Lung Cancer (Tables 59-5 and 59-6).[159,160] The newly proposed staging system is a product of the International Association for the Study of Lung Cancer Lung Cancer Staging Project, started in 1998, which put together an international database. The new staging system and TNM definitions further distinguish tumor size, downstage satellite nodules, and upstage malignant pleural effusions to be considered M1a or stage IV. Another proposed change will group lymph nodes in zones to aid in prognostic analysis.[160] These changes more accurately stage NSCLC and improve ability to determine prognosis.

The TNM staging system applies to anatomic staging only. Clinical staging using imaging modalities such as PET/CT is necessary to rule out M1 disease when pathological staging is not warranted. Clinical staging by PET/CT of the mediastinum is suggestive, however, not definitive, and a proper mediastinal lymph node dissection or mediastinoscopy is still the only way to truly stage the mediastinal lymph nodes.

### SMALL CELL LUNG CANCER

Small cell lung cancer is classified according to the Veterans Administration Lung Study Group definitions, and is defined as either limited stage or extensive stage disease. Limited stage disease is confined to a single hemithorax with or without contralateral mediastinal or supraclavicular lymph node involvement. This is generally the disease within a tolerable radiation port and can be treated with definitive intent. Extensive stage means that the disease has metastasized outside of the tolerable radiation port. The TNM staging is not consistently used as a staging system in SCLC, although at times clinicians have applied it.

## THERAPEUTIC APPROACHES AND NURSING CARE

Treatment of lung cancer is determined by the stage. Surgery, radiation, and chemotherapy or targeted therapies are the main staples of treatment, used either individually or in combination. A multidisciplinary approach is essential to managing and successfully treating lung cancer. Often, multimodality thoracic oncology programs and weekly conferences are held at institutions to discuss difficult cases as a group to get the opinions of pathologists, radiologists, radiation oncologists, thoracic surgeons, pulmonologists, nurses, and oncologists. Additional support staff include social workers, psychologists, a registered dietician, and pastoral care if needed. Nursing can be involved in many different roles at the first visit. A nurse navigator may initially speak with the patient on the phone to triage the patient to the appropriate doctors. The advanced practice nurse is often the first healthcare team member to see the patient and gather the history and physical exam. If the patient is eligible for a clinical trial, the study nurse may see the patient and screen them for a potential clinical trial. The infusion nurse may also evaluate the patient's venous access and perform teaching on the initial visit. Many different facets of oncology nursing improve the patient's experience through the journey of fighting lung cancer.

### SURGERY

Surgery is the preferred curative modality for early stage NSCLC. It is the treatment of choice for stage I and stage II NSCLC. Often a surgeon will start the procedure by performing a bronchoscopy to assess the lymph node status and tumor. Once this is completed, the surgeon then decides whether a mediastinoscopy is necessary to sample the mediastinal lymph nodes. If the mediastinal lymph nodes are negative, the surgeon removes the scope and proceeds to remove the lung tumor. Lung cancer surgery is a major surgical procedure that carries many more serious possible complications than other visceral surgeries. Patient selection and type of thoracotomy should be taken seriously into consideration as the procedure can have a significant impact on the patient's quality of life.[161]

A lobectomy, defined as the removal of the entire lobe of the lung, is considered the gold standard of definitive surgery for NSCLC. Even for a small tumor, lobectomy is considered the standard of care, with better survival outcomes likely because it is removing surrounding tissue as well as the lymph nodes contained in the lobe. Typically, the incision is a standard posterolateral thoracotomy or a muscle-sparing incision with the help of a videoscope.

Other surgical options are a wedge resection, segmentectomy, or pneumonectomy. A wedge resection or a segmentectomy, where part of the lobe is left behind, is not considered definitive surgery in NSCLC but is sometimes necessary in patients to preserve lung tissue. Other times, a wedge resection may be performed if the nodule is questionable and not known to be cancerous, although if the frozen section is positive for malignancy, the surgeon will most often do a completion lobectomy. If a wedge resection or segmentectomy is necessary, close margins present a risk of recurrence and radiation to the remaining lobe is sometimes recommended to prevent locoregional recurrence.[162]

A pneumonectomy is the removal of the entire lung. This is most often required in disease where either lymph nodes or the tumor is invading the right mainstem bronchus. A left-sided pneumonectomy is generally better tolerated than a right-sided pneumonectomy.[163] Particular attention is paid to the patient who has had neoadjuvant treatment for stage IIIA NSCLC. A right-sided pneumonectomy is a risky surgery in these patients; it carries a 23.9% mortality

**TABLE 59-5**

**Definitions for T, N, and M Descriptors**

| | |
|---|---|
| **T (Primary Tumor)** | |
| TX | Primary tumor cannot be assessed, or tumor proven by the presence of malignant cells in sputum or bronchial washings but not visualized by imaging or bronchoscopy |
| T0 | No evidence of primary tumor |
| Tis | Carcinoma in situ |
| T1 | Tumor less than or equal to 3 cm in greatest dimension, surrounded by lung or visceral pleura, without bronchoscopic evidence of invasion more proximal than the lobar bronchus (ie, not in the main bronchus)[a] |
| T1a | Tumor less than or equal to 2 cm in greatest dimension |
| T1b | Tumor > 2 cm but less than or equal to 3 cm in greatest dimension |
| T2 | Tumor > 3 cm but less than or equal to 7 cm or tumor with any of the following features (T2 tumors with these features are classified T2a if less than or equal to 5 cm)<br>Involves main bronchus, greater than or equal to 2 cm distal to the carina<br>Invades visceral pleura<br>Associated with atelectasis or obstructive pneumonitis that extends to the hilar region but does not involve the entire lung |
| T2a | Tumor > 3 cm but less than or equal to 5 cm in greatest dimension |
| T2b | Tumor > 5 cm but less than or equal to 7 cm in greatest dimension |
| T3 | Tumor > 7 cm or one that directly invades any of the following: chest wall (including superior sulcus tumors), diaphragm, phrenic nerve, mediastinal pleura, parietal pericardium; or tumor in the main bronchus (< 2 cm distal to the carina[a] but without involvement of the carina; or associated atelectasis or obstructive pneumonitis of the entire lung or separate tumor nodule(s) in the same lobe |
| T4 | Tumor of any size that invades any of the following: mediastinum, heart, great vessels, trachea, recurrent laryngeal nerve, esophagus, vertebral body, carina, separate tumor nodule(s) in a different ipsilateral lobe |
| **N (Regional Lymph Nodes)** | |
| NX | Regional lymph nodes cannot be assessed |
| N0 | No regional lymph node metastases |
| N1 | Metastasis in ipsilateral peribronchial and/or ipsilateral hilar lymph nodes and intrapulmonary nodes, including involvement by direct extension |
| N2 | Metastasis in ipsilateral mediastinal and/or subcarinal lymph node(s) |
| N3 | Metastasis in contralateral mediastinal, contralateral hilar, ipsilateral or contralateral scalene, or supraclavicular lymph node(s) |
| **M (Distant Metastasis)** | |
| MX | Distant metastasis cannot be assessed |
| M0 | No distant metastasis |
| M1 | Distant metastasis |
| M1a | Separate tumor nodule(s) in a contralateral lobe; tumor with pleural nodules or malignant pleural (or pericardial) effusion[b] |
| M1b | Distant metastasis |

*Notes*: [a]The uncommon superficial spreading tumor of any size with its invasive component limited to the bronchial wall, which may extend proximally to the main bronchus, is also classified as T1a.

[b]Most pleural (and pericardial) effusions with lung cancer are due to tumor. In a few patients, however, multiple cytopathological examinations of pleural (pericardial) fluid are negative for tumor, and the fluid is nonbloody and is not an exudate. Where these elements and clinical judgement dictate that the effusion is not related to the tumor, the effusion should be excluded as a staging element and the patient should be classified as M0.

*Source*: Data from Goldstraw P, Crowley J, Chansky K, et al.[159]

**TABLE 59-6**

**Descriptors, T and M Categories, and Stage Groupings**

| Sixth Edition T/M Descriptor | 7th Edition T/M | N0 | N1 | N2 | N3 |
|---|---|---|---|---|---|
| T1 (less than or equal to 2 cm) | T1a | IA | IIA | IIIA | IIIB |
| T1 (>2–3 cm) | T1b | IA | IIA | IIIA | IIIB |
| T2 (≤ 5 cm) | T2a | IB | **IIA** | IIIA | IIIB |
| T2 (>5–7 cm) | T2b | **IIA** | IIB | IIIA | IIIB |
| T2 (>7 cm) | T3 | **IIB** | **IIIA** | IIIA | IIIB |
| T3 invasion | T3 | IIB | IIIA | IIIA | IIIB |
| T4 (same lobe nodules) | T3 | **IIB** | **IIIA** | **IIIA** | IIIB |
| T4 (extension) | T4 | **IIIA** | **IIIA** | IIIB | IIIB |
| M1 (ipsilateral lung) | T4 | **IIIA** | **IIIA** | **IIIB** | **IIIB** |
| T4 (pleural effusion) | M1a | **IV** | **IV** | **IV** | **IV** |
| M1 (contralateral lung) | M1a | IV | IV | IV | IV |
| M1 (distant) | M1b | IV | IV | IV | IV |

*Note*: Cells in **bold** indicate a change from the sixth edition for a particular TNM category.

*Source*: Data from Goldstraw P, Crowley J, Chansky K, et al.[159]

rate from surgical complications and should be performed only in very select patients.[163]

Approaches to surgery are constantly evolving in order to improve postoperative complications and be minimally invasive. Video-assisted thoracoscopy (VATS) is an example of a minimally invasive procedure in which the surgeon can use a scope to view the chest cavity. The VATS lobectomy has been shown to be a safe procedure in patients over the age of 80, patients with marginal pulmonary function, and patients at risk for surgical complications following neoadjuvant treatment.[164] Due to the complicated nature and importance of proper pulmonary lymph node dissections, studies suggest that there are significantly improved patient outcomes when lung cancer surgeries are performed at teaching hospitals or high-volume centers by surgeons who are highly skilled in these procedures.[165]

Surgery for SCLC is controversial and plays a limited role. SCLC, when diagnosed, is usually at minimum locally advanced, given its aggressive nature. If SCLC is expected in a possible surgical case, it should be ruled out first before proceeding with surgery. The only prospective randomized trials evaluating the role of surgery in SCLC failed to show a benefit, whereas retrospective analyses and prospective nonrandomized trials showed longer disease-free survival and higher rates of long-term survival than did chemotherapy and radiation alone.[166]

## Complications and nursing management

Dyspnea and cough are very common symptoms associated with lung cancer surgery. With dyspnea, even at 4 months after surgery, some patients still experience a significant decrease in quality of life.[167] Type of procedure, preoperative lung function, and patient comorbidities should all be taken seriously when assessing the surgical patient. Many surgeons will require that a patient quit smoking prior to lung cancer surgery.

Acute pain or chronic pain can be a serious problem after thoracic surgery for lung cancer. Acute pain occurring within the first week after surgery must be well managed so that the patient can follow postoperative pulmonary exercises and avoid atelectasis. Usually in the postoperative setting, the patient will require a patient-controlled analgesic pump that is able to deliver on-demand IV pain medication via an IV or epidural route. There is also less postoperative pain in patients who have had an anterolateral thoracotomy vs a posterolateral approach, and there is less pain associated with lobectomy than pneumonectomy.[168] Chronic pain is the most common long-term side effect from lung cancer surgery.[169]

Cardiopulmonary side effects after surgery are also potentially serious. These side effects are also the ones that most commonly result in death postoperatively. Patients who are former or current smokers at the time of surgery are at a higher risk for respiratory- and cardiac-related deaths from surgery than nonsmokers.[170] Atrial arrhythmias such as atrial fibrillation often occur due to irritation to the vagus nerve. Beta-blockers are sometimes necessary for these patients for a few months postoperatively. Patients over the age of 70 also demonstrate a higher incidence of postoperative heart failure and should be closely monitored.[171]

## RADIATION

Radiation therapy (RT) utilizes sophisticated computer simulators to map out radiation fields to deliver the maximum tolerated dose. There are many different ways to deliver radiation to the patient with lung cancer. The most commonly used techniques in lung cancer are 3-dimensional conformal RT (3D-CRT) or 4-dimensional CRT (4D-CRT). The 3D-CRT technique allows for improved target definition and treatment planning and is considered the minimal standard of care for thoracic radiation.[172] The 4D-CRT technique employs PET/CT and permits organ motion to be observed and quantified, allowing for precise daily patient positioning to minimize target volumes.[173]

There is still controversy over the use of intensity-modulated RT (IMRT) in lung cancer patients. IMRT uses an increased number of beam angles, which can increase dose delivery to target areas; however, it also can increase toxicity to surrounding pulmonary tissue and warrants further study in lung cancer.[174] Image-guided RT is also being used in lung cancer treatment. Image-guided RT uses a linear accelerator equipped with a cone-beam CT scanner that can verify tumor position during treatment and narrow the therapy to spare normal tissues. Finally, proton-beam radiation is in the early stages of clinical trials in lung cancer, but preliminary data show that it may be effective in minimizing toxicity in early stage and locally advanced lung tumors.[175]

### Non-small cell lung cancer

Radiation has many roles in the treatment of lung cancer. In early stage NSCLC, it can be used in the postoperative setting to prevent recurrence in incomplete resection or as curative intent therapy for early stage disease in which the patient is inoperable due to comorbidities. In locally advanced disease, radiation can be utilized postoperatively for high-risk disease or combined with chemotherapy as definitive intent treatment in inoperable disease. In the metastatic setting of NSCLC, radiation is used as palliative treatment for pain management in patients with bone metastases or for lung masses causing hemoptysis, shortness of breath, or a postobstructive pneumonia.

Studies examining radiation in the adjuvant and neoadjuvant setting for patients with early stage NSCLC have failed to show a benefit over sugery alone.[176] Also, a meta-analysis of postoperative radiation showed increased adverse events for patients with completely resected NSCLC.[177] Therefore, adjuvant radiation therapy remains controversial, and high-risk patients should be discussed in a multidisciplinary group before treatment decisions are made.

Several trials have looked at sequential radiation and chemotherapy vs concurrent radiation and chemotherapy for the treatment of locally advanced NSCLC. The goal of treatment in locally advanced disease is to treat the tumor and much of the mediastinum to encompass the affected lymph nodes, aiming for curative intent treatment. Concurrent chemotherapy and radiation shows the best survival numbers and local control rates, provided the patient is able to tolerate the treatment.[178–180] Treatments are given as a regimen of 180 to 200 cGy fractions over 6 to 7 weeks, not exceeding 6000 cGy.

In metastatic disease, radiation is commonly used to palliate symptoms in bones or visceral organs. It is also the treatment of choice for brain metastases. Whole brain radiation (WBXRT) is often used as the technique because, even though there may be only 1 brain lesion, there is a high risk for others to develop. Another option is stereotactic radiosurgery, in which a neurosurgeon places a halo fixation device onto the patient's head and then delivers a high-dose radiation treatment precisely to the tumor, thus sparing other brain tissue. Stereotactic radiosurgery is a good option for patients who have had prior WBXRT and develop new brain metastases, or for patients with new brain metastases where there is concern to reduce the risk of side effects from WBXRT.

### Small cell lung cancer

In SCLC, radiation plays an important role in limited stage disease. It can be utilized as definitive treatment. Similar to NSCLC, concurrent chemotherapy and radiation suggests an improved survival advantage over sequential treatment.[181,182] Furthermore, when concurrent chemotherapy and radiation are administered, giving twice daily fractionated radiation offers improved survival over once daily radiation.[183] Prophylactic cranial irradiation (PCI) is radiation to the brain for prevention of brain metastases due to their prevalence in SCLC. It shows a significant improvement in 3-year survival rates among patients treated definitively with limited-stage SCLC.[184] More recent data have supported the use of PCI in extensive-stage SCLC in patients who are responding to treatment.[185] Although statistically significant, the data for PCI in extensive-stage SCLC are controversial and, given the very poor prognosis of this disease, each patient considered for this treatment must heavily weigh the risks and benefits.

### Complications and nursing management

Esophagitis is the most complicating side effect from thoracic radiation when the mediastinum is included in the field. Patients usually experience pain and dryness when trying to swallow food, and even liquids at times. It can be a dose-limiting side effect and can cause dehydration, many times necessitating hospitalization. Keys to nursing intervention are to assess patients frequently and implement treatment early. Pain management, usually with narcotics, often helps to facilitate swallowing. Topical preparations such as magic mouthwash and viscous lidocaine have limited efficacy because their potency is often diminished by the time the solution reaches the esophagus. Sucralfate liquid has also been used for prevention of worsening esophagitis and to facilitate healing, but it does little to improve the pain while on treatment. If severe esophagitis presents early in the radiation cycle, a temporary percutaneous endoscopic gastrostomy tube needs to be considered. It is important for nurses to perform a thorough assessment, including weight, diet recall with specific foods the patient is able to tolerate, and orthostatic blood pressures.

Radiation pneumonitis is an inflammatory response in the lungs due to radiation injury to the lung tissue. It presents as a delayed reaction to radiation anywhere from 2 weeks to 6 months after completion of the radiation course. This can be a serious event, occurring in up to 69% of patients, and can be severe in up to 25% of patients.[186] As patients often experience radiation pneumonitis after treatment, nurses will frequently receive a phone call from a patient complaining of shortness of breath and nagging cough. These patients should be brought into the office immediately for evaluation of pulmonary status and to rule out other respiratory complications. If radiation pneumonitis is suspected, steroids are the treatment of choice and are often effective almost immediately upon administration. If the pulse oximetry is unstable or the dyspnea is profoundly uncomfortable, inpatient admission may be necessary. Ongoing clinical trials are looking at dietary supplementation of flaxseed as a possible way to prevent radiation pneumonitis.

Fatigue, myelosuppression, and skin burns are other common side effects of radiation. Myelosuppression is often associated with patients who are receiving concurrent chemotherapy. The fatigue can be associated with anemia, poor nutritional intake secondary to esophagitis, or the radiation itself. Nurses may need to monitor blood work at intervals during radiation therapy to assess for myelosuppression, especially in asymptomatic patients. Skin burns are less common now, due to improvements in radiation techniques. Nurses need to educate patients about avoiding sun exposure and about moisturizing emollients to apply after they receive their daily radiation treatment.

## OTHER LOCAL THERAPIES

Photodynamic therapy (PDT), brachytherapy, and radiofrequency ablation (RFA) are current techniques being utilized and studied for local control therapy of lung cancer, especially when patients cannot take radiation for various reasons. PDT uses a photosensitizing agent, porfimer sodium (Photofrin), and laser application via bronchoscopy to destroy tumor through a photochemical reaction. The use of PDT postoperatively in high-risk surgeries is also undergoing clinical trials. However, patients undergoing treatment with PDT must avoid direct sunlight for a period of time to avoid severe sunburns after receiving the photosensitizing agent. Side effects include hemorrhage, scarring, fibrosis, and airway perforation.[187]

Brachytherapy is the use of radioactive seeds applied locally to lung tissue to deliver a high dose of radiation to a specific area. The seeds are placed directly during open thoracotomy; they are mounted on a mesh or placed with a syringe-type device that spaces the seeds specifically at intervals to deliver predetermined doses to projected areas.[188] Brachytherapy is indicated for incomplete resections, close margins, or sublobar resections to improve local recurrence rates.

Radiofrequency ablation is a thermal energy delivery system in which a needle electrode applies a high-frequency current supplied by a radiofrequency generator.[189] This technique is still fairly new to lung cancer and is clinically indicated for inoperable patients and for palliation of lung tumors or liver metastases. Side effects of RFA to lung tumors include risk of hemorrhage, pneumothorax, pneumonia, abscess, and damage to surrounding tissues.[189]

## CHEMOTHERAPY

Several chemotherapy and targeted agents are indicated for use in lung cancer (Table 59-7). Chemotherapy alone cannot cure lung cancer at any stage. Studies have shown survival benefits for chemotherapy in all stages of lung cancer, except for stage IA disease, where surgery alone is indicated. Chemotherapy in lung cancer can be used in combinations, as a single agent, or combined with radiation or surgery, or both. More recently, the addition of biotherapies to chemotherapy has shown survival advantages as well as maintenance therapy in metastatic disease.

Elderly patients have been historically underrepresented in clinical trials; however, many studies have shown retrospective analyses of these populations in the past 10 years. Special considerations for the elderly patient must take into account performance status, comorbidities, renal function, and living situations with support systems. These patients are at higher risk to develop dehydration and myelosuppression at a quicker rate than their younger counterparts; however, the fit elderly are able to tolerate platinum-based chemotherapy and have equal survival benefit.[190]

### Non-small cell lung cancer

Chemotherapy in NSCLC can be broken down into 3 major categories: adjuvant or neoadjuvant, combined modality

**TABLE 59-7**

| Chemotherapeutic and Targeted Agents Used in Lung Cancer |
|---|
| **Platinum Agents** |
| Cisplatin |
| Carboplatin |
| **Nonplatinum Agents** |
| Etoposide |
| Topotecan |
| Irinotecan |
| Gemcitabine |
| Pemetrexed |
| Paclitaxel |
| Docetaxel |
| Vinorelbine |
| Vincristine |
| Doxorubicin |
| Cyclophosphamide |
| Ifosfamide |
| **Targeted Agents** |
| Erlotinib |
| Cetuximab |
| Bevacizuimab |
| Gefitinib |

with radiation for locally advanced disease, and palliative for metastatic disease. Because there are many different agents available for use, a thorough medical history, as well as addressing the patient's goals of therapy, can help determine the best drug(s) to treat a patient according to the side effect profile.

Over the past 6 years, there have been several studies that have revealed a survival benefit for adjuvant (postoperative) chemotherapy in NSCLC.[191–193] There is no survival benefit with adjuvant chemotherapy in stage IA completely resected NSCLC; however, in stage IB to IIIA, cisplatin-based chemotherapy is indicated. A closer analysis of an adjuvant trial looking at stage IB patients discovered that patients with tumors smaller than 4.0 cm did not benefit from adjuvant chemotherapy, but that if the primary tumor was larger than 4.0cm, there was a statistically significant survival benefit, and chemotherapy continues to be indicated in that setting.[194] The survival benefit is small, with a recent meta-analysis of these studies showing an overall benefit of only 3% to 4%, with somewhere between 24 and 39 patients needing to be treated for just 1 patient to benefit.[195] Despite its increased toxicity profile, cisplatin is usually the cornerstone of therapy because it exhibits better response rates and a survival benefit over carboplatin.[196,197] Future study should include determining patient characteristics that would predict for benefit from adjuvant chemotherapy due to the minimal benefit and toxicities associated with treatment. Current clinical trials are asking whether adding targeted therapies to adjuvant chemotherapy will improve the 5-year survival rates.

Chemotherapy in stage III disease can be used as neoadjuvant to surgery, as an adjuvant to surgery as discussed previously, or in combination with radiation for definitive intent treatment. Neoadjuvant chemotherapy has been associated with a favorable long-term survival over surgery alone for stage III NSCLC.[198] One randomized study failed to show an improvement in overall survival; however, it did show a decrease in distant metastases in favor of the neoadjuvant chemotherapy arm, suggesting that neoadjuvant chemotherapy may treat micrometastatic disease in the preoperative setting of stage III disease.[199] Also, neoadjuvant chemotherapy for stage III NSCLC gives clinicians a chance to see whether the tumor will respond rather than metastasize on treatment, which implies that surgery would not benefit the patient with an aggressive, treatment-resistant tumor. A more aggressive approach may be chemotherapy given with radiation prior to surgery; however, the toxicity can delay surgery and produce severe surgical complications in dealing with radiated tissue.[199] These patients should be discussed within the multidisciplinary team to determine the best neoadjuvant strategy.

When a patient is deemed inoperable with stage IIIA disease or has stage IIIB NSCLC, chemotherapy is given in combination with radiation for curative intent treatment. There are several studies that have looked at giving chemotherapy and radiation either sequentially or in combination. There is a clear benefit to concurrent chemotherapy plus radiation over sequential chemotherapy and radiation.[200] Provided a patient has a good performance status and will be able to tolerate concurrent therapy, it is the preferred treatment. The regimen of choice tends to be controversial. Etoposide and cisplatin at systemic doses with daily radiation has shown the best survival data to date, with an American Society of Clinical Oncology 2008 updated median survival time of 25.9 months and a 3-year survival rate of 33.6%.[201] Subsequent trials looking at adding consolidation docetaxel or gefitinib after the initial concurrent therapy have both been negative and caused more toxicity with decreased survival.[202,203]

The other option for concurrent chemotherapy and radiation is weekly low-dose chemotherapy to provide a radiosensitizing effect. These trials have shown good efficacy, with sometimes a more favorable side effect profile than the full dose etoposide and cisplatin regimen.[204,205]

When weekly radiosensitizing doses of chemotherapy are given with radiation, it is usually recommended to add either induction or consolidation full-dose chemotherapy to provide some systemic control.

In the 1980s, clinicians were not sure that the risks and side effects with chemotherapy outweighed the benefit for a patient getting palliative chemotherapy for metastatic NSCLC. Currently, there are many chemotherapy regimens that have shown a clear survival advantage and improvement in quality of life, making chemotherapy a standard of care for these patients. A major pivotal trial in NSCLC was the ECOG 1594 trial, which placed 4 commonly used chemotherapy regimens up against each other to see which would emerge as the optimal regimen for frontline treatment.[206] Three arms used cisplatin, and 1 arm used carboplatin. Each arm combined either paclitaxel, gemcitabine, or docetaxel with a platinum. The outcome of this trial revealed that the 4 regimens were essentially equal when it comes to overall survival and response rates. The arm that utilized carboplatin instead of cisplatin had a more desirable toxicity profile, and therefore carboplatin became the cornerstone of first-line therapy for NSCLC in the US.

Another study confirmed the results of ECOG 1594, looking at platinum-based doublets and their tolerability and efficacy in NSCLC. It showed that taxanes in combination with carboplatin or cisplatin were tolerable and showed comparable response rates to other frontline therapies for metastatic NSCLC.[207] Since the ECOG 1594 study, there have been important trials looking at adding targeted agents to standard chemotherapy, which have improved outcomes. These will be discussed in the biotherapy section of this chapter. A recent study also gave another frontline treatment option for utilizing pemetrexed (Alimta) with a platinum.[208] A trial also looked at response by histology, showing greater efficacy for patients with adenocarcinoma responding better to the pemetrexed. These results will be further detailed in the personalized medicine section of this chapter. Giving more than 4 to 6 cycles of chemotherapy in the frontline setting usually leads to increased toxicity rather than clinical benefit, although continuance of maintenance with targeted therapy has shown improvement.[209]

After the patient develops disease progression on first-line treatment, second-line chemotherapy can be considered. Currently there are 3 drugs approved in this setting: pemetrexed, docetaxel, and erlotinib. Docetaxel is approved in both the first-line and second-line settings, depending on when the clinician decides it is most suitable for the patient. It was the first chemotherapeutic agent to get a second-line indication on the basis of 2 phase III clinical trials showing improvement over best supportive care or regimens containing vinorelbine or ifosfamide.[210,211] Pemetrexed gained approval in NSCLC for use in the second-line setting after its initial indication for malignant mesothelioma. In a head-to-head trial against docetaxel, there was equal efficacy, with a slightly improved or comparable toxicity profile.[212] It is an antifolate chemotherapy that requires daily folic acid supplementation, vitamin B12 injections every 9 weeks, and a steroid prep. It is generally well tolerated as a single agent, with minimal nausea and myelosuppression, provided the patient is compliant with the folate and B12 supplements. Finally, erlotinib is also indicated for second-line or third-line treatment of NSCLC. In a randomized phase III study of erlotinib vs best supportive care, erlotinib showed an improvement in overall survival at 2 months over best supportive care.[213] Erlotinib is a targeted therapy and will be discussed further in the biotherapy section of this chapter.

Chemotherapy in elderly populations or patients with an ECOG performance status of 2, with metastatic NSCLC, has been a topic of controversy, although clinical trials have shown that the fit elderly can tolerate it as well as benefit from it. A trial of 100 patients suggested that platinum-containing regimens are a feasible option with acceptable toxicity.[214] The study reported inferior survival among patients with a performance status of 0 to 1, but still a clinical benefit. Another trial, called the ELVIS study, looked at single-agent vinorelbine in patients over the age of 70 and found an acceptable toxicity profile with a modest, but statistically significant, improvement in overall survival and 1-year survival.[215] The elderly and performance status 2 populations can benefit from therapy but must be monitored closely due to their heightened risk for toxicity.

### Small cell lung cancer

Small cell lung cancer is very sensitive to chemotherapy, and it is important to initiate systemic chemotherapy as soon as possible. Response rates of 70% to 80% can be achieved in extensive stage disease, and up to 50% complete responses can be achieved with combination therapy in limited stage disease, often with symptom improvement.[216] But duration of the response is short, with relapsed disease having a median survival of only around 7 to 14 months.

If a patient ends up having surgery for limited stage disease, adjuvant chemotherapy is recommended due to the aggressive nature of SCLC. If there is disease in the lymph nodes, radiation should also be considered. If the disease is limited stage, appropriate treatment is combined chemotherapy and radiation for those who can tolerate it. Extensive stage SCLC should be treated with palliative chemotherapy, mostly using carboplatin-based regimens, which cause less toxicity than cisplatin. A study comparing etoposide and cisplatin with etoposide and carboplatin showed a comparable median survival time with less nausea, vomiting, and neurotoxicity in the carboplatin arm, but a greater amount of myelosuppression.[217]

A recent study compared the commonly used etoposide (VP-16) and cisplatin with irinotecan (Camptosar, CPT-11) and cisplatin, showing comparable efficacy with some difference in toxicity in the different arms.[218] Prior to this study, there had been a Japanese study showing improvement in survival for patients receiving irinotecan and cisplatin compared with etoposide and cisplatin.[219] This inconsistency in survival shows that lung cancer and pharmacogenomics may be different in certain countries and cultures.[218] Survival advantages have also been seen with a regimen of cyclophosphamide, doxorubicin, and etoposide, which in a European study was shown to be of equal efficacy to paclitaxel and carboplatin in extensive stage SCLC.[220] The paclitaxel and carboplatin arm revealed significantly less hematologic toxicity and febrile neutropenia.

Second-line chemotherapy or treatment when disease has relapsed has limited efficacy. The only FDA-approved therapy is topotecan (Hycamtin). A meta-analysis of topotecan studies in second-line treatment of SCLC reported an 18% response rate and median survival of 30 weeks.[221] Topotecan also now comes in an oral formulation, which has similar efficacy and less neutropenia.[222] Paclitaxel, irinotecan, gemcitabine, and docetaxel have also demonstrated response rates in relapsed SCLC.[216,223] Pemetrexed has been shown in multiple trials to be ineffective in the treatment of SCLC.[224,225]

In general, adding a third drug to the standard 2-drug regimen does not improve survival and increases toxicity for SCLC.[226] Maintenance therapy after induction chemotherapy is associated with a worse quality of life with no survival benefit.[227] To date, there is no evidence to add any biological therapies to chemotherapy; however, this is still under study.

### Complications and nursing management

Patients receiving chemotherapy for lung cancer suffer from common side effects of chemotherapy, often complicated by pulmonary comorbidities. Due to the aggressive nature of lung cancer, often these patients may experience more weight loss, anemia, and fatigue. Nursing management includes controlling nausea and vomiting and teaching patients about signs and symptoms of myelosuppression and febrile neutropenia. Many of these side effects are covered extensively in other chapters.

## BIOTHERAPY

Biotherapy, defined as targeted therapy, has been a critical part of numerous advances in the treatment of NSCLC. These therapies have significantly improved response rates and overall survival rates in NSCLC, and generally elicit fewer toxicities, such as myelosuppression and hair loss, although each has its own set of specific side effects. To date, targeted therapies have not been approved or shown benefit in SCLC; however, trials are ongoing.

One targeted agent in NSCLC is erlotinib (Tarceva). Erlotinib is a small-molecule EGFR tyrosine kinase inhibitor (TKI) and is orally available. As stated earlier, it is approved for second-line or third-line use in patients with NSCLC after failure of a platinum-based chemotherapy regimen. In 2 large randomized clinical trials, erlotinib combined with chemotherapy in the front-line setting failed to show an improvement in overall survival, and therefore, at this time, is relegated to chemotherapy-refractory disease.[228,229] Common side effects include rash and diarrhea, and in rare instances interstitial lung disease, which manifests as acute pulmonary inflammation, often requiring hospitalization and steroids. Targeting populations who exhibit an EGFR mutation has been at the forefront of research, with some of these patients demonstrating dramatic responses and long-term survival. This will be discussed further in the personalized medicine section of this chapter.

Bevacizumab (Avastin) is a VEGF receptor inhibitor. It is a fully humanized monoclonal antibody that targets and binds to the VEGF ligand, thus inhibiting new blood vessel formation to the tumor. In a randomized phase III trial looking at paclitaxel and carboplatin plus or minus bevacizumab, the bevacizumab arm showed a 2-month improvement in overall survival, with a median survival of 12.3 months.[230] This was the first study in NSCLC to show that a 3-drug regimen was better than 2 drugs, and the first study to quote a median survival for advanced stage disease of more than 1 year. The indication for bevacizumab is that it should be used in combination with front-line chemotherapy, and be continued as maintenance therapy after completion of 4 to 6 cycles of chemotherapy in order to continue VEGF inhibition and prolong progression-free survival. Possible side effects of bevacizumab include hypertension, proteinuria, impaired wound healing, risk of bleeding or hemoptysis, and risk for bowel perforation. Its use in the adjuvant setting is currently under investigation in a large cooperative group trial.

Cetuximab (Erbitux) is a large-molecule EGFR inhibitor in the form of a monoclonal antibody that has been shown to improve survival when combined with front-line chemotherapy in advanced NSCLC. In a phase III trial of 1125 patients with randomization to vinorelbine and cisplatin plus or minus cetuximab, the cetuximab arm showed an improvement in overall survival of 11.3 months, vs 10.1 months in the standard chemotherapy arm.[231] In order to receive cetuximab on this study, patients needed to have EGFR overexpression via immunohistochemistry of at least 1 tumor cell. It has not gained FDA approval at this time; however, it has attained a Medicare compendia listing based on these data and has been added to the National Comprehensive Cancer Network (NCCN) guidelines with certain qualifying criteria. Common side effects include rash, diarrhea, and magnesium wasting.

Gefitinib (Iressa) was the first targeted agent to gain FDA approval in NSCLC based on response rates; however, it was pulled from the market after a randomized phase III trial failed to show a survival advantage over placebo.[232] Gefitinib, like erlotinib, is an EGFR TKI, orally available, and can cause rash and diarrhea. Recently, it has gained an indication in the United Kingdom in NSCLC based on the INTEREST trial, a phase III, noninferiority study that showed a comparable survival between second-line docetaxel and gefitinib.[233] At this time, it is only available in the US if a patient was on it before the negative trial results were published and is still responding via radiological imaging.

There are many other targeted therapies in clinical trials for NSCLC. Vandetanib (Zactima, ZD6474, AstraZeneca, Wilmington, DE) is a dual inhibitor of both the VEGF pathway and the EGFR pathway. There are multiple phase II trials suggesting vandetanib concurrent with chemotherapy will be an effective treatment in NSCLC, and trials are ongoing.[234] Also, there are some promising data on combining targeted agents. Phase II data using erlotinib combined with bevacizumab imply it is a competitive treatment option with decreased toxicity, especially for selected populations of patients.[235] Once considered to be a potential treatment in NSCLC, sorafenib (Nexavar, BAY12–9566) in combination with chemotherapy has demonstrated unacceptable toxicity without disease improvement, and clinical trials with it have ceased in lung cancer.[236] There is continued interest and ongoing clinical trials looking for activity in lung cancer with COX-2 inhibitors, FTIs, and insulin growth factor receptor inhibitors, to name a few. Gene therapy and cancer vaccines are also being trialed in locally advanced disease or for patients with positive pleural effusions.

### PERSONALIZED MEDICINE

The goal of personalized medicine is to make better use of available therapies, thereby improving outcomes while minimizing toxicity. Personalized medicine in lung cancer requires learning about tumor tissue and searching for characteristics that predict prognosis and predict for response to treatment. A key example is the correlation between the EGFR mutation and response to EGFR TKIs. After a subpopulation of patients developed dramatic tumor reduction while on EGFR TKIs, researchers identified the common denominator to be a somatic mutation in the kinase domain of EGFR.[237] The most common clinical features of these patients were female gender, never smoking, Asian ethnicity, and adenocarcinoma histology, with the strongest being low or never smoking history. The mutation occurs in around 10% of the general population; however, in Asians the rate is about 25% to 50%.[238] A prospective trial looking at response rates and survival in EGFR mutation–positive patients receiving EGFR TKIs resulted in significantly improved response rates as well as overall survival.[239] Upon retrospective analysis of multiple EGFR TKI studies, these results have been verified, and therefore the NCCN has updated the guidelines to allow for consideration of frontline EGFR TKI use in patients demonstrating an EGFR mutation or a never-smoking history.

Another very important advancement in tailoring therapy for lung cancer is treating by histology. In a retrospective analysis of a large randomized phase III trial of gemcitabine and cisplatin vs pemetrexed and cisplatin in chemotherapy-naïve NSCLC patients, histology played a significant role in response rates.[208] Patients with adenocarcinoma or large cell histologies had a significant improvement in overall survival when treated with pemetrexed and cisplatin; conversely, patients with squamous histology had a significant survival advantage in the gemcitabine and cisplatin arm. This is the first chemotherapeutic trial to show a favorable response by histology and warrants meticulous attention to pathology reports and histological subtype.

In addition to predicting response to treatment, analyzing tissue to predict prognosis is a part of personalizing treatment. Scientists have started to identify gene signatures by indentifying common genes that are present in patients with long-term survival. One study indentified a 5-gene signature by using a decision-tree analysis that was closely associated with relapse-free and overall survival in patients with NSCLC.[155] Future directions are toward an algorithm for finding a genomic signature, validating it with a prospective trial, predicting metastasis and drug sensitivity, and then personalizing the treatment on the basis of these characteristics.[240] Although EGFR mutations may be associated with a better prognosis, it has been suggested that KRAS may have poorer clinical outcomes in lung cancer for patients treated with erlotinib and chemotherapy.[241] The best way to achieve large cohorts and validation is to collect as much tissue from lung cancer patients and manage a database of treatment response and survival data. Many large academic institutions with high volumes of patients have already started this important initiative.

## SYMPTOM MANAGEMENT AND SUPPORTIVE CARE

There are multiple symptoms of advanced lung cancer that nurses must be aware of and ready to manage. Symptoms such as pain, fatigue, cough, and dyspnea are common and are often seen in clusters. These often interfere with activities of daily living and determine performance status. Severity of presenting symptoms many times guides the ability to be aggressive with treatment and predicts prognosis. However, in 1 study, performance status did not play a large role in treatment decisions, whereas age and comorbidities played a significant role.[242] Common side effects of chemotherapy for lung cancer are nausea, vomiting, anemia, neutropenia, alopecia, and asthenia. With the addition of biological therapies, newer side effects such as a papulopustular rash, diarrhea, and hypertension are routine issues that nurses face. Many of these side effects will be addressed in others chapters.

## PAIN

Pain in advanced lung cancer is often a result of direct extension of the primary tumor or from extrathoracic metastases such as bone metastases. Pain medication such as narcotics or neuromodulators is the mainstay of treatment, often coupled with palliative radiation if applicable.[243] Treatment for lung cancer pain is usually focused on using long-acting narcotics in combination with short-acting narcotics for quick relief of breakthrough pain. Adding an NSAID or medications that treat neuropathic pain can be a good adjunctive treatment. Acupuncture and complementary therapies have often been good additions for pain relief.[244] Lytic bone lesions are often a source of pain associated with lung cancer. Bisphosphanates combined with external beam radiation have been associated with providing some pain relief.[245] Sometimes surgery is necessary to stabilize bones at risk for fracture. Back pain in a lung cancer patient must be taken seriously, and radiographic imaging should be performed to rule out spinal cord compression.

## FATIGUE

Patients may not necessarily realize they are feeling fatigue or that it is related to their diagnosis. Fatigue and pain are the most common and most distressing symptoms in adults receiving treatment for lung cancer.[102,246] Anemia can sometimes complicate the issue of fatigue. Treatment of anemia with erythropoietin stimulating agents in lung cancer has been controversial due to questionable results of large trials suggesting a possibility of decreased survival when targeting higher hemoglobin or treating nonchemotherapy patients.[247] For now, treatment of anemia is limited to patients with a hemoglobin level under 10 g/dL, and only patients who are receiving chemotherapy. Fatigue can also be the result of dehydration, anorexia, and depression. The use of psychostimulants has shown some promising results and warrants larger studies to show significant symptom improvement.

## DYSPNEA

Dyspnea is common in lung cancer patients, and 65% of patients will experience it at some point during the course of their disease.[248] There are numerous reasons a patient with lung cancer may experience dyspnea: hypoxia, airway obstruction, pleural effusion, comorbidities such as COPD, pulmonary toxicity from treatments such as radiation, rapidly progressing disease, and pulmonary embolism. However, an emergency room study showed that most patients with lung cancer were dyspneic as a result of their primary tumor.[249] When a nurse encounters a patient with lung cancer complaining of dyspnea, many things need to be taken into consideration. First and foremost, could the patient have a pulmonary embolism (PE)? Patients with lung cancer are at high risk for PE, and this is potentially life threatening, requiring immediate attention and anticoagulation. If there is an acute change in dyspnea, the patient must be ruled out for PE first by performing either a ventilation/perfusion (VQ) scan or a PE-protocol chest CT. When this is ruled out, other causes mentioned above may be contributing factors and need to be assessed.

Treatment of dyspnea is centered on determining cause. Oxygen supplementation has been shown to provide relief from dyspnea and insomnia and to improve quality of life in lung cancer patients, regardless of oxygenation status.[250] If a patient has end-stage lung cancer and is on a hospice program, oxygen can help with end-of-life dyspnea; however, for a patient not on a hospice program, usually insurance panels require a pulse oximetry of less than 88% to 90% on room air before the patient qualifies for supplemental oxygen.

Analgesics can also help manage dyspnea in 2 distinct ways. Pain can cause dyspnea and hyperventilation, so analgesics that relieve pain can help. Also, if a patient has dyspnea in the terminal stage, IV morphine can help by causing sedation.[243]

Bronchodilators can help if dyspnea seems related to COPD or asthma flares. Positioning for patients with orthopnea is a key mediator of dyspnea and can also help them to clear secretions. Assessing the patient for depression and anxiety can also lead to pharmacological management of these symptoms to improve shortness of breath or a panicky feeling. If the patient is found to have tumor obstruction or a pleural effusion, a pulmonary evaluation will help determine the need for a bronchoscopy or a thoracentesis for a pleural effusion. A more permanent catheter can be placed to allow frequent draining, or a talc pleurodesis can be performed to inhibit new fluid accumulation.

## COUGH

Cough can have many contributing factors, similar to those that cause dyspnea. About 15% of patients will develop hemoptysis, and up to 3% of patients develop fatal hemoptysis.[243] It is important that a patient report hemoptysis right away and undergo an evaluation by either the oncologist or the pulmonologist to quantify it and possibly perform bronchoscopy to cauterize bleeding vessels. Radiation is also often a useful technique to treat hemoptysis. However, a chronic cough without hemoptysis can be common in lung cancer patients and difficult to treat. Over-the-counter syrups can help, but opioids tend to offer the best relief, especially when added with the syrup. Benzonatate is a capsule that has a numbing effect in the throat and lungs to minimize chronic irritation and cough, and is a good option for patients who cannot tolerate opioids or need an additional medication. However, the nurse should be aware of a possible underlying infection, especially if it is a productive cough, that may require antibiotics. Physical exam, review of systems, including amount and color of the mucus, and vital signs can help make this diagnosis.

## CONCLUSION

In the past 5 years there have been great strides in the treatment of lung cancer. Newer chemotherapeutics, biologically targeted therapies, and advances in radiation technique have improved outcomes and have somewhat minimized toxicity. However, a screening tool has still not been established, and clinicians anxiously await the results of the NLST. Hopefully, smoking rates will continue to fall as more strategies are utilized for smoking prevention and cessation. Exciting research for newer and more diverse biological therapies will hopefully yield better and safer pharmacological therapies to improve the dismal survival rates of this disease.

## REFERENCES


1. American Cancer Society. *Cancer Facts and Figures 2009*. Atlanta, American Cancer Society; 2009.
2. Boyle P, Levin B. *World Cancer Report 2008*. International Agency for Research on Cancer (IARC), 2008; Lyon Cedex, France.
3. Wakelee HA, Chang ET, Gomez SL, et al. Lung cancer incidence in never smokers. *J Clin Oncol*. 2007; 25:472–478
4. American Cancer Society. *Cancer Facts and Figures 2000*. Atlanta, American Cancer Society; 2000.
5. National Cancer Institute. NCI SEER stat fact sheet, lung cancer. http://seer.cancer.gov/statfacts/html/lungb.html. Accessed November 1, 2009.
6. Subramanian J, Govindan R. Lung cancer in never smokers: a review. *J Clin Oncol*. 2007; 25:561–568.
7. Patel JD. Lung cancer in women. *J Clin Oncol*. 2005; 23:3212–3218.
8. Haiman CA, Stram DO, Wilkens LR, et al. Ethnic and racial differences in the smoking-related risk of lung cancer. *N Engl J Med*. 2006;354:333–342.
9. National Cancer Institute. NCI fact sheet, Cancer research funding http://www.cancer.gov/cancertopics/factsheet/NCI/research-funding. Accessed November 1, 2009.
10. Thun MJ, Lally CA, Flannery JT, Calle EE, Flanders WD, Heath Jr CD. Cigarette smoking and changes in histopathology of lung cancer. *J Natl Cancer Inst*. 1997; 89:1580–1586.
11. Peto R, Darby S, Deo H, Silcocks P, Whitley E, Doll R. Smoking, smoking cessation, and cancer in the UK since 1950: combination of national statistics with two case-control studies. *BMJ* 2000; 321:323–329.
12. Alberg AJ, Ford JG, Samet JM. Epidemiology of lung cancer. *Chest*. 2007;132:29S-55S.
13. Caraballo RS, Giovino GA, Pechacek TF, et al. Racial and ethnic differences in serum cotinine levels of cigarette smokers: Third National Health and Nutrition Examination Survey, 1988–1991. *JAMA*. 1998;280:135–139.
14. Perez-Stable EJ, Herrera B, Jacob P III, Benowitz NL Nicotine metabolism and intake in black and white smokers. *JAMA* 1998;280:152–156.
15. International Early Lung Cancer Action Program Investigators. Women's susceptibility to tobacco carcinogens and survival after diagnosis of lung cancer. *JAMA*. 2006;296:180–184.
16. Toyooka S, Toshihide T, Gazdar AF. The P53 gene, tobacco exposure, and lung cancer. *Hum Mutat*. 2003;21:229–239.
17. US Environmental Protection Agency. Radon: the health hazard with a simple solution. http://www.epa.gov/radon/. Accessed November 1, 2009.
18. Gray A, Read S, McGale P, Darby S. Lung cancer deaths from indoor radon and the cost effectiveness and potential policies to reduce them. *BMJ*. 2009;338:1–11.
19. Duckworth LT, Frank-Stromborg M, Oleckno WA, et al. Relationship of perception of radon as a health risk and willingness to engage in radon testing and mitigation. *Oncol Nurs Forum*. 2002;29:1099–1107.
20. Zielinski JM, Carr Z, Krewski D, Repacholi M. World Health Organization's International Radon Project. *J Toxicol Environ Health. Part A*. 2006;69:759–769.
21. Besaratinia A, Pfeifer GP. Secondhand smoke and human lung cancer. *Lancet Oncol*. 2008;9:657–666.
22. Boffetta P. Involuntary smoking and lung cancer. *Scand J Work Environ Health*. 2002;28(Suppl):30–40.
23. Taylor R, Cumming R, Woodward A, et al. Passive smoking and lung cancer: a cumulative meta-analysis. *Aust NZ J Public Health*. 2001;25:203–211.
24. Zhou W, Heist RS, Liu G, et al. Secondhand smoke exposure and survival in early-stage non-small cell lung cancer. *Clin Cancer Res*. 2006;12:7187–7193.
25. Asomaning K, Miller DP, Liu G, et al. Secondhand smoke, age of exposure, and lung cancer risk. *Lung Cancer*. 2008;61:13–20.
26. Nelson DI, Concha-Barrientos M, Driscoll T, et al. The global burden of selected occupational diseases and injury risks: methodology and summary. *Am J Ind Med*. 2005;48:400–418.
27. Bach PB, Ginsberg RJ. Epidemiology of lung cancer. In: Ginsberg RJ, ed. *American Cancer Society Atlas of Clinical Oncology: Lung Cancer*. Hamilton, ON, BC: Decker; 2002:1–10.
28. Hashibe M, Straif K, Tashkin DP, et al. Epidemiologic review of marijuana use and cancer risk. *Alcohol*. 2005;35:265–275.
29. Aldington S, Harwood M, Cox B, et al. Cannabis use and risk of lung cancer: a case-control study. *Eur Respir J*. 2008;31:280–286.
30. De Stefani E, Boffetta P, Ronco AL, et al. Nutrient patterns and risk of lung cancer: a factor analysis in Uraguayan men. *Lung Cancer*. 2008;61:283–291.
31. Wright ME, Park Y, Subar AF, et al. Intake of fruit, vegetables and specific botanical groups in relation to lung cancer risk in the NIH-AARP diet and health study. *Am J Epidemiol*. 2008;168:1024–1034.
32. Mahabir S, Schendel K, Dong YQ, et al. Dietary alpha-, beta-, gamma- and delta-tocopherols in lung cancer risk. *Int J Cancer*. 2008;123:1173–1180.
33. Goodman GE, Schaffer S, Omenn GS Chen C, King I. The association between lung and prostate cancer risk and serum micronutrients: results and lessons learned from beta-carotene and retinol efficacy trial. *Cancer Epidemiol Biomarkers Prev*. 2003;12:518–526.
34. Omenn GS, Goodman GE, Thornquist MD, et al. Risk factors for lung cancer and for intervention effects in CARET, the Beta-Carotene and Retinol Efficacy Trial. *J Natl Cancer Inst*. 1996;88:1550–1559.
35. Virtamo J, Pietinen P, Huttunen JK, et al. Incidence of cancer and mortality following alpha-tocopherol and beta-carotene supplementation: a post-intervention follow-up. *JAMA*. 2003;290:476–485.
36. Gallicchio L, Boyd K, Matanoski G, et al. Carotenoids and the risk of developing lung cancer: a systematic review. *Am J Clin Nutr*. 2008;88:372–383.
37. Clapp RW, Jacobs MM, Loechler EL. Environmental and occupational causes of cancer: new evidence 2005–2007. *Rev Environ Health*. 2008;23:1–37.
38. Beelan R, Hoek G, van den Brandt PA, et al. Long-term exposure to traffic-related air pollution and lung cancer risk. *Epidemiology*. 2008;19:702–710.
39. Shen M, Chapman RS, He X, et al. Dietary factors, food contamination and lung cancer risk in Xuanwei, China. *Lung Cancer*. 2008;61:275–282.

40. Bach PB, Kattan MW, Thornquist MD, et al. Variations in lung cancer risk among smokers. *J Natl Cancer Inst.* 2003;95:470–478.
41. Schwartz AG, Yang P, Swanson GM. Familial risk of lung cancer among nonsmokers and their relatives. *Am J Epidemiol.* 1996;144:554–562.
42. Travis LB, Gospodarowicz M, Curtis RE, et al. Lung cancer following chemotherapy and radiotherapy for Hodgkin's disease. *J Natl Cancer Inst.* 2002;94:182–192.
43. Santillan AA, Camargo CA Jr, Colditz GA. A meta-analysis of asthma and risk of lung cancer (United States). *Cancer Causes Control.* 2003;14:327–334.
44. Schabath MB, Delclos GL, Martynowicz MM, et al. Opposing effects of emphysema, hayfever, and select genetic variants on lung cancer risk. *Am J Epidemiol.* 2005;161:412–422.
45. US Department of Health and Human Services. *The Health Consequences of Involuntary Exposure to Tobacco Smoke: A Report of the Surgeon General.* Rockville, MD: U.S. Department of Health and Human Services, Public Health Service, Centers for Disease Control and Prevention, National Center for Chronic Disease Prevention and Health Promotion, Office on Smoking and Health; 2006.
46. Bal DG, Kizer KW, Felten PG, Mozar HN, Niemeyer D. Reducing tobacco consumption in California. Development of a statewide anti-tobacco use campaign. *JAMA.* 1990;264:1570–1574.
47. Lightwood JM, Dinno A, Glantz SA. Effect of the California Tobacco Control Program on personal health care expenditures. *PLoS Med.* 2008;5:e178.
48. Barnoya J, Glantz S. Association of the California tobacco control program with declines in lung cancer incidence. *Cancer Causes Control.* 2004;15:689–695.
49. King C, Siegel M. The master settlement agreement with the tobacco industry and cigarette advertising in magazines. *N Engl J Med.* 2001;345:504–511.
50. Centers for Disease Control and Prevention. Best practices for comprehensive tobacco control programs—2007. Atlanta (Georgia): US Department of Health and Human Services, Centers for Disease Control and Prevention, National Center for Chronic Disease Prevention and Health Promotion, Office on Smoking and Health. Available: http://www.cdc.gov/tobacco/stateandcommunity/best_practices/index.html. Accessed November 1, 2009.
51. Winterhalder RC, Hirsch FR, Kotantoulas GK, et al. Chemoprevention of lung cancer—from biology to clinical reality. *Ann Oncol.* 2004;15:185–196.
52. Akhmedkhanov A, Toniolo P, Zeleniuch-Jacquotte A, et al. Aspirin and lung cancer in women. *Br J Cancer.* 2002;87:49–52.
53. Vogel U, Christensen J, Wallin H, et al. Polymorphisms in genes involved in the inflammatory response and interaction with NSAID use or smoking in relation to lung cancer risk in a prospective study. *Mutat Res.* 2008;639:89–100.
54. Mahabir S, Forman MR, Barerra SL, et al. Joint effects of dietary trace metals and DNA repair capacity in lung cancer risk. *Cancer Epidemiol Biomarkers Prev.* 2007;16:2756–2762.
55. Zhou W, Park S, Liu G, et al. Dietary iron, zinc, and calcium and the risk of lung cancer. *Epidemiol.* 2005;16:772–779.
56. Hu J, Johnson K, Mao Y, et al. A case-control study of diet and lung cancer in northeast China. *Int J Cancer.* 1997;71:924–931.
57. Ebbert JO, Yang P, Vachan CM, et al. Lung cancer risk reduction after smoking cessation: observations from a prospective cohort. *J Clin Oncol.* 2003;21:921–926.
58. Fiore MC, Bailey WC, Cohen SJ, et al. *Treating Tobacco Use and Dependence. Quick Reference Guide for Clinicians.* Rockville, MD, U.S. Department of Health and Human Services, Public Health Service, October 2000.
59. Wong PW, White DA. Prevention and screening of lung cancer. In: Ginsberg RJ, ed. *American Cancer Society Atlas of Clinical Oncology: Lung Cancer.* Hamilton, ON, BC: Decker, 2002;11–22.
60. Rennard SI, Daughton DM. Nicotine replacement therapy: what are the options today? *J Respir Dis.* 1998;19:S20-S25.
61. Fiore MC, Smith SS, Jorenby DE, et al. The effectiveness of nicotine patch for smoking cessation: a meta-analysis. *JAMA.* 1994;27:1940–1947.
62. GlaxoSmithKline. Zyban® [package insert]. Research Triangle Park, NC. 2008, GlaxoSmithKline http://us.gsk.com/products/assets/us_zyban.pdf. Accessed November 1, 2009.
63. Gonzales D, Rennard SI, Nides M, et al. Varenicline, an alpha4beta2 nicotine acetylcholine receptor partial agonist, vs sustained-release bupropion and placebo for smoking cessation. *JAMA.* 2006;296:47–55.
64. Tonstad S, Tonnesen P, Hajek P, et al. Effect of maintenance therapy with varenicline on smoking cessation. *JAMA.* 2006;296:64–71.
65. Pfizer. Chantix® [package insert]. Pfizer Inc, Mission, KS. http://media.pfizer.com/files/products/uspi_chantix.pdf. Accessed November 1, 2009.
66. Zbikowski SM, Hapgood J, Barnwell SS, McAfee T. Phone and web-based tobacco cessation treatment: real-world utilization patterns and outcomes for 11,000 tobacco users. *J Med Internet Res.* 2008;10:e41.
67. Volpp KG, Troxel AB, Pauly MV, et al. A randomized, controlled trial of financial incentives for smoking cessation. *N Engl J Med.* 2009;360:699–709.
68. Gagnon F, Courchesne M, Levesque B, et al. Assessment of the effectiveness of radon screening programs in reducing lung cancer mortality. *Risk Analysis.* 2008;28:1221–1229.
69. US Environmental Protection Agency. Consumer guide to radon reduction. http://www.epa.gov/radon/pubs/consguid.html#testmean. Accessed November 1, 2009.
70. Cohen V, Khuri FR. Chemoprevention of lung cancer. *Curr Opin Pulm Med.* 2004;10:279–283.
71. Khuri FR, Cohen V. Molecularly targeted approaches to chemoprevention of lung cancer. *Clin Cancer Res.* 2004;10:4249s-4253s.
72. Merrick DT, Kittelson J, Winterhalder R, et al. Analysis of c-ErbB1/epidermal growth factor receptor and c-ErbB2/HER-2 expression in bronchial dysplasia: evaluation of potential targets for chemoprevention of lung cancer. *Clin Cancer Res.* 2006;12:2281–2288.
73. Lee JM, Yanagawa J, Peebles KA, et al. Inflammation in lung carcinogenesis: new targets for lung cancer chemoprevention and treatment. *Critl Rev Oncol/Hematol.* 2008;66:208–217.
74. Bach PB, Silvestri GA, Hanger M, Jett JR. Screening for lung cancer. *Chest.* 2007;132:69s-77s.
75. Karp DD, Thurer RL. Non-small cell lung cancer. In: Furie B, Cassileth PA, Atkins MB, Mayer RL, ed: *Clinical Hematology and Oncology: Presentation, Diagnosis, and Treatment.* Philadelphia, PA: Churchill Livingstone, 2003;958–982.
76. Giarelli E. To screen or not to screen: using spiral computerized tomography in the early detection of lung cancer. *J Clin Oncol Nurs.* 2002;6:223–224.
77. Henschke CI, Naidich DP, Yankelevitz DF, et al: Early Lung Cancer Action Project: initial findings on repeat screening. *Cancer.* 2001;92:153–159.
78. International Early Lung Cancer Action Program. Survival of patients with stage I lung cancer detected on CT screening. *N Engl J Med.* 2006;355:1763–1771.
79. Midthun DE, Jett JR. Update on screening for lung cancer. *Semin Respir Crit Care Med.* 2008;29:233–240.
80. National Cancer Institute. National Lung Screening Trial: what is NLST. http://www.cancer.gov/nlst/what-is-nlst. Accessed November 1, 2009.
81. Vachani A, Seijo L, Unger M, Sterman D. Bronchoscopy, transthoracic needle aspiration, and related procedures. In Fishman AP, Elias JA, Fishman JA, Grippi MA, Senior RM, Pack AI, ed. *Fishman's Pulmonary Diseases and Disorders,* 4th ed. China: The McGraw-Hill Companies;2008:629–648.
82. Shaipanich T, McWilliams A, Lam S. Early detection and chemoprevention of lung cancer. *Respirology.* 2006;11:366–372.
83. Haubinger K, Becker H, Stanzel F, et al. Autofluorescense bronchoscopy with white light bronchoscopy compared with white light bronchoscopy alone for the detection of precancerous lesions: a European randomized controlled muticentre trial. *Thorax.* 2005;60:496–503.
84. Edell E, Lam S, Pass H, et al. Detection and localization of intraepithelial neoplasia and invasive carcinoma using fluorescence-reflectance bronchoscopy: an international, multicenter trial. *J Thorac Oncol.* 2009;4:49–54.

85. Ross J. Biology of lung cancer. In Hass M, ed: *Contemporary Issues in Lung Cancer: A Nursing Perspective*. Sudbury, MA: Jones and Bartlett; 2003:11–23.
86. Zakowski MS. Pathology. In Ginsberg R,ed. *American Cancer Society Atlas of Clinical Oncology: Lung Cancer*. Hamilton, ON, BC: Decker; 2002:23–42.
87. Bambilla E, Travis WD, Colby TV, et al: The new World Health Organization classification of lung tumours. *Eur Respirat J*. 2001;18:1059–1068.
88. Franklin WA. Diagnosis of lung cancer: pathology of invasive and preinvasive neoplasia. *Chest*. 2000;117:80s-89s.
89. Rosti G, Bevilacqua G, Bidoli P, Portalone L, Santo A, Genestreti G. Small cell lung cancer. *Ann Oncol*. 2006;17:ii5-ii10.
90. Burger H, deb Bakker MA, Stoter G, et al. Lack of c-kit exon 11 activating mutations in c-kit/Cd117 positive SCLC tumor specimens. *Eur J Cancer*. 2003;39:793–799.
91. Pelosi G, Fraggetta F, Pasini F, Maisonneuve P, Sonzogni A, Iannucci A, et al. Immunoreactivity for thyroid transcription factor-1 in stage I non-small cell carcinomas of the lung. *Am J Surg Pathol*. 2001;25:363–372.
92. Comperat E, Zhang F, Perrotin C, Molina T, Magdeleinat P, Marmey B, et al. Variable sensitivity and specificity of TTF-1 antibodies in lung metastatic adenocarcinoma of colorectal origin. *Mod Pathol*. 2005;18:1371–1376.
93. Miettinen M, Sarlomo-Rikala M. Expression of calretinin, thrombomodulin, keratin 5, and mesothelin in lung carcinomas of different types: an immunohistochemical analysis of 596 tumors in comparison with epithelioid mesotheliomas of the pleura. *Am J Surg Pathol*. 2003;27:150–158.
94. Kargi A, Gurel D, Tuna B. The diagnostic value of TTF-1, CK5/6, and p63 immunostaining in classification of lung carcinomas. *Appl Immunohistochem Molecul Morphol*. 2007;15:415–420.
95. Downey P, Cummins R, Moran M, Gulmann C. If it's not CK 5/6 positive, TTF-1 negative, it's not a squamous cell carcinoma of the lung. *APMIS*. 2008;116:526–529
96. Dang TP, Carbone DP. Cancer of the lung. In: DeVita Jr. VT, Lawrence TS, Rosenberg SA, ed. *DeVita, Hellman, and Rosenberg's Cancer: Principles and Practice of Oncology 8th Edition*. Philadelphia, PA: Lippincott Williams & Wilkins; 2008;887–972.
97. Riva M, Landonio G, Arena O, et al. Pathophysiology, clinical manifestations and supportive care of metastatic brain cancer. *Forum* (Genova). 2001;11:4–26.
98. Ferrara N, Gerber HP, LeCouter J. The biology of VEGF and its receptors. *Nat Med*. 2003;9:669–676.
99. Rowinsky EK. The erbB family: Targets for therapeutic development against cancer and therapeutic strategies using monoclonal antibodies and tyrosine kinase inhibitors. *Annu Rev Med*. 2004;55:433–457.
100. Roskoski Jr R. The ErbB/HER receptor protein-tyrosine kinases and cancer. *Biochem Biophys Res Commun*. 2004;319:1–11.
101. Feinstein MB, Stover D. Clinical features and of lung cancer. In: Ginsberg R, ed. *American Cancer Society Atlas of Clinical Oncology: Lung Cancer*. Hamilton, ON, BC: Decker; 2002:43–55.
102. Kiteley CA, Fitch MI. Understand the symptoms experienced by individuals with lung cancer. *Can Oncol Nurs J*. 2006;16:25–30.
103. Ernst A, Thurer RL. Hemoptysis. In: Furie B, Cassileth PA, Atkins MB, Mayer RL, ed. *Clinical Hematology and Oncology: Presentation, Diagnosis, and Treatment*. Philadelphia, PA: Churchill Livingstone; 2003:106–114.
104. Boyar M, Raftopoulos H. Supportive care in lung cancer. *Hematol Oncol Clin North Am*. 2005;19:369–387.
105. Laurie SA, NG KK, Rosenzweig K, Ginsberg RJ. Treatment of local and locoregional non-small cell lung cancer. In: Ginsberg RJ, ed.: *American Cancer Society Atlas of Clinical Oncology: Lung Cancer*. Hamilton, ON, BC: Decker; 2002:101–119.
106. Swanson S, Batirel HF. Pleural effusion. In Furie B, Cassileth PA, Atkins MB, Mayer RL, ed. *Clinical Hematology and Oncology: Presentation, Diagnosis, and Treatment*. Philadelphia, PA: Churchill Livingstone; 2003:87–93.
107. Evans T, Lynch Jr TL, Superior vena cava syndrome. In: Furie B, Cassileth PA, Atkins MB, Mayer RL, ed. *Clinical Hematology and Oncology: Presentation, Diagnosis, and Treatment*. Philadelphia, PA: Churchill Livingstone; 2003:98–105.
108. Rice TW, Rodriguez RM, Light RW. The superior vena cava syndrome: clinical characteristics and evolving etiology. *Medicine*. 2006;85:37–42.
109. Tyson LB, Patient assessment. In: Houlihan NG, ed. *Site-Specific Cancer Series: Lung Cancer*. Pittsburg, PA: Oncology Nursing Society. 2004;35–44.
110. Beckles MA, Spiro SG, Colice GL, et al. Initial evaluation of the patient with lung cancer: symptoms, signs, laboratory tests, and paraneoplastic syndromes. *Chest*. 2003;123:97s-104s.
111. Joyce M, Schwartz S, Huhmann M. Supportive care in lung cancer. *Semin Oncol Nurs*. 2008;24:57–67.
112. Tyson LB, Paraneoplastic syndromes. In: Houlihan NG, ed. *Site-Specific Cancer Series: Lung Cancer*. Pittsburg, PA: Oncology Nursing Society. 2004;57–72.
113. Armstrong T, Paraneoplastic syndromes. In: Yarbro CH, Frogge MH, Goodman M, eds. *Cancer Nursing: Principles and Practice*. 6th ed. Sudbury, MA: Jones and Bartlett; 2005:809–824.
114. Ezzone SA. Syndrome of inappropriate antidiuretic hormone. In: Camp-Sorrell D, Hawkins RA, eds. *Clinical Manuel for the Oncology Advanced Practice Nurse*. Pittsburg, PA: Oncology Nursing Society; 2000:571–575.
115. Flounders JA. Syndrome of inappropriate antidiuretic hormone. *Oncol Nurs Forum*. 2003;30:E63-E70.
116. Dalmau J, Bataller L. Paraneoplastic neurologic syndromes: approaches to diagnosis and treatment. *Semin Neurol*. 2003; 23:215–224
117. Thomas L, Kwok Y, Edelman MJ. Management of paraneoplastic syndromes in lung cancer. *Curr Treat Opt Oncol*. 2004;5:51–62.
118. Knop CS. Lung cancer. In: Yarbro CH, Frogge MH, Goodman M, eds. *Cancer Nursing: Principles and Practice*. 6th ed. Sudbury, MA: Jones and Bartlett; 2005:1379–1413
119. Oken MM, Creech RH, Tormey DC, et al. Toxicity and response criteria of the Eastern Cooperative Oncology Group. *Am J Clin Oncol*. 1982;5:649–655.
120. Seidel HM, Ball JW, Dains JE, Benedict GW, eds. *Mosby's Guide to Physical Examination*. 4th ed. St. Louis, MO: Mosby; 1999:352–408.
121. Roth K, Nilson TIL, Hatlen E, et al. Predictors of long time survival after lung cancer surgery: a retrospective cohort study. *BMC Pulm Med*. 2008;8:22.
122. Poonyagariyagorn H, Mazzone PJ. Lung cancer: Preoperative pulmonary evaluation of the lung resection candidate. *Semin Respir Crit Care Med*. 2008;29:271–284.
123. Markos J, Mullan BP, Hillman DR, et al. Preoperative assessment as a predictor of mortality and morbidity after lung resection. *Am Rev Respir Dis*.1989;139:902–910.
124. Belda J, Cavalcanti M, Ferrer M, et al. Bronchial colonization and postoperative respiratory infections in patients undergoing lung cancer surgery. *Chest*. 2005;128:1571–1579.
125. Li R, Todd NW, Qiu, Qi, et al. Genetic deletions in sputum as diagnostic markers for early detection of stage 1 non-small cell lung cancer. *Clin Cancer Res*. 2007;13:482–487.
126. Petty TL. Sputum cytology for the detection of early lung cancer. *Curr Opin Pulm* Med. 2003;9:309–312.
127. Choi YD, Han CW, Kim JH, et al. Effectiveness of sputum cytology using Thinprep® method for evaluation of lung cancer. *Diagn Cytopathol*. 2008;36:167–171.
128. Toloza EM, Harpole L, Detterbeck F, McCrory DC. Invasive staging of non-small cell lung cancer. *Chest*. 2003;123:157S-166S.
129. Tournoy KG, Rintoul RC, van Meerbeeck JP, et al. EBUS-TBNA for the diagnosis of central parenchymal lung lesions not visible at routine bronchoscopy. *Lung Cancer*. 2009;63:45–49.

130. Wallace MB, Pascual JMS, Raimondo M, el al. Minimally invasive endoscopic staging of suspected lung cancer. *JAMA.* 2008;299:540–546.
131. Lee HS, Lee GK, Lee HS, et al. Real-time endobronchial ultrasound-guided transbronchial needle aspiration in mediastinal staging of non-small cell lung cancer. *Chest.* 2008;134:368–374.
132. Mountain CF, Dressler CM. Regional lymph node classification for lung cancer staging. *Chest.* 1997;111:1718–1723.
133. LeBlanc JK, Espada R, Ergun G. Non-small cell lung cancer staging techniques and endoscopic ultrasound: tissue is still the issue. *Chest.* 2003;123:1718–1725.
134. Akhurst T, Heelan R. Imaging work-up of lung cancer: Utility and comparison of computed tomography and FDG positron emission tomography. In: Ginsberg R, ed. *American Cancer Society Atlas of Clinical Oncology: Lung Cancer.* Hamilton, ON, BC: Decker; 2002:71–93.
135. MacDonald SLS, Hansell DM. Staging of non-small cell lung cancer: imaging of intrathoracic disease. *Eur J Radiol.* 2003;45:18–30.
136. CerfolioRJ, Bryant AS, Ohja B, Bartolucci AA. The maximum standard uptake values on positron emission tomography of a non-small cell lung cancer predicts stage, recurrence, and survival. *J Thorac Cardiovasc Surg.* 2005;130:151–159.
137. PETNET solutions. CMS medicare policies for PET documented in a National Coverage Decision, section 220.6, http://www.petscaninfo.com/zportal/portals/pat/my_pet_scan/insurance_coverage. Accessed November 1, 2009.
138. Miele E, Spinelli GP, Tomao F, et al. Positron Emission Tomography (PET) radiotracers in oncology-utility of 18F-Fluoro-deoxy-glucose (FDG)-PET in the management of patients with non-small cell lung cancer (NSCLC). *J Exp Clin Cancer Res.* 2008;27:52.
139. Bryant AS, Cerfolio RJ. The maximum standardized uptake values on integrated FDG-PET/CT is useful in differentiating benign from malignant pulmonary nodules. *Ann Thorac Surg.* 2006;82:1016–1020.
140. Pope RJE, Hansell DM. Extra-thoracic staging of lung cancer. *Eur J Radiol.* 2003;45:31–38.
141. Wisnivesky JP, Yankelevitz D, Henschke CI. The effect of tumor size on curability of stage I non-small cell lung cancers. *Chest.* 2004;126:761–765.
142. Riquet M, Foucault C, Berna P, et al. Prognostic value of histology in resected lung cancer with emphasis on the relevance of the adenocarcinoma subtyping. *Ann Thorac Surg.* 2006;81:1988–1995.
143. Kerr KM. Pulmonary adenocarcinomas: classification and reporting. *Histopathology.* 2009;54:12–27.
144. Guo X, Chen Y, Xu Z, et al. Prognostic significance of VEGF-C expression in correlation with COX-2, lymphatic microvessel density, and clinicopathologic characteristics in human non-small cell lung cancer. *Acta Biochimica et Biophysica Sinica.* 2009; 41:217–222.
145. Berghmans T, Paesmans M, Mascaux C, et al. Thyroid transcription factor 1-a new prognostic factor in lung cancer: a meta-anaylsis. *Ann Oncol.* 2006;17:1673–1676.
146. Ou S-H I, Zell JA, Ziogas A, Anton-Culver H. Low socioeconomic status is a poor prognostic factor for survival in stage I non-small cell lung cancer and is independent of surgical treatment, race, and marital status. *Cancer.* 2008;112:2011–2020.
147. Meert AP, Martin B, Delmotte P, et al. The role of EGFR expression on patient survival in lung cancer: a systematic review with meta-analysis. *Eur Respir J* 2002;20:975–981.
148. Shah L, Walter KL, Borczuk AC, et al. Expression of syndecan-1 and expression of epidermal growth factor receptor are associated with survival in patients with non-small cell lung carcinoma. *Cancer.* 2004;101:1632–1638.
149. Selvaggi G, Novello S, Torri V, et al. Epidermal growth factor receptor overexpression correlates with a poor prognosis in completely resected non-small cell lung cancer. *Ann Oncol.* 2004;15:28–32.
150. Brundage MD, Davies D, Mackillop WJ. Prognostic factors in non-small cell lung cancer: a decade of progress. *Chest.* 2002;122:1037–1057.
151. Hirsch FR, Spreafico A, Novello S. The prognostic and predictive role of histology in advanced non-small cell lung cancer: a literature review. *J Thorac Oncol.* 2008;3:1468–1481.
152. Giaccone G, Iacona RB, Fandi A, et al. Epidermal growth factor receptor analysis in chemotherapy-naïve patients with advanced non-small cell lung cancer treated with gefitinib or placebo in combination with platinum-based chemotherapy. *J Cancer Res Clin Oncol.* 2009;135:467–476.
153. Olaussen KA, Dunant A, Fouret P, et al. DNA repair by ERCC1 in non–small-cell lung cancer and cisplatin-based adjuvant chemotherapy. *N Engl J Med.* 2006;355:983–991.
154. Zheng Z, Chen T, Li X, et al. DNA syntheses and repair genes RRM1 and ERCC1 in lung cancer. *N Engl J Med.* 2007;356:800–808.
155. Chen HY, Yu SL, Chen CH, et al. A five-gene signature and clinical outcome in non-small cell lung cancer. *N Engl J Med.* 2007;356:11–20.
156. Petty RD, Nicolson MC, Kerr KM, et al. Gene expression profiling in non-small cell lung cancer: from molecular mechanisms to clinical application. *Clin Cancer Res.* 2004;10:3237–3248.
157. Komaki R. Combined treatment for limited small cell lung cancer. *Semin Oncol.* 2003;30:56–70.
158. Van Klaveren RJ, Kloover JS. Staging, staging procedures and prognostic factors. In: Hansen HH, ed. *Lung Cancer Therapy Annual 5.* London, UK, Informa UK Limited; 2006:63–91.
159. Goldstraw P, Crowley J, Chansky K, et al. The IASLC lung cancer staging project: proposals for the revision of the TNM stage groupings in the forthcoming (seventh) edition of the TNM classifications of malignant tumours. *J Thorac Oncol.* 2007;2:706–714.
160. Rusch VW, Asamura H, Wantanabe H, et al. A proposal for a new international lymph node map in the forthcoming seventh edition of the TNM classification for lung cancer. *J Thorac Oncol.* 2009;4:568–577.
161. Schulte T, Schniewind B, Dohrmann P, Kuchler T, Kurdow R. The extent of lung parenchyma resection significantly impacts long-term quality of life in patients with non-small cell lung cancer. *Chest.* 2009;135:322–329.
162. El-Sherif A, Fernando HC, Santos R, et al. Margin and local recurrence after sublobar resection of non-small cell lung cancer. *Ann Surg Oncol.* 2007; 14:2400–2405.
163. Martin J, Ginsberg RJ, Abolhoda A, et al. Morbidity and mortality after neoadjuvant therapy for lung cancer: the risks of right pneumonectomy. *Ann Thorac Surg.* 2001;72:1149–1154.
164. Shaw JP, Dembitzer FR, Wisnivesky JP, et al. Video-assisted thoracoscopic lobectomy: state of the art and future directions. *Ann Thorac Surg.* 2008;85:S705-S709.
165. Cheung MC, Hamilton K, Sherman R, et al. Impact of teaching facility status and high-volume centers on outcomes for lung cancer resection: an examination of 13,469 surgical patients. *Ann Surg Oncol.* 2008;16:3–13.
166. Szczesny TJ, Szczesny A, Shepherd FA, et al. Surgical treatment of small cell lung cancer. *Semin Oncol.* 2003;30:47–56.
167. Sarna L, Cooley ME, Brown JK, et al. Symptom severity 1 to 4 months after thoracotomy for lung cancer. *Am J Crit Care.* 2008;17:455–467.
168. Balduyck B, Hendriks J, Lauwers P, Van Schil P. Quality of life evolution after lung cancer surgery: A prospective study in 100 patients. *Lung Cancer.* 2007;56:423–431.
169. Cannon J, Win T. Long term quality of life after lung resection. *Thorac Surg Clin.* 2008;18:81–91.
170. Nakamura H, Haruki T, Adachi Y, et al. Smoking affects prognosis after lung cancer surgery. *Surg Today.* 2008;38:227–231.
171. Quinn KL. Managing patients through thoracic surgery. In: Haas M, ed. *Contemporary Issues in Lung Cancer: A Nursing Perspective.* Sudbury, MA, Jones and Bartlett; 2003:33–48.
172. Senan S, De Ruysscher D, Giraud P, Mirimanoff R, Budach V. Literature-based recommendations for treatment planning and execution in high-dose radiotherapy for lung cancer. *Radiother Oncol.* 2004;71:139–146.

173. Keall P. Four-dimensional computed tomography imaging and treatment planning. *Semin Radiat Oncol.* 2004;14:81–90.
174. Haasbeek CJA, Slotman BJ, Senan S. Radiotherapy for lung cancer: clinical impact of recent technical advances. *Lung Cancer.* 2009;64:1–8.
175. Mulcahy N. Proton-beam therapy reduces bone marrow toxicity in lung cancer patients. 2008 Chicago Multidisciplinary Symposium in Thoracic Oncology: Abstract 185. Presented November 14, 2008. http://www.medscape.com/viewarticle/583655. Accessed November 30, 2009.
176. Smythe WR, American College of Chest Physicians. Treatment of stage I non-small cell lung carcinoma. *Chest.* 2003;123:181S-187S.
177. PORT Meta-Analysis Trialists Group. Postoperative radiotherapy in non-small-cell lung cancer: Systematic review and meta-analysis of individual patient data from nine randomized controlled trials. *Lancet.* 1998;352:257–263.
178. Albain KS, Crowley JJ, Turrisi AT, et al. Concurrent cisplatin, etoposide, and chest radiotherapy in pathologic stage IIIB non-small cell lung cancer: a southwest oncology group phase II study, SWOG 9019. *J Clin Oncol.* 2002;20:3454–3460.
179. Sause W, Kolesar P, Taylor SI, et al: Final results of phase III trial in regionally advanced unresectable non-small cell lung cancer: Radiation Therapy Oncology Group, Eastern Cooperative Oncology Group, and Southwest Oncology Group. *Chest.* 2000;117:358–364.
180. Le Chevalier T, Arriagada R, Quoix E, et al: Radiotherapy alone versus combined chemotherapy and radiotherapy in nonresectable non-small cell lung cancer: First analysis of a randomized trial in 353 patients. *J Natl Cancer Inst.* 1991;83:417–423.
181. Takada M, Fukuoka M, Kawahara M, et al. Phase III study of concurrent vs sequential thoracic radiotherapy in combination with cisplatin and etoposide for limited-stage small-cell lung cancer: results of the Japan Clinical Oncology Group Study 9104. *J Clin Oncol.* 2002;20:3054–3060.
182. Park SK, Kim GH, Jeong SS, et al. The effects according to the timing of thoracic radiotherapy in limited stage small cell lung cancer. *Tuberc Respir Dis.* 1996;43:903–915.
183. Turrisi AT III, Kim K, Blum R, et al. Twice-daily compared with once-daily thoracic radiotherapy in limited small-cell lung cancer treated concurrently with cisplatin and etoposide. *N Engl J Med.* 1999;340:265–271.
184. Prophylactic Cranial Irradiation Overview Collaborative Group. Cranial irradiation for preventing brain metastases of small cell lung cancer in patients in complete remission. *Cochrane Database Syst Rev.* 2000; 4:CD002805.
185. Vachani C. Prophylactic cranial irradiation (PCI) in extensive stage small cell lung cancer (ES-SCLC) (EORTC 22993–08993. Presented at the annual meeting of the American Society for Therapeutic Radiotherapy and Oncology, October 2007 http://www.oncolink.com/conferences/article.cfm?c=3&s=47&ss=267&id=1690. Accessed November 30, 2009.
186. Inoue A, Kunitoh H, Sekine I, et al. Radiation pneumonitis in lung cancer patients: a retrospective study of risk factors and the long-term prognosis. *Int J Radiat Oncol Biol Phys.* 2001;49:649–655.
187. Inzeo D, Haughney A. Laser therapy in the management of lung cancer. *Clin J Oncol Nurs.* 2004;8:94–95.
188. Stewart AJ, Mutyala S, Holloway, CL, Colson YL, Devlin PM. Intraoperative seed placement for thoracic malignancyd. A review of technique, indications, and published literature. *Brachytherapy.* 2009;8:63–69.
189. Roy AM, Bent, C, Fotheringham, T. Radiofrequency ablation of lung lesions: practical applications and tips. *Curr Probl Diagn Radiol.* 2009;38:44–52.
190. Langer CJ. Neglected and underrepresented populations: elderly and performance status 2 patients with advanced stage non-small cell lung cancer. *Clin Lung Cancer.* 2006;7:S126-S137.
191. The International Adjuvant Lung Cancer Trial Collaborative Group. Cisplatin-based adjuvant chemotherapy in patients with completely resected non-small-cell lung cancer. *N Engl J Med.* 2004;350:351–360.
192. Winton T, Livingston R, Johnson D, et al. Vinorelbine plus cisplatin vs observation in resected non-small-cell lung cancer. *N Engl J Med.* 2005;352:2589–2597.
193. Douillard JY, Rosell R, De Lena M, et al. Adjuvant vinorelbine plus cisplatin versus observation in patients with completely resected stage IB-IIIA non-small-cell lung cancer (Adjuvant Navelbine International Trialist Association [ANITA]): A randomised controlled trial. *Lancet Oncol.* 2006;7:719–727.
194. Strauss GM, Herndon JE, Maddaus MA, et al. Adjuvant paclitaxel plus carboplatin compared with observation in stage IB non-small cell lung cancer: CALGB 9633 with the Cancer and Leukemia Group B, Radiation Therapy Oncology Group, and North Central Cancer Treatment Group Study Groups. *J Clin Oncol.* 2008;26:5043–5051.
195. Bria E, Gralla RJ, Raftopoulos H, et al. Magnitude of benefit of adjuvant chemotherapy for non-small cell lung cancer: Meta-analysis of randomized clinical trials. *Lung Cancer.* 2009;63:50–57.
196. Rosell R, Gatzmeir U, Betticher DC, et al. Phase III randomized trial comparing paclitaxel/carboplatin with paclitaxel/cisplatin in patients with advanced non-small cell lung cancer: a cooperative multinational trial. *Ann Oncol.* 2002;13:1539–1549.
197. Rodriguez J, Pawell J, Pluzanska A, et al. A multicenter randomized phase III study of docetaxel + cisplatin and docetaxel + carboplatin versus vinorelbine + cisplatin in chemotherapy naïve patients with advanced and metastatic non-small cell lung cancer. [Abstract 1252] *Pro Am Soc Clin Oncol.* 2001;20:314a.
198. Carretta A, Ciriaco P, Melloni G, et al. Results of surgical treatment after neoadjuvant chemotherapy for stage III non-small cell lung cancer. *World J Surg.* 2008;32:2636–2642.
199. Edelman MJ. Neoadjuvant chemotherapy and chemoradiotherapy for non-small cell lung cancer: current status and future prospects. *Exp Opin Pharmacother.* 2003;4:843–852.
200. Auperin A, Rolland E, Curran WJ, et al. Concomitant radiochemotherapy RT-CT versus sequential RT-CT in locally advanced non-small cell lung cancer (NSLCLC): a meta-analysis using individual patient data from randomized clinical trials. IASLC 2007;A1–05:S310.
201. Mina LA, Neubauer MA, Ansari RH, et al. Phase III trial cisplatin (P) plus etoposide (E) plus concurrent chest radiation (XRT) with or without consolidation docetaxel (D) in patients (pts) with inoperable stage III non-small cell lung cancer (NSCLC): HOG LUN 01–24/USO-023—Updated results. *J Clin Oncol* 26: 2008 (May 20 Suppl; abstr 7519).
202. Hanna N, Neubauer M, Ansari R, et al. Phase III trial of cisplatin (P) plus etoposide (E) plus concurrent chest radiation (XRT) with or without consolidation docetaxel (D) in patients (pts) with inoperable stage III non-small cell lung cancer (NSCLC): HOG LUN 01–24/USO-023. *J Clin Oncol* 2005;23(16S):7512.
203. Kelly K, Chansky K, Gaspar LE, et al. Updated analysis of SWOG 0023: a randomized phase III trial of gefitinib versus placebo maintenance after definitive chemoradiation followed by docetaxel in patients with locally advanced stage III non-small cell lung cancer. *J Clin Oncol* 2007;25(18S):7513.
204. Nakamura M, Koizumi T, Hayasaka M, et al. Cisplatin and weekly docetaxel with concurrent thoracic radiotherapy for locally advanced stage III non-small-cell lung cancer. *Cancer Chemother Pharmacol.* 2009;63:1091–1096.
205. Blackstock AW, Socinski MA, Bogart J, et al. Induction plus concurrent chemotherapy with high-dose (74 Gy) 3-dimensional thoracic radiotherapy in stage III non-small cell lung cancer (NSCLC): Preliminary report of the Cancer and Leukemia Group B (CALGB) 30105. *J Clin Oncol.* 2006;24(18S):7042.
206. Schiller JH, Harrington D, Belani CP, et al. Comparison of four chemotherapy regimens for advanced non-small cell lung cancer. *N Engl J Med.* 2002;346:92–98.
207. Fossella F, Pereira JR, von Pawel J, Pluzanska A, Gorbounova V, Kaukel E, et al. Randomized, multinational phase III study of docetaxel plus

platinum combinations versus vinorelbine plus cisplatin for advanced non-small-cell lung cancer: the TAX 326 Study Group. *J Clin Oncol* 2003;21:3016–3024.
208. Scagliotti GV, Parikh P, von Pawel J, et al. Phase III study comparing cisplatin plus gemcitabine with cisplatin plus pemetrexed in chemotherapy-naïve patients with advanced-stage non-small cell lung cancer. *J Clin Oncol.* 2008;26:3543–3551.
209. Socinski MA, Schell MJ, Peterman A, et al. Phase III trial comparing a defined duration of therapy versus continuous therapy followed by second-line therapy in advanced-stage IIIB/IV non-small cell lung cancer. *J Clin Oncol.* 2002;20:1335–1343.
210. Shepherd FA, Dancey J, Ramlau R, et al: Prospective randomized trial of docetaxel versus best supportive care in patients with non-small-cell lung cancer previously treated with platinum-based chemotherapy. *J Clin Oncol.* 2000;18:2095–2103.
211. Fossella FV, DeVore R, Kerr RN, et al: Randomized phase III trial of docetaxel versus vinorelbine or ifosfamide in patients with advanced non-small-cell lung cancer previously treated with platinum-containing chemotherapy regimens: The TAX 320 Non-Small Cell Lung Cancer Study Group. *J Clin Oncol.* 2000;18:2354–2362.
212. Hanna N, Shepherd FA, Fossella FV, et al. Randomized phase III trial of pemetrexed versus docetaxel in patients with non-small-cell lung cancer previously treated with chemotherapy. *J Clin Oncol.* 2004;22:1589–1597.
213. Shepherd FA, Rodrigues Pereira J, Ciuleanu T, et al. Erlotinib in previously treated non-small-cell lung cancer. *N Engl J Med.* 2005;353:123–132.
214. Langer C, Li S, Schiller J, Tester W, Rapoport BL, Johnson DH. Randomized phase II trial of paclitaxel plus carboplatin or gemcitabine plus cisplatin in eastern cooperative oncology group performance status 2 non-small-cell lung cancer patients: ECOG 1599. *J Clin Oncol.* 2007;25:418–423.
215. Gridelli C. The ELVIS trial: a phase III study of single-agent vinorelbine as first-line treatment in elderly patients with advanced non-small cell lung cancer. Elderly Lung Cancer Vinorelbine Italian Study. *Oncologist.* 2001;6:4s-7s.
216. Sandler AB. Chemotherapy for small cell lung cancer. *Semin Oncol.* 2003;30:9–25.
217. Kosmidis PA, Samantas E, Fountzilas G, Pavlidis N, Apostolopoulou F, Skarlos D. Cisplatin/etoposide versus carboplatin/etoposide chemotherapy and irradiation in small cell lung cancer: a randomized phase III study. Hellenic Cooperative Oncology Group for lung cancer trials. Semin Oncol. 1994;21:23–30.
218. Lara Jr PN, Natale R, Crowley J, et al. Phase III trial of irinotecan/cisplatin with etoposide/cisplatin in extensive-stage small-cell lung cancer: clinical and pharmacogenomic results from SWOG S0124. *J Clin Oncol.* 2009;27:2530–2535.
219. Noda K, Nishiwaki Y, Kawahara M, et al. Irinotecan plus cisplatin compared with etoposide plus cisplatin for extensive stage small cell lung cancer. *N Engl J Med.* 2002;346:85–91.
220. De Jong WK, Groen HJM, Koolen MGJ, et al. Phase III study of cyclophosphamide, doxorubicin, and etoposide compared with carboplatin and paclitaxel in patients with extensive disease small-cell lung cancer. *Eur J Cancer.* 2007;43:2345–2350.
221. Eckhardt J, Depierre A, Ardizzoni A, et al. Pooled analysis of topotecan (T) in the second-line treatment of patients (pts) with sensitive small cell lung cancer. *Proc Am Soc Clin Oncol.* 1997;16:1624 (abstr).
222. von Pawel J, Gatzemeier U, Pujol JL, et al. Phase II comparator study of oral versus intravenous topotecan in patients with chemosensitive small-cell lung cancer. *J Clin Oncol.* 2001;19:1743–1749.
223. Eckhardt JR. Second-line treatment of small-cell lung cancer. *Oncology.* 2003;17:181–188
224. Gronberg BH, Bremnes RM, Aasebo U, et al. A prospective phase II study: high-dose pemetrexed as second-line chemotherapy in small-cell lung cancer. *Lung Cancer.* 2009;63:88–93.
225. Jalal S, Ansari R, Govindan R, et al. Pemetrexed in second-line and beyond small cell lung cancer: A Hoosier Oncology Group phase II study. *J Thorac Oncol.* 2009;4:93–96.
226. Simon GR, Wagner H, American College of Chest Physicians. Small cell lung cancer. *Chest.* 2003;123:259s-271s.
227. Murren J, Glatstein E, Pass HI. Small cell lung cancer. In: DeVita, Jr, Hellman S, Rosenberg SA, eds. *Cancer: Principles and Practice of Oncology (6th ed).* Philadelphia,PA, Lippincott Williams & Wilkins; 2001:983–1018.
228. Gatzemeier U, Pluzanska A, Szczesna A, et al. Phase III study of erlotinib in combination with cisplatin and gemcitabine in advanced non–small-cell lung cancer: The Tarceva Lung Cancer Investigation Trial. *J Clin Oncol.* 2007; 25:1545–1552.
229. Herbst R, Prager D, Hermann R, et al. TRIBUTE: A phase III trial of erlotinib hydrochloride (OSI-774) combined with carboplatin and paclitaxel chemotherapy in advanced non–small-cell lung cancer. *J Clin Oncol.* 2005;23:5892–5899.
230. Sandler A, Gray R, Perry MC, et al. Paclitaxel–carboplatin alone or with bevacizumab for non–small-cell lung cancer. *N Engl J Med.* 355;2542–2550.
231. Pirker R, Pereira JR, Szczesna A, et al. Cetuximab plus chemotherapy in patients with advanced non-small-cell lung cancer (FLEX): an open-label randomized phase III trial. *Lancet.* 2009; 373: 1525–1531.
232. Thatcher N, Chang A, Parikh P, et al. Gefitinib plus best supportive care in previously treated patients with refractory advanced non-small cell lung cancer: results from a randomised, placebo-controlled, multicentre study (Iressa Survival Evaluation in Lung Cancer). *Lancet.* 2005;366:1527–1537.
233. Kim ES, Hirsh V, Mok T, et al. Gefitinib versus docetaxel in previously treated non-small-cell lung cancer (INTEREST): a randomised phase III trial. *Lancet.* 2008;372:1809–1818.
234. Natale RB. Dual targeting of the vascular endothelial growth factor receptor and epidermal growth factor receptor pathways with vandetinib (ZD6474) in patients with advanced or metastatic non-small cell lung cancer *J Thorac Oncol.* 2008; 3:S128-S130.
235. Herbst RS, Sandler A. Bevacizumab and erlotinib: a promising new approach to the treatment of advanced NSCLC. *Oncologist.* 2008;13:1166–1176.
236. Gridelli D, Maione P, Del Gaizo F, et al. Sorafenib and sunitinib in the treatment of advanced non-small cell lung cancer. *Oncologist.* 2007;12:191–200.
237. Sequist LV, Lynch TJ. EGFR tyrosine kinase inhibitors in lung cancer: an evolving story. *Annu Rev Med.* 2008;59:79–92.
238. Pham D, Kris MG, Riely GJ, et al. Use of cigarette-smoking history to estimate the likelihood of mutations in epidermal growth factor receptor gene exons 19 and 21 in lung adenocarcinomas. *J Clin Oncol.* 2006;24:1700–1704.
239. Sequist LV, Joshi VA, Jänne PA, et al. Response to treatment and survival of patients with non-small cell lung cancer undergoing somatic EGFR mutation testing. *Oncologist.* 2007;12:90–98.
240. Herbst RS, Lippman SM. Molecular signatures of lung cancer-toward personalized therapy. *N Engl J Med.* 2007;356:76–78.
241. Eberhard DA, Johnson BE, Amler LC, et al. Mutations in the epidermal growth factor receptor and in KRAS are predictive and prognostic indicators in patients with non-small-cell lung cancer treated with chemotherapy alone and in combination with erlotinib. *J Clin Oncol.* 2005;23:5900–5909.
242. de Rijke JM, Schouten LJ, ten Velde GPM, et al. Influence of age, comorbidity, and performance status on the choice of treatment for patients with non-small cell lung cancer; results of a population-based study. *Lung Cancer.* 2004;46:233–245.
243. Boyar M, Raftopoulos H. Supportive care in lung cancer. *Hematol Oncol Clin North Am.* 2005;19:369–387.
244. Shen J, Glaspy J. Acupuncture: evidence and implications for cancer supportive care. *Cancer Pract.* 2001;9:147–150.
245. Bloomfield DJ. Should bisphosphonates be part of the standard therapy of patients with multiple myeloma or bone metastases from other cancers? An evidence-based review. *J Clin Oncol.* 1998;16: 1218–1225.

246. Cooley ME, Short TH, Moriarty HJ. Symptom prevalence, distress, and change over time in adults receiving treatment for lung cancer. *Psychooncology.* 2003;12:694–708.
247. Wright JR, Ung YC, Julian JA, et al. Randomized, double-blind, placebo-controlled trial of erythropoietin in non-small-cell lung cancer with disease-related anemia. *J Clin Oncol.* 2007;26:1027–1032.
248. Kvale PA, Simoff M, Prakash UB; American College of Chest Physicians. Lung cancer. Palliative care. *Chest.* 2003;123:284S-311S.
249. Escalante CP, Martin CG, Elting LS, et al. Dyspnea in cancer patients. Etiology, resource utilization, and survival-implications in a managed care world. *Cancer.* 1996;78:1314–1319.
250. Ringbaek TJ, Viskum K, Lange P. Non-continuous home oxygen therapy: utilization, symptomatic effect and prognosis, data from a national register on home oxygen therapy. *Respir Med.* 2001;95:980–985.

CHAPTER

# 60

Sharon D. Manson, RN, MS, ACNP, Carlene Porter, RN, MSN, ACNP

# Lymphomas

## INTRODUCTION

Hodgkin's lymphoma (HL) and non-Hodgkin's lymphoma (NHL) constitute a diverse group of cancers of the immune system. Arising from a single malignant lymphoid clone, the lymphoma may be B cell, T cell, or natural killer (NK) cell in origin. It is thought that lymphomagenesis results from a genetic change or series of changes that allow the cell to evade programmed cell death (apoptosis) or to grow uncontrollably. The subtype of lymphoma and its degree of aggressiveness depend on the precise genetic changes and the stage of lymphocyte maturation at which these changes occurred. During the disease course, a lymphoma can acquire additional abnormalities that may change its aggressiveness and prognosis.

The Leukemia and Lymphoma Society predicts that there will be 74,490 new cases of lymphoma in the US in 2009, with 20,790 deaths being attributed to this disease.[1] NHL is expected to account for 65,980 of the cases, while the much rarer HL is predicted to account for 8,510 cases.[1] In the US, the incidence of lymphoma increases with age and tends to show a male predominance. Since the 1970s, the incidence of NHL has almost doubled. According to the National Cancer Institute (NCI)'s Surveillance, Epidemiology, and End Result (SEER) program,[2] the following subgroups have experienced a steady increase in NHL: young whites (age 15–24 years), older blacks (age ≥ 55 years), and females (age 25–54 years). Suspected reasons for these increases include a compromised immune system (eg, from human immunodeficiency virus [HIV] infection and the use of immunosuppressive drugs), environmental carcinogens, other infectious agents, and genetic predisposition. Unfortunately, the majority of people who will be diagnosed with lymphoma have no known risk factors.

## LYMPHOID TISSUES AND THE IMMUNE SYSTEM

The immune system is a highly integrated, complex mechanism that has evolved to help the body protect itself against invading microbes such as viruses, bacteria, fungi, and parasites. Another important function of the immune system is to differentiate "self-antigens" from "nonself," or foreign, antigens and to orchestrate specific and nonspecific measures to destroy the foreign antigens. The main organs of the immune system are scattered throughout the body and are referred to as the lymphatics or lymphoid tissues. Malignant lymphomas arise from these tissues.

The lymphoid tissues can be divided into primary and secondary lymphoid organs (Figure 60-1). The primary organs are represented by the bone marrow, where the lymphocytes originate, and the thymus, where T lymphocytes mature. The thymus is a large organ located in the mediastinum that grows rapidly in the first 2 years of life, grows more slowly through puberty, and then slowly involutes. Adipose and connective tissue replace thymic tissue, and the thymus shrinks in size. Once the maturation of T lymphocytes is complete, the lymphocytes migrate to the secondary lymphoid tissues through the circulation. B lymphocytes derive their name from the bone marrow and T lymphocytes from the thymus.

The lymph nodes, spleen, and mucosa-associated lymphoid tissues (MALTs) form the secondary lymphatics. The MALTs are clumps of lymphocytes that protect the respiratory and gastrointestinal epithelium. These tissues include the tonsils, adenoids, appendix, and Peyer's patches, which are found in the small intestine. Those tissues associated with the gut have been named gut-associated lymphoid tissues, and those associated with the bronchial tree are called bronchial-associated lymphoid tissues. Singular lymph nodules are found in and below the mucosa of the respiratory tract, the gastrointestinal tract, the urinary tract, and the vagina. The blood and the lymphatic vessels that transport lymphocytes can also be considered part of this system.

Extracellular fluid, known as lymph, is drained via the afferent lymphatics to the lymph nodes. This fluid also carries antigens from sites of infection to the lymph nodes. Lymph nodes are encapsulated, highly organized structures that facilitate lymphocyte maturation and differentiation. They are found scattered throughout the body in the neck, axilla, chest, abdomen, and groin (Figure 60-2). The lymph

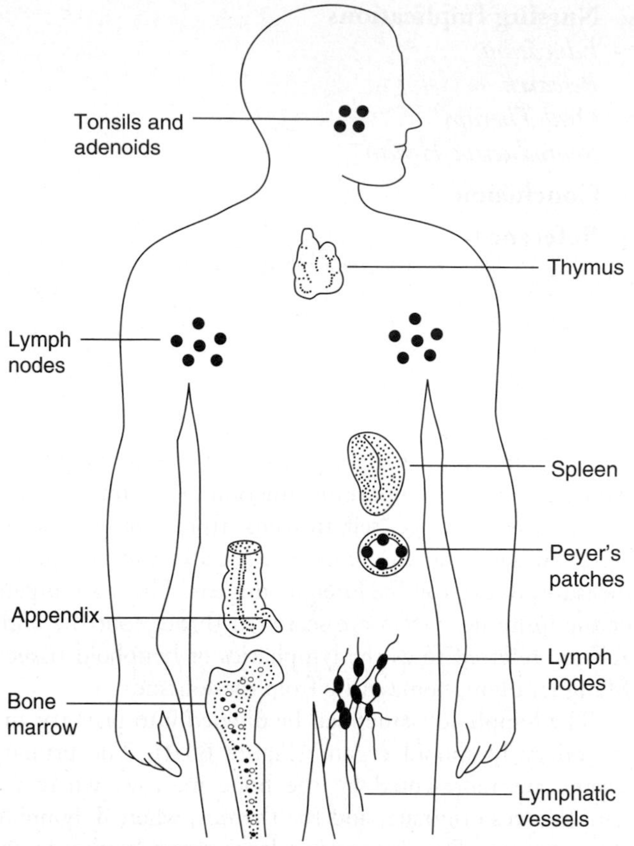


**FIGURE 60-1**

Organs of the immune system.

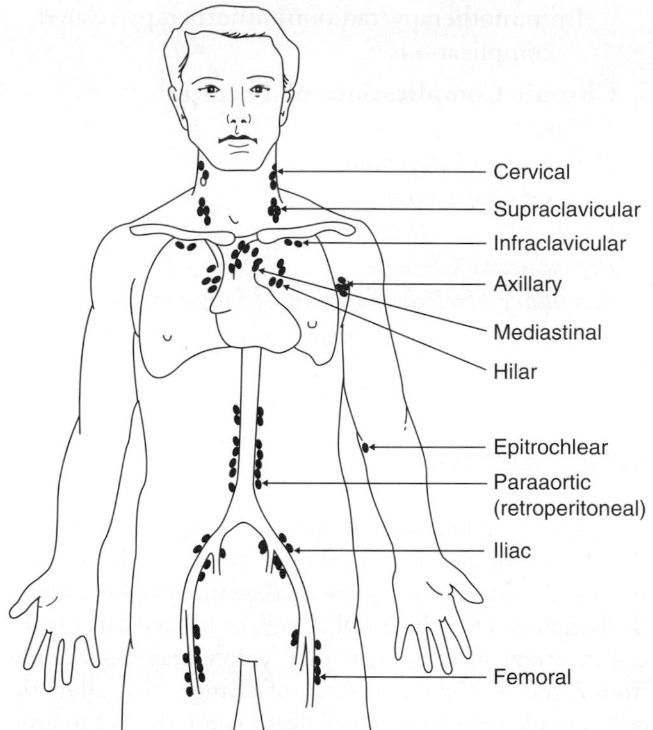


**FIGURE 60-2**

Major lymph node groups.

node has an outer cortex and an inner medulla. The cortex contains follicles comprising largely B lymphocytes and a small number of T cells that facilitate B-cell differentiation. Some follicles contain germinal centers and are called secondary follicles. Deeper paracortical areas selectively concentrate T lymphocytes and dendritic cells. The medulla contains strands of T and B lymphocytes, macrophages, and antibody-secreting plasma cells. The architecture of the lymph node can be seen in Figure 60-3.

Lymph leaves the lymph node through the efferent lymphatics in the medulla and is transported to the thoracic duct. This duct returns the lymph to the circulatory system through the left subclavian vein. The organization of the spleen is similar to that of a lymph node; however, antigens enter the spleen through the blood, not the lymph.

Lymphomas are preeminently a malignancy of the lymphocytes, and the process by which a lymphoid neoplasm is generated may be envisioned as a series of cellular changes in which a normal lymphoid cell (or cell clone) becomes refractory to the regulation of its differentiation and proliferation. The unregulated growth is due to genetic mutations, chromosomal translocations, deletions, and insertions of foreign genes into the cell. Translocations occur when genetic material from one chromosome becomes rearranged with another chromosome, altering the expression of adjacent genes. This alters the expression and function of the genes, disrupting control of cell growth. Genes that result in the development of cancer when their expression and function are altered are called oncogenes. Deletions result in a loss of genetic material in a particular gene, whereas insertions result in the addition of other genetic material into a particular chromosome. These alterations may also result in deficiencies of cell growth and function. Follicular lymphomas (FLs) are believed to be tumors of germinal center B cells in which the cells fail to undergo programmed death (apoptosis) because they have developed a chromosomal translocation. Translocations, deletions, and insertions may be identified microscopically when dividing cells (metaphases) are analyzed.

Once transformed, the new clone of malignant cells follows the behavior pattern of the stage at which lymphocyte alteration took place. For example, if the function of the maturing lymphocyte is secretion of an antibody protein, the tumor cells will continue to secrete the antibody, albeit in abnormal quantities. The neoplasms' tendency to mimic the normal cells' differentiation serves as the basis for their classification.

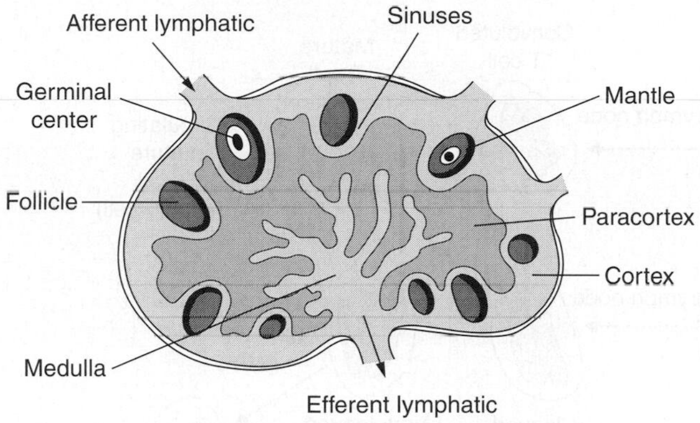


**B-CELL LYMPHOMAS**

*Follicle*
- Nodular lymphoma
- Large cell lymphoma
- Burkitt's lymphoma

*Germinal Center/Mantle Zone*
- Lymphocytic lymphoma
- Mantle zone lymphoma (intermediate differentiation)

*Medulla*
- Chronic lymphocytic leukemia
- Well-differentiated lymphocytic lymphoma
- Waldenström's macroglobulinemia

**T-CELL LYMPHOMAS**

*Paracortex*
- Perlpheral T-cell lymphoma
- Mycosis fungoides
- Sézary syndrome
- Acute lymphoblastic leukemia
- T-cell lymphoblastic lymphoma

*Miscellaneous Malignancies*

Sinus Region
- Malignant histiocytosis
- Kt-1 large cell lymphoma

**FIGURE 60-3**

Sites of lymphocyte transformation in the lymph node.

The association of certain malignancies with congenital or acquired immunodeficiency states and the bimodal distribution of cancer in the very young and the very old suggest that an immature or debilitated immune system predisposes an individual to developing neoplasia. Malignant lymphomas are strongly linked with congenital immunodeficiency disorders such as Wiskott-Aldrich syndrome, Klinefelter syndrome, and ataxia telangiectasia and in acquired diseases such as HIV infection. Patients who have had prior organ or stem cell transplantation are at higher risk for the development of lymphomas. The etiology of these posttransplant lymphoproliferative disorders is thought to be multifactorial, including immunosuppression (often drug-induced) and the presence of Epstein–Barr virus (EBV). EBV and other viruses have been implicated in the etiology of lymphoma. Likewise, some bacteria or the immunological response to the antigens found on the bacteria may contribute to the formation of malignant cells. This relationship has been best identified with the *Helicobacter pylori* bacterium. The chronic inflammatory process activated by many autoimmune diseases (eg, rheumatoid arthritis, systemic lupus erythematosus, and Sjögren's syndrome) and the immunosuppressive treatment of these disorders may predispose these individuals to lymphoma.

Lymphocytes, like other blood cell types, originate in the bone marrow from pluripotent stem cells. Pluripotent stem cells have the ability to self-replicate and differentiate into myeloid stem cells or lymphoid stem cells. Immature lymphocyte precursors arise from the commitment of the lymphoid stem cells. Subsequent maturation of these primitive cells leads to the development of mature T lymphocytes and B lymphocytes, as illustrated in Figure 60-4.

Lymphocytes are responsible for cellular and humoral immunity, which are both important immunological defenses. An early step in the differentiation of the maturing lymphocyte occurs when the cell is programmed either by the bone marrow (bursa equivalent) or the thymus to become a B lymphocyte or T lymphocyte. Plasma cells develop from B lymphocytes and produce circulating antibodies against foreign antigens upon exposure. These B lymphocytes serve as the basis of humoral immunity. Memory cells are also produced to establish long-lasting immunity. Cellular immunity consists of circulating T lymphocytes that have developed specificity against foreign antigens. T lymphocytes, when stimulated, will clone into subsets of cells that include cytotoxic, suppressor, helper, and memory T cells. These subsets work together to kill identified targets and to regulate the immune process. Although the humoral and cellular arms of the immune system are distinct entities, they have a high degree of interaction and together protect the host against foreign proteins.

Approximately 90% of lymphomas worldwide have a B-cell origin,[3] and most patients initially present with disease involving the lymph nodes or bone marrow and, to a lesser degree, the liver and spleen. Extranodal disease—either extension from a node or an isolated site—can be observed either at the time of diagnosis or during the course of the disease. If the extranodal involvement occurs as the

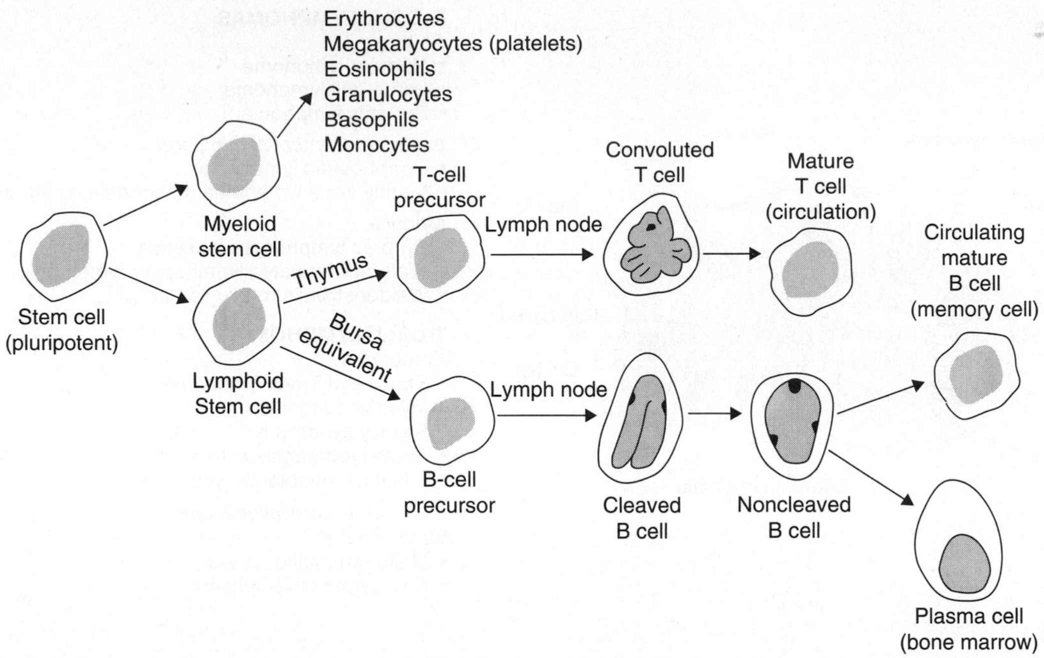


**FIGURE 60-4**

Maturation sequence of the lymphocyte.

only site of the lymphoma, it is called primary extranodal lymphoma. This condition can include tissues such as the central nervous system (CNS), eye, paranasal sinuses, skin, lung, pericardium, gastrointestinal tract, testicle, spleen, bone, bone marrow, genitourinary tract, and, rarely, the heart, salivary glands, adrenals, and thyroid.

Lymphomas with a T-cell origin are less frequently observed but often present with more aggressive features. They are known to be among the most aggressive of all hematological neoplasms, although variability is seen. T-cell lymphomas are often grouped with neoplasms that arise from NK cells. Mature T-lymphocyte malignancies arise from postthymic T cells. Because NK cells are closely related and share many properties, the 2 types of cancers are often considered together.

## DIAGNOSIS

The diagnosis of HL or NHL is made on the basis of biopsy and histopathology of the tumor. The clinical presentation and subsequent assessment of the patient are often quite similar between these 2 malignancies and lead to a staging work-up. In this section, the diagnostic evaluation will be discussed in general terms. Each pathologic subtype of lymphoma may have unique characteristics, which will be noted in the discussion of that specific disease entity.

## CLINICAL MANIFESTATIONS

Lymphadenopathy is the most common presentation in patients with lymphoma. It may be unilateral or bilateral. Characteristic nodes are nontender, firm, and rubbery. Some patients with HL report pain at involved lymph node sites with alcohol consumption. The size of the lymph node varies, as does the growth pattern. Patients may report a slow, insidious growth of the node or even a waxing and waning pattern. Patients with a more aggressive lymphoma may report rapid growth of the mass and spread to contiguous or noncontiguous nodes. Lymph nodes of the same region may coalesce, forming a fixed mass. In such a case, individual nodes may be impossible to distinguish and measure.

Hodgkin's lymphoma presents most commonly in the cervical and supraclavicular area nodes (55%–58%) and mediastinal nodes (59%), with involvement of axillary and inguinal nodes being reported in less than 15% of the patients. At diagnosis, 27% of patients have evidence of splenic involvement.[4] Mediastinal lymphadenopathy may be noted on routine chest x-ray, or complaints of cough and dyspnea may have led to a chest radiograph being performed.

Patients with NHL are more likely to present with extranodal disease. Approximately 25% to 50% of NHL cases show evidence of extranodal disease and may present with signs and symptoms related to its presence.

The liver or spleen may be involved in both HL and NHL. Related symptoms include pain, abdominal complaints, anorexia, early satiety, and even signs of bowel obstruction.

Lymphoma can occasionally infiltrate the skin. These lesions appear as red or purplish nodules, primarily in the head and neck region. Lytic bone lesions may be seen in the femurs, pelvis, vertebrae, ribs, and skull. Affected patients frequently complain of bone pain, which leads to the diagnosis of lymphoma. These lesions must be differentiated from bone metastasis, from solid tumors, and from the lytic lesions observed in multiple myeloma. On rare occasions, lymphomas may present as oncologic emergencies such as cardiac tamponade, superior vena cava syndrome, spinal cord compression, increased intracranial pressure, or sepsis. These presentations are often due to the growth of aggressive lymphomas resulting in obstruction of lymphatic or circulatory vessels. Solitary brain lymphomas are being reported with increasing frequency and are associated with AIDS or iatrogenic immunosuppression.[5] These mass lesions may result in headaches, seizures, and changes in mental status. Another common CNS manifestation is leptomeningeal spread, which results in cranial nerve palsies, meningeal irritation, and increased intracranial pressure. Replacement of the bone marrow by lymphoma can lead to a deficiency of the normal white blood cells (WBCs), red blood cells, and platelets, resulting in a picture similar to that seen with leukemia.

It is important to determine whether the patient has experienced night sweats, fever, or unintentional weight loss of more than 10% of body weight within 6 months of presentation. The presence of these "B" symptoms (2 of the 3 symptoms noted here) has an unfavorable prognostic significance. Patients with NHL are more likely than patients with HL to present with B symptoms, but these events have less prognostic significance in NHL. Other characteristic symptoms of lymphoma include generalized pruritus and fatigue, but the significance of these symptoms is unclear. Pruritus is found in as many as 30% of patients with HL prior to diagnosis.[6] Occasionally, patients with HL may complain of cyclical fevers, called Pel Ebstein fevers.

## BIOPSY

Few areas of pathology have evoked as much controversy and confusion as the classification of lymphoma. Nevertheless, following history and physical examination, pathologic diagnosis is required. A biopsy of the involved tissue is done to formulate the diagnosis of lymphoma. In most situations, morphology (the way the cell looks) and immunophenotyping (the markers identified on the tumor) done via flow cytometry are sufficient for diagnosis of the subtype of lymphoma. In addition, immunoglobulin and T-cell receptor gene rearrangements are often performed on the involved tissues.

Other studies include polymerase chain reaction for *BCL-1* (B-cell lymphoma) and *BCL-2*, immunohistochemistry studies, and cytogenetics. Cytogenetic studies assess for translocations, insertions, and deletions, which may be reflective of a particular subclassification of lymphoma or may have prognostic significance. Florescent in situ hybridization (FISH) is a method of analyzing large numbers of cells to assess for a particular genetic abnormality. This test may be employed if a specific type of lymphoma is suspected and can aid in the diagnosis or monitoring for disease status following treatment. All available data are utilized to define the disease, predict response, and refine treatment plans.

## STAGING

Accurate staging is critical in the management of patients with lymphoma. It directs the intensity of treatment and allows for less toxic therapy to be administered when minimal disease is present, decreasing the risk of secondary malignancies and improving quality of life. Clinical, pathologic, and radiographic data are utilized to determine the stage of disease. Staging laparotomy, considered controversial for years, is rarely indicated today. On rare occasions, surgery may be required to relieve an obstruction or to obtain pathologic diagnosis.

The Ann Arbor staging classification system was created for the staging of HL.[7] Although it is not optimal for the staging of NHL, it has been viewed for years as the gold standard. The Ann Arbor staging system identifies 4 specific stages on the basis of the number and location of lymph node regions or extranodal tissues determined to be involved. A modification of the Ann Arbor staging system was made to include the identification of those individuals with extranodal or splenic involvement. Bulky disease may also be noted by the subscript "x." Known as the Cotswold modification of the Ann Arbor system, it is outlined in Table 60-1.[8] The absence of B symptoms is denoted with an "A" after the appropriate stage; the presence of B symptoms is indicated with a "B."

## LABORATORY TESTS

Laboratory studies performed as initial staging include blood chemistries and a complete blood count. Elevations of the hepatic transaminase levels (aspartate transaminase and alanine transaminase) and, more specifically, an alkaline phosphatase level greater than twice the normal limit suggest liver involvement.[9] Fractionation of alkaline phosphatase may be useful in identifying the source of disease (ie, liver vs bone). Unfortunately, these laboratory findings are nonspecific and may be elevated without radiographic evidence of disease. Bone marrow involvement may result in a deficiency of the normal mature cells produced in

**TABLE 60-1**

**Cotswold Modification of Ann Arbor Staging System**

| Stage | Criteria |
|---|---|
| I | Involvement of a single lymph node region<br>or |
| $I_E$ | Involvement of a single extranodal organ or site |
| II | Involvement of two or more lymph node regions on the same side of the diaphragm<br>or |
| $II_E$ | Involvement of a contiguous extranodal organ or site |
| III | Involvement of lymph node regions on both sides of the diaphragm<br>or |
| $III_S$ | Involvement on both sides of the diaphragm including spleen<br>or |
| $III_E$ | Involvement on both sides of the diaphragm with a contiguous extranodal organ or site<br>or |
| $III_{ES}$ | Involvement on both sides of the diaphragm including the spleen and a contiguous extranodal organ or site |
| IV | Multiple or disseminated sites of disease; may involve multiple extranodal organs or sites with or without lymphatic involvement |

*Notes*: All cases should be subclassified with either "A" to indicate the absence of B symptoms or "B" to indicate the presence of B symptoms. Clinical staging (CS) is determined by history, physical examination, biopsy, and laboratory and radiographic tests. Pathologic staging (PS) is determined by biopsy of strategic sites and histopathological information.

the marrow, leading to anemia and thrombocytopenia. Leukocytosis is often noted at presentation or at other points of disease activity. Lymphopenia is found in 50% of individuals diagnosed with HL and is a poor prognostic factor. Eosinophilia may also be seen. The erythrocyte sedimentation rate is characteristically elevated in HL and may be used as a crude marker for disease activity. This test has been employed more commonly in Europe than in the United States.[9] The *BCL-2* gene, present in some lymphomas, corresponds to a poor response to chemotherapy and reduced survival. The tumor or the blood can be analyzed for the presence of this gene.

Due to patchy infiltration of lymphoma, bilateral bone marrow aspirate and biopsies are performed to assess for evidence of disease. Flow cytometry and cytogenetic studies are often done on the bone marrow specimens to further characterize the tumor.

## RADIOGRAPHIC TESTS

Computerized tomography (CT) scans of the chest, abdomen, and pelvis are completed at diagnosis to delineate sites of disease that may not be clinically evident. A CT scan or magnetic resonance imaging (MRI) scan of the brain may be performed as well as a lumbar puncture with analysis of the CNS, if symptoms dictate it. Gallium scans have historically been performed as part of staging of lymphomas. If the tumor is positive for gallium, this scan will detect areas of disease and may be used in follow-up to determine response.

Positron emission tomography (PET) scanning is a novel imaging technique that uses a radiolabeled glucose analog. The glycolytic activity is greater in tissues with metabolic activity. A higher uptake is observed in malignant tissues and, to a lesser degree, in areas of inflammation. PET scans appear to detect more disease sites above and below the diaphragm than gallium scans and have better sensitivity in detecting disease in the spleen. They may identify lymphomatous organ involvement that would otherwise not be documented by CT or MRI.[10,11] PET scanning typically results in the increase of the Ann Arbor stage, but rarely results in a change in treatment.[12] The reliability of PET scans in detecting malignant disease is greater than 90% in classical Hodgkin's disease (HD), diffuse B-cell lymphoma, FL, and mantle cell lymphoma (MCL). They are less reliable (50%-90% positive) in marginal zone or MALT lymphoma and small lymphocytic lymphoma (SLL).[11] Some lymphomas may have poor sensitivity to PET scanning. PET scans cannot replace bone marrow biopsies. A pooled analysis of 587 patients with lymphoma from 13 different studies reports only a sensitivity of 51%, with a specificity of 91%.[13] PET scans, like gallium scans, cannot quantify the dimensions of the tumor and may be used only as an adjunct to CT scanning. The cost and the limited number of PET scanning units may impact the use of this technology. The use of combination PET/CT scans is gaining popularity.

## INTERNATIONAL PROGNOSTIC INDEX

Sixteen institutions and cooperative groups in the US, Canada, and Europe participated in a project to develop a model for prognostic factors for patients with aggressive NHL.[14] Aggressive NHLs are those lymphomas that tend to grow rapidly and refer to intermediate-grade and high-grade lymphomas. Patients with aggressive NHL who were treated with similar regimens between 1982 and 1987 were evaluated for clinical and laboratory features that were predictive for overall survival (OS) and relapse-free survival. This analysis resulted in the development of an International Prognostic Index (IPI) based on age, stage of disease, serum lactate dehydrogenase (LDH), performance status, and number of extranodal disease sites. Four risk groups were identified, with 5-year survival rates of 73%, 51%, 43%, and 26%, respectively.[14] While the IPI was originally developed for NHL patients with aggressive tumors, it has since been analyzed with various types of lymphoma.[15] The model has been successful in identifying patients with high-risk and low-risk FL and other indolent, low-grade disease.[16–18] A working group in the Netherlands validated the IPI in low-grade, intermediate-grade, and high-grade lymphoma.[19] Table 60-2[20,21] details the IPI scoring.

# HODGKIN'S DISEASE

## HISTORICAL PERSPECTIVE

In 1832, Thomas Hodgkin, an English physician, described clinical data and postmortem findings of 7 patients with a relentlessly progressive, ultimately fatal, tumorous enlargement of the lymph nodes, liver, and spleen.[22] His recognition that these pathologic changes represented a primary proliferation inherent in the nodal tissues themselves rather than a reactive, inflammatory process was extremely important and insightful. Prior to that time, lymphomas often were mistaken for a common infectious disease, tuberculosis of the lymph nodes.

More than 3 decades after Hodgkin's paper was presented, Samuel Wilks rediscovered the original manuscript. After further clinical clarification and elaboration, he attached the eponym *Hodgkin's disease* to the phenomenon in 1865.[23] A review of the original tissues nearly 100 years later demonstrated that Hodgkin's cases actually represented examples of what we now call HD as well as NHL. All lymphomas were called HD until around the turn of the century, when the giant, multinucleated cells in the nodal material of HD patients were characterized by Reed[24] and Sternberg,[25] and their names have been associated with the pathognomonic cell of HL ever since. Subsequently, those lymphomas demonstrating the Reed-Sternberg cell were classified as HL and those in which the cell was absent were called lymphosarcoma or reticulum cell sarcoma and later NHL. Although the precise nature and origin of the Reed-Sternberg cell remain uncertain, it is believed that this cell is B cell in origin and useful in predicting prognosis. Lymphocytic malignancies that are similar in pathologic appearance behave differently depending on the presence or absence of this cell.

Today, diagnosis of HD requires 2 components. First, the presence of Reed-Sternberg cells must be documented. Second, the diagnostic cells must be identified within an appropriate cellular background that is composed of a polymorphous mixture of apparently normal inflammatory cells in various proportions.

## EPIDEMIOLOGY

Hodgkin's disease accounts for less than 1% of all new cancers in the Unites States and less than 15% of all lymphomas. Approximately 8510 new cases of HD were diagnosed in 2009.[1] Although a relatively uncommon disease, it has been among the most widely studied over the years and is considered among the most curable, with a 5-year survival of greater than 86%. There is a slightly higher incidence in males than in females over all age spans (3:2 ratio), but in childhood HL the relative incidence in males is even greater (7:4).[26]

In Western countries, HL has a bimodal age distribution. The rates rise through early life, peak in the third decade, and decline through age 45, at which time the incidence again increases. Geographic patterns have been identified in the 3 major age groups: children, young adults, and older adults. In childhood, mixed cellular HL is seen commonly in less developed countries. More favorable subtypes are seen in developed countries in young adulthood. Studies have supported the increased risk of HD in young adults with high socioeconomic status. High intelligence, higher education, small family size, early birth order, and single-family dwellings have all been identified as factors associated with higher risk.[27] There is a clear association between infectious exposure to EBV and HL. The EBV genome has been seen in about 40% of the Reed-Sternberg cells in patients with HL,[28] with a 3-fold increased risk in patients with a history of mononucleosis.

## ETIOLOGY

Many reports have suggested an infectious etiology of HL. B symptoms such as fever and chills, as well as leukocytosis and pathologic changes similar to a granulomatous process, support this theory. Clusters of reported cases have even led to the question of infectious transmission. Significant controversy remains regarding this hypothesis, and many believe that statistical analyses show that these cases likely occurred by chance.[29] Nevertheless, it is has clearly been

**TABLE 60-2**

**Prognostic Indices for Non-Hodgkin's Lymphoma**

| Clincal Feature | IPI Points | R-IPI[20] (For DLBC NHL) Points | FLIPI[21] Points |
|---|---|---|---|
| Age ≥ 60 years | 1 | 1 | 1 |
| LDH > Normal | 1 | 1 | 1 |
| ECOG status 2–4 | 1 | 1 | – |
| > 1 Extranodal sites | 1 | 1 | – |
| > 4 Nodal sites | — | – | 1 |
| Ann Arbor stage III or IV | 1 | 1 | 1 |
| Hemoglobin < 12g/dL | — | – | 1 |

*Add up points in appropriate column to determine number of risk factors*

| | IPI | R-IPI (For DLBC NHL) | FLIPI |
|---|---|---|---|
| 0 | Low | Very good | Low |
| 1 | Low | Good | Low |
| 2 | Low-intermediate | Good | Intermediate |
| 3 | High-intermediate | Poor | High |
| 4 | High | Poor | High |
| 5 | High | Poor | High |

**IPI**

| Risk Group | Complete Response (%) | 5 Year Relapse Free Survival (%) | 5 Year Overall Survival (%) |
|---|---|---|---|
| Low | 87 | 70 | 73 |
| Low-Intermediate | 67 | 50 | 51 |
| High-Intermediate | 55 | 49 | 43 |
| High | 44 | 40 | 26 |

**R-IPI[20]**

| Risk Group | 4 Year Progression Free Survivial (%) | 4 Year Overall Survival (%) |
|---|---|---|
| Very Good | 94 | 94 |
| Good | 80 | 79 |
| Poor | 53 | 55 |

**FLIPI[21]**

| Risk Group | 5 Year Overall Survival (%) | 10 Year Overall Survival (%) |
|---|---|---|
| Low | 91 | 71 |
| Intermediate | 78 | 51 |
| High | 53 | 36 |

documented that a prior history of mononucleosis with serologically confirmed EBV results in a 3-fold increased risk of HL in young adults. In developing countries, exposure to EBV occurs in early childhood. In several studies, 85% to 100% of pediatric patients diagnosed with HL had associated EBV exposure.[30,31] One study reported that HIV-infected individuals who developed HL had a high frequency of EBV with the Reed-Sternberg cells.[32]

Evidence supports a genetic basis for increased susceptibility to HL. It has been difficult to distinguish genetic influences from environmental factors in these situations, however, and both may contribute to the increased risk of developing lymphoma. There is a 7-fold increased risk for the development of HL in siblings of patients with known disease, with a higher incidence in same-sex siblings.[33]

Cytogenetic clonal abnormalities have been demonstrated in more than half of cases of HL studied. The most common breakpoints reported are similar to those found in NHL, which supports a lymphoid origin for HL. The various cytogenetic abnormalities identified suggest that genetic instability is a significant component of the etiology of HL.

## HISTOLOGICAL CLASSIFICATION AND PATIENT PRESENTATION

Two distinct disease entities make up HD: classical HL and nodular lymphocyte-predominant HL (NLPHL). These 2 lymphomas share the feature that only a minority of the involved tissues contain the Hodgkin and Reed-Sternberg cells, and the majority of the cells appear to be inflammatory and accessory cells. A distinction has been made between these entities because the epidemiology, clinical manifestations, natural history, immunophenotyping, genetics, and association with EBV differ for each.

In 1966, Lukes and Butler established a histological classification system for HL that appeared to correlate well with the known clinical characteristics of the disease. This system was later simplified into the Rye classification and has been widely used.[34] The World Health Organization (WHO) classification mimics the Rye classification, with the exception of the establishment of the nodular lymphocyte predominant HL category. The classical HLs represent the same 4 subclassifications noted in the Rye system: nodular sclerosis, mixed cellularity, lymphocyte rich, and lymphocyte depleted. Many differences in their clinical features and characteristics distinguish these subtypes, but all 4 variants share the same immunophenotyping.

### NODULAR LYMPHOCYTE-PREDOMINANT HODGKIN'S LYMPHOMA

Nodular lymphocyte-predominant Hodgkin's lymphoma accounts for only about 5% of all cases of HL. It affects predominantly males, and the most common age at diagnosis ranges from 30 to 50 years.[35] Most patients present with localized disease involving the cervical, axillary, or inguinal nodes. Only 5% to 20% of patients present with advanced disease. This subtype of HL if diagnosed at an early stage (I or II) is very responsive to therapy and rarely proves fatal. However, advanced stage disease has an unfavorable prognosis.

A small percentage of these patients will have transformation to large B-cell NHL. Morphologically, this monoclonal B-cell neoplasm has a nodular or nodular and diffuse distribution of lymphocytic and/or histiocytic Reed-Sternberg cell variants called L & H cells. Due to the appearance of these large cells, which have folded or multilobulated nuclei, they have also been called "popcorn" cells.[35] The cells phenotypically are positive for CD20, CD79a, BCL-6, and CD45 in nearly all cases.[36]

### CLASSICAL HODGKIN'S LYMPHOMA

The 4 histological types of classical HL account for 95% of all cases of HL.[35] The cervical lymph nodes are involved in 75% of cases; approximately 60% of cases involve mediastinal nodes. Involvement of axillary and paraaortic nodes is less common. The spleen is involved in about 20% of patients and the bone marrow in only 5%. Approximately half of the patients present with localized disease (stage I or II) and half with advanced disease (III or IV). B symptoms are reported to be present in approximately 40% of patients.

*Nodular sclerosis HL* is the most common subtype of HL, accounting for approximately 70% of all cases. The median age at presentation is 28 years, and this disease is unique in that it has no male or female predominance.[35] Mediastinal involvement is very common (approximately 80% of cases), and bulky disease is noted in half of the cases. Bulky mediastinal adenopathy is an adverse risk factor. The spleen is involved in about 10% of cases and the bone marrow in 3% of cases.[37,38] The majority of patients present with stage II disease, and B symptoms are noted in 40% of cases.[39] A nodular growth pattern consistent with classical HL is observed morphologically. Collagen bands surround at least 1 nodule, resulting in fibrosis and thickening of the lymph node capsule. The presence of the lacunar cell, a variant of the Hodgkin Reed-Sternberg cells, is observed, giving this tumor a unique appearance morphologically.[35] The prognosis for patients with nodular sclerosing HL is better than that for patients with mixed cellularity or lymphocyte-depleted subtypes.

*Mixed cellularity HL* represents 20% to 25% of classical HL. It is observed more commonly in patients with HIV infection and in developing countries. The median age at presentation is 37 years, and males account for 70% of cases.[35] Mixed cellularity HL presents more commonly as advanced stage disease, and B symptoms are common. Mediastinal lymph node involvement is uncommon, but the spleen and the bone marrow are involved in approximately 30% and 10% of cases, respectively.[35] Morphologically, the lymph node structure is obliterated. There is no thickening of the lymph node capsule, as is observed in nodular sclerosing HL. Typical Hodgkin Reed-Sternberg cells are found. The background cells are a mixture of cell types, including eosinophils, neutrophils, histiocytes, and plasma cells—hence the name mixed cellularity HL. The prognosis with mixed cellularity HL has historically been slightly worse than that with nodular sclerosis HL and better than that with lymphocyte-depleted HL. New treatment regimens, however, have minimized the differences in prognosis.

*Lymphocyte-rich classical HL* accounts for approximately 5% of all cases of HL. As with mixed cellularity HL, males account for 70% of the cases, but the median age at diagnosis for this variant is the highest of all subtypes of HL.[35] Most patients present with peripheral lymphadenopathy resulting in stage I or II disease. Mediastinal adenopathy and bulky disease are uncommon.[40] The morphology of the lymph node can appear as a nodular pattern or (uncommonly) a diffuse one.[41] Scattered Hodgkin Reed-Sternberg cells are present and small lymphocytes are abundant. Eosinophils and neutrophils are either absent or present in small numbers. Lymphocyte-rich classical HL is often difficult to distinguish morphologically from NLPHL, and immunophenotyping is critical to demonstrate the classical Hodgkin Reed-Sternberg cells.[41] Prognosis is slightly better than that for other subtypes of classical HL and similar to that for NLPHL. Relapse is less common than in NLPHL; if relapse occurs, however, prognosis is less favorable.[40,41]

*Lymphocyte-depleted HL* is the rarest of all subtypes of HL, accounting for less than 5% of all cases.[35] The median age at diagnosis is similar to that for most other forms of HL (37 years), with 75% of cases being found in males.[42] Like mixed cellularity HL, this subtype is more common in individuals with HIV and in developing countries. Peripheral lymphadenopathy is rarely seen. Disease is often found in the abdominal organs, retroperitoneal lymph nodes, and bone marrow. Diagnosis is usually made while the disease is in a more advanced stage with B symptoms present. Morphologically, the appearance of lymphocyte-depleted HL is quite variable, but there is generally a predominance of Hodgkin Reed-Sternberg cells and a paucity of lymphocytes in the background cells. Prognosis is now thought to be similar to that for other subtypes of HL, although patients with HIV often experience a more aggressive course.[42]

## TREATMENT MODALITIES

HL has one of the highest cure rates found among adult cancers, but only if appropriate and full-dose therapy is given on schedule. It is reported that more than 80% of patients can be cured with first-line therapy.[43] Treatment of this disease entails a balance of sufficient therapies to cure the disease but no more than is required to prevent unnecessary long-term consequences. This balance continues to inspire debate in the literature. It is important to understand the history of HL treatment, as some survivors have undergone various treatments that are no longer considered standard therapy. It is imperative to monitor these individuals for long-term side effects particular to their HL treatment.

HL must be staged carefully to determine appropriate therapy. In the past, a staging laparotomy and splenectomy were performed to definitively identify those patients with limited vs advanced disease. Curative radiation therapy was originally used as treatment. After World War II, a plethora of chemotherapy drugs became available and many were studied as single agents in HL. Eventually combinations of chemotherapy evolved and the mechlorethamine, vincristine, procarbazine, prednisone (MOPP) regimen was developed. Originally used as salvage therapy, it was later employed as first-line therapy. This combination therapy produced a 54% disease-free survival (DFS) rate at 20 years and has demonstrated effective long-term management of HL with systemic treatment.[44]

### RADIATION THERAPY

Prior to the 1960s, radiation therapy was the initial, and sometimes only, treatment for HL. When it was discovered that HL spread via contiguous lymph node chains, radiation for early stage disease often was given as extended field. This included 1 lymph node group beyond those that were positive. The 3 classic areas of radiation fields were the mantle, paraaortic, and pelvic regions (Figure 60-5). The mantle field consisted of the cervical, supraclavicular, infraclavicular, axillary, mediastinal, and hilar lymph node groupings. The paraaortic field included the spleen, if present. The pelvic field included the pelvic, inguinal, and femoral nodes. Subtotal lymphoid radiation encompassed all of the fields, while the extended field included the mantle and paraaortic regions. Finally, the inverted Y field consisted of the paraaortic region in addition to the pelvic area. Many vital organs fall within these fields, and blocks needed to be devised to provide organ protection. Therapy typically consisted of 3500 to 4400 cGy given to affected areas, with 3000 to 3500 cGy going to uninvolved areas.

Advances in radiotherapy have helped make these treatments less toxic, but this approach is still associated with significant long-term side effects. Currently, the extent and dose of radiation depend on the stage of disease as well as the residual tumor, if any, after combination chemotherapy. Alternatively, many centers use radiotherapy following completion of chemotherapy to sites of bulky disease.[27] Positron emission tomography results are now being taken into consideration in the determination of radiation therapy.

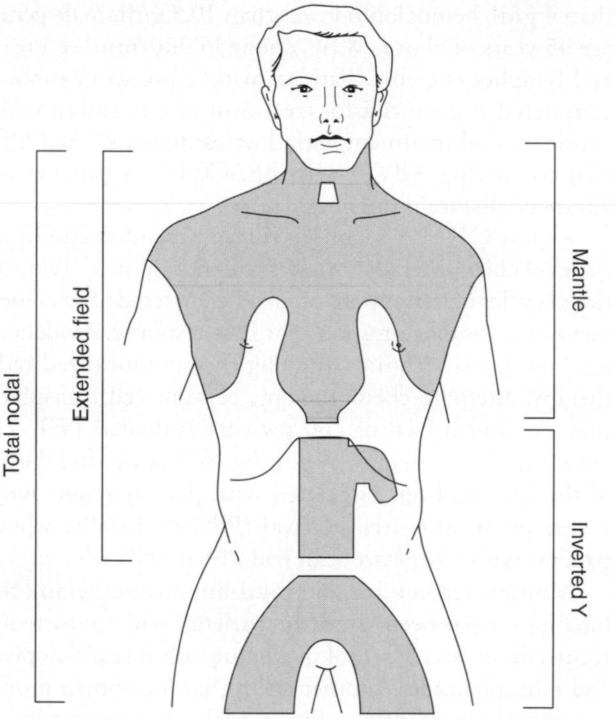


**FIGURE 60-5**

Standard radiation fields for Hodgkin's disease. Mantle—from mandible to diaphragm. Lungs, heart, spinal cord, and humeral heads are shielded. Inverted Y—from diaphragm to ischial tuberosities, including the spleen if not removed; spinal cord, kidneys, bladder, rectum, and gonads are shielded. Extended field—involves mantle zone and uppermost inverted Y zone; does not include the pelvic, inguinal, or femoral nodes. Total nodal—mantle zone and completed inverted Y zone.

## CHEMOTHERAPY

With the advent of effective combination chemotherapy, staging laparotomies with splenectomies have fallen by the wayside on the presumption that chemotherapy will clear any occult disease. Early stage HL is typically treated with 4 (sometimes fewer) cycles of combination chemotherapy followed by involved field radiation. Studies of treatment of early stage HL with combination chemotherapy and radiotherapy to sites of known disease compared with subtotal nodal radiotherapy demonstrated a statistically significant 10-year OS benefit to patients receiving combination chemotherapy and radiotherapy.[45]

More advanced disease is often treated with 6 to 8 cycles of combination chemotherapy. Radiation may or may not be given to sites of bulky disease. A study from Europe investigated the use of randomized involved field radiation for advanced disease. The researchers concluded that involved field radiation did not improve outcomes in patients who were in complete remission (CR) after combination therapy, but it was useful for those who were in partial remission (PR).[46] Typically, patients are restaged after 3 to 4 cycles of chemotherapy to gauge their response and to finalize the treatment plan.

Prior to 1960, chemotherapy agents were used only for palliative purposes. In 1964, MOPP combination chemotherapy was investigated and became the first treatment that cured patients with advanced disease.[47] Several years later, Italian researchers developed the doxorubicin, bleomycin, vinblastine, dacarbazine (ABVD) protocol. It was first considered to be a non–cross-resistant treatment for MOPP failures, but later proved to be superior in efficacy with less long-term toxicity than MOPP.[48] Table 60-3[49-52] describes the chemotherapy regimens used to treat HL. MOPP has fallen out of favor as standard treatment for HL due to the increased risk of azoospermia, ovarian

**TABLE 60-3**

**Common Combination Chemotherapy Regimens Used to Treat Hodgkin's Lymphoma**

| | |
|---|---|
| **ABVD**[50] | |
| Doxorubicin (Adriamycin) | 25 mg/m² IV days 1 and 5 |
| Bleomycin | 10 units/m² IV days 1 and 15 |
| Vinblastine | 6 mg/m² IV days 1 and 15 |
| Dacarbazine | 375 mg/m² days 1 and 15 |
| Cycle repeated every 28 days | |
| **Stanford V**[51] | |
| Mechlorethamine | 6 mg/m² IV day 1 |
| Doxorubicin | 25 mg/m² IV days 1 and 15 |
| Vinblastine | 6 mg/m² IV days 1 and 15 |
| Vincristine | 1.4 mg/m² (max 2 mg) IV days 8 and 22 |
| Bleomycin | 5 units/m² IV days 8 and 22 |
| Etoposide | 60 mg/m² IV days 15 and 16 |
| Prednisone | 40 mg PO every other day (*taper started with last cycle*) |
| Cycle repeated every 28 days. Check for dose changes in patients > 50 years | |
| *Prophylactic antibiotics, antivirals, and antifungals typically added followed by radiation therapy* | |
| **BEACOPP**[52] | |
| Bleomycin | 10 mg/m² IV day 8 |
| Etoposide | 100 mg/m² day IV days 1,2,3 |
| Cyclophosphamide | 650 mg/m² IV day 1 |
| Vincristine | 1.4 mg/m² (max 2 mg) IV day 8 |
| Procarbazine | 100 mg/m² PO days 1–7 |
| Prednisone | 40 mg/m² PO days 1–14 |
| Cycle repeated every 21 days | |

Many regional/institutional variations to these regimens exist.
Rituximab frequently added to regimens.
Some regimens require prophylactic antibiotics.

failure, myelodysplastic syndrome, and secondary malignancies associated with it. A randomized, multicenter trial compared a MOPP/ABV hybrid to ABVD, reporting results after 5 years. The 2 regimens appear to be equally effective, but the MOPP/ABV therapy is associated with increased pulmonary and hematological toxicity as well as an increased incidence of secondary leukemia.

Other combination therapies currently used include the 12-week Stanford V treatment (mechlorethamine, doxorubicin, vinblastine, vincristine, bleomycin, etoposide, and prednisone, or BEACOPP) and the European BEACOPP using cyclophosphamide, doxorubicin, etoposide, procarbazine, bleomycin, and vincristine as well as the escalated BEACOPP. The National Comprehensive Cancer Network (NCCN) guidelines identify the Stanford V treatment as an acceptable alternative to ABVD. It is important to note that Stanford V is designed as a combined-modality treatment. In the Stanford regimen, 85% of patients at Stanford received radiation following chemotherapy to initial tumor sites.[53] As mentioned earlier, ongoing debate in the literature focuses on the balance between cure and toxicity. The German Hodgkin's Lymphoma Study Group recommends that patients with advanced, high-risk disease receive aggressive treatment upfront, rather than multiple chemotherapy regimens, including stem cell transplant, at time of relapse.[43] These researchers report that standard BEACOPP is equivalent to cyclophosphamide, vincristine, procarbazine, prednisone (COPP/ABVD), but produces higher toxicities. Escalated BEACOPP, by comparison, appears to be more effective than either therapy.[54] Acute toxicities, including leukopenia, thrombocytopenia, anemia, infection, and nausea, as well as long-term concern regarding gonadal toxicity and risk of second malignancies, are significant. Elderly patients did not tolerate BEACOPP therapy, and 21% died of acute toxicity.[55] A trial comparing 6 to 8 cycles of ABVD to 4 cycles of escalated BEACOPP plus 4 cycles of standard BEACOPP in patients with advanced disease was performed. Radiation was given to those patients who had bulky disease or a residual mass. The intent was to readminister chemotherapy in treatment failures and then to treat with autologous stem cell transplantation. Initial reports show no difference in the 3-year OS. Freedom from progression was superior in the BEACOPP arm but toxicity was greater.[56] Increased-dose BEACOPP may be most useful in those with the highest-risk disease. Autologous stem cell transplantation following therapy with BEACOPP may be limited due to stem cell damage.

The NCCN has provided a list of unfavorable factors for early stage HL that have been identified from several study groups. These factors include bulky disease, an elevated erythrocyte sedimentation rate of 50 or above if asymptomatic, more than 3 sites of adenopathy or 2 or more extranodal sites, and B symptoms.[57] Hasenclever and Diehl have developed an International Prognostic Score for patients with advanced HL.[58] One point is given for albumin lower than 4 g/dl, hemoglobin lower than 10.5 g/dl, male gender, age 45 years or above, WBC count 15,000/$mm^3$ or greater, and lymphocytopenia. Patients with 4 points or more are considered at great risk for treatment failure and should be considered for treatment with dose-escalated BEACOPP. A trial comparing ABVD with BEACOPP in patients with advanced disease is ongoing.

Repeat CT/PET scanning is recommended after 2 to 4 cycles of chemotherapy to assess patient response. Two additional cycles of therapy are often administered after achievement of a complete response or best response. Evidence of residual disease requires ongoing therapy; localized radiotherapy, alternate chemotherapy, or stem cell transplantation. A clinical trial of 260 patients evaluated PET scans after 2 cycles of therapy. A positive PET scan after 2 cycles of therapy has been associated with poor outcome with a 2-year progression-free survival (PFS) of 12.8%, whereas patients with a negative scan had PFS of 95%.[59]

Multiple second-line and third-line chemotherapy combinations have been used for patients with persistent or recurrent disease. Many of these protocols include etoposide and iphosphamide. Another agent that has shown promise is gemcitabine. Multiple clinical trials are investigating the efficacy and safety of a monoclonal antibody targeted to CD30. CD30 positivity is a hallmark for HL. It is observed in nearly all HL (as well as anaplastic T-cell lymphomas) but has limited expression in normal tissues, making it an ideal agent to investigate.

## STEM CELL TRANSPLANT

Stem cell transplant remains a potentially curative option for relapsed HL with chemotherapy-sensitive disease. Over the past 20 years, it has been established as the most effective treatment for patients not cured by initial multidrug regimens. Candidates for stem cell transplant include patients who progress through initial treatment, those who respond to treatment but fail to achieve a complete response, and those who have early relapse within 12 months after treatment.[60] Second relapse after conventional treatment for first relapse is another indication for transplant.[61]

Two European clinical trials have failed to demonstrate an advantage for consolidative high-dose therapy with stem cell transplant over conventional treatment for patients with high-risk, advanced disease who achieved CR or PR after initial doxorubicin-based chemotherapy.[62,63] Despite the availability of high-dose therapy, prognosis remains poor for these patients, with an OS rate of 34% and a DFS rate of 29% at 10 years.[64] Two subsets of patients with a better prognosis have been identified: those who have relapsed at original lymph node sites that were not irradiated and those whose relapse occurred more than 1 year after completion of initial therapy. Patients receiving allogeneic (donor marrow) transplants are more likely to remain relapse free after transplant, but the increased morbidity and mortality of allogeneic transplants offset the benefits achieved by an allogeneic marrow source, and no survival advantage is seen. Negative prognostic factors for disease progression after stem cell transplant include chemotherapy resistance prior to transplant, advanced stage disease, and greater number of chemotherapeutic regimens prior to transplant.

## FUTURE DIRECTIONS

Many clinical trials are looking for a nontoxic agent or regimen that is effective against HL. As the biology of HL becomes better understood, it is hoped that new therapies will emerge. Targeted immunotherapy, an important adjuvant to treatment of NHL, is now being investigated in the management of HL. Preliminary data suggest that rituximab (anti-CD20 therapy) may have efficacy in some patients. A phase II study combining 6 weekly doses of rituximab with 6 cycles of ABVD demonstrated a 3-year event-free survival (EFS) of 85%.[65]

Important questions still need to be answered. How little therapy can be used and still cure low-risk, early stage disease? How much should we treat high-risk, advanced disease? What is the role of radiation therapy at all stages of disease? It is recommended that patients be offered enrollment in clinical trials to help answer these questions. Close follow-up for efficacy, acute toxicity, and long-term complications is necessary to discern the best options over the long term.

## PROGNOSIS

Hodgkin's disease has historically been among the most "curable" cancers. Patients with early stage disease (stages I and II) have a 10-year survival rate exceeding 80%. Negative prognostic factors were determined by an international consortium.[66] Seven factors associated with poor prognosis were identified: stage IV disease, male sex, age greater than or equal to 45 years, hemoglobin less than 10.5 g/dL, WBC count greater than or equal to 15,000/µl, lymphocyte count less than 800/µl or less than 6%, and albumin less than 4 g/dL. Eighty-four percent of patients with no high-risk factors were estimated to be free of disease at 5 years. The rates declined steadily in patients with risk factors; patients with 5 to 7 factors had an estimated PFS rate of 42%.[66]

# NON-HODGKIN'S LYMPHOMA

## HISTORICAL PERSPECTIVE

Non-Hodgkin's lymphoma encompasses a diverse group of neoplasms of the immune system involving B or T lymphocytes. Although these malignancies share many characteristics, they also reflect the diversity of their normal counterpart cells and exhibit a wide range of immunological and biological characteristics. No precise, universally accepted definition of NHL exists. Although many disease entities meet the criteria that have been proposed, others lurk in a nebulous area between benign lymphoproliferation and true malignancy. Furthermore, the classification of lymphoma has long been a controversial issue and continues to undergo change.

In the past, pathologists used a variety of terms (eg, giant follicle lymphoma, lymphosarcoma, and reticulum cell sarcoma) to categorize these tumors, and "pseudoleukemia" became a catch-all term for describing a host of conditions that exhibited lymphadenopathy and splenomegaly. Technological refinements have enabled pathologists and clinicians to classify NHL according to a number of individual determinants, including cytoarchitecture (follicular vs diffuse), cell size (small or large), nuclear characteristics (cleaved or noncleaved, convoluted or cerebriform), immunological origin (T-cell or B-cell lymphocytes), and maturity of the cell (precursor or mature). Today, the identity of the lymphoma is also determined with the aid of cytogenetic and immunological markers.

## EPIDEMIOLOGY

An estimated 74,490 new cases of NHL were diagnosed in 2009, accounting for approximately 89% of all lymphomas.[1] The incidence of lymphoma climbed rapidly during the 1970s and 1980s, nearly doubling the number of new cases. Better detection and diagnosis accounted for some of this increase. The climbing incidence of AIDS and AIDS-related NHL, as well as the expanding use of immunosuppressive treatments, accounted for a substantial portion of these cases. In the 1990s, the incidence rates stabilized, a trend that has been attributed to the decline in AIDS-related NHL. An estimated 20,790 deaths are expected to occur in 2009 due to NHL. The prognosis for NHL is highly variable, but the overall 5-year survival rate is approximately 69%.[1] Within the past 4 years, there has been a mild increase in the number of cases of NHL, with a mild drop in the number of deaths[67] related to NHL. The incidence of NHL increases with age, and is slightly higher in males than in females. A male younger than age 40 has a 1 in 763 chance of developing NHL, whereas a male aged 70 or older has a 1 in 60 chance. The incidence also increases with age in females: a 1 in 1,191 chance prior to age 40, and 1 in 73 for ages over 70.[67] The reduction in immune function during the aging process may help to explain the increasing rate of NHL. This theory is supported by other patients who are known to be at increased risk for the development of NHL: patients posttransplant who receive immunosuppressive therapy and those with HIV infection.

## ETIOLOGY

An increased incidence of lymphoma has been reported in individuals with exposure to toxins, such as chemists, farmers, and those working with rubber production, asbestos, and arsenic. Japanese survivors of the atomic bomb and patients receiving ionizing radiation for congenital disorders and HD also face increased neoplastic potential specifically related to NHL.[68,69] Other investigators report minimal or no risk associated with ionizing radiation and the risk of lymphoma.[70] Controversy has existed since 1975 over the risk associated with hair dyes. While many studies do not substantiate greater risk associated with the use of hair dyes, either personally or occupationally, a subset of individuals who use permanent dyes, dark in color, for prolonged periods (more than 20 years) may have an increased risk of lymphoma.[71] A European review reports a moderate increased risk for lymphoma in woman who use hair dye for personal use, particularly those who used dyes before 1980.[72]

Chromosomal abnormalities are common in NHL. Investigators have identified cytogenetic abnormalities in more than 90% of cases.[73] The impact of chromosomal translocations may be significant. For example, the translocation t(14:18)(q32;q21), which is commonly found in FL, results in overexpression of *BCL-2*. The accumulation of BCL-2 protein results in inhibition of apoptosis (programmed cell death).[74–77] Chromosomal translocations result in the activation of oncogenes and the inactivation of tumor suppressor genes. These alterations in the expression of genes affect normal cell function and regulation and are implicated in the process of malignant transformation.

Infectious agents have been implicated in the etiology of NHL as well as HL. The clearest evidence for this role is seen in the etiology of adult T-cell leukemia/lymphoma that arises in patients infected with human T-cell leukemia/lymphoma virus 1 (HTLV-1). Yet not all individuals who are exposed and infected with HTLV-1 develop lymphoma. There appear to be host factors, potentially genetic, that result in the transformation of normal lymphocytes to lymphoma. The greatest incidence of adult T-cell leukemia/lymphoma is found on an island of Japan. Ten to fifteen percent of the population of this island are found to have antibodies (signifying prior exposure) to HTLV-1. Other endemic areas include the Caribbean and southeastern US.

Epstein–Barr virus has also been implicated in the development of NHL, especially Burkitt's lymphoma (BL). Burkitt's lymphoma has been endemic in the "lymphoma belt" in central Africa. EBV is present in more than 95% of these cases.[78] Malaria is thought to play a role in the stimulation of lymphocytes that then undergo transformation; this disease is commonly seen in endemic areas of BL. Of note, EBV is present in only 20% of nonendemic cases of BL.[79]

There is clear evidence that *H. pylori*, a gram-negative bacillus that induces gastric ulceration, can result in MALT lymphoma of the stomach. In its early stages, it may be cured by eradication of the bacteria with antibiotics. It has also resulted in the development of large cell lymphomas in the gastric region, either de novo or due to transformation from a MALT lymphoma.

Immunosuppression has also been identified as a significant risk factor for the development of NHL. Clear evidence exists that individuals with primary (genetic) immunodeficiency states have a greater incidence of lymphoma. It has been estimated that 25% of these individuals will develop cancer during their lifetime, with more than 50% of those cases resulting in NHL.[80] Secondary exposure, generally associated with immunosuppressive therapy in the setting of organ transplantation, also is linked to a substantially greater risk for the development of NHL. Although the etiology is not entirely clear, it has been proposed that the immunosuppression and the chronic antigenic stimulation by the graft result in the lymphoma. A meta-analysis performed by Zintzras et al reported a 3.9-fold increased risk for the development of lymphoma in patients with rheumatoid arthritis, a 7.4-fold increased risk in patients with systemic lupus erythematosus, and an 18.8-fold increased risk in those with primary Sjögren's syndrome.[81]

## HISTOLOGICAL CLASSIFICATION SYSTEMS

### RAPPAPORT CLASSIFICATION

No malignancy has undergone more changes in terms of its classification system than NHL. The first widely accepted classification was proposed by Rappaport et al in 1956.[82] This system distinguished lymphomas on the basis of the pattern and growth within the lymph node (nodular or diffuse) and the degree of cytological differentiation of the predominant malignant cells. Tumors composed of cells similar in size and morphology to normal lymphocytes were denoted as "well differentiated," and those composed of irregularly shaped lymphocytes were referred to as "poorly differentiated." If the tumor cells were 2 to 3 times larger than small lymphocytes and had abundant cytoplasm, they were called histiocytes because of their resemblance to macrophages. Undifferentiated lymphomas were composed of intermediate-sized cells that failed to demonstrate evidence of either lymphoid or histiocytic origin. Mixed lymphomas were tumors formed by poorly differentiated lymphocytes and histiocytes.

### INTERNATIONAL WORKING FORMULA

A study funded by the NCI developed what was hoped to be the international standard for classifying lymphomas. The

International Working Formula was proposed in 1982, and was built upon the foundation of the Rappaport classification.[83] The term "histiocytic" was replaced by "large cell," and the histiocytic group was divided into large cell and immunoblastic large cell categories. This division created a split, with large cell disease falling into the intermediate grade and immunoblastic disease becoming the high grade. At that time, 6 different classifications systems were in use, making it impossible to analyze and compare results of clinical investigations using different systems. The International Working Formula proposed 3 major NHL categories: low-grade, intermediate-grade, and high-grade lymphomas. These categories were based on both clinical (response to treatment) and pathologic findings. Letter designations from A to J were assigned, corresponding roughly to aggressiveness of the disease and decreasing survival rates.

As a group, low-grade lymphomas have a long natural history, with an average survival of 9 years.[84] These diseases, however, show a relatively poor response to treatment, with few CRs, and are considered incurable. Low-grade lymphoma commonly affects the elderly. Patients tend to present with stage III or IV disease, and the bone marrow is often involved. During progression of the disease, the low-grade lymphoma will often become transformed into an intermediate-grade or high-grade lymphoma. At this time, the lymphoma becomes more aggressive and requires more intensive therapy.

Intermediate-grade lymphomas include B-cell neoplasms that present largely in adults, most often with nodal presentation. These subtypes frequently involve extranodal progression to the skin, bone, and gastrointestinal tract. These lymphomas are responsive to chemotherapy and curative therapy is possible. Although they demonstrate an intermediate aggressiveness, if left untreated they are often rapidly fatal.

High-grade lymphomas are highly aggressive and are B cell or T cell in origin. These malignancies exhibit rapid tumor growth and a high mitotic index. They may present in children or adults. Some subsets of high-grade lymphomas share many characteristics with acute leukemia. Affected patients require rapid diagnosis and treatment. If left untreated, high-grade lymphomas will frequently develop large lymph nodes, creating compression and obstruction of other organs and oncological emergencies. Despite the aggressive nature of these diseases, they are sensitive to treatment, and cure is possible.

### REVISED EUROPEAN–AMERICAN CLASSIFICATION OF LYMPHOID NEOPLASMS

The International Lymphoma Study Group met in 1994 and proposed the Revised European–American Classification of Lymphoid Neoplasms (REAL) system.[85] This classification system was constructed by integrating all known information about the tumor to define the lymphoma: morphology, immunophenotyping, genetics, etiology, epidemiology, and clinical features.[86] It relies on recognition of the cell of origin (T cell or B cell) and the stage of differentiation (precursor vs peripheral). The REAL system acknowledges that a distinct lymphoma subtype may vary in histological grade and clinical aggressiveness. The follicle center (follicular) lymphomas exemplify this point. Three grades of this disease entity have been identified: I (predominantly small cleaved), II (mixed small cleaved and large cell), and III (predominantly large cell). The International Working Formula, Rappaport, and REAL classification systems are compared in Table 60-4.

### WORLD HEALTH ORGANIZATION CLASSIFICATION

The World Health Organization (WHO) classification of hematopoietic and lymphatic tumors is the result of several years of discussions and consensus meetings, which began in 1995 and involved more than 50 hematopathologists from around the world. The classification of NHL is just 1 group of disease entities addressed. The WHO classification system is built upon the principles of the REAL classification system. As in the REAL system, the lymphoma is defined by its morphology, immunophenotype, and genetic and clinical features. The lineage of the cell and the cell of origin are important features. The cell of origin in many lymphoid neoplasms is determined at the stage of differentiation of the malignant cells seen in the tissues, not on the basis of the cell in which the initial transforming event occurred. Two categories of NHL are recognized: B-cell neoplasms and T-cell and NK-cell neoplasms. Lymphoid leukemias, both chronic and acute, as well as multiple myeloma and related disorders, are now categorized within the classification of NHL, as they are of T-cell or B-cell lineage, but discussion of these diseases will be minimal here as they are discussed in other chapters of this book. Characteristics and management of the more common subtypes of NHL as classified by the WHO system will be discussed, followed by a review of treatment modalities. Table 60-5 outlines the WHO classification for NHL.[87] The WHO classification for lymphoma is the most commonly used today. International experts reached a consensus that the treatment of lymphoid malignancies should be based on the specific lymphoma type, the grade, and clinical prognostic features. Groupings of lymphoma were not considered beneficial.[88]

## CHARACTERISTICS AND MANAGEMENT OF B-CELL NHL

### SMALL LYMPHOCYTIC LYMPHOMA/CHRONIC LYMPHOCYTIC LEUKEMIA

Small lymphocytic lymphoma (SLL)/chronic lymphocytic leukemia (CLL) is a neoplasm of small, round B cells found in the peripheral blood, bone marrow, and lymph nodes.

**TABLE 60–4**

**Non-Hodgkin's Lymphoma Nomencalture: Comparative Classifications**

| | Working Formulation | Rapport System | Real Classification[a] |
|---|---|---|---|
| | | **Low Grade** | |
| A | Small lymphocytic | Diffuse well-differentiated lymphocytic | Chronic lymphocytic leukemia |
| B | Follicular, small cleaved | Nodular, poorly differentiated lymphocytic | MALT[b] follicle center cell, follicular grade I |
| C | Follicular, mixed small cleaved, and large cell | Nodular, mixed lymphocytic and histiocytic | Follicle center cell, follicular grade II |
| | | **Intermediate Grade** | |
| D | Follicular, large cell | Nodular histiocytic | Follicle center cell, follicular grade III |
| E | Diffuse, small cleaved | Diffuse, poorly differentiated lymphocytic | Mantle cell[c] |
| F | Diffuse, mixed small and large | Diffuse, mixed lymphocytic and histiocytic | Follicle center cell, diffuse small cell<br>Large B cell rich in T cells |
| G | Diffuse large cell | Diffuse histiocytic | Diffuse large B cell |
| | | **High Grade** | |
| H | Immunoblastic large cell | Diffuse histiocytic | Diffuse large B cell |
| I | Lymphoblastic | Lymphoblastic | Precursor B lymphocytic |
| J | Small, noncleaved Burkitt's | Undifferentiated Burkitt's and non-Burkitt's | Burkitt's high-grade B cell, Burkitt's-like |

[a]The REAL classification separated B-cell and T-cell lymphomas. Most of the T-cell lymphomas are not shown here except for chronic lymphocytic leukemia.

[b]Mucosa-associated lymphoma tissue (MALT) tumors are extranodal indolent and usually follicular, but some were previously classified in groups A, B, C, E, and rarely F.

[c]Mantle cell tumors are defined by *BCL-l* overexpression and sometimes have a morphology similar to groups A, B, and F.

*Abbreviation*: REAL, Revised European-American Classification of Lymphoid Neoplasms.

*Source*: Data from Rappaport et al.[82]; National Cancer Institute[83]; and Pileri et al.[85]

By definition, CLL entails bone marrow and peripheral blood involvement and a lymphocyte count greater than 10 × $10^9$/L. Small lymphocytic lymphoma can be diagnosed without CLL if the morphology of the cells meets the criteria but the blood and bone marrow are not involved. Pathologically, it is considered to be the same disease at different stages. Historically, a monoclonal lymphocytosis of greater than 5 × $10^9$/L was required for the diagnosis of CLL, and this parameter continues to be used as a criterion by many clinicians. The proportion of prolymphocytes is usually small. Increasing proportions are associated with a more aggressive form of the disease. The pattern of malignant cells seen in the bone marrow may be described as nodular, interstitial, diffuse, or a combination of these. The nodular and interstitial patterns are usually associated with early disease. Advanced disease is associated with the interstitial pattern. The international NHL project reported that 91% of patients with SLL presented with stage III or IV disease; 72% had bone marrow involvement, almost all patients had generalized lymphadenopathy, and 30% had extranodal disease at diagnosis.[84]

Immunoglobulin gene rearrangements of both heavy-chain and light-chain variable regions are noted in SLL/CLL in 50% of patients. Approximately 80% of patients have abnormal karyotypes as determined by FISH analysis.[89] Deletion 13q14, trisomy 12, deletion 17p, and deletion 11q are the cytogenetic abnormalities most commonly noted. Those with deletion 13q14 more frequently have mutated variable genes, and those with trisomy 12 have predominantly unmutated genes. Malignant cells express immunoglobulin M (IgM) or IgM and IgD, CD5, CD19, CD23, and CD43. CD20 and CD22 also express weak activity. CD5 and CD23 markers are positive in SLL/CLL and negative in other B-cell lymphomas with the exception of MCL, which expresses CD5. The overexpression of Zap (zeta-chain-associated protein) 70, CD38, and unmutated immunoglobulin variable heavy gene has been associated with poorer prognosis.[90]

Small lymphocytic lymphoma/CLL accounts for 6.7% of cases of NHL.[91] The majority of patients are more than 50 years old, with a median age of 65 years. There is a male-to-female predominance of approximately 2:1. Many patients with CLL are asymptomatic at diagnosis,

**TABLE 60-5**

**WHO Classification of NHL**

**Precursor B-Cell and T-Cell Neoplasms**
Precursor B-lymphoblastic leukemia/lymphoblastic lymphoma (precursor B-cell acute lymmphoblastic leukemia)
Precursor T-lymphoblastic leukemia/lymphoblastic lymphoma (precursor T-cell acute lymphoblastic leukemia)

**Mature B-Cell Neoplasms**
Chronic lymphocytic leukemia/small lymphocytic lymphoma
B-cell prolymphocytic leukemia
Lymphoplasmacytic lymphoma
Splenic marginal zone lymphoma
Hairy cell leukemia
Plasma cell myeloma
Monoclonal gammopathy of undetermined significance (MGUS)
Solitary plasmacytoma of bone
Extraosseous plasmacytoma
Primary ameloidosis
Heavy-chain diseases
Extranodal marginal zone B-cell lymphoma of mucosa-associated lymphoid tissue (MALT lymphoma)
Nodal marginal-zone B-cell lymphoma
Follicular lymphoma
Mantle cell lymphoma
Diffuse large B-cell lymphoma
Mediastinal (thymic) large B-cell lymphoma
Intravascular large B-cell lymphoma
Primary effusion lymphoma
Burkitt's lymphoma/leukemia

**B-Cell Proliferations of Uncertain Malignant Potential**
Lymphatoid granulomatosis
Posttransplant lymphoproliferative disorder, polymorphic

**Mature T-Cell and NK Cell Neoplasms**
*Leukemic disseminated*
T-cell prolymphocytic leukemia
T-cell large granular lymphocytic leukemia
Aggressive NK cell leukemia
Adult T-cell leukemia/lymphoma
*Cutaneous*
Mycosis fungoides
Sézary syndrome
Primary cutaneous anaplastic large cell lymphoma
Lymphomatoid papulosis[a]
*Other extanodal*
Extranodal NK/T-cell lymphoma, nasal type
Enteropathy-type T-cell lymphoma
Hepatosplenic T-cell lymphoma
Subcutaneous panniculitis-like T-cell lymphoma
*Nodal*
Angioimmunoblastic T-cell lymphoma
Peripheral T-cell lymphoma, unspecified
Anaplastic large cell lymphoma
*Neoplasm of uncertain lineage and stage of differentiation*
Blastic NK lymphoma

[a]Not clinically considered a neoplastic disorder.
*Abbreviations*: NHL, non-Hodgkin's lymphoma; NK, natural killer; WHO, World Health Organization.

and a lymphocytosis is found on a routine complete blood count. Because the SLL subtype does not have a significant lymphocytosis, diffuse lymphadenopathy or lymph node masses' effects on normal organ function often lead to diagnosis. The spleen and liver are often enlarged, and extranodal disease is not uncommon. Patients may complain of fatigue. Autoimmune disorders are often observed, with the most common being autoimmune hemolytic anemia and idiopathic thrombocytopenia. Hypogammaglobulinemia is identified in 75% of patients at some point during their disease, contributing to an increased risk of infection.

Treatment is often deferred in early stage SLL/CLL unless there is an indication to treat. The following criteria have been identified as indications to treat: (1) patient eligibility for a clinical trial, (2) presence of autoimmune cytopenias, (3) recurrent infections, (4) significant symptomatology, (5) cytopenias, (6) massive bulky disease at presentation, (7) steady progression over at least 6 months, (8) lymphocyte number doubling in less than 12 months, and (9) patient preference.[92]

Single-agent therapy with a purine analog or alkylating agent may be administered or combination therapy may be initiated. It is recommended that anthracycline use be avoided in combination regimens unless the patient is unable to tolerate fludarabine therapy or other appropriate options. Fludarabine has been associated with higher response rates and longer PFS than anthracycline-containing regimens.[93] It has not, however, been shown to improve survival. Current acceptable combinations include CVP (cyclophosphamide, vincristine, prednisone) and CF (cyclophosphamide, fludarabine). Rituximab is often added to combination therapy. If the disease continues to progress, treatment options include purine analog for fludarabine-sensitive or fludarabine-naïve patients or alkylator-based therapy for fludarabine-resistant disease. Bendamustine has been recently approved by the Food and Drug Administration (FDA) for the treatment of CLL in first-line therapy or following treatment failure. Alemtuzumab may also be used in the elderly as first-line treatment or as second-line therapy following fludarabine failure. It appears to be particularly effective in patients with *p53* mutations and deletions.[94]

Although stem cell transplantation remains controversial, it may be utilized as a treatment option. Small numbers of patients appear in long-term follow-up to be cured of their disease following stem cell transplantation. Locoregional radiotherapy may be used for adenopathy that is localized and producing significant symptomatology.

Detection of minimal residual disease (MRD) following treatment is of growing interest in this disorder. Flow cytometry has been utilized to detect cells that co-express CD5 and CD19. Polymerase chain reaction for the identification of immunoglobulin heavy gene rearrangement appears to be a sensitive test for identifying MRD. In a study, patients without evidence of MRD who demonstrated a complete response following therapy with alemtuzumab had a longer time to treatment failure than those who were MRD positive.[95]

The clinical course for SLL/CLL is indolent (slow growing), but the disease is not considered curable. The median survival for patients with CLL reported by Dohner et al is 108 months.[96] They report 17p deletion being the strongest negative prognostic factor. Other negative prognostic factors found include advanced Binet stage, 11q deletion, advanced age, LDH elevation, and elevated WBCs. Other features associated with shortened survival include unmutated variable region of the immunoglobulin genes, presence of more than 20% Zap positivity, and higher than 30% CD38 expression. A 13q deletion has been associated with a favorable prognosis.[97] Transformation to a high-grade lymphoma is seen in as many as 15% of these individuals, and is known as Richter's syndrome. Although diffuse large B cells are most commonly associated with this disorder, patients treated with purine analogs may develop a lymphoma resembling HL.

## FOLLICULAR LYMPHOMA

Follicular lymphoma is a neoplasm of follicle center (germinal center) B cells. The neoplastic follicles are poorly defined due to the closely packed lymphocytes. The pattern is reported as follicular if more than 75% of cells are follicular, as follicular and diffuse if 25% to 75% are follicular, and as minimally follicular if less than 25% are follicular. Two types of cells are normally found in the follicle centers—centrocytes (small, cleaved follicle center cells) and centroblasts (large, noncleaved follicle center cells)—but centrocytes typically dominate. One of 3 possible grades is assigned on the basis of the number of centroblasts counted. Grade 1 has 0 to 5 centroblasts per high-power field (predominantly small cell), grade 2 has 6 to 15 centroblasts (mixed small and large cell), and grade 3 has more than 15 centroblasts (large cell). Grade 3 has also been subdivided into grade 3a, in which centrocytes are present, and grade 3b, in which solid sheets of centroblasts are observed.[98] Grades 1 and 2 tend to be indolent in nature, consistent with low-grade NHL; grade 3 is more aggressive, with a natural history similar to that of diffuse large cell NHL.

Follicular lymphoma accounts for approximately 45% of all cases of NHL in adults in the US.[99] This disease is the most frequent subtype of "low-grade" lymphoma observed. Follicular lymphoma is seen predominantly in adults and is characterized by a male-to-female ratio of 1:1.7 and a median age at diagnosis of 59 years. Patients often present with widespread disease. Approximately two thirds of cases involve stage III or IV lymphoma at diagnosis.[91] Diffuse adenopathy may be present, but patients are frequently asymptomatic.

The BCL-2 protein is commonly expressed in FL. Lai et al report that the incidence of BCL-2 expression ranges from 100% in grade 1 FL to 75% in grade 3 FL.[100] Because most low-grade lymphomas express BCL-2, it is not a useful tool for differentiating FL from other lymphoma subtypes but it can help differentiate neoplastic lymph nodes from reactive nodes. BCL-6 abnormalities can also be observed. The malignant cells are typically $CD10^{+}$, $CD23^{+/-}$, $Sig^{+}$, $CD5^{-}$, and $CD43^{-}$. B-cell-associated antigens are expressed, including CD19, CD20, CD22, and CD79a. Cytogenetic abnormalities are almost universally found in FL. The most common abnormality, t(14;18)(q32;q21), is associated with the rearrangement of the *BCL-2* gene, a hallmark of FL. This genetic abnormality does not appear to either positively or negatively impact prognosis.

Treatment of FL depends on the stage and grade of disease. Grade 1 and 2 disease is more indolent, with a median survival of 7 to 10 years, which has been relatively unchanged over the past several years despite increasing treatment options.[101] Observation—the "watch and wait" approach—is a valid option in select cases. Local radiotherapy to regions of disease is preferred, but immunotherapy and chemotherapy may also be administered in early stage FL. Rituximab has been demonstrated to increase overall response rates (ORRs), response duration, and PFS.[102,103] Therefore it is often given in combination with other therapies or as single therapy in the elderly or those who cannot tolerate other treatments. Stage III or IV disease or stage II with bulky abdominal disease may be treated if indicated. The NCCN recommends treatment if the patient has significant symptomatology, end-organ function is threatened, cytopenias are present due to the lymphoma, bulky disease is present, there has been steady progressive disease over the past 6 months, or the patient prefers it.[92] Due to the inability to cure this disease, participation in clinical trials is strongly advised.

Initial therapy for more advanced stage FL or transformed FL is usually combination therapy such as CHOP (cyclophosphamide, doxorubicin, vincristine, prednisone), CVP, or FND (fludarabine, mitoxantrone, dexamethasone) with rituximab. Localized radiotherapy may be added for locally symptomatic disease. The use of anthracyclines has resulted in improved survival, especially in grade III FL or FL transformed to diffuse large B-cell NHL.[98] If a complete or partial response is obtained, stem cell transplantation, participation in a clinical trial, or observation may be considered.

Radioimmunotherapy is an option if the patient shows no response or progressive disease. Two radioimmunoconjugates, Y-ibritumomab tiuxetan (Zevalin) and $^{131}I$-tositumomab (Bexxar), are approved in the US for the treatment of relapsed, refractory follicular NHL, with or without transformation. Bendamustine, a drug recently approved by the FDA for use in CLL, has demonstrated activity against FL and is recommended by the NCCN as an option for second-line or subsequent therapy.[57]

Maintenance therapy for the management of FL with rituximab has been under investigation, with mounting evidence to support its use. Ghielmini et al report that the administration of maintenance rituximab every 2 months for 4 doses following standard rituximab therapy increases overall EFS from 12 months to 23 months, and in chemotherapy-naive patients from 19 months to 36 months.[104] Van Oers et al performed a trial first randomizing patients with FL to receive CHOP or RCHOP (the addition of rituximab with CHOP). Those receiving CHOP alone had a PFS of 20.2 months, compared with 33.1 months with RCHOP. Those patients achieving a CR or PR were randomized a second time to rituximab maintenance (a dose every 3 months for 2 years) vs observation. Rituximab maintenance increased PFS from 14.9 months to 51.5 months in this group.[102]

Grade I and II FL, while indolent in nature, is generally not curable. Grade III disease is more aggressive, but its curative potential is similar to that for diffuse large cell NHL. Transformed disease is also aggressive and associated with rapid decline. Advanced stage patients with FL were treated with various Southwest Oncology Group (SWOG) chemotherapeutic regimens: CHOP, ProMACE-MOPP, and CHOP plus rituximab or I-tositumomab.[105] The 4-year PFS was 46%, 48%, and 61%, respectively, with an OS of 69%, 79%, and 91%. While this malignancy is chemotherapy-sensitive, multiple relapses are common, with response time decreasing as the number of therapies increases.

It has been reported that clinical factors identified in the IPI are as important as the grade in predicting outcome in FL.[14,91] In 1999, an international cooperative group developed the Follicular Lymphoma International Prognostic Index, commonly known by the acronym FLIPI. Adverse prognostic factors included in FLIPI are Ann Arbor stage III/IV disease, 5 or more nodal sites involved, serum LDH greater than normal, age of 60 years or older, and hemoglobin less than 12 g/dL. The good-risk group (36% of patients) had 0 or 1 negative prognostic factor; the intermediate-risk group (37% of patients) had 2 negative factors; and the poor-risk group (27% of patients) had 3 or more factors. The 10-year OS rates reported were 70.7%, 50.9%, and 35.5%, respectively.[106]

## MALT LYMPHOMA

MALT lymphoma, also known as maltoma, is an extranodal lymphoma of the mucosa-associated lymphoid tissues. Morphologically, the cells appear as heterogeneous, small B cells of various cell types. They include centrocyte-like cells known as marginal zone cells. The infiltrate of malignant cells is observed in the marginal zone of reactive B-cell follicles extending into the interfollicular region.

Eight percent of B-cell NHLs and 50% of primary gastric lymphomas are classified as MALT lymphoma.[91,107] It is primarily a disease of adults, with a median age at diagnosis of 61 years. The male-to-female ratio is 1:1.2. A higher incidence of gastric MALT lymphoma has been reported in northeast Italy. Chronic inflammatory states, frequently involving autoimmune disorders, often precede the development of MALT lymphoma. In addition, *H. pylori* infection has been strongly implicated in the development of gastric maltomas. Wotherspoon et al reported that *H. pylori* was found in more than 90% of gastric maltomas.[108] Others have reported a lower incidence. In any event, the rate of detection of *H. pylori* diminishes as the lymphoma evolves; indeed, there is an inability to detect the bacteria even when the patient is seropositive.

The gastrointestinal system is the most common site of disease, accounting for 50% of all MALT lymphomas. Of those cases, the stomach is involved in 85%.[107] When the intestine or colon is involved, patients typically are found to have a special subtype of MALT lymphoma known as immunoproliferative small intestine disease (IPSID), previously known as α-chain disease. IPSID is more commonly found in the Middle East, especially the Mediterranean area.[109] Other, less common sites of disease, in descending order of frequency, include the lung, head and neck, ocular adnexae, skin, thyroid, and breast.[110]

Patients frequently present with stage I or II disease. Overall, only 20% of patients have disease involving the bone marrow, but the incidence varies with the primary site of involvement. Gastric cases have a low frequency of marrow involvement, while cases of ocular adnexal and pulmonary origin have a higher incidence.[111] Multiple extranodal or nodal sites are uncommon, occurring in less than 10% of patients.[110] Even when multiple extranodal sites exist, they may not reflect the existence of disseminated disease and poorer prognosis, making the staging systems less useful in this lymphoma.

Malignant cells typically express IgM, although IgA or IgG may be observed. Light-chain restriction is noted in MALT lymphomas, which is significant because it differentiates between a MALT lymphoma and benign lymphoid infiltrations. Typical cells are $CD10^-$, $CD5^-$, $CD20^+$, $CD23^-$, $CD79a^+$, and $CD43^{+/-}$ (weak).[112] Cyclin D1 is negative and *BCL-2* follicles are negative. Immunoglobulin heavy-chain and light-chain rearrangement occurs. Two cytogenetic abnormalities are commonly observed in this subtype: trisomy 3 is found in 60% of cases and t(11:18)(q21;q21) is seen in 25% to 50% of cases. A t(11;18) alteration is a predictor for lack of disease response to antibiotic therapy.[113]

Patients with stage I extranodal gastric MALT lymphoma may receive currently accepted antibiotic therapy for *H. pylori* as sole treatment for their disease if they lack the previously noted translocation and test positive for *H. pylori*. If they are *H. pylori* negative or have stage II disease, antibiotic therapy may still be considered, or radiotherapy may be added to the treatment plan. Rituximab treatment is recommended if radiotherapy is contraindicated. Advanced stage disease is uncommon, but if more aggressive disease is noted, if the patient is experiencing significant symptomatology, or if gastrointestinal bleeding is present, treatment usually involves chemotherapy. Appropriate chemotherapy regimens are the same as those indicated for FL using alkylating agents or anthracycline-containing regimens, with or without regional radiotherapy. Failure to eradicate the *H. pylori* infection occurs in approximately 10% of cases, so an alternative antibiotic regimen is required.[114]

Serial endoscopies are recommended to follow the disease. Regression of the lymphoma may require several months, and chemotherapy is usually required only to treat recurrent or persistent disease. Regimens used to treat FL are often considered appropriate therapy for maltomas. Surgical resection of gastric MALT lymphoma is reserved for life-threatening disease.

Early stage nongastric MALT lymphomas are generally treated with surgical resection and local radiotherapy. Advanced stage disease is treated similarly to FL. The presence of diffuse large cell lymphoma, either primary gastric or coexistent with a MALT lymphoma, requires more aggressive management.

Mucosa-associated lymphoma tissue lymphomas are indolent and do not disseminate rapidly. Extranodal recurrences are more often observed. Prognosis does not seem to be affected by the existence of multiple extranodal sites or even bone marrow involvement.[111] This disease is sensitive to antibiotic therapy, and successful eradication of the *H. pylori* infection frequently leads to regression of the lymphoma. MALT lymphomas have demonstrated sensitivity to radiotherapy, often resulting in prolonged complete responses. Transformation to diffuse large B-cell lymphomas (DLBCLs) may occur, resulting in a need for more aggressive treatment.

## MANTLE CELL LYMPHOMA

Mantle cell lymphoma (MCL) is a relatively uncommon B-cell neoplasm consisting of small to medium-sized cells that resemble cleaved follicular center cells or centrocytes. A monoclonal lymphoid proliferation destroys the architecture of the lymph node. A nodular, diffuse, or mantle zone growth pattern is observed. It is uncommon for a true follicular growth pattern to be seen. Blastoid cell types and other variants have been identified.

Mantle cell lymphomas have strong surface IgM. The typical immunophenotyping is $CD20^+$, $CD5^+$, $CD3^-$, $CD10^-$, $CD23^-$ (or weakly positive), $CD43^+$, and *BCL-6* negative. $CD5^-$ cases do exist. These lymphomas tend to demonstrate a more indolent nature. All mantle cell lymphomas are *BCL-2* positive, and the vast majority express cyclin D1.[115]

Conventional cytogenetics demonstrate the t(11:14)(q13;q32) mutation between the immunoglobulin heavy-chain gene on chromosome 14 and the *BCL-1* gene on chromosome 11 in 70% to 75% of cases of MCL.[116,117] However, this translocation is virtually universal if FISH testing is performed to identify it.[118] Many other cytogenetic abnormalities have been reported in low frequencies. Some have been associated with variants of MCL, whereas others are associated with SLL/CLL.

Mantle cell lymphoma accounts for only 5% to 10% of all cases of NHL.[119] The median age of individuals at diagnosis is 60 years, and the disease shows a male-to-female predominance of 2:1. Although lymph nodes are most commonly involved, the spleen, liver, and bone marrow also have a high frequency of involvement. Hepatomegaly and splenomegaly are common findings on physical examination. Abnormalities of the peripheral blood, which may include a marked lymphocytosis, are seen in approximately 20% of patients. The most common extranodal sites reported include the gastrointestinal tract (about 30% of patients) and the Waldeyer's ring, found in the tonsils. Multiple lymphomatous polyposis, a disorder involving multiple lymphomatous lesions of the gastrointestinal tract, is usually a form of MCL.[120] Unfortunately, patients tend to present with advanced stage disease.

Many treatments for MCL have been tried, albeit with limited success. Clinical trials are therefore highly encouraged. Treatment, usually involving an alkylating agent either alone or with chemotherapeutic combinations such as CHOP, HyperCVAD, or EPOCH (etoposide, vincristine, doxorubicin, cyclophosphamide, and prednisone), is often undertaken if the patient does not participate in a clinical trial, although anthracyclines have not been proven to improve survival in randomized trials. Rituximab is frequently added to the chemotherapy regimen, as MCL is a $CD20^+$ lymphoma. Second-line therapies include agents such as bendamustine, bortezomib, and cladribine as a single agent that may be combined with rituximab. Combination protocols utilizing fludarabine are also indicated.

The disease course for mantle cell lymphoma is aggressive and cure is rare. Between 30% and 50% of patients will have a complete response, with a median duration of remission of 1 to 3 years. Median survival has been reported at 3 to 5 years.[121]

Adverse prognostic indicators include a high mitotic rate, blastoid variant, peripheral blood involvement, and trisomy 12.[122] There have been several studies of autologous stem cell transplantation as a strategy in the management of mantle cell lymphoma during consolidation, with mixed results. One supports superior PFS, but statistically significant increased survival has not been yet been demonstrated. Others show more promise.[123,124] Relapse is frequently seen following autologous transplantation and is thought to be associated with contamination of stem cells with circulating mantle cells.[119,125] Allogeneic stem cell transplant has been effective for young patients who have not been heavily pretreated, as toxicity is often prohibitive in relation to the allogeneic transplant.

## DIFFUSE LARGE B-CELL LYMPHOMA

Diffuse large B-cell lymphoma, the most common type of NHL, encompasses a diffuse group of large, neoplastic B lymphocytes with large nuclei. The predominant cell is either a large noncleaved cell or an immunoblast, or a mixture of both types of cells.

Destruction of the normal architecture of the involved lymph node occurs in a diffuse pattern. Multiple variants of DLBCL with different cytological features exist, but there is poor reproducibility among pathologists. No definitive immunophenotypic or genetic markers are available by which to distinguish the variants. Morphologic variants include centroblastic, immunoblastic, T-cell/histiocytic-rich, and anaplastic subtypes. Diffuse large B-cell lymphoma can occur de novo or it can represent transformation from a more indolent lymphoma. Lymphoma subtypes known to cause this transformation include SLL/CLL, FL, marginal-zone B-cell lymphoma, and nodular lymphocyte-predominant HL.

Diffuse large B-cell lymphomas frequently express pan-B-cell markers such as CD19, CD20, CD22, and CD79a, but they may not express all markers. Surface or cytoplasmic immunoglobulin can be observed in one half to two thirds of these malignancies, with IgM being the most frequently seen, and IgG and IgA encountered in decreasing incidence. Diffuse large B-cell lymphoma is typically $CD45^{-/+}$ and $CD3^{-}$; CD5, CD30, and CD10 may be expressed. Cyclin D1 is negative; it is a biomarker that distinguishes this subtype from blastoid variants of mantle cell lymphoma. CD5 and CD10 markers are typically not observed. The CD5 marker may be noted in de novo DLBCL but is not observed in transformed SLL/CLL.[126] Translocation of the *BCL-2* gene resulting in the t(14;18) mutation commonly observed in FL is noted in 20% to 30% of DLBCL,[127,128] and there is a high frequency of *BCL-6* positivity.[99] Heavy-chain and light-chain, immunoglobulin gene rearrangements as well as multiple cytogenetic abnormalities are commonly observed.

The International Lymphoma Conference evaluated lymphoma cases from 9 institutions, representing 8 countries. Diffuse large B-cell lymphoma was the subtype of NHL represented, accounting for 31% of all NHL.[129] These lymphomas may be noted in a wide range of individuals, including children, but the median age at diagnosis is 64 years. There is a slightly higher incidence in males. The incidence of DLBCL has been increasing over the past several years.[130] Immunodeficiency is a risk factor for this lymphoma, and in this setting may be associated with EBV infection.

Diffuse large B-cell lymphoma presents either as primary lymph node disease or at extranodal sites. Armitage reports that 71% of patients have extranodal involvement at presentation, with 18% of patients having the gastrointestinal tract involved and another 16% having bone marrow involvement.[129] The disease often grows rapidly and is symptomatic. Many patients present with disseminated, advanced stage disease. Disease may involve any organ. Without biopsy, the diagnosis of lymphoma may be missed. Lymphomas often have a much more favorable prognosis than the primary malignancy of the involved organ. Diffuse large cell lymphoma of the brain as the primary site of disease is being diagnosed with increased frequency. Mediastinal (thymic) large B-cell lymphoma is a subtype of DLBCL that arises in the mediastinum. Affected patients generally present with localized disease and symptoms related to large mediastinal masses. These masses may impinge on the superior vena cava, resulting in obstruction. Patients are typically young adult females.

Treatment of DLBCL usually involves a multidrug, anthracycline-based chemotherapy regimen, such as CHOP, which is administered for 3 to 8 cycles, depending on the stage and IPI. Historically, this therapy has been administered every 21 days. Trials to evaluate the efficacy of dose-dense CHOP, administered every 14 days, have been performed with conflicting results.[131,132] The number of cycles of CHOP may be decreased and locoregional radiotherapy administered to sites of involvement in nonbulky stage I or II disease. If radiotherapy is contraindicated, 6 to 8 cycles of chemotherapy may be administered. Rituximab has activity against this disease and is usually added to the chemotherapy regimen. A recent meta-analysis reviewed the efficacy of high-dose chemotherapy followed by stem cell transplantation compared with conventional therapy in frontline treatment of patients with DLBCL. In good-risk patients there was no added benefit seen in those receiving transplantation. The data were inconclusive in high-risk patients.[133] High risk patients may receive high-dose therapy with autologous stem cell transplantation as consolidation therapy. Significant research is now seeking to determine the best method of incorporating rituximab into the treatment plan. Radioimmunotherapy has been investigated in patients with transformed DLBCL (as well as relapsed or refractory low-grade FL). It has been suggested that $^{113}$Y-ibritumomab tiuxetan is more effective when given earlier in the course of this disease. Because hematological toxicity is the most significant toxicity, this treatment is recommended only when the patient has adequate bone marrow reserves and less than 25% of the marrow is involved with lymphoma.[134] Many different regimens are available for treatment failure. Peripheral blood stem cell transplantation has been effective for patients who have failed to obtain a complete response or have relapsed and should be considered if the patient is otherwise an appropriate candidate. Disease sensitivity to chemotherapy is the most important prognostic factor for the success of transplantation.[135,136]

Diffuse large B-cell lymphoma is aggressive but curable with appropriate multidrug chemotherapy. The IPI is strongly predictive of outcome in this disease. Disease-free survival rates are approximately 60% for patients with an IPI of 0 or 1, 35% for those with an IPI of 2 or 3, and 20% for those with an IPI of 4 or 5.[137] *BCL-2* overexpression has been associated with a higher incidence of relapse.[138] Conversely, the *BCL-6* translocation has been associated with a better prognosis.

## BURKITT'S LYMPHOMA

Burkitt's lymphoma is the most aggressive lymphoma, involving 100% of the cells in the cell cycle at any time. The malignancy is composed of monomorphic medium B cells and divides rapidly. Three variants of BL exist: endemic, sporadic, and immunodeficiency associated. Each of the variants demonstrates a different morphology and clinical history. Burkitt's lymphoma may also present as leukemia.

Endemic BL is found in Africa and Papua, New Guinea. It is the most common malignancy in childhood in these countries, occurring in a male-to-female ratio of 2:1 and with a peak age incidence of 4 to 7 years.[139,140] There appears to be a possible link between the climatic factors that are associated with malaria in the endemic regions. In addition, EBV is found in nearly all patients with endemic BL.[141] Multiple bacterial, viral, and parasitic infections (especially malaria) result in polyclonal B-cell activation and proliferation. Patients with malaria are noted to have defective EBV-specific T-cell immunity, which supports the development of lymphoma.[141]

Sporadic BL may be found throughout the world, affecting mainly children and young adults. It is rare in adults. It accounts for only 2% to 3% of all lymphomas in immunocompetent adults but is responsible for 30% to 50% of childhood lymphomas.[142] This variant of BL also has a higher incidence in males than in females (2:1 to 3:1 ratio), and the average age of adults at diagnosis is 30 years. There is an association with EBV infection, but it is observed in only 15% to 20% of patients with BL in Europe and North America. Low socioeconomic status and early EBV infection are associated with increased risk of EBV-positive BL. Between 50% and 70% of patients with these risk factors are EBV positive.[143]

Both the endemic and the sporadic forms of BL occur in immunocompetent hosts. Tumor growth is not related to malfunction of the individual's immunity. Rather, the BL cell is thought to escape immune rejection because cell factors resemble resting B cells. In contrast, immunodeficiency-associated BL is primarily seen in patients with HIV infection, but may be observed in other immunodeficiency states. It may be the initial AIDS-defining illness.[144] EBV is reported in 25% to 40% of immunodeficiency-associated BL.[144,145]

Burkitt's lymphoma commonly presents at extranodal sites. Patients with all 3 variants are at risk for CNS disease. In endemic disease, the jaw, orbit, or other facial bones are involved approximately 50% of the time. Other potentially affected sites include the small intestine, omentum, ovaries, kidneys, and breast. Most patients with sporadic BL present with abdominal masses. The ileocecal region is the most common site of involvement. Retroperitoneal masses may compress the spinal cord, resulting in sensory and motor loss. The ovaries, kidneys, and breasts may also be involved. Breast involvement is usually bilateral and is associated with the onset of puberty, pregnancy, or lactation. Lymph node involvement may occur but is more common in adults than children. A leukemic phase of this lymphoma may be observed, especially in patients with bulky disease. Rarely, patients present with bone marrow infiltration without other sites of disease. In such cases, the cells observed in the bone marrow resemble Burkitt cells. If more than 5% but less than 25% of the cells in the bone marrow are involved, the patient is classified as having stage IV BL. If the bone marrow has more than 25% infiltration, the condition may be classified as acute lymphocytic leukemia (ALL), L3, or Burkitt's leukemia. Both nodal disease and marrow involvement are more common in immunodeficiency-associated BL.

The morphology of classical BL is observed in endemic BL and most sporadic cases of BL, especially in children. The cells are medium in size and diffusely infiltrate the tissue. These cells have multiple mitotic figures suggestive of a high proliferative rate. Two variants may be observed: the BL variant with plasmacytoid differentiation and the atypical Burkitt/Burkitt-like variant. The BL variant with plasmacytoid differentiation lacks the monotonous morphology of the classical BL cells and most commonly arises in immunodeficiency states.[146] The atypical Burkitt/Burkitt-like variant is composed of cells similar to Burkitt cells except for their greater variety of nuclear size and shape. Diagnosis is dependent on a growth fraction of nearly 100% and evidence or strong suggestion of *MYC* translocation. Some individuals with BL or Burkitt-like lymphoma demonstrate a strong granulomatous reaction. It has been postulated that it may represent an immune response to the disease and is associated with an excellent prognosis.

B-cell-associated antigens are expressed on BL cells (CD19, CD20, CD22) as well as CD10, CD77, and *BCL6*. The cells are negative for CD5, CD23, TdT, and *BCL-2*. Blasts of BL presenting with a leukemic phase are consistent with a mature B cell, unlike precursor B-ALL (B-cell acute lymphocytic leukemia). Cells in the leukemic phase of BL are $CD34^-$ and usually $TdT^-$. CD45 is brightly expressed. Clonal rearrangements of the immunoglobulin heavy-chain and light-chain genes are seen. All cases have an *MYC* translocation, t(8;14), or, less commonly, t(2;8) or t(8;22). The *MYC* translocation plays a significant role in the pathology of this disease, increasing the rate of cell cycling, activating genes involved in apoptosis, and enhancing the lymphogenicity.[147,148] The *MYC* translocation is present in all BL variants, regardless of EBV status.

Patients typically present with rapidly growing, bulky disease. Elevated serum uric acid and LDH levels are commonly found due to the rapid cell turnover. Patients are at risk for tumor lysis syndrome (TLS) during institution of therapy and require close monitoring. Burkitt's lymphoma has a unique staging system developed by Murphy et al and modified by Magrath (Table 60-6).[149,150]

Both endemic and sporadic BL are extremely aggressive but potentially curable. Endemic BL is very sensitive to multidrug regimens. Treatment should be initiated as soon as possible because of the rapid doubling time of the tumor. Intensive regimens result in long-term EFS of 80%[151] of patients with BL. Children have a more favorable prognosis than adults. Negative prognostic indicators include stage IV disease (CNS or bone marrow involvement), unresected tumor larger than 10 cm, and an elevated serum LDH level. Relapse, if it occurs, is likely to take place within the first year of diagnosis. Relapse-free survival for 2 years is considered a cure.[149] Burkitt's leukemia is treated with very intensive regimens but for short durations. Regimens must include alkylating agents with an anthracycline and high-dose methotrexate. Traditional CHOP therapy, often prescribed for other lymphomas, is not adequate therapy for BL. Treatment is also considerably different from that for other subtypes of ALL; as a consequence, accurate diagnosis is essential. Intrathecal therapy is recommended for all patients, possibly with the exception of those with stage I disease. Methotrexate and cytarabine are often administered intrathecally, sometimes including systemic high-dose or moderate-dose methotrexate.

The use of radiotherapy to prevent CNS involvement is controversial in this disease. No clear evidence proves that it benefits patients without known disease involving the CNS. Clearly, there is an increased risk of neurotoxicity associated with the addition of cranial irradiation. Even without radiotherapy, intrathecal chemotherapy in addition to systemic high-dose cytarabine and methotrexate may increase neurotoxicity. With appropriate treatment, 80% to 90% of patients with BL survive.[152,153]

**TABLE 60-6**

**Staging System for Burkitt's Lymphoma**

| Stage | Definition |
|---|---|
| I | A single nodal or extranodal mass with the exclusion of the mediastinum or abdomen |
| II | A single extranodal tumor with regional lymph node involvement |
| | Two or more nodal areas on the same side of the diaphragm |
| | Two extranodal tumors with or without regional node involvement on the same side of the diaphragm |
| | Primary gastrointestinal tract tumor, with or without involvement of the mesenteric nodes only |
| IIA | Completely resected abdominal disease |
| III | Two single extranodal tumors on opposite sides of the diaphragm |
| | Two or more nodal areas above and below the diaphragm |
| | All mediastinal, pleural, or thymic tumors (primary intrathoracic tumors) |
| | All paraspinal or epidural tumors, regardless of other sites |
| | All extensive primary intraabdominal disease |
| IIIA | Localized but nonresectable abdominal tumors |
| IIIB | Widespread multiorgan abdominal disease |
| IV | Any of the above with initial central nervous system and/or bone marrow involvement < 25% |

Source: Data from Murphy and Hustu[149]; and Magrath et al.[150]

## AIDS-RELATED LYMPHOMA

AIDS-related lymphoma is discussed further in Chapter 45. Between 25% and 40% of patients with HIV eventually develop a malignancy. This is reported to be NHL in approximately 10% of cases.[154,155] The risk increases with time.[156] HIV does not seem to cause NHL, but rather the immune compromise due to the HIV infection appears to be a significant risk factor for this lymphoma's development.

The role of EBV in the development of these high-grade, aggressive lymphomas remains controversial. Levine et al reported that 68% of HIV-positive lymphoma patients had the EBV genome present, compared with 15% of HIV-negative patients.[157] Nearly all patients with primary CNS lymphoma and primary effusion lymphoma and 30% to 70% of patients with BL have experienced EBV infections.

Most of these malignancies are monoclonal B-cell neoplasms. Immunophenotyping is consistent with the histological subtype of lymphoma that develops. Immunoglobulin gene rearrangements are commonly observed, while the minority of T-cell cases have clonal rearrangement of the T-cell receptor genes. Numerous genetic abnormalities involving the *MYC* and *BCL-6* oncogenes as well as tumor suppressor genes are recognized in HIV-related lymphomas. Abnormalities of the *MYC* gene are observed in HIV-related BL, similar to other cases of BL. Similarly, rearrangements of *BCL-6* are observed in DLBCL, and mutations of the noncoding region of *BCL-6* can be detected in both DLBCL and BL. They represent the most common genetic alteration seen in HIV-related lymphoma.[157] Fifteen percent of cases demonstrate mutation of the *Ras* family proto-oncogenes. These mutations are unique to HIV-related lymphomas and are not normally found in lymphomas developing in immunocompetent hosts. Tumor suppressor gene mutations and deletions are observed in 50% to 60% of BL cases and 40% of DLBCL cases, leading to inactivation of this gene.[158]

Patients with HIV-associated lymphomas generally present with advanced stage and bulky disease. B symptoms are observed in 80% of individuals and often lead to diagnosis. These early symptoms may prompt a work-up for opportunistic infection. HIV-related lymphomas commonly present in extranodal sites such as the CNS (20%),[159] gastrointestinal tract (45%),[160] bone marrow (33%), lung (33%), and liver (33%).[161] Unusual sites of disease, such as the oral cavity, jaw, and body cavities, may be involved as well. These tumors often meet the criteria of plasmablastic lymphomas of the oral cavity. As localized tumors, they grow rapidly and have a high mitotic index. The myocardium, testes, rectum, anus, gallbladder fossa, skeletal muscle, skin, soft tissue, ear lobes, adrenals, and other organs have been reported as sites of involvement. Only one third of patients have lymph node disease at presentation. Serum LDH is elevated. Primary effusion lymphoma typically presents as either a pleural or peritoneal effusion. It can, however, occasionally present as a solid tumor mass, most commonly involving the gastrointestinal tract or soft tissue.[162]

A dilemma exists over treatment of AIDS-related lymphoma. Aggressive chemotherapy regimens are typically utilized to treat the high-grade disease that is manifested as BL. Due to the immunosuppression caused by the underlying HIV infection, patients with low CD4 counts often develop significant toxicity and a high incidence of opportunistic infections. Patients with minimal risk factors can usually tolerate full-dose chemotherapy. The coadministration of highly active coantiretroviral therapy (HAART) appears to negate the poor risk-prognostic factors associated with HIV. The risk of opportunistic infection and rate of survival approach those of patients with similar lymphomas without HIV.[163] Less aggressive treatment regimens, such as CHOP, with or without rituximab, may be used to treat DLBCL. Treatment is comparable to that given to patients without HIV infection. However prophylaxis of the CNS must be strongly considered for this population, however.[164] Although CNS lymphoma has been treated with radiotherapy or high-dose methotrexate, survival in affected patients is poor.

Treatment with RCHOP resulted in a complete response in 77% of patients with HIV and DLBCL, and a 2-year OS of 75% in those patients without adverse factors (CD4 count less than 100 cells/μL, prior AIDS, or a performance status less than 2). However, concern has been raised over the use of rituximab in patients with CD4 counts less than 50, as it has been associated with an increased incidence of opportunistic infections and death.[165] The 2-year survival is better in patients with BL than in those with DLBCL. Although primary effusion lymphoma responds poorly to treatment and has a poor prognosis, the worst prognosis is associated with primary CNS lymphoma. The level of immunosuppression is a significant indicator of prognosis and correlates well with the IPI. Negative independent prognostic indicators include age greater than 35 years, intravenous drug use, advanced stage disease (III or IV), and CD4 counts less than 100/mm$^3$. A multivariate analysis of prognostic factors was performed in 60 patients with newly diagnosed AIDS lymphoma. Four factors were associated with shorter survival: the diagnosis of AIDS made prior to the diagnosis of lymphoma, a low CD4 count, Karnofsky performance status less than 70%, and stage IV disease (with bone marrow involvement).[166] Primary CNS lymphoma may respond to radiotherapy, improving the patient's quality of life, but survival is in the range of 2 to 3 months.

## LYMPHOBLASTIC LYMPHOMA: PRECURSOR B-CELL OR T-CELL LYMPHOBLASTIC LEUKEMIA/LYMPHOMA

Sternberg first recognized lymphoblastic lymphoma (LL) in 1905, when a case of lymphoma of the mediastinum evolved into acute leukemia. At that time, this disease entity was known as Sternberg sarcoma. Lymphoblastic lymphoma—now classified by the WHO as precursor B-cell or T-cell lymphoblastic leukemia/lymphoma—has seen significant advances in therapy. In particular, recognition of low-risk and high-risk groups, as determined by cytogenetics and immunophenotyping, has permitted more specific therapeutic regimens.

The distinction between the terms "lymphoblastic leukemia" and "lymphoblastic lymphoma" is a blurry one. If the disease process presents with a mass lesion (nodal or extranodal) with minimal or no evidence of bone marrow and blood involvement, the term "lymphoma" is generally used. The cell of origin, either a precursor B lymphoblast or T lymphoblast, will further classify the disease. Precursor B-cell lymphoma accounts for approximately 10% to 20% of LL, and precursor T-cell lymphoma represents 80% to 90% of cases. Lymphoblastic lymphoma is rare in adults, accounting for only 2% of all cases of NHL, but represents one third to one half of all cases of pediatric lymphoma.[129,167] Precursor T-lymphoblastic lymphoma (T-LBL) is composed of small to medium-sized blasts. Morphologically, the cells look similar to those found in precursor B-lymphoblastic lymphoma (B-LBL). They diffusely infiltrate the lymph node and invade capsular and pericapsular tissues. Azurophilic granules may be observed in about 10% of B-LBL cases. Mitotic figures are generally more numerous in T-LBL. Immunophenotyping is required to distinguish these diseases. The lymphoblasts in T-LBL are positive for TdT and for CD7, CD5, CD2, and CD3. The presence of CD3 is considered specific to the T-cell lineage. Other markers may be variably expressed, including CD1a, CD4, and CD8. Findings are negative for CD10.

Abnormal cytogenetic findings have been reported in 60% of LL. The abnormalities are similar to those found in T-cell acute lymphocytic leukemia (T-ALL)[168] and support the belief that these diseases are different manifestations of the same disorder.[88] Certain translocations, such as t(9;17), however, have been identified only in patients with T-LBL. At this time, the cytogenetic changes in T-LBL do not have any significant prognostic relevance. Burkitt's lymphoma must be ruled out, particularly in children presenting with LL. In adults, the blastoid variant of mantle cell lymphoma is included in the differential diagnosis. Evidence of TdT rapidly distinguishes these other types of lymphoma.

The lymphoblasts in B-LBL are positive for TdT and are almost always positive for CD10 (CALLA), CD19, and CD24. A cytogenetic abnormality, t(4;11) (q21;q23), may be seen. These mutations often account for those cases that do not express CD10 and CD24. Cytogenetic abnormalities in B-cell acute lymphoblastic leukemia/lymphoma are classified into multiple groups. These groups have significant prognostic significance and influence treatment planning, especially in the pediatric populations. Groups with a good prognosis include individuals with hyperdiploidy (those with more than 2 sets of chromosomes) between chromosomes 59 and 65 and t(12;21) (p12;q22). Abnormalities including del(6q), del(9p), del(12p), hyperploidy less than 51, near triploidy, and near tetraploidy denote an intermediate risk. Groups with a poor prognosis include those that have t(9;22) (Philadelphia chromosome), t(4;11), t(1;19), and hypoploidy.[169] T-LBL is frequently found in adolescent males.

T-cell acute lymphocytic leukemia is frequently characterized by its presentation of a rapidly growing mass in the mediastinum (50% of cases), with associated pleural effusions. Other sites of involvement include peripheral lymph nodes, skin, liver, spleen, Waldeyer's ring, CNS, and gonads.[170]

Historically, LL was associated with a poor prognosis. Today, due to more aggressive treatment regimens stratified by prognostic features and the availability of CNS prophylaxis, it is considered among the most curable lymphomas. Intensive induction and consolidation regimens are used, similar or identical to leukemia regimens. Treatment regimens typically include higher doses of cyclophosphamide and an anthracycline, standard-dose vincristine and asparaginase, and intrathecal chemotherapy.[93] Adults with advanced age, high serum LDH levels, bone marrow involvement, and CNS involvement have a poorer prognosis.

B-lymphoblastic lymphoma is most commonly found in pediatric and young adult patients. Seventy-five percent of cases involve individuals who are younger than 18 years of age.[171] Although most patients with B-cell leukemia/lymphoma present with leukemia, a small number (approximately 10%) present without significant marrow involvement. The most frequent sites of involvement in this subtype are the skin (may manifest as multiple nodules), bone, soft tissue, and lymph nodes.[172] Mediastinal masses in B-LBL are rare, in contrast to T-LBL. Treatment is similar to that identified for T-LBL. There is a high remission rate in patients with B-LBL, and a high cure rate in disease that remains limited to lymph nodes. Allogeneic stem cell transplantation should be considered in disease reoccurrences. As treatment for LBL is aggressive, often impairing fertility, thus discussion about sperm banking and ovarian protection should take place. Negative prognostic indicators include a high WBC count, symptomatic CNS disease, and unfavorable cytogenetic abnormalities.

## POSTTRANSPLANT LYMPHOPROLIFERATIVE DISORDER

Postttransplant lymphoproliferative disorder (PTLD) is a lymphoma or lymphoid proliferation that develops due to immunosuppression in a recipient of a solid organ or peripheral blood (or bone marrow) stem cell transplant. The Cincinnati Transplant Tumor Registry reports that PTLDs account for 21% of all malignancies following organ transplant, compared with 5% of lymphomas in the general population.[173] These lymphomas have a high association with EBV infection (80% positive) and typically develop sooner after transplant than they do in EBV-negative cases.[174] The majority of PTLD cases that occur more than 5 years after transplant are EBV negative and are associated with a poorer outcome. Although PTLDs resulting in B-cell lymphomas are far more common, T-cell lymphomas represent approximately 12% to 14% of these lymphomas.

Posttransplant lymphoproliferative disease comprises a spectrum of disorders that range from early lesions with reactive plasmacytic hyperplasia or infectious mononucleosis-like disease to monomorphic B-cell or T-cell neoplasms or HL. Table 60-7 outlines the categories of PTLD. The early lesions seen in PTLD are characterized by a diffuse proliferation of plasma cells and immunoblasts that do not completely destroy the architecture of the affected lymph node or tissue, typically occurring 2 to 8 weeks after initiation of immunosuppression. Polyclonal B cells are observed with normal cytogenetics. Abnormal immunoglobulin gene rearrangements characteristic of malignant transformation are absent. These early lesions account for 55% of PTLDs, tend to occur in children and young adults, and are often EBV negative. They may regress spontaneously with withdrawal or reduction of the immunosuppression or they may progress to monomorphic or polymorphic PTLD.

Polymorphic PTLD consists of destructive lesions affecting immunoblasts, plasma cells, and lymphoid cells in 20% to 80% of cases, dependent on the report.[175] Unlike the early lesions, these lesions may efface the architecture of the lymph nodes or form destructive extranodal tumors. Cytogenetic abnormalities and immunoglobulin gene rearrangements are common. They are considered polymorphic because they demonstrate the full maturation

**TABLE 60-7**

**Categories of Posttransplant Lymphoproliferative Disease (PTLD)**

1. Early lesions
   Reactive plasmacytic hyperplasia
   Infectious mononucleosis-like
2. Polymorphic PTLD
3. Monomorphic PTLD
   B-cell neoplasms
      Diffuse large B-cell lymphoma
      Burkitt's/Burkitt-like lymphoma
      Plasma cell myeloma
      Plasmacytoma-like lesion
   T-cell neoplasms
      Peripheral T-cell lymphoma
      Other
4. Hodgkin's lymphoma and Hodgkin's-like lymphoma

of B cells. As with the early lesions, withdrawal or reduction of immunosuppressive agents is the treatment of choice, but it may lead to regression of the PTLD or progression to lymphoma. Monomorphic PTLDs have sufficient changes to diagnose lymphoma and express either B-cell or T-cell antigens. Although the majority of B-cell PTLDs are DLBCLs, BL may be diagnosed in a minority of cases. Plasma cell myeloma is uncommon, but is important in that it appears to be unresponsive to withdrawal of immunosuppression.[176,177]

Plasmacytoma-like PTLD is also rare, and its clinical behavior is not well studied. The extramedullary plasmacytomas occur in the gastrointestinal tract, lymph nodes, or other extranodal sites. Monomorphic T-cell lymphomas account for 12% to 14% of PTLD. A broad spectrum of T-cell neoplasms are reported. The development of T-cell PTLDs is generally longer than that for the B-cell PTLDs. Response to withdrawal or reduction of immunosuppression is less likely. Some reports have cited cases involving both HL and Hodgkin's-like lymphoma. Classical HL has been reported after allogeneic stem cell transplants with a sixfold increase over its expected frequency.[178]

The genetic features of PTLDs vary depending on the category of lesion found. The monomorphic B-PTLDs consistently demonstrate clonal immunoglobulin gene rearrangement, typically containing EBV genomes. Conversely, the monomorphic T-PTLDs demonstrate clonal T-receptor gene rearrangements, and only 25% have EBV genomes.

Fewer than 2% of organ transplant recipients develop PTLD, but the risk of lymphoma depends on the type of organ transplanted and the immunosuppressive regimen used to prevent rejection. The highest risk is associated with multiorgan transplantation (11%-33%), followed by the lung (2%-9%), the heart (2%-6%), the kidney (1%-3%), and the liver (1%-2%).[179] Lymphoproliferative cells can arise from either recipient cells or donor cells. Disease that arises from recipient cells tends to be more systemic and less responsive to withdrawal of immunosuppression. Tacrolimus is associated with a higher incidence of PTLD than cyclosporine.[180] Mycophenolate mofetil may have little or no risk.

Initial treatment of PTLDs is targeted at withdrawal of immunosuppression. Risk of organ rejection must be weighed into the plan, as rejection of a heart, liver, or lungs may lead to the patient's death. Immunosuppression withdrawal is often effective in managing early PTLDs and EBV-related PTLDs. If this is insufficient, chemotherapy and monoclonal antibodies may be incorporated into the treatment plan. Anecdotal cases of antiviral therapy successes exist.[181]

Allogeneic stem cell transplant recipients have a low overall risk of developing PTLD (less than 1%), but risk factors have been identified that may substantially increase the incidence in this group. In a study, more than 18,000 patients who underwent allogeneic bone marrow transplant at 235 centers throughout the world were followed for development of PTLD. The disease ultimately developed in 78 recipients. Of these cases, 82% arose within 1 year of transplant, the other 18% occurred between 1 and 8.6 years posttransplant. The peak incidence of PTLD development was during the third month posttransplant. Eighty-six percent of patients who had a confirmed PTLD died during the survey period; rapid disease progression was noted in this group. Nine patients with early PTLD were alive with a range of follow-up of 3 to 131 months (median 88 months).[182] Identified risk factors for early-onset PTLD (within 1 year) included receipt of T-cell-depleted marrow and use of antithymocyte globulin or human leukocyte antigen-mismatched or unrelated donor stem cells (but only with those who received T-cell-depleted marrow or ATG). Of the patients with 3 of these risk factors, 8.1% developed a PTLD. A weaker association was noted with acute or chronic graft-vs-host disease (GVHD), age greater than 50 years, and second transplantation.[183] The significance of these risk factors diminished after 1 year, and only extensive chronic GVHD was identified as a strong risk factor.

Clinical manifestations of PTLD vary depending on the immunosuppressive agent administered. Patients receiving azathioprine-based therapy tend to present with extranodal disease, whereas those receiving cyclosporine-based or tacrolimus-based regimens present with lymph node and gastrointestinal tract involvement. The time to diagnosis posttransplant also correlates to the immunosuppressant used, the type of allograft, and EBV status. The mean interval to the development of PTLD posttransplant is 48 months when azathioprine is used and 15 months with cyclosporine therapy.[184] The majority of PTLDs develop within 5 months of stem cell transplant, and new cases of the disease are relatively uncommon among survivors more than 1 year after transplant.[182] The median interval for the development of EBV-positive PTLD is 10 months, compared with 4 to 5 years for EBV-negative cases.[174,185]

Treatment of many PTLDs is often directed at reduction of the immunosuppressant. This treatment must be accomplished without rejection of the transplanted organ and control of GVHD in stem cell transplant recipients. It is often successful in early lesions and in children. Cases that fail to respond to withdrawal of immunosuppression require chemotherapy. The mortality among solid-organ transplant recipients who develop PTLD is high, with only 25% to 35% long-term survivors,[186] and among stem cell transplant recipients long-term survival is reported to range from 25% to 60%.[187] The use of rituximab is being investigated in these transplant patients. Choquet et al reported on 47 patients who failed immunosuppression withdrawal. Forty-four percent of patients treated with rituximab responded to treatment, and 12 complete responses were noted. Two thirds of these patients remained disease free at 1 year.[188] Curtis et al have reported that careful monitoring for EBV reactivation following bone marrow transplantation may provide warning of early PTLD development.[182] There have been rare case reports of successful autologous hematopoietic stem cell transplantation (HSCT) in patients with chemosensitive, relapsed PTLDs; however, most patients are not candidates for this therapy due to organ dysfunction, comorbid diseases, and chemotherapy resistance.[189]

## CHARACTERISTICS AND MANAGEMENT OF T-CELL NHL

### CUTANEOUS T-CELL LYMPHOMA

Cutaneous T-cell lymphomas (CTCL) encompass a group of lymphomas of T-cell origin that involve primarily the skin and affect other sites secondarily. The skin is the second most common extranodal site related to NHL, secondary only to the gastrointestinal tract. The subtypes of lymphoma that make up this group include mycosis fungoides (MFs), Sézary syndrome (SS), primary cutaneous anaplastic large cell lymphoma (ALCL), and lymphomatoid papulosis. Lymphomatoid papulosis is not clinically considered a neoplastic disease.

*Mycosis fungoides* is a mature T-cell lymphoma. It has no relationship to a fungal etiology but received its name because of the mushroom-like appearance of the malignant lesions.[190] Infiltration of the epidermis and dermis with small to medium-sized T cells results in the characteristic cutaneous patches/plaques. Mycosis fungoides is the most common of the CTCLs, but is still a rare disease, accounting for 0.5% to 3% of all cases of NHL. It is primarily a disease of the middle aged to elderly and strikes males twice as often as females.[191] Mycosis fungoides is a slow-growing disease. Although the etiology of this cutaneous lymphoma is unknown, some reports have implicated recreational or occupational exposure to some chemicals as an origin. These reports have been refuted by 2 studies, 1 based on the SEER program.[192] Whittemore et al hypothesize that chronic antigenic stimulation from contact allergens may be an initiating factor in the development of MF.[193] Patients may report a history of scaly skin lesions for years prior to diagnosis. The skin may be the only site of involvement for many years, with lesions initially seen on the trunk. The palms and soles may be either heavily involved or spared. These plaques usually become more generalized and eventually progress to tumor formation. At later stages, extracutaneous dissemination may occur involving the lymph nodes, liver, spleen, lungs, and blood. This spread is seen most frequently in patients who have developed cutaneous tumors (30%), compared with only 8% of those with limited plaques.[194] Involvement of bone marrow is rare. A simple clinical staging system has been developed for MF and is important in determining prognosis; Table 60-8 outlines this staging system.[195] The Mycosis Fungoides Clinical Grading System (MFCG) has proved to be an extremely useful tool in the management of patients with MF/SS and is the standard for the staging and classification of MF/SS patients today. The International Society for Cutaneous Lymphomas and the Cutaneous Lymphoma Task Force of the European Organization of Research and Treatment of Cancer have developed a much more involved staging system (see Table 60-9), which continues to go through revision, as reported by Olsen et al.[196] This staging system provides more detailed information incorporating cell biology, diagnosis, clinical characteristics, prognosis, and a standardized approach to the MF/SS to improve communication and clinical trials.

Lymph nodes are categorized when they become enlarged. Category I represents no involvement by MF, category II reflects early involvement, and category III entails massive involvement by MF. Clonal T cells are present occasionally in category I lesions, and in most category II

**TABLE 60-8**

**Clinical Staging System for Mycosis Fungoides**

| | |
|---|---|
| Stage I | Disease confined to the skin |
| Ia | Limited plaques/patches |
| Ib | Disseminated plaques/patches |
| Ic | Skin tumors |
| Stage II | Lymph nodes enlarged, but histologically uninvolved |
| Stage III | Lymph node involved documented histologically |
| Stage IV | Visceral dissemination |

*Source*: Data from Willemze et al.[195]

**TABLE 60-9**

**ISCL/EORTC Revision to the Classification of Mycosis Fungoides and Sézary Syndrome**

| | |
|---|---|
| **TNMB Stages** | |
| **Skin** | |
| T1 | Limited patches,[a] papules, and/or plaques[b] covering < 10% of the skin surface<br>May further stratify into T1a (patch only) vs T1b (plaque ± patch) |
| T2 | Patches, papules, or plaques covering ≥ 10% of the skin surface<br>May further stratify into T2a (patch only) vs T2b (plaque ± patch) |
| T3 | One or more tumors[c] (≥1 cm diameter) |
| T4 | Confluence of erythema covering ≥ 80% body surface area |
| **Node** | |
| N0 | No clinically abnormal peripheral lymph nodes[d]; biopsy not required |
| N1 | Clinically abnormal peripheral lymph nodes; histopathology Dutch grade 1 or NCI LN0–2 |
| N1a | Clone negative[e] |
| N1b | Clone positive[e] |
| N2 | Clinically abnormal peripheral lymph nodes; histopathology Dutch grade 2 or NCI LN3 |
| N2a | Clone negative[e] |
| N2b | Clone positive[e] |
| N3 | Clinically abnormal peripheral lymph nodes; histopathology Dutch grades 3–4 or NCI LN4; clone positive or negative |
| Nx | Clinically abnormal peripheral lymph nodes; no histological confirmation |
| **Visceral** | |
| M0 | No visceral organ involvement |
| M1 | Visceral involvement (must have pathology confirmation[f] and organ involvement should be specified) |
| **Blood** | |
| B0 | Absence of significant blood involvement: ≤ 5% of peripheral blood lymphocytes are atypical (Sézary) cells[g] |
| B0a | Clone negative[e] |
| B0b | Clone positive[e] |
| B1 | Low blood tumor burden: > 5% of peripheral blood lymphocytes are atypical (Sézary) cells but does not meet the criteria of B2 |
| B1a | Clone negative[e] |
| B1b | Clone positive[e] |
| B2 | High blood tumor burden: ≥ 1000/μL Sézary cells[g] with positive clone[e] |

[a]For skin, patch indicates any size skin lesion without significant elevation or induration. Presence/absence of hypo- or hyperpigmentation, scales, crusting, and/or poikiloderma should be noted.

[b]For skin, plaque indicates any size skin lesion that is elevated or indurated. Presence or absence of scales, crusting, and/or poikiloderma should be noted. Histological features such as folliculotropism or large-cell transformation (>25% large cells), $CD30^+$ or $CD30^-$, and clinical features such as ulceration are important to document.

[c]For skin, tumor indicates at least one 1 cm diameter solid or nodular lesion with evidence of depth and/or vertical growth. Note total number of lesions, total volume of lesions, largest size lesion, and region of body involved. Also note if histological evidence of large-cell transformation has occurred. Phenotyping for CD30 is encouraged.

[d]For node, abnormal peripheral lymph node(s) indicates any palpable peripheral node that on physical examination is firm, irregular, clustered, fixed, or 1.5 cm or larger in diameter. Node groups examined on physical examination include cervical, supraclavicular, epitrochlear, axillary, and inguinal. Central nodes, which are not generally amenable to pathologic assessment, are not currently considered in the nodal classification, unless used to establish N3 histopathologically.

[e]A T-cell clone is defined by PCR or Southern blot analysis of the T-cell receptor gene.

[f]For viscera, spleen and liver may be diagnosed by imaging criteria.

[g]For blood, Sézary cells are defined as lymphocytes with hyperconvoluted cerebriform nuclei. If Sézary cells are not able to be used to determine tumor burden for B2 then one of the following modified ISCL criteria along with a positive clonal rearrangement of the TCR may be used instead: (1) expanded $CD4^+$ or $CD3^+$ cells with CD4/CD8 ratio of 10 or more, (2) expanded $CD4^+$ cells with abnormal immunophenotype including loss of CD7 or CD26.

*Abbreviations*: EORTC, European Organization of Research and Treatment of Cancer; ISCL, International Society for Cutaneous Lymphomas; LN, lymph node; NCI, National Cancer Institute; TNMB, tumor, node, metastasis, blood.

*Source*: Data from Olsen et al.[196]

and III lesions. These clonal cells may be associated with an unfavorable outcome. Immunophenotyping is usually $CD2^+$, $CD3^+$, $CD5^+$, $CD4^+$, and $CD8^-$.[195] No specific cytogenetic abnormality is associated with MF, but numerous, complex karyotypes are present in advanced disease.

Treatment depends on the stage of disease. Phototherapy, topical chemotherapy, topical retinoids, radiotherapy, and occasionally systemic therapy are all used in the treatment of MF. Topical corticosteroids may be sufficient to relieve symptoms of early disease. This therapy does not provide long-term control, however, nor does it affect survival.

Phototherapy is performed by providing the patient with an oral photosensitizing drug (Psoralens), followed by ultraviolet light exposure (PUVA). Until the lesions clear, patients require treatment 2 to 3 times per week. Approximately 50% of patients will see the disease clear with phototherapy. The combination of PUVA with interferon has resulted in a complete response in as many as 80% of patients.[197] If clearance is achieved, a maintenance program is continued, with variable frequencies of treatment. Erythema and blistering are common acute side effects of PUVA. Cataract development and secondary skin malignancies are long-term concerns.

Topical chemotherapy is an effective but less intrusive therapy on the patient's lifestyle. Topical nitrogen mustard is the most common agent administered. There is no absorption of the drug, which limits the toxicity and the follow-up needed. The drug is generally mixed in a water or ointment base and applied daily until the lesions clear. The concentration of the nitrogen mustard may be altered depending on the response of the lesions and the patient's tolerance. Self-administration may be impossible, depending on the location of the lesions. The average time to clearance is approximately 6 months, and maintenance therapy is used for another 6 months.[190] A cutaneous hypersensitivity reaction develops in approximately 30% of patients receiving the aqueous solution and 5% receiving the ointment.[198] Desensitization has proved successful in overcoming this problem. Complete responses range from 50% to 70%, depending on the initial extent of skin involvement.[198,199] Only 10% to 15% of patients maintain a long-term complete response after discontinuation of the topical nitrogen mustard. Topical carmustine (bis-chloronitrosourea, BCNU) has also been utilized for this disease. Although the response rate is similar to that with nitrogen mustard, carmustine is systemically absorbed. Its toxicity is also greater and hematological monitoring is required.

Mycosis fungoides is very sensitive to radiotherapy, and ionizing irradiation is the most effective single-agent treatment for it. The delivery of 36 cGy in small fractions over 10 weeks to the skin is a standard approach.[200] Patients stand on a rotating platform during radiotherapy treatment. Electron therapy is more effective than photon therapy. Acute complications related to radiotherapy include erythema, desquamation, and temporary loss of hair and nails in the treatment fields. For 6 to 12 months, patients experience an inability to sweat. Similar to other treatments for MF, an increased risk of secondary skin malignancies exists. Complete response rates have been reported to be as high as 98% in patients with limited plaques and approximately 35% in patients with generalized erythroderma or skin tumors. However, only about half of these complete responders demonstrated long-term responses.[190]

Systemic chemotherapy such as doxorubicin or gemcitabine has limited value in the treatment of MF. Although multiple agents have been utilized, complete responses have been documented in only about 25% of cases, with limited durations. Only 10% to 20% of patients with MF require systemic treatment. Denileukin diftitox (Ontak) is a biological agent produced by genetically fusing protein from the diphtheria toxin to the interleukin 2 (IL-2) receptor. This biotherapeutic agent targets cells that express the CD25 component of the IL-2 receptor. Nearly 60% of patients with CTCLs have IL-2 receptors, and denileukin diftitox has demonstrated activity in this population of patients.[201] Acute hypersensitivity reactions have been reported in 69% of patients during or within the 24 hours of the denileukin diftitox infusion. These reactions were frequently associated with the first dose of a treatment cycle. In clinical trials, 27% of the patients developed vascular leak syndrome manifested by hypotension, edema, and hypoalbuminemia.[201] Because patients with CTCL are at risk for infection, and Ontak affects normal lymphocytes, patients must be monitored closely for this complication.

Prognosis depends on the extent of the MF. Limited disease generally has an excellent prognosis, and survival is not affected by the disease. Prognosis is poor in advanced stages of MF, however. Negative prognostic factors include age more than 60 years, skin tumors, extracutaneous dissemination, and elevated LDH. Transformation to a large T-cell lymphoma may be seen as a terminal event. Ulcerated tumors may develop a suprainfection. Sepsis is the leading cause of death in MF.

*Sézary syndrome* is often considered a variant of MF, but the clinical behavior is much more aggressive. This mature CTCL is characterized by erythroderma, lymphadenopathy, and malignant T lymphocytes in the blood. Sézary cells have the same morphology, immunophenotyping, and cytogenetic characteristics as the cells that infiltrate the epidermis.[202] SS is defined by the presence of $1000/mm^3$ or more of Sézary cells or increased $CD4^+$ cells with a CD4/CD8 ratio of 10 or above, $CD4^+$/CD7 ratio of 40% or above, or $CD4^+$/CD26 ratio of 30% or above, in addition to the presence of a clonal T-cell receptor gene rearrangement.[196] Despite the presence of neoplastic cells in the blood, the bone marrow is rarely involved. In advanced stages of disease, the visceral organs may be involved. Intense pruritus, cold intolerance, and skin pain are common complaints and can be very debilitating.

Sézary syndrome is an extremely rare disease and is found only in adults. There is a question of association of this disease with HTLV-1 infection. Morphologically, the cutaneous infiltrates are similar to those seen in MF. However, the density of dermal involvement and the extent of epidermal involvement may be significantly less, making diagnosis difficult. Topical use of corticosteroids may diminish the changes in the epidermis, further complicating diagnosis. The presence of neoplastic cells in the blood is the hallmark sign of SS. The size of these cells may be small, large, or a combination of both. Small cells are called Lutzner cells, and large cells are known as classical Sézary cells.[195] The immunophenotype of the malignant cells is typically $CD3^+$, $CD4^+$, $CD5^+$, $CD7^-$, and $CD8^-$. T-cell receptor gene rearrangement is found.[197]

Sézary syndrome is an aggressive disease. Treatment requires a systemic approach due to its disseminated nature. Chemotherapy may clear systemic disease or may prove useful in relief of symptoms. Common chemotherapy drugs used include liposomal doxorubicin and gemcitabine. Histone deacetylase inhibitors, such as depsipeptide and vorinostat, have demonstrated significant clinical responses, resulting in decreased erythema, pruritus, and number of circulating Sézary cells.[203] Alternative approaches, such as PUVA or topical nitrogen mustard, may be utilized, with or following systemic therapy. As in MF, denileukin diftitox[204] is indicated for refractory or relapsed SS that expresses the CD25 component of the IL-2 receptor.[201] Transformation to large T-cell lymphoma may be seen as a terminal event. Five-year survival rates are reported to be between 10% and 20%.[195]

*Primary cutaneous CD30-positive T-cell lymphoproliferative disorder (ALCL)* is a CTCL that consists of anaplastic large T-lymphoid cells, most of which are $CD30^+$.[195] This subtype of lymphoma must be distinguished from systemic ALCL with skin involvement. It is found primarily in adults and shows an increased incidence in males relative to females.

At diagnosis, nearly all patients have only skin involvement. Presentation commonly occurs with a solitary or localized skin lesion. Such lesions appear as a tumor, a nodule, or, uncommonly, a papule.[195] In approximately 20% of cases, multiple lesions or a lesion with satellites of tumor in surrounding tissues (multicentric) can be found. Dissemination to regional lymph nodes may occur, but involvement of other organs is rare.[202]

Morphologically, the features are similar to those of systemic ALCL. Giant cells and Reed-Sternberg-like cells are often numerous. The infiltrates are diffuse and may involve all layers of the dermis as well as the subcutaneous tissue. Cells usually express CD4 in addition to the T-cell antigens. More than 75% of the cells are $CD30^+$.[202] T-cell rearrangement is recognized in the majority of cases.

Partial or complete regression of the lesions of ALCL may occur, even without intervention. However, relapse is common. Dissemination, primarily to regional lymph nodes, occurs in approximately 10% of cases. It is seen more frequently in patients who present with multicentric disease. Treatment of limited disease is usually restricted to radiotherapy or surgical excision. Multidrug chemotherapeutic regimens such as CHOP, EPOCH, and HyperCVAD are withheld unless evidence of overt extracutaneous involvement is found. Cutaneous ALCL is considered indolent but incurable. The 5-year survival rate is approximately 90%.[205] Spontaneous regression of the disease has been identified as a positive prognostic factor, whereas extracutaneous disease is associated with a poorer outcome.

*Lymphomatoid papulosis* is a generally benign disorder characterized by the spontaneous appearance and regression of papules and/or nodules infiltrated with atypical T lymphocytes. This disorder is limited to the skin. Dissemination of the disease can occasionally occur, resulting in progression to lymphoma in 10% to 20% of patients.[195,205] Various lymphoma subtypes have been reported following lymphomatoid papulosis, including MF, cutaneous ALCL, and HL.

## ANAPLASTIC LARGE CELL LYMPHOMA

Anaplastic large cell lymphoma is a T-cell lymphoma accounting for 2% to 3% of adult and 10% to 20% of childhood lymphomas.[206] It is characterized by large lymphoid cells with abundant cytoplasm. These cells express CD30, also known as Ki-1 antigen. Most ALCLs express cytotoxic granule-associated proteins and are positive for ALCL kinase (ALK) protein. $ALK^+$ tumors are commonly seen in younger patients and are associated with a better clinical outcome. It is important to distinguish this subtype of NHL from cutaneous ALCL and from other NHL subtypes with anaplastic features.

Anaplastic large cell lymphoma is most commonly seen in younger patients. Patients with $ALK^+$ tumors present at a median age of onset of 34 years, compared with 54 years for those with $ALK^-$ disease. There is a male predominance to its incidence, especially during the second and third decades of life, for which the male-to-female ratio is reported to be 6.5:1.0. Patients who present with $ALK^-$ ALCL are often older, and this form of the disease demonstrates an almost even distribution between males and females.[207]

Between 50% and 70% of patients present with stage III to IV disease, and most report B symptoms. High fevers are common. Serum LDH is elevated in approximately 50% of cases.[208] Peripheral and/or abdominal lymph nodes often present with extranodal disease and bone marrow involvement. The skin (21%), bone (17%), soft tissue (17%), lung (11%), and liver (8%) are the most common extranodal sites of involvement.[209] The bone marrow is found to be involved in almost one third of cases when special stains are utilized to detect CD30 and ALK.[210] Bone marrow disease, however, is difficult to detect with morphological examination only due to the small number of scattered neoplastic cells.

Morphologically, considerable variability exists among cases of ALCL. However, all cases contain some cells with characteristic horseshoe or kidney-shaped nuclei; these cells are found in all variants of ALCL.[211] The cells are often large, with a larger cytoplasm than is observed in most lymphomas. When the architecture of the involved lymph node is only partially destroyed, the neoplastic cells grow within the sinus, resembling a metastatic tumor.

Several variants of ALCL have been identified, including a lymphohistiocytic variant found in 10% of cases and a small cell variant found in 5% to 10% of cases.[212] The lymphohistiocytic variant occurs when malignant cells are found with a large number of histiocytes. The numerous histiocytes often mask the neoplastic cells, making morphologic diagnosis difficult. Special stains and testing to identify CD30, ALK, and cytotoxic granule-associated proteins are important aids in diagnosing this variant of ALCL. The small cell variant features a predominant population of small to medium-sized neoplastic cells. Hallmark cells can always be found and are often seen in highest concentration around blood vessels.[211] When diagnosis is made without the use of specialized testing, this variant may be confused with peripheral T-cell lymphoma.

The large neoplastic cells are most strongly positive for CD30. Smaller cells may be negative or weakly positive. ALK is expressed in 60% to 85% of cases. ALK staining is extremely specific for ALCL. Other than ALCL, only rare cases of DLBCL express ALK. Clonal T-cell receptor rearrangement is seen in approximately 90% of ALCL cases. The ALK expression is due to genetic abnormalities of the *ALK* locus on chromosome 2. The most frequent and characteristic abnormality is a translocation between the *ALK* gene on chromosome 2 and the nucleophosmin gene on chromosome 5.[213] Translocations between the *ALK* gene on chromosome 2 and other genes on chromosomes 1, 2, 3, and 17 may also be seen.

Aggressive treatment regimens using anthracycline therapy, such as those used to treat patients with DLBCL, are appropriate for treatment of ALCL. Rituximab is effective if the disease is $CD20^+$/B cell in origin. Jagasia et al. reported on the outcome of 28 patients with peripheral T-cell lymphoma compared with that of 86 patients with DLBCL treated with autologous transplantation.[214] The 3-year OS was 69% for the peripheral T-cell lymphomas (PTLs), with an 86% OS for the 16-patient subset with ALCL; DLBCL had a 50% OS. Comparable to treatment with nontransplant therapy, the most important prognostic factor is ALK positivity, which is associated with a favorable outcome. The 7 patients with $ALK^+$ disease had an EFS of 100% at 3 years, and the $ALK^-$ patients had a 0% EFS. Negative prognostic factors other than ALK negativity include poor performance status, advanced age, elevated LDH, and poor IPI score. The various genetic translocations seem to lack prognostic significance. The 5-year survival rate is close to 80% in ALK-positive cases, compared with 40% in ALK-negative cases.[205]

## PERIPHERAL T-CELL LYMPHOMA, UNSPECIFIED

Peripheral T-cell lymphomas as a group account for 15% of lymphomas.[88] They are aggressive in nature. ALCL is discussed above; other lymphomas that belong to this group include angioimmunoblastic T-cell lymphoma, extranodal NK/T-cell lymphoma, nasal type, subcutaneous panniculitis-like T-cell lymphoma, enteropathy-type T-cell lymphoma, and hepatosplenic gamma/delta T-cell lymphoma. However, the largest subset of PTL is a group of heterogeneous, unspecified, mature T-cell neoplasms that lack the distinct characteristics for a specific diagnosis, identified as unspecified PTLs. The neoplastic cells are typically a combination of small and large atypical lymphocytes. Although some features of this group may lead the pathologist toward diagnosis of other specific T-cell subtypes, clear evidence of diagnosis is lacking and there is poor interobserver and intraobserver reproducibility.[215] Anaplastic large cell lymphoma, MF, SS, and other subtypes of NHL are identified as specific types of PTL.[216] T-cell antigens are generally observed on immunophenotyping. Most nodal disease is $CD4^+$ and $CD8^-$. Most large cell variants express CD30. Although ALCLs express cytotoxic granule-associated proteins, the unspecified PTLs rarely do so. Frequent cytogenetic abnormalities have been noted, but no consistent karyotypes have been associated with this group of malignancies.

Unspecified PTLs are common, representing 7% to 10% of all cases of NHL in the US. They are typically found in adults at a median age near 60, and patients frequently present with systemic disease.[217] Most patients present with generalized lymphadenopathy. Involvement of the bone marrow, liver, spleen, and extranodal tissues—especially the skin—is common. Leukemic presentation may be seen with malignant cells in the peripheral blood. B symptoms are usually present.[216,218] Other common manifestations include eosinophilia and pruritus. The disease is aggressive and relapses are common. Treatment is similar to that of DLBCL. With adequate treatment, this disease may be curable in some patients.

In an analysis of 92 cases of peripheral T-cell lymphoma by Arrowsmith et al, 28 patients (30%) had what the WHO classifies as an unspecified peripheral T-cell lymphoma.[217] The median age of this group was 57.5 years and the male-to-female ratio was 3:1. Two thirds of the patients presented with advanced (stage III/IV) disease, and 70% had either a low-intermediate or high-intermediate IPI. Twenty-three of the 28 patients received combination chemotherapy, with 74% achieving a CR. However, at 5 years, the estimated PFS was only 17%, with an estimated survival of 42%. It was suggested that many of these cases acted similarly to a low-grade lymphoma.[217] Another analysis by Lopez-Guillermo et al of 95 cases of unspecified PTL yielded a CR rate of 45% after treatment with an Adriamycin-containing regimen. Median survival was 20 months.[218] Others have reported 5-year failure-free survival rates of 10% to 30%.[219,220] Only stage and IPI have demonstrated significant prognostic value with PTLs.[218]

## TREATMENT MODALITIES

The treatment of NHL usually requires a multimodal approach to effect optimal results. This approach is determined by several key factors: histology of the tumor, stage of the disease, appropriate prognostic index score, and the physiological condition of the patient. These, in turn, help predict the curability of the tumor and guide treatment decisions. The WHO classification system encompasses a wide variety of lymphomas; some are indolent and may not need treatment for several years, whereas more aggressive disease may require immediate attention. Unlike HL, NHL is often widely disseminated at diagnosis. Treatment to cure NHL is often multimodal and can be toxic. New chemotherapeutic drugs and combinations are being developed, radiation therapy is becoming more precise, monoclonal antibodies are increasing therapy responses, transplant technology continues to evolve, and many new approaches are in clinical study. Even with the significant advances achieved in research and treatment, many people diagnosed with lymphoma will not be cured. Enrollment in a clinical trial should always be a consideration.

The NCCN is an organization of nationally recognized comprehensive cancer treatment centers. Experts in their fields belong to disease-specific panels and set forth nationally recognized guidelines for the diagnosis, staging, treatment, response to treatment, and long-term monitoring of malignancies. These guidelines are readily available online and are frequently updated to reflect the current accepted practices. They are a valuable resource and can be found online at http://www.nccn.org.

### CHEMOTHERAPY

Depending on the intent of the treatment, chemotherapy for NHL may consist of single-agent therapy or multidrug regimens. With indolent NHL, there exists a wide range of treatment options, including watchful waiting, radiation therapy, immunotherapy, chemotherapy, and combination therapy. Depending on the disease, stage, FLIPI, and patient characteristics, single-agent oral therapy or treatment with a purine analog may be offered. Patients may undergo combination chemotherapy with or without a stem cell transplant, or they may be enrolled in a clinical trial utilizing a novel agent.

In the more aggressive lymphomas, multidrug regimens are the standard of care. Several common regimens are listed in Table 60-10.[221–230] It must be stressed that variations of the same combination of chemotherapy agents may be in use at individual institutions or cooperative groups. A randomized study conducted by SWOG and the Eastern Cooperative Oncology Group (ECOG) compared standard CHOP therapy with third-generation combination therapies such as Pro-MACE-CytaBOM in aggressive NHL. With a 6-year follow-up, they concluded that there were no differences in response or survival rates, but that toxicity and cost were much higher with the newer therapies.[231] For B-cell lymphomas, the addition of rituximab is generally considered standard.

Most chemotherapy is myelotoxic. Growth factors may be used in conjunction with chemotherapy in an attempt to decrease the risk of febrile neutropenia, treatment delays, and transfusion requirements. The use of these agents must be tempered with care. Recently, research has implicated the use of erythroid-stimulating agents in thrombotic events and perhaps decreased effectiveness of chemotherapy.[232,233] Practice recommendations have changed frequently over the past few years. The most current recommendations for growth factors may be found in the NCCN clinical practice guidelines in oncology at http://www.nccn.org.

One must be vigilant to observe side effects. Given that patients are now living longer, latent effects of chemotherapy, such as myelodysplastic syndrome (MDS) and secondary malignancies, are becoming evident. Alkylating agents have been particularly implicated in the higher incidence of MDS, and treatment-related MDS is almost universally fatal.[234]

### RADIATION THERAPY

Unlike HL, NHL typically does not spread via contiguous lymph nodes. Radiation therapy is frequently combined with chemotherapy and is targeted to areas of bulky disease, but not to entire zones of lymph nodes as it is in HL. Rarely, for stage I indolent NHL, radiation may be used alone in a curative attempt. In the more aggressive lymphomas, radiation therapy may be added after completion of chemotherapy to sites of prior bulky disease in an attempt to increase cure or prolong responses. Symptomatic lymphadenopathy can be treated with palliative doses of radiation for local control.

### TARGETED THERAPY

In 1997, rituximab (Rituxan) became the first monoclonal antibody approved for cancer treatment. The mechanism for manufacturing monoclonal antibodies, which was devised in 1975 by Kohler and Milstein, involved making a hybridoma by fusing murine antibody-producing lymphocytes

**TABLE 60-10**

**Common Combination Regimens for the Treatment of Follicular and Diffuse Large Cell Lymphoma**

| | |
|---|---|
| **Follicular NHL** | |
| **CHOP**[221] | |
| Cyclophosphamide | 750 mg/m$^2$ day 1 |
| Doxorubicin | 50 mg/m$^2$ IV day1 |
| Vincristine | 1.4 mg/m$^2$ (max 2 mg) IV day 1 |
| Prednisone | 100 mg PO days 1–5 |
| *Cycle repeated every 21 days* | |
| **CVP**[222] | |
| Cyclophosphamide | 400 mg/m$^2$ IV days 1–5 |
| Vincristine | 1.4 mg/m$^2$ (max 2 mg) IV day 1 |
| Prednisone | 100 mg/m$^2$ PO days 1–5 |
| *Cycle repeated every 21 days* | |
| **FND**[223] | |
| Fludarabine | 25 mg /m$^2$ IV days 1–3 |
| Mitoxantrone (Novantrone) | 10 mg/m$^2$ IV day 1 |
| Dexamethasone | 20 mg PO days 1–5 |
| *Cycle repeated every 28 days* | |
| **FC**[224] | |
| Fludarabine | 20 mg/m$^2$ IV days 1–5 |
| Cyclophosphamide | 1000 mg/m$^2$ IV day 1 |
| *Cycle repeated every 21–28 days* | |
| **Diffuse Large Cell Lymphoma** | |
| **CHOP** (please see follicular above) | |
| **EPOCH**[225] | |
| Etoposide | 50 mg/m$^2$ IV continuous infusion days 1–4 |
| Prednisone | 60 mg/m$^2$ PO BID days 1–5 |
| Vincristine | 0.4 mg/m$^2$ IV continuous infusion days 1–4 |
| Cyclophosphamide | 750 mg/m$^2$ IV day 5 |
| Doxorubicin | 10 mg/m$^2$ IV continuous infusion days 1–4 |
| *Cycle repeated every 21 days* | |
| **ESHAP**[226] | |
| Etoposide | 40 mg/m$^2$ IV days 1–4 |
| Methylprednisolone | 500 mg IV days 1–4 |
| Cisplatin | 25 mg/m$^2$/day IV continuous infusion days 1–4 |
| Cytarabine | 2000 mg/m$^2$ IV day 4 |
| *Cycle repeated every 21 days* | |
| **DHAP**[227] | |
| Cisplatin | 100 mg/m$^2$ IV continuous infusion over 24 hours day 1 |
| Cytarabine | 2000 mg/m$^2$ IV over 3 hours every 12 hours ×2 doses; day 2 after completion of cytarabine |
| Dexamethasone | 40 mg PO/IV days 1–4 |
| *Cycle repeated every 21–28 days* | |
| **ICE**[228] | |
| Ifosfamide | 5000 mg/m$^2$ IV continuous infusion over 24 hours day 2 |
| Etoposide | 100 mg/m$^2$ IV days 1–3 |
| Carboplatin | AUC 5 IV day 2 |
| Mesna | 5000 mg/m$^2$ IV combined with ifosfamide |
| *Cycle repeated every 14 days* | |
| **Gem-Ox**[229] | |
| (Rituximab typical day 1) | 575 mg/m$^2$ IV day 1 |
| Gemcitabine | 1000 mg/m$^2$ IV day 2 |
| Oxaliplatin | 100 mg/m$^2$ IV day 2 |
| *Cycle repeated every 2 weeks* | |
| **MINE**[230] | |
| Mesna | 1330 mg/m$^2$ with ifosfamide days 1–3 and 500 mg /m$^2$ administered 4 hours after ifosfamide days 1–3 |
| Ifosfamide | 1330 mg/m$^2$ IV days 1–3 |
| Mitoxantrone | 8 mg/m$^2$ IV day 1 |
| Etoposide | 65 mg/m$^2$ IV days 1–3 |
| *Cycle repeated every 21 days* | |

with a myeloma cell line. This technique allowed large-scale production of specific monoclonal antibodies.[235] Monoclonal antibodies can be unconjugated (naked) or conjugated with radioisotopes or toxins. Although the first monoclonal antibodies were developed in mice, there are now other subtypes: chimeric (60% human, 40% murine), humanized (95% human, 5% murine), and fully human. Infusional toxicities and the duration of time the antibody remains in the bloodstream depend on its subtype of the monoclonal antibody. Typically, the less murine the antibody that is used, the lower the frequency of side effects and the longer it remains in circulation.[236]

*Rituximab* may be used alone or in conjunction with chemotherapy in the treatment of B-cell lymphomas. Premedication with acetaminophen and diphenhydramine is standard, and there should be easy access to emergency drugs and equipment. Rituximab often causes an infusional hypersensitivity reaction that may typically involve chills, fever, and rigors. These side effects are more common during the first infusion. If a reaction occurs, the drug is stopped and the symptoms are treated. Once the symptoms resolve, rituximab is restarted at a lower rate. Caution must be exercised in patients with high amounts of circulating lymphocytes such as those with CLL. They are at risk for life-threatening infusional reactions from cytokine release and tumor lysis.[237,238]

Early phase I/II studies of rituximab found that circulating B cells were promptly cleared and the effects lasted 3 to 6 months. In some patients, rituximab was still measurable in the blood several months after therapy completion.[239] The phase II pivotal trial used rituximab to treat relapsed, indolent disease. It reported an overall response rate (ORR) of 48%, but found that the response was delayed and occurred at a median of 50 days. Time to progression was 13 months. Patients with CLL or chemotherapy-resistant disease did not respond as well as chemosensitive patients.[240] Retreatment is possible in responding patients and can lead to a 40% response.[241]

Rituximab is also used in conjunction with chemotherapy. Coiffier and the the Groupe d'Etude des Lymphomes de l'Adulte in France explored the use of rituximab combined with CHOP chemotherapy in the treatment of diffuse large cell NHL in patients 60 to 80 years old. They found a significant difference in CR and improved EFS and OS rates at 2 years.[242] These results have been replicated in younger patients,[243] and the combination is now a standard first-line therapy. Many questions remain to be answered, however, and investigators are currently exploring the optimal dose and scheduling of rituximab, the role of maintenance rituximab, the usefulness of extended treatment, ways to combine rituximab with other monoclonal antibodies and therapies, and factors influencing rituximab sensitivity or resistance.

As experience with rituximab has grown it is now known that reactivation of hepatitis B may occur—sometimes up to 1 year after completion of therapy. It is common practice that all patients being considered for rituximab therapy be tested for hepatitis B-surface antigen/antibodies, core antigen/antibodies, and hepatitis e-antigen. Those who test positive should be evaluated for viral load and then be referred to a hepatologist/gastroenterologist prior to starting therapy.[244]

*Alemtuzumab (Campath-1H)* is a humanized monoclonal antibody that targets the CD52 antigen; it was approved by the FDA in 2001 for B-CLL. CD52 is found on the surface of most normal and malignant T and B cells, as well as on NK cells, macrophages, monocytes, and male reproductive system cells. Alemtuzumab has been used in the treatment of autoimmune disorders, solid organ transplants, graft-vs-host disease (GVHD), and both T-cell and B-cell malignancies, such as T-prolymphocytic leukemia and multiple myeloma.[245] In addition, it has been utilized in conditioning regimens for stem cell transplantation. It has, however, been used most often in the treatment of CLL. The pivotal trial for alemtuzumab was in fludarabine-resistant patients with CLL and showed a 33% response rate, with a time to progression of more than 9 months.[246] It is currently in use for first-line therapy with CLL and in fludarabine-refractory and del17 CLL.[244] This drug appears to have more of an effect in the blood, bone marrow, and spleen than in the lymph nodes.[247]

Alemtuzumab is typically given 3 times per week for a total of 12 weeks using an escalating dose. Infusion-related hypersensitivity reactions are common and pretreatment with acetaminophen and diphenhydramine is necessary. The drug may be given as a subcutaneous injection with less toxicity.[248] Because of its effect on many cells in the immune system, prolonged immunosuppression can occur that may last as long as 18 months and lead to opportunistic infections such as *Pneumocystis carinii.* Prophylaxis with trimethoprim/sulfamethizole, an antiviral agent, and an antifungal agent is indicated throughout the treatment and for at least 2 months after completion of this therapy.[249]

## Radioimmunotherapy

Although naked monoclonal antibodies have added much to the treatment of NHL, not all patients respond to them. Linking a radioactive molecule to a monoclonal antibody provides a number of advantages, as lymphoma cells are very radiosensitive, and cell kill does not have to depend on the presence of an intact immune system. Many different combinations of radionucleotides and monoclonal antibodies are being tested in a variety of cancerous and noncancerous diseases. Two radioconjugates currently on the market used for NHL, iodine-131 tositumomab (Bexxar) and ibritumomab tiuxetan (Zevalin), are both conjugated to a CD20 monoclonal antibody. These β-particle emitters lead to fatal DNA damage in both the cells they target via the CD20 antigen and cells in close proximity to them (the bystander effect).[250] Bexxar also emits γ-particles that can be used to determine dose.

Bexxar and Zevalin share many similarities, and both require a dedicated team to safely administer them. Physicians and nurses, along with nuclear medicine, radiation pharmacy, and radiation safety personnel, are needed. A "cold" antibody is first administered to deplete B cells in the peripheral blood; it has been shown to improve the distribution of the radioimmunotherapy (RIT) at the target sites. Depending on the drug, dosing is based on weight (Zevalin) or on gamma elimination of a test dose (Bexxar). Because it is important to clear the radiation from the body in a timely manner, the monoclonal antibody of both drugs is murine in derivation. Human antimouse antibodies and human antichimeric antibodies may be tested. Patients with high titers of these antibodies tend to respond poorly and can experience severe infusion reactions.[251]

Other safety issues important in patient selection are ensuring low tumor burden in the marrow and adequate marrow function. Patients who receive these drugs are at high risk for prolonged cytopenias and marrow dysfunction following treatment. Surrogate markers for marrow dysfunction are prior myeloablative therapy, external beam radiation to more than 25% of the marrow, failed stem cell harvest, a platelets count of less than 100,000/$mm^3$, an absolute neutrophil count of less than 1500/$mm^3$, and a hypocellular marrow (less than 15%). The marrow should be 25% or less involved with disease.[252] Depending on the drug, radiation safety precautions must occur for patients after therapy. For both drugs, body secretions are contaminated with radiation for about 1 week after dosing. Body fluids must be cleaned promptly, and condoms should be worn during sexual activity during this time. Because Bexxar is a gamma-emitter with a longer path length of radiation, patients must remain in semi-isolation for about 1 week. They need to avoid prolonged contact with others and avoid young children and pregnant women. In the US, radiation safety is regulated by both the state and federal governments. The Nuclear Regulatory Commission publishes regulations and guidelines that must be followed.

Because of the radiation, these drugs are myelotoxic. Peripheral blood count nadirs are more delayed and prolonged than with conventional chemotherapy. With Bexxar therapy in low-grade or transformed NHL, nadirs occur between 4 and 6 weeks and generally begin to recover by weeks 8 to 9. The incidence of grade III/IV hematological toxicity is 30% to 40%.[252]

Both Bexxar and Zevalin have produced remissions in 60% to 80% of patients with indolent NHL and relapsed/refractory disease. The results are even better in treatment-naïve patients, with 97% response rate and 63% complete response.[236] Many remissions are durable, and patients who relapse after Bexxar can still have a 56% response with repeat dosing.[252] Radioimmunotherapy is currently a recommended practice for first-line and second-line therapy for FLs. Investigations are ongoing in examining the use of RIT in a variety of B-cell lymphomas as well as its use as part of conditioning regimens in stem cell transplant.

## HEMATOPOIETIC STEM CELL TRANSPLANTATION

Hematopoietic stem cell transplantation (HSCT) is a viable treatment option for many patients with high-risk, resistant, or recurrent lymphoma. However, the use of HSCT remains controversial in first-line or low-risk to standard-risk disease due to the variable range of pathology represented by the term "lymphoma" and the risk of HSCT.

The NCCN has guidelines for HSCT at various stages of disease states or treatment (Table 60-11).[254] First-line treatment refers to the initial treatment intended to achieve remission; second-line treatment refers to treatment provided after first-line therapy fails. Consolidation therapy is administered following treatment that achieves a complete response and is intended to eliminate .

The role of transplantation as a treatment option is discussed in each specific section of this chapter. Here, a review of issues and concerns when HSCT is considered as a therapeutic option is provided:

- Mortality. The risk of death from short-term and long-term complications limits the use of transplantation, especially allogeneic (matched sibling) or unrelated transplant. This is of particular concern in patients with indolent disease, who may survive for many years with conventional treatment. Infection, GVHD, multiorgan failure, and secondary malignancies contribute to this risk.
- Disease Resistance. Stem cell transplantation has been shown in other diseases such as leukemia to be much

**TABLE 60-11**

| Indications for Stem Cell Transplantation in Lymphoma |
|---|
| del 17 q CLL/SLL |
| Mantle cell NHL—first line and second line consolidation |
| DLBC NHL—first line consolidation and second line treatment |
| Burkitt's NHL—relapsed disease |
| PTC NHL—first line consolidation |
| MF/SS—refractory disease or progression |

*Abbreviations*: CLL, chronic lymphocytic leukemia; del, deletion; DLBC, diffuse large B-cell lymphoma; MF, mycosis fungoides; NHL, non-Hodgkin's lymphoma; PTC, peripheral T-cell; SLL, small lymphocytic lymphoma; SS, Sézary syndrome.

*Source*: Data from National Comprehensive Cancer Network.[244]

more effective in patients with chemotherapy-sensitive disease. Conventional treatment options can be offered with less toxicity, which requires consideration of the ideal timing of HSCT to maximize survival and minimize toxicities. Patients with DLBCL are often offered HSCT if disease persists after initial therapy or with first relapse, and those with indolent lymphomas may receive multiple therapies prior to HSCT. HSCT is considered appropriate therapy for patients with chemotherapy-sensitive aggressive lymphomas if the bone marrow is negative. Salvage therapies may be used to demonstrate chemotherapy sensitivity and to minimize disease in patients being considered for transplant (see Table 60-10). Stem cell transplantation may also be used as first-line treatment in select patients with high-risk disease.

- Marrow Contamination. The high frequency of marrow and blood involvement in some types of lymphoma, such as FL, raises the concern of reinfusing contaminated cells in autologous stem cell transplantation. Success of treatment is dependent on the ability to "clean" marrow cells, either through systemic treatment of the recipient or through in vitro attempts to decontaminate the stem cells after collection from the patient. Systemic treatment involves the administration of chemotherapy. The addition of rituximab has significantly increased the in vivo clearing of viable tumor cells in the stem cell harvest; that is, administration of systemic rituximab decreases the number of tumor cells in the blood and bone marrow.[253]

Several studies support the use of anti–B-cell monoclonal antibodies (eg, rituximab) as a method of in vitro purging.[254,255] The Dana Farber Cancer Institute reported on 153 patients with advanced FL who received purging of the stem cells. Only 30% were in CR at harvest, but 8 years posttransplant, 42% maintain DFS, and 66% are alive. Those who achieved a complete response at time of harvest had a significantly longer CR.[255] Patients with aggressive lymphomas who relapse posttransplant are most likely to recur at sites of prior disease. Only one third relapse in new sites. This raises questions as to the involvement of contaminated marrow cells, and data suggest that patients with tumor-free marrow are less likely to relapse than those with evidence of disease.[256]

### Donor source

The ideal donor source must be considered. Patients with relapsed and refractory disease may be most appropriate to receive an allogeneic transplant. The European Bone Marrow Transplantation registry, however, reports no survival advantage to allogeneic transplants despite lower recurrence rates. The increased treatment-related mortality ranged from 20% to 50%.[257] Methods to decrease GVHD may improve morbidity but may negatively impact relapse of disease.

### Conditioning regimens

Several different conditioning regimens have been utilized for HSCT, including total body irradiation in addition to chemotherapy. The addition of rituximab has been studied in multiple ways: prior to mobilization chemotherapy, as part of the preconditioning chemotherapy, and as consolidation posttransplant.[258–260] These pilot studies look promising, but more evidence is required prior to developing conclusive standards. Nonmyeloablative HSCT, utilizing low-intensity conditioning therapies has been studied in NHL. Reduced-intensity therapies allow allogeneic transplantation to be utilized for patients not otherwise considered to be appropriate candidates: older patients and those with high risk or who were heavily pretreated. However, age over 50 and chemoresistance were identified as predictors of negative outcome.[261]

### Role of immunotherapy

The immune system seems to have an important role in the prevention and treatment of relapse following HSCT. There is clear evidence that GVHD also creates a graft-vs-tumor (GVT) effect, and subsequently a drop in relapse rate. Donor leukocyte infusions administered to enhance a GVT effect appear to result in disease response in the treatment of relapse posttransplant in subsets of patients with NHL.[261] These concepts have led to clinical trials evaluating the efficacy of the administration of immunotherapeutic agents. Fifty-six patients with HL and NHL were treated with a combination of IL-2 and interferon alpha for 4 weeks following transplant. Significant but tolerable toxicity was observed. Significantly higher survival (90% vs 46% at 48 months) as well as higher rates of CR (80% vs 53%) were observed as compared with historical data.[262] Holmberg et al reported on 20 patients who were treated with rituximab and IL-2 after autologous transplantation in a phase II trial. Toxicity was manageable, and 18 of 20 patients remain in remission, with a median follow-up of 55 months.[258] These pilot studies have generated interest and have led to randomized trials.

## NEW THERAPIES

With today's standard therapies, 50% or less of patients with advanced diffuse large cell lymphoma are cured; rarely are those with more than limited stages of low-grade NHL or CLL/SLL cured.[244] To compound the problem, many patients with NHL are older, have comorbidities, and/or have decreased marrow reserves from the myelotoxicity of treatment. Clearly, new approaches are needed. As we learn more about the biology and cellular activities of lymphoma cells, novel ways to fight the disease are becoming apparent. A chromosomal abnormality and adverse markers for a lymphoma are turning into areas for investigation. The therapies described here are in clinical trials either alone or in combination with approved treatments in an attempt to increase response and eventually cure rates.

## New chemotherapeutic agents

Bendamustine is a chemotherapy drug that has been recently FDA approved for first-line therapy in B-CLL as well as for second-line therapy in FL. It is a unique agent: it has the chemical structure of an alkylator and possesses a purine-like structure group.[263] It is being used alone or in combination in numerous trials in the management of NHL. A recent noninferiority trial comparing bendamustine plus rituximab with the standard RCHOP in indolent lymphomas was presented at the 2008 meeting of the American Society of Hematology. On a median 28 month follow-up, the ORRs were similar, with trends to less toxicity/fewer infections in the bendamustine plus rituximab group.[264]

Pentostatin is a purine analog with a purported lower incidence of myelosuppression and is active in CLL. It is undergoing comparisons to fludarabine-based regimens.[265]

## New anti-CD20 antibodies

Ofatumumab and veltuzumab are second-generation CD20 monoclonal antibodies currently in clinical trials for the management of NHL. They differ from rituximab by being humanized or fully human (thereby being less immunogenic). Ofatumumab is a fully human monoclonal antibody that binds to a different CD20 epitope (a site on an antigen recognized by antibodies) than rituximab. It is closer to the cell membrane and remains in place longer. It is felt to be a stronger activator of complement.[266] It has been tested in patients with follicular NHL, CLL, and rituximab-refractory NHL.[267,268] Veltuzumab, although targeting the same epitope on CD20 as rituximab, is humanized. In an early trial using this drug with relapsed NHL it was found to be effective at lower doses than rituximab.[269] Other CD20 monoclonal antibodies under development include AME-133, PRO131921, and GA-101.

## New monoclonal antibodies

New monoclonal antibodies used in the treatment of NHL include epratuzumab (anti-CD22), inotuzumab ozogamicin (CMC-544), galiximab (anti-CD80), SGN-40 (CD40), and HCD122 (CD40). CD20 is a well-known B-cell antigen targeted by the monoclonal antibody rituximab, but there are concerns that resistance to it may develop. As a consequence, other targets on B cells are under investigation for monoclonal antibody development. CD22 is an attractive target expressed in 60% to 80% of B-cell lymphomas. This transmembrane protein is internalized when it binds to antibody. It appears to be involved with numerous B-cell operations, including homing, intracellular adhesion, and receptor signaling thresholds.[270] Epratuzumab is a humanized monoclonal antibody targeted against CD22. Several human studies are looking at epratuzumab's use in naked form as well as conjugated with radiation molecules. Responses were seen in relapsed/refractory follicular and diffuse large cell lymphoma with the naked antibody. Toxicities were mild and no dose-limiting toxicities were observed.[270–272] An ongoing study is examining the use of epratuzumab in conjunction with RCHOP in frontline treatment for patients with DLBC NHL. An interim analysis reports a 95% ORR.[273]

Inotuzumab ozogamicin (CMC-544) is an anti-CD22 humanized monoclonal antibody attached to a toxin (calicheamicin). It is currently undergoing investigation in combination with rituximab in patients with rituximab-sensitive progressing follicular NHL and DLBCL NHL. Side effects include cytopenias.[274]

CD80 is another target under investigation. It is found on the surfaces of activated B cells and other antigen-presenting cells.[275] Unlike in normal B cells, CD80 is highly expressed on malignant B cells and is thought to lead to deregulated growth. The monoclonal antibody galiximab, which targets CD80, has been given as a continuous intravenous infusion over 7 days either alone or in combination with RCHOP. A phase II trial recently reported on the use of galiximab along with rituximab in patients with untreated follicular NHL.[276] It is also being studied in the relapsed/refractory HL population. Reported side effects are primarily infusion related in addition to fatigue.[276] It is currently undergoing phase III testing

CD40 is found on both B and T cells, and is implicated in cellular growth and differentiation. SGN-40 is a humanized anti-CD40 monoclonal antibody currently in trials for the treatment of B-cell NHL.[277] HD122 is fully human and is also in trial for a variety of malignancies, including CLL, multiple myeloma, and lymphoma.[278]

## Vaccine therapy: tumor-specific idiotype vaccines

On the surface of each B lymphocyte is a unique immunoglobulin molecule that is produced by shuffling of gene segments during the lymphocyte's development. B-cell lymphomas frequently express this unique molecule on all cells in the malignancy. Thus the individual with a B-cell lymphoma has an idiotype unique to his or her tumor cells—and a potential target for vaccine therapy. Upon vaccination, the immune system can prime T cells to reject the tumor. Anti-idiotype vaccines can be made via hybridoma technology or via dendritic cells. Trials of such vaccines are currently under way in human patients. Upon diagnosis, a piece of tumor is sent to the laboratory for idiotype amplification and vaccine manufacture. The patient is then given therapy to achieve an MRD state. The vaccine is attached to keyhole limpet hemocyanin and given to the patient on a set schedule, typically in conjunction with another drug, such as GM-CSF, that is used to prime the immune system. Despite promising phase I/II data, recently reported results of phase III trials have not been promising,[279] and the role of these vaccines in lymphoma therapy is still unanswered.

### T-cell adoptive immunotherapy

The role of some T lymphocytes in the immune system is to recognize self from nonself by the expression of intracellular peptides on the surface of cells in conjunction with class I and class II major histocompatibility complex (MHC) molecules. When nonself substances are identified an entire chain of events occurs to recruit the immune system to destroy the cell. T cells are an attractive idea for cancer therapy because they can be very specific in their mechanism of action as well as being self-replicating. It is known that lymphomas present many targets for the immune system, and research has shown that the infusion of specific T cells can be very effective in shrinking large cancers. However, the clinical results have been erratic, and technical difficulties in manufacturing viable and specific T cells persist.[280] This method of treatment remains in clinical trials, and as knowledge and technology advance it may be a very promising therapy.

### Proteasome inhibition

The ubiquitin-proteasome pathway regulates the breakdown of many intracellular proteins involved with cell homeostasis, proliferation, and apoptosis in both normal and cancer cells. This pathway is responsible for the control of key cell cycle regulatory activities such as the p53 protein, NF-κB system, and BCL-2.[281] Malignant cells are thought to be more sensitive to disruption of this pathway than are normal cells. Bortezomib (velcade) inhibits this pathway. First approved for the treatment of multiple myeloma, it is now an FDA-approved agent in the second-line treatment of peripheral T-cell NHL.[244] It is under investigation in other subtypes of NHL, both as a single agent and in combination therapy.[282] Its toxicities include fatigue, malaise, nausea, diarrhea, thrombocytopenia, and anemia. In a phase II trial in relapsed/refractory lymphoma, it produced a 53% response rate.[283]

### Fusion toxins

Denileukin diftitox is a fusion protein that combines a diphtheria toxin with an IL-2 sequence. It thereby targets the diphtheria toxin to IL-2 receptor-bearing cells, which include activated T cells, B cells, and macrophages. Denileukin diftitox is currently FDA approved for use in $CD25^+$ cutaneous T-cell lymphoma, but also shows promise in B-cell NHL. A phase II clinical trial from MD Anderson Cancer Center has demonstrated responses in diffuse large cell, mantle cell, and follicular NHL, with the median time to response occurring after 4 cycles. The acute infusion-related toxicities such as fever, rash, and hypotension were diminished secondary to premedication with corticosteroids.[284] Phase III trials of this drug are in progress.

### Folate analogue

Pralatrexate is a targeted folate analogue designed to preferentially accumulate within tumor cells, thereby preventing them from replicating. It is being tested in phase II trials in relapsed/refractory cutaneous T-cell NHL. It has been shown to induce rapid and durable responses. Cytopenias and mucositis were among the reported side effects.[285]

### Histone deacetylase inhibitors

Histones are a family of proteins located within the nucleus that are responsible for the "packaging" and transcription of DNA. Enzymes known as acetylases and deacetylases lead to changes in packaging and therefore the shape of the DNA. The shape/packaging of the DNA influences which genes are transcribed. Many cancers can alter the activity of these enzymes. Histone deacetylase (HDAC) inhibitors can restore some of this altered gene expression, restoring cell cycle regulation. Vorinostat is an HDAC inhibitor that is currently approved for use in refractory cutaneous T-cell NHL. It is also in trials for indolent NHL. An oral agent, its main side effects are fatigue, thrombocytopenia, neutropenia, and nausea/diarrhea. Hypercholesterolemia, hyperglycemia, and electrolyte disturbances have been seen.[203] Romidepsin is another HDAC being examined for use in refractory cutaneous T-cell NHL.[286]

### mTOR inhibitors

mTOR is an intracellular serine/threonine protein kinase that is a critical regulator of cell growth and proliferation. Mutations in this pathway leading to overexpression or aberrant expression have been implicated in many different types of cancer.[287] Blocking mTOR with inhibitors such as temsirolimus (CCI-779) or everolimus with an inhibitor is being studied in many different types of cancer, including lymphomas such as mantle cell NHL.

### Anti–vascular endothelial growth factors

Vascular endothelial growth factors (VEGFs) are responsible for blood vessel formation. Many patients with a variety to tumors have been shown to have high VEGF levels. Bevacizumab is a humanized monoclonal antibody against VEGF. Successful in a variety of solid organ cancers, it is now being studied in DLBC NHL.[288]

### Immune modulators

Immune modulators have been suggested to have many mechanisms of action, including antiproliferative effects, antiangiogenic properties, and T-cell function suppression. Lenalidomide is FDA approved for use in multiple myeloma and myelodysplastic syndrome, and it is now being studied in newly diagnosed as well as recurrent/refractory CLL.[289] The studies are demonstrating that lower than expected doses are required to increase toxicities, namely, cytopenias, tumor lysis, tumor flare, and sepsis. Lenalidomide is also associated with a tumor "flare," where the absolute lymphocyte count may rapidly increase from baseline before decreasing.[290] This drug is also being studied in relapsed/refractory mantle cell NHL.[291]

## ACUTE COMPLICATIONS OF THERAPY

Therapies used in the management of HL and NHL may result in various acute and chronic side effects. The precise complications of therapy depend on the subtype of lymphoma, tumor burden, treatment, and patient variances. The treatment team must be prepared to anticipate, prevent, and manage these toxicities in a timely manner. Preparation and education of the patient and family are critical to effective treatment.

### LYMPHOMA SUBTYPE AND TUMOR BURDEN

Both the subtype of lymphoma and the amount of tumor burden may impact anticipated complications. High-grade and intermediate-grade lymphomas may grow very quickly and lead to obstruction of vital organs or major blood vessels. Superior vena cava syndrome, spinal cord compression, and syndrome of inappropriate secretion of antidiuretic hormone are all possible. These may occur at diagnosis, prior to treatment, or during treatment.

High-grade and intermediate-grade lymphomas are typically very sensitive at least to initial courses of therapy. Patients are at risk for the development of TLS, particularly if the tumor burden is high. It is imperative to evaluate these patients prior to initiating treatment to formulate a plan for the prevention and early detection of TLS. Even though many lymphoma therapies may be given on an outpatient basis, some patients may require hospitalization with their initial treatment for aggressive hydration and close monitoring. Elevated pretreatment potassium, phosphorus, or uric acid levels may be useful in helping to predict those patients at risk for TLS.

### TREATMENT-RELATED COMPLICATIONS

#### Chemotherapy-related complications

Acute toxicities of chemotherapy agents vary widely, depending on the agent or combination of agents given as well as their doses. The most common acute side effects occur due to damage of the normal tissues of the gastrointestinal tract, hair, skin, bladder, kidneys, peripheral nervous system, and bone marrow. Emphasis on prevention and/or control, where possible, is important. It is imperative that patients and their families be taught the signs and symptoms of potential side effects so that they can be identified and reported in a timely manner to lessen their impact.

Bone marrow suppression, resulting in neutropenia and an increased risk of infection, is a recognized toxicity of aggressive combination chemotherapy. Neutropenia is the dose-limiting toxicity of many regimens that are used to treat patients with HL and NHL. Age, poor performance status, and increased intensity of chemotherapy doses are the major risk factors for neutropenia.[292] Because NHL is more common in elderly individuals (more than 60% of patients are older than age 60), the incidence of this complication is substantial. The use of colony stimulating factors and/or prophylactic antibiotics, antivirals, and antifungals should be considered. Neutropenic fever can be a life-threatening complication; thus it requires prompt intervention.

Bacterial infections are the most frequently encountered infections following chemotherapy for HL and NHL. Opportunistic infections from other organisms such as *Pneumocystis carinii* (protozoan), *Aspergillus* or *Candida* species (fungal), and cytomegalovirus and herpes (viral) may be seen in individuals treated with dose-intensive therapy. Other treatments that lead to prolonged neutropenia, that suppress cellular and humoral immunity, or that incorporate corticosteroids in the regimen result in the highest incidence of bacterial and opportunistic infections.

Anemia and thrombocytopenia may also be observed either directly related to the lymphoma or secondary to therapy. In addition, it is estimated that up to 60% of people with cancer may be iron deficient for a variety of reasons.[293] This severely impairs their ability to manufacture red blood cells. Iron studies with B12 and folate levels should be standard in the initial evaluation of patients with lymphoma. Supplementation with iron when necessary should occur. Erythropoiesis-stimulating agents such as epoetin alfa (Procrit) or darbepoetin (Aranesp) may be indicated for patients with anemia related to chemotherapy. Recent investigations into the use of these medications indicates that in certain cancers they may decrease the potential for cure as well as lead to an increased risk of blood clots.[294]

Peripheral neuropathies are common side effects with vinca alkaloids. Preexisting hypertension and diabetes mellitus have been identified as risk factors for the development of peripheral neuropathy during treatment.[295]

Neuropathies may also occur with thalidomide and bortezomib. There is a current phase II trial examining the role of acupuncture in patients who have developed peripheral neuropathies associated with bortezomib or thalidomide.[296] Constipation, severe enough to lead to obstruction, may also occur with these medications. Prevention and prompt intervention are necessary.

Acute myocardial injury may occur, and congestive heart failure may be observed as an acute or a chronic toxicity. Congestive heart failure may be precipitated by the use of aggressive hydration, corticosteroids, and anthracycline therapy. An analysis by Sonnen et al found that congestive heart failure was observed only in patients with prior heart disease.[295] The use of steroids as part of the chemotherapy regimen, or as part of the antiemetic regimen may result in transient hyperglycemia. This may be more pronounced in patients who are diabetic. Steroids have many effects on glucose metabolism, including inducing insulin resistance as well as promoting hepatic production of glucose. This often manifests itself as postprandial hyperglycemia.[297] Studies done in hospitalized nondiabetic patients who are hyperglycemic show decreased morbidity when blood sugars are controlled.[298,299] Oral hypoglycemics may not be useful in treating steroid-induced hyperglycemia due to their side effects and a long delay in their onset of action. Insulin may be considered for the hospitalized patient with steroid-induced hyperglycemia.[300]

### Radiation therapy-related complications

Radiation therapy may cause local or more generalized toxicities depending on the site being irradiated. Radiation to the neck or oral cavity is often associated with loss of taste, xerostomia, and dysphagia. Due to decreased saliva production, individuals who undergo such treatment are at increased risk for dental caries.

With mantle radiation all of the above oral problems with the addition of hair loss at the nape of the neck and acute radiation pneumonitis are possible. Pneumonitis may be clinically observed as early as 3 to 4 months following mantle radiotherapy.[301] Inverted Y-port irradiation usually results in anorexia, nausea, vomiting, diarrhea, and malaise. Because a large amount of active bone marrow is in the radiation field, myelosuppression may occur.

Localized radiation therapy to a specific lymph node or extranodal mass is often delivered at higher doses. As a consequence, local skin reactions may become a significant problem. In addition, toxicity to underlying or nearby organs may be more pronounced; for example, radiation of the cervical lymph node chain might result in severe mucositis and dysphagia. Total nodal irradiation may result in the previously mentioned side effects as well as pronounced suppression of bone marrow function.

The use of total-body irradiation is limited to myeloablative therapy followed by stem cell transplantation. The gastrointestinal tract and bone marrow are exquisitely sensitive to radiotherapy, and most acute side effects are related to toxicity of these organs. Stomatitis, esophagitis, gastritis, parotitis, nausea, vomiting, and diarrhea may be observed. The profound suppression of the bone marrow, resulting in aplasia, is a desired effect in this treatment.

### Immunotherapy/radioimmunotherapy-related complications

Immunotherapy including monoclonal antibodies and radioimmunotherapy (RIT) are frequently associated with infusion-related toxicities. Fever, chills, hypotension, dyspnea, hypoxia, and signs of hypersensitivity reactions are common side effects. The initial doses of agents such as rituximab, anti-CD52 monoclonal antibody (alemtuzumab), and denileukin diftitox are associated with the greatest risk of reaction. The frequency of reactions to rituximab has been associated with an elevated WBC count, number of circulating $CD20^+$ cells, and intensity of CD20 staining. Premedication with diphenhydramine and acetaminophen is standard with many of these agents, and close monitoring during the infusion is mandatory. Agents such as anti-CD52 monoclonal antibody therapy (alemtuzumab) suppress both humoral and cellular immunity, and opportunistic infections are well documented with their use.[302] Prophylaxis with antifungals, antivirals, and antibiotics is highly recommended.

With RIT, the radioisotope is typically attached to a less humanized monoclonal antibody so that the radiation clears the body more quickly. Although not common, patients may develop human antimouse antibodies or human antichimeric antibodies, particularly if they are being retreated. Human antimouse/antichimeric antibodies are typically tested for prior to administering these medications. Individuals testing positive may experience severe infusional reactions.[303] See Table 60-12 for a summary of common acute toxicities associated with lymphoma treatments.

## CHRONIC COMPLICATIONS OF THERAPY

Advances in the treatment of all lymphomas now mean that many patients face a future in which long-term survival is a reasonable expectation. It is imperative to continue to follow patients once their treatment is completed to screen for long-term complications and to intervene if necessary.

Common long-term complications (Table 60-13)[304–307] of lymphoma treatments include various organ toxicities, secondary malignancies,[308] myelodysplastic syndrome/acute myelogenous leukemia (AML),[309] and numerous quality of life issues such as fatigue[301] and impacts on sexuality/fertility and employability/insurability. Depending on the therapy and the target of past radiation, no organ system is

**TABLE 60-12**

**Common Acute Toxicities Associated With Lymphoma Treatments**

| Treatment | Toxicity |
|---|---|
| Radiation therapy | Local toxicity depending on radiation field[202]<br>Systemic toxicity such as bone marrow depression depending on volume of marrow irradiated; ie, inverted Y field or total nodal radiation |
| Anthracyclines | Congestive heart failure |
| Bleomycin | Pneumonitis<br>Anaphylaxis |
| Cyclophosphamide | Cardiomyopathy<br>Hemorrhagic cystitis |
| Steroids | Hyperglycemia[290]<br>Hypertension<br>Mood disturbances<br>Weight gain<br>Insomnia |
| Purine analogues | Immunosuppression |
| Vinca alkaloids | Constipation<br>Peripheral neuropathies[290] |
| Radioimmunotherapy | Cytopenias, particularly thrombocytopenia that is delayed in occurring and may be prolonged<br>Infusional toxicities<br>Radiation safety issues |
| Rituximab | Infusion-related toxicities: hypersensitivity<br>Tumor lysis syndrome |
| Alemtuzumab | Profound suppression of cellular and humoral immunity[297] |

exempt from the potential for chronic therapy-related problems. As lymphoma therapies continue to evolve, the long-term side effects of new treatments or new combinations remain unclear. Older patients, those with prior history of organ dysfunction, and those who received combination therapy are at highest risk.

Pediatric survivors of HL and childhood leukemias have provided substantial information regarding the long-term complications of their therapies. The Children's Oncology Group has developed the Long-Term Follow-Up program for childhood cancer survivors. It is available on the Internet (http://www.survivorshipguidelines.org) and provides chemotherapy-specific referenced guidelines for the long-term monitoring of patients treated with chemotherapy as children. It is not certain how this applies to patients who have received therapy as adults. The NCCN has provided guidelines for monitoring for late effects after 5 years that can be seen in Table 60-14.[257]

## FATIGUE

Fatigue is a subjective, common, and often underreported complaint among cancer survivors. Although the majority of research regarding long-term fatigue has been done in breast cancer survivors and following stem cell transplantation, some studies do exist in the lymphoma survivor population.[310] Fatigue may be multifactorial in nature and may be accompanied by other problems, such as pain, anemia, depression, or sleep problems.[311] Fatigue may be a sign of disease recurrence or it may be a sign of physical toxicities from prior therapy such as pneumonitis or heart failure. An analysis of 116 survivors of HD reported that pulmonary dysfunction—most commonly manifested by impairment of gas transfer—was highly associated with chronic fatigue.[301]

The NCCN provides recommendations regarding the evaluation of and interventions for cancer-related fatigue. It should be assessed, preferably on a 1 to 10 scale, with further investigations into disease status, organ function, anemia, comorbidities/medications, and other factors. Evidence-based interventions include advocacy for increased activity and psychosocial evaluation/treatment.[301]

## PULMONARY DYSFUNCTION

Lung injury from chemotherapy (particularly bleomycin) or radiation therapy to the lungs may result in pneumonitis, pulmonary fibrosis, and lung cancers. Higher doses of chemotherapy and larger radiation fields increase the risk.[312] It is recommended that patients who fit into these risk categories be screened at least annually for pulmonary symptoms and undergo chest x-ray or a chest CT scan.[57] Dyspnea, fatigue, and exercise intolerance are all common complaints with lung pathology. Patients should be encouraged to address controllable risk factors, for example smoking cessation and annual influenza vaccination.

## THYROID DYSFUNCTION

Thyroid dysfunction is a relatively common finding in the general population, with 2% of all people having a diagnosed hypothyroidism. The true incidence is likely much higher, as the condition often goes unrecognized. Subsets

**TABLE 60-13**

**Summary of Common Treatment-Related Long-Term Problems**

| Toxicity | Implicated Agent(s) | Action |
|---|---|---|
| Congestive heart failure | Anthracyclines: onset is early to decades after treatment; dose-related<br>Cyclophosphamide/Ifosphamide<br>Bevacizumab<br>Interferon<br>Interleukins<br>Radiation[304] | Evaluate total dose of anthracycline<br>Evaluate for hypertension: control if present<br>Evaluate for signs and symptoms of heart failure; if present, order work-up |
| Pneumonitis | Bleomycin[305]<br>Radiation to lung fields<br>Smokers are at highest risk | Advocate smoking cessation<br>Initiate yearly CXR/CT chest for screening<br>Be alert for the possibility of a secondary lung cancer<br>Bronchoalveolar lavage (if concern about lung cancer)<br>Annual influenza vaccine |
| Hypothyroidism | Thyroid in radiation field<br>Radioimmunotherapy | Routine thyroid function tests |
| Myeloid dysfunction | Chemotherapy<br>Radiation therapy | Annual blood tests<br>Monitor for infections |
| Cataracts | Total body irradiation | Annual ophthalmology evaluation |
| Infertility | Numerous chemotherapy regimens/ radiotherapy to gonads | Ideally discussed prior to treatments; sperm/embryos frozen if appropriate<br>Referral to reproductive endocrinologist: eg, Fertile Hope http://www.fertilehope.org |
| Premature menopause | Numerous chemotherapy regimens/ radiotherapy to gonads; more likely to occur when treatment given closer to natural menopause | Advocate calcium/vitamin D supplementation, weight bearing exercise, smoking cessation, and moderation of alcohol intake<br>Monitor bone density<br>Consider prophylactic measures to preserve bone and cardiac health<br>Referral to gynecologist/endocrinologist if experiencing sexual dysfunction |
| Neurocognitive changes | Chemotherapy<br>Radiation therapy | Monitor for occurrence<br>Refer for neurocognitive testing if appropriate |
| Secondary malignancies[306] | Radiation therapy<br>Combination chemotherapy | Initiate early screenings for breast cancer; if breasts within radiation fields, advocate for routine self breast exams<br>Monitor for symptoms of lung cancer if lungs within radiation fields; image if symptomatic<br>Advocate lifestyle changes such as smoking cessation |
| Therapy-related MDS/AML[307] | Exposure to alkylating agents and topoisomerase inhibitors | Monitor blood counts annually or more frequent if abnormal |

*Abbreviations*: AML, acute myelogenous leukemia; CT, computed tomography; CXR, chest x-ray; MDS, myelodysplastic syndrome.

**TABLE 60-14**

**NCCN Guidelines—Monitoring for Late Effects: 5 Years-Post-Treatment for Hodgkin's Lymphoma Survivors**

| | |
|---|---|
| Annual | History and physical, complete blood count, platelets, electrolytes<br>Thyroid-stimulating hormone if history of neck radiation<br>Lipid profile<br>Chest imaging for at-risk patients (those who received radiotherapy to lung fields)<br>Breast screening: initiate 8–10 years after therapy or at age 40 (whichever comes first) (The American Cancer Society recommends breast MRI for patients who received chest radiation between the ages of 10 and 30)<br>Influenza vaccine |
| As needed | Aggressive management of cardiovascular risk factors<br>Stress test/echocardiogram at 10 years post treatment<br>Pneumococcal vaccination every 5–7 years for those with splenectomy or splenic radiation<br>Counseling regarding health habits, psychosocial concerns, breast exams, increased skin cancer risk |

*Abbreviations*: MRI, magnetic resonance imaging; NCCN, National Comprehensive Cancer Network.

Source: Data from NCCN Clinical Practice Guidelines in Oncology.[57]

of patients treated for lymphoma are at greater risk for hypothyroidism. More than 50% of long-term survivors of HL who received mantle field radiation therapy eventually develop thyroid dysfunction and require synthetic supplementation.[313] Iodine 131 tositumomab therapy may result in hypothyroidism due to a high level of radiation-absorbed dose. Patients must receive thyroid-blocking agents prior to its administration and should be evaluated clinically and through laboratory assessment on an annual basis. It is recommended that patients be tested annually with a thyroid stimulating hormone (TSH) and thyroixine or free T4 blood tests.

## CARDIOVASCULAR TOXICITY

Pericarditis, accelerated coronary artery disease that may lead to myocardial infarction, and valvular dysfunction are potential major complications following radiation therapy for HL,[312,313] and for NHL if the heart is within the radiation field. Exposure to even a low dose of radiation may increase atherosclerotic changes 20 to 30 years later.[314] The incidence of coronary artery disease has been estimated to be 4% to 11% following radiation therapy for HL. The relative risk of fatal cardiovascular events after mediastinal irradiation for HL ranges between 2.2 and 7.2.[304] Ultimately, 76% of patients who receive mediastinal radiotherapy develop pericardial toxicity.[315] A retrospective review of patients who underwent mediastinal irradiation and then required valve replacement concluded that radiation injury was the major factor responsible for the development of mitral valve disease and was a contributing factor in aortic valve disease.[315] Chemotherapy regimens that include anthracyclines also result in an increased risk for cardiac damage. Anthracycline-related cardiotoxicity is dose related and cumulative. The risk of cardiotoxicity, secondary to doxorubicin therapy, substantially increases when the cumulative dose exceeds 550 mg/m$^2$. Between 6% and 10% of adults who received a total doxorubicin dose of 550 mg/m$^2$ reported signs of symptomatic congestive heart failure. Synergistic toxic effects on the myocardium have been reported in patients receiving radiation and doxorubicin.[315] Moser et al have identified that preexisting hypertension, young age at diagnosis, larger doses of radiation therapy to the lung fields, and the need for salvage therapy lead to an increased incidence of cardiovascular events.[305]

The NCCN recommends yearly evaluation for symptoms of heart failure as well as aggressive prevention and management of cardiovascular risk factors for long-term survivors of HL.[57] The American Society of Clinical Oncology also recommends these evaluations for NHL survivors.[316] It is important to remember that cardiovascular disease may appear earlier than among otherwise healthy members of a patient's cohort. It is recommended to begin stress testing/echocardiograms at about 10 years after treatment and to continue life-long monitoring.

## REPRODUCTIVE CHANGES

Reproductive changes will vary significantly with the therapy and the intensity of the treatment used as well as the age and pretreatment fertility status of the patient. With chemotherapy drugs, the alkylating agents tend to carry a higher risk of infertility, whereas agents such as vincristine and bleomycin carry a relatively low risk of infertility. The common therapies such as CHOP and ABVD tend not to render most patients sterile. An Israeli study examined a group of 36 women below age 40 receiving CHOP therapy for at least 6 cycles. About one half of the women developed amenorrhea during the course of treatment, but almost all resumed their menses within a few months after completion. Of the study subjects, 18 women were able to become pregnant.[316] Lee at al caution that the resumption of menses does not equate with fertility and that any cancer therapy may result in a decreased duration of fertility.[317] Total body irradiation, which is used as a conditioning regimen for stem cell transplantation, may result in sterility in both males and females. External beam radiation to the gonads carries a high risk of subsequent infertility. Premature menopause in women leads to an increased and earlier risk of bone loss.

Fertility preservation may be attempted in numerous ways, but the most effective methods are sperm banking and embryo cryopreservation. Due to the time required for embryo harvesting it is often difficult to offer women this method of fertility preservation, particularly if antineoplastic therapy needs to begin urgently. Small studies have examined the use of protective ovarian suppression in women, with conflicting results.[318,319] Reproductive counseling and procreative alternatives are essential components to consider for this patient population. This discussion should start as early as possible in the treatment of lymphoma. The American Society of Clinical Oncology has published recommendations regarding fertility preservation and initiating discussions regarding this issue prior to commencing treatment.[317]

### SECONDARY MYELODYSPLASIA AND MALIGNANCIES

Therapy for NHL and HL, like that for many cancers, is in itself potentially carcinogenic. As therapies improve and patients are living longer, MDS/AML as well as solid organ tumors have become apparent.[320] In fact, therapy-related cancers are the leading cause of mortality and morbidity in long-term HL survivors.[321]

Myelodysplastic syndrome is a group of disorders characterized by abnormal cell morphology in the bone marrow and a deficiency of normal blood cells in the peripheral blood.[322] Myelodysplastic syndrome may progress to AML. Exposure to alkylating agents and radiotherapy, as well as other toxins, is a risk factor for the development of MDS and AML. Dose intensity and advanced age are associated with a higher frequency of AML following treatment for lymphoma.[323] The risk of MDS and AML is increased following therapy for HL and NHL, especially when bone marrow/stem cell transplantation has been performed. The development of secondary AML typically occurs early, within a few years to 10 years after treatment for HL.[324,325] Myelodysplasia may precede the development of leukemia and is often characterized by unexplained anemia or thrombocytopenia. Cytogenetic findings often demonstrate abnormalities of chromosomes 5 and 7 in treatment-related secondary MDS and AML. This therapy-related MDS/AML carries a poor prognosis. At the Mayo Clinic, 64 patients with HL and 166 patients with NHL who underwent autologous stem cell transplantation were followed for evidence of MDS or AML. Of the 230 consecutive patients followed, 10 developed MDS or AML (incidence of 4.3%) at a median time of 40 months following transplant and 75 months from original lymphoma diagnosis. None of these patients survived.[326] Following radiation therapy, secondary cancers may be seen typically within the radiation portal. The most common secondary cancers are those of the breast and lung.

Radiation therapy-related breast cancer is the leading secondary solid tumor in women treated for HL. The risk is highest in women treated before the age of 25 years, and the cancer may take 15 to 20 years to develop.[327] Girls younger than age 15 years who receive mantle field irradiation have more than a 100-fold increased risk for the development of breast cancer; those 15 to 25 years old have a 20-fold increased risk; those 25 to 29 years old have a sevenfold increased risk; and those older than age 30 have no increased risk.[328] The NCCN's most recent guidelines recommend initiating breast MRI and mammography 8 to 10 years after therapy or at age 40 (whichever is first) for those women who were treated with radiation therapy between the ages of 10 and 30 years. Self-breast exam is also highly encouraged.[57]

Patients with lymphomas receiving radiation therapy that involves the lungs in the radiation portal have an increased risk of lung cancer. Lorigan reports a 2.6-fold to 7-fold increase in risk for HL patients treated with radiation therapy that included the lung.[329] Patients who smoked more than 10 pack-years after the diagnosis of HL was established have a sixfold increased risk of lung cancer compared with those who had less than a 1-pack-year history.[330] Malignant mesothelioma may also be a post-radiation therapy risk for patients treated for HL. DeBruin and her group report a 30-fold increased risk in 1122 five-year survivors of HL treated with radiation.[330] These data support the need for education of patients and close follow-up after therapy. It is recommended that patients be counseled regarding the NCCN *Clinical Practice Guidelines in Oncology—Hodgkin Disease/Lymphoma* (v.2.2009; available at http://www.nccn.gov). Healthy lifestyles should be advocated, and patients should have yearly chest imaging with a chest x-ray or CT scan.[57]

## NURSING IMPLICATIONS

The role of nursing in treating patients with lymphoma is immense. Lymphomas represent a broad category of malignancies that require a solid grasp of immunology to understand their pathogenesis and treatment. While a minority of people who present with aggressive lymphomas may have a short survival, typically this group of patients live for many years. It is both rewarding and challenging to work with patients and families in what may be a chronic illness.

## EDUCATION

Nurses play a key role in educating patients and their families with regards to their disease as well as treatment options. Patients and their families can differ widely in their educational background and understanding of the disease and its treatment. Explaining physiology and immunology in terms that each individual can understand is an art. It is crucial that patients and their families understand what is taught to them so that they can be informed and active participants in their care. Being familiar with a variety of lymphoma-specific resources in print and on the Internet, as well as local and national support groups, is important.

## RESEARCH

Many people with lymphoid malignancies will consider and/or be treated on research protocols. Nurses play an important role in explaining and demystifying research protocols so that patients and families can decide whether they wish to participate. The coordination of care and the monitoring of these patients are critical to their success. Whether the nurse is helping to conduct the specific trials or is present at the referring center, communication between nurses at these different centers contributes to patient safety and feelings of security.

Many of the new agents/regimens have shown increased time to PFS and DFS, but not necessarily a difference in OS. Nurses are and should be active in initiating quality of life measurements for these patients to help determine the risk/benefit ratio of these therapies.

## ORAL THERAPY

There has been a rise in oral therapies for lymphoma treatment. There are benefits and risks to the use of oral therapies. Nurses need to educate patients and their families about side effects and give specific guidelines for holding treatment. Close monitoring and follow-up are necessary when patients are taking oral cancer therapies. Patients may continue to take oral medications when it is not safe or may stop taking oral medications for a variety of reasons; thus monitoring understanding of medications and compliance is critical.

Patient compliance with oral therapy is a significant issue. Studies have confirmed that patients often forget to take their medications—even ones that treat their cancer. Nurses need to work with patients and families to develop patient-specific methods to ensure compliance and therefore the best chance for a good outcome. Asking "Are you taking your medications?" is not sufficient. A better approach is "Tell me how many doses you have missed in the past week." This acknowledges that missing medications occurs and allows for a more accurate assessment of delivered therapy.

Another issue with oral therapy is cost. Insurance companies and government plans have often not kept pace with the development of oral therapies. Coverage needs to be investigated, and correspondence with insurance companies is often required to try to obtain insurance coverage of these drugs. The cost of these new oral therapies can be thousands of dollars per month. It is important that the nurse be familiar with assistance plans offered by pharmaceutical companies.

## REPRODUCTIVE HEALTH

Although the incidence of lymphomas increases with age, many younger people are diagnosed and require treatment. The nurse needs to provide a comfortable forum to address sexuality for any age group as well as fertility preservation for those of reproductive age. It is important to have available local resources for egg and sperm banking as well as referral to reproductive endocrinologists. Although some lymphomas are aggressive and require immediate treatment, it is important to allow time for consideration of fertility preservation if possible.

## CONCLUSION

The diagnosis, classification, and treatment of HL and NHL have undergone significant changes over the past 5 years. The identification of immunological or cytogenetic markers is extremely important to the continued expansion of treatment options. Many treatment options now exist for the patient with lymphoma. Because many of the lymphomas are potentially curable malignancies, the acute and chronic toxicities of these treatments are important factors in decision making. Ideally, the use of targeted therapy will result in improved survival and decreased long-term toxicity.

## REFERENCES


1. Non-Hodgkin Lymphoma Facts & Statistics. The Leukemia & Lymphoma Society. http://www.leukemia-lymphoma.org. Accessed January 20, 2010.
2. National Cancer Institute Surveillance Epidemiology and End Results. Seer Data 1973–2006. http://www.cancer.gov. Accessed January 20, 2010.
3. Jaffe ES, Harris HL, Stein H, Campo E, Pileri SA, Swerdlow SH. Introduction and overview of the classification of the lymphoid neoplasms. In: Swerdlow SH, Campo E, Harris NL, et al, eds. *WHO Classification of Tumours of Haematopoietic and Lymphoid Tissue.* Lyon, France: ARC Press; 2008:158–166.
4. Mauch, PM, Kalish LA, Kadin M, et al. Patterns of presentation of Hodgkin disease: implications for etiology and pathogenesis. *Cancer.* 1993;71:2062–2070.

5. Schabet M. J Epidemiology of primary CNS lymphoma. *J Neurooncol.* 1999;43:199–201.
6. Moses S, Pruritis. *Am Fam Physician.* 2003;68:1135–1142, 1145–1146.
7. Carbone P, Kaplan H, Musshoff K. Report of the committee on the Hodgkin's disease staging. *Cancer Res.* 1971;31:1860–1861.
8. Lister TA, Crowther D, Sutcliffe SB, et al. Report of a committee convened to discuss the evaluation and staging of patients with Hodgkin's disease: Cotswolds meeting. *J Clin Oncol.* 1989;7:1630–1636.
9. Rosenberg SA, Cannellos GP. Hodgkin's disease. In: Cannellos GP, Lister TA, Sklar JL, eds. *The Lymphomas.* Philadelphia, PA: WB Saunders; 1998:305–331.
10. Golder W. Positive emission tomography and lymphoma therapy. *Oncologie.* 2001;24:496–498.
11. Friedberg JW, Chengazi V. PET scans in the staging of lymphoma: current status. *Oncologist.* 2003;8:438–447.
12. Podoloff DA, Advani RH, Allred C, et al. NCCN Task Force Report: Posiron emission tomography (PET)/computed tomography (CT) scanning in cancer. *J Natl Compr Canc Netw.* 2007;5:S1-S19.
13. Pakos EE, Fotopoulos AD, Ioannidis JP. 18F-FDG PET for evaluation of bone marrow infiltration in staging of lymphoma: a meta analysis. *J Nucl Med.* 2005;46:958–963.
14. Anonymous. A predictive model for aggressive non-Hodgkin's lymphoma: the International Non-Hodgkin's Lymphoma Prognostic Factors Project. *N Engl J Med.* 1993;329:987–994.
15. Ship MA. Prognostic factors in aggressive non-Hodgkin's lymphoma: who has "high-risk" disease? *Blood.* 1994;83:1165–1173.
16. Coiffier B, Bastion Y, Berger F, et al. Prognostic factors in follicular lymphomas. *Semin Oncol.* 1993;20:89–95.
17. Lopez-Guillermo A, Montserrat E, Rozman C. The International Prognostic Index (IPI) for large-cell lymphomas is also useful when applied to patients with low-grade lymphoma. [Abstract 59] Lugano, Switzerland, Fifth International Conference on Malignant Lymphoma 1993.
18. Bastion I, Coiffier B. Is the International Prognostic Index for aggressive lymphoma patients useful for follicular lymphoma patients? *J Clin Oncol.* 1994;12:1340–1342.
19. Hermans J, Krol ADG, van Groningen PHM, et al. International Prognostic Index for aggressive non-Hodgkin's lymphoma is valid for all malignancy grades. *Blood.* 1995;86:1460–1463.
20. Solal-Celigny P, Roy P, Colombat P, et al. Follicular lymphoma international prognostic index. *Blood.* 2004;104:1258–1265.
21. Sehn LH, Donaldson J, Chhanabhai M, et al. The revised international prognostic index (R-IPI) is a better predictor of outcome than the standard IPI for patients with diffuse large B-cell lymphoma treated with R-CHOP. *Blood.* 2007;109:1857–1861.
22. Hodgkin T. On some morbid appearances of the absorbent glands and spleen. *Med Chir Tran.* 1832;17:69–114.
23. Wilks S. Cases of enlargement of the lymphatic glands and spleen, or Hodgkin's disease. *Guys Hosp Rep.* 1865;11:56–67.
24. Reed DM. On the pathological changes in Hodgkin's disease, with especial reference to tuberculosis. *Johns Hopkins Hosp Rep.* 1902;10:133–196.
25. Sternberg C. Uber eine eigenartige unter dem Bilde der Pseukoleukamie verlaufende: tuberculose des lymphatischen apparates. *Z Heilkd.* 1898;19:21–90.
26. Horner MJ, Ries LAG, Krapcho M, et al. eds. *SEER Cancer Statistics Review*, 1975–2006, National Cancer Institute. Bethesda, MD, http://seer.cancer.gov/csr/1975_2006. Accessed March 7, 2010.
27. Horning S. Hodgkin's lymphoma. In: Abeloff MD, Armitage JO, Niederhuber JE, et al, eds. *Abeloff's Clinical Oncology* 4th ed. Philadelphia, PA: Churchill Livingstone; 2008:2253–2268.
28. Weiss LM, Strickler JG, Warnke RA, et al. Epstein–Barr viral DNA in tissues of Hodgkin's disease. *Am J Pathol.* 1987;129: 86–91.
29. Grufferman S, Cole P, Levitan TR. Evidence against transmission of Hodgkin's disease in high schools. *N Engl J Med.* 1979;18:1006–1011.
30. Ambinder RF, Browning P, Lorenza I, et al. Epstein–Barr virus and childhood Hodgkin's disease in Honduras and the United States. *Blood.* 1993;81:462–467.
31. Weinreb M, Day PJ, Niggli F. The consistent association between Epstein–Barr virus and Hodgkin's disease in children in Kenya. *Blood.* 1996;87:3828–2836.
32. Herndier BG, Sanchez HC, Chang KL, et al. High prevalence of Epstein–Barr virus in the Reed-Sternberg cells of HIV-associated Hodgkin's disease. *Am J Pathol.* 1993;142:1073–1079.
33. Grufferman S, Cole P, Smith PG, Lukes RJ. Hodgkin's disease in siblings. *N Engl J Med.* 1977;296:248–250.
34. Craver LF, Hall TC, Rappaport H, et al. Report of the nomenclature committee. *Cancer Res.* 1966;26:1311.
35. Popperma S, Swerdlow SH, Delsol G, et al. Nodular lymphocyte predominant Hodgkin lymphoma. In: Swerdlow SH, Campo E, Harris NL, et al, eds. *WHO Classification of Tumours of Haematopoietic and Lymphoid Tisses.* Lyon, France: ARC Press; 2008:323–325.
36. Pinkus GS, Said JW. Hodgkin's disease, lymphocyte predominance type, nodular—a distinct entity? Unique staining profile for L & H variants of Reed-Sternberg cells defined by monoclonal antibodies to leukocyte common antigen, granulocyte-specific antigen, and B-cell-specific antigen. *Am J Pathol.* 1985;118:1–6.
37. Diehl V, Franklin J, Sextro M, Mauch P. Clinical presentation and treatment of lymphocyte predominance Hodgkin's disease. In: Mauch P, Armitage JO, Diehl V, eds. *Hodgkin's Disease.* Philadelphia, PA: Lippincott, Williams & Wilkins; 1999:563–582.
38. Colby TV, Hoppe RT, Warnke RA. Hodgkin's disease: a clinicopathologic study of 659 cases. *Cancer.* 1982;49:1848–1858.
39. MacLennan KA, Bennett MH, Vaughan HB, et al. Diagnosis and grading of nodular sclerosing Hodgkin's disease: a study of 2190 patients. *Int Rev Exp Pathol.* 1992;33:27–51.
40. Diehl V, Sextro M, Franklin J, et al. Clinical presentation, course, and prognostic factors in lymphocyte-predominant Hodgkin's disease and lymphocyte-rich classical Hodgkin's disease: report from the European Task Force on Lymphoma Project on Lymphocyte-Predominant Hodgkin's Disease. *J Clin Oncol.* 1999;17:776–783.
41. Anagnostopoulos I, Hansmann ML, Franssila K, et al. European Task Force on Lymphoma Project on Lymphocyte Predominance Hodgkin Disease: histologic and immunohistologic analysis of submitted cases reveals 2 types of Hodgkin disease with a nodular growth pattern and abundant lymphocytes. *Blood.* 2000;96:1889–1899.
42. Kant JA, Hubbard SM, Longo DL, et al. The pathologic and clinical heterogeneity of lymphocyte-depleted Hodgkin's disease. *J Clin Oncol.* 1986;4:284–294.
43. Josting A, Wiedenmann S, Franklin J, et al. Secondary myeloid leukemia and myelodysplastic syndromes in patients treated for Hodgkin's disease: a report from the German Hodgkin's Lymphoma Study Group. *J Clin Oncol.* 2003;21:3440–3446.
44. Longo DL, Young RC, Wesley M, et al. Twenty years of MOPP therapy for Hodgkin's disease. *J Clin Oncol.* 1986;4:1295–1306.
45. Ferme C, Eghball H, Meerwaldt JH, et al. Chemotherapy plus involved-field radiation in early-stage Hodgkin lymphoma. *N Engl J Med.* 2007;357:1916–1927.
46. Aleman BMP, Raemaekers JM, Trelli U, et al. Involved field radiotherapy for advanced Hodgkin's lymphoma. *N Engl J Med.* 2003;348:2396–2406.
47. DeVita VT, Serpick AA, Carbone PP. Combination chemotherapy in the treatment of advanced Hodgkin's disease. *Ann Intern Med.* 1970;73:881–895.
48. Bonadonna G, Zucali R, Monfardini S, et al. Combination chemotherapy of Hodgkin's disease with adriamycin, bleomycin, vinblastine, and imidazole carboxamide versus MOPP. *Cancer.* 1975;36:252–259.
49. Duggan DB. Randomized comparison of ABVD and MOPP/ABV hybrid for the treatment of advanced Hodgkin's disease: report of an intergroup trial. *J Clin Oncol.* 2003;21:607–614.
50. Bonadonna G, Zucali R, Monfardini S, De Lena M, Uslenghi C. Combination chemotherapy of Hodgkin's disease with adriamycin, bleomycin, vinblastine, and imidazole carboximide versus MOPP. *Cancer.* 1975;3:252–259.

51. Bartlett NH. Brief chemotherapy, Stanford V, and adjuvant radiotherapy for bulky or advanced stage Hodgkin's disease. *J Clin Oncol.* 1995;13:1080–1088.
52. Diehl V. BEACOPP, a new dose-escalated and accelerated regimen is at least as effective as COPP/ABVD in patients with advanced stage Hodgkin's lymphoma. *J Clin Oncol.* 1998;16:3810–3821.
53. Horning SJ, Hoppe RT, Advani R, et al. Efficacy and late effects of Stanford V chemotherapy and radiotherapy in untreated Hodgkin's disease: mature data in early and advanced stage patients [abstract]. *Blood.* 2008;104:308a.
54. Diehl V, Franklin J, Pfreundschuh M, et al. Standard and increased dose BEACOPP chemotherapy compared with COPP-ABVD for advanced Hodgkin's disease. *N Engl J Med.* 2003;348:2386–2395.
55. Ballova V, Ruffer JU, Haverkamp H, et al. A prospectively randomized trial carried out by the German Hodgkin Study Group (GHSG) for elderly patients with advanced Hodgkins's disease comparing BEACOPP baseline and COPP-ABVD (study HD9elderly). *Ann Oncol.* 2005;16:124.
56. Gianni AM, Rambaldi A, Zinzni P, et al. Comparable 3-year outcome following ABVD or BEACOPP first-line chemotherapy plus preplanned salvage, in advanced Hodgkin lymphoma (HL): a randomized trial of Michelangelo, GITIL, and IIL cooperative groups. [Abstract 8506] *J Clin Oncol.* 2008;26.
57. NCCN Clinical Practice Guidelines in Oncology: Hodgkin Disease/ Lymphoma. V2–2009, http://www.nccn.org. Accessed January 20, 2010.
58. Haenclever D, Diehl V. A prognostic score for advanced Hodgkin's disease: international prognostic factors project on advanced Hodgkin's disease. *N Engl J Med.* 1998;339:1547–1549.
59. Gallamini A, Hutchings M, Rigacci L, et al. Early interim 2 (18F) fluoro-2-deoxy-d-glucose positron emission tomography is prognostically superior to international prognostic score in advanced-stage Hodgkin's lymphoma: a report from a joint Italian–Danish study. *J Clin Oncol.* 2007;25:3746–3752.
60. Bastion BP, Divine M, Nedellec G, et al. Analysis of prognostic factors after first relapse in Hodgkin's disease in 187 patients. *Cancer.* 1996;78:1293–1299.
61. Mink A, Armitage JO. High dose therapy in lymphomas: a review of the current status of allogeneic and autologous stem cell transplantation in Hodgkin's disease and non-Hodgkin's lymphoma. *Oncologist.* 2001;6:247–256.
62. Federico M, Bellei M, Brice P, et al. High-dose therapy and autologous stem-cell transplantation versus conventional therapy for patients with advanced Hodgkin's Lymphoma responding to front-line therapy. *J Clin Oncol.* 2003;21:2320–2325.
63. Proctor SJ, Mackie M, Dawson A, et al. A population-based study of intensive multi-agent chemotherapy with or without autotransplant for the highest risk Hodgkin's disease patients identified by the Scotland and Newcastle Lymphoma Group (SNLG) prognostic index. A Scotland and Newcastle Lymphoma Group study (SNLG HD III). *Eur J Cancer.* 2002;38:775–806.
64. Popat U, Hosing C, Saliba RM, et al. Prognostic factors for disease progression after high-dose chemotherapy and autologous hematopoietic stem cell transplantation for recurrent or refractory Hodgkin's lymphoma. *Bone Marrow Transplant.* 2004;33:1015–1023.
65. Wedgwood AR, Fanale MA, Fayad LE, et al. Rituximab + ABVD improves event-free survival (EFS) in patients with classical Hodgkin lymphoma in all International Prognostic Score (IPS) Groups and in patients who have PETpositive disease after 2–3 cycles of therapy. *Blood* 2007;110:71a.
66. Hasenclever D, Diehl V. A prognostic score for advanced Hodgkin's disease. International Prognostic Factors Project on Advanced Hodgkin's Disease. *N Engl J Med.* 1998;339:1506–1514.
67. American Cancer Society: Statistics for 2009. http://www.cancer.org. Accessed July 11, 2009.
68. Urba WJ, Longo DL. Lymphocytic lymphomas: epidemiology, etiology, pathology, and staging. In: Moosa AR, Schimpff SC, Robson MC, eds. *Comprehensive Textbook of Oncology.* Vol. 2, 2nd ed. Baltimore, MD: Williams and Wilkins; 1991:1268–1276.
69. Beebe GW, Kato H, Land C. Studies of the mortality of A-bomb survivors. Mortality and radiation dose. 1950–1974. *Radiat Res.* 1978;75:138–201.
70. Boice JJ. Radiation and non-Hodgkin's lymphoma. *Cancer Res.* 1992;52:5489S-5491S.
71. Thun MJ, Altekruse SF, Namboodiri MM, et al. Hair dye use and the risk of fatal cancers in U.S. women. *J Natl Cancer Inst.* 1994;86:210–215.
72. de Sangose S, Benavente Y, Nieters A, et al. Association between personal use of hair dyes and lymphoid neoplasms in Europe. *Am J Epidemiol.* 2006;164:47–55.
73. Yunis JJ, Oken MM, Theologides A, et al. Recurrent chromosomal defects are found in most patients with non-Hodgkin's lymphoma. *Cancer Genet Cytogenet.* 1984;13:17–28.
74. Ngan BY, Chen-Levy Z, Weiss LM, et al. Expression in non-Hodgkin's lymphoma of the bcl-2 protein associated with the t(14;18) chromosomal translocation. *N Engl J Med.* 1988;318:1638–1644.
75. Korsmeyer SJ. Bcl-2 initiates a new category of oncogenes: regulators of cell death. *Blood.* 1992;80:879–886.
76. Hockenbery D, Zutter M, Hickey W, et al. Bcl-2 protein is topographically restricted in tissues characterized by apoptotic cell death. *Proc Natl Acad Sci USA.* 1991;88:6961–6965.
77. McDonnell T, Deanne N, Platt F, et al. BCL-2 immunoglobulin transgenic mice demonstrate extended B-cell survival and follicular proliferation. *Cell.* 1989;57:79–88.
78. van den Bosch CA. Is endemic Burkitt's lymphoma an alliance between three infections and a tumour promoter. *Lancet Oncol.* 2004;5:738–746.
79. Levine EG, Arthur DC, Frizzera G, et al. Cytogenetic abnormalities predict clinical outcome in non-Hodgkin's lymphoma. *Ann Inten Med.* 1988;108:14–20.
80. Filipovich AH, Mathur A, Kamat D, et al. Primary immunodeficiencies: genetic risk factors for lymphoma. *Cancer Res.* 1992;52: 5465s-5467s.
81. Zintzaras E, Voulgarelis M, Moutsopolous HM. The risk of lymphoma development in auto-immune disorders. *Arch Intern Med.* 2005;165: 2337–2344.
82. Rappaport H, Winter WJ, Hick EB. Follicular lymphoma: a re-evaluation of its position in the scheme of malignant lymphomas, based on a survey of 253 cases. *Cancer.* 1956;9:792–821.
83. National Cancer Institute sponsored study of classification of non-Hodgkin's lymphomas: Summary and description of a working formulation for clinical usage. The Non-Hodgkin's Lymphoma Pathologic Classification Project. *Cancer.* 1982;49:2112–2135.
84. Kurtin PJ, Aboudola S. Small B-cell lymphomas. In: Hsi ED, ed. *Hematotopathology.* Philadelphia, PA: Elsevier; 2006:203–254.
85. Pileri SA, Leoncini L, Falini B. Revised European–American lymphoma classification. *Curr Opin Oncol.* 1995;7:401–407.
86. Harris NL, Jaffe ES, Kiebold J, et al. Lymphoma classification—from controversy to consensus: the REAL and WHO classification of lymphoid neoplasms. *Ann Oncol.* 2000;11:s3-s10.
87. Jaffe ES, Harris NL, Stein H, Vardiman JW, eds. *World Health Organization Classification of Tumours. Pathology and Genetics. Tumours of Haematopoietic and Lymphoid Tissues.* Lyon, France: ARC Press; 2001.
88. Harris NL, Jaffe ES, Diebold J, et al. World Health Organization Classification of neoplastic diseases of the hematolopoietic and lymphomid tissues: report of the clinical advisory committee meeting—Airlie house, Virginia, November 1997. *J of Clin Oncol,*1999;17:3835–3849.
89. Dohner H, Stilgenbauer S, Dohner K, et al. Chromosome aberrations in B-cell chronic lymphocytic leukemia: reassessment based on molecular cytogenetic analysis. *J Mol Med.* 1997;77:266–281.
90. Rassenti LZ, Huynh L, Toy TL, Chen L, Keating MJ, Gribben JG, et al. ZAP-70 compared with immunoglobulin heavy-chain gene mutation status as a predictor of disease progression in chronic lymphocytic leukemia. *N Engl J Med.* 2004;351:893–901.

91. Anonymous. A clinical evaluation of the International Lymphoma Study Group classification of non-Hodgkin's lymphoma. The Non-Hodgkin's Lymphoma Classification. *Blood.* 1997;89:3909–3918.
92. National Comprehensive Cancer Network: NCCN Clinical Practice Guidelines in Oncology. Non-Hodgkin's Lymphoma. *J Natl Compr Canc Netw.* 2004;2:284–336.
93. Leporrier M, Chevret S, Cozin B, et al. Randomized comparison of fludarabine, CAP, and CHOP in 938 previously untreated stage B and C chronic lymphocytic leukemia patients. *Blood.* 2001;98:2319–2325.
94. Lozanski G, Heerema NA, Flinn IW, et al. Alemtuzumab is an effective therapy for chronic lymphocytic leukemia with p53 mutations and deletions. *Blood.* 2004;103:3278–3281.
95. Moreton P, Kennedy DB, Rawstron AC, et al. Achieving a MRD negative response after alemtuzumab for CLL is the best predictor for prolonged survival. *Hematol.* 2003;102. Abstract 5290.
96. Dohner H, Stilgenbauer S, Benner A, et al. Genomic aberrations and survival in chronic lymphocytic leukemia. *N Engl J Med.* 2000;343:1910–1916.
97. Hsi E. The leukemias of mature lymphocytes. *Hemat Oncol Clin North Am.* 2009;23:843–871.
98. Nathwani BN, Harris NL, Weisenburger D, et al. Follicular lymphoma. In: Jaffe ES, Harris NL, Stein H, et al, eds. *World Health Organization Classification of Tumours. Pathology and Genetics. Tumours of Haematopoietic and Lymphoid Tissues.* Lyon, France: ARC Press; 2001:162–167.
99. Jaffe ES, Pittaluga S. The pathological basis for the classifications of lymphomas. In Hoffman R, Benz EJ, Shattil SJ, et al, eds. *Hematology: Basic Principles and Practice.* 5th Ed. Philadelphia, PA: Churchill Livingstone; 2009:282.
100. Lai R, Arber DA, Chang KL, et al. Frequency of bcl-2 expression in non-Hodgkin's lymphoma: a study of 778 cases with comparison of marginal zone lymphoma and monocytoid B-cell hyperplasia. *Mod Pathol.* 1988;11:864–869.
101. Fisher RI. Overview of non-Hodgkin's lymphoma: biology, staging, and treatment. *Semin Oncol.* 2003;30:3–9.
102. van Oers MH; Klasa R, Marcus RE, et al. Rituximab maintenance improves clinical outcome of relapsed/resistant follicular non-Hodgkin lymphoma in patients both with and without rituximab during induction: results of a prospective randomized phase 3 intergroup trial. *Blood.* 2006;108:3295–3301.
103. Hainsworth JD. Rituximab as first-line and maintenance therapy for patients with indolent non-Hodgkin's lymphoma: Interim follow-up of a multicenter phase II trial. *Semin Oncol.* 2002;29:25–29.
104. Ghielmini M, Schmitz SF, Cogliatti SB. Prolonged treatment with rituximab in patients with follicular lymphoma significantly increases event-free survival and response duration compared with the standard weekly × 4 schedule. *Blood.* 2004;103:4416–4423.
105. Fisher R, LeBlanc M, Press O W. New treatment options have changed the survival of patients with follicular lymphoma. *Hemat Malig,* 2005;23:8447–8452.
106. Solal-Celigny P. Follicular Lymphoma International Prognostic Project (FLIPP) [abstr 054]. *Ann Oncol.* 2002;13:18.
107. Radaszkiewicz T, Dragosics B, Bauer P. Gastrointestinal malignant lymphomas of the mucosa-associated lymphoid tissues: factors relevant to prognosis. *Gastroenterology.* 1992;102:1628–1638.
108. Wotherspoon AC, Ortiz-Hidaglgo C, Falzon MR, et al. *Helicobacter pylori*-associated gastritis and primary B-cell gastric lymphoma. *Lancet.* 1991;338:1175–1176.
109. Zucca E, Bertoni F, Stathis A, Cavalli F. Marginal zone lymphomas. *Hematol Oncol Clin North Am.* 2008;22:883–901.
110. Thieblemont C, Bastion Y, Berger F, et al. Mucosa-associated lymphoid tissue gastrointestinal and nongastrointestinal lymphoma behavior: analysis of 108 patients. *J Clin Oncol.* 1997;15:1624–1630.
111. Thieblemont C, Berger F, Dumontet C, et al. Mucosa-associated lymphoid tissue lymphoma is a disseminated disease in one third of 158 patients analyzed. *Blood.* 2000;95:802–806.
112. Isaacson PG, Chott A, Nakamura S, et al. Extranodal marginal zone lymphoma of mucosa-associated lymphoid tissue (MALT lymphoma). In: Swerdlow SH, Campo E, Harris NL, ed. *WHO Classification of Tumours of Haematopoietic and Lymphoid Tissues.* Lyon, France: WHO Press; 2008:214–217.
113. Liu H, Ruskon-Formestraux A, Lavergne-Slove A, et al. Resistance of t(11:18) positive gastric-mucosa-associated lymphoid tissue lymphoma to *Helicobacter pylori* eradication therapy. *Lancet.* 2001;357:39–40.
114. Foon KA, Fisher RI. Lymphomas. In: Beutler E, Coller BS, Lichtman MA, et al, eds. *Williams Hematology.* 6th ed. New York, NY: McGraw Hill; 2001:1237–1261.
115. De Boer CJ, Schurring E, Dreef E, et al. Cyclin D1 protein analysis in diagnosis of mantle cell lymphoma. *Blood.* 1995;86:2715–2723.
116. Vandenberge E, Wolf-Peeters C, van Den OJ, et al. Translocation (11;14): a cytogenetic anomaly associated with B-cell lymphomas of non-follicle centre cell lineage. *J Pathol.* 1991;163:13–18.
117. William ME, Swerdlow SH, Rosenberg CL, Arnold A. Chromosome 11 translocation breakpoints at the PRAD1/cyclin D1 gene locus in centrocytic lymphoma. *Leukemia.* 1993;7:241–245.
118. Vaandrager JW, Schuuring E, Zwikstra E, et al. Direct visualization of dispersed 11q13 chromosomal translocations in mantle cell lymphoma by multicolor DNA fiber fluorescence in situ hybridization. *Blood.* 1996;88:1177–1182.
119. Schmidt C, Dreyling M. Therapy of mantle cell lymphoma: current standards and future strategies. *Hematol Oncol Clin North Am.* 2008: 22:953–963.
120. Obriain DS, Kennedy MJ, Daly PA, et al. Multiple lymphomatous polyposis of the gastrointestinal tract. A clinicopathologically distinctive form of non-Hodgkin's lymphoma of B-cell centrocytic type. *Am J Surg Pathol.* 1989;13:691–699.
121. Dunleavy K, Wilson WH. Diagnosis and treatment of non-hodgkin lymphoma (aggressive). In: Hoffman R, Benz EJ, Shattil SJ, et al, eds. *Hematology: Basic Principles and Practice.* 5th ed. Philadelphia, PA: Churchill Livingstone; 2009:1298–1299.
122. Swerdlow SH, Berger F, Isaacson PI, et al. Mantle cell lymphoma. In: Jaffe ES, Harris NL, Stein H, et al, eds. *World Health Organization Classification of Tumours. Pathology and Genetics. Tumours of Haematopoietic and Lymphoid Tissues.* Lyon, France: ARC Press; 2001: 168–170.
123. Andersen NS, Pedersen L, Elonen E, et al. Primary treatment with autologous stem cell transplantation in mantle cell lymphoma: outcome related to remission pretransplant. *Eur J Haematol.* 2003;71:73.
124. Mangel J, Leitch HA, Connors JM, et al. Intensive chemotherapy and autologous stem-cell transplantation plus rituximab is superior to conventional chemotherapy for newly diagnosed advanced stage mantle-cell lymphoma: a matched pair analysis. *Ann Oncol.* 2004;15:283.
125. Khouri IF, Lee MS, Saliba RM, et al. Nonablative allogeneic stem-cell transplantation for advanced/recurrent mantle-cell lymphoma. *J Clin Oncol.* 2003;21:4407.
126. Matolcsy A, Chadburn A, Knowles DM, et al. De novo CD5-positive and Richter's syndrome-associated diffuse large B cell lymphomas are genotypically distinct. *Am J Pathol.* 1995;147:207–216.
127. Lossos I. Molecular pathogenesis of diffuse large B cell lymphoma. *J Clin Oncol.* 2005;23:6351–6357.
128. Niitsu N, Nakamine H, Hagiwara Y, et al. The t(1;3)(p34;q27)translocation: a nonrandom BCL6 rearrangement in diffuse large B cell lymphoma. *Ann Hematol.* 2008;87:151–153.
129. Armitage JO, Weisenburger DD. New approach to classifying non-Hodgkin's lymphomas: clinical features of the major histologic subtypes. *J Clin Oncol.* 1998;16:2780–2795.
130. Gatter KC, Warnke RA. Diffuse large B-cell lymphoma. In: Jaffe ES, Harris NL, Stein H, et al, eds. *World Health Organization Classification of Tumours. Pathology and Genetics. Tumours of Haematopoietic and Lymphoid Tissues.* Lyon, France: ARC Press; 2001:171–174.
131. Pfreundschuh M, Trumper L, Kloess M, et al. Two-weekly or 3-weekly CHOP chemotherapy with or without etoposide for the treatment of

elderly patients with aggressive lymphomas: results of the NHL-B2 trial of the DSHNHL. *Blood.* 2004;104:634–641.
132. Verdonck LF, Notenboom A, de Jong DD, et al. Intensified 12-week CHOP (I-CHOP) plus G-CSF compared with standard 24-week CHOP (CHOP-21) for patients with intermediate-risk aggressive non-Hodgkin lymphoma: a phase 3 trial of the Dutch-Belgian Hemato-Oncology Cooperative Group (HOVON). *Blood.* 2007;109:2759–2766.
133. Greb A, Bohlius J, Trelle S, et al. High dose chemotherapy with autologous stem cell support in first-line treatment of aggressive non-hodgkin lymphoma–results of a comprehensive meta-analysis. *Cancer Treat Rev.* 2007;33:338–346.
134. Gregory SA. Selecting patients for treatment with 90Y ibritumomab tiuxetan (Zevalin) [Review]. *Semin Oncol.* 2003;30:17–22.
135. Cortelazzo S, Rambaldi A, Rossi A, et al. Intensification of salvage treatment with high-dose sequential chemotherapy improves the outcome of patients with refractory or relapsed aggressive non-Hodgkin's lymphoma. *Br J Haematol.* 2001;114:333–341.
136. Hamlin PA, Zelenetz AD, Kewalramani T. Age-adjusted International Prognostic Index predicts autologous stem cell transplantation outcome for patients with relapsed or primary refractory diffuse large B-cell lymphoma. *Blood.* 2003;102:1989–1996.
137. Shipp MA, Harrington DP, Anderson JR, et al. A predictive model for aggressive NHL: the International Non-Hodgkin's Lymphoma Prognostic Factors Project. *N Engl J Med.* 1993;329:987–994.
138. Hill ME, MacLennan KA, Cunningham DC, et al. Prognostic significance of BCL-2 expression and bcl-2 major breakpoint region rearrangement in diffuse large cell non-Hodgkin's lymphoma: a British National Lymphoma Investigation Study. *Blood.* 1996;88:1046–1051.
139. Wright DH. Burkitt's lymphoma: a review of the pathology, immunology and possible aetiological factors. In: Sommers SC, ed. *Pathology Annual.* New York, NY: Appleton-Century-Crofts; 1971:337–363.
140. de Levale L. Diffuse large B-cell lymphomas and burkitts lymphoma. *Hematol Oncol Clin North Am.* 2009;23:791–827.
141. Mbulaiteye SM, Walters M, Engels A, et al. High levels of Epstein–Barr virus DNA in saliva and peripheral blood from Ugandan mother-child pairs. *J Infect Dis.* 2006;193:422–426.
142. Vinnecombe SJ, Reznek RH. Reticuloendothelial disorders: lymphomas. In: Dixon AK, ed. *Grainger and Allison's Diagnostic Radiology,* 5th ed. Edinburgh, UK: Churchill Livingstone; 2007:753.
143. Cavdar AO, Gozdasoglu S, Yavuz G, et al. Burkitt's lymphoma between African and American types in Turkish children. Clinical, viral (EBV), and molecular studies. *Med Pediatr Oncol.* 1993;21:36–42.
144. Raphael M, Gentihomme O, Tulliez M. Histopathologic features of high-grade non-Hodgkin's lymphomas in acquired immunodeficiency syndrome. The French Study Group of Pathology for Human Immunodeficiency Virus-Associated Tumors. *Arch Pathol Lab Med.* 1991;115:15–20.
145. Hamilton-Dutroit SJ, Raphael M, Audouin J. In situ demonstration of Epstein–Barr virus small RNAs (EBER 1) in acquired immunodeficiency syndrome-related lymphomas: correlation with tumor morphology and primary site. *Blood.* 1993;82:619–624.
146. Hui PK, Feller AC, Lennert K. High-grade non-Hodgkin's lymphoma of B-cell type. I. Histopathology. *Histopathology.* 1988;12:127–143.
147. Gaidano G, Ballerini P, Gong JZ, et al. p53 mutations in human lymphoid malignancies: association with Burkitt lymphoma and chronic lymphocytic leukemia. *Proc Natl Acad Sci USA.* 1991;88:5413–5417.
148. Yano T, Sander CA, Clark HM, et al. Clustered mutations in the second exon of the MYC gene in sporadic Burkitt's lymphoma. *Oncogene.* 1993;8:2741–2748.
149. Murphy SB, Hustu HO. A randomized trial of combined modality therapy of childhood non-Hodgkin's lymphoma. *Cancer.* 1980;45:630–637.
150. Magrath IT, Janus C, Edwards BK, et al. An effective therapy for both undifferentiated (including Burkitt's) lymphomas and lymphoblastic lymphomas in children and young adults. *Blood.* 1984;63:1102–1111.
151. Cairo MS, Spostos R, Perkins S, et al. Burkitt's and Burkitt-like lymphoma in children and adolescents: a review of the Children's Cancer Group Experience. *Br J Haematol.* 2003;120:660–670.
152. Weitzman S, Greenberg ML, Thorner P. Treatment of non-Hodgkin's lmphoma in childhood. In: Wiernik PH, Canellos GP, Kyle RA, et al, eds. *Neoplastic Disease of Blood.* 2nd ed. New York, NY: Churchill Livingstone; 1991:753–768.
153. Magrath IT. Burkitt's lymphoma. The small noncleaved cell lymphomas. In: Canellos GP, Lister TA, Sklar JL, eds. *The Lymphomas.* Philadelphia, PA: WB Saunders; 1998:423–437.
154. White DA. Pulmonary complications of HIV associated malignancies. *Clin Chest Med.* 1996;17:755–761.
155. Johnson CC, Wilcosky T, Kvale P, et al. Cancer incidence among an HIV-infected cohort. Pulmonary complications of HIV Infection Study Group. *Am J Epidemiol.* 1997;146:470–475.
156. Pluda JM, Venzon DJ, Tosato G, et al. Parameters affecting the development of non-Hodgkin's lymphoma in patients with severe human deficiency virus infection receiving antiretroviral therapy. *J Clin Oncol.* 1993;11:1099–1107.
157. Levine AM, Shibata D, Sullivan HJ, et al. Epidemiological and biological study of acquired immunodeficiency syndrome-related lymphoma in the County of Los Angeles: preliminary results. *Cancer Res.* 1992;52:5482s-5484s.
158. Martin A, Flaman JM, Frebourg T, et al. Functional analysis of the p53 protein in AIDS-related non-Hodgkin's lymphomas and polymorphic lymphoproliferations. *Br J Haematol.* 1998;101:311–317.
159. Kaplan LD, Straus DJ, Testa MA, et al. Low-dose compared with standard-dose m-BACOD chemotherapy for non-Hodgkin's lymphoma associated with human immunodeficiency virus infection. National Institute of Allergy and Infectious Diseases AIDS Clinical Trials Group. *N Engl J Med.* 1997;336:1641–1648.
160. Heise W, Arasteh K, Mostertz P, et al. Malignant gastrointestinal lymphomas in patients with AIDS. *Digestion.* 1997;58:218–224.
161. Klatt EC, Nichols L, Noguchi TT. Evolving trends revealed by autopsies of patients with the acquired immunodeficiency syndrome. 565 autopsies in adults with the acquired immunodeficiency syndrome, Los Angeles, Calif, 1982–1993 [corrected]. *Arch Pathol Lab Med.* 1994;118:884–890.
162. Mate JL, Navarro JT, Ariza A, et al. Oral solid form of primary effusion lymphoma mimicking plasmablastic lymphoma. *Hum Pathol.* 2004;35:632–635.
163. Rosenwald A, Wright G, Chan WC, et al. The use of molecular profiling to predict survival after chemotherapy for diffuse large-B-cell lymphoma. *N Engl J Med.* 2002;346:1937–1947.
164. Boue F, Gabarre J, Gisselbrecht C, et al. Phase II trial of CHOP plus rituximab in patients with HIV-associated non-Hodgkin's lymphoma. *J Clin Oncol.* 2006;24:4123–4128.
165. Kaplan LD, Lee JY, Ambinder RF, et al. Rituximab does not improve clinical outcome in a randomized phase III trial of CHOP with or without rituximab in patients with HIV-associated non-Hodgkin lymphoma: AIDS-Malignancies Consortium Trial 010. *Blood.* 2005;106:1538–1543.
166. Levine AM, Sullivan-Halley J, Pike MC, et al. HIV-related lymphoma: prognostic factors predictive of survival. *Cancer.* 1992;68:2466–2472.
167. Murphy SB. Classification, staging and end results of treatment of childhood non-Hodgkin's lymphomas: dissimilarities from lymphomas in adults. *Semin Oncol.* 1980;7:332–339.
168. Heerema NA, Sather HN, Sensel MG, et al. Frequency and clinical significance of cytogenetic abnormalities in pediatric T-lineage acute lymphoblastic leukemia: a report from the Children's Cancer Group. *J Clin Oncol.* 1998;16:1270–1278.
169. Harrison CJ, Moorman AV, Broadfield ZJ, et al. Three distinct subgroups of hypodiploidy in acute lymphoblastic leukaemia. *Br J Haematol.* 2004;125:552–559.
170. Brunning RD, Borowitz M, Matutes E, et al. Precursor T lymphoblastic leukaemia/lymphoblastic lymphoma (precursor T-cell acute

lymphoblastic leukaemia). In: Jaffe ES, Harris NL, Stein H, et al, eds. *World Health Organization Classification of Tumours. Pathology and Genetics. Tumours of Haematopoietic and Lymphoid Tissues.* Lyon, France: ARC Press; 2001:115–117.

171. Brunning RD, Borowitz M, Matutes E, et al. Precursor B lymphoblastic leukaemia/lymphoblastic lymphoma (precursor B-cell acute lymphoblastic leukaemia). In: Jaffe ES, Harris NL, Stein H, et al, eds. *World Health Organization Classification of Tumours. Pathology and Genetics. Tumours of Haematopoietic and Lymphoid Tissues.* Lyon, France: ARC Press; 2001:111–114.

172. Lin P, Jones D, Dorfman DM, Medeiros LJ. Precursor B-cell lymphoblastic lymphoma: a predominantly extranodal tumor with low propensity for leukemic involvement. *Am J Surg Pathol.* 2000;24:1480–1490.

173. Penn I. Cancers complicating organ transplantation. *N Engl J Med.* 1990;323:1767.

174. Nelson BP, Nalesnik MA, Bahler DW, et al. Epstein–Barr virus-negative posttransplant lymphoproliferative disorders: a distinct entity? *Am J Surg Pathol.* 2000;24:375–385.

175. Swerdlow SH, Webber SA, Chadburn A, Ferry JA. Posttransplant lymphoproliferative disorders. In: *WHO Classification of Tumours of Hematopoietic and Lymphoid Tissues*, 4th ed. Lyon, France: WHO Press; 2008:343–349.

176. Knowles DM, Cesarman E, Chadburn A, et al. Correlative morphologic and molecular genetic analysis demonstrates three distinct categories of posttransplantation lymphoproliferative disorders. *Blood.* 1995;85:552–565.

177. Chucrallah AE, Crow MK, Rice LE, et al. Multiple myeloma after cardiac transplantation: an unusual form of posttransplant lymphoproliferative disorder. *Hum Pathol.* 1994;25:541–545.

178. Said J. Immunodeficiency-related Hodgkin lymphoma and its mimics. *Adv Anat Pathol.* 2007;14:189–194.

179. Friedberg JW, Jessup M, Brennan D. Lymphoproliferative disorders following organ transplantation. In: Up To Date Online. 17.1. http://www.utdol.com. Accessed October 1, 2009.

180. Dharnidharka VR, Sullivan EK, Stablein DM, et al. Risk factors for posttransplant lymphoproliferative disorder (PTLD) in pediatric kidney transplantation: a report of the North American Pediatric Renal Transplant Cooperative Study (NAPRTCS). *Transplantation.* 2001;71:1065–1068.

181. Oertel SH, Ruhnke MS, Anagnostopoulos I, et al. Treatment of Epstein–Barr virus-induced posttransplantation lymphoproliferative disorder with foscarnet alone in an adult after simultaneous heart and renal transplantation. *Transplantation.* 1999;15:765–767.

182. Curtis RE, Travis LB, Rowlings PA, et al. Risk of lymphoproliferative disorders after bone marrow transplantation: a multi-institutional study. *Blood.* 1999;94:2208–2216.

183. Landgren O, Gilbert ES, Rizzo JD, et al. Risk factors for lymphoproliferative disorders after allogeneic hematopoietic cell transplantation. *Blood.* 2009;113:4992–5001.

184. Penn I. The changing pattern of post transplant malignancies. *Transplant Proc.* 1991;23:1101–1103.

185. Leblond V, Davi F, Dorent R, et al. Post transplant lymphoproliferative disorders not associated with Epstein–Barr virus: a distinct entity? *J Clin Oncol.* 1998;16:2052–2059.

186. Savage P, Waxman J. Posttransplantation lymphoproliferative disease. *QJM.* 1997;90:497–503.

187. Leblond V, Dhedin N, Mamzer Bruneel MF, et al. Identification of prognostic factors in 61 patients with posttransplantation lymphoproliferative disorders. *J Clin Oncol.* 2001;19:772–778.

188. Choquet S, Leblond V, Herbrecht R, et al. Efficacy and safety of rituximab in B-cell posttransplant lymphoproliferative disorders: results of a prospective multicentre phase II study. *Blood.* 2006;107:3053–3057.

189. Komrokji RS, Oliva JL, Zand M, et al. Mini-BEAM and autologous hematopoietic stem-cell transplant for treatment of posttransplant lymphoproliferative disorders. *Am J Hematol.* 2005;79:211–215.

190. Hoppe RT. Mycosis fungoides and other cutaneous lymphomas. In: Canellos GP, Lister TA, Sklar JL, eds. *The Lymphomas.* Philadelphia, PA: WB Saunders; 1998:495–506.

191. Macon WR. Peripheral T cell lymphomas. In: Hsi ED, Goldblum JR, ed. *Hematopathology.* 1st ed. Orlando, FL: Chrchill Livingstone; 2007:303–306.

192. Weinstock MA, Horm JW. Mycosis fungoides in the United States: increasing incidence and descriptive epidemiology. *JAMA.* 1988;260:42–46.

193. Whittemore AS, Holly EA, Lee IM, et al. Mycosis fungoides in relation to environmental exposures and immune response: a case control study. *J Natl Cancer Inst.* 1989;81:1560–1567.

194. van Doorn R, Van Haselen CW, Voorst Vader PC, et al. Myclosis fungoides: disease evolution and prognosis of 309 Dutch patients. *Arch Dermatol.* 2000;136:504–510.

195. Willemze R, Kerl H, Sterry W, et al. EORTC classification for primary cutaneous lymphomas: a proposal from the Cutaneous Lymphoma Study Group of the European Organization for Research and Treatment of Cancer. *Blood.* 1997;90:354–371.

196. Olsen E, Vonderheid E, Pimpnelli N, et al. Revisions to the staging and classification of mycosis fungoides and Sézary syndrome: a proposal of the International Society for Cutaneous Lymphomas (ISCL) and the Cutaneous Lymphoma Task Force of the European Organization of Research and Treatment of Cancer (EORTC). *Blood.* 2007;110:1713–1722.

197. Querfeld C, Guitart J, Kuzel TM, et al. Primary cutaneous lymphomas: a review with current treatment options. *Blood Rev.* 2003;17:131–142.

198. Hoppe RT, Abel EA, Deneau DG, et al. Mycosis fungoides: management with topical nitrogen mustard. *J Clin Oncol.* 1987;5:1796–1803.

199. Ramsay DL, Halperin PS, Zeleniuch-Jacquotte A. Topical mechlorethamine therapy for early stage mycosis fungoides. *J Am Acad Dermatol.* 1988;19:684–691.

200. Parker SRS, Bradley B. Treatment of cutaneous T-cell lymphoma/mycosis fungoides. *Dermatol Nurs.* 2006;18:566–570, 573–575.

201. Ligand Pharmaceuticals Inc. La Jolla, CA. Ontak package insert. 2003.

202. Weiss LM, Wood GS, Hu E, et al. Detection of clonal T-cell receptor gene rearrangements in the peripheral blood of patients with mycosis fungoides and dermatopathic lymphadenopathy. *N Engl J Med.* 1985;313:539–544.

203. Duvic M, Talpur R, Ni X, et al. Phase 2 trial of oral vorinostat (suberoylanilide hydroxamic acid, SAHA) for refractory cutaneous T-cell lymphoma (CTCL). *Blood.* 2007;109:31–39.

204. Piekarz RL, Robey R, Sandor V, et al. Inhibitor of histone deacetylation, depsipeptide (FR901228), in the treatment of peripheral and cutaneous T-cell lymphoma: a case report. *Blood.* 200;98:2865–2868.

205. Bekkenk MW, Geelen FA, Voorst Vader PC, et al. Primary and secondary cutaneous CD30+ lymphoproliferative disorders: a report from the Dutch Cutaneous Lymphoma Group on the long-term follow-up data of 219 patients and guidelines for diagnosis and treatment. *Blood.* 2000;95:3653–3661.

206. Delsol G, Jaffe ES, Falini B, et al. Anaplastic large cell lymphoma (ALCL) ALK-positive. In: Swerdlow SH, Campo E, Harris NL, et al, eds. *WHO Classification of Haematopoietic and Lymphoid Tissues.* 4th ed. Lyon, France: WHO Press; 2008:312–316.

207. Delsol G, Ralfkiaer E, Stein H, et al. Anaplastic large cell lymphoma. In: Jaffe ES, Harris NL, Stein H, et al, eds. *World Health Organization Classification of Tumours. Pathology and Genetics. Tumours of Haematopoietic and Lymphoid Tissues.* Lyon, France: ARC Press; 2001:230–235.

208. Longo DL. Malignancies of lymphoid cells (chapter). In: Fauci AS, Braunwald E, Kasper DL, et al. *Harrison's Principles of Internal Medicine*, 17e. http://www.accessmedicine.com/content.aspx?aID=2890045. Accessed August 14, 2009.

209. Brugieres L, Deley MC, Pacquement H, et al. CD30+ anaplastic large-cell lymphoma in children: analyses of 82 patients enrolled in two

consecutive studies of the French Society of Pediatric Oncology. *Blood.* 1998;92:3591–3598.

210. Fraga M, Brousset P, Schlaifer D, et al. Bone marrow involvement in anaplastic large cell lymphoma. Immunohistochemical detection of minimal disease and its prognostic significance. *Am J Clin Pathol.* 1995;103:82–89.
211. Benharroch D, Meguerian-Bedoyan Z, Lamant L, et al. ALK-positive lymphoma: a single disease with a broad spectrum of morphology. *Blood.* 1998;91:2076–2084.
212. Macon WR. Peripheral T-cell lymphomas. In: Hsi ED, Goldblum JR, ed. *Hematopathology.* 1st ed. Orlando, FL: Churchill Livingstone; 2006:283–310.
213. Wellman A, Otsuki T, Vogelbruch M, et al. Analysis of the t(2;5)(p23;q35) by RT-PCR in CD 30-positive anaplastic large cell lymphomas, in other non-Hodgkin's lymphomas of T-cell phenotype and in Hodgkin's disease. *Blood.* 1995;86:2321–2328.
214. Jagasia M, Morgan D, Goodman S, et al. Histology impacts the outcome of peripheral T-cell lymphomas after high dose chemotherapy and stem cell transplant. *Leuk Lymphoma.* 2004;45:2261–2267.
215. Hastrup N, Hamilton-Dutoit S, Ralfkiaer E, et al. Peripheral T-cell lymphomas: an evaluation of reproducibility of the updated Kiel classification. *Histopathology.* 1991;18:99–105.
216. Lee HF, Im FG, Goo FM, et al. Peripheral T-cell lymphoma: spectrum of imaging findings with clinical and pathologic features. *Radiographics.* 2003;23:7–26.
217. Arrowsmith ER, Macon WR, Kinney MC, et al. Peripheral T-cell lymphomas: clinical features and prognostic factors of 92 cases defined by the Revised European–American Lymphoma Classification. *Leuk Lymphoma.* 2003;44:241–249.
218. Lopez-Guillermo A, Cid J, Salar A, et al. Peripheral T-cell lymphomas: initial features, natural history, and prognostic factors in a series of 174 patients diagnosed according to the R.E.A.L. Classification. *Ann Oncol.* 1998;9:849–855.
219. Armitage J, Vose J, Weisenburger D. International peripheral T-cell and natural killer/T-cell lymphoma study: pathology findings and clinical outcomes. *J Clin Oncol.* 2008;26:4124–4130. Abstract.
220. Savage KJ, Chhanabhai M, Gascoyne RD, et al. Characterization of peripheral T-cell lymphomas in a single North American institution by the WHO classification. *Ann Oncol.* 2004;15:467–475.
221. McKelvey et al. Hydroxydaunomycin (adriamycin) combination chemotherapy in malignant lymphoma. *Cancer.* 1976;38:1484–1493.
222. Bagley CM Jr, Devita VT Jr, Bernard CW, Cannellos GP. Advanced lymphosarcoma: intensive cyclical combination chemotherapy with cyclophosphamide, vincristine, and prednisone. *Ann Inten Med.* 1972;76:227–234.
223. McLaughlin P, et al. Fludarabine, mitoxantrone, and dexamethasone: an effective new regimen for indolent lymphoma. *J Clin Oncol.* 1996;14:1262–1268.
224. Hochster H, Bendandi M, Gherlinzoni F, Merla E, Gozetti A, Tura S. Efficacy of cyclophosphamide (CYC) and fludarabine (FAMP) as first-line therapy of low-grade non-Hodgkin's lymphoma (NHL). *Blood.* 1994;84:383a.
225. Wilson WH, Bryant G, Bates S, et al. EPOCH chemotherapy: toxicity and efficacy in relapsed and refractory non-Hodgkin's lymphoma. *J Clin Oncol.* 1993;11:1573–1582.
226. Velasquez WS, McLauglin P, Tucker S, et al. ESHAP—an effective chemotherapy regimen in refractory and relapsing lymphoma: a 4-year follow-up study. *J Clin Oncol.* 1994;12:1169–1176.
227. Velasquez WS, Cabanillas F, Salvador P, et al. Effective salvage therapy for lymphoma with cisplatin in combination with high-dose ara-C and dexamethasone. *Blood.* 1988;71:117–122.
228. Moskowitz C, Bertino JR, Glassman JR, et al. Ifosfamide, carboplatin, and etoposide: a highly effective cytoreduction and peripheral blood progenitor cell mobilization regimen for transplant-eligible patients with non-Hodgkin's lymphoma. *J Clin Oncol.* 1999;17:3776–3785.
229. El Gnaoui T, Dupuis J, Belhadj K, et al. Rituximab, gemcitabine, and oxaliplatin: an effective salvage regimen for patients with relapsed or refractory B-cell lymphoma not candidates for high dose therapy. *Ann Oncol.* 2007;18:1363–1368.
230. Rodriguez MA, Cabanillas FC, Hagemeister FB, et al. A phase II trial of mesna, ifosfamide, mitozantrona, and etoposide for refractory lymphoma. *Ann Oncol.* 1995;6:609–611.
231. Fisher RI, Gaynor ER, Dahlberg S, et al. Comparison of standard regimen CHOP with three intensive chemotherapy regimens for advanced non-Hodgkin's lymphoma. *N Engl J Med.* 1993;328:1002–1006.
232. Rizzo JD, Somerfield MR, Hagerty KL, et al. American Society of Hemaotology/American Society of Clinical Oncology 2007 clinical practice guideline update on the use of epoetin and darbepoetin. *Blood.* 2008;111:25–41.
233. Rizzo JD, Somerfield MR, Hegerty KL, et al. Use of erythropoetin and darbepoetin in patients with cancer: 2007 American Society of Hematology/American Society of Clinical Oncology clinical practice guideline update. *J Clin Oncol.* 2008;26; 132–149.
234. Mudie NY, Swerdlow AJ, Higgins CD, et al. Risk of second malignancy after non-Hodgkin's lymphoma: a British Cohort Study. *J Clin Oncol.* 2006;24:107–108.
235. Forero A, LoBulio AF. History of antibody therapy for non-Hodgkin's lymphoma. *Semin Oncol.* 2003;30:1–5.
236. Press OS. Radioimmunotherapy for non-Hodgkin's lymphomas: a historical perspective. *Semin Oncol.* 2003;30:10–21.
237. Dillman RO, Hendrix CS. Unique aspects of supportive care using monoclonal antibodies in cancer treatment. *Support Cancer Ther.* 2003;1:38–48.
238. Plosker GL, Figgitt DP. Rituximab: a review of its use in non-Hodgkin's lymphoma and chronic lymphocytic leukaemia. *Drugs.* 2003;63:803–43.
239. Maloney DG, Liles TM, Czerwinski DK, et al. Phase I clinical trial using escalating single-dose infusion of chimeric anti-CD20 monoclonal antibody (IDEC-C2B8) in patients with recurrent B-cell lymphoma. *Blood.* 1994;84:2457–2466.
240. McLaughlin P, Grillo-Lopez AJ, Link BK, et al. Rituximab chimeric anti-CD20 monoclonal antibody therapy for relapsed indolent lymphoma: half of patients respond to a four-dose treatment regimen. *J Clin Oncol.* 1998;16:2825–2833.
241. Davis TA, Grillo-Lopez AJ, White CA, et al. Rituximab anti-CD20 monoclonal antibody therapy in non-Hodgkin's lymphoma: safety and efficacy of re-treatment. *J Clin Oncol.* 2000;18:3135–3143.
242. Coiffier B, LePage E, Briere J, et al. CHOP chemotherapy plus rituximab compared with CHOP alone in elderly patients with diffuse large-B-cell lymphoma. *N Engl J Med.* 2002;346:235–242.
243. Pfreundschuh M, Trumber L, Osterberg A, et al. CHOP-like chemotherapy plus rituximab versus CHOP-like chemotherapy alone in young patients with good prognosis diffuse large B cell lymphoma: a randomized controlled trial by the MabThera International Trial (MinT) Group. *Lancet Oncol.* 2006;7:379–391.
244. National Comprehensive Cancer Network (NCCN). *Clinical Practice Guidelines in Oncology. Non-Hodgkin's Lymphoma.* Rockledge, PA: NCCN; 2009. http://www.nccn.org. Accessed August 13, 2009
245. Leonard JP, Coleman M, Matthews JC, et al. Phase I/II trial of abratuzumab (humanized anti CD22 antibody) in non-Hodgkin's lymphoma. *J of Clin Oncol.* 2003;21:3051–3059.
246. Keating MJ, Byrd J, Rai K, et al. Multicenter study of CAM-PATH-1H in patients with chronic lymphocytic leukemia (B-CLL) refractory to fludarabine. *Blood.* 1999;94:705a.
247. Khorana A, Bunn P, McLaughlin P, et al. A phase II multicenter study of CAMPATH-1H antibody in previously treated patients with non-bulky non-Hodgkin's lymphoma. *Leuk Lymphoma.* 2001;41:77–87.
248. Lundin J, Kimby E, Bjorkholm M, et al. Phase II trial of subcutaneous anti-CD52 monoclonal antibody alemtuzumab (Campath-1H) as first-line treatment for patients with B-cell chronic lymphocytic leukemia (B-CLL). *Blood.* 2002;100:768–773.

249. Kennedy B, Rawstron A, Richards S, et al. CAMPATH-1H in CLL: immune reconstitution and viral infections during and after therapy. *Blood*. 2000;96:164a.
250. Vose JM, Chiu BC, Cheson BD, et al. Update of epidemiology and therapeutics for non-Hodgkin's lymphoma. *Hematology (Am Soc Hematol Educ Prog)*. 2002;1:241–262.
251. Witzig TE. Efficacy and safety of 90Y ibratumomab tiuxetan (Zevalin) radioimmunotherapy for non-Hodgkin's lymphoma. *Semin Oncol*. 2003;30:11–16.
252. Kaminski MS, Gregory SA, Fehrenbacher L, et al. Acute and delayed hematologic toxicities associated with Bexxar therapy are modest: overall experience in patients with low-grade or transformed low-grade non-Hodgkin's lymphoma (NHL). *Blood*. 2001;98:339a.
253. Magni M, Di Nicola M, Devizzi L, et al. Successful in vivo purging of CD34-containing peripheral blood harvests in mantle cell and indolent lymphoma: evidence for a role of both chemotherapy and rituximab infusion. *Blood*. 2000;96:864.
254. Bierman PJ, Sweetenham JW, Loberiza FR Jr, et al. Syngeneic hematopoietic stem-cell transplantation for non-Hodgkin's lymphoma: a comparison with allogeneic and autologous transplantation—The Lymphoma Working Committee of the International Bone Marrow Transplant Registry and the European Group for Blood and Marrow Transplantation. *J Clin Oncol*. 2003;21:3744–3753.
255. Freedman AS, Neuberg D, Mauch P, et al. Long-term follow-up of autologous bone marrow transplantation in patients with relapsed follicular lymphoma. *Blood*. 1999;94:3325.
256. Gribben JG, Freedman AS, Neuberg D, et al. Immunologic purging of marrow assessed by PCR before autologous bone marrow transplantation for B-cell lymphoma. *N Engl J Med*. 1991;325:1525–1533.
257. Chopra R, Goldstone AH, Pearce R, et al. Autologous versus allogeneic bone marrow transplantation for non-Hodgkin's lymphoma: A case-controlled analysis of the European Bone Marrow Transplant Group Registry data. *J Clin Oncol*. 1992;10:1690.
258. Holmberg LA, Maloney D, Bensinger W. Immunotherapy with rituximab/interleukin-2 after autologous stem cell transplantation as treatment for CD20+ non-Hodgkin's lymphoma. *Clinl Lymphoma Myeloma*. 2006;7:135–139.
259. Hosing C, Saliba RM, Korbling M, et al. High-dose rituximab does not negatively affect peripheral blood stem cell mobilization kinetics in patients with intermediate-grade non-Hodgkin's lymphoma. *Leuk Lymphoma*. 2006;47:1290–1294.
260. Rodriguez J. Should rituximab be used prior to autologous stem-cell transplantation for non-Hodgkin's lymphoma? *Nat Clin Pract Oncol*. 2005;2:74–75.
261. Robinson SP, Goldstone AH, Mackinnon S, et al. Chemoresistant or aggressive lymphoma predicts for a poor outcome following reduced-intensity allogeneic progenitor cell transplantation: an analysis from the Lymphoma Working Party of the European Group for Blood and Bone Marrow Transplantation. *Blood*. 2002;100:4310–4316.
262. Nagler A, Ackerstein A, Or R, et al. Immunotherapy with recombinant human interleukin-2 and recombinant interferon-alpha in lymphoma patients postautologous marrow or stem cell transplantation. *Blood*. 1997;89:3951.
263. Leoni LM, Bailey B, Reifert JB, et al. Bendamustine (Treanda) displays a distinct pattern of cytotoxicity and unique mechanistic features compared with other aylkylating agents. *Clin Cancer Res*. 2008;14: 309–317.
264. Rummel MJ, von Gruenhagen U, Niederle N, et al. Bendamustine plus rituximab versus CHOP plus rituximab in the first-line-treatment of patients with follicular, indolent, and mantle cell lymphomas: results of a randomized phase III study of the study group indolent lymphomas (StiL) [Abstract 2596]. *Blood*. 2008;111.
265. Lamanna N, Weiss MA. Pentostatin, cyclophosphamide, and rituximab show significant clinical activity in patients with previously untreated chronic lymphocytic leukemia. *Curr Oncol Rep*. 2007;9: 335–336.
266. Teeling JL, French RR, Cragg MS, et al. Characterization of new human CD20 monoclonal antibodies with potent cytolytic activity against non-Hodgkin lymphomas. *Blood*. 2004;104:1793–1800.
267. Hagenbeck A, Gadeberg O, Johnson P, et al. First clinical use of ofatumumab, a novel fully human anti CD20 monoclonal antibody in follicular lymphoma: the results of a phase 1/2 trial. *Blood*. 2008;111:5486–5495.
268. Coiffier B, Lepretre S, Pederson LM, et al. Safety and efficacy of ofatumomab, a fully human monoclonal anti CD20 antibody in patients with elapsed or refractory B cell chronic lymphocytic leukemia: A phase I/II study. *Blood*. 2008;111:1094–1100.
269. Morshhauser F, Leonard JP, Coiffier B, et al. Phase I/II results of a second generation humanized anti CD20 antibody, IMMU-106 (hA20) in NHL [Abstract 7530]. *J Clin Oncol*. 2006;24.
270. Siegal AB, Goldenberg DM, Cesano A, et al. CD22-directed monoclonal antibody therapy for lymphoma. *Semin Oncol*. 2003;30:457–464.
271. Leonard JP, Coleman M, Ketas JC, et al. Epratuzumab, a humanaized anti-CD22 antibody, in aggressive non-Hodgkin's lymphoma: phase I/II clinical trial results. *Clin Cancer Res*. 2004;10:5327–5334.
272. Strauss SJ, Morshhauser F, Rech J, et al. Multicenter phase II trial of immunotherapy with the humanized anti-CD22 antibody, epratuzumab, in combination with rituximab, in refractory or recurrent non-Hodgkin's lymphoma. *J Clin Oncol*. 2006;24:3880–3886.
273. Micallef IN, Maure J, Nikcerich DA, et al. A phase II study of epratuzumab and rituximab in combination with cyclophosphamide, doxorubicin, vincristine, and prednisone (ER-CHOP) in patients with previously untreated diffuse large B-cell lymphoma. *J Clin Oncol*. 2008;26:Abstract 8500.
274. Fayad L, Patel H, Verhoef F, et al. Safety and clinical activity of the anti-CD22 immunoconjugate inotuzumab ozogamicin (CMC-544) in combination with rituximab in folicular lymphoma or diffuse large B-cell lymphoma [abstr 261].*Blood*. 2008;112:103.
275. Leonard JP, Coleman M, Vose J, et al. Phase II study of oblimersen sodium (G3139) alone and with R-CHOP in mantle cell lymphoma [abstr 2276]. *Proc Am Soc Clin Oncol*. 2003;22:566.
276. Friedberg JW, Younes A, Fisher DC, et al. Durable responses in patients treated with Galiximab (anti CD80) in combination with rituximab for relapsed or refractory follicular lymphoma. Long-term follow-up of a phase II clinical trial. [Abstract 1004]. *Blood*. 2008;112.
277. Advani R, Forero-Torres A, Furman RR, et al. SGN-40 (anti huCD40 mAb) monotherapy induces durable objective responses in patients with relapses aggressive non-Hodgkin's lymphoma: evidence of antitumor activity from a phase I study. [Abstract 695]. *Blood*. 2006;108.
278. Long L, Patawaran M, Tong X, et al. Efficacy of an antagonistic anti CD40 monoclonal antibody, HCD122 (CHIR-12.12), in preclinical models of human non-Hodgkin's lymphoma and Hodgkin's disease. [Abstract 230]. *Blood*. 2006;108.
279. Freedman AS, Neelapau S, Nichols CR, et al. A placebo controlled phase III trial of patient specific immunotherapy with mitumprotimut-T (ID-KLA) and GM-CSF following rituximab in patients with CD20 positive follicular lymphoma. *J Clin Oncol*. 2009;27:3036–3043.
280. Riddell SR. Engineering antitumor immunity by T-Cell adoptive immunotherapy. *Hematology Am Soc Hematol Educ Program*. 2007; 2007:250–256.
281. Wang CY, Mayo MW, Korneluk RG, et al. NF-κB antiapoptosis: induction of TRAF1 and TRAF2 and c-IAP1 and cIAP2 to suppress capsase-8 activation. *Science*. 1998;281:1680–1683.
282. Leonard JP, Furman RR, Coleman M. Proteasome inhibition with bortezomib: a new therapeutic strategy for non-Hodgkin's lymphoma. *Int J Cancer*. 2006;119:971–979.
283. O'Connor OA, Wright L, Moskwitz C, et al. Promising activity of the proteosome inhibitor bortezomib (Velcade) in the treatment of indolent non-Hodgkin's lymphoma and mantle cell lymphoma. [Abstract 2346]. *Blood*. 2003;102.

284. Dang NH, Hagemeister FB, Pro B, et al. Phase II Study of Denileukin Diftitox for relapsed/refractory B-cell non-Hodgkin's lymphoma. *J Clin Oncol.* 2004;22:4095–4102.
285. O'Connor OA, Pro B, Pinter-Brown L, et al. PROPEL: A multi-center phase 2 open label study of Pralatrexate (PDX) with vitamin B12 and folic acid supplementation in patients with relapsed or refractory peripheral T-cell lymphoma. *Proc Am Soc Hematol.* 2008:261.
286. Kim YH, Reddy S, Kim EJ, et al. Romidepsin (depsipeptide) induces clinically significant responses in treatment-refractory CTCL: and international, multicenter study. [Abstract 123] *Blood.* 2007;110.
287. Witzig TE, Kaufman SH. Inhibition of the phosphatidylinositol 3-kinase/mamalian target of rapamycin pathway in hematologic malignancies. *Curr Treat Options Oncol.* 2006;7:285–294.
288. Ganjoo KN, Ac CS, Robertson MHJ, et al. Rituximab, bevacizumab and CHOP-(RA-CHOP) in untreated diffuse large cell lymphoma; safety, biomarkers, and pharmacokinetic analysis. *Leuk Lymphoma.* 2006;47:961–962.
289. Coleman M, Martin P, Ruan J, et al. The THRIL (thalidomide (T), rituximab (R), and lenalidomide (L)) regimen for chronic lymphocytic leukemia, small lymphocytic lymphoma, and mantle cell lymphoma, daily alternating ImiDs and rituximab maintenance. [Abstract 7079]. *J Clin Oncol.* 2008;26.
290. Ferrajoli A, O'Brien A, Weirda W, et al. Lenalidomide as initial treatment of elderly patients with chronic lymphocytic leukemnia (CLL). *Blood.* 2008;112. Abstract 45.
291. Zinzani PL, Witzig TE, Vose JH, et al. Efficacy and safety of lenalidomide oral monotherapy in patients with relpsed or refractory mantle cell lymphoma: results of an international study (NHL-003). *Blood.* 2008;112:262a.
292. Zelenetz AD: Risk models for chemotherapy-induced neutropenia in non-Hodgkin's lymphoma. *Oncology.* 2003;17:21–26.
293. Henry D, Dahl NV. Iron or vitamin B12 deficiency in anemic patients prior to erythropoiesis-stimulating agent therapy. *Commun Oncol.* 2007;4:95–101.
294. Bohlius J, LAngensiepen S, Schwarzer G, et al. Recombinent human erythropoietin and overall survival in cancer patients: results of a comprehensive meta-analysis. *J Natl Cancer Inst.* 2005;97:489–498
295. Sonnen R, Schmidt W-P, Kuse R, Schmitz N. Treatment results of aggressive B non-Hodgkin's lymphoma in advanced age con sidering comorbidity. *Br J Haematol.* 2002;119:634–639.
296. Acupuncture for chemo-induced peripheral neuropathy in multiple myeloma and lymphoma patients. http://Clinical trials.gov/ctz/show/NCT00891618. Accessed October 1, 2009.
297. Oyer DS, Shah A, Bettenhausen S. How to manage steroid diabetes in the patient with cancer. *J Support Oncol.* 2006;4:479–483.
298. Van den Berge G, Wilmer A, Hermans G, et al. Intensive insulin therapy in the medical ICU. *N Engl J Med.* 2006;354:449–461.
299. Furnary AP, Wu Y, Bookin SO. Effects of hyperglycemia and continuous intravenous insulin infusions on outcomes of cardiac surgical procedures: The Portland Diabetic Project. *Endocr Pract.* 2004;10:21–33.
300. Ellger B, Debeveye Y, Vanhorebeek I, et al. Survival benefits of insulin therapy in critical illness: impact of maintaining normogycemia versus glycemia-independent actions of insulin. *Diabetes.* 2006;55:1096–1105.
301. Knobel H, Loge JH, Lund MB, et al. Late medical complications and fatigue in Hodgkin's disease survivors. *J Clin Oncol.* 2001;19:3226–3233.
302. Pangalis GA, Dimopoulou MN, Angelopoulou MK, et al: Campath-1H (anti-CD52) monoclonal antibody therapy in lymphoproliferative disorders. *Med Oncol.* 2001;18:99–107.
303. Gordon LI, White CA, Leonard JP, et al. Zevalin radioimmunotherapy is associated with a low incidence of human anti-mouse antibody (HAMA) and human anti-Rituxan antibody (HACA) response (abstract) *Blood.* 2001;98:228B.
304. Adams MJ, Hardenbergh PH, Constine LS, Lipshultz SE. Radiation-associated cardiovascular disease. *Crit Rev Oncol-Hematol.* 2003;45:55–75.
305. Moser EC, Noordijk EM, van Leeuwan FE, et al. Long-term risk of cardiovascular disease after treatment for aggressive non-Hodgkin's lymphoma. *Blood.* 2006;107:2912–2919.
306. Sleijfer S. Bleomycin-induced pneumonitis. *Chest.* 2001;120:617.
307. Bhatia S. Secondary malignancies: What, When, Why, in Whom? NCCN Clinical Practice Forum. 2008. http:///www.medscape.com/viewarticle/581683. Accessed October 1, 2009.
308. Okines A, Thompson CS, Radstone CR, et al. Second primary malignancies after treatment for malignant lymphoma. *Br J Cancer.* 2005;93:418–424.
309. Karp JE, Sarkodee-Adoo CB. Therapy related acute leukemia [abstract]. *Clin Lab Med.* 2000;20:71–79.
310. Ruffer JU, Fletcher H, Tralls O, et al. Fatigue in long-term survivors of Hodgkin's lymphoma; a report from the German Hodgkin Lymphoma Study Group (GHSG). *Eur J Cancer.* 2003;39:2179–2186.
311. NCCN Clinical Practice Guidelines in Oncology. Cancer-Related Fatigue. V1.2009, http://www.nccn.org. Accessed October 1, 2009.
312. Carver JR, Shapiro CL, Ng A, et al. American Society of Clinical Oncology clinical evidence review on the ongoing care of adult cancer survivors: cardiac and pulmonary late effects. *J Clin Oncol.* 2007;25:3991–4008.
313. Cosset JM, Henry-Amar M, Pellae-Cosset B, et al. Pericarditis and myocardial infarctions after Hodgkin's disease therapy at the Institute of Gustave-Roussy. *Int J Radiat Oncol Biol Phys.* 1992;21:447–449.
314. Basavaraju SR, Easterly CE. Pathophysiological effects of radiation on atherosclerosis development and progression, and the incidence of cardiovascular complications. *Am Assoc Phys Med.* 2002;29:2391–2403.
315. Handa N, McGregor CGA, Danielson TA, et al. Coronary artery bypass grafting in patients with previous mediastinal radiation therapy. *J Thorac Cardovasc Surg.* 1999;117:1136–1143.
316. Elis A, Tevet a, Yerushalmi R, et al. Fertility status among women treated for aggressive non-Hodgkin's lymphoma. *Leuk Lymphoma.* 2006; 47:623.
317. Lee SJ, Schover LR, Partridge AH, et al. American Society of Clinical Oncology recommendations on fertility preservation in cancer patients. *J Clin Oncol.* 2006;24:2917–2931.
318. Blumenfeld Z, Avivi I, Linn S, et al. Prevention of irreversible chemotherapy-induced ovarian damage in young women with lymphoma by a gonadotropin releasing hormone agonist in parallel to chemotherapy. *Hum Reprod.* 1996;11:1620–1625.
319. Waxman JH, Ahmend R, Smith D, et al. Failure to preserve fertility in patients with Hodgkin's disease. *Cancer Chemother Pharmacol.* 1987;19:159–162.
320. Travis LB. Evaluation of the risk of therapy-associated complications in survivors of hodgkin lymphoma. *American Society of Hematology Education Program Book.* 2007;1:192–196.
321. Aleman BM, van dem Belt-Dusebout AW, Klokman WJ, et al. Long-term cause-specific mortality of pateints treated for Hodgkin's disease. *J Clin Oncol.* 2003;21:3431–3439.
322. Mudie NY, Swerdlow AJ, Higgins CD, et al. Risk of second malignancy after non-Hodgkin's lymphoma: A British cohort study. *J Clin Oncol.* 2006;24:1568–1574.
323. Sacchi S, Marcheselli L, Bari A, et al. Secondary malignancies after treatment for non-Hodgkin indolent lymhpoma: a 16-year follow-up study. *Haematologica.* 2008;93:372–380.
324. Mauch PM, Kalish LA, Marcus KC, et al. Second malignancies after treatment for laparotomy staged IA-IIIB Hodgkin's disease. *Blood.* 1996;87:3625.
325. Friedberg JW. Secondary malignancies after therapy of indolent non-Hodgkin's lymphoma. *Haematologica.* 2008;93:336–338.
326. Howe R, Micaleff INM, Inwards DJ, et al. Secondary myelodysplastic syndrome and acute myelogenous leukemia are significant

complications following autologous stem cell transplantation for lymphoma. *Bone Marrow Transplant.* 2003;32:317–324.
327. Bhatia S, Yasui Y, Robison LL, et al. High risk of second malignant neoplasms continues with the extended follow-up of childhood Hodgkin's disease: report from the late effects study group [Abstract]. *J Clin Oncolo.* 2003;21:4386–4394. .
328. Hancock SL, Tucker MA, Hoppe RT. Breast cancer after treatment. *J Natl Cancer Inst.* 1993;85:25–31.
329. Lorigan R, Radford J, Howel A, et al. Lung cancer after treatment for Hodgkin's lymphoma: a systematic review [Abstract]. *Lancet Oncol.* 2005;6:773–779.
330. De Bruin ML, Sparidans J, van't Veer MB, Noordijk EM, Louwman MWJ, Zijlstra JM, et al. Breast cancer risk in female survivors of Hodgkin's lymphoma: Lower risk after smaller radiation volumes. *J Clin Oncol.* 2009;27:4239–4246.

CHAPTER

61

*Joseph D. Tariman, APRN-BC, OCN®,*
*Beth Faiman, RN, MSN, APRN-BC, AOCN®*

# Multiple Myeloma

## INTRODUCTION

Multiple myeloma (MM) is a B-cell malignancy of the plasma cells. Its three hallmarks include the presence of a serum or urine monoclonal immunoglobulin, monoclonal plasmacytosis, and bony lytic lesions.[1] Cells are usually responsive to radiotherapy and chemotherapy, but relapse is inevitable. The need for novel therapeutic agents that can prolong and improve overall survival (OS) has remained high.[2]

Major advances have been seen in approaches to management of patients with MM in the past decade. Innovative approaches in high-dose chemotherapy (HDC), the use of bisphosphonates, the discovery of a novel proteasome inhibitor, bortezomib (Velcade, Millennium Pharmaceutical, Inc., Cambridge, MA), liposomal doxorubicin, and the development of lenalidomide (Revlimid, Celgene Corporation, Summit, NJ), an immunomodulatory drug (IMiD), are among the most encouraging breakthroughs in therapeutics.[3] In addition, latest developments in magnetic resonance imaging (MRI) and positron emission tomography (PET) scans, immunology, cytogenetics, molecular biology, and gene microarray expression profiling have also contributed to a significant understanding of MM.[4–6] A sequential approach in targeting not only the MM cells but also their microenvironment, using novel biologically based therapeutic agents alone or in combination with conventional chemotherapy, has shown that drug resistance can be overcome and better survival can be achieved.[7,8]

## EPIDEMIOLOGY

In the general population, MM accounts for 1% of all malignancies and approximately 10% of all hematologic malignancies.[3] Within the United States, it represents approximately 14% of all hematologic malignancies and is the second most common of all hematologic malignancies, after non-Hodgkin's lymphoma. In 2009, it is estimated that 20,580 men and women (11,680 men and 8900 women) will be diagnosed with and 10,580 men and women will die of myeloma.[9] A male predominance in incidence is noted, with a male-to-female ratio of 3:2, although African American females have a higher incidence than Caucasian males in the United States. More than 55,000 patients in the United States are living with myeloma. The peak occurrence of MM is among people in their 50s and 70s.[9] The reported increase in incidence during the past several decades in the United States is probably due to increased availability and use of medical facilities for the elderly and improved diagnostic techniques, rather than a true increase in incidence.[10]

Age and race are among the demographic factors that have been shown to have a consistent relationship with MM. Persons affected by MM are often elderly, with a median age at diagnosis of 66 years. Thirty-eight percent of patients are 70 years or older and 2% are younger than 40 years.[10] The disease affects African Americans twice as much as Caucasian Americans. MM is one of the leading causes of cancer death among African Americans. The black-white differential in incidence has been found to be substantially related to socioeconomic status.[11] Worldwide incidence of MM is relatively low among Asian and Hispanic populations.

The OS and management of MM has significantly changed in the past few years, particularly with the advent of novel therapeutic agents and aggressive symptom management. Although there are several clinical trials that have demonstrated improved survival in the past few years, the overall 5-year relative survival rate for males and females during the period 1996–2004, from 17 SEER geographic areas was 34.9%.[9] Racial differences continue to be noted in the 5-year relative survival rate for MM, but more important to note would be improved response rates and survival within the past decade. In a recent study published by the group at Mayo Clinic, patients diagnosed in the past decade had a median OS of 44.8 months vs those diagnosed before past decade (29.9 months).[12] This is a 50% improvement in OS independent of prognostic factors. In addition, those patients less than 65 years of age had an OS of 60 months, suggesting the diagnosis of MM is being transitioned into a chronic state with improved life expectancy in the past few years.[12]

## ETIOLOGY

The cause of MM is unknown. Although several epidemiological studies have been conducted, no single cause is directly associated with the pathogenesis of MM. In 1997, human herpes virus 8 (HHV-8), also called as Kaposi's sarcoma-associated human virus (KSHV), was reported to be present in dendritic cells of patients with MM,[13] but its role in the pathogenesis of MM remains controversial. No case-control and cohort studies have supported a consistent relationship of this virus in the majority of patients with MM. Further epidemiological studies, serologic data, and polymerase chain reaction assays did not implicate KSHV in the pathogenesis of MM.[14]

There are a few reports of a possible link between human immunodeficiency virus and MM.[15–17] Also, patients with acquired immune deficiency syndrome have a higher risk of developing MM compared with the normal population.[17] Conversely, little evidence suggests that chronic antigenic stimulation (ie, exposure to viruses) plays a role in myeloma pathogenesis.[18] Despite extensive epidemiological studies, the etiology of MM remains unclear.

## RISK FACTORS

Despite recent advances in clarifying the biological mechanisms of MM, there are no established risk factors other than male gender, increasing age, African American ethnicity, positive family history of lymphatohematopoietic cancer and monoclonal gammopathy of undetermined significance (MGUS).[19] The most recognized and most common risk factor for the development of MM is the presence of MGUS, a common precursor to MM. Patients with MGUS have a MM incidence rate of approximately 1.5%, and approximately 62% of patients will never progress to MM requiring active therapy.[20] Patients with MGUS should be monitored with routine laboratory and radiographic studies to assess for the progression to MM. There is also a risk that these patients may progress to other lymphoproliferative or B-cell disorders, such as Waldenstrom's macroglobulinemia, AL amyloidosis, or lymphoma.[21] As with MM, the etiology of MGUS just remains unknown.

Several risk factors have been identified in association with MM. An emerging area of research is the role of obesity in MM. Obesity is more prevalent in the African American population, and this may help explain some of the increased incidence of myeloma.[19,22] Other risk factors include high doses of ionizing radiation;[12,19] occupational exposures such as agricultural exposure, which includes fuels and pesticides;[23] diesel exhaust;[24] metal working;[25,26] working in the paint industry;[27] and employment in the leather[28] and textile industries.[29]

Employment in the petroleum industry does not increase an individual's risk of developing MM, but one recent study utilizing geographic information system analysis determined that there is a slight increase in risk among people who reside near a large chemical waste dump.[30] No association has been found between a history of asbestos exposure and MM[24,31] except in one report.[32] Diagnostic x-rays have a negligible impact, if any, on one's risk of developing MM.[33] Benzene exposure is also not a likely risk factor for developing MM.[34] The risk of having familial MM is relatively small, although an increased incidence of MM in certain families has been reported. One study reported 17 families had affected members in 2 or more generations, and 8 families had 2 or more affected members in a single generation. This observational study of 39 patients may provide insight into risk factors and future genetic descriptions.[35,36]

In most of the studies to date, some of the risk factors mentioned previously lacked the criteria of strength of association, consistency of association, and exposure risk relationship. It is fair to say that in the vast majority of patients, no obvious explanation for the occurrence of the disease is available at this time.

## PREVENTION, SCREENING, AND EARLY DETECTION

In the absence of known causative agents, identified tumor markers, or definitive diagnostic tests, the ability to apply prevention and early detection strategies to MM remains elusive. MM should be suspected when a patient presents with bone pain in which lytic lesions are discovered on radiographic films. An increase in serum total protein or presence of M-protein in the serum or urine, new-onset renal failure without an obvious cause, or hypercalcemia strongly suggests the diagnosis of MM, and a comprehensive diagnostic work-up must be performed.[37]

## PATHOPHYSIOLOGY

New insights into the pathophysiology of MM have been reported. Recent findings support the hypothesis that MM pathogenesis involves genetic and molecular defects in the early development of malignant plasma cells.[38–40] The nonrandom, recurrent nature of chromosomal abnormalities in myeloma suggests that they play a role in disease pathogenesis. One study reported that translocation of immunoglobulin heavy-chain (IgH) locus (14q32) and deletion of chromosome 13 were found in 75% and 45% of patients with plasma cell disorders, respectively, and were not randomly distributed but rather interconnected.[41] In contrast to certain hematologic malignancies such as chronic myelogenous leukemia, no single genetic anomaly has been implicated in the pathogenesis of MM.

The initial transformation is thought to occur in a postgerminal center (earliest stage of cell) B-lineage cell, carrying a somatically hypermutated IgH gene.[39] This plasmablastic (stem cell of plasma cell) cell colonizes the bone marrow, propagates clonally (originating from one cell), and then differentiates into a slowly proliferating myeloma cell population, all under the influence of specific cell adhesion molecules such as intracellular adhesion and vascular adhesion molecules and cytokines such as interleukin 6 (IL-6).[42] Cytogenetic analysis of myeloma cells frequently demonstrates multiple mutations and chromosomal aberrations. The most common cytogenetic abnormality found in MM involves the dysregulation of proto-oncogenes by rearrangement with the IgH locus of the plasma cell, commonly called translocation of IgH locus,[41,43] which could be among the earliest genetic events.[39] Translocation of IgH locus and deletion of chromosome 13 can be determined by using the fluorescent in situ hybridization technique during bone marrow biopsy. Researchers also found that there is high correlation between deletion of chromosome 13 in these patients and their immunological status and clinical presentation, which may also be useful in determining prognosis.

Aberrant expression of antiapoptotic oncogenes such as *bcl-2*, *bcl-x1*, and fibroblast growth factor receptor 3 (FGFR-3) has been identified in MM as well. Researchers believe that plasma cells are likely to require a mitogenic signal (a signal inducing the nucleus of the cell to divide, resulting into two nuclei) to promote malignancy. A study demonstrated that disease progression in patients with MM is associated with a concurrent alteration in the expression of both oncogenes and tumor suppressor genes, supporting the existence of a genetic abnormality in MM.[44] Another study showed that deletion of the *TP53* gene predicted resistance to chemotherapy, highlighting its importance in the MM disease process.[45] There is high interest in studying the molecular and cytogenetic alterations in MM, but the precise causes of these abnormalities remain largely unknown.[46]

A good understanding of the nature of plasma cells, the immunoglobulins secreted by plasma cells, features of the malignant clone, and changes induced by the bone marrow microenvironment could lead to better understanding of the pathophysiology of MM. Plasma cell development originates in the bone marrow, then progresses through a number of sequential stages defined primarily by the status of the immunoglobulin rearrangements.[47] Most circulating B lymphocytes are naïve cells that have not been exposed to an activating antigen. Their life span is about 1 week in the absence of antigenic activation. Plasma cells are derived from B lymphocytes that have been activated by antigenic stimuli.[48] Because a plasma cell is derived from the B lymphocyte, it has been thought to be the identifiable malignant cell in MM; MM is therefore considered a B-cell malignancy of the plasma cell.

Immunoglobulins or antibodies constitute the humoral immune response to a foreign antigen. They are secretory products of plasma cells, and each immunoglobulin molecule has 2 heavy and 2 light chains. The 5 types of heavy chains are denoted by the Greek letters $\mu$, $\delta$, $\gamma$, $\alpha$, and $\varepsilon$. The type of heavy chain present determines the class of the immunoglobulin: IgM, IgD, IgG, IgA, or IgE, respectively. The 2 types of light chains are denoted by the Greek letters $\kappa$ (kappa) and $\lambda$ (lambda). Each heavy-chain immunoglobulin molecule has either a $\kappa$ or a $\lambda$ subtype of light chain in association with one of the types of heavy chain (ie, IgG kappa or IgG lambda).

Because MM is a neoplastic clonal process, the malignant cells and the secreted immunoglobulins are either kappa- or lambda-restricted. Because only two types of immunoglobulin expressions are possible, this restriction readily enables determination of clonality. To determine clonality, one may perform immunohistochemistry staining of the plasma cell population during bone marrow biopsy. Most patients with MM have more than 10% plasma cells in the bone marrow, with an average of 30% to 40%,[48] and most of these cells are present in sheets or aggregates. It is important to note how much of the plasma cell population has either kappa or lambda restriction during immunohistochemistry staining to distinguish normal (polyclonal) from abnormal (monoclonal) plasma cells. Monoclonal plasma cells can express only either kappa or lambda restriction in immunohistochemistry studies.

The monoclonal proliferation of plasma cells produces a homogeneous immunoglobulin fraction detectable in the serum (heavy-chain protein) and/or urine (light-chain protein), called myeloma protein or M-spike. Bone destruction due to the production of osteoclastic factors by the malignant plasma cells is the most characteristic feature of the disease, and bone pain is the predominant presenting symptom.[49] Although most patients have serum proteins with or without associated urinary proteins, 20% of affected individuals have only urinary proteins (Bence-Jones protein [BJP] or light-chain protein). Even though an excessive amount of immunoglobulin is being produced, these immunoglobulins are unable to effectively produce the antibodies required for maintaining humoral immunity, thereby placing patients with MM at higher risk for infections. Immunofixation (the most sensitive test for M-protein) of the serum and urine shows M-protein in 97% of patients diagnosed with myeloma and only 3% are nonsecretory (no detectable M-protein).[10,50] Individuals who present with bone pain, numerous lytic lesions in their skeletal survey, hypercalcemia, and low blood counts with no detectable M-protein either in blood or urine most likely have a nonsecretory type of MM (monoclonal plasma cells are not producing the homogenous immunoglobulin).

## ROLE OF CYTOKINES

Cytokines are believed to play a major role in the pathogenesis and pathophysiological changes of myeloma cells. Cytokines are extracellular signaling molecules that activate a cascade of intracellular pathways and that regulate growth and differentiation of cells. These growth factors bind to specific cell-surface receptors, thereby establishing communication between malignant precursors and their environment.[51]

Plasma cell proliferation in MM is influenced by cytokines and certain biological variables. Plasma cells produce IL-6, a major proliferative cytokine for malignant plasma cells, and vascular endothelial growth factor (VEGF), one of the most important cytokines for angiogenesis.[48,51] In addition, myeloma cells express IL-1$\beta$ and tumor necrosis factor alpha (TNF-$\alpha$), which are potent osteoclast-activating factors (OAF). Notably, IL-6 does not induce proliferation of normal B lymphocytes or normal plasma cells, but rather has a significant proliferative and antiapoptotic effect on myeloma cells that confers resistance to conventional chemotherapy.[52] Although controversy surrounds the exact source of IL-6 in myeloma, some evidence suggests both autocrine (stimulates the myeloma cells itself for the production of growth factor) and paracrine (stimulates other cells that are closest to the myeloma cells) production. IL-6 mediation of paracrine myeloma cell growth is supported by observations that bone marrow stromal cells (BMSC) are the major source of IL-6 in myeloma. Studies have also found that freshly isolated myeloma cells cultured without exogenous IL-6 rapidly stop proliferating[53] and that adhesion of myeloma cells to BMSC upregulates IL-6 secretion by BMSC.[54]

VEGF is also expressed by plasma cells and is a potent angiogenic cytokine.[55] Studies have shown that bone marrow angiogenesis is increased in MM and has prognostic value. Normal plasma cells do not produce IL-1β, whereas plasma cells from almost all MM patients produce it.[48] This aberrant production of IL-1β can induce the expression of genes for IL-6, colony-stimulating factors,[48] and various adhesion molecules, as well as mediate IL-6 production by BMSC.[56] IL-1β has potent OAF activity, and it may be the predominant factor responsible for the development of osteolytic lesions in myeloma as well as the receptor activator of nuclear factor-κB (RANK) ligand (RANKL)–osteoprotegerin–RANK system, and inhibitors of Wnt signaling.[57,58]

Several other cytokines are implicated in the development of bone disease (lytic lesions) in patients with MM. Besides IL-6 and other members of the gp130 cytokine family, osteoclast-stimulating factors (OSF) or bone-resorbing activity has been detected in the supernatants of both myeloma cell lines and fresh patient cells; macrophage inflammatory protein 1-alpha (MIP-1α) has also been found to induce osteoclast formation.[59]

Granulocyte-macrophage colony-stimulating factor (GM-CSF), IL-3, stem cell factor (SCF), TNF-α, hepatocyte growth factor, insulin-like growth factors 1 and 2 (IGF-1 and -2),[60–62] and VEGF are all potential myeloma growth factors. All have been shown to stimulate growth or specific intracellular signaling events of myeloma cells or cell lines in vitro.[63,64]

Interferon-alpha (IFN-α) is another cytokine that has been used in patients with myeloma because of its antiproliferative action, but clinical data have shown variable responses to it. This variation may be due to the dual role played by IFN-α in cytokine growth inhibition and proliferation. A study involving cell cycle regulatory genes revealed that differential induction of cyclin D2 and $p19^{INK4D}$ may be one of the key mechanisms underlying these variable responses.[65]

IL-10 is also a growth factor for myeloma cells, increasing the proliferation of malignant plasma cells.[66] This IL increases the responsiveness of some myeloma cells to IL-11 (one of the cytokines responsible for the development of bone lesions in myeloma patients) by upregulating the expression of IL-11 receptors.[67]

Recent advances in our understanding of the complex cytokine interactions between tumor cells and their microenvironment have already resulted in the development of novel therapeutic agents. Further research leading to a better understanding of the roles played by cytokines in the pathogenesis of MM may soon open up even more therapeutic targets, adding more potent and selective treatments in the armamentarium against MM (Table 61-1).

**TABLE 61-1**

**Cytokines Under Investigation in the Pathogenesis of Multiple Myeloma**

| | |
|---|---|
| Interleukin 1β (IL-1β) | Insulin-like growth factor 1 and 2 (IGF-1 and -2) |
| Interleukin 3 (IL-3) | Vascular endothelial growth factor (VEGF) |
| Interleukin 6 (IL-6) | Osteoclast-stimulating factor (OSF) |
| Viral IL-6 | Hepatocyte growth factor (HGF) |
| Interleukin 10 (IL-10) | Leukemia inhibitory factor (LIF) |
| Interleukin 11 (IL-11) | Granulocyte-macrophage colony-stimulating factor (GM-CSF) |
| Alfa-interferon | Granulocyte colony-stimulating factor (G-CSF) |
| Oncostatin M (OSM) | Tumor necrosis factor (TNF)<br>Tumor growth factor-β (TGF-β) |

## CLINICAL MANIFESTATIONS

Bone pain, particularly in the back and chest, is present at diagnosis in more than two-thirds of patients with myeloma and is the most predominant presenting symptom.[37] Other symptoms at presentation may include anemia, uremia, recurrent infection, and, less commonly, hypercalcemia, hyperviscosity, polyneuropathy, and spinal cord compression.[49] In most patients presenting with symptomatic disease, the classic triad of MM, consisting of multiple lytic bone lesions, high serum M-protein, and extensive bone marrow plasmacytosis (>30%), is present.

Some individuals with MM may have a long prodromal, indolent, or asymptomatic period (Durie-Salmon or International Staging System [ISS] stage 1), which can also be termed "smoldering myeloma." Many of these patients do not need primary treatment because they can do well for many months to years before the disease progresses. Patients should be initially observed; if their disease progresses to stage II or higher, then they should be treated according to the guidelines for advanced MM.[50] Disease progression is defined as a sustained 25% or greater increase in serum or urine M-protein or development of new sites of lytic disease or hypercalcemia.[50,68]

### SKELETAL INVOLVEMENT

Destructive, painful osteolytic lesions are one of the major clinical manifestations of myeloma.[49] In fact, patients who respond to chemotherapy may still have progression of skeletal disease, and recalcification of osteolytic lesions is slow and rare.[69] This bone destruction could lead to pathological fractures, spinal cord compression, hypercalcemia, bone pain, and loss of height (if the vertebral spine is affected).[70] These complications are major causes of morbidity and mortality in patients with MM. The osteolytic lesions in MM are due to rapid bone turnover, wherein increased osteoclastic bone resorption is not accompanied by a comparable increase in bone formation. A recent report has found an association between the myeloma cell production of DKK1, an inhibitor of osteoblast differentiation, and the presence of lytic bone lesions in patients with MM.[71]

Conventional radiography (metastatic skeletal survey, to include axial skeleton and large cortical bones) reveals osteolytic lesions, osteopenia, or fractures in 80% of patients with MM at diagnosis, and has been found to be more sensitive than MRI as well for disease classification.[37,72] Comparative studies have repeatedly shown that conventional radiographic surveys can detect more lytic lesions than bone scanning.[73] Bone scan is usually negative in MM. For this reason, radiographic studies continue to be used almost universally in the initial evaluation and widely in the follow-up of patients with myeloma. Subsequent follow-up skeletal surveys during and after treatment help determine worsening of myeloma status based on the occurrence of new lytic lesions and/or increases in their size. One disadvantage of this simple test is its lack of sensitivity, particularly in determining response to treatment.[74]

In cases of equivocal response to treatment, MRI can supplement conventional radiographs. It offers clinicians an additional tool not only for determining response to treatment, but also for assessing the extent of the disease and detecting disease progression in patients with no measurable M-protein.[74,75] Likewise, MRI is useful in patients with suspected cord compression and solitary plasmacytoma of the spine,[50] and in patients with MM who have bone pain but no abnormalities found on the radiographs.[37] The use of whole-body Fluorine-18 fluorodeoxyglucose positron emission tomography ($^{18}$F-FDG PET) scan in myeloma is controversial. FDG is an analog of glucose that is radiolabeled with the positron-emitting radionuclide $^{18}$F. Metabolically active cells take up and phosphorylate FDG, which is not further metabolized, but remains trapped within the cell. The resulting intracellular accumulation of FDG is then imaged with PET. Typically, high levels of uptake are seen in tumor cells, with increased rates of metabolism compared with normal tissue. PET is routinely used in other types of cancer, such as lymphoma. This technique may be effective at distinguishing between active and inactive myeloma at various time points, such as after stem cell transplantation and in extramedullary plasmacytomas (EMP),[76] yet reimbursement remains an issue and this is not considered standard of care for all MM patients at this time.

## INFECTION

Infection plays an important role in the morbidity and mortality associated with MM.[77] Fever caused by viral and bacterial infections is the presenting symptom in about 10% of patients with MM. The incidence of infection in patients with MM is 15 times higher than in normal individuals,[49] and approximately 70% of patients will die from infection.[77] The predominant pathogens isolated from patients with MM are bacterial in nature, which reflects the defect in humoral immunity seen in myeloma. This defect is demonstrated in the reduction of polyclonal immunoglobulin (the immunoglobulins produced by myeloma cells are monoclonal and defective) synthesis and a failure to make antibody responses post immunization.[77]

*Streptococcus pneumoniae* and *Haemophilus influenzae* are the most frequently isolated bacteria during the early course of the disease, and the respiratory and urinary tracts are common sites of infection. Other infections occurring later during the course of the disease may involve gram-negative organisms and *Staphylococcus aureus*. This biphasic pattern of bacterial infections in patients with MM is related to the stage of the disease,[78] treatment modalities such as high-dose therapy and transplantation leading to neutropenia, high-dose corticosteroids, and the use of central venous catheters.[49]

Systemic, fungal, protozoal, and mycobacterial infections are uncommon in patients with MM. The only viral infection that has been consistently reported in patients with myeloma is herpes zoster.[77] Prophylactic use of antiviral agents is recommended particularly in post-transplant patients or other severely immunocompromised patients. Impairment of T-cell function is commonly seen in MM, although it is clinically not as important as the B-cell deficiency.[49] The intensive corticosteroid therapy found in regimens such as vincristine, doxorubicin, and dexamethasone (VAD) or high-dose pulsed dexamethasone suppresses T-cell function markedly, and there are incidental reports of *Pneumocystis carinii* infections.[77] Prophylactic use of antibiotic agents such as the trimethoprim/sulfamethoxazole combination may prove highly useful in preventing these opportunistic infections.[49]

## BONE MARROW INVOLVEMENT

Approximately two-thirds of patients with MM have anemia at presentation.[10] It is usually normocytic, normochromic, and clinically manifested by fatigue and weakness. This problem is typically associated with depressed erythropoietin levels due to an inadequate erythropoietin response to anemia. Other contributing factors to the development of anemia include impaired availability of storage iron and overproduction of cytokines such as IL-1, IL-6, and TNF-α that can inhibit erythropoiesis. Determining the level of endogenous erythropoietin may help to select patients who may benefit from treatment with recombinant erythropoietin. A recent study reported that anemia in patients with MM is related to a pathogenetic mechanism whereby malignant plasma cells express very high levels of apoptogenic receptors, which triggers apoptosis of immature erythroblasts. This persistent erythroblast cytotoxicity within the bone marrow leads to progressive destruction of the erythroid matrix.[79]

As myeloma cells infiltrate the bone marrow or if the patient is treated with systemic chemotherapy, both qualitative and quantitative defects in neutrophil and platelet function can occur. Impaired serum opsonic activity (release of a substance that renders microbes more vulnerable to being engulfed by phagocytes) in the neutrophils of patients with MM can result in a quantitative defect in the function of circulating neutrophils. Decreased platelets can be attributed to M-protein's effect on clotting factors or to nonspecific coating of platelets with immunoglobulins resulting in platelet dysfunction and bleeding. Leukopenia usually occurs in very advanced disease or after chemotherapy.[80]

## RENAL INSUFFICIENCY

Multiple myeloma is frequently associated with renal dysfunction. In addition, it has been shown that the presence of renal failure indicates a higher tumor burden and consequently more aggressive disease.[81] Patients who are diagnosed with renal insufficiency should be treated aggressively because reversal of renal insufficiency results in survival outcomes similar to those for patients who have normal renal function at diagnosis. The reported incidence of renal disease at presentation or during the course of MM ranges from 20% to 60%. Most renal disease is found in patients who produce excess light chains and IgD myeloma. These groups include patients with cast nephropathy, renal tubular dysfunction (acquired Fanconi syndrome), amyloidosis, and light-chain deposition disease (LCDD). A spectrum of renal syndromes, including proteinuria, progressive renal failure, acute renal failure (ARF), and various acid-base and electrolyte disorders, may be seen in patients with MM.[82]

Cast nephropathy or myeloma kidney is the most common histological diagnosis found in refractile tubular casts surrounded by multinucleated giant cells located in the distal and collecting tubules.[83] These large, dense, tubular casts could lead to the formation of precipitates in the tubules that might obstruct or rupture the tubular epithelium. Tubulo-interstitial damage may appear as flattened tubular cells, varying degrees of degeneration with necrosis, and denudation of the tubular basement membrane, leading to tubulo-epithelial cell atrophy and interstitial fibrosis.[82]

Light-chain deposition disease (LCDD) occurs in 5% to 10% of patients with myeloma. It is characterized by the deposition of light chains in the kidney and other vital organs (liver, heart, peripheral nerves).[82] The primary renal presentation involves elevated serum creatinine and nephrotic range proteinuria in 25% of the cases. Symptomatic management of these patients with correction of volume depletion and hypercalcemia, plus chemotherapy for control of the underlying malignancy, may improve renal function in as many as 50% of cases.[82] LCDD in the proximal tubules of the kidney can cause tubular dysfunction with an acquired Fanconi syndrome. Fanconi syndrome is a generalized disorder of proximal tubular transport dysfunction, leading to urinary excretion of amino acids, glucose, bicarbonate, uric acid, phosphate, potassium, and low-molecular-weight proteins.[84] The presence of hypophosphatemia, hypokalemia, hypouricemia, and a normal anion gap metabolic acidosis point to the possibility of Fanconi syndrome. Glycosuria in a patient with normal serum glucose may be also seen. LCDD has a poor prognosis. Apart from age, prognostic factors that have been identified include degree of renal insufficiency at presentation affecting the renal prognosis, underlying hematological disorder, and extrarenal LC deposition affecting the patient prognosis. Dialysis is worth performing in uremic LCDD patients.[85]

Primary (AL) amyloidosis can occur in as many as 10% of patients with myeloma. It results from tissue infiltration with immunoglobulin light chains. In contrast, secondary amyloidosis (AA protein) is commonly associated with chronic infectious, inflammatory, immune, genetic, and neoplastic disorders. AL amyloidosis is most commonly associated with IgD myeloma and light-chain disease.[86] Patients with AL amyloidosis present with renal impairment and proteinuria often in the nephrotic range (> 3.5 g/24 hours). Renal insufficiency was observed in approximately 50% of patients, while proteinuria was seen in 90% of cases at diagnosis of myeloma with coexisting amyloidosis.[82] Coexisting amyloidosis in patients with MM is a strong adverse prognostic factor, and treatment-related mortality with autologous stem cell transplant (ASCT) remains high.[87]

Acute renal failure (ARF) is a common feature of MM, and as many as half of patients with MM have potentially reversible and quick identifiable factors.[82] Dehydration, hypercalcemia, and infection are the most important precipitating factors, and are found in 50% to 95% of patients with myeloma-associated renal failure.[49] Dehydration leads to decreased renal perfusion, resulting in prerenal azotemia. In addition, enhanced reabsorption of fluids in response to fluid depletion results in an increased concentration of paraproteins in the distal tubules, promoting aggregation and cast formation. Hypercalcemia, by contrast, can cause dehydration due to osmotic diuresis induced by the high serum calcium level, hypercalcemia-induced emesis, and nephrogenic diabetes insipidus.[82] Hypercalcemia can also cause a decrease in the glomerular filtration rate (GFR) secondary to renal vasoconstriction and alteration in the glomerular permeability coefficient. Lastly, hypercalcemia may increase the toxicity of light chains by increasing the aggregability of BJP and Tamm–Horsfall protein (THP).[82] BJPs are immunoglobulin light chains synthesized by plasma cells independently of heavy chains that combine in the endoplasmic reticulum to form immunoglobulin molecules. When excess light chains are synthesized, they escape into circulation and appear in the urine as light-chain proteins or BJPs.[88] BJPs and THPs are components of casts in patients with cast nephropathy secondary to myeloma.[82] Infections such as bacteremia without hemodynamic compromise or full-blown sepsis can decrease renal perfusion, resulting in acute tubular necrosis (ATN).

Other reversible factors producing ARF include nephrotoxic antibiotics like aminoglycosides and amphotericin B, acyclovir, nonsteroidal anti-inflammatory drugs (NSAIDs), radiographic contrast, hyperuricemia, and tumor lysis syndrome. Aminoglycosides and amphotericin B can cause ATN, while acyclovir can cause acute interstitial nephritis, ATN, and obstruction secondary to tubular deposition of crystals.[82] Nonsteroidal anti-inflammatory drugs (NSAIDs) block the production of vasodilatory prostaglandins, cause a reduction in renal blood flow and GFR, and can lead to ARF. Several reports cite the risk of ARF due to NSAIDs intake in patients with MM, and the use of these drugs should be avoided in such individuals.[89,90] The contrast agents with high protein binding commonly used in the 1950s and 1960s were predisposed to precipitate and obstruct tubular fluid flow, leading to increased incidence of contrast-induced ARF.[82] Consequently, the use of contrast agents that could potentially damage the kidney should be minimized. Hyperuricemia results from rapid cell turnover, especially after chemotherapy, or tumor lysis syndrome after combination chemotherapy or HDC with hematopoietic stem cell transplantation (HSCT). Aggressive hydration, alkalinization of urine, and allopurinol are helpful in addressing this condition. Hemodialysis may be considered in patients with severe hyperuricemia who become oliguric.[82]

Relative to plasmapheresis, conflicting evidence as to its efficacy exists, and this technique remains controversial in an attempt to reverse renal failure in patients with MM. Patients with heavy chain disease (such as IgG, IgM, or IgA types of myeloma), and those with hyperviscosity syndromes, may benefit, yet additional randomized controlled trials (RCTs) are required to determine its efficacy, when to initiate therapy, and other supportive measures to consider.[88] Dialysis may be indicated if the patient's GFR is critically low, if they are experiencing difficulty managing serum electrolyte levels, or if uremia becomes an issue.

Careful evaluation for potentially reversible factors in patients with MM who present with or develop renal insufficiency is critical. Treatment should be directed toward preventing or correcting the factor that contributed to the renal insufficiency and reducing the concentration and/or risk for the precipitation of light-chain proteins in the renal tubules.

In the past, patients with MM who developed renal insufficiency were considered to have a worse prognosis. Today, due to advances in intensive supportive therapy, OS is not dramatically changed by the presence of renal failure but rather is determined by the response of the underlying disease to chemotherapy regardless of kidney function.[82]

## METABOLIC SYNDROMES

Hypercalcemia may be observed in 20% to 30% of patients with MM, but a high proportion of patients with hypercalcemia may be totally asymptomatic.[49] The severity of signs and symptoms will vary depending on the degree of hypercalcemia. Typical symptoms include polydipsia (increased thirst), nausea, constipation, irritability, confusion, and precoma. As described earlier, hypercalcemia can precipitate renal insufficiency through multiple mechanisms and must be reversed quickly to prevent serious, permanent kidney damage.

Hyperuricemia is frequently found in patients with MM and is related to a combination of factors, including high tumor cell turnover, tumor cell kill, and impairment of renal function.[91] Symptomatic hyperuricemia (gout) is rare, but prophylaxis is indicated, because a raised serum uric acid may contribute to renal impairment.[49] Usually, the really symptomatic patient is dehydrated and has a severely impaired renal function. Uric acid–induced nephropathy is caused by the precipitation and crystallization of uric acid in the distal tubules, where the urine pH is low and the concentration of uric acid is high. Aggressive hydration, alkalinization of urine, allopurinol, and hemodialysis may be instituted as indicated.

Other uncommon metabolic disturbances associated with MM that have been reported include hyperviscosity and hyperammonemia. The latter is manifested as central nervous system symptoms such as somnolence and precoma. Hyperviscosity syndrome is rare, occurring in 2% to 6% of patients with MM. It can occur in individuals with IgM myeloma (< 0.01% of all MM cases), and occasionally in those with IgA and IgG MM. This syndrome is caused by a high concentration of macroglobulins (eg, IgA and IgM immunoglobulins) that increase serum viscosity and result in vascular sludging. Symptoms usually appear when the relative serum or plasma viscosity exceeds 5 (normal range, 1.4–1.8 cp).[92] The most common sign of hyperviscosity is hemorrhagic diathesis resulting in gingival and mucosal bleeding, ecchymosis, and epistaxis.[49] Ophthalmic changes, such as visual disturbances, diplopia, and retinal abnormalities, are also common. Neurological signs include headache, dizziness, vertigo, drowsiness, coma, and seizures. Vascular sludging may also occur in the kidney, further compromising renal perfusion and increasing the risk of renal insufficiency. Other symptoms related to hyperviscosity may include malaise and cardiac insufficiency. Plasmapheresis is an effective—albeit temporary—measure for patients in whom rapid reduction in the concentration of circulating macroglobulins is deemed essential, such as those with ARF.[92] Conflicting evidence exists regarding its efficacy; thus, this technique remains controversial. Additional RCTs are required to determine its efficacy.[93] Effective tumor kill is necessary to eventually decrease the circulating macroglobulins produced by plasma cells, thereby decreasing serum viscosity.[82] When the patient's GFR is critically low or they are experiencing difficulty managing electrolyte levels, or when they become uremic, dialysis may be indicated.

### NEUROLOGICAL INVOLVEMENT

The most well-known and dramatic presenting symptom of MM is the sudden onset of paraplegia due to spinal cord compression.[94] Signs of spinal cord compression on examination were found in 12% of newly diagnosed patients with myeloma. Other studies reported incidence of presentation with neurological symptoms at a lower rate, less than 5%.[49] Additional neurological complications include cauda equina syndrome, radicular pain, peripheral neuropathy, and cranial nerve palsies usually due to local encroachment by tumor cells near the exit foraminae of the skull floor. A careful neurological history and examination are done at presentation and during follow-up, so that early signs of cord compression will be recognized and adequately treated.

Peripheral neuropathy associated with MM at diagnosis is rare with an incidence rate of less than 5% in patients with overt MM.[95] In most patients with MM, it is a late complication. The axonal, mixed sensorimotor symptoms are usually symmetrical, distal, mild, and progressive. Peripheral neuropathy may or may not be associated with amyloid deposits in the nerves.[52] Its exact mechanism is unknown, but it may be related to paraprotein, weight loss, or other metabolic or toxic factors associated with the malignancy.[95] In some cases, hyperviscosity syndrome has been identified as a causative factor; other studies have shown that neuropathy could be related to an autoimmune mechanism, with the IgM monoclonal antibody being directed at peripheral nerve antigens. There is no known effective treatment for peripheral neuropathy associated with MM. In particular, removing the paraprotein by plasmapheresis has no consistent effect on the neuropathy.[50]

Neuropathic symptoms developing during therapy may result from administration of drugs such as vincristine, cisplatin, thalidomide, and bortezomib.[96–98] Neuropathy arising from treatment is considered chemotherapy-induced peripheral neuropathy (CIPN). Pharmacological agents (eg, mild analgesics, opioids, tricyclic antidepressants, and anticonvulsants) and nonpharmacological agents (eg, capsaicin cream, exercise, relaxation techniques, transcutaneous electronic nerve stimulation, and occupational therapy) may be helpful in alleviating chemo-induced peripheral neuropathy.[96]

## ASSESSMENT

Patient and family history are obtained during the initial visit. Clinicians should look for any history of MGUS, as it is a well-known predisposing factor for MM. It is also important to obtain a work history, because certain occupational exposures predispose individuals to developing MM. Family history should be assessed for any occurrence of MM among the patient's relatives.

The most common physical finding related to MM is pallor. The liver and spleen are palpable in a minority of patients. Mental status changes such as disorientation, decreased level of consciousness, or coma can be related to hypercalcemia, hyperviscosity syndrome, or renal insufficiency.[49] Limitations in range of motion, inability to bear weight, loss of height, or abnormal curvature of the spine may be seen on initial presentation or later in the disease course and could be related to bone disease associated with MM. Routine chemistry laboratory values may be significant for elevations in blood urea nitrogen (BUN), creatinine, uric acid, and calcium. Serum and urine protein electrophoresis (SPEP) may reveal monoclonal spikes. Immunofixation, which is more sensitive than electrophoresis, can confirm specific, small residual monoclonal protein; this technology is particularly helpful in identifying the presence of abnormal immunoglobulin in the hyposecretory type of myeloma.[80]

Less than 5% of all MM patients will present with solitary plasmacytomas of bone (SPB) or EMP. Solitary plasmacytomas of bone are tumors that may present affixed to bone at diagnosis or throughout the course of the disease. Extramedullary (nonbony) plasmacytomas are rare but may be found late in the disease course. They may appear as large, purplish, subcutaneous masses, or an area of soft tissue swelling.[37] Definitive radiotherapy with curative intent may result in disease free survival of 30% with EMP and up to 60% with SPB. Solitary plasmacytomas without evidence of systemic myeloma elsewhere at diagnosis may carry a favorable prognosis.[99]

True nonsecretors comprise between 1% and 5% of all myeloma patients, and are often misdiagnosed or undiagnosed because of the absence of a monoclonal protein in the serum or urine. In some cases, severe complications from myeloma, such as pathological fracture, may have already occurred before the patient with nonsecretory myeloma is diagnosed. It is also important that a 24-urine specimen for urine protein electrophoresis and urine immunofixation be checked during the initial work-up to assess for urine M-spike and to identify the specific monoclonal light chain, respectively. Twenty percent of myeloma cases have urinary light-chain proteins only (kappa- or lambda-type MM), which may not be detectable by serum protein electrophoresis.[100]

In 2001, an automated immunoassay was found to be effective in detecting trace amounts of serum-free light chains (sFLC) in patients with nonsecretory myeloma. In 19 out of 28 patients who were studied, increased concentrations of either kappa or lambda sFLC were detected. In 6 of those patients, elevations in sFLC correlated with disease progression.[100] Two separate measurements are used, one to quantify the presence of elevated kappa- or lambda-free light chains, and a ratio between the two types may be also effective to determine clonality. Serum-free light chains can be identified in most patients with nonsecretory myeloma and may be helpful in identifying the presence of myeloma, or determining disease progression. Overall treatment and prognosis is thought to be the same for conventionally diagnosed secretory and nonsecretory myeloma.[101] The National Comprehensive Cancer Network (NCCN) recommends specific laboratory tests as part of a MM diagnostic work-up (Table 61-2).[50] Some tests may be needed in most patients, including plasma cell labeling index (PCLI), popularized by the Mayo Clinic, to identify the fraction of the myeloma cell that is proliferating; C-reactive protein, a surrogate marker for IL-6; lactic acid dehydrogenase (LDH), which can serve as a measure of tumor burden in lymphoma-like or plasmablastic myeloma; cytogenetic tests, to detect chromosomal abnormalities—particularly deletions—which may suggest a worse prognosis; and bone marrow flow cytometry, used to quantify the number of phenotypically abnormal plasma cells and help confirm the diagnosis. Useful in diagnosing and monitoring monoclonal gammopathies, the sFLC assay should be considered for all patients with plasmacytomas and nonsecretory MM. Additional tests under some circumstances include MRI for suspected spinal cord compression or SPB; computerized tomography (CT) scan or PET scan for the evaluation of extradural extraosseous plasmacytomas; serum viscosity if hyperviscosity is suspected; tissue biopsy through fine-needle aspiration to confirm the presence of plasmacytomas; evaluation of the erythropoietin level or hemoglobin to help determine the necessity of erythropoietin therapy; and bone marrow immunohistochemistry to confirm the clonality of the plasma cells.

**TABLE 61-2**

**Diagnostic Work-up for Multiple Myeloma**

| Tests | Purpose |
|---|---|
| Bone marrow aspirate/biopsy | Check percentage of plasma cells |
| Serum protein electrophoresis (SPEP) | Check for the presence of serum M-protein |
| Quantitative immunoglobulins | Identify specific elevated immunoglobulin level |
| Serum immunofixation electrophoresis (SIFE) | Identify specific monoclonal immunoglobulin |
| Serum chemistry | Check for evidence of hypercalcemia, renal dysfunction |
| Complete blood count | Check for evidence of anemia, thrombocytopenia |
| 24-Hour urine for urine protein electrophoresis (UPEP) | Check for urine M-protein (Bence-Jones protein) |
| Serum free light chain assay | Measures kappa or lambda light chain and $\kappa/\lambda$ ratio |
| Urine immunofixation electrophoresis (UIFE) | Identify specific monoclonal light-chain ($\kappa$ or $\lambda$) immunoglobulin |
| Skeletal survey | Check for osteolytic lesions |
| Plasma cell labeling index | Check for proliferative rate of plasma cells, prognostication purpose |
| Beta-2 microglobulin | Prognosis |
| Magnetic resonance imaging | Check for occult osteolytic lesions, spinal cord compression |

## PROGNOSTIC FACTORS

A number of negative prognostic factors (Table 61-3)[102] have been identified in the literature in patients who have been treated with conventional chemotherapy, defined as treatment that has been validated and routinely offered outside clinical trial. As these prognostic factors were identified during conventional therapy, the roles of prognostic factors need to be reassessed in the context of high-dose therapy[102] and new targeted therapies.

Several attempts have been made to combine prognostic factors with disease staging, and as a result, a new staging system for MM has emerged. Through a collaborative effort among 20 research institutions internationally, the international prognostic index (IPI) for MM[103] was introduced in 2002 to supersede the Durie-Salmon system introduced in 1975. Clinical and laboratory data were gathered on 10,750 previously untreated, symptomatic myeloma patients from 17 institutions internationally. Serum $\beta_2$-microglobulin and serum albumin values provided a validated and reproducible three-stage classification system, regardless of age, standard therapy, or previous autotransplantation.[103] The Durie-Salmon staging system remains widely utilized, but the new ISS is becoming more popular among community

**TABLE 61-3**

**Negative Prognostic Factors in Multiple Myeloma**

| |
|---|
| Older age |
| High labeling index |
| High lactic acid dehydrogenase (LDH) |
| High beta-2 microglobulin ($\beta_2$M) |
| High C-reactive protein (CRP) |
| Chromosomal aberration |
| Abnormal cytogenetics—t(4;14), t(14;16), deletion of chromosome 13 |
| Poor immune status |
| Poor performance status |
| Refractory to induction chemotherapy |
| Plasmacytosis (> 50%) in the bone marrow |
| High level (> 20%) of circulating plasma cells (plasma cell leukemia) |

physicians because of its ease of use and wide applications during clinical trials.

One reason for studying prognostic factors is to identify high-risk groups so that the patient treatment can be adapted to the expected outcome. Among the prognostic factors identified, the initial $\beta_2$M level appears to be more accurate, as its prognostic value has been shown in a number of clinical trials with conventional chemotherapy and confirmed in studies on autologous transplantation. Cytogenetics may emerge as an important prognostic factor for the future. Likewise, the combination of $\beta_2$M and cytogenetics might help to define therapeutic strategies. Patients with low $\beta_2$M and without unfavorable cytogenetics could benefit from intensive strategies with autologous transplantation, while new approaches are needed for patients with high $\beta_2$M and/or unfavorable cytogenetics.[7]

## DIAGNOSTIC CRITERIA

Several diagnostic systems are used to diagnose and classify patients with plasma cell dyscrasias, including the Durie-Salmon, Kyle and Greipp, and British Columbia Cancer Agency (BCCA) systems.[49] The BCCA criteria were thought by most clinicians to be the easiest to use since they require just one of the following for diagnosis: presence of a paraprotein in serum or urine, lytic bone lesions, or bone marrow plasma cell infiltrate in excess of 10% of the cells present.[49] The Durie and Salmon diagnostic criteria are widely used in the US because a number of parameters included in other diagnostic systems have not yet been validated by large multicenter trials and are not easily accessible in the majority of hematology–oncology clinics.[102]

The diagnosis of MM can be confirmed utilizing the Durie and Salmon diagnostic criteria, which are divided into two categories: "major" and "minor." In most cases, one major criterion plus one minor criterion are sufficient to diagnose myeloma (Table 61-4). In patients who satisfy the diagnostic criteria for MM, the Durie-Salmon clinical staging system is commonly applied to determine the stage of disease based on the presence or absence of bone lesions, anemia, hypercalcemia, and paraproteinemia levels.

More recently, confirmation of a myeloma diagnosis in patients with active or symptomatic disease can be made if three criteria are met. These criteria include monoclonal plasma cells in the bone marrow > 10% and/or presence of a biopsy-proven plasmacytoma, monoclonal protein present in the serum and/or urine, and myeloma-related organ dysfunction (1 or more myeloma-related organ dysfunction). The 4 major types of myeloma-related organ dysfunction may be acknowledged by the "CRAB" acronym. Patients will meet the "CRAB" criteria for active myeloma, as evidenced by increased blood calcium levels (> 10.5 mg/L or upper limit of normal), renal insufficiency (serum creatinine > 2 mg/dL), anemia (Hgb < 10 g/dL or 2 g < normal) or bone lesions, including compression fractures, lytic lesions, or widespread osteoporosis.[104]

## CLASSIFICATION AND STAGING

The Durie-Salmon clinical staging system for MM has been the most widely used system in the US. This simple and reproducible system is based on easily accessible data. However, its usefulness in MM prognostication has been demonstrated only in the context of conventional chemotherapy, and has not been confirmed in the context of autologous transplantation.[102] This staging system incorporates both the Durie-Salmon system proposed in 1975 and the labeling index proposed by Durie and associates in the 1980s.[105,106] It integrates both clinical and laboratory findings associated with MM.

In 1980, Durie and associates identified a process to quantitate the total-body myeloma cell mass.[106] This number is calculated by dividing the total-body M component synthetic rate per myeloma cell. In examining a large series of individuals with MM, the authors identified three stages of the disease. Stage I disease, or low cell mass, consists of $<0.6 \times 10^{12}$ cells/m$^2$. Stage II disease, or intermediate cell mass, reflects $>0.6$ to $1.2 \times 10^{12}$ cells/m$^2$. Stage III disease, or high cell mass, consists of $>1.2 \times 10^{12}$ cells/m$^2$.

Further staging is done based on renal status at the time of diagnosis. Group A includes individuals with a normal renal function (creatinine level <2.0 mg/dL), and group B includes individuals with evidence of renal dysfunction (creatinine level >2.0 mg/dL).

**TABLE 61-4**

**Diagnostic Criteria: Durie and Salmon**

**Myeloma**

| Major Criteria | Minor Criteria |
|---|---|
| 1. Plasmacytoma on-tissue biopsy | a. Bone marrow plasmacytosis with 10%–30% plasma cells |
| 2. Bone marrow plasmacytosis with 30% plasma cells | b. Monoclonal globulin spike present, but lower levels than defined in the major criteria |
| 3. Monoclonal globulin spike (M-protein) on SPEP: IgG > 3.5 g/dL, IgA > 2.0 g/dL, light-chain excretion on UPEP ≥ 1 g/24 hours in the absence of amyloidosis | c. Lytic bone lesions |
| | d. Normal IgM > 50 mg/dL, IgA > 100 mg/dL, or IgG > 600 mg/dL |

The diagnosis of myeloma requires a minimum of one major criterion and one minor criterion (although 1 + a is not sufficient) or three minor criteria that must include a + b

**Indolent Myeloma**

Criteria for myeloma with the following limitations:

a. Absent or only limited bone lesions (≤ 3 lytic lesions), no compression fractures
b. Stable paraprotein levels: IgG level < 700 mg/dL, IgA <500 mg/dL
c. No symptoms or associated disease features: Karnofsky performance status > 70%, hemoglobin >10 g/dL, normal serum calcium, normal serum creatinine, no infections
d. Plasma cell labeling index ≤ 0.5%

*Source*: Data from Lokhorst.[49]

Other attempts have been made to simplify the staging system for MM. The simple staging system developed by Southwest Oncology Group (SWOG) is based on two common measures with prognostic significance in MM: serum $\beta_2$M and serum albumin. The proponents of the SWOG staging system believe that this scheme could provide an alternative to Durie-Salmon staging for patients with previously untreated MM based on easily obtained laboratory measures.[107] These two simple parameters have been successfully adapted in the ISS staging system (see Table 61-5).

**TABLE 61-5**

**International Staging System for Multiple Myeloma**

| Stage | Criteria | Median Survival |
|---|---|---|
| Stage I | Serum β2-microglobulin < 3.5 mg/L<br>Serum albumin ≥ 3.5 g/dL | 62 months |
| Stage II | Not stage I or stage III<br>2 possibilities:<br>Serum β2-microglobulin < 3.5 mg/L but serum albumin < 3.5 g/dL<br>Serum β2-microglobulin 3.5 to < 5.5 mg/L irrespective of serum albumin level | 44 months |
| Stage III | Serum β2-microglobulin ≥ 5.5 mg/L | 29 months |

*Source*: Reprinted with permission from from Greipp et al.[103] 

## THERAPEUTIC APPROACHES AND NURSING CARE

### PRIMARY CONVENTIONAL TREATMENT (PATIENTS INELIGIBLE FOR TRANSPLANT)

Conventional chemotherapy is defined by the NCCN guidelines as therapy where the safety and efficacy have been validated and, as a result, the therapy is routinely offered outside the context of a clinical trial. It is classified into three categories: primary, salvage, and maintenance. Primary conventional therapies utilized in MM are outlined in Table 61-6.[50]

Not all patients who fulfill the minimal criteria for diagnosis of MM should be treated.[38] Individuals with indolent, asymptomatic, or smoldering MM should be observed initially for months and may do well without treatment over many years.[50] No evidence indicates that early treatment of patients with asymptomatic MM offers an OS advantage.[50] A review of RCTs with a parallel design that compared

**TABLE 61-6**

**Treatment Options for Patients With Multiple Myeloma**

| **Primary Induction Therapy for Transplant Candidates** |
| --- |
| Vincristine/doxorubicin/dexamethasone (VAD) |
| Dexamethasone |
| Thalidomide/dexamethasone (TD) |
| Liposomal doxorubicin/vincristine/dexamethasone (DVD) |
| Lenalidomide/dexamethasone (LD) |
| Bortezomib/dexamethasone |
| Bortezomib/doxorubicin/dexamethasone |
| Bortezomib/thalidomide/dexamethasone |
| **Primary Induction Therapy for Nontransplant Candidates** |
| Melphalan/prednisone (MP) |
| Melphalan/prednisone/thalidomide (MPT) |
| Melphalan/prednisone/bortezomib (MPB) |
| Vincristine/doxorubicin/dexamethasone (VAD) |
| Dexamethasone |
| Thalidomide/dexamethasone (TD) |
| Liposomal doxorubicin/vincristine/dexamethasone (DVD) |
| **Maintenance Therapy** |
| Steroids (50 mg prednisone every other day) |
| Thalidomide |
| Interferon |
| **Salvage Therapy** |
| Repeat primary induction therapy (if relapse at >6 months) |
| Bortezomib ± dexamethasone |
| Bortezomib/liposomal doxorubicin |
| Lenalidomide ± dexamethasone |
| Cyclophosphamide ± VAD |
| High-dose cyclophosphamide |
| Thalidomide ± dexamethasone (consider prophylactic anticoagulation) |
| DT-PACE (consider prophylactic anticoagulation) |
| Dexamethasone |

*Source*: Data from the NCCN Clinical Practice Guidelines v2.2008.[50]

early vs deferred treatment of patients with early-stage MM, based on the Durie-Salmon staging system, concluded that early treatment of early-stage MM inhibits disease progression and may reduce vertebral compression, but no significant effects on response rates or OS were seen.[108]

When disease progression is evident, as demonstrated by a sustained 25% or greater increase in M-protein in serum or urine, or by development of new sites of lytic disease or hypercalcemia, treatment should be started immediately.[50] Exposure to myelotoxic agents (alkylating agents—ie, mustards such as melphalan and cyclophosphamide, and nitrosureas such as carmustine or lomustine) and pelvic irradiation should be limited to avoid compromising the stem cell reserve prior to stem cell harvest in patients who may be candidates for transplant.[50,109] Systemic therapy is the preferred initial approach to symptomatic MM. The use of radiation therapy (RT) in this disease should be limited to discrete lesions, because it does not benefit the patient with systemic disease and could further deplete the bone marrow reserve.

If the individual is 70 years of age or younger, or in excellent physiological health status, the clinician should discuss the possibility of autologous stem cell transplantation.[37] Ideally, the hematopoietic stem cells should be collected before the patient is exposed to alkylating agents. High-dose chemotherapy followed by ASCT has been recommended by the NCCN myeloma panel as a primary treatment in patients with symptomatic MM, with the consensus being based on high level evidence.[50]

In patients with symptomatic MM who are older than 70 years of age or in younger patients in whom transplant is not feasible, intermittent systemic oral melphalan and prednisone (MP) combination therapy has been the first-line choice for the past three decades.[37,110,111] Numerous regimens have been tested in an attempt to improve mean survival from the time of diagnosis, but none has proved superior to systemic oral MP until the advent of several novel therapeutic agents, which will be described later.[112] After three decades of anticipated benefits of combination chemotherapy, not a single combination regimen appears to be better than MP.[109] In 1998, the Myeloma Trialists' Collaborative Group conducted an overview of MM clinical trials, which included data on 6623 patients entered in 27 trials worldwide. The group declared MP and combination therapy to be of comparable effectiveness, although the response to combination therapy may occur more rapidly.[113] This group's findings supported an earlier meta-analysis of 18 clinical trials, which suggested that there was no survival difference between the 2 approaches, either overall or within any patient subgroup.[109,114]

## Melphalan and prednisone

Prior to the advent of HDC with or without stem cell rescue, the MP oral regimen was the most frequent treatment for newly diagnosed MM.[115] Its response rate ranges from 50% to 60%, and the mean survival rate with this regimen is 24 to 36 months.[116] The survival rates at 5 and 10 years are 25% and 8%, respectively. Standard MP chemotherapy consists of melphalan 8 mg/day for 7 days and prednisone

20 mg 3 times daily for the same 7 days every 6 weeks.[38] It can also be given as melphalan 8 mg/m$^2$ daily for 4 consecutive days, and prednisone 60 mg/m$^2$ daily by mouth, also for 4 consecutive days.

Oral melphalan must be taken on an empty stomach, at least 2 hours before meals, or 3 hours after eating, because food reduces its absorption by at least 50%; in contrast, prednisone needs to be taken with meals. Patients may take an $H_2$ histamine receptor antagonist to prevent the gastric distress associated with steroids. White blood cells and platelets are checked every 3 weeks after beginning each cycle of therapy. The dosage of melphalan must be adjusted until modest mid-cycle cytopenia occurs.[37] If the serum creatinine level is more than 2 mg/dL, the dose of melphalan should be reduced by 25% to prevent severe myelosuppression. If cytopenias do not occur, the dose of melphalan should be increased in a stepwise escalation by 2 to 3 mg/m$^2$.[37,109]

Unless the disease progresses rapidly, at least three courses of MP should be given before therapy is discontinued because delayed responses are common. An objective response may not be seen for 6 to 12 months or even longer in some patients. If the pain is alleviated and no evidence of progressive disease is present (no increase in serum or urine M-protein, no new bone lesions, no hypercalcemia), the regimen should be continued.

The relative importance of the two active agents in the MP regimen has been debated because of conflicting results when using either the MP combination or intermittent melphalan alone. Analysis has clearly shown the usefulness of steroids by correlating survival with prednisone dose intensity and not with the total melphalan dose.[117] In general, corticosteroids as part of primary treatment of MM demonstrate high activity in plasma cells, with concomitant sparing of normal hematopoietic elements. Corticosteroids may increase the speed of response without added myelosuppression while improving the well-being of patients.[109] Older individuals who are at risk for infectious or gastrointestinal complications must be monitored closely.

### Bortezomib, melphalan, and prednisone

Bortezomib, formerly known as PS-341, is a novel, first-in-class agent that inhibits the 26S proteasome (simply called "the proteasome").[118] The mechanism of action of this proteasome inhibitor in MM has been described, and its potential effects in myeloma and other types of cancer are outlined in Table 61-7.[119] A trial comparing bortezomib, melphalan, and prednisone to melphalan and prednisone alone, called the VISTA trial, included 682 elderly patients over the age of 65 years (median age 71 years), with newly diagnosed myeloma and ineligible for a stem cell transplant. The combination of bortezomib, melphalan, and prednisone (VMP) demonstrated superiority to MP for time-to-event end points, including time to progression (TTP) (median 24.0 months vs 16.6 months), OS, and time to subsequent therapy. In addition to response, the side effects were well tolerated. These results led to the Food and Drug Administration (FDA) approval of VMP for patients not candidates for stem cell transplantation.[120]

**TABLE 61-7**

| Potential Effects of Bortezomib in Cancer |
|---|
| Induce cancer cell apoptosis |
| Limit tumor survival, growth, spread, and angiogenesis |
| Affect cellular signals involved in resistance to standard chemotherapies |
| Affect ability of myeloma cells to interact with bone marrow microenvironment |

Patients on bortezomib therapy should be closely monitored for any adverse effects. Failure to assess for them and lack of appropriate early interventions may jeopardize the patient's health. Peripheral neuropathy needs close monitoring, and appropriate dose reduction based on patient's degree of neuropathy is recommended. Monitoring of complete blood counts before each dose and weekly chemistries are done to check for any electrolyte imbalance and creatinine abnormality.[98] Transfusion support and use of growth factors may be clinically indicated. Grade 4 hematological toxicities will require dose reduction, and the dose is usually withheld until it returns to the grade 2 level (based on National Cancer Institute toxicity criteria) with or without transfusion and/or use of growth factors. Antidiarrheals and antiemetics may be used as clinically indicated. Oncology nurses play a vital role in the assessment and monitoring of these adverse effects and in initiating immediate interventions before serious health problems or irreversible damage occur.[121]

### Vincristine, doxorubicin, and dexamethasone (VAD) therapy

Infusional VAD came into use in the early 1980s, when it was developed at the M.D. Anderson Cancer Center in Houston, Texas. The reported response rate in these classic studies in chemotherapy-naïve patients with MM is approximately 60% to 80% with a 10% to 15% complete remission (CR) response rate.[122,123] When VAD was compared with standard alkylating agent-based therapies, researchers found no obvious survival benefit in the VAD arm.[124] Clinically, the VAD regimen followed by bortezomib may be preferable for patients in whom rapid tumor control is desired, such as those with hypercalcemia, renal failure, or widespread painful bone lesions. It is especially indicated in patients with plasma cell leukemia (myeloma associated with > 20% circulating plasma cells), because standard alkylating agents are ineffective in such cases.[125] VAD and bortezomib is also useful in patients with renal failure because none of its components are excreted through the renal system and dose adjustments are not necessary. No more than 3 courses of VAD are usually needed to confirm partial response (50% reduction of M-protein) or resistance to this regimen.[123] Monitoring the total dose of doxorubicin and treating patients to a maximum tolerated dose of 450 mg/m$^2$ are typical.

The major drawbacks of this regimen are the side effects associated with high-dose steroids, particularly among elderly patients, who may have more steroid-related toxicity,[126] and the need for central intravenous (IV) access monitoring for signs and symptoms of steroid toxicity (eg, severe dyspepsia, fluid and sodium retention, corticosteroid myopathy, acute pancreatitis, insulin-dependent hyperglycemia, and steroid psychosis) is important. Patient and family education will include signs and symptoms of steroid-induced gastritis; if these persist or worsen (including nausea and vomiting with or without hematemesis), the clinician is usually contacted to prevent serious complications such as gastric ulceration and bleeding.

Elderly patients require close monitoring, particularly those with concurrent diseases such as congestive heart failure, because steroid-associated sodium and water retention can exacerbate symptoms.[126] Monitoring the patient for weight gain and peripheral edema on a daily basis will help in detecting pulmonary crackles and compromise. Instructing the patient to report to the clinician any weight gain greater than 5 pounds in 1 day is also important. Individuals with preexisting diabetes require close monitoring for signs and symptoms of steroid-induced hyperglycemia. Teaching patients how to monitor blood sugar and when to report side effects to the clinician are important aspects of treatment. Home care visits by a registered nurse may be initiated to monitor blood pressure, blood sugar level, and other steroid-related side effects, as clinically indicated. Dose reductions or change of treatment regimen may be required in patients who develop steroid-related psychosis, when side effects become more pronounced, and when the risks outweigh the benefits of treatment.

VAD produces much less myelosuppression than do other alkylating agent combinations, and it may be conveniently used in cases presenting with neutropenia or thrombocytopenia secondary to bone marrow infiltration.[109] In some patients, prolonged thrombocytopenia and granulocytopenia may be observed and require a reduction in the dose of doxorubicin. If the doxorubicin cannot be administered due to prolonged bone marrow suppression, the entire cycle may be delayed for 1 week and therapy resumed once the platelet count exceeds 50,000/mm$^3$ and the absolute neutrophil count (ANC) exceeds 750/mm$^3$. Hepatic toxicity characterized by a bilirubin level greater than 2.0 mg/dL requires reduction or discontinuation of both doxorubicin and vincristine, depending on the severity. If the bilirubin level is greater than 5.0 mg/dL, both doxorubicin and vincristine should be discontinued.

Newer regimens have attempted to address steroid doses and cumulative toxicity in recent years, and the use of pegylated liposomal doxorubicin (PLD), which is a nonvesicant, avoids the inherent risks (extravasation of a vesicant) that result from the use of central venous catheters, and the treatment regimen appears to be effective and well tolerated as first-line treatment. PLD has replaced adriamycin in the VAD regimen, which is given on day 1 of a 28-day cycle as a 90-minute infusion and a reduced dose of dexamethasone (40 mg po) is given on days 1 to 4 of a monthly cycle. The reduced intensity and dose of steroids attempt to address concerns of high-dose steroid-related side effects, which may negatively affect quality of life, yet not compromise overall response. Patients receiving the PLD regimen have experienced less steroid toxicity and achieved similar response rates as compared to the VAD regimen.[127]

### High-dose pulsed dexamethasone

High-dose pulsed dexamethasone (D) is another primary treatment regimen in patients with MM, offering response and survival rates that are similar to those achieved with other standard regimens, such as VAD.[128] Steroids, in general, are effective in treating myeloma because they induce apoptosis and promote myeloma cell death by inhibiting activity of IL-6, a growth factor for myeloma.[129] Dexamethasone alone could be an alternative regimen for VAD, and it provides the convenience of oral administration. It is usually dosed at 40 mg on days 1 to 4, 9 to 12, and 17 to 20 with a 1-week break (28-day cycle) or 2-week break (35-day cycle). Because dexamethasone is not associated with myelosuppression, this agent is indicated when radiotherapy is needed for the treatment of painful bone lesions, and it may be the primary treatment of choice in the occasional patient who presents with pancytopenia.[109]

Although effective at inducing remissions in patients with newly diagnosed and relapsed MM, the duration of response when using steroids alone is not sustained. In addition, multiple body systems can be adversely affected by the use of steroids, which can negatively impact the physical, social, and psychological functioning of patients. Decreased quality of life and reduced adherence to the treatment plan may result from these negative effects. Education regarding the side effects of steroids, and prompt reporting to the nurse or caregiver may warrant intervention and improve outcomes.[130]

Prophylactic antacids or proton pump inhibitors and anti-infectives are usually given to prevent the gastrointestinal side effects common with steroids. Steroid-induced myopathy may result in lower extremity weakness in high doses, and with long-term use. Hyperglycemia is also a common side effect in patients with impaired fasting glucose or preexisting diabetes; therefore, blood glucose levels should be closely monitored. Insomnia and hyperactivity may result from steroid use, as well as personality changes. Given these common side effects, recent studies have suggested that the toxicities associated with high-dose steroids may outweigh the benefits to myeloma cell death, and high-dose steroids should be avoided in combination with certain novel agents in the front-line setting such as lenalidomide[131] and in elderly patients, if possible.[132]

### Interferon plus conventional chemotherapy

Interferon was introduced into the treatment of patients with MM more than 2 decades ago,[133] but its role is still not clearly defined. It has been added to standard chemotherapy in previously untreated patients with myeloma because it has antitumor activity and because it may have a different mechanism of action from conventional chemotherapeutic regimens.[134] The specific mechanisms of action employed by IFNs (alpha, beta, and gamma) have not been clearly elucidated, but they may have direct antitumor effects through induction of apoptosis and indirect effects mediated through the host, inhibition of angiogenesis, or immunomodulation.[135] A meta-analysis of trials of IFN therapy in patients with MM revealed a 6% higher response rate and a 6-month prolongation of the recurrence-free interval for the IFN-α containing induction regimens.[136] This report lacked compelling data to support the addition of IFN-α to standard alkylating agent regimens; however, the minor benefits, if any, should be weighed against possible bone marrow or systemic toxicities and the cost.[109]

The toxicities associated with IFN-α require thorough assessment and consistent interventions to manage side effects. They may include flu-like syndrome, anorexia, progressive fatigue, depression, hepatotoxicity, thrombocytopenia, granulocytopenia, neurological, and renal/metabolic toxicity.[135] A patient on IFN-α needs close monitoring by the clinician for evidence of IFN toxicity so that appropriate dose reduction can be initiated in a timely manner. The dose reduction schedule and plan to discontinue IFN-α depend on the patient's response to the severity of the toxicity. Nurses play a key role in assessing and grading treatment-related toxicities and in assisting patients and their families in managing side effects.

Many attempts have been made to define the role of IFNs in the treatment of MM so that they may be utilized to maximum effect. Controversy continues regarding the in vitro studies showing that, under various conditions, IFN-α can either stimulate or inhibit the growth and proliferation of myeloma cells. Overall, the IFNs' use appears beneficial, and IFN-α currently plays a role as part of standard myeloma treatment, mostly as maintenance therapy and not with standard alkylating agent regimens.[135] The role of IFNs in improving OS in patients with MM remains equivocal.

## PRIMARY TREATMENT (PATIENTS ELIGIBLE FOR TRANSPLANT)

### Thalidomide and dexamethasone

During the past decade, there has been an increased knowledge of the complexity of the bone marrow microenvironment. How MM cells evolve has provided us with several therapeutic options in terms of combining older, standard-of-care therapies with newer therapies. These may include newer drug combinations such as thalidomide and dexamethasone, lenalidomide and dexamethasone, and bortezomib and dexamethasone, but the first to be discussed here will be thalidomide and dexamethasone (TD).

Thalidomide re-entered the oncology clinical setting in 1998. Since then, it has demonstrated significant activity against relapsed and refractory MM and currently, in the newly diagnosed setting.[137] Several studies confirmed the finding that thalidomide has antitumor properties against relapsed and refractory multiple MM, with response rates averaging 30% to 35% (minimal response of less than 50% reduction of M-protein was not included).[138–140] The median duration of response is approximately 8 to 9 months. Individual responses were maintained from as little as 2 months up to more than 30 months.[141]

The exact mechanism of the antineoplastic action of thalidomide is unclear. Researchers believe that angiogenesis inhibition, immunomodulation, and cytokine modulation, individually or in combination, likely underlie the drug's antitumor activity. The mechanisms of action of thalidomide are outlined in Table 61–8.[142]

The most common reported side effects of thalidomide are constipation, somnolence, and fatigue. Fairly common to least common side effects include peripheral neuropathy, skin rash, and deep-vein thrombosis.[97] In addition, thalidomide is highly teratogenic. Clinicians and patients must strictly adhere to the STEPS (System for Thalidomide Education and Prescribing Safety) program.[143] Therapeutic anticoagulation may be also essential during thalidomide therapy in newly diagnosed patients,[144,145] and when the drug

**TABLE 61-8**

| Mechanisms of Action of Thalidomide |
|---|
| Inhibition of angiogenesis |
| Inhibition of TNF-α |
| Inhibition of cyclooxygenase-2 (COX-2) |
| Downregulation of IL-6 |
| Inhibition of TNF-α-induced interleukin-8 (IL-8) |
| Increased IL-10 |
| Enhancement of Interleukins (IL-4, IL-5, and IL-12) |
| Stimulatory effect on T-cell activity |

is combined with cytotoxic chemotherapy such as doxorubicin, cyclophosphamide/dexamethasone/etoposide/cisplatin (CDEP), and dexamethasone, thalidomide, cisplatin, doxorubicin, cyclophosphamide, and etoposide (DT-PACE), given that deep vein thrombosis incidence was reported to be higher.[146]

The optimal dose and duration of treatment with thalidomide for patients with relapsed or refractory MM remain unknown, but most clinicians use a maximum 200 mg daily dose to prevent severe peripheral neuropathy. Various titrations and dosing have been employed. Furthermore, a reasonable approach for use of thalidomide in MM is to initiate therapy at 50 to 100 mg nightly and escalate the dose every 2 weeks in 50 to 100 mg increments as tolerated.

Several trials have demonstrated the clinical benefit of thalidomide in newly diagnosed patients with MM. Thalidomide has emerged as a very effective oral agent in the treatment of myeloma either alone, in maintenance after stem cell transplantation, or in combination with other therapies. In a phase III trial among newly diagnosed MM patients, each were randomized to thalidomide plus dexamethasone (Arm A) and 235 patients to placebo plus dexamethasone (Arm B). Patients randomized to therapy in Arm A received 50 mg of oral thalidomide daily, which was escalated to 100 mg on day 15, and to 200 mg from day 1 of cycle 2. Oral dexamethasone 40 mg was given on days 1 to 4, 9 to 12, and 17 to 20 of a 28-day treatment cycle. Patients in Arm B received placebo instead of thalidomide, and dexamethasone as in Arm A. The combination of thalidomide and dexamethasone resulted in better overall response rates than dexamethasone alone, and a longer median TTP.[147] Venous thromboembolism (VTE) complications were higher with the combination of thalidomide and dexamethasone than dexamethasone alone, but overall, the treatment was very well tolerated. On the basis of these results, the trial was halted early, patients were unblinded and given the option of transitioning to thalidomide (if they were only receiving dexamethasone). FDA approval of TD was granted for first-line treatment of patients with MM in 2006.

Although TD provides an effective regimen in patients with newly diagnosed MM, the combination of TD may not be optimal for patients over the age of 70. A recent study compared MP to TD. Patients receiving TD noted more neuropathy, deep-vein thrombosis, and psychological toxicity and a higher rate of early treatment discontinuation, despite a better initial response to therapy with improvement in the myeloma parameters. In addition, those patients receiving TD had a shorter OS than those receiving MP, although more hematological toxicity was seen in patients who had received MP. This suggests that high doses of dexamethasone alone or in combination with other therapies may not be well tolerated in the older adult population as also mentioned previously.[148]

## Autologous stem cell transplantation

The efficacy of HDC and ASCT is well established in MM and both are considered effective first-line treatments for patients with MM.[149] HDC has been used for more than 10 years for the treatment of MM, either alone or with ASCT. HDC with ASCT treatment has improved remission rates, event-free survival, and OS in patients with MM compared to conventional chemotherapy,[150] but there is currently an ongoing debate as to whether or not to utilize this approach upfront or further on in therapy. This procedure is suitable for patients younger than 70 years without significant comorbid conditions and for selected older patients. Alkylating agents, such as regimens containing melphalan, should not be administered to newly diagnosed patients with MM to avoid damage to stem cells. Patients who have received standard treatment for less than 1 year and/or a total melphalan dose of less than 200 mg/m$^2$ retain a good chance of mobilizing sufficient numbers of stem cells to provide for ASCT.[149] A large French study reported that although OS was not influenced by the time of ASCT, the early-transplant group had superior event-free survival, which suggests that transplantation should be considered as the initial therapy.[151] However, since this study was performed, newer therapeutic agents have emerged, and some suggest to be at least as effective an option as transplant. Therefore, the timing of ASCT continues to be debated, as to whether it should be incorporated into the initial plan at diagnosis, or if it should be delayed until relapse. Ongoing studies are being performed to address these questions.

One trial comparing single ASCT to tandem transplant, consisting of 231 previously treated patients with MM, may suggest that a percentage of patients benefit from two transplants. In this study, patients were randomized to ASCT or double ASCT. The 10-year event-free survival in this total therapy trial was 15% and OS 33%, suggesting the superiority of transplant in a subgroup of patients with myeloma. Further analysis of these patients had shown that those who failed to achieve a 90% reduction in the serum M-protein benefited from the second transplant, but those that did not achieve this reduction showed no benefit from the second transplant. Many additional studies are evaluating the role of transplant and especially with the novel therapeutic agents, the timing of the transplant is under debate.[152]

Given the excellent response to ASCT in younger patients, who are considered eligible, several studies have attempted to determine whether older adults with myeloma should undergo HDC or a standard approach. Advanced age has been a poor prognostic factor in several, conventional chemotherapy trials in patients with myeloma, with a median survival of less than 3 years, even after adjusting for major variables such as comorbidities and general health status. Some groups believe that some older adults may have a poor response to general treatment, partly because of less intensive doses of chemotherapy. One study evaluated 159 patients with myeloma, older than 70 years, from 1992 to 1999. Lower transplant-related doses of IV melphalan were better tolerated than in the higher-dose group, and transplant-related mortality was less in the lower-dose group.[153] Reduced-dose melphalan also was found to be better than the previous standard of care, oral melphalan, in the Italian Study Group.[154]

In a study comparing melphalan, prednisone, and thalidomide (MPT) vs MP and autologous stem cell transplantation in myeloma, patients were randomized to MP, MPT, or melphalan 100 mg/m$^2$ IV as part of transplantation. Patients randomized to the MPT regimen had fewer adverse events and improved OS vs the transplantation group and showed improved progression-free survival, suggesting that MPT is superior to autologous transplantation for older adults with myeloma, and transplant may not be beneficial.[154]

*Induction chemotherapy.* Today, there are several options as to what the optimal preparative regimen for myeloma should consist of to induce a remission. Chemotherapy is an option, and historically has consisted of VAD as the primary preparative regimen. Described in 1986, this has been the gold standard for induction regimens and remains a favorite among many because it produces a rapid response and causes less damage to bone marrow progenitor cells than other available regimens. Patients receiving the PLD regimen have experienced less steroid toxicity and achieved similar response rates as compared to the VAD regimen.[127] Vincristine, doxorubicin, melphalan, and prednisone (VAMP) or VAMP plus weekly cyclophosphamide (C-VAMP)[155] may be an alternative that provides an enhanced response without affecting cumulative toxicity or compromising subsequent stem cell collection. A vincristine, melphalan, cyclophosphamide, and prednisone (VMCP)/vincristine, carmustine, doxorubicin, and prednisone (VBAP) with IFN-α regimen has also been utilized as induction therapy to produce remission prior to stem cell collection and transplantation.[156] (See Table 61-9.)[157] Dexamethasone, thalidomide, cisplatin, doxorubicin, cyclophosphamide, and etoposide may be also utilized as an induction therapy before ASCT, especially in patients with high-risk characteristics such as those with high LDH or chromosome 13 abnormality, and in those patients who are refractory to standard therapy. C-VAMP, VMCP, and DT-PACE are currently being replaced by less cumbersome regimens such as thalidomide and dexamethasone, bortezomib and dexamethasone, or bortezomib, thalidomide, and dexamethasone.[50]

The combination of thalidomide and dexamethasone has provided an alternative to infusional VAD as induction therapy in autotransplantation and is now, in many centers, being considered the standard of care. One study reported promising results using thalidomide and dexamethasone as induction therapy in transplant-candidate patients who were newly diagnosed with MM.[144] A lower incidence of major complications and an absence of stem cell collection problems among this group of patients were also reported. A similar study reported thalidomide and dexamethasone to be a possible alternative induction regimen.[145] Both of these studies demonstrated that the use of thalidomide in combination with dexamethasone in newly diagnosed patients with symptomatic myeloma can induce a high frequency of response, rapid onset of remission, low incidence of serious irreversible toxicities, and no substantial effect on stem cell collection. An earlier study on the use of thalidomide plus dexamethasone with doxorubicin in patients with

**TABLE 61-9**

**Treatment Schema of European Bone Marrow Transplant Trial in Multiple Myeloma**

| **Conventional Treatment—VMCP/BVAP[a]** | |
|---|---|
| **VMCP** | |
| Vincristine | 1 mg IV; day 1 |
| Melphalan | 5 mg/m$^2$ PO; days 1–4 |
| Cyclophosphamide | 110 mg/m$^2$ PO; days 1–4 |
| Prednisone | 60 mg/m$^2$ PO; days 1–4 |
| **BVAP** | |
| Vincristine | 1 mg IV; day 1 |
| Carmustine | 30 mg/m$^2$ IV; day 1 |
| Doxorubicin | 30 mg/m$^2$ IV; day 1 |
| Prednisone | 60 mg/m$^2$ PO; days 1–4 |
| Recombinant alfa-interferon (3 million U/m$^2$ SQ 3 times/week from cycle 9 until relapse) | |
| **High-Dose as Above** | |
| Autologous bone marrow was collected after cycle 4 (200 million nucleated cells/kg body weight) | |
| All patients received between 4 and 6 cycles VMCP/BVAP; if their WHO (World Health Organization) performance status was < 3 and a transplant facility was available, the individual was transplanted | |
| Preparative regimen: Melphalan 140 mg/m$^2$ Total-body irradiation (8 Gy 4 fractions over 4 days with no lung shields | |
| Unpurged autologous bone marrow was readministered | |
| Alfa-interferon was administered from cycle 9 until relapse; after bone marrow transplantation hematologic recovery occurred (granulocyte count > 1500/mm$^3$; platelet count > 75,000/mm$^3$) | |

[a]Alternating cycles (every 3 weeks for 12 months; total 18 cycles).
*Source*: Data from Attal et al.[156]

untreated, symptomatic myeloma reported similar findings.[158] Thromboembolic events were reported but patients receiving therapeutic doses of warfarin or low-molecular-weight heparin did not experience thrombotic episodes.[145]

In order to determine the best induction regimen prior to stem transplantation, a RCT with at least 6 treatment groups (VAD, Dexamethasone, Thal/Dex, Bortezomib and Dexamethasone, Bortezomib/Thal/Dex, etc.) would be required and patients from all treatment groups must undergo ASCT. Whether this type of RCT is feasible, given the current healthcare system in the US, remains questionable and the answer to this question of best induction regimen may remain elusive.

*Collection of peripheral blood stem cells.* In general, collection and cryopreservation of blood stem cells should be initiated as soon as the best possible response is confirmed (reduction of M-protein from baseline).[109] The use of another chemotherapeutic agent prior to stem cell collection and cryopreservation is a common practice (chemo-mobilization) to further reduce tumor burden. Use of growth factor alone (ie, granulocyte colony-stimulating factor [GCSF] or granulocyte-macrophage colony-stimulating factor [GM-CSF]) without chemotherapy prior to stem collection to mobilize stem cells (G-mobilization) may be used in a selected group of patients. Older age adversely affects CD34+ cell yield even with limited premobilization therapy, indicating that early collection is especially important in elderly patients.[159] Sequential administration of VAD followed by high-dose cyclophosphamide and consolidated by the combination of etoposide, dexamethasone, cytarabine, and cisplatin (EDAP) has improved the CR rate and allowed for the collection of an adequate number of stem cells to support two autologous transplants.[160] Other chemomobilization regimens include high-dose cyclophosphamide and CDEP.

Purging (removal of lingering malignant plasma cells) with monoclonal antibodies or 4-hydroperoxycyclophosphamide and positive selection of CD34+ progenitor cells (myeloma cells do not express the CD34 antigen) has been performed to obtain tumor-free stem cells and improve the response rate and OS. A long-term follow-up of a randomized study[161] showed no survival benefit from CD34+ selection. Thus, the benefits of purging and positive selection of stem cells remain questionable.[149]

*Conditioning regimen.* High-dose melphalan appears to be the most active conditioning regimen and is considered the standard method for ablating the bone marrow of patients with MM. Other combination regimens containing busulfan or etoposide proved to be complex and showed no obvious additional benefit.[149] High-dose melphalan at 200 mg/m$^2$ given in 1 dose or at 100 mg/m$^2$ on 2 consecutive days followed by reinfusion of stem cells 24 hours after the completion of melphalan administration is commonly utilized in clinical practice.

The reinfusion of stem cells 24 hours after high-dose melphalan administration is safe based on pharmacokinetic studies suggesting that the terminal half-life of melphalan ranges from 50 to 170 minutes.[149] The dose of melphalan is sometimes reduced depending on the age of the patient (ie, age > 70 years) and presence of comorbid conditions. A reduced dose of melphalan at 140 mg/m$^2$ is commonplace in the elderly patient population to avoid high mortality.[153,162]

In the past, age older than 65 years and comorbid conditions such as renal compromise were considered negative factors in the selection of transplant candidates. Recently, studies have shown that neither of these factors is an important adverse parameter affecting the outcome following high-dose therapy and autologous transplantation.[163–167] These reports have led to an increase in the number of older patients who are deemed eligible for ASCT for the treatment of MM.[109]

A number of studies have shown that the attainment of a complete response is an independent favorable prognostic factor for OS and event-free survival after HDC.[149] Several other variables have been found to be predictive of prognosis in patients undergoing high-dose therapy. These include high tumor burden (based on M-protein and plasma cells in the marrow), chromosomal aberrations, abnormal karyotype (cytogenetic abnormality), high $\beta_2$M at the time of initial presentation, and duration of standard therapy prior to high-dose therapy.[149] Gender is the only patient factor that has prognostic significance; age was found to be a nonsignificant factor, except in patients with renal failure.[166] Response to previous therapy was once thought to be a poor prognostic factor[149] but recent reports have contradicted this conclusion, so patients who showed a lack of response to induction therapy should not be disqualified from undergoing ASCT.[168]

*Long-term sequelae.* Patients with MM who underwent ASCT may develop secondary acute myeloid leukemia (AML) or myelodysplastic syndrome (MDS).[149,169,170] One study reported that these complications were seen exclusively in patients treated with conventional-dose alkylating agent chemotherapy.[170] The actuarial 5-year probabilities of developing cytogenetic MDS and combined cytogenetic MDS-MM are 5% and 10%, respectively. It is also possible that this high rate of myelodysplastic changes results from undergoing 2 ASCTs in comparison with a single transplant.[149] Another study reported that prolonged duration of pretransplant chemotherapy was the most important risk factor for the development of MDS, followed by older age and a low number of infused CD34+ cells.[171] Reported risks for treatment-related malignancies range between 1.3-fold and 20-fold higher in patients with MM in comparison to the general public. Clearly, monitoring patients with MM for evidence of acute leukemia and treatment-related MDS is crucial. As patients with MM continue to undergo intensive regimens requiring transplant support, clinicians will need to incorporate attention to the risk for the development of AML and MDS into the informed consent process, the ongoing management, and the long-term follow-up of these patients.

In the controversial field of myeloma disease management, HDC with ASCT seems to be an approach with tangible benefits such as longer OS.

## MAINTENANCE THERAPY

The role of maintenance therapy in patients with MM remains controversial. It is usually initiated following induction remission therapy (conventional chemotherapy)[153] or 8 to 12 weeks after HDC with ASCT.[172]

### Interferon

The role of IFN-α as maintenance therapy in patients with MM has been well studied.[135] Unfortunately, IFN-α treatment trials in MM have yielded discordant results regarding response rate, maintenance duration, and survival times. Despite the fact that these studies have shown conflicting results, most investigators suggested that the role of IFN-α in the management of patients with MM is mainly as maintenance therapy to prolong the plateau phase of remission.[135]

### Steroids

Steroids play a significant role as single agents or in combination with chemotherapy as induction remission treatment for myeloma. Studying their role as maintenance therapy, therefore, has merit. The use of alternate-day prednisone 50 mg as an effective maintenance treatment for patients with MM who achieve a response to induction chemotherapy has been reported.[173]

### Thalidomide

The combination of thalidomide and pamidronate may show improved progression-free survival. In a French myeloma intergroup study, patients were randomized to maintenance after ASCT with thalidomide, pamidronate, and thalidomide, or no maintenance. When compared with the 2 arms (no maintenance and pamidronate alone), although the OS was similar among the 3 arms, 56% of the patients receiving thalidomide and pamidronate had a progression-free survival advantage at 3 years.[174]

## CONVENTIONAL AND NOVEL THERAPIES FOR RELAPSED AND REFRACTORY MYELOMA

At least one-third of patients with MM fail to respond to induction chemotherapy and those who initially achieve remission even with HDC may eventually relapse and require additional treatment.[175] Patients with MM treated with HDC and HSCT are considered to have disease progression when the serum or urine paraprotein has increased by 25%.[176] Patients with relapsed myeloma are usually divided into 2 groups: drug-resistant and relapsing. The drug-resistant group has the poorest overall prognosis, and only a few respond to alternative treatments.[177] For simplicity, refractory myeloma indicates disease unresponsive to the most recent therapy administered. Patients with refractory MM are usually encouraged to participate in clinical trials.

For treatment of patients with relapsed MM, therapeutic agents typically include the same drugs used in initial induction therapy. The appropriate therapy for a given situation depends on the nature of the disease, age, organ function, prior treatment, availability of stem cell donors, and access to novel agents. Broadly, these options include bortezomib, thalidomide and thalidomide-based therapies, high-dose dexamethasone, HDC with ASCT, allogeneic HSCT, combination chemotherapy such as etoposide-based regimens, and novel/investigational agents.[178,179]

Approximately 40% of patients with resistant and relapsing MM may achieve second remission with glucocorticoids[177] and 40% to 50% of patients with relapsing MM respond to VAD.[180] Second-line combination chemotherapy regimens (primarily including alkylating agents) may help a small percentage of patients: 8% of resistant patients, 22% of refractory patients, and a slightly higher percentage of patients receiving doxorubicin-based regimens may respond, but the duration of second response may be less than 1 year.[177]

### Lenalidomide and dexamethasone

Lenalidomide, a structural analogue of thalidomide, belonging to a class of drugs called immunomodulatory agents that carry a different side effect profile from many existing chemotherapy agents. This drug has shown efficacy in relapsed and refractory patients with myeloma. The FDA has approved the combination of lenalidomide and dexamethasone for relapsed and refractory patients with MM, after a pooled analysis of patients randomized to lenalidomide 25 mg po days 1 to 21 of a 28-day cycle with dexamethasone 40 mg orally days 1 to 4, 9 to 12, and 17 to 20 of a 28-day cycle, vs dexamethasone alone. Pooled analysis of data consisting of over 700 patients in 48 North American and 51 European sites showed an improved TTP for patients receiving lenalidomide and dexamethasone vs dexamethasone alone (11.1 months vs 4.7 months, respectively), and a survival advantage (29.6 months vs 20.5 months).[180,181] Lenalidomide is administered orally, at a dose of 25 mg daily, for 1 to 21 days out of a 28-day cycle, and is given in combination with dexamethasone 40 mg orally days 1 to 4, 9 to 12, and 17 to 20 of a 28-day cycle.[180,182] Common nonhematological toxicities include fatigue and constipation, and hematological toxicities include anemia, leukopenia, and thrombocytopenia. Myelosuppression is very common and may require dosage reductions; therefore, blood counts must be monitored every 2 weeks for the first 3 months of therapy, and at least monthly thereafter. Growth colony-stimulating factors for neutropenia and erythropoeisis stimulating agents for symptomatic anemia may be administered as supportive care.[183]

### Bortezomib

Multiple options are available in the management of relapsed and refractory MM, but few RCT data are available to guide clinicians regarding what approach to take first. A systematic review of randomized studies in MM concluded that the overall quality of the body of evidence for myeloma management was poor and has ample room for improvement.[150] These findings support the recommendation that the best management of any cancer patient occurs in clinical trials and patient participation should therefore be encouraged.[50] In clinical trials, patients with relapsed and refractory MM treated with bortezomib had a longer TTP and had shown higher response rates than those treated with dexamethasone alone.[184]

Newer trials are evaluating different combinations, and one trial looked at the combination of bortezomib and PLD. This regimen has been approved by the FDA for treatment of relapsed and refractory myeloma, based on results from the DOXIL-MMY-3001, which was a large, international study consisting of 646 patients previously treated for their myeloma, using a steroid-free regimen. Patients were randomized to either PLD 30 mg/m$^2$ day 4 of the treatment cycle, and bortezomib 1.3 mg/m$^2$ days 1, 4, 8, and 11 or bortezomib alone. Treatment was given every 21 days. The results showed that the combination of PLD and bortezomib resulted in a 45% risk reduction of experiencing disease progression over bortezomib alone.[184] Also, the median TTP in the bortezomib only group was improved from 6.5 months to 9.3 months for the PLD plus bortezomib combination. Side effects of thrombocytopenia, and neutropenia were only slightly higher in the group receiving PLD and bortezomib vs bortezomib alone, and grade 3 hand-foot syndrome (erythema and pain in hands and feet) was only 6%.[185] This suggests the combination to be well tolerated, and superior to bortezomib alone in patients with relapsed MM.

## RADIATION THERAPY

Radiation therapy (RT) has long been recognized as an important therapeutic option to palliate symptoms associated with MM. Approximately 70% of patients will eventually benefit from this therapy.[177] MM is considered a disseminated disease with evidence of distant organ involvement at the time of diagnosis requiring systemic combination chemotherapy, rather than focal treatment such as radiation. In rare instances (fewer than 5% of cases), the disease may be localized and present as a SPB (approximately 70% of cases) or EMP (approximately 30% of cases). On biopsy, the individual's bony lesion will show evidence of plasma cells. Bone marrow aspiration and biopsy, peripheral counts including blood counts, and serum chemistry will be unremarkable and show no evidence of other organ involvement. The diagnosis of osseous plasmacytoma, defined as a plasmacytoma emanating from bone without other evidence of disease, requires a thorough evaluation to rule out the presence of systemic disease, because many patients presumed to have solitary plasmacytomas are eventually found to have occult disease.[186] MRI of the spine may be very useful in these conditions.[50]

Radiation therapy of a solitary plasmacytoma in doses of 40 Gy or more demonstrates local control rates of 88% to 100% in osseous sites and 80% to 100% in soft tissue sites.[186] These data support the contention that MM is an extremely radiosensitive malignancy. The NCCN recommends delivering doses of 45 Gy or more to involved field in both osseous and tissue plasmacytomas. For soft tissue plasmacytoma, surgery may be required plus CT or MRI every 6 months for 2 cycles, then as clinically indicated. Follow-up and surveillance in osseous plasmacytoma includes quantitative immunoglobulin tests plus quantification of M-protein after RT, complete blood counts, differential assessment, platelets, bone survey annually or for symptoms, bone marrow biopsy as clinically indicated, and M-protein measurement every 3 to 6 months as clinically indicated.[50]

The outcome following RT for a SPB or an EMP should be discussed thoroughly with the patient and family. Nearly all patients presenting with SPB will progress to myeloma, with a median myeloma-free interval of approximately 10 years with adequate local therapy. Because true solitary plasmacytoma is a rare event,[186] it is important that patients understand the need for continued follow-up and surveillance. Solitary plasmacytoma of bone has higher risk of conversion of 54% at 10 years after adequate treatment, compared with a conversion rate of 11% for patients with EMP.[187] Moreover, patients presenting with SPB have a poorer prognosis following progression to myeloma than do patients with EMP. The disappearance of M-protein following RT of SPB has been found to be a significant prognostic indicator.[188]

In MM, just as in solitary plasmacytoma, RT is a very effective palliative modality for symptomatic osseous or extramedullary manifestations. Palliative RT for MM must be individualized. The palliative regimen of 30 Gy given in 10 fractions, which is commonly used to treat metastatic lesions, may not be appropriate for all patients. Lower doses of 10 to 20 Gy will produce palliation in the majority of patients, while allowing for retreatment in those few in whom it is required. Higher total doses may be recommended in 2 situations: neurological compromise from tumor impingement on the spinal cord or cranial nerve and involvement of weight-bearing bones with impending pathological fracture. In these cases, it is recommended that higher doses of 30 to 40 Gy be given in standard fractionation (usually 2 Gy per fraction) to obtain the best probability of durable reversal of symptoms in the former case and tumor eradication and bone healing in the latter.[186]

### Hemibody irradiation

Hemibody irradiation has been used in patients with advanced or refractory MM because of the disseminated nature and radiosensitivity of myeloma. However, it is rarely used today because of its toxicities and equivocal therapeutic benefit.[189] In this technique, a single dose of radiation (500–800 cGy) is administered to a large body area at one time. This approach allows the potential treatment of both halves of the body sequentially using doses that are higher than could be delivered with total-body irradiation. It can provide pain relief in 24 to 48 hours, and this time frame is taken into consideration by clinicians when ordering and administering narcotic analgesics to manage pain. Treatment fields include the upper hemibody field—head to the fourth lumbar vertebrae; the mid-body field—the abdomen and pelvis from the top of the diaphragm to the obturator foramina; and the lower hemibody—the torso below the iliac crest and extending to the ankles. Complications may be significant particularly in patients receiving upper-half-body irradiation and may include pnuemonitis, infection or sepsis, pancytopenia, bleeding, and treatment-related death.[189] Patient education is very important regarding the potential side effects depending on the field of treatment. Proper coordination and administration of premedications such as corticosteroids, antiemetics, and narcotic analgesics is important to maintain the patient's comfort and facilitate compliance with the plan of treatment.

## BISPHOSPHONATES

Bisphosphonates are potent inhibitors of osteoclast-mediated bone resorption and accumulate in the mineralized bone matrix, making it more resistant to dissolution by osteoclasts. Moreover, bisphosphonates directly inhibit the osteolytic activity of osteoclasts and reduce their survival. They have been shown to provide supportive benefits to MM patients with lytic bone disease.[190]

Pamidronate, a second-generation amino-bisphosphonate, has been evaluated in a randomized, double-blind trial focusing on advanced MM.[191] Bone pain and analgesic requirements were significantly reduced in the pamidronate group. The total number of skeletal events and episodes of hypercalcemia was reduced by half. Pamidronate is currently used at a dose of 90 mg once a month in a 2-hour IV infusion indefinitely; long-term use with this agent has been shown to be safe and efficient.[192] In comparison with ibandronate, pamidronate was found to be superior in reducing osteoclast activity, bone resorption, IL-6, and possibly tumor burden in MM.[193]

A more potent third-generation bisphosphonate, zoledronic acid (Zometa, Novartis Pharmaceutical Corporation, East Hanover, NJ), has proven superior to pamidronate in the treatment of hypercalcemia and skeletal metastasis.[194] Also, preclinical studies have demonstrated that this agent has a direct antitumor activity in myeloma cells.[195] Zoledronic acid is currently used at a dose of 4 mg once a month in a 15- to 30-minute IV infusion, indefinitely. Although concerns over the nephrotoxicity of zoledronic acid have arisen,[190] one study reported that in patients with mildly to moderately reduced renal function, dosage adjustment of zoledronic acid is likely not necessary.[196] Both zoledronic acid and pamidronate can reduce the risk of vertebral, wrist, and hip fractures by 30% to 50%.[197] Zoledronic acid is contraindicated in patients who have renal impairment and patients who are experiencing fluid and electrolyte imbalance. As with pamidronate, its prolonged use seems to be well tolerated and safe.[192,198]

Common side effects from IV bisphosphonates include bone pain, nausea, fatigue, fever, vomiting, diarrhea, and myalgia.[198] Supportive care measures include assessing for dehydration, measurement of electrolyte level, and administration of antiemetics, antipyretics, antidiarrheals, and analgesics as clinically indicated.[199] Chemistry results are usually reviewed before IV bisphosphonate administration, and serum creatinine is monitored on a regular basis. An increase in creatinine of 0.5 mg/dL in patients with normal baseline and of 1.0 mg/dL in patients with abnormal baseline creatinine would require the dose to be held until the creatinine returns to within 10% of the baseline value. Patients who are receiving any bisphosphonate therapy for malignant bone disease are instructed to take daily calcium (500 mg) and vitamin D (400 IU) supplements.[199]

Osteonecrosis of the jaw (ONJ) has also been associated with long-term use of bisphosphonates, such as pamidronate and zoledronic acid, at a rate of between 2% for less than a year of therapy and 12% with continuing therapy depending on the series.[183] Patients may present with various stages of infection, from a nonhealing dental extraction, gingival swelling, pain, purulent discharge, or even an exposed area of bone. Antibiotics are indicated in the management of ONJ and are oftentimes an effective treatment option. Patients receiving or considering bisphosphonate therapy should be made aware of the risk of ONJ, be advised to avoid invasive dental procedures and maintain good oral health, and be monitored regularly for ONJ by their dental and oncology healthcare professionals.[183]

The American Society of Clinical Oncology (ASCO) has published clinical practice guidelines for the use of bisphosphonates in the prevention and treatment of lytic bone disease in patients with MM. The committee has recommended IV pamidronate or zoledronic acid only for the prevention of skeletal related events (SRE). The superiority of one agent relative to the other cannot be definitively established. As a consequence, the choice between pamidronate and zoledronic acid will depend on balancing the higher cost of zoledronic acid, with its shorter, more convenient infusion time (15 minutes), against the lower cost of pamidronate, with its longer infusion time (2 hours).[190]

As the duration of therapy may impact the incidence of ONJ, ASCO has also suggested that when using bisphosphonates in the prevention of SREs, caution must be exercised. Patients with demonstrated bone disease should receive monthly bisphosphonates for a period of 2 years and if the patient remains in stable disease, consideration should be given toward stopping bisphosphonate use, or increasing the interval of administration to prevent long-term side effects of bisphosphonate therapy.[200]

## VERTEBRAL COMPRESSION FRACTURES

Patients sustaining vertebral compression fractures as a result of secondary osteoporosis and vertebral body collapse, or from myelomatous lesions themselves, may benefit from medical as well as surgical intervention. In addition to open repair and reconstruction to stabilize the spine, two minimally invasive techniques may be used to treat spinal vertebral compression fractures.

Balloon kyphoplasty and vertebroplasty are minimally invasive surgical techniques that are useful in reducing painful vertebral compression fractures.[201] By using a percutaneous approach and with the guidance of fluoroscopy, immediate pain relief has been demonstrated by both techniques in several clinical trials. Although, at this time, no randomized, controlled clinical trial suggests that one technique is more effective than the other; both can be successful for pain control. Exercise and aquatic therapy, which is effective in strengthening the muscular network to support the spine, decrease the risk of deep-vein thrombosis and pneumonia, and maintain optimal functioning, should be suggested to all patients.[201]

## INVESTIGATIONAL NOVEL THERAPEUTIC AGENTS

### Lenalidomide and dexamethasone in newly diagnosed patients

Lenalidomide has been widely studied in newly diagnosed MM in phase III randomized, controlled clinical trials.[202] In a pivotal trial, patients with symptomatic and untreated MM who were eligible to participate in this study were randomized to 1 of 2 arms, both containing dexamethasone in either high or low doses. Arm A consisted of lenalidomide 25 mg days 1 to 21 of a 28-day cycle plus high-dose dexamethasone therapy consisted of 40 mg/day on days 1 to 4, 9 to 12, and 17 to 20 every 28 days (LD). Arm B received lenalidomide 25 mg/day by mouth on days 1 to 21 every 28 days and low-dose dexamethasone therapy consisted of 40 mg/day on days 1, 8, 15, and 22 every 28 days (Ld). Patients were treated for four 28-day cycles after which further treatment was based on response, and those with a complete or partial response (CR or PR) and were eligible for stem cell transplant proceeded to transplant. The results of this study were impressive. One- and 2-year survival rates for the Ld group were better than the LD group meaning that patients receiving low-dose dexamethasone in combination with lenalidomide did better and had less toxicities. In addition, subgroup analysis of patients younger than 65 years of age and in those ≥ 65 years of age showed that this was the group that had the most benefit from lower doses of steroids again suggesting that the toxicity of high-dose dexamethasone in patients may not be worth the risk of side effects and their complications.[203] On the basis of the preponderance of phase III randomized, clinical trial data and the efficacy of the regimen, the NCCN guidelines suggest that this combination be considered as induction therapy for patients eligible for stem cell transplant.

## SYMPTOM MANAGEMENT AND NURSING CARE

During the course of their disease, patients with MM experience a number of complications that occur secondary to the widespread immunological, hematological, and hormonal/cytokine abnormalities seen in this disorder. These problems include infections, hypercalcemia, anemia, pain, and fractures. Nursing interventions are directed toward addressing these clinical issues, which in some cases, could be fatal. Rice and Sheridan have identified some aspects of care for the patient with MM that may have a significant impact on the medically underserved and underrepresented minority—namely, pain, polypharmacy, renal insufficiency, transfusion dependency, and HDC with ASCT. These authors have suggested specific nursing actions and collaboration with other disciplines to address these clinical issues.[204] In planning the nursing care, the entire treatment team must be knowledgeable about the patient's prognosis. It is also critical to include the patient and family when discussing therapeutic goals and treatment options. Goals may include intensive treatment, preventing or delaying life-threatening complications, prolonging disease-free survival, palliation, or end-of-life care. Regardless of the goal, a symptom management approach to nursing care with a review of systems is useful in organizing assessment and interventions (Table 61-10).[205]

**TABLE 61-10**

**Nursing Care of the Patient with Multiple Myeloma**

| System | Signs and Symptoms | Patient Education |
|---|---|---|
| Neuromuscular | Pain (acute/chronic) | Pain control measures |
| | Hypercalcemia | Signs and symptoms of hypercalcemia |
| | Hyperviscosity syndrome | Signs and symptoms of hyperviscosity |
| | Spinal cord compression | Immediate reporting of signs and symptoms of cord compression |
| | Pathological fracture | Prevention of pathological fractures |
| | Depression | Counseling and cognitive strategies |
| Immunosuppression | Anemia | Exercise and energy conservation activities |
| | Neutropenia | Prevention of infection |
| | Thrombocytopenia | Avoiding contact with individuals with known infection |
| | | Prevention of bleeding |
| | | Self-administration of prescribed hematopoietic growth factors |
| Respiratory | Pneumonia | Prevention of pooling of pulmonary secretions |
| | | Increase gas exchange |
| | | Use of incentive spirometer |
| | | Strict adherence to antibiotic treatment |
| Gastrointestinal | Constipation | Preventive measures |
| | | Change in fluid and dietary intake; exercise |
| Genitourinary | Renal insufficiency | Increase fluid intake |
| | | Avoidance of nephrotoxic drugs |
| | | Recognition of signs of urinary tract infection |

## SKELETAL SYMPTOMS

Bone pain is one of the most common symptoms of MM and is caused mainly by bone lesions. Other causes of pain in patients with MM include nerve or root compression, post-herpetic neuralgia and unrelated causes.[206] The degree of pain may vary from moderate to severe in intensity. The pain can be acute, characterized by a specific trauma and lasting less than 6 months in duration, or chronic, having no specific obvious initiation point and occurring over a protracted period. Optimal pain control is essential in maintaining satisfactory quality of life. One study found that pain and mood disturbance were significant predictors of quality of life in patients with MM.[207]

Oncology nurses play a significant role in facilitating an ongoing, adequate pain assessment and effective management. Specific nursing interventions for pain include assessment and documentation of the individual's severity of pain (0–10 scale), proper positioning of affected limbs, use of supports and braces (cervical collar, back brace, sling) to prevent additional stress on bones, and consultation with physical or occupational therapists. Effective pain control is possible in patients with MM utilizing the WHO pain treatment ladder, a 3-step treatment plan that has been widely used for the treatment of tumor pain.[208] The use of a clinical algorithm may also assist the nurse in identifying bone metastases and managing clinical sequelae, such as pain.[209] Pain management should incorporate nonpharmacological therapies such as aromatherapy, massage, heat, cold, relaxation, and immobilization as necessary.[210]

## NEUROLOGICAL SYMPTOMS

Mental status changes can be an initial sign of hypercalcemia, hyperviscosity syndrome, or drug toxicity. Any change in mental status requires careful assessment to determine its etiologic factors so that appropriate treatment can be promptly initiated. When hypercalcemia occurs, adequate IV hydration (3–6 L daily) is started immediately. Patients who are at risk of developing hypercalcemic crisis may require calcitonin for rapid reduction of calcium levels. The use of saline replenishment and bisphosphonates such as pamidronate or zoledronic acid has become the standard of treatment for hypercalcemia.[211,212] Corticosteroids, which are part of most chemotherapy regimens for the treatment of myeloma, inhibit bone resorption to some degree: they also exert an inhibitory effect on intestinal calcium absorption. They are often used as part of the combination therapy of hypercalcemia.[206] Hyperviscosity syndrome requiring plasmapheresis in myeloma is rare but may be indicated if symptomatic hyperviscosity occurs. Effective tumor kill is necessary to correct both hypercalcemia and hyperviscosity. The nursing plan should include prevention of injury and maintenance of patient safety.

Patients on bortezomib or thalidomide therapy should be closely monitored for any adverse effects, particularly peripheral neuropathy. Failure to assess for them and lack of appropriate early interventions may jeopardize the potential therapeutic benefits from bortezomib or thalidomide and compromise patient's long-term outcomes. Peripheral neuropathy screening at the start of therapy followed by close monitoring and appropriate dose reduction of current treatment regimen based on patient's degree of neuropathy are critical to prevent severe neuropathy.[213]

## PSYCHOSOCIAL ISSUES

Depression, anxiety, and insomnia, are but a few of the psychological responses that patients may exhibit in response to their disease and treatment.[214,215] Listening, cognitive restructuring, assisting with problem solving, giving information in small amounts, and expressing care and concern are among the strategies that oncology nurses can employ to assist patients in the adaptation to their cancer diagnosis. It is reasonable to experience and show genuine sadness about a patient's situation. Mood disturbances are more severe in patients with MM than in other cancers and objectively affect their quality of life.[207] Because MM is an incurable disease with a median survival of 3 to 5 years, it places a significant psychological burden on patients, especially the elderly. Oncology nurses play a vital role in ensuring that patients receive the optimal psychological support necessary to promote their well-being and overall quality of life. Information about support groups and MM organizations is beneficial when patients and families desire it (Table 61-11). These organizations provide individual and group support, as well as written materials describing the disease and its treatment. Many of these organizations can be accessed via the Internet.

**TABLE 61-11**

**Patient Education Support Services**

| Counseling and Support | Patient Resources |
|---|---|
| Bone Marrow Transplant Family Support Network<br>P.O. Box 845<br>Avon, CT 06001<br>800–826-9376 | American Cancer Society (ACS)<br>1599 Clifton Road, NE<br>Atlanta, GA 30329–4251<br>404–329-7623 (patient services)<br>800-ACS-2345<br>*http://www.cancer.org* |
| Cancer Care, Inc.<br>275 Seventh Avenue<br>New York, NY 10001<br>212–712-8354<br>*http://www.cancercare.org* | International Myeloma Foundation (IMF)<br>2129 Stanley Hills Drive<br>Los Angeles, CA 90046<br>800–452-CURE<br>*http://www.myeloma.org* |
| National Coalition for Cancer Survivorship (NCCS)<br>1010 Wayne Avenue, Suite 505<br>Silver Spring, MD 20910<br>301–650-8868 | Leukemia Society of America (LSA)<br>600 Third Avenue<br>New York, NY 10016<br>212–573-8484<br>800–955-4LSA<br>*http://www.leukemia.org* |
| | Multiple Myeloma Research Foundation (MMRF)<br>3 Forest Street<br>New Canaan, CT 06840<br>203–972-1250<br>*http://www.multiplemyeloma.org* |

## PROTECTIVE MECHANISMS

Infection, particularly of bacterial origin, is the leading cause of death in patients with MM. Their susceptibility to infection stems mainly from granulocytopenia and deficiencies in humoral and/or cellular immunity. Non-neutropenic patients are at risk due to impaired antibody formation following antigenic stimulation, and prompt identification of symptoms that may suggest active infection is critical. Gram-positive–encapsulated organisms typically affecting the sinus and respiratory tracts are common. For recurrent life-threatening infections, passive immunity with IV immunoglobulin (IVIG) may be required. IVIG promotes passive immunity and is indicated in patients with myeloma who have hypogammaglobulinemia. Even in the event that a patient with myeloma may have an overproduction of dysfunctional IgG, and the laboratory value of serum IgG may be elevated (or fall within the normal range), patients still may derive benefit.[216]

Guidelines for the care of neutropenic patients are also aimed at the early recognition and prevention of infection. Prophylactic use of antibiotics during the first 3 months of induction chemotherapy based on institutional protocol may be initiated to prevent pneumococcal infections.[217]

Routine use of hematopoietic colony-stimulating factors as an adjunct therapy for the treatment of uncomplicated fever and neutropenia is not generally recommended because it has little impact on disease-free and OS.[218] However, clinicians may use poor performance status and advanced form of cancer as risk factors when assessing patients prior to ordering hematopoietic growth factors for primary prophylaxis of febrile neutropenia after myelosuppressive therapy.[202] While many antimyeloma therapies may place patients at an increased risk of infection, bortezomib has been shown most recently to carry an increased risk of herpes zoster especially in combination with steroids such as dexamethasone. The use of acyclovir or valacyclovir prophylaxis in patients receiving bortezomib may decrease the incidence of shingles.[219] Shingles are lesions that begin as an itchy, vesicular rash that typically follows a dermatome, or nerve root. If the virus travels to the nerve root, pain may result that can be particularly debilitating. It is highly important to note that although the zoster vaccine was recently approved by the U.S. FDA, the vaccine is contraindicated in immunosuppressed individuals. This is a live, attenuated vaccine and may reactivate in patients without an intact immune system.[219] The Centers for Disease Control and Prevention (CDC) urge older adults to receive an annual influenza vaccine, yet as many as 40% of older patients may not develop immunity after receiving the influenza vaccine. Vaccines against pneumococcus also are less effective in patients with MM, yet the CDC still recommends that the vaccine be administered once after the age of 60. As patients with myeloma have an altered immune system, even a small amount of benefit derived from the vaccine outweighs the associated risks and costs; therefore, vaccinations are recommended for older adults as well as patients with myeloma.[220]

Blood product support will consist mainly of packed red blood cells and platelet transfusions. The clinical use of hematopoietic growth factors in the prevention of febrile neutropenia after myelosuppressive therapy, in the treatment of anemia in cancer patients receiving chemotherapy, in patients undergoing peripheral blood progenitor cell (PBPC) collection, and in patients receiving bone marrow or stem cell transplant, is now well established as supportive therapy in managing individuals with MM.[217,221–224]

The supportive care of cancer patients with anemia, thrombocytopenia, and neutropenia is well documented in the nursing literature. Guidelines for the care of patients with anemia, infection, and bleeding are provided in this book in Chapters 23, 28, and 29, respectively.

## RESPIRATORY SYMPTOMS

The respiratory system is the most frequent site of infection in patients with MM. As a result, nursing care is directed toward teaching patients and their families about ways to decrease pooling of pulmonary secretions and increase gas exchange (eg, coughing and deep breathing exercises, use of incentive spirometers, avoiding contact with individuals who show signs and symptoms of upper respiratory tract infection). Patient and family instructions—for example, immediate notification of the healthcare team when the patient develops fever, cough, sore throat, and sputum production—are important. Vaccination with live organisms is contraindicated in patients with MM due to their defective humoral immunity and exposure to others who may have received live organism vaccines should be avoided (ie, children immunized with oral polio and measles/mumps/rubella vaccines). All patients with MM, and in particular those older than age 65, should be immunized with a single dose of the 23-valent pneumococcal vaccine.[225]

## GASTROINTESTINAL SYMPTOMS

Constipation is a problem experienced by many patients with MM, especially the elderly. It usually results from decreased activity or lack of exercise due to bone pain/pathological fractures, dehydration, opioids analgesic use, spinal cord compression, or use of vinca alkaloids. Although not a life-threatening problem, constipation can influence nutritional intake, comfort, and quality of life.[226] Nursing management includes assessment of past and present bowel habits, increasing dietary fiber, adequate hydration, use of a stool softener, judicious use of mild laxatives, encouraging the patient to increase his or her physical activity, facilitating home-based exercise therapy,[227] and patient and family education.

## GENITOURINARY SYMPTOMS

Renal insufficiency can be exacerbated as a result of the primary disease, fluid and electrolyte abnormalities (hyperuricemia, hypercalcemia), dehydration, or infection that could lead to renal failure. The NSAIDs frequently employed in the treatment of bone pain have been associated with the development of ARF in patients with MM.[228] Amphotericin B and acyclovir can also be nephrotoxic and should be used cautiously or avoided in patients with MM unless no other alternatives are available.[229–231] When ARF occurs, nursing care is directed toward reversing renal insufficiency. Prevention and immediate intervention in case of known reversible causes such as infection, dehydration, hypercalcemia, hyperuricemia, and use of nephrotoxic drugs should be one of the goals of care. Patients require close monitoring for early signs and symptoms of urinary tract infection (eg, fever, dysuria, frequency, urgency). Patient and family education directed toward recognition of these signs and symptoms is important, and prompt reporting of such events to the healthcare team is crucial.

## CONCLUSION

New treatments that have been developed to target the MM cell, the MM cell-host interaction, and the bone marrow microenvironment to overcome drug resistance are now widely used in patients with MM. These include bortezomib, liposomal doxorubicin, and IMiDs, such as lenalidomide. Better understanding of the biology of myeloma cells and the bone marrow microenvironment has led to the development of these novel agents. Both these drugs initially entered the relapsed and/or refractory setting, but have now moved to the front-line setting. Numerous clinical trials are under way to identify their exact roles in the management of patients with MM, particularly in patients with known high-risk factors.

Two sequential autologous transplants (tandem transplantation) have been used in an attempt to improve response rates and survival in patients with MM. The evidence suggests that those who did not achieve a very good response from the first transplant would highly benefit from a second tandem transplant. Thus, tandem ASCT is recommended to those patients who have responded to the first ASCT but are not in CR or near-CR.[232] For those patients with high-risk features defined by chromosomal abnormalities (usually involving chromosomes 11 and 13) and high $\beta_2$M levels, novel therapies should be offered as an option during induction therapy.

Despite its curative potential, allogeneic transplantation had been used sparingly in MM until recently because of poor results.[233] The factors responsible for the poor outcomes are related to the underlying disease, the patient's condition, and the treatment regimen, including supportive therapy: advanced Durie-Salmon stage, extensive prior therapy, high $\beta_2$M, high LDH, long diagnosis-transplant interval, low albumin, prior autograft, refractory disease, and renal dysfunction. It is also believed that poor patient selection (eg, including patients with poor performance status and terminal disease) has contributed to the poor results.[233] The role of nonmyeloablative transplantation is currently being investigated in MM management because of its lower mortality rate and possible therapeutic benefit.

Several other biologically based therapeutic agents are currently under preclinical and clinical investigation for MM. These include NF-κB inhibitor (PS1145), 2-methoxyestradiol (2ME2), tyrosine kinase inhibitor (PTK787), histone deacetylase inhibitor (NVPLAQ824), farnesyl transferase inhibitor (R115777), carfilzomib, pomalidomide, and osteoprotegerin (OPG).[234–245] One promising agent that is now currently in phase III clinical trial is tanespimycin, a novel heat shock protein inhibitor, which shows significant activity against MM.[246]

The past decade has witnessed dramatic improvements in the overall response rates for patients with MM. Therapeutic options have increased, patient outcomes have improved, and further insight has been gained into the biology and genetics of MM.[7] With the advent of novel agents, clinicians are optimistic that the patient's OS will continue to improve in the future. ASCT using high-dose melphalan as a conditioning regimen is now considered standard therapy for myeloma, at least for younger patients.[7,247] Evidence-based guidelines that address the initial work-up, ongoing surveillance, and supportive care of patients with MM have been established by NCCN and could guide clinical practice, clinical trials, and areas for future nursing research.[50]

We are also witnessing increasing utilization of new technologies and biologically based novel therapeutics.[234] The use of tumor- and host-directed nongenocidal therapies (ie, glucocorticoids, bisphosphonates, anti-IL-6, proteasome inhibitors, immunomodulatory agents) may be important adjuncts in effecting a traditional cure or a return to a chronic benign state akin to MGUS or smoldering myeloma.[7] The role of immunotherapy in MM remains under investigation, and it is hoped that future strategies will further improve OS of patients with MM.[248] Systematic application of cytogenetics and molecular genetics, especially gene expression profiling, may soon aid in a molecular classification of MM.[6,249,250]

The nursing care of patients with MM and their families offers the nurse an opportunity to interact with patients who are experiencing both acute and chronic sequelae of the disease. Nursing care can have a direct effect by ensuring early recognition of complications and management of treatment-related toxicity. Patient and family education regarding the disease, conventional and novel treatment, and early recognition of signs and symptoms of complications can contribute to an overall improvement in quality of life. Nurses play important roles not only as direct caregivers, but also as patient advocates and educators. It is imperative that they keep abreast of the recent changes and advances related to MM. Promising areas for nursing research include clinical demonstration projects that produce evidence that specific nursing interventions enhance patients' quality of life and event-free and OS.[251]

## REFERENCES


1. Kyle RA, Rajkumar SV. Treatment of multiple myeloma: an emphasis on new developments. *Ann Med.* 2006;38:111–115.
2. Tariman JD. Understanding novel therapeutic agents for multiple myeloma. *Clin J Oncol Nurs.* 2003;7:521–528.
3. Kyle RA, Rajkumar SV. Multiple myeloma. *Blood.* 2008;111:2962–2972.
4. Shaughnessy, JD Jr, Barlogie B. Interpreting the molecular biology and clinical behavior of multiple myeloma in the context of global gene expression profiling. *Immunol Rev.* 2003;194:140–163.
5. Weininger M, Lauterbach B, Knop S, et al. Whole-body MRI of multiple myeloma: comparison of different MRI sequences in assessment of different growth patterns. *Eur J Radiol.* 2009;69:339–345.
6. Claudio JO, Masih-Khan E, Stewart AK. Insights from the gene expression profiling of multiple myeloma. *Curr Hematol Report.* 2004; 3:67–73.

7. Barlogie B, Shaughnessy J, Tricot G, et al. Treatment of multiple myeloma. *Blood.* 2004;103:20–32.
8. Anderson KC. Moving disease biology from lab to the clinic. *Cancer.* 2003;97(suppl 3):796–801.
9. Jemal A, Siegel R, Ward E, et al. Cancer statistics, 2009. *CA: Cancer J Clin.* 2009;59:225–249.
10. Kyle RA, Gertz MA, Witzig TE, et al. Review of 1027 patients with newly diagnosed multiple myeloma. *Mayo Clin Proc.* 2003;78:21–33.
11. Baris D, Brown LM, Silverman DT, et al. Socioeconomic status and multiple myeloma among US blacks and whites. *Am J Public Health.* 2000;90:1277–1281.
12. Kumar SK, Rajkumar SV, Dispenzieri A, et al. Improved survival in multiple myeloma and the impact of novel therapies. *Blood.* 2008;111:2516–2520.
13. Rettig MB, Ma HJ, Vescio RA, et al. Kaposi's sarcoma-associated herpes virus infection of bone marrow dendritic cells from multiple myeloma patients. *Science.* 1997;276:1851–1854.
14. Tarte K, Klein B. The role of viruses in the pathogenesis of plasma cell disorders. In: Mehta J, Singhal S, eds. *Myeloma*. London: Martin-Dunitz; 2002:39–51.
15. Yee TT, Murphy K, Johnson M, et al. Multiple myeloma and human immunodeficiency virus-1 (HIV-1) infection. *Am J Hematol.* 2001;66:123–125.
16. Pantanowitz L, Dezube BJ. Editorial comment: multiple myeloma and HIV infection—causal or casual coincidence? [comment]. *AIDS Reader.* 2003;13:386–387.
17. Grulich AE, Li Y, McDonald A, et al. Rates of non-AIDS-defining cancers in people with HIV infection before and after AIDS diagnosis. *AIDS.* 2002;16:1155–1161.
18. Morgan GJ, Davies FE, Linet M. Myeloma aetiology and epidemiology. *Biomed Pharmacother.* 2002;56:223–234.
19. Alexander DD, Mink PJ, Adami H, et al. Multiple myeloma: a review of the epidemiologic literature. *Int J Cancer.* 2007;120:40–61.
20. Kyle RA, Therneau TM, Rajkumar SV, et al. A long-term study of prognosis in monoclonal gammopathy of undetermined significance. *N Engl J Med.* 2002;346:564–569.
21. Kyle RA, Rajkumar SV. Plasma cell disorders. In: Goldman L, Ausiello D, eds. *Cecil Textbook of Medicine.* 22nd ed. Philadelphia, PA: W.B. Saunders; 2004:1184–1195.
22. Benjamin M, Reddy S, Brawley OW. Myeloma and race: a review of the literature. *Cancer Metastasis Rev.* 2003;22:87–93.
23. Lee WJ, Hoppin JA, Blair A, et al. Cancer incidence among pesticide applicators exposed to alachlor in the Agricultural Health Study. *Am J Epidemiol.* 2004;159:373–380.
24. Lee WJ, Baris D, Jarvholm B, et al. Multiple myeloma and diesel and other occupational exposures in Swedish construction workers. *Int J Cancer.* 2003;107:134–138.
25. Fritschi L, Siemiatycki J. Lymphoma, myeloma and occupation: results of a case-control study. *Int J Cancer.* 1996;67:498–503.
26. Costantini AS, Miligi L, Kriebel D, et al. A multicenter case-control study in Italy on hematolymphopoietic neoplasms and occupation. *Epidemiology.* 2001;12:78–87.
27. Lundberg I, Milatou-Smith R. Mortality and cancer incidence among Swedish paint industry workers with long-term exposure to organic solvents. *Scand J Work Environ Health.* 1998;24:270–275.
28. Mikoczy Z, Schutz A, Hagmar L. Cancer incidence and mortality among Swedish leather tanners. *Occup Environ Med.* 1994;51:530–535.
29. Miligi L, Seniori Costantini A, Crosignani P, et al. Occupational, environmental, and life-style factors associated with the risk of hematolymphopoietic malignancies in women. *Am J Ind Med.* 1999;36:60–69.
30. Speer SA, Semenza JC, Kurosaki T, et al. Risk factors for acute myeloid leukemia and multiple myeloma: a combination of GIS and case-control studies. *J Environ Health.* 2002;64:9–16.
31. Satin KP, Bailey WJ, Newton KL, et al. Updated epidemiological study of workers at two California petroleum refineries, 1950–95. *Occup Environ Med.* 2002;59:248–256.
32. Raffn E, Lynge E, Juel K, et al. Incidence of cancer and mortality among employees in the asbestos cement industry in Denmark. *Br J Ind Med.* 1989;46:90–96.
33. Hatcher JL, Baris D, Olshan AF, et al. Diagnostic radiation and the risk of multiple myeloma (United States). *Cancer Causes Control.* 2001; 12:755–761.
34. Sonoda T, Nagata Y, Mori M, et al. Meta-analysis of multiple myeloma and benzene exposure. *J Epidemiol.* 2001;11:249–254.
35. Lynch HT, Watson P, Tarantolo S, et al. Phenotypic heterogeneity in multiple myeloma families. *J Clin Oncol.* 2005;23:685–693.
36. Hemminki K, Li X, Czene K. Familial risk of cancer: data for clinical counseling and cancer genetics. *Int J Cancer.* 2004;108:109–114.
37. Kyle RA. Diagnosis and treatment of multiple myeloma in the elderly. *Clin Geriat.* 2002;10:47–56.
38. Saez B, Martin-Subero JI, Guillen-Grima F, et al. Chromosomal abnormalities clustering in multiple myeloma reveals cytogenetic subgroups with nonrandom acquisition of chromosomal changes. *Leukemia.* 2004;18:654–657.
39. Seidl S, Kaufman H, Drach J. New insights into the pathophysiology of multiple myeloma. *Lancet Oncol.* 2003;4:557–564.
40. Debes-Marun CS, Dewald GW, Bryant S, et al. Chromosome abnormalities clustering and its implications for pathogenesis and prognosis in myeloma. *Leukemia.* 2003;17:427–436.
41. Avet-Loiseau H, Facon T, Grosbois J, et al. Oncogenesis of multiple myeloma: 14q32 and 13q chromosomal abnormalities are not randomly distributed, but correlate with natural history, immunological features, and clinical presentation. *Blood.* 2003;99:2185–2191.
42. Kastrinakis NG, Gorgoulis VG, Foukas PG, et al. Molecular aspects of multiple myeloma. *Ann Oncol.* 2000;11:1217–1228.
43. Avet-Loiseau H, Li JY, Facon T, et al. High incidence of translocations t(11;14)(q13;q32) and t(4;14)(p16;q32) in patients with plasma cell malignancies. *Cancer Res.* 1998;58:5640–5645.
44. Pope B, Brown R, Luo XF, et al. Disease progression in patients with multiple myeloma is associated with a concurrent alteration in the expression of both oncogenes and tumor suppressor genes and can be monitored by the onco-protein phenotype. *Leuk Lymphoma.* 1997;25:545–554.
45. Elnenaei MO, Gruszka-Westwood AM, A'Hernt R, et al. Gene abnormalities in multiple myeloma: the relevance of TP53, MDM2, and CDKN2A. *Haematologica.* 2003;88:529–537.
46. Elnenaei MO, Hamoudi RA, Swansbury J, et al. Delineation of the minimal region of loss at 13q14 in multiple myeloma. *Genes Chromosomes Cancer.* 2003;36:99–106.
47. Rudin CM, Thompson CB. B-cell development and maturation. *Semin Oncol.* 1998;25:435–446.
48. Rajkumar SV, Greipp PR. Plasma cells and immunoglobulins. In: Mehta J, Singhal S, eds. *Myeloma*. London: Martin Dunitz;2002:3–23.
49. Lokhorst H. Clinical features and diagnostic criteria. In: Mehta J, Singhal S, eds. *Myeloma*. London: Martin Dunitz; 2002:151–168.
50. National Comprehensive Cancer Network (NCCN). NCCN 2008 multiple myeloma clinical practice guidelines in oncology. In: *The Complete Library of NCCN Clinical Practice Guidelines in Oncology* [CD-ROM]. Rockledge, PA: National Comprehensive Cancer Network;2008.
51. Anderson KC. Targeted therapy of multiple myeloma based upon tumor-microenvironmental interactions. *Exp Hematol.* 2007;35:155–162.
52. Hideshima T, Nakamura N, Chauhan D, et al. Biologic sequelae of interleukin-6 induced P13-K/Akt signaling in multiple myeloma. *Oncogene.* 2001;20:5991–6000.
53. Zhang XG, Klein B, Bataille R. Interleukin 6 is a potent myeloma cell growth factor in patients with aggressive multiple myeloma. *Blood.* 1989;74:11–13.
54. Chauhan D, Uchiyama H, Akbarali Y, et al. Multiple myeloma cell adhesion-induced interleukin-6 expression in bone marrow stromal cells involves activation of NF-κB. *Blood.* 1996;87:1104–1112.
55. Dankbar B, Padro T, Mesters RM, et al. VEGF is expressed by myeloma cells and stimulates IL-6 secretion by microvascular endothelial and marrow stromal cells. *Blood.* 1998;92(suppl 1):681a.

56. Lauta VM. A review of the cytokine network in multiple myeloma: diagnostic, prognostic, and therapeutic implications. *Cancer.* 2003; 97:2440–2452.
57. Yeh HS, Berenson JR. Myeloma bone disease and treatment options. *Eur J Cancer.* 2006;42:1554–1563.
58. Roux S, Mariette X. The high rate of bone resorption in multiple myeloma is due to RANK (Receptor activator of nuclear factor-κB) and RANK ligand expression. *Leuk Lymphoma.* 2004;45:1111–1118.
59. Abe M, Hiura K, Wilde J, et al. Role for macrophage inflammatory protein (MIP)-1alpha and MIP-1beta in the development of osteolytic lesions in multiple myeloma. *Blood.* 2002;100:2195–2202.
60. Tai YT, Podar K, Catley L, et al. Insulin-like growth factor-1 induces adhesion and migration in human multiple myeloma cells via activation of beta1-integrin and phosphatidylinositol 3-kinase/AKT signaling. *Cancer Res.* 2003;63:5850–5858.
61. Mitsiades CS, Mitsiades N, Poulaki V, et al. Activation of NF-kappaB and upregulation of intracellular anti-apoptotic proteins via the IGF-1/Akt signaling in human multiple myeloma cells: therapeutic implications. *Oncogene.* 2002;21:5673–5683.
62. Qiang Y-W, Yao L, Tosato G, et al. Insulin-like growth factor I induces migration and invasion of human multiple myeloma cells. *Blood.* 2004; 103:301–308.
63. Hideshima T, Chauhan D, Schlossman R, et al. The role of tumor necrosis factor alpha in the pathophysiology of human multiple myeloma: therapeutic applications. *Oncogene.* 2001;20:4519–4527.
64. Podar K, Tai YT, Davies FE, et al. Vascular endothelial growth factor triggers signaling cascades mediating multiple myeloma cell growth and migration. *Blood.* 2001;98:428–435.
65. Arora T, Jelinek DF. Differential myeloma cell responsiveness to interferon-alpha correlates with differential induction of p19INK4D and cyclin D2 expression. *J Biol Chem.* 1998;273:11799–11805.
66. Klein B, Tarte K, Jourdan M, et al. Survival and proliferation factors of normal and malignant plasma cells. *Int J Hematol.* 2003;78:106–113.
67. Otsuki T, Yata K, Sakaguchi H, et al. IL-10 in myeloma cells. *Leuk Lymphoma.* 2002;43:969–974.
68. Blade J. Criteria for disease progression. *Br J Haematol.* 1998;102: 1115–1123.
69. Berenson JR. Bone disease in myeloma. In: Mehta J, Singhal S, eds. *Myeloma.* London: Martin Dunitz; 2002:97–117.
70. Berenson JR. Advances in the biology and treatment of myeloma bone disease. *Semin Oncol.* 2002;29(suppl 6):11–16.
71. Tian E, Zhan F, Walker R, et al. The role of the Wnt-signaling antagonist DKK1 in the development of osteolytic lesions in multiple myeloma. *N Engl J Med.* 2003;349:2483–2494.
72. Lecouvet F, Malghem J, Michaux L. Skeletal survey in advanced multiple myeloma: radiographic versus MR imaging survey. *Br J Haematol.* 1999;106:35–39.
73. Roodman, GD. Skeletal imaging and management of bone disease. *Hematol Am Soc Hematol Educ Program.* 2008;313–319.
74. Angtuaco EJC, Fassas ABT, Walker R, et al. Multiple myeloma: clinical review and diagnostic imaging. *Radiology.* 2004;231:11–23.
75. Tariman JD. Clinical applications of magnetic resonance imaging (MRI) in patients with multiple myeloma. *Clin J Oncol Nurs.* 2004;8:317–318.
76. Durie BGM, Waxman A, D'Agnolo A, et al. Whole-body 18F-FDG PET identifies high-risk myeloma. *J Nucl Med.* 2002;43:1457–1463.
77. Kelleher P, Chapel H. Infections: principles of prevention and therapy. In: Mehta J, Singhal S, eds. *Myeloma.* London: Martin Dunitz;2002:223–239.
78. Savage DG, Lindenbaum J, Garrett TJ. Biphasic pattern of bacterial infection in multiple myeloma. *Ann Intern Med.* 1982;96:47–50.
79. Silvestris F, Tucci M, Quatraro C, et al. Recent advances in understanding the pathogenesis of anemia in multiple myeloma. *Int J Hematol.* 2003;78:121–125.
80. San Miguel JF, Almeida J, Orfao A. Laboratory investigations. In: Mehta J, Singhal S, eds. *Myeloma.* London: Martin Dunitz;2002:243–268.
81. Pandit SR, Vesole DH. Management of renal dysfunction in multiple myeloma. *Curr Treat Options Oncol.* 2003;4:239–246.
82. Shaver-Lewis MJ, Shah SV. The kidney in plasma cell disorders. In: Mehta J, Singhal S, eds. *Myeloma.* London: Martin Dunitz; 2002:203–221.
83. Chim CS, Li FK, Chan KW. Cast nephropathy in multiple myeloma. *Haematologica.* 2004;89:EIM08.
84. Messiaen T, Deret S, Mougenot B, et al. Adult Fanconi syndrome secondary to light chain gammopathy. Clinicopathologic heterogeneity and unusual features in 11 patients. *Medicine (Baltimore).* 2000;79:135–154.
85. Pozzi C, D'Amico M, Fogazzi GB, et al. Light chain deposition disease with renal involvement: clinical characteristics and prognostic factors. *Am J Kidney Dis.* 2003;42:1154–1163.
86. Sinclair D. IgD myeloma: clinical, biological and laboratory features. *Clin Lab.* 2002;48:617–622.
87. Mollee PN, Wechalekar AD, Pereira DL, et al. Autologous stem cell transplantation in primary systemic amyloidosis: the impact of selection criteria on outcome. *Bone Marrow Transplant.* 2004;33:271–277.
88. Gertz MA. Managing myeloma kidney. *Ann Intern Med.* 2005; 143:835–837.
89. Guo X, Nzerue C. How to prevent, recognize, and treat drug-induced nephrotoxicity. *Cleve Clin J Med.* 2002;69:289–290, 293–294, 296–297.
90. Perazella MA. Drug-induced renal failure: update on new medications and unique mechanisms of nephrotoxicity. *Am J Med Sci.* 2003;325:349–362.
91. Fuente N, Mane JM, Barcelo R, et al. Tumor lysis syndrome in a multiple myeloma treated with thalidomide. *Ann Oncol.* 2004;15:537.
92. Mehta J, Singhal S. Hyperviscosity syndrome in plasma cell dyscrasias. *Semin Thromb Hemost.* 2003;29:467–471.
93. Clark WF, Stewart AK, Rock GA, et al. Plasma exchange when myeloma presents as acute renal failure. *Ann Intern Med.* 2005;143:777–784.
94. Yeshurun M, Laporte JP, Lesage S, et al. Spinal cord compression of dual etiology, multiple myeloma and spinal tuberculosis. *Leuk Lymphoma.* 2002;43:427–428.
95. Gorson KC, Ropper AH. Neuropathy in plasma cell disorders. In: Mehta J, Singhal S, eds. *Myeloma.* London: Martin Dunitz; 2002: 185–201.
96. Marrs J, Newton S. Updating your peripheral neuropathy "know-how." *Clin J Oncol Nurs.* 2003;7:299–303.
97. Tariman JD. Thalidomide: current therapeutic uses and management of its toxicities. *Clin J Oncol Nurs.* 2003;7:143–147.
98. Tariman JD, Lemoine C. Bortezomib. *Clin J Oncol Nurs.* 2003; 7:687–689.
99. Weber DM. Solitary bone and extramedullary plasmacytoma. 2005. http://asheducationbook.hematologylibrary.org/cgi/content/full/2005/1/373. Accessed August 10, 2008.
100. Drayson M, Tang LX, Drew R. Serum free light-chain measurements for identifying and monitoring patients with nonsecretory multiple myeloma. *Blood.* 2001;97:2900–2902.
101. Shaw GR. Nonsecretory plasma cell myeloma—becoming even more rare with serum free light-chain assay: a brief review. *Arch Pathol Lab Med.* 2007;130:1212–1215.
102. Harousseau JL, Moreau P. Prognostic factors in myeloma. In: Mehta J, Singhal S, eds. *Myeloma.* London: Martin Dunitz; 2002:169–183.
103. Greipp PR, San Miguel J, Durie BGM, et al. International staging system for multiple myeloma. *J Clin Oncol.* 2005;23:3412–3420.
104. Durie BG, Kyle RA, Belch A, et al. Myeloma management guidelines: a consensus report from the Scientific Advisors of the International Myeloma Foundation. *Hematol J.* 2003;4:379–398.
105. Durie BG, Salmon SE. A clinical staging system for multiple myeloma: correlation of measured myeloma cell mass with presenting clinical features, response to treatment and survival. *Cancer.* 1975;36:842–854.
106. Durie BG, Salmon SE, Moon TE. Pretreatment tumor mass cell kinetics and prognosis in multiple myeloma. *Blood.* 1980;55:364–372.

107. Jacobson JL, Hussein MA, Barlogie B, et al. Southwest Oncology Group. A new staging system for multiple myeloma patients based on the Southwest Oncology Group (SWOG) experience. *Br J Haematol.* 2003;122:441–450.
108. He Y, Wheatley K, Clark O, et al. Early versus deferred treatment for early stage multiple myeloma. *Cochrane Database System Rev.* 2003;1:CD004023.
109. Zomas A, Dimopoulos MA. Conventional treatment of myeloma. In: Mehta J, Singhal S, eds. *Myeloma.* London: Martin Dunitz; 2002:313–326.
110. Anderson KC, Hamblin TJ, Traynor A. Management of multiple myeloma today. *Semin Hematol.* 1999;36:3–8.
111. Rajkumar SV, Gertz MA, Kyle RA, et al. Current therapy for multiple myeloma. *Mayo Clin Proc.* 2002;77:813–822.
112. Hjorth M, Holmberg E, Rodjer S, et al. Survival in conventionally treated younger (<60 years) multiple myeloma patients: no improvement during two decades. Nordic Myeloma Study Group (NMSG). *Eur J Haematol.* 1999;62:271–277.
113. Myeloma Trialists' Collaborative Group. Combination chemotherapy versus melphalan plus prednisone as treatment for multiple myeloma: an overview of 6633 patients from 27 randomized trials. *J Clin Oncol.* 1998;16:3832–3842.
114. Gregory WM, Richards MA, Malas JS. Combination chemotherapy versus melphalan and prednisone in the treatment of multiple myeloma: an overview of published trials. *J Clin Oncol.* 1992;10:334–342.
115. Sonneveld P, Segeren CM. Changing concepts in multiple myeloma: from conventional to high-dose treatment. *Eur J Cancer.* 2003;39:9–18.
116. Bataille R, Harousseau JL. Multiple myeloma. *N Engl J Med.* 1997;336:1657–1664.
117. Palmer M, Belch A, Hanson J, et al. Dose intensity analysis of melphalan and prednisone in multiple myeloma. *J Natl Cancer Inst.* 1988;80:414–418.
118. Adams J. The proteasome: structure, function, and role in the cell. *Cancer Treat Rev.* 2003;29(suppl 1):3–9.
119. Adams J. Potential for proteasome inhibition in the treatment of cancer. *Drug Discov Today.* 2003;8:307–315.
120. San Miguel JF, Schlag R, Khuageva NK, et al. Bortezomib plus melphalan and prednisone for initial treatment of multiple myeloma. *N Engl J Med.* 2008;359:906–917.
121. Colson K, Doss DS, Swift R, et al. Bortezomib, a newly approved proteasome inhibitor for the treatment of multiple myeloma: nursing implications. *Clin J Oncol Nurs.* 2004;8:473–480.
122. Samson D, Gaminara E, Newland A, et al. Infusion of vincristine and doxorubicin with oral dexamethasone as first-line therapy for multiple myeloma. *Lancet.* 1989;2:882–885.
123. Alexanian R, Barlogie B, Tucker S. VAD-based regimens as primary treatment for multiple myeloma. *Am J Hematol.* 1990;33:86–89.
124. Monconduit M, Menard JF, Michaux JL, et al. VAD or VMBCP in severe multiple myeloma: The Groupe d'Etudes et de Recherche sur le Myelome (GERM). *Br J Haematol.* 1992;80:199–204.
125. Ataergin S, Arpaci F, Kaya A, et al. VAD combination chemotherapy followed by bortezomib may be an effective treatment in secondary plasma cell leukemia. *Am J Hematol.* 2006;81:987–988.
126. Gautier M, Cohen HJ. Multiple myeloma in the elderly. *J Am Geriatric Soc.* 1994;42:653–664.
127. Hussein MA, Baz R, Srkalovic G, et al. Phase 2 study of pegylated liposomal doxorubicin, vincristine, decreased-frequency dexamethasone and thalidomide in newly diagnosed and relapsed-refractory multiple myeloma. *Mayo Clin Proc.* 2006;81:889–895.
128. Alexanian R, Dimopoulos MA, Delasalle K, et al. Primary dexamethasone treatment of multiple myeloma. *Blood.* 1992;80:887–890.
129. Alexanian R, Dimopoulos MA, Delasalle K, Barlogie B. Primary dexamethasone treatment of multiple myeloma. *Blood.* 1992;80:887–890.
130. Faiman B, Bilotti E, Mangan PA, et al. Steroid-associated side effects in patients with multiple myeloma: consensus statement of the IMF Nurse Leadership Board. *Clin J Oncol Nurs.* 2008;12(suppl 3): 53–63.
131. Rajkumar SV, Jacobus S, Callander N, et al. Randomized trial of lenalidomide plus high-dose dexamethasone versus lenalidomide plus low-dose dexamethasone in newly diagnosed myeloma (E4A03), a trial coordinated by the Eastern Cooperative Oncology Group: analysis of response, survival, and outcome with primary therapy and with stem cell transplant. [Abstract 8504] *J Clin Oncol.* 2008;(May 20 suppl).
132. Facon T, Mary JY, Pégourie B, et al. Dexamethasone-based regimens versus melphalan-prednisone for elderly multiple myeloma patients ineligible for high-dose therapy. *Blood.* 2006;107:1292–1298.
133. Mellstedt H, Aahre A, Bjorkholm M, et al. Interferon therapy in myelomatosis. *Lancet.* 1979;2:697.
134. Quesada JR, Alexanian R, Hawkins M, et al. Treatment of multiple myeloma with recombinant alpha-interferon. *Blood.* 1986;67:275–278.
135. Sirohi B, Treleaven J, Powles R. Role of interferon. In: Mehta J, Singhal S, eds. *Myeloma.* London: Martin Dunitz;2002:383–396.
136. Wheatley K. A meta-analysis of trials of interferon as therapy for myeloma. Abstract book of the VIIth International Multiple Myeloma Workshop 973;1999.
137. Singhal S, Mehta J, Desikan R, et al. Antitumor activity of thalidomide in refractory multiple myeloma. *N Engl J Med.* 1999;341:1565–1571.
138. Yakoub-Agha I, Attal M, Dumontet C, et al. Thalidomide in patients with advanced multiple myeloma: a study of 83 patients—report of the Intergroupe Francophone du Myelome (IFM). *Hematol J.* 2002;3:185–192.
139. Kyle RA, Rajkumar SV. Therapeutic application of thalidomide in multiple myeloma. *Semin Oncol.* 2001;28:583–587.
140. Barlogie B, Tricot G, Anaissie E. Thalidomide in the management of multiple myeloma. *Semin Oncol.* 2001;28:577–582.
141. Durie B, Stepan D. Low dose thalidomide alone and in combination: long term follow-up. *Blood.* 2001;98:163a (abstract 688).
142. Singhal S, Mehta J. Thalidomide in cancer. *Biomed Pharmacother.* 2002;56:4–12.
143. Zeldis JB, Williams BA, Thomas SD, et al. S.T.E.P.S.: a comprehensive program for controlling and monitoring access to thalidomide. *Clin Ther.* 1999;21:319–330.
144. Rajkumar SV, Hayman S, Gertz MA, et al. Combination therapy with thalidomide plus dexamethasone for newly diagnosed myeloma. *J Clin Oncol.* 2002;20:4319–4323.
145. Weber D, Rankin K, Gavino M, et al. Thalidomide alone or with dexamethasone for previously untreated multiple myeloma. *J Clin Oncol.* 2003;21:16–19.
146. Zangari M, Barlogie B, Thertulien R, et al. Thalidomide and deep vein thrombosis in multiple myeloma: risk factors and effect on survival. *Clin Lymphoma.* 2003;4:32–35.
147. Rajkumar SV, Hussein M, Catalano J, et al. A randomized, double-blind, placebo-controlled trial of thalidomide plus dexamethasone versus dexamethasone alone as primary therapy for newly diagnosed multiple myeloma. *Blood.* 2006;108(11):abstract 795. http://abstracts.hematologylibrary.org/cgi/content/abstract/108/11/795. Accessed July 27, 2008.
148. Ludwig H, Tothova E, Hajek R, et al. Thalidomide-dexamethasone vs. melphalan-prednisone as first line treatment and thalidomide-interferon vs. interferon maintenance therapy in elderly patients with multiple myeloma. *Blood.* 2007;110:Abstract 529. http://abstracts.hematologylibrary.org/cgi/content/abstract/110/11/529. Accessed July 27, 2008.
149. Singhal S. High-dose therapy and autologous transplantation. In: Mehta J, Singhal S, eds. *Myeloma.* London: Martin Dunitz;2002:327–347.
150. Kumar A, Loughran T, Alsina M, et al. Management of multiple myeloma: a systematic review and critical appraisal of published studies. *Lancet Oncol.* 2003;4:293–304.
151. Fermand JP, Ravaud P, Chevret S, et al. High-dose therapy and autologous peripheral blood stem cell transplantation in multiple myeloma: upfront or rescue treatment? Results of a multi-center sequential randomized clinical trial. *Blood.* 1998;92:3131–3136.

152. Barlogie B, Tricot GJ, van Rhee F, et al. Long-term outcome results of the first tandem autotransplant trial for multiple myeloma. *Br J Haematol.* 2006;135:158–164.
153. Badros A, Barlogie B, Siegel E, et al. Autologous stem cell transplantation in elderly multiple myeloma patients over the age of 70 years. *Br J Haematol.* 2001;114:600–607.
154. Palumbo A, Triolo T, Argentino C, et al. Dose-intensive melphalan with stem cell support (MEL100) is superior to standard treatment in elderly myeloma patients. *Blood.* 1999;94:1248–1253.
155. Raje N, Powles R, Kulkarni S, et al. A comparison of vincristine and doxorubicin infusional chemotherapy with methylprednisolone (VAMP) with the addition of weekly cyclophosphamide (C-VAMP) as induction treatment followed by autografting in previously untreated myeloma. *Br J Haematol.* 1997;97:153–160.
156. Attal M, Harousseau JL, Stoppa AM, et al. A prospective randomized trial of autologous bone marrow transplantation and chemotherapy in multiple myeloma. Intergroupe Francais du Myelome. *N Engl J Med.* 1996;335:91–97.
157. Lee CK, Barlogie B, Munshi N, et al. DTPACE: an effective, novel combination chemotherapy with thalidomide for previously treated patients with myeloma. *J Clin Oncol.* 2003;21:2732–2739.
158. Osman K, Frank R, von Hassel M, et al. Thalidomide, Adriamycin, and dexamethasone as initial therapy in patients with multiple myeloma [abstract #P227]. VIIIth International Myeloma Workshop, Banff, Canada; 2001.
159. Morris CL, Siegel E, Barlogie B, et al. Mobilization of CD34+ cells in elderly (>/= 70 years) with multiple myeloma: influence of age, prior therapy, platelet count and mobilization regimen. *Br J Haematol.* 2003;120:413–423.
160. Barlogie B, Jagannath S, Vesole D, et al. Superiority of tandem transplantation over standard therapy for previously untreated multiple myeloma. *Blood.* 1997;89:789–793.
161. Vescio R, Schiller G, Stewart AK, et al. Multicenter phase III trial to evaluate CD34(+) selected versus unselected autologous peripheral blood progenitor cell transplantation in multiple myeloma. *Blood.* 1999;93:1858–1868.
162. Badros A, Barlogie B, Siegel E, et al. Results of autologous stem cell transplantt in multiple myeloma patients with renal failure. *Br J Haematol.* 2001;114:822–829.
163. Siegel DS, Desikan KR, Mehta J, et al. Age is not a prognostic variable with autotransplants in multiple myeloma. *Blood.* 1999;93:51–54.
164. Terpos E, Apperley JF, Samson D, et al. Autologous stem cell transplantation in multiple myeloma: improved survival in non-secretory multiple myeloma but lack of influence of age, status at transplant, previous treatment and conditioning regimen. A single center experience in 127 patients. *Bone Marrow Transplant.* 2003;31:163–170.
165. Magagnoli M, Castagna L, Balzarotti M, et al. Feasibility and toxicity of high-dose therapy (HDT) supported by peripheral blood stem cells in elderly patients with multiple myeloma and non-Hodgkin's lymphoma: survey from a single institution. *Am J Hematol.* 2003;73:267–272.
166. Badros A, Barlogie B, Siegel E, et al. Results of autologous stem cell transplant in multiple myeloma patients with renal failure. *Br J Haematol.* 2001;114:822–829.
167. Sirohi B, Powles R, Mehta J, et al. The implication of compromised renal function at presentation in myeloma: similar outcome in patients who receive high-dose therapy: a single-center study of 251 previously untreated patients. *Med Oncol.* 2001;18:39–50.
168. Singhal S, Powles R, Sirohi B, et al. Response to induction chemotherapy is not essential to obtain survival benefit from high-dose melphalan and autotransplantation in myeloma. *Bone Marrow Transplant.* 2002;30:673–679.
169. Govindarajan R, Jagannath S, Flick JT, et al. Preceding standard therapy is the likely cause of MDS after autotransplant for multiple myeloma. *Br J Haematol.* 1996;95:349–353.
170. Saso R, Kulkarni S, Powles R, et al. Secondary MDS/AML in patients treated for myeloma. *Blood.* 1998;92(suppl 1):455a.
171. Drach J, Ayers D, Govindarajan R, et al. MDS-associated cytogenetic abnormalities (CGA) in both hematopoietic and neoplastic cells after autotransplants (AT) in 868 patients with multiple myeloma (MM). *Blood.* 1998;92(suppl 1):97a.
172. Santos ES, Goodman M, Byrnes JJ, et al. Thalidomide effects in the post-transplantation setting in patients with multiple myeloma. *Hematology.* 2004;9:35–39.
173. Berenson JR, Crowley JJ, Grogan TM, et al. Maintenance therapy with alternate-day prednisone improves survival in multiple myeloma patients. *Blood.* 2002;99:163–168.
174. Attal M, Harousseau JL, Leyvraz S, et al. Maintenance treatment with thalidomide after autologous transplantation for myeloma: first analysis of a prospective randomized study of the Intergroupe Francophone du Myelome (IFM 99 02). *ASH Annual Meeting Abstracts.* 2004;104:535.
175. Kyle RA. Multiple myeloma, macroglobulinemia, and the monoclonal gammopathies. *Cur Pract Med.* 1999;2:1131–1137.
176. Samson D. Criteria for evaluating disease response and progression in patients with multiple myeloma treated by high-dose therapy and hematopoietic stem cell transplantation. *Br J Haematol.* 1998;102:1115–1123.
177. Munshi NC, Tricot G, Barlogie B. Plasma cell neoplasms. In: De-Vita VT, Hellman S, Rosenberg SA, eds. *Principles and Practice of Oncology.* 6th ed. Philadelphia: Lippincott-Raven; 2001:2465–2493.
178. Singhal S, Mehta J. Treatment of relapsed and refractory multiple myeloma. *Curr Treat Opts Oncol.* 2003;4:229–237.
179. Zaidi AA, Vesole DH. Multiple myeloma: an old disease with new hope for the future. *CA Cancer J Clin.* 2001;51:273–285.
180. Weber D, Chen C, Niesvizky R, et al. Lenalidomide plus dexamethasone for relapsed multiple myeloma in North America. *N Engl J Med.* 2007;357:2133–2142.
181. Dimopoulos M, Spencer A, Attal M, et al. Lenalidomide plus dexamethasone for relapsed multiple myeloma. *N Engl J Med.* 2007; 357:2123–2132.
182. Doss D. Advances in oral therapy in the treatment of myeloma. *Clin J Oncol Nurs.* 2006;10:514–520.
183. Faiman B. Clinical updates and nursing considerations for patients with multiple myeloma. *Clin J Oncol Nurs.* 2007;11:831–840.
184. Richardson PG, Sonneveld P, Schuster MW, et al. Bortezomib or high dose dexamethasone for relapsed multiple myeloma. *N Engl J Med.* 2005;352:2487–2498.
185. Orlowski RZ, Nagler A, Sonneveld P, et al. Randomized phase III study of pegylated liposomal doxorubicin plus bortezomib compared with bortezomib alone in relapsed or refractory multiple myeloma: combination therapy improves time to progression. *J Clin Oncol.* 2007;25:3892–3901.
186. Shrieve DC. The role of radiotherapy. In: Mehta J, Singhal S, eds. *Myeloma.* London: Martin Dunitz;2002:367–381.
187. Bolek TW, Marcus RB, Mendenhall NP. Solitary plasmacytoma of bone and soft tissue. *Int J Radiat Oncol Biol Phys.* 1996;36:329–333.
188. Liebross RH, Ha CS, Cox JD, et al. Solitary plasmacytoma: outcome and prognostic factors following radiotherapy. *Int J Radiat Oncol Biol Phys.* 1998;41:1063–1067.
189. Hu K, Yahalom J. Radiotherapy in the management of plasma cell tumors. *Oncology (Williston Park).* 2000;14:101–108, 111.
190. Berenson JR, Hillner BE, Kyle RA, et al. American Society of Clinical Oncology clinical practice guidelines: the role of bisphosphonates in multiple myeloma. *J Clin Oncol.* 2002;20:3719–3736.
191. Berenson JR, Lichtenstein A, Porter L, et al. Efficacy of pamidronate in reducing skeletal events in patients with advanced multiple myeloma. *N Engl J Med.* 1996;334:488–493.
192. Ali SM, Esteva FJ, Hortobagyi G, et al. Safety and efficacy of bisphosphonates beyond 24 months in cancer patients. *J Clin Oncol.* 2001;19:3434–3437.

193. Terpos E, Viniou N, de la Fuente J, et al. Pamidronate is superior to ibandronate in decreasing bone resorption, interleukin-6 and beta 2-microglobulin in multiple myeloma. *Eur J Haematol.* 2003; 70:34–42.
194. Major P, Lortholary A, Hon J, et al. Zoledronic acid is superior to pamidronate in the treatment of hypercalcemia of malignancy: a pooled analysis of two randomized, controlled clinical trials. *J Clin Oncol.* 2001;19:558–567.
195. Derenne S, Amiot M, Barille S, et al. Zolendronate is a potential inhibitor of myeloma cell growth and secretion of IL-6 and MMP-1 by the tumoral environment. *J Bone Mineral Res.* 1999;14:2048–2056.
196. Skerjanec A, Berenson J, Hsu C, et al. The pharmacokinetics and pharmacodynamics of zoledronic acid in cancer patients with varying degrees of renal function. *J Clin Pharmacol.* 2003;43:154–162.
197. Body JJ. Zoledronic acid: an advance in tumour bone disease therapy and a new hope for osteoporosis. *Exp Opin Pharmacother.* 2003;4:567–580.
198. Rosen LS, Gordon D, Kaminsky M, et al. Long-term efficacy and safety of zoledronic acid compared with pamidronate disodium in the treatment of skeletal complications in patients with advanced multiple myeloma or breast carcinoma: a randomized, double blind, multicenter, comparative trial. *Cancer.* 2003;98:1735–1744.
199. Maxwell C, Swift R, Goode M, et al. Advances in supportive care of patients with cancer and bone metastasis: nursing implications of zoledronic acid. *Clin J Oncol Nurs.* 2003;7:403–408.
200. Kyle RA, Yee GC, Somerfield MR, et al. American Society of Clinical Oncology 2007 clinical practice guideline update on the role of bisphosphonates in multiple myeloma. *J Clin Oncol.* 2007;25:2464–2472.
201. Faiman B. Balloon kyphoplasty and metastatic cancer: a case presentation. *Oncol Nurs News.* 2007;1:7–9.
202. Lacy M, Gertz M, Dispenzieri A, et al. Lenalidomide plus dexamethasone (Rev/Dex) in newly diagnosed myeloma: response to therapy, time to progression, and survival. *Blood.* 2006;108(11):abstract 798. http://abstracts.hematologylibrary.org/cgi/content/abstract/108/11/798. Accessed February 20, 2010.
203. Rajkumar SV, Jacobus S, Callander N, et al. Randomized trial of lenalidomide plus high-dose dexamethasone versus lenalidomide plus low-dose dexamethasone in newly diagnosed myeloma (E4A03), a trial coordinated by the Eastern Cooperative Oncology Group: analysis of response, survival, and outcome with primary therapy and with stem cell transplant. [Abstract 8504] *J Clin Oncol.* 2008(May 20 suppl).
204. Rice D, Sheridan CA. Nursing care of patients with multiple myeloma: a paradigm for the needs of special population. *Clin J Oncol Nurs.* 2001;5:89–93.
205. Bertolotti P, Bilotti E, Colson K, et al. Management of side effects of novel therapies for multiple myeloma: consensus statements developed by the International Myeloma Foundation's Nurse Leadership Board. *Clin J Oncol Nurs.* 2008;12(suppl 3):9–12.
206. Ludwig H, Fritz E. Supportive therapy. In: Mehta J, Singhal S, eds. *Myeloma.* London: Martin Dunitz; 2002:397–412.
207. Poulos AR, Gertz MA, Pankratz VS, et al. Pain, mood disturbance, and quality of life in patients with multiple myeloma. *Oncol Nurs Forum.* 2001;28:1163–1172.
208. World Health Organization. WHO's pain relief ladder. http://www.who.int/cancer/palliative/painladder/en/. Accessed March 31, 2009
209. Struthers C, Mayer D, Fisher G. Nursing management of the patient with bone metastasis. *Semin Oncol Nurs.* 1998;14:199–209.
210. Fellowes D, Barnes K, Wilkinson S. Aromatherapy and massage for symptom relief in patients with cancer. *Cochrane Database Syst Rev.* 2004;002287.2.
211. Body JJ. Dosing regimens and main adverse events of bisphosphonates. *Semin Oncol.* 2001;28(suppl 11):49–53.
212. Major PP, Coleman RE. Zoledronic acid in the treatment of hypercalcemia of malignancy: Results of the International Clinical Development Program. *Semin Oncol.* 2001;28(suppl 3):17–24.
213. Tariman JD, Love G, McCullagh E, Sandifer S. Peripheral neuropathy associated with novel therapies in patients with multiple myeloma: consensus statement of the IMF Nurse Leadership Board. *Clin J Oncol Nurs.* 2008;12(suppl 3):29–36.
214. Blade J, Rosinol L. Complications of multiple myeloma. *Hematol Oncol Clin North Am.* 2007;21:1231–1246.
215. Redeker NS, Lev EL, Ruggiero J. Insomnia, fatigue, anxiety, depression, and quality of life of cancer patients undergoing chemotherapy. *Sch Inq Nurs Pract.* 2000;14:275–290, discussion 291–298.
216. Malpas JS, Bergsagel DE, Kyle R, Anderson K. Eds. *Myeloma Biology and Management.* 3rd ed. Philadelphia, PA: Saunders; 2004.
217. Miceli T, Colson K, Gavino M, et al. Myelosuppression associated with novel therapies in patients with multiple myeloma: consensus statement of the IMF Nurse Leadership Board. *Clin J Oncol Nurs.* 2008;12(suppl 3):13–20.
218. Ozer H, Armitage JO, Bennett CL, et al. ASCO 2000 update of recommendations for the use of hematopoietic colony-stimulating factors: evidence-based, clinical practice guidelines. *J Clin Oncol.* 2000;18:3558–3585.
219. Chanan-Khan A, Sonneveld P, Schuster M, et al. Analysis of varicella zoster virus reactivation among bortezomib-treated patients in the APEX study. *Blood.* 2006;108:Abstract 3535. http://abstracts.hematologylibrary.org/cgi/content/abstract/108/11/3535. Accessed February 20, 2010.
220. Kroger A, Atkinson W, Marcuse E, Pickering L. Centers for Disease Control and Prevention. Recommendations of the Advisory Committee on the Immunization Practices. 2006. http://www.cdc.gov/mmwr/preview/mmwrhtml/rr5515a1.htm. Accessed February 20, 2010.
221. Rizzo JD, Lichtin AE, Woolf SH, et al. Use of epoetin in patients with cancer: evidence-based clinical practice guidelines of the American Society of Clinical Oncology and the American Society of Hematology. *J Clin Oncol.* 2002;20:4083–4107.
222. Desikan KR, Barlogie B, Jagannath S, et al. Comparable engraftment kinetics following peripheral blood stem cell infusion mobilized with granulocyte colony stimulating factor with or without cyclophosphamide in multiple myeloma. *J Clin Oncol.* 1998;16:1547–1553.
223. Alegre A, Diaz-Mediavilla J, San Miguel J, et al. Autologous peripheral blood stem cell transplantation for multiple myeloma: a report of 259 cases from the Spanish Registry. Spanish Registry for Transplant in MM (Grupo Espanol de Trasplante Hematopoyetico-GETH) and PETHEMA. *Bone Marrow Transplant.* 1998;21:133–140.
224. Weaver CH, Zhen B, Schwartzberg LS, et al. Phase I-II evaluation of rapid sequence tandem high-dose melphalan with peripheral blood stem cell support in patients with multiple myeloma. *Bone Marrow Transplant.* 1998;22:245–251.
225. MMWR. Prevention of pneumococcal disease: recommendations of the Advisory Committee on Immunization Practices (ACIP). *MMWR Recomm Rep.* 1997;46:1–24.
226. Lynch MP. *Oncology Nursing Essentials.* New York, NY: Professional Publishing Group;2002:112.
227. Coleman EA, Coon S, Hall-Barrow J, et al. Feasibility of exercise during treatment for multiple myeloma. *Cancer Nurs.* 2003;26:410–419.
228. Vonkeman HE, van de Laar MA. Nonsteroidal anti-inflammatory drugs: adverse effects and their prevention. *Semin Arthritis Rheum.* 2008 Sep 27 [Epub ahead of print].
229. Brincat S, Hilton R. Prevention of acute kidney injury. *Br J Hosp Med (Lond).* 2008;69:450–454.
230. Taber SS, Mueller BA. Drug-associated renal dysfunction. *Crit Care Clin.* 2006;22:357–374.
231. Izzedine H, Launay-Vacher V, Deray G. Antiviral drug-induced nephrotoxicity. *Am J Kidney Dis.* 2005;45:804–817.
232. Attal M, Harousseau JL, Facon T, et al. Single versus double autologous stem-cell transplantation for multiple myeloma. *N Engl J Med.* 2003;349:2495–2502.

233. Mehta J. Allogeneic hematopoietic stem cell transplantation in myeloma. In: Mehta J, Singhal S, eds. *Myeloma*. London: Martin Dunitz;2002:349–365.
234. Anderson KC. Novel therapies for multiple myeloma. *Br J Haematol.* 2003;120:10–17.
235. Mooberry SL. New insights into 2-methoxyestradiol, a promising antiangiogenic and antitumor agent. *Curr Opin Oncol.* 2003; 15:425–430.
236. Chauhan D, Catley L, Hideshima T, et al. 2-Methoxyestradiol overcomes drug resistance in multiple myeloma cells. *Blood.* 2002;100:2187–2194.
237. Lin B, Podar K, Gupta D, et al. The vascular endothelial growth factor receptor tyrosine kinase inhibitor PTK787/ZK222584 inhibits growth and migration of multiple myeloma cells in the bone marrow microenvironment. *Cancer Res.* 2002;62:5019–5026.
238. Catley L, Weisberg E, Tai YT, et al. NVP-LAQ824 is a potent novel histone deacetylase inhibitor with significant activity against multiple myeloma. *Blood.* 2003;102:2615–2622.
239. Santucci R, Mackley PA, Sebti S, et al. Farnesyl transferase inhibitors and their role in the treatment of multiple myeloma. *Cancer Control.* 2003;10:384–387.
240. Ochiai N, Uchida R, Fuchida S, et al. Effect of farnesyl transferase inhibitor R115777 on the growth of fresh and cloned myeloma cells in vitro. *Blood.* 2003;102:3349–3353.
241. Alsina M, Fonseca R, Wilson EF, et al. The farnesyl transferase inhibitor Zanestra is well tolerated, induces stabilization of disease and inhibits farnesylation and oncogenic/tumor survival pathways in patients with advanced multiple myeloma. *Blood Online.* 2004. DOI 10.1182/Blood-2003-08-2764.
242. Mitsiades CS, Mitsiades NS, McMullan CJ, et al. Transcriptional signature of histone deacetylase inhibition in multiple myeloma: biological and clinical applications. *Proc Natl Acad Sci USA.* 2004;101:540–545.
243. Vanderkerken K, De Leenheer E, Shipman C, et al. Recombinant osteoprotegerin decreases tumor burden and increases survival in murine model of multiple myeloma. *Cancer Res.* 2003;63:287–289.
244. Streetly MJ, Gyertson K, Daniel Y, et al. Alternate day pomalidomide retains anti-myeloma effect with reduced adverse events and evidence of in vivo immunomodulation. *Br J Haematol.* 2008;141:41–51.
245. Kuhn, DJ, Chen Q, Voorhees PM, et al. Potent activity of carfilzomib, a novel, irreversible inhibitor of the ubiquitin-proteasome pathway, against preclinical models of multiple myeloma. *Blood.* 2007; 110:3281–3290.
246. National Institute of Health. A study of tanespimycin (KOS-953) in patients with multiple myeloma in first relapse (TIME-1). http://clinicaltrials.gov/ct2/show/NCT00546780. Accessed February 20, 2010.
247. Attal M, Harousseau JL, Facon T, et al. Double autologous transplantation improves survival of multiple myeloma patients: final analysis of a prospective randomized study of the Intergroupe Francophone du Myelome (IFM 94). *Blood.* 2002;100:5a (Abstract 7).
248. Yi Q. Immunotherapy in multiple myeloma: current strategies and future prospects. *Expert Rev Vaccines.* 2003;2:391–398.
249. Zhan F, Hardin J, Kordsmeier B, et al. Global gene expression profiling multiple myeloma, monoclonal gammopathy of undetermined significance, and normal bone marrow plasma cells. *Blood.* 2002;99:1745–1757.
250. Bumm K, Zheng M, Bailey C, et al. CGO: utilizing and integrating gene expression microarray data in clinical research and data management. *Bioinformatics.* 2002;18:327–338.
251. Skeel RT. Measurement of outcomes in supportive oncology. In: Weissman DE, ed. *Principles and Practices of Supportive Oncology.* Philadelphia, PA: Lippincott-Raven; 1998:875–888.

CHAPTER 62

Virginia R. Martin, MSN, RN, AOCN®

# Ovarian Cancer

## INTRODUCTION

Remarkable progress has been made in the understanding and management of ovarian cancer. It is now known that there is a genetic basis for hereditary ovarian cancer and screening efforts can target those at high risk; the roles of cytoreductive surgery and accurate staging of the disease are now well defined; and effective adjuvant chemotherapy treatment is available for advanced disease. Yet considerable work remains before the origin and biology of the disease are completely elucidated and, more important, before specific and sensitive tests to detect the disease in its early curable stages can be developed. For years ovarian cancer has been characterized as a "silent killer." This label has been largely dispelled by women affected by the disease. Patients with ovarian cancer have found a powerful voice through coalition and advocacy groups, which speak out for research funding and other issues. The National Ovarian Cancer Coalition has launched a national education program to raise awareness and encourage a public dialogue about the symptoms and risk factors for ovarian cancer called "Break the Silence." The Ovarian Cancer National Alliance (OCNA) mission is to conquer ovarian cancer by uniting individuals and organizations in a national movement. Both organizations helped support and endorse a consensus statement in June 2007 that outlined symptoms that were more likely to occur in women with ovarian cancer than in the general population.

## EPIDEMIOLOGY

Ovarian cancer is the most lethal of the gynecologic cancers. Its incidence is about one-half that of endometrial cancer; however, its mortality rate in the Western world exceeds that of cervical and endometrial cancers combined. In 2009, 21,550 new cases were predicted in the United States and 14,600 deaths.[1] This disease accounts for only 3% of all cancer cases in women but, more notably, is the fifth leading cause of cancer death in women. Over a lifetime, 1 in every 72 women will develop ovarian cancer. The lifetime risk of this disease in the general population is 1.8%; unfortunately, three-fourths of those individuals will have advanced disease at diagnosis.[2] Ovarian cancer occurs primarily in women ages 40 to 70. The mean age of occurrence is 63, but the mean age of diagnosis for women with a family history is 54.[3] The incidence of ovarian cancer is highest in women between the ages of 45 and 85 (see Table 62-1).[4]

Ovarian cancer has a wide variation in international incidence rates, with the highest rates found in North America, Scandinavia, and Eastern Europe. The lowest incidence is in Japan and in developing countries. Caucasians develop ovarian cancer slightly more frequently than African Americans. During the period from 1987 to 2004, ovarian cancer incidence declined at a rate of 0.9% per year.[1]

**TABLE 62-1**

**SEER Incidence of Ovarian Cancer by Age**

| Incidence, % | Age |
|---|---|
| 1.3 | Under age 20 |
| 3.4 | 20–34 |
| 7.9 | 35–44 |
| 19.0 | 45–54 |
| 21.8 | 55–64 |
| 20 | 65–74 |
| 19.2 | 75–84 |
| 7.4 | ≥ 85 |

*Source*: Surveillance, Epidemiology, and End Results.[4]

## ETIOLOGY

Hormonal, environmental, and genetic factors all play roles in the development of ovarian cancer. The major risk and preventive factors for ovarian cancer are summarized in Table 62-2. The factors that attract the most attention are those that are related to hormonal and reproductive issues.

### REPRODUCTIVE AND HORMONAL

The ovaries are located in the pelvis lateral to the uterus, and slightly posterior and caudal to the fallopian tubes (Figure 62-1).[5] Due to endocrine stimulation, the ovaries change size, shape, position, and histology during the monthly menstrual cycle and during their lifetime.[5] The ovary is surrounded by a single layer of peritoneal mesothelium. As the epithelium transforms, it becomes more differentiated which is in contrast to other malignancies. The epithelium can differentiate to a cell type found in the mullerian tract including fallopian tube, uterus, cervix, and ovarian stroma.[6,7] It is postulated that most ovarian cancers develop from the surface epithelium or postovulatory inclusion cysts that are subjected to exposure of hormones or cytokines.[6,8] Primary peritoneal and fallopian tube cancers have similar profiles to ovarian cancer and are considered variations of ovarian cancer. Recent pathological examination of ovarian cancer cases suggests that a percentage of ovarian cancers higher than expected may actually have a fallopian origin with metastasis to the ovary.[9]

The monthly ovulatory cycle in women and its effects on the ovarian epithelium are the focus of the hormonal etiology. Three hypotheses have been proposed to explain the basis of ovarian cancer: the incessant ovulation theory, excessive gonadotropin stimulation, and inflammation.

**TABLE 62-2**

**Risk Factors and Preventive Factors in Ovarian Cancer**

| Risk Factors | Preventive Factors |
|---|---|
| Nulliparity | Parity |
| Use of infertility drugs | Lactation |
| Pelvic inflammatory disease | Oral contraceptives |
| Low serum gonadotropin | Tubal ligation |
| Use of talc | Oophorectomy |
| Family history of breast or ovarian cancer | |
| Living in industrialized Western countries | |
| Being of Jewish descent | |

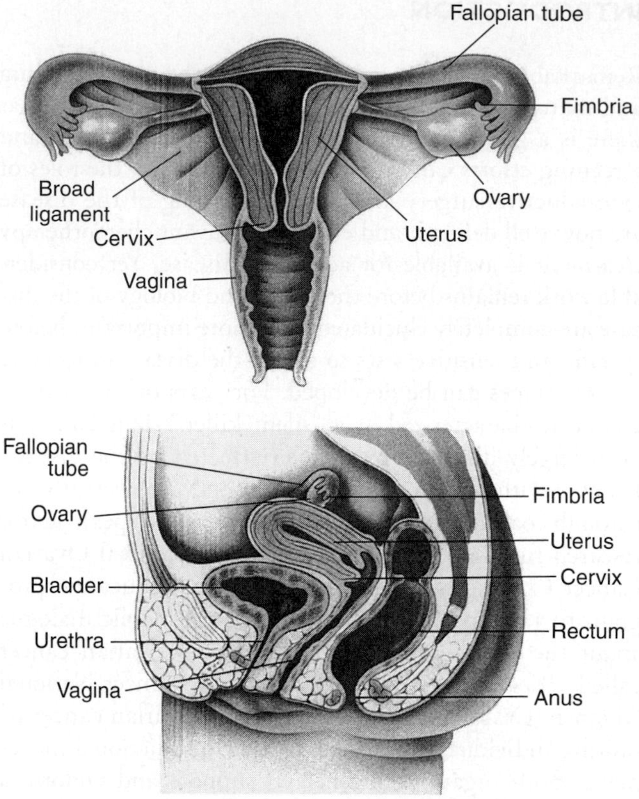


**FIGURE 62-1**

Female reproductive system. The ovaries are located deep in the pelvis, which makes it difficult to detect ovarian cancer at an early stage. Reprinted with permission from Eriksson and Frazier.[5]

The classic incessant ovulation hypothesis postulates that the uninterrupted cell division and regeneration of the ovarian epithelium provides an opportunity for mutation and malignant transformation without pregnancy-induced rest periods, which contributes to neoplasia of the ovary.[10] Some laboratory experiments have supported this theory by showing that higher ovulatory activity is associated with more inclusion cysts and other changes in the surface of the ovary.[11] Studies of the ovaries of women with significant family histories have reported more changes in the surface epithelium compared to control ovaries.[12] This theory is supported by epidemiological data indicating that the risk of ovarian cancer is inverse to the following circumstances that suppress ovulation: the use of oral contraceptives, breast-feeding (especially long term), and the number of pregnancies.

The gonadotropin theory postulates that the ovarian epithelium repeatedly invaginates throughout life to form clefts and inclusion cysts within the ovary. Inclusion cysts are postulated to occur when surface cells of the ovary find their way into the stroma (or connecting tissue) and become trapped. It suggests that, under excessive gonadotropin stimulation of the ovarian stroma by follicle-stimulating hormone (FSH) and by lutenizing hormone (LH) may place the cells of the epithelium at risk for proliferation and eventually malignant transformation.[6] The risk of infertile women using fertility drugs led researchers to this hypothesis; however, further studies have been inconsistent in this association and suggest instead that the condition of infertility is responsible for the increased risk.[9,13]

Ness and Cottreau[13] suggest that inflammation may have a role in disease development. Inflammation may help explain the increased risk associated with environmental factors, and inflammatory agents or conditions may increase risk by inducing cytokines, prostaglandins, and other stress responses that may be mutagenic. The exact cause of ovarian cancer remains unknown; these theories present mechanisms that may be involved in the role of carcinogenesis, but suggest multiple processes instead of 1 are more likely associated with the etiology. In addition, a recent study presents a possible 2-way pathway model of ovarian cancer carcinogenesis. These authors postulate that high-grade malignancies are rapidly growing, relatively chemosensitive, and without a precursor lesion; whereas, low-grade tumors grow more slowly, are less responsive to chemotherapy, and share malignant characteristics with low-malignant potential (LMP) neoplasms.[6]

## Parity, infertility, and lactation

Pregnancy has been associated with a protective effect in ovarian cancer risk. The highest risk women for developing ovarian cancer are the nulliparous women since these women tend to have more ovulatory cycles. There is a 6% increase in risk of ovarian cancer for each full ovulation year a woman experiences.[14,15] Infertility and its association with an increased risk for ovarian cancer remains controversial and unclear. Theories postulate that high circulating levels of gonadotropin and growth factor roles such as insulin-like growth factor may promote the development of ovarian cancer.[14] In addition, treatment for infertility with ovulation-induction agents has been studied as a possible causative factor but at this time risk has not been noted to be increased in women who had taken these agents.[14,16] Endometriosis, a common cause of infertility, has been linked to an increased risk of ovarian cancer. A possible theory is that these implants grow when local estradiol and inflammatory mediators are increased and this promotes angiogenesis, extracellular disintegration, cell proliferation, and abnormal apoptosis all of which may be a factor in the promotion of ovarian cancer.[17] Evidence also suggests that pelvic inflammatory disease, which may result in infertility, may stimulate proliferation of the surface epithelium of the ovary and increase the risk for those women.[18] Lactation is known to suppress ovulation in some women, and pregnancy with lactation appears protective. The protection from lactation is especially significant in nonmucinous types of ovarian cancer and the increased length of time of breast-feeding correlates with a decreased risk (18 months or greater providing the most protection).[19]

### Exogenous hormones

The use of oral contraceptives gives long-term protection against ovarian cancer; the longer they are used the greater the reduction in risk.[20] These authors found after collating 45 epidemiological studies that the use of contraceptives was estimated to reduce ovarian cancer incidence from 12 per 1000 to 8 per 1000 and mortality from 7 per 1000 to 5 per 1000.[20] There is not one clear recommendation on how long to take the pill or on which pill to use; however, it does appear that the protective effect lasts long after the pill has been discontinued.[21] These authors also noted that although estrogen doses in oral contraceptives have decreased over the years, there was no variation in the risk.[20] The protection mechanism is not well understood but there is evidence that the progestins are the most protective component of the oral contraceptives.[22] They may work by suppressing ovulation or by increasing cell death of abnormal ovarian cells. Carriers of the *BRCA1/BRCA2* mutations and the use of oral contraceptives were found to have a 38% risk reduction in long-term users of oral contraceptives in an international pooled analysis.[23] Some studies have shown a modest increase in the risk of ovarian cancer or ovarian cancer mortality with postmenopausal estrogen use, whereas other studies have not.[24–26]

### Endogenous hormones

Women with low serum gonadotropin levels (FSH and LH) are at an increased risk of ovarian cancer, as are women with high androstenedione and dehydroepiandrosterone (DHEA) levels.[27] Furthermore, women with a history of polycystic ovary syndrome and elevated androstenedione levels may be at increased risk of developing ovarian cancer.[28] Women with endometriosis experience a variety of hormone and immunological abnormalities and are thus at increased risk, as are women with more total ovulatory cycles in their lifetime.[29] Women who have more ovulatory cycles are at higher risk for having p53-positive tumors if they develop ovarian cancer, which lends support to the theory that a higher number of ovulatory cycles may lead to increased DNA damage.[30]

A tubal ligation or hysterectomy physically interrupts the utero-ovarian circulation, thereby decreasing the risk of developing epithelial ovarian cancer, especially endometrioid tumors.[31] It appears that because the route from the vagina to the ovaries is disrupted, exposure to exogenous toxins is likely to be diminished. The role of hormones in the etiology of ovarian cancer likely reflects a composite of factors. For example, among younger women with fewer menstrual cycles, aside from a family history, exposure to androgens may be the dominant factor; among older women, continuous uninterrupted ovulation and the greater number of menstrual cycles may be the most critical factor.[18]

## ENVIRONMENTAL

Industrialized countries, with the exception of Japan, have a higher incidence of ovarian cancer, which suggests the as-yet-unproven conclusion that environmental factors are somehow related to the etiology of ovarian cancer. Multiple dietary influences have been studied, however, and the results are not clear. Overweight and obesity have been linked to many cancers, ovarian cancer included, and obesity has been linked to an increase in mortality in ovarian cancer as well as other cancers. Galactose metabolism has been proposed as a risk factor for ovarian cancer based on data showing that galactose is toxic to oocytes. Galactosemic women have premature menopause and increased gonadotropin levels. One study[32] has supported this theory; others have not.[33,34] The American Cancer Society, the American Heart Association, and the American Diabetes Association have established healthy guidelines for preventing cancer, cardiovascular disease, and diabetes in response to the high proportion of overweight and obese Americans (Table 62-3).[35]

Increased activity and vigorous physical exercise may increase the number of anovulatory cycles, which may provide a protective effect against ovarian cancer. However, in direct contrast to this finding, women reporting regular leisure physical activity have a 1.5-fold greater risk, and women who exercise vigorously (more than 4 times per week) have been found to have a 2.5-fold greater risk of developing ovarian cancer.[36] Daly and Obrams[18] theorize that the rigorous activity has a negative effect on

**TABLE 62-3**

**Diet and Physical Activity Guidelines for Preventing Cancer, Cardiovascular Disease, and Diabetes**

| Diet | Physical Activity |
|---|---|
| Choose at least 5 servings of fruits and vegetables daily | Moderate exercise at least 30 minutes on 5 or more days per week |
| Choose whole-grain carbohydrates | |
| Limit: saturated fat, alcohol, and refined carbohydrates | |

circulating estrogen feedback and produces increased serum gonadotropins.

Cosmetic talc use in dusting the perineum, in feminine hygiene sprays, or on sanitary napkins, condoms, or diaphragms has also been suggested as a possible risk. A significant association between the use of talcum powder and the risk of developing ovarian cancer was not demonstrated even with prolonged exposure.[37] In the Nurses Health Study, no association was found between using talc and ovarian cancer incidence.[38] A recent review concluded that mechanistic, pathology, and animal model studies have not found evidence for a carcinogenic effect, and these data collectively do not indicate that cosmetic talc causes ovarian cancer.[39]

More research in the area of exercise, diet, and other potential environmental factors related to ovarian cancer is needed before final conclusions can be drawn.

## GENETICS

Of all the factors associated with increased risk of ovarian cancer, nothing alters the magnitude of risk, besides increasing age, than a family history of ovarian cancer.[18] Five to 10 percent of all ovarian cancers are due to an inherited predisposition of an altered gene. The number of family members with ovarian cancer defines the individual's degree of risk. If 1 family member has ovarian cancer, there is a 2-fold to 3-fold increased risk, leading to a lifetime risk of 4% to 5%.[40] If 2 or more family members have the disease, the lifetime risk increases to 7%.[40]

Families with multiple members with ovarian or breast cancer may exhibit a hereditary syndrome related to mutations in the *BRCA1* or *BRCA2* genes. *BRCA1* is located on chromosome 17 and is a tumor suppressor gene whose normal function is to inhibit the development of cancer. Mutations in this gene destroy its protective function and increase the chance of developing breast or ovarian cancer. A second breast cancer susceptibility locus on the long arm of chromosome 13q is the *BRCA2* gene.[41,42] *BRCA2* is associated with ovarian cancer, breast cancer, prostate cancer, head and neck cancer, malignant melanoma, and pancreatic cancer. Mutations in *BRCA1* and *BRCA2* are responsible for the hereditary breast/ovarian cancer syndrome (HBOC). Hereditary breast/ovarian cancer syndrome syndrome accounts for 85% of hereditary ovarian cancers.[5] Characteristics of the hereditary breast and ovarian cancer syndrome include multiple family members in the same lineage affected with breast and/or ovarian cancer; younger than typical age of onset (<50 years); more than 1 primary cancer in an individual; autosomal dominant pattern of inheritance; and male breast cancer.[21] Women with mutations of the *BRCA1* gene have up to a 45% lifetime risk of developing ovarian cancer, whereas the risk approaches 23% in *BRCA2* mutation carriers.[43] BRCA-1-associated ovarian cancer occurs at a younger age, median age at diagnosis mid-forties, whereas BRCA-2-associated ovarian cancers occur later, median age 63.[43] Women of Ashkenazi Jewish descent are a special population at risk and have *BRCA1* and *BRCA2* mutations that are carried by 1 in 40 women, as compared to by 1 carrier in 280 women in the general population.[44,45] Serous adenocarcinomas are part of the phenotype of *BRCA* germ-line mutation ovarian malignancies; mucinous and borderline tumors are not.[46]

Another 10% of hereditary ovarian cancers are attributed to alterations in DNA mismatch repair genes (*hMLH1*, *hMSH2*, *hMSH6*, and *PMS2*). Hereditary nonpolyposis colorectal cancer (HNPCC) or the family cancer syndrome known as Lynch II is the identified high-risk group.[47,48] The criteria for HNPCC include colon cancer in >3 relatives, one of whom is a first-degree relative of the other 2; colon cancer in at least 2 generations; 1 or more colon cancers diagnosed <50 years of age; and extracolonic cancers may be associated: ovary, uterine, stomach, kidney, biliary tract. Carriers of HNPCC-related gene alteration have a 9% to 12% lifetime risk of developing ovarian cancer.[49]

Families with either of these hereditary syndromes should be referred for cancer risk assessment counseling by professionals with training in cancer genetics. A national directory of trained genetic professionals can be found at http://www.cancer.gov/search/genetics_services. Commercial genetic testing is available and often covered by insurance.

## PREVENTION, SCREENING, AND EARLY DETECTION

The ovaries are located anatomically deep in the pelvis (see Figure 62-1), which is one reason why it is difficult to detect ovarian cancer at an early stage. An ovarian tumor can grow undiscovered until it becomes large and is detected on pelvic exam. Along with the pelvic exam, serum tumor markers and ultrasonography may be useful for screening in certain circumstances. Overall, however, these tests fail to detect ovarian cancer at an earlier, more curable stage. Neither ultrasound nor the CA-125 tumor marker has been shown to reduce morbidity or mortality of the disease, and neither is specific or sensitive enough to be recommended for general population screening.[50] The Prostate, Lung, Colorectal, and Ovarian screening trial has randomized 155,000 men and women to a screening or control arm and is ongoing in the United States studying both incidence and mortality rates. The UK Collaborative Trial of Ovarian Cancer Screening invited over 1 million women to participate and successfully recruited and enrolled 202,638 women to a randomized controlled trial to assess the impact of screening on mortality for ovarian cancer. Both trials have completed the enrollment part of the trial but continue to gain mature data and results of screening will not be known for some time.

Current research on potential new screening modalities is ongoing. New markers are being studied either alone or in combination with ultrasonography and proteomic screening with mass spectroscopy is a new area of research that holds promise.

## PELVIC EXAMINATION

An annual physical exam, including a pelvic examination with bimanual rectovaginal exam, is part of routine health care for women. The palpation of the ovaries during this exam is not established as a useful screening procedure for ovarian cancer. Pap smear should be performed during the exam, although this test does not provide valuable screening information in this disease. The size of the ovaries in premenopausal women can change. Palpation of a pelvic mass on pelvic exam is abnormal in postmenopausal women and is an indication for a diagnostic ultrasound.

## CA-125

CA-125 is a tumor antigen that is commonly elevated in ovarian cancer. Eighty percent or more of women with epithelial ovarian cancers have been found to have serum CA-125 titers greater than 35 U/mL, whereas just 1% of healthy women have serum CA-125 titers at this level.[51] However, population screening studies found that only 50% of primary ovarian carcinomas confined to the ovary (stage I) are associated with elevated CA-125 levels.[52] Serum CA-125 determinations, while encouraging, are not sufficiently sensitive or specific enough to recommend them as a single test for population screening, particularly for premenopausal women.[52] Therefore, CA-125 is not helpful in the screening of the general population, although 75% to 90% of women diagnosed with ovarian cancer will have an elevated CA-125 level.[51] An elevated CA-125 level in asymptomatic women may indicate the presence of cancer; if the CA-125 level is normal in women with an ovarian mass, however, it does not rule out ovarian cancer. This level can be elevated in multiple benign or other malignant diseases (Table 62-4).[53]

The rate of change of the CA-125 level over time appears to be a more specific screening method. A large prospective study in postmenopausal women with 2 or more longitudinal measurements of the CA-125 level found an improvement in sensitivity for the detection of ovarian cancer.[54] This finding led to the development of the Risk of Ovarian Cancer Algorithm (ROCA). It is currently being studied in a multicenter trial where high-risk women have the blood test performed every 3 months.[49,50]

If the CA-125 level is elevated prior to diagnosis, it is an important indicator of early treatment failure during frontline therapy. Further, this biomarker is of proven value in confirmation of disease relapse, and its measurement during treatment can serve as a tool to evaluate response to therapy.[55]

**TABLE 62-4**

| Conditions Associated With an Increased CA-125 Level |
|---|
| Ovarian cancer |
| Endometriosis |
| Fibroids |
| Hemorrhagic ovarian cysts |
| Menstruation |
| Pelvic inflammatory disease (acute) |
| Pregnancy (first trimester) |
| Acute pancreatitis |
| Colitis |
| Chronic active hepatitis |
| Cirrhosis |
| Diverticulitis |
| Pericarditis |
| Renal disease (serum creatinine > 2.0 mg/dl) |
| Polyarteritis nodosa |
| Sjogren syndrome |
| Systemic lupus erythematosus |
| Other malignancies: bladder, breast, endometrium, lung, liver, non-Hodgkin's lymphoma, pancreas |

*Source*: Reprinted with permission from Rosenthal and Jacobs.[53]

## ULTRASONOGRAPHY

Although transabdominal ultrasound provides information on the characteristics of an ovarian mass and the presence or absence of ascites, it does not provide a definitive diagnosis. Ultrasound is unable to differentiate between a benign, functional, or malignant mass.

The transabdominal method has been replaced by the transvaginal method, which allows a closer evaluation of the ovaries via a probe placed in the vagina. Transvaginal ultrasound (TVS) permits superior visualization with shorter examination times, more comfort, and greater patient acceptance. Although color Doppler imaging is sometimes used with ultrasound to measure the blood flow patterns in ovarian vessels, the early enthusiasm for the addition of color Doppler imaging has not been supported.[56] Annual TVS was performed on 25,327 asymptomatic women from 1987 to 2005. TVS was found to have an 85% sensitivity, 98.7% specificity on the 364 women with persisting ovarian tumors.[57] This study concludes that TVS performed annually was associated with a decrease in disease stage at detection, but it was not effective in detecting ovarian cancers in women who had normal ovarian volume.[57]

## PROTEOMICS

Proteomic screening is one of the more sensitive and specific screening tests expected to be used in the future for ovarian cancer detection. Proteomics, the study of protein patterns in the blood, documents the consequences of genetic changes, including protein mutation, rearrangement, loss, amplification, or silencing of genes.[58] In June 2008, LabCorp announced the availability of a new serum-based diagnostic test for ovarian cancer called OvaSure. The study results reported a 99% accuracy with 6 protein markers to detect early-stage ovarian cancer.[58] The 6 biomarkers used in the study were leptin, prolactin, osteoporin, insulin-like growth factor II, macrophage inhibitory factor, and CA-125 in a multiplex immunoassay. The release of this test and the results it is based on are biased according to US Food and Drug Administration and need clinical validation. The Society of Gynecologic Oncologists issued a statement that it is their opinion additional research is needed to validate the test's effectiveness. Therefore at this time there remains no currently available test to detect ovarian cancer in its earliest and most curable stages.

Routine screening with pelvic examination, CA-125, and ultrasound is not recommended for the general population. However, intensive screening using a combination of the methods available should be used for women with familial or hereditary risk factors. These women should be referred for cancer risk assessment by professionals with specialized training in cancer genetics. Pedigree analysis, linkage studies, and/or DNA testing are done to determine genetic risk.[48] The process of determining genetic risk begins with information about the availability of DNA testing. Genetic counseling is mandatory prior to DNA testing and at the time of disclosure of the findings. It is the clinician's role to provide detailed information regarding the inheritance and natural history of ovarian cancer as well as advantages and limitations of genetic testing, surveillance, and management strategies. If a patient does not have an increased genetic risk based on the DNA testing, then she should return to the general population screening recommendations.

For those women with a defined risk profile, one of the following is recommended: increased surveillance, surgical prophylaxis, pharmacologic interventions (chemoprevention), or lifestyle changes. Screening and surveillance with baseline and interval multiple serum tumor markers and pelvic TVS are recommended for women at high risk. The National Comprehensive Cancer Network (NCCN) has published screening guidelines with criteria for identifying women with HBOC. The screening measures include an annual pelvic exam and TVS, plus a CA-125 level on an annual or semi-annual basis starting at age 25 to 35. Prophylactic oophorectomy should be considered on a case-by-case basis.[49] The International Collaborative Group on HNPCC have published the following guidelines for screening: (1) colonoscopy starting at age 20 to 25, repeat every 2 years to age 35, then annually; (2) annual endometrial curettage beginning at age 30; and (3) ovarian cancer screening with TVS, Doppler color blood flow, and serum CA-125 annually after the age of 30.[49]

Women should be counseled to eat a balanced diet, restrict fat and carbohydrate intake, and maintain a reasonable weight. High-risk women may also elect to take medicine to suppress ovulation or consider prophylactic oophorectomy at the completion of childbearing. Elective removal of the ovaries is an option chosen by women at high risk with increasing frequency. Bilateral salpingoophorectomy (BSO) surgery in women with *BRCA 1* mutation affords a risk reduction of 85% to 96%.[59] Counseling is indicated as the risk is not reduced by 100% and there is a 5% risk of primary peritoneal cancer after oophorectomy. Breast cancer risk is also reduced by BSO in *BRCA1/BRCA2* carriers by 50%.[59] It is important to note that the fallopian tubes should always be removed since occult cancers are found in the tubes following this surgery. The decision to have this surgery for women of this young age group is not an easy decision. Premenopausal women will experience an abrupt surgical menopause with hot flashes, vaginal dryness, urinary tract infections, loss of libido, joint pains, and possibly osteoporosis. A multidisciplinary team at a comprehensive cancer center developed a resource for women considering the surgery that provides a thorough examination of the pros and cons and expected and possible side effects. This resource is available free by emailing surgerybook@fccc.edu.

Video laparoscopy is a method to examine the undersurfaces of the diaphragm, the peritoneum, serosal surfaces, and the pelvic contents. Members of families that have autosomal dominant hereditary cancer syndrome are encouraged to participate in studies to detect early precancerous and cancerous changes in their ovaries through programs that test and evaluate the screening methods now available.[46]

In the past, it was recommended that women in families vulnerable to HBOC and HNPCC syndrome take combined estrogen–progestin oral contraceptives before plans for conception and between pregnancies.[47] Oral contraceptives have since been linked to an increased risk for breast cancer among younger women, so it is no longer recommended for the HBOC syndrome families. Oral contraceptives are recommended for HNPCC families not genetically at risk for breast cancer.[47] Other agents in chemoprevention pilot studies include retinoids, progestational agents, and COX-2 inhibitors.

Women with hereditary ovarian cancer are usually diagnosed at an earlier age (early 40s and younger) than women with sporadic ovarian cancer. The mean age for developing ovarian cancer in HBOC families is 51 years, compared to 43 years for HNPCC syndrome.[48] The youngest age observed was 26 years for HBOC, and 24 years for HNPCC syndrome.[48] For these reasons, genetic counseling of high-risk females should begin in their teenage years.

At present, the recommendations for the general population state that any woman older than age 18 should see a physician yearly for a thorough physical examination that should include a bimanual rectovaginal examination. With the tests currently available, routine screening for ovarian cancer is not recommended.[40] Asymptomatic women may consider discussing with their practitioner the use of oral contraceptives and tubal ligation for increased protection. Although a very personal decision, another method of risk reduction is parity.

## PATHOPHYSIOLOGY

### BIOLOGY

The molecular events that underlie ovarian cancer development remain to be discovered. Although the exact mechanism of transformation is not clear, ovarian cancer appears to arise from a multistep process that entails the accumulation of mutations in multiple combinations of genes.[60] The normal ovarian epithelial cell has mechanisms that control its growth and differentiation. Cancer development involves alterations in many specific genes, including protooncogenes, tumor suppressor genes, and DNA repair genes. Ovarian cancer has demonstrated defects in genes such as *AKT, EGFR, ERBB2, RAS, PIK3CA, MYC, DOC-2l BAB2*, y-synuclein (*SNCG*), and *TP53*.[11,61] Penetration of the tumor cells through the basement membrane is a prerequisite for metastatic disease. The combination of genetic changes that determine the malignant phenotype, with its ability to invade and metastasize, accounts for the lethality of the disease.

The most common type of ovarian cancer is the epithelial type, which accounts for 90% of the disease. Germ cell or sex-cord stromal cell tumors constitute the majority of nonepithelial tumors. Ovarian tumors range from benign, to tumors of LMP, to invasive cancer. Epithelial cancer is further classified according to its behavior—either as borderline or invasive—and the cell type. Serous or mucinous types are the most common classifications of epithelial tumors. The epithelial type originates from the cells on the surface of the germinal epithelium or the mesothelium of the ovary. The remaining tumors arise from the germ or stromal cells. Germ cells are precursors of the ova; the most common type of malignancy is dysgerminoma. Sex-cord stromal cells secrete hormones and connect the different components of the ovary together; the most common tumor is the granulosa cell tumor.

Metastasis in epithelial ovarian cancer can often occur by direct extension. The malignancy penetrates the capsule of the ovary and invades the structures next to it. It can also spread by lymphatic dissemination, most frequently the pelvic or aortic lymph nodes. Rarely it spreads by blood-borne metastases. The continuous circulation of the peritoneal fluid in the peritoneal cavity facilitates the widespread dissemination of the malignant cells. This process may be referred to as peritoneal seeding. Disease spreads to the liver, diaphragm, bladder, or intestines by this route (Figure 62-2).[62]

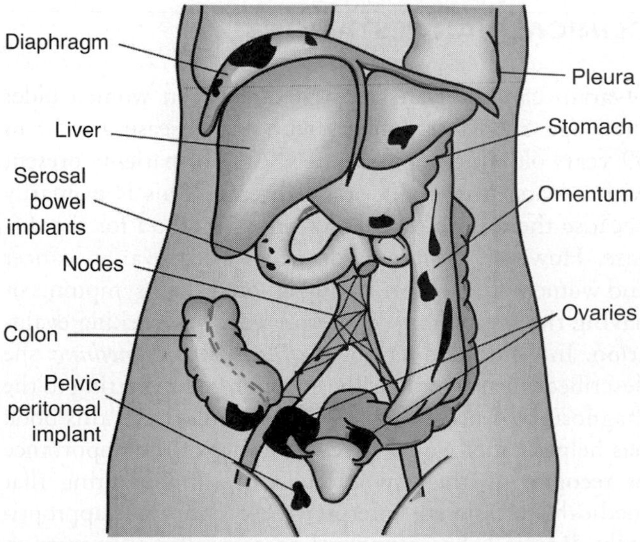


**FIGURE 62-2**

Typical sites of metastases.

*Source*: Adapted with permission from DiSaia.[62]

## PROGNOSTIC FACTORS

In terms of patient characteristics, age and performance status correlate with outcome. A patient with a good performance status (Easter Cooperative Oncology Group [ECOG] 0-2) is more likely to respond to treatment and experience less toxicity and a better outcome.[63–65] In a classic study that is true today, the Gynecology Oncology Group (GOG) reported age as a prognostic variable in 2000 patients participating in 6 trials.[66] Patients older than age 69 had a poorer survival compared to those younger than age 50. Histological subtypes and grades are significant, clear cell, and mucinous. Poorly differentiated tumors have the worst prognosis. The volume of disease after surgery is also significant: the more disease, the poorer the prognosis. The standard prognostic indicators are subjective and far from sufficient to predict prognosis. Abnormalities of oncogenes, such as *p53*, *MYC*, *RAS*, *ERB-2*, and tumor suppressor genes, have been reported to have prognostic importance; likewise, the expression of certain growth factors may be associated with poor prognosis.[67] The prognostic significance of *p53* mutations and overexpression was examined in 125 patients and *p53* alterations were found to be common. A mutation in *p53* was associated with a short-term survival benefit.[67] Other prognostic factors under investigation include DNA ploidy, proliferation activity (S-phase fraction), tumor markers, flow cytometry, and factors regulating transformation and growth.[68] It is still too early to completely understand the significance of these findings related to the development of ovarian cancer or the progression of the disease and to apply the findings to clinical practice.

## CLINICAL MANIFESTATIONS

Ovarian cancer occurs most frequently in women older than age 50. Most patients with the disease are 50 to 59 years old, and approximately 70% of patients present with advanced-stage III or IV disease. This is primarily because there is no reliable screening method for the disease. However, symptoms do occur with ovarian cancer and women often report having ignored their symptoms or having the symptoms misinterpreted when seeking evaluation. In Gilda Radner's book, *It's Always Something*, she described the frustrations she encountered in getting to the diagnosis of ovarian cancer.[69] The popularity of this book has helped other women become aware of the importance of recognizing their symptoms early and insisting that medical professionals interpret these symptoms appropriately. Research has supported that specific symptoms in conjunction with their frequency and duration were useful identifying women with ovarian cancer.[70] In 2007, the Gynecologic Cancer Foundation, Society of Gynecologic Oncologists, and American Cancer Society released an Ovarian Symptom Consensus Statement highlighting symptoms that occur more frequently in women with ovarian cancer than the general population. The symptoms include bloating, pelvic or abdominal pain, difficulty eating or feeling full quickly, and urinary symptoms (urgency or frequency) (Table 62-5). The recommendation is that women who experience these symptoms for more than a few weeks to see their healthcare provider for a pelvic exam. Even though the presence of these symptoms do not represent a step forward in screening for the disease, awareness of symptoms is best and the diagnosis at a potentially earlier stage may lead to an improvement in survival.

## ASSESSMENT

During a physical assessment, the most important finding is the presence of an ovarian mass. A mass is considered suspicious if it is immobile and painless, if it is irregular, if there is bilateral ovarian involvement, or if any other mass is found on exam.[5] In premenopausal women, enlarged ovaries are common due to functioning ovarian cysts or benign ovarian cysts. It is common practice for the physician to observe an ovarian mass through several menstrual cycles because it may typically regress in 1 to 3 cycles. If the mass measures 8 cm or less on exam, observation is indicated. If the mass is greater than 10 cm or enlarges beyond 5 cm while under observation, further evaluation is indicated.[5] A physician may also prescribe oral contraceptives for these patients, expecting the mass to disappear. Masses that persist need investigation, including a CA-125 and a TVS. Ultrasound should reveal if the mass has irregular borders, presence of solid components with papillary projections, or bilateral involvement or multiple dense irregular septae. If any of these characteristics are present, a malignancy is suspected.[5]

After these studies document an abnormality, a computerized tomography (CT) scan of the abdomen and

**TABLE 62-5**

| Ovarian Cancer Symptoms |
|---|
| Bloating |
| Pelvic or abdominal pain |
| Difficulty eating or feeling full quickly |
| Urinary symptoms (urgency or frequency) |

*Note*: Women with persistent symptoms that represent a change from normal and are noticed almost daily for more than a few weeks should see a doctor, preferably a gynecologist.

The frequency of the symptoms and the number of the symptoms are key factors.

pelvis with oral and intravenous (IV) contrast is ordered to assess the entire area. Particular attention is paid to the lymph nodes in the retroperitoneal and para-aortic areas. A barium enema or colonoscopy may be ordered if cancer is present or suspected or if the patient has symptoms. A chest x-ray, mammogram, and a baseline CA-125 complete the metastatic work-up prior to surgery. The patient should be referred to a gynecologic oncologist. Research has demonstrated that patients experience increased disease-free and overall survival when a gynecologic oncologist is part of the management team.[71–73]

## CLASSIFICATION AND STAGING

The more than 30 types of ovarian cancer are classified by their cells of origin. The World Health Organization (WHO) and the International Federation of Gynecology and Obstetrics (FIGO) histologic classification is presented in Table 62-6.[74] This classification system reflects the cell type, the location of the tumor, and the degree of malignancy.

Ovarian cancer is a surgically staged disease and the FIGO staging system is used universally (Table 62-7).[75] FIGO stage is the most important prognostic variable—hence the need for rigorous surgical staging. Table 62-8[76] outlines survival based on FIGO stage.[77] Surgery provides the tissue for diagnosis, the surgeon assesses the extent of disease, and maximum cytoreduction is the goal. Studies have shown the amount of disease remaining after surgery inversely correlates with survival and the goal of cytoreductive surgery is to have no residual disease greater than 1 cm left behind as defined by the GOG.[78–80] Two studies have provided evidence that challenges this definition of optimal

**TABLE 62-6**

| World Health Organization Classification of Malignant Ovarian Tumors |
|---|
| **Common Epithelial Tumors** |
| **Malignant Serous Tumors** |
| Adenocarcinoma, papillary, papillary cystadenocarcinoma |
| Surface papillary carcinoma |
| Malignant adenofibroma, cystadenofibroma |
| **Malignant Mucinous Tumors** |
| Adenocarcinoma, cystadenocarcinoma |
| Malignant adenofibroma, cystadenofibroma |
| **Malignant Endometrioid Tumors** |
| Carcinoma |
| — Adenocarcinoma |
| — Adenoacanthoma |
| — Malignant adenofibroma, cystadenofibroma |
| Endometrioid stromal sarcomas |
| Mesodermal (müllerian) mixed tumors; homologous and heterologous |
| Clear cell (mesonephroid) tumors, malignant carcinoma, and adenocarcinoma |
| Brenner tumors, malignant |
| Mixed epithelial tumors, malignant |
| Undifferentiated carcinoma |
| Unclassified |
| **Sex-Cord Stromal Tumors** |
| **Granulosa–Stromal Cell Tumors** |
| Granulosa cell tumor |
| Tumors in the thecoma-fibroma group |
| Fibroma |
| Unclassified |
| **Androblastomas: Sertoli-Leydig Cell Tumors** |
| Well differentiated |
| Tubular androblastoma, Sertoli cell tumor (tubular adenoma of Pick) |
| Tubular androblastoma with lipid storage, Sertoli cell tumor with lipid storage (folliculoma lipidique of Lecene) |
| Sertoli-Leydig tumor, hilus cell tumor of intermediate differentiation |
| Poorly differentiated (sarcomatoid) with heterologous elements |
| Gynandroblastoma |
| Unclassified |
| **Lipid (Lipoid) Cell Tumors** |
| **Germ Cell Tumors** |
| Dysgerminoma |
| Endodermal sinus tumor |
| Embryonal carcinoma |
| Polyembryoma |
| Choriocarcinoma |
| Teratomas |
| — Immature |
| — Mature dermoid cyst with malignant transformation |
| — Monodermal and highly specialized |
| — — Struma ovarii |
| — — Carcinoid |
| — — Struma ovarii and carcinoid |
| — — Others |
| — Mixed forms |
| **Gonadoblastoma** |
| Pure |
| Mixed with dysgerminoma or other form of germ cell tumor |

**TABLE 62-7**

**Staging for Ovarian Cancer: International Federation of Obstetrics and Gynecology**

| Stage | Description |
|---|---|
| Stage I | Growth limited to the ovaries |
| Stage IA | Growth limited to one ovary, no ascites; no tumor on the external surface, capsule intact |
| Stage IB | Growth limited to both ovaries, no ascites; no tumor on the external surface, capsules intact |
| Stage IC[a] | Tumor stage IA or IB but with tumor on the surface of one or both ovaries, with capsule ruptured, with ascites present containing malignant cells, or with positive peritoneal washings |
| Stage II | Growth involving one or both ovaries with pelvic extension |
| Stage IIA | Extension or metastases to the uterus or tubes |
| Stage IIB | Growth involving one or both ovaries with pelvic extension |
| Stage IIC[a] | Tumor either stage IIA or IIB with tumor on the surface of one or both ovaries, with capsules ruptured, with ascites present containing malignant cells, or with positive peritoneal washings |
| Stage III | Tumor involving one or both ovaries with peritoneal implants outside the pelvis or positive retroperitoneal or inguinal nodes; superficial liver metastases equal stage III; tumor limited to the true pelvis but with histologically verified malignant extension to small bowel or omentum |
| Stage IIIA | Tumor grossly limited to the true pelvis with negative nodes but with histologically confirmed microscopic seeding of abdominal peritoneal surfaces |
| Stage IIIB | Tumor of one or both ovaries with histologically confirmed implants of abdominal peritoneal surfaces, none exceeding 2 cm diameter; nodes negative |
| Stage IIIC | Abdominal implants greater than 2 cm in diameter, or positive retroperitoneal or inguinal nodes |
| Stage IV | Growth involving one or both ovaries with distant metastases; if pleural effusion is present, there must be positive cytologic test results to allot a case to stage IV; parenchymal lower metastases equals |

[a] To evaluate the impact on prognosis of the different criteria for allotting cases to stage IC or IIC, it would be of value to know whether rupture of the capsule was spontaneous or caused by the surgeon, and what the source of malignant cells detected was—peritoneal washings or ascites.

**TABLE 62-8**

**Five-Year Survival of Patients With Ovarian Cancer**

| Stage | Five-Year Survival (%) |
|---|---|
| I | 85 |
| II | 60 |
| III | 30 |
| IV | 18 |

*Source*: Data from Partridge et al.[76]

cytoreduction, survival was highest among women with no macroscopic disease or with small volume disease (less than 0.5 cm).[81,82] At this time the GOG definition has not been changed.

Although histological subtype is important to determine, only clear cell and mucinous types of tumors are of independent prognostic significance. Grade is more important prognostically than histological subtype, although there is no universally accepted grading system. Well-differentiated tumors are grade 1, moderately differentiated tumors are grade 2, and poorly differentiated tumors are grade 3.

As the tumor grade increases, the survival rate decreases within each cell type. Grade is especially important in determining treatment. For example, grade 1 and 2 tumors need no further therapy.[83] Numerous studies have shown a high degree of intraobserver and interobserver variability associated with grading. Pathologists are interested in developing a more quantitative and reproducible grading system, such as molecular markers or DNA cytometry.[84]

A newer grading system that is reproducible, simple, and useful for all histological subtypes and clinical stages of ovarian cancer has been developed.[85] With the new system, tumors are graded on architectural patterns, nuclear pleomorphism, and mitotic activity. The tumor grades correlate with survival in early and advanced disease for all histological cell types except clear cell.[85] Staging, however, is commonly documented using the FIGO staging system that was revised in 1987 (see Table 62-7).[75] Surgical staging during cytoreductive surgery provides the basis of treatment decisions for ovarian cancer.

## THERAPEUTIC APPROACHES AND NURSING CARE

### SURGERY

Surgery is the mainstay of treatment in ovarian cancer. The aim of surgery is to provide a definitive diagnosis, determine the exact stage, and remove as much tumor as possible so as to improve survival and relieve symptoms. The

National Institutes of Health (NIH) consensus conference concluded that aggressive efforts at maximal cytoreduction are important because minimal residual tumor is associated with improved survival.[40] The surgical procedures used include total abdominal hysterectomy, BSO, peritoneal cytology, omentectomy, scraping of the undersurface of the right diaphragm, multiple peritoneal biopsies, pelvic and para-aortic lymph node sampling, and multiple random biopsies. A vertical midline incision from the symphysis pubis to above the umbilicus is essential. The goal is to leave no tumor greater than 1 cm (ie, optimally debulked disease).

A gynecologic surgical oncologist is specially trained to perform ovarian cancer surgery. Gynecologic oncologists are concerned about adequate surgical staging in ovarian cancer and achieving an optimal cytoreduction depends in part on the judgment, aggressiveness, and experience of the surgeon.[86] In a study of 785 women diagnosed with stage I or II ovarian cancer, only 10% of the women received optimal debulking surgery according to the NIH treatment guidelines.[87] The study revealed that women older than age 65 typically received incomplete surgical staging compared with those younger than 65.[87] When performed by those optimally trained to provide complete surgical cytoreduction, surgery is associated with a significant increase in survival.[88]

The gynecologic surgeon should discuss with the patient and family the goals of surgery, potential outcomes, and complications. Surgery is the initial approach to treatment in stages I to III of ovarian cancer. Surgical debulking is more controversial in stage IV disease. In a study by Curtin and associates,[89] optimal debulking resulted in a 40-month median survival in stage IV patients vs an 18-month median survival in those suboptimally debulked. There is an apparent survival benefit for women with stage IV disease who are aggressively debulked. This approach is supported by the NIH consensus conclusions, which stress the importance of aggressive surgical debulking.[40]

Surgery has a role at other times in the ovarian disease process. Procedures can include secondary cytoreductive surgery, second-look surgery, laparoscopic surgery, and palliative surgery. When cytoreductive surgery is not possible initially at diagnosis, it should be considered in patients who have not had progressive disease after 3 to 5 cycles of chemotherapy.[90]

Secondary cytoreductive surgery used at time of relapse is an approach whose value is unknown at this time. Second-look surgery, or exploratory surgery at the end of primary treatment, remains controversial. It is not appropriate for stage I and II disease but remains an option for stage III and IV disease. The patient with stage III or IV disease who had cytoreductive surgery followed by standard chemotherapy and is in a complete remission with a normal CA-125 and a negative CT scan is a potential candidate for second-look surgery that is recommended within the context of a clinical trial. The goal would be to explore the entire abdomen and pelvis and do a series of biopsies to provide the most accurate assessment of the response to induction chemotherapy. Unfortunately, a negative second-look surgery does not mean the patient is cured. In fact, negative second-look surgery may be followed by relapse in as many as 50% of patients.[91] In addition, if a patient is found to have disease at second-look surgery, the treatment available at this time is not effective in obtaining a cure.[91,92] No prospective randomized trials have confirmed any benefit from second-look surgery, and it is not routinely recommended outside of a clinical trial.

Laparoscopic surgery is not standard practice but is an acceptable alternative in a research setting.[93] Controversy exists because this type of surgery may facilitate rupture of the ovarian mass and studies have documented the adverse effects of rupture in patients with early-stage ovarian cancer.[94,95] Neoadjuvant chemotherapy treatment prior to surgery continues to be investigated, especially in stage IV disease. The goal of neoadjuvant therapy is to shrink the tumor so that debulking surgery will be more effective.

In recurrent disease, surgery has a role in promoting the patient's comfort. Patients who develop a recurrence following a long disease-free interval may benefit from a secondary debulking. Surgery is often effective in the palliative setting—for example, when a bowel obstruction occurs from peritoneal carcinomatosis. Surgery is an important treatment component in improving a patient's quality of life and providing relief of adverse symptoms in the palliative setting.

## TREATMENT OF EPITHELIAL OVARIAN CANCER

### Early-stage disease

Once surgery has been performed, patients with early-stage (I and II) disease are further classified into the low-risk (favorable) category or the high-risk (unfavorable) category based on grade, cytology, presence or absence of ascites, differentiation of the tumor, rupture of the capsule, or growth outside the ovaries (Table 62-9).[96] Early-stage, low-risk (IA, IB, well or moderately well differentiated) patients require no further treatment after a comprehensive staging surgery.[83] Their 5-year survival rate is greater than 90%.[83]

The recurrence rate for high-risk patients is 25% to 30%. Vergote and colleagues[97] reported on an analysis of 1000 high-risk patients with early-stage disease and established that the 4 most important risk factors for this group were degree of differentiation, FIGO stage (IA or IB), rupture of the capsule, and age.

The perspective on treatment for the high-risk group began to evolve with a GOG trial of 81 patients randomized to melphalan vs observation that resulted in 5-year survival rates of 91% and 98%, respectively, and defined the

**TABLE 62-9**

**Classification of Risk of Early-Stage Ovarian Cancer**

| Favorable or Low Risk | Unfavorable or High Risk |
|---|---|
| Stage IA or IB disease with well- or moderately well-differentiated tumor | Stage IA or IB with poorly differentiated tumor<br>All stage II |
| No ascites | Ascites |
| No tumor on external surface of the ovary | Tumor on external surface of ovary |
| Negative peritoneal cytology | Positive peritoneal cytology |
| Growth confined to ovaries | Growth outside the ovaries<br>Ruptured capsule |

*Source*: Adapted with permission from Ozols et al.[96]

good-prognosis patients who required no further therapy.[80] High-risk (IC, high-grade IA2 or IB2, II), early-stage disease has a 25% to 40% recurrence rate, and the role of immediate treatment and the type of therapy remains controversial. Those in the high-risk group have a 30% to 40% risk of relapse and a 25% to 30% chance of dying within the first 5 years after surgery.[98] When a high-risk group was treated with therapy in a trial randomizing them to either melphalan or p32, an intraperitoneal (IP) radioisotope, the result was an equivalent 5-year survival rate of 80% in both arms.[83] Melphalan's risk of a second malignancy and severe myelosuppression eliminated this drug from further trials and p32 was the preferred treatment. The high-risk patients were then randomized in the next set of trials to IP p32 vs cisplatin and cyclophosphamide (CP). Because p32 was difficult to administer and bowel complications occurred, the standard treatment became a platinum-based regimen for the high-risk group. The 10-year incidence of recurrence was 35% for the patients receiving p32 and 28% for the patients receiving CP.[99] Patients had a lower cumulative recurrence rate with CP, but no significant difference in survival was found. The authors concluded that platinum-based therapy was the preferred adjuvant treatment.[99]

Cisplatin and CP were replaced with carboplatin and paclitaxel after the results of the GOG-111 trial. A recently completed GOG trial looked at whether 3 cycles vs 6 cycles of this regimen was significant. The conclusion from this study was that 6 cycles is associated with a 5% reduction in absolute probability of the cancer recurring within 5 years.[100] This reduction was not statistically significant and 6 cycles were noted to be more toxic.[100] European investigators reported the result of an Adjuvant Chemotherapy in Ovarian Neoplasm Trial (ACTION) trial that compared early-stage optimally debulked patients who were observed vs received adjuvant treatment and reported both progression-free survival and overall survival rates as similar (83% vs 80% and 87% vs 89%)[101] The current GOG trial is studying 3 cycles of carboplatin and paclitaxel, at standard doses, followed by observation, versus 24 weekly injections of paclitaxel at 40 mg/m$^2$. This study is investigating a theory that the weekly dose of paclitaxel may have antiangiogenic properties and markers of angiogenesis are being collected. It is reasonable to conclude based on the data that the standard of care in the management of high-risk early-stage disease should include the administration of platinum-based chemotherapy. Until mature survival data is reported patients are offered somewhere between 3 and 6 cycles depending on clinical factors. Markman poses a strong argument that in the absence of contraindications to receiving a full 6 cycle course of treatment because of, for example, excessive emesis or significant neuropathy, women should be treated similarly as women with advanced disease.[102] If a patient has a stage Ia or b or stage II tumor of LMP, no adjuvant chemotherapy is recommended.

## Advanced disease

***Front-Line Treatment.*** Advanced-stage disease is routinely managed with a combination of surgery and postoperative chemotherapy. Ovarian cancer is a chemosensitive disease and it was established early in the treatment of the disease that a 2 drug regimen was superior to single agent therapy. In the early 1980s, the standard of care included the combination of CP and doxorubicin. The platinum compounds were introduced into cancer treatment around this same time and quickly found to be active in ovarian cancer and added to the 2 drug standard regimen. The benefit of the drug doxorubicin to CP and cisplatin was modest and did not justify the added toxicity so the standard of care became CP and a platinum compound (either cisplatin or carboplatin) until the 1990s. The early 1990s saw the development of a new class of drugs, the taxanes. The first drug from this group to be used in clinical trials, paclitaxel, was very active in women with advanced recurrent ovarian cancer.[103] Due to the drug's activity in recurrent disease, it was quickly included in clinical trials as initial therapy to be compared to the standard combination at that time, cisplatin and CP.

Several pivotal clinical trials occurred in the mid-1990s. First, in the GOG-111 trial, standard CP and cisplatin combination therapy was compared to paclitaxel and cisplatin. The paclitaxel arm, there was improvement in response rate of 73% vs 60% for the standard therapy.[104] A large clinical trial that confirmed these findings was titled "OV-10," and involved the Ovarian Group from Canada and Europe. The treatment arms consisted of CP and cisplatin vs paclitaxel and cisplatin; paclitaxel was given at 175 mg/m$^2$ over 3 hours, a change from the GOG-111 protocol. Similar to the GOG-111 results, the response rate was significantly improved in the paclitaxel arm, 59% vs 45% for the CP arm, and the complete clinical response rates were 41% and 27%, respectively.[105]

The GOG trial compared the cisplatin/paclitaxel combination with paclitaxel alone and cisplatin alone. Although no significant difference in median overall survival was noted between the 3 arms, cisplatin alone or in combination yielded superior response rates and progression-free survival.[106] The second and third International Collaborative Ovarian Neoplasm group studies (ICON-2, ICON-3) have provided further insight. ICON-2 compared carboplatin to CP, doxorubicin, and cisplatin (CAP) and found no difference in survival between the 2 groups.[107] The CAP arm was more toxic. ICON-3 compared carboplatin vs carboplatin and paclitaxel vs carboplatin plus paclitaxel with CAP. A total of 2074 patients were enrolled. The follow-up at 51 months did not show any difference in overall survival between the 3 arms of the trial.[108] Some of the challenges in interpreting this study are that it recruited a wide range of patient types (stages I-IV), 46% of patients had tumor bulk greater than 2 cm, 30% had absent or microscopic disease, and 55% had poorly differentiated disease.[109] In all of these studies, some patients did cross over and receive a taxane. As these data mature, they may offer an opportunity for review and refinement of current treatment guidelines.

Today the standard for ovarian cancer treatment with chemotherapy is a platinum compound and paclitaxel for first-line treatment. Clinical guidelines have been published to support the use of this regimen.[110] Three trials have now been completed using carboplatin/paclitaxel compared to cisplatin/paclitaxel.[111–113] The GOG-158 trial studied debulked stage III patients and compared cisplatin and paclitaxel (R1) vs carboplatin and paclitaxel (R2). Patients were randomized to second-look surgery or no second-look surgery at the time of enrollment. The results showed no difference in median overall survival (48.8 months for R1 vs 56.7 months for R2) and no difference in progression-free survival or overall survival in the second-look surgery patients vs the no second-look surgery patients.[114] The researchers concluded that carboplatin/paclitaxel is not less effective than cisplatin/paclitaxel, carboplatin/paclitaxel is less toxic and easier to administer, and second-look surgery does not influence recurrence-free survival.[113] Two more studies confirmed this result by comparing carboplatin/paclitaxel vs cisplatin/paclitaxel and found no difference in progression-free survival or overall survival between the treatment arms.[111,112] The conclusion drawn from these studies is that the carboplatin/paclitaxel combination is the preferred regimen because it is equally effective, less toxic, and easy to administer in the outpatient setting.

Docetaxel has been studied as a single-agent therapy, in combination with the platinum drugs, and as front-line therapy in ovarian cancer; it demonstrated activity in all settings.[115–117] Docetaxel also has activity in paclitaxel-resistant ovarian cancer. A recent trial compared docetaxel/carboplatin with paclitaxel/carboplatin and found no significant difference between the regimens in terms of response or median progression-free survival.[117] The toxicity profiles are different, however: docetaxel/carboplatin produces more myelosuppression, whereas paclitaxel/carboplatin is associated with more peripheral neuropathy. All of these studies have supported the use of docetaxel as an alternative to paclitaxel in front-line therapy.

The definition of the most effective carboplatin dose (area under the curve, or AUC 7.5 or lower), the optimal number of platinum-based cycles of therapy, and the value of combined versus sequential therapy with taxanes are all questions that remain unanswered.

Activity with bevacizumab in phase II trials in recurrent ovarian cancer produced positive results. In 1 study there was an overall response rate of 21% and in a second study 24%.[118] These results led to the development of a front-line phase III trial underway currently. The schema is presented in Table 62-10. Carboplatin and paclitaxel is being compared to carboplatin, paclitaxel, and bevacizumab. Both of these arms of the trial will be followed with 14 months of placebo. The third arm is carboplatin, paclitaxel, and bevacizumab followed by maintenance bevacizumab. This trial is about halfway to its accrual goal and expected to complete accrual in 2010.

Paclitaxel administration poses several nursing challenges, the most significant of which is hypersensitivity reactions. Prevention of the hypersensitivity reaction involves a premedication regimen, including dexamethasone, given orally the evening before and morning of treatment or intravenously immediately before treatment. Most patients who have hypersensitivity reactions experience itching, shortness of breath, a tightness in the chest, and perhaps back pain. In such cases, the infusion is stopped immediately and routine anaphylactic measures are employed. The infusion may be restarted at half the rate. Olson and associates[119] found that in the case of paclitaxel hypersensitivity,

**TABLE 62-10**

| Schema for Current Front-Line GOG Trial for Ovarian Cancer |
|---|
| Optimal or suboptimal stage III or IV epithelial ovarian or primary peritoneal cancer, no prior therapy are randomized to 1 of 3 arms: |
| Arm I: carboplatin/paclitaxel × 6 cycles + concurrent placebo × 6 cycles + placebo for 15 months |
| Arm II: carboplatin/paclitaxel × 6 cycles + concurrent bevacizumab × 6 cycles + placebo for 15 months |
| Arm III: carboplatin/paclitaxel × 6 cycles + concurrent bevacizumab + bevacizumab for 15 months |

rapid retreatment was safe and cost-effective. Platinum hypersensitivity reactions are also seen with ovarian cancer treatment. Hypersensitivity arises most frequently with subsequent treatment for recurrent disease and after primary therapy with platinum agents as compared to initial treatment with paclitaxel. The theory of the exact mechanism responsible for this sensitivity is not clear, it is postulated that the reaction occurs in individuals secondary to a gradual developing allergy to metallic platinum.[120] This author suggests careful considerations in the decision to continue treatment with a platinum-based regimen following carboplatin hypersensitivity such as the severity of the reaction and the strong evidence of platinum responsive disease.[120]

To summarize, the majority of women with clinically curable ovarian cancer will receive primary debulking surgery and combination chemotherapy. The overall 10-year survival rate for ovarian cancer is approximately 20%; therefore, continued efforts must be directed at improving the results obtained with primary therapy.[121] The phase III clinical trial now under way may help define a new standard regimen for ovarian cancer if the progression-free interval and overall survival found in it are improved. Until results are improved with current standard treatment, research continues with new agents specifically biological agents in ovarian cancer.

## Strategies to improve outcomes of primary therapy

*Maintenance therapy.* Once a patient has completed primary therapy and achieves a complete remission, there is controversy regarding the role of maintenance therapy. In reviewing the results of a GOG trial, it was found that approximately 90% of patients achieve a clinical complete remission after standard chemotherapy; however, the median time to progression was 22 months and median overall survival was 57.4 months.[113]

Maintenance or consolidation therapy is commonly used to decrease the relapse rate and increase survival. Such therapy in women who achieve a clinical complete response has been studied using high-dose therapy with stem cell transplant, IP therapy, administration of the radioactive isotope of phosphorous ($^{32}P$), hormone therapy, whole-abdominal radiotherapy, or prolonged administration of single-agent chemotherapy. Biological agents have also been used but neither interferon-alpha nor a metalloproteinase inhibitor has had an effect on survival. A monoclonal antibody (oregovomab) was studied vs a placebo and showed a negative result, but this antibody continues to be studied in a subset of patients.[122] Interest in maintenance therapy has intensified due to the results of a study evaluating 12 monthly cycles of single-agent paclitaxel compared to 3 monthly cycles following primary therapy; the former regimen provided improved progression-free survival (28 months vs 21 months).[123] However, no overall difference in survival was reported and the trial was stopped early. The GOG has a study open that randomizes patients in complete clinical remission to no further therapy, 12 cycles of paclitaxel, or 12 cycles of paclitaxel poliglumex with survival as the primary endpoint. Controversy surrounds the issue of maintenance therapy, as its additional toxicity cannot be underestimated. At this time no maintenance therapy has improved survival and is not the established standard of care. Ideally, future studies will include research on quality of life, symptom control, and survival factors.

*Intraperitoneal therapy.* Intraperitoneal therapy allows for uniform distribution of the drug in the peritoneal cavity. Also the drugs administered via the IP route will also enter the systemic circulation and achieve a 50% to 75% uptake of IV administration exposure via the lymphatic channels or by passive diffusion. Dose intensity remains an important concept and if drugs infuse into the tumor directly there may be a pharmacological advantage. Because ovarian cancer is predominantly confined to the abdomen, there has been a great deal of interest in pursuing the IP method of drug administration. IP therapy has been investigated as consolidation therapy after a negative second-look laparotomy, as second-line treatment for resistant disease, and as first-line therapy in ovarian cancer. Numerous phase I and II trials over the past 4 decades have studied single agents including methotrexate, fluorouracil doxorubicin, carboplatin, cisplatin, and paclitaxel.

Cisplatin is the drug most frequently used in IP therapy in ovarian cancer. There have been 3 phase III clinical trials that have reached similar conclusions regarding IP chemotherapy in ovarian cancer. A GOG/Southwest Oncology Group (SWOG) trial enrolled optimal stage III patients with no tumor larger than 2 cm. These patients received IP or IV cisplatin (100 mg/m$^2$) and IV CP (600 mg/m$^2$).[124] More than 600 women participated, and the complete response rate for IP therapy was 47% compared to an IV rate of 36%; overall median survival was 49 months vs 41 months, respectively. A subsequent GOG trial randomized patients to 6 months of IV cisplatin (75 mg/m$^2$) and paclitaxel 135 mg/m$^2$ over 24 hours vs 2 doses of carboplatin (AUC = 9) followed by 6 cycles of IP cisplatin (100 mg/m$^2$) and IV paclitaxel 135 mg/m$^2$ over 24 hours.[125] There were statistically significant differences in progression-free survival (28 months vs 22 months) and overall survival (63 vs 52 months).[125] A third randomized trial examined first-line therapy of IV paclitaxel (135 mg/m$^2$ for 24 hours day 1) plus IP cisplatin (100 mg/m$^2$ day 2) and IP paclitaxel (60 mg/m$^2$ day 8) vs the control arm of cisplatin (75 mg/m$^2$) plus paclitaxel (135 mg/m$^2$ for 24 hours) every 21 days in 415 patients. Forty-two percent of patients randomized to the IP arm completed all 6 cycles of therapy compared to 83% in the IV arm.[126] Most patients in both arms ended up completing 6 cycles of therapy by crossing over and getting standard therapy if unable to finish IP therapy. Reasons for discontinuation of the IP treatment included catheter complications, toxicity, and noncatheter-related issues. There was a statistically significant improvement in progression-free survival associated with the IP therapy (23.8 vs 18.3 months) and an improvement in overall survival in the IP arm (65.6 months vs 49.7 months).[126] This study result led to a clinical announcement being issued by the National Cancer Institute in January 2006 recommending that women with stage III ovarian cancer who undergo optimal surgical cytoreduction be considered for IP therapy.

Intraperitoneal consolidation therapy with platinum-based drugs has been used in patients with low volume stage III disease following complete remission after platinum-based standard chemotherapy. The trials results did not show significance for improvement in progression-free survival or overall survival.[122]

In conclusion, IP therapy has shown an ability to improve progression-free or overall survival in multiple clinical trials. The therapy also produces significant toxicity. Women with optimally debulked disease should be given the information about IP therapy results and offered the option of treatment using this strategy or offered to participate in IP clinical trials.

*New combinations of existing cytotoxic drugs.* The most recently reported phase III GOG intergroup trial included 4 experimental arms to evaluate the addition of 3 new drugs (topotecan, gemictabine, and PEG-liposomal doxorubicin) using 2 different strategies for drug administration (sequential doublets and triplet combinations) and compared all arms to the standard control treatment (paclitaxel and carboplatin). All 5 arms of this study produced similar progression-free and overall survival rates. The conclusion from this study was that none of these new agents added to the standard paclitaxel and carboplatin regimen.[127]

*Novel agents.* Many new novel chemotherapeutic agents and biological agents are being developed and tested in ovarian cancer (Tables 62-11 and 62-12). Novel chemotherapeutic agents include new platinum drugs, new taxanes, other tubulin inhibitors, and DNA-binding drugs.[128] Biological agents include both monoclonal antibodies and small molecule drugs. Bevacizumab as previously mentioned is the most well-studied and active agent to date.

*Second-line treatment.* Ovarian cancer is highly responsive to initial chemotherapy. In fact over 90% of women with optimally debulked stage III disease will achieve a complete response and of those 75% will recur. Of the women with suboptimal disease stage III and IV, about 50% will achieve a complete response and greater than 90% will recur.[113] Hence the magnitude of the clinical problem in ovarian cancer. The therapeutic goals shift in recurrent ovarian cancer. The disease is no longer curable but chronic.

A serological relapse may be the first evidence of recurrent disease. An elevated level of the tumor marker CA-125 is predictive of a recurrence of ovarian cancer. The median time for CA-125 to become elevated is 2 to 4 months prior to obvious symptoms or definitive clinical disease progression. Thus, a rising CA-125 level has clouded the definition of time of recurrence because the patient often does not have clinically detectable disease. No evidence indicates that immediate chemotherapy is beneficial in recurrence. A European randomized trial currently underway may provide evidence as to whether delaying chemotherapy until clinical relapse is detrimental.[129] This trial is a phase III trial comparing the benefits of early administration of chemotherapy based on the CA-125 assay alone vs delaying treatment until there is clinical or radiological evidence of disease recurrence. Patients follow this tumor marker closely, however, and they usually want treatment as soon as it is elevated. A rising CA-125 level is definitely associated with increased stress in patients. Other patterns of recurrence include a localized recurrence, disseminated IP disease, or extraperitoneal metastasis.

**TABLE 62-11**

| Chemotherapy Agents Utilized in the Treatment of Recurrent Ovarian Cancer |
|---|
| Altretamine |
| Carboplatin or cisplatin |
| Docetaxel |
| Epirubicin |
| Etoposide |
| Gemcitabine |
| Ifosfamide |
| Liposomal doxorubicin |
| Paclitaxel |
| Tamoxifen |
| Topotecan |
| Vinorelbine |
| Pemetrexed |
| Epothliones |
| TLK 286 |
| Trabectidin |
| Irinotecan |

**TABLE 62-12**

**New Biological Agents Being Investigated in Ovarian Cancer**

| |
|---|
| Bevacizumab |
| Erlotinib |
| Gelfitinib |
| Cetuximab |
| Laptinib |
| Pertuzumab |
| Enzastaurin |
| Tratuzumab |
| Imatinib |
| Sorafenib |
| Oregovomab |
| Bortezomib |
| CI-779 |
| AMG-706 |
| SAHA |
| VEGF-trap |
| Tipifarnib |
| AZD2281 |

**TABLE 62-13**

**Classification of Recurrent Ovarian Cancer**

| | |
|---|---|
| Platinum sensitive | Disease free interval greater than 6 months |
| Platinum resistant | No response to platinum or a duration of response less than 6 months following completion of therapy |

As discussed previously, secondary cytoreduction may be considered at time of relapse. There is no established clinical benefit and patients who should not undergo secondary cytoreduction include those patients with a short disease-free interval; IP carcinomatosis; ascites; or drug-resistant disease.

Patients with recurrent disease are classified as platinum sensitive or platinum resistant (Table 62-13). In treatment of recurrence, the drug-sensitive patients have a high response rate to drugs used in the initial regimen and the longer the treatment-free interval, the higher the chance of response when recurrence is treated.[130] The most appropriate treatment choice until recently was single agent carboplatin. Two more recent phase III randomized trials have changed the treatment of choice. Each trial compared a combination carboplatin-based regimen to carboplatin alone. In the first trial platinum plus a taxane was compared to platinum drug alone. The second trial compared carboplatin plus gemcitabine to carboplatin alone. Both trials results reported the combination regimens had an improvement in progression-free and overall survival was improved in the paclitaxel and carboplatin regimen.[131,132] Comparing the toxicity profiles the carboplatin and paclitaxel regimen had a 20% incidence in grade 2 to 3 neuropathy compared to 1% in the carboplatin alone arm. There was no difference in neuropathy reported in the gemcitabine and carboplatin compared to carboplatin alone trial but there was significant bone marrow suppression in the combination regimen.[131,132] The toxicity profile helps the clinician with making the treatment decisions. For example, if the patient had experienced neuropathy in the first-line treatment and still had lingering effects, the gemcitabine and carboplatin regimen would be a more appropriate choice.

Platinum-resistant disease treatment is a different discussion. There is no one definitive answer for the optimal second-line treatment in this patient group. Rather clinicians should consider the side effects of treatment, the impact of a particular drug on the ability to deliver other antineoplastic agents in the future, convenience, cost, or a possible hospitalization.[133] This is particularly important when there will be an extended period of treatment necessary as there is in this disease. There are a large number of agents with at least modest activity to choose from for second-line platinum-resistant treatment (Table 62-11). No data exist to support one agent over another but recent phase III trials results support the use of an active agent over an inactive agent.[134] In addition, extended survival (over 1 year) is a realistic possibility even in the presence of platinum-resistant disease.[135] The likelihood of benefit must be weighed against the toxicity of the treatment. The patients most likely to benefit from second-line treatment include those with small-volume disease, good performance status, a long treatment-free interval, serous histology, and a small number of sites of disease. Some critical parameters when choosing a treatment for recurrent disease include prior response, toxicity of prior treatment, quality of life, toxicity profile, age, comorbid illness, extent of disease, cost, and patient preference. The standard approach is to treat the patient for 2 to 3 cycles and then reevaluate the patient to determine whether there has been a clinical benefit before continuing. If no response occurs, an alternative regimen is selected. Palliative support is used through the end stages of the disease.

*Hormone therapy.* Tamoxifen has been studied in this disease extensively both as a single agent and in combination with chemotherapy. About 10% of treated patients exhibit a response.[102] An alternative approach to a rising CA-125 without evidence of disease may be to use tamoxifen, a nontoxic but active drug, until clinical evidence of disease recurrence emerges.[110,136,137] Many clinicians feel that there is no reason to start chemotherapy in a patient with a serological marker of recurrence as long as the patient is asymptomatic, has a normal pelvic exam, and is without evidence of definitive disease recurrence. Tamoxifen has also been used as a maintenance approach after completion of chemotherapy and in the treatment of recurrent ovarian cancer.[102] Other hormonal agents studied include leuprorelin, high-dose progesterone, and letrozole.

*New emerging therapies.* Small molecule inhibitors, monoclonal antibodies, antisense therapy, and gene therapy are all being evaluated in ovarian cancer (Table 62-12). The family of epidermal growth factor receptors (EGFRs), therapies targeted at the vascular endothelial growth factor (VEGF), DNA methylation, and alpha-folate receptor agents are the furthest along in clinical development.

The most studied target for therapy is EGFR, which is expressed in 30% to 70% of epithelial ovarian cancers.[11] Receptor function can be inhibited by blocking the binding of ligand to the receptor by a monoclonal antibody (pertuzumab and trastuzumab) or by inhibition of the enzyme activity of the receptor tyrosinase kinase with small molecules (gefitinib, erlotinib, or CI-1033).[128] Pertuzumab and transtuzumab trials produced response rates of 4% and 7% and stable disease in 7% and 39%.[138,139] Erlotinib, gefitinib, and CI-1033 produced response rates of 6%, 3%, 0%; however, there was stabilization of disease in 44% of patients treated with erlotinib, 15% with gefitinib, and 50% with CI-1033.[140–142] Response is only part of the result with these new agents. Schilder et al[141] noted that EGFR-expressing tumors had longer progression-free survival and objective response was associated with mutation in EGFR.

Bevacizumab is currently the most active biological agent in ovarian cancer. Four studies demonstrate activity with ovarian cancer and bevacizumab treatment either in combinations or as a single agent. Response rates from 15.9% to 35% were reported with careful observation of toxicity also noted.[118,143–145] Bowel perforation has been observed in 5% to 10% of patients with ovarian cancer treated with this agent but also noted is that these patients had extensive intra-abdominal disease at the time of treatment.[143] As stated previously, clinical trials are underway to evaluate bevacizumab in combination with chemotherapy as primary treatment in ovarian cancer. Vascular endothelial growth factor plays a key role in ascites formation in ovarian cancer. Research conducted with an antibody against VEGF in preclinical murine models bearing human ovarian carcinoma xenografts prevented and even reversed ascites formation.[146]

Decitabine, a demethylating agent, is under investigation in combination with carboplatin in patients with recurrent ovarian cancer.[128] The alpha-folate receptor is of interest in ovarian cancer because of the high rate of overexpression. A monoclonal antibody (MORAb-003) and a thymidylate synthase inhibitor (BGC945) targeting the alpha-folate receptor are under investigation.[147,148]

The poly ADP ribose polymerase (PARP) inhibitors are another group of targeted therapy agents. PARP is an enzyme involved in DNA repair. The PARP inhibitors are selectively toxic to tumors without any functioning BRCA genes. A phase I trial using a PARP inhibitor, AZD 2281, in patients with BRCA platinum-resistant and refractory ovarian cancer reported 14 partial responses and 8 stable disease results with mild toxicity.[149] More clinical trials are underway with this agent.

These new forms of therapy remain in the early stages of research. Clearly, the presence of a target on a tumor by itself may not be sufficient for drugs to have activity. There may be a subset of patients in whom the target has a critical biological role in the growth of the cancer, and this group is most likely to benefit from targeted therapy. New tools that will allow highly specific tumor profiling such as genomic microarray and proteomic analysis will help facilitate the selection of those patients who are most likely to benefit from these techniques.[150]

## INTRAPERITONEAL CHEMOTHERAPY

The drugs ordered will be directly administered in to the abdominal cavity via a catheter. Peritoneal access is accomplished with either an implantable port or a tenckhoff catheter. The GOG workshop on IP therapy recommended the Bard 9.6 French silicone venous access port with a single lumen (Potter, GOG Web site: http://gog.org). Suggestion was also made to implant this device at the time of surgery. Contraindications for placing the catheter or port include no abdominal infection present, preexisting peripheral neuropathy, malnutrition, adhesive disease in the abdomen, gastrointestinal dysfunction, massive ascites, hypovolemia, or abnormal renal function.[151] The most ideal patient is one with low or no volume disease after debulking surgery.

Getting started involves writing the policy and procedures for the treatment and a standard of care. Some excellent sources for getting started are listed in Table 62-14.[152,153] The procedure for administration via the PORT is presented in Table 62-15.[152,154,155] Remember to keep the patient informed and comfortable during the procedure. Administration via the tenchkoff catheter is a similar procedure with the following differences: the entire procedure is sterile, skin care must be given around the catheter

**TABLE 62-14**

**Resources for Getting Started With Intraperitoneal Therapy Procedures and Standards**

CJON article by Almadrones L, Hydzik C. April 2007

CJON article by Marin et al.[167] December 2007

GOG Web site, GOG Nursing Manual, http://www.gog.org

Oncology Nursing Society, http://www.ons.org

Society of Gynecologic Nurse Oncologists, http://www.sgno.org

insertion site during the procedure and a sterile dressing applied, use of a clamp and cap on the catheter, and fluid may be drained at the start of the procedure. To drain the fluid, the catheter is attached to a drainage bag and the peritoneal contents are drained. If there is more than 600 cc's of fluid or the appearance of the fluid is abnormal, the physician should be notified.[154] Nursing interventions during the procedure include explaining about the chemotherapy side effects, instructing the patient on the signs and symptoms of infection, monitoring blood counts and electrolytes, assessing for pain or any discomfort, and observing for fluid overload symptoms.[152–154] Catheter-related issues can be a primary reason for discontinuation of therapy. Thirty-four percent of patients in Armstrong et al[126] study discontinued IP therapy because of catheter-related problems. It is important to trouble shoot and manage catheter complications. Table 62-16 outlines management of some frequent catheter complications.

**TABLE 62-15**

**Administration Procedure for IP Therapy via PORT**

- Use EMLA on site 1 hour before procedure
- Patient should lie flat, instruct patient to wear comfortable loose clothes and empty bladder before procedure
- Obtain vital signs
- Verify PORT location
- Use sterile technique, wear PPE: gown, gloves, mask
- Access PORT with 19 or 20 gauge noncoring right angle Huber needle either 1" or 1.5"
- Preflush with 10 to 20 mL of normal saline to determine patency. No blood return is expected.
- Some institutions use heparin flush, many do not
- Look for leakage, ease of flow, subcutaneous infiltration or discomfort
- Apply transparent dressing
- Connect and anchor IP tubing and begin infusion, do not use infusion pump, flows by gravity
- Infusion solution can be warmed to 37°C
- Flush port at end of procedure with 10 to 20 mL normal saline
- De-access, apply a pressure dressing

*Note*: Patient can turn from side to side for 15 minutes to one hour starting with infusion and continuing up to one hour post. Monitor vital signs during turning as ordered.

*Abbreviation*: IP, intraperitoneal; PPE, personal protective equipment.

*Source*: Data from Potter and Held-Warmkessle[151]; Hydzik[153]; and Marin et al.[154]

Unfortunately, the majority of patients with advanced ovarian cancer will have a recurrence of their disease. Nurses are critical caregivers during this final phase of care. Ovarian cancer, which is usually spread throughout the abdomen, can cause dysfunction in many different organ systems. Women often present with a multitude of gastrointestinal complaints at diagnosis, and these symptoms may continue or reoccur during treatment or recurrence. Metastases can appear in any organ and site; the most frequently occurring metastatic sites include the intestines, liver, diaphragm, or lungs. Complications identified at the end of life in women with ovarian cancer include fatigue or weakness (75%), nausea and vomiting (71%), constipation (49%), edema of the extremities

**TABLE 62-16**

**Troubleshooting Catheter Complications**

**Slow Infusion Rate**
Check for kinks in tubing, increase height of bag, irrigate port or catheter, check needle placement

**Inflow Failure**
Catheter kinks, fibrin blood in catheter, catheter migration, tumor progression
Irrigate before and after drug administration, reposition patient, check catheter placement with dye study, TPA instillation for 2 to 4 hours and retry

**Exit Site Infection**
Prevent by maintaining aseptic technique, culture exudates, administer antibiotic as ordered, site care
Leakage of chemotherapy
Check needle for dislodgement, PORT separation from catheter
Stop infusion, provide skin care at site, follow hazardous drug spill procedure

**Outflow Failure (Tenckhoff Catheter only)**
Fibrin sheath formation likely, reposition, flush

*Source*: Adapted with permission from Marin et al.[154]

(44%), and anemia (34%).[156] The major problems that nurses confront in caring for women with advanced recurrent disease include ascites (28%), intestinal obstruction (12%), malnutrition (9%), pleural effusion (10%), and bladder obstruction (3%).[156] Several of these potential problems are discussed here along with relevant nursing management strategies.

## PRIMARY TREATMENT OF OTHER OVARIAN TUMORS

### Ovarian germ cell tumors

Ovarian germ cell tumors are uncommon making up about 5% of all ovarian tumors and occur in women in their teens and twenties.[157] These tumors arise form the primordial germ cells of the ovary and can be benign or malignant. The critical distinction to make during diagnosis is between dysgerminoma tumors and nondysgerminoma tumors (all others). Dysgerminoma is analogous to seminoma and is a radiosensitive tumor; it may be associated with pregnancy. The signs and symptoms of germ cell tumors include abdominal pain and a palpable pelvic or abdominal mass. Some 85% of patients have both an abdominal mass and abdominal pain at presentation.[158] The acute abdominal pain is usually caused by rupture, hemorrhage, or torsion of the ovarian mass.[157] Abdominal distention, fever, and vaginal bleeding are less common signs and symptoms. An abnormal HCG or alphafetoprotein level, or both, may be found, and the level of the marker CA-125 may be elevated. The staging system used for germ cell tumors is identical to that employed for epithelial ovarian cancer.

Initial treatment is surgery for both definitive diagnosis and treatment. A vertical midline incision is made, and the type of surgical procedure depends on the findings when the abdomen is explored. All attempts will be made to save the uterus and the other ovary if 1 goal is to preserve childbearing. At a minimum, it is important to remove the tumor and inspect the entire peritoneal cavity. Any suspicious lesions should be biopsied. If metastatic disease is present, cytoreductive principles apply as in epithelial ovarian cancer.

Treatment after surgery for nondysgerminoma includes 3 cycles of bleomycin, etoposide, and platinum (BEP) chemotherapy starting within 7 to 10 days postoperatively. Dysgerminoma patients will have the same chemotherapy but only if their disease stage is greater than IA. Patients with stage IA are followed with observation only. Most cases of dysgerminoma are curable and have a good prognosis. A small percentage of patients do recur and usually within 12 to 24 months of primary diagnosis. Radiotherapy is effective in dysgerminomas and is considered although loss of fertility may be a result. Chemotherapy regimen POMB-ACE (vincristine, bleomycin, cisplatin, etoposide, actinomycin, and CP) can be considered for recurrent disease.

### Sex-cord stromal tumors

Sex-cord stromal tumors arise from the sex cords or ovarian stroma and constitute 5% to 8% of ovarian malignancies. These tumors consist of granulosa and theca cells as well as Sertoli and Leydig cells; the most common type is granulosa cell. Granulosa cell tumors are low grade but have the potential to recur and metastasize and often secrete estrogen or testosterone. Women with sex-cord stromal tumors are typically younger than age 40. The symptoms include irregular periods in premenopausal women and vaginal bleeding in postmenopausal women. Granulosa cell tumors can be associated with endometrial hyperplasia. Sertoli-Leydig tumors are low-grade malignancies that occur usually in the third or fourth decade of life. These tumors present with signs of virilization due to androgen production.

The staging process for sex-cord stromal tumors is the same as for epithelial tumors, a surgical staging process. If the disease is diagnosed early, treatment consists of surgery alone. The surgical procedure depends on the extent of the tumor, the age of the patient, and whether the desire for fertility preservation is important. If chemotherapy is indicated, it is usually a combination such as BEP or cisplatin, bleomycin, and vinblastine. A GOG trial with these drugs showed a 37% response rate.[159] Prognosis is good, with a 5-year disease-free rate of 85% to 90%.[51] The majority of these tumors are diagnosed early, but advanced and recurrent disease may be found and granulosa cell tumors can recur 5 to 30 years after diagnosis.[160]

### Ovarian cancer of low-malignant potential

Epithelial tumors account for 90% of all ovarian cancers. Of the epithelial tumors, 10% to 15% will have LMP or be borderline tumors or atypical proliferating epithelial tumors. Borderline or LMP designation means that although the cells of the tumor appear malignant, the cells have not invaded the underlying tissue. These tumors tend to occur in younger patients, in earlier stages, and have an excellent overall survival rate of 80% to 90%.[161,162] These are intermediate tumors, between cystadenomas and frankly invasive disease. Lu and colleagues[163] found that bilateral and advanced borderline tumors were multifocal in origin, whereas epithelial ovarian cancer is unifocal. In 1971, FIGO called this group LMP; in 1973, WHO labeled it borderline tumors.[164,165]

The surgical procedure and staging for LMP ovarian cancer are similar to those for epithelial ovarian cancer. Overall, the most important characteristic to note is that these tumors are not invasive. Surgery alone cures the majority, and adjuvant therapy is not indicated.

### Extraovarian peritoneal carcinoma

Primary peritoneal carcinomas are characterized by their diffuse involvement of the peritoneal surfaces with a neoplasm appearing identical to papillary serous carcinoma but without a primary ovarian tumor. This disease can occur in women with intact ovaries or after an oophorectomy. The tumors are frequently advanced at presentation. Surgical cytoreductive surgery is less successful due to the diffuseness of the metastasis. The tumors are sensitive to platinum-based therapy after surgery.

## SYMPTOM MANAGEMENT AND SUPPORTIVE CARE

Nursing care and support of patients with ovarian cancer occurs in 3 major phases: (1) during surgical therapy, (2) during chemotherapy, and (3) during advanced disease. The nurse plays critical roles in delivery and management of care, in patient education, as an advocate for the patient, and for emotional support.

In the first phase of care, nursing care focuses on the patient's preparation for surgery, the acute postoperative period and prevention of postsurgical complications, and the psychosocial support for a cancer diagnosis. Initially, the nurse will explain the plan with the patient and emphasize the prevention of possible postoperative complications (Table 62-17). Preadmission testing is done, and the patient is given a bowel prep to cleanse the bowel entirely prior to surgery. The family must be educated about the operative procedure itself and the length of time it takes. Tools that outline care help increase the nurse's efficiency and decrease costs by providing specific outcomes to follow. Discharge instructions start at the preoperative phase and preparation of the expectations postoperatively will provide the patient with the knowledge and support. Monitoring temperature, signs and symptoms of infection, taking analgesics as directed, following strategies to prevent constipation, maintaining nutrition and hydration and gradually increasing activity are all part of the discharge instructions. The diagnosis and surgical intervention phase usually covers 5 to 7 days in the hospital and a short recuperative break before the next phase of treatment, chemotherapy. However, many clinicians administer the first course of treatment during the postoperative period.

**TABLE 62-17**

| Common Problems Following Laparotomy for Tumor Debulking |
|---|
| Bleeding/hemorrhage |
| Thromboembolic event |
| Infection/sepsis |
| Fluid and electrolyte imbalance |
| Atelectasis/pneumonia |
| Bowel dysfunction |
| Bladder dysfunction |

The second phase of nursing care targets the chemotherapy treatment plan. The nursing care focus is mainly one of education and information regarding the treatment regimen, and support and assessment for potential problems from chemotherapy toxicities. The specifics of nursing care in this phase depend on the treatment administered to the patient. The current standard for chemotherapy involves a taxane and a platinum compound. Possible side effects include alopecia, an allergic reaction, myelosuppression, nausea, vomiting, arthralgias, and myalgias. If woman receives information about side effects of treatment and ways to mange those side effects, she is more likely to successfully reduce physical and emotional distress from treatment effects.[166] Nurses provide vital links to patients by performing telephone triage roles in the ambulatory or office setting for questions, problems, or support during this phase of care. Special attention needs to be focused on the administration of chemotherapy directly in the abdomen since this method requires standards of care and procedures.

### ASCITES

One-third of women with ovarian cancer will present with ascites at diagnosis; two-thirds will have ascites present at their death. The parietal peritoneum lines the abdominopelvic wall, the diaphragm, and the visceral peritoneum that covers the abdominal organs and encloses the peritoneal cavity. Peritoneal fluid is normally present in a small volume to constantly lubricate the cavity and prevent abdominal organs from adhering to abdominal walls; 80% of this fluid is drained by the lymphatic system.[167,168] Ascites occurs when the fluid produced is greater than the amount of fluid cleared, usually caused by tumor obstructing the diaphragmatic or abdominal lymphatic channels or the tumor itself producing excessive fluid.[168,169] A fluid increase of greater than 500 mL produces symptoms that include weight gain, abdominal bloating, feeling full after small meals, indigestion, peripheral edema, altered bowel habits, inability to bend or sit upright, and lack of appetite. Early symptoms of ascites may progress if no intervention is instituted to eliminate its source. Profound ascites will have a devastating effect on the individual's ability to function. Gastrointestinal function, nutrition, ambulation, breathing, sleeping, and psychosocial sequelae are all affected by this condition. Nursing assessment could reveal any or all of the following physical findings: shiny or tense abdominal skin, everted umbilicus, diminished bowel sounds, dullness over flank area, or midabdomen tympany.[170,171] The presence of ascites in the abdomen may create a compression phenomenon that could contribute to bowel obstruction.

A diagnosis of ascites is confirmed with an abdominal flat plate x-ray or abdominal ultrasound. Paracentesis is used most often to remove the fluid without altering the hemodynamic equilibrium of the peritoneum. Blood chemistries should be drawn—specifically, serum protein, potassium, and sodium—and the ascitic fluid may be sent for gross inspection, cytology, cell count, chemistries, and microbiology. Paracentesis is a temporary measure. Unless the underlying reason for fluid accumulation is addressed, the ascitic fluid will recur.

An approach for fluid removal is peritoneovenous shunting, which is used infrequently. Peritoneovenous shunting entails placement of a continuous shunt that rechannels ascites fluid from the peritoneal cavity to the superior vena cava and eventually into the venous circulation. The shunt consists of a length of tubing, one end of which is placed in the peritoneal cavity; the other is tunneled subcutaneously and inserted into the superior vena cava.[171] The fluid flows upward into the superior vena cava via a 1-way valve that opens with each inhalation as the IP pressure increases and the intrathoracic pressure decreases.[168,172] Shunt malfunctions such as kinking or occlusion, pulmonary edema from rapid intravascular infusion of large quantities of fluid, disseminated intravascular coagulation, infection, and pulmonary embolus are all potential complications of this procedure. Shunting is reserved for untreatable disease and is appropriate if the time for reaccumulation of ascites is less than 1 month. It is usually reserved for those patients with a reasonable life expectancy where symptom relief is anticipated.[173] Mild diuretics are often prescribed but are usually not effective in diminishing ascites fluid.

Nursing care includes educating the patient to notify the physician or nurse when fluid starts to reaccumulate by measuring weight daily or abdominal girth daily or weekly. A bowel regimen may be needed to relieve constipation. Nursing care is aimed at relieving symptoms associated with ascites and minimizing further accumulation of the fluid. Instruct the patient to alternate activity with rest periods in an effort to conserve energy. Encourage the patient to lay on her left side with her feet elevated to alleviate pressure on the internal organs, improve vascular return from the lower extremities, facilitate lymphatic flow, and improve diuresis. Ascites can make it physically uncomfortable to eat, so consuming small frequent snacks or meals is suggested. An adequate protein intake and calories are needed to help increase low serum albumin levels. Families should offer calorie-rich beverages and encourage adequate fluids, especially after the paracentesis procedure, to restore fluid and electrolyte balance. Fluid restrictions may be imposed in some circumstances to minimize ascites reaccumulation. Ascites affects self-esteem, body image, and the ability to function. Assisting patients to take an active part in the management of ascites will lessen anxiety and help restore control.

## INTESTINAL OBSTRUCTION

The incidence of bowel obstruction is reported between 5.5% and 42% of patients with ovarian cancer.[174] With more advanced-stage disease, there is a higher probability of obstruction. Tumor or adhesions may cause extrinsic compression of the bowel. Obstruction can involve either the small or large intestine, can be acute or chronic, and can be partial or complete. Signs and symptoms depend on the location of the obstruction and are summarized in Table 62-18.[170]

When obstruction occurs, the bowel responds by increasing the force of peristalsis and attempting to move the bowel contents beyond the obstruction, so the first sounds are hyperactive bowel sounds.[175] After some time the bowel tires and the peristalsis process slows. Hypoactive bowel sounds are then present.[175] A bowel obstruction with ovarian cancer most frequently tends to be an insidious process that progresses over weeks to months. An acute presentation of obstruction, such as perforation, is a rare complication. Accumulation of fluid in the bowel near the obstruction, increased gas from swallowed air, and overgrowth of bowel flora can all contribute to the compression problem.[172]

**TABLE 62-18**

**Signs and Symptoms of Intestinal Obstruction**

| Location | Signs and Symptoms |
|---|---|
| Small intestine | Colicky pain<br>Vomiting<br>Severe dehydration<br>Minimal or absent distention |
| Lower small intestine | Less acute presentation<br>Moderate vomiting<br>Dehydration<br>Some distention<br>Lack of feces or flatus<br>Severe electrolyte imbalances |
| Large intestine | Insidious<br>Pronounced distention<br>Lack of feces or flatus<br>Overflow diarrhea<br>Vomiting |

*Source*: Data from Martin.[170]

The most common presenting symptom is colicky abdominal pain. Abdominal distention usually occurs once the obstruction is established. Stools gradually become more infrequent and vomiting can occur with small bowel obstruction. If intestinal strangulation with ischemia is found, fever, rebound tenderness, and leukocytosis may be present.[172] A diagnosis is made based on presenting signs, physical findings, and a flat and upright x-ray film of the abdomen. The film will reveal dilated loops of bowel, increased gas and fluid accumulation, and multiple air–fluid levels.[172,175] Further testing might include a barium swallow with small bowel follow-through or a barium enema, an endoscopy, or a CT scan. A thorough assessment of the patient by the nurse includes evaluation for pain or abdominal tenderness, fever, distention, nausea, vomiting and quality of emesis, bowel pattern, history, bowel sounds, peritoneal signs, and fluid status.[172,174]

Medical treatment consists of relieving the distention, correcting the fluid imbalances, and removing the source of obstruction. Initial treatment may involve decompression of the bowel with a nasogastric tube or long intestinal tube or venting gastrostomy tube or simple bowel rest for 24 to 48 hours without oral intake. A retrospective chart review of 24 patients' records was done to examine the effectiveness of managing a bowel obstruction with a percutaneous endoscopic gastrostomy (PEG) tube. Seventy-five percent of the patients did not have nausea or vomiting at discharge, 92% resumed a clear liquid diet, 83% were discharged from the acute care setting, and 70% did not require readmission.[176] The PEG tube intervention effectively palliated the obstruction in these patients with advanced ovarian cancer. Intravenous fluids are administered simultaneously, if needed. Analgesics, antiemetics, anticholinergics, antihistamines, and somatostatin analogs are prescribed to manage pain, nausea, and vomiting, and to reduce gastrointestinal secretions. If no significant improvement occurs, surgery is considered. Intestinal stenting using colonic stents may provide a nonsurgical alternative for relief of the obstruction.

Decisions about surgery for advanced cancer are always difficult. Quality of life considerations and potential complications after surgery are significant factors that must be weighed against possible gains, because as many as one-third of patients with a bowel obstruction will develop another bowel obstruction from their advanced disease.[177] On the other side, the mortality rate from an ischemic bowel is 30% and patients who develop perforation, peritonitis, or bowel strangulation will likely require emergency surgery.[178] As part of an assessment for surgery, certain prognostic factors should be considered: the patient's age, tumor burden, nutritional status, and ability to tolerate additional chemotherapy after surgery to prevent further recurrence.[5] Surgery may involve lysis of the adhesions or a bypass procedure with a proximal diverting colostomy or ileostomy if the obstruction is in the colon. The goals of surgical intervention are to alleviate the obstruction, remove ischemic and necrotic tissue, prevent gangrene, and prevent sepsis.

Long-term medical management for patients who are not surgical candidates is achieved with placement of a gastrostomy tube. A gastrostomy tube is comfortable and patients can maintain adequate hydration by consuming small, low-residue fluid meals. In addition, total parental nutrition (TPN) may be initiated for temporary or permanent nutritional supplement. In advanced ovarian cancer, conservative management of a bowel obstruction through restricted oral intake is indicated and can be achieved while the patient is at home. Patients are instructed to begin taking small amounts of clear liquids after several hours of bowel rest and slowly advance their diet as tolerated. A low fiber diet may be indicated because of profound narrowing of the small or large intestine.

## MALNUTRITION

Anorexia and cachexia both lead to malnutrition.[179,180] The anorexia–cachexia syndrome can be caused by a bowel obstruction or dysfunction; excessive protein or fluid loss from the bowel; gastrointestinal symptoms such as nausea, vomiting, diarrhea, or early satiety; complications of chemotherapy; or psychological factors.[5] Appetite and the ability to eat are closely linked to a patient's quality of life.[181] It is important to understand that the meaning of being able to eat is more significant than the nutritional or biological loss of food.[182] Unfortunately, the anorexia–cachexia symptom progresses as the ovarian cancer progresses.

Weight loss in patients with cancer can influence both response to therapy and duration of survival.[181] In an ECOG analysis of 3047 patients with cancer on 9 treatment protocols, median survival was significantly shorter for patients with weight loss compared with patients with no weight loss.[183] Patients should be evaluated first for reversible causes of decreased appetite, such as xerostomia and depression. Symptoms contributing to weight loss can include nausea, vomiting, diarrhea, fatigue, dyspnea, pain, and taste changes.[184]

Anorexia–cachexia syndrome is a major concern for nurses because its impact on patients is tremendous, coupled with disease and treatment side effects, physical weakness, fatigue, altered physical appearance, and loss of control over everyday life. The greater the degree of weight loss and malnutrition, the greater the degree of functional deficit and the higher the risk of complications.[185] In addition, anorexia is most distressing to patients and their family members because those who have prepared the food may feel that they—not the food—are being rejected; as a consequence, tremendous struggles can develop over eating.[173]

An assessment of anorexia–cachexia involves subjective and objective measures including a food diary, daily weight measurements, tools to assess nutritional status and appetite, and blood tests. Severe weight loss is defined as an involuntary loss of more than 10% of usual body weight in 6 months or a 5% loss of usual body weight in 1 month; it is associated with poorer outcomes.[186,187] Early intervention is essential. The oral route of intervention is preferred because it is known that significant atrophy of intestinal villi occurs within days of decreased enteral stimulation.[178] Provide information on maintaining a well-balanced, high-calorie diet, enlist the help of a dietitian, and use nutritional supplements. Instruction includes tips on enhancing the flavor of foods, attention to the likes and dislikes of the patient, and avoiding foods with disturbing odors or tastes. Management of symptoms interfering with appetite may also be necessary.

Pharmacologic intervention for anorexia–cachexia include corticosteroids, appetite stimulants, metoclopramide, or cannabinoids. Corticosteroids may produce short-term improvements in appetite but are associated with adverse effects. Megestrol acetate demonstrated a dose-related benefit on appetite, caloric intake, body weight gain, and sensation of well-being with an optimal dose of 400 to 800 mg/day orally.[188–190]

A study of megesterol acetate vs dronabinol vs combination therapy found 75%, 49%, and 66% appetite increases, respectively.[191] Megesterol alone was the superior approach and had an improvement on the patients' quality of life.[193] Newer agents being studied include drugs to increase muscle mass, omega-3 fatty acids, growth hormones, and anticytokine therapies.[192] Nurses should assess food intake every 4 weeks and allow 8 to 12 weeks for weight gain. Successful intervention for anorexia–cachexia must focus on both the physiological and psychological factors influencing the development of the problem.

If adequate calories cannot be consumed by mouth, then nutritional support via the enteral route may be necessary. Enteral tube placement, such as a PEG tube (percutaneous endoscopically placed gastrostomy or jejunostomy tube), is an option. Total parental nutrition should be reserved for those patients who are undergoing aggressive surgery, chemotherapy, or radiotherapy with severe gastrointestinal toxicity, or severely malnourished patients who are receiving active therapy. The difficult decision to initiate TPN must be made with the consensus of the entire medical team regarding its ethical appropriateness for a given patient.

## LYMPHEDEMA

In ovarian cancer, lymphedema usually arises secondary to an obstruction or blockage of the lymph system caused by tumor or trauma to the lymphatic channels.[193] The dominant site for lymphedema in ovarian cancer is in the lower extremities because of blockage of the pelvic or inguinal lymph nodes. In the early stages of obstruction, compensatory mechanisms such as collateral lymphatic flow are activated, but often they prove insufficient and excessive accumulation of a protein-rich fluid in the tissue spaces ensues. Patients experience discomfort or pain, a fullness or heaviness of the extremity, numbness, weakness, and limited mobility. Clothing becomes increasingly tight and ambulation more difficult. Assessment is usually by patient self-report and measurement of the swollen limb. The current methods for assessing the extent of the lymphedema in the extremity are water displacement, circumferential measurements, calculation of the volume using the formula for a truncated cone, biometric impedance analysis, and comparative circumferential measurements.[194] CT scan or magnetic resonance imaging (MRI) can confirm a diagnosis of lymphedema and provide measures to characterize the degree of involvement: mild (stage I), moderate (stage II), or severe (stage III).[195] Management of lymphedema is related to the primary treatment of the cancer. With systemic chemotherapy, the lymph node involvement will shrink and the fluid will subsequently drain.

The stages of lymphedema, a description of the swollen limb's appearance and physical findings, and treatment are found in Table 62-19. Complex decongestive physiotherapy is a 5-part regimen critical to successful management of lymphedema. It consists of skin care, manual lymphatic drainage (MLD), bandaging the affected limbs, exercises, and wearing a compression garment.[196] The mainstay of symptomatic lymphedema treatment is MLD performed by a physical therapist trained in lymphedema management. MLD entails light stimulation of the dermal lymphatomes and the lymphatic vessels; it is not to be confused with deep massage, which concentrates on the muscles.[195,197] By stimulating the lymphatic vessels, a therapist is able to redirect the protein-rich fluid around the affected area and increase the reabsorption of lymphatic fluid. Compression therapy is applied at the end of the 1-hour session, wrapping the extremity with a low-pressure stretch bandage while carefully distributing pressure in a distal-to-proximal direction.[197] Patients are also instructed to perform exercises to increase flexion of the muscle, which creates resistance against the bandage to stimulate additional lymphatic flow. Patients are treated daily for 4 to 5 weeks during the initial phase. Maintenance therapy frequency is determined by the patient's response and the therapist's judgment. Compression garments should be worn continuously between treatments. Meticulous instructions regarding skin care are a component of the therapy plan, because skin of the edematous limb is at risk for breakdown and infection. If MLD no longer helps, gradient pressure pneumatic pumps may be prescribed. The pumps require a 2 hour daily commitment and should be provided by a company that requires therapists and home counseling in conjunction with the treatment.

Limitations of mobility are difficult for patients to deal with because many people try to maintain their normal

**TABLE 62-19**

**Management of Lymphedema**

| Stages of Lymphedema | Findings | Treatment |
|---|---|---|
| Stage I (reversible) | Skin smooth, textured<br>Pitting edema<br>2–3 cm difference between limb circumference<br>Limb feels heavy, throbbing | Elevate extremity<br>Compression garment<br>Massage<br>Physical therapy |
| Stage II (chronic, does not reverse spontaneously) | Limb is swollen<br>Edema, *not* pitting<br>Skin stretched, shiny<br>Tissue soft<br>3–5 cm difference in limb circumference | Same as stage I; if ineffective begin complex decongestive physiotherapy |
| Stage III (severe) | Extreme increase in swelling until the limb is column shaped, *not* pitting<br>Hand or foot massively swollen<br>Skin dark or purple colored<br>Skin stretched, tissue firm<br>Rough textured<br>Lymph leaks directly through the skin<br>> 5 cm difference in limb circumference | Aggressive treatment<br>May use gradient<br>Pneumatic pressure<br>Pump therapy<br>Pain management |

*Source*: Data from Martin.[170]

activities despite progressive disease. Diuretics are of limited benefit in the treatment of edema due to advanced disease. The nurse needs to engage women in protecting their legs from infection or trauma, provide nursing care that includes educating women about the early signs and symptoms of lymphedema, and provide information on how to access specialists early so that effective management can be initiated.[198] Lower limb lymphedema has an impact on appearance, mobility, finances, and self-image in many women.[198]

## PLEURAL EFFUSION

Pleural effusions are an accumulation of fluid in excess of the normal 25 mL of fluid within the intrapleural space.[199] Approximately 25% to 30% of patients with metastatic ovarian cancer develop pleural effusions.[5,200] They develop when the flow of pleural fluid from the parietal pleura to the visceral pleura is interrupted by tumor. The effusion may be exudate or transudate in nature. Two major pathophysiological processes are associated with exudative effusion: an inflammatory process and neoplastic disease. Dyspnea caused by the accumulating effusion is the most commonly reported symptom.[199,201,202] Sharp pleuritic chest pain, if present, may or may not be accompanied by a pleural rub.[199,201] Other symptoms associated with a pleural effusion include fever (if inflammatory), dry irritating cough, and hypoxia.[199] Effusions are diagnosed by a posterior, anterior, and lateral chest x-ray. On physical exam, findings include decreased breath sounds and dullness to percussion, most often in the lung base.

Once the diagnosis of pleural effusion is made, a thoracentesis may be required to remove the excess fluid if it is causing significant impairment. An ultrasound is often used to locate the fluid for removal during a thoracentesis. The patient must be prepared for the procedure and its possible complications, which include pain, infection, pneumothorax, and pulmonary edema. The nurse must observe for any pain or discomfort, increased respiratory rate or dyspnea, increased pulse rate, vertigo, or uncontrollable cough during the procedure.[5] The fluid is removed and sent for diagnostic studies. A chest x-ray is performed after the procedure to rule out a pneumothorax. The fluid will usually rapidly reaccumulate in 4 to 5 days, unless the underlying cause of the problem, the ovarian cancer, is effectively treated with systemic chemotherapy.

The Pleurx pleural catheter is a treatment option that allows patients to be treated on an outpatient basis for weeks or months.[203] The catheter is a 66-cm, 15.5-French, flexible silicone catheter that is surgically inserted into the pleural space and held in place by a polyester cuff. It remains in place and the family members are taught how to drain it on an intermittent basis. Another tunneled catheter choice is the Aspira pleural drainage system. The Pleurx or Aspira systems offer more comfort, less infection, and tend to provide the patient with more control, being taught to drain intermittently. Pigtail catheters are also inserted and attached to a drainage bag, usually short-term use of this type of system is preferred.

Insertion of a chest tube or thoracostomy and the addition of a sclerosing agent or pleurodesis may also be performed if pleural fluid reaccumulates. The sclerosing procedure requires hospitalization; the chest tube is inserted at the bedside and the tube is connected to suction for several days. As the drainage diminishes, the pleural space is obliterated using a sclerosing agent to prevent the fluid reaccumulation. In women whose effusion cannot be adequately drained or in whom the lung does not reexpand, but who have a reasonable life expectancy, open pleurodesis or a pleuroperitoneal shunt may be considered.[172]

The severe dyspnea caused by a pleural effusion can be controlled in sedentary patients who have advanced disease with oxygen and/or opioids.[172] Opioids decrease the intensity of dyspnea and the sense of respiratory effort.[204] Morphine, hydromorphone, and fentanyl are all used and can be given via any route. The use of nebulized opioids can assist with dyspnea. By providing information concerning palliative measures to manage this distressing side effect, the nurse can help lessen anxiety, because pleural effusion is an undeniable indicator of disease progression. Relaxation exercises are helpful in decreasing anxiety and may include guided imagery, progressive relaxation with controlled breathing, listening to relaxing music, mild massage, and range-of-motion exercises.[205] Exercises to help with breathlessness include sitting upright and leaning forward, leaning over a table, or resting elbows on knees to promote lung expansion and help the patient breathe easier.[205] Patients must modify their activities of daily living and plan frequent rest periods for increased support.

## STRESS AND SUPPORT

The prevalence of psychological distress in women with ovarian cancer is reported in multiple studies to be in the range of 23% to 67%.[206] Clinicians need to be aware that anxiety and depression in patients with ovarian cancer appear related to the patients' physical symptom experiences and degree of empathetic support the patients perceived from their informal caregivers. Lower levels of anxiety and depression in women with end stage ovarian cancer were noted if caregivers had empathetic behavior towards them.[154] Evidence exists that women with ovarian cancer suffer high levels of psychological distress due to a high rate of disease recurrence and low cure rate.[156,207,208] Ovarian cancer survivors report significant quality of life concerns across the dimension of physical, psychological, social, and spiritual well-being.[206] The 10 most frequently mentioned concerns for women who responded to a mailed survey included recurrence, death or dying, getting the cancer under control or being cancer free; managing treatment side effects; running out of drugs or options for treatment; severe pain or neuropathy; husband or family being left alone; financial or employment issues; quality of life issues; future chemotherapy or radiation treatment.[206] These concerns outline for nurses important areas for nursing intervention in clinical practice. High rates of anxiety and depression have been noted during chemotherapy treatment and high distress levels continue for one-third of long-term survivors.[209,210] Guidozzi[210] found significant psychological distress in patients that impaired physical function. For these distressed women, relief came from psychological counseling and support and improvement in their physical symptoms. Women who experienced pain and fatigue lost the ability to enjoy life, engage in normal relationship activities, and maintain employment status.[211] Fox and Lyon[208] studied 76 women who had completed treatment or on treatment and found depression and fatigue a symptom cluster in ovarian cancer. The nursing implication is that this symptom cluster impacts quality of life and interventions to target the symptoms would have potential impact in altering outcomes for these patients.[208] Increased family stress arose from anxiety about the diagnosis and treatment, sexual changes, and fears about prognosis. Women reported problems with pain, appetite, fatigue, and finances that had a significant impact on their quality of life, and these symptoms worsened as the disease progressed.[209,212]

Positive changes have also been reported about the way some women have changed after the diagnosis. A new appreciation of life and adoption of a "live for the moment" philosophy have been reported.

One qualitative study describing the concerns of women with ovarian cancer found increased distress because of the compressed time frame in which to confront life-threatening issues.[213] The group expressed overwhelming feelings of helplessness and uncertainty while facing mortality and redefining goals and expectations. Another study examined 21,806 letters, cards, and e-mails reflecting correspondence between ovarian cancer survivors and the editor of an ovarian cancer newsletter between 1994 and 2000. These authors identified major themes during all phases of the disease trajectory. Unique psychological factors found included the women experienced profound isolation living with ovarian cancer; they contended with anxiety resulting from the genetic association of the disease and fear for their daughters more often than fear for themselves; and the stress of living with periods of recurrence created considerable stress and uncertainty.[214] The investigators hope to use the coping strategies identified in this study to build interventions that healthcare providers can use to assist women with ovarian cancer.[214]

Because ovarian cancer is a disease that commonly recurs, research looking at the time period after primary therapy and during disease recurrence has added to the knowledge base of the disease. The continual monitoring of the CA-125 level serves as a constant reminder of the potential for recurrence. Hamilton[215] noted that women identified their CA-125 levels as evidence of disease status and that their emotions were governed by the value of the marker.

In another study, 263 women returned surveys eliciting important issues associated with ovarian cancer. The respondents included 93 women who had experienced recurrent disease and 170 who had not. A greater proportion of the women with recurrent disease reported bowel problems, fear of dying, pain, problems getting around, and feelings of self-blame.[216] Overall, women with recurrent disease reported experiencing more problems since diagnosis than those without recurrent disease.[216] A particular concern raised in this study was that a significant proportion of women felt they had not received adequate help for the problems they experienced. Two specific areas of inadequate assistance were difficulties with bowels and sexual function.[216] These women perceived nurses as being helpful to them, thereby creating opportunities for nurses to provide more support.

In another study, 18 women with ovarian cancer were interviewed and identified the following major challenges: living with uncertainty, lack of control, fear of the unknown, the stigma of cancer, and facing death.[217] These authors outline the implications of their findings for nursing practice: family-centered care to help deal with the adjustments in roles and relationships; a sensitivity to financial issues; the ability to express fears and anxieties about death; and assistance in planning for the future.[217] As these women faced recurrent disease, 4 primary themes surfaced: waiting for recurrence, facing the diagnosis of recurrence, managing treatment-related concerns, and attempting to regain control.[211] More important, these women described changed communication with their healthcare providers when recurrent disease was found. They felt increased hopelessness as a result of their perception that the provider was not listening to their symptoms and had no treatment options to present.[211] The message these patients received was that symptom management rather than prolongation of life had become the goal, and this caused them distress.

Twelve women living with recurrent ovarian cancer were interviewed to deepen the understanding of how the recurrence of ovarian cancer was experienced and lived through by the women.[207] Findings showed that women's daily life had markedly changed. The women described feelings of alienation from both themselves and others and a feeling that they were living in limbo. Dialogue, counseling, information, and education may help support these women achieve the highest possible level of well-being.[207]

Finally, studying women without active disease has yielded additional information. In 1 study, 200 women who had ovarian cancer, were without evidence of active disease, and were not on treatment for at least 2 years, were surveyed. Most respondents reported good physical, psychological, social, and spiritual health. However, the cancer experience did have a detrimental effect (57% reported) on the women's sex lives.[218] Nurses therefore have an opportunity to educate these women about their sexual health.

Patient support groups offer another way to provide emotional support to patients with ovarian cancer. In a support group for patients with ovarian cancer, over a 2-year period 30 women discussed 2 consistent themes: "fate vs freedom" (the struggle to face the real possibility of dying vs the freedom to enjoy life) and "despair vs hope" (the struggle to give in to loss, pain, and dejection vs maintaining optimism).[219] Struggling with these existential issues stood out as the most important therapeutic factor in this support group.

Information gained from surveys and interviews of patients with ovarian cancer, provides nurses with valuable insight into the experience of living with this disease. Nurses can help patients understand the information and meaning of monitoring for disease recurrence and provide more sensitive communication about their treatment options. They play key roles in helping women with ovarian cancer by providing both physical and emotional care during the disease trajectory and improving quality of life.

## PATIENT RESOURCES

Following the path established by the successful breast cancer and AIDS advocacy groups, ovarian cancer now has a public voice. The OCNA, formed in 1997, is an organization with a mission of uniting organizations and individuals in the fight to overcome ovarian cancer. The National Ovarian Cancer Coalition (NOCC) was founded by a group of ovarian cancer survivors in April 1995. It now has more than 2000 members and 23 state chapters. The mission of NOCC is to raise awareness about ovarian cancer and to promote education about the disease. The alliance and coalition succeeded in having September 1998 designated as the first National Ovarian Cancer Awareness Month. President Clinton designated September 13 to 19, 1998, as the first Ovarian Cancer Awareness Week. Ovarian Cancer National Alliance held the initial national advocacy conference on ovarian cancer called "Silent No More" in September 1998, with other founding partner and member organizations. The national agenda for OCNA is to conquer ovarian cancer by uniting individuals and organization to a national movement. The organization is now 10 years old and presents a national agenda for ovarian cancer. The goals are to advance ovarian cancer research, improve healthcare practice for ovarian cancer across the continuum of care, and expand the national advocate movement for ovarian cancer. Included in those goals are specific objectives such as doubling the total federal funding devoted to ovarian cancer research (currently estimated at $125 million annually); increase the enrollment of women on clinical trials, increase awareness of risk factors and symptoms of ovarian cancer, and unite the organization with a focus on ovarian cancer into a collaborative national force.

The Web sites http://www.ovarian.org and http://www.ovariancancer.org offer a multitude of information and include a chat forum and an "Ask the Experts" page. Other general information resources include the American Cancer Society, National Cancer Institute Cancer Information Service; Society of Gynecologic Oncologists; Gilda Radner Familial Ovarian Cancer Registry; and Gynecologic Cancer Foundation Information Hotline. Resources focusing on support include Cancer Care; National Coalition for Cancer Survivorship; Gilda's Club; SHARE; and the Wellness Community. Addresses, phone numbers, and Internet addresses are provided in Table 62-20.

A new diagnosis of an unfamiliar disease prompted one woman to launch her own network of support. She was desperate to talk with another woman like herself, specifically a survivor, which led to the birth of a newsletter titled Conversations, for women fighting ovarian cancer.[220] Conversations started with a circulation of 10, but has grown considerably over the last 10 years. Unfortunately, the editor lost her battle with ovarian cancer in 2003, but her family has continued to produce the newsletter for other women with ovarian cancer. The newsletter is filled with tips for dealing with treatment side effects and the latest clinical trials available for patients seeking

**TABLE 62-20**

**Resources for Ovarian Cancer Information**

| | |
|---|---|
| National Ovarian Cancer Coalition (NOCC)<br>500 NE Spanish River Boulevard, Suite 14<br>Boca Raton, FL 33431<br>888-OVARIAN<br>*http://www.ovarian.org* | Marsha Rivkin Ovarian Cancer Research Center<br>1221 Madison Street<br>Seattle, WA 98104<br>206-215-6200<br>800-328-1124<br>*http://www.marsharivkin.org* |
| National Ovarian Cancer Alliance<br>910 17th Street NW. Suite 413<br>Washington, DC 20006<br>202-331-1332<br>*http://www.ovariancancer.org* | National Ovarian Cancer Association<br>27 Park Road<br>Toronto, Canada<br>877-413-7970<br>*http://www.ovariancanada.org* |
| Women's Cancer Network<br>c/o Gynecologic Cancer Foundation<br>401 N. Michigan Avenue<br>Chicago, IL 60611<br>312-644-6610<br>*http://www.wcn.org* | Ovarian Cancer Research Fund<br>One Pennsylvania Plaza, Suite 1610<br>New York, NY 10119<br>800-873-9569<br>*http://www.ocrf.org* |
| CancerCare, Inc.<br>275 Seventh Avenue<br>New York, NY 10001<br>800-813-HOPE<br>*http://www.cancercare.org* | SHARE: Self-Help for Women with Breast or Ovarian Cancer<br>1501 Broadway, Suite 1720<br>New York, NY 10036<br>212-719-1204<br>*http://www.sharecancersupport.org* |
| Gilda Radner Ovarian Cancer Familial Registry<br>Roswell Park Cancer Institute<br>Elm and Carlton Streets<br>Buffalo, NY 14263<br>800-OVARIAN<br>*http://www.ovariancancer.com* | FORCE: Facing Our Risk of Cancer Empowerment<br>954-255-8732<br>*http://www.facingourrisk.org* |
| | Gilda's Club<br>888-445-3248<br>*http://www.gildasclub.org* |
| Conversations!<br>The Newsletter for Those Fighting Ovarian Cancer<br>PO Box 7948<br>Amarillo, TX 79114–7948<br>806-355-2565<br>*http://www.ovarian-news.com* | The Blanton-Davis Ovarian Cancer Researching Program<br>800-392-1611<br>*http://www.mdanderson.org* |

treatments. The address for subscribing to this newsletter is PO Box 7948, Amarillo, TX 79114-7948.

## CONTINUITY OF CARE

Because no effective screening methods for ovarian cancer exist, this disease is often discovered in its late stages. Continuity of care during the long and chronic course of treating ovarian cancer is an area warranting concentration by the nurse. The trajectory of primary treatment and then management of the complications in advanced disease are often centered in the outpatient or home setting. The acute phase of care in an inpatient setting usually occurs during the early phase of the disease treatment or briefly during a crisis of treatment or advanced disease. Nurses are in the key position to educate patients on the prevention and control of the side effects from treatment or disease progression so that their quality of life can be maintained. The plan for continuity of care must include seamless access to necessary care as needs arise, and information must flow between caregivers irrespective of their practice settings.

Ambulatory and office nurses are critical links to support and guide patients with ovarian cancer. For example, the patient typically uses self-care measures to monitor the reaccumulation of ascites fluid and the nurse is informed when weight gain or discomfort reaches an unacceptable level. The nurse consults with the physician and a plan is developed to relieve the existing problem. In other instances, surgical intervention for a partial intestinal obstruction may not be possible in an advanced disease case. It is then the nurse who helps the patient and family cope with the problem until the end of life.

Addressing emotional needs is as important a component of nursing care as managing symptoms. Helping the patient and family cope with the end of life is central to the role and skills of the oncology nurse. Dealing with anxiety and depression and preventing feelings of abandonment or despair are a few of the psychosocial needs of both the patient and family during the final stages of the disease. Involvement of the hospice team when appropriate will add support at a critical phase of need for the patient and family. At each phase and step along the trajectory of ovarian cancer care, collaboration between healthcare team members, the patient, and the family is critical.

## FUTURE TRENDS

The 5-year survival rate for ovarian cancer has improved from 37% in 1975 to 1977 to 45% in 1996 to 2003.[1] Ovarian cancer is now considered and managed as a chronic disease. Much still remains to be discovered regarding its development, the exact pathogenesis remains unclear although it is believed to be a multistep process. Two gene mutations have been identified in hereditary forms of the disease but how their discovery fits together with nonhereditary ovarian cancer is not yet known.[221] Several identified factors may increase an individual's risk, and attention has turned to identifying molecular markers (genomic and proteomic) to improve the predictive value of screening.[221] Symptoms, although nonspecific, have been identified and when recognized early may lead to detection and improved survival. Future directions for treatment of ovarian cancer include research aimed at screening and prevention, finding a molecular basis for ovarian cancer, identifying high-risk individuals, and targeted therapy with molecular profiling. Chemotherapy will continue to have a major role in the treatment of ovarian cancer in the future, with clinical trials helping to establish the regimen of choice. Subsequent trials will combine chemotherapy with molecular-targeted biological agents as initial treatment for patients with ovarian cancer. New targeted therapy in ovarian cancer appears particularly promising. The current treatment regimens induce a state where minimal disease is present. In this situation the newer therapies may be at their most effective, and they may ultimately be continued as maintenance therapy to prevent or delay recurrences.[221] Drug resistance mechanisms and pharmacological techniques to reverse the resistance are also major areas of clinical research.

Nursing research has made gains in increasing our knowledge base about living with ovarian cancer and some of the most important challenges faced by patients. Ovarian cancer is particularly difficult due to its advanced stage at diagnosis, the repetitive cycles of aggressive treatment with little respite, and the dismal survival statistics that serve as a constant reminder of the disease's seriousness to patients. Patients need to be assessed more thoroughly and given more information throughout the treatment trajectory. Support group referrals may be particularly helpful.[222] Nurses are key in improving awareness of the disease so that education is available and no delay in diagnosis occurs. The chronic nature of ovarian cancer challenges providers to balance quality of life issues with treatment toxicities.[222] The healthcare team will continue to be challenged to keep pace as new treatments for ovarian cancer enter the clinical arena and new patient care strategies unfold. The nurse on the healthcare team has the opportunity to make an invaluable contribution.

## REFERENCES

1. Jemal A, Siegel R, Ward E, et al. Cancer statistics 2009. *CA Cancer J Clin.* 2009;59:225–249.
2. Surveillance, Epidemiology, and End Results Program. *SEER Cancer Statistics Review, 1975–2001.* Bethesda, MD: National Cancer Institute; 2004.
3. Piver MS. Hereditary ovarian cancer. *Gynecol Oncol.* 2002;85:9–17.

4. Surveillance, Epidemiology, and End Results. SEER Stat Fact Sheets, Ovary. http://seer.cancer.gov/statfacts/html/ovary.html. Accessed January 12, 2010.
5. Eriksson JH, Frazier SR. Epithelial cancers of the ovary and fallopian tube. In: Moore GJ, ed. *Women and Cancer: A Gynecologic Oncology Nursing Perspective.* Sudbury, MA: Jones and Bartlett; 1997:205–256.
6. Landen C, Birrer M, Sood A. Early events in the pathogenesis of epithelial ovarian cancer. *J Clin Oncol.* 2008;46:995–1005.
7. Narora H. Developmental patterning in the wrong context: the paradox of ovarian cancers. *Cell Cycle.* 2005;4:1033–1035.
8. Auersperg N, Wong A, Choi K, et al. Ovarian surface epithelium: biology, endocrinology, and pathology. *Endocr Rev.* 2001;22:255–288.
9. Brinton L, Lamb E, Moghiss K, et al. Ovarian cancer risk after the use of ovulation stimulating drugs. *Obstet Gynecol.* 2004;103:1194–1203.
10. Fathalla MF. Incessant ovulation: a factor in ovarian neoplasia? *Lancet.* 1971;2:163.
11. Ozols RF, Bookman MA, Connolly DC, et al. Focus on epithelial ovarian cancer. *Cancer Cell.* 2004;5:19–24.
12. Schlosshauer PW, Coeh CJ, Penault–Liorca F, et al. Prophylactic oophorectomy: a morphologic and immunohistochemical study. *Cancer.* 2003;98:2599–2606.
13. Ness RB, Cottreau C. Possible role of ovarian epithelial inflammation in ovarian cancer. *J Natl Cancer Inst.* 1999;91:1459–1467.
14. Vo C, Carney ME. Ovarian cancer hormonal and environmental risk effect. *Obstet Gynecol Clin North Am.* 2007;34:687–700, viii.
15. Purdie DM, Bain CJ, Siskind V, et al. Ovulation and risk of epithelial ovarian cancer. *Int J Cancer.* 2002;104:228–232.
16. Mahdavi A, Pejovic T, Nezhat F. Induction of ovulation and ovarian cancer: a critical review of the literature. *Fertil Steril.* 2006;85:819–826.
17. Ness RB. Endometriosis and ovarian cancer: thoughts on shared pathophysiology. *Am J Obstet Gynecol.* 2003;189:280–294.
18. Daly M, Obrams GI. Epidemiology and risk assessment for ovarian cancer. *Semin Oncol.* 1998;25:255–264.
19. Danforth KN, Tworger SS, Hecht JL. Breastfeeding and risk of ovarian cancer in two prospective cohorts. *Cancer Causes Control.* 2007;18:517–523.
20. Franco E, Duarto–Franco E. Oral contraceptives and ovarian cancer. *Lancet.* 2008;371:277–278.
21. Martin V, Cherry C. Ovarian cancer. In: Dow K, ed. *Nursing Care of Women with Cancer.* St Louis, MO: Mosby Elsevier; 2006:96–119.
22. Modugno F. Ovarian cancer and polymorphisms in the androgen and progesterone receptor gene: a huge review. *Am J Epidemiol.* 2004;155:217–224.
23. Whittemore A, Balise RR, Pharoah PD, et al. Oral contraceptive use and ovarian cancer risk among carriers of BRCA1 or BRCA2 mutations. *Br J Cancer.* 2004;91:1911–1915.
24. Anderson GL, Judd HL, Kaunitz AM, et al. Effects of estrogen plus progestin on gynecologic cancers and associated diagnostic procedures: the women's health initiative randomized trial. *JAMA.* 2003;290:1739–1748.
25. Coughlin SS, Giustozzi A, Smith SJ, et al. A meta–analysis of estrogen replacement therapy and risk of epithelial ovarian cancer. *J Clin Epidemiol.* 2000;53:367–375.
26. Sit AS, Modugno F, Weissfeld JL, et al. Hormone replacement therapy formulations and risk of epithelial ovarian carcinoma. *Gynecol Oncol.* 2002;86:118–123.
27. Helzlsouer KJ, Alberg AJ, Gordon GB, et al. Serum gonadotropin and steroid hormones and the development of ovarian cancer. *JAMA.* 1995;274:1926–1930.
28. Schildkraut J, Schwingl PJ, Bastos E, et al. Epithelial ovarian cancer risk among women with polycystic ovarian syndrome. *Obstet Gynecol.* 1996;88:554–559.
29. Brinton LA, Gridley G, Persson I, et al. Cancer risk after a hospital discharge of endometriosis. *Am J Obstet Gynecol.* 1997;176:572–579.
30. Schildkraut JM, Bastos E, Berchuck A. Relationship between lifetime ovulatory cycles and overexpression of mutant p53 in epithelial ovarian cancer. *J Natl Cancer Inst.* 1997;89:932–938.
31. Tung KH, Goodman MT, Wu AH, et al. Reproductive factors and epithelial ovarian cancer risk by histologic type: a multiethnic case–control study. *Am J Epidemiol.* 2003;158:629–638.
32. Cramer DW, Muto MG, Reichardt JK, et al. Characteristics of women with a family history of ovarian cancer. I. Galactose consumption and metabolism. *Cancer.* 1994;74:1309–1317.
33. Risch HA, Jain M, Marrett LD, et al. Dietary lactose intake, lactose intolerance, and the risk of ovarian cancer in southern Ontario (Canada). *Cancer Causes Control.* 1994;5:540–548.
34. Herrinton LJ, Weiss NS, Beresford SA, et al. Lactose and galactose intake and metabolism in relation to the risk of epithelial ovarian cancer. *Am J Epidemiol.* 1995;141:407–416.
35. Eyre H, Kahn R, Robertson R. Preventing cancer, cardiovascular disease, and diabetes: a common agenda for the American Cancer Society, the American Diabetes Association, and the American Heart Association. *CA Cancer J Clin.* 2004;54:190–207.
36. Mink PJ, Folsom AR, Sellers TA, et al. Physical activity, waist–to–hip ratio, and other risk factors for ovarian cancer: a follow–up study of older women. *Epidemiology.* 1996;7:38–45.
37. Cramer DW, Liberman RF, Titus–Ernstoff L, et al. Genital talc exposure and risk of ovarian cancer. *Int J Cancer.* 1999;81:351–356.
38. Gertig DM, Hunter DJ, Cramer DW, et al. Prospective study of talc use and ovarian cancer. *J Natl Cancer Inst.* 2000;92:249–252.
39. Muscat JE, Huncharek MS. Perineal talc and ovarian cancer: a critical review. *Eur J Cancer Prev.* 2008;17:139–146.
40. National Institutes of Health Consensus Development Conference Statement. Ovarian cancer: screening, treatment, and follow–up. *Gynecol Oncol.* 1994;55:S4–S14.
41. Wooster R, Neuhausen SL, Mangion J, et al. Localization of a breast cancer susceptibility gene, BRCA2, to chromosome 13q12–13. *Science.* 1994;265:1088–2090.
42. Wooster R, Bignell G, Lancaster J, et al. Identification of the breast cancer susceptibility gene BRCA2. *Nature.* 1995;378:789–792.
43. Pavelka JC, Li AJ, Karlan BY. Hereditary ovarian cancer–assessing risk and prevention strategies. *Obstet Gynecol Clin North Am.* 2007;34:651–655.
44. Struewing JP, Abeliovich D, Peretz T, et al. The carrier frequency of the BRCA1 185delAG mutations is approximately 1 percent in Ashkenazi Jewish individuals. *Nat Genet.* 1995;11:198–200.
45. Abeliovich D, Kaduri L, Lerer I, et al. The founder mutations in 185delAG and 5382insC in BRCA1 and 617delIT in BRCA2 appear in 60% of ovarian cancer and 30% of early–onset breast cancer patients among Ashkenazi women. *Am J Hum Genet.* 1997;60:505–514.
46. Reedy M, Gallion H, Fowler JM, et al. Contribution of BRCA 1 and BRCA 2 to familial ovarian cancer: a gynecologic oncology group study. *Gynecol Oncol.* 2002;85:255–259.
47. Lynch HT, Casey MJ, Shaw TG, et al. Hereditary factors in gynecologic cancer. *Oncologist.* 1998;3:319–338.
48. Lynch HT, Casey MJ, Lynch J, et al. Genetics and ovarian carcinoma. *Semin Oncol.* 1998;25:265–280.
49. Cherry C, Vacchiano SA. Ovarian cancer screening and prevention. *Semin Oncol Nurs.* 2002;18:167–173.
50. Modugno F. Ovarian cancer and high–risk women symposium presenters: ovarian cancer and high–risk women—implications for prevention, screening, and early detection. *Gynecol Oncol.* 2003;91:15–31.
51. Bast R, Klug T, St John E, et al. A radioimmunoassay using a monoclonal antibody to monitor the course of epithelial ovarian cancer. *N Engl J Med.* 1993;309:883–887.
52. Bast RC, Xu FJ, Yu YH, et al. CA 125: the past and the future. *Int J Biol Markers.* 1998;13:179–187.
53. Rosenthal A, Jacobs I. Ovarian cancer screening. *Semin Oncol.* 1998;25:315–323.

54. Skates SJ, Menon U, MacDonald N, et al. Calculation of the risk of ovarian cancer from serial CA–125 values for preclinical detection in postmenopausal women. *J Clin Oncol.* 2003;21:206–210.
55. Rustin GJS, Nelstrop AE, McClean P, et al. Defining response of ovarian carcinoma to initial chemotherapy according to serum CA 125. *J Clin Oncol.* 1996;14:1545–1551.
56. Shy K, Dubinsky T. Is color Doppler ultrasound useful in diagnosing ovarian cancer? *Clin Obstet Gynecol.* 1999;42:902–915.
57. van Nagell JR Jr, DePriest PD, Ueland FR, et al. Ovarian cancer screening with annual transvaginal sonography. *Cancer* 2007;109:1887–1896.
58. Visintin I, Feng Z, Longton G, et al. Diagnostic markers for early detection of ovarian cancer. *Clin Cancer Res.* 2008;14:1065–1072.
59. Schwartz M, Kaufman E, Peshkin BN, et al. Bilateral prophylactic oophorectomy and ovarian cancer screening following BRCA1/BRCA2 mutation testing. *J Clin Oncol.* 2003;21:4034–4041.
60. Bast RC Jr, Boyer CM, Jacobs I. Cell growth regulation in epithelial ovarian cancer. *Cancer.* 1993;71:1597–1601.
61. Prowse A, Frolov A, Godwin AK. The genetics of ovarian cancer. In: Ozols RF, ed. *American Cancer Society Atlas of Clinical Oncology.* Hamilton, Ontario: BC Decker; 2003:49–82.
62. DiSaia PJ. Diagnosis and management of ovarian cancer. *Hosp Pract.* 1987;22:235–250.
63. Omura GA, Brady MF, Homesley HD, et al. Long term follow up and prognostic factor analysis in advanced ovarian carcinoma: the Gynaecological Oncology Group experience. *J Clin Oncol.* 1991;9:1138–1150.
64. van Houwelingen JC, ten Bokkel Huinink W, van der Burg ATM, et al. Predictability of the survival of patients with ovarian cancer. *J Clin Oncol.* 1989;7:769–773.
65. Voest EE, van Houwelingen JC, Nejit JP. A meta–analysis of prognostic factors in advanced ovarian cancer with median survival and overall survival measured with the log (relative risk) as main objectives. *Eur J Cancer Clin Oncol.* 1989;28A:1328–1330.
66. Thigpen T, Brady MF, Omura GA, et al. Age as a prognostic factor in ovarian carcinoma: the Gynaecological Oncology Group experience. *Cancer.* 1993;71(suppl):606–614.
67. Havrilesky L, Darcy KM, Hamdan H, et al. Prognostic significance of p53 mutation and p53 overexpression in advanced epithelial ovarian cancer: a Gynecologic Oncology Group study. *J Clin Oncol.* 2003;21:3814–3825.
68. van der Zee AGT, Hollema H, Suurmeijer AJH, et al. Value of p–glycoprotein, glutathione s–transferase pi, c–erbB–2, and p53 as prognostic factors in ovarian carcinomas. *J Clin Oncol.* 1995;13:70–78.
69. Radner G. *It's Always Something.* New York: Avon Books; 1989.
70. Goff B, Mandel L, Drescher C, et al. Development of an ovarian cancer symptom index. *Cancer.* 2007;109:221–227.
71. Mayer AR, Chambers SK, Graves E, et al. Ovarian cancer staging: does it require a gynecologic oncologist? *Gynecol Oncol.* 1992;47:223–227.
72. Nguyen HN, Averette HE, Hoskins W, et al. National survey of ovarian carcinoma. Part V. The impact of physicians' specialty on patients' survival. *Cancer.* 1993;72:3663–3670.
73. Eisenkop SM, Spirtos NM, Montag TW, et al. The impact of subspecialty training on the management of advanced ovarian cancer. *Gynecol Oncol.* 1992;47:203–209.
74. Scully RE. Tumors of the ovary and maldeveloped gonads. In: Rosai J, Sobun LH, eds. *Atlas of Tumor Pathology.* Washington, DC: Armed Forces Institute; 1998:340–358.
75. International Federation of Gynecology and Obstetrics. Changes in definition of clinical staging for carcinoma of the cervix and ovary. *Am J Obstet Gynecol.* 1987;156:263–264.
76. Partridge EE, Phillips JL, Menck HR. The National Cancer Database report on ovarian cancer treatment in the United States hospitals. *Cancer.* 1996;78:2239–2246.
77. Friedlander ML. Prognostic factors in ovarian cancer. *Semin Oncol.* 1998;25:305–314.
78. Griffiths CT, Parker LM, Fuller AF. Role of cytoreductive surgery in the management of advanced ovarian cancer. *Cancer Treat Rep.* 1979;63:235–240.
79. Hogberg T, Carstensen J, Simonsen E. Treatment results and prognostic factors in a population–based study of epithelial ovarian cancer. *Gynecol Oncol.* 1993;48:38–49.
80. Eisenkop S, Nalick R, Teng N. Peritoneal implant excision or ablation during cytoreductive surgery. The impact on survival. *Gynecol Oncol.* 1993;45:97(abstr).
81. Chi Ds, Ramirez PT, Teitcher JB, et al. Prospective study of the correlation between postoperative computed tomography scan and primary surgeon assessment in patients with advanced ovarian, tubal, and peritoneal carcinoma reported to have undergone primary surgical cytoreduction to residual disease 1 cm or less. *J Clin Oncol* 2007;5: 4946–4951.
82. Winter WE III, Maxwell GL, Tian C, et al. Tumor residual after surgical cytoreduction in prediction of clinical outcome in stage IV epithelial ovarian cancer: a Gynecologic Oncology Group Study. *J Clin Oncol* 2008;26:83–89.
83. Young RC, Walton L, Ellenberg SS, et al. Adjuvant therapy in stage I and II epithelial ovarian cancer. Results of two prospective randomized trials. *N Engl J Med.* 1990;322:1021–1027.
84. Bertelson K, Holund B, Anderson E. Reproducibility and prognostic value of histologic type and grade in early epithelial ovarian cancer. *Int J Gynecol Cancer.* 1993;3:72–79.
85. Shimizu Y, Kamai S, Amada S, et al. Toward the development of a universal grading system for ovarian epithelial carcinoma. *Cancer.* 1998;82:893–901.
86. Mann WJ, Chalas E, Valea FA. Initial surgical management of epithelial ovarian cancer. Up to date. http://www.uptodate.com. Accessed September 28, 2009.
87. Munoz KA, Harlan CC, Trimble EL. Patterns of care for women with ovarian cancer in the United States. *J Clin Oncol.* 1997;15: 3408–3415.
88. Mutch DG. Surgical management of ovarian cancer. *Semin Oncol.* 2002;29(suppl 1):3–8.
89. Curtin JP, Malik R, Venkatraman ES, et al. Stage IV ovarian cancer: impact of surgical debulking. *Gynecol Oncol.* 1997;18:161–163.
90. duBois A, Quinn M, Thigpen T, et al. 2004 Consensus statements on the management of ovarian cancer: final document of the 3rd International Gynecologic Cancer Intergroup Ovarian Cancer Consensus Conference (GCIG OCCC 2004). *Ann Oncol.* 2005;(suppl 8):7–12.
91. Rubin SC, Hoskins WJ, Hakes TB, et al. Recurrence after negative second look laparotomy for ovarian cancer: analysis of risk factors. *Am J Obstet Gynecol.* 1988;159:1094–1098.
92. Nicoletto MO, Tumolo S, Talamini R, et al. Surgical second look in ovarian cancer: a randomized study in patients with laparoscopic complete remission—a Northeastern Oncology Cooperative Group—Ovarian Cancer Cooperative Group Study. *J Clin Oncol.* 1997;15: 994–997.
93. Boente MP, Chi DS, Hoskins WJ. The role of surgery in the management of ovarian cancer: primary and interval cytoreductive surgery. *Semin Oncol.* 1998:326–334.
94. Webb MJ, Decker DG, Mussey E, et al. Factors influencing the survival in stage I ovarian cancer. *Am J Obstet Gynecol.* 1973;116:222–228.
95. Purola E, Nieminim U. Does rupture of cystic cancer during operation influence the prognosis? *Ann Chir Gynaecol.* 1968;57:615–617.
96. Ozols RF, Rubin SC, Thomas G, et al. Epithelial ovarian cancer. In: Hoskins WJ, Perez CA, Young RC, eds. *Principles and Practices of Gynecologic Oncology.* 2nd ed. Philadelphia, PA: Lippincott–Raven; 1997:919–986.
97. Vergote I, DeBrabanter J, Fyles A, et al. Prognostic importance of degree of differentiation and cyst rupture in stage I invasive epithelial ovarian carcinoma. *Lancet.* 2001;357:176–182.
98. Young RC, Pecorelli S. Management of early ovarian cancer. *Semin Oncol.* 1998;25:335–339.

99. Young RC, Brady MF, Nieberg RK, et al. Adjuvant treatment for early ovarian cancer: a randomized phase III trial of intraperitoneal 32P or intravenous cyclophosphamide and cisplatin—a Gynecologic Oncology Group study. *J Clin Oncol.* 2003;21:4350–4355.
100. Bell J, Brady M, Young R, et al. Randomized phase III trial of three versus six cycles of adjuvant carboplatin and paclitaxel in early stage epithelial ovarian carcinoma: a Gynecologic Oncology Group study. *Gynecol Oncol.* 2006;102:432–439.
101. Trimbos J, Vergote I, Bolis G, et al. Impact of adjuvant chemotherapy and surgical staging in early–stage ovarian carcinoma: European Organisation for research and treatment of cancer–adjuvant chemotherapy in ovarian neoplasm trial. *J Natl Can Inst.* 2003;95:113–125.
102. Markman M. Pharmaceutical management of ovarian cancer. *Drugs.* 2006;68:771–789.
103. Trimble EL, Adams JD, Vena D, et al. Paclitaxel for platinum–refractory ovarian cancer: results from the first 1,000 patients registered to National Cancer Institute Treatment Referral Center 9103. *J Clin Oncol.* 1993;11:2405–2410.
104. McGuire WP, Hoskins WJ, Brady MR, et al. Cyclophosphamide and cisplatin compared with paclitaxel and cisplatin in patients with stage III and IV ovarian cancer. *N Engl J Med.* 1996;334:1–6.
105. Piccart MJ, Bertelsen K, James K, et al. Randomized intergroup trial of cisplatin–paclitaxel vs cisplatin–cyclophosphamide in women with advanced epithelial ovarian cancer: three year results. *J Natl Cancer Inst.* 2000;92:699–708.
106. Muggia FM, Braly PS, Brady MF, et al. Phase III randomized study of cisplatin vs paclitaxel vs cisplatin and paclitaxel in patients with suboptimal stage III or IV ovarian cancer: a Gynecologic Oncology Group study. *J Clin Oncol.* 2000;18:106–115.
107. ICON (International Collaborative Ovarian Neoplasm Group). ICON 2: randomized trial of single agent carboplatin against three–drug combination of CAP (cyclophosphamide, doxorubicin, and cisplatin) in women with ovarian cancer. *Lancet.* 1998;352:1571–1576.
108. ICON (International Collaborative Ovarian Neoplasm Group). Paclitaxel plus carboplatin versus standard chemotherapy with either single–agent carboplatin or cyclophosphamide, doxorubicin, and cisplatin in women with ovarian cancer. The ICON 3 randomized trial. *Lancet.* 2002;360:505–515.
109. McGuire WP, Markman M. Primary ovarian cancer chemotherapy: current standards of care. *Br J Cancer.* 2003;89(suppl 3):S3–S8.
110. Ozols RF. Ovarian cancer practice guidelines. *Oncology.* 1997;11:95–105.
111. Neijt JP, Engelholm SA, Tuxen MK, et al. Exploratory phase III study of paclitaxel and cisplatin versus paclitaxel and carboplatin in advanced ovarian cancer. *J Clin Oncol.* 2000;18:3084–3092.
112. duBois A, Luck HJ, Meier W, et al. Cisplatin/paclitaxel vs carboplatin/paclitaxel in ovarian cancer. An update of an Arbeitsgemeinschaft Gynakologie (AGO) Study Group trial. *Proc Am Soc Clin Oncol.* 1999;18:A1374(abstr).
113. Ozols RF, Bundy BN, Greer BE, et al. Phase III trial of carboplatin and paclitaxel compared with cisplatin and paclitaxel in patients with optimally resected stage III ovarian cancer: a Gynecology Oncology Group study. *J Clin Oncol.* 2003;21:3194–3200.
114. Bookman MA, Greer BE, Ozols RF. Optimal therapy of advanced ovarian cancer: carboplatin and paclitaxel vs cisplatin and paclitaxel (GOG 158) and an update on GOG0 182–ICON5. *Int J Gynecol Cancer.* 2003;13:735–740.
115. Rose PG. Chemotherapy for newly diagnosed and relapsed advanced ovarian cancer. *Semin Oncol Nurs.* 2003;19(suppl 2):25–35.
116. Vasey P; for Scottish Gynaecological Cancer Trials Group. Preliminary results of the SCOTROC trial: a phase III comparison of paclitaxel–carboplatin (PC) and docetaxel–carboplatin (DC) as first–line chemotherapy for stage Ic–IV epithelial ovarian cancer (EOC). *Proc Am Soc Clin Oncol.* 2001;20:202a(abstr 804).
117. Vasey PA; for Scottish Gynaecological Cancer Trials Group. Survival and long–term toxicity results of the SCOTROC study: docetaxel–carboplatin (DC) vs paclitaxel–carboplatin (PC) in epithelial ovarian cancer (EOC) [abstract 804]. *Proc Am Soc Clin Oncol.* 2002;21:202a:804(abstr).
118. Burger R, Sill M, Monk B, et al. Phase II trial of bevacizumab in persistent or recurrent epithelial ovarian cancer or primary peritoneal cancer: a Gynecologic Oncology Group study. *J Clin Oncol.* 2007;25:5180–5186.
119. Olson JK, Sood AK, Sorosky JI, et al. Taxol hypersensitivity: rapid retreatment is safe and cost effective. *Gynecol Oncol.* 1998;68:25–28.
120. Markman M. The dilemma of carboplatin–associated hypersensitivity reactions in ovarian cancer management. *Gynecol Oncol.* 2007;107:163–165.
121. Choi M, Fuller CD, Thomas CR Jr, et al. Conditional survival in ovarian cancer: results from the SEER Dataset 1998–2001. *Gynecol Oncol.* 2008;109:203–209.
122. Ozols R. Systemic therapy for ovarian cancer: current status and new treatments. *Semin Oncol.* 2006;33(suppl 6):S3–S11.
123. Markman M. Role of intraperitoneal chemotherapy in the front–line setting. *J Clin Oncol.* 2003;21:134s–148s.
124. Alberts DS, Liu PY, Hannigan EV, et al. Intraperitoneal cisplatin plus intravenous cyclophosphamide versus intravenous cisplatin plus intravenous cyclophosphamide for stage III ovarian cancer. *N Engl J Med.* 1996;335:1950–1955.
125. Markman M, Bundy BN, Alberts DS, et al. Phase III trial of standard–dose intravenous cisplatin plus paclitaxel versus moderately high–dose carboplatin followed by intravenous paclitaxel and intraperitoneal cisplatin in small–volume stage III ovarian carcinoma: an intergroup study of the Gynecologic Oncology Group, Southwestern Oncology Group, and Eastern Cooperative Oncology Group. *J Clin Oncol.* 2001;19:1001–1007.
126. Armstrong D, Bundy B, Wenzel L, et al. Intraperitoneal cisplatin and paclitaxel in ovarian cancer. *N Engl J Med.* 2006;354:34–43.
127. Bookman M; for the Gynecologic Cancer Intergroup GOG–182–ICON5. 5–Arm phase III randomized trial of paclitaxel and carboplatin versus combinations with gemcitabine and pegylated liposomal doxorubicin or topotecan in patients with advanced epithelial ovarian or primary peritoneal carcinoma [abstract 5002]. *J Clin Oncol.* 2006;24(suppl 18):256a.
128. Bukowski R, Ozols R, Markman M. The management of recurrent ovarian cancer. *Semin Oncol.* 2007;34(suppl):S1–S15.
129. Gaducci A, Cosio S. Surveillance of patients after initial treatment of ovarian cancer. *Crit Rev Oncol Hematol.* 2009;71:43–52.
130. Markham M. Second–line chemotherapy of epithelial ovarian cancer. *Expert Rev Anticancer Ther.* 2003;3:31–36.
131. The ICON and AGO Collaborators. Paclitaxel plus platinum–based chemotherapy versus conventional platinum–based chemotherapy in women with relapsed ovarian cancer: the ICON4/AGO–OVAR 2.2 trial. *Lancet.* 2003;361:2099–2106.
132. Pfisterer J, Plante M, Vergote I, et al. Gemcitabine plus carboplatin compared with carboplatin in patients with platinum–sensitive recurrent ovarian cancer: an intergroup trial of the AGO–OVAR, the NCIC, CTG, and the EORTC GCG. *J Clin Oncol.* 2006;24:4699–4707.
133. Markman M. Unresolved issues in the chemotherapeutic management of gynaecologic malignancies. *Semin Oncol.* 2006;33(suppl):S33–S38.
134. Vergote I, Finkler N, delCampo J, et al. Single agent canfosfamide versus pegylated doxorubicin or topotecan in 3rd line treatment of platinum refractory or resistant ovarian cancer: phase 3 study results. *J Clin Oncol.* 2006;25:966.
135. Markman M, Webster K, Zanotti K, et al. Survival following the documentation of platinum and taxane–resistance in ovarian cancer: a single institution experience involving multiple phase 2 trials. *Gynecol Oncol.* 2004;93:699–701.
136. Markman M, Iseminger K, Hatch KD, et al. Tamoxifen in platinum–refractory ovarian cancer. A Gynecologic Oncology Group ancillary report. *Gynecol Oncol.* 1996;62:4–6.

137. van der Velden J, Gitsch G, Wain GV, et al. Tamoxifen in patients with advanced epithelial ovarian cancer. *Int J Gynecol Cancer.* 1995;5:301–305.
138. Gordon M, Matei D, Aghajania C, et al. Clinical activity of pertuzumab (rhuMAB 2C4) a HER dimerization inhibitor, in advanced ovarian cancer. Potential predictive relationship with tumor HER2 activation status. *J Clin Oncol.* 2006;24:4324–4332.
139. Bookman M, Darcy K, Clarke–Pearson D, et al. Evaluation of monoclonal humanized anti–HER2 antibody, trastuzumab, in patients with recurrent or refractory ovarian or primary peritoneal carcinoma with overexpression of HER2: a phase II trial of the Gynecologic Oncology Group. *J Clin Oncol.* 2003;21:283–290.
140. Gordon A, Finkler N, Edwards R, et al. Efficacy and safety of erlotinib HCl, an epidermal growth factor receptor (HER1/EGFR) tyrosine kinase inhibitor, in patients with advanced ovarian carcinoma: results from a phase II multicenter study. *Int J Gynecol Cancer.* 2005;15:785–792.
141. Schilder R, Sill M, Chen X, et al. Phase II study of gefitinib in patients with relapsed or persistent ovarian or primary peritoneal carcinoma and evaluation of epidermal growth factor receptor mutations and immunohistochemical expression: a gynaecologic Oncology Group study. *Clin Cancer Res.* 2005;11:5539–5548.
142. Campos S, Hamid O, Seiden M, et al. Multicenter randomized phase II trial of oral CI–1033 for previously treated advanced ovarian cancer. *J Clin Oncol.* 2005;23:5597–5604.
143. Cannistra SA, Matulonis UA, Penson RT, et al. Phase II study of bevacizumab in patients with platinum resistant ovarian cancer or peritoneal serous cancer. *J Clin Oncol.* 2007;25:5180–5186.
144. Wright JD, Hagemann A, Rader JS, et al. Bevacizumab combination therapy in recurrent platinum–refractory, epithelial ovarian carcinoma: a retrospective analysis. *Cancer.* 2006;107:83–89.
145. Garcia AA, Hirte H, Fleming G, et al. Phase II clinical trial of bevacizumab and low–dose metronomic oral cyclophosphamide in recurrent ovarian cancer: a trial of California, Chicago and Princess Margaret Hospital Phase II consortia. *J Clin Oncol.* 2008;26:76–82.
146. Hu L, Hofmann J, Zaloudak C, et al. Vascular endothelial growth factor immunoneutralization plus paclitaxel markedly reduces tumor burden and ascites in athymic mouse model of ovarian cancer. *Am J Pathol.* 2002;161:1917–1924.
147. Parker N, Turk M, Westrick E, et al. Folate receptor expression in carcinomas and normal tissues determined by a quantitative radioligand binding assay. *Anal Biochem.* 2005;338:284–293.
148. Konner J, Ahmed S, Gerst N, et al. Phase I study of MORAb–003, a humanized anti–folate receptor–alpha monoclonal antibody, in platinum resistant ovarian cancer. *J Clin Oncol.* 2006;24:262s.
149. Fong P, Boss D, Carden C, et al. AZD2281 (KU–0059436) a PARP (poly ADP–ribose polymerase) inhibitor with a single agent anticancer activity in patients with BRCA deficient ovarian cancer: results for a phase I study. *J Clin Oncol.* 2008;26:5510(abstr).
150. Sawiris GP, Sherman–Baust CA, Becker KG, et al. Development of a highly specialized cDNA array for the study and diagnosis of epithelial ovarian cancer. *Cancer Res.* 2002;62:2923–2928.
151. Potter K, Held–Warmkessle J. Intraperitoneal chemotherapy for women with ovarian cancer: nursing care and considerations. *Clin J Oncol Nurs.* 2008;12:265–271.
152. Almadrones L. Evidence based research for intraperitoneal chemotherapy in epithelial ovarian cancer. *Clin J Oncol Nurs.* 2007;11:211–216.
153. Hydzik C. Implementation of intraperitoneal chemotherapy for the treatment of ovarian cancer. *Clin J Oncol Nurs.* 2007;11:221–225.
154. Marin K, Oleszewski K, Muehlbauer P. Intraperitoneal chemotherapy: implications beyond ovarian cancer. *Clin J Oncol Nurs.* 2007;11:881–889.
155. Anderson N, Hacker E. Fatigue in women receiving intraperitoneal chemotherapy for ovarian cancer: a review of contributing factors. *Clin J Oncol Nurs.* 2008;12:445–456.
156. Herrinton L, Neslund–Dudas C, Rolnick S, et al. Complications at the end of life in ovarian cancer. *J Pain Symptom Manage.* 2007;34:237–243.
157. Williams SD. Ovarian germ cell tumors: an update. *Semin Oncol.* 1998;25:407–413.
158. Dorgio O, Berek J. Overview of germ cell tumors of the ovary. Up to date. http://www.uptodate.com. Accessed January 12, 2010.
159. Homesley HD, Bundy BN, Hurteau JA, et al. Bleomycin, etoposide, and cisplatin combination therapy of ovarian granulose cell tumors and other stromal malignancies: a Gynecologic Oncology Group study. *Gynecol Oncol.* 1999;72:131–137.
160. Door A. Less common gynecologic malignancies. *Semin Oncol Nurs.* 2002;18:207–222.
161. Aure JC, Hoeg K, Kolstad P. Clinical and histologic studies of ovarian carcinoma. Long term follow up of 990 cases. *Obstet Gynecol.* 1971;37:1–9.
162. Trimble CL, Trimble EL. Management of epithelial ovarian tumors of low malignant potential. *Gynecol Oncol.* 1994;55:552–561.
163. Lu KH, Bell DA, Welch WR, et al. Evidence for multifocal origin of unilateral and advanced human serous borderline ovarian tumors. *Cancer Res.* 1998;58:2328–2330.
164. Ingelman–Sandberg A. Classification and staging of malignant tumours of the female pelvis. *Acta Obstet Gynecol Scand.* 1971;50:1–7.
165. Serov SF, Scully RE, Solun LH. Histologic typing of ovarian tumours. In: *International Histologic Classification of Tumours No. 9.* Geneva: World Health Organization; 1973.
166. Ferrell BR, Dow KH, Leigh S, et al. Quality of life in long–term cancer survivors. *Oncol Nurs Forum.* 1995;22:915–922.
167. Walczak JR, Heckman CS. Ascites. In: Yarbro CH, Frogge MH, Goodman M, eds. *Cancer Symptom Management.* 2nd ed. Sudbury, MA: Jones and Bartlett; 1999:405–415.
168. Collins CA. Ascites. *Clin J Oncol Nurs.* 2001;5:43–45.
169. Puls LE, Duniho T, Hunter JE, et al. The prognostic implication of ascites in advanced–stage ovarian cancer. *Gynecol Oncol.* 1996;61:109–112.
170. Martin VR. *Managing Symptoms Associated with Ovarian Cancer, Negotiating Optimal Ovarian Cancer Care: A Clinician's Guide* (Monograph). Bala Cynwyd, PA: Meniscus Educational Institute; 1999:18–26.
171. Kraemer K, Lynch MP. Ascites. In: Preston FA, Cunningham RS, eds. *Clinical Guidelines for Symptom Management in Oncology.* New York: Clinical Insights Press; 1998:115–119.
172. Kelvin JF, Scagliola J. Metastases involving the gastrointestinal system. *Semin Oncol Nurs.* 1999;14:187–198.
173. Abrahm JL. Promoting symptom control in palliative care. *Semin Oncol Nurs.* 1998;14:95–109.
174. Murphy–Ende K. Bowel obstruction. *Clin J Oncol Nurs.* 2000;4:291–293.
175. Waldman AR. Bowel obstruction. *Clin J Oncol Nurs.* 2001;5: 281–286.
176. Jolicoeur L, Faught W. Managing bowel obstruction in ovarian cancer using a percutaneous endoscopic gastrostomy (PEG) tube. *Can Oncol Nurs J.* 2003;13:212–219.
177. Chang AE, August DA. Acute abdomen, bowel obstruction, and fistula. In: Abeloff MD, Armitage JO, Lichter AS, et al, eds. *Clinical Oncology.* New York, NY: Churchill Livingstone; 1995:583–597.
178. Summers RW, Lu CC. Approach to the patient with ileus and obstruction. In: Yamada T, ed. *Textbook of Gastroenterology.* 2nd ed. Philadelphia, PA: Lippincott; 1995:796–812.
179. Rust DM. Anorexia and cachexia. In: Yasko JM, ed. *Management of Symptoms Associated with Chemotherapy.* Bala Cynwyd, PA: Meniscus Health Care Communications; 1998:35–54.
180. Grant MM, Rivera LM. Anorexia, cachexia, and dysphagia: the symptom experience. *Semin Oncol Nurs.* 1995;11:266–271.
181. Cunningham R, Bell R. Nutrition in cancer: an overview. *Semin Oncol Nurs.* 2000;16:90–98.

182. Gwilliam B, Bailey C. The nature of terminal malignant bowel obstruction and its impact on patients with advanced cancer. *Int J Palliat Nurs.* 2001;7:474–481.
183. Dewys WD, Begg C, Lavin PT, et al. Prognostic effect of weight loss prior to chemotherapy in cancer patients. *Am J Med.* 1980;69:491–497.
184. Grant M, Kravits K. Symptoms and their impact on nutrition. *Semin Oncol Nurs.* 2000;16:113–121.
185. Levy MH, Rosen SM, Ottery FD, et al. Supportive care in oncology. *Curr Probl Cancer.* 1992;16:335–385.
186. American Society for Parental and Enteral Nutrition. Standards for nutrition support: hospitalized patients. *Nutr Clin Pract.* 1995;10:208–219.
187. Ottery FD. Supportive nutrition to prevent cachexia and support quality of life. *Semin Oncol.* 1995;22(suppl 3):98–111.
188. Loprinzi CL, Schaid DJ, Dose AM, et al. Body–composition changes in patients who gain weight while receiving megesterol acetate. *J Clin Oncol.* 1993;11:152–154.
189. Oster MH, Enders SR, Samuels SJ, et al. Megesterol acetate in patients with AIDS and cachexia. *Ann Intern Med.* 1994;121:400–408.
190. Loprinzi CL, Michalak JC, Schaid DJ. Phase three evaluation of four doses of megesterol acetate as therapy for patients with cancer anorexia and/or cachexia. *J Clin Oncol.* 1993;11:762–767.
191. Jatoi A, Windschitl HE, Loprinzi CL, et al. Dronabinol versus megesterol acetate versus combination therapy for cancer–associated anorexia: a North Central Cancer Treatment Group study. *J Clin Oncol.* 2002;20:567–573.
192. Bloch A. Nutrition support in cancer. *Semin Oncol Nurs.* 2000;16:122–127.
193. Joyce M, Cunningham RS. Metastases that interfere with circulation. *Semin Oncol Nurs.* 1998;14:230–239.
194. Brown J. A clinically useful method for evaluating lymphedema. *Clin J Oncol Nurs.* 2004;8:35–38.
195. Ascherl P. Lymphedema. *Soc Gynecol Oncol Nurs J.* 1998;8:9–11.
196. Kalinowski BH. Lymphedema. In: Yarbro CH, Frogge MH, Goodman M, eds. *Cancer Symptom Management.* 2nd ed. Sudbury, MA: Jones and Bartlett; 1999:457–486.
197. Cutter K, Atkins B. Freedom from lymphedema. *Soc Gynecol Oncol Nurs J.* 1996;6:11–13.
198. Ryan M, Stainton MC, Jaconelli C, et al. The experience of lower limb lymphedema for women after treatment for gynecologic cancer. *Oncol Nurs Forum.* 2003;30:417–423.
199. Shuey KM. Heart, lung, and endocrine complications of solid tumors. *Semin Oncol.* 1994;10:177–188.
200. Rubin SC, Sutton GP. *Ovarian Cancer.* New York, NY: McGraw–Hill; 1993:361–373.
201. McCoy AM, Mierzewski A. Acute oncologic disorders. In: Kinney MR, Packa DR, Dunbar SB, eds. *AACN's Clinical Reference for Critical Care Nursing.* 3rd ed. St Louis, MO: Mosby; 1993:1077–1097.
202. Harwood KV. Dyspnea. In: Yarbro CH, Frogge MH, Goodman M, eds. *Cancer Symptom Management.* 2nd ed. Sudbury, MA: Jones and Bartlett; 1999:45–57.
203. Brobacher S, Gobel BH. Use of the Pleurx pleural catheter for the management of malignant pleural effusions. *Clin J Oncol Nurs.* 2003;7:35–38.
204. Wickham R. Dyspnea: recognizing and managing an invisible problem. *Oncol Nurs Forum.* 2002;29:925–933.
205. Smith EL. Pulmonary metastasis. *Semin Oncol Nurs.* 1998;14:178–186.
206. Ferrell B, Cullinane C, Ervin K, et al. Perspectives on the impact of ovarian cancer: women's views of quality of life. *Oncol Nurs Forum.* 2005;32:1143–1149.
207. Eckwall E, Ternestedt B, Sorbe B, et al. Recurrence of ovarian cancer–living in limbo. *Cancer Nurs.* 2007;30:270–277.
208. Fox S, Lyon D. Symptom clusters and quality of life in survivors of ovarian cancer. *Cancer Nurs.* 2007;30:354–361.
209. Kornblith AB, Thaler HT, Wong G, et al. Quality of life of women with ovarian cancer. *Gynecol Oncol.* 1995;59:231–242.
210. Guidozzi F. Living with ovarian cancer. *Gynecol Oncol.* 1993;50:202–207.
211. Howell D, Fitch MI, Deane KA. Impact of ovarian cancer perceived by women. *Cancer Nurs.* 2003;26:1–9.
212. Lakusta CM, Atkinson MJ, Robinson JW, et al. Quality of life in ovarian cancer patients receiving chemotherapy. *Gynecol Oncol.* 2001;81:490–495.
213. Powell L, Midler A, Steiner A. Concerns of women with ovarian cancer: a qualitative investigation. *Quality Life Res.* 1998;6:92–101.
214. Ferrell B, Smith SL, Cullinane CA, et al. Psychological well being and quality of life in ovarian cancer survivors. *Cancer.* 2003;98:1061–1071.
215. Hamilton AB. Psychological aspects of ovarian cancer. *Cancer Invest.* 1999;17:335–341.
216. Fitch MI, Gray RE, Franssen E. Women's perspective regarding the impact of ovarian cancer. *Cancer Nurs.* 2000;23:359–366.
217. Howell D, Fitch MI, Deane KA. Women's experience with recurrent ovarian cancer. *Cancer Nurs.* 2003;26:10–17.
218. Stewart DE, Wong F, Duff S, et al. What doesn't kill you makes you stronger: an ovarian cancer survivor survey. *Gynecol Oncol.* 2001;83:537–541.
219. Sivesind D, Baile WF. An ovarian cancer support group. *Cancer Pract.* 1997;5:247–251.
220. Melancon C. From victim to victor: a personal perspective of ovarian cancer. *Quality Life Res.* 1996;4:78–81.
221. Ozols RF. Future directions in the treatment of ovarian cancer. *Semin Oncol.* 2002;29(suppl 1):32–42.
222. Martin VR. Ovarian cancer. *Semin Oncol Nurs.* 2002;18:174–183.

CHAPTER 63

*Mary B. Hodgin MS, CMSRN*

# Pancreatic Cancer

## INTRODUCTION

Pancreatic cancer accounts for 3% of new cancer cases each year in the United States as well as worldwide.[1] The current estimate of 42,500 new cases of pancreatic cancer each year has stabilized since the end of the twentieth century. There are 35,240 deaths from pancreatic cancer annually in the United States.[1,2] The disease has a poor prognosis and is considered by many to be one of the deadliest malignancies. Fewer than 24% of affected individuals survive 1 year after diagnosis, and the overall 5-year survival rate is only 5%.[1] The majority of pancreatic cancers are metastatic at the time of diagnosis. Surgical resection offers the best possibility for cure, with the 5-year survival rate approaching 15 to 25% when it is performed at specialized major medical institutions.[3–5]

Pancreatic cancer is one of the most difficult tumors to detect or diagnose because of the anatomical location of the pancreas. It is also difficult to treat due to the biological nature of the tumor. Its onset is insidious, with signs and symptoms that occur late, are vague and misleading, and mimic other diseases. The individual with pancreatic cancer typically will ignore the initial signs and symptoms or rely on self-treatment for months until jaundice or other prominent and intolerable signs appear.

Recent advances in basic science and improved technology have provided a better understanding of the pathogenesis and clinical management of cancer of the pancreas.[6,7] It is hoped that a growing understanding of the biology and molecular genetics and the influence of growth factors on the progression of pancreatic cancer will provide opportunities for advances in prevention, earlier tumor detection, and more effective and novel therapies.

## EPIDEMIOLOGY

The demographics of pancreatic cancer have been widely investigated (Table 63-1). Age is the strongest risk factor for pancreatic cancer, with the peak incidence occurring between the ages 60 and 80.[8] Pancreatic carcinoma incidence is slightly higher in men than in women.[2] The incidence rate is 30% to 40% higher in African American men. Persons of Ashkenazi Jewish heritage have a higher risk of pancreatic cancer related to germ-line mutations.[9,10] Geography has been considered a possible risk factor. The incidence rates of pancreatic cancer are highest in Western and industrialized countries, and lowest in underdeveloped nations. Studies have been inconclusive regarding the risk of pancreatic cancer and socioeconomic status and migrant status.[11]

**TABLE 63-1**

**Risk Factors for Pancreatic Cancer**

| | |
|---|---|
| **Demographic Factors** | Advancing age<br>Black race<br>Male gender<br>Jewish religion<br>Geography |
| **Environmental Factors** | Tobacco<br>Radiation |
| **Dietary Factors** | Carbohydrate<br>Cholesterol<br>Meat<br>Salt<br>Dehydrated food<br>Fried food<br>Refined sugar<br>Soybeans<br>Nitrosamines |
| **Occupational Factors** | Chemists<br>Coal gas workers<br>Metal industries<br>Aluminum milling<br>Leather tanning<br>Textile industry<br>Building trades<br>Transportation<br>Butchers<br>Flour industry<br>Ethylene chlorhydrin<br>Halogenated hydrocarbons<br>Chlorinated water<br>DDT |
| **Host Factors** | Diabetes<br>Chronic pancreatitis<br>Genetic syndromes |

### ETIOLOGY

Numerous environmental factors may be associated with increased risk of pancreatic cancer, including personal cigarette smoking, environmental tobacco smoke (tobacco smoke exposure), and chemical exposures. It has been estimated that tobacco smoking contributes to the development of 20% to 30% of pancreatic cancers.[9,12,13] The strongest associations with cigarette smoking and pancreatic cancer were found when the pack-years smoked occurred within the previous 15 years. Environmental tobacco smoke contains the same toxins, irritants, and carcinogens as cigarettes and is known to cause cancer in humans. At this time, the exact contribution of environmental tobacco smoke to the development of pancreatic cancer has not been characterized, but it is thought to have a definite association, especially in persons with a lower education level.[14] Exposure to radiation has also been investigated as a risk for pancreatic carcinogenesis. Persons irradiated in infancy for skin hemangioma have been reported to have an increased risk of pancreatic cancer.[15]Many epidemiological studies have examined the role of diet and pancreatic cancer, but the relationship remains unclear.[13] A number of studies have reported an association between pancreatic cancer and increasing ingestion of carbohydrate, cholesterol, meat, salt, dehydrated food, fried food, refined sugar, soybeans, and nitrosamines. The studies do not support an association with pancreatic cancer and excess intake of dietary fat or beta-carotene.[13] A decreased risk or perhaps a protective effect has been reported for fiber, vitamin C, fruits, vegetables, preservative-free foods, raw foods, and the use of pressure cooking and microwave cooking.[11]

Obesity as a risk factor for pancreatic cancer suggests that energy balance may play an important role in pancreatic carcinogenesis.[8] High body mass index, increased weight, and a low level of physical activity, all increase the risk of pancreatic cancer.[16]

Numerous studies have examined certain occupational exposures. Cancer of the pancreas has been reported to occur among chemists, and coal gas workers, and among individuals working in metal industries, aluminum milling, and the leather tanning industry. There have been reports of increased risk associated with exposure to welding materials, paint thinners, refuse and detergents, and floor cleaning agents, as well as petroleum products. Butchers, transportation workers, and workers in flour mills where pesticides were used more frequently than in other segments of the industry are occupations considered to be a possible risk. Workers exposed to DDT during the manufacturing process were at risk. Those workers exposed during production of ethylene chlorhydrin, halogenated hydrocarbons, and consumption of chlorinated water have also been implicated between exposure and disease.[17,18]

A meta-analysis of the relationship between diabetes and the development of pancreatic cancer confirmed that the relative risk in persons who have had diabetes for 5 years is double the risk of persons without diabetes. Diabetes may be an early symptom of pancreatic cancer as the tumor itself can destroy pancreatic parenchyma, causing pancreatitis and diabetes.[13]

Peptic ulcer surgery and cholecystectomy have also been linked to pancreatic cancer. The initial symptoms of pancreatic cancer can mimic biliary tract disease, which in turn may lead to cholecystectomy and subsequent discovery of pancreatic cancer.

## GENETICS

With advances in the understanding of human genetics, it is now known that cancer of the pancreas is a disease of acquired and inherited mutations in cancer-causing genes. The development of cancer of the pancreas has been associated with the activation of the oncogene, *K-ras*, the inactivation of multiple tumor suppressor genes, and DNA mismatch repair.[19] Mutant *K-ras* is found in approximately 95% of pancreatic adenocarcinomas.[7] Specifically, the *p16* tumor suppressor gene is inactivated in approximately 95% of pancreatic cancers. The second most important tumor suppressor gene is *p53*, which is inactivated in 70% of pancreatic cancers.[7] The *DPC4* (deleted in pancreatic cancer on locus 4) gene is specific for pancreatic cancer and is inactivated in approximately 50% of pancreatic cancers.[20] The *BRCA2* gene is inactivated in only 7% of pancreatic cancers, but is noteworthy because the mutations in *BRCA2* associated with pancreatic cancer are inherited mutations.[21]

*K-ras* is the most frequently activated oncogene in pancreatic cancer. More than 95% of pancreatic cancers harbor activating mutations in *K-ras*, and most of these mutations affect codon 12 of the gene, although codon 13 or 61 can also be affected.[22]

The DNA mismatch repair genes are the last group of cancer-causing genes that have been found to play a role in the development of pancreatic cancer. When these DNA repair genes, sometimes called caretaker genes, do not function appropriately, errors in DNA replication are not repaired.[22] Approximately 4% of pancreatic cancers have been found to contain genetic alterations in DNA mismatch repair genes. This subgroup of cancers may arise through a pathway separate from that of the usual ductal carcinomas and therefore may have a more favorable prognosis.[22,23]

Cancer of the pancreas has been shown to cluster within families. Two broad groups of familial aggregation of pancreatic cancer exist: those associated with known syndromes and those without such an association.[24] Six genetic syndromes are associated with an increased risk of developing pancreatic cancer. These syndromes account for less than 10% of the familial aggregation of pancreatic cancer (see Table 63-2).

Hereditary pancreatitis is a rare disease characterized by recurrent episodes of severe epigastric pain and hyperamylasemia, with an onset usually before age 10. Individuals

**TABLE 63-2**

| Genetic Syndromes Predisposing an Individual to Pancreatic Cancer |
|---|
| Hereditary pancreatitis |
| Hereditary nonpolyposis colorectal cancer (HNPCC) |
| Familial breast cancer (linked to *BRCA2* tumor suppressor gene) |
| Familial atypical multiple mole melanoma syndrome (FAMMM) |
| Ataxia–telangiectasia syndrome |
| Peutz–Jeghers syndrome |

affected with this disease are at increased risk for the development of pancreatic pseudocysts, pancreatic exocrine insufficiency, chronic pancreatitis, diabetes mellitus, and a 50-fold increased risk of pancreatic cancer.[25]

Hereditary nonpolyposis colorectal cancer (HNPCC) can predispose some families to the development of pancreatic cancer, but the contribution of this syndrome to the number of individuals with pancreatic cancer appears to be small.[25] Familial breast cancer with germ-line mutations in the *BRCA2* gene are the most common mutations in persons with hereditary pancreatic cancer.[26] *BRCA2* has been found to be associated not only with an increased risk of breast cancer but also cancer of the ovary, prostate, colon, and pancreas.[21,27,28]

Familial atypical multiple mole melanoma (FAMMM) syndrome is characterized by multiple nevi, atypical nevi, and multiple melanomas. The gene responsible for the FAMMM syndrome is the *p16* tumor suppressor gene.[29,30] There is a 12 to 20-fold increase in the risk of pancreatic cancer associated with this genetic syndrome.[31]

The ataxia-telangiectasia syndrome is associated with disabling cerebellar ataxia, oculocutaneous telangiectasia, and humoral and cellular immune deficiencies. The *ATM* gene is responsible for this syndrome, and individuals who carry this genetic mutation are also at increased risk of leukemia, lymphoma, and cancer of the breast, ovary, biliary tract, stomach, and pancreas.[19]

Peutz-Jeghers syndrome is characterized by hamartomatous polyps of the gastrointestinal tract, and by melanin deposits on the lips and around and inside the mouth. Affected individuals are at an increased risk of developing multiple cancers and have a 100 fold greater incidence of pancreatic cancer than expected.[28] The gene responsible for this syndrome has been found on a region of chromosome 19p.[32]

Studies of families without a genetic syndrome in which an aggregation of pancreatic carcinoma exists, help researchers understand the genetic alterations associated with the development of cancer of the pancreas. A recent analysis of familial pancreatic tumor data looked at similarities and differences between familial and sporadic cases. There was no difference in the age at which pancreatic cancer was diagnosed between the 2 groups of cases, with both groups having a mean age at diagnosis of 65 years.[19]

### GROWTH FACTORS

Various growth factors and their receptors are important in the regulation of pancreatic cancer cell growth. Overexpression of specific growth factors and their receptors may contribute to the biological aggressiveness of pancreatic cancer.[33]

The epidermal growth factor receptor (EGFR) binds a family of peptides that includes epidermal growth factor (EGF), transforming growth factor alpha (TGF-α), heparin-binding EGF-like growth factor, amphiregulin, betacellulin, and epiregulin. These growth factors may all contribute to pancreatic cell growth. Overexpression of EGFR has been linked to enhanced metastatic potential and increased tumor invasiveness.[34]

The transforming growth factor beta (TGF-β) polypeptide family has been implicated in the development of pancreatic cancer. Overexpression of TGF-β enhances tumor development by promoting tumor angiogenesis, altering the extracellular array/matrix, and enhancing adhesiveness that facilitates tumor metastasis.[33] Overexpression of TGF-β has been associated with a shorter postoperative survival or worse prognosis in individuals with pancreatic adenocarcinoma.[35]

The fibroblast growth factor (FGF) family consists of many polypeptide growth factors that have an affinity for heparin, which results in changes in cell differentiation and tissue repair.[36] A current hypothesis suggests that certain FGF signaling pathways in the earliest stages of cell development may lead to pancreatic cancer.[37] The insulin-like growth factor I (IGF-I) is also overexpressed in pancreatic cancer cells and enhances the growth of those cells.[36,38] Targeting these receptors and molecular pathways gives researchers a better understanding of the cellular environment in which pancreatic cancer thrives.[36]

Other analyses that illuminate genetic alterations in pancreatic cancer-causing genes are karyotyping, comparative genomic hybridization (CGH), and allelotyping. Karyotyping can help to identify specific chromosomes lost or gained in pancreatic cancer. Comparative genomic hybridization has been used to screen for gains or losses of chromosomal material within the tumor DNA. Allelotyping has allowed for improved precision in identifying genetic material. Examination of pancreatic adenocarcinomas has revealed high frequencies of losses at specific chromosome arms.[39]

## PREVENTION, SCREENING, AND EARLY DETECTION

Prevention of pancreatic cancer will require definitive identification of factors demonstrated to cause or place individuals at a high risk of developing this disease. Then reduction or elimination of these risk factors may prevent cancer of the pancreas. It is an insidious disease with little known about the best treatment, much less the cause.

The general hypothesis currently being tested is that adenocarcinoma of the pancreas represents a multistep disease involving progressive, acquired genetic rearrangements in cancer-causing genes. These mutations are detectable in stool, duodenal fluid, pancreatic juice samples, bile, and blood, and they may become an accurate screening marker for pancreatic cancer to easily detect persons at risk.[39] An ideal approach would be the use of an imaging test along with molecular markers of neoplastic disease to diagnose a benign, dysplastic precancerous lesion, or an early, localized cancer.[9]

## PATHOPHYSIOLOGY

Pancreatic cancer is most commonly an adenocarcinoma that originates from the cells lining the pancreatic duct. Tumors of the pancreas develop in both the endocrine and the exocrine parenchyma (see Table 63-3). Approximately 90% of tumors arise from the exocrine pancreas, which contains 2 major types of epithelium: acinar and ductal. The acinar cells of the pancreas produce digestive enzymes, whereas the cells lining the pancreatic duct are responsible for the secretion of fluid and electrolytes and the conveyance of pancreatic juice to the duodenum.

### CELLULAR CHARACTERISTICS

Adenocarcinomas of the pancreas usually are whitish yellow, hard, nodular, poorly defined, firm masses surrounded by dense reactive fibrous tissue that often obstruct and dilate the distal common bile duct and pancreatic ducts. Tumors may vary from well differentiated to undifferentiated, and exhibit variable gland formation, irregular cell size, and variable nuclear changes. Because of the tumor's infiltrative nature, visualizing the complete extent of the disease is difficult. Many ductal adenocarcinomas of the pancreas infiltrate into vascular spaces, lymphatic spaces, and perineural spaces, which can be appreciated only on microscopic examination.

### PRECURSORS TO DUCTAL ADENOCARCINOMA

Lesions in the small pancreatic ducts frequently are first found on histological examination in resected pancreatic specimens. These lesions are now referred to as Pancreatic Intraepithelial Neoplasms (PanINs). Precursor lesions may progress from flat duct lesions (PanIN-1A), to papillary duct lesions without atypia (PanIN-1B), to papillary duct lesions with atypia (PanIN-2), and finally to carcinoma in situ of the pancreas (PanIN-3)[40] (see Figure 63-1).[41] The lesions occur equally in both men and women in their 60s to 70s and can be found anywhere throughout the pancreas.[9]

Mucinous cystic neoplasms (MCNs) can be precursors of infiltrating ductal adenocarcimonas of the pancreas. These tumors differ from PanINs in that they are grossly visible and do not involve the ducts of the pancreas. It is important to differentiate MCNs from ductal adenocarcinomas, as MCNs have a better prognosis.[42] These neoplasms are found mostly in women in their 40s to 50s and can be located in the body or tail of the pancreas.[9]

Intraductal papillary mucinous neoplasms (IPMNs) are grossly visible tumors that grow in the large ducts of the pancreas and have varying degrees of atypia.[43] They occur with approximately equal frequency in both sexes in their 60s to 70s; they are found mostly in the head of the pancreas but can infiltrate throughout the entire pancreas.[9] Patients with IPMNs usually have favorable outcomes after resection, but metastases can occur if carcinoma in situ is found.[43,44]

Adenosquamous carcinoma of the pancreas is a rare variant of ductal adenocarcinoma that shows both glandular (adeno) and squamous differentiation. This variation is more common in individuals who have received previous chemotherapy or radiation therapy. The biological behavior of adenosquamous carcinoma is the same as that of the typical ductal adenocarcinomas. Adenosquamous carcinoma has an especially poor prognosis.[45]

A small percentage of pancreatic cancers are classified as acinar cell carcinomas, which have a distinct histological

**TABLE 63-3**

| **Pathology of Exocrine Pancreatic Cancer** |
|---|
| **Solid tumors** |
| Ductal adenocarcinoma |
| Adenosquamous carcinoma |
| Acinar cell carcinoma |
| Giant cell carcinoma |
| **Cystic tumors** |
| Serous cystic neoplasms |
| Mucinous cystic neoplasms |
| Intraductal papillary mucinous neoplasms (IPMN) |
| Solid and cystic papillary neoplasms (Hamoudi tumor) |

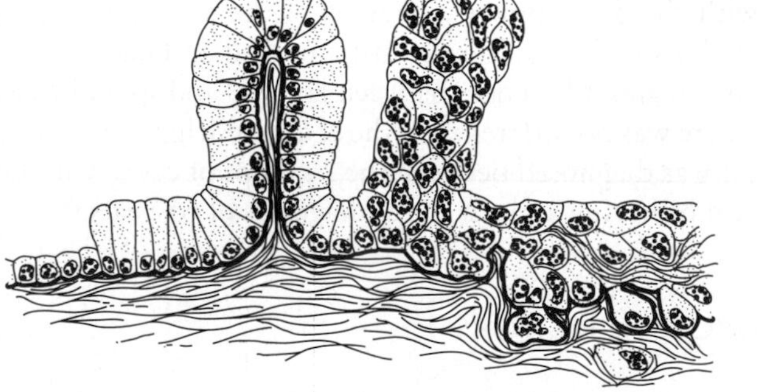

**FIGURE 63-1**

Progression from normal duct epithelium (left) to low-grade pancreatic intraepithelial neoplasia (PanIN) to high-grade PanIN to infiltrating cancer (right). (Artwork by Jennifer L. Parsons.)

*Source:* Used with permission from Wilentz RE, Hruban RH. Pathology of cancer of the pancreas. *Surg Oncol Clin North Am.* 1998;7:47.[41]

appearance and an unusual clinical presentation. Most individuals with acinar cell carcinoma have biliary or gastrointestinal obstruction because of the tumor. Individuals with acinar cell carcinoma fare slightly better than those with ductal adenocarcinoma.[46,47]

Giant cell carcinoma accounts for approximately 5% of primary nonendocrine pancreatic malignancies. Giant cell carcinomas arise with equal frequency in the head, body, and tail regions of the pancreas. These pancreatic carcinomas are associated with a poorer prognosis than ductal adenocarcinomas.[41]

Cystic neoplasms of the pancreas, arising from the exocrine pancreas, are classified as either benign serous cystadenomas, potentially malignant mucinous cystadenomas, or malignant cystadenocarcinomas. Most serous cystic neoplasms are benign, and the prognosis for individuals with resected mucinous cystadenomas is excellent.[41]

Solid and cystic papillary neoplasms of the pancreas, also called *Hamoudi tumors*, occur primarily in women in their third and fourth decades of life. These tumors have solid, cystic, and papillary components when viewed microscopically. Most individuals are cured after surgical resection.[47] Pancreaticoblastoma is a neoplasm that occurs primarily in children younger than 15 years of age. The survival rate for patients with resected pancreaticoblastomas is relatively good.[48]

The most common tumor sites that may metastasize to the pancreas are breast, lung, colorectal, melanoma, and renal cell carcinoma. Systemic neoplasms such as leukemia and lymphoma can involve the pancreas. The pancreas may be the presenting site for these cancers. Most pancreatic lymphomas are non-Hodgkin's lymphomas.[39] Pancreatic lymphomas are rare, but early recognition is important because of their dramatic response to chemotherapy.[49]

Endocrine or islet cell tumors constitute the remainder of pancreatic malignant tumors. These uncommon tumors account for approximately 5% of all pancreatic neoplasms. Many islet cell tumors secrete excessive hormones, resulting in significant clinical manifestations. Nonfunctional islet cell tumors do not produce obvious clinical manifestations and are usually detected because of their space-occupying characteristics or as an incidental finding.[50]

Islet cell tumors arise from the endocrine parenchyma. They usually occur as small, well-circumscribed, reddish-orange tissue that rarely extends beyond the pancreas. On microscopy, islet cell tumors are well vascularized and encapsulated, usually compressing adjacent parenchyma. Fibrosis and calcification may be seen. Malignant islet cell tumors are difficult to distinguish because they closely resemble normal islet cells and retain secretory or synthetic functions. The presence of metastases is the most reliable criterion for establishing malignancy.[51] Chapter 50 presents a more detailed discussion of endocrine tumors.

## PROGRESSION OF DISEASE

Tumors of the head of the pancreas are those arising to the right of the left border of the superior mesentric vein. The uncinate process is part of the head of the pancreas. Tumors of the body of the pancreas are those arising between the left border of the superior mesenteric vein and the left border of the aorta. Tumors of the tail of the pancreas are those arising between the left border of the aorta and the hilum of the spleen.

Pancreatic cancer arises in the head, neck, or uncinate process of the pancreas in 60% to 70% of cases. About 15% of tumors develop in the body and tail of the gland, and the remaining 20% diffusely involve the entire gland[8,39] (Figure 63-2).

Tumors in the head of the gland are often detected at a small size (2–3 cm). The bile duct is invaded early in the course of the disease, causing obstruction of the distal common bile duct. This obstruction accounts for easily recognized symptoms, such as jaundice, which enable detection of smaller tumors. Extension beyond the pancreas is the rule rather than the exception. Ductal adenocarcinomas usually infiltrate into vascular, perineural, and lymphatic spaces. These tumors tend to invade local structures, such as the duodenum and retroperitoneum, either directly or along the course of autonomic nerves of the celiac plexus. Some degree of perineural invasion is present in 90% of cases. The portal or superior vein may also be invaded. Venous invasion or encasement by tumor growth may result in obstruction, thrombosis, ascites, and portal hypertension. Vascular encasement and neural infiltration can contribute to severe back pain. Involvement of the mesenteric vessels may preclude resection of these tumors.[39]

In the body and tail of the pancreas, tumors often reach sizes larger than 5 cm before they produce symptoms. Tumors of the body and tail of the pancreas can invade the splenic vein, resulting in thrombosis and gastric varices.[9]

At the time of detection, the tumor may be fixed to tissues behind the pancreas or to the vertebral column. The tumor may directly invade surrounding organs, such as kidney, spleen, or diaphragm. Invasion of the celiac nerve plexus may account for unrelenting pain. Other sites of local invasion, which tends to occur later, include the superior mesenteric and splenic arteries, transverse colon, stomach, kidneys, and left adrenal gland.[9] Obstruction of the portal vein and tributaries can lead to portal hypertension and esophageal varices.

Characteristically, tumors of the pancreas grow slowly, with late signs and symptoms of pathology. At the time of diagnosis, 90% of cases have perineural invasion, 70% to 80% have lymphatic spread, 50% have venous involvement, and 20% to 25% have duodenal invasion. The liver, peritoneum, and regional lymph nodes are the most commonly involved structures.[52] Supraclavicular nodes (Virchow nodes) may be involved more frequently with carcinoma

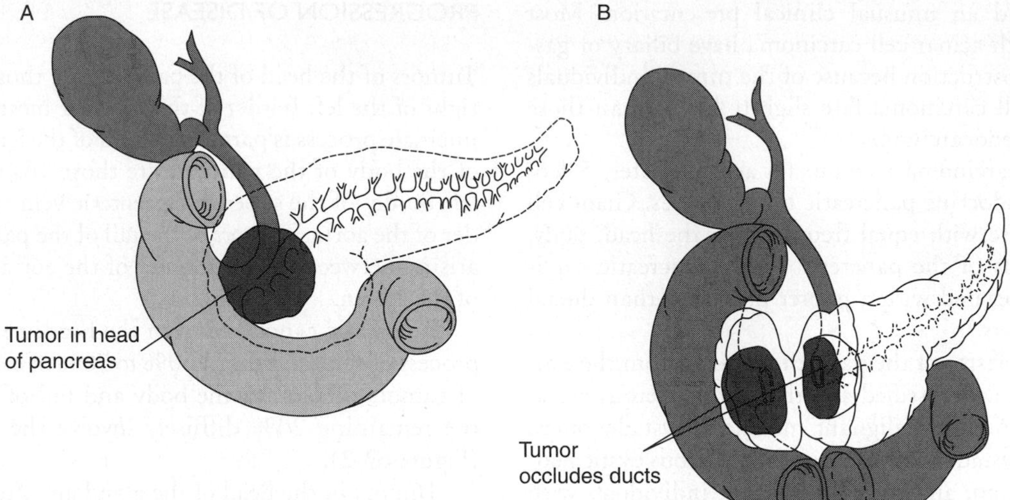


**FIGURE 63-2**

Pancreatic cancers originate in the duct and when they are located in the head of the pancreas (A) they will occlude the distal common bile duct (B). Note the proximity of the pancreatic duct and common bile duct, explaining the characteristic cut-off on cholangiography at the "knee" of the distal bile duct.

*Source*: Used with permission from Bastidas VA, Neiderhuber JE. Pancreas. In: Abeloff MD, Armitage JD, Lichter AS, Neiderhuber JE, eds. Clinical Oncology. New York: Churchill Livingstone; 1995:1373–1403.[59]

of the body and tail of the pancreas. Metastatic deposits reach the liver through the portal bloodstream or lymphatics. Peritoneal seeding by metastatic deposits also occurs.[9] The frequency of lymph node metastasis correlates with the size of the primary tumor.[53,54]

## CLINICAL MANIFESTATIONS

The early signs and symptoms of pancreatic cancer are vague, nonspecific, and gradual, which often contributes to a delay in diagnosis by both the individual and the physician. Specific symptoms usually develop late and only after invasion or obstruction of a nearby structure. Careful assessment and extensive inquiry into the character, onset, duration, and modulators of presenting signs and symptoms is important. Manifestations of disease differ according to the location of the tumor (see Table 63-4). A clinical suspicion of pancreatic cancer must be high to identify the presence of a tumor. Individuals who have resectable pancreatic cancer tend to present with few symptoms.

Weight loss and clinical wasting are classic symptoms of cancer of the pancreas, particularly when the tumor is located in the head of the gland. Initially, the weight loss may not cause concern and may be attributed to gastric maladies. As the cancer advances, significant weight loss is common and often accelerated by pain, anorexia, flatulence, nausea, and vomiting. Duodenal obstruction, with nausea and vomiting, is a late manifestation of pancreatic cancer. Tumor involvement of the pancreas prevents

**TABLE 63-4**

**Clinical Manifestations of Cancer of the Pancreas**

| Location of Tumor | Stage | Clinical Manifestation |
|---|---|---|
| Head | Early | Weight loss<br>Jaundice<br>Pain<br>Anorexia<br>Diarrhea<br>Weakness<br>Indigestion<br>Depression |
| Body | Late | Palpable mass<br>Severe pain<br>Early satiety<br>Indigestion<br>Vomiting<br>Weight loss |
| Tail | Late | Severe pain<br>Indigestion<br>Anorexia<br>Weight loss<br>GI bleeding<br>Splenomegaly |

secretions of the digestive pancreatic enzymes and may diminish insulin production. Malabsorption can lead to diarrhea, constipation, steatorrhea, and muscle weakness.[9] New onset diabetes may be the first clinical feature in 10%

to 20% of individuals.[8,24] The onset of glucose intolerance in an elderly person with vague gastrointestinal symptoms should alert the clinician to the possibility of pancreatic cancer in a person with previously controlled diabetes. Metabolic disturbances such as hyperglycemia, glycosuria, and hypoalbuminemia may occur.

A combination of factors probably causes the weight loss associated with pancreatic cancer. An increase in resting energy expenditure, a decrease in consumption of calories, and fat malabsorption exist in individuals with this disease.[55]

Pain is often vague and nonspecific. A dull, intermittent, diffuse, upper abdominal or back discomfort is initially experienced by most individuals. The discomfort may be attributed to other causes such as indigestion or gaseous distention. The discomfort or pain may become more distinctive. It may progress to continuous midepigastric pain and frequently radiates to the back flanks or right upper quadrant of the abdomen, often becoming most pronounced during the evening or night. It may be colicky, dull, or vague. The intensity of the pain is affected by activity, eating, and posture. The pain is often ameliorated when the individual sits or leans forward, called *proning*, or lies in the fetal position on their right side with both knees drawn up to the chest.[56] The pain can be caused by invasion of the tumor into the splanchnic plexus and retroperitoneum, as well as by obstruction of the pancreatic duct.

Pain is a more prevalent symptom in individuals who have tumors in the body and tail of the pancreas. These tumors are larger at presentation and are located in the retroperitoneum, which contributes to nerve involvement, resulting in pain. Although intractable pain is associated with pancreatic cancer, seldom is it an early manifestation. Recent studies suggest that less than one-third of individuals with cancer of the pancreas report moderate to severe pain. Epigastric pain radiating to the back or flank pain usually indicates invasion of splanchnic nerves or compression of organs and is suggestive of advanced disease.[57]

Acute pancreatitis may be the presenting sign of a pancreatic neoplasm. It is caused by the partial obstruction of the pancreatic duct. Consideration must be given to the diagnosis of a pancreatic tumor in patients who are initially seen with pancreatitis, especially when there is no obvious cause for acute pancreatitis, such as gallstones or alcohol abuse.[39,58]

## HEAD OF PANCREAS

When carcinoma involves the head of the pancreas, the signs and symptoms often appear earlier than with a tumor in the body or tail of the pancreas (Figure 63-2).[57,59] A classic triad of symptoms is seen in individuals with cancer of the head of the pancreas: jaundice, pain, and weight loss.

Jaundice, caused by obstruction of the distal common bile duct as it passes through the head of the pancreas, is the presenting symptom in most cases of cancer of the head of the pancreas. Regardless of whether jaundice is the initial symptom or follows the onset of pain, it is the symptom that invariably causes individuals to seek medical attention. Jaundice accompanied by abdominal pain is far more common than painless jaundice. Obstructive jaundice leads to severe pruritus; dark, tea-colored urine; and clay-colored (acholic) stools. Jaundice does not necessarily indicate extensive disease and unresectability.

Other symptoms are less common and nonspecific. They include weakness, food intolerance, and anorexia. Two unusual symptoms are depression and superficial thrombophlebitis. Depression and anxiety may be part of the initial presentation of pancreatic cancer, independent of pain and other somatic symptoms. These symptoms predate the diagnosis of a pancreatic tumor by as much as 43 months before physical symptoms appear.[60] A triad of depression, anxiety, and feelings of impending doom was first described in 1931.[61] The increased incidence of depression in pancreatic cancer is 2 to 3 times greater than that seen in individuals with other intra-abdominal malignancies.[60] This triad may indicate the presence of hormonal neuroendocrine agents in pancreatic cancer that circulate and target the central nervous system. Another theorem is that pancreas cancer cells stimulate or produce substances which inhibit the activity of serotonin or that T lymphocytes cause nonmetastatic tissue damage in the brain.[62] A multidisciplinary approach can identify and treat these patients who have the highest mean score for anxiety and depression.[63]

Trousseau syndrome is a thrombolytic condition affecting many patients with cancer. In an autopsy study conducted in 2006, researchers found that the prevalence of patients with pancreatic cancer and pulmonary embolism (PE) was 48% as compared to 23% for the general population.[64] The study further reports that after controlling for confounding variables, patients with pancreatic cancer also have the greatest risk of a thomboembolytic event, 2 times more likely to have a PE than other patients with cancer.

## BODY OF PANCREAS

Tumors in the body of the pancreas produce signs and symptoms late in the disease process, making early detection virtually impossible. By the time it is brought to the attention of a clinician, the tumor may be large enough to palpate. Severe epigastric pain usually is the predominant symptom. The individual may experience intense epigastric pain 3 to 4 hours after a meal, caused by the space-occupying tumor displacing the stomach or by encroachment at the ligament of Treitz. The pain often is excruciating and accompanied by vomiting. Relief is brought about by sitting up, leaning forward (proning), or lying on the right side with both knees drawn up to the chest (fetal position). Cancer located in the body and tail of the pancreas produces more pain and weight loss than lesions in the head of the pancreas.[39] There is no jaundice with tumors of the body and tail of the pancreas. An enlarged spleen may be found on palpation, caused by tumor pressing on the splenic vein and resulting in splenic vein thrombosis and splenomegaly.

### TAIL OF PANCREAS

Cancer in the tail of the pancreas has the most silent and insidious progression of disease. Individuals with such a carcinoma may complain of left upper quadrant abdominal pain, generalized weakness, vague indigestion, anorexia, and unexplained weight loss. Metastatic disease is usually present when cancer in the tail of the pancreas is diagnosed. Upper gastrointestinal bleeding, splenomegaly, and signs of portal hypertension and ascites may result from thrombosis of the portal system or extensive liver damage.

In advanced carcinoma of the pancreas, hepatomegaly and a palpable gallbladder (Courvoisier sign) may also be found. There may be evidence of cachexia, muscle wasting, and a nodular texture of the liver consistent with metastatic disease. Other physical findings that serve as markers in disseminated tumor include left supraclavicular adenopathy (Virchow node), periumbilical lymphadenopathy (Sister Mary Joseph nodes), and drop metastases in the pelvis encircling the perirectal region (Blumer's shelf).[39]

## ASSESSMENT

### PATIENT AND FAMILY HISTORY

Careful attention to an individual's presenting symptoms and risk factors as well as a heightened awareness of the possibility of pancreatic cancer by the clinician are important. Eliciting a family history of pancreatic cancer or related genetic syndromes could help to detect genetic abnormalities, perhaps aid in surveillance, and provide better prophylactic treatments for family members at risk in the future.

### PHYSICAL EXAMINATION

Physical examination of the pancreas is virtually impossible because it is an inaccessible organ, lying behind the stomach and in front of the vertebral column. It has been called the *hermit organ* because of its hidden location in the abdomen. Few signs are evident on presentation except in those individuals presenting with obstructive jaundice. A palpable liver is the most common finding on physical exam in 30% to 50% of individuals. A hard, well-defined mass that is palpable in the left upper quadrant of the abdomen is found in individuals presenting with lesions in the body and tail of the pancreas but is uncommon in lesions in the head of the pancreas. Any finding of lymphadenopathy on physical examination may warrant a lymph node biopsy.

### DIAGNOSTIC STUDIES

A number of diagnostic studies are available to assist in the identification of pancreatic cancer, to accurately define the extent of disease, to direct appropriate therapy, and to avoid unnecessary interventions in a cost-efficient fashion (Table 63-5). If definitive diagnosis cannot be made with these studies, diagnostic laparoscopy may be necessary, with exploratory laparotomy being performed as a last resort.

As the knowledge base of the molecular genetic abnormalities in pancreatic cancer accumulates, the importance of specific oncogenes, tumor suppressor genes, and genome maintenance genes will be elucidated and may play a role in the staging of the disease.

#### Diagnostic procedures

Ultrasonography (US) of the abdomen can be used as an initial diagnostic test when pancreatic cancer is suspected, especially for lesions in the head of the pancreas. It is a marginal study for visualization of the body, tail, and uncinate process of the pancreas. US can detect intrahepatic and extrahepatic bile duct obstruction, a pancreatic mass, liver metastases larger than 1 cm in diameter, and ascites. It is not sensitive in defining local nodal spread or involvement of the major blood vessels in the area.[65] This imaging modality has largely been replaced by computerized tomography (CT).

A high-quality spiral or helical multidetector CT with three-dimensional reconstruction using thin-cut examination is the noninvasive diagnostic and staging procedure of choice for the jaundiced individual with a suspected pancreatic malignancy. Multidetector CT incorporates dual-phase imaging in both the arterial and venous phases of enhancement.[66] CT is superior in defining the level of obstruction. It can also demonstrate the presence of a pancreatic mass and enlarged lymph nodes adjacent to the pancreas, as well as detect liver metastases, local vascular invasion, or thrombosis. Likewise, CT is more accurate in the diagnosis of unresectability. CT findings that indicate the tumor is unlikely to be resected for cure include liver metastases, ascites, vascular invasion, and tumor spread to adjacent retroperitoneal structures.

Pancreatic cancer usually appears as a hypoechoic mass that differs in consistency from the normal surrounding tissue. The use of intravenous iodine contrast enhances the imaging of the pancreas and liver. Both venous- and arterial-phase imaging is necessary for the most complete evaluation of the pancreas and its adjacent structures. Improved CT imaging has diminished the role of visceral angiography and

**TABLE 63-5**

**Techniques for Assessment of Cancer of the Pancreas**

| Imaging | Laboratory | Tumor Markers | Surgery |
|---|---|---|---|
| Ultrasound | Total bilirubin | CA 19–9 | Laparoscopy |
| Computerized tomography | Alkaline phosphatase | CA 494 | Percutaneous fine-needle aspiration biopsy |
| Magnetic resonance imaging | Gamma glutamyl transpeptidase | CA 50 | |
| Cholangiography | Alanine aminotransferase (ALT) | DU-PAN-2 | |
| Endoscopic | Aspartate aminotransferase (AST) | CA 125 | |
| Percutaneous | Hemoglobin | CA 72–4 | |
| Angiography | Hematocrit | Span-1 | |
| Endoscopic ultrasound | Albumin | | |
| Positive emission tomography | Total protein | | |
| Magnetic resonance cholangiopancreatography | PT, aPTT<br>Glucose | | |

endoscopic retrograde cholangiopancreatography (ERCP) in the diagnosis and staging of cancers of the pancreas.

Recent advances in magnetic resonance imaging (MRI), including high-resolution imaging and magnetic resonance cholangiopancreatography (MRCP), have led to an improved quality of MRI for diagnosing and staging pancreatic cancer. Although CT is usually more cost-effective and less time-consuming, MRI may be used if CT is inconclusive.[67] It may also be used if the patient has a contraindication to CT, such as an allergy to iodine contrast. Positron emission tomography (PET) is a newer technique that may provide additional imaging of the pancreas. Major indications for MRI and PET include the detection of small neoplasms, characterization of metastatic disease, and particularly differentiation between pancreatic carcinoma and chronic pancreatitis.[68] There is evidence to suggest that the use of enhanced PET combined with CT increases sensitivity of detecting tumors of less than 1 cm and also improves diagnosis of metastatic disease.[69,70] Because of their limited availability and higher cost, MRI and PET continue to play complementary roles to CT in the evaluation of pancreatic malignancies.[71,72]

Cholangiography is indicated in the evaluation of the jaundiced individual to define the site of biliary obstruction, by either the endoscopic or the percutaneous approach. Using ERCP, both biliary and pancreatic ductal systems can be visualized. In addition to delineating the site of obstruction, biopsy specimens for cytological analysis can be obtained. A diagnostic ERCP may be important if the differential diagnosis includes chronic pancreatitis and clinical deterioration. In most cases of pancreatic carcinoma, the pancreatic ductal system will be obstructed with the finding of a long, irregular stricture in an otherwise normal pancreatic duct—a finding not usually seen in pancreatitis. ERCP may be most useful to evaluate the nonjaundiced individual with vague gastrointestinal symptoms in whom an early nonobstructing cancer is suspected or in the person with obstructive jaundice presumed to have pancreatic cancer but in whom no mass is evident on CT.[73]

The percutaneous transhepatic cholangiographic (PTC) approach to the biliary tree is technically easier if a dilated biliary tree is present. It is most helpful in defining the proximal biliary system in cases of bile duct cancer (cholangiocarcinoma). PTC with percutaneous transhepatic biliary drainage (PTBD) is usually reserved for those individuals who fail endoscopic biliary drainage and need palliation of obstructive jaundice.

Preoperative angiography is performed selectively to determine vascular invasion and to delineate the important vascular anomalies that might alter the operative approach. The study may also be done when the CT scan suggests vascular abnormalities or in persons who have undergone previous operative palliation or chemoradiation. Assessment of the vascular anatomy may be difficult because of previous operation or radiation-induced scar formation.[39] Modern CT with three dimensional reconstruction and MRI, including magnetic resonance angiography (MRA), can now assess any vessel involvement and have replaced angiography in the staging of pancreatic tumors.[67]

Endoscopic ultrasonography (EUS) is useful in staging pancreatic tumors because it can establish the size of the tumor, its extension into adjacent structures, local and regional nodal involvement, and any vascular involvement such as the celiac axis, superior mesenteric artery, and mesenteric venous structures. It is most useful in the detection of small pancreatic lesions, smaller than 3 cm, which may not be visualized on CT or ERCP. EUS has also been found to be superior to both dynamic, nonspiral CT and MRI for staging pancreatic tumors. This technique is useful in the assessment of the pancreas in the case of failed ERCP, or in the evaluation of ductal structures seen at ERCP with a brush cytology sample that tests negative for malignancy. The development of EUS-guided fine-needle aspiration is a safe and effective approach for confirming the diagnosis of a pancreatic malignancy.[74]

Laparoscopy and direct visualization are best used for staging cancer of the pancreas particularly when other imaging methods have failed. Laparoscopic examination allows direct visualization of intra-abdominal contents and can identify hepatic and peritoneal metastases not visualized by other modalities. Biopsy of metastatic peritoneal, or omental lesions, or liver implants can be performed at the same time. Enlarged lymph nodes can also be sampled with needle biopsy. Laparoscopic ultrasound has also been used for the detection of metastases not seen on the surface of the liver, vascular invasion, or deep lymph node involvement. This minimally invasive procedure can help prevent an unnecessary laparotomy for diagnosis and staging of pancreatic cancer, particularly in individuals with advanced disease and limited survival prospects. Laparoscopy can be performed as an outpatient procedure, or it may be done as an initial procedure at the time of proposed resection to evaluate for resectability.[75] Peritoneal washings at the time of laparoscopy have detected micrometastases in individuals who had no other evidence of metastatic spread. This finding predicted advanced disease in which the individual would not benefit from aggressive surgical therapy.[76]

Percutaneous fine-needle aspiration biopsy (FNAB) of pancreatic tumors is useful in selected individuals, especially when guided by CT or US. This technique is safe and reliable, but it is not indicated in individuals who are candidates for resection or surgical palliation. FNAB may not be useful in potentially resectable tumors because a negative result cannot exclude malignancy, and it is the smaller and more curable tumors that are most likely to be missed by the needle.[9] Some reports have noted neoplastic cells seeding along the tract of the needle, raising concerns regarding tumor dissemination within the abdominal cavity.[77] The pancreas is a vascular organ with a rich lymphatic network. Unnecessary manipulation can disseminate a cancer that already has a high propensity for local invasion and vascular permeation.[78] FNAB is primarily used in individuals with unresectable cancer based on preoperative staging in whom nonoperative palliation is appropriate. The results of the biopsy may then help to direct palliative chemoradiation therapy. This technique is also useful in individuals with cancer in the head of the pancreas who are not surgical candidates and for whom neoadjuvant protocols are being considered. FNAB may be most useful in individuals whose clinical presentation and imaging studies do not suggest pancreatic adenocarcinoma. Uncommon pancreatic malignancies may be treated differently after diagnosis by FNAB, such as pancreatic lymphoma, which is best managed with chemotherapy, and pancreatic islet cell carcinoma may need further testing and consideration for aggressive surgery for tumor debulking.[79]

## Laboratory tests

Routine laboratory tests are generally within the normal range in the setting of pancreatic cancer, except for those individuals presenting with obstructive jaundice. Increased serum total bilirubin, alkaline phosphatase, gamma glutamyl transpeptidase, and often elevated levels of hepatic aminotransaminases are found. Normochromic anemia and hypoalbuminemia may reflect chronic neoplastic disease and its nutritional sequelae. When liver function test abnormalities occur in individuals with cancer of the body and tail of the pancreas, it usually indicates metastatic disease with liver involvement. Coagulation parameters should be checked in persons with deep jaundice because prolonged absence of bile from the gastrointestinal tract leads to malabsorption of fat-soluble vitamins and decreased production of vitamin K-dependent clotting factors.[39]

New-onset diabetes mellitus may be found in an individual with elevated glucose levels, which may or may not be controlled with oral hyperglycemic agents. A pancreatic problem should be investigated in an individual with previously controlled diabetes who exhibits any unexplained changes in glucose control.

## Tumor markers

No serum tumor marker is sufficiently sensitive or specific to be considered cost-effective and 100% reliable for screening of pancreatic cancer. Instead, a wide variety of serum tumor markers have been proposed for use in the diagnosis and follow-up of pancreatic carcinoma. The carbohydrate antigen 19–9 (CA 19–9) is tumor associated, not tumor specific, and has been a useful tool in the diagnosis and management of individuals with pancreatic cancer. Several factors can influence interpretation of CA 19–9. These include reference value, positive Lewis blood phenotype, jaundice, and prior use of interferon.[80,81] There is a lack of consensus concerning a useful reference value for the diagnosis of carcinoma of the pancreas. A reference value of CA 19–9 greater than 90 U/mL reaches an accuracy of 85% for diagnosis; the accuracy improves to 95% with a level greater than 200 U/mL.[82] CA 19–9 is not produced by individuals who lack the Lewis antigen (5%–10% of the Western population). Jaundice in an individual can cause a false increase in serum levels of CA 19–9. In addition, interferon significantly elevates CA 19–9 levels.[83]

CA 19–9 has not proved useful as a screening test, as levels are normal in early stage, potentially curable tumors. Use of CA 19–9 measurements combined with US, CT, or ERCP improves diagnostic accuracy. Elevated levels may help differentiate benign diseases from pancreatic cancer. After resection of pancreatic cancer, CA 19–9 levels fall. The antigen may then prove useful for prognosis and follow-up surveillance for tumor recurrence. A recent retrospective study suggests that CA 19–9 level >353 U/mL correlates with high sensitivity and specificity for unresectable pancreatic cancer.[84] This biomarker is used to monitor response to treatment, as increasing levels of CA 19–9 reflect progression of disease. Stable or declining levels of CA 19–9 are associated with a stable tumor burden and an improved prognosis.[85]

Several other tumor markers have been evaluated, either alone or in combination, as ways to screen for pancreatic cancer but thus far have not proved as reliable as CA 19–9 in the disease's diagnosis and monitoring. The use of molecular genetic markers as a mechanism for screening for genetic abnormalities in individuals with pancreatic cancer continues to evolve.

## CLASSIFICATION AND STAGING

The goal when staging cancer of the pancreas is to select the optimal treatment for each individual with minimal risks in a cost-effective manner. The aim is to determine whether the individual has potentially resectable disease, locally advanced disease, or metastatic disease, because therapeutic options and ultimate prognosis differ in each case. The definition of "resectability" can vary and reflects both the expertise and philosophy of the individual surgeon and institution.[86]

The staging of pancreatic carcinoma is based on the tumor-node-metastasis (TNM) system. Four stages have been described for use in the diagnosis of exocrine cancer of the pancreas by the American Joint Committee on Cancer (AJCC; see Table 63-6).[87] These parameters represent the most important factors influencing resectability and prognosis of exocrine tumors of the pancreas.

**TABLE 63-6**

**AJCC TNM Staging for Exocrine Pancreas Cancer**

**Primary Tumor (T)**

TX Primary tumor cannot be assessed

T0 No evidence of primary tumor

Tis Carcinoma in situ

T1 Tumor limited to pancreas and 2 cm or less in greatest dimension

T2 Tumor limited to pancreas and more than 2 cm in greatest dimension

T3 Tumor extends beyond pancreas but does not involve celiac axis or superior mesentery artery

T4 Tumor invades the celiac or the superior mesentery artery (unresectable primary tumor)

**Regional Lymph Nodes (N)**

NX Regional lymph nodes cannot be assessed

N0 No regional lymph node metastasis

N1 Regional lymph node metastasis

**Distant Metastasis (M)**

MX Distant metastasis cannot be assessed

M0 No distant metastasis

M1 Distant metastasis

**Stage Grouping**

| | | | |
|---|---|---|---|
| Stage 0 | Tis | N0 | M0 |
| Stage IA | T1 | N0 | M0 |
| Stage IB | T2 | N0 | M0 |
| Stage IIA | T3 | N0 | M0 |
| Stage IIB | T1-T3 | N1 | M0 |
| Stage III | T4 | Any N | M0 |
| Stage IV | Any T | Any N | M1 |

## THERAPEUTIC APPROACHES AND NURSING CARE

Every individual diagnosed with cancer of the pancreas should be carefully evaluated prior to initiation of any therapy. An individual must also be adequately prepared physiologically and psychologically before undergoing any therapy. Historically, the poor prognosis of individuals with pancreatic cancer has caused many clinicians to have a dismal outlook and thus be reluctant to treat the disease aggressively. However, recent reports on surgical outcomes are encouraging,[88,89] and the overall perspective on the disease appears to be changing.

Surgery, radiotherapy, and chemotherapy are the principal treatment modalities used for pancreatic cancer. Surgical resection remains the best therapeutic option, even though few individuals are cured. Most surgical procedures are palliative as unresectable pancreatic cancer predominates. Only about 15% to 20% of malignancies of the head of the pancreas are resectable and potentially curable at surgery.[5] The 3-year and 5-year survival rates after resection of the head of the pancreas are only 32% and 15%, respectively.[5] Survival rates improve favorably if the patient is younger than 65 at diagnosis.[5] The resection and survival rates for tumors in the body and tail of the pancreas are much lower.

Available therapeutic interventions include surgery, usually in combination with radiation therapy, and chemotherapy with single agents or a combination of agents for either cure or palliation. Various regimens of chemotherapeutic agents alone or combinations of agents with or without radiation therapy are also used for nonoperative cancer of the pancreas. Experimental vaccines and drugs that target the genes involved with pancreatic cancer are being investigated and may soon be a routine part of multimodal therapies.[90] Palliation for longer periods is usually achieved with combined modalities.

Once a diagnosis has been made, the extent of the tumor involvement established, and complete assessment of the individual's physical status made, a treatment plan will be presented to the individual. If surgery is an option, the patient's physical ability to undergo general anesthesia and a major abdominal operation must be considered; advanced age is not necessarily a negative factor.[91] Nutritional status, hematological status, liver function, concomitant disease, and skill of the principal clinicians all contribute to the choice of therapy.

Prior to surgery, a biliary stent to alleviate jaundice may be placed through the obstructing lesion by either the endoscopic or the percutaneous approach. Current studies suggest that the use of routine preoperative biliary stenting leads to an increase in postoperative surgical complications including increased incidence of pancreatic fistula formation, biliary contamination, and wound infections.[92,93] In selected individuals with severe malnutrition, sepsis, and/or correctable medical conditions, or in whom there is a time delay before surgery for preoperative chemoradiation therapy, preoperative biliary drainage may be useful.[93,94] Theoretically, the internal drainage of biliary secretions may provide an immunological advantage, leading to decreased perioperative complications of sepsis. An endoscopic stent or a percutaneously placed biliary stent can be used in the operative management of individuals with pancreatic cancer either for resection or for palliation. An ERCP with stent placement is performed under conscious sedation, and the person can be discharged the same day. Antibiotics are usually administered intravenously as prophylaxis against cholangitis due to manipulation within the biliary tract. The benefit of an internal stent for drainage is that there is no external tube to manage. The individual needs to be taught the signs and symptoms of possible complications of the stent, such as recurrent jaundice and cholangitis (shaking chills and fever). Any manifestation of these signs or symptoms needs to be reported to the health care provider immediately, as the individual may be prone to bacteremia and sepsis.

The individual having a PTC with placement of a PTBD stent needs to be taught about the procedure as well as the care and management of the external biliary stent. This interventional radiological procedure is performed under conscious sedation. An internal-external stent is placed. Prophylactic antibiotics are given to prevent biliary sepsis. Individuals are usually monitored for 24 hours to assess patency of the stent and to ensure bile drainage. Initially, the biliary stent is attached to a bile bag, for external drainage, to allow the obstructed biliary tree to decompress. The bile bag is then removed, and the biliary stent is capped off with a one-way valve to allow internal drainage and the free flow of bile into the bowel.

Care of a percutaneously placed biliary stent to maintain a properly functioning tube is an important aspect of patient teaching. Signs and symptoms of any complications—such as fever, chills, recurrent jaundice, bleeding at the exit site or through the biliary stent, dislodgment of the catheter from its original site, or inability to flush the stent—must be reported immediately to the health care provider to prevent problems. Teaching protocols are important for consistent and correct information. Written instructions given to the individual as a handout or a video to take home may be helpful.[95,96]

Cure is the objective if the tumor is small, localized, and not fixed to other structures, and if there is no evidence of regional or distant metastases. Complete resection of the tumor will be performed and supplemented with adjuvant therapy.

Control or palliation is the goal of therapy if the tumor is unresectable or has metastasized to regional or distant nodes or to other organs. Unfortunately, approximately 90% of all cases of pancreatic carcinoma are diagnosed as unresectable.[97] For some individuals, operative palliation for obstructive jaundice or gastric outlet obstruction may be indicated for optimal long-term management. Other treatments aimed at relieving devastating symptoms may include radiotherapy, chemotherapy, percutaneous pain block, percutaneous or endoscopic biliary decompression to relieve obstruction and pressure, and gastric decompression for gastric outlet obstruction. Nutritional supplementation to achieve adequate total protein levels helps to decrease surgical risk, puts the individual in a better metabolic state for having any treatment modality, and increases the patient's overall well-being.

It is important to understand the individual's goal and plan for therapy, method of family coping, and pattern of communication. When all members of the health care team, along with the patient, agree upon a course of treatment, communication is enhanced and issues or problems can be identified and addressed. Illness has a special meaning to each person. Living with cancer of the pancreas and dealing with the knowledge that the disease has a poor prognosis, regardless of what treatment is undertaken, can create many unforeseen problems. Comprehensive education about diagnostics and modes of therapy, along with physical and emotional support to the patient with a new diagnosis of pancreatic carcinoma, is the hallmark of nursing care.

## SURGERY

Surgical resection of pancreatic cancer remains the best therapeutic option and the only opportunity for cure. Most surgical procedures for this disease are palliative. Only about 10% to 20% of carcinomas of the head of the pancreas are resectable and potentially curable at surgery. The survival rate for individuals with tumors in the body and tail is much lower. There is limited prospective research evaluating surgical procedures for cancer of the pancreas.

Recent reports from institutions with large series of patients have reported increasing survival periods following resection and operative mortality rates that have decreased to less than 5%.[89,98–101] Decreased complications are attributed to refinements in surgical technique, anesthesia, critical care, and preoperative and postoperative care. Other reasons for the improvements in surgical outcome include the operations being performed by surgeons who are experienced in the surgical management of pancreatic carcinoma, concentration of patients in centers of excellence, and improved methods to diagnose and treat complications.[102] Most surgical results report collective overall outcomes; however, individuals with small (less than 2 cm) tumors have 5-year survival rates of 30%, and survival rates increase for those with no residual disease or without lymphatic involvement.[5,100] The crux of the problem is late detection of pancreatic tumors. Until advances in early detection and diagnosis are made, curative surgery will be limited to very few candidates and palliative measures will continue as the mainstay of therapy.

When cure is the objective, the surgical approach most frequently used for neoplasms of the head of the pancreas is a pancreaticoduodenectomy (Whipple procedure). Total pancreatectomy may be performed for tumor involving the entire gland, tumor that extends across the neck and body of the gland, or when the pancreatic remnant is too soft and friable to allow a safe pancreatic-enteric anastomosis. An extended or radical pancreaticoduodenectomy has also been performed as an alternative or modification of the original regional pancreatectomy. Regional pancreatectomy has been found to have higher morbidity and mortality rates, with no improvement in survival over the standard pancreaticoduodenectomy.[4] Controversy exists regarding the advantages, disadvantages, and long-term results of each operation[8] (see Table 63-7).[6] Data from prospective randomized studies comparing standard vs radical pancreaticoduodenectomy in individuals have been evaluated and there is no difference in outcomes. Surgical intervention is individualized based on disease process.

Despite sophisticated preoperative staging methods, many individuals with adenocarcinoma of the head of the pancreas that preoperatively appears to be resectable are ultimately found to have metastatic or locally invasive disease. During surgical exploration, it is possible to encounter local spread of tumor into adjacent major vascular structures (portal vein, superior mesenteric vein, superior mesenteric artery, or abdominal aorta). The tumor can encase and grow into these vessels, precluding surgical resection. The tumor may also have metastasized to the liver or peritoneal surfaces. If unresectable or metastatic disease is discovered, surgical palliation can be used to treat or prevent the major symptoms of obstructive jaundice, duodenal obstruction, and pain.

### Pancreaticoduodenectomy (Whipple procedure)

The Whipple procedure is the most commonly performed operation for carcinoma of the head of the pancreas (Figure 63-3A). The classic Whipple procedure[103] includes resection of the distal stomach, gallbladder, distal common bile duct, head of the pancreas, and duodenum. Gastrointestinal continuity is restored by anastomosing the common bile duct and the remaining pancreas to the jejunum proximal to the gastrojejunostomy. Some surgeons anastomose the remaining pancreas to the back of the stomach because they believe it is safer and decreases the potential for pancreatic fistula formation.[104] The gastrojejunostomy is performed to allow alkaline bile and pancreatic juices to enter the jejunum before acidic gastric secretions.[105] This step decreases the potential for ulceration at the gastrojejunostomy. The distal gastrojejunostomy also reduces reflux of intestinal contents into the bile duct and pancreas. The risk of ulceration has been greatly reduced by the use of postoperative prophylactic acid antisecretory agents such as $H_2$-receptor antagonists and proton pump inhibitors.

A modification of the original or classic Whipple procedure, called a *pylorus-preserving pancreaticoduodenectomy*, is preferred by some surgeons (Figure 63-3B). This procedure preserves the entire stomach, including the pylorus, and a small cuff of proximal duodenum. It has the advantage of maintaining a normal gastric reservoir and environment, thereby avoiding potential nutritional problems associated with the classic Whipple procedure such as weight loss, dumping syndrome, diarrhea, and anastomotic ulcer at the gastrojejunostomy site. This procedure requires less time and is technically easier to perform.[106] Delayed gastric emptying that may occur following this operation generally resolves over time with conservative treatment (gastric decompression, parenteral or enteral nutrition, and prokinetic agents). Erythromycin, a motilin agonist, also has been prescribed to improve gastric emptying after surgery.[8] Concern has arisen that the pylorus-preserving pancreaticoduodenectomy may not be an adequate cancer operation because of the limited surgical margins and inadequate removal of lymph nodes in the area draining the cancer, which may compromise cure.

**TABLE 63-7**

**Comparison of Types of Pancreatic Resections for Malignancy**

| | Indications | Tissues Removed | Potential Advantages | Potential Disadvantages |
|---|---|---|---|---|
| Classic pancreaticoduodenectomy (Whipple) | Periampullary or localized carcinoma of head, neck, or uncinate process of pancreas | Head, neck, and uncinate process<br>Duodenum<br>Gastric antrum and pylorus<br>Common bile duct<br>Gallbladder<br>Lymph nodes in pancreaticoduodenal groove | Pancreatic remnant may prevent diabetes and malabsorption<br>Better cancer operation compared with pylorus preservation | Partial pancreatic resection may leave residual tumor in body or tail of gland<br>Issue of multicentricity<br>Dumping syndrome secondary to loss of pylorus<br>Nutritional problems<br>Leak at pancreatic anastomosis |
| Pylorus-preserving pancreaticoduodenectomy (Whipple) | Periampullary or localized carcinoma of head, neck, or uncinate process of pancreas | Head, neck, and uncinate process<br>Duodenum (except most proximal portion)<br>Common bile duct<br>Gallbladder<br>Lymph nodes in pancreaticoduodenal groove | Pancreatic remnant may prevent diabetes and malabsorption<br>Normal gastric reservoir<br>Less disruption of digestion compared with classic Whipple<br>Reduced marginal ulceration at duodenojejunostomy | Partial pancreatic resection may leave residual tumor in body or tail of gland<br>Leak at pancreatic anastomosis<br>Delayed gastric emptying |
| Extended or radical pancreaticoduodenectomy | Periampullary or localized carcinoma of head, neck, or uncinate process of pancreas | Head, neck, and uncinate process<br>Duodenum<br>Gastric antrum and pylorus<br>Common bile duct<br>Gallbladder<br>Extensive lymph node and retroperitoneal tissue dissection<br>Vascular resection may be included | Extensive regional nodal dissection<br>Pancreatic remnant may prevent diabetes and malabsorption<br>Better cancer operation? | Partial pancreatic resection may leave residual tumor in body or tail of gland<br>Leak at pancreatic anastomosis<br>Dumping syndrome secondary to loss of pylorus<br>Nutritional problems<br>Chylous leak<br>Longer operation with potential for increased blood loss and complications |
| Total pancreaticoduodenectomy (may be classic or pylorus-preserving) | Diffuse carcinoma of entire gland or a multicentric tumor | Entire pancreas<br>Duodenum<br>Gastric antrum and pylorus<br>Common bile duct<br>Gallbladder<br>Spleen<br>Peripancreatic nodes<br>Lymph nodes in pancreaticoduodenal groove | Excision of entire pancreas may remove multifocal tumor<br>More complete peripancreatic nodal dissection<br>No pancreatic enteric anastomosis | Insulin-dependent diabetes and complete exocrine absence<br>Need for insulin and enzyme replacement<br>Postsplenectomy state |
| Distal pancreatectomy | Carcinoma localized to body or tail of gland | Distal pancreas<br>Spleen<br>Peripancreatic lymph nodes | Pancreatic remnant may prevent diabetes and malabsorption<br>No pancreatic or biliary enteric anastomosis | Limited resection may leave residual tumor<br>Postsplenectomy state |

*Source:* Reprinted with permission from Sauter PK, Coleman J. Pancreatic cancer: a continuum of care. *Semin Oncol Nurs.* 1999;15:36–47.[6]

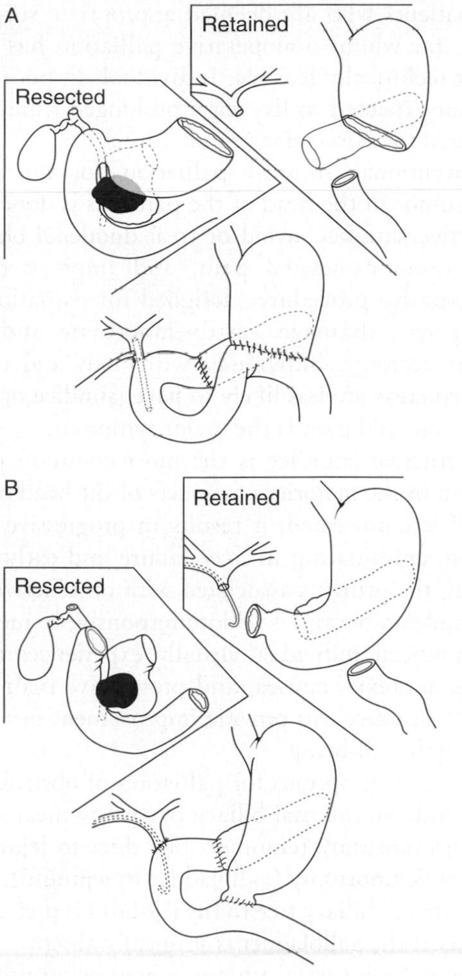


**FIGURE 63-3**

Classic pancreaticoduodenectomy (**A**) and pylorus-preserving pancreaticoduodenectomy (**B**) showing the resected specimens, the structures retained, and one method of reconstruction by way of pancreaticojejunostomy. (Reprinted with permission from Yeo CJ, Cameron JL. The pancreas. In: Hardy JD, ed. *Hardy's Textbook of Surgery*, ed 2. Philadelphia, PA: Lippincott-Raven; 1998:695–725.[103])

Studies have shown that pylorus preservation appears to be associated with no consistent adverse sequelae, and it has equivalent survival and quality of life as compared to classic pancreaticoduodenectomy.[99,101,107,108]

Pancreatic fistula and delayed gastric emptying are the most common serious complications after a pancreaticoduodenectomy. The pancreas, attached to the jejunum, is technically the most difficult of the anastomoses. If it does not heal properly, a pancreatic fistula may develop. Although fistulae and leaks were previously associated with significant mortality because pancreatic juices eroded into major blood vessels, the incidence and severity of pancreatic anastomotic leaks appear to have decreased with improved surgical technique, intravenous nutritional support, modern antibiotics, and appropriate wound drainage systems.[91,108] Intraabdominal infection, gastrointestinal bleeding, wound infection, diabetes, and pancreatic exocrine insufficiency occur less frequently[106,109,110] (see Table 63-8).

**TABLE 63-8**

| Complications After Pancreaticoduodenectomy |
|---|
| Pancreatic fistula |
| Delayed gastric emptying |
| Wound infection |
| Intraabdominal abscess |
| Hemorrhage |
| Diabetes |
| Pancreatic exocrine insufficiency |

It is important for the nurse to know exactly what surgical procedure was performed so as to know what to assess from various drains and tubes placed at the time of surgery. Bile duct-to-jejunum anastomosis may be stented with a preoperatively placed percutaneous transhepatic biliary stent to ensure decompression of the jejunum and to allow the free flow of bile. This stent also provides direct access into the biliary tree postoperatively to assess for an anastomotic leak, obstruction, or stricture. Likewise, wound drains may be placed adjacent to the pancreatic and biliary anastomoses to enable rapid assessment of bile or pancreatic juice leakage or bleeding. The use of various feeding tubes placed at the time of surgery depends on the preference of the surgeon.

Nutritional assessment is important to establish that the person has adequate protein and calories for wound healing. Most individuals will receive postoperative adjuvant therapy; therefore, good nutritional status, along with physical and psychological readiness, are essential. Immediate postoperative pain management can be successfully provided by intravenous or epidural patient-controlled analgesia (PCA).

## Extended (radical) pancreaticoduodenectomy

This operation consists of a pancreaticoduodenectomy or sometimes a total pancreatectomy, along with an extensive retroperitoneal lymph node and soft tissue resection. Resection of the superior mesenteric vein, portal vein, or superior mesenteric artery may also be performed. The extended pancreaticoduodenectomy has been advocated by some Japanese and European researchers because lymph node involvement is an important prognostic factor in individuals with carcinoma of the head of the pancreas. No published prospective randomized studies demonstrate a consistent survival advantage for individuals undergoing extended pancreaticoduodenectomy.[4,39,97]

### Total pancreatectomy

A total pancreatectomy entails an en bloc resection of the distal stomach, duodenum, gallbladder, and distal common bile duct, along with the entire pancreas, spleen, and a wide margin of peripancreatic tissue including lymph nodes. It eliminates the problem of residual tumor at the margins of the pancreas, tumor spillage when the pancreas is divided, and pancreatic fistula. This operation has shown no reduction in mortality or morbidity and no evidence of any increase in survival when it is performed routinely.[9] Individuals who have a total pancreatectomy develop pancreatic endocrine and exocrine insufficiency and become brittle diabetics with glucose levels that may be difficult to control. Pancreatic enzyme supplementation is necessary for a lifetime. This operation is usually reserved for selected cases, particularly when there is evidence of tumor throughout the entire pancreas or when the pancreas is considered to be unsafe for anastomosis. Reasons for an unsafe anastomosis are that the pancreas is too soft and friable, or acute edematous pancreatitis develops during surgery after manipulation of the gland.[9]

### Distal pancreatectomy

In rare cases, tumors of the body and tail of the pancreas are detected early enough to be considered curable. A distal pancreatectomy with a splenectomy is performed in these patients. The prognosis is poor, with few patients surviving for more than 2 years. Lesions of the body and tail rarely cause gastrointestinal obstructive symptoms and as a result are not recognized until the tumor has become unresectable.[111,112] Most individuals with adenocarcinomas of the body or tail of the pancreas are unresectable and survive for only a short period. The only change in the management of these individuals has been a diminished need for exploratory laparotomy to establish tissue diagnosis. The use of laparoscopy and FNAB to determine metastatic or unresectable disease spares these individuals an unnecessary laparotomy.[9]

### Palliative procedures

Only about 10% of individuals with pancreatic cancer are resectable for cure at the time of presentation. Therefore, palliation of symptoms to maximize quality of life is the primary goal for most patients who are not curable.[111] These individuals present challenging management problems because optimal palliation of symptoms may be difficult. Obstructive jaundice, duodenal obstruction, and pain are the symptoms most frequently requiring aggressive intervention using operative and nonoperative techniques.[9] Management can be tailored to the individual's clinical presentation, prognosis, and overall medical condition.[111] A choice must be made between operative and nonoperative palliation. Operative palliation is used for those patients who are deemed appropriate surgical candidates, for whom nonoperative palliation has failed, or was not technically feasible. Individuals in poor health or those not expected to live for a prolonged time should be considered for nonoperative palliation.[9]

Conventional surgical palliation for an individual with a tumor in the head of the pancreas is done to relieve obstructive jaundice, avoid or treat duodenal obstruction, relieve tumor-associated pain, and improve quality of life. Operative procedures designed for palliation include biliary-enteric drainage, gastrojejunostomy, and chemical splanchnicectomy. Individuals with body and tail lesions of the pancreas are less likely to have jaundice or duodenal obstruction, and pain is the major symptom.

Obstructive jaundice is the most common presenting symptom in the majority of cancers of the head of the pancreas. If left untreated, it results in progressive liver dysfunction, culminating in liver failure and early death. In addition, the pruritus associated with obstructive jaundice can be unbearable and is seldom responsive to medications. The jaundiced individual usually experiences alterations in taste, anorexia, nausea, and progressive malnutrition.[39] Relief of jaundice can provide improvement in an individual's overall well-being.

The surgical options for palliation of obstructive jaundice include an internal biliary bypass by means of a choledochojejunostomy (common bile duct to jejunum) or a cholecystojejunostomy (gallbladder to jejunum). Bypass of the obstructed biliary tree to the jejunum is preferred and is necessary if the gallbladder is surgically absent.

Minimally invasive surgery is now being used for palliation of biliary and duodenal obstruction with laparoscopic cholecystojejunostomy and gastrojejunostomy.[113] The preliminary results have shown technical success, low morbidity, and satisfactory outcomes. Palliative pancreaticoduodenectomy for tumor debulking may also offer some advantages to those individuals with seemingly unresectable disease. This major operation would be performed on selected patients considered to have low perioperative morbidity and mortality.[114]

Nonoperative palliation of obstructed jaundice by either percutaneous or endoscopic drainage methods is also effective. Placement of a stent through the area of biliary obstruction facilitates the free flow of bile. Compared with operative decompression, a biliary stent reduces the length of initial hospitalization, is associated with lower complication rates, and lower procedure-related mortality, and is significantly less expensive.[39]

Endoscopically placed biliary stents offer an advantage over the percutaneous technique, with fewer procedure-related complications and better patient acceptance. The major complication is stent occlusion associated with recurrent jaundice and sepsis. This problem can require stent replacement every 3 to 4 months or sooner. Prolonged stent patency is now being achieved with the use of large-diameter, expandable metallic stents. These stents appear to remain patent for a time that closely approximates the length of survival of the individual.[115] Endoscopic stents are also preferred for individuals with ascites to prevent the external leakage of ascites and avoid being a portal for infection.

Percutaneous biliary drainage is indicated when endoscopic biliary drainage is unsuccessful and with recurrent jaundice following surgical bypass.[116] An internal-external drainage stent is placed by an interventional radiologist. The biliary stent requires daily maintenance by the individual or caregiver—in particular, daily stent flushing and dressing of the stent entry site. The presence of the external stent serves as a constant reminder to the patient of the disease. Bile leakage around the stent, skin irritation, stent dislodgment, and stent occlusion may occur. In individuals with ascites, leakage of ascitic fluid around the stent almost always occurs and is difficult to control. Because all stents placed within the biliary tree eventually will occlude, percutaneous biliary stents are exchanged approximately every 3 months to prevent development of stent obstruction, recurrent jaundice, or cholangitis. This exchange can be easily performed as an outpatient procedure. Complications related to percutaneous biliary drainage include transient bacteremia or sepsis, hemobilia, and bile peritonitis.

Duodenal obstruction occurs in a significant number of individuals when unresectable disease progresses. Obstruction from cancer in the head of the pancreas typically occurs at the duodenal C loop, causing nausea and vomiting. A large tumor in the body or tail of the pancreas will usually obstruct the junction of the duodenum and jejunum at the ligament of Treitz.[117] A retrocolic gastrojejunostomy can be performed to treat or prevent gastric outlet obstruction. The procedure, when implemented as a prophylactic measure and combined with a biliary bypass, has been shown to be of value as the individual's morbidity or mortality is not increased when gastrojejunostomy is performed as either a therapeutic or a prophylactic measure.[118] If the patient is not a surgical candidate because of recurrent tumor or is in the terminal stage of disease, duodenal obstruction can be alleviated by placement of a percutaneous endoscopic gastrostomy (PEG) decompression tube. This tube is not used for feeding, but it is effective in relieving gastric distention and may improve the comfort of the individual in the terminal stages of the disease.

Endoscopically placed metallic stents within the native duodenum at the site of tumor infiltration or at the site of an obstructed gastrojejunostomy have provided an alternative nonoperative option for individuals with malignant duodenal obstruction. This novel approach continues to be assessed as an appropriate palliative management device to allow the patient to resume enteral nutrition until death.[119]

Pain is the most significant symptom for individuals with pancreatic cancer. For many patients, pain is poorly managed and remains so until death. The severity and persistence of pain correlate with the stage of the disease. For most individuals with pancreatic cancer who are not surgical candidates, the appropriate use of oral agents can successfully manage pain.[120] Chemical splanchnicectomy (alcohol nerve block) is an alternative therapy available to those patients who do not benefit from oral analgesia or who cannot tolerate oral intake due to gastric outlet obstruction. It is performed using a spinal needle to inject alcohol on each side of the aorta at the level of the celiac axis (Figure 63-4).[121] Percutaneous celiac nerve block, with either fluoroscopic or CT guidance, can be performed to reduce pain and to decrease the need for oral narcotics. Nerve blocks can be done as an outpatient procedure or at the time of surgery for those individuals undergoing a palliative operation. Percutaneous nerve blocks can be repeated in individuals when previous blocks have subsequently worn off. Orthostatic hypotension is the most common complication after the block. Intraoperative injection of alcohol into the celiac nerves has been shown to both relieve pain and prevent the development of pain. Improvement in pain control is associated with prolonged survival and enhanced quality of life.[121,122]

Another modality used for control of pain due to unresectable pancreatic cancer is external beam radiation

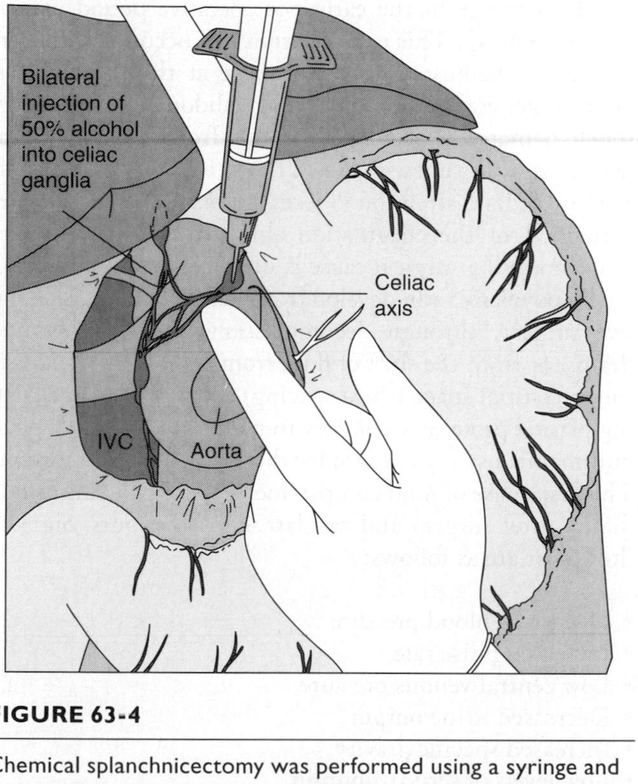


**FIGURE 63-4**

Chemical splanchnicectomy was performed using a syringe and a 20- or 22-gauge spinal needle. Solution (20 mL) was injected on each side of the aorta at the level of the celiac axis. (Used with permission from Lillemoe KD, Cameron JL, Kaufman HS, et al. Chemical splanchnicectomy in patients with unresectable pancreatic cancer: a prospective randomized trial. *Ann Surg.* 1993;217:447–457.[121])

therapy.[39] Finally, transthoracic splanchnicectomy and endoscopic chemical splanchnicectomy with the aid of US guidance have been performed to relieve pain due to unresectable pancreatic cancer in selected individuals.[122]

## Postoperative care

Postoperative medical and nursing management of individuals who undergo pancreatic resection is critical for reducing surgical morbidity and mortality. Careful assessment, anticipatory management, and complete patient and family teaching will greatly enhance recovery and rehabilitation.[122,123] Hemorrhage, hypovolemia, and hypotension pose the greatest threats in the immediate postoperative period.

Following a pancreatic resection, individuals may be admitted to an intensive care unit, where hemodynamic monitoring is performed. Stabilizing and maintaining fluid requirements are essential. Careful attention is given to signs of bleeding, security and patency of wound drains, and pain management. Pain management can be achieved with opiates delivered by intravenous or epidural PCA. Following endotracheal extubation, aggressive pulmonary toilet is needed to reduce the risk of respiratory problems. Ideally, patients should be out of bed and sitting in a chair within a few hours following extubation.

Hemorrhage in the early postoperative period can be life-threatening. This complication can occur from failure of surgical hemostasis, from leakage at the anastomosis, or from generalized coagulopathy. Abdominal distention, shock, hematemesis, bloody drainage from gastrointestinal decompression tubes, wound drains, or bloody stool warrant immediate attention. Successful management requires correction of the coagulation abnormalities and prompt reoperation if a surgical cause is suspected.

Hypovolemia can develop from fluids lost during extensive surgery, through decompression tubes and wound drains, or from the shift of fluid from the vascular space to the interstitial space (third spacing). Low levels of circulating plasma proteins secondary to malnutrition and hypoalbuminemia usually account for the third spacing syndrome. The first phase of fluid compartment shifting begins immediately after surgery and can last 48 to 72 hours. Signs of fluid shift are as follows:

- Decreased blood pressure
- Increased pulse rate
- Low central venous pressure
- Decreased urine output
- Increased specific gravity
- Low levels of serum albumin
- Hemoconcentration

When the plasma protein is replaced and levels return to normal, fluid reabsorption follows. Urine output will dramatically increase and will greatly exceed intake. The individual is closely monitored for signs of circulatory overload. The reabsorption phase will reach equilibrium within 24 to 48 hours.

Hypotension is a potential postoperative complication that is believed to result from severance of the sympathetic nerve fibers of the mesenteric complex. Vital signs and urine output should be monitored frequently to detect alterations. Vasopressor drugs and liberal intravenous fluids may be administered.

Pulmonary complications following surgery usually result from immobility and inadequate lung expansion secondary to pain and splinting. In addition, those individuals who are malnourished and protein deficient are susceptible to pneumonia. The importance of vigorous pulmonary hygiene and early ambulation cannot be overemphasized. Parenteral nutrition may also be needed to correct nutritional deficiencies.

Careful attention is given to wound drains for any sudden change in amount, color, or consistency of drainage. Abdominal wound drains are observed for evidence of bile or clear pancreatic juice that would suggest anastomotic leakage. Pancreatic juice that changes color to milky or brown with a foul odor suggests a pancreatic fistula. Although used in the past, recent studies show that the somatostatin analog, octreotide, administered postoperatively, does not provide any substantial benefit in reducing the incidence of postoperative complications.[4,124] Parenteral nutrition may be initiated when the patient is NPO, to rest the pancreas and allow a pancreatic fistula to heal.

Prolonged ileus and delayed gastric emptying are other potential complications. These problems can generally be resolved by taking a conservative approach with nasogastric suction, maintenance of parenteral or enteral nutrition, and use of prokinetic agents, such as metoclopramide, or a motilin agonist, such as erythromycin.[125] The surgical incision must be examined routinely for any signs of infection, as this complication can be synergistic with a pancreatic fistula or delayed gastric emptying.[109]

Following resection of the pancreas, exocrine and endocrine functions will be temporarily or permanently altered, depending on the amount of viable pancreatic tissue remaining. In the immediate postoperative period, laboratory tests are useful for monitoring protein, fat, and glucose levels. Prior to discharge, the patient and family must become familiar with and be able to recognize the signs and symptoms of exocrine and endocrine abnormalities such as hyperglycemia, hypoglycemia, steatorrhea, stupor, and lethargy, especially in those patients who have undergone a total pancreatectomy.

Endocrine function, the secretion of insulin, and the production of glucagon may be altered after a pancreatic resection. Usually, a nondiabetic individual will not develop diabetes after a pancreaticoduodenectomy (occurring in less than 10% of cases).[126] Individuals who have a total pancreatectomy will develop significant hyperglycemia and are usually managed in the immediate postoperative period with an insulin drip infusion. Endocrinology consultants should be contacted soon after surgery to assist with glucose management and insulin adjustment, particularly when the patient is taking oral foods and fluids. During the immediate postoperative period when the patient remains NPO, serum glucose levels are monitored every 4 hours, and a sliding-scale insulin dose is administered as needed. Basal nutritional and correctional insulin requirements, as well as carbohydrate management comprise a comprehensive approach to maintaining a stable serum blood glucose level. These patients generally require only moderate amounts of insulin and are not prone to ketoacidosis. However, they are particularly brittle and readily develop life-threatening hypoglycemia. Maintaining tight glucose control is now advocated for postoperative and lifelong management. Discharge teaching and home therapy programs—including self-administration of insulin, knowledge of signs and symptoms of hyper- or hypoglycemia, diabetic diet, meticulous hygiene, and the importance of routine follow-up with an endocrinologist or a medical physician for diabetes management—are the same as for individuals with diabetes. Inability to control glucose levels may indicate recurrence of disease.

Alteration of exocrine function by removal of pancreatic tissue can result in a malabsorption syndrome characterized by an inability to use ingested forms of fat and protein. The caloric requirements of the individual following surgery exceed 3000 calories per day; therefore, adequate nutritional intake is essential to recovery. Oral ingestion of food is the best means of maintaining essential nutrients, but ileus or delayed gastric emptying may prohibit this mode. Parenteral or enteral alimentation may be necessary to replace calories lost as a result of the surgically induced malabsorption of fats and proteins until the individual can be advanced to an oral diet. Pancreatic enzymes are replaced with oral enzyme supplements, which contain lipase, amylase, and trypsin. The most frequently used forms are pancreatin and pancrelipase. Pancreatin and pancrelipase supplements are made from extracts of porcine or bovine pancreas enriched with bile salts and plant and fungal enzymes. The usual therapeutic dose is 2 to 4 tablets with each meal and 1 to 2 tablets with a fatty snack. The enzymes are taken with or during the meal.[127] It may require several adjustments before the most appropriate dosage for each person is determined, because eating patterns and individual responses vary.[128]

When the patient is able to tolerate food, several small feedings consisting of foods that are low in fat and high in carbohydrates and protein are tolerated better than large meals. Restrictions include overindulgence (which places a great demand on the pancreas), caffeine, and alcohol. It is advantageous for the clinical dietitian to consult with the patient to select the most agreeable diet plan based on individual needs and lifestyle. The patient and family should be instructed on how to monitor the individual's tolerance to the diet and pancreatic enzyme replacement therapy. Stool should be examined daily for the characteristic signs of steatorrhea: frothy, floating, foul-smelling stool with greasy, fat particles floating in the water, crampy abdominal pain, or bloating. If these characteristics are observed, they should be reported to the healthcare provider for dietary and/or pancreatic enzyme dosage adjustment.[127] The individual should be informed that steatorrhea will decrease but may not be eliminated.

## CHEMOTHERAPY

Because most individuals present with unresectable cancer of the pancreas and are already in a debilitated state, benefit from antineoplastic therapy is unlikely. Individuals with pancreatic cancer exhibit precarious physiological conditions, which makes it difficult to differentiate the side effects of therapy from the natural progression of the disease. Response to therapy is also difficult to evaluate.

Although the only curative therapy for pancreatic cancer is surgical resection, most studies document high rates of both local recurrence and distant metastases.[54,97,129] The benefit of using adjuvant combined chemotherapy and radiation therapy after surgical resection for pancreatic cancer was first demonstrated by the Gastrointestinal Tumor Study Group (GITSG).[130] Radiation therapy is directed at the region from which the tumor was resected or where the greatest tumor burden lies; chemotherapy addresses the smaller or microscopic residual tumor. With the recent surge in interest in treatments for cancer of the pancreas, the role of multimodality therapy for patients with potentially resectable pancreatic cancer continues to evolve. Many different combinations of chemotherapeutic agents and radiation therapy are being investigated. Adjuvant therapy is now recommended for all individuals after resection for pancreatic cancer.

### Neoadjuvant therapy

Trials exploring neoadjuvant chemoradiation were prompted by the observation of a prolonged recovery in some patients after pancreaticoduodenectomy, leading to a delay or cancellation of adjuvant therapy. This approach has both advantages and disadvantages. However, there are no objective data from recent randomized trials demonstrating superior survival results.[131–133]

### Treatment for locally advanced pancreatic cancer

Locally advanced pancreatic cancer is defined as arterial involvement, or superior mesenteric artery, or superior mesenteric-portal vein confluence occlusion. These patients are deemed unresectable due to invasion of the portal or mesenteric vessels even in the absence of metastatic disease. Studies have examined patients with locally unresectable pancreatic cancer who received neoadjuvant chemoradiation followed by surgery but suggest that it is unlikely to convert a locally, advanced, unresectable pancreatic cancer to a resectable one.[134] There is also some evidence that significantly elevated CA19–9 levels may have some predictive value related to survival or recurrence after treatment in this subset of patients.[135] Intraoperative electron beam radiation (IOERT) has been used in an attempt to enhance local-regional control achieved by conventional external beam radiation and chemotherapy. No significant improvement in long-term survival was found using IOERT.[136]

## Treatment of metastatic and recurrent disease

Minimal success has been achieved in identifying effective chemotherapy for metastatic pancreatic cancer. The median survival for patients with metastatic disease remains less than 9 months. Chemotherapy with 5-fluorouracil (5-FU) intravenous, or Xeloda (PO) remains the most widely used regimen in pancreatic cancer.[137] There is recent evidence to suggest that adjuvant 5-FU administered with folinic acid may also improve survival.[132]

Gemcitabine has been studied in patients with locally advanced and metastatic pancreatic cancer.[138] Gemcitabine is a cytotoxic agent that was developed specifically for patients with advanced-stage disease. Clinical benefit response was the objective of treatment with this new drug rather than measuring tumor shrinkage. Clinical benefit response is a novel approach to assess the clinical effectiveness of gemcitabine based on marked improvement in pain control, analgesic consumption, and performance status. Prolonged survival was a secondary benefit. Gemcitabine is usually well tolerated, with a relatively mild toxicity profile. Studies have shown that gemcitabine confers a modest survival advantage as compared to treatment with 5-FU.[139] The results of these trials helped gemcitabine to become accepted as first-line therapy for patients with advanced or metastatic pancreatic carcinoma in the US.

Both gemcitabine and 5-FU are now standard therapy as single agents for the treatment of metastatic and recurrent disease. More recent studies have incorporated gemcitabine into combined modality therapy. Other combination partners with gemcitabine under investigation include the antimetabolite 5-FU, the topoisomerase-I inhibitor irinotecan, the taxane docetaxel, the platinum agent oxaliplatin, the multitargeted antifolate pemetrexed, the farnesyl transferase inhibitor R115777, the anti-*HER2/NEU* antibody trastuzumab, the EGF inhibitor cetuximab, and bevacizumab a monoclonal antibody.[34] Combined modality approaches with gemcitabine and radiation are also under investigation.[140]

## Small-molecule therapy

Matrix metalloproteinases (MMPs) are a family of enzymes capable of degrading the components of the extracellular matrix. A high concentration of MMP enzymes has been detected in tumors, and the enzymes are considered to be important in invasion, angiogenesis, and metastasis. Matrix metalloproteinase inhibitors (MMPIs) bind to and inactivate MMPs. Marimastat, the first of the new class of MMPIs, is an oral agent that has been investigated in patients with advanced pancreatic cancer. Initial results did not establish marimastat as a treatment option for patients with unresectable disease when the drug was compared to gemcitabine.[34,141] Important conclusions of recent studies suggested that marimastat should be further investigated in patients with nonoperable, nonmetastatic pancreatic cancer, or for use adjuvantly as a maintenance therapeutic.[34,142]

Pancreatic cancer arises from cells exhibiting a complex, multiple genetic aberrant state; in addition, selective genes are known to be involved in some sporadic and heritable tumors.[143] Potential therapeutic targets are the oncogene and tumor suppression gene pathways involved in the neoplastic transformation of the pancreas. The *K-ras* oncogene is one of the mutated genes most frequently found in pancreatic cancer, which makes it an attractive target. Targeting *ras* by using farnesyl-transferase inhibitors is 1 strategy being explored.[34,144] Tumor suppressor genes being investigated include *p53, p16, DPC4,* and *BRCA2*; DNA mismatch repair genes (*MLH1* and *MSH2*) and mitochondrial DNA mutations are also under study.[134]

A large number of growth factors and their receptors are overexpressed in pancreatic cancer, including EGF and fibroblast growth factor (FGF) and their receptors (EGFRs and FGFRs) and ligands. Inhibitors of these new targeted compounds are being studied, including members of the erbB family, HER1 (or EGFR) and HER2.[134]

Inhibitors of angiogenesis, also called antiangiogenetic agents, are another group of compounds offering promise in cancer research. These drugs block angiogenesis, the development of new blood cells. Solid tumors cannot grow beyond the size of a pinhead (1–2 $mm^3$) without causing the formation of new blood vessels to supply the nutritional needs of the tumor. Blocking the development of new blood vessels ensures that oxygen and nutrients are not supplied to the tumor, thereby preventing the continued growth and spread of the tumor. Vascular endothelial growth factor (VEGF) is upregulated in pancreatic cancer[145]; TPN-470, derived from the fungus *Aspergillus*, has been found to have antiangiogenic properties[146]; and angiostatin, a peptide fragment of plasminogen, and endostatin, a fragment from collagenase,[147] are novel agents being studied for their effect on pancreatic carcinoma.

## New therapeutic approaches for systemic disease

Treatment strategies have been developed in an attempt to modulate or interrupt growth factors and signal transduction pathway. Perillyl alcohol is a nontoxic, naturally occurring substance that may enhance tumor apoptosis by increasing the ability of tumor cells to activate and respond to TGF-β.[148] In pancreatic cancer cell lines, perillyl alcohol causes a 3- to 10-fold increase in apoptosis. Rodent experiments showed these same responses.[149]

## IMMUNOTHERAPY

Immunotherapy of pancreatic cancer is an exciting therapeutic approach that focuses on activating the patient's immune system in an attempt to eradicate malignancy. Novel treatment strategies that capitalize on gene transfer technology have become possible through recent developments in molecular biology. Modern gene therapeutics, incorporating the use of recombinant DNA technology and more efficient gene delivery systems, have led to the development of new anticancer protocols.

Immunotherapeutic strategies that use recombinant DNA technology constitute the largest group of anticancer gene therapies. Immunotherapy has the potential to provide an alternative systemic treatment for adenocarcinoma of the pancreas. Having such an option is an important consideration in the treatment of pancreatic cancer as most individuals with pancreatic cancer present with locally unresectable or metastatic disease. Even for those individuals who have surgery that removes all evidence of gross disease, most will die of locally recurrent or metastatic disease within 5 years, and almost all eventually die as a direct result of their disease. Any effective treatment regimen against pancreatic cancer must address both its aggressive local growth and its propensity to metastasize.[150]

Immunotherapy has an advantage over chemotherapy and radiation because it can act specifically against the tumor without causing normal tissue damage. Vaccines are a form of immunotherapy. Pancreatic cancer vaccines have been developed using the whole tumor cell as the antigen source because it is not known which proteins expressed by pancreatic cancers are recognized by the immune system. Research is currently studying the genetic modification of pancreatic tumor cells to better present their tumor antigens to the immune system, which it is hoped will result in potent activation of a systemic antitumor immune response. In addition, tumor-associated antigens mixed with defined adjuvant therapy administered systemically are being developed that will result in new and more potent vaccines. Antigen-based vaccines may eliminate the need for the genetic manipulation of tumor cells.[85]

A phase I trial of an allogenic GM-CSF-secreting tumor vaccine for pancreatic cancer was assessed in patients with stage I, II, or III carcinoma of the pancreas. The vaccine was found to be safe and lacked treatment-related toxicity; it produced improvements in systemic antitumor immunity as measured by increased postvaccination delayed-type hypersensitivity responses against autologous tumors.[151] Reported results using this vaccine in an adjuvant setting show improved survival rates.[34] Another vaccine study evaluated the benefit of a vaccine which is delivered intramuscularly to activate the production of antibodies to gastrin, a hormone shown to increase proliferation of human pancreatic cancer cells.[34] Although gastrin antibodies increased, there was no clinically significant difference in survival in patients receiving the vaccine.[34] Results of a vaccine using irradiated pancreatic cancer cell line which was transduced to express granulocyte-macrophage colony-stimulating factor (GM-CSF) show promise in the postoperative adjuvant setting when used with chemotherapy and radiation. Research is ongoing.[34]

The effects of gene therapy and vaccine strategies on survival in individuals with pancreatic cancer are currently unknown. Immunotherapy has the potential to provide a mechanism of antitumor activity that may be integrated with surgery, chemotherapy, and radiation therapy.

## RADIATION THERAPY

Radiation therapy has been used for both palliation and curative therapy of pancreatic cancer. Directed radiation to the pancreas is difficult because of the limited radiation tolerance of adjacent organs in the upper abdomen, including the kidney, liver, stomach, small bowel, and spinal cord. The technique typically used to treat pancreatic cancer is external beam radiotherapy. Newer techniques, such as conformal radiation and intensity-modulated radiation therapy, have the advantage of being able to precisely localize the radiation dose to the target volume while reducing the dose to critical structures.[152] Stereotactic radiotherapy, often referred to as Cyberknife, delivers therapy with very precise control of organ movement to minimize contact with nearby structures. At this time there is no data to support its use in pancreatic cancer treatment outside of the clinical trial setting.[153] More specialized methods of radiotherapy have been employed as well, such as intraoperative radiotherapy and brachytherapy, but no benefit over external beam irradiation has been found.[136,154]

The use of radiation-sensitizing agents is now being studied. Preliminary data demonstrate that gemcitabine may be a potent radiation sensitizer of human pancreatic cancer cells. It appears that DNA synthesis is prolonged in tumor cells as compared with normal tissues when gemcitabine is combined with irradiation.[155] For those individuals with unresectable pancreatic cancer, radiation therapy may palliate symptoms of local disease, especially pain.[156] Other radiosensitizing chemotherapy agents being investigated include capecitabine, which is more convenient than infusional 5-FU; cyclooxygenase-2 (COX-2) inhibitors, as there is a high degree of overexpression of COX-2 in pancreatic cancer; paclitaxel; and cisplatin.[157,158] Tumor necrosis factor alpha (TNFα), is being investigated as a facilitator of radiation therapy by sensitizing pancreatic cancer cells to apoptosis. Using the tumor necrosis factor-related apoptosis–inducing ligand (TRAIL) and gemcitabine with radiation shows promise in development of a novel strategy in pancreatic cancer treatment.[159]

Newer combinations and techniques of administering radiation therapy and chemotherapy may provide better local control and survival for patients with resectable and locally unresectable disease. The development of more promising neoadjuvant and adjuvant therapies, such as combining chemoradiation with immunotherapy, may further enhance survival of individuals with pancreatic cancer.

## SYMPTOM MANAGEMENT AND NURSING CARE

The individual who has undergone surgery for pancreatic cancer usually dies of locally recurrent disease and/or metastatic disease. The most common harbingers of imminent death are recurrence of pain, jaundice from obstruction or intrahepatic metastases, and development of ascites. These symptoms require symptomatic or palliative treatment. Likewise, the individual who is diagnosed with advanced cancer of the pancreas, either locally or due to metastases, may present with the following:

- Pain
- Obstructive jaundice, which can lead to intrahepatic abscess
- Infection
- Ascites
- Liver failure
- Hemorrhage
- Malnutrition from bowel obstruction
- Anorexia
- Early satiety
- Cachexia
- Nausea and vomiting
- Change in bowel habits (constipation or diarrhea)
- Dyspnea

The goal of palliative therapy is to reduce the debilitating symptoms of the disease and to improve the quality of remaining life. This is best accomplished by treating the individual with respect to his or her wishes and not just treating the tumor.[160]

Relief of pain is a primary objective, particularly in advanced disease. The pain syndrome associated with cancer of the pancreas is usually related to the anatomical location of the tumor in the organ and subsequent impingement on other structures: tissues, blood vessels, bile or pancreatic ducts, or body organs. The complex nerve fibers and ganglions that affect the pancreas and related organs and structures contribute to the pain associated with pancreatic cancer.[161] Pain associated with tumors in the head of the pancreas may be due to pancreatitis. Tumors located in the body and tail of the pancreas often present later, are larger, and tend to cause pain by invading the stomach, retroperitoneum, and nerves.

The nature of pain will evolve and change throughout the progression of the disease. Treatment approaches must address the current, specific complaints of pain using all available modalities. Eliminating the source of the pain is the first objective, as in bile duct decompression or relief of duodenal obstruction. The most effective approach to pain therapy in individuals with advanced disease is to prevent the pain from peaking by routinely administering the selected relief measures. Oral, parenteral, or transdermal opiates, sedatives, nerve blocks, relaxation therapy, and proper positioning may provide pain relief. The administration of continuous subcutaneous opiate infusions by means of a PCA pump has the advantage of delivering analgesics to individuals with impaired gastrointestinal function and for whom oral analgesics are not appropriate. The pump can also provide optimal analgesia in those patients who develop a bowel obstruction and are not able to take food or liquids by mouth. Radiotherapy in combination with chemotherapy has also been used to reduce pain. Concomitant use of analgesics, celiac nerve blocks, and radiotherapy should be considered as palliative treatments. An aggressive pain treatment plan should be devised and started immediately. The goal of pain management should be to permit an acceptable level of functioning and to allow the individual to die as free of pain as possible.[162] Continuous pain assessment facilitated by good communication and trust between the individual and the clinician is necessary for effective pain management.

Nutritional status affects an individual's quality of life in regard to self-image, ability to perform activities of daily living, and overall life satisfaction. An individual's ability to socialize and interact with friends and family is affected by his or her ability or desire to eat. Malnutrition, cachexia, muscle weakness, and fatigue all contribute to depression, causing a cycle of difficulties.[163] Reduced activity and bedrest lead to constipation and more muscle wasting.[164,165]

Nutritional support may pose a difficult problem as a result of the obstructive nature of advanced pancreatic cancer. Supportive nutritional efforts for individuals undergoing active treatment can decrease complications, shorten hospital stays, reduce costs, and improve patients' sense of well-being. Oral feedings should be maintained as long as the individual can meet caloric requirements. Frequent, small feedings and supplemental mixtures may be tolerated better than larger meals. Administering antiemetics prior to eating may assist in controlling nausea and vomiting. Metoclopramide, megestrol acetate, and cannabinoids are some of the pharmacological agents used to manage anorexia by stimulating the appetite.[166,167] Many individuals with pancreatic cancer complain of sensory changes that interfere with food intake. The sense of smell may be profoundly affected. Sensitivity to food odors as well as aversions to perfumes and soaps can also occur. Serving food cold instead of hot may be helpful in decreasing the aroma. Cooking odors can be minimized by using covered pots, boiling bags, or a kitchen fan. Taste changes are common, particularly complaints that food has a metallic taste. The use of plastic eating utensils and non-metal cooking containers can help alleviate this problem. The use of parenteral nutrition in end-stage disease is controversial due to the high cost, high risk of complications, and lack of proven benefit.[166,167]

If the patient is diagnosed with a bowel obstruction, the cause must be elicited. Bowel obstruction can derive from a mechanical or a functional problem. Immediate management consists of nasogastric suction for control of nausea and large-volume emesis along with hydration by intravenous fluids. Bowel obstruction caused by tumor may necessitate the placement of a gastric tube—either surgically or endoscopically—for decompression. Removal of a nasogastric tube and allowing small amounts of liquids by mouth are the most humane course after a gastrostomy tube has been placed. Metallic expandable stents may be used successfully in a large percentage of patients as a palliative measure to maintain the duodenal opening and allow unobstructed flow through this part of the small bowel.[168] Somatostatin has also been used in treating individuals with bowel obstruction, as it reduces intestinal secretions and the dose can be titrated to control the volume of secretions. Prokinetic agents should not be used in patients with known bowel obstruction.

Opiate-induced bowel obstruction must also be considered. This complication can be avoided by the aggressive use of laxatives and an established bowel regimen along with appropriate education of the individual and family for symptoms suggestive of bowel obstruction: pain, nausea, vomiting, abdominal distention, and change in bowel elimination.

The cause of constipation can usually be delineated by a careful bowel history and abdominal examination. Prevention of opioid-induced constipation can best be accomplished by the use of an established bowel program.[169] Diarrhea is associated with tumors in the head of the pancreas; its management depends on identifying the cause. Malabsorption may result from steatorrhea and pancreatic exocrine insufficiency. Lactose intolerance may also be seen. Treatment consists of a diet high in protein and carbohydrate and replacement of pancreatic enzymes.

Individuals with cancer of the pancreas frequently have liver involvement, resulting in abdominal distention from malignant ascites. The treatment is difficult, but symptom control can be accomplished with the careful use of diuretics. Spironolactone and furosemide can reduce ascites, improve the person's comfort, and decrease the need for paracentesis.[160] Dyspnea may result not directly from the tumor itself but rather from disease complications, as seen in an individual with ascites and a diminished lung capacity. Patients with dyspnea from pancreatic cancer will have a shortened survival.

Jaundice due to bile duct obstruction or liver damage is a debilitating symptom that occurs in the majority of individuals with pancreatic cancer. It causes severe pruritus and dry skin. The individual should be instructed to use soap sparingly, preferably using mild soaps and oil-based lotions, calamine lotion, or cocoa butter, or to bathe in sodium bicarbonate to relieve pruritus.

Palliation of obstructive jaundice can be provided utilizing endoscopic or percutaneous procedures. Insertion of internal biliary stents by endoscopy can relieve jaundice and its concomitant symptoms. Percutaneously placed internal-external biliary stents also can provide relief of jaundice. The stent and insertion site must receive daily care and stent flushing. Unrelieved biliary obstruction can cause recurrent infection in the biliary tree as well as lead to liver abscess that can cause pain and sepsis. Liver abscesses are treated by percutaneous insertion of a drain and intravenous antibiotics.

Jaundice that is not relieved by biliary decompression is usually a sign of liver failure. Liver failure results in progressive weakness, lethargy, encephalopathy, and eventual coma with imminent death of the individual. Renal failure usually occurs as the liver fails (hepatorenal failure). Patients are more prone to coagulation problems and bleeding as the liver continues to fail. Hemorrhage may also occur from metastatic tumor eroding into blood vessels in the liver or local tumor eroding into nearby vessels. Affected individuals may die of massive internal hemorrhage.

Almost 90% of individuals with pancreatic cancer die within a year of their diagnosis. The course of the disease can be rapid. Patients should be assured that many treatments can be used aggressively to maintain their comfort and independence for as long as possible. They should be encouraged to inform their healthcare providers of any discomfort, or medical, or psychological problems they are experiencing. Timely referral to a palliative care service and hospice can have significant beneficial impact on the total care of the patient and on the home-based caregiver.[170]

Whatever the course of treatment chosen by the individual, both physiological and psychological preparation is necessary. By discerning patterns of family support, coping, and communication, the nurse can adopt a teaching style that suits the individual. Listening is vital to good communication, to understand and be sensitive to the patient's needs. Education by the nurse can increase compliance as well as prepare the individual and family for side effects of both the disease and its treatment. The nurse is the constant figure of hope, understanding, and support through all of the diagnostic tests, from the time the patient is told of the diagnosis of cancer of the pancreas, continuing through whatever treatment modalities are performed as the disease progresses, assisting with symptom management, and helping the individual and his or her family in the terminal stages of the disease.

The individual with terminal pancreatic cancer can be cared for at home by family or a caregiver with hospice support. The hospice nurse assists the patient and the caregiver in the terminal stages of the disease by educating them about what to expect and helping to manage symptoms. Individuals in the terminal stage of pancreatic cancer may not wish to eat, may become extremely cachectic, and may have decreased or no urine output as hepatorenal failure ensues. Helping the family—and especially the caregiver—to deal with the eventuality of the disease is a primary nursing concern.

## FUTURE TRENDS

Molecular genetics will play an increasingly important role in targeted therapy for pancreatic carcinoma. Knowledge of genetic alterations in individual tumors may allow selection of optimal therapeutic strategies for individual patients. Genetic aberrations include copy number changes, tumor suppressor genes, caretaker genes, mitochondrial DNA mutations, and proteomic abnormalities.[10] Because of these highly sophisticated genetics discoveries, scientists are developing targeted therapies interrupting the cancer signaling pathways.[34] These pathways determine disease growth and metastasis; interrupting these pathways slows disease progression. Molecular detection of oncogene and tumor suppressor gene mutations may find application in the form of screening tests for pancreatic adenocarcinoma, at least in high-risk populations.

Nanotechnology is emerging as an important aspect in treatment options. Because the toxicity levels of most chemotherapeutic agents produce patient symptoms before completion of therapy, and because the bioavailability of these medications is reduced, administering these agents requires an innovative approach. In one study, chemotherapeutic agents, targeted for specific cell sites, are administered using gold nanoparticles as the delivery agent for the targeted chemotherapeutic drug.[171] These drugs can be delivered by actively using targeting agents or by using passive methods related to permeability and absorption.[22] The results of this study show promise for the use of nanoparticles for the delivery of chemotherapeutic agents for pancreatic cancer.

Immunotherapy represents an exciting therapeutic approach that opens new perspectives in the treatment of pancreatic cancer. One study using adjuvant vaccine showed an increased survival rate when used in addition to chemotherapy and radiation therapy.[34] Although promising, data is limited and research is ongoing.

About 40% of patients are able to tolerate a second line of treatment if there is tumor recurrence. There is no standard of treatment for this select group of patients.[172]

Chemoprevention is a promising area of investigation targeted at pancreatic disease prevention. Understanding the molecular pathways in the disease process enables researchers to use a variety of agents to interrupt the cascade. Several compounds have been shown to reduce the risk of pancreatic cancer in certain groups. A recent study identified a correlation between aspirin, NSAIDS and other COX-2 inhibitors and reduction of relative risk of developing pancreatic cancer.[173] Most epidemiological cancer studies identify smoking as a significant risk factor. Therefore any reduction in smoking may lead to decrease in the incidence of pancreatic cancer. Researchers are investigating long acting forms of somatostatins as potential chemopreventive agents. Researchers are investigating tamoxifen as an antiproliferative agent against tumor growth.[173] Selective estrogen receptor modulators (SERMs) show promise also as a potential chemoprotective agent. Studies show inverse correlation between estrogen levels and carcinogenesis, and tumor growth rate in rats. Antiandrogen therapy is also part of the broader hormonal implication in pancreatic carcinogenesis. Tea polyphenols from green and black tea, known as catechins, have antioxidant properties. Investigation is underway to determine their relationship to apoptosis and reduction of carcinogenesis.[149] More randomized controlled trials are needed to support the efficacy of these agents and their chemoprotective properties.

Advances in prevention and screening for pancreatic cancer lie on the horizon. Innovations continue to emerge in diagnostic studies as well as in surgery, chemotherapy, and radiation therapy. Preliminary analysis of SEER data shows the potential benefit of neoadjuvant chemotherapy and radiation treatment in increasing survival periods for both resectable and locally advanced patients.[131] Combined modalities will continue to be employed as treatment for pancreatic cancer. Multidisciplinary collaboration and communication among all healthcare providers, including oncology nurses, will ensure optimal care for patients with pancreatic carcinoma.

Much research is now being done on all aspects of pancreatic cancer. Discoveries in the field of molecular genetics hold promise for earlier detection. The ability to predict tumor biology and subsequently customize the treatment of patients with pancreatic cancer brings hope for improved survival. New vaccines aimed at activating an individual's immune system to fight his or her cancer are currently being developed and tested.

Superior outcomes have been reported for high volume centers incorporating a multidisciplinary approach to evaluation and treatment. Adjuvant chemotherapy and radiation therapy should be considered in patients with successfully resected pancreatic cancer. Combined modality treatment with chemotherapy and radiation should be considered for locally advanced, unresectable tumors.

Many advances have been made in the management of pancreatic cancer in the past several decades. Emerging techniques in the fields of surgery, radiation therapy, chemotherapy, and immunotherapy offer hope for greater locoregional control, improved survival, and enhanced quality of life for these patients. New modalities, therapies and combinations of therapies provide patients with pancreatic cancer the opportunity to move through various phases of treatment providing bridging mechanisms until the next novel approach is available. Ongoing opportunity for treatment has the potential to make pancreatic cancer a chronic disease allowing the patient to maintain quality of life. All patients with pancreatic cancer should be encouraged to enter clinical trials of new therapies.

## REFERENCES


1. Jemal A, Siegel R, Ward E, et al. Cancer statistics. *CA Cancer J Clin.* 2009;59:225–249.
2. American Cancer Society. *Cancer Facts and Figures 2009.* Atlanta, GA: Author; 2009.
3. Rosemurgy A, Cowgill A, Coe B, et al. Frequency with which surgeons undertake pancreaticoduodenectomy continues to determine length of stay, hospital charges and in-hospital mortality. *J Gastrointest Surg.* 2008;12:442–449.
4. Ujiki MB, Talamonti MS. Guidelines for the surgical management of pancreatic adenocarcinoma. *Semin Oncol.* 2007;34:311–320.
5. Garcea G, Dennison AR, Pattenden CJ, Neal CP, Sutton CD, Berry DP. Survival following curative resection for pancreatic ductal adenocarcinoma. A systematic review of the literature. *J Pancreas (online).* 2008;9:99–132.
6. Sauter PK, Coleman J. Pancreatic cancer: a continuum of care. *Semin Oncol Nurs.* 1999;15:36–47.
7. Goggins M. Identifying molecular markers for the early detection of pancreatic neoplasia. *Semin Oncol.* 2007;34:303–310.
8. Binkley CE, Simeone DM. Pancreatic cancer. In: Johnson L, Gerwin TA. eds. *Encyclopedia of Gastroenterology.* Vol. 1. San Diego, CA: Elsevier; 2004:41–48.
9. Yeo TP, Hruban RH, Leach SD, et al. Pancreatic cancer. *Curr Probl Cancer.* 2002;26:176–275.
10. Hariharan D, Saied A, Kocher HM. Analysis of mortality rates for pancreatic cancer across the world. *HPB.* 2008;10:58–62.
11. Gold EB, Goldin SB. Epidemiology of and risk factors for pancreatic cancer. *Surg Oncol Clin North Am.* 1998;7:67–91.
12. Lowenfels AB, Maisonneuve P. Environmental factors and risk of pancreatic cancer. *Pancreatology.* 2003;3:1–8.
13. Hart AR, Kennedy H, Harvey I. Pancreatic cancer: a review of the evidence on causation. *Clin Gastroenterol Hepatol.* 2008;6:275–282.
14. Stamatakis K, Brownson R, Luke D. Risk factors for exposure to environmental tobacco smoke among ethnically diverse women in the United States. *J Women's Health Gend Based Med.* 2002;11:45–51.
15. Dondon MG, Vathaire F, Shamsaldin A, et al. Cancer mortality after radiotherapy for a skin hemangioma during childhood. *Radiother Oncol.* 2004;72:87–93.
16. Michaud DS, Giocannucci E, Willett WC, et al. Physical activity, obesity, height, and the risk of pancreatic cancer. *JAMA.* 2001;286:921–929.
17. Ojajarvi J, Partanen T, Ahlbom A, et al. Occupational exposures and pancreatic cancer: a meta-analysis. *Occup Environ Med.* 2000;57:316–324.
18. Michaud DS. Epidemiology of pancreatic cancer. *Minerva Chirurgica.* 2004;59:99–111.
19. Hruban RH, Petersen GM, Ha PK, et al. Genetics of pancreatic cancer. From genes to families. *Surg Oncol Clin North Am.* 1998;7:1–23.
20. Hahn SA, Schutte M, Hogue ATMS, et al. *DPC4*, a candidate tumor suppressor gene at human chromosome 18q211. *Science.* 1996;271:350–353.
21. Goggins M, Schutte M, Lu J, et al. Germline BRCA2 gene mutations in patients with apparent sporadic pancreatic carcinomas. *Cancer Res.* 1996;56:5360–5364.
22. Feldmann G, Maitra A. Molecular genetics of pancreatic ductal adenocarcinomas and recent implications for translational efforts. *J Mol Diagn.* 2008;10:111–122.
23. Goggins M, Offerhaus GJ, Hilgers W, et al. Pancreatic adenocarcinomas with DNA replication error (RER+) are associated with wild-type K-ras and characteristic histopathology. Poor differentiation, a syncytial growth pattern, and pushing borders suggest RER+. *Am J Pathol.* 1998;152:1501–1507.
24. Chari ST. Detecting early pancreatic cancer: problems and prospects. *Semin Oncol.* 2007;34:284–294.
25. Hahn SA, Bartsch DK. Genetics of hereditary pancreatic carcinoma. *Clin Lab Med.* 2005;25:117–133.
26. Breast Cancer Linkage Consortium. Cancer risks in BRCA2 mutation carriers. *J Natl Cancer Inst.* 1999;91:1310–1316.
27. Phelan CM, Lancaster JM, Tonin P, et al. Mutation analysis of the BRCA2 gene in 49 site-specific cancer families. *Nat Genet.* 1996;13:120–122.
28. Canto MI. Screening and surveillance approaches in familial pancreatic cancer. *Gastrointest Endosc Clin N Am.* 2008;18:535–553.
29. Lynch HT, Fusaro RM, Lynch JF, Brand R. Pancreatic cancer and the FAMMM syndrome. *Familial Cancer.* 2008;7:103–112.
30. Lynch HT, Brand RE, Hogg D, et al. Phenotypic variation in eight extended CDKN2A germline mutation familial atypical multiple mole melanoma-pancreatic carcinoma-prone families: the familial atypical mole melanoma-pancreatic carcinoma syndrome. *Cancer.* 2002;94:84–96.
31. Jaffee E, Hruban R, Canto M, Kern S. Focus on pancreatic cancer. *Cancer Cell.* 2002;2:25–28.
32. Hemminki A, Tomlinson I, Markie D, et al. Localization of a susceptibility locus for Peutz-Jeghers syndrome to 19p using comparative genomic hybridization and targeted linkage analysis. *Nat Genet.* 1997;15:87–90.
33. Kroc M. Role of growth factors in pancreatic cancer. *Surg Oncol Clin North Am.* 1998;7:25–41.
34. Ko AH. Future strategies for targeted therapies and tailored patient management in pancreatic cancer. *Semin Oncol.* 2007;34:354–364.
35. Friess H, Yamanaka Y, Buchler M, et al. Enhanced expression of transforming growth factor beta isoforms in human pancreatic cancer correlates with decreased survival. *Gastroenterology.* 1993;105:1846–1856.
36. Korc M. Pancreatic cancer-associated stroma production. *Am J Surg.* Oct 2007;194(4 suppl 1):S84–S87.
37. Nomura S, Yoshitomi H, Takano S, et al. FGF10/FGFR2 signal induces cell migration and invasion in pancreatic cancer. *B J Cancer.* 2008;99:305–313.
38. Bergmann U, Funatomi H, Yokoyama M, et al. Insulin-like growth factor I overexpression in human pancreatic cancer: evidence for autocrine and paracrine roles. *Cancer Res.* 1995;55:2007–2011.
39. Yeo CJ, Cameron JL. Pancreatic cancer. *Curr Prob Surg.* 1999;36:57–152.
40. Hruban RH, Adsay NV, Albores-Saavedra J, et al. Pancreatic intraepithelial neoplasia (PanIN): a new nomenclature and classification system for pancreatic duct lesions. *Am J Surg Pathol.* 2001;25:579–586.
41. Wilentz RE, Hruban RH. Pathology of cancer of the pancreas. *Surg Oncol Clin N Am.* 1998;7:43–65.
42. Wilentz RE, Albores-Saavedra J, Zahurak M, et al. Pathologic examination accurately predicts prognosis in mucinous cystic neoplasms of the pancreas. *Am J Surg Path.* 1999;23:1320–1327.
43. Ogawa H, Itoh S, Ikeda M, Suzuki K, Naganawa S. Intraductal papillary mucinous neoplasm of the pancreas: assessment of the likelihood of invasiveness with multisection CT. *Radiology.* 2008;248:876–888.
44. Sohn TA, Yeo CJ, Cameron JL, et al. Intraductal papillary mucinous neoplasms of the pancreas: an increasingly recognized clinicopathologic entity. *Ann Surg.* 2001;234:313–322.

45. Smoot RL, Zhang L, Sebo TJ, Que FG. Adenosquamous carcinoma of the pancreas: a single-institution experience comparing resection and palliative care. *J Am Coll Surg.* 2008;207:368–370.
46. Chiou YY, Chiang JH, Hwang JI, et al. Acinar cell carcinoma of the pancreas: clinical and computed tomography manifestations. *J Comput Assist Tomogr.* 2004;28:180–186.
47. Mortenson MM, Katz MHG, Tamm EP, et al. Current diagnosis and management of unusual pancreatic tumors. *Am J Surg.* 2008; 196:100–113.
48. Kataria R, Bhatnagar V, Agarwala S, et al. Clinical course and management of pancreaticoblastoma in children. *Trop Gastroenterol.* 1998;19:67–69.
49. Boni L, Benevento A, Dionigi G, et al. Primary pancreatic lymphoma. *Surg Endosc.* 2002;16:1107–1108.
50. Chun J, Doherty GM. Pancreatic endocrine tumors. *Curr Opin Oncol.* 2001;13:52–56.
51. Somogyi L, Mishra G. Diagnosis and staging of islet cell tumors of the pancreas. *Curr Gastroenterol Rep.* 2000;2:159–164.
52. Vogel I, Kalthoff H, Henne-Bruns D, et al. Detection and prognostic impact of disseminated tumor cells in pancreatic carcinoma. *Pancreatology.* 2002;2:79–88.
53. Lillemoe KD. Current management of pancreatic carcinoma. *Ann Surg.* 1995;221:133–148.
54. Schnelldorfer T, Ware AL, Sarr MG, et al. Long-term survival after pancreaticoduodenectomy for pancreatic adenocarcinoma: is cure possible? *Ann Surg.* 2008;247:456–462.
55. Barber MD. Cancer cachexia and its treatment with fish oil-enriched nutritional supplementation. *Nutrition.* 2001;17:751–755.
56. Ventafridda GV, Caraceni AT, Sbanotto AM, et al. Pain treatment in cancer of the pancreas. *Eur J Surg Oncol.* 1990;16:1–6.
57. Shin EJ, Canto MI. The clinical assessment of pancreatic cancer. In: Beger HG, Matsuno S, Cameron JL. eds. *Diseases of the Pancreas: Current Surgical Therapy.* New York, Berlin, Heidelberg: Springer; 2008:527–540.
58. Goldacre MJ, Wooten CJ, Yeates D, Seagroatt V, Collier J. Liver cirrhosis, other diseases, pancreatitis and subsequent cancer: record linkage study. *Eur J Hepatol Gastroenterol.* 2008;20:384–392.
59. Bastidas VA, Neiderhuber JE. Pancreas. In: Abeloff MD, Armitage JD, Lichter AS, et al, eds. *Clinical Oncology.* New York: Churchill Livingstone;1995:1373–1403.
60. Makrilia N, Indeck B, Syrigos K, Saif MW. Depression and pancreatic cancer: a poorly understood link. *JOP.* 2009;10:69–76.
61. Yaskin JD. Nervous symptoms at earliest manifestations of cancer of the pancreas. *JAMA.* 1931;96:1664–1668.
62. Zilikis N, Dervenis C. Psychosomatic aspects of pancreatic cancer. *Pancreatology.* 2003;3:273–275.
63. Zabora J, Brintzenhofeszoc, K, Curbow B, Hooker C, Piantadosi S. The prevalence of psychological distress by cancer site. *Psycho-Oncology.* 2001;10:19–28.
64. Ögren M, Bergqvist D, Wåhlander K, Erikssom H, Sternby NH. Trousseau's syndrome—what is the evidence?: a population-based autopsy study. *Thromb Haemost.* 2006;95:541–545.
65. Brand RE, Matamoros A. Imaging techniques in the evaluation of adenocarcinoma of the pancreas. *Dig Dis.* 1998;16:242–252.
66. Horton KM. Multidetector CT and three-dimensional imaging of the pancreas. State of the art. *J Gastrointest Surg.* 2002;6:126–128.
67. Bluemke DA, Fishman EK. CT and MR evaluation of pancreatic cancer. *Surg Oncol Clin N Am.* 1998;7:103–124.
68. Reinhold C. Magnetic resonance imaging of the pancreas in 2001. *J Gastrointest Surg.* 2002;6:133–135.
69. Schick V, Franzius C, Beyna T, et al. Diagnostic impact of $^{18}$F-FDG PET-CT evaluating solid pancreatic lesions vs endosonography, endoscopic retrograde cholangio-pancreatography with intraductal ultrasonography and abdominal ultrasound. *Eur J Nucl Med Mol Imaging.* 2008;35:1775–1785.
70. Strobel K, Heinrich S, Bhure U, et al. Contrast-enhanced $^{18}$F-FDG PET/CT: 1–Stop-shop imaging for assessing the resectability of pancreatic cancer. *J Nucl Med.* 2008;49:1408–1412.
71. Mortele KJ, Ji H, Ros P. CT and magnetic imaging in pancreatic and biliary tract malignancies. *Gastrointest Endosc.* 2002;56:S206–S212.
72. Alazraki N. Imaging of pancreatic cancer using fluorine-18 fluorodeoxyglucose positron emission tomography. *J Gastrointest Surg.* 2002;6:136–138.
73. Hawes RH. Diagnostic and therapeutic uses of ERCP in pancreatic and biliary tract malignancies. *Gastrointest Endosc.* 2002;56:S201-S205.
74. Wiersema MJ. Endoscopic ultrasonography. *J Gastrointest Surg.* 2002; 6:129–132.
75. Conlon KC, Minnard EA. The value of laparoscopic staging in upper gastrointestinal malignancy. *Oncologist.* 1997;2:10–17.
76. Fernandez-del Castillo C, Warshaw AL. Laparoscopic staging and peritoneal cytology. *Surg Oncol Clin North Am.* 1998;7:135–142.
77. Rashleigh-Belcher HJ, Russell RC, Lees WR. Cutaneous seeding of pancreatic carcinoma by fine-needle aspiration biopsy. *Br J Radiol.* 1986;59:182–183.
78. Moosa AR, Gamagami PA: Diagnosis and staging of pancreatic neoplasms.Surg Clin North Am 75;871–890, 1995.
79. Centeno BA. Fine needle aspiration biopsy of the pancreas. *Clin Lab Med.* 1998;18:401–427.
80. Ritts RE, Pitt HA. CA 19–9 in pancreatic cancer. *Surg Oncol Clin North Am.* 1998;7:93–101.
81. Parsons CM, Sutcliffe JL, Bold RJ. Preoperative evaluation of pancreatic adenocarcinoma. *J Hepatiobiliary Pancreat Surg.* 2008;15:429–435.
82. Forsmark CE, Lambiase L, Vogel SB. Diagnosis of pancreatic cancer and prediction of unresectability using tumor-associated antigen CA 19–9. *Pancreas.* 1994;9:731–734.
83. Fabris C, Basso D, Piccoli A, et al. Role of local and systemic factors in increasing serum glycoprotein markers of pancreatic cancer. *J Med.* 1991;22:145–146.
84. Zhang S, Wang Y, Sun C, Lu Y, Wu L. Clinical value of serum CA19–9 levels in evaluating resectability of pancreatic carcinoma. *World J Gastroenterol.* 2008;14:3750–3753.
85. Koom WS, Seong J, Kim YB, Pyun HO, Song SY. CA19–9 as a predictor for response and survival in advanced pancreatic cancer patients treated with chemoradiotherapy. *Int J Radiat Oncol Biol Phys.* 2008;72(1 supp 1):S261–S262.
86. Yeo CJ. Pancreatic cancer: 1998 update. *J Coll Surg.* 1998;187:429–442.
87. Greene FL, Page DL, Fleming ID, et al. *AJCC Cancer Staging Manual.* 6th ed. New York: Springer; 2002:157–164.
88. Yeo CJ, Cameron JL, Sohn A, et al. Six hundred fifty consecutive pancreaticoduodenectomies in the 1990s: pathology, complications, and outcomes. *Ann Surg.* 1997;226:248–260.
89. Yeo CJ, Sohn TA, Cameron JL, et al. Periampullary adenocarcinoma: analysis of 5-year survivors. *Ann Surg.* 1998;227:821–831.
90. Jaffee EM, Schutte M, Gossett J, et al. Development and characterization of cytokine-secreting pancreatic adenocarcinoma vaccine from primary tumors for use in clinical trials. *Cancer J Sci Am.* 1998;4:194–203.
91. Sohn TA, Yeo CJ, Cameron JL, et al. Should pancreaticoduodenectomy be performed in octogenarians? *J Gastrointest Surg.* 1998;2:207–216.
92. Sohn, TA, Yeo CJ, Cameron JL, Pitt HA, Lillemoe KD. Do preoperative biliary stents increase postpancreaticoduodenectomy complications? *JOGS.* 2000;4:258–267.
93. Velanovich V, Kheibek T, Khan M. Relationship of postoperative complications from preoperative biliary stents after pancreaticoduodenectomy. A new cohort analysis and meta-analysis of modern studies. *JOP (online).* 2009;10:24–29.
94. Sewnath ME, Karsten TM, Prins MH, Rauws EJ, Obertoop H, Gouma DJ. A meta-analysis on the efficacy of preoperative biliary drainage for tumors causing obstructive jaundice. *Ann Surg.* 2002;236:17–27.
95. Heslin MJ, Brooks AD, Hochwald SN, et al. A preoperative biliary stent is associated with increased complications after pancreaticoduodenectomy. *Arch Surg.* 1998;133:149–154.
96. Povoski SP, Karpeh MS, Conlon KC, et al. Preoperative biliary drainage: impact on intraoperative bile cultures and infectious morbidity and mortality after pancreaticoduodenectomy. *J Gastrointest Surg.* 1999; 3:496–505.

97. Franko J, Greer JB, Moran CM, Khalid A, Moser AJ. Multimodality therapy for pancreatic cancer. *Gastroenterol Clin N Am.* 2007;36: 391–411.
98. Sohn TA, Yeo CJ, Cameron JL, et al. Resected adenocarcinomas of the pancreas—616 patients: results, outcomes, prognostic indicators. *J Gastrointest Surg.* 2000;4:567–579.
99. Yeo CJ, Cameron JL, Sohn TA, et al. Pancreaticoduodenectomy with or without extended retroperitoneal lymphadenectomy for periampullary adenocarcinoma: comparison of morbidity and mortality and short-term outcome. *Ann Surg.* 1999;229:613–624.
100. Cohen SJ, Pinover WH, Watson JC, et al. Pancreatic cancer. *Curr Treat Options Oncol.* 2000;1:375–386.
101. Yeo CJ, Cameron JL, Lillemoe KD, et al. Pancreaticoduodenectomy with or without distal gastrectomy and extended retroperitoneal lymphadenectomy for periampullary adenocarcinoma, part 2: randomized controlled trial evaluating survival, morbidity and mortality. *Ann Surg.* 2002;236:355–378.
102. Sosa JA, Bowman HM, Gordon TA, et al. Importance of hospital volume in the overall management of pancreatic cancer. *Ann Surg.* 1998;228:424–438.
103. Karanicholas PJ, Davies E, Kunz R, et al. The pylorus: take it or leave it? systematic review and meta-analysis of pylorus-preserving versus standard Whipple pancreaticoduodenectomy for pancreatic or periampullary cancer. *Ann Surg Oncol.* 2007;14:1825–1834.
104. Pikarsky AJ, Muggia-Sullam M, Eid A, et al. Pancreaticogastrostomy after pancreaticoduodenectomy: a retrospective study of 28 patients. *Arch Surg.* 1997;132:296–299.
105. Yamamoto J, Shimamura Y, Nakahara H, et al. Simple technique for pancreaticogastrostomy and the histological findings of pancreaticogastric anastomosis. *Arch Surg.* 1997;132:785–788.
106. Yeo CJ. Pylorus-preserving pancreaticoduodenectomy. *Surg Oncol Clin North Am.* 1998;7:143–156.
107. Nyugen TC, Sohn TA, Cameron JL, et al. Standard versus radical pancreaticoduodenectomy for periampullary adenocarcinoma: a prospective, randomized trial evaluating quality of life in pancreaticoduodenectomy survivors. *J Gastrointest Surg.* 2003;7:1–11.
108. Yeo CJ. The Whipple operation: is a radical resection of benefit? *Adv Surg.* 2003;37:1–25.
109. Yeo CJ. Management of complications following pancreaticoduodenectomy. *Surg Clin North Am.* 1995;75:913–924.
110. Halloran CM, Ghaneh P, Bosommet L, et al. Complications of pancreatic cancer resection. *Dig Surg.* 2002;19:138–146.
111. Sohn TA, Lillemoe KD. Surgical palliation of pancreatic cancer. *Adv Surg.* 2000;34:249–271.
112. Freelove R, Walling AD. Pancreatic cancer: Diagnosis and management. *Am Fam Physician.* 2006;73;485–492.
113. Burdiles R, Rossi RL. Laparoscopy in pancreatic and hepatobiliary cancer. *Surg Oncol Clin N Am.* 2001;10:531–555.
114. Lillemoe KD, Cameron JL, Yeo C, et al. Pancreaticoduodenectomy. Does it have a role in the palliation of pancreatic cancer? *Ann Surg.* 1996;223:718–728.
115. Baron TH, Mallery JS, Hirota WK, et al. The role of endoscopy in the evaluation and treatment of patients with pancreaticobiliary malignancy. *Gastrointest Endosc.* 2003;58:643–649.
116. Arguedas MR, Heudebert GH, Stinnett AA, et al. Biliary stents in malignant obstructive jaundice due to pancreatic carcinoma: a cost-effective analysis. *Am J Gastroenterol.* 2002;97:898–904.
117. Sohn TA, Lillemoe KD, Cameron JL, et al. Surgical palliation of unresectable periampullary adenocarcinoma in the 1990s. *J Am Coll Surg.* 1999;188:658–669.
118. Lillemoe KD, Cameron JL, Hardacre JM, et al. Is prophylactic gastrojejunostomy indicated for unresectable periampullary cancer? A prospective randomized trial. *Ann Surg.* 1999;230:322–330.
119. Das A, Sivak MV. Endoscopic palliation for inoperable pancreatic cancer. *Cancer Control.* 2000;7:452–457.
120. Levy MH. Pharmacologic treatment of cancer pain. *N Engl J Med.* 1996;335:1124–1132.
121. Lillemoe KD, Cameron JL, Kaufman HS, et al. Chemical splanchnicectomy in patients with unresectable pancreatic cancer. A prospective randomized trial. *Ann Surg.* 1993;217:447–457.
122. Lillemoe KD. Palliative therapy for pancreatic cancer. *Surg Oncol Clin N Am.* 1998;7:199–216.
123. Coleman J. Supportive management of the patient with pancreatic cancer: role of the oncology nurse. *Oncology.* 1996;10(suppl):23–24.
124. Zeng Q, Zhang Q, Han S, et al. Efficacy of somatostatin and its analogues in prevention of postoperative complications after pancreaticoduodenectomy: a meta-analysis of randomized controlled trials. *Pancreas.* 2008;36:18–25.
125. Yeo CJ, Barry MK, Sauter PK, et al. Erythromycin accelerates gastric emptying after pancreaticoduodenectomy. A prospective, randomized, placebo-controlled trial. *Ann Surg.* 1998;218:229–238.
126. Doty JE, Fink AS, Meyer JH. Alterations in digestive function caused by pancreatic disease. *Surg Clin North Am.* 1989;69:447–465.
127. Ottery F. Supportive nutritional management of the patient with pancreatic cancer. *Oncology.* 1996;10(suppl):26–32.
128. Held-Warmkessel J, Volpe H, Waldman AR. Treatment for pancreatic cancer. *Clin J Oncol Nurs.* 1998;2:127–134.
129. Mulcahy MF. Adjuvant therapy for pancreas cancer: advances and controversies. *Semin Oncol.* 2007;34:321–326.
130. Gastrointestinal Tumor Study Group. Further evidence of effective adjuvant combined radiation and chemotherapy following curative resection of pancreatic cancer. *Cancer.* 1987;59:2006–2010.
131. Stessin AM, Meyer JE, Sherr DL. Neoadjuvant radiation is associated with improved survival in patients with resectable pancreatic cancer: an analysis of data from the surveillance, epidemiology and end results (SEER) registry. *Int J Radiat Biol Phys.* 2008;72:1128–1133.
132. Ghaneh P, Smith R, Tudor-Smith C, Raraty M, Neoptolemos JP. Neoadjuvant and adjuvant strategies for pancreatic cancer. *Eur J Surg Oncol.* 2007;34:297–305.
133. Kim HJ, Czischke K, Brennan MF, Conlon KC. Does neoadjuvant chemoradiation downstage locally advanced pancreatic cancer? *J Gastrointest Surg.* 2002;6:763–769.
134. Akerele CE, Rybalova I, Kaufman HL, et al. Current approaches to novel therapeutics in pancreatic cancer. *Invest N Drugs.* 2003;21:113–129.
135. Brown KM, Siripurapu V, Davidson M, et al. Chemoradiation followed by chemotherapy before resection for borderline pancreatic adenocarcinoma. *Am J Surg.* 2008;195:318–321.
136. Crane CH, Beddar AS, Evans DB. The role of intraoperative radiotherapy in pancreatic cancer. *Surg Oncol Clin North Am.* 2003;12: 965–977.
137. Glimelius B, Hoffman K, Sjoden PO, et al. Chemotherapy improves survival and quality of life in advanced pancreatic and biliary cancer. *Ann Oncol.* 1996;7:593–600.
138. Casper ES, Green MR, Kelsen DP, et al. Phase II trial of gemcitabine (2,2 -difluorodeoxycytidine) in patients with adenocarcinoma of the pancreas. *Invest N Drugs.* 1994;12:29–34.
139. Burris HA, Moore MJ, Andersen J, et al. Improvements in survival and clinical benefit with gemcitabine as first-line therapy for patients with advanced pancreas cancer: a randomized trial. *J Clin Oncol.* 1997;15:2403–2413.
140. Haller DG. Future directions in the treatment of pancreatic cancer. *Semin Oncol.* 2002;29:31–39.
141. Bramhall SR, Rosemurgy A, Brown PD, et al. Marimastat as first-line therapy for patients with unresectable pancreatic cancer: a randomized trial. *J Clin Oncol.* 2001;19:3447–3455.
142. Hess KR, Abbruzzese JL. Matrix metalloproteinase inhibition of pancreatic cancer: matching mechanism of action to clinical trial design. *J Clin Oncol.* 2001;19:3445–3446.
143. Mangray S, King TCL. Molecular pathobiology of pancreatic adenocarcinoma. *Front Biosci.* 1998;3:D1148-D1160.

144. Adjei A. Blocking oncogenic Ras signaling for cancer therapy. *J Natl Cancer Inst.* 2001;93:1062–1074.
145. Jayson GC, Mulatero C, Ranson M, et al. Anti-VEGF antibody HuMV833: an EORTC biological treatment development group phase 1 toxicity, pharmacokinetic and pharmacodynamic study. *Proc Am Soc Clin Oncol.* 2001;20:4a(abstract 14).
146. Kudelka AP, Verschraegen CF, Edwards CL, et al. A phase 1 study of TNP-470 administered to patients with advanced squamous cell cancer of the cervix. *Clin Cancer Res.* 1997;3:1501–1505.
147. Wolff RA. Novel therapies for pancreatic cancer. *Cancer J.* 2001;7: 3349–3358.
148. Ariazi EA, Satomi Y, Ellis MJ, et al. Activation of the transforming growth factor beta signaling pathway and induction of cytostasis and apoptosis in mammary carcinomas treated with anticancer agent perillyl alcohol. *Cancer Res.* 1999;59:1917–1928.
149. Doucas H, Garcea G, Neal CP, Manson MM, Berry DP. Chemoprevention of pancreatic cancer: a review of the molecular pathways involved and evidence for the potential for chemoprevention. *Pancreatology.* 2006;6:429–439.
150. Clary BM, Lyerly HK. Gene therapy and pancreatic cancer. *Surg Oncol Clin North Am.* 1998;7:217–237.
151. Jaffee EM, Hruban RH, Biedrzycki B, et al. Novel allogeneic granulocyte-macrophage colony-stimulating factor-secreting tumor vaccine for pancreatic cancer: a phase I trial of safety and immune activation. *J Clin Oncol.* 2001;19:145–156.
152. Pennerthy DR, Rich TA, Adams RB. Postoperative adjuvant therapy for pancreatic cancer. *Semin Oncol.* 2003;21:256–260.
153. Crane CH, Varadhachary G, Pisters PWT, Evans DB, Wolff RA. Future chemoradiation strategies in pancreatic cancer. *Semin Oncol.* 2007;34:335–346.
154. Abrams RA. Adjuvant therapy for pancreatic adenocarcinoma. *J Gastrointest Surg.* 2001;5:6–7.
155. Li D, Xie K, Abbruzzese JL. Pancreatic cancer. *Lancet.* 2004;363: 1049–1057.
156. Dobelbower RR, Battle JA. Radiotherapy. In: Howard JM, Idezuki Y, Ihse I, Prinz RA, eds. *Surgical Diseases of the Pancreas.* 3rd ed. Baltimore, MD: Williams and Wilkins;1998:587–595.
157. Rich TA, Shepard R. COX-2 inhibitors as radiation sensitizers for upper GI tract cancers: esophagus, stomach, and pancreas. *Am J Clin Oncol.* 2003;26:S110–S113.
158. Tsai JY, Iannitti DA, Safran H. Combined modality therapy for pancreatic cancer. *Semin Oncol.* 2003;30(suppl 9):71–79.
159. Karikari CA, Roy I, Tryggestad E, et al. Targeting the apoptotic machinery in pancreatic cancers using small-molecule antagonists of the X-linked inhibitor of apoptosis protein. *Mol Cancer Ther.* 2007;6:957–966.
160. Walsh D. Palliative management of the patient with advanced pancreatic cancer. *Oncology.* 1996;10:40–44.
161. Alter CL. Palliative and supportive care of patients with pancreatic cancer. *Semin Oncol.* 1996;23:229–240.
162. Moynihan TJ. Use of opioids in the treatment of severe pain in terminally ill patients—dying should not be painful. *Mayo Clin Proc.* 2003;78:1397–1401.
163. Padilla GV. Psychological aspects of nutrition and cancer. *Surg Clin North Am.* 1986;66:1121–1135.
164. Palesty JA, Dudrick SJ. What we have learned about cachexia in gastrointestinal cancer? *Dig Dis.* 2003;21:198–213.
165. Tisdale MJ. Loss of skeletal muscle in cancer: biochemical mechanisms. *Front Biosci.* 2001;6:D164-D174.
166. Watanabe S, Bruera E. Anorexia and cachexia, asthenia and lethargy. *Hematol Oncol Clin North Am.* 1996;10:189–206.
167. Albrecht JT, Canada TW. Cachexia and anorexia in malignancy. *Hematol Oncol Clin North Am.* 1996;10:791–800.
168. Yim HB, Jacobson BC, Saltzman JR, et al. Clinical outcome of the use of enteral stents for palliation of patients with malignant upper GI obstruction. *Gastrointest Endosc.* 2001;53:329–332.
169. McNicol E, Horowicz-Mehler N, Fisk RA, et al. management of opioid side effects in cancer-related and chronic noncancer pain: a systematic review. *J Pain.* 2003;4:231–256.
170. Ellison NM, Chevlen E, Still CD, et al. Supportive care for patients with pancreatic adenocarcinoma: symptom control and nutrition. *Hematol Oncol Clin North Am.* 2002;16:105–121.
171. Patra CR, Bhattacharya R, Wang E, et al. Targeted delivery of gemcitabine to pancreatic adenocarcinoma using cetuximab as a targeting agent. *Cancer Res.* 2008;68:1970–1978.
172. O'Reilly EM, Abou-Alfa GK. Cytotoxic therapy for advanced pancreatic adenocarcinoma. *Semin Oncol.* 2007;34:347–353.
173. Wolff RA. Chemoprevention for pancreatic cancer. *Int J Gastrointest Cancer.* 2003;33:27–41.

CHAPTER 64

*Meredith Wallace Kazer, PhD, APRN, A/GNP-BC, Ashley Somerset Harmon, MSN, APRN, ANP-BC*

# Prostate Cancer

## EPIDEMIOLOGY

Each year, thousands of men are diagnosed with prostate cancer. Prostate cancer is the most commonly diagnosed solid tumor in US males and the second leading cause of cancer-related deaths[1] and 85% of all prostate cancers are diagnosed in men older than 65 years. With the widespread adoption of prostate-specific antigen (PSA) screening, 58% of men older than 50 years were screened in 2003, an increase of 17% from 2000.[2,3] Prostate-specific antigen screening was largely responsible for the initial increase in the number of newly diagnosed patients. With the new availability of PSA testing in 1986, large numbers of men were diagnosed. As time passed, the pool of potential patients dwindled and fewer men were potentially diagnosable; as a consequence, the incidence of disease fell.[4] Prior to 1990, the death rate from prostate cancer was on the rise.[5] The death rate from prostate cancer fell from 28.56 to 26.56 deaths per 100,000 men in the years 1990 to 2003.[6] Possible causes underlying this trend include screening over the prior 20 years, improved documentation of cause of death, changes in treatment modalities, and diagnosis of disease at an earlier, more treatable stage.[5] The current increased incidence may be related to the increasing age and size of the population and ongoing screening efforts.

African American males have the highest incidence of prostate cancer with a mortality rate twice that for Caucasian males.[6] Racial and ethnic groups living in the US with a lower prostate cancer incidence include men of Korean descent, for whom prostate cancer ranked as the fifth most common cause of cancer. Japanese men who emigrate to the US have a similar incidence of prostate cancer as compared to Caucasian men living in the US, even though Japanese men living in Japan have the world's lowest incidence of prostate cancer.[7]

Prostate cancer is a major health problem throughout the world. Countries with incidence rates similar to the US may be found within North America and northeastern Europe, but the disease is rare in countries within Asia and South America.[2,3] The risk of prostate cancer continues to rise throughout the world even in countries characterized by a relatively low risk of prostate cancer.

## ETIOLOGY

The cause of prostate cancer is unknown. Risk factors have been identified and relate primarily to lifestyle, age, and heredity.

Lifestyle factors include nutrition and exposure to carcinogens. Fat consumption appears to be related to the risk of the development of prostate cancer or the diagnosis at an advanced stage.[8] Diets higher in animal fat may alter the hormonal environment and predispose a man to an increased cancer risk.[9] Beef and butter are high in α-linolenic acid, and increased consumption of this essential fatty acid may increase the risk of prostate cancer.[10] Reducing one's consumption of animal fats and increasing the consumption of fiber may reduce the risk of prostate cancer.[11] Obesity may contribute to the higher incidence of prostate cancer among African American men.[12]

Soy products contain elevated levels of phytoestrogens that have been hypothesized to play a role in the reduced prostate cancer rates in Asia but the data supporting this concept are limited.[13] Tomatoes and tomato products may reduce the risk of prostate cancer[14] as may the consumption of beans, lentils, and peas. More research is needed on the relationship between these foods and prostate cancer carcinogenesis.

The relationship between vitamins and risk of prostate cancer is being investigated in preclinical and clinical trials. Vitamin E is an antioxidant, proapoptotic, antiproliferative agent being studied in combination with selenium for the prevention of prostate cancer. Selenium is a trace element found in plants and in the animals that eat the plants grown in soil containing selenium. Prostate antioxidant enzymes contain selenium, which suggests that this element may play a role in disease prevention.[15] Vitamin D is metabolized by the body to the active form of the vitamin called calcitriol, which inhibits cancer cell growth and induces apoptosis. Weekly high-dose calcitriol is being studied in combination with chemotherapy for the treatment of metastatic prostate cancer with promising results. Beta-carotene (a vitamin A precursor) and retinol (vitamin A) may play roles in prostate cancer as well. Vitamin A is an essential fat-soluble vitamin that promotes normal cellular growth. More study of the role of these antioxidant and nutritional supplements is needed, as a recent study failed to demonstrate an association between several of these components and prostate cancer.[15]

Exposure to carcinogens such as chlorinated pesticides and methyl bromide, smoking, and heavy alcohol abuse may play a role in prostate cancer development.[16] Further research is needed into the roles that diet, animal fat, fiber, vitamins, and trace elements play in prostate carcinogenesis.

The use of bilateral vasectomy for birth control was studied extensively during the early 1990s and was initially thought to increase the risk of prostate cancer. However, this hypothesis has now been disproven and vasectomy is not considered a risk factor for prostate cancer development. Sexual activity has been studied as a possible etiological factor, along with infection with gonorrhea and having multiple female sexual partners.[17]

Prostate cancer is predominantly a disease of the older male. Before age 50, clinically evident prostate cancer is rare. The incidence after age 50 increases on a yearly basis to reach approximately 1000 cases per 100,000 males aged 65 to 69.[18] By age 80 to 84, the incidence per 100,000 males is greater than 3000. Prostate cancer in younger men often behaves in a more aggressive manner.

Hereditary prostate cancer (HPC) is defined as familial clustering of prostate cancer in 1 to 3 family members with the disease and early disease onset.[19] Familial prostate cancer (FPC) refers to a clustering of prostate cancer within families,[19] 10% to 20% of all patients with prostate with cancer having a family history of the disease.[20] Hereditary prostate cancer accounts for approximately 8% to 9% of prostate cancer diagnoses by age 85 and 43% of cases diagnosed in men younger than age 55.[21] A study of 4112 men with prostate cancer indicated that while genetic factors may influence the development of prostate cancer, especially in men with a first-degree relative, the effect of heredity on prognosis is minimal.[22] Also, family history is a greater risk factor for patients younger than age 55 than it is for older patients (70–85 years), and for African American and Caucasian men than for Asian American men.

African American males have the highest incidence of prostate cancer in the world[23] averaging more than a 50% higher incidence and poorer survival rates than Caucasians.[24] Multiple factors may cause this higher incidence, including higher prevalence of high-grade prostatic intraepithelial neoplasia (PIN), a possible cancer precursor, and the reluctance of African American males to participate in screening programs.[25] Generally poor attitudes held about the healthcare system by African American males represent an additional barrier to the health care. African American males have more advanced tumors at the time of diagnosis, and their tumors may follow a more aggressive course.[26] It was thought that when patients have equal access to the same healthcare system, the survival rates for both groups would be similar. This was supported by Wyatt et al,[27] who did not find race to be associated with mortality in their study of 379 men with prostate cancer. However, the time of diagnosis, treatment, and cancer stage, which could be influenced by race, impacted survival in this study. Surveillance, Epidemiology and End Results (SEER) program data found that PSA testing has altered the incidence, survival, and mortality rates of prostate cancer, such that the rates are now similar for Caucasian and African American males.[28]

Testosterone levels are regulated by the hypothalamus and the anterior pituitary gland. The hormones from these glands cause the testicles to produce testosterone. The enzyme 5-alpha-reductase in the prostate converts testosterone into dihydrotestosterone (DHT), which has a potent direct effect on prostate development[29] Research into the influence of hormones on prostate cancer development has been inconclusive. Men without androgens do not develop prostate cancer. A study comparing tissue samples of African American and Caucasian men with prostate cancer revealed that testosterone levels were similar among the 2 groups. However, African American men had higher levels of androstenedione (ASD) and sex hormone-binding globulin (SHBG) than Caucasian men. Higher levels of SHBG may activate the androgen receptor resulting in higher testosterone.[29] Additional research on circulating testosterone levels did not support the finding that high levels of testosterone promoted cancer growth.[30]

Multiple genetic changes may play a role in the development of prostate cancer, the development of PIN, the incidence of localized disease, and a tumor's metastatic potential. The change from androgen dependence to androgen independence is associated with additional genetic alterations. Changes occur in oncogene expression, deletion of chromosome arms, suppression of apoptosis activation of oncogenes, and inactivation of tumor suppressor genes. Variants of the human genes are found in high-risk patients with prostate cancer and may help explain the higher incidence of prostate cancer in various high risk groups. Chromosome abnormalities have been discovered, including changes in the X chromosome and on chromosomes 8, 17, and 20.[31] It is thought that multiple genetic changes are needed for the development of prostate cancer, similar to the situation in other solid tumors; at least 9 changes have been found in the *HPC1* gene.[32]

## PREVENTION, SCREENING, AND EARLY DETECTION

As the etiology of prostate cancer is unknown, specific recommendations regarding prevention of the disease cannot be made. Rather, based on the known risk factors, several suggestions can be put forth. Consuming a low-fat, high-fiber diet may reduce the risk of developing prostate cancer. Maintaining normal weight for height would also seem reasonable. Obtaining vitamins and trace minerals from vegetable sources and avoiding known carcinogens such as cigarette smoke may also reduce one's risk of prostate cancer. Participating in screening would be another important intervention.

The Prostate Cancer Prevention Trial (PCPT) opened to enrollment in 1993 and closed in 1996 after 18,882 men without prostate cancer were randomized. The men received either placebo or 5 mg finasteride daily for 7 years. Finasteride is a 5-alpha-reductase inhibitor that interferes with the formation of DHT.[33] Each year, the participants underwent digital rectal exam (DRE) and analysis of PSA using a cutoff of 3 ng/mL as the maximum level. Seven years later, at the end of the drug intervention, the men had prostate biopsies performed if their PSA level was greater than 4.0 ng/mL or if an abnormality was found on DRE.[33] Although there was a 24.8% reduction in prostate cancer prevalence over the 7-year period in the finasteride group, the men in the finasteride group with prostate cancer were more likely to have more aggressive prostate cancer as indicated by higher Gleason scores (7–10) than the men in the placebo group with prostate cancer (37% vs

22.2%). Side effects observed more commonly in the finasteride group included reduced libido, erectile dysfunction (ED), reduced volume of ejaculate, and gynecomastia. The placebo group experienced more symptoms related to an enlarged prostate such as urgency, frequency, retention, and urinary tract infections. Finasteride is the first agent that has demonstrated the ability to reduce the risk of prostate cancer development, although multiple questions remain unanswered regarding its use.[33]

Vitamin E and selenium were investigated in a prostate cancer prevention trial,[34] indicating a significant reduction in prostate cancer risk among men in the study who took these supplements. The risk reduction was not supported in men who had higher dietary intake of these antioxidants. The most significant risk was seen among smokers in the sample.

Screening for prostate cancer involves the use of DRE, PSA level, and, if appropriate, evaluation of the gland using transrectal ultrasound (TRUS). Digital rectal exam involves palpation of the prostate gland. The posterior and lateral glandular tissue is evaluated by the examiner's finger. DRE is the most commonly performed screening exam for prostate diseases and assists in evaluating for lesions, texture, and symmetry of the gland. Limitations of DRE include its failure to locate tumors in the anterior and midline of the prostate. However, with a positive predictive value of 72% for a diagnosis of prostate cancer, DRE is recommended as part of an annual physical exam for men beginning at age 50 who are expected to live 10 years or more.[35]

Men considered to be at high risk for prostate cancer are those who have relatives diagnosed with prostate cancer before age 65. Those with higher risk factors, such as African American men, should begin screening at a younger age (45), and those with the highest risk factors (more than 1 first-degree relative with prostate cancer) should begin at age 40.[36] Ongoing follow-up after the first screening is dependent of the PSA result. It is also important that the man being screened is educated as to the risks vs the benefits of screening.

PSA is a serine protease, a member of the kallikrein family, that is found in prostate luminal epithelial cells.[37] The protein occurs in higher concentrations within the prostate gland than in the blood. A barrier of 3 tissue layers separates the blood and the PSA found in prostate ducts. Anything that destroys this natural tissue barrier allows PSA to enter the bloodstream, where it can be collected and evaluated in a laboratory. Procedures that can falsely elevate PSA levels, such as biopsy, urethral instrumentation, sexual intercourse, catheterization, and possibly rectal examination, should be avoided prior to obtaining PSA blood specimens. However, no definitive wait time has been established. Saw palmetto, a nutraceutical that is promoted widely for management of urinary symptoms related to prostatic hypertrophy, has not been shown to impact PSA secretion or serum PSA levels.[38]

The androgen receptor controls PSA production.[39] The normal reference range for PSA is 0 to 4 ng/mL. Serial PSA levels provide more valuable information than a single reading. Relying on a single value of PSA greater than 4 ng/mL for performing biopsies on men of all ages will miss a number of clinically significant prostate cancers,[39] because not all men with prostate cancer secrete enough PSA to raise the level. The human prostate gland continues to grow in the adult male after the completion of puberty. As the prostate increases in size, the PSA level also increases. For this reason, benign prostatic hyperplasia (BPH) tissue can be expected to produce a higher serum concentration of PSA both in the absence and presence of prostate cancer. Conditions other than prostate cancer can also give rise to elevated PSA levels. Age and racial background should be considered in the interpretation of PSA values.[40]

Of course, PSA tests are not infallible. Approximately 25% of cancers do not secrete PSA, and an elevated PSA level does not guarantee that a man has cancer. Additional diagnostic tests using PSA have been developed to more clearly identify men with prostate cancer and avoid unnecessary biopsies in those who do not have cancer.

Cancerous prostate cells and normal prostate cells produce the same amount of PSA. Total PSA includes free PSA (fPSA) and conjugated (unbound) PSA. Conjugated PSA is bound to alpha[1]-antichymotrypsin, and this level is higher in patients with prostate cancer. Free PSA has been evaluated for its ability to enhance differentiation of benign and malignant disease. Free PSA levels are lower in patients with prostate cancer than in patients without prostate cancer.[37] Studies have determined that fPSA is useful in reducing the number of biopsies in men with PSA ranges of 4 to 10 ng/mL.[37] For cancer detection, lower percentages of fPSA (%fPSA) as a percentage of total PSA may predict prostate cancer.[41] Small[42] reports that fPSA less than 25% warrant further diagnostics. Patients with higher percentages of fPSA are more likely to have benign disease, whereas those with lower percentage of fPSA need to undergo biopsy to assess for cancer.[41]

PSA density (PSAD) describes the ratio of serum PSA to prostate volume as determined by TRUS.[37] A PSAD level exceeding 0.15 ng/mL is indicative of prostate cancer (sensitivity of 72%, specificity of 95%).[37] PSA velocity describes how much PSA values increase over time. An increase of 0.75 to 0.80 ng/mL per year is significant in men with a PSA value of less than 10 ng/mL[37] and may be useful in identifying cancers. As noted earlier, finasteride (a 5-alpha-reductase inhibitor used to treat BPH) reduces PSA levels by 50%. Thus, a PSA level of 2 ng/mL (half the concentration that would normally prompt biopsy) should be used when screening for prostate cancer in men who are taking finasteride.[43]

A subject of recent debate is the issue of whether the threshold for PSA values should be lowered to increase the specificity and sensitivity of PSA testing. In one clinical trial focusing on PSA testing, a large number of prostate cancers were missed in men both older and younger than 60.[44] Even though PSA has been available as a diagnostic test for more than 15 years, its use is still being studied extensively in clinical trials.

TRUS is used to follow up abnormal DRE or elevated PSA levels. The test can evaluate prostate volume and identify suspicious areas of 5 mm or larger for biopsy.[45] In this imaging study, an ultrasound probe is inserted into the rectum and can reveal hypoechoic areas and other abnormalities in the prostate. Needle biopsies of suspicious areas are then obtained under ultrasonic guidance. Three additional directed biopsies from each lobe of the prostate are routinely obtained.

No area of cancer research continues to be as hotly debated as the issue of whether mass public screenings to detect prostate cancer are justified. The number of clinically significant cancers diagnosed at an early stage by PSA screening has increased.[46] Finnish researchers reported on the 8975 men in their arm of the European Randomized Study of Screening for Prostate Cancer. Using a prospective randomized clinical trial format, 5975 men served as controls and 3707 men were asked to participate in the study of which 75% (2781) agreed. The men were screened using PSA testing. If the PSA level was 4 ng/mL or higher, they were referred to an urologist, if the PSA level was 3 to 4 ng/mL, they were offered DRE. Additional screening included TRUS and biopsy. Biopsy was repeated every 3 months if the initial work-up for cancer was negative. There were 56 cancers (2%) in the PSA-screened group and 21 cancers (0.32%) in the control group. The tumors identified in the PSA-screened group were more aggressive than those in the control group.[46]

In another study of PSA screening, 1116 patient records were reviewed to determine whether there was a relationship between PSA levels and treatment decisions for prostate cancer and also to determine the impact of PSA progression on later treatment decisions. The study found that age was the strongest predictor of surgery and radiation treatments for first-line treatment of prostate cancer, followed by PSA levels. Higher PSA levels predicted hormone therapy, followed by age. PSA progression significantly predicted the initiation of subsequent treatment for prostate cancer recurrence.[47] This study underscores the continuing role of PSA in making both initial and subsequent treatment decisions for prostate cancer.

Additional clinical trials are needed to validate the benefits of screening across age groups. However, given the potential risk for overtreatment for prostate cancer, the US Preventive Services Task Force[48] recommends against PSA screening in men aged 75 and older. The report reveals that, while, several large-scale clinical trials are currently under way in both the US and Europe, the current evidence shows minimal risk of aggressive disease and fails to reveal a survival benefit for prostate diagnosis in the age 75 and older age group. The American Cancer Society (ACS) initiated a review of their guidelines in 2007. Currently ACS recommends annual PSA screening beginning at the age of 50. ACS continues to recommend that males of sub-Saharan African descent with a first-degree relative diagnosed younger than age 65, because of their higher risk of prostate cancer, should be encouraged by nurses to participate in annual prostate cancer screening provided by their family physicians beginning at age 45. Those men who have first-degree relatives with prostate cancer should also be educated regarding the need to participate in prostate screening at the age of 40.[36]

The cost of screening to both the individual and society cannot be ignored. From a financial perspective, do the dollars spent on screening prolong life or prevent unnecessary deaths? Currently no research trials can answer the question of whether prostate cancer screening is cost-effective or not.[48] Screening identifies not only clinically important cancers that require treatment but also clinically insignificant prostate cancers that may not shorten survival or threaten the patient's life. The individual needs to understand that treatment may not influence survival and may cause important side effects including ED and incontinence.

## PATHOPHYSIOLOGY

The prostate gland, which is approximately the size of an inverted, triangularly shaped walnut, sits beneath the bladder and anterior to the rectum. The section of the urethra that passes through the prostate is known as the *prostatic urethra*. Draining into the prostatic urethra are the prostatic ducts. Prostatic fluid drains into the prostatic ducts from the glandular elements of the prostate. This fluid aids in the fertilization process.

The prostate gland is composed of 3 major sections: the central zone, the peripheral zone, and the transitional zone. The larger peripheral zone that surrounds the central zone is the most common site for cancer.[49]

The prostate is well vascularized. Its major blood supply originates from the inferior vesicle artery.[49] Venous drainage occurs through the inferior hypogastric venous system and the presacral prevertebral venous plexus; lymphatic drainage occurs via the external and internal iliac groups and obturator lymph nodes. These nodes and lymphatics then drain into the common iliac and preaortic lymph nodes.

### CELLULAR CHARACTERISTICS

The vast majority (95%) of prostate cancers are adenocarcinomas. Of the 5% of prostate cancers that are not adenocarcinomas, greater than 90% are transitional cell carcinomas. Rarely, squamous cell carcinoma—the third most common type—may occur. All prostate cancers arise from glandular epithelial cells.[50]

Epithelial cells proceed through a variety of stages on their way to becoming malignant. As already mentioned, premalignant changes in prostate tissue are termed PIN.[50] PIN is further categorized as low or high grade[50] and may be present for 10 or more years before cancer is diagnosed. Currently, it is not possible to determine whether PIN will evolve into cancer in a particular patient, but high-grade PIN is considered a risk factor for prostate cancer.[51] High-grade PIN should be further evaluated for the presence of invasive cancer; on rebiopsy, the incidence of prostate cancer increases over time.[50]

Prostate tissue specimens are subjected to a type of pathological scoring based on cellular architecture known as the Gleason score. The majority of the tumor is occupied by cells with 1 type of histological feature that is given a number (grade) of 1 to 5 based on the severity of the cellular changes. The lower numbers are assigned to cellular patterns that are similar to prostatic tissue (well differentiated). The higher numbers designate cellular patterns that look less like normal prostatic tissue (poorly differentiated).[42] This primary number is added to a secondary number, which reflects the second most common type of cellular structure using the same grading format. The sum of the 2 numbers gives the total Gleason score. Not all studies utilize the summed format. Tumors graded 1 to 3 are considered well differentiated, whereas those graded 4 or 5 are considered poorly differentiated carcinomas. When the entire prostate gland is available for pathological review, the volume of tissue and the Gleason grade may be able to predict the presence of extracapsular spread and lymph node metastases. When the Gleason grade is 4 to 5 (poorly differentiated), the risk of nodal metastases increases when the volume of cancer increases.[42]

Prostate cancers can also be divided into those that are clinically important (significant) and those that are clinically unimportant. Clinically, important cancers include features such as large tumor volume; Gleason grade 3 to 5 (moderate to poor differentiation); an invasive, proliferative pattern of growth, elevated PSA level; and origination in the peripheral zone. These cancers threaten the patient's life because they progress to fatal metastatic cancers. Cancers that do not threaten the patient's life are termed indolent and considered clinically unimportant. These indolent cancers, which constitute about 30% of men aged 50 years and older and 60% to 70% of men older than age 80[52] are small with a Gleason grade of 1 to 2 (well differentiated), are noninvasive in their pattern of growth, do not elevate the PSA level, originate in the transitional zone, and tend to fail to progress into invasive metastatic cancers.[53] Patients with low Gleason score tumors require follow-up on a regular basis to monitor the status of the tumor, monitor for any progression of the disease, and determine whether therapy should be initiated.

### PROGRESSION OF DISEASE

Prostate cancer is generally characterized by a slow pattern of growth. The tumor grows locally along tissue planes such as the prostatic capsule and may penetrate through junctional areas of the capsule that include the bladder neck, ejaculatory ducts, and prostatourethral area. Cancers of the prostate apex and base are more likely to have spread beyond the capsule due to inherent structural weaknesses in these areas. Perineural invasion may accompany capsular invasion. Surrounding structures such as the bladder may be involved with tumor growth. When lymphatic metastases occur, they may involve the obturator, presacral, presciatic, internal, and external iliac nodes. After lymph node metastases, the next most commonly involved metastatic site is the bone, especially the lumbar spine, pelvis, femur, and skull. The cancer cells spread to these distant sites via the bloodstream after gaining access to the Batson plexus of presacral veins. Other distant sites of metastasis include the lungs, bladder, and liver.

## CLINICAL MANIFESTATIONS

Prostate cancer is usually asymptomatic in its early stages. As the disease progresses, patients may present with urinary tract obstructive symptoms similar to BPH, such as frequency, incomplete bladder emptying, hesitancy, nocturia, and urgency especially if the tumor lies in the central zone or near the urethra. The closer the proximity of the tumor to the urethra, the more likely it is to produce symptoms of bladder outlet obstruction. Symptoms may be abrupt in their onset but otherwise are similar to those seen with BPH. Other symptoms may include a change in erectile capability.

Advanced prostate cancer may be evidenced by the appearance of urethral obstruction caused by ureterovesical junction compression by tumor or nodal metastases. Hydronephrosis can then ensue, threatening the function of the associated kidney. Back pain may reveal the presence of vertebral body metastases with the potential for spinal cord compression. In addition, local pain may occur due to the presence of the cancer in the prostate gland and invasion into surrounding structures, as well as referred pain to the legs and abdomen. Bone pain can be problematic and is related to the presence of additional skeletal metastases. The hip, legs, neck, shoulders, and ribs are the next most common areas to be affected. Additional symptoms related to advanced prostate cancer growth include weight loss, rectal obstruction from local growth, coagulation deficits related to the release of procoagulant into the bloodstream from the prostate cancer cells, hypercalcemia, leg edema from nodal metastases, and pancytopenia from marrow metastases. In the past, patients often presented to the physician with symptoms of advanced disease, including back and hip pain or inability to void. It is now uncommon for patients to present with these symptoms of advanced disease without a prior diagnosis of prostate cancer.

## ASSESSMENT

### PATIENT AND FAMILY HISTORY

Nursing assessment of patients at risk for or with a diagnosis of prostate cancer should begin by questioning the patient about past medical problems or prior diagnoses of prostate disorders. The presence of a prostate cancer diagnosis in first- and second-degree relatives should be ascertained, and exposure to potential prostate carcinogens or risk factors needs to be determined.

The nurse should evaluate the patient's voiding pattern and ask whether the patient has problems with dysuria, frequency, nocturia, hematuria, and other signs of bladder outlet obstruction (Table 64-1).[54]

### PHYSICAL EXAMINATION

The patient is examined for evidence of local and distant metastases. Early prostate cancer does not usually produce symptoms. The pelvic and suprapubic areas should be percussed and palpated for bladder distention. A postvoid residual measurement may be ordered by the physician or nurse practitioner to evaluate the volume of residual urine in the bladder. Inguinal nodes are assessed, and the patient is queried regarding bone pain, specifically back pain. If back pain is present, the patient is questioned about signs of spinal cord compression, such as numbness, tingling, and other indications of sensory loss, motor weakness, or bowel or bladder incontinence.[55] Other potential areas of pain include the rectum and local pelvic area. The patient is asked for information about any pain medications he has been using, their effectiveness, and side effects. The patient's legs should be examined for edema and its severity and for indications of deep-vein thromboses, such as unilateral leg edema, pain, local heat, and redness. The skin should be checked for petechiae and ecchymoses. The patient is weighed and asked how much weight he has lost since the illness began.

### DIAGNOSTIC STUDIES

Once a presumptive diagnosis of prostate cancer is made, the patient will have a PSA level drawn and a DRE performed if these tests have not previously been ordered. As stated earlier, PSA levels often reflect the amount of the patient's disease. Thus, samples may be drawn before and after therapeutic interventions and then periodically to monitor the status of the cancer. Additional blood tests include serum chemistries, including calcium, liver function tests, blood urea nitrogen (BUN), creatinine, and complete blood count (CBC). A urine analysis is performed and a chest x-ray is completed. Magnetic resonance imaging (MRI) scans of the abdomen and pelvis may be done to evaluate local and nodal metastasis and to determine the proper treatment for the patient. A bone scan is frequently performed to evaluate bone pain and may be carried out as part of the staging workup. TRUS is used to assist in evaluating the extent of localized prostate cancer[56] and in guiding prostate biopsies. In patients who are being considered for curative surgery and who have a Gleason score greater

**TABLE 64-1**

**Questions Useful in Assessing Urinary Symptoms Associated With Prostate Cancer and Other Urological Disorders**

| Symptom | Assessment |
|---|---|
| Dysuria | Does the patient have difficulty initiating urination? If so, how often? |
| | Does the patient have difficulty maintaining or ending the urine stream? |
| | Does the patient need to apply pressure to the bladder to initiate urination? |
| | Does dribbling occur at the end of urination? |
| | Is there pain on urination? If so, how does the pain feel? Does it persist or is it intermittent? |
| | Are there bladder spasms? |
| Frequency | How often does the patient need to urinate? What is the volume of each voiding? |
| | Does the patient void and then need to void again a few minutes later? |
| | Is there a reduction in the urine volume produced? |
| Nocturia | How many times does the patient get out of bed each night to urinate? |
| | Is there incontinence at night? |
| Hematuria | Is there blood in the urine? Clots? |
| | What is the color of the urine? |
| Other | Does the urine have an odor? |
| | Is particulate matter present in the urine? |
| | When did the patient void most recently? |
| | Can the patient feel his bladder through the abdominal wall? |
| | Is there flank pain? |
| | How many urinary tract infections has the patient had in the last 12 months? |
| | Has there been a change in the strength of penile erections? |

*Source*: Data from Degler, MA.[54]

than 7 ng/mL, a laparoscopic pelvic lymph node dissection may be performed to evaluate the presence of nodal metastasis. One study examined 1091 men who had a radical retropubic prostatectomy performed, 695 of whom had a bilateral pelvic lymph node dissection.[57] A PSA level of 15 ng/mL or higher, or a Gleason grade of 4 to 5 on 4 or more of the biopsy specimens, or a Gleason grade of 4 to 5 as the predominant architecture on the pathology specimen predicted lymph node metastasis.

### PROGNOSTIC INDICATORS

Prostate-specific antigen levels may reflect the extent of disease and the amount of cancer found in the prostate gland. They increase in a logarithmic fashion with the patient's stage of disease. PSA levels are used to assess the effectiveness of treatment and to monitor the patient for disease recurrence. Unfortunately, not all prostate cancers produce PSA, so other diagnostic studies—such as MRI, computerized tomography (CT) scan, or ProstaScint scan—may be needed to monitor disease status. Baseline blood levels are obtained before and after treatment and usually are monitored every 3 months after treatment for 1 year and then every 6 to 12 months. Levels greater than 80 ng/mL reflect a large disease burden and, often, metastatic cancer.

After undergoing primary therapy for any stage of prostate cancer, an increasing PSA level reflects disease activity. After undergoing curative resection for prostate gland-confined cancer, PSA levels should be undetectable.

When external beam radiation therapy is used to treat prostate cancer, PSA levels should be normal 3 to 18 months after completion of therapy. Failure of PSA to normalize often reflects persistent disease. For all of these reasons, PSA is a highly useful tool for the monitoring of disease response to therapy and monitoring the patient for cancer relapse.

## CLASSIFICATION AND STAGING

Two commonly used staging systems for prostate cancer are the American Urologic Association (AUA) system, which was originally developed by Whitmore and then updated by Jewett, and the tumor node metastasis (TNM) system (Table 64-2) developed by the American Joint Committee on Cancer (AJCC).[58] Table 64-3 presents the Gleason grading system and the Jewitt staging system.

Small cancers found on transurethral resection of the prostate for BPH are often asymptomatic and are staged as A. When the cancer involves less than 1 lobe of the gland, it is considered B1 disease. B2 cancer involves both lobes of the prostate. After the cancer has invaded into or beyond the prostate capsule, stage C disease is present. With metastases to distant sites, the patient has stage D cancer. Survival is stage dependent. The 10-year survival rate for patients with stage A disease is 95%; for stage B is 80%; for stage C is 60%; for stage D (nodal metastases) is 40%; and for stage D (distant metastases) is 10%.

## THERAPEUTIC APPROACHES AND NURSING CARE

Treatment options available for a particular patient are based on patient preference, PSA level, age, life expectancy, general medical condition, tumor grade (Gleason score), tumor volume (stage), potential treatment complications, and risk of relapse. A patient may be offered watchful waiting (periodic observation), surgery, radiation therapy, combination therapy, hormonal manipulation, chemotherapy, or investigational drugs administered in a clinical trial setting.

### ACTIVE SURVEILLANCE, WATCHFUL WAITING, OR PERIODIC OBSERVATION FOR EARLY-STAGE PROSTATE CANCER

Prostate cancer is often a slow-growing disease and recent research has focused on identifying those tumors that require treatment and those that would benefit from an active surveillance approach. Active surveillance (formerly known as watchful waiting) has been an option for prostate cancer management for many years. Yet, the wide availability and improved effectiveness of curative treatments for prostate cancer have resulted in a substantial underutilization of this management option, with only 10.2% of clinically appropriate prostate cancers undergoing this management option.[59] However, all available therapeutic modalities for localized prostate cancer (radical prostatectomy, external beam radiotherapy, brachytherapy, cryotherapy, hormone therapy, and chemotherapy) entail significant risk of adverse effects such as sexual dysfunction, urethral strictures, urinary incontinence, and bowel problems.[60] Dall'Era et al[61] report that the increased use of PSA testing have resulted in overdetection rates ranging between 27% and 56%. Cooperberg et al[62] state that "A significant proportion of men with prostate cancer may be over-diagnosed, in the sense that diagnosis may not improve their lifespan or quality of life. However, the extent to which over-diagnosis represents a true problem relates to the consistency with which diagnosis leads invariably to active treatment" ([62] p. 8125).

For men with low-volume, nonpalpable, early-stage prostate tumors, active surveillance is an alternative to surgery or radiation therapy. In other words, men make the decision to actively monitor their disease with the knowledge that treatment remains an option.[63] Candidates for active surveillance

**TABLE 64-2**

**American Joint Committee on Cancer Staging for Prostate Cancer**

**Definition of TNM**

***Primary Tumor (T)***

*Clinical*

| | |
|---|---|
| TX | Primary tumor cannot be assessed |
| T0 | No evidence of primary tumor |
| T1 | Clinically inapparent tumor not palpable nor visible by imaging |
| T1a | Tumor incidental histological finding in 5% or less of tissue resected |
| T1b | Tumor incidental histological finding in more than 5% of tissue resected |
| T1c | Tumor identified by needle biopsy (eg, because of elevated PSA) |
| T2 | Tumor confined within prostate[a] |
| T2a | Tumor involves one-half of 1 lobe or less |
| T2b | Tumor involves more than one-half of 1 lobe but not both lobes |
| T2c | Tumor involves both lobes |
| T3 | Tumor extends through the prostate capsule[c] |
| T3a | Extracapsular extension (unilateral or bilateral) |
| T3b | Tumor invades seminal vesicle(s) |
| T4 | Tumor is fixed or invades adjacent structures other than seminal vesicles bladder neck, external sphincter, rectum, levator muscles, and/or pelvic wall |

*Pathological (pT)*

| | |
|---|---|
| pT2[d] | Organ confined |
| pT2a | Unilateral involving one-half of 1 lobe or less |
| pT2b | Unilateral involving more than one-half of 1 lobe but not both lobes |
| pT2c | Bilateral disease |
| pT3 | Extraprostatic extension |
| pT3a | Extraprostatic extension[e] |
| pT3b | Seminal vesicle invasion |
| pT4 | Invasion of bladder, rectum |

***Regional Lymph Nodes (N)***

*Clinical*

| | |
|---|---|
| NX | Regional lymph nodes cannot be assessed |
| N0 | No regional lymph node metastasis |
| N1 | Metastasis in regional lymph node or nodes |

*Pathological*

| | |
|---|---|
| pNX | Regional nodes not sampled |
| pN0 | No positive regional nodes |
| pN1 | Metastases in regional node(s) |

*Distant Metastasis (M)*[b]

| | |
|---|---|
| MX | Distant metastasis cannot be assessed (not evaluated by any modality) |
| M0 | No distant metastasis |
| M1 | Distant metastasis |
| M1a | Nonregional lymph node(s) |
| M1b | Bone(s) |
| M1c | Other site(s) with or without bone disease |

**Stage Grouping**

| | | | | |
|---|---|---|---|---|
| Stage I | T1a | N0 | M0 | G1 |
| Stage II | T1a | N0 | M0 | G2, 3–4 |
| | T1b | N0 | M0 | Any G |
| | T1c | N0 | M0 | Any G |
| | T1 | N0 | M0 | Any G |
| | T2 | N0 | M0 | Any G |
| Stage III | T3 | N0 | M0 | Any G |
| Stage IV | T4 | N0 | M0 | Any G |
| | Any T | N1 | M0 | Any G |
| | Any T | Any N | M1 | Any G |

[a]Tumor found in 1 or both lobes by needle biopsy, but not palpable or reliably visible by imaging, is classified as T1c.
[b]When more than 1 site of metastasis is present, the most advanced category is used, pM1c is most advanced.
[c]Invasion into the prostatic apex or into (but not beyond) the prostatic capsule is not classified as T3, but as T2.
[d]There is no pathological T1 classification.
[e]Positive surgical margin should be indicated by an R1 descriptor (residual microscopic disease).

are usually men who are 65 and older with low-grade and stage disease, and low, stable PSA values. Active surveillance is defined as initial surveillance of prostate cancer followed by active treatment if the tumor progresses to the extent that quality or quantity of life is affected.

There have been a number of studies that have researched outcomes of men undergoing active surveillance and some that have compared active surveillance patient outcomes to aggressive treatment modalities. In a pivotal study, Klotz[64] analyzed the survival data of 299 men with low-risk prostate cancer over the age of 70. Inclusion criteria for the study were prostate cancer stage T ≤ 2a with PSA values <10 ng/ml and Gleason scores ≤6. He found that the median time to disease progression (measured by PSA doubling time (PSA-DT)) was 7 years and that 35% of participants had no sign of disease progression at 10 years. Moreover, even in the population with significant PSA-DT, active surveillance remained an option. Median follow-up at 55 months revealed that 60% of the total sample remained on active surveillance. At 8 years the study revealed a 99% disease-specific survival rate. This indicates the potential clinical applicability of active surveillance for patients with low grade and stage disease.

Hardie et al[65] followed a small sample ($n$ = 80) of men with localized prostate cancer undergoing the active surveillance management approach. Participants in the study had clinical stage T1/T2 cancer with PSA values < 20 ng/ml.

**TABLE 64–3**

**Comparison of the Gleason Grading and Whitmore-Jewett Staging Systems for Clinically Localized Prostate Cancer**

**Gleason Grading System**

Prostate cancers often have areas with different grades.
The grades from the two most common cancer cell patterns are added together in a combined *Gleason score.*

For example, if the most common pattern is grade 4 and the second most common pattern is grade 3, then the combined Gleason score is 4 + 3 = 7. If there is only one pattern within the tumor, the combined Gleason score can be as low as 1 + 1= 2 or as high as 5 + 5=10.

| | |
|---|---|
| Low-grade | Combined scores of 2 to 4<br>Well-differentiated. |
| Intermediate-grade | Combined scores of 5 to 6<br>Moderately-differentiated. |
| High-grade | Combined scores of 7 to 10<br>Poorly-differentiated. |

**Jewett Staging System (Modified)**

| | |
|---|---|
| Stage A1 | Tumor ≤ 5%, Gleason score ≤ 4 |
| Stage A2 | Tumor > 5%, Gleason score > 4 |
| Stage B1 | Palpable, < 1 lobe, ≤ 1.5 cm |
| Stage B2 | Palpable, both lobes, > 1.5 cm |
| Stage C1 | ECE, negative margins |
| Stage C2 | ECE, positive margins |
| Stage C3 | Seminal vesicle involvement |
| Stage D1 | Microscopic pelvic lymph node involved |
| Stage D2 | Disease outside pelvis |

*Abbreviations*: ECE, extracapsular extension; M, metastasis; N, node; PIN, prostatic intraepithelial neoplasia; PSA, prostate-specific antigen; T, tumor, TRUS, transrectal ultrasonography.

Participants' ages were not reported. The authors used a longitudinal approach and followed patients every 6 months, gathering data on PSA levels, clinical characteristics conversion to other treatments. At median follow-up time of 42 months, 80% of patients remained in active surveillance and none had died of prostate cancer. This study illustrates the indolent nature of prostate cancer and its potential applicability for men with the appropriate clinical characteristics.

Dall'Era et al[61] conducted a study of 321 patients with prostate cancer with a mean age of 63.4 years undergoing active surveillance. Criteria for the study were stage T1/T2a cancer with PSA values < 10 and Gleason scores < 6. Median follow-up time was 3.6 years. At the median follow-up time, 13% of the sample had converted to active surveillance without any clinical evidence of disease progression. The median time to active treatment for men with clinical indicators of disease progression was 3 years. This underscores the potential for remaining in active surveillance for a period of time after diagnosis, affording increased-life years free from common treatment adverse effects.

Men who undergo active surveillance live every day with the knowledge that they have cancer in their bodies and the associated uncertainty as to whether this cancer will grow, spread, and kill them. In a recent qualitative report by Wallace and Storms[66] on the needs of men with prostate cancer, one focus group participant stated, "The word cancer is followed closely in my mind with death." Moreover, research has found that when men are asymptomatic or experience only occasional signs that the cancer is present, their uncertainty about the state of cancer is intense.[67] Except for biannual PSA readings, men have no clinical markers to indicate disease symptomatology, and thus may incorrectly attribute physical changes associated with aging to disease progression.[67] Other men, who experience no physical discomfort, find it hard to believe that the cancer exists. Patients need help to manage the uncertainty of living with cancer.[67] Men without education and support may experience emotional distress such as depression or choose to undergo unnecessary aggressive therapy.[62]

Nursing care for patients undergoing active surveillance focuses heavily upon psychosocial support and education to help patients to live with prostate cancer. Patients should be encouraged to follow-up with their healthcare providers for PSA testing and evaluation of disease progression approximately every 6 months. Psychosocial and educational nursing interventions can help patients to transform prostate cancer from an aggressive cancer with the potential to result in an early death into a chronic disease, similar to diabetes or hypertension, which requires periodic monitoring, management, and evaluation. Wallace and Bailey[68] are currently testing a Web-based uncertainty management program designed to help men manage the uncertainty associated with living with prostate cancer as a chronic illness.

## SURGERY

### Transurethral resection of the prostate

Prostate cancer is not cured by transurethral resection of the prostate (TURP). Rather, the procedure is used to treat symptoms of bladder outlet obstruction. In some patients, it provides pathological evidence that a cancer, previously unsuspected, is present. Using a transurethral resectoscope and electrocautery, the hypertrophic prostate is removed in pieces called *chips*. The procedure is performed under spinal anesthesia or general anesthesia with the patient in the dorsal lithotomy position. Potential immediate postoperative complications include clot retention, bleeding, and infection. The bladder is kept as free of blood and clots as possible using continuous saline irrigation through a 3-way indwelling catheter. Bladder spasms can be problematic, and patients may require analgesics and antispasmodics. After the bleeding decreases, bladder irrigation is discontinued. As the urine becomes more normal in appearance, the catheter is removed. Rarely, patients may have difficulty initiating urination after catheter removal and may require recatheterization.

Nursing management includes preoperative education about routine aspects of anesthesia, such as coughing, deep breathing, and early ambulation. The patient needs to know that he will have a catheter after surgery and that bladder irrigation will continue for approximately 24 hours or less. Pain management approaches using oral and rectal medications are discussed. The patient must drink large volumes of fluid, such as water, to promote urine formation. Accurate recording of intake and output is required until discharge. Large amounts of fluid may be absorbed through the cut prostatic capillaries during surgery, resulting in volumetric overload. This phenomenon, known as the TUR syndrome, may occur in the first 24 hours postoperatively. Transurethral resection syndrome is uncommon, and not thought to be a significant risk in current TURP procedures.[69] As a result of fluid shifts, electrolyte disturbances and hypoosmolality may precipitate neurological and hypovolemic symptoms.[70] Supportive therapy is used to manage the patient. The nurse must monitor the patient for changes in mental status and cardiac and renal function.

The patient also needs to be aware that late complications, such as incontinence, ED, and bladder neck contraction requiring urethral dilation, may occur. Patients may have problems with recurrent bladder outlet obstruction; approximately 5% of men need to undergo repeat TURP. Table 64-4 presents an overview of the management of the TURP patient.

### Radical prostatectomy

Radical prostatectomy involves removal of the prostate gland, ejaculatory ducts, seminal vesicles, and possibly the lymph nodes. This procedure is usually performed on patients staged with T1 or T2 disease.[42] With T3 disease, it may be more difficult to obtain tumor-free margins. The patient should be informed preoperatively by the physician about the potential for postoperative incontinence and ED. Incrocci[71] reports that the rates of ED following radical prostatectomy range between 7% and 72%. Risk factors identified for the development of postoperative incontinence include age older than 65, development of anastomotic stricture, and stage T1a or T1b disease. Persistent incontinence requires urological evaluation for bladder neck contracture, stricture, bladder dysfunction, or sphincter dysfunction.

The autonomic nerves that control erectile function lie next to the prostate. Surgery may damage or sever these nerves. However, the right, left, or both neurovascular bundles may be preserved using newer nerve-sparing procedures (see Figure 64-1). With this nerve-sparing procedure, it is possible to retain potency; however, there will be no prostatic fluid and, therefore, no emission and ejaculation. This approach is recommended for patients with stage T1 or T2 disease who are eligible to undergo radical prostatectomy. Factors that promote sexual function after surgery include age younger than 50, stage of disease, and preservation of neurovascular bundles. In younger men (age 50 and younger), lower stage and surgical procedure were the factors associated with potency. Pharmacological prophylaxis with oral erectile agents early after these procedures can enhance the recovery of erectile function after surgery.[72] When 1 bundle is intact in patients younger than 50, potency is preserved. In patients older than age 70, only 22% will regain potency postoperatively, even if both neurovascular bundles are spared. If disease is more advanced and there is involvement of the prostatic capsule or seminal vesicles at the time of surgery, resection may involve removal of or damage to the nerves. In the patients with stage B2

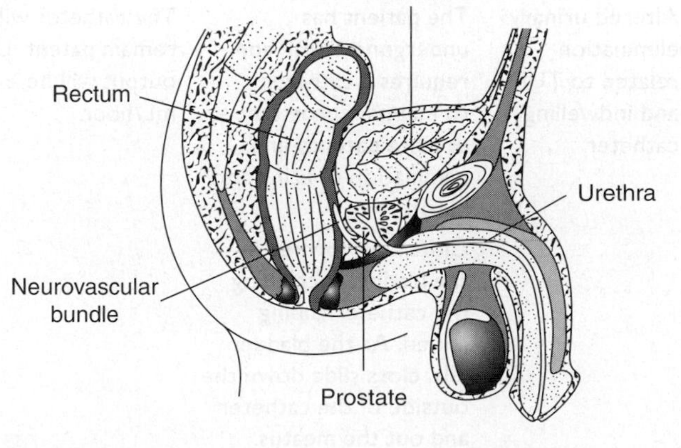


**FIGURE 64-1**

Prostate anatomy.

**TABLE 64-4**

**Nursing Management of the Patient Undergoing a TURP**

| Nursing Diagnosis | Etiology | Outcome | Nursing Management |
|---|---|---|---|
| Knowledge deficit, surgery | Lack of prior experience with surgery. | Patient will verbalize an understanding of preoperative and postoperative course | 1. Assess patient's understanding of cancer diagnosis, planned surgery to remove obstructing section of prostate gland around prostatic urethra compressing urethra and impeding release of urine from the bladder, expected outcome that patient will be able to void with reduced difficulty, potential complications of surgery including incontinence.<br>2. Educate patient regarding<br>• Care of indwelling catheter<br>• Continuous bladder irrigation (CBI)<br>• Drinking fluids<br>• Ambulating first postoperative day<br>• Coughing and deep breathing<br>• Pain management with belladonna and opium suppositories for bladder spasms, oral narcotics for pain<br>• Signs/symptoms of urinary tract infection (UTI) to report to physician after surgery—pain, burning, frequency, hematuria<br>• Need to notify physician after discharge of inability to void, continued incontinence, bright red urine, numerous clots, chills, fever, decreased stream size and force |
| Incontinence | The urinary sphincter may be injured during surgery—may persist up to 3 months in elderly. | The patient will be able to manage incontinence. | 1. Methods for managing incontinence (see Table 64-6). |
| Indwelling catheter care | The patient is unable to void after indwelling catheter is removed postoperatively and requires recatheterization and discharge home with indwelling catheter. | The patient will demonstrate the skills necessary to maintain an indwelling catheter at home | 1. Educate patient to<br>• Wash around urinary meatus with soap and water, rinse, and dry the area twice daily.<br>• Utilize leg bag during day, how to attach, disconnect, empty, and cleanse bag to maintain a clean environment inside the equipment.<br>• Utilize straight drainage at night, how to cleanse bag to maintain a clean environment inside the equipment<br>• Maintain a clean bag environment by rinsing the equipment, washing it with soapy water, rinsing well, and allowing it to air dry. |
| Altered urinary elimination related to TURP and indwelling catheter | The patient has undergone TURP and requires a catheter to maintain prostate urethra patency and elimination of urine and blood.<br>Clots have formed in the bladder, occluding the catheter/tubing lumen. As the bladder fills, clots slide down the outside of the catheter and out the meatus. | The catheter will remain patent. Urine output will be $\geq$ 30 mL/hour. | 1. Maintain accurate I&O.<br>2. Empty urinary drainage bag when two-thirds full.<br>3. Maintain CBI at rate to keep urine clear using NSS 3 L irrigation bags. Do not allow bags to empty. Keep NSS running at all times to maintain pink-colored drainage. CBI is usually discontinued after 24 hours.<br>4. Monitor for clots in the tubing, monitor for clot retention with subsequent bleeding around the catheter. Assess for bladder distention. Notify physician of clot retention. Irrigate Foley catheter manually with saline until free of clots. Do not forcefully irrigate catheter—notify surgeon.<br>5. Maintain IV fluids at prescribed rate of infusion.<br>6. Encourage fluid intake, usually 2000 mL/24 hour.<br>7. Maintain catheter tubing patency by unkinking tubing.<br>8. One to 2 days postoperatively, the catheter is removed. Accurately measure the first and each subsequent voiding until discharge. Notify physician if patient does not void in 8 hour. |

(Continued)

**TABLE 64-4**

**Nursing Management of the Patient Undergoing a TURP (*Continued*)**

| Nursing Diagnosis | Etiology | Outcome | Nursing Management |
|---|---|---|---|
| Bleeding related to TURP | The prostate is highly vascularized. Cauterization during the surgery does not seal all the bleeding capillaries, therefore bleeding occurs in the postoperative period. | The patient will have prompt recognition of and immediate intervention for increased bleeding. Bleeding will decrease daily. | 1. Monitor hemoglobin and hematocrit values. Notify physician of ≥1 g reduction in hemoglobin.<br>2. Maintain traction with tape on catheter applied during surgery to assist in control of venous bleeding in prostatic bed.<br>3. Monitor color of urine. There should be a noted reduction in the amount of blood in the urine daily. If increased blood is present, notify physician.<br>4. Do not remove water from overfilled indwelling catheter balloon, as this helps to control bleeding.<br>5. Do not remove indwelling catheter until physician orders its removal. Premature removal may result in bleeding.<br>6. Monitor for bladder distention, which increases bleeding by pulling on capillaries. |
| Potential for infection related to surgery and indwelling catheter | The presence of an indwelling catheter may promote bladder infection. The patient has undergone surgery under general anesthesia and may develop postoperative atelectasis, which may develop into pneumonia. | The patient will not develop a fever or other sign of infection | 1. Encourage coughing and deep breathing q 1 hour.<br>2. Use aseptic technique when emptying drainage bag and attaching new bladder irrigation bags.<br>3. Perform meatal care twice daily with soap and water.<br>4. Maintain catheter patency. Observe for clots, chips of tissue, mucus that can obstruct catheter lumen. Keep catheter and tubing straight and free of kinks. Keep drainage bag off floor. Hang with hook from bed.<br>5. Notify physician of temperature ≥38.5°C, tachycardia, tachypnea, decreased BP, other signs of infection.<br>6. Obtain urine, blood, or other cultures as prescribed. |
| Altered comfort related to pain, bladder spasms, or both | Pain or bladder spasms may be due to surgery, bladder distention, infection, clots, or the catheter balloon. | The patient will verbalize an acceptable level of analgesia. | 1. Assess quantity, quality, and duration of pain.<br>2. Check for bladder distention, kinked tubing, free flowing drainage. Palpate bladder after turning off CBI. Restart CBI if patient not distended. Otherwise, notify physician.<br>3. Administer prescribed narcotic for pain.<br>4. Administer belladonna and opium suppository, oxybutynin, or propantheline for bladder spasms.<br>5. Gently irrigate indwelling catheter if prescribed. Never force irrigation fluid—notify physician.<br>6. Remind patient not to tug or pull at the catheter. If the patient should pull out the catheter, notify physician immediately. |
| Potential for urethral stricture formation related to surgery | The urethra may heal with stricture formation if catheter is removed prematurely. | The patient will have a patent urethra. | 1. The catheter is never to be removed without a physician's order.<br>2. Monitor for signs of stricture, such as small urine stream, straining to void, and difficulty voiding. |
| Potential for urinary retention after catheter removed. | The patient is not able to void after catheter is removed. | The patient will not develop urinary retention. | 1. The patient should void when he feels the urge and not wait, as this may produce urinary distention, which may cause retention. |

(*Continued*)

**TABLE 64-4**

**Nursing Management of the Patient Undergoing a TURP (*Continued*)**

| Nursing Diagnosis | Etiology | Outcome | Nursing Management |
|---|---|---|---|
| Constipation related to antispasmodics used to manage bladder spasms | Anticholinergic drugs cause constipation.<br>Straining can cause bleeding. | The patient will have an easy bowel movement. | 1. Administer stool softeners/laxatives to reduce constipation and promote easy colon evacuation.<br>2. Educate patient not to strain on bowel movement. |
| Potential for altered fluid and electrolyte balance | Fluid balance and electrolyte alterations occur during surgery. | The patient will have prompt recognition of signs and symptoms of altered fluid and electrolyte balance. | 1. Monitor electrolytes, BUN, creatinine. Notify physician of abnormal results.<br>2. Assess patient for changes in mental status, vital signs, tremor, vomiting, headache.<br>3. Monitor patient for change in renal or cardiac function. |

*Abbreviation*: TURP, transurethral resection of the prostate.

or C disease in the previously mentioned study, 51% had 1 bundle left intact.[72] Age again becomes important, with men younger than 50 regaining potency and older patients having a reduced likelihood of potency.

Incontinence and ED can place a heavy burden on male patients and their families. Increasingly, research is addressing concerns related to quality of life. Compared with normal age-matched men living in the same location, men who have undergone treatment for localized prostate cancer are more likely to have problems related to sexual, urinary, or bowel function. Quality of life issues may be amenable to nursing interventions, such as patient education, and nurses need to accept responsibility for the assessment, management, and evaluation of these patient concerns. Yoshimasa et al[73] studied 151 men who had undergone radical prostatectomy ($n$ = 70) or brachytherapy ($n$ = 81) for prostate cancer to determine the impact of treatment on quality of life issues such as urinary and sexual function. Men treated with radical prostatectomy reported lower urinary and sexual function and more sexual bother, even in men who had undergone the nerve sparing procedures ($n$ = 30).

Preoperative nursing care is similar to that provided to patients undergoing other surgical procedures of the abdomen and pelvis. Many patients undergoing radical prostatectomy will be older than age 50, and special attention should be paid to the patient's comorbid factors such as cardiopulmonary status. Additional routine preoperative care includes administering a bowel preparation to evacuate the colon, starting prescribed intravenous therapy, and ensuring that the patient eats or drinks nothing after midnight. Elderly patients should understand that they may have longer postoperative recovery times.

Intraoperatively, the prostate and its surrounding structures are removed via a perineal or retropubic incision. One or more drains may be placed during surgery, and frequent dressing changes may be required to control drainage, reduce bacterial growth, and reduce the risk of skin maceration and resultant infection. The nurse must monitor incision and drainage sites for infection.

Depending on the surgical approach and degree of intraoperative findings, such as disease greater than expected, the patient may be immobilized on the operating room table for several hours and is thus at risk for the usual postoperative complications. The nurse needs to encourage coughing, deep breathing, use of analgesics, and moving around in bed to promote lower extremity venous return to the heart. Compression stockings are typically used in the postoperative period to reduce the risk of thrombophlebitis and potentially fatal pulmonary embolus. In the presence of thrombophlebitis or suspected/proven pulmonary emboli, anticoagulant therapy is initiated with a heparin bolus and a heparin drip is started or low molecular weight heparin is used.

An indwelling urinary catheter is placed in the operating room and will remain in place postoperatively. Attention is needed to reduce the risk of infection with thorough hand washing, use of aseptic technique when emptying the drainage bag, and monitoring the catheter for patency. In addition to maintaining the indwelling catheter, the nurse must monitor the amount of hematuria.

In the initial postoperative period, a nasogastric tube may be placed to control gastric distention and remove gastric secretions. Management includes monitoring the type and amount of drainage, providing mouth care to promote oral comfort, and maintaining tube patency. Drains will collect serosanguineous drainage postoperatively. A sudden increase in the amount of drainage, the presence of increased bleeding, or the appearance of urine in the drains requires prompt physician notification.

Postoperatively, it is crucial that the patient maintain a urine output of greater than 30 mL/hr. In addition to monitoring for hematuria and clots, maintaining a patent catheter and ensuring an accurate intake and output, the nurse should assess the bladder for urinary retention and administer parenteral fluids. Also, the catheter taped to the patient's upper leg must be maintained securely to avoid catheter movement and tugging on the newly anastomosed urethra. The catheter provides support to the healing urethra and must not be removed without a physician's order.

Bladder spasms can be annoying and painful. They may be caused by kinking of the catheter, bladder distention, or the catheter itself. Bladder spasms are commonly managed by administering antispasmodics such as oxybutynin and, if not contraindicated, belladonna and opium (B&O) suppositories.

Hematuria is common during the first 24 hours after surgery. Frank bleeding and clots are abnormal and require physician notification. Frequent monitoring of vital signs is needed to assess the patient for signs of excess blood loss and temperature elevation, which may indicate a wound or urinary tract infection.

The patient is discharged with an indwelling catheter and needs to be educated in meatal care, attachment of a leg drainage bag, change to a straight drainage bag at bedtime, cleaning technique, and signs of urinary tract infection that would require physician notification. After the catheter is removed 2 to 3 weeks postoperatively, incontinence may be a problem for days, weeks, or months. A variety of management options are available. Simple devices, such as penile clamps or incontinence pads, may be suggested. Reducing the volume of fluid consumed after dinner may control problems with nighttime incontinence. Frequent emptying of the bladder (eg, every hour) may provide a patient with enough control over his incontinence that he finds occasional incontinence tolerable. Instructing the patient to use Kegel exercises to strengthen the muscles also may prove beneficial.

Incontinence is a problem not only for patients undergoing prostate surgery but also for many other adults. The problem is so severe that the Agency for Health Care Policy and Research released urinary incontinence guidelines in 1992.[74] The guidelines provide an in-depth discussion of incontinence and its management (Table 64-5).

An additional burden placed on postprostatectomy men is the development of altered sexuality.[75] See Chapter 36 for an in-depth discussion of sexual dysfunction and suggestions for nursing management. Table 64-6 presents helpful hints for starting sexual activity after prostate surgery.

A rising PSA level after surgery indicates biochemical (PSA) failure of the disease to respond to treatment and evidence of prostate cancer recurrence.[76] Morris et al[76] report on a study of 49 clinical oncologists to determine their opinions regarding treatment for patients with rising PSA after treatment for prostate cancer. Ninety-three percent of those surveyed recommended salvage radiotherapy in asymptomatic postradical prostatectomy patients. Respondents varied on the PSA threshold for initiating treatment in these asymptomatic patients and on treatment choices for those with undetectable PSAs.

## Cryosurgery

Primary cryotherapy has been an approved therapeutic treatment method for men with localized prostate cancer that is stage T2b or lower, with a Gleason score <9 or a PSA <8 ng/mL.[77] Cryotherapy, also referred to as cryosurgery or cryoablation was approved by the AUA as a therapy for prostate cancer in 1996 and as a Medicare approved treatment in 1999. The procedure involves freezing the malignant cells in the prostate gland, causing cellular death. The cells are frozen through gas induced via needles forming ice balls. The needles are inserted via the perineum and guided by TRUS. The procedure is generally done in 2 cycles to enhance ablation of cells. Cryosurgery may be done under general or regional anesthesia and is generally completed as an outpatient procedure.

Since the approval of cryotherapy, research has sought to improve the procedure to lessen associated adverse effects such as ED and incontinence, while improving ability to destroy malignant cells. When the process of cryosurgery was initially researched, the process involved freezing the prostate tissue with liquid nitrogen-based systems and resulted in a 60% to 90% disease specific survival rate at 5 years. The procedure now involves argon gas to freeze cells instead of liquid nitrogen. Newer cryosurgery techniques are capable of generating apoptosis, also known as gene regulated cell death, and the introduction of cytokines during the procedure has the potential to increase immunity to tumors. The emergence of ultrathin needles and changes in cryotherapy techniques have decreased the morbidity of this procedure and improved outcomes resulting in an undetectable PSA levels.[78]

Salvage cryotherapy is an increasingly considered procedure for disease recurrence after radiation, indicated by a rising PSA and confirmed by biopsy. In the past, these patients were generally candidates for hormonal and palliative treatments. However, in the absence of metastatic disease, cryosurgery may be performed in patients with a life expectancy of greater than 10 years.

New developments in cryosurgical techniques have reduced adverse treatment side effects substantially. However, ED continues to be a problematic outcome among men undergoing cryosurgery. The rates of ED following primary cryosurgery are between 80% and 90% and rise to 95% to 100% following salvage cryoablation.[78] Moreover, the ED related to this procedure extends years after surgery with only 13% of patients reporting full recovery of sexual function 3 years after the procedure. Urinary incontinence

## TABLE 64-5

### Assisting Patients to Manage Urinary Incontinence after Prostate Surgery

After prostate surgery, continence is maintained by the external urinary sphincter. This striated urethral sphincter prevents urinary leakage after prostate surgery. Damage to the muscle controlling the sphincter or damage to its nerve supply can result in postoperative incontinence. The retropubic approach to prostatectomy may result in a lower rate of incontinence by avoiding injury to the cavernous nerves of the pelvic plexus. After radical prostatectomy, 92% of patients achieve urinary control, 8% experience stress incontinence, and 6% wear 1 or fewer incontinence pads per day. Approximately 1% of men are incontinent after a TURP.

**Evaluation**

Diagnostic studies are performed to evaluate incontinence after a history and physical exam are performed. Cystourethroscopy is used to evaluate the integrity of the external urinary sphincter under direct visualization. A voiding cystourethrogram looks for anatomical abnormalities, while urodynamic studies evaluate physiology.

**Management**

Diapers, liners—these devices absorb urine. There are a variety available. Liners are useful for light to moderate incontinence. Adult diapers are needed for heavy urine loss. All devices should be changed frequently to avoid odor and skin maceration. Fungal infections can occur, and in summer, diapers can be hot and uncomfortable. Cost can become a factor when absorbent products need to be changed frequently; for people with a limited income, this can be a financial burden. Bulky items may be noticed under clothing.

Drip collectors—the penis is placed inside the collector, which is worn underneath clothing in a garment holder designed to hold the disposable collecting device.

Condom catheters—latex and nonlatex self-adhesive condom-shaped external urine collecting device. Problems include adhesive loss, skin breakdown, and urinary tract infections. The skin needs to be cleansed daily and monitored daily for irritation and infection. Available in single use and reusable models.

Indwelling catheters—closed sterile system that includes a catheter with a retaining water-filled balloon inserted into the urethra attached to a collection bag. Often left in place after surgery, these devices require daily cleansing and skin care to reduce the risk of infection and skin necrosis. They are not useful for long-term management of incontinence unless no other approach is successful.

Penile clamps—external urethral compressive device that occludes the urethra to reduce incontinence. The position of the clamp must be changed every 3 hours to prevent skin necrosis. Other complications include pain, edema, penile and urethral erosion, and urethral obstruction. Inflatable compression cuff band placed around penis and held in place with velcro. Inflated air bladder in band compresses urethra. Complications include tissue damage from compression. Bladder needs to be deflated every 3 hr.

Ostomy pouch—useful for a small or retracted penis. Clip the hair around where the adhesive is applied and attach pouch to a collection bag.

Fluid restriction—the patient who experiences incontinence mostly at night should restrict fluids after dinner to reduce the bladder urine volume and thus the risk of incontinence. Otherwise, 2 quarts of fluids per day are encouraged.

Timed voiding—at predetermined intervals, the patient empties the bladder. To develop a schedule, the patient needs to keep a diary for 3 or 4 days to identify times of incontinence. A schedule is then developed for the patient to void prior to the times identified as being at risk for incontinence.

Kegel exercises—the pelvic floor muscles are crucial to maintaining continence. These muscles can be strengthened with exercise. The exercise consists of contracting the pelvic floor muscles by squeezing the pubococcygeus muscle. Squeezing this muscle closes the urethra. The abdominal, pelvic, and thigh muscles must not be contracted during the exercises. Contracting the muscles involved in a bowel movement by pulling them in and holding for 10 seconds, followed by a 10-second rest, and repeated 30 to 80 times a day for a minimum of 6 weeks, can result in better bladder control.

Biofeedback—used in conjunction with Kegel exercises and timed voiding, biofeedback helps the patient become attuned to his physiology.

Instruments help the person learn about bladder control.

Bladder dysfunction (detrusor instability)—symptoms include frequency, urgency, urge incontinence. Treatment includes fluid restriction and medications:

**Anticholinergics**

Propantheline—blocks bladder contractions, dose 7.5 mg to 30 mg 3 to 5 times per day; cost—inexpensive; effect—may reduce incontinence in as many as 53% of patients; side effects—urinary retention, dry mouth, blurred vision, nausea, constipation, confusion, drowsiness. Hyoscyamine is a newer drug.

Oxybutynin—also relaxes smooth muscle, dose 2.5 to 5 mg 3 to 4 times per day; effect—may reduce incontinence in as many as 56% of patients; side effects—dry skin, blurred vision, nausea, constipation.

**Muscarinic Receptor Antagonist**

Tolterodine—dose 2 mg 2 times per day PO—muscarinic receptor antagonist, new drug—expensive, lower incidence of dry mouth, better tolerated and as effective as oxybutynin.

**Antidepressants**

Imipramine—anticholinergic properties, dose 10 to 25 mg 1 to 3 times per day; side effects—rare; effect—as many as 77% of patients may have reduced incontinence.

Sphincter incompetence—symptoms include dribbling and stress incontinence. Treatment includes alpha-adrenergic agonist drugs and surgery. The drugs increase sphincter resistance:

Phenylpropanolamine—dose 50 mg twice per day; effect—as many as 45% of patients are drier; side effects—nausea, dry mouth, rash, itching, restlessness, insomnia.

Surgery—goal is urethral compression. Artificial urinary sphincter—useful in patients with normal detrusor function and an incompetent sphincter and after failure of previously discussed methods.

Approximately 80% of patients treated will be dry or almost dry requiring no incontinence pads. Complications include infection, device malfunction, bleeding, erosion of cuff site, and urethral injury. Injections of collagen or polytetrafluoroethylene may be useful in patients who are not surgical candidates.

*Abbreviation*: TURP, transurethral resection of the prostate.

**TABLE 64-6**

**Helpful Hints for Men Starting Sexual Activity after Prostate Surgery**

With removal of the prostate, men may notice changes in their sexual functioning. Some men and their partners benefit from understanding these changes and learn how to adapt to them. Beginning with some definitions of the changes, methods of ways to adapt to these changes will be described.

Erection—stiff penis due to increased blood flow

Potency—ability to cause vaginal penetration

Orgasm—sexual climax or pleasure with ejaculation of semen

Semen—mixture of sperm, prostate secretions, and seminal vesicle fluid

Sperm—reproductive cells produced by testes

Radical prostatectomy—removal of prostate, seminal vesicles, and surrounding tissues to remove cancer. With removal of the prostate and seminal vesicles, the ejaculate will be reduced and may be retrograde into the bladder resulting in a dry ejaculation. The urine will become cloudy from the sperm. Orgasms may still occur without ejaculation but with the contractions that occur as part of ejaculation. Impotency can result from surgery or radiation therapy. This can be partial or complete inability to obtain an erection. Some men will regain potency postoperatively, especially those younger than age 50.

Nerve-sparing radical prostatectomy—depending on the size and location of the tumor, the surgeon spares one or both nerve bundles responsible for an erection. In the majority of men younger than 50 potency returns after wound healing occurs and all edema from the surgery subsides. This can take up to 2 years. Older men, over age 70, will probably not regain an erection.

Orgasms after prostate surgery may be weaker but are rarely completely absent. Alternative methods of obtaining pleasure need to be pursued if there is impotency.

To begin sexual activity after prostate surgery, wound healing must be complete; therefore, the urologist's permission is needed. This may occur 6 weeks to 3 months after surgery. Open, honest discussion of sexual issues with one's physician, nurse, and partner will help explore avenues of sexuality not previously considered. Open communication with the partner is the cornerstone of sexual recovery. Explore alternative methods of pleasure such as kissing, stroking, cuddling, massage, gentle rubbing, and fondling. Consider sexual counseling with a therapist if open discussion with the partner and other methods of pleasure are not successful. Couples need to understand that there is more to sexuality and pleasure than penis–vagina intercourse. The intimacy that develops between 2 partners who love each other will permit exploration. Beginning exploration produces trust and more intimacy that promotes the desire to find ways to pleasure the partner that may not have been previously considered. Failure to communicate desires and needs to one's partner is the greatest barrier to regaining sexual relations. It must also be understood that cancer of the prostate cannot be transmitted during sex or in the sperm. Cancer of the prostate is not a sexually transmitted disease.

Alternative methods of obtaining an erection include external and internal devices. Men in stable relationships with a previously good sex life are the best candidates. However, many of these couples have been able to substitute other sexual activity if erections are not able to penetrate the vagina.

**External Devices**

Suction apparatus—vacuum erection device fits over the penis and air is removed by pumping it out with the device. Blood flows into the penis, making it rigid. A band is placed at the base of the penis to prevent blood from leaving the penis after the device is removed. After intercourse, the band is removed. (First-line therapy)

Injections of drugs into the spongy penile tissue increase blood flow to the area and produce an erection. Side effects include penile fibrosis and priapism. Drugs include prostaglandin E (alprostadil) and papaverine. (second-line therapy)

Drug-impregnated pellets that are placed into the urethra also produce an erection. Side effects include hypotension, urethral pain and burning, penile pain, and dizziness. (Second-line therapy)

**Internal Devices (Implanted Penile Prostheses)**

Semirigid—a variety of devices are available. The rod is placed in the spongy tissue of the penis but away from the urinary sphincter so that voiding is not affected. Heavy athletic undergarments will conceal the crotch bulge. Many of the devices available have a metal core that allows the device to be bent upward for sexual activity and downward for everyday activities. (Third-line therapy)

Self-containing prosthesis, semirigid—a self-contained device with a pump behind the head of the penis that is pumped to fill the rod with fluid from a reservoir. As the rod fills, an erection is produced. After sexual activity, a release valve drains the fluid back into the reservoir.

Many of these devices can be placed under local anesthesia. Semirigid rods are the most commonly implanted penile prostheses. Success rates run about 95% for semirigid devices. (Third-line therapy)

Medication—eg. sildenafil 100 mg PO 1 hr prior to sexual activity. Effective in men with both neurovascular bundles intact. Less effective in unilateral or non-nerve-sparing surgery. Taken as needed 30–60 min prior to sexual activity. Other agents include vardenafil and tadalafil.

Side effects include flushing, indigestion, headache, color vision abnormalities. Contraindications—nitrates. Deaths have been reported in men taking both medications. May cause shock, myocardial infarction, or severe hypotension. (First-line therapy)

related to cryotherapy is between 8% and 9%, which is lower than that seen among radical prostectomy patients. New nerve sparing cryotherapy techniques currently being researched have significantly improved rates of ED, but are still considered experimental at this time.

Nursing care for cryosurgery patients includes preoperative teaching regarding the bowel preparation and home care of indwelling or suprapubic urinary drainage catheter. Postoperative care includes monitoring vital signs, intake and output (I&O), administering intravenous (IV) fluids, assessing the urinary catheter drainage, and pain management. Sequential compression stockings may be used to promote venous return. Ambulation is promoted on the first postoperative day. The patient must drink large amounts of fluid each day (2.5 L) and report signs of infection to the physician after discharge. Home care may be needed to assist with bladder retraining and care of the catheter, which may remain in place for 3 weeks to allow for urethral healing.

### Laparoscopic prostatectomy

Laparoscopic prostatectomy is a new surgical procedure developed in Europe that entails the removal of the prostate gland and associated structures, including the seminal vesicles and pelvic lymph nodes, which are removed first.[79] The procedure is performed under general anesthesia with the patient in a pronounced lithotomy position with the hips above the shoulders. An indwelling urinary drainage catheter is placed before the surgery begins. The abdomen is filled with carbon dioxide gas, and trochars are inserted into the gas-distended abdominal cavity through 5 stab wounds. The insertion of the instrumentation and removal of the organs occur through the wounds. A TV screen monitor is used to view the internal organs by means of 1 instrument. Robotics are used to hold the instruments.[80] The urethral anastomosis is seen under magnification. A bag is passed through a trocar, the removed organs are placed inside the bag, and then the bag and contents are removed from the body. A drain is placed and the incisions are sutured.

Preoperative care includes patient education and routine care of the general anesthesia patient undergoing abdominal and pelvic surgery. Postoperative care includes monitoring for infection and bleeding, volume and type of wound drainage, care of the indwelling urinary catheter, monitoring of urine output, administration of antibiotics and parenteral fluids, and compression stockings. Because the patient has been immobilized in the lithotomy position, he is at risk for the hazards of immobility, including cardiopulmonary and venous thromboembolic complications. Ileus can be a postoperative complication, so the gastrointestinal system needs ongoing monitoring. The integrity of the indwelling urinary catheter must not be compromised, as it supports the urethral anastomotic site. Lab work and vital signs are monitored. Pain is managed with parenteral narcotics and antispasmodics (eg, oxybutynin) are used for bladder spasms.[81] The patient is not allowed any food or fluids and is kept on bed rest during the day of surgery. On the first postoperative day, the patient is gotten out of bed, switched to oral analgesics, and taught to care for and manage the indwelling urinary catheter at home.

Candidates for laparoscopic prostatectomy include patients with T1b-T2b disease.[79] Side effects and complications include the need to perform an open radical prostatectomy, bleeding, arterial injury, rectal injury, nerve damage, ileus, leaking anastomosis, uroma, myocardial infarction, infection, and urinary retention.[79] Advantages of the procedure include less pain, reduced risk of ED and incontinence due to magnification of the operative site with increased visibility, less blood loss, fewer blood transfusions, and fewer indwelling catheter days.[82] A disadvantage is the surgeon learning curve—operative times become shorter as the individual surgeon performs the procedure more often. Cancer outcomes appear to be similar between laparoscopic prostatectomy and open radical prostatectomy.[82] However, because laparoscopic prostatectomy is a new surgical procedure, there is no long-term patient follow-up and no prospective randomized clinical trials comparing the outcomes of the 2 approaches.

## RADIATION THERAPY

External beam radiation therapy may be administered in curative doses to treat men with early prostate cancer (T1, T2) confined to the gland itself. Radiation therapy is an option if a patient wishes to avoid surgery or is not a surgical candidate due to preexisting medical problems. There is no evidence that either radiation therapy or surgery is superior in treating early-stage disease (T1a-T2b).[83] As yet, no randomized trials have been completed to compare surgery and radiation therapy in patients with the same stage of disease.[83] Radiation therapy may also be used for locally advanced stage T3 or T4 disease.[42] The dose of radiation administered ranges from 73 to 77 Gy over 7 to 8 weeks and depends on tumor size, PSA level, Gleason score, and number of core biopsies positive for cancer.[84] Factors predicting postradiation treatment failure are the pre- and postradiation PSA levels and tumor characteristics.[76]

Conventional radiation therapy uses 3-dimensional conformal radiation therapy to plan the treatment field and deliver the radiation using 5 to 8 beams that are administered at different angles to spare normal tissues from radiation.[84] Intensity-modulated radiation therapy (IMRT) is the current state-of-the-art method for administering therapy. Using computer simulation, the area to be treated is identified; working in reverse, the number of beams and the intensity required to achieve the desired dose are determined.

Radiation therapy also can be administered adjuvantly in the postoperative setting after radical prostatectomy. Indications often prompting use of such therapy include positive surgical margins, "close" surgical margins, and seminal vesicle involvement.[76] Patients who relapse after prostatectomy may also benefit from radiation therapy.[76] Radiation is also useful in managing complications of advanced prostate cancer, including hematuria, urinary obstruction, urethral obstruction, and pelvic pain. Patients who experience disease recurrence after radiation therapy may be eligible to receive additional treatment with brachytherapy.[76]

Side effects of radiation therapy may include fatigue, urinary frequency and dysuria, ED, urinary incontinence, diarrhea, and rectal bleeding.[85] Diarrhea can be problematic, as part of the colon and rectum lie within the radiation field. The patient needs dietary counseling at the initiation of therapy. Teaching includes the need to consume a low-residue diet and management of diarrhea through regulation of the quantity of fiber consumed. Antidiarrheals, such as loperamide HCl, may be used to control diarrhea. Severe diarrhea may require opioid therapy.

The skin in the perineal area is thin and easily damaged by radiation therapy. Skin integrity is maintained through frequent perineal care, including gentle washing of the rectal area with soap and water after each bowel movement and applying a radiation-approved gel such as Natural Care Gel (Bard Patient Care Division) or a cream after treatment. All gels and creams should be washed off before treatment each day. The patient needs to avoid ointments and products that are difficult to remove until radiation therapy is completed. Silver sulfadiazine cream may be useful in promoting wound healing after radiation is completed.

Symptoms of radiation cystitis can be managed through the use of urinary antispasmodics such as oxybutynin, urinary analgesics such as phenazopyridine, alpha1 blockers such as tamsulosin, frequent voiding, and management of urinary tract infections with antibiotic therapy. Fluids should be consumed in large volumes and caffeine should be avoided.

Altered sexual functioning probably is related to damage to the blood supplying the corpora cavernosa.[86] Potency is maintained in 20% to 80% of patients receiving radiation[87] and may be related to age, with older men being at greater risk of impotency. Erectile dysfunction begins months to years after completion of therapy. Cigarette smoking may have a negative effect on potency. Diabetes, hypertension, and heart disease are also known to decrease potency.[88]

Proctitis and rectal bleeding require medical management, including sigmoidoscopy, fulguration of bleeding vessels, and hydrocortisone enemas. Blood transfusions may be required if bleeding causes the hemoglobin to drop to 8 g/dL. Urethral strictures from inflammation are managed with periodic dilation or transurethral incision of the stenosis. Repeated dilation may be needed. The incidence of urinary complications from radiation therapy is related to the dose of radiation delivered.

## BRACHYTHERAPY

Prostatic brachytherapy involves the placement of radioactive seeds directly into the prostate. Iodine-125 and palladium-103 seeds are frequently used as the sources of radiation. In brachytherapy, a high dose of radiation is delivered to a smaller volume of tissue, with reduced doses being delivered to surrounding normal structures such as the bladder and rectum. Implants may be permanent or temporary. With the patient under general anesthesia and in the lithotomy position, a template is placed on the perineal area and needles are inserted into the target tissue. Radioactive seeds are left in place. Patients with early-stage disease may be offered brachytherapy as a single-modality therapy, or it can be used in locally advanced disease as a boost to the primary therapy.[85] In patients with local relapse, brachytherapy may be employed as salvage therapy.[89]

After insertion of the source, the principles of time, distance, and shielding should be utilized because iodine-125 emits gamma radiation. Side effects include discomfort from the needle and seed insertion, proctitis, dysuria, hematuria for 24 hours, and, in rare cases, infection. Urine should be strained to locate any dislodged radioactive seeds if required by state or local ordinances or laws. Routine predischarge instructions for patients with permanent implants include teaching the patient to avoid close contact with children and pregnant women. A condom must be worn during sexual intercourse (when permitted by the physician) following implantation in case a radioactive seed is lost during intercourse. In this way, the seed can be safely retrieved. Radiation safety precautions as determined by the radiation safety officer must be followed by the patient and his family members. Palladium-103 has a shorter half-life than iodine-125 and therefore produces fewer urinary and rectal side effects.

## HORMONAL THERAPY

Advanced prostate cancer is frequently managed by altering the patient's hormonal status. Tumors comprise a heterogeneous population of cells. Three different cell populations constitute both normal and malignant prostate tissues: androgen dependent, androgen sensitive, and androgen independent. When the androgen source is eliminated from androgen-dependent cells, they die, and the androgen-sensitive cells no longer divide. In contrast, androgen-independent cells do not respond to the loss of hormones and continue to grow.

The adrenal gland also produces hormones, which will continuously support hormone-independent cells and account for about 40% of the intraprostatic testosterone.

The vast majority of androgen is produced by the testes. Androgen secretion is dependent on luteinizing hormone–releasing hormone (LHRH) released from the hypothalamus. LHRH stimulates the pituitary gland to produce luteinizing hormone (LH), which in turn stimulates the testes to produce testosterone (androgen). The goal of hormone therapy for prostate cancer is to reduce the level of circulating androgens to castration levels, causing the death of androgen-dependent cells and inhibiting the growth of androgen-sensitive cells, thereby reducing tumor size.[85] Although hormonal manipulation is not curative therapy, it can provide many patients with symptom control and palliation.

Both surgical and medical approaches are used to reduce serum testosterone levels. The oldest method is bilateral orchiectomy.[85] With this procedure, testosterone levels are reduced quickly because 90% to 95% of testosterone production is eliminated with removal of the testicles.[85]

Estrogen administration blocks LHRH and LH, resulting in reduced testosterone secretion. The estrogen diethylstilbestrol is rarely used as treatment for prostate cancer. The potential for cardiovascular side effects makes estrogen therapy less favored given the newer therapies available, which include LHRH agonists and antiandrogens. An estrogen compound is also found in estramustine, an oral antineoplastic.

LHRH agonists initially increase testosterone levels, but after several days of therapy testosterone levels fall to castration level. The surge of testosterone production after initiation of an LHRH agonist is called a flare. During a flare, patients need to be aware that symptoms can worsen and require prompt medical intervention. Pain may increase as well as symptoms of bladder outlet obstruction. Serious complications include spinal cord compression. Flutamide, an antiandrogen, may be administered prior to the initiation of an LHRH agonist to reduce the flare. Antiandrogens prevent the binding of testosterone to receptors on prostate cells.[90] Three antiandrogens are commercially available: flutamide, bicalutamide, and nilutamide. All have the side effect of hepatotoxicity. Liver function tests need to be monitored prior to the initiation of therapy, 1 month after therapy begins, and then every 3 months.

Combining antiandrogenic therapy with an LHRH agonist, such as leuprolide or goserelin, is called combined androgen blockade (CAB). When a patient is a suitable candidate for hormonal manipulation, combination therapy is an often-used treatment option. However, a meta-analysis of CAB studies failed to demonstrate that CAB was superior to castration alone in terms of prolonging survival.[91] Hormonal manipulation may also be used with radiation therapy in patients with T2 to T3 disease.[90] Compared to radiation alone, patients receiving hormonal manipulation and radiation therapy have better local, distant, and PSA outcomes.

LHRH antagonists also cause castration levels of testosterone to develop. One agent, abarelix, is commercially available and is administered by intramuscular injection. It works by blocking LH and follicle-stimulating hormone (FSH) production and causes testosterone levels to fall without producing a flare.[92] Side effects include allergic reactions, increased values on liver function tests, reduced hemoglobin and hematocrit, and adverse effects on the gastrointestinal and central and peripheral nervous systems. This agent is useful in patients who should not experience a tumor flare with LHRH agonists.

All hormonal manipulations have the potential to produce side effects. The ones most commonly encountered include hot flashes, fatigue, ED, and decreased libido.[85] Osteoporosis and bone metastasis are of significant concern in this patient population and may affect pain levels and the patient's quality of life. Metastatic lesions may develop due to concurrent osteoblastic and osteoclastic activity in sites of bone metastasis, so that the patient experiences an increase in both bone loss and bone formation. The new bone formed is not deposited at sites of bone loss, however. Osteoporosis in men on androgen ablative therapy results from increased loss of bone mineral density.[93] Risk factors for osteoporosis in men on a LHRH agonist taken either alone or in combination with an antiandrogen include Caucasian race and slender build.[94] Prior to starting hormonal therapy, a bone mineral density test should be performed and then repeated periodically. The patient should receive dietary counseling regarding calcium and vitamin D supplements.[94] Physical activity should be initiated following a consultation with a physical therapist. Patient education includes instructing the patient to remove throw rugs and other objects that could precipitate falling, install safety devices in the bathroom, and avoid activities that could result in bone injury.

Bisphosphonates interfere with osteoclast function and increase bone strength. Zoledronic acid, a bisphosphonate, reduces skeletal-related events in patients with metastatic prostate cancer.[95] Clinical trials are needed to determine whether zoledronic acid can prevent bone metastasis, osteoporosis, or both in men with advanced prostate cancer.

Patients on hormonal therapy may have problems with altered self-esteem, loss of libido, and loss of sexual potency that may present a crisis for the patient and his sexual partner. Sensitive discussions allowing verbalization of feelings are encouraged before and during treatment.

Leuprolide and goserelin injections are administered parenterally every 3 to 4 months. Leuprolide acetate is given as a depot intramuscular injection available in a prefilled syringe. Special instructions are provided by the manufacturer for mixing the drug and diluent. This agent is also available as an injectable "gel" given subcutaneously and as a 1-year implanted pump. Goserelin is a pellet given as a subcutaneous injection into abdominal fat.

An analysis of the Cancer of the Prostate Strategic Urologic Endeavor (CaPSURE) database of 7045 men was undertaken to determine time to treatment failure in men who received primary androgen deprivation therapy (PADT) for prostate cancer. A total of 993 of the men in the database (14.1%) had received PADT. These patients had higher disease risk as classified by more comorbidities, higher PSA levels and more advanced disease as indicated by Gleason and T-scores. Men who received PADT were also older and of lower socioeconomic status and less educated. Five-year evaluations of the sample indicated that 67.3% of the sample continued on PADT and 13.8% had undergone an additional treatment option, such as radical prostatectomy, radiation, or cryotherapy. Mortality of the sample revealed that 4.1% had died of prostate cancer and 19% had died of other causes.[96]

Hormone-refractory prostate cancer may respond to the withdrawal of flutamide. Discontinuing flutamide in 36 patients who were receiving flutamide plus an LHRH agonist resulted in 10 patients having reduced PSA levels and improved clinical symptoms. Suppression of adrenal androgens can be achieved with ketoconazole. Ketoconazole and hydrocortisone combination therapy may be tried, or hydrocortisone may be used as a single agent given that it lowers testosterone levels. Both high-dose (400 mg tid) and low-dose (200 mg tid) ketoconazole with hydrocortisone (10 mg bid) may be effective, with fewer side effects arising with the lower-dose ketoconazole regimen.[97] One study enrolled 28 patients with progressive prostate cancer after antiandrogen withdrawal and castration levels of testosterone. The participants received high-dose ketoconazole with hydrocortisone until disease progression occurred, at which time the dose of ketoconazole was increased to the high-dose level. Of the 28 patients, 13 demonstrated lower PSA levels (> 50%) with a median duration of response of at least 30 weeks (range 36–53 weeks). Toxicities noted included hepatotoxicity and depression. Side effects included nausea, dry skin, and fatigue.[97]

## CHEMOTHERAPY

For a patient with hormone-refractory prostate cancer (HRPC), antineoplastic therapy may be an option. Over the past several years, research has produced several drug regimens that can enhance the quality of life of patients with HRPC. Until recently, none of these drug combinations has improved survival. Pirtskhalaishvili et al[85] discuss the use of estramustine, mitoxantrone, taxanes, and suramin as chemotherapeutic agents that are currently being used to treatment hormone refractory prostate cancer. Further research and clinical trials evaluating the response rates are needed. PSA results can be reduced by these drug effects without evidence of a corresponding reduction in tumor size and therefore should be used with caution as means of evaluating tumor response in drug trials. Clarification of outcomes, including PSA values need to be clearly established with respect to partial and complete responses and the length of time the response needs to be maintained in addition to how frequently blood levels are evaluated. Likewise, soft tissue disease and bone metastases may not reflect response to treatment, as patients may not have adequate disease to measure on a CT scan and bone disease is slow to demonstrate response on a bone scan.

Estramustine is a nornitrogen mustard conjugated with estradiol that demonstrates antimitotic and antimicrotubule activity.[85] Side effects include nausea, vomiting, breast tenderness, gynecomastia, and clotting problems. Paclitaxel is a taxane that demonstrates antimitotic activity. Side effects include peripheral neuropathy, neutropenia, edema, fatigue, myalgia, and arthralgia.[98] Estramustine and paclitaxel have different but additive mechanisms of action. Docetaxel is another taxane with antimitotic activity. Its side effects include increased liver function tests, neutropenia, stomatitis, fatigue, anemia, hyperglycemia, edema, and infection.[99] Both paclitaxel and docetaxel have been combined with estramustine in the treatment of HRPC.[100] Partial response rates for docetaxel and estramustine combination therapy range from 16% to 66% and for paclitaxel and estramustine combination therapy range from 27% to 46%.[100] Survival has not been affected by any of the regimens, even though these combinations show activity in the management of HRPC.[85]

The efficacy of docetaxel and estramustine vs mitoxantrone and prednisone has been investigated in a cooperative group phase III trial. Patients were randomized to receive 280 mg of estramustine (tid 1 hour before meals or 2 hours after) on days 1 to 5 and 60 mg/m$^2$ docetaxel on day 2.[101] Dexamethasone 20 mg tid (total dose 60 mg) was given the evening of day 1 prior to docetaxel. Of the eligible patients, 338 received estramustine and docetaxel (plus dexamethasone) and 336 received mitoxantrone (12 mg/m$^2$) plus prednisone (5 mg orally bid) on day 1. Cycles were repeated every 21 days. Doses of docetaxel or mitoxantrone were increased after cycle 1 if patients did not develop grade 3 or 4 toxicities. Two years into the study, the patients on the arm containing estramustine also started taking aspirin 325 mg plus warfarin 2 mg each day as prophylaxis against the vascular side effects due to estramustine. Eligible patients showed evidence of progressive metastatic HRPC on bone scan, by PSA, or by bidimensional measurable disease. Patients were stratified by the type of disease progression and severity of bone pain. Antiandrogens and bisphosphonates were stopped at least 4 weeks prior to starting therapy. Serious adverse events were more common in the docetaxel plus estramustine arm ($P$ <0.001). They included cardiovascular side effects, nausea and vomiting, infection, metabolic problems, and neurotoxicites. Patients in the docetaxel plus estramustine arm had improved survival (17.5 months) compared to the mitoxantrone plus prednisone arm (15.6 months, $P = 0.02$). In addition, the docetaxel arm had a 20% lower mortality rate.

In another study comparing docetaxel and mitoxantrone reported by Tannock and colleagues,[102] all patients received 5 mg oral prednisone bid beginning on day 1. Eligible patients had HRPC with evidence of disease progression. Antiandrogen therapy was stopped at least 4 weeks prior to therapy. Patients were stratified by pain severity and performance status. The standard therapy arm was mitoxantrone 12 mg/m$^2$ on day 1 IV every 21 days. There were 2 docetaxel arms. One arm was 75 mg/m$^2$ IV over 1 hour every 21 days; the other was 30 mg/m$^2$ IV weekly for 5 weeks followed by 1 week off therapy (6-week cycles). Side effects were more common in the docetaxel arms (neutropenia, peripheral edema, and cutaneous changes) whereas there were more cardiac side effects in the mitoxantrone arm. Patients in the docetaxel every 21 days arm had a median survival greater than the weekly docetaxel arm or the mitoxantrone arm (18.9 months vs 17.4 months vs 16.5 months). The docetaxel patients also had better pain control.

These 2 docetaxel-based studies are the first chemotherapy studies to demonstrate a survival advantage in patients with progressive HRPC. Hopefully, these results will translate into practice changes in community settings and that future studies will continue to build on this beginning success. Docetaxel-based therapy should now be considered the new standard against which other chemotherapy regimens will be compared.

## SYMPTOM MANAGEMENT AND SUPPORTIVE CARE

Patients with advanced prostate cancer may experience a number of symptoms requiring nursing management. Problems include cachexia from weight loss, bone pain, spinal cord compression (SCC), fractures of long bones, leg or scrotal edema, coagulation disorders, and bladder or urethral obstruction.

Bone pain management includes a thorough assessment of the pain's location, onset, duration, and precipitating and alleviating factors. Analgesics useful in the management of bone pain include nonsteroidal anti-inflammatory drugs (NSAIDs) and narcotics, including opioids. Routine long-acting narcotics supplemented by immediate-release, short-acting narcotics constitute a useful regimen. Doses are titrated to achieve maximal analgesia with minimal side effects. Expected narcotic side effects include constipation that requires management with routine laxatives and stool softeners. Additional side effects may include dry mouth, nausea, vomiting, and sedation. NSAID side effects include gastric distress, dizziness, and drowsiness. Higher doses produce more side effects but without enhancing analgesia. Other agents useful in the management of bone pain include the radionuclides strontium-89 and samarium-153.[103] Myelosuppression is the dose-limiting toxicity with these agents. Zoledronic acid is FDA approved for use in the management of patients with HRPC and at least 1 bone metastasis. This bisphosphonate reduces skeletal pain and skeletal-related events and plays a role in the management of patients with HRPC.[104] Radiation therapy is also effective in the management of bone pain.

All patients with bone metastasis are at risk for SCC. Prompt diagnosis and intervention are required to reduce the risk of permanent disability. Patients with SCC frequently experience back pain. This pain may have a radicular component, with the pain encircling the chest or abdomen. Leg weakness, sensory changes, and alterations in bowel or bladder function may be present. Diagnosis of SCC is made by MRI or myelogram. Treatment includes the use of pain management, dexamethasone, external bracing, radiation therapy, and, in selected cases, surgery.[105] Nursing management focuses on preserving function, promoting restoration of lost function, and assisting the patient to adapt to changes in his ability to perform activities of daily living while monitoring for changes in neurological functioning.

Leg and scrotal edema are distressing symptoms produced by advanced prostate cancer. A deep-vein thrombosis (DVT) must always be considered as a potential cause of unilateral or bilateral leg edema. Additional causes include lymphedema and medical conditions such as hypoalbuminemia or fluid overload. Elevation of the affected area may be useful but is often difficult to maintain. Compression therapy, exercise, skin care, and diuretics are all used in the management of lymphedema.[106]

In addition to DVT, patients with advanced prostate cancer may develop disseminated intravascular coagulation (DIC), which is characterized by the consumption of clotting factors and platelets resulting in concurrent hemorrhage and clotting. Patients experience bleeding from multiple body areas, abnormal laboratory results, and clotting throughout the body. Nursing management includes frequent assessment of all body systems, administration of blood products, IV fluids, and medications, and monitoring of laboratory results.

Bladder outlet obstruction evidenced by the inability to void may be managed by intermittent or indwelling urinary bladder catheterization, TURP, or urethral stent. Urethral stents or percutaneous nephrostomy tubes are used in the treatment of urethral obstructions. Nursing management includes monitoring for infection and bleeding and educating the patient about catheter care.

Gradually, as the disease progresses and symptoms worsen, patients will find that they are less able to perform their usual activities of daily living. A palliative care team approach is useful in managing the progressive symptoms associated with advancing prostate cancer. A hospice referral provides optimal end-of-life care.

## CONCLUSION

As the incidence and prevalence of prostate cancer continue to rise, it is imperative that nurses—particularly those in advanced nursing practice roles—become active in early detection programs that target high-risk individuals, especially African American males. Participation in public education programs in the workplace will further demonstrate the nurse's role as educator and patient advocate. Helping families to understand the controversies involved in the management of prostate cancer continues to be a nursing priority.

## REFERENCES


1. American Cancer Society. *American Cancer Society. Cancer Facts and Figures 2008.* Atlanta, GA: American Cancer Society; 2008.
2. American Cancer Society. *Cancer Facts and Figures 2005.* Atlanta, GA: American Cancer Society. http://www.cancer.org/downloads/STT/CAFF2005f4PWSecured.pdf. Accessed November 1, 2009.
3. American Cancer Society. *Cancer Facts and Figures for African Americans (2007–2008).* Atlanta, GA: American Cancer Society; 2007.
4. Hoffman RM, Stone SN, Espey D, Potosky AL. Differences between men with screening-detected versus clinically diagnosed prostate cancers in the USA. *BMC Cancer.* 2005;5:27.
5. Collin SM, Martin RM, Metcalfe C, et al. Prostate-cancer mortality in the USA and UK in 1975–2004: an ecological study. *Lancet Oncol.* 2008;9:445–452.
6. Jemal A, Siegel R, Ward A, Murray T, Xu J, Thun MJ. Cancer statistics. *CA: Cancer J Clin.* 2007;57:43–66.
7. Kurahashi N, Sasazuki S, Iwasaki M, Inoue M, Tsugane S; for the JPHC Study Group. Green tea consumption and prostate cancer risk in Japanese men: a prospective study. *Am J Epidemiol.* 2008;168:119.
8. Jones RA, Underwood SM, Rivers BM. Reducing prostate cancer morbidity and mortality in African American men: issues and challenges. *Clin J Oncol Nurs.* 2007;11:865–872.
9. Boyle P, Severi G, Giles GG. The epidemiology of prostate cancer. *Urol Clin North Am.* 2003;30:209–217.
10. De Stefani E, Deneo-Pellegrini H, Boffetta P, et al. α-Linolenic acid and risk of prostate cancer: a case-control study in Uruguay. *Cancer Epidemiol Biol Prev.* 2000;9:335–338.
11. Doyle C, Kushi LH, Byers T, et al. The 2006 Nutrition, Physical Activity and Cancer Survivorship Advisory Committee. American Cancer Society. Nutrition and physical activity during and after cancer treatment: an American Cancer Society guide for informed choices. *CA: Cancer J Clin.* 2006;56:323–353.
12. Amling CL, Riffenburgh RH, Sun L, et al. Pathologic variables and recurrence rates as related to obesity and race and men with prostate cancer undergoing radical prostatectomy. *J Clin Oncol.* 2004;22:1–7.
13. Crawford ED. Epidemiology of prostate cancer. *Urology.* 2003;62(suppl 6A):3–12.
14. Chan JM, Holick CN, Leitzmann MF, et al. Diet after diagnosis and the risk of prostate cancer progression, recurrence and death (United States). *Cancer Causes Control.* 2006;17:199–208.
15. Kenfield SA, Chang ST, Chan JM. Diet and lifestyle interventions in active surveillance patients with favorable-risk prostate cancer. *Curr Treat Options Oncol.* 2007;8:173–196.
16. Chang ET, Hedelin M, Adami HO, Gronberg JH, Balter KA. Alcohol drinking and risk of localized versus advanced and sporadic versus familial prostate cancer in Sweden. *Cancer Causes Control.* 2005;16:275–284.
17. Huang WY, Hayes R, Pfeiffer R, et al. Sexually transmissible infections and prostate cancer risk. *Cancer Epidemiol Biomarkers Prev.* 2008;17:2374–2381.
18. Gronberg H. Prostate cancer epidemiology. *Lancet.* 2003;361:859–864.
19. Wakefield CE, Meiser B, Gaff CL, et al. Issues faced by unaffected men with a family history of prostate cancer: a multidisciplinary overview. *J Urol.* 2008;180:38–46.
20. Roehl KA, Loeb S, Antenor JA, Corbin N, Catalona WJ. Characteristics of patients with familial versus sporadic prostate cancer. *J Urol.* 2006;176:2438.
21. Verhage BAJ, Baffoe-Bonnie AB, Baglietto L, et al. Autosomal dominant inheritance of prostate cancer: a confirmatory study. *Urology.* 2001;57:97–101.
22. Kupelian PA, Reddy CA, Reuther AM, Mahadevan A, Ciezki JP, Klein EA. Aggressiveness of familial prostate cancer. *J Clin Oncol.* 2006;24:3445–3450.
23. Hsieh K, Albertsen PC. Populations at high risk for prostate cancer. *Urol Clin North Am.* 2003;30:669–676.
24. Jemal A, Thomas A, Murray T, et al. Cancer statistics, 2002. *CA: Cancer J Clin.* 2002;52:23–47.
25. Sakr WA, Partin AW. Histological markers of risk and the role of high-grade prostatic intraepithelial neoplasia. *Urology.* 2001;57(suppl 4A): 115–120.
26. Thompson IM, Ankerst DP, Chi C, et al. Assessing prostate cancer risk: results from Prostate Cancer Prevention Trial. *J Natl Cancer Inst.* 2006;98:529–534.
27. Wyatt RB, Sanchez-Ortiz RF, Wood CG, Ramirez E, Logothetis C, Pettaway CA. Prognostic factors for survival among caucasian, African-American and Hispanic men with androgen-independent prostate cancer. *J Natl Med Assoc.* 2004;96:1587–1593.
28. Chu KC, Tarone RE, Freeman JP. Trends in prostate cancer mortality among black men and white men in the United States. *Cancer.* 2003;97:1507–1516.
29. Mohler JL, Gaston KE, Moore DT, et al. Racial differences in prostate androgen levels in men with clinically localized prostate cancer. *J Urol.* 2004;171(6 pt 1):2277–2280.
30. Stattin P, Lumme S, Tenkanen L, et al. High levels of circulating testosterone are not associated with increased prostate cancer risk: a pooled prospective study. *Int J Cancer.* 2004;108:418–424.
31. Schaid DJ. The complex genetic epidemiology of prostate cancer. *Hum Mol Genet.* 2004;13(spec 1):R103-R121.
32. Silva APM, Salim ACM, Bulgarelli A, et al. Identification of 9 novel transcripts and two RGSL genes within the hereditary prostate cancer region (HPC1) at 1q25. *Gene.* 2003;310:49–57.
33. Thompson IM, Goodman PJ, Tangen CM, et al. The influence of finasteride on the development of prostate cancer. *N Engl J Med.* 2003;349:215–224.
34. Weinstein SJ, Wright ME, Pietinen P, et al. Serum alpha-tocopherol and gamma-tocopherol in relation to prostate cancer risk in a prospective study. *J Natl Cancer Inst.* 2005;97:396–399.
35. Ng TK, Vasilareas D, Mitterdorfer AJ, Maher PO, Lalak A. Prostate cancer detection with digital rectal examination, prostate-specific antigen, transrectal ultrasonography and biopsy in clinical urological practice. *BJU Int.* 2005;95:545–548.
36. Smith JA Jr, Chan RC, Chang SS, et al. A comparison of the incidence and location of positive surgical margins in robotic assisted laparoscopic radical prostatectomy and open retropubic radical prostatectomy. *J Urol.* 2007;178:2385–2389.
37. Gretzer MB, Partin AW. PSA markers in prostate cancer detection. *Urol Clin North Am.* 2003;30:677–686.
38. Comhaire F, Mahmoud A. Preventing diseases of the prostate in the elderly using hormones and nutriceuticals. *Aging Male.* 2004;7: 155–169.
39. Balk SP, Ko Y-J, Bubley GJ. Biology of prostate-specific antigen. *J Clin Oncol.* 2003;21:383–391.
40. Smith RA, Cokkinides V, Eyre HJ. American Cancer Society guidelines for the early detection of cancer, 2004. *CA: Cancer J Clin.* 2004;54:41–52.
41. Finne P, Auvinen A, Määttänen L, et al. Diagnostic value of free prostate-specific antigen among men with a prostate-specific antigen level of <3.0mug per liter. *Eur Urol.* 2008;54:362–370.

42. Small E. Prostate cancer. In: Goldman L, Ausiello D. *Cecil Medicine.* 23rd ed. Philadelphia, PA: Saunders Elsevier Publishing Company; 2008. 1516–1519.
43. Nadler RB. Effect of finasteride on prostate-specific antigen. *Lancet Oncol.* 2007;8:4–5.
44. Punglia RS, D'Amico AV, Catalona WJ, et al. Effect of verification bias on screening for prostate cancer by measurement of prostate-specific antigen. *N Engl J Med.* 2003;349:335–342.
45. Pinthus JH, Pacik D, Ramon J. Diagnosis of prostate cancer. *Recent Results Cancer Res.* 2007;175:83–99.
46. Isola J, Auvinen A, Poutiainen M, et al. Predictors of biological aggressiveness of prostate specific antigen screening detected prostate cancer. *J Urol.* 2001;165:1569–1574.
47. Unger HA, Kane RD, Fox KM, et al. Relative importance of PSA in prostate cancer treatment. *Urol Oncol.* 2005;23:238–245.
48. Lin K, Kenneth Lin, Robert Lipsitz, et al. Benefits and harms of prostate-specific antigen screening for prostate cancer: an evidence update for the US Preventive Services Task Force. *Ann Intern Med.* 2008;149: 192–199.
49. Brooks JD. Anatomy of the lower urinary tract and male genitalia. In: Retik AB, Vaughan ED, Wein AJ, et al, eds. *Campbells' Urology.* 8th ed. Philadelphia, PA: Saunders; 2002:41–80.
50. Bostwick DG, Junqu J, Schlesinger C. Contemporary pathology of prostate cancer. *Urol Clin North Am.* 2003;30:181–207.
51. Moore CK, Karikehalli S, Nazeer T, Fisher HA, Kaufman RP Jr, Mian BM. Prognostic significance of high grade prostatic intraepithelial neoplasia and atypical small acinar proliferation in the contemporary era. *J Urol.* 2005;173:70–72.
52. Gray M, Sims T. Prostate cancer: prevention and management of localized disease. *Nurse Pract.* 2006;31:14–31.
53. Epstein JI. What's new in prostate cancer disease assessment in 2006? *Curr Opin Urol.* 2006;16:146–151.
54. Degler MA: Assessment of renal and urinary tract function. In: Smeltzer SC, Bare BG, eds. *Brunner and Suddarth's Textbook of Medical-Surgical Nursing* ed 10. Philadelphia, Lippincott, Williams & Wilkins, 2004: 1250–1270.
55. Wilkes. GM: Spinal cord compression. In: Yarbro CH, Frogge MH, Goodman M, eds. *Cancer Symptom Management* ed 3. Sudbury, MA, Jones and Bartlett, 2004: 359–371.
56. Hanson KA. Diagnostic tests and tools in the evaluation of urologic disease: part II. *Urol Nurs.* 2003;23:405–414.
57. Naya Y, Babaian RJ. The predictors of pelvic lymph node metastasis at radical retropubic prostatectomy. *J Urol.* 2003;170:2306–2310.
58. Carroll PR, Lee KL, Fuks ZY, et al: Cancer of the prostate. In: DeVita VT, Hellman S, Rosenberg SA, eds. *Cancer: Principles and Practice of Oncology* ed 6. Philadelphia, Lippincott, Williams & Wilkins, 2001: 1418–1479.
59. Cooperberg MR, Broering JM, Kantoff PW, Carroll PR. Contemporary trends in low risk prostate cancer: risk assessment and treatment. *J Urol.* 2007;178:S14–S19.
60. Wilt TJ, Partin MR. Prostate cancer intervention. Involving the patient in early detection and treatment. *Postgrad Med.* 2003;114:43–50.
61. Dall'Era MA, Cooperberg MR, Chan J, et al. Active surveillance for early-stage prostate cancer—Review of the current literature. *Cancer.* 2008;112:1650–1659.
62. Cooperberg MR, Moul JW, Carroll PR. The changing face of prostate cancer. *J Clin Oncol.* 2005;23:8146–8151.
63. Bailey DE, Wallace M, Mishel MH. Watching, waiting and uncertainty in prostate cancer. *J Clin Nurs.* 2007;16:734–741.
64. Klotz LH. Active surveillance for good risk prostate cancer: rationale, method, and results. *Can J Urol.* 2005;12:521–524.
65. Hardie C, Parker C, Norman A, et al. Early outcomes of active surveillance for localized prostate cancer *BJU Int.* 2005;95:956–960.
66. Wallace M, Storms S. The needs of men with prostate cancer. *Appl Nurs Res.* 2007;20:181–187.
67. Bailey DE, Mishel MH, Belyea M, Stewart JL, Mohler J. Uncertainty intervention for watchful waiting in prostate cancer. *Cancer Nurs.* 2004; 27:339.
68. Wallace M, Bailey DE. Out of the black box: Expansion of a theory-based intervention to self-manage the uncertainty associated with active surveillance [AS] for prostate cancer. *Res Theor Nurs Pract.* 2010;24 in press.
69. Rajbabu K, Dudderidge T, Barber N, Walsh K, Muir G. Evaluation of ideal irrigation fluid in "Greenlight" photoselective vapourization of the prostate. *Prostate Cancer Prostatic Dis.* 2007;10:101–103.
70. Chambers A. Transurethral resection syndrome—it does not have to be a mystery. *AORN J.* 2002;75:156–170.
71. Incrocci L. Radiation therapy for prostate cancer and erectile (dys)function: the role of imaging. *Acta Oncol.* 2005;44:673–678.
72. Briganti A, Salonia A, Gallina A, et al. Management of erectile dysfunction after radical prostatectomy in 2007. *World J Urol.* 2007;25:143–148.
73. Yoshimasa JO, Junichi H, Tomohiro F, Yoshinari I, Masato F. Radical prostatectomy versus high-dose rate brachytherapy for prostate cancer: effects on health-related quality of life. *BJU Int.* 2005;95:43–47.
74. Urinary Incontinence Guideline Panel. *Urinary Incontinence in Adults: Clinical Practice Guidelines.* AHCPR Publication No. 92–0038. Rockville, MD: Agency for Health Care Policy and Research; 1992.
75. Athanasiadis L, Papaharitou S, Salpiggidis G, et al. Educating physicians to treat erectile dysfunction patients: development and evaluation of a course on communication and management strategies. *J Sex Med.* 2006;3:47–55.
76. Morris SL, Parker C, Huddart R, Horwich A, Dearnaley D. Current opinion on adjuvant and salvage treatment after radical prostatectomy. *Clin Oncol.* 2004;16:277–282.
77. Mouraviev V, Polascik TJ. Update on cryotherapy for prostate cancer in 2006. *Curr Opin Urol.* 2006;16:152–156.
78. Shinohara K. Prostate cancer: cryotherapy. *Urol Clin North Am.* 2003;30:725–736.
79. Guillonneau B, Vallancien G. Laparoscopic radical prostatectomy: the Montsouris technique. *J Urol.* 2000;163:1643–1649.
80. Miller J, Smith A, Kouba E, Wallen E, Pruthi RS. Prospective evaluation of short-term impact and recovery of health related quality of life in men undergoing robotic assisted laparoscopic radical prostatectomy versus open radical prostatectomy. *J.Urol.* 2007;178(3 Pt 1): 854–858.
81. Bickert D, Frickel D. Laparoscopic radical prostatectomy. *AORN J.* 2002;75:762–782.
82. Rassweiller J, Seemann O, Schulze M, et al: Laparoscopic versus open radical prostatectomy: a comparative study at a single institution. *J Urol.* 2003;169:1689–1693.
83. Klein EA, Kupelina PA. Localized prostate cancer: radiation or surgery? *Urol Clin North Am.* 2003;30:315–330.
84. Pollack A, Horwitz EM, Movsas B, et al. Mindless or mindful? Radiation oncologists' perspectives on the evolution of prostate cancer treatment. *Urol Clin North Am.* 2003;30:337–349.
85. Pirtskhalaishvili G, Hrebinko TL, Nelson JB. The treatment of prostate cancer. *Cancer Prac.* 2001;9:295–306.
86. Akbal C, Tinay I, Simsek F, Turkeri LN. Erectile dysfunction following radiotherapy and brachytherapy for prostate cancer: pathophysiology, prevention and treatment. *Int Urol Nephrol.* 2008;40:355–363.
87. Siegel T, Moul JW, Spevak M, et al. The development of erectile dysfunction in men treated for prostate cancer. *J Urol.* 2002;165:430–435.
88. Morley JE, Tariq SH. Sexuality and disease. *Clin Geriatr Med.* 2003;19: 563–573.
89. Beyer C. Salvage brachytherapy after external-beam irradiation for prostate cancer. *Oncology.* 2004;18:151–158.
90. Hellestedt BA, Pienta KJ. The current state of hormonal therapy for prostate cancer. *CA: Cancer J Clin.* 2002;52:154–179.
91. Prostate Cancer Trialists' Collaborative Group. Maximal androgen blockade in advanced prostate cancer: an overview of randomised trials. *Lancet.* 2000;355:1491–1498.

92. Koch M, Steidle C, Brosman S, et al. An open-label study of abarelix in men with symptomatic prostate cancer at high risk of treatment with LHRH agonists. *Urology.* 2003;62:877–882.
93. Berruti A, Dogliotti L, Tucci M, et al. Metabolic bone disease induced by prostate cancer: rationale for the use of bisphosphonates. *J Urol.* 2001;166:2023–2031.
94. Oefelein MG, Ricchuiti V, Conrad W, et al. Skeletal fracture associated with androgen suppression induced osteoporosis: the clinical incidence and risk factors for patients with prostate cancer. *J Urol.* 2001;166:1724–1728.
95. Smith MR. Bisphosphonates to prevent skeletal complications in men with metastatic prostate cancer. *J Urol.* 2003;170:S55-S58.
96. Kawakami J, Cowan JE, Elkin EP, et al. Androgen-deprivation therapy as primary treatment for localized prosate cancer. *Cancer.* 2006;106:1708–1714.
97. Harris KA, Weinberg V, Bok RA, et al. Low dose ketoconazole with replacement doses of hydrocortisone in patients with progressive androgen independent prostate cancer. *J Urol.* 2002;168:542–545.
98. Trivedi C, Redman B, Flaherty LE, et al. Weekly 1-hour infusion of paclitaxel. *Cancer.* 2000;89:431–436.
99. Picus J, Schultz M. Docetaxel (Taxotere) as monotherapy in the treatment of hormone-refractory prostate cancer: preliminary results. *Semin Oncol.* 1999;26:14–18.
100. Obasaju C, Hudes GR. Paclitaxel and docetaxel in prostate cancer. *Hematol/Oncol Clin North Am.* 2001;15:525–544.
101. Petrylak DP, Tangen CM, Hussain MHA, et al. Docetaxel and estramustine compared with mitoxantrone and prednisone for advanced refractory prostate cancer. *N Engl J Med.* 2004;351:1513–1520.
102. Tannock IF, de Wit R, Berry WR, et al. Docetaxel plus prednisone or mitoxantrone plus prednisone for advanced prostate cancer. *N Engl J Med.* 2004;351:1502–1512.
103. Kampen WU, Fischer M. Pain palliation using unsealed radionuclides [in German]. *Schmerz.* 2008;22:699–705.
104. Clarke NW. The management of hormone-relapsed prostate cancer. *BJU Int.* 2003;92:860–868.
105. Chen TC. Prostate cancer and spinal cord compression. *Oncology.* 2001;15:841–854.
106. Cheville AL, McGarvey CL, Petrek JA, et al. Lymphedema management. *Semin Radiat Oncol.* 2003;13:290–301.

CHAPTER

# 65

*Laura S. Wood, RN, MSN, OCN®*

# Renal Cancer

- **Introduction**
- **Epidemiology**
- **Etiology**
- **Prevention, Screening, and Early Detection**
- **Pathophysiology**
- **Clinical Manifestations**
- **Assessment**
- **Classification and Staging**
- **Therapeutic Approaches and Nursing Care**
  - *Surgery*
  - *Targeted Therapy*
  - *Immunotherapy*
  - *Radiation*
  - *Chemotherapy*
  - *Symptom Management and Supportive Care*
- **Conclusion**
- **References**

## INTRODUCTION

Renal cancer accounts for approximately 3% of all cancers. Renal cancers include adenocarcinomas; transitional cell tumors of the renal pelvis, ureter, and urethra; and Wilms' tumor, which occurs in children. Differences between the types of renal cancers are related to molecular events leading to oncogenesis as well as the epithelial site targeted by these events, and reflect the disparate clinical course of renal cancer and its variable prognosis.[1] Advances in detection and therapeutic management of kidney cancer are discussed here, providing the oncology nurse with a basis for the care and management of the person diagnosed with this cancer.

## EPIDEMIOLOGY

Cancer of the kidney and renal pelvis are a heterogeneous group of diseases. Renal cancer incidence and death rates continue to rise steadily, with an estimated 57,760 new cases and 12,980 deaths in the United States in 2009, and a male-to-female ratio of 2:1.[2,3] Renal cancer is the third most common genitourinary malignancy. Its incidence rises steadily between the ages of 25 and 79, and reaches a peak between ages 40 and 70. The incidence of kidney cancer rose steadily between 1975 and 1995, increasing by 2.3% among Caucasian men, 3.9% among African American men, 3.1% among Caucasian women, and 4.3% among African American women.[4] This trend was confirmed by a comprehensive review of data in the Surveillance, Epidemiology, and End Results (SEER) program from 1973 to 1998.[5] Advances in diagnostic imaging has led to the detection of an increasing number of localized and regionally advanced renal masses with a significantly lower stage and grade, but has not led to a decrease in the incidence of patients presenting with advanced disease.[6,7]

Five-year relative survival rates have slowly improved to approximately 66.5% for patients with all stages of disease, 89.9% for patients with localized disease, 61.3% for patients with regional disease, 9.9% for patients with stage IV disease, and 35.5% for patients with unstaged disease.[2,3] Increased understanding of the molecular pathogenesis of renal cell carcinoma (RCC) and the development of targeted therapies demonstrating significant improvements in progression-free survival (PFS) should lead to improved survival for patients diagnosed with renal cancer.

## ETIOLOGY

Renal cell carcinoma arises from the proximal renal tubular epithelium. It occurs in sporadic, inherited, and noninherited forms, with 75% to 80% of cases having a clear cell histology. Although many potential risk factors have been associated with renal cancer, strong associations have not been found, partly because RCC is a relatively rare disease and many associations fall short of statistical significance. Cigarette use, obesity, and hypertension or its medications have been associated with an increased risk of renal cancer. The combined effect of obesity and hypertension poses a greater risk for women compared to men. Several hereditary forms of renal cancer have been identified, including von Hippel-Lindau (VHL) disease, tubular sclerosis, hereditary clear cell, hereditary papillary syndromes, and hereditary renal oncocytoma.[8] Associations have been made between sickle cell anemia and collecting duct carcinoma, and between end-stage renal disease and both clear cell and papillary type renal cancers. Genetic alterations associated with renal cancer have been studied with inconsistent results. Interpretation of the clinical value of some genetic alterations is challenging because of the difficulty in separating chromosomal changes of tumor initiation and proliferation compared to those occurring secondary to tumor growth.[9]

von Hippel-Lindau disease is a familial multiple-cancer syndrome in which the affected person has a predisposition to a variety of malignancies, including clear cell renal carcinoma, renal cysts, and other tumors. Clear cell renal carcinomas are characterized by abnormalities in chromosome 3, whereas VHL disease is not associated with papillary tumors. Individuals with VHL disease inherit a germ-line mutation that inactivates one of the VHL suppressor genes located on chromosome 3p25. Malignancies result when the remaining VHL allele is inactivated, and unregulated cell growth occurs.[10] Individuals present with multifocal or bilateral disease at an earlier age, often between 35 and 50 years, with a higher incidence being noted in males. The VHL mutations, which are seen in 60% to 70% of clear cell renal carcinomas, result in aggressive biologic behavior and increased tumor vascularity.

## PREVENTION, SCREENING, AND EARLY DETECTION

Renal carcinoma is characterized by a lack of early warning symptoms and variability of presenting symptoms that do not appear directly related to the kidney. This cancer is generally curable only when it is localized and amenable to surgical resection; approximately one-third of patients present with synchronous metastasis, and approximately 50% of patients surgically resected will develop metastatic disease. von Hippel-Lindau disease is an autosomal dominant inherited disorder resulting in the potential to develop multiple types of cancer. Periodic clinical screening may benefit those who are clinically affected with VHL, individuals who carry the VHL gene mutation but do not have clinical manifestations, and family members who are at genetic risk for inheriting VHL.[11] Screening may also be beneficial in patients with end-stage renal disease, acquired renal cystic disease, hereditary papillary renal cancer, tuberous sclerosis, and autosomal dominant polycystic kidney disease.[12]

Epidemiological studies identifying potential relationships between occupational, dietary, and environmental exposure and the development of sporadic renal cancer may provide direction for risk-reduction and prevention strategies. Increases in renal cancer in patients who are obese and those with tobacco exposure may provide insight regarding relative environmental risk, increasing with amount of exposure and decreasing relative to time since exposure.[13–16] Advising patients regarding weight loss and tobacco cessation are important, further progress in the prevention of renal cancer requires studies to explore the mechanisms of tumorigenesis in these individuals and determination whether such tumors have unique biological features.[17]

## PATHOPHYSIOLOGY

The pathophysiology of RCC represents the extreme heterogeneity of these tumors. The accumulation of germ-line or somatic mutations in critical gain-of-function or loss-of-function genes has been associated with the clonal evolution of most histological phenotypes of RCC.[18] Because of the diversity in tumor types and the variability in the clinical progression of each type, a revised classification for renal neoplasms was developed in 1997 (Table 65-1).[19] Advances in pathological techniques including electron microscopy, immunohistochemistry, molecular genetics, and cytogenetics have led to the recognition of multiple histological subtypes of renal cancer with associated clinical, histopathological, and prognostic characteristics.[20]

Most RCCs are solid, with sinusoidal vessels that create a highly vascular tumor. Renal tumors are found most frequently in the superior pole, ranging from 3 to 15 cm in size, and averaging 7 cm. They may invade the renal capsule and perirenal fat, becoming large enough to fill the entire retroperitoneum.[21] Tumors have a tendency to invade the renal vein and inferior vena cava with potential for tumor thrombus extension above the level of the hepatic vein and ultimately into the right atrium requiring detailed surgical planning.[22,23] Advances in surgical techniques have made possible extensive surgical resection of both tumor and inferior vena caval thrombi.

Clear cell RCC accounts for 70% of renal cancers. It is sporadic, unilateral, and unifocal, and usually presents during the sixth or seventh decade of life.[24,25] The cytoplasms of these tumors consist of mixtures of cells with clear and granular cytoplasms, and occasionally a pure clear or granular carcinoma. Clear cell tumors are characterized by alveolar nests and sheets of cells that have a delicate branching vasculature that can facilitate histological diagnosis of metastatic lesions.[20,26] Papillary tumors account for 7% to 14% of renal cancers and have a unique tumor pattern, in which cells aggregate in papillae supplied by a single fibrovascular stalk.[20] Papillary renal masses are typically unilateral, but may present as bilateral or multifocal lesions; and include an autosomal dominant hereditary form characterized by late onset with bilateral and multiple tumors.[27] In the absence of distant metastatic disease at diagnosis, the presence of lymph node metastasis appears to reflect a more indolent disease course, whereas presence of inferior vena cava tumor thrombus represents a more aggressive malignancy compared to clear cell renal cancer.[28] Chromophobe tumors account for approximately 5% of renal cancers, are spherical, well-circumscribed, and often arise from cells of the renal cortex.[20] Chromophobe RCC may have an indolent course, although those cancers with a sarcomatoid component behave more aggressively.[25] Oncocytomas represent 7% to 10% of renal neoplasms, occur in the seventh decade of life, are benign tumors, and are not graded. Collecting duct carcinoma (Bellini duct carcinoma) are rare tumors, accounting for 1% of renal neoplasms; they arise within the collecting ducts of the renal medulla and have an aggressive course.[19] Medullary renal carcinomas tend to affect young African-Americans, originate in the renal medulla, may be associated with a sickle cell trait, and have an aggressive course.[20] Clinical presentation is highly variable including flank pain, hematuria, palpable mass, urinary tract infection, or renal abscess and is associated with distinct immunohistochemical features, including epithelial markers, CAM 5.2, and epithelial membrane antigen.[29,30]

Grading of renal tumors is based on nuclear size, irregularity of the nuclear membrane (shape), and nucleolar prominence, which can be used to characterize the clinical behavior of tumors and serves as a prognostic factor.[22] Nuclear grade classifies cells from grades 1 to 4, with Fuhrman grade 4 tumors having a larger nucleus, a more irregular shape, and a more aggressive behavior, and being associated with a shorter survival.[24] Renal cancer metastasizes via the circulatory and lymphatic systems, involving the retroperitoneal lymph nodes, lungs, liver, bone, muscle, and brain. The most common sites of metastasis involve the lungs, pulmonary and retroperitoneal lymph nodes, liver, and bone. Paraneoplastic syndromes occur in renal cancer and may be the initial

**TABLE 65-1**

**Classification of Epithelial Tumors Arising in the Renal Parenchyma**

| Malignant Tumors |
|---|
| • Conventional (clear cell) RCC<br>• Papillary RCC<br>• Chromophobe RCC<br>• Collecting duct carcinoma ("Bellini duct carcinoma")<br>• Medullary carcinoma |

*Abbreviation*: RCC, renal cell carcinoma.

**TABLE 65-2**

| Paraneoplastic Syndromes |
|---|
| • Hypercalcemia |
| • Erythrocytosis |
| • Thrombocytosis |
| • Anemia |
| • Anorexia |
| • Fever/night sweats |
| • Hypertension |
| • Cachexia |
| • Polyneuromyopathy |
| • Amyloidosis |

symptoms that lead to the diagnosis of renal cancer. These syndromes, which result from biologically active substances or hormones released by the malignant tumor, occur in 10% to 14% of renal cancer patients (Table 65-2).

## CLINICAL MANIFESTATIONS

Renal carcinoma is characterized by diverse symptoms, many of which may be unrelated to the kidney mass. The classic diagnostic triad of gross hematuria, costovertebral pain, and a flank mass is estimated to occur in only 10% to 20% of patients. Additional presenting symptoms include weight loss, anorexia, or symptoms arising from metastatic sites and paraneoplastic syndromes. The lung is the most common site of metastatic disease in renal cancer (in approximately 50% of cases), while other sites of metastasis include the retroperitoneal lymph nodes, liver, bone, adrenal gland, and brain. Renal cancer metastasizes to other sites as well, including the pancreas, abdominal and pelvic muscles, diaphragm, and skin. Asymptomatic brain metastasis may be identified during diagnostic work-up or pretreatment staging studies, with symptomatic disease being diagnosed at any time during the disease. Lytic disease occurs in approximately 30% of patients, emphasizing the importance of early assessment and intervention to reduce the potential for significant functional impairment and morbidity.

Spontaneous regression of metastatic RCC occurs in a small percentage of patients, most often in those individuals with good-risk prognostic criteria and minimal disease, although the immunologic process occurring in such cases is unclear. Spontaneous regression occurs in 3% to 5% of patients with metastatic disease following nephrectomy or during periods of observation.

## ASSESSMENT

Diagnosis of RCC includes the exclusion of other malignant or nonmalignant processes, including benign inflammatory abscesses or pyelonephritis; hematomas within the structure of the kidney; various pseudotumors; and various cystic masses including benign cysts, polycystic kidney, cystic dysplastic kidney, and hydronephrosis. Incidental detection of renal tumors has resulted from increased use of imaging, including ultrasound, computed tomography (CT) scan, and magnetic resonance imaging (MRI) for nonrenal symptoms.[25,26] Patients diagnosed with RCC detected incidentally often have tumors which are smaller, have a lower grade and disease stage than those presenting with symptoms associated with the disease.[31] These patients have a better prognosis and have a higher 5-year cancer-specific survival than those with symptomatic disease.[31]

A detailed review of symptoms, family history, and current physical exam will assist in determining appropriate radiology procedures to be completed. Intravenous urography is often the initial diagnostic procedure done to evaluate nonspecific symptoms including flank pain or hematuria; it assesses the urothelial tract.[26] Ultrasound is a noninvasive procedure that can differentiate between cystic and solid masses. Doppler ultrasound procedures can further evaluate the vascularity of a renal mass and assess the renal vein and inferior vena cava for the presence of tumor thrombus.[26] Computed tomography scans provide highly sensitive imaging, including scans obtained both before and after administration of intravenous contrast. Magnetic resonance imaging may be used in patients in whom intravenous ionic contrast is contraindicated due to allergy. Demonstration of "enhancement" or increased density on CT scan or an increase in signal intensity on MRI after intravenous contrast is given is indicative of increased vascularity associated with a renal mass. Arteriography, venography, and multiphase renal helical CT scan provide information concerning the relationship of the tumor to the collecting system and adjacent normal parenchyma, involvement of anatomical structures within the kidney, and the renal and tumor vascular supply; data essential for preoperative planning and intraoperative management of renal lesions.[32,33] Multiphase imaging includes noncontrast arterial scans that detect calcifications and allow quantification of enhancement on the postcontrast scans, arterial-phase scans that depict the arterial anatomy and perform CT angiography, corticomedullary scans that provide information on the vasculature of the renal mass and kidney, nephrographic scans which are the most sensitive for detecting and characterizing lesions, and excretory phase images that evaluate the renal collecting system and ureters.[34] Three-phase renal CT imaging also provides data for three-dimensional volume rendering in a video format that enhances preoperative and intraoperative planning and management for nephron-sparing surgical procedures.[32] An inferior venacavogram can further delineate the presence and extent of tumor thrombus involvement of the vena cava. Histological confirmation of RCC can be obtained from ultrasound or CT-guided biopsy procedures. F-18 fluorodeoxyglucose positron emission tomography

(FDG-PET) imaging provides information regarding the presence of metastatic lesions and may reduce the need for biopsy procedures.[28]

The prognosis for individuals with RCC takes into account several variables, including grade, tumor histology, TNM staging, and various prognostic groupings. Important prognostic indicators include the TNM staging at diagnosis, tumor histology, tumor grade, and Eastern Cooperative Oncology Group (ECOG) performance status.[24,35] Recent analysis has provided new information regarding prognostic indicators for previously untreated patients with renal carcinoma (Table 65-3), previously treated patients with renal carcinoma (Table 65-4), and patients treated with vascular endothelial growth factor (VEGF)-targeted therapies (Table 65-5).[36–40] Five criteria (Karnofsky performance status (KPS), lactate dehydrogenase, hemoglobin, calcium, and nephrectomy status) were used to retrospectively analyze survival in 670 previously untreated patients, demonstrating 3-year survival rates of 31% for patients in the favorable-risk group (no risk factors), 7% for the intermediate-risk group (1 to 2 risk factors), and 0% for the poor-risk group (3 or more risk factors).[36] Analysis of another group of previously untreated patients identified similar criteria, with the additional criteria related to the number of sites of metastatic disease (fewer than 2 sites or more than 2 sites).[37] The median overall survival in 353 previously untreated patients studied was 14.9 months, with a 32.2-month median survival for patients having a favorable risk (fewer than 2 risk factors), 17.6-month median survival for the intermediate-risk group (3 to 5 risk factors), and 8.8-month median survival for the poor-risk group (more than 5 risk factors).[38]

Three prognostic factors were identified in a group of 251 previously treated patients to categorize them into 3 different groups.[39] Using a multivariate survival analysis, KPS, corrected calcium, and hemoglobin were identified as prognostic factors. Patients with zero factors are considered to have a favorable prognosis with a median survival of 22.1 months. Patients with 1 factor are considered to have an intermediate prognosis with a median survival of 11.9 months, and those with 2 or 3 factors have a poor prognosis with a median survival of 5.4 months.[39] Recently approved therapies for RCC target the VEGF and have significantly changed the prognosis for patients. Clinical features associated with outcome were identified in a review of 120 patients including time from diagnosis to current treatment < 2 years, baseline platelet count > 300 K/μL, baseline neutrophil count > 4.5 K/μL, baseline corrected serum calcium <8.5 mg/dL or > 10.0 mg/dL, and ECOG performance status > 0.[40] Patients with 0 to 1 factors have a favorable prognosis with a median progression-free survival (PFS) of 20.1 months, those with 2 factors have an intermediate prognosis with a median PFS of 13 months, and those with > 3 factors have a poor prognosis with a median PFS of 3.9 months.[40] Further studies in untreated and treated patients with renal cancer will provide additional information relevant to determining appropriate therapeutic strategies and evaluation of outcomes for new anticancer agents.

**TABLE 65-3**

**Prognostic Factors in Untreated, Advanced Renal Carcinoma**

- KPS < 80%
- LDH > 1.5 × upper limit of normal
- Hemoglobin < lower limit of normal
- Corrected serum calcium > 10 mg/dL
- Absence of prior nephrectomy
- Metastasis-free interval
- Number of sites of metastatic disease

*Abbreviations*: KPS, Karnofsky performance status; LDH, low-density lipoprotein cholesterol.

**TABLE 65-4**

**Prognostic Factors in Previously Treated Advanced Renal Carcinoma**

| | |
|---|---|
| • KPS | • < 80% |
| • Corrected serum calcium | • > 10 mg/dL |
| • Hemoglobin | • ≤ 13.0 mg/dL (males)<br>or<br>• ≤ 11.5 mg/dL (females) |

*Abbreviation*: KPS, Karnofsky performance status.

## CLASSIFICATION AND STAGING

Renal carcinoma has been previously classified according to the Robson classification system for RCC staging, but this system does not sufficiently differentiate stages that might have substantially different prognoses.[41] The fifth edition of the American Joint Committee on Cancer's TNM system altered staging criteria to mirror the improved results attained with the contemporary management of renal cancer.[42] The TNM staging system differentiates between

**TABLE 65-5**

**Prognostic Factors in Patients Treated With VEGF-Targeted Therapy**

- Time from diagnosis to current treatment < 2 years
- Baseline platelet count > 300 K/μL
- Baseline neutrophil count > 4.5 K/μL
- Baseline corrected calcium < 8.5 mg/dL or > 10.0 mg/dL
- ECOG status > 0

*Abbreviations*: ECOG, Eastern Cooperative Oncology Group; VEGF, vascular endothelial growth factor.

**TABLE 65-6**

**TNM Staging of Renal Carcinoma**

| | | | |
|---|---|---|---|
| **Primary Tumor (T)** | | | |
| TX | Primary tumor cannot be assessed | | |
| T0 | No evidence of primary tumor | | |
| T1 | Tumor 7 cm or less in greatest dimension limited to the kidney | | |
| T2 | Tumor more than 7 cm in greatest dimension limited to the kidney | | |
| T3 | Tumor extends into major veins or invades the adrenal gland or perinephric tissues, but not beyond Gerota's fascia | | |
| T3a | Tumor invades the adrenal gland or perinephric tissues but not beyond Gerota's fascia | | |
| T3b | Tumor grossly extends into the renal vein(s) or vena cava below the diaphragm | | |
| T3c | Tumor grossly extends into the renal vein(s) or vena cava above the diaphragm | | |
| T4 | Tumor invades beyond Gerota's facia | | |
| **Regional Lymph Nodes (N)**[a] | | | |
| NX | Regional lymph nodes cannot be assessed | | |
| N0 | No regional lymph node metastases | | |
| N1 | Metastasis in a single regional lymph node | | |
| N2 | Metastasis in more than one regional lymph node | | |
| **Distant Metastasis (M)** | | | |
| MX | Distant metastasis cannot be assessed | | |
| M0 | No distant metastasis | | |
| M2 | Distant metastasis | | |
| **Stage Grouping** | | | |
| Stage I | T1 | N0 | M0 |
| Stage II | T2 | N0 | M0 |
| Stage III | T1 | N1 | M0 |
| | T2 | N1 | M0 |
| | T3a | N0 | M0 |
| | T3a | N1 | M0 |
| | T3b | N0 | M0 |
| | T3b | N1 | M0 |
| | T3c | N0 | M0 |
| | T3c | N1 | M0 |
| Stage IV | T4 | N0 | M0 |
| | T4 | N1 | M0 |
| | Any T | N2 | M0 |
| | Any T | Any N | M1 |

[a]Laterality does not affect the N classification.

*Source:* Data from American Joint Committee on Cancer, American Cancer Society, American College of Surgeons.[43]

tumor size, local invasion, vena caval involvement, regional lymph node status, and distant metastasis (Table 65-6).[43] The optimal breakpoint in tumor size for defining localized tumor stage remains controversial, as recent studies demonstrate prognostic differences between small tumors (3–4 cm) and larger tumors (4–7 cm).[44,45]

## THERAPEUTIC APPROACHES AND NURSING CARE

### SURGERY

Nephrectomy has long been the mainstay of treatment for renal carcinoma, but advances in surgical procedures have reduced the need for radical nephrectomy and potential surgical complications. Minimally invasive nephron-sparing surgery preserves functioning of renal parenchyma, with potentially comparable outcomes demonstrated when long-term data are analyzed.[46–48] Procedures include laparoscopic partial or radical nephrectomy (Figures 65-1 and 65-2), probe ablation (cryotherapy or radiofrequency ablation [RFA]), and noninvasive ablation (high-intensity, focused ultrasound), all of which are associated with shorter hospital stays and fewer complications. Laparoscopic partial nephrectomy procedures demonstrate comparable surgical outcomes with minimally invasive techniques.[49,50] Laparoscopic renal cryoablation is appropriate for small (<4 cm) exophytic lesions located away from the collecting system. Laparoscopic radical nephrectomy is appropriate for T1 to T3a N0 M0 lesions without perirenal, lymphatic, or vascular extension. Complications include hemorrhage, ureteral injury, urinary leakage, hematoma, hematuria, incisional hernia, and infection. Long-term follow-up of

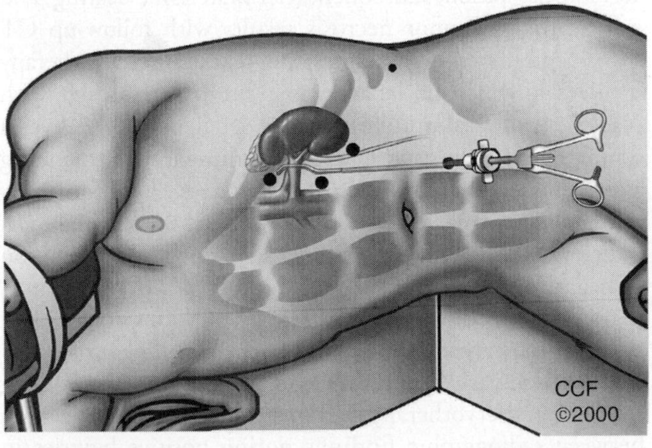


**FIGURE 65-1**

Transperitoneal technique for laparoscopic partial nephrectomy. (Reprinted with the permission of The Cleveland Clinic Center for Medical Art & Photography © 2008. All Rights Reserved.)

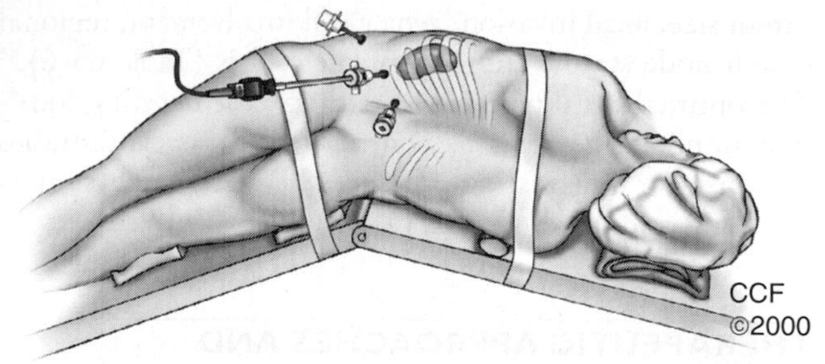


**FIGURE 65-2**

Retroperitoneal technique for laparoscopic partial or radical nephrectomy.

*Source*: Reprinted with the permission of The Cleveland Clinic Center for Medical Art & Photography © 2008. All Rights Reserved.

116 patients undergoing radical nephrectomy demonstrated similar 5-year overall survival, cancer-specific survival, and recurrence-free survival for 63 patients who underwent laparoscopic radical nephrectomy compared to 53 patients who underwent open radical nephrectomy procedures.[51] Elevations in serum creatinine, chronic renal insufficiency were similar for both groups, and no port site recurrences were noted in the laparoscopic group.[51] Nursing care includes monitoring for signs and symptoms of postoperative complications, patient education regarding wound care, and preparation for discharge and home recovery.

Thermal ablation provides an alternative to surgical excision of renal masses for certain situations including elderly patients and those with comorbidities who are not good candidates for partial or radical nephrectomy procedures. Radiofrequency ablation is performed as an outpatient procedure and involves the placement of needle electrodes into the tumor mass to deliver an alternating current that generates ionic agitation, subsequent frictional tissue heating, and cell death.[52,53] Tumor necrosis results with follow-up CT scans demonstrating nonenhancing scar tissue. Cryotherapy involves an open or laparoscopic surgical approach with placement of a cryoprobe into the renal mass to deliver a double freeze-thaw cycle with the resulting iceball extending approximately 1 cm beyond the tumor's edge.[54] Cryotherapy of renal masses results in decreased blood loss, reduced morbidity, and faster recovery, although histologic confirmation of negative margins is not possible.[54,55] Radiographic imaging at 3 and 6 months and intermittent biopsy of residual tissue at the cryosite provide appropriate follow-up for this minimally invasive procedure. Follow-up data are evolving for RFA and cryotherapy demonstrating mixed correlation between radiographic findings noting positive biopsies in both enhancing and nonenhancing imaging; emphasizing the importance on stringent selection criteria, rigorous follow-up, and identification of patients who may require a secondary salvage procedure.[56–58]

Cytoreductive nephrectomy prior to or following systemic therapy can prolong survival and delay disease progression for many patients. Lack of response to systemic treatment, avoidance of symptoms attributable to the primary tumor, and studies which demonstrate improvements in survival when nephrectomy is done prior to systemic treatment all support the role of cytoreductive nephrectomy.[59,60] A combined analysis of 2 prospective randomized trials comparing cytoreductive nephrectomy plus interferon (IFN) α-2b vs IFN-α-2b alone in 331 patients with metastatic renal cancer demonstrated a median survival of 13.6 months for patients who had nephrectomy followed by IFN compared to 7.8 months, representing a 31% decrease in the risk of death ($P = 0.002$).[60]

Resection of metastatic disease following immunotherapy or targeted therapy appears to be safe and may result in a significant disease-free period for patients who have a good performance status and minimal disease burden.[61–63] Prospective clinical trials involving treatment with targeted therapies in renal cancer are ongoing with careful attention to risk-benefit ratio, clinical outcomes, quality-of-life assessment, and long-term follow-up.

Follow-up care for patients after nephrectomy includes surveillance reflecting the stage of disease at diagnosis. Patients with stage I disease should be monitored yearly with a physical exam and blood studies. Those with stage II disease should be monitored yearly with a physical exam, blood studies, chest x-ray, and CT scans every 2 years. Patients with stage III disease will typically be monitored every 6 months with blood studies, chest x-ray, and CT scans for several years, with the interval between procedures increasing after 2 years. Those with stage IV disease will be monitored every 2 to 3 months during treatment to assess the effectiveness and appropriateness of treatment.

Nursing care of patients hospitalized for surgery includes patient and family education, support, and coordination of care. Discharge planning focuses on skin, wound and postoperative drain care, maximization of nutritional intake, effective pain management, and follow-up care. The goal is to minimize the incidence and severity of postoperative complications and ensure timely initiation of systemic therapy for patients with metastatic disease. More detailed information regarding nursing care of the surgical patient can be found in Chapter 11.

## TARGETED THERAPY

Significant advances in the treatment of RCC have occurred over the past 5 years leading to the FDA approval of 5 agents, with several more progressing through the clinical trial process. Sorafenib (Nexavar, Bayer & Onyx Pharmaceuticals, Emeryville, CA) was approved in December 2005; sunitinib malate (Sutent, Pfizer, La Jolla, CA) was approved in January 2006; temsirolimus

(Torisel, Wyeth Pharmaceuticals, Philadelphia, PA) was approved in May 2007; everolimus (Afinitor, Novartis Pharmaceuticals, East Hanover, NJ) was approved in March 2009; and bevacizumab (Avastin, Genentech Inc., South San Francisco, CA) in combination with IFN-α was approved in July 2009. The development of targeted therapy in renal cancer has resulted from significant gains in understanding the molecular biology of RCC, and the role of mutation or inactivation of the VHL tumor suppressor gene. Patients with the dominantly inherited VHL disease develop multiple bilateral renal masses in addition to other tumors.[64] VHL somatic mutations or VHL gene allele deletions occur in approximately 60% of sporadic clear cell renal cancers, rendering the gene transcriptionally inactive.[64,65] The VHL gene product (pVHL) targets the hypoxia-inducible factor (HIF) for proteosome degradation in the presence of oxygen. Hypoxic cells or those lacking pVHL, the VHL protein does not bind to HIF-α resulting in the accumulation of high levels of HIF which activates the transcription of a variety of genes including VEGF, platelet-derived growth factor, and transforming growth factor α.[66] In sporadic clear cell renal cancer, the loss of the VHL gene leads to VEGF overexpression which drives tumor angiogenesis making inhibition of VEGF and downstream signaling a therapeutic target in RCC (Figure 65-3).[65]

Sorafenib is an oral multikinase inhibitor of RAF-1, VEGFR-1, VEGFR-2, VEGFR-3, PDGFR-a, Flt-3, and c-KIT resulting in the inhibition of tumor angiogenesis and tumor-cell proliferation (Figure 65-4).[67] A phase III, randomized, double-blind, placebo-controlled trial of 903 patients refractory to front-line therapy, which began in 2003 demonstrated a PFS of 5.5 months compared to 2.8 months.[68] Based on the statistical benefit of sorafenib over placebo, the study was unblinded and crossover was permitted from placebo to sorafenib in May 2005. The median overall survival for patients randomized to sorafenib was 17.8 months, compared to 14.3 months for the placebo group, and the drug received FDA approval for the treatment of advanced RCC in December 2005.[68] A phase II randomized trial of sorafenib vs IFN-α as front-line therapy in 189 patients with advanced clear cell carcinoma demonstrated no difference between the PFS for the sorafenib patients (5.7 months) vs the IFN patients (5.6 months).[69] Common side effects experienced by patients treated with sorafenib included diarrhea, fatigue, hand–foot skin reaction, and hypertension.[70] See hyperkeratosis related to sorafenib (Color plate 10).

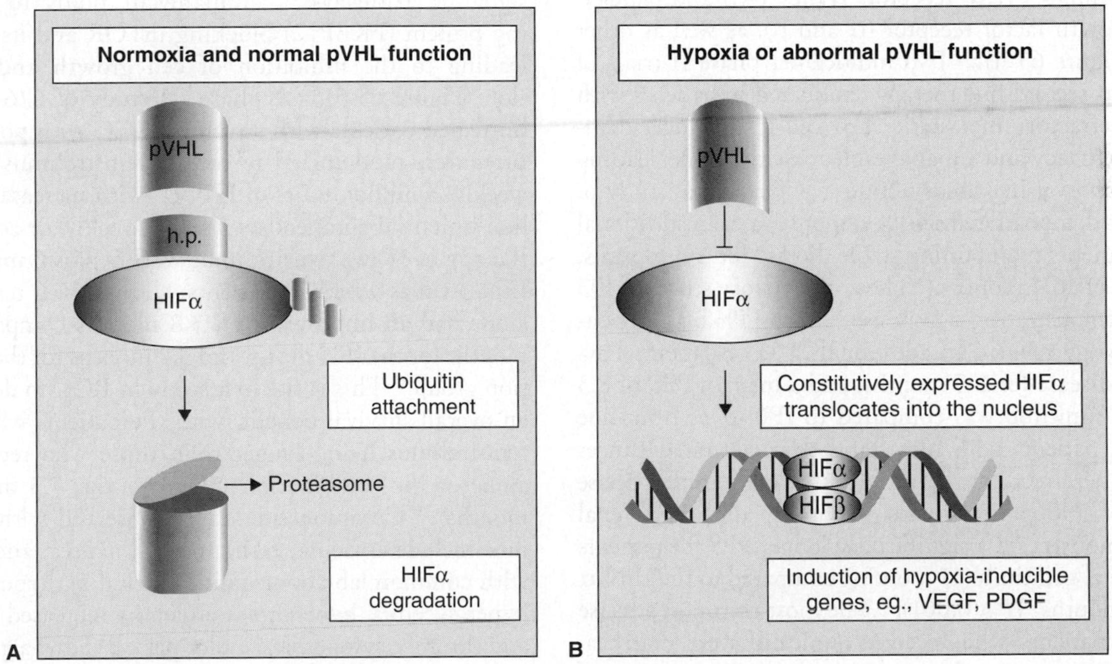


**FIGURE 65-3**

**(A)** In normoxic cells (normal oxygen tension) and clear cell renal cancer cells with normal VHL gene function, the von Hippel-Lindau protein gene product (pVHL) binds hypoxia-inducible factor-α (HIF-α) leading to ubiquitination and degradation in the proteasome. **(B)** In hypoxic cells and clear cell renal cancer cells with abnormal VHL function, pVHL does not bind to HIF-α leading to transcription of hypoxia-inducible genes, including VEGF and PDGF.

*Source:* Rini and Small.[65] Reprinted with permission. 

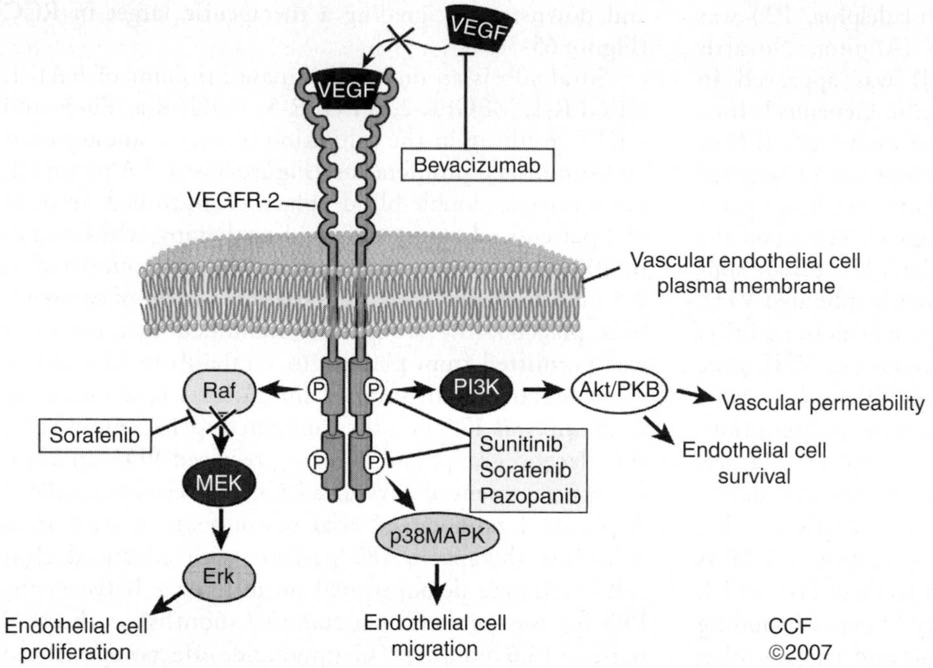


**FIGURE 65-4**

VEGF targets and anti-VEGF therapeutic strategies. Sunitinib and sorafenib are small molecule tyrosine kinase inhibitors which decrease VEGF and other downstream targets and intracellular kinase pathways inhibiting cell proliferation and angiogenesis. Bevacizumab binds and neutralizes biologically active isoforms of VEGF reducing the number of VEGF ligands available to bind to VEGFR-2, thus inhibiting downstream signaling and angiogenesis.

*Source*: Reprinted with the permission of The Cleveland Clinic Center for Medical Art & Photography © 2008. All Rights Reserved.

Sunitinib malate is a multikinase inhibitor that specifically inhibits VEGF receptors (types 1–3) and platelet-derived growth factor receptor (α and β), as well as other kinases (Figure 65-4).[71] Two multicenter phase II trials of sunitinib as second-line therapy conducted in patients with cytokine-refractory metastatic clear cell renal cancer demonstrated efficacy and a manageable toxicity profile, leading to FDA approval in January 2006.[72,73] The initial study of 63 patients demonstrated a 40% response rate, an additional 27% of patients maintaining stable disease for ≥ 3 months, and a PFS of 16.4 months.[72] The confirmatory study of 103 patients demonstrating a response rate of 34% by independent radiology review, an additional 29% of patients having stable disease for ≥ 3 months, and a median PFS of 8.3 months.[73] Sunitinib was compared to IFN-α as front-line therapy in patients with metastatic clear cell renal cancer following nephrectomy. A multicenter randomized phase III trial of 750 patients with previously untreated renal cancer demonstrated a significantly longer PFS for patients who received sunitinib (11 months) compared to the IFN-α group (5 months) ($P < 0.001$).[74] The most common adverse events by patients who received sunitinib were diarrhea, fatigue nausea, stomatitis, vomiting, hypertension, and hand–foot syndrome.[74] See Color Plate 9 for acral erythema due to sunitinib. The most common laboratory abnormalities in the sunitinib arm were leucopenia, neutropenia, anemia, increased creatinine, and thrombocytopenia.[74]

Temsirolimus is an inhibitor of mammalian target of rapamycin (mTOR), which is an important regulator of cell proliferation, cell growth, cell survival, and is implicated in multiple tumor-promoting intracellular signaling pathways.[75,76] Rapamycin binds to FK binding protein (FKBP12) blocking mTOR and its functions, leading to the inhibition of cell growth and proliferation (Figure 65-5).[77] A phase III study of 626 previously untreated patients with advanced RCC with poor-risk features were randomized to receive temsirolimus 25 mg IV weekly, 3 million units of IFN-α (with increase to 18 million units) subcutaneously 3 times weekly, or combination therapy of 15 mg temsirolimus weekly plus 6 million units IFN 3 times weekly.[78] Patients who received temsirolimus alone had an improved PFS 3.8 months compared to 1.9 months for the IFN group and 3.7 months for the combination group.[78] This is the first study in RCC to demonstrate an overall survival benefit, with the patients who received temsirolimus living longer than those who received IFN alone or the combination (10.9 months, 7.3 months, 8.4 months).[78] Common side effects observed with temsirolimus include asthenia, rash, anemia, nausea, and anorexia; with common lab abnormalities including hyperlipidemia, hyperglycemia, hypercholesterolemia, increased creatinine, and thrombocytopenia.[78] Color plate 8 shows a grade 3 rash due to temsirolimus. Temsirolimus received FDA approval for the treatment of advanced RCC in May 2007.

Everolimus (Afinitor), Novartis, East Hanover, NJ) is an oral mTOR pathway inhibitor which disrupts the growth, division, and metabolism of cancer cells (Figure 65-5).[79] Everolimus was evaluated in a double-blind, placebo-controlled trial of 410 patients who had failed VEGFr-TKI therapy for metastatic renal cancer. Everolimus

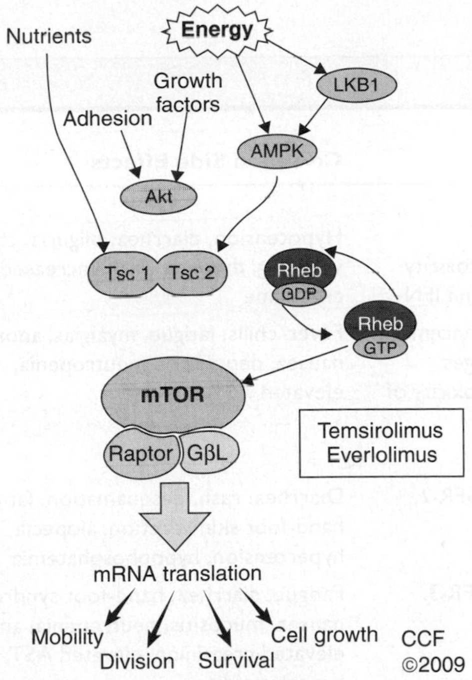


**FIGURE 65-5**

mTOR targets and anti-mTOR therapeutic strategies. The mammalian target of rapamycin (mTOR) is an important regulator of cell proliferation, growth, and survival. Temsirolimus and everolimus inhibit mTOR resulting in reduced levels of hypoxia-inducible factor, VEGF, and other proteins necessary for tumor cell progression and survival.

*Source*: Reprinted with the permission of The Cleveland Clinic Center for Medical Art & Photography © 2008. All Rights Reserved.

demonstrated a PFS of 4.0 months vs 1.9 months ($P < 0.001$).[80] Everolimus was approved by the FDA for the treatment of patients with advanced RCC after failure of treatment with sunitinib or sorafenib in March 2009.

Bevacizumab (Avastin, Genentech, South San Francisco, CA) binds with the VEGF ligand, blocking one of the key signals for tumor angiogenesis (Figure 65-4), and has demonstrated efficacy in combination with IFN-α in several clinical trials in clear cell renal cancer. The combination of Bevacizumab with IFN-α demonstrated a superior response rate compared to IFN alone in 2 randomized studies of patients with previously untreated RCC.[81,82] These studies provide additional support for the benefit of bevacizumab in renal cancer demonstrated in earlier studies and led to the FDA approval of bevacizumab in combination with IFN-α for the treatment of metastatic RCC.[81–84]

Ongoing clinical trials involving approved and investigational agents as sequential therapy and in combination with other cytokines or targeted therapy will provide clinicians with valuable information on the efficacy, risks, and benefits of the ever expanding armamentarium available for patients with RCC.

The recent approval of several targeted therapies for RCC allows patients to receive most treatments on an outpatient basis, and in many cases allows self-administration with limited planned interaction with oncology team members for ongoing assessment and intervention of side effects before they become moderate to severe in nature, potentially having a negative impact on efficacy and quality of life (see Table 65-7).[85–93] Patient education must include information on drug formulation, dosing, potential drug interactions, potential side effects, and their assessment and management. Emphasis on the early notification regarding the development of side effects will allow early intervention, ongoing assessment and evaluation of interventions, allowing patients to receive the maximal benefit of therapy while minimizing the severity of side effects, and the resulting negative impact on efficacy, outcome, and quality of life. Side effects associated with oral anti-VEGF therapies include fatigue, gastrointestinal, dermatological, and cardiac effects. Nursing care includes detailed assessment of fatigue, which has been defined as a persistent subjective sense of tiredness related to cancer or cancer treatment that interferes with usual functioning.[94] Detailed review of disease-related symptoms, comorbid conditions, and concurrent medications at the initiation of treatment provides oncology clinicians a baseline for assessment of side effects and impact on patient functionality and quality of life.

Gastrointestinal side effects include diarrhea, nausea, vomiting, taste changes, anorexia, and weight loss. Patients with disease-related nausea, vomiting, anorexia, or weight loss should be seen in the clinic every 2 weeks during the first few cycles of therapy to allow for frequent clinical assessment and intervention. Patients who experience nausea, vomiting, or diarrhea should have laboratory tests done to monitor electrolytes and renal function, administering IV fluids, and antiemetics as clinically appropriate.[95] Diarrhea is common with sorafenib and sunitinib and may require frequent assessment and adjustment of interventions including dietary modifications, loperamide, diphenoxylate hydrochloride and atropine sulfate, and the use of bulking agents.[95,96] Continued diarrhea associated with worsening fatigue, hypotension, or dehydration may require intravenous hydration, treatment interruption, and/or dose modification.

Dermatological side effects include dry skin, rash, pruritis, callus formation, flat blister formation, and possible desquamation. Refer to the 3 color plates here as well. These side effects may range from mild to severe requiring treatment interruption and dose modification, and the onset of symptoms varies greatly.[96–98] Nursing assessment should include a timeline regarding the initiation of therapy and the onset of dermatological side effects, and include assessment of area involved (anatomical location), type of dermatological reaction (rash, blisters, calluses), color changes (acral erythema, blanching), symptoms associated with the reaction (pruritis,

**TABLE 65-7**

**Therapeutic Options in Renal Cell Carcinoma**

| Class | Route of Administration | Mechanism of Action | Common Side Effects |
|---|---|---|---|
| **Immunotherapy** | | | |
| Interleukin-2 (aldesleukin [Proleukin]) | IV, SC | Activation of cellular immunity, enhancement of lymphocyte cytotoxicity, induction of LAK cells, NK cells, and IFN-γ | Hypotension, diarrhea, oliguria, chills, vomiting, dyspnea, rash, increased creatinine |
| Interferon | SC | Immunomodulatory activities, enhancement of phagocytic activity of macrophages, augmentation of the specific cytotoxicity of lymphocytes for target cells | Fever, chills, fatigue, myalgias, anorexia, nausea, depression, neutropenia, elevated AST |
| **Targeted Therapy** | | | |
| Sorafenib (Nexavar) | PO | Inhibits RAF, Flt-3, VEGFR-1, VEGFR-2, VEGFR-3, VEGFR-4 | Diarrhea, rash, desquamation, fatigue, hand-foot skin reaction, alopecia, hypertension, hypophosphatemia |
| Sunitinib (Sutent) | PO | Inhibits VEGFR-1, VEGFR-2, VEGFR-3, PDGFR-α, PDGFR-β, c-kit, Flt-3 | Fatigue, diarrhea, hand-foot syndrome, nausea, mucositis, neutropenia, anemia, elevated creatinine, elevated AST, ALT, hypothyroidism |
| Temsirolimus (Torisel) | IV | Inhibits mTOR resulting in reduced levels of HIF-1 a, HIF-2 a, and VEGF | Asthenia, rash, mucositis, nausea, edema, anemia, thrombocytopenia, neutropenia, hyperglycemia, elevated total cholesterol, elevated triglycerides, elevated creatinine |
| Everolimus | PO | Inhibits mTOR leading to inhibition of cell growth and proliferation, angiogenesis, cancer cell metabolism (bioenergetics) | Stomatitis, fatigue, diarrhea, anorexia, hypercholesterolemia, hypertriglyceridemia, hyperglycemia, elevated creatinine |
| Bevacizumab (Avastin) | IV | Binds to VEGF, prevents the interaction of VEGF to its receptors (Flt-1 and KDR) on the surface of endothelial cells leading to reduction in microvascular growth | Hypertension, proteinuria, hemorrhage, delayed wound healing |
| Pazopanib (Votrient) | PO | Inhibits VEGFR-1, VEGFR-2, VEGFR-3, PDGFR-α and -β, FGFR-1 and -3, c-kit, and others. | Elevated AST, ALT, diarrhea, hyperglycemia, hypertension, hair color changes, leukopenia, elevated bilirubin, neutropenia, thrombocytopenia |

*Abbreviations*: ALT, alanine aminotransferase; AST, aspartate aminotransferase; IFN-γ, interferon-gamma; IV, intravenously; LAK, lymphokine-activated killer; NK, natural killer; SC, subcutaneously; PO, orally; PDGFR, platelet derived growth factor receptor; VEGF, vascular endothelial growth factor; VEGFR, vascular endothelial growth factor receptor.

pain, swelling), presence of desquamation, presence of drainage, and impact on functional status. Patients should be instructed to apply emollients several times daily at the initiation of therapy, with increased application or the addition of other topical products based on dermatological side effects. Findings from a 2008 forum of international medical oncologists, dermatologists, and nurses provides a detailed review of the oral multikinase inhibitors, and the incidence, clinical features, assessment, and management strategies to date.[99]

Cardiac side effects associated with sorafenib or sunitinib include hypertension and rare but serious arrhythmias, thrombotic events, and decreased left ventricular ejection fraction (LVEF). Hypertension is also a common side effect associated with bevacizumab therapy. Hypertension requires close monitoring and is generally easy to manage, while the more serious cardiac events can have a significantly negative impact on current therapy and consideration of future therapeutic interventions. Recent history of thrombotic event, cardiac ischemia, or uncontrolled hypertension may be considered contraindications for treatment with an oral or intravenous anti-VEGF therapy. Hypertension should be closely monitored with initiation or escalation of antihypertensive therapy for systolic blood pressure >150 mm Hg and diastolic blood pressure readings >90 mm Hg. Patients should be given instructions regarding the frequency of blood pressure assessments, diary sheets for recording assessments, and guidelines when to call their oncology provider with changes in their blood pressure readings. Early clinical assessment and intervention will enhance effective control preexisting and treatment-related hypertension allowing patients to maximize the potential for efficacy with minimal cardiac risk. Based on the potential effect of CYP3A4 inhibitors and the lack of available data from clinical studies, dihydropyridones, such as amlodipine and nifedipine, are the preferred class of calcium-channel blockers to be used to treat hypertension associated with sorafenib therapy.[100]

mTOR inhibitors are associated with several unique side effects including elevated glucose, cholesterol, and triglycerides, in addition to hypersensitivity reactions associated with the infusion and rare but potentially life-threatening development of interstitial lung disease. It is important for nurses to monitor patients for these side effects which are not seen with sorafenib and sunitinib.[101,102] Diphenhydramine 25 to 50 mg should be administered prior to each infusion of temsirolimus, with the initial infusion being administered over 60 minutes. Subsequent infusions can be administered over 30 minutes if tolerated.[103] Patients should be monitored for flushing, hives, or complaints of chest pain, shortness of breast, or wheezing which may be associated with hypersensitivity reactions associated with temsirolimus.[101,102] Interruption of the infusion and the administration of antihistamines, corticosteroids, and oxygen therapy as indicated. Premedication with higher doses of antihistamines and/or corticosteroids, and a 60-minute infusion may allow patients to receive additional therapy without infusion-related reactions.

Bone marrow and organ function should be monitored based on the specific therapy in addition to consideration of each patient's clinical status. Myelosuppression associated with sunitinib can cause treatment interruption, delay the initiation of subsequent cycles of treatment, and may lead to dose reduction if neutropenia or thrombocytopenia is significant. For patients receiving temsirolimus, treatment should be held for significant neutropenia, thrombocytopenia, or renal impairment, with consideration of initiation of adjustment of hypoglycemic or lipid-lowering medications as indicated.

## IMMUNOTHERAPY

Cytokine therapy continues to be an option for systemic treatment of metastatic renal cancer based on its ability to stimulate various immune effector cells, including T cells and natural killer (NK) cells, to react to the tumor (see Table 65-7). Aldesleukin (interleukin-2 [IL-2]) is the only FDA-approved therapy for metastatic renal cancer in the US. High-dose intravenous IL-2 has demonstrated a 15% overall response rate; a 7% complete response rate and an 8% partial response rate, both of which are durable; and a median survival of 16.3 months.[104] A 3-arm study of high-dose IV, low-dose IV, and low-dose SC IL-2 found a higher response rate in the high-dose arm, but no difference in survival.[83] A recent retrospective review of 16 patients who received high-dose IL-2 following sorafenib or sunitinib demonstrated unexpected and severe cardiac toxicities demonstrating the potential for increased toxicities in patients receiving IL-2 following antiangiogenic therapy and suggests the need for careful patient selection and additional examination of the potential risks associated with sequential therapy in metastatic renal cancer.[105]

Nursing care of patients receiving IL-2 or IFN focuses on effective management of toxicities, in the hospital or the outpatient setting. Side effects vary according to the dose, route of administration, and duration of therapy, but may include chills, fever, subcutaneous injection site reactions, fluid retention and capillary leak syndrome, and organ toxicities that are generally reversible. Clinical pathways have been established that provide detailed nursing assessments, interventions, and patient education strategies.[106] IFN-α, -β, and -γ remain investigational therapies but provide additional options in clinical trials or for off-label use. The patient receiving high-dose IL-2 requires careful assessment and monitoring for cardiopulmonary toxicities including pulmonary edema, hypoxia, cardiac arrhythmia, and temporary renal impairment, which may require the use of vasopressor support. IL-2 and IFN-α therapy is associated with "constitutional symptoms," including chills, fever, myalgias, and arthralgias, which are typically managed with the use of acetaminophen and anti-inflammatory agents. Nursing care includes patient education for subcutaneous injection and management of side effects including chills, fever, fatigue, taste changes, and anorexia.

## RADIATION

Radiation in renal cancer focuses on symptom management, with occasional use in the initial management of the disease. Palliative radiation for patients with lytic metastasis provides both pain relief and structural stabilization. It may be given following orthopedic surgery, including bone stabilization using rods or pins, and joint replacement for metastatic disease. Palliative radiation is used for pulmonary metastasis and lymphadenopathy causing obstruction, providing relief of cough and postobstructive pneumonia. Surgical intervention prior to radiation for spinal cord compression may improve functional outcome.

The treatment of brain metastasis is best accomplished using a multidisciplinary approach involving neurosurgeons, radiation oncologists, and neuroradiologists in addition to the patient's medical oncologist. Treatment considerations include surgical resection, stereotactic radiosurgery, and whole brain radiotherapy; and should consider the status of the systemic disease, tumor type, KPS, patient's neurological status, number and location of lesions, and the presence of leptomeningeal disease.[107] Surgical resection leads to immediate elimination of a mass compressing surrounding brain structures or causing blockage of the CSF flow, and removal of the source of perifocal edema; and is particularly useful for patients with large (>3 cm) lesions.[107] Stereotactic radiosurgery provides a high dose of radiation to a localized brain tumor volume in a single session with minimal radiation exposure to adjacent tissues and structures.[108] These options provide superior levels of tumor control within the brain resulting in overall survival becoming increasingly dependent on the status of the patient's systemic disease. Whole-brain radiation is appropriate for patients who have disease progression following local intervention, have large tumors, or experience extensive metastasis.[109,110]

### CHEMOTHERAPY

Renal cell carcinoma is generally chemoresistant. Agents including vinblastine, floxuridine, 5-fluorouracil, and gemcitabine have been investigated for its treatment and have demonstrated response rates of 5% to 10%.[111–113] Research continues to define the multidrug resistance observed in kidney cancer, the role of p-glycoprotein and glutathione *S*-transferase, and use of combination strategies.

### SYMPTOM MANAGEMENT AND SUPPORTIVE CARE

Comprehensive care of the patient with renal carcinoma results from detailed assessment of disease-related symptoms, prompt intervention, and ongoing evaluation of medical and nonmedical interventions. Patients may develop complex symptoms that often overlap with toxicities associated with treatment, and they often require a multidisciplinary approach for effective management (Table 65-8). Pain management includes the use of narcotic analgesic agents, radiation, surgery, and bisphosphonate therapy for bone metastasis to reduce the incidence of skeletal-related events. Early diagnosis and intervention will minimize the severity and neurofunctional sequelae of spinal cord compression associated with lytic vertebral involvement. Physical therapy and rehabilitation services will assist patients with neurological impairments to return home, providing guidance to patients and family members regarding modifications to the home setting to facilitate patient safety while maximizing functional abilities. Erythrocytosis is rare, and phlebotomy should be considered for a hematocrit greater than 55 g/dL. Management of complex disease-related gastrointestinal symptoms will allow patients to tolerate anticancer therapies that might otherwise result in dose modification or discontinuation in treatment. Collaboration with palliative care specialists provides opportunities for coordination of multiple modalities so as to enhance therapeutic outcomes, ultimately improving quality of life.

**TABLE 65-8**

**Symptoms Associated With Renal Cancer**

- Pain
  - Tumor compression
  - Bone metastasis
  - Nerve root compression
- Gastrointestinal
  - Nausea
  - Vomiting
  - Anorexia
  - Constipation
  - Diarrhea
- Neurologic
  - Fatigue
  - Depression
  - Confusion due to brain metastasis
  - Impaired mobility due to bone metastasis or fracture
- Hematological
  - Anemia
  - Erythrocytosis
  - Thrombocytosis

## CONCLUSION

Treatment options for renal cancer have changed dramatically over the past 5 years with the FDA approval of 5 targeted therapies. Sorafenib, sunitinib, temsirolimus, everolimus, and bevacizumab in combination with IFN-$\alpha$ are the result of understanding the molecular biology of the disease, and signaling pathways that promote tumor progression and vascular development. Renal carcinomas are highly vascular tumors, and targeting VEGF and its associated pathways provides an approach to reduce the development or delay the progression of metastatic disease. Understanding the role of mTOR in renal cancer and the development of therapies to inhibit the mTOR pathway provide additional therapeutic strategies to treat RCC. Continued efforts in the identification, development, and clinical application of tumor antigens, tumor markers, and pathways involved in tumor progression will provide valuable information in the diagnosis and management of RCC.

## REFERENCES

1. Uzzo RG, Cairns P, Al-Saleem T, et al. The basic biology and immunobiology of renal cell carcinoma: considerations for the clinician. *Urol Clin North Am.* 2003;30:423–436.

2. Jamal A, Siegel R, Ward E, et al. Cancer statistics, 2009. *CA: Cancer J Clin.* 2009;59:225–249.
3. Surveillance, Epidemiology, and End Results: Kidney Cancer. http://seer.cancer.gov/statfacts/html/kidpr.html. Accessed August 30,2009.
4. Chow WH, Devesa SS, Warren JL, et al. The rising incidence of renal cell cancer in the United States. *JAMA.* 1999;281:1628–1631.
5. Hock LM, Lynch J, Balaju KC. Increasing incidence of all stages of kidney cancer in the last 2 decades in the United States: an analysis of surveillance, epidemiology and end results Program data. *J Urol.* 2002;167:57–60.
6. Russo P. Renal cell carcinoma: presentation, staging, and surgical treatment. *Semin Oncol.* 2000;27:160–176.
7. Tsui KH, Shvarts O, Smith RB, et al. Renal cell carcinoma: prognostic significance of incidentally detected tumors. *J Urol.* 2000;163:426–430.
8. Enquist D, Zambrano N, Zbar B, et al. Molecular genetics of renal cell carcinoma. In: Bukowski RM, Novick AC, eds. *Renal Cell Carcinoma: Molecular Biology, Immunology, and Clinical Management.* Totowa, NJ: Humana Press; 2000:79–92.
9. Rini BI, Vogelzang NJ. Prognostic factors in renal carcinoma. *Semin Oncol.* 2000;27:213–220.
10. Hwang JJ, Uchio EM, Linehan WM, et al. Hereditary kidney cancer. *Urol Clin North Am.* 2003;30:831–842.
11. Middelton L, Lessick M. Inherited urologic malignant disorders: nursing implications. *Urol Nurs.* 2003;23:15–29.
12. Cohn EB, Campbell SC. Screening for renal cell carcinoma. In: Bukowski RM, Novick AC, eds. *Renal Cell Carcinoma: Molecular Biology, Immunology, and Clinical Management.* Totowa, NJ: Humana Press; 2000:93–110.
13. Van Dijik BA, Schouten LJ, Kiemeney LA, et al. Vegetable and fruit consumption and risk of renal cell carcinoma: results from the Netherlands cohort study. *Int J Cancer.* 2005;117:648–654.
14. Bjorge T, Treli S, Engeland A. Relation of height and body mass index to renal cell carcinoma in two million Norwegian men and women. *Am J Epidemiol.* 2004;160:1168–1176.
15. Rashidkhani B, Akesson A, Lindblad P, et al. Major dietary patterns and risk of renal cell carcinoma in a prospective cohort of Swedish women. *J Nutr.* 2005;135:1757–1762.
16. Rashidkhani B, Lindblad P, Wolk A. Fruits, vegetables and risk of renal cell carcinoma: a prospective study of Swedish women. *Int J Cancer.* 2005;113:451–455.
17. Rini BI, Campbell SC, Rathmell WK. Renal cell carcinoma. *Curr Opin Oncol.* 2006;18:289–296.
18. Uzzo RG, Cairns P, Al-Saleem T, et al. The basic biology and immunobiology of renal cell carcinoma: considerations for the clinician. *Urol Clin North Am.* 2003;30:423–436.
19. Reuter VE, Presti JC. Contemporary approach to classification of renal epithelial tumors. *Semin Oncol.* 2000;27:124–137.
20. Hattab EM, Cheng L, Eble JN. Neoplams of the kidney. In: Zhou M, Magi-Galluzzi C, Goldblum JR, eds. *Genitourinary Pathology.* Philadelphia, PA: Churchill Livingstone Elsevier: 2007:281–340.
21. Levin HS, Myles JL. The pathology of renal neoplasms. In: Bukowski RM, Novick AC, eds. *Renal Cell Carcinoma: Molecular Biology, Immunology, and Clinical Management.* Totowa, NJ: Humana Press; 2000:15–38.
22. Pantuck AJ, Zisman A, Belldegrun A. Basic biology and clinical behavior of renal cell carcinoma. In: Belldegrun A, Ritchie AWS, Figlin RA, et al, eds. *Renal and Adrenal Tumors: Biology and Management.* New York: Oxford University Press; 2003:81–89.
23. Lam JS, Belldegrun AS, Pantuck AJ. Long-term outcomes of the surgical management of renal cell carcinoma. *J Urol.* 2006;24:255–266.
24. Tsui K, Shvarts O, Smith RB, et al. Prognostic indicators for renal cell carcinoma: a multivariate analysis of 643 patients using the revised 1997 TNM staging criteria. *J Urol.* 2000;163:1090–1095.
25. Israel GM, Bosniak MA. Renal imaging for diagnosis and staging of renal cell carcinoma. *Urol Clin North Am.* 2003;30:499–514.
26. Hilton S. Imaging of renal cell carcinoma. *Semin Oncol.* 2003;27:150–159.
27. Margulis V, Tamboli P, Matin SF, et al. Analysis of clinicopathologic predictors of oncologic outcome provides insight into the natural history of surgically managed papillary renal cell carcinoma. *Cancer.* 2008;112:1480–1488.
28. Majhail NS, Urbain JL, Albani JM, et al. F-18 fluorodeoxyglucose positron emission tomography in the evaluation of distant metastases from renal cell carcinoma. *J Clin Oncol.* 2003;21:3995–4000.
29. Swartz MA, Karth J, Schneider DT, et al. Renal medullary carcinoma: clinical, pathologic, immunohistochemical, and genetic analysis with pathogenic implications. *Urology.* 2002;60:1083–1089.
30. Baig MA, Lin YS, Rasheed J, et al. Renal medullary carcinoma. *J Nat Med Assoc.* 2006;98:1171–1174.
31. Tsui KH, Shvarts O, Smith RB, et al. Renal cell carcinoma: prognostic significance of incidentally detected tumors. *J Urol.* 2000;163:426–430.
32. Derweesh IH, Herts B, Novick AC. Three-dimensional image reconstruction for preplanning of renal surgery. *Urol Clin North Am.* 2003;30:515–528.
33. Dyer R, DiSantis DJ, McClennan BL. Simplified imaging approach for evaluation of the solid renal mass in adults. *Radiology.* 2008;247:331–343.
34. Coll DM, Smith RC. Update on radiological imaging of renal cell carcinoma. *BJU Int.* 2007;99:1217–1222.
35. Russo P. Renal cell carcinoma: presentation, staging, and surgical treatment. *Semin Oncol.* 2000;27:160–176.
36. Motzer RJ, Mazumdar M, Bacik J, et al. Survival and prognostic stratification of 670 patients with advanced renal cell carcinoma. *J Clin Oncol.* 1999;17:2530–2540.
37. Mekhail TM, Abou-Jawde RM, Merhi GB, et al. Validation and extension of the Memorial Sloan-Kettering prognostic factors model for survival in patients with previously untreated metastatic renal cell carcinoma. *J Clin Oncol.* 2005;23:832–841.
38. Elson P. Prognostic factors in advance renal cell carcinoma. In: Belldegrun A, Ritchie AWS, Figlin RA, et al, eds. *Renal and Adrenal Tumors: Biology and Management.* New York: Oxford University Press: 2003:186–194.
39. Motzer RJ, Bacik J, Schwartz LH, et al. Prognostic factors for survival in previously treated patients with metastatic renal cell carcinoma. *J Clin Oncol.* 2004;22:454–463.
40. Choueiri TK, Garcia JA, Elson P, et al. Clinical factors associated with outcomes in patients with metastatic clear-cell renal cell carcinoma treated with vascular endothelial growth factor-targeted therapy. *Cancer.* 2007;110:543–550.
41. Pantuck AG, Zisman A, Belldegrum AS. The changing natural history of renal cell carcinoma. *J Urol.* 2001;166:1611–1623.
42. Leibovich BC, Pantuck AJ, Matthew HT, et al. Current staging of renal cell carcinoma. *Urol Clin North Am.* 2003;30:481–497.
43. American Joint Committee on Cancer, American Cancer Society, American College of Surgeons. Kidney cancer. In: *AJCC Cancer Staging Handbook.* Philadelphia, PA: Lippincott-Raven; 2002.
44. Hafez KS, Fergany AF, Novick AC. Nephron sparing surgery for localized renal cell carcinoma: impact of tumor size on patient survival, tumor recurrence and TNM staging. *J Urol.* 1999;162:1930–1933.
45. Zisman A, Pantuck AH, Chao D, et al. Reevaluation of the 1997 TNM classification for renal cell carcinoma: T1 and T2 cutoff point at 4.5 rather than 7 cm better correlates with clinical outcome. *J Urol.* 2001;166:54–58.
46. Gill IS. Minimally invasive nephron-sparing surgery. *Urol Clin North Am.* 2003;30:551–579.
47. Margulis V, Tamboli P, Jacobsohn KM, Swanson DA, Wood CG. Oncological efficacy and safety of nephron-sparing surgery for selected patients with locally advanced renal cell carcinoma. *BJU Int.* 2007;100:1235–1239.
48. Weight CJ, Fergany AF, Gunn PW, et al. The impact of minimally invasive techniques on open partial nephrectomy: a 10-year single institutional experience. *J Urol.* 2008;180:84–88.

49. Gill IS, Desai MM, Kaouk JH, et al. Laparoscopic partial nephrectomy for renal tumor: duplicating open surgical techniques. *J Urol.* 2002;167:469–476.
50. Gill IS, Matin SF, Desai MM, et al. Comparative analysis of laparoscopic versus open partial nephrectomy for renal tumors in 200 patients. *J Urol.* 2003;170:64–68.
51. Colombo JR, Haber GP, Jelovsek JE, et al. Seven years after laparoscopic radical nephrectomy: oncologic and renal functional outcomes. *Urology.* 2008;71:1149–1154.
52. Gillams AR. The use of radiofrequency in cancer. *Br J Cancer.* 2005;92: 1825–1929.
53. Locklin JK, Wood BJ. Radiofrequency ablation: a nursing perspective. *Clin J Oncol Nurs.* 2005;9:346–349.
54. Gill IS, Novic AC, Meraney AM, et al. Laparoscopic renal cryoablation in 32 patients. *Urology.* 2000;56:748–753.
55. Schwartz BF, Rewcastle JC, Powell T, et al. Cryoablation of small peripheral renal masses: a retrospective analysis. *Urology.* 2006;68(suppl 1A):14–18.
56. Weight CJ, Kaouk JH, Hegarty NJ, et al. Correlation of radiographic imaging and histopathology following cryoablation and radio frequency ablation for renal tumors. *J Urol.* 2008;179:1277–1283.
57. Davol PE, Fulmer BR, Rukstalis DB. Long-term results of cryoablation for renal cancer and complex renal masses. *Urology.* 2006;68(suppl 1A): 1–6.
58. Matin SF, Ahrar K. Nephron-sparing probe ablation therapy: long-term outcomes. *Curr Opin Urol.* 2008;18:150–156.
59. Wood CG. The role of cytoreductive nephrectomy in the management of metastatic renal cell carcinoma. *Urol Clin North Am.* 2003;30:581–588.
60. Flanigan RC, Mickisch G, Sylvester R, et al. Cytoreductive nephrectomy in patients with metastatic renal cancer: a combined analysis. *J Urol.* 2004;171:1071–1076.
61. Margulis V, Matin SF, Tannir N, et al. Surgical morbidity associated with administration of targeted molecular therapies before cytoreductive nephrectomy or resection of locally recurrent renal cell carcinoma. *J Urol.* 2008;180:94–98.
62. Wood GC. Multimodal approaches in the management of locally advanced and metastatic renal cell carcinoma: combining surgery and systemic therapies to improve patient outcomes. *Clin Cancer Res.* 2007;13(suppl 2):697s–702s.
63. Rini BI, Campbell SC. The evolving role of surgery for advanced renal cell carcinoma in the era of molecular targeted therapy. *J Urol.* 2007; 177:1978–1984.
64. Gnarra JR, Tory K, Weng Y, et al. Mutations of the VHL tumour suppressor gene in renal carcinoma. *Nat Genet.* 1994;7:85–90.
65. Rini BI, Small EJ. Biology and clinical development of vascular endothelial growth factor-targeted therapy in renal cell carcinoma. *J Clin Oncol.* 2005;23:1028–1043.
66. Kaelin WG. The von Hippel-Lindau tumor suppressor gene and kidney cancer. *Clin Cancer Res.* 2004;10(suppl):6290s–6295s.
67. Wihelm SM, Carter C, Tang L, et al. BAY 43–9006 exhibits broad spectrum oral antitumor activity and targets the RAF/MEK/ERK pathway and receptor tyrosine kinases involved in tumor progression and angiogenesis. *Cancer Res.* 2004;64:7099–7109.
68. Escudier B, Eisen T, Stadler WM, et al. Sorafenib in advanced clear-cell renal-cell carcinoma. *N Engl J Med.* 2007;356:125–134.
69. Szczylik C, Demkow T, Staehler M, et al. Randomized phase II trial of first-line treatment with sorafenib versus interferon in patients with advanced renal cell carcinoma: final results. *J Clin Oncol.* 2007;25(18s Part I of II):Abstract #5025.
70. Bayer. Sorafenib Package Insert. West Haven, CT: Bayer Pharmaceuticals Corporation; 2009.
71. Mendel DB, Laird AD, Xin X, et al. In vivo antitumor activity of SU11248, a novel tyrosine kinase inhibitor targeting vascular endothelial growth factor and platelet-derived growth factor receptors. *Clin Cancer Res.* 2003;9:327–337.
72. Motzer RJ, Michaelson MD, Redman BG, et al. Activity of SU11248, a multitargeted inhibitor of vascular endothelial growth factor receptor and platelet-derived growth factor receptor, in patients with metastatic renal cell carcinoma. *J Clin Oncol.* 2006;24:1–8.
73. Motzer RJ, Rini BI, Bukowski RM, et al. Sunitinib in patients with metastatic renal cell carcinoma. *JAMA.* 2006;295:2516–2524.
74. Motzer RJ, Hutson TE, Tomczak P, et al. Sunitinib versus interferon alfa in metastatic renal-cell carcinoma. *N Engl J Med.* 2007;356:115–124.
75. Huang S, Houghton PJ. Targeting mTOR signaling for cancer therapy. *Curr Opin Pharmacol.* 2003;3:371–377.
76. Rini BI. Temsirolimus, an inhibitor of mammalian target of rapamycin. *Clin Cancer Res.* 2008;14:1286–1290.
77. Dutcher JP. Mammalian target of rapamycin. *Clin Cancer Res.* 2004; 10(suppl.):6382s–6387s.
78. Hudes G, Carducci M, Tomczak P, et al. Temsirolimus, interferon alfa, or both for advanced renal-cell carcinoma. *N Engl J Med.* 2007;356: 2271–2281.
79. O'Donnell AO, Faivre S, Burris HA, et al. Phase I pharmacokinetic and pharmacodynamic study of the oral mammalian target of rapamycin inhibitor Everolimus in patients with advanced solid tumors. *J Clin Oncol.* 2008;26:1588–1595.
80. Motzer RJ, Escudier B, Oudard S, et al. RAD001 versus placebo in patients with metastatic renal cell carcinoma (RCC) after progression on VEGFr-TKI therapy: results from a randomized, double-blind, multicenter phase III study. *J Clin Oncol.* 2008;26(18s part II of II): LBA5026.
81. Escudier B, Pluzanska A, Koralewski P, et al. Bevacizumab plus interferon alfa-2a for the treatment of metastatic renal cell carcinoma: a randomised double-blind phase III trial. *Lancet.* 2007;320:2103–2111.
82. Rini BI, Halabi S, Rosenberg JE, et al. Bevacizumab plus interferon alfa compared with interferon alfa monotherapy in patients with metastatic renal cell carcinoma: CALGB 90206. *J Clin Oncol.* 2008;26: 5422–5428.
83. Yang JC, Haworth L, Sherry RM, et al. A randomized trial of bevacizumab, an anti-vascular endothelial growth factor antibody, for metastatic renal cancer. *N Engl J Med.* 2003;349:427–434.
84. Bukowski RM, Kabbinavar FF, Figlin RA, et al. Randomized phase II study of erlotinib combined with bevacizumab compared with bevacizumab alone in metastatic renal cell cancer. *J Clin Oncol.* 2007;25: 4536–4541.
85. Interleukin-2 (Proleukin Aldesleukin for injection) package insert. East Hanover, NJ: Novartis Pharmaceuticals Corp.; June 2007.
86. Intron A (Interferon alfa-2b, recombinant for injection) package insert. Kenilworth, NJ: Schering-Plough; June 2008.
87. Pazopanib (Votrient) package insert. GlaxoSmithKline., Research Triangle Park, NC. October 2009.
88. Avastin (Bevacizumab for intravenous use) package insert. South San Francisco, CA: Genentech BioOncology; November 2008.
89. Bukowski RM, Kabbinavar FF, Figlin RA, et al. 2008. Randomized phase II study of erlotinib combined with bevacizumab compared with bevacizumab alone in metastatic renal cell cancer. *J Clin Oncol.* 25: 4536–4541.
90. Kay A, Motzer R, Figlin R, et al. Updated data from a phase III randomized trial of everolimus (RAD001) vs. PBO in metastatic renal cell carcinoma (RCC). *2009 Genitourinary Cancers Symposium*: Abstract 278.1
91. Sorafenib (Nexavar) package insert. Emeryville, CA: Bayer Healthcare Pharmaceuticals, Onyx Pharmaceuticals; 2009.
92. Sunitinib (Sutent) package insert. New York, NY: Pfizer Pharmaceuticals; 2008.
93. Temsirolimus (Torisel) package insert. Philadelphia, PA: Wyeth Pharmaceuticals Inc.; 2008.
94. Newton S. Fatigue: principles of symptom management. In: Newton S, Hickey M, Marrs J, eds. *Mosby's Oncology Nursing Advisor: A Comprehensive Guide to Clinical Practice.* St. Louis, MO: Mosby, Elsevier; 2009.
95. Wood LS. Managing the side effects of sorafenib and sunitinib. *Commun Oncol.* 2006;3:558–562.
96. Wood LS, Manchen B. Sorafenib: a promising new targeted therapy for renal cell carcinoma. *Clin J Oncol Nurs.* 2007;11:649–656.

97. Esper P, Gale D, Muehlbauer P. What kind of rash is it? Deciphering the dermatologic toxicities of biologic and targeted therapies. *Clin J Oncol Nurs.* 2007;11:659–666.
98. Robert C, Soria JC, Spatz A, et al. Cutaneous side effects of tyrosine kinase inhibitors and blocking antibodies. *Lancet.* 2005;6:491–500.
99. Lacouture ME, Wu S, Robert C, et al. Evolving strategies for the management of hand-foot skin reaction associated with the multitargeted kinase inhibitors sorafenib and sunitinib. *Oncologist.* 2008;13:1001–1011.
100. Wu S, Chen J, Kudelka A, et al. Incidence and risk of hypertension with sorafenib in patients with cancer: a systematic review and meta-analysis. *Lancet.* 2008;9:117–123.
101. Moldawer NP, Figlin R. Renal cell carcinoma: the translation of molecular biology into new treatments, new patient outcomes, and nursing implications. *Oncol Nurs Forum.* 2008;35:699–708.
102. Moldawer NP, Wood LS. Temsirolimus for advanced renal cell carcinoma: expanding nursing interventions and expertise in novel therapies. *Kidney Cancer J.* 2007;5:118–130.
103. Wyeth Pharmaceuticals. Temsirolimus (TORISEL) package insert. Philadelphia, PA: Wyeth Pharmaceuticals; 2007.
104. Fisher RI, Rosenberg SA, Sznol M, et al. High-dose aldesleukin in renal cell carcinoma: long-term survival update. *Cancer J.* 1997;3(suppl 1): S1–S4.
105. Schwarzberg T, Regan MM, Liu V, et al. Retrospective analysis of interleukin-2 therapy in patients with metastatic renal cell carcinoma who had received prior antiangiogenic therapy. *J Clin Oncol.* 2008;26(15s part I of II):5044.
106. Mavroukakis SA, Muehlbauer PM, White RL, et al. Clinical pathways for managing patients receiving Interleukin 2. *Clin J Oncol Nurs.* 2001;5:207–217.
107. Vogelbaum MA, Suh JH. Resectable brain metastases. *J Clin Oncol.* 2006;24:1289–1294.
108. Sheehan JP, Sun MH, Kondziolka D, et al. Radiosurgery in patients with renal cell carcinoma metastasis to the brain: long-term outcomes and prognostic factors influencing survival and local control. *J Neurosurg.* 2003;98:342–349.
109. Cannady SB, Cavanaugh KA, Lee SY, et al. Results of whole brain radiotherapy and recursive partitioning analysis in patients with brain metastases from renal cell carcinoma: a retrospective study. *Int J Radiat Oncol Biol Phys.* 2004;58:253–258.
110. Sheehan JP, Sun MH, Kondziolka D, et al. Radiosurgery in patients with renal cell carcinoma metastasis to the brain: long-term outcomes and prognostic factors influencing survival and local tumor control. *J Neurosurg.* 2003;98:342–349.
111. Amato RJ. Chemotherapy for renal cell carcinoma. *Semin Oncol.* 2000:27:177–186.
112. Milowsky MI, Nanus DM. Chemotherapeutic strategies for renal cell carcinoma. *Urol Clin North Am.* 2003;30:601–609.
113. Stadler WM, Halabi S, Rini B, et al. A phase II study of gemcitabine and capecitabine in metastatic renal cancer: a report of Cancer and Leukemia Group B Protocol 90008. *Cancer.* 2006;107:1273–1279.

CHAPTER 66

*Suzanne M. Mahon, RN, DNSc, AOCN®, APNG,*
*Susan Germann Yackzan, RN, MSN, AOCN®, ARNP*

# Skin Cancer

## INTRODUCTION

The skin is a large and very visible organ that serves both protective and aesthetic functions. Historically, these visible characteristics have served as indicators of social status and class. Until the second decade of the 20th century, smooth, pale skin was valued as an indication of belonging to the more wealthy, leisure class. Those who worked as laborers and field hands had darker skin, tanned from exposure to the sun. During this century, outdoor leisure activities have become associated with a higher social status.[1,2] This change in perception has led more people to seek tanned, bronze-colored skin. The increased exposure to ultraviolet radiation (UVR), either natural or artificial, may also be one of the biggest factors contributing to the rise in the incidence of skin cancer. Unfortunately, scientific knowledge about the carcinogenic and aging effects of UVR is relatively recent and attitudes have yet to change.[1]

The term *skin cancer* is utilized to describe several types of malignancies that occur in the skin. Basal cell carcinoma (BCC) and squamous cell carcinoma (SCC) are often combined and described as nonmelanoma skin cancer (NMSC). Malignant melanoma (MM) is usually addressed separately because of the differences in this malignancy when compared to NMSC in terms of treatment and prognosis. Most MMs are cutaneous; however, unusual presentations in the eye and viscera may occur. This chapter will focus on the cutaneous skin cancers.

Oncology nurses can have a significant impact on the morbidity and mortality associated with NMSC and MM. As educators, they can influence the public to practice primary and secondary prevention strategies. As clinicians, they can perform risk assessments and screening examinations to promote early detection of malignancies, ensure appropriate management of biopsies, administer therapies safely, manage symptoms, and provide appropriate psychosocial care. As researchers, they can improve strategies for education, management of symptoms, and knowledge acquisition through clinical trials.

## EPIDEMIOLOGY

The incidence of skin cancer continues to grow both in the United States and throughout the world. Skin cancers account for approximately one-third of all diagnosed cancers.[3] In the US alone, the American Cancer Society (ACS) estimates that approximately 1 million cases of the highly curable BCCs and SCCs are detected annually.[4] Of the NMSCs, cases of BCC predominate over SCC by about 5 to 1 in males and 10 to 1 in females.[5] Accurate figures on the incidence of these NMSCs are difficult to obtain, as many countries do not register these malignancies. In addition, these lesions are often removed in primary care practices and are treated without laboratory verification of the clinical diagnosis.[3,5] It is clear, however, that the incidence of these cancers has increased over the last few decades and that the increased incidence of NMSC is related to cumulative sun-exposure behaviors.[6]

Melanoma has been established as a medical diagnosis since the time of Hippocrates and was known as a black tumor (melas meaning black and oma meaning tumor).[7] The annual incidence of this more serious form of skin cancer, is estimated at 68,720 new cases in 2009 according to the ACS.[4] The annual incidence of MM has risen steadily from 1 in 1500 persons in 1930 to 1 in 75 persons in 2000, as shown in Figure 66-1.[8] For men, the lifetime risk of developing melanoma is 1 in 41; for women, the risk is 1 in 61.[4] Males have a higher risk of developing melanoma on the head, neck or trunk when compared to females.[9] A Caucasian individual is 20 times more likely to develop melanoma than an African American.[2,3]

From a public health perspective, it is vital to improve global awareness of MM. MM accounts for 3% of all skin cancers and 65% of all cancer deaths.[4] Better means are needed to identify high-risk persons and to detect MM early; more specific targeted therapies to treat MM are also needed. The incidence of MM continues to rise with age, as a consequence, lifetime prevention and early detection strategies are critical to decrease the morbidity and mortality associated with MM (Figure 66-1 and 66-2).[2,4,8]

Clearly, the dramatic rise in MM is real and not due to artifact. MM incidence is increasing worldwide at a faster rate than the incidence of any other cancer.[2,3] This trend is associated with increased morbidity, mortality, and rising healthcare costs. In Australia, direct healthcare costs for skin cancer are about $22 per person per year and exceed the expenditures for any other cancer.[10] In the United States, an estimated $740 million is spent treating MM.[10] In Australia, the lifetime risk for developing MM is 1 in 24 for men and 1 in 32 for women. This worldwide increase is not due to better surveillance techniques. Rather, is hypothesized that the increase in MM incidence is related to the fact that people are going outdoors more often than in the past and are exposing themselves not only to sunlight but also increasingly to artificial ultraviolet radiation (UVR).[2,10]

The mortality rate from the highly curable BCCs and SCCs is approximately 2940 persons per year according to ACS estimates.[4] These deaths are largely preventable, as most NMSCs are visible for long periods of time prior to metastasis. An estimated 8650 persons die annually from MM.[4] Although multiple factors influence survival, thickness of the tumor has been shown to be the most important factor across multiple studies.[2] The decreasing mean thickness of MMs at the time of diagnosis has resulted in an overall increased survival for localized MM, from about 50% in the 1950s to almost 90% in 2000. Note, however, that the absolute number of thicker MMs has also increased. The mortality rate from MM continues to increase, albeit not at the same rate as the emergence of new cases[4,8] (see Figures 66-1 and 66-2).

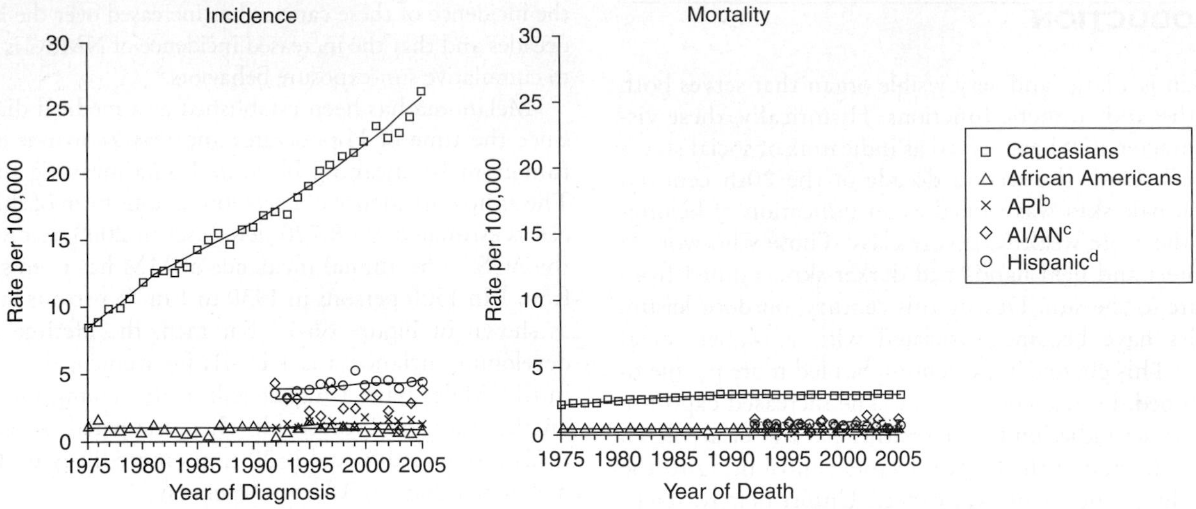


**FIGURE 66-1**

SEER incidence and US death rates,[a] melanoma of the skin, both sexes. Joinpoint analyses for Caucasians and African Americans from 1975–2005 and for Asian/Pacific Islanders, American Indians/Alaska Natives, and Hispanics from 1992–2005.

*Note*: Incidence data for Asian/Pacific Islanders, American Indians/Alaska Natives and Hispanics are from the SEER 13 Areas (SEER 9 Areas, San Jose-Monterey, Los Angeles, Alaska Native Registry and Rural Georgia). Mortality data are from US Mortality Flies, National Center for Health Statistics, CDC

[a]Rates are age-adjusted to the 2000 US Std Population (19 age groups – census P26–1103).
Regression lines are calculated using the Joinpoint Regression Program Version 3.3.1, April 2009, National Cancer Institute. Joinpoint analyses for Caucasians and African Americans during the 1975–2005 period allow a maximum of 4 joinpoints. Analyses for other ethnic groups during the period 1992–2005 allow a maximum of 3 joinpoints.
[b]API = Asian/Pacific Islander.
[c]AI/AN = American Indian/Alaska Native. Rates for American Indian/Alaska Native are based on the CHSDA (Contract Health Service Delivery Area) counties.
[d]Hispanic is not mutually exclusive from Caucasians, African Americans, Asian/Pacific Islanders and American Indians/Alaska Natives. Incidence data for Hispanics are based on NHIA and exclude cases from the Alaska Native Registry. Mortality data for Hispanics exclude cases from Connecticut, Maine, Maryland, Minnesota, New Hampshire, New York, North Dakota, Oklahoma and Vermont.

*Source*: Incidence data for Caucasians and African Americans are from SEER 9 areas (San Francisco, Connecticut, Detroit, Hawaii, Iowa, New Mexico, Seattle, Utah, Atlanta).[8]

## ETIOLOGY

The etiology of skin cancer is multifactorial in nature. The likelihood that an individual might develop skin cancer during his or her lifetime depends on both constitutional factors and environmental exposures. Constitutional factors include the genotypic and phenotypic characteristics of an individual.[3] Different skin cancers are associated with different risk factors (Table 66-1).[2,3,11,12]

### GENOTYPIC FACTORS

Skin color is one of the most important genotypic features that places a person at risk for developing skin cancer. MM is very rare in African Americans.[2,12,13] Persons with light or fair complexion have a tendency to freckle or burn easily are at higher risk. The development of melanocytic nevi in childhood is strongly related to characteristics of pigmentation associated with poor sun tolerance.[2,12]

The epidermis of African Americans has been shown to have a natural sun protection factor (SPF) of 13.4, with the melanin in the epidermis filtering twice as much ultraviolet B (UVB) as the epidermis of a white person.[2,12] This protection, however, is not complete, and both NMSC and MM can develop in African Americans. SCC is the most frequently seen skin cancer in African Americans. BCCs in African Americans are almost always pigmented. Furthermore, as many as 67% of MMs in the African American population arise in nonsun-exposed skin such as on the palmer and plantar surfaces and even the mucous membranes. African Americans have proportionately greater percentages of the acral lentiginous type of MM and also tend to have poorer prognoses than do whites with MM.

Large congenital melanocytic nevi are also considered a significant risk factor associated with the development of MM and are estimated to occur in 1% of newborns.[2,14,15] This increase in risk has been reported to range from 0% to 42%. In most studies, the larger the nevus, the higher

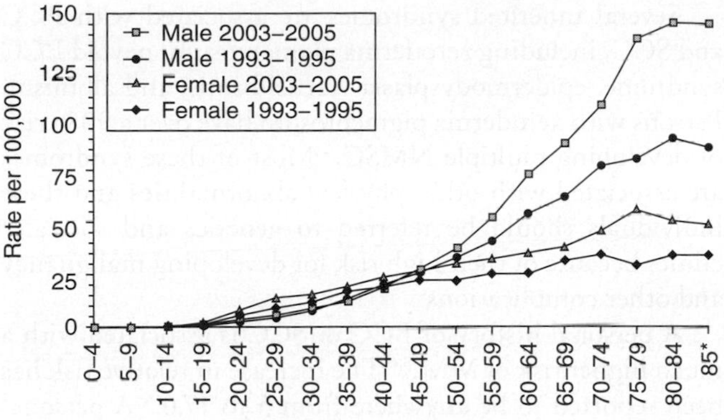


**FIGURE 66-2**

Melanoma of the skin: SEER incidence 1993–1995 vs 2003–2005 Caucasian by age and sex.

*Source*: Reprinted from Ries et al.[8]

the lifetime risk.[2,16] Surgical removal of these large nevi is thought to decrease but not eliminate these individuals' risk for developing MM because approximately 50% of the MMs arise in extracutaneous sites. Therefore lifetime screening is important.

The number of melanocytic nevi (moles) is correlated with risk. This includes common acquired nevi, atypical nevi, and dysplastic nevi.[2,14] On the basis of nevus numbers and especially dysplastic nevi, clinicians can identify individuals at high risk for developing MM and implement aggressive screening and intervention programs. Approximately one-third of MMs arise from preexisting nevi.[2] The total number of moles is an indicator of risk; persons with over 100 nevi have a relative risk of 7.6 compared to persons with 10 or fewer moles.[2] Persons with ten to twenty moles have a relative risk of 4.67.[9,17] The total surface area of the nevi also influences risk.

Dysplastic nevi may develop throughout life and show clinical features similar to normal moles and MMs (see Color Plates 11 and 12). These features include a size greater than 6 to 8 mm, irregular borders, variable pigmentation, and irregular surface characteristics. The identification of truly dysplastic nevi is more difficult to perform clinically than many epidemiologists realize, however, and in most cases requires a pathologic diagnosis.[14] Dysplastic nevi occur in approximately 10% of the general population, but the risk of progression to MM is not clear in this group.[2,12] The clinical importance of dysplastic nevi lies in their association with the risk of melanoma. The age-adjusted incidence of melanoma is approximately 15 times higher among persons with dysplastic nevi as compared to members of the general population. Similarly, risk is higher for a second malignancy in persons already diagnosed with MM and dysplastic nevi.[18]

Another important genotypic feature is family history. Approximately 10% of patients with MM describe a history of an affected family member.[2,12] People who have a

**TABLE 66-1**

**Risk Factors for Skin Cancer**

| Risk Factor | Risk Factor for NMSC | Risk Factor for MM |
|---|---|---|
| Actinic keratoses[a] | + | + |
| Arsenic ingestion (well water, insecticides, medical) | + | |
| Chronic exposure to tar, soot, shale, or petroleum | + | |
| Cigarette or pipe smoking | + | |
| Congenital nevus | | + |
| Family history of melanoma[a] | | + |
| Geographic area where childhood was spent | + | + |
| History of NMSC in a first-degree relative | + | |
| History of 3 or more blistering sunburns before the age of 20 years[a] | + | + |
| Immunosuppression | + | + |
| Increasing age | + | + |
| Ionizing radiation (therapeutic or occupational) | + | |
| Large number of dysplastic nevi | | + |
| Large number of melanocytic nevi | | + |
| Male gender | + | + |
| Personal history of BCC | + | + |
| Personal history of MM | + | + |
| Personal history of SCC | + | + |
| Red or blond hair[a] | + | + |
| Scar related to heat burn, chemical burn | + | |
| Skin color | + | + |
| Tendency to freckle, especially on the upper back area[a] | + | + |
| Three or more years of outdoor summer jobs during teenage years[a] | + | + |
| Xeroderma pigmentosum | | + |

*Note*: [a]The presence of any 1 or 2 of these factors increases a person's risk for the development of MM 3-fold, and 3 or more of these factors increases the risk almost 20-fold. *Abbreviations*: BCC, basal cell carcinoma; MM, malignant melanoma; NMSC, nonmelanoma skin cancer; SCC, squamous cell carcinoma.

*Source*: Data from Cummins et al,[2] American Cancer Society,[3] US Preventive Services Task Force,[11] and Markovic et al.[12]

family history of MM and/or dysplastic nevi, or who have a large number of nevi themselves, are at a very high risk (+100-fold increase) of developing MM over their lifetime.[2] Persons with a history of melanoma in a first-degree relative have twice the risk of developing MM than those without a family history.[12] A hereditary predisposition to MM is sometimes associated with an earlier age of onset.[11] Sex distribution between males and females is usually about equal to those without a hereditary predisposition to MM.[11] In general, individuals with a hereditary predisposition to MM have malignancies that are clinically and histopathologically similar to those without such a family history.[19] Hereditary melanoma should be suspected in patients with a family history of pancreatic cancer or astrocytoma.[12,20] Patients from these families are, however, often diagnosed with thinner lesions and generally have a better prognosis. This better outcome may be related to heightened awareness and increased surveillance. A second primary MM does develop in 17% to 20% of patients from these families who survive their first MM.[20,21]

As research continues based on sequencing from the Human Genome Project, it is likely that more skin cancer susceptibility loci will be identified, for which genetic testing will ultimately become available. To date, a susceptibility gene has been clearly linked to CDKN2A (*p16*).[2,12] Germ-line mutations in CDKN2A have been found in 20% to 40% of families in which at least 3 first-degree relatives are affected by melanoma and are the most common genetic abnormality associated with hereditary melanoma.[2,12] A *CDK4* mutation is found more rarely.[12] This particular mutation may be more prevalent in the Australian population.[20] There are 2 models in development and sometimes used in clinical practice by geneticists to predict the risk of having a mutation in CDKN2A. These are the MELPREDICT and GenoMEL models.[22,23]

The tumor suppressor gene *p16* is involved in the regulation of cell growth. It regulates cell proliferation by inhibiting the CDK4 cell cycle protein kinase; thus, mutations in *p16* that disrupt function lead to unregulated cell growth.[11,12] An understanding of the genetics of MM is just beginning. It is speculated that a genetic predisposition to MM may be present on a number of genes that interact to increase risk or protect against the development of MM.[20] Because penetrance may be variable, the gene or genes may not be expressed consistently.[21] It is also thought that the gene is transmitted in an autosomal dominant fashion, but the impact of environmental factors on the subsequent development of MM is not fully understood.[11,20] Therefore, even though the location of one or more susceptibility genes is now known, the usefulness of genetic testing is not completely clear. Genetic testing is commercially available for some CDKN2A mutations, although the clinical usefulness is not completely clear.[20] As genetic testing becomes available and the ramifications of testing are better understood, a number of education and counseling issues will emerge.

Several inherited syndromes are associated with BCC and SCC, including zeroderma pigmentosum, nevoid BCC syndrome, epidermodysplasia verruciformis, and albinism. Persons with xeroderma pigmentosum have over a 90% risk of developing multiple NMSC.[6] Most of these syndromes are associated with other physical abnormalities and these individuals should be referred to genetics and specialty clinics because of their high risk for developing malignancy and other complications.

A personal history of BCC or SCC is associated with a much higher risk of MM.[3,6] The increase in relative risk has been reported to be anywhere from 3 to 17.0.[6] A personal history of a NMSC is associated with a much higher risk of developing a second NMSC, especially in persons with a history of significant sun exposure.

The importance of the immune system in controlling skin cancers, particularly MM, is not completely understood.[2,10] Persons with chronic immunosuppression are at higher risk for developing MM.[12] Renal transplant recipients may have a 4-fold increased risk for developing MM.[2,12] The risk may be as much as 8 times higher in persons who have been successfully treated for cancers such as lymphoma. Evidence suggests that certain HPV infections including HPV 8 and HPV 38 may be found in up to 38% of persons with NMSC.[6]

Age itself is a risk factor for both NMSCs and MMs (see Figure 66-2).[2,5] It is difficult to separate the interaction of age and other genetic factors from cumulative exposure to sunlight.

## ENVIRONMENTAL FACTORS

Frequent and prolonged exposure to UVR over a period of years will induce cellular changes in human skin. Sun exposure adds up on a daily basis in everyday activities including walking back and forth from the car. Most individuals underestimate the cumulative effect of this exposure.[7,24] Ultraviolet radiation can act as an initiator, a promoter, a cocarcinogen, and an immunosuppressive agent.[10] Episodic high exposure resulting in sunburn, especially when it occurs in childhood, may be critical.[2,12,16] Skin cancer risk begins at an early age. It is estimated that 80% of total lifetime UVR exposure occurs before age 20.[1] Risk is also higher in child athletes who repeatedly expose their skin to UVR.[25]

Two adverse consequences are associated with UVR exposure. First, it leads to direct tissue and cellular damage. Second, exposure to UVR results in local and systemic immunosuppression.[3,12] The effects of UVR are both acute and chronic.[2,12] Acute changes include sunburn and discomfort. Chronic effects include photoaging, premalignant and malignant growths, and immunosuppression.[5,26] Immunosuppression is a significant risk factor for the development of both NMSC and melanoma.[6]

Recent evidence has addressed the beneficial effects of UVR and has become a controversy when educating the public about skin cancer prevention. UVR is essential for the body's production of Vitamin D. Casual exposure to UVR of the arms, face, and hands is adequate to insure normal levels of Vitamin D.[1] When providing public education it is important to emphasize that the negative effects of UVR outweigh the positive ones; Vitamin D can be supplemented with dietary measures.

Solar keratoses, which are a direct result of chronic sun exposure, are major risk factors for both NMSC and MM.[16] Persons with actinic keratoses have an increased risk for developing NMSC; about 10% will go on to develop a malignancy from these UVR-induced lesions.[6] Data suggest that NMSCs are associated with cumulative sun exposure, whereas MM is associated with short, intense episodes of sun exposure, especially those involving sunburns.[2,12] A history of severe and painful sunburn, especially repeated sunburn, is associated with upper extremity melanoma.[9] Exposure to sunlight is the only environmental factor consistently linked to MM in most studies.[2,3,27] The exact link between sunlight exposure and risk of MM is not completely clear, but is probably a causal relationship that includes a complex relationship between UVR-induced genetic changes, dose-response, latent period, body site, and other unknown factors.[2,28]

Risk of MM has also been linked to parity and hormonal factors. This association has been reported variably over time. Recent evidence suggests that risk might be slightly lower in women with early parity and multiple births. Most epidemiologists still believe that lifestyle factors that influence UVR exposure are associated with more substantial risk.[29]

The location of one's residence may also influence risk of developing SCC and MM.[30] There appears to be an inverse relationship between increasing latitude and MM mortality. The closer a person lives to the equator, the higher the risk. For every decrease in latitude of 2°, there is an associated 10% increase in the death rate from MM.[3,12] Persons who live in the US with a medium or high UV index (6 or more) have an increased risk for developing SCC, and a slightly higher risk for developing BCC.

Some occupations may be associated with a higher risk of developing MM.[12,24] It is estimated that at least 8% of the US workers are continually exposed to UVR during the workday and a large portion of these workers do not take adequate steps to protect themselves including the use of hats, clothing, and sunscreen.[31]

An association between high-paying jobs and MM may be due to confounding factors in recreational patterns rather than occupational choice.[11] Persons who earn a higher salary and are employed in typical white-collar occupations may be at higher risk for developing MM than those who have more chronic occupational outdoor exposure to UVR.[3,5] These risks may be related to the fact that persons from this socioeconomic group have the financial means to travel to sunny climates on vacation, where they intermittently expose themselves to intense UVR resulting in sunburn, especially those associated with pain and blistering. This is probably related to the combination of reflected UVR from disturbed water and the cooling effect of water, which leads to a false sense of security. The same is true of cloudy days. Clouds give a false sense of security that is similar to the cooling effect of the water because clouds reduce the warming sensation of the sun. Intermittent, intense, rather than cumulative exposure may be associated with increased risk for MM, whereas cumulative exposure is associated with increased risk of NMSC.[12] Another reason for the higher rate of MMs and NMSCs in this socioeconomic group is that people in these occupations may have better health insurance, a higher awareness of health issues, and ultimately better detection of lesions.[2,11]

High sun exposure at certain times of life confers higher risks for developing different types of skin cancer. Early sun exposure, particularly in childhood and adolescence, is associated with a much higher risk for developing BCC and is estimated to confer a 10-fold elevated risk for developing SCC.[6] Sun exposure in the 10 years prior to diagnosis may be important in accounting for many cases of SCC and is associated with a 2.5-fold increased risk when compared to those without this exposure.[5]

Sun exposure during childhood and adolescence also seems to have a substantial influence on the risk of developing MM.[2] Approximately 80% of lifetime sun exposure occurs before the age of 18 years. During this time, melanocytes may be more sensitive to the sun, resulting in alteration of their DNA and possibly leading to the formation of unstable moles that have a greater potential to become malignant. Sunlight exposure and blistering sunburns during youth may be more intense than those incurred later in life because of the recreation patterns of children.[2,12] Continued exposure in adulthood increases the risk for NMSC. For MM, the risk seems to increase with intermittent sun exposure on areas of skin only occasionally exposed.[12] Obtaining an accurate history of sun exposure is difficult, and clinicians should anticipate that individuals often grossly underestimate their sun exposure.[27,32,33]

The ocular structures can also be affected by UVR.[16] Repeated and prolonged exposure of the conjunctiva will lead to thickening and hypervascularity. There also appears to be a positive correlation between increased cataract formation, decreased latitude, increased UVB, and total sunlight exposure.[10,16]

Ultraviolet radiation includes radiation wavelengths ranging from 200 nm to more than 18,000 nm.[2,26] Damage to the skin comes from UVR in the 200 to 400 nm range. Several types of UVR occur in this range. The 2 that have been studied the most in relation to the development of NMSC and MM are ultraviolet A (UVA) and ultraviolet B (UVB). UVA are longer waves (320–400 nm), resulting in deeper skin penetration. It is estimated that 55% to 62% of UVA penetrates the dermis.[10] Although UVA carries significant risks, the risks of skin cancer are probably greatest in association with UVB.[10] UVB waves are the shortest (220–290 nm), make up about 5% of the sunlight striking the earth, and are probably the most biologically important component of UVR from the sun. Of UVB that reaches the skin, 85% is absorbed primarily in the epidermis, with only 10% to 15% being transmitted to the deeper dermal layers.[10] UVB has a greater intensity in the summer than in the winter, at midday than in morning or late afternoon, in places closer to the equator, and at high altitudes. Sand, snow, concrete, and water can reflect as much as 85% to 87% of UVB, thus intensifying exposure.[10,12] Ultraviolet C (UVC) is largely blocked by the ozone layer.[30] The physiological effects of UVA and UVB on the skin are different and are summarized in Table 66-2.[2,3,12]

Erythema associated with sunburn is due to excessive UVB. The minimal erythema dose (MED) is the amount of UVR necessary to cause the skin to change to shades of red or pink. MED is highly variable and depends on an individual's skin type, skin thickness, amount of melanin in the skin, and whether the UVR is short or long wave.[16] The erythema results from an increase in blood flow to the affected skin that begins about 4 hours after exposure, with peak erythema occurring 8 to 24 hours after exposure. The appearance of the erythema suggests that a threshold of UV damage has been reached sufficient to activate prostaglandin and other inflammatory pathways.

Wavelengths of UVR that produce the largest amount of erythema are also the most efficient at producing pyrimidine dimers. The inference is that the wavelengths that produce maximum erythema are most likely to be the wavelengths that produce the maximum number of carcinogenic mutations.

Two types of tanning occur in response to UVR exposure. Immediate tanning is a transient grayish, brown discoloration of the skin induced by UVA. It begins during exposure and is maximal at the end of exposure. Immediate tanning lasts a few hours to about 36 hours after exposure. Delayed tanning occurs 48 to 72 hours following UVR exposure, peaks in 7 to 10 days, and can persist for several days to months.[6,34]

Photodamage (dermatoheliosis) is a spectrum of skin changes affecting the epidermis and the dermis. It includes the formation and growth of flat, brown spots on the skin

**TABLE 66-2**

**Effects of Ultraviolet Light on the Skin**

| Effect | UVA (320–400 nm) | UVB (290–320 nm) |
|---|---|---|
| Immediate pigment darkening (usually fades within a few hours) due to photo-oxidation of melanin already in epidermis | Yes | Not as evident |
| Number of functioning melanocytes | No change | Increased number |
| Photosensitivity reactions | May occur quickly | May occur |
| Delayed tanning (occurs 36–72 hours after exposure) | Yes | Yes |
| Production of vitamin D from cholesterol precursors in the skin | None | Yes |
| Site of absorption | 55% in dermis | Primarily the epidermis; 10%–15% in dermis |
| Radiant heat | Little to none | Moderate to large amount |
| Sunburn | Seldom evident except after large doses | May occur very quickly |
| Thickening of the stratum corneum | No | Yes |
| Carcinogen | Potentiates the effects of UVB | Yes |
| Distribution of melanosomes | Within dendrites of melanocytes only in basal cell layer | Within keratinocytes throughout the epidermis |
| Photoaging | Yes | Yes |
| Etiologic cause of NMSC | Role not completely clear | Yes |
| Pathological changes in the dermis | Yes | Yes |

*Abbreviations*: NMSC, nonmelanoma skin cancer; UVA, ultraviolet light A; UVB, ultraviolet light B.

*Source*: Data from Cummins et al,[2] American Cancer Society,[3] and Markovic et al.[12]

(solar lentiges), fine and deep wrinkling, blackheads, telangiectasias, a yellow, sallow color to the skin, and loss of elasticity.[5,6,12] These changes can be prevented by the consistent and adequate application of sunscreen.[33] In some teenagers, the message that UVR promotes photodamage, may be a more effective means of encouraging protection from UVR.[1]

Stratospheric ozone depletion may also be a causative factor associated with both NMSC and MM.[30] Ozone depletion may lead to increased terrestrial UVB levels for many populations. It has been estimated that for every 1% decrease in ozone, there is a 2% increase in UVB penetration to the earth. This increased UVB penetration is predicted to result in an additional 1% to 4% increase per year in NMSC.[12] It has also been estimated that for each 1% decrease in the amount of ozone, MM incidence increases about 1%.[6,34]

Other environmental risk factors for the development of NSCC include exposure to ionizing radiation, phototherapy with psoralens, exposure to polycyclic hydrocarbons, and arsenic ingestion.[5,24] Photosensitizing agents have also been associated with the development of skin cancer, as well as premature skin aging, reduced immunity, blood vessel damage, and allergic reactions.[6,33] Photosensitivity is defined as a chemically induced change in the skin that renders an individual unusually sensitive to light. Rashes, sunburn, or other adverse effects may occur from exposure to UVR of an intensity or duration that would not normally affect that individual. Many medications contain photosensitizing agents, including antihistamines, oral contraceptives and estrogen, nonsteroidal and anti-inflammatory drugs, phenothiazines, psoralens, sulfonamides, sulfonylureas, thiazide diuretics, tetracylcines, tricyclic antidepressants, many chemotherapeutic agents, antiparasitic drugs, and oral hypoglycemics.[6,12] Persons who are taking a photosensitizing medication need to reduce UVR exposure whenever possible.

## CALCULATING MELANOMA RISK

Many individuals want to know what their lifetime risk of developing MM is and often knowledge of increased risk will motivate individuals to engage in primary skin cancer prevention practices. The NCI has a Web site in which individuals can use to calculate their absolute risk for developing MM at http://www.cancer.gov/melanomarisktool. This tool is based on a variety of risk factors and is constantly being updated.[35] Patients may need some assistance from a healthcare provider to understand what absolute risk implies, but there is information about the significance of the risk factor as well as suggested primary and secondary prevention measures.

## PREVENTION

The United States is beginning to develop strong public policy recommendations and initiatives to address skin cancer incidence, morbidity, and mortality by focusing on primary and secondary prevention measures. Primary and secondary prevention are both important in regard to skin cancer. Primary prevention strategies are the steps taken to keep the malignancy from developing. In the case of skin cancer, these efforts include properly applying sunscreen, wearing protective clothing, and decreasing UVR exposure. Public education programs are an excellent means of addressing these primary prevention strategies. Secondary prevention efforts include attempts to detect skin cancer early in asymptomatic persons. Tertiary prevention seeks to minimize the long-term consequences of cancer treatment and the detection of additional primary skin cancers early. Table 66-3 provides an overview of primary and secondary prevention strategies for both NMSCs and MMs and appropriate patient education points.

## PRIMARY PREVENTION

### Public policy

The Healthy People 2010 Guidelines (http://www.health.gov/healthypeople/Document/html) aim to decrease the US mortality rate from MM from 2.8 deaths per 100,000 persons to 2.5 deaths per 100,000 persons during the next 10 years.[36] The Guidelines also seek to increase the proportion of people using skin cancer primary prevention strategies, which include at least one of the following protective measures: avoiding the sun between 10 AM and 4 PM, wearing sun-protective clothing, using sunscreen with an SPF of 15 or higher, and decreasing or avoiding UVR exposure. Approximately 47% of the US population age 18 and older currently use at least one of the measures; the goal is to increase this proportion to 75%. To make the Healthy People 2010 guidelines become a reality, increased efforts to implement primary, secondary, and tertiary skin cancer prevention are needed. An interim analysis suggests that significant progress has been made in some areas as the age-adjusted proportion of adults aged 18 years and older who took protective measures (eg, use of sunscreens) against sun exposure to reduce the risk of skin cancer increased from 59% in 2000 to 71% in 2005. The target is 85%.[36]

### Public education programs

Public education programs need to include not only information about skin cancer and reducing UVR exposure, but also a behavioral component that ensures long-term adaptation of healthy behaviors.[37,38] All public education programs and health messages are most successful if they reflect regional and individual differences as well as the social context of culture and/or ethnicity.[3,11]

To reap the most benefits, public education programs need to be started early in a child's life, with the goal of

**TABLE 66-3**

**Primary and Secondary Prevention for Skin Cancer**

| Strategy | Patient Education | Strengths | Limitations |
|---|---|---|---|
| Risk assessment (secondary prevention) | Define and interpret individual risks for developing skin cancer | Patients who understand their personal risk for developing skin cancer may be more motivated to practice prevention strategies | Time-consuming<br>Patient must be motivated to assist with and try to understand assessment<br>Requires skilled healthcare providers |
| Reduce UVR exposure (primary prevention) | Decrease sun exposure between 10 AM and 3 PM<br>Instruction that UVR is present on cloudy days<br>Infants 6 mo of age and younger should not have direct UVR exposure | Decrease carcinogen exposure | Personal practices may be difficult to change |
| Avoid use of indoor tanning devices (primary prevention) | Large amounts of UVA are potentially carcinogenic<br>Tanned skin is not healthy; rather, it is a sign of injured skin<br>Use of indoor tanning devices may lead to premature aging of skin and cataract formation | Large source of carcinogen exposure that can be avoided | Personal practices may be difficult to change; many people believe they look healthier with a tan |
| Use chemical sunscreens correctly and consistently (primary prevention) | Use an SPF of at least 15–20 that is waterproof<br>Apply a test dose to check for allergies<br>Apply liberally (about an ounce for an adult in a swim suit) to all exposed skin surfaces 15–30 min prior to sun exposure<br>Reapply sunscreen every 90 min and more frequently after towelling off | When used correctly, sunscreen will block most of the UVB exposure and a variable amount of UVA | Some consider sunscreens expensive and inconvenient to use<br>Many people do not apply products prior to exposure, apply them in inadequate amounts, and do not reapply when indicated, thereby limiting the effectiveness of the agents<br>Personal practices may be difficult to change; many people believe they look healthier with a tan<br>May not apply on children younger than 6 months of age |
| Apply zinc oxide (a physical block) to sun-exposed areas (primary prevention) | Apply a visible, liberal coat to sun-exposed areas<br>Block is effective as long as a visible coat is seen on skin | Excellent for areas with a tendency to burn such as the nose, backs of ears<br>Is more waterproof than chemical sunscreens | Unsuitable to be applied to all sun-exposed areas because of the amount of product necessary |
| Wear protective clothing (primary prevention) | Protective clothing with a tighter weave can provide an effective physical block against UVR<br>Shirts with sleeves and hats with wide brims provide more protection | Provides a means to directly reduce direct UVR to skin surfaces<br>Relatively inexpensive<br>Easy to apply | Patients may forget to wear hats or not see the benefits of protective clothing as worth the effort |
| Take extra precaution to reduce UVR exposure when taking photosensitizing medications (primary prevention) | Teach patients about classes of photosensitizing medications and the need for extra protection | Reduces severe sunburns and UVR exposure | Patients may forget to take precautions or underestimate the dangers of photosensitizing medications |

*(Continued)*

**TABLE 66-3**

**Primary and Secondary Prevention for Skin Cancer (Continued)**

| Strategy | Patient Education | Strengths | Limitations |
|---|---|---|---|
| Practice monthly skin self-examination (secondary prevention) | Demonstrate technique on the patient<br>Point out any potential problems that require extra monitoring<br>Teach patients to perform in a well-lit area and to pay attention to hard-to-see areas as well sun-exposed areas | Inexpensive<br>Can be done in privacy of own home<br>Patient may be able to note an early interval change | Patients often forget to do examination or do not see the value of self-examination<br>Some areas of body may be difficult for patient to adequately examine<br>Patients may lack confidence in ability to detect a change |
| Annual professional examination (secondary prevention) | Opportunity to review many primary prevention strategies<br>Teach skin self-examination<br>Detect lesions that may not be immediately obvious to the patient | May detect subtle, early changes in lesions | May result in removal of borderline lesions<br>Dependent on the skill of the examiner<br>Most cost-effective in higher-risk patients; cost-effectiveness in the general population is not known |

*Abbreviations*: SPF, sun protection factor; UVA, ultraviolet light A; UVB, ultraviolet light B; UVR, ultraviolet radiation.

having the individual adopt attitudes and practices that minimize UVR exposure. A number of such programs have demonstrated that even preschoolers can learn and practice behaviors that reduce UVR exposure.[16,3,36,39] The Centers for Disease Control and Prevention (CDC) has released Guidelines for School Programs to Prevent Skin Cancer.[39] These guidelines include the establishment of policies that reduce UVR exposure, establishment of safe environments, provision of health education for students and staff, involvement of the family, incorporation with other school services, and periodic evaluation.

Evidence suggests that to get children to change their practices and attitudes, their parents must first adopt more healthy behaviors.[40] Despite educational programs and knowledge about the dangers of exposure to UVR, many individuals fail to practice primary prevention strategies.[39] Some believe that fear of skin cancer is not a deterrent to sun-seeking behaviors and that until it becomes culturally acceptable to have untanned skin in the US, there will not be a major decrease in MM and NMSC incidence and mortality rates. Some groups advocate that public messages should try to change this social norm and emphasize the photoaging effects of excessive UVR exposure. Presently, 25 states have imposed laws that limit and restrict teen access to indoor tanning.[26]

Surprisingly, even the offspring of health professionals diagnosed with melanoma are slow to adopt recommended skin cancer prevention strategies.[41] Data from the Nurses' Health Study suggests that this population reports frequent sunburns, suboptimal sunscreen use, and high rates of indoor tanning, despite a 2- to 8-fold increase in NMSCs and a significantly higher risk of MM.[41] The researchers suggest that at the time of diagnosis, parents and their offspring need to clearly be reminded of the benefits of adopting skin cancer prevention practices regardless of previous habits. Another research group also reported that even after a diagnosis of MM, 27% of persons still had a positive or neutral attitude toward tanning and still had many unprotected episodes of exposure to UVR.[42]

Short-term goals for primary prevention programs should include an increase in knowledge about the importance of sun protection and a decreased desire for a suntan.[3,12] Until these goals are achieved, primary prevention strategies will not be implemented effectively.

Medium-term goals for primary prevention programs should include an increased use of hats, clothing, shade, and sunscreens that result in a decreased number of sunburns.[3,12] Truly effecting these changes in behavior so that they are practiced from childhood through adulthood can be very complicated and difficult to accomplish.

Ultimately, the long-term goals for primary prevention programs (which may not be evident for decades) include a decrease in the incidence of NMSC and MM as well as a decrease in mortality, especially from MM. Because most cases of BCC and SCC are induced by natural or artificial sources of UVR, primary prevention may be theoretically possible.[2,5,12] The exact role of UVR in the development of MM is not as clear, although it is speculated that primary prevention strategies remain important for this disease.

Some progress has been made in improving skin cancer prevention practices.[32] In 2004, 69% of adolescents reported being sunburned during summer, which was not dramatically changed from 72% in 1998. During the same time the proportion of youth who reported using sunscreen regularly increased modestly from 31% in 1998 to 39% in 2004. There were few changes in other sun protection measures reported in this study. The authors conclude that current public policy measures in the United States are a beginning, but have not been sufficient to have a major impact on overall sun protection in youth.[32]

Programs in Australia suggest that public health programs can be effective. Recent data shows that 90% of children attending childcare or elementary school consistently use a 30+ SPF sunscreen and have lower nevi counts.[43] Significant progress has also been made with using hats and dense weave clothing because of public policy.[43,44]

In the United States, 25 states have laws mandating some type of education or skin cancer prevention programs in schools.[3] Early findings from an evaluation of the US Environmental Protection Agency's Sunwise program shows that the program could save up to 45 million dollars annually.[45] For every dollar spent on the program between \$1.95 and \$4.02 could be saved on medical costs and lost productivity attributed to skin cancer.

## Sunscreens

There are 2 types of sunscreens: chemical sunscreens that provide protection by absorbing UVR and physical sunscreens that block UVR from reaching the skin. Chemical sunscreens have been available since the 1920s with the introduction of para-aminobenzoic acid (PABA) based sunscreens.[2] The importance of sunscreen should not be underestimated as they have clearly been shown to prevent sunburn and regular use can retard or prevent the development of skin changes.[2] Educating the public about sunscreens is more complicated than it appears. Controversies continue regarding the labeling, application, and effectiveness of these agents.

*Chemical sunscreens.* The primary goal of protecting the skin from UVR is not just to avoid a sunburn. Incremental damage occurs with each exposure to UVR regardless of whether there is clinical evidence of erythema.[6] It is impractical and impossible to think that humans can avoid sun exposure completely; therefore prevention with sunscreens and other protective clothing is necessary.

Epidemiological studies suggest that recent UVR exposure may be more important than cumulative UVR exposure. Thus, even older individuals and those with high cumulative sun-exposure histories can benefit from sunscreen use by preventing the promoting influence of recent sun exposure and by avoiding new initiating mutations. Sunscreen clearly reduces further actinic damage in patients with such damage when used consistently and adequately. These results can be evident in as little as 2 years.[5,38]

The risks and benefits of sunscreen use for children under the age of 6 months are unknown and most advocate against use or UVR exposure for this group.[46] For all children greater than 6 months of age, the recommendation is a liberal application of water-resistant, child-safe broad spectrum sunscreen (UVA and UVB). Effectiveness is increased if the sunscreen is applied 30 minutes before exposure and reapplied every 120 minutes, especially after swimming or heavy perspiration.[46,47] Children and younger individuals benefit by avoiding the initiating mutations caused by UVR. It has been estimated that regular use of sunscreens (at least SPF 15) to the face, ears, neck, and upper extremities during the first 18 years of life could lead to a 78% reduction in the lifetime incidence of BCC and SCC.[5] There is good evidence that when sunscreens are applied on a daily basis and adequately applied that there is a significantly decreased risk for developing actinic keratoses and SCC in particular.[48,49] There appears to be a reduction in BSC but the exact reduction is not clear.[49]

A national population-based telephone survey conducted by the ACS reported that among youth on sunny days, 32% report wearing sunglasses, 21% report wearing long pants, 22% report staying in the shade, and 31% report applying sunscreen.[50] Current usage of sunscreen may be as high as 39%.[32] In Australia, the use of sunscreens—a default option to be used only when other measures do not provide sufficient protection—is supported by clinical studies, which have recently reported that sunscreen use has been associated with a statistically significant reduced risk for MM.[12] The AAD recommends that patients be educated that the first defense against skin cancer is avoiding midday sun and using protective clothing when outdoors. Sunscreen should be used as an adjunct to other primary prevention measures.[2,12]

Sunscreens are rated or classified by their sun protection factor (SPF). The SPF numbers that appear on a sunscreen's label refer to the product's ability to absorb, reflect, or scatter UVB. No uniformly acceptable standardized method currently exists to measure a sunscreen's ability to provide protection from UVA. UVA has a longer wavelength than UVB, which allows it to penetrate deeper into the skin.

Selection of a chemical sunscreen is a personal decision and is motivated by SPF number, cost, and other cosmetic influences. Up to 19% of individuals can have a reaction to a chemical sunscreen, so trial on a small area of the body is recommended.[46]

Chemical sunscreens are designed to be applied generously to all exposed skin. Depending on the chemicals used, a laboratory SPF can range from 2 to 60. Sunscreens are rated for their UVR absorption under strict and ideal laboratory conditions. In a laboratory, a sunscreen with an SPF of 15 will absorb 92% of UVB, an SPF of 30 will absorb 96.7% of UVB, and an SPF of 40 will absorb 97.5% of UVB.[46] The effectiveness of a particular sunscreen agent is affected by an individual's body site of application, degree of normal skin color, thickness of the epidermis, time of day, time of year, cloud cover, ozone levels, reflection, and UVR scatter. A sunscreen of SPF-15 is adequate if it is applied in the amount of 2 $mg/cm^2$.[46] Because most consumers typically apply less sunscreen than is used in laboratories to establish the SPF number, the actual SPF protection is often 20% to 50% of the number on the label.[51]

Chemical sunscreens of sufficient SPF can substantially limit or prevent DNA damage and pyrimidine dimer formation. They contain one or more chemicals in a carrier base—either a gel, lotion, cream, or ointment. Some formulations are clear; others are available in milky or colored formulations. An estimated $3.7 billion is spent each year on sunscreen products worldwide.[45]

Chemical sunscreens usually contain a variety of products that protect primarily against UVB and, to a lesser extent, against UVA. Ideally a sunscreen should be cosmetically pleasant, nontoxic, equally effective against UVA and UVB, water resistant, and have a high SPF.[52] Until 1989, sunscreens could only block UVB; the formulations currently available still only block a small amount of UVA. Organic absorbers include PABA esters, camphor derivatives, salicylates, and cinnamates that absorb primarily UVB.[53] Parsol 1789 absorbs the longer UVA rays. Other UVA absorbers include benzophenones, anthranilates, and dibenzoyl methanes. In 2006, the FDA approved the use of mexoryl as an agent that provides adequate protection against UVA.[52] Each family has a different absorption spectrum, so these agents are used in combination to provide broader protection.

The US Food and Drug Administration (FDA) requires sunscreen manufacturers to comply with product labeling regulations, including providing information on UVA protection.[54] In response to epidemiological evidence suggesting that use of higher-SPF sunscreens can lead to consumer overconfidence and thus increased UVR exposure, the FDA has also recommended a cap on SPF claims greater than 30 so that such agents would be labeled as 30+. The AAD has further recommended that labels should include directions on how often to reapply sunscreen, how resistant it is to water, and how thickly to apply it. Sunscreens designated as "waterproof" may not, in fact, be completely waterproof. This designation requires merely that the sunscreen retain its waterproof effectiveness for 80 minutes of immersion. Consequently, the FDA has changed the label wording from "waterproof" to "very water resistant."

Most healthcare professionals recommend an SPF of at least 15 but preferably an SPF of 30, and consider the patient's formulation preference (eg, gel, lotion).[3] Ideally, a broad-spectrum sunscreen should be used to block some UVA as well as UVB. Water-resistant sunscreens are usually preferred.

Many patient education points need to be emphasized regarding application of sunscreen.[12] To permit maximum absorption, sunscreens need to be applied 15 to 30 minutes before exposure, liberally (at least 1 ounce for an adult) and uniformly, and then should be allowed to dry. Products that are applied too thinly or rubbed vigorously into the skin will not provide the indicated protection. The technique of application greatly affects the effectiveness of the sunscreen product. In general, sunscreens should be reapplied every 90 minutes. Eyelids are commonly not covered to avoid skin irritation or stinging. Another facial area commonly missed is the ear. Sunscreen is now available in lipstick form to protect the lips. These products should also be applied liberally and reapplied frequently like chemical sunscreens.

When providing education about sunscreens, nurses need to instruct patients on how to read a label. One approach is to give samples to the patient, or examples of different agents with different labels for this education. It teaches the patient in a realistic setting how to be a better consumer and make good choices. Education must also include information about SPF, waterproof labeling, and ways to correctly apply and reapply the sunscreen. Most important, education should emphasize that sunscreen is an adjunct to other means to ultimately reduce UVR exposure.

When used properly, sunscreens with a high SPF are clearly effective in preventing sunburn.[38,45,53] Data are much more controversial as to whether sunscreen prevents BCC and MM, leading the International Agency for Research on Cancer (IARC) to state that sunscreens should not be the first choice for skin cancer prevention and should not be used as the sole means of sun protection.[53] In other words, sunscreen should not be used as a means to extend exposure to the sun. Current trends suggest, however, that may be the very thing that is happening.[12] The benefits of sunscreen should not be completely dismissed. Australians and Hawaiian Caucasians, who have some of the highest per capita uses of sunscreens, exhibit decreased incidence of MM, which is also related to other effective means of reducing UVR. The only real way to know the benefits of sunscreen with more certainty would be to conduct a prospective randomized study, with some participants using sunscreen and others not using sunscreen. Because it is not feasible and is unethical to conduct such a trial, the controversy about sunscreen will continue.[54]

***Physical sunscreens.*** Physical sunscreens physically block UVR from reaching the dermis and epidermis. These preparations contain molecules such as zinc oxide, talc, or titanium dioxide in an ointment base. They are considered inorganic chemical absorbers.[38] These sunscreens are available in white and neon colors and flesh tones. Physical sunscreens are effective and useful in protecting selected areas of the body such as the nose, cheeks, ears, and shoulders if applied thickly. The recent availability of physical sunscreens in bases that are cosmetically appealing (including titanium dioxide) has increased the use of these agents.[53] They are also sometimes combined with chemical sunscreens to create a more broad-spectrum product.

## Protective clothing

The effectiveness of hats and shirts as a primary prevention measure should not be underestimated. A brim size of 10 cm can lead to a reduction of 73% of UVR exposure to the head and neck.[12]

The weave of the material used in hats and clothing is very important. In general, synthetic materials provide better protection against UVA than cotton materials. Densely woven material provides a reflective barrier to UVR. An 85% polyester child size short-sleeved T-shirt provides the same protection abainst UVR as a sunscreen with an SPF of 5 to 10.[55] Clothes designed to cover the most skin provide the most protection. In general, synthetic materials provide better protection against UVA than cotton materials. Darker materials provide more protection.

Most clothes such as hats and summer wear offer an SPF of 2 to 6.5, although sun-protective clothing is available that offers an SPF of up to 30.[2,10] Clothing with an ultraviolet protection factor (UPF) is also available. This rating differs from an SPF rating, which is a measurement of sunburn or reddening time. The UPF provides information about the relative amount of UVR that penetrates the fabric and reaches the skin. The density of the fabric is the major determinant of UPF.[55] At this time, fabric UPF is not regulated by the FDA, but the Federal Trade Commission (FTC) carefully monitors advertising claims. The 3 classification categories for UPF are "good UVR protection" (UPF of 15–24), "very good UVR protection" (UPF of 25–39), and "excellent UVR protection" (UPF of 40–50+).[55] In some cases, fabrics may be treated with optical brighteners or chemical absorbers to increase UVR protectiveness before they are sold. Once purchased, clothes can be treated with detergents that contain optical brighteners to improve or retain UVR absorption. Spray-on treatments can also be used to increase UPF and last through repeated washings.

Nurses can educate patients about ways to assess the effectiveness of fabric as a sun protectant. This is a very important means to reduce UVR exposure that is consistently underestimated. Sunscreens should be used as an adjunct to sun exposed areas not protected by adequate clothing.[55] A simple test of efficacy is to hold the material up to strong light and see whether it casts a dense shadow or whether it is easy to distinguish objects through the shadow.[16] Nurses should also educate patients that virtually all garments lose about one-third of their sun-protective ability when wet.[55]

Protection of the ocular structures is also important. Some sunglasses can offer protection against both UVA and UVB.[45,47] Consumers need to be instructed to read labels correctly and carefully before purchasing sunglasses to assure that they actually offer UVR protection. The label should state "blocks 99% of UVR." Some manufacturers state "UVR up to 400 nm," which is equivalent to 100% UVR absorption. The color and degree of darkness do not provide any information about the ability of the lenses to block UVR. Detailed patient handouts from the American Optometric Association are available at http://www.aoa.org/documents/SunglassShoppingGuide0805.pdf.

## Reducing UVR exposure

The best way to reduce the incidence of skin cancer is to reduce UVR exposure. Public policy may be one of the most important ways to ultimately achieve the goal of decreasing UVR exposure. UVR exposure comes from both outdoor exposure and artificial sources. There is a need to educate both individuals and the public as a whole about ways to reduce this exposure in places where children play. Key targets for policy development and public education include schools, camps, sporting events, other outdoor events, parks, pools, and workplaces.

The recent availability of sunless tanning agents may have some impact on UVR exposure. Most of these agents contain dihydroxyacetone and provide a safe way to achieve a tanned skin appearance without UVR exposure. Early studies suggest that the use of these agents may not change reported outdoor sun exposure or sunscreen use, but the agents may be associated with a self-reported decreased in UVR tanning bed use.[56] Because of this early research, some believe that healthcare providers should advocate the use of sunless tanning agents to decrease tanning bed use.

*Outdoor exposure.* Approximately 60% of the total UVB exposure is received from 10 AM to 2 PM When possible, avoiding prolonged exposure during this time is recommended. Shade from trees and canopies can further reduce this exposure.[5]

In the United States, the National Weather Service (NWS) has developed an ultraviolet index (UVI) as one part of a national program of public education about the dangers of UVR.[30] The UVI accounts for time of day, cloud cover, haze, ozone concentrations, latitude, and altitude.[30] The public is informed by television and radio news and by newspapers of the day's solar ultraviolet intensity rating (a scale of 0 (minimal) to 10+ (very high)) and is given instructions on how to decrease UVR exposure. The long-term effectiveness of this program is not yet known, but it has been useful for epidemiological studies.[3,30]

In Australia, schools have "no hat, no play" policies that restrict children who do not have hats from playing outdoors.[3,36] Sunscreen is provided at public places, and many towns have installed shade cloths over play structures and pools in parks and community centers. A shade cloth, which is relatively simple to install, can reduce sun exposure by 60%.[16] Shade produced by trees can substantially reduce UVR. Note that the higher the canopy is from the ground, the more opportunity there is for scattered UVR to reach people under the shelter. Efforts in countries such as the US are much less extensive. In one survey, only 36% of child care centers had shade in more than half of the play area, and only 56% of the centers in another survey had implemented adequate sun protection policies.[16,36]

*Artificial UVR exposure.* Indoor tanning represents a relatively new area that public education programs need to target. Preliminary evidence suggests that there is an increase in MM risk for persons who regularly use artificial sources of UVA.[39] People who use artificial tanning expose their skin to 2.5-fold and 1.5-fold greater chances of developing SCC and BCC, respectively.[26,57,58]

Every day, more than 1 million Americans use tanning parlors that are largely unregulated. This $5 billion business features over 40,000 salons in the United States.[56] The FDA and the FTC share responsibilities in the regulation of sunlamps and tanning devices but regulation of this industry is complicated and not well regulated.[9,11] The FDA enforces regulations concerning labels on the devices; the FTC investigates false, misleading, and deceptive advertising claims about the devices. When these agencies determine that device labels do not comply with the regulations or that advertisements are not truthful, they may take corrective action. The FDA has the authority to remove products from the market. A few states include an active inspection program to make sure that beds emit the stated amount of UVR and enforce laws that limit or prohibit minors from using the facilities, but the indoor tanning industry remains largely unregulated.[26]

The most frequent users of artificial UVR exposure are adolescents and young adults, especially women. The UVA from these tanning parlors often amounts to 5 times more UVA per time unit than solar UVA.[12,56] Indoor tanning beds typically emit approximately 95% UVA and 5% UVB, which the parlors market as a "safe tan" because sunburning seldom occurs.[58] In reality, there is no known benefit from exposure to artificial UVA, and tanning actually represents the body's response to injury. Artificial tanning can substantially damage the skin, cause premature aging, cause loss of elasticity, and has been linked to ocular melanoma.[39,58]

Chemoprevention is a new area of research in MM prevention. An effective chemopreventive agent will prevent or significantly delay the development of MM Research suggests that the Ras pathway genes are important in the development of sporadic MM and that statins not only target Ras signaling but may have antiapoptotic and antiangiogenic effects.[59] Other agents being explored in animal trials include green tea and the flavonoid genistein.[59]

## SECONDARY PREVENTION

Early detection of BCC and SCC is important to prevent the disfiguring effects of these tumors and their treatment. Early detection of MM is an approach to control that, if used effectively and consistently, can have a relatively rapid impact on decreasing the mortality rate from this disease.[2,3] This approach is taken by most nations when implementing a public health control and awareness program for MM, even though the evolution of MM is not completely understood and it may not be completely preventable.[3–5] Recent evidence suggests that there has been a significant shift to the diagnosis of earlier stage melanoma in the past decade, although gains in decreasing the mortality have not been as great.[60] Table 66-4 provides an overview of approaches to screening. There are inherent strengths and weakness associated with each approach, so providers who design screening programs need to select one that is consistent with the goals of the program and the resources of the providers and their institution and the best means to approach skin cancer screening is still not completely clear.[11]

Skin cancer secondary prevention strategies are often defined as case finding, screening, and surveillance. Case finding is the incidental detection of cancer during a routine physical examination or visit to a healthcare professional for an unrelated medical problem. Skin cancer screening is the systematic cutaneous examination of a selected population, often from one geographic region, with individuals selected on the basis of age, sex, or other features. Screening may also be confined to those known to be at increased risk for skin cancer. Surveillance is the ongoing examination of individuals at regular intervals of 3 to 6 months for the development of new or changing lesions that might be early skin cancer. It may include photography of suspicious lesions. Presently there are no evidence-based guidelines for secondary skin cancer prevention.

### Screening programs

A panel sponsored by the American Association of Dermatologists (AAD) and the CDC identified skin cancer control issues as a priority.[2] Early detection of MM is critical because there is a direct correlation between tumor thickness and mortality. Screening should lead to the detection of thinner lesions. MM meets the criteria for a disease amenable to screening because it is a serious disease that is becoming increasingly common, it has an asymptomatic period, an available screening tool exists, and the disease can be detected and treated early. The panel concluded that primary care providers need to assume a major responsibility for skin cancer detection. These healthcare providers have an excellent opportunity either as part of a total physical examination or during focused examinations to assess for suspicious lesions and to refer for further evaluation when appropriate.

Data suggest, however, that total skin examinations are infrequently performed and documented in the primary care setting.[3,36] First, primary care physicians do not consistently examine the entire skin surface. Patients who are most likely to receive a skin examination from a primary care provider are those who request such an examination. Although managed care promotes health promotion and wellness services, in reality fewer patients may receive a total skin examination on a regular basis unless there is a clearly defined program directed toward screening, education, and prevention.[36,61]

The effectiveness of screening programs also reflects the skill of the provider performing the screening examination. This is the primary rationale of the US Preventive Services Task Force which does not recommend for or against routine skin cancer screening by dermatologists.[11,62] In general, dermatologists and health professionals with special training in detecting skin lesions are better able to diagnose MM

**TABLE 66-4**

**Approaches to Screening for Skin**

| Approach | Characteristics | Strengths | Limitations |
|---|---|---|---|
| Skin self-examination | Regular (usually monthly) examination of all skin surfaces | Note interval changes<br>Convenient<br>Inexpensive | Patients often forget to do examination<br>Some areas of body may be difficult for patient to adequately examine<br>Patients may lack confidence in ability to detect a change |
| Opportunistic screening (case finding) | Sporadic examination of patients who present for other health reasons | Earlier detection of lesions that patient may be unaware of | Dependent on the skill of the health provider<br>All skin surface areas may not be examined |
| Professional skin examination | Annual examination of all skin surfaces by a trained health professional with the goal of detecting skin cancers early | Trained professional may be able to detect a subtle sign or change<br>Examination is focused on finding early changes or skin cancers<br>Safe; noninvasive<br>Usually includes an extensive educational component on ways to prevent skin cancer | Dependent on the skill of the health provider<br>May result in increased removal of borderline lesions |
| Mass screening | Regular population-based screening of asymptomatic patients at a defined clinical site on a specific date | Large numbers of persons may be examined in a relatively short period of time<br>Trained professionals may be able to detect a subtle sign or change<br>Examination is focused on finding early changes or skin cancer | Dependent on the skill of the healthcare provider<br>May result in increased removal of borderline lesions<br>May be difficult to ensure patients with suspicious lesions receive adequate follow-up |
| Surveillance | Regular examination (usually every 3–6 months) of patients with a high risk of developing skin cancer<br>May include medical photography of suspicious lesions | Earlier detection of tumors<br>Usually includes an extensive educational component on ways to prevent skin cancer | May result in increased removal of borderline lesions<br>More expensive |
| Genetic testing | DNA studies to determine whether a patient who has a hereditary predisposition to malignant melanoma carries susceptibility genes | More accurately select patients who will benefit from intense surveillance<br>Usually includes extensive education on ways to reduce the risk of developing malignant melanoma | Expensive<br>Patient may be psychologically disturbed by the results<br>Results may be inconclusive<br>A negative test does not mean the patient may not go on to develop malignant melanoma<br>Results do not tell if, when, or where the patient will go on to develop malignant melanoma |

than primary care providers.[2,12] Over the last 4 decades, there has been a gradual improvement in the diagnostic accuracy of dermatologists in detecting MM. A common criticism of skin self-examination is that people will be burdening the medical system with benign lesions, although research has not substantiated this criticism.[2] It is also important to note that a total skin examination and skin self-examination detect NMSCs. The high prevalence of these types of skin cancers suggests that a total skin examination will result in a higher yield of positive finds than screening of any other organ system. A properly conducted skin examination may be considered time-consuming by some, although it can be performed effectively in approximately 7 minutes.[3] A risk assessment and total skin examination will identify persons at increased risk for developing NMSC and MM who may benefit from increased and more intensive surveillance. Often, these individuals can be referred to special clinics for pigmented lesions where intensive surveillance and education services are available.

While dependent on the population screened, rates of suspected melanoma in mass screening, case finding, and population-based screening range from 0 to 9 per 100 persons screened, with the most common findings between 1 and 3 cases per 100 population. Embarrassment remains a barrier to patients requesting or seeking a full-skin examination, especially if the examiner is of the opposite gender.[63] Rates of confirmed melanoma and melanoma in situ are commonly in the range of 1 to 4 per 1000 persons screened. In total, 1% to 5% of screened patients are confirmed to have NMSC.[61] The AAD has promoted free skin cancer education and screening programs in the United States since 1985 through the Melanoma Monday and the Melanoma Awareness Month campaigns, which are aimed at the early detection of melanoma and to improve recognition of early lesions.[60] Screenings have averaged nearly 100,000 persons per year since 1990 and represent the largest dermatological mass screening program in the country.

When skin cancer screening programs are designed, provisions for diagnostic and treatment services for those with positive screens need to be made available. Of great concern is the disposition of persons who have a positive screen.[3] Ultimately, the goal of such programs is that patients follow through with the recommended care. The utility and justifiability of any screening program depend on the extent to which those individuals with a positive screen can be followed and treated. If the financial resources necessary for such follow-up care and treatment are not included in the total budget for such screening programs, they will not achieve this goal.

Although dermatologists may have the most expertise in recognizing melanoma, their practice is often limited to persons at high risk for developing the disease.[61] Many melanomas do not occur in individuals with a family history or those with dysplastic nevi or fair skin. Thus, if early detection efforts are limited to this population, the overall impact to the population at large will be limited. To date, no randomized trials or case-controlled studies have examined whether screening by clinicians is associated with improved clinical outcomes such as reduced morbidity and mortality from skin cancer.[16,61] Increased awareness of the signs and symptoms of NMSCs and MM by the public and primary care providers is resulting in improved detection of these lesions.[60] Educating primary care providers who often have the most access to patients about appropriate referral strategies remains a challenge as it probably represents one of the most effective means to detect these malignancies early. Some speculate that earlier treatment as a result of screening improves outcomes.[20]

### Screening checklist

In clinical practice, decisions must be made regarding when to refer patients for further evaluation of suspicious skin lesions. Ideally, a screening checklist should detect abnormalities, without over-referring for benign lesions. There are few risk prediction models or screening checklists for MM. Most have been devised to make decisions for referral when screening for skin cancer. The most common checklist is the American ABCDE system. In this system, A stands for asymmetry, B stands for border irregularity, C stands for color irregularity, D stands for diameter greater than 6 mm, and E stands for evolving or elevation.

## PATHOPHYSIOLOGY

### NORMAL SKIN STRUCTURES

The skin is the largest organ of the body and is responsible for vital functions such as protection from injury, maintenance of homeostasis, and regulation of temperature. Skin consists of the epidermis and the dermis overlying the subcutaneous tissue layer or hypodermis (Figure 66-3). The epidermis is composed of stratified or layered epithelial cells, the majority of which are keratinocytes that are replaced every 14 to 30 days. The 4 layers of keratinocytic cells are named for their morphology and position: the stratum corneum (outermost layer), the stratum lucidum, the stratum granulosum, and the stratum spinosum.[64] Beneath these 4 layers is the stratum germinativum, or germinative layer consisting of basal cells that undergo mitosis in response to growth-stimulating signals. Following mitosis, the newly produced cells are outwardly displaced from the germanitive layer and move toward the superficial layers. As they do so, they lose their nuclei and thus their proliferative ability and they begin to manufacture keratin. Upon reaching the stratum corneum, the epithelial cells are flat, dead cells filled with keratin.

In the stratum germinativum, basal cells grow in a single column attached to a basement membrane. Other cells that may be present in the epidermis include Langerhans cells, Merkel cells and melanocytes. *Melanocytes* are derived from the neural crest in embryology. Most migrate to the hair follicles and skin, but melanocytes also populate the mucous membranes, uveal tract, meninges, and the inner ear.[65] MMs arise from melanocytes.

Epidermal melanocytes possess dendrites that contact keratinocytes in more superficial layers of the epidermis. This relationship, termed the epidermal melanin unit, consists of several keratinocytes for each melanocyte. In response to UVR exposure, melanosomes are produced

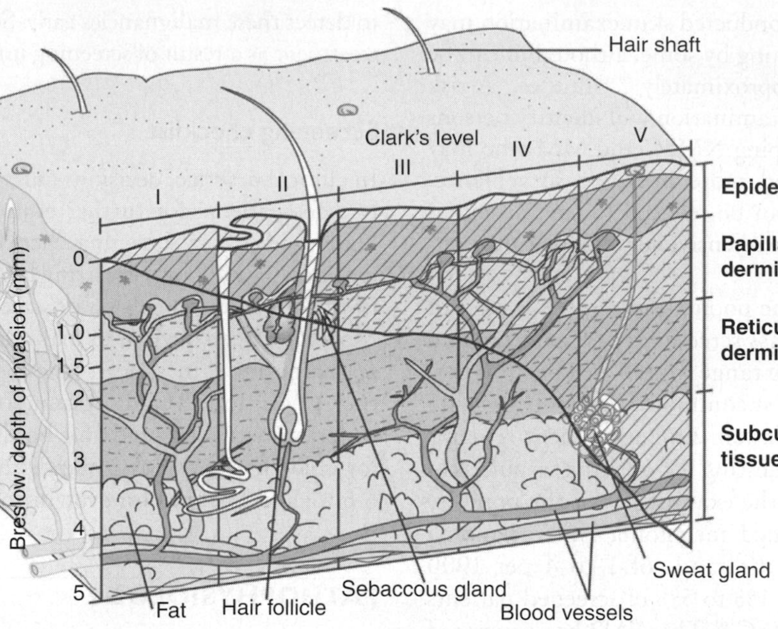


**FIGURE 66-3**

Anatomy of the skin demonstrating Clark's and Breslow's staging criteria.

and transferred through melanocyte dendrites to the neighboring keratinocytes. Melanosomes synthesize melanin, a substance that helps protect the skin cells by absorbing UVR. Melanin is also the primary skin pigment. Persons with darker pigmented skin have similar melanocyte density as those with lighter skin, but their melanocytes have darker, larger melanosomes that are more dispersed among the keratinocytes. Lighter skinned individuals have smaller melanosomes present in clusters among keratinocytes.[66]

Lying beneath the epidermis and connecting to the dermis is a basement membrane known as the dermal-epidermal junction. This area serves to connect the epidermis and dermis but also serves as a barrier to the passage of some cells and molecules.[66]

Immediately beneath the basement membrane lies the second layer of the skin, the dermis. This supportive, connective tissue network contains the vascular and lymphatic vessels, nerves, glands, hair follicles, and collagen-producing fibroblasts that give the skin much of its strength.[67] The dermis is also divided into 2 layers distinguished largely by the organization of the cells, nerves and vascular vessels, and connective tissue. The upper layer is known as the *papillary dermis* because it forms projections (papilla) into the epidermis. It is usually no more than 2 times the thickness of the epidermis. The lower layer, the *reticular dermis*, lies beneath the papillary dermis and is composed primarily of bundles of collagen. The reticular dermis lies above the hypodermis, a layer of subcutaneous fat and fascia that attaches the dermis to underlying structures.[64]

## MALIGNANT CHANGE

### Nonmelanoma skin cancers

*Basal cell carcinoma.* This is a result of malignant transformation in the nonkeratinizing cells that originate in the basal layer of the epidermis. The cell of origin is not defined but is known to resemble basal cells. BCCs may become locally invasive, rarely metastasize, and usually contain both epidermal and dermal components within the tumor. BCCs transplanted beyond the skin without dermal tissue usually do not survive.[68] This may explain the usual slow-growing, nonmetastatic nature of BCCs.

*Squamous cell carcinoma.* This is a tumor of the epidermis that arises from malignant transformation of keratinocytes. It can occur anywhere on the skin or mucous membranes where there is squamous epithelium and may arise from actinic keratosis or Bowen disease precursor lesions.[69] Unlike BCC, SCC can rapidly progress to local tissue destruction by filling the epidermis, invading the dermis, and then infiltrating other tissues.[67] SCC has the potential to metastasize depending largely on the location, depth, and size of the tumor. Metastases from SCC are more likely with larger and deeper cutaneous lesions, lesions of the lips, and lesions in scars.[69] Organ transplant patients and patients on immunosuppressive medications are at increased risk for the development of SCC. When SCC develops in this setting it is often more aggressive and carries an increased risk of metastasis and mortality.[70]

### Malignant melanoma

Most MM occurs in cutaneous sites after malignant transformation of melanocytes. Melanomas that lack pigment are described as amelanotic and account for approximately 1% of MM cases.[71] The initial site of MM is known as the *primary tumor.* MM may also occur in any melanocyte-containing tissue, including the meninges, the mucosa of the gastrointestinal (GI) and respiratory tracts, the uveal tract, and the vagina. MM arise from preexisting nevi in approximately 30% of cases and from apparently healthy skin in approximately 70% of cases.[72]

Most MMs exhibit 2 growth phases: radial and vertical. In the radial phase, cells grow in a radial fashion from the primary site and do not metastasize. This phase may continue for an extended period of time in superficial spreading, lentigo maligna and acral lentiginous MMs, or it may be of very short duration or absent as in nodular MM. As the MM enters a vertical growth phase, cells invade down into and through the dermis and have the potential to metastasize. MM tend to recur or metastasize in the stepwise manner of local recurrence, regional metastasis, and distant metastasis.[70,71]

Local recurrence is the reappearance of MM close to the primary site. The definition of local recurrence may be limited to recurrence within the scar or may include recurrence within 5 cm of the scar. Local recurrence is presumed to represent failure to totally excise the primary tumor. Intransit or satellite metastases may occur anywhere between the primary tumor site and the regional lymph nodes. They are thought to represent tumor emboli that were in the lymph channels draining the primary lesion and are a poor prognostic finding.[71,73]

Regional lymph node metastasis may present as a clinically palpable lump or may be identified after either sentinel lymph node sampling or lymph node dissection. Regional lymph node metastases are one of the most important predictors of survival, with positive nodes being highly predictive of visceral metastasis.

MM metastases can occur in any organ or tissue. The more common initial sites for metastases are subcutaneous tissue and lymph nodes. Distant metastatic locations include the lungs, liver, brain, and GI tract. Distant metastases can occur in other sites as well. Subcutaneous, lymph nodes and pulmonary metastases are associated with better prognosis than metastases to the central nervous system or liver. Around 50% of patients with other metastatic sites will eventually develop brain metastases.[70–72]

In approximately 2% to 5% of cases, MM may present as metastatic disease from an unknown primary site. In approximately 60% of these cases, the metastatic disease involves the lymph nodes; the rest involve distant sites such as skin/subcutaneous tissue, the lung, or the brain.[72] Patients who present with lymph node involvement with an unknown primary tumor have similar survival to those with a known primary tumor and lymph node involvement. Median survival is similar for those with unknown primary sites and visceral metastases as compared to those with known primary sites and visceral metastases.

## CLINICAL MANIFESTATIONS

Skin cancers have a wide variety of clinical presentations and signs and symptoms (Table 66-5). Tables 66-6 and 66-7 outline many of the common clinical characteristics of both NMSCs and MMs.[2,5,12,64,74–76] Many of these characteristics are shared among the malignancies and are difficult to distinguish with the naked eye. The signs and symptoms of different types of skin cancers can vary. SCCs seem to be difficult to diagnose clinically.[3,12] BCCs have more distinctive features, facilitating their clinical diagnosis. Distinguishing between dysplastic nevi and true MM can prove very challenging. MM often presents on the lower extremities in women and on the trunk in men. The classic signs in a preexisting nevus include darkening or irregular color, increasing size, nodularity, ulceration, pruritus, and bleeding. A biopsy is necessary to determine the histopathological characteristics of these different malignancies and to provide guidance for further treatment and follow-up recommendations.

**TABLE 66-5**

**Signs and Symptoms of Skin Cancer**

| Nonmelanoma Skin Cancer | Malignant Melanoma |
|---|---|
| Nonhealing sore or ulcer | New pigmented nevus |
| Scaling red or pink patch that does not heal | New unpigmented nevus |
| Enlarging pink papule or nodule | A nevus that is asymmetrical |
| New nodule with or without scaling, erosion, ulceration, or crusting | A preexisting lesion that has developed notched or faded borders |
| Pearly papule with telangiectasia | A preexisting lesion that has developed irregular borders |
| | An unusual or prominent nevus that stands out from the rest of the nevi on the body |
| | A nevus that is persistently itching, tender, or bleeding |
| | A nevus that has grown in size or is greater than 6 mm |
| | A nevus that has changed in color or has multiple colors |
| | A preexisting nevus that has a change in surface (elevation, erosion, crusting, ulceration) |

**TABLE 66-6**

**Characteristics of Premalignant and Nonmalignant Melanoma Skin Cancers**

| Type | Characteristics | Location | Other Features |
|---|---|---|---|
| Actinic keratosis | Raised red papule or patch with roughened surface | Light-exposed surfaced such as face, dorsum of hand, bald scalp<br>May occur on trunk | Premalignant lesions with variable degrees of dysplasia<br>Increased risk for NMSC |
| Actinic chelilitis | Well-defined white patches (leukoplakia) | Lips, especially the lower lips<br>Usually seen in men age 40–70 | Range from epidermal dysplasia to invasive squamous cell carcinoma |
| Bowen's disease | Solitary lesion usually a well-defined, slightly raised red plaque with an adherent scale | Predominantly on the legs, backs of hands, finger, and face<br>May occur on non-sun-exposed areas | Carcinoma in situ with full-thickness dysplasia<br>When Bowen's disease occurs on non-sun-exposed areas it is associated with an increased frequency of internal malignancy |
| Paget's disease | Solitary red, slightly raised well-defined plaque | Nipple and areola | Epidermis is infiltrated by variable numbers of large cells |
| Squamous cell carcinoma | Nodule or ulcer<br>May have a crusted surface | Sun-exposed areas including ears, lower lips, backs of hands, forearms | Grows more rapidly than BCC<br>Well- to poorly differentiated variants. |
| Basal cell—rodent ulcer | Small papule that subsequently ulcerates<br>Ulcer margin is well-defined and slightly raised with rolled, pearl-colored margin<br>Most common skin cancer | Face | Locally invasive<br>Rarely metastasized<br>Accounts for 70%–75% of BCC |
| Basal cell—cystic type | Central part of tumor does not break down until late in evolution | Face, especially the inner canthus of the eye | Often not detected early because it is mistaken for a benign cyst<br>Accounts for about 5% of BCC |
| Basal cell—pigmented | Features similar to rodent ulcer except margins are heavily pigmented | Usually the face | Often misdiagnosed as malignant melanoma<br>Accounts for 1%–3% of BCC |
| Basal cell—morphoeic type | Begins as a slightly elevated plaque | Usually the face | Often misdiagnosed because it spreads insidiously<br>Accounts for 2%–4% of BCC |
| Basal cell—superficial | Red plaque with adherent scale<br>Slightly raised, minute, well-defined margin that is rolled, pearly, and has telangiectasia | Usually the trunk | After a number of years it may become invasive<br>Accounts for 13%–15% of BCC |
| Basal cell—nevus syndrome (Gorlin's syndrome) | Multiple lesions<br>Multisystem disorder | Presence of palmar and planter pits | Dominantly inherited<br>Begins in childhood |

*Abbreviation*: BCC, basal cell carcinoma.

*Source*: Data from Rudolph Zelac[71]; Wolff et al[75]; and Habif.[76]

**TABLE 66-7**

**Characteristics of Malignant Melanoma Skin Cancers**

| Type | Characteristics | Location | Other Features |
|---|---|---|---|
| Dysplastic nevus syndrome | Large number of atypical nevi with irregular margins and variable pigmentation | Sun-exposed and non-sun-exposed areas | Increased risk of developing MM<br>May be sporadic or have a hereditary predisposition |
| Congenital nevus | May be giant or small<br>Present at birth or shortly after birth | May occur anywhere on the body | Giant congenital nevus is rare, occurring in about 1 of 20,000 births, with a lifetime risk of malignant transformation of 2%–40%<br>Small congenital nevus occurs in 1 of 100 births; lifetime risk of malignant transformation is not known |
| Lentigo maligna (Hutchinson freckle) | Flat, pigmented lesion that gradually enlarges<br>Light tan to brown or black with irregular notched borders | Usually on the face, neck, or arms of the elderly | Begins as MM in situ and may take 5–50 years to become invasive<br>Usually occurs in the seventh decade of life<br>Accounts for 5% of MM<br>3 times more common in females |
| Superficial spreading malignant melanoma | Slightly raised lesion with an irregular border and variable, unevenly distributed pigmentation with shades of red, blue, brown, purple, and black | May be found anywhere on the body but usually on the upper back of men and women and the lower extremities of females | Most common of the MMs (about 70%–75%)<br>With early diagnosis the 5-year survival rate approaches 95%<br>Long phase of horizontal growth prior to vertical growth and metastasis<br>Usually occurs in the fifth decade of life<br>Equally common in men and women |
| Acral lentinginous malignant melanoma | Initially the lesion is flat with irregular margins and pigmentation, but rapidly becomes raised and nodular | Soles, palms of hands, nailbeds, and oral mucosa | Early vertical growth and rapid metastasis<br>May occur in Asians and blacks<br>Accounts for 5%–10% of MM |
| Nodular malignant melanoma | Lesion is raised, nodular, and sometimes ulcerated<br>Borders are irregular and color variegated<br>Occasionally the tumor has no apparent visible pigmentation (amelanotic MM) | May occur on any part of the body, but most commonly on the legs and trunk | Does not seen to have a horizontal growth phase; grows vertically quickly with metastasis<br>Twice as common in men<br>Usually occurs in the fifth decade of life |

*Source*: Data from Cummins et al[2]; Markovic et al[12]; Habif[76]; Fleming.[77]

## ASSESSMENT

### PATIENT AND FAMILY HISTORY

A risk assessment is the first step in any secondary prevention or cancer screening program. Assessment should include all of the factors identified in Table 66-1. In particular, it is important to try to obtain an accurate history of sun exposure. This includes quantifying information about severe sunburns (especially in childhood), occupational history, use of indoor tanning devices, and overall cumulative exposure. In reality, it is very difficult to quantify lifetime exposure to UVR.[12]

The history should also include a family history with particular emphasis on the number of cases of NMSCs, MMs (including specific pathology when available), dysplastic nevus syndrome, and other genetic diseases such as Gorlin syndrome or xeroderma pigmentosum. Those patients who have a hereditary predisposition to developing MM may benefit from in-depth education about the physiology of the skin, genetic transmission, and the benefits of employing more sophisticated screening techniques such as medical photography. Information about the benefits and limitations of genetic testing should be presented. Such information should also be communicated with primary care providers. In addition, information about primary prevention strategies and chemoprevention should be provided when available. Written reminders for follow-up screening examinations at more frequent intervals may motivate the patient to comply with the screening recommendations. Patients from these families often need reassurance. They need to understand that primary prevention efforts may prevent or delay the onset of the malignancy and that regular, thoughtful screening may result in the detection of lesions at an earlier stage, when treatment is most effective.

Finally, the assessment should include detailed information about any lesions that have been removed in the past. Particular attention should be given to determining whether the patient has had any of the following lesions: dysplastic nevi, congenital melanocytic nevi, actinic keratosis, Bowen's disease, solar keratoses, BCC, SCC, or MM. In some cases, pathology reports must be ordered to provide a more accurate assessment and to ultimately provide better screening recommendations.

It is important to communicate to the patient that an accurate risk assessment provides more appropriate screening recommendations. It is also important for the patient to understand that the presence or absence of risk factors is not an absolute guarantee that he or she will or will not go on to develop malignancy. The risk assessment offers an opportunity to teach the patient about appropriate primary prevention strategies.[12] It also presents offers an opportunity to correct misconceptions about risk and offer reassurance about the benefits of early detection and primary prevention.

Once the assessment is complete, screening recommendations can be discussed in light of the individual's specific risks. Patients with higher risk profiles will need screening more often than annually and may possibly need medical photography. Follow-up after screening examinations is important, regardless of whether the screen was positive. It includes written communication to the patient and primary care provider(s) about the outcome of the screening and primary prevention recommendations. This includes information about the interval when screening should be repeated.

Before beginning the physical examination, it is important to determine whether the patient has noted any change in a lesion or if the patient has any concerns about a lesion. If such a history is elicited, further information should be obtained about any changes in size, shape, color, or other physical characteristics and when these changes were noted (see Table 66-5).

## PHYSICAL EXAMINATION

### Technical aspects

The mainstay for the early detection of both NMSC and MM is the physical examination. Clearly, the number of both NMSCs and MMs detected is greatly increased when the examiner focuses on that particular task and has a working knowledge of the different types of skin lesions (see Tables 66-6 and 66-7) as well as the signs and symptoms of skin cancer (see Table 66-5). Diagnostic methods that rely on inspection alone are 60% to 80% effective in identifying MM.[12] Primary care providers need to be aware of high-risk persons and high-risk anatomical sites, as only 20% of MMs occur on sun-exposed body surfaces, in contrast to 85% of NMSCs.[61] Those who practice in the pediatric setting need to emphasize primary prevention strategies.

To be effective, the examination should be carried out in a well-lit room and include all skin surfaces. Dermatological visual diagnosis is a skill that must be practiced to increase proficiency and appears to be based more on visual pattern recognition than on mastery of complex rules of logic.[61]

The physical examination of the skin should be performed systematically. The areas to be assessed are the same as those covered in a skin self-examination. The patient should be taught the importance of and rationale for a total skin examination. All concealing cosmetics should be removed. To make the patient as comfortable as possible, only one area of the skin should be exposed at a time.

The lighting in the room should be carefully selected. Ideally, a total skin examination would be conducted in daylight, but this is impractical. A combination of incandescent and fluorescent light is probably best. Fluorescent light accentuates blue to yellow colors and incandescent light brings out red colors. Their combination can help bring out the wide range of colors sometimes seen in skin cancers. Tangential lighting will aid in the recognition of subtle elevations.[76]

During the examination, all findings should be carefully documented on an anatomical chart. Characteristics to be documented include location, color(s), size (measured in millimeters), border characteristics, and presence or absence of elevation, telangiectasias, crusting, or ulceration. If the patient is being seen for follow-up screening, the anatomical chart from the most recent examination should be used for comparison to determine whether any characteristics of the lesions have changed.

Photography of lesions allows the clinician to accurately document the location and clinical characteristics for future reference. Total body photography is very important to assist in the identification of early MM in patients with dysplastic nevus syndrome. It usually requires about 24 different views.[74,75] In some cases, measuring tapes may be placed on the skin prior to photography to assess for changes in size.

Dermoscopy (epiluminescence microscopy, incident light microscopy, or surface microscopy) may be used as an adjunct to the physical examination in some clinical practices. Dermoscopy involves the application of a liquid, usually immersion oil to the surface of a lesion followed by examination. The oil eliminates some of the light reflection of skin and allows structures and colors of the skin to be visualized Examination is aided by the use of various tools such as hand-held dermatoscopes or computerized equipment that may include digital cameras. This procedure may aid in the early detection of MM by assisting in distinguishing malignancy from benign pigmented skin lesions.[77,78]

### Physical characteristics of lesions

Most BCCs begin as a small, firm, well-demarcated, dome-shaped papule (see Color Plate 13 and Table 66-6). A wide range of colors may be present, from pearly white to pink to red. Telangiectasias may or may not be present on the surface. Some lesions will have scaling plaques. As lesions progress, the center usually ulcerates and the borders develop a raised or rolled appearance.

The physical characteristics of SCC may not be as distinct (see Table 66-6). SCC often begins as a red, raised, firm papule. Crusting and ulceration is often seen (see Color Plate 14). It is not uncommon for the patient to report that the lesion is tender or painful.

A wide range of clinical characteristics may be noted in MM (see Table 66-7). It is often difficult to distinguish a dysplastic nevus from an MM. Within the different classifications of MM, a range of clinical characteristics may be observed (see Color Plates 15–18). Physical characteristics include asymmetrical, faded, or jagged borders; 2 or more colors in a lesion or a lesion that is a different color than the rest of the pigmented lesions on a patient; diameter greater than 5 mm; nodular surface characteristics; and bleeding or ulceration. MM may present with noncharacteristic features. Attention to the critical element of the patient's report of any skin change is essential.[72]

## DIAGNOSTIC STUDIES

Biopsy of the suspicious lesion is necessary for histological examination. On occasion, the lesion may be so small that boundaries of excision are much the same as they would be for a biopsy. In this circumstance, the entire diagnostic and treatment phases may be carried out in one step. This is only prudent for small lesions when the lesion and disease-free margin can be obtained.

Biopsies can be accomplished using several techniques: punch, shave saucerization, and incisional or excision elliptical biopsies. Although BCCs may be biopsied using any of those techniques, SCCs and lesions suspected of being MM—especially pigmented lesions—should be biopsied only using methods that remove the necessary tissue for complete dermatopathological examination so that lesions may be correctly staged. Incisional or punch biopsies should be taken from the most elevated portion of the lesion and from the darkest portion of a flat lesion.[74] Potential complications from biopsies include infection, bleeding, hyperpigmentation, hypopigmentation, adhesions, scarring, and problems with wound closure.

In some situations, immunohistochemistry (IHC) techniques must be used to assist with pathology study of the specimen. Biopsies that contain spindle cells, melanocytes without obvious characteristics of MM, or poorly differentiated specimens may require IHC techniques, for example. S-100, HMB-45, and MART-1 are molecules used in IHC review. S-100 is a calcium-channel-binding protein expressed in nearly all MMs. HMB-45 and MART-1 are markers for melanocytic-derived cells.[79,80]

A baseline chest x-ray may be part of the diagnostic workup for primary cutaneous MM. Additional diagnostic studies may be necessary if regional or distant disease is suspected. Lymph node sampling is recommended for most MM patients with primary lesions at least 1 mm in thickness, those who present with clinical lymphadenopathy, and those who present with other negative prognostic features. Lymph node sampling for lesions less than 1 mm may also be considered in those who present with negative prognostic features.[81,82] Blood tests such as complete blood count (CBC) and lactate dehydrogenase (LDH) may be performed. Liver scans or ultrasound may be indicated for persistent elevations in LDH to rule out liver metastases.[82]

Additional studies may include computerized tomography (CT) scans, bone scans, magnetic resonance imaging (MRI), positron emission tomography (PET) scans, and CT-PET studies.[73] More extensive work-up is necessary if patients complain of symptoms related to other body systems. For example, because MM may metastasize to the GI tract, patients with MM and GI symptoms should have further studies to rule out metastases.

## PROGNOSTIC INDICATORS

### Nonmelanoma skin cancers

BCC is usually slow-growing. Complete excision of a primary BCC suggests a 95% cure rate, and complete excision using Mohs surgery may further increase this percentage.[83] Primary lesions that are large and involve underlying structures, although rare, are more likely to have metastasized, in which case the prognosis is poorer. Extensive local invasion from BCC may cause significant cosmetic defects depending on the anatomical location of the lesion. For metastatic lesions, the 1-year survival rate is less than 20%; the 5-year survival rate is 10%.[83]

The course of SCC ranges along a continuum from slow-growing, locally invasive tumors to rapidly growing, widely invasive ones.[84] Overall, the 5-year survival rate for SCC is 90% and its metastatic rate is 3% to 6%. Dermal invasion and vertical tumor thickness are important prognostic indicators. Risk factors for recurrence and metastasis are related to the cause, location, treatment, morphological characteristics of the tumor, and immunocompetent status of the patient. SCC arising in areas of skin that have been irradiated or burned

**TABLE 66-8**

**Prognostic Factors for Malignant Cutaneous Melanoma by Stage**

| Stage | Factors | Prognostic Effect |
|---|---|---|
| I and II | Melanoma thickness | Worse prognosis with increasing thickness |
| | Ulceration | Increased risk of metastasis and decreased survival rates with ulceration |
| | Level of invasion (TI lesions only) | Worse prognosis with increasing level of invasion |
| III | Regional lymph nodes (macroscopic or microscopically positive) | Worse prognosis with increasing number of positive lymph nodes |
| | Ulceration | Increased risk of metastasis and decreased survival rates with ulceration |
| | Intralymphatic metastasis | Worse prognosis when present |
| IV | Location of metastasis | Worse prognosis with visceral vs extremity metastases; metastasis to the lung has an intermediate prognosis |
| | LDH | Worse prognosis with LDH elevation (measured by 2 or more values at least 24 hours apart) |

*Abbreviation*: LDH, lactate dehydrogenase.

*Source*: Data from Balch et al.[85]

have a higher metastatic rate (20% and 18%, respectively). SCC arising in areas of sun-damaged skin rarely metastasize, although SCC of the lower lip has a metastatic rate of approximately 15%. SCC originating in the oral mucosa, on the penis, and on the vulva tend to be more invasive at diagnosis and also have a higher rate of metastases.[83]

### Malignant melanoma

The prognosis of MM varies widely with the extent of disease and with consideration of several prognostic factors. In general, patients with in situ or very small (1.0 mm or smaller) lesions with favorable prognostic factors have almost a 90% ten-year survival rate, while patients with metastatic disease at presentation have a 10-year survival rate of less than 16%.[85] Prognostic factors are important in MM. Those that have been included in the revised staging system for MM are outlined in Table 66-8.[85] In the metastatic setting, elevation of serum LDH is the most predictive factor of decreased survival.[86] Additional prognostic factors have been suggested (Table 66-9)[72,85,87,88] and continue to be studied.

**TABLE 66-9**

**Additional Prognostic Factors for Cutaneous Malignant Melanoma**

| Factor | Prognostic Effect |
|---|---|
| Age | Better prognosis with younger age |
| Gender | Improved survival in females |
| Evidence of regression | Suggested better prognosis |
| Tumor site | Better prognosis with extremity lesions; worse prognosis with lesions on the hands and feet, acral lesions and intermediate-thickness lesions on the back, posterior arm, posterior neck, and scalp |
| Host immune response | Better prognosis with presence of tumor-infiltrating lymphocytes |
| Vascular invasion | Predictor of nodal metastasis |
| Mitotic rate | Worse prognosis with greater mitotic rate (number of mitoses/$mm^2$ in specimen) |
| Number of metastatic sites | Worse prognosis with increasing number of sites |
| Presence of respectable, solitary metastases | Better prognosis |
| Presence of serum S100B protein in stage IV disease | Worse prognosis when elevated |
| Overexpression of $NCOA_3$ in primary tumor | Reduced survival |

*Source*: Data from Paek et al[72]; Balch et al[85]; Zettersten et al[87]; and Retsas and Mastrangelo.[88]

## CLASSIFICATION AND STAGING

### NONMELANOMA SKIN CANCERS

Clinical staging is accomplished by inspection and palpation of lesions and involved lymph nodes plus imaging studies of any underlying bony structures.[89] Pathological staging is accomplished by the examination of completely resected tumors and lymph nodes. The TNM categories for both clinical and pathological classifications of NMSC are the same and are grouped as stages I-IV (Table 66-10). The histological grade of specimens is described as grades 1 to 4. G1 is a well-differentiated tumor, G2 is a moderately well-differentiated tumor, G3 is a poorly differentiated tumor, and G4 is an undifferentiated tumor. GX denotes a grade that cannot be assessed.

**TABLE 66-10**

**American Joint Committee on Cancer Staging for Nonmelanoma Skin Cancers**

| | |
|---|---|
| Stage 0 (Tis-N0-M0) | • Carcinoma in situ<br>• No regional lymph node or distant metastasis |
| Stage I (T1-N0-M0) | • Tumor 2 cm or less in greatest dimension<br>• No regional lymph node or distant metastasis |
| Stage II (T2-N0-M0 or T3-N0-M0) | • Tumor more than 2 cm but no more than 5 cm in greatest dimension (T2) or tumor more than 5 cm in greatest dimension (T3)<br>• No regional lymph node or distant metastasis |
| Stage III (T4-N0-M0 or any T-N1-M0) | • Tumor invades deep extradermal structure (ie, cartilage, skeletal muscle, or bone) or any tumor size with regional lymph node metastasis |
| Stage IV (any T-any N-M1) | • Any tumor size, any regional lymph node metastasis, and distant metastasis |

*Source*: Data from Greene et al.[89]

## MALIGNANT MELANOMA

Clinical staging of MM is based on biopsy results, clinical examination, and radiological procedures. Biopsied lesions may be described using either of 2 systems: Clark's level or Breslow's measurement (see Figure 66-3). Clark's level describes the lesion based on the depth of invasion into the dermis and subcutaneous fat. Level I (in situ) lesions do not penetrate the basement membrane. Level II lesions extend through the basement membrane and into the papillary dermis. Level III lesions reach into the reticular/papillary junction, Level IV lesions invade the reticular dermis, and level V lesions extends into the subcutaneous fat. The thickness of the dermis may vary depending on the anatomical site and individual differences and may affect the accuracy of Clark's level. The success of this method of microstaging depends on the examiner's ability to correctly interpret the microscopic anatomy of the skin.[71] The level of invasion is correlated to the metastatic potential of the lesion.

Tumor thickness is described by the Breslow method. The lesion is measured and defined as the distance from the epidermis to the deepest identifiable layer of contiguous MM cells.[71] Measurements are reported in millimeters.

Surgical staging should follow in all cases for which surgery will offer a clinical benefit. Depending on the extent of disease, surgical staging may include excision, sentinel lymph node biopsy, or lymph node dissection.

The American Joint Committee on Cancer (AJCC) has revised the MM staging system to incorporate research-proven prognostic factors and to organize subsets of patients by expected outcomes.[85] Several changes can be noted from the previous system: use of Clark's level for stage I MM only, inclusion of ulceration as a determinant of T and N staging, designation of satellite metastases as an N category, movement of lesions larger than 4.0 mm from stage IIIA to IIC, addition of the number of nodal metastases and metastatic tumor burden as N determinants, separation of lung metastasis into a distinct M category, and incorporation of sentinel lymph node sampling results (Table 66-11).[85,89] It is important not to confuse stage with Clark's level, both of which are reported in Roman numerals.

# THERAPEUTIC APPROACHES AND NURSING CARE

Initial treatment of both NMSC and MM relies on biopsy and histopathological evaluation of the suspicious lesion. In the case of MM, removal of the entire lesion for histopathological evaluation is the method of choice. This approach enables the pathologist to most accurately assess the primary lesion and prognostic indicators that will guide definitive treatment.

## NONMELANOMA SKIN CANCERS

Complete removal of the lesion, including tumor-free margins, is the goal of treatment. Treatment choices depend on the tumor type, size, location, and extent of disease. Skin cancers usually begin as small, locally invasive lesions that can be easily removed via a variety of methods with minimal morbidity. Extensive or recurrent skin cancer, however, may require complex surgical or radiation therapy, may be more expensive and difficult to treat, and has a less certain outcome. Treatments for NMSC include surgical excision, curettage and electrodessication (C&E), Mohs micrographic surgery, cryosurgery, radiation therapy, and chemotherapy. Surgical excision and Mohs micrographic surgery yield a complete specimen that can be examined by a pathologist. Laser removal, cryosurgery, and C&E should be used only when the diagnosis is certain and the lesion is small, as they will not produce a specimen for histopathological diagnosis and evaluation for free margins.

### Surgery

Surgical excision with tumor-free margins is the goal for most lesions. Primary closure or repair with skin graft or flaps usually produces good cosmetic results.[83] BCCs with tumor present in the lateral margins at the time of surgical excision may result in recurrence in approximately one-

**TABLE 66-11**

**AJCC Cancer Stage Grouping for Cutaneous Melanoma Pathological Staging**

| Stage | T | N | M | Criteria |
|---|---|---|---|---|
| 0 | Tis | N0 | M0 | In situ melanoma |
| IA | T1a | N0 | M0 | ≤ 1.0 mm without ulceration and Clark's level II/III |
| IB | T1b | N0 | M0 | ≤ 1.0 mm with ulceration or Clark's level IV/V |
| | T2a | N0 | M0 | .01–1.0 mm without ulceration |
| IIA | T2b | N0 | M0 | .01–1.0 mm with ulceration |
| | T3a | N0 | M0 | 1.01–4.0 mm without ulceration |
| IIB | T3b | N0 | M0 | 1.01–4.0 mm with ulceration |
| | T4a | N0 | M0 | > 4.0 mm without ulceration |
| IIC | T4b | N0 | M0 | > 4.0 mm with ulceration |
| IIIA | T1–4a | N1a | M0 | Primary without ulceration, 1 microscopic[a] node |
| | T1–4a | N2a | M0 | Primary without ulceration, 2–3 microscopic[a] nodes |
| IIIB | T1–4b | N1a | M0 | Primary with ulceration, 1 microscopic[a] node |
| | T1–4b | N2a | M0 | Primary with ulceration, 2–3 microscopic[a] nodes |
| | T1–4a | N1b | M0 | Primary without ulceration, 1 macroscopic[b] node |
| | T1–4a | N2b | M0 | Primary without ulceration, 1 macroscopic[b] node |
| | T1–4a/b | N2c | M0 | Primary with or without ulceration, intransit metastasis without positive nodes |
| IIIC | T1–4b | N1b | M0 | Primary with ulceration, 1 macroscopic[b] node |
| | T1–4b | N2b | M0 | Primary with ulceration, 2–3 macroscopic[b] nodes |
| | Any T | N3 | M0 | Any size primary, 4 or more nodes, or matted nodes, or intransit metastasis/ satellite(s) with positive nodes |
| IV | Any T | Any N | M1a | Distant skin, subcutaneous, or nodal metastasis with normal LDH |
| | Any T | Any N | M1b | Lung metastases with normal LDH |
| | Any T | Any N | M1c | All other visceral metastases with normal LDH or any distant metastasis with elevated LDH |

[a]Micrometastases diagnosed after sentinel or elective lymphadenectomy.
[b]Macrometastases defined as clinically detectable nodal metastases confirmed by therapeutic lymphadenectomy or nodal metastases exhibiting gross extracapsular extension.
*Abbreviation*: LDH, lactate dehydrogenase.
*Source*: Data from Balch et al[85]; and Greene et al.[89]

third of cases.[67] These recurrences usually present early and can often be surgically excised again. Positive deep BCC margins may result in deep, sometimes delayed recurrences at the tumor site and invasion of other structures.

Surgical excision may be recommended for SCC occurring within radiation fields. Further radiation therapy may be limited in those cases due to the exposure limits of normal tissue. SCCs should be removed with margins of 3 to 5 mm.[83] Margins of 6 mm are recommended for large tumors (>3 cm), invasive tumors, and those on high-risk areas (scalp, ears, nose, eyelids, or lips). Surgical excision is often the treatment of choice for SCC overlying bone and cartilage and for SCC occurring in scars, ulcers, and sinuses.[83]

*Curettage and electrodesiccation.* Curettage and electrodesiccation involves the use of heat to cut tissue. It is fast, efficient, and relatively inexpensive but relies significantly on the expertise of the operator.[69] Curettage and electrodessication may be useful in the removal of distinct, superficial BCCs. SCCs that are small, well differentiated, and are in situ lesions may also be removed in this manner. After the tumor is anesthetized, a sharp curette is used to scoop out the gelatinous carcinoma. Bleeding is stopped, and the perimeter of tissue is destroyed by using electrocautery or electrodessication. The wound is explored again with a curette to ensure complete removal of the lesion. Two or three cycles of curettage followed by electrodessication may be used.[70]

*Mohs micrographic surgery.* This procedure is often used for tumors that carry a high risk of recurrence or metastasis, are large, have indistinct margins, were incompletely excised and are in a location where excision with wide margins of healthy skin removal would be surgically or cosmetically unacceptable.[69,81] With this procedure, the tumor is excised under local anesthesia using horizontal frozen sections that are microscopically examined during the surgery (Figure 66-4). Any margins of areas with residual tumor can continue to be selectively excised while normal tissues are preserved, until clear margins are obtained. For removal of primary BCC, Mohs offers up to a 99% chance for complete removal without recurrence.[81]

*Cryosurgery.* Cryosurgery is the use of freezing temperatures to destroy tissue. It may follow shave excisions. A cryogen such as carbon dioxide, nitrous oxide, or liquid nitrogen must be used. The cryogen can be swabbed or sprayed on the lesion. Another method involves the use of a cryoprobe. It is cooled and then applied to the lesion for seconds or minutes. The deepest part of the tumor must reach at least –50°C during freezing. Cryosurgery for SCC may be used to treat superficial tumors and carcinoma in situ.[83] Cryosurgery may also be used to treat BCC in some cases such as limited, circumscribed lesions. More than one free-thaw cycle may be required and care must be taken to destroy subclinical disease.[70]

## Radiation therapy

Radiation therapy (RT) may be useful in treating both BCC and SCC lesions. Patients who are poor surgical candidates, elderly, or frail may still be able to undergo RT. RT for BCC lesions smaller than 5 cm in diameter may achieve good results, but lesions larger than 5 cm have higher recurrence rates when treated with RT alone.[83] Because SCCs have a tendency to follow embryonal planes of closure, tumors may invade deeply and not be amenable to cure by other treatments. Radiation therapy can penetrate through tissue and help destroy deeper tumors.[69] In both tumor types, doses between 4000 and 6000 cGy are often used and can be fractionated so as to decrease side effects. Treatment planning is based on the location and size of the lesion. Due to the risk of side effects to normal tissue, RT is rarely recommended for lesions overlying areas of bone or cartilage.[83] For recurrent skin cancers previously treated with RT, further radiation may not be an option due to poor vascularization and exposure limits of normal tissue in the field.

## Chemotherapy and biotherapy

Topical and intralesional fluorouracil (5-FU) has been used to treat BCCs. Topical applications are usually prescribed twice a day for several weeks for small, superficial tumors in patients who are unable to tolerate other treatments. Recurrence in patients treated with 5-FU is higher than that in patients treated with other therapies.[83] Intralesional 5-FU has been used in nodular lesions. Intralesional interferon has been used as an investigational treatment for both BCCs and SCCs.

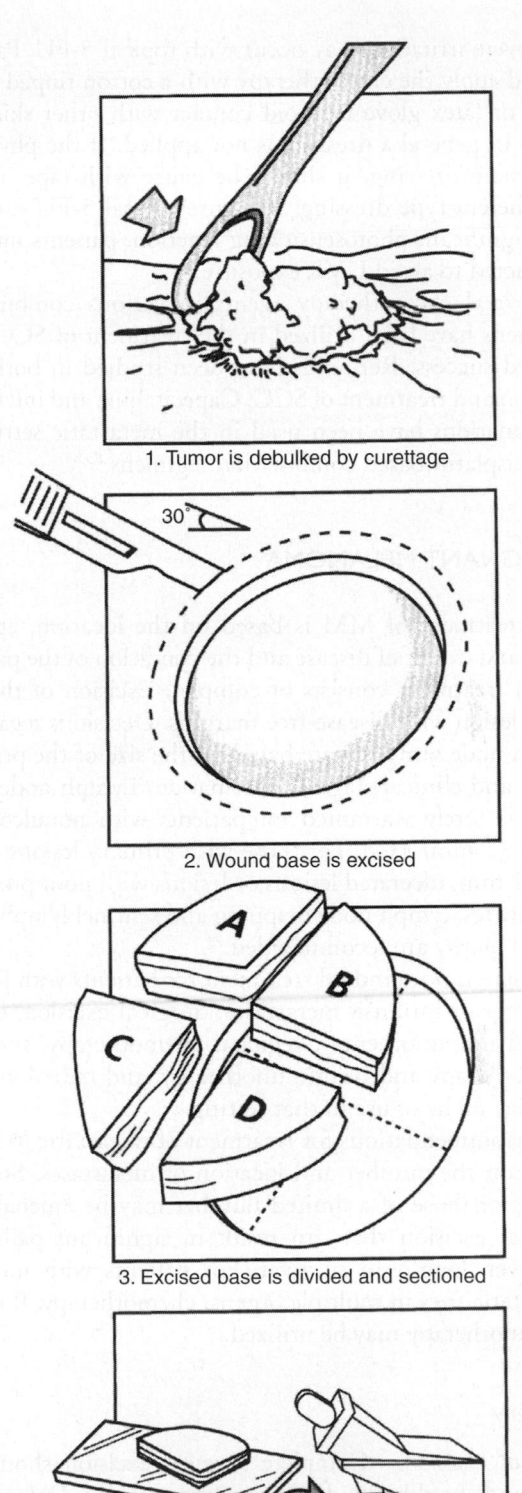

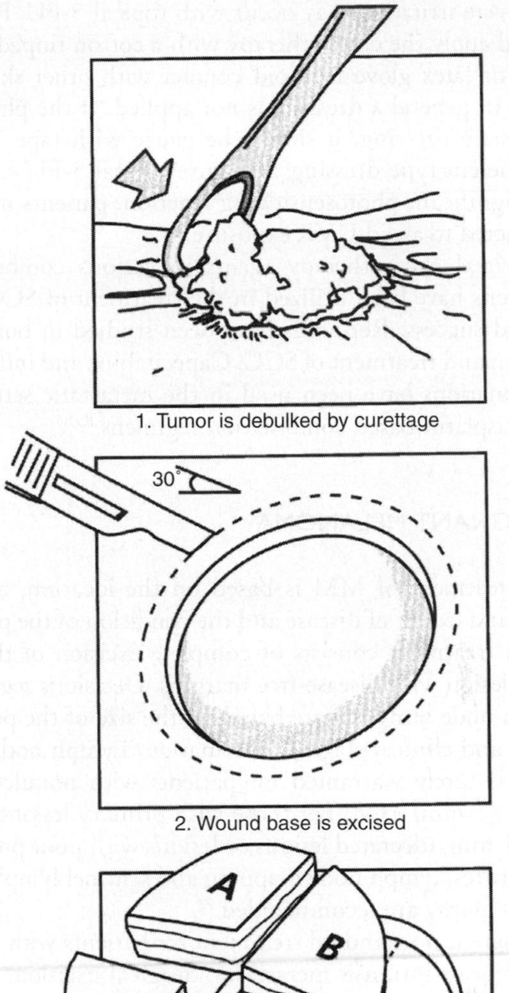


1. Tumor is debulked by curettage
30°
2. Wound base is excised

3. Excised base is divided and sectioned
4. Each section is examined for residual tumor

**FIGURE 66-4**

**Mohs' micrographic surgical technique.**

Severe irritation may occur with topical 5-FU. Patients should apply the chemotherapy with a cotton tipped applicator or latex glove to avoid contact with other skin surfaces. In general a dressing is not applied. If the physician requests a dressing, it should be gauze with tape instead of adherent-type dressings. Because topical 5-FU can lead to a significant photosensitizing reaction, patients must be instructed to avoid UVR exposure.

Several chemotherapy agents in various combination regimens have been utilized in the treatment of SCC with limited success. Retinoids have been studied in both prevention and treatment of SCC. Capecitabine and interferon combinations have been used in the metastatic setting as have cisplatin-based combination regimens.[83,84]

## MALIGNANT MELANOMA

The treatment of MM is based on the location, appearance, and extent of disease and the condition of the patient. Initial treatment consists of complete excision of the primary lesion with disease-free margins. Decisions regarding lymph node sampling are based on the size of the primary lesion and clinical staging information. Lymph node sampling is rarely warranted for patients with nonulcerated, thin (≤1 mm) MM. For those with primary lesions larger than 1 mm, ulcerated lesions or lesions with poor prognostic features, lymph node mapping and sentinel lymph node (SLN) biopsy are recommended.[73]

There is no standard treatment for patients with locally recurrent or intransit metastases. Surgical excision, intralesional immunotherapy, regional chemotherapy, systemic chemotherapy and/or immunotherapy, and radiation therapy may all be of use in that setting.

Recommendations for treatment of metastatic MM are based on the number and location of metastases. Solitary lesions or those of a limited number may be amenable to surgical excision that can result in significant palliation and even long-term survival. For patients with multiple metastatic sites in multiple organs, chemotherapy, RT, and immunotherapy may be utilized.

### Surgery

*Surgical excision.* Complete surgical excision should be wide and should include disease-free margins. Defects can usually be repaired by primary closure, although skin flaps may be necessary. The surgical margin size has been the subject of much controversy. In the past, margins of 3 to 5 cm were advocated for lesions of all sizes. Margin size has been the subject of several studies and practice standards currently allow for smaller margins with smaller tumors although discussion continues in this area. Excision of lesions larger than 4 mm should include skin and underlying adipose tissue. No improvements have been gained from the continuance of the excision through muscle fascia.[90] Amputation of the digit at the interphalangeal joint is necessary for subungual MM, and larger lesions may require more proximal amputation. Ear MMs may be successfully excised using a wedge excision and reconstruction without ear amputation.[71] Lesions on the face or vital structures may be excised with more limited margins depending on the situation. The use of Mohs micrographic surgery for MM is controversial but has been used for low-risk, thin MM on the face.[71,90]

*Lymph node dissection.* Lymph node dissection (LND) remains a controversial issue in the treatment of MM. The observation of the usual stepwise progression of melanoma from primary lesion to regional and then distant spread has been the basis for the use of LND. Elective lymph node dissection (ELND) is the removal of regional lymph nodes in the absence of clinical evidence of spread of disease. Theoretically, ELND should eliminate the most likely source of metastasis and translate into a survival advantage. Previous retrospective studies have shown that as many as 80% of patients with limited-stage MM who underwent ELND had uninvolved lymph nodes at the time of surgical excision of the primary tumor. Recommending ELND would, therefore, subject a large percentage of patients to an unnecessary procedure with potential complications and no benefit.[71] ELND has been largely abandoned in favor of sentinel lymph node biopsy.

Complete lymph node dissection (CLND) should be performed when lymph nodes are found to be positive by physical examination or by sentinel lymph node biopsy.[72] Infection, seroma, and nerve dysfunction are all potential side effects of lymphadenectomy. Lymphedema may also occur. Incidence of lymphedema after CLND varies by surgical location. Lymphedema has been reported in 4.6% of axillary CLND and 31.5% of groin CLND.[91]

*Lymphatic mapping and sentinel lymph node biopsy.* Lymphatic mapping and SLN biopsy is a minimally invasive technique used to identify and sample regional lymph nodes. With this procedure, the first or "sentinel" lymph node(s) draining a primary MM lesion can be identified and sampled. If the SLN biopsy is negative, further lymph node dissection is not currently recommended. If the SLN is positive, a regional lymph node dissection is recommended.[92]

Lymphoscintigraphy may first be used to identify the draining basin and therefore improve the identification of the sentinel lymph node(s). Extremity lesions usually drain into regional lymph basins in either the axilla or the groin. Trunk, head, and neck lesions may flow to more than one lymph node basin. In lymphoscintigraphy, radiolabeled substances are injected preoperatively into the site of the primary MM. Hand-held gamma probes are used to pick up the tracer and identify the location of the draining nodes.[71,73,81] The skin is marked to identify the location of the SLN. This procedure can identify the regional lymph node basins at risk for metastases but cannot determine the presence or absence of metastases.

Lymphatic mapping of the SLN can be accomplished by the injection of a tracer substance such as vital blue dye or a radiocolloid.[71] An incision is made over the identified lymph node basin. As the injected blue dye first stains the lymphatic channel and then stains the draining lymph nodes, SLNs can be identified. The SLN can be correctly identified in 95% of cases by using the combination of dye and radiolabeled substance.[73] These nodes can then be excised and examined by frozen or permanent section analysis.[71,90]

Allergic reactions to isosulfan blue dye used in the SLN biopsy procedure are rare but have been reported.[91] The incidence of wound infection, seroma, and necrosis following sentinel lymph node biopsy is less than 6%.[81,91] The most frequent complication is hematoma or seroma formation.[91,93] Incidence of lymphedema varies by surgical site. Results of a study of complications in patients enrolled in the Sunbelt Melanoma Trial showed a 0.3% rate of lymphedema in patients who had axillary SLN biopsy and in 1.5% of patients with groin SLN biopsy procedures.[91]

*Surgery for site-specific metastasis.* Surgical excision of satellite or intransit metastases can be an option. Patients with small numbers of lesions and slow-growing lesions may be candidates for such excision.[71,72] Metastatic disease may be present in patients with in-transit metastases. Before surgical treatment is recommended for intransit metastases, a thorough work-up for metastatic disease is recommended.[73]

Unlike many other types of cancer, surgical resection of metastatic sites has resulted in significant long-term survival advantage in some patients. Careful patient selection for these procedures is important. Patients with small numbers of metastases in few sites are the optimal candidates [73,90] Surgical resection of metastases is not usually considered a good option for those whose anticipated survival is imminently short.[90] Resection of metastatic disease in soft tissue and skin, lung, liver and the gastrointestinal tract have been reported.[73] Complete resection of metastastic sites can result in 5-year survival rates of approximately 20%.[86] Surgery may also be considered for palliation of symptoms. Resection of GI metastases may relieve bowel obstructions, for example.

## Chemotherapy

*Single-agent chemotherapy.* Since the 1970s, dacarbazine (DTIC) has been the standard of comparison for all other antineoplastic agents used to treat MM. In patients with soft tissue metastases, overall response rates as high as 20% have been documented with single-agent DTIC.[86] Subcutaneous, lymph node, and pulmonary metastases are the most likely to respond to DTIC, but the therapy has been largely ineffective against visceral, bone, and brain metastases.[94] Complete remissions are rare, and the median duration of response has been 4 to 6 months.[94] Side effects of DTIC vary with the dose and may include mild hematological toxicity, nausea and vomiting, photosensitivity, and liver toxicity.

Temozolomide is a prodrug. At physiological pH, it transforms to the active metabolite of DTIC. Because temozolomide can cross the blood-brain barrier, the potential exists for its use as a treatment of brain metastases. In clinical studies comparing DTIC with temozolomide in patients with metastatic melanoma, similar response rates and overall survival resulted for both agents. Regression of brain lesions in 25% of patients in a phase II study of temozolomide was noted.[94]

*Combination regimens.* Regimens including several different combination chemotherapies have been the subject of clinical trials, sometimes showing modest improvement over single-agent DTIC. Three of the most widely used combination regimens include: BOLD, Dartmouth, and the CVD regimens. The BOLD regimen includes bleomycin, vincristine (Oncovin), lomustine, and DTIC. The Dartmouth or CBDT regimen includes cisplatin, BCNU, DTIC and tamoxifen. The CVD regimen includes cisplatin, vinblastine and DTIC.[95] A phase II Dartmouth regimen trial noted an encouraging response rate of 40%.[95] However, no improvement in overall survival was noted when compared to single-agent DTIC and the therapy causes significant toxicity.[94] Few phase III randomized trials have been completed with these combination regimens; for those that have been completed, no survival advantage has been shown against single-agent DTIC.[72,94] Clinical use of combination regimens should be prescribed cautiously and with definite patient outcomes in mind. Toxicities may be greatly increased with combination regimens. Clinical trials in the use of combination regimens for the treatment of MM should be encouraged.[95]

Temozolomide presents new opportunities for combination chemotherapy regimens. Thalidomide, docetaxel and cisplatin have been studied in combination with temolozomide.[95]

The combination of immunotherapy agents with chemotherapy regimens has also been the subject of investigation. Interferon alfa (IFN-α) and interleukin 2 (IL-2) added to chemotherapy regimens have been particularly promising but need further study. The toxicity of these regimens can be significant.[72,95]

Dose intensification with and without stem cell support is another area of investigation in the treatment of MM. There is some indication that MM has a dose responsive nature with a few chemotherapeutic agents, particularly cisplatin.

*Regional chemotherapy.* When a relatively confined area is the target of treatment, regional rather than systemic administration of chemotherapy may be a therapeutic avenue. With this approach, systemic side effects can be diminished or avoided and higher concentrations of drugs can be delivered to the tumor site. Liver metastases from MM, for example, may be treated by intrahepatic infusion of chemotherapy with or without chemoembolization. One regional approach to treatment for intransit metastases in the extremities, known as isolated limb perfusion (ILP), is usually combined with hyperthermia. Arterial inflow and venous outflow vessels in the targeted area are isolated and cannulated, and collateral circulation of the area is interrupted. Venous blood is collected from the cannulated veins, pumped through an oxygenated extracorporeal circuit, warmed, and then pumped back through the cannulated artery. Tissue temperatures are monitored during the procedure. After completion of the perfusion, an electrolyte solution is used as a rinse, cannulas are removed, and vessels are repaired.[73]

Chemotherapy can be injected into the blood at several points in the ILP procedure, increasing the exposure of the tumor to the chemotherapy. Single agent melphalan is the most commonly used chemotherapy with regional perfusion, although other agents such as nitrogen mustard, cisplatin, tumor necrosis factor, and IL-2 have also been employed. Combinations of these agents have been studied as well. Overall response rates for these therapies have been as high as 65% with complete remission rates of 44%.[95] Acute local tissue reactions are possible and are graded based on their severity.[96] Despite the attempts to contain the chemotherapy to the targeted area, some systemic effects of the drugs may occur, as evidenced by severe hypotension in 10% of patients and a reaction similar to adult respiratory distress syndrome (ARDS) in 16% of patients receiving melphalan.[96]

Isolated limb infusion is a newer, less invasive and less toxic technique. Access to the circulation is gained by percutaneous radiological techniques. Extracorporeal circulation is established and a tourniquet is used around the proximal limb. Chemotherapy is infused and circulated but at lower doses than those used in isolated limb perfusion. More chemotherapy will distribute into the systemic circulation with this procedure as compared to isolated limb perfusion.[73]

## Radiation therapy

Radiation therapy may be of use in the treatment of MM, although it is rarely the primary mode of therapy for this disease. Exceptions include cases involving patients who cannot undergo surgery because of physical limitations or patients whose lesions are not amenable to surgery. An example might be a case of extensive facial LMM requiring extensive reconstruction in an elderly person.[97] Radiation therapy may serve as an adjuvant treatment when combined with surgical resection for patients with lesions at particularly high risk of recurrence, including primary lesions larger than 4 mm, positive surgical margins, locally recurrent disease, multiple positive lymph nodes, and lymph nodes with extracapsular extension.[92,97] In those cases, RT would follow surgical excision. This therapy may also be useful for palliation of symptoms of metastases such as bone pain, obstruction, and spinal cord compression. Approximately 60% to 70% of patients with brain metastases exhibit improved performance status after receiving RT.[92]

## Immunotherapy

The potentially immunoresponsive nature of MM has been suggested by both clinical and histopathological observations. Clinically, MM has a highly variable nature. The course of the disease may wax and wane over time. In less than 1% of patients, spontaneous regressions have been observed.[98] In addition, there is some evidence of increased incidence of MM in immuncompromised individuals, which points to a host immune response. Lymphoid infiltrates are frequently found on histopathological examination of MM specimens, suggesting an activated host response that occurs directly at the tumor site.[82]

Immunotherapy is an active area of research in the treatment of MM. Several agents, given either alone or in combination, have been examined. In many cases, these agents are used with chemotherapy in combined modality regimens. The 2 areas of greatest promise focus on the use of immunotherapy as adjuvant treatment for high-risk patients with surgical resection and for treatment of patients with metastatic disease. In either case, it is most effective as a treatment for patients with small tumor burden. As opposed to chemotherapy, the maximal effect from immunotherapy may not be seen until after 3 to 4 months of treatment, but the responses may be more durable.[98]

Immunotherapy of MM may be broadly classified as either specific or nonspecific. Specific immunotherapy agents target the tumor selectively; monoclonal antibody therapy is an example. Nonspecific immunotherapy agents (eg, interferon) stimulate the immune system as a whole.

*Interferon.* Interferon (IFN) is thought to both directly affect malignant cells and indirectly affect them by augmenting and stimulating the host immune response. In addition, low dose IFN therapy may have antiangiogenic properties.[86] IFN has been found to have synergistic activity with several chemotherapy agents and with other immunotherapy agents. It may be administered by subcutaneous, intravenous, and intralesional routes. Responses to IFN in the metastatic setting have been noted including durable remissions. Soft tissue or pulmonary metastases are more likely to respond.[82]

In the adjuvant setting for high-risk patients with resected disease, systemic therapy has not been helpful with the exception of IFN. A study by the Eastern Cooperative Oncology Group (EST1684) was the pivotal trial introducing this strategy. In this study, intensive intravenous

IFN (20 MU/m$^2$/day) was administered to patients for 1 month followed by subcutaneous IFN (10 MU/m$^2$ 3 times per week) for 11 months. Considerable toxicity was experienced with this regimen. Fifty percent of subjects required dose adjustments in the first month, and more than 50% required such adjustments during the final 11 months.[99] However, a significant increase in relapse-free survival was demonstrated and a trend toward increased overall survival was observed.[99] After a median follow-up of 7 years, this regimen has been shown to significantly prolong overall survival (OS) and disease-free survival (DFS). The 5-year relapse-free survival rate was 37% in patients who received high-dose IFN, compared to 26% in the observation group. The 5-year OS rate was 47% in the treatment group vs 36% in the control group.[94,100] A subsequent trial (E1690) used a 3-arm design to compare the EST1684 high-dose IFN regimen with low-dose IFN over 2 years against a control group. A DFS advantage was noted in the high-dose IFN group but no OS advantage was seen, bringing into question the use of high-dose IFN.[94,101] Several confounding variables were noted with this study, however.[94,100,101] Later analyses have shown that high-dose IFN therapy offers a benefit in relapse-free survival but no significant difference in OS.[102] Clinical trials continue in an attempt to discern whether lower doses of IFN or alternate administration schedules can achieve similar or better results and to further define the use of this therapy.[94,101,103]

High-dose IFN therapy is associated with significant toxicities.[104] Patient and family education, consistent assessment, early intervention and supportive care strategies are important. Patients may experience flu-like symptoms including fever, chills, malaise, anorexia and fatigue. Symptoms may range along a continuum from mild to life-threatening. Myelosuppression and liver toxicity are also seen with high dose IFN regimens. Most toxicities are reversible with dose interruption. After resolution, restarting IFN at a reduced dose is often successful. The flu-like symptoms may be managed symptomatically with supportive medications such as acetaminophen, diphenhydramine, and antiemetics. Neuropsychiatric events have also been noted as a result of high dose IFN.[100]

Contraindications to high dose IFN therapy include those with poor performance status, those who are pregnant or lactating, and those who have an autoimmune disease, immunosuppression, significant liver disease, severe neuropsychiatric disease, myelosuppression or a life threatening infection. High dose IFN should be used with caution in patients with diabetes mellitus, and in those with compromised cardiovascular, pulmonary and renal systems.[100]

Maintenance phase IFN may also cause toxicity. Flu-like symptoms may be worse at the beginning of the week or may increase over the course of the week. They may become better over time or become cumulative and more significant as time goes on. Dose reductions may be employed in this setting as well. Close and continued follow-up is important throughout this therapy. If the patient is stable, a recommended follow-up schedule may be monthly during maintenance for at least 3 months then every 3 months.[100,104]

Low dose IFN therapy has also been studied in the adjuvant setting. These regimens are associated with less toxicity. Improvements in OS with these regimens have not been realized although improvements in relapse free survival were seen while patients were receiving treatment.[100,102]

*Interleukin-2.* The therapeutic effect of interleukin-2 (IL-2) is brought about by stimulation of the immune system rather than direct cytotoxicity to MM cells. In the presence of IL-2, natural killer cells are activated to form lymphokine activated killer (LAK) cells, which have been shown to lyze MM cells. IL-2 may also cause damage to cells by generating nitric oxide.[87]

Clinical trials of IL-2 have employed different dosage ranges and administration routes. High-dose therapy (up to 720,000 IU/kg) given by intravenous bolus has resulted in response rates in up to 16% of patients.[105] High-dose IL-2 therapy may cause significant, life-threatening toxicities including capillary leak syndrome, respiratory distress, and hypotension, necessitating intensive monitoring and administration by expert clinicians.[71,105] Studies of IL-2 have also included combination therapies of IL-2 with lymphokine activated killer (LAK) cells, IL-2 with TILs, IL-2 plus IFN, and chemo/biotherapy combination regimens.[71,82,93,105]

*Bacille Calmette-Guérin.* Bacille Calmette-Guérin (BCG) is a nonspecific immunotherapy agent used to treat MM. It may be administered intralesionally or as an epilesional scarification.

Prior to treatment with BCG, purified protein derivative (PPD) skin tests are administered to assess the patient's prior sensitization to mycobacterial antigens. Individuals who are PPD positive are at risk for acute and life-threatening hypersensitivity reactions following BCG administration. Doses of BCG are adjusted based on the patient's PPD status, his or her immunocompetence, and the strain of BCG used.

*Monoclonal antibodies.* Antigens can be targeted for treatment with monoclonal antibodies and are an area of study in MM.[105] A recent advance is the development of antibody therapy against cytotoxic T lymphocyte antigen 4 (CTLA-4). CTLA-4 is a surface protein on T lymphocytes that suppresses the immune response. Two monoclonal antibodies, ipilimumab and tremelimumab (previously known as ticilimumab) can block CTLA-4, removing suppression and allowing activation of T cells. Clinical trials with these agents are ongoing. Commonly reported adverse events in trials with both agents include colitis/diarrhea and dermatitis. Pruritis and fatigue have also been reported.

*Vaccines.* MM vaccines are a form of specific, active immunotherapy. They are manufactured using a variety of techniques and may contain autologous antigens (from the patient's own tumor). More commonly, allogeneic preparations of antigens derived from multiple MM cell lines are used. A more recent development has allowed for the development of cell-lysate vaccines. Vaccinia melanoma oncolysate is prepared by infecting melanoma cells with vaccinia virus, lysing the cells, and collecting the resulting cell lysate. Immunogenicity is enhanced by using the vaccinia virus in these vaccines.[98] Other types of vaccines are also available, including DNA and RNA vaccines and dendritic cell vaccines. Melanoma vaccines are given to stimulate the immune system, causing it to actively seek out and destroy MM cells.

Few conclusions can be made about vaccine therapy for MM even after many years of study. Most studies have taken place in the adjuvant setting. Seven phase III vaccine trials have been conducted. Benefit has only been shown in 2 of the trials and only in subsets of patients.[102] Choice of the most effective MM antigen remains elusive as does the optimal method of immunization. A way to consistently test in vitro response is also undefined.[106]

*Targeted Agents.* As with other tumor types, interruption of signal transduction pathways and angiogenesis may result in clinical benefit as a treatment for MM. Sorafenib and oblimersen sodium have been studied in combination chemotherapy regimens in advanced MM.[93,95] Lenalidomide and the matrix mataloproteinase primomastat have shown some promise in studies.[95]

## CONCLUSION

The management of patients with skin cancer provides many challenges for oncology nurses. A number of subspecialty disciplines are often involved, including prevention and detection specialists, dermatologists, and surgical, medical, and radiation oncologists. In addition, treatment of these cancers may involve the services of other specialists such as geneticists, dermatopathologists, vascular surgeons, and immunologists. Oncology nurses often assume the responsibility of communicating to the patient what the role of each of these specialists is in the patient's care and providing clarification about treatment. Communication and documentation between these disciplines is vital to ensure a positive outcome for the patient.

There is much still to be learned about skin cancer. Given that this disease's incidence is increasing at an alarming rate, much work remains to be done in the areas of public education and awareness of prevention. The biggest gains in decreasing the morbidity and mortality associated with skin cancer will come from the prevention of the disease. Because the skin is a highly visible organ, these malignancies lend themselves to early detection. Programs staffed by qualified practitioners could be an important means of reducing the morbidity and mortality associated with both NMSC and MM. Treatment of early lesions is relatively straightforward and usually effective, but further research is needed to improve the outcomes with recurrence and second primary tumors. Especially in the case of MM, treatment is often unsuccessful and new therapies are needed. Genetics represent a promising area of research, and much remains to be learned about both the genetic predisposition for these cancers and the use of gene therapy as a targeted treatment for them.

## REFERENCES

1. Maselis TJ, Vandaele M, De Boulle K. Behaviour and motives of adolescents towards skin cancer. *Eur J Cancer Prev.* 2005;14:83–84.
2. Cummins DL, Cummins JM, Pantle H, Silverman MA, Leonard AL, Chanmugam A. Cutaneous malignant melanoma. *Mayo Clin Proc.* 2006;81:500–507.
3. American Cancer Society. *Cancer Prevention Facts and Figures—2008.* Atlanta, GA: American Cancer Society; 2008.
4. American Cancer Society. *Cancer Facts and Figures—2009.* Atlanta, GA; American Cancer Society; 2009.
5. Albert RA, Weinstock MA. Keratinocyte carcinoma. *CA: Cancer J Clin.* 2003;53:292–302.
6. Boukamp P. Non-melanoma skin cancer: what drives tumor development and progression? *Carcinogenesis.* 2005;26:1657–1667.
7. Yoder LH. Be sun safe! Understand skin cancer prevention and detection. *MEDSURG Nursing.* 2005;14:254–256.
8. Ries LAG, Melbert D, Krapcho M, et al, eds. *SEER Cancer Statistics Review, 1975–2005.* Bethesda, MD: National Cancer Institute. http://seer.cancer.gov/csr/1975_2005. Accessed September 29, 2009.
9. Cho E, Rosner BA, Colditz GA. Risk factors for melanoma by body site. *Cancer Epidemiol Biomarkers Prev.* 2005;14:1241–1244.
10. Losina E, Rochelle P, Walensky MD, et al. Visual screening for malignant melanoma: a cost-effectiveness analysis. *Arch dermatol.* 2007; 143:21–28.
11. US Preventive Services Task Force. Counseling to prevent skin cancer: recommendations and rationale of the US Preventive Services Task Force. *MMWR Recomm Rep.* 2003;52:13–17.
12. Markovic SN, Erickson LA, Rao RD, et al; Melanoma study group of the Mayo Clinic Cancer Center. Malignant melanoma in the 21st century, part 1: epidemiology, risk factors, screening, prevention, and diagnosis. *Mayo Clin Proc.* 2007;82:364–380.
13. Bellows CF, Belafsky P, Fortgang IS, Beech DJ. Melanoma in African Americans: trends in biological behavior and clinical characteristics over two decades. *J Surg Oncol.* 2001;78:10–16.
14. Naeyaert JM, Brochez L. Dysplastic nevi. *N Engl J Med.* 2003; 349:2233–2240.
15. Bermejo JL, Hemminki K. Familial risk of cancer shortly after diagnosis of the first familial tumor. *J Natal Cancer Inst.* 2005;97:1575–1579.
16. Emmons KM, Condit GA. Preventing excess sun exposure: it is time for a national policy. *J Natal Cancer Inst.* 2001;91:1164–1165.
17. Schaffer JV. Pigmented lesions in children: when to worry. *Curr Opin Pediatr.* 2007;19:430–440.
18. Bardia A, Pittelkow MR, Rao RD. Risk of multiple primary melanomas. *JAMA.* 2006;295:1516.
19. Bishop DT, Demenais F, Goldstein AM, et al. Geographical variation in the penetrance of CDKN2A mutations for melanoma. *J Natl Cancer Inst.* 2002;94:894–903.
20. Goldstein AM, Chan M, Harland M, et al. Lund Melanoma Study Group, Melanoma Genetics Consortium (GenoMEL). Features associated with germline CDKN2A mutations: a GenoMEL study of

melanoma-prone families from three continents. *J Med Genet.* 2007;44: 99–106.
21. Pollock PM, Trent JM. The genetics of cutaneous melanoma. *Clin Lab Med.* 2000;20:667–690.
22. Niendorf KB, Goggins W, Yang G, et al. MELPREDICT: a logistic regression model to estimate CDKN2A carrier probability *J Med Genet.* 2006;43:501–506.
23. Goldstein AM, Chan M, Harland M, et al. Features associated with germline CDKN2A mutations: a GenoMEL study of melanoma-prone families from three continents. *J Med Genet.* 2007;44:99–106.
24. Suarez B, Lopez-Abente G, Martinez C, et al. Occupation and skin cancer: the results of the HELIOS-I multicenter case-control study. *BMC Public Health.* 2007;7:180.
25. Wiggs WP. Playing it safe in the sun: primary prevention of skin cancer for sun-exposed athletes. *Dermatol Nurs.* 2007;19:555–560.
26. Whitworth A. Legislators combat melanoma, restrict teen tanning. *J Natl Cancer Inst.* 2006;98:1594–1596.
27. Veierod MB, Parr CL, Lund E, Hjartaker A. Reproducibility of self-reported melanoma risk factors in a large cohort study of Norwegian women: a randomized controlled trial. *Melanoma Res.* 2008;18:1–9.
28. Li C, Hu Z, Liu Z, et al. Polymorphisms in the DNA repair genes XPC, XPD, and XPG and risk of cutaneous melanoma: a case-control analysis. *Cancer Epidemiol Biomarkers Prev.* 2006;15:2526–2532.
29. Kaae J, Andersen A, Boyd HA, Wohlfahrt J, Melbye M. Reproductive history and cutaneous malignant melanoma: a comparison between women and men. *Am J Epidemiol.* 2007;1165:1265–1270.
30. Qureshi AA, Laden F, Colditz GA, Hunter DJ. Geographic variation and risk of skin cancer in US women: differences between melanoma, squamous cell carcinoma, and basal cell carcinoma. *Arch Intern Med.* 2008;168:501–507.
31. Glanz K, Buller DB, Saraiya M. Reducing ultraviolet radiation exposure among outdoor workers: state of the evidence and recommendations. *Environ Health.* 2007;6:22.
32. Cokknides V, Weinstock M, Glanz K, Albano J, Ward E, Thun M. Trends in sunburns, sun protection practices, and attitudes toward sun exposure protection and tanning among US adolescents, 1998–2004. *Pediatrics.* 2006;118:853–864.
33. Karagas M, Zens MS, Nelson HH, et al. Measures of cumulative exposure from a standardized sun exposure history questionnaire: a comparison with histologic assessment of solar skin damage. *Am J Epidemiol.* 2007;165:719–726.
34. Yamaguchi Y, Takahashi K, Zmudzka BZ, et al. Human skin responses to UV radiation: pigment in the upper epidermis protects against DNA damage in the lower epidermis and facilitates apoptosis. *FASEB J.* 2006;20:1486–1488.
35. Fears TR, Guerry IV D, Pfeiffer RM, et al. Identifying individuals at high risk of melanoma: a practical predictor of absolute risk. *J Clin Oncol.* 2006;24:3590–3596.
36. Centers for Disease Control and Prevention and National Institutes of Health. Healthy people 2010: readers guide. http://www.healthypeople.gov/Document/HTML/Volume1/ReadersGuide.htm. Accessed September 29, 2009.
37. Stone VB, Parker V, Quarterman M, et al. The relationship between skin cancer knowledge and preventive behaviors used by parents. *Dermatol Nurs.* 1999;11:411–424.
38. Dennis LK, Freeman LEB, VanBeek MJ. Sunscreen use and the risk of melanoma: a quantitative overview. *Ann Intern Med.* 2003;139:966–978.
39. Glanz K, Saraiya M, Wechsler H. Guidelines for school programs to prevent cancer. *MMWR.* 2002;51:1–20.
40. Olson AL, Gaffney C, Starr P, Gibson JJ, Cole BF, Dietrich AJ. SunSafe in the middle school years: a community-wide intervention to change early-adolescent sun protection. *Pediatrics.* 2007;119:e247–e256.
41. Geller AC, Brooks DR, Colditz GA, Koh HK, Frazier AL. Sun protection practices among offspring of women with personal or family history of skin cancer. *Pediatrics.* 2006;117:e688–e694.
42. Lee TK, Brazier AS, Shoveller JA, Gallagher RP. Sun-related behavior after a diagnosis of cutaneous malignant melanoma. *Melanoma Res.* 2007;17:51–55.
43. Harrison SL, Buettner PG, Maclennan R. The North Queensland "Sun-Safe Clothing" study: design and baseline results of a randomized trial to determine the effectiveness of sun-protective clothing in preventing melanocytic nevi. *Am J Epidemiol.* 2005;161:536–545.
44. English DR, Milne E, Jacoby P, Giles-Corti B, Cross D, Johnston R. The effect of a school-based sun protection intervention on the development of melanocytic nevi in children: 6-year follow-up. *Cancer Epidemiol Biomarkers Prev.* 2005;14:977–980.
45. Kyle JW, Hammitt JW, Lim HW, et al. Economic evaluation of the US Environmental Protection Agency's SunWise Program: sun protection education for young children. *Pediatrics.* 2008;121:e1074–e1084.
46. Meurer LN, Jamieson B, Thurman C. Clinical inquiries: what is the appropriate use of sunscreen for infants and children? *J Fam Pract.* 2006;55:437, 440, 444.
47. Kullavanijaya P, Lim HW. Photoprotection. *J Am Acad Dermatol.* 2005;52:937–958; 959–962.
48. Gallagher RP. Sunscreens in melanoma and skin cancer prevention. *CMAJ.* 2005;173:244–245.
49. van der Pols JC, Williams GM, Pandeya N, Logan V, Green AC. Prolonged prevention of squamous cell carcinoma of the skin by regular sunscreen use. *Cancer Epidemiol Biomarkers Prev.* 2006;15:2546–2548.
50. Cokkinides VE, Johnston-Davis K, Weinstock M, et al. Sun exposure and sun-protection behaviors and attitudes among US youth, 11–18 years of age. *Prev Med.* 2001;33:141–151.
51. Mayer JA. Promoting skin cancer prevention counseling by pharmacists. *Am J Public Health.* 2000;88:1096–1099.
52. D'Souza G, Evans GR. Plastic Surgery Educational Foundation Technology Assessment Committee. Mexoryl: a review of an ultraviolet a filter. *Plast Reconstr Surg.* 2007;120:1071–1075.
53. Vainio H, Miller AB, Bianchini F. An international evaluation of the cancer-preventive potential of sunscreens. *Int J Cancer.* 2000;88: 838–842.
54. Gottlieb N. Sunscreen: bodies of research remain to be covered. *J Natl Cancer Inst.* 2000;92:637–638.
55. Bauer J, Buttner P, Wiecker TS, Luther H, Garbe C. Effect of sunscreen and clothing on the number of melanocytic nevi in 1,812 German children attending day care. *Am J Epidemiol.* 2005;161:620–627.
56. Sheehan DJ, Lesher JL Jr. The effect of sunless tanning on behavior in the sun: a pilot study. *South Med J.* 2005;98:1192–1195.
57. Karagas MR, Stannard LA, Mott MJ. Use of tanning devices and risk of basal cell and squamous cell skin cancer. *J Natl Cancer Inst.* 2002;94:224–226.
58. American Academy of Dermatology. Position Statement on Indoor Tanning. http://www.aad.org/Forms/Policies/Uploads/Ps/Ps-Indoor%20Tanning%2011-16-09/Pdf. Accessed December 27, 2009.
59. Demierre MF. What about chemoprevention for melanoma? *Curr Opin Oncol.* 2006;18:180–184.
60. Halpern AC, Lieb JA. Early melanoma diagnosis: a success story that leaves room for improvement. *Curr Opin Oncol.* 2007;19:109–115.
61. Weinstock MA. Early detection of melanoma. *JAMA.* 2000; 284:886–889.
62. Lane JE, Dalton RR, Sangueza OP. Cutaneous melanoma: detecting it earlier, weighing management options. *J Fam Pract.* 2007;56:18–28.
63. Federman DG, Kravetz JD, Ma F, Kirsner RS. Patient gender affects skin cancer screening practices and attitudes among veterans. *South Med J.* 2008;101:513–518.
64. Chu DH. Development and structure of skin. In: Wolff K, Goldsmith LA, Katz SI, et al, eds. *Dermatology in General Medicine, vol 1.* 7th ed. New York, NY: McGraw-Hill; 2008:57–73.
65. Park H, Pongpudpunth M, Lee J, et al. Biology of melanocytes. In: Wolff K, Goldsmith LA, Katz SI, et al, eds. *Dermatology in General Medicine, vol 1.* 7th ed. New York, NY: McGraw-Hill; 2008:591–608.
66. Thibodeau GA, Patton KT, eds. Skin and its appendages. In: *Anatomy and Physiology.* 6th ed. St. Louis, MO: Mosby Elsevier; 2007:193–224.

67. Vargo N. Basal cell and squamous cell carcinoma. *Semin Oncol Nurs.* 2003;19:12–21.
68. Lang PG, Maize Sr. JC. Basal cell carcinoma. In: Rigel DS, Friedman RJ, Dzubow LM, et al, eds. *Cancer of the Skin.* Philadelphia, PA: Elsevier Saunders; 2005:101–132.
69. Grossman D, Leffell DJ. Squamous cell carcinoma. In: Wolff K, Goldsmith LA, Katz SI, et al, eds. *Dermatology in General Medicine, vol 1.* 7th ed. New York, NY: McGraw-Hill; 2008:1028–1036.
70. Aasi SZ, Leffell DJ. Cancer of the skin. In: DeVita VT, Hellman S, Rosenberg SA, eds. *Cancer Principles and Practice of Oncology, vol 2.* 7th ed. Philadelphia, PA: Lippincott Williams and Wilkins; 2005:1717–1744.
71. Morton DL, Essner R, Kirkwood JM, et al. Malignant melanoma. In: Kufe DW, Bast RC Jr, Hait WN, et al, eds. *Cancer Medicine.* 7th ed. Ontario: BC Decker; 2006:1644–1662.
72. Paek SC, Sober AJ, Tsao H, et al. Cutaneous melanoma. In: Wolff K, Goldsmith LA, Katz SI, et al, eds. *Dermatology in General Medicine, vol 1.* 7th ed. New York, NY: McGraw Hill; 2008:1134–1157.
73. Blazer DG, Sondak VK, Sabel MS. Surgical therapy of cutaneous melanoma. *Semin Oncol.* 2007;34:270–280.
74. Rudolph R, Zelac DE. Squamous cell carcinoma of the skin. *Plast Reconstr Surg.* 2004;114:82e–94e.
75. Wolff K, Johnson RA, Suurmond D. *Fitzpatrick's Color Atlas and Synopsis of Clinical Dermatology.* 5th ed. New York, NY: McGraw-Hill; 2005.
76. Habif TH. *Clinical Dermatology: A Color Guide to Diagnosis and Therapy.* 4th ed. St. Louis, MO: Mosby; 2004.
77. Fleming MG. Digital dermoscopy. *Dermatol Clin.* 2001;19:359–367.
78. Johr RH, Argenziano G, Zalaudek I. The use of dermoscopy in the diagnosis of skin cancer. In: Rigel DS, Friedman RJ, Dzubow LM, et al, eds. *Cancer of the Skin.* Philadelphia, PA: Elsevier Saunders; 2005:433–448.
79. Liu V, Mihm MC. Pathology of malignant melanoma. *Surg Clin North Am.* 2003;83:31–60.
80. Lamb LA, Halpern AC, Hwu WJ. Diagnosis and management of stage I/II melanoma. *Semin Oncol Nurs.* 2003;19:22–31.
81. Faries MB, Morton DL. Surgery and sentinel lymph node biopsy. *Semin Oncol.* 2007;34:498–508.
82. Lotze MT, Kirkwood JM. Melanoma and other tumors of the skin. In: Kirkwood JM, Lotze MT, Yasko JM, eds. *Current Cancer Therapeutics.* 4th ed. Philadelphia, PA: Current Medicine; 2001:205–213.
83. Neel VA, Sober AJ. Other skin cancers. In: Kufe DW, Pollock RE, Weichselbaum RR, et al, eds. *Cancer Medicine, vol 2.* 5th ed. Baltimore, MD: BC Decker; 2003:1997–2013.
84. Weinberg AS, Ogle CA, Shim EK. Metastatic cutaneous squamous cell carcinoma: an update. *Dermatol Surg.* 2007;33:885–899.
85. Balch CM, Buzaid AC, Soong SJ, et al. Final version of the American Joint Committee on Cancer Staging System for Cutaneous Melanoma. *J Clin Oncol.* 2001;19:3635–3648.
86. Pippas A, Reintgen DS. The treatment of disseminated melanoma. In: Rigel DS, Friedman RJ, Dzubow LM, et al, eds. *Cancer of the Skin.* Philadelphia, PA: Elsevier Saunders; 2005:655–659.
87. Zettersten E, Shaikh L, Ramirez R, Kashani-Sabet M. Prognostic factors in primary cutaneous melanoma. *Surg Clin North Am.* 2003;83:61–76.
88. Retsas S, Mastrangelo MJ. Reflecting on the 2001 American Joint Committee on Cancer Staging System for Melanoma. *Semin Oncol.* 2007;34:491–497.
89. Greene FL, Page DL, Fleming ID, et al, eds. *AJCC Cancer Staging Handbook.* 6th ed. New York, NY: Springer; 2002.
90. Essner R. Surgical treatment of malignant melanoma. *Surg Clin North Am.* 2003;83:109–156.
91. Wrightson WR, Wong SL, Edwards MJ, et al. Complication associated with sentinel lymph node biopsy for melanoma. *Ann Surg Oncol.* 2003;10:676–680.
92. Hollis G, Recio A, Schuchter L. Diagnosis and management of high-risk and metastatic melanoma. *Semin Oncol Nurs.* 2003;19:32–42.
93. Tawbi HA, Kirkwood JM. Management of metastatic melanoma. *Semin Oncol.* 2007;34:532–545.
94. Brown CK, Kirkwood JM. Medical management of melanoma. *Surg Clin North Am.* 2003;83:283–322.
95. Anderson CM. Systemic therapy for advanced melanoma. In: Perry M, ed. *The Chemotherapy Source Book.* 4th ed. Philadelphia, PA: Lippincott Williams and Wilkins; 2008:305–310.
96. Eggermont A, van Geel AN, deWilt J, tenHagen T. The role of isolated limb perfusion for melanoma confined to the extremities. *Surg Clin North Am.* 2003;83:371–384.
97. Ballo MT, Ang KK. Radiation therapy for malignant melanoma. *Surg Clin North Am.* 2003;83:323–342.
98. Kadison AS, Morton DL. Immunotherapy of malignant melanoma. *Surg Clin North Am.* 2003;83:343–370.
99. Kirkwood JM, Strawderman MH, Ernstoff MS, et al. Interferon alfa-2b adjuvant therapy of high-risk resected cutaneous melanoma: the Eastern Cooperative Oncology Group trial EST1684. *J Clin Oncol.* 1996;14:7–17.
100. Moschos SJ, Kirkwood JM. Adjuvant therapy for cutaneous melanoma. In: Rigel DS, Friedman RJ, Dzubow LM, et al, eds. *Cancer of the Skin.* Philadelphia, PA: Elsevier Saunders; 2005:641–654.
101. Agarwala SS, Kirkwood JM. Update on adjuvant interferon therapy for high-risk melanoma. *Oncology.* 2002;16:1177–1187.
102. Shah GD, Chapman PB. Adjuvant therapy of melanoma. *Cancer J.* 2007;13:217–222.
103. Eggermont AMM, Gore M. Randomized adjuvant therapy trials in melanoma: surgical and systemic. *Semin Oncol.* 2007;34:509–515.
104. Kirkwood JM, Bender C, Agarwala S, et al. Mechanisms and management of toxicities associated with high-dose interferon alpha-2b therapy. *J Clin Oncol.* 2002;20:3703–3718.
105. Cebon J, Gedye C, John T, et al. Immunotherapy of advanced or metastatic melanoma. *Clin Adv Hematol Oncol.* 2007;5:994–1006.
106. Chapman PB. Melanoma vaccines. *Semin Oncol.* 2007;34:516–523.

CHAPTER

67

Marcia Mickle, RN, MSN, ACNP, AOCN®

# Stomach Cancer

## INTRODUCTION

Stomach cancer remains one of the most prevalent cancers worldwide and is a leading cause of cancer deaths annually.[1] Diagnosing stomach cancer early, as with most other cancers, improves survival including possible cure for those diagnosed as Stage I. Improved surgical techniques and ongoing research into identifying genetic features for improved tumor response to chemotherapy and targeted therapy may contribute to better outcomes. Environmental factors that are contributing to a decline in stomach cancer incidence in the US and other developing countries include better eradication of *Helicobacter pylori* (*H. Pylori*), improvement in diet with an increase in consumption of fruits and vegetables, less reliance on salted and preserved foods, and an increase in screening for stomach cancer.[1]

## EPIDEMIOLOGY

Stomach cancer was the fourth most common cancer in the world in 2007 (following lung, breast, colon and rectum) and was the second leading cause of death from cancer in men and the fourth leading cause of death from cancer in women worldwide.[1,2] Nearly 70% of the cases of stomach cancer were diagnosed in developing countries.[1] Approximately 800,000 people died from stomach cancer worldwide in 2007.[1] The incidence of stomach cancer in the US and in other developed countries has fallen dramatically over the past 50 to 70 years, as has the number of deaths attributable to stomach cancer.[3] In the 1930s, stomach cancer was the most common cause of cancer death in the US. By 2008, it dropped to become the 14th most common cancer death, and the 16th most common cancer in the US.[4] The incidence of stomach cancer varies depending on the area of the stomach. There is a 10% incidence in the cardia, 10% in the body or fundus of the stomach, 2% to 3% in the greater curvature, 25% in the lesser curvature, and approximately 50% in the pyloric or distal stomach.[5] The incidence of stomach cancer related to location in the stomach are shown in Figure 67-1.

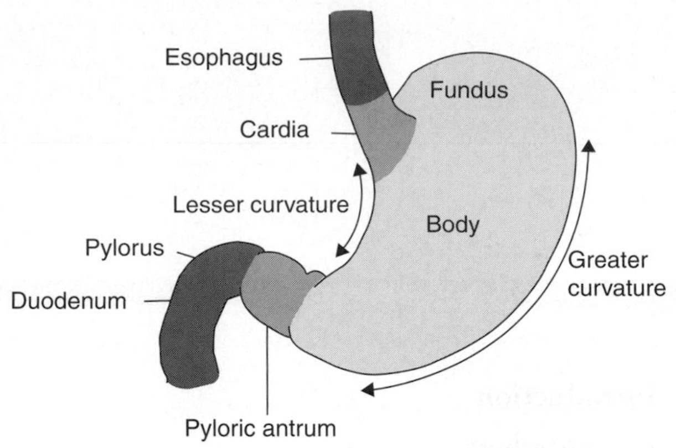


**FIGURE 67-1**

Incidence of stomach cancer according to location in the stomach: 10% incidence in the cardia, 10% in the body or fundus of the stomach, 2% to 3% in the greater curvature, 25% in the lesser curvature, and approximately 50% in the pyloric or distal stomach.

*Source*: Data from Boucher et al.[5]

Internationally, Japan and Korea have the highest incidence of stomach cancer in the world.[3] Noncardia stomach cancer has high incidence rates in East Asia, eastern Europe, and Central and South America. Low incidence rates are seen in South Asia, North and East Africa, North America, Australia, and New Zealand.[3] Statistics show that age-standardized incidence rates in males in Yamagata, Japan, are 95.5/100,000, compared with an incidence of 7.5/100,000 in white males in the US. Females have a similar ratio, but at a 50% lower incidence.[6] These geographic variances become more evenly distributed throughout the world for cancers of the stomach cardia. However, tumors of the stomach cardia are only about 5% of the total cases of stomach cancer in males in Japan, whereas they make up about 39% of total stomach cancer cases in white males in the US. Overall, the incidence of stomach cardia cancer in the US and other developed countries has risen five- to sixfold in the last 30 years. Tumors in this location now account for nearly 50% of all stomach cancers in men in the US and in the United Kingdom.[3] There is a substantial migration effect seen in individuals moving from a high-risk area such as Japan or Korea to a low-risk area such as the US.[7] These individuals may adopt an intermediate risk between that of their native country and that of their new country, but succeeding generations will acquire a risk level approximating that of the new country. Also, these migration effects may be dependent on the age of the individual at the time of migration. This, then, gives rise to the environment playing a key role in risk variations.[2]

The distribution of stomach cancer also varies according to age, sex, and ethnicity. In general, the incidence of stomach cancer rises progressively with age, with the peak incidence occurring between 50 and 70 years.[3,6,8] There is a significant male to female ratio in stomach cardia cancer predominance of 5:1, whereas in noncardia stomach cancer the ratio is about 2:1.[1,3,6] The prevalence of stomach cardia cancer is 2:1 in Caucasians compared with African Americans, but noncardia tumors are more prevalent, with an approximate ratio of 3:1 for African Americans compared with Caucasians. Also, lower socioeconomic status and living in developing countries are associated with an increased incidence of noncardia stomach cancer. However, there is a trend that the risk for cardia stomach cancer is relatively higher among the professional classes.[3,6]

## ETIOLOGY

Several risk factors are associated with the development of stomach cancer. The variation of incidence according to changes in geographic location over time and the migratory effect suggest that environmental or lifestyle factors are major contributors to the etiology of this disease.[3] *Helicobacter pylori*, a common bacterial infection worldwide that colonizes the stomach, is the strongest risk factor for the development of stomach cancer.[9] A high prevalence of *H. pylori* infection is seen in countries with high rates of stomach cancer. Declining rates of noncardia stomach cancer in developed countries parallel the decline in those countries of *H. pylori* infection.[3] In 1994, the International Agency for Research on Cancer classified *H. pylori* as a carcinogen in humans.[3,6] *H. pylori* is a gram-negative bacillus that colonizes the stomach and may be the most common chronic bacterial infection worldwide.[3] *H. pylori* infection leads to the development and progression of chronic gastritis. The infection likely triggers the sequence from chronic gastritis to gastric atrophy, intestinal metaplasia, dysplasia, and finally gastric (stomach) adenocarcinoma.[3,6] This development appears to be secondary to a sequence of events that leads to hyposecretion of acid. *H. pylori* is mainly acquired during early childhood, usually through oral ingestion, with the infection persisting throughout life. Factors such as low income, poor education, living conditions with poor sanitation, and overcrowding influence the prevalence of this infection.[3,10] It is estimated that approximately 59% of cases of stomach cancer in developing countries can be attributed to *H. pylori* infection and 63% of cases in developed countries.[1] Uemura et al. conducted a prospective study of 1,526 Japanese participants, 1,246 of whom were *H. pylori*-positive. Of these positive patients, 2.9% developed stomach cancer. None of the 280 *H. pylori*-negative patients in this study cohort developed stomach cancer.[11] Cancer risks from this bacterium are likely due to differences in strains of *H. pylori* and the host inflammatory response. *H. pylori* strains with *cytotoxin-associated gene-A (cagA)* are associated with an increased risk of intestinal stomach carcinoma, as opposed to *negative cagA* strains.[3,6,12] It has been reported that about 60% of *H. pylori* strains in the Western countries are *cagA*+, whereas, in Japan, nearly 100% are *cagA*+. Other host factors that may contribute to the increased risk of stomach cancer include genetic polymorphisms of the *interleukin-1B* (*IL-1B*) and *interleukin-1RN* (*IL-1RN*) genes leading to high levels of expression of these proinflammatory cytokines.[3,9,13]

Diet and nutrition, although no longer considered the most important factor for risk of stomach cancer or for its decline in frequency, does continue to play a major role in stomach cancer development.[14,15] A diet rich in fresh fruits and vegetables has been shown to have an inverse relationship with the development of stomach cancer.[3] In contrast, diets that include high salt intake and high intake of smoked foods, salted meat or fish, and pickled vegetables are associated with increased risk for stomach cancer.[3,9]

The polyphenols in green tea have been shown in animal studies to have antitumor and anti-inflammatory effects.[3] Polyphenols have antioxidant activities and have the ability to inhibit nitrosation, which has been implicated as an etiological factor in the development of stomach cancer.[3] Various case-control studies have shown a relationship between green tea consumption and a reduction in the risk of stomach cancer; however, recent prospective studies have found no protective effect with the consumption of green tea against the risk of stomach cancer.[3]

Smoking continues to be considered a risk factor for the development of stomach cancer, but what role it plays, or how close the association is, continues to be unclear.[1,2,6] Most studies that have shown a positive correlation between smoking and stomach cancer have found a less than two-fold increased relative risk, and the association relative to anatomic site or histological type lacks evidence.[6] Alcohol does not appear to contribute to the etiology of stomach cancer.[3,14]

It is estimated that 5% to 10% of stomach cancers are due to primary hereditary factors. Several autosomal-dominant inherited syndromes predispose individuals to stomach cancer. Hereditary nonpolyposis colon cancer (HNPCC) syndrome, also known as Lynch syndrome (LS), is secondary to germline mutations in mismatch repair genes such as *mutL homolog 1* (*MLH1*), *mutL homolog 2* (MLH2), *melanocyte-stimulating hormone* (*MSH*), *postmeiotic segregation increased 1* (*PMS1*), or *postmeiotic segregation increased 2* (*PMS2*). HNPCC is mainly associated with colorectal and endometrial cancer, and to a lesser degree, stomach cancer.[16,17] It is estimated that approximately 11% of individuals with a family history of HNPCC syndrome develop stomach cancer, with approximately 79% being of the intestinal type and having the same natural history as sporadic (nonhereditary) stomach cancer.[16] Peutz-Jeghers syndrome (PJS) characterized by hamartomatous polyps of the gastrointestinal (GI) tract, is associated with mutations in *serine/threonine kinase 11* (*STK11*).The risk of developing other cancers in individuals with PJS syndrome, including stomach cancer, falls within the range of benefiting from surveillance.[16] Some subsets of Li-Fraumeni syndrome caused by a germline mutation in tumor protein 53 (TP53) are associated with a predisposition to stomach cancer. Familial adenomatous polyposis (FAP) syndrome in families of Japanese and Korean descent appear to lead to an increased risk of developing a stomach cancer resulting from a transformation of fundic gland polyps into adenocarcinomas. However, there does not appear to be an appreciable risk of the development of stomach cancer in FAP-affected individuals in Western countries.[16]

Hereditary diffuse gastric cancer (HDGC) is an autosomal dominant inherited syndrome. Approximately 40% of families with HDGC have a mutation in the *E-cadherin* gene, also known as the *CDH1* tumor suppressor gene. It is thought that this mutation has an approximately 70% to 80% penetrance.[16,18] This means that carriers of the *CDH1* gene mutation have a 60% to 70% cumulative risk of developing diffuse stomach cancer by age 75 and a 75% to 85% cumulative risk by age 80.[18,19] Familial association with stomach cancer has been known for about 200 years—especifically in the case of Napoleon Bonaparte's family. He succumbed to stomach cancer, and several other members of his family, including his father, grandfather, brother, and 3 sisters, are reported to have died of stomach cancer, some at young ages.[16,18]

The hereditary syndromes and family aggregation appear more often in the diffuse-type stomach cancer. The increased risk for relatives of patients with diffuse-type gastric cancer is 7.0-fold compared with only a 1.4-fold increased risk for relatives of patients with intestinal-type cancer.[18,20]

## PREVENTION, SCREENING, AND EARLY DETECTION

The prevention of stomach cancer is divided into 2 main areas: moderating environmental factors and eradicating *H. pylori* infection. The large variation seen among geographic locations and migration studies show that stomach cancer is preventable in a majority of cases.[21,22] The availability of fresh fruits and vegetables with the development of modern refrigeration has led to increased consumption and may be a contributing factor to the decline of stomach cancer in developed countries over the past several decades.[6] The specific nutrients in fresh fruits and vegetables that confer this protection are unclear, but they may include vitamins C (ascorbic acid) and E (alpha-tocopherol, carotenoids, eg, beta-carotene) and selenium. Vitamin C levels are shown to be decreased in *H. pylori*–infected individuals. Vitamin C is a free radical scavenger; it can reduce the formation of N-nitroso compounds that are potentially carcinogenic. In animal studies, a synergistic relationship appears to be associated with dietary salt and nitroso compounds in stomach carcinogenesis. A study by Correa et al,[23] a controlled chemoprevention trial in a province of Colombia, showed that dietary supplementation with ascorbic acid and beta-carotene resulted in regression of precancerous stomach lesions. This benefit may be related to the cohort being from a high-risk population. In contrast, for low-risk populations, Jacobs et al,[24] in a prospective study in a US cohort, found little association between the use of vitamin C, vitamin E, or multivitamin supplements and the risk of stomach cancer mortality. The authors did not evaluate incidence of stomach cancer in this study, based on the assumption that with low rates overall of greater than 5-year survival, risk factors for incidence would likely be similar to associations of risk factors with stomach cancer mortality. Given the inconclusiveness of most studies, the protective role of ascorbic acid supplementation or other vitamin intake remains unclear.[6,25]

Prevention of stomach cancer through eradication of *H. pylori* infection is difficult as there is a long latency period between the time *H. pylori* bacteria are acquired and the development of mucosal changes or malignancy.[22,26] *H. pylori* is believed to be acquired in infancy or early childhood. Large trials that would include recruiting infected individuals who might be randomized to placebo certainly raise ethical considerations, and the required follow-up period would be long and could be prohibitive. Wong et al.[27] conducted a large randomized controlled trial with 1630 healthy individuals who were carriers of *H. pylori*. Each was randomized to either placebo or *H. pylori* eradication therapy. Over a 7.5 year follow-up, there was no overall difference in the incidence of stomach cancer between the 2 groups. In a subgroup analysis, those individuals in the active treatment group who had no endoscopic evidence of mucosal atrophy or intestinal metaplasia on entrance to the study did have a significant reduction in the risk of stomach cancer. This information may indicate that there is a point of no return in the pathogenesis of stomach adenocarcinoma, despite the eradication of *H. pylori*, or that these premalignant mucosal changes are no longer dependent on *H. pylori* as the driving force behind the further progression to carcinoma.[22,28] *H. pylori* remains the single most important environmental factor in developing noncardia stomach cancer and, to a lesser degree, cardia stomach cancer. Thus the prevention of acquisition of *H. pylori*, or the early eradication of the infection, remains a primary focus in the prevention of stomach cancer. *H. pylori* eradication rates of up to 90% can be achieved with effective therapy; thus a potential reduction in the number of stomach cancers by 20% to 30% in middle-aged adults in high-risk populations would be considered an effective preventive measure.[28]

The early detection and diagnosis of stomach cancer is vital to obtain a positive outcome. Early stomach cancer is a potentially curable disease, with a 5-year survival rate approaching 90%.[29] However, mass screening and early detection programs in the US remain limited as a result of the low incidence of this disease. In high-risk populations, such as Japan, nationwide mass screening programs have been in place for the past 50 years. Screening programs in Japan and among other high-risk Asian populations use barium swallow radiographs to identify abnormalities, which lead to more detailed barium radiographs and then to endoscopy as indicated. Case-control studies in high-risk areas have shown a 40% to 60% decrease in mortality from stomach cancer in those who have been screened; however, data from prospective studies are more inconsistent.[29–31]

For low-incidence populations, it is important to identify individuals who are at high risk by incorporating factors such as older age, family history of stomach cancer, *H. pylori* status, and other possible genetic factors and entering them into surveillance programs.[22] Patients identified as carriers of the HDGC mutation gene *CDH1* can be offered risk-reducing endoscopic surveillance or total gastrectomy.[32] Endoscopic surveillance should preferably be conducted in a center experienced with HDGC, and by the same specialist with each endoscopic evaluation. A study by Rogers et al.[19] evaluated asymptomatic high-risk families for *CDH1* mutation screening. Patients who were positive for the mutation gene went on for extensive preoperative screening and evaluation. Eight patients were identified with the mutation gene; only 1 had endoscopy biopsy-proven carcinoma prior to resection. All resected specimens were macroscopically normal, but microscopically all showed invasive diffuse (signet ring cell) adenocarcinoma. This study evaluated the location of the signet ring cells and may shed light on areas of concentration for biopsy among future *CDH1* mutation carriers undergoing routine surveillance biopsies who are reluctant to have or are delaying risk-reducing total gastrectomies.[19]

## PATHOPHYSIOLOGY

### CELLULAR CHARACTERISTICS

Histologically, 95% of stomach cancers are adenocarcinomas. The remaining 5% are leiomyosarcomas, lymphomas, carcinoids, squamous cancers, or other rare types.[33] The adenocarcinomas are classified into 4 subcategories: papillary, tubular, mucinous, or signet ring carcinomas.

Several classification systems are used to define stomach cancer. The Borrmann classification system is based on gross appearance and describes 4 types: type I is polypoid, type II is fungating, type III is ulcerated, and type IV is infiltrative.[34] Types I and II are often classified together and described as protruding. Type III is described as penetrating. Type IV is subdivided into superficial spreading (the tumor may spread along the mucosa and infiltrate superficially within the wall of the stomach) and linitis plastica (infiltration of the tumor into the stomach wall with a fibrous reaction causing a rigid leather bottle-appearing stomach). An addition to this classification by gross appearance is miscellaneous or mixed, where the tumor shows characteristics of 2 or more types.[35] On the basis of this classification system, the protruding tumors tend to have a better prognosis than the spreading tumors as they become symptomatic at an earlier stage of the disease.[35,36]

The Lauren classification system, which is probably the most widely used, classifies stomach tumors on the basis of patterns of local invasion by histological feature. There are 3 types of stomach tumors in this classification system: intestinal, diffuse, and mixed. The intestinal type, also called the epidemic form, is composed of cohesive neoplastic cells that form glands and tubular structures, and is often associated with precancerous lesions, gastric atrophy, and intestinal metaplasia. Most distal cancers are intestinal type, associated with *H. pylori* infection, and its incidence is declining.[8,34] Diffuse type, or endemic form, tumors are scattered neoplastic cells that invade individually, with minimal intercellular cohesion, leading to submucosal spread and contiguous spread of the carcinoma to the peritoneum. The diffuse type is most often associated with proximal tumors, is more common in younger patients with no history of gastritis, has increased in incidence worldwide, and tends to have a worse prognosis than distal tumors.[8,33,37]

### PROGRESSION OF DISEASE

Stomach tumors can spread to adjacent structures, the lymphatic system, the peritoneal surface, and other distant sites. The mode of spread is through the local invasive properties of the tumor, through the lymphatic system, or by hematogenous dissemination. Local spread to adjacent structures can be through radial intramural spread and also by deep invasion through the wall to involve the adjacent structures.[36] This extension through the gastric serosa can involve the omentum, spleen, adrenal gland, diaphragm, liver, pancreas, or colon. The ulcerative and polypoid types of stomach cancer tend to spread through the gastric wall and involve the serosa and draining lymph nodes. The diffuse type spreads through the submucosa and muscularis. Distant metastases can affect any organ: 40% involve the liver; 40% involve the lung, which may be lymphangitic; 10% involve the peritoneum, and often the Virchow node (a left supraclavicular lymph node), Irish node (left axillary lymph node), and Sister Joseph nodule (umbilicus). Other sites of tumor spread (10%) include sclerotic bone metastases, carcinomatous meningitis, the ovaries (Krukenberg tumor), or the rectal shelf in men (Blumer shelf).[33,36]

## CLINICAL MANIFESTATIONS

Stomach cancer is frequently diagnosed at an advanced stage, as symptoms are often vague or nonexistent in the early stages. Symptoms such as dyspepsia are nonspecific and may initially be treated as a peptic ulcer or dismissed altogether. Later, when the disease has advanced, weight loss of more than 10% is reported in as many as 80% of patients with stomach cancer. These patients tend to have a significantly shorter survival than those without weight loss.[36,38] Other, nonspecific symptoms include anorexia, fatigue, and epigastric discomfort. The ability of the stomach and abdomen to distend may be a reason for the delay in awareness of these symptoms. Signs of advanced disease may include gastrointestinal (GI) bleeding, abdominal distension secondary to ascites, bowel obstruction, palpable Virchow node or Irish node, and palpable Krukenberg tumor.[39] Paraneoplastic manifestations involving the skin can be present, such as acanthosis nigricans or the new appearance of seborrheic keratoses (a sign of Leser-Trélat).[8,33]

The type of symptoms is related to the classification of the stomach tumor, as it also usually relates to location. Those tumors located in the proximal stomach predominately cause dysphagia, whereas those located in the mid or distal stomach may have symptoms of nausea, vomiting, and early satiety, often related to diffuse-type stomach cancer resulting from loss of distensibility of the gastric wall.[29,36,40]

## ASSESSMENT

The patient presenting with symptoms suggestive of stomach cancer must undergo a complete history and physical. The exam must also include serum studies, including complete blood count, metabolic panel, and hepatic panel. Checking the blood for serum tumor markers is not well established. Approximately only one third of patients with primary stomach cancer will have an elevated carcinoembryonic antigen (CEA) level.[36,37] The sensitivity of CEA for stomach cancer is low, but when elevated it does generally indicate a correlation with the stage of the disease. Also checking other tumor markers along with CEA, including carbohydrate antigen 19–9 (CA 19–9) or carbohydrate antigen 50 (CA 50), may increase the sensitivity. Other studies suggest that an elevated beta-human chorionic gonadotropin (β-HCG) and cancer antigen 125 (CA-125) may indicate the tumor burden and the aggressiveness of the tumor.[36] HER 2 is receiving interest as a tumor marker in stomach cancer and may possibly provide another effective chemotherapy agent in some types of stomach cancer.[41] Visualization of the stomach and proximal portion of the duodenum via esophagogastroeuodenoscopy (EGD) and other imaging is required for complete workup.

### PATIENT AND FAMILY HISTORY

A complete patient history (including a nutrition and social history) and family history is required. Questions to evaluate the extent of the symptoms are important. Important questions include the onset, location, and associated symptoms that the individual is experiencing and the factors that aggravate or alleviate the symptoms. The patient's nutritional status should be explored, including typical oral intake (food and fluids); assess amounts, frequency, calories, and supplements. Changes in appetite or dietary habits may provide clues to the potential for stomach cancer. Questions related to weight are critical, including current weight, typical weight, and any weight loss. More specific questions should then be asked related to each symptom. Has the dysphagia had a gradual onset? Do you get full after eating certain types of foods, or is it related to foods in general? Do liquids cause as much of the feelings of fullness as foods? Do you have nausea and vomiting associated with types of foods or with the feelings of fullness? Has the pain been gradually increasing to be constant? Do you have heartburn? Does eating or drinking make the pain better or worse? Are you having any bowel issues, such as constipation, diarrhea, blood in the stools, or dark or tarry colored stools? Do you feel like your abdomen is larger and bloated even though you have lost weight?

### PHYSICAL EXAMINATION

A complete physical exam is needed in assessing the patient for stomach cancer. Special attention should be paid to assessing the left supraclavicular nodal basin and the left axillary nodal basin and to palpating around the umbilicus for nodules. The liver should be palpated for enlargement. A pelvic exam can reveal an ovarian mass, and a rectal exam can reveal fullness in the anterior shelf. These findings can help establish primary vs metastatic disease.

### DIAGNOSTIC STUDIES

An esopagogastroduodenoscopy (EGD) evaluation is an essential diagnostic tool for establishing a stomach cancer diagnosis.[37] This procedure provides a direct visualization of the gastric mucosa and allows for brushings and multiple biopsies for histological analysis. A minimum of 4 biopsies is the standard, and up to 6 biopsies can assure a near 100% diagnostic accuracy for stomach cancer.[37] Advanced endoscopic techniques can provide further evaluation of a stomach tumor to establish the depth of tumor invasion and allow for more accurate tumor staging. The endoscopic ultrasound (EUS) can also evaluate local lymph node involvement. The accuracy of this procedure is about 80%; thus it is an important tool that supplements preoperative evaluation.[8] Accurate staging provides prognostic information and can help with appropriate treatment strategies. The double-contrast barium swallow is a noninvasive procedure that can help detect mucosal changes and polypoid lesions, nondistensible lesions, and ulcerative areas; however, it is limited in its inability to perform biopsies or lymph node evaluation.

Endoscopic evaluation may also be used for the detection of *H. pylori*, an important etiological factor for many stomach cancers. The biopsy specimen is subjected to the rapid urease test that detects the presence of urease, which is not a normal gastric finding. Carbon-labeled breath testing indirectly detects the presence of urease and can be a noninvasive method to detect *H. pylori*. The early eradication of *H. pylori* is a preventive measure for stomach cancer in high-risk populations. Patients who are noted on endoscopy to have ulcerative lesions that do not respond after 6 to 8 weeks of proton pump inhibitor therapy should return for repeat EGD and repeat biopsies.

Computerized tomography (CT) is used as part of the standard workup for stomach cancer, including scanning of the chest, abdomen, and pelvis. It is noninvasive and can be used to assess for the degree of penetration of the tumor through the gastric wall (especially T2 or greater lesions with modern multiphase CT imaging) and to identify perigastric lymphadenopathy, peritoneal disease, and intra-abdominal visceral metastatic disease, such as liver metastasis or an ovarian mass. If metastatic disease is detected, the invasive EUS procedure for accurate tumor staging would likely not be indicated.

Positron emission tomography (PET) whole body evaluation is becoming a more standard part of the diagnostic evaluation of primary GI cancers as well as recurrent disease. However, with stomach cancer, only about 60% to 70% of primary tumors are found to be PET positive.[36] It is thought that glucose transporter-1, an important transporter of fluorodeoxyglucose (FDG) into tumor cells, is not present in many common subtypes of stomach cancer, such as signet ring cell and mucinous adenocarcinoma. This could contribute to false-negative PET imaging. There is consideration and ongoing evaluation that stomach cancers that are PET avid and do contain glucose transporter-1 may be associated with decreased overall survival.[36]

Laparoscopic evaluation is increasingly being used as a diagnostic tool for stomach cancers that appear on initial evaluation to be resectable; whereas CT imaging and PET imaging may not be able to detect occult peritoneal or liver metastasis. A highly skilled laparoscopy operator can identify these occult lesions and prevent a patient from undergoing gastric tumor resection when metastatic disease is present. Peritoneal lavage is also done at the time of laparoscopy for cytologic analysis.[35,40]

## CLASSIFICATION AND STAGING

The current method used for staging of stomach cancer is that of the American Joint Committee on Cancer (AJCC), using the tumor, node, distant metastasis (TNM) classification. Primary tumor (T) is based on depth of invasion. T2 has been subdivided into T2a and T2b, depending on (1) invasion into the muscularis propria or (2) invasion into the subserosa. This further delineation does not, however, change the location of T2 lesions in the overall staging categories. A lesion remains a T2 with extension into gastric ligaments or omentum if there is no visceral peritoneum perforation; if there is, then it is a T3 lesion. Direct extension to the duodenum or esophagus is classified by depth of invasion at its greatest point identified. Intra-abdominal lymph node groups, including hepatoduodenal, retropancreatic, mesenteric, and para-aortic designated as N3 or N4, are considered metastatic or advanced-stage disease.[8] See Table 67-1[42] for TNM definitions and disease stage.

## PROGNOSIS

Prognosis related to stomach cancer depends largely on the stage of the disease. Unfortunately, only a minority of

**TABLE 67-1**

**TNM Staging of Stomach Cancer**

| | |
|---|---|
| **Primary Tumor (T)** | |
| TX | Primary tumor cannot be assessed |
| T0 | No evidence of primary tumor |
| Tis | Carcinoma in situ: intraepithelial tumor without invasion of the lamina propria |
| T1 | Tumor invades lamina propria or submucosa |
| T2 | Tumor invades muscularis propria or subserosa |
| T2a | Tumor invades muscularis propria |
| T2b | Tumor invades subserosa |
| T3 | Tumor penetrates serosa (visceral peritoneum) without invasion of adjacent structures |
| T4 | Tumor invades adjacent structures |
| **Regional Lymph Nodes (N)** | |
| NX | Regional lymph node(s) cannot be assessed |
| N0 | No regional lymph node metastasis |
| N1 | Metastasis in 1–6 regional lymph nodes |
| N2 | Metastasis in 7–15 regional lymph nodes |
| N3 | Metastasis in > 15 regional lymph nodes |
| **Distant Metastasis (M)** | |
| MX | Distant metastasis cannot be assessed |
| M0 | No distant metastasis |
| M1 | Distant metastasis |

(Continued)

**TABLE 67-1**

**TNM Staging of Stomach Cancer (*Continued*)**

| **Stage Grouping** | | | |
|---|---|---|---|
| 0 | Tis | N0 | M0 |
| IA | T1 | N0 | M0 |
| IB | T1 | N1 | M0 |
| | T2a/b | N0 | M0 |
| II | T1 | N2 | M0 |
| | T2a/b | N1 | M0 |
| | T3 | N0 | M0 |
| IIIA | T2a/b | N2 | M0 |
| | T3 | N1 | M0 |
| | T4 | N0 | M0 |
| IIIB | T3 | N2 | M0 |
| IV | T4 | N1–3 | M0 |
| | T1–3 | N3 | M0 |
| | Any T | Any N | M1 |

| **Histological Grade (G)** | |
|---|---|
| GX | Grade cannot be assessed |
| G1 | Well differentiated |
| G2 | Moderately differentiated |
| G3 | Poorly differentiated |
| G4 | Undifferentiated |

| **Residual Tumor (R)** | |
|---|---|
| RX | Presence of residual tumor cannot be assessed |
| R0 | No residual tumor |
| R1 | Microscopic residual tumor |
| R2 | Macroscopic residual tumor |

patients present with early-stage disease that is amenable to resection and cure or prolonged survival. In the US, approximately 25% of individuals with stomach cancer present with localized disease, 30% with regional disease, and 35% with distant metastatic disease.[4] Only about 18% of patients with stomach cancer are long-term survivors; patients with stage 0 or IA disease have cure rates of up to 90% after surgery alone.[8,33,43] The prognosis for stage II through stage IV ranges from around 30% to as little as 3%.[8] Overall 5-year survival for stomach cancer is approximately 5% to 15%.[35] If the tumor is confined to the mucosa or submucosa, survival can extend to 80%; however, with local node involvement survival decreases to 20% to 40%. Widespread disease is usually fatal within 1 year.[35] Other factors that contribute to a poor prognosis include the following: age, proximal location, weight loss of more than 10% at diagnosis, linitis plastica, high-grade or undifferentiated tumors, 4 or more lymph nodes involved, aneuploid tumors, and elevations in epidermal growth factor/P-glycoprotein.[8]

## THERAPEUTIC APPROACHES AND NURSING CARE

### SURGERY

Surgical resection remains the treatment of choice for patients with locoregional stomach cancer. In the US, approximately 66% of patients with stomach cancer present with Stage III or greater disease.[44] Patients with stage I, II, or III disease may be candidates for surgical resection if there is minimal nodal involvement. The approach to appropriate resection is a thorough diagnostic workup. Patients found to have metastatic disease, such as liver lesions or peritoneal deposits on imaging or occult metastases on laparoscopy, can avoid an unnecessary laparotomy and resection. A planned laparoscopy as a separate staging procedure prior to definitive treatment planning has the disadvantage of putting the patient through additional risks and costs if the tumor is resectable, but it does allow for additional staging information from peritoneal washings and cytology results. On the other hand, proceeding from laparoscopy to laparotomy and resection does not allow for discussion of findings with the patient or with multidisciplinary teams to evaluate therapeutic options, including neoadjuvant therapy.[36,44]

Location and stage of the stomach tumor determine the type of surgical procedure. Subtotal gastrectomy is the preferred procedure for tumors located in the proximal cardia and for distal lesions, provided the cardioesophageal junction or fundus is not involved. A proximal gastrectomy is usually associated with increased morbidity as a result of increases in postoperative complications and a decrease in overall quality of life, as well as an increased morbidity.[8] Choices of approach for proximal stomach tumors include a transabdominal approach and a combined thoracic and abdominal approach. The latter procedure is termed a transhiatal esophagectomy. A subtotal gastrectomy for tumors located in the middle or distal stomach is called a Billroth I or Billroth II procedure. The Billroth I procedure, or gastroduodenostomy, joins the upper stomach back to the duodenum after a subtotal gastrectomy. The Billroth I procedure involves a limited amount of resection, and thus generally produces a lower cure rate than a more extensive surgery. The Billroth I procedure is generally done when patients are debilitated and cannot tolerate more extensive or longer surgery. The Billroth II is a wider resection that removes 75% of the stomach and connects the stomach to the jejunum (end to side), the middle portion of the small intestine after subtotal gastrectomy (Figure 67-2).[46]

In 3 small prospective randomized trials comparing total gastrectomy to subtotal gastrectomy for distal stomach cancer it was found that overall morbidity, mortality, and cancer outcome were comparable.[47–49] Thus, a gastric-preserving surgical approach is the preferred method for distal stomach tumors that can be resected with 5 cm clear margins macroscopically and no residual tumor microscopically (R0), which may minimize symptoms of fullness, weight loss, and need for supplementation with vitamin B12.[36]

A total gastrectomy is the surgical option for a diffuse-type tumor or one that arises in the body of the stomach and extends to within 6 cm of the cardia or presents with linitis plastica.[36] The treatment goal with either subtotal or total gastrectomy is to have negative surgical margins (R0), utilizing intraoperative frozen section analysis of proximal and distal margins to assess achievement of this goal.[36]

Debate remains about the number of lymph nodes that need to be dissected to adequately stage the disease and to determine whether a certain level of lymphadenectomy is therapeutic for the patient.[36] The Japanese consider an extended lymphadenectomy, D2, as standard, whereas in the West there remains debate.[39,50–52] A D1 dissection involves the nodes along the greater and lesser omenta and the perigastric lymph nodes, which is the minimum considered to achieve a cure.[40] A D2 lymphadenectomy is a D1 plus resection of nodes along the hepatic, left gastric, celiac, and splenic arteries. Studies in the United Kingdom and the Netherlands have shown increased morbidity and mortality perioperatively, with no overall survival benefit, with a greater than D1 resection.[40,53] The recommendation for TNM pathological staging is to have a minimum of 15 to 16 nodes removed and examined.[39,54–56]

Palliative surgery is considered when the patient presents with pain, bleeding, or obstruction; although mortality from the procedure can approach 25% to 50%, there appears to be a twofold increase in mean survival.[8] Other surgical debates remain involving the recommendations for partial pancreatectomy and splenectomy at the time of gastrectomy.[36,56]

Postoperative nursing care for patients undergoing gastric resection, total or subtotal, includes monitoring for postsurgical complications such as bleeding, anastomotic leak, infection, pneumonia, and poor wound healing. Patients initially are fed intravenously or with a nasojejunal tube, but as liquids and foods are introduced the nurse monitors closely for signs of aspiration, bezoar formation (a bolus of food blocking the gastric outlet), or dumping syndrome. A bezoar formation may be resolved with the use an enzyme substance such as papain or may require an endoscopy for mechanical removal.[58]

Dumping syndrome is a shock-like state that occurs when undigested food "dumps" into the small intestine. Gastric resection (Billroth I or Billroth II or total gastrectomy) may result in alterations in fundic tone, pyloric mechanisms, and duodenal feedback, as well as a decrease in gastric acid and enzymatic and hormonal secretions. Dumping syndrome can have 2 components, GI and vasomotor symptoms. The GI symptoms that are common to dumping syndrome include abdominal cramping, early satiety, nausea and vomiting, and severe diarrhea. The vasomotor symptoms, which may be overlooked, include dizziness, palpitations, flushing, and diaphoresis.[59]

Malnutrition, which may likely have been a presurgical condition of the patient, continues to be an issue after gastric resection. Iron deficiency anemia, vitamin B12 deficiency, edema, hypoalbuminemia, and decreased level of activity can be signs of malnutrition if 3 or more are present.[60] Close monitoring and having a dietician involved with the patient's care are essential to improving a patient's nutritional status.

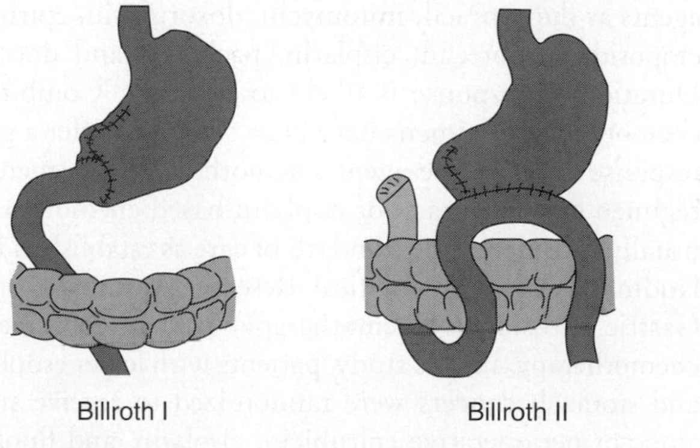


**FIGURE 67-2**

**Billroth I and Billroth II procedure**. The Billroth I procedure involves a limited amount of resection. The Billroth II is a wider resection that removes 75% of stomach. Used with permission from Stomach cancer. In: Livstone EM, reviewer. Merck Manual; 2007. http://www.mercksource.com/pp/us/cns/cns_merckmanualhome.jsp. January 1, 2010.

## RADIATION THERAPY

The use of radiation therapy alone in the management of stomach cancer is for the palliation of symptoms such as pain, persistent bleeding, and obstruction related to bulky tumors. Although curative resection offers the best chance for long-term survival, survival rates after resection vary from 10% to 50% depending on the nodal stage of the disease at the time of resection. Recurrence rates remain high despite resections with no residual disease. Adjuvant therapy addresses this issue of recurrence. Radiation therapy in combination with chemotherapy (CRT) has become the standard adjuvant therapy for resected stomach cancer in the US since the landmark study by the Gastric Cancer Intergroup (Intergroup 0116) results were published. In this study, patients who had undergone an R0 (no residual tumor) resection with curative intent, stage Ib to stage IV without known metastatic disease, were randomized to either post-surgery observation or post-surgery CRT. The combination arm received 1 cycle of fluorouracil (5FU) and leucovorin, followed by 5 weeks of radiation therapy with fluorouracil and leucovorin given on the first 3 days of radiation therapy and on the last 4 days of radiation therapy. This was followed by 2 more cycles of fluorouracil and leucovorin. Results at a median follow-up of 5 years showed a median survival of 36 months in the CRT group and 27 months in the surgery-alone group. The 3-year survival rates were 50% in the combination group and 41% in the observation group. Local recurrence was improved in the combination arm, at 19%, and was 29% in the surgery-alone group.[61] Since this landmark trial, a successor adjuvant trial is ongoing comparing a triplet regimen of epirubicin, cisplatin, and fluorouracil (ECF), along with fluorouracil-based CRT, with the treatment arm of the above trial, fluorouracil and leucovorin.

Radiation therapy in combination with chemotherapy in the neoadjuvant setting is supported by clinical trials such as the Radiation Therapy Oncology Group 9904 (RTOG 9904) trial, a phase II trial in which patients were treated with 2 cycles of induction, fluorouracil, leucovorin, and cisplatin followed by combination radiation therapy with continuous infusion fluorouracil and weekly paclitaxel, then proceeding to resection.[61] Results of this trial were consistent with a previous trial of the same regimen, but without the weekly paclitaxel in the combination cycle. The RTOG 9904 study reported a 26% pathological complete response (pCR), compared with 30% pCR in the earlier trial.[62] Neoadjuvant therapy is directed toward downstaging the tumor and improving the rate of obtaining an R0 resection, which in turn may provide an improvement in overall survival. Neoadjuvant treatment offers the potential opportunity to assess tumor sensitivity to a chemotherapeutic regimen and may increase the total amount of systemic chemotherapy that patients are able to receive. Often, in the postoperative adjuvant setting, less than anticipated systemic therapy is given secondary to a prolonged surgical recovery, compromised nutritional status, and the toxicities associated with chemotherapy.[37,39] Neoadjuvant therapy can help identify those patients with high-risk tumors who may progress through therapy, thus avoiding a futile resection. The radiation field can be more precisely identified in the neoadjuvant setting than in the postoperative adjuvant setting, potentially improving the accuracy and effectiveness of the radiation.[39,62,63]

Whether radiation therapy occurs preoperatively or postoperatively, the patient with stomach cancer must be managed with optimal nutrition in mind. As previously noted, the patient with stomach cancer is likely to have nutritional deficits at the time of diagnosis, and the toxicities of radiation therapy will make maintaining or improving nutritional status a challenge. Radiation therapy can cause nausea, vomiting, diarrhea, gastritis, and abdominal cramping. The postoperative patient may have a jejunostomy tube for enteral feeding that will facilitate maintaining nutrition. Nursing plays a key role in the ongoing assessment of radiation toxicities and nutritional status for the patient with stomach cancer who is receiving radiation therapy. The dietician is a key component of the interdisciplinary team to manage and assess the patient's nutritional status.

## CHEMOTHERAPY

Chemotherapy is the treatment modality for those patients who present with disseminated disease or residual disease after primary resection (likely in combination with radiation therapy), and for those whose disease recurs after definitive therapy. Stage IV disease is noncurative, and treatment is palliative. Studies comparing best supportive care with a chemotherapy regimen in patients with advanced disease showed a consistent survival advantage to those who received systemic therapy. Without treatment, patients had only a median 3- to 5-month survival. With treatment, patients in these studies showed a 7.5- to 12-month survival.[64–66]

Single-agent chemotherapy regimens for stomach cancer show a response rate of 10% to 25% and include such agents as fluorouracil, mitomycin, doxorubicin, epirubicin, etoposide, irinotecan, cisplatin, paclitaxel and docetaxel. Duration of response is likely to be short. Combination chemotherapy regimens have been shown to offer a greater response than single-agent chemotherapy treatment.[52] A regimen of fluorouracil or cisplatin-based chemotherapy is usually considered the standard of care as established by the landmark MAGIC (Medical Research Council Adjuvant Gastric Infusional Chemotherapy) trial for perioperative chemotherapy. In this study, patients with lower esophageal and stomach cancers were randomized to receive surgery alone or perioperative epirubicin, cisplatin, and fluorouracil. Results showed a median, 5-year, and progression-free survival favoring the treatment arm; 24 months, 36%, and 19 months, respectively, for the patients in the treatment arm compared with 20 months, 23%, and 13 months for patients in the control arm.[39,53]

Although the regimens of ECF or docetaxel, cisplatin, and fluorouracil (DCF) are considered the standard regimens for advanced stomach cancer, combinations with irinotecan or oxaliplatin have shown at least equal effectiveness. Toxicity profiles related to these drugs are sometimes the limiting factor. Significant diarrhea can be debilitating and life-threatening with irinotecan. Oxaliplatin toxicities include acute and chronic peripheral neuropathy, nausea and vomiting, and myelosuppression. In the Randomized ECF for Advanced and Locally Advanced Esophagogastric Cancer 2 (REAL 2) trial, patients with advanced stomach cancer were randomized to receive epirubicin, cisplatin, fluorouracil; epirubicin, cisplatin, capecitabine (an oral prodrug of fluorouracil); epirubicin, oxaliplatin, fluorouracil; or epirubicin, oxaliplatin, capecitabine. The substitution of capecitabine for fluorouracil and oxaliplatin for the cisplatin demonstrated noninferiority (study objectives were comparable).[53,67] Phase II studies with irinotecan in combination with cisplatin or infusional fluorouracil, or both, in patients with advanced untreated stomach cancer or as second-line therapy for advanced stomach cancer have shown objective responses.[68,69] S-1, a novel fluoropyrimidine derivative composed of tegafur (a flurouracil prodrug), has been shown to be effective in adjuvant therapy and in advanced stomach cancer in studies conducted in Japan. The S-1 plus cisplatin vs S-1 alone for first-line treatment of advanced gastric cancer (SPIRITS) trial randomized patients with advanced stomach cancer to receive S-1 alone or in combination with cisplatin. Results showed an improved response rate in the combination arm; prolonged median overall survival was 13 months in the combination arm, compared with 11 months for the S-1 alone arm. At this time, S-1 remains unavailable for commercial use in the US.[39,44,70]

The efficacy of current chemotherapy regimens for the treatment of stomach cancer is less than optimal, with best response rates of less than 50% and a median overall survival of around 12 months; thus, understanding the biology of stomach cancer is key to developing new chemotherapy drugs or novel approaches for directed therapy.[39] Immunotherapy, epidermal growth factor receptor (EGFR) inhibitors, and angiogenesis inhibitors are under investigation and are the components of current clinical trials. Nursing care for the patient with stomach cancer receiving chemotherapy includes close monitoring for fluorouracil toxicities such as stomatitis or cardiac arrhythmias; changes in doses or discontinuation of the drug may be indicated. Other monitoring in patients receiving chemotherapy regimens that suppress the bone marrow will include management of anemia that may already be present secondary to the patient's current disease status or to having had a partial or total gastrectomy.

## SYMPTOM MANAGEMENT AND SUPPORTIVE CARE

Patients presenting with stomach cancer often have had a significant decline in their overall physical well-being, as the symptoms of early stomach cancer are usually benign and it is not until the disease has advanced that patients are aware of symptoms. The progression of the disease in the advanced stage or with recurrent metastatic disease is often rapid. Nursing care involves not only the physical well-being of the patient, to help optimize nutritional status, maintain functional status, and provide support for complications such as gastric obstruction, but also evaluation and support of the emotional health of these individuals. Patients who are diagnosed and treated for early-stage stomach cancer with resection will need ongoing evaluation for anemia and may need vitamin B12,[71] folic acid, and iron replacement. This may require monthly vitamin B12 injections. Also, patients with stomach cancer who have not been resected and have stable disease may also need vitamin B12 replacement if their stomach is not functioning adequately. Osteoporosis, osteopenia, and osteomalacia in postgastrectomy patients may be treated or prevented with vitamin D and calcium supplements.[71]

The information that patient and families need to absorb once the diagnosis of stomach cancer has been made can be overwhelming. Nursing can intervene by educating the patient and family about the selected treatment and the expected and potential side effects and outcomes. Establishing goals toward end-of-life care is part of the nursing assessment that may occur at the time of diagnosis or upon failure of treatment regimens.

## CONCLUSION

The overall incidence of stomach cancer has declined in the US and Western countries; however, the incidence of proximal stomach cancer continues to rise. Developing preventive screening measures on a large scale remains infeasible given the overall low incidence of stomach cancer in the US. Surgical resection is the only curative treatment for patients with early-stage disease. Despite this, the 5-year survival rate remains poor. Unfortunately, the median survival for advanced, unresectable stomach cancer remains dismal, with median survival of less than 1 year. Continued research into understanding and identifying the natural history of the disease and to better define distinct subtypes may lead to targeted therapy options and to understanding specific tumor types and their response to current chemotherapy regimens.

## REFERENCES

1. Garcia M, Jemal A, Ward EM, et al. Global Cancer Facts & Figures 2007. American Cancer Society. Available at http://www.cancer.org/downloads/STT/Global_Facts_and_Figures_2007_rev2.pdf. Accessed January 1, 2010.
2. Parkin DM, Bray F, Ferlay J, Pisani P. Global cancer statistics, 2002. *CA Cancer J Clin.* Mar-Apr 2005;55:74–108.

3. Crew KD, Neugut AI. Epidemiology of gastric cancer. *World J Gastroenterol.* Jan 21, 2006;12:354–362.
4. Jemal A, Siegel R, Ward E, et al. Cancer statistics, 2008. *CA Cancer J Clin.* 2008;58:71–96.
5. Gastric cancer. In: Mills EJ, ed. *Handbook of Medical-Surgical Nursing.* 4th ed. Philadelphia: Lippincott Williams & Wilkins; 2006:312.
6. Kelley JR, Duggan JM. Gastric cancer epidemiology and risk factors. *J Clin Epidemiol.* Jan 2003;56:1–9.
7. Alberts SR, Cervantes A, van de Velde CJ. Gastric cancer: epidemiology, pathology and treatment. *Ann Oncol.* 2003;14(Suppl 2):ii31-ii36.
8. Saif MW. Gastric cancer. In: Abraham J, Gulley JL, Allegra CJ, eds. *Bethesda Handbook of Clinical Oncology.* 2nd ed. Philadelphia: Lippincott Williams & Wilkins; 2005:73–90.
9. Cabebe EC, Mehta VK. Gastric cancer: Medscape; 2008. http://emedicine.medscape.com/article/278744-overview. Accessed January 1, 2010.
10. Calam J, Baron JH. ABC of the upper gastrointestinal tract: pathophysiology of duodenal and gastric ulcer and gastric cancer. *BMJ.* 2001;323:980–982.
11. Uemura N, Okamoto S, Yamamoto S, et al. Helicobacter pylori infection and the development of gastric cancer. *N Engl J Med.* Sept 13, 2001;345:784–789.
12. Yamaoka Y, Kato M, Asaka M. Geographic differences in gastric cancer incidence can be explained by differences between Helicobacter pylori strains. *Intern Med.* 2008;47:1077–1083.
13. Kamangar F, Cheng C, Abnet CC, Rabkin CS. Interleukin-1B polymorphisms and gastric cancer risk—a meta-analysis. *Cancer Epidemiol Biomarkers Prev.* Oct 2006;15:1920–1928.
14. Lambert R, Parkin DM. Gastric cancer: epidemiology, screening, surveillance, and prevention. In: Kelsen DP, Daly JM, Kern SE, Levin B, eds. *Gastrointestinal Oncology: Principles and Practice.* 2nd ed. Philadelphia: Lippincott Williams & Wilkins; 2008:231–244.
15. Varadhachary GR, Ajani JA. Gastric cancer. *Clin Adv Hematol Oncol.* 2005;3:118–124.
16. Lynch HT, Grady W, Suriano G, Huntsman D. Gastric cancer: new genetic developments. *J Surg Oncol.* 2005;90:114–133; discussion 133.
17. Watson P, Vasen HF, Mecklin J-P, et al. The risk of extra-colonic, extra-endometrial cancer in the Lynch syndrome. *Int J Cancer.* 2008;123:444–449.
18. Barber M, Fitzgerald RC, Caldas C. Familial gastric cancer—aetiology and pathogenesis. *Best Pract Res Clin Gastroenterol.* 2006;20: 721–734.
19. Rogers WM, Dobo E, Norton JA, et al. Risk-reducing total gastrectomy for germline mutations in E-cadherin (CDH1): pathologic findings with clinical implications. *Am J Surg Pathol.* Jun 2008;32:799–809.
20. Bernini M, Barbi S, Roviello F, et al. Family history of gastric cancer: a correlation between epidemiologic findings and clinical data. *Gastric Cancer.* 2006;9:9–13.
21. Rozen P. Cancer of the gastrointestinal tract: early detection or early prevention? *Eur J Cancer Prev.* Feb 2004;13:71–75.
22. Lochhead P, El-Omar EM. Gastric cancer. *Br Med Bull.* 2008; 85:87–100.
23. Correa P, Fontham ET, Bravo JC, et al. Chemoprevention of gastric dysplasia: randomized trial of antioxidant supplements and anti-helicobacter pylori therapy. *J Natl Cancer Inst.* Dec 6, 2000;92:1881–1888.
24. Jacobs EJ, Connell CJ, McCullough ML, et al. Vitamin C, vitamin E, and multivitamin supplement use and stomach cancer mortality in the Cancer Prevention Study II Cohort. *Cancer Epidemiol Biomarkers Prev.* 2002;11:35–41.
25. Fock KM, Talley N, Moayyedi P, et al. Asia-Pacific consensus guidelines on gastric cancer prevention. *J Gastroenterol Hepatol.* 2008;23:351–365.
26. Sung J. Early gastric cancer: diagnosis, treatment and prevention. *Eur J Gastroenterol Hepatol.* Aug 2006;18:817–819.
27. Wong BC, Lam SK, Wong WM, et al. Helicobacter pylori eradication to prevent gastric cancer in a high-risk region of China: a randomized controlled trial. *JAMA.* Jan 14, 2004;291:187–194.
28. Cheung TK, Wong BC. Treatment of Helicobacter pylori and prevention of gastric cancer. *J Dig Dis.* Feb 2008;9:8–13.
29. Suzuki H, Gotoda T, Sasako M, Saito D. Detection of early gastric cancer: misunderstanding the role of mass screening. *Gastric Cancer.* 2006;9:315–319.
30. Leung WK, Wu MS, Kakugawa Y, et al. Screening for gastric cancer in Asia: current evidence and practice. *Lancet Oncol.* Mar 2008;9:279–287.
31. Kunisaki C, Ishino J, Nakajima S, et al. Outcomes of mass screening for gastric carcinoma. *Ann Surg Oncol.* Feb 2006;13:221–228.
32. Giarelli E. Prophylactic gastrectomy for CDH1 mutation carriers. *Clin J Oncol Nurs.* 2002;6:161–162.
33. Alberts S, Goldberg R. Gastric cancer. In: Casciato DA, ed. *Manual of Clinical Oncology.* 5th ed. Philadelphia: Lippincott Williams & Wilkins; 2004:189–195.
34. Shah M, Rathkopf D, Schwartz G. Gastric cancer. In: Boyiadzis M, Lebowitz P, Frame J, Fojo T, eds. *Hematology-Oncology Therapy.* New York: McGraw-Hill; 2007:135–143.
35. Stomach cancer. In: Livstone EM, reviewer. Merck Manual; 2007. http://www.mercksource.com/pp/us/cns/cns_merckmanualhome.jsp Accessed January 1, 2010.
36. Pisters PWT, Kelsen DP, Tepper JE. Cancers of the gastrointestinal tract: Section 3. Cancer of the stomach. In: DeVita VT, Lawrence TS, Rosenberg SA, eds. *Devita, Hellman & Rosenberg's Cancer: Principles & Practice of Oncology.* 8th ed. Philadelphia: Lippincott Williams & Wilkins; 2008:1043–1079.
37. Al-Refaie WB, Abdalla EK, Ahmad SA, Mansfield PF. Gastric cancer. In: Feig BW, Berger DH, Fuhrman GM, eds. *M.D. Anderson Surgical Oncology Handbook.* Philadelphia: Lippincott Williams & Wilkins; 2006:205–240.
38. Dewys WD, Begg C, Lavin PT, et al. Prognostic effect of weight loss prior to chemotherapy in cancer patients. Eastern Cooperative Oncology Group. *Am J Med.* Oct 1980;69:491–497.
39. Khushalani NI. Cancer of the esophagus and stomach. *Mayo Clin Proc.* 2008;83:712–722.
40. Yao JC, Pisters PWT, Crane C, Ajani JA. Gastric cancer. In: Ajani JA, Curley SA, Janjan NA, Lynch PM, eds. *M.D. Anderson Cancer Care Series: Gastrointestinal Cancer.* New York: Springer; 2005:219–231.
41. Gravalos C, Jimeno A. HER2 in gastric cancer: a new prognostic factor and a novel therapeutic target. *Ann Oncol.* Sept 2008;19:1523–1529.
42. *AJCC Cancer Staging Atlas.* 1st ed. New York: Springer Science+Business Media; 2006.
43. Greaves M, Markowitz A, Gerdes H. Gastric cancer: staging systems and techniques. In: Kelsen DP, Daly JM, Kern SE, Levin B, Tepper JE, van Cutsem E, eds. *Gastrointestinal Oncology: Principles and Practice.* Philadelphia: Lippincott Williams & Wilkins; 2008:275–282.
44. Phan AT, Yao JC, Allam SR, Ajani JA. Upper gastrointestinal malignancies. In: Kantarjcan HM, Wolff RA, Koller CA, eds. *M.D. Anderson Manual of Medical Oncology.* New York: McGraw-Hill; 2006.
45. Alexander R, Kelsen DG, Tepper JC. Cancer of the stomach. In: DeVita VT, Hellman S, Rosenberg SA, eds. *Principles and Practice of Clinical Oncology.* 5th ed. Philadelphia: Lippincott-Raven; 1997:1021–1050.
46. Dorland's Medical Dictionary for Healthcare Consumers. http://www.mercksource.com/pp/us/cns/cns_hl_dorlands_split.jsp?pg=/ppdocs/us/common/dorlands/dorland/nine/000950803.htm. Accessed January 4, 2009.
47. Bozzetti F, Marubini E, Bonfanti G, Miceli R, Piano C, Gennari L. Subtotal versus total gastrectomy for gastric cancer: five-year survival rates in a multicenter randomized Italian trial. Italian Gastrointestinal Tumor Study Group. *Ann Surg.* Aug 1999;230:170–178.
48. Gouzi JL, Huguier M, Fagniez PL, et al. Total versus subtotal gastrectomy for adenocarcinoma of the gastric antrum. A French prospective controlled study. *Ann Surg.* Feb 1989;209:162–166.
49. Robertson CS, Chung SC, Woods SD, et al. A prospective randomized trial comparing R1 subtotal gastrectomy with R3 total gastrectomy for antral cancer. *Ann Surg.* Aug 1994;220:176–182.

50. Bonenkamp JJ, Hermans J, Sasako M, et al. Extended lymph-node dissection for gastric cancer. *N Engl J Med*. Mar 25, 1999;340:908–914.
51. Cuschieri A, Fayers P, Fielding J, et al. Postoperative morbidity and mortality after D1 and D2 resections for gastric cancer: preliminary results of the MRC randomised controlled surgical trial. The Surgical Cooperative Group. *Lancet*. Apr 13, 1996;347(2007):995–999.
52. Cuschieri A, Weeden S, Fielding J, et al. Patient survival after D1 and D2 resections for gastric cancer: long-term results of the MRC randomized surgical trial. Surgical Co-operative Group. *Br J Cancer*. Mar 1999;79:1522–1530.
53. Blaszkowsky LS. Gastric cancer. In: Chabner BA, Lynch TJ, Longo DL, eds. *Harrison's Manual of Oncology*. New York: McGraw-Hill; 2008:395–401.
54. Part III—Digestive System, Chapter 10. Stomach. Greene FL, Fritz AG, Balch CM, et al, eds. *AJCC Cancer Staging Handbook*. 6th ed. New York, NY: Springer-Verlag; 2002: http://online.statref.com.ezproxy.galter.northwestern.edu/document.aspx?fxid=73&docid=1. Accessed February 10, 2010.
55. Barbour AP, Rizk NP, Gonen M, et al. Lymphadenectomy for adenocarcinoma of the gastroesophageal junction (GEJ): impact of adequate staging on outcome. *Ann Surg Oncol*. Feb 2007;14:306–316.
56. Karpeh MS, Leon L, Klimstra D, Brennan MF. Lymph node staging in gastric cancer: is location more important than number? An analysis of 1,038 patients. *Ann Surg*. Sep 2000;232:362–371.
57. Goldfaden D, Orringer MB, Appelman HD, Kalish R. Adenocarcinoma of the distal esophagus and gastric cardia. Comparison of results of transhiatal esophagectomy and thoracoabdominal esophagogastrectomy. Abstract. *J Thorac Cardiovasc Surg*. Feb 1986;91:242–247.
58. O'Connor KG: Stomach cancer. In: Yarbro CH, Frogge MH, Goodman M, eds. *Cancer Nursing Principles and Practice*. 6th ed. Sudbury, MA: Jones and Bartlett; 2005:1617–1629.
59. Blackwood H, ed. Clinical Q & A. *Bariatric Nurs Surg Patient Care*. 2008;3:167–170.
60. O'Donnell K. Case study: malnutrition following gastric bypass. *Bariatric Nurs Surg Patient Care*. 2006;1:251–254.
61. Macdonald JS, Smalley SR, Benedetti J, et al. Chemoradiotherapy after surgery compared with surgery alone for adenocarcinoma of the stomach or gastroesophageal junction. *N Engl J Med*. Sept 6, 2001;345:725–730.
62. Ajani JA, Winter K, Okawara GS, et al. Phase II trial of preoperative chemoradiation in patients with localized gastric adenocarcinoma (RTOG 9904): quality of combined modality therapy and pathologic response. *J Clin Oncol*. Aug 20, 2006;24:3953–3958.
63. Ajani JA, Mansfield PF, Janjan N, et al. Multi-Institutional Trial of Preoperative Chemoradiotherapy in patients with potentially resectable gastric cancer. *J Clin Oncol*. 2004;22:2774–2780.
64. Wagner AD, Grothe W, Haerting J, Kleber G, Grothey A, Fleig WE. Chemotherapy in advanced gastric cancer: a systematic review and meta-analysis based on aggregate data. *J Clin Oncol*. Jun 20, 2006;24:2903–2909.
65. Murad AM, Santiago FF, Petroianu A, Rocha PR, Rodrigues MA, Rausch M. Modified therapy with 5-fluorouracil, doxorubicin, and methotrexate in advanced gastric cancer. *Cancer*. Jul 1, 1993;72:37–41.
66. Pyrhonen S, Kuitunen T, Nyandoto P, Kouri M. Randomised comparison of fluorouracil, epidoxorubicin and methotrexate (FEMTX) plus supportive care with supportive care alone in patients with non-resectable gastric cancer. *Br J Cancer*. Mar 1995;71:587–591.
67. Cunningham D, Starling N, Rao S, et al. Capecitabine and oxaliplatin for advanced esophagogastric cancer. *N Engl J Med*. Jan 3, 2008;358:36–46.
68. Ajani JA, Baker J, Pisters PW, et al. CPT-11 plus cisplatin in patients with advanced, untreated gastric or gastroesophageal junction carcinoma: results of a phase II study. *Cancer*. Feb 1, 2002;94:641–646.
69. Park SH, Nam E, Park J, et al. Randomized phase II study of irinotecan, leucovorin and 5-fluorouracil (ILF) versus cisplatin plus ILF (PILF) combination chemotherapy for advanced gastric cancer. *Ann Oncol*. Apr 2008;19:729–733.
70. Sakuramoto S, Sasako M, Yamaguchi T, et al. Adjuvant chemotherapy for gastric cancer with S-1, an oral fluoropyrimidine. *N Engl J Med*. Nov 1, 2007;357:1810–1820.
71. Radigan AE. Post-gastrectomy: managing the nutrition fall-out. *Nutr Issues Gastroenterol*. June 2004;Series #18:63–75.

CHAPTER 68

*Eric Zack, RN, MSN, ACNP-BC, AOCN®*

# Testicular Germ Cell Cancer

## INTRODUCTION

Testicular germ cell tumors (GCTs) account for 98% of all testicular malignancies and are the most common solid malignancy in men age 15 to 35.[1] Approximately 8400 new cases of testicular cancer will be diagnosed in the US and 380 men will die of their disease in 2009.[2] Approximately 95.9% of patients with a newly diagnosed GCT will be cured of their disease.[3] A direct correlation exists between early diagnosis, successful intervention, and lower cancer staging at the time of presentation. The optimal management of patients with a GCT usually requires an interdisciplinary approach by medical, surgical, and (in the case of seminoma) radiation oncologists.

## EPIDEMIOLOGY

Testicular cancer accounts for approximately 1% of all male cancers. For unknown reasons, an increased worldwide incidence of testicular cancer has been observed in the past 30 years, primarily in industrialized regions such as North America, Europe, and Oceania (geographical/geopolitical region consisting of islands in the Pacific Ocean and near vicinity).[4] Norway and Denmark have the highest incidence rates in the world most notably doubling in the past 50 years.[5] Testicular cancer in African Americans and Asians is rare. However, recent information gleaned from the Surveillance and Epidemiological End Results (SEER) program showed that although incidence rates in the US have plateaued, racial differences especially among African Americans have showed the greatest increase in annual percentage change.[6] Although the disease can occur at any age, it most frequently affects men aged 15 to 35. Testicular cancer occurs less frequently in adolescents, with an increased incidence being noted after age 40 and again after age 60.

Germ cell tumors are composed of seminomatous and nonseminomatous cell types. The different types of testicular tumors and their descriptions are noted in Table 68-1. Seminomas arise from the seminiferous epithelium and are the most common singular cell type, but mixed GCTs are even more common and are treated similarly like nonseminomas. True seminomas do not differentiate, but rather they retain germ cell characteristics. Classic seminomas usually occur in men aged 40 to 50 years, whereas spermatocytic seminomas generally occur in men aged 60 or older. Testicular GCTs typically present at a later stage in men 60 years and older and although most are seminomas, several nonseminoma morphologies have been identified.[7] Nonseminomatous tumors are classified into 4 subtypes: teratomas, embryonal tumors, choriocarcinomas, and yolk-sac tumors.[2] Any seminoma associated with an increased alpha-fetoprotein (AFP) level is considered to be a nonseminomatous tumor.

**TABLE 68-1**

**Types and Descriptions of Testicular Cancer**

**Germ cell tumors (GCTs)** majority occur in cells that make sperm

- **Seminoma**
- **Nonseminoma**
  - Teratoma
  - Embryonal carcinoma
  - Choriocarcinoma
  - Yolk-sac tumors

**Stromal cell tumors** occur in cells in other parts of the testicle such as in cells that make hormones

**Secondary testicular tumors** occur from other types of cancer that have spread to the testicles from other parts of the body

In addition to GCTs, stromal cell tumors occur rarely, developing from the supportive structures of the testicle. Furthermore, secondary testicular tumors can result from metastases from different primary organ malignancies such as renal cell carcinoma and mesothelioma but also from lymphoma, multiple myeloma, and some acute leukemias.

Fewer than 10% of all GCTs arise outside the gonads termed extragonadal nonseminomatous GCTs. These rare tumors occur (in descending order) most frequently in the retroperitoneum, mediastinum, and pineal gland and connote a poorer prognosis than a primary testicular cancer.[8]

## ETIOLOGY

The exact cause of GCT is unknown, although several risk factors have been suggested for the development of this malignancy. These risk factors include prior history of testicular cancer, cryptorchidism, genetics, family history, environmental and dietary factors, and hormones.

Men who develop a GCT in 1 testis are 500 times more likely than the normal male population to develop testicular cancer in the contralateral testis.[9,10] This phenomenon occurs in approximately 2% to 5% of males diagnosed with testicular cancer as a cumulative risk during the 25 years after initial diagnosis.[11] Synchronous presentation of bilateral testicular cancer is uncommon and should suggest an infiltrative process resulting from secondary cancers such as leukemia or lymphoma.

Cryptorchidism (undescended testes) is associated with a 20- to 40-fold increased risk of developing testicular GCTs compared to that of the normal male population and has occurred in approximately 10% of all cases.[2] Controversies exist as to the best age at which to perform the surgery, if the surgery is necessary to fully prevent GCTs, and if cryptorchidism is directly implicated in the development of GCTs.[2] However, orchiopexy (an operation to mobilize an undescended testes, bring it into the scrotum, and attach it so that it does not retract) before puberty has been shown to reduce the risk for GCTs, and when the surgery is performed between the ages of 6 months and 2 years old, the risk is substantially reduced.[12–15] In some cases of cryptorchidism, a tumor is discovered in the scrotum while not the testes.[16]

Twenty-five different hereditary disorders have been reported in patients who developed testicular cancer. Under these circumstances, other urogenital abnormalities were often present, possibly implicating hereditary etiologies to some degree in the development of testicular cancer.[17] Klinefelter's syndrome, a rare genetic disorder occurring in men and boys who possess 1Y and 2X chromosomes, is associated with an increased incidence of some GCTs.[18,19] Down's syndrome has also been associated in the development of GCTs.[20]

A familial tendency for the development of testicular germ cell cancer has been reported. One such report suggests a 10-fold increase in risk for development of GCT in male siblings of patients with testicular cancer, with a 4-fold increase in risk for father–son transmission.[21] A study using data from the past 75 years of the Swedish Family-Cancer database revealed that testicular cancer had the highest risk of familial clustering among other cancers.[22] Furthermore, twins were found to have a 30% increase in risk of testicular GCTs.[23]

Racial differences have also been identified in terms of incidences of testicular GCTs. In the US, Caucasians after puberty have a 5 to 10 times greater risk of developing testicular GCTs than African American men.[2] Asian and African men have the lowest risk, while Hispanic men possess a risk level between that of Asian and non-Hispanic Caucasians. However, new findings analyzed from the SEER program concerning prepubertal boys depicted Asian/Pacific Islander boys more likely to have testicular GCTs than Caucasians.[24]

Environmental concerns, such as exposure to diethylstilbestrol (DES), have been widely studied. To date, no strong evidence links exposure in utero to the development of testicular cancer. However, some studies have associated persistent organochlorine pesticides as endocrine-disrupting chemicals with increased incidences of testicular GCTs.[25] Environmental exposure to polyvinyl chloride has been weakly linked to testicular cancer development.[26] In addition, boys born to women exposed to phthalates (compounds that make vinyl soft and flexible) during pregnancy have an increased risk of cryptorchidism, hypospadias, testicular cancer, and spermatogenic dysfunction collectively termed testicular dysgenesis syndrome (TDS).[27]

Strong evidence supports hormonal etiologies—primarily estrogen exposure during male development—as contributing to the development of testicular cancer. Recently there has been an explosion of research into endocrine disruptors that may cause TDS. Nausea during pregnancy is related to increasing maternal estrogen levels and has been associated with testicular GCT risk.[28] This mechanism of elevated estrogen exposure in utero is thought to promote testicular GCTs later in life after puberty when spermatogenesis accelerates through a membrane-mediated protein kinase A.[29] Another risk factor may relate to low sperm count in some men.[30]

A hormone-linked condition called gynecomastia, the most common benign breast condition in men, has been weakly associated with testicular GCTs.[31] However, it is not well understood whether gynecomastia contributes to the development of GCTs or results from the hormone imbalances caused by some GCTs. Syndrome X also called metabolic syndrome in the literature describes a cluster of symptoms that include hypertension, elevated triglycerides, reduced high-density lipoprotein (HDL), and obesity.[32] This metabolic syndrome may possibly have a weak association in the development of testicular GCTs, but more likely may develop later after chemotherapy and/or radiation treatments.

Other possible etiologies have been postulated. Infection with human immunodeficiency virus (HIV) has been shown to be associated with an increased risk for the development of testicular cancer.[33] Researchers believe that GCTs develop due to impaired immune function and surveillance. To date, no substantial data have proved a direct viral etiology. Dietary links have not been well established, although consumption of vitamin E has been associated with fewer seminoma cases.[34] Research investigating body type, age at puberty, and dairy consumption as risk factors have yielded inconsistent findings with only height being weakly associated with seminoma risk.[35,36] Low and excessive birth weight have also been linked with risk for testicular GCTs.[37,38]

Conversely, research studies have failed to prove that men who have received vasectomies have an increased risk of developing testicular GCTs as compared to men in the general population.[39] Testicular microlithiasis has been studied in terms of incidence rates for testicular GCTs, but conflicting findings are cited in numerous studies.[40–43] Smoking and exposure to smoke in utero have had inconsistent findings.[44–46] Cellular or cordless phones were also disproved as being possibly linked to testicular GCTs.[47]

## PREVENTION, SCREENING, AND EARLY DETECTION

Testicular self-examination (TSE), not unlike breast self-examination (BSE), should be performed routinely. Given the nature of testicular GCTs, early diagnosis can lead to a more favorable outcome. Cure rates are highest for early-stage disease but decrease with more advanced disease.[48] Unfortunately, there exist many barriers to TSE in men, particularly in diverse populations such as African Americans whose stage at diagnosis is typically higher due to differences in cultural perceptions of malignancy, understanding of screening, education, and access to healthcare.[49,50]

Given that testicular GCTs are the most common malignancies among men aged 15 to 35, testicular exams should be performed by the healthcare provider when accessible and taught to these men to perform on themselves monthly.[51] Moreover, healthcare providers can enhance screening behaviors in men through communication, relationship building, patient education, and consideration for privacy and modesty.[52] Special attention for those with learning disabilities may require an alternate learner be selected and educated on testicular examination such as a caregiver, partner, or parent.[53] Additionally, healthcare providers need to educate themselves more fully to boost their confidence in promoting healthy screening behavior in younger men.[54] One tool that has been established in many physician and nurse training institutions includes a PowerPoint lecture, reading materials, video, and an artificial male model named "Zack" upon which to practice physical examinations and to teach male patients the proper technique.[55]

Educational programs beginning during the individual's teens should incorporate specific instructions on how to perform TSE. One study found that college students had limited knowledge of risk factors and screening recommendations for testicular cancer.[56] Testicular self exams should be performed after a warm shower/bath when the scrotum is relaxed and abnormalities can be more easily identified. While standing, each testicle should be examined for lumps, swelling, and any changes by rolling the testicle between the thumb and fingers. Any abnormality particularly on the front or side of either testicle should be reported to a healthcare provider immediately. Both the American Cancer Society (ACS) and the National Cancer Institute (NCI) provide pamphlets explaining testicular cancer and TSE.

Certain physical characteristics in men should alert healthcare providers to the potential for development of testicular GCTs and the need to offer screening. These characteristics include the known risk factors for developing testicular GCT.[57] For example, it is imperative that all males who present with gynecomastia be screened for testicular cancer.[58,59] It was once thought that men who are overly physically active in their youth possessed a higher incidence of testicular cancer; however, new findings have revealed no correlation.[60] Patients in their second or third decade of life who initially presented with seminoma are more likely to develop a second GCT later in their fourth or fifth decade of life and should be followed more closely.[61]

Massive screening campaigns for testicular cancer in asymptomatic adolescent and adult males have not been deemed economically feasible by the NCI, the ACS, and the US Preventive Services Task Force because of the rarity of this disease and lack of evidence to improve outcomes.[62,63] Nonetheless, public awareness through education is important. Given the shifting incidence rates in terms of race specifically in certain minorities, educational materials may prove more beneficial to that specific target group when pamphlets are designed with culturally relevant pictures, scenes, words, and activities such as ones used for native Hawaiians.[64]

## PATHOPHYSIOLOGY

As mentioned earlier, GCTs are classified into 2 histological categories: seminomas and nonseminomas. Upon diagnosis, these testicular GCTs can be monitored with specific tumor markers. Some tumor markers that are commonly used in assessing testicular cancer are outlined in Table 68-2.[65] Alpha-fetoprotein and beta-human chorionic gonadotropin (B-hCG) are the 2 most useful tumor markers in testicular cancer care.[66] Teratomas are benign tumors that do not secrete markers.

Germ cell tumors, similar to other cancers, start with the transformation of a single cell and evolve from its subsequent abnormal growth pattern. They are believed to be

**TABLE 68-2**

**Common Serum Tumor Markers**

| Marker | Tumor |
|---|---|
| AFP | NSGCT (50%–60%) |
| B-hCG | Choriocarcinoma (100%)<br>Embryonal tumor (80%)<br>Pure seminoma (10%–25%) |
| LDH isoenzyme | Advanced or large-volume disease<br>Advanced pure seminoma |
| PLAP | NSGCT |
| GCAP | Seminoma |
| Inhibin-alpha | Leydig cell tumor |

*Abbreviations*: AFP, alpha-fetoprotein; B-hCG, beta-human chorionic gonadotropin; GCAP, germ cell-specific alkaline; LDH, lactate dehydrogenase; NSGCT, nonseminomatous germ cell tumor; PLAP, placental alkaline phosphatase.

*Source*: Data from Lee et al.[65]

more responsive to chemotherapy (and, in the case of seminoma, to radiation therapy) because of their fast tumor cell doubling time. More than 90% of GCTs will arise in the testicle. The spread of these cancers is generally predictable, with the initial spread occurring to the retroperitoneal lymph nodes and not to the contralateral testes. Once spread has occurred to the lymphatics, vascular spread follows. The lungs are the most common distant organ affected by this pattern of invasion.

Current research has identified a genetic mapping region that has been consistently linked to gains in the short arm of chromosome 12 (12p) given that all testicular GCTs, including seminomas, nonseminomas, and carcinoma in situ (CIS), become aneuploid.[67–69] In addition, 2 distinct regions on the long arm of chromosome 17 (17q) have been identified that show elevated expression of genes attributed to extra copies in the pathogenesis of about half of all testicular GCTs.[70]

## CLINICAL MANIFESTATIONS

The most common presenting symptom of testis cancer is a hard, painless, pea-sized swelling or enlargement of the testis. This symptom is often ignored because many men may attribute this finding to recent trauma. Painful enlargement occurs in 30% to 50% of patients and is often due to local hemorrhage within the tumor and, therefore, should not be discounted.[71] Table 68-3 describes the local, metastatic, and hormonal presenting symptoms of testicular tumors. The most common metastatic site for testicular GCTs is the lungs, which correlates with the late presenting features. In the case of painful scrotal enlargement, diagnosis of testicular cancer may be delayed as a result of initially being treated for epididymitis or testicular torsion since these conditions occur more frequently than testicular GCTs. Other testicular conditions may need to be investigated such as spermatoceles, varicoceles, and hydroceles (sacs filled with sperm, blood, and water respectively.)

**TABLE 68-3**

**Presenting Symptoms Associated With Testicular Cancer**

| | |
|---|---|
| Local effects | Painless lump<br>Testicular ache/discomfort<br>Enlargement or firmness of testis<br>Heaviness of scrotum<br>Asymmetry<br>Dull ache in lower abdomen or groin<br>Sudden collection of fluid in scrotum |
| Metastatic effects | Back pain (para-aortic lymphadenopathy)<br>Breathlessness or hemoptysis (pulmonary metastasis)<br>Chest pain<br>Coughing |
| Hormonal effects | Breast growth<br>Tender or swollen breasts<br>Reduced or loss of sex drive<br>Growth of hair on face and/or body before puberty |

## ASSESSMENT

### PATIENT AND FAMILY HISTORY

A thorough patient and family history are important components for establishing a plan of care. Patient histories of cryptorchidism, epididymitis, gynecomastia, back pain, and infertility should all be noted, as should a history of testicular cancer in the past given the 500-fold increase in risk. In addition, individuals who have Down's syndrome, Klinefelter's syndrome, or HIV infection are at a greater risk for developing testicular GCTs. Other individuals who may have been exposed to testicular feminization, such as those with syndrome X (metabolic syndrome), are also at greater risk for testicular cancers.[32] Family histories of male patients (brothers, father, grandfathers, and uncles) should be taken into account as well.

### PHYSICAL EXAMINATION

A physical examination should incorporate a careful inspection of the scrotum. A mass that cannot be separated from the testis indicates a need for further evaluation, as do irregularities of tissue or nodularities. The epididymis is located in the back of the scrotum and will normally possess a spongy texture. A thorough assessment will pay close attention to symmetry of the testicles, their size, body hair growth, and lung sounds. It is normal for one testicle to hang lower in the scrotum than the other. Lymph nodes should be examined, especially the abdominal and supraclavicular lymph nodes. In general, adenopathy is not observed in the absence of prior surgical violation of the scrotum. Breasts should also be examined for gynecomastia.

### DIAGNOSTIC STUDIES

Two-dimensional (2-D) ultrasonography (US) with a high-frequency transducer has become the imaging modality of choice for examination of the scrotum.[72] This technology can identify suspicious masses suspect of GCTs and differentiate those between other conditions of the testicle such as torsion, trauma, and epididymo-orchitis with reliability and accuracy.[73] However, US is unable to determine whether a testicular mass is malignant. Transillumination of the mass may reveal a hydrocele. Approximately 20% of patients with GCTs will have an associated hydrocele. Seminomatous masses will appear hypoechoic when compared to adjacent tissue, whereas nonseminomatous masses may have an echo pattern that is hypoechoic, hyperechoic, or isoechoic. Recent research has supported that 3-D US proved better than traditional 2-D US in characterization of scrotal lesions, but may not be cost effective.[74]

Suspicious masses discovered on US should be followed up with the most important diagnostic test for testicular GCTs, a radical inguinal orchiectomy (RIO) (a surgical procedure that removes the affected testicle and spermatic cord). This diagnostic procedure also serves a vital therapeutic role in that the primary site of cancer is removed. It is generally performed in the physician's surgical suite with local anesthesia through an incision in the lower abdomen just below the belt line on the affected side. Tissue samples are then sent to a pathologist who confirms the diagnosis with an array of microscopic and assay tests. A fine-needle biopsy or transcrotal-approach orchiectomy of the testicular mass is contraindicated because of an increased risk of local recurrence or metastatic spread of disease to inguinal lymph nodes. The entire testicle in question has to be removed. Conversely, in the case of surveillance in a testicular cancer survivor in an attempt to diagnose early-stage GCTs such as testicular intraepithelium neoplasms (TINs), multiple biopsies are recommended from 1 particular surgical incision site as they may safely increase detection rates.[75]

Serum tumor markers such as AFP and/or B-hCG are elevated in approximately 85% of nonseminomatous GCTs.[76] Beta-human chorionic gonadotropin is the most commonly elevated tumor marker in testicular GCTs. These 2 molecules are so sensitive and specific to the testis that the American Joint Committee on Cancer (AJCC) has incorporated them into their overall staging guidelines. Moreover, the presence of these markers allow for detection of subclinical disease. The lactate dehydrogenase (LDH) isoenzyme level is frequently elevated in patients with advanced disease. Other tests may include bone scintigraphy, which has gained radiologists' confidence because it seems to be more sensitive in detecting the spread of GCT diseases.[77] Scintigraphy is a radiopharmaceutic procedure that utilizes a gamma camera to detect the amount of gamma-emitting substance that has gathered in a particular organ, tissue, or system.

Chest x-rays are valuable in determining whether a patient has gross metastases. If the chest x-ray is normal, a chest computerized tomography (CT) scan is warranted to rule out metastases within the lung or mediastinum.[78] Magnetic resonance imaging (MRI) plays an important role in determining metastatic spread of testicular GCT into abdominal organ sites and bones.[79,80] However, MRI is more typically utilized later during the follow-up period for evaluating treatment and monitoring for recurrence after surgery.[81] Positron emission tomography (PET) scans have become more useful recently but potentially carry a high false-positive rate besides being more expensive.[82] Brain CT or MRI may also be warranted if other metastases are suspected.

### PROGNOSTIC INDICATORS

The extent of disease and histology at the time of diagnosis determine the stage of disease and prognosis. Moreover, the percentage of embryonal carcinoma and vascular invasion appear to be the most significant prognosticators for GCTs based on the current data.[83] Virtually all patients with stage I (testis alone) or II (testis and retroperitoneal lymph nodes) seminomatous and nonseminomatous tumors should survive their disease. Approximately 70% of patients with testicular GCTs will present with stage I (local) disease or stage II (regional) disease.[84] The remaining patients present with stage III, disseminated disease characterized by hematologic spread to the lung, liver, bone, brain, or supradiaphragmatic region.

Patients with low serum markers or no evidence of pulmonary or mediastinal disease have an excellent prognosis. Those with low levels of tumor markers and/or limited disease will have a strong chance of cure if treated appropriately. Most patients with disseminated testicular cancer fall into the minimal or moderate disease category at the time of their diagnosis, which is associated with a greater than 90% cure rate with cisplatin-based combination chemotherapy. Prognosis is closely correlated with increased stage of disease and tumor burden.

## CLASSIFICATION AND STAGING

Several systems exist for the classification and staging of testicular cancer and have often been institution dependent. The AJCC has developed the staging guide for testis tumors that most physicians in the world follow today[85] (Table 68-4). Furthermore, the International Germ Cell Collaborative Group developed a prognostication system in 1997 that has remained the standard and was recently verified to be applicable to a population-based cohort (Table 68-5).[86–89] Survival rates for each category have also been provided.

**TABLE 68-4**

**AJCC Testicular Cancer Staging**

**Primary tumor (T)**

TX: The primary tumor cannot be assessed

T0: There is no evidence of primary tumor

Tis: Carcinoma in situ (noninvasive cancer cells)

T1: The tumor has not spread beyond the testicle and the narrow tubules next to the testicles where sperm undergo final maturation (epididymis). Cancer cells are not found inside blood vessels or lymph vessels next to the tumor. The cancer may have grown through the inner layer surrounding the testicle (tunica albuginea) but not the outer layer covering the testicle (tunica vaginalis)

T2: Similar to T1 except that the cancer has spread to blood or lymph vessels near the tumor, or the tunica vaginalis

T3: The tumor invades the spermatic cord (which contains blood vessels, lymph vessels, nerves, and the vas deferens)

T4: The tumor invades the skin surrounding the testicles (scrotum)

**Regional lymph nodes (N)**

NX: Regional (nearby) lymph nodes cannot be assessed

N0: No spread to regional lymph nodes is seen on x-rays

N1: There is spread to at least 1 lymph node, but no lymph node is larger than 2 cm (about 3/4 inch) in any dimension

N2: There is spread to at least 1 lymph node that is larger than 2 cm but is not bigger than 5 cm (2 inches) in any dimension

N3: There is spread to at least 1 lymph node that is larger than 5 cm in any dimension

If the lymph nodes were taken out during surgery, there is a slightly different classification:

pNX: Regional (nearby) lymph nodes cannot be assessed

pN0: There is no spread to regional lymph nodes

pN1: There is spread to 1–5 lymph nodes, with no lymph node larger than 2 cm (about 3/4 inch) across in greatest dimension

pN2: There is spread to at least 1 lymph node that is bigger than 2 cm but not larger than 5 cm; or spread to more than 5 lymph nodes that aren't bigger than 5 cm; or the cancer is growing out the side of the lymph node

pN3: There is spread to at least 1 lymph node that is bigger than 5 cm

**Distant metastasis (M)**

MX: Distant metastasis cannot be assessed

M0: There is no distant metastasis (no spread to lymph nodes outside the area of the tumor or other organs, such as the lungs)

M1: Distant metastasis is present

M1a: The tumor has metastasized to distant lymph nodes or to the lung

M1b: The tumor has metastasized to other organs, such as the liver, brain, or bone

**Serum tumor markers (S)**

| | LDH (U/liter) | HCG (mIU/ml) | AFP (ng/ml) |
|---|---|---|---|
| SX | Marker studies not available or not performed | | |
| S0 | Normal | Normal | Normal |
| S1* | < 1.5 × Normal | < 5000 | < 1000 |
| S2+ | 1.5–10 × Normal | 5000–50,000 | 1000–10,000 |
| S3+ | > 10 × Normal | > 50,000 | > 10,000 |

* = All markers must be in the stated range to be S1.
+ = Only one marker needs to be in the stated range to be S2 and S3.
*Abbreviations*: AFP, alpha-fetoprotein; HCG, human chorionic gonadotropin; LDH, lactate dehydrogenase.

**TABLE 68-4 CONTINUED**

**Stage grouping**

Using the TNM staging system, the descriptions of the tumor, lymph nodes, metastasis, and serum markers are combined in a process called stage grouping to assign a stage using Roman numerals.

| Stage | T | N | M | S |
|---|---|---|---|---|
| Stage 0 | Tis (in situ) | N0 | M0 | S0 |
| Stage I | T1–T4 | N0 | M0 | SX |
| Stage IA | T1 | N0 | M0 | S0 |
| Stage IB | T2–T4 | N0 | M0 | S0 |
| Stage IS | Any T | N0 | M0 | S1–S3 |
| Stage II | Any T | N1–N3 | M0 | SX |
| Stage IIA | Any T | N1 | M0 | S0–S1 |
| Stage IIB | Any T | N2 | M0 | S0–S1 |
| Stage IIC | Any T | N3 | M0 | S0–S1 |
| Stage III | Any T | Any N | M1 | SX |
| Stage IIIA | Any T | Any N | M1a | S0–S1 |
| Stage IIIB | Any T | N1–N3 | M0 | S2 |
| | Any T | Any N | M1a | S2 |
| Stage IIIC | Any T | N1–N3 | M0 | S3 |
| | Any T | Any N | M1a | S3 |
| | Any T | Any N | M1b | Any S |
| Recurrent | Cancer has come back after treatment | | | |

*Source*: Data from the National Cancer Institute[84]; American Joint Committee on Cancer.[85]

## THERAPEUTIC APPROACHES AND NURSING CARE

### NONSEMINOMA TUMORS

Nonseminomatous germ cell tumors (NSGCTs) account for about 60% of all GCTs and serve as an extraordinary example of how a multidisciplinary approach may ensure successful cancer management.[2] Early-stage disease primarily is approached surgically. Subsequent stages are treated with cisplatin-based chemotherapy with possible postsurgical resection of remaining tumor. The advent of cisplatin-based combination chemotherapy has dramatically affected the treatment of advanced disease. This success has, in turn, influenced the treatment of patients with earlier-stage disease. Stage I and early-stage II disease can be managed well with primary surgery, but other options for selected patients are emerging. A discussion of the management of patients with NSGCTs follows.

#### Stage I

Stage I germ cell testis cancer is defined in Table 68-4 as disease that is confined to the testis. The choice for management for stage I NSGCT is one of the most controversial topics in urologic oncology. A retroperitoneal lymph node dissection (RPLND) following a RIO has been the time honored approach to the treatment of testicular cancer confined to the testis. Recently, another viable option, consisting of surveillance after RIO without further treatment, has been offered to these men in particular those without vascular invasion.[90,91] Both options offer a long-term cure rate of 97% up to 100%, and the treatment selected is ultimately the patient's decision.[92,93]

The rationale for surgery is well grounded. RPLND in low-volume testis cancer is useful for staging because approximately 30% of patients with clinical stage I testis cancer, in fact, have pathological stage II disease.[94] Surgery alone provides cure in approximately 100% of patients with pathological stage I and 70% of pathological stage

**TABLE 68-5**

**International Germ Cell Consensus Prognostic Classification**

| Nonseminoma Tumors | Seminoma |
|---|---|
| **Good Prognosis** | |
| Testis/retroperitoneal primary<br>*and*<br>No nonpulmonary visceral metastases<br>*and*<br>Good markers—all of AFP < 1000 ng/mL, B-hCG < 5000 IU/L, and LDH < 1.5 × upper limit of normal<br>*56% of non-seminomas*<br>*5 year PFS 89%*<br>*5 year survival 92%* | Any primary site<br>*and*<br>No nonpulmonary visceral metastases<br>*and*<br>Normal AFP, any B-hCG, any LDH<br>*90% of seminomas*<br>*5 year PFS 82%*<br>*5 year survival 86%* |
| **Intermediate Prognosis** | |
| Testis/retroperitoneal primary<br>*and*<br>No nonpulmonary visceral metastases<br>*and*<br>Intermediate markers—any of AFP ≥ 1000 ng/mL and ≤ 10,000 ng/mL or B-hCG ≥ 5000 IU/L or LDH ≥ 1.5 and ≤ 10 × upper limit of normal<br>*28% of non-seminomas*<br>*5 year PFS 75%*<br>*5 year survival 80%* | Any primary site<br>*and*<br>Nonpulmonary visceral metastases<br>*and*<br>Normal AFP, any B-hCG, any LDH<br>*10% of seminomas*<br>*5 year PFS 67%*<br>*5 year survival 72%* |
| **Poor Prognosis** | |
| Mediastinal primary<br>*or*<br>Nonpulmonary visceral metastases<br>*or*<br>Poor markers—any of: AFP > 10,000 ng/mL or B-hCG > 50,000 IU/L<br>*or*<br>LDH > 10 × upper limit of normal<br>*16% of non-seminomas*<br>*5 year PFS 41%*<br>*5 year survival 48%* | No patients classified as poor prognosis |

*Abbreviations:* AFP, alpha-fetoprotein; B-hCG, beta-human chorionic gonadotropin; LDH, lactate dehydrogenase; PFS, progression-free survival.

*Source:* Data from the National Cancer Institute[84]; International Germ Cell Cancer Collaborative Group[87] Murphy et al.[88]; van Dijk et al.[89]

II testis cancer with minimal chance of local recurrence.[95] Newer techniques have advanced RPLND in 2 major ways—nerve-sparing and laparoscopic procedures vs open RPLND. Nerve-sparing RPLND offers conventional surgery with strict emphasis on protecting all nerves, including those responsible for antegrade ejaculation, the major risk to fertility after surgery in these men. In addition, laparoscopic RPLND offers similar success rates with fewer scars and faster recovery time.[96] However, controversy exists with this procedure because only until recently has laparoscopic RPLND been compared to conventional open RPLND in long-term studies despite being utilized by surgeons as a result of the demand voiced by male patients.[97] Both procedures have now been deemed comparable in relation to long-term outcomes.[98]

RPLND typically offers excellent postoperative results, but success largely depends on high volume and experience of the surgeon in dealing with early-stage NSGCTs.[99] Hemorrhage and vascular injury are the most commonly reported complications.[100] Emphasis on improved management of NSGCTs has recently focused on identifying high-risk patient populations in an effort to base treatment decisions on a correlation between histological types of NSGCT and more aggressive disease requiring a more aggressive surgical approach. For example, patients with stage I embryonal carcinoma are at higher risk for developing metastatic disease (perhaps more than 80%) and therefore may be offered RPLND instead of surveillance.[101,102] Metastasis in stage I embryonal carcinoma rarely occurs to distant organs, but may be found in the retroperitoneum.[103] The likelihood of micrometastatic disease in the near lymph structures is greater in these patients, so the benefits of RPLND may begin to outweigh the risks in such cases.[104]

Teratomas, although benign, are the other type of stage I NSGCT that tends to recur more readily after chemotherapy. RPLND is used to remove the teratoma and often confers physical symptom relief for the patient.

Surveillance may be the preferred option for a man who has stage I NSGCT with a histological type other than carcinoma or teratoma. Because cisplatin-based chemotherapy will most likely cure this patient in the case of progressing disease or relapse, this option is gaining acceptance. Selection for surveillance must be considered carefully for individuals with stage I testicular cancer. Individuals must have normal serum AFP and B-hCG following RIO, plus normal x-rays and scans. Meticulous follow-up consisting of monitoring currently identified serum tumor markers and CT scans can detect relapse while avoiding the morbidity that can occur in RPLND.[105] In 1 study, approximately 80% of relapses of NSGCT occurred in the first year, increasing to 95% within 5 years from the start of the surveillance period.[106] None of these patients died of their disease or the treatment.

Men who have high-risk stage I NSGCT may also opt for 1 cycle of adjuvant chemotherapy consisting of bleomycin, etoposide, and cisplatin (BEP) in place of RPLND. One cycle of BEP was found to be just as effective with less toxicity than 2 cycles in this group.[107] Results of a long-term study showed minimal side effects and comparable outcomes.[108] Furthermore, a randomized phase III multicenter trial recently showed superiority of BEP over RPLND.[109]

### Pathological stage IIA/B

As described in Table 68–4, metastasis to the retroperitoneal lymph nodes signifies pathological stage II disease with either microscopic (IIA or nonbulky disease) or gross (IIB or bulky disease) involvement. More than one-third of patients with stage II disease will not harbor metastatic disease.[110] However, the risk of relapse is not uncommon and adjuvant chemotherapy is generally offered. Virtually all of these patients will be cured with 3 or 4 cycles of chemotherapy depending on the stage at time of recurrence. Significant improvements in relapse rates have been observed with adjuvant cisplatin-based chemotherapy—usually consisting of BEP—after complete resection of stage II disease. Indeed, this treatment has prevented relapse in nearly 100% of men diagnosed with testicular cancer. Without adjuvant chemotherapy, relapse rates are higher, but overall survival is unchanged.[111]

Surveillance after RPLND, rather than immediate postoperative chemotherapy, is another option for patients with pathological stage II disease. The obvious benefits of not having chemotherapy are that the 70% of patients who are cured by surgery are spared the experience as well as the long-term toxicities associated with such therapy.

### Clinical stage IIB

Individuals who have a nonpalpable (smaller than 3 cm in transverse diameter) abdominal mass visualized on CT scan typically will have RPLND with complete resection followed by either observation or adjuvant chemotherapy. For patients with bulkier disease, primary chemotherapy is indicated. In patients who achieve a clinical complete remission, no further therapy is indicated. If a residual mass is present following 3 or 4 cycles of BEP, surgical resection via RPLND should be performed. Although the mortality is low, the morbidity associated with RPLND is acceptable in these cases.[112] The surgical finding in such cases may be necrosis (40%-45%), teratoma (40%-45%), or cancer (10%). In patients who are found to have cancer in the resected residual specimen, 2 additional cycles of etoposide and cisplatin (EP) should be administered.

### Stage III/disseminated disease

A palpable mass with lymph nodes larger than 5 cm or involvement of more than 5 lymph nodes is designated as stage IIC disease. Abdominal disease of this magnitude will rule out initial surgical resection. Metastasis above the diaphragm or involvement of visceral organs, brain, or bone is classified as stage III disease. Chemotherapy is the preferred choice in this situation to reduce tumor burden before any other interventions are considered. Approximately 70% of men who initially present with stage III disease will be cured with conventional cisplatin-based chemotherapy.[84] Following chemotherapy, RPLND with complete resection of all residual masses confers a long-term disease-free survival of 95%.[113,114] The remainder will require surgical interventions also known as metastectomies if surgically feasible to rid the body of isolated metastatic disease that correlates with CT scan findings, as in the cases of pulmonary, mediastinal, and brain nodules.[115,116] If surgery cannot be safely performed, radiation treatments could be considered as an alternative. In men who present with advanced or bulky disease, chemotherapy—most often BEP—is the mainstay of treatment.

Table 68-6 describes currently employed testicular cancer chemotherapy regimens. These chemotherapy regimens should always be given on schedule, generally every 3 weeks, regardless of myelosuppression, in view of the typically rapid tumor cell doubling time. Likewise, cytokines are used when indicated to avoid dose reductions and treatment delays. Because cisplatin is not myelosuppressive, it is rarely necessary to reduce the dose or delay treatment. Special circumstances, such as in the case of severe renal and/or pulmonary disease, may occasionally eliminate bleomycin as an option because of safety concerns. Nonetheless, these individuals should receive 4 cycles of EP.

**TABLE 68-6**

| Testicular Germ Cell Cancer Chemotherapy Regimens |
|---|
| **Adjuvant Chemotherapy** |
| Bleomycin 30 units IV weekly for 8 weeks |
| Cisplatin 20 mg/m² IV daily for 5 days |
| Etoposide 100 mg/m² IV daily for 5 days every 28 days for 2 cycles |
| **Disseminated Disease Chemotherapy** |
| Etoposide 100 mg/m² IV daily for 5 days (days 1–5) + Cisplatin 20 mg/m² IV daily for 5 days for 4 cycles administered at 21-day intervals |
| *OR* |
| Etoposide 100 mg/m² IV daily for 5 days, |
| Cisplatin 20 mg/m² IV daily for 5 days, |
| + Bleomycin 30 units IV weekly on days 1, 8, 15 for 3 cycles administered at 21-day intervals |
| If a previously untreated patient is at intermediate or poor risk, then BEP for 4 cycles (not 3 as noted previously) |
| **Salvage Chemotherapy** |
| Ifosfamide 1.2 g/m² IV daily for 5 days |
| Mesna 400 mg/m² IV every 8 hours for 5 days |
| + Cisplatin 20 mg/m² IV daily for 5 days |
| + either vinblastine 0.11 mg/kg body weight IV on days 1 and 2, or etoposide 75 mg/m² IV daily for 5 days |
| *OR* |
| Paclitaxel 250 mg/m² IV day 1 followed by ifosfamide 1.5 g/m² IV and cisplatin 25 mg/m² IV daily on days 2 to 5 |
| Mesna 500 mg/m² IV before and then 4 and 8 hours after each ifosfamide dose |
| Each is administered every 21 days for 4 cycles |
| **Relapsed (Marker Positivity, with or without Radiographic Evidence of Disease)** |
| ABMT |
| High-dose chemotherapy (carboplatin and etoposide) with ABMT or peripheral stem cell rescue |
| Some patients would receive 1 to 2 cycles of either BEP or VEP prior to ABMT |

*Abbreviation*: ABMT, autologous bone marrow transplant; BEP, bleomycin, etoposide, and cisplatin.

## SEMINOMAS

Seminomas account for approximately 40% of all testicular GCTs.[2] With the use of effective chemotherapy and radiation therapy, the overall cure rate for all stages exceeds 90%.[117] Unlike nonseminomatous testicular tumors, 80% of seminomas present as clinical stage I disease.[118] Seminomas are known to be exquisitely sensitive to radiotherapy. Both stage I and stage IIA/B disease are treated with external beam irradiation. Chemotherapy is the primary treatment of bulky stage IIC and disseminated disease. The management following chemotherapy remains controversial.

### Stage I and stage IIA/B

Several management options consisting of adjuvant radiotherapy, surveillance, and adjuvant chemotherapy are available for stage I seminomas after RIO.[119] Typically, radiotherapy is offered due to its overwhelming success in curing these patients at upwards of 96% and higher.[120] Oncology radiologists will determine the amount of radiation divided into daily fractions that are delivered over a predetermined period of time. Higher doses of radiation are prescribed when more spread of disease is evident in the surrounding lymph nodes. Both anterior and posterior fields are treated. The area of treatment includes the paracaval and para-aortic nodes extending superiorly to the level of T10/11 and extending inferiorly to include the bilateral common iliac and the ipsilateral external iliac nodes. If the scrotum has been incised at the time of orchiectomy, if tumor spill has occurred, or if positive margins are present, the radiation field may be extended to include the ipsilateral hemiscrotum. More frequently, if an inguinal approach to orchiectomy was utilized, the scrotum, contralateral testis, and urinary bladder are shielded to limit scatter irradiation.

Although surveillance may be an option following orchiectomy for stage I seminoma, excellent results with minimal side effects and morbidity make radiation the treatment of choice. Nonetheless, a small risk of secondary malignancy is associated with radiotherapy; this risk should be taken into account but not overrated when compared to the long-term costs of surveillance.[121] One long-term study expressed about 9% rate in developing a secondary malignancy following radiotherapy which was higher than expected.[122] Furthermore, radiation to the anterior portion of the mediastinum at depths of 3 cm can lead to cardiac morbidity.[123] Oligospermia or azoospermia may occur as a result of radiation even when appropriate radiation shields are employed. Spermatogenesis recovery is dose dependent, but generally resumes a few months later. Patients with stage I and IIA/B disease who are treated with radiation therapy have a 98% and greater than 93% chance of cure, respectively (survival past 5 years without evidence of disease).[124] Minor reductions in radiation doses and volumes (treatment fields) and their effects on long-term secondary malignancies have been investigated in randomized clinical trials.[117]A reduction in dose from 30 Gy over 15 fractions to 20 Gy over 10 fractions in a randomized clinical trial revealed a relapse rate of only 0.7% compared to typically 3% thus allowing men to return to work sooner and potentially suffer fewer long term consequences.[125] Moreover, radiotherapy, when combined with reduced portals, yielded excellent control rates, minimal acute toxicity, and no late toxicity, making it the first-line treatment for patients with early-stage seminomas.[126]

Surveillance in men with stage I seminoma, however, does carry risks. Men who were diagnosed before 36 years of age were found to have an increased risk of relapse and should be reserved for those who can be followed up closely.[127] In addition, men who were under surveillance in British Columbia showed a 5 year relapse-free rate of 78% and a 5 year disease-free survival rate of 96%.[128] More than 80% of postorchiectomy patients can safely avoid further treatment unless relapse occurs.[129]

Adjuvant chemotherapy with 1 or 2 cycles of single-agent carboplatin has been investigated as an alternative to adjuvant radiotherapy or surveillance for stage I seminomas.[130] This alternative treatment option proved highly effective and was well tolerated.[131] In addition, 2 cycles of adjuvant EP proved comparable to carboplatin.[132] More recently, nerve-sparing RPLND was investigated in stage I and IIA seminoma with promising results in place of radiotherapy. All men were free of disease after 56 months of follow-up.[133]

### Stage IIC

Treatment of bulky, localized retroperitoneal disease is controversial. Both chemotherapy and radiation therapy are effective after RIO. Radiotherapy alone provides a cure for 30% to 60% of patients with stage IIC disease.[118] However, a direct correlation exists between the volume of disease and the anticipated cure rate with radiotherapy. Individuals who present with large abdominal masses (larger than 10 cm) have a high relapse rate when treated with radiation alone. On the one hand, postorchiectomy radiation to areas where disease had been identified, such as in the mediastinum, significantly decreased the likelihood of relapse in stage IIA, IIB, and IIC seminomas.[134] On the other hand, men with bulky retroperitoneal disease (larger than 5 cm) who were treated with radiotherapy alone had recurrent disease outside the treatment field, altering the current recommendations to offer chemotherapy as first-line treatment.[135] Besides the risk of recurrence, men who have been treated with radiation therapy to the mediastinum have a higher incidence of death related to cardiac disease.[136] Salvage chemotherapy consisting of ifosfamide and cisplatin may be sufficient for control.[137]

### Stage III/disseminated disease

Initial radiotherapy for metastasis to distant sites and bulky abdominal masses produces poorer survival rates when compared to cisplatin-based chemotherapy regimens. Given the nature of GCTs in advanced stages, when extranodal involvement and spread to distant organs such as the bone, lung, liver, or central nervous system (CNS) are evident, combination chemotherapy using BEP is generally prescribed for 3 to 4 cycles. Management of residual disease following chemotherapy remains controversial.

## STROMAL CELL TUMORS (SERTOLI AND LEYDIG CELL TUMORS)

Stromal cell tumors originate from the supporting structures of the testicle such as adipose and spermatic cord tissues. These tumor types rarely occur and are often benign. Standard treatment consisting solely of RIO typically cures the patient.[2] Radiation and chemotherapy are usually not effective for these tumors.

## SALVAGE CHEMOTHERAPY

The present emphasis in the treatment of disseminated, poor-risk, or relapsed disease is the exploration of cisplatin-intense regimens and the incorporation of innovative new agents. Clinical trials attempt to improve upon our understanding forging a way to better therapies using chemotherapy combinations that include etoposide, ifosfamide, cisplatin, vinblastine, and bleomycin (VIP/VeB) among others. Etoposide, ifosfamide, and cisplatin (VIP) plus carboplatin supplied an overall 5 year survival rate of 75% in relapsed testicular GCTs.[138] VIP plus high-dose carboplatin and etoposide successfully granted 43% of men a 3-year progression-free period.[139] Paclitaxel, gemcitabine, and oxaliplatin have also been investigated achieving 51% response.[140] Docetaxol, ifosfamide, and cisplatin were also studied in 1 case of relapsed disease with promising results.[141] Paclitaxel and gemcitabine have shown similar results of long-term disease-free survival.[142] Topoisomerase I inhibitor agents have proven useful in chemorefractory GCTs using a combination of irinotecan, paclitaxel, and oxaliplatin (IPO) followed by high-dose topotecan.[143]

### SURGICAL SALVAGE

Individuals with persistently elevated serum markers, indicative of viable disease following salvage chemotherapy, have not usually been considered surgical candidates because of the presumed systemic nature of their disease. However, after conventional treatment some men may show evidence of persistent localized tumors on CT scan and would benefit from surgical resection. Salvage surgeries should be performed at centers with significant experience with GCT management, as studies have shown that incomplete resection of residual masses may occur in more than 30% of cases.[144] In addition, careful preoperative planning and intraoperative judgment are necessary to reduce the potential for serious vascular complications.[145]

### HIGH-DOSE CHEMOTHERAPY WITH RESCUE

Approximately 25% of individuals with advanced, poor-risk, testicular GCTs will not be cured with current treatment modalities.[146] These patients with cisplatin-refractory disease require a more aggressive approach consisting of combination high-dose chemotherapy with peripheral stem cell rescue, surgery, and sometimes radiation to cure or, at minimum, control their disease. High-dose chemotherapy utilizing carboplatin and etoposide followed by peripheral stem cell transplantation (PSCT) is a safe and effective treatment option for men with aggressive or progressive disease allowing more than 46% of men disease-free after 37 months.[147] Furthermore, patients with poor-prognosis diseases often will fail on conventional chemotherapy but may benefit from dose-intensive protocols using these newer agents with or without PSCT as first-line therapy.[148]

### NURSING CARE

The time of diagnosis and initiation of treatment are stressful. Education must begin early. Careful explanations of the nature of the disease, its treatment, goals of therapy, and side effects are essential.[149] Information must be provided and reinforced at various intervals along the treatment continuum. The patient's and family's anxiety levels may be elevated from perceived and real threats of mortality, alterations in life roles, and issues related to sexual identity, all of which require specialized attention. Consistent evaluations of the patient and family knowledge deficits are necessary to provide effective educational interventions.

#### Surgery

A RIO is performed as an outpatient procedure for both diagnostic and therapeutic purposes—to establish a histological diagnosis and to remove the tumor. Nursing interventions should focus on postoperative teaching regarding pain management, activity level, and incisional wound care. Patients and family members need to learn how to change the dry, sterile dressing and how to recognize and report signs of infection and unusual bleeding. Men need to understand that neither sexual function nor fertility will be impaired or changed as a result of the orchiectomy. However, alterations in body image may result. Supportive interventions may be indicated to improve coping.

Care of the individual undergoing an RPLND, outside of the fertility issues, is similar to other abdominal surgeries. Paralytic ileus, a common side effect of abdominal surgery, may be prolonged for 2 to 4 days after RPLND depending on the extent of the abdominal resection performed and the length of time under anesthesia. Men are started on a clear liquid diet the day before surgery and undergo bowel preparation usually consisting of ingesting magnesium citrate or a full mechanical bowel preparation. A nasogastric tube is placed during surgery and remains in place until normal bowel sounds are present. After auscultation of normal bowel sounds, a clear liquid diet will be initiated, advancing to a regular diet as tolerated. Sufficient pain management interventions are necessary after the surgery and persist for several days.

#### Fertility

The traditional bilateral RPLND results in the loss of antegrade ejaculation, thus producing infertility from subsequent retrograde ejaculation. New, more refined techniques for RPLND have focused on preserving the nerves responsible for antegrade ejaculation and hence maintaining fertility in this population. With the advent of laparoscopic RPLND, fewer scars exist and less time is required to fully recover. Nevertheless, RPLND remains an important component of treatment for GCTs because it can eliminate any micrometastatic disease in the nearby surrounding lymph tissue, as predicted spread has been defined. The ability to experience a normal orgasm is not impaired because of RPLND.

Sperm banking prior to initiation of treatment may be an option depending on the stage of disease and sperm count at diagnosis. Because treatment of GCTs may include a combination of surgery, radiation, or chemotherapy, as well as the inherent risks for secondary malignancies such as leukemia, it is difficult to predict which men given different potential treatment options will develop fertility problems.[150,151] In addition, long-term hormonal treatment may reduce gonadal function.[152] It is therefore necessary to offer sperm banking to all men in this situation. When successful, sperm banking allows men who will probably be cured of their disease to establish pregnancies with assisted reproductive techniques.[153] Nearly all semen samples collected from adolescents proved to be potentially useful in this regard.[154] On the downside, sperm banking can take weeks to obtain sufficient viable sperm. Men need to understand the risks of treatment delay, the cost of sperm collection and storage, and the potential costs of reproductive assistance such as in vitro fertilization if needed.[155] Because of the aggressive nature of the disease, sperm banking may not be a viable option for some men due to their urgent need for therapy.

New techniques have been identified that enable testicular sperm extractions (TESE) synchronously with RIO followed with gamete cryopreservation in the most difficult of cases.[156] Furthermore, a system for long-term cryopreservation remains to be perfected given the increasing number of testicular cancer survivors.[151]

Testicular implants should be offered to all men who undergo RIO and supplied sufficient counseling about the advantages and disadvantages of having a prosthesis.[157] Men tend to experience more satisfaction with their prosthesis when they are given a choice when contemplating cosmetic issues such as size and elliptical shape. It is important to share information that the remaining testicle will likely grow somewhat in size to compensate in making sperm (if possible) and testosterone and to adjust the size of the prosthesis slightly. Also, a second surgery is required similar to that of the original RIO to insert and secure the implant, thus prompting many men to forego the procedure. Finally, adequate time should be allowed for men to consider their options given their situation.[157]

### Radiation

The resultant toxicities of abdominal radiotherapy for testicular cancer are less severe now than in the past due to lower effective doses, improved equipment, and computerized axial tomographic planning. Problematic sequelae may include diarrhea, fatigue, nausea, fertility issues, myelosuppression, and occasionally bladder irritation, peptic ulcers, and lymphedema.

*Gastrointestinal complications.* Radiation to the abdominal and pelvic regions can cause diarrhea. Individuals should be instructed to manage radiation-associated diarrhea with a low-residue diet and over-the-counter antidiarrheals, but to seek medical attention if diarrhea continues despite these interventions. Prescriptive antidiarrheal medication is often required to manage this side effect. A low-residue diet is designed to reduce the amount of fiber in the intestinal tract by restricting indigestible carbohydrates such as milk products, high-fat-content foods, fruits and vegetables with seeds or skins, and high-fiber breads.

Unlike with radiation administered to other parts of the body, nausea and vomiting are not unusual with the first radiotherapy treatment for testicular cancer. Oral antiemetics consisting of a serotonin (5HT-3) antagonist and a steroid administered 1 hour prior to the radiotherapy treatment and as needed has been found to be effective in controlling the associated mild nausea and vomiting.[158] Light meals prior to treatment should be encouraged. Radiation to the brain is necessary with metastatic disease and can be associated with significant CNS toxicity including seizures, hemiparesis, cranial neuropathies, headaches, blindness, dementia, and ataxia.[159] New technologies such as the gamma knife (stereotactic radiation) have improved outcomes and reduced toxicity greatly.[160]

*Myelosuppression.* Radiation to the para-aortic lymph nodes and the pelvis often produces myelosuppression. Weekly complete blood counts with differential and platelets are monitored. Acute complications are uncommon. Information should be provided on the importance of seeking medical assistance for fever when neutropenia is present. Instruction should be provided to avoid medication that could potentially mask a fever. Patients should be told to call the physician's office if bruising or unusual bleeding occurs, as they could be a sign of thrombocytopenia, although transfusion is rarely performed. Also, individuals should be made aware that fatigue can occur, is generally short lived, and could interfere with normal daily activities.[161] Pacing, prioritizing, and allowing frequent rest periods between activities will help patients cope with treatment related fatigue.

### Chemotherapy

Side effects resulting from chemotherapy are drug and dose dependent and must be managed accordingly. The extent of disease and history of prior therapy should also be taken into account. A thorough review of each medication's side-effect profile is necessary to successfully manage the patient's individual responses. Knowledge and experience in dealing with chemotherapy strengthen the nurse's ability to maximally assist each patient through his treatment continuum. Table 68-7 identifies the major side effects caused by common chemotherapeutic agents and their associated nursing interventions.[8,87,162] Potential side effects include nausea and vomiting, constipation, myelosuppression, nephrotoxicity, hemorrhagic cystitis, integumentary changes, reproductive changes, neurological changes, pulmonary complications, fatigue, and body image changes. Other chemotherapeutic

**TABLE 68-7**

**Nursing Care and Educational Needs of Patients Receiving Chemotherapy for Testicular Cancer**

| Problem | Drug(s) | Nursing Interventions |
|---|---|---|
| Nausea/vomiting | Cisplatin<br>Ifosfamide | • Administer prophylactic antiemetics with 5HT-3 antagonist, NK-1 antagonist, dexamethasone, and/or lorazepam<br>• Write down schedule for antiemetics regimen<br>• Encourage and maintain adequate fluid intake<br>• Consider supplemental IV hydration<br>• Consider the use of music and relaxation therapy |
| Constipation | Vinblastine<br>Etoposide | • Assess bowel function<br>• Encourage fluids and high-fiber diet<br>• Instruct patient to report significant bowel changes<br>• Administer stool softeners and laxatives if patient is prone to constipation |
| Myelosuppression | Ifosfamide<br>Vinblastine<br>Etoposide | • Monitor complete blood count<br>• Instruct patient to report signs of infection, fever, bleeding, shortness of breath, severe weakness, tachycardia<br>• Instruct patient to avoid crowds and individuals with active infections. Encourage frequent hand-washing<br>• Monitor incisions, wounds, catheter, sites for infection<br>• Obtain blood and urine cultures, chest x-ray prior to administering antibiotics<br>• Administer antibiotics as prescribed |
| Nephrotoxicity | Cisplatin<br>Ifosfamide | • Monitor serum electrolytes, creatinine, and BUN daily. Monitor daily weights and intake and output.<br>• Provide aggressive pre- and posthydration and increase oral intake<br>• Avoid aminoglycosides for the treatment of granulocytopenic fever when receiving cisplatin |
| Hemorrhagic cystitis | Ifosfamide | • Obtain urinalysis daily; if > 10 RBCs per high-powered field, alert physician and hold drug<br>• Provide aggressive pre- and posthydration and instruct patient to increase oral intake<br>• Administer Mesna, a uroprotectant, as directed |
| Integumentary changes | Ifosfamide<br>Bleomycin<br>Etoposide | • Prepare patient for hair loss, reinforcing its temporary nature. Protect exposed scalp from sun and cold<br>• Alert patient regarding skin hyperpigmentation and nail changes |
| Reproduction | Cisplatin<br>Etoposide<br>Bleomycin<br>Ifosfamide<br>Vinblastine | • Arrange for sperm banking if possible prior to chemotherapy<br>• Reinforce that ejaculation/impotence will not change<br>• Inform patients of azoospermia for at least 12 months with normal spermatogenesis returning in 50% of men within 2 years. Those treated with 3 to 4 cycles of BEP are at higher risk for persistent semen abnormalities. |
| Neurological changes | Cisplatin<br>Vinblastine<br>Bleomycin | • Instruct reporting of numbness and tingling of hands and feet (ie, Raynaud phenomenon)<br>• Inform patients to wear gloves and dress warmly in cold weather<br>• Instruct patients to report hearing changes<br>• Obtain baseline and serial audiometry for high-risk patients (ie, > 50 years, total dose of > 400 mg cisplatin, abnormal renal function) |
| Pulmonary complications | Bleomycin | • Assess for bibasilar rates, inspirational lag, and cough<br>• Evaluate men at high risk for fibrosis (ie, smokers, decreased renal function, previous chest irradiation, and >450 units of bleomycin) |
| Body image changes | | • Encourage patient to verbalize feelings about hair loss and changes in appearance<br>• Teach patient self-care activities related to body image disturbance<br>• Reinforce any attempts to attend to the body part<br>• Reinforce any verbalizations of feelings about actual or perceived loss<br>• Provide consultation with hair stylist or barber |

*Abbreviations*: BEP, bleomycin, etoposide, and cisplatin; BUN, blood urea nitrogen; RBCs, red blood cells.

*Source*: Data from Zack[8]; Poirier et al[87]; and Oncology Nursing Society.[162]

agents that have been investigated and show clinical efficacy against testicular GCTs include the following: vincristine, gleevec, methotrexate, paclitaxel, cyclophosphamide, carboplatin, gemcitabine, actinomycin D, and thiotepa.[163] Side effects of these agents should be reviewed before their administration.

Acute tumor lysis syndrome is a rare complication of chemotherapy directly caused by the rapid destruction of tumor cells (testicular cancer cells with a high tumor burden in this case) shortly after the initiation of treatment.[164] This oncological emergency occurs when lysed cell particles consisting of certain electrolytes and uric acid flood the bloodstream and overwhelm the kidneys. Renal failure results when uric acid particles crystallize and create obstructions in the distal tubules and collecting ducts. In addition, elevated serum levels of potassium and phosphorus can cause serious cardiac, neurological, and gastrointestinal toxicities.

Acute pulmonary complications can occur primarily when bleomycin is used in the chemotherapeutic regimen. Bleomycin is an antibiotic that possesses antitumor activity and plays a major role in curing patients with testicular GCTs.[165] Pulmonary fibrosis is correlated with increasing doses of bleomycin to a maximum lifetime dose of 400 mg or 400 units.[166] Furthermore, men who have poor renal function or who are 40 years and older have higher incidences of pulmonary toxicity.[167] Pulmonary fibrosis may lead to respiratory failure or death. Pulmonary function tests are often followed closely in men who have received bleomycin at some point in their treatment. Furthermore, men who have been treated with bleomycin in the past should always share that information with their surgeon when planning for general anesthesia with any procedure.

Nausea and vomiting are likely to occur in men being treated with cisplatin since it is the strongest emetogenic chemotherapeutic agent that all others are compared to. Similar to radiation protocol, nausea and vomiting control can be achieved well with a 5HT-3 antagonist and a steroid.[158] Dopamine antagonists, lorazepam, and neurokinin-1 antagonists may also prove beneficial. Acute electrolyte disturbances frequently occur and indirectly result from the side effects of chemotherapy such as nausea, vomiting, and diarrhea. In contrast, cisplatin may directly cause magnesium wasting and in effect increase the risk of seizures in susceptible patients.[168] Frequent monitoring of magnesium and other critical electrolytes is necessary, and supplementation is required to avoid potential complications in organ systems that depend on specific electrolyte therapeutic ranges.

#### Sanctuary sites

In advanced testis cancer, CNS and the contralateral testicle are the most common sanctuary sites for malignancy.[114,169] Isolated cerebral metastases occurring after successful chemotherapy are curable.[170] Because of the blood–brain barrier, most chemotherapeutic agents cannot penetrate the structures of the brain. Therefore, other aggressive measures are taken, including stereotactic radiotherapy, whole-brain radiation, and even surgical resection, in an attempt to cure the patient. Occult CNS metastases should be suspected if, in the presence of chest or abdominal radiological remission following therapy, new elevations or persistent tumor markers are present. In this situation, CT scans and MRI, of the brain should be obtained even in the absence of clinical symptoms.

It has been suggested that it is unlikely that chemotherapy penetrates the testicle because of the blood–testis barrier.[171] This barrier functions to prevent germ cells from encountering harmful influences and contains 3 components: capillaries and Sertoli cells, an efflux pump with P glycoprotein, and an immunological barrier consisting of FAS ligand on Sertoli cells. FAS ligand plays an important role in the maintenance of immune privilege by killing invading inflammatory cells.

Normally, the testis primary tumor is surgically resected prior to treatment. In the presence of advanced disseminated disease and positive tumor markers, however, chemotherapy may be initiated prior to a tissue diagnosis. At the completion of chemotherapy, the involved testis is removed. Whenever markers remain elevated following removal of the involved testicle (in the absence of radiographic evidence of disease), a second testis primary tumor should be investigated.

## SYMPTOM MANAGEMENT AND SUPPORTIVE CARE

### DISEASE PROGRESSION

Testicular GCTs arise from 1 cell, typically possess a fast cell doubling time, and can metastasize to distant sites in a matter of several months to years if left undiagnosed and untreated. The risk of metastasis is lowest for teratoma and highest for choriocarcinoma with all others posing an intermediate risk. Generally, the tumor inside the testicle will continue to grow with associated fluid accumulation and begin to cause local symptoms as discussed in the "Clinical Manifestations" section. As time passes, GCT cells spread via the spermatic cord and the associated lymphatic and circulatory systems to reach distant sites that include, but are not limited to, the retroperitoneal lymph nodes, the lungs, liver, bone, and brain. Here, GCTs acquire access to a blood supply for nutrition and waste removal purposes to support continued and unregulated growth and invasion. Testicular GCTs can become the cause of death in men because of their metastatic properties, but seldom do as a result of improved treatments.

## QUALITY OF LIFE AND PSYCHOSOCIAL ISSUES

Quality of life (QOL) and psychosocial issues have become important areas for nursing and medical research. As a consequence of the excellent cure rates for testicular GCTs, emphasis has now shifted in terms of optimizing the QOL in these men post-treatment. The incidence of depression and anxiety in these patients is lower than that in patients diagnosed with different malignancies, but remains slightly higher than the incidence in the general population.[172–175] Smoking behaviors have been linked to depression in studies after therapy.[176] In addition, cancer related fatigue (CRF) contributes to a poor QOL with multiple psychological and somatic health problems that need to be addressed routinely during follow-up.[177] Consequently, job strain, work engagement, nor work changes over a 2 to 6-year period of time took place for the majority of survivors.[178–180] Cancer-related stress in the form of fear with real or perceived threats in their current or future lives may require psychosocial intervention to strengthen coping skills.[181] Supervised high-intensity strength training has been shown to improve QOL, muscle strength, and cardiopulmonary function in cancer survivors.[182]

Preserving fertility in this population greatly impacts QOL. Awareness and sensitivity to the individual's and family's educational needs and initiating appropriate interventions to provide for psychosocial adjustment to the real or possible fertility changes will promote coping and acceptance. In addition, men who underwent treatment and received information pertaining to their disease, treatment, and useful coping skills reported satisfactory QOL scores by maintaining body image and controlling side effects.[183] However, in men who underwent a 3-day chemotherapy regimen consisting of BEP, reports identified excess gastrointestinal toxicities and tinnitus as having a detrimental effect on QOL.[184] Nursing interventions need to focus on controlling any and all disease- and chemotherapy-related symptoms that occur so as to maximize QOL and help these men complete their treatment regimens without delay.

## FOLLOW-UP CARE AND SURVIVORSHIP

Because most men survive more than 5 years after the diagnosis of testicular GCT, follow-up care and survivorship issues need to be addressed. Follow-up care starts shortly after treatment and ultimately needs to become incorporated into lifelong strategies that promote healthy behaviors, maintenance, and well-being. This period is critical because therapy-related toxicities may occur at any time post-treatment, even several decades later in life. Follow-up typically involves frequent physical assessments, monitoring of serum tumor markers, and CT scans at defined intervals.

Some specific health problems that have been observed in this population include late effects of chemotherapy such as secondary primary cancers, cardiovascular sequelae, metabolic syndrome, gonadal toxicity, neurotoxicity, and pulmonary sequelae.[185] Two forms of acute leukemia up to 30 years post-treatment posed an elevated risk thought to be caused by cisplatin.[186,187] Surprisingly, trace levels of cisplatin can be detected in both plasma and urine of testicular cancer survivors almost 20 years after treatment.[188,189] Moreover, treatment with cisplatin confers a higher-than-normal risk for long-term nephrotoxicity and hearing impairment.[190–192] The risk for a second solid tumor malignancy was also elevated after radiation.[187,193]

Cardiovascular sequelae is comprised of elevated serum markers of chronic inflammatory and endothelial dysfunction after radiation and atherogenic lipid changes and metabolic syndrome after chemotherapy.[194] Metabolic syndrome includes insulin insensitivity, central obesity dyslipidemia, and hypertension and is reliably prognosticated by low serum testosterone levels.[195] Furthermore, common consequences post-treatment can involve premature endocrine hypogonadism reducing fertility and possibly causing erectile dysfunction.[152,196] If testosterone needs to be supplemented, careful consideration and screening for invasive breast cancer in these men should ensue.[197]

Sensory neuropathy consistent with a stocking-glove distribution occurred commonly after cisplatin therapy.[198] Vascular toxicities in the form of Raynaud's disease have been observed in cured patients and are suspected to be caused by chemotherapeutic agents, specifically bleomycin.[190] This phenomenon is characterized by transient episodes of vasoconstriction of the digital arteries that lead to fluctuations in color, warmth, and pain.[190] Occurrences range dramatically, but when present, Raynaud's disease may become long-lasting (eg, more than 10 years post-treatment). Bleomycin induced pneumonitis (BIP) may occur during or usually after treatment causing respiratory distress and requires prompt treatment with steroids.[199]

Late relapse occurs in 2% to 3% of men who have been diagnosed and successfully treated for GCTs in the past.[200] Patients who initially present with a high tumor burden and the presence of teratomatous components within the primary testicular cancer have a higher likelihood of developing a late disease relapse.[201] Most patients with advanced seminomas after relapse have a poor prognosis despite further treatment.[202] The vast majority of relapses are discovered in the retroperitoneum and occur within the first 2 years following therapy and become exceedingly rare once a patient is 5 years post-treatment.[200] For this reason, close follow-up strategies generally cease after the 5-year mark, except in the cases of patients presenting with metastatic NSGCT.[203] There do exist some case reports of late relapse occurring more than 20 years after treatment.[204] Most institutions now propose 35 years of follow-up since secondary malignancies can occur up to this point and have become the leading cause of death in testicular cancer survivors.[205] Interestingly, lifelong follow-up is generally recommended for anyone who has been diagnosed with any other form of cancer.

Several national organizations offer information and assistance programs for survivorship as well as other disease-related concerns. The following list includes major organizations, their associated Web sites, and their telephone numbers:

American Cancer Society: www.cancer.org, (800) 227–2345
Lance Armstrong Foundation: www.laf.org, (512) 236–8820
National Cancer Institute: www.cancer.gov, (800) 422–6237
National Coalition for Cancer Survivorship: www.canceradvocacy.org, (877) 622–7937
National Comprehensive Cancer Network: www.ncnn.org

## CONCLUSION

Current research in testicular GCTs has focused on several aspects of the disease. Identifying the testicular cancer genome is one area that may offer insight into improved treatment modalities through identification of chromosomal abnormalities and gene expression profiling.[70,206] Countless studies are actively investigating the complexities of molecular genetics involved with signal transferring, stem cell markers, transcription factors, and nucleotide polymorphisms in both human and animal models. Angiogenesis and tumorigenesis are other topics being actively funded and researched.[207] The information gained from these studies may explain why some tumors show resistance to current pharmaceutical therapies. Researchers may eventually suggest ways to manipulate specific signal pathways so as to overcome drug resistance.[208] One groundbreaking example resulting from genetic research highlights a defective mismatch repair pathway that leads to the microsatellite instability thought to be responsible for cisplatin drug resistance.[209] Microsatellite instability is a type of genetic error that results when the cell's DNA mismatch repair system fails to correct damaged DNA strands, thereby allowing stretches of DNA to hook up with the wrong partner.

Despite the many advancements brought by research, testicular cancer continues to be responsible for the deaths of many men. This disease, unlike many other malignancies, has the true potential to offer 100% cure if resources became more widely available.[210] As a result of ongoing education and greater public awareness, TSEs could significantly lessen its death toll.[211] These efforts would single out testicular GCTs as an excellent illustration of control that other malignancies could model as new research sheds light on them.

Although testicular cancer is a rare and devastating disease to the young population it affects, it is also one of the most highly curable malignancies. Testicular self-examination remains the best available tool for early diagnosis and treatment. Most males today can be successfully treated, with adverse side effects being vastly reduced compared to those produced by the therapy available 20 years ago. The high cure rate of testicular cancer can be attributed to dedicated clinical researchers and interdisciplinary team who utilize combination modalities such as surgery, chemotherapy, radiation therapy, and bone marrow transplantation in the treatment of testicular cancer. Researchers continue to look for new ways to improve current treatment modalities and to reduce morbidity and mortality.

## REFERENCES


1. Weir HK, Thun MJ, Hankey BF, et al. Annual report to the nation on the status of cancer, 1975–2000, featuring the uses of surveillance data for cancer prevention and control. *J Natl Cancer Inst.* 2003;95:1276–1299.
2. American Cancer Society. *Cancer Facts and Figures 2009.* Atlanta, GA: American Cancer Society; 2009.
3. Sokoloff MH, Joyce GF, Wise M; Urologic Diseases in America Project. Testis cancer. *J Urol.* 2007;177:2030–2041.
4. Huyghe E, Matsuda T, Thonneau P. Increasing incidence of testicular cancer worldwide: a review. *J Urol.* 2003;170:5–11.
5. Oldenburg J, Lehne G, Fossa SD. Testicular cancer[in Norwegian]. *Tidsskr Nor Laegeforen.* 2008;128:457–460.
6. Holmes L Jr, Escalante C, Garrison O, et al. Testicular cancer incidence trends in the USA (1975–2004): plateau or shifting racial paradigm? *Public Health.* 2008;122:862–872.
7. Berney DM. Staging and classification of testicular tumours: pitfalls from macroscopy to diagnosis. *J Clin Pathol.* 2008;61:20–24.
8. Zack E. Testicular germ cell cancer. In: Yarbro CH, Frogge MH, Goodman M, eds. *Cancer Nursing: Principles and Practice.* 6th ed. Sudbury, MA: Jones and Bartlett; 2005:1630–1646.
9. Montie J. Carcinoma in situ of the testis and bilateral carcinoma. *Urol Clin North Am.* 1993;20:127–132.
10. Dieckmann K, Boeckman W, Brosig W, et al. Bilateral testicular germ cell tumors. *Cancer.* 1986;51:1254–1258.
11. Fossa SD, Chen J, Schonfeld SA, et al. Risk of contralateral testicular cancer: a population-based study of 29,515 US men. *J Natl Cancer Inst.* 2005;97:1056–1066.
12. Butenandt O. Cryptorchism. Treatment should be finished by age 2 [in German]. *MMW Fortschr Med.* 2007;149:14; author reply 14.
13. Pettersson A, Akre O, Richiardi L, Ekbom A, Kaijser M. Maternal smoking and the epidemic of testicular cancer—a nested case-control study. *Int J Cancer.* 2007;120:2044–2046.
14. Walsh TJ, Dall'Era MA, Croughan MS, Carroll PR, Turek PJ. Prepubertal orchiopexy for cryptorchidism may be associated with lower risk of testicular cancer. *J Urol.* 2007;178:1440–1446; discussion 1446.
15. van der Horst HJ, de Gier RP, de Jong TP, van den Hoek J, Callewaert PR, Feitz WF. The undescended testis: arguments in favour of early treatment, provided retractile testis and acquired non-scrotal testis have been excluded [in Dutch]. *Ned Tijdschr Geneeskd.* 2008;152:253–258.
16. Bani-Hani KE, Matani YS, Bani-Hani IH. Cryptorchidism and testicular neoplasia. *Saudi Med J.* 2003;24:166–169.
17. Lutke Holzik MF, Sijmons RH, Sleijfer DT, et al. Syndromic aspects of testicular carcinoma. *Cancer.* 2003;97:984–992.
18. Yoshida T, Takao T, Tsujimura A, Tomita H, Aozasa K, Okuyama A. Testicular epidermoid cyst in Klinefelter's syndrome. *Int J Urol.* 2006;13:478–480.
19. Ogawa Y, Yoshida H. Klinefelter syndrome [in Japanese]. *Nippon Rinsho.* 2004;62:327–332.
20. Hsiung Stripp DC, Vaughn D, Van Arsdalen K, et al. Three cases of advanced seminoma and Down's syndrome: a possible association. *Am J Clin Oncol.* 2003;26:197–199.

21. Rapley E. Susceptibility alleles for testicular germ cell tumour: a review. *Int J Androl.* 2007;30:242–250; discussion 250.
22. Hemminki K, Sundquist J, Lorenzo Bermejo J. Familial risks for cancer as the basis for evidence-based clinical referral and counseling. *Oncologist.* 2008;13:239–247.
23. Neale RE, Carriere P, Murphy MF, Baade PD. Testicular cancer in twins: a meta-analysis. *Br J Cancer.* 2008;98:171–173.
24. Walsh TJ, Davies BJ, Croughan MS, Carroll PR, Turek PJ. Racial differences among boys with testicular germ cell tumors in the United States. *J Urol.* 2008;179:1961–1965.
25. McGlynn KA, Devesa SS. Re: Nguyen MM, Ellison LM: Testicular cancer patterns in Asian American males: an opportunity for public health education to impact outcomes. *Urology.* 2005;66:606–609.
26. Ohlson CG, Hardell L. Testicular cancer and occupational exposures with a focus on xenoestrogens in polyvinyl chloride plastics. *Chemosphere.* 2000;40:1277–1282.
27. Chen GR, Dong L, Ge RS, Hardy MP. Relationship between phthalates and testicular dysgenesis syndrome. *Zhonghua Nan Ke Xue.* 2007;13:195–200.
28. Sonke GS, Chang S, Strom SS, Sweeney AM, Annegers JF, Sigurdson AJ. Prenatal and perinatal risk factors and testicular cancer: a hospital-based case-control study. *Oncol Res.* 2007;16:383–387.
29. Bouskine A, Nebout M, Mograbi B, Brucker-Davis F, Roger C, Fenichel P. Estrogens promote human testicular germ cell cancer through a membrane-mediated activation of extracellular regulated kinase and protein kinase A. *Endocrinology.* 2008;149:565–573.
30. Jacobsen R, Bostofte E, Engholm G, et al. Risk of testicular cancer in men with abnormal semen characteristics: cohort study. *BMJ.* 2000;321:789–792.
31. Olsson H, Bladstrom A, Alm P. Male gynecomastia and risk for malignant tumours—a cohort study. *BMC Cancer.* 2002;2:26.
32. Fukui M. Testicular cancer and syndrome X. *Lancet.* 2001;358:242.
33. Goedert JJ, Purdue MP, Mograbi B, Brucker-Davis F, Roger C, Fenichel P. Risk of germ cell tumors among men with HIV/acquired immunodeficiency syndrome. *Cancer Epidemiol Biomarkers Prev.* 2007;16:1266–1269.
34. Bonner MR, McCann SE, Moysich KB. Dietary factors and the risk of testicular cancer. *Nutr Cancer.* 2002;44:35–43.
35. McGlynn KA, Sakoda LC, Rubertone MV, et al. Body size, dairy consumption, puberty, and risk of testicular germ cell tumors. *Am J Epidemiol.* 2007;165:355–363.
36. Bjorge T, Tretli S, Lie AK, Engeland A. The impact of height and body mass index on the risk of testicular cancer in 600,000 Norwegian men. *Cancer Causes Control.* 2006;17:983–987.
37. Michos A, Xue F, Michels KB. Birth weight and the risk of testicular cancer: a meta-analysis. *Int J Cancer.* 2007;121:1123–1131.
38. Ahlgren M, Wohlfahrt J, Olsen LW, Sorensen TI, Melbye M. Birth weight and risk of cancer. *Cancer.* 2007;110:412–419.
39. Peterson HB. Sterilization. *Obstet Gynecol.* 2008;111:189–203.
40. DeCastro BJ, Peterson AC, Costabile RA. A 5-year follow-up study of asymptomatic men with testicular microlithiasis. *J Urol.* 2008;179:1420–1423; discussion 1423.
41. Sanli O, Kadioglu A, Atar M, Acar O, Nane I. Grading of classical testicular microlithiasis has no effect on the prevalence of associated testicular tumors. *Urol Int.* 2008;80:310–316.
42. Shichijo T, Sakamoto H, Saito K, Ogawa Y, Yoshida H, Kushima M. Relevance of testicular microlithiasis to the testicular carcinoma in situ in the contralateral testicle [in Japanese]. *Nippon Hinyokika Gakkai Zasshi.* 2007;98:541–546.
43. Parenti GC, Zago S, Lusa M, Campioni P, Mannella P. Association between testicular microlithiasis and primary malignancy of the testis: our experience and review of the literature.- *Radiol Med.* 2007;112:588–596.
44. Srivastava A, Kreiger N. Cigarette smoking and testicular cancer. *Cancer Epidemiol Biomarkers Prev.* 2004;13:49–54.
45. Pettersson A, Richiardi L, Nordenskjold A, Kaijser M, Akre O. Age at surgery for undescended testis and risk of testicular cancer. *N Engl J Med.* 2007;356:1835–1841.
46. Kaijser M, Akre O, Cnattingius S, Ekbom A. Maternal lung cancer and testicular cancer risk in the offspring. *Cancer Epidemiol Biomarkers Prev.* 2003;12:643–646.
47. Hardell L, Carlberg M, Ohlson CG, Westberg H, Eriksson M, Hansson Mild K. Use of cellular and cordless telephones and risk of testicular cancer. *Int J Androl.* 2007;30:115–122.
48. Huyghe E, Mazerolles C, Moran C, et al. Synchronous epidermoid cyst and mature teratoma of the testis: an unusual association. *Urol Int.* 2007;78:364–366.
49. Wynd CA. Testicular self-examination in young adult men. *J Nurs Scholarsh.* 2002;34:251–255.
50. Gajendran VK, Nguyen M, Ellison LM. Testicular cancer patterns in African American men. *Urology.* 2005;66:602–605.
51. Cook N. Testicular cancer: testicular self-examination and screening. *Br J Nurs.* 2000;9:338–343.
52. Dube CE, Fuller BK, Rosen RK, Fagan M, O'Donnell J. Men's experiences of physical exams and cancer screening tests: a qualitative study. *Prev Med.* 2005;40:628–635.
53. Peate I, Maloret P. Testicular self-examination: the person with learning difficulties. *Br J Nurs.* 2007;16:931–935.
54. Brenner JS, Hergenroeder AC, Kozinetz CA, et al. Teaching testicular self-examination: education and practices in pediatric residents. *Pediatrics.* 2003;111:e239-e244.
55. Taylor JS, Dube CE, Pipas CF, et al. Teaching the testicular exam: a model curriculum from "A" to "Zack." *Fam Med.* 2004;36:209–213.
56. Daley CM. College students' knowledge of risk and screening recommendations for breast, cervical, and testicular cancers. *J Cancer Educ.* 2007;22:86–90.
57. Stephenson AJ, Bosl GJ, Motzer RJ, Bajorin DF, Stasi JP, Sheinfeld J. Nonrandomized comparison of primary chemotherapy and retroperitoneal lymph node dissection for clinical stage IIA and IIB nonseminomatous germ cell testicular cancer. *J Clin Oncol.* 2007;25:5597–5602.
58. Daniels IR, Layer GT. Testicular tumours presenting as gynaecomastia. *Eur J Surg Oncol.* 2003;29:437–439.
59. Hassan HC, Cullen IM, Casey RG, Rogers E. Gynaecomastia: an endocrine manifestation of testicular cancer. *Andrologia.* 2008;40:152–157.
60. Cook MB, Graubard BI, Quraishi SM, et al. Genetic variants in the 8q24 locus and risk of testicular germ cell tumors. *Hum Genet.* 2008;123:409–418.
61. Che M, Tamboli P, Ro JY, et al. Bilateral testicular germ cell tumors: 20-year experience at M.D. Anderson Cancer Center. *Cancer.* 2002;95:1228–1233.
62. Moul JW. Timely diagnosis of testicular cancer. *Urol Clin North Am.* 2007;34:109–117; abstract vii.
63. Shaw J. Diagnosis and treatment of testicular cancer. *Am Fam Physician.* 2008;77:469–474.
64. Kulukulualani M, Braun KL, Tsark JU. Using a participatory four-step protocol to develop culturally targeted cancer education brochures. *Health Promot Pract.* 2008;9:344–355.
65. Lee F, Hamid R, Arya M, et al. Testicular cancer: current update and controversies. *Hosp Med.* 2002;63:615–620.
66. Duffy MJ. Clinical uses of tumor markers: a critical review. *Crit Rev Clin Lab Sci.* 2001;38:225–262.
67. Looijenga LH, Zafarana G, Grygalewicz B, et al. Role of gain of 12p in germ cell tumour development. *Apmis.* 2003;111:161–171; discussion 172–173.
68. McIntyre A, Gilbert D, Goddard N, Looijenga L, Shipley J. Genes, chromosomes and the development of testicular germ cell tumors of adolescents and adults. *Genes Chromosomes Cancer.* 2008;47:547–557.
69. Abbosh PH, Zhang S, Maclennan GT, et al. Germ cell origin of testicular carcinoid tumors. *Clin Cancer Res.* 2008;14:1393–1396.
70. Skotheim RI, Monni O, Mousses S, et al. New insights into testicular germ cell tumorigenesis from gene expression profiling. *Cancer Res.* 2002;62:2359–2364.
71. Wilson JP, Cooksey G. Testicular pain as the initial presentation of testicular neoplasms. *Ann R Coll Surg Engl.* 2004;86:284–288.

72. Dogra VS, Gottlieb RH, Oka M, Rubens DJ. Sonography of the scrotum. *Radiology*. 2003;227:18–36.
73. Wittenberg AF, Tobias T, Rzeszotarski M, Minotti AJ. Sonography of the acute scrotum: the four Ts of testicular imaging. *Curr Probl Diagn Radiol*. 2006;35:12–21.
74. Elwagdy S, Razmy S, Ghoneim S, Elhakim S. Diagnostic performance of three-dimensional ultrasound extended imaging at scrotal mass lesions. *Int J Urol*. 2007;14:1025–1033.
75. Kliesch S, Thomaidis T, Schutte B, et al. Update on the diagnostic safety for detection of testicular intraepithelial neoplasia (TIN). *Apmis*. 2003;111:70–74; discussion 75.
76. Perkins G, Slater E, Sanders G, Prichard J. Serum tumor markers. *Am Fam Physician*. 2003;68:1075–1082.
77. Braga FJ, Arbex MA, Haddad J, et al. Bone scintigraphy in testicular tumors. *Clin Nucl Med*. 2001;26:117–118.
78. Bramley R. The role of chest X-ray and computed tomography thorax in the surveillance of testicular tumours. *Clin Oncol (R Coll Radiol)*. 2003;15:441–442.
79. Sterpy MD, Tiutin LA. Role of MRI tomography in testicular cancer. *Vopr Onkol*. 2003;49:323–327.
80. Froehner M, Aikele P, Beuthien-Baumann B, Kittner T, Oehlschlaeger S, Wirth MP. Magnetic resonance imaging of bone metastases in patients with nonseminomatous germ cell tumors. *Urol Oncol*. 2007;25:201–206.
81. Corral DA, Varma DG, Jackson EF, et al. Magnetic resonance imaging and magnetic resonance angiography before postchemotherapy retroperitoneal lymph node dissection. *Urology*. 2000;55:262–266.
82. Hinz S, Schrader M, Kempkensteffen C, et al. The role of positron emission tomography in the evaluation of residual masses after chemotherapy for advanced stage seminoma. *J Urol*. 2008;179:936–940; discussion 940.
83. Heidenreich A, Srivastava S, Moul JW, et al. Molecular genetic parameters in pathogenesis and prognosis of testicular germ cell tumors. *Eur Urol*. 2000;37:121–135.
84. National Cancer Institute. Testicular cancer treatment (PDQ): *http://www.cancer.gov/cancertopics/pdq/treatment/testicular/healthprofessional* Accessed December 28. 2009.
85. American Joint Committee on Cancer. *The AJCC Cancer Staging Manual*. 6th ed. Chicago, IL; New York: Springer-Verlag; 2002.
86. International Germ Cell Cancer Collaborative Group. International Germ Cell Consensus Classification: a prognostic factor based staging system for metastatic germ cell cancers. *J Clin Oncol*. 1997;15:594–603.
87. Poirier S, Rawl S. Testicular germ cell cancer. In: Yarbro CH, Frogge MH, Goodman M, eds. *Cancer Nursing Practice and Principles*. 5th ed. Sudbury, MA: Jones and Bartlett; 2000:1494–1510.
88. Murphy EM, Douglas J, Thompson K, Wood L. Application of the International Germ Cell Consensus Classification to the Nova Scotia population of patients with germ cell tumours. *Can Urol Assoc J*. 2009;3:120–124.
89. van Dijk M, Steyerberg E, Habbema J. Survival of non-seminomatous germ cell cancer patients according to the IGCC classification: An update based on meta-analysis. *Eur J Cancer*.2006; 42(7):820–826.
90. Ondrus D, Ondrusova M, Hornak M, Matoska J. Nonseminomatous germ cell testicular tumors clinical stage I: differentiated therapeutic approach in comparison with therapeutic approach using surveillance strategy only. *Neoplasma*. 2007;54:437–442.
91. Groll RJ, Warde P, Jewett MA. A comprehensive systematic review of testicular germ cell tumor surveillance. *Crit Rev Oncol Hematol*. 2007;64:182–197.
92. Choueiri TK, Stephenson AJ, Gilligan T, Klein EA. Management of clinical stage I nonseminomatous germ cell testicular cancer. *Urol Clin North Am*. 2007;34:137–148; abstract viii.
93. Albers P. Management of stage I testis cancer. *Eur Urol*. 2007;51:34–43; discussion 43–44.
94. Donahue JP, Thornhill JH, Foster RS, et al. Retroperitoneal lymphadenectomy for clinical stage A testis cancer (1965 to 1989): modifications of technique and impact on ejaculation. *J Urol*. 1993;149:237–243.
95. Valdevenito Sepulveda JP, Merhe Nieva E, Valdevenito Sepulveda R, et al. Reduced retroperitoneal lymphadenectomy for clinical stage I non seminomatous germ cell testicular cancer [in Spanish]. *Arch Esp Urol*. 2007;60:245–254.
96. Nielsen ME, Lima G, Schaeffer EM, et al. Oncologic efficacy of laparoscopic RPLND in treatment of clinical stage I nonseminomatous germ cell testicular cancer. *Urology*. 2007;70:1168–1172.
97. Finelli A. Laparoscopic retroperitoneal lymph node dissection for nonseminomatous germ cell tumors: long-term oncologic outcomes. *Curr Opin Urol*. 2008;18:180–184.
98. Neyer M, Peschel R, Akkad T, et al. Long-term results of laparoscopic retroperitoneal lymph-node dissection for clinical stage I nonseminomatous germ-cell testicular cancer. *J Endourol*. 2007;21:180–183.
99. Leisinger HJ, Donohue JP. The role of retroperitoneal surgery in testis cancer. *Crit Rev Oncol Hematol*. 2002;44:71–80.
100. Kenney PA, Tuerk IA. Complications of laparoscopic retroperitoneal lymph node dissection in testicular cancer. *World J Urol*. 2008;26:561–569.
101. Sweeney CJ, Hermans BP, Heilman DK, et al. Results and outcome of retroperitoneal lymph node dissection for clinical stage I embryonal carcinoma—predominant testis cancer. *J Clin Oncol*. 2000;18:358–362.
102. Porcaro AB, Zecchini Antoniolli S, Novella G, et al. Histopathologic risk factors in patients with non-seminomatous germ tumors of the testis in clinical stage 1. Retrospective study of 75 patients [in Italian]. *Arch Ital Urol Androl*. 2001;73:177–180.
103. Pohar KS, Rabbani F, Bosl GJ, et al. Results of retroperitoneal lymph node dissection for clinical stage I and II pure embryonal carcinoma of the testis. *J Urol*. 2003;170:1155–1158.
104. Foster R, Bihrle R. Current status of retroperitoneal lymph node dissection and testicular cancer: when to operate. *Cancer Control*. 2002;9:277–283.
105. Roeleveld TA, Horenblas S, Meinhardt W, et al. Surveillance can be the standard of care for stage I nonseminomatous testicular tumors and even high-risk patients. *J Urol*. 2001;166:2166–2170.
106. Daugaard G, Petersen PM, Rorth M. Surveillance in stage I testicular cancer. *Apmis*. 2003;111:76–83; discussion 83–85.
107. Gilbert DC, Norman AR, Nicholl J, Dearnaley DP, Horwich A, Huddart RA. Treating stage I nonseminomatous germ cell tumours with a single cycle of chemotherapy. *BJU Int*. 2006;98:67–69.
108. Westermann DH, Schefer H, Thalmann GN, Karamitopoulou-Diamantis E, Fey MF, Studer UE. Long-term followup results of 1 cycle of adjuvant bleomycin, etoposide and cisplatin chemotherapy for high risk clinical stage I nonseminomatous germ cell tumors of the testis. *J Urol*. 2008;179:163–166.
109. Albers P, Siener R, Krege S, et al. Randomized phase III trial comparing retroperitoneal lymph node dissection with one course of bleomycin and etoposide plus cisplatin chemotherapy in the adjuvant treatment of clinical stage I nonseminomatous testicular germ cell tumors: AUO trial AH 01/94 by the German Testicular Cancer Study Group. *J Clin Oncol*. 2008;26:2966–2972.
110. Albers P, Siener R, Kliesch S, et al. Risk factors for relapse in clinical stage I nonseminomatous testicular germ cell tumors: results of the German Testicular Cancer Study Group Trial. *J Clin Oncol*. 2003;21:1505–1512.
111. Jones RH, Vasey PA. Part I: testicular cancer—management of early disease. *Lancet Oncol*. 2003;4:730–737.
112. Thijssens K, Vaneerdeweg W, Schrijvers D, et al. Retroperitoneal lymph node dissection as adjuvant therapy in the treatment of nonseminomatous testicular cancer. *Acta Chir Belg*. 2003;103:599–602.
113. Heidenreich A, Thuer D, Polyakov S. Postchemotherapy retroperitoneal lymph node dissection in advanced germ cell tumours of the testis. *Eur Urol*. 2008;53:260–272.
114. Fizazi K, Oldenburg J, Dunant A, et al. Assessing prognosis and optimizing treatment in patients with postchemotherapy viable

nonseminomatous germ-cell tumors (NSGCT): results of the sCR2 international study. *Ann Oncol.* 2008;19:259–264.
115. Kesler KA. Surgical techniques for testicular nonseminomatous germ cell tumors metastatic to the mediastinum. *Chest Surg Clin North Am.* 2002;12:749–768.
116. Horvath LG, McCaughan BC, Stockle M, et al. Resection of residual pulmonary masses after chemotherapy in patients with metastatic non-seminomatous germ cell tumours. *Intern Med J.* 2002;32:79–83.
117. Bauduceau O, Souleau B, Le-Moulec S, et al. Radiotherapy in stage I testicular seminoma: retrospective study and review of literature. *Cancer Radiother.* 2003;7:386–394.
118. Roth B, Nichols C, Einhorn L. Neoplasms of the testis. In: Frei E, Holland J, Bast R, et al. *Cancer Medicine.* vol 2. 3rd ed. Philadelphia, PA: Lea and Febiger; 1993:1592–1619.
119. Warde P, Specht L, Horwich A, et al. Prognostic factors for relapse in stage I seminoma managed by surveillance: a pooled analysis. *J Clin Oncol.* 2002;20:4448–4452.
120. Garcia-Serra AM, Zlotecki RA, Morris CG, Amdur RJ. Long-term results of radiotherapy for early-stage testicular seminoma. *Am J Clin Oncol.* 2005;28:119–124.
121. Warde P, Gospodarowicz MK, Panzarella T, et al. Long term outcome and cost in the management of stage I testicular seminoma. *Can J Urol.* 2000;7:967–972; discussion 973.
122. Fatigante L, Ducci F, Campoccia S, et al. Long-term results in patients affected by testicular seminoma treated with radiotherapy: risk of second malignancies. *Tumori.* 2005;91:144–150.
123. Majewski W, Majewski S, Maciejewski A, Kolosza Z, Tarnawski R. Adverse effects after radiotherapy for early stage (I,IIa,IIb) seminoma. *Radiother Oncol.* 2005;76:257–263.
124. Guden M, Ulutin C, Goktas S. Analyses of 98 seminoma cases: a review article. *Int Urol Nephrol.* 2001;33:529–531.
125. Jones WG, Fossa SD, Mead GM, et al. Randomized trial of 30 versus 20 Gy in the adjuvant treatment of stage I testicular seminoma: a report on Medical Research Council Trial TE18, European Organisation for the Research and Treatment of Cancer Trial 30942 (ISRCTN18525328). *J Clin Oncol.* 2005;23:1200–1208.
126. Classen J, Schmidberger H, Meisner C, et al. Radiotherapy for stages IIA/B testicular seminoma: final report of a prospective multicenter clinical trial. *J Clin Oncol.* 2003;21:1101–1106.
127. Yang GY, Li B, Wagner TD, Donohue KA, Flaherty L, Kuettel MR. Long-term outcome of stage I seminoma. *Am J Clin Oncol.* 2007;30:205–210.
128. Tyldesley S, Voduc D, McKenzie M, Duncan G, Liu M, Wu D. Surveillance of stage I testicular seminoma: British Columbia Cancer Agency Experience 1992 to 2002. *Urology.* 2006;67:594–598.
129. Chung P, Warde P. Surveillance in stage I testicular seminoma. *Urol Oncol.* 2006;24:75–79.
130. Porcaro AB, Antoniolli SZ, Schiavone D, et al. Management of clinical stage I testicular pure seminoma. Report on 42 patients and review of the literature. *Arch Ital Urol Androl.* 2002;74:77–80.
131. Steiner H, Holtl L, Wirtenberger W, et al. Long-term experience with carboplatin monotherapy for clinical stage I seminoma: a retrospective single-center study. *Urology.* 2002;60:324–328.
132. Bamias A, Aravantinos G, Deliveliotis C, et al. Two cycles of etoposide/cisplatin cured all patients with stage I testicular seminoma: risk-adapted protocol of the Hellenic Cooperative Oncology Group. *Urology.* 2007;70:1179–1183.
133. Mezvrishvili Z, Managadze L. Retroperitoneal lymph node dissection for high-risk stage I and IIA seminoma. *Int Urol Nephrol.* 2006;38:615–619.
134. Zagars GK, Pollack A. Radiotherapy for stage II testicular seminoma. *Int J Radiat Oncol Biol Phys.* 2001;51:643–649.
135. Fleshner N, Warde P. Controversies in the management of testicular seminoma. *Semin Urol Oncol.* 2002;20:227–233.
136. Zagars GK, Ballo MT, Lee AK, et al. Mortality after cure of testicular seminoma. *J Clin Oncol.* 2004;22:640–647.
137. Patel MI, Motzer RJ, Sheinfeld J. Management of recurrence and follow-up strategies for patients with seminoma and selected high-risk groups. *Urol Clin North Am.* 2003;30:803–817.
138. Hartmann JT, Gauler T, Metzner B, et al. Phase I/II study of sequential dose-intensified ifosfamide, cisplatin, and etoposide plus paclitaxel as induction chemotherapy for poor prognosis germ cell tumors by the German Testicular Cancer Study Group. *J Clin Oncol.* 2007;25:5742–5747.
139. Lorch A, Beyer J, Bokemeyer C. Germ-cell tumors. *N Engl J Med.* 2007;357:1772–1773; author reply 1773–1774.
140. Bokemeyer C. Bleomycin in testicular cancer: will pharmacogenomics improve treatment regimens? *J Clin Oncol.* 2008;26:1783–1785.
141. Kume H, Kakutani S, Tomita K, Kitamura T. Salvage combination chemotherapy with docetaxel, ifosfamide and cisplatin (DIP): successful treatment of a case with metastatic testicular immature teratoma. *Jpn J Clin Oncol.* 2008;38:143–145.
142. Einhorn LH. Role of the urologist in metastatic testicular cancer. *J Clin Oncol.* 2007;25:1024–1025.
143. Shamash J, Powles T, Mutsvangwa K, et al. A phase II study using a topoisomerase I-based approach in patients with multiply relapsed germ-cell tumours. *Ann Oncol.* 2007;18:925–930.
144. Flechon A, Bompas E, Biron P, Droz JP. Management of postchemotherapy residual masses in advanced seminoma. *J Urol.* 2002;168:1975–1979.
145. Sexton WJ, Wood CG, Kim R, et al. Repeat retroperitoneal lymph node dissection for metastatic testis cancer. *J Urol.* 2003;169:1353–1356.
146. May M, Georgieva G, Gunia S, Peter N, Steinhauer HB, Hoschke B. High-dose chemotherapy with transplantation of autologous stem cells in advanced germ-cell poor-risk testicular tumors. *Urologiia.* 2007;2:58–63.
147. Papiani G, Einhorn LH. Salvage chemotherapy with high-dose carboplatin plus etoposide and autologous peripheral blood stem cell transplant in male pure choriocarcinoma: a retrospective analysis of 13 cases. *Bone Marrow Transplant.* 2007;40:235–237.
148. Jones RH, Vasey PA. Part II: testicular cancer—management of advanced disease. *Lancet Oncol.* 2003;4:738–747.
149. Higgs D. The patient with testicular cancer: nursing management of chemotherapy. *Oncol Nurs Forum.* 1990;17:243–246.
150. Spermon JR, Kiemeney LA, Meuleman EJ, et al. Fertility in men with testicular germ cell tumors. *Fertil Steril.* 2003;79(suppl 3):1543–1549.
151. Suzuki K, Matuzaki J, Hattori Y, et al. Semen cryopreservation for patients with malignant or non-malignant disease: our 14-year experience [in Japanese]. *Hinyokika Kiyo.* 2007;53:539–544.
152. Kiserud CE, Magelssen H, Fedorcsak P, Fossa SD. Gonadal function after cancer treatment in adult men [in Norwegian]. *Tidsskr Nor Laegeforen.* 2008;128:461–465.
153. Agarwa A. Semen banking in patients with cancer: 20-year experience. *Int J Androl.* 2000;23(suppl 2):16–19.
154. Bahadur G, Ling KL, Hart R, et al. Semen quality and cryopreservation in adolescent cancer patients. *Hum Reprod.* 2002;17: 3157–3161.
155. Girasole CR, Cookson MS, Smith JA Jr, Ivey BS, Roth BJ, Chang SS. Sperm banking: use and outcomes in patients treated for testicular cancer. *BJU Int.* 2007;99:33–36.
156. Descombe L, Chauleur C, Gentil-Perret A, Aknin-Seifer I, Tostain J, Levy R. Testicular sperm extraction in a single cancerous testicle in patients with azoospermia: a case report. *Fertil Steril.* 2008;90:443, e1-e4.
157. Chapple A, McPherson A. The decision to have a prosthesis: a qualitative study of men with testicular cancer. *Psychooncology.* 2004;13:654–664.
158. Einhorn LH, Brames MJ, Dreicer R, Nichols CR, Cullen MT Jr, Bubalo J. Palonosetron plus dexamethasone for prevention of chemotherapy-induced nausea and vomiting in patients receiving multiple-

day cisplatin chemotherapy for germ cell cancer. *Support Care Cancer.* 2007;15:1293–1300.

159. Doyle DM, Einhorn LH. Delayed effects of whole brain radiotherapy in germ cell tumor patients with central nervous system metastases. *Int J Radiat Oncol Biol Phys.* 2008;70:1361–1364.
160. Nicolato A, Ria A, Foroni R, et al. Gamma knife radiosurgery in brain metastases from testicular tumors. *Med Oncol.* 2005;22:45–56.
161. Fleer J, Sleijfer DT, Hoekstra HJ, Tuinman MA, Hoekstra-Weebers JE. Prevalence, changes in and correlates of fatigue in the first year after diagnosis of testicular cancer. *Anticancer Res.* 2005;25: 4647–4653.
162. Polovich M, White JM, Kelleher LO, eds. *Chemotherapy and Biotherapy Guidelines and Recommendations for Practice.* 2nd ed. Pittsburgh, PA: Oncology Nursing Society; 2005.
163. Raghavan D. Testicular cancer: maintaining the high cure rate. *Oncology (Huntingt).* 2003;17:218–228; discussion 228–229, 234–235, passim.
164. Pentheroudakis G, O'Neill VJ, Vasey P, et al. Spontaneous acute tumour lysis syndrome in patients with metastatic germ cell tumours. Report of two cases. *Support Care Cancer.* 2001;9:554–557.
165. Kawai K, Akaza H. Bleomycin-induced pulmonary toxicity in chemotherapy for testicular cancer. *Expert Opin Drug Saf.* 2003;2:587–596.
166. Uzel I, Ozguroglu M, Uzel B, et al. Delayed onset bleomycin-induced pneumonitis. *Urology.* 2005;66:195.
167. O'Sullivan JM, Huddart RA, Norman AR, Nicholls J, Dearnaley DP, Horwich A. Predicting the risk of bleomycin lung toxicity in patients with germ-cell tumours. *Ann Oncol.* 2003;14:91–96.
168. van de Loosdrecht AA, Gietema JA, van der Graaf WT. Seizures in a patient with disseminated testicular cancer due to cisplatin-induced hypomagnesaemia. *Acta Oncol.* 2000;39:239–240.
169. Classen J, Dieckmann KP. Malignant germ cell tumor of the contralateral testis after radiotherapy for testicular intraepithelial neoplasia. *J Urol.* 2001;166:630–631.
170. Crabb SJ, McKendrick JJ, Mead GM. Brain as sanctuary site of relapse in germ cell cancer patients previously treated with chemotherapy. *Clin Oncol (R Coll Radiol).* 2002;14:287–293.
171. Bart J, Groen HJ, van der Graaf WT, et al. An oncological view on the blood-testis barrier. *Lancet Oncol.* 2002;3:357–363.
172. Fossa SD, Dahl AA, Loge JH. Fatigue, anxiety, and depression in long-term survivors of testicular cancer. *J Clin Oncol.* 2003;21:1249–1254.
173. Trask PC, Paterson AG, Fardig J, et al. Course of distress and quality of life in testicular cancer patients before, during, and after chemotherapy: results of a pilot study. *Psychooncology.* 2003;12:814–820.
174. Siafaka V, Hyphantis TN, Alamanos I, et al. Personality factors associated with psychological distress in testicular cancer survivors. *J Pers Assess.* 2008;90:348–355.
175. Dahl AA, Haaland CF, Mykletun A, et al. Study of anxiety disorder and depression in long-term survivors of testicular cancer. *J Clin Oncol.* 2005;23:2389–2395.
176. Shinn EH, Basen-Engquist K, Thornton B, Spiess PE, Pisters L. Health behaviors and depressive symptoms in testicular cancer survivors. *Urology.* 2007;69:748–753.
177. Orre IJ, Fossa SD, Murison R, et al. Chronic cancer-related fatigue in long-term survivors of testicular cancer. *J Psychosom Res.* 2008;64:363–371.
178. Gudbergsson SB, Fossa SD, Ganz PA, Zebrack BJ, Dahl AA. The associations between living conditions, demography, and the "impact of cancer" scale in tumor-free cancer survivors: a NOCWO study. *Support Care Cancer.* 2007;15:1309–1318.
179. Berg Gudbergsson S, Fossa SD, Dahl AA. Is cancer survivorship associated with reduced work engagement? A NOCWO study. *J Cancer Surviv.* 2008;2:159–168.
180. Gudbergsson SB, Fossa SD, Dahl AA. A study of work changes due to cancer in tumor-free primary-treated cancer patients. A NOCWO study. *Support Care Cancer.* 2008;16:1163–1171.
181. Fleer J, Hoekstra HJ, Sleijfer DT, Tuinman MA, Hoekstra-Weebers JE. The role of meaning in the prediction of psychosocial well-being of testicular cancer survivors. *Qual Life Res.* 2006;15:705–717.
182. De Backer IC, Van Breda E, Vreugdenhil A, Nijziel MR, Kester AD, Schep G. High-intensity strength training improves quality of life in cancer survivors. *Acta Oncol.* 2007;46:1143–1151.
183. Caffo O, Amichetti M, Tomio L, et al. Quality of life after radiotherapy for early-stage testicular seminoma. *Radiother Oncol.* 2001;59:13–20.
184. Fossa SD, de Wit R, Roberts JT, et al. Quality of life in good prognosis patients with metastatic germ cell cancer: a prospective study of the European Organization for Research and Treatment of Cancer Genitourinary Group/Medical Research Council Testicular Cancer Study Group (30941/TE20). *J Clin Oncol.* 2003;21:1107–1118.
185. Gospodarowicz M. Testicular cancer patients: considerations in long-term follow-up. *Hematol Oncol Clin North Am.* 2008;22:245–255, vi.
186. Howard R, Gilbert E, Lynch CF, et al. Risk of leukemia among survivors of testicular cancer: a population-based study of 42,722 patients. *Ann Epidemiol.* 2008;18:416–421.
187. Richiardi L, Pettersson A, Akre O. Genetic and environmental risk factors for testicular cancer. *Int J Androl.* 2007;30:230–240; discussion 240–241.
188. Gietema JA, Meinardi MT, Messerschmidt J, et al. Circulating plasma platinum more than 10 years after cisplatin treatment for testicular cancer. *Lancet.* 2000;355:1075–1076.
189. Gerl A, Schierl R. Urinary excretion of platinum in chemotherapy-treated long-term survivors of testicular cancer. *Acta Oncol.* 2000; 39:519–522.
190. Chaudhary UB, Haldas JR. Long-term complications of chemotherapy for germ cell tumours. *Drugs.* 2003;63:1565–1577.
191. Oldenburg J, Kraggerud SM, Brydoy M, Cvancarova M, Lothe RA, Fossa SD. Association between long-term neuro-toxicities in testicular cancer survivors and polymorphisms in glutathione-s-transferase-P1 and -M1, a retrospective cross sectional study. *J Transl Med.* 2007;5:70.
192. Biro K, Noszek L, Prekopp P, et al. Characteristics and risk factors of cisplatin-induced ototoxicity in testicular cancer patients detected by distortion product otoacoustic emission. *Oncology.* 2006;70:177–184.
193. Servagi-Vernat S, Langlois-Jacques C, Bontemps P, Clero E, Bosset JF, Danzon A. Risk of second cancer after germinal cell testicular cancer: study from the data of Doubs cancer registry. *Bull Cancer.* 2007;94:721–726.
194. Wethal T, Kjekshus J, Roislien J, et al. Treatment-related differences in cardiovascular risk factors in long-term survivors of testicular cancer. *J Cancer Surviv.* 2007;1:8–16.
195. Spark RF. Testosterone, diabetes mellitus, and the metabolic syndrome. *Curr Urol Rep.* 2007;8:467–471.
196. Wiechno P, Demkow T, Kubiak K, Sadowska M, Kaminska J. The quality of life and hormonal disturbances in testicular cancer survivors in Cisplatin era. *Eur Urol.* 2007;52:1448–1454.
197. Thomas SR, Evans PJ, Holland PA, Biswas M. Invasive breast cancer after initiation of testosterone replacement therapy in a man—a warning to endocrinologists. *Endocr Pract.* 2008;14:201–203.
198. Krarup-Hansen A, Helweg-Larsen S, Schmalbruch H, Rorth M, Krarup C. Neuronal involvement in cisplatin neuropathy: prospective clinical and neurophysiological studies. *Brain.* 2007;130:1076–1088.
199. von Rohr L, Klaeser B, Joerger M, Kluckert T, Cerny T, Gillessen S. Increased pulmonary FDG uptake in bleomycin-associated pneumonitis. *Onkologie.* 2007;30:320–323.
200. Ehrlich Y, Baniel J. Late relapse of testis cancer. *Urol Clin North Am.* 2007;34:253–258; abstract x-xi.
201. Kuczyk MA, Bokemeyer C, Kollmannsberger C, et al. Late relapse after treatment for nonseminomatous testicular germ cell tumors according to a single center-based experience. *World J Urol.* 2004;22:55–59.
202. Bompas E, Flechon A, Biron P, et al. Management of advanced seminoma: retrospective study of 96 patients. *Bull Cancer.* 2002;89: 877–885.

203. Shahidi M, Norman AR, Dearnaley DP, et al. Late recurrence in 1263 men with testicular germ cell tumors. Multivariate analysis of risk factors and implications for management. *Cancer*. 2002;95:520–530.
204. Kohei N, Kinoshita H, Kamoto T, Terai A, Kakehi Y, Ogawa O. Late relapse of testicular cancer 21 years after first complete remission: a case report. [In Japanese] *Hinyokika Kiyo*. 2008;54:39–42.
205. Travis LB, Fossa SD, Schonfeld SJ, et al. Second cancers among 40,576 testicular cancer patients: focus on long-term survivors. *J Natl Cancer Inst*. 2005;97:1354–1365.
206. Skotheim RI, Lothe RA. The testicular germ cell tumour genome. *Apmis*. 2003;111:136–150; discussion 50–51.
207. Jones A, Fujiyama C, Turner K, et al. Angiogenesis and lymphangiogenesis in stage 1 germ cell tumours of the testis. *BJU Int*. 2000;86:80–86.
208. Jones RH, Vasey PA. New directions in testicular cancer; molecular determinants of oncogenesis and treatment success. *Eur J Cancer*. 2003;39:147–156.
209. Mayer F, Gillis AJ, Dinjens W, et al. Microsatellite instability of germ cell tumors is associated with resistance to systemic treatment. *Cancer Res*. 2002;62:2758–2760.
210. Boyle P. Testicular cancer: the challenge for cancer control. *Lancet Oncol*. 2004;5:56–61.
211. Whiteford A, Wordley J. Raising awareness and detection of testicular cancer in young men. *Nurs Times*. 2003;99:34–36.

CHAPTER 69

*Karen Oleszewski, RN, MS, AOCN®*

# Vulvar and Vaginal Cancer

- **Introduction**
- **Vulvar Cancer**
  - *Epidemiology*
  - *Etiology*
  - *Prevention and Screening*
  - *Pathophysiology*
    - Cellular characteristics
    - Progression of disease
  - *Clinical Manifestations*
  - *Assessment*
    - Patient and family history
    - Physical examination
    - Diagnostic studies
    - Prognostic indicators
  - *Classification and Staging*
  - *Therapeutic Approaches and Nursing Care: VIN*
  - *Therapeutic Approaches and Nursing Care: Invasive Disease*
    - Surgery
    - Radiation therapy
    - Chemotherapy
  - *Symptom Management and Supportive Care*
    - Advanced/recurrent disease
  - *Future Trends*
- **Vaginal Cancer**
  - *Epidemiology*
  - *Etiology*
  - *Prevention and Screening*
  - *Pathophysiology*
    - Cellular characteristics
    - Progression of disease
  - *Clinical Manifestations*
  - *Assessment*
    - Patient and family history
    - Physical examination
    - Diagnostic studies
    - Prognostic indicators
  - *Classification and Staging*
  - *Therapeutic Approaches and Nursing Care: VAIN*
  - *Therapeutic Approaches and Nursing Care: Invasive Disease*
    - Radiation therapy
    - Surgery
    - Chemotherapy
  - *Symptom Management and Supportive Care*
    - Advanced/recurrent disease
  - *Future Trends*
- **Conclusion**
- **References**

## INTRODUCTION

Approximately 5740 females in the United States were expected to be diagnosed with vaginal or vulvar cancer in 2009, and an estimated 1,670 deaths were expected to occur from these cancers in the same year.[1] Even though vulvar and vaginal cancers occur infrequently, nursing care for these women is very challenging. These cancers usually affect older, postmenopausal women. Treatment with surgery and radiation therapy (RT) will typically affect sexuality, and many women will face some degree of change in their body image. Nurses need to understand normal female genital anatomy because it is often affected or altered by treatment. Nurses play a vital role in the health care team by helping women to cope with changes in sexual functioning.

Vulvar and vaginal cancers are frequently preceded by a preinvasive intraepithelial neoplasia, and both can be curable if diagnosed in the early stages. Close follow-up care and education for women with preinvasive disease are crucial for early detection and to prevent progression to invasive disease.

## VULVAR CANCER

### EPIDEMIOLOGY

Vulvar carcinoma accounts for 3% to 5% of all gynecological cancers and 1% of all cancers in women and is identified as 1 of the 12 cancers that rose in incidence between 1992 and 1998.[2] The definition of vulvar cancer frequently includes both vulvar cancer and carcinoma in situ, also called vulvar intraepithelial neoplasia (VIN) III. Similar to cervical cancer, vulvar cancer can be preceded by a preinvasive intraepithelial neoplasia of the vulvar tissue. Vulvar intraepithelial neoplasia is the term used to denote epithelial abnormalities of the vulva. The increases in the incidence of invasive vulvar cancer and of in situ vulvar carcinoma have occurred at different rates over the past 30 years, with a dramatic increase in the incidence of in situ of 411%, but only a 20% increase in invasive cancer.[3] The risk of developing invasive and in situ vulvar carcinoma is distributed differently across different age groups. Invasive vulvar cancer risk increases as a woman ages, typically with presentation occurring in the seventh decade, when comorbidity is common, whereas the risk for developing in situ vulvar cancer increases until the age of 40 to 49 years and then decreases.[4–6] The small increase in incidence of invasive carcinoma of the vulva, even as the overall number of cases of preinvasive disease increases, may suggest that the etiological factors for VIN and invasive carcinoma are different, that diagnostic procedures have improved, or that treatment of VIN is effective in preventing invasive disease.[6,7]

### ETIOLOGY

The etiology of vulvar cancer has been only partially elucidated and may be multifactorial. Even the relationship of VIN to invasive vulvar disease remains unclear and controversial. Recent evidence has shown that vulvar cancer consists of separate diseases, the first is human papillomavirus (HPV)-related and the second is not.[8]

The first type is caused by the HPV, most commonly HPV type 16, and is associated with VIN.[9] HPV infection has been found in 70% to 80% of women with VIN, but concomitant occurrence of HPV infection decreases to 10% to 50% in women with invasive disease.[10] HPV-positive tumors have a higher incidence among cigarette smokers than nonsmokers and are more commonly found in younger women, women who had their first sexual intercourse at a young age, and those who have had multiple sexual partners. HPV lesions tend to be multifocal in nature.

The second type of vulvar cancer more often affects older women who generally have a history of vulvar inflammation or lichen sclerosis. Their tumors are usually unifocal, well-differentiated, and keratinizing[4,11] (Table 69-1).

Since the 2 types of invasive vulvar cancer differ in epidemiology, clinical presentation, histopathology, and molecular profile, the presence of 2 different types of precursor legions has been inferred. New VIN terminology has been suggested by the International Society for the Study of Vulvovaginal Disease (ISSVD), consisting of VIN usual type (undifferentiated) and VIN differentiated type.[10,12]

Research has shown that the *p53* tumor suppressor gene may play a role in the etiology of squamous cell vulvar carcinoma. This gene has shown several key regulatory

**TABLE 69-1**

**Two Subsets of Women With Squamous Cell Carcinoma of the Vulva**

| | Type I | Type II |
|---|---|---|
| Age | 35–55 years | 55–85 years |
| Associated with HPV infection | Yes | No |
| Pre-existing disease | VIN | Lichen sclerosis, vulvar inflammation |
| Multifocal lesions | Yes | No |
| Histopathology of tumor | Poorly differentiated, nonkeratinizing | Well differentiated, keratinizing |

*Abbreviations*: HPV, human papillomavirus; VIN, vulvar intraepithelial neoplasia.

functions, which include cell growth, cell proliferation, and apoptosis. Studies have shown that *p53* mutations are more commonly seen in HPV-negative vulvar carcinomas that affect older women.[13,14] Other research has shown p16 protein, a cyclin-dependent kinase (cdk) inhibitor, is expressed in vulvar carcinomas and their precursors.[15]

In addition to HPV infection, risk factors for vulvar cancer include a history of genital warts, multiple sexual partners, preinvasive cervical cancer, and smoking. A history of chronic vulvar disease and previous malignancies of the lower genital tract is also seen in women with vulvar cancer. Preliminary reports suggest that chronic immunosuppression may play an important role in development of this cancer. Individuals who have undergone organ transplants or individuals who are infected with the human immunodeficiency virus (HIV) may have an increased risk of vulvar cancer.[5] Angiogenesis, the development of new blood vessels from existing vasculature, may play a role in the transition from VIN to invasive cancer. In a small study, vascular endothelial growth factor (VEGF) was not found in normal tissue, whereas it was present in 6% of the VIN specimens and in 92% of the vulvar cancer specimens. Ongoing research into angiogenesis will be important to determine how it contributes to the development of vulvar cancer and ultimately the impact of potential antiangiogenic therapies on the treatment of the premalignant vulvar disease.[16,17,18] Table 69-2 summarizes the risk factors and prevention measures for this cancer.

## PREVENTION AND SCREENING

Vulvar cancer is a rare disease. Currently there is no systematic screening available. Detection relies on the presence of vulvar symptoms and the knowledge of the health care provider inspecting the vulva.[12] Women should be encouraged to perform a vulvar self-examination on a monthly basis.[3] Screening for vulvar cancer should be performed when a woman has a Papanicolaou (Pap) smear done. Careful examination of the vulva is critical. Screening should focus on women who smoke, women with HPV infection, and women who have other preinvasive disease of the cervix, vagina, or perianal area. Nurses are excellent resources to help educate women (especially older women) that a regular pelvic examination following American Cancer Society (ACS) guidelines is crucial. They can also teach women about performing vulvar self-examination, avoiding exposure to HPV, and the negative effects of smoking.

Faced with a disease whose incidence is rising and whose median age is decreasing, women who are diagnosed with VIN or vulvar cancer at an early stage can benefit. Optimal management for a patient presenting with a suspicious lesion is a biopsy in order to provide an accurate and definitive diagnosis, thereby avoiding any delays in initiating appropriate therapy.[9,19] With early detection, treatment morbidity is often decreased because physicians may be able to perform less radical surgery to eradicate the disease.[20] Accurate diagnosis can offer improved response rates with appropriate interventions. In addition, early detection remains crucial because the disease can have a significant impact on a woman's sexuality, particularly in its advanced stages.[13,21]

**TABLE 69-2**

**Vulvar Cancer: Risk Factors and Preventive Measures**

| Risk Factors | Preventive Measures |
|---|---|
| Human papillomavirus | Pap smear per ACS guidelines |
| Herpes simplex virus type 2 | Routine vulvar self-examination |
| History of smoking | Stop smoking |
| Multiple sexual partners | Limit number of sexual partners |
| Immunosuppression | Use barrier contraception |
| Chronic vulvar disease | |
| Previous malignancies of the lower genital tract | |
| Age > 60 years | |

*Abbreviation*: ACS, American Cancer Society.

## PATHOPHYSIOLOGY

### Cellular characteristics

The vulva includes the mons pubis, the labia majora and minora, the clitoris, the vestibule of the vagina, and the Bartholin glands. The mons pubis is the pad of fat anterior to the pubis symphysis and is covered by hair-bearing skin. The labia majora extends posterior from the mons into the vaginal opening. The labia minora consists of small folds of skin that lie between the labia majora and divides anteriorly to envelop the clitoris. The vestibule is the area into which the vagina opens. The bulbs of the vestibule are erectile tissue on each side of the vaginal opening. The vulva is surrounded by a network of lymphatics, and keratinized squamous epithelium covers the vulva.[22]

Histologically, squamous cell carcinoma accounts for more than 90% of all primary vulvar neoplasms. The remaining 10% of vulvar neoplasms include malignant melanoma, sarcoma, basal cell, adenocarcinoma, and Bartholin gland. On physical exam, the lesion is usually raised and may be fleshy, ulcerated, leukoplakic, or warty in appearance. Discoloration of the vulva with red or white pigmentation can be seen.[23]

### Progression of disease

Vulvar intraepithelial neoplasia was introduced in 1986 to medical terminology, deriving its nomenclature from the cervical intraepithelial neoplasia (CIN) 3-grade system. The diagnosis of VIN was made histologically on the basis of the degree of dysplasia and the depth of changes to the epithelium, ranging from VIN I to VIN III. Due to its simplicity and consistency with CIN, it was widely accepted by all major organizations that deal with vulvar disease. Since its inception, the concept of a continuum in the progression of VIN I to invasive cancer has not been supported. In 2004, the ISSVD revised its classification of VIN by eliminating VIN I and combining VIN II and III into the same category, defined simply as VIN usual type. VIN usual type has 2 histological subtypes, basaloid or warty, and the usual type is more frequently diagnosed than the differentiated type. It presents as a distinct lesion with sharp margins. Lesions are usually elevated and have a rough surface, similar to a wart. Since usual-type VIN is often multifocal, the vulva perineum and perianal areas should be carefully inspected for other lesions. These usual lesions are HPV related and less prone to develop into invasive cancer. The second category of VIN is the differentiated type. These lesions are less common and typically HPV negative, have an irregular shape with roughened surface, and may show areas of erosion. These lesions show the highest potential to progress to invasive cancer.[10,12] Table 69-3 summarizes the 2 classifications systems used for VIN.

Although primary disease can develop anywhere on the vulva, approximately 60% to 70% of tumors arise on the labia majora and labia minora. Other primary sites include the clitoris (15%) and perineum (10%). Approximately 10% of cases are too extensive to determine the primary site, and 5% of cases will be multifocal. Vulvar cancer usually remains a localized disease with well-defined margins.[22]

The most common routes of metastatic spread are through direct extension, lymphatic embolization, or less commonly by hematogenous spread. Direct extension to adjacent structures may be seen in advanced stages, including the vagina, urethra, and anus. At diagnosis, the overall incidence of positive lymph nodes is approximately 30%. Lymphatic spread of vulvar cancer usually follows a predictable pattern. From the superficial inguinal lymph nodes, the tumor usually spreads to the deep inguinal/femoral nodes and then to the pelvic lymph nodes[13,24] (Figure 69-1). Tumors involving the midline can metastasize to the groin nodes on both sides. Early-stage tumors rarely metastasize to the contralateral lymph nodes.[7,25] Hematogenous spread occurs late in advanced stages of vulvar cancer and is rare in the absence of lymph node metastases. Distant metastases are uncommon at initial presentation. More often, distant metastases are seen in recurrent vulvar cancer, with the most common site being the lung.[9,24]

**TABLE 69-3**

**Comparison of ISSVD VIN Terminology**

| 1986 Classification | 2004 Classification |
|---|---|
| VIN I | (Eliminated) |
| VIN 2<br>VIN 3 | VIN–usual type[a] (undifferentiated)<br>• warty<br>• basaloid<br>• mixed (warty/basaloid) |
| VIN–differentiated | VIN–differentiated |

[a]In 1986 VIN 2 and VIN 3 were separate classifications, In 2004, VIN 2 and VIN 3 were combined to be VIN-usual type with the three subtypes.

*Abbreviations*: ISSVD, International Society for the Study of Vulvovaginal Disease; VIN, vulvar intraepithelial neoplasia.

## CLINICAL MANIFESTATIONS

The symptoms of VIN and invasive vulvar carcinoma are variable and insidious. The majority of women with VIN are asymptomatic. If systems exist, they may complain of vulvar pruritus, irritation, or presence of a lesion. Less common presenting symptoms include vulvar bleeding, discharge, or dysuria. As many as 20% of women with vulvar cancer are asymptomatic, with lesions being detected in more than 50% of patients only during routine pelvic examination. The most common symptoms are a vulvar lump or mass, often with a long history of pruritus.[24,27] The incidence of signs and symptoms of vulvar cancer is shown in Table 69-4.

Delay in diagnosing a woman with vulvar cancer may occur because women themselves have little to no genital education. A woman may be too embarrassed to seek medical assistance due to the intimate area of the body, or cultural taboos may prevent speaking about female genitalia. As a result, the woman may have symptoms for 2 to 16 months before seeking medical attention.[26] A delay in definitive treatment may occur because symptomatic topical treatment for vulvar lesions can continue for 12 months or longer before the lesion is biopsied for definitive diagnosis, or because the health care provider fails adequately to assess a woman reporting symptoms of vulvar irritation.[12,28]

## ASSESSMENT

Vulvar intraepithelial neoplasia and vulvar cancer is an orphan disease. A variety of health care providers in different specialties such as dermatologists, gynecologists, general practitioners, and colposcopists are involved in the diagnosis and treatment of vulvar disease. With varying levels of education and clinical experience, a lack of uniform approach may contribute to a delay in

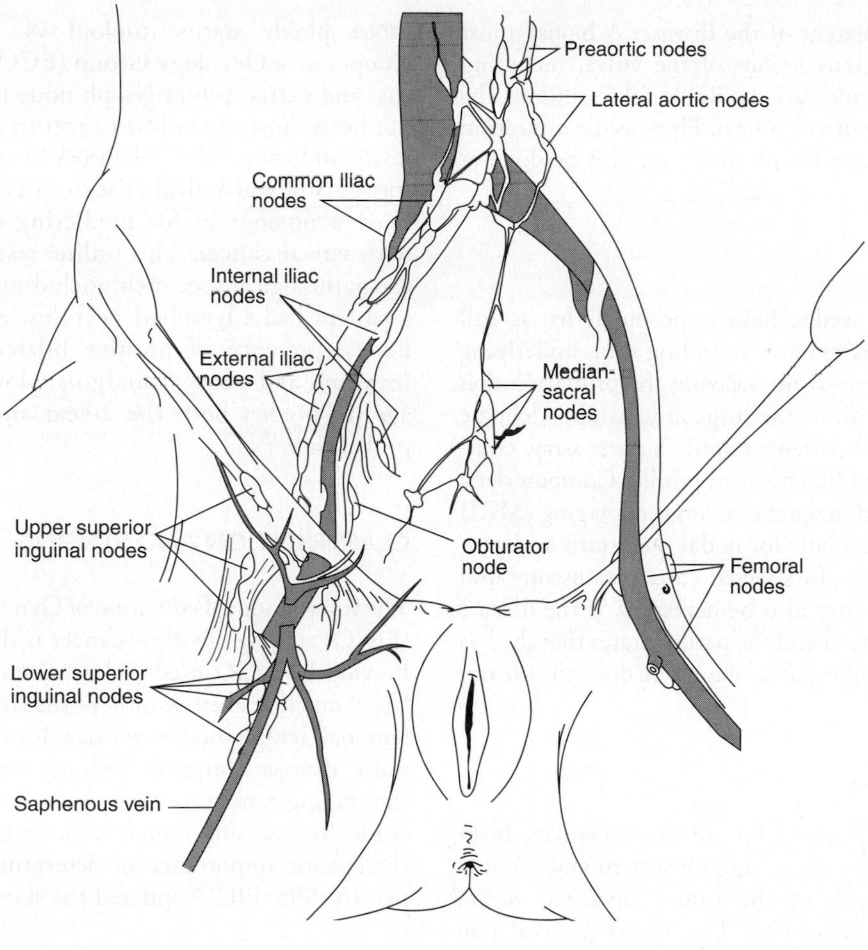


**FIGURE 69-1**

Inguinofemoral lymph nodes.

*Source*: Reprinted with permission from Hacker NF. Surgery for malignant tumors of the vulva. In: Gershenson DM, DeCherney AH, Curry SL, Brubaker L, eds. *Operative Gynecology.* 2nd ed. Philadelphia, PA: Saunders; 2001:237–261.[24]

**TABLE 69-4**

**Signs and Symptoms of Vulvar Cancer**

| Signs and Symptoms | % |
|---|---|
| Pruritus | 45 |
| Mass | 45 |
| Pain | 23 |
| Bleeding | 14 |
| Ulceration | 14 |
| Dysuria | 10 |
| Discharge | 8 |

diagnosis. In more than 50% of patients, there is a delay, either by the patient or the doctor, of more than 1 year before the diagnosis is made. Fortunately, vulvar cancer is indolent, progresses slowly, and metastasizes late in its course.[27,28]

## Patient and family history

Women with VIN and invasive cancer should have a complete history that includes the duration and severity of signs and symptoms. They may have a history of a previous malignancy in the lower genital tract, so detailed questioning about gynecological history is warranted. Because cigarette smoking and multiple sexual partners are risk factors, a smoking and sexual history should be taken. A family history related to cancer is important; however, having a history of vulvar cancer in the family is not a potential risk factor.

## Physical examination

Careful inspection of the vulva during routine gynecological examination is imperative because this practice remains the most productive diagnostic measure. Because the neoplasia is often multifocal, the entire vulva, perineum, and perianal area should be evaluated. Lymph nodes in the groin should be palpated. A Pap smear should be done to rule out synchronous cervical cancer. Colposcopic examination may help define the extent of the disease. A biopsy must be done of all suspicious lesions of the vulva, including pigmented areas and ulcerations. Table 69-5 outlines the indications for biopsy of vulva nevi. Fine-needle aspiration biopsy of any suspicious lymph node can also be done at this time.[23,30]

### Diagnostic studies

Diagnosis requires a wedge biopsy specimen that is full thickness and includes some surrounding skin, underlying dermis, and connective tissue. Leaving the primary lesion in situ is preferred to allow the surgeon to attain adequate surgical margins.[24] All patients require a chest x-ray, complete blood count, and biochemical profile. Computerized tomography (CT) and magnetic resonance imaging (MRI) are used to evaluate patients for nodal metastasis and possible distant metastasis. In selected cases, cystoscopy and proctosigmoidoscopy may also be necessary. If the disease is thought to be advanced and the patient states that she has pelvic pain, skeletal radiographs should be done to rule out bone metastasis.[22]

### Prognostic indicators

The major prognostic factors for vulvar cancer have been incorporated into the current staging system and include tumor diameter, depth of the tumor invasion, nodal spread, and distant metastasis.[9] The 5-year survival rate for vulvar cancer is correlated with stage of disease and nodal involvement. Lymph node status is the single best indicator of survival. Prognostic indicators for lymph nodes include whether the nodal spread is bilateral or unilateral, the number of positive nodes, the volume of tumor in the metastasis, and the extent or level of spread in the lymphatic system. In women with negative nodes, the 5-year survival rate is as high as 90%, but falls to 50% in patients with positive nodes. In addition to nodal status, tumors that show evidence of HPV infection have a better prognosis. HPV-negative tumors are correlated with a higher risk of recurrence and death rate from vulvar cancer than HPV-positive tumors.[31] Other independent prognostic variables for overall survival include DNA ploidy status (diploid vs. aneuploid), Eastern Cooperative Oncology Group (ECOG) performance status, and extracapsular lymph node involvement. Age has not been shown in vulvar cancer to be a significant prognostic indicator.[24,26,27] The ISSVD and European College for the Study of Vulval Disease (ECSVD) recently developed a nomogram for predicting outcome in patients with vulvar cancer. This online resource uses data from the pathological specimen, including tumor size, whether a patient had a lymphadenectomy, number of metastatic nodes, presence of positive bilateral nodes, depth of invasion, and surgical margins, along with the patient's age, to predict both the 2-year and 5-year relapse-free probability.[32]

**TABLE 69-5**

**Indications for Biopsy of Vulva Nevi**

Changes in:
- Color: especially brown to black
- Elevation of a lesion: raised, thickened, or nodular
- Surface area of lesion
- Surface: smooth to scaly or ulcerated
- Sensation: itchy or tingling

## CLASSIFICATION AND STAGING

The International Federation of Gynecology and Obstetrics (FIGO) staging of vulvar cancer is shown in Table 69-6.[33] Previously, FIGO used a clinical staging system that was based on clinical evaluation of the tumor size and palpable regional lymph nodes, with a limited search for metastatic disease. Surgical findings were incorporated into the staging system in 1988 due to the limited accuracy of clinically assessing lymph nodes and the prognostic and therapeutic importance of determining lymph node status. In 1995, FIGO updated the staging system to include

**TABLE 69-6**

**FIGO Staging of Vulvar Cancer**

| Stage | Clinical Findings |
|---|---|
| 0 | Carcinoma in situ |
| I | Tumor confined to the vulva, < 2 cm largest dimension<br>No nodal metastasis |
| II | Tumor confined to the vulva, > 2 cm largest dimension<br>No nodal metastasis |
| III | Tumor of any size with<br>• Adjacent spread to urethra, vagina, or anus, or<br>• Unilateral regional lymph node metastasis |
| IVA | Tumor invades upper urethra, bladder mucosa, rectal mucosa, pelvic bone, or bilateral regional lymph node metastasis |
| IVB | Any distant metastasis, including pelvic lymph nodes |

*Abbreviation*: FIGO, International Federation of Gynecology and Obstetrics.

a subclassification of stage I. In stage I and stage II disease, the tumor is confined to the vulva and/or perineum and all lymph nodes are negative. In stage III disease, the tumor has spread to adjacent areas of the urethra and/or the vagina, perineum, and anus. Unilateral regional lymph node metastasis is present. Stage IV disease consists of a tumor that has invaded the upper urethra, bladder mucosa, rectal mucosa, or pelvic bone, bilateral regional lymph node metastasis, or presence of distant metastasis, including pelvic lymph nodes.[7,9,27]

## THERAPEUTIC APPROACHES AND NURSING CARE: VIN

The therapeutic approach to VIN is still a challenge, and some controversy exists about the appropriate treatment for patients with VIN. Although a large number of treatment options are available for VIN, none of the treatments provides an ideal solution. The ideal treatment for VIN would foremost prevent progression of the lesion to cancer and relieve symptoms, as well as prevent recurrences, exclude microscopic disease, and prevent disfiguring surgery. At present, no treatment exists that fulfills all of these criteria. Individualized surgery remains the treatment modality of choice.[18] In the past, a total vulvectomy was done for the management of VIN. Due to the morbidity, decreasing median age of women with VIN, and the disfiguring "castration-like" self-image associated with this radical surgery, a more conservative surgical approach is usually undertaken. This approach helps maintain the sexual function of the vulva and may help women avoid the adverse physical and psychological effects of more extensive surgery. The type of surgery chosen depends upon factors related to the patient, such as symptoms, comorbid diseases, performance status, age, and ability to follow up, as well as factors related to the lesion, such as VIN type, size, location, and involvement of hair-bearing areas. The different techniques used include excision, electrosurgery, and laser therapy. A wide local excision is best for unifocal or lateral lesions with at least a 5 mm disease-free margin. This allows pathological assessment to rule out invasive disease and achieves a 90% cure rate.[3,12,19,34,35]

For multicentric disease, a skinning vulvectomy (Figure 69-2)[24] is performed in which the vulvar skin is excised while conserving the fat, muscle, and glands below the skin. A split-thickness skin graft reconstruction from the thigh or buttock is performed. This procedure gives an optimal cosmetic and functional result. A skinning vulvectomy with skin graft may not be an option for elderly or debilitated women, due to the requirement of prolonged bed rest (6–7 days) to allow healing of the skin graft. The potential for morbidity in these women is increased. As an alternative a simple vulvectomy can be performed. Ultimately, the patient's wishes must be taken into account regardless of the age of the patient.[35,36]

Laser therapy, either by laser excision or laser vaporization, is also considered to be a treatment of choice for many patients, especially those with multifocal disease. Laser excision requires more experience and expertise than vaporization and provides a surgical specimen. Cure rates are comparable to those of surgical excision. In contrast, laser vaporization destroys the tissue, not allowing histological evaluation, and cure rates may be slightly inferior to surgical excision, probably due to the undertreatment of cryptic invasive disease.[12,34–36] The advantages of laser treatments are outpatient management, sparing effect on surrounding tissue, and minimal scarring with good cosmetic and functional results. However, the procedures can result in painful ulcers and require several sequenced treatments. Healing time can be prolonged.[37,38]

Photodynamic therapy (PDT), a relatively new technique, uses a systemic or topical application of photosensitizing compound that accumulates preferentially in neoplastic tissue. The affected area is then exposed to nonthermal

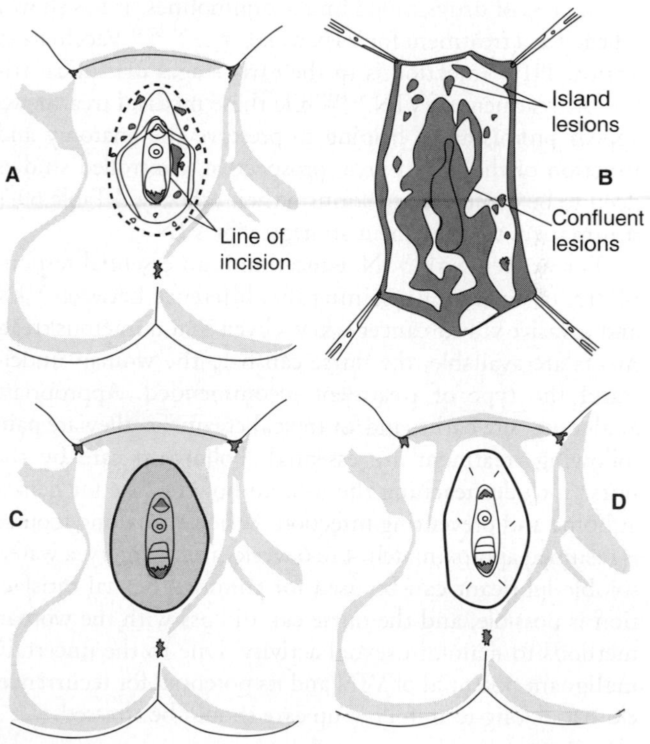


**FIGURE 69-2**

Skinning vulvectomy and skin graft. **A**, Excise all areas of involvement en bloc. **B**, Lesions may be isolated or confluent. **C**, Preserve all subcutaneous tissue as the graft bed. **D**, Suture the skin graft to the graft bed. Reprinted with permission from Stehman FB. Invasive cancer of the vulva. In: DiSaia PJ, Creasman WT, eds. *Clinical Gynecologic Oncology*. 7th ed. St. Louis, MO: Mosby; 2007:235–264.[27]

light, and oxygen-induced cell death results. Photodynamic therapy is appropriate for unifocal nonpigmented lesions. It has the advantages of not causing ulceration or scarring and of a short healing time, with only a few side effects, including erythema and pain.[12,19,34,39] Cavitational ultrasonic surgical aspiration (CUSA) is another promising treatment for VIN. This treatment uses ultrasound to cause cavitations of the superficial vulvar skin, which is then aspirated through a tube and collected as a specimen. The procedure is rapid and healing is faster than with laser surgery, with excellent cosmesis.[36,40] While both PDT and CUSA have many advantages, they may not allow for assessment of adequate margins.

Medical treatment options for VIN vary and remain suboptimal, with response rates around 40%. Topical treatments are an attractive strategy, as they can be applied by the patient and efficacy easily monitored. Systemic chemotherapy with 5-fluorouracil (5-FU) and bleomycin has been investigated, with inconsistent response rates and sometimes severe side effects. Immunotherapy, such as dinitrochlorobenzene (DNCB) and interferons, have been used to promote a localized immune response. The most promising immune response modifier is imiquimod, a compound from a new class of drugs called imidazoquinolines. It has shown efficacy as a treatment for VIN usual type.[12,34,41] Vaccination against HPV infection is in the early stages of clinical trials for treatment of VIN.[42] While these medical treatments appear promising in helping to preserve the anatomy and function of the vulvar area, prospective, controlled studies need to be completed to confirm their efficacy.[23] Table 69-7 summarizes the treatment strategies for VIN.

For women with VIN, education is an essential responsibility of nursing. Explaining the difference between VIN and invasive vulvar cancer is key. Given that numerous treatments are available, the nurse can help the woman understand the type of treatment recommended. Appropriate analgesics, sitz baths, and/or topical creams to alleviate pain following treatment are essential. Follow-up care by the nurse includes teaching the woman how to care for herself at home and preventing infection. When sexual intercourse is resumed approximately 4 to 6 weeks after surgery, a water-soluble lubricant can be used for comfort. Sexual satisfaction is possible, and the nurse can discuss with the woman methods to maintain sexual activity. Due to the uncertain malignant potential of VIN and its potential for recurrence, close and long-term follow-up care should be stressed.

**TABLE 69-7**

**Treatment Strategies For VIN**

| Strategy | Treatment |
|---|---|
| Surgical | Local excision |
| | Laser excision |
| | CUSA |
| | Superficial vulvectomy |
| Medical | |
| Destructive | Laser ablation |
| | PDT |
| Chemotherapy | 5-FU |
| | Bleomycin |
| Immunotherapy | DNCB |
| | Interferons |
| | Imiquimod |
| Vaccination | Prophylactic |
| | Therapeutic |
| Other | Retinoids |
| | Cidofovir |
| | Indole-3-carbinol |

*Abbreviations*: CUSA, cavitational ultrasonic surgical aspiration; DNCB, dinitrochlorobenzene; PDT, photodynamic therapy; VIN, vulvar intraepithelial neoplasia.

## THERAPEUTIC APPROACHES AND NURSING CARE: INVASIVE DISEASE

### Surgery

Modern management of vulva cancer requires an experienced, multidisciplinary team approach. The standard treatment for women with operable cancer of the vulva has been en bloc radical vulvectomy (labia majora, labia minor, clitoris, and perineal body) and bilateral dissection of the groin and pelvic nodes. With this therapy, 5-year survival rates for stage I and stage II disease are approximately 90%.[27] The rationale behind the radical "butterfly" surgery was to remove the lesion, the inguinofemoral lymph nodes, and the lymphatics in between.[28] Over the past 20 years, several factors have led to modification of this standard treatment: the occurrence of disease in younger women with smaller tumors, the concern for postoperative morbidity and long-term hospitalization, and increasing awareness of psychosexual concerns following radical vulvectomy.[24] Surgery has evolved to an individualized and conservative approach for each patient.[9] Today, many surgeons have abandoned the en bloc approach and perform the nodal dissections through separate groin incisions (Figure 69-3). Studies have attested to the reduced morbidity associated with separate groin incisions without increasing recurrence rates.[28,44] In the absence of clinical suspicion of groin node involvement, on the contralateral side, unilateral lymphadenectomy may be sufficient in patients with a small, lateralized tumor. The emphasis is on performing the most conservative operation consistent with cure of

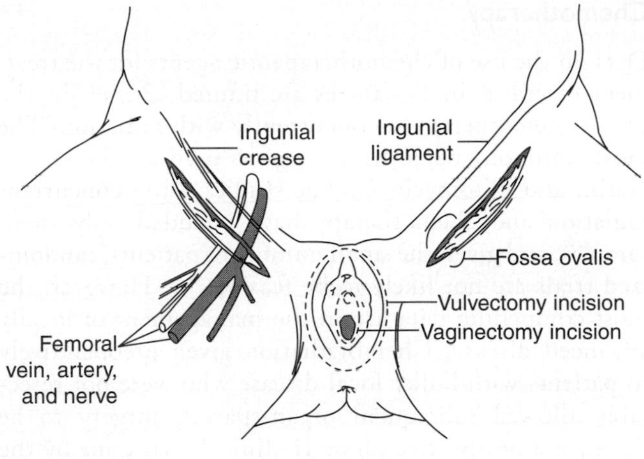


**FIGURE 69-3**

Vulvectomy and bilateral groin dissection through 3 separate incisions.

*Source*: Reprinted with permission from Hacker NF. Surgery for malignant tumors of the vulva. In: Gershershon DM, DeCherney AH, Curry SL, Brobaker L, eds. *Operative Gynecology.* 2nd ed. Philadelphia, PA: Saunders; 2001:237–261.[24]

the disease. The obvious advantages to a more conservative individualized approach is retention of the uninvolved vulva, less operative morbidity, and fewer late complications.[9]

Most stage I carcinomas of the vulva can be treated with wide local excision alone, assuring a 1 to 2 cm margin of normal tissue, because the risk of nodal spread is small. For larger and more invasive tumors, ipsilateral inguinofemoral lymphadenectomy or postoperative radiation is recommended. For patients with midline lesions, bilateral node dissections using separate groin incisions are recommended.[9] To further reduce the postoperative morbidity associated with groin dissections, the sentinel lymph node (SLN) procedure is being studied. In this procedure, the SLN is defined as the first node that would receive lymphatic drainage from a lesion site. An SLN without tumor implies absence of lymph node metastasis. The 2 techniques commonly used to identify the SLN are peritumor injection of isosulfan blue dye and injection of a radioactive tracer with lymphoscintigraphy. Preoperative injection of the tracer allows identification of the number and location of SLNs. Blue dye injection allows intraoperative mapping of the lymphatics. Once the SLNs are identified and removed, the pathologist can determine whether there is evidence of metastatic disease. If the SLN is negative, removal of additional lymph nodes is unnecessary,[28,45,46] reducing postoperative morbidity. A multicenter observational study on SLN procedure in 403 patients reported that women with a negative SLN had a low groin recurrence rate, excellent survival, and minimal treatment-related morbidity. The Gynecologic Oncology Group (GOG) is currently conducting a similar study of SLN procedure and initial results are expected in the spring of 2009. Clinical experience stresses the importance of a highly skilled multidisciplinary team approach to SLN.[47]

Stage II vulvar cancer may require more extensive surgery, which usually involves a radical vulvectomy to obtain adequate tumor-free margins. A more conservative resection can be done if surgical margins of at least 1 cm are obtained. The local recurrence rate for women with T2 tumors with radical local excision is identical to that for women with T1 tumors.[26]

In stage III disease, the tumor has spread to the urethra, vagina, anus, or lymph nodes in the inguinal area. Radical vulvectomy and bilateral inguinofemoral lymphadenectomy is recommended, along with a partial resection of a portion of the distal urethra or vagina if these organs are involved. Combined-modality treatment consisting of radiotherapy or chemoradiation with surgery is increasingly being used and studied as a means to eradicate disease with function-sparing surgery.[9,48,49]

Women with stage IV disease may require pelvic exenteration in addition to a radical vulvectomy if the bladder or rectum is involved. A total pelvic exenteration removes the vagina, uterus, ovaries, fallopian tubes, bladder, and rectum. Patients will have a urinary conduit and colostomy. A neovagina is usually constructed. While the 5-year survival rate for this surgery is approximately 50%, many complications may follow, including high psychological morbidity. Women should be carefully selected for this surgery. This radical surgery is often inappropriate for elderly women. For women with locally advanced disease, a combined approach of chemotherapy and radiation to shrink the tumor, followed by surgery, has improved survival and reduced morbidity. Treatment of patients with stage IVB disease, where the tumor is fixed to the bone or distant metastasis has occurred, should be considered palliative and mainly consists of radiotherapy or chemoradiation.[9,26,23,50]

The major immediate complication after radical surgery is groin wound infection and breakdown. With the use of the separate incision approach for nodal resection, the incidence of wound breakdown decreased to about 44%; with an en bloc operation, it was reported to be as high as 85%. Major wound breakdown occurs in about 14% of patients. With proper debridement and wound care, the groin area can granulate and reepithelialize within a few weeks. Wet-to-dry dressings are usually recommended. Whirlpool therapy is also effective for areas of extensive breakdown.[22,23] Other early postoperative complications include urinary tract infection, deep-vein thrombosis, seromas in the femoral triangle, pulmonary embolism, myocardial infarction, and hemorrhage.

The major late complication of radical surgery is chronic leg edema, which has been reported to occur in as many as

69% of women; the incidence in women who have a modified radical operation decreases to 28% to 39%. The use of elastic stockings is recommended for 12 months after surgery to facilitate development of collateral pathways for lymph drainage. Low-dose prophylactic, antibiotic therapy has also been shown to decrease lymphedema. Recurrent cellulitis of the leg occurs in about 10% of women and usually responds to antibiotics. Urinary stress incontinence and genital prolapse occurs in about 10% of patients and may require corrective surgery. Introital stenosis can lead to dyspareunia and may require a vertical relaxing incision.[23,24,26,44,51]

### Radiation therapy

The role of RT in the management of carcinoma of the vulva is increasing, and the indications for its use continue to evolve. To reduce the need for extensive radical surgery, this treatment is being used more often in combination with surgery. At present, radiation is indicated preoperatively in patients with advanced disease who would require pelvic exenteration. It is also clearly indicated postoperatively to treat pelvic lymph nodes and groins in women with 2 micrometastases or 1 macrometastasis or extracapsular spread.[50] An evolving role for radiation is postoperatively for women who have undergone a resection of the primary lesion and are considered at high risk for recurrence due to involved or close surgical margins. Although no prospective trials have been completed, reduced local recurrence rates have been reported when women receive postoperative irradiation.[9] Another possible role for RT is a primary therapy for patients with small primary tumors, particularly clitoral or preclitoral lesions where resections would have significant psychological consequences.[24] While the use of RT has decreased local recurrence rates, a GOG randomized phase III trial showed that groin irradiation cannot replace groin node dissection.[51]

Patients who receive external radiation to the vulva can develop severe erythema, moist desquamation, and swelling. Measures for managing these reactions include application of topical ointments, frequent sitz baths, and exposure to air.[50] Maintaining skin integrity and management of pain and discomfort are the aims of nursing care.

Radiation cystitis may also occur with radiation treatment of the pelvis. In such cases, appropriate antibiotic therapy and antispasmodics are indicated to provide relief of symptoms. The woman should also be encouraged to increase her fluid intake.[52]

Severe late radiation effects, such as vulvar fibrosis, telangiectasis, atrophy, or even necrosis, may occur. To prevent severe radiation effects, the total dose for postoperative RT is 4500 to 5000 cGy if there is no macroscopic residual disease. Higher doses of radiation (6000 to 7000 cGy) can be given to known areas of gross residual tumor. When chemotherapy is used in combination with RT, the maximum dose is usually 6500 cGy.[50]

### Chemotherapy

Data on the use of chemotherapeutic agents for the treatment of vulvar malignancies are limited. Primarily, the use of chemotherapy is concurrently with radiation. The most common chemotherapy agents used are 5-FU, cisplatin, and mitomycin C. The studies using concurrent radiation and chemotherapy have included only small samples, and given the small number of patients, randomized trials are not likely to be feasible.[53,54] However, the most compelling data are in the management of locally advanced disease. Chemoradiation given preoperatively to patients with bulky local disease who were not resectable allowed subsequent organ-sparing surgery to be done. In a prospective phase II clinical trial done by the GOG, patients were given 2 cycles of cisplatin and 5-FU concurrent with radiation. Only 2 of the 71 patients had unresectable disease after the chemoradiation and only 3 patients required a urinary conduit or colostomy.[55] Chemotherapy with RT is usually well tolerated by most women. Chemotherapy alone has been used primarily as salvage therapy in locally advanced or recurrent vulvar cancer. Responses are approximately 56%, with a 1-year survival rate of 32%.[56]

## SYMPTOM MANAGEMENT AND SUPPORTIVE CARE

### Advanced/recurrent disease

About 80% of recurrences of vulvar cancer will develop within the first 2 years after initial treatment, a fact that demands initial close follow-up. Patients with fewer than 3 positive nodes generally have a low incidence of recurrence, whereas high recurrence rates are correlated with more than 3 positive nodes.[36,57] More than half of the recurrences are local and occur in close proximity to the original lesion. In many instances, local recurrences can be successfully treated using wide local excision with adequate tumor-free margins. For treatment of advanced recurrent disease, pelvic exenteration may be an option for selected women. For recurrent vulvar cancer, the 5-year survival rate is 38% to 50%. Distant recurrence is difficult to treat and is associated with a poor prognosis. A combination of radiation and chemotherapy may be used as a palliative treatment measure in metastatic disease.[7] The most active agents are cisplatin, methotrexate, cyclophosphamide, bleomycin, and mitomycin C. Response rates are low, and survival rates at 5 years are only 8%.[7,23,36]

For the woman with advanced recurrent vulvar cancer, the physical symptoms can be distressing. The tumor can become very large, disfiguring, foul-smelling, and painful. With a comprehensive assessment of the pain, an appropriate and effective pain management regimen can be developed. If the tumor becomes ulcerated, care should be taken to prevent infection. Meticulous skin care is important. Leg edema may become a problem for the woman with positive, enlarged lymph nodes. Elastic stockings are usually recommended. Massage and exercise of the legs may also help relieve discomfort. Skin care of the legs is essential to prevent infection and cellulitis. Moisturizing the skin can help.

Along with the physical symptoms, the patient and her family may be at risk for ineffective coping. The nurse and health care team can help the patient and family manage the many debilitating changes of advanced disease. Nurses in the hospital can make appropriate referrals to home care or hospice care. Continual education and reassurance can facilitate effective coping mechanisms to allow the patient to live as fully as possible.

Among women who are cured of their disease by vulvectomy, sexual dysfunction is significant. Women report disturbances in body image leading to hypoactive sexual disorder and aversion disorder. Depression was a common underlying problem in these women. Nurses can help by promoting open discussions about sexual concerns and function after vulvar surgery, since discussion of these issues is often not initiated by the patient. Patients may need education and reassurance that sexual activity is safe and will not lead to recurrence of the cancer or spread the cancer to their partner. Unfortunately, no established tools have been developed to identify sexual dysfunction following vulvectomy. A pilot study of 41 women who underwent vulvectomy identified as risk factors advanced age, depression, and worsening GOG performance status. This finding may help nurses identify women at risk who would benefit from more intensive preoperative and postoperative sexual counseling. Individualized sexual and reproductive counseling may be needed. Maintaining a list of qualified professional counselors helps facilitate a referral for women with significant problems.[58] Nurses, by providing expert knowledge, are in a vital position to address these sensitive issues.

## FUTURE TRENDS

For vulvar cancer prevention, an HPV vaccine has been approved for use by the FDA to help prevent infection with some types of HPV. Gardasil protects against HPV types 6, 11, 16, and 18. The vaccine was designed to lower the risk of cervical cancer, but recent studies have shown it also helps prevent VIN and vulvar cancers caused by HPV 16 and 18.[59,60] Additional HPV vaccines for prophylactic as well as therapeutic use are being developed and tested.[59] A phase II study has completed enrollment at the National Cancer Institute (NCI) for women with recurrent or metastatic vulvar cancer with an HPV 16 vaccine. The vaccine attempts to produce an immune reaction to the parts of the virus (E6 and E7 proteins) that specifically contribute to the abnormal growth of cancer cells.[60]

Other strategies being investigated to prevent cancer of the vulva include topical treatments for women with VIN. Currently, the antineoplastic activity of the topical application of the fungicide ciclopirox is being studied as chemoprevention for women with VIN. Cidofovir, an acyclic nucleoside phosphonate that induces apoptosis in HPV-infected cells, is being tested as a topical application. The first trial of 10 patients showed 4 complete responders, 3 partial responders, and 3 patients who failed therapy.[61] Retinoids, a derivative of vitamin A with antiproliferative properties, are being tested as a topical application. A study of 16 patients treated with 13-cis-retinoic acid reported 50% complete responders with manageable side effects.[62] Indole-3-carbinol (I3C), an FDA-approved nutritional supplement available in capsule or powder form, has been shown to be anticarcinogenic and antiestrogenic. Early studies have shown a significant improvement in symptomatology and vulvoscopic appearance.[42,63]

Future trends in the management of vulvar cancer seek to focus on a more individualized approach, multimodality therapy, and a better understanding of the psychosexual adjustment of patients. Clinical trials are seeking to define the best way of combining neoadjuvant radiation and chemotherapy with surgery to reduce the need for extensive surgery. The goal of these trials is to shrink the tumor initially so that a less radical surgery can be performed. The use of multimodality therapy will not only preserve organ function but also will likely extend the lives of women with vulvar cancer. One such study is currently being conducted by the GOG. Protocol 0205 is a phase II trial of RT and weekly cisplatin for women with locally advanced squamous cell carcinoma of the vulva. The objective is to determine the complete clinical and pathological response to this therapy when used as the primary treatment, as well as the toxicity of this combined modality.[64] Results of the GOG trial of SLN identification are eagerly awaited to help define the role of pelvic lymphadenectomy in vulvar cancer. In the management of side effects from surgery, a GOG study recently reported results. The GOG 0195 study looked at the use of Tisseel VH Fibrin sealant to reduce drainage after inguinal lymph node dissection. This phase III clinical trial randomized patients following dissection to the application of Tisseel sealant to the inguinal wound base or to the closure of the wound. The results of 137 evaluable patients showed no difference in the development of lymphedema between the 2 treatment arms.[44] One area of need in vulvar cancer is proven systemic therapy for women with distant metastasis or recurrence. Due to the fact that vulvar cancer is a rare disease, the feasibility of large prospective randomized clinical trials is limited. International collaborative groups need to join forces in order to conduct these trials.

## VAGINAL CANCER

### EPIDEMIOLOGY

Primary carcinoma of the vagina represents only 1% to 3% of all gynecological malignancies. The incidence of invasive vaginal cancer is approximately 1 case in 100,000 women. In contrast to other gynecologic organs, the vaginal tissue rarely undergoes malignant transformation. The vagina is often a site of metastasis or direct extension from tumors originating in other genital sites or from extragenital sites. Only when the primary site of tumor growth is in the vagina should the disease be classified as vaginal carcinoma.[7,65,66]

Primary invasive vaginal cancer is associated with advanced age. The peak incidence occurs in women aged 70 to 79 years, with more than 50% of the cases occurring between the seventh and ninth decades. It is rare that women younger than age 40 are diagnosed with vaginal cancer. In contrast, the peak incidence for clear cell adenocarcinoma of the vagina, which is associated with maternal use of diethylstilbestrol (DES), occurs in women aged 15 to 22.[66]

Vaginal intraepithelial neoplasia (VAIN) can precede a diagnosis of vaginal cancer, just as cancer of the cervix and vulva can be preceded by CIN and VIN, respectively. Vaginal intraepithelial neoplasia is much less common than CIN or VIN. However, its incidence is climbing and the mean age at diagnosis has decreased to 30 years of age.[35] Several factors contribute to the increase in diagnosis of VAIN: increased clinical awareness, improved screening tests, and an absolute increase in incidence. The natural history of VAIN is not well understood and has not been prospectively studied. Like vulvar cancer, the degree to which a continuum exists, from mild dysplasia to an invasive cancer, has not been established.[35,65] While exact numbers are not known, estimates put the incidence of women with VAIN progressing to invasive carcinoma at 3% to 7%.[7]

### ETIOLOGY

There is an association between HPV, in particular HPV types 16 and 18, and vaginal cancer. HPV DNA has been found in more than 60% to 65% of women with vaginal cancer and in about 80% of cases of VAIN.[66–68] A history of in situ or invasive cervical cancer at least 5 years earlier is seen in approximately one third of women who develop vaginal cancer. Prior RT for cervical cancer or abdominal hysterectomy for benign or malignant disease may also be predisposing factors for primary vaginal carcinoma. Chronic vaginal irritation or traumas such as tampon use, coitus, or chronic pessary use have been suggested to contribute to vaginal cancers. Other risk factors include smoking, 5 or more sexual partners, sexual intercourse before age 17, genital warts, and low socioeconomic status.[66,68,69] See Table 69-8 for risk factors and prevention measures.

**TABLE 69-8**

**Vaginal Cancer: Risk Factors and Preventive Measures**

| Risk Factors | Preventive Measures |
|---|---|
| HPV | Pap smear per ACS guidelines<br>HPV vaccine |
| Maternal use of DES | Frequent monitoring by HCP |
| Chronic vaginal irritation | Decrease use of pessaries, tampons |
| Smoking | Smoking cessation treatment |
| Genital warts | Use of barrier protection |
| Sexual practices (> 5 sexual partners or age of first intercourse < 17 years) | |
| History of in situ or invasive cervical cancer > 5 years ago | |
| Prior RT to lower genital tract | |
| Abdominal hysterectomy | |
| Age > 60 years | |

*Abbreviations*: ACS, American Cancer Society; DES, diethylstilbestrol; HCP, healthcare provider; HPV, human papillomavirus; RT, radiation therapy.

Since 1971, the study of clear cell adenocarcinomas of the vagina has focused on young women who were exposed to DES in utero during the first 16 weeks of the pregnancy and have demonstrated a significantly higher incidence of vaginal cancer. Diethylstilbestrol was used in the management of diabetic pregnancies, threatened abortion, and other high-risk obstetric problems. From the late 1940s to 1970, an estimated 2 million pregnant women received DES. The risk of developing vaginal cancer in women who were exposed to DES in utero is estimated to be about 1 in 1,000 up to age 35 with the peak age of diagnosis at 19.[43,70] The oldest reported DES-exposed patient was 52 years old.[71] The incidence of DES-associated vaginal cancer is expected to decrease as the population of women exposed to DES ages. There have been several cases of older women with a history of in utero DES exposure who developed non-clear cell adenocarcinoma of the vagina. These vaginal cancers were more advanced than the clear cell adenocarcinoma.[71] Vaginal adenosis, the presence of glandular epithelium in the vagina, occurs in 45% of DES-exposed women, and 25% of these women have structural abnormalities of the uterus, cervix or vagina. While no direct relationship has been established, the adenosis may be a precursor to clear cell adenocarcinoma.[43,65] Also, recent studies suggest DES-exposed women may have an increased risk of developing breast cancer after age 40.[72] Given these increased risks of developing cancer, long-term surveillance of DES-exposed women is warranted.

## PREVENTION AND SCREENING

Routine screening is not cost effective, given the low incidence of vaginal cancer. However, women should be encouraged to have a Pap smear following the ACS guidelines. At the time the Pap smear is done, inspection of the vagina should be performed. Because women who have had cervical cancer, vulvar cancer, hysterectomy for benign disease, and exposure to DES before birth have a higher incidence of vaginal cancer, it is recommended that a Pap smear for vaginal cancer be performed yearly and continued, even in women older than 70 years.[69] For women who have a history of VAIN, follow-up should include colposcopy as a part of every examination.[69] Prevention of vaginal cancer is best accomplished through avoiding any known risk factors, such as HPV infection, and finding and treating any vaginal precancers. Nurses play an important role in educating patients about the importance of following guidelines for preventive medical care and decreasing risky sexual behavior.

## PATHOPHYSIOLOGY

### Cellular characteristics

The vagina originates at the cervix and terminates at the hymeneal ring. The vagina is lined throughout by nonkeratinized, stratified squamous epithelium and responds to estrogen stimulation. Embryologically, the upper two thirds of the vagina develops separately from the lower one third. The upper two thirds grows downward and shares its blood supply and lymphatic drainage with the cervix. The lower one third of the vagina grows upward and shares its blood supply and lymphatic system with that of the vulva. The lymphatics drain to the inguinal and femoral nodes (see Figure 69-1). The bladder is positioned anterior to the vagina. The rectum and anus are posterior to the vagina[73] (Figure 69-4).

Vaginal intraepithelial neoplasia lesions tend to be multifocal and are best seen using a colposcope and acetic acid application. The lesions most often involve the upper third of the vagina. Generally, the vascular changes are not striking with VAIN. Some authors have described the lesions as having a pink-blush appearance or slightly granular texture, while others have noted the lesions to be white and mosaic with sharp borders.[36,74] Squamous cell carcinoma accounts for 80% to 90% of all vaginal cancers. Other histological types include adenocarcinoma (6%), melanoma (3%), sarcoma (3%), and rarely small cell. Invasive lesions may be red, white, or gray in color and have an ulcerated appearance.[7]

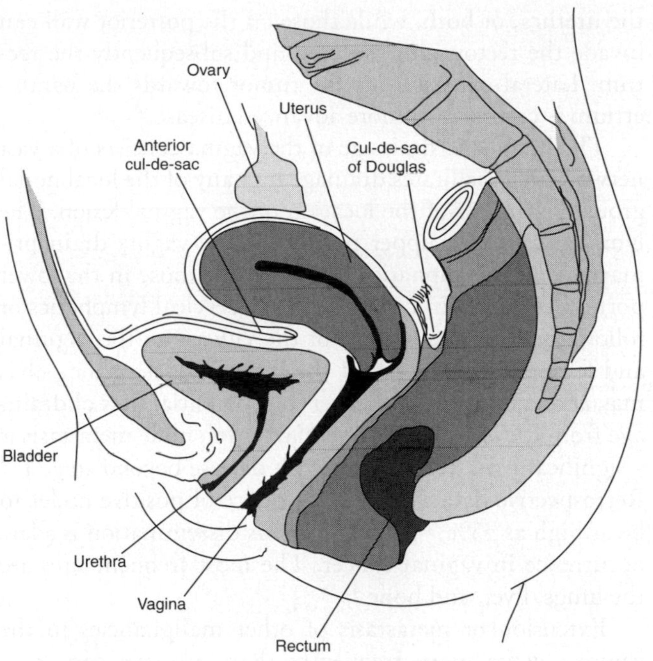


**FIGURE 69-4**

Sagittal section of the female pelvis.

*Source*: Reprinted with permission from Bengton JM. The vagina. In: Ryan KJ, Berkowitz RS, Barbieri RL, eds. *Kistner's Gynecology Principles and Practice*. St. Louis, MO: Mosby; 1996:80–93.[92]

### Progression of disease

Similar to vulvar and cervical disease, diagnosis of VAIN is made histologically, using the 3-grade nomenclature, ranging from VAIN I to VAIN III. VAIN I describes mild dysplasia that involves approximately one third of the epithelium. VAIN I has been found to be HPV-induced without evidence that it progresses. VAIN II describes moderate dysplasia that involves one half to two thirds of the thickness. VAIN III describes severe dysplasia or carcinoma in situ and is considered a premalignant lesion. High-grade VAIN lesions usually occur in tandem with high-grade CIN lesions.[35]

Vaginal cancers occur most commonly in the upper third of the vagina, and the lesions are equally distributed on the posterior, anterior, and lateral walls. The tumors may exhibit an exophytic or fungating polypoid appearance, while others appear ulcerative and infiltrating in their pattern of growth. The tumor may spread along the vaginal wall to involve the cervix or vulva. If the cervix is involved, the tumor is considered a primary cervical lesion.[68]

Vaginal cancer spreads by 3 routes: direct extension to the pelvic soft tissues and adjacent organs, lymphatic dissemination to the inguinofemoral and pelvic nodes, and hematogenous spread to distant organs. Most often vaginal cancer spreads by direct extension: a lesion on the anterior wall can penetrate into the vesicovaginal septum or the urethra, or both, while those on the posterior wall can invade the rectovaginal septum and subsequently the rectum. Lateral extension of the tumor towards the parametrium is common in more advanced disease.[68]

The lymphatic drainage of the vagina consists of a vast network that facilitates drainage into any of the local nodal groups regardless of the location of the vaginal lesion. The lymphatics in the upper portion of the vagina drain primarily via the lymphatics of the cervix; those in the lower portion either drain cephalad to the cervical lymphatics or follow the drainage pattern of the vulva into the inguinal and femoral nodes.[22] All of the lymph nodes of the pelvis may at one time or another serve as potential sites of drainage from the vagina.[66,73] Regional lymph node metastasis is a significant risk for patients with disease beyond stage I.[68] Retrospective data show the incidence of positive nodes to be as high as 35%.[65] Hematogenous dissemination is a late occurrence in vaginal cancer. The most frequent sites are the lungs, liver, and bone.[43]

Extension or metastasis of other malignancies to the vagina occurs more frequently than primary cancer of the vagina. Spread of cervical cancer to the vagina is the most common, but cancers of the vulvar, endometrium, ovary, urethra, bladder, rectum, and malignant trophoblastic disease may also spread or metastasize to the vaginal area.[7,65,66]

## CLINICAL MANIFESTATIONS

Most patients with VAIN are asymptomatic, and in patients with vaginal cancer 10% to 20% will be asymptomatic. An abnormal Pap smear may be the diagnostic event that initiates the search for a definitive diagnosis. The most frequent initial symptom of invasive vaginal cancer is painless vaginal bleeding, following coitus or menopause. Patients may also experience vaginal discharge or a palpable mass. Urinary symptoms such as pain and frequency are seen at an earlier stage of disease than with cervical cancer. This is due to the tumor being lower in the vagina and causing pressure on the bladder. Tumors developing on the posterior vaginal wall may produce rectal symptoms such as tenesmus, constipation, or blood in the stool.[65–67] Pelvic pain is a relatively late symptom and may be due to an extension of the disease beyond the vagina.[68]

## ASSESSMENT

### Patient and family history

All women should have a complete history regarding the duration and severity of their signs and symptoms. For some women, a primary vaginal cancer may actually be a second pelvic cancer. A detailed history of the previous cancer and its treatment are necessary. Information about a woman's exposure to HPV should be obtained. Because exposure to DES in utero is a major risk factor for developing vaginal cancer, all women should be questioned about their mother's possible use of DES. Vaginal cancer does not have a known genetic predisposition.

### Physical examination

Clinical diagnosis of a primary, metastatic, or recurrent vaginal neoplasm is made by careful visual examination of the cervix and vagina and a bimanual exam. It is important that the speculum be rotated and removed slowly so a small lesion is not overlooked. This examination helps determine the location, number, and size of the lesions. Colposcopy with application of acetic acid is valuable for identifying all the lesions and for performing directed biopsies of abnormal vaginal areas. Examination under anesthesia (EUA) may be warranted in order to conduct a thorough exam, especially in elderly women or in women where vaginal stenosis is present. For women who have stenosis, a short course of topical estrogen prior to the colposcopy or EUA can foster epithelial maturation to aid in the identification of areas for biopsy. Biopsies of lesions are necessary for definitive diagnosis. Negative biopsies of the cervix are necessary to rule out cervical cancer and confirm the diagnosis of primary vaginal carcinoma.[7] This information is essential for planning appropriate therapeutic management.[7,68,74]

### Diagnostic studies

Once a diagnosis of vaginal cancer is made it is important to determine whether there is any evidence of local or distant spread of the disease. All patients should have a chest x-ray, complete blood count, and biochemical profile. Patients whose tumors involve the anterior wall should have a cystoscopy and ureteroscopy, and those with tumors involving the posterior wall should have a proctoscopy. An intravenous pyelogram (IVP), barium enema, or skeletal films may be used in selected cases. Additional imaging such as a MRI, CT or positron emission tomography (PET)/CT is helpful in determining the extent of disease, although it is not allowed by FIGO guidelines to clinically stage a patient.[66,68]

### Prognostic indicators

Prognostic factors for patients with vaginal cancer have not been well established due to the rarity of the disease. Clinical stage is the most important prognostic indicator in vaginal cancer. A better prognosis is associated with early diagnosis, small tumor burden, and negative nodal involvement. The impact of histological grade and type, as well as location of the tumor, on prognosis has been controversial. Several studies indicate a poor prognosis with a higher grade of squamous cell carcinoma, as well as lesions on the posterior wall. Age at the time of diagnosis has been stated to be among the most important prognostic factors by several investigators. However, performance status, rather than chronological age, is likely a better reflection of the tolerance of women to aggressive multimodality treatments.[7,65]

## CLASSIFICATION AND STAGING

Staging for vaginal cancer is a clinical staging system, and FIGO criteria allow only certain diagnostic tests, along with the clinical examination, to determine the extent of the disease. Guidelines prohibit information from MRI, CT, lymphangiography, or surgery to be used to stage the patient. However, these imaging procedures aid in assessing for local invasion of the lymph nodes or distant metastasis and help to plan the patient's therapeutic treatment. The FIGO staging of vaginal cancer is shown in Table 69-9. The FIGO guidelines also state that any patient with tumor involvement of the cervix or vulva should be classified as primary cervical or primary vulvar carcinoma.[68]

The classification of vaginal lesions as stage I or II is somewhat subjective. Thin exophytic tumors tend to be classified as stage I, and thick, infiltrating tumors tend to be classified as stage II. A subclassification of stage II into stages IIA and IIB was proposed by Perez and Camel,[75] but has not demonstrated prognostic significance or been adopted into the staging system. Stage III disease has extended onto the pelvic side wall, and in stage IV, the disease has extended beyond the true pelvis. The FIGO staging does not specify the stage of patients with nodal involvement. So for patients with clinically palpable inguinal lymph nodes, the recommendations are somewhat ambiguous. The American Joint Committee on Cancer assigns patients with positive inguinal lymph nodes to stage III.[66,68] Retrospective review of multiple studies has shown the overall 5-year survival rate for all stages of squamous cell vaginal carcinoma to be 0% to 65%. The survival rates are 64% to 90% for patients with stage I disease, 31% to 80% for those with stage II disease, 0% to 79% for those with stage III disease, and 0% to 12% for those with stage IV disease.[7,65,68] Subjectivity in accurately determining the spread of disease by clinicians may account for the wide range of stage distributions, as well as the wide range of survival rates seen in each stage.[43] Modifications to the staging system to allow pathological or clinical TNM staging have been suggested.[66]

The overall survival rate in patients with adenocarcinoma is 80%. This relatively high rate may be related to the fact that females exposed to DES in utero have been followed closely due to their risk for developing adenocarcinoma and are often diagnosed with early-stage disease. However, in comparison to squamous cell carcinoma, clear cell adenocarcinoma has a greater tendency to recur late and to develop metastases in distant sites.[70]

**TABLE 69-9**

**FIGO Staging of Vaginal Cancer**

| Stage | Clinical Findings |
|---|---|
| 0 | Carcinoma in situ |
| I | Limited to vaginal wall |
| II | Involves the subvaginal tissue; has not extended to the sidewall |
| III | Extension to the sidewall |
| IV | Extension beyond the true pelvis or involvement of bladder or rectal mucosa |
| | Bullous edema as such does not permit a case to be allotted to stage IV |
| IVA | Spread to adjacent organs, or extension beyond the true pelvis, or both |
| IVB | Spread to distant organs |

*Abbreviation*: FIGO, International Federation of Gynecology and Obstetrics.

## THERAPEUTIC APPROACHES AND NURSING CARE: VAIN

Management of VAIN disease is controversial. There are a wide variety of treatment options, both surgical and medical, with advantages and disadvantages to each. Treatment options include local excision, loop electrosurgical excision procedure (LEEP), topical applications of estrogens or chemotherapy, intracavity brachytherapy, colpectomy, or vaginectomy. The degree of VAIN and the existence of a single focus or multiple foci, along with the location and size of the lesions, are factors considered in determining treatment options. Age and general health of the woman are also important considerations.[68,76] Women with VAIN I often do not require any treatment. The lesions may regress spontaneously, and due to their multifocal pattern will often recur quickly after attempts at ablative therapy. Women with VAIN II may be treated with observation, topical estrogen, or topical 5-FU cream.[66] 5-FU cream produces chemoinflammation and chemoulceration that adequately treats the VAIN; however, care must be taken to ensure direct contact with the entire lesion and to avoid contact with the vulva.[77]

Patients should be instructed by the nurse to coat the vulva with white petroleum and to use a small tampon or cotton ball at the introitus to help prevent leakage. If douching after the dwell period of the medication is prescribed, the nurse can instruct the women on proper technique, as well as the importance of adherence to the treatment regimen.[36]

VAIN II lesions that are unifocal or clustered can be managed with LEEP, and lesions that are multifocal with laser ablation.[78] Patients will often experience a watery discharge for 2 to 3 weeks after laser therapy. VAIN III lesions are more likely to be premalignant, and local excision is an excellent method to treat small upper-vaginal lesions. In patients who have had a previous hysterectomy, either for benign or malignant disease; prior pelvic radiation; or previous treatment for VAIN where the lesions are in the upper third of the vagina, the treatment of choice may be partial vaginectomy.[74,78] For diffuse, multifocal lesions, ablation using $CO_2$ laser treatment is the primary therapy of choice. The surgeon is able to control the depth of destruction, which is important due to the close proximity of the vagina to the bladder and rectum and the potential for injury to occur.[78–80] With laser therapy one fourth to one third of patients will require a second treatment to achieve long-term control.[81] Since there is a 25% risk of underlying invasive disease, many practitioners are favoring partial vaginectomy over laser therapy.[68] Recently, treatment with chemosurgery has been described. Patients apply 5-FU cream for several nights prior to a partial vaginectomy.[76] If the VAIN involves multiple sites, which includes the lower third of the vagina, laser vaporization can be combined with an upper vaginectomy. For disease that is multifocal and has multiple lesions and is recurrent, or in poor surgical candidates, the treatment may be irradiation of the vagina with high-dose brachytherapy. Treatment is usually delivered via a plastic vaginal cylinder loaded with cesium. Patents may experience vaginitis and in rare cases rectal bleeding.[66,82]

Recurrence rates with any of these methods vary and are based on retrospective reviews, but generally are reported to be very low.[66] Nursing care of the woman varies depending on the treatment used. All these treatments can affect sexual function to some degree. Keeping open lines of communication and helping women to cope is a vital part of the nurse's role.

## THERAPEUTIC APPROACHES AND NURSING CARE: INVASIVE DISEASE

Due to the rarity of vaginal cancer, there is no consensus as to its proper management. Therefore it is important to individualize therapy on the basis of the stage of the disease, the site of vaginal involvement, history of prior surgery and radiation, and the importance of maintaining a functional vagina.[83]

### Radiation therapy

Radiation therapy is the most widely used treatment modality for all stages of vaginal cancer. Despite its acceptance, optimal RT for each stage is not well defined in the literature and can include an integration of teletherapy (ie, external beam radiation therapy, EBRT) and brachytherapy (intracavitary brachytherapy, ICB, and/or interstitial brachytherapy, ITB).[50,68] Intracavitary brachytherapy involves the use of vaginal cylinders that are loaded with a radioactive source such as cesium or iridium and inserted into the vagina. The labia are usually sutured closed to keep the cylinder in place. Interstitial brachytherapy involves placement of either a temporary or permanent radioactive source. A temporary implant is achieved using a vaginal obturator and hollow guides of various lengths that are "afterloaded" with iridium. The placement of a tandem loaded with cesium through the center of the obturator allows the combination of ITB and ICB. A permanent implant involves the use of a perineal template to distribute the radioactive seeds equally, usually gold or iodine.[50,68] The principles of radiation for vaginal cancer also include treating the regional lymph nodes when there is a risk of nodal involvement. Recently, intensity-modulated radiotherapy (IMRT) has been introduced to the treatment planning protocols for vaginal cancer. Intensity-modulated radiotherapy is a novel approach to the planning and delivery of radiation. It provides the ability to conform the dose to the shape of the target in 3 dimensions, sparing the nearby normal tissue. This may lower the complication rate for patients. Intensity-modulated radiotherapy is also a means to escalate doses to the tumor to achieve better control of disease and to improve the chance of cure.[50,65,84]

Radiation therapy for patients who have stage I small (<2 cm), superficial tumors is with brachytherapy alone. A fractionated dose of 6000 to 7000 cGy to the whole vaginal mucosa is usually administered. For women with larger (>2cm) stage I or stage II tumors, the recommendation is a combination of EBRT, dosed at 4000 to 5000 cGy, followed by ICB or ITB, or both.[50,65]

In stage III or IV disease, a combination of EBRT and brachytherapy is recommended. A total dose of 7000 to 8500 cGy of EBRT and ICB to the pelvis is usually given. In women with positive nodes or in whom the tumor has invaded the lower third of the vagina, the groin area is included in the treatment field. Typically, 4000 to 5000 cGy is delivered by EBRT, and brachytherapy, either by ICB or ITB, or both, provides the boost to reach the total dose.[66] Women with stage III or IV vaginal tumors have a high recurrence rate, and to enhance the RT, radiosensitizers such as cisplatin or 5-FU may be given concurrently.[50] To date neoadjuvant chemotherapy prior to RT has no established role. In general, radiation treatment provides good tumor control with limited morbidity.[50,83] Recently, a retrospective series, from a single institution, reported that pretreatment and on-treatment hemoglobin levels and a history of prior hysterectomy were clinically significant prognostic factors for disease outcome. Patients who had a normal hemoglobin prior to treatment and maintained a normal hemoglobin level during treatment had improved pelvic control and disease-specific survival. Women who had a prior hysterectomy had a better outcome as well.[85]

Early treatment effects, either during or shortly after the RT, include acute cystitis, urethritis, and proctitis, as well as mucosal effects such as edema, erythema, moist desquamation, and mucositis, with or without ulceration. The intensity and duration of these symptoms will vary depending upon the patient's age, hormonal status, RT dose, and personal hygiene. Most symptoms resolve spontaneously within 2 to 3 months after completing therapy.[68] However, the desquamation of the skin from RT can be distressing to the patient. Educating the woman about meticulous skin care is imperative (Table 69-10). Soaks, air exposure, and the application of corticosteroid or antibiotic cream can help prevent a skin infection. For acute radiation vaginitis, the women can be instructed to douche daily with a diluted hydrogen peroxide/water mixture for up to 2 to 3 months after treatment.[68]

Late effects of RT include vaginal atrophy, fibrosis, and stenosis. Vaginal stenosis occurs with the greatest frequency, and regular vaginal dilation is recommended to maintain vaginal health and good sexual function. This can be achieved through frequent intercourse or, for patients who are not sexually active, the regular use of a vaginal dilator with water-soluble lubricants. The use of prescribed topical estrogen cream starting 2 weeks post RT helps stimulate epithelial regeneration and aids in minimizing functional loss.[50]

More serious complications include ulceration with necrosis that can lead to fistula formation (rectovaginal, vesicovaginal, or urethrovaginal), urethral or rectal stricture, small bowel obstruction, and hemorrhage. The patient should be closely monitored for these complications.[50]

**TABLE 69-10**

**Skin Care of the Woman Receiving Radiation to the Lower Pelvis**

- Wash the treated area with a mild soap; use warm water, not hot
- Do not rub skin dry; pat skin with a towel; try to keep the skin free from moisture
- Do not apply creams, lotions, or powder to the treated area
- Do not shave skin
- If skin becomes reddened, tell your nurse or physician; application of corticosteroid or antibiotic cream may be indicated; apply medicated cream after the daily dose of radiation

Fortunately, these complications develop in only a small percentage of women.[82] Retrospective analysis of serious complications post RT showed 2 factors that correlated with their development: FIGO stage and smoking history.[83] Women should be encouraged to stop smoking. The nurse can educate the patient of the risks associated with smoking and assist the patient in accessing resources to effectively stop smoking.

## Surgery

Surgery in the management of vaginal cancer has a limited role, mainly due to the radicality necessary to achieve negative surgical margins.[43] However, for a carefully selected group of women, surgery may be an option.[7] In patients who present with stage I disease in the upper posterior vagina, a radical hysterectomy, partial vaginectomy, and bilateral pelvic lymphadenectomy can be performed.[43,68] Surgery in patients who present with stage I disease in the lower third of the vagina would require the addition of a vulvovaginectomy and dissection of inguinofemoral nodes in order to achieve negative margins.[68] In younger women who wish to preserve reproductive, as well as sexual, function, a more conservative surgery has been piloted. The surgery consists of a radical tumorectomy with pelvic lymphadenectomy. In the 4 patients who had the conservative surgery, at 51, 45, 21, and 9 month follow-up time, respectively, all patients were regularly menstruating, sexual active, and clinically free of disease.[86]

For patients with stage IVA disease a primary pelvic exenteration is a treatment option if they are medically fit.[87] Unfortunately, the pelvic exenteration will be aborted in 25% of cases, because more advanced disease will be found during the exploratory laparotomy.[68] If completed, a pelvic exenteration results in both long-term functional changes and body image changes. With radical vaginectomy or pelvic exenteration, reconstruction of a vagina (ie, the creation of a neovagina) is done for patients who wish to continue vaginal intercourse. Postoperatively these women must be encouraged to continue regular intercourse or to use vaginal dilators, along with topical estrogen, to maintain adequate function of the neovagina.[67] Open communication between the nurse and the patient about sexual concerns is essential. For any patient who receives surgery, extensive preoperative counseling, postoperative care, and rehabilitation are necessary.

## Chemotherapy

For patients who have metastatic or recurrent vaginal cancer, or if surgery or RT cannot be utilized, chemotherapy may be an option. Chemotherapeutic agents used for the treatment of vaginal cancer include cisplatin, 5-FU, mitomycin C, and epirubicin.[65] In a phase II GOG study with 26 patients who had progressive or recurrent disease, cisplatin was given every 3 weeks. There was minimal activity in patients with squamous cell carcinoma. A study by Long and colleagues, using methotrexate, vinblastine, doxorubicin, and cisplatin for advanced or recurrent vaginal cancer, reported 3 patients who had a complete response of short duration. This regimen was found to be toxic, especially when used as salvage therapy after failure of RT.[88] Very few studies have addressed the role of chemotherapy to treat vaginal cancer; hence most of the data used for chemotherapy management have been extrapolated from carcinoma of the cervix, because the natural history, histology, and risk factors are similar to those for vaginal cancer.[65,89] The use of chemoradiation for advanced stage disease using cisplatin or 5-FU as a radiosensitizer has been proposed due to its utility in cervical cancer.[66] More research is needed to better define the role of chemotherapy in vaginal cancer.

## SYMPTOM MANAGEMENT AND SUPPORTIVE CARE

### Advanced/recurrent disease

Women who are treated for their early-stage vaginal cancer have high disease control rates approaching 80% to 90%, whereas women with stage III or IV vaginal cancer are reported to have a recurrence rate as high as a 50%.[68,83] More than 80% of women who develop recurrent disease will have pelvic recurrences, which usually appear within 2 years of primary treatment.[65] Distant sites of metastasis usually occur later, and are less frequently seen. Long-term survival for women with extrapelvic recurrence is poor. Overall, the 1-year survival rate for women with recurrence is reported at 12%.[82]

Optimal therapy for patients with recurrent disease is based on whether the primary goal is curative salvage or palliation. Therefore a careful evaluation for regional and distant metastasis by physical exam and imaging studies is required. A triad of symptoms—sciatic pain, leg edema, and hydronephrosis—is indicative of disease that has spread to the pelvic sidewall. Patients who did not receive prior RT and have an isolated pelvic recurrence can be managed with a combination of EBRT, brachytherapy, and concurrent chemotherapy.[68] Effective salvage therapy for patients with locally recurrent disease in a previously irradiated area who have no evidence of metastatic disease may be a radical surgery, usually a pelvic exenteration. Palliative therapy consists of radiation, chemotherapy, or chemoradiation. Response rates and long-term survival rates for these women with chemotherapy are low.[65]

The complications seen in advanced vaginal cancer depend on the location of the tumor. In tumors located anteriorly, the woman may experience urinary problems such as hematuria and urinary tract infections. Palliative radiotherapy can reduce hematuria from an ulcerating lesion. In addition to this RT, the patient may need continuous bladder irrigation to decrease the bleeding. Repeated urinary tract infections may be indicative of fistula formation and the patient may experience urinary incontinence, dysuria, and painful bladder spasms. For some women, surgery might be the best treatment choice to close the fistula.[83] For women who are too ill or when the tumor is too extensive, symptomatic treatment with appropriate antibiotics and antispasmodics is used. For larger draining fistulas, a urinary-vaginal prosthesis can be used to divert the drainage and to maintain the woman's skin integrity.[50]

If the tumor grows posteriorly, blood in the stool and constipation may occur. For mild constipation, the use of stool softeners and laxatives may be all that is necessary. If complete obstruction occurs, surgery or RT is usually warranted. A rectovaginal fistula can cause distressing fecal incontinence. If the fistula is small, measures to keep the stool well formed may help the healing process. The use of vaginal tampons can help to control fistula discharge. For larger fistulas, a simple loop colostomy should be considered to provide relief of symptoms.[83]

## FUTURE TRENDS

Establishing strong, evidence-based recommendations for the treatment of invasive vaginal cancer is problematic because it is such a rare disease. The ability to do randomized clinical trials is unlikely, and most future progress will likely come from single institution studies and retrospective analysis. Whenever possible, patients with vaginal cancer should be treated in a tertiary facility that has a well-established multidisciplinary team with experience in treating this disease. Not only may this be beneficial to the patient, but more experience can be gained in the management of this disease.

A continuing area of research for vaginal cancer centers on the role of HPV in vaginal cancer. Similar to cervical cancer prevention, the use of HPV vaccines may help to reduce the incidence of vaginal cancer or in the treatment of VAIN. Protein expression patterns in vaginal cancer reveal an abnormality of chromosome 3q in 70% of vaginal cancers. More research on the role this plays in vaginal cancer development might lead to a better treatment. In addition, this study also found vaginal and cervical carcinomas were relatively homogeneous in their gene expression, indicating similar carcinogenic pathways.[89] This may help support the extrapolation of data from cervical cancer, where more research has been done, to guide the treatment of vaginal cancer. Recent published data examined the use of F-18 fluorodeoxyglucose (FDG) PET in carcinoma of the vagina. In this study, 23 patients with vaginal cancer underwent both a CT of the abdomen and pelvis and an FDG-PET. The abilities of the procedures to detect the primary tumor and lymph node metastasis were compared. The FDG-PET detected 100% of primary tumors, compared with CT detecting 43%. The FDG-PET also detected twice as many patients with abnormal lymph nodes than CT. The most promising aspect of FDG-PET is a noninvasive method to detect lymph node metastasis and to tailor radiation fields, perhaps decreasing the number of women with recurrent disease.[90] Similar to vulvar carcinoma, SLN detection is also being investigated as a new minimally invasive technique to detect lymph node metastasis.[91] Research that could better define the role of chemotherapy as well as chemoradiation for vaginal cancer is being studied in hope of being able to preserve anatomy and function. There are also studies under way to determine the most effective way to combine external beam radiation and brachytherapy to decrease damage to normal tissue.

The offspring (ie, third generation) of DES daughters and sons are beginning to reach the age when relevant health problems can be studied. The potential risks associated with DES exposure in the third generation are being carefully monitored.

The majority of women with vaginal cancer are treated with RT. The radiation oncology nurse must address changes in body image, alteration in sexuality, and coping mechanisms with the woman. With half the patients with vaginal cancer over the age of 70, the probability of hospitalization or the need for home health care is high. The RT nurse can play a key role in helping facilitate communication between care settings.

## CONCLUSION

While the emphasis is on individualized treatment for the woman who is diagnosed with vulvar or vaginal cancer, the treatment may be aggressive and potentially disfiguring. Multimodal treatment has led to decreased recurrence rates. Effective communication across health care disciplines is necessary to achieve a successful and comprehensive approach for the patient. Nurses must consider the social, sexual, financial, and spiritual needs of all of these patients. To further improve the quality of care for women with vulvar or vaginal cancer, more nursing research on the management of treatment-related symptoms and care of the patient with advanced disease is essential. Nurses are also in the best position to address barriers to screening and to educate women to follow the ACS guidelines for obtaining regular Pap smears. If detected early, vulvar and vaginal cancers have high cure rates.

## REFERENCES

1. American Cancer Society. http://www.cancer.org. Accessed January 1, 2010.
2. Howe HL, Wingo PA, Thun MJ, et al. Annual Report to the nation on the status of cancer (1973 through 1998), featuring cancers with recent increasing trends. *J Natl Cancer Inst.* 2001;93:824–842.
3. Joura EA, Losch A, Haider-Angeler MG, et al. Trends in vulvar neoplasia. Increasing incidence of vulvar intraepithelial neoplasia and squamous cell carcinoma of the vulva in young women. *J Reprod Med.* 2000;45:613–615.
4. Jones RW. Vulvar intraepithelial neoplasia: current perspectives. *Eur J Gynaecol Oncol.* 2001;22:393–402.
5. Jones RW, Rowan DM, Stewart AW. Vulvar intraepithelial neoplasia: aspects of the natural history and outcome in 405 women. *Obstet Gynecol.* 2005;106:1319–1326.
6. Judson PL, Habermann EB, Baxter NU, et al. Trends in the incidence of invasive and in-situ vulvar carcinoma. *Obstet Gynecol.* 2006;107:1018–1022.
7. Eifel PJ, Berek JS, Thigpen JT. Cancer of the cervix, vagina, and vulvar. In: Devita VT, Hellman S, and Rosenberg SA, eds. *Cancer: Principles and Practice of Oncology.* 8th ed. Philadelphia, PA: Lippincott-Raven; 2008: 46–72.
8. Sutton BC, Allen RA, Moore WE, Dunn ST. Distribution of human papillomavirus genotypes in invasive squamous carcinoma of the vulva. *Mod Pathol.* 2008;21:345–354.
9. Moore DH, Koh WJ, McGuire WP, Wilkinson EJ. Vulva. In: Hoskins WJ, Perez CA, Young RC, et al, eds. *Principles and Practice of Gynecologic Oncology.* 4th ed. Philadelphia, PA: Lippincott, Williams & Wilkins; 2005:665–705.
10. Scurry J, Wilkerson E. Review of terminology of precursors of vulvar squamous cell carcinoma. *J Low Genit Tract Dis.* 2006;10:161–169.
11. Canavan TP, Cohen D. Vulvar cancer. *Am Fam Physician.* 2002;66:1269–1274.
12. Preti M, Van Seters M, Sideri M, Van Beurden M. Squamous vulvar intraepithelial neoplasia. *Clin Obstet Gynecol.* 2005;48:845–861.
13. Odunsi K, Petrovic T, Anderson ML, Chambers SK. Molecular biology of gynecologic cancers. In: Devita VT, Hellman S, and Rosenberg SA, eds. *Cancer: Principles and Practice of Oncology.* 8th ed. Philadelphia, PA: Lippincott-Raven; 2008:1488–1496.
14. Rosenthal AN, Hopster D, Ryan A, et al. Immunohistochemical analysis of p53 in vulvar intraepithelial neoplasia and vulvar squamous cell carcinoma. *Br J Cancer.* 2003;88:251–256.
15. Santos M, Montagut C, Mellado B, et al. Immunohistochemical Staining for p16 & p53 in Premalignant and Malignant Epithelial Lesions of the Vulva. *Int J Gynecol Pathol.* 2004;23:206–214.
16. Joura EA. Epidemiology, diagnosis and treatment of vulvar intraepithelial neoplasia. *Curr Opin Obstet Gynecol.* 2002;14:39–43.
17. Bamberger ES, Perrett CW. Angiogenesis in benign, pre-malignant and malignant vulvar lesions. *Anticancer Res.* 2002;22:3853–3865.
18. Saravanamuthu J, Reed WM, St George D, et al. The role of angiogenesis in vulvar cancer, vulvar intra epithelial neoplasia and vulvar lichen sclerosus as determined by microvessel density analysis. *Gynecol Oncol.* 2003;89:251–258.
19. Todd RW, Luesley DM. Medical management of vulvar intraepithelial neoplasia. *J Low Genit Tract Dis.* 2005;9:206–212.
20. Tyring SK. Vulvar squamous cell carcinoma: guidelines for early diagnosis. *Am J Obstet Gynecol.* 2003;189:S17-S23.
21. Cardosi RJ, Bomalaski JJ, Hoffman MS. Diagnosis and management of vulvar and vaginal intraepithelial neoplasia. *Obstet Gynecol Clin North Am.* 2001;28:685–702.
22. Chi DS, Mychalczak B, Hoskins WJ. Cancer of the vulvar and vagina. In: Bland KI, Daly JM, Karakouis CP, eds. *Surgical Oncology—Contemporary Principles and Practices.* New York, NY: McGraw Hill; 2001:852–882.
23. Hacker NF. Vulvar cancer. In: Berek JS, Adashi EY, Hillard PA, eds. *Gynecology.* 12th ed. Philadelphia, PA: Lippincott, Williams & Wilkins; 2007:1231–1260.
24. Hacker NF. Surgery for malignant tumors of the vulva. In: Gersherson DM, DeCherney AH, Curry SL, Brubaker L, eds. *Operative Gynecology.* 2nd ed. Philadelphia, PA: Saunders; 2001:237–261.
25. Dhar KK, Woolas RP. Changes in the management of vulval cancer. *Best Pract Res Clin Obstet Gynaecol.* 2003;17:529–542.

26. Holschneider CH, Berek IS. Vulvar cancer. In: Berek JS, ed. *Novak's Gynecology.* 14th ed. Philadelphia, PA: Lippincott, Williams & Wilkins; 2007:1549–1580.
27. Stehman FB. Invasive cancer of the vulva. In: DiSaia PJ, Creasman WT, eds. *Clinical Gynecologic Oncology.* 7th ed. St. Louis, MO: Mosby; 2007:235–264.
28. deHullu JA, VanderZee AGT. Surgery and radiotherapy in vulva cancer. *Crit Rev Oncol Hematol.* 2006;60:39–58.
29. Margessen LJ. Vulvar disease pearls. *Dermatol Clin.* 2006;24:145–155.
30. August CZ, Ganji M, Froula E. Misdiagnosis of high-grade vulvar intraepithelial neoplasia (VIN III) as mild cervical intraepithelial neoplasia (CIN I) on Papanicolaou tests. *Arch Pathol Lab Med.* 2003;127:68–70.
31. Rouzier R, Morice P, Haie-Meder C, et al. Prognostic significance of epithelial disorders adjacent to invasive vulvar carcinoma. *Gynecol Oncol.* 2001;81:414–419.
32. Rousier R, Preti M, Haddad B, Martin B, Micheletti L, Paneil BJ. Development and validation of a nomogram for predicting outcome of patients with vulvar cancer. *Obstet Gynecol.* 2006;107:672–677.
33. Sideri M, Jones RW, Wilkerson ET, et al. Squamous vulvar intraepithelal neoplasia: 2004 modified terminology, ISSVD Vulvar Oncology Subcommittee. *J Reprod Med.* 2005;50:807–810.
34. Hamilton CA, Berek JS. Vulvar pre-malignant and malignant disorders: non-surgical and minimally invasive options. In: Arici A, Seli E, eds. *Non-Invasive Management of Gynecologic Disorders.* London, UK: Informa Health Care; 2008:271–282.
35. Campion MJ. Preinvasive disease. In: Berk JS, Hacker NF, eds. *Practical Gynecologic Oncology.* 4th ed. Philadelphia, PA: Lippincott; 2005 :265–336.
36. Creasman WT. Preinvasive disease of the vagina and vulva and related disorders. In: DiSaia PT, Creasman WT, eds. *Clinical Gynecologic Oncology.* 7th ed. St. Louis, MO: Mosby; 2007:37–54.
37. Sideri M, Spinaci L, Spolti N, et al. Evaluation of $CO_2$ laser excision or vaporization for the treatment of vulvar intraepithelial neoplasia. *Gynecol Oncol.* 1999;75:277–281.
38. Penna C, Fallani MG, Fambrini M, et al. $CO_2$ laser surgery for vulvar intraepithelial neoplasia. Excisional, destructive and combined techniques. *J Reprod Med.* 2002;47:913–918.
39. Fehr MK, Hornung R, Degen A, et al. Photodynamic therapy of the vulvar and vaginal condyloma and intraepithelial neoplasia using topically applied 5-aminolevuline acid. *Lasers Surg Med.* 2002;30:273–279.
40. Miller BE. Vulvar intraepithelial neoplasia treated with cavitational ultrasonic surgical aspiration. *Gynecol Oncol.* 2002;85:114–118.
41. Todd RW, Etherington IJ, Luesley DM. The effects of 5% imiquimod cream on high-grade vulval intraepithelial neoplasia. *Gynecol Oncol.* 2002;85:67–70.
42. Snoeck R. Papillomavirus and treatment. *Antiviral Res.* 2006;71:181–191.
43. Hacker NF. Vaginal cancer. In: Berek JS, Hacker NF, eds. *Practical Gynecologic Oncology.* 4th ed. Philadelphia, PA: Lippincott, Williams & Wilkins; 2005:585–601.
44. Carlson J, Kauderer J, Walker JL, et al. A randomized phase III trial of VH fibrin sealant to reduce lymphedema after inguinal lymph node dissection: a Gynecologic Oncology Group study. *Gynecol Oncol.* 2008;110:76–82.
45. Gotlieb WH. The assessment and surgical management of early-stage vulvar cancer. *Best Pract Res Clin Obstet Gynaecol.* 2003;17: 557–569.
46. Sliutz G, Reinthaller A, Lantzsch T, et al. Lymphatic mapping of sentinel nodes in early vulvar cancer. *Gynecol Oncol.* 2002;84:449–452.
47. VanderSee AG, Oonk MH, DeHullu IA, Ansink AC, Vergote I. Sentinel node dissection is safe in the treatment of early-stage vulvar cancer. *J Clin Oncol.* 2008;26:884–889.
48. Hoffman MS. Squamous-cell carcinoma of the vulva: locally advanced disease. *Best Pract Res Clin Obstet Gynaecol.* 2003;17:635–647.
49. Blake P. Radiotherapy and chemotherapy for carcinoma of the vulva. *Best Pract Res Clin Obstet Gynaecol.* 2003;17:649–661.
50. Russell, AH. Vulvar and vaginal carcinoma. In: Gunderson LL, Teppe JE, eds. *Clinical Radiation Oncology.* Philadelphia, PA: Churchill Livingstone; 2007:1385–1422.
51. Stetman F, Bundy B, Thoma G, et al. Groin dissection versus radiation in carcinoma of the vulva: a Gynecologic Oncology Group Study. *Int J Radiat Oncol Biol Phys.* 1992;24:39.
52. Door A. Less common gynecologic malignancies. *Semin Oncol Nurs.* 2002;18:207–222.
53. Cunningham MJ, Goyer RP, Gibbons SK, et al. Primary radiation, cisplatin, and 5-fluorouracil for advanced squamous carcinoma of the vulva. *Gynecol Oncol.* 1997;66:258–261.
54. Kim RY, Alvarez RD, Omura GA. Advances in the treatment of gynecologic malignancies. Part 1: cancers of the cervix and vulva. *Oncology.* 2002;11:1510–1517.
55. Moore DH, Thomas GM, Montana GS, et al. Preoperative chemoradiation for advanced vulvar cancer: a phase II study of the Gynecologic Oncology Group. *Int J Radiat Oncol Biol Phys.* 1998;42:79–85.
56. Wagenaar HC, Colombo N, Vergote I, et al. Bleomycin, methotrexate, and CCNU in locally advanced or recurrent inoperable, squamous-cell carcinoma of the vulva: an EORTC Gynaecological Cancer Cooperative Group Study. *Gynecol Oncol.* 2001;81:348–354.
57. Rouzier R, Haddad B, Plantier F, et al. Local relapse in patients treated for squamous cell carcinoma: incidence and prognostic value. *Obstet Gynecol.* 2002;100:1159–1167.
58. Green MS, Naumann RW, Elliott M, et al. Sexual dysfunction following vulvectomy. *Gynecol Oncol.* 2000;77:73–77.
59. American Cancer Society. What's new in vulvar cancer research and treatment? http://www.nlm.nih.gov/medlineplus/vulvarcancer.html. Accessed October 1, 2009.
60. National Institutes of Health. http://www.clinicaltrials.gov. Accessed October 1, 2009.
61. Tristram A, Frander A. Clinical responses to Cidofovir applied topically to women with high grade vulval intraepithielal neoplasia. *Gynecol Oncol.* 2005;99:652–655.
62. Markowska J, Janik P, Wise E, Ostrowski J. Leukoplakia of the vulva locally treated by 13-CIS-retonic acid. *Neoplasma.* 1987;34:33–36.
63. Naik R, Nixon S, Lopes A, et al. A randomized phase II trial of indole-3-carbinol in the treatment of vulvar intra-epithelial neoplasia. *Int J Gynecol Cancer.* 2006;16:786–790.
64. Gynecologic Oncology Group. http://www.gog.org. Accessed October 1, 2009.
65. Slomovitz BM, Colemna RL. Invasive cancer of the vagina and urethra. In: DiSaia PJ, Creasman WT, eds. *Clinical Gynecologic Oncology.* 7th ed. St. Louis, MO: Mosby; 2007:265–281.
66. Eifel PJ, Berek JS, Markman MA. Cancer of the cervix, vagina and vulva. In: Devita VT, Hellman S, and Rosenberg SA, eds. *Cancer: Principles and Practice of Oncology.* 8th ed. Philadelphia, PA: Lippincott-Raven; 2008:1521–1528.
67. Bidus MA, Elkas JC. Vaginal cancer. In: Berek JS, ed. *Novak's Gynecology.* 14th ed. Philadelphia, PA: Lippincott, Williams & Wilkens; 2007:1403–1456.
68. Cardenes HR, Roth LM, McGuire WP, et al. Vagina. In: Hoskins WI, Perez CA, Young RC, et al. *Gynecologic Oncology.* 4th ed. Philadelphia, PA: Lippincott, Williams & Wilkins; 2005:707–742.
69. American Cancer Society. Can vaginal cancer be prevented? http://www.nlm.nih.gov/medlineplus/vaginalcancer.html. Accessed October 1, 2009.
70. Herbst AL, Anderson S, Hubby MM, et al. Risk factors for the development of diethylstilbestrol-associated clear cell adenocarcinoma: a case-control study. *Am J Obstet Gynecol.* 1986;154:814–822.
71. DeMars LR, Van Le L, Huang I, et al. Primary non-clear-cell adenocarcinoma of the vagina in older DES-exposed women. *Gynecol Oncol.* 1995;58:389–392.
72. Palmer JR, Wise LA, Hatch EE, et al. Prenatal diethylstilbestrol exposure at the risk of breast cancer. *Cancer Epidemiol Biomarkers Prev.* 2006;15:1509.

73. Entman SS, Graves CR, Jarnagin BK, Rao GG. Gynecologic surgery. In: Sabiston DC, Lyerly HK, eds. *Textbook Surgery: The Biological Basis of Modern Surgical Practice.* 15th ed. Philadelphia, PA: Saunders; 2008:2201–2235.
74. Wright TC. Pathogenesis and diagnosis of preinvasive lesions of the lower genital tract. In: Hoskins WJ, Perez CA, Young RC, et al, eds. *Principles and Practices of Gynecologic Oncology.* 4th ed. Philadelphia, PA: Lippincott, Williams & Wilkins; 2005:627–644.
75. Perez CA, Camel HM, Galakatos AE, et al. Definitive irradiation in carcinoma of the vagina: long term evaluation of results. *Int J Radiat Oncol Biol Phys.* 1988;15(6):1283–1290.
76. Indermaur MD, Martino MA, Fiorica JV, Roberts WS, Hoffman MS. Upper vaginectomy for the treatment of vaginal intraepithelial neoplasia. *Am J Obstet Gynecol.* 2005;193:577–581.
77. Rome RM, England PG. Management of vaginal intraepithelial neoplasia: a series of 132 cases with long-term follow-up. *Int J Gynecol Cancer.* 2000;10:382–390.
78. Massad LS. Outcomes after diagnosis of vaginal intraepithelial neoplasia. *J Low Genit Tract Dis.* 2008;12:16–19.
79. Campagnutta E, Parin A, DePiero G, et al. Treatment of vaginal intraepithelial neoplasia (VAIN) with the carbon dioxide laser. *Clin Exp Obstet Gynecol.* 1999;26:127–130.
80. Yalcin OT, Rutherford TJ, Chambers SK, et al. Vaginal intraepithelial neoplasia: treatment by carbon dioxide laser and risk factors for failure. *Eur J Obstet Gynecol Reprod Biol.* 2003;106:64–68.
81. Diakomanolis E, Stefanidis K, Rodolakis A, et al. Vaginal intraepithelial neoplasia: report of W2 cases. *Eur J Gynaecol Oncol.* 2002;23:457–459.
82. Chyle V, Zagars GK, Wheeler JA, et al. Definitive radiotherapy for carcinoma of the vagina: outcome and prognostic factors. *Int J Radiat Oncol Biol Phys.* 1996;35:891–905.
83. Frank SJ, Jhingran A, Levenback C, Eifel PJ. Definitive radiation therapy for squamous cell carcinoma of the vagina. *Int J Radiat Oncol Biol Phys.* 2005;62:138–147.
84. Leibe SA, Fuks Z, Zelefsky MJ. Intensity-modulated radiotherapy. *Cancer J.* 2002;8:164–171.
85. Tran PT, Su Z, Lee P, et al. Prognostic factors for outcomes and complications for primary squamous cell carcinoma of the vagina treated with radiation. *Gynecol Oncol.* 2007;105:641–649.
86. Cutillo G, Cignini P, Gianbeppi G, et al. Conservative treatment of reproductive and sexual function in young woman with squamous carcinoma of the vagina. *Gynecol Oncol.* 2006;103:234–237.
87. Tjalma WA, Monaghan JM, Lopes AB, et al. The role of surgery in invasive squamous carcinoma of the vagina. *Gynecol Oncol.* 2001;81:360–365.
88. Long HJ III, Rayson S, Podratz KC, et al. Long-term survival of patients with advanced/recurrent carcinoma of the cervix and vagina after neoadjuvant treatment with methotrexate, vinblastine, doxorubicin, and cisplatin with or without the addition of molgramostim, and review of the literature. *Am J Clin Oncol.* 2002;25:547–551.
89. Hellman K, Alaiya AA, Schedvins K, Stenberg W, Hellstrom AC, Aver G. Protein expression patterns in the primary carcinoma of the vagina. *Br J Cancer.* 2004;91:319–326.
90. Lamoreaux WT, Grigsby PW, Dehdashti F, et al. FDG-PET evaluation of vaginal carcinoma. *Int J Radiat Oncol.* 2005;62:733–737.
91. VanDam P, Sonnemans H, Van Dam PJ, et al. Sentinel node detection in patients with vaginal carcinoma. *Gynecol Oncol.* 2004;92:89–92.
92. Bengton JM. The vagina. In: Ryan KJ, Berkowitz RS, Barbieri RL, eds. *Kistner's Gynecology Principles and Practice.* St. Louis, MO: Mosby; 1996:80–93.

# PART VII

# Dimensions of Cancer Survivorship

CHAPTER 70

Victoria Wochna Loerzel, PhD, RN, OCN®
Karen Meneses, PhD, RN, FAAN

# Cancer Survivorship: A Critical Aspect of Care

## INTRODUCTION

Survival rates from cancer have steadily increased over the past 30 years. Improved survival is the result of multiple factors, including changes in our basic understanding about the disease, growth of translational research to practice, changes in dose-limiting treatment toxicities, development of new targeted therapies, increased screening and early detection activities, enhanced rehabilitation and support interventions, and changes in sociocultural factors.[1,2] We have likewise witnessed a change in the long-term and late effects of cancer requiring a larger perspective on cancer survivorship. The Institute of Medicine (IOM) Report entitled "From Cancer Patient to Cancer Survivor: Lost in Transition" outlines the essential components of survivorship care as follows: prevention of recurrent and new cancers, surveillance of cancer, interventions for late effects of cancer, and coordination among specialists providing care to cancer survivors.[3] Oncology nursing has as its ultimate goal to enhance the length and quality of survival of all cancer survivors. The purpose of this chapter is to (1) provide an overview of cancer survivorship, (2) describe the historical perspective of cancer survivorship, (3) explore psychosocial management of cancer survivors, and (4) describe future challenges in cancer survivorship and cancer survivorship research.

## OVERVIEW OF CANCER SURVIVORSHIP

The most recent cancer survivorship figures, compiled by the National Cancer Institute (NCI) as of January 2004, show that there are 10.8 million persons living with a history of cancer in the US.[4] The Office of Cancer Survivorship (OCS) at the NCI has the following definition of a cancer survivor: "an individual is a survivor from the time of diagnosis through the balance of his or her life."[4] The caregivers and family members are secondary survivors because they are also touched by the experience of cancer in a family member or loved one.

The population of cancer survivors is increasing, with 65% of adults surviving 5 years and 75% of children surviving beyond 10 years after their diagnosis. Fourteen percent of all survivors alive today were diagnosed more than 20 years ago. Of the 24,040 households in the 1992 National Health Interview Survey, 63% of respondents had a cancer diagnosis more than 5 years and 10% had a cancer diagnosis more than 25 years.[5]

Demographic trends show that cancer survivors in the future will be older and more ethnically diverse. First, both males and females are now older at the time of diagnosis—ages 68 and 67 years, respectively.[2] This trend, coupled with the growing elderly population in the US, which is expected to double from 1.3 million to 2.6 million by 2050, suggests that cancer rates in the elderly will also double.[6] Second, we can expect a racially and ethnically diverse population. Hispanics will account for 25% of the US population by 2050, while African Americans, Asian Americans, and Native Americans combined are projected to constitute an additional 25% of the population in that year.[7]

In the past, "unwarranted pessimism" has been prevalent in the treatment of older patients with cancer. Although uncertainty exists about the value of cancer treatment in older patients, Saltzstein and Behling[8] surprisingly found that survival among older patients is not affected for up to 10 years after treatment. The authors used data from the NCI's Surveillance, Epidemiology, and End Results (SEER) program.[9] For the period 1973 to 1998, they located 37,318 records of individuals of age 90 and older and then compared their records with those of 2 other age groups, 0 to 69 and 70 to 89. The results showed that relative survival data for all 3 age groups were similar after the first year of diagnosis. The largest number of deaths occurred during the first year after diagnosis, particularly within the first 4 months after diagnosis. Once past the first year postdiagnosis, patients 90 years of age and older did well compared to their younger counterparts. The oldest patients will benefit from treatment as much as younger ones within the first year. Thus, older age alone may not be a contraindication for treatment.

## LATE EFFECTS IN CANCER SURVIVORS

Although children and adults with a history of cancer are living longer, there is a growing body of evidence demonstrating long-term and late physiological effects such as secondary cancers; cognitive changes; cardiac dysfunction; respiratory late effects; infertility and sexual dysfunction; psychosocial late effects such as depression, anxiety, uncertainty, isolation, and altered body image; social late effects such as changes in interpersonal relationships, health and life insurance issues, and financial burden; and existential issues such as changes in life purpose and meaning, and spiritual effects.[10] These effects may be acute, meaning that they are short-lived and time-limited; long-term, meaning that they persist for various periods of time even after treatment ends; or late, meaning that they occur months or years after treatment. The long-term and late effects are of greatest consequence to long-term cancer survivors. Chapter 71 discusses the physical late effects of cancer. This chapter focuses on quality of life (QOL) in relationship to psychosocial late effects in adult cancer survivors.

### QUALITY OF LIFE AND CANCER SURVIVORS

Quality-of-life issues for long-term cancer survivors differ from the problems faced at the time of diagnosis and treatment.[11] Zebrack[12] provided an excellent and comprehensive overview of the literature on QOL and cancer survivors. He discussed the differences in the meaning of QOL, as this definition has changed over the past 30 years. In the 1970s, QOL research showed that how people survive is just as critical as how long they survive. Quality-of-life research in the 1980s examined the relationship between psychosocial effects of cancer (eg, psychological, behavioral, and environmental factors) in relationship to causes of cancer. The predominant conceptual framework was the stress-coping paradigm. Studies identified individuals at high risk for poor psychosocial adjustment, with clinical interventions being designed to help buffer or prevent these effects. In the 1990s, studies continued to focus on problems of adjustment and psychological distress, with less attention being paid to personal growth and well-being.[12] By the late 1990s, however, the focus on the positive psychosocial outcomes of resilience, hardiness, enhanced appreciation for life, and spiritual growth helped counterbalance the negative psychosocial effects of cancer and survivorship.[12] The 21st century data focus on psychosocial issues influencing long-term cancer survivors. The next section profiles the psychosocial late effects commonly seen in cancer survivors.

## PSYCHOSOCIAL LATE EFFECTS IN CANCER SURVIVORS

### FEAR OF RECURRENCE

Regardless of the type of cancer and its stage at diagnosis, fears—and more often fears of recurrence—can play a profound role in cancer survivorship and QOL. This topic has been reported extensively in the literature.[13–18] While recurrence in breast cancer survivors has received the majority of the attention,[19–22] recurrence in other cancer populations such as head and neck cancer,[14] prostate cancer,[13] and gynecological cancer[16,20] have recently been studied. Overall, few studies have focused on interventions for cancer survivors who have fear of recurrence. There are different levels of fear of recurrence. Vickberg[19] reported that the majority of women in her study had moderate levels of fear related to breast cancer recurrence. These include fears of death, further treatment such as chemotherapy, pain, difficult emotions, potential for progression of disease, loss of a breast with mastectomy, and suffering of family members. At the same time, several women identified certain life circumstances that had more impact than the potential for recurrence. For example, family issues, such as the health of a spouse or child, and other personal chronic conditions could take precedence over their own fear of recurrence. Interestingly, cancer stage, time since diagnosis, and type of surgery were not related to fears of recurrence.[21]

Breast cancer survivors also identified "triggers" of their fear of recurrence: being around other people newly diagnosed with cancer or hearing about cancer, attending support groups where women discussed more aggressive treatment, and second-guessing their own conservative treatment choices. In addition, survivors became more fearful in situations where cancer or recurrence could be detected, such as follow-up mammography and testing, or when they felt something new or different in their breasts.[16,19]

Wenzel and colleagues[16] note high QOL in their population of early-stage ovarian cancer survivors. Although the participants reported fears of recurrence, a second cancer diagnosis, and future diagnostic tests, 43% of their sample members stated that they had no current survivorship concerns. A notable aspect of this study, according to the authors, was that many participants reported having a positive attitude concerning their diagnosis and showed signs of growth and resilience as a result of their cancer experience.

Fear of recurrence influences the family's QOL as well. Caregivers report fear of recurrence for their family members. Other shared concerns include treatment distress, concerns over future diagnostic tests, and uncertainties about the future. Mellon and Northouse[15] found a direct relationship between family members' fear of recurrence and the family's QOL.

### DEPRESSION

Depression can manifest itself as sadness, depressed mood, insomnia, and fatigue in the cancer survivor. Overall, studies have demonstrated a depression rate between 0% and 58% in cancer survivors.[23] Depression is highly associated with a diagnosis of oropharyngeal, pancreatic, breast, and lung cancer. Lower rates have been noted in survivors of lymphoma, colon, and gynecological cancers.[23] Patients who have depression at the end of their treatment are more likely to report poorer QOL and more anxiety 6 months after treatment.[24] Depression and psychological distress in the cancer survivor may lead to poor adjustment and QOL as survivors attempt to transition their lives back to a new normal. One factor that may influence depression is the occurrence of intrusive thoughts. Cancer-related intrusive thoughts have been linked with poor psychological adjustment and QOL. Lewis et al[25] examined the link among cancer-related intrusive thoughts, QOL, and perceived social support. For women who reported high levels of social support, intrusive thoughts did not affect their QOL. However, a significant relationship was identified between cancer-related thoughts and poor QOL among women having low levels of social support. Matsuoka et al[26] further noted that intrusive thoughts and psychological adjustment persisted several years after diagnosis in cancer survivors.

Deimling and colleagues[27] explored physiological effects, psychological distress, and post-traumatic stress in cancer survivors. While acute symptoms from treatment may decline, the persistence of late and long-term physiological sequelae contribute to psychological distress. These long-term physiological effects may include lymphedema among breast cancer survivors, urinary changes in prostate cancer survivors, elimination problems in colorectal cancer survivors, and persistent dry mouth among head and neck cancer survivors.

Depression is not uncommon in the presence of late physiological effects. Deimling et al[27] found that distress was directly related to current illness symptoms, regardless of whether it was related to cancer. Individuals who continued to experience cancer-related long-term effects as well as new conditions had higher levels of depression and post-traumatic stress characteristics. Sarna et al[28] also noted a relationship between the number of comorbid conditions that lung cancer survivors experienced and their perception of QOL. The more comorbid conditions reported by participants, the poorer they rated their QOL. These results show the need for nurses and other oncology providers to acknowledge that those patients who continue to have cancer-related symptoms, even many years after treatment, are at risk for depression and psychological distress related to their current condition and may benefit from counseling.

## MEANING AND APPRAISAL

A positive aspect of long-term survivorship is the appraisal of the cancer experience and finding meaning in the experience. Many survivors find meaning in their illness through spirituality and a connection between the mind, body, and spirit.[29] Long-term survivors have had an opportunity to reflect about their cancer experience, and their appraisal can be either positive or negative. For some survivors, appraisal and meaning of illness may result in a new identity and social role.[30] Having cancer involves incorporating the experience into a sense of self and may change the way survivors view themselves. This view continues for the rest of the survivor's life. Zebrack[30] described the cancer survivor as being on a trajectory that starts with diagnosis, continues through a treatment trajectory, and then moves into a survivor trajectory. Each of these trajectories has its own experiences and challenges, and each can influence the sense of self, appraisal of the cancer experience, and perceived QOL. Bowman and colleagues[31] examined how survivors viewed the cancer experience over time and noted that appraisal of the experience changed with the passage of time. Many survivors believed that having cancer was both a stressful life event and "just part of living." Older survivors demonstrated a less stressful appraisal of the cancer experience. As the appraisal of the illness changes over time, coping may be affected in relation to perceived threats that may appear. This may, in turn, affect QOL. Threats that may be related to the cancer experience include concerns regarding employment or insurability, reproductive limitations, and reminders of the cancer experience such as follow-up tests.[30]

In studying breast cancer survivors 1 year after their diagnosis, Stanton and colleagues[32] found that women who coped by actively accepting their diagnosis had a more positive adjustment over time, whereas women who used the coping style of avoidance had greater fears of recurrence. Acceptance of the diagnosis may enable women to take an active approach toward their treatment and recovery, assisting in their adaptation to the disease.

Vachon[33] outlines several approaches to survivorship representing both positive and negative coping strategies. For some people, cancer is considered a nonissue; these people plan to return to their normal lives after treatment. Others minimize and deny the problem of cancer. Denial may result in not attending appropriate follow-up visits with healthcare providers as people try to get on with their normal lives. Still other individuals see surviving cancer as a strong part of their self-concept. Some view the experience as positive, using their experiences constructively by working as an individual advocate or as a member of a cancer group such as a support group or by becoming involved with the American Cancer Society (ACS). Other people allow their lives to revolve around the fact that they had cancer and focus on the suffering they have experienced. These patients may even be hesitant to give up their illness role. Many others see cancer as a turning point in their lives and seize the opportunity to reflect on their lives and mull over future directions. Recently, Vachon[29] provided an excellent overview of meaning, spirituality, and wellness in cancer survivorship. Essentially, as healthcare providers, we need to focus more on the whole person in survivorship, not simply on the late effects of treatment, in order to promote wellness. By recognizing the importance of the mind, body, and spirit connection, nurses are able to help develop interventions to assist survivors in finding meaning in their illness. Ferrell and colleagues[34] have also focused on spirituality and cancer survivors. Ovarian cancer survivors used their spirituality to cope, find meaning in their diagnosis, provide consolation during difficult times, and as a source of hope. In addition, spirituality allowed them to appraise their illness and see positive changes.

Whatever the evaluation, cancer has a profound impact on the lives of cancer survivors and their families. Having an understanding of patients' differing perspectives and experiences of the illness can give oncology nurses and healthcare providers the appropriate knowledge necessary to assist survivors through the experience while also assisting them to find meaning in the illness. Familiarizing nurses and healthcare professionals with the emotional and psychological aspects of illness and survivorship can facilitate interventions to assist patients in lessening distress and achieving good QOL.

In January 2004, the IOM[35] issued a report examining the psychosocial needs of women with breast cancer. Breast cancer survivors were chosen because they represent the largest group of cancer survivors and have been studied extensively. According to this report, strong data from clinical trials show that psychosocial interventions assist women with breast cancer in experiencing a better QOL; however, these measures have not been widely integrated into routine cancer care. The report recommends incorporating psychosocial services into treatment plans as an integral part of high-quality cancer care. The information contained in the report is also seen as having value in other patient populations, not just with breast cancer survivors.[36] In addition, the report urges professional organizations such as the Oncology Nursing Society, the National Cancer Institute, the American Cancer Society, and the American Society of Clinical Oncology to focus on the psychosocial needs of patients and to provide resources to meet the needs of patients on both national and local levels. Further research is needed to determine the benefits of specific interventions and the most effective way to deliver the intervention to the patient.

In summary, the vast majority of research concerning QOL, psychosocial clinical issues, and research-based interventions has been conducted in breast cancer survivors. While a few reports focus on cancer survivors in general, there is little diversity in the QOL literature. Thus, there is a great need to study cancer survivors who are dealing with other diagnoses and who might have different QOL issues related specifically to their disease and treatment. Further research concerning disease specific QOL issues might enable interventions to be designed to improve QOL for all cancer survivors.

## SPECIAL POPULATIONS OF CANCER SURVIVORS

### RURAL CANCER SURVIVORS

While a growing body of evidence demonstrates the positive and negative aspects of survivorship, these data have been obtained primarily from urban dwellers. We have few data on rural cancer survivorship, as the majority of rural research has focused on screening and prevention activities. What we do know is that rural cancer survivors report feeling poorly treated by the healthcare system and voice a strong desire for increased support and educational services.[37] A few investigators have identified positive aspects of rural cancer survivorship.[38,39]

A review of the literature on rural cancer shows that the few available studies have focused on psychosocial unmet needs after treatment. Wilson and colleagues[37] conducted focus groups with 128 cancer survivors in rural Washington state communities and explored ways to improve services to breast cancer survivors. Survivors, particularly those with advanced-stage disease, reported both positive and negative outcomes. They reported feeling poorly treated by the healthcare system and voiced a strong desire for increased support and educational services. According to the investigators, rural breast cancer survivors also needed more emotional support after the end of treatment. Braun et al[40] conducted focus groups to examine rural and urban perspectives of Native Hawaiian survivors' concerns in survivorship. Obstacles to survival included a lack of insurance, out-of-pocket costs, delayed diagnosis, and transportation issues.[40] Survival-supportive factors included personal advocacy.

Burman and Weinert[41] examined interpersonal relationships, self-image, healthcare interactions, and occupational concerns of rural men and women with cancer or with family members who had cancer. In their study, they used a mail survey that was sent to rural areas in the northern Rocky Mountain region. The sample included 294 people with cancer and 294 family caregivers in Montana. Fifty-two percent were women, and almost all were Caucasian. Results showed that women were more likely than men to report relationship problems and lack of support. People with cancer, as compared with caregivers, were more likely to report feeling alone and to say that other people avoided them and were afraid to talk to them. Men with cancer were more likely than women with cancer and caregivers to feel that their job security was threatened. However, only a small percentage of all participants felt discriminated against at work.

Burman and Weinert[42] further explored differences in cancer fears and perceptions of cancer treatment among 4 rural groups: men with cancer, men caregivers, women with cancer, and women caregivers ($N = 590$). The 4 groups differed in their cancer fears. Approximately half of the participants feared pain, nausea, body disfigurement, and sexual problems from cancer. More than two-thirds were worried about finances and decreases in QOL. They expressed more worries about separation from loved ones than worries about death.

While the few studies of rural cancer survivors emphasized the negative aspects of the illness experience, Rogers-Clark[38] found that resilience was a unique strength among rural women with breast cancer. Her findings suggest that "rurality" in the context of health and illness must be considered as a multifaceted dimension, with resources to support cancer survivors building on the existing strengths in rural communities. Similarly, Winstead-Fry and Schultz[43] found that rural residents in 2 northeastern rural states had higher QOL scores on the FACT-G compared with urban dwellers. Curran and Church[39] found that a pilot project to facilitate a self-help peer support group network using audio teleconferencing was very useful with rural breast cancer survivors.

Very few interventions are available for rural cancer survivors. Meneses and colleagues[44] reported the outcomes of a pilot study examining the feasibility of a psychoeducational support program for 53 rural breast cancer survivors. The intervention consisted of face-to-face education and support, telephone follow-up, and support. A cancer survivorship plan for self-monitoring of short- and long-term effects of therapy, psychosocial needs, and cancer surveillance were incorporated into the support and education program. The investigators found that rural breast cancer survivors can derive benefit from participating in a post-treatment survivorship care plan. Moreover, the feasibility of the intervention program would be greatly enhanced by telephone-mediated intervention delivery.

## MINORITIES AND CANCER

Tremendous cancer disparities in access to care, treatment, and survivorship services exist among racial and ethnic minorities. Data on minorities and cancer from the ACS indicate that African Americans develop cancer at a later stage and die earlier compared with any other racial or ethnic group.[45] Death rates for African American males is 37% higher as compared with Caucasian males. Likewise, death rates for African American females are 17% higher compared with Caucasian females.

Hispanics have a lower incidence of cancers combined with the exception of uterine cervix, liver, and stomach cancers.[45] Liver cancers are twice as high in both Hispanic men and women compared with non-Hispanic Caucasians. Asian Americans and Pacific Islanders have a lower incidence of most cancers with the exception of liver and stomach cancers.

The causes of cancer disparities among minorities are complex and often interrelated to socioeconomic status, income, education, standard of living, access to care, and quality of care.[45] In general, cancer disparities exist with racial and ethnic minorities in receiving quality cancer services in prevention, early detection, treatment, and follow-up. Inadequate health insurance, cultural and language barriers exist for minority cancer survivors. Poverty is a major confounder with 25% of African Americans and 22% of Hispanic/Latinos living below the poverty line compared with 11% of Caucasians.

Very few data are available to help determine the most favorable interventions to support minority cancer survivors. McInnes and colleagues[46] reported the perceptions of cancer-related information among cancer survivors. They surveyed 778 cancer survivors 3, 6, or 11 years post-treatment.[46] The investigators found that among the 462 respondents, African American cancer survivors and those who had low incomes reported more problems obtaining needed information about support groups, and long-term side effects.

## ELDERLY AND CANCER SURVIVORSHIP

Cancer is a disease of aging. More than 55% of all cancer diagnoses and 69.9% of cancer-related mortalities occur in individuals age 65 and older. At 10 years, 53.2% of these older persons will still be surviving with their cancer.[47] Older people are about to experience a population explosion. By the year 2030, it is expected that 1 in 5 people will be aged 65 or older. This age group is expected to double in number by 2050 to 88.5 million individuals. In addition, the number of people age 85 and older will triple by 2050 to include approximately 19 million individuals.[48] Given these statistics, it is fair to calculate that older persons will represent a very large group of cancer survivors.

Research involving older cancer survivors has been traditionally limited, but is now beginning to emerge. Deimling and colleagues[49] report that 26% to 44% older long-term cancer survivors experience cancer-related worries. These worries include fear of recurrence, a new cancer, future diagnostic tests, and symptoms that might indicate a recurrence. This cancer-related worry correlates with higher depression.

Physical and functional status has been studied in older cancer survivors. Elderly female cancer survivors report more functional limitations within 2 years of their diagnosis compared to older women without cancer. Women most affected had diagnoses of hematological cancer or lymphoma, kidney or urinary cancer, and lung cancer. Women with melanoma, colorectal, and endometrial cancers were the least affected. Women with breast cancer only reported slightly more limitations compared to women without breast cancer. Overall, these limitations improved over time and there were few differences in limitations between cancer survivors and women never diagnosed with cancer at 5 years.[50]

Keating and colleagues[51] compared the physical and mental health of cancer survivors, age 55 and older, to older persons who never had cancer. Findings indicate that older cancer survivors report more problems with arthritis, lung disease, heart conditions, pain, obesity, and incontinence compared to older people without a history of cancer. They were also less likely to report having very good or excellent health and more likely to report functional limitations. Interestingly, older cancer survivors reported similar mental health, levels of depression, and cognitive changes as those who never had a diagnosis of cancer. Rao and colleagues[52] provide an excellent summary of physical and psychological effects of treatment on the older cancer survivor and surmise that older survivors are more at risk for late physical and psychological effects from their treatment because of other coexisting conditions and normal declines in function status due to aging.

It is important to recognize that older cancer survivors may have different concerns and needs compared to younger cancer survivors. Interventions for older survivors have not been thoroughly developed, but evidence indicates that interventions designed to improve QOL-related issues, may have a different effect in older survivors. Loerzel and colleagues[53] reported that a psychoeducational support intervention that was previously successful in improving QOL in breast cancer survivors[54] did not improve QOL in older patients. Data shows that older breast cancer survivors experience a natural decline in QOL in the first year after treatment. The intervention designed to improve QOL, did not improve QOL, but instead slowed the decline of QOL.

Until recently, older cancer survivors have been overlooked in research. Given the number of older cancer survivors that are expected over the next 40 years, it is imperative to include older populations in research studies to discover and examine their unique survivorship needs. In addition, it is crucial to develop appropriate interventions specifically for older cancer survivors who may not respond to interventions that are effective in younger populations.

## CANCER SURVIVORSHIP CARE PLANNING

Cancer is considered a chronic condition that requires long-term disease surveillance and health promotion activities. In addition, the growing number of cancer survivors requires an additional model of health promotion long term. Until the IOM Report, published in 2006 and the subsequent follow-up of the workshop focusing on implementing cancer survivorship care planning in 2007, there were few adult models of cancer survivorship and virtually no models for survivorship care planning.[55] The Survivorship Care Plan, as outlined in the IOM Report, identified the following key elements that must be included in Survivorship Care Planning:

- Diagnosis and staging
- Treatment and treatment toxicities
- Short- and long-term effects of therapy
- Late-toxicity monitoring
- Surveillance for recurrence or second cancers
- Psychosocial and vocational needs
- Preventive behaviors/interventions.

However, widespread implementation of the survivorship care plans has not yet been realized. Many issues arise in terms of who is in the best position to create and implement the care plan, how will the care plan be delivered, and whether specialized adult cancer survivorship clinics would be most advantageous. For example, Hewitt and colleagues[56] conducted focus group and interviews with cancer survivors, nurses, primary care physicians, and oncologists to gain a perspective on post-treatment cancer care. They found that while cancer survivors reported satisfaction with post-treatment follow-up care, their psychosocial needs were not met. In general, while physicians acknowledged the value of survivorship care plans, nurses were in an ideal position to create and implement the survivorship plan.[56]

Ganz and colleagues,[57] in a review of the literature on cancer survivors, concluded that nurses have a vital role in implementing and delivering treatment summaries and cancer survivorship care plans.

## HEALTH PROMOTION AMONG CANCER SURVIVORS

### NUTRITION AND EXERCISE

Cancer survivors may benefit from additional health promoting behaviors. Long-term disease-free cancer survivors are interested in weight management through physical activity and healthy nutritional choices, and smoking cessation programs. The ACS recommendations for nutrition and physical activity during and after cancer treatment include maintaining a healthy weight throughout life, adopting a physically active lifestyle, and consuming a healthy diet that emphasizes plant sources.[58] Table 70-1 summarizes these recommendations.

In general, data support the combined use of good nutrition and exercise and resistance training for cancer survivors. A diet rich in vegetables, fruits, whole grains, and low-fat dairy products combined with exercise to preserve or increase lean muscle mass is recommended. Evidence suggests that weight gain post-treatment is associated with an increased risk of breast cancer recurrence. Thus, the need to maintain a healthy diet coupled with exercise takes on stronger importance for breast cancer survivors.[59,60]

Vallance and colleagues[61] examined the long-term effects of using pedometers and print materials on changes in physical activity in breast cancer survivors participating in a 3-month behavior change intervention. A sample of 377 breast cancer survivors were randomly assigned to a

**TABLE 70-1**

**Recommendations for a Health-Promoting Lifestyle**

- Physical activity may be beneficial for people with advanced cancer by increasing appetite and reducing constipation and fatigue.
- A standard multivitamin and mineral supplement in amounts equivalent to 100% of the daily value can help survivors meet their nutrient needs. Supplements that contain high levels of folic acid or antioxidants may be harmful during cancer treatment.
- A vegetarian diet may have health-promoting features, but no direct evidence indicates that it can prevent cancer recurrence. Survivors who eat a vegetarian diet need to ensure adequate nutrient intake.
- Alcohol can have positive and negative effects, increasing the risk of new cancers in survivors while reducing the risk of heart disease.

*Source:* Data from Doyle et al.[58]

standard public-health recommendation, a step pedometer, or a combination of the 2 interventions. Primary endpoint was self-reported moderate/vigorous physical activity minutes per week. The investigators found 10% attrition and concluded that print materials combined with pedometers may be an important strategy for increasing physical activity among breast cancer survivors.

Toles and Demark-Wahnefried[62] conducted a systematic review of reports on diet and cancer survivorship. Data continue to mount regarding the importance of weight management, and healthful diet using a plant-based, low-saturated-fat diet helps to improve overall health and promote disease-free survival in cancer survivors. The authors further suggest that nurses are well positioned to guide cancer survivors about the importance of weight management and healthful diets.

### SMOKING CESSATION

When patients with cancer smoke, they may be at increased risk for reduced survival, recurrence, and development of secondary cancers. Higher rates and longer duration of symptoms occurring during treatment (eg, loss of taste, dry mouth, impaired pulmonary function, and mucositis) are noted in patients with lung, head, and neck cancers who continue to smoke after treatment. Thus, smoking cessation during and after treatment is a high priority.[63]

Lifestyle choices of cancer survivors may influence their risk of late cardiac and pulmonary damage. Emmons and colleagues[64] examined smoking behavior among 5-year survivors in the Childhood Cancer Survival Study (CCSS) cohort. They found that 28% of patients reported ever smoking and 17% reported current smoking. While these figures are lower than the corresponding rates in the general population, they need to be reduced because of the greater risk of secondary cancers in this population. Factors that were related to the relative risk of smoking initiation included older age at cancer diagnosis, lower household income, less education, not having a pulmonary-related cancer treatment, and not having had brain radiation.

In a follow-up study, the same investigators describe baseline data collection for the Partnership for Health, a smoking cessation intervention for smokers in the CCSS.[65] Initial results showed that smokers had an average of 14 cigarettes per day, 53.2% were nicotine dependent, and 58% had made at least 1 attempt to quit smoking. Smoking behaviors were related to age at cancer diagnosis and perceived vulnerability to smoking-related illnesses.

Another study[66] evaluated the effectiveness of a nurse-managed smoking cessation intervention based on the Agency for Health Care Policy and Research's (AHCPR) smoking cessation guidelines. Subjects in the intervention group received a nurse-delivered, AHCPR-based smoking cessation intervention that included face-to-face and phone follow-up contact beginning with the first preoperative clinic consultation. The investigators found that smokers diagnosed with lung cancer wanted to quit smoking and may benefit from an intensive smoking cessation intervention implemented at the time of diagnosis.

Smoking prevention or cessation to reduce tobacco-related cardiac and pulmonary disease is another important area of health promotion for cancer survivors. Unfortunately, many young cancer survivors are not taught about the adverse health effects of smoking and the increased risks to themselves posed by smoking after cancer treatment. Smoking behaviors are related to age at cancer diagnosis and the perception that survivors are vulnerable to smoking-related illnesses. Strategies to help patients with cancer quit smoking include assessing smoking status and the survivors' readiness to quit; providing brief, supportive messages consistently over time; offering or referring patients to appropriate resources; and providing continued follow-up. In addition, the AHCPR and ACS smoking cessation guidelines can be used effectively with cancer survivors.

## SOCIAL ISSUES

### RETURNING TO WORK

The IOM's Report, "From Cancer Patient to Cancer Survivors: Lost in Transition" has made several recommendations that address employment- and insurance-related concerns of cancer survivors.[3] The IOM urges employers and other groups to eradicate discrimination of cancer survivors by working with survivors who may have short- or long-term effects from cancer that affect the survivors ability to work.

The Americans with Disabilities Act (ADA), enacted by Congress in 1990, protects individuals with disabilities, including cancer survivors, from workplace discrimination. Organizations with at least 15 employees must comply with the ADA guidelines. Cancer survivors must disclose their diagnosis to their employer to be protected by the ADA. The act also provides protection for cancer survivors when they apply for a job. In particular, it prohibits a potential employer from asking questions about an individual's health history or current health status during an interview. Cancer survivors are not required to disclose a cancer history. However, when a cancer survivor is hired and must undergo a physical examination, it is prudent to disclose one's cancer history. In companies with over 50 employees, the Family and Medical Leave Act provides the opportunity for cancer survivors to take up to 12 weeks of unpaid leave within a 12 month period to manage their own illness.[67]

In addition, the IOM is urging policy makers to ensure access to affordable and appropriate health insurance. These recommendations acknowledge the cancer survivors ability to transition from illness to survivorship and resume near-normal lives after treatment. In addition, the report acknowledges the survivors right to work, even with limitations related to their cancer. Due to improvements in early detection, screening, and treatment of cancer, it is not uncommon for cancer survivors to continue to work during treatment or return to work shortly after treatment is completed. However, working through or after treatment is difficult for survivors who are plagued with long-term side effects or lingering symptoms. At this time, employment issues receive little research attention, and issues encountered by survivors who return to work remain understudied.[68,69]

Available employment- or work-related research focuses on survivors of breast, prostate, and colorectal cancers. For those survivors that stopped working, approximately 78.4% to 92% returned to work within 2 years after treatment was completed.[70–72] Absences from work varied. Approximately 85% to over 90% of breast cancer survivors have reported being absent from work for more than a week due to having breast cancer.[70,73] These absences averaged from 6 to 7.5 months in duration.[70,73] Another study reported that breast cancer survivors missed an average of 44.5 days from work while prostate cancer survivors missed an average of 27 days from work.[74] More than 93% of breast cancer survivors and 82% of prostate cancer survivors missed at least 1 day due to their diagnosis.[74]

Longitudinal studies suggest that 6 months after diagnosis was a difficult time for many working survivors. Compared to cohorts without a history of cancer, both breast cancer and prostate cancer survivors were less likely to be working at 6 months after diagnosis. However, by 12 and 18 months, cancer survivors had the same rate of unemployment as the control groups.[75]

Factors that delayed return to work have also been examined. These include age, low income, being female, African American, partnered, lower educational level, receiving chemotherapy, life expectancy of less than 2 years, union membership, blue collar or service workers, working part time, new cancer events, and attaching less value to work.[71,72,76] Factors that aided returning to work included flexible work schedules, being able to manage side effects, support from coworkers and encouragement from their healthcare providers, and financial need.[68,77,78] Factors that hindered return to work included coworkers' ignorance about cancer and resultant side effects, physical issues such as fatigue, emotional issues and lack of support, being advised not to return to work from healthcare team, not wanting or needing to, or developing new attitudes towards work.[68,71,77,78]

Once back at work, survivors report adjustments to workload and work schedules many of which were voluntary and supported by their employer. More than 50% of survivors report reducing the number of hours worked each week. The reduction ranged from 3.3 hours to up to 7 hours per week.[72,75] Changes in work roles included less supervision of others, reduction in the number of jobs, and changing jobs or industry.[72] Some survivors did report avoiding changing jobs for fear of losing workplace insurance.[72]

## ADVOCACY

Survivorship is an ever-changing process for the cancer survivor. Reflecting on their own cancer experience and experiences of others may encourage some survivors to become advocates for others. The National Coalition for Cancer Survivorship (NCCS; http:/ /www.canceradvocacy.org/advocacy/) defines advocacy as a continuum. It can begin with self-advocacy, as the patient with cancer or a family member becomes an active participant in care. Many survivors find they become a peer advocate for others as the unofficial designated community "authority" on cancer and help others through the experience when they or a family member has been diagnosed with cancer. Support groups also create a forum for cancer survivors to advocate for one another. Many survivors benefit from hearing the experiences of others in similar situations.[79]

Advocacy can also be seen at the community level in support groups or as survivors share their experiences with friends. Also at the community level, many survivors volunteer in hospitals or cancer support organizations. Others participate in research studies or cancer awareness events such as "fun runs" and other sporting events.[79] In addition, advocacy can be found at the state and federal levels. Organizations such as the NCCS serve as the voice of cancer survivors and caregivers, assisting in the legislative process and promoting public-policy decisions that affect people with cancer. Approximately 300 organizations participate in organized efforts to effect changes and to make sure that the needs and concerns of cancer survivors are met.[79] Table 70-2 lists some Internet resources of interest to cancer survivors.

Nurses and other healthcare professionals are also in a position to be advocate partners by promoting educational programs for cancer survivors and their families and by helping to empower survivors to be advocates for themselves and make the best possible care decisions.[80] Through the involvement of special-interest groups (SIGs) such as the Oncology Nursing Society's Survivorship SIG and through the literature, nurses can learn about and support survivorship issues.

## CANCER SURVIVORSHIP RESEARCH

The NCI definition of cancer survivorship research encompasses the "physical, psychosocial, and economic sequelae of cancer diagnosis and its treatment among both pediatric and adult survivors of cancer."[81] Cancer survivorship

**TABLE 70-2**

**Internet Resources for Cancer Survivors**

- American Cancer Society provides general information for patient and survivors. 800-ACS-2345 or http://www.cancer.org
- ACS's Cancer Survivors Network provides online support and discussion for survivors. http://csn.cancer.org
- Childhood Cancer Survivors: http://www.patientcenters.com/survivors
- National Cancer Institute Office of Cancer Survivorship: dccps.nci.nih.gov/ocs/follow.html. NCI has a publication called "Facing Forward: Life after Cancer Treatment" that is available at http://www.cancer.gov/cancerinfo/life-after-treatment.
- National Coalition for Cancer Survivorship: 800-828-7866 or http://www.canceradvocacy.org. The Cancer Survival Toolbox consists of audiocassettes with basic guidelines to help navigate through survivorship and an Essential Care Resource Guide. The toolkit and the guide are available at the NCCS Web site.
- OncoChat is an online peer support for patients, families, and friends at http://www.oncochat.org/.
- Susan G. Komen Breast Cancer Foundation: 972-885-9600 or http://www.komen.org. It provides information specific to breast cancer survivors.
- Beyond the Cure: Information for survivors of childhood cancers. http://www.beyondthecure.org/
- Lance Armstrong Foundation provides cancer support for survivors. http://www.livestrong.org
- National Cancer Institute provides information for survivors about concerns after treatment and survivorship research. http://dccps.nci.nih.gov/ocs/

research programs focus on (1) chronic and late effects of cancer and its treatment; (2) intervention research; (3) healthy lifestyle and behaviors; (4) benefit finding and post-traumatic growth; and (5) impact on the family.[81]

Cancer survivorship research represents a major area of research opportunity. The majority of survivorship grants, to date, have focused on breast cancer, with a limited number targeting other high-incidence cancers such as prostate, colorectal, lung, and gynecologic cancers. A small but very important part of the NCI survivorship portfolio targets family research

The ACS conducted 2 studies of cancer survivors (SCS).[82] The first study was a longitudinal design to identify and survey survivors 1, 7, and 12 years postdiagnosis to identify predictors of QOL. The second study used a cross-sectional design of 3 survivor cohorts 3, 6, and 11 years postdiagnosis. Data were collected from 25 cancer registries that oversampled both African American and Hispanic survivors. Recruitment was 34% with more than 19% ethnically and racially diverse participants. These SCS provide important insights into the issues of ascertainment, sampling, and recruitment of cancer survivors.

## CONCLUSION

Survival rates from cancer have steadily increased over the past 35 years. The growing number of cancer survivors presents a tremendous opportunity for clinical practice, education, and research. Cancer survivors are living longer, but their long-term survival is tempered by the prospect of late effects. At the same time, these individuals are eager to learn ways to improve their health through physical activity and nutrition and to monitor their progress through cancer surveillance. This chapter provided an overview of the historical perspective of cancer survivorship, explored late psychosocial effects, described lifestyle and behavior changes for cancer survivors, and explored future challenges in cancer survivorship research.

## REFERENCES

1. Dow KH. Challenges and opportunities in cancer survivorship research. *Oncol Nurs Forum*. 2003;30:455–469.
2. Rowland JH, Aziz N, Tesauro G, et al. The changing face of cancer survivorship. *Semin Oncol Nurs*. 2001;17:236–240.
3. Institute of Medicine and National Research Council. *From Cancer Patient to Cancer Survivor: Lost in Transition*. Washington, DC: National Academies Press; 2006.
4. National Cancer Institute. Fact sheet on cancer survivorship. http://dccps.nci.nih.gov/OCS/ocs_factsheet.pdf. Accessed October 1, 2009.
5. Hewitt M, Breen N, Devesa S. Cancer prevalence and survivorship issues: analyses of the 1992 National Health Interview Survey. *J Natl Cancer Inst*. 1999;91:1480–1486.
6. Simmonds MA. Cancer statistics, 2003: further decrease in mortality rate, increase in persons living with cancer. *CA: Cancer J Clin*. 2003;53:5–26.
7. Aziz N, Rowland J. Cancer survivorship research among ethnic minority and medically underserved groups. *Oncol Nurs Forum*. 2001;29:788–801.
8. Saltzstein SL, Behling CA. 5- and 10-year survival in cancer patients aged 90 and older: a study of 37,318 patients from SEER. *J Surg Oncol*. 2002;81:113–117.
9. *SEER Cancer Incidence Public-Use Database, 1973–1998* (CDROM) [computer program]. Bethesda, MD: National Cancer Institute, DCCPS, Cancer Surveillance Research Program, Cancer Statistics Branch; April 2001.
10. Pollack LA, Greer GE, Rowland JH, et al. Cancer survivorship: a new challenge in comprehensive cancer control. *Cancer Causes Control*. 2005;16(suppl 1):51–59.
11. Dow KH, Ferrell BR, Haberman MR, Eaton L. The meaning of quality of life in cancer survivorship. *Oncol Nurs Forum*. 1999;26:519–528.
12. Zebrack BJ. Cancer survivors and quality of life: a critical review of the literature. *Oncol Nurs Forum*. 2000;27:1395–1401.
13. Hart SL, Latini DM, Cowan JE, Carroll PR. Fear of recurrence, treatment satisfaction, and quality of life after radical prostatectomy for prostate cancer. *Support Care Cancer*. 2008;16:161–169.
14. Humphris G, Ozakinci G. The AFTER intervention: a structured psychological approach to reduce fears of recurrence in patients with head and neck cancer. *Br J Health Psychol*. 2008;13:223–230.
15. Mellon S, Northouse LL. Family survivorship and quality of life following a cancer diagnosis. *Res Nurs Health*. 2001;24:446–459.
16. Wenzel LB, Donnelly JP, Fowler JM, et al. Resilience, reflection, and residual stress in ovarian cancer survivorship: a gynecologic oncology group study. *Psychooncology*. 2002;11:142–153.

17. Northouse LL, Schafer JA, Tipton J, et al. The concerns of patients and spouses after the diagnosis of colon cancer: a qualitative analysis. *J Wound Ostomy Continence Nurs.* 1999;26:8–17.
18. Ganz PA. Psychological and social aspects of cancer. *Oncology.* 2008;22:642.
19. Vickberg SM. Fears about breast cancer recurrence: interviews with a diverse sample. *Cancer Pract.* 2001;9:237–243.
20. Hodgkinson K, Butow P, Fuchs A, et al. Long-term survival from gynecologic cancer: psychosocial outcomes, supportive care needs and positive outcomes. *Gynecol Oncol.* 2007;104:381–389.
21. Vickberg SM. The concerns about recurrence scale (CARS): a systematic measure of women's fears about the possibility of breast cancer recurrence. *Ann Behav Med.* 2003;25:16–24.
22. Lyons MA, Jacobson SS, Prescott B, et al. Women's experiences during the first year following diagnosis of breast cancer. *Southern Online J Nurs Res.* 2002;3:26.
23. Massie MJ. Prevalence of depression in patients with cancer. *J Natl Cancer Inst Monogr.* 2004;32:57.
24. Deshields T, Tibbs T, Fan M, Taylor M. Differences in patterns of depression after treatment for breast cancer. *Psychooncology.* 2006;15:398–406.
25. Lewis JA, Manne SL, DuHamel KN, et al. Social support, intrusive thoughts, and quality of life in breast cancer survivors. *J Behav Med.* 2001;24:231–245.
26. Matsuoka Y, Nakano T, Inagaki M, et al. Cancer-related intrusive thoughts as an indicator of poor psychological adjustment at 3 or more years after breast surgery: a preliminary study. *Breast Cancer Res Treat.* 2002;76:117–124.
27. Deimling GT, Kahana B, Bowman KF, et al. Cancer survivorship and psychological distress in later life. *Psychooncology.* 2002;11:479–494.
28. Sarna L, Padilla G, Holmes C, et al. Quality of life of long-term survivors of non-small cell lung cancer. *J Clin Oncol.* 2002;20:2920–2929.
29. Vachon MLS. Meaning, spirituality, and wellness in cancer survivors. *Semin Oncol Nurs.* 2008;24:218–225.
30. Zebrack B. Cancer survivor identity and quality of life. *Cancer Pract.* 2000;8:238–242.
31. Bowman KF, Deimling GT, Smerglia V, et al. Appraisal of the cancer experience by older long-term survivors. *Psychooncology.* 2002;12:226–238.
32. Stanton AL, Danoff-Burg S, Huggins ME. The first year after breast cancer diagnosis: hope and coping strategies as predictors of adjustment. *Psychooncology.* 2002;11:93–102.
33. Vachon ML. The meaning of illness to a long-term survivor. *Semin Oncol Nurs.* 2001;17:279–283.
34. Ferrell BR, Smith SL, Juarez G, Melancon C. Meaning of illness and spirituality in ovarian cancer survivors. *Oncol Nurs Forum.* 2003;30:249–257.
35. Hewitt M, Herdman R, Holland J, eds. *Meeting Psychosocial Needs of Women with Breast Cancer.* Washington, DC: Institute of Medicine and National Research Council, The National Academies Press; 2004.
36. Tuma RS. IOM: psychosocial care in breast cancer improves quality of life, but more attention required. *Oncol Times.* 2004;26:7–8.
37. Wilson SE, Andersen MR, Meischke H. Meeting the needs of rural breast cancer survivors: what still needs to be done? *J Womens Health Gend Based Med.* 2000;9:667–677.
38. Rogers-Clark C. Living with breast cancer: the influence of rurality on women's suffering and resilience. A postmodern feminist inquiry. *Austral J Adv Nurs.* 2003;20:34–39.
39. Curran VR, Church JG. A study of rural women's satisfaction with a breast cancer self-help network. *J Telemed Telecare.* 1999;5:47–54.
40. Braun K, Mokuau N, Hunt G, et al. Supports and obstacles to cancer survival for Hawaii's native people. *Cancer Pract.* 2002;10:192–200.
41. Burman ME, Weinert C. Concerns of rural men and women experiencing cancer. *Oncol Nurs Forum.* 1997;24:1593–1600.
42. Burman ME, Weinert C. Rural dwellers' cancer fears and perceptions of cancer treatment. *Pub Health Nurs.* 1997;14:272–279.
43. Winstead-Fry P, Schultz A. Psychometric analysis of the functional assessment of cancer therapy-gene ral (FACT-G) scale in a rural sample. *Cancer.* 1997;79:2446–2452.
44. Meneses K, McNees P. Effectiveness of Psychoeducational Support Interventions on Quality of Life among Rural Breast Cancer Survivors. Birmingham, AL: *Proc Southern Nurs Res Soc*; 2008. [Abstract 290].
45. American Cancer Society. Cancer facts and figures. http://www.cancer.org/downloads/STT/2008CAFFfinalsecured.pdf. Accessed October 1, 2009.
46. McInnes DK, Cleary P, Stein K, et al. Perceptions of cancer-related information among cancer survivors: a report from the American Cancer Society's studies of cancer survivors. *Cancer.* 2008;113:1471–1479.
47. SEER. SEER statfact sheet. http://seer.cancer.gov/statfacts/html/all.html. Accessed December23, 2009.
48. US Census Bureau. An older and more diverse nation by midcentury. http://www.census.gov. Accessed December 23, 2009.
49. Deimling GT, Bowman KF, Sterns S, Wagner LJ, Kahana B. Cancer-related health worries and psychological distress among older adult, long-term cancer survivors. *Psychooncology.* 2006;15:306–320.
50. Sweeney C, Schmitz KH, Lazovich D, Virnig BA, Walace RB, Folsom AR. Functional limitations in elderly female cancer survivors. *J Natl Cancer Inst.* 2006;98:521–529.
51. Keating NL, Norredam M, Landrum MB, Huskamp HA, Meara E. Physical and mental health status of older long-term cancer survivors. *J Am Geriatr Soc.* 2005;53:2145–2152.
52. Rao AV, Demark-Wahnefried W. The older cancer survivor. *Crit Rev Oncol Hematol.* 2006;60:131–143.
53. Loerzel VW, McNees P, Powel LL, Su X, Meneses K. A longitudinal descriptive study of quality of life in older women with early stage breast cancer in the first year of post-treatment survivorship. *Oncol Nurs Forum.* 2008;35:924–932.
54. Meneses KD, McNees P, Loerzel VW, Su X, Zhang Y, Hassey LA. Transition from treatment to survivorship: effects of a psychoeducational intervention on quality of life in breast cancer survivors. *Oncol Nurs Forum.* 2007;34:1007–1016.
55. Institute of Medicine. *Implementing Cancer Survivorship Care Planning: Summary Workshop.* Washington, DC: National Academies Press; 2007.
56. Hewitt ME, Bamundo A, Day R, Harvey C. Perspectives on post-treatment cancer care: qualitative research with survivors, nurses and physicians. *J Clin Oncol.* 2007;25:2270–2273.
57. Ganz P, Casillas J, Hahn E. Ensuring quality care for cancer survivors: implementing the survivorship care plan. *Semin Oncol Nurs.* 2008;24:208–217.
58. Doyle C, Kushi L, Byers T, et al. Nutrition and physical activity during and after cancer treatment: an American Cancer Society guide for informed choices. *CA: Cancer J Clin.* 2006;56:323–353.
59. Thomson C, Rock C, Giuliano A, et al. Women's healthy eating and living study. *Eur J Nutr.* 2005;44:18–25.
60. Alfano C, Smith A, Irwin M, et al. Physical activity, long-term symptoms, and physical health-related quality of life among breast cancer survivors: a prospective analysis. *J Cancer Surviv.* 2007;1:116–128.
61. Vallance J, Courneya K, Plotnikoff R, Yasui Y, Mackey J. Randomized controlled trial of the effects of print materials and step pedometers on physical activity and quality of life in breast cancer survivors. *J Clin Oncol.* 2007;25:2352–2359.
62. Toles M, Demark-Wahnefried W. Nutrition and the cancer survivor: evidence to guide oncology nursing practice. *Semin Oncol Nurs.* 2008;24:171–179.
63. Demark-Wahnefried W, Pinto BM, Gritz ER. Promoting health and physical function among cancer survivors: potential for prevention and questions that remain. *J Clin Oncol.* 2006;24:5125–5131.
64. Emmons K, Li FP, Whitton J, et al. Predictors of smoking initiation and cessation among childhood cancer survivors: a report from the childhood cancer survivor study. *J Clin Oncol.* 2002;20:1608–1616.

65. Emmons KM, Butterfield RM, Puleo E, et al. Smoking among participants in the childhood cancer survivors cohort: the partnership for health study. *J Clin Oncol.* 2003;21:189–196.
66. Browning KK, Ahijevych KL, Ross P, et al. Implementing the Agency for Health Care Policy and Research's smoking cessation guideline in a lung cancer surgery clinic. *Oncol Nurs Forum.* 2000;27:1248–1254.
67. Short PF, Vargo MM. Responding to employment concerns of cancer survivors. *J Clin Oncol.* 2006;24:5138–5141.
68. Pryce J, Munir F, Haslam C. Cancer survivorship and work: symptoms, supervisor response, co-worker disclosure and work adjustment. *J Occup Rehab.* 2007;17:83–92.
69. Taskila T, Lindbohm ML. Factors affecting cancer survivors' employment and work ability. *Acta Oncol.* 2007;46:446–451.
70. Lauzier S, Maunsell E, Drolet M, et al. Wage losses in the year after breast cancer: extent and determinants among Canadian women. *J Natl Cancer Inst.* 2008;100:321–332.
71. Sanchez KM, Richardson JL, Mason HRC. The return to work experiences of colorectal cancer survivors. *AAOHN J.* 2004;52:500–510.
72. Steiner JF, Cavender TA, Nowels CT, et al. The impact of physical and psychosocial factors on work characteristics after cancer. *Psychooncology.* 2008;17:138–147.
73. Drolet M, Maunsell E, Mondor M, et al. Work absence after breast cancer diagnosis: a population-based study. *CMAJ.* 2005;173:765–771.
74. Bradley CJ, Oberst K, Schenk M. Absenteeism from work: the experience of employed breast and prostate cancer patients in the months following diagnosis. *Psychooncology.* 2006;15:739–747.
75. Bradley CJ, Neumark D, Luo Z, Schenk ML. Employment and cancer: findings from a longitudinal study of breast and prostate survivors. *Cancer Invest.* 2007;25:47–54.
76. Drolet M, Maunsell E, Brisson J, Brisson C, Masse B, Deschenes L. Not working 3 years after breast cancer: predictors in a population-based study. *J Clin Oncol.* 2005;23:8305–8312.
77. Nachreiner NM, Dagher RK, McGovern PM, et al. Successful return to work for cancer survivors. *AAOHN J.* 2007;55:290–295.
78. Kennedy F, Haslam C, Munir, Pryce F. Returning to work following cancer: a qualitative exploratory study into the experience of returning to work following cancer. *Eur J Cancer Care.* 2007;16:17–25.
79. Zebrack B. An advocate's perspective on cancer survivorship. *Semin Oncol Nurs.* 2001;17:284–287.
80. Clark EJ, Stovall EL. Advocacy: the cornerstone of cancer survivorship. *Cancer Pract.* 1996;4:239–244.
81. NCI. Research focus areas. http://dccps.nci.nih.gov/ocs/research_areas.html. Accessed October 1, 2009.
82. Smith T, Stein K, Mehta C, et al. The rationale, design and implementation of the American Cancer Society's studies of cancer survivors. *Cancer.* 2007;109:1–12.

CHAPTER 71

*Wendy Landier, RN, MSN, CPNP, CPON®, Sonia Smith, RN, MSN, ACNP-BC*

# Late Effects of Cancer Treatment

## INTRODUCTION

There are currently 11.4 million cancer survivors in the United States,[1] and 66% of adults and 80% of children currently diagnosed with cancer will survive at least 5 years.[2] Breast and prostate cancer survivors are the most numerous, with breast cancer survivors representing 23% of all cancer survivors, and prostate cancer survivors representing an additional 20%. The remaining cancer survivor population is made up of colorectal cancer survivors (10%), survivors of gynecological cancers (9%), hematological malignancies (8%), cancers of the urinary tract (7%), melanoma (7%), thyroid cancer (4%), and other cancers (11%) (Figure 71-1).[3] Recent improvements in cancer treatment and supportive care have resulted in a growing population of cancer survivors. Many cancer survivors today are living several decades beyond their diagnosis. While 66% of cancer survivors in the United States today are alive 5 or more years following their diagnosis, 30% have survived 10 or more years, and nearly 10% are alive 25 or more years following diagnosis (Figure 71-2).[1] Most cancer survivors today are expected to live for an extended period with a cancer history.[3]

As more and more patients become long-term cancer survivors, it is becoming evident that some patients are developing late complications related to their cancer treatment.[5] These long-term consequences of cancer treatment may affect the survivor's physical, psychological, and social well-being. It is therefore important for nurses to be aware of the potential late complications of treatment and of the resources needed to address the specialized ongoing needs of cancer survivors. This chapter will provide an overview of the late effects following cancer treatment in adulthood and will highlight late effects in the 2 largest groups of cancer survivors—survivors of breast and prostate cancer. In addition, key aspects of survivorship care, including development of survivorship care plans, will be addressed.

## OVERVIEW OF LATE EFFECTS FOLLOWING CANCER TREATMENT

### MEDICAL LATE EFFECTS

Many cancer treatments are associated with adverse physiological sequelae that may persist following treatment or that may first become evident weeks, months, or even years after completion of treatment. The risk of medical late effects related to cancer treatment for an individual patient depend on multiple factors, such as the specific therapies that the patient received, including therapeutic agents and cumulative doses, as well as the patient's age, health status, genetic predisposition, acute treatment-related complications, lifestyle factors, and comorbid conditions.[5]

Medical late effects of cancer therapy can potentially affect all body systems and may result from any of the major treatment modalities, including chemotherapy, radiation therapy, surgery, biotherapy, and hematopoietic stem cell transplant. Examples of late complications include anthracycline-associated cardiomyopathy,[6,7] radiation-related hypothyroidism,[8,9] and lymphedema as a consequence of surgical lymph node dissection.[10,11] A summary of potential late medical complications related to cancer therapy is presented in Table 71-1.[5,12,16]

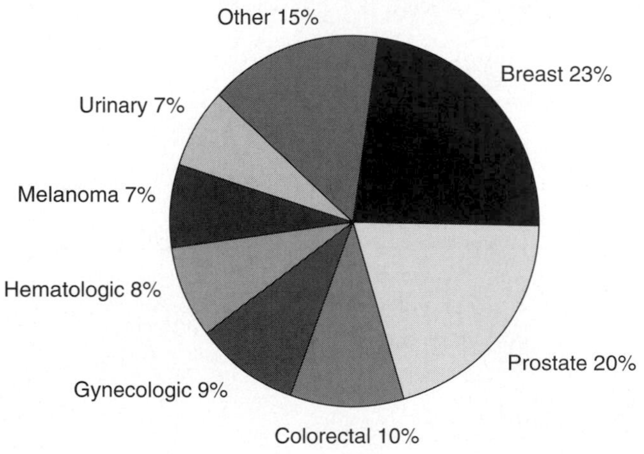


**FIGURE 71-1**

Cancer survivors by site (estimated persons alive in the United States diagnosed with cancer on January 1, 2006; $N$ = 11.4 M survivors).

*Source:* Data from American Cancer Society.[3]

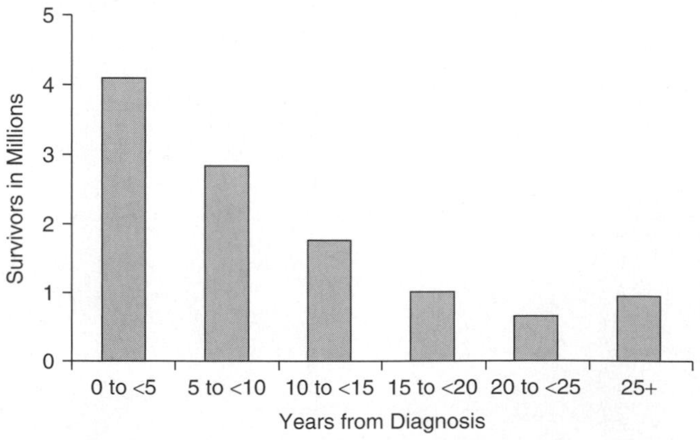


**FIGURE 71-2**

Cancer survivors by time from diagnosis (estimated number of persons alive in the United States diagnosed with cancer on January 1, 2006; $N$ = 11.4 million survivors).

*Source:* Data from Horner et al.[1]

**TABLE 71-1**

**Potential Late Effects of Selected Cancer Treatments by Organ System With Associated Monitoring**

| Organ System | Therapeutic Exposures: Chemotherapy | Radiation Therapy | Surgery | HSCT | Potential Late Effect(s) | Screening |
|---|---|---|---|---|---|---|
| Psychosocial | Any | Any | Any | Any | Depression, anxiety, posttraumatic stress disorder, limitations in health care access, alterations in body image | Psychosocial assessment |
| Ocular | Corticosteroids<br>Busulfan<br>Tamoxifen | Head/brain<br>TBI | Neurosurgery | Chronic GVHD | Cataracts, glaucoma<br>Crystal deposition of the retina (tamoxifen)<br>Retinopathy, optic nerve injury/atrophy<br>Ocular nerve palsy (surgery)<br>Xerophthalmia (radiation, GVHD) | Ophthalmology evaluation |
| Auditory | Platinum chemotherapy | Head/brain | | | Tinnitus<br>Sensorineural hearing loss<br>Conductive hearing loss<br>Eustachian tube dysfunction<br>Vestibular dysfunction/balance problems | Audiological evaluation |
| Dental | | Head/brain<br>Neck | | Chronic GVHD | Xerostomia<br>Periodontal disease<br>Dental caries | Dental exams |
| Cardiovascular | Anthracyclines<br>Trastuzumab<br>High-dose cyclophosphamide<br>Mitomycin<br>Platinum agents | Thorax | | | Congestive cardiomyopathy<br>Congestive heart failure<br>Electrical/conductive system disease<br>Pericardial disease/restrictive cardiomyopathy<br>Coronary artery disease<br>Valvular heart disease<br>Dyslipidemia (related to platinum agents) | EKG<br>Echocardiogram<br>MUGA |
| Respiratory | Bleomycin<br>Busulfan<br>Nitrosureas | Head/neck<br>Thorax<br>TBI | Head/neck surgery<br>Pulmonary lobectomy | Chronic GVHD | Upper airway sequelae<br>Pulmonary fibrosis<br>Interstitial pneumonitis<br>Restrictive/obstructive lung disease<br>Fatigue | PFT<br>CXR |

(Continued)

**TABLE 71-1**

**Potential Late Effects of Selected Cancer Treatments by Organ System With Associated Monitoring (*Continued*)**

| | Therapeutic Exposures | | | | | |
|---|---|---|---|---|---|---|
| **Organ System** | **Chemotherapy** | **Radiation Therapy** | **Surgery** | **HSCT** | **Potential Late Effect(s)** | **Screening** |
| Breast | | Thorax<br>Axilla<br>TBI | | | Radiation-induced breast cancer | Mammogram<br>Breast MRI |
| Gastrointestinal | | Head/neck<br>Abdominal<br>Pelvic | Head/neck surgery<br>Laparotomy<br>Colorectal surgery<br>Ostomy<br>Pelvic/spinal surgery | HSCT with chronic GVHD | Chronic enterocolitis<br>Diarrhea<br>GI tract strictures/fibrosis/vasculitis<br>Adhesions/fistulae/obstruction/perforation/herniae<br>Impaired swallowing<br>Anorexia<br>Impaired nutritional intake<br>Impaired gastrointestinal motility<br>Vomiting<br>Constipation<br>Impaired absorption of nutrients<br>Fecal incontinence<br>Subsequent malignancy (eg, colon cancer) | Colonoscopy |
| Hepatic | Antimetabolites | Abdominal | | HSCT | Hepatic dysfunction<br>VOD<br>Hepatic fibrosis, cirrhosis<br>Cholelithiasis<br>Iron overload (HSCT)<br>Hepatitis (related to blood product transfusions) | Liver function tests<br>Ferritin<br>Hepatitis serologies |
| Renal | Platinum agents<br>Ifosfamide<br>Methotrexate<br>Bisphosphonates<br>Nitrosureas<br>Calcineurin inhibitors (for GVHD) | Abdominal (including kidney)<br>TBI | Nephrectomy | HSCT with GVHD | Glomerular toxicity<br>Tubular dysfunction<br>Renal insufficiency<br>Hypertension<br>Radiation nephritis<br>Chronic kidney disease | Renal function tests<br>Urinalysis |

| | | | | | | |
|---|---|---|---|---|---|---|
| Bladder | Cyclophosphamide | Pelvic (including prostate and bladder)<br>Lumbar-sacral spine | Spinal surgery<br>Cystectomy<br>Prostatectomy | | Hemorrhagic cystitis<br>Bladder fibrosis<br>Dysfunctional voiding<br>Incontinence<br>Neurogenic bladder<br>Bladder malignancy | Urinalysis |
| Sexual/reproductive (males) | Alkylating agents<br>Androgen deprivation (hormonal) therapy | Hypothalamic-pituitary<br>Pelvic<br>Prostate<br>Testicular<br>TBI | Pelvic/spinal surgery<br>Orchiectomy<br>Prostatectomy | | Hypogonadism<br>Infertility<br>Erectile/ejaculatory dysfunction | FSH, LH<br>Testosterone<br>Semen analysis |
| Sexual/reproductive (females) | Alkylating agents<br>Tamoxifen<br>Aromatase inhibitors<br>Lupron | Hypothalamic-pituitary<br>Pelvic<br>Ovarian<br>Lumbar-sacral spine<br>TBI | Oophorectomy | Chronic GVHD | Premature menopause<br>Infertility<br>Uterine vascular insufficiency<br>Vaginal fibrosis/stenosis<br>Sexual dysfunction | FSH, LH<br>Estradiol |
| Endocrine/metabolic | Corticosteroids | Hypothalamic-pituitary<br>Neck (thyroid)<br>Pancreas | Thyroidectomy<br>Surgery involving the hypothalamus or pituitary<br>Surgery involving the pancreas | | Hypothyroidism<br>Adrenal insufficiency<br>Growth hormone deficiency<br>Impaired glucose tolerance<br>Thyroid nodules/cancer<br>High radiation doses<br>Hyperprolactinemia<br>Central adrenal insufficiency<br>Gonadotropin deficiency<br>Hyperthyroidism | Free T4<br>TSH<br>8:00 A.M. serum cortisol |
| Neurocognitive | Methotrexate (high dose IV, IT)<br>Cytarabine (high dose IV)<br>Adjuvant chemotherapy for breast cancer | Head/brain<br>TBI | Neurosurgery | | Neurocognitive deficits (executive function, attention, memory, processing speed, visual motor integration) | Neurocognitive testing |
| Central nervous system | Methotrexate (high dose IV, IT)<br>Cytarabine (high dose IV) | High radiation doses to head/brain/neck | Neurosurgery | | Leukoencephalopathy<br>Motor and sensory deficits<br>Cerebrovascular complications (stroke, moyamoya disease (certain arteries in the brain are constricted), occlusive cerebral vasculopathy)<br>Radiation-induced brain tumor<br>Seizures | |

(Continued)

**TABLE 71-1**

**Potential Late Effects of Selected Cancer Treatments by Organ System With Associated Monitoring (*Continued*)**

| | Therapeutic Exposures | | | | | |
|---|---|---|---|---|---|---|
| **Organ System** | **Chemotherapy** | **Radiation Therapy** | **Surgery** | **HSCT** | **Potential Late Effect(s)** | **Screening** |
| Peripheral nervous system | Vincristine<br>Vinblastine<br>Platinum agents<br>Taxanes<br>Bortezomib<br>Thalidomide<br>Oxaliplatin | High-dose radiation to brachial or lumbosacral plexus | Spinal surgery | | Peripheral sensory neuropathy (eg, paresthesias, dysesthesias, sensory loss)<br>Peripheral motor neuropathy (eg, weakness, foot drop)<br>Plexopathies | |
| Lymphatic | | Radiation involving lymphatic channels | Breast cancer surgery<br>Melanoma excision<br>Pelvic lymph node dissection<br>Axillary lymph node dissection | | Lymphedema | |
| Musculoskeletal | Corticosteroids<br>Methotrexate<br>Androgen deprivation therapy<br>Aromatase inhibitors | Pelvic/gonadal | Surgical castration<br>Bilateral oophorectomy<br>Gastrectomy | HSCT | Osteopenia/osteoporosis | DEXA scan |
| | | | Amputation<br>Limb-sparing procedures | | Functional changes<br>Postsurgical phantom pain | |
| | | | | HSCT with chronic GVHD | Joint contractures | |
| | Corticosteroids<br>Bisphosphonates | High-dose radiation to jaw | | HSCT | Osteonecrosis<br>Myopathy (proximal muscle weakness) | MRI of affected area |
| | Chemotherapy for breast and ovarian cancers | | | | Post-chemotherapy rheumatism syndrome | |
| | | All fields | | | Atrophy, deformity, fibrosis, fractures<br>Secondary benign or malignant neoplasms | X-ray of affected area |

| | | | | | | |
|---|---|---|---|---|---|---|
| Dermatologic | | All areas | | Chronic GVHD | Dysplastic nevi<br>Vitiligo<br>Scleroderma<br>Nail dysplasia<br>Alopecia<br>Skin cancer | |
| Hematologic | Anthracyclines<br>Epipodophyllotoxins<br>Aklylating agents<br>Stem cell priming with etoposide | | | Autologous transplantation for non-Hodgkin's or Hodgkin's lymphoma | Acute myeloid leukemia<br>Myelodysplastic syndrome (associated with alkylating agents) | CBC with differential |
| Immunologic | | Abdomen, left upper quadrant, spleen (high doses) | Splenectomy | Chronic active GVHD | Life-threatening infection related to functional or anatomic asplenia | |

*Abbreviations*: CBC, complete blood count; CXR, chest x-ray; DEXA, dual energy x-ray absorptiometry; EKG, electrocardiogram; FSH, follicle stimulating hormone; GI, gastrointestinal; GVHD, graft-vs-host disease; Gy, gray; HSCT, hematopoietic stem cell transplant; IT, intrathecal; IV, intravenous; LH, luteinizing hormone; MRI, magnetic resonance imaging; MUGA, multigated acquisition scan; PFT, pulmonary function testing; TBI, total body irradiation; TSH, thyroid stimulating hormone; VOD, veno-occlusive disease.
*Source*: Data from Miller and Triano[5]; Aziz[12]; the Children's Oncology Group[13]; Tichelli and Socie[14]; Ganz[15]; and Stricker and Jacobs.[16]

Of note, as cancer survivors age, new problems may be identified over time, and these late effects may represent the interaction of previous treatment and normal aging. In addition, the potential long-term effects of many of the newer agents used in contemporary cancer treatment, such as monoclonal antibodies and small molecule inhibitors, are currently unknown and may become evident over time.[5]

## PSYCHOSOCIAL LATE EFFECTS

The period following completion of active cancer treatment carries with it the risk for late adverse psychosocial sequelae. Many survivors experience significant fear related to potential cancer recurrence, which may manifest as a constant sense of worry and foreboding.[17] This "recurrence anxiety" is generally most intense during the first year following treatment and generally diminishes over time, but may resurface periodically at times of health surveillance or when unusual somatic symptoms occur.[18] Although the majority of cancer survivors experience depressed mood or acute stress reactions during the course of their treatment, intense psychological distress generally resolves within the first 2 years following diagnosis, and most cancer survivors do not go on to experience long-term psychological distress.[19] However, cancer survivors appear to be at higher risk for depression and anxiety than those who have never had cancer.[20,21]

Survivors at highest risk for psychological difficulties include those with chronic physical health problems and those with chronic pain.[20] In addition, survivors with visible manifestations of their cancer treatment, such as urinary incontinence related to prostate cancer, disfigurement and speech or swallowing difficulties related to head and neck cancer, or other alterations in body image, may be reluctant to engage in social activities, placing them at risk for social isolation.[22] However, not all survivors experience adverse psychosocial consequences related to their cancer treatment. For some, the challenge of cancer sets the stage for posttreatment psychological growth and acknowledgement of a deeper appreciation for life as a result of the cancer experience.[18,23]

In addition to facing psychological challenges following completion of therapy, cancer survivors may experience financial and employment-related difficulties. A recent meta-analysis of more than 20,000 cancer survivors determined that cancer survivors were more likely to be unemployed than healthy controls, and survivors of breast and gastrointestinal cancers were found to be at highest risk of unemployment.[24]

Long-term sequelae of cancer treatment may differ depending on the patient's age and life stage at diagnosis and treatment. Younger patients in their reproductive years may be affected by concerns regarding loss of fertility, stressors related to employment (eg, missed work days), financial issues related to treatment, and planning for an uncertain future. Older patients must often cope with multiple comorbidities related to aging, as well as social challenges, such as retirement, fixed income, physical frailty, suboptimal nutrition, death of peers, social isolation, and limited access to care.[12]

A psychosocial evaluation is a valuable component of care for cancer survivors. Survivors with anxiety, depression, or other psychological difficulties and survivors experiencing distress as a result of problems with employment, finances, or other psychosocial concerns should be referred for professional services with a mental health professional or social services provider in order to optimize well-being and quality of life. Not all survivors require professional mental health services. Survivors with mild symptoms may benefit from educational materials explaining common emotional symptoms related to the cancer experience, support groups, or telephone counseling.[18,20]

## IDENTIFYING LATE EFFECTS IN CANCER SURVIVORS

Regular monitoring for late complications of cancer treatment is important in order to permit early identification of problems, provide for early intervention, and promote preventive strategies (eg, smoking cessation, weight control) aimed at reducing the risk of developing late complications. Currently, there is no consensus regarding routine follow-up care for adult cancer survivors[25]; however, the Children's Oncology Group has developed systematic risk-based follow-up guidelines for childhood cancer survivors. (*Long-Term Follow-Up Guidelines for Survivors of Childhood, Adolescent, and Young Adult Cancers*, [http://www.survivorshipguidelines.org]).[13,26] In addition, the European Group for Blood and Marrow Transplantation, the Center for International Blood and Marrow Transplant Research, and the American Society of Blood and Marrow Transplantation have developed joint guidelines for survivors of hematopoietic cell transplantation (*Recommended Screening and Preventive Practices for Long-term Survivors after Hematopoietic Cell Transplantation*).[27]

The American Society of Clinical Oncology (ASCO) expert panel has released recommendations for the posttreatment follow-up of breast[28] and colorectal cancer[29] survivors; however, these guidelines are limited to recommendations for disease surveillance and do not offer guidance regarding monitoring for therapy-related complications. A task force within ASCO has been assigned to develop guidelines on topics related to survivorship care, including fertility preservation,[30] and surveillance for second malignancies, cardiac late effects, osteoporosis, and other reproductive health effects.[31]

Most current models for cancer follow-up care focus on disease surveillance. However, because long-term complications develop as a result of therapeutic intervention (ie, chemotherapy, radiation therapy, surgery, hormonal therapy), a model for long-term follow-up that is driven by screening for exposure-related adverse events and targeted health promotion may be more advantageous in delivering optimal follow-up care. Important components of follow-up care include surveillance for cancer recurrence, identification of therapy-related medical and psychosocial late effects, facilitation of rehabilitation and reintegration into normal activities, maintenance of general health, implementation of health-promotion strategies, and provision of a written survivorship care plan.[25,32–35] Several recent reviews provide additional guidance aimed at directing more comprehensive posttreatment follow-up care for cancer survivors.[14,22,36–39]

Long-term follow-up evaluations should generally include a detailed history and physical examination, with special attention to body areas and organs at risk for toxicity from the cancer treatment. Additional monitoring beyond the history and physical examination, such as radiographic evaluation of bone density (eg, dual energy X-ray absorptiometry[DEXA scan]) for survivors at risk for osteopenia or osteoporosis,[40] should be done as indicated on the basis of the specific treatment that each patient received and the associated risk for late effects, taking into consideration the patient's age, general health status, comorbidities, and genetic risk factors. Screening evaluations that have been suggested for detecting late complications in cancer survivors are presented in Table 71-1.

## LATE EFFECTS IN SPECIFIC POPULATIONS OF CANCER SURVIVORS

### BREAST CANCER SURVIVORS

Breast cancer is currently the most commonly diagnosed noncutaneous cancer in women in the US. There are currently approximately 2.5 million breast cancer survivors in the US, representing 43% of all female cancer survivors.[1] Although the vast majority of breast cancer survivors are female, breast cancer incidence in males is about 1 per 100,000, and male breast cancer survivors require specialized consideration of their unique follow-up needs.[41] The median age at diagnosis of breast cancer is currently 61 years of age; 10.5% of women with breast cancer are diagnosed between the ages of 35 and 44, 22.5% between the ages of 45 and 54, 23.7% between the ages of 55 and 64, 19.6% between the ages of 65 and 74, and 21.7% at age 75 or older.[1] Approximately 60% of women who are diagnosed with breast cancer today have localized disease, 33% have regional spread beyond the primary site or to the lymph nodes, and 5% have metastatic disease at diagnosis.[1] Five-year relative survival rates are currently 98.3% for localized disease, 83.5% for regional disease, and 23.3% for metastatic disease.[1] Understanding the unique late effects facing breast cancer survivors is therefore important in order to provide appropriate medical follow-up care for this rapidly growing population of survivors.

Contemporary treatment for breast cancer is complex and multimodal, requiring the involvement of multiple health care providers, including surgeons, radiation oncologists, medical oncologists, and oncology nurses. Treatment may include a variety of procedures, such as breast-conserving surgery, mastectomy, sentinel node biopsy, axillary lymph node dissection, breast reconstruction, chemotherapy (neoadjuvant or adjuvant), targeted therapy (eg, trastuzumab), radiation therapy, and endocrine therapy. Unfortunately, breast cancer treatment may result in late effects that can adversely impact health and quality of life. Sequelae may include persistent postsurgical pain,[42] lymphedema,[11,43] restricted arm motion or weakness, premature menopause, infertility,[44] menopausal symptoms,[45] fatigue,[46] mood disorders, sexual dysfunction, alteration in body image, impaired cognitive performance,[47,48] bone loss,[40] disease recurrence, development of contralateral breast cancer, and development of uterine cancer in women taking tamoxifen.[49] Rare but serious sequelae include secondary leukemia and cardiac complications.[6,36,50] The risk of late complications varies depending on each patient's age at diagnosis, stage of disease, treatment received, health status, comorbidities, and genetic predisposition. Follow-up care should include surveillance for recurrence, monitoring and intervention for therapy-related sequelae, and psychosocial support.[25,36,37]

#### Surgical sequelae

Complications related to breast cancer surgery are dependent on the surgical approach used. Lymphedema may occur following mastectomy or axillary node dissection, and occurs an average of 20% to 30% of the time, with rates ranging from 10% to nearly 50%.[22] In a cohort of patients treated with mastectomy and complete axillary node dissection in the 1970s, 20 years after surgery, 49% of patients reported lymphedema; 77% of those patients noted the onset within 3 years of surgery, with the remainder developing lymphedema at a rate of 1% per year.[43] Among patients who have undergone sentinel lymph node biopsy alone, the incidence of lymphedema has been reported to be as low as 3%,[11] with a 17% incidence among patients having an initial sentinel lymph node biopsy followed by axillary dissection. About 30% of women after surgery for breast cancer complain of phantom pain, numbness, or decreased movement in the arm[51]; these problems have been reported to persist up to 5 years following the surgical procedure.[42] In addition, patients who have undergone axillary lymph node resection may experience persistent pain, particularly if they have also received radiation therapy to the axillary area.[22]

### Sequelae related to radiation therapy

Cardiotoxicity related to radiation therapy for the treatment of breast cancer has been reported in patients who received therapy with older radiation techniques.[52] A recent study indicated that women treated with more contemporary radiation therapy techniques dating from the 1980s, particularly those who received radiation therapy to the internal mammary lymph node chains and to the left chest wall, may be at increased risk for cardiovascular disease and that this risk may not become manifest until 10 or more years following treatment.[53] The risk of cardiotoxicity is increased for patients receiving higher cumulative doses of doxorubicin (240 mg/m$^2$ or greater) in combination with radiation therapy.[52]

### Sequelae related to chemotherapy and endocrine therapy

Premature menopause is an issue for younger women with breast cancer.[54] Almost all women will develop amenorrhea during adjuvant chemotherapy; some of these women will go on to develop ovarian failure, while others may resume their menstrual cycles but remain at risk for premature menopause. Younger women with therapy-induced menopause are at higher risk for severe vasomotor symptoms (hot flashes) and sexual dysfunction.[55]

Menopausal symptoms may be related to premature onset of menopause in younger women, as well as endocrine therapy (eg, tamoxifen, aromatase inhibitors) in women of all ages. Symptoms may include hot flashes, night sweats, vaginal dryness or discharge, dyspareunia, mood swings, weight gain, and sexual dysfunction.

The risk of bone loss increases with age. While tamoxifen may protect against bone loss, treatment with aromatase inhibitors may exacerbate this problem.[56] Additional risk factors for bone loss include treatment-induced menopause, family history of osteoporosis, and body weight less than 70 kg.[40]

Cardiovascular toxicity in women who are treated for breast cancer may include left ventricular dysfunction leading to congestive heart failure after anthracycline chemotherapy or trastuzumab,[6] or thromboembolic events and hyperlipidemia related to endocrine therapy.[52] Women taking tamoxifen are at increased risk for pulmonary embolism.[22]

Cognitive dysfunction, sometimes referred to as "chemo brain," has been reported in up to 30% of patients treated with adjuvant chemotherapy for breast cancer.[57] Symptoms may include problems with concentration, forgetfulness, distractibility, and a general lack of mental sharpness ("mental fogginess").[47] However, recent concern has been expressed regarding the considerable variability in study results and the subtlety of findings to date. Further research is needed in order to better identify and define the neurocognitive deficits associated with adjuvant therapy for breast cancer and to identify risk factors associated with development of this complication.[48]

### Long-term follow-up care for breast cancer survivors

Optimal long-term follow-up for breast cancer survivors should address specific physical and psychosocial needs of this population. Care should include surveillance for recurrence of the primary cancer and secondary malignancies (therapy-related, or occurring as a result of genetic predisposition), assessment of genetic susceptibility to cancer and the potential need for genetic screening (for early detection or prevention of subsequent cancers in the patient or family members), monitoring and intervention for disease-related and treatment-related sequelae, and psychosocial follow-up and support.[22]

Current literature supports the importance of surveillance for recurrence following a diagnosis of breast cancer[22,28,38,58] and the need to address physiological alterations, psychosocial problems, therapy-related complications, secondary malignancies, genetic counseling, and testing as indicated, on the basis of the needs of each survivor.[22,38,49,59] Attention to age and life stage is important in planning follow-up care for breast cancer survivors, as some issues relevant to younger survivors (eg, fertility) may differ from those relevant to older survivors (eg, comorbid conditions related to aging).[12]

## PROSTATE CANCER SURVIVORS

Prostate cancer is the most commonly diagnosed noncutaneous cancer in American males. Currently there are 2.1 million prostate cancer survivors in the US, representing 45% of all male cancer survivors.[60] The median age at diagnosis for cancer of the prostate is currently 68 years of age, and 86.1% of men diagnosed with prostate cancer are between the ages of 45 and 74.[60] In more than 90% of cases, patients are diagnosed with asymptomatic, clinically localized prostate cancer, and 5-year relative survival rates for localized prostate cancer now approach 100%.[60] During the past 25 years, survival rates for all stages of prostate cancer combined have increased from 69% to 99%; the relative 10-year survival rate is now 91%, and 15-year survival is now 76%.[1]

The advent of prostate-specific antigen (PSA) screening has led to an increase in the number of younger men undergoing treatment for prostate cancer.[61] These patients are often better informed of the many treatment options and consequently more likely to request a second opinion. The patient and his family will select from state-of-the art treatment for prostate cancer, including minimally invasive radical prostatectomy (MIRP) such as laparoscopic radical prostatectomy (LRP) and robotic-assisted laparoscopic prostatectomy (RALP);[62] as well as improved methods for precise delivery of radiotherapy, such as helical TomoTherapy, intensity modulated radiotherapy (IMRT), and brachytherapy. Androgen deprivation (hormonal) therapy (ADT) and watchful waiting may also be considered.

Unfortunately, prostate cancer and the therapy required for its treatment can result in a multitude of physical and psychosocial challenges impacting health and quality of survivorship.[63,64] Examples of long-term sequelae include urinary complications (incontinence, urinary leakage, obstructive or irritative voiding symptoms, and stricture), sexual dysfunction (loss of libido, erectile dysfunction [ED], and possible alteration in penile morphology),[65–68] bowel complications (fecal incontinence, proctitis, enteritis), disease recurrence, psychological effects (anxiety, depression, mood swings), vasomotor symptoms, osteopenia and osteoporosis, and risk for developing metabolic syndrome, cardiovascular disease, insulin resistance, and subsequent malignancies.[38,39,69–75] The risk of these sequelae varies for individual men according to the stage of their disease and treatment received.[38]

Every treatment for prostate cancer has the potential to affect quality-of-life domains associated with sexual, urinary, bowel, and hormonal function. Intensity modulated radiotherapy offers the potential to deliver higher radiation doses to the prostate without greater gastrointestinal toxicity and with a decrease in rectal bleeding compared with conventional 3-dimensional conformal radiation therapy (3D-CRT) using the higher conformal dose.[76] While data with MIRP and nerve-sparing preservation are encouraging in mitigating the adverse sexual and urinary side effects, long-term follow-up data are needed to delineate the oncologic outcomes and long-term side effects of these surgical approaches.[62,63,73,77,78] The high survival rates coupled with typically long survival periods following prostate cancer treatment raise issues for patients and their families regarding optimizing their quality of life. Due to the potential impact of therapy-related sequelae on quality of life in men who have undergone treatment for prostate cancer, optimal long-term follow-up must incorporate care that addresses both the physical and psychosocial needs of prostate cancer survivors.

Follow-up care for prostate cancer should include surveillance for recurrence of the primary cancer, monitoring and intervention for disease-related and therapy-related sequelae, and psychosocial follow-up and support.[25,39] Current literature supports the importance of surveillance for recurrence following prostate cancer,[38,39,69,79] as well as the need to address therapy-related complications and psychosocial problems for each survivor on the basis of individual needs.[25,38,39]

### Sexual dysfunction

Sexual health is the experience of the ongoing process of physical, psychological, and sociocultural well-being related to sexuality.[80] With increased screening and consumer awareness, the median age of men diagnosed with prostate cancer has declined in recent years. In men who have undergone radical prostatectomy (RP), erectile dysfunction is a long-term and sometimes permanent side effect that must be confronted, even when maximal cavernous nerve-sparing techniques are applied.[81] Studies of sexual health outcomes after RP have consistently shown a significant correlation between sexual function and quality of life.[82–85]

Men who have undergone RP have a higher incidence of sexual dysfunction than age-matched controls.[86–88] Nerve-sparing procedures have improved postoperative potency rates, yet anecdotal complaints of penile size loss are increasingly reported.[89,90] Penile morphology may change following non-nerve-sparing prostatectomy or nerve-sparing prostatectomy, and changes appear to be more severe in patients with the greatest degree of ED. Penile rehabilitation (reviewed next) may provide long-term functional improvement; however, the current evidence is insufficient to show that rehabilitation stops morphological changes or loss of penile length.[67,91,92]

Rates of impotence (defined as erections insufficient for intercourse) have been reported to range from 14% to 87% in men assessed 10 months to 2 years following RP,[85,93] with the lowest rates of impotence reported in large medical centers with experienced surgeons who use nerve-sparing procedures.[81,93,94] Patient age, degree of cavernosal nerve sparing during surgery, cancer stage, and associated vascular comorbidities are all factors impacting postoperative potency.[65,95] Radiation treatment frequently leads to a steady decline in erectile function, thereby significantly impacting potency.[96] Postprostatectomy sequelae for ED may be related to surgical trauma (neural and vascular injury), psychosocial factors (depression, anxiety, and relationship circumstances), and comorbidities (eg, cardiovascular disease, diabetes).[25,38,39]

*Management of sexual dysfunction.* Permanent ED remains an important issue in prostate cancer survivors, and ED has a significant impact on health-related quality of life. The complete loss of sexual functioning as a result of RP has led medical professionals to develop programs for erectile rehabilitation.[81,97] This new concept for improving erectile outcome stemmed from the idea that early induced blood flow to the penis may facilitate the return of natural erectile function.[80,98] The American Urological Association has developed evidence-based guidelines to assist in treatment decision making regarding ED in men with localized prostate cancer and recommends that interventions be implemented in a stepwise fashion, with the likelihood for efficacy balanced against increasing invasiveness and risk.[94,99] Oral treatment with phosphodiesterase type 5 inhibitors (PDE5-Is) currently represents first-line treatment. Second-line treatments include the use of vasoactive medications and the external vacuum device (vacuum erection device). Vasoactive medications include the intraurethral suppository alprostadil and intracavernosal injections (ICIs) (alprostadil and vasoactive drug mixtures), and are believed to improve cavernous oxygenation, thereby limiting the development of hypoxia-induced tissue damage.[100] The external vacuum device works by generating a negative pressure leading to penile engorgement. Although efficacy rates and overall acceptance of intraurethral, intracavernosal, and vacuum erection devices are high, long-term compliance has been problematic, leading to high dropout rates. Reasons for dissatisfaction include poor treatment response, adverse side effects, and patient complaints that treatments lack spontaneity.[81] Third-line treatment is surgical implantation of penile prostheses, and is reserved for patients who do not respond to ICI or in whom ICI is not an acceptable form of treatment.[101]

## Urinary dysfunction

*Incontinence.* Problems with urinary control following RP have been widely reported, with incontinence rates ranging from 3% to 74% for RP, 0% to 61% for interstitial prostate brachytherapy, and 0% to 73% for external beam radiotherapy.[94] Most surgically treated men will experience transient urinary incontinence.[21,87,93,94] Postoperative outcomes for improved continence are multifactorial and depend on preoperative functions. Factors influencing outcome include age, surgical preservation of neurovascular bundles, absence of anastomotic stricture, preservation of the functional urethral length, eversion of the bladder neck, and smaller prostate volume.[65] Urinary control problems can range from less than total control to complete incontinence. Although most men experience improvement in their symptoms over time, some men have persistent urinary control problems. Symptoms persisting 2 or more years following surgery are likely to be permanent.[73]

*Other urinary sequelae.* Bladder neck contracture may occur as a late complication in a small minority of patients who undergo prostatectomy regardless of surgical approach.[102,103] Irritative voiding symptoms such as urinary frequency and urgency, and obstructive symptoms such as straining and decreased urine flow, may increase shortly after external beam therapy, yet will return to pretreatment levels by 1 to 2 years after treatment.[73]

*Management of urinary dysfunction.* For many patients, urinary incontinence can be a devastating complication of RP. Evaluation and management of non-obstructive post-prostatectomy urinary incontinence should include urodynamics and cystoscopy to address the possible reason for the dysfunction. Studies have demonstrated that early treatment has a significant positive impact on the return of urinary continence, with persistent improvements in the first 18 months after prostate surgery.[103,104]

Urinary incontinence due to sphincter insufficiency should be treated with early intervention involving physical therapy and biofeedback. Kegel exercises should be taught and reinforced after Foley catheter removal.[105] Patients with urinary incontinence due to sphincter insufficiency can be offered noninvasive treatment options such as condom catheters or urethral clamps. Injection of collagen into the periurethral space will increase sphincter competence, reducing leakage of urine. With this procedure more than 50% of men become continent; however, the effects are not long term. The best results for severe incontinence are obtained via placement of an artificial urinary sphincter (AUS).[104] Litwiller et al[106] reported 90% patient satisfaction with the artificial sphincter for postprostatectomy incontinence. Irritative and obstructive symptoms following radiation therapy may be improved with medications. Most men receive alpha-blockers, such as tamsulosin or terazosin,[107] or anticholinergics for several weeks during and after radiation therapy for the management of prostate cancer. As symptoms decrease, these medications are gradually withdrawn.[65]

## Bowel-related complications

Bowel dysfunction has been reported following RP; the incidence varies and depends on surgical methods.[65,102] Patients who receive radiation therapy are more likely to develop bowel dysfunction than those who undergo surgical treatment for prostate cancer. Typically 25% to 50% of men who receive external beam radiation therapy report long-term problems with bowel function, particularly diarrhea, bowel urgency, fecal incontinence, hemorrhoids,[86,94] and general decline in bowel function.[108] The most severe dysfunction generally occurs within the first 4 to 6 months following radiation treatment, with some function recovered by 3 years, thereafter often resolving slowly, reflecting some recovery of functional loss.[65,109] The majority of mild to moderate symptoms are treated effectively with simple dietary changes, especially increase in fiber intake, hydrocortisone suppositories, or foam application to the rectal area.[65]

### Hormonal-related complications

Androgen deprivation (hormonal) therapy is commonly used for patients for whom definitive treatment with surgery or radiation is not possible or acceptable. ADT is used routinely in conjunction with definitive radiation therapy in patients with high-risk clinically localized disease, locally advanced disease, or metastatic disease.[73,94] Androgen deprivation can be achieved with bilateral orchiectomy (surgical castration) or medical castration (luteinizing hormone–releasing hormone [LH-RH] agonists), antiandrogen (androgen blockade), or combined androgen blockade (CAB) (LH-RH agonist plus an antiandrogen).

Men who receive ADT may experience a constellation of symptoms and physical sequelae potentially impacting their long-term health. Sequelae associated with LH-RH agonists include diminished or absent libido, ED, vasomotor symptoms, fatigue, weight gain, depression, and decreased bone mineral density.[64,110] Sequelae associated with antiandrogen therapy include gynecomastia, nipple tenderness, liver toxicity, and gastrointestinal problems (abdominal pain, diarrhea, constipation, nausea, vomiting, and anorexia).[111–113] Additional symptoms and physical sequelae associated with hormonal therapy for prostate cancer may include adverse body composition (such as decreased lean body mass), insulin resistance, diabetes, cardiovascular disease, dyslipidemia,[65,114,115] mood swings, anxiety, insomnia, problems with memory and concentration, perceptions of decreased masculinity, decreased body hair, testicular atrophy, anemia, weakness, and sarcopenia (loss of skeletal muscle mass).[112]

***Osteopenia and osteoporosis.*** Men who receive ADT are at risk for potentially debilitating complications related to decreased bone mineral density, which may lead to adverse skeletal events. The bone loss associated with ADT for prostate cancer is accelerated over that associated with normal aging.[113] Strategies to improve bone mineral density include proper nutrition, healthy lifestyle (smoking cessation, moderate alcohol intake: for most men this means 2 or fewer alcoholic drinks per day), and regular weight-bearing and resistance exercises.[113,116,117] The National Institutes of Health recommends dietary calcium intake for adults age 50 and older at 1200 to 1500 mg/day,[116] and the National Osteoporosis Foundation recommends supplemental vitamin D intake at 800 to 1000 IU daily.[118] Bisphosphonate therapy may also be indicated for men with bone metastasis related to prostate cancer and for those with ADT treatment–related osteoporosis.[73,113]

***Other hormonal-related sequelae.*** Androgen deprivation therapy and orchiectomy result in profound hypogonadism.[116] The resultant decrease in testosterone due to ADT may lead to changes in body composition, hyperlipidemia, insulin resistance, metabolic syndrome, and coronary artery disease.[74,75,115,119] Health care professionals should routinely monitor patients treated with ADT for signs and symptoms of metabolic syndrome, diabetes, osteoporosis, and coronary artery disease, and should counsel these patients regarding healthy lifestyle choices.[114,119]

Fatigue as a result of prostate cancer treatment is often multifactorial and may significantly impact quality of life.[120] Increased rates of fatigue have been reported in men receiving ADT.[45] Changes in body composition, particularly decreased lean body mass, may contribute to treatment-related fatigue that may be associated with depression[121] or anemia.[122]

## OTHER CANCER SURVIVOR POPULATIONS

Late effects of therapy for other populations of cancer survivors, including those surviving colorectal cancer, head and neck cancers, gynecological malignancies, renal, bladder, or testicular cancers, lung cancer, and hematological malignancies, are specific to the types of therapy received.[16,123] Therefore, the follow-up needs of these survivors may differ widely. For example, a survivor of colorectal cancer may be at risk for issues related to bowel function, including bowel obstruction related to surgical adhesions, difficulties with adjustment to ostomy care, persistent radiation-related diarrhea, and incontinence or sexual dysfunction related to surgery or radiation therapy.[22] In contrast, a survivor of a hematological malignancy whose treatment involved allogeneic hematopoietic stem cell transplant may be at risk for problems related to graft-vs-host disease, such as functional asplenia with its attendant risk for life-threatening infection.[27] In addition to providing monitoring and intervention for potential therapy-related late effects, surveillance for cancer recurrence is an integral part of the follow-up plan for cancer survivors. Table 71-2 summarizes potential late effects and surveillance strategies for the most common types of adult cancers.

## SECONDARY MALIGNANCIES IN CANCER SURVIVORS

Some cancer survivors are at increased risk for secondary malignancies as a result of previous exposure to radiation

**TABLE 71-2**

**Potential Late Effects and Surveillance Strategies for the Most Common Types of Adult Cancers**

| Cancer Type | Common Late Effects | Common Disease Surveillance Strategies |
|---|---|---|
| Bladder cancer | Incontinence<br>Impotence | Cystoscopy<br>Urinary cytology |
| Breast cancer | Lymphedema<br>Restricted arm motion or weakness<br>Premature menopause<br>Menopausal symptoms<br>Cognitive dysfunction<br>Bone loss<br>Cardiovascular toxicity<br>Therapy-related myelodysplasia or leukemia<br>Alteration in body image | Clinical breast exam<br>Mammography |
| Cervical cancer | Incompetent cervix<br>Infertility | Pelvic exam<br>Pap smears |
| Colorectal cancer | Bowel dysfunction<br>Fecal incontinence<br>Chronic diarrhea<br>Bladder dysfunction<br>Sexual dysfunction | Colonoscopy<br>CEA |
| Endometrial cancer | Infertility<br>Sexual dysfunction | Pap smear<br>CA-125 |
| Head/neck cancers | Speech difficulties<br>Dysphagia<br>Dental caries<br>Mandibular dysfunction<br>Problems with body image related to disfigurement | CT scans<br>Chest x-ray<br>Endoscopy<br>Dental exam |
| Hodgkin's lymphoma | Fatigue<br>Cardiac dysfunction<br>Pulmonary dysfunction<br>Hypothyroidism<br>Radiation-related secondary malignancies (eg, breast, thyroid)<br>Life-threatening infection (in splenectomized patients) | CT/PET scans<br>X-ray<br>Tumor markers (eg, LDH, ESR) |
| Leukemia | Cognitive dysfunction (related to cranial radiation)<br>Infertility<br>Cardiac dysfunction (related to anthracyclines)<br>Avascular necrosis<br>Bone loss<br>Peripheral neuropathy | CBC |

| | | |
|---|---|---|
| Lung cancer | Dyspnea and pulmonary impairment<br>Cognitive dysfunction (related to prophylactic cranial radiation)<br>Fatigue<br>Post-thoracotomy pain syndrome | Chest x-ray<br>CT scans |
| Non-Hodgkin's lymphoma | Cognitive dysfunction (related to cranial radiation)<br>Infertility<br>Cardiac dysfunction (related to anthracyclines)<br>Avascular necrosis<br>Bone loss<br>Peripheral neuropathy | CT/PET scans |
| Ovarian cancer | Infertility<br>Ototoxicity<br>Nephrotoxicity<br>Peripheral neuropathy | Pelvic exam<br>CA-125 |
| Prostate cancer | Sexual dysfunction<br>Urinary incontinence<br>Bowel dysfunction<br>Hormonal-related sequelae | PSA |
| Testicular cancer | Gonadal toxicity<br>Peripheral neuropathy<br>Nephrotoxicity<br>Cardiovascular toxicity | Tumor marker (eg, hCG, AFP)<br>Chest x-ray |

*Abbreviations*: AFP, alpha fetoprotein; CA-125, cancer antigen 125; CBC, complete blood count; CEA, carcinoembryonic antigen; CT, computerized tomography; ESR, erythrocyte sedimentation rate; hCG, human chorionic gonadotropin; LDH, lactate dehydrogenase; Pap, Papanicolaou; PET, positron emission tomography; PSA, prostate specific antigen.
*Source*: Data from Kattlove and Winn[22]; Ganz[123]; and Fischer.[136]

therapy or chemotherapeutic agents during treatment for their primary malignancy. The risk of individual cancer survivors developing secondary malignancies varies and is dependent on such factors as gender, hormonal status, age at time of initial cancer treatment, cumulative dose of radiation, type of chemotherapy received and its cumulative dose, time since initial cancer treatment, exposure to environmental carcinogens, immune status, and genetic predisposition.[124]

Breast cancer survivors may develop contralateral breast cancer, sarcoma, and cancers of the skin, lung, and esophagus as a result of radiation exposure during their primary treatment.[125–127] Patients treated with alkylators (eg, cyclophosphamide) or topoisomerase II inhibitors (eg, anthracyclines, taxanes) are at risk for development of therapy-related leukemia and myelodysplasia. Although this complication is rare, the risk increases with age and affects nearly 2 out of every 100 breast cancer survivors age 65 and older.[128] Women taking tamoxifen are also at increased risk for endometrial cancer and pulmonary embolism.[22]

Men with prostate cancer who received treatment with radiation are also at risk for secondary malignancies, particularly those who received treatment at a younger age. Radiation-related secondary malignancies may include bladder cancer, colorectal cancer, and sarcomas within the treatment field.[129] Patients treated with external beam radiation therapy for prostate cancer have an almost 2-fold greater risk of developing acute myeloid leukemia than patients treated with prostatectomy.[130] The risk of developing a secondary malignancy is also increased when radiation is delivered at higher doses, and secondary cancers associated with radiation therapy most commonly occur 10 or more years following treatment.[129,131,132]

Patients who received total body irradiation during the conditioning regimen for hematopoietic stem cell transplant are at increased risk for a variety of secondary malignancies, including solid tumors, thyroid cancers, and cancers of the skin and brain.[27,133] The risk of secondary cancers in patients treated for other malignancies depends on the specific treatment received.

## PROVIDING CLINICAL CARE FOR CANCER SURVIVORS

Follow-up care for cancer survivors should address the following areas: (1) surveillance for disease recurrence, (2) monitoring and intervention for therapy-related sequelae impacting physical or psychosocial domains, (3) assessment of genetic susceptibility to cancer, if indicated, and (4) prevention strategies.[22,25,59] In addition, health maintenance and health-promotion strategies (eg, smoking cessation, weight management, vaccines) are an important aspect of health care for all cancer survivors and should be incorporated into the follow-up plan. The overall goal is to provide a coordinated plan for ongoing care, including primary prevention of further morbidity (ie, health promotion), early detection of new health problems (ie, screening for adverse events), and intervention and rehabilitation for identified health problems (ie, restoration of function, prevention of disease-related complications).

### MODELS OF SURVIVORSHIP CARE DELIVERY

Survivorship care in oncology was pioneered in the realm of pediatric oncology, and pediatric oncology survivorship programs were initially based almost exclusively in academic pediatric oncology programs.[134] As pediatric survivors began to age, their follow-up care was often transitioned into adult oncology programs or to community-based care, with mixed success. Challenges related to care transition have included lack of knowledge regarding the needs of cancer survivors among community-based providers and the complexity of care required by certain subgroups of survivors.

Over time, a variety of models for survivorship care have been developed in order to meet the needs of various groups of survivors and institutions in diverse geographic regions. The Children's Oncology Group has developed its *Long-Term Follow-Up Program Resource Guide*[135] to assist institutions in establishing and enhancing survivorship services for pediatric cancer survivors; however, much of the information is applicable to adult survivorship programs. This resource guide, available for downloading at http://www.survivorshipguidelines.org, includes information regarding challenges and barriers to survivorship care delivery, program funding and reimbursement, care delivery models, incorporation of survivorship research into clinical programs, patient advocacy issues, and samples and templates of clinical forms.

Currently in the United States, most patients continue to see their oncologist following completion of treatment for disease-related surveillance,[136] but other important domains of care (eg, general preventive health care, treatment of other medical problems, screening for other cancers) are often not addressed during the oncologic follow-up.[137] Current literature suggests that specialized survivorship programs or shared care models (sharing between oncology-focused providers and primary care providers) may better meet the sometimes complex follow-up needs of cancer survivors.[138,139] Communication is pivotal to the shared care process, and development of a written follow-up plan for each survivor is an integral part of a successful survivorship program.[134]

## HEALTH PROMOTION IN CANCER SURVIVORSHIP CARE

The period following completion of cancer treatment has been described as a "teachable moment"[140]—a time when the life-threatening nature of the illness may create a window of opportunity during which survivors may be ready to modify their health and lifestyle behaviors in order to optimize their future health status. Therefore, all cancer survivors should receive information regarding health-promotion strategies. Guidance regarding general age-appropriate health-promotion strategies (such as immunizations) should be provided according to the recommendations of the American Academy of Family Physicians[141] or the US Preventive Services Task Force,[142] and survivors should be encouraged to work with their primary health care providers to optimize management of any comorbid conditions, such as diabetes, in order to maximize overall health.

Health counseling should include information regarding cancer risk reduction, such as smoking cessation or avoidance[143] and the risks of sun exposure, and information regarding proper nutrition,[144] physical activity,[145] and psychological health.[146] In addition, survivors should be taught methods for early detection of subsequent cancers, including self breast or skin examinations. Patients who received radiation should be advised of the importance of surveillance for and early detection of subsequent radiation-related malignancies. Routine cancer screening examinations, such as colon cancer screening, pelvic examinations, and Papanicolaou (Pap) smears, should be recommended according to current guidelines, such as those of the American Cancer Society[147] or the US Preventive Services Task Force.[148,149] More frequent screening may be indicated for individual survivors on the basis of risk related to specific diagnostic and treatment-related variables, as well as personal and family history and genetic predisposition.

## THE ROLE OF THE NURSE IN SURVIVORSHIP CARE

Nurses are uniquely positioned to take a leading role in cancer survivorship care. Two major foci of nursing care are health promotion and symptom management, both of which are major components of survivorship care. In addition, nurses are adept at planning and coordinating care, and these are essential elements of survivorship care. Therefore, nurses often take the lead when it comes to planning and delivering oncology survivorship care, and may serve as care coordinators and program directors; advanced practice nurses may also serve as direct survivorship care providers.[135]

## THE SURVIVORSHIP CARE PLAN

### CARE PLANNING FOR CANCER SURVIVORS

An important component of follow-up care includes patient education designed to assist cancer survivors in understanding their diagnosis and treatment history and to emphasize the importance of cancer survivors providing this information to health care personnel who may be unfamiliar with their medical history. All cancer survivors should be provided with a written summary of their cancer treatment and recommendations for follow-up care, known as a "survivorship care plan."[33,150] Key components of the survivorship care plan include (1) details regarding the survivor's diagnosis and treatment (diagnostic workup results, tumor characteristics, dates of treatment, therapeutic exposures, and contact information for key care providers) and (2) a follow-up plan for care beyond cancer treatment (plan for surveillance, signs and symptoms of recurrence, potential late effects, genetic implications, preventive strategies, referrals, and resources).[34] An example of a written survivorship care plan is shown in Figure 71-3.

### HEALTH EDUCATION FOR CANCER SURVIVORS

In addition to the survivorship care plan, targeted education regarding specific health problems related to treatment should be provided according to the individual needs of survivors. Written materials to supplement health counseling, such as those available from the American Cancer Society (http://www.cancer.org), the National Cancer Institute (http://dccps.nci.nih.gov/ocs/resources.html), the US Preventive Services Task Force (http://www.ahrq.gov/CLINIC/uspstfix.htm), and the National Institute on Aging (http://www.nia.nih.gov/HealthInformation/Publications/) should be provided to survivors as appropriate.

## RESOURCES

A growing body of resources to assist in implementing cancer survivorship care has emerged over the past decade. An array of resources is available to guide public policy, educate survivors, and assist health care providers in developing programs and survivorship care plans. An annotated summary of a selection of currently available resources is provided in Table 71-3.

City of Hope
1500 East Duarte Road, Duarte, CA 91010

City of Hope Prostate Cancer Survivorship Clinic
**Treatment Summary and Survivorship Care Plan**

**PATIENT INFORMATION**

| | | |
|---|---|---|
| Patient name: Doe, John | | Medical Record Number: 123456 |
| Patient DOB: 1/1/1940 | Age: 69 | Patient phone: (555) 111-2222 |
| Urologist name: James Smith, M.D. | | Primary Care Provider Mary Jones, M.D. |
| Support contact name: Doe, Janet | | |
| Support contact relationship: Spouse | | Support contact phone: (555) 111-2233 |

**CLINICAL INFORMATION**

Diagnosis date 11/29/2006
Symptoms/signs: Elevated PSA, obstructive voiding symptoms, irritative voiding symptoms
Pre-treatment PSA: 7.19 ng/ml
Prostate Biopsy Result: Adenocarcinoma of the prostate
Gleason score at biopsy: 3+3=6
Androgen or hormonal deprivation therapy prior to surgery: None

Clinical Staging

| Test (if applicable) | Date | Findings |
|---|---|---|
| CT Scan | N/A | |
| Bone Scan | 12/1/06 | No evidence of metastatic disease |
| MRI | N/A | |

Family history of Prostate Cancer: Brother had prostate cancer
Major co-morbid conditions: Hypertension, hypercholesterolemia, non-insulin dependent diabetes mellitus
Tobacco use: Yes, past (If current, cessation counseling provided?: N/A)

**TREATMENT**

| | |
|---|---|
| Surgery Date: | 12/30/2006 |
| Hospital | City of Hope |
| Surgeon | James Smith, M.D. |
| Surgical procedure | Robotic-assisted laparoscopic radical prostatectomy |
| Nerve sparing procedure | Bilateral nerve sparing procedure |
| Lymph node Dissection: | No lymph node dissection |
| Blood Transfusion: | No |

| | |
|---|---|
| Pathologic (pT) stage: Pt2c<br>pT2a : Unilateral, involving one-half of one lobe or less<br>pT2b : Unilateral, involving more than one-half of one lobe but not both lobes<br>pT2c : Involves both lobes | pN stage: NX<br>NX: Regional lymph nodes were not assessed<br>NO: No regional node metastasis |
| M stage: MO<br>MX: Distant metastasis not evaluated by any modality<br>MO: No distant metastasis | Gleason Score at Surgery: 3+3=6<br>Margins: Negative |

**FIGURE 71-3**

Sample treatment summary and survivorship care plan.

*Source*: Center for Cancer Survivorship, City of Hope.

City of Hope

City of Hope Prostate Cancer Survivorship Clinic

## Treatment Summary and Survivorship Care Plan

| Treatment-related hospitalization required: | Ongoing side effects related to treatment: |
|---|---|
| No | Good return of urinary and erectile function |

**FOLLOW-UP AND SURVIVORSHIP CARE**

| Follow-up care | When/How Often? | Coordinating Provider |
|---|---|---|
| Urology survivorship clinic visits | Every six months for 5 years, then yearly. | Jane Jones, NP |
| PSA testing | Every six months for 5 years, then yearly | Jane Jones,NP |
| Primary Care Visits | As needed for routine screening, disease prevention, and management of co-morbidities | Patient |

| Last PSA result: | ng/ml | Date: | Lab: City of Hope |
|---|---|---|---|
| Undetectable | <0.1 | 1/7/2007 | |
| Undetectable | <0.1 | 7/2/2007 | |
| Undetectable | <0.1 | 1/8/2008 | |
| Undetectable | <0.1 | 7/22/2008 | |

Potential late effects of treatment: *See Survivorship Care Plan*

***Call your treating Urologist or go to the nearest Emergency Department if you are unable to urinate***

| UROLOGY TEAM MEMBER CONTACTS | SURVIVORSHIP CARE PROVIDER CONTACTS |
|---|---|
| **Urologist:** | **Provider:** |
| Name: Dr. James Smith | Name: Jane Jones, Nurse Practitioner |
| Contact Info: (555) 111-2333 | Contact Info: (555) 111-3333 |
| | |
| **NP/PA:** | **Clinical Research Assistant** |
| Name: Robert Johns, Nurse Practitioner | Name: Susan Smith, CRA |
| Contact Info: (555) 111-2333 | Contact Info: (555) 111-3334 |

| SPECIFIC HEALTH CARE RECOMMENDATIONS PROVIDED | REFERRALS PROVIDED |
|---|---|
| <u>Prevention and Wellness</u><br>**National Institute of Health:**<br>Exercise and Physical Activity: Getting Fit For Life<br>Good Nutrition: It's a Way of Life<br>Cancer Facts for People Over 50<br>High Blood Pressure<br>Diabetes in Older People<br>**City of Hope:**<br>Reducing Prostate Cancer Risk- The Nutritional Connection<br>Eat Your Way to a Healthier Heart!<br>**Department of Health And Human Services:**<br>Influenza and Pneumococcal Vaccine Guidelines<br>Hepatitis A and B Vaccine Guidelines<br>Shingles Vaccine<br><u>Screening</u><br>**American Cancer Society:**<br>Colorectal Cancer Prevention | Referral to gastroenterology for colorectal cancer screening |

**FIGURE 71-3** *(Continued)*

**TABLE 71-3**

**Cancer Survivorship Resources**

| Category | Organization | Item | Description | Availability |
|---|---|---|---|---|
| Patient Education and Advocacy | American Cancer Society | Cancer Survivors Network | Discussion boards and chat rooms for cancer survivors | http://csn.cancer.org |
| | American Society of Clinical Oncology | Cancer.Net Web site | Web site with links to information regarding late effects and survivorship, and templates for cancer treatment summaries and survivorship care plans | http://www.cancer.net/patient/Survivorship |
| | Association of Cancer Online Resources (ACOR) | Survivorship Issues Discussion Group | Discussion groups for issues related to cancer survivorship | http://www.acor.org |
| | Cancer*Care* | Cancer*Care* Web site | Access to telephone counseling, educational workshops, referrals to community resources, and assistance with financial challenges | http://www.cancercare.org |
| | Fertile Hope | Fertile Hope Web site | Information regarding fertility preservation options for cancer patients | http://www.fertilehope.org |
| | Lance Armstrong Foundation | Livestrong Web site | Survivor stories, on-line support, advocacy information | http://www.livestrong.org |
| | National Coalition for Cancer Survivors (NCCS) | NCCS Web site | Resources and publications for survivors, including the Cancer Survival Toolbox | http://www.canceradvocacy.org |
| | Office of Cancer Survivorship (National Cancer Institute) | NCI OCS Web site | Information for cancer survivors, caregivers, and advocates | http://cancercontrol.cancer.gov/ocs/resources.html |
| | Oncology Nursing Society | Survivorship Patient Resource Area | Annotated Web page with links to survivorship resources for patients | http://www.ons.org/patientEd/Psychosocial/survivorship.html |
| Professional Resources | Centers for Disease Control and Prevention | Cancer Survivorship Web Page | Cancer survivorship fact sheets, links to data sources, links to resources, downloadable copy of the *National Action Plan for Cancer Survivorship* | http://www.cdc.gov/cancer/survivorship |
| | Office of Cancer Survivorship (National Cancer Institute) | NCI OCS Web site | Access to information regarding late effects of cancer treatment, clinical practice guidelines, and data from the Childhood Cancer Survivor Study | http://cancercontrol.cancer.gov/ocs/resources.html |
| | President's Cancer Panel | Living Beyond Cancer: Finding New Balance | Report addressing cancer survivorship issues across the lifespan | http://deainfo.nci.nih.gov/advisory/pcp/pcp03–04rpt/Survivorship.pdf |

| | | | | |
|---|---|---|---|---|
| Survivorship Care Plans | Institute of Medicine | Fact Sheet on Post-Treatment Care Planning | Overview of essential elements of cancer survivorship care plans | http://www.iom.edu/CMS/28312/4931/30869/30879.aspx |
| | Journey Forward | Care Plan Builder | Downloadable program for creating customizable electronic care plans for patients | http://www.journeyforward.org |
| | University of Pennsylvania/OncoLink/Lance Armstrong Foundation | Livestrong Care Plan | Interactive care plan development tool customized to diagnosis and treatment; available in English and Spanish | http://www.oncolink.com/oncolife |
| Follow-Up Guidelines | American Society of Clinical Oncology (ASCO) | Clinical Practice Guidelines | Fertility preservation guideline; clinical follow-up guidelines for specific cancer sites | http://www.asco.org |
| | Children's Oncology Group | Long-Term Follow-Up Guidelines | Downloadable copy of the *Long-Term Follow-Up Guidelines for Survivors of Childhood, Adolescent, and Young Adult Cancers* | http://www.survivorshipguidelines.org |
| | National Comprehensive Cancer Network (NCCN) | NCCN Clinical Practice Guidelines in Oncology | Guidelines for cancer treatment and follow-up by site<br>Detection, prevention, and risk-reduction guidelines<br>Supportive care guidelines | http://www.nccn.org |
| Survivorship Program Development | Children's Oncology Group | Long-Term Follow-Up Program Resource Guide | Guide for development and enhancement of survivorship programs for childhood cancer survivors | http://www.survivorshipguidelines.org |

## CONCLUSION

As the population of cancer survivors continues to grow, survivorship care that provides survivors with information regarding their diagnosis, treatment, and potential physical and psychosocial therapy-related late effects, along with a written plan for follow-up care, will assist in empowering survivors to take an active role in their health. This type of high-quality survivorship care has the potential to enhance surveillance for disease recurrence and increase awareness of and monitoring for late complications, potentially leading to earlier intervention and improved health outcomes for today's cancer survivors.

## REFERENCES


1. Horner MJ, Ries LAG, Krapcho M, et al, eds. *SEER Cancer Statistics Review, 1976–2006*. Bethesda, MD: National Cancer Institute, based on November 2008 SEER data submission; 2009.
2. Jemal A, Siegel R, Ward E, Hao Y, Xu J, Thun MJ. Cancer statistics, 2009. *CA: Cancer J Clin.* 2009;59(4):225–249.
3. American Cancer Society. *Cancer Facts and Figures 2008*. Atlanta, GA: American Cancer Society; 2008.
4. Rowland JH. Cancer survivorship: rethinking the cancer control continuum. *Semin Oncol Nurs.* 2008;24:145–152.
5. Miller KD, Triano LR. Medical issues in cancer survivors—a review. *Cancer J.* 2008;14:375–387.
6. Singal PK, Iliskovic N. Doxorubicin-induced cardiomyopathy. *N Engl J Med.* 1998;339:900–905.
7. Simmons A, Vacek JL, Meyers D. Anthracycline-induced cardiomyopathy. *Postgrad Med.* 2008;120:67–72.
8. Bhandare N, Kennedy L, Malyapa RS, Morris CG, Mendenhall WM. Primary and central hypothyroidism after radiotherapy for head-and-neck tumors. *Int J Radiat Oncol Biol Phys.* 2007;68:1131–1139.
9. Illes A, Biro E, Miltenyi Z, et al. Hypothyroidism and thyroiditis after therapy for Hodgkin's disease. *Acta Haematol.* 2003;109:11–17.
10. Tsai RJ, Dennis LK, Lynch CF, Snetselaar LG, Zamba GK, Scott-Conner C. The risk of developing arm lymphedema among breast cancer survivors: a meta-analysis of treatment factors. *Ann Surg Oncol.* 2009;16:1959–1972.
11. Sener SF, Winchester DJ, Martz CH, et al. Lymphedema after sentinel lymphadenectomy for breast carcinoma. *Cancer.* 2001;92:748–752.
12. Aziz NM. Late effects of cancer treatments. In: Ganz PA, ed. *Cancer Survivorship: Today and Tomorrow.* New York: Springer; 2007:54–76.
13. Children's Oncology Group. *Long-Term Follow-Up Guidelines for Survivors of Childhood, Adolescent, and Young Adult Cancers,* Version 3.0. Arcadia, CA: Children's Oncology Group; 2008.
14. Tichelli A, Socie G. Considerations for adult cancer survivors. *Hematology Am Soc Hematol Educ Program.* http://asheducationbook.hematologylibrary.org/content/vol2005/issue1/ 2005:516-522.
15. Ganz PA. Monitoring the physical health of cancer survivors. a survivorship focused medical history. *J Clin Oncol.* 2006;24:5105–5111.
16. Stricker CT, Jacobs LA. Physical late effects in adult cancer survivors. *Oncology (Williston Park).* 2008;22(8 Suppl Nurse Ed):33–42.
17. Lobb EA, Joske D, Butow P, et al. When the safety net of treatment has been removed: Patients' unmet needs at the completion of treatment for haematological malignancies. *Patient Educ Couns.* 2009;77(1):103–108.
18. Boyle DA. Survivorship. In: Carroll-Johnson RM, Gorman L, Bush NJ, eds. *Psychosocial Nursing Care along the Cancer Continuum.* 2nd ed. Pittsburgh, PA: Oncology Nursing Society; 2006:25–51.
19. Stanton AL. Psychosocial concerns and interventions for cancer survivors. *J Clin Oncol.* 2006;24:5132–5137.
20. Recklitis CJ, Sanchez-Varela V, Bober S. Addressing psychological challenges after cancer: a guide for clinical practice. *Oncology (Williston Park).* 2008;22(11 Suppl Nurs Ed):11–20.
21. Krupski TL, Litwin MS. Medical and psychosocial issues in prostate cancer survivors. In: Ganz PA, ed. *Cancer Survivorship: Today and Tomorrow.* New York: Springer; 2007:145–153.
22. Kattlove H, Winn RJ. Ongoing care of patients after primary treatment for their cancer. *CA Cancer J Clin.* 2003;53:172–196.
23. Manne S, Ostroff J, Winkel G, Goldstein L, Fox K, Grana G. Posttraumatic growth after breast cancer: patient, partner, and couple perspectives. *Psychosom Med.* 2004;66:442–454.
24. de Boer AG, Taskila T, Ojajarvi A, van Dijk FJ, Verbeek JH. Cancer survivors and unemployment: a meta-analysis and meta-regression. *JAMA.* 2009;301:753–762.
25. Hewitt M, Greenfield S, Stovall E, eds. *From Cancer Patient to Cancer Survivor: Lost in Transition.* Washington, DC: National Academies Press; 2006.
26. Landier W, Bhatia S, Eshelman DA, et al. Development of risk-based guidelines for pediatric cancer survivors: the children's oncology group long-term follow-up guidelines from the children's oncology group late effects committee and nursing discipline. *J Clin Oncol.* 2004;22:4979–4990.
27. Rizzo JD, Wingard JR, Tichelli A, et al. Recommended screening and preventive practices for long-term survivors after hematopoietic cell transplantation: joint recommendations of the European Group for Blood and Marrow Transplantation, the Center for International Blood and Marrow Transplant Research, and the American Society of Blood and Marrow Transplantation. *Biol Blood Marrow Transplant.* 2006;12:138–151.
28. Khatcheressian JL, Wolff AC, Smith TJ, et al. American Society of Clinical Oncology 2006 update of the breast cancer follow-up and management guidelines in the adjuvant setting. *J Clin Oncol.* 2006;24:5091–5097.
29. Desch CE, Benson AB, 3rd, Somerfield MR, et al. Colorectal cancer surveillance: 2005 update of an American Society of Clinical Oncology practice guideline. *J Clin Oncol.* 2005;23:8512–8519.
30. Lee SJ, Schover LR, Partridge AH, et al. American Society of Clinical Oncology recommendations on fertility preservation in cancer patients. *J Clin Oncol.* 2006;24:2917–2931.
31. Ganz PA. A teachable moment for oncologists: cancer survivors, 10 million strong and growing! *J Clin Oncol.* 2005;23:5458–5460.
32. Gilbert SM, Miller DC, Hollenbeck BK, Montie JE, Wei JT. Cancer survivorship: challenges and changing paradigms. *J Urol.* 2008;179:431–438.
33. Ganz PA, Casillas J, Hahn EE. Ensuring quality care for cancer survivors: implementing the survivorship care plan. *Semin Oncol Nurs.* 2008;24:208–217.
34. Earle CC. Failing to plan is planning to fail: improving the quality of care with survivorship care plans. *J Clin Oncol.* 2006;24:5112–5116.
35. Haylock PJ, Mitchell SA, Cox T, Temple SV, Curtiss CP. The cancer survivor's prescription for living. *Am J Nurs.* 2007;107:58–70; quiz 71.
36. Hayes DF. Clinical practice. Follow-up of patients with early breast cancer. *N Engl J Med.* 2007;356:2505–2513.
37. Hurria A, Hudis C. Follow-up care of breast cancer survivors. *Crit Rev Oncol Hematol.* 2003;48:89–99.
38. Sunga AY, Eberl MM, Oeffinger KC, Hudson MM, Mahoney MC. Care of cancer survivors. *Am Fam Physician.* 2005;71:699–706.
39. Yao SL, Dipaola RS. An evidence-based approach to prostate cancer follow-up. *Semin Oncol.* 2003;30:390–400.
40. Hillner BE, Ingle JN, Chlebowski RT, et al. American Society of Clinical Oncology 2003 update on the role of bisphosphonates and bone health issues in women with breast cancer. *J Clin Oncol.* 2003;21: 4042–4057.
41. Giordano SH, Cohen DS, Buzdar AU, Perkins G, Hortobagyi GN. Breast carcinoma in men: a population-based study. *Cancer.* 2004;101: 51–57.

42. Baron RH, Fey JV, Borgen PI, Stempel MM, Hardick KR, Van Zee KJ. Eighteen sensations after breast cancer surgery: a 5-year comparison of sentinel lymph node biopsy and axillary lymph node dissection. *Ann Surg Oncol.* 2007;14:1653–1661.
43. Petrek JA, Senie RT, Peters M, Rosen PP. Lymphedema in a cohort of breast carcinoma survivors 20 years after diagnosis. *Cancer.* 2001;92:1368–1377.
44. Partridge AH, Ruddy KJ. Fertility and adjuvant treatment in young women with breast cancer. *Breast.* 2007;16(Suppl 2):S175-S181.
45. Stein KD, Jacobsen PB, Hann DM, Greenberg H, Lyman G. Impact of hot flashes on quality of life among postmenopausal women being treated for breast cancer. *J Pain Symptom Manage.* 2000;19:436–445.
46. Stone P, Richards M, A'Hern R, Hardy J. A study to investigate the prevalence, severity and correlates of fatigue among patients with cancer in comparison with a control group of volunteers without cancer. *Ann Oncol.* 2000;11:561–567.
47. Burstein HJ. Cognitive side-effects of adjuvant treatments. *Breast.* 2007;16(Suppl 2):S166-S168.
48. Castellon SA, Silverman DH, Ganz PA. Breast cancer treatment and cognitive functioning: current status and future challenges in assessment. *Breast Cancer Res Treat.* 2005;92:199–206.
49. Burstein HJ, Winer EP. Primary care for survivors of breast cancer. *N Engl J Med.* 2000;343:1086–1094.
50. Ganz PA, Hahn EE. Implementing a survivorship care plan for patients with breast cancer. *J Clin Oncol.* 2008;26:759–767.
51. Duncan MA, Lotze MT, Gerber LH, Rosenberg SA. Incidence, recovery, and management of serratus anterior muscle palsy after axillary node dissection. *Phys Ther.* 1983;63:1243–1247.
52. Shapiro CL, Recht A. Side effects of adjuvant treatment of breast cancer. *N Engl J Med.* 2001;344:1997–2008.
53. Hooning MJ, Botma A, Aleman BM, et al. Long-term risk of cardiovascular disease in 10-year survivors of breast cancer. *J Natl Cancer Inst.* 2007;99:365–375.
54. Bines J, Oleske DM, Cobleigh MA. Ovarian function in premenopausal women treated with adjuvant chemotherapy for breast cancer. *J Clin Oncol.* 1996;14:1718–1729.
55. Ganz PA. Breast cancer, menopause, and long-term survivorship: critical issues for the 21st century. *Am J Med.* 2005;118(Suppl 12B): 136–141.
56. Howell A, Cuzick J, Baum M, et al. Results of the ATAC (Arimidex, Tamoxifen, alone or in combination) trial after completion of 5 years' adjuvant treatment for breast cancer. *Lancet.* 2005;365:60–62.
57. Schagen SB, van Dam FS, Muller MJ, Boogerd W, Lindeboom J, Bruning PF. Cognitive deficits after postoperative adjuvant chemotherapy for breast carcinoma. *Cancer.* 1999;85:640–650.
58. Carlson RW, Allred DC, Anderson BO, et al. Breast cancer. Clinical practice guidelines in oncology. *J Natl Compr Canc Netw.* 2009;7:122–192.
59. Emens LA, Davidson NE. The follow-up of breast cancer. *Semin Oncol.* 2003;30:338–348.
60. Ries LAG, Melbert D, Krapcho M, et al, eds. *SEER Cancer Statistics Review, 1975–2005.* Bethesda, MD: National Cancer Institute, based on November 2007 SEER data submission; 2008.
61. Catalona WJ, Smith DS, Ratliff TL, et al. Measurement of prostate-specific antigen in serum as a screening test for prostate cancer. *N Engl J Med.* 1991;324:1156–1161.
62. Badani KK, Kaul S, Menon M. Evolution of robotic radical prostatectomy: assessment after 2766 procedures. *Cancer.* 2007;110:1951–1958.
63. Hu JC, Nelson RA, Wilson TG, et al. Perioperative complications of laparoscopic and robotic assisted laparoscopic radical prostatectomy. *J Urol.* 2006;175:541–546; discussion 546.
64. National Cancer Institute. Prostate cancer treatment (PDQ) health professional version. http://www.nci.nih.gov/cancertopics/pdq/treatment/prostate/HealthProfessional. Accessed November 1, 2009.
65. Michaelson MD, Cotter SE, Gargollo PC, Zietman AL, Dahl DM, Smith MR. Management of complications of prostate cancer treatment. *CA Cancer J Clin.* 2008;58:196–213.
66. Klein LT, Miller MI, Buttyan R, et al. Apoptosis in the rat penis after penile denervation. *J Urol.* 1997;158:626–630.
67. Fraiman MC, Lepor H, McCullough AR. Changes in penile morphometrics in men with erectile dysfunction after nerve-sparing radical retropubic prostatectomy. *Mol Urol.* 1999;3:109–115.
68. McCullough AR, Levine LA, Padma-Nathan H. Return of nocturnal erections and erectile function after bilateral nerve-sparing radical prostatectomy in men treated nightly with sildenafil citrate: subanalysis of a longitudinal randomized double-blind placebo-controlled trial. *J Sex Med.* 2008;5:476–484.
69. Scher HI, Leibel SA, Fuks Z, Cordon-Cardo C, Scardino PT. Cancer of the prostate. In: DeVita Jr. VT, Hellman S, Rosenberg SA, eds. *Cancer Principles and Practice of Oncology.* Philadelphia, PA: Lippincott Williams & Wilkins; 2005:1192–1259.
70. Brenner DJ. Induced second cancers after prostate-cancer radiotherapy: no cause for concern? *Int J Radiat Oncol Biol Phys.* 2006;65: 637–639.
71. Chun TY. Coincidence of bladder and prostate cancer. *J Urol.* 1997;157:65–67.
72. Thompson CA, Shanafelt TD, Loprinzi CL. Andropause: symptom management for prostate cancer patients treated with hormonal ablation. *Oncologist.* 2003;8:474–487.
73. Mohler J, Eastham JA, Hauke RJ, Kawachi MH, Sandler H, Shrieve DC. Prostate cancer, V.1.2008. *NCCN Clinical Practice Guidelines in Oncology.* Fort Washington, PA: National Comprehensive Cancer Network; 2008.
74. Keating NL, O'Malley AJ, Smith MR. Diabetes and cardiovascular disease during androgen deprivation therapy for prostate cancer. *J Clin Oncol.* 2006;24:4448–4456.
75. Smith MR, Finkelstein JS, McGovern FJ, et al. Changes in body composition during androgen deprivation therapy for prostate cancer. *J Clin Endocrinol Metab.* 2002;87:599–603.
76. O'Connor KM, Fitzpatrick JM. Side-effects of treatments for locally advanced prostate cancer. *BJU Int.* 2005;97:22–28.
77. Wei JT, Dunn RL, Marcovich R, Montie JE, Sanda MG. Prospective assessment of patient reported urinary continence after radical prostatectomy. *J Urol.* 2000;164(3 Pt 1):744–748.
78. Sanda MG, Dunn RL, Michalski J, et al. Quality of life and satisfaction with outcome among prostate-cancer survivors. *N Engl J Med.* 2008;358:1250–1261.
79. American Cancer Society. What's new in prostate cancer research and treatment? http://www.cancer.org/docroot/CRI/content/CRI_2_4_6X_Whats_New_in_Prostate_Cancer_Research_and_Treatment_36.asp?rnav=cri. Accessed November 1, 2009.
80. World Association for Sexology. Proceedings of a regional consultation convened by Pan American Health Organization and World Health Organization, 2000; Antigua, Guatemala.
81. Burnett AL. Erectile dysfunction following radical prostatectomy. *JAMA.* 2005;293:2648–2653.
82. Litwin MS, Hays RD, Fink A, et al. Quality-of-life outcomes in men treated for localized prostate cancer. *JAMA.* 1995;273:129–135.
83. Bradley EB, Bissonette EA, Theodorescu D. Determinants of long-term quality of life and voiding function of patients treated with radical prostatectomy or permanent brachytherapy for prostate cancer. *BJU Int.* 2004;94:1003–1009.
84. Perez MA, Meyerowitz BE, Lieskovsky G, Skinner DG, Reynolds B, Skinner EC. Quality of life and sexuality following radical prostatectomy in patients with prostate cancer who use or do not use erectile aids. *Urology.* 1997;50:740–746.
85. Wu AK, Cooperberg MR, Sadetsky N, Carroll PR. Health related quality of life in patients treated with multimodal therapy for prostate cancer. *J Urol.* 2008;180:2415–2422; discussion 2422.
86. Fowler FJ, Jr, Barry MJ, Lu-Yao G, Roman A, Wasson J, Wennberg JE. Patient-reported complications and follow-up treatment after radical prostatectomy. The National Medicare Experience: 1988–1990 (updated June 1993). *Urology.* 1993;42:622–629.

87. Potosky AL, Davis WW, Hoffman RM, et al. Five-year outcomes after prostatectomy or radiotherapy for prostate cancer: the prostate cancer outcomes study. *J Natl Cancer Inst.* 2004;96:1358–1367.
88. Smith DS, Carvalhal GF, Schneider K, Krygiel J, Yan Y, Catalona WJ. Quality-of-life outcomes for men with prostate carcinoma detected by screening. *Cancer.* 2000;88:1454–1463.
89. Gontero P, Galzerano M, Bartoletti R, et al. New insights into the pathogenesis of penile shortening after radical prostatectomy and the role of postoperative sexual function. *J Urol.* 2007;178:602–607.
90. Briganti A, Fabbri F, Salonia A, et al. Preserved postoperative penile size correlates well with maintained erectile function after bilateral nerve-sparing radical retropubic prostatectomy. *Eur Urol.* 2007;52:702–707.
91. Mulhall J, Land S, Parker M, Waters WB, Flanigan RC. The use of an erectogenic pharmacotherapy regimen following radical prostatectomy improves recovery of spontaneous erectile function. *J Sex Med.* 2005;2:532–540, discussion 540–532.
92. User HM, Hairston JH, Zelner DJ, McKenna KE, McVary KT. Penile weight and cell subtype specific changes in a post-radical prostatectomy model of erectile dysfunction. *J Urol.* 2003;169:1175–1179.
93. Walsh PC, Marschke P, Ricker D, Burnett AL. Patient-reported urinary continence and sexual function after anatomic radical prostatectomy. *Urology.* 2000;55:58–61.
94. American Urological Association. *Guideline for the Management of Clinically Localized Prostate Cancer: 2007 Update.* Linthicum, MD: American Urological Association; 2007.
95. Kendirci M, Bejma J, Hellstrom WJ. Update on erectile dysfunction in prostate cancer patients. *Curr Opin Urol.* 2006;16:186–195.
96. Raina R, Agarwal A, Goyal KK, et al. Long-term potency after iodine-125 radiotherapy for prostate cancer and role of sildenafil citrate. *Urology.* 2003;62:1103–1108.
97. Hatzimouratidis K, Burnett AL, Hatzichristou D, McCullough A, Montorsi F, Mulhall J. Phosphodiesterase type 5 inhibitors in post-prostatectomy erectile dysfunction: a critical analysis of the basic science rationale and clinical application. *Eur Urol.* 2009;55:334–347.
98. Montorsi F, McCullough A. Efficacy of sildenafil citrate in men with erectile dysfunction following radical prostatectomy: a systematic review of clinical data. *J Sex Med.* 2005;2:658–667.
99. American Urological Association. *Management of Erectile Dysfunction: An Update.* Linthicum, MD: American Urological Association; 2007.
100. Montorsi F, Guazzoni G, Strambi LF, et al. Recovery of spontaneous erectile function after nerve-sparing radical retropubic prostatectomy with and without early intracavernous injections of alprostadil: results of a prospective, randomized trial. *J Urol.* 1997;158:1408–1410.
101. Lue TF, Giuliano F, Montorsi F, et al. Summary of the recommendations on sexual dysfunctions in men. *J Sex Med.* 2004;1:6–23.
102. Salomon L, Sebe P, De la Taille A, et al. Open versus laparoscopic radical prostatectomy: part I. *BJU Int.* 2004;94:238–243.
103. Schraudenbach P, Bermejo CE. Management of the complications of radical prostatectomy. *Curr Urol Rep.* 2007;8:197–202.
104. Mariotti G, Sciarra A, Gentilucci A, et al. Early recovery of urinary continence after radical prostatectomy using early pelvic floor electrical stimulation and biofeedback associated treatment. *J Urol.* 2009;181:1788–1793.
105. Manassero F, Traversi C, Ales V, et al. Contribution of early intensive prolonged pelvic floor exercises on urinary continence recovery after bladder neck-sparing radical prostatectomy: results of a prospective controlled randomized trial. *Neurourol Urodyn.* 2007;26:985–989.
106. Litwiller SE, Kim KB, Fone PD, White RW, Stone AR. Post-prostatectomy incontinence and the artificial urinary sphincter: a long-term study of patient satisfaction and criteria for success. *J Urol.* 1996;156:1975–1980.
107. Elshaikh MA, Ulchaker JC, Reddy CA, et al. Prophylactic tamsulosin (Flomax) in patients undergoing prostate 125I brachytherapy for prostate carcinoma: final report of a double-blind placebo-controlled randomized study. *Int J Radiat Oncol Biol Phys.* 2005;62:164–169.
108. Potosky AL, Legler J, Albertsen PC, et al. Health outcomes after prostatectomy or radiotherapy for prostate cancer: results from the Prostate Cancer Outcomes Study. *J Natl Cancer Inst.* 2000;92:1582–1592.
109. Hamilton AS, Stanford JL, Gilliland FD, et al. Health outcomes after external-beam radiation therapy for clinically localized prostate cancer: results from the Prostate Cancer Outcomes Study. *J Clin Oncol.* 2001;19:2517–2526.
110. Potosky AL, Reeve BB, Clegg LX, et al. Quality of life following localized prostate cancer treated initially with androgen deprivation therapy or no therapy. *J Natl Cancer Inst.* 2002;94:430–437.
111. Iversen P. Quality of life issues relating to endocrine treatment options. *Eur Urol.* 1999;36(Suppl 2):20–26.
112. Kumar RJ, Barqawi A, Crawford ED. Preventing and treating the complications of hormone therapy. *Curr Urol Rep.* 2005;6:217–223.
113. Prostate Cancer Foundation. *Report to the Nation on Prostate Cancer: Focus on Advanced Disease.* Santa Monica, CA: Prostate Cancer Foundation; 2004.
114. Kintzel PE, Chase SL, Schultz LM, O'Rourke TJ. Increased risk of metabolic syndrome, diabetes mellitus, and cardiovascular disease in men receiving androgen deprivation therapy for prostate cancer. *Pharmacotherapy.* 2008;28:1511–1522.
115. Braga-Basaria M, Dobs AS, Muller DC, et al. Metabolic syndrome in men with prostate cancer undergoing long-term androgen-deprivation therapy. *J Clin Oncol.* 2006;24:3979–3983.
116. Smith MR. Osteoporosis during androgen deprivation therapy for prostate cancer. *Urology.* 2002;60(3 Suppl 1):79–85; discussion 86.
117. National Institute of Arthritis and Musculoskeletal and Skin Diseases. Bone resource page. http://www.niams.nih.gov/Health_Info/Bone/default.asp. Accessed November 1, 2009.
118. National Osteoporosis Foundation. *Clinician's Guide to Prevention and Treatment of Osteoporosis.* Washington, DC: National Osteoporosis Foundation; 2008.
119. Saylor PJ, Smith MR. Metabolic complications of androgen deprivation therapy for prostate cancer. *J Urol.* 2009;181:1998–2006; discussion 2007–1998.
120. Vogelzang NJ, Breitbart W, Cella D, et al. Patient, caregiver, and oncologist perceptions of cancer-related fatigue: results of a tripart assessment survey. The Fatigue Coalition. *Semin Hematol.* 1997; 34(3 Suppl 2):4–12.
121. Stone P, Richards M, A'Hern R, Hardy J. Fatigue in patients with cancers of the breast or prostate undergoing radical radiotherapy. *J Pain Symptom Manage.* 2001;22:1007–1015.
122. Strum SB, McDermed JE, Scholz MC, Johnson H, Tisman G. Anaemia associated with androgen deprivation in patients with prostate cancer receiving combined hormone blockade. *Br J Urol.* 1997; 79:933–941.
123. Ganz PA, ed. *Cancer Survivorship: Today and Tomorrow.* New York: Springer; 2007.
124. Zablotska LB, Matasar MJ, Neugut AI. Second malignancies after radiation treatment and chemotherapy for primary cancers. In: Ganz PA, ed. *Cancer Survivorship: Today and Tomorrow.* New York: Springer; 2007:225–233.
125. Boice JD, Jr, Harvey EB, Blettner M, Stovall M, Flannery JT. Cancer in the contralateral breast after radiotherapy for breast cancer. *N Engl J Med.* 1992;326:781–785.
126. Inskip PD, Stovall M, Flannery JT. Lung cancer risk and radiation dose among women treated for breast cancer. *J Natl Cancer Inst.* 1994;86:983–988.
127. Rubino C, de Vathaire F, Diallo I, Shamsaldin A, Le MG. Increased risk of second cancers following breast cancer: role of the initial treatment. *Breast Cancer Res Treat.* 2000;61:183–195.
128. Muss HB, Berry DA, Cirrincione C, et al. Toxicity of older and younger patients treated with adjuvant chemotherapy for node-positive breast cancer: the Cancer and Leukemia Group B Experience. *J Clin Oncol.* 2007;25:3699–3704.

129. Brenner DJ, Curtis RE, Hall EJ, Ron E. Second malignancies in prostate carcinoma patients after radiotherapy compared with surgery. *Cancer.* 2000;88:398–406.
130. Ojha RP, Thertulien R, Zhou Y, Fischbach LA. Prostate cancer treatment and risk of acute myeloid leukemia in a population-based prospective cohort. *J Clin Oncol.* 2008;26(15 Suppl):5073.
131. Baxter NN, Tepper JE, Durham SB, Rothenberger DA, Virnig BA. Increased risk of rectal cancer after prostate radiation: a population-based study. *Gastroenterology.* 2005;128:819–824.
132. Boorjian S, Cowan JE, Konety BR, et al. Bladder cancer incidence and risk factors in men with prostate cancer: results from Cancer of the Prostate Strategic Urologic Research Endeavor. *J Urol.* 2007;177: 883–887, discussion 887–888.
133. Curtis RE, Rowlings PA, Deeg HJ, et al. Solid cancers after bone marrow transplantation. *N Engl J Med.* 1997;336:897–904.
134. McCabe MS, Jacobs L. Survivorship care: models and programs. *Semin Oncol Nurs.* 2008;24:202–207.
135. Landier W, ed. *Establishing and Enhancing Services for Childhood Cancer Survivors: Long-Term Follow-Up Program Resource Guide.* Arcadia, CA: Children's Oncology Group; 2007.
136. Fischer DS. *Follow-Up of Cancer: A Handbook for Physicians.* 4th ed. Philadelphia, PA: Lippincott-Raven; 1996.
137. Oeffinger KC, McCabe MS. Models for delivering survivorship care. *J Clin Oncol.* 2006;24:5117–5124.
138. Cheung WY, Neville BA, Cameron DB, Cook EF, Earle CC. Comparisons of patient and physician expectations for cancer survivorship care. *J Clin Oncol.* 2009;27:2489–2495.
139. Nekhlyudov L. "Doc, should I see you or my oncologist?" A primary care perspective on opportunities and challenges in providing comprehensive care for cancer survivors. *J Clin Oncol.* 2009;27:2424–2426.
140. Demark-Wahnefried W, Aziz NM, Rowland JH, Pinto BM. Riding the crest of the teachable moment: promoting long-term health after the diagnosis of cancer. *J Clin Oncol.* 2005;23:5814–5830.
141. American Academy of Family Physicians. Summary of Recommendations for Clinical Preventive Services. October 2009. http://www.aafp.org/online/etc/medialib/aafp_org/documents/clinical/CPS/rcps08-2005.Par.0001.File.tmp/Oct2009RCPSwithedits.pdf Accessed November 25, 2009.
142. US Preventive Services Task Force. Guide to clinical preventive services. 2008. http://www.ahrq.gov/clinic/pocketgd.htm. Accessed November 1, 2009.
143. de Moor JS, Elder K, Emmons KM. Smoking prevention and cessation interventions for cancer survivors. *Semin Oncol Nurs.* 2008;24:180–192.
144. Toles M, Demark-Wahnefried W. Nutrition and the cancer survivor: evidence to guide oncology nursing practice. *Semin Oncol Nurs.* 2008;24:171–179.
145. Schwartz AL. Physical activity. *Semin Oncol Nurs.* 2008;24:164–170.
146. Andrykowski MA, Lykins E, Floyd A. Psychological health in cancer survivors. *Semin Oncol Nurs.* 2008;24:193–201.
147. Smith RA, Cokkinides V, Brawley OW. Cancer screening in the United States, 2009: a review of current American Cancer Society guidelines and issues in cancer screening. *CA Cancer J Clin.* 2009;59:27–41.
148. US Preventive Services Task Force. Screening for skin cancer: US Preventive Services Task Force recommendation statement. *Ann Intern Med.* 2009;150:188–193.
149. US Preventive Services Task Force. Screening for colorectal cancer: US Preventive Services Task Force recommendation statement. *Ann Intern Med.* 2008;149:627–637.
150. Earle CC, Schrag D, Woolf SH, Ganz PA. The survivorship care plan: what, why, how, and for whom. In: Ganz PA, ed. Cancer Survivorship: Today and Tomorrow. New York: Springer; 2007:287–293.

CHAPTER 72

*Laurel Northouse, PhD, RN, FAAN, Lixin Song, PhD, RN*

# Family and Caregiver Issues

## INTRODUCTION

The stress of cancer spreads from patients to family members like a stone dropping in a pond. Family members who are primary caregivers often report as much distress as patients, and in some cases even more.[1] Although cancer is not in the bodies of the family members, it is in their lives and it can affect all aspects of their quality of life. Family caregivers need information and emotional support, but these needs are not being addressed in healthcare settings in a systematic way.

To draw greater attention to the needs of family caregivers and ways to help them, this chapter addresses 4 major areas. First, the chapter discusses the importance of helping family members to meet their needs. Second, the chapter provides a theoretical framework for understanding the effects of cancer on patients and patients' caregivers. Third, we discuss the effects of cancer on the quality of life of patients and family members—namely, their emotional, social, physical, spiritual, and financial well-being. Fourth, the chapter concludes with assessment and intervention strategies that can be used to address the needs of patients and their family members.

## WHY HELP FAMILIES OF PATIENTS WITH CANCER?

There are several key reasons why families of patients with cancer need our help. First, families are the bedrock of chronic care in the US. There are over 44 million informal family caregivers in the US who provide unpaid care to people with chronic illnesses such as cancer.[2] Patients with cancer are leaving the hospital sicker and sooner than ever before, and their long-term care is most often provided in the home by family caregivers. Family caregivers assume multiple roles: they help patients to make treatment decisions, carry out skilled nursing tasks (ie, dressing changes, medication administration), and provide emotional support to patients on an ongoing basis. It is essential that nurses develop effective partnerships with family caregivers to provide seamless care as patients transition from hospital to home, and as they receive long-term care in outpatient, community-based settings.

A second reason to help family members is that the patient's illness can affect all aspects of life of the family members. Family members have sometimes been referred to as "copatients" or "cosufferers" because of the concurrent effect that cancer has on their lives as well as on the lives of patients. Because cancer affects the well-being of patients and family members, both persons have a legitimate need for information and support from health professionals. Too often, however, the needs of family members are overlooked as health professionals direct nearly all of their attention toward the patients.

Third, as burden of care increases, family caregivers report a decrease in their own physical and mental health, and also a decrease in their ability to care for the patient.[3] In order for family members to maintain their important caregiving role, they need assistance from nurses and other health professionals to reduce their burden and to maintain their own well-being. Some professionals believe that without help, the caregiver today may become the patient tomorrow.

Fourth, family caregivers are the "first responders" to changes in the patient's health status in community settings. One major task for family caregivers is to monitor patients who receive aggressive, multimodal cancer treatments in outpatient settings. These treatments can cause many treatment-related symptoms and toxicities.[4] Family caregivers are expected to manage and monitor patients for symptoms, and promptly report any changes in the patient's condition to healthcare professionals.[5,6] In a sense, family caregivers are "the eyes" of healthcare professionals in home settings. Based on the observations and assessments made by family caregivers, health professionals may adjust the dose of a patient's treatment or prescribe a supplemental medication to address treatment-related toxicities.

A fifth reason to help family members is because they lack preparation for the complex care that they are expected to provide. Family caregivers are seldom prepared for their important role, and they perceive little help and support from healthcare professionals on a routine basis.[7] Research indicates that when family caregivers feel more prepared or confident in their caregiving role, they themselves experience less fatigue, confusion, and depression.[8] Furthermore, when patients are cared for by family caregivers who feel more prepared for their role, patients have better symptom management and higher mental health.[9]

## BARRIERS TO HELPING FAMILIES OF PATIENTS WITH CANCER

In spite of the importance of family caregivers, there are barriers that can limit family members' ability to obtain information and support from nurses and other health professionals. The most common barrier is the time constraints that exist in healthcare settings. Health professionals, especially nurses, face an increase in patients with more complex conditions and a decrease in nursing personnel; both factors leave less time for them to assist family caregivers. Nurses are often evaluated by recordable and quantifiable patient-centered tasks that they complete per shift, rather than by the care they provide to family members.[10] In order to manage time demands and to fulfill their patient-centered role expectations, nurses often believe that they do not have time to address the needs of family members.

A second barrier is the lack of clarity about who is responsible for helping family members within the healthcare system. Although various professionals espouse the importance of helping families and the value of family-centered care, in reality there is little accountability for who will intervene to help family caregivers. Most family members lack a strong advocate in healthcare settings who will take responsibility for addressing family members' needs as an integral component of quality healthcare delivery.

A third barrier is the lack of value placed on the contribution of the family to the care of a patient. From anecdotal reports, some healthcare professionals view families as a burden rather than as a resource. Family members are viewed at times as getting in the way of or taking time away from the nurse's ability to deliver care to the patient. The value of developing an effective working alliance with family caregivers is often not appreciated or is undervalued by healthcare professionals.

Fourth, the lack of effective professional–family communication in healthcare settings is also a barrier. Professional–family communication is often limited in healthcare settings, and as a result, nurses often make assumptions about families' needs, wishes, and abilities based on nurses' subjective opinions rather than on direct communication with the family.[11] Discussing feelings about the diagnosis, options for treatment, and worries about the illness are not simple, straight-forward information-sharing tasks. Rather, they are more complex behaviors that require an understanding of effective interpersonal and family communication. Research has shown that healthcare providers often receive limited training in effective interviewing and counseling skills[12,13] and are uneasy discussing cancer-related psychosocial issues. As a result, many professionals involved in cancer care prefer to focus primarily on technical tasks, and distance themselves from psychological and social concerns experienced by family members.

Fifth, a lack of cultural sensitivity to the values of various families can also be a barrier. Healthcare professionals in western cultures such as the US place a high priority on "patient autonomy" and less priority on family-based, collective decision-making that are often found in other cultures. In many cultures, the family assumes the responsibility for making treatment decisions on the patient's behalf.[14,15] Cultural values and behaviors are the key variables in the process of coping with cancer and cancer-related issues (eg, suffering and death) for patients and their families,[14] and require that professionals have a broad understanding of these values in order to provide culturally sensitive care.

## A THEORETICAL PERSPECTIVE

### STRESS AND COPING THEORY

*Stress and Coping Theory*[16] provides a useful framework for understanding the effects of illness on patients with cancer and their family caregivers. Although the theory was originally developed from an individually-oriented perspective, in recent years the theory was adapted to explain the effects of illness on both patients and their family members.[17] More specifically, elements of family systems theory were integrated into the stress-coping model to indicate that both patients and family members go through the stress-coping process, and their individual responses to the illness affect one another.

Figure 72-1 illustrates the model and identifies the main components of the model. It also illustrates how these components are related to one another. As indicated in Figure 72-1, there are 3 major components of the model: antecedents, mediators, and outcomes. Antecedents are baseline characteristics of patients and/or family caregivers that are evident prior to or at the time of diagnosis. There are 3 types of antecedent characteristics: personal (such as age, education, and gender), social (such as family support or relationships), and illness (such as type of cancer or stage of cancer). As shown in Figure 72-1, personal, social, and illness characteristics affect patients' and caregivers' appraisal of an illness or the caregiving associated with it. Appraisal and coping resources affect one another, and they both have a direct effect on the quality of life outcomes of patients and family members. In addition, as shown in the model, the quality of life of patients' and family members' influence one another.

This model helps nurses and other health professionals determine how and where to intervene with patients and caregivers. According to this model, most intervention takes place in the middle of the model to reduce the negative appraisal of illness and caregiving, and to enhance coping resources. For example, as nurses provide patients and family members with information, support, ways to reduce stress, manage symptoms, and ways to cope with the illness, the patients' and caregivers' negative appraisals decrease, their coping resources increase, and the outcome: their quality of life improves.

In the model, antecedents are considered to be factors that influence how people appraise and cope with the illness, but they are not typically factors that can be changed

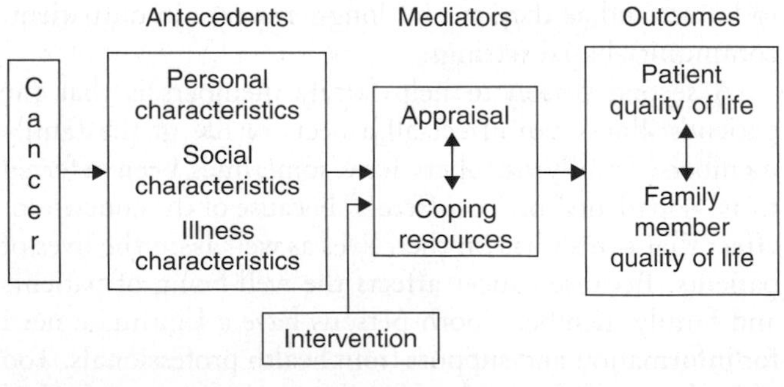


**FIGURE 72-1**

Stress-coping theoretical framework.

by interventions. For example, it is not possible to change a person's age or type of cancer, but we can take into consideration that age (eg, being a younger patient) or type of cancer (eg, lung cancer) may influence their appraisals of the illness or caregiving. These antecedent characteristics, however, can be used to tailor interventions to the specific characteristics of patients and family members. For example, a nurse may adapt or tailor information about sexuality and provide information about fertility to younger couples rather than to older couples beyond child-bearing age.

Theoretical models are useful. They can help us understand how patients' and family members' may respond to an illness and how we can help them. Effective interventions are not simply random behaviors or just good ideas. Interventions are more likely to be effective if they are derived from a theoretical perspective. The combination of Stress-Coping Theory and Family Systems Theory are useful for understanding how patients with cancer and family members cope with illness, and the influence their lives have on one another.

## EFFECT OF CANCER ON THE QUALITY OF LIFE OF FAMILY MEMBERS

The focus of this section of the chapter is on how cancer affects the quality of life in patients with cancer and their family members. According to the research, cancer affects the quality of life of family members in 5 major areas: emotional, social, physical, spiritual, and financial. The specific effects in each of these areas will be addressed to underscore the many ways in which family members are affected by the patient's cancer.

### EMOTIONAL WELL-BEING

Most of the research on the impact of cancer on family members has been conducted on emotional well-being. Hagedoorn and colleagues conducted a meta-analysis of 43 studies on the emotional effects of cancer on patients and their spouses.[18] From their analysis, they found that a significant reciprocal relationship existed between the level of emotional distress reported by patients with cancer and their spouses. They concluded that couples facing cancer react as an "emotional system" rather than as isolated individuals.[18] The investigators also found that the emotional distress reported by patients with cancer and their spouses was significantly higher than the distress reported by couples not dealing with cancer. These important findings were based on studies with patients with various types of cancer who were at both early and later stages of the illness. This meta-analysis provides rationale for including spouses or family caregivers in programs of care.

Longitudinal studies have been conducted to answer the question, "How long does the emotional distress last in patients with cancer and their family members?" Research indicates that emotional distress and adjustment problems extend over time. Figure 72-2 illustrates the difference in adjustment problems reported by women with breast cancer and women with benign breast disease and their husbands, starting at the time of diagnosis and extending to 1 year later. As illustrated by the solid lines, both women with breast cancer and their husbands report significantly more problems than do women with benign breast disease and their husbands (dotted lines) during the first year following diagnosis. Studies indicate that emotional distress is higher during the first 12 to 18 months following diagnosis, and gradually deceases over time.[19,20] Studies conducted with long-term cancer survivors and their family members report that there are no negative effects on their emotional well-being or overall quality of life 3 years following diagnosis, if survivors remain cancer-free or in remission.[21,22]

#### Fear of recurrence

Even though emotional distress decreases over time, patients and family members still have worries about the cancer. A universal concern of cancer survivors and their family members is the fear that the cancer will recur. Fear of recurrence is not a sign of poor coping or hypochondrias, as some professionals used to think. Rather, it is the response to having

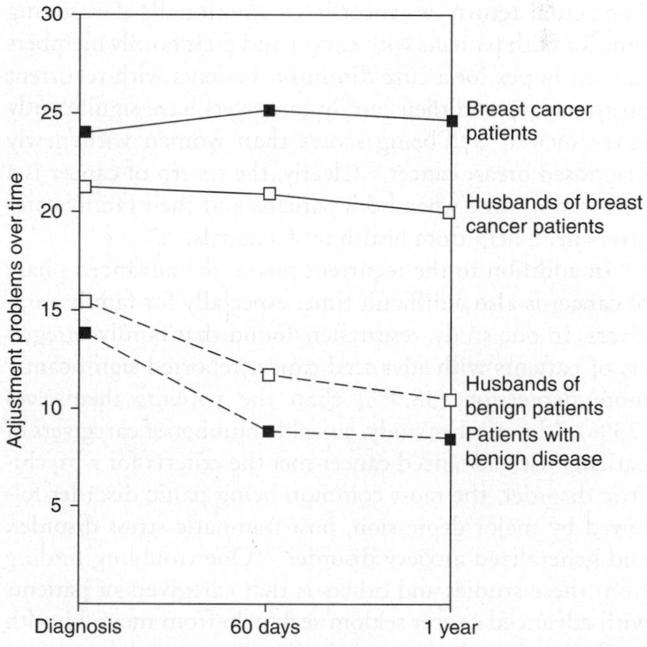


**FIGURE 72-2**

Trajectories of emotional adjustment problems.

been diagnosed with a potentially life-threatening illness that can have remissions and exacerbations, like any other chronic illness. Although fear of recurrence was thought of primarily as a patient concern, research indicates that fear of recurrence is also a concern of family members.[23,24] Furthermore, research indicates that there is a significant relationship between the fear reported by patients and their family caregivers.[25] Patients with a higher fear of recurrence typically have family members who also have a higher fear of recurrence.

Some studies indicate that family caregivers have significantly more fear than cancer survivors.[23,25] Although this may seem somewhat surprising, there may be reasons why family members have more fear of recurrence. Some family members hide their fears because they do not want to worry the patient. Hiding fears, however, prevents family members from getting the help they need to reduce their own fears. Family members often have less direct communication with professionals, which limits family members' ability to obtain information or to get answers to their questions, which could reduce their fears. Although the exact reason is not known, it is clear that both survivors and their family caregivers worry about the cancer recurring. Some research indicates that survivors and family caregivers who have more fear of recurrence are younger, dealing with many other stressors in addition to the cancer (eg, child care issues, employment problems), and have less positive meaning associated with the illness.[25]

### Recurrent and advanced cancer

The actual return of cancer is an emotionally devastating time for both patients with cancer and their family members as their hopes for a cure diminish. Patients with recurrent breast cancer and their family caregivers have significantly lower mental well-being scores than women with newly diagnosed breast cancer.[17] Clearly, the return of cancer is a devastating time when both patients and their family caregivers need help from health professionals.

In addition to the recurrent phase, the advanced phase of cancer is also a difficult time, especially for family caregivers. In one study, researchers found that family caregivers of patients with advanced cancer reported significantly more depression (38.9%) than the patients themselves (23%).[26] In another study, a sizable number of caregivers of patients with advanced cancer met the criteria for a psychiatric disorder, the most common being panic disorder followed by major depression, post-traumatic stress disorder, and generalized anxiety disorder.[27] One troubling finding from these studies and others is that caregivers of patients with advanced cancer seldom seek help from mental health professionals to deal with their own distress and depression. For example, in one study, fewer than half of the caregivers who had a psychiatric disorder ever obtained help from a mental health professional.[27] Furthermore, depressed caregivers were less likely than depressed patients to use any form of mental health treatment to deal with their depression.[28] These studies document the enormous effect that advanced cancer has on the emotional well-being of caregivers, and that more interventions need to be targeted to caregivers of patients with advanced cancer because the caregivers are less likely than patients to seek help for their own mental health problems.

### Effects on children's emotional well-being

Although most studies focus on the effects of the patient's cancer on the adult family caregiver, there is a small body of research that indicates children feel the effects of their parent's illness as well. In general, most young children, adolescents, and young adults of a parent with cancer are well-adjusted. Yet, a significant number of these children are at risk for moderate-to-high levels of emotional distress and behavioral problems.[29,30]

Researchers have found that children's responses vary by developmental age. In one of the most extensive investigations of children of patients with cancer, Lewis and colleagues reported that younger children of patients with cancer experience some negative behavioral or emotional problems based on reports from both parents and the children themselves.[31,32] Compared to younger children, research indicates that adolescents and young adults report more difficulty dealing with a parent's cancer.[30] For example, symptoms of anxiety and depression are higher for adolescents and young adults whose parent is ill than for younger children.[30] The findings are mixed about whether male or female adolescents are more affected by the parent's illness. One study found that adolescent girls report higher symptoms of anxiety and depression than adolescent boys.[30] However, a more recent study that compared school-aged children and adolescents (age 8–16) of patients with breast cancer and their matched healthy classmates, found that sons, rather than daughters, of mothers with breast cancer were seen by teachers and peers as more socially sensitive and isolated than comparison peers.[33] Although more research is needed on gender differences, these findings identified adolescents as a highly vulnerable group because of their parents' cancer.

Existing research also has provided evidence about factors that have a major effect on children's emotional well-being. For example, disease and treatment factors of the parental cancer (eg, advanced stage, poor prognosis, worse functional impairment, recurrence, and more intensive treatment regimes) have been associated with various outcomes in children and adolescents, such as more behavior problems, lower self-esteem, less social competence, more stress, and higher anxiety and depression.[34,35] Interestingly, some researchers also have reported that children of parents with more severe complications of their illnesses had better outcomes,[36] suggesting that parental cancer may help children to develop more resilience in some situations. Maternal factors (eg, maternal mood and adjustment) have been associated with less emotional distress in children, and family factors (eg, more open communication and family expressiveness) have been associated with better outcomes in adolescents.[37,38]

## SOCIAL WELL-BEING

Cancer can have an effect on the social well-being of patients with cancer and their family members. For many years, people often assumed that the effects of breast cancer and the treatment for it would cause major problems in couples' marital relationships. However, over the years this assumption has turned out to be false. Instead of drawing couples apart, the illness draws most couples closer together as they learned to appreciate one another more and to value their time together.[39] Studies that compared the marital satisfaction scores of couples who are coping with cancer with the scores of couples without cancer, have found no significant difference in their martial satisfaction scores on well-established instruments.[40,41] While a small number of couples do separate or divorce after a partner is diagnosed with cancer, these couples typically had preexisting marital problems that were evident prior to the cancer diagnosis.

### Communication issues

Although divorce is not common, there are strains that can create stress in the couples' marital relationships. One area of strain pertains to couples' difficulty communicating about the cancer. Some patients and their family caregivers have different preferences or needs about discussing the illness, and these differences can hinder their communication. Another difficulty related to effective communication is that some family members think it is "unhealthy" to express worries about cancer. In one study, husbands of patients with breast cancer thought discussing the cancer would hinder their wives' adjustment and possibly lead to a recurrence of her cancer.[42] Also, the use of criticism among patients and their family members can hinder effective communication about the illness. When patients or family members criticize one another as they are trying to cope with cancer, it creates tension in their relationships and blocks effective communication about the illness.[43]

The concept of "protective buffering" has been used to describe problems that occur in the communication between patients with cancer and their family caregivers. Protective buffering is defined as hiding worries and denying concerns in an effort to avoid disagreement.[44] Protective buffering is an interpersonal process that involves limiting one's own expression of emotion about threatening topics in an attempt to avoid upsetting a partner. It involves setting up a protective barrier by one or both partners as a way to hide feelings they think may be upsetting to the other partner (Figure 72-3). The use of protective buffering by either patients or their partners has been related to increasing the emotional distress of both persons, and to a decrease in marital satisfaction.[45,46] Mismatched communication (ie, one partner wants to talk but the other partner withdraws) also is associated with higher distress and lower relationship satisfaction in partners.[43]

Research indicates that couples with better communication (eg, use direct communication instead of hiding concerns) report higher marital satisfaction and better quality of life, primarily because expressiveness and self-disclosure are major determinants of marital intimacy.[45] Further, couples who are able to share information about cancer and its consequences, as well as their thoughts and feelings, have better adjustment, enhanced cohesion and intimacy, and lower mood disturbance.[47–52] Research indicates that sharing information and concerns helps healthy partners to gain a better understanding of the patients' physical and emotional needs, which subsequently decreases the strain on the caregiver.[53,54]

### Sexuality and fertility

Social well-being can also be affected by changes in intimacy and fertility associated with cancer treatments. For

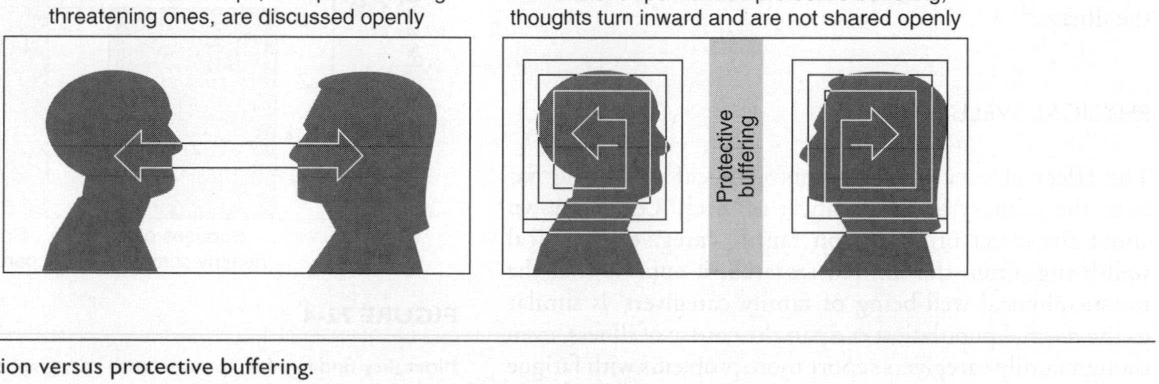
In effective relationships, all topics including threatening ones, are discussed openly
In relationships that use protective buffering, thoughts turn inward and are not shared openly
Protective buffering

**FIGURE 72-3**

Open communication versus protective buffering.

example, sexual expression among women with breast cancer can be hindered by women's concerns about disfigurement due to breast surgery.[55] Although some husbands want to reassure their wives that the surgical incision does not bother them or their sexual feelings for their wives, these husbands avoid the topic because they are unsure about how to discuss it. Men with prostate cancer often experience erectile dysfunction following a prostatectomy or a loss of libido as a result of hormone treatments. These treatments affect sexual relationships with their wives or partners and can hinder their social well-being.

Certain treatments for cancer can also cause fertility problems for couples. This is especially the case for younger couples who had planned to start a family or add to their family. Although there are more options today for young survivors and their partners to use sperm banks or to consider adoption, these decisions are not easy for young couples who often have considerable uncertainty about their future and about the long-term health of the cancer survivors. Both sexuality and fertility issues are discussed in previous chapters on cancers of the reproductive organs, but are mentioned briefly in this section because they can have an effect on couples' interpersonal and social well-being.

### Changes in family roles and relationships

A cancer diagnosis can also create disruption in usual family roles and relationships. Because of the interdependence of family members, when one family member becomes ill, other family members often take on some of the household or family roles of the ill person.[56] Although many families are able to negotiate these role changes on a temporary basis, over time these role changes become more difficult as family caregivers become overloaded. Trying to maintain some equity or the give-and-take between partners can become an issue as couples try to manage changes brought on by the cancer.[57] Some family caregivers feel angry when they perceive that they are getting very few benefits from their caregiving role. On the other hand, patients with cancer can feel guilty when they are getting many benefits from the role of a patient, and are not contributing equally to the relationship. Clearly, dealing with role changes is another aspect of social well-being that may be altered by the illness.[58]

## PHYSICAL WELL-BEING

The effect of cancer on patients' physical well-being has been the primary focus in cancer research. Less is known about the effect of cancer on family caregivers' physical well-being. From the limited research, it appears that the overall physical well-being of family caregivers' is similar to the normal population early in the course of illness, even though family caregivers report more problems with fatigue and cognitive function (eg, concentration) than noncaregivers.[28] In one study, researchers examined the amount of fatigue reported by a large sample of caregivers of patients with cancer ($N = 248$) and found that 45% of the caregivers had mild fatigue, 25% had moderate fatigue, and 28% had severe fatigue.[59] Higher fatigue was associated with providing more hours of care.

Family caregivers who experience high levels of caregiver burden and ongoing caregiver strain, are at the greatest risk of developing physical health problems of their own.[2,60,61] For example, Schulz and colleagues conducted a study on the effects of caregiving on the health of spousal caregivers of cardiac patients. Spouses who experienced strain rated their own health lower, used more prescription medications, and had a greater risk of mortality than spouses without strain.[60,61] These investigators compared 4 groups of spouses of cardiac patients who had various limits in their activities of daily living (ADL). The 4 groups were (1) spouses of partners with no limits (control group), (2) spouses of partners with limits but required no help, (3) spouses of partners with limits who needed help, but it caused no caregiver strain on the spouses, and (4) spouses of partners with limits, who needed help, and whose spouse experienced caregiver strain. Four years later, spouses of partners who reported caregiver strain had a 63% greater risk of death themselves than did spouses of partners who had no limits (control condition) (see Figure 72-4). Possible explanations for the greater mortality in spouses who reported caregiver strain were that they had insufficient time to rest, engage in self-care, or carry out other health-related activities that may have maintained their own health.

It is important to remember that caregivers often have preexisting health problems of their own which can be

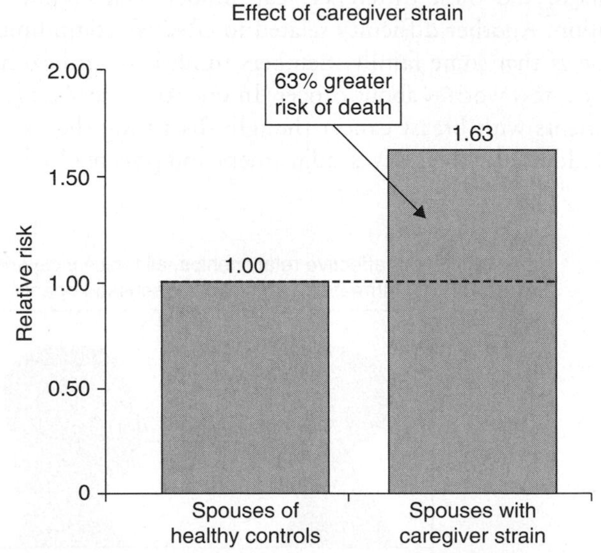


**FIGURE 72-4**

Mortality findings for spouses with caregiver strain.

negatively affected by the stress of caregiving. Research indicates that approximately 30% to 50% of the family caregivers of patients with cancer have reported chronic health problems of their own, such as heart disease, hypertension, and arthritis.[62,63] These preexisting health problems may be exacerbated by the stress of caregiving, especially as the caregiving burden or the strain increases and extends over time. Because caregivers are likely to place patients' needs above their own, caregivers have less time to spend on their own health promotion activities such as exercise or cancer screening, which over time may have negative consequences. Nurses and other health professionals need to encourage caregivers to maintain their own health as they provide care for their ill family member.

## SPIRITUAL WELL-BEING

Another important dimension of quality of life pertains to spiritual well-being. This refers to the meaning and purpose that people find in the challenges they face, such as coping with cancer. Both patients with cancer and their family caregivers seek meaning as they try to understand why the cancer occurred and how they will make sense of it. Studies indicate that the more that patients and family caregivers can reframe an illness as positive, the better they are able to cope with the illness and maintain their quality of life.[63–65]

Following the diagnosis of cancer, patients and family members often reevaluate their priorities and the way they are spending their time. For example, individuals who have been working long hours, 7 days a week, may decide to change that pattern and spend more time with partners, children, or grandchildren. Other families become more aware of the fragility of life and decrease their drive for material things.[62] Families also report a greater reliance on their spiritual faith to help them cope with the uncertainty they feel about the future.

## FINANCIAL WELL-BEING

Cancer creates a substantial financial burden that affects the quality of life of patients with cancer and their family caregivers, and society as a whole.[66] From 1995 to 2004, the overall costs of treating only cancer increased by 75% to approximately 72 billion dollars a year.[67] In addition to this soaring cost, over 44 million people in the US are currently uninsured or underinsured. For those families with insurance, they still have to pay many out-of-pocket expenses for medications and treatments that are not covered by their insurance (eg, oral medicines commonly used to treat cancers of the breast and prostate). Financial problems also increase when patients have physical disabilities that cause interruptions in patients' employment. Compared to healthy people, cancer survivors tend to have more lost days from work, are less able to work, or have more restrictions in the kind and amount of work they can perform because of their health problems.[68]

A national survey found that 44% of the families dealing with a devastating illness reported great economic hardship, 31% lost most or all of their family savings, and 29% reported the loss of a major source of income. Families of younger, poorer, and more functionally dependent patients were more likely to report loss of most or all of the family's savings.[69] African American and Hispanic caregivers were likely to experience more economic disruption of various types compared with Caucasians.[2]

Economic disruptions also occur because of disruptions in the lives of family caregivers. Estimates indicate that 20% to 77% of the family caregivers miss work or quit jobs to provide care.[69,70] Many caregivers arrive at work late, leave early, or take time off during the day to provide care. At times, caregivers need to take a leave of absence from work, change from full-time to part-time employment, or switch to less demanding jobs. Some family caregivers need to relocate to geographical areas closer to the patient to accommodate caregiving responsibilities.[71] These changes can affect caregivers' ability to maintain their usual employment, and create further financial hardships for families.

While the informal care provided by family members is unpaid, its value to society has been estimated at $305 billion annually.[72] In spite of the enormous contribution of family caregivers to the national budget, the government support for family caregiving is limited. The Family Medical Leave Act of 1993 guarantees only unpaid leave to care for a seriously ill spouse, son, daughter, or parent. Furthermore, only a few states allow those eligible for Medicaid's personal care benefit to receive a cash allowance to purchase their own care and hire friends or family to provide care.[73]

In view of the limited support available to help families and the financial changes associated with cancer treatment and caregiving, it is clear that their financial well-being is affected a great deal by the illness.

## PRACTICAL STRATEGIES FOR HELPING PATIENTS AND FAMILY MEMBERS

This section of the chapter addresses strategies that nurses and other health professionals can use to help patients and family members to cope with the multiple effects of cancer and to maintain their quality of life. The section begins by identifying assessment issues and describing ways to screen patients and family members for emotional distress. Next, interventions that health professionals can use to help patients and family members are described, such as (1) promoting family communication and mutual support, (2) providing information, (3) encouraging an optimistic outlook, (4) teaching self-monitoring and stress reduction, and (5) promoting effective coping and healthy lifestyle behaviors.

## ASSESSMENT ISSUES

### Assessment questions

Nurses and other healthcare professionals need to assess and periodically reevaluate the needs and resources of patients and their families in order to tailor interventions for them. The assessment process does not need to be long and time consuming, but rather can be guided by several key questions. It is often helpful to start by asking, Who is the primary family caregiver who will be helping the patient to manage the illness? Some family members do not label themselves as "caregivers" if the patient is fairly independent, and it may help to clarify that the family caregiver is anyone who provides emotional support or physical care to the patient without pay on an ongoing basis. Other assessment questions are included in Table 72-1. These are only a few of the kinds of questions that can be used to assess the family. By conducting a brief assessment, the nurse will begin to form a partnership to help family members as well as patients cope with the illness.

### Assessing distress

Another important assessment issue is determining which patients and their family members are experiencing more psychological distress than others. Assessing distress has been identified as an important component of comprehensive cancer care.[74,75] Distress has been identified as the "sixth vital sign"[76] because it is so common among patients and family members facing a new diagnosis of cancer or a long-standing illness.[41,77–79] Distress refers to unpleasant feelings (such as powerlessness, sadness, uncertainty, fear, depression, anxiety, and panic) that affect people's thoughts and behaviors, and that interfere with their ability to cope with cancer.[74] Studies indicate that the incidence of emotional distress ranges from 35% to 45% in patients,[77] and from 41% to 62% in family members.[80]

There are a number of factors that can influence patients' or family members' levels of distress (see Table 72-2). These include demographic factors such as younger age,[81] female gender,[82–85] low family income, and being a minority.[86,87] In addition, a pile-up of other concerns in the lives of patients and their family members can deplete their resources and increase their vulnerability to experiencing more distress.[88,89]

There are also a number of cancer-related factors that can contribute to distress in patients with cancer and their family members. These include having a more advanced stage of cancer, more aggressive type of cancer (ie, lung or pancreatic), more symptoms,[80,81,90] greater functional impairment,[91–93] and a prior history of physical or mental health problems.[94–96]

In recent years, the Distress Thermometer has been used as a brief screening tool to assess distress and to determine which patients are in need of more intensive interventions than others to reduce their distress (see Chapter 26) which depicts the Distress Thermometer. Distress Thermometer is a single-item, self-report measure of psychological distress. Scores range from 0 to 10, with 10 indicating extreme distress. Respondents are instructed to circle the number on the Distress Thermometer that best describes how much distress they feel that day and over the past week. A problem list is also included with the Distress Thermometer to help identify the possible reasons for the distress, such as practical, family, emotional, spiritual, or physical concerns.[74] Although the screening tool was originally developed primarily for patients, researchers have found that it can also

**TABLE 72-1**

| Assessment Questions for Family Caregivers |
|---|
| Who is the primary family caregiver? |
| What effect is the illness having on you or other family members? |
| How confident are you to provide emotional or physical care? |
| How well are the patient and family members communicating about the illness? |
| How are you managing the stress that caregivers often experience? |
| What support is available to you and your family? |
| What kind of information or help do you need to cope with the illness? |

**TABLE 72-2**

| Factors Influencing Patients' or Family Members' Levels of Distress |
|---|
| Age |
| Gender |
| Family income |
| Ethnicity |
| Psychosocial concerns |
| Stage or phase of the illness |
| Type of cancer |
| Symptoms |
| Functional impairment |
| History of physical and mental health problems |

accurately assess distress in family members.[97] A score of 4 or 5 has been identified as the cut-off score for identifying whether patients or family members are experiencing increased distress.[98] Data from a series of studies have shown that Distress Thermometer has satisfactory validity and reliability, and it also is an effective screening tool that can be easily implemented in clinical settings.[83,98,99]

Although screening measures such as the Distress Thermometer are not used routinely in healthcare settings, their use is likely to increase. As healthcare resources decline, professionals will increasingly want to screen patients and their family members to determine who is in most need of limited healthcare resources.

## INTERVENTIONS TO HELP PATIENTS AND FAMILY MEMBERS

In addition to assessing patients and family members, there are practical interventions that nurses and other health professionals can use to assist them. Various strategies are described in the following section.

### Promote family communication and mutual support

Effective communication among care providers, patients, and their family members can improve care and relieve suffering. Ways to improve communication include (1) fostering effective professional communication with patients and their family members, and (2) facilitating intrafamily communication or communication between patients and their family members.

*Professional Communication With Patients and Family Members.* Nurses and other health professionals communicate with patients with cancer and their family members in a variety of ways and some ways are more effective than others. There are 3 patterns of communication that occur between professionals, patients, and family members: privileged communication, filtered communication, and balanced communication (see Figure 72-5).[100]

Privileged communication occurs when there is direct communication between the professional and family members, but the patient is left out of the interaction (see Figure 72-5). This type of communication pattern was more common in the early 1960s when professionals did not disclose the cancer diagnosis to patients. For example, in 1961, Oken[101] reported that 90% of the physicians did not tell patients with cancer their diagnoses. Instead, family members were often given this information so they could do financial planning or get business matters in order before the death of the patient. Family members were thought of as "healthy" and able to hear the truth, while patients were viewed as "sick" and unable to

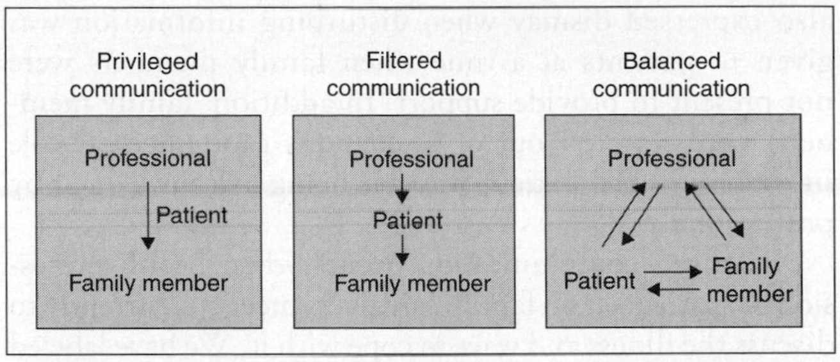


**FIGURE 72-5**

Communication patterns.

cope with the knowledge that they had cancer. Although this practice no longer exists, at times subtle remnants of privileged communication are still evident. For example, when professionals give more details about the patient's illness or life expectancy to family members than to patients, privileged communication is operating. There are negative effects to this type of professional–family communication. It hinders more open professional–patient communication and it can also disrupt patient–family communication. Privileged communication sends the message that difficult topics are too threatening and should not be openly discussed. It also fosters protective buffering and avoidant communication between patients and family members which hinders adjustment to illness as discussed earlier in the chapter.

Filtered communication occurs when information is transmitted from professional to patient, but there is no direct communication between professionals and family members; all or most of the information that family members receive is filtered through the patient (see Figure 72-5). This pattern of communication is similar to the "telephone game," in which one person whispers a message to another, who passes it to another, and so on. By the end of the game, the message the last person receives seldom resembles the initial message sent. This pattern of communication is still common in busy healthcare settings as professionals, in an attempt to be efficient, try to send information to family members by way of the patient.

There are a number of problems with filtered communication. One problem is that family members can receive incomplete or inaccurate information from patients, especially if patients are hard of hearing, highly anxious, or have memory problems. Another problem is that family members lack direct communication with health professionals, which hinders them from getting their own questions answered and their fears allayed. Furthermore, in a qualitative study, family caregivers reported they felt marginalized when they were left out of discussions that took place between patients and providers, especially in situations in which the patient expressed a desire for the caregiver to be involved in the dialogue.[102] Family members also expressed dismay when disturbing information was given to patients at a time when family members were not present to provide support. In addition, family members who were left out of discussions thought their role in caring for the patient was not being acknowledged by professionals.[102]

Balanced communication occurs when health professionals, patients, and family caregivers meet concurrently to discuss the illness and ways to cope with it. We have labeled this pattern of communication as balanced because it allows communication to and from all participants; no one is left out (see Figure 72-5). It allows for an open exchange of information and direct feedback from one person to another. Each person gains a greater understanding of the perceptions of the others and it also increases patients' and family members' satisfaction with care. Research indicates that when professionals make more of an effort to talk with family members and to include them in discussions, they reported feeling more positive about their communication with health professionals,[102] and they perceived less stress associated with the illness.[103]

There is also some evidence that when nurses meet jointly with patients with cancer and their family caregivers, it facilitates intrafamily communication. For example, in a recent clinical trial, patients with prostate cancer and their spouse caregivers were randomly assigned to (1) a family-based intervention program in which they met with a nurse to discuss the illness or (2) usual standard care (control condition). Patients and their spouses who received the family intervention reported more open communication with one another about the illness than couples who did not receive the intervention.[104] Patients and spouses who received the intervention also reported that it was easier to discuss their concerns in the presence of a supportive nurse, who facilitated their conversation about difficult topics, and who also answered any questions either of them had.

Professional-patient–family communication also is facilitated when professionals provide information in layman terms,[105] and when professionals avoid using patronizing, insensitive, or impersonal behaviors which are barriers to effective communication.[102] Further, communication can be improved when professionals demonstrate warmth and they attend to the emotional needs of both patients and their family members.[12] Finally, communication is enhanced when professionals "model" effective communication by demonstrating open, honest, respectful, and supportive communication while interacting with patients and their family members.

*Facilitating Patient–Family Communication.* There are also a number of strategies that nurses and other health professionals can use to facilitate communication between patients and their family members. These strategies are outlined in Table 72-3. One strategy is to encourage patients and family members to work as a "team" to manage the effects of the illness. It is important for them to know that each of them is affected in some way by the illness (eg, emotionally, financially) as discussed earlier in the chapter, and that by coming together and by providing one another with support that they will be able to work more effectively. Second, it is important to encourage patients and family members to share rather than hide their concerns, and to avoid protective buffering, which was discussed earlier in the chapter (see Figure 72-2). By sharing concerns, patients and family members will have a better understanding of one another's feelings, and be able to support each other more effectively. It is useful, however, to let patients and family members know that open communication does not mean they have to "tell everything" to one another; it is acceptable for them to have private thoughts of their own.[106] Also, open communication does not mean "dumping" feelings on the other person in an indiscriminate, cathartic way.[106] Rather, it means sharing feelings in an open, direct, and thoughtful manner. Fourth, it is helpful for patients and family members to avoid criticizing one another as it is detrimental to maintaining supportive relationships. Fifth, some families have preexisting problems that developed prior to the cancer diagnosis, and these can get in the way supporting one another. If possible, it is helpful when professionals encourage family members to set aside those differences or past hurts, at least temporarily, so that they can help one another through the stress of cancer. Those families who are not able to move beyond the preexisting problems may need additional guidance from a social worker or counselor so that past issues do not drain family resources, which are needed for dealing with the illness. While encouraging patients and spouses to discuss their feelings, professionals can also emphasize the importance of being sensitive to each other, being good listeners, and showing affection to one another.

**TABLE 72-3**

| Examples of Strategies Professionals Can Use to Promote Patient–Family Communication |
|---|
| Encourage patients and family members to |
| Work as a "team" |
| Share feelings rather than hide them (avoid protective buffering) |
| Recognize you do not have to share everything, but can have private thoughts of your own |
| Share feelings in a thoughtful manner rather than "dumping" your feelings |
| Set aside previous problems and help each another through the stress of illness |

## Provide information

Information is important to patients and their family members because it increases their knowledge and reduces their uncertainty about the illness. Information also facilitates their understanding of the illness's trajectory, and it enables them to plan for transitions from one phase of illness to another.

Nurses and other healthcare professionals can provide information to patients and their families through a variety of approaches. These include encouraging spouses or other key family members to attend clinic appointments or consultation sessions so they can get direct, first-hand information. In large families or extended families, 1 or 2 key family members can be identified to attend appointments with the patient, and Web-based blogs such as Care Pages can be used to keep other family members informed. It is also helpful when patients or family members bring a list of questions to clinic visits so they can get specific questions answered before leaving the office. Many outpatient offices have designated telephone lines that patients and family members can use to contact nurses with additional questions.

Information can also be provided through different media. Flyers, pamphlets, videos, and other media are commonly used to distribute information. There is also an increasing number of Web sites available through major organizations such as the American Cancer Society or the National Cancer Institute where patients and family members can get information about a specific kind of cancer and usual treatments for it. Many of these Web sites also provide information on ways to manage symptoms and side-effects of treatments (see Table 72-4).

In addition, there are general Web sites that have been established to help family caregivers (see Table 72-5). These Web sites are not cancer-specific, but provide general information to family caregivers dealing with a variety of chronic illnesses. Although patients and family members value information, some want more information than others. At times, they can be overwhelmed by too much information and become anxious. Thus, it is important to determine how much and what kind of information they want and to tailor information (eg, pamphlets) to their specific needs.

**TABLE 72-4**

**Examples of Useful Cancer-Related Web Sites**

| Name of Organization | Web Site |
|---|---|
| American Cancer Society | http://www.cancer.org |
| National Cancer Institute | http://www.cancer.gov/cancertopics/caring-for-the-caregiver |
| Lance Armstrong Foundation | http://www.livestrong.org |
| Cancer care | http://www.cancercare.org |
| The Cancer Information Network | http://thecancer.net/ and http://www.caringtoday.com/caregiver-wellbeing |

## Encourage optimistic outlook

Another way that nurses and other professionals can help patients with cancer and their family members is by encouraging them to maintain an optimistic outlook during the cancer experience. The ability to stay optimistic or hopeful has been associated with lower distress and a higher quality of life in both patients with cancer and their family caregivers.[89] Optimism is not a false sense of hope or denial. It is a realistic appraisal of a person's illness or situation with a belief that they will be able to cope and experience some positive outcomes from the experience. Even patients with advanced cancer and their families can maintain an optimistic outlook when a cure is not possible. Instead of focusing solely on a cure, they can hope for other outcomes, such as an extended remission, better pain control, and the ability to enjoy meaningful activities with family and friends.

The term "post-traumatic growth" has been used to characterize positive outcomes that can accompany or follow a serious illness such as cancer.[107] Post-traumatic growth occurs when patients with cancer and their family members

**TABLE 72-5**

**Examples of Useful Web Sites for Family Caregivers**

| Name of Organization | Web Site |
|---|---|
| Strength for Caring | http://www.strengthforcaring.com |
| National Family Caregivers Association | http://www.nfcacares.org |
| The Family Caregiver Web | http://www.familycaregiverweb.com |
| National Family Caregiver Support Program | http://www.agingcarefl.org/caregiver/NationalSupport |
| Caring Connections | http://www.caringinfo.org/AboutUs.htm |
| Family Caregiver Alliance | http://www. caregiver.org |
| Family Caregiving 101 | http://www.familycaregiving101.org |
| Family Caregiver Online | http://www.familycaregiversonline.com |
| Family Caregiver Support Network | http://www.caregiversupportnetwork.org |

are able to move through a difficult or traumatic experience and obtain positive changes as a result of it. Research has shown the ability to engage in positive reframing is related to higher post-traumatic growth in patients with cancer and their families.[108,109] On the other hand, a constantly negative view of the illness, and the inability to find positive meaning in the illness, has been associated with lower quality of life and increased fear of cancer recurrence for both cancer survivors and their family caregivers.[25,110]

Nurses and other healthcare professionals can help patients with cancer and their families to maintain optimistic outlooks in several ways. First, it is helpful to assess patients' and family members' level of optimism by asking each of them to rate how optimistic they feel about the illness on a scale from 0 (low) to 10 (high). We have used this brief assessment in our own work with families[104] and found that it enables nurses to determine each person's level of optimism, and compare them. Second, it can be helpful for nurses to encourage them to "reframe" the illness as an opportunity for personal growth or positive outcomes (eg, greater appreciation of their family) rather than as a totally negative, overwhelming experience. Third, optimism can be contagious, and it is helpful when nurses encourage patients with cancer and their family members to surround themselves with people who will help them to maintain hope. Some family members and friends are more pessimistic and are not able to provide encouragement and hope. It is important for patients with cancer and their family members to recognize who will be more hopeful and to spend time with them. Fourth, professionals can help patients and families to set realistic, short-term goals that they can accomplish. By setting realistic expectations, patients and families can regain a sense of control and feel more optimistic about their ability to manage the illness. Finally, it is important for professionals to tell patients and their family members that it is not realistic for them to feel optimistic all of the time. There will be times when they will experience sadness or a loss of hope. Encourage them to accept these feelings as a normal part of the cancer experience, but also continue to find ways to restore and maintain their hope.

### Teach stress reduction

There are a variety of stress-reduction techniques that healthcare professionals can teach patients with cancer and their families. First, meditation and relaxation are good stress-reduction techniques, which involve sitting motionlessly, breathing evenly and deeply, and focusing thoughts on a peaceful phrase, sound, or image. Patients and their caregivers can learn to contain their thoughts and settle their minds by practicing these activities regularly. Patients and families can also use relaxation tapes or CDs to direct their deep breathing and visualization. Keeping a diary or journal is another common therapeutic technique that can be soothing and meditative. It provides a means for sorting out and clarifying what a person is feeling so that they can gain a better understanding of themselves and their situations. It also provides a way for them to vent their feelings that may be difficult to express in conversations with others.

Exercise is also considered a powerful stress-reduction technique for patients and families. Research has shown that regular exercise can help maintain physical fitness, prevent disease, and facilitate better management of stress, depression, and anxiety.[111–113] Exercise can promote neurotransmitters in the brain and boost endorphins, reduce levels of the stress hormone cortisol, release muscle tension, and promote better sleep.[114] Exercise can also provide distraction by shifting the focus away from unpleasant thoughts to body movements. It can also boost self-confidence by making one feel a sense of command over his or her body and life. Research suggests that even small amount of activity (eg, as little as 10 or 15 minutes at a time) can improve mood, while 30 minutes of exercise a day for at least 5 days a week can significantly improve mental well-being.[115]

Religion and prayers also reduce stress and induce a sense of calm. By appealing to a higher power, patients and families remove themselves from the mire of daily routines and see their struggles as part of a larger picture or universal plan. In addition, praying also involves meditation, slow rhythmic breathing, and the repetition of well-known phrases or chants, so that it can create a relaxed state.

### Encourage effective coping and healthy lifestyle behavior

It is important for patients and their families to develop effective coping strategies and healthy lifestyle behaviors to deal with the demands of cancer. There are 2 major types of coping strategies: active and avoidant. Active coping refers to strategies such as use of emotional support, positive reframing, acceptance, and planning. Avoidant coping refers to strategies such as denial, behavioral disengagement, and use of alcohol and drugs.[116] For the most part, use of active coping strategies is associated with higher psychological well-being, whereas use of avoidant strategies is associated with poorer psychological well-being.[117,118]

There are a number of strategies that nurses and other professionals can use to encourage effective coping. One strategy is to teach them about the types of coping and encourage them to use active rather than avoidant coping to deal with problems associated with the illness. It also may be helpful for them to know that acceptance is an active coping strategy, and it is one of the most common strategies used by patients with cancer and their family caregivers to deal with a cancer diagnosis.[117] By accepting the illness and the caregiving that may be required, patients and caregivers can direct their energy toward managing changes brought about by the illness, rather than denying or avoiding them.

It also helps to encourage patients and family members to avoid negative coping strategies or unhealthy lifestyle behaviors. In the face of cancer, some people adopt negative coping behaviors such as smoking, drinking too much alcohol, and using drugs to relax. Patients and family members need to understand that self-medicating with alcohol or drugs may provide them with an easy or temporary escape from the stress, but will not restore their emotional balance. These negative coping strategies can also lead to other problems.

It is also important to encourage patients, and especially family caregivers to obtain emotional support. A number of studies have found that family caregivers receive less support than patients with cancer, even though their levels of emotional distress are similar.[119] Research indicates that even when the caregiving burden is relatively light, family members can feel deprived and depleted when others are not interested in their emotional reactions and do not provide support.[7,120] Support groups are an effective means of obtaining support. They can provide a forum for patients and families to share how they feel in a similar situation. Support groups also allow them to compare and contrast their experiences and also to learn from others. In recent years, there are more online support groups that patients and family can use to share their stories and obtain assistance.

Family caregivers who provide daily care need encouragement to obtain tangible support from others. When cancer is diagnosed initially, family members often promise to help one another with caregiving responsibilities. However, as time passes and some family members go back to their own personal and family responsibilities, the care for the patient often falls on one family member, typically the patient's spouse or adult daughter. Primary caregivers need to utilize support from others so they can withstand the strain of caregiving over time. Caregivers also need to learn to delegate caregiving tasks to other interested relatives so that the burden of caregiving is shared by others.

As the demands of illness extend over time, patients and family need to try to continue enjoyable activities in their lives so that the illness and treatments do not consume their lives. Professionals need to encourage them to take "time off" from focusing on the illness and to engage in restorative activities, such as going out with friends or spending time outdoors in nature. Caregivers feel guilty when they take time out of their caregiving role to participate in enjoyable activities outside of the home. Nurses need to encourage caregivers to take time to do things for themselves as a way to reduce the stress of caregiving; this will allow them to continue in their caregiving role without becoming burned out.

Nurses and other health professionals also need to encourage patients and family members to adopt healthy lifestyles to maintain their own physical and mental well-being. Healthy lifestyles can increase resistance to stress and strengthen their physical and emotional health. Exercise, as discussed earlier can play a key role in reducing and preventing stress. Eating a healthy diet is also critical because well-nourished bodies are in a better condition to weather the stress associated with illness and caregiving. Finally, patients and caregivers need to engage in cancer prevention and health screening activities (eg, cholesterol, colorectal and breast cancer screening) so that problems can be detected in a timely manner.

## CONCLUSION

The diagnosis of cancer and its treatment pose a major challenge to patients and their families, and it affects all aspects of their quality of life. Nurses and other health professionals can play a key role in helping both patients and their family members to manage the effects of illness by utilizing effective professional-patient-family communication with them, providing them information, encouraging an optimistic outlook, teaching them ways to reduce stress, and encouraging them to use effective coping strategies and healthy lifestyle behaviors. Helping families through family-centered care is an integral part of oncology care.

## REFERENCES


1. Kornblith AB, Herr HW, Ofman US, Scher HI, Holland JC. Quality of life of patients with prostate cancer and their spouses. The value of a database in clinical care. *Cancer*. 1994;73:2791–2802.
2. National Alliance for Caregiving. *Caregiving in the US*. Bethesda, MD: National Alliance for Caregiving; 2004.
3. National Alliance for Caregiving. *Evercare Study of Caregivers in Decline*. Bethesda, MD: National Alliance for Caregiving; 2006.
4. Schumacher KL, Stewart BJ, Archbold PG, Caparro M, Mutale F, Agrawal S. Effects of caregiving demand, mutuality, and preparedness on family caregiver outcomes during cancer treatment. *Oncol Nurs Forum*. 2008;35:49–56.
5. Bakas T, Lewis RR, Parsons JE. Caregiving tasks among family caregivers of patients with lung cancer. *Oncol Nurs Forum*. 2001;28: 847–854.
6. Ferrario SR, Zotti AM, Massara G, Nuvolone G. A comparative assessment of psychological and psychosocial characteristics of cancer patients and their caregivers. *Psychooncology*. 2003;12:1–7.
7. Given BA, Given CW, Kozachik S. Family support in advanced cancer. *CA: Cancer J Clin*. 2001;51:213–231.
8. Sherwood PR, Given BA, Given CW, et al. The influence of caregiver mastery on depressive symptoms. *J Nurs Scholarsh*. 2007;39:249–255.
9. Campbell LC, Keefe FJ, McKee DC, et al. Prostate cancer in African Americans: relationship of patient and partner self-efficacy to quality of life. *J Pain Symptom Manage*. 2004;28:433–444.
10. Walker E, Dewar BJ. How do we facilitate carers' involvement in decision making? *J Adv Nurs*. 2001;34:329–337.
11. Casey A. Partnership nursing: influences on involvement of informal carers. *J Adv Nurs*. 1995;22:1058–1062.
12. Hack TF, Degner LF, Parker PA, et al. The communication goals and needs of cancer patients: A review. *Psychooncology*. 2005;14: 831–845.

13. Greene MG, Adelman RD. Physician-older patient communication about cancer. *Patient Edu Counsel.* 2003;50:55–60.
14. Mystakidou K, Parpa E, Tsilila E, Katsouda E, Vlahos L. Cancer information disclosure in different cultural contexts. *Support Care Cancer.* 2004;12:147–154.
15. Searight HR, Gafford J. Cultural diversity at the end of life: issues and guidelines for family physicians. *Am Fam Physician.* 2005;71: 515–522.
16. Lazarus RS, Folkman S. *Stress, Appraisal, and Coping.* New York, NY: Springer Publishing Company; 1984.
17. Northouse LL, Mood D, Kershaw T, et al. Quality of life of women with recurrent breast cancer and their family members. *J Clin Oncol.* 2002;20:4050–4064.
18. Hagedoorn M, Sanderman R, Bolks HN, Tuinstra J, Coyne JC. Distress in couples coping with cancer: a meta-analysis and critical review of role and gender effects. *Psychol Bull.* 2008;134:1–30.
19. Hoskins CN. Adjustment to breast cancer in couples. *Psychol Rep.* 1995;77:435–454.
20. Northouse L. A longitudinal study of the adjustment of patients and husbands to breast cancer. *Oncol Nurs Forum.* 1989;16:511–516.
21. Gritz ER, Wellisch DK, Siau J, Wang HJ. Long-term effects of testicular cancer on marital relationships. *Psychosomatics.* 1990;31: 301–312.
22. Mellon S. Comparisons between cancer survivors and family members on meaning of the illness and family quality of life . *Oncol Nurs Forum.* 2002;29:1117–1125.
23. Matthews BA, Baker F, Spillers RL. Family caregivers and indicators of cancer-related distress. *Psychol Health Med.* 2003;8:45–56.
24. Walker BL. Adjustment of husbands and wives to breast cancer. *Cancer Prac.* 1997;5:92–98.
25. Mellon S, Kershaw TS, Northouse LL, Freeman-Gibb L. A family-based model to predict fear of recurrence for cancer survivors and their caregivers. *Psychooncology.* 2007;16:214–223.
26. Braun M, Mikulincer M, Rydall A, Walsh A, Rodin G. Hidden morbidity in cancer: spouse caregivers. *J Clin Oncol.* 2007;25:4829–4834.
27. Vanderwerker LC, Laff RE, Kadan-Lottick NS, McColl S, Prigerson HG. Psychiatric disorders and mental health service use among caregivers of advanced cancer patients. *J Clin Oncol.* 2005;23:6899–6907.
28. Bishop MM, Beaumont JL, Hahn EA, et al. Late effects of cancer and hematopoietic stem-cell transplantation on spouses or partners compared with survivors and survivor-matched controls. *J Clin Oncol.* 2007;25:1403–1411.
29. Birenbaum LK, Yancey DZ, Phillips DS, Chand N, Huster G. School-age children's and adolescents' adjustment when a parent has cancer. *Oncol Nurs Forum.* 1999;26:1639–1645.
30. Compas BE, Worsham NL, Epping-Jordan JE, et al. When mom or dad has cancer: markers of psychological distress in cancer patients, spouses, and children. *Health Psychol.* 1994;13:507–515.
31. Lewis FM. Psychosocial transitions and the family's work in adjusting to cancer. *Semin Oncol Nurs.* 1993;9:127.
32. Lewis FM, Ellison ES, Woods NF. The impact of breast cancer on the family. *Semin Oncol Nurs.* 1985;1:206.
33. Vannatta K, Grollman JA, Noll RB, Gerhardt CA. Impact of maternal breast cancer on the peer interactions of children at school. *Psychooncology.* 2008;17:252–259.
34. Compas BE, Worsham NL, Ey S, Howell DC. When mom or dad has cancer: II. Coping, cognitive appraisals, and psychological distress in children of cancer patients. *Health Psychol.* 1996;15:167–175.
35. Siegel K, Mesagno FP, Karus D, Christ G, Banks K, Moynihan R. Psychosocial adjustment of children with a terminally ill parent. *J Am Acad Child Adolesc Psychiatry.* 1992;31:327–333.
36. Visser A, Huizinga GA, Hoekstra HJ, van der Graaf WT, Gazendam-Donofrio SM, Hoekstra-Weebers JE. Emotional and behavioral problems in children of parents recently diagnosed with cancer: a longitudinal study. *Acta Oncologica.* 2007;46:67–76.
37. Wagner BM, Compas BE. Gender, instrumentality, and expressivity: moderators of the relation between stress and psychological symptoms during adolescence. *Am J Community Psychol.* 1990;18:383–406.
38. Huizinga GA, Visser A, van der Graaf WT, Hoekstra HJ, Hoekstra-Weebers JE. The quality of communication between parents and adolescent children in the case of parental cancer. *Ann Oncol.* 2005;16:1956–1961.
39. Dorval M, Guay S, Mondor M, et al. Couples who get closer after breast cancer: frequency and predictors in a prospective investigation. *J Clin Oncol.* 2005;23:3588–3596.
40. Ganz PA, Rowland JH, Desmond K, Meyerowitz BE, Wyatt GE. Life after breast cancer: understanding women's health-related quality of life and sexual functioning. *J Clin Oncol.* 1998;16:501–514.
41. Northouse LL, Templin T, Mood D. Couples' adjustment to breast disease during the first year following diagnosis. *J Behav Med.* 2001;24:115–136.
42. Lichtman RR, Taylor SE, Wood JV. Social support and marital adjustment after breast cancer. *J Psychosoc Oncol.* 1987;5:47–74.
43. Manne S, Ostroff J, Norton TR, Fox K, Goldstein L, Grana G. Cancer-related relationship communication in couples coping with early stage breast cancer. *Psychooncology.* 2006:15: 234–247.
44. Coyne J, Smith D. Couples coping with a myocardial infarction: a contextual perspective on wives' distress. *J Pers Soc Psychol.* 1991;61:404–412.
45. Hagedoorn M, Kuijer RG, Buunk BP, DeJong GM, Wobbes T, Sanderman R. Marital satisfaction in patients with cancer: does support from intimate partners benefit those who need it the most? *Health Psychol.* 2000;19:274–282.
46. Manne SL, Norton TR, Ostroff JS, Winkel G, Fox K, Grana G. Protective buffering and psychological distress among couples coping with breast cancer: the moderating role of relationship satisfaction. *J Fam Psychol.* 2007;21:380–388.
47. Walker BL. Psychosocial correlates of adjustment to breast cancer in marital dyads. *Doctoral Dissertation,* The University of Texas at Austin. 1989.
48. Oh S, Meyerowitz BE, Perez MA, Thornton AA. Need for cognition and psychosocial adjustment in prostate cancer patients and partners. *J Psychosoc Oncol.* 2007;25:1–19.
49. Giese-Davis J, Hermanson K, Koopman C, Weibel D, Spiegel D. Quality of couples' relationship and adjustment to metastatic breast cancer. *J Fam Psychol.* 2000;14:251–266.
50. Pistrang N, Barker C. The partner relationship in psychological response to breast cancer. *Soc Sci Med.* 1995;40:789–797.
51. Gotcher JM. Interpersonal communication and psychosocial adjustment. *J Psychosoc Oncol.* 1992;10:21–39.
52. Gotcher JM. Well-adjusted and maladjusted cancer patients: an examination of. communication variables. *Health Communication.* 1995;7:21–33.
53. Badr H, Carmack Taylor CL. Social constraints and spousal communication in lung cancer. *Psychooncology.* 2006;15:673–683.
54. Hinton J. An assessment of open communication between people with terminal cancer, caring relatives, and others during home care. *J Palliat Care.* 1998;14:15–23.
55. Shands ME, Lewis FM, Sinsheimer J, Cochrane BB. Core concerns of couples living with early stage breast cancer. *Psychooncology.* 2006;15:1055–1064.
56. Vess JD, Moreland JR, Schwebel AI. An empirical assessment of the effects of cancer on family role functioning. *J Psychosoc Oncol.* 1985;3:1–16.
57. Kuijer RG, Buunk BP, Ybema JF, Wobbes T. The relation between perceived inequity, marital satisfaction and emotions among couples facing cancer. *Br J Soc Psychol.* 2002;41(pt 1):39–56.
58. Zahlis EH, Shands ME. Breast cancer demands of the illness on the patient's partner. *J Psychosoc Oncol.* 1991;9:75–93.
59. Jensen S, Given B. Fatigue affecting family caregivers of cancer patients. *Support Care Cancer.* 1993;1:321–325.

60. Schulz R, Beach SR. Caregiving as a risk factor for mortality: the caregiver health effects study. *JAMA.* 1999;282:2215–2219.
61. Schulz R, Newsom J, Mittelmark M, Burton L, Hirsch C, Jackson S. Health effects of caregiving: the caregiver health effects study: an ancillary study of the cardiovascular health study. *Ann Behav Med.* 1997;19:110–116.
62. Hilton BA. Issues, problems, and challenges for families coping with breast cancer. *Semin Oncol Nurs.* 1993;9:88–100.
63. Mellon S, Northouse LL, Weiss LK. A population-based study of the quality of life of cancer survivors and their family caregivers. *Cancer Nurs.* 2006;29:120–131.
64. Morse SR, Fife B. Coping with a partner's cancer: adjustment at 4 stages of the illness trajectory. *Oncol Nurs Forum.* 1998;25:751–760.
65. Germino BB, Fife BL, Funk SG. Cancer and the partner relationship: what is its meaning? *Semin Oncol Nurs.* 1995;11:43–50.
66. Yabroff KR, Bradley CJ, Mariotto AB, Brown ML, Feuer EJ. Estimates and projections of value of life lost from cancer deaths in the United States. *J Natl Cancer Inst.* 2008;100:1755–1762.
67. National Cancer Institute. Costs of cancer care: US National Institutes of Health. Bethesda, MD: National Cancer Institute; 2007.
68. Yabroff KR, Lawrence WF, Clauser S, Davis WW, Brown ML. Burden of illness in cancer survivors: findings from a population-based national sample. *J Natl Cancer Inst.* 2004;96:1322–1330.
69. Covinsky KE, Goldman L, Cook EF, et al. The impact of serious illness on patients' families. SUPPORT investigators. Study to understand prognoses and preferences for outcomes and risks of treatment. *JAMA.* 1994;272:1839–1844.
70. Grunfeld E, Coyle D, Whelan T, et al. Family caregiver burden: results of a longitudinal study of breast cancer patients and their principal caregivers. *CMAJ.* 2004;170:1795–1801.
71. Hanratty B, Holland P, Jacoby A, Whitehead M. Financial stress and strain associated with terminal cancer a review of the evidence. *Palliat Med.* 2007;21:595–607.
72. Houser AN, Gibson MJ. *Valuing the Invaluable: The Economic Value of Family Caregiving, 2008 Update.* Washington, DC: AARP Public Policy Institute; 2008.
73. Wage and Hour Division. *The Family and Medical Leave Act of 1993.* Washington, DC: US Department of Labor, Employment Standards Administration, Wage and Hour Division. http://www.dol.gov/whd/regs/compliance/whdfs28.pdf; 2008.
74. National Comprehensive Cancer Network. *Distress: Treatment Guidelines For Patients.* Fort Washington, PA: National Comprehensive Cancer Network; 2005.
75. National Cancer Institute. *Supportive Care.* Bethesda, MD: National Cancer Institute; 2006.
76. Bultz BD, Carlson LE. Emotional distress: the sixth vital sign—future directions in cancer care. *Psychooncology.* 2006;15:93–95.
77. Zabora J, Brintzenhofeszoc K, Curbow B, Hooker C, Piantadosi S. The prevelance of psychosocial distress by cancer site. *Psychooncology.* 2001;10:19–28.
78. Cameron JI, Franche RL, Cheung AM, Stewart DE. Lifestyle interference and emotional distress in family caregivers of advanced cancer patients. *Cancer.* 2002;94:521–527.
79. Northouse LL, Templin T, Mood D, Oberst MT. Couples' adjustment to breast cancer and benign breast disease: a longitudinal analysis. *Psychooncology.* 1998;7:37–48.
80. Dumont S, Turgeon J, Allard P, Gagnon P, Charbonneau C, Vezina L. Caring for a loved one with advanced cancer: determinants of psychological distress in family caregivers. *J Palliat Med.* 2006;9:912–921.
81. Parker PA, Baile WF, Moor CD, Cohen L. Psychosocial and demographic predictors of quality of life in a large sample of cancer patients. *Psychooncology.* 2003;12:183–193.
82. Hagedoorn M, Buunk BP, Kuijer RG, Wobbes T, Sanderman R. Couples dealing with cancer: role and gender differences regarding psychological distress and quality of life. *Psychooncology.* 2000;9:232–242.
83. Jacobsen PB, Donovan KA, Trask PC, et al. Screening for psychologic distress in ambulatory cancer patients. *Cancer.* 2005;103:1494–1502.
84. Hopwood P, Stephens RJ. Depression in patients with lung cancer: prevalence and risk factors derived from quality-of-life data. *J Clin Oncol.* 2000;18:893–903.
85. Tuinstra J, Hagedoorn M, Van Sonderen E, et al. Psychological distress in couples dealing with colorectal cancer: gender and role differences and intracouple correspondence. *Br J Health Psychol.* 2004;9:465–478.
86. Carlson LE, Angen M, Cullum J, et al. High levels of untreated distress and fatigue in cancer patients. *Br J Cancer.* 2004;90:2297–2304.
87. Powe BD, Hamilton J, Hancock N, et al. Quality of life of African American cancer survivors. A review of the literature. *Cancer.* 2007;109:435–445.
88. Turner J, Kelly B, Swanson C, Allison R, Wetzig N. Psychosocial impact of newly diagnosed advanced breast cancer. *Psychooncology.* 2005;14:396–407.
89. Northouse LL, Caffey M, Deichelbohrer L, et al. The quality of life of African American women with breast cancer. *Res Nurs Health.* 1999;22:449–460.
90. Northouse LL, Mood D, Montie JE, et al. Living with prostate cancer: patients' and spouses' psychosocial status and quality of life. *J Clin Oncol.* 2007;25:4171–4177.
91. Kurtz ME, Kurtz JC, Stommel M, Given CW, Given B. Predictors of depressive symptomatology of geriatric patients with lung cancer—a longitudinal analysis. *Psychooncology.* 2002;11:12–22.
92. Brown DJ, McMillan DC, Milroy R. The correlation between fatigue, physical function, the systemic inflammatory response, and psychological distress in patients with advanced lung cancer. *Cancer.* 2005;103:377–382.
93. Roth RS, Lowery JC, Davis J, Wilkins EG. Quality of life and affective distress in women seeking immediate versus delayed breast reconstruction after mastectomy for breast cancer. *Plast Reconstr Surg.* 2005;116:993–1002.
94. Bennett KK, Compas BE, Beckjord E, Glinder JG. Self-blame and distress among women with newly diagnosed breast cancer. *J Behav Med.* 2005;28:313–323.
95. Green HJ, Pakenham KI, Headley BC, Gardiner RA. Coping and health-related quality of life in men with prostate cancer randomly assigned to hormonal medication or close monitoring. *Psychooncology.* 2002;11:401–414.
96. Millar K, Purushotham AD, McLatchie E, George WD, Murray GD. A 1-year prospective study of individual variation in distress, and illness perceptions, after treatment for breast cancer. *J Psychosom Res.* 2005;58:335–342.
97. Zwahlen D, Hagenbuch N, Carley MI, Recklitis CJ, Buchi S. Screening cancer patients' families with the distress thermometer (DT): a validation study. *Psychooncology.* 2008;17:959–966.
98. Gil F, Grassi L, Travado L, Tomamichel M, Gonzalez JR. Use of distress and depression thermometers to measure psychosocial morbidity among southern European cancer patients. *Support Care Cancer.* 2005;13:600–606.
99. Özalp E, Cankurtaran ES, Soygür H, Geyik PÖ, Jacobsen PB. Screening for psychological distress in Turkish cancer patients. *Psychooncology.* 2006;16:304–311.
100. Northouse LL, Northouse PG. *Health Communication—Strategies For Health Professionals.* Stamford, CT: Appleton & Lange; 1998.
101. Oken D. What to tell cancer patients. A study of medical attitudes. *JAMA.* 1961;175:1120–1128.
102. Kimberlin C, Brushwood D, Allen W, Radson E, Wilson D. Cancer patient and caregiver experiences: communication and pain management issues. *J Pain Symptom Manage.* 2004;28:566–578.
103. Gionta DA, Harlow LL, Loitman JE, Leeman JM. Testing a mediational model of communication among medical staff and families of cancer patients. *Struc Equation Modeling.* 2005;12:454.

104. Northouse L, Mood D, Kershaw T, et al. Effects of a family intervention on men with prostate cancer and their spouses. *Oncol Nurs Forum.* 2007;34:176–177.
105. Fried TR, Bradley EH, O'Leary JR, Byers AL. Unmet desire for caregiver-patient communication and increased caregiver burden. *J Am Geriatr Soc.* 2005;53:59–65.
106. Hilton BA. Family communication patterns in coping with early breast cancer. *West J Nurs Res.* 1994;16:366–388.
107. Calhoun LG, Tedeschi RG. *Facilitating Posttraumatic Growth: A Clinician's Guide.* Mahwah, NJ: Lawrence Erlbaum Associates Publishers; 1999.
108. Manne S, Ostroff J, Winkel G, Goldstein L, Fox K, Grana G. Posttraumatic growth after breast cancer: patient, partner, and couple perspectives. *Psychosom Med.* 2004;66:442–454.
109. Thornton AA, Perez MA. Posttraumatic growth in prostate cancer survivors and their partners. *Psychooncology.* 2006;15:285–296.
110. Sarna L, Brown JK, Cooley ME, et al. Quality of life and meaning of illness of women with lung cancer. *Oncol Nurs Forum.* 2005;32: E9-E19.
111. Knobf MT, Insogna K, DiPietro L, Fennie C, Thompson AS. An aerobic weight-loaded pilot exercise intervention for breast cancer survivors: bone remodeling and body composition outcomes. *Biol Res Nurs.* 2008;10:34–43.
112. Knobf MT, Musanti R, Dorward J. Exercise and quality of life outcomes in patients with cancer. *Semin Oncol Nurs.* 2007;23:285–296.
113. Carmack CL, Boudreaux E, Amaral-Melendez M, Brantley PJ, de Moor C. Aerobic fitness and leisure physical activity as moderators of the stress-illness relation. *Ann Behav Med.* 1999;21:251–257.
114. Jonsdottir IH. Special feature for the Olympics: effects of exercise on the immune system: neuropeptides and their interaction with exercise and immune function. *Immunol Cell Biol.* 2000;78:562–570.
115. Physical Activity Guidelines Steering Committee. *Physical Activity Guidelines for Americans.* Washington, DC: US Department of Health and Human Services; 2008.
116. Kershaw T, Northouse L, Kritpracha C, Schafenacker A, Mood D. Coping strategies and quality of life in women with advanced breast cancer and their family caregivers. *Psychol Health.* 2004;19:139–155.
117. Manne S. Couples coping with cancer: Research issues and recent findings. *J Clin Psychol Med Settings.* 1994;1:317.
118. Holland KD, Holahan CK. The relation of social support and coping to positive adaptation to breast cancer. *Psychol Health.* 2003;18:15–29.
119. Northouse LL. Social support in patients' and husbands' adjustment to breast cancer. *Nurs Res.* 1988;37:91–95.
120. Arora NK, Finney Rutten LJ, Gustafson DH, Moser R, Hawkins RP. Perceived helpfulness and impact of social support provided by family, friends, and health care providers to women newly diagnosed with breast cancer. *Psychooncology.* 2007;16:474–486.

CHAPTER

73

Elizabeth Johnston Taylor, PhD, RN

# Spiritual Responses to Cancer

## INTRODUCTION

> You get something that's going to impact your life like this (cancer) and, it's sad—but it's true, you turn back to God. You start going back to church, praying more. You realize you may be meeting your maker. You want to be on your best behavior . . . . It's part of human nature to do that. I think it's done by everybody and it's true. It's sad that's what has to happen to get us to be a better person and to think along those lines, but that's what it does.

This statement from a 65-year-old gentleman living with advanced melanoma poignantly describes a pervasive experience among persons living with cancer. When diagnosed with cancer, individuals inevitably become more aware of their personal vulnerability and mortality. Heightened spiritual awareness is a typical response to this threat to self. The cancer experience not only prompts spiritual questions, struggles, and triumphs, but may also inspire continued or renewed use of spiritual resources for coping. Because the spirit is an innate and influential aspect of being human, it is valuable for nurses to consider how spiritual responses to cancer might affect the illness experience. Likewise, nurses will do well to consider how best to support spiritual health, given that "No cure that fails to engage our spirit can make us well."[1(pp30–32)]

This chapter reviews recent research that describes spiritual responses across the cancer continuum. The spiritual perspectives of patients with cancer, family caregivers, and oncology nurses are discussed. The chapter concludes with a brief discussion of fundamental skills that nurses must practice to provide care that nurtures the spiritual health of patients and their family members. First, however, it is necessary to define what spirituality is and examine why it is important to address in oncology nursing care.

## DEFINITIONS

Before a discussion using the easily misunderstood terms of *spirituality* and *religiosity* proceeds, the terms must be defined. *Spirituality* refers to that dimension of being human that motivates meaning-making and self-transcendence—or intra-, inter-, and transpersonal connectedness.[2] In nursing literature that defines related terms such as spiritual distress, need, or well-being; one will find spirituality described as an integrating energy, a life principle, an innate human quality.[3] Spirituality prompts individuals to make sense of their universe and to relate harmoniously with self, nature, and others—including any god(s), as conceptualized by each person. Recently, doubt has been cast on the assumed all-inclusiveness of this broad and "elastic" conceptualization of spirituality[4–6]; for instance, numerous authors have argued that spirituality is a Western and Judeo-Christian concept that fails to appreciate the naturalistic perspectives of atheists, humanists, hedonists, and other nontheists. Such criticism highlights the need for nurses to recognize how their worldviews—whether of a secular, nonreligious, or religious orientation—inevitably affect their practice, theory, and research.[7]

In contrast to spirituality, *religiosity* often is viewed as a narrower concept in the nursing literature.[3,8] Religion is a representation and expression of spirituality. A religion offers an individual a specific worldview and an explanation that seeks to provide answers to the questions of ultimate meaning; it also may recommend how one is to live harmoniously with self, others, nature, and god(s). Such explanations and recommendations are presented in a religion's belief system (eg, myths/stories, doctrines, dogmas) and are remembered and appreciated with rituals and other religious practices or observances. One's religion may or may not be of an institutional nature. Although the vast majority of Americans reported in 2008 that religion was important to them, 6% did not believe in a God or universal spirit/higher power.[9]

Those studying the interrelatedness of spirituality and health are increasingly recognizing spirituality and religion (often conflated as "religiousness/spirituality" [R/S]) as a multidimensional concept. Numerous instruments are now available to measure these various aspects of R/S. For example, most of the recent health research investigating spirituality in the context of cancer has explored religious coping (especially the impact of negative vs positive religious coping),[10] spiritual well-being (SWB) (measured by existential and religious dimensions),[11] and how patients' specific beliefs (eg, their image of God) contributes to adjustment.[12,13] These approaches to studying R/S demonstrate more precise thinking about the concept compared to those of several years ago that often only measured religious affiliation and service attendance, or measured R/S in terms of its being intrinsic or extrinsic (now debated as culturally insensitive).

## WHY ADDRESS SPIRITUALITY?

Health psychologist Park[14] offers a beginning framework for explaining how R/S affects health. Everyone has a "meaning system" or means for interpreting and reacting to life experiences. This meaning system is composed of beliefs, goals, and a sense of meaning and purpose in life. Religions provide worldviews, which essentially are meaning systems. The pathways which may explain the contribution of R/S to physical and mental health include:

- R/S creates a sense of meaning, and meaning in life is related to psychological and physical well-being.
- Social support, which is inherent in affiliating with a religion, is linked with health—especially when experienced within a faith community.
- Body sanctification or pursuing a lifestyle that appreciates the sacredness of one's body or health (eg, viewing

one's body as a "temple," observing proscriptions against alcohol, illicit drugs, smoking, nonmarital sex, eating certain foods), assumedly contributes to better health.
- Health locus of control, or how one believes self, others, chance, or God control their health, may have an impact then on health behaviors.
- Gratitude, hope, optimism, and compassion may contribute to a sense of meaningfulness and social connection, which as discussed above appear to enhance well-being.
- Health behaviors such as prayer and meditation, in addition to the religious proscriptions mentioned above, appear to have stress-buffering effects which can also contribute to health.
- Positive religious coping and other aspects of religion that produce a positive affect also appear to have a stress-buffering effect.

Although there is much room for systemic study of these proposed mechanisms whereby R/S may mediate health, there is enough empirical evidence to date to suggest these are possible pathways. Given this, it is evident that nurses appreciate how spirituality manifests and influences the cancer experience.

## SPIRITUALITY THROUGHOUT THE CANCER EXPERIENCE

Empirical research investigating spirituality in the context of health has grown exponentially over the past two decades; much of it investigates the spirituality of persons living or dying with cancer.[3] This recent research exploring spirituality and cancer is showing a strong trend toward using more sophisticated approaches. That is, more conceptually precise measurements are employed, and more rigorous designs are followed (eg, controlling for pertinent variables prior to statistically analyzing between groups, using a longitudinal design). Also, there is an increase in the number of non-American studies exploring spirituality among patients with cancer. While in the past much of this research focused on women (especially those with breast cancer), some recent research provides evidence about the spirituality of men with prostate cancer. The research in this area continues to seek to describe and understand the spiritual responses of persons newly diagnosed, actively living with cancer or in treatment, surviving, and dying from cancer. A few studies have explored how spirituality may influence the decision-making process involved in cancer screening and prediagnostic experiences of cancer. Following is a summary of research from the past decade that provides evidence about spirituality during different phases of the cancer experience.

### CANCER SCREENING AND PREDIAGNOSIS

The impact of spiritual beliefs and religiosity on cancer screening continues to receive scanty attention from researchers. It is arguable that the research exploring the interface of religion and culture for cancer screening among African Americans is an exception.[15–17] However, even for this ethnic group, there is much to learn about how R/S contributes to cancer screening adherence. However, past studies suggest that religion may play a significant role in cancer screening practices, especially among women.[18]

Results from a large nationally representative survey study ($N = 6055$) of noninstitutionalized elders provides strong evidence that both religious denominational affiliation and holding religion to be very important predict preventative health behavior.[19] Along with other preventative health practices, this study examined how religiosity contributed to whether an elder sought cancer screening (ie, prostate, breast, cervical). Findings indicate that religiosity predicted preventative care among the very religious women, but not men. Still, religious men were at least twice likely to have prostate screenings than were their nonreligious counterparts.

A few researchers have recognized that a fatalistic attitude toward cancer does occur in some cultural groups and presumably affects what one believes about cancer screening and how one treats cancer. Fatalism essentially reflects one's worldview, or personal philosophical framework that is shaped largely by spirituality. A fatalistic attitude is illustrated by comments such as "My cancer is God's will, so there is nothing I can do about it." The belief that God determines whether one will die or be cured of cancer is strong among African Americans; among low and middle-income African Americans especially, women are fearful, fatalistic, and silent about breast cancer.[20] Holt and colleagues[21] observed a strong active and passive spiritual locus of control [ie, believing God empowers individuals to take care of themselves (active) vs believing that control rests with God (passive)] among 1227 African American women surveyed about mammography. Although the study used weak instrumentation, the findings indicated that God orientation among black women may be associated with perceiving more barriers and fewer benefits to mammography, which in turn influences mammography utilization. These attitudes presumably contribute to African American women's tendency to delay their visits to healthcare centers for cancer screening and treatment and, therefore, they have higher mortality rates for breast cancer compared to American women of European descent.

Religiosity, for an African American woman, however, is not always antagonistic toward cancer screening. From a Grounded Theory study of African American women about mammography screening perspectives, Fowler[17] observed not only fears and fatalistic beliefs, but also that religious beliefs and supports greatly influenced these informants' decision-making process. That is, religious scriptures' stories of strong women taking charge inspired these women to take charge of their own health. Also, these women understood from their scriptures body sanctification. Although these scriptural influences affirmed mammography, religious belief also led these informants to submit such decision making to their higher power. As one participant said, "I count on the Lord 100% . . . . I walk by faith and not by sight."

Pakistani researchers[22] found that 53% of women recently diagnosed with breast cancer delayed seeking medical help; 15% reported using various spiritual therapies in attempts to rid themselves of the breast lump. This study raises the question of who else might use spiritual "therapies" in an attempt to cure cancer prior to seeking health care. Indeed, as will be discussed later in this chapter, "spiritual therapies" (eg, prayer) constitute some of the most frequently used complementary and alternative medicines (CAMs).[23]

## DIAGNOSIS

Over 30 years ago, Weisman and Worden[24] described the first 100 days after a diagnosis of cancer as an "existential plight." Subsequently, very little research has focused on the spiritual responses to the diagnostic phase. Because receiving the diagnosis of cancer is typically devastating or unsettling at best, it is likely that it can be a time of petitionary prayer or invocations of magic, questions about the nature of God, or calls for support from a spiritual community.

The diagnostic phase usually includes the process of determining how to treat the cancer. A case study of one woman's decision making after a diagnosis of leukemia identified spirituality as a factor contributing to this challenging process.[25] Shannon-Dorcy and Wolfe[25] noted that spiritual questions arise, such as "Where is God in the midst of this?"; "Does my faith answer questions or create them?"; and "Do I use my spirituality to help me make decisions?" A qualitative study revealed that patients with cancer may pray about these decisions; they bring to God the questions of which physician and which treatment plan, and ask for providential guidance.[26] A phenomenological study of 20 Turkish women receiving an excisional breast biopsy found that alongside fears and need for information, these women prayed.[27] All 20 informants reported after they palpated their lump, that they prayed "it would not be something bad."

Four studies provide insight about how the role of faith in God influences diagnostic decision making. Silvestri and colleagues[28] surveyed 100 patients with advanced lung cancer, their caregivers, and 257 medical oncologists about how they would rank factors that influence treatment decisions. All three groups ranked the doctor's recommendation highest. For patients and their family members, the second most important factor to consider while making a treatment decision was "faith in God." It is interesting to note that the physicians ranked this factor lowest (seventh).

In a study of 218 patients designed to determine why African Americans infrequently join clinical trials, Advani and colleagues[29] found that a belief in God, along with low income and education, predicted unwillingness to participate in a cancer clinical trial. A qualitative study of 29 Canadian men who had refused conventional treatment for prostate cancer in lieu of CAM noted spiritual beliefs to play a key role in these participants' decision making.[30] Many of these men, although few belonged to a specific faith tradition, believed they possessed a divine energy and pursued spiritual practices to promote healing. In contrast, a team of researchers at a major medical institution conducting phase I clinical trials observed that patients with advanced cancer enrolling in these trials were no different from nontrial participants with regard to spirituality or religious problem solving style.[31] These just-as-spiritual patients placed their trust in both God and Western medicine.

These findings suggest that nurses involved in helping patients with cancer treatment decision making will do well to recognize and support those patients for whom "faith in God" is a salient decision-making factor. For example, the patient could be encouraged to consult with clergy or chaplains, or to explore "How does my faith guide me now?" Lack of such support may bring about an outcome that is unsatisfactory.

## LIVING WITH CANCER

Often individuals living with cancer have a heightened spiritual awareness.[30,32–34] This heightened awareness of personal spirituality may manifest itself as spiritual or existential distress or increased SWB.[34] The spiritual aspects of living with cancer that have received the most extensive and rigorous study recently will be reviewed; these include meaning-making, spiritual coping, and SWB/existential well-being (EWB), and quality of life (QOL). This section, however, opens with a review about the spiritual needs of patients with cancer to set the stage.

### Spiritual needs

Regardless of whether patients experience spiritual distress, spiritual needs are an inherent part of living.[3] As early as 1983, typologies of spiritual needs of patients with cancer were described; subsequently, researchers have identified the myriad of spiritual needs.[35] A qualitative study of 28 patients with cancer and family caregivers identified 7 categories of spiritual needs, which encompass those observed by previous researchers.[35] These categories included:

- Needs associated with relating to an Ultimate Other (eg, "God"). For example, the need "get right" with God, or realize that "Something out there is looking after you."

- Need for positivity, gratitude, and hope, such as "keeping a positive attitude" and "not taking life for granted."
- Need to give and receive love from other persons, such as wanting to make the world a better place and protecting one's family from knowing you suffer.
- Need to review spiritual beliefs, often initiated by wondering if one's religious beliefs are correct, or by asking "why?" questions.
- Need for meaning and finding purpose, such as "getting past asking, why me?" and remembering that there are others worse off.
- Religious needs, such as to have quiet time and space, pray, read scripture, worship (eg, by watching a religious program on television).
- Need to prepare oneself for death, for example, by balancing thoughts about death with hoping for health.

Using a questionnaire based on the above categories of spiritual need, Taylor[36] surveyed 156 patients with cancer and 68 family caregivers to determine the prevalence of these needs and related factors. The most important spiritual needs of these participants were being positive, loving others, finding meaning, and relating to God. Those rated as least important were the need to ask "why?" questions and prepare for dying. Greater spiritual need was found among patients (or the family caregivers of those) who were inpatients, perceived the cancer was incurable, and were religious.

## Search for meaning

The spiritual needs of persons living with cancer are not only varied, but often deeply painful and distressing. The search for meaning, or the yearning to make sense of a senseless disease and suffering, can plague many patients.[37] Inner questions that may be discomforting to voice (or thought to be forbidden by religion) may include "Why do bad things happen, especially since I was good?" and "Why me? Why now?" The search for meaning can include an attempt to attribute causality (what caused the cancer), selective incidence (why a certain person got it), blame (what is responsible), or significance (positive meanings of an ultimate nature). The search for meaning often brings one's religious beliefs to the forefront.[38]

Research has described the difference between the process of searching for meaning, and the outcomes of having searched.[39,40] For example, a qualitative study of 9 women with ovarian cancer identified "finding meaning in life" as the core category in the data.[41] Finding meaning involved self-reflection, reappraisal of life, and development of new short-term life goals. Although patients can get "stuck" attempting to find meaningfulness in having cancer (28% in a study of 60 women surviving breast cancer), many are able to ascribe positive meanings in a way that is spiritually transformative.[42] A qualitative study of 24 women with breast cancer described the process and outcomes of transforming the tragedy of cancer.[40] The outcomes included reevaluating and reprioritizing personal values; reconsidering the direction and mission of life; having a sense of urgency, intentionality, and immediacy about life; appreciating profoundly with joy the gifts of life and nature; having a more intense spiritual awareness; and becoming more self-respectful or self-aware.

Recent studies have explored how meaning (and its constituent parts, variously defined) contributes to the well-being of patients with cancer.[43–45] Simonelli and colleagues[43] found meaning in life functioned as a mediator explaining a relationship between physical sequelae and depression among 260 gynecological cancer survivors. That is, more physical distress was related to lower sense of meaning in life, which was related to depression. Park and fellow researchers[44] also tested whether meaning making mediated psychological adjustment among 172 cancer survivors. They observed that survivors who did experience posttraumatic growth, did find life meaningful, and were able to restore for themselves a sense that the world was just, showed better adjustment. This group of researchers also found that life meaning was a significant factor contributing to whether a cancer survivor changed health behaviors (ie, diet, exercise, sleep, and stress management).[44] Dutch researchers[45] have likewise studied how meaning in life (ie, satisfying worldview or framework and goal fulfillment) contributes to well-being. In a study of 354 testicular cancer survivors, 60% reported they experienced a more positive outlook on life since their diagnosis. After controlling for significant factors, life meaning was found to predict mental health, happiness, social function, and distress caused by cancer.

Although much of the research describing this process of searching for meaning has been qualitative, recent research has used rigorous designs and quantitative methods. While much of the research on meaning and cancer has studied only women with breast cancer, more recent studies have included mixed samples and even samples of men only. In concert, these studies provide strong and consistent evidence that the sense of meaning of a patient with cancer plays a key role in psychosocial adjustment.

## Spiritual or religious coping

Spiritual or religious coping, often described in terms of "strategies" or "resources," appears to be an important mechanism that often promotes adaptation for patients with cancer and their families.[10,46] R/S coping has been defined in a variety of ways, including beliefs and practices (especially prayer). Thuné-Boyle and colleagues[10] speculated that R/S coping may function by helping patients to maintain self-esteem, offer meaningfulness, and provide comfort and hope.

Several studies have documented the pervasive use of specifically religious beliefs and practices among persons living with cancer.[45,48] For example, in a survey of 108 women with various stages of gynecological cancer, 76% reported religion to be important, and 49% indicated they had become more religious since their diagnosis.[41] A study of 73 women diagnosed within the past 3 months indicated that religious beliefs were considered very helpful in coping with treatment (mean of 7.8 on scale of 1–9).[48] A qualitative study of 143 Hawaiian patients with cancer offers reasons for why patients use their religious beliefs and practices to cope with illness.[47] Tatsumura and colleagues[47] noted that spiritual resources not only supported treatment or cure, but also provided the possibility of treatment or cure, and were used simply because they were part of the patients' lives.

Research on R/S coping has been greatly influenced by the Pargament's[49] conceptualization, which recognizes the potential positive, as well as negative effects of R/S coping. That is, negative coping is exemplified by thinking one's cancer is a punishment, that church or God has abandoned, that God may not be all loving or powerful as once thought. Positive coping is illustrated by perceiving that God is present, helpful, and loving. Koffman and coresearchers[38] observed not only positive and negative implications from religious beliefs among British patients with cancer, but also guarded or ambivalent perspectives.

Several studies have investigated the impact of R/S coping (especially whether it is negative or positive) on emotional and physical health outcomes in patients with cancer. Tarakeshwar and colleagues[50] investigated how negative and positive R/S predicted QOL among 170 patients with advanced cancer. They found positive religious coping predicted better overall QOL; conversely, negative coping contributed to worse QOL. They also noted that non-whites and females reported more positive coping than did their counterparts.

Similarly, Gall and colleagues[12,51] have studied how the image of God, or perceived relationship with God, has an impact on general well-being of a patient with cancer. In a study of 93 women with breast cancer, Gall's team[12] found that negative images of God and religious salience correlated with emotional distress as expected, prediagnostically and 6 months postsurgery. However, path analyses showed these indicators of spirituality to have an impact on distress only cross-sectionally, but not over time. They concluded that women, who may not be very religious prior to cancer and try to mobilize their R/S to cope, may experience struggles and doubts that lead to greater distress. In a small study of prostate cancer survivors ($N = 34$), Gall found relationship with God to be a significant predictor of physical, social, and emotional function.[51]

A couple of studies have been used to investigate how R/S coping relates to physical distress. A longitudinal study of 94 myeloma patients undergoing stem cell transplantation revealed that post-transplant physical well-being was predicted by baseline R/S coping.[52] Negative R/S coping prior to transplantation predicted post-transplant emotional distress (including anxiety and depression) and transplant-related concerns. A German longitudinal study explored whether patients with head-and-neck cancer with "a belief giving [them] comfort" (their indicator of religious coping) was related to overall QOL.[53] This research team observed that believers reported less pain and other side effects, fear of death, and anxiety, than nonbelievers ($N = 66$).

It may be this dichotomous nature of R/S coping that explains why a systematic review of 17 research studies on the topic found discrepant results.[10] Although the majority (7) of these studies observed R/S coping beneficial for patients with cancer, 3 found negative effects and 7 studies obtained results Thuné-Boyle and colleagues characterized as neutral. Examining R/S coping as positive or negative appears to provide further clarity in an area of substantial promise.

Several studies of CAM used by persons with cancer have documented the frequency and perceived helpfulness of prayer and other R/S coping strategies or "therapies."[23,47,54–56] The CAM options that appear most to reflect spirituality and religiosity include prayer (personal and from others), "spiritual healing," church-related activities, personal faith, counseling with religious leader, scripture reading, attending religious services and other spiritual ceremonies, indigenous healing, meditation, spiritual imagery, spending time where spiritual energy is felt, and help from ancestors.[23,30] Culture and spirituality may be factors that predict CAM use. Of interest here, Jones and colleagues[55] found that most of the 14 African American men surviving cancer in their qualitative study were leery of CAMs other than prayer. Hsiao's research team[55] noted that considerably religious participants were less likely than nonreligious cancer survivors to use non-R/S CAMs, while considerably spiritual participants were more likely to use non-R/S CAMs than those describing themselves as nonspiritual.

Prayer is a common CAM.[23] Data from the 2002 US National Health Interview Survey found that 68.5% of the 2262 cancer survivors reported having prayed for their health.[57] Prayer was used more by women, African Americans, and married survivors. A study of breast cancer survivors revealed 81% ($N = 175$) prayed.[58] The women who prayed throughout their illness construed more benefit from having cancer and had higher SWB than those who did not pray. Quality of life and psychological well-being and social support, however, were not different between these 2 groups of women. A study of 30 patients with cancer found that for some persons with cancer, the intensity and frequency with which they pray increased since being diagnosed with cancer.[26] These informants prayed for many things, including both physical concerns (especially pain and distressing symptoms) and spiritual concerns ("Why?"). While some denied petitioning God for a cure, others prayed for healing in a vague way or for "God's will." A secondary analysis of these data revealed that beliefs about prayer can also contribute to spiritual distress, such as questions about why God does not "answer" or whether God exists.[59]

### Spiritual well-being and quality of life

The past 20 years have seen numerous studies examining the relationship between SWB and QOL. Research ranking the various components of QOL including SWB, typically show that persons living with cancer typically rank SWB second highest in importance, after physical QOL.[60] Whether spirituality is measured as EWB or some other aspect of spirituality, study findings are generally consistent in showing SWB to be strongly and positively correlated with overall QOL.[60,61] Fisch and colleagues,[62] for example, found that more than half of 163 patients with noncurable cancer receiving therapies in an ambulatory care clinic had high SWB and that spiritual QOL correlated with overall QOL ($r = 0.56$, $P < 0.0001$).

Indeed, SWB and EWB have been observed to be significant, unique predictors of overall QOL.[11,63] Furthermore, EWB (a more generic meaningfulness) has been shown to be distinct from religious well-being (RWB), and impacts cancer survivors' QOL differently—that is, more substantially—than does RWB. Edmondson and colleagues[11] argue that RWB, when studied alongside EWB, may conceal the strong impact of EWB on QOL. Although recent methodologically robust research indicates SWB predicting overall QOL after controlling for pertinent variables, a decade old study of good size ($N = 142$ women with breast cancer) suggested that SWB may not predict QOL much, once adjustment style and demographic factors are controlled.[64] More research can be anticipated in this area, and it is likely to ascertain just how SWB contributes to QOL.

Many studies have documented relationships between SWB and more specific variables. For example, SWB is correlated with fighting spirit, optimism, physical, and mental health. Spiritual well-being has also been shown to be negatively correlated with depression, anxiety, pain level, demands of illness, boredom/purposelessness, helplessness/hopelessness, and negative moods.[11,4,65]

Although most studies examining SWB and QOL remain cross-sectional, one well-designed investigation explored the longitudinal impact of cancer on SWB and other domains of QOL. Andrykowski and colleagues[66] conducted telephone interviews with 662 recipients of stem cell transplants, an average of 6.7 years post-transplant and matched healthy comparison group to collect data about spiritual, physical, social, and psychological aspects of QOL. Results indicated that for all aspects of QOL, except spiritual, the transplant survivors faired worse than the controls. SWB (ie, measured as post-traumatic growth), however, was significantly greater for the survivors, suggesting that even amidst the negative long-term sequelae, positive spiritual growth continues for many survivors.

Together, these research findings demonstrate SWB is a salient contributor to health-related QOL. It is also an important dimension of QOL from the patient perspective. This evidence raises questions about how SWB can be enhanced or nurtured, and if such nurture can promote QOL.

## DYING WITH CANCER

Dying entails facing an unknown, the loss of self, the desire to leave a legacy, the yearning to know that life—and death—possess purpose, and many other experiences that are inherently spiritual. Williams observed from a meta-analysis of 11 qualitative studies providing evidence about the spiritual perspectives of the dying (most of which involved a sample of patients with cancer) that spirituality is fundamentally important to the work of dying.[67] This meta-analysis identified the following themes:

- Spiritual despair (alienation, loss of self, dissonance)
- Spiritual work (forgiveness, self-exploration, search for balance)
- Spiritual well-being (connection, self-actualization, consonance)

A couple of dated quantitative studies provide documentation that patients near the end of life rank spiritual concerns extremely high. Greisinger and colleagues[68] found 92% to 99% of 120 patients rated spiritual and existential concerns as extremely or very important. Steinhauser and collaborators[69] reported that seriously ill patients ($N = 340$, many with cancer) ranked "coming to peace" and prayer along with other psychosocial concerns often described as spiritual needs (eg, not being a burden) among the top ranked factors important at the end of life. Indeed, in a study of 100 patients with lung cancer using content analysis of written open-ended responses to questions ascertaining what is a good death, found having a peaceful death to be 1 of 4 primary themes.[70]

Several studies have explored spirituality in relation to QOL in the context of terminal cancer.[60] Two studies measuring various domains of QOL found SWB to rank highest among samples of hospice patients.[71,72] McClain and colleagues[73] observed that SWB functioned to protect patients with terminal cancer against end-of-life despair. They found SWB to have moderately strong inverse relationships with the desire for a hastened death, hopelessness, and suicidal ideation.

Two studies have investigated how spirituality or religiosity influence end-of-life decisions for persons with an advanced cancer.[74,75] Both research teams found that R/S coping was associated with greater desire for life-sustaining measures (eg, CPR). True and colleagues[74] also observed that participants who believed in divine intervention were less apt to have an advanced directive. These corroborating results underscore how spiritual beliefs influence decision making throughout the cancer experience.

## CAREGIVER PERSPECTIVES

Although the experience of living with cancer in one's body is challenging, if not traumatizing, the experience of caring for someone with cancer is difficult as well. Family and nurse caregivers alike witness the challenges and inevitably have their own spiritual responses to watching life with cancer.

### FAMILY CAREGIVER PERSPECTIVES

Being the family caregiver can be an emotionally and physically exhausting role. Family caregivers' spiritual questions may include "Why does my loved one have to suffer?"; "Where can I get my need for love filled when all I do is give care?"; and "What did I do to deserve this?" Harrington and colleagues[76] documented that spiritual needs, alongside informational needs, were ranked as most important by 55 family caregivers. Findings from three studies suggest there may be little difference between the spiritual needs of patients with cancer and those of their family caregivers.[35,36,77]

It is likely, however, that family caregivers may receive less spiritual nurture than do their loved ones with cancer. Two descriptive Scandinavian studies[78,79] indicate that nurses attend to patients' spiritual needs more than to family members'. Bishop and colleagues[80] surveyed 133 spouses and partners of stem cell transplant recipients nearly 7 years after their loved one's transplant, and found that their stressors (eg, fatigue, depression, loneliness, sleep, and sexual problems) continued—even as they did for cancer survivors. However, the one factor that was significantly different between the patients and partners was the degree of posttraumatic growth. That is, the spouses and partners shared all the turmoil, but without the benefit of personal growth and transformation (which the patients did experience).

Spirituality is a resource for this stressful caregiving role.[81] This likely explains why family caregivers' sense of meaningfulness and SWB are associated with emotional health.[82,83] "Prayer or putting trust in God"—examples of spiritual resources— were identified by Steele and Fitch[84] as a coping strategy used and found effective by hospice family caregivers ($N = 18$). The import and nature of the relationship a caregiver has with God, however, may influence this coping and QOL.[85–87] For example, among 125 family caregivers of hospice patients, Mickley and colleagues[86] found that those who viewed God as apathetic or unfair were more anxious, were more depressed, and perceived less purpose in life. Abernethy and colleagues[87] found that the relationship between religious coping and depression among 156 spouses of patients with lung cancer was significant but not linear; that is, those who used moderate amounts of religious coping were less depressed than those who used either high or low amounts of such coping.

### ONCOLOGY NURSE PERSPECTIVES

Inherent in oncology nursing is sharing with care recipients the profound and humbling experiences of life, both the sacred and the profane. This role can be burdensome and draining; at the same time, it can be a privilege. A survey of 813 hospice and oncology nurses revealed that most acknowledged that working with cancer-care recipients had influenced their own spirituality either a great deal (65%) or somewhat (24%).[88] While working with patients influences nurses, it is also true that hospice and oncology nurses' personal spirituality and religiousness influence if and how spiritual care is delivered to care recipients. Taylor and colleagues[89] found that self-reported spirituality and attitudes about spiritual care were predictors of how frequently and how comfortably cancer nurses provided spiritual care. Similarly, studies of Israeli[90] and Swedish[91] oncology nurses indicate that personal spirituality, as well as training in providing spiritual care, influence attitudes toward spiritual caregiving.

Several studies provide insight about what oncology nurses think constitutes spiritual care.[92–94] Spiritual care was described by 29 oncology nurses in a phenomenological study as being "about developing caring relationships through fostering connections to promote spiritual comfort and well-being."[94(p.690)] Essential qualities a nurse must possess were identified as receptivity (ie, true presence, being fully there for the patient); humanity (ie, being authentically who one is); competency (ie, providing proper care for the body is requisite to spiritual care); and positivity (ie, exuding positive and healing energy).[94] A survey of 181 clinicians reported the following categories of spiritual caregiving: verbally communicating about spiritual or religious concerns, involving spiritually supportive others in patient care, facilitating or initiating prayer, attending to family, providing or suggesting religious materials, being therapeutically present, touching, and conveying a benevolent attitude.[92] When Kristeller and colleagues[93] surveyed 267 oncology nurses, they found that 47% viewed themselves as the primary professional responsible for addressing spiritual distress. These respondents identified the following interventions for spiritual needs: suggesting patients seek help (11%), giving an educational brochure (7%), informing clients of local resources (27%), discussing an issue in depth (39%), and making a referral (37%).

## PROVIDING SPIRITUAL CARE

Given that persons with cancer and their family members often use spiritual coping strategies and that SWB contributes to adjustment and QOL, it follows that nurses should support these coping strategies and nurture SWB in ways that are patient-centered and ethical. Although this idea is accepted and promoted in nursing practice and education, little evidence exists regarding what patients desire in terms of nurses providing spiritual care. When Taylor[95] interviewed 28 patients and family members living with cancer about what spiritual care they might want from a nurse, some responded that they would not want or expect it, while others stated "it depends" or were enthusiastic about receiving spiritual care. It is possible that like others with serious illness, patients with cancer and their loved ones receive and are generally satisfied with spiritual care primarily from family or friends.[96]

When Balboni and colleagues[75] surveyed 230 persons with advanced cancer about whether their spiritual needs were addressed, 72% responded that these needs were minimally or not at all supported by the healthcare system. Another study demonstrated that when patients with cancer perceive their spiritual needs are not being met, their satisfaction with care and rating of the quality of care is lower.[97] These findings suggest that although many patients want and seek spiritual support, they may not always expect it from a nurse. An oncology nurse, therefore, must conduct a spiritual assessment that includes questions such as "How can we nurses best support your spiritual health?" Taylor's findings also indicate that a patient may not be receptive to spiritual care from a nurse unless some degree of rapport and respectful relationship are established first.[95,98]

## ORGANIZATIONAL APPROACHES

Although most discussions of spiritual care describe how a nurse can provide care on a one-to-one basis, other approaches to spiritual care have been provided by cancer care institutions. For example, a cancer center in Ohio has instituted measures designed to nurture the spirit, including a healing garden on the premises (which includes a waterfall, labyrinth, and lush landscaping).[99] Wellness Centers across the US offer a myriad of experiences that support the spirit of patients with cancer and their family members. These often include classes such as yoga, journal writing, meditation, and dream analysis. Others have created weekends of renewal (eg, Healing Odyssey Retreats[100]), spiritual events,[101] or support groups[102–104] that include spiritual nurturing for patients or family members. While most hospitals maintain a chapel, some hospital chaplaincy departments have also instituted unique approaches that provide spiritual care to oncology patients as well as others, such as mobile carts with spiritually edifying tapes, books, and other resources. Churches, especially those serving African American communities, have collaborated with nurses to promote cancer screening and health promotion activities.[105]

## INDIVIDUAL APPROACHES

Although not a spiritual care specialist, the nurse can be a spiritual care generalist. A nurse must possess basic spiritual assessment skills, be able to provide fundamental spiritual care such as presencing and empathic listening, and be able to make referrals to diverse spiritual care experts when unable to address spiritual needs adequately. Experts who nurses may consult, or to whom they can make referrals, include chaplains, clergy, folk healers, lay ministers, spiritual directors, parish nurses, mental health professionals with sensitivity toward spirituality, or others with knowledge about various spiritual practices such as meditation. Sometimes, however, family and friends may be the persons best suited to meet the patient's spiritual needs.[3]

Many persons with cancer do want their physicians to inquire about their spirituality and possibly address spiritual concerns.[97,106–108] There is, however, little information about patients' receptivity toward nurses addressing spiritual matters. Roughly half of 156 patients with cancer and 68 family caregivers surveyed wanted spiritual care from a nurse, while the other half did not.[109] The spiritual care nursing interventions that generated the greatest enthusiasm among these respondents were those that allowed for personal spiritual development in an independent way (eg, help to have quiet times, tell me about spiritual resources) and humor (ie, help me laugh, bring me humorous things). In contrast, the lowest-ranked items were interventions that involved approaching a patient in a personal way, with nontraditional methods for spiritual nurturing, and even inferring a hierarchal position in the nurse-patient relationship (ie, help me to think about my dreams, teach me about ways to draw or write about my spirituality, talk about difficulties of praying when sick). Generally, interventions that were less intimate, commonly used, and not overtly religious found the most approval.[109]

### Assessment

Before any spiritual care generalist or specialist can provide appropriate care, a spiritual assessment is necessary. A two-tiered approach to spiritual assessment is recommended for nurses.[3] Because it is impossible, if not inappropriate, to conduct a thorough spiritual assessment on every patient, an initial assessment of patient spirituality should glean basic information about spiritual care requirements and function as a screening tool for spiritual distress. Taylor suggested the following components for this initial spiritual assessment: general spiritual status (eg, "How are your spirits now?"); spiritual needs (eg, "What kinds of spiritual concerns bother you most?"); and spiritual resources (eg, "What do you think might help you with these concerns? In what ways can members of your healthcare team boost your spirits?"). Steinhauser and colleagues[110] tested the validity of the question "Are you at peace?" among terminally ill patients and found it to be strongly related to spirituality and QOL. They conclude the question can be a "brief gateway" for assessing patient spirituality. An alternative to interviewing patients is a paper-and-pencil questionnaire about spirituality that may be appropriate for patients who are capable of reading and writing (see Table 73-1).[3]

**TABLE 73-1**

**Patient Spiritual Self-Assessment Form**

Often when people confront health challenges, they become more aware of their spirituality. For some, spiritual ways of thinking or living are especially helpful when health concerns emerge. For others, spiritual questions or doubts arise. This form will guide you to think about spiritual issues. After completing it, you may choose to keep it or give it to your nurse, who may want to share it with other healthcare professionals who will be caring for you.

NAME: ______________________________

ROOM NUMBER: ______________

Place an "X" on the lines to show the answer that comes closest to describing your feelings.

Recently, my spirits have been . . .

______________________________

Awful | Low | Okay | Good | Great

In general, I see myself as . . .

______________________________

Not at all spiritual | A little spiritual | Somewhat spiritual | Fairly spiritual | Very spiritual

In general, I see myself as . . .

______________________________

Not at all religious | A little religious | Somewhat religious | Fairly religious | Very religious

What can a nurse do that would help to nurture or boost your spirits? (Check all that apply.)

—— Spend quiet time with you
—— Have prayer with you
—— Help you meditate
—— Allow time and space for your private prayer or meditation
—— Let you know nurse(s) are praying privately for you

—— Read spiritually helpful literature to you
—— Bring art or music to you that nurtures your spirit
—— Bring you literature that you feel is spiritually helpful

—— Help you to stay connected to your spiritual community
—— Help you to observe religious practices

—— Listen to your thoughts about certain spiritual matters
—— Help you to remember how you have grown from previous difficult life experiences
—— Help you to tell your life story
—— Help you to face painful questions, doubts, or suffering

—— Just be with you, not necessarily talking with you
—— Just show a genuine and personal interest in you

I would also like help in boosting my spirits from:

—— My friends and family
—— Other healthcare professionals
—— My own clergy or spiritual mentor
—— Other clergy or spiritual leader
—— A chaplain at this institution

What would you like your nurse to know about your prayer or meditation beliefs and practices?

______________________________

______________________________

______________________________

What literature, art, or music nurtures your spirit?

______________________________

______________________________

How can the nurse assist you with religious practices or fellowship?

______________________________

______________________________

What spiritual matters would you like to talk about most?

______________________________

______________________________

In what other ways can the nurse help to boost your spirits?

______________________________

______________________________

If there is anyone in particular you would like to meet with for spiritual fellowship, please so state. If there is someone you would like us to contact for you, please share what contact information you know:

______________________________

______________________________

______________________________

*Source*: Reprinted with permission from Taylor EJ. *Spiritual Care: Nursing Theory, Research, and Practice*. Upper Saddle River, NJ: Prentice Hall; 2002.[3]

The second tier of assessment can occur when the nurse observes a need for detailed assessment. For example, if a patient remarks, "Sometimes I wonder if God hears me, because He's not answering me," the nurse will support spiritual health if further assessment is conducted. In this case, the nurse would query the patient about prayer experience and beliefs about relating to God. Assessment questions could include the following: "Tell me more about how you believe God hears and answers people." (Note the use of language that mirrors the patient's wording.) "How are you finding that illness affects your praying?" (Note the nonthreatening and nonbiasing tone.) "At times like these, exploring doubts can help to build faith. Could we do anything to assist you in this process?" (Assess not only what the problem is, but also what intervention would be acceptable.) The spiritual assessment not only provides data with which to determine appropriate interventions, but also functions to provide care. Prompting patients to consider their spirituality in this way often allows them to begin an internal journey toward spiritual healing.

### Empathic listening and presencing

The two skills that are probably the most fundamental to providing spirit-nurturing care are empathic listening and presencing. Because more detailed information about these "interventions" can be found elsewhere,[3,111,112] a brief review will suffice here. Four levels of empathic listening have been identified: (1) listening intellectually; (2) listening intellectually and emotionally; (3) listening intellectually, emotionally, and physically; and (4) listening intellectually, emotionally, physically, and spiritually. A holistic listener, one who listens at this fourth level, is a "holy" listener.[3] Key components of empathic listening to promote spiritual health are striving to hear all aspects of patients' message, recognizing your inner response, and helping patients to listen to the self who is speaking and make sense of what they have heard. While empathically communicating with patients with cancer, it is important to follow their cues regarding how intimate or deep they want to talk. Kvale's qualitative study with 20 Danish patients illustrates how sometimes they do not want to talk with a nurse about difficult feelings.[113] Talking with patients about their "normal" life, hobbies, and families may be the most spiritually healing topic.

In a classic discussion about presencing, Pettigrew[114] delineated the components of presence as vulnerability and silence, invitation, and privilege. Willingness to "just" be with a patient in pain is extremely difficult. Nurses can easily escape this discomfort by literally avoiding patients in pain or by "hid[ing] behind the facade of professionalism or the technology or traditions of [their] role."[114(p.505)] Indeed, *being* with patients in pain can be avoided by engaging in *doing*. Being present to a patient therefore requires vulnerability, presence in a helpless situation. Being present to someone in pain also challenges the developed and practiced instinct to say "the right thing." Because words are often inadequate to comfort, nurses must learn to share silence. Likewise, because suffering is so private, nurses must never force their presence upon an individual. Indeed, Pettigrew posits that it is a privilege to be present for and with persons who suffer.

### Fostering positive meaning

Perhaps the most pressing spiritual need for those with cancer, according to several studies cited earlier, is the need to create positive meanings—to transform the tragedy and experience spiritual growth. Although the research suggests that it may happen without professional intervention for many patients, it also indicates that some individuals may get "stuck" searching and experience spiritual distress ruminating about "why" questions. Taylor[3] identified some specific strategies nurses can employ to assist persons searching for meaning:

- Encourage resiliency (eg, assist individuals to remember how previous traumatic life events were surmounted, help patients to find an inspirational role model who similarly made good from bad circumstances).
- Encourage disclosure, remembering that one must encounter the darkness of this process before passing through it (eg, "What kinds of questions are you finding yourself wondering about?" or "Who suffers with you?").
- If the patient is ready, prompt a movement toward asking "Wherefore?" instead of "Why?" (eg, ask the individual questions like "What are some of the good things that have come out of your illness experience?" or "What sorts of lessons has this taught you?" or "What have you learned about yourself?").
- Avoid inappropriate responses such as imposing your beliefs about why cancer happens or avoidance and minimizing strategies like "It's God's will."
- Facilitate meaning-making activities (eg, have individuals get involved with altruistic work such as volunteering or dedicating themselves to a social, religious, scientific, or other cause).

With any attempts to promote positive meaning, the nurse must remember that only the patient can ascribe the meaning. This positive meaning cannot be forced; it cannot be fed.

### Supporting spiritual or religious coping

After assessment, the nurse may determine that religious beliefs or practices need to be supported. Prayer is likely the most frequent religious practice benefiting from support. Other religious beliefs and practices may need to be respected or incorporated in the plan of care. Guidelines for ethically participating in spiritual practices with patients are essential to follow. The following are guidelines developed by an ethicist and nurse:

- First, try to understand the patient's spiritual needs, resources, and preferences
- Employ religious practices with permission; respect the patient's expressed wishes
- Do not prescribe or push religious beliefs or practices
- Strive to understand your own spiritual beliefs and needs, before addressing others'
- When it is appropriate to employ religious practices with patients, do so in a manner that is authentic and in harmony with your spiritual beliefs.[115]

Although these guidelines were developed to guide nurses wondering whether praying with patients was ethical, the guidelines can be applied to any religious practice as well.

*Prayer.* Because many persons with cancer use prayer, oncology nurses may need to support patients' prayer practices. Many patients may even appreciate a nurse praying with or for them.[116] Although two-thirds of 1 oncology nurse sample ($N$ = 181) reported praying privately for their patients,[92] many nurses may feel discomfort with the idea of praying with patients. Tips for praying with patients follow:

- Determine whether it would be ethical to pray with a patient.[116] Ask whether the patient wants it. Reflect on whether you have an improper, hidden agenda in your offer to pray.
- Assess the patient's desire for this intervention with a question such as "Many people at times like this want someone to pray with them. Would you feel comfortable with me praying with you?" Make sure the patient will be comfortable declining any offer.
- Assess the type of prayer experience from which the patient would benefit. Introverts may prefer a shared time of silence. Others may prefer a conversational or ritual style of prayer. If petitionary prayer is preferred, inquire for what the patient desires prayer so that it can be included. (Styles of prayer are further described in Taylor's text on spiritual caregiving.)
- Pray by acknowledging the realities of the patient's current situation and feelings.
- Remember that the patient may also want to pray for the nurse. This can be a very spiritually intimate experience and the nurse should be prepared to receive this gift graciously.
- Know that prayer with a patient can be a springboard for further spiritual caregiving. Do not use prayer as an avoidance strategy to bring premature closure to an uncomfortable conversation.[3,116]

Although a nurse may not share the religious beliefs of the patient, these tips assume that the nurse's spiritual beliefs overlap in some fundamental way with those of the patient. For example, they both accept that there is an Ultimate Other with whom they can interact through prayer.

*Religious beliefs and practices.* Although a nurse is unlikely to have extensive knowledge about diverse religions, a broad appreciation for the general tenets of the basic world religions will be helpful. Some of the religious peculiarities that can affect cancer care are summarized in Table 73-2 For more information, the reader is referred to texts on spiritual care[3,117] or a handbook of religion.

On occasion, a patient's spiritual beliefs may create conflict with the healthcare team, which is trying to benevolently impose the best of healthcare. For example, a Jehovah's Witness with leukemia may refuse a blood transfusion. The oncology nurse can play a pivotal role in creating a resolution between the conflicting parties. Taylor[118] adapted anthropologist Kleinman's steps to managing conflicting cultural values, as follows:

1. Assess the patient's "model" that determines the approach to explaining illness and choosing a response to it (eg, What do you think has caused your illness [or distressed your spirit]? What do you think your sickness does to you [spiritually]? How does it work? What do you think are the best things to do for your illness [or spiritual health]? What [spiritual] concerns has your illness caused you? What do you do about them?)
2. Explain simply to the patient your model and beliefs about etiology (or meaning) and how best to respond to (or cope with) this illness.
3. Openly discuss with patients how your model differs from theirs. Objectively discuss how your different cultural backgrounds and spiritual beliefs contribute to the contrast in models.
4. Encourage the patient to ask questions about your model.
5. Support individual beliefs and practices that are healthful (from your perspective).
6. Accommodate patient beliefs and practices that are neither helpful nor harmful.
7. Change and provide alternatives for patient beliefs and practices that are harmful without trying to change the underlying belief system, if possible. Engage family member(s) and religious clergy as therapeutic allies.

## CONCLUSION

Recent research about the experience of living with cancer documents that spiritual responses to the illness affect both adjustment and overall QOL. Personal spiritual factors, such as degree of faith development and perceptions about God, likely contribute to how healthy the adjustment is. It is expedient—even vital—that oncology nurses provide

**TABLE 73-2**

**Selected Religious Beliefs and Practices Pertinent to Cancer Care**

| Religion | Selected Beliefs and Practices |
|---|---|
| Amish | Unless employed by non-Amish employer, will not have health insurance. Will rely on personal/family savings and Amish community resources. Extended family very involved during illness. |
| Baha'i | Cremation and embalming prohibited (unless civic law or exemption directs otherwise). |
| Buddhist | Health-related decisions (eg, medical treatment, euthanasia, organ donation) are based on ultimate goal of Enlightenment (eg, attainment of wisdom, truth, peace): if outcome allows continued pursuit of Enlightenment, it is encouraged. After death, reincarnated unless Enlightenment is attained. |
| Catholic, Roman | "Sacrament of the Sick" is a ritual for all those who seek healing (not just for time of death). Lay ministers may bring Holy Communion to the sick. Ordinary (but not extraordinary) means for preserving life are an obligation. |
| Christian Science | Illness results from imperfect understanding of God's spiritual creation. Cure comes with prayer and spiritual regeneration. Seek assistance with healing from church-approved practitioners and nurses. Generally avoid medical procedures and therapies. |
| Latter-Day Saints (Mormons) | May wear temple garments under clothing. Church offers strong social support network (including a Relief Society). Ordinance for the sick involves anointing and prayer. Use only King James version of Bible. |
| Hinduism | Reincarnation occurs after death. Eating meat is forbidden, especially beef. Cremation is common. |
| Islam | Ablutions and ritual prayer five times every day (facing Mecca) part of "pillars of faith." Eat no pork. Burial is compulsory and procedure is specified; should occur as soon as possible after death. Modesty (remaining covered) is critically important for women, especially in the presence of men. |
| Jehovah's Witness | Blood and blood products are forbidden. Giving blood would be "medical rape." Blood volume expanders, hematopoietic agents, and blood-conserving equipment are used. Reading Jehovah's Witness version of Bible can comfort and bring spiritual healing. |
| Judaism | Practices vary widely among Orthodox, Conservative, and Reform branches. Observant Jews keep Shabbat (observe Friday sunset to Saturday sunset as a holy day) and refrain from specified activities of work. Refrain from medical/surgical procedures on Shabbat unless life is threatened. Dietary law proscribes never eating pork, certain fowl, and sea foods; never mixing meat and dairy foods at same meal; and eating only ritually slaughtered meats. After death; ritual washing, no embalming, undelayed burial, family "sitting shiva" for 7 days to mourn and receive social support. |
| Native American | Illness may result from natural or supernatural causes. Often use native healing practices and consult a medicine man. May disbelieve in efficacy of Western medicines and refuse blood. |
| Orthodox, Eastern | May request Holy Communion, confession, or anointing. Shave males only if necessary. May oppose autopsy, embalming, or cremation. |
| Seventh-Day Adventist | Observe Sabbath. Often vegetarian and refrain from caffeine and tobacco. Hypnotism viewed negatively. May request ritual anointing. |

Many religious traditions observe fasts; ill persons, however, are exempted from observing these fasts. Many religions discourage or forbid use of alcohol and narcotics, but support their use for the medically ill. Religions that have restrictions on autopsies and biopsies permit them for medical or legal reasons. Most religions oppose euthanasia.

*Source*: Reprinted with permission from Taylor EJ. Spirituality, culture, and cancer care. *Semin Oncol Nurs*. 2001;17:197–205.[113]

care that recognizes these personal spiritual variables and promotes SWB. Although many approaches to spiritual caregiving are possible, the most effective care may be dependent on a spiritually sensitive and aware nurse who creates a spiritually healing environment through a therapeutic use of self in a respectful nurse–client relationship.

## REFERENCES

1. Mattison D. The forgotten spirit: integration of spirituality in health care. *Nephrol News Issues*. 2006;20:30–32.
2. Reed PG. An emerging paradigm for the investigation of spirituality in nursing. *Res Nurs Health*. 1992;15:349–357.

3. Taylor EJ. *Spiritual Care: Nursing Theory, Research, and Practice.* Upper Saddle River, NJ: Prentice Hall; 2002.
4. McSherry W, Cash K. The language of spirituality: an emerging taxonomy. *Int J Nurs Studies.* 2004;41:151–161.
5. Paley J. Spirituality and secularization: nursing and the sociology of religion. *J Clin Nurs.* 2008;17:175–186.
6. Paley J. Spirituality and nursing: a reductionist approach. *Nurs Philos.* 2008;9:3–18.
7. Pesut B. A reply to "Spirituality and nursing: a reductionist approach" by John Paley. *Nurs Philos.* 2008;9:131–137.
8. Indinopulus TA, Wilson BC, eds. *What Is Religion? Origins, Definitions, and Explanations.* Boston, MA: Brill; 1998.
9. Newport F. *Belief in God Far Lower in Western U.S.* July 28, 2008. http://www.gallup.com/poll/109108/Belief-God-Far-Lower-Western-US.aspx. Accessed September 30, 2009.
10. Thuné-Boyle IC, Stygall JA, Keshtgar MR, Newman SP. Do religious/spiritual coping strategies affect illness adjustment in patients with cancer? *Soc Sci Med.* 2006;63:151–164.
11. Edmondson D, Park CL, Blank TO, Fenster JR, Mills MA. Deconstructing spiritual well-being: existential well-being and HRQOL in cancer survivors. *Psychooncology.* 2008;17:161–169.
12. Gall TL, Kristjansson E, Charbonneau C, Florack P. A longitudinal study on the role of spirituality in response to the diagnosis and treatment of breast cancer. *J Behav Med.* 2009;32:174–186.
13. Edmondson D, Park CL, Chaudoir SR, Wortmann JH. Death without God: religious struggle, death concerns, and depression in the terminally ill. *Psychol Sci.* 2008;19:754–758.
14. Park CL. Religiousness/Spirituality and health: a meaning systems perspective. *J Behav Med.* 2007;30:319–328.
15. Abernethy AD, Magat MM, Houston TR, Arnold HL Jr, Bjorck JP, Gorsuch RL. Recruiting African-American men for cancer screening studies: applying a culturally based model. *Health Educ Behav.* 2005; 32:441–451.
16. Underwood SM, Powell RL. Religion and spirituality: influence and health/risk behavior and cancer screening behavior of African Americans. *ABNF J.* 2006;17:20–31.
17. Fowler BA. Social processes used by African American women in making decisions about mammography screening. *J Nurs Scholarsh.* 2006; 38:247–354.
18. Taylor EJ. Spiritual responses to cancer. In Yarbro CH, Frogge MH, Goodman M, eds. *Cancer Nursing: Principles and Practice.* 6th ed. Sudbury, MA: Jones and Bartlett; 2005:1713–1726.
19. Reindl Benjamins M, Brown C. Religion and preventative health care utilization among the elderly. *Soc Sci Med.* 2004;58:109–118.
20. Gullatte MM, Phillips JM, Gibson LM. Factors associated with delays in screening of self-detected breast changes in African-American women. *J Natl Black Nurses Assoc.* 2006;17:45–50.
21. Holt CL, Clark EM, Kreuter MW, et al. Spiritual health locus of control and breast cancer beliefs among urban African American women. *Health Psychol.* 2003;22:294–299.
22. Malik IA, Gopalan S. Use of CAM results in delay in seeking medical advice for breast cancer. *Eur J Epidemiol.* 2003;18:817–822.
23. Taylor EJ. Spiritual complementary therapies in cancer care. *Semin Oncol Nurs.* 2005;21:159–163.
24. Weisman AD, Worden JW. The existential plight in cancer: significance of the first 100 days. *Int J Psychiatr Med.* 1976;7:1–15.
25. Shannon-Dorcy K, Wolfe V. Decision-making in the diagnosis and treatment of leukemia. *Semin Oncol Nurs.* 2003;19:142–149.
26. Taylor EJ, Outlaw FH. Use of prayer among persons with cancer. *Holist Nurs Pract.* 2002;16:46–60.
27. Demir F, Donmez YC, Ozsaker E, Diramali A. Patients' lived experiences of excisional breast biopsy: a phenomenological study. *J Clin Nurs.* 2008;17:744–751.
28. Silvestri GA, Knittig S, Zoller JS, Nietert PJ. Importance of faith on medical decisions regarding cancer care. *J Clin Oncol.* 2003;21: 1379–1382.
29. Advani AS, Atkeson B, Brown CL, et al. Barriers to the participation of African-American patients with cancer in clinical trials: a pilot study. *Cancer.* 2003;97:1499–1506.
30. White M, Verhoef M. Cancer as part of the journey: the role of spirituality in the decision to decline conventional prostate cancer treatment and to use complementary and alternative medicine. *Integr Cancer Ther.* 2006;5:117–122.
31. Daugherty CK, Fitchett G, Murphy PE, Peterman MH, Banik DM, Tartaro J. Trusting God and medicine: spirituality in advanced cancer patients volunteering for clinical trials of experimental agents. *Psychooncology.* 2005;14:135–146.
32. Hamrick N, Diefenbach MA. Religion and spirituality among patients with localized prostate cancer. *Palliat Support Care.* 2006;4:345–355.
33. Fitch MI. Needs of patients living with advanced disease. *Can Oncol Nurs J.* 2005;15:230–242.
34. Gould J, Wilson S, Grassau P. Reflecting on spirituality in the context of breast cancer diagnosis and treatment. *Can Oncol Nurs J.* 2008;18:34–46.
35. Taylor EJ. Spiritual needs of cancer patients and family caregivers. *Cancer Nurs.* 2003;26:260–266.
36. Taylor EJ. Prevalence of spiritual needs among cancer patients and family caregivers. *Oncol Nurs Forum.* 2006;33:729–735.
37. Taylor EJ. Whys and wherefores: adult patient perspectives of the meaning of cancer. *Semin Oncol Nurs.* 1995;11:32–40.
38. Koffman J, Morgan M, Edmonds P, Speck P, Higginson IJ. "I know he controls cancer": the meanings of religion among Black Caribbean and White British patients with advanced cancer. *Soc Sci Med.* 2008;67:780–789.
39. Park CL, Edmondson D, Fenster JR, Blank TO. Meaning making and psychological adjustment following cancer: the mediating roles of growth, life meaning, and restored just-world beliefs. *J Consult Clin Psychol.* 2008;76:863–875.
40. Taylor EJ. Transformation of tragedy among women surviving breast cancer. *Oncol Nurs Forum.* 2000;27:781–788.
41. Bowes DE, Tamlyn D, Butler LJ. Women living with ovarian cancer: dealing with an early death. *Health Care Women Int.* 2002;23:135–148.
42. Carpenter JS, Brockop DY, Andrykowski MA. Self-transformation as a factor in the self-esteem and well-being of breast cancer survivors. *J Adv Nurs.* 1999;29:1402–1411.
43. Simonelli LE, Fowler J, Maxwell FL, Andersen BL. Physical sequelae and depressive symptoms in gynecologic cancer survivors: meaning in life as a mediator. *Ann Behav Med.* 2008;35:275–284.
44. Park CL, Edmondson D, Fenster JR, Blank TO. Positive and negative health behavior changes in cancer survivors: a stress and coping perspective. *J Health Psychol.* 2008;13:1198–1206.
45. Fleer J, Hoekstra HJ, Sleijfer DT, Tuinman MA, Hoekstra-Weebers JE. The role of meaning in the prediction of psychosocial well-being of testicular cancer survivors. *Qual Life Res.* 2006;15:705–717.
46. Weaver AJ, Flannelly KJ. The role of religion/spirituality for cancer patients and their caregivers. *Southern Med J.* 2004;97:1210–1214.
47. Tatsumura Y, Maskarinec G, Shumay DM, et al. Religious and spiritual resources, CAM, and conventional treatment in the lives of cancer patients. *Altern Ther Health Med.* 2003;9:64–71.
48. Ebright PR, Lyon B. Understanding hope and factors that enhance hope in women with breast cancer. *Oncol Nurs Forum.* 2002;29:561–568.
49. Pargament KI. *The Psychology of Religion and Coping.* New York: Guilford; 1997.
50. Tarakeshwar N, Vanderwerker LC, Paulk E, Pearce MJ, Kasl SV, Prigerson HG. Religious coping is associated with the quality of life of patients with advanced cancer. *J Palliat Med.* 2006;9:646–657.
51. Gall TL. Relationship with God and the quality of life of prostate cancer survivors. *Qual Life Res.* 2004;13:1357–1368.
52. Sherman AC, Plante TG, Simonton S, Latif U, Anaissie EJ. Prospective study of religious coping among patients undergoing autologous stem cell transplantation. *J Behav Med.* 2009;32:118–128.
53. Becker G, Momm F, Xander C, et al. Religious belief as a coping strategy: an exploratory trial in patients irradiated for head-and-neck cancer. *Strahlenther Onkol.* 2006;182:270–276.

54. Hsiao AF, Wong MD, Miller MF, et al. Role of religiosity and spirituality in complementary and alternative medicine use among cancer survivors in California. *Integr Cancer Ther.* 2008;7:139–146.
55. Jones RA, Taylor AG, Bourguignon C, et al. Complementary and alternative medicine modality use and beliefs among African American prostate cancer survivors. *Oncol Nurs Forum.* 2007;34:359–364.
56. Gerson-Cwilich R, Serrano-Olvera A, Villalobos-Prieto A. Complementary and alternative medicine (CAM) in Mexican patients with cancer. *Clin Transl Oncol.* 2006;8:200–207.
57. Ross LE, Hall IJ, Fairley TL, Taylor YJ, Howard DL. Prayer and self-reported health among cancer survivors in the United States, National Health Interview Survey, 2002. *J Altern Complement Med.* 2008;14: 931–938.
58. Levine EG, Aviv C, Yoo G, Ewing C, Au A. The benefits of prayer on mood and well-being of breast cancer survivors. *Support Care Cancer.* 2009;17:295–306.
59. Taylor EJ, Outlaw FH, Bernardo T, et al. Spiritual conflicts of cancer patients who pray. *Psychooncology.* 1999;8:386–394.
60. Taylor EJ. Spiritual quality of life. In: King CR, Hinds PS, eds. *Quality of Life: From Nursing and Patient Perspectives.* 2nd ed. Sudbury, MA: Jones and Bartlett; 2003:93–116.
61. Leak A, Hu J, King CR. Symptom distress, spirituality, and quality of life in African American breast cancer survivors. *Cancer Nurs.* 2008;31:E15–E21.
62. Fisch MJ, Titzer ML, Kristeller JL, et al. Assessment of quality of life in outpatients with advanced cancer: the accuracy of clinician estimations and the relevance of spiritual well-being—a Hoosier Oncology Group Study. *J Clin Oncol.* 2003;21:2754–2759.
63. Whitford HS, Olver IN, Peterson MJ. Spirituality as a core domain in the assessment of quality of life in oncology. *Psychooncology.* 2008;17:1121–1128.
64. Cotton SP, Levine EG, Fitzpatrick CM, et al. Exploring the relationships among spiritual well-being, quality of life, and psychological adjustment in women with breast cancer. *Psychooncology.* 1999;8:429–438.
65. Inman A, Kirsh KL, Passik SD. A pilot study to examine the relationship between boredom and spirituality in cancer patients. *Palliat Support Care.* 2003;1:143–151.
66. Andrykowski MA, Bishop MM, Hahn EA, et al. Long-term health related quality of life, growth, and spiritual well-being after hematopoietic stem-cell transplantation. *J Clin Oncol.* 2005;23:599–608.
67. Williams AL. Perspectives on spirituality at the end of life: a meta-summary. *Palliat Support Care.* 2006;4:407–417.
68. Greisinger AJ, Lorimor RJ, Aday L, et al. Terminally ill cancer patients: their most important concerns. *Cancer Pract.* 1997;5:147–154.
69. Steinhauser KE, Christakis NA, Clipp EC, McNeilly M, McIntyre L, Tulsky JA. Factors considered important at the end of life by patients, family, physicians, and other care providers. *JAMA.* 2000;284: 2476–2482.
70. Hughes T, Schumacher M, Jacobs-Lawson JM, Arnold S. Confronting death: perceptions of a good death in adults with lung cancer. *Am J Hosp Palliat Care.* 2008;25:39–44.
71. Thomson JE. The place of spiritual well-being in hospice patients' overall quality of life. *Hospice J.* 2000;15:13–27.
72. McMillan SC, Weitzner M. How problematic are various aspects of quality of life in patients with cancer at the end of life? *Oncol Nurs Forum.* 2000;27:817–823.
73. McClain CS, Rosenfeld B, Brietbart W. Effect of spiritual wellbeing on end-of-life despair in terminally ill cancer patients. *Lancet.* 2003;361:1603–1607.
74 True G, Phipps EJ, Braitman LE, Harralson T, Harris D, Tester W. Treatment preferences and advance care planning at end of life: the role of ethnicity and spiritual coping in cancer patients. *Ann Behav Med.* 2005;30:174–179.
75 Balboni TA, Vanderwerker LC, Block SD, et al. Religiousness and spiritual support among advanced cancer patients and associations with end-of-life treatment preferences and quality of life. *J Clin Oncol.* 2007;25:555–560.
76. Harrington V, Lackey NR, Gates MF. Needs of caregivers of clinic and hospice cancer patients. *Cancer Nurs.* 1996;19:118–125.
77. Mellon S. Comparisons between cancer survivors and family members on meaning of the illness and family quality of life. *Oncol Nurs Forum.* 2002;29:1117–1125.
78. Kuuppelomaki M. Spiritual support for families of patients with cancer: a pilot study of nursing staff assessments. *Cancer Nurs.* 2002;25: 209–218.
79. Strang S, Strang P, Ternestedt BM. Existential support in brain tumour patients and their spouses. *Support Care Cancer.* 2001;9:625–633.
80. Bishop MM, Beaumont JL, Hahn EA, et al. Late effects of cancer and hematopoietic stem-cell transplantation on spouses or partners compared with survivors and survivor-matched controls. *J Clin Oncol.* 2007;25:1403–1411.
81. Petrie W, Logan J, DeGrasse C. Research review of the supportive care needs of spouses of women with breast cancer. *Oncol Nurs Forum.* 2001;28:1601–1607.
82. Ferrell BR, Ervin K, Smith S, et al. Family perspectives of ovarian cancer. *Cancer Pract.* 2002;10:269–276.
83. Strang S, Strang P. Spiritual thoughts, coping and "sense of coherence" in brain tumour patients and their spouses. *Palliat Med.* 2001;15:127–134.
84. Steele RG, Fitch MI. Coping strategies of family caregivers of home hospice patients with cancer. *Oncol Nurs Forum.* 1996;23:955–960.
85. Germino BB, Mishel MH, Belyea M, et al. Uncertainty in prostate cancer: ethnic and family patterns. *Cancer Pract.* 1998;6: 107–113.
86. Mickley JR, Pargament KI, Brant CR, et al. God and the search for meaning among hospice caregivers. *Hospice J.* 1998;13:1–17.
87. Abernethy AD, Chang HT, Seidlitz L, et al. Religious coping and depression among spouses of people with lung cancer. *Psychosomatics.* 2002;43:456–463.
88. Highfield MEF, Taylor EJ, Amenta MO. Preparation to care: the spiritual care education of oncology and hospice nurses. *J Hospice Palliat Nurs.* 2000;2:53–63.
89. Taylor EJ, Highfield MF, Amenta MO. Predictors of oncology and hospice nurses spiritual care perspectives and practices. *App Nurs Res.* 1999;12:30–37.
90. Musgrave CF, McFarlane EA. Israeli oncology nurses' religiosity, spiritual well-being, and attitudes toward spiritual care: a path analysis. *Oncol Nurs Forum.* 2004;31:321–327.
91. Lundmark M. Attitudes to spiritual care among nursing staff in a Swedish oncology unit. *J Clin Nurs.* 2006;15:863–874.
92. Taylor EJ, Amenta MO, Highfield MF. Spiritual care practices of oncology nurses. *Oncol Nurs Forum.* 1995;22:31–39.
93. Kristeller JL, Zumbrun CS, Schilling RF. "I would if I could"; how oncology nurses address spiritual distress in cancer patients. *Psychooncology.* 1999;8:451–458.
94. Carr T. Mapping the processes and qualities of spiritual nursing care. *Qual Health Res.* 2008;18:686–700.
95. Taylor EJ. Nurses caring for the spirit: patients with cancer and family caregiver expectations. *Oncol Nurs Forum.* 2003;30:585–590.
96. Hanson LC, Dobbs D, Usher BM, Williams S, Rawlings J, Daaleman TP. Providers and types of spiritual care during serious illness. *J Palliat Med.* 2008;11:907–914.
97. Astrow AB, Wexler A, Texeira K, He MK, Sulmasy DP. Is failure to meet spiritual needs associated with cancer patients' perceptions of quality of care and their satisfaction with care? *J Clin Oncol.* 2007;25:5753–5757.
98. Taylor EJ. Client perspectives about nurse requisites for spiritual caregiving. *Appl Nurs Res.* 2007;20:44–46.
99. Abdallah-Baran R. Nurturing spirit through complementary cancer care. *Clin J Oncol Nurs.* 2003;7:468–470.
100. Rutledge DN, Raymon NJ. Changes in well-being of women cancer survivors following a survivor weekend experience. *Oncol Nurs Forum.* 2001;28:85–91.

101. Dann NJ, Higby DJ, Mertens WC. Can a cancer program-sponsored spiritual event meet with acceptance from patients and other attendees? *Integr Cancer Ther.* 2005;4:230–235.
102. Coward DD. Facilitation of self-transcendence in a breast cancer support group: II. *Oncol Nurs Forum.* 2003;30:291–300.
103. Rummans TA, Clark MM, Sloan JA, et al. Impacting quality of life for patients with advanced cancer with a structured multidisciplinary intervention: a randomized controlled trial. *J Clin Oncol.* 2006;24: 635–642.
104. Coward DD, Kahn DL. Resolution of spiritual disequilibrium by women newly diagnosed with breast cancer. *Oncol Nurs Forum.* 2004;31:E24-E31.
105. Campbell MK, Hudson MA, Resnicow K, Blakeney N, Paxton A, Baskin M. Church-based health promotion interventions: evidence and lessons learned. *Annu Rev Public Health.* 2007;28:213–234.
106. Hart A, Kohlwes RJ, Deyo R, et al. Hospice patients' attitudes regarding spiritual discussions with their doctors. *Am J Hosp Palliat Care.* 2003;20:135–139.
107. Miller BE, Pittman B, Strong C. Gynecologic cancer patients' psychosocial needs and their views of the physician's role in meeting those needs. *Int J Gynecol Cancer.* 2003;13:111–119.
108. Frick E, Riedner C, Fegg MJ, Hauf S, Borasio GD. A clinical interview assessing cancer patients' spiritual needs and preferences. *Eur J Cancer Care.* 2006;15:238–243.
109. Taylor EJ, Mamier I. Spiritual care nursing: what cancer patients and family caregivers want. *J Adv Nurs.* 2005;49:260–267.
110. Steinhauser KE, Voils CI, Clipp EC, Bosworth HB, Christakis NA, Tulsky JA. "Are you at peace?": one item to probe spiritual concerns at the end of life. *Arch Intern Med.* 2006;166:101–105.
111. Burkhardt MA, Nagai-Jacobson MG. *Spirituality: Living Our Connectedness.* Albany, NY: Delmar; 2002.
112. Taylor EJ. *What Do I Say? Talking with Patients about Spirituality.* Philadelphia, PA: Templeton; 2007.
113. Kvale K. Do cancer patients always want to talk about difficult emotions? A qualitative study of cancer inpatients communication needs. *Eur J Oncol Nurs.* 2007;11:320–327.
114. Pettigrew J. Intensive nursing care: the ministry of presence. *Crit Care Nurs Clin North Am.* 1990;2:503–508.
115. Winslow GR, Winslow BW. Examining the ethics of praying with patients. *Holist Nurs Pract.* 2003;17;170–177.
116. Taylor EJ. Prayer's clinical issues and implications. *Holist Nurs Pract.* 2003;17:179–188.
117. Mauk KL, Schmidt NK. *Spiritual Care in Nursing Practice.* Philadelphia, PA: Lippincott, Williams & Wilkins; 2004.
118. Taylor EJ. Spirituality, culture, and cancer care. *Semin Oncol Nurs.* 2001;17:197–205.

# PART VIII

# Palliative Care and End of Life

CHAPTER

74

Peg Esper, MSN, MSA, RN, ANP-BC, AOCN®

# Principles and Issues in Palliative Care

*This journey called "life" can become the most difficult to navigate as it nears its end. What a privilege it is to help another find their way.*

Peg Esper

## INTRODUCTION

The science of oncology continues to advance. Even so, cancer continues to claim the lives of more than 562,000 people in the United States each year.[1] Despite improvements in the treatment of individuals with a cancer diagnosis, the need for improved palliative care continues.

Palliative care is a concept that has been defined with some degree of ambiguity. As more efforts have been concentrated in this area, various groups have struggled over the continuum of care to be encompassed by this term. How does palliative care differ from hospice care or end-of-life care or supportive care—or does it?

The differences in how these concepts are applied vary based on the geographical and cultural frameworks from which they are applied. The term *supportive care* has often had a *treatment-focused* correlative encompassing those measures taken to support the patient during active therapy. These measures may include interventions such as growth factor administration, blood transfusions, and antiemetics. More recently, supportive care has taken on some of the psychosocial and spiritual components of care. It typically is identified as having its endpoint at the time of patient death.[2]

*Hospice care*, particularly in the United States, has been identified primarily in legalistic fashion and, because of governmental definition, as being a "time-specific" point in the care of terminally ill individuals. This term is derived from the Latin word *hospitium*, which in its medieval roots referred to a place of shelter or rest and implied what we now refer to as "hospitality." Those who were acutely ill were cared for in *hospitals*, and those with illnesses for which no cure existed were cared for in *hospices*.[3] More traditionally, hospice care places the patient and family at the center of an interdisciplinary model of caring for individuals in the final stages of an illness.[4]

Places the patient at the center of care.
Acknowledges dying as a normal part of life.
Seeks to provide relief from symptoms that cause distress.
Provides care that does not hasten or postpone death.
Offers support to family following the patient's death.

**FIGURE 74-1**

Goals of palliative care.

The World Health Organization has defined *palliative care* as "an approach that improves the quality of life of patients and their families facing the problems associated with life-threatening illness, through the prevention and relief of suffering by means of early identification and impeccable assessment and treatment of pain and other problems, physical, psychosocial and spiritual."[5] Palliative care begins with the initial identification of an incurable illness and concludes as the illness ends in death and bereavement. Its fundamental precept is that the goals of care are patient directed and quality oriented. Palliative care follows a design that neither hastens nor prolongs death, but allows individuals to "live with their illness" as long as possible prior to "dying from it" (Figure 74-1). The relationship between these 3 models of care is overlapping and occasionally the subject of debate (Figure 74-2).

## HISTORICAL PERSPECTIVES

The word "palliative" has its origin in the Latin word *pallium*, meaning "a cloak." When discussing palliative care, one refers to the *covering* of the effects of illness rather than addressing the actual cause of the illness. Palliation provides protection from the internal and external threats to the individual precipitated by the disease and its treatment.

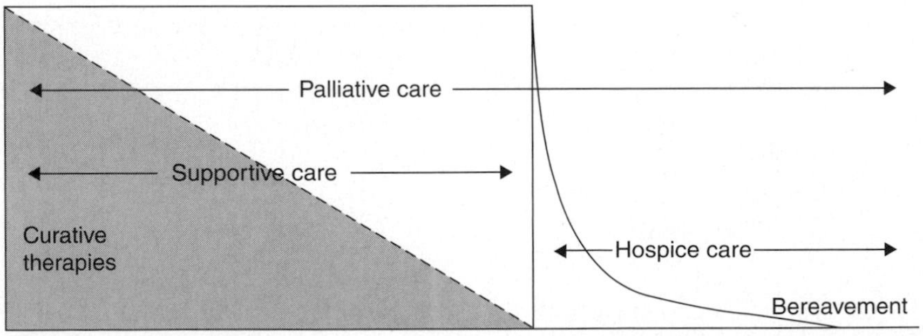


**FIGURE 74-2**

Overlap of concepts related to care of individuals with a terminal diagnosis.

The provision of care with the same intent as what we now refer to as palliative care is not unique to the past few decades. Reference to this type of treatment for the sick can be found dating back to the 4th century AD and before. Hostels for those with incurable illnesses such as leprosy were among those early efforts in palliative care.[3]

Modern-day palliative care acknowledges the tremendous efforts of a number of individuals, but specifically the contributions of Jeanne Garnier, John Bonica, Dame Cicely Saunders, Elisabeth Kubler-Ross, and, more recently, proponents of palliative care such as Russell Portenoy, Eduardo Bruera, Robert Twycross, and Ira Byock. Saunders describes her passion for the care of the dying as stemming from her interactions with a patient who died of cancer in the late 1940s when she was a nurse. A surgeon recognized her interest in learning more about pain management and symptom control and persuaded her to go to medical school, which she did at age 33. Her continued practice in this area led to the founding of the first modern hospice—St. Christopher's Hospice, in a London suburb in 1967.[6]

It was just 2 years later that Kubler-Ross published *On Death and Dying.* This book represented the culmination of more than 500 interviews with dying patients in which she theorized that there were 5 stages to the process of death and dying. Kubler-Ross was one of the first people to promote the concept of dying at home and letting patients have a choice in decisions related to their own care at the end of life.[7] Balfour Mount opened the first hospital-based palliative care service at the Royal Victoria Hospital at McGill University in Montreal in 1975. It was the first institution to include research and education in the area of symptom management.[8]

Interest in hospice care was growing in the US as well. An early leader in the US movement was Florence Wald, the dean of the Yale University graduate nursing program. Wald and Saunders met in 1963 when Saunders was a guest lecturer at the Yale School of Medicine. This meeting ultimately led to Wald opening the New Haven Hospice, which provided home care, in 1974.[3] Over the next 30 years, governmental efforts specific to hospice and end-of-life care received various levels of support (Table 74-1). In September of 2006, the American Board of Medical Specialties recognized Hospice and Palliative Medicine as an official medical subspecialty.

**TABLE 74-1**

**Hospice-Related Legislative Activity, 1972–2000**

| Legislative Activity | |
|---|---|
| 1972 | Elisabeth Kubler-Ross testifies before the US Senate Special Committee on Aging. She supports helping patients and families remain in their homes for terminal care. |
| 1979 | The HCFA evaluates the cost-effectiveness of hospice care using 26 hospice programs across the country. |
| 1982 | Medicare hospice benefit is introduced in the Tax Equity and Fiscal Responsibility Act of 1982. |
| 1984 | Hospice accreditation by JCAHO begins. |
| 1986 | Medicare hospice benefit made permanent by Congress. |
| 1989 | Omnibus Budget Reconciliation Act of 1989 ties reimbursement increases to the annual increase in the hospital market basket. |
| 1993 | Hospice becomes a nationally guaranteed benefit under the healthcare reform proposal during the Clinton administration. |
| 1996 | Bills introduced in the Senate and House of Representatives seek to improve the Medicare hospice benefit. |
| 1997 | Legislation passed by Congress prohibits taxpayer dollars from funding physician-assisted suicide. This same year, Oregon voters pass the "Death with Dignity Act" for the second time, sanctioning physician-assisted suicide in that state. |
| 1999 | HCFA releases the Hospice Cost Report. |
| 2000 | Hospice rate increase approved by Congress. |

*Abbreviations*: HCFA, Health Care Financing Administration; JCAHO, Joint Commission on Accreditation of Healthcare Organizations (currently known as The Joint Commission).

## MODELS OF PALLIATIVE CARE

The goals of palliative care remain constant despite the model of care being used. Five precepts of palliative care were identified as part of a multimillion-dollar, multiple-year campaign named *Last Acts.* The mission of Last Acts, which was funded by the Robert Wood Johnson Foundation, was to promote improvements in care and caring near the end of life. These 5 precepts were identified by the Palliative Care Committee of Last Acts as key areas for humane and technically competent end-of-life care[9]:

- Respecting patient goals, preferences, and choices
- Comprehensive caring
- Utilizing the strengths of interdisciplinary resources
- Acknowledging and addressing caregiver concerns
- Building systems and mechanisms of support.

The particular models of care utilized are determined largely by the population being served and by the associated facility and geographical constraints identified. In the broad sense, these models can be divided into inpatient and outpatient services. They include the following elements[10–12]:

- Dedicated inpatient palliative care unit
- Consultation service within the acute care setting
- Combined consultative service with designated inpatient beds
- Combined hospital/palliative care unit (with or without a community-based hospice program)
- Outpatient palliative care clinic
- Community-based hospice program
- Nursing home palliative care

## INPATIENT SERVICES

Palliative care can be provided within the confines of the acute care setting. In this model, there may be a designated unit managed by a team of specialists in palliative care including physicians, nurses, therapists, social workers, and other caregivers. The design of the unit allows for great flexibility in visitation and participation in care by family and friends of the individual. Admission to an inpatient palliative care unit generally results from an exacerbation of symptoms that require more intensive management to control or offers a means of providing respite care to overburdened caregivers.[13,14] Funding of such units is often a limiting factor for institutions, as is their ability to designate an entire unit for this type of service. Beds are typically at a premium in most hospital settings and the lower per diem rate for palliative services may be perceived as economically disadvantageous for an institution.

Inpatient palliative care can also be provided across all units of an inpatient facility with the support of a consultative team. The team in this model will often include anesthesiologists, radiologists, and possibly a consultant from an outpatient palliative care program; as well as physicians, nurses, and social workers who have specialized expertise in palliative care. In this model, patients admitted to any inpatient unit can benefit from a consultation from the palliative care team.[15,16] Upon evaluation, recommendations from the team may be either accepted or the team may jointly participate in management of the patient with the medical service requesting the consultation. Limitations of a palliative consultation service include the absence of specially trained staff providing around-the-clock care for the patient. Limitations may also arise due to the physical structure of the units on which care is provided. There may be little or no room for multiple family members to be present and participate in the patient's care. The condition of roommates may prohibit flexibility in established visiting hours. A benefit of this model, however, is that specialist consultation can be made available to patients throughout the facility and, in effect, may broaden the reach of palliative care services across multiple specialty units.[8,15,17] A financial benefit can be seen with the use of hospital palliative care consultation services as they have demonstrated an ability to help decrease length of stay for patients, as well as cost savings through the coordination of care and avoidance of transfers to the intensive care unit (ICU) to manage symptoms.[6]

A combination of the 2 aforementioned models may also exist. A small number of designated palliative care beds may be provided on a particular unit for those patients needing various levels of intense symptom management. A consultative team remains available for those patients throughout the institution who have palliative care needs to be addressed by the team. This is frequently a very workable model for facilities that do not have the ability to devote an entire unit to palliative care patients, but would benefit from having "swing beds" that can be assigned to a unit where staff have an identified interest and additional education in the clinical management of these patients. This model of care may or may not be associated with a community-based hospice program.[8,15,16]

## OUTPATIENT SERVICES

Ambulatory palliative care clinics may exist within the scope of services provided by an established ambulatory care clinic. These clinics primarily serve as symptom management clinics. Visits may be based on preset appointments for the ongoing management of problems such as cachexia or lymphedema, or they may be scheduled for urgent care needs outside of regularly scheduled physician appointments. These clinics may be staffed by physicians or advanced practice nurses who have additional expertise in palliative care. Once again, revenue to justify providing this service within an ambulatory care clinic may be a limitation in utilizing this model.

Palliative day care centers are not as popular in the US, but have found more widespread use in the United Kingdom. These centers allow a small number of patients (generally 10–15) to attend the center during the day to provide both respite for caregivers and a social break for patients. Patients have access to medical support in the day care center as well as services such as manicures, massages, and hairstyling.[17] Palliative care focused *Rapid Response Teams* and *Respite Care Teams* are also unique to the United Kingdom. Rapid Response Teams go into the home to provide urgently needed care and stay until the crisis is resolved. Such a team is typically contacted by a terminally ill patient's family physician to respond to an acute need. Respite Care Teams take over the care of patients for a couple of hours daily to provide relief for caregivers.[12,18]

Probably the best known and most widely employed model of palliative care in the United States is the home hospice model of care. In its purest form, this model functions as an interdisciplinary team providing quality, compassionate care at the end of life. Hospice care places an emphasis on managing a patient's pain and symptoms, and provides psychosocial/spiritual support to the patient and their family using the expertise of a team of professionals and volunteers.[19] Care is provided on a 24-hour, 7-day-a-week availability basis.

Much to the consternation of most palliative care providers, hospice care in the US has been defined more by government regulations than by the scope of services provided. The interdisciplinary team is made up of physicians, nurses, social workers, and counselors. The patient's own primary physician may also be a member of the team. Four levels of hospice care exist based on Medicare hospice regulations; they are outlined in Table 74-2.[20] The establishment of a Medicare hospice benefit has placed a number of regulations on hospice care: an expected prognosis of 6 months or less; patient's decision to choose hospice care rather than curative therapy for their illness; and enrollment in an accredited Medicare hospice program. Additional requirements that the individual hospice program may apply can specify that a primary caregiver be present in the home, and that patients agree to a "do not resuscitate" status. Those patients without Medicare coverage may have hospice home care coverage through their third-party insurance provider or may agree to pay out-of-pocket for services.[21,22]

**TABLE 74-2**

**Levels of Hospice Care (Medicare Hospice Regulations)**

| Level of Care | Description |
|---|---|
| **Mandated Services** | |
| Routine home care | Care typically provided in the patient's home with hospice staff providing the full scope of services. |
| Continuous home care | More intensive care in the home requiring skilled nursing for at least 8 of 24 hours per day. Typically used for acute symptom management to prevent the need for hospitalization. |
| Respite care | Patients are transferred to an inpatient facility to give caregivers a break from the physical and emotional stresses of caring for a terminally ill individual. |
| Inpatient care | Admission to an inpatient facility when acute problems require medical and nursing management (limitations on days exist). |
| **Optional Services (Funding Not Provided by Medicare)** | |
| Residential care | Care provided in an inpatient setting for patients who are unable to meet their own self-care needs and for whom caregivers are either not able or available to do so for them. Skilled care should not be required to qualify for this level of care. |
| Day care | Patients are taken to a day care site where planned activities, meals, socialization, and supervision are available. |
| Extended caregiver services | In-home respite care offers shifts of nursing assistance to patients to substitute for or supplement caregivers. |

*Source*: Data from Kitzes, Sehmoll, and Dixon.[20]

Hospice home care has typically been viewed as the final trajectory of an incurable illness, and there are those in the field who have difficulty with the current overlapping of the terms "palliative" and "hospice." Those who embody the ideals of the modern hospice movement, however, expand the initially limited scope of hospice care from management of terminal symptoms to an approach that seeks to address the multidimensional plethora of issues concerning patients and their caregivers.[23]

Hospices are also forming partnerships with hospitals in an effort to promote a more seamless continuum of care for patients. This collaboration allows hospitals to benefit from the expertise of hospices in providing end-of-life care and maintaining high levels of satisfaction among patients and families. It allows hospices to gain greater exposure to the hospital setting, thereby engendering a greater appreciation for the intricacies of caring for the acutely terminally ill. Ultimately, patients probably stand to gain the most from such partnerships, as they receive more specialized care within the inpatient setting that can transfer into the home setting in a more streamlined fashion. Much work remains, however, if we are to address the multitude of regulatory and revenue-related issues pertaining to this model of care.[24]

Another combined effort being seen on a much more frequent basis is the "bridge"-type program for home care and hospice. Patients who do not fully meet the requirements for hospice eligibility or who are reluctant to sign on to a hospice benefit with their insurance provider can receive traditional home care from an agency that has the joint accreditation for both standard and hospice home care. Patients can transition within the same organization to hospice home care as their condition warrants. Many times the staff of these agencies will maintain the care of patients on both sides of the "bridge." This allows patients to have the benefit of receiving home care from nurses, who have palliative care skills, earlier in their care and then to enjoy the continuity of caregivers as they enter into a more terminal stage of their illness.[21]

## EXTENDED CARE SERVICES

An anticipated 8.5 million individuals will be over the age of 85 in the year 2050. This will likely result in an increase in individuals with chronic illness residing in long-term care facilities. A study conducted in 2004 by Miller and Han found that only 9% of nursing homes in the US had special programs and trained staff for hospice and palliative/end-of-life care.[25] These patients with chronic illnesses often have similar needs but may or may not receive specialized palliative care. There is a growing trend at this time for hospices to contract with long-term care facilities to allow for cooperative efforts. Such liaisons should prove beneficial for patients as well as the long-term care facility and hospice organizations.[20,26] Challenges to the provision of quality palliative care in long-term care facilities have been identified and include issues related to staffing shortages, lack of physician presence, and inability to recognize terminal states in patients.[23]

## BARRIERS TO PROVIDING QUALITY PALLIATIVE CARE

The incentive for taking a harder look at how end-of-life and palliative care are provided in this country had one of its most poignant moments, when the report of the Study to Understand Prognoses and Preferences for Outcomes and Risks of Treatments (SUPPORT) was released in 1995.[27,28] This report, funded by the Robert Wood Johnson Foundation, heralded the shortcomings in the care of hospitalized patients related to end-of-life care and set the stage for a nationwide evaluation of how palliative care is provided. The results of this study provided a number of disturbing findings.[27]

- Only 47% of physicians knew that their patients did not want cardiopulmonary resuscitation (CPR).
- Approximately 46% of do-not-resuscitate orders were written within 2 days of death.
- Intensive care unit stays of 10 days or more were noted for 38% of patients who died.
- Family members of conscious patients who died in the hospital reported that 50% of patients experienced moderate to severe pain at least half the time.

While this study was never intended to unmask such a deficit in the provision of end-of-life care, it became the cornerstone for further research and initiatives to determine what went wrong and how to correct the problem.

A number of barriers to providing quality palliative care persist. These barriers overlap to some degree, but have been divided into 5 categories: access to care, economics, patients, families, and professionals (Figure 74-3). While each will be discussed for its own merit, the barriers are typically not found in isolation from one another.

### ACCESS TO CARE

Issues surrounding access to care are not unique to the palliative care environment, but are often an overlooked barrier to quality care in this setting. The lack of access to palliative care can be related to social as well as geographical factors. Minority groups, such as African Americans, are already known to experience inadequate access to health care in general. African Americans have higher

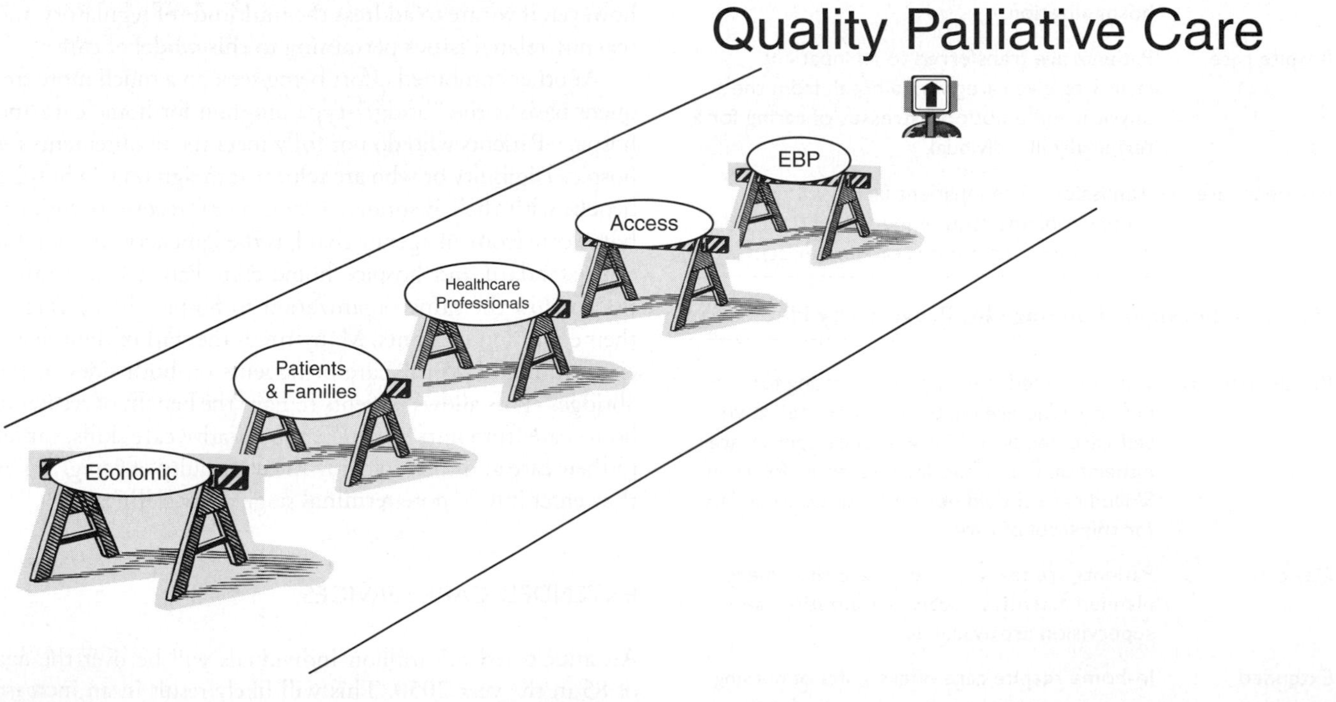


**FIGURE 74-3**

Barriers to quality palliative care.

Abbreviation: EBP, evidence-based practice.

cancer incidence and mortality rates than Caucasians. While African Americans make up approximately 14% of the total population, they make up only 7% of hospice patients.[19, 28,29] This disparity holds true for other vulnerable populations.[19,30,31] The reasons underlying this issue are multifactorial, but need further exploration. Specific cultural barriers for these populations are discussed later in this chapter.

The lack of palliative care resources in low socioeconomic and rural areas is another factor that limits access to palliative care. Resources, both in personnel and arising from economic constraints, restrict the availability of palliative care services in these areas.[28,32]

## ECONOMICS

A diagnosis of cancer is no longer necessarily synonymous with a "death sentence." The advent of new therapies and new technologies has enabled individuals to receive multiple therapies and often experience longer remissions prior to a determination being made that further attempts at cure are futile. While most would agree that philosophically this is a positive advancement, from an economic perspective, it has placed a considerable drain on an already-overstressed healthcare system. Few data are available regarding how to accurately calculate cost-effectiveness ratios in palliative care.[33]

Questions are also posed about whether multiple successive treatments have any impact on quality or quantity of life for individuals with an advanced cancer diagnosis and how this potential overuse of resources should be handled.[34] Throughout the treatment period, patients are in need of various degrees of palliative support. While physicians may hesitate to make treatment decisions based on the costs of two equally effective therapies, it may be wise for them to do so before the decision is made for them due to increased government restrictions on prescribers.[34] Technology can be used in an appropriate way to provide a higher quality of palliative care for patients. The challenge becomes finding the balance between those technologies that aid in comfort vs those that only induce more pain and suffering.[35] For instance, subjecting a patient, who has a radiation insensitive tumor, to come in daily for radiation therapy is likely a poor choice of technology.

Patients in the United States fall into 1 of the 3 categories: the insured, the underinsured, and the uninsured. A single patient may move between these categories during the course of illness based on his or her disease trajectory. Many patients are employed when they receive a cancer diagnosis. As they begin to explore treatment options, concerns are often expressed about maintaining healthcare coverage by their employers. This issue can have a significant impact not only on the patient, but also for the entire family when the patient is the insurance carrier for the family. Patients making the transition between treatments being provided with curative intent and those with palliative intent face unique economic issues. The changeover for these patients to a Medicare benefit (specifically Medicare disability insurance) may mean a loss of coverage for office visits and for prescription coverage prior to initiation of the Medicare hospice benefit. The subsequent financial strain on patients can be overwhelming when coupled with the stresses already induced by their diagnosis and treatment. In contrast, patients who elect to transfer into a home hospice program may be required to forgo some expensive palliative strategies. This is due to the hospice program's inability to financially offset the costs of such therapies as part of the per diem received from Medicare and other third-party payers.[36] For instance, patients who have achieved optimal control of pain by using a specific long-acting analgesic such as a fentanyl patch may be told that enrollment into a particular home hospice program requires that they switch to another agent that is part of that hospice's contracted pharmaceutical formulary. Only if they have documented evidence that the new agent is ineffective can they go back to the original treatment. Those unwilling to change may be asked to pay for the prescription out-of-pocket.

Palliative care is no longer limited to administration of morphine. As research in the area of symptom management continues, the use of newer therapies to improve symptoms and quality of life such as antiemetics and other analgesics has increased almost logarithmically. The cost of these therapies, however, has increased substantially, turning optimal pain and symptom management into a significant challenge for patients and healthcare providers alike. The cost of palliative care services is also affected by the location where that care is delivered. The SUPPORT study[27] depicted the inadequacies of the end-of-life care being provided in the intensive care unit (ICU). Resource allocation in the ICU involves modalities such as renal dialysis, anti-endotoxin therapy, and thromboplastin administration. Ethical issues may clash with economic issues as decisions regarding patient condition and appropriateness of resource utilization are made, as well as who should be making those decisions.[33]

Limited research currently exists on the cost-effectiveness of moving some of the higher-technology services provided in the hospital setting to the home setting. It may be reasonable to provide palliative measures such as intravenous hydration and analgesia in the home setting with home care nursing support. Other studies have attempted to demonstrate the cost-effectiveness of providing palliative or supportive care services earlier in the course of treatment for terminal illnesses. For example, the staff may initiate home care services as patients begin what is felt to be palliative therapies for advanced cancer. The staff is educated in the intricacies of therapeutic cancer treatment but also have expertise in palliative symptom management. Their efforts help to bridge the movement of patients from acute care to palliative care and diminish feelings of abandonment perceived by patients and families.[37]

## PATIENT AND FAMILY BARRIERS

The patient and family barriers to quality palliative care can be grouped under the general headings of "lack of knowledge" and "fear." With attention to these barriers, great strides can be made in the quality of the dying experience.

Patients and their families may start with a lack of basic knowledge about palliative care. Even more fundamental is the recognition that the patient is the central controlling force in care. Misconceptions related to what palliative care involves can lead to patients not seeking this support or, in worse scenarios, refusing support made available to them.[38]

Misunderstandings may also emerge regarding how insurance benefits are handled. Patients and families who are not familiar with the Medicare hospice benefit may have concerns that they will have no insurance coverage if they participate in hospice care.[39] Patients and families should be referred to social workers or other personnel who can assist them with insurance issues. Those patients who have established strong bonds with their physician and healthcare team may also be reluctant to enter a hospice program for fear that their care will be managed by a new group of healthcare workers with whom they have not developed a trusting relationship. In fact, hospice care encourages the participation of and continued management by the referring physician. Those physicians and nurses who maintain responsibility for their patients even as they enter hospice care should make this continuity of care very clear to patients and families when they begin discussions concerning referral.

Another major way in which patients become barriers to quality palliative care is the absence of advance directives. Advance directives are intended to provide very specific instructions regarding the medical care that an individual would want to receive if unable to express his or her wishes at a future date.[40] Advance directives may be either written or verbal and include documents such as a living will and durable power of attorney. A living will is a type of advance directive that describes the specific types of care that should and should not be used in particular situations. The durable power of attorney for health care identifies a specific person who the individual trusts to make these types of decisions in the event that the appointing person becomes incapable of doing so.[36] Advance directives do more than merely state whether the patient wants to be resuscitated. They should encompass a range of scenarios that are possible in the event of an illness that incapacitates the patient and leaves the individual unable to express his or her desires.[41]

In 1991, the Patient Self-Determination Act (PSDA) was passed. This act requires that patients be informed on admission that they have the right to refuse or accept medical treatment and to specify in advance what their wishes are.[42] Thus advance directives can encompass patient preferences pertaining to issues such as CPR, use of invasive procedures, intubation, nutritional support provided by non-oral means, and transfusions. The expression of these desires in advance can decrease patients' concerns over what may happen to them if they are in a state that prevents their direct decision making. It also decreases potential guilt feelings of family members who are left to make these decisions in the absence of knowing specifically what type of care is desired by the individual.[43]

Documentation in some form, however, is critical in trying to assure that the patient's desires are followed. The absence of this documentation can lead to conflicts between the healthcare team and the patient's family as well as among family members. Rules governing advance directives may vary from state to state. State-specific advance directives are available online through the Partnership for Caring Web site (http://www.caringinfo.org/stateaddownload).

Patients bring many fears with them into the healthcare arena. In the case of minority patients such as those of African American descent, there are historical events. A general mistrust of the healthcare system has been shared by many African Americans as a result of the atrocities that took place as part of the National Public Health Service Syphilis Study at Tuskeegee Institute. Discussions surrounding palliative or hospice care may be interpreted as withholding of the best medical treatment.[28,29,44,45] This same mistrust exists in many minority groups, who question whether their best interests are being taken into consideration as part of care planning.

Patient fears are also well documented pertaining to their reporting of pain and other symptoms. Concerns that lead to underreporting, specifically of pain, can involve a number of factors. Patients often fear addiction to pain medication and, as a result, will give inaccurate representations of pain scores.[46] For some patients, admitting that they have pain or other symptoms related to their illness forces them to abandon their denial of the extent of their disease.[47] At the most basic level, the patient's fear of death may block communication in discussing it. Some patients fear that just the act of discussing their death may hasten it.[48]

All members of the healthcare team have a responsibility to assess for patient-related barriers to care and implement approaches to address them. The importance of open communication cannot be overstressed. Only when open exchange of information and an atmosphere of trust exist can these barriers be broken down.

## PROFESSIONALS AS BARRIERS

Recent research has uncovered a number of roadblocks to successful palliative care that pertain to healthcare professionals. These barriers include inadequate knowledge related to palliative care, lack of cultural awareness and sensitivity, difficulty with issues related to death and dying, and delays in referral for hospice services.

A survey was conducted in 1998 by the American Society of Clinical Oncology to evaluate experiences of US oncologists in end-of-life care. A key finding of this survey was the identification of a lack of formal training in palliative care.[49] This theme carried over to nurses, who identified an overall lack of formal preparation in dealing with a number of end-of-life topics.[50] The issue led to sentinel research on end-of-life content found in medical and nursing textbooks conducted by Ferrell and colleagues[51] and Rabow and colleagues,[52] which has prompted a major education initiative. Their studies demonstrated that the end-of-life content in both medical and nursing textbooks was extremely limited. Physicians and nurses have typically lacked the basic preparation needed to manage patients at the end-of-life. Much of what has been learned has been gleaned via "on-the-job training."

Based on these studies, programs have now been developed in medicine and nursing to provide education for healthcare professionals in palliative care. The End-of-Life Nursing Education Consortium (ELNEC) was a 3-year project that began in February 2000 and was funded with grants from the Robert Wood Johnson Foundation. Through this "train the trainer" program, nurse educators in all 50 states have received training through ELNEC.[53] The ELNEC curriculum has now been expanded with specific foci in pediatric palliative care, critical care, oncology, and geriatrics. The core content is divided into 9 modules (Figure 74-4). Education in Palliative and End-of-Life Care (EPEC) began as a project, funded by the Robert Wood Johnson Foundation, American Medical Association, and the National Institute of Health, for the education of physicians in the critical clinical competencies needed for quality end-of-life care.[54] The stated mission for EPEC is now *to educate all healthcare professionals on the essential clinical competencies in palliative care.*[55] Both programs have also broadened education to involve international audiences. The need for culturally competent care is not unique to palliative care, but inattention as to how it impacts those with a terminal diagnosis will severely limit the effectiveness of healthcare providers. Even practitioners with the purest motives may unintentionally disregard cultural aspects of care as they care for individuals outside of their own culture. It is predicted that by 2050, over half of Americans will identify with a specific ethnic minority group.[56] The concept of culture, however, is much broader than an individual's race or ethnicity; it encompasses a multitude of personal variables such as age, gender, religious preferences, socioeconomic status, and educational background.[57] There is a tendency to become ethnocentric as we provide care to individuals. Unfortunately, this can create barriers in the way in which patients and families communicate with the healthcare team. Differences may arise between what is considered to be traditional medical practice and what the patient wants to have done. Individuals who are made to feel that their beliefs and practices are not valued will be less likely to share essential information that can influence the quality of their care.[57,58]

| ELNEC modules |
|---|
| Nursing care at the end of life |
| Pain management |
| Symptom management |
| Ethical/legal issues |
| Cultural considerations in end-of-life care |
| Communication |
| Grief, loss, bereavement |
| Achieving quality care at the end of life |
| Preparation and care for the time of death |

**FIGURE 74-4**

End-of-Life Nursing Education Consortium (ELNEC) modules.

In our society's efforts to wage a "war on drugs," there has been an increase in "opioidphobia" on the part of patients, but more importantly on the part of healthcare providers, including both doctors and nurses. Despite the efforts of state Cancer Pain Initiatives to recognize pain as a fifth vital sign, pain medications are being withheld from individuals due to fear of patients becoming addicted or "selling" their narcotics on the street.[17] Education of healthcare professionals on pain and symptom management principles is essential. While mandates such as the Joint Commission on Accreditation of Healthcare Organizations (JCAHO) standards for pain management[59] are wonderful from a broad institutional perspective, the fears that exist in individuals who are responsible for care must be addressed. Nurses have admitted withholding doses of morphine out of concern that they would cause too much respiratory depression and actually provoke a patient's death.[50] It is critical that nurses take the lead in removing this barrier. There are no symptoms that should be endured solely because the patient is "terminal."

Another significant barrier to quality care stems from difficulties in discussing issues related to death. Patients admitted to an acute care facility in a crisis situation who are then found to have a terminal prognosis may be cared for by hospital staff who are unable to communicate this information to the patient and their family due to their own lack of comfort with the prognosis. Patients may have to endure unnecessary procedures and lose valuable time with family members as a result.[60] The dichotomy of inciting death vs allowing death may lead to paralysis in making decisions that can have an enormous impact on the quality of death. As caregivers, each of us must reflect on the issues we may have with our own mortality. It is nearly impossible to discuss concerns related to the patient's death and the dying process if that is the ground where we ourselves fear to tread. The pinnacle of quality palliative care is reached through open and honest communication with patients.[17]

Difficulties in discussing end-of-life issues with patients and families can result in delays in referral to hospice care. While 70% of Americans state that they want to die at home, only 25% actually do so. Most states in the US have less than optimal use of hospice services, with only 38.5% of deaths in 2006 including a hospice stay (median length of stay 20.6 days).[19] The causes underlying this trend are likely to be multifactorial. Physicians may be unaware that they can continue to follow their patients after enrollment into a hospice program and, as a result, may have a sense of abandoning them, which prevents earlier referral. Members of the acute healthcare team may not have an appreciation for the depth of services provided by hospice, leading to impediments in discussing these services with patients and families.[61–63]

## LACK OF EVIDENCED-BASED INTERVENTIONS

Providing quality palliative care is best accomplished when there is a combination of research based evidence, clinical expertise, patient preferences, and values. This combination is the essence of evidence-based practice.[64] There have been ongoing efforts in improving evidence-based practice in palliative care, but challenges arise from the uniqueness and the associated ethical and moral issues, which are cited, in using standard randomized trials in this patient population.[65] While work is ongoing in hospice populations, quality measures for palliative care are also being established for patients in critical care.[66]

## ETHICAL AND LEGAL ISSUES IN PALLIATIVE CARE

The 4 ethical principles guiding clinical practice—autonomy, nonmaleficence, beneficence, and justice—must also be utilized in the practice of palliative care.[17,67] *Autonomy* refers to the process of helping patients make the decisions that are right for them.[68] Nurses are in the position to advocate for patients. It is our responsibility to ensure that patients have the knowledge they need to weigh the pros and cons of proposed treatment decisions. It also means making a concerted effort to allow patients to control as many aspects of their care as possible.

*Nonmaleficence* in palliative care involves avoiding practices that will do harm to the individual. An example of harm would be ordering inappropriate diagnostic tests that cause discomfort but have no real clinical merit.[69] Inappropriate care could also entail withholding pain medication for a patient in pain. The opposite of this would be *beneficence,* which seeks to help the patient while balancing the benefits against the risk of harm. Turning a patient to prevent skin breakdown seems like a reasonable activity unless the patient is imminently dying and has widespread bony metastasis causing severe pain with any movement.

*Justice* refers to the distribution of resources in a fair and reasonable way. How should healthcare dollars be spent? Should more funding be devoted to research in palliative care? Should a patient with a terminal diagnosis receive care that is comprehensive but devoid of the more expensive tests? How are staffing assignments made in relation to high-acuity patients receiving end-of-life care?[70]

How these principles are applied in physician-assisted suicide and euthanasia is the subject of continued debate. Active euthanasia has been defined as "the direct administration of a lethal agent to the patient by another party with a merciful intent."[71] In 1994, the state of Oregon passed the Death with Dignity Act, a legislative effort that allows physician-assisted suicide.[72] These measures should not be confused with terminal sedation and the withholding or discontinuation of life-sustaining therapy. The latter is typically employed in palliative care as a means of providing dignity to a patient when there is believed to be no chance for recovery.[73] This practice gained extensive media coverage as the family of Karen Ann Quinlan fought to gain the right to remove her from a respirator following a respiratory arrest in 1975 that left Quinlan in a permanent vegetative state.[74] Terminal sedation is a means of palliating symptoms that have become refractory to all other measures and that may ultimately have the unforeseen side effect of death.[75] Unfortunately, there are times when conflict occurs between good clinical judgment, ethics, and the law. It is important that healthcare professionals have an understanding of what is fact and what is myth so as to provide optimal care.[76] Proponents of palliative care are hopeful that increased efforts and success in providing quality end-of-life care will eliminate the need for physician-assisted suicide as an alternative.

## CHALLENGES FOR THE FUTURE OF PALLIATIVE CARE

Whenever a major need is identified in a society, multiple groups inevitably begin to independently try to meet that need. The same has been true of palliative care. Since the SUPPORT data[27] were released and the inadequacies of care in this area were identified, a number of local and national efforts have sought to address these issues.

While this movement has in general been very positive, it has also resulted in disagreements about what the issues are and what the best approaches to deal with them by those who deem themselves to be experts in the field. This section of the chapter addresses a number of issues that will help shape the future of palliative care, including consistency in practice, research efforts, and outcome measures.

## CONSISTENCY IN PRACTICE

Determining how to provide consistency in the delivery of care is a daunting task. It is frequently attempted via the use of policy, nationally accepted standards of practice, and the formation of consensus panels. Standards for specialization in a given field are often addressed by means of specialty certification.

*Scope and Standards of Hospice and Palliative Nursing Practice* provide guidelines on nursing care delivered in the palliative care setting. This text is useful in formulating programmatic planning and evaluation and in the development of individual state guidelines.[77] The Hospice and Palliative Nurses Association (HPNA) was originally formed in 1987 (at that time it was called the Hospice Nurses Association) as an organization to promote excellence in hospice nursing practice. Out of that organization came what is now known as the National Board for the Certification of Hospice and Palliative Nurses (NBCHPN). Certification in the palliative care specialty for nurses is currently provided through this board for registered nurses and nursing assistants.[78] In 2003, the first certification for advanced practice nurses in palliative care was offered through the joint efforts of HPNA and the American Nurses Credentialing Center (ANCC).[79] A specialty for physicians practicing in palliative care exists through the American Board of Hospice and Palliative Medicine, which was formed in 1995.[80]

On a more global level, the goal of the National Consensus Project for Quality Palliative Care (NCP; http://www.nationalconsensusproject.org) is to improve the delivery of palliative care in the United States by developing clinical practice guidelines by voluntary consensus. The steering committee for this project was formed following a 2001 national leadership conference in New York City. Three organizations (American Academy of Hospice and Palliative Medicine, Hospice and Palliative Nurses Association, and the National Hospice and Palliative Care Organization) continue as members of a consortium with the following purpose: The purpose of the National Consensus Project for Quality Palliative Care is to promote the implementation of Clinical Practice Guidelines that ensure care of consistent and high quality, and that guide the development and structure of new and existing palliative care services.[81]

## RESEARCH ISSUES IN PALLIATIVE CARE

The paucity of data available in the area of palliative care has a multifactorial etiology. Frequently cited as a barrier to research in palliative care is the concern that patients at the end-of-life are too vulnerable and that it is not ethical to place them in a position where they can be exploited.[82] The concern with vulnerability is associated with decreased decision-making capability and volunteerism. Patients in the palliative setting, however, are not unique to this threat and researchers must use strategies to determine if the patient is capable of making an informed decision to participate in research efforts. A fear that patients will volunteer to participate in research because of a closeness established with the researcher or solely out of desperation is also not unique to this population. Phase I clinical studies can be said to offer the same risk for patients.[83] Other ethical issues arise from conflicts relating to investigators as they attempt to wear the hats of both researcher and clinician. For instance, if the nurse researcher identifies that an intervention in one group of patients has an enormous benefit for symptom management and the other group of patients continues to experience suffering while receiving another intervention, what should be done? These are difficult, but not unanswerable, questions. Research design must take the potential for such issues into consideration prior to study implementation.[84]

Another identified concern is that the risks and benefits of research in the palliative care setting are more difficult to determine. The risk of a terminally ill patient responding to interview questions for 15 minutes may appear minimal on a superficial level, but may be intolerable for a patient who feels that it takes away precious time with his or her loved ones.[83] Additional study is clearly needed that focuses on the identification of what patients and families view to be the risks and benefits associated with research in the hospice and palliative care setting.

## OUTCOME MEASUREMENT

It is critical to rethink the traditional concept of outcome measurement when application is made to palliative care. This creates another exigency in advancing this science. While the anticipated outcome is not resolution of the illness, the assorted maladies seen concomitantly are appropriate targets on which to focus. Recent data have shown that over the past 25 years, hospice is the fastest growing benefit in the Medicare program (though less than 3% of all Medicare expenditures).[6] Enrollment in the Medicare Hospice benefit has been shown to decrease overall Medicare expenditures incurred during the last year of life.[85] Reports of economic outcomes of palliative care remain limited. Studies have suggested, however, that clinical outcomes of palliative care were maintained by nurses coordinating care with a 40% cost savings.[86] Outcomes pertaining to the provision of palliative care that have been discussed in the literature include patient and family satisfaction, quality of life, relief of symptoms, provider continuity, comfortable dying, self-determined life closure, and effective grieving.[87,88]

Critical in outcome measurement is making sure that the focus is on areas that the patient and family believe to be important. Measures of patient satisfaction have been criticized because this area remains difficult to both quantify and define. There are also a number of inconsistencies across studies regarding patient satisfaction.[89] Additional work is required to substantiate the results in a meaningful way.

Quality of life questionnaires have been used more frequently over the past decade as a multidimensional approach in the evaluation of care. Quality of life essentially becomes the primary goal in end-of-life care. A number of instruments have been developed that are specific for the palliative care population (Table 74-3).[90–95] Another resource is available through the Center for Gerontology and Health Care Research at Brown University. The *Toolkit of Instruments to Measure End of Life Care (TIME)* provides an annotated bibliography of instruments currently available to measure quality of care at the end-of-life and is available online (http://www.chcr.brown.edu/pcoc/toolkit.htm). In determining how to measure quality of care, consideration must be given to the purpose of measurement, the patient population involved, the timing of the measurement, the source of the information, and the setting in which care is to be measured.[96] Some criticism has focused on the use of measurement instruments that attempt to evaluate excessive numbers of outcomes, as their psychometric utility may be compromised.[97]

An Institute of Medicine report entitled *Describing Death in America* reviewed the data related to quality assessment in the months just prior to death. This report indicated that there are wide gaps between what we should know and what we actually know. It recommended several initiatives to address the problem.[98]

**TABLE 74-3**

**Quality of Life Instruments for Palliative Care**

| Instrument | Brief Description |
|---|---|
| Missoula-Vitas Quality of Life Index[90] | 25-item survey validated in a hospice setting; covers 5 domains, including spirituality |
| McGill Quality of Life Questionnaire[91] | 17-item questionnaire including 5 subscales that measure physical well-being, physical symptoms, psychological symptoms, existential well-being, and support |
| FAMCARE[92] | 20-item scale that measures family satisfaction with health care provided to the patient and to them |
| Life Evaluation Questionnaire[93] | 45-item questionnaire evaluating aspects not measured by existing surveys; 5 domains covered include appreciation of life, contentment, resentment, social interaction, and freedom vs restrictions |
| McMaster Quality of Life Scale[94] | 32-item questionnaire measuring 4 domains from patient's perspective |
| After-Death Bereaved Family Member Interview[95] | Retrospective telephone-administered survey with bereaved family members; 7 domains included; full instrument contains 133 questions; shortened and adapted for specific sites of care (hospice, hospital, nursing home) |

## CONCLUSION

Progress continues in collective efforts to advance the practice of palliative care in the US and around the world. Major sources of funding have been allocated by the government and charitable organizations such as the Robert Wood Johnson Foundation, which have supported efforts to identify and address the inadequacies associated with end-of-life care reported in the literature. Efforts must continue in the provision of evidence-based care as well as addressing ongoing concerns related to access to palliative care in minority populations, providing palliative care in nontraditional settings such as critical care units, and establishing financial outcomes that can be utilized in evaluating the Medicare Hospice Benefit.

## REFERENCES

1. American Cancer Society. *Cancer Facts and Figures 2009*. Atlanta American Cancer Society, 2009.
2. Senn HJ, Glaus A. Supportive care in cancer—15 years thereafter. *Support Care Cancer.* 2002;10:8–12.
3. Bennahum DA. The historical development of hospice and palliative care. In: Forman WB, Kitzes JA, Anderson RP, et al, eds. *Hospice and Palliative Care.* Sudbury, MA: Jones and Bartlett; 2003:1–12.
4. Moore CD. Caregiver issues. In: Esper P, Kuebler K. *Palliative Practices from A to Z for the Bedside Clinician.* Pittsburgh, PA: ONS Press; 2008:59.
5. World Health Organization. *What Is Palliative Care?* http://www.who.int/cancer/palliative/definition/en/. Accessed February 10, 2010.
6. Connor SR. Development of hospice and palliative care in the United States. *OMEGA.* 2007–2008;56:89–99.
7. National Hospice and Palliative Care Organization. Hospice and Palliative Care—History of Hospice Care. http://www.nhpco.org/i4a/pages/index.cfm?pageid=3285. Accessed October 1, 2009.
8. Enborg P. Dr Ina Cummings and Palliative Care in Canada. http://section15.ca/features/ideas/2007/10/19/palliative_care/. Accessed December 26, 2009.

9. Fins JJ, Renes LC, Schumacher JD, et al. *On the Road From Theory to Practice: Progressing Toward Seamless Palliative Care Near the End-of-Life.* Washington, DC: Last Acts; 2003. http://www.lastacts.org. Accessed February 10, 2010.
10. Center to Advance Palliative Care. http://www.capc.org/building-a-hospital-based-palliative-care-program/designing/characteristics//. Accessed February 10, 2010.
11. von Gunten CF, Martinez J. Hospice and palliative care. http://www.galter.northwestern.edu/geriatrics/. Accessed February 10, 2010.
12. Abu-Saad HH. Palliative care: an international view. *Patient Educ Couns.* 2000;41:15–22.
13. Twycross R. *Introducing Palliative Care.* 4th ed. Oxford: Radcliffe Medical Press; 2003.
14. Santa-Emma PH, Roach R, Gill MA, et al. Development and implementation of an inpatient acute palliative care service. *J Palliat Med.* 2002;5:93–100.
15. Ross K, Mathis S, Brockopp D. Developing a successful palliative care service in an acute care setting. *JONA.* 2008;38:282–286.
16. Stephens S. Hospital-based palliative care-cost-effective care for patients with advanced disease. *JONA.* 2008;38:143–145.
17. Twycross RG. Palliative care: an international necessity. *J Pain Palliat Care Pharmacother.* 2002;16:61–80.
18. Faull C, Woof R. *Palliative Care: An Oxford Core Text.* Oxford, UK: Oxford University Press; 2002.
19. National Hospice and Palliative Care Organization. NHPCO Facts and Figures. http://www.nhpco.org/files/public/Statistics_Research/NHPCO_facts_and_figures.pdf. Accessed February 10, 2010.
20. Kitzes JA, Sehmoll BL, Dixon CE. Hospice/palliative care settings. In: Forman WB, Kitzes JA, Anderson RP, et al, eds. *Hospice and Palliative Care.* Sudbury, MA: Jones and Bartlett; 2003:47–55.
21. Billings JA. Definitions and models of palliative care. In: Berger AM, Portenoy RK, Weissman DE, eds. *Principles and Practice of Palliative Care and Supportive Oncology.* Philadelphia, PA: Lippincott, Williams & Wilkins; 2002:635–646.
22. Eustler NE, Martinez JM. The interdisciplinary team. In: Forman WB, Kitzes JA, Anderson RP, et al, eds. *Hospice and Palliative Care.* Sudbury, MA: Jones and Bartlett; 2003:13–33.
23. Miller SC, Teno JM, Mor V. Hospice and palliative care in nursing homes [review]. *Clin Geriatr Med.* 2004;20:717–734.
24. National Hospice and Palliative Care Organization and the Center to Advance Palliative Care. Hospital-hospice partnerships in palliative care: creating a continuum of service. http://www.capc.org/palliative-care-across-the-continuum/hospital-hospice/Hospital-Hospice-Partnerships.pdf. Accessed February 10, 2010.
25. Miller SC, Han B. End-of-life care in US nursing homes: nursing homes with special programs and trained staff for hospice or palliative/end-of-life care. *J Palliat Med.* 2008;11:866–877.
26. Zerzan J, Stearns S, Hanson L. Access to palliative care and hospice in nursing homes. *JAMA.* 2000;284:2489–2494.
27. SUPPORT Study Investigators. A controlled trial to improve care for seriously ill hospitalized patients: SUPPORT. *JAMA.* 1995;274:1591–1598.
28. O'Mahony S, McHenry J, Snow D, Cassin C, Schumacher D, Selwyn PA. A review of barriers to utilization of the Medicare hospice benefits in urban populations and strategies for enhanced access. *J Urban Health.* 2008;85:281–288.
29. Payne R. Palliative care for African Americans and other vulnerable populations: access and quality issues. In: Foley KM, Gelband H, eds. *Improving Palliative Care for Cancer.* Washington, DC: National Academy Press; 2001:153–160.
30. Krakauer EL, Crenner C, Fox K. Barriers to optimum end-of-life care for minority patients. *J Am Geriatr Soc.* 2002;50:182–190.
31. McCarthy EP, Burns RB, David RB, et al. Barriers to hospice care among older patients dying with lung and colorectal cancer. *J Clin Oncol.* 2003;21:728–735.
32. Lipman AG. Calls for improved cancer symptom control…and some responses. *J Pain Palliat Care Pharmacother.* 2003;17:71–76.
33. Pronovost P, Angus DC. Economics of end-of-life care in the intensive care unit. *Crit Care Med.* 2001;29:N46-N51.
34. Lynn J, O'Mara A. Reliable, high-quality, efficient end-of-life care for cancer patients: economic issues and barriers. In: Foley KM, Gelband H, eds. *Improving Palliative Care for Cancer.* Washington, DC: National Academy Press; 2001:65–95.
35. Tinnelly K, Kristjanson LJ, McCallion A, Cousins K. Technology in palliative care: steering a new direction or accidental drift? *Int J Palliat Nurs.* 2000;6:495–500.
36. Pace JC, Mann C. Palliative Care. In: Kuebler KK, Esper P, eds. *Palliative Practices from A-Z for the Bedside Clinician, 2nd ed.* Pittsburgh, PA: Oncology Nursing Society; 2008:211–15.
37. Abelson R. A chance to pick hospice, and still hope to live. *New York Times.* February 10, 2007. http://www.nytimes.com/2007/02/10/business/10hospice.html. Accessed October 1, 2009.
38. Davis MP, Kuebler KK. Palliative and end-of-life perspectives. In Kuebler KK, Heidrich DE, Esper P. *Palliative and End-of-Life Care—Clinical Practice Guidelines.* St Louis, MO: Saunders; 2007:19–32.
39. Longaway D. Death education and family support. In: Forman WB, Kitzes JA, Anderson RP, et al, eds. *Hospice and Palliative Care.* Sudbury, MA: Jones and Bartlett; 2003:13–33.
40. Leland JV, Schonwetter RS. Hospice. In: Berger AM, Portenoy RK, Weissman DE, eds. *Principles and Practice of Palliative Care and Supportive Oncology.* Philadelphia, PA: Lippincott, Williams & Wilkins; 2002:647–652.
41. Feeg VD, Elebiary D. Exploratory study on end-of-life issues: barriers to palliative care and advance directives. *Am J Hosp Pall Med.* 2005;22:119–124.
42. Balus ME. Palliative care: ethics and the law. In: Berger AM, Portenoy RK, Weissman DE, eds. *Principles and Practice of Palliative Care and Supportive Oncology.* Philadelphia, PA: Lippincott, Williams & Wilkins; 2002:902–914.
43. Gomez D. Advance directives and CPR. In: Kinzbrunner BM, Weinreb NJ, Policzer JS, et al, eds. *20 Common Problems in End-of-Life Care.* New York, NY: McGraw-Hill Medical Publishing; 2002:297–311.
44. Freimuth VS, Quinn SC, Thomas SB, et al. African Americans' views on research and the Tuskegee Syphilis Study. *Soc Sci Med.* 2001;52:797–808.
45. Shavers VL, Lunch CF, Burmeister LF. Knowledge of the Tuskegee study and its impact on willingness to participate in medical research studies. *J Natl Med Assoc.* 2000;92:563–572.
46. Esper P. Pain management in patients with advanced malignancies. *Home Health Consultant.* 2000;7:11–18.
47. Murphy-Ende K. Barriers to palliative and supportive care. *Nurs Clin North Am.* 2001;36:843–853.
48. Heidrich DE, Esper P. Pain. In: Kuebler KK, Heidrich DE, Esper P, eds. *Palliative and End-of-Life Care—Clinical Practice Guidelines.* St. Louis, MO: Saunders; 2007:447–479.
49. Gelband H. Professional education in palliative and end-of-life care for physicians, nurses, and social workers. In: Foley KM, Gelband H, eds. *Improving Palliative Care for Cancer.* Washington, DC: National Academy Press; 2001:277–310.
50. Ferrell BR, Virani R, Grant M, et al. Beyond the Supreme Court decision: nursing perspective on end-of-life care. *Oncol Nurs Forum.* 2000;27:445–455.
51. Ferrell BR, Grant M, Virani R. Strengthening nursing education to improve end-of-life care. *Nurs Outlook.* 1999;47:252–256.
52. Rabow MW, Hadie GE, Fair JM, McPhee SJ. End-of-life care content in 50 textbooks from multiple specialties. *JAMA.* 2000;283:771–778.
53. American Association of Colleges of Nursing. *ELNEC Project, 2003.* http://www.aacn.nche.edu/ELNEC/. Accessed February 10, 2010.
54. NHPCO. Hospice statistics and research. http://www.nhpco.org/i4a/pages/Index.cfm?pageid=3274. Accessed October 1, 2009.
55. EPEC. http://www.epec.net/EPEC/Webpages/index.cfm. Accessed February 10, 2010.
56. US Minorities Will Be the Majority by 2042, Census Bureau Says Report sees quicker growth, more diversity; Hispanics fastest-growing

group. http://www.america.gov/st/diversity-english/2008/August/20080815140005xlrennef0.1078106.html. Accessed October 1, 2009.
57. Mazanec P, Tyler MK. Cultural considerations in end-of-life care: how ethnicity, age, and spirituality affect decisions when death is imminent. *Am J Nurs.* 2003;103:50–58.
58. Crawley LM, Marshall PA, Lo B, et al. Strategies for culturally effective end-of-life care. *Ann Intern Med.* 2002;136:673–679.
59. Phllips D. JCAHO pain management standards are unveiled. *JAMA.* 2000;284:726–733.
60. Seymour JE. Negotiating natural death in intensive care. *Soc Sci Med.* 2000;51:1241–1252.
61. Ogle K, Mavis B, Want T. Hospice and primary care physicians: attitudes, knowledge, and barriers. *Am J Hosp Palliat Care.* 2003;20:41–51.
62. Ogle KS, Mavis B, Wyatt GK. Physicians and hospice care: attitudes, knowledge, and referrals. *J Palliat Med.* 2002;5:85–92.
63. Davies B, Sehring SA, Partridge JC, et al. Barriers to palliative care for children: perceptions of pediatric healthcare providers. *Pediatrics.* 2008;121;282–288.
64. DiCenso A, Guyatt G, Ciliska D. *Evidence-Based Nursing: A Guide To Clinical Practice.* St. Louis, MO: Mosby; 2005.
65. Eaton LH. Introduction to evidence-based practice. In: Esper P, Kuebler K, eds. *Palliative Practices from A to Z for the Bedside Clinician.* 2nd ed. Pittsburgh, PA: ONS Press; 2008:xv-xix.
66. Mularski RA, Curtis R, Billings A, et al. Proposed quality measures for palliative care in the critically ill: a consensus from the Robert Wood Johnson Foundation Critical Care Workgroup. *Crit Care Med.* 2006;34:S404-S411.
67. Beauchamp TL, Childress JF. *Principles of Biomedical Ethics.* 5th ed. New York: Oxford University Press; 2001.
68. Hermsen MA, ten Have HAMJ. Moral problems in palliative care practice: a qualitative study. *Med Health Care Philos.* 2003;6:263–273.
69. Weinreb NJ. Diagnostic tests and invasive procedures. In: Kinzbrunner BM, Weinreb NJ, Policzer JS, et al, eds. *20 Common Problems in End-of-Life Care.* New York: McGraw-Hill Medical Publishing; 2002:329–364.
70. Coveney A. Ethical issues surrounding advanced disease. In: Kuebler KK, Heidrich DE, Esper P. *Palliative and End-of-Life Care—Clinical Practice Guidelines.* 2nd ed. St Louis, MO: Saunders; 2007:63–74.
71. Supanich BA. Palliative care and physician-assisted death. In: Berger AM, Portenoy RK, Weissman DE, eds. *Principles and Practice of Palliative Care and Supportive Oncology.* Philadelphia, PA: Lippincott, Williams & Wilkins; 2002:891–901.
72. Barnard D. Ethical issues in hospice care. In: Forman WB, Kitzes JA, Anderson RP, et al, eds. *Hospice and Palliative Care.* Sudbury, MA: Jones and Bartlett; 2003:87–101.
73. Neumann JL. Ethical issues confronting oncology nurses. *Nurs Clin North Am.* 2001;36:827–841.
74. McKeever L. Legal issues in hospice and palliative care. In: Forman WB, Kitzes JA, Anderson RP, et al, eds. *Hospice and Palliative Care.* Sudbury, MA: Jones and Bartlett; 2003:103–117.
75. McHale HK. Terminal sedation. In: Kuebler KK, Esper P, eds. *Palliative Practices from A-Z for the Bedside Clinician.* Pittsburgh, PA: Oncology Nursing Society; 2002:231–234.
76. Meisel A, Snyder L, Quill T. Seven legal barriers to end-of-life care: myths, realities, and grains of truth. *JAMA.* 2000;284:2495–2501.
77. Hospice and Palliative Nurses Association. *Scope and Standards of Hospice and Palliative Nursing Practice.* Washington, DC: American Nurses Association; 2007.
78. National Board for Certification of Hospice and Palliative Nurses. http://www.nbchpn.org. Accessed October 1, 2009.
79. American Nurses Credentialing Center. http://nursingworld.org/ancc/. Accessed February 10, 2010.
80. American Board of Hospice and Palliative Medicine. http://www.abhpm.org/. Accessed October 1, 2009.
81. The National Consensus Project for Quality Palliative Care. http://www.nationalconsensusproject.org/. Accessed February 10, 2010.
82. Lee S, Kristjanson L. Human research ethics committees: issues in palliative care research. *Int J Palliat Nurs.* 2003;9:13–18.
83. Casarett DJ, Karlawish HT. Are special ethical guidelines needed for palliative care research? *J Pain Symptom Manage.* 2000;20:130–139.
84. Fine PG. Maximizing benefits and minimizing risks in palliative care research that involves patients near the end-of-life. *J Pain Symptom Manage.* 2003;25:S53-S62.
85. Taylor DH, Ostermann J, Van Houtven CH, Tulsky JA, Steinhauser K. What length of hospice use maximizes reduction in medical expenditures near death in the US Medicare program? *Soc Sci Med.* 2007;65:1466–1478.
86. Payne SK, Coyne P, Smith TJ. The health economics of palliative care. *Oncology.* 2002;16:801–808.
87. Merriman MP. Measuring outcomes and quality of life. In: Kinzbrunner BM, Weinreb NJ, Policzer JS, et al, eds. *20 Common Problems in End-of-Life Care.* New York: McGraw-Hill Medical Publishing; 2002:73–88.
88. National Hospice Workgroup. http://www.nhwg.org/. Accessed February 10, 2010.
89. Aspinal F, Addington-Hall J, Hughes R, Higginson IJ. Using satisfaction to measure the quality of palliative care: a review of the literature. *J Adv Nurs.* 2003;43:533–534.
90. Byock IR, Merriman MP. Measuring quality of life for patients with terminal illness: the Missoula-VITAS quality of life index. *Palliat Med.* 1998;12:231–244.
91. Cohen SR, Mount BM, Strobel MG, et al. The McGill Quality of Life Questionnaire: a measure of quality of life appropriate for people with advanced disease. A preliminary study of validity and acceptability. *Palliat Med.* 1995;9:207–219.
92. Ringdal GI, Jordhoy MS, Kaasa S. Measuring quality of palliative care: psychometric properties of the FAMCARE scale. *Qual Life Res.* 2003;12:167–176.
93. Salmon P, Manzi F, Valori RM. Measuring the meaning of life for patients with incurable cancer: the life evaluation questionnaire (LEQ). *Eur J Cancer.* 1996;32A:755–760.
94. Sterkenburg C. A reliability and validity study of the McMaster Quality of Life Scale (MQOLS) for a palliative population. *J Palliat Care.* 1996;12:18–25.
95. Teno JM, Clarridge B, Casey V, et al. Validation of toolkit after-death bereaved family member interview. *J Pain Symptom Manage.* 2001;22:752–758.
96. Donaldson MS, Field MJ. Measuring quality of care at the end of life. *Arch Intern Med.* 1998;158:121–128.
97. Kaasa S, Loge JH. Quality of life in palliative care: principles and practice. *Palliat Med.* 2003;17:11–20.
98. Institute of Medicine. *Describing Death in America, 2003.* http://www.nap.edu/books/0309087252/html/. Accessed December 26, 2009.

CHAPTER 75

Judith A. Paice, PhD, RN, FAAN

# Care During the Final Days of Life

## INTRODUCTION

Many people living with a cancer diagnosis will ultimately die of their disease. Because of their strong training in symptom control, oncology nurses are uniquely prepared to care for those patients who are in their final days of life. Furthermore, oncology nurses understand the psychological and spiritual distress expressed by these patients and their families and are able to address these concerns. Oncology nurses often have long-term relationships with these patients and their loved ones, thus providing continuity of care during what can be a very stressful time.

To be equipped to provide this care, oncology nurses must be aware of the common symptoms experienced during the final days of life, as well as the appropriate assessment and management of these symptoms. Although many dying patients have few symptoms, and most of these can be easily managed, difficult situations can arise that can complicate the dying process. Well-trained oncology nurses can ensure a peaceful death for these patients, ultimately improving the experience for the patient as well as for all the loved ones in attendance during this process. Finally, as societal changes have moved death out of the home and into institutions, many people have little understanding of the dying process. Oncology nurses must provide education for patients and their family members to alleviate fear and foster the relationship work that may take place during this time.

## SYMPTOMS DURING THE FINAL DAYS OF LIFE

### PREVALENCE OF SYMPTOMS

Certain symptoms are common during the final days of life, although their prevalence and other characteristics have not been extensively investigated. In a study of patients with colon and lung cancer during the last three days of life, pain was prevalent in more than 40%, while delirium occurred in more than 25% of these patients.[1] Noisy breathing ("rattle"), pain, and urinary dysfunction were the most common symptoms of 200 patients, most with cancer, during the last 48 hours of life.[2] In a study of patients dying in long-term care facilities (some with cancer), pain, noisy breathing, dyspnea, and delirium were common during the final days of life.[3] Studies of patients in various stages of the dying process who had been referred to palliative care services, many of whom had cancer, affirm the prevalence of these symptoms. These studies and others assert that the most common symptoms are pain, anorexia, constipation, weakness, rattle, dyspnea, cough, and delirium.[4–7]

Children also experience an increased symptom burden during the final days of life. In a study of 30 children, more than half with cancer, the mean number of symptoms was 11.1 during the last week of life.[8] In another study of children who died from cancer, pain, fatigue, and dyspnea were the most common symptoms during the final days of life, and 89% suffered "a lot" or "a great deal" from at least one symptom.[9] Unfortunately, many centers treating children with cancer do not yet have palliative care services.[10]

Two "roads" to death have been described.[11] The "usual death" includes a continuum where patients become sleepy and withdrawn, lethargic, and obtunded, gradually progressing to coma and death. The "difficult death"is one where the patient develops confusion and restlessness, followed by hallucinations, delirium, myoclonus, seizures, and eventually, coma and death.[11,12] The degree to which patients travel each of these roads is not known, yet even if less common, clinicians need to be prepared to manage the disturbing "difficult death."

Thus, a wide range of symptoms are common during the final stages of life. Oncology nurses with knowledge and skills regarding palliative care can effectively manage these symptoms, reducing the prevalence of the "difficult death" and ultimately relieving distress experienced by patients and their families. Furthermore, oncology nurses can educate family caregivers providing assistance to loved ones in the home to reduce symptom distress.[13] This chapter addresses those symptoms commonly seen in the final days of life. For a complete review of symptoms common in those with cancer at other times during the disease trajectory, see Part IV, Cancer Symptom Management, Chapters 25–36.

### MANAGEMENT OF SPECIFIC SYMPTOMS

#### Pain

Pain is common throughout the cancer continuum, yet is particularly prevalent toward the end of life. The assessment and management of pain are thoroughly discussed in Chapter 27, and the strategies offered are pertinent to individuals during the final days of life. Unique aspects of pain control at the end of life include assessment in the cognitively impaired, delivery of drugs when the oral route is no longer feasible, and concerns by family and professionals that opioids hasten death.

*Assessment of pain.* Assessment of pain in the final days of life may be complicated when the patient is no longer able to report the intensity or presence of pain. In nonverbal patients, examine the brow for tightening or furrowing.[11] Treat the pain empirically and reassess. If the furrowed brow becomes smooth, assume that the patient was in pain and continue treatment. If the brow remains furrowed, consider other causes of discomfort, such as impaction, a distended bladder, or spiritual concerns. Standardized assessment tools that have been found to be valid and reliable in patients with cancer who are cognitively impaired are currently being tested. Family members can be of some assistance, but studies demonstrate that they consistently overestimate the intensity of symptoms of their loved ones.[14]

*Routes of administration.* Many routes of administration are available when patients can no longer swallow, including transdermal, transmucosal (including sublingual and buccal), rectal, vaginal, topical, epidural, and intrathecal delivery (see Table 75-1). In a study of patients with cancer at 4 weeks, 1 week, and 24 hours before death, the oral route of opioid administration was continued in 62%, 43%, and 20% of patients, respectively.[20] Intermittent subcutaneous injections and intravenous or subcutaneous infusions were most commonly used when patients were no longer able to swallow.[15]

Preexisting enteral feeding tubes can be used to access the gut when patients can no longer swallow. The rectum, stoma, or vagina also can be used to deliver medication, although thrombocytopenia or painful lesions preclude the use of these routes. Nurses must assess for the possibility that family members may have physical or cultural barriers to delivering medications by these routes. Transdermal delivery of fentanyl, as well as buccal or sublingual administration of this opioid, are other useful alternatives.[21]

Parenteral administration includes subcutaneous and intravenous delivery (intramuscular opioid delivery is inappropriate and not indicated at any time, but particularly during end of life). The intravenous route provides rapid drug delivery but requires vascular access, occasionally a problem for patients in the final days of life. Subcutaneous boluses have a slower onset (approximately 30 minutes) and lower peak effect when compared with intravenous boluses.[16] Subcutaneous infusions may include up to 10 mL/hour (although most patients absorb 2 to 3 mL/hour with the least difficulty).[17,18]

Epidural or intrathecal routes of delivery allow the administration of several analgesic agents, including opioids, local anesthetics, and/or $\alpha_2$-adrenergic agonists (such as clonidine). A randomized controlled trial demonstrated benefit of an implantable drug delivery system for patients with cancer experiencing pain.[19] Although an external epidural catheter may be placed to assist in intractable pain control during the final days of life, implanted devices should not be initiated at this time.

**TABLE 75-1**

**Routes of Administration During the Final Days of Life**

| Route | Considerations |
|---|---|
| Enteral administration via tubes | • Caution when using long-acting opioid "sprinkles" to avoid plugging small lumen tubes |
| Oral (buccal, sublingual, transmucosal) | • Possible even in last days of life<br>• Liquid placed sublingually or buccally is absorbed via the gastrointestinal tract |
| Parenteral | • IM route not indicated |
| • Intravenous | • Vascular access may be complicated in home environment due to need for complex technology (yet delivery is ensured) |
| • Subcutaneous | • Subcutaneous infusion is a useful alternative |
| Rectal/stomal/vaginal | • Not recommended in patients with thrombocytopenia or rectal lesions<br>• May be physically difficult for family members to place |
| Spinal<br>• Epidural<br>• Intrathecal | • Allows administration of other agents such as local anesthetics<br>• May increase level of care due to high-tech nature of equipment |
| Transdermal | • Ease of administration, yet may be difficult to titrate for patient with rapidly changing pain |

*Source:* Data from van den Beuken-van Everdingen et al[15]; the American Pain Society[16]; Nelson et al[17]; Watanabe et al[18]; and Smith et al.[19]

*Opioids and time of death.* Family members and clinicians express great fear that they will hasten the patient's death through the use of opioids. In fact, many family members and less experienced nurses have commented that they do not want to be the one to give the "last dose" of opioid. These fears may lead to undertreatment of pain during the dying process. There will always be a last dose of opioid. Furthermore, the literature does not support the concern that opioids hasten death.[22] In an analysis of 17 studies employing opioids at the end of life, patterns of delivery, dose, type of opioid, and survival were examined.[23] None of the five studies that explored the effect of opioids on survival found any association.[24] This finding also is consistent with sedative use and survival.[25] The implication for oncology nurses is that patients can obtain good control of pain and other symptoms through appropriate titration of opioids. Because of this lack of association, the often cited (and frequently misunderstood) "doctrine of double effect" is not relevant to opioids and care delivered at the end of life.[23] The Hospice and Palliative Nurses Association has a position statement on the Ethics of Opiate Use Within Palliative Care that is an important resource for oncology nurses (http://www.hpna.org).

## Myoclonus

Myoclonus, characterized by sudden, uncontrollable, and nonrhythmic jerking, usually of the extremities, is relatively uncommon at the end of life, with one recent study describing a prevalence of 3.5%.[26] However, this neuroexcitatory toxicity of opioids can be devastating when it occurs.[27]

Given in high doses, opioids, including morphine, hydromorphone, methadone,[28] meperidine,[29] and transdermal fentanyl[30,31] may result in myoclonus.[32] Patients may first present with nocturnal myoclonus, and thus nurses should be attuned to early identification of this syndrome, particularly in patients receiving high doses of opioids.[33]

Specifically, neuroexcitatory metabolites of the opioids have been implicated in the development of opioid-induced myoclonus.[32,34] The best studied of these metabolites are morphine-3-glucuronide and hydromorphone-3-glucuronide.[35,36] Serum and cerebrospinal fluid levels of these metabolites are elevated in patients receiving morphine for cancer and nonmalignant pain, particularly individuals with renal dysfunction.[37,38] However, metabolites alone do not explain the etiology of myoclonus, as other opioids with no known metabolites have also been shown to produce myoclonus.[39]

Hyperalgesia may also occur as a result of metabolite accumulation. In this case, patients will report increased pain with additional doses of the opioid. The first response by well-meaning clinicians is often to increase the opioid dose. This generally results in greater pain, with potential progression to delirium and possibly seizures.

Other reported causes of myoclonus include electrolyte disturbances, beta-lactam antibiotics, tricyclic and newer antidepressants, surgery to the brain,[40] placement of an intrathecal catheter,[41] AIDS dementia,[42] hypoxia,[43] chlorambucil,[44] and a rare paraneoplastic syndrome called opsoclonus-myoclonus that occurs in fewer than 1% of people with cancer.[45]

Assessment includes asking the patient and his or her family about a jerking sensation, particularly in the extremities. A physical exam will reveal jerking of the extremities that is uncontrolled by movement or other activities. Jerking can also be elicited by single or repeated tapping of an isolated muscle group.

Unfortunately, strategies to relieve myoclonus have not been well studied, particularly at the end of life. If the patient is receiving opioids, the primary treatment includes changing the opioid, reducing the dose when possible, and adding a benzodiazepine[27,46,47] (see Table 75-2). Rotation to another opioid is the primary treatment of myoclonus, particularly if the patient is receiving higher doses and has renal dysfunction.[27,48] Calculate the equianalgesic dose, using standardized tables, and reduce by 25% to 50% to account for cross-tolerance between agents.[49] Pain reassessment is critical as opioids are rotated, since equianalgesic conversions are approximations and wide variability exists. Methadone has been used as an alternative agent with success,[37] although titration must be done slowly to avoid adverse effects. Furthermore, myoclonus has been reported with methadone use.[28] Other strategies include adding adjuvant analgesics, with the goal of reducing the overall opioid dose. Of the benzodiazepines, clonazepam is most frequently recommended, although its use is limited during the final days of life by the absence of a parenteral formulation. Other benzodiazepines, including lorazepam and midazolam, are also recommended and available in parenteral forms.[27,50] The antispasmodic baclofen has been used to treat myoclonus due to intraspinal opioid administration.[51]

As was mentioned earlier, opioid-induced myoclonus can progress to seizures. When more severe neurotoxicities occur, the opioid dose should be reduced by at least 50% or more.[46] Naloxone is not effective in reversing this toxicity. If seizures occur, first- and second-line therapies include phenytoin and benzodiazepines, such as diazepam or lorazepam.[52] If seizures are refractory to treatment, or if they advance to status epilepticus, then midazolam, barbiturates, or propofol may be indicated (see Table 75-3).[47,53] Midazolam has a fairly rapid onset and short duration and can be given subcutaneously, intravenously, orally, bucally, sublingually, or rectally. Furthermore, particularly important in the end-of-life period, when numerous medications are given, the only known drug incompatibility for midazolam is with corticosteroids, particularly betamethasone, dexamethasone, and methylprednisolone.[47] The standard dose of phenobarbital in the management of seizures is 20 mg/kg intravenous infusion, with a maximum rate of 50 to 100 mg/minute. The recommended dose of propofol to treat refractory status epilepticus is 1 to 2 mg/kg via intravenous injection over 5 minutes, then starting a continuous intravenous infusion of 2 to 10 mg/kg per hour.[47]

**TABLE 75-2**

**Management of Myoclonus**

**1. Rule Out Potential Causes**
- Opioids, metoclopramide, and chlorambucil are the most common pharmacological causes
- Nonpharmacological causes include hypoxia, AIDS dementia, surgery to the brain, and paraneoplastic syndrome

**2. Rotate the Opioid**
- Calculate the equianalgesic dose of the existing opioid, using a standard table
- Convert to another opioid, based on the patient's past experiences with these medications
- Reduce the dose by 25%–50% to account for cross-tolerance
- Reassess frequently, as these equivalents are only a guide; there is significant variation in response among individuals

**3. Reduce the Dose of the Opioid by**
- Adding adjuvant analgesics
- Considering interventional therapies

**4. Add a Benzodiazepine**
- Clonazepam 0.5 mg orally twice daily, and increase upward
- Midazolam 0.5 mg intravenous or subcutaneous if unable to swallow, and titrate upward

*Source*: Data from Mercadante[27]; the End of Life/Palliative Education Resource Center[46]; and Golf et al.[47]

**TABLE 75-3**

**Management of Seizures**

**Assessment**

Consider reversible causes, including

- Hypoglycemia
- Metabolic conditions (eg, hyponatremia hypercalcemia, hypoxia, withdrawal from opioids, benzodiazepines, or alcohol)

**Management**

***Pharmacological***

- Lorazepam 1–2 mg intravenous or 4 mg rectally (alternatives include rectal diazepam available in suppository or rectal gel)
- Phenytoin 18 mg/kg intravenous over 30 min (monitor for bradycardia and hypotension); if able to swallow, 300 mg orally every 2–3 hrs for 3 doses, followed by 300 mg/day (alternatives, include fosphenytoin)

*If ineffective:*

- Phenobarbital 20 mg/kg intravenous infusion; maximum rate 50–100 mg/min
- Midazolam 0.5 mg/kg/hr with upward titration (can be given subcutaneously, intravenously, orally, bucally, sublingually, or rectally)
- Propofol 1–2 mg/kg intravenous loading dose, followed by infusion of 2–10 mg/kg/hr (incompatible with most other drugs; contraindicated in patients with egg allergies or soya lecithin hypersensitivity)
- Lidocaine infusions 1–2 mg/kg/hr intravenous

***Nonpharmacological***

- Pad side rails with pillows
- Provide calm, soothing, and safe environment
- Instruct family and caregivers not to place items in mouth

*Source:* Data from Golf et al[47]; Eisele et al[50]; Stayer et al[52]; and Lowenstein and Alldredge.[53]

**TABLE 75-4**

**Causes of Dyspnea**

**Cancer-Related Causes (Direct or Indirect)**

Anemia
Ascites
Cachexia
Electrolyte abnormalities
Hepatomegaly
Pericardial effusion
Pleural effusion
Pneumonia
Superior vena cava syndrome
Tracheal esophageal fistula
Tumor, either primary or metastatic

**Treatment-Related Causes**

Surgery
Radiation
Chemotherapy

**Causes Unrelated to Cancer or Its Treatment**

Anxiety
Arrhythmias
Asthma
Cardiac ischemia
Chronic obstructive pulmonary disease
Congestive heart failure
Neuromuscular disorders (eg, amyotrophic lateral sclerosis, multiple sclerosis)
Pneumothorax
Obesity

Nursing interventions include safety measures such as padding around the bed rails and assistive devices if the patient is ambulatory. Interventions designed to reduce fatigue are critical, including the provision of a relaxing and calm environment.

## Dyspnea

Dyspnea is a common symptom in people diagnosed with cancer. Often described as shortness of breath or air hunger, this symptom shares many attributes with pain in that self-report is the only reliable strategy for assessment. Laboratory values (eg, oxygen saturation) do not necessarily correlate with the intensity of the symptom, and opioids are the primary treatment for both dyspnea and pain. As with pain, patients may be reluctant to report the presence of dyspnea. As a result, oncology nurses must routinely ask patients about this symptom.

Although dyspnea can occur in a variety of cancer diagnoses and throughout the disease trajectory, this symptom is more common in those with advanced lung or breast cancer.[4,54] Other risk factors for dyspnea include ascites, congestive obstructive pulmonary disease (COPD), and pneumonia (see Table 75-4). Furthermore, 50% of patients with lung cancer experienced dyspnea in one study, and anxiety and fatigue were associated with this symptom.[55] However, it is important to note that the National Hospice Study determined that approximately one-quarter of patients reporting dyspnea had no underlying cardiopulmonary pathology.[56] Dyspnea also is extremely common in children who die from cancer, occurring in more than 80% of the patients.[9] In general, dyspnea occurs when there is either an increase in respiratory effort necessary to overcome obstruction or restrictive disease (eg, tumor or pleural effusions), an increase in the amount of respiratory muscles required to maintain adequate breathing (eg, neuromuscular weakness or cachexia), or an increase in ventilatory need (eg, hypercapnia, metabolic acidosis).[57]

Because of its prevalence during the final days of life, and because of the distress it causes patients, screening for and assessment of dyspnea is critical. Patients can be asked to rate their level of dyspnea at rest and during activity using a 0 to 10 scale, where 0 equals “no breathlessness” and

10 indicates the "worst possible breathlessness." Patients often use phrases such as "I cannot get enough air," "I feel tightness in my lungs," or "I feel as if I am drowning."[58,59] A thorough assessment of dyspnea should include past medical history, smoking history, exposure to occupational hazards that may affect pulmonary function, and past medication use, as well as cancer treatments. Questions that incorporate the psychosocial and spiritual domains of the individual's life might include "What does this symptom mean to you?" and "What effect does this have on your daily life?"[60] Assessment of fatigue, anxiety, depression, and other symptoms is important so these can be addressed appropriately.

Physical examination, with attention to auscultation and percussion of the lung fields, can assist in identifying the underlying cause of dyspnea. Diagnostic evaluation may also be helpful; however, in the final days of life, the goals of care should always be considered when ordering these tests. For example, pneumonia may potentially be treatable with antibiotics, leading to relief of shortness of breath.[61] Yet this treatment may not be consistent with the patient's goals of care. Furthermore, CT scans, arterial blood gases, and pulmonary function tests do not provide useful information about the patient's dyspnea and are unlikely to reveal treatable causes of this symptom at this time in the patient's life.[62] In addition, conducting these tests will likely result only in pain and discomfort for the patient, as well as reducing time spent with loved ones. An important nursing consideration is that although continuous pulse oximetry is widely available on most oncology units, patients and family members often focus on the monitor. This serves only to exacerbate existing fear and anxiety and yields little meaningful information during the final days of life. Therefore, reliance upon pulse oximetry should be minimal.[60]

During the final days of life, the goal of dyspnea management is to lessen the sensation of breathlessness. Opioids are the first-line therapy in relieving dyspnea.[57,63–65] Opioids decrease the intensity of dyspnea, regardless of the underlying pathophysiology, without causing respiratory depression.[57,63] Very low doses of an opioid administered on an as-needed basis are generally very effective in patients with mild to moderate dyspnea who have previously not been taking opioids. Despite the fears of some healthcare professionals and family members, opioids have not been shown to produce respiratory depression in patients with dyspnea.[66] Individuals with more persistent or severe dyspnea, or those patients currently using opioids for pain relief, may require higher doses.[60] As with pain control, titrate the dose as needed to provide relief, and develop a plan to prevent opioid-induced side effects, particularly constipation. A stimulant laxative and stool softener, administered nightly and increased as needed, will reduce straining necessary to produce a bowel movement, which can exacerbate dyspnea.

The route of opioid administration does not seem to correlate with relief of dyspnea, and thus oral, parenteral, and transdermal routes can all be effective. A controversial delivery method is nebulized opioids for control of dyspnea. The rationale for administering opioids via nebulizer is based on the presence of opiate receptors within the lung. Delivering the drug directly to the lung might provide relief while preventing systemic side effects of the opioids.[67] However, although uncontrolled clinical trials and case reports described benefits of using this technique,[68] controlled trials have not confirmed these positive results.[57,64,69,70]

Other treatment options in relieving dyspnea include benzodiazepines to treat the anxiety that often is associated with dyspnea, but only after using opioids to manage the primary symptom. Initial doses should be low and titrated upward as indicated. Glucocorticoids or bronchodilators can relieve bronchospasm, although bronchodilators should be used cautiously due to their potential to cause anxiety and worsen dyspnea. In patients with pleural effusions, thoracentesis may provide relief.[71]

Supplemental oxygen may be useful, but only in the face of hypoxemia. In general, oxygen is no more effective than room air in reducing the sensation of dyspnea in those patients with relatively normal oxygenation.[54,70,72,73] Nursing interventions include providing a cool fan blowing on the patient's face and repositioning the patient so he or she is sitting upright. Nurses may also recommend and guide patients in the use of cognitive behavioral therapies that have been shown to be effective in relieving dyspnea, including relaxation, breathing control exercises, and psychosocial support.[74] The use of behavioral therapies requires patient involvement, which in many cases may be difficult during the final days of life due to cognitive changes or extreme weakness. Complementary therapies, such as acupuncture and acupressure, may also be of benefit in relieving dyspnea, although controlled studies are needed.[75]

## Anxiety

Anxiety is common during the final days of life and is highly correlated with other symptoms, such as unrelieved pain and dyspnea.[76] Thus, a thorough assessment of anxiety includes screening for these and other symptoms, as well as a complete review of current pharmacological therapies. Medications commonly used in palliative care can contribute to the sense of anxiety, including corticosteroids, neuroleptics (eg, metoclopramide), bronchodilators, antihistamines, digitalis, and occasionally benzodiazepines (which can cause a paradoxical reaction in elderly patients). The nurse should also consider the patient's risk for withdrawal from alcohol, opioids, benzodiazepines, and nicotine, which can also produce agitation.[77] Other factors to be considered include hypoxia, pulmonary embolus, sepsis, hypoglycemia, thyroid abnormalities, and heart failure, as well as certain tumors, including pheochromocytomas and some pancreatic cancers. During the final days of life, spiritual or existential distress, as well as fear of the unknown, can manifest as anxiety.

The pharmacological management of anxiety often includes benzodiazepines, particularly lorazepam, as it has a short duration of action and generally produces fewer adverse effects. A common initial dosage is 0.5 to 2 mg orally 3 to 4 times daily, with upward titration as needed. Lorazepam can be placed sublingually, which is useful when patients have difficulty swallowing, or given parenterally as a bolus or infusion. Haloperidol is frequently used for short-term management of severe anxiety and as an antipsychotic (as discussed in the section on delirium), with the initial dosage starting at 0.5 to 1 mg orally twice daily.[76]

Nurses should foster frank discussion of the patients' fears in a supportive environment. Relaxation strategies, such as massage, audiotapes/CDs, breathing exercises, and guided imagery, may also alleviate anxiety if the patient is able to participate at this time.[78,79] Consultation with psychology, social work, chaplains, and others can be useful.

## Delirium

Delirium is common during the final days of life and includes altered perception, impaired memory, emotional lability, hallucinations, incoherent speech, and disorientation to time, place, and person.[3,80,81] These symptoms may be misdiagnosed as anxiety or depression, particularly when mild or in the early stages. Common causes of delirium at the end of life include medications, such as opioids, corticosteroids, benzodiazepines, and adjuvant analgesics, as well as metabolic changes resulting from hypercalcemia and hyperglycemia, sepsis, central nervous system involvement by tumor, encephalopathy, and other organ system failure.[82–84]

Careful assessment includes a review of the onset and character of symptoms with family members and caregivers. Standardized tests of cognition frequently used in clinical practice, such as the Mini-Mental Status Exam, can help to determine the degree of impairment. Delirium has been characterized as two subtypes, including hyperactive and hypoactive. Signs and symptoms of hyperactive delirium include agitation, hyperarousal, hallucinations, and delusions. Withdrawal from benzodiazepines or alcohol can result in this type of delirium. Hypoactive delirium leads to lethargy and withdrawal and is more commonly related to encephalopathies and organ system failure.[85]

Treatment includes reversing the underlying cause whenever possible. Pharmacological therapy includes haloperidol, an agent that blocks dopamine. Low doses (0.5–1 mg) can be given orally, intravenously, rectally, or subcutaneously. Risperidone and olanzapine are also used, risperidone is not available parenterally and olanzapine is limited to intramuscular injections.[86] Benzodiazepines such as lorazepam have been found to worsen delirium and cognitive impairment and, therefore, are not recommended.

Nursing management includes fostering a safe, quiet environment, respecting the patient's experience, and supporting family members.[87] Keep the patient's room well lit during the day, with visible clocks. At night, dim the lights and minimize interruptions to sleep, as a normal pattern of waking and sleeping is believed to help prevent disorientation. Reality orientation is no longer considered beneficial in actively hallucinating patients. In fact, correcting the patient's perceptions may only increase anxiety and agitation. Rather, speak in a calm, relaxed tone, ask questions gently, and offer support. Also, be open to comments by dying patients about "going home" or seeing loved ones who have previously died. These are common behaviors seen during the dying process and are very beautifully described by Callanan and Kelley in the book *Final Gifts*.[88]

## Terminal secretions

Excessive respiratory tract secretions, often called "death rattle" or "rattle," are common during the last hours of life. Although not likely painful to the patient, these secretions are extremely disturbing to professionals, family members, and other loved ones in attendance during this time.[89] This may be due in part to the meaning of this symptom, as terminal secretions are a strong indicator that the patient is actively dying. Studies indicate that terminal secretions typically occur within 16 to 57 hours before death, often preceding other symptoms such as cyanosis.[90–92] The prevalence of terminal secretions varies greatly (ranging from 23% to 50%), likely as a result of practice variations, particularly in relation to hydration.[91] In people with cancer, risk factors for the development of terminal secretions include neoplasms of the brain and lung, as well as pulmonary infection, or edema.[90,93]

Two categories of secretions have been identified. Type I originates from salivary secretions and appears to respond well to anticholinergic and other drying agents, with more than 90% of patients obtaining relief.[91] Type II originates in the bronchi and is likely due to pulmonary pathology, such as infection, tumor, fluid retention, or aspiration. These secretions do not seem to respond well to treatment.[91]

Few studies have explored the most effective pharmacological treatment of terminal secretions, and therefore, treatment is often empiric (see Table 75-5).[94–96] Hyoscine (scopolamine) is available in transdermal and parenteral formulations. Originally released to reduce motion sickness, the scopolamine patch (Transderm Scop) is available in the US in a 1.5 mg dose that is changed every 3 days. If 2 patches are ineffective, a continuous intravenous or subcutaneous scopolamine infusion is started.[91] The infusion is often started at 50 micrograms/hour, with doubling of the dose every hour until the secretions are reduced, to a maximum dose of 200 to 300 micrograms/hour. Glycopyrrolate 0.2 mg (Robinul) with upward titration to relieve the noisy breathing is another option.[97] Other agents reported to reduce these secretions include atropine 0.4 mg subcutaneously every 15 minutes as needed or hyoscyamine (Levsin) 0.125 to 0.25 mg orally

**TABLE 75-5**

**Management of Terminal Secretions**

- Atropine 0.4 mg subcutaneous every 15 min until relief
- Scopolamine transdermal patch 1.5 mg
  - Increase to 2 patches after 24 hrs
  - If inadequate relief, begin scopolamine infusion 50 μg/hr intravenous or subcutaneous and double every hour to a maximum dose of 200–300 μg/hr
- Glycopyrrolate 1–2 mg orally or 0.1–0.2 mg intravenous or subcutaneous every 4 hrs as needed or 0.4–1.2 mg continuous infusion
- Hyoscyamine 0.125–0.25 mg orally every 4 hrs
- Stop or reduce parenteral or enteral fluids
- Diuretics may reduce overhydration
- Reposition to avoid accumulation of fluid

*Source*: Data from Callanan and Kelley[88]; Wildiers and Menten[91]; Kass and Ellershaw[92]; Morita et al[93]; Bennett et al[94]; Spiess and Scott[95]; and Back et al.[97]

every 4 hours. Because most patients cannot swallow at this time, the oral liquid can be placed sublingually.

Parenteral and enteral fluids contribute to respiratory secretions and should be discontinued whenever possible. If this is not feasible, the volume should be minimized to less than 500 mL in 24 hours. When patients have received large amounts of fluid, often during resuscitation efforts, diuretics may be useful in reducing the excess volume. Nursing measures such as altering the patient's position in bed may reduce pooling of secretions and the resultant rattle. Although suctioning may seem an appropriate intervention, this technique often elicits gagging and can be painful for patients. In those rare cases when suctioning is necessary, soft catheters should be used to suction only the oral cavity. Family members may require education, particularly if they request that suctioning be performed.

## GENERAL CHANGES AS DEATH NEARS

In addition to the symptoms just described, patients will develop weakness, fatigue, and anorexia. Nausea and vomiting may also occur. Patients may become incontinent of urine or feces. Greater assistance with the activities of daily living and hygiene will be required, until total care must be provided. Family members require additional support as they witness their loved ones dying.

Patients' lack of interest in food or fluids is particularly distressing to loved ones, as nutrition holds such meaning of nurturance in our culture.[12] Family members may inadvertently try to force patients to eat or drink, leading to aspiration or to discomfort for the patient. Some loved ones may demand the placement of intravenous lines, total parenteral nutrition, or tube feedings, expressing fears that we are "starving" their loved one to death. Tube feeding does not prolong survival (with the possible exception of those with amyotrophic lateral sclerosis) and actually may increase the risk of aspiration. In fact, in several studies of patients with advanced cancer, tube feedings may actually have decreased survival.[98] Other data support the lack of suffering or discomfort associated with dehydration, thus negating the need for hydration.[99] Oncology nurses must be aware of these findings to support patients and family as they are faced with difficult decisions regarding artificial nutrition and hydration. The Hospice and Palliative Nurses Association has developed a position paper, "Withholding and/or Withdrawing Life-Sustaining Therapies," that can be accessed at http://www.hpna.org.

Spiritual suffering is not uncommon as patients review their lives and reflect on their meaning. This appraisal can raise feelings of guilt, regret, or sadness. Oncology nurses can provide comfort simply through their presence, allowing the patient to express these thoughts in a nonjudgmental environment.[100] Rituals are useful for some, and consults with chaplains, social workers, or other team members can be beneficial.

As the dying process progresses, patients will become more withdrawn and less interactive with loved ones and caregivers. They may develop decreased perfusion in their extremities, leading to coolness, mottling, and a bluish cast to the skin. Changes in breathing, with periods of apnea, may also occur. Family members and loved ones often question whether they should leave the bedside, hoping to be present at the time of death. Because prognostication is so difficult, it is important to avoid giving a specific time frame. One helpful communication strategy that can be used throughout the disease process is to give a range of time, such as "hours to days," "days to weeks," or "weeks to months." Family members also need to be cautioned that some patients wait for loved ones to leave the room to die, sparing them the pain of witnessing their death, so that the timing of death can be very unpredictable.

## AFTER-DEATH CARE

After-death care includes preparing the body so that loved ones can see the patient in as natural a state as possible. Cleaning and redressing the patient, as well as removing tubes and equipment, assists family members in developing a less painful memory of their loved one, fostering a healthy bereavement process. Cultural practices need to be considered. For example, Jewish and Muslim families may refuse autopsies, on the belief that the body belongs to God or Allah and must remain whole, even in death.[101,102] In Islam, a male patient can be cared for only by another male, and in Buddhism, the body should not be moved for several hours, to allow the spirit to leave without becoming confused.[103] Family members can provide guidance, and chaplains may be consulted.

Oncology nurses may offer to assist family members and friends with phone calls and notification. Some may need time to adjust to the death before making these calls, yet others may find healing and comfort in telling the story to those who were important to the patient.

Oncology nurses who are knowledgeable regarding the physical changes that occur in those who are actively dying, as well as the emotional and cultural needs of the patient and family, can greatly affect the final hours of life for those in their care. They can also significantly improve the memories of loved ones witnessing this death, fostering the bereavement process.

## DIFFICULT SITUATIONS

### SUDDEN DEATH

Although excellent symptom control and attention to psychosocial and spiritual concerns generally provide relief, for some the dying process can be quite difficult. These difficult situations can include sudden death from events such as hemorrhage, or intractable symptoms including pain, dyspnea, nausea, and vomiting.

A particularly difficult death may be due to sudden, fatal hemorrhage.[104] For patients with hematological malignancies, bleeding from any orifice, such as the mouth, nose, eyes, rectum, urethra, or vagina can be due to thrombocytopenia or other coagulopathies.[105] Sudden death also may involve massive hemoptysis due to pulmonary or aerodigestive tumors or external hemorrhage from carotid involvement by tumor.[106] These scenarios are frightening to patients and family members. Rapid sedation using parenteral benzodiazepines is warranted. Offer a comforting environment through calm communication, reassuring the patient that he or she will not be left alone, covering wounds or secretions with dark towels, cleansing the area frequently, and rapidly disposing of soiled linens to reduce offensive odors.[107] A standing order for these types of unexpected events, particularly in patients at risk, may be helpful to ensure rapid management.

### PALLIATIVE SEDATION

Palliative, or controlled sedation at the end of life is an important option for patients with intractable pain, dyspnea, delirium, and suffering.[108] In one study, 16% of patients in an inpatient palliative care unit required treatment to relieve symptoms that resulted in sedation to a level of unresponsiveness.[109] In other studies, as many as 15% to 30% of dying patients may require this therapy.[110,111] In children, the most common indications for palliative sedation were pain as well as for seizures in those with brain tumors.[112] However, this approach is not without controversy. Some fear hastened death or believe this practice is the same as assisted suicide.[113] The general recommendation is to reserve palliative sedation to those who have hours to days of life.[114] To mediate these concerns and provide a guide to clinicians, the Hospice and Palliative Nurses Association has developed a position paper that addresses these concerns, "Palliative Sedation at the End of Life."[115]

Education and informed consent of the patient (if possible) and family is essential. They should understand the benefits and risks of initiating therapy and should never feel coerced into making a decision. A Do Not Resuscitate order should be discussed and, if desired, should be in place, and discussions regarding other life-prolonging therapies (such as dialysis or implanted defibrillators) should occur.[113] A team approach is critical, along with consultation from pain and palliative care specialists and, in some circumstances, the ethics team.[114]

The literature describing specific agents used to provide sedation at the end of life is largely anecdotal and refers to a wide variety of drugs, including opioids, neuroleptics, benzodiazepines, ketamine (a dissociative anesthetic), barbiturates, and propofol.[53,82,116,117] Because there are no randomized, controlled clinical trials, guidelines for drug selection do not exist, and therefore, the choice of agent is often empirical.

Regardless of the drug selected, titration is necessary to provide relief from intractable symptoms, followed by ongoing therapy to maintain the desired effect. The depth of sedation necessary to control symptoms varies greatly, so that a few patients may retain consciousness. Once adequate relief is obtained, ongoing monitoring is determined by the goal of care. If the goal of care is to ensure comfort until death, vital signs or other indicators may be taken infrequently. However, comfort care of the patient and family remains critical. Turning, cleansing, massaging, or other measures that provided relief prior to sedation, should continue. Family members require support during this time as they observe their loved one being alive but unable to respond. Chaplains and social workers should be consulted prior to beginning this therapy to assist in decision making and support.

Each agent used to provide palliative sedation has different side effects. Haloperidol is particularly useful for the patient with delirium at the end of life and can be given by the oral, subcutaneous, or intravenous routes. The oral or parenteral starting dose is generally 0.5 mg and can be increased to as much as 5 mg/hour continuous infusion.

Benzodiazepines, such as lorazepam or midazolam, produce sedation and can treat neurotoxicity related to opioids. Both have short half-lives. Lorazepam can be given orally, sublingually, or intravenously (starting at 0.5–5 mg every hour), while midazolam can be given parenterally (starting with a loading dose of 0.5 mg or higher). Benzodiazepines can produce paradoxical reactions, including increased agitation, particularly in the elderly.[113]

Barbiturates have been used for decades, yet their long half-lives complicate their administration. In addition, their lack of analgesic efficacy and their numerous incompatibilities make their use more complicated. Pentobarbital can be given rectally (usual starting dose 60–200 mg) or via the intravenous route (with a usual loading dose of 2 to 3 mg/kg and 1 to 2 mg/kg per hour continuous infusion). Phenobarbital can be given by subcutaneous or intravenous routes, with a loading dose of 200 mg followed by 0.5 mg/kg/hour.[113]

Propofol is an anxiolytic, antiemetic, anticonvulsant, and anesthetic. Although generally used in the operating room, propofol can provide relief of intractable symptoms, such as pain, myoclonus, and seizures.[53] Usual starting doses begin at 2.5 mcg/kg/minute, titrating every 10 minutes.[113] Patients allergic to lipids should not be given propofol, and the solution is not compatible with other compounds. There is no literature at this time regarding the safety of subcutaneous infusion.[53]

Parenteral administration of ketamine may be useful for some patients with refractory pain at the end of life. Ketamine is a potent analgesic at low doses and a dissociative anesthetic at higher doses.[118] It has been reported to relieve intractable pain and, in some cases, results in a significant decrease in the dose of opioids and sedatives, allowing the patients to interact with loved ones. However, ketamine can produce rapidly developing tolerance and hallucinations, dysphoria, or nightmares that may occur with higher doses and with drug accumulation.[119,120] Haloperidol can be used to treat the hallucinations, and scopolamine may be needed to reduce the excess salivation seen with this drug.

The oncology nurse should investigate whether institutional policies exist regarding palliative sedation. If not, an interdisciplinary team must develop such policies and educate colleagues throughout the institution regarding this type of care.[116] For more information regarding palliative sedation, access the Web site at http://www.eperc.mcw.edu.

## PATIENT AND FAMILY EDUCATION

The patient and family are the center of care, particularly during the final days of life. Patients may be aware that they are dying, and honest communication is needed between patient, family, and clinicians. Education and open communication help build trust and empower the patient and family regarding end-of-life decision making. Patients and family may fear the dying process. Many people in our society have never witnessed death and, therefore, need explicit guidance regarding the physical and emotional changes that occur during this time. Assess the family's level of understanding regarding their loved one's condition, as well as their readiness to discuss these issues. Caregiver fatigue and stress may preclude the ability to fully comprehend complex medical information, and repetition may be indicated. Written materials and role modeling, provided in an unhurried manner, are essential. Assist families to be involved in the care of their loved one, if appropriate, as this facilitates coping after death. Family meetings help ensure that consistent information is provided and heard by all present. These meetings may need to be repeated as the patient's condition changes or as the family is gradually able to assimilate the information. All of these interventions ease the dying process for the patient and support bereavement in loved ones.

## CONCLUSION

Oncology nurses are well prepared to provide care to patients with cancer facing the end of life. Because of their long-term relationships with these patients and their loved ones, oncology nurses can provide continuity of care during what can be a very stressful time. To be equipped to provide end-of-life care, oncology nurses must be aware of the common physical, psychological, and spiritual symptoms experienced during the final days of life, as well as the appropriate assessment and management of these symptoms. Oncology nurses can ensure a peaceful death for these patients, ultimately improving the experience for the patient as well as all the loved ones in attendance during this process. By being present and educating patients and families, nurses can help alleviate fear and can foster the relationship work that may take place during this time period. This care relieves the patient's distress and facilitates the bereavement process of family and loved ones. The Oncology Nursing Society, in conjunction with the Association of Oncology Social Work, have developed a position statement that describes the need for improved end-of-life care (see http://www.ons.org/Publications/positions/EndOfLifeCare.shtml). This statement provides a guide to oncology nurses working to improve the needs of patients and their family members at this most important time of life.

## REFERENCES


1. McCarthy EP, Phillips RS, Zhong Z, et al. Dying with cancer: patients' function, symptoms, and care preferences as death approaches. *J Am Geriatr Soc.* 2000;48:S110–S121.
2. Lichter I, Hunt E. The last 48 hours of life. *J Palliat Care.* 1990;6:7–15.
3. Hall P, Schroder C, Weaver L. The last 48 hours of life in long-term care: a focused chart audit. *J Am Geriatr Soc.* 2002;50:501–506.
4. Potter J, Hami F, Bryan T, et al. Symptoms in 400 patients referred to palliative care services: prevalence and patterns. *Palliat Med.* 2003;17:310–314.
5. Teunissen SC, Wesker W, Kruitwagen C, de Haes HC, Voest EE, de Graeff A. Symptom prevalence in patients with incurable cancer: a systematic review. *J Pain Symptom Manage.* 2007;34:94–104.
6. Doorenbos AZ, Given CW, Given B, Verbitsky N. Symptom experience in the last year of life among individuals with cancer. *J Pain Symptom Manage.* 2006;32:403–412.
7. McMillan SC, Small BJ. Symptom distress and quality of life in patients with cancer newly admitted to hospice home care. *Oncol Nurs Forum Online.* 2002;29:1421–1428.

8. Drake R, Frost J, Collins JJ. The symptoms of dying children. *J Pain Symptom Manage.* 2003;26:594–603.
9. Wolfe J, Grier HE, Klar N, et al. Symptoms and suffering at the end of life in children with cancer. *N Engl J Med.* 2000;342:326–333.
10. Johnston DL, Nagel K, Friedman DL, Meza JL, Hurwitz CA, Friebert S. Availability and use of palliative care and end-of-life services for pediatric oncology patients. *J Clin Oncol.* 2008;26:4646–4650.
11. Education for Physicians on End-of-life Care Project (EPEC). http://www.epec.net. Accessed September 30, 2009.
12. Furst CJ, Doyle D. The terminal phase. In: Doyle D, Hanks G, Cherny N, et al, eds. *Oxford Textbook of Palliative Medicine.* 3rd ed. Oxford: Oxford University Press; 2004:1119–1133.
13. McMillan SC, Small BJ. Using the COPE intervention for family caregivers to improve symptoms of hospice homecare patients: a clinical trial. *Oncol Nurs Forum Online.* 2007;34:313–321.
14. McMillan SC, Moody LE. Hospice patient and caregiver congruence in reporting patients' symptom intensity. *Cancer Nurs.* 2003;26:113–118.
15. van den Beuken-van Everdingen MH, de Rijke JM, Kessels AG, Schouten HC, van Kleef M, Patijn J. Prevalence of pain in patients with cancer: a systematic review of the past 40 years. *Ann Oncol.* 2007;18:1437–1449.
16. American Pain Society. *Principles of Analgesic Use in the Treatment of Acute Pain and Cancer Pain.* 5th ed. Glenview, IL: Author; 2003.
17. Nelson KA, Glare PA, Walsh D, et al. A prospective, with in-patient, crossover study of continuous intravenous and subcutaneous morphine for chronic cancer pain. *J Pain Symptom Manage.* 1997;13:262–267.
18. Watanabe S, Pereira J, Hanson J, et al. Fentanyl by continuous subcutaneous infusion for the management of cancer pain: a retrospective study. *J Pain Symptom Manage.* 1998;16:323–326.
19. Smith TJ, Staats PS, Deer T, et al. Randomized clinical trial of an implantable drug delivery system compared with comprehensive medical management for refractory cancer pain: impact on pain, drug-related toxicity, and survival. *J Clin Oncol.* 2002;20:4040–4049.
20. Coyle N, Adelhardt J, Foley KM, et al. Character of terminal illness in the advanced cancer patient: pain and other symptoms during the last four weeks of life. *J Pain Symptom Manage.* 1990;5:83–93.
21. Portenoy RK, Taylor D, Messina J, Tremmel L. A randomized, placebo-controlled study of fentanyl buccal tablet for breakthrough pain in opioid-treated patients with cancer. *Clin J Pain.* 2006;22:805–811.
22. Portenoy RK, Sibirceva U, Smout R, et al. Opioid use and survival at the end of life: a survey of a hospice population. *J Pain Symptom Manage.* 2006;32:532–540.
23. Sykes N, Thorns A. The use of opioids and sedatives at the end of life. *Lancet Oncol.* 2003;4:312–318.
24. Thorns A, Sykes N. Opioid use in last week of life and implications for end-of-life decision-making. *Lancet.* 2000;356:398–399.
25. Sykes N, Thorns A. Sedative use in the last week of life and the implications for end-of-life decision making. *Arch Intern Med.* 2003;163:341–344.
26. Ross JR, Riley J, Taegetmeyer AB, et al. Genetic variation and response to morphine in cancer patients: catechol-O-methyltransferase and multidrug resistance-1 gene polymorphisms are associated with central side effects. *Cancer.* 2008;112:1390–1403.
27. Mercadante S. Pathophysiology and treatment of opioid-related myoclonus in cancer patients. *Pain.* 1998;74:5–9.
28. Sarhill N, Davis MP, Walsh D, et al. Methadone-induced myoclonus in advanced cancer. *Am J Hosp Palliat Care.* 2001;18:51–53.
29. Kaiko RF, Foley KM, Grabinski PY, et al. Central nervous system excitatory effects of meperidine in cancer patients. *Ann Neurol.* 1983;13:180–185.
30. Han PK, Arnold R, Bond G, et al. Myoclonus secondary to withdrawal from transdermal fentanyl: case report and literature review. *J Pain Symptom Manage.* 2002;23:66–72.
31. Bruera E, Pereira J. Acute neuropsychiatric findings in a patient receiving fentanyl for cancer pain. *Pain.* 1997;69:199–201.
32. Hagen N, Swanson R. Strychnine-like multifocal myoclonus and seizures in extremely high-dose opioid administration: treatment strategies. *J Pain Symptom Manage.* 1997;14:51–58.
33. Thwaites D, McCann S, Broderick P. Hydromorphone neuroexcitation. *J Palliat Med.* 2004;7:545–550.
34. Hemstapat K, Monteith GR, Smith D, et al. Morphine-3-glucuronide's neuro-excitatory effects are mediated via indirect activation of N-methyl-d-aspartic acid receptors: mechanistic studies in embryonic cultured hippocampal neurones. *Anesth Analg.* 2003;97:494–505.
35. Smith MT. Neuroexcitatory effects of morphine and hydromorphone: evidence implicating the 3-glucuronide metabolites. *Clin Exper Pharmacol Physiol.* 2000;27:524–528.
36. Wright AW, Mather LE, Smith MT. Hydromorphone-3-glucuronide: a more potent neuro-excitant than its structural analogue, morphine-3-glucuronide. *Life Sci.* 2001;69:409–420.
37. Sjogren P, Thunedborg LP, Christrup L, et al. Is development of hyperalgesia, allodynia and myoclonus related to morphine metabolism during long-term administration? Six case histories. *Acta Anaesthesiol Scand.* 1998;42:1070–1075.
38. Lee MA, Leng ME, Tiernan EJ. Retrospective study of the use of hydromorphone in palliative care patients with normal and abnormal urea and creatinine. *Palliat Med.* 2001;15:26–34.
39. Gong QL, Hedner J, Bjorkman R, et al. Morphine-3-glucuronide may functionally antagonize morphine-6-glucuronide induced antinociception and ventilatory depression in the rat. *Pain.* 1992;48:249–255.
40. Nishigaya K, Kaneko M, Nagaseki Y, et al. Palatal myoclonus induced by extirpation of a cerebellar astrocytoma: case report. *J Neurosur.* 1998;88:1107–1110.
41. Ford B, Pullman SL, Khandji A, et al. Spinal myoclonus induced by an intrathecal catheter. *Mov Disord.* 1997;12:1042–1045.
42. Maher J, Choudhri S, Halliday W, et al. AIDS dementia complex with generalized myoclonus. *Mov Disord.* 1997;12:593–597.
43. Werhahn KJ, Brown P, Thompson PD, et al. The clinical features and prognosis of chronic posthypoxic myoclonus. *Mov Disord.* 1997;12:216–220.
44. Wyllie AR, Bayliff CD, Kovacs MJ. Myoclonus due to chlorambucil in two adults with lymphoma. *Ann Pharmacother.* 1997;31:171–174.
45. Pranzatelli MR, Tate ED, Kinsbourne M, et al. Forty-one year follow-up of childhood-onset opsoclonus-myoclonus-ataxia: cerebellar atrophy, multiphasic relapses, and response to IVIG. *Mov Disord.* 2002;17:1387–1390.
46. End of Life/Palliative Education Resource Center. Fast Fact and Concept #58: Neuroexcitatory effects of opioids: treatment. http://www.eperc.mcw.edu/fastFact/ff-58.htm. Accessed September 30, 2009.
47. Golf M, Paice JA, Feulner E, et al. Refractory status epilepticus. *J Palliat Med.* 2004;7:85–88.
48. Mercadante S, Bruera E. Opioid switching: a systematic and critical review. *Cancer Treat Rev.* 2006;32:304–315.
49. Indelicato RA, Portenoy RK. Opioid rotation in the management of refractory cancer pain. *J Clin Oncol.* 2002;20:348–352.
50. Eisele JH Jr, Grigsby EJ, Dea G. Clonazepam treatment of myoclonic contractions associated with high-dose opioids: case report. *Pain.* 1992;49:231–232.
51. Chang BS, Lowenstein DH. Epilepsy. *N Engl J Med.* 2003;349:1257–1266.
52. Stayer C, Tronnier V, Dressnandt J, et al. Intrathecal baclofen therapy for stiff-man syndrome and progressive encephalomyelopathy with rigidity and myoclonus. *Neurology.* 1997;49:1591–1597.
53. Lowenstein DH, Alldredge BK. Status epilepticus. *N Engl J Med.* 1998;338:970–976.
54. Bruera E, Schmitz B, Pither J, et al. The frequency and correlates of dyspnea in patients with advanced cancer. *J Pain Symptom Manage.* 2000;19:357–362.
55. Henoch I, Bergman B, Gustafsson M, Gaston-Johansson F, Danielson E. Dyspnea experience in patients with lung cancer in palliative care. *Eur J Oncol Nurs.* 2008;12:86–96.
56. Reuben DB, Mor V. Dyspnea in terminally ill cancer patients. *Chest.* 1986;89:234–236.
57. Ripamonti C. Management of dyspnea in advanced cancer patients. *Support Care Cancer.* 1999;7:233–243.

58. O'Driscoll M, Corner J, Bailey C. The experience of breathlessness in lung cancer. *Eur J Cancer Care.* 1999;8:37–43.
59. Bausewein C, Booth S, Higginson IJ. Measurement of dyspnoea in the clinical rather than the research setting. *Curr Opin Support Palliat Care.* 2008;2:95–99.
60. Thomas JR, von Gunten CF. Management of dyspnea. *J Support Oncol.* 2003;1:23–34.
61. Dudgeon DJ, Kristjanson L, Sloan JA, et al. Dyspnea in cancer patients: prevalence and associated factors. *J Pain Symptom Manage.* 2001;21:95–102.
62. Mosenthal AC, Lee KF. Management of dyspnea at the end of life: relief for patients and surgeons. *J Am Coll Surg.* 2002;194:377–386.
63. LeGrand SB, Khawam EA, Walsh D, et al. Opioids, respiratory function, and dyspnea. *Am J Hospice Palliat Care.* 2003;20:57–61.
64. Viola R, Kiteley C, Lloyd NS, Mackay JA, Wilson J, Wong RK. Supportive Care Guidelines Group of the Cancer Care Ontario Program in Evidence-Based Care. The management of dyspnea in cancer patients: a systematic review. *Support Care Cancer.* 2008;16:329–337.
65. Qaseem A, Snow V, Shekelle P, et al; for the Clinical Efficacy Assessment Subcommittee of the American College of Physicians. Evidence-based interventions to improve the palliative care of pain, dyspnea, and depression at the end of life: a clinical practice guideline from the American College of Physicians. *Ann Int Med.* 2008;148:141–146.
66. Clemens KE, Quednau I, Klaschik E. Is there a higher risk of respiratory depression in opioid-naive palliative care patients during symptomatic therapy of dyspnea with strong opioids? *J Palliat Med.* 2008;11:204–216.
67. Zebraski SE, Kochenash SM, Raffa RB. Lung opioid receptors: pharmacology and possible target for nebulized morphine in dyspnea. *Life Sci.* 2000;66:2221–2231.
68. Farncombe M, Chater S, Gillin A. The use of nebulized opioids for breathlessness: a chart review. *Palliat Med.* 1994;8:306–312.
69. Foral PA, Malesker MA, Huerta G, et al. Nebulized opioids use in COPD. *Chest.* 2004;125:691–694.
70. Ben-Aharon I, Gafter-Gvili A, Paul M, Leibovici L, Stemmer SM. Interventions for alleviating cancer-related dyspnea: a systematic review. *J Clin Oncol.* 2008;26:2396–2404.
71. Brubacher S, Gobel BH. Use of the pleurx pleural catheter for the management of malignant pleural effusions. *Clin J Oncol Nurs.* 2003;7:35–38.
72. Booth S, Wade R. Oxygen or air for palliation of breathlessness in advanced cancer. *J R Soc Med.* 2003;96:215–218.
73. Uronis HE, Abernethy AP. Oxygen for relief of dyspnea: what is the evidence? *Curr Opin Support Palliat Care.* 2008;2:89–94.
74. Bredin M, Corner J, Krishnasamy M, et al. Multicentre randomised controlled trial of nursing intervention for breathlessness in patients with lung cancer. *BMJ.* 1999;318:901–904.
75. Pan CX, Morrison RS, Ness J, et al. Complementary and alternative medicine in the management of pain, dyspnea, and nausea and vomiting near the end of life: a systematic review. *J Pain Symptom Manage.* 2000;20:374–387.
76. Payne DK, Massie MJ. Anxiety in palliative care. In: Chochinov HM, Breitbart W, eds. *Handbook of Psychiatry in Palliative Medicine.* New York: Oxford University Press; 2000:63–74.
77. Bruera E, Moyano J, Seifert L, et al. The frequency of alcoholism among patients with pain due to terminal cancer. *J Pain Symptom Manage.* 1995;10:599–603.
78. Buckman RA. Breaking bad news: the S-P-I-K-E-S strategy. *Commun Oncol.* 2005;2:138–142.
79. Stephenson NL, Weinrich SP, Tavakoli AS. The effects of foot reflexology on anxiety and pain in patients with breast and lung cancer. *Oncol Nurs Forum.* 2000;27:67–72.
80. Lawlor PG, Gagnon B, Mancini IL, et al. Occurrence, causes, and outcome of delirium in patients with advanced cancer: a prospective study. *Arch Intern Med.* 2000;160:786–794.
81. Lawlor PG, Bruera ED. Delirium in patients with advanced cancer. *Hematol Oncol Clin North Am.* 2002;16:701–714.
82. Fainsinger RL, Waller A, Bercovici M, et al. A multicentre international study of sedation for uncontrolled symptoms in terminally ill patients. *Palliat Med.* 2000;14:257–265.
83. Gaudreau JD, Gagnon P, Roy MA, Harel F, Tremblay A. Opioid medications and longitudinal risk of delirium in hospitalized cancer patients. *Cancer.* 2007;109:2365–2373.
84. Gaudreau JD, Gagnon P, Harel F, Roy MA, Tremblay A. Psychoactive medications and risk of delirium in hospitalized cancer patients. *J Clin Oncol.* 2005;23:6712–6718.
85. Breitbart W, Gibson C, Tremblay A. The delirium experience: delirium recall and delirium-related distress in hospitalized patients with cancer, their spouses/caregivers, and their nurses. *Psychosomatics.* 2002;43:183–194.
86. Breitbart W, Tremblay A, Gibson C. An open trial of olanzapine for the treatment of delirium in hospitalized cancer patients. *Psychosomatics.* 2002;43:175–182.
87. Namba M, Morita T, Imura C, Kiyohara E, Ishikawa S, Hirai K. Terminal delirium: families' experience. *Palliat Med.* 2007;21: 587–594.
88. Callanan M, Kelley P. *Final Gifts: Understanding the Special Awareness, Needs, and Communications of the Dying.* New York: Bantam Books; 1992.
89. Wee B, Coleman P, Hillier R, Holgate S. Death rattle: its impact on staff and volunteers in palliative care. *Palliat Med.* 2008;22:173–176.
90. Morita T, Tsunoda J, Inoue S, et al. Risk factors for death rattle in terminally ill cancer patients: a prospective exploratory study. *Palliat Med.* 2000;14:19–23.
91. Wildiers H, Menten J. Death rattle: prevalence, prevention and treatment. *J Pain Symptom Manage.* 2002;23:310–317.
92. Kass RM, Ellershaw J. Respiratory tract secretions in the dying patient: a retrospective study. *J Pain Symptom Manage.* 2003;26:897–902.
93. Morita T, Tsunoda J, Inoue S, et al. Contributing factors to physical symptoms in terminally-ill cancer patients. *J Pain Symptom Manage.* 1999;18:338–346.
94. Bennett M, Lucas V, Brennan M, et al. Using anti-muscarinic drugs in the management of death rattle: evidence-based guidelines for palliative care. *Palliat Med.* 2002;16:369–374.
95. Spiess JL, Scott SD. Anticholinergic agents for the treatment of "death rattle" in patients with myasthenia gravis. *J Pain Symptom Manage.* 2003;26:684–686.
96. Wee B, Hillier R. Interventions for noisy breathing in patients near to death. *Cochrane Database Syst Rev.* 2008;(1):CD005177.
97. Back IN, Jenkins K, Blower A, et al. A study comparing hyoscine hydrobromide and glycopyrrolate in the treatment of death rattle. *Palliat Med.* 2001;15:329–336.
98. Ersek M. Artificial nutrition and hydration: clinical issues. *J Hospice Palliat Nurs.* 2003;5:221–230.
99. Huang ZB, Ahronheim JC. Nutrition and hydration in terminally ill patients: an update. *Clin Geriatr Med.* 2000;16:313–325.
100. Ferrell BR, Coyle N. The nature of suffering and the goals of nursing. *Oncol Nurs Forum Online.* 2008;35:241–247.
101. Salahi H, Ghahramani N, Malek-Hosseini SA, et al. Religious sanctions regarding cadaveric organ transplantation in Iran. *Transplant Proc.* 1998;30:769–770.
102. Rappaport ZH, Rappaport IT. Brain death and organ transplantation: concepts and principles in Judaism. *Adv Exp Med Biol.* 2004;550:133–137.
103. Hardacre H. Response of Buddhism and Shinto to the issue of brain death and organ transplant. *Camb Q Healthc Ethics.* 1994;3:585–601.
104. Black M, Graham DI. Sudden unexplained death in adults. *Curr Top Pathol.* 2001;95:125–148.
105. Enck RE. Dying from hematological cancers. *Am J Hospice Palliat Care.* 2002;19:79–80.
106. Whedon MB. Revisiting the road not taken: integrating palliative care into oncology nursing. *Clin J Oncol Nurs.* 2002;6:27–33.

107. Ferrell BA. *ELNEC: Promoting Palliative Care in Oncology Nursing.* Duarte, CA: City of Hope; 2004. http://www.aacn.edu/e/nec/index.htm. Accessed March 10, 2009.
108. Rietjens JA, van Zuylen L, van Veluw H, van der Wijk L, van der Heide A, van der Rijt CC. Palliative sedation in a specialized unit for acute palliative care in a cancer hospital: comparing patients dying with and without palliative sedation. *J Pain Symptom Manage.* 2008;36:228–234.
109. Fainsinger R, Miller MJ, Bruera E, et al. Symptom control during the last week of life on a palliative care unit. *J Palliat Care.* 1991;7:5–11.
110. Cowan JD, Palmer TW. Practical guide to palliative sedation. *Curr Oncol Rep.* 2002;4:242–249.
111. Cowan JD, Walsh D. Terminal sedation in palliative medicine: definition and review of the literature. *Support Care Cancer.* 2001;9:403–407.
112. Postovsky S, Moaed B, Krivoy E, Ofir R, Ben Arush MW. Practice of palliative sedation in children with brain tumors and sarcomas at the end of life. *Pediatr Hematol Oncol.* 2007;24:409–415.
113. Lynch M. Palliative sedation. *Clin J Oncol Nurs.* 2003;7:653–657, 667.
114. de Graeff A, Dean M. Palliative sedation therapy in the last weeks of life: a literature review and recommendations for standards. *J Palliat Med.* 2007;10:67–85.
115. Hospice and Palliative Nurses Association. HPNA Position Statement: Palliative Sedation; 2008. http://www.hpna.org. Accessed September 30, 2009.
116. Braun TC, Hagen NA, Clark T. Development of a clinical practice guideline for palliative sedation. *J Palliat Med.* 2003;6:345–350.
117. Hanks-Bell M, Paice J, Krammer L. The use of midazolam hydrochloride continuous infusions in palliative care. *Clin J Oncol Nurs.* 2002;6:367–369.
118. Hocking G, Cousins MJ. Ketamine in chronic pain management: an evidence-based review. *Anesth Analg.* 2003;97:1730–1739.
119. Bell RF, Eccleston C, Kalso E. Ketamine as adjuvant to opioids for cancer pain: a qualitative systematic review. *J Pain Symptom Manage.* 2003;26:867–875.
120. Fitzgibbon EJ, Viola R. Parenteral ketamine as an analgesic adjuvant for severe pain: development and retrospective audit of a protocol for a palliative care unit. *J Palliat Med.* 2005;8:49–57.

# PART IX

# Professional Issues for the Cancer Nurse

CHAPTER

76

Janet S. Fulton, PhD, RN, ACNS-BC

# The Advanced Oncology Practice Nurse

## INTRODUCTION

Our understanding of cancer pathology, diagnosis, treatment, and care has grown steadily since the 1971 creation of the National Cancer Institute. Oncology nursing has evolved as a specialty along with the increasing knowledge and care options generated by a national agenda. Oncology advanced practice nurses (OAPNs)—clinical nurse specialists (CNSs) and nurse practitioners (NPs)—continue to extend and expand oncology nursing practice to meet the opportunities and challenges of cancer care. Oncology advanced practice nurses work in a variety of settings, with all types of cancer patient populations, and across the continuum of care from prevention and screening to palliative and end-of-life care. OAPNs serve as direct care providers, consultants, clinical leaders, care coordinators, educators, and entrepreneurs. This chapter discusses OAPN roles as CNSs and NPs and describes educational preparation, regulation, certification, clinical practice, and future opportunities and challenges for CNSs and NPs in the practice of advanced oncology nursing.

## ADVANCED PRACTICE NURSING DEFINED

The American Nurses Association (ANA) defines an advanced practice nurse as a registered nurse (RN) with advanced specialized clinical knowledge and skills for providing health care.[1] Advanced practice nurses hold graduate degrees, master's or doctorate, and build on the role of generalist RN with increased depth and breadth of knowledge, increased ability to synthesize data, and increased ability to deliver complex interventions. Advanced practice nurses have significant role autonomy.[1] The terms "advanced practice nurse" and "advanced practice registered nurse" often are used interchangeably; however, advanced practice registered nurse (APRN) is used by the ANA to designate an RN license as foundational to the advanced practice role.

Advanced practice registered nurse is an umbrella term covering 4 distinct advanced practice roles: CNS, NP, nurse midwife and nurse anesthetist.[1] A role is defined as a distinct function or set of functions, also called role competencies. The knowledge and skills needed to attain role competencies and perform in a designated functional role are obtained through formal academic preparation. Professional nursing organizations develop functional role competencies to communicate to the public and others the practice expectations of providers in the role. Each of the 4 advanced practice roles has unique role competencies developed by its respective professional organization. Academic curricula are designed to achieve role competencies. Each functional role achieves different outcomes because each role has unique competencies; however, each advanced practice role is built on the generalist education of RN, and all graduate nursing curricula satisfy a core of similar graduate content: theory, research, leadership, ethics, and policy; thus, overlapping knowledge and skill is common among the 4 advanced practice roles.[1] It is in the practice of each role—competencies and outcomes—that distinctions among the roles are most discernible.

Lack of clarity about the differences among the advanced practice functional roles has persisted, especially involving CNS and NP roles. Among the contributions to role confusion is a common practice of labeling professional behaviors such as collaboration and advanced skill sets such as consultation as "subroles." The CNS functional role in particular was initially described as a composite of subroles: care provider, consultant, collaborator, educator, and researcher.[2,3] In 1998, the National Association of Clinical Nurse Specialists (NACNS) conducted a comprehensive study of CNS role functions and abandoned the conceptual view of CNS practice as several subroles, instead creating a practice framework with 3 domains.[4] All advanced practice nurses are expected to demonstrate professional behaviors and skills in direct client care, consultation, collaboration, research, education, and leadership. Defining the CNS functional role by these skills is confusing and is being abandoned in favor of the 3-domains framework, to be discussed later in this chapter.

All APRNs share similar foundational knowledge, skills, and professional behaviors. Application may be different depending on specialty population, care setting, or intervention. For example, a CNS providing education to patients and families about bone marrow transplant procedures is using knowledge and skill in patient education while practicing in a CNS functional role. Likewise, a pediatric NP educating school health nurses about a childhood immunization program is using knowledge and skills in peer education while practicing in an NP functional role. However, the measurable outcomes in each of these examples are different, reflecting the different focus of each role.

Defining the focus of each advanced practice role has been challenging. Nurse midwife and nurse anesthetist roles each serve a distinct target patient population, are associated with a circumscribed area of knowledge, and in practice are not easily confused with each other or with CNS or NP roles. Distinguishing between CNS and NP has been problematic. Moore[5] stated that CNSs are focused on nursing models, while NPs are strongly focused on the medical model. This distinction between models of practice has been used over the years; however, it fails to explain fully differences between CNS and NP practice because each discipline—nursing and medicine—uses many different models to guide practice. Nonetheless, practice differences between CNSs and NPs can be observed. The following excerpts are used to demonstrate differences between CNSs and NPs in practice focus.

. . .

Three staff nurses were in conversation after their shift was over. Mia said, "His wife was angry and said she was going to sue the oncologist and the hospital. I didn't know what to do."

"So what did you do?" asked Frances.

"I called the CNS," replied Mia. "She's great when it comes to dealing with angry families." She added, "I think I'll ask the CNS if we can discuss the topic of managing angry families at our next journal club meeting."

Anna joined the conversation. "Have you seen the policy on reporting medication errors? Are they trying to fire nurses who make even one mistake?"

Mia replied, "I thought so at first too, but then I talked to the CNS. She is going to explain the policy and reporting process to us tomorrow at the change-of-shift report."[6]

. . .

One busy day in the chemotherapy infusion center, Nancy, an oncology staff nurse, listens to Mr. Smith complain about a cough, sore throat, and runny nose. Prior to chemotherapy administration, Nancy asks Katherine, the oncology nurse practitioner, to evaluate Mr. Smith to determine whether they can proceed with chemotherapy. Katherine completes a thorough physical exam and then provides a plan of care to relieve the symptoms.[7,p.1]

Katherine describes the oncology patient population she cares for as patients that have either a stable, chronic condition, an exacerbation of a chronic problem, or an acute problem that needs to be addressed, as well as patients receiving preventative care.[7,p.3]

. . .

In the examples, the CNS and NP role functions are distinguishable from each other and from the staff nurse role functions. The CNS's contributions are direct, as seen in the intervention with a family, and indirect by supporting and guiding bedside care givers. The NP's contributions are direct and focused on individual patients. Does this mean that CNSs don't assess patient symptoms and NPs don't support other care providers? No. But it does illustrate the unique focus of each role. Here is how each author summed up the role.

. . .

CNS practice involves direct care of patients, such as managing new equipment, while supporting nursing staff at the bedside with one-to-one teaching. It involves helping families deal with anger that often results when they learn that disease has progressed. They mentor nurses on managing complex care demands and personal feelings. The CNS role involves leadership for journal clubs and other forums that promote scholarship in practice. The CNS is someone who can interface with the system on behalf of nurses so that errors can be reported in a blameless culture and is someone who can facilitate interdisciplinary collaboration even in the most challenging of circumstances. The CNS is an expert care provider, a resource for nurses, a boundary spanner for system issues.[6,p.2]

. . .

NPs provide comprehensive care independently or in collaboration with a physician or group practice, depending on the individual state's board of nursing regulation. Examining, assessing, diagnosing, prescribing, ordering, and interpreting diagnostic tests, teaching and counseling are just a few examples of the multiple components of an ONP practice. Primary, secondary, and tertiary preventative care, as well as therapeutic care, may be performed. ONPs can practice in acute, primary, or long-term care settings, hospice, home care, or in the community, providing health care for people with or at risk for developing cancer.[7,p.3]

. . .

The CNS role pushes out the boundary of nursing practice, expanding and extending nursing to address newly emerging needs of nursing care and improving nursing interventions for established health concerns. CNSs practice largely in a domain historically viewed as nursing, and there has been little pushback from other disciplines or regulatory bodies. The NP role is also pushing the boundary of nursing practice, expanding and extending nursing into a domain historically identified with physician practice. Figure 76-1 illustrates the roles of CNS and NP expanding and extending the boundaries of nursing. NPs, by pushing the boundary into space historically occupied by physicians in primary care, more often experience considerable pushback over statutory and regulatory authority. Medicine was the first health care profession to be licensed, and licensing language in most if not all states granted physicians practice broad authority for "health." As time has marched on, the practice of primary care has been moving from physicians to NPs. At present, it is more accurate to say that NP

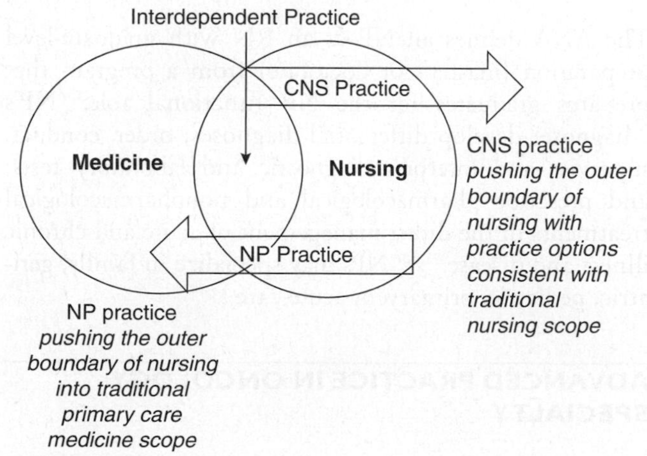


**FIGURE 76-1**

Schema depicting clinical nurse specialist (CNS) and nurse practitioner (NP) practices expanding nursing practice in different directions.

*Source:* Copyright © 2009 Janet S. Fulton. Printed with permission.

practice is focused on the practice of primary care rather than "the medical model." NPs are prepared with primary care knowledge and skills, as the above examples illustrate.

Nursing and medicine, while distinct in legal scope and regulation, in practice also have interdependent practice elements, as shown in Figure 76-1. Interdependent practice is illustrated in the example of a physician prescribing an intravenous fluid, and leaving the decisions for type of intravenous device and placement site, as well as physical placement of the device, to a nurse. Another example in the interdependent domain is the management of a central venous access line, a medical device for which nurses exercise independent judgment in determining care interventions and teaching and coaching patient and family in self-care. Advanced practice nurses and nurse researchers have generated a body of scientific evidence to support practice decisions involving central line management, demonstrating significant contributions to the scientific literature and standards for clinical care in this area of interdependent practice.

### CLINICAL NURSE SPECIALIST DEFINED

The ANA defines a CNS as an RN with graduate-level preparation (master's or doctorate) from a program that prepares graduates for the CNS functional role.[1] CNSs are "clinical experts in evidence-based nursing practice with a specialty area, treating and managing the health concerns of patients and populations."[1,p.15] CNS specialty practice may focus on individuals, populations, settings, type of care, type of problem, or diagnostic system subspecialty.[1,8]

### NURSE PRACTITIONER DEFINED

The ANA defines an NP as an RN with graduate-level preparation (master's or doctorate) from a program that prepares graduates for the NP functional role.[1] NP's "diagnose; develop differential diagnoses; order, conduct, supervise and interpret diagnostic and laboratory tests; and prescribe pharmacological and nonpharmacological treatments in the direct management of acute and chronic illness and disease."[1,p.16] NPs may specialize in family, geriatric, pediatric, primary, or acute care.[1]

## ADVANCED PRACTICE IN ONCOLOGY SPECIALTY

The Oncology Nursing Society (ONS) used the term "oncology advanced practice nurses" to include both CNS and NP functional roles and defined an OAPN as "a licensed registered nurse with a master's or doctoral degree who was educated in a school of nursing that offers either a graduate program in oncology nursing or graduate-level courses with oncology nursing theoretical and clinical components."[9,p.3] The first advanced oncology nursing credential offered by the Oncology Nursing Certification Corporation (ONCC) did not distinguish between a CNS and an NP; both roles took the same examination and earned the same credential, AOCN®. Subsequent role delineation studies conducted by the certification corporation led to development of 2 separate credentials, AOCNS® and AOCNP®.

In 2005, the ONS convened a panel with representation from national nursing organizations with interest in advanced practice registered nursing education, oncology nursing practice, and certification. This panel developed practice competencies for both ONPs and oncology CNSs (OCNSs).[10,11] Developing competencies for advanced oncology nursing practice by functional role was a milestone. Competencies drive curricula. With competencies in hand, educators can design graduate programs, courses, and program activities to help students develop the expected level of competency. Further, certification mechanisms, whether written examination or other mechanism, should validate knowledge consistent with established practice competencies for each role; thus, role competencies support certification.

### ONCOLOGY CLINICAL NURSE SPECIALIST PRACTICE FRAMEWORK

The OCNS practice competencies are organized in a framework composed of 3 domains and constructed by the NACNS to describe CNS practice regardless of specialty.[8] The domains are referred to as spheres of influence and are (1) patient/client, (2) nurses and nursing practice, and (3) organizations/systems. Further, NACNS states that CNS specialty practice should be imbedded in specialty knowledge, specialty standards of practice, and specialty competencies (Figure 76-2). For OCNSs, specialty oncology practice is defined by the OCNS practice competencies,[11] standards of oncology nursing practice,[9] and oncology specialty knowledge.[12]

The patient/client domain, or sphere of influence, is foundational to all OCNS practice.[11] The client may be an individual, family, group, or community.[8] In this client sphere, OCNSs assess, diagnose, and manage illness and risk behaviors. Illness is defined as symptoms and functional problems.[8] OCNSs design, deliver, and evaluate innovative, cost-effective, quality interventions for illness problems and risk behaviors amenable to nursing interventions in the specialty of cancer care.[8,11] By focusing on problems amenable to nursing interventions, OCNSs help achieve and improve nursing-sensitive patient outcomes (NSPOs).[11]

In the nurses and nursing practice domain, OCNSs advance nursing practice by leading, behavior-modeling, coaching, and supporting the practice of staff nurses and nursing personnel in direct care giver roles. OCNSs influence nursing care by updating oncology nursing standards and unit-based norms of practice and by developing and

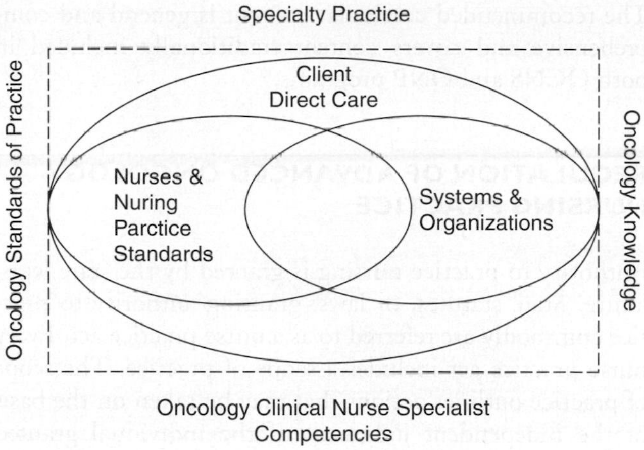


**FIGURE 76-2**

Clinical nurse specialist (CNS) practice conceptualized as 3 interacting domains of competencies and actualized in specialty oncology practice, and grounded in knowledge and practice standards.

*Source:* Copyright © 2009 Janet S. Fulton. Printed with permission.

implementing evidence-based policies, procedures, protocols, best practice models, and guidelines.[11] In the organizations/systems domain, OCNSs articulate the contributions of oncology nursing care and act as advocates for professional nursing in the system. OCNSs provide leadership, knowledge, and skills to remove system barriers and promote oncology nursing best practice for achieving quality, cost-effective outcomes. OCNSs lead nursing and interprofessional groups in designing and implementing innovative patient, family, and community-level care programs that address cancer care across the continuum of care and in multiple settings.[8,11]

Each domain in the framework described by NACNS includes competencies in assessment (identifying and defining problems), diagnosis (outcome identification and planning), and intervention (developing and testing solutions and evaluation of effects).[8] The ONS OCNS practice competencies adapted the NACNS framework to address the specialty care demands of an oncology patient population. The complete list of OCNS competencies is in Appendix A.[11]

## ONCOLOGY NURSE PRACTITIONER PRACTICE FRAMEWORK

The ONP practice framework is consistent with the practice framework described for primary care NP practice.[13] This primary care framework was developed by the National Organization of Nurse Practitioner Faculties in partnership with American Association of Colleges of Nursing.[13] It comprises 7 domains and is focused on the client as an individual and the delivery of care to individuals. Appendix B is a complete list of ONP competencies organized in this 7-domain framework.[10] The domains and a brief description are:

Health promotion, health protection, and disease prevention and treatment (direct health services involving synthesis of theoretical, scientific, and contemporary clinical knowledge for the management of health and illness states for the purpose of health promotion, health protection, and disease prevention and treatment)

Nurse practitioner–patient relationship (includes personal, collegial, and collaborative interactions to enhance effectiveness of patient care and the importance of interpersonal transactions in achievement of therapeutic patient outcomes)

Teaching/coaching function (ability to impart knowledge and associated psychomotor skills to patients, and to interpret and individualize therapies thorough activities of advocacy, modeling and tutoring)

Professional role (advancing the profession and enhancing direct care and management, a commitment to implementing, preserving, and evolving the NP role)

Negotiating health care delivery systems (managing and negotiating health care delivery systems, addresses handling situations to achieve improved health outcomes for patients, communities, and systems through overseeing and directing delivery of clinical services within an integrated system of health care)

Monitoring and assuring quality in health care practice (consultation, collaboration, continuing education, certification, and evaluation, as well as monitoring one's own practice and engaging in peer and systems review)

Caring for diverse populations (providing culturally competent care, delivering care with respect to cultural, and spiritual beliefs and making health care resources available to patients from diverse cultures)

## ONCOLOGY ADVANCED PRACTICE NURSING EDUCATION

Oncology advanced practice nurses—CNSs and NPs—are prepared with a graduate degree in nursing, either master's or doctorate. An advanced practice nurse specializing in oncology is expected to be educated in a designated graduate oncology program or in one that includes graduate-level courses with oncology nursing theoretical and clinical components in the curriculum.[9] OAPNs are educationally prepared to meet the specialized physiological and psychological needs of patients throughout the continuum of care, including cancer prevention and detection, cancer diagnosis and treatment, rehabilitation, survivorship, and end-of-life care.[10,11]

Early in the development of oncology nursing as a specialty, the American Cancer Society (ACS) helped delineate standards for graduate nursing education. The first standards for graduate oncology nursing education were published by the ACS in 1979 and titled *Master's Degree with a Specialty in Cancer Nursing: Curriculum Guide and Role Definition*.[14] The second and third editions, *The Master's Degree with a Specialty in Advanced Practice Oncology Nursing*, were published in 1986 and 1994, as joint efforts between ACS and ONS. In 2003, ONS released the fourth edition, including both competencies for graduates and course content for curricula. A framework for OAPN practice was not discussed; however, the categories of competencies identified were clinical practice, education, consultation, collaboration, systems, professional roles, research and outcomes evaluation, program development, and leadership. The 2003 competencies have been replaced by the newer role-specific competencies for CNSs and NPs published by ONS in 2008 and 2007, respectively, using the contemporary frameworks for CNS and NP practice.

The standards for oncology education at the advanced level address resources needed to deliver content, curriculum guidelines, faculty preparation, the teaching-learning process, and student outcomes. Criteria for achieving each standard are provided and include principles, norms, and performance behaviors. The current standards for oncology advanced practice level education are listed in Table 76-1. Course content includes clinical practice, ethical and legal aspects of oncology practice, education, consultation, collaboration, system, role competency, research and outcomes evaluation, program development, and leadership.[15] The most detailed section is clinical practice, which recommends content in advanced pathophysiology, cancer epidemiology, advanced health assessment, principles of disease treatment, principles of management across the continuum of care, advanced pharmacology and therapeutics, clinical therapeutics, and theories and models for clinical practice. The recommended curricular content is general and comprehensive and covers content traditionally included in both OCNS and ONP programs.[15]

## REGULATION OF ADVANCED ONCOLOGY NURSING PRACTICE

Authority to practice nursing is granted by the state legislature. State statutes, or laws, granting authority to practice commonly are referred to as a nurse practice act. Every nurse practice act includes a scope of practice. The scope of practice outlines actions that may be taken on the basis of the independent judgment of the individual granted authority to practice. Regulations, developed to enact the law, are established by state regulatory boards such as the board of nursing and have the force of law. Regulations are required to be within the scope of the law: regulations may not enlarge or restrict the intent of the statute. Each state has a regulatory board vested with authority by the state legislature to enact the nurse practice act.[16]

### LEVELS OF REGULATION

Regulation occurs at 1 of 4 levels from least to most restrictive. The levels are designation/recognition, registration, certification, and licensure. Designation/recognition, the least restrictive, is recognition of credentials by a state's regulatory board. Registration involves placing names on an official state roster. Neither of these mechanisms involves an inquiry into the competence of the individual. Certification involves title protection; only those persons who meet requirements are permitted to use a title such as CNS or NP. To obtain state-issued certification, applicants meet predetermined requirements. Licensure is the most restrictive form of regulation. Through licensure the government

**TABLE 76-1**

**Oncology Advanced Practice Education Standards**

| | |
|---|---|
| Standard I: Faculty | The faculty is prepared academically and clinically to teach masters-level oncology nursing |
| Standard II: Resources | Clinical and educational resources are adequate to achieve graduate program objectives related to oncology nursing |
| Standard III: Curriculum | Specialized knowledge, skills, and attitudes required for the implementation of oncology nursing at the advanced practice level are included in the curriculum |
| Standard IV: Teaching–Learning Process | Teaching–learning theories are applied to the development, implementation, and evaluation of learning experiences related to oncology nursing practice |
| Standard V: Student Outcomes | Graduate-level nursing education program graduates assume responsibilities for oncology nursing commensurate with their educational preparation and experience |

*Source:* Data from Oncology Nursing Society.[12]

grants exclusive permission to practice. Licensure includes a unique scope of practice. Licensure also allows the grantor, such as the board of nursing, to take disciplinary action for violation of laws or rules.[17] Regulation through licensure is a mechanism for assuring the public that a licensed individual has achieved minimal competence to practice.[1]

## THE RELATIONSHIP BETWEEN LEGAL AND PROFESSIONAL REGULATION

Like all professions, nursing is autonomous and therefore responsible for ensuring that its members act in the public interest. Society entrusts self-regulation to professions in ensuring public access to needed services. Nursing regulates itself by defining practice, providing research to support and advance practice, establishing a system for education, establishing systems for the delivery of nursing services, and providing quality monitoring mechanisms such as a code of ethics, standards of practices, structures for peer review, and a system for credentialing.[1]

Professions establish standards; standards define expectations of the professional role that all members must practice. Standards are authoritative statements describing responsibilities and reflecting values and priorities. Standards are written in measurable terms and define accountability to the public. Standards of practice apply to the care provided to clients, whereas standards for practice describe behaviors in the professional role.[1] Standards of practice include assessment, diagnosis, outcome identification, planning, implementation, and evaluation. Several themes span nursing practice, including providing culturally and ethnically appropriate care, maintaining a safe environment, educating patients about healthy behaviors, ensuring continuity of care, and communicating effectively.[1] Standards of practice describe competent care. Standards may also differentiate between minimum levels of competency and excellence in practice. Standards for practice include behaviors and activities related to education, collegiality, ethics, research, professional development, evaluation of care, resource utilization, and other professional behaviors appropriate for the level of provider, client, and care setting.[1] Standards developed by professional organizations provide the legal basis for judging care competency and professional behavior in a court of law. Specialty practice standards are developed by specialty nursing organizations. The ONS, as the professional nursing society for the specialty of nursing cancer care, has established standards for advanced practice oncology nursing.[9]

Governmental oversight is imposed on professions that could cause harm to the public if practiced by a person who does not have the abilities (practice competencies) to deliver services competently. Legal definitions of nursing practice need to encompass the profession's definition, be general enough to allow for the dynamic nature of an evolving practice, and be specific enough to differentiate nursing from other statutorily regulated health professions.[1] The professional nursing community guides content of a nurse practice act and shepherds it through the legislature. Rules and regulations evolve from the law and serve as guidelines for issuing licensure and other authority to practice to protect the public safety.

## AUTHORITY TO PRACTICE AS AN ADVANCED PRACTICE NURSE

Legal recognition to practice as an OAPN varies by state. All states require an advanced practice nurse to hold an unrestricted license to practice as an RN. All states recognize NPs; 35 states recognize CNSs.[18] Some states recognize CNSs and NPs through title protection; some through licensure. States may issue a second license, a certificate or other written document based on review of a candidate's credentials. States may simply state the necessary credentials and not issue a document to the individual or even keep a roster of advanced practice nurses in the state.

To address licensure inconsistencies among states, the Nurse Licensure Compact was created. The compact is a mutual recognition model of nurse licensure allowing nurses to have a single license and to practice in other states subject to each state's practice laws and regulations.[19] At present, 23 of 50 states are members of the RN compact.[20] The APRN Compact, also a mutual recognition model, was created in 2000 to promote access to advanced practice nursing care within states and across state lines. To participate in the APRN Compact, a state must first be a member state in the RN Compact. Only 3 states have passed laws authorizing the states to join the APRN Compact.[21] The compact as a legal mechanism for resolving licensing inconsistencies among states has been criticized and is not endorsed by the ANA.[22,23]

The advanced practice community in the US is engaged in developing universal recommendations for state-level regulation for advanced practice nurses. This collaborative effort involving professional nursing organizations, professional certification bodies, educators, and regulators has arrived at several foundational pillars important for all for advanced practice nurses. The initiative has been labeled LACE to signify the interwoven nature of *licensure* (authority to practice as an advanced practice nurse), *accreditation* (recognition of academic programs meeting educational standards in preparing advanced practice nurses), *certification* (professional recognition of an individual's practice competencies), and *education* (curricular standards and criteria for academic-degree-granting programs).[24] The initiative has been endorsed by many professional organizations representing advanced practice nurses.

Whether remaining states adopt the RN or APRN Compact or whether states adopt the LACE initiative recommendations remains to be seen. Adoption of either initiative will proceed state by state following each state's procedures for changing rules and regulations governing nursing practice. OAPNs should monitor their state board for opportunities to become involved in any changes in advanced practice regulation.

## Certification

Professional certification is defined by the American Board of Nursing Specialties (ABNS) as the formal recognition of specialized knowledge, skills, and experience demonstrated by achievement of standards identified by a nursing specialty to promote optimal health outcomes.[25] Professional certification is voluntary and awarded by a nongovernmental agency; it is not a state-issued license to practice. Professional nursing certification assures the public that a nurse has met eligibility criteria to earn a specific credential and has earned recognition by demonstrating minimum competency in the specialty. Specialty standards change over time to reflect state of knowledge for practice in the specialty; thus, the public can be assured that nurses obtaining and maintaining specialty certification are current in specialty practice.

Many different specialty certifications are available for nurses at both the basic specialty and advanced specialty levels. In 1991, the ABNS was created to address criticism about variations in nursing certification programs across different organizations. The ABNS is analogous to the American Board of Medical Specialties and other professional boards that certify individuals to practice in circumscribed specialty areas of practice. ABNS maintains standards to which certifying nursing organizations are expected to adhere, and it accredits specialty nursing certification programs.[5,25]

The ONCC is a professional organization that offers certification. It has several types of certification at both the basic and advanced levels of practice in the specialty of oncology nursing, summarized in Table 76-2. All ONCC certification options meet ABNS standards for nursing specialty certification. In addition, ONCC is accredited by the National Commission for Certifying Agencies (NCCA), demonstrating compliance with the NCCA's *Standards for the Accreditation of Certification Programs,* which were the first standards for professional certification programs developed by the industry.

In the 1990s, many states began changing regulations to recognize advanced practice nursing roles. States began asking for validation of advanced role-specific competency and accepted professional certification at the advanced level as evidence of practice competency. The original advanced oncology nursing credential was the AOCN® and was available to both CNSs and NPs. Subsequent role delineation study identified role competency differences between

**TABLE 76-2**

**Oncology Nursing Certification Options Available From the Oncology Nursing Certification Corporation (http://www.oncc.org)**

| Credential | Description |
|---|---|
| Oncology Certified Nurse: OCN® | Validates a nurse's knowledge for competent practice at the basic level within the specialty of oncology nursing |
| Certified Pediatric Oncology Nurse: CPON® | Validates a nurse's knowledge for competent practice at the basic level within the specialty of pediatric oncology nursing |
| Certified Pediatric Hematology/Oncology Nurse: CPHON *Coming in 2010* | This new certification will validate basic level knowledge within the specialty of both pediatric oncology and hematology |
| Advanced Certified Oncology Nurse: AOCN® *Certification Renewal Only* | Validates a nurse's knowledge for competent practice at the advanced level within the specialty of oncology certified nursing |
| Advanced Oncology Certified Nurse Practitioner: AOCNP® | Validates a nurse's knowledge for competent practice at the advanced level in the NP role within the specialty of oncology nursing |
| Advanced Oncology Clinical Nurse Specialist: AOCNS® | Validates a nurse's knowledge for competent practice at the advanced level in the CNS role within the specialty of oncology nursing |
| Certified Breast Care Nurse: CBCN | Validates a nurse's knowledge to practice competently in breast care<br>Breast care practice may include nursing practice along the entire continuum of breast care, from prevention to detection, diagnosis and treatment, survivorship, and end of life care |

OCNS and ONP practice, and the certification validation process was split into 2 role-specific certifications. At present, OCNS and ONP are distinct certifications. The current eligibility criteria for the advanced OCNS and ONP credentials are as follows:

*Eligibility criteria for AOCNS® certification*

I. Current, active, unrestricted RN license at the time of application and examination
II. A master's or higher degree in nursing from an accredited institution
III. A minimum of 500 hours of supervised clinical practice in an advanced practice role in oncology nursing. These hours may be obtained within the graduate educational program or following graduation from the program.

*Eligibility criteria for AOCNP® certification*

I. Current, active, unrestricted RN license at the time of application and examination
II. A master's or higher degree in nursing from an accredited institution
III. Successful completion of an accredited NP program
IV. A minimum of 500 hours of supervised clinical practice as an ONP. These hours may be obtained within the NP program or following graduation from the program.

The NP eligibility criteria stipulate that a candidate must have graduated from an accredited NP program, whereas the CNS eligibility criteria do not stipulate graduation from a program that prepares CNSs. Both pros and cons are associated with not requiring CNS eligibility requirements to stipulate graduation from a CNS master's program. Pro arguments include being able to award the credential to CNS graduates from older programs that may not have been designated CNS, and being able to include CNSs successfully practicing in the role for many years regardless of graduate preparation. Con arguments include awarding the credential to persons not adequately prepared for the role, so future role delineation studies will be influenced by those not prepared in the role competencies, distorting the OCNS role. The ONCC is aware of the pro and con arguments and carefully monitors candidates for CNS certification (Cindy Miller Murphy, personal communication, May 2008).

## Prescriptive authority

Prescriptive authority for advanced oncology practice nurses is regulated at the state level but also involves the Drug Enforcement Administration (DEA), where prescriptive authority includes controlled substances. The scope of prescriptive authority varies from state to state. Some states grant total independence for CNSs and NPs, including in regard to controlled substances; others grant dependent authority, meaning that a CNS or NP must prescribe under the supervision of a licensed physician. Some states offer prescriptive authority to NPs only; some grant prescriptive authority to CNSs only in the specialty of mental health, and some states offer all CNSs prescriptive authority along with an opt-out choice. Most states specify educational requirements for advanced practice nurses seeking prescriptive authority. The level of detail varies greatly in rules or regulations about educational specifications.

All states have some scope of prescriptive authority for NPs;[26] not all states offer prescriptive authority to CNSs (Jo Ellen Rust, personal communication, March 2009). The Pearson Report, published yearly, provides detailed state-by-state information about prescriptive authority for NPs.[26] No such database yet exists for CNSs. Many states and certifying bodies require documentation of pharmacology continuing education for license or certification renewal.

Where optional prescriptive authority is available, many CNSs elect to opt out due to the expense of education and insurance requirements when they have no intent or need to prescribe pharmaceuticals. However, CNSs do need and seek authority to prescribe durable medical equipment separate from authority to prescribe pharmaceutical agents. Authority to prescribe durable medical equipment is consistent with the CNS practice focus on interventions to manage functional problems.

In states where advanced practice nurses prescribe controlled substances, DEA registration numbers are required. The DEA has established a midlevel practitioner registration category under which advanced practice nurses, physician assistants, and others are given DEA registration numbers. These numbers begin with the letter M to allow responsible parties in the controlled-substance distribution chain to contact state officials to verify authority to prescribe. DEA registration allows a wide variety of acts, including purchasing, storing, administering, dispensing, and prescribing controlled substances.[5] An OAPN may engage in only those activities authorized by the state that issues the authority to prescribe controlled substances. Many states restrict controlled-substance prescriptive authority for advanced practice nurses to schedules III-V, which can be a barrier to practice and interfere with patients receiving adequate pain control with schedule II narcotics.

## Credentialing and privileging

Credentialing and privileging are hospital-organization-specific activities to ensure that professionals in the organization are competent to practice and are practicing within the legal scope of the professional license.[27] Credentialing and privileging are related but separate activities; both are mandated by the Joint Commission.[28] Credentialing is the process of assessing and validating the qualification of a licensed independent provider of patient care services on the basis of an evaluation of the provider's licensure, education, experience, current competence, and ability to perform requested privileges.[29] The purpose is to ensure that the provider's credentials are consistent with the position's responsibilities and that applicants are prepared to provide the services implied by the credential competently and safely. Collecting and verifying providers' credentials is usually designated to a department such as human resources. Privileging is a process by which the governing body of a health care organization grants authorization to providers for specific patient care services based on qualifications identified in the credentialing process.[29] Privileging involves developing a list of services to be provided and matching services with credentials. Services included on the privileging list must be consistent with the state's scope of practice for the role, and privileges must specify collaborative agreements or other restrictions consistent with state regulations for the advanced practice role. The applicant's ability to perform requested privileges should be included in the evaluation, including a review of physical or health-related problems that could affect practice, and the National Practitioner Data Bank is queried for any reports against the applicant.[29] Peer recommendations are required and should address an applicant's clinical knowledge and abilities, interpersonal skills, and professionalism. On the basis of the information provided, the governing board of the agency decides to grant, limit, or deny privileges.

Organizations should have written policies and procedures for reviewing applicants, and these should reflect a peer review process by nurses. In addition to peer review, the chief nursing officer should review the application. Regardless of the specific procedures, credentialing and privileging for nurses should be reflected in an organization's written policies and procedures for reviewing credentials and assessing competency for privileging.[29] Magnet Accreditation standards require documentation of the chief nursing officer's participation in the credentialing and privileging process for nurses, which is seen as a measure of nursing's autonomy within the organization.[30]

## ECONOMICS AND ADVANCED ONCOLOGY PRACTICE

In a growing climate of cost consciousness in health care, OAPNs must become savvy in both reimbursement for services provided and cost-avoidance related to better resource utilization and improved management of expensive outlier cases. NPs typically provide direct patient care that can be linked to billable services, whereas CNSs typically provide services that reflect cost-avoidance. Both OAPN roles can impact the bottom line.

### REIMBURSEMENT FOR SERVICES

Reimbursement for direct patient care is provided through federal and state programs such as Medicare and Medicaid or through private insurers, including health maintenance organizations and preferred provider organizations. Medicare is a federal insurance program for the elderly and disabled and is administered by Centers for Medicare and Medicaid Services. Medicare has 2 parts: part A, or hospital insurance, covers inpatient hospital services and some home health care; part B, known as supplemental medical insurance, covers services of physicians and other providers including advanced practice nurses (CNSs and NPs).

Medicaid is also a federal program administered by the states to provide health care to low-income individuals and families, the elderly, and the disabled. Each state establishes its own Medicaid rules within federal guidelines. Medicaid also reimburses advanced practice nurses. The rules for reimbursement specific to advanced practice nurses are complicated, vary from payer to payer, and are set according to state and federal laws.

For inpatient care, OAPNs are paid directly by the hospital organization, with salary costs considered part of the operational expenses of the organization. Hospital organizations subsidize the nonreimbursable activities of their employees through reimbursement for services by providers able to bill directly.[31] Under the Balanced Budget Act of 1997, CNSs and NPs working in ambulatory care settings such as clinics or private practices can bill Medicaid directly. To bill directly a CNS or NP must be an RN, be authorized to perform services in the state, be certified by the American Nurses Credentialing Center or comparable certifying agency, and hold a master's degree in nursing.[32] The Balanced Budget Act of 1997 specifies that direct payment to CNSs and NPs should be equal to 80% of the lesser of either the actual charge or 85% of the fee schedule amount for the same service if provided by a physician. For services provided in a hospital outpatient department, payment is made to that department both for the professional services and for the facility component of the hospital outpatient department.

Requirements, if any, for physician collaboration related to reimbursement are defined by state regulations. In states without collaboration regulations, CNSs and NPs need to indicate a clinical collaborative relationship for dealing with patient care problems outside their scope. In these states, CNSs and NPs bill directly for services as well as for ancillary services provided to a patient by staff working under the advanced practice nurse supervision. To bill Medicare directly, an OAPN must obtain a federal provider identification number (PIN). To obtain a PIN, contact a local Medicare carrier or Social Security office. To obtain a Medicaid PIN, contact the state Medicaid office within the state health department.

In situations where a CNS or NP is employed by a physician, the physician can bill 100% of the Medicare fee for services provided by an OAPN, called "incident-to services," provided the physician is present (in the office or suite) where services are provided, the patient has been previously seen by a physician and has a medical plan of care, the patient does not present with a new problem, services are consistent with those commonly provided in the physician's office, and the physician's presence is documented. Medicare fraud can be charged if all incident-to-billing requirements are not met.

Private insurers do not have standard policies or procedures for advanced practice nurse billing and reimbursement. Each insurance company can establish its own policies, and many do not issue rules regarding advanced practice nurse credentialing, collaboration, billing, or reimbursement. A CNS or NP interested in obtaining reimbursement from a private insurer needs to investigate the insurer's requirements.

## COST-AVOIDANCE

Cost-avoidance is defined as fiscal savings related to direct or indirect activities that avoid or reduce expenses associated with patient care services while maintaining or improving clinical outcomes. Savings are identified in the hospital organization's budget as costs that were not incurred due to change(s) in service(s), including type of service, level of provider, shift in care setting, new programs, or other changes. Cost-avoidance initiatives begin by identifying a potential or actual recurring problem in a group of patients. Following problem analysis, an alternative strategy is implemented. Cost-effective alternatives may include an innovative care strategy, a targeted education program for patients or staff, or work redesign for more effective use of resources. Cost-avoidance has resulted from clinical programs that improve diabetic patient self-care management,[33] support heart failure patients in the home,[34] screen high-risk patients for methicillin-resistant *Staphylococcus aureus*,[35] implement bundled interventions for ventilated patients,[36] and manage wounds via telehealth directed interventions.[37] Inpatient cardiac care costs were reduced by shifting care of less acutely ill patients from the coronary care unit to the telemetry unit.[38]

Emphasizing prevention, early intervention, and programs for self-care management for patients can reduce costs and improve outcomes by eliminating or minimizing costs associated with symptoms and treatment side effects. Emphasizing early identification of problems may result in increased but less costly outpatient visits, and early interventions can reduce both severity and cost of complications. Increasing demands on oncology patients to provide complex care in the home have not kept up with programs to support patients and families to develop the knowledge and skills necessary for self-care. Patients and families may lack resources to manage in the home. Community resources may not be available, and when they are available, patients may lack ability to access the community resources. Patients lacking ability to care for themselves in the home adequately and appropriately are admitted to expensive inpatient care when problems are exacerbated. For example, inability to manage nausea with pharmacological and nonpharmacological interventions can lead to costly inpatient treatment of dehydration. OAPNs can work together to develop patient and family self-care programs, to monitor self-care, and to reduce the severity and cost of complications.

OAPN's should be in the habit of questioning the cost of patient services and programs. Capturing revenue data generated from reimbursement may be easier than capturing cost-avoidance. However, OAPNs should consider cost implications of all the dimensions of practice and work with fiscal staff in hospital organizations to capture cost-avoidance revenue data.

## IMPLEMENTING ADVANCED ONCOLOGY NURSING PRACTICE: WORKING COLLABORATIVELY

After a decade or more of debate about the similarities and differences between CNSs and NPs, the distinction remains blurred. The language used to describe the roles often overlaps, and areas of distinction are poorly articulated. Good models and case examples of CNSs and NPs working collaboratively and highlighting the strengths of each role for the improvement of patient outcomes are lacking. For discussion purposes, let's go back to the CNS and NP examples discussed at the beginning of the chapter and create a scenario of collaboration. The setting is *All City Hospital*, a large public hospital with 2 inpatient oncology units, a medical unit, a surgical unit, and a large oncology outpatient service with multiple specialty clinics for diagnostic, treatment, and follow-up services. Katherine, an ONP, is a clinic employee assigned to work with the breast cancer service. Angie and Peggy are the staff nurses in the breast clinic. Barbara is the OCNS assigned to outpatient services, and she works closely with Robert, an OCNS assigned to the inpatient units. Mia, Frances, Anna, and Lorraine are staff nurses working on the medical oncology unit.

On a typical day in the breast clinic, staff nurses Angie and Peggy will complete a brief focused assessment and help prepare patients for physical examination. NP Katherine sees patients with stable disease and those with acute problems. Angie asks Peggy whether she has noticed an increase in the number referrals to Katherine to evaluate patients with elevated temperatures. Peggy agrees and discusses with Katherine. Katherine begins a medical record review of patients seen for problems related to fever and finds a moderate increase over the same 6 month time period in the previous 2 years.

NP Katherine calls CNS Barbara and they discuss the audit finding. Barbara and Katherine recall an administrative decision that consolidated the All City Hospital breast clinic services with *Neighborhood Clinic*, resulting in an increase in older, low-income patients with lower literacy levels. They conclude that the hospital's teaching materials are not appropriate for older patients with low literacy levels. The solution is to create new, more targeted materials including print and audiovisual options. CNS Barbara agrees to organize a work group to update education materials. Outpatient staff nurse Peggy agrees to serve on the work group. Patient education materials are used by inpatient and outpatient units, so Barbara contacts CNS Robert, who suggests that inpatient staff nurses Mia and Lorraine be invited to participate. Barbara asks staff nurse Peggy to chair the work group; she declines, citing lack of experience. To support Peggy's professional development, Barbara agrees to co-chair with Peggy. Barbara provides direction and support for Peggy, gradually giving her more independence as her confidence grows. The work group reviews the literature, research, and other evidence on best practice in educational materials for low-literacy older adults. New teaching materials are drafted; NP Katherine and staff nurse Angie from the outpatient clinic and CNS Robert and staff nurses Amy and Frances from the inpatient units evaluate the new materials. Feedback is reviewed and changes are made. Staff nurses Mia and Peggy agree to lead a pilot evaluation of the new materials. Robert guides staff nurse Mia in conducting the pilot evaluation in the inpatient setting. Barbara coaches staff nurse Peggy through the hospital procedure for approval of new education materials, including preparing a budget and obtaining necessary fiscal approvals. The new education materials are completed and implemented in both inpatient and outpatient areas. After 6 months, NP Katherine again conducts a chart audit and finds increasing numbers of patient visits and calls to the breast clinic for fever-related complications. NP Katherine and CNS Barbara conduct a cost analysis. NP Katherine determines the fiscal outcomes of her services seeing increased patients in clinic: revenue generated. CNS Barbara calculates the cost savings for patients treated early in clinic and therefore not admitted for expensive inpatient care: cost-avoidance. As a result of innovative targeted teaching materials and early outpatient intervention, billable revenue was increased and costly inpatient admissions were avoided. And, largely because of what she learned working on the task group, staff nurse Peggy was promoted to Level II in the nursing governance clinical ladder program.

This simplistic fictional scenario is offered as an example of OCNSs and ONPs working together to improve patient outcomes. It was necessary to create an example of OCNS–ONP collaboration because none could be found in the literature. Models of collaboration are needed to demonstrate the synergistic impact of OAPNs working together for improved clinical and fiscal outcomes.

## CHALLENGES FOR THE FUTURE

The ONS defined an advanced oncology practice nurse as "a licensed registered nurse with a master's or doctoral degree who was educated in a school of nursing that offers either a graduate program in oncology nursing or graduate-level courses with oncology nursing theoretical and clinical components."[9,p.3] While the ONS recommends OCNSs and ONPs be prepared in oncology-specific curricula, oncology-specific graduate programs are limited. The first graduate-level oncology-specific program was opened in 1968 at the University of Pittsburgh.[39] The number of graduate programs in oncology continued to grow through the first half of the 1990s; since then there has been a steady decline.[39] A 1993 assessment identified 42 oncology graduate programs; a follow-up 1999 survey found 31 programs.[40,41] Currently, more than 330 master's degree programs are accredited by the Commission on Collegiate Nursing Education or by the National League for Nursing Accrediting Commission.[42] Searching Peterson's guide to nursing programs found only 6 oncology-focused graduate programs for either CNSs or NPs. The American Association of Colleges of Nursing enrollment data for advanced practice programs, reported by type of certification the graduate is eligible to obtain, lists 16 programs preparing graduates for OCNS certification.[43] Under NP programs, ONP is not listed, suggesting no programs are preparing graduates for ONP certification.[43] Two combined CNS/NP programs report preparing graduates for either OCNS certification or adult NP certification, and 1 program reported preparing students for either the OCNS certification or the acute care NP.[43]

While the total number of programs is unclear, it is clear that the overall number of advanced oncology program options has greatly decreased over the past 15 years. Oncology NP practice emanates predominantly from a primary care focus and is concentrated in direct care of individual patients, and role implementation varies widely by type of setting and type of cancer or cancer treatment. OCNS practice, in addition to focusing on care of individuals, includes supporting nurses and nursing staff to provide evidence-based nursing care and remove system barriers to achieving best practice. CNS role implementation also varies widely. While variation in practice is to be expected, the lack of oncology graduate programs has resulted in CNSs and NPs being prepared without oncology specialty knowledge and leaving acquisition of advanced oncology knowledge to continuing education and on-the-job training. Lacking a standard for oncology education, it is difficult to know whether practice variations represent adaptation of a core set of knowledge and skills in a unique setting or gaps in practice competency.

Ten years ago Mooney[39] noted that the emerging faculty shortage was threatening the growth of oncology nursing as a specialty. The faculty shortage is now critical, and little has been done to safeguard oncology education programs.

No comprehensive report of the number of graduate-level oncology programs has been conducted in recent years, and no systematic assessment of current graduate curricula could be found in the literature. With so few oncology graduate programs, CNSs and NPs are prepared in broad, non-oncology content areas, such as adult or pediatric, creating a new generation of CNSs and NPs who are not academically prepared in oncology content. This situation not only threatens oncology advanced practice; it suppresses the pipeline for future oncology faculty and oncology researchers.

The ONCC offers an OCNS and ONP exam. Periodic role delineation studies capture the actual practice of these roles, which helps ensure that the certification examination measures appropriate role knowledge and practice skills. With fewer CNSs and NPs prepared in oncology programs, future role delineation studies will be capturing an actual practice that may not be comprehensive or may not sufficiently reflect a preferred standard of advanced oncology knowledge or skill. Basing future certification examinations on the actual practice of persons underprepared to practice in oncology specialty may become self-defeating.

The release of the role-specific oncology practice competencies provides opportunity to update and reconfigure the standards for advanced oncology education. One recommendation is to split the educational standards into core knowledge and role application. Core knowledge is baseline knowledge for all OAPNs, including cancer epidemiology, pathophysiology, physical assessment, epidemiology, and cancer treatment modalities. Application knowledge is role specific and related to the functional practice competencies associated with each role. Such a strategy would conserve educational resources while promoting adequate preparation in both oncology advanced practice roles.

Multiple challenges exist in the regulatory arena. While LACE is intended to clarify the path to advanced practice recognition by states, it is far from finalized. Under the LACE initiative, advanced practice nurses must earn a graduate degree (master's or doctorate), and the degree program curriculum must prepare graduates for 1 of the 4 functional advanced practice roles. CNSs have always been educated with a minimum of a master's degree; however, many NPs were prepared with in postbaccalaureate certificate programs and a few of these programs remain. A final conversion of these certificate programs will need to be completed.

Professional certification has long been emphasized for NP programs, even prior to moving NP education to the master's level. For CNSs, certification programs were not emphasized, and until recently certification was a credential of excellence in practice, not validation of entry-level competencies as it is presently. Under LACE, certification eligibility criteria will stipulate that candidates show proof of graduation from a program that prepared them in a functional role consistent with the certification credential; thus, NPs will need to demonstrate proof of graduation from an NP program, and CNSs will likewise show proof of graduation from a CNS program. A considerable number of CNSs graduated from master's programs not specifically labeled CNS. The CNS track was often the clinical option in a graduate curriculum that also offered education or supervision/administration options. Graduates of these older CNS programs may have difficulty where certification eligibility requirements stipulate "CNS" be identified on the academic transcript. CNSs prepared in programs not labeled CNS should explore certification options and seek certification soon.

The LACE model specifies that specialty population be linked to functional role preparation. Specialty populations considered for regulatory purposes in the model include family (across the lifespan), adult and gerontology, neonatal, pediatrics, women's/gender-related, and mental health.[24] Under the LACE model, CNSs and NPs would be regulated to practice in a role and specialty population. For example, an adult CNS would be restricted by regulation to providing services to adults only, and likewise a pediatric NP would be restricted to pediatric patient services only. Specialties such as oncology would not be considered at the regulatory level. An adult CNS specializing in oncology would provide oncology services to adults only. If the adult CNS decided to specialize in diabetes, he or she would be able to switch specialty with no regulatory barriers; however, if the adult CNS decided to provide services to pediatric patients, regulation would demand he or she complete an educational program as a pediatric CNS.

Under the LACE model, oncology is not a specialty population for regulatory purposes. Graduate programs will prepare CNSs and NPs for specialty populations such as adult and pediatric; after obtaining a degree and certification in the role and population, CNSs and NPs may elect to practice in the specialty of oncology nursing. Considering the lack of oncology-focused graduate programs, the LACE model presents additional challenges to the adequate education and development of OAPNs.

## CONCLUSION

OCNSs and ONPs practice in a variety of settings across the continuum of care, providing unique services to persons with cancer and their families. Nationally recognized definitions for OCNSs and ONPs are in place. Under the leadership of the ONS, CNS and NP oncology specialty practice competencies were developed to communicate practice expectations to individuals and the public and to guide education and practice. Separate OCNS and ONP certification options are available to document practice competencies. OAPNs are an important part of the health care team, making valuable contributions to improved patient outcomes.

The future holds several challenges for OAPNs. The oncology nursing community will need to consider carefully the implications of the current educational and regulatory initiatives. The LACE model does not recognize oncology as a population for regulatory purposes; thus, CNSs and NPs will be first prepared in a program that focuses on family, adult, neonatal, pediatrics, women's/gender-related, and mental health. Oncology CNS and NP certifications will become a second certification after an initial role and population certification. Advanced oncology academic preparation will no longer be a "first-line" option, creating greater concerns about the adequacy and completeness of OAPNs' oncology knowledge and skill. In addition, the faculty shortage is decreasing the pool of those educationally and clinically prepared to teach advanced oncology courses. Innovative options are needed to promote oncology education and advanced oncology practice competency.

Research is needed to better understand the implications of changes on OAPN practice and to point the way to the future. Research exploring CNS and NP practice outcomes is needed. Differences between CNS and NP practice roles should be identified through research, and research-supported models of collaborative CNS and NP practice should be designed. Up-to-date information is needed about graduate-level educational programs for advanced oncology practice. The linkage among practice competencies, certification examination items, and education standards for CNSs and NPs needs to be explored.

OCNSs and ONPs provide much-needed services to cancer patients and their families. With all the changes and challenges, OAPNs working together as partners will continue to advance the specialty of oncology nursing.

## REFERENCES


1. American Nurses Association. *Nursing Scope and Standards of Practice.* Washington, DC: American Nurses Association; 2004.
2. American Nurses Association. *The Role of the Clinical Nurse Specialist.* Kansas City, MO: American Nurses Association; 1986.
3. Sparacino PSA, Cooper DM. The role components. In: Sparacino PSA, Cooper DM, Minarik PA, eds. *The Clinical Nurse Specialist: Implementation and Impact.* Norwalk, CT: Appleton & Lange; 1990:11–40.
4. Baldwin KM, Lyon BL, Clark AP, Fulton J, Dayhoff N. Developing clinical nurse specialist competencies. *Clin Nurse Spec.* 2007;21:297–303.
5. Moore S. The oncology advanced practice nurse. In: Yarbro CH, Frogge MH, Goodman M, eds. *Cancer Nursing: Principles and Practice.* Sudbury, MA: Jones and Bartlett; 2005:1759–1776.
6. Fulton JS. So, do I really want to make a difference? In: Fulton JS, Wickline MM, eds. *So, You Want to Be an Oncology Clinical Nurse Specialist?* Pittsburgh, PA: Oncology Nursing Society; 2008:1–13.
7. Biedrzycki BA. So, what does an oncology nurse practitioner do? In: Vogel WH, ed. *So, You Want to Be an Oncology Nurse Practitioner?* Pittsburgh, PA: Oncology Nursing Society; 2007:1–9.
8. National Association of Clinical Nurse Specialists. *Statement on Clinical Nurse Specialist Practice and Education.* 2nd ed. Harrisburg, PA: National Association of Clinical Nurse Specialists; 2004.
9. Oncology Nursing Society. *Statement on the Scope and Standards of Advanced Practice Nursing in Oncology.* 3rd ed. Pittsburgh, PA: Oncology Nursing Society; 2003a.
10. Oncology Nursing Society. *Oncology Nurse Practitioner Competencies.* Pittsburgh, PA: Oncology Nursing Society; 2007. https://ons.org/media/ons/docs/publications/npcompentencies.pdf. Accessed December 30, 2009.
11. Oncology Nursing Society. *Oncology Clinical Nurse Specialist Competencies.* Pittsburgh, PA: Oncology Nursing Society; 2008. https://ons.org/media/ons/docs/publications/cnscomps.pdf Accessed December 30, 2009.
12. Oncology Nursing Society. *Standards of Oncology Nursing Education: Generalist and Advanced Practice Levels.* 3rd ed. Pittsburgh, PA: Oncology Nursing Society; 2003.
13. National Organization of Nurse Practitioner Faculties. *Nurse Practitioner Primary Care Competencies in Specialty Areas: Adult, Family, Gerontological, Pediatric, and Women's Health.* Washington, DC: National Organization of Nurse Practitioner Faculties; 2002.
14. Jacobs LA, Scarpa R, Lester J, Smith J. Oncology nursing as a specialty: The education, scope and standards for advanced practice nursing in oncology. *Oncol Nurs Forum.* 2004;31:507–509.
15. Oncology Nursing Society. *The Master's Degree with a Specialty in Advanced Practice Oncology Nursing.* 4th ed. Pittsburgh, PA: Oncology Nursing Society; 2003b.
16. Lyon BL. What to look for when analyzing clinical nurse specialist statutes and regulations. *Clin Nurse Spec.* 2002a;16:33–34.
17. Lyon BL. The regulation of clinical nurse specialist practice: issues and current developments. *Clin Nurse Spec.* 2002b;16:239–241.
18. Goudreau KA. What clinical nurse specialists need to know about the consensus model for advanced practice registered nurse regulation. *Clin Nurse Spec.* 2009;23:50–51.
19. National Council of State Boards of Nursing. https://www.ncsbn.org/nlc.htm. Accessed February 25, 2010.
20. National Council of State Boards of Nursing. *Participating States in the NLC.* https://www.ncsbn.org/158.htm. Accessed February 25, 2010.
21. National Council of State Boards of Nursing. *APRN Compact.* https://www.ncsbn.org/917.htm. Accessed February 25, 2010.
22. Gaffney T. The regulatory dilemma surrounding interstate practice. *Online J Issues Nurs.* 1999. http://www.nursingworld.org/MainMenuCategories/ANAMarketplace/ANAPeriodicals/OJIN/TableofContents/Volume41999/No1May1999/RegulatoryDilemma.aspx. Accessed February 25, 2010.
23. Glazer G. Legislative column: "Legislative and policy issues related to interstate practice: board position statement." *Online J Issues Nurs.* 1999. http://www.nursingworld.org/MainMenuCategories/ANAMarketplace/ANAPeriodicals/OJIN/Columns/Legislative/BoardPositionStatement.aspx. Accessed February 25, 2010.
24. Consensus Model for APRN Regulation: Licensure, Accreditation, Certification and Education. 2008. https://www.ncsbn.org/7_23_08_Consensue_APRN_Final.pdf. Accessed February 25, 2010.
25. American Board of Nurse Specialties. 2009. http://www.nursingcertification.org/. Accessed February 25, 2010.
26. Pearson LJ. The Pearson report. *Am J Nurse Pract.* 2009;13:8–82.
27. Madic KS, Hravanak M, McCartney S. Credentialing for nurse practitioners: an update. *AACN Clin Issues: Adv Pract Acute Crit Care.* 2005;16:16–22.
28. Joint Commission. *Comprehensive Accreditation Manual.* Oakbrook Terrace, IL: Joint Commission; 2009.
29. Sendelbach S. Navigating the privileging and credentialing process. In: Duffy M, Dresser S, Fulton J, eds. *Clinical Nurse Specialist Toolkit: A Guide for the New Clinical Nurse Specialist.* New York, NY: Springer; 2009:159–162.
30. American Nurses Credentialing Center. *The Magnet Recognition Program.* Silver Spring, MD: American Nurses Credentialing Center; 2005.
31. O'Brien JM. How nurse practitioners obtained provider status: lessons for pharmacists. *Am J Health Syst Pharm.* 2003;60:2301–2307.

32. Miller M, Snyder M, Lindeke LL. Nurse practitioners: current status and future challenges. *Clin Excell Nurse Pract*. 2005;9:162–169.
33. Wilhide C, Hayes, JR, Farah, JR. Impact of behavioral adherence on clinical improvement and functional status in a diabetes disease management program. *Dis Manag*. 2008;11:169–175.
34. Anderson JH. Impact of using nursing presence in a community heart failure program. *J Cardiovasc Nurs*. 2007;22:89–94.
35. Clancy M, Graepler A, Douglas I, Johnson J, Price CS. Active screening in high-risk units is an effective and cost-avoidant method to reduce the rate of methicillin-resistant *Staphylococcus aureus* infection in the hospital. *Infect Control Hosp Epidemiol*. 2007;27:1009–1017.
36. Hampton D, Norton J. A model for qualifying quality initiatives in intensive care. *J Nurs Care Qual*. 2006;21:70–77.
37. Specht JKP, Wakefield B, Flanagan, J. Evaluating the cost of one telehealth application connecting an acute and long-term care setting. *J Gerontol Nurs*. 2001;27:34–39.
38. Servais SH. Nursing resource applications through outcome based nursing practice. *Nurs Econ*. 1991;9:171–179.
39. Mooney KH. Oncology nursing education: peril and opportunities in the new century. *Semin Oncol Nurs*. 2000;16:25–34.
40. Brown JK, Hinds P. Assessing master's programs in oncology nursing. *Oncol Nurs Forum*. 1993; 20:1425–1433.
41. Survey of graduate programs in oncology nursing. *Oncol Nurs Forum*. 1999;26:1373–1380.
42. Dracup K. The nursing school adviser: master's programs. http://www.petersons.com/nursing/articles/masters.asp?sponsor=1. Accessed February 25, 2010.
43. Fang D, Tracy C, Bednash GD. *2008–2009 Enrollment and Graduations in Baccalaureate and Graduate Programs in Nursing*. Washington, DC: American Association of Colleges of Nursing; 2009.

## APPENDIX A: ONCOLOGY CLINICAL NURSE SPECIALIST PRACTICE COMPETENCIES

### I. PATIENT/CLIENT DOMAIN/SPHERE OF INFLUENCE

In this sphere, which is foundational to the other 2 spheres, the OCNS uses knowledge and skills to assess, diagnose, and manage illness (symptoms and functional problems) and risk behaviors in patients with a past, current, or potential diagnosis of cancer. To improve NSPOs for patients with cancer, the OCNS demonstrates knowledge, skills, and behavior in the design, delivery, and evaluation of innovative, cost-effective, quality interventions for illness problems and risk behaviors amenable to nursing interventions. By focusing on problems amenable to nursing interventions, the OCNS achieves improved NSPOs.

### ASSESSMENT OF HEALTH STATUS

I. Obtains a relevant health history for patients with a past, current, or potential diagnosis of cancer, which includes a review of systems and the evaluation of the presence or absence of manifestations of cancer and cancer treatment.
II. Uses evidence-based practice guidelines and assessment tools for evaluating patients with a past, current, or potential diagnosis of cancer.
III. Performs a relevant cancer risk assessment for
   a. The community at large
   b. At-risk populations
   c. Patient with a past, current, or potential diagnosis of cancer.
IV. Obtains comprehensive information related to risk, diagnosis, or past experience with cancer.
V. Assesses patients' personal and family history of cancer and the need for genetic counseling and/or testing.
VI. Performs a physical assessment of patients with cancer that includes an evaluation of manifestations related to cancer and cancer treatment.
VII. Assesses the impact of physical comorbidities on cancer symptoms and response to treatment.
VIII. Assesses for common signs and symptoms indicating the presence of cancer, disease progression, or recurrence.
IX. Assesses for signs and symptoms of oncological emergencies in high-risk patients.
X. Conducts a pharmacological assessment, including over-the-counter medications, prescription drugs, nutritional supplements, and other complementary, alternative, and integrative therapies, to identify any potential interactions with cancer therapeutics.
XI. Assesses the risks of polypharmacy to the patient's health and treatment plan.
XII. Performs a comprehensive assessment of functional status and ability to perform routine activities of daily living.
XIII. Assesses for presence of psychological comorbidities, past and present coping skills, and the psychosocial impact of the cancer experience, including emotional distress and grief.
XIV. Assesses for risk of sexual or fertility-related problems or issues in patients with a past, current, or potential diagnosis of cancer, including the impact on relationships.
XV. Assesses developmental, cultural, ethnic, racial, spiritual, gender, and socioeconomic variations in symptom presentation or illness experience of patients with cancer.
XVI. Assesses educational needs related to a past, current, or potential diagnosis of cancer and cancer treatment.
XVII. Assesses the roles, tasks, and stressors of individuals, support systems, and caregivers and their ability to manage the cancer experience.
XVIII. Assesses the need for changes in equipment or other products based on evidence, clinical outcomes, and cost effectiveness to improve outcomes for patients with cancer.
XIX. Identifies the need for new or modified methods or tools to better assess patients with a past, current, or potential diagnosis of cancer.
XX. Analyzes data from target groups and populations to design new programs to improve patient outcomes.
XXI. Documents assessment findings to facilitate coordination of care among health care providers.

### DIAGNOSIS OF HEALTH STATUS AND PLAN OF CARE

I. Develops differential diagnoses of cancer-related problems and risk factors for patients, with a focus on manifestations of cancer and cancer treatment.
II. Diagnoses physical and psychosocial problems based on knowledge of symptoms, functional status, risk factors, or developmental processes.
III. Plans for the management of cancer and cancer treatment-related symptoms.
IV. Integrates interventions into the plan of care to prevent, remediate, modify, or resolve expected and unexpected outcomes in patients with cancer.
V. Integrates pharmacological and nonpharmacological treatment modalities into the plan of care.
VI. Contributes to a comprehensive plan of care as patients transition from active treatment to long-term survivorship or end-of-life care.

VII. Integrates long-term evaluation and management of late effects of treatment into the plan of care.
VIII. Provides information about clinical trials and research studies for which patients may be eligible.
IX. Incorporates appropriate patient care technology into the plan of care for patients with cancer.
X. Documents the cancer-specific plan of care and intended patient outcomes to facilitate communication among health care team members.
XI. Contributes to the resolution of anticipated ethical conflicts that may arise in the care of patients with a past, current, or potential diagnosis of cancer.

## INTERVENTIONS

I. Facilitates an interprofessional and evidence-based approach to the management of patients with a past, current, or potential diagnosis of cancer across the continuum of care.
II. Uses evidence-based interventions for patients that target cancer-related risk reduction.
III. Refers patients to other health care providers for further evaluation as appropriate.
IV. Facilitates transitions between health care settings to provide continuity of care.
V. Integrates nursing interventions into an interprofessional plan of care to improve NSPOs for patients with cancer.
VI. Uses system and community resources that improve the delivery of care for patients with a past, current, or potential diagnosis of cancer.
VII. Provides anticipatory guidance and education to assist patients in coping with the diagnosis of cancer and its potential or expected outcomes.
VIII. Addresses comorbid conditions when implementing cancer treatment.
IX. Initiates appropriate interventions for patients experiencing an oncological emergency.
X. Uses an ethical framework in all aspects of patient care to assist patients with cancer on issues related to the care and management of symptoms, advance directives, and palliative and end-of-life care.
XI. Facilitates palliative and end-of-life care for patients with cancer in collaboration with patients and other members of the interprofessional health care team.

## EVALUATION

I. Identifies methods to evaluate outcomes of nursing interventions for patients with a past, current, or potential diagnosis of cancer.
II. Evaluates clinical effectiveness, patient responses, efficiency, cost effectiveness, and ethical considerations of interventions for patients with a past, current, or potential diagnosis of cancer.
III. Monitors progress toward targeted outcomes for patients with a past, current, or potential diagnosis of cancer and facilitates modifications as needed.
IV. Evaluates the overall effect of interventions on patients, based on synthesis of data.
V. Documents patient care outcomes in a reportable manner.
VI. Evaluates the use of new or modified methods or tools to assess patients with a past, current, or potential diagnosis of cancer.
VII. Evaluates the use of innovative or modified interventions for the care of patients with a past, current, or potential diagnosis of cancer.

## NURSE AND NURSING PRACTICE SPHERE OF INFLUENCE

In this sphere, the OCNSs advance nursing practice and improve NSPOs by updating and improving norms and standards of oncology nursing practice. The OCNS provides leadership, knowledge, skills, and behavior modeling that influence nursing practice. The OCNS also influences the development of evidence-based policies, procedures, and protocols, as well as best practice models and guidelines.

## ASSESSMENT

I. Identifies methods to assess outcome trends related to oncology nursing practice within and across units of care and practice settings.
II. Assesses outcome trends related to oncology nursing practice within and across units of care and practice settings.
III. Assesses knowledge, skills, and practice competencies of nurses and nursing personnel to advance the practice of oncology nursing, using tools and instruments when available.
IV. Identifies needed changes in processes of care, therapeutic approaches, equipment, or other products based on evidence to improve oncology nursing practice.
V. Assesses the influence of nursing practice on desirable and undesirable outcomes for patients with a past, current, or potential diagnosis of cancer.
VI. Analyzes barriers and facilitators to quality nursing practice and positive NSPOs for patients with a past, current, or potential diagnosis of cancer, within or across settings.
VII. Assesses collaboration and communication of the interprofessional cancer care team.
VIII. Analyzes role conflicts or confusion and seeks information that leads to resolution.

## DIAGNOSIS, OUTCOMES IDENTIFICATION, AND PLANNING

I. Monitors oncology nursing practice to identify desirable and undesirable outcomes.
II. Determines aspects of oncology nursing practice that require change, improvement, or maintenance based on available evidence.
III. Plans strategies to overcome barriers and facilitate changes in oncology nursing practice, including the implementation of new programs, products, and devices.
IV. Analyzes the clinical, human resource, and fiscal implications of implementing programs, products, and devices into oncology nursing practice.
V. Plans educational programs that target the needs of staff to improve oncology nursing practice and outcomes for patients with a past, current, or potential diagnosis of cancer based on available evidence.

## INTERVENTION

I. Develops new, evidence-based solutions to existing cancer-related care issues.
II. Incorporates evidence-based information into oncology nursing to improve NSPOs.
III. Mentors nurses to critique and apply evidence to oncology nursing practice.
IV. Implements innovative interventions that improve NSPOs.
V. Develops oncology-related policies, procedures, standards, and guidelines based on available evidence.
VI. Implements interventions that improve oncology nursing care related to complex patient care problems that are consistent with system resources and evidence.
VII. Implements strategies to overcome barriers to implementation of new programs, products, and devices that affect oncology nursing practice.
VIII. Implements educational programs, based on assessed needs of staff, to improve oncology nursing practice and patient outcomes.
IX. Mentors nursing staff to develop and implement innovative, cost-effective programs of care for patients with a past, current, or potential diagnosis of cancer.
X. Mentors nurses to acquire new skills, maintain skills, and develop nursing careers in oncology.
XI. Creates a nursing practice environment that stimulates self-learning and reflective practice.

## EVALUATION

I. Evaluates methods used to implement improvements in the nursing care of patients with a past, current, or potential diagnosis of cancer.
II. Evaluates the effects of changes in oncology nursing practice on patient and staff outcomes.
III. Documents outcomes of changes in oncology nursing practice in an accessible, reportable manner.
IV. Disseminates outcomes of changes in oncology nursing practice to diverse internal and external stakeholders.

## PROFESSIONAL ROLE

I. Promotes life-long learning and evidence-based practice, by self and others, to improve the care of patients with a past, current, or potential diagnosis of cancer.
II. Participates in community and professional organizations that influence cancer care and support the role of the OCNS.
III. Demonstrates effective communication skills with patients, nurses, and interprofessional groups.
IV. Contributes to the oncology knowledge base of the health care community through activities such as community outreach, involvement in professional organizations, presentations, publications, and participation in research.
V. Maintains professional competence and credentials appropriate to the CNS role and the oncology specialty.
VI. Disseminates knowledge required to care for patients with a past, current, or potential diagnosis of cancer to other health care workers and caregivers through peer education, staff development, mentoring, and preceptor experiences.
VII. Translates research findings and other evidence for other health care professionals to improve the care of patients with a past, current, or potential diagnosis of cancer.
VIII. Participates in clinical and nursing research to promote positive outcomes for patients with cancer.

## ORGANIZATION/SYSTEMS SPHERE

In this sphere, the OCNS influences health care organizations and systems by articulating the contributions of oncology nursing care and acts as an advocate for professional nursing. To improve NSPOs for patients with cancer, the OCNS provides leadership, knowledge, and skills to influence changes in systems that promote oncology nursing best-practice for the improvement of quality, cost-effective outcomes. The OCNS leads nursing and interprofessional groups to implement innovative patient care programs that address patient needs across the full continuum of care.

## ASSESSMENT OF HEALTH STATUS

I. Performs system assessments to identify organizational structures and functions that affect oncology nursing practice and outcomes.
II. Assesses system variables, such as professional climate, organizational culture, finances, regulatory requirements, and external demands that influence oncology nursing practice and outcomes.
III. Analyzes facilitators and barriers to oncology nursing practice within and external to the organization/system.
IV. Analyzes system-wide variations in oncology nursing practice.

## DIAGNOSIS, OUTCOMES IDENTIFICATION, AND PLANNING

I. Analyzes barriers and facilitators to achieving desired outcomes of cancer care programs.
II. Diagnoses variations in organizational culture, such as values, beliefs, or attitudes, that can affect oncology outcomes.
III. Analyzes the impact of legislative and regulatory policies on oncology nursing practice.

## INTERVENTION

I. Develops system-level policies that can be generalized across different oncology units and settings, populations, or specialty services.
II. Leads nursing and interprofessional groups that address issues related to cancer care.
III. Implements evidence-based patient care programs that address issues affecting patients across the continuum of cancer care.
IV. Participates in the development of interprofessional standards of practice and evidence-based guidelines for oncology care.
V. Collaborates with stakeholders to foster the adoption of oncology practice innovations.
VI. Implements strategies to reduce system-level barriers to changes in oncology nursing practices and cancer-related programs of care.
VII. Implements processes to sustain evidence-based changes in oncology nursing practice, cancer programs of care, and clinical innovation.
VIII. Participates in legislative and regulatory initiatives to advance the health care of the public across the cancer continuum.
IX. Promotes the use of information systems to improve cancer care across settings.

## EVALUATION

I. Evaluates system-level clinical and fiscal outcomes of oncology products, devices, and patient care processes.
II. Uses organizational structure and processes to provide feedback regarding effectiveness of oncology nursing practice.
III. Evaluates the effectiveness of interprofessional communication in meeting identified outcomes of cancer care programs.
IV. Evaluates organizational policies for the ability to support and improve outcomes of cancer care programs.
V. Uses the results of system-level evaluations to make process or structural changes, including policy, procedure, or protocols affecting oncology nursing practice across settings.
VI. Evaluates the impact of oncology nursing interventions on human and fiscal resources.
VII. Documents the evaluation of the impact of OCNS practice on the organization in a measurable and reportable manner.
VIII. Disseminates to stakeholders the impact of OCNS practice on system-wide and nursing practice outcomes.

## APPENDIX B: ONCOLOGY NURSE PRACTITIONER COMPETENCIES

### HEALTH PROMOTION, HEALTH PROTECTION, DISEASE PREVENTION, AND TREATMENT

#### Assessment of Health Status

These competencies describe the role of the ONP in assessing all aspects of the patient's health status, including for purposes of health promotion, health protection, and disease prevention. The ONP uses evidence-based clinical practice guidelines when available to guide screening activities, identify health promotion needs, and provide anticipatory guidance and counseling, addressing environmental, lifestyle, and developmental issues.

I. Obtains and documents a comprehensive health history for patients with a past, current, or potential diagnosis of cancer.

II. Uses evidence-based practice guidelines and assessment tools for evaluating patients with a past, current, or potential diagnosis of cancer.

III. Performs a relevant cancer risk assessment for:
- general populations
- at-risk populations
- newly diagnosed patients with cancer
- cancer survivors.

IV. Obtains comprehensive information related to risk, diagnosis, and past experience with cancer.

V. Performs and documents complete, system-focused, symptom-specific physical examinations for patients.

VI. Performs a physical assessment of patients with cancer that includes a comprehensive review of systems and evaluation of manifestations and toxicities related to cancer and its treatment.

VII. Assesses actual or potential late effects of cancer and its treatment (eg, second malignant neoplasms, cardiomyopathy, pulmonary dysfunction) in cancer survivors.

VIII. Assesses the impact of physical comorbidities on cancer symptoms and response to treatment.

IX. Identifies the relationship between normal physiology and specific system alterations produced by cancer and cancer treatment.

X. Assesses symptoms commonly seen in patients with cancer (eg, fatigue, pain, nausea, vomiting).

XI. Assesses for common signs and symptoms related to disease progression or recurrence.

XII. Assesses patients who are at high risk for signs and symptoms of oncological emergencies.

XIII. Performs a comprehensive assessment of nutritional status in patients with a current or past diagnosis of cancer.

XIV. Conducts a pharmacological assessment, including over-the-counter medications, prescription drugs, nutritional supplements, and other complementary, alternative, and integrative therapies, to identify and correct any potential interactions with cancer therapeutics.

XV. Assesses the risks of polypharmacy to the patient's health.

XVI. Performs a comprehensive assessment of functional status and the impact on activities of daily living, including but not limited to the following domains:
- psychological
- role
- social
- cognitive
- physical.

XVII. Assesses for the presence of psychological comorbidities (eg, anxiety/depression, substance use), past and present coping skills, and the psychosocial impact of the cancer experience.

XVIII. Assesses concerns and issues related to sexual function, sexual well-being, and fertility of patients with a past, current, or potential diagnosis of cancer, including the impact on relationships.

XIX. Assesses developmental, ethnic, spiritual, racial, socioeconomic, and gender variations in symptom presentation or illness experience of patients with cancer.

XX. Assesses the roles, tasks, and stressors of individuals, families, and caregivers and their ability to manage the illness experience (eg, resources, support services, equipment, transportation, child care, anxiety, depression).

XXI. Assesses patients' ability to navigate the complex health care system and the barriers to continuity, coordination, and communication among multiple care providers.

### DIAGNOSIS OF HEALTH STATUS

The ONP is engaged in the diagnosis of health status. This diagnostic process includes critical thinking, differential diagnosis, and the integration and interpretation of various forms of data:

I. Orders screening, diagnostic, and surveillance examinations or tests.

II. Demonstrates knowledge of technical skills needed to perform diagnostic procedures to confirm or rule out health problems (eg, bone marrow aspirations, spinal taps, skin biopsies).

III. Performs an initial interpretation of laboratory studies and diagnostic tests, including but not limited to chest x ray or electrocardiogram.

IV. Reviews diagnostic and laboratory study results to confirm or rule out health problems.
V. Demonstrates knowledge of atypical presentations of cancer.
VI. Demonstrates understanding of the principles of cancer staging.
VII. Collaborates with relevant health care team members and gathers additional information for further differential diagnosis and problem identification.
VIII. Diagnoses common episodic, acute, and chronic physical problems in patients with a past or current diagnosis of cancer.
IX. Diagnoses acute and chronic conditions that may result in rapid physiological deterioration or life-threatening instability, including oncological emergencies.
X. Identifies the need for screening for common late effects in cancer survivors (eg, infertility, cardiomyopathy).
XI. Reformulates diagnoses based on new or additional assessment data.
XII. Determines the impact of comorbidities on the prognosis and treatment of patients with cancer.
XIII. Diagnoses acute and chronic psychological complications (eg, anxiety, depression, substance abuse) and their influence on the patient's psychological state.
XIV. Documents diagnoses and problems to facilitate identification and initiation of the treatment plan and outcome evaluation.
XV. Demonstrates knowledge of diagnostic and procedural coding documentation requirements.

## PLAN OF CARE AND IMPLEMENTATION OF TREATMENT

The objectives of planning and implementing therapeutic interventions are to return the patient to a stable state and to optimize the patient's health. These competencies describe the ONP's role in managing the patient, minimizing physical and psychological complications, and maximizing the patient's health potential.

### Plan of care

I. Collaborates with the multidisciplinary team, patient, family, and caregivers to formulate a comprehensive plan of care for patients with cancer, including appropriate health education, health promotion and health maintenance, rehabilitation, and palliative care.
II. Plans for the management of common cancer-related episodic, acute, and chronic problems.
III. Plans for the management of cancer and cancer treatment-related symptoms (eg, pain, nausea/vomiting, neuropathies, infection).
IV. Integrates evidence-based, nonpharmacological treatment modalities into the plan of care.
V. Plans therapeutic interventions to restore or maintain an optimal level of functioning.
VI. Establishes a comprehensive plan of care as patients transition from active treatment to cancer survivorship or end-of-life care.
VII. Plans for long-term evaluation and management of late effects of treatment.
VIII. Coordinates care with attention to resource availability, accessibility, quality, and cost-effectiveness.
IX. Coordinates care within a context of functional status, cultural considerations, spiritual needs, family or caregiver needs, and ethical principles.
X. Demonstrates awareness of appropriate clinical trials and research studies for which patients may be eligible and assists in recruiting patients as appropriate.
XI. Incorporates patients' developmental learning needs and preferences in planning patient and family teaching.
XII. Documents the plan of care and intended outcomes to ensure that interventions will be implemented as planned.

### Implementation

I. Uses evidence-based strategies in the management of patients across the continuum of care (ie, prevention, early detection, diagnosis, treatment, rehabilitation, survivorship, and end-of-life care).
II. Monitors and manages the effects of cancer and cancer treatment.
III. Provides anticipatory guidance to assist patients and families in coping with the illness and its potential or expected outcomes.
IV. Considers comorbid conditions when implementing cancer treatment.
V. Treats episodic, acute, and chronic health problems.
VI. Initiates appropriate treatments and referrals for patients experiencing an oncological emergency (eg, disseminated intravascular coagulation, superior vena cava syndrome, spinal cord compression).
VII. Implements interventions to support patients who have a rapidly deteriorating physiological condition, including the application of basic and advanced life support and other invasive interventions or procedures to regain physiological stability.
VIII. Educates and supports patients in self-care strategies.
IX. Refers patients to other health care providers for further evaluation as appropriate.
X. Refers patients and families to appropriate support services.
XI. Facilitates transitions between health care settings to provide continuity of care.

XII. Uses an ethical framework in all aspects of patient care to assist patients, families, and other. caregivers on issues related to the care and management of symptoms, advance directives, and palliative and end-of-life care.
XIII. Coordinates palliative and end-of-life care in collaboration with patients, families, caregivers, and other members of the multidisciplinary health care team.
XIV. Evaluates the effectiveness of interventions and revises the plan of care as appropriate.
XV. Determines the impact of cancer treatment and its side effects and long-term effects on patient outcomes.

## NURSE PRACTITIONER–PATIENT RELATIONSHIP

Competencies in this area demonstrate the personal, collaborative, and therapeutic approach, which enhances the effectiveness of the ONP's patient care. These competencies speak to the critical importance of interpersonal transactions as they relate to patient outcomes.

I. Establishes caring relationships with patients, families, and other caregivers to facilitate coping with sensitive issues.
II. Facilitates patient and family decision making regarding complex treatment, symptom management, and end-of-life care.
III. Assists patients with cancer and their families in preparing for and coping with grief and bereavement.

## TEACHING/COACHING FUNCTION

These competencies describe the ONP's teaching function, which is to impart knowledge and skills for self-care to the patient. The coaching function involves the skills of advocacy, support, and reinforcement.

I. Develops interventions with patients and families that are consistent with patients' physiological and psychological needs and values.
II. Uses age-appropriate learning principles in patient, family, and caregiver education.
III. Educates patients, families, caregivers, and the community about cancer risk, screening, and early detection.
IV. Uses evidence-based information to help patients with cancer and their families to make informed decisions.
V. Provides information to patients and families to facilitate adherence to cancer treatment, supportive care, and follow-up.
VI. Educates patients and families about expected and potential adverse effects and costs (as appropriate) of prescribed pharmacological and nonpharmacological treatments and interventions.
VII. Educates cancer survivors regarding their risk for long-term effects of cancer and its treatment (eg, second malignant neoplasm, skin cancer, cardiopulmonary complications).
VIII. Facilitates patient decision making by explaining treatment alternatives and potential outcomes, including the option of discontinuing active cancer treatment while optimizing supportive care.
IX. Educates patients and families on the risks and benefits of alternative, integrative, and complementary therapies, including possible adverse interactions with standard and investigational cancer therapies.

## PROFESSIONAL ROLE

These competencies describe the varied role of the ONP, specifically related to advancing the profession and enhancing direct care and management. The ONP demonstrates a commitment to the implementation, preservation, and evolution of the ONP role.

I. Builds collaborative, interdisciplinary relationships to provide optimal care to patients with cancer.
II. Promotes life-long learning and evidence-based practice while continually acquiring knowledge and skills needed to improve patient care.
III. Recognizes the importance of participation in community and professional organizations that influence cancer care and support the role of the ONP.
IV. Contributes to the knowledge base of the health care community through community outreach, involvement in professional organizations, presentations, publications, and participation in research.
V. Maintains professional competence and credentials appropriate to the role and specialty.
VI. Disseminates knowledge required to care for patients with cancer to other health care workers and caregivers through peer education, staff development, mentoring, and preceptor experiences.
VII. Translates research findings and other evidence for other health care professionals to improve the care of patients with cancer.
VIII. Promotes the role of the ONP and its significance in improving patient outcomes to the health care team, third-party payers, regulators, legislators, and the public.
IX. Participates in clinical and nursing research to promote positive outcomes for patients with cancer and their caregivers.
X. Advocates within the health care system and policy arenas for the health needs of patients with cancer.

## NEGOTIATING HEALTH CARE DELIVERY SYSTEMS

These competencies describe the ONP's role in achieving improved health outcomes for patients, communities, and systems by overseeing and directing the delivery of clinical services within an integrated system of health care.

I. Assists patients with cancer and their families and caregivers to negotiate health care delivery systems.
II. Creates and enhances positive, health-promoting environments that maintain a climate of dignity and privacy for patients with cancer.
III. Identifies aspects of the health care system that create barriers to comprehensive cancer care and long-term care for cancer survivors.
IV. Incorporates knowledge of payment and reimbursement systems and financial resources into the plan of care for patients with cancer.
V. Documents clinical services provided in accordance with reimbursement regulations and guidelines.
VI. Adheres to institutional, state, and federal laws and regulations related to the care of patients with cancer.
VII. Refers patients to appropriate local, state, and national patient-support resources.

## MONITORING AND ENSURING THE QUALITY OF HEALTH CARE PRACTICE

These competencies describe the ONP's role in ensuring quality of care through consultation, collaboration, continuing education, certification, and evaluation. The monitoring function of the role also is addressed relative to the monitoring of one's own practice, as well as by engaging in interdisciplinary peer and systems review.

I. Applies evidence-based practice using quality improvement strategies in providing care to patients with cancer.
II. Promotes an environment for ethical decision making and patient advocacy for patients with cancer.
III. Participates in the design and implementation of evidence-based protocols and processes of care to improve outcomes for patients with cancer (eg, decreasing medication errors, reducing infection rate, pain management).
IV. Uses internal resources (eg, ethics committee, risk management, legal department) and external resources (eg, professional organizations, government officials, community agencies) to facilitate the resolution of moral and ethical issues.
V. Identifies research questions based on recurrent problems related to the care of patients with a potential, actual, or previous diagnosis of cancer.
VI. Advocates for patient/family rights to make decisions regarding durable power of attorney, advance directives, and related issues.

## CARING FOR DIVERSE POPULATIONS

These competencies describe the ONP's role in providing competent care to diverse populations with respect to culture, race, ethnicity, religion, spirituality, gender, or lifestyle.

I. Recognizes the diversity among patients, families, caregivers, and the community that influences patient decisions and outcomes of care.
II. Recognizes the impact of provider and institutional cultural biases on cancer care.
III. Recognizes the potential limitations of assessment methods and tools in a diverse population.
IV. Incorporates resources that meet the diverse needs of patients into the planning and delivery of care.
V. Educates professional and lay caregivers to provide care with attention to individual diversity for patients with cancer.

Reprinted with permission, ONS.[10]

CHAPTER

77

*Lisa C. Schulmeister, MN, APRN-BC, OCN®, FAAN*

# Legal Issues

## INTRODUCTION

A major goal of oncology nursing practice is the safe delivery of patient care. Many mechanisms exist to help ensure that this goal will be met, such as federal laws, state licensing requirements for professional nursing practice, technological advancements (eg, safer medical equipment), institutional procedures (eg, use of health information technology), and personal practices (eg, double-checking medications). However, because health care is a complex system of people and processes, risk is inherent in its delivery.

Oncology nurses practice in high-risk environments. Patients with cancer are often weak, fatigued, and mobility-impaired, thus increasing their risk of injury from falls. Most cancer treatments, such as chemotherapy, biotherapy, and radiation therapy, are based on individual rather than standardized dosing, and the potential for dosing or delivery errors is high. Some patients receive chemotherapy or monoclonal antibody treatments that can cause anaphylaxis or infusion-related reactions, so these patients are at risk for life-threatening adverse events. In addition, vesicant chemotherapy agents have the potential to cause severe tissue necrosis if they extravasate. Patient harm, and even death, can potentially result from medical errors and events. Legal action can also ensue.

Litigation involving oncology nurses may be prompted by patient falls, medication errors, hypersensitivity and infusion-related reactions, and vesicant chemotherapy extravasations, as well as other situations, such as failure to monitor a patient, privacy and confidentiality violations, inappropriate triage or management of patient-reported complaints, and undertreatment of pain. Oncology nurses play a key role in preventing these errors and adverse events.

## PATIENT SAFETY

Patient safety received increased attention following the publication of the Institute of Medicine's (IOM) report *To Err Is Human: Building a Safer Health System* in 2000, which closely examined the problem of medical errors and estimated that they cause 44,000 to 98,000 deaths per year in the US.[1] Although this report prompted a significant increase in the number of patient safety initiatives and publications,[2] some safety experts assert that patient safety remains an elusive goal.[3] As recently as 2008, it was estimated that more than 10% of deaths from medical errors were preventable and could have been avoided.[4]

Medical errors can occur when the wrong plan is used to achieve an aim (error in planning), a planned action is not completed (error of omission), or an action is performed incorrectly (error of execution or commission). Medical errors are costly, preventable adverse events and include errors associated with medication or treatment administration, healthcare-acquired infections, restraint-related injuries, falls, burns, and pressure sores.[5–7] A subset of adverse events, termed sentinel events, are defined as unexpected occurrences that result in death or serious physical or psychological risk or injury not present on admission or related to the natural course of illness or underlying condition.[8] Events categorized as sentinel events by The Joint Commission include medication errors, rape or patient suicide in a healthcare facility, hemolytic transfusion reactions, wrong-site or wrong-patient surgery, and infant abduction or discharge to the wrong family.[9]

In 2001, the IOM identified potential solutions to the problem of medical errors and recommended a redesign of the US healthcare system in *Crossing the Quality Chasm: A New Health System for the 21st Century*. In order to provide continuous, customized care, with patients in control of their care, the IOM advocates organizational support for change, evidence-based healthcare delivery, the use of information technology, and the alignment of legislative and payment policies with quality improvement in health care.[10]

In December 2004, the Institute for Healthcare Improvement (IHI) launched its "100,000 Lives" campaign to prevent 100,000 unnecessary deaths. More than 3000 hospitals (representing 75% of all US hospital beds) implemented evidence-based life saving interventions that included rapid response teams, medication reconciliation, and use of guidelines to prevent pneumonia, surgical site and central line infections. In 2006, IHI announced that the campaign had surpassed its goal and had saved 122,300 lives.[11]

In 2003, The Joint Commission issued national patient safety goals and recommendations. The goals have been updated annually and are now delineated by practice setting; for example, there are specific goals for hospitals, ambulatory care, home care, etc. (see Table 77-1).[12]

Despite the growing body of knowledge of risk-reduction strategies, adverse events still occur and may result in patient harm and legal action. While many of these events, such as patient falls and medication errors, are not unique to the practice of oncology nursing, some errors and events are specific to oncology nursing practice, such as chemotherapy medication errors, chemotherapy-induced hypersensitivity reactions, monoclonal antibody infusion-related reactions, and vesicant extravasations.

## CHEMOTHERAPY MEDICATION ERRORS

The incidence and severity of chemotherapy medication errors are unknown. Sometimes these errors, especially those involving lethal overdoses of chemotherapy, prompt litigation and are publicized in the media. For example, in 1999, newspapers reported that a patient with testicular cancer died after receiving a 4-fold overdose of cyclophosphamide,

**TABLE 77-1**

**Joint Commission National Patient Safety Goals and Recommendations for Hospitals for 2009**

| Goal | Key Recommendations |
|---|---|
| Improve patient identification procedures | Use at least 2 patient identifiers other than room or chair number. |
| Improve communication | Develop institutional procedures to standardize processes, such as creating a list of prohibited abbreviations and delineating procedures for verbal orders and timely reporting of critical test results. |
| Improve the safety of using medications | Limit the number of different drug concentrations in stock, manage "look-alike, sound-alike" medications, improve medication labeling, and develop procedures to reduce harm from anticoagulation therapy. |
| Reduce the risk of health care-associated infections | Adhere to hand hygiene guidelines, institute procedures to prevent multi-drug resistant organism infections, and prevent central-line associated bloodstream and surgical site infections. |
| Accurately and completely reconcile medications across the continuum of care | Compare current and newly ordered medications, communicate medications to the next provider, and provide reconciled medication lists to patients. |
| Reduce the risk of patient harm from falls | Implement a fall reduction program. |
| Encourage patients' active involvement in their own care as a patient safety strategy. | Develop a system for patient and family reporting of safety concerns. |

*Source*: Data from Joint Commission.[12]

and the family agreed to a $7.9 million settlement with the hospital.[13]

Chemotherapy medication errors often are reported only internally and are not reported to national medication error reporting programs or published in the literature. The low external error reporting rate, reported to be 3% in one study,[14] is attributable to several factors, such as fear of employer punishment, coworker disapproval, concern that a lawsuit may be filed, feelings of guilt and inadequacy, and lack of awareness of the process for externally reporting errors. In addition, there is a prevailing perception that medication errors causing minimal or no harm do not need to be reported externally.[15,16]

Chemotherapy medication errors include incorrect preparation, wrong drug, dose errors (including under- and overdosing), incorrect administration time or route, and chemotherapy administered to the wrong patient.[14] Examples of these errors include mix-ups caused by similar drug names (eg, cisplatin administered instead of carboplatin, which caused 3 patient deaths reported in a review of 469 fatal medication errors)[17] or "look-alike" vial labels, dose miscalculations (eg, underdosing that occurred when 1 day's dose of cladribine was administered over 1 week, which resulted in 2 patients with hairy-cell leukemia not responding to treatment,[18] and overdosing that occurred when a nurse thought she had used five 10-mg vials of vinorelbine to prepare a 50-mg dose but inadvertently used two 50-mg and three 10-mg vials),[19] mistakes in interpreting orders (eg, infusion of doxorubicin and vincristine over 1 day instead of 4 days),[20] and lack of patient understanding (eg, oral chemotherapy dose for 1 week taken all at 1 time).

Many of these errors are preventable. Education is paramount so that individuals who prescribe, prepare, handle, and administer chemotherapy are well-informed about the drugs' properties, toxicities, cumulativedoses, and effects. The environment in which chemotherapy is prepared and administered needs to be uncluttered and nondistracting. The individuals involved in these processes need to be focused, have resources such as up-to-date references available at the point of care, and strictly adhere to principles of practice (eg, the "five rights" of medication administration) and institutional procedures. Applicable risk-reduction strategies include not storing chemotherapy drugs with similar names or labels side by side, being familiar with the generic and trade names of chemotherapy agents, triple-checking dose calculations and checking doses against reference sources such as the treatment protocol, clearly labeling the route of administration, verifying patient identity, clarifying unclear orders, and dispensing 1 course of oral chemotherapy at a time. Several publications describe additional strategies that can be used to prevent chemotherapy medication errors.[21–24]

Chemotherapy medication errors can result in various actions. Employers may initiate remedial actions (eg, staff education) or disciplinary actions (eg, termination of employment). State licensing boards may take action and mandate staff education and institutional procedural improvements, or may revoke or restrict professional licensure. Patients and their families may initiate legal action following chemotherapy medication errors, especially those associated with patient injury, and sometimes file criminal charges against healthcare providers as well. For example, a review of 17 lethal medication errors that occurred in the United Kingdom from 1970 to 1999 describes 2 incidents involving cases in which vincristine for intravenous use was erroneously administered intrathecally, and the physicians involved were charged with manslaughter.[25]

Being well-informed about the chemotherapy administration process, adhering to institutional procedures, employing risk-reduction strategies, and openly communicating with patients and other staff members are key strategies for reducing the likelihood that a chemotherapy medication error will be made and legal action will ensue.

## HYPERSENSITIVITY AND INFUSION-RELATED REACTIONS

Hypersensitivity, defined as an unexpected reaction with signs and symptoms not consistent with known toxicity of the drug,[26] may be experienced by patients when they receive asparaginase, bleomycin, taxanes, platinum compounds, and monoclonal antibodies. The severity of these reactions can range from mild symptoms, such as urticaria and rash, to life-threatening dyspnea and bronchospasm. The incidence of severe reactions is <5%, provided patients receive recommended premedication, are closely monitored during the infusion, and there is prompt intervention if symptoms occur.[27] Although severe reactions do not often occur, they may be fatal and may prompt legal action.

Asparaginase is an enzyme derived from *Escherichia coli* (*E. coli*) or *Erwinia* that is primarily used to treat acute lymphoblastic leukemia. Its risk of hypersensitivity when administered intravenously is well known and is estimated to occur in 20% to 30% of patients. Test dosing (0.1 mL of a 20 units/mL dilution of drug given intradermally) is advocated, and educating the patient about the risk of hypersensitivity and the importance of reporting early symptoms of this reaction is essential.[26] However, skin testing is not standardized in clinical practice, and reactions have occurred in patients with negative skin tests, so the drug needs to be administered in a facility that is capable of treating anaphylaxis. The drug is often given intramuscularly or subcutaneously; these routes of administration are associated with a lower reaction rate. Patients sensitive to asparaginase may need to undergo desensitization, switch from the *E. coli* form to the *Erwinia* product, or change to the polyethylene glycolated (PEG) form of the drug, pegaspargase, which is better tolerated, especially when given intramuscularly.[28,29]

Bleomycin is another agent with hypersensitivity potential. Reactions can occur in any patient receiving the drug, but they occur more often in patients with lymphoma during or after the first or second dose of the drug. Symptoms of a bleomycin-induced hypersensitivity reaction include hypotension, tachycardia, wheezing, confusion, and facial edema. In some settings, test dosing (0.5–1 unit administered intravenously or intradermally) is performed on all patients scheduled to receive bleomycin, and in other settings, only patients with lymphoma are test-dosed.[30] Both asparaginase and bleomycin increase leukotriene production, which is thought to explain the etiology of hypersensitivity to these agents, since leukotriene activation of the mast cells causes febrile and inflammatory responses, including anaphylactic reactions.[31]

Paclitaxel is an agent that induces a hypersensitivity reaction in 1% to 10% of patients.[30] Docetaxel, another taxane, induces hypersensitivity in about 2% of patients.[26] It is unclear if reactions occur because of sensitivity to these agents or to excipients added to solubilize these agents (eg, Cremophor EL in paclitaxel and polysorbate-80 in docetaxel).[26] All patients require pretreatment with steroids and antihistamines before *each dose* of either drug.[26] Reactions may be mild (dyspnea, hypotension) to severe (angioedema, tachycardia, chest pain). Some patients experiencing mild reactions to paclitaxel are rechallenged with paclitaxel infusing at a lower rate,[30] some are switched to docetaxel, which is tolerated by most patients who have had reactions to paclitaxel,[26] and some have required treatment using a desensitization protocol in order to receive subsequent infusions of paclitaxel.[32] Desensitization should only be performed in settings where staffing levels allow for close patient monitoring (preferably, a nurse remains with the patient during desensitization) and resuscitation equipment and personnel are immediately available.[33]

Another agent, and one that is sometimes administered concurrently with paclitaxel, is carboplatin. Carboplatin typically causes hypersensitivity in 16% to 27% of patients after multiple cycles of the drug have been administered.[34–36] Patients with ovarian cancer appear to be at a higher risk of developing hypersensitivity, which may be attributed to prolonged carboplatin exposure.[37] Clinical features of carboplatin-induced hypersensitivity include diffuse rash, tachycardia, dyspnea, wheezing, facial swelling, and chest tightness.[35,36] Some patients become hypotensive while others become hypertensive. In half of the patients, the reaction develops after 50% or more of the carboplatin has been infused.[35] Reactions are treated by stopping the infusion and administering steroids, antihistamines, benzodiazepines, nebulized beta-agonists, and/or vasopressors.[38] Some patients may require oxygen administration and intravenous hydration.[39] Patients who have had a hypersensitivity reaction to a platinum agent will often have a repeat reaction with rechallenge, and pretreatment with steroids or antihistamines has not prevented these reactions.[26] Skin-testing protocols, such as the use of a 0.02-mL intradermal injection of an undiluted aliquot of the planned carboplatin dose 1 hour before each course of the drug, have been developed to help predict which patients are hypersensitive to carboplatin.[40] Desensitizing carboplatin infusion regimens may be required for patients with moderate to severe carboplatin hypersensitivity.[41,42] Subsequent treatment with cisplatin, using a cisplatin desensitization protocol, has also been successful for patients who cannot continue carboplatin because of an allergic reaction to the drug.[43,44]

Initial reports of oxaliplatin hypersensitivity reactions were low; however, more recent data suggest that their incidence is similar to that of the earlier generation platinum compounds (eg, carboplatin). Hypersensitivity reactions range from mild flushing to life-threatening anaphylaxis. Following mild reactions, patients may be reexposed to oxaliplatin after administering immunosuppressants (eg, high-dose corticosteroids and histamine antagonists). Patients with a history of moderate to severe hypersensitivity to oxaliplatin are usually not reexposed to the drug and receive alternative treatment, although there are anecdotal reports of successful desensitization to oxaliplatin.[45]

The monoclonal antibodies alemtuzumab, cetuximab, gemtuzumab, panitumumab, rituximab, tositumomab, and trastuzumab have the potential to cause rare but life-threatening anaphylaxis. Mouse antibodies that are used in the production of monoclonal antibodies are foreign substances and may stimulate anaphylaxis. The fusion protein denileukin diftitox also has the potential to cause acute hypersensitivity reactions.

Infusion reactions are common when alemtuzumab is administered, and premedication is required to prevent them. Common symptoms include fever and chills (80%), nausea (60%), rash (50%), and hypotension (16%). Infusion reactions usually resolve after a week of treatment. Premedications, including acetaminophen and diphenhydramine, are often prescribed, and the dose of alemtuzumab is escalated during treatment (started at 3 mg and gradually increased as tolerated to 10 mg and then 30 mg).[46]

Mild infusion-related reactions, including chills, fever, and dyspnea, occur in 23% of patients who receive single-agent cetuximab and in 16% who receive this agent in conjunction with irinotecan. About 3% of patients experience severe cetuximab infusion-related reactions characterized by the rapid onset of airway obstruction, rash, and hypotension. Most of these infusion-related reactions occur on the first day of initial dosing and patients in the middle south of the US (particularly in Tennessee and North Carolina) appear to be at a higher risk for reaction than patients in other regions.[47] Premedication with 50 mg diphenhydramine IV is recommended; however, a recent observational study suggests that premedication may not be necessary after the second infusion of cetuximab if patients did not develop any symptoms during the first 2 infusions.[48] Patients who experience mild to moderate infusion-related reactions should have the rate of infusion reduced by 50%, and those who experience severe infusion reactions usually do not receive further therapy with this agent.[30,49–51] There are anecdotal reports of patients continuing cetuximab despite infusion reactions; these patients are given corticosteroids and are closely monitored in intensive care units.[52]

Gemtuzumab ozogamicin is a monoclonal antibody conjugated to the cytotoxic antibiotic calicheamicin. Patients receiving this agent for the first time often experience a postinfusion syndrome that occurs within 24 hours and is characterized by chills and fever (60%), nausea and vomiting (35%), and headache (12%). It resolves with supportive therapy of acetaminophen, diphenhydramine, and fluids. Patients are less likely to experience this postinfusion syndrome with subsequent treatments and are typically premedicated with acetaminophen and diphenhydramine prior to treatment.[30,53]

Panitumumab is an epidermal growth factor receptor antagonist. Severe infusion reactions, characterized by bronchospasm and hypotension, occurred in approximately 1% of all patients in clinical trials and no deaths have been reported to occur. Panitumumab infusions should be immediately stopped if an infusion reaction occurs, and, depending on the severity or persistence of the reaction, may need to be discontinued.[54]

Infusion-related reactions occur in about 80% of patients receiving the first dose of rituximab and 40% of patients receiving subsequent infusions. Fever and chills commonly occur, and other symptoms include nausea, headache, and throat irritation. Reactions generally occur within 30 minutes to 2 hours of the start of the first infusion and resolve when the infusion is slowed or interrupted and supportive care (eg, diphenhydramine, acetaminophen, fluids) is provided. Initial infusions of rituximab are started at 50 mg/hour. If tolerated, the rate is escalated in 50 mg/hour increments every 30 minutes to a maximum of 400 mg/hour. Subsequent infusions, if the patient tolerated the first infusion well, are initiated at 100 mg/hour and increased by 100 mg/hour increments at 30-minute intervals to a maximum of 400 mg/hour as tolerated.[30,55]

Treatment with tositumomab and iodine-131 tositumomab is dual action (immunotherapy with a monoclonal antibody and radiotherapy with iodine-131). Rare but potentially life-threatening reactions during the 2-step treatment may occur. The first step, the dosimetric step, is followed 7 to 14 days later by the therapeutic step. Approximately 8% of patients experience fever and/or chills during the infusion and require a 50% reduction in the infusion rate. Infusions are interrupted if severe infusion-related reactions occur.[30]

Infusion reactions to trastuzumab consist of a symptom complex of fever and chills, rash, dyspnea, and hypotension. Severe reactions may be characterized by bronchospasm, hypoxia, and anaphylaxis and may be fatal. Reactions have been reported to occur during or immediately following the initial infusion of trastuzumab. If patients experience dyspnea or hypotension during trastuzumab infusion, the trastuzumab should immediately be discontinued and supportive care (eg, corticosteroids, epinephrine, bronchodilators, oxygen) should be initiated. Discontinuation of trastuzumab may need to be considered for patients with severe reactions. Patients with mild to moderate infusion reactions may be able to resume treatment when premedicated with antihistamines and/or corticosteroids; however, while some patients tolerated subsequent infusions, others had recurrent infusion reactions despite premedication.[56]

Denileukin diftitox, a recombinant protein containing diphtheria toxin fragments and interleukin-2, can cause acute hypersensitivity reactions. In clinical trials, 69% of patients experienced a hypersensitivity reaction during or within 24 hours of the infusion. Most reactions occur during the first day of dosing of each treatment cycle and are characterized by hypotension (50%), back pain (30%), dyspnea (28%), and rash (25%).[30,57]

Patient injury has occurred, and litigation has been initiated, when patients who were treated with agents with known hypersensitivity potential, but who were not premedicated when premedication was indicated or not test-dosed when test dosing was indicated, experienced a hypersensitivity or infusion-related reaction. Legal actions also have been filed when reactions occurred but were not promptly recognized or properly treated.

Risk-reduction measures include educating staff about chemotherapy agents and side effects, using appropriate test-dose or premedication procedures, immediately stopping an infusion if a hypersensitivity reaction is suspected, being prepared for emergencies (eg, having oxygen, medications, etc, available), issuing standing orders to administer emergency medications, having written policies on emergency management procedures, educating patients regarding the risk of hypersensitivity and its symptoms, and closely monitoring patients during chemotherapy and administration of monoclonal antibodies (including monitoring and recording vital signs when indicated).[58] With both paclitaxel and carboplatin, patients with a prior history of systemic hypersensitivity to medications or environmental causes (eg, bee stings) were noted to be at increased risk for experiencing allergic reactions to these agents.[59] Therefore, nurses also need to obtain an allergy history when assessing patients scheduled to receive chemotherapy agents that have the potential for hypersensitivity.

## VESICANT EXTRAVASATION

A number of vesicant chemotherapy agents cause extensive damage if they extravasate out of the vein into the tissue. Extravasation may occur with peripherally administered vesicants, as well as vesicants administered via indwelling central venous access devices, such as percutaneously placed central venous catheters and implanted ports. Peripheral extravasations may occur following inaccurate device placement, vein damage, patient movement, and other factors. Catheter rupture or fracture, or backtracking of the vesicant along the catheter because of thrombus formation at the catheter tip can cause extravasations from central venous catheters. Port-related extravasations can occur from perforation of the superior vena cava, incomplete needle placement, needle dislodgment, thrombus formation, catheter fracture, and catheter/portal septum separation.[60]

Extravasation-related injuries may resolve with time and symptomatic management or if untreated, may be extensive, in some cases requiring surgery and skin grafting. Extensive injury often delays or prevents cancer treatment, may cause functional impairment of the affected body part, renders the patient vulnerable to infection, and may cause related problems, such as the patient's inability to perform daily activities. Consequently, the physical and emotional impact of an extensive extravasation injury may prompt legal action. Although extravasation is a known risk of vesicant administration, patients may allege that the nurse administering the vesicant was negligent. The circumstances surrounding the administration of the vesicant are closely examined to ascertain whether the nurse deviated from the institution's procedures or the level of care that nurses in similar situations would provide. For instance, administering a vesicant through a device that lacks a blood return, without taking further action to verify placement and patency, deviates from safe practice. A case example is an account of an implanted port lacking a blood return that was used to administer vesicant chemotherapy. The nurse's rationale for using the port despite a lack of blood return or other evidence of placement and patency was that the port was newly inserted. Although an anterior-posterior chest x-ray was interpreted as showing the port's catheter tip in good position, the catheter had perforated the superior vena cava, and an intrathoracic extravasation subsequently occurred. The patient became septic and died. The family filed a malpractice claim, which was settled for nearly $500,000.[61]

The best defense against claims of negligence related to extravasation injuries is to prevent them from occurring to the extent possible, to detect them quickly should they occur, and to intervene promptly. Guidelines and recommendations for vesicant administration, such as those published by the Oncology Nursing Society (ONS),[62] and institutional policies should guide vesicant administration and extravasation management. Vesicants should never be administered without evidence of proper device placement and patency.[63] Clinical resources, such as experienced staff members, along with institutionally defined procedures for using declotting agents and radiological studies, should be used to evaluate devices with questionable placement or patency. Patients receiving vesicants need close monitoring during vesicant administration and should be instructed regarding actions to take, such as not moving the arm during peripheral vesicant administration, and signs and symptoms to report. Patients need to be informed that extravasation is a risk of vesicant administration, and they should be reminded of this risk with each course of treatment. Nurses should document ease of device insertion (when applicable), number of attempts to insert the device, detailed location of the device, assessment of the device and patient during the infusion, and the patient's response. If an extravasation occurs or is suspected, the vesicant should be stopped immediately and institutional policies for managing extravasations initiated. The area involved should be measured and promptly and appropriately treated. Totect (dexrazoxane for injection), the only FDA-approved treatment for anthracycline extravasation treatment, must be administered as soon as possible and within 6 hours of the extravasation.[64] Antidotes for other types of extravasations, such as local injection of sodium thiosulfate for nitrogen mustard extravasation and hyaluronidase for plant alkaloid extravasation, may be given in accordance with institutional protocols.[65] Patients who receive extravasation treatment need to be instructed to observe the extravasation area for redness, blistering, and skin sloughing. Close follow-up of the patient for the next several days, and possibly weeks, along with referral to a plastic or hand surgeon, may be needed if skin necrosis occurs.[63,65]

## RESPONDING TO ERRORS AND ADVERSE EVENTS

When an error contributes to or causes an injury, patients and their families are entitled to a prompt explanation of how the event occurred and its short- and long-term effects. Patients and family members should receive an honest, compassionate explanation of the error and the treatment or remedies that are available. They should be informed that the event and the factors contributing to the event will be investigated so that action can be taken to reduce the likelihood of similar events occurring in the future.[66] Truthful and complete disclosure is the healthcare provider's only appropriate ethical response to a medical error or adverse event.[67]

It is unknown whether full disclosure influences malpractice liability (eg, whether a lawsuit is filed or not);[68] however, legal action is sometimes initiated by patients or their families in an effort to obtain information about what happened when they perceive that healthcare providers are withholding or concealing information. The patient's perception of lack of communication or poor communication is frequently the impetus for filing a lawsuit.[69]

A systems approach is advocated for investigating and responding to errors and adverse events. The basic premise of a systems approach is that humans are fallible and errors are to be expected. Errors are viewed as consequences of an ineffective system.[70] A systems approach represents the philosophical belief that it was not the nurse who failed, but rather the system.

A root cause analysis (RCA) is the process of defining the underlying cause of an event and involves repeatedly asking why an event occurred. An RCA is a retrospective evaluation of an incident that considers several perspectives, including, in most instances, that of the patient and family. The goal of this analysis is to identify the many factors that contribute to an error. After an incident occurs, a particular action or omission of action may at first appear to be the cause of the incident; however, closer analysis often reveals a cascade of events and a multitude of contributing factors.[71,72] The Joint Commission requires hospitals to conduct RCAs of adverse events as part of its accreditation program, and encourages reporting these events. In addition, many states mandate adverse event reporting.[73] Medical errors and adverse events should be reported internally and externally to appropriate agencies as soon as possible following the incident (see Figure 77-1).

A procedure that often is used in conjunction with RCAs is failure mode and effects analysis (FMEA), which proactively identifies potential problems within systems or processes. An FMEA can be conducted after an RCA to identify other potential problems related to the system under scrutiny, or can be performed independently to prevent errors. For instance, FMEA can be used proactively to examine high-risk areas, such as chemotherapy prescribing, dispensing, and administering.[74]

Food and Drug Administration (FDA) MedWatch program provides an online voluntary reporting form to report serious adverse events potential and actual medical product errors, and product quality problems associated with the use of FDA-regulated drugs, biologics, devices and dietary supplements. Phone 800-FDA-1088. http://www.accessdata.fdagov/scripts/medwatch/medwatch_online.cfm.

Instiutute for Safe Medication Practices (ISMP) Medication Errors Reporting Program (MERP), operated by the United States Pharmacopeia (USP) in cooperation with ISMP, is a confidential national voluntary reporting program that collects information about medication errors provides analysis of the system causes of these errors, and disseminates recommendations to healthcare providers. Phone 800-FAIL-SAF(E) (800–324-5723). http://www.ismp.org/pages/meden_usa.html.

United States Pharmacopeia (USP) Medication Errors Reporting Program, operated in cooperation with ISMP, is an FDA MedWatch partner. Phone 800–23 ERROR (800–233-7767). http://secure.usp.org/patientsafety/reporting/merform.html.

The Joint Commission provides tools for conducting a root cause analysis and a self-report form to describe and report sentinel events occuring in healthcare facilities: http://www.jcaho.org/accredited+organizations/hospitals/sentinel+events/forms+and+tools/index.htm.

**FIGURE 77-1**

Sources for reporting medical errors and adverse events.

When a medical error or an adverse event occurs, even in organizations that purport to embrace a systems approach to examining those events, a subtle undercurrent to assign some degree of blame to the individual involved may occur. A survey of 1400 hospitals conducted by the American Hospital Association, Health Research and Education Trust, and Institute for Safe Medication Practices found that only 46% of respondents reported full confidence that error-reduction strategies at their institutions targeted the system and not the individual. Only 23% indicated that they felt they could openly report and discuss errors without undue embarrassment or fear of reprisal.[75] The implication of this study's findings is that despite the widespread promotion of a systems-based approach to reducing medication error, truly nonpunitive environments are not yet the norm. It also has been recognized that the individual involved in a medical error is the "second victim" of the error. Unconditional sympathy and support for this individual is needed but often not provided by coworkers and supervisory staff after a medical error occurs.[76]

## RISK MANAGEMENT

The healthcare delivery system has been compared to the aviation industry because of their similar complex environments, extensive use of technology, and the potential for human error. Consequently, many risk-management procedures used in health care are modeled after those used in aviation, including proactively examining environmental, organizational, individual, team, and patient factors that can cause or contribute to the occurrence of medical errors and close calls (often termed "near misses"). Error prevention is based on understanding the nature and extent of potential errors, changing the conditions that can induce errors, determining behaviors that prevent or mitigate errors, and training personnel.[77–79]

Institutions can conduct periodic self-assessments of their error prevention programs. These programs should demonstrate evidence of organizational commitment, utilize clearly delineated policies and procedures, include staff education (both initial and ongoing), and contain detailed assessment parameters specific to the area being assessed. For instance, medication error prevention may include assessing environmental factors such as storage, dispensing, and administration areas; organizational factors such as the prescription, preparation, and administration processes; individual and team factors such as education and information resources; and patient factors such as patient education and partnership.

Although a variety of specific strategies have been advocated by safety experts (see Table 77-2),[80–113] concepts integral to risk reduction in health care include the need to simplify and standardize, proactively examine systems, educate for safety, train for teamwork, and create and support a culture of safety.[114] In an organizational culture of safety, it is recognized that humans are fallible and that errors will occur even in a perfect system. The imperfection of human performance is accepted and workplace modifications are made to reduce the likelihood of human error.[115] Examples include "smart" computerized infusion pumps,[116] computerized prescriber order entry systems with integrated clinical decision support,[117] and standardization, such as stocking only one concentration of high-risk medications (eg, heparin).[118]

In order to foster a culture of safety, effective leadership must be present, team building needs to be emphasized, and quality improvement objectives must align with the institution's core values.[119] An additional error prevention strategy is to design jobs for safety by considering length of work hours, workload, staffing ratios, and so forth. Staffing issues also encompass insufficient staffing and the use of inexperienced staff, floating and temporary staff, and unlicensed assistive personnel.

Some safety experts recommend developing a strategic plan for safety. To formulate short- and long-term goals, the plan should assess the institution's internal processes and capabilities. The goals should be measurable to allow tracking of progress and allow for modification as needed, be compatible with the organization's culture, and be able to remain applicable over the long term despite anticipated changes in the organization and healthcare delivery. External influences should be examined, including the current and projected economy, reimbursement patterns, trends in technology, applicable laws, regulatory and accreditation requirements, the legal climate, and healthcare trends such as staffing shortages.[120]

## COMPLAINTS AND LITIGATION

Although the prevailing philosophy of examining medical errors has changed from one of "naming, blaming, and shaming"[70] to a nonpunitive systems approach, the desire to find fault continues in the legal arena. Legal action following a medical error or adverse event is intended to identify and punish those perceived to be at fault.

Formal complaints are sometimes filed with state licensing boards. Licensing boards are charged with protecting the public by licensing and regulating healthcare providers under their jurisdiction. They also investigate complaints filed against healthcare providers by patients, their family members, or the general public to determine whether the healthcare providers violated state practice acts. Professional practice acts enumerate the infractions that could result in disciplinary actions such as formal reprimands or consent orders to restrict or revoke licensure. In many states, licensing boards have the right to (and usually do) publish the circumstances of a consent order in local newspapers. Licensing boards are also required to disclose adverse actions to the National Practitioner Data Bank.

**TABLE 77-2**

**Risk Management Strategies Applicable to Oncology**

| Action | Examples |
|---|---|
| Use automated systems and information technology[80–88] | Automated dispensing machines, electronic communication and medical records, computerized physician order entry, computerized medication administration records, computerized clinical decision support systems, personal data assistants, bar coding, use of robots |
| Reduce complexity[89–93] | Minimize and standardize stock inventory, use one type or brand of equipment (eg, infusion pumps), streamline procedures, simplify systems, unify the prescribing vocabulary, and use generic rather than trade names for medications |
| Include constraints in systems[92,94,95] | Restrict actions that can result in error (eg, avoid use of abbreviations, delineate who can order and administer chemotherapy, etc.), remove concentrated electrolytes from patient-care areas, use automated medication ordering systems with alerts for higher-than-standard doses |
| Utilize human resources[94,96–101] | Require pharmacist verification of order entry, have pharmacists and nurses on rounding teams, place advanced practice nurses in clinical decision support roles, involve patients in the treatment verification process, create a patient safety committee, utilize medical librarians to obtain information |
| Educate healthcare providers[102,103] | Provide formal instruction on safety in schools of nursing, hospital teaching rounds, and conferences; perform comprehensive orientation of new employees; offer ongoing staff education programs; encourage and reward specialty certification |
| Monitor patients closely and promote continuity of care[104–108] | Ensure adequate patient/staff ratios; employ qualified staff; have an appropriate skill mix of personnel; conduct change-of-shift rounds and reports in patients' rooms; use reliable, well-maintained equipment; provide alarm and alerting mechanisms when indicated (eg, call bells, bed alarms, etc.) |
| Optimize infection control practices[108,109] | Comply with CDC hand hygiene and infection control recommendations, monitor personnel and the environment, use proper medical device sterilization and environmental disinfection |
| Periodically assess procedures, risks, and emergency preparedness[97,110,111] | Self-assess or have policies and procedures externally reviewed: update as needed. Identify high-alert medications and high-risk procedures, conduct mock emergency drills |
| Improve communication[112] | Delineate who is "in charge" during medical emergencies, identify channels of communication, communicate openly and honestly with patients and their families, fully disclose medical errors and adverse events |
| Implement voluntary, nonpunitive error reporting[113] | Identify what to report, such as actual events and near misses, delineate staff involvement, educate staff, provide positive reinforcement, promote accountability, support culture of learning from mistakes instead of hiding or minimizing them |

*Abbreviation*: CDC, Centers for Disease Control and Prevention.

Patients and/or their families sometimes retain legal counsel to explore filing a lawsuit against healthcare providers when they perceive that an injury has occurred as a result of negligence or malpractice. Lawsuits alleging patient injury following medication errors, vesicant chemotherapy extravasations, chemotherapy-induced hypersensitivity reactions, and other events often specifically name the nurses involved and may include others, such as supervisory personnel. Plaintiffs (the parties initiating the lawsuit) typically allege incorrect or improper actions (acts of commission) but also may sue for injuries related to acts of omission, such as failure to monitor a patient. Litigation can be physically and emotionally draining for the nurses involved, and costly. Jury awards in medical malpractice cases often exceed $1 million.[121]

The documentation of an error or event is scrutinized when a lawsuit is filed. It has been said that "if it wasn't charted, it wasn't done" and that "the palest ink is better than the best memory." Although the primary purpose of documentation is to provide communication among the healthcare team, it also provides a legal record of the care rendered to a patient. It is essential that documentation in medical records be accurate. Inaccurate, incomplete, or contradictory documentation creates confusion for healthcare providers, increases legal liability, and decreases the credibility of healthcare providers, especially when medical record entries are scrutinized in the courtroom.

Defensive administrative strategies to reduce the risk of litigation include appropriate and adequate staffing, use of qualified healthcare providers, extensive staff education and close supervision, clear role delineation, open communication, and truthful documentation.

## PRIVACY PROTECTION

When the US Congress enacted the Health Insurance Portability and Accountability Act (HIPAA) of 1996, it mandated regulations to protect the privacy, security, and confidentiality of health information. Title II of HIPAA, the Privacy Rule, became effective on April 14, 2001, and provides comprehensive protections against inappropriate or unintended disclosure of personal health information. Provisions of the Privacy Rule include patient control of the use of health information, patients' rights to review and amend their health information, standards limiting the disclosure of health information, requirements for patients to be informed of providers' health information disclosure policies, and penalties for noncompliance with the law. The Privacy Rule applies to personally identifiable health information in any form, communicated electronically, on paper, or verbally by healthcare providers, health plans, and healthcare clearinghouses. However, the rule does not preempt state laws that provide more stringent privacy protection. Therefore, in some areas, healthcare providers need to comply with multiple layers of federal and state law.[122–125]

The specific procedures used to protect patients' privacy vary by institution but generally involve not posting patients' names or health information in public or prominent places, such as large wipe-off boards in nurses' stations or hallways, using "sign-in" procedures that promote privacy, such as covering names of patients who have already signed in, maintaining medical records in secure locations, and using password-protected computer access. In addition, healthcare providers cannot sell or provide patients' names and addresses to product or pharmaceutical manufacturers. Under the Privacy Rule, patients are given information about the law and the healthcare providers' privacy practices and are able to specifically stipulate how their health information will be used.

The HIPAA privacy rule has had both positive and negative effects on the release of patient information by healthcare facilities. There have been unintended consequences, such as difficulty in enrolling patients in clinical research studies,[126] as well as breaches in confidentiality and integrity of personal health information.[127] A major concern is the protection of sensitive patient information in an era of electronic communication and information systems.[128]

## TELEPHONE AND ELECTRONIC COMMUNICATION

Nurses routinely place follow-up telephone calls to patients and receive calls from patients when questions or concerns arise. Telephone triage and advice provides education and social support, and promotes continuity of care.[129] Because nurses cannot physically assess patients they must rely on their interviewing skills in order to obtain information. Protocol-driven and computer-supported telephone advice systems are increasingly being used to help ensure appropriateness and consistency of information provided.[130,131]

Verbal and "hard copy" (eg, paper) communication, including facsimile transmissions, are increasingly being replaced by electronic communication. Electronic mail, Web sites, cellular phone text messaging, and document-imaging technology are being used to improve the speed and accuracy of communication among healthcare providers. These technologies also are beginning to be used by healthcare providers when they communicate with patients.[132–134] Guidelines for clinical use of electronic mail include using electronic communication only for nonurgent matters, delineating what types of requests will be permitted (eg, appointment scheduling, prescription refills, test results), establishing a set turnaround time for messages received, and developing an explicit privacy policy for electronic communication.[135]

## PAIN MANAGEMENT

In recent years, the undertreatment of pain has received media attention and in some cases has prompted litigation and state licensing board action. Despite the existence of guidelines for cancer pain management,[136] nearly half of all patients with cancer-related pain are undertreated.[137] Inadequate pain management occurs frequently and has been attributed to healthcare providers' lack of knowledge, inappropriate concerns about opioid side effects and addiction, focus on disease treatment rather than symptom management, and other factors.[137]

Physicians have been cited for negligent pain management. For instance, a physician was disciplined by a state board of medical examiners in 1999 after he used acetaminophen to treat an elderly man's cancer-related pain. In another case, a jury found a nurse liable for failure to medicate and control pain in a patient dying of cancer. The nurse withheld the prescribed opioid analgesics and substituted a placebo instead. In a case involving inadequate pain management experienced by an elderly patient with cancer, the patient's family alleged elder abuse as well as medical malpractice, and the case went to trial as an elder abuse charge. A jury awarded the family $1.5 million.[138]

Nurses are liable for the undertreatment of pain. They need to be proactive in managing pain effectively and protecting themselves from lawsuits claiming inappropriate or inadequate pain management. The ONS position on cancer pain management lists several statements that can be used to guide practice and assist in institutional policy development. For example, ONS states that placebos should not be used to assess or manage cancer pain, determine if the pain really exists, or be used in the diagnosis of other disorders often associated with pain.[139]

Nurses should treat a patient's level of pain as the "fifth vital sign"; use the World Health Organization's analgesic ladder, which serves as a basis for the Agency for Healthcare Policy and Research's pain management guidelines, to assess and treat pain; individualize the pain treatment to the patient; and advocate for treatment modification as needed in order to effectively control pain.[140] Nurses also play an important role in implementing state pain initiatives that enhance the knowledge and skills of healthcare providers, support institutional change, and stress the importance of patient and family involvement in effective pain control.[141]

## CONCLUSION

Oncology nurses are instrumental in promoting patient safety. Strategies for ensuring safety include implementing national safety recommendations and adhering to principles of practice and institutional policies. A high-risk area of practice is chemotherapy administration, since the potential exists for chemotherapy medication errors, hypersensitivity reactions, and vesicant extravasations. Other areas of liability include documentation, privacy, electronic communication, and pain management. By employing risk-management strategies, nurses can reduce the risk of legal action and, more importantly, deliver safe patient care.

## REFERENCES


1. Kohn LT, Corrigan JM, Donaldson MS, eds. *To Err Is Human: Building a Safer Health System*. Washington, DC: National Academies Press; 2000.
2. Stelfox HT, Palmisani S, Scurlock C, et al. The "To Err is Human" report and the patient safety literature. *Qual Saf Health Care.* 2006; 15:174–178.
3. Leape LL, Berwick DM. Five years after "To Err is Human": what have we learned? *JAMA.* 2005;293:2384–2390.
4. Creagh H. More than 10% of hospital deaths could be avoided, conference is told. *BMJ.* 2008;336:852.
5. Kanjanarat P, Winterstein AG, Johns TE, et al. Nature of preventable adverse drug events in hospitals: a literature review. *Am J Health Syst Pharm.* 2003;60:1750–1759.
6. Kellogg VA, Havens DS. Adverse events in acute care: an integrative literature review. *Res Nurs Health.* 2003;31:398–408.
7. Lassetter JH, Warnick ML. Medical errors, drug-related problems, and medication errors: a literature review on quality of care and cost issues. *J Nurs Care Qual.* 2003;18:175–181.
8. Radtke K. Take the fear out of sentinel events. *Nurs Manage.* 2003;34: 24–25.
9. The Joint Commission. Sentinel Event Statistics. Updated through September 2009. http://www.jointcommission.org/SentinelEvents/Statistics/. Accessed January 18, 2010.
10. Committee on Quality of Healthcare in the United States, Institute of Medicine. *Crossing the Chasm: A New Health System for the 21st Century.* Washington, DC: National Academies Press; 2001.
11. Wachter RM, Pronovost PJ. The 100,000 lives campaign: a scientific and policy review. *Jt Comm J Qual Patient Saf.* 2006;32:631–633.
12. Joint Commission. 2009 National patient safety goals. http://www.jointcommission.org/PatientSafety/NationalPatientSafetyGoals/. Accessed October 27, 2009.
13. Associated Press. Fatal dosage costs hospital millions. *Times Picayune.* September 10, 1999:A6.
14. Schulmeister L. Chemotherapy medication errors: descriptions, severity, and contributing factors. *Oncol Nurs Forum.* 1999;26:1033–1042.
15. Crawford SY, Cohen MR, Tafesse E. Systems factors in the reporting of serious medication errors in hospitals. *J Med Syst.* 2003;27:543–551.
16. Wakefield DS, Wakefield BJ, Uden-Holman T, et al. Understanding why medication administration errors may not be reported. *Am J Med Qual.* 1999;14:81–88.
17. Phillips J, Beam S, Brinker A, et al. Retrospective analysis of mortalities associated with medication errors. *Am J Health Syst Pharm.* 2001;58:1835–1841.
18. Golde DW, Jakubowiak A, Caggiano J, et al. Cladribine underdosing in hairy-cell leukemia: a cause for apparent response failure. *Leuk Lymphoma.* 2002;43:365–367.
19. Institute for Safe Medication Practices. Cancer patients deserve the safest practices, regardless of where they are treated. *ISMP Med Saf Alert.* 2003;8:3.
20. Waddell JA, Coleman TA. Clinical response to unintended infusion of doxorubicin and vincristine over one instead of four days. *Am J Health Syst Pharm.* 2000;57:1242–1244.
21. Bartel SB. Safe practices and financial considerations in using oral chemotherapeutic agents. *Am J Health Syst Pharm.* 2007;64(9 suppl 5): S8-S14.
22. Bates DW. Preventing medication errors: a summary. *Am J Health Syst Pharm.* 2007;64(suppl 9):S3-S9.
23. Jacobson JO, Polovich M, McNiff KK, et al. American Society of Clinical Oncology/Oncology Nursing Society chemotherapy administration safety standards. *J Clin Oncol.* 2009; 27: 5469–5475.
24. Schulmeister L. Preventing chemotherapy errors. *Oncologist.* 2006;11: 463–468.
25. Ferner RE. Medication errors that have led to manslaughter charges. *BMJ.* 2000;321:1212–1216.
26. Shepherd GM. Hypersensitivity reactions to chemotherapeutic drugs. *Clin Rev Allergy Immunol.* 2003;24:253–262.
27. Lenz HJ. Management and preparedness for infusion and hypersensitivity reactions. *Oncologist.* 2007;12:601–609.
28. Dinndorf PA, Gootenberg J, Cohen MH, et al. FDA drug approval summary: pegaspargase (oncaspar) for the first-line treatment of children with acute lymphoblastic leukemia (ALL). *Oncologist.* 2007;12:991–998.
29. Graham ML. Pegaspargase: a review of clinical studies. *Adv Drug Deliv Rev.* 2003;55:1293–1302.
30. Wilkes GM, Ingwersen K, Barton-Burke M, eds. *Oncology Nursing Drug Handbook.* Subdury, MA: Jones and Bartlett; 2008.
31. Geuenich S, Haberl C, Egger D, et al. Induction of leukotriene production by bleomycin and asparaginase in mast cells in vitro and in vivo. *Biochem Pharmacol.* 1998;55:447–453.
32. Markman M, Kennedy A, Webster K, et al. Paclitaxel-associated hypersensitivity reactions: experience with the gynecologic oncology programs of the Cleveland Clinic Cancer Center. *J Clin Oncol.* 2000;18:102–105.
33. Castells, M. Rapid desensitization of hypersensitivity reactions to chemotherapy agents. *Curr Drug Saf.* 2006;1:243–251.
34. Markman M, Zanotti K, Peterson G, et al. Expanded experience with an intradermal skin test to predict for the presence or absence of carboplatin hypersensitivity. *J Clin Oncol.* 2003;21:4611–4614.
35. Markman M, Kennedy A, Webster K, et al. Clinical features of hypersensitivity reactions to carboplatin. *J Clin Oncol.* 1999;17:1141.
36. Polyzos A, Tsavaris N, Kosmas C, et al. Hypersensitivity reactions to carboplatin administration are common but not always severe: a 10-year experience. *Oncology.* 2001;61:129–133.

37. Navo M, Kunthur A, Badell ML, et al. Evaluation of the incidence of carboplatin hypersensitivity reactions in cancer patients. *Gynecol Oncol.* 2006;103:608–613.
38. Robinson JB, Singh D, Bodurka-Bevers DC, et al. Hypersensitivity reactions and the utility of oral and intravenous desensitization in patients with gynecologic malignancies. *Gynecol Oncol.* 2003;82: 550–558.
39. Winkeljohn D, Polovich M. Carboplatin hypersensitivity reactions. *Clin J Oncol Nurs.* 2006;10:595–598.
40. Zanotti KM, Rybicki LA, Kennedy AW, et al. Carboplatin skin testing: a skin-testing protocol for predicting hypersensitivity to carboplatin chemotherapy. *J Clin Oncol.* 2001;19:3126–3129.
41. Markman M, Hsieh F, Zanotti K, et al. Initial experience with a novel desensitization strategy for carboplatin-associated hypersensitivity reactions. *J Cancer Res Clin Oncol.* 2004;130:25–28.
42. Rose PG, Fusco N, Smrekar M, et al. Successful administration of carboplatin in patients with clinically documented carboplatin hypersensitivity. *Gynecol Oncol.* 2003;89:429–433.
43. Jones R, Ryan M, Friedlander M. Carboplatin hypersensitivity reactions: re-treatment with cisplatin desensitization. *Gynecol Oncol.* 2003; 89:112–115.
44. Ottaiano A, Tambaro R, Greggi S, et al. Safety of cisplatin after severe hypersensitivity reactions to carboplatin in patients with recurrent ovarian carcinoma. *Anticancer Res.* 2003;23:3465–3468.
45. Hewitt MR, Sun W. Oxaliplatin-associated hypersensitivity reactions: clinical presentation and management. *Clin Colorectal Cancer.* 2006; 6:114–117.
46. Berlex Laboratories. Campath (alemtuzumab) prescribing information. http://www.campath.com. Accessed October 27, 2009.
47. O'Neil BH, Allen R, Spigel DR, et al. High incidence of cetuximab-related infusion reactions in Tennessee and North Carolina and the association with atopic history. *J Clin Oncol.* 2007;25:3644–3648.
48. Chung CH. Managing premedications and the risk for reactions to infusional monoclonal antibody therapy. *Oncologist.* 2008;13:725–732.
49. Wilkes F. Managing drug infusion reactions: focus on cetuximab monoclonal antibody therapy. *Clin J Oncol Nurs.* 2008;12:530–532.
50. ImClone Systems, Bristol-Myers Squibb. Erbitux (cetuximab) prescribing information. http://www.erbitux.com. Accessed October 27, 2009.
51. Needle MN. Safety experience with IMC-C225, an anti-epidermal growth factor receptor antibody. *Semin Oncol.* 2002;29(5 suppl 14):55–60.
52. Melichar B, Cerman J, Malirova E. Successful management of infusion reaction accompanying the start of cetuximab therapy. *Support Care Cancer.* 2007;15:445–449.
53. Wyeth Laboratories. Mylotarg (gemtuzumab ozogamicin) prescribing information. http://http://www.wyeth.com/products?page=2&letters=all&fromLetters=all Accessed October 27, 2009.
54. Amgen. Vectibix (panitumumab) prescribing information. http://www.vectibix.com/pdfs/misc/vectibix_pi.pdf. Accessed October 27, 2009.
55. Genentech, IDEC Pharmaceuticals Corp. Rituxan (rituximab) prescribing information. http://www.rituxan.com. Accessed October 27, 2009.
56. Genentech. Herceptin (trastuzumab) prescribing information. http://www.gene.com/gene/products/information/pdf/herceptin-prescribing.pdf. Accessed October 27, 2009.
57. Ligand Pharamceuticals. ONTAK (denileukin difitox) prescribing information. http://http://www.eisai.com/pdf_files/Final%20Ontak%20PI%20PLR%2017OCT2008.pdf Accessed October 27, 2009.
58. Carney PH, Ollom CL. Infusion reactions triggered by monoclonal antibodies treating solid tumors. *J Infus Nurs.* 2008;31:74–83.
59. Markman M, Zanotti K, Kulp B. Relationship between a history of systematic allergic reactions and risk of subsequent carboplatin hypersensitivity. *Gynecol Oncol.* 2003;89:514–516.
60. Schulmeister L, Camp-Sorrell D. Chemotherapy extravasation from implanted ports. *Oncol Nurs Forum.* 2000;27:531–538.
61. Schulmeister L. A complication of vascular access device insertion: a case study and review of subsequent legal action. *J Intraven Nurs.* 1998;21:197–202.
62. Polovich M, White JM, Kelleher LO, eds. *Chemotherapy and Biotherapy Guidelines and Recommendations for Practice.* 2nd ed. Pittsburgh, PA: Oncology Nursing Society; 2005.
63. Schulmeister L. Managing vesicant extravasations. *Oncologist.* 2008; 13:284–288.
64. Schulmeister L. Totect: a new agent for treating anthracycline extravasation. *Clin J Oncol Nurs.* 2007;11:387–395.
65. Schulmeister L. Extravasation management. *Semin Oncol Nurs.* 2007; 23:184–190.
66. National Patient Safety Foundation. Talking to patients about health care injury. *Focus Patient Safety.* 2001;4:3.
67. Banja JD. Disclosing medical error: how much to tell. *J Healthc Risk Manag.* 2003;23:11–14.
68. Kachalia A, Shojania KG, Hofer TP, et al. Does full disclosure of medical errors affect malpractice liability? *Jt Comm J Qual Saf.* 2003; 29:503–511.
69. Wissow LS. Communication and malpractice claims-where are we now? *Patient Educ Couns.* 2004;52:3–5.
70. Reason J. Human error: models and management. *BMJ.* 2000;320: 768–770.
71. Gluck PA. Root cause analysis studies incidents to reveal system failures. *Focus Patient Safety.* 2003;6:1–5.
72. Vincent C, Taylor-Adams S, Chapman EJ, et al. How to investigate and analyse clinical incidents: Clinical Risk Unit and Association of Litigation and risk management protocol. *BMJ.* 2000;320:777–781.
73. National Academy of Sciences. *Patient Safety: Achieving a New Standard for Care.* Washington, DC: National Academies Press; 2003.
74. Sheridan-Leos N, Schulmeister L, Hartranft S. Failure mode and effect analysis: a technique to prevent chemotherapy errors. *Clin J Oncol Nurs.* 2006;10:393–398.
75. Smetzer J. Pathways for medication safety project background: ISMP survey pinpoints weaknesses in medication practices. Pathways for Medication Safety. http://http://www.medpathways.info/medpathways/tools/content/phasetwo.pdf Accessed October 27, 2009.
76. Wu AW. Medical error: the second victim. *BMJ.* 2000;320:726–727.
77. Barach P, Small SD. Reporting and preventing medical mishaps: lessons from non-medical near miss reporting systems. *BMJ.* 2000;320: 759–763.
78. Cohoon BD. Learning from near misses through reflection: a new risk management strategy. *J Healthc Risk Manag.* 2003;23:19–25.
79. Helmreich RL. On error management: lessons from aviation. *BMJ.* 2000;320:781–785.
80. Bates DW, Gawande AA. Improving safety with information technology. *N Engl J Med.* 2003;348:2526–2534.
81. Chung K, Choi YB, Moon S. Toward efficient medication error reduction: error-reducing information management systems. *J Med Syst.* 2003; 27:553–560.
82. Foote SO, Coleman JR. Medication administration: the implementation process of bar-coding for medication administration to enhance medication safety. *Nurs Econ.* 2008;26:207–210.
83. Gray MD, Felkey BG. Computerized prescriber order-entry systems: evaluation, selection, and implementation. *Am J Health Syst Pharm.* 2004;61:190–197.
84. Kaushal R, Shojania KG, Bates DW. Effects of computerized physician order entry and clinical decision support systems on medication safety: a systematic review. *Arch Intern Med.* 2003;163:1409–1416.
85. Larrabee S, Brown MM. Recognizing the institutional benefits of bar-code point-of-care technology. *Jt Comm J Qual Saf.* 2003;29: 345–353.
86. Mahoney CD, Berard-Collins CM, Coleman R, et al. Effects of an integrated clinical information system on medication safety in a multi-hospital setting. *Am J Health Syst Pharm.* 2007;64:1969–1977.
87. McMahan R. Operationalizing MTM through the use of health information technology. *J Manag Care Pharm.* 2008;14(2 suppl):S18-S21.
88. Whiting SO, Gale A. Computerized physician order entry usage in North America: the doctor is in. *Healthc Q.* 2008;11:94–97.

89. Adamson AJ. Infusion devices: characteristics, limitations and risk management. *Nurs Stand.* 2003;17:45–52.
90. Hoffman J, Prouix S. Medication errors cause by confusion of drug names. *Drug Safety.* 2003;26:445–452.
91. Keselman A, Patel VL, Johnson TR, et al. Institutional decision-making to select patient care devices: identifying venues to promote patient safety. *J Biomed Inform.* 2003;36:31–44.
92. Nolan TW. System changes to improve patient safety. *BMJ.* 2000; 320:771–773.
93. Schwab M, Oetzel C, Morike K, et al. Using trade names: a risk factor for accidental drug overdose. *Arch Intern Med.* 2002;162:1065–1066.
94. George D, Austin-Bishop N. Error rates for computerized order entry by physicians versus nonphysicians. *Am J Health Syst Pharm.* 2003;60:2250–2252.
95. Karch AM. Looks can be deceiving: use caution when using abbreviations. *Am J Nurs.* 2003;103:73.
96. Awe C, Lin SJ. Patient empowerment model to prevent medication errors. *J Med Syst.* 2003;27:503–517.
97. Cohen HS. Developing a patient safety committee: one hospital's experience. *Focus Patient Safety.* 2003;6:6–7.
98. Gandhi TK, Graydon-Baker E, Barnes JN, et al. Creating an integrated patient safety team. *Jt Comm J Qual Saf.* 2003;29:383–390.
99. Kucukarsian SH, Peters M, Mlynarek, et al. Pharmacists on rounding teams reduce preventable adverse drug events in hospital general medicine units. *Arch Intern Med.* 2003;138:2014–2018.
100. Rucker NL. "Risk, respect, responsibility": educational strategies to promote safe medication use. *J Med Syst.* 2003;27:519–530.
101. Williams L, Zipperer L. Improving access to information: librarians and nurses team up for patient safety. *Nurs Econ.* 2003;21:199–201.
102. Papastrat K, Wallace S. Teaching baccalaureate nursing students to prevent medication errors using a problem-based learning approach. *J Nurs Educ.* 2003;42:459–464.
103. Pierluissi E, Fischer MA, Campbell AR, et al. Discussion of medical errors in morbidity and mortality conferences. *JAMA.* 2003;290:2838–2842.
104. Hyun S, Bakken S, Douglas K, et al. Evidence-based staffing: potential roles for informatics. *Nurs Econ.* 2008;26:151–158, 173.
105. Moore C, Wisnivesky J, Williams S, et al. Medical errors related to discontinuity of care from an inpatient to outpatient setting. *J Gen Intern Med.* 2003;18:646–651.
106. Sasichay-Akkadechanunt T, Scalzi CC, Jawad AF. Relationship between nurse staffing and patient outcomes. *J Nurs Admin.* 2003;33:478–485.
107. Stone PW, Tourangeau AE. Measuring nursing services in patient safety research. *Appl Nurs Res.* 2003;16:131–132.
108. Cozad A, Jones RD. Disinfection and the prevention of infectious disease. *Am J Infect Control.* 2003;31:243–254.
109. Zanni GR. Hand hygiene: more than just hands. *Consult Pharm.* 2008;23:434–444.
110. ECRI. Medication safety: self assessment questionnaire. *Healthc Risk Contr.* 2003;1(SAQ 31):1–24.
111. Smetzer JL, Vaida AJ, Cohen MR, et al. Findings from the ISMP Medication Safety Self Assessment for hospitals. *Jt Comm J Qual Saf.* 2003;29:586–597.
112. Rosenstein AH, O'Daniel M. A survey of the impact of disruptive behaviors and communication defects on patient safety. *Jt Comm J Qual Patient Saf.* 2008;34:464–471.
113. Clancy CM. New patient safety organizations lower roadblocks to medical error reporting. *Am J Med Qual.* 2008;23:318–321.
114. Schulmeister L. Risk-reduction strategies. *Sentinel Events Toolkit.* Pittsburgh, PA: Oncology Nursing Society; 2002.
115. Dennison RD. Creating an organizational culture for medication safety. *Nurs Clin North Am.* 2005;40:1–23.
116. Keohane CA, Hayes J, Saniuk C, et al. Intravenous medication safety and smart infusion systems: lessons learned and future opportunities. *J Infus Nurs.* 2005;28:321–328.
117. Durieux P, Trinquart L, Colombet I, et al. Computerized advice on drug dosage to improve prescribing practice. *Cochrane Database Syst Rev.* 2008;16:CD002894.
118. Amalberti R, Auroy Y, Berwick D, et al. Five system barriers to achieving ultrasafe health care. *Ann Intern Med.* 2005;142:756–764.
119. Cohen MM, Eustis MA, Gribbins RE. Changing the culture of patient safety: leadership's role in health care quality improvement. *Jt Comm J Qual Saf.* 2003;29:329–335.
120. American Hospital Association, Health Research & Education Trust, Institute for Safe Medication Practices. Creating an organization-specific strategic plan for medication safety. http://www.medpathways.info/medpathways/tools/content/1_3.pdf. Accessed October 27, 2009.
121. Nepps ME. The basics of medical malpractice: a primer on navigating the system. *Chest.* 2008;134:1051–1055.
122. Blechner B, Butera A. Health Insurance Portability and Accountability Act of 1996 (HIPAA): a provider's overview of new privacy regulations. *Conn Med.* 2002;66:91–95.
123. Gostin LO. National health insurance information privacy: regulations under the Health Insurance Portability and Accountability Act. *JAMA.* 2001;285:3015–3021.
124. Maddox PJ. HIPAA: Update on rule revisions and compliance requirements. *Nurs Econ.* 2002;20:88–92.
125. Office for Civil Rights, Department of Health and Human Resources. Standards for privacy of individually identifiable health information: final rule. *Fed Reg.* 2002;67:53181–53273.
126. Nosowsky R, Giordano TJ. The Health Insurance Portability and Accountability Act of 1995 (HIPAA) privacy rule: implications for clinical research. *Annu Rev Med.* 2006;57:575–590.
127. Collmann J, Cooper T. Breaching the security of the Kaiser Permanente internet patient portal: the organizational foundations of information security. *J Am Med Inform Assoc.* 2007;14:239–243.
128. Houser SH, Houser HW, Shewchuk RM. Assessing the effects of the HIPAA privacy rule on release of patient information by healthcare facilities. *Perspect Health Inf Manag.* 2007;4:1.
129. Omery A. Advice nursing practice: on the quality of the evidence. *J Nurs Adm.* 2003;33:353–360.
130. Marklund B, Strom M, Mansson J, et al. Computer-supported telephone nurse triage: an evaluation of medical quality and costs. *J Nurs Manag.* 2007;15:180–187.
131. McNeil C. Skilled telephone triage programs streamline symptom management. *Oncology.* 2007;21(2 suppl nurse ed.):42–44.
132. Pelletier AL, Sutton GR, Walker RR. Are your patients ready for electronic communication? *Fam Pract Manag.* 2007;14:25–26.
133. Scherger JE. Online communication with patients: making it work. *Fam Pract Manag.* 2004;11:73–74.
134. Simonian AI. Medication order communication using fax and document-imaging technologies. *Am J Health Syst Pharm.* 2008;15:570–573.
135. Kane B, Sands D. Guidelines for the clinical use of electronic mail with patients. *J Am Med Inform Assoc.* 1998;5:104–111.
136. National Comprehensive Cancer Network. NCCN Clinical practice guidelines in oncology: adult cancer pain. Vol 1. 2008. http://www.nccn.org/professionals/physician_gls/PDF/pain.pdf. Accessed October 27, 2009.
137. Deandrea S, Montanari M, Moja L, et al. Prevalence of undertreatment in cancer pain. A review of published literature. *Ann Oncol.* 2008;19:1985–1991.
138. Frank-Stromborg M, Christensen A. A serious look at the undertreatment of pain: part I. *Clin J Oncol Nurs.* 2001;5:235–236.
139. Oncology Nursing Society. Cancer pain management. 2006. http://ons.org/publications/positions/CancerPainManagement.shtml. Accessed October 27, 2009.
140. Frank-Stromborg M, Christensen A. The undertreatment of pain: a liability risk for nurses. *Clin J Oncol Nurs.* 2000;4:41–44.
141. Dahl JL, Bennett ME, Bromley MD, et al. Success of the state pain initiatives: moving pain management forward. *Cancer Pract.* 2002;10(suppl 1):S9–S13.

# Index

Note: Page numbers followed by *f* and *t* denote figures and tables, respectively.

## A

## B

## D

## F

## G

## H

## M

## N

## O

## Q



## R

## U



## V